INTERNATIONAL DICTIONARY OF MEDICINE AND BIOLOGY

INTERNATIONAL DICTIONARY OF MEDICINE AND BIOLOGY

IN THREE VOLUMES

Volume II

A WILEY MEDICAL PUBLICATION
JOHN WILEY & SONS
New York • Chichester • Brisbane • Toronto • Singapore

R
610.3
I 61

Cover design by Wanda Lubelska

Library of Congress Cataloging-in-Publication Data

Main entry under title:

International dictionary of medicine and biology

  (A Wiley medical publication)
  Includes index.
  1. Medicine—Dictionaries. 2. Biology—
Dictionaries. I. Becker, E. Lovell (Ernest Lovell),
1923–   . II. Landau, Sidney I. III. Series.
[DNLM: 1. Biology—dictionaries. 2. Dictionaries,
Medical. W 13 I615]

R121.I58   1986   610'.3'21   85-16867
ISBN 0-471-01849-X

Printed in the United States of America

10 9 8 7 6 5 4 3 2 1

F

F **1** Symbol for the unit, farad. **2** Chemical symbol for the element, fluorine. **3** Symbol for phenylalanine. **4** Symbol for variance ratio.

F. **1** Fahrenheit (scale). **2** visual field. **3** French (cathether size). See under FRENCH SCALE. **4** formula.

F₁ A symbol used in genetics for the hybrid progeny resulting from the first mating of two organisms that differ by at least one phenotypic trait; the first filial generation.

F₂ A symbol used in genetics for the progeny resulting from the mating of two members of the first filial generation; the second filial generation.

°F Symbol for the unit, degree Fahrenheit.

f **1** Symbol for femto-: used with SI units. **2** Symbol for the unit, fors. **3** frequency.

F Symbol for (1) Faraday constant, expressed in coulombs per mole; (2) force, expressed in newtons; (3) magnetomotive force, expressed in amperes; (4) free energy.

f Symbol for the quantities (1) frequency, expressed in hertz; (2) focal length, expressed in meters.

FA **1** fluorescent antibody (fluorescein-labeled antibody). **2** femoral artery. **3** Fanconi's anemia. **4** fluorescent assay.

Fab [from *Fragment, antigen-binding*] See under FAB FRAGMENT.

fabella [L *fab(a)* a bean + *-ella*, diminishing suffix] A small sesamoid of bone or fibrocartilage frequently occurring in the lateral head of the gastrocnemius muscle.

fabellae Plural of FABELLA.

Faber [Knud Helge *Faber*, Danish physician, 1862–1956] Faber's anemia, Faber syndrome. See under IRON DEFICIENCY ANEMIA.

fabism FAVISM.

fabrication **1** CONFABULATION. **2** Conscious and willful distortion of the truth; lying.

Fabricius [Girolamo *Fabricius* ab Aquapendente, Italian anatomist and embryologist, 1533–1619] See under BURSA.

Fabry [Johannes *Fabry*, German physician, 1860–1930] Fabry's disease, diffuse angiokeratoma of Fabry, Fabry syndrome. See under ANGIOKERATOMA CORPORIS DIFFUSUM.

face [French (from L *facies* shape, form, face), face] The front, or anterior, aspect of the head from the top of the forehead to the point of the chin; facies.

adenoid face ADENOID FACIES.

bony face FACIES OSSEA CRANII.

bovine face FACIES BOVINA.

cow face FACIES BOVINA.

cushingoid face MOON FACE.

dish face FACIES SCAPHOIDEA.

frog face Broadening and flattening of the nose, imparting to the face a froglike appearance.

hatchet face MYOPATHIC FACIES.

hippocratic face FACIES HIPPOCRATICA.

hippopotamus face The facial appearance produced by hyperplasia of the gingiva.

mask face MASKLIKE FACE.

masklike face The expressionless, unblinking facial appearance typical of parkinsonism. Also called *mask face, Parkinson's facies*.

moon face The round face characteristic of Cushing syndrome, with prominent fatty deposits in the temporal fossae and the cheeks. Also called *cushingoid face, cushingoid facies, moon facies*.

face-bow A device attached to the teeth or occlusal rims for recording the position of the hinge axis and transferring it to an articulator.

adjustable axis face-bow A face-bow with condyle rods adjustable in the vertical plane. Also called *kinematic face-bow*.

kinematic face-bow ADJUSTABLE AXIS FACE-BOW.

face-lift A plastic operation to eliminate or greatly decrease wrinkles and sagging of the soft tissues covering the face and neck, thus producing a more youthful appearance. Also called *melocervicoplasty, face-lift operation*.

faceometer An instrument used in the measurement of the face.

facet [French *facette* (dim. of *face* face) a little face] A small, smooth, flat surface, often rounded, on a hard structure, such as bone.

acromial facet FACIES ARTICULARIS ACROMIALIS CLAVICULAE.

anterior articular facet of axis FACIES ARTICULARIS ANTERIOR AXIS.

anterior articular facet of talus FACIES ARTICULARIS CALCANEA ANTERIOR TALI.

anterior calcaneal facet **1** FACIES ARTICULARIS CALCANEA ANTERIOR TALI. **2** FACIES ARTICULARIS TALARIS ANTERIOR CALCANEI.

anterior costal facet FACIES ARTICULARIS TUBERCULI COSTAE.

anteromedial articular facet of talus Either facies articularis calcanea anterior tali or facies articularis talaris anterior calcanei. An outmoded and incorrect term.

articular facet A small, smooth surface located on a bone at the site of articulation with another structure and covered with articular cartilage.

articular facet of anterior arch of atlas FOVEA DENTIS ATLANTIS.

articular facets for rib cartilages INCISURAE COSTALES STERNI.

auricular facet of iliac bone FACIES AURICULARIS OSSIS ILII.

auricular facet of sacrum FACIES AURICULARIS OSSIS SACRI.

circular articular facet of atlas FOVEA DENTIS ATLANTIS.

clavicular facet INCISURA CLAVICULARIS STERNI.

costal articular facet Any of three facets: (1) fovea costalis inferior; (2) fovea costalis superior; (3) fovea costalis processus transversus.

costal facets of sternum   INCISURAE COSTALES STERNI.

costal facet of transverse process   FOVEA COSTALIS PROCESSUS TRANSVERSUS.

fibular articular facet of tibia   FACIES ARTICULARIS FIBULARIS TIBIAE.

inferior articular facet of atlas   FACIES ARTICULARIS INFERIOR ATLANTIS.

inferior costal facet   FACIES ARTICULARIS TUBERCULI COSTAE.

internal malleolar facet of tibia   FACIES ARTICULARIS MALLEOLI TIBIAE.

lateral external facet of patella   The lateral facet of the articular surface of the patella which articulates with the lateral slope of the patellar surface of the femur in extension of the knee and with the lateral condyle in extreme flexion. An outmoded term.

lateral internal facet of patella   The medial facet of the articular surface of the patella which articulates with the medial slope of the patellar surface of the femur in extension of the knee. The medial part of the medial facet articulates with the medial condyle of the femur in extreme flexion. An outmoded term.

lateral malleolar facet of talus   FACIES MALLEOLARIS LATERALIS TALI.

lateral facets of sternum   INCISURAE COSTALES STERNI.

Lenoir's facet   A narrow articular facet on the medial edge of the patella for the lateral margin of the medial condyle of the femur in extreme flexion.

locked facets of spine   A dislocation of the zygapophyseal joints, with complete overlapping of the joint surfaces. It most commonly occurs in the cervical spine.

medial malleolar facet of talus   FACIES MALLEOLARIS MEDIALIS TALI.

middle articular facet of talus   FACIES ARTICULARIS CALCANEA MEDIA TALI.

middle facet of patella   The central, ridged portion and adjacent part of the medial facet of the articular surface of the patella. It does not come into contact with the medial condyle of the femur in extreme flexion of the knee but faces the intercondylar fossa. An outmoded term.

posterior articular facet of talus   FACIES ARTICULARIS CALCANEA POSTERIOR TALI.

posterior calcaneal facet   Either facies articularis calcanea posterior tali or facies articularis talaris posterior calcanei.

posterior costal facet   FACIES ARTICULARIS CAPITIS COSTAE.

posterior medial facet of calcaneus   FACIES ARTICULARIS TALARIS MEDIA CALCANEI.

prestyloid facet of fibula   A small, rough, triangular or semilunar surface that is situated on the anterior margin of the apex of the head of the fibula and on the anterior part of the head of the fibula. It provides attachment for the fibular collateral ligament and, laterally, the tendon of insertion of the biceps femoris muscle. An outmoded term.

squatting facet   An adventitious articular facet found on the anterior aspect of the lower end of the tibia, with a reciprocal facet on the neck of the talus. It is found in individuals who habitually adopt a squatting position.

sternal articular facet of clavicle   FACIES ARTICULARIS STERNALIS CLAVICULAE.

superior articular facet of atlas   FACIES ARTICULARIS SUPERIOR ATLANTIS.

superior costal facet   FACIES ARTICULARIS CAPITIS COSTAE.

superior costal facet of vertebra   FOVEA COSTALIS SUPERIOR.

facet for tubercle of rib   FOVEA COSTALIS PROCESSUS TRANSVERSUS.

wear facet   A flattened polished surface of a tooth produced by grinding contact between occluding surfaces.

facetectomy   [FACET + -ECTOMY]   Excision of an articular facet.

facial   Pertaining to the face.

facies

facies   [L, shape, form, face]   **1** [NA] The face.   **2** [NA] A surface of a structure, organ, or part of the body.   **3** A facial expression.

facies abdominalis   A grimace associated with colicky abdominal pain.

acromegalic facies   The enlarged face characteristic of acromegaly, with increased length (due chiefly to lengthening of the maxilla), prominent frontal bosses, prominent zygomas, prognathism, increased size of the nose and ears, and an overall aspect of increased mass.

adenoid facies   The facial expression often observed in children with nasal obstruction resulting from adenoid hypertrophy and characterized by mouth breathing and a vacant, dull expression. Also called *adenoid face.*

facies anterior antebrachii   REGIO ANTEBRACHIALIS ANTERIOR.

facies anterior brachii   REGIO BRACHIALIS ANTERIOR.

facies anterior corneae   [NA] The broad, elliptical, outer surface of the cornea which is covered by epithelium and faces the eyelids. Also called *anterior surface of cornea.*

facies anterior cruris   REGIO CRURALIS ANTERIOR.

facies anterior dentium premolarium et molarium   The mesially directed surface of premolar and molar teeth.

facies anterior femoris   REGIO FEMORALIS ANTERIOR.

facies anterior glandulae suprarenalis   [NA] The anterior, or ventral, surface of the adrenal gland, that of the right being in contact with the inferior vena cava and the bare area of the liver, while that of the left is related to the stomach through the omental bursa, and to the pancreas and splenic artery directly. Also called *anterior surface of suprarenal gland.*

facies anterior iridis   [NA] The outer surface of the iris which faces the cornea, forms part of the posterior wall of the anterior chamber of the eye, and extends from the pupillary border to its junction with the ciliary body. It comprises the annulus iridis major and annulus iridis minor and presents delicate, sinuous radiations caused by blood vessels shining through it. It is covered by the endothelium of the anterior chamber in infancy. Also called *anterior surface of iris, anterior limiting layer of iris.*

facies anterior lateralis humeri   [NA] The anterolateral surface of the humerus, extending between the anterior and lateral margins, presenting the deltoid tuberosity and a groove for the radial nerve, and providing partial attachment for the brachialis muscle.

facies anterior lentis   [NA] The outer surface of the lens which faces the anterior chamber of the eye and is in contact with the pupillary margin of the iris. It is covered by a single layer of epithelium which is bounded by the capsule. Also called *anterior surface of lens.*

facies anterior maxillae   [NA] The surface of the body of maxilla that is directed anterolaterally. Its medial margin forms the nasal notch, which ends anteroinferiorly in the anterior nasal spine, and laterally it is separated from the infratemporal surface by the zygomatic process. Superiorly, the infraorbital margin separates it from the orbital surface, and just below the margin is the infraorbital foramen. Above the incisor teeth its surface shows the incisive and canine fossae.

facies anterior medialis humeri [NA] The anteromedial surface of the humerus, situated between the anterior and medial margins. Its upper third forms the floor of the intertubercular sulcus where the latissimus dorsi muscle is inserted, while near its middle the coracobrachialis muscle is inserted, and the rest of the surface provides partial origin for the brachialis muscle. Also called *anteromedial surface of humerus.*

facies anterior palpebrarum [NA] The outer surface of the eyelids, which is formed by skin and meets the posterior surface at the free margin of each eyelid. There the thin skin is continuous with the palpebral conjunctiva. Also called *anterior surface of eyelids.*

facies anterior pancreatis [NA] The slightly concave surface of the pancreas that lies between the anterior and superior margins and faces anterosuperiorly to come into contact with the posteroinferior surface of the stomach through the omental bursa. Also called *anterior surface of pancreas.*

facies anterior partis petrosae ossis temporalis [NA] The somewhat triangular anterior, or superior, surface of the petrous part of the temporal bone that forms part of the floor of the middle cranial fossa. Posterior to its apex, its major features include the trigeminal impression, grooves for the greater and the lesser petrosal nerves, the arcuate eminence, and the roof of the tympanic cavity. Also called *facies anterior pyramidis ossis temporalis.*

facies anterior patellae [NA] The convex anterior surface of the patella, marked by longitudinal striations and foramina of nutrient vessels, over which fibers of the common tendon of the quadriceps femoris muscle are prolonged into the ligamentum patellae. It is separated from the skin by a bursa.

facies anterior prostatae [NA] The convex anterior surface that extends from the base to the apex of the prostate and lies behind the pubic symphysis from which it is separated by the prostatic and vesical venous plexuses and some fat and areolar tissue. Superiorly it is attached to the pubic bones by the puboprostatic ligaments, and inferiorly the urethra pierces it near the apex.

facies anterior pyramidis ossis temporalis FACIES ANTERIOR PARTIS PETROSAE OSSIS TEMPORALIS.

facies anterior radii [NA] The anterior surface of the radius, situated between the anterior and the interosseous margins and providing attachment on the proximal two-thirds for the origin of the flexor pollicis longus muscle, and in the distal third for the insertion of the pronator quadratus muscle. The nutrient foramen is just below the proximal third. Also called *facies volaris radii.*

facies anterior renis [NA] The convex surface of the kidney that faces anterolaterally and has different relations to organs and vessels on the two sides. On the right side it is covered by peritoneum where it is related to the liver and coils of small intestine, but is bare against the suprarenal gland, descending part of the duodenum, and right colic flexure. On the left side, it is covered by peritoneum where it is related to the stomach, spleen, jejunum, and left colic flexure, but it is bare in relation to the body of the pancreas, the splenic vessels, and left suprarenal gland. Also called *anterior surface of kidney.*

facies anterior ulnae [NA] The anterior surface of the ulna, situated between the anterior and the interosseous margins and grooved in its proximal three-fourths for the origin of the flexor digitorum profundus muscle, while distally it is narrow and convex for the origin of the pronator quadratus muscle. The nutrient foramen is just below the proximal third. Also called *facies volaris ulnae.*

facies anterolateralis cartilaginis arytenoideae [NA] The convex, irregular anterolateral surface of the arytenoid cartilage, crossed sinuously from the apex to the vocal process by the arcuate crest, separating the fovea triangularis above from the fovea oblongata below.

facies articulares inferiores vertebrarum The oval, concave surfaces on the inferior articular processes of the vertebrae that are directed inferiorly, anteriorly and, often, medially. Also called *inferior articular sinus of vertebrae* (outmoded).

facies articulares superiores vertebrarum The flat surfaces on the superior articular processes of the vertebrae that are directed superiorly, posteriorly, and laterally in a plane slightly anterior to that of the inferior articular surfaces.

facies articularis acromialis claviculae [NA] The smooth, oval articular surface at the lateral end of the clavicle, directed laterally and downward for the articular surface of the acromion. The capsule of the acromioclavicular joint is attached to its margin. Also called *acromial articular surface of clavicle, acromial facet.*

facies articularis acromialis [NA] The small, oval articular surface on the medial border of the acromion of scapula for the acromial articular surface of the clavicle.

facies articularis anterior axis [NA] The small, oval facet on the anterior surface of the dens of the axis vertebra for articulation with the fovea dentis on the posterior surface of the anterior arch of atlas. Also called *anterior articular facet of axis, facies articularis anterior epistrophei, anterior articular process of axis, anterior articular sinus of axis* (outmoded).

facies articularis anterior calcanei FACIES ARTICULARIS TALARIS ANTERIOR CALCANEI.

facies articularis anterior epistrophei FACIES ARTICULARIS ANTERIOR AXIS.

facies articularis arytenoidea cartilaginis cricoideae [NA] An oval, convex articular facet on each superolateral aspect of the posterior surface at the upper border of the cricoid cartilage that articulates with the base of the arytenoid cartilage.

facies articularis calcanea anterior tali [NA] A small, oval articular facet on the plantar aspect of the head of talus that rests on the plantar calcaneonavicular ligament and on the anterior articular surface on the upper aspect of the calcaneus. Also called *anterior calcaneal facet, anterior articular facet of talus.*

facies articularis calcanea media tali The elongated, convex middle calcaneal facet on the inferomedial aspect of the articular head of talus that articulates with the sustentaculum tali of the calcaneus. Also called *middle articular facet of talus.*

facies articularis calcanea posterior tali [NA] The concave, oblong articular surface set transversely across the inferior surface of the body of talus for articulation with a corresponding articular surface on the superior surface of the calcaneus in the subtalar joint. Also called *posterior articular facet of talus.*

facies articularis capitis costae [NA] The articular surface on the head of a rib that is divided by a crest into two convex facets that articulate with the bodies of two adjacent vertebrae. The articular surfaces of the heads of the first, tenth, eleventh, and twelfth ribs are usually not divided. Also called *facies articularis capituli costae, posterior costal facet, superior costal facet.*

facies articularis capitis fibulae [NA] The circular articular surface on the medial side of the head of fibula that is directed anterosuperiorly for the lateral condyle of the tibia in the tibiofibular joint. Also called *facies articularis capituli fibulae.*

facies articularis capituli costae FACIES ARTICULARIS CAPITIS COSTAE.

facies articularis capituli fibulae FACIES ARTICULARIS CAPITIS FIBULAE.

facies articularis carpi radii [NA] The concave, quadrilateral articular surface at the distal extremity of the radius, divided by a small vertical ridge so that the medial quadrangular portion articulates with the lunate bone and the lateral triangular portion articulates with the scaphoid bone. Also called *carpal articular surface of radius.*

facies articularis cartilaginis arytenoideae [NA] A small articular surface on the concave base of the arytenoid cartilage for articulation with a facet on the superolateral aspect of the posterior surface of the cricoid cartilage.

facies articularis cuboidea calcanei [NA] The concavoconvex, quadrangular anterior surface of the calcaneus that articulates with the cuboid bone to form the calcaneocuboid joint. Also called *cuboid articular surface of calcaneus.*

facies articularis fibularis tibiae [NA] The flat, circular articular surface on the posterolateral aspect of the lateral condyle of tibia, directed posteroinferiorly for the head of the fibula to form the tibiofibular joint. Also called *fibular articular facet of tibia.*

facies articularis fossae mandibularis FACIES ARTICULARIS OSSIS TEMPORALIS.

facies articularis inferior atlantis The circular and slightly hollowed surface on the inferior aspect of the lateral mass of the atlas, facing medially and downward to articulate with a similar superior articular facet on the axis in the lateral atlantoaxial joint. Also called *inferior articular fovea of atlas, fovea articularis inferior atlantis, inferior articular facet of atlas, inferior articular fossa of atlas, inferior articular pit of atlas.*

facies articularis inferior tibiae [NA] The smooth, quadrangular surface, wider in front than behind and concave anteroposteriorly, on the inferior aspect of the distal extremity of the tibia, and articulating with the body of the talus. Medially it is continuous with the malleolar articular surface. Also called *inferior articular surface of tibia.*

facies articularis malleoli fibulae [NA] The anterosuperior part of the medial surface of the lateral malleolus of fibula, triangular-shaped and convex and articulating with the lateral side of the talus. Also called *lateral malleolar fovea of fibula, fovea of lateral malleolus.*

facies articularis malleoli tibiae [NA] The smooth lateral surface of the medial malleolus of tibia that articulates with the medial side of the talus. It is continuous with the inferior articular surface of tibia. Also called *internal malleolar facet of tibia.*

facies articularis media calcanei FACIES ARTICULARIS TALARIS MEDIA CALCANEI.

facies articularis navicularis tali [NA] The oval and convex anterior part of the large articular surface on the head of the talus, for articulation with the navicular bone.

facies articularis ossis temporalis [NA] The anterior, articular portion of the mandibular fossa, oval and deeply concave and formed by the squamous part of temporal bone, extending anteriorly onto the articular tubercle and articulating with the articular disk of the temporomandibular joint. Also called *facies articularis fossae mandibularis.*

facies articularis ossium Any articular surface of a bone; a joint surface.

facies articularis patellae [NA] The upper part of the posterior surface of the patella, divided into two angulated surfaces by a vertical ridge, the lateral surface being broader and deeper than the medial, both of which articulate with the respective condyles of the femur. The ridge, also covered with hyaline cartilage, articulates with a corresponding groove on the patellar surface of the femur.

facies articularis posterior axis [NA] A smooth, grooved surface on the posterior aspect of the dens of axis that abuts against the transverse ligament of the atlas. Also called *facies articularis posterior epistrophei.*

facies articularis posterior calcanei FACIES ARTICULARIS TALARIS POSTERIOR CALCANEI.

facies articularis posterior epistrophei FACIES ARTICULARIS POSTERIOR AXIS.

facies articularis sternalis claviculae [NA] The somewhat triangular surface on the sternal end of the clavicle, directed inferomedially to articulate with the clavicular notch of the manubrium sterni through the interposed articular disk attached to the superior margin of the surface. Also called *sternal articular facet of clavicle.*

facies articularis superior atlantis [NA] The elongated, bean-shaped, concave articular facet on the superior surface of each lateral mass of the atlas for articulation with a corresponding convex occipital condyle in the atlanto-occipital joint on each side. Also called *fovea articularis superior atlantis, superior articular pit of atlas, superior articular surface of atlas, superior articular facet of atlas, superior articular fossa of atlas, condyloid fossa of atlas, superior articular sinus of atlas* (outmoded), *glenoid cavity of atlas* (outmoded).

facies articularis superior tibiae [NA] The expanded, oval articular surface on the proximal extremity of the tibia, subdivided by a median nonarticular intercondylar area into medial and lateral articular surfaces for the condyles of the femur. Also called *condyloid surface of tibia, superior articular surface of tibia.*

facies articularis talaris anterior calcanei [NA] The most anterior of the three articular surfaces on the superior aspect of the calcaneus that articulate with three corresponding facets on the overlying talus. The small, oval facet is located at the junction of the sustentaculum tali with the anterior portion of the calcaneus. Also called *anterior talar articular surface of calcaneus, facies articularis anterior calcanei, anterior calcaneal facet.*

facies articularis talaris media calcanei [NA] The middle facet of the three articular surfaces on the superior aspect of the calcaneus that articulate with three corresponding facets on the overlying talus. It is larger than the anterior facet, behind which it is located on the sustentaculum tali. Also called *middle talar articular surface of calcaneus, facies articularis media calcanei, posterior medial facet of calcaneus.*

facies articularis talaris posterior calcanei [NA] The most posterior of the three articular surfaces on the superior aspect of the calcaneus that articulate with three corresponding facets on the overlying talus. Large and oval, it is located in the center of the superior surface, separated from the middle facet by the sulcus calcanei. Also called *posterior talar articular surface of calcaneus, facies articularis posterior calcanei.*

facies articularis thyroidea cartilaginis cricoideae [NA] A circular articular facet facing posterolaterally on the cricoid cartilage, at the junction of the arch with the lamina, for articulation with the inferior horn of the thyroid cartilage on each side. Also called *eminentia lateralis cartilaginis cricoideae* (outmoded).

facies articularis tuberculi costae [NA] A small, raised, oval facet on the medial portion of the tubercle of a rib for articulation with the transverse process of the numerically corresponding vertebra. Also called *anterior costal facet, inferior costal facet.*

facies auricularis ossis ilii [NA] The rough, ear-shaped surface at the anteroinferior end of the sacropelvic surface of the ilium that articulates with the auricular surface of the sacrum in the sacroiliac joint. Also called *facies auricularis ossis ilium, auricular facet of iliac bone.*

facies auricularis ossis ilium FACIES AURICULARIS OSSIS ILII.

facies auricularis ossis sacri [NA] The ear-shaped articular surface on the upper part of the lateral surface of the lateral portion of the sacrum that articulates with the auricular surface of the ilium in the sacroiliac joint. Its position corresponds to the costal elements of the first, second, and third sacral segments.

Also called *lateral articular surface of sacral bone* (outmoded), *auricular plane of sacral bone, auricular facet of sacrum.*

facies bovina   A cowlike facial appearance owing to orbital hypertelorism. It is seen in cases of the Crouzon syndrome. Also called *bovine face, cow face.*

facies brachialis anterior   REGIO BRACHIALIS ANTERIOR.

facies brachialis posterior   REGIO BRACHIALIS POSTERIOR.

facies buccalis dentis   The buccally directed surface of a posterior tooth.

facies cerebralis   The internal surface, adjacent to the brain, of any cranial bone.

facies cerebralis alae magnae   FACIES CEREBRALIS ALAE MAJORIS.

facies cerebralis alae majoris   [NA] The concave inner surface of the greater wing of the sphenoid bone, forming part of the middle cranial fossa and supporting the anterior part of the temporal lobe of cerebrum. Among the numerous foramina piercing it are the foramen rotundum, foramen ovale, and foramen spinosum. Also called *facies cerebralis alae magnae.*

facies cerebralis ossis frontalis   FACIES INTERNA OSSIS FRONTALIS.

facies cerebralis ossis parietalis   FACIES INTERNA OSSIS PARIETALIS.

facies cerebralis partis squamosae ossis temporalis   [NA] The concave internal surface of the squamous part of the temporal bone, its depressions corresponding to the convolutions of the temporal lobe and its grooves being formed by branches of the middle meningeal vessels. Also called *facies cerebralis squamae temporalis.*

facies cerebralis squamae temporalis   FACIES CEREBRALIS PARTIS SQUAMOSAE OSSIS TEMPORALIS.

facies colica lienis   FACIES COLICA SPLENIS.

facies colica splenis   [NA] The flattened impression on the lateral extremity of the visceral surface of the spleen which is related to the left colic flexure and phrenicocolic ligament. Also called *colic impression of spleen, colic surface of spleen, facies colica lienis.*

facies contactus dentis   [NA] A tooth surface directed toward an adjacent tooth in the same dental arch.

facies convexa cerebri   FACIES SUPEROLATERALIS CEREBRI.

facies costalis pulmonis   [NA] The convex outer surface of each lung. It corresponds to the inner surface of the thoracic wall and is in contact with the costal pleura. Also called *costal surface of lung.*

facies costalis scapulae   [NA] The triangular concave surface of the scapula that faces anteromedially toward the thorax and forms the subscapular fossa, the surface of which is ridged for the attachment of tendinous intersections of the subscapularis muscle. Near the medial margin is a longitudinal ridge for attachment of the serratus anterior muscle. Also called *anterior surface of scapula, costal surface of scapula.*

facies cubitalis anterior   REGIO CUBITALIS ANTERIOR.

facies cubitalis posterior   REGIO CUBITALIS POSTERIOR.

cushingoid facies   MOON FACE.

facies diaphragmatica cordis   [NA] The inferior surface of the heart, separated from the sternocostal surface by the right margin and resting on the central tendon and part of the left muscular portion of the diaphragm, from which it is separated by the pericardium. It comprises mostly the left ventricle and some of the right ventricle which are separated from the base by the coronary sinus. Also called *diaphragmatic surface of heart.*

facies diaphragmatica hepatis   [NA] The extensive convex surface of the liver, which is related to the diaphragm and is divided into anterior, posterior, right, and superior parts. Also called *diaphragmatic surface of liver, parietal surface of liver.*

facies diaphragmatica lienis   FACIES DIAPHRAGMATICA SPLENIS.

facies diaphragmatica pulmonis   [NA] The concave, semilunar inferior surface of each lung which rests on the diaphragm and is separated from it by pleura. The diaphragm separates this surface of the right lung from the right lobe of the liver and that of the left lung from the left lobe of the liver, the fundus of the stomach, and the spleen. Also called *diaphragmatic surface of lung.*

facies diaphragmatica splenis   [NA] The convex, and largest, surface of the spleen. It is directed superiorly and posterolaterally to the left and is related to the inferior surface of the diaphragm that separates it from the left pleura and lung and the ninth through eleventh ribs. Also called *diaphragmatic surface of spleen, facies diaphragmatica lienis.*

facies digitales dorsales manus   [NA] The posterior, or dorsal, surfaces of the fingers.

facies digitales ventrales manus   [NA] The anterior, or palmar, surfaces of the fingers. Also called *facies volares digitorum manus, facies ventrales digitorum manus.*

facies distalis dentis   [NA] A distally directed surface of a tooth.

facies dolorosa   The drawn appearance of the face of an individual suffering pain.

facies dorsales digitorum pedis   The superior, or dorsal, surfaces of the toes.

facies dorsalis antebrachii   REGIO ANTEBRACHIALIS POSTERIOR.

facies dorsalis ossis sacri   [NA] The triangular and markedly convex posterior surface of the sacrum, ridged by the median, intermediate, and lateral sacral crests, perforated by four dorsal sacral foramina on either side, and providing origin for the erector spinae and multifidus muscles. At its base are two superior articular processes, and at its apex is the sacral hiatus bounded by the cornua. Also called *posterior surface of sacrum.*

facies dorsalis radii   FACIES POSTERIOR RADII.

facies dorsalis scapulae   FACIES POSTERIOR SCAPULAE.

facies dorsalis ulnae   FACIES POSTERIOR ULNAE.

facies externa ossis frontalis   [NA] The convex, smooth outer surface of the frontal bone, marked by the frontal eminence on each side, and occasionally by a remnant of the frontal, or metopic, suture centrally. Also called *facies frontalis ossis frontalis, outer table of frontal bone* (outmoded).

facies externa ossis parietalis   [NA] The convex, smooth outer surface of the parietal bone, crossed transversely below the center by the superior and the inferior temporal lines, above which is the bulge of the parietal eminence. Also called *facies parietalis ossis parietalis.*

facies facialis dentis   FACIES VESTIBULARIS DENTIS.

facies fibularis cruris   FACIES LATERALIS CRURIS.

facies frontalis ossis frontalis   FACIES EXTERNA OSSIS FRONTALIS.

facies gastrica lienis   FACIES GASTRICA SPLENIS.

facies gastrica splenis   [NA] The broad and deeply concave area on the visceral surface of the spleen. It is directed anterosuperiorly and medially and is related to the posterior surface of the stomach through the greater sac of the peritoneum. Near its lower margin is the fissure for the hilum of the spleen. Also called *gastric surface of spleen, facies gastrica lienis, gastric impression of spleen.*

facies glutea ossis ilii   [NA] The outer surface of the ala of ilium, convex anteriorly and concave posteriorly, divided into four areas by posterior, inferior, and anterior gluteal lines, the upper three areas being for attachments of the gluteus maximus, medius, and minimus muscles. Also called *dorsum ilii, external iliac fossa* (outmoded).

facies hepatica   The drawn facial expression and appearance of a person with a chronic disorder of the liver, usually characterized as sunken eyes and cheeks, a sallow complexion with dilated capillaries, and spider angiomata.

facies hippocratica A facial appearance associated with impending death. It is characterized by dull, sunken eyes; hollow temples and cheeks; and drooping lower jaw. Also called *hippocratic face*.

Hutchinson's facies The appearance of congenital syphilis, including frontal bony prominence, sunken bridge of the nose, and deformed peg-shaped incisor teeth.

facies inferior cerebri [NA] The basal surface of the cerebrum. Also called *basis encephali, basis cerebri, base of brain.*

facies inferior hemispherii cerebelli The inferior surface of the cerebellar hemispheres in the posterior cranial fossa.

facies inferior hemispherii cerebri The basal cerebral surfaces lying upon the anterior and middle cranial fossae and the tentorium cerebelli. Also called *base of cerebrum.*

facies inferior hepatis An outmoded term for FACIES VISCERALIS HEPATIS.

facies inferior linguae [NA] The inferior surface of the freely mobile body of the tongue that faces the floor of the mouth. It is covered by thin, smooth mucous membrane that forms the frenulum in the midline, on each side of which the lingual vein produces an elevation between it and the plica fimbriata.

facies inferior pancreatis [NA] The narrow surface of the body of the pancreas which faces inferiorly and is covered with peritoneum of the posteroinferior layer of the transverse mesocolon. It is related to the duodenojejunal flexure, jejunum, and left colic flexure. Also called *inferior surface of pancreas.*

facies inferior partis petrosae ossis temporalis [NA] The inferior surface of the petrous part of the temporal bone, forming an irregular section of the external surface of the base of skull, the main features of which are, anteroposteriorly, the circular opening of the carotid canal, the deep depression of the jugular fossa, the styloid process, and the stylomastoid foramen. There are numerous foramina and grooves for nerves and vessels, as well as attachments of muscles and fascia. Also called *facies inferior pyramidis ossis temporalis, basilar part of temporal bone* (outmoded).

facies inferior pyramidis ossis temporalis FACIES INFERIOR PARTIS PETROSAE OSSIS TEMPORALIS.

facies inferolateralis prostatae [NA] The convex inferolateral surface on each side of the prostate, related to the superior surface of the levator ani muscle, from which it is separated by the fibrous tissue forming the prostatic sheath and containing the prostatic plexus of veins.

facies infratemporalis maxillae [NA] The convex surface of the maxilla facing laterally and posteriorly and forming the anterior wall of the infratemporal fossa. It is separated from the anterior surface by the zygomatic process and a vertical ridge extending down to the alveolar arch at the first molar tooth. At the posteroinferior angle is the prominent maxillary tuberosity, above which is a smooth surface forming the anterior boundary of the pterygopalatine fossa, and near the middle are two or three foramina for the posterior superior alveolar nerves and vessels. Also called *infratemporal surface of maxilla.*

facies interlobaris pulmonis [NA] The surface of each lobe of the lung which faces either the oblique or the horizontal fissure. Also called *interlobar surface of lung.*

facies interna ossis frontalis [NA] The concave internal surface of the frontal bone, divided in the midline by the longitudinal groove of superior sagittal sinus, below which is the frontal crest terminating at the foramen cecum. On each side are digitate impressions of the convolutions of the frontal lobes. There are small vascular furrows, and near the parietal margin are depressions of arachnoid granulations. Also called *facies*

cerebralis ossis frontalis, inner table of frontal bone (outmoded), *frontal fossa.*

facies interna ossis parietalis [NA] The concave internal surface of the parietal bone, having light digitate impressions and marked vascular grooves produced by the middle meningeal vessels. Along the superior margin is part of the groove of the superior sagittal sinus, adjacent to which are pits for arachnoid granulations. Also called *facies cerebralis ossis parietalis.*

facies intestinalis The surface of any organ, such as the uterus, that faces or is in contact with the intestines.

facies intestinalis uteri [NA] The convex posterior surface of the uterus adjacent to the intestine.

facies labialis dentis The labially directed surface of an anterior tooth.

facies laterales digitorum manus The outer, or lateral, surfaces of the fingers along which digital vessels and nerves course. Also called *facies radiales digitorum manus* (outmoded), *margines radiales digitorum manus, radial margins of fingers.*

facies laterales digitorum pedis The outer, or lateral, surfaces of the toes along which the digital vessels and nerves course. Also called *margines laterales digitorum pedis* (outmoded).

facies lateralis brachii The outer, or lateral, surface of the arm between the acromial angle and the elbow joint.

facies lateralis cruris The outer, or lateral, surface of the leg extending from the knee joint to the lateral malleolus. Also called *facies fibularis cruris.*

facies lateralis dentium incisivorum et caninorum The distally directed surface of incisor and canine teeth.

facies lateralis femoris The outer, or lateral, surface of the thigh, flattened due to the presence of the iliotibial tract.

facies lateralis fibulae [NA] The surface between the anterior and the posterior margins of the fibula, twisted and often deeply grooved for the origin of the peroneus longus on the proximal two-thirds and that of the peroneus brevis on the distal two-thirds.

facies lateralis ossis zygomatici [NA] The convex outer surface of the zygomatic bone on which is located the zygomaticofacial foramen and which provides for the origin of both zygomatic muscles. Also called *facies malaris ossis zygomatici.*

facies lateralis ovarii The surface of the lateral portion of the ovary which faces the lateral pelvic wall. An obsolete term.

facies lateralis radii [NA] The convex outer surface of the radius on which the supinator muscle is inserted proximally and the pronator teres muscle near the middle. It is smooth distally where it is crossed by the radial extensors of the forearm and by the abductor pollicis longus and extensor pollicis brevis muscles.

facies lateralis testis [NA] The convex, smooth lateral surface of the testis situated between the anterior and posterior borders and invested by the visceral layer of tunica vaginalis. Near the upper pole the appendix testis may be attached.

facies lateralis tibiae [NA] The lateral surface of the tibia lying between the anterior and the interosseous margins and providing attachment on its proximal two thirds for the tibialis anterior muscle. Also called *external border of tibia.*

leonine facies The nodulation, thickening, and fissuring of facial skin in lepromatous leprosy that imparts a lionlike appearance. Also called *leontiasis* (obsolete), *facies leontina, facies leprosa.*

facies leontina LEONINE FACIES.

facies leprosa LEONINE FACIES.

facies lingualis dentis [NA] A lingually directed surface of a tooth.

facies lunata acetabuli [NA] The horseshoe-shaped articular portion of the acetabulum, deficient inferiorly and on which the femur articulates in the hip joint. The synovial membrane is attached to its medial margin, and the acetabular labrum to its lateral edge. Also called *articular surface of acetabulum.*

facies malaris ossis zygomatici FACIES LATERALIS OSSIS ZYGOMATICI.

facies malleolaris lateralis tali [NA] The lateral surface of the body of the talus, having a large triangular facet for articulation with the lateral malleolus and terminating inferiorly in the lateral process. Also called *lateral malleolar facet of talus.*

facies malleolaris medialis tali [NA] The medial surface of the body of the talus, the upper part of which has a horizontal, comma-shaped surface covered with cartilage, continuous with the superior surface, for articulation with the medial malleolus of tibia, while the lower part has numerous vascular foramina and gives attachment to deep fibers of the medial collateral ligament of the ankle joint. Also called *medial malleolar facet of talus.*

Marshall Hall's facies The facies seen in hydrocephalus, characterized by broadening of the forehead with increased prominence of the frontal bones, giving the face a triangular appearance.

facies masticatoria dentis A tooth surface which is directed towards the opposing dental arch.

facies maxillaris alae majoris [NA] A small area on the anteroinferior aspect of the greater wing of the sphenoid bone, located at the base of the lateral lamina of the pterygoid process and forming part of the posterior wall of the pterygopalatine fossa, where it is perforated by the foramen rotundum. Also called *facies sphenomaxillaris alae magnae.*

facies maxillaris laminae perpendicularis ossis palatini [NA] The irregular lateral surface of the perpendicular plate of the palatine bone, divided by a vertical groove that superiorly forms the medial wall of the pterygopalatine fossa and inferiorly becomes the greater palatine sulcus, which is converted into a canal by a similar groove on the nasal surface of the maxilla articulating with it. The portion anterior to the groove overlaps the orifice of the maxillary sinus, while that posterior to the groove articulates with the maxilla and the pterygoid process. Also called *facies maxillaris partis perpendicularis ossis palatini* (outmoded).

facies maxillaris partis perpendicularis ossis palatini An outmoded term for FACIES MAXILLARIS LAMINAE PERPENDICULARIS OSSIS PALATINI.

facies mediales digitorum manus The medial surfaces of the fingers along which digital vessels and nerves course. Also called *facies ulnares digitorum manus, margines ulnares digitorum manus* (outmoded), *ulnar margins of fingers.*

facies mediales digitorum pedis The medial surfaces of the toes along which digital vessels and nerves course. Also called *margines mediales digitorum pedis* (outmoded).

facies medialis brachii The inner, or medial, surface of the arm from the apex of the axilla to the elbow joint.

facies medialis cartilaginis arytenoideae [NA] The narrow, flat medial surface of each arytenoid cartilage, covered by mucous membrane and lying parallel to each other, forming the intercartilaginous part of the rima glottidis between their lower margins.

facies medialis cerebri [NA] The median surface of the cerebral cortex facing the midline of the sagittal sulcus and underlying the falx cerebri. Also called *facies medialis hemispherii cerebri.*

facies medialis cruris The inner, or medial, surface of the leg between the knee and the ankle joints. Also called *facies tibialis cruris.*

facies medialis dentium incisivorum et caninorum The mesially directed surface of incisor and canine teeth.

facies medialis femoris The inner, or medial, surface of the thigh.

facies medialis fibulae [NA] The surface of the fibula between the anterior and interosseous margins, very narrow proximally but broad distally, providing origin for the extensor digitorum longus, peroneus tertius, and extensor hallucis longus muscles.

facies medialis hemispherii cerebri FACIES MEDIALIS CEREBRI.

facies medialis ovarii [NA] The rounded medial surface of the ovary, largely overlapped by the fimbriated end of the uterine tube and the mesosalpinx and partly related to a loop of intestine.

facies medialis pulmonis FACIES MEDIASTINALIS PULMONIS.

facies medialis testis [NA] The convex, smooth medial surface of the testis, invested by the visceral layer of the tunica vaginalis and situated between the anterior and posterior borders of the testis. It faces the opposite testis but is also directed anteriorly and inferiorly to some degree.

facies medialis tibiae [NA] The medial surface of tibia, lying between the medial and anterior margins and receiving the tendons of insertion of the sartorius, gracilis, and semitendinosus muscles on its broad proximal end. Most of it is convex and subcutaneous, the distal end being crossed obliquely by the great saphenous vein.

facies medialis ulnae [NA] The smooth, rounded medial surface of the ulna that gives attachment to part of the origin of the flexor digitorum profundus muscle on the proximal two-thirds. Distally it is subcutaneous.

facies mediastinalis pulmonis [NA] The medial concave surface of each lung, related to the mediastinum and containing the hilum of the lung. Anterior to the hilum is the cardiac impression, larger and deeper on the left than on the right lung. Above and behind the hilum of the left lung, the arch of the aorta and descending thoracic aorta are related, respectively, while on the right side are the azygos vein and esophagus, respectively. Also called *mediastinal surface of lung, medial surface of lung, facies medialis pulmonis, pars mediastinalis faciei medialis pulmonis* (outmoded).

facies mesialis dentis [NA] A mesially directed surface of a tooth.

mitral facies The highly colored, slightly cyanotic flush over the malar region in patients with long-standing mitral stenosis. Also called *mitrotricuspid facies.*

mitrotricuspid facies MITRAL FACIES.

mongolian facies Facial abnormalities in the Down syndrome, such as slanted palpebral fissures, small ear lobules, irregular alignment of teeth, and large tongue or lips.

moon facies MOON FACE.

myasthenic facies The facial appearance in myasthenia gravis, characterized usually by bilateral ptosis, drooping and expressionless facial muscles, and, when the patient smiles, a typical myasthenic grimace.

myopathic facies Any of the facial appearances seen in myopathy. The two most characteristic abnormalities of facial appearance are seen in facioscapulohumeral muscular dystrophy, where the affected individual cannot close the eyes and there is a pouting appearance of the lips (tapir mouth), and in dystrophia myotonica, in which there is hollowing of the temporal fossae, bilateral ptosis and a lugubrious expression. Also called *hatchet face.*

myxedematous facies The appearance of the face associated with myxedema, showing a yellowish pallor and puffiness, particularly around the eyes, and producing a general impression of lethargy and sluggishness.

facies nasalis laminae horizontalis ossis palatini [NA] The smooth, concave upper surface of the horizontal plate of the palatine bone that forms the posterior part of the floor of the nasal cavity. Also called *facies nasalis partis horizontalis ossis palatini.*

facies nasalis laminae perpendicularis ossis palatini [NA] The medial surface of the perpendicular plate of the palatine bone that presents the ethmoidal and conchal crests separating three depressions that form part of the walls of the superior, middle, and inferior meatus of the nose. Also called *facies nasalis partis perpendicularis ossis palatini.*

facies nasalis maxillae [NA] The nasal surface of the maxilla that helps to form the lateral wall of the nasal cavity. Posterior to it is a large, irregular gap, or hiatus, leading into the maxillary sinus, just anterior to which is the downward sloping lacrimal groove. More anteriorly on the smooth surface is the conchal crest, above which is the wall of the atrium of the middle meatus, while below is the inferior meatus.

facies nasalis partis horizontalis ossis palatini FACIES NASALIS LAMINAE HORIZONTALIS OSSIS PALATINI.

facies nasalis partis perpendicularis ossis palatini FACIES NASALIS LAMINAE PERPENDICULARIS OSSIS PALATINI.

facies occlusalis dentis [NA] The occlusally directed surface of a posterior tooth.

facies orbitalis alae magnae FACIES ORBITALIS ALAE MAJORIS.

facies orbitalis alae majoris [NA] The quadrilateral anteromedial surface of the greater wing of the sphenoid bone that forms the posterior part of the lateral wall of the orbit. The inferior margin is the posterolateral border of the inferior orbital fissure while its medial margin is the lower border of the superior orbital fissure. Also called *facies orbitalis alae magnae, orbital border of sphenoid bone, orbital surface of sphenoid bone.*

facies orbitalis maxillae [NA] A triangular surface of the maxilla that forms most of the floor of the orbit, which is traversed by the infraorbital groove and canal. Anteriorly it forms the infraorbital margin, and its posterior border forms part of the anterior margin of the inferior orbital fissure. Its medial border presents the lacrimal notch, just lateral to which is the origin of the inferior oblique muscle of the orbit.

facies orbitalis ossis frontalis [NA] The concave, smooth orbital surface of the frontal bone forming most of the roof of the orbital cavity, its anterior edge being the supraorbital margin, just posterior to which on the lateral side is the fossa for the lacrimal gland, while the trochlear fovea, or spine, is on the medial side. On its internal, or cerebral, aspect are impressions produced by the gyri on the inferior surface of the frontal lobe of the cerebrum. Also called *orbital fossa.*

facies orbitalis ossis zygomatici [NA] The concave orbital surface of the zygomatic bone that takes part in the formation of the lateral wall of the orbit, on which are located the zygomatico-orbital foramina. Also called *orbital process of the zygomatic bone* (outmoded).

facies ossea cranii The bony skeleton of the face. Also called *bony face.*

facies palatina laminae horizontalis ossis palatini [NA] The inferior surface of the horizontal plate of the palatine bone, forming the posterior one-fourth of the hard palate with the corresponding surface of the opposite bone, their medial borders meeting at the median palatine suture. Near its posterior margin is the crista palatina for attachment of the tensor veli palatini muscle. Also called *facies palatina partis horizontalis ossis palatini* (outmoded).

facies palatina partis horizontalis ossis palatini An outmoded term for FACIES PALATINA LAMINAE HORIZONTALIS OSSIS PALATINI.

paralytic facies The facial appearance resulting from unilateral or bilateral paralysis of the facial muscles. When unilateral, the eye on the affected side cannot be closed and the affected corner of the mouth droops in comparison with the other side.

facies parietalis ossis parietalis FACIES EXTERNA OSSIS PARIETALIS.

Parkinson's facies MASKLIKE FACE.

facies patellaris femoris [NA] The trochlear surface between and continuous with the articular surfaces of the condyles of the femur anteriorly, for articulation with the patella. It lies in front of the intercondylar fossa, and is separated from the tibial surfaces of the condyles by a shallow, oblique groove on each side. Also called *patellar fossa of femur, trochlea of femur* (outmoded), *patellar incisure of femur* (outmoded).

facies pelvica ossis sacri [NA] The concave anterior surface of the sacrum, directed anteroinferiorly and forming part of the posterior wall of the pelvic cavity. Four central transverse ridges indicate the lines of fusion between the five sacral vertebrae, at the extremities of which are four pelvic sacral foramina on each side. The bars of bone between these foramina represent costal elements fused to the vertebrae. Also called *anterior surface of sacrum.*

facies plantares digitorum pedis The inferior, or plantar, surfaces of the toes.

facies poplitea femoris [NA] The triangular area at the lower end of the posterior surface of the femoral shaft, located between the medial and lateral supracondylar lines that come together at the apex of this area as the linea aspera. This surface forms the upper part of the floor of the popliteal fossa, a pad of fat separating it from the popliteal artery. Also called *planum popliteum femoris, popliteal plane of femur, popliteal triangle of femur.*

facies posterior antebrachii REGIO ANTEBRACHIALIS POSTERIOR.

facies posterior brachii REGIO BRACHIALIS POSTERIOR.

facies posterior cartilaginis arytenoideae [NA] The concave, triangular posterior surface of the arytenoid cartilage, covered by the transverse arytenoid muscle.

facies posterior corneae [NA] The posterior surface of the cornea which faces the anterior chamber of the eye and is lined by the posterior limiting lamina and the endothelium of the anterior chamber. At its periphery it meets the iris at the iridocorneal angle. Also called *posterior surface of cornea.*

facies posterior cruris REGIO CRURALIS POSTERIOR.

facies posterior dentium premolarium et molarium The distally directed surface of premolar and molar teeth.

facies posterior femoris REGIO FEMORALIS POSTERIOR.

facies posterior fibulae [NA] The large surface between the interosseous and posterior margins of the fibula, divided longitudinally into two in its upper two-thirds by the medial crest for the attachment of an intermuscular septum that separates the tibialis posterior muscle arising on its medial side and the soleus and flexor hallucis longus muscles from its posterior side.

facies posterior glandulae suprarenalis [NA] The surface of the suprarenal gland which is directed posteromedially and is related to the diaphragm on each side. Also called *posterior surface of suprarenal gland.*

facies posterior hepatis An outmoded term for PARS POSTERIOR FACIEI DIAPHRAGMATICAE HEPATIS.

facies posterior humeri [NA] The dorsal surface of the humerus lying between the lateral and medial margins, divided into two by the oblique, shallow groove of the radial nerve that runs from superomedial to inferolateral across the middle third. Above the groove is the linear origin of the lateral head of the triceps muscle, while the large, triangular area below it provides origin for the medial head of the triceps muscle.

facies posterior iridis [NA] The surface of the iris which forms the anterior wall of the posterior chamber of the eye and rests against the anterior surface of the lens near the pupil. It is covered with a double layer of heavily pigmented epithelium, or the iridial portion of the retina, the outer, or anterior, layer of which becomes differentiated into smooth muscles, namely, the sphincter pupillae and the dilator pupillae. Also called *posterior surface of iris.*

facies posterior lentis [NA] The posterior surface of the lens which rests in the hyaloid fossa of the vitreous body. At its periphery some of the zonular fibers are attached. Also called *posterior surface of lens.*

facies posterior palpebrarum [NA] The internal surface of the eyelids which faces the eyeball and is covered by the conjunctiva. At its free margin, where it is continuous with the anterior surface of each eyelid, are the openings of the tarsal glands which are embedded in the tarsal plate deep to the conjunctiva. Also called *posterior surface of eyelids.*

facies posterior pancreatis [NA] The flattened posterior surface of the body of the pancreas. It has no peritoneal covering and is related posteriorly to the aorta and origin of the superior mesenteric artery, the left suprarenal gland, left kidney, and renal vein. It is separated from these structures by the splenic vein which runs along it from left to right. Above the vein, near the superior margin, is the splenic artery. Also called *posterior surface of pancreas.*

facies posterior partis petrosae ossis temporalis [NA] The surface of the petrous part of the temporal bone, forming the anterior part of the posterior cranial fossa. Among its prominent features are the opening of the internal acoustic meatus, behind which is the slitlike opening of the aqueduct of vestibule, while between and superior to these orifices is a depression, the subarcuate fossa. Also called *facies posterior pyramidis ossis temporalis.*

facies posterior prostatae [NA] The convex posterior surface of the prostate separated from the lower part of the rectum by the prostatic sheath and the rectovesical septum. The ejaculatory ducts pierce it superiorly in a depression that divides the surface into a smaller upper area that is part of the median lobe and a larger lower area that is subdivided into the right and left lobes by a median furrow.

facies posterior pyramidis ossis temporalis FACIES POSTERIOR PARTIS PETROSAE OSSIS TEMPORALIS.

facies posterior radii [NA] The posterior surface of the radius lying between the interosseous and the posterior margins, the upper part of which gives origin to the abductor pollicis longus muscle proximally and the extensor pollicis brevis distally, while the lower part is only covered by the extensor pollicis longus and brevis muscles. Also called *facies dorsalis radii.*

facies posterior renis [NA] The surface of the kidney which faces posteromedially, is devoid of peritoneum, and is related to the posterior abdominal wall. The upper part lies against the diaphragm, which separates it from the pleura, while the lower part lies against the psoas major muscle, the quadratus lumborum muscle, and the transversus abdominis muscle from medial to lateral side. Also called *posterior surface of kidney.*

facies posterior scapulae [NA] The convex posterior surface of the scapula, divided by the somewhat horizontal spine of scapula into a small supraspinous fossa for the supraspinatus muscle and a larger infraspinous fossa for the infraspinatus muscle. The surface is separated from the lateral margin by a thick, rounded vertical ridge. Also called *dorsal surface of scapula, posterior surface of scapula, dorsum of scapula, facies dorsalis scapulae.*

facies posterior tibiae [NA] The posterior surface of the tibia lying between the interosseous and medial margins and subdivided by two ridges—the oblique soleal line for the attachment of the soleus and popliteus muscles, the latter covering the area above the line, and a longitudinal ridge below the line, medial to which the flexor digitorum longus muscle arises and lateral to which the tibialis posterior muscle arises. The distal third of the surface is covered by tendons and vessels.

facies posterior ulnae [NA] The posterior surface of the ulna lying between the interosseous and the posterior margins and divided into three areas by an oblique line running from the posterior margin to the posterior extremity of the radial notch and by a vertical ridge that divides the area below the oblique line into medial and lateral parts. Also called *facies dorsalis ulnae.*

Potter facies A combination of facial features consisting of orbital hypertelorism, low-set ears, receding chin, and a flat nose, characteristically seen in a newborn infant with bilateral renal agenesis or other severe renal malformations. Also called *renal agenesis facies.*

facies pulmonalis cordis [NA] The convex left surface of the heart, formed mainly by the left ventricle and partly by the left atrium and producing the cardiac impression on the medial surface of the left lung. Also called *pulmonary surface of heart, left border of heart* (outmoded), *left margin of heart* (outmoded).

facies radiales digitorum manus FACIES LATERALES DIGITORUM MANUS.

renal agenesis facies POTTER FACIES.

facies renalis glandulae suprarenalis [NA] The concave inferolateral surface of each suprarenal gland which lies against the superior extremity of its corresponding kidney. It is separated from the kidney by some fibroareolar tissue. Also called *renal surface of suprarenal gland, basis glandulae suprarenalis, inferior margin of suprarenal gland.*

facies renalis lienis FACIES RENALIS SPLENIS.

facies renalis splenis [NA] The slightly concave area on the lower part of the visceral surface of the spleen which rests posteromedially against the superolateral part of the rounded anterior surface of the left kidney and, occasionally, the adjacent suprarenal gland. It is separated from the hilum and gastric surface of the spleen by a longitudinal ridge. Also called *renal surface of spleen, facies renalis lienis.*

facies sacropelvica ossis ilii [NA] The posterior part of the medial aspect of the ilium, located behind and below the iliac fossa. It is subdivided into three areas posteroanteriorly: the iliac tuberosity, a rough area just below the posterior part of the iliac crest mainly for the attachment of the interosseous and dorsal sacroiliac ligaments; the auricular surface; and the pelvic surface, lying between the inferior margin of the auricular surface and the superior margin of the greater sciatic notch and forming part of the wall of pelvis minor. Also called *sacropelvic surface of ilium.*

facies scaphoidea A face that appears concave in profile, due to a protruding forehead, depressed nose and upper jaw, and a prominent chin. Also called *dish face, dishface deformity.*

facies sphenomaxillaris alae magnae FACIES MAXILLARIS ALAE MAJORIS.

facies sternocostalis cordis [NA] The anterior surface of the heart, facing anterosuperiorly and to the left and formed partly by the right atrium above and to the right and mainly by the ventricles, two-thirds by the right and one-third by the left. It is separated from the body of the sternum and the related costal cartilages by the pericardium and the anterior margins of the pleurae and lungs. Also called *sternocostal surface of heart.*

facies superior hemispherii cerebelli The rostral, superior face of the cerebellum, consisting essentially of those portions rostral to the horizontal cerebellar fissure.

facies superior hepatis An outmoded term for PARS SUPERIOR FACIEI DIAPHRAGMATICAE HEPATIS.

facies superior trochleae tali [NA] The broad upper surface of the talus, widest anteriorly, convex anteroposteriorly, and concave from side to side, that articulates with the inferior articular surface of the tibia in the ankle joint. Also called *superior surface of talus.*

facies superolateralis cerebri [NA] The outer convex surface of the cerebral hemispheres underlying the calvaria. Also called *facies convexa cerebri.*

facies symphyseos ossis pubis   FACIES SYMPHYSIALIS.

facies symphysialis   [NA] The elongated, oval medial surface of the body of the pubis that articulates with the opposite pubis in the symphysis pubis. Also called *facies symphyseos ossis pubis, symphysial surface of pubis.*

tabetic facies   Bilateral ptosis with compensatory wrinkling of the forehead seen in some cases of advanced tabes dorsalis.

facies temporalis alae magnae   FACIES TEMPORALIS ALAE MAJORIS.

facies temporalis alae majoris   [NA] The convex outer, or lateral, surface of the greater wing of the sphenoid bone, divided by the horizontal infratemporal crest into a large upper part, a portion of the temporal fossa, and a small lower part, a portion of the wall of the infratemporal fossa. Also called *facies temporalis alae magnae.* ● Some textbooks refer to the upper part as the temporal surface, and to the lower part as the infratemporal surface of the greater wing of sphenoid bone.

facies temporalis ossis frontalis   [NA] A small concave area posterior to the temporal line on the lateral aspect of the frontal bone that helps to form the wall of the temporal fossa. Also called *semicircular plane of frontal bone* (outmoded), *temporal surface of frontal bone.*

facies temporalis ossis zygomatici   [NA] A small concave area facing posteromedially on the zygomatic bone, the posterior part of which extends upwards on the frontal process to form the anterior boundary of the temporal fossa. A backward extension on the medial part of the temporal process helps to form the lateral wall of the infratemporal fossa. The surface has a foramen for the zygomaticotemporal nerve.

facies temporalis partis squamosae   [NA] The large, convex anterior portion of the outer surface of the squamous part of the temporal bone that participates in the posterior part of the wall of the temporal fossa. Also called *facies temporalis squamae temporalis, semicircular plane of squama temporalis* (outmoded).

facies temporalis squamae temporalis   FACIES TEMPORALIS PARTIS SQUAMOSAE.

facies tibialis cruris   FACIES MEDIALIS CRURIS.

typhoid facies   The facial appearance characteristic of typhoid fever, marked by moderate flushing, lustrous and sunken eyes, a vacant, apathetic expression, and ashen color. Also called *facies typhosa.*

facies typhosa   TYPHOID FACIES.

facies ulnares digitorum manus   FACIES MEDIALES DIGITORUM MANUS.

facies urethralis penis   [NA] The inferior surface of the penis, in apposition with the scrotum and opposite to the dorsal aspect of the penis.

facies ventrales digitorum manus   FACIES DIGITALES VENTRALES MANUS.

facies vesicalis uteri   [NA] The normally flattened anterior surface of the body of the uterus, in apposition with the urinary bladder from which it is separated by the vesicouterine excavation, or peritoneal pouch.

facies vestibularis dentis   [NA] A tooth surface directed toward the vestibule of the oral cavity. Also called *facies facialis dentis.*

facies visceralis hepatis   [NA] The surface of the liver that faces inferiorly and posteriorly and is covered by peritoneum, except over the fossa for the gallbladder, at the porta hepatis, and in the fissure for ligamentum teres. It is divided into the right, left, and quadrate lobes, which are closely related to adjacent abdominal organs, such as the right kidney, stomach, transverse colon, gallbladder, and duodenum. Also called *visceral surface of liver, inferior surface of liver, facies inferior hepatis* (outmoded).

facies visceralis lienis   FACIES VISCERALIS SPLENIS.

facies visceralis splenis   [NA] The medial surface of the spleen. It faces the abdominal organs and is divided into facies colica, facies gastrica, and facies renalis, which are related to the left colic flexure, the stomach, and the left kidney, respectively. The hilum of the spleen is situated on the gastric surface. Also called *facies visceralis lienis, visceral surface of spleen.*

facies volares digitorum manus   FACIES DIGITALES VENTRALES MANUS.

facies volaris antibrachii   An outmoded term for REGIO ANTEBRACHIALIS ANTERIOR.

facies volaris radii   FACIES ANTERIOR RADII.

facies volaris ulnae   FACIES ANTERIOR ULNAE.

---

facilitation   [L *facilitas* (from *facilis* easy to do, easy, from *facere* to make, do) easiness, readiness + -ATION]   The neural process of enhancing or promoting synaptic events or reflex actions whereby the sum of separate inputs is additive.

associative facilitation   That process by which one association, already established, makes it easier to form another association to one of its elements. Thus, having already established an association between moon and June, an association between moon and spoon (or June and spoon) would be facilitated.

proprioceptive neuromuscular facilitation   The use of proprioceptive stimuli and reflex patterns to enhance contraction or relaxation of muscles.

facilitation of reflexes   REINFORCEMENT OF REFLEXES.

social facilitation   The stimulatory effect on an individual resulting from having others of the species present. The others reinforce proper behavior and performance of an individual, especially in a social species such as man.

Wedensky's facilitation   The additive effect of an appropriately timed sequence of electric shocks, resulting in greater amplitude of muscle contraction than with a single shock of the same strength.

facilitatory   Producing or promoting facilitation.

facility   [L *facilitas* (from *facilis* easy to do, easy, from *facere* to make, do + -itas -ITY) readiness, easiness]   A physical plant, along with its equipment and supplies, in which services are provided.

extended care facility   An inpatient health care facility providing skilled nursing and related services for long-term stays not appropriate to community hospitals.

health care facility   The physical plant, along with its equipment and supplies, in which health care services are provided.

intermediate care facility   A health care facility that provides inpatient care that is less complex or sophisticated than that of a general or community hospital or a skilled nursing facility but which is required by patients needing long-term institutionalization because of their mental or physical condition.

skilled nursing facility   An inpatient health care facility which provides care for patients that do not require the services of a community hospital but do require nursing care due to injury, disability, or mental health problems.

facing   The visible tooth-colored part of a combined metal/nonmetal crown or unit of a prosthesis.

facio-   [L *facies* face]   A combining form denoting the face.

faciobrachial   Relating to or affecting the face and the arm.

faciocephalalgia   [FACIO- + CEPHAL- + -ALGIA]   Pain in the face, head and neck. An imprecise and outmoded term.

faciocervical   Relating to or affecting the face and the neck.

faciolingual   Relating to or affecting the face and the tongue.

facioplasty   [FACIO- + -PLASTY]   Any plastic operation on the face.

facioplegia FACIAL PARALYSIS.

facioscapulohumeral Pertaining to or affecting the face, the scapula, and the arm.

factitious Not occurring naturally; artificial or contrived.

factor

factor [L (from *fact(us)*, past part, of *facere* to make, do + *-or* -OR), a maker, doer] Any agent or element which helps to produce a result, as in an enzyme reaction, blood coagulation, or hormonal change.

factor I FIBRINOGEN. • The I in this term represents the roman numeral for 1, not the letter I.

factor II PROTHROMBIN.

factor III A rarely used term for THROMBOPLASTIN.

factor IV The calcium present in plasma. A seldom used term.

factor V The coagulation factor that, when activated, is the cofactor of factor Xa in the formation of prothrombinase. Also called *labile factor* (obsolete), *proaccelerin, accelerator globulin, cofactor V, accelerator factor.*

factor VI The original designation for activated factor V (accelerin). This term is no longer applied to any coagulation factor.

factor VII A plasma coagulation factor intermediate in the clotting cascade. It dominates the "extrinsic" coagulation pathway. Also called *stable factor, proconvertin, serum prothrombin conversion accelerator* (outmoded), *kappa factor, cothromboplastin.*

factor VIII A plasma coagulation factor whose inherited deficiency is responsible for classic hemophilia (lack of factor VIII: C) or von Willebrand's disease (lack of factor VIII R: Ag). It is deficient in acute disseminated intravascular coagulation. Also called *antihemophilic factor, antihemophilic factor A, hemophilic factor A, platelet cofactor I, thromboplastic plasma component, antihemophilic globulin* (original term).

factor VIII:c The coagulant moiety of the factor VIII complex, having a molecular weight of about 250 000. This is primarily deficient in classic hemophilia.

factor VIII:CAg The plasma protein that normally has factor VIII:C coagulant activity. Patients with or without hemophilia who develop anti-factor VIII antibodies do so against factor VIII:CAg.

factor VIIIR:Ag The noncoagulatnt portion of factor VIIIR:Ag, which is necessary for platelets to adhere to damaged endothelium. This accounts for the long bleeding time in patients with von Willebrand's disease, who have a deficiency of this factor. This factor must also be present in adequate amounts in order for the antibiotic ristocetin to clump platelets. Also called *Willebrand factor, transhemophilin, ristocetin cofactor, ristocetin factor, factor VIII T.*

factor VIII T FACTOR VIIIR:AG.

factor IX A plasma coagulation factor that may be deficient on an inherited basis (hemophilia B), or an acquired basis (vitamin K deficiency). Also called *plasma thromboplastin component, Christmas factor, platelet cofactor II, autoprothrombin II, antihemophilic factor B, hemophilic factor B.*

factor X A vitamin K-dependent plasma coagulation factor. When activated (factor Xa) it combines with activated factor V (factor Va) plus calcium and phospholipid to form the prothrombinase complex. Also called *Stuart factor, Prower factor, Stuart-Prower factor, autoprothrombin I.*

factor XI A plasma coagulation factor that forms the bridge between the activation factors, such as factor XII, and the hemophilic factors, factors IX and VIII. Deficiency of factor XI causes a bleeding tendency. Also called *plasma thromboplastin antecedent, antihemophilic factor C, hemophilic factor C.*

factor XII One of the activation factors initiating the intrinsic coagulation pathway. There is no bleeding diathesis when this factor is deficient. Also called *Hageman factor, glass factor.*

factor XIII An enzyme of blood plasma that cross-links strands of fibrin monomers, thus creating a mesh of polymerized fibrin and stabilizing the blood clot. Also called *fibrin stabilizing factor, fibrinase, fibrinoligase, Laki-Lorand factor.*

accelerator factor FACTOR V.

accessory food factor Any vitamin.

activated clotting factors Products with clotting activity generated from the inactive plasma clotting proteins during the coagulation process. The inactive proteins have been assigned Roman numerals, and the active products have an *a* appended. Thus proaccelerin is factor V and accelerin is factor Va.

activation factor Any of three plasma coagulation factors that, when activated, initiate the intrinsic clotting cascade. They are factor XII, prekallikrein (Fletcher factor), and high-molecular weight kininogen (Fitzgerald factor). Bleeding does not result from deficiencies of these factors. Also called *contact activation factor.*

alpha factor The estrogen hormones secreted during the first, or follicular, phase of the ovarian cycle. An obsolete term.

amplification factor 1 The ratio of output voltage to input voltage in the operation of an electronic or other amplifier, or one of its components. In a pulse amplifier this factor is equal to the voltage at the peak of an output pulse divided by that at the peak of the corresponding input pulse. 2 See under GAS-AMPLIFICATION FACTOR.

anabolism-promoting factor An agent that increases protein utilization and facilitates the growth and repair of tissues.

animal protein factor VITAMIN B_{12}.

antiachromotrichia factor PANTOTHENIC ACID.

antiacrodynia factor VITAMIN B_6.

antialopecia factor INOSITOL.

antianemia factor VITAMIN B_{12}.

antiberiberi factor THIAMIN.

anti-black-tongue factor NIACIN.

anticanities factor PANTOTHENIC ACID.

antidermatitis factor of chicks PANTOTHENIC ACID.

antidermatitis factor of rats VITAMIN B_6.

anti-egg-white factor BIOTIN.

anti-gray-hair factor PANTOTHENIC ACID.

antihemophilic factor FACTOR VIII.

antihemophilic factor A FACTOR VIII.

antihemophilic factor B FACTOR IX.

antihemophilic factor C FACTOR XI.

antihemorrhagic factor VITAMIN K.

anti-insulin factor Any circulating substance or process opposing the action of insulin through any mechanism. An imprecise usage.

antineuritic factor THIAMIN.

antinuclear factor ANTINUCLEAR ANTIBODY.

antipellagra factor NIACIN.

antirachitic factor VITAMIN D.

antiscorbutic factor VITAMIN C.

antisterility factor VITAMIN E.

antistiffness factor A factor once believed to be necessary to prevent stiffness of the wrist which was then followed by emaciation and death in animals. When unrefined molasses, raw cream, or unheated cane juice, each of which contained the factor, were fed to an animal, none of the symptoms appeared. The factor was never isolated. An outmoded term.

antixerophthalmia factor VITAMIN A.

antixerotic factor VITAMIN A.

area comparability factor   A number by which to multiply the crude rate (birth rate, death rate, etc.) of a local population in order to allow direct comparison with the corresponding rate of a standard (e.g., the national), population free from the influence of differences in the age-sex structure of the populations being compared.

atrial natriuretic factor   A heart atrial extract which produces marked natriuresis and diuresis when injected into rats. A synthetic form has been produced.

factor B   The component of the alternative complement pathway that is the homolog of C2 in the classical pathway. It is the zymogen of a complex serine protease. Factor B complexes with C3b in the presence of magnesium ions and is then cleaved by factor D to give rise to two products, Ba and C3b,Bb, the latter being the C3-converting enzyme of the alternative complement pathway.

backscatter factor   The ratio of the exposure or of the absorbed dose at a point on the surface of a patient or phantom to the exposure or absorbed dose due to primary photons only.

bacteriocinogenic factor   BACTERIOCINOGEN.

basophil chemotactic factor   A lymphokine that stimulates migration of basophils.

basophil chemotaxis augmentation factor   A lymphokine that stimulates and augments migration of basophils.

Be blood factor   Be^a is a red cell antigen, recently demonstrated to belong to the Rh system.

bed-use factor   The average number of patients using each hospital bed during a given period, a measure of the intensity of use of hospital beds. It is the ratio of the number of discharges and deaths in the period to the number of beds available on average daily during the period. A British usage.

beta factor   The hormone (progesterone) secreted during the second or secretory phase of the ovarian cycle. An obsolete term.

biotic factor   The ecological or environmental effect of a living organism or assemblage of organisms.

Bittner milk factor   MOUSE MAMMARY TUMOR VIRUS.

bone factor   A hypothetical factor intended to account for individual differences in resistance to bone resorption in chronic peridontitis.

bugger factor   A correction factor improperly applied to an instrumental reading to achieve a more nearly correct result. A slang expression. See also CORRECTION FACTOR.

buildup factor   In a beam of high energy x rays or gamma rays the ratio of the peak absorbed dose to the surface absorbed dose.

cabbage factor   GLUCOSINOLATE PROGOITRIN.

calibration factor   **1** A multiplier applied to the numerical reading of an instrument to convert a quantity with one physical dimension to a more informative one, for example counts per second to millicuries of radioactivity.   **2** An incorrect term for CORRECTION FACTOR.

CAMP factor   A product of group B streptococci, seen when streptococci are grown on a blood agar plate near a hemolytic strain of *Staphylococcus aureus*. The factor enlarges the zone of β-hemolysis that surrounds the streaked colonies of *S. aureus*.

Castle's factor   INTRINSIC FACTOR.

chemotactic factor   A chemical agent that induces chemotaxis.

chick antipellagra factor   PANTOTHENIC ACID.

chick growth factor   STREPTOGENIN.

chick growth factor S   STREPTOGENIN.

Christmas factor   FACTOR IX.

citrovorum factor   FOLINIC ACID.

clearing factor   LIPOPROTEIN LIPASE.

clone-inhibiting factor   A factor that is produced by activated lymphocytes and that can be shown to have either cytotoxic or growth inhibitory effects on target cells in a tissue culture, particularly tumor cells.

clumping factor   Surface-bound coagulase of *Staphylococcus aureus*, which causes clumping in plasma by reaction with fibrinogen.

C3 nephritic factor   An autoantibody present in the plasma of some patients with membranoproliferative glomerulonephritis who have low plasma complement activity. The autoantibody has specificity for the C3b,Bb complex of the alternative pathway of complement activation, and it stabilizes the system for enzymatic cleavage of C3 to C3a and C3b.

coagulation factors   Any of the plasma proteins in the coagulation cascade plus calcium and thromboplastin.

colicin factor   COLICINOGEN.

colony stimulating factor   A lymphokine that enhances erythrocyte colony formation or growth in tissue culture media.

conglutinogen-activating factor   FACTOR I.

contact activation factor   ACTIVATION FACTOR.

cord factor   6,6′-Dimycolyl trehalose, a component of the cell envelope of *Mycobacterium tuberculosis* that promotes virulence and serpentine growth.

correction factor   A multiplier, either greater or less than unity, applied to an erroneous instrumental reading to achieve a result more nearly correct. Such a multiplier must be derived from sound experimental evidence. Otherwise it is known vernacularly as a bugger factor. Also called *calibration factor* (incorrect).

corticotropin releasing factor   An older term for CORTICOTROPIN RELEASING HORMONE. Abbreviation: CRF

coupling factors   Substances which allow, or restore, mitochondrial oxidation to bring about phosphorylation so that adenosine triphosphate can again be produced, especially in mitochondria in which these processes have been uncoupled.

cow manure factor   VITAMIN B$_{12}$.

factor D   A serine protease of molecular weight 25 000 daltons which occurs in fully active form in plasma and is an essential component of the alternative pathway of complement activation. It cleaves Fb when this protein is bound to C3b.

decapacitation factor   A factor that prevents capacitation of spermatozoa, such that the ability of spermatozoa to fertilize an ovum is impaired.

decay accelerating factor   An erythrocyte membrane protein which functions as a control protein of the complement system. It accelerates the decomposition of C4b,2b, the C3-converting enzyme of the classical pathway, into its components. Decay accelerating factor is absent on the abnormal erythrocytes of patients with paroxysmal nocturnal hemoglobinuria.

density-dependent factor   A population control factor, such as food availability, that exerts influence in direct relationship to population density.

density-independent factor   A population control factor, such as a flood or other natural disaster, whose influence does not depend on the size of the population.

depolarization factor   The process of decreasing the membrane potential of a cell by any course in which the absolute potential value becomes less negative.

Duran-Reynals factor   HYALURONIDASE.

duty factor   Pulse duration multiplied by pulse repetition frequency. For example, in ultrasonography the pulse duration of 1 μs and a pulse repetition frequency of 2000 pulses/s yields a low duty factor of 0.002.

edaphic factor   A physical or chemical feature of a site, soil, microclimate, etc., that influences the distribution of an organism.

elongation factor   One of several cytoplasmic proteins that function cyclically during each addition of an amino acid in polypeptide chain elongation. In bacteria EFTu complexes with aminoacyl-tRNA and GTP to form a ternary complex that binds to the ribosome in the recognition step. EFTu·GDP is released and then interacts with EFTs, which leads to replacement of the GDP by GTP. EFG, complexed with GTP, participates in the translocation step in chain elongation, and it is released after hydrolysis of the GTP. In eukaryotic systems similar factors are called EF-1 and EF-2.

eluate factor   VITAMIN B$_6$.

encephalitogenic factor   A peptide fraction isolated from myelin basic protein derived from cerebral white matter. When injected with Freund's adjuvant into animals it can produce experimental allergic encephalomyelitis.

eosinophil chemotactic factor   A lymphokine that, when activated by immune complexes, attracts blood eosinophils to sites of inflammation.

epidermal growth factor   A protein substance, extracted from submaxillary glands of male mice, which when administered to immature mice induces more rapid eyelid opening, eruption of teeth, and growth of epidermal structures. Larger doses may inhibit these processes.

erythropoietic stimulating factor   ERYTHROPOIETIN.

essential food factors   Substances that are required by the body to sustain life but which cannot be synthesized by the body and so must be supplied exogenously by the diet. Such substances include linoleic acid, the vitamins and minerals, and the essential amino acids, specifically tryptophan, phenylalanine, lysine, threonine, valine, methionine, leucine, and isoleucine. Histidine is an essential amino acid during childhood.

extrinsic factor   VITAMIN B$_{12}$.

F factor   A particular plasmid that codes efficiently for transfer of itself, and also of the bacterial chromosome, by conjugation. This plasmid is the one with which bacterial conjugation was discovered in *Escherichia coli*. It is unusually efficient because it lacks a gene, present in most conjugative plasmids, that represses the transfer operon. Also called *F plasmid, F agent, fertility factor.*

fertility factor   1 F FACTOR. 2 Any conjugative plasmid.

fibrin stabilizing factor   FACTOR XIII.

filtrate factor   PANTOTHENIC ACID.

Fletcher factor   The original term for PREKALLIKREIN. ● *Fletcher* was the name of the family in which an inherited deficiency of this factor was discovered.

follicle stimulating hormone releasing factor   FOLLICLE STIMULATING HORMONE RELEASING HORMONE. Abbreviation: FSHRF

F-prime factor   An F factor that has incorporated specific host genes and thus mediates their high-frequency transfer by conjugation.

Fy factor   The gene responsible for expressing the red cell phenotype Fy(a-b-) which is commonly found in blacks and rarely in whites. The Fy factor is so named because it is part of the Duf*fy* blood group.

G factor   G FACTOR OF SPEARMAN.

galactagogue factor   1 Any agent stimulating the flow of milk. 2 An obsolete term for PROLACTIN.

galactopoietic factor   An outmoded term for PROLACTIN.

gas-amplification factor   A ratio for a given ionizing event in a Geiger-Müller tube that is operating under conditions where avalanche ionization can occur: the total number of ions collected by the anode divided by the number of primary ions causing the avalanche. The factor may be 10^8.

gastric intrinsic factor of Castle   INTRINSIC FACTOR.

general factor   G FACTOR OF SPEARMAN.

glass factor   FACTOR XII.

gonadotropin releasing factor   GONADOTROPIN RELEASING HORMONE. Abbreviation: GnRF

growth factor   1 Any factor essential to skeletal or somatic growth, such as vitamin D, minerals, or the growth hormone. 2 A substance that is required for or that enhances growth of a particular microbe. Most growth factors are nutrients utilized by the cell, but some, as albumin or starch, are protective, acting by binding toxic compounds, especially soap, in the medium.

growth hormone inhibitory factor   SOMATOSTATIN.

growth hormone releasing factor   GROWTH HORMONE RELEASING HORMONE.

G factor of Spearman   A unitary factor said to underlie performance scores earned on virtually all tests of mental ability and to contribute to and be responsible for the tendency for all cognitive measures to be positively related. Individuals are held to possess this general factor of mental ability in varying amounts, and it is to this ability to reason, to perceive relationships, and to educe correlates from them that reference is made when speaking of the individual's intelligence. Also called *G component, general ability, general factor, G factor.*

factor H   1 BIOTIN. 2 One of the control proteins of the complement system. Factor H binds to C3b and allows its cleavage by factor I.

Hageman factor   FACTOR XII.

hemophilic factor A   FACTOR VIII.

hemophilic factor B   FACTOR IX.

hemophilic factor C   FACTOR XI.

HLA factor   HLA ANTIGEN.

H factor of Lewis   The substances liberated into the skin after rubbing with a blunt instrument as part of the triple response of Lewis. It was presumed by Lewis, probably correctly, to be histamine with or without other pharmacologically active substances.

host factor   An attribute or statistical characteristic associated with a likelihood of developing a given disease, such as a cancer of a particular body site.

human factor IX complex   1 A fraction prepared from the supernatant plasma after precipitating human antihemophilic globulin. It is a concentrated mixture of coagulation factors II, VII, IX, and X, and it is used to treat bleeding episodes in patients with hemophilia B. 2 A fraction prepared from the supernatant plasma after precipitating human antihemophilic globulin. It is a concentrated mixture of coagulation factor II, VII, IX, and X, and it is used to treat bleeding episodes in patients with hemophilia B.

hyperglycemic factor   An imprecise term for GLUCAGON.

hyperglycemic-glycogenolytic factor   An outmoded term for GLUCAGON.

factor I   One of the control proteins of the complement system. It is a serine protease occurring in fully active form in plasma which cleaves C3b to iC3b. This reaction is of central importance in the control of the alternative complement pathway. Factor I will also cleave iC3b to C3c and C3dg; and C4b to C4c and C4d. All factor I cleavage requires the substrate to be bound to a substrate modifying protein. Also called *C3b inactivator, conglutinogen-activating factor.* ● The *I* in this term represents the letter I, not the roman numeral.

IgG rheumatoid factor   Immunoglobulin G with antibody activity against the Fc portion of a normal immunoglobulin G molecule.

IgM rheumatoid factor   The classic rheumatoid factor, consisting of an immunoglobulin M molecule with antibody activity directed against the Fc portion of a normal immunoglobulin G molecule.

initiation factor   One of several protein factors that participate in the initiation step in protein synthesis and then are released from the ribosome as it moves on into chain elongation. Bacteria have three initiation factors (IF-1, IF-2, IF-3). Eukaryotic cells have a larger number.

insulin-antagonizing factor   1 An outmoded term for GLU-

CAGON. **2** Any nonhormonal insulin antagonist, such as a fatty acid.

intermediate lobe inhibiting factor MELANOCYTE STIMULATING HORMONE INHIBITORY HORMONE.

intrinsic factor A glycoprotein of molecular weight in the order of 50 000 which is produced by normal gastric parietal cells. It dimerizes when it combines with vitamin B_{12} to give a complex consisting of two molecules of intrinsic factor and two molecules of vitamin B_{12}. In this form B_{12} is permitted to enter ileal mucosal cells. Deficiency of intrinsic factor impairs the absorption of B_{12}. This is common in old people. Also called *gastric intrinsic factor of Castle, Castle's factor.*

kappa factor **1** A large, complex particle composed of DNA, RNA, and protein, occurring in the cytoplasm of certain strains of paramecia. Strains having kappa particles produce toxic materials which kill sensitive strains of paramecia. **2** FACTOR VII.

labile factor An obsolete term for FACTOR V.

***Lactobacillus bulgaricus* factor** An outmoded term for FOLIC ACID.

***Lactobacillus casei* factor** An outmoded term for FOLIC ACID.

lactogenic factor An outmoded term for PROLACTIN.

Laki-Lorand factor FACTOR XIII.

LE factor ANTINUCLEAR ANTIBODY.

LE cell factor ANTINUCLEAR ANTIBODY.

letdown factor An outmoded term for PROLACTIN.

lethal factor LETHAL ALLELE.

leukocyte migration inhibition factor A lymphokine that inhibits migration of polymorphonuclear leukocytes.

leukopenic factor A hypothetical substance postulated to occur in inflammatory conditions as a result of cell death, and causing reduction in number of blood leukocytes. Endotoxin, derived from bacterial cell walls, is a well-defined leukopenic factor.

limiting factor A scarce chemical substance or physical environmental factor whose availability determines the potential for growth in an organism.

liver factor A factor in liver that was found to cause remissions of pernicious anemia. Its purified form is vitamin B_{12}.

liver filtrate factor PANTOTHENIC ACID.

LLD factor VITAMIN B_{12}.

lupus erythematosus factor ANTINUCLEAR ANTIBODY.

luteinizing hormone releasing factor GONADOTROPIN RELEASING HORMONE. Abbreviation: LHRF, LRF

lymph node permeability factor A substance derived from extracts of lymph nodes having the capacity to increase the permeability of vessels. Abbreviation: LNPF

lymphocyte-activating factor INTERLEUKIN-1.

lymphocytosis-promoting factor A protein product of *Bordetella pertussis* that stimulates lymphocyte production and may be responsible for other toxic effects.

macrophage-activating factor A lymphokine that enhances phagocytic, bactericidal, and tumoricidal activities of macrophages.

macrophage chemotactic factor A lymphokine that stimulates migration of macrophages.

macrophage migration inhibition factor MIGRATION INHIBITION FACTOR.

maturation factor Any substance, real or hypothetical, which can cause differentiation or maturation of a cell.

mauve factor A substance excreted in urine that creates a mauve-pink spot following chromatography. Although it was once thought to be a marker for schizophrenia, possibly representing dimethoxyphenylethylamine, the theory has not been corroborated and the pink spot is considered to be a diet-related artifact.

melanocyte inhibiting factor MELATONIN.

melanocyte stimulating hormone inhibiting factor MELANOCYTE STIMULATING HORMONE INHIBITORY HORMONE.

melanocyte stimulating hormone release inhibiting factor MELANOCYTE STIMULATING HORMONE INHIBITORY HORMONE.

melanocyte stimulating hormone releasing factor MELANOCYTE STIMULATING HORMONE RELEASING HORMONE. Abbreviation: MSHRF

melanophore-spreading factor MELANOPHORE-STIMULATING FACTOR.

melanophore-stimulating factor An old name for the peptide hormone of the intermediate lobe of the pituitary of amphibians, having the property of inducing the spreading of dermal melanin-containing cells, the melanophores with consequent darkening of the skin. An outmoded term. Also called *melanophore-spreading factor.*

migration inhibition factor A protein of approximately 70 000 daltons released from sensitized lymphocytes and which inhibits the mobility of macrophages. Also called *macrophage migration inhibition factor.* Abbreviation: MIF

milk factor MOUSE MAMMARY TUMOR VIRUS.

mitogenic factor A substance that stimulates transformation, DNA synthesis, and mitosis in immunocompetent lymphocytes.

modifying factor MODIFYING GENE.

mouse antialopecia factor INOSITOL.

mouse mammary tumor factor MOUSE MAMMARY TUMOR VIRUS.

mullerian duct inhibiting factor MULLERIAN REGRESSION FACTOR.

mullerian regression factor A protein hormone secreted by the Sertoli cells of the fetal testis. The hormone induces the normal involution of the embryonic mullerian duct structures in the male. Also called *mullerian duct inhibiting factor.*

multiple factors Two or more genetic loci, the individual actions of which cannot be separated from their cooperative action in producing a recognizable character.

myocardial depressant factor A circulating substance thought to be responsible for an inadequate cardiac response during resuscitation after some severe burns or shock. Its nature and even its existence are controversial.

necrotizing factor A poorly characterized factor, probably representing one or more of the known toxins of staphylococci, capable of causing tissue and cell necrosis. An obsolete term.

nerve growth factor A specific protein which causes cells of embryonic spinal ganglia to send out axons. Snake venom and submaxillary salivary glands of mice contain very potent nerve growth factors.

neutrophil chemotactic factor A lymphokine that stimulates migration of neutrophils.

osteoclast activating factor A lymphokine that stimulates osteoclasts thus causing resorption of bone.

Passovoy factor An activation factor acting in the vicinity of factor XI in the coagulation cascade.

pellagra-preventive factor NIACIN.

plasma prothrombin conversion factor Factors VII and X, once thought to be a single factor. An obsolete term.

plasma thromboplastin factor Any intrinsic coagulation plasma factor that promotes acceleration of the conversion of prothrombin to thrombin. Three such factors are recognized: factors VIII, IX, and XI.

platelet factor Any of several substances that are primarily located within platelets or on their surface membranes and that contribute to coagulation by affecting platelet aggregation, adhesion, or retraction, or accelerate conversion of prothrombin to thrombin. Adsorbed substances are not considered platelet factors. Seven platelet factors are recognized. ● Whereas coagulation factors are assigned Roman numerals, platelet factors are assigned Arabic numerals 1–7.

platelet activating factor   Acetyl glyceryl ether phosphorylcholine, a substance released by neutrophils, monocytes, mast cells, and basophils that causes platelets to aggregate and release β-thromboglobulin, 5-hydroxytryptamine, and platelet factor 4.

platelet derived growth factor   A heat-stable protein having a molecular weight of 13 000, which is contained in the α-granules of platelets. It stimulates proliferation of smooth-muscle cells in tissue culture.

prolactin inhibiting factor   PROLACTIN INHIBITORY HORMONE. Abbreviation: PIF

prolactin releasing factor   PROLACTIN RELEASING HORMONE. Abbreviation: PRF

Prower factor   FACTOR X.

quality factor   A number which relates the relative biologic effect of different types of radiation and is used in the field of radiation protection. The International Commission on Radiological Protection has assigned the quality factor values of from 1 to 20, depending on the linear energy transfer, defined in terms of the collision stopping power. Multiplying the absorbed dose in rads by the quality factor gives the dose in rems. Symbol: Q

R factor   Any of a large group of plasmids characterized by the presence of genes that cause resistance to various antimicrobial agents, mostly by coding for enzymes that inactivate the agent. Factors are classified in terms of incompatibility group or in terms of their pattern of resistance genes. Also called *resistance factor, R plasmid.* See also FERTILITY INHIBITION.

rat acrodynia factor   PYRIDOXINE.

reducing factor   VITAMIN C.

relaxing factor   An outmoded term for RELAXIN.

releasing factor   RELEASING HORMONE.

resistance factor   R FACTOR.

resistance transfer factor   The part of a resistance plasmid, sometimes found alone, that codes for its own replication and machinery of conjugation. Combined with R-determinants, which code for enzymes that inactivate various antimicrobial agents, it becomes a resistance factor (R factor). Abbreviation: RTF

Reynals factor   HYALURONIDASE.

Rh factor   RH ANTIGEN.

Rhesus factor   RH ANTIGEN.

rheumatoid factor   An immunoglobulin, usually pentameric IgM but sometimes monomeric IgM or IgG, that is defined by its reactivity with the Fc portion of IgG. Rheumatoid factor is commonly present in the serum of patients with rheumatoid arthritis.

factor rho   The transcription termination factor, which promotes release of RNA polymerase from DNA. Its deficiency in mutants results in suppression of operon polarity.

risk factor   In epidemiology, an attribute or circumstance associated with an enhanced risk of developing or of dying from a specific disease.

ristocetin factor   FACTOR VIIIR:AG.

factor S   BIOTIN.

safety factor   A numerical factor applied to the apparent safety level of an activity as determined by experimental, epidemiologic, or other scientific means, or from experience. The factor, which may, for example, be two, ten, or one hundred, is designed to give an adequate margin of safety to allow for possible unknown ill effects and cases of personal idiosyncrasy or sensitivity.

scale factor   The ratio of the size of a display to the real size of the object or variable displayed.

secretor factor   1 A genetically-determined agent responsible for the secretion in body fluids of water-soluble A, B, or H substances, corresponding to the ABO type of the individual.

Individuals who inherit the factor are secretors, those lacking it are nonsecretors. 2 SECRETOR.

separation factor   A factor used in the calculation of infant mortality rates to ensure that the numerator (infant deaths) and the denominator (live births) correspond at least approximately when both relate to a calendar year. The factor takes account of the fact that a proportion of the infants that die in any one year were born in the year previous. Separation factors become important in practice only when birth rates are changing rapidly.

serum accelerator factor   A proposed coagulation accelerator found in serum. It may be related to serum thrombotic accelerator.

sex factor   CONJUGATIVE PLASMID.

sigma factor   One of the subunits of bacterial DNA-directed RNA polymerase. It binds to the rest of the enzyme and enables it to bind to a promoter site in DNA while diminishing its affinity for the rest of the DNA. The sigma factor functions only during the initiation of a new RNA chain, after which it is released and recycled to another RNA polymerase.

skin factor   BIOTIN.

skin reactive factor   A lymphokine that causes local cutaneous inflammatory reactions.

somatotropin-releasing factor   GROWTH HORMONE RELEASING HORMONE.

specific macrophage arming factor   A lymphokine that causes macrophages to be cytotoxic for tumor cells.

spreading factor   HYALURONIDASE.

stable factor   FACTOR VII.

Stuart factor   FACTOR X.

Stuart-Prower factor   FACTOR X.

sulfation factor   An outmoded term for SOMATOMEDIN.

T-cell growth factor   INTERLEUKIN-2.

T-cell replacing factor   A lymphokine that augments antiheterologous erythrocyte plaque-forming cell responses.

termination factor   TERMINATION SEQUENCE.

thyroid stimulating hormone releasing factor   THYROTROPIN RELEASING HORMONE. Abbreviation: TSH-RF

thyrotoxic complement-fixation factor   One of several abnormal proteins found in the serum of patients with Graves disease. Its presence provides support for an autoimmune basis of this type of hyperthyroidism.

thyrotropin releasing factor   THYROTROPIN RELEASING HORMONE. Abbreviation: TRF

tissue plasminogen factor   TISSUE PLASMINOGEN ACTIVATOR.

transfer factor   1 An activity found in the dialysate of leukocyte extracts from subjects who show delayed hypersensitivity to an antigen which is claimed to confer, when injected into other human subjects who are believed not to have encountered the antigen concerned, the specific delayed hypersensitivity to that antigen. 2 Single breath carbon monoxide diffusing capacity per unit lung volume. A British term. • Transfer factor is calculated and expressed in the American literature as the carbon monoxide diffusing capacity (DCO) divided by the calculated alveolar volume at which the test is performed (D/V).

transfer factor II   TRANSLOCASE.

transforming factor   A fragment of bacterial DNA which is capable of being integrated into the genome of a recipient bacterium. The term applies especially to type transformation in the pneumococcus, which was the initial observation of this phenomenon.

transmethylation factor   CHOLINE.

transmission factor   The ratio of the radiation intensity behind a protective barrier or other material to the radiation intensity at the surface.

tumor-angiogenesis factor   A substance produced by cancer cells which stimulates nearby blood vessels to grow into the tumor.

tumor cell migration inhibition factor   A lymphokine that inhibits migration of tumor cells.

tumor necrosis factor   A naturally occurring substance that causes necrosis of tumor cells.

factor V   NICOTINAMIDE ADENINE DINUCLEOTIDE.   • The *V* in this term represents the letter V, not the roman numeral.

vascular permeability factor   A lymphokine that increases vascular permeability and induces inflammatory reactions.

vascular tissue factor   TISSUE PLASMINOGEN ACTIVATOR.

virulence factor   **1** Any genetic variable that affects virulence of a microbe or virus.   **2** Any feature whose elimination may have a large effect, such as formation of a capsule, of a toxin, or of a surface molecule required for adherence. Also called *aggressin* (obsolete).

factor W   BIOTIN.

Willebrand factor   FACTOR VIIIR:AG.

windchill factor   A measure of air temperature adjusted for the chilling effect that wind produces on an exposed skin surface. The strength of the wind, air temperature, and humidity affect the determination of windchill factor. Also called *windchill*.

factor X   A heat-stable factor found in blood and required for growth by *Haemophilus influenzae*. Since its discovery it has been identified as hemin.   • The *X* in this term represents the letter X, not the roman numeral.

XYZ factor   A poorly defined factor, isolated from tumor cells, which upon injection into experimental animals renders the host more susceptible to a subsequent transplant of the same tumor.

Y factor   PYRIDOXINE.

yeast eluate factor   PYRIDOXINE.

yeast filtrate factor   PANTOTHENIC ACID.

---

factorial   For any given positive integer *n:* the product, written *n*!, of the first *n* positive integers. Thus, factorial 4, or 4!, is equal to $4 \times 3 \times 2 \times 1$, or 24. By convention, $0! = 1$.

facultative   **1** Able to live under more than one set of conditions, as in the case of certain organisms which can adapt to either a parasitic or nonparasitic existence, or which can grow either anaerobically or aerobically. Compare OBLIGATE.   **2** Characterized by the capacity to operate or function in adapting to particular circumstances, as homosexuality in response to conditions where it is accepted and no heterosexual object is available, as in prisons.

faculty   [L *facult(as)* (from *facilis* easy, skillful) power, ability, faculty + -Y] Any demonstrated ability to perform a given act.   • Historically, this term was used by those who sought to describe the activities of the mind by the action and interaction of posited mental powers, such as memory, reason, imagination, or will. As this doctrine is now discredited, use of the term is avoided.

fusion faculty   The ability of the brain to synthesize the stimuli from the two eyes into a single binocular image.

FAD   flavin adenine dinucleotide.

faecalith   A British spelling for FECALITH.

faeces   A British spelling for FECES.

faex   [L (gen. *faecis*), the dregs or lees of a liquid, esp. wine, brine of pickles]   **1** A sediment or other material at the bottom of a solution.   **2** YEAST.

faex medicinalis   A yeast that was once used in certain patent medicines.

faex medicinalis sicca   A tablet form of yeast used as a supplemental source of the B complex vitamins.

Faget   [Jean Charles *Faget*, French physician, 1818–1884]   Fa-

get sign. See under FAGET'S LAW.

fagicladosporic acid   One of a number of fungal toxins produced by *Cladosporium epiphyllum*. It usually occurs in soybeans and dried beans.

fagopyrism   A primary photosensitivity disease, mainly of sheep and cattle, caused by the ingestion of *Fagopyrum esculentum* (buckwheat), which induces photosensitization when the animal is exposed to sunlight. Clinically, the main features are intense irritation, initially of the skin, followed by edematous swelling and serous exudation. Parts of the body, as the ears and muzzle, where the hair covering is light, are most affected. Also called *buckwheat poisoning*.

Fagopyrum   A genus of plants that contain a photodynamic agent which, when eaten by animals, can cause photosensitization.

Fahr   [Theodor *Fahr*, German neurologist, 1877–1945]   See under DISEASE.

Fahraeus   [Robin Sanno *Fahraeus*, Swedish pathologist and anatomist, 1888–1968]   **1** Fahraeus-Lindqvist effect. See under EFFECT.   **2** Fahraeus reaction, Fahraeus test. See under ERYTHROCYTE SEDIMENTATION.

Fahrenheit   [Daniel Gabriel *Fahrenheit*, German-Dutch physicist, 1689–1736]   **1** Degree Fahrenheit. See under DEGREE.   **2** See under THERMOMETER.

fail-safe   Describing a circuit or system that fails in a way that prevents harm or destruction. An example of a fail-safe device is a mechanism on an anesthesia machine which will automatically shut off the delivery of nitrous oxide to a patient whenever the oxygen supply falls below a safe level.

failure   [French *faillir* (inf. used as verb or substantive; from L *fallere* to deceive, from Gk *sphallein* to make to fall, foil, disappoint) to make a default; a failing]   A condition or instance of not functioning or not functioning adequately.

acute anuric renal failure   Acute renal failure with no urine output. This is rare, but is most likely to develop in complete urinary obstruction, acute glomerulonephritis, bilateral cortical necrosis, and vascular disorders.

acute congestive heart failure   Heart failure of sudden onset associated with congestion of the lungs and systemic veins.

acute nonoliguric renal failure   ACUTE POLYURIC RENAL FAILURE.

acute oliguric renal failure   Sudden renal excretory failure characterized by oliguria of less than 400 ml per 24 hours and rapidly increasing azotemia. Correctable causes include urinary tract obstruction, decreased renal blood flow and glomerular filtration rate associated with decreased extracellular and intravascular volumes, and transient hypotension. The most common cause of acute renal failure is hypotension after trauma, burns, or surgical shock. Other causes include nephrotoxins, acute glomerular diseases, acute interstitial disease, acute intravascular hemolysis, and acute renal vascular disorders such as embolus, thrombosis, vasculitis, and bilateral cortical necrosis. In approximately half of the cases the etiology is difficult to establish.

acute polyuric renal failure   Acute renal failure characterized by urinary output greater than 1 liter per 24 hours. This is most common in acute renal failure due to drugs and anesthetic agents. Also called *acute nonoliguric renal failure*.

acute renal failure   Sudden decrease of kidney function usually manifested by oliguria or rarely anuria.

backward heart failure   Heart failure attributable to a rise in filling pressure of the heart and a consequent rise in venous pressure: a mechanism proposed as the major cause of the manifestations of congestive heart failure. Compare FORWARD HEART FAILURE.

biventricular failure Cardiac failure involving both right and left ventricles.

chronic renal failure Permanent renal damage of multiple causation from varying degrees of renal dysfunction to retention of metabolic products.

congestive heart failure Heart failure manifested by congestion of the lungs if the left ventricle is involved, or by peripheral venous engorgement, hepatomegaly, and edema if the right ventricle has failed. Abbreviation: CHF

forward heart failure Heart failure attributable to low cardiac output. It is proposed that the manifestations of congestive heart failure, such as pulmonary edema, hepatomegaly, and peripheral edema, are the consequence of low cardiac output and therefore of inadequate renal blood flow, leading to retention of sodium and water. Compare BACKWARD HEART FAILURE.

glycerol-induced acute renal failure A frequently studied experimental model of acute renal failure following intramuscular injection of glycerol, characterized by acute hemolysis, myoglobinemia, and blood volume decrease due to the osmotic effect of glycerol. The use of intravenous 20% glycerol in the treatment of cerebral edema in man has rarely been complicated by hemoglobinuria and acute renal failure.

heart failure Inability of the heart to meet the circulatory needs of the body, or meeting those needs only at the expense of excessively high venous pressures. Also called *cardiac insufficiency.*

hepatic failure A syndrome that results from massive necrosis of liver cells and marked by the inability of the liver to perform such synthetic and metabolic functions as bilirubin metabolism or synthesis of coagulation factors II, V, VII, IX, and X. It is manifested by progressive jaundice, fluid retention, hypoglycemia, and encephalopathy, and has a very high mortality rate.

high output heart failure Failure of the heart to meet the needs of the body in spite of a higher than normal cardiac output, as seen in thyrotoxicosis, anemia, beriberi, and Paget's disease.

high output renal failure Acute renal failure characterized by the kidney's inability to concentrate urine, thus producing normal or supranormal volumes of urine. Because urine output is normal or increased, the condition may be misdiagnosed. Recovery can be expected if the condition is diagnosed and treated.

kidney failure RENAL FAILURE.

left heart failure LEFT-SIDED HEART FAILURE.

left-sided heart failure Heart failure in which the manifestations are related to failure of the left ventricle or high pressure in the left atrium. Also called *left heart failure.*

left ventricular heart failure Left-sided heart failure due to a failure of the left ventricle. Also called *left ventricular insufficiency.*

liver failure See under HEPATIC FAILURE.

low output heart failure Cardiac failure in which inadequate cardiac output is a major feature.

metabolic failure A local or general failure of metabolic processes.

pacemaker failure Failure of a natural or artificial pacemaker to stimulate the heart.

peripheral circulatory failure Failure of the circulation as a consequence of inadequate peripheral vascular function. See also SHOCK.

prerenal failure Renal failure due to decreased renal blood flow and glomerular filtration rate, associated with shock, volume depletion, congestive heart failure, or renal artery obstruction. Except for the last, prerenal failure is readily reversible by appropriate therapy.

primary adrenocortical failure ADDISON'S DISEASE.

pump failure Cardiac failure as a result of inadequate pumping function of the heart.

renal failure Acute or chronic decrease in renal function associated with uremic symptoms, due to any cause. Lesser degrees of renal function impairment usually are termed renal insufficiency. Also called *kidney failure.*

respiratory failure Failure of the respiratory system to maintain normal tensions of oxygen or carbon dioxide in the arterial blood.

right heart failure RIGHT-SIDED HEART FAILURE.

right-sided heart failure Heart failure due to failure of the right ventricle or an excessively high pressure in the right atrium. Also called *right heart failure.*

right ventricular heart failure Right-sided heart failure due to malfunction of the right ventricle. Also called *right ventricular insufficiency.*

secondary adrenocortical failure SECONDARY ADRENOCORTICAL INSUFFICIENCY.

secondary glandular failure Deficiency of a hormone secreted by a particular gland owing to absence of stimulation by the hormone of another gland. Secondary hypogonadism, for example, results from anterior pituitary gonadotropin insufficiency.

template failure A failure of the template of DNA or RNA to be correctly replicated, transcribed, or translated, thus interfering with a cell's ability to synthesize functional proteins, considered as one explanation of cellular aging.

faint [Middle English *feint*, from Old French *feint*, past part. of *feindre* to fain, dissimulate, from L *fingere* to touch] SYNCOPE.

fainting A sudden loss of consciousness due to transient global diminution of cerebral blood flow.

Fajersztajn [J. *Fajersztajn*, Austrian neurologist, flourished late 19th–early 20th centuries] Fajersztajn's test. See under FAJERSZTAJN'S CROSSED SCIATIC SIGN.

falcate FALCIFORM.

falces Plural of FALX.

falcial 1 Pertaining to a falx. 2 Sickle-shaped.

falciform Sickle-shaped. Also *falcular, falcate.*

falcula FALX CEREBELLI.

falcular FALCIFORM.

fallacy A false idea or assumption.

ecological fallacy The assumption that because a statistical association exists at one level of aggregation it must also exist at a lower level. This assumption is false. Thus, although the incidence of a disease may be positively associated with a given environmental factor when data at, say, state level are compared, the association may be positive, absent, or even negative when data for individual patients are analyzed.

Fallopio [Gabriele *Fallopio*, Italian anatomist, 1523–1562] 1 Foramen of Fallopio. See under HIATUS CANALIS NERVI PETROSI MAJORIS. 2 Canalis facialis fallopii. See under CANALIS FACIALIS. 3 Ligament of Fallopius. See under LIGAMENTUM INGUINALE. 4 Fallopian valve. See under VALVA ILEOCECALIS.

Fallot [Étienne Louis Arthur *Fallot*, French physician, 1850–1911] 1 See under PENTALOGY, TRILOGY. 2 Fallot's disease, Fallot syndrome, Fallot's tetrad. See under TETRALOGY.

fallout Fine radioactive dust or other material projected into the atmosphere by a nuclear explosion and later resettling to earth.

Falls [Harold Francis *Falls*, U.S. opththalmologist and geneticist, born 1909] Rundles-Falls syndrome. See under HEREDITARY SIDEROBLASTIC ANEMIA.

falsification A deliberate misrepresentation of the truth.

retrospective falsification The addition of false details to a memory that is otherwise true, usually to bring it into accord with one's wishes or desires.

Falta [Wilhelm *Falta*, Austrian physician, born 1875] **1** See under TRIAD. **2** Kahn-Falta sign. See under SIGN.

falx [L (gen. *falçis*), a scythe, sickle] (*plural* falces) **1** A sickle-shaped structure or tissue. **2** Either the falx cerebri or the falx cerebelli.

aponeurotic falx FALX INGUINALIS.

falx aponeurotica FALX INGUINALIS.

falx cerebelli [NA] A fold of dura mater lying in the midsagittal plane, separating the two cerebellar hemispheres. Also called *falx of cerebellum, mediastinum cerebelli, falcula, falciform process of cerebellum.*

falx of cerebellum FALX CEREBELLI.

falx cerebri A midline fold of dura mater situated superiorly in the midsagittal plane that separates the two cerebral hemispheres. Also called *falx of cerebrum, mediastinum cerebri* (seldom used), *falciform process of cerebrum.*

falx of cerebrum FALX CEREBRI.

inguinal falx FALX INGUINALIS.

falx inguinalis [NA] The conjoint tendon of the transverse and internal oblique muscles of the abdomen, arching over the spermatic cord in the male and the round ligament of the uterus in the female and descending behind the superficial inguinal ring to its insertion on the crest and the pecten of the pubis, while it fuses medially with the anterior lamina of the rectus sheath. Occasionally the lateral fibers are continuous with the interfoveolar ligament. Also called *conjoint tendon, conjoined tendon, tendo conjunctivus, falciform aponeurosis of rectus abdominis muscle* (outmoded), *inguinal falx, aponeurotic falx, falx aponeurotica, falciform process of rectus abdominis muscle* (outmoded). See also HENLE'S LIGAMENT.

falx ligamentosa An outmoded term for PROCESSUS FALCIFORMIS LIGAMENTI SACROTUBERALIS.

ligamentous falx An outmoded term for PROCESSUS FALCIFORMIS LIGAMENTI SACROTUBERALIS.

falx septi VALVULA FORAMINIS OVALIS.

fames [L, hunger] HUNGER.

familial **1** Of or pertaining to the family. **2** Affecting more members of a family than would be predicted on the basis of mere chance.

family [L *familia* (gen. *familiae*; old gen. *familias* following *pater* father etc.; from *famulus* a servant, slave, akin to Gaelic *feumail* useful) the slaves belonging to one master, one's whole property, a family] **1** A social group, especially a human social group, comprising parents and their offspring and sometimes other relatives. **2** A biological taxonomic group ranking above the genus and below the order.

biologic family In demography, the group comprising a couple and their children. A seldom used term.

broken family A family that has been disrupted by separation or divorce. A popular usage.

extended family A group related by blood or marriage, extending over three or more generations, and including collateral relatives, their spouses, and offspring to an extent varying according to custom and mores in different cultures.

form-family See under FORM.

Jukes family A family descended from five sisters from New York State that was studied by the sociologist and penal reformer R.L. Dugdale in the 1870s. Many family members were described as criminals, paupers, or feeble-minded. Dugdale, who assigned the pseudonym Jukes to the family, ascribed these defects to such environmental influences as malnutrition, illiteracy, and congenital infections. Later authors distorted the data and ignored Dugdale's conclusions by promulgating genetic causes for the so-called defects. The Jukes family became a prototype for hereditarians seeking negative eugenic solutions to societal problems.

Kallikak family A family from New Jersey sired by a Revolutionary War soldier and studied by H.H. Goodard in 1912. In one branch of the family, descended from an illegitimate son, more than one quarter of the relatives were described as feebleminded, illegitimate, prostitutes, or alcoholics. The legitimate branch contained relatives described as intelligent and respectable. The study was cited by hereditarians in support of negative eugenic solutions to societal problems, particularly low intelligence.

nuclear family A family unit comprising the father, mother, and their unmarried children. Also called *family nucleus.*

family-centered Pertaining to health care processes that focus on patients or clients in their family setting, or on the family as a unit.

family romance The fantasy that one is the child of people other than one's own parents.

famine [Middle English and Old or Middle French, from presumed Vulgar L *famina* hunger, from L *fames* hunger, famine] Severe hunger and starvation occurring as a result of a widespread drastic shortage of food.

fan [Old English *fann*, from L *vannus* a winnowing fan]

Dunham's fans DUNHAM'S TRIANGLES.

macular fan A fanlike or stellate area of lipoidal deposits in the macula area of the retina occurring as a consequence of severe papilledema or as a result of other abnormal vascular permeability. Also called *macular star.*

FANA fluorescent antinuclear antibody.

Fanconi [Guido *Fanconi*, Swiss pediatrician, born 1892] **1** Wissler-Fanconi syndrome. See under SYNDROME. **2** Fanconi syndrome, Fanconi's disease. See under CONGENITAL HYPOPLASTIC ANEMIA. **3** De Toni-Fanconi syndrome, de Toni-Debré-Fanconi syndrome, Debré-de Toni-Fanconi syndrome, Fanconi's disease. See under FANCONI SYNDROME. **4** Lignac-Fanconi syndrome. See under NEPHROGENIC CYSTINOSIS. **5** Fanconi's pancytopenia. See under FANCONI'S ANEMIA. **6** Lignac-Fanconi disease. See under CYSTINOSIS.

fang [Middle English *fang* a thing seized, from root of Old English *fon, fōn* to seize; akin to German *fangen* to take] **1** A large canine tooth of carnivores used for seizing prey. **2** An enlarged hollow tooth of venomous snakes used for injecting poison. **3** A root of a tooth.

fango See under FANGO THERAPY.

Fannia [Gk *phanos* (adj.) light, bright; as substantive, a lamp, lantern + -IA] A genus of flies of the family Muscidae. The larvae of some species cause myiasis and pseudomyiasis in humans.

Fannia canicularis The lesser housefly. It is largely black with yellow markings on the sides of the abdomen, and is more slender than the common housefly. It is thought to cause intestinal myiasis in Europe, though feces may actually be contaminated in the environment. Also called *Anthomyia canicularis.*

Fannia scalaris The latrine fly, larger than *F. canicularis* and differentiated from it by having two rather than three stripes on the adult thorax. It lays its eggs on human and animal excrement more frequently than on decaying vegetable material. Also called *Anthomyia scalaris.*

fanning The spreading movement of the second to the fifth toes seen on eliciting the plantar reflex in patients with an extensor plantar response (Babinski's sign).

Fansidar An antimicrobial agent consisting of a fixed combination of pyrimethamine and sulfadiazine and effective in the prevention of chloroquine-resistant malaria. A proprietary name.

fantascope [Gk *phanta(sma)* an image presented to the mind + -SCOPE] RETINOSCOPE.

fantasy A group of symbols synthesized into a unified story by the secondary process of the ego; an imagining. Also called *phantasia*. Also *phantasy*.

beating fantasy A fantasy that oneself or another, often a child, is being whipped.

forced fantasy In psychiatry a technique whereby the therapist directs a patient whose associations lack significant affect. The patient is urged to fabricate or guess about memories and the affects that accompanied the actual event.

Fantus [Bernard *Fantus*, U.S. pharmacologist, 1874–1940] See under ANTIDOTE.

Farabeuf [Louis Hubert *Farabeuf*, French surgeon, 1841–1910] See under SAW, AMPUTATION, TRIANGLE.

farad [after Michael *Faraday*, English chemist and physicist, 1791–1867] The special name for the SI derived unit of capacitance, the capacitance of a capacitor between the plates of which there appears a difference of electric potential of one volt when it is charged by a quantity of electricity of one coulomb; 1 farad = 1 coulomb/1 volt. Symbol: F

Faraday [Michael *Faraday*, English chemist and physicist, 1791–1867] **1** Cage, constant. **2** Faraday's laws. See under LAW.

faraday [after Michael *Faraday*, English physicist, 1791–1867] A unit of quantity of electricity, the quantity that will deposit one mole of monovalent ion from a conducting solution, equal to 9.648 456 coulombs per mole. • Originally a *faraday* was that quantity that would deposit one kilogram equivalent of silver from a conducting solution.

faradic Of or relating to the asymmetric alternating current used in faradism.

faradimeter An instrument for measuring faradic current.

faradipuncture The application of therapeutic faradic electrical currents to the body, using needle electrodes. Also called *faradopuncture*.

faradism The therapeutic application of faradic current used principally for the stimulation of muscles and nerves. Also called *faradization*.

galvanic faradism The combination of constant galvanic current with surging faradic current for therapy.

general faradism The application of surging faradic current to the main muscles of the arms, legs, and trunk to treat obesity.

surging faradism A gradually increasing and decreasing faradic current obtained by varying a series resistance in the circuit.

faradization FARADISM.

faradize To subject to, or to treat with, a faradic current; to treat by faradism.

faradocontractility [FARAD + *o* + *contractility*] The ability of muscle to respond to an alternating electric current.

faradomuscular Denoting the effect of an alternating current in exciting muscle.

faradonervous Pertaining to or resulting from faradic stimulation of a nerve. A seldom used term.

faradopalpation The use of faradic stimulation to identify cutaneous or subcutaneous trigger zones. An obsolete term.

faradopuncture FARADIPUNCTURE.

faradotherapy Therapy using a faradic current.

Farber [Sidney *Farber*, U.S. pathologist, 1903–1973] **1** See under TEST. **2** Farber's disease. See under LIPOGRANULOMATOSIS.

farcinoma [French *farcin* farcy + -OMA. See FARCY.] A granulomatous, tumorlike swelling, as that seen in glanders, called, in the aggregate, farcy buds.

farcy [French *farcin* (from L *farciminum* a disease of horses, from *farcire* to fill up, stuff, from Gk *phrassein* to block up, make full) a contagious disease of horses in which the nasal fossae are inflamed] A form of glanders characterized by subcutaneous ulcerative lesions and thickening of the superficial lymphatics with formation of nodules (farcy buds). The disease is believed to follow inoculation through breaks in the skin.

button farcy A form of farcy characterized by tubercular nodules on the trunk and extremities.

cattle farcy A chronic, suppurative disease of the skin and superficial lymphatics of cattle, caused by *Nocardia farcinica*.

farcy pipes Dilated lymphatic vessels, particularly of the limbs, that form in the cutaneous form of glanders (farcy).

farfara [L, coltsfoot] The dried leaves of the herb *Tussilago farfara* of the Compositae family. An infusion made from it relieves bronchitis.

farina [L (from *far* corn or grain of any kind), meal, flour] **1** A meal or flour made from cereal grains. **2** A starchy food usually prepared from wheat.

farinaceous [L *farin(a)* meal, flour + English *-aceous*, adjectival suffix denoting characterized by] Containing starch, such as flour.

farinometer [L *farin(a)* meal, flour + *o* + -METER] An instrument used to determine the gluten content of flour.

farnesol $C_{15}H_{25}OH$. 3,7,11-trimethyldodeca-2,6,10-trien-1-ol. A terpene alcohol with *trans* configuration of the 2 and 6 double bonds and containing three isoprene units. It occurs in plants. Its diphosphate (pyrophosphate) is an intermediate in the biosynthesis of sterols and many terpenes.

farnesyl pyrophosphate The ester of diphosphoric acid with farnesol. It is formed by elimination of diphosphate from a molecule of dimethylallyl pyrophosphate and two molecules of isopentenyl pyrophosphate. It is an intermediate in the biosynthesis of sterols, via squalene, and of various terpenes.

farnoquinone An obsolete term for MENAQUINONE.

Farr [William *Farr*, English medical statistician, 1807–1883] See under LAW.

Farre [Arthur *Farre*, English obstetrician and gynecologist, 1811–1887] Farre's white line. See under LINE.

Farre [John Richard *Farre*, English physician, 1775–1862] Farre's tubercles. See under TUBERCLE.

farrow [Middle English *farwen* to give birth (to pigs), from Old English *fearh* a young pig] **1** To give birth to a litter of pigs. **2** A litter of pigs.

farsighted [*far* + *sighted* (having sight)] HYPEROPIC.

farsightedness HYPEROPIA.

fasc. *fasciculus* (L, bundle).

fascia

fascia [L, a bandage, band, woman's girdle] (*plural* fasciae) A layer or sheet of connective tissue composed mainly either of loose areolar tissue or compactly arranged collagen fibers and found subcutaneously investing or separating muscles and various structures and organs of the body. It may be a simple, single sheet or complex and multilayered, and is usually divided into superficial fascia, immediately beneath the skin, and deep fascia.

Abernethy's fascia FASCIA ILIACA.

alar fascia of pharynx A sheet of fascia extending medially from the carotid sheath to the pharyngeal part of the buccopharyngeal fascia, fusing with it along the posterior median line of the pharynx from the base of the skull to the level of the seventh cervical vertebra and also attaching to the transverse processes of the cervical vertebrae. Also called *sagittal septa of Charpy.*

anal fascia   FASCIA DIAPHRAGMATIS PELVIS INFERIOR.

anoscrotal fascia   An outmoded term for FASCIA PERINEI SUPERFICIALIS.

antebrachial fascia   FASCIA ANTEBRACHII.

fascia antebrachii   [NA] The deep fascia of the forearm investing the muscles and sending septa between them. It is firmly attached to the posterior margin of ulna and the posterior surface of olecranon, and is continuous proximally with brachial fascia and distally with deep fascia of the hand. It is strengthened by transverse, longitudinal, and oblique fibers attached to certain bony parts and to tendons, especially at the wrist where it is thickened to form the extensor retinaculum posteriorly and the palmar carpal ligament and the flexor retinaculum anteriorly. Also called *antebrachial fascia, deep fascia of forearm, fascia of forearm.*

anterior interosseous fascia   The fascial expansion on the anterior surface of the palmar interosseous muscles.

anterior longitudinal fascia   LIGAMENTUM LONGITUDINALE ANTERIUS.

aponeurotic fascia   DEEP FASCIA.

fascia of arm   FASCIA BRACHII.

fascia axillaris   [NA] A dome-shaped fibrous membrane that stretches across the base of the pyramidal-shaped axilla between the lower borders of the pectoralis major and latissimus dorsi muscles, continuous laterally with the brachial fascia and medially with fascia over the serratus anterior muscle. Because the clavipectoral fascia is attached to it by the suspensory ligament of axilla, the axillary fascia is raised during elevation of the arm, producing the hollowing of the armpit. It is pierced by the axillary tail of the mammary gland, lymphatics, and the intercostobrachial nerve. Also called *axillary fascia.*

axillary fascia   FASCIA AXILLARIS.

bicipital fascia   APONEUROSIS MUSCULI BICIPITIS BRACHII.

brachial fascia   FASCIA BRACHII.

fascia brachii   [NA] The deep fascia investing the muscles of the arm, continuous proximally with the axillary fascia and that of the muscles of the shoulder, and distally with the antebrachial fascia. It is anchored to the distal half of the humerus by the medial and lateral intermuscular septa, to the epicondyles, and to the posterior surface of olecranon. It is pierced by nerves and vessels, the largest being the basilic vein. Also called *brachial fascia, fascia of arm, deep fascia of arm.*

buccinator fascia   An outmoded term for FASCIA BUCCO-PHARYNGEALIS.

buccopharyngeal fascia   FASCIA BUCCOPHARYNGEALIS.

fascia buccopharyngealis   [NA] The thin layer of fibrous tissue surrounding the constrictor muscles of the pharynx, extending anteriorly to cover the buccinator muscle and blending superiorly with the pharyngobasilar fascia. Inferiorly it extends forwards to blend with the pretracheal fascia and the sheath of the thyroid gland. Also called *buccopharyngeal fascia, buccinator fascia* (outmoded), *peripharyngeal fascia* (outmoded).

Buck's fascia   FASCIA PENIS PROFUNDA.

bulbar fascia   VAGINA BULBI.

fascia bulbi tenoni   An outmoded term for VAGINA BULBI.

fascia of Camper   The superficial, or fatty, layer of the superficial fascia of the lower third of the anterior abdominal wall, becoming continuous over the inguinal ligament with the superficial fascia of the thigh, while more centrally it extends into the penis as its superficial fascia, while in the female it continues into the labia majora. In the penis it loses its fat and continues into the scrotum, where it develops a few dartos muscle fibers. Occasionally it fuses with the deep layer (Scarpa's fascia) in the penis and scrotum.

cervical fascia   FASCIA CERVICALIS.

fascia cervicalis   [NA] The deep fascia investing the neck and extending around and between muscles, vessels, and viscera as fibrous sheets and sheaths. Deep to the superficial fascia and platysma, it roofs the anterior triangle of the neck, surrounds the sternocleidomastoid muscle, roofs the posterior triangle, encloses the trapezius muscle, and becomes continuous with the ligamentum nuchae. Superiorly it is attached to the inferior margin of mandible, ascending to form the masseteric fascia and parotid fascia before attaching to, among others, the zygoma, the mastoid process, and the superior nuchal line. Inferiorly it attaches to the clavicle and the manubrium sterni. More deeply in the neck, it forms the pretracheal fascia, prevertebral fascia, stylomandibular ligament, and the carotid sheath. Also called *cervical fascia, fascia colli, fascia of neck, fascia propria colli, proper fascia of neck.*

cervical visceral fascia   LAMINA PRETRACHEALIS FASCIAE CERVICALIS.

fascia cinerea   GYRUS FASCIOLARIS.

clavipectoral fascia   FASCIA CLAVIPECTORALIS.

fascia clavipectoralis   [NA] A strong sheet of connective tissue between the subclavius and pectoralis minor muscles, deep to the pectoralis major and attached to the first rib medially and the coracoid process of scapula laterally, the latter part often being designated the costocoracoid ligament, or membrane. Superiorly it splits around the subclavius to attach to the clavicle, and inferiorly it splits around the pectoralis minor to rejoin below it and continue inferiorly to fuse with the axillary fascia. The fascia above pectoralis minor is pierced by lymphatics, the cephalic vein, the lateral pectoral nerve, and thoracoacromial vessels. Also called *fascia coracoclavicularis, coracoclavicular fascia, clavicoracoaxillary aponeurosis, coracocostal fascia, clavipectoral fascia, costocoracoid fascia* (outmoded), *costocoracoid membrane.*

clavipectoroaxillary fascia   The suspensory ligament of the axilla and the clavipectoral fascia considered as a unit. An outmoded term.

fascia clitoridis   [NA] The dense fibrous tissue surrounding the body of the clitoris and continuous with the suspensory ligament. The fascia is not as clearly demarcated as that of the penis. Also called *fascia of clitoris.*

fascia of clitoris   FASCIA CLITORIDIS.

Cloquet's fascia   SEPTUM FEMORALE.

Colles fascia   FASCIA PERINEI SUPERFICIALIS.

fascia colli   FASCIA CERVICALIS.

fasciae of colon   An outmoded term for TAENIAE COLI.

Cooper's fascia   FASCIA CREMASTERICA.

coracoclavicular fascia   FASCIA CLAVIPECTORALIS.

fascia coracoclavicularis   FASCIA CLAVIPECTORALIS.

coracocostal fascia   FASCIA CLAVIPECTORALIS.

costocoracoid fascia   An outmoded term for FASCIA CLAVIPECTORALIS.

cremasteric fascia   FASCIA CREMASTERICA.

fascia cremasterica   A sheet of loosely arranged fasciculi of the cremaster muscle joined together by loose connective tissue, extending from the superficial inguinal ring down the spermatic cord to the testis and lying between the external and the internal spermatic fasciae. Also called *cremasteric fascia, Cooper's fascia, Scarpa sheath.*

cribriform fascia   FASCIA CRIBROSA.

fascia cribrosa   [NA] The deep layer of superficial fascia that covers the saphenous opening in the fascia lata femoris, continuous with the margins of the opening and with the femoral sheath and pierced by the great saphenous vein, branches of the femoral artery, and lymph vessels. These perforations create a sievelike appearance. Also called *cribriform fascia, Hesselbach's fascia, cribriform plate, cribriform lamina* (outmoded), *cribriform membrane.*

crural fascia   FASCIA CRURIS.

fascia cruris   [NA] The investing deep fascia of the leg, continuous with the fascia lata and attached superiorly to the patella, ligamentum patellae, condyles of tibia, and head of fibula, and inferiorly to the malleoli and the back of the calcaneus. It is adherent to periosteum on the subcutaneous medial surface of the tibia, and from its deep surface arise muscles, the anterior and posterior crural intermuscular septa, and the deep transverse fascia of the leg. Around the ankle it is reinforced to form the superior and inferior extensor retinacula, the flexor retinaculum, and the peroneal retinacula. Also called *crural fascia, crural aponeurosis, fascia of leg, tibial fascia* (outmoded), *tendinous sheath of leg* (outmoded), *crural sheath.*

fascia cruris profunda   An outmoded term for DEEP TRANSVERSE FASCIA OF LEG.

Cruveilhier's fascia   FASCIA PERINEI SUPERFICIALIS.

dartos fascia of scrotum   TUNICA DARTOS.

deep fascia   Compact connective tissue sheets that invest muscles and form intermuscular septa between them, become thickened around joints to form retinacula over tendons, vessels and nerves, ensheath certain vessels or nerves, fuse with periosteum over bone, or form osseofibrous channels or fibrous sheaths over tendons, and may invest certain organs and glands. Also called *aponeurotic fascia.*

deep fascia of anterior region of forearm   A transverse intermuscular septum deep to the flexor digitorum superficialis muscles. It is more marked in the distal half of the forearm and separates the superficial from the deep digital flexor muscles.

deep fascia of arm   FASCIA BRACHII.

deep fascia of back   FASCIA THORACOLUMBALIS.

deep cervical fascia   FASCIA NUCHAE.

deep dorsal fascia   FASCIA THORACOLUMBALIS.

deep dorsal fascia of the foot   A very thin aponeurosis that covers the dorsal surface of the metatarsal bones and the interosseous muscles.

deep fascia of forearm   FASCIA ANTEBRACHII.

deep fascia of penis   FASCIA PENIS PROFUNDA.

deep perineal fascia   An outmoded term for MEMBRANA PERINEI.

deep fascia of perineum   An outmoded term for MEMBRANA PERINEI.

deep fascia of thigh   FASCIA LATA FEMORIS.

deep transverse fascia of leg   A broad, transverse, intermuscular septum that extends from the medial margin of the tibia to the posterior margin of the fibula and lies between the superficial and the deep muscles of the back of the leg. Also called *fascia cruris profunda* (outmoded).

Denonvilliers fascia   SEPTUM RECTOVESICALE.

fascia dentata hippocampi   GYRUS DENTATUS.

dentate fascia   GYRUS DENTATUS.

Dupuytren's fascia   APONEUROSIS PALMARIS.

fascia diaphragmatis pelvis inferior   [NA] The thin layer of fascia that lines the inferior surface of the levator ani and coccygeus muscles on each side, as well as the medial wall of the ischiorectal fossa. It is continuous superiorly with the obturator fascia and the upward extension of the sheath of pudendal canal, and inferiorly with the fasciae of the sphincter ani externus and sphincter urethrae muscles. Anteriorly it is attached to the ischiopubic rami, while posteriorly it attaches to the anococcygeal ligament and the coccyx. Also called *ischiorectal fascia, ischiorectal aponeurosis* (obsolete), *inferior fascia of pelvic diaphragm, anal fascia, superficial perineal aponeurosis, inferior layer of pelvic diaphragm.*

fascia diaphragmatis pelvis superior   [NA] The fascia lining the superior, or pelvic, surface of the levator ani and coccygeus muscles on each side, blending medially with the visceral pelvic fascia. From its anterior attachment at the back of the symphysis pubis it follows the attached origin of levator ani, blending with the obturator fascia, to the ischial spine where it fuses with the fascia covering the coccygeus muscle and with the tendinous insertion of the pubococcygeus muscle. Along its line of attachment from pubis to ischial spine is the tendinous arch of pelvic fascia. Also called *superior fascia of pelvic diaphragm, rectal fascia, aponeurosis of superior surface of levator ani muscle, superior perineal aponeurosis, superior layer of pelvic diaphragm.*

fascia diaphragmatis urogenitalis inferior   MEMBRANA PERINEI.

fascia diaphragmatis urogenitalis superior   The layer of superficial fascia that was once believed to separate the sphincter urethrae muscle from the prostate gland. It is now known that this layer does not, in fact, exist. Also called *middle perineal fascia, deep layer of triangular ligament, puboischiadic ligament of prostate gland* (outmoded), *deep layer of urogenital diaphragm.*

dorsal fascia of foot   FASCIA DORSALIS PEDIS.

dorsal fascia of hand   FASCIA DORSALIS MANUS.

fascia dorsalis manus   [NA] The deep fascia on the back of the hand, continuous with the antebrachial fascia and split around the extensor tendons on the hand, fusing with the tendons on the back of the fingers. At the medial and lateral borders of the hand it is attached to the fifth and first metacarpals, where it is continuous with the hypothenar and thenar fascia respectively. Also called *dorsal fascia of hand.*

fascia dorsalis pedis   [NA] A thin fascial membrane continuous with fascia cruris at the inferior extensor retinaculum and extending to the dorsum of the toes where it forms fibrous sheaths for the extensor tendons. At the medial and lateral margins of the foot it is continuous with the plantar fascia. A thin sheet adheres to each dorsal interosseous muscle and to the extensor digitorum brevis muscle. Also called *dorsal fascia of foot.*

endoabdominal fascia   FASCIA TRANSVERSALIS.

endopelvic fascia   FASCIA ENDOPELVINA.

fascia endopelvina   The areolar connective tissue between and investing the pelvic viscera, continuous with extraperitoneal tissue and condensed in places into membranes, ligaments and folds, such as the uterosacral, lateral cervical, uterovesicular, pubovesical, and puboprostatic ligaments. The fascia is continuous with that between the broad ligament of the uterus, and in both sexes fuses with the superior fascia of pelvic diaphragm where the viscera pass through the latter. The fascia also surrounds the internal iliac vessels and their main branches. It includes the tela subserosa of the viscera and of the walls of the pelvis. Also called *endopelvic fascia.*

endothoracic fascia   FASCIA ENDOTHORACICA.

fascia endothoracica   [NA] The thin layer of loose connective tissue that lines the internal surface of the thoracic cavity, lying outside the parietal pleura and fusing with the periosteum of the ribs and sternum. It is continuous posteriorly with the thoracic part of the prevertebral fascia, superiorly with the cervical prevertebral fascia and the scalene fascia along the first rib, and inferiorly with the transversalis fascia through the aortic opening in the diaphragm and the lumbocostal arches. Also called *endothoracic fascia, extrapleural fascia.*

fascia of extensor digitorum brevis   A thin aponeurotic layer that covers the extensor digitorum brevis muscle, the dorsal vessels, and the deep peroneal nerve in the foot. It is deep to the long extensor tendons and attached laterally to the lateral margin of the foot and medially to the fascia dorsalis pedis and the tendon of the extensor hallucis longus muscle. An outmoded term.

external cervical fascia   LAMINA SUPERFICIALIS FASCIAE CERVICALIS.

external spermatic fascia   FASCIA SPERMATICA EXTERNA.

extraperitoneal fascia FASCIA EXTRAPERITONEALIS.

fascia extraperitonealis [NA] The layer of fascia external to the parietal peritoneum and deep to the abdominal and pelvic walls. It varies in quantity and may contain fat in different areas, such as around the kidney. In some areas, such as behind the linea alba, it may be dense, causing the peritoneum to adhere to the wall. In others it may be very loose, permitting organs to distend it. Also called *subperitoneal fascia, extraperitoneal fascia, fascia subperitonealis.*

extrapleural fascia FASCIA ENDOTHORACICA.

femoral fascia FASCIA LATA FEMORIS.

fibroareolar fascia TELA SUBCUTANEA.

fascia of forearm FASCIA ANTEBRACHII.

Gerota's fascia FASCIA RENALIS.

gluteal fascia Fascia lata that descends as a dense layer from the iliac crest over the gluteus medius muscle to the upper margin of the gluteus maximus muscle. There it splits into two layers, one superficial to the gluteus maximus and one deep to it. At the lower border of the muscle they reunite. Posteriorly it is attached to the sacrum and the coccyx. The deep layer gives off a lamella which extends between the gluteus medius and minimus muscles.

fascia of Godman The prolongation of the pretracheal fascia into the superior mediastinum.

Hesselbach's fascia FASCIA CRIBROSA.

fascia of Hunter's canal A dense fibrous aponeurosis that forms the roof of the adductor canal, extending across the femoral vessels and saphenous nerve from the vastus medialis to the adductor longus and magnus muscles and lying deep to the sartorius muscle.

hypogastric fascia FASCIA PELVIS.

hypothenar fascia The thin medial part of the palmar aponeurosis that covers the hypothenar muscles and becomes continuous medially with the fascia on the dorsum of the hand and laterally with the central part of the aponeurosis.

iliac fascia 1 FASCIA ILIACA. 2 ARCUS ILIOPECTINEUS.

fascia iliaca [NA] The fascia covering the psoas and iliacus muscles. It is especially thick in the inguinal region, where it is firmly adherent to the internal aspect of the inguinal ligament and the transversalis fascia lateral to the femoral vessels, and forms the arcus iliopectineus. The psoas portion is continuous laterally with the anterior layer of thoracolumbar fascia above the iliac crest, and with the iliac portion below the crest, while medially it is attached to the lumbar vertebrae, intervertebral disks, and the ala of the sacrum. The iliac portion is attached laterally to the iliac crest, and medially to the iliac portion of linea terminalis. Inferiorly the fused iliac and psoas portions continue with the iliopsoas muscle to its femoral insertion. Behind the femoral vessels it helps to form the pectineal fascia. Also called *iliac fascia, Abernethy's fascia.* ● In some texts, the iliac and psoas portions are described separately as the iliac fascia and psoas fascia.

fascia iliopectinea ARCUS ILIOPECTINEUS.

iliopectineal fascia ARCUS ILIOPECTINEUS.

inferior fascia of pelvic diaphragm FASCIA DIAPHRAGMATIS PELVIS INFERIOR.

infundibuliform fascia An outmoded term for FASCIA SPERMATICA INTERNA.

fascia of insertion APONEUROSIS OF INSERTION.

intercolumnar fascia An outmoded term for FASCIA SPERMATICA EXTERNA.

intermediate fascia of the serrated muscles A semitransparent fibrous membrane situated between the two serratus posterior superior muscles on the back. The transverse fibers are reinforced by three tendinous bundles opposite the sixth, seventh, and eighth ribs. It represents the fibrous remains of the middle part of the spinocostal or posterior serratus muscle found in certain mammals and corresponds, in humans, to the two serratus posterior muscles.

internal abdominal fascia FASCIA TRANSVERSALIS.

internal spermatic fascia FASCIA SPERMATICA INTERNA.

interpterygoid fascia A layer of fibrous tissue that is situated between the medial and lateral pterygoid muscles in a superoinferior, mediolateral, and anteroposterior plane. Superiorly it is attached to the base of the skull medial to the foramen ovale while its posterior margin constitutes the sphenomandibular ligament. It is fused inferiorly with the superficial lamina of the sheath of the medial pterygoid muscle, whereby it becomes attached to the mandible. It is pierced by vessels and nerves to the tensor veli palatini, tensor tympani, and medial pterygoid muscles. An outmoded term.

investing fascia APONEUROSIS OF INVESTMENT.

ischioprostatic fascia MEMBRANA PERINEI.

ischiorectal fascia FASCIA DIAPHRAGMATIS PELVIS INFERIOR.

lacrimal fascia The thick anterior layer of the periorbita that extends from the lacrimal crest of the maxilla to the crest of the lacrimal bone, forming the roof of the fossa for the lacrimal sac and separating the sac from the medial palpebral ligament anteriorly and from the lacrimal part of musculus orbicularis oculi posteriorly.

fascia lata femoris [NA] The deep fascia investing the hip and thigh regions, thin medially and posteriorly and thick and strong laterally, where it forms the iliotibial tract. It provides intermuscular septa in the gluteal region as well as the medial, lateral, and posterior septa in the thigh where they are anchored to the linea aspera and separate the extensor, adductor, and flexor groups of muscles. Superiorly it is attached to the inguinal ligament, iliac crest, sacrotuberous ligament, ischial tuberosity, back of sacrum and coccyx, and the ischiopubic ramus, while inferiorly it is attached to the condyles of femur and tibia, the patella, and the head of fibula, where it is strengthened by tendinous extensions. Also called *femoral fascia, deep fascia of thigh, fascia of thigh, femoral aponeurosis, vagina femoris* (outmoded), *fascia lata of thigh.*

fascia lata proper The lateral portion of the fascia lata that encloses the tensor fasciae latae and forms the iliotibial tract. An outmoded term.

fascia lata of thigh FASCIA LATA FEMORIS.

fascia of leg FASCIA CRURIS.

lumbar fascia FASCIA THORACOLUMBALIS.

lumbodorsal fascia FASCIA THORACOLUMBALIS.

fascia lumbodorsalis FASCIA THORACOLUMBALIS.

fascia lunata The deep fascia lining and arching over the ischioanal fossa and comprising the inferior fascia of pelvic diaphragm and either the obturator fascia below the arcus tendineus musculus levator ani or an upward extension of the sheath of pudendal canal. The latter blends with the inferior fascia and attaches to the falciform process of sacrotuberous ligament.

masseteric fascia FASCIA MASSETERICA.

fascia masseterica [NA] A layer of deep cervical fascia that spreads upwards from the inferior and posterior margins of the mandible to cover and attach to the masseter muscle, while superficially it forms the parotid fascia investing the gland. At the anterior margin of the mandibular ramus it is continuous with the pterygoid fascia, while superiorly it is attached to the zygomatic arch and may be continuous with the temporal fascia. Also called *masseteric fascia.* ● Some texts consider it to be an extension of the parotid fascia.

middle perineal fascia FASCIA DIAPHRAGMATIS UROGENITALIS SUPERIOR.

middle fascia of pharynx An outmoded term for FASCIA PHARYNGOBASILARIS.

fasciae musculares bulbi [NA] Tubular fibrous sheaths of the bulbar muscles which thicken and fuse with the vagina bulbi where it is pierced by each of the muscles. Proximally they thin out and fuse with the perimysium and may form expansions such as the medial and lateral check ligaments. Also called *muscular fasciae of eye, fasciae musculares oculi.* (outmoded).

fasciae musculares oculi An outmoded term for FASCIAE MUSCULARES BULBI.

muscular fasciae of eye FASCIAE MUSCULARES BULBI.

fascia of nape FASCIA NUCHAE.

fascia of neck FASCIA CERVICALIS.

fascia nuchae [NA] The investing fascial layer of the deep muscles at the back of the neck, including a series of membranes attached to it that surround groups of deep muscles. It is attached to the tips of the transverse processes of cervical vertebrae where it is continuous with the prevertebral fascia. Posteriorly and medially it fuses with ligamentum nuchae. Inferiorly it is continuous with fascia thoracolumbalis, and superiorly it attaches to the skull below the superior nuchal line. Also called *nuchal fascia, fascia of nape, deep cervical fascia.*

nuchal fascia FASCIA NUCHAE.

obturator fascia FASCIA OBTURATORIA.

fascia obturatoria [NA] That part of the parietal pelvic fascia that covers the internal surface of the obturator internus muscle. It fuses with the periosteum around the edges of the obturator foramen except superiorly where it attaches to the obturator membrane, forming a boundary of the obturator canal, and becomes continuous with iliac fascia. Below the tendinous arch, it becomes the lateral wall of the ischioanal fossa and forms the pudendal canal. Posteriorly it leaves the pelvic cavity with the muscle and the two gemellus muscles to their insertion. Also called *obturator fascia.*

orbital fasciae FASCIAE ORBITALES.

fasciae orbitales [NA] The tissues connecting and supporting the various contents of the orbit, including the periorbita, septum orbitale, fasciae musculares, vagina bulbi, and corpus adiposum orbitae. Also called *orbital fasciae.*

palmar fascia APONEUROSIS PALMARIS.

palpebral fascia SEPTUM ORBITALE.

fascia palpebralis An outmoded term for SEPTUM ORBITALE.

parietal pelvic fascia FASCIA PELVIS PARIETALIS.

parietal fascia of pelvis FASCIA PELVIS PARIETALIS.

parotid fascia FASCIA PAROTIDEA.

fascia parotidea [NA] An extension, forward of the investing layer of the deep cervical fascia, from the anterior border of the sternocleidomastoid muscle that splits and invests the parotid gland. The superficial part then extends anteriorly to form the masseteric fascia and attach to the zygomatic arch, while the deep layer fuses with the fascia of the posterior belly of the digastric muscle, attaches to the styloid process, and forms the stylomandibular ligament. Also called *parotid fascia.*

fascia parotideomasseterica Fascia parotidea and fascia masseterica together.

fascia pectinea An extension of the iliac fascia behind the femoral vessels, attaching to the pecten pubis where it is continuous with the deep layer of fascia lata that forms the inferomedial margin of the saphenous opening and turns upwards and laterally behind the femoral vessels and in front of the pectineus muscle to attach to the pecten pubis. Also called *Cowper's ligament, pubic fascia, pectineal fascia.*

pectineal fascia FASCIA PECTINEA.

pectoral fascia FASCIA PECTORALIS.

fascia pectoralis [NA] The thin membrane that invests the pectoralis major muscle, continuous at its lower border with the axillary fascia and attached medially to the sternum and superiorly to the clavicle. It is continuous laterally with the fascia of the deltoid muscle and inferiorly with the fascia over the

serratus anterior muscle and the external oblique muscle of abdomen. Also called *pectoral fascia.*

pelvic fascia FASCIA PELVIS.

pelviprostatic fascia An outmoded term for FASCIA PROSTATAE.

fascia pelvis [NA] The overall fascial sheaths of the pelvis, comprising the parietal pelvic fascia, visceral pelvic fascia, and endopelvic fascia. Also called *pelvic fascia, hypogastric fascia.*

fascia pelvis parietalis [NA] The fascia lining the inner walls of the pelvis, including the muscles passing from the pelvic cavity to the gluteal region, namely, obturator internus and piriformis, as well as the muscles of the pelvic diaphragm on both superior and inferior aspects. Also called *parietal layer of pelvic fascia, parietal fascia of pelvis, parietal pelvic fascia, parietal part of pelvic fascia.*

fascia pelvis visceralis [NA] The fascia that surrounds the various organs and vessels of the pelvis, comprising the endopelvic fascia of specific viscera and the fascia associated with the pelvic peritoneum. Also called *visceral pelvic fascia, visceral fascia of pelvis, visceral layer of pelvic fascia, visceral part of pelvic fascia.*

fascia penis FASCIA PENIS PROFUNDA.

fascia penis profunda [NA] The condensed deep layer of the superficial fascia of the penis, continuous proximally and superiorly with the membranous layer of the superficial fascia of the anterior abdominal wall, and inferiorly with the tunica dartos of the scrotum and the membranous layer in the urogenital triangle where it encloses the crura and the bulb of penis and is joined to the perineal membrane and the perineal body. In the body of the penis it forms a firm sheath around the corpora cavernosa and the corpus spongiosum and separates the deep dorsal vessels and the tunica albuginea from the subcutaneous areolar tissue. Distally it is firmly attached at the collum glandis. Dorsally and proximally it is continuous with the fundiform and suspensory ligaments. Also called *deep fascia of penis, fascia penis, Buck's fascia.*

fascia penis superficialis [NA] The subcutaneous loose areolar tissue surrounding the penis, devoid of fat and continuous proximally and superiorly with the fatty layer of the superficial fascia of the anterior abdominal wall, and inferiorly with the tunica dartos of the scrotum. Distally it fuses with the deep fascia at the collum glandis. Also called *superficial fascia of penis.*

fascia perinei superficialis [NA] The superficial fascia of the perineum, separated into a superficial, fatty layer and a deeper, membranous layer continuous with similar layers on the anterior abdominal wall. The fatty layer becomes the superficial fascia of the penis and the tunica dartos in the scrotum. It is continuous posteriorly with the perianal subcutaneous areolar tissue and laterally with the superficial fascia of the thighs. In the ischioanal fossa it develops a pad of fat. The membranous layer forms the deep fascia of the penis and is continuous with the tunica dartos in the scrotum, whereas in the urogenital triangle it is attached to the margins of the ischiopubic rami over the crura of the penis as far posteriorly as the ischial tuberosities. Centrally it is attached to the lower, posterior margin of the perineal membrane and the perineal body. The arrangement is modified in the female to accommodate the vagina. Also called *superficial fascia of perineum, Colles fascia, Cruveilhier's fascia, superficial perineal fascia, anoscrotal fascia* (outmoded), *fascia superficialis perinei* (outmoded). • *Nomina Anatomica* does not distinguish between the fatty and membranous layers. Strictly, though, Colles fascia designates the membranous layer, and Cruveilhier's fascia the fatty layer.

fasciae of the perineum The fasciae of the muscles and tissues of the perineum, namely the membrana perinei, fascia perinei superficialis, and fascia pelvis.

perirenal fascia   FASCIA RENALIS.

peripharyngeal fascia   An outmoded term for FASCIA BUC-COPHARYNGEALIS.

pharyngobasilar fascia   FASCIA PHARYNGOBASILARIS.

fascia pharyngobasilaris   [NA] The fibrous layer of the wall of the pharynx situated between the mucous and muscular layers, thick superiorly where it is attached to the base of the skull and adjacent structures where the pharyngeal muscle fibers are absent and becoming thinner as it descends. It is supported posteriorly by the pharyngeal raphe, which provides attachment for the pharyngeal constrictor muscles. Also called *pharyngobasilar fascia, pharyngobasilar aponeurosis, pharyngeal aponeurosis, aponeurosis pharyngis* (outmoded), *aponeurosis pharyngobasilaris* (outmoded), *pharyngeal plate* (outmoded), *pharyngobasilar coat, middle fascia of pharynx* (outmoded), *pharyngobasilar tunic, pharyngeal tunic, pharyngobasilar membrane.*

fasciae of the pharynx   The fascial layers related to the muscles of the pharynx, namely the fascia buccopharyngealis, fascia pharyngobasilaris, raphe pharyngis, raphe pterygomandibularis, and the alar fascia of the pharynx.

phrenicopleural fascia   FASCIA PHRENICOPLEURALIS.

fascia phrenicopleuralis   [NA] A flimsy layer of endothoracic fascia that binds the diaphragmatic pleura to the superior surface of the diaphragm. Also called *phrenicopleural fascia.*

plantar fascia   APONEUROSIS PLANTARIS.

popliteal fascia   An extension of fascia cruris over the popliteal fossa where it is strengthened by transverse fibers and pierced by the small saphenous vein.

posterior longitudinal fascia   LIGAMENTUM LONGITUDINALE POSTERIUS.

pretracheal fascia   LAMINA PRETRACHEALIS FASCIAE CERVICALIS.

prevertebral fascia   LAMINA PREVERTEBRALIS FASCIAE CERVICALIS.

fascia prevertebralis   LAMINA PREVERTEBRALIS FASCIAE CERVICALIS.

proper fascia of neck   FASCIA CERVICALIS.

fascia propria colli   FASCIA CERVICALIS.

fascia propria cooperi   An outmoded term for FASCIA SPERMATICA INTERNA.

fascia prostatae   Visceral fascia of the pelvis that ensheathes the prostate gland and its capsule, continuous anteriorly with the puboprostatic ligaments and inferiorly with the fascia on the deep aspects of the transversus perinei profundus and the sphincter urethrae muscles. It contains the prostatic plexus of veins embedded in connective tissue which separates it anteriorly and at the sides from the capsule. Laterally it is continuous with the lateral puboprostatic ligaments, while posteriorly it is separated from the rectum by the rectovesical septum. Also called *fascia of prostate, pelviprostatic fascia* (outmoded), *pelviprostatic capsule* (outmoded), *basal pelviprostatic ligament, sheath of prostate, pelviprostatic capsular ligament* (outmoded).

fascia of prostate   FASCIA PROSTATAE.

psoas fascia   The fascia covering the psoas muscle. Also called *fascia psoatis.*

fascia psoatis   PSOAS FASCIA.

pterygotemporal-maxillary fascia   A fibrous band situated lateral to the upper part of the pterygobasilar fascia. It is attached superiorly to the greater wing of the sphenoid bone in front of the upper part of the lateral lamina of the pterygoid process. It overlaps the mandibular nerve as it emerges below the foramen ovale and separates it from the lateral pterygoid muscle. An outmoded term.

pubic fascia   FASCIA PECTINEA.

fascia of quadratus lumborum muscle   The anterior layer of the thoracolumbar fascia which covers the quadratus lumborum muscle anteriorly. It is attached medially to the anterior surfaces of the transverse processes of the lumbar vertebrae and inferiorly to the iliolumbar ligament and the adjacent part of the iliac crest, while superiorly it forms the lateral lumbocostal arch. Laterally it fuses with the middle and posterior layers to form the common lamella of the thoracolumbar fascia.

rectal fascia   FASCIA DIAPHRAGMATIS PELVIS SUPERIOR.

rectoabdominal fascia   An outmoded term for VAGINA MUSCULI RECTI ABDOMINIS.

rectovaginal fascia   SEPTUM RECTOVAGINALE.

rectovesical fascia   SEPTUM RECTOVESICALE.

renal fascia   FASCIA RENALIS.

fascia renalis   [NA] A sheath of condensed fibroareolar tissue that surrounds the kidney and perirenal fat. It is connected to the fibrous capsule of the kidney by fibrous bands that pierce the perirenal fat. It consists of an anterior and a posterior layer, which are fused at the lateral margin of the kidney. Medially, the anterior layer thins and merges with the connective tissue of the aorta and inferior vena cava, whereas the posterior layer fuses with the psoas fascia. In addition, fibrous tissue binds the two layers to each other medially around the renal vessels. Superiorly the two layers fuse above the suprarenal glands and blend with the diaphragmatic fascia, while inferiorly the layers remain separate and cover the ureter. Also called *renal fascia, perirenal fascia, Gerota's fascia, perinephric sheath* (outmoded), *fibrous sheath of kidney.*

retrorectal fascia   A layer of fibroareolar tissue posterior to the rectum and separating it from the pelvic wall. An outmoded term.

Richet's fascia   A fold of subperitoneal fascia surrounding the ligamentum teres hepatis as it pierces the fibers of the transversus abdominis muscle.

scalene fascia   MEMBRANA SUPRAPLEURALIS.

Scarpa's fascia   The deep or membranous layer of the superficial fascia in the lower part of the anterior abdominal wall. Inferiorly it is attached to the fascia lata in a straight line lateral to the pubic tubercles, whereas between them it is continuous with the membranous layer of the superficial fascia of the perineum.

semilunar fascia   APONEUROSIS MUSCULI BICIPITIS BRACHII.

Sibson's fascia   MEMBRANA SUPRAPLEURALIS.

fascia between soleus and gastrocnemius muscles   An insignificant layer of intermuscular fascia between the aponeurotic posterior surface of the soleus muscle and the deep surface of the medial and lateral gastrocnemius muscles. An outmoded term.

fascia spermatica externa   [NA] A tubulosaccular sheath that forms the outermost covering layer of the spermatic cord and testis. It is composed of fibrous tissue that extends down from the margins of the superficial inguinal ring in the aponeurosis of the external oblique muscle of the abdomen and the overlying fascia. Also called *external spermatic fascia, intercolumnar fascia* (outmoded).

fascia spermatica interna   [NA] A tubulosaccular sheath forming the innermost covering layer of the spermatic cord and testis and being a prolongation of the transversalis fascia at the deep inguinal ring, thereby surrounding the structures passing through the ring and along the inguinal canal. Also called *internal spermatic fascia, infundibuliform fascia* (outmoded), *fascia propria cooperi* (outmoded), *tunica vaginalis communis testis et funiculi spermatici* (outmoded), *common sheath of testis and spermatic cord* (outmoded).

stylopharyngeal fascia   The fascial connection between the buccopharyngeal fascia on the lateral wall of the larynx and the fascia surrounding the muscles and ligaments that are attached to the styloid process. An outmoded term.

subcutaneous fascia   TELA SUBCUTANEA.

subperitoneal fascia 1 FASCIA EXTRAPERITONEALIS. 2 TELA SUBSEROSA PERITONEI.

fascia subperitonealis FASCIA EXTRAPERITONEALIS.

fascia subscapularis The thin membranous layer attached to the total circumference of the subscapular fossa of the scapula, and providing origin from its deep surface to some fibers of the subscapularis muscle. Also called *subscapular aponeurosis.*

subvesical fascia A poorly differentiated pelvic fascia between the base of the urinary bladder and the anterior wall of the vagina.

superficial fascia TELA SUBCUTANEA.

fascia superficialis TELA SUBCUTANEA.

superficial fascia of penis FASCIA PENIS SUPERFICIALIS.

fascia superficialis perinei An outmoded term for FASCIA PERINEI SUPERFICIALIS.

superficial perineal fascia FASCIA PERINEI SUPERFICIALIS.

superficial fascia of perineum FASCIA PERINEI SUPERFICIALIS.

superior fascia of pelvic diaphragm FASCIA DIAPHRAGMATIS PELVIS SUPERIOR.

superior fascia of urogenital fascia See under SPATIUM PERINEI PROFUNDUM.

fascia supraspinata The fascial covering and partial origin of the supraspinatus muscle, attached to the edges of the supraspinous fossa and the spine of the scapula. It is thick medially but thinner under the coracoacromial ligament. Also called *supraspinous aponeurosis.*

fascia of Tarin GYRUS DENTATUS.

fascia tarini GYRUS DENTATUS.

temporal fascia FASCIA TEMPORALIS.

fascia temporalis [NA] A fibrous sheet covering the temporalis muscle and attached superiorly to the superior temporal line of the parietal bone and the temporal line of the frontal bone. Inferiorly it splits into two layers, the more superficial of which is attached to the lateral border and the deep one to the medial border of the zygomatic arch. Between the layers is some fat and small nerves and vessels. Also called *temporal fascia, temporal aponeurosis.*

fascia of Tenon VAGINA BULBI.

thenar fascia The thin fibrous lateral part of the palmar aponeurosis that covers the thenar muscles and is continuous laterally with the fascia on the dorsum of the hand and medially with the central portion of the aponeurosis.

fascia of thigh FASCIA LATA FEMORIS.

fascia thoracolumbalis [NA] The fascia covering the deep muscles of the back of the trunk and continuous superiorly with the nuchal fascia. In the thoracic region it separates the vertebral extensors from the more superficial muscles to the shoulder girdle and upper limb, and is attached laterally to the angles of the ribs and medially to the spines of vertebrae. In the lumbar region there are three layers of fascia that fuse lateral to the quadratus lumborum muscle into a common lamella from which arise parts of transversus abdominis and internal oblique muscles. The posterior layer covers the erector spinae muscle and is attached to the spines of lumbar and sacral vertebrae and their supraspinous ligaments, while the origin of the latissimus dorsi muscle blends with it to form the lumbar aponeurosis. The middle layer, between the erector spinae and quadratus lumborum, is attached to the tips of the transverse processes of lumbar vertebrae, while the anterior layer anterior to the quadratus lumborum is attached medially to the anterior surfaces of those transverse processes and inferiorly to the iliac crest and iliolumbar ligament. The anterior layer blends with the fascia transversalis and psoas fascia. Also called *thoracolumbar fascia, fascia lumbodorsalis, lumbodorsal fascia, deep dorsal fascia, deep fascia of back, vertebral aponeurosis, lumbar aponeurosis, lumbar fascia.*

thoracolumbar fascia FASCIA THORACOLUMBALIS.

thyrolaryngeal fascia An outmoded term for LAMINA PRETRACHEALIS FASCIAE CERVICALIS.

tibial fascia An outmoded term for FASCIA CRURIS.

fascia of Toldt 1 The subperitoneal fascial layer posterior to the ascending colon (the right fascia of Toldt) and the descending colon (the left fascia of Toldt). It results from the fusion of the parietal peritoneum with the peritoneum covering corresponding parts of the colon or, when present, their mesocolon. 2 A fixation of fascial layers behind the body of the pancreas that is continuous with the fascia of Treitz.

fascia transversalis [NA] The layer of connective tissue between the extensive internal surface of the transversus abdominis muscle and the subperitoneal fascia, the right and left sides fusing behind the linea alba. It is continuous superiorly with the diaphragmatic fascia, posteriorly with the anterior layer of the thoracolumbar and psoas fasciae, while inferiorly it is attached to the iliac crest and the posterior edge of the inguinal ligament, where it is continuous with the iliac fascia. It is also attached to pecten pubis behind the conjoint tendon, helping to form the pectineal ligament. It forms the anterior wall of the femoral sheath. Also called *transverse fascia, internal abdominal fascia, endoabdominal fascia.*

transverse fascia FASCIA TRANSVERSALIS.

fascia of Treitz A layer of fascia that is situated behind the head of the pancreas and separates it from structures on the posterior abdominal wall, namely the right crus of the diaphragm, abdominal aorta, inferior vena cava, and right renal vein.

triangular fascia of abdomen LIGAMENTUM REFLEXUM.

triangular fascia of Macalister An outmoded term for MUSCULUS PYRAMIDALIS.

triangular fascia of Quain LIGAMENTUM REFLEXUM.

Tyrrell's fascia SEPTUM RECTOVESICALE.

umbilical prevesical fascia UMBILICOVESICAL FASCIA.

umbilicovesical fascia The deeper layer of the transversalis fascia and its continuation along the anterior surface of the bladder that forms the dorsal boundary of the retropubic space. An outmoded term. Also called *umbilical prevesical fascia.*

fascia of urogenital trigone DIAPHRAGMA UROGENITALE.

visceral pelvic fascia FASCIA PELVIS VISCERALIS.

visceral fascia of pelvis FASCIA PELVIS VISCERALIS.

volar fascia APONEUROSIS PALMARIS.

Waldeyer's fascia 1 The visceral pelvic fascia surrounding the pelvic part of the ureter. An outmoded term. 2 A sheath of vesical muscle fibers extending about 5 mm up the supravesical part of the ureter. It is probably the additional outer layer of longitudinal muscle fibers observed in the lower part of the ureter. An outmoded term.

---

fasciae Plural of FASCIA.

fasciagram [FASCIA + -GRAM] A radiograph of fasciae obtained with the use of air injected as a contrast medium.

fasciagraphy [FASCIA + -GRAPHY] Radiographic examination of fasciae obtained with the use of air injected as a contrast medium.

fascial Pertaining to fascia.

fasciaplasty [FASCIA + -PLASTY] A plastic operation on a fascia, usually utilizing plication. Also called *fascioplasty.*

fascicle [L *fasciculus,* dim. of *fascis* a bundle of wood, rods, twigs, reeds, or straws] 1 A group of nerve fibers coursing in the same direction and often subserving a similar function. 2 FASCICULUS. 3 A condensed or close cluster, as of flowers or pine needles.

gracile fascicle FASCICULUS GRACILIS MEDULLAE SPINALIS.

longitudinal fascicles of cruciform ligament FASCICULI LONGITUDINALES LIGAMENTI CRUCIFORMIS ATLANTIS.

fascicular 1 Pertaining to a fasciculus. 2 FASCICULATED.

fasciculated Arranged in clusters or bundles. Also *fascicular*.

fasciculation [*fascicul(us)* + -ATION] Spontaneous contraction of bundles of skeletal muscle fibers resulting in a localized twitching or flickering which can be seen under the skin or a mucous membrane but does not produce movement at a joint. Compare FIBRILLATION. Also called *muscular tremor*.

benign fasciculation Fasciculation usually in the calf muscles or first interosseous space, less often in other muscles, which is benign and of no pathologic significance. Benign coarse fasciculation is a prominent feature of one form of myokymia.

fasciculi Plural of FASCICULUS.

fasciculitis [*fascicul(us)* + -ITIS] Inflammation limited to a few fascicles, usually of a nerve.

fasciculitis optica An outmoded term for OPTIC NEURITIS.

fasciculus

fasciculus [L (dim. of *fascis* a bundle, packet), a little bundle or packet] (*plural* fasciculi) [NA] A bundle of muscle, nerve, or connective tissue fibers. Also called *fascicle*.

fasciculus aberrans of Monakow TRACTUS RUBROSPINALIS.

fasciculus acusticus An incorrect and obsolete term for STRIAE MEDULLARES VENTRICULI QUARTI.

fasciculus anterior proprius flechsigi The fasciculi proprii, intersegmental axons, bordering the gray matter of the spinal ventral horn running in the anterior funiculus.

anterior pyramidal fasciculus TRACTUS CORTICOSPINALIS VENTRALIS.

fasciculus anterolateralis superficialis Gowersi TRACTUS SPINOCEREBELLARIS VENTRALIS.

fasciculus arcuatus FASCICULUS LONGITUDINALIS SUPERIOR CEREBRI.

fasciculus atrioventricularis [NA] A slender bundle of cardiac muscle fibers specially differentiated to conduct impulses for the contraction of cardiac muscle. It commences at the atrioventricular node in the lower part of the interatrial septum and passes subendocardially through the right trigonum fibrosum to reach the interventricular septum, ventral to which it divides into a right and a left crus, or limb. Each passes down either side of the septum to branch out to the walls of the ventricles. Also called *atrioventricular bundle, A-V bundle, bundle of His, Kent-His bundle, bundle of Stanley Kent, His band, Gaskell's bridge* (outmoded), *ventriculonector, atrioventricular band, auriculoventricular band* (outmoded).

fasciculus of Burdach FASCICULUS CUNEATUS BURDACHI.

calcarine fasciculus A short bundle of association fibers lying beneath the calcarine sulcus and reciprocally connecting the upper and lower banks.

central tegmental fasciculus TRACTUS TEGMENTALIS CENTRALIS.

cerebellospinal fasciculus An imprecise term for TRACTUS SPINOCEREBELLARIS DORSALIS.

fasciculus cerebellospinalis An imprecise term for TRACTUS SPINOCEREBELLARIS DORSALIS.

fasciculus cerebrospinalis anterior TRACTUS CORTICOSPINALIS VENTRALIS.

fasciculus cerebrospinalis lateralis TRACTUS CORTICOSPINALIS LATERALIS.

fasciculus circumolivaris pyramidalis A bundle of axons coursing from the surface of the medullary pyramid, over the inferior olivary protuberance, and into the pons.

crossed pyramidal fasciculus TRACTUS CORTICOSPINALIS LATERALIS.

cuneate fasciculus of Burdach FASCICULUS CUNEATUS BURDACHI.

cuneate fasciculus of medulla oblongata FASCICULUS CUNEATUS MEDULLAE OBLONGATAE.

cuneate fasciculus of spinal cord FASCICULUS CUNEATUS MEDULLAE SPINALIS.

fasciculus cuneatus FASCICULUS CUNEATUS BURDACHI.

fasciculus cuneatus burdachi The fasciculus cuneatus medullae spinalis, along with its rostral continuation, the fasciculus cuneatus medullae oblongatae. Also called *fasciculus cuneatus, cuneate fasciculus of Burdach, fasciculus of Burdach, Burdach's tract, column of Burdach*.

fasciculus cuneatus medullae oblongatae [NA] The rostral continuation of the cuneate fasciculus of the spinal cord, overlying the cuneate nucleus of the medulla oblongata. Also called *cuneate fasciculus of medulla oblongata, funiculus cuneatus medullae oblongatae* (outmoded), *funiculus cuneatus Burdachi* (outmoded), *cuneate funiculus*.

fasciculus cuneatus medullae spinalis [NA] The axonal bundle forming the lateral portion of the posterior (dorsal) column and constituting the largest demarcated fascicle of myelinated fibers in the spinal cord. It is composed chiefly of large ascending axons arising from spinal ganglion cells of the cervical and upper thoracic levels that terminate in the cuneate nucleus (Burdach's nucleus) of the medulla oblongata. It also contains ascending axons from neurons of the spinal dorsal horn and a few descending interfascicular axons. Also called *cuneate fasciculus of spinal cord*.

diagonal fasciculus of rhomboid muscle An occasional muscle fasciculus that extends obliquely on the deep surface of the rhomboideus major muscle from the upper part of its origin to the distal part of its insertion. An outmoded term.

direct pyramidal fasciculus TRACTUS CORTICOSPINALIS VENTRALIS.

dorsal longitudinal fasciculus FASCICULUS LONGITUDINALIS DORSALIS.

dorsolateral fasciculus TRACTUS DORSOLATERALIS.

fasciculus dorsolateralis TRACTUS DORSOLATERALIS.

fasciculus exilis A variant of the origin of the flexor pollicis longus muscle, consisting of some fasciculi attaching to the medial epicondyle of humerus or to the coronoid process of ulna.

extrapyramidal motor fasciculus An outmoded and imprecise term for TRACTUS RUBROSPINALIS.

fastigiobulbar fasciculus An efferent bundle of cerebellar fibers emerging from the fastigial nucleus via the uncinate fasciculus (of Russell) arching around the superior cerebellar peduncle. Fibers from the rostral fastigial nucleus are uncrossed, sweep ventromedially, and terminate in the vestibular nuclei and dorsomedial parts of the pontine and medullary reticular formation. The larger, crossed component arises from the caudal fastigial nucleus and terminates in the medullary lateral reticular nucleus and perihypoglossal nucleus.

fibrous fasciculus of biceps muscle APONEUROSIS MUSCULI BICIPITIS BRACHII.

Flechsig's fasciculus Either fasciculus anterior proprius flechsigi or fasciculus lateralis proprius flechsigi.

Flechsig's fasciculi FASCICULI PROPRII.

fasciculus of Foville STRIA TERMINALIS.

fasciculus of Goll FASCICULUS GRACILIS MEDULLAE SPINALIS.

fasciculus of Gowers TRACTUS SPINOCEREBELLARIS VENTRALIS.

fasciculus gracilis 1 FASCICULUS GRACILIS MEDULLAE SPINALIS. **2** FASCICULUS GRACILIS MEDULLAE OBLONGATAE.

fasciculus gracilis Golli FASCICULUS GRACILIS MEDULLAE SPINALIS.

fasciculus gracilis medullae oblongatae The rostral continuation of the spinal fasciculus gracilis medullae spinalis, overlying and penetrating the nucleus gracilis in the medulla oblongata. Also called *fasciculus gracilis, funiculus gracilis* (outmoded), *funiculus gracilis medullae oblongatae, posterior pyramid of medulla oblongata.*

fasciculus gracilis medullae spinalis A slender axonal bundle forming the medial segment of the posterior (dorsal) column. It is composed largely of long ascending axons from spinal ganglion cells of the lower thoracic, lumbar, and sacral levels of the spinal cord that terminate in the gracile nucleus of the medulla oblongata. It also contains ascending axons from posterior horn neurons, and a sector of interfascicular axons. Also called *fasciculus gracilis, gracile fascicle, fasciculus gracilis Golli, fasciculus of Goll, column of Goll, tract of Goll.*

gyral fasciculus The subcortical association fibers running between gyri of the cerebral cortex.

inferior longitudinal fasciculus of cerebrum FASCICULUS LONGITUDINALIS INFERIOR CEREBRI.

interfascicular fasciculus FASCICULUS INTERFASCICULARIS.

fasciculus interfascicularis The descending axonal branches of the medial division of the spinal nerve dorsal roots situated between the fasciculi gracilis and cuneatus of the cervical and thoracic spinal cord. It also contains some descending axons from the dorsal horn. Also called *comma tract of Schultze, bundle of Schultze* (obsolete), *fasciculus semilunaris, interfascicular fasciculus, comma tract, Schultze's tract, semilunar tract.*

lateral cerebrospinal fasciculus TRACTUS CORTICOSPINALIS LATERALIS.

fasciculus lateralis plexus brachialis A major component of the brachial plexus formed proximally by the joining of anterior divisions of the superior and middle trunks, in its course giving rise to the lateral pectoral nerve, and splitting distally into a lateral component of the median nerve and the musculocutaneous nerve. It carries axons of C_{4-7} segmental levels. Also called *lateral cord of brachial plexus, lateral cord.*

fasciculus lateralis proprius flechsigi The fasciculi proprii, intersegmental axons, bordering the lateral ventral horn of the spinal cord in the lateral funiculus.

lateral pyramidal fasciculus TRACTUS CORTICOSPINALIS LATERALIS.

fasciculus lenticularis The bundle of fibers emerging from the globus pallidus of the lenticular nucleus, continuing below the zona incerta in the dorsal part of the ansa lenticularis, and entering the H field of Forel to form the fasciculus thalamicus. Also called *field H_2 of Forel.* See also H FIELDS OF FOREL.

longitudinal fasciculi of colon An outmoded term for TAENIAE COLI.

longitudinal fasciculi of cruciform ligament FASCICULI LONGITUDINALES LIGAMENTI CRUCIFORMIS ATLANTIS.

fasciculi longitudinales Collectively, the several longitudinal fiber tracts of the central nervous system.

fasciculi longitudinales ligamenti cruciformis atlantis [NA] Thick, longitudinal bundles of ligamentous fibers that extend from the anterior margin of the foramen magnum to the posterior surface of the body of the axis vertebra. In between, they blend with the transverse ligament of the atlas, forming the cruciform ligament. Also called *longitudinal fasciculi of cruciform ligament, longitudinal fascicles of cruciform ligament.*

fasciculi longitudinales pontis The axonal bundles in the ventral pons arising from the cerebral cortex and constituting the corticonuclear and corticopontine components of the pyramidal tract. Also called *fasciculi longitudinales pyramidales pontis.*

fasciculi longitudinales pyramidales pontis FASCICULI LONGITUDINALES PONTIS.

fasciculus longitudinalis dorsalis A small bundle of axons consisting principally of descending axons from the medial and periventricular hypothalamus to the mesencephalic central gray and the dorsal tegmental nucleus. Also called *dorsal longitudinal fasciculus, Schütz bundle, tract of Schütz, periventricular tract, periependymal tract.*

fasciculus longitudinalis inferior cerebri The grossly delimited large myelinated bundle of association fibers coursing along the inferior horn of the lateral ventricle, reciprocally connecting the temporal and occipital lobes and including most of the geniculocalcarine tract. Also called *inferior longitudinal fasciculus of cerebrum, inferior longitudinal bundle.*

fasciculus longitudinalis medialis A prominent myelinated bundle, close to the midline and below the central gray matter, extending from the upper mesencephalon to the upper cervical levels of the spinal cord. It consists largely of axons from the vestibular nuclei ascending to the abducens, trochlear, and oculomotor nuclei and descending to motoneurons innervating the neck musculature. Also called *medial longitudinal fasciculus, posterior longitudinal fasciculus, medial longitudinal bundle, posterior longitudinal bundle.*

fasciculus longitudinalis medialis medullae oblongatae The portion of the fasciculus longitudinalis medialis within the medulla oblongata, coursing rostrally from the vestibular nuclei and caudally to motoneurons of the accessory nerve.

fasciculus longitudinalis medialis pontis The portion of the fasciculus longitudinalis medialis within the pons, chiefly innervating the motor nuclei of extraocular muscles. Also called *fasciculus teres* (outmoded).

fasciculus longitudinalis superior cerebri [NA] The poorly demarcated, longitudinally directed, lateral bundle of cortical association fibers reciprocally connecting the frontal, temporal, parietal, and occipital lobes. Also called *fasciculus arcuatus, superior longitudinal fasciculus of cerebrum, superior longitudinal bundle.*

fasciculus of Lower TUBERCULUM INTERVENOSUM.

maculary fasciculus A bundle of fibers in the optic nerve, derived from ganglion cells that radiate from the macula lutea of the retina.

mamillotegmental fasciculus The tract connecting the mamillary nuclei of the hypothalamus with the dorsal and ventral tegmental nuclei (of Gudden).

mamillothalamic fasciculus FASCICULUS MAMILLOTHALAMICUS.

fasciculus mamillothalamicus The myelinated axon bundle extending between the hypothalamic mamillary nuclei and the anterior nuclei of the thalamus. Also called *fasciculus of Vicq d'Azyr, fasciculus thalamomamillaris, mamillothalamic fasciculus, thalamomamillary bundle, bundle of Vicq d'Azyr, tractus mamillothalamicus, tract of Vicq D'Azyr, mamillothalamic tract.*

fasciculus marginalis ventralis The ventral fasciculus containing the tectospinal and vestibulospinal tracts. An outmoded term.

fasciculus medialis plexus brachialis In the brachial plexus, a cord formed by the anterior division of the inferior trunk (C_8 and T_1). It gives rise to the medial pectoral, medial brachial, and medial antebrachial cutaneous nerves, and as terminal branches, the ulnar nerve and the medial root of the median nerve. Also called *medial cord of brachial plexus.*

fasciculus medialis telencephali MEDIAL FOREBRAIN BUNDLE.

medial longitudinal fasciculus FASCICULUS LONGITUDI-NALIS MEDIALIS.

median triangular fasciculus FASCICULUS TRIANGULARIS.

Meynert's fasciculus FASCICULUS RETROFLEXUS.

Monakow's fasciculus TRACTUS RUBROSPINALIS.

fasciculus obliquus crucis cerebri A fiber bundle passing from the lateral part of the cerebral peduncle obliquely backward and medialward across the peduncle to enter the interpeduncular fossa at the pontine gray and tegmentum.

fasciculus obliquus pontis An indistinct bundle of fibers on the ventral pontine surface running obliquely lateral and caudal from the anteromedial portion of the pons.

fasciculus occipitofrontalis inferior The deep part of the fasciculus uncinatus, connecting the cortex of the frontal and occipital lobes. Also called *inferior occipitofrontal bundle.*

fasciculus occipitofrontalis superior A bundle of association fibers connecting frontal and occipital gyri coursing within the fasciculus subcallosus.

occipitothalamic fasciculus A seldom used term for RADIA-TIO OPTICA.

olivary fasciculus The fibers forming the external surface of the inferior olive. An outmoded term.

oval fasciculus FASCICULUS SEPTOMARGINALIS.

fasciculus pedunculomamillaris An ascending axonal bundle arising in the midbrain dorsal and ventral tegmental nuclei that projects mainly upon the lateral mamillary nucleus, with some fibers ascending in the medial forebrain bundle.

perpendicular fasciculus A vertical bundle of cortical association fibers interconnecting regions of the temporal, parietal, and occipital lobes.

fasciculi pontis longitudinales The numerous bundles of myelinated, principally descending fibers running in the rostrocaudal axis of the pons. Also called *longitudinal fibers of pons.*

posterior longitudinal fasciculus FASCICULUS LONGITUDI-NALIS MEDIALIS.

posterior longitudinal fasciculus of medulla oblongata The portion of the fasciculus longitudinalis dorsalis within the medulla oblongata.

fasciculus posterior plexus brachialis The posterior nerve cord of the brachial plexus. It is formed by posterior divisions of the superior, middle, and inferior trunks of C_5 through C_8 or T_1, giving rise to the subscapular, thoracodorsal, axillary, and radial nerves. Also called *posterior cord of brachial plexus, posterior cord.*

fasciculus precommissuralis Interhemispheric axons rostral to the anterior commissure of the cerebrum.

prerubral fasciculus STRIORUBRAL TRACT.

proper fasciculi of cord FASCICULI PROPRII.

fasciculi proprii Intersegmental ascending and descending axonal bundles of the spinal cord lying superficial to the gray matter of the anterior, lateral, and posterior funiculi. Also called *Flechsig's fasciculi, ground bundles of Flechsig, proprius bundles of spinal cord, proper fasciculi of cord, basis bundles* (outmoded), *fundamental bundles* (obsolete), *spinospinal tracts, lateral intersegmental tract.*

fasciculi pyramidales medullae oblongatae FIBRAE PY-RAMIDALES MEDULLAE OBLONGATAE.

fasciculus pyramidalis anterior TRACTUS CORTICOSPINALIS VENTRALIS.

fasciculus pyramidalis lateralis TRACTUS CORTICOSPINALIS LATERALIS.

fasciculus retroflexus [NA] A myelinated bundle of nerve fibers which have their neuronal cell bodies in the habenular nuclei of the epithalamus and which terminate in the ipsilateral interpeduncular nucleus of the mesencephalon. It is the largest efferent pathway from the habenula, and in its course it passes through the rostromedial part of the red nucleus. Also called

tractus habenulointerpeduncularis, habenulointerpeduncular tract, Meynert's tract, Meynert's bundle, Meynert's fasciculus, habenulopeduncular tract (incorrect), *fibers of Meynert.*

fasciculus of Rolando The elevated portion of the fasciculus cuneatus, overlying the bulge of the nucleus cuneatus in the medulla oblongata. Also called *funiculus of Rolando.*

fasciculus rotundus A seldom used term for TRACTUS SO-LITARIUS.

fasciculus semilunaris FASCICULUS INTERFASCICULARIS.

septomarginal fasciculus FASCICULUS SEPTOMARGINALIS.

fasciculus septomarginalis [NA] The myelinated, descending axons in the lumbar dorsal column near the posterior septum that in the sacral cord form a superficial, median triangular zone, the fasciculus triangularis. Also called *septomarginal fasciculus, oval bundle of Flechsig, oval area of Flechsig, septomarginal tract, tract of Bruce and Muir, Bruce's tract, Hoche's tract, oval fasciculus.*

solitary fasciculus TRACTUS SOLITARIUS.

subcallosal fasciculus FASCICULUS SUBCALLOSUS.

fasciculus subcallosus A thin bundle of axons on the ventricular surface of the angle formed by the corpus callosum and the internal capsule. It is thought to contain fibers extending from the frontal motor cortex to the caudate nucleus, and cortical association fibers connecting the frontal, temporal, and occipital lobes. There is ambiguity about whether it includes the tapetum of the corpus callosum and the fasciculus occipitofrontalis superior. Also called *subcallosal bundle, subcallosal fasciculus.*

sulcomarginal fasciculus FASCICULUS SULCOMARGINALIS.

fasciculus sulcomarginalis A lamina of descending dorsal root fibers running in the anteromedial funiculus of the spinal cord along the margin of the anterior fissure. Also called *sulcomarginal fasciculus, sulcomarginal tract.*

superior longitudinal fasciculus of cerebrum FASCICULUS LONGITUDINALIS SUPERIOR CEREBRI.

fasciculus teres An outmoded term for FASCICULUS LONGI-TUDINALIS MEDIALIS PONTIS.

thalamic fasciculus FASCICULUS THALAMICUS.

fasciculus thalamicus The myelinated bundle of axons entering the rostral portion of the thalamic ventral nuclear group dorsal to the zona incerta via the H field of Forel. These axons originate primarily in the globus pallidus and the dentate and red nuclei, course through the fasciculus lenticularis (field H_2), and terminate principally in the rostral nuclei of the ventral thalamic nuclear group. Also called *field H_1 of Forel, thalamic fasciculus.* See also H FIELDS OF FOREL.

fasciculus thalamomamillaris FASCICULUS MAMILLOTHAL-AMICUS.

transverse fasciculi of palmar aponeurosis FASCICULI TRANSVERSI APONEUROSIS PALMARIS.

transverse fasciculi of plantar aponeurosis FASCICULI TRANSVERSI APONEUROSIS PLANTARIS.

fasciculi transversi aponeurosis palmaris [NA] The transverse fibers on the deep aspect of the palmar aponeurosis that thicken to form strong ligamentous bands in the webs of the fingers, closing the gaps between the more superficial longitudinal bands to the fingers. Also called *transverse fasciculi of palmar aponeurosis, transverse bundles of palmar aponeurosis.*

fasciculi transversi aponeurosis plantaris [NA] Well-marked transverse bundles of fibers that close the gaps between the longitudinal digital bands of the plantar aponeurosis at the webs of the toes. Also called *transverse fasciculi of plantar aponeurosis.*

triangular fasciculus FASCICULUS TRIANGULARIS.

fasciculus triangularis [NA] A group of descending fibers in the dorsal columns of the lumbosacral spinal cord that consists in large part of intersegmental connections. Also called *median* *triangular fasciculus, triangular fasciculus, Gombault-Philippe triangle, tract of Philippe-Gombault, triangular tract of Philippe-Gombault, median root zone.*

fasciculus of Türck   TRACTUS CORTICOSPINALIS VENTRALIS.

unciform fasciculus   FASCICULUS UNCINATUS.

uncinate fasciculus   FASCICULUS UNCINATUS.

fasciculus uncinatus   A bundle of frontotemporal association fibers extending between the orbitofrontal region to the uncus and parahippocampal gyrus. Also called *uncinate fasciculus, unciform fasciculus, uncinate bundle.*

uncrossed pyramidal fasciculus   TRACTUS CORTICOSPINALIS VENTRALIS.

fasciculus ventrolateralis superficialis   TRACTUS SPINOCEREBELLARIS VENTRALIS.

fasciculus of Vicq d'Azyr   FASCICULUS MAMILLOTHALAMICUS.

---

fasciectomy [*fasci(a)* + -ECTOMY]   Excision of the fascia, such as of the fascia lata.

fasciitis [*fasci(a)* + -ITIS]   Inflammation of a fascia. Also called *fascitis, fibrofascitis,.*

eosinophilic fasciitis   Fasciitis of unknown cause, usually chronic, accompanied by marked increase in blood eosinophils.

necrotizing fasciitis   A rapidly advancing soft-tissue infection that moves along fascial planes causing disruption of the fascial blood supply. It is usually caused by a synergistic infection of two bacterial species and can be fatal if not surgically treated.

nodular fasciitis   A benign soft tissue growth typically developing rapidly in the upper extremities, trunk, or neck of young adults. It can be easily confused with a sarcoma because of its infiltrative margins and rapid growth in relation to a fascia. Microscopically, it consists of a reactive proliferation of myofibrasts in a loose, myxoid matrix. Also called *pseudosarcomatous fibromatosis, subcutaneous pseudosarcomatous fibromatosis.*

perirenal fasciitis   IDIOPATHIC RETROPERITONEAL FIBROSIS.

proliferative fasciitis   A benign soft tissue growth very similar to nodular fasciitis, from which it can be differentiated by the presence of large, basophilic cells resembling rhabdomyoblasts, or ganglion cells. It tends to affect patients older than 45 and involves the skeletal muscles of the shoulder, thorax, and thigh.

pseudosarcomatous fasciitis   A benign but rapidly progressive fibroblastic growth extending from superficial fascia into subcutaneous fat or muscle. High cellularity and mitotic activity simulate sarcoma.

fascination   The mastery of a factor in the environment through imitation, a form of identification observable in infants.

fasciodesis [*fasci(a)* + *o* + -DESIS]   An operation in which a fascia is anchored to bone or cartilage.

Fasciola [L (dim. of *fascia* a bandage, band, woman's girdle), a little bandage or swath]   A genus of large digenetic flukes of the class Trematoda. They are parasitic in the liver of herbivorous animals and, infrequently, of humans.

Fasciola gigantica   The giant liver fluke, a trematode found primarily in herbivores and occasionally in humans in Africa, Asia, Australasia, and Hawaii. It is similar in appearance to *F. hepatica* but larger and without an apical cone. Human infection is usually acquired by eating raw watercress contaminated by sheep feces. Adult flukes inhabit bile ducts which become distended and thick-walled. Sheep are more susceptible than cattle to the damaging effects of migration of flukes through the liver parenchyma. Severe anemia and death can occur. Praziquantel is the treatment of choice.

Fasciola hepatica   The sheep liver fluke, a common trematode found in sheep, cattle, goats, horses, other animals including,

though rarely, humans. Various species of snails of the genus *Lymnaea* serve as first intermediate hosts. The cercariae leave the snail, encyst on vegetation, and are ingested by the final host. In heavy infections extensive damage to the liver by migrating immature flukes causes severe hemorrhage, anemia, and even death. Adult flukes inhabit the bile ducts which become greatly thickened, fibrosed, and distended. Also called *Distoma hepaticum* (obsolete).

Fasciola heterophyes   HETEROPHYES HETEROPHYES.

Fasciola magna   A former name for FASCIOLOIDES MAGNA.

fasciola [L (dim. of *fascia* a bandage), a little bandage or swath]   A small strip or band of nerve fibers.

fasciola cinerea cinguli   GYRUS FASCIOLARIS.

fasciola dentata   GYRUS DENTATUS.

fasciolae   Plural of FASCIOLA.

fasciolar   **1** Denoting the gyrus fasciolaris.   **2** Pertaining to a fasciola.

Fascioletta ilocana   ECHINOSTOMA ILOCANUM.

fascioliasis   Infection with flukes of the genus *Fasciola*, especially *F. hepatica*.

Fasciolidae [*Fasciol(a)* + -IDAE]   A family of large, leaf-shaped distomous digenetic flukes that are parasitic in mammals. It includes the genera *Fasciola, Fascioloides,* and *Fasciolopsis,* which can infect animals and humans.

Fascioloides   A genus of flukes in the family Fasciolidae.

Fascioloides magna   A liver fluke whose natural hosts are elk, deer, and moose. It infests cattle, sheep, goats, and other herbivores in North America and Europe.

fascioloidiasis [*Fascioloid(es)* + -IASIS]   The clinical condition in animals infested with liver flukes of the genus *Fascioloides*. In cattle the worms are enveloped in heavy closed cysts that may occlude the bile ducts, though little inflammation occurs. In sheep the worms continue to migrate in the liver parenchyma and the host is frequently killed.

fasciolopsiasis   Infection with flukes of the genus *Fasciolopsis*.

Fasciolopsis [*fasciol(a)* + *o* + OPSIS]   A genus of large flukes in the family Fasciolidae. Besides *F. buski,* it contains *F. fuelleborni,* which has been found in humans in India and Egypt, and *F. rathouisi,* found in humans in China.

Fasciolopsis buski   A species found in the small intestine of humans, pigs, and other mammals in eastern and southeastern Asia. In heavy infections, the flukes cause nausea, diarrhea, and malabsorption. Intermediate hosts include the snail genera *Planorbis* and *Segmentina,* which release cercariae that develop into the infective metacercariae on water chestnuts and other aquatic vegetation. Also called *Distoma buski* (obsolete).

fascioplasty   FASCIAPLASTY.

fasciorrhaphy [*fasci(a)* + *o* + -RRHAPHY]   An operation involving suturing of a fascia or of an aponeurosis. Also called *aponeurorrhaphy.*

fascioscapulohumeral   Pertaining to the scapula, the humerus, and related fascia.

fasciotomy [*fasci(a)* + *o* + -TOMY]   Incision in the fascia that invests muscles, usually performed to release pressure on the invested muscles, nerves, and blood vessels, especially in the forearm or calf.

fascitis   FASCIITIS.

fast¹ [Old English *fæst*, akin to German *fest* firm, fast]   **1** Securely fastened; immobilized.   **2** Resistant to dissolution or decolorization.

fast²   **1** To abstain from food, usually for a set period or on a set schedule.   **2** A period of abstention from food.

fast-fatiguable   Denoting the fast-contracting, fatigue-susceptible type of motor unit.

fast-glycolytic Denoting the fast-contracting, glycolysis-dependent, fatigue-susceptible type of motor unit or muscle fiber.

fastidious In microorganisms, having complex growth requirements.

fastigial Denoting the nucleus fastigii or fibers emanating from it.

fastigiobulbar Denoting nerve fibers from the cerebellar fastigial nucleus to the pons.

fastigium [L (from *fastus* elevation), roof, slope] The peak of the roof of the fourth ventricle of the brain, formed by the angle of union between the superior medullary velum and the nodulus cerebelli.

fast-oxidative-glycolytic Denoting motor units or muscle fibers that are fast-contracting, fatigue-resistant, and capable of utilizing both oxidative and glycolytic pathways for the energy used in contraction.

fat [Old English *fætt* (noun, adj.)] Any of class of naturally occurring neutral organic compounds formed by ester bonds between three fatty acid molecules and one molecule of glycerol. They are insoluble in water, soluble in ether, and combustible. Fats are distinguished from oils in that fats are solid at 20°C and lower temperatures. Fats are rich in energy (9.3 kcal/g) and are stored in cells and tissues.

body fat That portion of the body that consists of fat. It represents about 14% of the body weight of a man of ideal body composition and about 28% of a woman. However, the ratio of body fat to body weight varies widely among normal subjects.

bound fat In a cell, a lipid component that is not demonstrable with conventional fat stains. Also called *masked fat*.

brown fat INTERSCAPULAR GLAND.

chyle fat An emulsion of fat within the lymphatic system.

depot fat Body stores of triglyceride fat. Usually found in limited areas, such as the abdominal wall, it constitutes the main energy reserve.

masked fat BOUND FAT.

milk fat The fat contained in milk, making up 45% of the calories of whole cow's milk. It is composed predominantly of long-chain saturated fatty acids and includes 14 mg of cholesterol per 100 g.

molecular fat Intracellular fat within numerous minute vacuoles.

neutral fat A fat composed entirely of triglyceride esters, containing no free fatty acids.

perirenal fat CAPSULA ADIPOSA RENIS.

wool fat LANOLIN.

yellow fat The usual type of adipose tissue, as distinguished from the brown fat characteristic of the interscapular gland.

fatal [L *fatal(is)* (from *fatum* fate, destiny, natural death, from *fatum*, neut. sing. of *fatus*, past part. of *fari* to say; + *-alis* -AL) pertaining to fate, fatal] Causing death.

fatality [Late L *fatalitas* (from L *fatal(is)* pertaining to fate, fatal, decreed + *-itas* -ITY, from *fatum* fate, destiny) an event or condition decreed by fate] 1 A death, especially one resulting from a specific disease, trauma, or other misfortune. 2 In medical statistics, the probability of an illness proving fatal, expressed as a percentage; fatality rate.

case fatality FATALITY RATE.

fate The ultimate state of development normally achieved by any embryonic cell or region of an early embryo. See also FATE MAP.

potential fate Collectively, the possible fates of a cell or group of cells or of a part or even whole region of an embryo. The prospective fate is chosen from among the possible fates. Also called *prospective potency*.

prospective fate The development normally achieved by a part or region of an embryo, assuming no external interference is involved to modify the normal course of events. Also called *prospective significance*.

fathom [Old English *fæthm* (from L *patere* to be open, akin to *pandere* to stretch, extend, open, akin to Gk *petannynai* to spread, stretch out) the length of two arms outstretched, a unit of length] A unit of length equal to six feet, used especially for measuring depth of sea; 1.8288 meter. An obsolete unit.

fatigability The condition of being subject to fatigue; tendency to tire or become exhausted.

fatigue [French (from L *fatigare* to weary, tire), weariness] A state of weariness of mind and body following prolonged or excessive exertion or prolonged sensory stimulation. It results in loss of capacity to respond to stimulation.

auditory fatigue Decreased response to a steady state tone or noise. The subject perceives the sound as diminishing in loudness.

battle fatigue COMBAT NEUROSIS.

combat fatigue COMBAT NEUROSIS.

emotional fatigue A reaction to stress characterized by neurasthenia. Also called *nervous exhaustion*.

flying fatigue 1 Combat neurosis occurring in pilots. 2 JET LAG.

industrial fatigue Fatigue caused by prolonged or excessive work and exacerbated by monotony or by exposure to extreme conditions, as of heat and cold. It may lead to lowered output, mistakes, and accidents.

operational fatigue COMBAT NEUROSIS.

stance fatigue A state of weariness or exhaustion produced by prolonged standing.

stimulation fatigue A rise in the threshold of response to electrical stimulation in a nerve or nerve fiber as a result of prior repetitive stimulation.

fatty Composed of, resembling, or associated with fat: used particularly of chemical compounds whose molecules contain long chains of methylene groups. Thus fatty alcohols are long-chain alcohols, derivable by reduction of fatty acids.

fatty acid Any acid of formula $CH_3-[CH_2]_n-COOH$. Such acids occur in biologic material, particularly as esters in fats and phospholipids.

cyclopropane fatty acids A class of fatty acids formed by bacteria by addition of a methylene group across a double bond. They are more stable than unsaturated fatty acids, from which they are formed, especially in the stationary phase.

essential fatty acid Any of the interconvertible polyunsaturated fatty acids required in the diet and not made in mammals, such as linoleic acid.

free fatty acids Fatty acids that are not esterified, e.g. as fat or as phospholipid. Thus the albumin-bound fatty acid of the blood is included, since its binding to albumin is noncovalent.

nonesterified fatty acid A fatty acid in free form, in contrast with acyl groups in fats. It may, however, be noncovalently bound to a protein, as to serum albumin.

polyunsaturated fatty acids Monobasic aliphatic acids containing only carbon, hydrogen, and oxygen. They are made up of an alkyl radical attached to the carboxyl group and have more than one double bond. They fall into several groups: linoleic series with two double bonds between carbon atoms 9 and 10 and 12 and 13 (Δ 9 and 12) and general formula $C_nH_{2n}-COOH$, linolenic series with three double bonds (Δ 9, 12, and 15) and general formula $C_nH_{2n-5}COOH$, fatty acids with four double bonds (Δ 5, 8, 11, and 14), such as arachidonic acid, and general formula $C_nH_{2n-7}COOH$, and those with five double bonds such as clupanodonic acid. Good sources are certain vegetable oils such as peanut, cottonseed, corn, sunflower, and safflower. They have a blood cholesterol lowering effect but increase the requirement for vitamin E.

fatty-acid synthase complex The enzyme complex responsible for the biosynthesis of fatty acid from acetyl-CoA, malonyl-CoA, and NADPH. It has several active centers, on which condensation and reduction reactions occur.

fauces [L, the gullet, pharynx, throat, a narrow passage, mouth; used in pl. *fauces* only, except for ablative sing. *fauce*] [NA] The narrowed space and surrounding structures between the oral cavity and the pharynx. It includes the isthmus and arches of the fauces, as well as the tonsillar fossa and the palatine tonsil. Also called *vestibule of pharynx* (outmoded), *throat.* Adjective: faucial.

Fauchard [Pierre *Fauchard*, French dentist, 1678–1761] Fauchard's disease. See under CHRONIC PERIODONTITIS.

faucial Pertaining to the fauces.

fauna [after Late L *Fauna* sister or wife of Faunus a nature god; adopted by Linnaeus as a parallel to Flora] **1** The composite animal community of a given area or period. **2** A descriptive listing of the animals of an area or period.

fauntail A tuft of long, fine hair in the lumbosacral region that usually overlies a defect, as that in diastematomyelia.

faunula [dim. of FAUNA] An animal population confined to a small area such as the intestine, a fecal pellet, or the like.

Faust [Ernest Carroll *Faust*, U.S. parasitologist, flourished 20th century] See under METHOD.

faute de mieux A situation in which a same-sex partner is acceptable because there is no opposite-sex partner. Such situations often occur in prisons or military installations.

Fauvel [Supice Antoine *Fauvel*, French physician, 1813–1884] Fauvel's granules. See under GRANULE.

faveolar Pertaining or belonging to a faveolus.

faveolate [New L *faveol(us)*, dim. of L *favus* honeycomb + -ATE] Having a pitted surface.

faveoli Plural of FAVEOLUS.

faveolus [New L, dim. of L *favus* honeycomb] **1** A small depression or pit. **2** ALVEOLUS.

favic Having the character of favus. • The term is usually applied to a fungal mycelium that grows in a branched pattern, such as *Trichophyton schoenleinii,* the cause of favus.

favid [*fav(us)* + -ID] A dermatophytid reaction provoked by an infection (favus) due to *Trichophyton schoenkeinii.* Also *favide.*

favide FAVID.

faviform Resembling a honeycomb.

favism Severe hemolytic anemia that follows ingestion of fava beans in some persons with glucose-6-phosphate dehydrogenase deficiency (Mediterranean variant). Also called *Baghdad spring anemia* (seldom used), *fabism.*

Favre [Maurice Jules *Favre*, French physician, 1876–1954] **1** Favre-Racouchot syndrome. See under NODULAR ELASTOSIS OF THE SKIN. **2** Durand-Nicolas-Favre disease, maladie de Nicolas et Favre, Nicolas-Favre disease, Favre-Durand-Nicolas disease. See under LYMPHOGRANULOMA VENEREUM. **3** Gamna-Favre bodies. See under MIYAGAWA BODIES.

favus [L, honeycomb] A disease of the hair follicle which results in a cup-shaped crust (scutula). If the crust is removed, an oozing, red lesion will be exposed. In most instances the agent of this disease is *Trichophyton schoenleinii.*

favus circinatus An oozing crusty type of ringworm in which the lesion is considerably larger and generally circular.

favus of fowl A dermatomycosis caused by *Trichophyton megnini (T. gallinae, Achorion gallinae),* usually affecting the comb of chickens and occasionally of turkeys and other birds, the comb becoming covered with a white crust. In severe cases other parts of the head and even the body can be affected. Other animals, including man, can also be infected by *T. megnini.* Also called *tinea galli, whitecomb.*

favus of the glabrous skin TINEA GLABROSA.

favus herpetiformis A ringworm affecting mice, caused by *Trichophyton terrestre.* Also called *mouse favus, favus murium.*

mouse favus FAVUS HERPETIFORMIS.

favus murium FAVUS HERPETIFORMIS.

faxen-psychosis [German *Faxen* buffoonery + PSYCHOSIS] BUFFOONERY PSYCHOSIS.

Fazio [E. *Fazio,* Italian physician, 1849–1902] **1** Fazio-Londe atrophy. See under ATROPHY. **2** Fazio-Londe syndrome, Fazio-Londe disease. See under INFANTILE PROGRESSIVE BULBAR PALSY.

Fc See under FC FRAGMENT.

fc Symbol for the obsolete unit, foot candle.

FCA Freund's complete adjuvant.

F-Cortef A proprietary name for fludrocortisone.

FD **1** focal distance. **2** fatal dose (lethal dose).

Fd See under FD FRAGMENT.

FDA Food and Drug Administration.

FD & C Federal Food, Drug and Cosmetic: used to designate approved food colorings, such as coal-tar colors.

FDNB fluoro-2,4-dinitrobenzene.

F-duction A gene transfer from a donor bacterium to a recipient in which a piece of donor DNA is incorporated into the F plasmid and is transferred by conjugation. The modified plasmid is called F′ (F-prime). Also called *sexduction.*

Fe Symbol for the element, iron.

fear [Middle English *fer,* from Old English *fær* peril, sudden attack, akin to German *(ge)fahr* danger] A strong, primitive emotional reaction to a specific danger that exists or is perceived, characterized subjectively by feelings of unpleasantness and agitation, and behaviorally by postures and movements to bring about escape or concealment. Fear responses are dependent on the action of diencephalic centers in the brain, and are accompanied by widespread physiologic changes in the body mediated by the sympathetic nervous system, such as sweating or a rapid heartbeat.

guilty fear Fear that one's misdeeds will bring drastic punishment, often a core symptom in obsessive patients.

Feather [Norman *Feather,* English physicist, born 1904] See under ANALYSIS.

feather [Old English *fether,* akin to German *Feder* feather] A light horny epidermal outgrowth forming part of the plumage of a bird. It is typically composed of a hard tubelike quill at the epidermis tapering distally into a thin tube, the rachis, bearing a series of barbs which are arranged as a sheet on each side of the shaft.

contour feather Any feather that forms part of the visible external body surface of a bird.

flight feather Any of the large feathers of the wings and tail of a bird that support it during flight.

feature Any characteristic element, as of a structure, condition, or appearance.

feb. dur. *febre durante* (L, while the fever lasts).

febre [Portuguese, fever] Fever.

febre maculosa A Brazilian term for FLEA-BORNE TYPHUS.

febricant PYROGEN.

febricide ANTIPYRETIC.

febricity [Med L *febricit(as)* (irreg. from L *febris,* fever + -itas -ITY) having a fever + -Y] The condition of having a fever.

febricula [L, dim. of *febris* fever] A short-lived and mild fever of indefinite cause.

febriculose [*febricul(a)* + -OSE¹] Mildly feverish.

febriculosity [*febriculos(e)* + -ITY]   Mild feverishness.

febrifacient   **1** Fever-producing.   **2** A febrifacient agent.

febriferous   FEBRILE.

febrific   FEBRILE.

febrifugal   ANTIPYRETIC.

febrifuge   ANTIPYRETIC.

febrile [Med L *febril(is)* (from L *febris* fever) pertaining to fever] Of or characterized by fever. Also *pyretic, pyrexial, febriferous, febrific, feverish.*

febris [L, a burning, fever]   FEVER.

  febris endemica roseola   DENGUE.

  febris entericoides   PARENTERIC FEVER.

  febris melitensis   MALTA FEVER.

  febris quintana   TRENCH FEVER.

  febris recurrens   RELAPSING FEVER.

  febris rubra   SCARLET FEVER.

  febris sudoralis   UNDULANT FEVER. See under BRUCELLOSIS.

  febris undulans   UNDULANT FEVER. See under BRUCELLOSIS.

  febris uveoparotidea   HEERFORDT SYNDROME.

  febris wolhynica   TRENCH FEVER.

fecal   Of or relating to feces.

fecalith   A solid mass of fecal material found in the colon or identified as a radiopaque object on an abdominal radiograph; a fecal calculus. Also called *coprolith, stercolith, stercorolith* (seldom used).

fecaloid   Bearing a resemblance to feces.

fecaloma [FECAL + -OMA]   STERCOROMA.

fecaluria [FECAL + -URIA]   The presence of feces in the urine, associated with a fistula between the colon or rectum and the bladder.

feces [Middle English, pl. of *fece, fex,* from L *faex,* pl. *faeces,* dregs or lees of wine, sediment]   The excreta expelled from the anus, consisting of undigested material, bacteria, mucosal cells, and mucus.

  feces cruentae   Bloody feces; fecal material containing blood. See also MELENA, HEMATOCHEZIA.

Fechner [Gustav Theodor *Fechner,* German psychologist, 1801–1887]   **1** See under FRACTION, LAW.   **2** Weber-Fechner law. See under LAW.

feculent   Fecal or foul; filthy.

fecundability   The probability that a woman who is neither pregnant nor in postpartum amenorrhea will conceive during a given menstrual cycle.

fecundate [L *fecundat(us),* past part. of *fecundare* (from *fecundus* fruitful, fertile) to fertilize, make fruitful]   To fertilize; to make fertile.

fecundatio [Late L (from L *fecundatus,* past part. of *fecundare* to fertilize, make fruitful; from *feo,* root of FETUS), a making fecund]   FERTILIZATION.

  fecundatio ab extra   Pregnancy which occurs in the absence of penile penetration into the vagina.

fecundation [L *fecundatus,* past part. of *fecundare* (from root *feo* of *fetus*) to make fertile or fruitful]   FERTILIZATION.

  artificial fecundation   ARTIFICIAL INSEMINATION.

fecundity [L *fecunditas* (from *fecundus* fruitful, fertile, from *fere* to bring forth) fruitfulness, fertility. Compare *fetus.*]   In demography, the ability to conceive; reproductive potential as distinguished from reproductive performance (fertility).

Fede [Francesco *Fede,* Italian physician, 1832–1913]   Fede's disease, Riga-Fede disease. See under FRENAL ULCER.

Federici [Cesare *Federici,* Italian physician, 1832–1892]   See under SIGN.

fee / contingency fee   A payment based or conditioned on future occurrences or conclusions, or on the results of services to be performed: used primarily in malpractice litigation for attorney fee payment.

  dispensing fee   The fee charged by a pharmacist for filling a prescription.

  fee for service   A method of charging or paying for health care services whereby the provider bills or is reimbursed a defined amount for each service.

feeblemindedness   An older term for MENTAL RETARDATION.

feedback   In a system, the return of a fraction of the output to the input for use in regulation.

  alpha feedback   A type of relaxation training in which the subject receives information about his electroencephalogram and learns under what conditions alpha waves, characteristic of relaxed and peaceful wakefulness, are produced.

  delayed auditory feedback   Interference with a subject's hearing of his own speech, typically by using special headphones that impose a delay of 200 to 300 milliseconds on the transmission of the sound. In the ordinary person such a delay produces marked distortion in speech, while in some schizophrenic patients the delay has remarkably little effect on speech patterns. Abbreviation: DAF

  negative feedback   A process in which the output of a system acts upon the input to decrease its action. For example, increased circulating hormone causes decreased hormone production.

  positive feedback   A process in which the output of a system acts upon the input to reinforce its action. For example, placing a microphone near a loudspeaker reinforces the undesirable sustained oscillations in a public-address system.

feeder   A container with a spout to facilitate feeding infirm or recalcitrant individuals.

feeding   The process of taking or giving food.

  artificial feeding   The feeding of an infant by any means other than suckling at the breast.

  breast feeding   The nourishment of an infant by the act of suckling; the obtaining of breast milk by sucking at the mother's breast. The infant controls its own intake which reduces the possibility of overfeeding. The composition of the milk is normally such as to satisfy completely the infant's nutrient needs.

  demand feeding   Giving nourishment to a child when he signals he is hungry, typically by crying, rather than feeding according to a rigidly imposed schedule.

  drip feeding   INTRAVENOUS FEEDING.

  extrabuccal feeding   The giving of nutrients by some method other than by the mouth.

  forced feeding   Administration of nutritive substance either against the recipient's will or in quantities which exceed those required to satisfy the appetite. Also called *forcible feeding.*

  forcible feeding   FORCED FEEDING.

  intravenous feeding   The intravenous administration of five or ten percent glucose solutions with electrolytes and vitamins. Because of the inability to provide sufficient calories to meet the needs of undernourished or hypermetabolic patients and to provide the patient with adequate amino acids, it can only be used for a short period. Long-term intravenous feeding requires total parenteral feeding or hyperalimentation which provides the patient with all the essential nutrients. Also called *drip feeding, drip treatment.*

  nasal feeding   The taking in of food through a tube inserted into the stomach via the nose.

  sham feeding   **1** An experimental procedure in which food is chewed and swallowed but is then diverted to the exterior by way of an esophageal fistula in order to prevent it from entering the stomach.   **2** An experiment in which food is chewed but is expectorated rather than swallowed.

  tube feeding   The supplying of nutrients through a tube placed in the stomach by way of the nostril, pharynx, and esophagus or through a tube inserted into the stomach or jejunum at operation. Gastrostomy and jejunostomy feedings are only used when it is not possible to pass an intragastric tube or when there is gross disease of the stomach, respectively. Feeds are usually presented every four hours in a volume of 250 ml followed by 50 ml of water to rinse the tube. Distasteful medicines may also be administered through a tube.

feeling **1** Any conscious state containing some elements not obviously referable to the immediate environment. **2** The subjective aspect of affective or emotional experience; an awareness of one's mood or of a particular emotional reaction.

feelings of estrangement A sense of being apart from people and outer reality because external objects seem unfamiliar or unreal. Feelings of estrangement are frequent in dissociative states and certain types of schizophrenia and affective disorders. Such feelings may take the form of nihilistic delusions. Also called *feelings of unreality.*

feeling of incompleteness A sense that something is lacking in one's makeup, or sensations of emptiness and loneliness. Such feelings are reported to be frequent in borderline personality.

feelings of inferiority Doubts about one's worth, value, or ability to achieve and perform.

negative feeling Any feeling in the range of dislike, hostility, anger, hate, or vengeance. Such feelings are commonly related to the aggressive drive.

positive feeling Any feeling in the range of like, affection, love, caring, or protection. Such feelings are commonly related to the sexual drive.

feelings of unreality FEELINGS OF ESTRANGEMENT.

Feer [Walther Emil *Feer*, Swiss pediatrician, 1864–1955] Swift-Feer disease. See under PINK DISEASE.

fee-splitting The sharing of a fee by two or more individuals. Sometimes a provider will share a fee in exchange for a referral but this may be considered unethical.

feet Plural of FOOT.

Fegeler [Ferdinand *Fegeler*, German dermatologist, flourished 20th century] See under SYNDROME.

Fehleisen [Friedrich *Fehleisen*, German-born U.S. physician, 1854–1924] Fehleisen streptococcus. See under *STREPTOCOCCUS PYOGENES.*

Fehling [Hermann Christian von *Fehling*, German chemist, 1812–1885] Fehling's test. See under FEHLING SOLUTION.

Feichtiger [H. *Feichtiger*, German physician, flourished mid-20th century] Ullrich-Feichtiger syndrome. See under SYNDROME.

Feil [Andre *Feil*, French physician, born 1884] **1** Klippel-Feil sign. See under SIGN. **2** Klippel-Feil syndrome. See under SYNDROME. **3** Klippel-Feil malformation. See under MALFORMATION.

Feiss [Henry O. *Feiss*, U.S. orthopedic surgeon, flourished 20th century] See under LINE.

fel BILE.

Feldberg [Wilhelm Siegmund *Feldberg*, German-born British physiologist, born 1900] Dale-Feldberg law. See under LAW.

Feldman [Harry Alfred *Feldman*, U.S. epidemiologist, born 1914] Sabin-Feldman dye test. See under TEST.

Feleky [Hugó von *Feleky*, Hungarian urologist, 1860–1932] See under INSTRUMENT.

Felicola A genus of biting lice of the family Trichodectidae. It includes the species *F. subrostratus,* a common parasite of cats.

Felix [Arthur *Felix*, Czech bacteriologist, 1887–1956] **1** Felix-Weil reaction, Weil-Felix reaction. See under WEIL-FELIX TEST. **2** See under VACCINE.

Felix [Jules *Felix*, French physician, 1838–1912] Felix Vi serum. See under SERUM.

Fell [George Edward *Fell*, U.S. physician, 1850–1918] Fell-O'Dwyer method. See under METHOD.

fellatio [New L (from *fellatus*, past part. of *fellare* to suck, akin to English *feminive*)] Oral stimulation of the penis. Also called *irrumation.*

fellifluous Characterized by ample flow of bile.

felo-de-se [Med L and L, suicide, from Med L *felo* villain, felon + L *de* of + *se* oneself (ablative case)] The act of suicide, especially when committed by one having no predisposing mental disorder. An obsolete term.

felon [French *félon* (origin uncertain; possibly akin to Gaelic *feallan*, a traitor from Low L *felo* a crime, from L *fel* gall, anything bitter, bitterness, akin to *bilis* bile, wrath) disloyal, traitorous] A suppurating abscess or infection of the distal phalanx of the finger.

bone felon A felon involving subperiosteal bone and causing necrosis.

deep felon A felon located deep within a structure such as the bone cortex or subcutaneous tissue.

subcutaneous felon A felon that involves tissues below the skin surface.

subcuticular felon A felon that arises between the dermis and the epidermis. Also called *subepithelial felon, superficial felon.*

subepithelial felon SUBCUTICULAR FELON.

subperiosteal felon A felon involving the periosteum.

superficial felon SUBCUTICULAR FELON.

thecal felon A felon involving a synovial sheath. Also called *thecal whitlow.*

felony [See FELON.] A very serious crime defined by legal statute and most commonly punished by imprisonment in a penitentiary. Adjective: felonious.

Felton [Lloyd Derr *Felton*, U.S. pathologist, 1885–1953] See under SERUM, UNIT.

feltwork Any layer of densely interwoven nerve fibers.

Kaes feltwork BEKHTEREV'S LAYER.

Felty [Augustus Roi *Felty*, U.S. physician, born 1895] See under SYNDROME.

female [Middle English, altered by the influence of *male* from Old French *femelle* female, from L *femella*, dim. of *femina* a female, woman] **1** Of or pertaining to the sex that in animals produces ova and brings forth young. **2** An individual of the female sex, as a woman.

genetic female **1** A human possessing a normal female karyotype, 46,XX. **2** In any species, an individual possessing the karyotype that is usually present in the female. **3** A female pseudohermaphrodite in which the karyotype is 46,XX. The gonads are ovaries, a uterus is present, and the external genitalia are virilized or ambiguous. An outmoded term.

feminine [Old French *feminin* feminine, from L *femininus* female, from *femin(a)* a woman + *-inus*, combining form denoting belonging to] Of or relating to the female sex; having the qualities characteristic of women.

femininity The state of being feminine; possession of the normal characteristics of women.

feminism An older term for FEMINIZATION.

mammary feminism A seldom used term for GYNECOMASTIA.

feminization [L *femin(a)* a female + *-iz(e)* + *-ATION*] **1** The development in the male of secondary sex characters of a female, as regression of masculine body hair and assumption of feminine body contour. Also called *effemination, effeminacy* (imprecise), *feminism* (older term), *eviration.* **2** Normal development of secondary sex characters in the female.

testicular feminization A condition that prevents both embryologic and postnatal androgen-dependent development. It is due to a defective or absent cellular androgen receptor, the genetic locus for which is on the X chromosome. The phenotype in the affected hemizygote includes the absence of the ovaries, uterus, and tubes; inguinal or abdominal testes; a vagina and female external genitalia; female habitus and breast development; the absence of virilization;. Also called *testicular feminization syndrome, Morris syndrome* (seldom used), *Goldberg-Maxwell syndrome* (seldom used), *androgen insensitivity syndrome.*

feminize 1 To induce the development of female secondary sex characters in the female. **2** To promote the development of female secondary sex characters in the male.

feminizing 1 Inducing female qualities, especially female secondary sex characters. **2** Inducing feminization by excessive secretion of estrogens.

feminonucleus [L *femin(a)* a female, woman + *o* + NUCLEUS] FEMALE PRONUCLEUS.

femme [French (from L *femina* woman, female), woman]
sage femme MIDWIFE.

femora Plural of FEMUR.

femoral Pertaining or belonging to the femur or the thigh.

femoroarticular Denoting a bony part articulating with the femur or the process of articulating with the femur.

femorocele [*femor(al)* + *o* + -CELE¹] FEMORAL HERNIA.

femoroiliac Pertaining to the femur and the ilium.

femoropopliteal Pertaining to the femur and the popliteal space.

femoropretibial Pertaining to the thigh and the anterior crural region.

femorotibial Pertaining to the femur and the tibia.

femto- [Danish *femten* fifteen] A combining form denoting 10^{-15}: used with SI units. Symbol: f

femtogram [FEMTO- + GRAM] A unit of mass or weight equal to 10^{-15} gram. Symbol: fg

femtoliter [FEMTO- + LITER] A unit of volume or capacity equal to 10^{-15} liter; 10^{-18} cubic meter; 10^{-12} cubic centimeter. Symbol: fl

femtometer [FEMTO- + METER] A unit of length equal to 10^{-15} meter. Symbol: fm

femtomole An amount of substance equal to 10^{-15} mole. Symbol: fmol

femur [L, the thigh] (*plural* femora) **1** [NA] The long bone of the thigh, extending from the hip joint to the knee joint; the proximal bone in the hindlimb of vertebrates. Also called *thigh bone, femoral bone.* **2** [NA] The thigh; regio femoralis.
pilastered femur A femur with an unusually prominent linea aspera.

fenbencillin PHENBENICILLIN.

Fendt [Heinrich *Fendt*, German physician, flourished early 20th century] Sarcoid of Spiegler-Fendt. See under BENIGN LYMPHOCYTOMA CUTIS.

fenestra [L (akin to Gk *phainein* to bring to light, show), a window] (*plural* fenestrae) **1** In anatomy, an opening between two chambers or spaces, usually in the wall between them; a window. **2** Any opening resembling a window, as in some plaster casts, surgical drapes, or surgical instruments.

fenestra choledocha The opening into the duodenum made by the common bile duct and the pancreatic duct.

fenestra of cochlea FENESTRA COCHLEAE.

fenestra cochleae [NA] A small, rounded, recessed opening in the medial wall of the tympanic cavity, located behind and below the fenestra vestibuli, under cover of the projecting edge of the promontory and communicating with scala tympani of the cochlea from which it is separated by the secondary tym-

panic membrane. Also called *fenestra of cochlea, round window, fenestra rotunda* (outmoded), *cochlear window, porta labyrinthi* (outmoded).

fenestra ovalis An outmoded term for FENESTRA VESTIBULI.

puboischiadic fenestra A large opening in the pelvic girdle of a turtle. It develops beneath the origin of the obturator muscle and separates the pubis and the ischium, turning the pelvic girdle into a tripartite structure.

fenestra rotunda An outmoded term for FENESTRA COCHLEAE.

fenestra vestibuli [NA] A small oval opening located posterosuperior to the promontory on the medial wall of the tympanic cavity and communicating with the vestibule of the internal ear. It has the base of the stapes covering it and fixed by the annular ligament to its margin. Also called *oval window, fenestra ovalis* (outmoded), *vestibular window.*

fenestrae Plural of FENESTRA.

fenestrate [L *fenestr(a)* a window + -ATE] To create one or more openings in (tissue).

fenestrated Perforated by one or more openings, as tissue.

fenestration [*fenestr(a)* + -ATION] **1** FENESTRATION OPERATION. **2** The establishment of a fistulous opening (fenestra) usually to bypass some obstruction. **3** A condition in which one or more abnormal communications, usually congenital, exist between compartments of the body, as, for example, between the aorta and pulmonary artery. A rare usage.

alveolar plate fenestration FENESTRATION OF ALVEOLAR PROCESS.

fenestration of alveolar process A circumscribed opening in the alveolar bone over the root of a tooth. If the opening is not circumscribed it is called a dehiscence. Also called *alveolar plate fenestration.*

aortopulmonary fenestration AORTICOPULMONARY WINDOW.

tracheal fenestration The making of an opening in the anterior wall of the trachea, as in tracheostomy.

fennel *Foeniculum vulgare*, a herbaceous plant of the Umbelliferae family. The dried ripe fruit yields a volatile oil which contains anethole, fenchone, and pinene as its principal constituents. The oil is an aromatic carminative, and it is used to mask unpleasant medicinal tastes.

fenoprofen calcium $C_{30}H_{26}CaO_6 \cdot 2H_2O$. α-Methyl-3-phenoxybenzeneacetic acid calcium dihydrate. It is used as an analgesic and anti-inflammatory agent.

fentanyl $C_{22}H_{28}N_2O$. *N*-Phenyl-*N*-[1-(2-phenylethyl)-4-piperidinyl]propanamide, a narcotic analgesic with actions that resemble those of morphine. It is used therapeutically for the same purposes as morphine and has the same addicting potential. It is given intravenously or intramuscularly.

fentanyl citrate $C_{28}H_{36}N_2O_8$. *N*-Phenyl-*N*-[1-(2-phenylethyl)-4-piperidinyl]-propanamide citrate, a potent analgesic that is related to the synthetic phenylpiperidine derivatives. Its effects are like those of morphine, but its duration of action is shorter than meperidine or morphine. It is administered parenterally, and chronic use can lead to addiction.

fenugreek *Trigonella foenumgraecum*, an herb of the Leguminosae family that has been used for medicinal purposes.

Fenwick [Edwin Hurry *Fenwick*, English physician, 1856–1944] Fenwick-Hunner ulcer. See under HUNNER'S ULCER.

Fenwick [Samuel *Fenwick*, English physician, 1821–1902] Fenwick's disease. See under ATROPHIC GASTRITIS.

-fer [L *ferre* to bear] A combining form meaning one that bears.

feral [Med L *feral(is)* (from L *fer(a)* a wild beast + -*alis* -AL) wild, untamed] **1** Existing in the wild state: said of an undomesticated animal. **2** Characterized by reversion to the wild state: said of a domestic animal.

fer-de-lance [French (from L *ferrum* iron + French *de* of + L *lancea* spear), spearhead]   The venomous snake *Bothrops atrox* of the family Viperidae.

Féréol [Louis Henri Felix *Féréol*, French physician, 1825–1891]   **1** Féréol's nodes. See under RHEUMATIC NODULES.   **2** Féréol-Graux paralysis, Féréol-Graux palsy. See under PARALYSIS.

Fergon   A proprietary name for ferrous gluconate.

Ferguson-Smith [John *Ferguson-Smith*, English dermatologist, flourished 20th century]   Ferguson-Smith type epithelioma. See under SELF-HEALING SQUAMOUS EPITHELIOMA.

Fergusson [Sir William *Fergusson*, Scottish surgeon, 1808–1877]   Fergusson's incision. See under WEBER-FERGUSSON INCISION.

ferment [French (from L *fermentum* for *fervimentum* leaven, yeast, from *fervere* to be boiling hot, ferment + -*mentum* -scment), agent causing fermentation]   **1** An obsolete term for ENZYME.   **2** To undergo or bring about fermentation.

fibrin ferment   An obsolete term for THROMBIN.

glycolytic ferment   Any enzyme involved in the digestion of glucose or other simple sugars.

fermentable   Capable of being used as a substrate by an organism in anaerobic catabolism.

fermentation [FERMENT + -ATION]   The anaerobic catabolism of organic substances by organisms, usually microorganisms. In contrast to respiration, the final electron acceptors for the oxidation of organic substrates are also organic. Reduced end-products thus accumulate. Also called *zymosis, zymolysis, zymohydrolysis.*

acetone-butanol fermentation   *N*-BUTANOL FERMENTATION.

alcoholic fermentation   The breakdown of sugars to ethanol and carbon dioxide as performed by yeast.

amino acid fermentation   Any of a variety of fermentations, prominent in putrefaction and in cheese manufacture, that oxidize one amino acid and reduce another.

butanediol fermentation   A fermentation that yields, via the glycolytic pathway, the nonacidic products butanediol and its oxidation product, acetoin. It is characteristic of *Enterobacter* species and is used to differentiate this genus from coliforms. Also called *butylene glycol fermentation.*

n-butanol fermentation   A bacterial fermentation (e.g., in clostridia and bacteroides) that yields principally *n*-butyric acid, acetone, and *n*-butanol ($CH_3CH_2CH_2CH_2OH$), via head-to-tail condensation of two acetyl groups. Also called *butyric fermentation, acetone-butanol fermentation.*

butylene glycol fermentation   BUTANEDIOL FERMENTATION.

butyric fermentation   *N*-BUTANOL FERMENTATION.

formic fermentation   MIXED ACID FERMENTATION.

heterolactic fermentation   A fermentation in which C atoms 4,5,6 of hexose are converted to lactic acid and atoms 1,2,3 to carbon dioxide and acetic acid (or alcohol).

homolactic fermentation   The dissimilation of glucose ($C_6H_{12}O_6$) to two molecules of lactic acid ($C_3H_6O_3$) as sole product. This process occurs in many types of bacteria, such as those responsible for the souring of milk, in plants, and in animal muscle starved of oxygen.

lactic fermentation   The conversion of sugar into lactic acid by fermentation, characteristically carried out by the lactic acid bacteria. Lactic fermentation may be heterofermentative or homofermentative, the two types being important in classifying lactic acid bacteria. Animal cells deprived of oxygen also perform this process.

methane fermentation   The fermentation characteristic of *Methanobacterium*, which reduces CO_2 to CH_4 and H_2O at the expense of H_2, methanol, or ethanol.

mixed acid fermentation   A fermentation, characteristic of

Escherichia coli and many other Enterobacteriaceae, that yields primarily acetic acid and formic acid which is often converted to H_2 and CO_2. In this fermentation, the acetic acid is formed via acetyl CoA, which can generate ATP, thus yielding more energy per mole of sugar than the lactic or the ethanolic fermentation. Also called *formic fermentation.*

propionic fermentation   The process of breakdown of sugars by bacteria, especially *Propionibacterium*, in which propionic acid is produced, together with some acetic acid and either succinic acid or carbon dioxide. In Swiss cheese, these organisms use the lactic acid formed by other organisms as carbon source, converting it to propionic and acetic acids with the liberation of carbon dioxide. The propionic acid contributes to the flavor while the carbon dioxide is responsible for the holes in the cheese.

stormy milk fermentation   Fermentation that involves clotting with entrapment of gas bubbles in a milk-containing medium. It is characteristic of the clostridia of gas gangrene.

Fermi [Claudio *Fermi*, Italian physician, born 1862]   See under VACCINE.

Fermi [Enrico *Fermi*, Italian-born U.S. physicist, 1901–1954]   Fermi-Dirac statistics. See under STATISTICS.

fermi [after Enrico *Fermi*, Italian-born American physicist, 1901–1954]   A unit of length, used especially in nuclear physics, equal to 10^{-15} meter. Symbol: fm

fermion [after Enrico *Fermi*, Italian-born U.S. physicist, 1901–1954 + *mes(on)*]   Any of a group of mesons assumed to conform to Fermi-Dirac statistics.

fermium   A synthetic radioactive element of the actinide series, having atomic number 100. Fermium 257, discovered in 1954, is produced by neutron bombardment of plutonium. Ten isotopes are known. Fermium 257 has the longest half-life, 80 days. Symbol: Fm

fern [Middle English, from Old English *fearn*]   Any of the seedless plants that comprise the class Filicophytina. They have large leaves with veins of vascular tissue.

male fern   ASPIDIUM.

ferning   CERVICAL MUCUS ARBORIZATION.

-ferous [L *ferre* to bear]   A combining form meaning bearing, producing.

Ferrata [Adolfo *Ferrata*, Italian physician, 1880–1946]   Ferrata cell. See under HEMOHISTIOBLAST.

ferrate   An anion with irons as the central atom, such as hexacyanoferrate(III), i.e. $Fe(CN)_6^{3-}$.

Ferraton [Louis *Ferraton*, French surgeon, born 1860]   Perrin-Ferraton disease. See under SNAPPING HIP.

ferredoxin   Any of a class of iron-sulfur compounds found in photosynthetic and anaerobic bacteria and photosynthetic plants, where they serve as electron carriers with very low redox potentials.

Ferrein [Antoine *Ferrein*, French surgeon and anatomist, 1693–1769]   **1** Ferrein's cord. See under PLICA VOCALIS.   **2** Ferrein's ligament. See under LIGAMENTUM LATERALE ARTICULATIONIS TEMPOROMANDIBULARIS.   **3** Ferrein's canal. See under RIVUS LACRIMALIS.   **4** Ferrein's tubules. See under TUBULE.   **5** Pyramid of Ferrein. See under PARS RADIATA LOBULI CORTICALIS RENIS.   **6** Ferrein's vasa aberrantia. See under VAS.   **7** See under FORAMEN.

ferri- [L *ferrum* iron]   A combining form denoting iron, especially iron(III).

ferric [L *ferr(um)* iron + -IC]   Denoting compounds containing iron in the Fe(III) state.

ferric ammonium citrate   IRON AND AMMONIUM CITRATE.

brown ferric ammonium citrate   A preparation of ferric ammonium citrate containing 16.5–18.5% iron used in the treatment of iron deficiency anemia.

green ferric ammonium citrate A hydrated form of ferric ammonium citrate with about 15 percent, by weight, ferric iron. It is green, is in the form of transparent scales or a powder, and is very soluble in water. It is used as a hematinic agent to treat iron deficiency anemia. Also called *iron citrate green*.

ferric ammonium sulfate IRON AND AMMONIUM SULFATE.

ferric citrate A mixture of ferric iron and citric acid in an indefinitely defined composition. It is in the form of solid red transparent scales or a brown powder which is soluble in water. It is used as a source of iron to treat iron-deficiency anemia. Also called *iron citrate*.

ferric glycerophosphate $C_9H_{21}Fe_2O_{18}P_3$. Solid orange-to-yellow transparent scales or powder which are soluble in water. It is used as a hematinic agent. Also called *iron glycerophosphate*.

ferric hydroxide with magnesium oxide $Fe_2O_3 \cdot 3H_2O$. Ferric hydroxide, mixed with a suspension of magnesium oxide. It has been alleged to be an antidote for arsenic poisoning.

ferric hypophosphite $FeH_6O_6P_3$. A white or gray-white powder which is soluble in water. It has been used as a hematinic agent. Also called *iron hypophosphite*.

ferric phosphate $FePO_4 \cdot 4H_2O$. A yellowish compound, insoluble in water, that is used in feeds and fertilizers and as a food supplement, especially to enrich breads.

ferric pyrophosphate $Fe_4O_{21}P_6$. A bioavailable form of iron that is used as a hematinic.

ferric sodium edetate Ferric monosodium ethylenediaminetetracetate, a chelated preparation of iron(III) used in the treatment of iron deficiency anemia.

ferricyanide The ion $Fe(CN)_6^{3-}$, and salts that contain it. It is a mild oxidizing agent, and is systematically and increasingly called hexacyanoferrate(III).

ferriheme HEME.

ferrihemochrome Any respiratory pigment containing iron(III).

ferrihemoglobin METHEMOGLOBIN.

ferriporphyrin Any porphyrin containing iron(III).

ferriprotoporphyrin **1** Any protoporphyrin containing iron(III). **2** An incorrect term for HEMIN.

Ferrissia A genus of snails in the family Ancylidae, a worldwide group having limpet-shaped shells. Several species serve as first intermediate hosts of trematodes.

Ferrissia tenuis A species reported as a probable intermediate host of *Schistosoma haematobium* near Bombay, India, though this report has been questioned by many authorities.

Ferris Smith [*Ferris Smith*, U.S. otolaryngologist, born 1884] **1** See under TECHNIQUE. **2** Ferris Smith technique. See under MULTIPLE PARTIAL EXCISIONS.

ferritin A protein constituting a storage form of iron in liver and other tissues. It consists of an outer shell of 24 molecules of a protein of mass 18.5 kDa, surrounding a crystalline region of iron(III), largely as its hydroxide, which may be filled to a variable extent. When completely filled, the ferritin contains 23% iron. This gives it high electron density, a property used in the technique of ferritin labeling.

ferro- [L *ferrum* iron] A combining form denoting iron, especially iron(II).

ferrochelatase The enzyme (EC 4.99.1.1) responsible for heme synthesis by catalyzing the reaction of protoporphyrin with iron(II) to yield heme with displacement of two hydrogen ions. This is a step in the biosynthesis of hemoglobin. Also called *heme synthetase*.

ferrocholinate $C_{11}H_{24}FeNO_{11}$. A mixture of equal molar concentrations of choline dihydrogen citrate and ferric hydroxide

or ferrous carbonate. It is used as a hematinic agent. Also called *iron choline citrate*.

ferrocyanide The ion $Fe(CN)_6^{4-}$, and salts that contain it. It is a mild reducing agent, and is systematically and increasingly called hexacyanoferrate(II).

ferroelectric Denoting crystalline materials in which an external electric field can create a permanent electric polarization, much as an external magnetic field creates a permanent magnet.

ferrography [FERRO- + -GRAPHY] A method of treating a sample of synovial fluid with a solution rich in magnetic ions and exposing it to a magnetic field which sorts out breakdown products by size and structure.

ferrokinetics The changes undergone by elemental iron in the body in the course of its absorption, distribution, metabolism, and excretion.

Ferrolip A proprietary name for ferrocholinate.

ferrotherapy Treatment with iron or iron compounds.

ferrous [L *ferrum* iron + -OUS] Denoting compounds containing iron, particularly in the Fe(II) state.

ferrous arsenate IRON ARSENATE.

ferrous fumarate $C_4H_2FeO_4$. A bioavailable powder of iron used as a hematinic agent. It is prepared by mixing ferrous sulfate and sodium fumarate.

ferrous gluconate $C_{12}H_{22}FeO_{14}$. A bioavailable form of iron that is used as a hematinic and as a food coloring and flavoring agent. Also called *iron gluconate*.

ferrous iodide $FeI_2 \cdot 5H_2O$. A deliquescent compound of iron used in tonic syrups. Also called *iron iodide*.

ferrous lactate $(CH_3CHOHCOO)_2Fe \cdot 3H_2O$. A compound of iron used in the treatment of iron deficiency anemia. Also called *iron lactate*.

ferrous sulfate $FeSO_4 \cdot 7H_2O$. Bluish green crystals or granules that are a very commonly used form of iron in medical tonics and for the treatment of iron deficiency anemia. Also called *copperas, green vitriol, iron protosulfate, iron sulfate*.

ferrous sulfate $FeSO_4$. An iron salt used therapeutically as a hematinic. As a source of iron it is used as a food supplement.

dried ferrous sulfate $FeSO_4 \cdot H_2O$. A gray powder of ferrous sulfate that has less water of crystallization. It is used for the same purposes as the more hydrated form.

ferruginous Containing iron.

ferrule [L *viriola* (dim. of *viria* a bracelet, influenced in Old French and Med L by L *ferrum* iron) a small bracelet] A metal band encircling the end of a root as in a collar crown.

Ferry [Erwin Sidney *Ferry*, U.S. physicist, 1868–1956] Ferry-Porter law. See under LAW.

fertile [L *fertil(is)* fruitful, fertile] Capable of producing offspring.

fertility [L *fertilitas* (from *fertilis* fruitful, fertile, from *ferre* to bear) fruitfulness] **1** The condition of being fertile; capacity to conceive and bear offspring. Also called *uberty* (seldom used). **2** In demography, reproductive performance as distinguished from reproductive capacity or fecundity. **3** The influence of births on population change.

cohort fertility The number of births to a group of women who all belong to the same cohort, the cohort being usually defined by reference to the year of birth of the women.

completed fertility The number of births to a cohort of women all of whose members have completed their reproductive period.

duration-specific fertility The fertility of women married for a stated duration, expressed as the number of legitimate live births to women married for a given number of years per 1000 women of reproductive age married for the same number of years.

effective fertility　REPRODUCTION PROBABILITY.

excess fertility　SUPERFECUNDITY.

fertilization [L *fertilis* fruitful, fertile + -IZE + -ATION]　The process of union of a sperm and an ovum in order to form a zygote in either animals or plants. In man, fertilization takes place usually in the outer third of the uterine tube shortly after ovulation. One spermatozoon penetrates the zona pellucida of the ovum and then enters the ovum itself to form the male pronucleus. This soon joins the female pronucleus of the ovum to provide the nucleus of the zygote with the diploid number of chromosomes. The process of fertilization is the normal means of stimulation of development of a single-celled ovum into an individual of a particular species. See also PARTHENOGENESIS.

cross fertilization　The fertilization of a gamete of one organism by a gamete from another organism, as distinguished from self-fertilization.

double fertilization　Fertilization, characteristic of angiosperms, in which a diploid zygote results from the fusion of an egg and a sperm while a triploid endosperm nucleus is produced by the fusion of a second sperm with two polar nuclei.

external fertilization　Union of a sperm and an ovum to form a zygote outside the body of the female.

internal fertilization　Union of a sperm and an ovum to form a zygote inside the body of the female.

fertilization in vitro　The union of an ovum and a sperm under laboratory conditions.

fertilization in vivo　The natural occurrence of fertilization in the female genital tract.

fertilizin　A substance associated with the plasma membrane of the ovum of some species, which is capable of agglutinating and binding spermatozoa of the same species to the ovum. In the sea urchin, it has been characterized as a glycoprotein with a molecular weight in the region of 300 000.

ferv.　*fervens* (L, boiling).

fervescence [L *fervescens*, pres. part. of *fervescere* (from *fervere* to boil, burn) to begin to boil or be hot]　An increase in body temperature above normal; fever.

fescue [Middle English *festu*, from Old French *festu* (from L *festuca* a stalk, straw) a piece of straw]　**1** *FESTUCA*.　**2** FESCUE LAMENESS.

fester [Middle English *fester, festre*, from Middle French *festre* sore, from L *fistula* a pipe, reed, ulcer]　**1** A suppurating ulcer.　**2** To become inflamed and suppurate superficially.

festinant [L *festinans*, gen. *festinantis*, pres. part. of *festinare* to hasten]　Hastening; accelerating: used especially of the characteristic gait of those afflicted by parkinsonism, in which increasingly rapid steps are taken.

festination [L *festinatio* (from *festinatus*, past part. of *festinare* to hurry) a hurrying]　FESTINATING GAIT.

festoon [French *feston* (from Italian *festone* festoon, from *festa* a holyday feast, from Vulgar L *festa* feast) a garland]　**1** One of the segments found on the posterior submarginal border of the dorsum of certain hard ticks, consisting of rectangular divisions separated by grooves in the edge of the dorsum.　**2** GINGIVAL FESTOON.

gingival festoon　**1** The curved shape of the gingival margin.　**2** A simulation of this in a prosthesis.　**3** A thickening and rounding of the gingival margin caused by inflammation. Also called *festoon*.

McCall's festoon　A gingival festoon thought to be caused by occlusal trauma.

Festuca　A genus of grass, of which one species, *F. arundinacea*,

contains a toxin that causes lameness in cattle. Also called *fescue*.

fetal [*fet(us)* + -AL]　Of or relating to a fetus. For humans, the fetal stage of intrauterine development extends from the ninth week of pregnancy until term.

fetalism [FETAL + -ISM]　Persistence of a fetal character into postnatal life, as may occur in the vascular system. See also FETALIZATION.

fetalization　A theory proposed to account for the alleged occurrence of fetal features in the adult, as shown during anthropogenesis. It was propounded by L. Bolk, Dutch anatomist, from 1922–26. Man was represented as a fetal ape because of such features as lack of pigmentation, absence of hair, shape of auricle and mandible, persistence of sutures, position of the foramen magnum, and others. Also called *Bolk's retardation theory*.　● The theory was not accepted and is not tenable today because of modern genetic and hormonal explanations. However, the term *fetalism* is still occasionally used to describe persistence of a fetal character into postnatal life.

fetation [*fet(us)* + -ATION]　Fetal growth and development taking place inside the uterus.

fetch　**1** To place computer data and instructions in registers in preparation for execution.　**2** Designating that portion of a computer cycle during which fetching is done.

feti-　FETO-.

feticide [FETI- + -CIDE]　The killing or destruction of a fetus, usually by artificial means.

fetid [L *foetid(us)* stinking, fetid]　Having an offensive odor. Also *graveolent* (obsolete).

fetish [French *fétiche* (from Portuguese *feitiço*, as adjective artificial, as noun a charm, from L *facticius*, also *factitius* artificial) an object venerated as an idol]　A body part or material thing, associated with the love object, whose presence is necessary for the subject's sexual excitement. The fetish may totally replace the need for the love object itself. Also called *idolum* (obsolete).

fetishism [FETISH + -ISM]　A paraphilia consisting of the preferred or obligatory use of an object (fetish) in order to achieve sexual excitement. Also called *idolomania*.

foot fetishism　Fetishism in which the foot or shoe is the preferred object. Also called *rétifism*.

fetishist [FETISH + -IST]　A person whose sexual excitement depends on a fetish.

fetlock [Middle English *fitlok, fetlak*, prob. from *fet* feet + *lok* lock, from *lokke*, from Old English *loc* a twist]　**1** A tuft of hair that grows from the posterior aspect of the metacarpophalangeal and metatarsophalangeal joints of the horse.　**2** The general area comprised by the metacarpophalangeal and metatarsophalangeal joints of the horse.　**3** The metacarpophalangeal and metatarsophalangeal joints of the horse.

feto- [L *fetus* or *foetus*, past part. of *fere* to bring forth]　A combining form meaning fetus, fetal. Also *feti-, foeti-, foeto-*.

fetoamniotic [FETO- + AMNIOTIC]　Relating to both the fetus and the amnion.

fetoglobulin　FETOPROTEIN.

fetography [FETO- + -GRAPHY]　Radiographic examination of a fetus *in utero*.

fetologist [*fet(o)-* + -OLOGIST]　A specialist in fetology.

fetology [FETO- + -LOGY]　The scientific study of the fetus.　● The study of the fetus is often considered to be part of embryology, but *fetology* is still used when a distinction is necessary between study of the embryo and study of the fetus.

fetomaternal　Pertaining to the relationship between the fetus and the mother.

fetometry [FETO- + -METRY]　Measurement of the fetus. The term usually applies to skull diameters.

roentgen fetometry The measurement of fetal head size by roentgenographic methods.

fetopathy [FETO- + -PATHY] Any morbid state or condition in a fetus *in utero*, or, by extension, in a newborn infant. It may be of developmental, infectious, inflammatory, or traumatic origin.

fetoplacental [FETO- + PLACENTAL] Pertaining to the relationship between the fetus and placenta.

fetoprotein One of a number of proteins found in fetal blood. α-fetoprotein is the fetal equivalent of albumin. It is produced in adults by hepatomas and certain teratomas for which its presence is a marker. α-fetoprotein is immunosuppressive and may play some part in the immunosuppression associated with tumors that secrete it. β- and γ-fetoproteins are associated with various neoplasms in the adult. Also called *fetoglobulin.*

fetor [L *foetor* foul smell, stench] A strong, offensive smell or stench.

fetor ex ore A rarely used term for FETOR ORIS.

fetor hepaticus A unique sweet, musty smell of the breath which may occur in patients with severe hepatocellular disease. Its exact cause it not known. Also called *liver breath.*

fetor oris Foul breath. The cause may be apparent, such as disease within the mouth (dental caries, severe ulcerative stomatitis, ulceromembranous pharyngitis etc.) or the nose (ozena, malignant disease etc.) but frequently defies diagnosis. Also called *halitosis, fetor ex ore* (rarely used), *ozostomia, bromopnea* (outmoded), *stomatodysodia.*

fetoscope [FETO- + -SCOPE] **1** An instrument utilized to detect and measure the fetal heartbeat. **2** An instrument utilized to visualize a fetus through transabdominal insertion of the device into the amniotic cavity.

fetoscopy [FETO- + -SCOPY] The direct visualization of a fetus using a fetoscope.

fetotoxic [FETO- + TOXIC] **1** Characteristic of an agent that is toxic to the fetus; that is, to the conceptus after completion of organogenesis. **2** Descriptive of toxic effects on the conceptus at any time during intrauterine life. These effects are not limited to lethality but also may include malformation and intrauterine growth retardation. Compare EMBRYOTOXIC.

fetuin A serum lipoprotein (α-fetoprotein) in the blood and on lymphocyte membranes of fetal animals.

fetus [L (past part. of *fere* to bring forth), brought forth; as substantive, a producing, procreating, offspring] The unborn child or offspring while still in the uterus during the later part of gestation and after the time of appearance of the major systems and parts during the embryonic period. A fetus displays the beginnings of adult features of the species and the fetal period is principally one of growth. A human embryo becomes a fetus at about the end of the eighth week after fertilization.

fetus acardius A fetus or newborn infant lacking a heart.

fetus amorphus AMORPHUS.

fetus anideus ANIDEUS.

calcified fetus LITHOPEDION.

fetus compressus FETUS PAPYRACEUS.

harlequin fetus A fetus or newborn, often premature, infant with the most severe form of ichthyosis vulgaris. The keratin layer of the skin is so thickened as to interfere with vital functions. The multidirectional cracks in the skin produce a harlequin pattern of diamond-shaped, grayish brown plaques. In addition, the face, hands, and feet may be malformed. The condition is transmitted as a recessive trait and is incompatible with survival for more than a few hours or days. Also called *ichthyosis fetus.*

ichthyosis fetus HARLEQUIN FETUS.

fetus in fetu FETAL INCLUSION.

mummified fetus LITHOPEDION.

paper-doll fetus FETUS PAPYRACEUS.

papyraceous fetus FETUS PAPYRACEUS.

fetus papyraceus The remains of a dead twin which during intrauterine development died and was pressed flat against the uterine wall by the living twin. Also called *fetus compressus, paper-doll fetus, papyraceous fetus.*

parasitic fetus PARASITIC TWIN.

fetus parasiticus PARASITIC TWIN.

retroperitoneal fetus in fetu A conjoined twin situated outside the peritoneum, usually on the posterior abdominal wall, of the host fetus. Although retroperitoneal, it is covered by an amniotic sac and protrudes forward into the peritoneal cavity of the host. The parasitic twin may contain organs and limbs with some vertical axis symmetry, and it is removable with good prognosis during infancy of the host.

fetus sanguinolentus A partially macerated dead fetus that has darkened to approximately the color of clotted blood.

sireniform fetus SIRENOMELUS.

sirenoform fetus SIRENOMELUS.

Feulgen [Robert Joachim *Feulgen*, German biochemist, 1884–1955] Feulgen procedure, Feulgen's test, Feulgen reaction. See under METHOD.

Feulgen-positive [after Robert *Feulgen*, German biochemist, 1884–1955 + *positive*] Describing any cytologic structure that stains as a result of the Feulgen method: used especially in reference to DNA.

fever

fever [L *febris* a burning, fever] **1** An increase of body temperature above normal. Also called *fire, febris.* **2** Any state of ill health in which an elevated body temperature is a primary symptom. For defs. 1 and 2 also called *pyrexia, pyrexy.*

abenteric typhoid fever A form of typhoid fever in which it was thought that the intestinal tract was not involved. An outmoded term.

abortus fever Brucellosis in humans caused by *Brucella abortus.* It is generally contracted from cattle or cow's milk.

absorption fever Fever occurring in the first 12 hours following labor and delivery. An older term.

Aden fever DENGUE.

adynamic fever Low-grade fever in patients who are generally weak or asthenic. An imprecise and outmoded term. Also called *asthenic fever.*

African coast fever EAST COAST FEVER.

African hemorrhagic fever EBOLA VIRUS DISEASE.

African swine fever An acute, highly contagious, systemic disease of swine caused by an unclassified virus. The signs and lesions resemble those of hog cholera. Differentiation from the latter is made by laboratory tests. In 1957 it spread from Africa to some countries of southern Europe. It does not occur in the United States. Also called *warthog disease.*

African tick fever A tick-borne endemic relapsing fever caused by the spirochete *Borrelia duttoni,* transmitted by *Ornithodoros moubata.* Also called *Dutton's relapsing fever, Dutton's disease.*

fever and ague An obsolete term for MALARIA.

algid pernicious fever Malaria accompanied by symptoms of collapse. An obsolete term.

Andaman A fever Leptospirosis caused by a strain of *Lep-*

tospira icterohaemorrhagiae first isolated in the Andaman Islands.

anginoid scarlet fever A particularly severe form of scarlet fever, now rarely encountered, characterized by acute septic pharyngitis often spreading to the larynx and sometimes leading to ulceration and necrosis of the fauces and soft palate. Cellulitis of the neck with suppuration of the cervical lymph nodes may occur, and death may ensue from profound toxemia or bacteremia. Also called *scarlatina anginosa* (older term), *scarlatina septica* (older term), *angina phlegmonosa* (obsolete).

aphthous fever FOOT-AND-MOUTH DISEASE.

apyretic typhoid fever A form of typhoid fever in which the temperature remains nearly normal.

Archibald's fever An illness considered to be caused by organisms of the *Bacterium cloacae* group, found in the Sudan. It seems more likely that this was a form of salmonellosis. It is characterized by fever, drowsiness, and sometimes delirium. An outmoded term.

Argentinian hemorrhagic fever An acute, severe disease caused by the Junín virus, an arenavirus contracted from the urine of infected rodents, and marked by fever, chills, lymphadenopathy, headache, myalgia, leukopenia, shock, hemorrhagic, neurologic manifestations, and renal involvement. Also called *mal de rastrojos, Junín fever, South American hemorrhagic fever.*

artificial fever INDUCED FEVER.

aseptic fever Fever that accompanies an aseptic wound and that is brought on by the absorption of noninfected but injured tissue.

Assam fever KALA-AZAR.

asthenic fever ADYNAMIC FEVER.

auric fever A toxic reaction to gold, characterized by dermatitis which is expressed as erythema, urticaria, or rash. Temporary nephritis with albuminuria may sometimes occur. Blood dyscrasias such as leukopenia, agranulocytosis, and thrombopenia have also been reported.

Australian Q fever Q FEVER.

Australian tick fever NORTH QUEENSLAND TICK TYPHUS.

autumn fever 1 NANUKAYAMI. 2 SEVEN-DAY FEVER.

Bangkok hemorrhagic fever DENGUE HEMORRHAGIC FEVER.

barbeiro fever CHAGAS DISEASE.

biduotertian fever Tertian malaria in which paroxysms of fever are nearly continuous resulting from infection by two broods of parasites, with merozoite release occurring on alternate days.

biliary fever of dogs CANINE BABESIOSIS.

biliary fever of horses EQUINE BABESIOSIS.

bilious fever A febrile illness characterized by bilious vomiting. An obsolete term.

bilious fever of cattle ANAPLASMOSIS.

black fever 1 ROCKY MOUNTAIN SPOTTED FEVER. 2 KALA-AZAR.

blackwater fever An acute intravascular hemolysis associated with maglignant tertian malaria, caused by *Plasmodium falciparum*. The urine becomes dark brown or black. It may occur as a single crisis in which more than half the circulating erythrocytes are hemolyzed intravenously, or repeated smaller crises may occur. The disease is frequently fatal. It occurs mainly among foreigners in malarial countries, who have previously had attacks of malignant tertian malaria inadequately treated by quinine. Quinine often precipitates an attack, but its etiologic role is still unclear. The disease is quite unusual where newer synthetic antimalarial drugs are used. Also called *hemolytic malaria, melanuric fever, West African fever, canebrake yellow fever* (rarely used).

blue fever ROCKY MOUNTAIN SPOTTED FEVER.

Bolivian hemorrhagic fever Hemorrhagic fever caused by the Machupo virus (an arenavirus), clinically similar to Argentinian hemorrhagic fever, with involvement of hematopoietic, cardiovascular, renal, clotting, and central nervous systems. There is 10–20 percent mortality. Also called *South American hemorrhagic fever.*

bouquet fever DENGUE.

boutonneuse fever A tick-borne disease caused by *Rickettsia conorii*, widespread in the Mediterranean, Africa, and India. It is characterized by an initial necrotic skin lesion (tache noire), headache, muscle pain, and a skin rash covering the entire body, including palms of hands and soles of feet. Also called *Mediterranean fever, Marseilles fever, Olmer's disease, Conor and Bruch disease, escarronodulaire, Mediterranean exanthematous fever, Mediterranean tick fever, eruptive Mediterranean fever, exanthematic fever of Marseille, South African tick-bite fever, tickbite fever, fièvre boutonneuse, fièvre exanthématique de Marseille.*

bovine infectious petechial fever A disease of cattle in Kenya, caused by a rickettsial-like organism, *Cytoectes ondiri*, which is transmitted by biting insects. It is characterized by hemorrhages of the mucous membranes, fever, and diarrhea. Severe conjunctivitis and proptosis may occur, and death may result in one to three days. Also called *Ondiri disease.*

brain fever Meningitis, encephalitis, or any other febrile illness involving the brain. A popular usage.

brass-founders' fever METAL-FUME FEVER.

Brazilian fever ROCKY MOUNTAIN SPOTTED FEVER.

Brazilian spotted fever ROCKY MOUNTAIN SPOTTED FEVER.

breakbone fever DENGUE.

Brisbane fever Q FEVER.

bulam fever PYM'S FEVER.

Bullis fever A mild disease characterized by fever, leukopenia, postorbital and occipital headache, and lymphadenitis. It is thought to be caused by a species of *Rickettsia* and transmitted by the Lone Star tick (*Amblyomma americanum*). Also called *Texas tick fever, Lone Star fever.* ● It was given its name following an epidemic originating at Camp Bullis, Texas, in 1942.

burdwan fever KALA-AZAR.

Bushy Creek fever FORT BRAGG FEVER.

Bwamba fever A mild, febrile disease of viral origin which resembles yellow fever and occurs in central Africa, particularly Uganda. There are many strains of the virus, which is transmitted by *Anopheles gambiae*. Headache and backache are the main symptoms, which usually subside in 5–7 days. ● The name is derived from *Bwamba* forest in the western province of Uganda.

cachectic fever KALA-AZAR.

cachexial fever KALA-AZAR.

Cameroon fever MALARIA.

camp fever EPIDEMIC LOUSE-BORNE TYPHUS.

canebrake yellow fever A rarely used term for BLACKWATER FEVER.

canefield fever Leptospirosis occurring among canefield workers, caused principally by *Leptospira interrogans* serovar *australis*.

canicola fever Leptospirosis of dogs caused by *Leptospira interrogans* of the serotype *canicola* and usually transmitted to man by means of the urine of infected dogs. In the early stages of the disease, dogs have a fever and general signs of a severe systemic illness. Icterus and diarrhea may develop. The organism localizes in the kidneys where it causes initially severe, acute inflammation. If recovery occurs, chronic nephropathy ensues. Also called *canine leptospirosis, Stuttgart disease, Stuttgart dog plague, dog plague, canine typhus* (imprecise).

carapata fever GARAPATA DISEASE.

carbuncular fever ANTHRAX.

Carter's fever A form of relapsing fever caused by *Borrelia carteri* and occurring in Asia.

cat fever FELINE VIRAL ENTERITIS.

cat-bite fever **1** An infectious disease caused by *Pasteurella multocida* and spread to humans by the bite of a cat. An abscess forms at the site of injury. Also called *cat-bite disease*. **2** An incorrect term for CAT-SCRATCH DISEASE.

cat-scratch fever CAT-SCRATCH DISEASE.

Cavite fever A denguelike fever found in Cavite naval station in Manila Bay.

Central Asian hemorrhagic fever A tick-borne hemorrhagic fever due to the Congo virus (a togavirus) and reported in Kazakhstan and Uzbekistan. It is thought to be transmitted by the tick *Hyalomma anatolicum*. Also called *Uzbekistan hemorrhagic fever*.

Central European tick-borne fever The central European subtype of tick-borne encephalitis. See under TICK-BORNE ENCEPHALITIS.

cerebrospinal fever CEREBROSPINAL MENINGITIS.

cesspool fever TYPHOID FEVER.

Chagres fever **1** A form of falciparum malaria once prevalent near the Chagres River in Panama. An obsolete usage. Also called *Panama fever*. **2** A fever caused by the Chagres virus, an arbovirus endemic in Panama.

Charcot's fever INTERMITTENT HEPATIC FEVER.

Charcot's intermittent fever INTERMITTENT HEPATIC FEVER.

chikungunya fever CHIKUNGUNYA.

childbed fever An older term for PUERPERAL FEVER.

Choix fever ROCKY MOUNTAIN SPOTTED FEVER.

coastal fever SCRUB TYPHUS. • The term refers to endemic areas on the coast of Queensland, Australia.

Colombian tick fever ROCKY MOUNTAIN SPOTTED FEVER.

Colombo fever PARATYPHOID FEVER.

Colorado fever COLORADO TICK FEVER.

Colorado tick fever A febrile illness of man caused by an orbivirus (Colorado tick fever virus) and transmitted by *Dermacentor andersoni* ticks from small rodents. The disease occurs only in the region where the tick resides, i.e. in the Rocky Mountains and westward, with the majority of cases reported in Colorado. The signs and symptoms are nearly identical to those of Rocky Mountain spotted fever, although there is usually no rash. Developing 3–6 days after the infecting tick bite, the disease is characterized by high fever (biphasic in 50% of cases), chills, myalgia, severe headache, nausea and vomiting, ocular and abdominal pain, and, in a majority of cases, leukopenia. The virus is erythrocyte-associated and persists in the blood for two weeks to two months after onset of illness. Also called *Colorado fever, mountain tick fever, mountain fever*.

Congolian red fever FLEA-BORNE TYPHUS.

continued fever CONTINUOUS FEVER.

continuous fever An unremitting fever. Also called *continued fever, synochus, synocha*.

Corsican fever MALARIA.

cotton-mill fever A condition characterized by chills, nausea, and vomiting which occurs in some workers when they are first exposed to cotton dust or when they return to work after a prolonged absence. It lasts only a few days and seldom recurs. The cause is thought to be an endotoxin from Gram-negative bacteria contaminating the cotton. It also occurs in persons exposed to other vegetable dusts, such as hemp. Also called *mill fever*.

Crimean hemorrhagic fever A hemorrhagic fever caused by a virus of the Crimean-Congo group of the Bunyaviridae and transmitted principally by the tick *Hyalomma marginatum*, which occurs in the Crimea and the lower Don and Volga river valleys.

cyclic fever A fever that recurs regularly.

Cyprus fever MALTA FEVER.

dandy fever DENGUE.

date fever DENGUE.

deer-fly fever TULAREMIA.

deer hemorrhagic fever A hemorrhagic disease of deer, similar to bluetongue of sheep, occurring in the eastern and central parts of the United States. It is caused by an orbivirus.

dehydration fever Rise of body temperature in the newborn on the second to fifth day of life, when the combination of a high room temperature and low fluid intake reduces the insensible evaporation from the lungs and heat loss in the breath. Also called *inanition fever, exsiccation fever*.

dengue fever DENGUE.

dengue hemorrhagic fever A form of dengue characterized by hemorrhagic manifestations. It often occurs in epidemics in large urban centers in Asia, and is associated with a substantial mortality rate (50 percent or more), especially in children. Thrombocytopenia, concurrent hemoconcentration, and circulatory failure (dengue hemorrhagic shock syndrome), probably mediated by immunopathologic mechanisms, are important features of the disease. Intensive care with fluid replacement, blood transfusion, and administration of corticosteroids plays a part in management. Also called *hemorrhagic dengue, Bangkok hemorrhagic fever, Philippine hemorrhagic fever, Thai hemorrhagic fever*.

desert fever COCCIDIOIDOMYCOSIS.

digestive fever An obsolete term for DIETARY INDUCED THERMOGENESIS.

diphasic milk fever The central European subtype of tick-borne encephalitis. See under TICK-BORNE ENCEPHALITIS.

double quartan fever Malaria in which paroxysms of fever occur on two days in succession followed by an interval of one day. An obsolete term. Also called *quartana duplex*.

double quotidian fever Malaria characterized by two paroxysms of fever daily. An obsolete term.

drug fever An elevated body temperature brought about by the administration of a drug. These reactions are not uncommon from vaccines, some antibiotics, and antineoplastic agents. Usually the effect is over when medication is stopped.

Dumdum fever KALA-AZAR.

dust fever UNDULANT FEVER. See under BRUCELLOSIS.

Dutton's relapsing fever AFRICAN TICK FEVER.

East Coast fever A serious and economically important theileriasis of cattle, principally in eastern Africa, caused by *Theileria parva*, which parasitizes erythrocytes. Mortality is high. The signs include high fever and swollen lymph nodes. It is transmitted by ticks of the genera *Rhipicephalus* and *Hyalomma*. Also called *Rhodesian tick fever, Rhodesian fever, amakebe, coastal fever, cattle anemia, African coast fever, Rhodesian red water*.

elephantoid fever Fever and lymphangitis associated with the early stages of elephantiasis in human filariasis. A rarely used term. Also called *muma fever (Samoan), filarial fever*.

endemic relapsing fever See under RELAPSING FEVER.

English sweating fever A disease marked by profuse sweating and fever that occurred in England in the Middle Ages. It is thought to have been an epidemic of influenza. Also called *anglicus sudor*.

enteric fever A febrile illness caused by bacteria of the genus *Salmonella*; typhoid fever or paratyphoid fever.

entericoid fever PARENTERIC FEVER.

ephemeral fever **1** A mild viral disease of cattle in Australia, Asia, and Africa. The course is usually short and recovery is spontaneous. Also called *three-day sickness, stiff sickness* (popular). **2** Any fever of brief duration.

epidemic catarrhal fever An outmoded term for INFLUENZA.

epidemic hemorrhagic fever An acute infectious disease seen in northeastern Asia, caused by the Hantaan virus and transmitted by field rodents. The disease is characterized by fever, purpura, vascular damage, renal failure, prostration, and shock. Also called *epidemic hemorrhagic disease, Far Eastern hemorrhagic fever, Korean hemorrhagic fever, Korean fever, Manchurian hemorrhagic fever, Korin fever, Kokka disease, Songo fever, Nidoko disease, epidemic nephrosonephritis, nephrosonephritis* (rarely used).

equine biliary fever EQUINE BABESIOSIS.

equine swamp fever EQUINE INFECTIOUS ANEMIA.

eruptive fever Any fever accompanied by a skin eruption. Also called *exanthematous fever.*

eruptive Mediterranean fever BOUTONNEUSE FEVER.

essential fever Any fever of unknown origin.

etiocholanolone fever An episodic fever due to periodic elevations of plasma 5β-androstane (etiocholanolone).

exanthematic fever of Marseille BOUTONNEUSE FEVER.

exanthematous fever ERUPTIVE FEVER.

exsiccation fever DEHYDRATION FEVER.

falciparum fever FALCIPARUM MALARIA.

familial Mediterranean fever A hereditary disease found in persons of Mediterranean origin, consisting of episodic fever, arthritis, serositis, and sometimes complicated by amyloidosis. Also called *Armenian disease, familial paroxysmal peritonitis.*

famine fever **1** RELAPSING FEVER. **2** TYPHUS.

Far Eastern hemorrhagic fever EPIDEMIC HEMORRHAGIC FEVER.

fatigue fever A fever that follows violent and/or prolonged exercise.

filarial fever ELEPHANTOID FEVER.

flood fever SCRUB TYPHUS.

fog fever BOVINE ATYPICAL INTERSTITIAL PNEUMONIA.

food fever Fever with gastrointestinal disturbances lasting from several days to several weeks and thought to be the result of food poisoning.

Fort Bragg fever Leptospirosis, presumably due to *Leptospira autumnalis,* characterized by fever and a pretibial rash. Also called *Bushy Creek fever, pretibial fever.*

foundrymen's fever METAL-FUME FEVER.

Gambian fever An irregular, recurrent, febrile condition lasting from one to four days, with from two to five days between relapses, and characterized by rapid pulse and breathing, and enlargement of the spleen. It is caused by the presence of *Trypanosoma gambiense,* the agent of Gambian trypanosomiasis, in the bloodstream.

Gibraltar fever MALTA FEVER.

glandular fever INFECTIOUS MONONUCLEOSIS.

goat fever **1** Brucellosis caused by *Brucella melitensis* and contracted typically from goats or goat's milk; Malta fever. Also called *goat's milk fever, fièvre caprine.* **2** LECHUGUILLA POISONING.

goat's milk fever GOAT FEVER.

Guáitara fever OROYA FEVER.

Hankow fever Schistosomiasis due to *Schistosoma japonicum.*

harvest fever A type of leptospirosis characterized by conjunctivitis, vomiting, diarrhea, abdominal pains, stupor, and fever. Occurring principally among field workers during harvest, it is caused by *Leptospira interrogans* serovar *grippotyphosa.* Also called *erntefieber.*

Hasami fever Mild leptospirosis caused by *Leptospira autumnalis* or a similar leptospiral agent and occurring in Japan, especially in the Hasami district of Nagasaki Prefecture. Also called *hasamiyami.*

Haverhill fever An illness characterized by fever, chills, an erythematous eruption, headache, and arthritis. One causative agent is *Streptobacillus moniliformis,* which has been recovered from raw milk believed to be contaminated by rats. First identified in Haverhill, Massachusetts in 1926, it occurs in epidemics and in isolated cases. Also called *streptobacillary fever, epidemic arthritic erythema, erythema arthriticum epidemicum.* See also RAT-BITE FEVER.

hay fever Allergic rhinitis due to pollen hypersensitivity and therefore seasonal. In the United States, ragweed pollen is the usual allergen and August and September the season, whereas in the United Kingdom, grass pollens are most often incriminated and the season runs from the end of May until the middle of July. Also called *seasonal nasal allergy, pollen coryza* (seldom used), *summer catarrh* (rarely used), *autumnal catarrh, corasthma* (obsolete), *Bostock's catarrh* (obsolete), *June cold* (popular).

hectic fever A fever characterized by wide swings in temperature which recur daily.

hematuric bilious fever *Plasmodium falciparum* malaria associated with hematuria. A rarely used term.

hemoglobinuric fever BLACKWATER FEVER.

hemorrhagic fever A category of infectious diseases of diverse viral origin characterized generally by fever, myalgia, headache, capillaritis, and hemorrhagic manifestations often followed by focal inflammation and necrosis. The mortality rate among those suffering from these fevers ranges from 10 to 50 percent. Hemorrhagic fevers include Argentinian hemorrhagic fever, Bolivian hemorrhagic fever, Crimean hemorrhagic fever, African hemorrhagic fever, Omsk hemorrhagic fever, Kyasanur forest disease, Ebola virus disease, Marburg disease, yellow fever, hemorrhagic dengue, and epidemic hemorrhagic fever.

herpetic fever Infection of the mucous membranes of the mouth and lips and surrounding skin with herpes simplex virus, usually herpes simplex virus type 1, associated with fever, chills, and, occasionally, sore throat.

Herxheimer's fever HERXHEIMER REACTION.

hospital fever EPIDEMIC LOUSE-BORNE TYPHUS.

hyperpyrexial fever Any fever that is associated with a very high body temperature.

icterohemorrhagic fever ICTERIC LEPTOSPIROSIS.

Ikwa fever TRENCH FEVER.

Ilheus fever A febrile disease, sometimes with encephalitis, of eastern Brazil and other parts of South and Central America, caused by the Ilheus virus (a flavivirus).

inanition fever DEHYDRATION FEVER.

induced fever Fever caused deliberately by procedures such as the application of heat or the administration of a pyrogen. Also called *artificial fever.*

intermittent fever Any fever characterized by recurrent episodes of elevated temperature occurring between periods of normal temperature.

intermittent hepatic fever An intermittent fever, usually septic or hectic, caused by episodes of biliary tract infection and obstruction as a result of gallstones. Also called *Charcot's fever, Charcot's intermittent fever.*

intermittent malarial fever INTERMITTENT MALARIA.

inundation fever SCRUB TYPHUS.

island fever SCRUB TYPHUS.

Izumi fever A febrile exanthematic disease of unknown etiology that occurs in Japan.

Jaccoud's dissociated fever Meningitis and fever in association with a slow and irregular pulse. It was originally observed in cases of tuberculous meningitis. An obsolete term.

jail fever EPIDEMIC LOUSE-BORNE TYPHUS.

Japanese flood fever SCRUB TYPHUS.

Japanese river fever SCRUB TYPHUS.

jungle fever A term used in the East Indies for FALCIPARUM MALARIA.

jungle yellow fever Yellow fever endemic among primates in African and Central and South American forests which is occasionally transmitted to humans by infected treetop-breeding mosquitoes, usually of the genus *Aedes*, but *Haemogogus* and *Sabethes* may also be responsible. Also called *sylvan yellow fever*.

Junín fever ARGENTINIAN HEMORRHAGIC FEVER.

kagami fever INFECTIOUS MONONUCLEOSIS.

kedani fever SCRUB TYPHUS.

Kenya fever KENYA TYPHUS.

Kew Gardens fever RICKETTSIALPOX.

Kew Gardens spotted fever RICKETTSIALPOX.

Kinkian fever SCHISTOSOMIASIS JAPONICA.

Kinkiang fever SCHISTOSOMIASIS JAPONICA.

Korean fever EPIDEMIC HEMORRHAGIC FEVER.

Korean hemorrhagic fever EPIDEMIC HEMORRHAGIC FEVER.

Korin fever EPIDEMIC HEMORRHAGIC FEVER.

Kyoto fever A kind of nanukayami or seven-day fever seen in the vicinity of Kyoto, Japan.

Lassa fever A highly communicable, hemorrhagic fever caused by the Lassa virus (an arenavirus) and occurring principally in west Africa, where it is endemic or hyperendemic. It has also been reported from Zimbabwe and South Africa. Rodents (especially *Mastomys natalensis*) constitute the only known reservoir of infection, and the disease is spread from person to person by multiple routes. It ranges in severity from a mild infection to a fatal multisystem illness and is characterized by fever, diarrhea, myalgia, severe pharyngitis, headache, epigastric and chest pain, vomiting, and cough. In fatal cases, hypovolemia, hypotension, pleural effusion, ascites, and pulmonary edema may develop. Virologic studies and a complement fixation test are of value in diagnosis. Hospital outbreaks have produced the highest mortality rates. Strict isolation is essential. Ribavirin when administered intravenously appears to be a promising treatment. Injection of human convalescent serum has been used for therapy, but its efficacy is not known.

lechuguilla fever LECHUGUILLA POISONING.

lemming fever 1 An epidemic disease of lemmings, probably tularemia, that causes high mortality, possibly associated with overcrowding among the rapidly breeding animals. 2 In man an infectious disease in Norway, thought to be attributable to contamination of drinking water by the excreta and drowned bodies of lemmings infected with *Francisella tularensis*.

lent fever TYPHOID FEVER.

leprotic fever The fever which characterizes the early stage of leprosy and is a part of the lepra reaction.

Levant fever A fever of possible malarial origin which is endemic in the Levantine states of the eastern Mediterranean (Syria, Lebanon, Israel, Jordan). An obsolete term.

Lone Star fever BULLIS FEVER.

louse-borne relapsing fever A spirochetal disease, spread by lice, characterized by alternating fevers and apyrexial episodes. It is caused by *Borrelia recurrentis*. Distibution is widespread in Africa, Asia, and South America.

lung fever PULMONARY FEVER.

macular fever 1 Any febrile disease characterized by a macular cutaneous eruption. 2 An obsolete term for TYPHUS.

malarial fever MALARIA.

malignant fever 1 EPIDEMIC LOUSE-BORNE TYPHUS. 2 FALCIPARUM MALARIA.

malignant catarrhal fever A usually acute, viral disease of cattle, characterized by a mucopurulent inflammation of the upper respiratory tract, as well as keratitis and encephalitis. Also called *malignant catarrh of cattle, malignant head catarrh*.

malignant tertian fever FALCIPARUM MALARIA.

Malta fever Brucellosis in humans caused by *Brucella melitensis*. It is common on Mediterranean islands and coastal areas but is also widely distributed elsewhere. Also called *febris melitensis, melitensis, Cyprus fever, Gibraltar fever, Maltese fever, Neapolitan fever, rock fever, mountain fever, Mediterranean phthisis, Mediterranean fever, melitensis septicemia*.

Maltese fever MALTA FEVER.

Manchurian fever A disease occurring in Manchuria that resembles typhus or typhoid fever.

Manchurian hemorrhagic fever EPIDEMIC HEMORRHAGIC FEVER.

Marseilles fever BOUTONNEUSE FEVER.

marsh fever MALARIA.

Mediterranean fever 1 MALTA FEVER. 2 BOUTONNEUSE FEVER.

Mediterranean Coast fever A theileriasis of cattle similar to East Coast fever but somewhat less severe, caused by *Theileria annulata* and transmitted by *Hyalomma* ticks. It is a widespread serious disease in north Africa, southeastern Europe, and southern USSR, and parts of Asia.

Mediterranean exanthematous fever BOUTONNEUSE FEVER.

Mediterranean tick fever BOUTONNEUSE FEVER.

Mediterranean yellow fever An outmoded term for ICTERIC LEPTOSPIROSIS.

melanuric fever BLACKWATER FEVER.

metabolic fever A fever caused by a disturbance of the heat-regulating mechanism of the body, a condition seen in some metabolic disorders. It may be associated with dehydration or an electrolyte imbalance.

metal-fume fever A condition caused by exposure to zinc fumes in the smelting of zinc ores, in galvanizing or welding, in cutting galvanized iron, etc. Inhaled zinc oxide destroys cells in lung alveoli, producing proteins which are absorbed and cause malaise, shivering, fever, and muscular pains. Recovery is almost always complete within 24 hours. Metal fumes other than zinc may also cause this condition. Also called *brass-founders' ague, spelter-workers' ague, welders' ague, zinc-smelters' ague, brass chill, braziers' chill, spelters' chill, zinc chill, brass-founders' disease, braziers' disease, brass-founders' fever, foundrymen's fever, spelters' fever, zinc-fume fever, brass poisoning, spelter shakes, zinc-poisoning tremor, Monday fever*.

Meuse fever TRENCH FEVER.

Mexican spotted fever ROCKY MOUNTAIN SPOTTED FEVER.

Miana fever MIANEH FEVER.

Mianeh fever A form of relapsing fever present in Iran and other parts of the Middle East. It is caused by *Borrelia persica* and commonly characterized by eye complications and jaundice. Though spread by a tick, it is considered clinically distinct from the classical tick-borne and louse-borne relapsing fevers. There may be a high death rate. Also called *Persian relapsing fever, Miana disease, Mianeh disease*. Also *Miana fever*.

milk fever 1 Fever occurring in women during the immediate postpartum period and associated with the onset of lactation. A seldom used term. Also called *galactopyra*. 2 PARTURIENT PARESIS.

mill fever COTTON-MILL FEVER.

miniature scarlet fever A rare reaction following immunization with a scarlet fever prophylactic containing a toxin of *Streptococcus pyogenes* and characterized by a generalized scarlatiniform rash, malaise, nausea, and vomiting.

mite fever SCRUB TYPHUS.

Monday fever 1 METAL-FUME FEVER. • This term is based on the fact that workers lose their tolerance to zinc fumes during a weekend break and the fever occurs on Mondays. 2 An incorrect term for BYSSINOSIS. • There are respiratory symptoms at the beginning of the work week, but, except among new workers, there is no fever.

monoleptic fever Any fever which is continuous, in contrast to one which occurs in two or more paroxysms (polyleptic).

Mossman fever A febrile disease occurring in sugar cane cutters in Australia. It was formerly thought to be caused by *Leptospira australis* but is probably a rickettsial infection, perhaps a form of scrub typhus. • The name is derived from the *Mossman* district of north Queensland, Australia.

mountain fever 1 MALTA FEVER. 2 COLORADO TICK FEVER. 3 ROCKY MOUNTAIN SPOTTED FEVER.

mountain tick fever COLORADO TICK FEVER.

mud fever Leptospirosis caused by *Leptospira interrogans* serovar *grippotyphosaro*, occurring principally among workers in flooded fields or other muddy workplaces. Also called *slime fever*. See also SCHLAMMFIEBER, HARVEST FEVER.

muma fever A Samoan term for ELEPHANTOID FEVER.

Murchison-Pel-Ebstein fever PEL-EBSTEIN FEVER.

nanukayami fever NANUKAYAMI.

Neapolitan fever MALTA FEVER.

neurogenic fever Pyrexia occurring in disorders of the central nervous system, not due to infection but to a disturbance of brain centers responsible for temperature control.

night-soil fever TYPHOID FEVER.

nine-mile fever Q FEVER.

north Queensland tick fever NORTH QUEENSLAND TICK TYPHUS.

Omsk hemorrhagic fever A hemorrhagic fever occurring seasonally or epidemically in southwestern Siberia and caused by a tick-borne flavivirus. The disease is characterized by fever, headache, bronchopneumonia, hemorrhagic and encephalitic manifestations, and, rarely, shock.

O'nyong-nyong fever An acute epidemic disease that occurs in Uganda and Kenya, caused by a mosquito-borne alphavirus and characterized by fever, lymphadenitis, arthritis, and rash. An epidemic affecting 5 million people occurred in northern Uganda in 1959.

Oroya fever The acute, febrile phase of bartonellosis. Also called *Guáitara fever*. See also BARTONELLOSIS. • A severe epidemic occurred among laborers in 1870 during construction of the railway between Lima and La Oroya, a mining center in the high Andes.

Pahvant Valley fever TULAREMIA.

paludal fever MALARIA.

Panama fever CHAGRES FEVER.

papatasi fever SANDFLY FEVER.

pappataci fever SANDFLY FEVER. • *Pappataci* is the Italian word for sandfly.

papular fever A febrile illness with a papular eruption and joint pain. An obsolete term.

paramalta fever Any febrile illness resembling Malta fever but not caused by *Brucella melitensis*. Also called *paramelitensis fever, paraundulant fever*.

paramelitensis fever PARAMALTA FEVER.

paratyphoid fever Enteric fever caused by *Salmonella* serotypes other than *S. typhi*, especially *S. paratyphi, S. schottmuelleri* (formerly *S. paratyphi* B), and *S. hirschfeldii* (formerly *S. paratyphi* C). The clinical features of the disease are essentially identical with those of typhoid fever, but paratyphoid fever is usually a milder illness than typhoid. Also called *Brion-Kayser disease, Schottmüller's disease, Colombo fever, paratyphoid*.

paraundulant fever PARAMALTA FEVER.

parenteric fever A febrile illness which has the characteristics of typhoid or paratyphoid fever but which is not caused by *Salmonella* organisms. Also called *entericoid fever, febris entericoides*.

parrot fever PSITTACOSIS.

Pel-Ebstein fever Recurrent episodes of fever that persist for several days, separated by afebrile intervals that last for several days to a few weeks. Pel-Ebstein fever is a manifestation of Hodgkin's disease. Also called *Murchison-Pel-Ebstein fever, Pell-Ebstein pyrexia, Pel-Ebstein symptom*.

periodic fever 1 Recurrent episodes of fever interspersed with periods of wellness. It is a feature of several syndromes, including familial Mediterranean fever, an autosomal recessive trait. 2 A specific, rare autosomal dominant condition of idiopathic fever in otherwise well individuals.

Persian relapsing fever MIANEH FEVER.

petechial fever CEREBROSPINAL MENINGITIS.

Pfeiffer's glandular fever INFECTIOUS MONONUCLEOSIS.

pharyngoconjunctival fever An epidemic, febrile illness caused primarily by adenovirus types 3, 4, 7, 14, and 21 and usually affecting school-age children. It is characterized by fever, pharyngitis resembling that seen in streptococcal infections, and, in about 35–50% of cases, conjunctivitis. Accompanying symptoms may include myalgia, headache, chills, and dizziness.

Philippine hemorrhagic fever DENGUE HEMORRHAGIC FEVER.

phlebotomus fever SANDFLY FEVER.

pinta fever ROCKY MOUNTAIN SPOTTED FEVER. • *Pinta fever* should not be confused with *pinta*, the name of a treponemal skin disease.

pneumonic fever PULMONARY FEVER.

polka fever DENGUE.

polyleptic fever RELAPSING FEVER.

polymer fume fever A disorder with symptoms similar to those of metal-fume fever, caused by exposure to fumes emitted during the burning of polymers such as Teflon or paratetrafluoroethylene. Also called *Teflon shakes, Teflon fever*.

Pomona fever Leptospirosis caused by *Leptospira pomona* and occurring mostly in hogs and cattle. The disease is spread to humans by contact with the urine of an infected animal, usually through scratches or abrasions of the skin. In adult animals infection is often asymptomatic but young animals may become acutely ill with jaundice, hemolytic anemia, and hemoglobinuria. Late abortions and neonatal deaths may also occur.

porcelain fever An obsolete term for URTICARIA.

Potomac fever ACUTE EQUINE DIARRHEAL SYNDROME. • The term is named after the *Potomac* River, which flows between Maryland and Virginia, the region where this disorder occurs.

pretibial fever FORT BRAGG FEVER.

prison fever EPIDEMIC LOUSE-BORNE TYPHUS.

protein fever Any fever caused by the injection of a protein material into the body. An obsolete term.

puerperal fever Endometritis, often associated with septicemia, following childbirth or abortion. The infection is usually due to streptococci but occasionally is caused by *Mycoplasma hominis* or *Ureaplasma urealyticum*. In the preantibiotic era this disease was associated with a high death rate. Also called *childbed fever* (older term), *puerperal sepsis, puerperal septicemia, lechopyra*.

pulmonary fever Any febrile illness characterized by inflammation of the lung with consolidation; pneumonia. Also called *pneumonic fever, lung fever*.

Pym's fever A febrile illness, probably yellow fever, which was observed on the small island of Bulama off the coast of West Africa. Also called *bulam fever*.

pythogenic fever TYPHOID FEVER.

Q fever A globally distributed infectious disease caused by the rickettsia *Coxiella burnetii* and first observed in Brisbane, Australia. It is usually transmitted to man from cattle, sheep, and goats when aerosolized particles containing the infectious agent are inhaled. Manifestations include fever, headache, myalgia, and pneumonia. The disease is most prevalent in areas where cattle, sheep, and goats are raised. Also called *Australian Q fever, Brisbane fever, nine-mile fever.* • The disease was designated Q fever in the original report in 1937 "until further knowledge should allow a better name." Though further knowledge was soon forthcoming, the nonce designation has prevailed.

quartan fever MALARIAE MALARIA.

Queensland coastal fever SCRUB TYPHUS.

Queensland tick fever NORTH QUEENSLAND TICK TYPHUS.

quintan fever TRENCH FEVER.

quintana fever TRENCH FEVER.

quotidian fever Fever recurring daily, as in some types of malaria.

rabbit fever TULAREMIA.

rat-bite fever A febrile infectious disease acquired through the bite of a rat or other rodent or, rarely, through ingestion of contaminated milk. There are two forms of the disease: sodoku (spirillary fever), caused by *Spirillum minus* and occurring most often in Japan, and Haverhill fever (streptobacillary fever), caused by *Streptobacillus moniliformis* and occurring most commonly in the United States. Fever, chills, localized lymphangitis and lymphadenitis, and a characteristic rash are seen in both forms of the disease. Half of the cases of Haverhill fever also exhibit a nonsuppurative migrating polyarthritis. Also called *rat-bite disease, morbus morsus muris.*

recurrent fever RELAPSING FEVER.

red fever **1** DENGUE. **2** FLEA-BORNE TYPHUS.

red fever of Congo FLEA-BORNE TYPHUS.

redwater fever An outmoded term for BOVINE BABESIOSIS.

relapsing fever One of a group of acute febrile diseases occurring worldwide and caused by arthropod-borne spirochetes of the genus *Borrelia.* Epidemic relapsing fever is caused by *V. recurrentis,* has a person-to-person cycle, and is transmitted by the human body louse. Endemic relapsing fever is caused by various *Borrelia* species and is transmitted by ticks of the genus *Ornithodoros.* The disease is characterized by alternating febrile and afebrile episodes, each lasting two to nine days, with recurrence and abatement of symptoms. A petechial rash, conjunctival infection and hepatosplenomegaly may be present. Diagnosis is made from blood films. Tetracycline, and less frequently, erythromycin are used in treatment. Herxheimer reactions are common. Mortality rates of up to 70 percent have been reported in untreated patients, but with adequate treatment mortality may be reduced to 5 percent. Also called *febris recurrens, famine fever, polyleptic fever, recurrent fever, typhinia, kimputu (An African term).*

remittent fever Fever in which the temperature fluctuates significantly in the course of a day but is still above normal at its lowest point.

rheumatic fever An acute, self-limited, febrile disease occurring as a sequela to a group A streptococcal pharyngeal infection and affecting children and young adults. The disease is characterized by fever and nonsuppurative inflammation of the heart, joints, subcutaneous tissue, and central nervous system. Myocardial and valvular damage may result, particularly if there are recurrent attacks of the disease. Also called *inflammatory rheumatism, polyarthritis rheumatica acuta, rheumapyra, rheumatopyra, active rheumatic heart disease.*

Rhodesian fever EAST COAST FEVER.

Rhodesian tick fever EAST COAST FEVER.

rice-field fever Leptospirosis contracted by rice-field workers.

Rift Valley fever An acute, infectious, febrile disease caused by a bunyavirus and transmitted by *Culex* and *Aedes* mosquitoes and by contact with infected tissues. The incubation period is 3–6 days. It occurs in eastern, western, and southern Africa and in Egypt. It affects man as well as sheep, cattle, goats, camels, antelope, and rodents. Hepatic necrosis is a consistent finding. In severe cases there is encephalitis, retinitis, and hemorrhagic

fever. A vaccine is available. Mortality from the disease is approximately 10–15 percent. Also called *enzootic hepatitis.*

Rio Grande fever Brucellosis caused by *Brucella melitensis,* contracted by humans from goats in Texas; goat fever. An outmoded term.

river fever of Japan SCRUB TYPHUS.

Robles fever A disease occurring in Belize, causing irregular fever and mild general symptoms and lasting from two weeks to three months. • It is not related to Robles disease (onchocerciasis).

rock fever MALTA FEVER.

Rocky Mountain spotted fever An acute, febrile illness caused by *Rickettsia rickettsii* and transmitted by various ticks, the usual vectors in the United States being *Amblyomma americanum, Dermacentor variabilis,* and *Dermacentor andersoni.* Sudden onset of fever, headache, and myalgia occur within a few days of the infective tick bite and a characteristic macular, petechial rash appears first on the extremities and spreads centripetally. Widely distributed in the western hemisphere, the disease is known by a variety of regional names. Also called *spotted fever, Brazilian spotted fever, Brazilian fever, Colombian tick fever, Tobia fever (Colombian), Choix fever, Mexican spotted fever, São Paulo fever, São Paulo typhus, exanthematic typhus of São Paulo, pinta fever, fiebre manchada, Colorado fever, black fever, blue fever, mountain fever, blue disease.*

Roman fever A severe type of falciparum malaria previously common in the city of Rome and the Roman Campagna which surrounds the city.

rose fever **1** An outmoded term for ALLERGIC RHINITIS. **2** An outmoded term for ROSE COLD.

Ross River fever Epidemic polyarthritis first described in or around the Ross River Valley in Australia, and caused by a specific alphavirus.

Russian headache fever Fever and headache associated with tick-borne flaviviruses, such as Omsk hemorrhagic fever virus and tick-borne encephalitis viruses.

Russian intermittent fever TRENCH FEVER.

Sakushu fever A type of seven-day epidemic fever, probably leptospiral, occurring in the autumn in Japan, especially in Okayama Prefecture.

Salonica fever A form of trench fever which occurred during World War I among the allied troops in Greece.

sandfly fever A febrile illness caused by a bunyavirus transmitted by the sandfly *Phlebotomus papatasii.* The disease occurs endemically in the Mediterranean region, the Middle East, and central Asia, and sporadically elsewhere. It is characterized by a three-day fever, headache, conjunctivitis, leukopenia, and malaise. Also called *phlebotomus fever, pappataci fever, papatasi fever, dog disease, three-day fever, summer influenza of Italy* (outmoded).

San Joaquin fever COCCIDIOIDOMYCOSIS.

São Paulo fever ROCKY MOUNTAIN SPOTTED FEVER.

scarlet fever An acute, contagious illness which results from infection, usually of the pharynx, with group A β-hemolytic streptococci which elaborate erythrogenic toxin. The disease most commonly affects the pharynx but may follow streptococcal infections of wounds or the birth canal. It is characterized by fever, acute exudative pharyngitis, tonsilitis (or endometritis in the case of puerperal infection), a red enanthem, and a scarlet red exanthem which is followed by extensive desquamation. In the antibiotic era, severe forms of the disease are rarely seen. Certain other bacteria, for example staphylococci, may occasionally produce erythrogenic toxins and so give rise to a syndrome resembling scarlet fever. Also called *scarlatina, febris rubra, canker rash.*

septic fever Elevation of body temperature, commonly to

40°C or more, due to the presence of bacteria or bacterial toxins in blood.

seven-day fever **1** NANUKAYAMI. **2** Any of various forms of anicteric leptospirosis or similar diseases occurring in Japan, such as Hasami fever or Sakushu fever. **3** A denguelike fever occurring in India at the end of summer. For defs 1, 2, and 3 also called *autumn fever*. • The term is imprecise and may apply to diverse febrile illnesses including dengue.

shank fever TRENCH FEVER.

sheep fever Heartwater in sheep.

shinbone fever TRENCH FEVER.

ship fever EPIDEMIC LOUSE-BORNE TYPHUS.

shouten fever DENGUE.

Singapore fever TROPICAL EAR.

slime fever MUD FEVER.

snail fever SCHISTOSOMIASIS.

solar fever **1** DENGUE. **2** SUNSTROKE.

Songo fever EPIDEMIC HEMORRHAGIC FEVER.

South African tick-bite fever BOUTONNEUSE FEVER.

South American hemorrhagic fever **1** ARGENTINIAN HEMORRHAGIC FEVER. **2** BOLIVIAN HEMORRHAGIC FEVER.

spelters' fever METAL-FUME FEVER.

spirillar fever SODOKU.

spirillary fever SODOKU.

spirillum fever SODOKU.

splenic fever ANTHRAX.

spotted fever **1** ROCKY MOUNTAIN SPOTTED FEVER. **2** Any of various other tick-borne rickettsioses characterized by cutaneous eruptions, such as boutonneuse fever, north Queensland tick typhus, or Siberian tick typhus.

sthenic fever A fever characterized by a high temperature, strong pulse, hot dry skin, and delirium.

stiffneck fever **1** DENGUE. **2** CEREBROSPINAL MENINGITIS.

streptobacillary fever HAVERHILL FEVER.

sulfonamide fever A toxic reaction to sulfonamides. The symptoms include fever, anemia, leukopenia, dermatitis, and nephritis, the last being due to the precipitation of crystals in the collecting tubules of the kidney.

Sumatran mite fever SCRUB TYPHUS.

sun fever DENGUE.

swamp fever EQUINE INFECTIOUS ANEMIA.

sweat fever MILIARIA.

swine fever The British term for HOG CHOLERA.

sylvan yellow fever JUNGLE YELLOW FEVER.

Teflon fever POLYMER FUME FEVER.

tertian fever VIVAX MALARIA.

tetanoid fever CEREBROSPINAL MENINGITIS.

Texas fever An outmoded term for BOVINE BABESIOSIS.

Texas tick fever BULLIS FEVER.

Thai hemorrhagic fever DENGUE HEMORRHAGIC FEVER.

therapeutic fever The induced fever used in fever therapy.

thermic fever HEATSTROKE.

thirst fever A fever associated with dehydration.

three-day fever SANDFLY FEVER.

thyroid fever The high fever often encountered in thyroid crisis.

tibialgic fever TRENCH FEVER.

tick fever Any of various human and animal diseases caused by organisms found at some stage in the blood and transmitted by a tick vector. Examples include tick-borne relapsing fever, tick-borne encephalitis, bovine babesiosis, East Coast fever, Colorado tick fever, and Rocky Mountain spotted fever and some other viral and rickettsial diseases.

tickbite fever BOUTONNEUSE FEVER.

tick-borne relapsing fever A spirochetal disease, spread by ticks, characterized by alternating fevers and apyrexial episodes.

It is caused by several species of *Borrelia*, especially *B. duttoni*. Distribution is widespread in Africa, Asia, the Middle East, and central and South America.

Tobia fever A Colombian term for ROCKY MOUNTAIN SPOTTED FEVER.

Tokushima fever INFECTIOUS MONONUCLEOSIS.

Transcaucasian fever A form of Mediterranean Coast fever occurring beyond the Caucasus, caused by *Theileria annulata*.

traumatic fever A fever resulting from the hypermetabolism induced by injury or burns. Although the traumatic origin is readily recognized, an infectious cause should always be sought. Also called *traumatopyra* (seldom used).

trench fever A louse-borne relapsing fever caused by *Rochalimaea quintana* (formerly *Rickettsia quintana*). The disease was epidemic in Europe during the First World War. It is characterized by paroxysms of fever, chills, headache, myalgia (especially of the back and legs), and a rash on the trunk. Also called *quintan fever, Meuse fever, shank fever, tibialgic fever, shinbone fever, Volhynia fever, Wolhynia fever, His disease, His-Werner disease, Werner-His disease, van der Scheer's fever, febris quintana, febris wolhynica, Russian intermittent fever, Ikwa fever, quintana fever*.

triple quartan fever Intermittent quartan malaria with nonsynchronous cycles of fever resulting in daily paroxysms. An obsolete term. Also called *quartana triplex*.

trypanosome fever TRYPANOSOMIASIS.

tsutsugamushi fever SCRUB TYPHUS.

twelve-day fever of Nigeria A febrile illness marked by a rash and lasting a week or more, associated with mild albuminuria. It resembles dengue and typhus.

typhoid fever An acute, febrile illness caused by *Salmonella typhi* and usually acquired as a result of ingesting contaminated water or food. The disease may occur in epidemic form and is characterized by headache, chills, myalgia, diarrhea, bacteremia, abdominal distention, and splenomegaly. Characteristic rose-colored spots appear in the early stages of some cases. In severe cases prostration, intestinal perforation, and hemorrhage may occur. A vaccine is available. Also called *enterotyphus, pythogenic fever, cesspool fever, lent fever, night-soil fever, typhia, typhoid*.

typhus fever TYPHUS.

undulant fever Brucellosis in humans. Also called *Bruce's septicemia, febris undulans, febris sudoralis, dust fever*.

urban fever A form of tropical typhus, usually flea-borne, occurring in urban areas.

urban yellow fever The classical or urban cycle of human yellow fever transmitted by *Aedes aegypti*.

urinary fever A fever caused by a urinary tract infection.

urticarial fever SCHISTOSOMIASIS JAPONICA.

uveoparotid fever HEERFORDT SYNDROME.

Uzbekistan hemorrhagic fever CENTRAL ASIAN HEMORRHAGIC FEVER.

vaccinal fever Fever occurring subsequent to vaccination.

valley fever COCCIDIOIDOMYCOSIS.

van der Scheer's fever TRENCH FEVER.

vivax fever VIVAX MALARIA.

Volhynia fever TRENCH FEVER.

war fever EPIDEMIC LOUSE-BORNE TYPHUS.

West African fever BLACKWATER FEVER.

West Nile fever A mild fever resembling dengue, caused by a group B arbovirus which has antigenic similarities to the Japanese B, Murray B Valley, and St. Louis encephalitis viruses. The natural reservoir probably exists in birds. It is spread by many species of *Culex* mosquitoes, some *Anopheles*, and one *Mansonia* species. It is also spread by ticks, such as *Argas hermanni* in Egypt, or several *Ornithodoros* species in the USSR. The virus has been isolated in Africa, India, the USSR, and the

Middle East. Also called *West Nile encephalitis*.

Whitmore's fever   MELIOIDOSIS.

Wolhynia fever   TRENCH FEVER.

wound fever   A fever resulting from a bacterial infection within a wound.

Yangtze Valley fever   SCHISTOSOMIASIS JAPONICA.

yellow fever   An infectious disease caused by a flavivirus of the togavirus family, transmitted between humans by the *Aedes aegypti* mosquito (urban yellow fever) and from animals to humans by various species of mosquitoes (jungle or sylvan yellow fever). The disease is endemic in tropical areas of Central and South America and Africa. The reservoir of infection may be in man (urban cycle) or in animals (sylvan or jungle cycle), especially primates. The disease is characterized by jaundice, fever, chills, headache, gastrointestinal hemorrhage, and albuminuria. In fatal cases, liver histology establishes the diagnosis. Control of the disease depends on destruction of the vector. Vaccines are available. The attenuated 17D strain is given subcutaneously and renders excellent protection for ten years. There is no specific treatment for the disease. Also called *yellow jack* (popular), *amarillic typhus* (outmoded).

Zika fever   An acute degenerative disease of the central nervous system, involving especially the hippocampus, which occurs in Africa and Malaysia. The presentation and clinical picture resemble dengue. It is caused by a flavivirus first isolated from monkeys and from the mosquito *Aedes africanus*, which appears to be the insect vector, in the Zika forest of Uganda.

zinc-fume fever   METAL-FUME FEVER.

---

feverish   FEBRILE.

Fevold [Harry Leonard *Fevold*, U.S. biochemist, born 1902] See under TEST.

FF   filtration fraction.

FFT   flicker fusion threshold.

fg   Symbol for the unit, femtogram.

FGT   female genital tract.

f.h.   *fiat haustus* (L, let a draught be made).

fi⁺   Denoting a plasmid, especially an R factor, that represses conjugation mediated by an F factor in the same cell.

fi⁻   Denoting an R factor that does not repress conjugation mediated by an F factor in the same cell.

FIA   Freund's incomplete adjuvant.

fiat   Let there be made, as used in prescription writing.

fiber

fiber [L *fibra*. See FIBRA.]   1 An elongated, tapering, sclerenchyma cell of a vascular plant. The cell wall may or may not be lignified, and the cell may or may not have a living protoplast at maturity.   2 FIBRA.

Ia fiber   PRIMARY AFFERENT.

Ib fiber   GROUP IB FIBER.

A fibers   All peripheral myelinated axons, originally defined as the "A" elevation of the compound action potential, thus constituting the fastest conducting nerve fibers. Each subdivision, α–δ, can be further defined in terms of sensory and motor functional categories as well as axonal diameter.

α-fiber α-EFFERENT.

accelerating fiber   ACCELERATOR FIBER.

accelerator fiber   A sympathetic nerve fiber that, when stim-

ulated, increases the heart rate. Also called *augmentor fiber, accelerating fiber, cardiac accelerator fiber, cardioacceleratory fiber*.

accessory fiber   1 A fiber of the ciliary zonule that is not attached to the lens capsule directly. Also called *auxiliary fiber*. 2 An unmyelinated or fine myelinated nerve fiber that enters the center of a pacinian, paciniform, or Ruffini corpuscle alongside the major axon of innervation. It is possibly of sympathetic origin.

adrenergic fibers   Sympathetic nerve fibers for which norepinephrine or epinephrine serve as synaptic transmitter.

afferent fiber   A nerve fiber conducting towards a nucleus or center. Also called *centripetal fiber, sensory fiber*.

alveolar fiber   A collagen fiber of the periodontal membrane which is attached to alveolar bone.

alveolar crest fiber   A collagen fiber of the periodontal membrane which is attached to the crest of the alveolar bone. Also called *crestal fiber*.

anastomosing fibers   Nerve fibers extending between fascicles of peripheral nerve trunks or dorsal rootlet bundles. Also called *anastomotic fibers*.

anastomotic fibers   ANASTOMOSING FIBERS.

anterior external arcuate fibers   FIBRAE ARCUATAE EXTERNAE VENTRALES.

apical fiber   A collagen fiber of the periodontal membrane which connects the apex of the root to the fundus of its socket.

archiform fibers   FIBRAE INTERCRURALES.

arcuate fibers   1 Collectively, the various fascicles of arcuate fibers in the brainstem, including the fibrae arcuatae internae, fibrae arcuatae externae ventrales, and fibrae arcuatae externae dorsales.   2 FIBRAE ARCUATAE CEREBRI.

arcuate fibers of cerebrum   FIBRAE ARCUATAE CEREBRI.

argentaffin fiber   A nerve fiber that can be stained by silver solutions without the addition of an external reducing agent. Also called *argentophil fiber, argentophilic fiber*.

argentophil fiber   ARGENTAFFIN FIBER.

argentophilic fiber   ARGENTAFFIN FIBER.

argyrophilic fiber   A nerve fiber that can be stained by silver solutions only in the presence of an external reducing agent.

asbestos fibers   Degenerated cartilaginous fibers that have calcified. An obsolete term.

association fibers   The nerve fibers connecting different regions of the cerebral cortex within the same hemisphere. They consist of short association fibers that curve beneath each sulcus, connecting adjacent gyri, and long association fibers that interconnect different lobes.

augmentor fiber   ACCELERATOR FIBER.

auxiliary fiber   ACCESSORY FIBER.

axial fiber   The axonal core of a nerve fiber exclusive of its sheaths.

B fibers   Myelinated nerve fibers of up to 3 μ diameter and conduction rates of up to 15 m/sec. They occur primarily in autonomic nerves as preganglionic fibers.

β-fiber β-EFFERENT.

basilar fibers   Compact bundles of birefringent fibrils embedded in ground substance, forming the middle layer of the basilar membrane of the cochlear duct and arranged in a network in the zona arcuata and in straight, thick fibers in the zona pectinata. They spread out in the spiral ligament. Also called *auditory strings*.

Bergmann's fibers   Glial processes of specialized astrocytes (Bergmann cells) in the molecular layer of the cerebellar cortex that extend through that layer to the pia.

Berneheimer's fibers   A band of nerve fibers extending from the dorsal optic tract to the subthalamic nucleus (nucleus of Luys), unconfirmed in experimental studies of the optic tract axonal trajectory.

β motor fiber   β-EFFERENT.

fibers of Bogrov   Nerve fibers that pass from the optic tract to the thalamus.

bone fibers   Collagen fibers that connect a tendon, ligament, fascia, or periosteum to underlying bone. Also called *Sharpey's fibers*.

Brücke's fibers   FIBRAE MERIDIONALES MUSCULI CILIARIS.

bulbospiral fibers   A group of cardiac muscle fibers that run a spiral course in the walls of the atria and ventricles of the heart.

Burdach's fibers   Axons of the fasciculus cuneatus medullae oblongatae (column of Burdach) terminating in the nucleus cuneatus (nucleus of Burdach's column).

C fibers   Unmyelinated, slowly-conducting axons of the peripheral nervous system, usually found in small bundles ensheathed by a single Schwann cell. They constitute the majority of autonomic axons, and also innervate a variety of deep and cutaneous sense organs including nociceptors, thermoreceptors, and sensitive mechanoreceptors.

capsular fibers   Nerve fibers of the cerebral internal capsule. An imprecise usage.

cardiac accelerator fiber   ACCELERATOR FIBER.

cardiac depressor fiber   A cholinergic nerve fiber that supplies the heart and causes a fall in cardiac output and a drop in blood pressure.

cardiac pressor fiber   A sympathetic nerve fiber that supplies the heart and, when stimulated, causes an increase in cardiac output and a rise in blood pressure.

cardioacceleratory fiber   ACCELERATOR FIBER.

cemental fiber   A collagen fiber which is incorporated into cementum.

centripetal fiber   AFFERENT FIBER.

cerebrospinal fibers   FIBRAE CORTICOSPINALES.

chief fibers   Those fibers of the ciliary zonule that are attached to the lens capsule. They are supported by accessory fibers which are attached to them at various angles. An outmoded term. Also called *principal fibers, main fibers, white fibers*.

cholinergic fiber   An axon that releases the neurotransmitter acetylcholine at its synaptic terminals.

chromatic fiber   A threadlike fiber or chromatin observed in the early mitotic nucleus.

chromosomal fiber   CHROMOSOMAL SPINDLE FIBER.

chromosomal spindle fiber   A fiber which is visible microscopically during prometaphase to telophase of cell division and which extends from the centrosome to the centromere (actually the kinetochore) of each chromosome. The structure of the spindle and the composition of the fibers vary among organisms, but all contain microtubules and help orchestrate segregation of daughter chromosomes. Also called *chromosomal fiber, traction fiber, chromosomal microtubule, half-spindle fiber, kinetochore microtubule*.

cilioequatorial fibers   Those fibers of the ciliary zonule that are attached to the equator of the lens. An outmoded term.

cilioposterocapsular fibers   The fine curved fibers of the ciliary zonule that are attached to the posterior surface of the lens capsule. An outmoded term.

circular fiber   A collagen fiber of the gingiva which encircles a tooth.

circular fibers of ciliary muscle   FIBRAE CIRCULARES MUSCULI CILIARIS.

circular fibers of eardrum   Circularly arranged fibers that form the deep part of the fibrous connective tissue layer of the eardrum. They are maximal at the periphery and sparse centrally.

climbing fibers of cerebellum   Myelinated axons emanating from the inferior olivary complex and extending through the cerebellar granular layer, where they climb along the extensive tree of Purkinje neuron dendrites, contacting the smooth dendritic branches and forming powerful excitatory synapses. Collaterals also contact cerebellar stellate, basket, and Golgi cells.

collagen fiber   The predominant type of connective tissue fiber, synthesized from tropocollagen subunits by fibroblasts. The individual fibers have a characteristic periodicity of 64 nm when examined by electron microscopy. Also called *white fiber*.

collateral fibers of Winslow   An outmoded term for FIBRAE INTERCRURALES.

commissural fibers   1 Nerve fibers that cross the midline to connect symmetric, homotopic zones of the cerebral cortex via the corpus callosum and anterior commissure. 2 Nerve fibers that cross the midline to connect symmetric zones throughout the brain and spinal cord.

cone fibers   The fibers that extend from either side of the retinal cone bodies or cells. Stout, smooth inner fibers that resemble axons descend from the bodies of all cones to the middle zone of the outer plexiform layer, where they end in the club-shaped cone pedicles. Their lengths and course vary according to the region of the retina. The short, outer fibers extend from the cell body in the outer fovea and resemble dendrites physiologically.

conjunctival fibers   Nerve fibers from the trigeminal nerve that supply the conjunctival membrane. The opthalmic division deals with the upper half and the maxillary branch with the lower half.

continuous fiber   CONTINUOUS SPINDLE FIBER.

continuous spindle fiber   A fiber visible microscopically during prometaphase to telophase of cell division which extends between the two poles of the spindle apparatus and which does not terminate at a chromosome kinetochore. Also called *continuous fiber, interzonal fiber*.

Corti's fibers   PILLARS OF CORTI.

corticobulbar fibers   FIBRAE CORTICONUCLEARES.

corticofugal fiber   An axon that emanates from a neuron cell body within the cerebral or cerebellar cortex and enters the underlying white matter.

corticonuclear fibers   FIBRAE CORTICONUCLEARES.

corticopetal fiber   An axon entering the cerebral or cerebellar cortex from the underlying white matter and terminating in the cortical neuropil.

corticopontine fibers   FIBRAE CORTICOPONTINAE.

corticorubral fibers   The sparse nerve fibers arising in the cerebral cortex and descending in the internal capsule to the region of the red nucleus.

corticospinal fibers   FIBRAE CORTICOSPINALES.

corticostriate fibers   Corticofugal fibers that are derived in large numbers from neurons in nearly all regions of the cerebral cortex and that project to the striatum (caudate nucleus and putamen). Some corticostriate fibers project to the ipsilateral striatum, while others cross in the corpus callosum and project to the contralateral striatum.

corticothalamic fibers   FIBRAE CORTICOTHALAMICAE.

crestal fiber   An alveolar crest fiber.

dark fiber   TYPE I MUSCLE FIBER.

fibers of Darkschewitsch   Nerve fibers derived from neurons in the nucleus of Darkschewitsch that course in the posterior commissure but whose precise terminations are not well known.

daughter fiber   One of the muscle fibers formed by the splitting of a single parent fiber.

dendritic fibers   The branching processes of neurons.

dentinal fiber   An obsolete term for ODONTOBLASTIC PROCESS.

dentinogenic fibers   KORFF'S FIBERS.

dentogingival fiber   A collagen fiber which passes from the cementum at the neck of a tooth into the gingiva.

dentoperiosteal fiber   A collagen fiber which passes from the neck of a tooth across the alveolar crest and into the periosteum on the vestibular and lingual surfaces of the alveolar bone.

depressor fiber   A cholinergic nerve fiber that causes vasodilatation and results in a lowering of blood pressure.

dietary fiber   The structural parts of plant foods such as fruits, vegetables, grains, nuts, and beans. It includes the coatings, such as the bran around brown rice or whole wheat, and the networks throughout a plant, as in celery, carrots, and sweet potatoes. Fiber is that part of ingested plant material which is not broken down and digested in the human gastrointestinal tract. Because it is not digested, dietary fiber has no caloric value, however, the nutrients bound to some fibers, such as the B vitamins in bran, are released during digestion and are therefore beneficial. There are several different forms of indigestible fiber substances found in foods, including cellulose and hemicellulose, two fibers common to all plants, and pectin, found mainly in fruits. Although some are fully or partially digestible, vegetable gums are classified as dietary fiber by some scientists. Lignin found in most plants, particularly in overmatured vegetables, is not carbohydrate but functions as other plant tubers. A low fiber dietary intake is thought to be associated with constipation, diverticulitis, colon cancer, gallbladder disease, and appendicitis.

Dieters fibers   STILLING'S FIBERS.

dorsal arcuate fibers   FIBRAE ARCUATAE EXTERNAE DORSALES.

dorsal external arcuate fibers   FIBRAE ARCUATAE EXTERNAE DORSALES.

efferent fiber   An axon emanating from a neural center containing its neuron cell body. ● The term is largely used to denote motor pathways.

elastic fibers   Connective tissue fibers that display considerable flexibility. They branch and rejoin freely, forming a network and imparting a yellowish tinge to the tissue when present in quantity. They are found in the skin, the walls of larger blood vessels, and the ligamenta flava of the neck. Also called *yellow fibers*.

enamel fibers   An obsolete term for ENAMEL PRISMS.

endogenous fibers   Axons derived from cell bodies in the local gray matter, especially in the spinal cord. Also called *intrinsic fibers*. Compare EXOGENOUS FIBERS.

epicritic fibers   Axons believed to subserve acute perception and the discrimination of minimal tactile stimulus variation.

exogenous fibers   Axons derived from distant cell bodies, especially axons from spinal ganglia innervating neurons in the spinal gray matter. Also called *extrinsic fibers*. Compare ENDOGENOUS FIBERS.

external arcuate fibers   FIBRAE ARCUATAE EXTERNAE.

extrafusal muscle fiber   Any skeletal muscle fiber other than the modified intrafusal fibers within muscle spindles.

extrinsic fibers   EXOGENOUS FIBERS.

fastigioperiventricular fibers   Fascicles arising in the fastigial nucleus which leave the anterior cerebellar peduncle to enter the periventricular gray and the dorsal nucleus of the raphe.

flocculo-oculomotor fibers of Wallenberg-Klimoff   Fascicles passing from the cerebellar flocculus to the oculomotor nuclei.

frontopontine fibers   TRACTUS FRONTOPONTINUS.

fusimotor fiber   γ-EFFERENT.

γ-fiber   γ-EFFERENT.

geminal fiber   A fiber of the pyramidal tract believed to bifurcate with one branch descending on each side of the spinal cord. A seldom used term.

Gerdy's fibers   Fibers of ligamentum metacarpeum transversum superficiale.

giant fiber   GIANT AXON.

gingival fiber   A collagen fiber which is an intrinsic component of the gingiva or which enters it from adjacent structures.

Goll's fibers   Nerve fibers extending from the nucleus gracilis (nucleus of Goll's column) to the cerebellar vermal cortex.

fibers of Gratiolet   RADIATIO OPTICA.

Gratiolet's radiating fibers   RADIATIO OPTICA.

gray fibers   FIBERS OF REMAK.

group I fiber   One of the largest sensory fibers in cutaneous or muscle nerves, having a diameter of 12–22 μ and a conduction rate of 72–130 m/sec. They supply the primary endings of muscle spindles, tendon organs, and to a lesser degree other mechanoreceptors.

group Ia fiber   PRIMARY AFFERENT.

group Ib fiber   **1** A large, myelinated axon leading from the sensory terminal in a tendon organ.   **2** Such an axon, along with the sensory terminal itself. Also called *Ib afferent, Ib fiber, tendon organ afferent*.

group II fiber   **1** In mammalian nerves, a myelinated fiber of intermediate diameter, i.e., of 6–12 μm, with variation according to species. It may arise in one of several types of sensory receptors, as in the secondary ending of a muscle spindle.   **2** SECONDARY AFFERENT.

group III fiber   One of the smallest, unmyelinated sensory fibers in cutaneous and muscle nerves, having a diameter of 1–7 μ and a conduction rate of 6–30 m/sec. They supply nociceptive, blood-vessel, and hair-follicle receptors.

half-spindle fiber   CHROMOSOMAL SPINDLE FIBER.

Herxheimer's fibers   HERXHEIMER SPIRALS.

heterodesmotic fibers   Myelinated axons connecting two dissimilar zones of neuropil, such as thalamocortical fibers.

homodesmotic fibers   Myelinated axons connecting similar structures, such as those of the corpus callosum connecting homotopic cortical fields.

horizontal fiber   A collagen fiber which runs at right angles to the long axis of a tooth between the cervical cementum and the alveolar bone.

IF fiber   INTRAFUSAL MUSCLE FIBER.

impulse-conducting fiber   PURKINJE'S FIBER.

inhibitory fibers   Axons whose synaptic action on neuron somata, dendrites, and axons suppresses membrane excitatory events to produce a reduction in membrane potential change and/or the rate of impulse discharge.

interciliary fibers   The short fibers of the ciliary zonule that are located between the ciliary processes and join the longer fibers so as to serve as supports. An outmoded term.

intercolumnar fibers   FIBRAE INTERCRURALES.

intercrural fibers   FIBRAE INTERCRURALES.

internal arcuate fibers   FIBRAE ARCUATAE INTERNAE.

internuncial fibers   Axons connecting neurons, especially neurons intrinsic to the same nuclear group or cortical field.

interzonal fiber   CONTINUOUS SPINDLE FIBER.

intrafusal fiber   INTRAFUSAL MUSCLE FIBER.

intrafusal bag fiber   INTRAFUSAL MUSCLE FIBER.

intrafusal muscle fiber   One of the specialized muscle fibers in a muscle spindle. In mammals, three distinct types of fibers are distinguished within each spindle by their ultrastructural, histochemical, and contractile characteristics. They are all striated, and have a concentration (or bag) of nuclei at their mid-length. They receive innervation from dynamic fusimotor fibers and are responsible for the dynamic component in stretch sensitivity of the spindle primary ending. Also called *intrafusal fiber, IF fiber, intrafusal bag fiber*.

intrinsic fibers   ENDOGENOUS FIBERS.

isotropic fiber   I BAND.

itinerant fibers   Efferent fibers coursing from the cerebral cortex to the brain stem and spinal cord. A seldom used term.

James fiber   A postulated accessory atrioventricular bundle that has been suspected of causing some anomalies in readings on the electrocardiogram.

Korff's fibers Channels between odontoblasts which occur during the initial formation of dentin and which resemble corkscrew-shaped fibers when stained with silver. Also called *dentinogenic fibers*.

Kühne's fiber MUSCLE SPINDLE.

lattice fibers Fibers, such as collagen fibers, arranged in the form of a lattice, as determined by light or electron microscopy.

Lenhossek's fibers STILLING'S FIBERS.

fibers of lens FIBRAE LENTIS.

light fibers Fibers which do not take a histopathologic stain deeply.

long fiber of brachialis A branch of the radial nerve that arises in front of the lateral intermuscular septum just above the elbow joint and supplies the lateral part of the brachialis muscle. An outmoded term.

longitudinal fibers of pons FASCICULI PONTIS LONGITUDINALES.

Luschka's fibers The anteriormost fibers of the levator ani muscle, which insert into the perineal body of the female.

Mahaim fibers That part of the atrioventricular bundle that supplies the base of the ventricular septum. An obsolete term.

main fibers CHIEF FIBERS.

mantle fiber CHROMOSOMAL SPINDLE FIBER.

Mauthner's fiber One of several types of giant nerve fibers found in the central nervous system of lower vertebrate and invertebrate forms. The Mauthner fibers are derived from a pair of Mauthner neuron cell bodies located in the lower brainstem, one on each side of the midline, in many species of fish and amphibians. Dendrites extend from the Mauthner neuron cell body laterally and ventrally and receive impulses from vestibular, acoustic, cerebellar and trigeminal sources, while the Mauthner fibers cross the midline and descend to the caudal end of the spinal cord, providing a fast-conducting pathway to motoneurons that supply the tail muscles. The Mauthner fiber is an essential part of a reflex mechanism that allows these animals a rapid motor reaction to vibratory and other startling stimuli.

medullated fibers MYELINATED FIBERS.

meridional fibers of ciliary muscle FIBRAE MERIDIONALES MUSCULI CILIARIS.

fibers of Meynert FASCICULUS RETROFLEXUS.

Monakow's fibers TRACTUS RUBROSPINALIS.

mossy fiber Myelinated afferent axons to the cerebellar cortex terminating broadly in the granular layer, where they form numerous complex glomerular synaptic arrangements.

motor fiber An efferent axon, arising from a motoneuron in the anterior horn of the spinal cord or a motor nucleus in the brain stem, that innervates several skeletal muscle fibers, constituting a motor unit.

Müller's fibers Complex supporting neuroglial elements with oval nuclei and cell bodies in the middle zone of the inner nuclear layer from which long vertical processes extend radially through most of the thickness of the retina between the two limiting membranes and form the internal limiting membrane. Dendritic processes spread horizontally into the plexiform layers and form a network around the bodies of cells in the nuclear and ganglion cell layers. The cell bodies of the radial fibers have recesses and projections which fit around and support bodies of the neighboring nerve cells. Also called *sustentacular fibers, retinal gliocytes*.

muscle fiber The single unit of an intact muscle, composed of one or more muscle cells. Also called *myofiber* (seldom used).

myelinated fibers Axons whitish in appearance due to their covering of myelin. These fibers correspond to the A group of the compound action potential, denoting the fastest impulse-conducting elements. Also called *medullated fibers*.

myelinated nerve fiber A nerve fiber within either the central or peripheral nervous system. It is enclosed by a multilaminar coat formed from the cell membrane of an oligodendroglial cell or a Schwann cell.

naked fiber An unencapsulated sensory nerve ending that lacks either a myelin sheath or Schwann cell covering.

Nélaton's fibers Circular smooth muscle fibers forming a part of a transverse fold in the rectum.

nerve fiber 1 AXON. 2 The axon with its Schwann sheath, which forms myelin around some axons; the individual unit of a nerve trunk, subdivided into myelinated and unmyelinated fibers.

neuroglial fiber A fibrillar structure in the cytoplasm of a neuroglial cell.

30 nm fiber The electron microscopic appearance of native, condensed, chromatin with a fiber diameter of about 30 nm. Histone H1 is responsible for packing nucleosomes into the regular, repeating array that constitutes this fiber. Also called *30 nm chromatin fiber, condensed chromatin*.

30 nm chromatin fiber 30 NM FIBER.

nonmedullated fibers UNMYELINATED FIBERS.

nuclear bag fiber An intrafusal fiber distinguished by relatively large size and a cluster of as many as 100 nuclei at the midlength. Two types, bag$_1$ and bag$_2$, differing markedly in histochemical, ultrastructural, and contractile characteristics, are usually present in a mammalian muscle spindle.

nuclear chain muscle fiber An intrafusal fiber in mammalian muscle spindles characterized by a chain of nuclei at midlength, extremely fast contraction, and innervation by static fusimotor fibers.

oblique fiber A collagen fiber of the periodontal membrane whose attachment to cementum is situated more apically than its attachment to bone.

oblique fibers of stomach FIBRAE OBLIQUAE GASTRICAE.

odontogenic fibers Collagen fibers of the matrix of dentin which are produced by odontoblasts. An outmoded term.

olfactory fibers NERVI OLFACTORII.

olivocerebellar fibers TRACTUS OLIVOCEREBELLARIS.

orbiculoanterocapsular fibers Those fibers of the ciliary zonule that extend to the capsule on the posterior surface of the lens and lie close to the vitreous body. An outmoded term.

orbiculociliary fibers Fibers of the ciliary zonule that extend between and beyond the ciliary processes to become continuous with the basement membranes of the superficial layer of epithelial cells over the orbiculus ciliaris. An outmoded term.

orbiculoposterocapsular fibers Long fibers of the ciliary zonule that are continuous with the vitreous membrane. An outmoded term.

osteocollagenous fibers Collagen fibers that develop in osteoid and become part of the bone matrix.

osteogenetic fibers The collagen fibers within osteoid around which bone mineralization occurs. Also called *osteogenic fibers*.

osteogenic fibers OSTEOGENETIC FIBERS.

oxytalan fiber A dense connective-tissue fiber.

pale muscle fiber TYPE II MUSCLE FIBER.

pallidohypothalamic fibers Efferent axons that arise in the globus pallidus and project to the ventromedial nucleus of the hypothalamus.

pallidothalamic fibers See under LENTICULOTHALAMIC TRACT.

palliopontine fiber TRACTUS CORTICOPONTINUS.

parent fiber A muscle fiber which, through longitudinal division (splitting), gives rise to two or more separate fibers.

perforating fibers A connective tissue collagen fiber that passes through the cortex of a bone.

periventricular fibers FIBRAE PERIVENTRICULARES.

pilomotor fibers The unmyelinated nerve fibers supplying the arrector muscles of the hair follicles.

postcommissural fibers   **1** Axons of the descending column of the fornix that course behind the anterior commissure and terminate in the mamillary nuclei of the hypothalamus.   **2** Axons caudal to any commissure. An obsolete term.

posterior arcuate fibers   FIBRAE ARCUATAE EXTERNAE DORSALES.

postganglionic fibers   Peripheral nerve axons that emanate from sympathetic and parasympathetic ganglia and innervate viscera, glands, and smooth muscle.

precollagenous fibers   An obsolete term for RETICULAR FIBERS.

precommissural fibers   **1** Axons in the descending column of the fornix that course rostral to the anterior commissure and terminate in the septal nuclei.   **2** Axons rostral to any commissure. An obsolete term.

preganglionic fibers   Autonomic axons in peripheral nerves that emanate from cell bodies within the spinal cord or brain stem and terminate in peripheral sympathetic and parasympathetic ganglia.

pressor fiber   A sympathetic nerve fiber that causes vasoconstriction and a corresponding rise in blood pressure.

primitive fiber   An obsolete term for AXON.   • The term was applied in the early 1800s to an axon as seen in a teased preparation of a nerve.

principal fibers   **1** CHIEF FIBERS.   **2** Collagen fibers in the periodontal ligament, attaching the root of a tooth to the bone of the socket. Arranged in bundles, they follow a wavy course and can be grouped as oblique, apical, horizontal, crestal, and transseptal fibers.

projection fibers   Axons which emanate from a circumscribed neuronal aggregate and which can be traced to a specific distant structure, such as the thalamocortical projection fibers. Also called *projection tract.*

protopathic fibers   According to the system devised by Sir Henry Head, peripheral sensory fibers responsible for a "lower order" of sensibility, especially pain, temperature, and "crude touch".

Prussak's fibers   Connective tissue fibers connecting the apex of the lateral process of the malleus with the margins of the tympanic notch bounding the flaccid part of the tympanic membrane.

Purkinje's fiber   One of the cardiac muscle cells that are modified for rapid conduction of the excitatory impulse from the atrioventricular node to the ventricular muscle. Also called *impulse-conducting fiber.*

pyramidal fibers of medulla oblongata   FIBRAE PYRAMIDALES MEDULLAE OBLONGATAE.

radiating fibers of anterior chondrosternal ligaments   LIGAMENTA STERNOCOSTALIA RADIATA.

radiating fibers of eardrum   The superficial portion of the fibrous connective tissue of the eardrum, which consists of fibers radiating outward from the handle of the malleus.

radicular fibers   FILA RADICULARIA NERVORUM SPINALIUM.

ragged-red muscle fibers   The disorganized type I muscle fibers seen in histochemically stained sections in cases of mitochondrial myopathies.

Rasmussen's nerve fibers   OLIVOCOCHLEAR BUNDLE OF RASMUSSEN.

red muscle fiber   TYPE I MUSCLE FIBER.

Reissner's fiber   The highly refractile rod extending along the central canal of the spinal cord in primitive vertebrates, believed to be involved in neurosecretory function. In Amphioxus, it originates in the infundibular organ.   • It was first described in the cord of Petromyzon by Ernst Reissner in 1860.

fibers of Remak   Unmyelinated postganglionic axons of the sympathetic nervous system. Also called *gray fibers.*

reticular fibers   Small, connective-tissue fibers identifiable

with a silver stain. Also called *precollagenous fibers* (obsolete).

reticuloreticular fibers   RETICULORETICULAR TRACT.

Retzius fiber   PHALANGEAL PROCESS OF DEITER CELL.

ring fibers   RINGBINDEN.

Ritter's fiber   One of a number of fibers lying between the rods and cones of the retina. It was believed to be an optic nerve fiber, but now it is considered to be an artifact.

rod fibers   Smooth protoplasmic threads of uniform thickness and varying length that connect the rod processes to the cell bodies in the retina. Physiologically, the outer fibers resemble dendrites while the inner fibers resemble axons.

Rolando's fibers   FIBRAE ARCUATAE EXTERNAE.

Rosenthal fibers   Eosinophilic masses found in the cytoplasm of astrocytes. They are elongated, carrot-shaped, dense, and homogeneous, and show positive PTAH staining. Associated with advanced, long-standing gliosis, they are seen in such conditions as Alexander's disease, syringomyelia, and juvenile pilocytic astrocytoma.

Sappey's fibers   Smooth muscle fibers in the medial and lateral check ligaments of the eyeball.

Schroeder's fibers   STILLING'S FIBERS.

secondary fiber   SECONDARY AFFERENT.

secretomotoric fibers   Postganglionic, parasympathetic axons the electrical stimulation of which results in secretory activity, such as that elicited by the vasodilator fibers to the submandibular salivary gland. Also called *secretomotor nerves, secretory nerves, secretory fibers.*

secretory fibers   SECRETOMOTORIC FIBERS.

sensory fiber   AFFERENT FIBER.

Sharpey's fibers   BONE FIBERS.

short association fibers   Nerve fibers connecting adjacent gyri in the cerebral cortex.

skeletofusimotor fiber β-EFFERENT.

spinal parasympathetic fibers   Neurons homologous to parasympathetic fibers which were thought to synapse in the dorsal root ganglia with secondary neurons that innervated skeletal muscle fibers.   • The hypothesis has been discredited, and the term is of historical interest only.

spindle fiber   Any of the microtubules which form the spindle shaped structure between the poles during mitosis and meiosis, especially those extending from pole to pole (continuous spindle fibers), or those which extend from the centrosome to the centromere (chromosomal spindle fibers).

Stilling's fibers   Axonal bundles of the formatio reticularis medullae oblongatae. Also called *Lenhossek's fibers, Dieters fibers, Schroeder's fibers.*

striated muscle fiber   A muscle cell in which the actin and myosin filaments are arranged in a structured pattern. Microscopy reveals a series of transverse bands or stripes across the length of the cells. Such striations can be seen in both cardiac muscle and skeletal muscle. Also called *rhabdium* (obsolete).

sustentacular fibers   MÜLLER'S FIBERS.

sympathetic fibers   Axons of the peripheral sympathetic nervous system.

T fiber   An axon that branches at right angles, giving rise to two separate axons extending in opposite directions. This form is typical of axonal bifurcations in sensory ganglion cells.

thalamocortical fibers   FIBRAE CORTICOTHALAMICAE.

thalamostriate fibers   THALAMOSTRIATE RADIATION.

Tomes fiber   ODONTOBLASTIC PROCESS.

traction fiber   CHROMOSOMAL SPINDLE FIBER.

transilient fibers   Short association fibers that connect one gyrus with another not immediately adjacent. Also called *U fibers.*

transseptal fiber   A collagen fiber which passes across the interdental septum of alveolar bone and unites the roots of adjacent teeth.

transverse fibers of pons FIBRAE PONTIS TRANSVERSAE.

type I muscle fiber A skeletal muscle fiber that is predominantly concerned with slow, tonic contractions. Such fibers contain abundant myoglobin, mitochondria, and oxidative enzymes, yet lack phosphatase enzymes. Also called *red muscle fiber, dark fiber*.

type II muscle fiber A skeletal muscle fiber that is predominantly concerned with rapid contractions. Such fibers contain abundant glycogen and phosphatase enzymes but are relatively lacking in mitochondria and oxidative enzymes. Also called *pale muscle fiber*.

U fibers TRANSILIENT FIBERS.

ultraterminal fiber The final unmyelinated branch of a myelinated axon before it expands to form a synaptic enlargement, such as the motor endplate.

unmyelinated fibers Axons lacking a myelin sheath. In peripheral nerves, they are surrounded by Schwann cytoplasm, with several axons per Schwann cell. In the central nervous system, they form bundles lacking a glial sheath. Also called *nonmedullated fibers, unmyelinated axons*.

varicose fibers Axons displaying variations in diameter along their length in the form of bulges or varicosities. They are often a consequence of postmortem changes.

vasoconstrictor fibers Nerve fibers the stimulation of which causes constriction of blood vessels.

vasodilatory fibers Nerve fibers the stimulation of which causes dilatation of blood vessels.

ventral external arcuate fibers FIBRAE ARCUATAE EXTERNAE VENTRALES.

von Monakow's fibers TRACTUS RUBROSPINALIS.

Weissmann's fibers Fibers of the muscle spindle.

white fiber COLLAGEN FIBER.

white fibers CHIEF FIBERS.

yellow fibers ELASTIC FIBERS.

zonular fibers FIBRAE ZONULARES.

---

fibercolonoscope [FIBER + COLONOSCOPE] An instrument for examining the colon that utilizes fiberoptics.

fibergastroscope [FIBER + GASTROSCOPE] An instrument for examining the stomach that utilize fiberoptics. Also called *gastric fiberscope*.

fiberglass Glass spun in thin fibrous form. It is increasingly used in industry to replace asbestos as an insulating material. It can cause skin irritation, and it possibly affects the respiratory tract. Unlike asbestos exposure, there is no definite evidence that workers exposed to fiberglass risk lung cancer or mesothelioma.

fiber-illuminated Illuminated by fiberoptics.

fiberoptic Of or pertaining to fiberoptics.

fiberoptics [FIBER + OPTICS] A bundle of parallel thin transparent glass or plastic fibers individually clad with material having a lower index of refraction. The fibers transmit light by total internal reflection. A fiberoptic endoscope bends around corners and transmits images from internal organs to the exterior.

fiberscope [FIBER + -SCOPE] A flexible instrument used for internal examination that utilizes fiberoptic bundles. Also *fibrescope*.

gastric fiberscope FIBERGASTROSCOPE.

Fibiger [Johannes Andreas Grib *Fibiger*, Danish pathologist, 1867–1928] Fibiger's tumor. See under SPIROPTERA CARCINOMA.

fibr- FIBRO-.

fibra [L, a fiber, filament; in pl. the entrails of an animal] (*plural*

fibrae) A long, threadlike strand of nerve, muscle, or connective tissue. Also called *fiber*.

fibrae annulares Either pars annularis vaginae fibrosae digitorum manus or pars annularis vaginae fibrosae digitorum pedis.

fibrae arcuatae cerebri [NA] Short arc-shaped bundles of association fibers running through the white matter underlying the cerebral cortex, connecting adjacent gyri. Also called *fibrae propriae, arcuate fibers of cerebrum, arcuate fibers*.

fibrae arcuatae externae [NA] Axons that arise from the arcuate nuclei of the medullary pyramid and run laterally on the surface of the medulla oblongata into the inferior cerebellar peduncle. Also called *external arcuate fibers, Rolando's fibers*.

fibrae arcuatae externae anteriores FIBRAE ARCUATAE EXTERNAE VENTRALES.

fibrae arcuatae externae dorsales [NA] Fascicles of fibers arising in the accessory cuneate nucleus that enter the cerebellum by way of the inferior cerebellar peduncle on the same side. They comprise the fibers in the cuneocerebellar pathway, and transmit afferent proprioceptive impulses from the cervical spinal segments that serve the upper limb. The fibers course to the medulla by way of the fasciculus cuneatus. Also called *fibrae arcuatae externae posteriores, posterior arcuate fibers, dorsal arcuate fibers, dorsal external arcuate fibers*.

fibrae arcuatae externae posteriores FIBRAE ARCUATAE EXTERNAE DORSALES.

fibrae arcuatae externae ventrales [NA] Fascicles of fibers that arise in the arcuate nuclei located in the ventromedial aspect of the medulla oblongata. Emerging from the ventral median fissure, these fibers course laterally, dorsally, and superiorly over the surface of the medulla to reach the posterior spinocerebellar tract, which they accompany to the cerebellum by way of the inferior cerebellar peduncle. Also called *anterior external arcuate fibers, fibrae arcuatae externae anteriores, ventral external arcuate fibers*.

fibrae arcuatae internae [NA] Axons that arise in the nuclei gracilis and cuneatus and course in a lateroventral arc to form the midline decussation of the medial lemniscus, which terminates principally in the ventral nuclear group of the thalamus. Also called *internal arcuate fibers*.

fibrae cerebello-olivares TRACTUS OLIVOCEREBELLARIS.

fibrae circulares musculi ciliaris [NA] A sphincteric band of muscle fibers of the ciliary muscle situated internal to the meridional fibers near the base of the iris and close to the periphery of the lens. Also called *circular fibers of ciliary muscle, Müller's muscle, Rouget's muscle*.

fibrae corticonucleares [NA] Axons arising broadly from the cerebral cortex, and in primates principally from the precentral gyrus, that join corticospinal (pyramidal tract) axons in their course through the internal capsule and cerebral peduncles, and then disperse to innervate various somatic motor nuclei of the midbrain, pons, and medulla oblongata. Also called *corticobulbar fibers, corticonuclear fibers*.

fibrae corticopontinae Axons that arise in the cerebral cortex and descend in the internal capsule and cerebral peduncles together with axons destined to form the pyramidal tracts, but which terminate in various nuclei of the pons. Also called *corticopontine fibers*.

fibrae corticoreticulares Axons that arise from the cerebral cortex and descend together with corticospinal fibers to terminate on neurons of the pontine and medullary reticular formation.

fibrae corticospinales [NA] Corticospinal axons arising broadly from the cerebral cortex, and in primates principally from the precentral gyrus. These axons descend through the internal capsule, cerebral peduncles, mesencephalon, and pons, and enter the medullary pyramids before descending into the white matter of the spinal cord. Also called *corticospinal fibers, cerebrospinal fibers.*

fibrae corticothalamicae Large numbers of corticofugal nerve fibers, derived from neuronal cell bodies located in specific regions of the cerebral cortex, that project to the several thalamic nuclei. Also called *corticothalamic fibers, thalamocortical fibers.*

fibrae intercrurales [NA] Arched transverse fibers of the aponeurosis of the external oblique muscle of the abdomen that pass upward and toward the midline, reinforcing the junction of the crura at the apex of the superficial inguinal ring. Also called *intercrural fibers, collateral fibers of Winslow* (outmoded), *intercolumnar fibers, archiform fibers.*

fibrae lentis [NA] Elongated bands of curved fibers that constitute the substance of the lens of the eye. Young fibers close to the surface have nuclei and narrow serrated edges which interdigitate, forming concentric laminae, while the ends of the fibers meet at the sutures. Older fibers in the dense inner portion of the lens lose their nuclei. The fibers extend from the sutures on the anterior surface to those on the posterior surface, but they do not extend from pole to pole. Also called *fibers of lens.*

fibrae meridionales brückei An outmoded term for FIBRAE MERIDIONALES MUSCULI CILIARIS.

fibrae meridionales musculi ciliaris [NA] The outermost fibers of the ciliary muscle which run posteriorly in a longitudinal direction from the pectinate ligament into the stroma of the choroid. There many of them end by branching. Also called *meridional fibers of ciliary muscle, fibrae meridionales brueckei* (outmoded), *Brücke's fibers, tensor muscle of the choroid.*

fibrae obliquae gastricae [NA] The oblique muscle fibers that form the innermost layer of the tunica muscularis of the stomach, being internal to the circular layer. They are strongly developed around the cardiac orifice from which they extend downward on the anterior and posterior surfaces of the body of the stomach almost parallel to the lesser curvature. Also called *fibrae obliquae ventriculi, oblique fibers of stomach, Gavard's muscle.*

fibrae obliquae ventriculi FIBRAE OBLIQUAE GASTRICAE.

fibrae periventriculares Axons within the central gray matter surrounding the third and fourth ventricles and cerebral aqueduct that are believed to originate in the hypothalamus and terminate in the thalamus, midbrain tectum, pontine and medullary reticular formation, and raphe nuclei. A partially myelinated bundle is segregated ventromedially, forming the dorsal longitudinal fasciculus (of Schütz), which runs in the subependymal portion of the central gray, terminating partly on surrounding neurons and partly on the dorsal tegmental nucleus. Also called *periventricular fibers.*

fibrae pontis profundae The deep internal axons of the fibrae pontis transversae.

fibrae pontis superficiales The more superficial axons of the fibrae pontis transversae.

fibrae pontis transversae Axons that arise in the pontine nuclei and course laterally in the ventral pons, where most cross the midline to form the middle cerebellar peduncles. Also called *transverse fibers of pons.*

fibrae propriae FIBRAE ARCUATAE CEREBRI.

fibrae pyramidales medullae oblongatae Axons within the pyramidal tract surrounding the midline at the base of the medulla oblongata. Also called *pyramidal fibers of medulla oblongata, fasciculi pyramidales medullae oblongatae.*

fibrae zonulares [NA] Fine, elastic filaments that arise from the surface of the epithelium of the ciliary body as far back as the ora serrata and especially from the corona ciliaris and extend to the equatorial region of the lens of the eye. Through their attachments, the ciliary muscle produces changes in the curvature of the lens during accommodation. Collectively they form the zonula ciliaris. Also called *zonular fibers.*

fibrae Plural of FIBRA.

fibration [FIBR- + -ATION] **1** The organizational pattern of a fibrous structure. **2** The process of forming fibers.

fibre A British spelling for FIBER.

dietary fibre A British spelling for DIETARY FIBER.

fibremia FIBRINEMIA.

fibrescope FIBERSCOPE.

fibriform Having the shape of a fiber.

fibril [New L *fibrilla* (dim. of L *fibra* a fiber, filament) a little fiber, a little filament] A small fiber or a component of a fiber. Also called *fibrilla, microfibril.*

Alzheimer fibril INTRANEURAL FIBRILLARY TANGLE.

axial fibrils The organs of locomotion in spirochetes, arising near each terminus of the helical protoplasmic cylinder and each extending between that body and the outer envelope.

border fibrils BRUSH BORDER.

collagen fibrils Fibrils made of collagen.

cytoplasmic fibrils Fine filaments within the cytoplasm of cells, including thin filaments of actin, various intermediate filaments, and thick filaments of myosin.

dentinal fibril **1** ODONTOBLASTIC PROCESS. **2** A collagen fiber of the matrix of dentin. An outmoded term.

Ebner's fibrils Collagen fibers in dentin and cementum. An obsolete term.

fibroglia fibrils FIBROGLIA.

muscle fibril MYOFIBRIL.

muscular fibril MYOFIBRIL.

nerve fibril NEUROFIBRIL.

side fibril of Golgi The branch of a sensory axon at its T-shaped junction extending towards the sensory ganglion cell.

Tomes fibril ODONTOBLASTIC PROCESS.

young collagen fibrils Fine collagen fibers that form at the surface of fibroblasts as a result of the condensation of tropocollagen molecules secreted by the cells.

fibrilla FIBRIL.

fibrillae Plural of FIBRILLA.

fibrillar Characteristic of or resembling a fibril. Also called *fibrillary.*

fibrillary FIBRILLAR.

fibrillate [See FIBRILLATION.] **1** To undergo a spontaneous and uncoordinated twitching of a single muscle fiber. **2** FIBRILLATED.

fibrillated Composed of fibrils. Also *fibrillate.*

fibrillation [New L *fibrilla* (dim. of *fibra* a fiber, filament) a little fiber, a little filament + -ATION] Spontaneous contraction of single muscle fibers which can be recorded electromyographically and which is usually a manifestation of denervation, with wallerian degeneration of at least some motor axons. It initially appears three weeks after division of the motor nerve fibers and may persist for as long as the active process of denervation continues. Fibrillation cannot be observed through the skin but may in rare cases be visible in the tongue. Also called *fibrillary contraction.* Compare FASCICULATION.

atrial fibrillation An arrhythmia, characterized by total disorganization of atrial electrical activity, in which multiple wavelets course in a chaotic fashion across the atrium. Impulses are conducted in a random fashion to the ventricles causing ventricular activity which is quite irregular and usually fast. Also called *auricular fibrillation, ataxia cordis* (obsolete), *delirium cordis.*

auricular fibrillation ATRIAL FIBRILLATION.

ventricular fibrillation An arrhythmia characterized by totally disorganized ventricular electrical activity, associated with a clinical picture of cardiac arrest. Abbreviation: VF

fibrilloblast An outmoded term for ODONTOBLAST.

fibrillogenesis [New L *fibrill(a)* a little fiber or filament + *o* + GENESIS]   The formation of fibrils.

fibrillolysis   The process of destruction and degradation of fibrils.

fibrillolytic   Capable of destroying fibrils.

fibrin [*fibr(a)* + -IN]   The protein responsible for the formation of a blood clot. It is formed from plasma fibrinogen following removal of anionic peptides by the proteolytic plasma enzyme thrombin.

    canalized fibrin   A fibrin thrombus through which new vascular channels have been established.

    gluten fibrin   Fibrin obtained from the seeds of various plants that forms a tough, horny mass when dry. Also called *vegetable fibrin.*

    stroma fibrin   Fibrin presumed to have arisen from the stroma of blood cells.

    vegetable fibrin   GLUTEN FIBRIN.

fibrinase   FACTOR XIII.

fibrinemia   The presence of formed fibrin in the blood. Also called *fibremia.*

fibrinocellular   Consisting of cells within a fibrin network.

fibrinogen   The precursor of fibrin in clot formation. It is a plasma glycoprotein of about 340 000 daltons, consisting of three pairs of subunits (designated α, β, and γ). Thrombin induces clotting by the conversion of fibrinogen to fibrin monomer. The monomers then polymerize to form a clot. Also called *factor I.*
• The variant listed above refers to the roman numeral for 1, not the letter.

    human fibrinogen   A preparation of fibrinogen obtained from human blood and given therapeutically for the treatment of hypofibrinogenemia.

fibrinogenesis   The formation of fibrin.

fibrinogenic [FIBRIN + *o* + -GENIC]   Of or relating to the formation of fibrin.

fibrinogenolysis   The destruction of fibrinogen by action of an enzyme such as plasmin.

fibrinogenolytic   Related to or causing fibrinolysis.

fibrinogenopenia   HYPOFIBRINOGENEMIA. Adjective: fibrinogenopenic.

fibrinogenous   Forming or containing fibrinogen.

fibrinoid [FIBRIN + -OID]   Homogeneous, eosinophilic, acellular material resembling fibrin, typically seen in the wall of blood vessels when there is increased endothelial permeability, as in necrotizing vasculitis.

    canalized fibrinoid   Fibrinoid material with a canalized structure, found on the chorionic plate in late pregnancy. See also LANGHANS STRIA.

    placental fibrinoid   The fibrin and fibrinoid material which, from early in normal human pregnancy, is found between maternal and fetal tissues and is also related to syncytial villi. This material may prevent escape of placental transplantation antigens to the mother.

fibrinoligase   FACTOR XIII.

fibrinolysin   An obsolete term for PLASMIN.

fibrinolysis   The digestion of fibrin, usually by action of an enzyme such as plasmin that is normally present in plasma or by a bacterial enzyme such as streptokinase. Fibrinolysis is usually accompanied by fibrinogenolysis.

fibrinolytic   Of, relating to, or producing fibrinolysis.

fibrinopenia   An imprecise term for HYPOFIBRINOGENEMIA.

fibrinopeptide   One of the peptides released by thrombin from the N terminus of two of the three chains of fibrinogen to produce fibrin. Each has several negative charges.

fibrinoplastin   An obsolete term for THROMBIN. Adjective: fibrinoplastic.

fibrinopurulent   An exudate composed of fibrin and pus. Typically seen in the early stages of the acute inflammatory response, when exudation predominates over suppuration.

fibrinoscopy [FIBRIN + *o* + -SCOPY]   The use of observations about the consistency, appearance, and dissolution of fibrin in the blood or body fluids. A rarely used term.

fibrinose   A proteolytic digestion product of fibrin. An outmoded term.

fibrinous   Like or related to fibrin.

fibrinuria [*fibrin(ogen)* + -URIA]   Excretion of fibrinogen or its products in the urine. This is an indication of glomerular damage, usually severe.

fibro- [L *fibra* fiber]   A combining form meaning fiber, fibrous tissue. Also *fibr-.*

fibroadenia   Atrophy and fibrous replacement of lymphoid tissue. An obsolete term.

fibroadenoma [FIBRO- + ADENOMA]   A benign tumor containing proliferating glandular and stromal components. It is typically found in the female breast. Also called *adenoma fibrosum.*

    fibroadenoma of the breast   A benign tumor with epithelial and stromal components, the latter predominating.

    cellular intracanalicular fibroadenoma   CYSTOSARCOMA PHYLLODES.

    giant fibroadenoma   CYSTOSARCOMA PHYLLODES.

    intracanalicular fibroadenoma   A fibroadenoma of the breast in which the proliferating stroma compresses, elongates, and distorts the glandular elements. Also called *intracanalicular myxoma, intracanalicular papilloma.*

    periacinar fibroadenoma   PERICANALICULAR FIBROADENOMA.

    pericanalicular fibroadenoma   A benign fibroadenoma of the breast in which the stromal component proliferates in a relatively regular manner around the glandular elements, leading to less distortion than in the intracanalicular form. Also called *periacinar fibroadenoma.*

fibroadenosis   A state characterized by numerous fibroadenomas of the breast.

fibroadipose   FIBROFATTY.

fibroangiolipoma [FIBRO- + ANGIO- + LIPOMA]   A benign tumor with fibrous, vascular, and adipose elements.

fibroangioma [FIBRO- + ANGIOMA]   An angioma containing much fibrous tissue. • *Sclerosing hemangioma* is more commonly used when a vascular tumor appears to be undergoing involution and fibrosis.

    nasopharyngeal fibroangioma   An inaccurate term for JUVENILE ANGIOFIBROMA.

fibroareolar   Having the quality of being both fibrous and areolar.

fibroatrophy   Atrophy of the parenchymal cells of an organ with an accompanying increase in fibrous connective tissue.

fibroblast [FIBRO- + -BLAST]   **1** A connective-tissue cell, usually large and spindle-shaped, with an oval, pale-staining nucleus, and cytoplasmic processes at the ends. The cell functions in the production of fibers and amorphous ground substance. **2** An undifferentiated connective tissue cell which differentiates into chondroblasts, collagenoblasts, and osteoblasts. For defs. 1 and 2 also called *inocyte, phorocyte, phoroblast.*

    contractile fibroblast   MYOFIBROBLAST.

fibroblastic   Relating to or characterized by the presence of fibroblasts.

fibroblastoma [FIBRO- + BLASTOMA]   **1** A tumor of fibroblasts. An outmoded term. **2** An outmoded term for FI-

BROMA. **3** An outmoded term for FIBROSARCOMA.

meningeal fibroblastoma FIBROUS MENINGIOMA.

fibrocalcareous Both fibrous and calcareous; characterized by fibrosis and calcification.

fibrocalcific Formed largely from connective tissue fibers and impregnated with calcium salts.

fibrocarcinoma [FIBRO- + CARCINOMA] SCIRRHOUS CARCINOMA.

fibrocartilage [FIBRO- + CARTILAGE] FIBROCARTILAGO.

fibrocartilage of the auricle CARTILAGO AURICULAE.

basal fibrocartilage BASILAR CARTILAGE.

basilar fibrocartilage SYNCHONDROSIS SPHENO-OCCIPITALIS.

circumferential fibrocartilage Fibrocartilage that surrounds a joint.

connecting fibrocartilage Fibrocartilage joining two bones as in a synchondrosis. Also called *spongy fibrocartilage.*

cotyloid fibrocartilage LABRUM ACETABULARE.

diarthrodial fibrocartilage SYNOVIAL FIBROCARTILAGE.

elastic fibrocartilage Fibrocartilage in which the connective tissue fibers are primarily of the yellow elastic type. Also called *yellow fibrocartilage, yellow cartilage, reticular cartilage, elastic cartilage.*

external semilunar fibrocartilage MENISCUS LATERALIS ARTICULATIONIS GENUS.

glenoid fibrocartilage That part of the fibrocartilaginous palmar and plantar ligaments that is attached to the bases of the proximal phalanges of the digits, providing grooves for the passage of the flexor tendons. Their deep surfaces form parts of the articular facets for the heads of the metacarpal and metatarsal bones, and they are lined by synovial membrane. In the thumb and great toe the grooves articulate with sesamoid bones. An outmoded term.

interarticular fibrocartilage DISCUS ARTICULARIS.

internal semilunar fibrocartilage MENISCUS MEDIALIS ARTICULATIONIS GENUS.

intervertebral fibrocartilages DISCI INTERVERTEBRALES.

intra-articular fibrocartilage DISCUS ARTICULARIS.

semilunar fibrocartilages Meniscus lateralis and meniscus medialis articulationis genus.

spongy fibrocartilage CONNECTING FIBROCARTILAGE.

sternoclavicular fibrocartilage DISCUS ARTICULARIS ARTICULATIONIS STERNOCLAVICULARIS.

stratiform fibrocartilage Fibrocartilage found outside the joint spaces in and around tendon sheaths.

synovial fibrocartilage White fibrocartilage that either occurs circumferentially, as in the labrum glenoidale and labrum acetabulare, or forms an articular disk. An outmoded term. Also called *diarthrodial cartilage, diarthrodial fibrocartilage.*

white fibrocartilage A fibrocartilage in which the connective tissue fibers are primarily of the collagenous type.

yellow fibrocartilage ELASTIC FIBROCARTILAGE.

fibrocartilagines Plural of FIBROCARTILAGO.

fibrocartilaginous Pertaining to or composed of fibrocartilage.

fibrocartilago [FIBRO- + CARTILAGO] Cartilage in which the matrix of the chondrocytes, or cartilage cells, consists mainly of bundles of dense white fibrous tissue, or collagen. Transitional between cartilage and connective tissue, it combines toughness with elasticity, and occurs in such tissues as intervertebral and articular disks, labrum acetabulare, and labrum glenoidale. Also called *stratified cartilage, fibrocartilage.*

fibrocartilago basalis BASILAR CARTILAGE.

fibrocartilago basilaris SYNCHONDROSIS SPHENO-OCCIPITALIS.

fibrocartilagines intervertebrales DISCI INTERVERTEBRALES.

fibrocartilago navicularis A triangular, fibrocartilaginous facet on the superior surface of the plantar calcaneonavicular ligament that supports a facet medial to the anterior calcaneal articular surface on the plantar aspect of the head of the talus.

fibrocaseous Having both a fibrous and necrotic, cheeselike appearance.

fibrocavitary A lesion comprised of abscess cavities surrounded by dense fibrosis, characteristic of chronic pulmonary tuberculosis.

fibrocellular Formed largely from connective tissue fibers and cells, with a minimum of intercellular matrix.

fibrocementoma [FIBRO- + CEMENTOMA] CEMENTIFYING FIBROMA.

fibrochondritis Inflammation of fibrocartilage.

fibrochondroma CHONDROFIBROMA.

fibrochondro-osteoma [FIBRO- + CHONDRO- + OSTEOMA] An osteochondroma with a prominent fibrous component.

fibrochondro-osteosarcoma [FIBRO- + CHONDRO- + OSTEOSARCOMA] An osteosarcoma containing cartilaginous and fibrous components. An obsolete term.

fibrocollagenous Consisting of collagen fibers.

fibrocongestive Characteristic of the diffuse atrophy and fibrosis in an organ subject to chronic vascular congestion, as in congestive splenomegaly.

fibrocyst [FIBRO- + CYST] **1** A cyst surrounded by fibrous tissue. **2** A fibroma with cysts.

fibrocystic Containing fibrous and cystic components.

fibrocystoid Resembling a fibrocystic lesion.

fibrocystoma [FIBRO- + CYSTOMA] A fibroma containing cysts. An obsolete term.

fibrocyte A mature connective-tissue cell. The cytoplasm is less abundant and less basophilic than the cytoplasm of a fibroblast.

fibrocytogenesis The formation of fibrocytes.

fibrodysplasia MYOSITIS OSSIFICANS PROGRESSIVA.

fibrodysplasia ossificans multiplex progressiva FIBRODYSPLASIA OSSIFICANS PROGRESSIVA.

fibrodysplasia ossificans progressiva The progressive deposition of heterotopic bone in connective tissue throughout the body, especially in skeletal muscle, tendons, and ligaments. It results in calcified subcutaneous masses, immobility, and death from respiratory compromise. Congenital hallux valgus should arouse suspicion of this disorder. While an autosomal dominant trait, most cases are sporadic and reproduction is markedly limited by the condition. Also called *fibrodysplasia ossificans multiplex progressiva.*

renal artery fibrodysplasia An occlusive condition of the renal arteries, characterized pathologically by exuberant ingrowth of smooth muscle cells and fibroblasts. The condition is characterized by multiple stenoses with interspersed aneurysmal dilatations and may cause renovascular hypertension or diminished renal function.

fibroelastic Composed of connective tissue of both fibrous and elastic nature.

fibroelastosis [FIBRO- + ELASTOSIS] A form of scar tissue in which there is deposition of elastic as well as fibrous tissue. It is commonly seen in the endocardium, among other sites.

fibroelastosis cordis ENDOMYOCARDIAL FIBROELASTOSIS.

endocardial fibroelastosis A disorder characterized by thickening of the endocardium with the presence of elastic and collagenous fibers. Primary endocardial fibroelastosis occurs as a lone feature, particularly involving the left ventricle. Secondary fibroelastosis occurs in association with disorders in which the left ventricle is dilated, such as ventricular septal defect or persistent ductus arteriosus. Also called *subendocardial sclerosis*.

endomyocardial fibroelastosis Congenital thickening of the ventricular mural endocardium with subendocardial changes in the myocardium, mainly evidenced by excessive amounts of fibrous and elastic tissue. Cardiac valves are usually thickened and may be malformed. Some studies suggest a viral etiology. Also called *fibroelastosis cordis*.

fibroenchondroma An enchondroma containing fibrous elements.

fibroendothelioma [FIBRO- + ENDOTHELIOMA] A tumor with fibrous and endothelial components.

fibroepithelioma [FIBRO- + EPITHELIOMA] A tumor with fibrous and epithelial components.

  premalignant fibroepithelioma A skin tumor in which cords of basal cells surround islands of fibrous stroma. It is considered to be a form of basal cell carcinoma. Also called *premalignant fibroepithelial tumor*.

fibrofascitis [FIBRO- + *fasc(ia)* + -ITIS] FASCIITIS.

fibrofatty Containing both fibrous and adipose components. Also *scleroadipose, fibroadipose*.

fibrofibrous FIBROUS.

fibrogenesis The process of synthesizing collagen reticulin or elastic fibers.

  fibrogenesis imperfecta ossium A rare disorder of bone, caused by a defect in the collagen, that is characterized by multiple fractures and osteoporosis. It resembles osteogenesis imperfecta, but it usually presents in adult life.

fibrogenic Causing the formation of fibrous tissue. Also *fibroplastic*.

fibroglia [FIBRO- + GLIA] Fine connective tissue fibrils attached to the external aspect of a fibroblast after the secretion of tropocollagen molecules by the cell. Also called *fibroglia fibrils*.

fibroglioma [FIBRO- + GLIOMA] A glioma containing fibrous tissue. An obsolete term.

fibrohemothorax Hemothorax which had led to accumulation of fibrous tissue in the pleural cavity.

fibroid [FIBR- + -OID] LEIOMYOMA.

fibroidectomy [FIBROID + -ECTOMY] The surgical excision of a dense fibrous mass or masses, especially a uterine fibromyoma or leiomyoma. Also called *fibromectomy*.

fibroin A fibrous protein forming silk fibers and the fibers of spiders' webs. It is a 206-residue polypeptide, lacking some of the common amino acids, and glycine, alanine, tyrosine and serine make up over 75% of its residues.

fibrokeratoma A benign keratotic outgrowth, usually from the region of a finger joint. It is probably a response to trauma.

fibrolaminar Formed from layers of connective tissue fibers.

fibroleiomyoma [FIBRO- + LEIOMYOMA] A leiomyoma with a prominent fibrous component.

fibrolipoma [FIBRO- + LIPOMA] A lipoma containing mature fibrous tissue. It is most common in the skin, where it is usually pedunculated. Also called *fibroma molle, soft fibroma, lipofibroma, lipoma fibrosum*.

fibroliposarcoma [FIBRO- + LIPOSARCOMA] A liposarcoma with a prominent fibrous component.

fibrolymphoangioblastoma [FIBRO- + LYMPHO- + ANGIO- + BLASTOMA] A lymphangioma containing abundant fibrous tissue.

fibroma [FIBR- + -OMA] A benign tumor composed of fibroblasts forming collagen. It can occur in a variety of tissues. Also called *fibroblastoma* (outmoded), *fibrocellular tumor, fibroid tumor, fibroplastic tumor, fibrous tumor, desmocytoma*.

  ameloblastic fibroma A benign jaw tumor with odontogenic epithelium embedded in cellular mesodermal tissue that resembles dental papilla but without odontoblasts. It usually occurs in the mandible of children.

  calcified fibroma A fibroma containing calcifications.

  fibroma cavernosum A fibroma with numerous dilated blood-filled channels. A rarely used term.

  cementifying fibroma A jaw tumor containing cellular fibrous tissue with small basophilic masses of cementumlike tissue. It usually occurs in the mandible of adults. Also called *fibrocementoma*.

  chondromyxoid fibroma A benign tumor characterized by lobulated areas of spindle-shaped or stellate cells with abundant myxoid or chondroid intercellular material, separated by zones of more cellular tissue rich in spindle-shaped or rounded cells with a varying number of multinucleated giant cells of different sizes. Large pleomorphic cells may be present and can result in confusion with chondrosarcoma. This type of lesion is usually situated in the metaphyseal region of a long bone, particularly the upper tibia, and produces an expansion of part of the cortex. Lesions of the tarsal and metatarsal bones are not infrequent. The patients are adolescents or young adults, and males and females are affected in equal numbers.

  fibroma of the choroid A benign choroidal mass composed of connective tissue.

  concentric fibroma A leiomyoma surrounding the uterine cavity.

  fibroma cutis A fibroma in the skin.

  cystic fibroma A fibroma containing cysts.

  fibroma durum A fibroma made firm by the presence of dense mature collagen. Also called *hard fibroma, sclerotic fibroma*.

  endoneural fibroma NEUROFIBROMA.

  fibroma fungoides MYCOSIS FUNGOIDES.

  hard fibroma FIBROMA DURUM.

  irritation fibroma An overgrowth of fibrous tissue at the margin of a denture which has been abrading the mucosa for a long time. It is not a true tumor.

  juvenile nasopharyngeal fibroma An inaccurate term for JUVENILE ANGIOFIBROMA.

  fibroma molle FIBROLIPOMA.

  fibroma mucinosum A fibroma with mucinous degeneration.

  multiple fibroma NEUROFIBROMATOSIS.

  myxoid fibroma FIBROMYXOMA.

  fibroma myxomatodes FIBROMYXOMA.

  nasopharyngeal fibroma An inaccurate term for JUVENILE ANGIOFIBROMA.

  nonossifying fibroma A lesion of growing children in the metaphyseal regions of long bones, in which bone is replaced by fibrous tissue containing giant cells, hemosiderin pigment, and lipid-laden histiocytes. Also called *metaphyseal fibrous defect, nonosteogenic fibroma*.

  nonosteogenic fibroma NONOSSIFYING FIBROMA.

  odontogenic fibroma A fibroma occurring in the jaws and containing strands or islands of epithelial cells. Also called *fibrous odontoma*.

  ossifying fibroma An encapsulated neoplasm, mainly of the jaws, that consists of fibrous tissue containing varying amounts of metaplastic bone and mineralized masses that have rounded outlines and few entrapped cells. Although the lesional tissue may be indistinguishable from fibrous dysplasia, it is an encapsulated growth that behaves as a benign neoplasm. Also called *fibro-osteoma, osteofibroma*.

  osteogenic fibroma OSTEOBLASTOMA.

  papillary fibroma A fibroma with papillary projections.

  parasitic fibroma A leiomyoma which detaches from the

uterus, finds a new growth site on the peritoneum, and acquires an alternate blood supply.

fibroma pendulum A pedunculated fibroma.

periapical fibroma A fibroma occurring adjacent to the apex of a vital tooth. In some cases it develops into a cementoma.

periungual fibroma A fibrous nodule that develops beneath the nail folds in cases of tuberous sclerosis. It is a pathognomic feature of the disease. Also called *Koenen's tumor.*

rabbit fibroma SHOPE FIBROMA.

recurrent digital fibroma One of a group of disorders of connective tissue in which flesh-colored nodules form on the extensor aspects of the terminal phalanges of the fingers and toes in infants. There is a tendency to recurrence. Spontaneous regression occurs in two to three years. There is abundant normal collagen in the lesions and spindle-shaped cells containing small round intracytoplasmic bodies. The cause is unknown. Also called *digital fibromatosis, infantile digital fibromatosis.*

fibroma sarcomatosum FIBROSARCOMA.

sclerotic fibroma FIBROMA DURUM.

senile fibroma CUTANEOUS FIBROUS POLYP.

Shope fibroma A naturally occurring cutaneous fibroma in wild cottontail rabbits (*Sylvilagus*). It is caused by a poxvirus. Also called *rabbit fibroma.*

soft fibroma FIBROLIPOMA.

submucous fibroma A fibroma developing beneath a mucous membrane and usually projecting into the overlying lumen.

telangiectatic fibroma A fibroma containing dilated blood vessels. A rarely used term. Also called *angiofibroma.*

fibroma of the testis A benign growth of the testicular tunica which may occur as a solitary, large ovoid tumor or as multiple nodules. Calcification may occur. On palpation, it resembles a bunch of grapes.

fibroma thecocellulare xanthomatodes THECOMA.

fibroma xanthoma FIBROUS HISTIOCYTOMA.

fibromatogenic [*fibromat(a)*, pl. of FIBROMA, + *o* + -GENIC] Causing fibromas to form.

fibromatoid [*fibromat(a)*, pl. of FIBROMA, + -OID] Resembling a fibroma.

fibromatosis [*fibromat(a)*, pl. of FIBROMA + -OSIS] A group of tumorlike lesions of fibrous tissue, characterized by active proliferation, and including keloid, nodular fasciitis, palmar, penile, plantar, abdominal, and aggressive fibromatoses, and fibromatosis colli.

aggressive fibromatosis A locally invasive tumorlike proliferation of fibrous tissue.

fibromatosis colli A fibrous proliferation in the sternocleidomastoid muscle, typically occurring in children. It can be bilateral. Contraction of the affected muscle may lead to torticollis.

congenital generalized fibromatosis A very rare and usually rapidly fatal congenital disease in which there is an overgrowth of fibrous tissue in the subcutaneous tissues, myocardium, the lungs, the liver, and the intestines.

digital fibromatosis RECURRENT DIGITAL FIBROMA.

fibromatosis gingivae GINGIVAL FIBROMATOSIS.

gingival fibromatosis A fibrous enlargement of the gingiva, which may be idiopathic or hereditary. The deciduous and permanent dentition may be affected, eruption delayed or prevented and teeth displaced. Another type develops in the posterior regions of the jaws, with eruption of the permanent molar teeth. Also called *elephantiasis gingivae, hereditary gingival enlargement, idiopathic gingival enlargement, fibromatosis gingivae, idiopathic gingival enlargement, keloid of gums* (outmoded).

infantile digital fibromatosis RECURRENT DIGITAL FIBROMA.

palmar fibromatosis Fibromatosis originating in the palmar

aponeuroses and leading to Dupuytren's contracture.

plantar fibromatosis A form of fibromatosis orginating in the plantar aponeuroses and leading to progressive contracture of the toes. Also called *Dupuytren's disease of the foot.*

pseudosarcomatous fibromatosis NODULAR FASCIITIS.

sebaceous fibromatosis The presence of sebaceous hypertrophy and fibrosis. If the condition becomes chronic, it will progress to rhinophyma.

subcutaneous pseudosarcomatous fibromatosis NODULAR FASCIITIS.

fibromatosis ventriculi LINITIS PLASTICA.

fibromatous Relating to or characterized by fibromas.

fibromectomy FIBROIDECTOMY.

fibromembranous Formed as a membrane with a high fibrous component.

fibromuscular Pertaining to or comprising fibrous tissue and muscular tissue.

fibromyitis An obsolete term for FIBROMYOSITIS.

fibromyoma [FIBRO- + MYOMA] LEIOMYOMA.

fibromyoma uteri LEIOMYOMA UTERI.

fibromyomectomy [FIBRO- + MYOMECTOMY] The surgical excision of a dense fibromuscular mass or masses.

fibromyositis Nonspecific inflammation and fibrous replacement of skeletal muscle. Also called *fibromyitis* (obsolete), *inomyositis* (obsolete).

fibromyotomy [FIBRO- + MYOTOMY] A surgical procedure in which an incision is made into one or more fibromuscular masses.

fibromyxolipoma MYXOLIPOMA.

fibromyxoma [FIBRO- + MYXOMA] A tumor composed of fibrous and myxomatous tissue. Also called *myxofibroma, myxoid fibroma, fibroma myxomatodes, myxoinoma, myxoma fibrosum.*

fibromyxosarcoma [FIBRO- + MYXO- + SARCOMA] A sarcoma composed of fibrous and myxomatous elements. Also called *fibrosarcoma myxomatodes.*

fibronectin A protein of the extracellular matrix. It assists cells, especially fibroblasts, to adhere to each other. Fibroblasts derived from tumors produce less fibronectin than do normal ones.

fibroneuroma [FIBRO- + NEUROMA] A benign neoplasm occurring in a peripheral nerve and containing both fibrous and neural elements.

fibroneurosarcoma [FIBRO- + NEURO- + SARCOMA] **1** A malignant neoplasm occurring in a peripheral nerve and containing both fibrous and neural elements. **2** MALIGNANT SCHWANNOMA.

fibronuclear Composed of nucleated fibers.

fibro-odontoma [FIBRO- + ODONTOMA] AMELOBLASTIC FIBRO-ODONTOMA.

ameloblastic fibro-odontoma A tumor resembling an ameloblastic fibroma but containing dentine and enamel. Also called *ameloblastic odontoma, fibro-odontoma.*

fibro-osteoma [FIBRO- + OSTEOMA] OSSIFYING FIBROMA.

fibro-osteosarcoma [FIBRO- + OSTEOSARCOMA] An osteosarcoma with a prominent fibrous component.

fibropapilloma [FIBRO- + PAPILLOMA] **1** A papilloma with a prominent fibrous tissue component. • The term is poor as it emphasizes the stroma but does not describe the epithelial component, as transitional or squamous, of what is basically an epithelial tumor. **2** Irritation hypoplasia caused by chronic cheek biting. An inaccurate term.

fibroplasia [FIBRO- + -PLASIA] The formation of fibrous tissue.

intimal fibroplasia A form of fibromuscular disease of the renal arteries characterized by stenosis related to segmental circumferential fibrous changes in the internal elastic membrane, usually in children and young adults. The condition can be unilateral or bilateral. If the elastic is disrupted, dissecting aneurysms may develop. Hypertension is a common complication, which may be corrected by vascular surgery or nephrectomy.

medial fibroplasia A form of fibromuscular disease of the renal arteries, usually bilateral, characterized by fibrous hyperplasia of the media with microaneurysms which produce a "string-of-beads" appearance on an arteriogram. The condition usually occurs in women from 30 to 50 years of age, and is complicated by hypertension. It may be corrected by surgery.

myointimal fibroplasia A thickening of a damaged vessel's inner lining that follows an episode of trauma, such as vascular surgery. The thickening is brought about by the exuberant ingrowth of fibroblasts and smooth muscle cells. See under FIBROMUSCULAR DISEASE.

retrolental fibroplasia The end stage of oxygen-induced retinopathy of prematurity, in which the detached retina and a mass of fibrovascular tissue lie just behind the lens. Also called *Terry syndrome*.

subadventitial fibroplasia A form of fibromuscular disease of the renal arteries, characterized by deposition of collagen in the outer media, usually in women from 20 to 40 years of age. The renal artery, especially on the right, usually is severely stenosed with resultant hypertension, which can be corrected surgically.

fibroplastic FIBROGENIC.

fibroplate DISCUS ARTICULARIS.

fibropolypus A structure with the shape of a polyp and composed exclusively of fibrous tissue. An obsolete term.

fibropsammoma [FIBRO- + PSAMMOMA] A tumor containing fibrous tissue and psammoma bodies. An obsolete term.

fibroreticulate Pertaining to or comprising a network of fibers.

fibrosarcoma [FIBRO- + SARCOMA] A malignant tumor of fibroblastic cells. The histologic appearance is chiefly of interlacing, densely cellular fascicles of spindle cells, often forming a herringbone pattern. Reticulin fibers are closely related to the tumor cells. Collagen production is a constant feature. No other form of cellular differentiation should be present. Mitoses are usually frequent. Pleomorphism may be marked. Metastasis is chiefly by the bloodstream. Also called *fibroblastoma* (outmoded), *fibroma sarcomatosum, fibroblastic sarcoma*.

ameloblastic fibrosarcoma A malignant odontogenic neoplasm similar to the ameloblastic fibroma but in which the stromal component shows the features of a sarcoma. Also called *ameloblastic sarcoma*.

Earle L fibrosarcoma An experimentally transmissible fibrosarcoma, derived from an explant of subcutaneous tissue of mice of the C3H strain and grown in a medium containing 20-methylcholanthrene.

fibrosarcoma myxomatodes FIBROMYXOSARCOMA.

fibrosarcoma of the nerve sheath MALIGNANT SCHWANNOMA.

odontogenic fibrosarcoma A very rare fibrosarcoma arising from odontogenic tissue.

fibrosarcoma phyllodes CYSTOSARCOMA PHYLLODES.

renal fibrosarcoma An uncommon malignant tumor which arises from the renal capsule. Growth may be rapid, although many such tumors are encapsulated.

fibrosclerosis Advanced fibrosis where most fibroblasts have been replaced by dense collagen.

multifocal fibrosclerosis Sclerosis occurring in multiple areas, as in retroperitoneal fibrosis.

fibrose To form fibrous tissue; to scar.

fibroserous Pertaining to a structure composed of fibrous tissue elements and having a serous surface.

fibrosing Inducing formation of fibrous tissue.

fibrosis [FIBR- + -OSIS] The deposition of collagen, usually in the form of a scar but also in the interstitium, surrounding parenchymal cells. It occurs in the healing stage of inflammation when restoration of normal anatomic integrity is not possible.

African endomyocardial fibrosis ENDOMYOCARDIAL FIBROSIS.

arteriocapillary fibrosis Fibrosis, stenosis, and occlusion by thrombosis of small arterioles and capillaries, especially associated with syphilis and tuberculosis.

arteriocapillary fibrosis of Gull and Sutton An obsolete term for GULL-SUTTON DISEASE.

bauxite pulmonary fibrosis BAUXITE PNEUMOCONIOSIS.

cardiac fibrosis MYOCARDIAL FIBROSIS.

fibrosis chorioideae corrugans An irregular contour of the ocular fundus resulting from postinflammatory scarring.

condensation fibrosis The apparent focal increase in fibrous tissue in an organ due to the necrosis and resorption of parenchyma and subsequent approximation of the surviving stroma.

congenital hepatic fibrosis An idiopathic congenital fibrosis of the liver, usually accompanied by bile ductular proliferation within the fibrotic bands. Also called *congenital hepatic cirrhosis*.

cystic fibrosis An autosomal recessive disorder characterized by a decreased pancreatic exocrine function that leads to maldigestion, decreased mucociliary transport with chronic sinopulmonary infections, and abnormal sweat gland function which causes high electrolyte concentrations. It is usually diagnosed in infancy on account of meconium ileus or failure to thrive, or in early childhood because of pulmonary infections. Mild variants may escape detection until adulthood. The effects of the disorder include sterility, deafness, and intraocular damage. The worst effects are seen in the bronchial tree, where the infected, viscid secretions cannot be eliminated and chronic bronchopneumonia leads to death in childhood, adolescence, or early adult life. Survival has been extended through aggressive treatment until the third decade on average. It is the most common lethal condition in Caucasian children, with a heterozygote frequency of 1 in 40. Also called *cystic fibrosis of pancreas, mucoviscidosis, viscidosis, fibrocystic disease of pancreas, congenital pancreatic steatorrhea* (older term).

cystic fibrosis of pancreas CYSTIC FIBROSIS.

desquamative interstitial pulmonary fibrosis A form of fibrosis of the lungs in which alveolar lining cells are found within the alveoli.

diatomaceous earth fibrosis DIATOMITE FIBROSIS.

diatomite fibrosis Silicosis caused by exposure to diatomaceous earth. Also called *diatomaceous earth fibrosis*. See also DIATOMACEOUS EARTH PNEUMOCONIOSIS.

diffuse interstitial pulmonary fibrosis Widespread accumulation of fibrous tissue in alveolar walls and interstitial tissues of the lungs. Also called *interstitial pneumonia, cirrhosis of the lung* (obsolete), *pulmonary cirrhosis*.

endocardial fibrosis ENDOMYOCARDIAL FIBROSIS.

endomyocardial fibrosis A form of restrictive cardiomyopathy characterized by pronounced thickening of the endocardium and adjacent myocardium by dense fibrous tissue. The fibrosis involves the ventricles and sometimes extends to the atrioventricular valves, particularly the mitral valve. The condition is endemic in Africa and its etiology is unknown. Also called *endocardial fibrosis, African endomyocardial fibrosis, subendocardial sclerosis*.

glomerular fibrosis The presence of collagen in the glomerular mesangial region, segmental scars, or in fibrous crescents.

Small deposits of collagen can be seen only on electron microscopy, but larger amounts are demonstrable on light microscopy.

graphite fibrosis A pneumoconiosis caused by exposure to graphite in mining and processing. It can lead to progressive and disabling disease. Also called *graphitosis.*

hepatic fibrosis Fibrosis in the liver, usually the result of previous inflammation and a necessary component of hepatic cirrhosis.

hepatolienal fibrosis HEPATOSPLENIC FIBROSIS.

hepatosplenic fibrosis Fibrosis of the liver and spleen resulting in poor parenchymal function. Also called *hepatolienal fibrosis.*

idiopathic retroperitoneal fibrosis Fibrosis of the peritoneal tissue, resulting at times in compression of the great vessels and the ureters. Also called *retroperitoneal fibrosis, periureteritis plastica, Ormond's disease, perirenal fasciitis.*

mediastinal fibrosis Fibrosis occurring within the mediastinum and often compressing the mediastinal structures. Also called *fibrous mediastinitis, indurative mediastinitis.*

myocardial fibrosis Fibrosis of the myocardium, usually as a result of infarction, cardiomyopathy, or congestive heart failure. Also called *cardiac fibrosis.*

neoplastic fibrosis PROLIFERATIVE FIBROSIS.

panmural fibrosis Diffuse fibrous scarring of the wall of an organ such as the heart. A seldom used term.

panmural fibrosis of the bladder CHRONIC INTERSTITIAL CYSTITIS.

perimuscular fibrosis A form of fibromuscular dysplasia characterized by smooth muscle proliferation and fibrosis of the outer media of arteries, especially the carotid vessels. It may lead to stenosis and hypotension. Also called *subadvential fibrosis.* See also FIBROMUSCULAR DISEASE.

perisaccular fibrosis Fibrosis around the endolymphatic sac such as might interfere with its postulated role in the pressure regulation of the endolymphatic system. Such fibrosis has been considered as a possible factor in cases of Menière's disease and is the theoretical basis for the different operations to decompress the saccus.

periureteric fibrosis Retroperitoneal fibrosis causing ureteric obstruction.

pipestem fibrosis SYMMERS PIPESTEM FIBROSIS.

pleural fibrosis The presence of abnormal amounts of fibrous tissue in the pleura.

pluriglandular fibrosis An outmoded term for PANHYPOPITUITARISM.

postfibrinous fibrosis Organization and fibrosis of a fibrinous exudate.

progressive massive fibrosis An advanced form of pneumoconiosis in which simple pneumoconiosis progresses to form one or more masses of fibrous tissue intermingled with dust, usually located in the upper part of the lung. Its cause is unknown, but it is probably related to dust burden and possibly to an immunologic process. It occurs in coal miners and has been described as a complication of other pneumoconioses. Also called *complicated pneumoconiosis, collagenous pneumoconiosis.*

proliferative fibrosis Excessive production of fibrous elements that continues after the stimulus has ceased. Also called *neoplastic fibrosis.*

pulmonary fibrosis The accumulation of abnormal quantities of fibrous tissue in the lung. Also called *pneumonocirrhosis* (obsolete), *pneumosclerosis* (obsolete).

renal fibrosis The presence of collagen anywhere in the kidney, involving glomeruli or the interstitium of the cortex, medulla, or capsule. Fibrosis of the renal cortex can occur in almost any renal disease, but is especially common in nephrosclerosis, chronic glomerulonephritis, and interstitial nephritis.

replacement fibrosis The replacement of damaged tissue with fibrous scar as wound healing progresses.

retroperitoneal fibrosis IDIOPATHIC RETROPERITONEAL FIBROSIS.

root sleeve fibrosis Fibrosis of the dural covering of the spinal nerves and/or nerve roots as they pass through the intervertebral foramina.

subadventitial fibrosis PERIMUSCULAR FIBROSIS.

Symmers fibrosis SYMMERS PIPESTEM FIBROSIS.

Symmers clay pipestem fibrosis SYMMERS PIPESTEM FIBROSIS.

Symmers pipestem fibrosis Periportal and perilobular fibrosis of the liver in schistosomiasis, occurring in response to trapped embolic eggs and egg products of schistosomes, especially *Schistosoma mansoni.* This condition results in characteristic, grossly observable accumulations of white fibrotic tissue. Also called *Symmers clay pipestem fibrosis, pipestem fibrosis, Symmers fibrosis.*

fibrosis uteri Thickening and coarsening of the myometrium caused by an increase in collagenous fibrous tissue in the uterus.

fibrositis [New L *fibros(us)* (from L *fibr(a)* fiber, filament + *-osus* -OSE) fibrous + -ITIS] A condition of uncertain cause characterized by diffuse myalgia, sometimes with trigger points. Some authorities feel this is a psychological illness, others regard it as physiologic. Also called *intramuscular fibrositis, rheumatoid myositis.*

intramuscular fibrositis FIBROSITIS.

fibrositis ossificans progressiva MYOSITIS OSSIFICANS PROGRESSIVA.

traumatic fibrositis A nonspecific inflammation of fibrous tissue caused by single or multiple traumatic episodes, resulting in painful, tender areas and joint motion limitations or muscle weakness.

fibrosplenomegaly Splenomegaly with fibrosis.

congestive fibrosplenomegaly CHRONIC CONGESTIVE SPLENOMEGALY.

fibrothorax Fibrosis of the pleural space, often causing adhesion of the pleural surfaces, seen as opacified hemithorax on chest radiograph. Thick, nonexpansile fibrous tissue may lead to restriction of lung motion. Also called *pachypleuritis.*

fibrotic Characterized by fibrosis.

fibrotuberculosis FIBROSING TUBERCULOSIS.

fibrous Characterized by, composed of, or resembling fibers. Also *fibrofibrous.*

fibrovascular Formed primarily from connective tissue fibers with a good supply of blood vessels.

fibroxanthoma [FIBRO- + XANTHOMA] FIBROUS HISTIOCYTOMA.

fibula [L, for *figibula* (from stem of *figere* to fasten, fix) a clasp, buckle, brace, pin] [NA] The slender lateral, or outer, bone of the leg, articulating with the tibia superiorly and taking part in the ankle joint inferiorly. It is less important than the tibia as a weightbearing bone. Also called *calf bone, fibular bone, perone, canna minor* (outmoded), *paracnemis* (outmoded), *paracnemidion* (outmoded).

fibular Pertaining or belonging to the fibula. Also *peroneal, fibularis.*

fibularis [New L, from L *fibul(a)* a clasp, buckle, brace, pin + *-aris* -AR] [NA] FIBULAR.

fibulation INFIBULATION.

fibulocalcaneal Pertaining to the fibula and the calcaneus.

fibulocalcaneus An occasional muscle fascicle that arises from the lower third of the shaft of the fibula, passes beneath flexor retinaculum, and inserts into either quadratus plantae or flexor digitorum longus tendon.

-fic [L *-fic(us)*, combining from denoting doing, making, from *facere* to do, make] A combining form meaning making or causing.

-fication [L *-ficatio*, gen. *-ficationis* (from *facere* to make), a suffix denoting a making] A suffix denoting the process of making.

Fichera [Gaetano *Fichera*, Italian physician, 1880–1935] See under TREATMENT.

ficin A cysteine proteinase (EC 3.4.22.3) found in the fig genus *Ficus*. The thiol group of a cysteine residue at its active site performs nucleophilic attack on the carbonyl group of the bond to be split, and hence its activity is destroyed by reagents for thiol groups, such as *N*-ethylmaleimide.

Fick [Adolf Eugen *Fick*, German physician, 1829–1901] **1** See under METHOD, HALO, PHENOMENON, VEIL. **2** Fick's first law of diffusion. See under LAW. **3** Fick formula. See under PRINCIPLE.

ficosis [L *fic(us)* a fig + -OSIS] SYCOSIS.

fiction / autarchic fiction The child's belief that he or she is omnipotent.

fictive Denoting a functionally meaningful pattern of motor activity, as in a decerebrate animal, initiated by the administration of a pharmacologic agent or electrical stimulation of some nervous structure. It is generally applied to repetitive motor activity, such as chewing, scratching, or ambulation.

fidelity [L *fidel(itas)* (from *fidel(is)* faithful, from *fides* faith + *-itas* -ITY) fidelity] The degree to which an electronic system accurately reproduces at its output the desired input signal.

fidicinales An outmoded term for MUSCULI LUMBRICALES MANUS.

fiebre [Spanish, fever] Fever.

fiebre manchada 1 A Mexican term for FLEA-BORNE TYPHUS. **2** A Spanish term for ROCKY MOUNTAIN SPOTTED FEVER.

fiebre petequial A Colombian term for FLEA-BORNE TYPHUS.

Fiedler [Carl Ludwig Alfred *Fiedler*, German physician, 1835–1921] **1** Fiedler's myocarditis. See under ACUTE ISOLATED MYOCARDITIS. **2** Fiedler's disease. See under ICTERIC LEPTOSPIROSIS.

field 1 An area or surface that can be seen or defined, as in function or extent. **2** In microscopy, the area which can be viewed at one time with a particular lens system. **3** The space surrounding a charged particle or other force-creating body, throughout which the force is effective.

address field The portion of a computer instruction that specifies the source or destination of data in the memory.

adversive field Any region of the cerebral cortex which upon stimulation causes turning of the head and eyes and sometimes of the body toward the opposite side.

auditory field The primary auditory receptive area of the cerebral cortex.

binocular field The area that can be seen with both eyes simultaneously. This excludes the 30° temporal monocular field of each eye.

card field In computer data processing, a set of corresponding columns on a punch card used to store similar data on successive cards.

centrocecal area of field See under AREA.

Cohnheim's fields Myofibrillar areas seen in cross-section of muscle fiber.

field of consciousness That which is being experienced at a given moment and of which the individual is aware.

cribriform field of vision A visual field containing many scotomata.

deaf field A rarely used term for AURAL SCOTOMA.

developmental field MORPHOGENETIC FIELD.

electromagnetic field 1 The field by means of which electrically charged bodies interact. **2** A region in which there exists electric and/or magnetic fields.

electrostatic field The region surrounding a charged body or particle throughout which another charged body will experience a force of attraction or repulsion.

far field 1 That region of the field where the angular field distribution is independent of distance. **2** In ultrasound, the region of the sound beam beyond the distance r^2/λ where r is the radius of the transducer and λ is the wavelength. It is the region of the sound beam in which the beam diameter increases as the distance from the transducer increases. Also called *Fraunhofer zone, far zone.*

field of fixation The extent of excursion, measured in degrees, of which the eye is capable in the various directions of gaze.

Flechsig's field MYELINOGENETIC FIELD.

Forel's field H FIELDS OF FOREL.

free field A field in a homogeneous isotropic medium free of boundaries or in which the effects of boundaries are negligible.

frontal adversive field FRONTAL EYE FIELD.

frontal eye field The region of the cerebral cortex of the frontal lobe, corresponding approximately to area 8 of Brodmann, from which adversive (nonconjugate) eye movements can be elicited by electrical stimulation. Also called *eye area, frontal adversive field.*

H fields of Forel An H-shaped configuration of myelinated fibers as seen on coronal section of the prerubral portion of the cerebrum. It is comprised of a ventral stratum of incoming fibers from the lenticular nucleus (fasciculus lenticularis) and a dorsal layer of emergent fibers (fasciculus thalamicus), which together embrace the zona incerta and merge medially as the ansa lenticularis. Also called *area Foreli, Forel's field.*

field H_1 of Forel FASCICULUS THALAMICUS.

field H_2 of Forel FASCICULUS LENTICULARIS.

high-power field The portion of a microscope slide visible under a high-power objective lens. It is the basis for quantifying discrete objects.

individuation field A localized region within a developing embryo which is influenced by the presence of a single modifying substance or organizer. The organizer has the ability to rearrange the regional structure of both itself and the adjacent tissue so that they form part of an integrated embryo.

Krönig's field KRÖNIG'S AREA.

low-power field The portion of a microscope slide seen when a low-magnification objective lens system is used. It serves as a unit of areal measure for calculating the concentration of discrete objects.

magnetic field A condition in a region of space in the neighborhood of a magnet or of an electric current, characterized by the existence of a torque on a test magnet.

mesobranchial field MESOBRANCHIAL ZONE.

morphogenetic field The region of an embryo which is generally larger than its main derivatives, out of which definite structures, such as organs, normally develop. Also called *developmental field.*

myelinogenetic field Any fiber pathways or tracts in the central or peripheral nervous system in which the process of myelination is taking place or about to take place. Also called *Flechsig's field.*

near field 1 That region of the field between the antenna and the far field. **2** In ultrasound, the region of the beam within a distance of r^2/λ where r is the radius of the transducer and λ is the wavelength. It is the region of a beam in which the beam diameter decreases as the distance from the transducer increases. Also called *Fresnel zone, near zone.*

occipital eye field The cerebral cortex surrounding the calcarine fissure, including striate (area 17) and peristriate fields (areas 18 and 19), the electrical stimulation of which elicits conjugate eye movements towards the opposite side.

parietal adversive field   The area of the parietal lobe of monkeys lying rostral to the lunate sulcus from which adversive eye movements can be elicited by electrical stimulation.

perceptual field   The totality of all aspects of the external world of which the individual is aware at a given moment. The sensory field, created by sense organ reactivity to actual objects in the outer world, interacts with the mental set of the individual and with the effects of prior experience so that what is perceived is an active process and not a mere registration of stimuli reaching the sense organs. The perceptual field may include illusory or distorted subjective elements, departing significantly from the objective facts of the environment.

prefrontal eye field   FRONTAL EYE FIELD.

primary nail field   The earliest sign of the development of the nail as a flattened plate on the terminal phalanx of a finger or toe.

receptive field   1 The area of skin or deeper structures capable upon adequate stimulation of exciting a discharge in a sensory axon, nerve, root, or rootlet. It represents the extent of ramification of the axons.   2 SENSITIVE AREA.

septic field   An area of land that is used for irrigation by a sewage effluent.

spiral field   A variable extent of the visual field due to functional factors such as hysteria. If the order of presentations of the test object is in a regular circumferential sequence, a progressive functional constriction of the field will result in plotting a border that is shaped like a decreasing spiral.

subicular fields   The cytoarchitectonically defined cortex of the hippocampal gyrus, lateral to the hippocampus proper and medial to the rhinal fissure. It is sometimes subdivided into subiculum, presubiculum, and prosubiculum and is often considered a part of the hippocampus distinct from the CA fields.

surplus field   The remaining portion of the visual field on the side of an incomplete hemianopsia.

tactile field   An area concerned with touch sensation within which it is not possible to distinguish two stimuli applied simultaneously.

treatment field   In radiation therapy, the area of the body to which a treatment is administered.

field of vision   VISUAL FIELD.

visual field   The area that is visible to an eye at a given position. Also called *field of vision*.

Wernicke's field   1 The myelinated fibers traversing the lateral posterior and pulvinar nuclei of the thalamus.   2 The cortical field comprising Wernicke's area in the posterior superior temporal gyrus, including the supramarginal and angular gyri. This area is believed to be a speech center.

field-dependent   Characterizing those persons whose interpretation of events occurring within their perceptual field is strongly governed by cues supplied by the surrounding frame of reference. Such individuals, when attempting to adjust to a true vertical a luminous rod viewed in a darkened room, are more influenced by the position of a surrounding luminous square which is also slightly tilted than are field-independent subjects, who reposition the rod in a way less influenced by the immediate embedding context.

Fielding   [George Hunsley *Fielding*, English anatomist and ophthalmologist, 1801–1871]   Fielding's membrane, membrana versicolor of Fielding. See under TAPETUM.

Fiessinger   [Noel *Fiessinger*, French physician, 1881–1946]   1 Fiessinger-Leroy-Reiter syndrome. See under REITER SYNDROME.   2 Fiessinger-Rendu syndrome. See under STEVENS-JOHNSON SYNDROME.

fièvre   [French, fever]   Fever.

fièvre boutonneuse   BOUTONNEUSE FEVER.

fièvre caprine   GOAT FEVER.

fièvre exanthématique de Marseille   BOUTONNEUSE FEVER.

FIGLU   formiminoglutamic acid.

figuratum   [L, neut. of *figuratus*, past part. of *figurare* to form, mold]   Figured: said of skin that is marked by geometrically shaped lesions.

figure   [L *figura* (akin to *fingere* to shape, mold, fashion) a form, shape, figure]   1 A shape or outline.   2 An amount or a number representing it.   3 A person taken to be representative of a type or role.

achromatic figure   MITOTIC APPARATUS.

chromatic figure   The pattern formed by the chromosomes during mitosis or meiosis. Also called *nuclear figure*.

comparative mortality figure   The number of deaths that would have occurred in a given group, such as an occupational or socioeconomic group, if the group were the same in number and age-sex distribution as a standard population in which 1000 deaths had occurred.

fortification figure   TEICHOPSIA.

Gottschaldt figures   A series of relatively simple geometric figures hidden within more complete figures. They are used to examine the perception of form.

mitotic figure   MITOTIC APPARATUS.

myelin figure   A lysosome that contains a laminated structure composed of incompletely digested cytoplasmic membranes. Also called *myelinoid body*.

nuclear figure   CHROMATIC FIGURE.

Purkinje's figures   The images cast by a thin network of blood vessels that supply the retina and are interposed between the sensitive cells and the incoming light. These figures may become visible under certain special conditions.

Stifel's figure   A white spot upon a dark background, intended for demonstration of the physiologic blind spot.

Zöllner's figures   An optical illusion in which parallel lines seem to converge or diverge because of angled background lines.

fila   Plural of FILUM.

filaceous   FILAMENTOUS.

filament   [L *filamentum* (from *filare* to spin, from *filum* a thread + *-mentum* -MENT) a small thread]   A long, threadlike structure. Ordinary bacteria may form filaments when a mutation, or an inhibitor such as a borderline concentration of penicillin, impairs cell division but not cell growth. Some actinomycetes, sheathed bacteria, and fungi form filaments naturally. Also called *filamentum*.

acrosomal filament   A thin, stiff filament projecting from the head of the spermatozoon, formed by elongation of a central part of the acrosome. It plays a part in penetration of the ovum at fertilization. Also called *perforatorium* (obsolete).

actin filament   One of the smaller of the two types of myofilament that can be demonstrated in skeletal muscle by electron microscopy. They are attached at one end to the Z band and the other ends interdigitate with the myosin filaments.

axial filament   AXONEME.

gill filament   A fingerlike projection from the gill arch, occurring in fishes, cephalopods, and gastropods.

intermediate filament   One of the fibrous components of the cytoskeleton of a cell. Such filaments are approximately 10 nm in diameter and are intermediate in size between microfilaments and the large filaments such as myosin.

linin filament   The threadlike achromatic material which forms a network in the nucleus of a cell. The chromatin appears as granules along the filaments.

root filaments of spinal nerves   FILA RADICULARIA NERVORUM SPINALIUM.

spermatic filament   A short segment at the end of the tail of a spermatozoon, characterized by lack of a sheath and with irregular arrangement and extent of the axial fibrile.

terminal filament FILUM TERMINALE.

terminal filament of spinal dura mater FILUM DURAE MATRIS SPINALIS.

transverse filament A narrow (2 nm) protein fiber extending perpendicular to and between the central and lateral elements in the synaptonemal complex.

filamenta Plural of FILAMENTUM.

filamentation [FILAMENT + -ATION] A shape change manifested by bacilli growing in adverse conditions, as in the presence of antibodies or antibiotics, wherein normal, short, rod-shaped forms change to elongated threadlike forms. Also called *thread reaction.*

filamentous Forming or consisting of filaments. Also *filaceous.*

filamentum FILAMENT.

Filaria [See FILARIA.] A genus of secernentean (phasmidian) nematodes of the superfamily Filarioidea, family Filariidae. The genus formerly included all of the filarial worms with microfilariae, but these have been assigned to families such as Onchocercidae, Dirofilariidae, and Dipetolonematidae in the superfamily Onchocercoidea. Only a few species, chiefly mustelid parasites, remain as true members of the genus, the related cattle filariae being assigned to the genus *Parafilaria.*

Filaria bancrofti WUCHERERIA BANCROFTI.

Filaria conjunctivae A species of parasite found in the eye, and possibly identical with *Dirofilaria conjunctivae* of horses, asses, and occasionally humans. Human infections referred to this species have caused cystlike tumors of the eye, nose, arm, and mesentery in Europe, India, the Soviet Union, and Thailand. These may well have been caused by *D. repens,* a parasite of dogs. The American cases may be from parasites of wild animals, such as *D. tenuis* of raccoons or *D. scaphiceps* of rabbits. Also called *Filaria palpebralis.*

Filaria demarquayi MANSONELLA OZZARDI.

Filaria diurna LOA LOA.

Filaria equina SETARIA EQUINA.

Filaria extraocularis LOA LOA.

Filaria hominisoris A species of uncertain identification reported to have been found in the mouth of a child.

Filaria immitis DIROFILARIA IMMITIS.

Filaria juncea MANSONELLA OZZARDI.

Filaria labialis A species reported to have been found in a pustule of the lip. Its identification is uncertain but it is probably an animal parasite.

Filaria lentis LOA LOA.

Filaria loa LOA LOA.

Filaria magalhaesi A species similar to *Wuchereria bancrofti,* found in Brazil in the left ventricle of a cadaver. It has also been considered to be a species of *Dirofilaria.*

Filaria malaya BRUGIA MALAYI.

Filaria medinensis DRACUNCULUS MEDINENSIS.

Filaria nocturna WUCHERERIA BANCROFTI.

Filaria oculihumani LOA LOA.

Filaria ozzardi MANSONELLA OZZARDI.

Filaria palpebralis FILARIA CONJUNCTIVAE.

Filaria philippinensis Filaria in the Philippines. Most, if not all, cases are caused by *Brugia malayi* and *Wuchereria bancrofti.*

Filaria recondita DIPETALONEMA RECONDITUM.

Filaria sanguinis hominis WUCHERERIA BANCROFTI.

Filaria streptocerca MANSONELLA STREPTOCERCA.

Filaria taniguchii A species reported in Japan from a human lymphatic gland. The identification is uncertain.

Filaria volvulus ONCHOCERCA VOLVULUS.

filaria [L *filum* thread + -ARIA] (*plural* filariae) Any nematode in the suborder Filarina (including the superfamilies Filarioidea

and Onchocercoidea) but especially any onchocercid nematode that has microfilariae parasitic in the blood or tissues of the host.

Bancroft's filaria A filarial nematode of the species *Wuchereria bancrofti.*

Brug's filaria A filarial nematode of the species *Brugia malayi.*

filariae Plural of FILARIA.

filarial Of or pertaining to filariae.

filariasis [*Filari(ia)* + -IASIS] Infection with filarial nematode worms, common in many tropical and subtropical regions, especially west Africa, India, southeast Asia, and South America. Adult worms live in the lymphatics, skin, connective tissue, or serous membranes, producing live embryos (microfilariae). *Wuchereria bancrofti* and *Brugia malayi* are associated with lymphatic obstruction, which may result in elephantiasis and chyluria. *Onchocerca volvulus* causes river blindness, rashes, and subcutaneous nodules. *Loa loa* is responsible for Calabar swellings. *Dracunculus medinensis* (the guinea worm) causes dracontiasis. Other species are less pathogenic. Inflammation and lymphatic obstruction may continue after the death of the worms. Also called *wagaga (Fijian), wanganga (Fijian).*

Bancroft's filariasis Infection with *Wuchereria bancrofti.* Also called *bancroftian filariasis, bancroftiasis, bancroftosis.*

bancroftian filariasis BANCROFT'S FILARIASIS.

Brug's filariasis MALAYAN FILARIASIS.

Malayan filariasis A filarial infection caused by *Brugia malayi* and transmitted by *Mansonia* and *Anopheles* mosquitoes. The disease occurs in Malaysia, Borneo, Indonesia, India, and much of southeast Asia. It is characterized by lymphatic obstruction and lymphangitis as occur in *Wuchereria bancrofti* infections. The swelling, however, is usually more distal and is usually confined to the arms below the elbows and to the legs below the knees. Also called *filariasis malayi, Brug's filariasis.*

filariasis malayi MALAYAN FILARIASIS.

Ozzard's filariasis Infection with *Mansonella ozzardi* filariae.

periodic filariasis Filariasis in which microfilariae are found in the bloodstream only during certain periods in the daily cycle. For example, *Loa loa* is diurnal, while certain strains of *Wuchereria bancrofti* and *Brugia malayi* are nocturnal. This periodicity is usually attributable to the insect vector's biting habits.

filariasis of the spermatic cord A chronic inflammation of the tissues of the spermatic cord following lymphatic obstruction chiefly by the filarial worms *Wuchereria bancrofti* or *Brugia malayi.*

Filariata [*Filari(a)* + -ATA] The filarial worms and their allies, considered by some to represent a separate suborder in the nematode order Spirurida containing the superfamilies Filarioidea and Spiruroidea. More recent classifications place these and eight other superfamilies in the suborder Spirurina.

filaricidal [*filari(a)* + *-cid(e)* + -AL] Destructive to filariae.

filaricide An agent that destroys filariae.

filariform [*filari(a)* + -FORM] **1** Resembling small nematode worms such as filariae; hairlike or threadlike. **2** Pertaining to filariform larvae, the third or infective larval stage of many nematodes, such as the skin-invading stage of hookworm or *Strongyloides* larvae.

Filarioidea [*Filari(a)* + New L *-oidea*, from L *-oid(es)* -OID + *-ea,* neut. pl. of *-eus* English *-eous*] A superfamily of nematodes that are parasitic in the tissues, blood, or body cavities of many vertebrate animals including man. It is generally considered to include *Filaria, Parafilaria, Acanthocheilonema, Dipetalonema, Dirofilaria, Loa, Mansonella, Onchocerca, Wuchereria,* and *Brugia.* In some classifications, the superfamily Filarioidea includes only the family Filariidae with only the genera *Filaria* and *Parafilaria* of medical or veterinary interest, while the other genera (possessing microfilariae) are placed in a separate super-family, Onchocercoidea, in the family Onchocercidae.

filarious 1 Pertaining to or due to filariae. 2 Infected with filariae.

Filaroides [FILARIA + L -*oïdes*, suffix denoting resembling] A genus of strongyle nematodes with the male bursa rudimentary or absent. They are found in the trachea, lungs, and bronchi of carnivores and primates. Nine species are known in the genus which in some classifications is placed in a distinct family, Filaroididae, but in others is placed in a subfamily, Filaroidinae in the family Metastrongylidae.

Filaroides milksi A species found in bronchi, bronchioles, and alveoli of striped skunks and dogs in the United States. It causes small white nodules of no pathologic importance in the pulmonary parenchyma.

Filaroides osleri A cosmopolitan nematode found in small nodules usually at the junction of the trachea and bronchi of dogs and other canids. The disease produced is chronic and characterized by a cough, but is not often fatal.

Filatov [Nils Feodorovich *Filatov*, Russian pediatrician, 1847–1902] 1 Filatov's treatment. See under COMBY-FILATOV TREATMENT. 2 Filatov-Dukes disease. See under EXANTHEM SUBITUM. 3 Filatov's disease. See under INFECTIOUS MONONUCLEOSIS.

Filatov [Vladimir Petrovich *Filatov*, Russian ophthalmologist, 1875–1956] 1 See under OPERATION. 2 Filatov flap. See under TUBED FLAP. 3 Filatov-Gillies tubed pedicle. See under PEDICLE.

Fildes [Paul Gordon *Fildes*, English bacteriologist, born 1882] See under ENRICHMENT, LAW.

file [Old English *fil, feol*] Any of various instruments having a hard, ridged surface that can be applied abrasively to another surface to cut, smooth, or polish it.

gold file A file used for removing surplus gold from the margin of a gold restoration.

Hedström file A root canal file with rasplike teeth.

Hirschfeld-Dunlop file A file used in periodontal treatment for the removal of calculus.

root canal file A fine tapering wire with a fine-pitch thread, used to scrape the sides of root canals. It is held in the fingers and used with a push-pull action.

filial Pertaining to offspring with respect to the parental generation.

filicism [*fili(xic a)c(id)* + -ISM] Poisoning from ingestion of an extract of the male fern, *Dryopteris filix-mas*, containing filixic acid.

filiform Having the form of a filament; threadlike.

filigree [earlier *filigrain*, also *filigreen*, from French *filigrane* (from Italian *filigrana* filigree, from L *fili*, gen. of *filum* thread, + *granum* grain) lacelike silver work] An open arrangement of fine silver or stainless steel wire.

Filipovitch [Casimir *Filipovitch*, Polish physician, flourished 1870] Filipovitch sign. See under PALMOPLANTAR SIGN.

filixic acid A mixture of related substances derived from male fern. It has been used as an anthelmintic.

filix mas ASPIDIUM.

filler / paste filler A fine tapering wire with medium-pitch thread, used to feed paste into root canals. It is used in a handpiece and acts in the manner of an Archimedean screw. Also called *lentula, lentulo plugger*.

fillet 1 LEMNISCUS. 2 To surgically remove a bone so that only soft tissue remains, such as removing a phalanx in order to correct the deformity in a toe.

filling 1 The act of putting into a prepared cavity or root canal a material that acts as a substitute for the lost tooth substance.

2 The finished restoration produced by filling.

combination filling A tooth filling composed of layers of different filling materials.

complex filling COMPOUND FILLING.

composite filling A filling made with a mixture of a setting resin and siliceous particles.

compound filling A filling which involves more than one surface of a tooth, such as a mesio-occlusal filling. Also called *complex filling*.

contour filling A dental filling shaped to restore the original outline of the tooth.

direct filling A filling created by placing a plastic material into the cavity, where it sets.

immediate root filling A root canal filling placed immediately following pulpectomy.

indirect filling A filling created by taking an impression and making a model of the prepared cavity. The restoration is then prepared to fit the model, usually in cast gold, and is subsequently cemented into the prepared cavity.

nonleaking filling A dental filling with good adaptation to walls of the cavity, preventing ingress of moisture or bacteria.

overhanging filling A filling with excess material at the margin.

permanent filling A definitive filling; not a temporary or treatment filling.

postresection filling A root canal filling placed after an apicoectomy, usually from the apical end of the root canal. Also called *retrograde filling, retrofilling, retrograde amalgam*.

retrograde filling POSTRESECTION FILLING.

root canal filling The filling of the root canal of a nonvital tooth with inert material. The primary objective is to seal the apical foramen.

silicate filling A filling made of silicate cement.

treatment filling A temporary filling placed without removing all the caries.

film [Middle English *filme*, from Old English *filmen, fylmen* membrane, akin to Gk *pelma* sole of the foot or shoe and to Old English *fell* skin] 1 A thin coating or layer. 2 A roll or sheet of material coated with an emulsion to render it light-sensitive or sensitive to other forms of radiant energy for producing photographs, roentgenograms, or other visual records.

absorbable gelatin film A substitute membrane made of gelatin, which is absorbed by the body as a new membrane forms.

baseline film A roentgenogram which is used as a reference for comparison with subsequent similar roentgenograms of the same area.

bite-wing film 1 A packeted intraoral film with a central tab which is held between the upper and lower teeth in order to make a bite-wing radiograph. Also called *interproximal film*. 2 BITE-WING RADIOGRAPH.

double-emulsion film Radiographic film with an emulsion on each side.

fibrin film A substitute membrane made of human fibrin, usually used to repair defects in the dura.

fixed blood film A peripheral blood smear which has been dried and treated with histologic fixatives.

interproximal film BITE-WING FILM.

lateral cephalometric head film A radiograph of the head taken from the lateral aspect using a standardized and reproducible technique to obtain maximal mensural identity between the skull and its radiographic image.

nonscreen film Radiographic film intended for use without intensifying screens.

occlusal film 1 OCCLUSAL RADIOGRAPH. 2 The film used in making an occlusal radiograph.

panoramic x-ray film 1 A specially shaped film used in making a panoramic radiograph. **2** PANORAMIC RADIOGRAPH.

periapical film **1** A small packeted film used for intraoral radiography. **2** PERIAPICAL RADIOGRAPH.

plain film A roentgenogram done without the use of any radiopaque contrast material, often taken preliminary to examination with a contrast medium.

port film A roentgenogram, usually made with the radiation source for treatment, to demonstrate the size, shape, and location of the area being treated.

postevacuation film A roentgenogram obtained after evacuation of barium in barium contrast studies of the intestine.

precorneal film The tear film upon the corneal surface.

preliminary film SCOUT FILM.

scout film A plain film taken prior to radiologic examination with contrast medium, such as in intravenous urography or barium enema. Also called *preliminary film, survey radiograph*.

spot film A rapid-exposure roentgenogram taken during fluoroscopy.

stripping film A film, used for autoradiography, having a sensitive photographic emulsion which can be stripped from a prepared matrix, the emulsion being applied directly to the section of the radionuclide-containing specimen for exposure and later developed.

sulfa film An obsolete dressing for burns made from sulfadiazine, sulfanilamide, and methyl cellulose.

x-ray film A very thin flexible transparent sheet of plastic, e.g., cellulose acetate, coated on one side or both sides with a radiant-energy sensitive emulsion, used in radiology. The term is used for both nonexposed and exposed film.

Filobasidiella neoformans The perfect state or teleomorph of the yeastlike fungus *Cryptococcus neoformans*.

filopod FILOPODIUM.

filopodia Plural of FILOPODIUM.

filopodium [*fil(um)* + *o* + -POD + L -*ium*, nuet. noun suffix] (*plural* filopodia) A slender, hyaline pseudopodium largely composed of ectoplasm that is seen in certain free-living amebas. The pseudopodia often anastomose, fuse locally, and form thin sheets of cytoplasm. Also called *filopod*.

filopressure [*fil(um)* + *o* + *pressure*] Temporary pressure on a blood vessel by means of a ligature.

filovaricosis [L *fil(um)* a thread + *o* + VARICOSIS] The presence of abnormal areas of swelling or enlargement along the length of a nerve or nerve fiber.

filter [French *filtre* (from Italian *filtro* a filter, from Late Med L *filtrum* a filter, from German *Filt* felt) a filter] **1** A device that traps particles suspended in a fluid (liquid or gas) that is passed through it. Also called *colatorium*. **2** A device or material through which a mixture of penetrating radiations can pass, but which selectively absorbs some components (usually those with lower energy, or longer wavelength) more than others, thus "purifying" the transmitted beam. X-ray filters are used for this purpose in radiology, and similar filters are sometimes used in nuclear medicine to suppress unwanted scattered radiation. Wave filters (acoustic and electrical) similarly pass some of the incident frequencies while attenuating others. They may be "high-pass," "low-pass," or "band-pass" according to the frequencies transmitted with little attenuation. Analogous spatial filters similarly pass or suppress spatial frequencies in the processing of scintigraphs and other images for computation or display.

acoustic filter An acoustic or electroacoustic device by which specified components of complex tonal sound or noise are permitted to pass through while the other frequencies are filtered out.

band-pass filter A component of an electronic amplifying system, designed to pass a desired range of frequencies while attenuating undesired noise above and below this range. This improves the signal-to-noise ratio. Also called *filter-band pass*.

band-stop filter A filter that rejects a band of frequencies and passes higher and lower frequencies.

barrier filter A filter used in fluorescence microscopy to protect the eye of the viewer from exposure to light of the wavelengths that excite the fluorochrome.

Berkefeld filter BERKEFELD CANDLE.

biologic filter A bed of coarse filter material such as rock or clinker presenting a large surface area on which sewage is oxidized by the action of aerobic organisms. Also called *bacteria bed*.

Chamberland filter CHAMBERLAND CANDLE.

Coors filter A flat filter of unglazed porcelain, used to prepare bacteria-free filtrates.

excitation filter A filter used in fluorescence microscopy that restricts the light reaching the specimen to only those wavelengths capable of exciting the fluorochrome.

Gooch filter A filter made by pouring a suspension of asbestos fibers into a small vessel (Gooch crucible) with holes in its base while suction is being applied to this crucible, used in gravimetric analysis.

gravity filter An appliance or installation for the purification of a fluid such as drinking water using gravitational force through a porous medium.

Greenfield filter A caval interruption device that is designed to be inserted transvenously, either through the jugular or femoral route, into the inferior vena cava. There it remains permanently to block thrombi from embolizing to the central pulmonary circulation.

high-pass filter A component of an electronic amplifying system designed to pass desired high frequencies while attenuating undesired noise below a selected cutoff frequency. This improves the signal-to-noise ratio.

intermittent sand filter A sand filter through which sewage is passed intermittently to prevent the sand from becoming waterlogged and to allow air to penetrate, thus encouraging the oxidation of organic matter.

low-pass filter A component of an electronic amplifying system, designed to pass desired low frequencies while attenuating all undesired noise above a selected cutoff frequency. This improves the signal-to-noise ratio.

mechanical filter A filter of porous material through which a liquid is forced rapidly to remove gross particles.

membrane filter A filter of graded porosity, usually made of nitrocellulose. It may be used to sterilize media, to prepare culture filtrates, and to enumerate bacteria in dilute suspensions, as in water bacteriology, by collection on the filter followed by its incubation in contact with the surface of a solid medium.

Millipore filter A proprietary name for A device used to filter parenteral feeding solutions as they are given intravenously.

notch filter A filter that rejects a narrow band of frequencies and passes higher and lower frequencies.

percolating filter A bed of stones or clinker over which partly treated sewage trickles and is thus exposed to the action of aerobic organisms. Also called *trickling filter*.

pollen filter A device designed to remove pollen from the air.

pressure filter A device for removing solid or liquid particles from a gas, or solid particles from a liquid, by passage through a porous filter medium, assisted by an increase in pressure on one side of the medium, a decrease in pressure on the other, or a combination of both.

rapid sand filter A sand filter through which water is passed under pressure to increase the speed of filtration.

roughing filter A filter composed of coarse material designed to remove the larger particles from turbid water, thus preventing clogging during subsequent sand filtration. Also called *scrubbing filter.*

scrubbing filter   ROUGHING FILTER.

Seitz filter   A bacterial filter consisting of a pad of asbestos.

sintered glass filter   A bacterial filter composed of a layer of fine glass particles fused into a porous mass.

slow sand filter   A sand and gravel filter through which water is passed slowly during treatment. The water is purified mainly by microorganisms growing on the sand particles at or near the surface of the filter.

smoke filter   An instrument for measuring the concentration of smoke in the atmosphere. A predetermined volume of air is passed through a white filter paper and the darkness of the stain on the filter paper is measured colorimetrically. Smoke thus sampled is the permanently suspended matter. The validity of this measurement depends on the optical properties of the smoke sampled.

sprinkling filter   A percolating filter over which partly treated sewage is sprayed.

Thoraeus filter   A filter consisting primarily of tin, usually about 0.44 mm, backed by 0.25 mm Cu and 1.0 mm Al, used to harden the beam in high-voltage radiation therapy.

trickling filter   PERCOLATING FILTER.

ultraviolet filter   A filter that only transmits light rays of the ultraviolet range. It is used in microscopy, spectrophotometry, photography, and in the excitation of fluorescence.

umbrella filter   A filter in the shape of an umbrella placed in the inferior vena cava to prevent pulmonary embolism.

wedge filter   A filter of graduated thickness, used to cause a progressive decrease in the dose rate across a radiation beam.

Wood's filter   A glass that contains 9 percent nickel oxide and only transmits light that exceeds 365 nm. It is used in the Wood's lamp with ultraviolet light.

filterable   Small enough in particle size to pass through a filter of a given pore size. Also *filtrable.*

filtering / perceptual filtering   The ability to differentiate between figure and ground, between the important and the insignificant, and thereby to ignore the mass of stimuli that are impinging continuously on the organism and attend to those that are related to its current objectives, long-term goals, or survival. Defective perceptual filtering is characteristic of many psychotic patients and of schizophrenics in particular.

filtrable   FILTERABLE.

filtrate   [Late Med L *filtratus* (past part. of *filtrare* to filter, from *filtrum* a filter, from German *Filt* felt) filtered]   That portion of a solution that passes through a filter.

bacterial filtrate   The filtrate from a bacterial culture which has been passed through a filter fine enough to retain the bacterial cells.

Folin's protein-free filtrate   A preparation of blood serum from which proteins have been removed by precipitation with sodium tungstate and sulfuric acid, with the resulting chocolate brown semisolid material removed by filtration through filter paper.

glomerular filtrate   The ultrafiltrate of plasma formed across the glomerular capillary wall. All diffusible solutes of plasma appear in the glomerular filtrate in the same concentration as in plasma, corrected for Donnan's equilibrium.

filtration   [FILTER + -ATION]   **1** Separation of particulate matter from solution by passage through a filter.   **2** Sterilization of fluids by passage through a membrane or other filter with fine enough pores to retain all bacteria.   **3** The interposition of a radiation-absorbing material that allows only a selective range of wavelengths to pass through.

centrifugal filtration   A means to enhance filtration by the application of centrifugal force.

gel filtration   See under GEL FILTRATION CHROMATOGRAPHY.

glomerular filtration   The ultrafiltration of solutes from the blood across the glomerular capillary basement into the Bowman space.

inherent filtration   The filtration that is inevitably present in a radiation source, such as the glass envelope of an x-ray tube, or the material encapsulating a radioactive source.

nasal filtration   The removal of particulate matter and bacteria in the air as it passes through the nose. The majority of the particles are trapped by the mucous film blanketing the nasal mucosa which is moved into the nasopharynx by the activity of the cilia.

pressure filtration   Filtration by means of a pressure filter.

sand filtration   **1** A method of treating water to render it fit for drinking.   **2** A method sometimes used for the final treatment of a sewage effluent before discharge.

vacuum filtration   The use of a vacuum to enhance the passage of liquid through a filter, thereby improving the separation of solids from the liquid.

filtratometer   A device used for obtaining and measuring filtrates of gastric or enteric fluids.

filtros   [Italian *filtro* a filter + English pl. *-s.* See FILTER.]   A plate containing minute holes through which air is bubbled to aerate sewage during activated sludge treatment.

filtrum   PHILTRUM.

Merkel's filtrum   FILTRUM VENTRICULI.

filtrum ventriculi   A shallow, vertical furrow between the corniculate cartilage and the cuneiform cartilage in the posterior part of the aryepiglottic fold. Inferiorly it is continuous with the sinus of the larynx. An outmoded term. Also called *Merkel's fossa, Merkel's filtrum.*

filum   [L (akin to *pilus* a hair, *pellis* the skin of a beast, *vellus* wool, fleece, and *villus* a long hair, shaggy hair), a thread, fiber] (*plural* fila) A threadlike structure.

fila anastomotica nervi acustici   The nerve filaments extending between the seventh and eighth nerve roots.

fila coronaria   The tendon of the conus arteriosus.

filum durae matris spinalis   [NA] The slender, connective-tissue continuation of the filum terminale of the spinal cord, forming the coccygeal ligament, which fuses with the posterior periosteal surface of the coccyx. Also called *filum of spinal dura mater, terminal filament of spinal dura mater.*

fila lateralia pontis   An obsolete term for TAENIA PONTIS.

fila olfactoria   NERVI OLFACTORII.

fila radicularia   FILA RADICULARIA NERVORUM SPINALIUM.

fila radicularia nervorum spinalium   The threadlike filaments of the dispersed axonal bundles of the dorsal and ventral roots of the spinal cord. Also called *root filaments of spinal nerves, fila radicularia, radicular fibers.*

filum of spinal dura mater   FILUM DURAE MATRIS SPINALIS.

filum terminale   [NA] The slender, threadlike prolongation of the conus medullaris of the spinal cord. It extends downward to the fundus of the dural sac at the level of the second sacral vertebra, where it penetrates the dura and fuses with the filum of the dura mater to form the coccygeal ligament, which in turn fuses with the periosteum of the posterior surface of the coccyx. The rostral portion contains a prolongation of the central canal, but this is composed mostly of pial connective tissue. Also called *terminal filament, central ligament of spinal cord* (obsolete).

fimbria   [L, a fringe, thread, fiber] (*plural* fimbriae)   **1** A fringelike structure; a fringed border or edge.   **2** Collectively, the very fine filamentous projections from the surface of cells or bacteria. The individual filaments usually have a diameter of .01 μm or less and a length of 1–2 μm. Also called *fringe, lacinia* (outmoded).

fimbriae of fallopian tube FIMBRIAE TUBAE UTERINAE.

fimbria hippocampi [NA] A narrow band of fibrous white matter (myelinated axons), which form the fornix, situated on the medial ventricular surface of the hippocampus. Also called *fimbria of hippocampus, corpus fimbriatum hippocampi*.

fimbria of hippocampus FIMBRIA HIPPOCAMPI.

ovarian fimbria FIMBRIA OVARICA.

fimbria ovarica [NA] The longest and most grooved of the fimbriae tubae uterinae, lying along the free border of the mesosalpinx as far as the tubal end of the ovary. Also called *fimbriated extremity of fallopian tube, ovarian fimbria, infundibulo-ovarian ligament*.

fimbriae of tongue PLICA FIMBRIATA.

fimbriae tubae uterinae [NA] A number of irregular, fingerlike processes extending from the circumference of the expanded abdominal end, or infundibulum, of the uterine tube. They are lined by a mucous membrane thrown into longitudinal folds continuous with those in the infundibulum. Also called *fimbriae of uterine tube, morsus diaboli* (outmoded), *fimbriae of fallopian tube*.

fimbriae of uterine tube FIMBRIAE TUBAE UTERINAE.

fimbrial **1** Pertaining to a fimbria. **2** FIMBRIATED.

Fimbriaria [*fimbri(a)* + -ARIA] A genus of tapeworms (family Hymenolepididae) that are parasitic in ducks, geese, and other anseriform birds. It is unusual in that it possesses a pseudoholdfast organ consisting of a flangelike extension of the anterior end of the worm, the scolex being reduced to a minute structure at the tip of the worm which is often lost.

Fimbriaria fasciolaris A common tapeworm of domestic and wild fowl. It has a modified anterior end, the pseudoscolex, which replaces the reduced, remnant terminal scolex. It inhabits the small intestine but has no significant effects on the host.

fimbriate Fringed; bearing fimbriae.

fimbriated Possessing fimbriae or fringelike processes; fringed. Also *fimbrial, fimbriatum*.

fimbriation **1** The process of forming fimbriae. **2** The condition of having fimbriae or a fringed border.

fimbriatum FIMBRIATED.

fimbriectomy [*fimbri(a)* + -ECTOMY] Amputation of the fimbria of the fallopian tube for purposes of sterilization.

fimbriocele [*fimbri(a)* + *o* + -CELE[1]] A vaginal herniation of the fimbriae of the oviduct.

fimbriodentate Denoting the fimbria of the fornix and the underlying dentate gyrus from which it is separated by a groove (fimbriodentate sulcus).

fimbrioplasty [*fimbri(a)* + *o* + -PLASTY] The surgical freeing of the fimbria of an ovarian tube when obstruction is present.

fin [Middle English, from Old English *finn*] A thin winglike or paddlelike projection from the body of an aquatic animal, which functions in locomotion and guidance of the organism.

anal fin A median ventral fin located posterior to the anus of most fishes.

caudal fin The tail fin of an aquatic vertebrate, usually providing the primary force for locomotion.

dorsal fin A fin located on the dorsal surface of an aquatic organism, such as a fish or amphibian.

pectoral fin One of the paired, anterior, lateral fins of a fish, associated with the pectoral girdle.

pelvic fin One of the paired posterior, lateral fins of fishes, associated with the pelvic girdle. Also called *ventral fin*.

ventral fin PELVIC FIN.

finch Any of a diverse group of small birds belonging to the family Fringillidae.

Darwin's finches An isolated gene pool of finches of the Galapagos Islands that, in the absence of competition, evolved into species able to exploit the diverse niches available.

Finckh [Johann *Finckh*, German psychiatrist, born 1873] Finckh's test. See under PROVERBS TEST.

finder A microscope slide that has been marked out in numbered squares in order to facilitate the locating of a given point on the slide.

Findley [Francis McRae *Findley*, U.S. surgeon, born 1898] See under OPERATION.

finger [Old English] Any one of the five digits of the hand.

baseball finger MALLET FINGER.

bayonet fingers Deformation of the fingers consisting of palmar flexion of the distal phalanges of the index and middle fingers, with hyperextension and subluxation of the middle phalanges and flexion of the first. This condition is sometimes seen in hemiplegic patients, with contractures in the spastic muscles. A seldom used term.

bolster fingers A chronic infection of the nail fold caused predominately by *Candida albicans* and often coexisting with Staphylococcae and occasionally with Gram-negative organisms.

clubbed finger A bulbous enlargement of the terminal segment of the finger. It is seen in infants and children with various diseases of the thoracic organs, particularly with certain congenital heart diseases, or it may be inherited. There is no constant osseous change in the terminal phalanx, but the surrounding fibrous tissue proliferates excessively. Also called *drumstick finger, hippocratic finger, digitus hippocraticus*.

dead finger WHITE FINGER.

drop finger MALLET FINGER.

drumstick finger CLUBBED FINGER.

first finger POLLEX.

giant finger MACRODACTYLY.

hammer finger MALLET FINGER.

hippocratic finger CLUBBED FINGER.

index finger INDEX.

insane finger Whitlow in residents of mental asylums, due usually to poor hygiene within the institution. An outmoded term.

lock finger A finger with bony or fibrous ankylosis.

Madonna fingers The delicate, slender fingers characteristic of acromicria.

mallet finger A flexion deformity of the terminal phalanx of the finger provoked by striking the dorsum of the finger tip. It is caused by the complete or partial rupture of the extensor tendon to the terminal phalanx or by the avulsion of its bony insertion. It can be passively, but not actively, corrected. Also called *baseball finger, drop finger, hammer finger, digitus malleus*.

middle finger DIGITUS MEDIUS.

ring finger DIGITUS ANNULARIS.

sausage fingers The thickened fingers characteristic of acromegaly.

snapping finger TRIGGER FINGER.

spade fingers The thickened, square-tipped fingers of acromegaly, due mainly to an increase in soft tissue.

spider finger ARACHNODACTYLY.

spring finger **1** TRIGGER FINGER. **2** A finger that resists the extremes of flexion or extension.

stuck finger TRIGGER FINGER.

trigger finger A deformity of the finger in which the digit becomes stuck in flexion at the proximal interphalangeal joint. The condition is due to entrapment of the flexor tendon at the entrance of the fibrous flexor sheath. Also called *stuck finger, snapping finger, spring finger, digitus recellens*.

tulip fingers A distinctive clinical syndrome of hyperkeratosis, scaling, and fissuring of the fingertips that is common among those whose occupation involves handling tulip bulbs.

vibration-induced white fingers See under VIBRATION DISEASE.

washerwoman's fingers Shriveled fingers caused by extreme dehydration, as seen in the terminal stages of cholera.

waxy finger Cyanotic mottling and numbness of the fingers due to impaired circulation, as seen in the Raynaud syndrome.

webbed fingers A slight degree of syndactyly in which adjacent fingers are joined by a fold of skin of greater distal extent than is usually seen. There is no union of fibrous or osseous elements. Also called *palmature.*

white finger A condition characterized by numbness and blanching of the fingers, especially in workers who use vibrating hand tools such as pneumatic hammers and chain saws in cold environments. It constitutes an occupational variant of Raynaud's syndrome. Also called *dead finger, digitus mortuus, doigt mort.*

windswept fingers The appearance of the fingers in cases of ulnar drift.

fingerdrop One of the results of radial (musculospiral) nerve paralysis characterized by inability to extend the fingers at the metacarpophalangeal joints. It is often associated with wristdrop and other evidences of radial nerve paralysis depending on the level of the nerve lesion.

fingernail The unguis that covers the distal aspect of the terminal phalanx of the finger.

fingerprint **1** The transferred impression of the dermatoglyphic pattern of the distal phalangeal volar surface of a finger or thumb, formed by intentional or chance contact of the distal phalanx with a surface that will retain the impression. Also called *dactylogram.* **2** The result of an analytic technique capable of distinguishing between or separating similar compounds, such as the final position on a chromatographic plate of individual peptides from a mixture of peptides subjected to two-dimensional paper chromatography.

chance fingerprints Fingerprints left unintentionally when contact of ridged skin is made with a surface that retains the dermatoglyphic pattern, such as fingerprints on a polished surface where the deposited perspiration and oily skin secretions leave ridge impressions. Also called *trace fingerprints.*

latent fingerprints Chance fingerprints which are invisible or barely visible. Enhancement techniques, such as dusting the suspected surface with powder or exposing it to iodine fumes, are required to detect their presence.

record fingerprints Fingerprints made by applying ink or other suitable staining material to the volar surfaces of the distal phalanges and rolling each fingertip across an assigned space on a white card or paper. They are used for identification and comparison purposes.

trace fingerprints CHANCE FINGERPRINTS.

fingerstall A thimble-shaped device fabricated of leather, plastic, or rubber material and used to protect fingers.

Finkeldey [Wilhelm *Finkeldey*, German pathologist, flourished 20th century] Warthin-Finkeldey cell. See under CELL.

Finney [John Miller Turpin *Finney*, U.S. surgeon, 1863–1942] Finney's operation. See under PYLOROPLASTY.

Finochietto [Enrique *Finochietto*, Argentinian surgeon, 1881–1948] See under STIRRUP.

Finsen [Jon Constant *Finsen*, Icelandic physician, born 1826] Daae-Finsen disease. See under DISEASE.

Finsen [Niels Ryberg *Finsen*, Danish physician, 1860–1904] **1** See under TREATMENT, LIGHT, LAMP, APPARATUS. **2** Finsen rays. See under RAY.

Finzi [Neville Samuel *Finzi*, English radiotherapist, born 1881] Finzi-Harmer operation. See under OPERATION.

fire [Old English *fȳr*; akin to Gk *pyr* fire] **1** FEVER. **2** ERYSIPELAS.

Saint Anthony's fire ERGOTISM.

St. Francis fire ERYSIPELAS.

firedamp A colorless, odorless gas, composed mainly of methane (more than 60%), nitrogen, and carbon dioxide, that occurs naturally in coal mines. Although it has no physiologic action on its own it creates a hazard as a simple asphyxiant. It is inflammable and gives rise to the risk of explosion in mines. Also *fire damp.*

first aid See under AID.

Fischer [Emil Hermann *Fischer*, German chemist, 1852–1919] See under FORMULA.

Fischer See under KARL FISCHER.

Fischer [Louis *Fischer*, Austrian-born U.S. pediatrician, 1864–1945] See under SIGN.

fish [Middle English, from Old English *fisc*, akin to L *piscis* fish] (*plural* fish, fishes) An aquatic vertebrate of the superclass Pisces. Fish are poikilothermic, have gills, and generally are covered with scales. • The plural form *fishes* is preferred when referring to species.

bony fishes Any of the fish in the class Osteichthyes, characterized by having a bony skeleton.

cartilaginous fishes Any of the fishes in the class Chondrichthyes, characterized by having a skeleton composed of cartilage. The sharks and rays are included in this group.

ganoid fishes Those fishes, such as garpikes and sturgeons, having rhombic scales composed of a layer of ganoin over a layer of lamellate bone.

torpedo fish A member of the family of electric rays, Torpedinidae. The electric organ is used for research on acetylcholine receptor function.

Fishberg [Arthur Maurice *Fishberg*, U.S. physician, born 1898] Fishberg's method. See under FISHBERG CONCENTRATION TEST.

Fisher [Miller *Fisher*, U.S. physician, born 1910] Miller Fisher syndrome. See under FISHER SYNDROME.

Fisher [Ronald Aylmer *Fisher*, English statistician and geneticist, 1890–1962] Fisher test, Fisher-Yates test. See under FISHER'S EXACT TEST OF PROBABILITY (at *test*).

fishing In laboratory usage, the picking of single colonies from a culture with a needle or toothpick.

fishmeal Surplus fish, waste from filleting, and fish considered unfit for human consumption that is dried and powdered. Fishmeal is an excellent source of protein used for animal feeds. After removal of its natural odor, it is considered palatable enough for human consumption. It contains 70% protein of biologic value 75. It comes as white fishmeal, used in animal feeds, and in an oily form, used in fertilizers.

fishpox [FISH + POX] A cutaneous, poxlike disease of fish, caused by a herpesvirus.

Fiske [Cyrus Hartwell *Fiske*, U.S. biochemist, born 1890] Fiske and Subbarow method. See under METHOD.

fissile [L *fissil(is)* (from *fiss(us)*, past part. of *findere* to cleave, divide + *-ilis* -ILE) capable of being cleaved or divided] **1** FISSIONABLE. **2** Capable of being cleaved along natural planes of cleavage.

fission [L *fissio* (from *fissus*, past part. of *findere* to cleave, cut; interchangeable with *scindere* to cut, tear, divide, from Gk *schizein* to split, cleave) a cleaving, dividing] The act of splitting or breaking apart, as an atomic nucleus or the nucleus of a cell.

binary fission Asexual reproduction by the splitting of a cell by nuclear division (karyokinesis) followed by cytoplasmic separation (cytokinesis) to form two new cells of equal size, a common method of reproduction of various protists.

bud fission GEMMATION.

cellular fission CYTOKINESIS.

charged-particle fission Nuclear fission brought about by bombardment with charged particles, most commonly protons, deuterons, or alpha particles.

multiple fission A series of nuclear divisions followed by the division of the body of the cell into an equal number of parts, each with a daughter nucleus, as is seen in the asexual reproduction of sporozoa (schizogony), or the result of sexual fusion (sporogomy). A specialized form of multiple fission is called endopolygeny, in which daughter cells form within their cell membranes in the cytoplasm of the mother cell rather than at the periphery. Compare SIMPLE FISSION.

nuclear fission The splitting of a heavy nucleus into two roughly equal parts, with the release of large amounts of energy. A few naturally occurring nuclides undergo spontaneous fission, but ordinarily fission will not occur unless the nucleus can absorb external neutrons or gamma photons, thus causing instability. Fission of a given nuclide leads to any of a variety of pairs of daughter nuclides rather than just a prespecified pair.

simple fission The division of the cell nucleus followed by division of the body of the cell into two equal parts; binary fission. Compare MULTIPLE FISSION.

fissionable Capable of undergoing nuclear fission. Also *fissile.*

fissiparity [L *fissi(o)* a cleaving, dividing + L *par(ere)* to beget, bring forth young + -ITY] Reproduction by fission. An older term.

fissiparous Reproducing by fission. An older term.

Fissipedia [New L, variant of *Fissipeda* a suborder of carnivores, irreg. from Late L *fissipes*, gen. *fissipedis*, cloven-footed, from L *fiss(us)*, past part. of *findere* to cleave, split + *i* + New L *-peda*, neut. pl. combining form from L *pes*, gen. *pedis*, foot] The suborder of the mammalian order Carnivora comprising the terrestrial carnivores. It includes several families of advanced predatory types, such as the Canidae, Ursidae, Mustelidae, and Felidae. Compare PINNIPEDIA.

fissula [Late L, dim. of L *fissum* cleft, fissure] A small cleft or fissure.

fissula ante fenestram An oblique, slitlike space through the lateral wall of the internal ear that is filled with a strip of connective tissue extending from the vestibule immediately in front of the fenestra vestibuli to the mucoperiosteum of the tympanic cavity near the processus cochleariformis. It is considered to be an appendage of the perilymphatic labyrinth. Also called *Cozzolino's zone.*

fissura [Late L (from *fiss(us)*, past part. of *findere* to cleave, cut + -*ura* -URE), fissure, cleft, groove] (*plural* fissurae) A furrow, groove, or cleft, especially a deep fold separating gyri in the cerebral cortex; sulcus. Also called *fissure.* • Though close in meaning, *fissura* usually denotes a deeper, and *sulcus* a more shallow furrow.

fissura antitragohelicina [NA] A deep notch in the auricular cartilage separating the cauda helicis posteriorly from the antitragus anteriorly. Also called *antitragohelicine fissure, posterior fissure of auricle.*

fissura calcarina SULCUS CALCARINUS.

fissurae cerebelli [NA] Major grooves separating the corpus cerebelli into lobes and lobules.

fissura cerebri lateralis Sylvii SULCUS LATERALIS CEREBRI.

fissura choroidea The linear evagination of the choroid plexus along the walls of the lateral ventricles. Also called *Schwalbe's fissure.*

fissura collateralis SULCUS COLLATERALIS.

fissura dentata SULCUS HIPPOCAMPI.

fissura hippocampi SULCUS HIPPOCAMPI.

fissura horizontalis cerebelli The horizontal fissure separating the ansiform lobule of the hemispheres into the rostral crus I (superior semilunar lobule) and caudal crus II (inferior semilunar lobule). Medially, it separates the folium vermis from the tuber vermis. Also called *sulcus horizontalis cerebelli, great horizontal fissure, horizontal fissure of cerebellum.*

fissura horizontalis pulmonis dextri [NA] A short, deep horizontal cleft that extends from the anterior margin of the right lung to the hilum, where it meets the oblique fissure and separates the superior from the middle lobe. Also called *horizontal fissure of right lung.*

fissura in ano ANAL FISSURE.

fissura ligamenti teretis [NA] A fissure of variable depth on the visceral surface of the liver. It extends from a notch on the inferior margin to the left extremity of the porta hepatis, where it meets the fissure for ligamentum venosum. It separates the quadrate lobe from the left lobe and lodges the ligamentum teres of the liver. Also called *fissure for ligamentum teres, fissure of round ligament, umbilical fissure* (outmoded), *fossa venae umbilicalis* (outmoded), *fossa umbilicalis hepatis* (outmoded), *fossa for ligamentum teres.*

fissura ligamenti venosi [NA] A deep groove on the posterior part of the diaphragmatic surface of the liver that separates the caudate lobe from the left lobe and contains the two layers of the lesser omentum. Inferiorly it reaches the left extremity of the porta hepatis, where it meets the fissure for ligamentum teres. In its depths is the ligamentum venosum, the fibrous cordlike remnant of the fetal ductus venosus, which is attached below to the left umbilical portion of the left branch of the portal vein and superiorly either to the left hepatic vein or to the inferior vena cava. Also called *fissure for ligamentum venosum.*

fissura longitudinalis cerebri The largest and deepest cerebral fissure, separating the two cerebral hemispheres. Also called *superior longitudinal sulcus, longitudinal fissure, longitudinal fissure of cerebrum, intercerebral fissure.*

fissura mediana anterior FISSURA MEDIANA ANTERIOR MEDULLAE SPINALIS.

fissura mediana anterior medullae oblongatae The continuation of the median fissure of the ventral spinal cord into the medulla oblongata, where it becomes more shallow. Also called *anterior median fissure of medulla oblongata, fissura mediana ventralis medullae oblongatae.*

fissura mediana anterior medullae spinalis The deep midline fissure parting the ventral spinal cord throughout its length. Also called *fissura mediana anterior, sulcus medianus, anterior median fissure of spinal cord, anteromedian groove of spinal cord, Haller's line* (obsolete), *sulcus ventralis medullae spinalis.*

fissura mediana posterior medullae oblongatae SULCUS MEDIANUS POSTERIOR MEDULLAE OBLONGATAE.

fissura mediana ventralis medullae oblongatae [NA] FISSURA MEDIANA ANTERIOR MEDULLAE OBLONGATAE.

fissura obliqua pulmonis [NA] A long, deep cleft that extends from the costal to the mediastinal surface of each lung and from a point below the apex on the posterior margin obliquely through the hilum to the inferior margin close to its junction with the anterior margin. It separates the superior and inferior lobes in the left lung and the inferior lobe from the superior and middle lobes in the right lung. Also called *oblique fissure of lung.*

fissura orbitalis inferior [NA] The cleft at the apex of the orbit between the lateral and inferior walls. It is bounded laterally and posteriorly by the inferior margin of the orbital surface of the greater wing of the sphenoid bone, and anteriorly and medially by the orbital process of the palatine bone and the posterior margin of the orbital surface of the maxilla. It serves as a communication between the orbit and the pterygopalatine fossa medially and the infratemporal fossa laterally. Through it pass the maxillary nerve, the infraorbital vessels, and connections between the ophthalmic veins and the pterygoid venous plexus. Also called *inferior orbital fissure, inferior sphenoidal fissure* (outmoded), *sphenomaxillary fissure* (outmoded).

fissura orbitalis superior [NA] An oblique, narrow cleft at the apex of the orbit between the lateral wall and roof. Its long axis is directed medially, posteriorly, and inferiorly. It lies between the greater and lesser wings of the sphenoid bone and connects the orbit with the middle cranial fossa. It transmits numerous structures including the ophthalmic, oculomotor, trochlear, and abducent nerves and the ophthalmic veins. Also called *superior orbital fissure, superior sphenoidal fissure* (outmoded), *sphenoidal fissure* (outmoded), *foramen lacerum anterius* (outmoded), *anterior lacerate foramen* (outmoded).

fissura parieto-occipitalis SULCUS PARIETO-OCCIPITALIS.

fissura petro-occipitalis A cranial fissure extending caudally from the foramen lacerum between the basioccipital and the posterior and inferior borders of the petrous portion of the temporal bone. Also called *occipital fissure, petrobasilar fissure, petro-occipital fissure, petrospheno-occipital suture of Gruber* (outmoded).

fissura petrosquamosa A superficial cranial fissure following the line of fusion of the petrous and squamous portions of the temporal bone. Also called *petrosquamous fissure, petrosquamous suture.*

fissura petrotympanica [NA] The medial part of the tympanosquamous fissure in the mandibular fossa of the temporal bone, situated between the inferiorly projecting anterolateral edge of the tegmen tympani and the tympanic part of the temporal bone. It transmits the chorda tympani from the tympanic cavity, the anterior tympanic branch of the maxillary artery, and part of the anterior ligament of the malleus. In the tympanic cavity the fissure opens just above the flaccid part of the tympanic membrane and contains the anterior process of the malleus. Also called *petrotympanic fissure, glaserian fissure, tympanic fissure, tympanosquamous fissure, pterygotympanic fissure* (outmoded).

fissura posterolateralis cerebelli The first fissure to appear in the development of the cerebellum, separating the corpus cerebelli from the flocculonodular lobe. Also called *floccular fissure.*

fissura prima cerebelli The primary cerebellar fissure, separating the anterior from the posterior lobe. It extends laterally into the hemispheres from behind the culmen, separating the culmen and declive medially and the posterior and superior semilunar lobules laterally. Also called *superior anterior fissure, primary fissure.*

fissura pterygoidea INCISURA PTERYGOIDEA.

fissura pterygomaxillaris [NA] The V-shaped cleft between the back of the maxilla and the pterygoid process of the sphenoid bone through which the infratemporal fossa communicates medially with the pterygopalatine fossa, giving passage to the maxillary nerve and the terminal part of the maxillary artery. Also called *pterygomaxillary fissure, pterygopalatine fissure.*

fissura pudendi RIMA PUDENDI.

fissura secunda cerebelli [NA] A fissure, located on the anterior surface of the cerebellum, that separates the pyramis and uvula portions of the cerebellar vermis. Also called *secondary fissure.*

fissura spheno-occipitalis The fissure filled with cartilage in the synchondrosis spheno-occipitalis before it is ossified. Also called *spheno-occipital fissure, basilar fissure, occipitosphenoidal fissure.*

fissura sphenopetrosa [NA] The slit between the petrous part of the temporal bone and the lateral portion of the posterior margin of the greater wing of sphenoid, just medial to the sphenoidal spine. The fissure is filled with fibrocartilage, forming

a synchondrosis. Also called *angular fissure, petrosphenoidal fissure, sphenopetrosal fissure.*

fissura transversa cerebelli The transverse indentation between the nodulus and the cerebellar peduncles. Also called *transverse fissure of cerebellum.*

fissura transversa cerebri [NA] The cleft separating the corpus callosum and fornix from the underlying diencephalon rostrally and the cerebellum caudally, where the fissure is occupied by the tentorium cerebelli. The fissure contains a double layer of pia, the lower portion of which forms the invaginated tela choroidea of the third ventricle. Also called *fissure of Bichat, cerebral fissure of Bichat, great fissure of cerebrum, great transverse fissure of cerebrum, transverse fissure of cerebrum.*

fissura tympanomastoidea [NA] A slit usually located on the inferior aspect of the skull lateral to the base of the styloid process and between the tympanic part and the mastoid process of the temporal bone. Opening into the fissure is the mastoid canaliculus. Also called *tympanomastoid fissure, petromastoid fissure, auricular fissure of temporal bone.*

fissura tympanosquamosa [NA] A transverse fissure between the tympanic and the squamous parts of the temporal bone, observed externally in the mandibular fossa. It is relatively wide in the infant but in the adult narrows to a slit into which the anterolateral edge of the tegmen tympani turns downward, dividing the medial part of the fissure into the petrosquamous fissure anteriorly and the petrotympanic fissure posteriorly. Also called *tympanosquamous fissure, squamotympanic fissure, anterior tympanosquamous fissure.*

fissurae Plural of FISSURA.

fissural Pertaining to a fissure.

fissuration [*fissur(e)* + -ATION] The formation of furrows or fissures, especially in the cerebral and cerebellar cortices during the development of gyri and folia respectively.

fissure

fissure [L *fissura.* See FISSURA.] FISSURA.

adoccipital fissure A variable sulcus extending from the parieto-occipital sulcus into the caudal precuneus.

Ammon's fissure HIPPOCAMPAL FISSURE.

amygdaline fissure A variable groove near the cerebral temporal pole extending toward the uncus.

anal fissure A mucosal tear of the anus. Also called *fissura in ano, Allingham's ulcer.*

angular fissure FISSURA SPHENOPETROSA.

anterior median fissure of medulla oblongata FISSURA MEDIANA ANTERIOR MEDULLAE OBLONGATAE.

anterior median fissure of spinal cord FISSURA MEDIANA ANTERIOR MEDULLAE SPINALIS.

anterior paracentral fissure A transverse fissure in the frontal lobe motor cerebral cortex approximately parallel to the sulcus centralis and forming the rostral limit of the precentral gyrus.

anterior tympanosquamous fissure FISSURA TYMPANOSQUAMOSA.

antitragohelicine fissure FISSURA ANTITRAGOHELICINA.

ape fissure An obsolete term for SULCUS LUNATUS.

fissure of aqueduct of vestibule APERTURA EXTERNA AQUEDUCTUS VESTIBULI.

arciform fissure HIPPOCAMPAL FISSURE.

arcuate fissure A major fissure of the monkey brain that passes laterally from the medial margin of the cerebrum and demarcates the frontal eye field anteriorly from motor areas behind.

auricular fissure of temporal bone FISSURA TYMPANOMASTOIDEA.

azygos fissure A fissure in the right upper lung field which separates an accessory lobe, the azygos lobe, from the remainder of the right upper lobe. The fissure contains four rather than two layers of pleura (two visceral and two parietal), and an elliptic density representing the azygos vein can often be seen somewhere along the course of the fissure.

basal fissure DECIDUAL FISSURE.

basilar fissure FISSURA SPHENO-OCCIPITALIS.

basisylvian fissure In the human brain, the portion of the sulcus lateralis cerebri (sylvian fissure) extending down from the temporal lobe toward the orbital surface of the frontal lobe.

fissure of Bichat FISSURA TRANSVERSA CEREBRI.

branchial fissures BRANCHIAL CLEFTS.

Broca's fissure Branches of the sulcus lateralis cerebri of the inferior frontal lobule associated with Broca's motor speech area on the left hemisphere of humans.

Burdach's fissure The hidden circumferential cleft that separates the insula from the operculum.

calcarine fissure SULCUS CALCARINUS.

callosal fissure SULCUS CORPORIS CALLOSI.

callosomarginal fissure SULCUS CINGULI.

central fissure SULCUS CENTRALIS CEREBRI.

cerebral fissures SULCI CEREBRI.

cerebral fissure of Bichat FISSURA TRANSVERSA CEREBRI.

fissures of cerebrum SULCI CEREBRI.

cervical fissure An epithelially lined opening on the side of the neck that is a persistent remnant of one of the embryonic branchial grooves. It may be the external termination of either a sinus tract or a fistula connecting with the pharynx.

choroid fissure A fissure present in the brain of the human embryo from the third month. It arches upwards and backwards from the interventricular foramen on the medial aspect of the telencephalon. It marks the invagination of the medial wall of the developing hemisphere by vascular tissue which will constitute the choroid plexus of the lateral ventricle. Also called *fetal fissure.*

choroidal fissure of eye A cleft on the inferior aspect of the embryonic optic vesicle continuing on to the optic stalk, resulting from the original invagination of the optic vesicle also involving its under side. The tips of the cleft close during the seventh week in human development. Also called *optic fissure, fetal fissure of optic cup.*

Clevenger's fissure SULCUS TEMPORALIS INFERIOR.

collateral fissure SULCUS COLLATERALIS.

corneal fissure An apparent groove in the scleral margin in which the cornea fits and which is created by the sclera encroaching more upon the cornea anteriorly than posteriorly. An outmoded term. Also called *rima cornealis, corneal cleft.*

craniofacial fissure In comparative anatomy, a vertical fissure dividing the mesethmoid, or median cranial, bone of vertebrates.

crucial fissure An obsolete term for CRUCIATE SULCUS.

decidual fissure A space of cleft developing in the decidua basalis toward the end of pregnancy. Also called *basal fissure.*

dentate fissure SULCUS HIPPOCAMPI.

fissure of ductus venosus A fissure on the inferior aspect of the developing liver. The depression becomes deeper as the liver grows and is the fissure of the ductus venosus. When the ductus venosus closes after birth and becomes a fibrous remnant it lies in a deep cleft lying between the left lobe and the caudate lobe of the liver then called the fissure for ligamentum venosum. Also called *fissure of the venous ligament, fossa ductus venosi, fossa of ductus venosus, fossa chordae ductus venosi.*

Duverney's fissures INCISURAE CARTILAGINIS MEATUS ACUSTICI.

Ecker's fissure SULCUS OCCIPITALIS TRANSVERSUS.

enamel fissure A cleft in the surface of the crown of a tooth produced by a localized deficiency of enamel.

entorbital fissure An inconstant sulcus on the base of the human frontal lobe lying between the orbital and olfactory sulci.

ethmoid fissure An outmoded term for MEATUS NASI SUPERIOR.

fetal fissure CHOROID FISSURE.

fetal fissure of optic cup CHOROIDAL FISSURE OF EYE.

floccular fissure FISSURA POSTEROLATERALIS CEREBELLI.

genitovesical fissure A groove between the genital cord and the bladder of the fetus which in the female becomes the excavation between the uterus and the bladder.

glaserian fissure FISSURA PETROTYMPANICA.

fissure of glottis RIMA GLOTTIDIS.

great fissure of cerebrum FISSURA TRANSVERSA CEREBRI.

great horizontal fissure FISSURA HORIZONTALIS CEREBELLI.

great transverse fissure of cerebrum FISSURA TRANSVERSA CEREBRI.

Henle's fissures The slitlike spaces between anastomosing cardiac muscle fibers, containing a delicate endomysium with capillaries and lymphatics. An outmoded term.

hippocampal fissure 1 In a human embryo of about two months, a longitudinal fissure with an inferior concavity extending from the interventricular foramen to the temporal lobe. Also called *Ammon's fissure, arciform fissure.* **2** SULCUS HIPPOCAMPI.

fissure of hippocampus SULCUS HIPPOCAMPI.

horizontal fissure of cerebellum FISSURA HORIZONTALIS CEREBELLI.

horizontal fissure of right lung FISSURA HORIZONTALIS PULMONIS DEXTRI.

inferior orbital fissure FISSURA ORBITALIS INFERIOR.

inferior sphenoidal fissure An outmoded term for FISSURA ORBITALIS INFERIOR.

inferofrontal fissure SULCUS FRONTALIS INFERIOR.

intercerebral fissure FISSURA LONGITUDINALIS CEREBRI.

intercotyledonary fissures Fissures or grooves which separate the cotyledons on the maternal aspect of the placenta.

interparietal fissure SULCUS INTRAPARIETALIS.

intratonsillar fissure FOSSA SUPRATONSILLARIS.

lacrimal fissure SULCUS LACRIMALIS.

lateral cerebral fissure SULCUS LATERALIS CEREBRI.

lateral fissure of cerebrum SULCUS LATERALIS CEREBRI.

left hepatic fissure An intrahepatic plane that functionally separates the left lateral segments drained by the left hepatic veins from the left medial segments drained by the intermediate hepatic veins. The plane corresponds externally to a line between the right and left anatomical lobes of the liver. An outmoded term.

left portal fissure An intrahepatic plane that is situated transversely in the left lobe to the left of the fissure for ligamentum teres and fissure for ligamentum venosum. It separates the superior from the inferior parts of the left lateral segment. It lies in the line of the course of the left hepatic vein.

fissure for ligamentum teres FISSURA LIGAMENTI TERETIS.

fissure for ligamentum venosum FISSURA LIGAMENTI VENOSI.

linguogingival fissure A fissure on the lingual surface of an upper incisor tooth extending from the lingual fossa towards the root.

longitudinal fissure FISSURA LONGITUDINALIS CEREBRI.

longitudinal fissure of cerebellum VALLECULA CEREBELLI.

longitudinal fissure of cerebrum FISSURA LONGITUDINALIS CEREBRI.

mandibular fissures Grooves present in the lower part of the embryonic face where the mandibular arches come together in the midline and where they are in contact with the maxillary processes.

maxillary fissure A groove posterior to the maxillary hiatus that is converted into the greater palatine canal by the perpendicular plate of the palatine bone. An outmoded term.

fissure of Monro SULCUS HYPOTHALAMICUS.

oblique fissure of lung FISSURA OBLIQUA PULMONIS.

occipital fissure FISSURA PETRO-OCCIPITALIS.

occipitosphenoidal fissure FISSURA SPHENO-OCCIPITALIS.

optic fissure CHOROIDAL FISSURE OF EYE.

oral fissure RIMA ORIS.

palatine fissure An oblique groove at the base of and behind the inferior angle of the hiatus of the maxillary sinus into which the maxillary process of the palatine bone fits. An outmoded term.

fissure of palpebrae RIMA PALPEBRARUM.

palpebral fissure RIMA PALPEBRARUM.

Pansch's fissure SULCUS INTRAPARIETALIS.

parafloccular fissure The indentation between the flocculus and paraflocculus of the cerebellum.

parieto-occipital fissure SULCUS PARIETO-OCCIPITALIS.

parietosphenoid fissure INCISURA PARIETALIS OSSIS TEMPORALIS.

paroccipital fissure The caudal portion of the sulcus interparietalis extending towards the occipital lobe of the cerebrum. An obsolete term.

petrobasilar fissure FISSURA PETRO-OCCIPITALIS.

petromastoid fissure FISSURA TYMPANOMASTOIDEA.

petro-occipital fissure FISSURA PETRO-OCCIPITALIS.

petrosphenoidal fissure FISSURA SPHENOPETROSA.

petrosquamous fissure FISSURA PETROSQUAMOSA.

petrotympanic fissure FISSURA PETROTYMPANICA.

portal fissure PORTA HEPATIS.

postcentral fissure SULCUS POSTCENTRALIS.

posterior fissure of auricle FISSURA ANTITRAGOHELICINA.

posterior median fissure of medulla oblongata SULCUS MEDIANUS POSTERIOR MEDULLAE OBLONGATAE.

posterior median fissure of spinal cord SULCUS MEDIANUS POSTERIOR MEDULLAE SPINALIS.

posterior petrosquamous fissure A vestige of a segment of the petrosquamous fissure that is visible on the external surface of the temporal bone at the union of the mastoid process and the squamous part of the temporal bone. It is directed anteriorly and downwards from the parietal notch to the anterior border of the mastoid process. An outmoded term.

posterolateral fissure SULCUS POSTEROLATERALIS CEREBELLI.

postlingual fissure The superior, transverse cerebellar fissure separating the lingula from the lobus centralis.

postlunate fissure The superior, transverse cerebellar fissure between the lunate and ansiform lobule.

postpyramidal fissure The fissure separating the cerebellar pyramis from the tuber vermis.

postrhinal fissure The caudal continuation of the rhinal fissure, separating the posterior entorhinal cortex from the occipital neocortex. A seldom used term.

precentral fissure SULCUS PRECENTRALIS.

preculminative fissure An outmoded term for SULCUS POSTCENTRALIS.

precuneal fissure A variable fissure in the rostral cuneus of the cerebrum.

prepyramidal fissure The fissure separating the cerebellar pyramis and uvula.

presylvian fissure The rostral continuation of the sulcus lateralis cerebri.

primary fissure FISSURA PRIMA CEREBELLI.

pterygoid fissure INCISURA PTERYGOIDEA.

pterygomaxillary fissure FISSURA PTERYGOMAXILLARIS.

pterygopalatine fissure FISSURA PTERYGOMAXILLARIS.

pterygopalatine fissure of palatine bone SULCUS PALATINUS MAJOR OSSIS PALATINI.

pterygotympanic fissure An outmoded term for FISSURA PETROTYMPANICA.

pudendal fissure RIMA PUDENDI.

fissure of pudendum RIMA PUDENDI.

retrotonsillar fissure A deep fissure on the inferior surface of the cerebellar hemisphere anterior to the biventral lobule and posterior to the tonsil of the cerebellum. It is continuous with the anterior part of the sulcus valleculae, which also bounds the tonsil.

rhinal fissure **1** The sulcus or fissure which demarcates the olfactory cortex or rhinencephalon from adjacent regions of the cerebral surface. In the human brain it lies lateral to the uncus. Also called *rhinal sulcus.* **2** SULCUS RHINALIS.

right hepatic fissure **1** An intrahepatic plane which functionally separates the liver segments drained by the right hepatic veins from those drained by the intermediate hepatic veins. Although the line of demarcation is not clear, as a particular segment is drained by more than one hepatic vein, it has been placed to the right of the right portal fissure. An outmoded term. **2** A caudolateral extension in the liver substance from the right margin of the porta hepatis. It contains vessels and ducts and is filled with connective tissue.

right portal fissure An intrahepatic anteroposterior plane that separates the anterior and posterior segments of the right lobe from the paramedian or middle segment of the right lobe. It follows the course of the right hepatic vein. An outmoded term.

fissure of Rolando SULCUS CENTRALIS CEREBRI.

fissure of round ligament FISSURA LIGAMENTI TERETIS.

sagittal portal fissure An intrahepatic plane that extends through the fossa for the gallbladder to the left side of the fossa for the inferior vena cava. It divides the liver into right and left functional lobes, according to the distribution of the right and left hepatic vessels and bile ducts. It passes along the course of the intermediate hepatic vein.

sagittal fissure of liver FOSSA SAGITTALIS SINISTRA HEPATIS.

Santorini's fissures INCISURAE CARTILAGINIS MEATUS ACUSTICI.

Schwalbe's fissure FISSURA CHOROIDEA.

sclerotomic fissure Loosening of cells which occurs transitorily to subdivide each sclerotomic segment into a cranial and a caudal half around the notochord and which becomes incorporated in the perichordal disk.

secondary fissure FISSURA SECUNDA CEREBELLI.

simian fissure An obsolete term for SULCUS LUNATUS.

sphenoidal fissure An outmoded term for FISSURA ORBITALIS SUPERIOR.

sphenomaxillary fissure **1** An outmoded term for FISSURA ORBITALIS INFERIOR. **2** An outmoded term for FOSSA PTERYGOPALATINA.

spheno-occipital fissure FISSURA SPHENO-OCCIPITALIS.

sphenopetrosal fissure FISSURA SPHENOPETROSA.

squamotympanic fissure FISSURA TYMPANOSQUAMOSA.

subfrontal fissure SULCUS FRONTALIS INFERIOR.

subsylvian fissure **1** The posterior branch of the sulcus lateralis cerebri. **2** A variable posterolateral fissure on the base of the frontal lobe. An obsolete term.

subtemporal fissure A variable fissure in the inferior temporal gyrus.

superficial petrosal fissure   HIATUS CANALIS NERVI PETROSI MAJORIS.

superior anterior fissure   FISSURA PRIMA CEREBELLI.

superior orbital fissure   FISSURA ORBITALIS SUPERIOR.

superior petrosquamous fissure   A segment of the petrosquamous fissure that is visible on the endocranial surface of the temporal bone at the junction of the squamous and petrous parts. An outmoded term.

superior sphenoidal fissure   An outmoded term for FISSURA ORBITALIS SUPERIOR.

supertemporal fissure   SULCUS TEMPORALIS SUPERIOR.

supraorbital fissure   An outmoded term for INCISURA SUPRAORBITALIS.

sylvian fissure   SULCUS LATERALIS CEREBRI.

fissure of Sylvius   SULCUS LATERALIS CEREBRI.

tentorial fissure   That portion of the sulcus collateralis above the tentorial notch. An obsolete term.

tracheopharyngeal fissure   An outmoded term for LARYNGOTRACHEAL GROOVE.

transtemporal fissure   A variable, short, transverse fissure on the lateral temporal lobe.

transverse fissure   PORTA HEPATIS.

transverse fissure of cerebellum   FISSURA TRANSVERSA CEREBELLI.

transverse fissure of cerebrum   FISSURA TRANSVERSA CEREBRI.

transverse occipital fissure   SULCUS OCCIPITALIS TRANSVERSUS.

tympanic fissure   FISSURA PETROTYMPANICA.

tympanomastoid fissure   FISSURA TYMPANOMASTOIDEA.

tympanosquamous fissure   1 FISSURA TYMPANOSQUAMOSA. 2 An outmoded term for FISSURA PETROTYMPANICA.

umbilical fissure   An outmoded term for FISSURA LIGAMENTI TERETIS.

urogenital fissure   RIMA PUDENDI.

fissure of the venous ligament   FISSURE OF DUCTUS VENOSUS.

vestibular fissure of the cochlea   A slitlike gap between the free edge of the projecting osseous spiral lamina and the tip of the secondary spiral lamina that projects inwards from the outer wall of the lower part of the first turn of the bony cochlea.

fissure of the vestibule   RIMA VESTIBULI.

zygal fissure   An H-shaped configuration produced by a transverse fissue linking two parallel cerebral fissures.

zygomaticosphenoid fissure   SUTURA SPHENOZYGOMATICA.

fistula

fistula [L (akin to Gaelic *fead* to whistle and Gk *physan* to blow, puff, with breath or bellows, from *physa* bellows), a whistle, pipe, reed, fistula, sinuous ulcer, water pipe] (*plural* fistulas, fistulae) An abnormal communication between two normally unconnected structures, body cavities, or the surface of the body.

abdominal fistula   A communicating tract between an abdominal organ and the external surface of the abdomen.

alveolar fistula   ALVEOLAR SINUS.

anal fistula   A fistula with one end opening onto the mucosal epithelium of the anus or nearby skin. Also called *perirectal fistula, hedrosyrinx.*

antral fistula   A communication that is surgically fashioned between the maxillary antrum and the nasal passages. It is created to facilitate drainage in cases of chronic sinusitis.

aortocaval fistula   A communication that develops between the aorta and the inferior vena cava, usually between the infrarenal aorta and vena cava because of an aortic aneurysm. It may occasionally occur as a result of penetrating abdominal trauma.

aortoduodenal fistula   See under AORTOENTERIC FISTULA.

aortoenteric fistula   A communication that develops between the aorta and the gastrointestinal tract. It is most common between the proximal suture line of an aortic prosthesis and the nearby duodenum (referred to as an aortoduodenal fistula), forming as a consequence of a pseudoaneurysm at the suture line. It may rarely develop primarily between an aortic aneurysm and the overlying bowel.

arteriovenous fistula   An abnormal communication between an artery and a vein, allowing shunting of blood from the arterial system. It may either result from trauma or be congenital.

fistula auris congenita   Preauricular sinus.

biliary fistula   An abnormal communication between the gallbladder or other part of the biliary tree and another cavity or the cutaneous surface of the body.

fistula bimucosa   An abnormal passage both ends of which open on mucosal surfaces.

blind fistula   An abnormal passage arising on an internal organ or the skin and ending in a cul-de-sac. Also called *incomplete fistula.*

branchial fistula   An abnormal passage representing persistence of the embryonic branchial system of arches, grooves, and pouches. The position of the fistula depends upon which of the four arches and associated grooves and pouches have persisted. In all instances the embryonic pharynx or one of its derivatives communicates with the exterior through a persistent external groove or fissure on the side of the face or neck. Also called *cervicoaural fistula.*

Brescia-Cimino fistula   RADIOCEPHALIC FISTULA.

bronchobiliary fistula   A fistula between a bronchus and intrahepatic bile ducts. It may be a complication of trauma or hepatic abscesses with transdiaphragmatic extension into the chest.

bronchoesophageal fistula   An abnormal communication between a bronchus and the esophagus allowing aspiration of esophageal contents into the lungs. This type of fistula may occur in association with an erosive tumor involving either of these structures. Also called *esophagobronchial fistula.*

bronchopleural fistula   An abnormal communication between a bronchus and the pleural cavity. Also called *pleurobronchial fistula.*

caroticocavernous fistula   A rupture of the intracavernous portion of the internal carotid artery, allowing arterial blood to pass directly into the venous sinus. It usually results either from trauma or from aneurysmal rupture. Also called *carotid-cavernous fistula.*

carotid-cavernous fistula   CAROTICOCAVERNOUS FISTULA.

cerebrospinal fluid fistula   A fistula, caused by injury or disease or complicating surgical procedures on the ear, nose or paranasal sinuses, by which cerebrospinal fluid escapes from the ear or nose or, having passed via the nasopharynx, is swallowed.

cervical fistula   A branchial fistula representing abnormal persistence of the epithelial tissues of the second, third, or fourth embryonic branchial arch, which connects the pharynx with the exterior. The external opening is on the side of the neck, as opposed to being on the face anterior to the auricle. Also called *fistula colli congenita.*

cervicoaural fistula   BRANCHIAL FISTULA.

fistula cervicovaginalis laqueatica   A fistulous communication between the uterine cervix and the vagina.

cholecystoduodenal fistula   A communication between the gallbladder and the duodenum resulting from chronic irritation and inflammation of the gallbladder and adjacent duodenal wall, a complication of severe cholecystitis. Large gallstones may pass through the fistula into the duodenum and be carried distally where they may cause intestinal obstruction. This condition may be diagnosed by radiographic evidence of intrabiliary air.

chylous fistula A fistula resulting in an external leakage of chyle as a result of injury to the abdominal lymphatics, especially the cisterna magna.

fistula cibalis An outmoded term for ESOPHAGUS.

fistula colli congenita CERVICAL FISTULA.

colocutaneous fistula A fistula between colon and skin.

coloileal fistula A fistula between colon and ileum.

colonic fistula A fistula with one end opening into the colon.

colovaginal fistula A fistula between colon and vagina.

complete fistula A pathological communication between two sites, one end of which may open to a mucosal or cutaneous surface.

congenital fistula of the auricle PREAURICULAR SINUS.

congenital preauricular fistula PREAURICULAR SINUS.

congenital rectourethral fistula CONGENITAL URETHRO-RECTAL FISTULA.

congenital urethrorectal fistula A congenital anomaly resulting from incomplete separation of the rectum from the posterior urethral segment of the bladder, permitting passage of urine through the rectum and feces through the urethra. Also called *congenital rectourethral fistula.*

fistula corneae A corneal perforation that remains open and continues to leak aqueous humor.

craniosinus fistula A fistula between the subarachnoid space of the brain and one of the paranasal sinuses, allowing the flow of cerebrospinal fluid into the nose.

dental fistula A fistula between the apical region of a tooth and the gingival mucosa which may drain pus from an apical abscess. Also called *gingival fistula.*

duodenal fistula A fistula with one end opening into the duodenum.

Eck's fistula A shunt performed in an experimental animal between portal circulation and the vena cava, with ligation of the portal vein close to the liver.

Eck's fistula in reverse Anastomosis of the portal vein to the inferior vena cava with ligation of the vena cava above the anastomosis. Through this arrangement, all blood from the lower body is routed through the hepatic circulation.

enterocutaneous fistula A fistula between the small or large intestine and the abdominal skin.

enterovaginal fistula A fistula between the vagina and an adjacent portion of intestine, usually the rectum.

enterovesical fistula A fistula between the urinary bladder and an adherent portion of intestine.

esophagobronchial fistula BRONCHOESOPHAGEAL FISTULA.

esophagotracheal fistula TRACHEOESOPHAGEAL FISTULA.

external fistula A fistula between an internal organ and the skin, generally accompanied by inflammation and drainage to the outside.

fecal fistula A fistula between the lumen of the distal intestine and the abdominal skin which discharges feces to the outside. This type of fistula can be a sequel of any process that results in intestinal perforation, such as diverticulitis, regional enteritis, carcinoma, radiation damage, or the passage of a foreign body. Also called *intestinal fistula, stercoral fistula.*

frontal sinus fistula A fistula in the fronto-orbital region leading into the frontal sinus. It occasionally persists at the site of drainage of frontal sinus suppuration or of frontal sinus mucocele. It can occur, though rarely, as the result of trauma or of surgical excision.

gastric fistula An abnormal passage through the abdominal wall communicating the lumen of the stomach with the outside.

A surgically created passage (gastrostomy) is often created for feeding purposes.

gastrocolic fistula A fistula between the stomach and the colon. It is usually a complication of gastric surgery for peptic ulcer, or it may result from neoplastic invasion.

gastroduodenal fistula A fistula between stomach and duodenum.

gastrojejunal fistula An abnormal communication between the stomach and the jejunum. It may develop as a complication of marginal ulcer following surgery for peptic ulcer.

gingival fistula DENTAL FISTULA.

hepatic fistula A fistula between the liver and another structure.

horseshoe fistula An anal fistula forming a semicircular tract communicating at both extremities with the surface of the perianal skin.

fistula in ano A fistulous tract in close proximity to the anus that opens to the surface of the skin and may communicate with the rectum.

incomplete fistula BLIND FISTULA.

internal fistula A fistula between two internal, generally hollow, organs.

intestinal fistula FECAL FISTULA.

lacrimal fistula An abnormal communication between the lacrimal duct or sac and the external skin of the periorbital area.

lacteal fistula A fistula between a lactiferous duct and the periareolar skin of the breast.

fistula of lip A very rare hereditary defect at the margin of the lower lip, consisting of a small pit 5–25 mm long. It is usually bilateral and is associated with other deformities, such as clefts.

lymphatic fistula An abnormal communication with a lymphatic vessel allowing drainage of lymph out of the lymphatic system. This type of fistula is often congenital and found in the neck.

Mann-Bollman fistula An artificial communication produced surgically for experimental purposes: a segment of intestine is isolated, the proximal end is sutured to the abdominal wall and the distal end is anastomosed side to side to the proximal jejunum or duodenum. Due to intrinsic peristalsis, there is minimal leakage through the abdominal wall, and food as well as other substances can be administered directly through the abdominal orifice.

mediastinobronchial fistula A fistula between a bronchus and the mediastinal cavity. It may be a complication of lung resection in which the bronchial stump leaks into the mediastinum.

mucus fistula DRY COLOSTOMY.

oroantral fistula An abnormal communicating passage between the maxillary sinus and the oral cavity, occurring most commonly in the region of the first or second molar teeth following surgical manipulation of that area or infection of the maxillary sinus.

orofacial fistula A communication between the inside of the mouth and the surface of the face, usually in the region of the cheek.

oronasal fistula A fistula between the interior of the mouth and the nose, usually through the hard palate. The causes include neoplastic and granulomatous ulceration and certain surgical procedures, sometimes for the relief of such diseases. Rarely, accidental trauma may be responsible.

parietal fistula An abnormal passage through the abdominal or thoracic wall that either ends blindly or communicates with some external structure.

perilymph fistula A fistula between the periotic compartment of the inner ear and the middle ear, permitting the escape of perilymph into the tympanic cavity. It occurs usually in the oval window region as a complication of stapedectomy.

perirectal fistula   ANAL FISTULA.

pharyngeal fistula   An abnormal, often congenital passage communicating the pharynx with the skin of the neck.

pilonidal fistula   PILONIDAL SINUS FISTULA.

pilonidal sinus fistula   A sinus tract developed in the subcutaneous tissues of the intergluteal fold that opens to the outside at a point located from four to five cm posterior to the anus. Seen most commonly among young white males with straight black hair, this lesion is a giant cell foreign body reaction to inverted hairs that lodge in the dermis in skin folds subject to irritation and inflammation. These sinuses frequently become infected, causing chronic suppuration and requiring surgical removal. Also called *pilonidal fistula*.

pleurobronchial fistula   BRONCHOPLEURAL FISTULA.

pleurocutaneous fistula   A communication between the pleural cavity and the skin.

preauricular fistula   Preauricular sinus.

pulmonary fistula   A pathological communication between the thoracic wall and the underlying lung.

radiocephalic fistula   An anastomosis of the radial artery and cephalic vein at the wrist. It is usually created to bring about the development of large venous channels in the forearm of subjects who require vascular access for hemodialysis. Also called *Brescia-Cimino fistula*.

rectovaginal fistula   An abnormal communication between the rectum and vagina often resulting in serious infections of the vaginal mucosa ascending to the cervix.

rectovesical fistula   An abnormal communication between the urinary bladder and the rectum often resulting from tumor invasion. It causes severe cystitis and the presence of gas and feces in the urine.

salivary fistula   An abnormal communication from a salivary duct allowing drainage of saliva to the outside or into the oral cavity through a newly formed passage.

spermatic fistula   A fistula communicating with either the seminal ducts or the testicular parenchyma.

stercoral fistula   FECAL FISTULA.

submental fistula   A form of salivary fistula connecting a salivary duct with a cutaneous opening below the chin.

Thiry's fistula   An artificially produced isolation of a segment of intestine for the purpose of collecting intestinal juice for experimental use. The procedure generally involves isolation of a loop of intestine, attachment of one end to the abdominal wall for drainage, and occlusion of the other end.

Thiry-Vella fistula   An isolated loop of intestine, one end of which is closed and the other exteriorized through the abdominal wall. It is used to study intestinal secretions.

thoracic fistula   A fistula through the thoracic wall that communicates with the pulmonary parenchyma or a loculated portion of the pleural cavity.

tracheoesophageal fistula   A communication between the esophagus and trachea. It is a life-threatening condition that can be either congenital or acquired. As a congenital condition it occurs almost always in association with congenital esophageal atresia, and in acquired cases it is usually a complication of esophageal carcinoma, the result of the misuse of cuffed tracheostomy tubes, or, rarely, due to the presence of impacted esophageal foreign bodies. Also called *esophagotracheal fistula*.

umbilical fistula   A fistula between the intestine and umbilicus resulting from patency of the vitello-intestinal duct after birth. When the umbilical cord is cut, an open intestinal fistula is formed. Intestinal obstruction resulting from evagination and prolapse of intestinal loops through the fistula is a serious and life-threatening complication.

urachal fistula   An abnormal communication between the urachus and other internal structures, most commonly the rectum.

Rarely, the fistula is between the urachus and the bladder, resulting in escape of urine through the umbilicus.

ureterocervical fistula   An abnormal communication between the cervix and the ureter.

urinary fistula   An abnormal communication of the urinary tract with other internal structures allowing drainage of urine from the system and predisposing to ascending urinary tract infections.

uterovesical fistula   An abnormal communication between the uterus and the urinary bladder.

Vella's fistula   An isolated loop of intestine, both ends of which are exteriorized through the abdominal wall. It is used to study intestinal secretions.

vesical fistula   Any abnormal communication of the urinary bladder with other structures.

vesicoabdominal fistula   A fistula between the urinary bladder and the abdominal skin.

vesicocolonic fistula   An abnormal communication between the urinary bladder and the colon.

vesicoenteric fistula   An abnormal communication between the urinary bladder and the intestinal tract.

vesicointestinal fistula   An abnormal communication between the urinary bladder and the intestine.

vesicorectal fistula   An abnormal communication between the urinary bladder and the rectum.

vesicoumbilical fistula   A fistulous connection between the urinary bladder and the umbilicus, representing persistence of the embryonic continuity between the cloaca and the allantois. The fistula courses through the urachus and allows urine to escape at the umbilicus.

vesicovaginal fistula   An abnormal communication between the urinary bladder and the vagina, often resulting from erosion by advanced carcinoma of the cervix.

vitelline fistula   A persistence of the embryonic vitelline duct between the terminal ileum and the umbilicus, allowing fecal material to escape at the umbilicus.

---

fistulae   Plural of FISTULA.

fistulation   FISTULIZATION.

fistulatome [FISTULA + -TOME]   A surgical instrument used to incise a fistula.

fistulectomy [*fistul(a)* + -ECTOMY]   A surgical procedure in which a fistula or extra-anatomic communication is removed. Also called *syringectomy*.

fistulization   The formation of an abnormal communication between two structures, one of which is usually a hollow organ or cavity. Also called *fistulation*.

fistulization of the eyeball   The surgical creation of an artificial channel for escape of the aqueous humor from the eye, a therapy for glaucoma.

fistulize   **1** To make (a fistula) surgically. **2** To develop a fistula, as by a disease process.

fistuloenterostomy   A surgical operation for repair of a biliary or pancreatic fistula, in which a permanent connection is established between the fistula and the small intestine and the abnormal opening is closed.

fistulography [*fistul(a)* + *o* + -GRAPHY]   Radiographic examination of a fistulous tract after injecting it with an opaque contrast medium through its external orifice.

fistulotomy [*fistul(a)* + *o* + -TOMY]   A surgical incision into a fistula. Also called *syringotomy*.

fistulous   Pertaining to the presence of a fistula.

fit [Old English *fitt* a strife]   **1** An epileptic seizure. ● *Fit* in this sense is still used in Britain as a neutral, descriptive term without pejorative connotation, but in the United States and Canada it is outmoded in medical contexts. The disparaging connotations associated with its nonmedical uses have imparted an unintended judgmental quality to the word even in medical contexts. Thus, in the U.S. and Canada, *seizure* and *convulsion* are preferred, whereas in Britain all three terms are considered equivalent. Usage in South Africa, Australia, and New Zealand accords with that of the United Kingdom. **2** Accuracy of adaptation of a dental restoration to its site.

ague fit A chill followed by a fever, as in a malarial attack. A popular usage.

cerebellar fit TONIC FIT.

jacksonian fit An attack of focal epilepsy. • See note at FIT.

tetanoid fit An obsolete term for TONIC EPILEPSY.

tonic fit An attack of tonic epilepsy. Also called *cerebellar fit.* • See note at FIT.

uncinate fit UNCINATE ATTACK.

visual fits Any attack of focal epilepsy accompanied or preceded by hallucinations or other visual phenomena. • See note at FIT.

fitness Good health or physical condition.

darwinian fitness The capability of an organism for transmitting its genome to progeny relative to the average capability of the population or to some reference genotype. Also called *adaptive value.*

genetic fitness The capability of an organism for transmitting its genome to progeny.

physical fitness The capacity of the body to perform, especially in terms of voluntary movement.

fitness to plead See under COMPETENCY TO STAND TRIAL.

reproductive fitness The capability of an organism for reproducing, usually relative to the population average. Also called *survival value.*

Fitz [Reginald Heber *Fitz*, U.S. physician 1843–1913] Fitz syndrome. See under LAW.

Fitz Gerald [William Henry Hope *Fitz Gerald*, U.S. physician, 1872–1939] Fitz Gerald method, Fitz Gerald treatment. See under ZONE THERAPY.

Fitz-Hugh [Thomas *Fitz-Hugh*, Jr., U.S. physician, 1894–1963] Curtis and Fitz-Hugh syndrome. See under SYNDROME.

fix In microscopy, to preserve and render suitable for sectioning and staining.

fixate To direct the gaze of (the eye) at a particular point (fixation point).

fixation [Med L *fixatio* (from L *fix(us)*, past part. of *figere* to fix, fasten, affix + *-atio* -ATION) an act of fixing or fixating] **1** The act of directing vision at a given point. **2** Persistence of libidinal or aggressive cathexis at an infantile level to a greater than usual degree, thereby constituting a focus for subsequent regression and expression of neurotic conflicts. Also called *psychic inertia.* **3** In genetics, the attainment of a given allele of a gene frequency of 1.0, either by drift or by selection. Also called *fixing.* **4** In chemistry, the formation of a stable compound. **5** The preservation of tissue for microscopic analysis, usually by immersion in a substance, as alcohol, that quickly kills and hardens it. **6** The act of immobilizing fragments of fractured bone, as with pins or screws.

alexin fixation An obsolete term for COMPLEMENT FIXATION.

arch bar fixation A method of holding the upper teeth firmly in occlusion with the lower teeth, used in the treatment of fractures of the jaws. Narrow strips of malleable metal, having small hooks attached at intervals, are wired to the outside of each dental arch, and the hooks of the upper arch bar are connected to those of the lower with rubber bands or wires.

autotrophic fixation **1** The fixation of energy from the sun into organic form by a plant. **2** The synthesis of organic compounds by a primary producer.

binocular fixation Simultaneous observation of the object of regard by foveas of both eyes.

biphase external pin fixation The substitution of the metal bar of an external fixator with the more versatile acrylic cement following reduction of a fracture.

complement fixation The removal of components of complement from serum by reaction with immune complexes, antibody-coated cells or bacteria, or other material that activates complement. Also called *fixation phenomenon, Moreschi phenomenon, Gengou phenomenon, Bordet-Gengou phenomenon, alexin fixation* (obsolete), *Bordet and Gengou reaction, fixation reaction, complement fixation reaction.* See also COMPLEMENT FIXATION TEST.

elastic band fixation **1** Any fixation of small parts using elastic bands. **2** Immobilization of facial fractures accomplished by placing wires around the teeth and holding the jaws together with elastic bands. **3** A dynamic splint, usually used to position the fingers, using elastic bands.

external pin fixation A method of securing the fractured parts of the mandible using metal pins which penetrate the skin and underlying tissues and are fixed into the bone. The outer ends are linked together with metal bars.

false associated fixation Observation of the object of regard by a nonmacular area with an eye suffering from suppression amblyopia.

father fixation An inordinate attachment to one's father.

freudian fixation The abnormal persistence of libidinal or aggressive cathexis on an object or stage of early development.

intermaxillary fixation MAXILLOMANDIBULAR FIXATION.

internal fixation The maintenance of a fracture reduction by the application of bone plates, screws, pins, wires, or any other means involving a surgical implant.

intramedullary fixation A method of maintaining fracture reduction and stabilization in a long bone in which a metal rod is inserted in the medullary canal of the bone across the fracture site.

intraosseous fixation A method of securing the fractured parts of the mandible or maxilla by means of wires, pins, plates, or screws, which are covered by the tissues after being put in place.

maxillomandibular fixation **1** A method of securing the fractured parts of the maxilla or mandible by pulling the opposing teeth towards each other with wire and elastics, so that the uninjured jaw supports the injured. **2** The fixing of the normal jaws together by means of wires as a treatment for obesity. Also called *intermaxillary fixation.*

mother fixation An inordinate attachment to one's mother.

nasomandibular fixation A method of securing the fractured mandible, especially when both jaws are edentulous, using a Gunning splint which is fixed to the mandible by means of circummandibular wiring and to the maxilla by intraosseous wiring through the nasal process of the maxilla.

nitrogen fixation One of the phases of the nitrogen cycle in nature in which molecular nitrogen, N_2, is transformed into nitrates and ammonia. This fixation may be chemical, biologic, or electrical. The chemical process involves transformation into ammonia, followed by conversion of this into ammonium sulfate, urea, cyanamide, and nitrate. The biologic process occurs only in prokaryotes. It is rapid in certain blue-green bacteria (cyanobacteria) and in *Rhizobium* and *Azobacter* species, but it also occurs in many other species, including *Klebsiella*. The electrical process occurs in thunderstorms when ammonium nitrate is synthesized and is found dissolved in rain water.

parent fixation An inordinate attachment to one or both parents.

postural fixation A method of correcting a bone or joint deformity by the use of slings and splints.

reflex ocular fixation The normal mechanism whereby the eyes fix upon and follow a moving object.

Roger Anderson pin fixation A method of immobilization of fractures by means of pins driven into the bone from the surface. It was developed in 1936 and used extensively during World War II.

skeletal fixation The immobilization of a part or joint in which metal wires or pins are placed directly through bone and are then attached to external traction devices.

fixation of tissues The use of chemical substances such as formalin and glutaraldehyde to preserve the structure of tissues and cells for histologic and ultrastructural study.

visual fixation The alignment of an eye with the object of regard.

fixative [L *fixus* (past part. of *figere* to fix, fasten, affix) fixed, fastened + -IVE] A chemical agent used in the preparation of a histologic specimen to maintain the essential structure of its constituent elements. Various substances are used for this, such as formaldehyde, which cross-links proteins and renders them insoluble.

aldehyde fixative A histologic fixative that utilizes aldehyde groups to crosslink with lysine residues, thereby stabilizing protein molecules in tissues. Widely used aldehyde fixatives include formaldehyde and glutaraldehyde.

Bouin's fixative BOUIN'S FLUID.

dental fixative DENTURE FIXATIVE.

denture fixative A substance used to improve the adhesion of a denture, especially a full upper denture. It is commonly supplied as a powder (tragacanth) which becomes adhesive when wet, but also occasionally as a paste. Also called *dental fixative*.

glutaraldehyde fixative 1 A fixative used in specimen preparation for electron microscopy, consisting of a 4% solution of glutaraldehyde dissolved in phosphate or cacodylate buffer together with calcium chloride. It is the best general fixative for this purpose, and does not simultaneously stain the tissue. 2 A fixative used in preparation and sterilization of heterograft or allograft cardiac valves.

Helly's fixative HELLY'S FLUID.

Kaiserling's fixative KAISERLING'S FLUID.

lanthanum permanganate fixative A fixative solution used in electron microscopy in which lanthanum and potassium permanganate clearly demonstrate the cell membranes but preserve less well such intracytoplasmic structures as ribosomes.

Maximow's fixative A solution used to prepare tissue for microscopic sectioning. It is a variation of Zenker's fluid.

Palade's fixative A fixative solution, suitable for electron microscopy, that contains osmium tetroxide dissolved in veronal acetate buffer.

paraformaldehyde fixative A fixative solution for use in electron microscopy that contains methanol-free formaldehyde and provides a high standard of tissue preservation.

potassium permanganate fixative A fixative solution for electron microscopy that is based on potassium permanganate.

Rhodin's fixative An isotonic solution for electron microscopy that contains osmium tetroxide dissolved in veronal acetate buffer.

Schaudinn's fixative A solution containing mercuric chloride, alcohol, and acetic acid, used to fix smears for cytologic examination.

Susa fixative A fixative solution based on formol sublimate, with the addition of small quantities of glacial acetic acid and trichloracetic acid to balance the tendency of mercuric chloride

to cause shrinkage of tissues. Also called *Susa fixing fluid, Heidenhain's liquid.*

van Gehuchten's fixative A rapid fixative solution that contains acetic acid, chloroform, and alcohol. Also called *Carnoy's fluid.*

Zenker's fixative ZENKER'S FLUID.

Zenker-formol fixative HELLY'S FLUID.

fixator A rarely used term for ANTIBODY.

fixedness / functional fixedness A lack of flexibility in problem solving in which the individual, having once used an element in one way, later finds it difficult to perceive or to use it in any other way.

fixing FIXATION.

fixity [Med L *fixitas* (from L *fix(us)*, past part. of *figere* to fix, fasten + -*itas* -ITY) an affixing, making fast] Engagement of the fetal head during labor.

fl Symbol for the unit, femtoliter.

fl. fluid.

flabby Characterized by a loss of form and shape, as in a body that undergoes an increase in adipose tissue along with an underuse of muscle.

flabellum [L (from *flabrum* a breeze), a fan] The fanlike array of myelinated fibers in the corpus striatum. An obsolete term.

flaccid Characterized by flaccidity.

flaccidity The property of being soft and relaxed.

Flack [Martin William *Flack*, English physiologist, 1882–1931] Flack's node, Keith-Flack node, sinuatrial node of Keith and Flack. See under NODUS SINUATRIALIS.

flag / sweet flag CALAMUS.

flagella Plural of FLAGELLUM.

flagellantism [L *flagellans*, gen. *flagellantis*, pres. part. of *flagellare* to whip + -ISM] A type of sadism in which the individual derives sexual stimulation from whipping someone or from being whipped. Also called *flagellomania.*

flagellar Pertaining to a flagellum or to organisms possessing flagella.

Flagellata [*flagell(um)* + -ATA] A former name for MASTIGOPHORA.

flagellate [*flagell(um)* + -ATE] 1 Having one or more flagella. 2 An organism having one or more flagella, especially a protozoan of the subphylum Mastigophora. 3 To whip; to subject to flagellation, often implying that the action is a requisite part of the sexual arousal pattern of the beater.

collared flagellate CHOANOFLAGELLATE.

flagellated Having one or more flagella.

flagellation 1 A form of massage in which the trunk or limb is tapped rapidly with the fingers. 2 The whipping or beating of another or oneself as a means of sexual gratification. 3 The formation or arrangement of flagella.

flagelliform Shaped like a flagellum.

flagellin A protein of molecular mass 53 kDa. It is the constituent of the helical filament of a bacterial flagellum.

flagellomania FLAGELLANTISM.

flagellosis [*flagell(ate)* + -OSIS] An infection with flagellate protozoa.

flagellospore An obsolete term for ZOOSPORE.

flagellula An obsolete term for ZOOSPORE.

flagellum [L (dim. of *flagrum*, a whip, scourge, from *fligere* to beat, dash down), a whip, scourge] (*plural* flagella) 1 In protozoa, a locomotor organelle found in all Mastigophora and in intermediate forms of certain amebas and sporozoans. It is the definitive structure of flagellates. It is a filamentous cytoplasmic projection with a central axial filament or axoneme composed of a central and nine peripheral fibrils. The flagellum arises from a basal body. **2** In bacteria, a filament consisting of a helical chain of molecules of a single protein (flagellin) attached by a hooklike sheath to a basal body embedded in the wall and membrane. Locomotion is caused by rotation.

tinsel flagellum A featherlike structure which aids the motility of a zoospore.

whiplash flagellum A simple (as opposed to multiple or complex) organelle of locomotion of a zoospore.

Flagyl A proprietary name for metronidazole.

flail Capable of abnormal mobility, as of a joint, or paradoxical mobility, as of the chest wall following injury.

Flajani [Giuseppe *Flajani*, Italian surgeon, 1741–1808] **1** See under OPERATION. **2** Flajani's disease. See under EXOPHTHALMIC GOITER.

flame [French *flamme* (from L *flamma* a flame, blaze) luminous appearance of combustion] **1** The gaseous material that results from a rapid chemical reaction between a combustible material and oxygen or other oxidizing agent, usually in the form of an ascending cone that gives off energy as heat and light. **2** To expose noncombustible material to a flame for purposes of heat sterilization. **3** To expose combustible material to a flame for purposes of photometric analysis.

capillary flame STORK BITE.

manometric flame A gas flame whose height and characteristics vary with the patterns of gas flow that are determined by changing sound waves.

flange [Possibly from Old French *flangir* to bend, turn] A projecting edge, especially one providing guidance or serving as a means of attachment.

buccal flange The buccal part of a denture flange.

denture flange The part of a denture base that extends into the vestibule of the mouth or into the alveololingual sulcus.

labial flange The labial part of a denture flange.

lingual flange The lingual part of a denture flange.

flank [Middle English *flanke*, from Old French *flanc* flank, from Germanic presumed *hlanka* flank, hip] The side of the trunk between the lowest rib and the iliac crest; latus.

flap

flap [Middle English *flappe*] **1** In reconstructive surgery, one to several associated tissue layers dissected and transferred to a nearby site with an intact blood supply, or separated and transplanted to a distant site, with revascularization through anastomoses of recipient and donor arteries and veins. Also called *surgical flap*. **2** PEDICLE GRAFT. **3** ASTERIXIS.

Abbe flap A cross-lip flap, usually for reconstructing the upper lip. The triangular flap from the central part of the donor lip is rotated through 180 degrees as a small pedicle and sutured into the defect in the other lip. Also called *Abbe lip flap*.

Abbe lip flap ABBE FLAP.

abdominal flap A flap fashioned from the tissues of the abdominal wall.

acromiocervical flap A flap fashioned from the skin and subcutaneous tissues of the shoulder and neck.

acromiopectoral flap A flap fashioned from the skin and subcutaneous tissues of the shoulder and anterior chest wall.

advancement flap SLIDING FLAP.

amputation flap A skin flap used to cover the stump left after the amputation of an extremity.

arterial flap AXIAL FLAP.

arterialized flap AXIAL FLAP.

axial flap A pedicled skin flap which has its blood supplied entirely by a known artery and vein which are in the pedicle and which traverse the flap. Also called *arterialized flap, arterial flap, axial pattern flap*.

axial pattern flap AXIAL FLAP.

axilloabdominal flap THORACOEPIGASTRIC FLAP.

biceps femoris muscle flap A flap consisting of the entire biceps femoris muscle on the back of the thigh. It can cover defects of the trochanter, ischium, and perineum.

biceps femoris myocutaneous flap A biceps femoris muscle flap with the addition of a segment of the overlying skin.

bilobed flap A pedicled flap consisting of a larger tongue and a smaller tongue of tissue, both based on a single stem and the whole somewhat V-shaped. After surgical excision of a lesion not far from the larger tongue, the latter is rotated into the defect to cover it, while the smaller tongue is rotated into the donor defect from the larger tongue. The donor defect from the smaller tongue is closed by undermining the edges and bringing them together with sutures. Also called *Zimany's bilobed flap*.

bipedicle flap A flap devised with a soft tissue attachment at either end, thereby enhancing the vascular supply. Such flaps rarely die but they cannot be moved as far as a single pedicle flap. Also called *double pedicle flap, bridge flap*.

Björk flap A rectangular flap from the anterior tracheal wall, hinged downwards and stitched to the lower lip of the skin incision so as to facilitate the introduction of the tube in tracheostomy.

bone flap A reflected plate of the cranium hinging on attached temporal muscle. Also called *osteoplastic flap*.

brachial flap Any flap fashioned from the tissues of the arm.

breast flap Any flap fashioned from the tissues of the breast.

bridge flap BIPEDICLE FLAP.

buccal flap A flap from the mucosa of the internal surface of the cheek used to cover defects after ablative surgery in the oral and pharyngeal regions. Also called *cheek flap*.

caterpillar flap A tubed flap which is moved end-over-end in stages, usually at intervals of about three weeks, to achieve transfer to a distant recipient site.

cellulocutaneous flap SKIN FLAP.

cervical flap Any flap fashioned from the tissues of the neck.

cervical apron flap A rectangular flap fashioned from the skin and subcutaneous tissue of the neck and based on the inferior border of the mandible. It is turned under the mandibular border and into the mouth for the closure of intraoral defects.

cervicofacial flap Any flap fashioned from tissues of both the face and neck.

cheek flap BUCCAL FLAP.

composite flap Any flap, other than a skin flap, containing a considerable quantity of two or more tissues, as an osteocutaneous flap or a myocutaneous flap. Also called *compound flap*.

compound flap COMPOSITE FLAP.

coronal flap A flap created to obtain surgical exposure of the bones of the naso-orbital region without leaving facial scars. A skin incision is made transversely in the scalp in the area of the coronal suture, and the flap of scalp and forehead tissues are reflected forward and downward. At the completion of the operation the flap is returned to its original position.

cross-arm flap A skin flap which is transferred directly from one arm to the hand or forearm of the other arm.

cross-finger flap A flap that is fashioned from the tissues of one finger and transferred to an adjacent finger.

cross-leg flap A flap raised on one leg and transferred to the other. Such flaps require several weeks of immobilization while the new blood supply becomes established.

cross-lip flap A flap for repairing a defect in one lip raised from the other and rotated across the mouth on a pedicle containing the coronary (labial) blood vessels. The pedicle is divided after three weeks, by which time the flap can be expected to have acquired an adequate blood supply from the receiving lip.

cross-thigh flap   A flap fashioned from the tissues of one thigh and transferred to the opposite thigh.

de-epithelized skin flap   A skin flap from which the epidermis has been removed, thus permitting permanent burial of the flap beneath the skin. Also called *dermal flap*.

delayed flap   A pedicled skin flap which is prepared before transfer by a series of operation at intervals of seven or more days so as to divest the flap of a portion of its normal blood supply and augment the blood supply coming through the pedicle. The procedure is used most frequently in the preparation of random flaps.

deltopectoral flap   An axial flap taken from the skin and subcutaneous tissues of the anterior chest wall and the front of the shoulder. Its blood supply comes from the internal mammary artery.

dermal flap   DE-EPITHELIZED SKIN FLAP.

dermis-fat flap   A de-epithelized skin flap with the retention of subcutaneous fat.

direct flap   A skin flap which is elevated from its donor area and applied to the recipient area in the same operation, without any intervening procedure. Also called *immediate transfer flap*.

distant flap   A skin flap transferred from a donor area to a distant recipient site, as in a caterpillar flap, a jump flap, or an Italian flap.

dorsalis pedis flap   An axial flap receiving its blood supply from the dorsalis pedis artery, and fashioned from the skin and subcutaneous tissue on the top of the foot.

double-end flap   A tubed flap elevated with an intact pedicle at each end, somewhat resembling a suitcase handle.

double pedicle flap   BIPEDICLE FLAP.

eave flap   A method of deepening the helical sulcus of the ear. The lateral superior skin of the ear is elevated as a broad flap based at the superior free border of the ear. The under surface is then skin-grafted, and the overall effect resembles the eaves of a roof.

envelope flap   A mucoperiosteal flap made in the gum by incising horizontally, as along the free gingival margin, then undermining through this incision in the plane between the bony alveolus and the mucoperiosteal cover. No vertical incisions are made.

Estlander flap   A cross-lip flap for repairing a defect in the lateral part of one lip with a flap raised from the vermilion border of the other and rotated so that the pedicle becomes the new commissure.

fan flap   **1** A flap taken from the cheek for reconstruction of the upper or lower lip. The flap resembles a fan in shape. **2** Any fan-shaped flap.

Filatov flap   TUBED FLAP.

forehead flap   A flap of forehead skin and subcutaneous tissue based on the superficial temporal artery, used in plastic reconstruction within the mouth or of the lateral wall of the oropharynx. Also called *temporal flap*.

free flap   A skin flap or composite flap having no continuous pedicle or tether between the donor and recipient sites. After being completely elevated, as an island flap, on a long stalk of its nourishing artery and vein(s), the base of the stalk is severed and the flap is transferred to the distant recipient site, where it is revascularized by anastomosing its artery and vein(s) to comparable isolated vessels in the new site. Also called *microvascular free graft*.

free bone flap   A segment of cranium, unattached to muscle, removed in surgical exposure of the brain and replaced as the wound is closed.   • Its designation as a flap is a misnomer.

French flap   SLIDING FLAP.

Gillies flap   TUBED FLAP.

Gillies up-and-down flap   A flap fashioned from tissues of the forehead and used in reconstruction of the nose.

groin flap   An axial flap fashioned from tissues centered over the inguinal crease and receiving its blood supply from branches of the femoral artery and vein.

hinge flap   TURNOVER FLAP.

immediate transfer flap   DIRECT FLAP.

Indian flap   A skin flap from the forehead used for partial or total reconstruction of the nose.   • This flap was described about 900 B. C. in the Sushruta Samhitá of ancient India. Many modifications have been developed since that time.

intercalated flap   One of two adjacent flaps which can be transposed, as in a Z-plasty.

interpolated flap   A flap inserted between two or more structures.

island flap   A flap, usually a skin flap, which is completely raised so that it remains attached to the donor area only by the long pedicle of its nourishing artery and vein(s). In order to be transferred to another site, a subcutaneous tunnel is created between the donor and recipient sites. The flap is put through the tunnel, keeping the nourishing vessels intact. Also called *island graft* (incorrect).

Italian flap   A pedicled skin flap from the arm, used for partial or total reconstruction of the nose. After the arm flap is raised on its pedicle, the forearm is brought over the scalp, the head is rotated slightly toward the arm, and the flap is sutured in place in the nasal defect. Also called *Tagliacozzi flap*.

jump flap   A skin flap which is raised at a distant donor site and attached to a carrier, usually the wrist, and later, sometimes in stages, detached from the donor area and brought by the carrier to the recipient site. Jump flaps may be tubed or may be kept flat as in an open jump flap. Also called *jump graft* (incorrect).

kineplastic flap   A flap used in a kineplasty.

Langenbeck flap   VON LANGENBECK'S BIPEDICLED MUCOPERIOSTEAL FLAP.

latissimus dorsi muscle flap   A flap consisting of the entire latissimus dorsi muscle or a portion thereof. Its blood supply is provided by the thoracodorsal artery.

lingual flap   A flap consisting of a lengthwise portion of the tongue, between 20 to 40 percent, based posteriorly and used to reconstruct defects of the floor of the mouth and alveolus as well as buccal defects following ablative surgery. Also called *tongue flap*.

lining flap   Any flap used in plastic surgery to line the inside of a hollow structure such as the nose or mouth.

liver flap   Asterixis in hepatic encephalopathy.

local flap   A flap having its donor area contiguous or very near to the recipient site.

median flap   **1** Any flap taken from a sagittal part of the body. **2** An Indian forehead flap or any of its modifications.

Millard island flap   A method of lengthening the palate wherein a mucoperiosteal island flap from the anterior palate, receiving its blood supply from the greater palatine artery, is inserted, with the mucosa on the nasal side, between the hard and soft palates.

Monks-Esser island flap   A flap fashioned from an island of hair-bearing scalp and utilized in the reconstruction of an eyebrow. The flap receives its blood supply from the anterior branches of the superficial temporal artery and vein.

mucomuscular flap   A flap incorporating muscle and the overlying mucous membrane.

mucoperiosteal flap   A flap of mucous membrane with underlying periosteum taken from bone of the hard palate.

muscle flap   A pedicle graft consisting entirely of muscle.

musculocutaneous flap   MYOCUTANEOUS FLAP.

myocutaneous flap A flap consisting of a muscle, usually in its entirety, together with all the overlying tissue, including the skin. Also called *musculocutaneous flap*.

nasal pedicled flap A pedicled skin flap used to repair the nose in cases where the defect is too large to repair with a free graft or a local flap.

nasolabial flap A flap fashioned from the tissues in the vicinity of the nasolabial fold.

neurovascular flap An axial flap with its sensory nerves retained intact.

neurovascular island flap An island flap with its sensory nerves kept intact.

omental flap See under OMENTAL GRAFT.

open jump flap A jump flap which is not tubed.

osteocutaneous flap A composite flap consisting of a segment of bone with an overlying skin flap and all the intervening tissues. It may be pedicled or free.

osteoperiosteal flap A bone flap which retains the adjacent or overlying periosteum.

osteoplastic flap BONE FLAP.

pectoral muscle flap A flap consisting of the entire pectoralis muscle or a portion thereof. Its major blood supply is from branches of the thoracoacromial artery and vein.

pedicle flap An incorrect term for PEDICLE GRAFT.

pericoronal flap Gingiva overlying but not attached to the crown of a partially erupted tooth.

pharyngeal flap 1 A flap raised from the posterior pharyngeal wall, as in a palatopharyngoplasty. 2 Any flap from the pharynx.

pocket flap A skin flap made by making a single straight incision, then undermining a pocket under the skin to one side of the incision.

random flap A skin flap with its blood supply coming from a number of small and unidentified vessels, often running in various directions, rather than from a single and known main artery with its accompanying veins. Also called *random pattern flap*.

random pattern flap RANDOM FLAP.

rope flap TUBED FLAP.

rotation flap A local flap for which the tissue is advanced into its new position by rotating the tissue about an axis in the center of the flap.

sandwich flap A flap consisting of two flaps placed back to back.

scalp flap Any flap fashioned from the tissues of the scalp.

scalping flap A flap consisting of a temporarily elevated scalp which is used as a carrier for the forehead or small segments of the hair-bearing scalp that are utilized in the reconstruction of the nose or eyebrows. When its use as a carrier is complete, it is returned to its original position.

sickle flap A narrow curved axial flap taken from the temple, and with its blood supply received from the anterior branch of the superficial temporal artery and vein. It is used to transfer portions of the scalp and/or forehead to other areas of the face.

skin flap A flap consisting of the entire thickness of the skin plus part or all of the subjacent subcutaneous fat. Also called *cellocutaneous flap*.

sliding flap A skin flap designed and elevated adjacent to a defect and then, taking advantage of the stretchability of the skin, pulled over the defect and sutured in place. This flap is usually applicable only to small defects. Also called *advancement flap*, *French flap*.

split thickness flap In periodontal surgery, a flap of epithelium and connective tissue which does not include the periosteum.

subcutaneous flap A flap consisting entirely of subcutaneous tissue.

subcutaneous pedicle flap TUNNEL FLAP.

surgical flap FLAP.

Tagliacozzi flap ITALIAN FLAP.

temporal flap FOREHEAD FLAP.

tensor fasciae latae muscle flap A flap consisting of the entire tensor fascia latae muscle or a portion thereof. Its vascular pedicle is the lateral circumflex femoral artery.

thoracoabdominal flap A flap fashioned from the tissues of both the abdominal and chest walls.

thoracoabdominal tubed flap A tubed flap that has been fashioned from a thoracoabdominal flap.

thoracobrachial flap A flap that has been fashioned from the tissues of both the chest wall and the arm.

thoracoepigastric flap A flap, usually superiorly based, that is fashioned from the combined tissues of the lateral chest wall and the anterior abdominal wall. Also called *axilloabdominal flap*.

tongue flap 1 LINGUAL FLAP. 2 Any flap fashioned from the tongue.

transposition flap A flap that is moved at an angle in order to reach the recipient site. The movement is around a vertical axis located in the base of the flap.

trapdoor flap A flap, roughly square in shape and left attached on one border, that consists of an elevated segment of skin and subcutaneous tissue. It is created to obtain surgical exposure and is returned to its original position after completion of the operation.

tube flap TUBED FLAP.

tubed flap A flap created by making two long, parallel cuts through the skin and subcutaneous tissue, undermining the area between the incisions, then suturing the two skin edges of the flap together, with the epidermis facing outward, to make a rope, or tube, of the skin and subcutaneous tissue. Also called *tube flap*, *tubed pedicle flap*, *Filatov flap*, *Gillies flap*, *rope flap*, *double-end graft* (incorrect), *Gillies graft* (incorrect), *rope graft* (incorrect), *tube graft* (incorrect).

tubed pedicle flap TUBED FLAP.

tunnel flap A long, rectangular, skin flap in which the pedicle is denuded of all contiguous epidermis, and the flap is then passed through a subcutaneous tunnel to the recipient site so that the denuded pedicle lies in the tunnel and the skin-covered portion emerges on the other side to cover the original defect. Also called *subcutaneous pedicle flap*.

turnover flap A flap in which the axis of rotation lies along the length of its base, thus causing the surface of the flap to be inverted and to lie adjacent to its original position. It is a type often used as a lining flap. Also called *hinge flap*.

von Langenbeck's bipedicled mucoperiosteal flap A flap used in closure of a complete cleft of the palate, consisting of the entire thickness of oral mucosa and periosteum on one side of the hard palate from front to back. The anterior pedicle contains the incisive artery and vein and the posterior pedicle contains the major palatine artery and vein. Also called *Langenbeck flap*.

V-Y flap A V-shaped flap that is elongated to cover a greater area of tissue. The flap, which is at first triangular, is undermined and then pulled so that the area is then sutured in the shape of a Y.

Z-flap A flap consisting of two triangular flaps formed from a Z-shaped incision that has been made through the skin and subcutaneous tissues. The two flaps are rotated and then interchanged, which serves to rotate the axis of tension, originally

along the central limb of a the Z-shaped incision, by 90 percent.
Zimany's bilobed flap BILOBED FLAP.

---

flare [Middle English *fleare*] **1** The visible reflection of light from the aqueous or vitreous humors made turbid by a pathologic amount of protein present because of breakdown of the blood-aqueous barrier. Flare is recognized by biomicroscopic observation of the path of a sharply focused beam of light. **2** The eccentric deposition of soot, unburned powder, and metal shavings and thermal burning of the skin on one side of a short-range, gunshot entrance wound. Also called *flip*.

aqueous flare Visibility of the slit lamp beam as it passes through aqueous humor containing plasma proteins due to a defect of the blood-eye barrier.

flare of the nostrils ALAE NASI.

flash [Middle English *flaschen*] The flange of surplus material surrounding a dental cast which is made in a two-part mold. It prevents complete closure of the flask.

welders' flash WELDERS' CONJUNCTIVITIS.

flashback An involuntary recurrence of some aspect of a hallucinatory experience or perceptual distortion days or even weeks after taking the hallucinogenic drug which produced it and without further ingestion of the substance. Such experiences are often negative in tone, and a reaction of fear and anxiety to their unexpected and unbidden occurrence is common.

flashblindness See under BLINDNESS.

flask [French *flacon* (from Low L *flasco* or *flasca*, akin to Italian *fiasco* bottle or *fiasca* flask, flagon and to German *Flasche* bottle, flask, possibly of Teutonic origin or from Gk *phlaskeion* a flask covered with plaited willow twigs) a bottle with stopper] **1** A narrow-mouthed, usually glass container, often with a rounded or expanded lower portion, that is used for storage and manipulation of fluids. **2** A metal box or cylinder that is used to contain investment material when making a mold, as for a denture.

Carrel flask A flask used in tissue culture. The elongated neck may be slanted from the vertical at any angle from a slight deviation to a right angle.

casting flask A flask for use with refractory investment in casting with molten metal. Also called *casting ring, refractory flask, retaining ring*.

crown flask A small flask used for making a dental crown.

denture flask A large flask used for making a denture.

Dewar flask VACUUM FLASK.

Erlenmeyer flask A glass laboratory flask with a broad base, cone-shaped body, and a relatively short neck.

refractory flask CASTING FLASK.

swan-neck flask A flask with a long, sinuous neck that allows air but not particulate matter, such as contaminated dust, to enter. • Pasteur used such a flask to show that a sterile medium contained therein remained sterile, thus refuting the belief that spontaneous generation occurred.

vacuum flask A double-walled glass container, often with silvered surfaces. An evacuated space between the two walls provides thermal insulation between the contents of the flask and the environment. Also called *Dewar flask*.

volumetric flask A flask with a relatively large body and a slender, elongated neck marked to denote a precise quantity of liquid that the container holds.

flasking The act of investing a pattern within a flask.

flat **1** Lacking irregularities or curvature: said of a surface, or of a line on a graph. **2** Lacking resonance: said of auscultatory sounds. **3** Somewhat lower than a standard or intended pitch: said of musical tones.

optical flat A surface, usually glass or quartz, ground to deviate from a true plane surface by no more than 0.05 μm.

Flatau [Edward *Flatau*, Polish neurologist, 1869–1932] **1** See under LAW. **2** Redlich-Flatau syndrome. See under REDLICH'S ENCEPHALOMYELITIS. **3** Flatau-Schilder disease. See under SCHILDER'S DISEASE.

Flateau [Edward *Flateau*, Polish neurologist, 1869–1932] Flateau's disease. See under SCHILDER'S DISEASE.

flatfoot TALIPES PLANUS.

rocker-bottom flatfoot A congenitally malformed foot in which a congenital dislocation of the talonavicular joint results in a convex contour to the sole. It may be associated with the chromosomal defect of autosomal trisomy, especially of 13–15 and 18. Also called *rocker-bottom foot, congenital convex club foot, convex foot, rocker-bottom deformity*.

spastic flatfoot A painful variety of flatfoot which is believed to result from spasm of the peroneal muscles with consequent partial eversion of the foot. Also called *spasmodic talipes planus, talipes spasmodicus*.

static flatfoot The stabilized, fixed loss of the normal longitudinal arch of the foot.

traumatic flatfoot The loss of the normal longitudinal arch of the foot following an injury.

flatness A lack of resonance; a quality of sound heard on percussion of airless tissues.

flattening In psychiatry, the leveling, impoverishment, or dulling of emotional reactivity.

flatulence [French, irreg. from L *flatus*, past part. of *flare* to blow, breathe] The presence of an excessive amount of gas in the stomach or intestine.

flatulent Affected with or characterized by flatus or flatulence.

flatus [L, substantive from *flatus*, past part. of *flare* to blow, breathe] **1** Gas generated in the stomach or the intestinal tract. **2** Gas expelled from the intestinal tract.

flatus vaginalis Audible expulsion of gas from the vagina.

flatworm Any worm belonging to the phylum Platyhelminthes.

flav- FLAVO-.

flavacidin AMYLPENICILLIN SODIUM.

flavanoid Any of the 2-phenyl derivatives of chroman, usually any of those not possessing a 4-oxo group. They are related to many flower pigments. Compare FLAVONOID.

flavanone A 4-oxo-2-phenylchroman, one of the flavonoids found in flower pigments. It normally carries hydroxyl and methoxyl groups on both its aromatic rings.

flavedo [New L, from L *flavus* yellow, yellowish, gold-colored, red, reddish] Yellowness. An obsolete term.

flavescent [L *flavescens*, gen. *flavescentis*, pres. part. of *flavescere* (from *flavus* yellow) to grow or become yellow] Becoming yellow.

flavianic acid $C_{10}H_6N_2O_8S$. A naphthol derivative used to precipitate arginine and histidine in protein hydrolysis. As the sodium or potassium salt, it is used in tissue stains.

flavicin AMYLPENICILLIN SODIUM.

flavin Any of a few compounds that contain the tricyclic nucleus dimethylisoalloxazine, which consists of dimethylbenzene fused to a pterin ring. In its oxidized, quinonoid form it is yellow. Most natural flavins are combined forms of riboflavin.

flavin adenine dinucleotide A prosthetic group of many oxidizing enzymes, which can exist in oxidized or reduced forms. It consists of a diphosphate residue, esterified with adenosine on one phosphorus and riboflavin on the other.

flavin mononucleotide Riboflavin 5'-phosphate, the prosthetic group of some enzymes. Also called *isoalloxazine mononucleotide, riboflavin phosphate, riboflavin mononucleotide, vitamin B₂ phosphate.*

flavivirus [*flav(o)-* + *i* + VIRUS]　Any of a large group of RNA viruses (formerly group B arboviruses) belonging to the genus *Flavivirus*, family Togaviridae. These viruses produce a variety of febrile systemic syndromes and meningoencephalitis in humans.

flavo- [L *flavus* yellow]　A combining form meaning yellow. Also *flav-*.

Flavobacterium [FLAVO- + BACTERIUM]　A genus of Gram-negative, mostly nonmotile bacilli, found in nature, that form yellow to red pigmented colonies, and that ferment so slowly that they are often mistaken for nonfermenters (especially for pseudomonads). *F. meningosepticum* often causes serious illness in the newborn.

flavodoxin　Any of a class of electron carriers containing flavin mononucleotide and having a very low redox potential. They are formed instead of ferredoxin by many bacteria, especially in media low in Fe^{2+}.

flavokinase　RIBOFLAVIN KINASE.

flavone　One of the flavonoids, the 2,3-dehydro derivative of a flavanone.

flavonoid　Any of the 2-phenyl derivatives of chroman, usually possessing a 4-oxo group, found in flower pigments. They are formed from cinnamic acid. Compare FLAVANOID.

flavonol　A 3-hydroxy derivative of a flavone.

flavoprotein　A yellow protein containing a flavin as prosthetic group.

flavor　1 A distinctive taste. The olfactory sense as well as the gustatory sense contributes to the sensation of flavor.　2 To impart a flavor to; especially, in pharmacology, to disguise the taste of by admixing additives: used of medicines taken orally.

flavoxate hydrochloride　$C_{24}H_{26}ClNO_4$. 3-Methyl-4-oxo-2-phenyl-4*H*-1-benzopyran-8-carboxylic acid 2-piperidinoethyl ester hydrochloride, an anticholinergic drug with local anesthetic and analgesic properties. It is also capable of relaxing smooth muscles. it is administered orally for urinary tract pain and discomfort from inflammation of the bladder and urinary tract components.

flax / spurge flax　MEZEREUM.

flaxseed　LINSEED.

flay　To tear away strips of skin and subcutaneous tissues by repetitive blows, as in whipping.

fld.　fluid.

fl dr　1 Symbol for the unit, fluid dram.　2 Symbol for the obsolete unit, fluid drachm.

flea [Middle English *fle, flee*, from Old English *flēah, flēa*, akin to German *fliehen* to flee]　A dorsoventrally flattened, wingless, ectoparasitic insect of the order Siphonaptera equipped with an extraordinarily developed jumping third pair of legs, mouth parts adapted for sucking blood, smooth body segments with posteriorly directed ctenoid or comblike hairs, and extremely complex genitalia. Some 1500 species are known ectoparasites of warmblooded animals, particularly rodents. Many species attack man and are carriers of a number of diseases such as plague and typhus, and many species are intermediate hosts of helminths of birds and mammals.

　Asiatic rat flea　A flea of the species *Xenopsylla cheopis*; the oriental rat flea.

　burrowing flea　A flea of the species *Tunga penetrans*; a chigoe.

　cat flea　A flea of the species *Ctenocephalides felis*.

　cavy flea　A flea of the species *Rhopalopsyllus cavicola*.

　chigger flea　CHIGOE.

　chigoe flea　CHIGOE.

　common flea　A flea of the species *Pulex irritans*.

　common rat flea　A flea of the species *Nosopsyllus fasciatus*.

　dog flea　A flea of the species *Ctenocephalides canis*.

　European rat flea　A flea of the species *Nosopsyllus fasciatus*.

　hen flea　A flea of the genus *Ceratophyllus*, especially *C. gallinae*.

　human flea　A flea of the species *Pulex irritans*.

　Indian rat flea　A flea of the species *Xenopsylla astia*.

　jigger flea　CHIGOE.

　mouse flea　A flea of the species *Leptopsylla segnis*.

　oriental rat flea　A flea of the species *Xenopsylla cheopis*.

　rat flea　Any of several species of fleas found as ectoparasites of rats, some of which are involved in transmission of plague, including *Xenopsylla cheopis, X. brasiliensis,* and *X. astia*.

　sand flea　CHIGOE.

　squirrel flea　A flea of the species *Hoplopsyllus anomalus*.

　sticktight flea　A flea of the species *Echidnophaga gallinacea*.

　suslik flea　Any of a number of species of fleas found on Russian ground squirrels.

　tropical hen flea　A flea of the species *Echidnophaga gallinacea*; the sticktight flea.

　tropical rat flea　A flea of the species *Xenopsylla cheopis*.

　water flea　A popular term for COPEPOD.

fleam [Middle English *fleme*, from Middle French *flieme* a lancet, ultimately from Gk *phlebotomon* (from *phleps*, gen. *phlebos*, a vein + *-tomon*, combining form from *temnein* to cut) a vein cutting]　An instrument for lancing gums or for bloodletting.

Flechsig [Paul Emil *Flechsig*, German neurologist, 1847–1929]　1 Ground bundles of Flechsig. See under BUNDLE.　2 Flechsig's areas. See under AREA.　3 See under FASCICULUS.　4 Flechsig's fasciculi. See under FASCICULI PROPRII.　5 Flechsig's tract. See under TRACTUS SPINOCEREBELLARIS DORSALIS.　6 Flechsig's myelogenetic law. See under MYELOGENETIC LAW.　7 Oval area of Flechsig, oval bundle of Flechsig. See under FASCICULUS SEPTOMARGINALIS.　8 Fasciculus anterior proprius Flechsigi, fasciculus lateralis proprius Flechsigi. See under FASCICULUS.　9 Flechsig's territories. See under FLECHSIG'S PRIMORDIAL ZONES.　10 Flechsig's field. See under MYELINOGENETIC FIELD.

fleck / Michel's flecks　Atrophic areas of the iris, as may result from granulomatous infection.

　tobacco flecks　An obsolete term for GAMNA-GANDY BODIES.

fleckfieber [German (from *Fleck* spot, blemish + *Fieber* fever), spotted fever]　EPIDEMIC LOUSE-BORNE TYPHUS.

flection　FLEXION.

fledge [Middle English *flegge* old enough to fly, from Old English *(un)flycge* (un)fledged, from the root of English *fly*]　1 To acquire the ability to fly.　2 To care for (a bird) until it develops flight feathers and can fly.

fleece　A neural fiber network.

　fleece of Stilling　The lattice of myelinated axons surrounding the dentate nucleus of the cerebellum.

Fleischer [Richard *Fleischer*, German physician, 1848–1909]　1 Fleischer-Strümpell ring. See under FLEISCHER KERATOCONUS RING.　2 Kayser-Fleischer ring. See under RING.　3 See under VORTEX.

Fleischmann [Friedrich Ludwig *Fleischmann*, German anatomist, flourished 19th century]　See under FOLLICLE.

Fleischmann [Gottfried *Fleischmann*, German anatomist, 1777–1853]　1 See under HYGROMA.　2 Fleischmann's bursa. See under BURSA SUBLINGUALIS.

Fleischner [Felix *Fleischner*, German-born U.S. radiologist and physician, born 1893]　1 Fleischner lines. See under LINE.　2 See under DISEASE.

Flemming [Walther *Flemming*, German anatomist, 1843–1905] **1** Intermediate body of Flemming. See under BODY. **2** Flemming center. See under GERMINAL CENTER. **3** Flemming's liquid, Flemming solution. See under FLEMMING'S FIXING FLUID.

flesh [Old English *flæsc*; akin to German *Fleisch* flesh] **1** The muscular tissues of the body. **2** The soft outer tissues of the animal body, including the muscles.

goose flesh Skin in which piloerection has taken place as a reaction to cold or emotion. Also called *cutis anserina, goose skin, horrida cutis* (obsolete), *gooseflesh, goose bumps.*

live flesh MYOKYMIA.

proud flesh 1 GRANULATION TISSUE. **2** Exuberant granulation tissue that has overgrown the boundaries and contours of the wound where it was formed.

fletcherism [after Horace *Fletcher*, U.S. dietician, 1849–1919.] The thorough chewing of solid foods and the drinking of liquids in very small sips.

flex To bend or limb or other body part at a joint. Compare EXTEND.

flexibilitas FLEXIBILITY.

flexibilitas cerea A characteristic of catalepsy in which the patient allows bending of the limbs or body into a particular posture or attitude which is maintained for inordinate periods of time. Also called *cerea flexibilitas, waxy flexibility.*

flexibility The property of being flexible.

waxy flexibility FLEXIBILITAS CEREA.

flexible Capable of bending without breaking. Also *flexile.*

flexile FLEXIBLE.

fleximeter An instrument for measuring the angle of flexion of a joint.

flexion [L *flexio* (from *flexus*, past part. of *flectere* to bend, turn) a bending, winding] The movement of parts of the body, usually around an axis which is transverse or obliquely transverse. It usually results in a diminution of the angle between two ventral surfaces. Also *flection.*

lateral flexion The act of bending to the right or left.

lateroflexion flexion Flexion of the fetal head to one side of the body as a normal process during labor.

mass flexion A general contraction of flexor musculature, such as occurs when a mass reflex is triggered in the chronic spinal patient.

plantar flexion Movement of the ankle and tarsal joints in which the dorsum of the foot moves away from the anterior (cranial) aspect of the tibia or, in the forelimb of a quadruped, from the radius. After plantar flexion the foot or toes are said to be extended downward in the direction of the sole. Also called *plantiflexion.* Compare DORSIFLEXION.

posterior flexion The approximation of the two sides of a joint posteriorly. An outmoded term. Also called *postexion* (outmoded). • The term is sometimes incorrectly used by clinicians when referring to movements of the vertebral column as extension or hyperextension is taking place.

universal flexion Flexion of the fetal parts onto the body as a normal process during labor.

Flexner [Simon *Flexner*, U.S. pathologist, 1863–1946] **1** See under SERUM. **2** Flexner's dysentery. See under BACILLARY DYSENTERY. **3** Flexner-Jobling carcinosarcoma. See under CARCINOSARCOMA.

flexor [New L, from L *flex(us)*, past part. of *flectere* to bend + *-or* -OR] A muscle that produces an approximation of the movable part on one side of a joint to the fixed side to a varying degree. In general, the approximation results in a forward movement of the movable part except in the lower limb, where, in the case of the knee, ankle, and toe joints, it produces a posterior movement of the movable part. Compare EXTENSOR.

flexor carpi ulnaris brevis An occasional accessory muscle of the forearm which arises from the distal part of the anterior surface of the ulna and is inserted into the hamate bone, pisiform bone, abductor digiti minimi muscle, or the the proximal end of the fifth metacarpal bone. Also called *ulnocarpeus* (outmoded).

flexura [L (from *flexus*, past part. of *flectere* to bend, bow, turn, akin to *plectere* to braid, intertwine, from Gk *plekein* to twine, twist; + *-ura* -URE), a bending, winding, turning] An angulation or bend, usually in a structure or organ. Also called *flexure.*

flexura coli dextra [NA] The bend between the terminal part of the ascending colon and the beginning of the transverse colon. It is situated below the right lobe of the liver and anterior to the inferolateral part of the anterior surface of the right kidney. Also called *right flexure of colon, right colic flexure, hepatic flexure of colon, flexura hepatica coli* (outmoded), *right angle of colon* (outmoded).

flexura coli sinistra [NA] The acute bend between the termination of the transverse colon and the commencement of the descending colon. It is situated in the left hypochondriac region, inferior to the lateral extremity of the spleen and tail of the pancreas and anterior to the left kidney. It is attached to the diaphragm by the phrenicocolic ligament. Also called *left flexure of colon, left colic flexure, flexura lienalis coli* (outmoded), *splenic flexure of colon, left angle of colon* (outmoded).

flexura duodeni inferior [NA] The bend between the descending part and the horizontal part of the duodenum. It is situated at the right side of the lower border of the third lumbar vertebra and of the inferior vena cava. Also called *inferior flexure of duodenum, inferior angle of duodenum.*

flexura duodeni superior [NA] The acute bend between the superior part and the descending part of the duodenum, which is usually located below the neck of the gallbladder. Also called *superior flexure of duodenum, superior angle of duodenum.*

flexura duodenojejunalis [NA] The sharp bend between the end of the ascending part of the duodenum and the commencement of the jejunum, which is situated at the level of the upper border of the second lumbar vertebra. It is fixed posteriorly by the suspensory muscle of the duodenum and is related to the body of the pancreas superiorly and the transverse colon and mesocolon anteriorly. Also called *duodenojejunal flexure, duodenojejunal angle.*

flexura hepatica coli An outmoded term for FLEXURA COLI DEXTRA.

flexura lienalis coli An outmoded term for FLEXURA COLI SINISTRA.

flexura perinealis recti [NA] The sharp backward bend of the terminal part of the rectum at the anorectal junction. Also called *perineal flexure of rectum.*

flexura sacralis recti [NA] The anteroposterior curvature of the upper part of the rectum. It has its concavity directed anteriorly. Also called *sacral flexure of rectum.*

flexura sigmoidea An outmoded term for COLON SIGMOIDEUM.

flexurae Plural of FLEXURA.

flexural Pertaining to a flexure.

flexure [L *flexura.* See FLEXURA.] FLEXURA.

basicranial flexure PONTINE FLEXURE.

caudal flexure The ventral curvature which develops at the hind end of an embryo and ends in the tail. Also called *sacral flexure.*

cephalic flexure In the embryo, a flexure (concave below) on the inferior aspect of the cranial extremity of the closed neural tube at the level of the midbrain. Also called *mesencephalic flexure, cranial flexure, mesencephalic arch, head bend.*

cerebral flexure CERVICAL FLEXURE.

cervical flexure An encephalic flexure of the embryo, the first to appear, at the junction of the rhombencephalon and the spinal cord. Also called *cerebral flexure, nuchal flexure, neck bend.*

cranial flexure CEPHALIC FLEXURE.

dorsal flexure The curvature that develops ventrally in the thoracic region of the developing embryo.

duodenojejunal flexure FLEXURA DUODENOJEJUNALIS.

encephalic flexure Any of three flexures that appear in the developing neural tube as a result of unequal growth of its different parts. Two are concave ventrally (cephalic and cervical flexures), one is convex ventrally (pontine).

hepatic flexure of colon FLEXURA COLI DEXTRA.

iliac flexure of colon An outmoded term for COLON SIG-MOIDEUM.

inferior flexure of duodenum FLEXURA DUODENI INFE-RIOR.

left colic flexure FLEXURA COLI SINISTRA.

left flexure of colon FLEXURA COLI SINISTRA.

lumbar flexure The anteriorly convex curvature of the lumbar region of the vertebral column.

mesencephalic flexure CEPHALIC FLEXURE.

nuchal flexure CERVICAL FLEXURE.

perineal flexure Ventral curvature in the embryo where the back sweeps round to the perineum.

perineal flexure of rectum FLEXURA PERINEALIS RECTI.

pontine flexure An encephalic flexure of the embryo which develops in the rhombencephalon between the metencephalon and the myelencephalon. Also called *basicranial flexure, varolian bend.*

right colic flexure FLEXURA COLI DEXTRA.

right flexure of colon FLEXURA COLI DEXTRA.

sacral flexure CAUDAL FLEXURE.

sacral flexure of rectum FLEXURA SACRALIS RECTI.

sigmoid flexure of colon An outmoded term for COLON SIG-MOIDEUM.

splenic flexure of colon FLEXURA COLI SINISTRA.

subpubic flexure of urethra An outmoded term for PRE-PUBIC ANGLE OF URETHRA.

superior flexure of duodenum FLEXURA DUODENI SUPE-RIOR.

flicker [Middle English *flikeren,* from Old English *flicorian* to move the wings, akin to *flacor* flying, L *plangere* to beat, strike noisily] The quality of visual sensation produced by a rapid and regular intermittance of a stimulus within the visual field.

Flieringa [Henri Johan *Flieringa,* Dutch ophthalmologist, born 1891] See under RING.

flight / flight of ideas Rapid speech with the speaker switching from one topic to another, as in manic states. Also called *topical flight.*

flight into disease The conversion of a mental conflict into physical symptoms, as seen in neurotic disorders.

flight into health TRANSFERENCE CURE.

topical flight FLIGHT OF IDEAS.

flimmerskotoma [German *flimmer(n)* to glisten, glitter + Gk *skotōma* dizziness with darkening of vision, from *skotoren* to darken, blind] A shimmering visual field defect, as may occur in the aura of migraine.

Flint Flint's murmur. See under AUSTIN FLINT MURMUR.

Flint [Austin *Flint,* Jr., U.S. physiologist, 1836–1915] Flint's arcade. See under ARTERIAE ARCUATAE RENIS.

flip FLARE.

float [partly Middle English *flote,* from Old English *flota* a ship and *flot* the sea; partly Middle English *floten* to float, from Old English *flotian* to float] **1** An instrument for filing or rasping the molar teeth of a horse. **2** To file or rasp the molar teeth of a horse.

floaters [*float* + -ER] An apparent visual opacity perceived as drifting in suspension in front of the eye. This is due to the presence of an opacity in the posterior portion of the vitreous humor, a position from which a shadow can be cast upon the retina. Floaters may represent benign embryologic remnants or acquired pathologic changes within the vitreous humor. Also called *flocci volitantes.*

floating **1** Unattached; free or partly free, as the lowest two pairs of ribs, whose anterior ends are not connected to the cartilages above. **2** Being or capable of being displaced from its normal position, as a kidney.

floc [L *floc(cus)* a lock or pile of wool] The fluffy, woolly, or lumpy precipitates that result when an antigen and antibody unite in a flocculation reaction. A popular usage.

flocci volitantes FLOATERS.

floccilegium [L *flocci,* gen. of *floccus* a tuft of wool + -*legium,* combining form from *leg(ere)* to pick up + -*ium,* neuter noun suffix] CARPHOLOGY.

floccillation [L *flocc(us)* a tuft of cotton + -*ill(us),* masc. diminishing suffix + English -ATION] CARPHOLOGY.

floccose Having a woolly appearance: used especially of the outer surface of a mushroom.

floccular [*floccul(us)* + -AR] **1** Of or relating to the fluffy, woolly or lumpy precipitates that develop after some antigen-antibody reactions. **2** Pertaining to the flocculus of the cerebellum.

flocculation [*floccul(e)* + -ATION] The formation of fluffy, woolly, or lumpy precipitates following the combination of an antibody with colloidally suspended particulate antigens. This immunologic reaction is often performed to detect bacterial antibodies.

Ramon flocculation A means of quantifying antitoxin potency, in which the end point is the speed of flocculation produced by the test antitoxin, as compared with that of a standardized antitoxin.

floccule [L *flocculus.* See FLOCCULUS.] One of the fluffy or tuftlike precipitates formed during flocculation.

flocculent **1** Precipitated from a fluid as fluffly lumps. **2** Growing in loose aggregates in a liquid medium, as bacteria. **3** Appearing as a tuft, similar to cotton or wool: said of part of a fungus.

flocculi Plural of FLOCCULUS.

flocculonodular Denoting the flocculonodular lobe of the cerebellum.

flocculoreaction An antigen-antibody reaction in which the end point is flocculation.

flocculus [Late L (dim. of L *floccus* a lock or pile of wool), a small lock or pile of wool] (*plural* flocculi) [NA] A downward-hanging, semidetached lobule at the lower extremity of each cerebellar hemisphere, continuous with the nodulus of the vermis. Also called *nucleus nervi pneumogastrici* (obsolete), *floccular process.*

accessory flocculus The small, lateral, lobular extension of the cerebellar flocculus. Also called *paraflocculus, secondary flocculus, flocculus secondarii.*

flocculus secondarii ACCESSORY FLOCCULUS.

secondary flocculus ACCESSORY FLOCCULUS.

Flocks [Milton *Flocks,* U.S. ophthalmologist, born 1914] Harrington-Flocks test. See under TEST.

Flood [Valentine *Flood,* Irish surgeon, 1800–1847] See under LIGAMENT.

flooding Prolonged exposure of the phobic subject to the very object or situation he fears, as a form of therapy.

floor [Middle and Old English *flor*, akin to L *planus* level, flat] The inferior, or lowest, surface of any cavity or hollow organ; the surface joining the lowest parts of the walls of any space, area, or organ.

jugular floor of tympanic cavity PARIES JUGULARIS CAVITATIS TYMPANICAE.

floor of orbit PARIES INFERIOR ORBITAE.

flop / Colombo flop An obsolete term for DECK LEGS.

flora [L *Flora* goddess of flowers. See FLORES.] **1** The plants of a particular geographical area or period of time. **2** A list of plants growing in a certain locality. **3** The total microbial population of a localized region, as of the intestinal tract or the skin.

intestinal flora The highly mixed bacterial population in the feces. The intestinal contents are anaerobic, and the facultative organisms that can grow on aerobic plates, consisting largely of Enterobacteriaceae, are in fact usually greatly outnumbered by obligate anaerobes (bacteroids).

oral flora The microorganisms normally resident in the oral cavity.

resident flora Those microbial species that permanently colonize the skin or other regions of an individual. The constituent species vary with the age of the subject.

transient flora Microbial species that are occasionally isolated from normal skin or other regions of an individual but do not become established as permanent members of the flora.

Floraquin A proprietary name for diiodohydroxyquin.

Florence [Albert *Florence*, French physician, 1851–1927] See under REACTION, TEST, REAGENT.

flores [L, pl. of *flos* flower] **1** The blossoms of a plant. **2** The floral form assumed by certain substances after sublimation.

floret [Middle English *flouret, flourette*, from Old French *florete*, dim. of *flor* flower, from L *flos* flower] Any of the individual small flowers, especially in the grasses and composites, that make up the dense, composite form of inflorescence.

florid [L *florid(us)* (from *flos*, gen. *floris*, a flower) flowery, blooming, bright-colored] **1** Bright red, as a skin lesion. **2** Fully represented or developed, as the symptoms of a disease.

Floridin A proprietary name for fuller's earth.

Florinef A proprietary name for fludrocortisone.

Floropryl A proprietary name for isoflurophate.

Florschütz [Georg *Florschütz*, German physician, born 1859] See under FORMULA.

floss [earlier *flosh*, from Old French *floche* (from L *floccus* a lock of wool) a light heap of wool] To clean the teeth with dental floss.

dental floss A fine untwisted thread used for cleaning interdentally. It was originally made of silk, but now nylon is used.

waxed floss Dental floss in which the fibers are bound together with wax.

flour A powdery substance produced by milling wheat and other grains. Occupational exposure to flour and to its additives and contaminants can cause dermatitis and asthma.

Flourens [Marie Jean Pierre *Flourens*, French physiologist, 1794–1867] See under THEORY.

flow [L *fluere* (akin to *pluere* to rain and Gk *plynein* to wash) to flow] **1** The movement of a fluid or the course of such movement. **2** A measure of the quantity or rate of the movement of a fluid, as of blood through the vessels or of air in inspiration into the lungs.

axoplasmic flow The physiologic movement of protein molecules along an axon. Fast and slow rates of flow have been described and studied using radioactively labeled substances.

cerebral blood flow The volume of blood that passes through vessels of the brain in a given period, usually measured between the carotid artery and jugular vein.

effective pulmonary blood flow Pulmonary blood flow available for gas exchange.

effective renal blood flow Blood flow calculated by dividing the effective renal plasma flow by unity minus the hematocrit ratio.

effective renal plasma flow The plasma flow that perfuses the renal parenchyma, approximately 90 percent of total renal plasma flow. The remaining 10 percent is presumed to perfuse the supporting tissues of the kidney. It is measured by the clearance method, using agents such as *p*-amino hippurate (PAH) at such low plasma concentrations that all of the agent is removed during one passage through the kidney.

gene flow The transfer of genes between distinct populations of the same species through mating. It may influence allele frequency and evolution. Also called *gene spread*.

inspiratory triggering flow INSPIRATORY TRIGGERING PRESSURE.

laminar flow **1** A directional flow of air in a controlled environment with the use of fan and filter, used to decrease contamination by airborne bacteria. **2** A type of flow by liquids in tubes in which successive cylindrical layers of fluid move with decreasing velocity as one proceeds from the axis of flow to the wall of the tube. Cohesive forces between the wall and the liquid limit the movement of an infinitesimally thin layer of fluid at the periphery but the movement of inner layers of fluid upon one another is related to the viscosity of the fluid.

maximal midexpiratory flow The greatest flow of air generated during the midpart of a forced exhalation.

peak expiratory flow The greatest flow rate attained during a forced exhalation: a measure of airway obstruction.

regional cerebral blood flow Blood flow which can be measured in different regions of the cerebrum.

renal blood flow TOTAL RENAL BLOOD FLOW. Abbreviation: RBF

storm water flow An additional flow of water resulting from heavy rain. The potential for such increased volume must be considered in the planning of sewage or drainage disposal schemes.

total renal blood flow Blood flow to the entire kidney. Also called *renal blood flow*.

Flower [Sir William Henry *Flower*, English surgeon and anatomist, 1831–1899] **1** Flower's bone. See under EPIPTERIC BONE. **2** Flower's index. See under DENTAL INDEX.

flower A part of a higher plant that is modified for reproduction and bears one or more pistils or carpels, or one or more stamens, or both.

flower of paradise CATHA.

passion flower *Passiflora incarnata*, a twining plant of the Passifloraceae family. The dried flowering tops of the plant contain harman, and they are used in the preparation of a sedative and analgesic. Also called *passiflora, maypop*.

flowers [French *fleur* (from L *flos*, gen. *floris*, flower) flower] The form of a drug or chemical obtained by sublimation.

Dalmatian insect flowers PYRETHRUM.

insect flowers PYRETHRUM.

pyrethrum flowers PYRETHRUM.

flowmeter [FLOW + -METER] An instrument for measuring the rate at which a volume of liquids or gases is moving within a closed hydraulic system. Examples include instruments which measure rate of blood flow within arteries and veins, and rate of gas flow within the airways. Also called *stromuhr*.

continuous wave Doppler flowmeter DOPPLER FLOWMETER.

Doppler flowmeter A blood flowmeter that continuously transmits ultrasound into a vessel. Reflected ultrasound has a

Doppler frequency shift that is proportional to blood cell velocity. An acoustic output provides information on blood velocity, while a recorder indicates blood flow averaged across the cross-section. Also called *continuous wave Doppler flowmeter.*

dry flowmeter   A flowmeter which measures gas flow quantitatively. A bobbin is placed in a tapered tube attached to the source of gas, and as the gas is released the bobbin will rise.

electromagnetic flowmeter   A device measuring blood flow based upon the voltage created by blood moving through a magnetic field.

pulsed Doppler flowmeter   A blood flowmeter that transmits pulses of ultrasound into the vessel. Reflected ultrasound has a Doppler frequency shift that is proportional to blood cell velocity. It displays velocity versus radial position as it changes with time.

rotameter flowmeter   ROTAMETER.

sight-feed flowmeter   A crude flowmeter which indicates gas flow by the progressive escape of gas bubbles downward from openings in a tube immersed in water.

floxuridine $C_9H_{11}FN_2O_5$. 2'-Deoxy-5-fluorouridine. An antineoplastic drug that is an analogue of fluorouracil. It is used in the treatment of carcinomas and is given by intra-arterial infusion. Abbreviation: FUDR

fl oz   Symbol for the unit, fluid ounce.

flu   A popular term for INFLUENZA.

intestinal flu   A viral infection of the gastrointestinal tract usually resulting in emesis or diarrhea.

Flucort   A proprietary name for flumethasone.

flucrylate $C_7H_6F_3NO_2$.   2,2,2-Trifluoro-1-methylethyl-2-cyanoacrylate. A tissue adhesive used in surgical procedures.

flucytosine $C_4H_4FN_3O$. 5-Fluorocytosine. An antifungal agent employed in the treatment of serious fungal infections from *Candida* and *Cryptococcus* organisms.

fludrocortisone $C_{23}H_{31}FO_6$.   21-(Acetyloxy)-9α-fluoro-11β17α-dihydroxy-pregn-4-ene-3,20-dione. A synthetic corticosteroid possessing both glucocorticoid and mineralcorticoid activities. It is used as a replacement therapy in mineralcorticoid insufficiency and in congenital adrenocortical hyperplasia. Also called *fluohydrisone, fluohydrocortisone.*

fludrocortisone acetate $C_{23}H_{31}FO_6$ The acetate ester form of fluorocortisone. It is used as an anti-inflammatory drug, with uses and actions like those of hydrocortisone and deoxycortisone.

fluence   [French, adaptation of L *fluens*, pres. part. of *fluere* to flow]   INTEGRAL NEUTRON FLUX.

energy fluence   In radiation dosimetry, the sum of the energies of all the particles which enter a sphere of unit cross-sectional area.

flufenamic acid $C_{14}H_{10}F_3NO_2$. 3'-Trifluoromethyldiphenylamine-2-carboxylic acid. It is used as an anti-inflammatory agent and as an analgesic.

flügelplatte   [German *Flügel* a wing, fin, blade + *Platte* plate]   ALAR LAMINA.

fluid   [French *fluide* (from L *fluidus* flowing, fluid) fluid (adj.)]   **1** Capable of flowing, as a liquid or gas.   **2** A fluid substance; a liquid or gas.

Altmann's fluid   A fixative solution, comprising potassium dichromate and osmium tetroxide, that is used for the demonstration of all cytologic structures except chromosomes. Also called *Altmann's liquid.*

amniotic fluid   The fluid that accumulates in the amnion, in human embryos from the twelfth day. It increases in quantity until it surrounds the embryo and then the fetus, except at the point of attachment of the umbilical cord. The amount decreases slightly after the seventh month in human pregnancy and about one liter is present at term. Initially it resembles blood plasma in composition but it becomes diluted as pregnancy advances, presumably due to the addition of fetal urine. The fluid probably derives mostly from the fetal membranes and the fetus, but maternal factors may play a part. It contains desquamated fetal epithelial cells and may also in some mammals contain shed lanugo and partially calcified, precociously erupted, deciduous teeth. The fluid may be drawn off by the procedure of amniocentesis. Also called *liquor amnii, aqua amnii, waters* (older term).

ascitic fluid   The serous fluid found in the peritoneal cavity in ascites. It is usually composed of water, proteins in a concentration of 1 to 2 g/100 ml, and other solutes found in the plasma.

body fluid   Any liquid component of the body.

Bouin's fluid   A solution of picric acid, formaldehyde, and acetic acid used as a fixative for detailed nuclear study and the preservation of glycogen. In recent years it has been used extensively for renal biopsy material. Also called *Bouin's fixative, Bouin solution.*

Brodie fluid   A fluid used in the Warburg's apparatus, composed of sodium chloride, sodium choleate, a dye such as Evans blue or acid fuchsin, and water.

Carnoy's fluid   VAN GEHUCHTEN'S FIXATIVE.

cerebrospinal fluid   LIQUOR CEREBROSPINALIS.

crevicular fluid   GINGIVAL FLUID.

culture fluid   The fluid separated from a culture by filtration.

decalcifying fluid   Any solution that removes calcium from tissues and leaves organic constituents intact for sectioning.

Delafield's fluid   A fixative solution that contains osmic acid, chromic acid, acetic acid, and alcohol. It is suitable for delicate histologic material.

diluting fluid   Any fluid added to blood or other biological specimens to reduce the concentration of constituents to be enumerated or measured, and thus bring the constituents into a concentration range suitable for analysis.

Ecker's fluid   REES-ECKER SOLUTION.

extracellular fluid   Any fluid not contained within the cell membrane, such as plasma, interstitial fluid, and joint fluid, and fluid within body cavities or pleural or pericardial spaces.

extravascular fluid   Any fluid not contained within the vascular system, generally excluding intracellular fluid but including interstitial fluid and fluid within body cavities.

Flemming's fixing fluid   A widely used cytological fixative, containing osmium tetroxide, chromic acid, and glacial acetic acid. Also called *Flemming's liquid, Flemming solution.*

follicular fluid   The fluid which surrounds the maturing oocyte within the ovarian follicle and which is partially exuded with the oocyte at ovulation. Its origin is not clearly understood and primary, secondary and tertiary types of fluid have been described which vary in consistency and viscosity as the follicle enlarges. Also called *liquor folliculi.*

formol-Müller fluid   ORTH SOLUTION.

Gendre's fluid   A histologic fixative containing picric acid, acetic acid, and formaldehyde. It is excellent for the preservation of glycogen.

gingival fluid   A flow of clear fluid, not pus, from the gingival sulcus or periodontal pocket. It contains a large number of substances derived from the subgingival plaque, the gingival tissues, and the interaction between these two. It also contains large numbers of polymorphonuclear leukocytes. In perfect gingival health there is no flow. In chronic gingivitis and chronic periodontitis the rate of flow varies with the degree of inflammation, and the measurement of the flow is used in periodontal research as an indication of the degree of inflammation present. Also called *crevicular fluid, gingival exudate.*

Helly's fluid   A fixative solution comprising mercuric chloride, potassium dichromate, and formaldehyde with the addition of sodium sulfate for osmotic purposes. It is an excellent cytoplasmic fixative that is used particularly for delicate tissues and in situations where cytoplasmic details are important. Also called *Helly's fixative, Zenker-formol fixative.*

interstitial fluid   Body fluid contained within the spaces between cells, excluding intracellular fluid, intravascular fluid, and fluid contained within body cavities. Also called *tissue fluid, intercellular lymph, tissue lymph* (outmoded).

intracellular fluid   Fluid contained within a cell.

intraocular fluid   HUMOR AQUOSUS.

Kaiserling's fluid   A sequential fixative designed for the preservation of gross anatomical and pathological specimens for exhibition in museums. Initial fixation is provided by a formaldehyde solution buffered with potassium salts to a neutral pH. Color restoration is achieved by immersion in ethyl alcohol. The specimen is then mounted in a third solution containing glycerol and sodium acetate with thymol added as a preservative. Also called *Kaiserling's fixative, Kaiserling solutions.*

labyrinthine fluid   An outmoded term for PERILYMPHA.

Mitchell's fluid   A fluid used in an obsolete treatment for pulmonary tuberculosis consisting of sodium chloride, bromine, hydrochloric acid, and water which has been acted on by an electric current.

Müller's fluid   A simple fixative that contains potassium dichromate with sodium sulfate added for osmotic purposes. It has been used particularly for its mordanting properties in relation to tissues from the central nervous system.

non-newtonian fluid   A fluid whose viscosity changes with the gradient of rate of flow. Solutions of fibrous macromolecules are examples, the alignment of the molecules with the flow diminishing the viscosity.

otic fluid   An outmoded term for ENDOLYMPHA.

Parker's fluid   A fixative solution composed of alcohol and formaldehyde.

Pasteur's fluid   A liquid medium once used for growing filamentous fungi and yeasts. It consisted of ammonium tartrate, cane sugar, and ashed yeast cells in water. Also called *Pasteur's liquid.*

pericardial fluid   The small amount of fluid in the pericardial cavity that facilitates movement of the heart within the pericardium. Also called *liquor pericardii, aqua pericardii, pericardial serum.*

periotic fluid   An outmoded term for PERILYMPHA.

Piazza's fluid   A reagent used to coagulate blood *in vitro*, consisting of an aqueous solution of ferric and sodium chlorides.

puncture fluid   Any fluid obtained from a body cavity through a hollow needle.

Rees and Ecker diluting fluid   REES-ECKER SOLUTION.

Rossman's fluid   A general histologic fixative containing picric acid and formaldehyde.

saline fluid   SALINE.

Scarpa's fluid   An outmoded term for ENDOLYMPHA.

Schaudinn's fluid   A rapidly penetrating histologic fixative containing mercuric chloride, ethyl alcohol, and acetic acid. It has also been used for exfoliative cytology.

seminal fluid   SEMEN.

serous fluid   A clear, watery fluid produced within the body, especially in body cavities or in sterile abscesses. Also called *serofluid.*

Susa fixing fluid   SUSA FIXATIVE.

synovial fluid   SYNOVIA.

Thoma's fluid   A strong decalcifying solution composed of nitric acid in alcohol. Also called *Thoma's liquid.*

tissue fluid   INTERSTITIAL FLUID.

transcellular fluid   That part of the extracellular fluid volume that is derived from the intracellular volume by active transport across cell membranes.

ventricular fluid   The cerebrospinal fluid that is found within the ventricles of the brain.

von Behring's fluid   TULASE.

Waldeyer's fluid   A decalcifying fluid containing palladium chloride and hydrochloric acid.

Zenker's fluid   A fixative solution that contains mercuric chloride, potassium dichromate, and glacial acetic acid. It provides for excellent preservation of cell cytoplasm. Also called *Zenker's fixative, Zenker solution.*

fluidextract   A liquid preparation of a drug dissolved in alcohol in a concentration such that one milliliter of the solution contains the extracted material from one gram of the drug source. Also called *fluidextractum, liquid extract.* Also *fluid extract.*

fluidextractum   FLUIDEXTRACT.

fluidglycerates   Preparations that contain 50 percent glycerin by volume with no alcohol in the formulation. Such a preparation is made equivalent to a fluidextract, as 1 ml of solution contains the material extracted from 1 g of the crude drug.

fluidism   HUMORALISM.

fluidity / libidinal fluidity   The mobility of the energy available to the libido. This energy can be transferred from one developmental level to another or from one object to another.

fluidounce   See under FLUID OUNCE.

fluidrachm   See under FLUID DRACHM.

fluidram   See under FLUID DRAM.

fluigram [*flui(d)* + GRAM]   A unit of capacity or volume equal to one cubic centimeter; one milliliter. An obsolete unit.

fluke [Old English *flōc*]   **1** A parasitic flatworm of the class Trematoda; a trematode. There are over 4000 species of flatworms of the class Trematoda. Also called *fluke worm.* **2** A flatfish, as the flounder. **3** The lateral expansion of the tail of a whale.

blood fluke   A trematode worm that inhabits blood vessels of vertebrates; a member of the family Schistomatidae (superfamily Schistosomatoidea).

bronchial fluke   A fluke of the species *Paragonimus westermani.*

cat liver fluke   A fluke of the species *Opisthorchis felineus.*

Chinese liver fluke   A fluke of the species *Clonorchis sinensis.* Also called *oriental fluke.*

digenetic fluke   **1** A member of the trematode order (or subclass in other systems) Digenea. **2** A fluke having two stages of reproduction, asexual in the larval form and sexual in the adult form.

Egyptian intestinal fluke   A fluke of the species *Heterophyes heterophyes.*

human lung fluke   A fluke of the species *Paragonimus westermani.*

intestinal fluke   Any of various trematodes that parasitize the intestine of man and other hosts. Examples include *Fasciolopsis buski, Echinostoma, Fasciolopsis, Gastrodiscoides, Heterophyes, Metagonimus,* and *Watsonius.*

lancet fluke   A fluke of the species *Dicrocoelium dendriticum.*

liver fluke   Any of various trematode worms that infect the liver and biliary system of their definitive host. Examples are *Fasciola hepatica, Clonorchis sinensis, Opisthorchis* spp., and *Dicrocoelium* spp.

lung fluke   A trematode worm that parasitizes the lung of its host, such as *Haematoloechus* of frogs or *Paragonimus westermani* of humans.

oriental fluke   CHINESE LIVER FLUKE.

rumen fluke   A trematode worm belonging to any of several species of *Paramphistomum* that parasitize the rumen of ruminants.

sheep liver fluke   A fluke of the species *Fasciola hepatica.*

flukicide [*fluk(e)* + *i* + -CIDE] A substance used to kill parasitic flukes.

flumen [L, a flowing or running of water, a river, stream] A stream.

flumina pilorum Groups of hair growing in the skin so as to produce hair tracts that slope in a common direction in specific regions, such as the hairs on the extensor surface of the forearms that are directed ulnarward. Also called *hair streams*.

flumethasone $C_{22}H_{28}F_2O_5$. 6α,9α-Difluoro-11β,17α,21-trihydroxy-16α-methylpregna-1,4-diene-3,20-dione. A synthetic glucocorticoid used primarily as a topical anti-inflammatory drug to treat skin conditions that respond to steroid therapy. It is usually given as the acetate or pivalate ester.

flumethasone pivalate $C_{27}H_{36}F_2O_6$. The pivalate (dimethylpropionate) ester through the C-21 position of the steroid. It has the same uses and properties as the parent drug.

flumina Plural of FLUMEN.

flunarizine hydrochloride $C_{26}H_{28}Cl_2F_2N_2$. 1-Cinnamyl-4-(di-p-fluorobenzhydryl)piperazine. The dihydrochloride salt form of flunarizine, used as a vasodilator.

fluo- FLUOR-.

fluocinoline acetonide $C_{24}H_{30}F_2O_6$. 6α,9α-Difluoro-11β,21-dihydroxy-16α,17α-isopropylidenedioxypregna-1,4-diene-3,20-dione. A synthetic glucocorticoid. It is used topically as an anti-inflammatory drug to treat dermatologic conditions that respond to steroid therapy.

fluocinonide $C_{26}H_{32}F_2O_7$. The 21-acetate ester of fluocinolone acetonide. It has the same anti-inflammatory and antipruritic properties as the parent drug and is used topically for steroid-responsive dermatoses.

fluohydrisone FLUDROCORTISONE.

fluohydrocortisone FLUDROCORTISONE.

fluor [L (from *fluere* to flow), a flow, flux] One of a class of solids that has the property of fluorescence, useful for detector construction.

fluor albus LEUKORRHEA.

plastic fluor A synthetic material that has the characteristic of emitting a flash of light as the result of an ionizing event within it.

fluor- [L *fluere* to flow] A combining form denoting the presence of fluorine in a chemical compound. Also *fluo-, fluori-, fluoro-*.

fluorapatite $Ca_{10}(PO_4)_6F_2$. The form of apatite in which fluorite ions replace the commoner hydroxide ions, the inorganic portion of bone made up largely of calcium phosphate or hydroxyapatite. Fluorapatite is formed in tooth enamel in the developmental and maturing stages and continues to be added to the enamel surface but at a declining rate as the tooth ages, ceasing when the tooth is completely mineralized. Fluorapatite serves to harden bone and makes teeth more resistant to caries.

fluorecin LEUCOFLUORESCEIN.

fluorescein $C_{20}H_{12}O_5$. An orange-red crystalline compound that produces a green fluorescence in an alkaline solution. As the isothiocyanate derivative it can be coupled to proteins, especially immunoglobulins, for use in immunofluorescence techniques. In a dilute solution as the sodium compound, it is used to detect ophthalmic lesions and to evaluate blood circulation. Also called *fluorescein dyes*.

fluoresceinuria [FLUORESCEIN + -URIA] Excretion of fluorescein in the urine after its intravenous injection, an outmoded test of renal function.

fluorescence [FLUOR + -escence, noun suffix from L -escentia denoting beginning] 1 Photoluminescence in which the initial state of the radiative transition is a singlet state. 2 Any photoluminescence in which the emission ceases within a fraction of a second upon cessation of the stimulating radiation. An imprecise usage. Compare PHOSPHORESCENCE.

natural fluorescence AUTOFLUORESCENCE.

nonspecific fluorescence Fluorescence spontaneously present in a preparation, not resulting from an attachment of a fluorochrome-labeled specific antibody or reagent.

x-ray fluorescence Emission of characteristic x rays from an atom as a result of the absorption of higher energy radiation.

fluorescent Exhibiting or capable of exhibiting fluorescence.

fluorescin The reduced form of fluorescein. The sodium salt is comparable to the sodium salts of fluorescein, and the bromine derivative is the parent compound of eosin.

fluori- FLUOR-.

fluoridate [back formation from *fluoridation*, from *fluorid(e)* + -ATION] To adjust the fluoride level in a water supply by the addition of fluoride.

fluoridation [FLUOR + -IDE[1] + -ATION] Adjustment of the fluoride level in a water supply by the addition or injection of a substance which will provide sufficient fluoride ions for the desired concentration to be attained for dental health and in particular, the reduction of caries. In temperate climates, the optimum level is approximately one part per million of fluoride ion.

fluoride F^-. The anion formed from fluorine, or a salt containing it.

topical fluoride An agent containing fluoride for application to the teeth to increase resistance to caries. It may be in the form of a solution, gel, paste, varnish, or mouthwash.

fluoridization 1 The addition of fluoride to foods or drinks, other than by means of the public water supply. 2 The topical applications of fluoride solution to the teeth.

fluoridize [*fluorid(e)* + -IZE] To add fluoride to or apply fluoride solution to (the teeth).

fluorine Element number 9, having atomic weight 18.9984. Fluorine is a member of the halogen family and it is the most electronegative and reactive of all elements, forming compounds even with the usually inert gases krypton, xenon, and radon. The valence is 1. In elemental form it is a pale yellow, corrosive gas. Both the gas and its compounds are very toxic. In trace amounts, however, it is possibly a constituent of teeth and bones, and it is known to be an essential factor in the growth of rats. Soluble fluoride is often introduced into drinking water supplies in order to increase the resistance to caries of developing teeth. Fluorine 19 is the sole stable isotope occurring in nature. Symbol: F

fluorine 18 A radioactive isotope of fluorine. Physical half-life is 1.86 hours. Symbol: ^{18}F

fluoro- FLUOR-.

fluoroacetic acid $F-CH_2-COOH$. A simple derivative of acetic acid found in some African plants. It is highly toxic because it is converted via fluoroacetyl-CoA into a fluorocitrate, which powerfully inhibits aconitase.

fluorocarbon One of a group of hydrocarbons in which some or all of the hydrogen has been substituted by fluorine. It is characterized by a low boiling point and chemical inertness, and it is used as a refrigerant fluid and in fire extinguishers and aerosol sprays. Also called *fluorinated hydrocarbon*.

fluorocardiogram The record made by fluorocardiography.

fluorocardiograph [FLUOR- + *o* + CARDIOGRAPH] An orthodiagram used for recording the size and shape of the heart.

fluorocardiography [FLUOR- + *o* + CARDIOGRAPHY] Orthodiagraphy of the heart.

fluorochrome A fluorescent substance used to impart fluorescence to a cell, tissue, or type of molecule in the tissue.

fluorochroming The attachment of a fluorescent compound

to a protein, usually as a marker for an immunoglobulin.

fluorocitric acid HOOC—CHF—C(OH)(COOH)—CH$_2$—COOH. One of the diastereoisomers of this compound is highly toxic because it inhibits aconitase and blocks the citric acid cycle. This diastereoisomer is formed, by a process that has been termed "lethal synthesis," from fluoroacetyl-CoA and oxaloacetate by citrate synthase.

9α-fluorocortisol A synthetic corticosteroid. The fluorine substitution is made because it inhibits activity little but inhibits catabolism more and so prolongs the activity of the compound.

fluorocyte A reticulocyte that exhibits red fluorescence due to its porphyrin content.

fluorodinitrobenzene Normally fluoro-2,4-dinitrobenzene, which is a reagent for amino groups, especially for the N-terminal residues of proteins, and also for lysine residues whose side chains are unsubstituted and therefore usually nutritionally available. The electron-withdrawing nitro groups enable fluoride ion to be displaced by the nucleophilic amino group. Also called *dinitrofluorobenzene*.

fluorography [FLUOR- + *o* + -GRAPHY] PHOTOFLUOROGRAPHY.

digital fluorography Fluorography in which the x-ray images are digitized so that they may be computer processed for contrast enhancement. See also DIGITAL SUBTRACTION ANGIOGRAPHY.

Fluoromar A proprietary name for fluroxene.

fluorometer An apparatus, no longer used, to measure the output of an x-ray tube.

fluorometholone C$_{22}$H$_{29}$FO$_4$. 9α-Fluoro-11β,17α-dihydroxy-6α-methyl-1,4-pregnadiene-3,20-dione. A glucocorticoid agent possessing anti-inflammatory activity. It may be applied topically to the skin in the form of a cream.

p-fluorophenylalanine An analogue of phenylalanine which can be incorporated into proteins in its place. The products formed may still be functional, but they are often less stable than the natural proteins.

fluorophosphate Phosphorofluoridate. Any of the anions and esters of (HO)$_2$P(F)=O. Simple dialkyl fluorophosphates, (RO)$_2$P(F)=O, are powerful inhibitors of cholinesterase and of serine proteinases. The nucleophilic group of each of these enzymes, which normally attacks the carbonyl group of the substrate, becomes phosphorylated by displacing fluoride from the inhibitor.

fluororoentgenography PHOTOFLUOROGRAPHY.

fluoroscope [FLUOR- + *o* + -SCOPE] Any apparatus which contains a fluorescent screen that absorbs x rays and produces a visible image which continuously shows the passage of x ray through an object. All modern fluoroscopes use some form of image amplifier, and most display the image on a television monitor. Also called *cryptoscope* (obsolete), *radioscope* (seldom used), *roentgenoscope*.

biplane fluoroscope A fluoroscope constructed so that examinations can be made either horizontally or vertically.

fluoroscopic Relating to fluoroscopy or use of the fluoroscope.

fluoroscopy Examination by a fluoroscope. Also called *cryptoscopy* (obsolete), *radioscopy*, *roentgenoscopy*, *actinoscopy* (obsolete), *umbrascopy* (outmoded).

fluorosis [FLUOR- + -OSIS] The long-term effects of the ingestion of excessive amounts of dietary fluoride. These may include chronic endemic dental fluorosis (mottled enamel) and osteosclerosis. Also called *darmous* (North African Arabic name).

chronic endemic dental fluorosis Mottled enamel caused by ingestion of excess fluoride from the water supply during the period of enamel formation.

dental fluorosis Mottled enamel from excess ingestion of fluoride from any source. Also called *dentes de Chiaie*.

fluorouracil C$_4$H$_3$FN$_2$O$_2$. 5-Fluoro-2,4(1H,3H)-pyrimidine-dione. A fluoro-substituted pyrimidine used as an antimetabolite by its conversion *in vivo* to the deoxynucleotide, a compound that inhibits thymidylate synthetase and inhibits DNA synthesis. It is used as an antineoplastic drug against colorectal carcinoma and some other types of cancer. It is administered intravenously. It is also used topically for the treatment of multiple actinic keratoses of the skin.

Fluothane A proprietary name for halothane.

fluoxymesterone C$_{20}$H$_{29}$FO$_3$. 9-α-fluoro-11β, 17β-hydroxy-17α-methylandrost-4-en-3-one. A white, crystalline powder, practically insoluble in water but soluble in alcohol. It is used for the same conditions as methyltestosterone, and is also given to cancer patients as an anabolic steroid.

fluphenazine dihydrochloride C$_{22}$H$_{28}$Cl$_2$F$_3$N$_3$OS. 4-[3-[2-(Trifluoromethyl)-10H-phenothiazin-10-yl]propyl]-1-piperazineethanol dihydrochloride. A piperazine phenothiazine derivative with the ability to prevent nausea from toxins, radiation treatment, and cytotoxic drugs. It is ineffective against motion sickness. It is also used as an antipsychotic tranquilizer. It is administered orally or intramuscularly.

fluprednisolone C$_{21}$H$_{27}$FO$_5$. A fluoridated prednisolone analogue with glucocorticoid and anti-inflammatory properties. Flupredisolone and its valerate salt are used for the management of allergic and arthritic disorders.

flurandrenolide C$_{24}$H$_{33}$FO$_6$. 6α-fluoro-11β,21-dihydroxy-16α,17-[(1-methylethylidene)bis-(oxy)]pregn-4-ene-3,20-dione. A synthetic glucocorticoid with anti-inflammatory actions. It is used in dermatologic conditions that respond to these agents. It also has antipruritic and vasoconstrictive properties.

flurazepam hydrochloride C$_{21}$H$_{25}$Cl$_3$FN$_3$O. C-Chloro-1-[2-(diethylamino)ethyl]-5-(*o*-fluorophenyl)-1,3-dihydro-2H-1,4-benzodiazepin-2-one dihydrochloride. It is used as a sedative and hypnotic and given orally.

fluroxene CH$_2$=CH—O—CH$_2$—CF$_3$. A slightly flammable, volatile liquid with a pungent odor, that is used as a general anesthetic. An obsolete term.

flush [alteration of *flux*, ultimately from L *fluxus* a flow, from *fluxus*, past part. of *fluere* to flow; influenced by Middle English *flusshen* to fly up suddenly, as a bird, by Old French *fluiss-*, stem of *fluir* to flow, and by Middle English *flashen* to flash, of onomatopoeic origin] **1** A reddening of tissue caused by vasodilatation. **2** To wash out or cleanse with a brisk flow of liquid, usually water.

atropine flush A reaction characterized by reddening and dryness of the skin over the face and neck regions. This is observed when atropine is given in overdose amounts.

breast flush Erythema or redness of the breast associated with lactation.

carcinoid flush The episodic flush, thought to be hormonally induced by vasoactive kinins or serotonin, occurring in patients with carcinoid syndrome.

flamingo flush SCHWARTZE SIGN.

harlequin flush HARLEQUIN COLOR CHANGE.

hectic flush The heightening of facial coloring associated with a rise in body temperature.

histamine flush A flushing of the face and upper trunk as a result of the sudden release of histamine from drugs or from the mast cells in some forms of mastocytosis.

limbal flush Hyperemia in the circumcorneal region, of importance because it usually indicates presence of a severe inflammation of the anterior portion of the eye.

mahogany flush A unilateral deep red flush sometimes seen in lobar pneumonia. An obsolete term.

malar flush A flush over the cheek bones.

menopausal flush Intermittent flushing and sweating due to vasodilatation accompanying estrogen withdrawal in the menopause.

fluspirilene $C_{29}H_{31}F_2N_3O$. 8-[4,4-Bis(*p*-fluorophenyl)butyl]-1-phenyl-1,3,8-triazaspiro[4,5]-decan-4-one. An antipsychotic agent occurring as a white crystalline solid. It is administered orally.

flutter A rapid vibrating or pulsating activity.

atrial flutter An arrhythmia in which atrial activation is occurring in a regular fashion at a rate between 260 and 320 per minute. It is probably the result of a reentrant circuit. Usually only a proportion of atrial impulses are conducted to the ventricles, most commonly as a 2:1 block with a ventricular rate of 130 to 160 per minute. Also called *auricular flutter, pure flutter.*

auricular flutter ATRIAL FLUTTER.

diaphragmatic flutter Rapid, rhythmic contractions of the diaphragm.

impure flutter An arrhythmia in which there appears at times to be organized atrial flutter while at other times it more closely resembles atrial fibrillation.

mediastinal flutter Rapid, rhythmic movements of the mediastinum in response to respiratory activity.

pure flutter ATRIAL FLUTTER.

ventricular flutter A form of ventricular tachycardia in which the ventricular rate is much faster than usual (in the neighborhood of 300 per minute), and which often degenerates into ventricular fibrillation.

flutter-fibrillation An arrhythmia which varies in appearance between atrial flutter and atrial fibrillation.

flux [L *fluxus* (from *fluxus,* past part. of *fluere* to flow) a flow, flowing] **1** An excessive discharge of fluid. **2** The movement of any vector quantity through an area, per unit time. Also called *fluxion.*

biliary flux Diarrhea with excessive amounts of bile; biliary diarrhea.

celiac flux FATTY DIARRHEA.

hepatic flux Diarrhea accompanying severe liver disease.

integral neutron flux The product of the flux of neutrons and the time, usually expressed in neutrons per square centimeter. Also called *fluence.*

luminous flux The rate of flow of radiant energy, expressed in lumens.

magnetic flux The lines of a magnetic field, measured as the integral over a specified surface of the component of magnetic induction (magnetic flux density), expressed in webers. Symbol: Φ

menstrual flux The blood and fluid of menstruation.

neutron flux The intensity of a neutron beam, expressed as the number of neutrons per second crossing a unit area.

substance flux The amount of substance excreted in urine divided by time, expressed in nanomoles per second.

fluxion FLUX.

fly [Old English *flēoge, flȳge*] Any winged insect of the order Diptera other than those called gnats, midges, or mosquitoes. The term is also used in the names of certain nondipteran insects such as caddis flies.

black fly BLACKFLY.

blackbottle fly A fly of the genus *Phormia.*

blow fly BLOWFLY.

bluebottle fly A fly of a metallic blue color in the genus *Calliphora.*

bot fly BOTFLY.

buffalo fly A horn fly, *Haematobia irritans exigua,* that attacks water buffalo and other domestic animals in the Oriental zoogeographic region and Australia.

caddis fly An insect of the order Trichoptera, whose freshwater aquatic larvae construct a characteristic tube, or caddis,

from which the head or legs can emerge for feeding or movement. The adults have membranous wings covered with hairs which, when shed, produce allergic symptoms in sensitized persons.

cheese fly A fly of the species *Piophila casei.*

crane fly A fly belonging to the dipteran family Tipulidae.

deer fly Any of various tabanid flies of the genus *Chrysops,* especially *C. discalis.*

drone fly A fly of the species *Eristalis tenax.*

dung fly A fly of the species *Sepsis violacea.*

eye fly A fly which hovers around or attacks the eye, such as *Siphunculina funicola.* See also HIPPELATES.

face fly A fly of the species *Musca autumnalis.*

filth fly A fly, such as *Musca domestica,* that feeds or breeds on garbage, feces, or the like.

flesh fly Any of various kinds of fly whose larvae feed on the living or necrotic flesh of vertebrates or cause myiasis, such as screwworm flies of the genera *Cochliomyia, Sarcophaga,* and *Wohlfahrtia* and blowflies of the genus *Calliphora.*

frit fly Any of various flies of the dipteran family Chloropidae.

fruit fly **1** A fly of the family Drosophilidae, such as *Drosophila melanogaster.* Also called *vinegar fly, pomace fly.* **2** A fly of the family Trypetidae (Tephritidae), such as *Ceratitis capitata,* the Mediterranean fruit fly.

gad fly See under GADFLY.

gold fly A fly of the species *Lucilia caesar.*

greenbottle fly A fly of a metallic green color of the genus *Lucilia* or the genus *Phaenicia.*

heel fly A fly of the genus *Hypoderma;* a warble fly.

horn fly A fly of the genus *Haematobia,* especially *H. irritans.*

horse fly HORSEFLY.

house fly HOUSEFLY.

hover fly A fly of the family Syrphidae, such as *Helophilus* or *Eristalis.*

lake fly A mayfly that swarms on the shores of lakes, especially *Hexagenia bilineata.*

latrine fly A fly of the species *Fannia scalaris.*

louse fly A bloodsucking ectoparasitic fly of the family Hippoboscidae, especially one of the genus *Hippobosca.*

mango fly MANGROVE FLY.

mangrove fly An African fly of the genus *Chrysops,* such as *C. dimidiata* or *C. silacea.* Also called *mango fly.*

moth fly Any of various nonbiting flies of the family Psychodidae, especially of the genus *Psychoda.*

nose fly The sheep nose botfly, *Oestrus ovis.* Also called *nostril fly.*

nostril fly NOSE FLY.

ox warble fly WARBLE FLY.

phlebotomus fly A sandfly of the genus *Phlebotomus.*

pomace fly FRUIT FLY.

Russian fly SPANISH FLY.

sand fly SANDFLY.

screwworm fly Any of various calliphorid or sarcophagid flies. See also SCREWWORM.

seroot fly A fly of the species *Tabanus ditaeniatus* or *T. fasciatus.*

snipe fly A fly of the family Rhagionidae or the family Athericidae.

soldier fly A fly of the family Stratiomyidae.

Spanish fly **1** A blister beetle of the species *Cantharis vesicatoria.* Also called *Russian fly.* **2** A popular term for CANTHARIDES.

stable fly A fly of the genus *Stomoxys,* especially one of the species *S. calcitrans.*

tick fly KED.

tsetse fly An African fly of the genus *Glossina,* which includes the vectors of African trypoanosomiasis. Also called *tsetse, tzetze*.

tumbu fly A fly of the species *Cordylobia anthropophaga*.

typhoid fly An obsolete term for HOUSEFLY.

vinegar fly FRUIT FLY.

warble fly A fly of the family Oestridae (or Hypodermatidae) whose larvae produce warbles in cattle and other domestic herbivores. The best-known species are *Hypoderma bovis* and *H. lineatum*. Also called *warble botfly, ox warble fly*.

flyway A major migratory route of birds.

f.m. *fiat mistura* (L, have a mixture made).

Fm Symbol for the element, fermium.

fm 1 Symbol for the unit, femtometer. 2 Symbol for the unit, fermi.

FMG foreign medical graduate.

FMN flavin mononucleotide.

fmol Symbol for the unit, femtomole.

foal [Middle English *fole*, from Old English *fola*] 1 A young horse of either sex. 2 To give birth: said of a mare.

foam / fibrin foam Fibrin derived from fractionation of human blood. It was formerly applied to bleeding surfaces to control oozing of blood, but its use is now obsolete.

focal [L *foc(us)* hearth, fireplace + -AL] Denoting or relating to focus; pertaining to the point of convergence of light rays originating from a common source by the action of dioptric power.

Fochier [Alphonse *Fochier*, French gynecologist, 1845–1903] Fochier's abscess. See under FIXATION ABSCESS.

foci Plural of FOCUS.

focil [Med L *focil(e)* a steel for striking fire] Any of the bones of either the forearm or the leg. Also called *focile*.

focile FOCIL.

focimeter A device for measuring the dioptric strength of a lens.

focus [L, hearth, fireplace] (*plural* foci) 1 The point at which rays of parallel light, heat, or sound intersect after reflection from a mirror or refraction from a lens. Also called *focal point*. 2 The source or central area, as of an infection or other pathologic process.

aplanatic focus A focus at which spherical aberration and circular coma are absent.

Assmann focus A localized inflammatory lesion, usually in the subapical region of the lung, which is an early phase of pulmonary tuberculosis. Also called *Assman's tuberculous infiltrate*.

conjugate focus Each of two points in an optical system such that each is the image point of the other regarded as object point.

epileptic focus 1 The totality of the neural tissue involved in a focal epileptic discharge. When the discharge spreads and ultimately becomes generalized, the term denotes that site in the brain from which the discharge originated. 2 In electroencephalography, localized spike or sharp wave discharges occurring between attacks in an epileptic patient. For defs. 1 and 2 also called *epileptogenic focus*.

epileptogenic focus EPILEPTIC FOCUS.

Ghon focus GHON TUBERCLE.

Küss-Ghon focus GHON TUBERCLE.

negative focus 1 The location of a virtual image in an optical system. 2 A focus on the same side of the lens as the object.

principal foci The location at which an optical system brings parallel light to a point.

real focus The location at which an optical system places a convergent image.

spike focus A recurring spike discharge in the electroenceph-

alogram usually indicative of a focus of epileptic discharge in the underlying brain.

virtual focus The location at which an optical system places a divergent image. Also called *point of dispersion*.

focusing / dioptric focusing The change in strength of the crystalline lens of the eye that permits clear vision to be achieved at various distances.

dynamic focusing Electronically changing the focal distance of a receiving transducer array so that it equals the distance to the propagating transmitted pulse.

electronic focusing Focusing an ultrasonic beam by electronic phasing of electrical pulses applied to the elements of a linear phased transducer array.

isoelectric focusing An electrophoretic technique in which migrating proteins are additionally characterized according to their isoelectric point. A pH gradient is established in the support medium and proteins migrate until they reach the pH zone that equals the isoelectric point of the individual molecule.

Foerster [Otfrid *Foerster*, Polish neurosurgeon, 1873–1941] See under SIGN.

foeti- FETO-.

foeto- FETO-.

foetor A British spelling for FETOR.

foetus A British spelling for FETUS.

fog [prob. from the Scandinavian] 1 A colloid system in which the dispersion medium is a gas and the dispersed particles are liquid. 2 A suspension of very small moisture droplets in the air. • By international meteorological agreement, the term *fog* is used scientifically when the horizontal visibility at the earth's surface is less than 1 km, while *haze* and *mist* describe lesser degrees of visual impairment.

advection fog A fog that forms in the lower levels of a warmer moist air mass as it moves over a colder surface.

evaporation fog A fog formed under conditions of cold stable air by rapid evaporation from an underlying surface of warm water.

frontal fog A fog that forms along an atmospheric front as a result of the mixing of two air masses.

ground fog A shallow fog lying near the surface of the ground.

high inversion fog A fog formed by the downward extension to ground level of a layer of stratus cloud formed under a temperature inversion.

ice fog A fog in which the reduced visibility is caused by tiny ice crystals suspended in the air.

mental fog CLOUDING OF CONSCIOUSNESS.

radiation fog Fog resulting from a cooling of the surface air following terrestrial radiation.

sea fog An advection fog forming over the sea.

Fogarty [Thomas J. *Fogarty*, U.S. thoracic surgeon, born 1934] See under CATHETER.

fogging The deliberate blurring of distance vision used as a technique for preventing unconscious accommodation when testing for refractive error by placing an excessively convex lens before the eye of a hypermetrope or an excessively concave lens before the eye of a myope.

fogo selvagem An endemic bullous disease found in South America and indistinguishable from nonendemic pemphigus foliaceus. Its localization to small endemic foci points to an infective cause. Also called *Brazilian pemphigus, South American pemphigus, wildfire pemphigus*.

foil [French *feuille* (from L *folium* a leaf) leaf] A very thin pliable sheet of metal. In dental usage foil often refers to gold foil or even a gold foil restoration.

activation foil A material used to measure a neutron flux or flux density by means of the radioactivity induced due to neutron capture in the foil. Also called *activation detector*.

adhesive foil   Tin foil made adhesive on one side with gum and used as a periodontal dressing.

cohesive gold foil   Pure gold foil which retains its natural property of cold-welding under pressure.

gold foil   An exceedingly thin foil of gold. If the gold is pure and is kept clean, the foil has the property of cold-welding to itself under pressure. It is used for dental restorations by adding small rolled-up pieces one at a time with considerable pressure. Also called *fibrous gold*.

invisible foil   LINGUAL APPROACH FOIL.

lingual approach foil   A gold foil restoration in an anterior tooth, made invisible from the labial aspect by preparing and filling the cavity from the lingual side. Also called *invisible foil*.

noncohesive gold foil   Gold foil which has been rendered noncohesive by adding impurities or by treating the surface.

platinized gold foil   Foil made from an alloy of gold and platinum.

platinum foil   Foil of pure platinum used as a foundation for making porcelain full crowns because of its high melting point.

Foix [Charles *Foix*, French neurologist, 1882–1927]   **1** Foix paramedian syndrome. See under MEDIAN MEDULLARY SYNDROME. **2** Marie-Foix sign. See under SIGN. **3** Marie and Foix maneuver. See under MANEUVER. **4** Foix-Alajouanine syndrome, Foix-Alajouanine disease. See under SUBACUTE NECROTIC MYELITIS.

folacin   An obsolete term for FOLIC ACID.

folate   Any of the various ionized forms of folic acid.

fold

fold   **1** An edge or margin produced by doubling a layer of a tissue or a structure over on itself. **2** A ridge formed by a flexure in a tissue or organ; plica.

adipose folds of pleura   PLICAE ADIPOSAE PLEURAE.

alar folds   PLICAE ALARES.

amniotic fold   Extraembryonic ectoderm with mesoderm that gives rise in many vertebrates to the amnion by folding together over the early embryo and fusing at junctions, thus closing off the amniotic cavity. The amnion of human embryos is not formed in this way but is the result of cavitation between the embryonic disk and the cytotrophoblast.

anterior mallear fold of mucous membrane of tympanum   PLICA MALLEARIS ANTERIOR MEMBRANAE TYMPANI.

anterior mallear fold of tympanic membrane   PLICA MALLEARIS ANTERIOR MEMBRANAE TYMPANI.

aryepiglottic fold   PLICA ARYEPIGLOTTICA.

aryepiglottic fold of Collier   An outmoded term for PLICA TRIANGULARIS.

arytenoepiglottidean fold   PLICA ARYEPIGLOTTICA.

avascular fold of Treves   PLICA ILEOCAECALIS.

axillary folds   Plica axillaris anterior and plica axillaris posterior.

bloodless fold of Treves   PLICA ILEOCAECALIS.

Brachet's mesolateral fold   MESOLATERAL FOLD.

bulboventricular fold   A fold or pleat in the developing heart tube between the bulbus cordis and the ventricle. It either atrophies or is absorbed as the proximal part of the bulbus is incorporated into the right ventricle. Also called *bulboventricular loop*.

caudal genital fold   An elevation on the posterior abdominal wall of an embryo, extending caudally from the caudal pole of

the gonad and containing the upper portion of the gubernaculum. Also called *inguinal fold, epigonal fold, gubernacular fold*.

caval fold   A ridge raised on the posterior abdominal wall of an embryo by the inferior vena cava where it passes to the posterior aspect of the liver.

cecal folds   PLICAE CAECALES.

cholecystoduodenocolic fold   CYSTICODUODENAL LIGAMENT.

ciliary folds   PLICAE CILIARES.

circular folds   PLICAE CIRCULARES.

circular folds of Kerckring   PLICAE CIRCULARES.

conjunctival fold   PALPEBRAL FOLD.

costocolic fold   LIGAMENTUM PHRENICOCOLICUM.

cranial genital fold   A ridge raised by connective tissue on the posterior abdominal wall of an embryo, stretching cranially from the upper pole of the gonad. It involutes to become the diaphragmatic ligament.

cutaneous folds of anus   Skin corrugations at the lower margin of the anal canal which are probably produced by the corrugator cutis ani muscle.

Douglas fold   **1** PLICA RECTOUTERINA. **2** LINEA ARCUATA VAGINAE MUSCULI RECTI ABDOMINIS.

Duncan's folds   The redundant appearance of the visceral peritoneum overlying a postpartum uterus. An older term.

duodenojejunal fold   PLICA DUODENALIS SUPERIOR.

duodenomesocolic fold   PLICA DUODENALIS INFERIOR.

epicanthal fold   PLICA PALPEBRONASALIS.

epicanthic fold   PLICA PALPEBRONASALIS.

epigastric fold   PLICA UMBILICALIS LATERALIS.

epigonal fold   CAUDAL GENITAL FOLD.

falciform fold of fascia lata   MARGO FALCIFORMIS HIATUS SAPHENUS.

false vocal fold   PLICA VESTIBULARIS.

fimbriated fold   PLICA FIMBRIATA.

fin fold   A median fold of tissue in the embryo of a primitive vertebrate, as a fish or an amphibian, which gives rise to a fin. The dorsal, caudal, and anal fins arise from a fin fold.

folds of the gallbladder   The epithelial lining of the gallbladder. Its numerous folds or rugae give it a honeycomb appearance.

gastric folds   PLICAE GASTRICAE.

gastropancreatic fold   PLICA GASTROPANCREATICA.

gastropancreatic folds of Huschke   The plica gastropancreatica and the plica hepatopancreatica.

genital fold   Either of a pair of posterior prolongations of mesoderm from the primitive streak, which skirt each side of the cloacal membrane to raise the surface ectoderm into folds extending from the genital tubercle. The folds give rise primarily to the labia minora. Also called *gonadal fold*.

glossoepiglottic folds   Plica glossoepiglottica mediana and plica glossoepiglottica lateralis.

gluteal fold   SULCUS GLUTEALIS.

gonadal fold   GENITAL FOLD.

gubernacular fold   CAUDAL GENITAL FOLD.

Guérin's fold   VALVULA FOSSAE NAVICULARIS.

Hasner's fold   PLICA LACRIMALIS.

head fold   See under HEAD AND TAIL FOLDS.

head and tail folds   A tucking under of the front and back of the embryonic disk so that the embryo is folded up ventrally along its longitudinal axis. This phenomenon, which in man occurs about the 21st day after fertilization, happens at the start of neurulation and marks the beginning of the processes which gradually delimit the embryo from its adnexa to which up until then it had been intimately related.

Heister's fold   PLICA SPIRALIS.

Hensing's fold   LIGAMENTUM PHRENICOCOLICUM.

hepatopancreatic fold   PLICA HEPATOPANCREATICA.

horizontal folds of rectum   PLICAE TRANSVERSALES RECTI.

hypogastric fold An outmoded term for PLICA UMBILICALIS MEDIALIS.

ileocecal fold PLICA ILEOCAECALIS.

ileocolic fold An outmoded term for PLICA CAECALIS VASCULARIS.

iliopectineal fold An outmoded term for ARCUS ILIOPECTINEUS.

iliopubic fold of Thompson A transverse band of thickened connective tissue that runs parallel to the inguinal ligament, reinforcing its posterior margin from close to the anterior superior iliac spine to the pubic tubercle. It is considered to be thickened transversalis fascia that is joined by the recurved aponeurotic fibers of the external oblique muscle. It is also attached to the fascia iliaca laterally and to Henle's ligament medially.

incudal fold PLICA INCUDIS.

inferior duodenal fold PLICA DUODENALIS INFERIOR.

infrapatellar fold PLICA SYNOVIALIS INFRAPATELLARIS.

infrapatellar synovial fold PLICA SYNOVIALIS INFRAPATELLARIS.

inguinal fold CAUDAL GENITAL FOLD.

interarticular fold of hip LIGAMENTUM CAPITIS FEMORIS.

interarytenoid fold PLICA INTERARYTENOIDEA.

interureteric fold PLICA INTERURETERICA.

iridial folds PLICAE IRIDIS.

ischial fold of Broca and Gery An extensive thickening of the parietal layer of pelvic fascia that descends in front of the anterior margin of the greater sciatic notch as far as the ischial spine and is limited by the fascial sheaths of the piriformis and obturator internus muscles. An outmoded term.

Jonnesco's fold PARIETOPERITONEAL FOLD.

junctional fold A ridge of cytoplasm of a muscle cell between the secondary clefts produced by infolding of the sarcolemma at a myoneural junction.

Juvara's fold PARIETOPERITONEAL FOLD.

Kerckring's folds of small intestine PLICAE CIRCULARES.

Kohlrausch folds PLICAE TRANSVERSALES RECTI.

labioscrotal fold GENITAL SWELLING.

lacrimal fold PLICA LACRIMALIS.

folds of large intestine PLICAE SEMILUNARES COLI.

fold of laryngeal nerve In the laryngopharynx, the elevated fold of mucous membrane overlying the internal branch of the superior laryngeal nerve.

lateral fold A fold at both the right and left sides of a young embryo which gradually constricts and cuts off the yolk sac.

lateral fold of Douglas Either the plica rectouterina or the sacrogenital fold.

lateral glossoepiglottic fold PLICA GLOSSOEPIGLOTTICA LATERALIS.

lateral nasal fold An elevation on the outer side of the nasal placode in the embryo. It gives rise to much of the ala or wing of the nostril.

lateral umbilical fold PLICA UMBILICALIS LATERALIS.

left gastropancreatic fold An outmoded term for PLICA GASTROPANCREATICA.

fold of the left vena cava PLICA VENAE CAVAE SINISTRAE.

longitudinal fold of duodenum PLICA LONGITUDINALIS DUODENI.

mammary fold 1 MAMMARY RIDGE. 2 The lower fold marking the line of attachment of the breast to the anterior chest wall.

Marshall's fold PLICA VENAE CAVAE SINISTRAE.

medial nasal fold An elevation on the medial side of each nasal placode in the embryo, which will, with its neighbor, give rise to the fleshy part of the nasal septum. Also called *globular process.*

medial umbilical fold PLICA UMBILICALIS MEDIALIS.

median glossoepiglottic fold PLICA GLOSSOEPIGLOTTICA MEDIANA.

median umbilical fold PLICA UMBILICALIS MEDIANA.

medullary fold NEURAL FOLD.

mesentericoparietal fold An outmoded term for PLICA ILEOCAECALIS.

mesolateral fold The right layer of the dorsal mesentery of the embryonic foregut that becomes isolated by the formation of the upper recess of the lesser sac, or vestibule, and forms the caval mesentery in which the upper segment of the inferior vena cava develops. Also called *Brachet's mesolateral fold.*

mesonephric fold MESONEPHRIC RIDGE.

metapleural fold A lateroventral fold of tissue found in cephalochordates. It grows ventrally and posteriorly over the gills as a protective covering.

middle glossoepiglottic fold PLICA GLOSSOEPIGLOTTICA MEDIANA.

middle umbilical fold PLICA UMBILICALIS MEDIANA.

mucobuccal fold The reflection of the alveolar mucosa of the upper and lower jaw onto the adjacent lips and cheeks, limiting the vestibule of the mouth above and below. An outmoded term. Also called *mucosobuccal fold, mucobuccal reflection.*

mucolabial fold The arched fold of mucous membrane extending from the gums to the inner surface of each lip. In the median plane it forms a raised fold, the frenulum.

mucosal fold PLICA MUCOSA.

mucosobuccal fold MUCOBUCCAL FOLD.

mucous fold PLICA MUCOSA.

mucous folds of rectum COLUMNAE ANALES.

nail fold A fold of skin around the nail.

nasal fold The medial and lateral elevated edges of the two olfactory pits in the embryo which contribute to the formation of the edges of the primitive anterior nares.

nasolabial fold SULCUS NASOLABIALIS.

nasopharyngeal fold PLICA SALPINGOPALATINA.

Nélaton's fold The most prominent of the transverse mucosal folds within the rectum. It is located at the junction of the middle and lower thirds. Also called *Nélaton sphincter.*

neural fold One of the two edges of the neural groove which rise high, fold over, and fuse to form the neural tube. Also called *medullary fold, neural ridge, medullary ridge.*

opercular fold A fold of connective tissue adhering the palatine tonsil to the palatoglossal arch.

palmate folds PLICAE PALMATAE.

palpebral fold Either fornix conjunctivae inferior or fornix conjunctivae superior. Also called *retrotarsal fold* (outmoded), *conjunctival fold.*

palpebronasal fold PLICA PALPEBRONASALIS.

pancreaticogastric fold PLICA GASTROPANCREATICA.

paraduodenal fold PLICA PARADUODENALIS.

parietocolic fold An outmoded term for LIGAMENTUM PHRENICOCOLICUM.

parietoperitoneal fold A fold of fetal peritoneum stretching from the left side of the ascending colon to the parietal peritoneum on the right. Also called *Jonnesco's fold, Juvara's fold.*

patellar synovial fold PLICA SYNOVIALIS INFRAPATELLARIS.

Pawlik's folds The proximal part of the columna rugarum anterior and its rugae vaginales, related to the trigone of the bladder anteriorly.

pharyngoepiglottic fold An outmoded term for PLICA GLOSSOEPIGLOTTICA LATERALIS.

pituitary folds DIAPHRAGMA SELLAE.

pleuroperitoneal fold A fold of parietal (somatopleuric) mesoderm semilunar in shape, which contributes, together with the septum transversum, to the formation of the diaphragm and its crura. Also called *pleuroperitoneal membrane, pleuroperitoneum.*

posterior mallear fold of tympanic membrane PLICA MAL-LEARIS POSTERIOR MEMBRANAE TYMPANI.

presplenic fold The angulated peritoneal reflection between the gastrosplenic and lienorenal ligaments towards the lower end of the spleen where it usually transmits some branches of the splenic artery. An outmoded term.

primitive fold One of the ridges flanking the primitive groove that extends axially along the surface of the primitive streak.

proximal nail fold A fold of skin around the proximal portion of the nail.

Rathke's folds Folds of mesoderm that unite to form the cloacal or urorectal septum which divides the urogenital sinus from the rectum in the embryo.

rectal folds PLICAE TRANSVERSALES RECTI.

rectouterine fold PLICA RECTOUTERINA.

rectovaginal fold A peritoneal fold that extends from the back of the posterior fornix of the vagina to the front of the rectum and forms the bottom of the rectouterine pouch. Also called *posterior ligament of uterus, plica rectovaginalis* (outmoded).

rectovesical fold SACROGENITAL FOLD.

retrotarsal fold An outmoded term for PALPEBRAL FOLD.

right gastropancreatic fold An outmoded term for PLICA HEPATOPANCREATICA.

Rindfleisch folds Crescentic folds in the serous pericardium around the ascending aorta.

sacrogenital fold A peritoneal fold that extends from the posterior surface of the urinary bladder to the sides of the rectum and the front of the sacrum, bounding the rectovesical pouch in the male. It corresponds in part with the rectouterine fold in the female. Also called *rectovesical fold, posterior ligaments of bladder of Morris, posterior false ligaments of bladder.*

salpingonasal folds Two mucosal folds that extend from the roof of the nasal cavity through the choanae into the superior wall of the pharynx as far as the opening of the auditory tube on each side. An outmoded term.

salpingopalatine fold PLICA SALPINGOPALATINA.

salpingopharyngeal fold PLICA SALPINGOPHARYNGEA.

Schultze's folds Folds of amnion at the point of attachment of the umbilical cord to the placenta. The folds were considered to be related to the regression of the yolk sac during the development of the human placenta.

folds of scrotum Transverse ridges of skin, both parallel and irregular, that extend laterally from the median raphe across the anterior and lateral surfaces of the scrotum. They are produced by the dartos muscle, the fibers of which are at right angles to the ridges.

semilunar fold PLICA SEMILUNARIS CONJUNCTIVAE.

semilunar folds of colon PLICAE SEMILUNARES COLI.

semilunar fold of conjunctiva PLICA SEMILUNARIS CONJUNCTIVAE.

semilunar fold of transversalis fascia LIGAMENTUM INTERFOVEOLARE.

serosal fold PLICA SEROSA.

serous fold PLICA SEROSA.

sexual fold GENITAL RIDGE.

sigmoid folds of colon PLICAE SEMILUNARES COLI.

spiral fold PLICA SPIRALIS.

spiral fold of cystic duct PLICA SPIRALIS.

stapedial fold PLICA STAPEDIS.

sublingual fold PLICA SUBLINGUALIS.

superior duodenal fold PLICA DUODENALIS SUPERIOR.

synovial fold PLICA SYNOVIALIS.

synovial fold of hip LIGAMENTUM CAPITIS FEMORIS.

tail fold See under HEAD AND TAIL FOLDS.

transverse mucosal fold of Schreiber A transverse mucosal fold encountered above the rectosigmoid junction about 32–35 cm from the anal orifice during rect osigmoid endoscopic examination. An outmoded term.

transverse palatine folds PLICAE PALATINAE TRANSVERSAE.

transverse folds of rectum PLICAE TRANSVERSALES RECTI.

transverse vesical fold PLICA VESICALIS TRANSVERSA.

Treves fold **1** PLICA ILEOCAECALIS. **2** PLICA CAECALIS VASCULARIS.

triangular fold PLICA TRIANGULARIS.

triangular fold of His PLICA TRIANGULARIS.

tubal folds of uterine tube PLICAE TUBARIAE TUBAE UTERINAE.

fold of the urachus PLICA UMBILICALIS MEDIANA.

urethral fold UROGENITAL RIDGE.

urogenital fold UROGENITAL RIDGE.

uterosacral fold PLICA RECTOUTERINA.

vaginal folds RUGAE VAGINALES.

vascular fold A peritoneal fold containing blood vessels.

vascular cecal fold PLICA CAECALIS VASCULARIS.

vascular fold of cecum PLICA CAECALIS VASCULARIS.

Vater's fold A prominent, hoodlike fold of mucous membrane that is situated proximal to the greater duodenal papilla and at the lower extremity of the plica longitudinalis in the descending part of the duodenum.

ventricular fold An outmoded term for PLICA VESTIBULARIS.

Veraguth's fold A fold of skin on the lateral third of the upper eyelid. It was believed to occur in melancholic states, yet it is commonly observed in normal, aging individuals. An obsolete term.

vestibular fold PLICA VESTIBULARIS.

vestigial fold of Marshall PLICA VENAE CAVAE SINISTRAE.

villous folds of stomach PLICAE VILLOSAE GASTRICAE.

vocal fold PLICA VOCALIS.

Foley [Frederic Eugene Basil *Foley*, U.S. urologist, 1891–1966] **1** Foley Y-type ureteropelvioplasty. See under FOLEY Y-PLASTY. **2** Catheter.

folia Plural of FOLIUM.

foliaceous Pertaining to, possessing, or resembling leaves. Also *foliated.*

foliated FOLIACEOUS.

folic acid Any of a number of compounds including pteroic acid and its conjugates with one or more molecules of glutamic acid. The glutamic residues are joined by acylation of the amino group of one by the γ-carboxyl of the next. Folic acid is a vitamin, since it is required in the form of tetrahydrofolate, produced by enzymic reduction, for carrying various one-carbon groups in metabolism. Deficiency leads to megaloblastic anemia. The richest dietary sources of folic acid are liver, kidneys, and fresh, dark green vegetables. Three quarters of the folic acid found in foods is in polyglutamyl forms. These forms are hydrolyzed to pteroylglutamic acid before intestinal absorption. Methyltetrahydrofolate is the principal form in the plasma and liver. Normal plasma levels are in the range of 6–20 μg/l. Deficiency is indicated at 3–6 μg/l. Recommended dietary allowance for adults is 400 μg. Also called *Lactobacillus bulgaricus factor* (outmoded), *Lactobacillus casei factor* (outmoded), *folacin* (obsolete). See also FOLATE TRAP.

folie [French (from L *follis* a leather ball, balloon), madness] **1** Acquired insanity. **2** Any psychologic abnormality.

folie à deux The simultaneous appearance of psychosis in two persons closely associated with one another. Also called *double insanity, simultaneous delusion.* See also SHARED DELUSION.

folie circulaire An outmoded term for ALTERNATING MANIC-DEPRESSIVE DISORDER.

folie communiquée SHARED DELUSION.

folie des grandeurs   DELUSION OF GRANDEUR.

folie des persécutions   Paranoia accompanied by delusions of persecution.

folie du doute   An obsessive-compulsive neurosis characterized by repeated checking to see if a mistake was made or to be sure something was done properly. Also called *doubting mania, checking compulsion, folie raisonnante, doubting insanity.*

folie du pourquoi   An obsessive-compulsive neurosis characterized by a repeated need to ask questions. Also called *questioning mania, Fragesucht.*

folie gemellaire   Psychosis occurring simultaneously in twins, a special form of folie à deux.

folie imitative   SHARED DELUSION.

folie imposée   SHARED DELUSION.

folie induite   SHARED DELUSION.

folie musculaire   Severe chorea.

folie raisonnante   FOLIE DU DOUTE.

Folin   [Otto *Folin*, Swedish-born U.S. biochemist, 1867–1934] **1** See under REACTION, TEST. **2** Folin's alkaline copper tartrate reagent. See under REAGENT. **3** Folin and Wu test. See under TEST. **4** Folin's protein-free filtrate. See under FILTRATE. **5** Folin and Svedberg method. See under METHOD.

folinic acid $C_{20}H_{23}N_7O_7$. 5-Formyl-5,6,7,8 tetra-hydropteroyl-L-glutamic acid. An active form of folic acid used in the treatment of megaloblastic anemia resulting from folic acid deficiency, as opposed to that arising from vitamin B_{12} deficiency. It is also used in other forms of folic acid deficiency, such as that arising from the chronic administration of folic acid antagonists. Also called *citrovorum factor, leucovorin.*

folium   [L (from Gk *phyllon* a leaf), a leaf]   (*plural* folia) [NA] A leaflike structure or part, as those in the cerebellum.

folium cacuminis   An obsolete term for FOLIUM VERMIS.

folia cerebelli   [NA] The extensive, parallel leaflike structures formed by the folds of cerebellar cortex. Also called *folia of cerebellum.*

folia of cerebellum   FOLIA CEREBELLI.

lingual folia   An outmoded term for PAPILLAE FOLIATAE.

folium vermis   [NA] The small superior portion of the cerebellar vermis lying between the tuber vermis and the declive. Also called *folium cacuminis.*

Folli   [Cecilio Folli (*Folius*), Italian anatomist, 1615–1660]   **1** Folius muscle. See under LIGAMENTUM MALLEI LATERALE.   **2** Processus anterior mallei Folii, process of Folius. See under PROCESSUS ANTERIOR MALLEI.

follicle   [L *folliculus.* See FOLLICULUS.]   A small, saclike depression. Also called *folliculus.*

aggregated follicles   FOLLICULI LYMPHATICI AGGREGATI.

aggregated lymphatic follicles of Peyer   PEYER'S PATCHES.

aggregated lymphoid follicles of vermiform appendix   A coalescence of lymphoid follicles in the wall of the vermiform appendix. Also called *folliculi lymphatici aggregati appendicis vermiformis, noduli aggregati processus vermiformis* (outmoded), *aggregated lymphatic nodules of appendix, noduli lymphatici aggregati appendicis vermiformis.*

anovular ovarian follicle   CORPUS ATRETICUM.

atretic follicle   CORPUS ATRETICUM.

atretic ovarian follicle   CORPUS ATRETICUM.

closed follicle   A completely closed sac or pouch.

dental follicle   **1** A mesenchymal condensation surrounding a tooth germ. **2** A fibrous envelope surrounding the crown of a tooth prior to its eruption through the oral mucosa. Also called *odontotheca.*

Fleischmann's follicle   A lymphatic nodule occasionally present in the oral mucosa over the genioglossus muscle.

gastric follicle   **1** LYMPHOID FOLLICLE OF STOMACH. **2** GLANDULA GASTRICA PROPRIA.

germinal follicle   GERMINAL CENTER.

graafian follicle   VESICULAR OVARIAN FOLLICLE.

hair follicle   The tube of epidermal cells at the base of which the hair matrix forms the hair shaft. Also called *folliculus pili, vagina pili* (outmoded).

intestinal follicles   GLANDULAE INTESTINALES.

laryngeal lymphatic follicles   NODULI LYMPHATICI AGGREGATI CAVITATIS LARYNGIS.

lenticular follicle   LYMPHOID FOLLICLE OF STOMACH.

Lieberkühn's follicles   GLANDULAE INTESTINALES.

lingual follicles   FOLLICULI LINGUALES.

lymphatic follicle   NODULUS LYMPHATICUS.

lymphatic follicles of tongue   FOLLICULI LINGUALES.

lymphoid follicle of stomach   A collection of normal and reactive lymphoid cells in the lamina propria of the stomach. It sometimes spills over into the submucosal layer. Also called *gastric follicle, lymphatic nodule of stomach, lenticular follicle, folliculus lymphaticus gastricus, nodulus lymphaticus gastricus, lenticular gland of stomach* (outmoded).

mature ovarian follicle   The ovarian follicle when fully developed and about to rupture at ovulation. Usually only one follicle reaches maturity during each reproductive cycle in the human female. It is then 15–18 mm in diameter. In polytocous mammals, several follicles reach maturity and ovulate simultaneously.

Montgomery's follicles   MONTGOMERY'S GLANDS.

nabothian follicles   NABOTHIAN CYSTS.

nasal mucous follicles   An outmoded term for GLANDULAE NASALES.

ovarian follicle   The egg-containing, fluid-filled sphere that develops in the ovary and ruptures at ovulation to liberate the ovum. It is also an endocrine gland, producing estrogens and giving rise after ovulation to a corpus luteum. It appears first as a primordial follicle with the oocyte surrounded by a single layer of flattened follicular cells, then by a single layer of cuboidal or columnar cells (and called a primary follicle). Follicles mature at intervals depending on the type of reproductive pattern in response to the follicle-stimulating hormone (FSH) from the anterior lobe of the pituitary. The epithelial covering becomes a many-layered membrana granulosa and a second outer covering is added, the theca interna. An antrum usually forms in the granulosa layer and fluid, liquor folliculi, accumulates as the follicle enlarges. The oocyte, usually a secondary oocyte by the stage of antrum formation, is surrounded by granulosa cells forming the corona radiata and is mounted eccentrically on the follicle wall on the cumulus oophorous. This stage is sometimes called a secondary or vesicular or graafian follicle. Only about 300 follicles mature and rupture at ovulation during a woman's reproductive life. The others degenerate at various stages of maturation by the process of follicular atresia.

palpebral follicles   An outmoded term for GLANDULAE TARSALES.

pilosebaceous follicle   An invagination of the epidermis that extends down to the hair root sheath and communicates with a sebaceous gland.

polyovular ovarian follicle   A follicle containing more than one oocyte. The condition has been reported in many mammalian types, including humans, but apart from some marsupials it is thought that polyovular follicles become atretic and do not give rise to multiple births.

primary follicle   A lymphoid follicle that has not received an antigenic stimulus.

primary ovarian follicle   An ovarian follicle at an early stage in its development succeeding that of the primordial follicle when the oocyte is surrounded by a single layer of cuboidal or columnar follicle cells. Also called *folliculus ovaricus primarius.*

primordial ovarian follicle   The earliest and smallest type of ovarian follicle, consisting of an oogonium or oocyte surrounded by a single layer of follicle cells. It is formed by the time of birth or just afterwards in most mammals by division of oogonia. Some 400 000 are present in each human ovary at birth. The number falls rapidly, due to atresia, to about half at puberty and none remains a few years after the menopause. Also called *folliculus ovaricus primordialis.*

sebaceous follicle A pilosebaceous unit in which the sebaceous gland is prominent.

secondary follicle 1 VESICULAR OVARIAN FOLLICLE. **2** An ovarian follicle at the stage of its development when it is enveloped by a stratified follicular epithelium and a developing follicular theca. Also called *folliculus ovaricus secundarius.* • See note at VESICULAR OVARIAN FOLLICLE. **3** A follicle which has developed a germinal center following antigenic stimulation.

solitary follicle A single rounded collection of lymphoid cells within a tissue or organ.

solitary lymphatic follicles of colon SOLITARY LYMPHOID FOLLICLES OF LARGE INTESTINE.

solitary lymphoid follicles of large intestine An isolated collection of normal and reactive lymphoid cells in the lamina propria of the large intestine. Also called *solitary lymphatic nodules of large intestine, folliculi lymphatici solitarii intestini crassi, noduli lymphatici solitarii intestini crassi, solitary lymphatic follicles of colon.*

splenic lymph follicles FOLLICULI LYMPHATICI SPLENICI.

follicle of Stannius A unit of lymphoid tissue in the wall of the bursa of Fabricius (cloacal bursa). It comprises a cortex and medulla.

tertiary follicle VESICULAR OVARIAN FOLLICLE. • See note at VESICULAR OVARIAN FOLLICLE.

thyroid follicle FOLLICULUS GLANDULAE THYROIDEAE.

follicle of thyroid gland FOLLICULUS GLANDULAE THYROIDEAE.

follicles of tongue FOLLICULI LINGUALES.

follicles of urethra The glandulae urethrales urethrae femininae and glandulae urethrales urethrae masculinae. An outmoded term.

vesicular ovarian follicle An ovarian follicle at the stage of its development when a fluid-filled cavity (antrum) appears. Also called *secondary follicle, tertiary follicle, graafian follicle, ovisac, Baer's vesicle, folliculus ovaricus vesiculosus.* See also OVARIAN FOLLICLE. • The Fifth Edition of Nomina Histologica (1983, based on the world congress held in Mexico City in 1980) defined the vesicular ovarian follicle as a tertiary follicle, and a secondary follicle as "a growing primary ovocyte enveloped by a stratified follicular epithelium and a developing follicular theca . . ." However, *secondary follicle* is well established as referring to the vesicular ovarian follicle.

folliclis An obsolete term for PAPULONECROTIC TUBERCULID.

follicular Pertaining to one or more follicles.

folliculi Plural of FOLLICULUS.

folliculitis [*follicul(us)* + -ITIS] Inflammation of one or more follicles. Also called *epifolliculitis* (obsolete).

folliculitis abscedens et suffodiens A burrowing, suppurating folliculitis of the scalp.

acneform folliculitis Folliculitis associated with the formation of comedones, as in acne vulgaris.

agminate folliculitis Inflammation of a cluster of contiguous follicles.

folliculitis barbae Folliculitis of the beard.

folliculitis cheloidalis KELOID ACNE.

conglomerate folliculitis KERION.

conglomerative pustular folliculitis KERION.

folliculitis cruris atrophicans Pustular folliculitis that leads to cicatricial alopecia of the lower leg. It occurs predominantly in males and in tropical climates.

folliculitis decalvans Folliculitis that results in alopecia.

folliculitis decalvans cryptococcica A scarring folliculitis of the scalp caused by a yeast species.

folliculitis decalvans of the glabrous skin Folliculitis leading to the destruction of follicles in parts of the body not bearing terminal hair.

folliculitis decalvans of Quinquaud An inflammatory destructive process characterized by follicular pustulation that leads to cicatricial alopecia.

folliculitis gonorrhoeica A gonococcal inflammation of Littre's glands. An obsolete term.

Gram-negative folliculitis A pustular or papular inflammation of the hair follicles due to infection with Gram-negative bacteria such as *Proteus.* This is a rare complication of the antibiotic treatment of acne vulgaris.

industrial folliculitis OIL ACNE.

keloidal folliculitis KELOID ACNE.

folliculitis keloidalis KELOID ACNE.

Malassezia folliculitis An uncommon pustular eruption of the skin of the upper trunk or face, thought by some to be a reaction to the *Malassezia* species of yeasts normally present in the hair follicles and sebaceous glands in these regions. Also called *Pityrosporum folliculitis.*

folliculitis nares perforans Inflammation of a hair follicle in the nasal vestibule, that progresses to abscess formation, the abscess discharging eventually through the skin adjacent to the nasolabial or nasobuccal sulcus.

folliculitis necrotica Folliculitis complicated by focal necrosis of the follicles and the surrounding tissue.

oil folliculitis OIL ACNE.

Pityrosporum folliculitis *MALASSEZIA* FOLLICULITIS.

pustular folliculitis Folliculitis with clinically evident pus formation.

pyococcal folliculitis PYOGENIC FOLLICULITIS.

pyogenic folliculitis Folliculitis caused by infection with staphylococci. Also called *pyococcal folliculitis.*

seborrheic folliculitis Folliculitis as a manifestation of seborrheic dermatitis.

folliculitis simplex SUPERFICIAL FOLLICULITIS.

superficial folliculitis Inflammation confined to the upper part of a follicle. Also called *folliculitis simplex.*

folliculitis ulerythematosa reticulata VERMICULATE ATROPHODERMA OF THE CHEEKS.

folliculitis varioliformis Folliculitis that leaves scars resembling those of smallpox lesions.

folliculoid Resembling a follicle.

folliculoma [*follicul(us)* + -OMA] GRANULOSA CELL TUMOR.

folliculoma lipidique A Sertoli cell tumor in which the tumor cells are distended with lipid.

folliculose 1 Resembling a follicle. **2** Marked by many follicles.

folliculosis [*follicul(us)* + -OSIS] The state of having excess numbers of follicles, such as lymph follicles.

folliculosis of the conjunctiva The presence of multiple small lymphoid follicles, usually more marked in the tarsal portion of the conjunctiva, often due to virus infections.

folliculus [L (dim. of *follis* a leather bag, esp. a pair of bellows), a little sack or bag] (*plural* folliculi) **1** FOLLICLE. **2** A spherical collection of cells which may contain a cavity.

folliculus glandulae thyroideae [NA] Any of the rounded, hollow cellular units that form the lobules of each lobe of the thyroid gland and consist of an outer layer of epithelial cells of varying size surrounding a space containing jelly-like colloid. Between the units is highly vascular connective tissue, as well as nerve fibers and lymphatics. The shape of the follicle cells vary with the activity of the gland, their secretions being hormones. Also called *thyroid follicle, follicle of thyroid gland.*

folliculi linguales [NA] Nodules of lymphoid tissue in the submucous layer of the pharyngeal part of the tongue that produce a number of bulgings on the surface and are collectively termed the lingual tonsil. Also called *lingual follicles, follicles of tongue, lymphatic follicles of tongue, follicular glands of tongue* (outmoded), *lenticular glands of tongue* (outmoded).

folliculi lymphatici aggregati   A group of lymphatic follicles. Also called *aggregate nodule, insulae of Peyer, aggregate glands, aggregated follicles, Peyer's glands, agminated glands, noduli lymphatici aggregati Peyeri* (outmoded), *intestinal tonsil* (outmoded), *tonsilla intestinalis* (outmoded).

folliculi lymphatici aggregati appendicis vermiformis AGGREGATED LYMPHOID FOLLICLES OF VERMIFORM APPENDIX.

folliculi lymphatici laryngei   NODULI LYMPHATICI AGGREGATI CAVITATIS LARYNGIS.

folliculi lymphatici lienales   An outmoded term for FOLLICULI LYMPHATICI SPLENICI.

folliculi lymphatici recti   Occasional solitary lymphatic follicles that are irregularly scattered in the mucous membrane of the rectum and that resemble those of the small intestine. Also called *noduli lymphatici solitarii recti.*

folliculi lymphatici solitarii intestini crassi SOLITARY LYMPHOID FOLLICLES OF LARGE INTESTINE.

folliculi lymphatici splenici [NA] Nodular localized enlargements of the sheaths of lymphatic tissue that surround the small arteriolar branches of the splenic arteries as far as their divisions into capillaries and form the white pulp of the spleen. Also called *malpighian bodies of spleen, malpighian corpuscles of spleen, malpighian glands, noduli lymphatici lienales malpighii* (outmoded), *splenic lymph follicles, splenic lymph nodules, acini lienales* (outmoded), *acini lienis* (outmoded), *malpighian nodules, folliculi lymphatici lienales* (outmoded), *splenic corpuscles.*

folliculus lymphaticus   NODULUS LYMPHATICUS.

folliculus lymphaticus gastricus   LYMPHOID FOLLICLE OF STOMACH.

folliculus lymphaticus solitarius intestinus tenuis SOLITARY LYMPHOID NODULE OF SMALL INTESTINE.

folliculus ovaricus primarius   PRIMARY OVARIAN FOLLICLE.

folliculus ovaricus primordialis   PRIMORDIAL OVARIAN FOLLICLE.

folliculus ovaricus secundarius   SECONDARY FOLLICLE. ● See note at VESICULAR OVARIAN FOLLICLE.

folliculus ovaricus vesiculosus   VESICULAR OVARIAN FOLLICLE.

folliculus pili   [NA] HAIR FOLLICLE.

Fölling [Ivar Asbjørn *Fölling*, Norwegian physician, born 1888] Fölling's disease. See under PHENYLKETONURIA.

following   In electroencephalography, a phenomenon in which repeated sensory stimuli, such as photic stimulation, cause cortical response patterns characterized by one response wave for each stimulus. This is sometimes described as "driving" the brain waves, so that the alpha rhythm varies in frequency according to the frequency of the stimulus or at a frequency that represents a harmonic of the latter.

follow-up   **1** Done or administered to a patient subsequent to the initial diagnosis or treatment, as *follow-up care.* **2** A follow-up measure or treatment.

Follutein   A proprietary name for human chorionic gonadotropin.

Foltz [Jean Charles Eugene *Foltz*, French ophthalmologist, 1822–1876] Valvule of Foltz. See under VALVE.

Folvite   A proprietary name for folic acid.

fomentation [Late L *fomentatio* (from *fomentatus*, past part. of

fomentare to foment, from *fomentum* poultice, from L *fovere* to warm) application of a poultice] **1** The use of hot, moist applications, especially to ease pain or reduce inflammation. **2** The hot, moist substance or material used in fomentation, such as a poultice.

fomes [L (from *fovere* to warm, keep warm, foster), tinder] (*plural* fomites) Any nonpathogenic substance or inanimate object other than food that is capable of harboring or transmitting pathogenic microorganisms. Fomes or fomites need not *actively* harbor or transmit, but must be *capable of* harboring or transmitting. Also called *fomite.*

fomite [L *fomit(is)*, gen. of FOMES. See FOMES.]   FOMES.

fomites   Plural of FOMES.

fons pulsatilis   ANTERIOR FONTANEL.

Fonsecaea   A genus of fungi which are among the several agents of chromomycosis.

fontactoscope [L *fons*, gen. *fontis*, spring water + Gk *act(is)* a ray, beam + *o* + -SCOPE]   An electroscope designed for measuring the radioactivity of water and gases.

Fontan [François *Fontan*, French thoracic surgeon, born 1929] See under OPERATION.

Fontana [Arturo *Fontana*, Italian dermatologist, 1873–1950] See under STAIN.

Fontana [Felice *Fontana*, Italian neurologist, 1730–1805] **1** Fontana's markings. See under MARKING. **2** Fontana spaces. See under SPATIA ANGULI IRIDOCORNEALIS.

fontanel [French *fontanelle* (dim. of *fontaine* fountain, from L *fontanus* pertaining to a spring or fountain, from *fons*, gen. *fontis*, a spring, fountain) a soft place in the skull preceding complete ossification]   FONTICULUS.

anterior fontanel   The fontanel located at the junction of the coronal, frontal, and sagittal sutures of a fetal or newborn skull. Also called *fonticulus quadrangularis, bregmatic fontanel, quadrangular fontanel, frontal fontanel, fonticulus frontalis major, fonticulus major, fonticulus anterior, fons pulsatilis, bregmatic space* (outmoded).

anterolateral fontanel   SPHENOIDAL FONTANEL.

bregmatic fontanel   ANTERIOR FONTANEL.

Casser's fontanel   MASTOID FONTANEL.

casserian fontanel   MASTOID FONTANEL.

Casserio's fontanel   MASTOID FONTANEL.

cranial fontanels   FONTICULI CRANII.

frontal fontanel   ANTERIOR FONTANEL.

Gerdy's fontanel   SAGITTAL FONTANEL.

lateral fontanels   Fonticulus sphenoidalis and fonticulus mastoideus.

mastoid fontanel   The fontanel located at the junction of the lambdoidal, occipitomastoid, and parietomastoid sutures of a fetal or newborn skull. Also called *fonticulus mastoideus, Casser's fontanel, casserian fontanel, Casserio's fontanel, posterolateral fontanel, posterotemporal fontanel.*

occipital fontanel   The fontanel located at the junction of the lambdoidal and sagittal sutures of the fetal or newborn skull. Also called *posterior fontanel, triangular fontanel, fonticulus minor, fonticulus occipitalis, fonticulus posterior, fonticulus triangularis.*

posterior fontanel   OCCIPITAL FONTANEL.

posterolateral fontanel   MASTOID FONTANEL.

posterotemporal fontanel   MASTOID FONTANEL.

quadrangular fontanel   ANTERIOR FONTANEL.

sagittal fontanel   A fontanel that occasionally occurs along the sagittal suture in a fetal or newborn skull. Also called *Gerdy's fontanel.*

sphenoidal fontanel   A fontanel located at the articulations of the parietal, frontal, sphenoidal, and temporal bones in the fetal or newborn skull. Also called *anterolateral fontanel, fonticulus sphenoidalis.*

supraoccipital fontanel   The membranous area in front of the cartilaginous precursor of the supraoccipital bone in the fetus.

triangular fontanel   OCCIPITAL FONTANEL.

fontanelle   FONTICULUS.

fonticuli   Plural of FONTICULUS.

fonticulus [L (dim. of *fons*, gen. *fontis*, a spring, fountain), a little spring or fountain]   An unossified area of the fibrous membrane that forms the fetal cranial vault before ossification begins, usually present for varying periods up to two years after birth, depending on the site. There are six main areas, one at each angle of the parietal bones, those in the median plane fusing into two areas. The membrane consists of the periosteum externally and the dura mater internally. Also called *fontanel, fontanelle.* See also FONTICULI CRANII.

fonticulus anterior   ANTERIOR FONTANEL.

fonticuli cranii   [NA] The unossified areas, occupied by membrane, in the developing human skull, found principally at the angles of the parietal bone, comprising the fonticulus anterior, fonticulus posterior, fonticulus sphenoidalis, and fonticulus mastoideus. Also called *cranial fontanels.*

fonticulus frontalis major   ANTERIOR FONTANEL.

fonticulus gutturis   An outmoded term for FOSSA SUPRACLAVICULARIS MINOR.

fonticulus major   ANTERIOR FONTANEL.

fonticulus mastoideus   MASTOID FONTANEL.

fonticulus minor   OCCIPITAL FONTANEL.

fonticulus occipitalis   OCCIPITAL FONTANEL.

fonticulus posterior   OCCIPITAL FONTANEL.

fonticulus quadrangularis   ANTERIOR FONTANEL.

fonticulus sphenoidalis   SPHENOIDAL FONTANEL.

fonticulus triangularis   OCCIPITAL FONTANEL.

food [Middle English *fode*, from Old English *fōda*, akin to Old English *fōdor* food, fodder and Gk *pateisthai* to feed on]   Any substance that can be used by the body to provide some essential nutrient and/or energy.

health food   Food that has been organically grown, i.e., without the use of inorganic fertilizers. Such food is eaten in its natural state without the addition of chemical additives such as artificial flavors, colorings, and preservatives. Such foods include unpolished rice, raw sugar, sea salt, and whole grain flour.

isodynamic foods   Two or more foods which when metabolized give rise to equal amounts of energy as measured in heat units.

predigested food   Food that is ingested after it has been partially digested in an artificial manner external to the body.

foot [Old English *fōt*, akin to L *pes*, gen. *pedis*, foot and to Gk *pous*, gen. *podos*, foot]   (*plural* feet)   **1** A unit of length equal to 1/3 yard; 0.3048 meter exactly. Symbol: ft **2** The distal end of the lower limb; pes.

athlete's foot   A popular term for TINEA PEDIS.

bifid foot   CLEFT FOOT.

broad foot   A broadening of the distal foot that is caused by the separation of the metatarsal heads and collapse of the transverse arch. Also called *metatarsus latus, talipes transversoplanus, splay foot, spread foot.*

burning feet   A form of nutritional sensory polyneuropathy of uncertain cause, but probably due to vitamin B deficiency, giving a severe burning sensation in the feet. Also called *hot feet, ignipedites.*   ● The phenomenon was first described in certain prisoner-of-war camps in the Far East in the Second World War.

buttress foot   PYRAMIDAL DISEASE.

cavus foot   A foot with a high longitudinal arch.

Charcot's foot   A deformity of the foot resulting from arthrop-

athy, consequent to neurologic lesions of tabes dorsalis.

claw foot   A foot deformity characterized by a high longitudinal arch, abnormal flexion of the interphalangeal joints, and hyperextension of the toes at the metatarsophalangeal joints. Also called *gampsodactyly, gampsodactylia.*

cleft foot   A developmental defect in which one or more of the three central digits are absent, as in lobster-claw deformity, or abnormally aligned with respect to other digits, so that the usual interdigital space extends into the metatarsal region. Also called *bifid foot, split foot.* See also LOBSTER-CLAW DEFORMITY.

club foot   TALIPES.

congenital convex club foot   ROCKER-BOTTOM FLATFOOT.

conventional prosthetic foot   A component of an artificial limb, shaped to resemble the human foot, and articulating with the shank of the artificial limb by a system of mechanical joints that permit ankle-foot motion.

 conventional foot of water   A unit of pressure equal to 304.8 conventional millimeters of mercury; $2.989\ 07 \times 10^3$ pascals; 2.989 07 kilopascals. Also called *foot of water.* Symbol: ftH_2O

convex foot   ROCKER-BOTTOM FLATFOOT.

cross foot   TALIPES VARUS.

crow's foot   A skin crease radiating from the lateral canthus of the eye. Also called *pes corvinus* (obsolete).

cubic foot   A unit of volume equal to a cube having sides of length one foot; 0.028 317 cubic meter; 28.317 liters. Symbol: ft^3

dancers' foot   Traumatic inflammation of the second and third metatarsal heads. The condition is quite painful and is usually associated with dancing.

dangle foot   FOOTDROP.

dangling foot   An obsolete term for FOOTDROP.

drop foot   FOOTDROP.

dropped foot   FOOTDROP.

end foot   The terminal expansion of an axon at the site of synaptic contact on the soma or dendrite of a neuron. Also called *bouton, bouton terminal, terminal bouton, terminal button, synaptic button, synaptic bouton, terminal knob, synaptic knob, terminal ending, end-bulb, neuropodium, neuropodion, clava terminalis* (rarely used).

end feet of Held   Distinctive, large terminal expansions of cochlear nerve synapses.   ● When first described, it was believed that neurofibrils extended across these contacts.

equinus club foot   TALIPES EQUINOVARUS.

fescue foot   FESCUE LAMENESS.

flat foot   Talipes planus. See also entries under FLATFOOT.

Friedreich's club foot   Pes cavus and other foot deformities occurring in Friedreich's disease.

fungus foot   MADURA FOOT.

hollow foot   TALIPES CAVUS.

Hong Kong foot   TINEA PEDIS.

hot feet   BURNING FEET.

immersion foot   Trench foot, especially when it occurs in temperatures above freezing.

foot lambert   A unit of luminance equal to the luminance of a uniform diffuser emitting one lumen per square foot, equal to 3.426 25 nit, 3.426 25 candela per square meter. Symbol: ft La

Madura foot   Mycetoma of the foot caused by *Actinomadura madurae* (formerly *Streptomyces madurae)* and found in India, northern Africa, Cyprus, and South America. Entry of the organism follows trauma. Multiple sinuses ultimately develop. Antifungal agents are sometimes effective, but amputation is frequently necessary. Also called *fungus foot.* See also MYCETOMA.

Morand's foot   An extremely rare malformation in which a foot has eight toes.

Morton's foot   MORTON'S NEUROMA.

mossy foot   An outmoded term for LYMPHOSTATIC VERRU-COSIS.

paralytic club foot   Pes cavus developing as a consequence of lower motor neuron paralysis of the long flexor and extensor muscles of the leg and of the intrinsic muscles of the foot.

foot pound   An incorrect term for FOOT POUND-FORCE. Symbol: ft·lb

foot poundal   A unit of work in the FPS system, equal to the work done when the point of application of one poundal is displaced through a distance of one foot in the direction of the force; 0.042 140 joule. An obsolete unit. Symbol: ft·pdl

foot pound-force (*plural* foot pounds-force) A unit of work equal to the work done when the point of application of one pound-force is displaced through a distance of one foot in the direction of the force; 1.355 82 joules. Also called *foot pound* (incorrect). Symbol: ft·lbf

reel foot   TALIPES.

rocker-bottom foot   ROCKER-BOTTOM FLATFOOT.

root foot   One of the fine digitations on the lower aspect of the basal cells of the epidermis.

SACH foot   An artificial ankle-foot component of a prosthesis, shaped like a human foot, with a solid, nonmovable articulation to the prosthetic shank and including a cushion heel that absorbs the impact of heel strike.   • SACH is an acronym formed from *single axis cushion heel.*

septic foot   Ischemic necrosis of the skin appendages of the foot that extends into the deep tissues along fascial planes. It is usually seen in diabetics and often requires emergency treatment by guillotine amputation.

shuffle foot   The shuffling gait associated with spastic weakness of the legs or with parkinsonism. An imprecise and outmoded term.

splay foot   BROAD FOOT.

split foot   CLEFT FOOT.

spread foot   BROAD FOOT.

square foot   A unit of area equal to 0.092 903 square meter; 929.03 square centimeters. Symbol: ft^2

strawberry rot foot   See under DERMATOPHILOSIS.

stump foot   TALIPES.

sucker foot   The terminal expansion of an astrocytic (glial) process on the basal lamina of a small blood vessel in the central nervous system. Also called *sucker apparatus* (seldom used), *vascular footplate, sucker process.*

tabetic foot   The flattened foot deformity resulting from the tarsal bone destruction seen in tabes dorsalis.

taut foot   The appearance of the foot when there is contracture of the calcaneal tendon and of the plantar flexors of the foot. This condition is thought sometimes to result from wearing shoes with high heels.

tip foot   TALIPES EQUINUS.

trench foot   The painful, vascular response of the feet to prolonged exposure to damp and cold, aggravated by physical inactivity. Such conditions were experienced by many soldiers in trench warfare in World War I. Signs include swelling and inflammation and, in the most severe cases, gangrene. Also called *water-bite.*

valgus club foot   TALIPES EQUINO VALGUS.

varus club foot   TALIPES EQUINOVARUS.

foot of water   CONVENTIONAL FOOT OF WATER.

weak foot   A precursory stage of flatfoot.

footboard   A board placed at the foot of a bed to prevent plantiflexion contractures.

foot-candle   An obsolete term for LUMEN PER SQUARE FOOT. Symbol: ftc, fc

footdrop   Plantar flexion of the foot caused by paralysis or paresis of the muscles of the anterior compartment of the leg,

making it impossible to dorsiflex the foot and leading to a high-stepping gait. Also called *dangling foot* (obsolete), *drop foot, dropped foot, dangle foot, ankle drop.*

foot-engine   A treadle-operated dental drilling machine.

foot lambert   See under FOOT.

footling [FOOT + -*ling*, adverbial suffix meaning manner or direction]   Pertaining to various forms of an incomplete breech presentation in which either one or both feet are presenting parts (footling breech presentation).

footplate   1 BASIS STAPEDIS. 2 PEDICEL.

vascular footplate   SUCKER FOOT.

footprint   The impression of the dermatoglyphic pattern, flexion creases, and secondary folds of the sole of the foot and the plantar aspects of the toes, made by applying ink to these surfaces and pressing them on paper. Footprints, like palmprints, are used chiefly as supplemental records for identification of newborn infants, and rarely in cases of criminal identification. Also called *ichnogram.*

forage [French, a drilling, piercing]   A surgical procedure involving a V-shaped incision of the prostate to treat hypertrophy and obstruction.

foramen

foramen [L (gen. *foraminis*; from *forare* to bore, pierce), a hole, opening] (*plural* foramina) An opening, perforation, or hole into or through a structure or tissue, particularly a bone.

accessory foramen   A foramen on the root of a tooth which opens into the root canal or pulp chamber in addition to the apical foramen.

accessory palatine foramina   An outmoded term for FORAMINA PALATINA MINORA.

foramina alveolaria maxillae   POSTERIOR SUPERIOR ALVEOLAR FORAMINA.

alveolar foramina of maxilla   POSTERIOR SUPERIOR ALVEOLAR FORAMINA.

anterior foramen cecum   A small median depression situated more or less deep to the apex of the substantia perforata interpeduncularis. An outmoded term.

anterior condyloid foramen   CANALIS HYPOGLOSSI.

anterior ethmoid foramen   FORAMEN ETHMOIDALE ANTERIUS.

anterior ethmoidal foramen   FORAMEN ETHMOIDALE ANTERIUS.

anterior lacerate foramen   An outmoded term for FISSURA ORBITALIS SUPERIOR.

anterior maxillary foramen   An obsolete term for MENTAL FORAMEN.

anterior palatine foramen   1 An outmoded term for FORAMEN INCISIVUM. 2 An outmoded term for FOSSA INCISIVA.

anterior sacral foramina   FORAMINA SACRALIA ANTERIORA.

anterior zygomatic foramen   FORAMEN ZYGOMATICOFACIALE.

aortic foramen   HIATUS AORTICUS.

apical foramen of tooth   An opening at or near the apex of the root of a tooth through which vessels and nerves enter and leave the pulp. Also called *foramen apicis dentis, pulpal foramen, foramen radicis dentis, root foramen.*

foramen apicis dentis   APICAL FORAMEN OF TOOTH.

arachnoid foramen   APERTURA MEDIANA VENTRICULI QUARTI.

Bartholin's foramen   An outmoded term for FORAMEN OB-TURATUM.

Bichat's foramen   An obsolete term for CISTERNA VENAE MAGNAE CEREBRI.

blind foramen of tongue   FORAMEN CAECUM LINGUAE.

foramen of Bochdalek   A seldom used term for HIATUS PLEU-ROPERITONEALIS.

Botallo's foramen   An obsolete term for FORAMEN OVALE.

Bozzi's foramen   An outmoded term for MACULA RETINAE.

foramen bursae omentalis majoris   An opening produced by the encroachment of the left gastropancreatic fold of the left gastric artery and the right gastropancreatic fold of the hepatic artery on the omental bursa so that it is divided into a superior and an inferior recess that communicate through the opening in the constriction. Also called *foramen of omental bursa*.

foramen caecum   [NA] Either foramen cecum linguae, foramen cecum ossis frontalis, or foramen cecum medullae oblongatae. Also *foramen cecum*.

foramen caecum linguae   [NA] A prominent median pit at the apex of the sulcus terminalis that separates the dorsum of the tongue into anterior and posterior parts. The pit is the site of the upper end of the thyroid diverticulum in the embryo. Also called *foramen cecum of tongue, Morgagni's foramen, glandular foramen of Morgagni* (outmoded), *glandular foramen of tongue* (outmoded), *Morand's foramen, blind foramen of tongue, ductus lingualis* (outmoded), *lingual duct* (outmoded), *meibomian foramen* (outmoded), *morgagnian foramen*. Also *foramen cecum linguae*.

foramen caecum ossis frontalis   [NA] An opening produced between the notch in the frontal crest and the notched base of the crista galli at the frontoethmoidal suture. Rarely, an emissary vein passes through it to connect the superior sagittal sinus with the nasal veins. Also called *cecal foramen, foramen cecum of frontal bone, frontoethmoidal foramen, cranionasal pore* (outmoded).

caroticoclinoid foramen   An occasional foramen produced by a bar of bone bridging the gap between the anterior and the middle clinoid processes of the sphenoid bone. It provides passage for the internal carotid artery when it leaves the cavernous sinus at the end of the carotid sulcus.

caroticotympanic foramina   CANALICULI CAROTICOTYM-PANICI.

foramen caroticum externum   The large circular opening on the inferior surface of the petrous part of the temporal bone for the internal carotid artery and its plexus of sympathetic nerves entering the carotid canal. Also called *external carotid foramen*.

foramen caroticum internum   The opening at the apex of the petrous part of the temporal bone where the internal carotid artery and its plexus of nerves exit the carotid canal to enter the cranial cavity. Also called *internal carotid foramen*.

carotid foramen   Either foramen caroticum externum or foramen caroticum internum.

cecal foramen   FORAMEN CAECUM OSSIS FRONTALIS.

foramen cecum   FORAMEN CAECUM.

foramen cecum of frontal bone   FORAMEN CAECUM OSSIS FRONTALIS.

foramen cecum linguae   Foramen caecum linguae.

foramen cecum medullae oblongatae   A small midline notch formed by the rostral termination of the anterior median fissure of the medulla oblongata and the caudal border of the pons. Also called *foramen cecum posterius, Schwalbe's foramen, foramen of Vicq d'Azyr, foramen cecum of Vicq d'Azyr, inferior foramen cecum* (outmoded).

foramen cecum posterius   FORAMEN CECUM MEDULLAE OB-LONGATAE.

foramen cecum of tongue   FORAMEN CAECUM LINGUAE.

foramen cecum of Vicq d'Azyr   FORAMEN CECUM MEDUL-LAE OBLONGATAE.

foramen centrale   A foramen in the apical turn of the bony cochlea that transmits filaments of the cochlear division of the vestibulocochlear nerve and is continuous with a canal that runs down the middle of the modiolus to its apex. An outmoded term.

cervical vertebral foramen   FORAMEN PROCESSUS TRANS-VERSI.

common interclinoid foramen   A rarely formed opening between bony bridges joining the anterior, middle, and posterior clinoid processes of the sphenoid bone.

conjugate foramen   A foramen produced by apposing notches at the junction of two bones, such as foramen caecum ossis frontalis.

foramen costotransversarium   A gap occupied by the costotransverse ligament between the posterior surface of the neck of a rib and the anterior aspect of the transverse process and pedicle of the corresponding vertebra. Also called *costotransverse foramen*.

costotransverse foramen   FORAMEN COSTOTRANSVERSAR-IUM.

cotyloid foramen   The opening formed deep to the transverse ligament as it spans the acetabular notch, giving passage to vessels and a nerve to the hip joint.

cribroethmoid foramen   FORAMEN ETHMOIDALE ANTERIUS.

dental foramina   Openings which transmit into the mandible or maxilla nerves and vessels supplying the teeth. An outmoded term.

foramen diaphragmatis sellae   The small opening in the diaphragma sellae covering the sella turcica that accommodates the stalk of the pituitary gland extending from the base of the hypothalamus. Also called *foramen of Pacchioni, pacchionian foramen*.

dorsal sacral foramina   FORAMINA SACRALIA POSTERIORA.

Duverney's foramen   FORAMEN OMENTALE.

ectepicondylar foramen   An opening in the ectepicondyle of the humerus through which a nerve and blood vessels pass. This foramen persists in certain turtles, lizards, and members of the genus *Sphenodon*.

emissary foramen   Any foramen in the skull through which an emissary vein passes, providing communication between dural venous sinuses and veins outside the skull.

entepicondylar foramen   A small opening in the entepicondyle of the humerus through which a nerve and blood vessels pass. This foramen is present in some primitive mammals.

epiploic foramen   FORAMEN OMENTALE.

foramen epiploicum   FORAMEN OMENTALE.

esophageal foramen   HIATUS ESOPHAGEUS.

ethmoidal foramina   FORAMINA ETHMOIDALIA.

foramen ethmoidale anterius   [NA] An opening near the anterior end of the frontoethmoidal suture at the junction of superior and medial walls of the orbit that transmits the anterior ethmoidal nerve and vessels. Also called *anterior ethmoidal foramen, anterior internal orbital canal, anterior ethmoid foramen, cribroethmoid foramen, ethmoidal sulcus of Gegenbaur* (outmoded).

foramen ethmoidale posterius   [NA] An opening near the posterior end of the frontoethmoidal suture at the junction of the superior and medial walls of the orbit that transmits the posterior ethmoidal nerve and vessels. Also called *posterior ethmoidal foramen, posterior ethmoid foramen, posterior internal orbital canal*.

foramina ethmoidalia   [NA] The foramen ethmoidale anterius and the foramen ethmoidale posterius considered together. Also called *ethmoidal foramina, orbital canals, ethmoidal canals*.

external auditory foramen   MEATUS ACUSTICUS EXTERNUS.

external carotid foramen FORAMEN CAROTICUM EXTERNUM.

external zygomatic foramen FORAMEN ZYGOMATICOFACIALE.

facial zygomatic foramen FORAMEN ZYGOMATICOFACIALE.

foramen of Fallopio HIATUS CANALIS NERVI PETROSI MAJORIS.

Ferrein's foramen HIATUS CANALIS NERVI PETROSI MAJORIS.

frontal foramen FORAMEN FRONTALE.

foramen frontale [NA] An occasional foramen, present in about 50 percent of humans, that is located on the supraorbital margin of the frontal bone just medial to the supraorbital notch or foramen. It transmits the supratrochlear artery and the medial branch of the supraorbital nerve and is formed by a small bar of bone bridging over the incisura frontalis. Also called *frontal foramen, medial frontal foramen.*

frontoethmoidal foramen FORAMEN CAECUM OSSIS FRONTALIS.

Galen's foramen The orifice of the anterior cardiac vein in the right atrium draining blood from the front of the right ventricle.

glandular foramina of Littre The orifices of the urethral glands in the mucous membrane of the urethra. An outmoded term.

glandular foramen of Morgagni An outmoded term for FORAMEN CAECUM LINGUAE.

glandular foramen of tongue An outmoded term for FORAMEN CAECUM LINGUAE.

great foramen FORAMEN MAGNUM.

greater ischiadic foramen FORAMEN ISCHIADICUM MAJUS.

greater palatine foramen FORAMEN PALATINUM MAJUS.

greater sciatic foramen FORAMEN ISCHIADICUM MAJUS.

great occipital foramen FORAMEN MAGNUM.

great sacrosciatic foramen FORAMEN ISCHIADICUM MAJUS.

Hartigan's foramen An occasional foramen which is stated to be present at the base of the transverse process of a lumbar vertebra but is rarely observed in adults.

hemal foramen An opening limited by the hemal arch. Also called *visceral foramen.*

Hyrtl's foramen PORUS CROTAPHITICOBUCCINATORIUS.

incisive foramen FORAMEN INCISIVUM.

foramen incisivum [NA] One of the lower openings of the four incisive canals that lead from the floor of the nasal cavity into the incisive fossa lying immediately behind the incisor teeth anteriorly in the median plane of the hard palate and transmitting the nasopalatine nerves. Also called *incisive foramen, incisor foramen, foramen of Stensen, nasopalatine foramen, anterior palatine canal, anterior palatine foramen* (outmoded).

incisor foramen FORAMEN INCISIVUM.

inferior foramen cecum An outmoded term for FORAMEN CECUM MEDULLAE OBLONGATAE.

inferior left foramen An outmoded term for HIATUS AORTICUS.

inferior maxillary foramen An outmoded term for FORAMEN OVALE ALAE MAJORIS.

inferior occipital foramen FORAMEN MAGNUM.

inferior zygomatic foramen FORAMEN ZYGOMATICO-ORBITALE.

infraorbital foramen FORAMEN INFRAORBITALE.

foramen infraorbitale [NA] The anterior opening of the infraorbital canal situated on the anterior surface of the body of the maxilla just below the inferior margin of the orbital opening and above the canine fossa. It transmits the infraorbital nerve and vessels. Also called *infraorbital foramen, suborbital foramen* (outmoded).

foramen infrapiriforme The space in the greater sciatic foramen below the piriformis muscle through which the inferior gluteal nerves and vessels leave the pelvis. A rarely used term.

innominate foramen A very small opening occasionally located posteromedial to foramen ovale in the greater wing of the sphenoid bone through which the small, or lesser, petrosal nerve may leave the skull to pass on to the otic ganglion.

interatrial foramen primum OSTIUM PRIMUM.

interatrial foramen secundum OSTIUM SECUNDUM.

internal auditory foramen PORUS ACUSTICUS INTERNUS.

internal carotid foramen FORAMEN CAROTICUM INTERNUM.

internal sacral foramina FORAMINA SACRALIA ANTERIORA.

internal zygomatic foramen of Arnold FORAMEN ZYGOMATICO-ORBITALE.

internal zygomatic foramen of Meckel FORAMEN ZYGOMATICOTEMPORALE.

intersacral foramina FORAMINA INTERVERTEBRALIA OSSIS SACRI.

interventricular foramen FORAMEN INTERVENTRICULARE.

foramen interventriculare [NA] The opening between one lateral ventricle and the third ventricle. It lies between the column of the fornix and the anterior end of the thalamus. Also called *foramen of Monro, foramen interventriculare Monroi, interventricular foramen, interventricular opening.*

foramen interventriculare Monroi FORAMEN INTERVENTRICULARE.

intervertebral foramen FORAMEN INTERVERTEBRALE.

foramen intervertebrale [NA] The passage formed by the apposition of the vertebral notches of two adjacent vertebrae, transmitting a spinal nerve and vessels. Also called *intervertebral foramen.*

foramina intervertebralia ossis sacri [NA] Four forked channels through which the four pairs of both pelvic and dorsal sacral foramina communicate with the sacral canal through its lateral wall. Also called *intervertebral foramina of sacrum, intersacral canals, intersacral foramina.*

intervertebral foramina of sacrum FORAMINA INTERVERTEBRALIA OSSIS SACRI.

foramen ischiadicum majus [NA] The large aperture of the greater sciatic notch of hip bone spanned by the sacrotuberous ligament and separated from the lesser sciatic foramen by the sacrospinous ligament. Passing through it are the piriformis muscle separating the superior gluteal vessels and nerves above it from the inferior gluteal vessels and nerves, internal pudendal vessels, and pudendal, sciatic, and other nerves below it. Also called *greater sciatic foramen, great sacrosciatic foramen, greater ischiadic foramen.*

foramen ischiadicum minus [NA] The small aperture of the lesser sciatic notch of hip bone spanned by the sacrotuberous ligament and separated from the greater sciatic foramen by the sacrospinous ligament. The bony surface is covered by cartilage over which pass the tendon of the obturator internus muscle and its nerve, while the internal pudendal vessels and pudendal nerve re-enter the pelvis through it from the greater sciatic foramen. Also called *lesser ischiadic foramen, lesser sciatic foramen, small sacrosciatic foramen.*

ischiopubic foramen FORAMEN OBTURATUM.

jugular foramen FORAMEN JUGULARE.

foramen jugulare [NA] An irregularly rounded and deep orifice on the base of the skull, usually larger on the right side, located at the posterior end of the petro-occipital suture and formed anteriorly by the jugular fossa of the petrous part of the temporal bone apposing, posteriorly, the jugular notch on the jugular process lateral to the condyle of the occipital bone. It is partially divided by the processus intrajugularis, lateral to which is the sigmoid sinus, while medial to it are, anteroposteriorly, the inferior petrosal sinus, the glossopharyngeal, vagus, and accessory nerves, and the internal jugular vein. The foramen is posterior to foramen caroticum externum and medial to the base of the styloid process. Also called *jugular foramen, foramen lacerum posterius* (outmoded), *posterior lacerate foramen* (outmoded).

foramen of Key and Retzius APERTURA LATERALIS VENTRICULI QUARTI.

foramen lacerum [NA] An opening with a serrated margin located at the base of the skull between the basilar part of the occipital bone, the junction of the body and greater wing of the sphenoid bone, and the apex of the petrous part of temporal bone. It is normally closed inferiorly by fibrocartilage on which the internal carotid artery rests as the artery leaves the foramen caroticum internum and bends upwards to the cavernous sinus. Also called *middle lacerate foramen, foramen lacerum medium, sphenotic foramen.*

foramen lacerum anterius An outmoded term for FISSURA ORBITALIS SUPERIOR.

foramen lacerum medium An outmoded term for FORAMEN LACERUM.

foramen lacerum posterius An outmoded term for FORAMEN JUGULARE.

foramina of Lannelongue The largest of the foramina venarum minimarum.

lateral foramen An opening on the side of the root of a tooth which leads into the root canal.

lateral incisive foramen The most lateral of several openings of the incisive canals into the incisive fossa posterior to the upper incisor teeth. It conducts the nasopalatine nerve and the terminal branch of the greater palatine artery. Also called *foramen of Stensen.*

lesser ischiadic foramen FORAMEN ISCHIADICUM MINUS.

lesser palatine foramina FORAMINA PALATINA MINORA.

lesser sciatic foramen FORAMEN ISCHIADICUM MINUS.

foramen of Luschka APERTURA LATERALIS VENTRICULI QUARTI.

foramen of Magendie APERTURA MEDIANA VENTRICULI QUARTI.

foramen magnum [NA] The largest cranial foramen, the midline opening of the occipital bones through which emerges the medulla oblongata extending caudally into the vertebral canal. Also called *great foramen, occipital foramen, inferior occipital foramen, foramen occipitale magnum, great occipital foramen.*

malar foramen FORAMEN ZYGOMATICOFACIALE.

foramen mandibulae MANDIBULAR FORAMEN.

mandibular foramen An opening on the medial surface of the ascending ramus of the mandible which transmits the inferior alveolar nerve and vessels. Also called *foramen mandibulae, foramen mandibulare, posterior maxillary foramen.*

foramen mandibulare MANDIBULAR FORAMEN.

mastoid foramen FORAMEN MASTOIDEUM.

foramen mastoideum [NA] A small opening behind the mastoid process of the temporal bone, near or on the occipitomastoid suture, for transmission of an emissary vein from the sigmoid sinus and a branch of the occipital artery to the dura mater. Its location is very variable. Also called *mastoid foramen.*

maxillary foramen HIATUS MAXILLARIS.

medial frontal foramen FORAMEN FRONTALE.

median incisive foramen One of two incisive foramina occasionally present and opening on the anterior and posterior walls of the incisive fossa of the bony palate. Also called *median incisor foramen, Scarpa's foramen.*

median incisor foramen MEDIAN INCISIVE FORAMEN.

medullary foramen FORAMEN VERTEBRALE.

meibomian foramen An outmoded term for FORAMEN CECUM LINGUAE.

mental foramen An opening on the lateral surface of the

mandible adjacent to the premolar teeth which transmits the mental nerve and vessels. Also called *foramen mentale, anterior maxillary foramen* (obsolete).

foramen mentale MENTAL FORAMEN.

middle lacerate foramen An outmoded term for FORAMEN LACERUM.

foramen of Monro FORAMEN INTERVENTRICULARE.

Morand's foramen FORAMEN CAECUM LINGUAE.

Morgagni's foramen 1 The occasional deficiency between the costal and sternal origins of the respiratory diaphragm, filled on each side with areolar tissue and transmitting the superior epigastric vessels and lymphatic vessels. Also called *pleuroperitoneal foramen, trigonum sternocostale* (outmoded), *morgagnian foramen, Larrey space, sternocostal triangle, Larrey's cleft.* **2** FORAMEN SINGULARE. **3** FORAMEN CAECUM LINGUAE.

morgagnian foramen 1 MORGAGNI'S FORAMEN. 2 FORAMEN SINGULARE. 3 FORAMEN CAECUM LINGUAE.

nasal foramina Small openings on the external, or facial, surface of the nasal bone for transmission of tributaries of the angular vein. Also called *foramina nasalia* (outmoded).

foramina nasalia An outmoded term for NASAL FORAMINA.

nasopalatine foramen FORAMEN INCISIVUM.

foramina nervosa laminae spiralis FORAMINA NERVOSA LIMBUS LAMINAE SPIRALIS OSSEAE.

foramina nervosa limbus laminae spiralis osseae [NA] Numerous openings on the tympanic lip of the limbus laminae spiralis osseae of the cochlear labyrinth for the transmission of the branches of the cochlear nerve to the spiral organ. Also called *foramina nervosa laminae spiralis, habenula perforata.*

foramen nutricium [NA] NUTRIENT FORAMEN.

nutrient foramen An aperture, perforation, or passage through the cortex of the bone that carries the blood vessels to the medullary space. Also called *foramen nutricium.*

obturator foramen FORAMEN OBTURATUM.

foramen obturatum [NA] A large, irregularly oval opening bounded above and laterally by the acetabulum and acetabular notch, anteromedially and posterolaterally by the pubis and ischium respectively, and anteroinferiorly by the ischiopubic ramus. Attached to its circumference is a fibrous membrane, except superiorly at the obturator canal. Also called *obturator foramen, thyroid foramen* (outmoded), *oval foramen of hip bone* (outmoded), *ischiopubic foramen, Bartholin's foramen* (outmoded).

occipital foramen FORAMEN MAGNUM.

foramen occipitale magnum FORAMEN MAGNUM.

olfactory foramen One of numerous foramina arranged in rows on the lamina cribrosa of the ethmoid bone through which pass filaments of the olfactory nerve.

foramen of omental bursa FORAMEN BURSAE OMENTALIS MAJORIS.

foramen omentale [NA] A short peritoneal canal between the omental bursa and the greater sac of abdominal peritoneum. It is bounded anteriorly by the right margin of the lesser omentum, inferiorly by the superior part of the duodenum, posteriorly by the inferior vena cava, and superiorly by the caudate process of liver. It is located just to the right of the midline. Also called *foramen epiploicum, epiploic foramen, foramen of Winslow, Duverney's foramen, aditus ad saccum peritonaei minorem* (outmoded), *hiatus of Winslow, porta of omentum* (outmoded), *porta omenti* (outmoded), *opening of omental bursa, opening to lesser sac of peritoneum, epiploic orifice.*

optic foramen 1 CANALIS OPTICUS. 2 An outmoded term for LAMINA CRIBROSA SCLERAE.

optic foramen of sclera LAMINA CRIBROSA SCLERAE.

optic foramen of sphenoid bone CANALIS OPTICUS.

foramen opticum ossis sphenoidalis An outmoded term for CANALIS OPTICUS.

orbital zygomatic foramen FORAMEN ZYGOMATICO-ORBIT-ALE.

orbitomalar foramen FORAMEN ZYGOMATICO-ORBITALE.

foramen ovale A valved communication between the right atrium and left atrium in the fetal heart. It is usually an obliquely elongated cleft bounded by the upper edge of the persisting part of the septum primum and by the lower edge of the septum secundum. The part of the septum primum that overlaps the cleft is called the valve of the foramen ovale. The foramen serves to direct oxygenated blood from the fetal inferior vena to the left atrium. It is obliterated shortly after birth in most individuals because increase in pressure in the left atrium closes the valve and fusion leaves a depression on the right side of the interatrial wall, called the fossa ovalis, lying inside the arched edge, or annulus ovalis, of the septum secundum. Not infrequently fusion is incomplete but the opening is small and possibly still valvular so that function is unimpaired. In a minority the opening remains unclosed in postnatal life and constitutes a patent foramen ovale. Also called *Botallo's foramen* (obsolete). See also OSTIUM PRIMUM, OSTIUM SECUNDUM.

foramen ovale alae majoris [NA] A large oval foramen near the middle of the posterior margin of the greater wing of the sphenoid bone between foramen rotundum anteriorly and foramen spinosum posterolaterally, transmitting the mandibular nerve to the infratemporal fossa along with the accessory meningeal artery and, occasionally, the lesser petrosal nerve. Also called *foramen ovale ossis sphenoidalis, oval foramen of sphenoid bone, inferior maxillary foramen* (outmoded), *foramen ovale basis cranii.*

foramen ovale basis cranii FORAMEN OVALE ALAE MAJORIS.

foramen ovale cordis OSTIUM SECUNDUM.

foramen ovale ossis sphenoidalis FORAMEN OVALE ALAE MAJORIS.

foramen ovale of Pacchioni An outmoded term for INCISURA TENTORII.

foramen ovale of Weitbrecht An opening between the superior and middle glenohumeral ligaments in the fibrous capsule of the shoulder joint that permits communication between its synovial membrane and the subtendinous bursa of the subscapularis muscle. An outmoded term.

oval foramen of fetus OSTIUM SECUNDUM.

oval foramen of hip bone An outmoded term for FORAMEN OBTURATUM.

oval foramen of sphenoid bone FORAMEN OVALE ALAE MAJORIS.

foramen of Pacchioni FORAMEN DIAPHRAGMATIS SELLAE.

pacchionian foramen FORAMEN DIAPHRAGMATIS SELLAE.

foramina palatina minora [NA] Two or more small openings piercing the pyramidal process of the palatine bone in each posterolateral angle of the bony palate behind the greater palatine foramina and transmitting the lesser palatine nerves and vessels from their canals. Also called *lesser palatine foramina, accessory palatine foramina.*

foramina of palatine tonsil FOSSULAE TONSILLARES TONSILLAE PALATINAE.

foramen palatinum majus [NA] The lower orifice of the greater palatine canal that opens on the posterolateral part of the bony palate just behind the palatomaxillary suture and transmits the greater palatine nerve and vessels. Also called *greater palatine foramen, posterior palatine foramen, pterygopalatine foramen* (outmoded), *sphenopalatine foramen* (outmoded).

foramina papillaria renis [NA] The numerous openings of the papillary ducts of Bellini on the summit of a renal papilla, forming the area cribrosa and discharging the urine into the minor calices. Also called *papillary foramina of kidney, foveolae papillae* (outmoded).

papillary foramina of kidney FORAMINA PAPILLARIA RENIS.

foramen parietale [NA] A small, round opening, occasionally absent on one or both sides, adjacent to the sagittal margin of the parietal bone near lambda and transmitting an emissary vein from the superior sagittal sinus.

patent foramen ovale The valvelike aperture in the interatrial septum which remains patent in some 25 percent of adults, as a result of failed fusion of the embryonic septum secundum in such manner as to close the foramen of the septum primum. Also called *acleistocardia.*

pleuroperitoneal foramen 1 MORGAGNI'S FORAMEN. 2 An incorrect term for HIATUS PLEUROPERITONEALIS.

posterior condyloid foramen CANALIS CONDYLARIS.

posterior ethmoid foramen FORAMEN ETHMOIDALE POSTERIUS.

posterior ethmoidal foramen FORAMEN ETHMOIDALE POSTERIUS.

posterior lacerate foramen An outmoded term for FORAMEN JUGULARE.

posterior maxillary foramen MANDIBULAR FORAMEN.

posterior palatine foramen FORAMEN PALATINUM MAJUS.

posterior sacral foramina FORAMINA SACRALIA POSTERIORA.

posterior superior alveolar foramina Openings on the infratemporal surface of the maxilla which transmit the posterior superior alveolar nerves and vessels. Also called *alveolar foramina of maxilla, foramina alveolaria maxillae.*

posterior zygomatic foramen FORAMEN ZYGOMATICOTEMPORALE.

postglenoid foramen A rarely-present small orifice in the tympanosquamosal fissure in front of the external acoustic meatus that transmits a communication between the anterior end of the petrosquamous sinus and the retromandibular vein.

primary interventricular foramen CHANNEL OF HALLER.

primitive interatrial foramen OSTIUM PRIMUM.

foramen primum OSTIUM PRIMUM.

foramen processus transversi [NA] A rounded opening that pierces the transverse process of the cervical vertebrae, through the upper six of which it transmits the vertebral artery, vein, and plexus of sympathetic nerves. Also called *cervical vertebral foramen, transverse foramen, vertebroarterial foramen, foramen transversarium, foramen vertebrarteriale.*

pterygoalar foramen PORUS CROTAPHITICOBUCCINATORIUS.

pterygopalatine foramen An outmoded term for FORAMEN PALATINUM MAJUS.

pulpal foramen APICAL FORAMEN OF TOOTH.

quadrate foramen An outmoded term for FORAMEN VENAE CAVAE.

foramen radicis dentis APICAL FORAMEN OF TOOTH.

foramen of Retzius APERTURA LATERALIS VENTRICULI QUARTI.

right foramen An outmoded term for FORAMEN VENAE CAVAE.

rivinian foramen An outmoded term for INCISURA TYMPANICA.

Rivinus foramen An outmoded term for INCISURA TYMPANICA.

root foramen APICAL FORAMEN OF TOOTH.

foramen rotundum FORAMEN ROTUNDUM OSSIS SPHENOIDALIS.

foramen rotundum ossis sphenoidalis [NA] A circular opening in the anteromedial part of the greater wing of the sphenoid bone, anterior to foramen ovale and inferomedial to the superior orbital fissure and conducting the maxillary nerve to the pterygopalatine fossa. Also called *superior maxillary fo-*

ramen, superior maxillary canal, foramen rotundum.

foramina sacralia anteriora [NA] Four pairs of large openings located at the ends of the transverse lines on the anterior, or pelvic, surface of the sacrum that are linked by the intervertebral foramina to the sacral canal, from which they transmit the ventral rami of the first four sacral nerves, arteries, and veins. Also called *foramina sacralia pelvina, anterior sacral foramina, internal sacral foramina, foramina sacralia pelvica.*

foramina sacralia dorsalia FORAMINA SACRALIA POSTERIORA.

foramina sacralia pelvina FORAMINA SACRALIA ANTERIORA.

foramina sacralia posteriora [NA] Four paired large openings on the posterior surface of the sacrum located between the intermediate sacral crest and articular tubercles medially, and the lateral sacral crest and transverse tubercles laterally. The intervertebral foramina link them with the sacral canal, from which they transmit dorsal rami of the first four sacral nerves, arteries, and veins. Also called *foramina sacralia dorsalia, posterior sacral foramina, dorsal sacral foramina.*

foramen of saphenous vein HIATUS SAPHENUS.

Scarpa's foramen MEDIAN INCISIVE FORAMEN.

Schwalbe's foramen FORAMEN CECUM MEDULLAE OBLONGATAE.

foramen secundum OSTIUM SECUNDUM.

foramen singulare [NA] An isolated foramen below and behind the inferior vestibular area, on the vertical plate of the fundus of the internal acoustic meatus. It transmits the nerve to the ampulla of the posterior semicircular duct of the internal ear. Also called *Morgagni's foramen, morgagnian foramen.*

foramina of smallest veins of heart FORAMINA VENARUM MINIMARUM CORDIS.

small sacrosciatic foramen FORAMEN ISCHIADICUM MINUS.

Soemmering's foramen An outmoded term for FOVEA CENTRALIS RETINAE.

sphenopalatine foramen 1 FORAMEN SPHENOPALATINUM. 2 An outmoded term for FORAMEN PALATINUM MAJUS.

foramen sphenopalatinum [NA] The foramen in the upper part of the medial wall of the pterygopalatine fossa, formed by the orbital process of the perpendicular plate of the palatine bone anteriorly, its sphenoidal process posteriorly and the body of the sphenoid bone above. Through it the fossa communicates with the nasal cavity posterior to the superior meatus, and transmits the nasopalatine and superior nasal nerves and the sphenopalatine vessels. Also called *sphenopalatine foramen.*

sphenotic foramen FORAMEN LACERUM.

spinal foramen FORAMEN VERTEBRALE.

foramen of spinal cord FORAMEN VERTEBRALE.

foramen spinosum [NA] A small, circular opening in the posterior angle of the greater wing of the sphenoid bone, situated posterolateral to the foramen ovale and anteromedial to the spine of the sphenoid on the infratemporal surface. It transmits the middle meningeal artery and the meningeal branch of the mandibular nerve to the middle cranial fossa. Also called *spinous foramen.*

spinous foramen FORAMEN SPINOSUM.

Spöndli's foramen A small, transient opening between the developing cartilages of the sphenoid and the ethmoid bones in the embryo.

foramen of Stensen 1 LATERAL INCISIVE FORAMEN. 2 FORAMEN INCISIVUM.

sternal foramen An inconstant foramen that occurs in the xiphoid process of the sternum.

stylomastoid foramen FORAMEN STYLOMASTOIDEUM.

foramen stylomastoideum [NA] An opening between the root of the styloid process and the anterior end of the mastoid notch on the inferior surface of the petrous part of the temporal

bone. It is the external opening of the facial canal and transmits the facial nerve, the stylomastoid branch of the posterior auricular artery and, occasionally, the auricular branch of the vagus nerve. Also called *stylomastoid foramen.*

suborbital foramen An outmoded term for FORAMEN INFRAORBITALE.

foramen subseptale OSTIUM PRIMUM.

superior left foramen An outmoded term for HIATUS ESOPHAGEUS.

superior maxillary foramen FORAMEN ROTUNDUM OSSIS SPHENOIDALIS.

superior zygomatic foramen An outmoded term for FORAMEN ZYGOMATICO-ORBITALE.

supraorbital foramen FORAMEN SUPRAORBITALE.

foramen supraorbitale [NA] The foramen at the junction of the medial and intermediate thirds of the supraorbital margin which is formed by bone or fibrous tissue bridging over the incisura supraorbitalis. It transmits the supraorbital nerve and vessels and has an opening in its floor for a diploic vein. Also called *supraorbital foramen, foramen supraorbitalis* (outmoded), *supraorbital sulcus* (outmoded).

foramen supraorbitalis An outmoded term for FORAMEN SUPRAORBITALE.

suprapiriform foramen A space above the piriformis muscle in the greater sciatic foramen through which the superior gluteal vessels and nerves leave the pelvis.

foramen of Tarin An outmoded term for HIATUS CANALIS NERVI PETROSI MAJORIS.

temporal zygomatic foramen FORAMEN ZYGOMATICOTEMPORALE.

temporomalar foramen FORAMEN ZYGOMATICOTEMPORALE.

thebesian foramina FORAMINA VENARUM MINIMARUM CORDIS.

foramina thebesii An outmoded term for FORAMINA VENARUM MINIMARUM CORDIS.

thyroid foramen 1 FORAMEN THYROIDEUM. 2 An outmoded term for FORAMEN OBTURATUM.

foramen thyroideum [NA] An occasional opening in the upper part of the lamina of the thyroid cartilage transmitting the superior laryngeal vessels and resulting from the incomplete fusion of the fourth and fifth branchial cartilages. Also called *thyroid foramen.*

tonsillar foramina Either fossulae tonsillares tonsillae palatinae or fossulae tonsillares tonsillae pharyngeae.

foramen transversarium FORAMEN PROCESSUS TRANSVERSI.

transverse foramen FORAMEN PROCESSUS TRANSVERSI.

transverse accessory foramen A small foramen frequently present in the transverse process of the sixth cervical vertebra, posterior to and smaller than the foramen processus transversi. It may transmit a vein and it is seldom present in other cervical vertebrae.

foramina of urethra An outmoded term for LACUNAE URETHRALES.

vena caval foramen FORAMEN VENAE CAVAE.

foramen venae cavae [NA] The highest of the three major openings in the respiratory diaphragm, situated at the junction of the right leaf with the middle part of its tendon and transmitting the inferior vena cava and some branches of the right phrenic nerve. Also called *vena caval foramen, vena caval hiatus, venous foramen* (outmoded), *quadrate foramen* (outmoded), *right foramen* (outmoded), *opening for vena cava, opening of inferior vena cava.*

foramina venarum minimarum cordis [NA] The minute orifices of the venae cardiacae minimae opening on the internal surface of the walls, especially the septal and right lateral, of the right atrium. Also called *foramina of smallest veins of heart,* *thebesian foramina, foramina thebesii* (outmoded), *Vieussens foramina, pores of Vieussens, foraminula of Lannelongue.*

foramen venosum A small opening, usually in the cortex of a bone, for the passage of a vein. An outmoded term.

venous foramen An outmoded term for FORAMEN VENAE CAVAE.

vertebral foramen FORAMEN VERTEBRALE.

foramen vertebrale [NA] The large space behind the body of a vertebra, bounded posteriorly and laterally by the vertebral arch, varying in shape in different parts of the vertebral column and containing mostly the spinal cord, meninges and associated vessels. Also called *medullary foramen, spinal foramen, spinal aperture, vertebral foramen, foramen of spinal cord.*

foramen vertebrarteriale FORAMEN PROCESSUS TRANS-VERSI.

vertebroarterial foramen FORAMEN PROCESSUS TRANS-VERSI.

foramen of Vesalius A small, inconstant opening in the greater wing of the sphenoid bone between the foramen rotundum and the foramen ovale, transmitting an emissary vein between the cavernous sinus and pterygoid plexus.

foramen of Vicq d'Azyr FORAMEN CECUM MEDULLAE OB-LONGATAE.

Vieussens foramina FORAMINA VENARUM MINIMARUM CORDIS.

visceral foramen HEMAL FORAMEN.

Weitbrecht's foramen An opening, variable in size and occurrence, in the fibrous capsule of the shoulder joint, situated between the superior and middle glenohumeral ligaments, through which the bursa under the tendon of the subscapularis muscle communicates with the joint cavity.

foramen of Winslow FORAMEN OMENTALE.

zygomaticofacial foramen FORAMEN ZYGOMATICOFA-CIALE.

foramen zygomaticofaciale [NA] The opening near the orbital margin on the lateral surface of the zygomatic bone for the zygomaticofacial nerve and vessels. Also called *zygomaticofacial foramen, malar foramen, anterior zygomatic foramen, external zygomatic foramen, facial zygomatic foramen, zygomaticofacial canal.*

zygomatico-orbital foramen FORAMEN ZYGOMATICO-OR-BITALE.

foramen zygomatico-orbitale [NA] Either of two openings on the oribtal surface of the zygomatic bone leading to two canals that terminate in the zygomaticofacial foramen and the zygomaticotemporal foramen. Also called *zygomatico-orbital foramen, superior zygomatic foramen* (outmoded), *orbital zygomatic foramen, internal zygomatic foramen of Arnold, inferior zygomatic foramen, orbitomalar foramen.*

zygomaticotemporal foramen FORAMEN ZYGOMATICOTEM-PORALE.

foramen zygomaticotemporale [NA] The opening on the temporal surface and near the base of the frontal process of the zygomatic bone for transmission of the zygomaticotemporal nerve and branch of lacrimal artery. Also called *zygomaticotemporal foramen, temporal zygomatic foramen, posterior zygomatic foramen, internal zygomatic foramen of Meckel, temporomalar foramen, zygomaticotemporal canal.*

---

foramina Plural of FORAMEN.

foraminal Pertaining to a foramen.

foraminated Possessing a foramen or foramina.

Foraminifera [L *foramen,* gen. *foraminis,* a hole, opening + -*fera,* neut. pl. of -*fer,* combining form denoting carrying] An order of protozoans in the superclass Rhizopoda, subphylum Sarcodina. These testate marine amebas with one or more chambers have pseudopodia that protrude through a central aperture or wall perforations. The test may be extremely complex and geometrically symmetrical and is usually composed of calcium carbonate. Sexual and asexual generations usually alternate, and commonly with flagellated gametes. Great masses of ocean bottom and rockbeds overlying oil deposits consist of accumulated foraminiferous tests. Also called *Foraminiferida.*

Foraminiferida FORAMINIFERA.

foraminiferous 1 Pertaining to or consisting of protozoans of the order Foraminifera. 2 Possessing foramina.

foraminotomy [*foramin(is),* gen. of L *foramen* a hole, opening + *o* + -TOMY] Enlargement of an aperture in the skull or the vertebra for passage of a nerve.

foraminulate Possessing a foraminulum or foraminula. Also *foraminulous, foraminulose.*

foraminulose FORAMINULATE.

foraminulous FORAMINULATE.

foraminulum A very small foramen.

foraminula of Lannelongue An outmoded term for FORAMINA VENARUM MINIMARUM CORDIS.

foration [L *forat(us),* past part. of *forare* to bore, pierce + -ION] TREPHINING.

forb [Gk *phorb(ē)* (from *pherbein* to feed, akin to Old English *biergan* to taste) pasture, food, fodder] Any herbaceous plant exclusive of the grasses and sedges.

Forbes [A. P. *Forbes,* U.S. physician, flourished mid-20th century] Forbes-Albright syndrome. See under SYNDROME.

Forbes [Gilbert Burnett *Forbes,* U.S. pediatrician, born 1915] Forbes disease. See under GLYCOGEN STORAGE DISEASE III.

force [French (from Low L *fortia* strength, from L *fortis* strong), power, strength] That influence which produces or tends to produce acceleration of a body.

catabiotic force The energy derived from the metabolism of food.

catabolic force Energy obtained from the conversion of complex substances to simpler compounds in living cells.

centrifugal force The force exerted on a body rotating around a fixed central axis, directed outward along the radius of the curving movement. Compare CENTRIPETAL FORCE.

centripetal force A force of both magnitude and direction that moves a body along a circular path directed radially toward the center of the circle formed by its motion. Compare CEN-TRIFUGAL FORCE.

chewing force MASTICATORY FORCE.

coercive force The magnetizing force at which the magnetic flux density is zero in a previously magnetized material.

condensing force The force used in dental condensation.

electromotive force The relative potential between two dissimilar electrodes in the same electrolyte. Abbreviation: EMF

extraoral force A force used for orthodontic movement having extraoral anchorage.

field forces Hypothetical forces which are thought to play a part in the individuation process during early embryonic development by means of which organizers influence adjacent cells and tissues. See also INDIVIDUATION FIELD.

G force A unit of force such that a body subjected to it would have the acceleration of gravity at sea level. G force is the unit of measurement for bodies undergoing the stress of acceleration.

London dispersion forces The same forces as van der Waals forces, but with the cause described in terms of the attraction between oscillating dipoles.

masticatory force The force exerted by the muscles of mastication. Also called *chewing force, biting strength.*

nuclear force The strongly attractive forces between protons and neutrons that prevent a nucleus from flying apart in spite of repulsion between protons. Also called *strong force.*

occlusal force The force applied to teeth by opposing teeth or interposed food. Also called *biting pressure, occlusal pressure.*

psychic force Mental energy generated by thinking and other psychologic processes. Also called *psychic energy, cathexis, psychokym* (obsolete).

radiation force The force exerted on a body by radiation incident on it.

force of recoil of the lung The force with which the lung, because of its inherent elasticity, tends to retract and lose volume when not held in contact with the thoracic wall.

reserve force A reserve of energy in excess of that required for normal function.

shearing force The stress existing between the bony skeleton and the skin overlying it when a patient, sitting propped up in bed, slides down and the skin continues to adhere to the surface with which it is in contact, i.e., the mattress. The stress causes disruption of blood vessels and body tissues and it predisposes the patient to the formation of a decubitus ulcer.

strong force NUCLEAR FORCE.

van der Waals forces Relatively weak forces of attraction between all molecules, due to interaction of oscillating electrical dipoles, even in molecules with no permanent dipoles. They were recognized from the equations of van der Waals for representing the deviation of behavior of actual gases from the ideal gas laws.

forceps

forceps [L (from *formus* hot + *-ceps*, from *captus*, past part. of *capere* to hold, seize; or possibly from *ferrum* iron + *-ceps*), a pair of tongs, pincers] **1** A surgical instrument that is used for grasping tissues or surgical materials. It may resemble scissors, with a locking mechanism at the handles to maintain a desired position, or it may look like tweezers. **2** Any tissue or fiber that assumes a forcipate or bowl-like shape. Adjective: forcipate, forcipal.

Adams forceps A powerful forceps with flattened oval-shaped blades for gripping the nasal septum in the Adams operation.

adenoid forceps Forceps with cupped or fenestrated blades for removing the adenoids or adenoid remnants left behind after the use of an adenoid curette or adenotome, or for excising a sample of a postnasal tumor as a biopsy specimen.

advancement forceps A surgical instrument for the treatment of strabismus by moving the tendon insertion of a rectus muscle forward upon the sclera.

alligator forceps Strong, toothed forceps, having a double clamp.

Allis forceps A tissue forceps with fine-toothed, incurved jaws, widely used in several branches of surgery.

alveolar forceps BONE FORCEPS.

forceps anterior FORCEPS MINOR.

Arruga's forceps A capsule forceps, used for grasping the lens capsule during cataract extraction.

Asch forceps A forceps for centralizing the displaced nasal septum in cases of fracture of the nose. The forceps are applied to the interior of the nose with one blade on either side of the septum.

attic-ridge forceps A small rongeur for removing the outer attic wall in middle-ear surgery.

aural forceps Any of a wide range of forceps designed or adapted for use in the treatment or surgery of the ear. Also called *ear forceps.*

axis-traction forceps Obstetrical forceps designed to exert traction in an axis corresponding to that of the lower maternal birth canal.

Bailey-Williamson forceps A modified version of the Elliot obstetrical forceps with fenestrated blades and with lengthened shanks which accentuate their cephalic curve.

Ballenger's forceps Curved, locking forceps which are a modification of volsella forceps, used in seizing the tonsil in tonsillectomy.

Barton forceps An obstetrical forceps utilized to exert traction on a fetal head in the occiput transverse position. It consists of a hinged anterior blade and a rigid posterior blade.

bayonet forceps Forceps shaped like a bayonet, commonly used in the treatment and surgery of the nose and ear. The object of the design is to prevent the fingers holding the forceps from obscuring a view of the tips of the forceps.

bone forceps Forceps with sharp curved beaks, meeting edge-to-edge, used for the removal of bone. Also called *alveolar forceps.*

bone-cutting forceps Plierlike forceps that are used to cut bone or cartilage.

bone-nibbling forceps Forceps used to remove small sections of bone or cartilage. Also called *gouge forceps.*

Brenner forceps A type of obstetrical forceps utilized in breech presentations.

broad-ligament forceps An instrument designed to grasp and expose the broad ligament of the uterus.

brossage forceps An obsolete eyelid forceps that was designed for use in the treatment of lids severely affected with trachoma.

bulldog forceps A small spring forceps, the jaws usually covered with rubber tubing, used for occluding blood vessels.

capsule forceps A surgical instrument for grasping the lens capsule during cataract extraction.

cartilage forceps Forceps used to extract cartilage in a surgical procedure.

chalazion forceps A surgical instrument for securing the everted eyelid during incision and curettage of a retention cyst of the meibomian gland. It is also used during removal of lesions from the lip or cheek.

Chamberlen forceps A forerunner of modern obstetrical forceps developed by four generations of English physicians, the Chamberlens, between 1600 and 1728. Their instrument was one of the first designed to save not only the mother's life but the infant's life as well.

cholecystectomy forceps Forceps used to facilitate the removal of a gallbladder.

cilia forceps An instrument for epilation of eyelashes.

clamp forceps Locking forceps that are used to compress arteries, the pedicle of a tumor, and the like.

clip forceps A forceps with specially designed jaws used for the placement of metal clips, as for the occlusion of blood vessels or approximation of the skin.

clip-compressing forceps Forceps designed to apply and compress surgical clips.

clot-breaking forceps Forceps with blades used to break up and remove blood clots in the bladder.

forceps of corpus callosum The forceps minor and forceps major of the corpus callosum.

craniotomy forceps A seldom used obstetrical instrument utilized to crush a fetal head in order to facilitate vaginal delivery.

crocodile forceps Any of a variety of forceps having elongated jaws with only the upper jaw being hinged. Light-weight forceps of this kind are commonly used in modern otologic surgery.

crushing forceps Forceps used to compress tissue.

DeLee forceps An obstetrical forceps similar to Simpson's forceps but consisting of longer shanks and modified handles.

dental forceps DENTAL EXTRACTING FORCEPS.

dental extracting forceps Forceps with curved beaks shaped to fit the roots of teeth. There is a large variety of design, often named after the tooth which the design fits, such as upper right molar forceps. Also called *dental forceps, extracting forceps*.

depilatory forceps EPILATING FORCEPS.

disk forceps A delicate surgical forceps used to remove the trephined scleral disk in a glaucoma filtering operation.

dissecting forceps Forceps used to separate and delineate tissues and organs. Also called *dissection forceps*.

dissection forceps DISSECTING FORCEPS.

double-action forceps A surgical scissorlike instrument that is constructed with two joints or hinges between the blades and handles. It is used for applying pressure to compress or divide tissues.

dressing forceps Forceps used for removing a dressing from a wound or dressings from a container with multiple dressings.

duck-bill forceps Any forceps the principal feature of which is jaws shaped like a duck's bill, that is, flatter and wider distally than at the base.

dural forceps A two-bladed surgical instrument having small teeth. It is used for grasping the dura mater.

ear forceps AURAL FORCEPS.

Elliot forceps Obstetrical forceps consisting of a rounded cephalic curve with fenestrated blades and overlapping of the shanks.

entropion forceps A surgical instrument used in operations for correcting positional defects of the eyelids.

epilating forceps An instrument used to pluck hair. Also called *depilatory forceps, tricholabion* (obsolete).

extracting forceps DENTAL EXTRACTING FORCEPS.

failed forceps The unsuccessful application of obstetrical forceps, usually due to cephalopelvic disproportion, incomplete cervical dilatation, or malposition of the fetal head.

fixation forceps Tweezerlike forceps with serrated tips that are used to stabilize tissues during operative procedures. Also called *rat-tooth forceps*.

Foster-Ballenger forceps A punch forceps with flattened blades, one fenestrated to receive the other, for cutting out portions of the septal cartilage in submucous resection of the nasal septum.

frontal-sinus forceps Bone-nibbling forceps designed for removing bone in operations on the frontal sinus.

galea forceps WILLETT FORCEPS.

Garrison's forceps LUIKART FORCEPS.

gland forceps Forceps used to grasp and manipulate a gland.

Good forceps An obstetrical forceps similar to Simpson's forceps.

gouge forceps BONE-NIBBLING FORCEPS.

Haig Ferguson forceps An obstetrical forceps similar in design to Simpson's forceps.

Hawks-Dennen forceps A modified version of Simpson's obstetrical forceps with the shanks bent backwards to form an exaggerated perineal curve in order to facilitate axis traction.

high forceps The application of obstetrical forceps to an unengaged fetal head, an application very rarely if ever utilized by modern-day obstetricians. Also called *inlet forceps*.

Hodge's forceps A type of obstetrical forceps.

inlet forceps HIGH FORCEPS.

insertion forceps POINT FORCEPS.

Jansen forceps 1 A cranked punch forceps designed for operations on the sphenoidal sinus. 2 A bayonet-shaped rongeur used in mastoid surgery.

Kazanjian forceps A forceps formerly used to cut off the nasal hump in some reduction rhinoplasties.

Kerrison forceps A tympanic rongeur designed to minimize the risk of injury to the facial nerve during mastoid surgery.

kidney-holding forceps Forceps used in renal surgery to grasp and support the kidney.

kidney-pedicle forceps Forceps for clamping the renal vessels.

Kielland forceps An obstetrical forceps primarily utilized for rotation with narrow, separated handles, a sliding lock, overlapping shanks, and a bayonet appearance of the blades and shanks due to a reversed pelvic curve.

Knapp's forceps TRACHOMA FORCEPS.

Kocher's forceps Forceps with teethlike projections for holding tissue during surgery or for compressing bleeding tissue.

Laborde's forceps A three-bladed tracheal dilator.

laminectomy forceps Forceps used to facilitate the removal of a posterior or vertebral arch.

laryngeal forceps Any one of a variety of forceps intended for use in the treatment or surgery of the larynx. Most of these instruments are designed for use while visualizing the larynx in a mirror. Because they are introduced through the mouth to reach a part, the axis of which is approximately at right angles to the axis of the mouth and at some distance from it, most of these lengthy forceps are characterized by having the tips of the forceps at approximately a right angle to the finger hold.

Levret's forceps An eighteenth-century obstetrical forceps, one of the first instruments to incorporate a pelvic curve. It was a forerunner of modern-day obstetrical forceps.

lion-jawed forceps Strong, long-handled, serrated forceps that are used to hold large pieces or shafts of bone.

lithotomy forceps Forceps used in extracting stones from the bladder.

lock forceps POINT FORCEPS.

low forceps The application of obstetrical forceps after the fetal head has reached the perineal floor and with the sagittal suture in the anteroposterior diameter of the maternal outlet. Also called *outlet forceps*.

Löwenberg's forceps Adenoid forceps with cupped ends and cutting edges.

Luc's forceps A stout forceps, with angled blades and cupped or, more often, fenestrated jaws of different shapes and sizes. They are widely used in nasal surgery, particularly in turbinectomy and for removing nasal polyps.

Luikart forceps An obstetrical forceps similar to the Tucker-McLean forceps with overlapping shanks with a sliding lock, handles similar to those on the Kielland forceps, and blades with an incomplete fenestration (pseudofenestration) on the cephalic side of the blades. Also called *Garrison's forceps*.

forceps major The interhemispheric fibers of the occipital cerebral cortex extending through the splenium of the corpus callosum. Also called *forceps posterior*.

McKenzie forceps Forceps designed for the application of neurosurgical clips.

median forceps MID FORCEPS.

mid forceps The application of obstetrical forceps after engagement of the fetal head but prior to meeting the criteria for low forceps. Also called *median forceps, low-plane forceps*.

mid-plane forceps MID FORCEPS.

forceps minor The interhemispheric fibers of the frontal cerebral cortex extending through the genu of the corpus callosum and coursing forward. Also called *forceps anterior*.

mosquito forceps Small delicate forceps for holding tissue.

mouse-tooth forceps A surgical instrument having meshing teeth used for grasping tissue.

nasal forceps Any one of a variety of forceps designed or adapted for use in the treatment or surgery of the nose.

Negus ligature forceps An artery forceps with backward

curving tips designed for use in tonsillectomy to facilitate the tying of ligatures around bleeding points in the tonsil bed. Also called *Negus tonsil artery forceps*.

Negus tonsil artery forceps   NEGUS LIGATURE FORCEPS.

nonfenestrated forceps   Obstetrical forceps in which the blades consist of solid metal without a window or fenestration.

obstetrical forceps   An instrument usually consisting of two blades, each connected to a handle by a shank and utilized to exert traction on a fetal head or to rotate the fetal head in order to facilitate vaginal delivery. Also called *cephalotractor* (older term).

O'Hara forceps   An obsolete instrument used for intestinal anastomosis.

Ostrom forceps   A backward cutting punch forceps designed for enlarging the antrostome forwards in intranasal antrostomy.

outlet forceps   LOW FORCEPS.

ovum forceps   A surgical forceps having blades with oval tips designed for removing tissue from the uterus following an incomplete abortion or at the time of a dilatation and curettage in search of an endometrial polyp.

pedicle forceps   Large flat-faced forceps that are used for grasping significant amounts of tissue.

Piper forceps   An obstetrical forceps with long shanks and a perineal curve. It is designed to be applied to an aftercoming head in order to facilitate the vaginal delivery of an infant in the breech presentation.

placenta forceps   A forceps usually consisting of fenestrated blades which are passed transcervically in order to grasp and extract placental tissue still lying within the uterine cavity.

point forceps   Fine forceps, with serrated or longitudinally grooved beaks, used for inserting points such as gutta-percha points into root canals. The beaks can be locked in the closed position. Also called *lock forceps, insertion forceps*.

forceps posterior   FORCEPS MAJOR.

punch forceps   **1** A forceps used to punch out a small sample of tissue for biopsy.   **2** A forceps used to punch out a hole, or holes, in a piece of cartilage during reconstructive surgery.

rat-tooth forceps   FIXATION FORCEPS.

rib-cutting forceps   Forceps designed to divide ribs.

roller forceps   TRACHOMA FORCEPS.

rongeur forceps   Bone cutting forceps that combine a rongeur-type cutting head with forceps handle and have a double fulcrum lever action to enhance mechanical power. They are used to remove small fragments of bone during an exposure procedure.

root-splitting forceps   Dental forceps with cutting blades for separating the roots of multirooted teeth.

rubber dam clamp forceps   Forceps with curved, ball-ended beaks, used for holding and opening rubber dam clamps. The beaks can be locked in the open position. Also called *clamp holder, rubber dam clamp holder*.

sequestrum forceps   Plierlike forceps with strong serrated locking teeth that are used to remove fragments of dead bone.

Simpson's forceps   An obstetrical forceps consisting of a long, tapered cephalic curve with fenestrated blades and parallel separated shanks.

sinus forceps   A forceps designed with narrow, tapered blades, used to gain entrance to or enlarge an abscess.

speculum forceps   Long-handled forceps designed to be used through a speculum.

sponge-holding forceps   SPONGE HOLDER.

spring forceps   Lightweight forceps with two opposable blades separated by spring tension.

strabismus forceps   A surgical instrument for securing the tendons of the extraocular muscles during operations for ocular misalignment.

suture forceps   NEEDLE HOLDER.

tenaculum forceps   Forceps having two blades, both of which

have a sharp hook, used for grasping and stabilizing tissues.

thumb forceps   TISSUE FORCEPS.

tissue forceps   Forceps having two fine-toothed blades, designed for gentle, nontraumatic manipulation of tissues. Also called *thumb forceps*.

tongue forceps   A forceps used to grasp and pull the tongue forward from the pharynx in order to overcome soft-tissue obstruction, as occurs in coma or seizures or during anesthesia. Also called *linguotrite* (obsolete).

torsion forceps   Forceps utilizing torsion or twisting to stop hemorrhaging of an artery.

towel forceps   TOWEL CLIP.

tracheal forceps   Long, fine forceps designed to reach into the trachea. They are used in direct laryngoscopy.

trachoma forceps   A surgical instrument fashioned with apposable rollers and used to express semifluid material from the eyelids. It was originally designed for treatment of trachomatous follicles. Also called *Knapp's forceps, roller forceps*.

tubular forceps   Long, slender forceps designed to be used through a speculum or a very limited incision.

Tucker-McLean forceps   A modified version of the Elliot obstetrical forceps with either semifenestrated or nonfenestrated blades and with lengthened shanks which accentuate their cephalic curve.

uterine forceps   A long, slender, curved instrument with blunted serrations, used to remove tissue or insert packing in the uterus.

volsella forceps   A long forceps with sharp teeth on the end, used in some gynecologic procedures to grasp tissues and apply torsion or traction. Also called *vulsellum forceps, vulsella, volsella, vulsellum*.

vulsellum forceps   VOLSELLA FORCEPS.

Walsham forceps   A forceps for correcting lateral deviation of the fractured nose. With one blade inside the nose and the other, surrounded by a piece of rubber tubing, outside, the fractured nasal bones are disimpacted and repositioned.

Willett forceps   An instrument formerly utilized to control hemorrhage from a placenta previa. A T-shaped clamp is attached transcervically to the fetal scalp and a 1–2 pound weight is applied to the clamp via a pulley in order to compress the low-lying placenta. It may also be of use in assisting the delivery of a dead fetus. Also called *Willett's clamp, galea forceps*.

Forchheimer [Frederick *Forchheimer*, U.S. physician, 1853–1913] Forchheimer spots. See under SPOT.

forcipal   **1** FORCIPATE.   **2** Serving the purpose of a forceps.

forcipate   Shaped like forceps. Also *forcipal*.

forcipital   Of or relating to forceps.

Forcipomyia   A genus of biting midges (family Ceratopogonidae). Members of the subgenus *Lasiohelea* feed on vertebrate blood. *F. (L.) taiwana* is a vicious man-biter in Taiwan. Several other man-biting species are found in the tropics.

forcipressure   A technique for arresting hemorrhage by compressing the artery with the forceps.

Fordyce [John Addison *Fordyce*, U.S. dermatologist, 1858–1925] **1** Fox-Fordyce disease. See under DISEASE. **2** Fordyce disease, Fordyce granules. See under FORDYCE SPOTS.

forearm   ANTEBRACHIUM.

forebrain [*fore* + *brain*]   PROSENCEPHALON.

forecast / population forecast   The outcome of calculations to indicate the future trends of a population given those assumptions regarding fertility, mortality, and migration most likely to be realized judging from the existing situation. A population forecast, unlike a population projection, is usually confined to the short term.

forefinger INDEX.

forefoot 1 An anterior foot of a quadruped. 2 The distal or anterior part of the human foot: used most often with respect to the fitting of shoes, prostheses, or the like.

foregilding The impregnation of fresh nerve fibers with gold chloride solution. The process is particularly suitable for the demonstration of nerve endings.

foregut The anterior portion of the embryonic intestine from which the pharynx, esophagus and stomach, and the proximal part of the duodenum and its derivatives will develop. Also called *cephalogaster, prosogaster, headgut, head gut.*

forehead The region of the face between the eyebrows and the hairline; frons.

bony forehead FRONS CRANII.

high forehead An unduly prominent or enlarged facial area or cranium above the eye.

olympian forehead OLYMPIC BROW.

forehead-plasty A plastic operation on the forehead, usually as an attempt to remove wrinkles.

foreign [Middle English *forein*, from Old French *forain* foreign, from Late L *foranus* foreign, on the outside, from L *foras* out of doors, from Old L *foras*, accus. pl. of *fora* door] In immunology, deriving from a source other than the subject's own tissues (self); being or relating to nonself.

forekidney PRONEPHROS.

Forel [Auguste Henri *Forel*, Swiss neurologist, 1848–1931] 1 Forel's decussation. See under DECUSSATION OF RUBROSPINAL TRACTS. 2 Area Foreli, Forel's field. See under H FIELDS OF FOREL. 3 Forel's commissure. See under SUPRAMAMILLARY DECUSSATION. 4 Field H_1 of Forel. See under FASCICULUS THALAMICUS. 5 Field H_2 of Forel. See under FASCICULUS LENTICULARIS.

foreleg 1 An anterior limb of a quadruped. 2 The distal part of the human leg, near the ankle: used most often with respect to the fitting of prostheses or the like.

foremilk COLOSTRUM.

forensic [L *forens(is)* pertaining to a forum where justice was publicly administered + -IC] Pertaining to or concerned with courts of justice or public debate.

foreplay The sexual activity which immediately precedes intromission and intercourse.

forepleasure [*fore-*, combining form denoting earlier in time + *pleasure*] Pleasure attained during pregenital sexuality, which is subordinate to mature genital sexuality and in the adult is largely confined to foreplay.

foreseeability of harm The ability to foresee or predict that a negligent act or the negligent failure to act would introduce a risk of injury or damage that would not otherwise have existed. In malpractice cases where negligence is charged, it must be proven that a reasonably prudent person would have been able to predict that a negligent act or omission would, in all probability, have resulted in injury or damage, and the injuries or damages can be directly related to the negligent act or omission.

foreskin PREPUTIUM PENIS.

hooded foreskin The appearance of the prepuce in hypospadias, when the prepuce only partially covers the glans penis.

forespore A region of increased refractility seen with the light microscope in bacteria beginning to form a spore. At this stage the electron microscope shows an invaginated double layer of cytoplasmic membrane surrounding a chromosome and associated cytoplasm.

forest [Med L (*silva*) *foresta* an unenclosed (wood)] An area of vegetation dominated by trees.

forestomach 1 Any one of the three food chambers in the digestive tract of ruminant animals immediately proximal to the abomasum or true stomach. They are the rumen, reticulum, and omasum. • The term is usually used in the plural, referring collectively to all three chambers. When a specific chamber is intended, the specific name for that chamber is used. 2 The anterior or nonglandular part of the stomach of the rat and mouse.

foretop That part of the mane of a horse which falls forward over the head.

forewaters [*fore* + *waters*] The portion of the amniotic membranes and the contained fluid which lies between the fetal head and the opening of the uterine cervix.

Forficula A genus of earwigs (order Dermaptera).

Forficula auricularia The common European earwig.

forgetting An inability to recall or recognize what has been earlier learned, or to perform an action once learned.

forging A defective gait of the horse, which may be observed when the horse is trotting. Forging consists of the toe of a rear foot striking the sole or undersurface of the shoe of the forefoot on the same side.

fork / face-bow fork A Y-shaped device for attaching a bite-rim or occlusal record to a face-bow. The arms of the Y are placed between the dental arches and the tail is attached to the face-bow by a fixable universal joint.

orbital fork The earliest sign of the orbit in the embryo, really only the forked bony outlines of the future orbit. Also called *furca orbitalis.*

replication fork The region in a DNA molecule where replication occurs. Before the fork there is one fiber of double-stranded parental DNA, and at the fork the two strands separate, each being copied and soon possessing a newly synthesized complementary strand. Also called *growing point.*

tuning fork A two-pronged instrument resembling a long U with a short stem attached to its base. For clinical purposes the stem has a disk-shaped foot. When the fork is tapped against a firm surface the prongs vibrate virtually at a single characteristic frequency depending on the length and mass of the fork. The tuning fork has been of immense historic and practical importance in the development of tests of hearing for different tones and in facilitating the diagnosis between conductive and sensorineural hearing loss. Low frequency tuning forks are also used in neurologic diagnosis to assess the subject's vibration sense.

form 1 Shape or configuration of an object or body. 2 When prefixed to a taxon, as in *form-genus* or *form-class*, denoting a grouping of organisms that lack a sexual reproductive stage: used especially in classifying the imperfect fungi.

accolé form A surface adherent form of *Plasmodium falciparum* in which the early stage trophozoite (ring form) appears to cling to the outside of the human red cell. Also called *appliqué form, appliqué.*

appliqué form ACCOLÉFORM.

boat form The form of a ring of six atoms in which two sides are parallel and the remaining two atoms are both on the same side of the plane formed by the parallel sides. It resembles a simple boat.

chair form The form of a ring of six atoms in which each side is parallel to the side opposite it, and any two opposite atoms are on opposite sides of the plane formed by the remaining four atoms. It resembles an easy chair. This is the predominant ring form of pyranose sugars, and it also occurs in steroids.

convenience form That factor, in the determination of the shape of a prepared tooth cavity, which takes into account the ease of access for the preparation of the cavity and for the insertion of the restoration.

envelope form The form of a ring of five atoms in which four are in a plane from which the fifth is displaced.

face form   The shape of the outline of the face viewed from the front.

growth form   ECOPHENE.

half-chair form   The form of a ring of six atoms in which five are in one plane and the sixth displaced from it. The chair form of a pyranose unit in a polysaccharide approaches the half-chair form in the transition state for hydrolysis.

involution forms   Irregularly shaped cells that appear in a culture after prolonged incubation in the stationary phase. An older term.

life form   An organism's characteristic shape, form, or appearance.

outline form   The shape of the margin of a prepared tooth cavity.

Raunkaier's life forms   A system of categorizing the life form of plants based upon the position of buds or other meristematic tissue in relation to the surface of the soil.

replicative form   The double-stranded form of viral DNA capable of replicating in a host cell. Many viruses of single-stranded nucleic acid direct the synthesis of a complementary strand to produce such a replicative form, which then multiplies in the cell.

resistance form   That factor in the determination of the shape of a prepared tooth cavity which takes into account the need to support the restoration against occlusal forces.

retention form   That factor in the determination of the shape of a prepared tooth cavity which takes into account the need for the restoration to be retained in the cavity.

sickle form   The crescent- or sausage-shaped gametocyte of *Plasmodium falciparum.*

skew form   The form of a ring of six atoms in which three adjacent atoms and the central atom of the remaining three are in a single plane, the other two atoms being displaced to opposite sides of it. A skew form is midway between two boat forms as one folds into the other.

trypanosomal form   An outmoded term for TRYPOMASTI-GOTE.

twist form   The form of a ring of five atoms in which no four atoms are in one plane. Its conformation may be defined by specifying the two atoms most displaced from the mean least-squares plane of the ring, and the sides to which they are displaced.

wax form   WAX PATTERN.

Z form   Z DNA.

-form [L *forma* (akin to Gk *morphē* form, shape) form, shape] A combining form meaning having the form or appearance of.

Formad [Henry F. *Formad*, U.S. physician, 1847–1892] See under KIDNEY.

formal   FORMALDEHYDE SOLUTION.

formaldehyde   H—CHO. Methanal. It is a highly reactive aldehyde, largely hydrated in water and easily reversibly polymerized. It is somewhat toxic and can be used to fix and preserve animal tissues.

formalin   An outmoded term for FORMALDEHYDE SOLUTION.

formamidase   KYNURENINE FORMAMIDASE.

formamide   H—CO—NH$_2$. The amide of formic acid. Since its melting point is 2°C, it is unusual among amides in being liquid at room temperature.

formant [L *formans*, gen. *formantis*, pres. part. of *formare* to form] A restricted band of relatively high acoustic energy in comparison with other harmonics or overtones. Its center frequency and the total number of formants depend on the characteristics of the resonating chamber related to the primary sound source. It is of particular importance in the acoustic phonetics of speech. The shape of the supraglottic part of the vocal tract is capable of considerable variation, with direct effects on its performance as a series of linked resonators, most clearly seen in the production of vowels.

format [L *format(us)* a forming, shaping] In a computer, the general form in which data appear on the input or output medium.

formate dehydrogenase   Any of several enzymes that convert formic acid into carbon dioxide with concomitant reduction of an oxidizing agent. The most important is involved in fermentation by most enteric bacteria, which convert glucose, via pyruvate, into acetyl-CoA and formic acid. The acetyl-CoA gives rise to ethanol and acetic acid, and this production of acid lowers the pH enough to induce formate dehydrogenase.

formatio [L (from *formatus*, past part. of *formare* to form, shape), a forming, shaping] 1 A nuclear region with ill-defined limits. 2 [NA] Any structure having a definite shape. Also called *formation.*

formatio alba   The myelinated portion of the central reticular formation of the spinal cord. An outmoded term.

formatio bulbaris   The gray matter of the olfactory bulb. An obsolete term.

formatio grisea   The outer, cellular portion of the central reticular formation of the spinal cord. An obsolete term.

formatio hippocampalis   HIPPOCAMPAL FORMATION.

formatio reticularis   [NA] Diffusely organized neural tissue consisting characteristically of a meshwork of both large and small neuronal cell bodies and their dendrites, axons, and branching collaterals found in the gray matter of the spinal cord, the central core region of the medulla oblongata, pons, and midbrain, and extending rostrally into the medial thalamus and hypothalamus. They exert profound effects upon all sensory and motor systems as well as the rest-activity cycle, i.e., sleep and wakefulness. Also called *reticular formation, reticular substance, substantia reticularis, reticular system.*

formatio reticularis medullae oblongatae   The diffuse, poorly circumscribed cell groups and fiber tracts of the medulla oblongata, interspersed among the main nuclei and tracts. Also called *medullary reticular formation, reticular formation of medulla oblongata.*

formatio reticularis medullae spinalis   The medial, intermediate portion of the spinal gray matter, consisting of scattered cell groups and fiber tracts. Also called *reticular formation of spinal cord.*

formatio reticularis mesencephali   The midbrain reticular formation, interposed between the substantia nigra and the periaqueductal gray matter. Also called *formatio reticularis pedunculi cerebri, reticular formation of mesencephalon.*

formatio reticularis pedunculi cerebri   FORMATIO RETICULARIS MESENCEPHALI.

formatio reticularis pontis   The nuclei and tracts located principally in the tegmentum of the pons, including the central tegmental reticular nucleus (nucleus dissipata), the superior central pontine tegmental nucleus (associated with the pneumotaxic center), and the medial and lateral ventral tegmental nuclei. Also called *reticular formation of pons.*

formatio vermicularis   The combined cerebellar tonsil and flocculus. An obsolete term.

formation [L *formatio.* See FORMATIO.] 1 The process of forming or developing. 2 The result of such a process; something formed. 3 FORMATIO.

Ammon's formation   HIPPOCAMPUS. • The term is named after *Ammon,* the ram-headed deity of ancient Egypt.

chiasma formation   The process during meiosis of chromosomal crossing over in which pairs of homologous chromosomes physically join at chiasmata.

coffin formation The histologic appearance of neuronophagia.

compromise formation The process of developing symptoms as substitutes for repressed conflicts. Also called *substitute formation, symptom formation.*

concept formation The cognitive operation of generating classes of stimuli with common properties, whether objects, events, or ideas. Abstracting the shared property is the first stage, followed by generalizing of that quality to all other appropriate objects, events, or ideas.

crater formation Interdental depressions in the gingiva and/or underlying bone, resulting from periodontal disease.

endochondral bone formation ENDOCHONDRAL OSSIFICATION.

hippocampal formation The fascia dentata, fornix, hippocampus, and subicular fields. An imprecise usage. Also called *formatio hippocampalis, gyrus hippocampi* (imprecise).

intracartilaginous bone formation ENDOCHONDRAL OSTEOGENESIS.

intramembranous bone formation The process of creating the structure of bone directly through osteoblastic activity in a noncartilaginous matrix.

medullary reticular formation FORMATIO RETICULARIS MEDULLAE OBLONGATAE.

palisade formation Cells arranged with their long axis in a parallel manner to give a picket fence effect. This formation typically occurs in neurilemmomas. A similar appearance can be seen around areas of necrosis in glioblastomas.

plant formation Plants existing together in a community within the same environment.

reaction formation An unconscious defense mechanism of the ego consisting of denying the presence of unacceptable infantile urges and therefore altering one's character and one's way of relating to the external world.

reticular formation FORMATIO RETICULARIS.

reticular formation of medulla oblongata FORMATIO RETICULARIS MEDULLAE OBLONGATAE.

reticular formation of mesencephalon FORMATIO RETICULARIS MESENCEPHALI.

reticular formation of pons FORMATIO RETICULARIS PONTIS.

reticular formation of spinal cord FORMATIO RETICULARIS MEDULLAE SPINALIS.

rouleaux formation The arrangement of erythrocytes in overlapping fashion, suggesting a stack of coins.

substitute formation COMPROMISE FORMATION.

symptom formation COMPROMISE FORMATION.

white reticular formation SUBSTANTIA RETICULARIS ALBA MEDULLAE OBLONGATAE.

formationes Plural of FORMATIO.

formative Having to do with the shaping or molding of the final product of any developmental process.

formboard [*form* + *board*] A performance test of nonverbal intelligence which requires fitting into insets appropriate blocks of different shapes, designs, or colors. The time taken, or errors made, or both, serve as score.

forme fruste (*plural* formes frustes) An incomplete or abortive form of a disease or anomaly.

forme tardive Late-appearing manifestations of a disease with variable age of onset and which is normally seen at a younger age. For example, epiloia (tuberose sclerosis) may present no serious symptoms until late in life.

form-genus See under FORM.

formic [L *formic(a)* an ant] **1** Of or relating to ants. **2** Relating to or derived from formic acid.

formic acid $H-COOH$. A weak acid (pK 3.7), that is colorless, corrosive, and harmful to the skin. It has the distinctive smell of ants, which secrete it. It is used as a reducing agent, and is miscible with water, alcohol, and ether. It can be formed from the metabolism of many biochemical compounds, such as serine or glycine, or by the oxidation of "one-carbon compounds," such as formaldehyde or methanol, which may be free or combined with tetrahydrofolic acid. However, the metabolically active forms are N^{10}- and N^5- formyl tetrahydrofolic acids, which are intermediates in the biosynthesis of purines.

formicant Describing or producing formication.

formication [L *formic(a)* an ant + -ATION] A sensation of insects creeping in or under one or more areas of the skin. It is most commonly reported in drug and alcohol abusers. Also called *crawling, Magnan sign, Magnan symptom.*

formiciasis [*formic (acid)* + -IASIS] Formic acid poisoning from ant bites.

Formicoidea [L *formic(a)* ant + *o* + New L *-idea,* neut. pl. form of Gk *-ideus,* patronymic suffix] A superfamily, in the order Hymenoptera, that includes all of the ants. In some classifications, the ants (family Formicidae) are placed in the superfamily Scolioidea.

formimino The group $HN=CH-$. This group is transferred to tetrahydrofolate during the catabolism of histidine.

N-formiminoglutamate $HN=CH-NH-CH(COOH)-$ CH_2-CH_2-COOH. The substance whose formula is shown and its ionized forms. It is an intermediate in the catabolism of histidine.

formiminonoglutamic acid $HN=CH-NH-CH(COOH)-CH_2-CH_2-COOH$. An intermediate in the breakdown of histidine, it transfers its formimino group to tetrahydrofolate.

formiminoglutamicaciduria The excessive urinary excretion of formiminoglutamic acid. It occurs in two distinct autosomal recessive inborn errors of metabolism: cyclodeaminase deficiency, in which patients are severely mentally retarded with cerebral cortical atrophy, and formiminotransferase deficiency, in which patients have variable but mild neurologic abnormalities.

formiminoglycine $H_2N^+=CH-NH-CH_2-COO^-$. A substance found as a metabolite in the breakdown of purines. It yields glycine by transferring its $H_2N^+=CH-$ group to tetrahydrofolate.

formiminotetrahydrofolate Tetrahydrofolate substituted on N-5 with the formimino group. It is derived from formiminoglutamate in histidine breakdown or from formiminoglycine in purine breakdown. It is metabolized to liberate ammonia with formation of 5,10-methenyltetrahydrofolate.

formiminotransferase Any enzyme that transfers the formimino group. Also called *transformiminase.*

Formin A proprietary name for methenamine.

forminitrazole $C_4H_3N_3O_3S$. A bacteriostatic agent that is used in the treatment of trichomoniasis vaginitis.

formol An aqueous solution of formaldehyde. An obsolete term.

formol saline A widely used general purpose fixative solution that contains 10 percent formaldehyde in physiologic saline.

formol sublimate A compound fixative composed of mercuric chloride and formaldehyde. It is a swift histological fixative that enhances subsequent staining.

formula [L (dim. of *forma* form, shape), a rule, form, order, condition] **1** A designation of the structure or composition of a chemical that uses symbols and signs to identify the structural characteristics. **2** The ingredients and directions that are to be combined for the preparation of a medicinal drug or application. **3** An algebraic or symbolic expression of a rule or concept.

acoustic formula Any mathematical formula used in the characterization of acoustic phenomena, such as the relation between sound pressure level and sound power level or between transmission loss and noise reduction.

Ambard's formula An outmoded estimate of renal function, of historical interest, based on measurement of urea in the blood and urine, but not based on the clearance principle. Also called *Ambard's coefficient, Ambard's constant, Ambard's equation, urea index, ureosecretory index, urea constant.*

Arneth's formula The proportions of segmented neutrophils, when classified by number of nuclear lobes. Also called *Arneth's count.*

Bazett formula A formula for correcting the Q-T interval for the effects of rate (where RR is the time interval between successive R waves):

$$QTc = \frac{QT \text{ sec}}{\sqrt{RR \text{ sec}}}.$$

Bernhardt's formula A formula once used to calculate the ideal weight in kilograms of an adult, in which the circumference of the chest and the height, both measured in centimeters, are multiplied. The product is then divided by 240.

Black's formula A formula formerly used to calculate the strength of an adult. The height in inches is subtracted from the weight in pounds and added to the chest circumference at full inspiration, in inches. A result exceeding 120 is rated very strong; 110–120, strong; 80–90, weak; less than 80, very weak.

Broca's formula A method formerly used for estimating the ideal weight of an adult, by which the height in centimeters, less 100, would equal the ideal weight in kilograms.

canonical formula A structural formula depicted with localized double or triple bonds although these are now known to be partly delocalized in the molecule represented.

Casper's formula A formula used in forensic medicine: the amount of putrefaction occurring in one week in a body exposed to air equals that amount occurring in two weeks in a body in water or the amount occurring in eight weeks in a body in soil. Putrefaction is assumed to occur at a set rate. The formula is used as a rule of thumb to assess the time of death in decaying or decomposing bodies. However, it is a useful approximation only in temperate climates.

chemical formula The representation of a molecule or ion by symbols for the elements. It may depict either composition or structure.

clearance ratio formula A formula basic to the evaluation of renal function, expressed as C = UV/P, where C = clearance in ml/min, U = concentration of a substance in urine, V = rate of urine flow in ml/min, and P = concentration of the substance in plasma. Concentration may be measured in terms of grams or moles per liter but must be the same units for urine and plasma results.

Cooke's formula A refinement of Arneth's formula, in which the lobes of neutrophil nuclei are regarded as unsegmented if connected by more than the narrowest thread of chromatin. Also called *Cooke's count, Cooke's index.*

Demoivre's formula The expectation of life of a person aged *x* years is equal to $2/3(80 - x)$ years.

dental formula A concise representation of the number of incisors, canines, premolars, and molars in the dentition of a particular animal.

diffusion formula A mathematical formula incorporating meteorological and other variables that predict the behavior of chimney plumes. It is used for determining probable ground levels of pollution under varying conditions.

digital formula A numerical expression of the relative lengths of the digits, both fingers and toes, indicating which digits are longer or shorter than others. A seldom used term.

Dreyer's formula A formula which relates vital capacity of the lungs to body surface area.

Du Bois formula A formula that relates the surface area of the body to the body weight and height: $O = W^{0.425} \times H^{0.725} \times 71.84$, where O = surface area in cm², W = weight in kg, and H = height in cm.

empirical formula The chemical formula of a substance if this gives only the ratio between the atoms present without giving the absolute number of each in the molecule.

extemporaneous formula A prescription for a medicinal preparation that must be prepared just before being dispensed and not taken from stock or off the shelf.

Fick formula See under FICK PRINCIPLE.

Fischer projection formula A formula representing the configuration of chiral centers of molecules. It shows all angles as right angles, because it views each chiral center from the direction such that the central atom is closer to the viewer than its bonds to the other atoms in the main chain of the compound (usually drawn vertically). The bonds to substituents (usually drawn horizontally) come towards the viewer.

Florschütz formula A formula once used to express the degree of overweight in an individual. The height, expressed in a given unit of measure, is subtracted from twice the abdominal circumference, as expressed in the same unit of measure. The resulting value, if less than five, indicates the degree of overweight, the value of five being the threshold for adiposity.

Gorlin formula A formula for calculating the area of a cardiac valve orifice: Valve area = blood flow ÷ K × 44.5 × $\sqrt{P1 - P2}$, (where valve area is in square centimeters, blood flow is in mm/sec during the time of valve opening, K is an empirical constant, and P1 and P2 are the mean pressures in mmHg on either side of the valve during the time it is open).

Guthrie's formula A formerly used method of estimating the ideal weight of an adult. The number of inches that the body height exceeds 5 feet is multiplied by 5.5 and then added to 110 to give a weight in pounds.

Hamilton-Stewart formula A formula for calculating cardiac output following the rapid injection of an indicator substance: F = i/CT (where F = blood flow in liters/min; *i*, the injected substance in mg; C, the average concentration of the injected substance during the primary curve; and T, the duration of the primary curve, i.e., the curve in which there is no recirculation of the injected substance).

Katz formula A seldom used formula for determining erythrocyte sedimentation rate: an average of the one-hour plasma column height and half of the two-hour plasma column height.

Mall's formula An outmoded way of estimating the age in days of an embryo up to 100 mm in length by calculating the square root of the crown-rump length in millimeters and multiplying by 100. It was later pointed out that the multiplication factor of 100 was inaccurate, 110 being the correct factor.

Meeh's formula An obsolete formula for estimating the surface area of the body that is based on the body weight.

official formula An approved and accepted formula that has been recognized and designated by a pharmacopeia or similar authoritative group.

paretic formula A formula for diagnosing general paresis using the colloidal gold test on cerebrospinal fluid. The results are positive if the color change is greatest in the first tubes in the series.

Pignet's formula A formula once used to rank the strength of an adult, in which the chest circumference during full inspiration, measured in centimeters, is added to the body weight in kilograms and then subtracted from the height in centimeters.

The remainder is categorized as follows: less than 10, very strong; 10–15, strong; 15–20, good; 20–25, medium; 25–30, weak; and greater than 30, very weak. Also called *Pignet standard.*

Poisson-Pearson formula   A formula for the percentage error in calculating the endemic index of malaria for a population given the spleen rate estimated from a sample and the size of the population under 15 years:

$$\frac{200}{n}\sqrt{\frac{2(n-x)}{n}}\sqrt{1-\frac{(n-1)}{(N-1)}},$$

where n is the size of the sample, x the number with enlarged spleens, N the size of the child population, and x/n is the estimated spleen rate.

resuscitation formula   Any of several solutions or mixtures of solutions used to restore the circulation following severe burns.

Rollier's formula   A formula used to increase progressively the ultraviolet dosage being applied to the body, to prevent excessive use of ultraviolet radiation.

structural formula   A formula showing the structure of a molecule by depicting the positions of atoms and the bonds between them.

vertebral formula   A numerical representation of the number of vertebrae usually found in the cervical, thoracic, lumbar, sacral, and coccygeal regions, namely, C 7, T 12, L 5, S 5, Co (or Cd) 4 = 33, for humans.

Vierordt-Meeh formula   A formula that relates the surface area of the body to the body weight and height: $O = mP^{2/3}$, where O = surface area, m= height, and P = weight.

formulary   **1** A listing of drugs, usually by generic name, and usually including all drugs available through a pharmacy or health care plan.   **2** A published collection of formulas used in compounding drugs. See also NATIONAL FORMULARY.

formulation / ALI formulation   AMERICAN LAW INSTITUTE FORMULATION.

American Law Institute formulation   "A person is not responsible for criminal conduct if at the time of such conduct as a result of mental disease or defect he lacks substantial capacity either to appreciate the wrongfulness of his conduct or to conform his conduct to the requirements of law." It was first adopted in 1966 by the Second Circuit U.S. Court of Appeals based on the case of the United States vs Brawner. Also called *American Law Institute rule, ALI formulation.*

formyl   The group H—CO—; the acyl group derived from formic acid.

formylation   The process of replacing a hydrogen atom by the formyl group.

N-formylmethionine $HCO—NH—CH(COOH)—[CH_2]_2—S—CH_3$. The acylated amino acid with which bacterial protein synthesis starts. It is produced as formylmethionyl-tRNA by formylation of one of the two forms of methionyl-tRNA, and is transferred on the ribosome onto the second residue of the protein being synthesized, releasing its tRNA.

formyltetrahydrofolate   Tetrahydrofolate formylated on N-5 or N-10. Each of these compounds is an intermediate in some biologic formylations. They can be derived by oxidation of methylenetetrahydrofolate as well as by direct formylation.

fornical   Pertaining or belonging to a fornix.

fornicate   Arched or vaulted; shaped like a fornix.

fornication   [Late L *fornicatio* (from *fornicatus,* past part. of *fornicari* to fornicate, from L *fornix,* gen. *fornicis,* an arch, vault, brothel) fornication]   Sexual intercourse involving an unmarried person.

fornicolumn   COLUMNA FORNICIS.

fornicommissure   COMMISSURA FORNICIS.

fornix   [L, a furnacelike ceiling, an arch, vault, brothel]   **1** Any archlike structure, or the concave recess produced by such a structure.   **2** FORNIX CEREBRI.

anterior fornix   PARS ANTERIOR FORNICIS VAGINAE.

cerebral fornix   FORNIX CEREBRI.

fornix cerebri   Large, paired myelinated tracts that emerge from the hippocampus, arch and fuse beneath the corpus callosum, and descend in separate columns to the septal region (precommissural fornix) and mamillary bodies (postcommissural fornix). It contains mainly efferent fibers arising from the subiculum and hippocampus, but numerous other afferent and efferent connections have been described. Also called *fornix of cerebrum, cerebral fornix, psalis* (outmoded), *cerebral trigone, trigonum cerebrale, fornix.*

fornix of cerebrum   FORNIX CEREBRI.

fornix of conjunctiva   Either the fornix conjunctivae superior or the fornix conjunctivae inferior.

fornix conjunctivae inferior   [NA] The line of reflection of the conjunctiva from the inner surface of the lower eyelid to the eyeball. Also called *inferior conjunctival fornix.*

fornix conjunctivae superior   [NA] The line of reflection of the conjunctiva from the inner surface of the upper eyelid to the eyeball. The excretory ductules of the lacrimal gland open into its lateral part. Also called *superior conjunctival fornix.*

fornix gastricus   FUNDUS GASTRICUS.

inferior conjunctival fornix   FORNIX CONJUNCTIVAE INFERIOR.

fornix of lacrimal sac   FORNIX SACCI LACRIMALIS.

lateral fornix   PARS LATERALIS FORNICIS VAGINAE.

fornix longus   The portion of the fornix cerebri bundle emerging from the hippocampus in its longitudinal course above the diencephalon, before forming the descending columns.

fornix pharyngis   [NA] The arched roof and adjacent posterior wall of the nasopharynx that is attached to the inferior surface of the basilar part of the occipital bone and the adjoining body of the sphenoid bone and related anteriorly to the nasal choanae. Its mucous membrane contains the pharyngeal tonsil. Also called *fornix of pharynx, vault of pharynx.*

fornix of pharynx   FORNIX PHARYNGIS.

posterior fornix   PARS POSTERIOR FORNICIS VAGINAE.

fornix sacci lacrimalis   [NA] The dome-shaped upper junction of the lateral and medial walls of the lacrimal sac which is situated above the level of the opening of the lacrimal canaliculi. Also called *fornix of lacrimal sac.*

fornix of the stomach   FUNDUS GASTRICUS.

superior conjunctival fornix   FORNIX CONJUNCTIVAE SUPERIOR.

fornix vaginae   [NA] The arched recess surrounding the vaginal portion of the uterine cervix at the upper end of the vagina. The continuous space is divided into pars anterior, pars lateralis, and pars posterior in relation to the walls of the vagina. Also called *fundus vaginae* (outmoded), *fundus of vagina, ampulla of vagina* (outmoded).

fornix ventricularis   FUNDUS GASTRICUS.

Foroblique   A telescopic lens used especially in cystoscopes. A trade name.

fors   A unit of acceleration equal to the standard acceleration of free fall; 9.806 65 meters per second squared. An obsolete unit. Symbol: f

Forsman   [Hans Axel *Forsman,* Swedish physician, born 1912]   Börjeson-Forsman-Lehmann syndrome. See under BÖRJESON SYNDROME.

Forssell   [Gosta *Forssell,* Swedish radiologist, 1876–1950]   See under SINUS.

Forssman   [John *Forssman,* Swedish pathologist, 1868–1947]   **1**

See under SYNDROME, ANTIBODY, SHOCK. **2** Forssman antigen-antibody reaction. See under REACTION. **3** Forssman's lipoid. See under ANTIGEN.

Förster [Carl Friedrich Richard *Förster*, German ophthalmologist, 1825–1902] **1** Förster's choroiditis, Förster's disease. See under AREOLAR CENTRAL CHOROIDITIS. **2** Förster's disease. See under DIPLEGIA. **3** See under UVEITIS, PHENOMENON.

Förster [Otfrid *Förster*, German neurologist, 1873–1941] Förster-Penfield operation. See under OPERATION.

Forthane A proprietary name for methylhexaneamine.

fortification ENRICHMENT.

FORTRAN [*for(mula) tran(slation)*] The most popular high-level scientific programming language designed for problems expressed in algebraic notation.

fosfomycin PHOSPHONOMYCIN.

Foshay [Lee *Foshay*, U.S. bacteriologist, 1896–1961] **1** Foshay's reaction. See under ERYTHEMATOUS-EDEMATOUS REACTION. **2** Foshay serum. See under ANTITULARENSE SERUM. **3** See under TEST.

fossa

fossa [L (from fem. of *fossus*, past part. of *fodere* to dig), a ditch, trench] (*plural* fossae) A trenchlike depression, hollow area, or recess.

acetabular fossa FOSSA ACETABULI.

fossa acetabuli [NA] The rough nonarticular portion above the acetabular notch forming the floor of the acetabulum. Also called *acetabular fossa, acetabular recess* (outmoded).

adipose fossae Spaces in the subcutaneous areolar tissue in the breast that contain varying amounts of fat, producing the contour of the breast.

amygdaloid fossa An outmoded term for FOSSA TONSILLARIS.

anconal fossa FOSSA OLECRANI.

anconeal fossa FOSSA OLECRANI.

antecubital fossa FOSSA CUBITALIS.

anterior condylar fossa A depression located anterosuperior to the occipital condyle into which the canalis hypoglossi opens. An outmoded term.

anterior cranial fossa FOSSA CRANII ANTERIOR.

anterior intercondylar fossa of tibia AREA INTERCONDYLARIS ANTERIOR TIBIAE.

fossa anthelicis [NA] The curved, vertical groove on the cranial surface of the auricular cartilage corresponding to the anthelix on the lateral surface. Also called *fossa of anthelix, periconchal sulcus* (outmoded).

fossa of anthelix FOSSA ANTHELICIS.

fossa articularis A depression on a bone lined by cartilage into which the extremity of another bone fits to form an articulation. An outmoded term.

articular fossa of mandible FOSSA MANDIBULARIS.

articular fossa for odontoid process of axis FOVEA DENTIS ATLANTIS.

articular fossa of temporal bone FOSSA MANDIBULARIS.

fossa of auditory canal A depression of variable depth which is situated at the junction of the medial surface of the tragus and the anterior wall of the external auditory meatus. In adults it may be occupied by hairs. An outmoded term.

fossa axillaris The pyramidal fossa between the upper part of the medial side of the arm and the lateral side of the upper

thorax. The anterior and posterior walls are mainly muscular; the apex, behind the middle third of the clavicle, communicates with the base of the neck; and the floor is formed of skin and fasciae that stretch between the lower borders of the anterior and posterior walls and is continuous medially with the thorax and laterally with the arm. It provides passage for the brachial plexus and axillary vessels between the upper limb and the neck and trunk, and it contains lymph nodes, fat, and connective tissue. Also called *maschale, axilla, axillary space, axillary fossa, armpit, arm pit, axil.*

axillary fossa FOSSA AXILLARIS.

fossa of Baréty A small fossa that is situated anterior and to the right of the junction of the superior vena cava and the right brachiocephalic vein. It is bounded medially by the trachea, arch of aorta, and brachiocephalic trunk; superiorly by the right subclavian artery, and inferiorly by the arch of the azygos vein. It is external to the mediastinal pleura and contains the right paratracheal lymph nodes. An outmoded term.

Biesiadecki's fossa FOSSA ILIACOSUBFASCIALIS.

Broesike's fossa PARAJEJUNAL FOSSA.

fossa caecalis An outmoded term for RECESSUS RETROCAECALIS.

fossa canina CANINE FOSSA.

canine fossa A shallow depression on the anterolateral surface of the maxilla, above and lateral to the canine eminence, which gives origin to the levator anguli oris muscle. Also called *fossa canina, maxillary fossa, suborbital fossa.*

fossa capitelli The saddle-shaped articular facet on the anterior surface of the body of the incus for articulation with the head of the malleus. An outmoded term.

fossa capitis femoris An outmoded term for FOVEA CAPITIS OSSIS FEMORIS.

fossa carotica An outmoded term for TRIGONUM CAROTICUM.

cerebellar fossa FOSSA CRANII POSTERIOR.

cerebral fossa Any of the following: 1) fossa cranii anterior; 2) fossa cranii media; 3) fossa cranii posterior.

fossa cerebri lateralis Sylvii FOSSA LATERALIS CEREBRI.

fossa chordae ductus venosi FISSURE OF DUCTUS VENOSUS.

Claudius fossa FOSSA OVARICA.

cochleariform fossa An outmoded term for SEMICANALIS MUSCULI TENSORIS TYMPANI.

fossa cochlearis of vestibule An outmoded term for RECESSUS COCHLEARIS VESTIBULI.

condylar fossa FOSSA CONDYLARIS.

fossa condylaris The depression behind each occipital condyle that receives the posterior margin of the superior facet of the atlas when the head is extended. Also called *condylar fossa, condyloid fossa, fossa condyloidea* (outmoded), *postcondyloid fossa, posterior condyloid fossa, postcondylar notch* (outmoded).

condyloid fossa FOSSA CONDYLARIS.

condyloid fossa of atlas FACIES ARTICULARIS SUPERIOR ATLANTIS.

fossa condyloidea An outmoded term for FOSSA CONDYLARIS.

condyloid fossa of mandible FOSSA MANDIBULARIS.

condyloid fossa of temporal bone FOSSA MANDIBULARIS.

coronoid fossa FOSSA CORONOIDEA HUMERI.

fossa coronoidea humeri [NA] An oval pit situated anteriorly and proximal to the trochlea of the humerus into which the coronoid process of ulna fits during flexion of the elbow joint. Also called *coronoid fossa of humerus, fossa of coronoid process, cubital fossa* (outmoded), *ulnar fossa, anterior supratrochlear fovea, fovea of coronoid process, greater anterior fovea of humerus, supratrochlear fovea of humerus, coronoid fossa.*

coronoid fossa of humerus FOSSA CORONOIDEA HUMERI.

fossa of coronoid process FOSSA CORONOIDEA HUMERI.

cranial fossa Either fossa cranii anterior, fossa cranii media, or fossa cranii posterior.

fossa cranii anterior [NA] The anterior of the three subdivisions of the internal cranial base, depressed to fit the rounded lower aspect of the frontal lobes of the cerebrum, and limited in front and on the sides by the frontal bone. The surface, or floor, is lined by dura mater and is formed by parts of the frontal, ethmoid, and sphenoid bones. Also called *anterior cranial fossa.*

fossa cranii media [NA] The irregular depression in the middle of the internal surface of the base of the cranium, situated at a lower level than the anterior fossa and consisting of a central and two lateral portions, bounded anteriorly by the posterior margins of the lesser wings of the sphenoid bone and the anterior margin of the sulcus chiasmatis and posteriorly by the superior margins of the petrous parts of the temporal bones and the dorsum sellae of the sphenoid bone between them. Laterally it merges with the lateral wall of the cranium on each side while the floor comprises the body and greater wings of the sphenoid bone and the anterior surfaces of the petrous parts of the temporal bones. On each side it lodges the temporal lobe of the cerebrum while in the center the hypophysis cerebri is contained. Also called *middle cranial fossa, temporal fossa, middle fossa, mesocranial fossa* (outmoded).

fossa cranii posterior [NA] The posterior, largest, and deepest depression of the internal surface of the irregular base of the cranium, bounded anteriorly by the dorsum sellae of the sphenoid bone, laterally by the superior margin of the petrous part of the temporal bone and the mastoid angle of the parietal bone, and posteriorly by the squamous part of the occipital bone below the transverse sinuses. The floor is constituted by the occipital bone, which supports the cerebellum posteriorly and the pons and medulla oblongata anteriorly. Also called *posterior cranial fossa, cerebellar fossa.*

crural fossa FEMORAL FOSSA.

Cruveilhier's fossa FOSSA SCAPHOIDEA OSSIS SPHENOIDALIS.

cubital fossa **1** FOSSA CUBITALIS. **2** An outmoded term for FOSSA CORONOIDEA HUMERI.

fossa cubitalis [NA] A triangular hollow in front of the elbow joint between the pronator teres muscle medially, the brachioradialis muscle laterally, and a base formed by an imaginary line between the humeral epicondyles. The floor is formed by the brachialis and supinator muscles, and it is roofed over by skin and fascia containing superficial veins, nerves, and lymphatics. Also called *cubital fossa, antecubital fossa, chelidon, triangle of elbow, antecubital space.*

fossa cystidis felleae An outmoded term for FOSSA VESICAE BILIARIS.

digastric fossa **1** FOSSA DIGASTRICA. **2** INCISURA MASTOIDEA OSSIS TEMPORALIS.

fossa digastrica [NA] A small rough pit on the base of the mandible on each side of the midline for the attachment of the anterior belly of the digastric muscle. Also called *digastric fossa, fossa musculi biventeris* (outmoded), *digastric fovea, digastric impression.*

digital fossa of femur FOSSA TROCHANTERICA.

fossa ductus venosi FISSURE OF DUCTUS VENOSUS.

fossa of ductus venosus FISSURE OF DUCTUS VENOSUS.

duodenal fossa Either recessus duodenalis inferior or recessus duodenalis superior.

duodenojejunal fossa **1** RECESSUS DUODENALIS SUPERIOR. **2** A deep peritoneal recess which is situated between the duodenojejunal junction and the root of the transverse mesocolon on the left of the abdominal aorta and below the pancreas. It lies behind a peritoneal fold formed by the left colic artery. Also called *mesocolic recess.*

epigastric fossa **1** FOSSA EPIGASTRICA. **2** FOSSA SUPRAVESICALIS.

fossa epigastrica A small depression on the anterior abdominal wall which is situated just below the xiphoid process in the epigastric region. Also called *epigastric fossa, fovea cardiaca* (outmoded), *scrobiculus cordis* (outmoded), *precordial depression.*

ethmoid fossa A groove on the cribriform plate of the ethmoid bone on each side of the crista galli occupied by the olfactory bulb and pierced by numerous foramina for filaments of the olfactory nerve. Also called *olfactory fossa, olfactory groove.*

fossa of eustachian tube An outmoded term for FOSSA SCAPHOIDEA OSSIS SPHENOIDALIS.

external iliac fossa An outmoded term for FACIES GLUTEA OSSIS ILII.

external inguinal fossa FOSSA INGUINALIS LATERALIS.

femoral fossa A small depression in the parietal peritoneum overlying the annulus femoralis and separated from the lower end of the lateral inguinal fossa by the medial end of the inguinal ligament. Also called *crural fossa, crural fovea, femoral fovea, inferior digital fossa, hiatus femoralis.*

floccular fossa The fossa subarcuata ossis temporalis in quadrupeds.

frontal fossa FACIES INTERNA OSSIS FRONTALIS.

fossa of gallbladder FOSSA VESICAE BILIARIS.

fossa of gasserian ganglion An outmoded term for IMPRESSIO TRIGEMINALIS OSSIS TEMPORALIS.

Gerdy's hyoid fossa An outmoded term for TRIGONUM CAROTICUM.

fossa glandulae lacrimalis [NA] A rounded, shallow depression situated on the anterolateral part of the orbital surface of the frontal bone and medial to the zygomatic process of the frontal bone. In it the orbital part of the lacrimal gland is lodged. Also called *fossa of lacrimal gland, lacrimal fossa, glandular fossa of frontal bone* (outmoded).

glandular fossa of frontal bone An outmoded term for FOSSA GLANDULAE LACRIMALIS.

glenoid fossa **1** CAVITAS GLENOIDALIS. **2** FOSSA MANDIBULARIS.

glenoid fossa of scapula CAVITAS GLENOIDALIS.

glenoid fossa of temporal bone FOSSA MANDIBULARIS.

glossoepiglottic fossa VALLECULA EPIGLOTTICA.

greater fossa of Scarpa TRIGONUM FEMORALE.

greater supraclavicular fossa TRIGONUM OMOCLAVICULARE.

Gruber's fossa GRUBER'S CUL-DE-SAC.

Gruber-Landzert fossa **1** RECESSUS PARADUODENALIS. **2** A superior duodenal recess that extends behind the duodenojejunal flexure.

harderian fossa An irregular depression in the orbit of some nonhuman animals in which the harderian gland is located.

Hartmann's fossa RECESSUS ILEOCECALIS INFERIOR.

fossa of head of femur FOVEA CAPITIS OSSIS FEMORIS.

fossa helicis An outmoded term for SCAPHA.

fossa hemielliptica An outmoded term for RECESSUS ELLIPTICUS VESTIBULI.

fossa hemispherica An outmoded term for RECESSUS SPHERICUS VESTIBULI.

hyaloid fossa FOSSA HYALOIDEA.

fossa hyaloidea [NA] A deep concavity on the front of the vitreous body against which the posterior surface of the lens fits. Also called *hyaloid fossa, lenticular fossa of vitreous body, lenticular fossa, patellar fossa* (outmoded).

hypogastric fossa FOSSA INGUINALIS MEDIALIS.

fossa hypophyseos An outmoded term for FOSSA HYPOPHYSIALIS.

hypophysial fossa FOSSA HYPOPHYSIALIS.

fossa hypophysialis [NA] The deep hollow in the center of the sella turcica of the sphenoid bone occupied by the hypophysis cerebri. The floor is perforated by foramina for blood vessels. Also called *hypophysial fossa, fossa hypophyseos* (outmoded), *pituitary fossa, sellar fossa, suprasphenoidal fossa.*

ileocolic fossa   RECESSUS ILEOCECALIS SUPERIOR.

iliac fossa   FOSSA ILIACA.

fossa iliaca [NA] The hollow anterior and superior part of the medial surface of the ilium, anterior to the sacropelvic surface and bounded above by the iliac crest and below by the arcuate line. It provides attachment for the iliacus muscle. Also called *iliac fossa, venter ilii* (outmoded), *internal iliac fossa* (outmoded).

iliacosubfascial fossa   FOSSA ILIACOSUBFASCIALIS.

fossa iliacosubfascialis   An occasional peritoneal recess located between the lateral border of the psoas major muscle and the iliac crest. Also called *Biesiadecki's fossa, iliacosubfascial fossa.*

fossa iliopectinea   The deep groove between the psoas major and iliacus muscles laterally and the pectineus and adductor longus muscles medially, in which the femoral vessels lie proximally in the femoral triangle. Also called *iliopectineal fossa, lesser fossa of Scarpa* (outmoded), *iliopectineal trigone.*

iliopectineal fossa   FOSSA ILIOPECTINEA.

fossa incisiva [NA] A funnel-shaped depression that is situated in the median plane of the bony palate just behind the incisor teeth. It contains the lower openings of the two lateral incisive canals in its lateral walls, one on each side, extending from the nasal cavity and providing passage for the nasopalatine nerves and the termination of the greater palatine arteries. In addition, the median anterior and posterior incisive foramina may be present and open in the depression in the midline, the left nasopalatine nerve then passing through the anterior foramen and the right nasopalatine nerve passing through the posterior foramen. Also called *incisive fossa, anterior palatine foramen* (outmoded), *palatine fossa* (outmoded), *incisive fossa of maxilla.*

incisive fossa   FOSSA INCISIVA.

incisive fossa of maxilla   **1** A small depression on the anterior surface of the maxilla above the lateral incisor tooth that gives origin to the depressor septi muscle. Also called *myrtiform fossa, fossa praenasalis, prenasal fossa.*   **2** FOSSA INCISIVA.

incudal fossa   FOSSA INCUDIS.

fossa incudis [NA] A small depression in the posteroinferior part of the epitympanic recess in which the short process of the incus is lodged, attached by ligamentous fibers. Also called *incudal fossa, fossa of incus.*

fossa of incus   FOSSA INCUDIS.

inferior articular fossa of atlas   FACIES ARTICULARIS INFERIOR ATLANTIS.

inferior costal fossa   FOVEA COSTALIS INFERIOR.

inferior digital fossa   FEMORAL FOSSA.

inferior duodenal fossa   RECESSUS DUODENALIS INFERIOR.

inferior duodenojejunal fossa   An occasional peritoneal recess that is situated in the duodenojejunal flexure and is limited anteriorly by a peritoneal fold extending from the ascending portion of the duodenum to the origin of the jejunum. It is open inferiorly and to the left.

inferior ileocecal fossa   RECESSUS ILEOCECALIS INFERIOR.

inferior fossa of omental sac   RECESSUS INFERIOR OMENTALIS.

infraclavicular fossa   FOSSA INFRACLAVICULARIS.

fossa infraclavicularis [NA] The triangular depression below the clavicle and between the superior border of the pectoralis major muscle and the anterior border of the deltoid muscle, containing the cephalic vein and the deltoid branch of the thoracoacromial artery. Also called *infraclavicular fossa, infraclavic-*

ular region, infraclavicular triangle, regio infraclavicularis (outmoded), *trigonum deltoideopectorale* (outmoded), *deltopectoral trigone* (outmoded), *Mohrenheim's fossa, Mohrenheim's space.*

infraduodenal fossa   An occasional small peritoneal recess situated just below the horizontal part of the duodenum.

fossa infraspinata [NA] The large triangular area formed by the inferior surface of the spine of the scapula and the posterior surface of the scapula below it. Most of the area is occupied by the origin of the infraspinatus muscle. Also called *infraspinous fossa, subspinous fossa, infraspinous region.*

infraspinous fossa   FOSSA INFRASPINATA.

infratemporal fossa   FOSSA INFRATEMPORALIS.

fossa infratemporalis [NA] An irregular space below and medial to the zygomatic arch, bounded anteriorly by the posterolateral, or infratemporal, surface of the maxilla, superiorly by the infratemporal surface of the greater wing of the sphenoid bone and a part of the squamous temporal bone, and medially by the lateral pterygoid lamina. Laterally it is only partly bounded by the ramus of the mandible, while behind and below it is open. Its roof is pierced by the foramen ovale and foramen spinosum in the greater wing of the sphenoid bone. The anterior and medial walls are united inferiorly but separated superiorly by the pterygomaxillary fissure, through which it communicates with the pterygopalatine fossa. It also communicates superiorly with the temporal fossa through the gap medial to the zygomatic arch, and anteriorly with the orbit through the inferior orbital fissure. Also called *infratemporal fossa, zygomatic fossa* (outmoded).

fossa inguinalis lateralis [NA] The depression in the parietal peritoneum that is lateral to the lateral umbilical fold formed by the inferior epigastric vessels on the inner surface of the anterior abdominal wall. The fossa is related to the deep inguinal ring inferiorly and corresponds to the saccus vaginalis in the embryo. Also called *lateral inguinal fossa, fovea inguinalis lateralis, lateral inguinal fovea, superior digital fossa* (outmoded), *external inguinal fovea, external inguinal fossa.*

fossa inguinalis medialis [NA] The depression in the parietal peritoneum that lies between the lateral umbilical fold formed by inferior epigastric vessels and the medial umbilical fold formed by the obliterated umbilical artery on the inner surface of the anterior abdominal wall. Also called *medial inguinal fossa, fovea inguinalis medialis, internal inguinal fovea, medial inguinal fovea, middle inguinal fovea, middle inguinal fossa, internal inguinal fossa, medial umbilical fossa, hypogastric fossa.*

fossa innominata   A shallow vertical groove that extends from the gap between the corniculate and cuneiform tubercles on the aryepiglottic fold to the sinus of the larynx behind the vestibular fold. An outmoded term. Also called *innominate fossa.*

innominate fossa   FOSSA INNOMINATA.

innominate fossa of auricle   An outmoded term for CAVITAS CONCHAE.

fossa for insertion of obliquus capitis superior muscle   An oval area for the insertion of the obliquus capitis superior muscle that is situated laterally between the superior and inferior nuchal lines of the occipital bone and lateral to the insertion of semispinalis capitis muscle. An outmoded term.

fossa for insertion of rectus capitis posterior major muscle   A small oval area for the insertion of the rectus capitis posterior major muscle that is situated laterally between the inferior nuchal line of the occipital bone and the foramen magnum and lateral to the insertion of the rectus capitis posterior minor muscle. An outmoded term.

fossa for insertion of rectus capitis posterior minor muscle   A small oval area for the insertion of the rectus capitis posterior minor muscle. It is situated medially between the inferior nuchal line of the occipital bone and the foramen magnum, lateral to the external occipital crest, and medial to the insertion of rectus capitis posterior major muscle. An outmoded term.

fossa for insertion of semispinalis capitis muscle A triangular area for the insertion of the semispinalis capitis muscle that is situated medially between the superior and inferior nuchal lines of the occipital bone and medial to and overlapping the obliquus capitis superior muscle insertion. An outmoded term.

intercondylar fossa of femur FOSSA INTERCONDYLARIS FEMORIS.

fossa intercondylaris femoris [NA] A deep notch separating the projecting cartilage-covered condyles of the femur posteriorly and providing attachment for the anterior and posterior cruciate ligaments of the knee joint on the opposed surfaces of the condyles and for the infrapatellar synovial fold anteriorly, while posteriorly the intercondylar line separates the notch from the popliteal surface of the femur. Also called *intercondylar fossa of femur, fossa intercondyloidea femoris* (outmoded), *popliteal incisure, fossa intercondylica, intercondyloid fossa, popliteal fossa of femur, intercondylar notch of femur, sinus condylarum femoris* (outmoded), *intercondylar notch.*

fossa intercondylica An outmoded term for FOSSA INTERCONDYLARIS FEMORIS.

intercondyloid fossa FOSSA INTERCONDYLARIS FEMORIS.

fossa intercondyloidea anterior tibiae AREA INTERCONDYLARIS ANTERIOR TIBIAE.

fossa intercondyloidea femoris An outmoded term for FOSSA INTERCONDYLARIS FEMORIS.

fossa intercondyloidea posterior tibiae AREA INTERCONDYLARIS POSTERIOR TIBIAE.

fossa intercruralis FOSSA INTERPEDUNCULARIS.

fossa intermesocolica transversa An occasional deep recessus duodenalis superior that extends transversely along the base of the transverse mesocolon. An outmoded term.

internal iliac fossa An outmoded term for FOSSA ILIACA.

internal inguinal fossa FOSSA INGUINALIS MEDIALIS.

interpeduncular fossa FOSSA INTERPEDUNCULARIS.

fossa interpeduncularis The midline depression between the cerebral peduncles, the site of the interpeduncular cistern. Also called *interpeduncular fossa, Tarin's fossa, fossa Tarini, fossa intercruralis, interpeduncular space, interpeduncular trigone, trigonum interpedunculare, interpeduncular recess.*

intersigmoid fossa RECESSUS INTERSIGMOIDEUS.

intertrochanteric fossa An irregular furrow medial to the intertrochanteric crest of the femur and continuous with the trochanteric fossa superiorly. A rarely used term.

intrabulbar fossa The dilated segment of the spongiose part of the male urethra in the bulb of the penis just beyond the perineal membrane.

ischioanal fossa FOSSA ISCHIOANALIS.

fossa ischioanalis [NA] The wedge-shaped space that is bounded medially by the inferior fascia of the pelvic diaphragm and the sphincter ani externus, laterally by the inner aspect of the ischial tuberosity and the obturator fascia, posteriorly by the sacrotuberous ligament and lower part of the gluteus maximus muscle, and anteriorly by the perineal membrane. The floor or base is formed by the skin of the perineum while the apex is roofed over by fascia arching between the medial and lateral walls. The space is filled by a pad of fat traversed by vessels and nerves, while the pudendal canal is situated along the lateral wall. Also called *ischiorectal fossa, ischioanal fossa, fossa ischiorectalis, perineal fossa* (outmoded), *Velpeau's fossa* (outmoded), *ischiorectal cavity, rectoischiadic cavity* (outmoded), *cavum rectoischiadicum, ischiorectal excavation, rectoischiadic excavation* (outmoded).

ischiorectal fossa FOSSA ISCHIOANALIS.

fossa ischiorectalis FOSSA ISCHIOANALIS.

Jobert's fossa A furrow formed between the distal part of the adductor magnus muscle anteriorly and the sartorius and gracilis muscles posteriorly when the knee is flexed and the thigh is rotated laterally.

fossa of Jonnesco 1 RECESSUS DUODENALIS SUPERIOR. **2** A peritoneal recess between the superior and the inferior duodenal folds on the left of the duodenojejunal flexure.

jugular fossa FOSSA SUPRACLAVICULARIS MINOR.

fossa jugularis An outmoded term for FOSSA SUPRACLAVICULARIS MINOR.

fossa jugularis ossis temporalis [NA] A deep, rounded depression behind the external opening of the carotid canal on the inferior aspect of the posterior portion of the petrous part of the temporal bone. It forms the anterior and lateral part of the wall of the jugular foramen and lodges the superior bulb of the internal jugular vein. The roof separates it from the tympanic cavity and in its lateral wall is the mastoid canaliculus. Also called *jugular fossa of temporal bone, fovea jugularis* (outmoded).

jugular fossa of temporal bone FOSSA JUGULARIS OSSIS TEMPORALIS.

lacrimal fossa 1 FOSSA GLANDULAE LACRIMALIS. **2** SULCUS LACRIMALIS. **3** FOSSA SACCI LACRIMALIS.

fossa of lacrimal gland FOSSA GLANDULAE LACRIMALIS.

fossa of lacrimal sac FOSSA SACCI LACRIMALIS.

Landzert's fossa RECESSUS PARADUODENALIS.

lateral fossa of brain FOSSA LATERALIS CEREBRI.

lateral fossa of cerebrum FOSSA LATERALIS CEREBRI.

lateral fossa of frenulum of prepuce LATERAL FOSSA OF PREPUTIAL SPACE.

lateral inguinal fossa FOSSA INGUINALIS LATERALIS.

fossa lateralis cerebri A slight depression that appears at the beginning of the fourth fetal month in the lateral surface of the cerebrum anterior and superior to the temporal pole. As the cortical lobes develop, the lateral cerebral fossa becomes submerged and overlapped by the opercula of the frontal, parietal, and temporal lobes. Its floor becomes the insula, and it opens toward the anterior perforated substance at the base of the cerebrum. Also called *vallecula sylvii, vallecula fossa sylvii, vallecula cerebri lateralis, sylvian fossa, fossa of Sylvius, lateral fossa of cerebrum, fossa occipitalis cerebralis* (obsolete), *fossa cerebri lateralis Sylvii, fossa lateralis cerebri, lateral fossa of brain.*

fossa of lateral malleolus FOSSA MALLEOLI LATERALIS.

lateral pharyngeal fossa RECESSUS PHARYNGEUS.

lateral fossa of preputial space Either of two shallow fossae that extend laterally from the frenulum preputii penis in the preputial space along the collum glandis penis. Also called *lateral fossa of frenulum of prepuce.*

fossa of lateral pterygoid muscle FOVEA PTERYGOIDEA MANDIBULAE.

lenticular fossa FOSSA HYALOIDEA.

lenticular fossa of vitreous body FOSSA HYALOIDEA.

lesser fossa of Scarpa An outmoded term for FOSSA ILIOPECTINEA.

lesser sigmoid fossa of ulna INCISURA RADIALIS ULNAE.

lesser supraclavicular fossa FOSSA SUPRACLAVICULARIS MINOR.

fossa for ligamentum teres FISSURA LIGAMENTI TERETIS.

fossa of little head of radius An outmoded term for FOVEA ARTICULARIS CAPITIS RADII.

fossa longitudinalis hepatis An outmoded term for FOSSA SAGITTALIS SINISTRA HEPATIS.

longitudinal fossae of right liver FOSSAE SAGITTALES DEXTRAE HEPATIS.

Luschka's fossa RECESSUS ILEOCECALIS SUPERIOR.

Malgaigne's fossa An outmoded term for TRIGONUM CAROTICUM.

fossa malleoli lateralis [NA] An oval depression at the lower end of the fibula behind the malleolar articular surface for the talus, pierced by many vascular foramina and attaching the posterior tibiofibular and posterior talofibular ligaments. Also called *fossa of lateral malleolus.*

mandibular fossa   FOSSA MANDIBULARIS.

fossa mandibularis   [NA] The deep, oval concavity, with its long axis directed posteromedially, at the root of the zygomatic process on the inferior surface of the squamous part of the temporal bone, for articulation with the mandibular condyle through the articular disk. The small nonarticular posterior wall of the fossa is formed by the temporal part of the temporal bone, anterior to which is the squamotympanic fissue. Also called *mandibular fossa, glenoid fossa, glenoid fossa of temporal bone, articular fovea of temporal bone* (outmoded), *articular fossa of mandible, articular fossa of temporal bone, condyloid fossa of mandible, condyloid fossa of temporal bone, glenoid cavity of temporal bone* (outmoded).

mastoid fossa of temporal bone   FOVEOLA SUPRAMEATICA.

maxillary fossa   CANINE FOSSA.

medial inguinal fossa   FOSSA INGUINALIS MEDIALIS.

medial umbilical fossa   FOSSA INGUINALIS MEDIALIS.

median fossa of lower lip   A median depression of variable size in the skin of the lower lip. Occasionally a tuft of hair grows at this site. An outmoded term.

mental fossa   An occasional median depression on the chin. An outmoded term.

Merkel's fossa   FILTRUM VENTRICULI.

mesentericoparietal fossa   An occasional peritoneal recess that is situated below the horizontal part of the duodenum and invaginates the adjacent base of the mesentery to the right. The large orifice is covered anteriorly by a fold of peritoneum formed by the superior mesenteric artery. It is more common in fetuses than in adults. Also called *Waldeyer's fossa.*

mesocranial fossa   An outmoded term for FOSSA CRANII MEDIA.

mesogastric fossa   An outmoded term for RECESSUS DUODENALIS SUPERIOR.

middle fossa   FOSSA CRANII MEDIA.

middle cranial fossa   FOSSA CRANII MEDIA.

middle inguinal fossa   FOSSA INGUINALIS MEDIALIS.

Mohrenheim's fossa   FOSSA INFRACLAVICULARIS.

fossa of Morgagni   FOSSA NAVICULARIS URETHRAE.

fossa musculi biventeris   An outmoded term for FOSSA DIGASTRICA.

mylohyoid fossa of mandible   An outmoded term for FOVEA SUBLINGUALIS.

myrtiform fossa   INCISIVE FOSSA OF MAXILLA.

nasal fossa   The space in the nasal cavity on each side of the median nasal septum that is further subdivided by the projections of the nasal conchae.

navicular fossa of Cruveilhier   An outmoded term for FOSSA SCAPHOIDEA OSSIS SPHENOIDALIS.

fossa navicularis urethrae   [NA] A dilated portion of the male urethra, flattened from side to side, within the glans penis. In its dorsal wall is a pitlike recess, lacuna magna. Also called *navicular fossa of male urethra, fossa navicularis urethrae morgagnii, fossa of Morgagni, terminal fossa* (outmoded), *crypt of Morgagni, fovea of Morgagni.*

fossa navicularis urethrae morgagnii   FOSSA NAVICULARIS URETHRAE.

fossa navicularis vestibuli vaginae   An outmoded term for FOSSA VESTIBULI VAGINAE.

navicular fossa of male urethra   FOSSA NAVICULARIS URETHRAE.

navicular fossa of sphenoid bone   An outmoded term for FOSSA SCAPHOIDEA OSSIS SPHENOIDALIS.

occipital fossa   Any of the four depressions on the internal surface of the squamous part of the occipital bone that are separated by the grooves for the transverse sinuses, extending laterally from the internal occipital protuberance, and by the sulcus of superior sagittal sinus and internal occipital crest, extending superiorly and inferiorly, respectively, from the protuberance. The upper two lodge the poles of the occipital lobes of the cerebrum while the lower two lodge the hemispheres of the cerebellum.

fossa occipitalis cerebralis   An obsolete term for FOSSA LATERALIS CEREBRI.

occlusal fossa   An irregular rounded depression on the occlusal surface of a tooth.

fossa olecrani   [NA] A deep oval depression on the posterior aspect of the condyle of the humerus above the trochlea, into which the tip of the olecranon process of ulna fits during extension of the elbow. Its floor is thin and may be perforated. Also called *olecranon fossa, anconal fossa, anconeal fossa, posterior fossa of humerus, posterior supratrochlear fossa.*

olecranon fossa   FOSSA OLECRANI.

olfactory fossa   ETHMOID FOSSA.

oral fossa   STOMODEUM.

orbital fossa   FACIES ORBITALIS OSSIS FRONTALIS.

oval fossa of heart   FOSSA OVALIS CORDIS.

fossa ovalis   1 FOSSA OVALIS CORDIS. 2 HIATUS SAPHENUS. 3 RECESSUS ELLIPTICUS VESTIBULI.

fossa ovalis cordis   [NA] An oval depression bounded by the prominent limbus fossae ovalis on the lower part of the interatrial septum in the right atrium, situated to the left of and above the opening of the inferior vena cava. Its floor represents the septum primum of the fetal heart. Also called *oval fossa of heart, fossa ovalis.*

fossa ovalis femoris   HIATUS SAPHENUS.

oval fossa of thigh   HIATUS SAPHENUS.

ovarian fossa   FOSSA OVARICA.

fossa ovarica   [NA] A peritoneum-lined depression occupied by the ovary on the lateral wall of the pelvis, bounded anteriorly by the obliterated umbilical artery, posteriorly by the internal iliac artery and the ureter, superiorly by the external iliac vessels, and inferiorly by the obturator vessels and nerve. Also called *ovarian fossa, Claudius fossa.*

fossae of Pacchioni   FOVEOLAE GRANULARES.

palatine fossa   An outmoded term for FOSSA INCISIVA.

paracecal fossa   An occasional variant of recessus retrocecalis in which the recess extends to one side of the cecum.

paraduodenal fossa   RECESSUS PARADUODENALIS.

paraduodenal venous fossa   An inconstant shallow peritoneal recess formed by a fold over the inferior mesenteric vein. It is situated between the superior and inferior duodenal recesses with which it may form a single large recess. It is one of several paraduodenal recesses described that have a low frequency and little significance. An outmoded term.

parajejunal fossa   An infrequently seen peritoneal recess that extends into the mesentery below the commencement of the jejunum. Also called *Broesike's fossa.*

pararectal fossa   A peritoneal recess that is situated on either side of the upper part of the rectum and varies in size with the fullness of the rectum. It contains the sigmoid colon on the left and the lower part of the ileum on the right.

paravesical fossa   FOSSA PARAVESICALIS.

fossa paravesicalis   [NA] A peritoneal depression on each side of the urinary bladder that is bounded medially by the lateral margin of the superior vesical surface and laterally by a raised fold of peritoneum covering the ductus deferens in the male and the round ligament of the uterus in the female. The degree of distension of the bladder determines the size and depth of the fossa. When the bladder is empty the fossa is crossed by the transverse vesical fold, when present. Posteriorly the fossa is separated from the pararectal fossa by peritoneal ridges formed by the internal iliac vessels and ureter as well as, in the female, the broad ligament of the uterus. Also called *paravesical fossa, obturator pouch, paracystic pouch, paravesical pouch.*

parietal fossa The deepest part of the concavity on the inner surface of the parietal bone of the skull. An outmoded term.

patellar fossa An outmoded term for FOSSA HYALOIDEA.

patellar fossa of femur FACIES PATELLARIS FEMORIS.

patellar fossa of tibia AREA INTERCONDYLARIS ANTERIOR TIBIAE.

perineal fossa An outmoded term for FOSSA ISCHIOANALIS.

petrosal fossa FOSSULA PETROSA.

fossa for petrosal ganglion An outmoded term for FOSSULA PETROSA.

pharyngeal fossa An occasional small depression in front of the pharyngeal tubercle on the inferior surface of the basilar portion of the occipital bone, indicating the site of the pharyngeal bursa.

piriform fossa RECESSUS PIRIFORMIS.

pituitary fossa FOSSA HYPOPHYSIALIS.

fossa of Poisson An outmoded term for RECESSUS DUODENALIS INFERIOR.

fossa poplitea [NA] A diamond-shaped area behind the knee joint, bounded superiorly by the semitendinosus and semimembranosus muscles medially and the biceps femoris muscle laterally, while inferiorly the medial wall is the medial head of the gastrocnemius and the lateral wall is the lateral head of the gastrocnemius and plantaris muscles. The floor is formed by the popliteal surface of femur, the oblique posterior ligament of knee joint, and the popliteus muscle and its fascia. The roof is the popliteal fascia pierced by the small saphenous vein. During flexion of the knee the boundaries and the hollow between them become obvious. Also called *popliteal fossa, popliteal cavity, popliteal space, poples, ham.*

popliteal fossa FOSSA POPLITEA.

popliteal fossa of femur FOSSA INTERCONDYLARIS FEMORIS.

popliteal fossa of tibia AREA INTERCONDYLARIS POSTERIOR TIBIAE.

postauditory fossa FOVEOLA SUPRAMEATICA.

postcondyloid fossa FOSSA CONDYLARIS.

posterior condyloid fossa FOSSA CONDYLARIS.

posterior cranial fossa FOSSA CRANII POSTERIOR.

posterior fossa of humerus FOSSA OLECRANI.

posterior intercondylar fossa of tibia AREA INTERCONDYLARIS POSTERIOR TIBIAE.

posterior supratrochlear fossa FOSSA OLECRANI.

fossa praenasalis INCISIVE FOSSA OF MAXILLA.

prenasal fossa INCISIVE FOSSA OF MAXILLA.

prescapular fossa A shallow concavity on the costal surface of the scapula opposite the attachment of the spine of scapula. A rarely used term. Also called *prespinous fossa.*

prespinous fossa PRESCAPULAR FOSSA.

fossa provesicalis An outmoded term for HARTMANN'S POUCH.

pterygoid fossa FOSSA PTERYGOIDEA OSSIS SPHENOIDALIS.

fossa pterygoidea ossis sphenoidalis [NA] The deep, elongated space separating the medial and lateral pterygoid laminae, open posteriorly and closed anteriorly by the fusion of the laminae and containing the medial pterygoid and tensor veli palatini muscles. Also called *pterygoid fossa of sphenoid bone, pterygoid fossa.*

pterygoid fossa of inferior maxillary bone An outmoded term for FOVEA PTERYGOIDEA MANDIBULAE.

pterygoid fossa of sphenoid bone FOSSA PTERYGOIDEA OSSIS SPHENOIDALIS.

pterygomaxillary fossa FOSSA PTERYGOPALATINA.

fossa pterygopalatina [NA] A small pyramidal space bounded anteriorly by the superomedial portion of the posterior surface of the maxilla, posteriorly by the root of the pterygoid process and the adjacent part of the greater wing of the sphenoid bone, medially by the upper portion of the perpendicular plate of the palatine bone, and laterally communicating with the infratemporal fossa through the pterygomaxillary fissure. Inferiorly the anterior and posterior walls meet at the opening of the greater palatine canal. The space also communicates anteriorly with the orbit through the inferior orbital fissure, and medially with the nasal cavity through the sphenopalatine foramen. The major contents comprise the maxillary nerve and vessels and the pterygopalatine ganglion and their branches. Also called *pterygopalatine fossa, sphenomaxillary fossa* (outmoded), *pterygomaxillary fossa, sphenomaxillary fissure.*

pterygopalatine fossa FOSSA PTERYGOPALATINA.

radial fossa 1 FOSSA RADIALIS HUMERI. 2 An outmoded term for AREA NERVI FACIALIS.

radial fossa of humerus FOSSA RADIALIS HUMERI.

fossa radialis humeri [NA] A small, shallow hollow lateral to the coronoid fossa and above the capitulum of the condyle of humerus into which the rim of the head of the radius fits during full flexion of the elbow joint. Also called *radial fossa of humerus, radial depression, fovea for head of radius, lesser anterior fovea of humerus, radial fossa.*

radial fossa of ulna An outmoded term for INCISURA RADIALIS ULNAE.

retrocecal fossa RECESSUS RETROCAECALIS.

retrocolic fossa A variant of recessus retrocaecalis in which there is incomplete fusion of the ascending colon with the parietal peritoneum, allowing a peritoneal recess to extend between the ascending colon and the posterior abdominal wall. It may contain the vermiform appendix.

retroduodenal fossa RECESSUS RETRODUODENALIS.

retromandibular fossa The wedge-shaped space behind the ramus of the mandible and in front of and below the external acoustic meatus, occupied mainly by the parotid gland. An outmoded term. Also called *fossa retromandibularis* (outmoded).

fossa retromandibularis An outmoded term for RETROMANDIBULAR FOSSA.

retromolar fossa A smooth, shallow depression at the base of the anterior surface of the coronoid process of the mandible.

retroureteric fossa A hollow area posterior to the trigonum vesicae. An outmoded term.

rhomboid fossa FOSSA RHOMBOIDEA.

fossa rhomboidea The diamond-shaped floor of the fourth ventricle forming the roof of the medulla oblongata and caudal pons. Also called *rhomboid fossa.*

Rosenmüller's fossa RECESSUS PHARYNGEUS.

fossa sacci lacrimalis [NA] The vertical depression on the anteromedial wall of the orbit that contains the lacrimal sac and its fascia and is formed by the lacrimal sulcus of the lacrimal bone and the frontal process of the maxilla. It is limited posteriorly by the posterior lacrimal crest. Also called *lacrimal groove, fossa of lacrimal sac, lacrimal fossa.*

fossae sagittales dextrae hepatis The longitudinal grooves on the visceral surface of the right lobe of the liver that are formed by the fossa vesicae biliaris and sulcus venae cavae. An outmoded term. Also called *longitudinal fossae of right liver.*

fossae sagittales hepatis The fossa sagittalis sinistra hepatis and the fossae sagittales dextrae hepatis considered together.

fossa sagittalis sinistra hepatis A longitudinal groove on the visceral surface of the left lobe of the liver which is formed by fissura ligamenti teretis anteriorly and fissura ligamenti venosi posteriorly. An outmoded term. Also called *sagittal fissure of liver, fossa longitudinalis hepatis* (outmoded).

scaphoid fossa 1 An outmoded term for SCAPHA. 2 An outmoded term for FOSSA TRIANGULARIS AURICULAE. 3 An outmoded term for FOSSA SCAPHOIDEA OSSIS SPHENOIDALIS.

fossa scaphoidea **1** An outmoded term for SCAPHA. **2** An outmoded term for FOSSA TRIANGULARIS AURICULAE. **3** An outmoded term for FOSSA SCAPHOIDEA OSSIS SPHENOIDALIS.

fossa scaphoidea ossis sphenoidalis [NA] A small, oval depression formed by the splitting of the upper end of the posterior margin of the medial pterygoid plate, lying at the upper end of the pterygoid fossa and providing attachment for part of the tensor veli palatini muscle. Also called *scaphoid fossa of sphenoid bone, navicular fossa of Cruveilhier* (outmoded), *navicular fossa of sphenoid bone* (outmoded), *fossa of eustachian tube* (outmoded), *fossa scaphoidea* (outmoded), *scaphoid fossa* (outmoded), *Cruveilhier's fossa.*

scaphoid fossa of sphenoid bone FOSSA SCAPHOIDEA OSSIS SPHENOIDALIS.

fossa scarpae major An outmoded term for TRIGONUM FEMORALE.

sellar fossa FOSSA HYPOPHYSIALIS.

semilunar fossa of ulna INCISURA TROCHLEARIS ULNAE.

sigmoid fossa SULCUS SINUS TRANSVERSI.

sigmoid fossa of temporal bone SULCUS SINUS SIGMOIDEI OSSIS TEMPORALIS.

sigmoid fossa of ulna INCISURA TROCHLEARIS ULNAE.

sphenoidal fossa An outmoded term for APERTURA SINUS SPHENOIDALIS.

sphenomaxillary fossa An outmoded term for FOSSA PTERYGOPALATINA.

splenic fossa of omental sac RECESSUS SPLENICUS.

fossa subarcuata ossis temporalis [NA] An irregular pit just below the superior petrosal sinus and posterosuperior to the internal acoustic meatus, situated on the posterior surface of the petrous part of the temporal bone and containing a small vein and a fold of dura mater. In fetal life the pit is large, containing the cerebellar flocculus and extending under the anterior semicircular canal. Also called *subarcuate fossa of temporal bone, subarcuate hiatus.*

subarcuate fossa of temporal bone FOSSA SUBARCUATA OSSIS TEMPORALIS.

subauricular fossa A small surface depression just below the auricle of the ear. An outmoded term.

subcecal fossa RECESSUS ILEOCECALIS INFERIOR.

fossa subinguinalis The shallow depression that overlies the base of the femoral triangle just below the groin.

sublingual fossa FOVEA SUBLINGUALIS.

submandibular fossa FOVEA SUBMANDIBULARIS.

submaxillary fossa An outmoded term for FOVEA SUBMANDIBULARIS.

subnasal fossa A small hollow on the anterior surface of the maxilla just below the anterior nasal spine. An outmoded term.

suborbital fossa CANINE FOSSA.

subpyramidal fossa An insignificant depression below the pyramid and behind the fenestra cochleae on the posteromedial wall of the middle ear.

subscapular fossa FOSSA SUBSCAPULARIS.

fossa subscapularis [NA] The major, central portion of the concave costal surface of the scapula, providing origin for the subscapularis muscle and ridged for attachment of tendinous intersections. Also called *subscapular fossa, venter scapulae* (outmoded).

subsigmoid fossa An occasional peritoneal space between the root of the sigmoid mesocolon and the mesocolon of the descending colon when the latter is present.

subspinous fossa FOSSA INFRASPINATA.

superior articular fossa of atlas FACIES ARTICULARIS SUPERIOR ATLANTIS.

superior costal fossa FOVEA COSTALIS SUPERIOR.

superior digital fossa An outmoded term for FOSSA INGUINALIS LATERALIS.

superior duodenal fossa RECESSUS DUODENALIS SUPERIOR.

superior ileocecal fossa RECESSUS ILEOCECALIS SUPERIOR.

superior fossa of omental sac RECESSUS SUPERIOR OMENTALIS.

superior retroduodenal fossa A rare variant of recessus retroduodenalis in which the pocket is situated behind the duodenojejunal flexure.

supinator fossa A small triangular hollow distal to the radial notch of the ulna and between the diverging proximal ends of the interosseous margin. The anterior part of the hollow receives the radial tuberosity during pronation, while the posterior part and the supinator crest posterior to it provide origin to part of the supinator muscle.

supraclavicular fossa Either the fossa supraclavicularis minor or the fossa supraclavicularis major.

fossa supraclavicularis major [NA] TRIGONUM ONOCLAVICULARE.

fossa supraclavicularis minor [NA] A small triangular space above and behind the clavicle between the sternal and the clavicular heads of origin of the sternocleidomastoid muscle. The area is roofed over by external cervical fascia. Also called *lesser supraclavicular fossa, Zang space, fovea jugularis* (outmoded), *fossa jugularis* (outmoded), *jugular fossa, fonticulus gutturis* (outmoded).

supracondyloid fossa An insignificant groove between the adductor tubercle and the medial epicondyle of the femur, for part of the origin of medial head of gastrocnemius muscle.

supramastoid fossa FOVEOLA SUPRAMEATICA.

suprasphenoidal fossa FOSSA HYPOPHYSIALIS.

fossa supraspinata [NA] The hollow formed by the superior surface of the spine of scapula and the posterior surface of scapula above it, the medial two thirds of which provides origin for the supraspinatus muscle. It is about one fourth the area of the infraspinous fossa. Also called *supraspinous fossa, supraspinous region.*

supraspinous fossa FOSSA SUPRASPINATA.

suprasternal fossa SUPRASTERNAL SPACE.

supratonsillar fossa FOSSA SUPRATONSILLARIS.

fossa supratonsillaris **1** [NA] A space above the palatine tonsil, especially obvious in the adult when the tonsil is diminished in size. **2** A horizontal semilunar cleft in the upper part of the palatine tonsil. Also called *intratonsillar cleft* (outmoded), *intratonsillar fissure.* For defs. 1 and 2 also called *supratonsillar fossa, supratonsillar recess.*

supravesical fossa FOSSA SUPRAVESICALIS.

fossa supravesicalis [NA] The depression in the parietal peritoneum between the median umbilical fold formed by the urachus and the medial umbilical fold formed by the obliterated umbilical artery on the internal surface of the anterior abdominal wall. The fossa is particularly obvious when the urinary bladder is empty. Also called *supravesical fossa, fovea supravesicalis peritonaei, supravesical fovea, urachal fossa* (outmoded), *interligamentous fovea of peritoneum* (outmoded), *epigastric fossa.*

sylvian fossa **1** FOSSA LATERALIS CEREBRI. **2** SULCUS LATERALIS CEREBRI.

fossa of Sylvius **1** FOSSA LATERALIS CEREBRI. **2** SULCUS LATERALIS CEREBRI.

Tarin's fossa FOSSA INTERPEDUNCULARIS.

fossa Tarini FOSSA INTERPEDUNCULARIS.

temporal fossa **1** FOSSA TEMPORALIS. **2** An outmoded term for FOSSA CRANII MEDIA.

fossa temporalis [NA] The space on the lateral side of the cranium bounded superiorly and posteriorly by the temporal line, laterally by the zygomatic arch, and anteriorly by the temporal surface of the zygomatic bone, while inferiorly it is continuous with the infratemporal fossa deep to the zygomatic arch. It is occupied by the temporalis muscle, which is attached to its floor. Also called *temporal fossa.*

terminal fossa An outmoded term for FOSSA NAVICULARIS URETHRAE.

tibiofemoral fossa A space palpable on each side of the apex of the patella between the femoral and tibial condyles, especially when the knee is flexed.

tonsillar fossa FOSSA TONSILLARIS.

fossa tonsillaris [NA] A triangular depression lodging the palatine tonsil between the palatoglossal and palatopharyngeal arches. Also called *tonsillar fossa, tonsillar sinus, sinus tonsillaris* (outmoded), *amygdaloid fossa* (outmoded), *sinus interarcualis* (outmoded).

fossa transversalis hepatis An outmoded term for PORTA HEPATIS.

transverse costal fossa FOVEA COSTALIS PROCESSUS TRANS-VERSUS.

fossa of Treitz RECESSUS DUODENALIS INFERIOR.

triangular fossa of auricle FOSSA TRIANGULARIS AURICU-LAE.

fossa triangularis auriculae [NA] A small triangular depression lying between the two diverging crura of the anthelix at its upper end. Also called *triangular fossa of auricle, fossa scaphoidea* (outmoded), *scaphoid fossa* (outmoded).

trochanteric fossa FOSSA TROCHANTERICA.

fossa trochanterica [NA] A deep pit on the concave medial surface of the curved posterosuperior part of the greater trochanter of femur into which the obturator externus muscle is inserted. Also called *trochanteric fossa, digital fossa of femur.*

trochlear fossa FOVEA TROCHLEARIS.

fossa trochlearis An outmoded term for FOVEA TRO-CHLEARIS.

ulnar fossa FOSSA CORONOIDEA HUMERI.

fossa umbilicalis hepatis An outmoded term for FISSURA LIGAMENTI TERETIS.

ungual fossa A small slit on the posterosuperior surface of the petrous part of the temporal bone. It is located 1 cm behind the internal auditory meatus and leads to the aqueduct of the vestibule.

urachal fossa An outmoded term for FOSSA SUPRAVESICALIS.

Velpeau's fossa An outmoded term for FOSSA ISCHIOANALIS.

fossa venae cavae An outmoded term for SULCUS VENAE CAVAE.

fossa venae umbilicalis An outmoded term for FISSURA LI-GAMENTI TERETIS.

fossa venosa An outmoded term for RECESSUS PARADUO-DENALIS.

fossa vesicae biliaris [NA] A shallow oval impression for the gallbladder on the visceral surface of the right lobe of the liver. It extends from the inferior margin of the liver to the right end of the porta hepatis and lies on the right of the quadrate lobe. It is usually not covered by peritoneum. Also called *fossa of gallbladder, fossa vesicae felleae, notch of gallbladder, fossa cystidis felleae* (outmoded), *vallecula ovata* (outmoded), *incisure of gallbladder.*

fossa vesicae felleae FOSSA VESICAE BILIARIS.

vestibular fossa FOSSA VESTIBULI VAGINAE.

fossa of vestibule of vagina FOSSA VESTIBULI VAGINAE.

fossa vestibuli vaginae [NA] A portion of the vestibule that forms a shallow depression between the frenulum of the labia minora and the vaginal orfice. Also called *vestibular fossa, fossa of vestibule of vagina, fossa navicularis vestibuli vaginae* (outmoded).

Waldeyer's fossa 1 MESENTERICOPARIETAL FOSSA. **2** Duodenal fossa; either recessus duodenalis superior or recessus duodenalis inferior.

zygomatic fossa An outmoded term for FOSSA INFRATEM-PORALIS.

fossae Plural of FOSSA.

Fossaria [*foss(a)* + -ARIA] A genus of freshwater pulmonate snails in the family Lymnaeidae. The shell is usually small (10 mm or less in height) with a smooth columella and without distinct spiral sculpture.

Fossaria cubensis The first intermediate host of the schistosome *Heterobilharzia americana,* of raccoons, nutria, rabbits, and dogs in Louisiana, and of the amphistome fluke *Paramphistomum microbothrium (Cotylophoron cotylophorum)* and the liver fluke *Fasciola hepatica* of sheep and cattle in Puerto Rico and Louisiana.

Fossaria parva A first intermediate host of the North American giant intestinal fluke, *Fascioloides magna,* of cattle, horse, sheep, and deer.

Fossaria truncatula A first intermediate host of the sheep liver fluke *Fasciola hepatica.*

fossette A small pit or depression; fossula.

fossil [L *fossil(is)* (from *foss(us)*, past part. of *fodere* to dig, + *-ilis* -ILE) dug up] The remains, impression, or other evidence of a plant or an animal of a former geologic age, especially parts that are petrified or converted to stone.

fossorial [Med L *fossori(us)* (from *fossor* a digger) suitable for digging + -AL] Adapted for burrowing or digging: said of an animal.

fossula [L (dim. of *fossa* a ditch, trench), a small ditch or trench] A small pit or depression.

fossula of cochlear window FOSSULA FENESTRAE COCH-LEAE.

fossula fenestrae cochleae [NA] The deep hollow posteroinferior to the promontory at the bottom of which is the fenestra cochleae in the medial wall of the middle ear. Also called *fossula of cochlear window, fossula of round window* (outmoded), *fossula rotunda* (outmoded), *pelvis rotunda* (outmoded).

fossula fenestrae vestibuli [NA] A depression situated posterosuperior to the promontory at the bottom of which is the fenestra vestibuli in the medial wall of the middle ear. Also called *fossula of vestibular window, fossula of oval window* (outmoded), *pelvis ovalis* (outmoded).

inferior costal fossa FOVEA COSTALIS INFERIOR.

fossula of oval window An outmoded term for FOSSULA FENESTRAE VESTIBULI.

fossula petrosa [NA] A small notch located on the inferior surface of the petrous portion of the temporal bone, located between the jugular fossa and the external orifice of the carotid canal. It lodges the inferior (or petrous) ganglion of the glossopharyngeal nerve, and nearby is located the canaliculus tympanicus through which courses the tympanic branch of the glossopharyngeal nerve on its way to the middle ear. Also called *petrous fossula, vallecula for petrosal ganglion, receptaculum ganglii petrosi, petrosal fossula, petrosal fossa, fossula of petrous ganglion, fossa for petrosal ganglion* (outmoded).

petrosal fossula FOSSULA PETROSA.

petrous fossula FOSSULA PETROSA.

fossula of petrous ganglion FOSSULA PETROSA.

fossula post fenestram An inconstant evagination of the connective tissue of the perilymphatic space into a hollow in the lateral wall of the internal ear immediately behind the vestibular window and between the latter and the nonampullated end of the lateral semicircular canal.

fossula rotunda An outmoded term for FOSSULA FENESTRAE COCHLEAE.

fossula of round window An outmoded term for FOSSULA FENESTRAE COCHLEAE.

superior costal fossula FOVEA COSTALIS SUPERIOR.

fossulae tonsillares tonsillae palatinae [NA] The pitlike openings of the deep, tubular tonsillar crypts on the medial surface of the palatine tonsil. Also called *tonsillar fossulae of palatine tonsil, foramina of palatine tonsil, crypts of palatine tonsil.*

fossulae tonsillares tonsillae pharyngeae FOSSULAE TONSILLARES TONSILLAE PHARYNGEALIS.

fossulae tonsillares tonsillae pharyngealis [NA] The surface openings of the cleftlike invaginations of diffuse lymphoid tissue in the pharyngeal tonsil. Also called *tonsillar fossulae of pharyngeal tonsil, fossulae tonsillares tonsillae pharyngeae, crypts of pharyngeal tonsil, sulci of pharyngeal tonsil.*

tonsillar fossulae of palatine tonsil FOSSULAE TONSILLARES TONSILLAE PALATINAE.

tonsillar fossulae of pharyngeal tonsil FOSSULAE TONSILLARES TONSILLAE PHARYNGEALIS.

fossula of vestibular window FOSSULA FENESTRAE VESTIBULI.

fossulae Plural of FOSSULA.

fossulate Having a small fossa or groove.

Foster Kennedy [Robert *Foster Kennedy*, U.S. neurologist, 1884–1952] See under SYNDROME.

Fothergill [John *Fothergill*, English physician, 1712–1780] **1** Fothergill's disease, Fothergill's neuralgia. See under TRIGEMINAL NEURALGIA. **2** Fothergill sore throat. See under THROAT.

Fothergill [William Edward *Fothergill*, English gynecologist, 1865–1926] **1** See under OPERATION. **2** Manchester-Fothergill operation, Fothergill-Donald operation. See under MANCHESTER OPERATION.

Fouchet [André *Fouchet*, French chemist and physician, born 1894] See under REAGENT.

foudroyant FULMINANT.

foulage [French (from *foul(er)* to press, tread upon, from L *fullo* a fuller, + *-age* -AGE), a pressing, treading upon] A form of massage using kneading motions to relax muscles that are in varying degrees of spasm.

foul brood A contagious disease of honey bees caused by *Bacillus alvei,* and a cause of serious economic and agricultural loss resulting from destruction of apiary colonies.

fouling In forensic medicine, the solid, black, circular zone of deposited soot surrounding the edges of skin or clothing caused by the passage of a projectile, as by the near contact or penetration of a bullet.

foundation [French *fondation* (from L *fundatus*, past part. of *fundare* to found, lay the bottom of) an act of founding or starting to build] The combination of tooth substance and restorative material such as cement, gold, or amalgam, made when the tooth substance itself is insufficient to make a satisfactory support for a full crown.

denture foundation STRESS-BEARING AREA.

medical foundation An organization of physicians, in the United States primarily, usually sponsored by a local medical society which is involved in certain activities such as peer review and sponsorship or operation of prepaid health care plans. Also called *foundation for medical care.*

foundation for medical care MEDICAL FOUNDATION.

founder [Middle English *foundren* to fall to the ground, from Old French *fondrer* to sink, from *fond* bottom, from L *fundus* bottom] LAMINITIS.

foundling [Middle English *foundeling*, from *founden*, past part. of *finden* to find + Middle and Old English *-ling*, suffix denoting small, young] An unidentified child, usually an infant, who has been found following abandonment by parents or guardians.

fourchette [French (dim. of *fourche* pitchfork, from L *furca*

fork), fork, fork-shaped object] FRENULUM LABIORUM PUDENDI.

Fourier [Jean Baptiste Joseph *Fourier*, French mathematician, 1768–1830] See under ANALYSIS.

Fourneau 190 [after Ernest François Auguste *Fourneau*, French chemist, 1872–1949] ACETARSOL.

Fourneau 309 [after E. F. A. *Fourneau*] SURAMIN.

Fourneau 710 [after E. F. A. *Fourneau*] $C_{17}H_{25}N_3O$. A quinoline antimalarial drug similar to primaquine and usually used in combination with other agents. It is reported to be very toxic to the central nervous system.

Fourneau 933 [after E. F. A. *Fourneau*] PIPEROXAN HYDROCHLORIDE.

Fournier [Jean Alfred *Fournier*, French dermatologist, 1832–1914] **1** Fournier's gangrene. See under FOURNIER'S DISEASE. **2** Fournier's exercises. See under EXERCISE. **3** See under TEST, SIGN, TREATMENT. **4** Fournier sign. See under SABER SHIN.

fovea

fovea [L (akin to *biber* beaver, possibly to *fodere* to dig), a pit, esp. for catching game] A small fossa, pit, or depression.

anterior supratrochlear fovea FOSSA CORONOIDEA HUMERI.

fovea articularis capitis radii [NA] A shallow, circular depression on the proximal end of the head of the radius for articulation with the capitulum of the humerus. Also called *fossa of little head of radius* (outmoded), *fovea of little head of radius, foveola radialis.*

fovea articularis inferior atlantis FACIES ARTICULARIS INFERIOR ATLANTIS.

fovea articularis superior atlantis FACIES ARTICULARIS SUPERIOR ATLANTIS.

articular foveae for rib cartilages INCISURAE COSTALES STERNI.

articular fovea of temporal bone An outmoded term for FOSSA MANDIBULARIS.

calcaneal fovea An outmoded term for SULCUS CALCANEI.

fovea capitis ossis femoris [NA] A small pit just posteroinferior to the middle of the head of the femur, not covered by cartilage and providing attachment for the ligament of head of femur. Also called *fovea of head of femur, fossa capitis femoris* (outmoded), *fossa of head of femur.*

fovea cardiaca 1 An outmoded term for FOSSA EPIGASTRICA. **2** INCISURA CARDIACA PULMONIS SINISTRI.

caudal fovea FOVEA INFERIOR.

fovea centralis FOVEA CENTRALIS RETINAE.

fovea centralis retinae [NA] The conical central depression in the macula retinae where the retina is very thin so that rays of light have free passage to the layer of photoreceptors, mostly cones. This is the area of most distinct vision to which the visual axis is directed. Also called *central fovea of retina, Soemmering's foramen* (outmoded), *fovea centralis.*

central fovea of retina FOVEA CENTRALIS RETINAE.

fovea of condyloid process FOVEA PTERYGOIDEA MANDIBULAE.

fovea of coronoid process FOSSA CORONOIDEA HUMERI.

fovea costalis inferior [NA] A hollowed articular facet near the inferior margin of the vertebral body and anterior to the vertebral notch of most thoracic vertebrae for articulation with the head of a rib. Also called *inferior costal fovea, inferior costal* *fossa, inferior costal fossula, inferior costal pit, inferior demifacet for head of rib, costal pit.*

fovea costalis processus transversus   [NA] A small hollow pit on the anterolateral surface of the transverse processes of most thoracic vertebrae for articulation with the tubercle of a rib to form a costotransverse joint. Also called *costal pit of transverse process, transverse costal fovea, transverse costal fossa, costal facet of transverse process, fovea costalis transversalis* (outmoded), *facet for tubercle of rib.*

fovea costalis superior   [NA] A hollowed articular facet, usually larger than the inferior fovea, located near the superior margin of the vertebral body anterior to the base of the pedicle of most thoracic vertebrae for articulation with the head of a rib. Also called *superior costal fovea, superior costal facet of vertebra, superior costal fossa, superior costal fossula, superior demifacet for head of rib.*

fovea costalis transversalis   An outmoded term for FOVEA COSTALIS PROCESSUS TRANSVERSUS.

costal foveae of sternum   INCISURAE COSTALES STERNI.

cranial fovea   FOVEA SUPERIOR.

crural fovea   FEMORAL FOSSA.

dental fovea of atlas   FOVEA DENTIS ATLANTIS.

fovea dentis atlantis   [NA] A rounded, concave facet on the posterior surface of the anterior arch of the atlas for articulation with the dens of the axis in the median atlantoaxial joint. Also called *dental fovea of atlas, fovea of tooth of atlas* (outmoded), *circular articular facet of atlas, articular fossa for odontoid process of axis, articular facet of anterior arch of atlas, middle sinus of atlas* (outmoded), *articular sinus of atlas* (outmoded), *anterior sinus of atlas* (outmoded).

digastric fovea   FOSSA DIGASTRICA.

fovea elliptica   RECESSUS ELLIPTICUS VESTIBULI.

external inguinal fovea   FOSSA INGUINALIS LATERALIS.

femoral fovea   FEMORAL FOSSA.

fovea of fourth ventricle   FOVEA INFERIOR.

foveae of fourth ventricle   The fovea inferior and the fovea superior.

glandular foveae of Luschka   An outmoded term for FOVEOLAE GRANULARES.

greater anterior fovea of humerus   FOSSA CORONOIDEA HUMERI.

fovea of head of femur   FOVEA CAPITIS OSSIS FEMORIS.

fovea for head of radius   FOSSA RADIALIS HUMERI.

fovea hemielliptica   An outmoded term for RECESSUS ELLIPTICUS VESTIBULI.

fovea hemispherica   An outmoded term for RECESSUS SPHERICUS VESTIBULI.

fovea inferior   A small indentation of the sulcus limitans in the floor of the fourth ventricle at the caudal end of the striae medullares. Also called *inferior fovea of floor of fourth ventricle, fovea of fourth ventricle, caudal fovea.*

inferior articular fovea of atlas   FACIES ARTICULARIS INFERIOR ATLANTIS.

inferior costal fovea   FOVEA COSTALIS INFERIOR.

inferior fovea of floor of fourth ventricle   FOVEA INFERIOR.

fovea inguinalis lateralis   FOSSA INGUINALIS LATERALIS.

fovea inguinalis medialis   FOSSA INGUINALIS MEDIALIS.

interligamentous fovea of peritoneum   An outmoded term for FOSSA SUPRAVESICALIS.

internal inguinal fovea   FOSSA INGUINALIS MEDIALIS.

fovea jugularis   1 An outmoded term for FOSSA JUGULARIS OSSIS TEMPORALIS.   2 An outmoded term for FOSSA SUPRACLAVICULARIS MINOR.

lateral inguinal fovea   FOSSA INGUINALIS LATERALIS.

lateral malleolar fovea of fibula   FACIES ARTICULARIS MALLEOLI FIBULAE.

fovea of lateral malleolus   FACIES ARTICULARIS MALLEOLI FIBULAE.

lesser anterior fovea of humerus   FOSSA RADIALIS HUMERI.

fovea of little head of radius   FOVEA ARTICULARIS CAPITIS RADII.

medial inguinal fovea   FOSSA INGUINALIS MEDIALIS.

middle inguinal fovea   FOSSA INGUINALIS MEDIALIS.

fovea of Morgagni   FOSSA NAVICULARIS URETHRAE.

fovea nuchae   A depression in the midline of the back of the neck just below the external occipital protuberance.

fovea oblonga cartilaginis arytenoideae   [NA] An oblong depression below the lower part of the arcuate crest on the anterolateral surface of the arytenoid cartilage that provides attachment for the vocalis and lateral cricoarytenoid muscles. Also called *oblong fovea of arytenoid cartilage, oblong pit of arytenoid cartilage.*

oblong fovea of arytenoid cartilage   FOVEA OBLONGA CARTILAGINIS ARYTENOIDEAE.

foveae palati   Two pits situated near the junction of hard and soft palates on either side of the midline.

fovea pharyngis   An outmoded term for RECESSUS PHARYNGEUS.

fovea of the pharynx   An outmoded term for RECESSUS PHARYNGEUS.

pterygoid fovea   FOVEA PTERYGOIDEA MANDIBULAE.

fovea pterygoidea mandibulae   [NA] The rough depression on the anteromedial aspect of the neck of the condylar process of the mandible for the attachment of lateral pterygoid muscle. Also called *pterygoid fovea, fovea pterygoidea processus condyloidei, fovea of condyloid process, pterygoid depression, pterygoid pit, pterygoid fossa of inferior maxillary bone* (outmoded), *fossa of lateral pterygoid muscle.*

fovea pterygoidea processus condyloidei   FOVEA PTERYGOIDEA MANDIBULAE.

fovea spherica   RECESSUS SPHERICUS VESTIBULI.

sublingual fovea   FOVEA SUBLINGUALIS.

fovea sublingualis   [NA] A smooth triangular depression above the anterior end of the mylohyoid line, posterolateral to the mental spine of the mandible and lodging the sublingual salivary gland. Also called *sublingual fossa, sublingual fovea, mylohyoid fossa of mandible* (outmoded).

submandibular fovea   FOVEA SUBMANDIBULARIS.

fovea submandibularis   [NA] An elongated shallow depression below the middle portion of the mylohyoid line and muscle on the inner surface of the body of the mandible which lodges the submandibular salivary gland and some submandibular lymph nodes. Also called *submandibular fossa, submandibular fovea, fovea submaxillaris* (outmoded), *submaxillary fossa* (outmoded).

fovea submaxillaris   An outmoded term for FOVEA SUBMANDIBULARIS.

fovea superior   A small indentation of the sulcus limitans in the fourth ventricle at the rostral end of the striae medullares. Also called *superior fovea of sulcus limitans, cranial fovea.*

superior costal fovea   FOVEA COSTALIS SUPERIOR.

superior fovea of sulcus limitans   FOVEA SUPERIOR.

supratrochlear fovea of humerus   FOSSA CORONOIDEA HUMERI.

supravesical fovea   FOSSA SUPRAVESICALIS.

fovea supravesicalis peritonaei   FOSSA SUPRAVESICALIS.

fovea of talus   SULCUS TALI.

fovea of tooth of atlas   An outmoded term for FOVEA DENTIS ATLANTIS.

transverse costal fovea   FOVEA COSTALIS PROCESSUS TRANSVERSUS.

fovea triangularis of arytenoid   FOVEA TRIANGULARIS CARTILAGINIS ARYTENOIDEAE.

fovea triangularis cartilaginis arytenoideae [NA] A triangular depression above the lower part of the arcuate crest on the anterolateral surface of the arytenoid cartilage that provides attachment for the vestibular ligament and lodges some mucous glands. Also called *triangular pit of arytenoid cartilage, triangular foveola, fovea triangularis of arytenoid.*

fovea trigemini A small depression in the rostral floor of the fourth ventricle lying anterolateral to the facial colliculus and overlying the motor and main sensory trigeminal nuclei.

trochlear fovea FOVEA TROCHLEARIS.

fovea trochlearis [NA] A small, shallow depression at the anteromedial angle of the roof of the orbital cavity just behind the medial end of the supraorbital margin for the attachment of the fibrocartilaginous trochlea of the superior oblique muscle. It is often occupied by the trochlear spine. Also called *trochlear fovea, trochlear fossa, fossa trochlearis* (outmoded).

---

foveate Having foveae; pitted.

foveation Pitting, as of the skin.

foveola [New L (dim. of FOVEA), a very small pit] (*plural* foveolae) **1** A small pit, fossa, or depression. **2** ALVEOLUS.

foveola coccygea [NA] A shallow dimple often present in the skin over the coccyx. It marks the point at which the embryonic neural tube made a caudal contact with the ectoderm. The dimple is created by a bundle of white fibrous tissue that extends from the tip of the last coccygeal vertebra to the skin. Also called *coccygeal foveola, postanal dimple, postanal pit.*

coccygeal foveola FOVEOLA COCCYGEA.

foveolae gastricae [NA] Slitlike furrows on the surface of the mucous membrane of the stomach into the bottoms of which the gastric glands open. Because of their large number, the mucosa has a honeycomb appearance. Also called *gastric pits, gastric foveolae of Frey, gastric pits of Frey.*

gastric foveolae of Frey FOVEOLAE GASTRICAE.

granular foveolae FOVEOLAE GRANULARES.

foveolae granulares [NA] A number of irregular depressions that are on the inner surface of the parietal bones on each side of the sagittal sulcus and are occupied by the arachnoid granulations. They increase in size and number with advancing age. Also called *granular foveolae, foveolae granulares pacchioni, pacchionian depressions, meningeal impression, impressio meningealis, glandular foveae of Luschka* (outmoded), *fossae of Pacchioni.*

foveolae granulares pacchioni An outmoded term for FOVEOLAE GRANULARES.

foveola palatina A small pit in the mucous membrane for the openings of a few mucous glands at the junction of the hard and soft palate. An outmoded term.

foveolae papillae An outmoded term for FORAMINA PAPILLARIA RENIS.

foveola radialis An outmoded term for FOVEA ARTICULARIS CAPITIS RADII.

foveola suprameatalis FOVEOLA SUPRAMEATICA.

foveola suprameatica [NA] A small pit that marks the center of the suprameatal triangle and is situated below the supramastoid crest and behind the suprameatal spine at the junction of the superior and posterior margins of the external acoustic meatus. Also called *foveola suprameatalis, mastoid fossa of temporal bone, postauditory fossa, supramastoid fossa.*

triangular foveola FOVEA TRIANGULARIS CARTILAGINIS ARYTENOIDEAE.

foveolae Plural of FOVEOLA.

foveolar Pertaining to a foveola.

foveolate Displaying foveolae.

Foville [Achille-Louis *Foville*, French physician, 1799–1878] **1** Fasciculus of Foville. See under STRIA TERMINALIS. **2** Foville superior syndrome, Foville's median syndrome. See under FOVILLE'S PEDUNCULAR SYNDROME. **3** Foville's inferior syndrome. See under FOVILLE SYNDROME.

Fowler [George Ryerson *Fowler*, U.S. surgeon, 1848–1906] See under INCISION, POSITION.

Fowler [Thomas *Fowler*, English physician, 1736–1801] Fowler solution. See under POTASSIUM ARSENITE SOLUTION.

fowlpox AVIAN POX.

Fox [George Henry *Fox*, U.S. dermatologist, 1846–1937] Fox-Fordyce disease. See under DISEASE.

Fox [Lewis *Fox*, U.S. periodontist, born 1903] **1** Fox scissors. See under SCISSORS. **2** Goldman-Fox knife. See under KNIFE.

foxfire [Middle English, from *fox* + *fire*] A phosphorescent glow emitted by moist, rotting wood and caused by cellulose-degrading fungal hyphae of *Omphalotus olearius.*

foxglove [Old English *foxes* fox's + *glōfa* glove] Any of various plants of the genus *Digitalis.*

Austrian foxglove DIGITALIS LANTANA LEAF.

purple foxglove A plant of the species *Digitalis purpurea.* See also DIGITALIS.

woolly foxglove DIGITALIS LANTANA LEAF.

FP Symbol for properdin.

f.p. **1** freezing point. **2** *fiat potio* (L, let a potion be made).

f. pil. *fiant pilulae* (L, let pills be made).

FPS Symbol for the foot-pound-second system of units.

fPt fasting patient.

FR **1** flocculation reaction. **2** fixed ratio.

F and R force and rhythm (of the arterial pulse).

Fr **1** Symbol for the element, francium. **2** Symbol for the obsolete unit, franklin.

fract. dos. *fracta dosi* (L, in divided doses).

fraction [L *fractio* (from L *fractus,* past part. of *frangere* to break, shatter) a breaking] A portion of a mixture obtained by a separation technique, as by centrifugation, distillation, or precipitation, and representing a discrete constituent of the mixture.

absorbed fraction The fraction of energy, radiated by an embedded radionuclide, that is absorbed within a specified volume of a living body or other absorbing mass.

blood plasma fraction HUMAN PLASMA PROTEIN FRACTION.

dried human plasma protein fraction Plasma protein fraction from which all water has been removed by dehydration or lyophilization. Also called *dried human plasma, blood-plasma powder.*

ejection fraction An index of the heart pumping function. It equals the proportion of total blood volume that is expelled from the heart with each heartbeat.

Fechner fraction A measure of contrast sensitivity of the eye, dB/B, where B is the brightness of a large field of view and dB the difference of brightness which is just distinguishable on a small area within that field.

filtration fraction The ratio of glomerular filtration rate to effective renal plasma flow. This represents the amount of effective renal plasma flow filtered at the glomerulus. In disease, the filtration fraction reflects relative change in effective renal plasma flow and glomerular filtration rate, being increased when the afferent glomerular arterioles are relatively constricted, as in hypertension and congestive heart failure, or decreased in glomerular diseases, as in acute glomerulonephritis and the nephrotic syndrome.

human plasma protein fraction Plasma pooled from several donors to which certain preservatives and salts are added so that it is isotonic and iso-oncotic with normal human plasma. The product is heat-treated at 60°C for 10 hours to eliminate viable hepatitis virus particles. Also called *blood plasma fraction, plasma fraction, pooled plasma.*

microsome fraction   A membrane-rich fraction obtained as the components of a tissue homogenate are separated with an ultracentrifuge. Most of the membranes are formed from Golgi complexes or from endoplasmic reticulum.

mole fraction   The amount of substance of a component (x) divided by the amount of substance of the mixture (all components of the system), expressed in mol/mol. Also called *substance fraction.* Abbreviation: molfr. Symbol: x_x

packing fraction   The mass defect per nucleon in the atom of a specified nuclide. The mass defect is the difference between the atomic weight (in amu) and the sum of the proton and neutron numbers.

plasma fraction   HUMAN PLASMA PROTEIN FRACTION.

plasma protein fraction   A sterile solution of selected plasma proteins obtained from the pooled plasma of adult blood donors. The preparation contains 4.5 to 5.5 g of protein per 100 ml, with albumin representing 83 to 90 percent of the protein; the rest is largely alpha and beta globulins. It is used for its oncotic properties, much the same as albumin solutions.

recombination fraction   RECOMBINATION FREQUENCY.

renal fraction of cardiac output   The ratio of renal blood flow to cardiac output, which in resting man is approximately 0.2. In congestive heart failure, blood flow is shunted away from the kidneys with a decrease in the renal fraction of cardiac output.

sampling fraction   SAMPLING RATIO.

soluble fraction   **1** The fraction that is soluble, as opposed to precipitated, in any fractionation.   **2** The cell cytoplasm in distinction from the organelles, such as mitochondria, that are suspended in it.

substance fraction   MOLE FRACTION.

volume fraction   Of a component of a system, the volume of the component divided by the volume of the system, expressed in l/l or m³/m³.

fractional   Constituting a fraction; partial.

fractionate   **1** To separate constituent materials into discrete portions or categories.   **2** To divide a quantity of radiation or other therapeutic intervention so as to administer small portions at timed intervals.

fractionation [FRACTION + -ATION]   **1** Separation of a mixture according to differences among the constituents in regard to some property, such as boiling point or solubility.   **2** In radiation therapy, the use of small doses of radiation given at intervals. Also called *dose fractionation, fractionated treatment, fractionated radiation, fractionation radiation.*

cell fractionation   A method used to separate various cellular components. The tissue or cells are homogenized and the homogenate is centrifuged to separate the particles on the basis of density and/or sedimentation velocity.

Cohn fractionation   The separation of plasma proteins by treatment of plasma with cold mixtures of water and ethanol in varying proportions. By this technique major plasma proteins are obtained in the following fractions: fibrinogen in fraction I, beta and gamma globulins in fractions II and III, alpha globulin in fraction IV, and albumen in fraction V. Also called *cold ethanol fractionation.*

cold ethanol fractionation   COHN FRACTIONATION.

dose fractionation   FRACTIONATION.

fractography   An examination, by light or electron microscopy, of fractured surfaces such as cells and membranes.

fracture

fracture [L *fractura* (from *fract(us)*, past part. of *frangere* to break, shatter + *-ura* -URE) a breaking]   **1** A break in the continuity of a structure such as bone, cartilage, or metal.   **2** A discontinuity in the mechanical strength of a structure.   **3** To cause to have a break in continuity.

abduction fracture   A fracture in which the distal part is displaced away from the midline.

adduction fracture   A fracture in which the distal part is displaced towards the midline.

agenetic fracture   A fracture that occurs spontaneously due to a defect in osteogenesis. A seldom used term.

anatomic neck fracture   A break through the collum anatomicum humeri.

apophyseal fracture   The avulsion of a small fragment of an apophysis or epiphyseal center. It is most often seen in growing children.

articular fracture   INTRA-ARTICULAR FRACTURE.

atrophic fracture   A fracture of an atrophic bone, occurring spontaneously or as a result of minimal trauma.

avulsion fracture   A bone fracture that is caused by the pulling away of a tendon, muscle, ligament, or joint capsule from the bone while taking with it a fragment of the bone.

Barton's fracture   A fracture-dislocation of the radius at the wrist joint.

basal skull fracture   A fracture, usually linear, through the bony floor of the skull. It may be clinically manifested by rhinorrhea, collection of blood on the deep side of the tympanic membrane, otorrhea, or the Battle sign.

basocervical fracture   A basal neck fracture of the femur at the junction with the trochanteric line.

bending fracture   GREENSTICK FRACTURE.

Bennett's fracture   A fracture-dislocation of the base of the first metacarpal bone that involves the carpo-metacarpal joint.

bent fracture   GREENSTICK FRACTURE.

birth fracture   Fracture of a fetal bone which occurs during the process of delivery.

blow-out fracture   A fracture through the floor of the orbit caused by a blow on the eye with a sudden increase in pressure of the orbital contents. Part of the orbital contents may become trapped in the fracture site, particularly the inferior rectus or inferior oblique muscles, resulting in diplopia on upward gaze.

boxers' fracture   A fracture through the neck of a metacarpal bone. It is usually seen on the first or fifth metacarpal and is marked by anterior displacement.

bucket-handle fracture   A splitting of the meniscus of the knee into a thin circumferential section and a larger remaining section, resembling a bucket with a handle.

bumper fracture   A comminuted, often bilateral, fracture of the upper tibia and fibula, caused by a motor vehicle striking a pedestrian, with the point of impact being immediately below the knee of the pedestrian. Also called *fender fracture.*

bursting fracture   An expansile comminuted fracture that usually occurs in the distal phalanx. Also called *tuft fracture.*

butterfly fracture   A comminuted fracture characterized by one large central fragment and two smaller adjacent fragments.

buttonhole fracture   A punched out, circular fracture caused by a gunshot wound.

capillary fracture   An undisplaced hairline fracture of bone as seen on a roentgenogram.

cementum fracture   The breaking away of cementum from the dentin of the root.

chauffeurs' fracture   REVERSE COLLES FRACTURE.

chip fracture   The separation of a small sheared-off fragment of bone adjacent to a joint space.

chisel fracture   The displacement of a fragment of the radial head.

cleavage fracture   A fracture of the lower end of the humerus that involves the cartilage and bone of the capitulum.

closed fracture   A fracture in which the overlying soft tissue and skin remain intact. Also called *subcutaneous fracture*.

closed skull fracture   Fracture of the skull with intact scalp.

Colles fracture   A fracture in which the lower end of the radius is displaced backwards and upwards to produce the silver-fork deformity. Avulsion of the ulnar styloid process usually takes place as well. Also called *silver-fork fracture*.

comminuted fracture   A fracture that results in numerous fragments.

comminuted skull fracture   Multiple fractures of the skull resulting in fragmentation of the bone.

complete fracture   A fracture in which the bone is completely broken across.

complicated fracture   A fracture accompanied by adjacent tissue or organ damage.

compound fracture   A fracture in continuity with the external environment through divided skin or mucous membrane. Also called *open fracture*.

compound skull fracture   Fracture of the skull accompanied by laceration of the overlying scalp. Also called *open skull fracture*.

compression fracture   A fracture of the calcaneus or a vertebral body that is usually produced by vertical forces associated with a fall from a height.

condylar fracture   A fracture through a condyle, usually that at the lower end of the humerus or femur.

congenital fracture   INTRAUTERINE FRACTURE.

contrecoup fracture   A linear fracture of the skull occurring on the side of the head opposite the direct blow.

cortical fracture   LINEAR FRACTURE.

cough fracture   A fracture, usually of the middle ribs, produced by excessive coughing.

craniofacial dysjunction fracture   LeFort III FRACTURE.

crush fracture   A fracture, usually produced by a blunt force, that results in multiple, depressed fragments.

deferred fracture   A fracture in the horse, usually of an upper limb bone, in which the fractured ends do not separate until some time after the traumatic incident.

dentate fracture   A fracture in which the opposing fragment surfaces are serrated and fit into each other.

depressed fracture   DEPRESSED SKULL FRACTURE.

depressed skull fracture   Fracture of the skull with inward displacement of fragments of bone. Also called *derby hat fracture, ping-pong fracture, depressed fracture*.

derby hat fracture   DEPRESSED SKULL FRACTURE.

diacondylar fracture   TRANSCONDYLAR FRACTURE.

diastatic skull fracture   Fracture of the skull resulting in separation of bone fragments.

direct fracture   A fracture that occurs at the point of injury.

dislocation fracture   See under FRACTURE-DISLOCATION.

displaced fracture   A fracture in which the fragments are separated and are not in alignment.

double fracture   A fracture at two points on the same bone. Also called *segmental fracture*.

Dupuytren's fracture   A fracture of the lower fibula complicated by a dislocation of the ankle joint.

Duverney's fracture   A fracture of the ilium that is directed from the anterior superior iliac spine.

fracture en coin   A v-shaped fracture.

endocrine fracture   A pathologic fracture through weakened bone produced by an endocrine disorder such as hyperparathyroidism or thyrotoxicosis.

fracture en rave   A transverse fracture of, but not across, a cortex surface.

epiphyseal fracture   The traumatic separation of the epiphyseal plate of a long bone, with or without a fracture involving the adjacent bone.

expressed skull fracture   Fracture of the skull with brain tissue squeezed out through the fracture site.

extracapsular fracture   A fracture in a bone that is adjacent to a joint but outside the attachment of the capsule. It is usually seen in the humerus or femur.

fatigue fracture   A fracture that occurs usually in the short bones of the foot when exposed to repeated or undue loading, such as in marching.

fender fracture   BUMPER FRACTURE.

fissure fracture   LINEAR FRACTURE.

freeze fracture   A procedure for preparing materials for observation with an electron microscope, in which materials are rapidly frozen and then fractured. The fracture of the ice occurs along natural structures, such as the membranes of cellular organelles, so that their structure can be revealed by electron microscopy of the fractured surface.

Galeazzi's fracture   A fracture of the lower end of the radius accompanied by dislocation of the ulna at the wrist.

Gosselin's fracture   A v-shaped fracture of the lower end of the tibia that involves the ankle joint.

greenstick fracture   An incomplete fracture, usually seen in children, in which only the convex side of the cortex is broken with bending of the bone. Also called *willow fracture, hickory-stick fracture, bending fracture, bent fracture*.

Guérin's fracture   LeFort I FRACTURE.

gutter fracture   A fracture of the skull characterized by a groove or channel caused by the passage of a high speed missile.

hairline fracture   A small fracture of bone without displacement. Also called *microfracture*.

hangman's fracture   A fracture through the base of the odontoid peg or through the pedicles of the second cervical vertebra, with or without the dislocation of the second upon the third cervical vertebra.

heat fractures   Artifactual fractures of the long bones and skull, found in burned bodies, occurring postmortem from heat. The fracture lines tend to be curved, and in the skull, they often radiate laterally from a common point located near the vertex.

hickory-stick fracture   GREENSTICK FRACTURE.

horizontal maxillary fracture   LeFort I FRACTURE.

idiopathic fracture   A pathologic break in a weakened bone without a known cause.

impacted fracture   A fracture in which the fragments are driven into each other with a resulting reestablishment of some stability.

incomplete fracture   A break or rupture of bone that does not involved the total bone segment or length. Also called *infracture, infraction*.

indirect fracture   A fracture, usually of the skull, that occurs at a site away from the traumatic force.

inflammatory fracture   A pathologic fracture of a bone that occurs through a lesion caused by osteitis or osteomyelitis.

intertrochanteric fracture   A fracture between the two trochanters of the upper femur.

intra-articular fracture   A fracture through a joint surface. Also called *articular fracture, intracapsular fracture*.

intracapsular fracture   INTRA-ARTICULAR FRACTURE.

intraperiosteal fracture   A fracture through the cortex that does not rupture the periosteum.

intrauterine fracture   A fracture of a fetal bone when the fetus is within the uterus, usually traumatic in origin. Also called *congenital fracture*.

joint fracture   A fracture within the joint capsule.

lacunar fracture of the skull   A fracture in which a fragment of a skull bone, circular oval, or elongated, is depressed below the level of the normal part of the skull bone.

lead pipe fracture   A crack, seen in young bones, in one cortex with bulging of the opposite cortex.

LeFort fracture   A fracture of the skull involving any or all of the maxillary, nasal, zygomatic, or orbital bones. Also called *midfacial fracture*.

LeFort I fracture   A midfacial fracture involving the maxilla. Also called *horizontal maxillary fracture, transverse maxillary fracture, Guérin's fracture*.

LeFort II fracture   A midfacial fracture in which the main fracture lines meet at the nasion. Also called *pyramidal fracture*.

LeFort III fracture   A fracture in which the facial bones are separated from the cranium. Also called *craniofacial dysjunction fracture, transverse facial fracture*.

linear fracture   A fracture extending down along the length of the bone. Also called *fissure fracture, cortical fracture*.

linear skull fracture   A fracture of the skull that is a single fissure or line.

Lisfranc's fracture   Multiple fractures across the midtarsal bones and the bases of the metatarsal bones.

longitudinal fracture   A fracture in the long axis of a long bone.

loose fracture   A fracture in which the bone ends are freely mobile and not in contact.

malar fracture   Fracture of the lateral part of the central third of the facial skeleton caused by a direct blow to the malar bone resulting usually in flattening of the cheek, epistaxis, gross swelling and bruising of the lower eyelid and, often, double vision.

mallet fracture   The avulsion of a dorsal fragment of the epiphysis of the terminal phalanx of the finger.

mandibular fracture   Fracture of the lower jaw.

march fracture   STRESS FRACTURE.

midfacial fracture   LeFort FRACTURE.

Monteggia's fracture   MONTEGGIA FRACTURE-DISLOCATION.

Moore's fracture   A fracture of the distal half of the radial shaft together with dislocation of the ulnar head and entrapment of the styloid process by the wrist ligaments.

multiple fracture   More than one fracture occurring in the same bone without communication between fracture points.

nasal fracture   Fracture of the bony nasal skeleton, commonly of the nasal bones alone but, in more severe cases, of the frontal processes of the maxillae also. The cartilaginous septum is frequently involved. The degree of deformity, extent of comminution, severity of epistaxis, and whether or not the fracture is compound depend on the force, direction, and nature of the blow causing the injury.

neoplastic fracture   Fracture occurring through a region of bone that has been weakened by the presence of a tumor.

neurogenic fracture   A fracture occurring through a bone that has become weakened owing to lack of function secondary to neurologic disease.

oblique fracture   A fracture of a long bone that runs obliquely to the long axis.

occult fracture   A symptomatic fracture that is not visible radiographically until callus formation or bone resorption is seen more than two weeks after the onset of symptoms.

open fracture   COMPOUND FRACTURE.

open skull fracture   COMPOUND SKULL FRACTURE.

panfacial fracture   An injury in which all of the facial bones have been fractured.

paratrooper fracture   A fracture of the ankle joint consisting of a fragment from the posterior articular margin of the tibia and of the medial or lateral malleolus.

parry fracture   MONTEGGIA FRACTURE-DISLOCATION.

pathologic fracture   A fracture that occurs through any bone weakened by a preexisting disease such as a tumor, osteoporosis, or osteomalacia. Also called *secondary fracture, spontaneous fracture, trophic fracture*.

perforating fracture   Any open fracture caused by a missile passing through a bone. Also called *puncture fracture*.

periarticular fracture   A fracture near to but not involving a joint.

pertrochanteric fracture   A fracture of the proximal femur involving the greater trochanter.

pillion fracture   A T-shaped fracture of the distal femur with posterior displacement of the condyles. It is caused by a blow to the flexed knee.

ping-pong fracture   DEPRESSED SKULL FRACTURE.

pond fracture   A fracture of the skull in which the line of fracture takes a circular form.

posterior element fracture   A fracture through the pedicles or facet joints of the vertebrae.

Pott's fracture   A fracture, usually oblique, of the lateral malleolus of the fibula, with an avulsion transverse fracture of the tibial medial malleolus. The hindfoot is outwardly displaced at the mortice of the ankle joint.

pressure fracture   A resorption and fracturing of bone due to an adjacent tumor.

puncture fracture   PERFORATING FRACTURE.

pyramidal fracture   LeFort II FRACTURE.

reverse Colles fracture   A fracture of the lower end of the radius in which the radial fragment is displaced anteriorly. It is usually caused by a direct blow to the dorsal aspect of the radius. Also called *Smith's fracture, chauffeurs' fracture*.

rosette fracture   A fracture of the skull in which the lines of fracture take a rosette form.

secondary fracture   PATHOLOGIC FRACTURE.

segmental fracture   DOUBLE FRACTURE.

shaft fracture   A fracture through or across the shaft of a long bone.

Shepherd's fracture   An avulsion or shear fracture of the posterior process of the talus.

silver-fork fracture   COLLES FRACTURE.

simple fracture   A closed fracture without significant soft tissue injury or displacement.

simple skull fracture   A fracture of the skull that is linear and closed.

Skillern's fracture   In children, a complete fracture of the lower end of the radius along with a greenstick fracture of the ulna.

skull fracture   A break in the continuity of the skull caused by trauma.

Smith's fracture   REVERSE COLLES FRACTURE.

spiral fracture   A fracture of a long bone that is spiral or helical in outline and is due to torsional force. Also called *torsion fracture*.

splintered fracture   A comminuted fracture in which the numerous fragments are thin and sharp.

spontaneous fracture   PATHOLOGIC FRACTURE.

sprain fracture   An avulsion fracture of a small piece of bone or cartilage with its attached ligament or tendon by a sudden force. Also called *strain fracture*.

sprinters' fracture   The avulsion of the anterior superior or inferior iliac spine of the ilium due to excessive muscle pull.

stellate fracture   A fracture resulting from a central impact of force, with the fracture lines radiating outward.

stellate skull fracture   A fracture of the skull having a star shape.

Stieda's fracture   A fracture through the medial condyle of the femur.

strain fracture   SPRAIN FRACTURE.

stress fracture   A fracture that results from repetitive strong forces in the shafts of weight-bearing long bones adjacent to muscle attachments, such as the tibia or fibula. It is often seen in runners or ballet dancers. Also called *march fracture, Deutschländer's disease.*

subcapital fracture   A fracture at the junction of the head and neck of the femur.

subcutaneous fracture   CLOSED FRACTURE.

subperiosteal fracture   A cortical crack without displacement or irregularity, suggesting that the periosteum is still intact.

subtrochanteric fracture   A transverse fracture at the junction of the femoral shaft and the lesser trochanter.

supracondylar fracture   A fracture above the lines of the condyles in either the humerus or the femur.

surgical neck fracture   A fracture line through the surgical neck of the humerus.

temporal bone fracture   Fracture of the skull involving the temporal bone. Eighty percent of such fractures involve the long axis of the petrous portion of the bone and are likely to be accompanied by bleeding into the tympanic cavity or bleeding from the ear together with impaired hearing of the conduction type. Transverse fractures of the petrous portion are likely to involve the inner ear, resulting in irreversible sensorineural deafness. This is a common injury, particularly in road accidents.

tibial plateau fracture   A fracture through one or both tibial plateaus, usually with downward or oblique displacement.

torsion fracture   SPIRAL FRACTURE.

transcervical fracture   An intracapsular fracture through the neck of the femur.

transcondylar fracture   A fracture through the intercondylar fossa of either the lower end of the humerus or the femur and separating the two condyles. Also called *Y and T fracture, diacondylar fracture.*

transverse fracture   A fracture across the longitudinal axis of the bone.

transverse facial fracture   LEFORT III FRACTURE.

transverse maxillary fracture   LEFORT I FRACTURE.

trimalleolar fracture   A fracture through both lateral and medial malleoli of the ankle joint as well as the posterior process of the tibia.

trophic fracture   PATHOLOGIC FRACTURE.

tuft fracture   BURSTING FRACTURE.

ununited fracture   A fracture in which the callus fails to unite the bone ends, resulting in abnormal mobility, i.e., a false joint.

vertebra plana fracture   A fracture through the plate of a vertebral body.

willow fracture   GREENSTICK FRACTURE.

Y and T fracture   TRANSCONDYLAR FRACTURE.

---

fracture-dislocation   A fracture or fractures associated with instability and disruption of articulating surfaces making up a joint.

Monteggia fracture-dislocation   A displaced fracture of the upper end of the ulnar shaft with dislocation of the radial head. Also called *Monteggia's fracture, parry fracture, Monteggia's dislocation.*

posterior fracture-dislocation   A fracture-dislocation, usually of the hip joint, in which the posterior margin has been sheared off by the dislocating femoral head. It can also be seen at the elbow joint, where the anterior margin of the ulnar coronoid process is sheared off by the humerus.

fradicin   A substance with antibiotic activity against some fungi. It is isolated from *Streptomyces fradiae.*

Fragesucht [German *Frage* a question + *Sucht* sickness] FOLIE DU POURQUOI.

fragiform [L *frag(um)* strawberry + *i* + -FORM] Resembling a strawberry in shape.

fragile   Characterized by fragility.

fragilitas [L (from *fragil(is)* fragile, from *frangere* to break, shatter + *-itas* -ITY), frailty, weakness] FRAGILITY.

fragilitas crinium   An abnormal fragility of the hair.

fragilitas ossium   OSTEOGENESIS IMPERFECTA.

fragilitas unguium   A brittleness of the nails.

fragility [L *fragilitas.* See FRAGILITAS.]   The likelihood of being damaged or destroyed. Also called *fragilitas.*

fragility of blood   ERYTHROCYTE FRAGILITY.

capillary fragility   Excessive liability of the capillaries to rupture, as in purpura.

erythrocyte fragility   The pattern of susceptibility of erythrocytes to hemolysis, when subjected to graduated hypotonic saline solutions. Also called *fragility of blood.*

hereditary fragility of bone   OSTEOGENESIS IMPERFECTA.

mechanical fragility   The ease with which erythrocytes are disrupted by shear stress.

osmotic fragility   The susceptibility of erythrocytes to lyse in hypotonic solutions of sodium chloride. Erythrocytes of normal blood exhibit very little lysis in NaCl solution of 0.5 g/dl concentration, whereas blood that contains spherocytes lyse at this or higher salt concentration. A test for osmotic fragility is used in the diagnosis of hereditary spherocytosis.

fragilocyte   SPHEROCYTE.

fragilocytosis   SPHEROCYTOSIS.

fragment [L *fragmentum* (from *frang(ere)* to break + -*mentum* -MENT) a piece broken off]   **1** A part detached or broken off. **2** One of the parts of an antibody molecule obtained by treatment with a proteinase. The two main fragments are Fab and Fc. Fab contains the antigen-binding site and comprises the complete light chain and about half the heavy chain of the immunoglobulin molecule. Fc comprises half the heavy chain and can be crystallized, since Fc molecules from different antibodies have identical structures.

fragment A   The smaller of the two fragments into which diphtheria toxin is split by various proteases. It is the enzymatically active moiety of the toxin and the part that enters the host cell.

fragment B   The larger of the two fragments of diphtheria toxin, which functions in binding the toxin to a host cell receptor.

Fab fragment   A fragment of the immunoglobulin molecule obtained following papain hydrolysis of the molecule. The Fab moiety has an approximate molecular mass of 45 000 daltons and consists of one light chain linked to the N-terminal portion of the contiguous heavy chain. Two Fab fragments are obtained from the hydrolysis of one 7 S immunoglobulin and each fragment contains one antibody combining site.

F(ab')₂ fragment   The major fragment of immunoglobulins obtained after pepsin digestion of the molecule. It has a molecular weight of 90 000 daltons and retains the two antibody combining sites but does not have the major Fc fragment. It is a useful tool in immunologic research, since it will not bind specifically to Fc receptor present on the surface of many tissue cells.

Fc fragment   A fragment of the immunoglobulin molecule which has a molecular weight of 45 000 daltons and is obtained following papain digestion of the molecule. Unlike papain digestion of immunoglobulins, this fragment contains no antibody combining sites but does retain its site for complement fixation and for binding to Fc receptors in tissues.

Fc′ fragment   The smaller molecular weight material following papain digestion of immunoglobulin molecules. It consists of a dimer of the C-terminal half of the two Fc fragments and has a molecular weight of 24 000 daltons. It has no antibody combining activity.

Fd fragment   The heavy chain fragment of the immunoglobulin molecule obtained after papain digestion. It contains both the constant and variable region of the heavy chain molecule. The variable region of the heavy chain is involved in the antibody combining site of immunoglobulins. Also called *Fd piece*.

fission fragment   Any daughter nuclide produced by a fission event. There are two daughters per fission, and they are not necessarily alike. The mass numbers from the fission of uranium 235, for example, range from 72 to a little over 160. Most fragments are radioactive. The amounts of each produced vary widely.

immunoglobulin fragment   Any of the various pieces of the immunoglobulin molecule, such as Fab, Fc, Fd, obtained after enzymatic digestion of the molecule.

one-carbon fragment   Any of the formyl, formimino, hydroxymethyl, and methyl groups, and their equivalents, carried on tetrahydrofolate and metabolically interconvertible. They are used in various biosyntheses, as that of purines.

papain fragment   Any of the various fragments of the immunoglobulin molecule obtained after papain digestion of the immunoglobulin.

Spengler's fragments   Small, spherical bodies found in the sputum of patients with pulmonary tuberculosis.

fragmentation [FRAGMENT + -ATION]   Gross disturbance in thinking because of lack of purposefulness in associations, which are often haphazard and illogical and incomprehensibly combined.

fragmentation of the myocardium   Transverse rupture of cardiac muscle fibers.

fraise [French, strawberry]   A hemispheric, fluted reamer for enlarging burr holes in the skull.

frambesia [New L, from French *framboise* raspberry, from the Germanic]   YAWS.

frambesia tropica   YAWS.

frambesiform [New L *frambesi(a)* (from French *framboise* raspberry, from the Germanic) yaws + -FORM]   Similar in appearance to the lesions of yaws.

frambesioma [*frambesi(a)* + -OMA]   An obsolete term for MOTHER YAW.

framboesia [See FRAMBESIA.]   YAWS.

frame   1 A rigid structure providing support or immobilization of the body and to which various traction systems can be affixed. **2** One in a sequence of two-dimensional images that combine to produce a picture over time, as in motion picture film, or in a third spatial dimension, as in ultrasound scanning.

Balkan frame   A frame consisting of overhead bars attached to a hospital-type bed to which can be attached suspension slings, traction units, and weight-resisted pulley systems. Also called *Balkan splint*.

Bradford frame   A heavy rectangular frame on which canvas is stretched to form a body splint for immobilizing the patient. It was originally designed for handling children with tuberculosis of the spine.

Deiters terminal frame   A platelike expansion at the free end of each of the phalangeal processes of the outer phalangeal cells of Deiters that ends on the reticular lamina and connects the cells of Deiters to the hair cells and the supporting cells of Hensen at the outer side of the spiral organ of Corti. An outmoded term.

Foster frame   A variant of the Stryker frame.

implant superstructure frame   The metal part of an implant superstructure.

occluding frame   A simple type of nonhinged articulator.

quadriplegic standing frame   A frame used to support a quadriplegic patient in a standing posture for physiological benefits.

rubber dam frame   A wire frame for holding a rubber dam in a stretched state while teeth are isolated from the mouth.

sampling frame   A complete inventory of the entities to be sampled in which each is separately identifiable such as an electoral roll or a list by name of persons admitted to a hospital.

Stryker frame   A rigid stretcher-type frame used to rotate a patient without active or passive motion of the patient's trunk and limbs.

suture frame   A rectangular, metal frame designed for attachment to a mouth gag, sometimes used in operations for the repair of cleft palate. It is provided with a means for retaining in an orderly way the long ends of a number of sutures until the surgeon is ready to cut them short.

trial frame   A spectacle frame designed to hold interchangeable optical lenses during an examination for refractive error.

unidentified reading frame   A nucleotide sequence, bounded by an initiation codon and a termination codon, that does not encode any known protein. Abbreviation: URF

frame shift   See under FRAME-SHIFT MUTATION.

framework   The metal part of a partial denture. Also called *skeleton of partial denture*.

scleral framework   The part of the iridocorneal angle adjacent to the sclera.

uveal framework   RETICULUM TRABECULARE SCLERAE.

Franceschetti [Adolphe *Franceschetti*, Swiss ophthalmologist, born 1896]   **1** Franceschetti syndrome, Franceschetti-Klein syndrome, Franceschetti-Zwahlen-Klein syndrome, Treacher Collins-Franceschetti syndrome. See under MANDIBULOFACIAL DYSOSTOSIS. **2** Franceschetti-Jadassohn syndrome. See under NAEGELI SYNDROME.

Francis [Edward *Francis*, U.S. bacteriologist, 1872–1957] Francis disease. See under TULAREMIA.

Francis [Thomas *Francis*, Jr., U.S. epidemiologist, 1900–1969] See under TEST.

Francisella tularensis   A very small, nonmobile, unencapsulated, aerobic, Gram-negative bacillus which causes tularemia. It has complex growth requirements, including a high concentration of a sulfhydryl compound, and it grows slowly and forms minute colonies. The organism is an intracellular parasite. It is transmitted to humans from rabbits and other wild animals by the deer fly, ticks, contact with animals, and ingestion of meat, the manifestations depending largely on the site of entry. The organism is dangerous in the laboratory. It can penetrate unbroken skin and a very small dose is infectious. Also called *Pasteurella tularensis* (obsolete).

francium   A radioactive element having atomic number 87. Its position in the periodic table identifies it as the heaviest of the alkali metals. About 20 very short-lived isotopes have been made synthetically. The only naturally occurring isotope is a decay product of actinium having mass number 223. No weighable amount has been isolated. It decays by emitting alpha particles and electrons and has a half-life of 22 minutes. Symbol: Fr

Francke [Karl Ernst *Francke*, German physician, 1859–1920] See under NEEDLE.

Franco [Pierre *Franco*, French surgeon, 1500–1561]   Franco's operation. See under SUPRAPUBIC CYSTOTOMY.

François [Jules *François*, Belgian ophthalmologist, flourished mid-20th century]   Hallermann-Streiff-François syndrome. See under HALLERMANN-STREIFF SYNDROME.

franghi   The Syrian term for SYPHILIS.   • The term is reserved for venereal syphilis.

frangula The dried bark of *Rhamnus frangula*. It is used as a cathartic. Also called *buckthorn bark, alder buckthorn.*

frangulic acid EMODIN.

Frank [Otto *Frank*, German physiologist, 1865–1944] **1** See under FRANK-STARLING CURVE. See under STARLING CURVE. **2** Frank-Starling mechanism. See under MECHANISM.

Frank [Rudolf *Frank*, Austrian surgeon, 1862–1913] Ssabanejew-Frank operation. See under FRANK'S OPERATION.

Franke [Felix *Franke*, German surgeon, born 1860] See under OPERATION.

Fränkel [Albert *Fränkel*, German physician, 1848–1916] See under SIGN.

Fränkel [Bernhard *Fränkel*, German laryngologist, 1836–1911] See under SPECULUM.

Fränkel [Henri *Fränkel*, French ophthalmologist, born 1864] Bordier-Fränkel sign. See under SIGN.

Frankenhäuser [Ferdinand *Frankenhäuser*, German gynecologist, 1832–1894] Frankenhäuser's ganglion. See under CERVICAL GANGLION OF UTERUS.

frankincense A gum resin obtained by incising the bark of *Boswellia carterii* and other species. It is a bitter drug and is used in fumigating powders.

Frankl-Hochwart [Lothar von *Frankl-Hochwart*, Austrian neurologist, 1862–1914] See under DISEASE.

Franklin [Benjamin *Franklin*, U.S. statesman and scientist, 1706–1790] **1** See under SPECTACLES. **2** Franklinic taste. See under TASTE. **3** Franklinic electricity. See under FRICTIONAL ELECTRICITY.

Franklin [Edward Claus *Franklin*, German-born U.S. physician, born 1928] Franklin's disease. See under GAMMA HEAVY-CHAIN DISEASE.

franklin [after Benjamin *Franklin,* American scientist, 1706–1790] The special name for the unit charge in CGS electrostatic units, the charge which exerts a force of one dyne on an equal charge at one centimeter, equal to 3.336×10^{-10} coulomb approximately. An obsolete unit. Symbol: Fr

franklinism [after Benjamin *Franklin*, American statesman, 1706–1790 + -ISM] FRICTIONAL ELECTRICITY.

franklinization [after Benjamin *Franklin*, U.S. statesman, scientist, and philosopher, 1706–1790 + *-iz(e)* + -ATION] The use of static electricity for treatment.

Fraser [G. R. *Fraser*, British geneticist, flourished 20th century] Fraser syndrome. See under CRYPTOPHTHALMIA-SYNDACTYLY SYNDROME.

fraternal [Med L *fraternal(is)* (from L *fratern(us)* pertaining to brother, from *frater* brother, + *-alis* -AL) pertaining to brothers] **1** Having a brotherly or sibling relationship. **2** Derived from separately fertilized ova: said of twins.

fratricide [L *frater*, gen. *fratris*, brother + -CIDE] **1** The killing of one's own brother or sister. **2** One who commits fratricide.

Fraunhofer [Joseph *Fraunhofer*, German physicist, 1787–1826] **1** Fraunhofer lines. See under LINE. **2** Fraunhofer zone. See under FAR FIELD.

fraxin $C_{16}H_{18}O_{10}$. A diuretic glycoside obtained from the bark of *Fraxinus excelsior*, European ash.

Frazier [Charles Harrison *Frazier*, U.S. surgeon, 1870–1936] Frazier-Spiller operation. See under OPERATION.

FRC functional residual capacity.

freckle [Middle English *frekel, frakel*, from the Scandinavian] A light brown pigmented macule that develops on light-exposed skin in a genetically predisposed subject. Also called *sunspot, macula solaris, lentigo aestiva.*

cold freckle A freckle on an area of skin not exposed to sunlight. An obsolete term.

Hutchinson's melanotic freckle A pigmented lesion of the malar region of the face containing abnormal melanocytes in the epidermis. The lesion can become a malignant melanoma. Also called *precancerous melanosis of Dubreuilh, lentigo maligna, Hutchinson's malignant lentigo, malignant lentigo.*

melanotic freckle See under HUTCHINSON'S MELANOTIC FRECKLE.

Fredet [Pierre *Fredet*, French surgeon, 1870–1946] Fredet-Ramstedt operation. See under PYLOROMYOTOMY.

free-end Supported only at one end: said of a base unit of a partial denture which is supported by teeth at one end only. A free-end saddle is a base extension.

free-living **1** Not parasitic; not metabolically dependent on another living organism. **2** Nonsessile; not permanently attached; motile.

Freeman [E. A. *Freeman*, English physician, flourished mid-20th century] Freeman-Sheldon syndrome, Freeman-Sheldon whistling face syndrome. See under WHISTLING FACE-WINDMILL VANE HAND SYNDROME.

freemartin [origin unknown] A female bovine animal whose twin is male. Usually, a freemartin has a hypoplastic uterus, vagina, and ovaries.

Freer [Otto Tiger *Freer*, U.S. surgeon, 1857–1932] See under ELEVATOR.

free-swimming Describing any aquatic organism which is not permanently attached to a surface and is thus able to swim about; free-living.

freeze / frame freeze Display of a single frame of a real-time sequence, as in ultrasound, to allow close examination of specific features of the image.

freeze-drying LYOPHILIZATION.

freeze-etching A method of forming a stable replica of a small particle for examination in an electron microscope. The particle is frozen in a block of ice, partially etched by warming, and subsequently coated with a shadowing technique to form the stable replica.

freeze-substitution A freezing technique that is used to facilitate the impregnation of embedding media into tissues prior to electron microscopy.

Frei [Wilhelm Siegmund *Frei*, German dermatologist, 1885–1943] **1** See under ANTIGEN, BUBO, TEST. **2** Frei's disease. See under LYMPHOGRANULOMA VENEREUM.

Freiberg [Albert Henry *Freiberg*, U.S. surgeon, 1869–1940] Freiberg's disease, Freiberg's infraction. See under KÖHLER SECOND DISEASE.

Frejka [Bedrich *Frejka*, Czech physician, born 1890] Frejka pillow. See under FREJKA PILLOW SPLINT.

fremitus [L (from *fremitus*, past part. of *fremere* to murmur, mutter, from Gk *bremein* to roar), a murmuring, roaring] A palpable vibration.

bronchial fremitus A fremitus felt over the chest due to passage of air through narrowed or distorted bronchi. Also called *rhonchal fremitus.*

pericardial fremitus A thrill due to pericardial friction. See also PERICARDIAL RUB.

pleural fremitus A fremitus felt over the chest due to friction between two pleural surfaces.

rhonchal fremitus BRONCHIAL FREMITUS.

subjective fremitus A fremitus perceived in one's own body, particularly that produced by phonation.

tactile fremitus A fremitus felt on palpation, especially of the chest.

tussive fremitus   A fremitus felt over the chest during coughing.

vocal fremitus   The fremitus felt on palpation of the chest during phonation. Abbreviation: VF

frena   Plural of FRENUM.

frenal   Pertaining to a frenum.

frenectomy [*fren(um)* + -ECTOMY]   A surgical procedure in which a frenum is excised.

frenetic [See PHRENETIC.]   PHRENETIC.

Frenkel [Heinrich S. *Frenkel*-Heiden, German neurologist, 1860–1931]   **1** Frenkel's treatment. See under FRENKEL'S EXERCISES. **2** See under SYMPTOM. **3** Frenkel's movements. See under MOVEMENT.

frenoplasty [*fren(ulum)* + *o* -PLASTY]   A plastic operation on a frenulum.

frenotomy [*fren(ulum)* + *o*+ -TOMY]   The surgical cutting of a frenum, usually of the lingual frenum for the correction of ankyloglossia.

frenula   Plural of FRENULUM.

frenulum [Late L (dim. of L *frenum* a bridle, bit, reins), a small bridle]   (*plural* frenula) A fold of mucous membrane or other tissue that prevents, controls, or limits the movements of an organ or part to which it is attached; a small frenum.

frenulum of anterior medullary velum   FRENULUM VELI MEDULLARIS SUPERIOR.

frenulum cerebelli   FRENULUM VELI MEDULLARIS SUPERIOR.

frenulum clitoridis   [NA] The small fold on the under-surface of the clitoris formed by the lower division of the anterior ends of the labia minora meeting under and uniting with the clitoris. Also called *frenulum of clitoris, crus glandis clitoridis*.

frenulum of clitoris   FRENULUM CLITORIDIS.

frenulum of duodenal papilla   A variable fold of mucous membrane that extends downward from the lower margin of the papilla duodeni major and is a continuation of the plica longitudinalis duodeni.

frenulum epiglottidis   An outmoded term for PLICA GLOSSOEPIGLOTTICA MEDIANA.

frenulum of Giacomini   GIACOMINI'S BAND.

frenulum of ileocecal valve   FRENULUM VALVAE ILEALIS.

frenulum of ileocolic valve   FRENULUM VALVAE ILEALIS.

frenulum of inferior lip   FRENULUM LABII INFERIORIS.

frenulum labii inferioris   [NA] The small raised fold of mucous membrane connecting the inner surface of the lower lip with the lower gum in the median plane. Also called *frenulum of inferior lip*.

frenulum labii superioris   [NA] The prominent raised fold of mucous membrane connecting the inner surface of the upper lip with the upper gum in the median plane. Also called *frenulum of superior lip*.

frenulum labiorum pudendi   [NA] The fold of skin joining the posterior ends of the labia minora across the midline and anterior to the posterior commissure. Also called *frenulum of pudendal labia, frenulum pudendi, fourchette, frenum of labia*.

frenulum linguae   [NA] The raised median, vertical fold of mucous membrane connecting the inferior surface of the tongue to the floor of the mouth. Also called *frenulum of tongue, frenum of tongue, lingual frenum, vinculum linguae* (outmoded), *glossodesmus* (seldom used), *sublingual ridge*.

frenulum linguae cerebelli   VINCULA LINGULAE CEREBELLI.

frenulum of Macdowel   An aponeurotic sheet spreading across the bicipital groove of the humerus from the tendon of insertion of the pectoralis major muscle. Also called *Macdowel's frenum*.

frenulum of Morgagni   FRENULUM VALVAE ILEALIS.

posterior meniscal frenulum of Poirier   A short, thick fibroelastic band of the posterior part of the fibrous capsule of the temporomandibular joint that is situated between the tympanosquamous fissure and the posterior edge of the articular disk. It limits the forward movement of the disk when the mouth is opened and pulls the disk back when it is closed. An outmoded term.

frenulum of prepuce of penis   FRENULUM PREPUTII PENIS.

frenulum preputii penis   [NA] A small median fold of skin on the urethral surface of the penis extending from the deep surface of the prepuce to the glans penis just behind the external urethral orifice. Also called *frenulum of prepuce of penis*.

frenulum of pudendal labia   FRENULUM LABIORUM PUDENDI.

frenulum pudendi   FRENULUM LABIORUM PUDENDI.

frenulum of superior lip   FRENULUM LABII SUPERIORIS.

frenulum of superior medullary velum   FRENULUM VELI MEDULLARIS SUPERIOR.

frenulum synoviale   Any one of the vincula tendinum. Also called *ligamentum vaginale* (outmoded).

frenulum of tongue   FRENULUM LINGUAE.

frenulum valvae ilealis   A ridge that is formed by the fused lips of the ileocecal valve. It runs laterally and downwards, demarcating the cecum from the ascending colon. Also called *frenulum of ileocecal valve, frenulum of ileocolic valve, frenulum valvae ileocecalis, frenula valvulae coli, frenulum of Morgagni, frenum of Morgagni, frenum of valve of colon*.

frenulum valvae ileocecalis   FRENULUM VALVAE ILEALIS.

frenula valvulae coli   FRENULUM VALVAE ILEALIS.

frenulum veli medullaris anterioris   FRENULUM VELI MEDULLARIS SUPERIOR.

frenulum veli medullaris superior   [NA] A band running from the rostral end of the superior medullary velum to the longitudinal groove between the inferior colliculi. Also called *frenulum of superior medullary velum, frenulum of anterior medullary velum, frenulum veli medullaris anterioris, frenulum cerebelli*.

frenum [L *frenum*, also *fraenum* a bridle, bit, reins]   (*plural* frenums, frena) A body structure that serves to restrain or check movement. Also called *bridle*.

buccal frenum   A fold of mucosa stretching from the cheek to the alveolar process in the canine region.

frenum of labia   FRENULUM LABIORUM PUDENDI.

labial frenum   A fold of mucosa stretching from the lip to the alveolar process between the central incisor teeth.

lingual frenum   FRENULUM LINGUAE.

Macdowel's frenum   FRENULUM OF MACDOWEL.

frenum of Morgagni   FRENULUM VALVAE ILEALIS.

frenum of tongue   FRENULUM LINGUAE.

frenum of valve of colon   FRENULUM VALVAE ILEALIS.

frenzy [Middle English *frenesie*, from Old French *frenesie* frenzy, from Med L *phrenesia* madness, from L *phrenesis* frenzy, madness, from Gk *phrenitis* (from *phrēn* the mind + -*itis* -ITIS) delirium of fever, frenzy]   Delirium induced by meningitis or by other acute cerebral conditions. An outmoded term. Also called *phrenism* (obsolete).

epileptic frenzy   An exceptionally rare epileptic manifestation, occurring either during a state of automatism or during postepileptic confusion in a patient with temporal lobe epilepsy, in which the patient manifests rage or may commit violent or aggressive acts. This diagnosis is in rare cases justified, though it is sometimes improperly invoked, especially in the case of those accused of murder, rape, or other violent crimes, who show EEG abnormalities. An older term. Also called *furor epilepticus, epileptic raptus, paroxysmal furor*.

frequency [L *frequentia* (from *frequens* repeated), frequency]   **1** In statistics, the number of occurrences of a given event or the number of observations falling within a given class. Also called *absolute frequency*. **2** The number of complete variations (cycles) of an electromagnetic or acoustic wave occurring in one second.

absolute frequency   FREQUENCY.

angular frequency   The frequency of a periodic phenomenon expressed as a rate of change of phase angle. $\omega = 2\pi f$ where ω is the angular frequency and f is the periodic repetition rate.

audio frequency   Sonic frequency in the audible range: between about 20 and 20 000 Hz for humans.

audio Doppler frequency   Doppler shift presented as audible sound.

center frequency   The dominant frequency present in an ultrasound pulse.

frequency of contractions   The recurrence of uterine contractions during labor in a given time period.

critical flicker fusion frequency   The slowest rate of stroboscopic presentation of a light at which the illumination is perceived as a constant and unvarying light. Also called *fusion frequency*.

cumulative frequency   The sum of the frequencies of successive values of a random variable below or up to a stated value.

cutoff frequency   The frequency of a system identified with the transition between those frequencies that pass through the system and those that are attenuated, and where the attenuation is 3 dB.

dominant frequency   In the electroencephalogram, the frequency, usually that of the alpha rhythm, which dominates the record.

electromagnetic frequency   The number of repetitions completed by a periodic electromagnetic quantity in unit time, expressed in hertz.

fusion frequency   CRITICAL FLICKER FUSION FREQUENCY.

gene frequency   In a defined population, the frequency of a specific allele at a given genetic locus.

high frequency   **1** A frequency that is high in comparison to a given standard such as the pitch frequency of middle C.   **2** A radio frequency in the range of 3 to 30 megahertz.

Larmor frequency   The frequency of precession of a rotator whose angular momentum is associated with a magnetic moment (as in the case of an electron or nucleus) when subjected to a magnetic field. See also LARMOR EQUATION.

low frequency   **1** A frequency low in comparison to a certain standard such as the pitch frequency of middle C.   **2** Radio frequency in the range of 30 to 300 kilohertz.

mutant frequency   The proportion of a particular mutant in a population. It depends not only on mutation rate but on the accumulation of the progeny of mutants arising in the culture.

nearest neighbor frequency   With reference to nucleic acids of a given organism, usually DNA, the relative frequency with which two nucleotides are adjacent.

projection frequency   The proportion of neurons in a circumscribed nucleus synaptically contacted by a given or average fiber projecting onto the nucleus, e.g., the percentage of motoneurons in a muscle's motor pool with which a primary spindle afferent makes contact.

radio frequency   A frequency in the range at which coherent electromagnetic radiation of energy is useful for communication purposes, roughly in the range 10 kilohertz to 100 gigahertz. Abbreviation: r.f.

recombination frequency   **1** The frequency of genetic recombination between two given syntenic loci. It is determined by dividing the number of individuals in a given sibship in whom recombination occurred by the total number of individuals. For loci sufficiently closely linked that multiple crossovers are infrequent, the recombination frequency is a measure of map distance.   **2** The frequency of transfer of a bacterial gene from a donor to a recipient.   **3** The frequency of crossover between two genetic markers in a merozygote.   **4** The frequency of recombination between markers in two viral genomes infecting the same cell. For defs. 1, 2, 3, and 4 also called *recombination fraction*. Abbreviation: RF

rectified radio frequency   A radio frequency signal which has been converted from alternating to direct current form.

relative frequency   In statistics, a frequency expressed as a proportion of the total number of events or of some other totality.

respiratory frequency   The rate of breathing, measured usually by the number of breaths per minute. Also called *ventilatory frequency*.

subsonic frequency   A frequency below the audible range.

ultrasonic frequency   Frequency of vibration above the audible range, especially in the range of 1 to 10 MHz.

ventilatory frequency   RESPIRATORY FREQUENCY.

Frerichs [Friedrich Theodore von *Frerichs*, German physician, 1819–1885]   See under THEORY.

freshening   The considerable enlargement of the mammary gland that occurs as parturition nears.   • The term is chiefly applied to cattle, sheep, and goats.

Fresnel [Augustin Jean *Fresnel*, French physicist, 1788–1827]   **1** Fresnel zone. See under NEAR FIELD.   **2** Fresnel zone plate. See under PLATE.

fresnel [after Augustin Jean *Fresnel*, French physicist, 1788–1827]   A unit of optical frequency used in spectroscopy, equal to 10^{12} hertz; one terahertz. An obsolete unit.

fressreflex   A primitive reflex composed of sucking, rooting, and chewing reflexes elicited by touching the lips or cheeks either of very young infants or of adults with advanced degenerative brain disease.

freta   Plural of FRETUM.

fretum [L, a place of passage, strait, channel]   In anatomy, a constriction, narrowing, or channel.

fretum halleri   CHANNEL OF HALLER.

Freud [Sigmund *Freud*, Austrian neurologist and psychiatrist, 1856–1939]   **1** See under FIXATION.   **2** Freud's theory. See under PSYCHOANALYTIC THEORY.

freudian [after Sigmund *Freud*, Austrian neurologist and psychiatrist, 1856–1939 + -*ian*, suffix denoting pertaining to]   Relating to concepts proposed by Freud in the development of his theories of psychoanalytic psychology and technique.

Freund [Jules Thomas *Freund*, U.S. immunologist, 1890–1960]   **1** See under ADJUVANT.   **2** Freund's incomplete adjuvant. See under ADJUVANT.   **3** Freund's complete adjuvant. See under ADJUVANT.

Freund [Wilhelm Alexander *Freund*, German surgeon, 1833–1918]   See under ANOMALY.

Frey [Heinrich *Frey*, Swiss histologist, born 1822]   Gastric foveolae of Frey, gastric pits of Frey. See under FOVEOLAE GASTRICAE.

Frey [Lucie *Frey*, Polish physician, 1852–1932]   Frey-Baillarger syndrome, Frey syndrome. See under AURICULOTEMPORAL SYNDROME.

Frey [Maximilian Ruppert Franz von *Frey*, Austrian-born German physician, 1852–1932]   Frey's hairs. See under HAIR.

Freyer [Peter Johnston *Freyer*, English surgeon, 1851–1921]   See under OPERATION.

FRF   follicle releasing factor.

friable [L *friabil(is)* (from *fri(are)* to break into small pieces + -*abilis* -ABLE) capable of being ground or broken into small pieces]   Easily broken up into discrete pieces, as a bacterial colony.

Fricke [Johann Karl Georg *Fricke*, German surgeon, 1790–1841]   See under BANDAGE.

Friderichsen [Carl *Friderichsen*, Danish pediatrician, born 1886] Waterhouse-Friderichsen syndrome. See under SYN-DROME.

Fridericia [Louis Sigurd *Fridericia*, Danish hygienist, born 1881] See under METHOD.

Friedenwald [Jonas Stein *Friedenwald*, U.S. ophthalmologist, 1897–1955] See under NOMOGRAM.

Friedländer [Karl *Friedländer*, German physician, 1847–1887] **1** Friedländer's bacillus. See under *KLEBSIELLA PNEUMONIAE*. **2** Friedländer's disease. See under ENDARTERITIS OBLITERANS. **3** Friedländer's pneumonia. See under *KLEBSIELLA* PNEU-MONIA.

Friedman [Emanuel A. *Friedman*, U.S. physician, born 1926] See under CURVE.

Friedman [Maurice Harold *Friedman*, U.S. physician, born 1903] Friedman-Lapham test, Friedman test. See under FRIEDMAN TEST.

Friedmann [Max *Friedmann*, German neurologist, 1858–1925] **1** Friedmann's complex, Friedmann syndrome, Friedmann's vasomotor syndrome. See under BOXERS' ENCEPHALOPATHY. **2** Friedmann's disease. See under NARCOLEPSY.

Friedreich [Nikolaus *Friedreich*, German physician, 1826–1882] **1** See under FOOT, PHENOMENON, SIGN. **2** Friedreich's ataxia, Friedreich's tabes. See under FRIEDREICH'S DISEASE.

Friend [Charlotte *Friend*, U.S. microbiologist, born 1921] See under VIRUS.

friente A dermatitis that occurs in forestry workers. It is possibly due to sensitization to plant smuts such as Basidiomycetes.

fright [Old English *fryhto, fyrhto*] The combination of surprise and fear that characterizes reaction to an unexpected danger.

stage fright Fear felt when one has to perform on stage. It may stem from a fear of forgetting one's lines.

frigidity [Late L *frigiditas* (from L *frigid(us)* cold + *-itas* -ITY) frigidity] Emotional coldness; unresponsiveness.

sexual frigidity Female psychosexual dysfunction that may reflect inhibited sexual desire, sexual excitement, or orgasm, or any combination thereof. The end result is failure to achieve orgasm through coitus. Also called *sexual anesthesia*.

frigolabile [L *frig(us)* cold (noun) + *o* + L *labil(is)* (from *lab(i)* to slip down, fall + *-ilis* -ILE) capable of slipping down or falling] Readily damaged by cold.

frigorie [French (from L *frigor(is)*, gen. of *frigus* coldness, cool air), a calorific unit] A unit of quantity of heat, used especially for extraction of heat in refrigeration engineering, equal to 10^3 calories; 4185.5 joules if the 15°C calorie is used; 4186.8 joules if the International Table calorie is used. Symbol: frigorie

frigorism Circulatory failure due to prolonged exposure to extreme cold.

frigostabile FRIGOSTABLE.

frigostable [L *frig(us)* cold (noun) + *o* + *stabil(is)* stable] Resistant to cold. Also *frigostabile*.

frigotherapy CRYOTHERAPY.

frill [possibly from Flemish *frul* frill, edge] The posterior iris pigment of neuroectodermal origin that is visible as a thin brown edge of the pupil.

iris frill IRIS COLLARETTE.

frina CUTANEOUS LEISHMANIASIS.

fringe [French *frange* (from L *fimbria* a thread, fiber, in sing., and often pl. *fimbriae* a fringe, hem, akin to *fibra* a fiber, filament) a fringe] FIMBRIA.

Adamson's fringe The fringe of parallel apical hyphae in a hair invaded *in vivo* by a ringworm fungus. When the advancing hyphae reach the incompletely keratinized tissue of the hair bulb, further progress is halted. The tips of the apical hyphae

may be seen through the microscope in longitudinal section to be forming a fringe in the shape of an inverted V.

subliminal fringe A region within a neuron pool from which no discharge of impulses takes place during weak stimulation of one or other of two afferent nerves but from which discharge of impulses does occur if the afferent nerves are stimulated simultaneously.

frit [French, past part. of *(faire) frire* to fry or from Italian *frit(to)* fried; from L *frigere* to roast, parch] **1** Fractured porcelain from which dental porcelain powders are made. **2** Semifused porcelain before glazing.

Fritsch [Heinrich *Fritsch*, German gynecologist, 1844–1915] Fritsch catheter. See under BOZEMAN-FRITSCH CATHETER.

frog [Middle English *frogge*, from Old English *frogga*] **1** Any of various tailless amphibians in the order Anura, having strong back legs for jumping. Frogs have smooth, moist, scaleless skin, and are customarily associated with a moist environment. The aquatic larval form is called a tadpole. **2** A triangular mass of horny tissue in the middle of the sole of the foot of a horse.

Fröhde [A. *Fröhde*, German chemist, flourished 19th century] See under REAGENT.

Fröhlich [Alfred *Fröhlich*, Austrian-born pharmacologist active in the United States, 1871–1953] Babinski-Fröhlich syndrome, Fröhlich's adiposogenital dystrophy. See under FRÖHLICH SYNDROME.

Frohn [Damianus *Frohn*, German physician, born 1843] See under REAGENT.

Froin [Georges *Froin*, French physician, born 1874] Nonne-Froin syndrome, Lépine-Froin syndrome. See under FROIN SYNDROME.

frolement [French *frôlement* a touching lightly in passing] **1** A type of massage using the palm of the hand to lightly stroke a body surface. **2** A rustling sound heard on ausculation of the chest, usually pericardial in origin.

Froment [Jules *Froment*, French physician, 1878–1946] **1** Froment's paper sign. See under NEWSPAPER SIGN. **2** See under SIGN. **3** Froment sign. See under ROGER'S COUNTER SIGN.

Frommann [Carl *Frommann*, German anatomist, 1831–1892] Frommann's lines. See under STRIATIONS OF FROMMANN.

Frommel [Richard Julius Ernst *Frommel*, German gynecologist, 1854–1912] **1** Frommel's disease, Chiari-Frommel disease, Frommel-Chiari syndrome. See under CHIARI-FROMMEL SYNDROME. **2** See under OPERATION.

frond **1** A fern leaf. **2** A large, compound leaf, such as that of a palm tree. **3** Any of the leaflike growths along the stipes of algae.

frondose [L *frondos(us)* (from *frons*, gen. *frondis*, leaf of a tree, branch or tree with leaves + *-osus* -OSE[1]) leafy] Bearing leaflike, tufted, or villous structures.

frons [L, the brow, forehead] The region of the face between the eyebrows and the hairline; forehead. Also called *brow*.

frons cranii [NA] The external surface of the frontal bone corresponding to the forehead. Also called *bony forehead, frons of cranium*.

frons of cranium FRONS CRANII.

wave front A continuous surface at which all vibratory motion has the same phase at a given instant.

frontad [*front* (forehead) + -AD] Toward the front or the frontal aspect.

frontal **1** FRONTALIS. **2** Pertaining to the front of the body.

frontalis [New L, frontal] **1** Pertaining to the frontal, or coronal, plane. **2** Pertaining to the frontal bone or the forehead. For defs. 1 and 2 also *frontal*.

frontipetal [L *frons*, gen. *frontis*, brow, forepart + -PETAL] Directed towards the front.

frontocerebellar   Denoting fiber tracts from the frontal cerebral cortex extending through the pons to the cerebellum. Also *frontopontocerebellar*.

frontoethmoid   Pertaining to the frontal and the ethmoid bones.

frontoethmoidectomy   EXTERNAL   FRONTOETHMOIDECTOMY.

external frontoethmoidectomy   An operation intended for the relief of chronic frontal sinusitis either alone or with ethmoidal disease, particularly when there are nasal polyps. A curved skin incision (Howarth's incision) is made medial to the inner canthus of the eye and the frontal sinus opened through its floor. The ethmoidal air cells are broken into through the medial wall of the orbit and exenterated, providing a pathway to drain the frontal sinus into the nose beneath the middle concha. There are many modifications known by the names of their advocates. Also called *frontoethmoidectomy*.

frontolacrimal   Pertaining to the frontal and the lacrimal bones.

frontomalar   FRONTOZYGOMATIC.

frontomaxillary   Pertaining to the frontal bone and the maxilla.

frontomental   Pertaining to the forehead or frontal bone and the chin.

frontonasal   Pertaining to the frontal and nasal bones or to the frontal sinus and nasal cavity. Also called *nasofrontal*.

frontonuchal   Pertaining to the frontal bone and the nape of the neck.

fronto-occipital   Pertaining to the frontal and occipital bones or to the forehead and the occiput.

fronto-orbital   Pertaining to the frontal bone and the orbital cavity.

frontoparietal   PARIETOFRONTAL.

frontopontine   Denoting the tractus frontopontinus (Arnold's bundle).

frontopontocerebellar   FRONTOCEREBELLAR.

frontosphenoid   Pertaining to the frontal and the sphenoid bones.

frontotemporal   Pertaining to the frontal and the temporal bones. Also *temporofrontal*.

frontotemporale   A craniometric point on the frontal bone situated on the temporal line at the point of minimal frontal breadth.

frontozygomatic   Pertaining to the frontal and zygomatic bones. Also called *frontomalar*.

Froriep [August Friedrich von *Froriep*, German anatomist, 1849–1917] **1** See under GANGLION, LAW. **2** Froriep induration. See under MYOSITIS FIBROSA.

Frost [William Adams *Frost*, English ophthalmologist, 1853–1935] **1** Frost-Lang operation. See under OPERATION. **2** See under SUTURE.

frost / uremic frost   Fine, white, crystalline powder on the skin of patients with uremia, secondary to increased urea excreted with sweat which has then evaporated. Also called *urinary sweat*.

frostbite   Tissue destruction resulting from exposure to low environmental temperature. The extent of damage is difficult to determine on first inspection. Also called *pagoplexia* (seldom used).

deep frostbite   Tissue destruction extending beyond the skin and involving subcutaneous tissues, muscle, and/or bone. Also called *third degree frostbite*.

superficial frostbite   Frostbite confined to the skin.

third degree frostbite   DEEP FROSTBITE.

froth [Middle English *froth*, *frothe*, from Old Norse *frotha* froth] Bubbles of foamy saliva issuing from the mouth in patients with either hysterical or epileptic attacks.

froth of drowning   The abundant white, occasionally blood-tinged, foamy liquid that exudes from the nose and mouth of drowning victims. The fluid is an admixture of mucus, proteins, and inhaled water. The finding of this frothy fluid in corpses recovered from water is a strong indication of drowning death.

frottage [French (from *frott(er)* to rub one body on another + -*age* -AGE), a rubbing of one body on another]   The obtaining of sexual gratification by rubbing against the sexual object.

frotteur [French, from *frott(er)* to rub one body against another + -*eur* -ER]   The sexually active person in frottage.

fructi-   FRUCTO-.

fructification [L *fructificatio* (from *fructificatus*, past part. of *fructificare* to bear fruit, from *fruct(us)* fruit + *i ro*+ -*ficare* English -*fy*, suffix denoting to make) a bearing fruit] **1** The process of producing fruit. **2** The formation of a fruiting body. **3** FRUITING BODY.

fructivorous   Existing on a diet composed of fruit. Also *frugivorous*.

fructo- [L *fructus* fruit]   A combining form denoting relationship to fructose, as in *phosphofructokinase*. Also *fructi-*.

fructofuranose [*fructo(se)* + *furanose*, from *furan* (from L *fur(fur)* bran + -*an(e)*, variant of -INE) + -OSE^2]   Fructose in its furanose form; a hemiacetal formed between its carbonyl group and O-5. This is only a minor form in solution, where the more stable 6-membered ring is favored, but occurs if O-6 is substituted (as in fructose 6-phosphate), and it predominates also in glycosides of fructose, such as sucrose.

fructofuranoside   A glycoside of fructose in the furanose form.

fructokinase   The enzyme (EC 2.7.1.4) that catalyzes the reaction of fructose with ATP to form ADP and fructose 1-phosphate. In animals, this is one of the ways in which fructose derived from the digestion of sucrose can enter metabolism. It is also a route for the assimilation of fructose by microorganisms.

fructopyranose   Fructose in its pyranose form; a hemiacetal formed between its carbonyl group and O-6. This form predominates in solution. The alternative fructofuranose form is commoner in glycosidically linked fructose.

fructose [L *fructus* (from *fructus*, past part. of *frui* to have the use or profit of, akin to *ferre* to bear) fruit + -*ose*, carbohydrate suffix esp. denoting sugar] CH_2OH—$[CHOH]_3$—CO—CH_2OH. A 6-carbon ketose sugar with the same configuration at its chiral atoms as that of glucose. It exists mainly in the pyranose form when uncombined. Its main occurrences are in combination as sucrose, and as phosphates, which are intermediates in several pathways of carbohydrate metabolism. It is the most rapidly absorbed simple sugar and is sweeter than sucrose. Also called *levulose* (outmoded).

fructose-bisphosphatase   The enzyme (EC 3.1.3.11) that catalyzes the hydrolysis of fructose 1,6-bisphosphate to fructose 6-phosphate and orthophosphate. It is allosterically controlled, being inhibited by AMP and activated by citrate. The progress of glycolysis depends on its being inactive, whereas gluconeogenesis requires its activity.

fructose 1,6-bisphosphate   Fructose carrying phosphate groups on O-1 and O-6. It is an intermediate in glycolysis, being formed from ATP and fructose 6-phosphate under the influence of phosphofructokinase, and also in gluconeogenesis, being formed by aldol condensation of triose phosphates. Also called *fructose 1,6-diphosphate, Harden-Young ester* (obsolete).

fructose 2,6-bisphosphate   The glycoside formed between fructose 6-phosphate and phosphoric acid. It stimulates phosphofructokinase and inhibits fructose-bisphosphatase, thereby stimulating glycolysis. In liver, its concentration falls in response to stimulation by glucagon.

fructose-bisphosphate aldolase The enzyme (EC 4.1.2.13) of the glycolytic pathway that catalyzes the interconversion of fructose 1,6-bisphosphate with glyceraldehyde 3-phosphate and glycerone phosphate (dihydroxyacetone phosphate), often simply known as aldolase. It is highly specific for glycerone phosphate, but catalyzes its condensation with a variety of aldehydes. Also called *aldolase*.

fructose 1,6-diphosphate FRUCTOSE 1,6-BISPHOSPHATE.

fructosemia The presence of fructose in blood. Also called *levulosemia*.

fructose 1-phosphate The product of fructokinase. It is an intermediate in the catabolism of fructose. A specific aldolase converts it in the liver into glyceraldehyde and dihydroxyacetone phosphate.

fructose 6-phosphate An intermediate in glycolysis. It is formed by the isomerization of glucose 6-phosphate and is a substrate for phosphofructokinase, which converts it into fructose 1,6-bisphosphate. It can also be formed, especially in adipose tissue, by phosphorylation of fructose with hexokinase.

fructosidase Any enzyme capable of liberating fructose, possibly substituted by other sugars, from glycoside linkage by hydrolysis.

fructoside Any compound containing fructose in glycosidic linkage, such as sucrose, which is β-D-fructofuranosyl-(2′1)-α-D-glucopyranoside.

fructosuria [*fructos(e)* + -URIA] The excretion of fructose in the urine.

  benign fructosuria A rare, asymptomatic, metabolic defect, apparently confined to Jewish people, in which an excess blood fructose level after meals is associated with fructosuria. The condition probably is due to a deficiency of hepatic fructokinase. Also called *essential fructosuria*.

  essential fructosuria BENIGN FRUCTOSURIA.

fructosyl The group formed by removing the 2-hydroxyl group from the furanose or, occasionally, pyranose form of fructose.

frugivorous FRUCTIVOROUS.

Frugoni [Cesare *Frugoni*, Italian physician, born 1881] See under SYNDROME.

fruit [Old French (from L *fructus* fruit, from *fructus* or *fruitus*, past part. of *frui* to have the use or profit of, akin to *ferre* to bear), fruit] In flowering plants, a mature ovary or group of ovaries that contains one or more seeds.

fruitarian [FRUIT + -ARIAN AS IN VEGETARIAN] One who lives on a diet consisting mainly of fruit.

fruitarianism [FRUITARIAN + -ISM] The consumption of a diet composed chiefly of fruit.

frumentum [L (from *fructus*, past part. of *frui* to have the use of fruit), corn or grain, esp. wheat or barley] GRAIN.

frust. *frustillatum* (L, in small pieces).

frustration [L *frustratio* (from *frustratus*, past part. of *frustrare* to deceive, frustrate, from *frustra* deceitfully, in vain) a deceiving, frustration] Lack or denial of gratification, as because of internal conflict or external circumstances; the thwarting of a desire.

frustule [L *frustul(um)* (dim. of *frustum* a piece of anything) a small piece] The siliceous cell wall of a diatom.

fry [Middle English *frie*, prob. a combining of Old Norse *frjo* offspring with Anglo-French *frei* offspring, from Old French *freier, frier* to spawn, from L *fricare* to rub] A recently hatched fish that still bears a yolk sac.

FSH follicle stimulating hormone.

FSHRF follicle stimulating hormone releasing factor (follicle stimulating hormone releasing hormone).

FSHRH follicle stimulating hormone releasing hormone.

ft Symbol for the unit, foot.

ft. *fiat* (L, let it be made).

ft² Symbol for the unit, square foot.

ft³ Symbol for the unit, cubic foot.

ftc Symbol for the obsolete unit, foot candle.

ftH₂O Symbol for the unit, conventional foot of water.

FTI free thyroxine index.

ft La Symbol for the unit, foot lambert.

ft·lb Symbol for the unit, foot pound.

ft·lbf Symbol for the unit, foot pound-force.

ft. mas. div. in pil. *fiat massa dividenda in pilulae* (L, let a mass be made, to be divided into pills).

ft·pdl Symbol for the obsolete unit, foot poundal.

ft. pulv. *fiat pulvis* (L, let a powder be made).

Fuadin A proprietary name for stibophen.

Fuchs [Ernst *Fuchs*, Austrian ophthalmologist, 1851–1930] **1** See under POSITION, ATROPHY, SIGN, COLOBOMA, DYSTROPHY. **2** Fuchs stomas. See under STOMA. **3** Dalen-Fuchs nodules. See under NODULE. **4** Fuchs syndrome. See under HETEROCHROMIC CYCLITIS. **5** Crypts of Fuchs. See under CRYPTS OF IRIS. **6** Fuchs dimples. See under DELLEN.

fuchsin [after Leonhard *Fuchs*, German physician and botanist, 1501–1566 + -IN] Any of several dyes or stains that impart a red or purple color. They may be either acid or basic.

  acid fuchsin A synthetic acid dye that is the sulfonated derivative of basic fuchsin. It is used in the van Gieson and Masson trichrome connective tissue stains. Also called *acid fuchsin stain, rubin*.

  basic fuchsin A biologic stain that is a mixture of pararosanilin, rosanilin, and magenta II. It is a powerful dye used in the Ziehl-Neelsen technique and is the main constituent of Schiff's reagent. Also called *aniline red, basic rubin, basic fuchsin stain, magenta, diamond fuchsin*.

  diamond fuchsin BASIC FUCHSIN.

  English fuchsin A synthetic basic dye that is closely related to basic fuchsin and contains roseine, rosanilin, and pararosanilin acetate.

  iron resorcin fuchsin A staining solution of ferric salt, resorcin, and basic fuchsin that is used to demonstrate the presence of elastic fibers in tissues.

fuchsinophil Denoting the affinity of a tissue structure for acidic or basic fuchsin. Also *fuchsinophilic, fuchsinophilous*.

fuchsinophilia The property of staining with either basic or acid fuchsin.

fuchsinophilic FUCHSINOPHIL.

fuchsinophilous FUCHSINOPHIL.

fucosan A polysaccharide formed of fucose residues. Although fucose is common in oligosaccharides, such as those of the blood group substances, polymers of it alone are rare, except in certain seaweeds.

fucose L-Fucose (6-deoxy-L-galactose). A substance that occurs widely in the carbohydrates of glycoproteins. It is produced as its GDP derivative from GDP-D-mannose by a series of reactions in which C-6 is deoxygenated and the centers at C-3 and C-5 are epimerized. D-Fucose is used experimentally as a noncatabolizable analogue of galactose.

fucoside A glycoside of fucose.

fucosidosis Either of two types of an autosomal recessive inborn error of glycoprotein degradation due to deficiency of the enzyme α-fucosidase. The two major clinical variants share mild coarsening of the facies, hepatosplenomegaly, mental retardation, and vacuolated lymphocytes. Type I is of infantile onset with frequent seizures. Type II is of childhood onset and causes the development of tortuous conjunctival vessels and angiokeratoma.

fucoxanthin $C_{40}H_{56}O_6$. The carotenoid pigment found in brown algae.

fucus   The dried thallus of the marine alga *Fucus vesiculosus*, bladderwrack, rockweed, or seawrack. It contains minute amounts of iodine and has been used to stimulate thyroid activity.

FUDR   floxuridine.

Fuerbringer   [Paul Walther *Fuerbringer*, German physician, 1849–1930]   See under LAW.

fugacity   [L *fugax*, gen. *fugacis* (from *fugere* to flee) flying swiftly, fleeting + -ITY]   A physical property of a gas, the quantity to which its chemical potential is related in the same way that chemical potential would be related to pressure for an ideal gas. It therefore approaches the actual pressure at low pressures, and is an idealized pressure.

-fuge   [L *fugare* to put to flight]   A combining form designating an agent that expels or rids of.

fugitive   [L *fugitiv(us)* (from *fugit(us)*, past part. of *fugere* to flee, vanish + -*ivus* -IVE) running away]   Existing briefly or changing rapidly, and therefore difficult to distinguish; fleeting, as a symptom.

fugu   The Japanese name for PUFFER.

fugue   [French (from Italian *fuga* flight, fugue in music, from L *fuga* a fleeing, flight, desire to escape, akin to Gk *phygē flight), a fugue in music, escape*]   A condition in which the subject takes leave of his usual activities and wanders about. Typically the individual suffers from amnesia for the period he is absent from his usual activities.

epileptic fugue   Prolonged epileptic automatism, lasting for several hours, and in rare cases for days, and occurring during a postepileptic confusional state, usually in cases of temporal lobe epilepsy.

hysterical fugue   An amnesic episode marked by loss of a sense of personal identity as a consequence of hysteria, usually in an effort to escape the stress of emotional conflict, and by the desertion of one's usual surroundings. The subject may wander briefly around his own neighborhood or travel over great distances for extended periods, with no subsequent memory of the episode. It has not been associated with demonstrable organic disorders, such as epilepsy.

Fukala   [Vincenz *Fukala*, Austrian ophthalmologist, 1847–1911] See under OPERATION.

fulcrum of the tooth   A hypothetical fulcrum about which a tooth rotates in a vertical plane when a lateral tilting force is applied to it, as in orthodontics. It is situated at approximately one third of the length of the root from the apex.

fulfillment / wish fulfillment   Gratification of an impulse or desire.

fulgurant   Piercing; intense. Also *fulgurating*.

fulgurate   To destroy (tissue) with a sparking electrode.

fulgurating   1 FULGURANT.   2 Of or relating to fulguration.

fulguration   [L *fulguratio* (from *fulguratus*, past part. of *fulgurare* to send lightning flashes, from *fulgur* lightning) a lightning flash]   A method of destroying tissue using a sparking, movable electrode.

Keating-Hart fulguration   See under KEATING-HART METHOD.

fulgurize   To treat (necrotic tissue) by fulguration.

fuliginous   [Late l *fuligin(osus)* (from L *fuligo*, gen. *fuliginis*, soot + -*osus* -OSE¹) sooty + -OUS]   Sooty in color.

Fülleborn   [Friedrich *Fülleborn*, German parasitologist, 1866–1933]   See under METHOD.

Fuller   [Eugene *Fuller*, U.S. urologist, 1858–1930]   See under OPERATION.

füllkörper   Degenerated glial cells. An obsolete term.

fulminant   [L *fulminans*, gen. *fulminantis*, pres. part. of *fulminare* to fulminate, strike with lightning]   Sudden and severe, as the onset of an illness; hyperacute. Also *fulminating, foudroyant*.

fulminating   FULMINANT.

fulminic acid $H—O—N^+\equiv C^-$. The hypothetical acid that is parent of organic compounds of the type R—O—NC. It polymerizes as it is formed, probably via the predominant tautomer $O^-—N^+\equiv C—H$. Its salts are highly unstable, and its mercury salt readily detonates and is used for that purpose.

fumarase   The original name for FUMARATE HYDRATASE.   • The name was changed because the ending -*ase* applied to the name of a substrate normally implies that the enzyme hydrolyzes that substrate. Fumarase catalyzes the reversible hydration of fumarate to malate.

fumarate hydratase   The enzyme (EC 4.2.1.2) that catalyzes the readily reversible *trans* addition of water to fumarate to form (*S*)-malate. This is a step in the citric acid cycle. Also called *fumarase (original name)*.

fumarate reductase (NADH)   The enzyme (EC 1.3.1.6) that catalyzes the reduction of fumarate to succinate with concomitant oxidation of NADH.

fumaric acid $HOOC—CH\equiv CH—COOH$. The isomer of butenedioic acid with *trans* configuration. It is an intermediate in the citric acid cyle, being made from succinic acid by dehydrogenation, and being converted into malic acid by addition of the elements of water.

fumaric hydrogenase   An outmoded term for SUCCINATE DEHYDROGENASE.

fumarine   PROTOPINE.

fumarylacetoacetic acid   (2*E*)-4,6-Dioxooct-2-endioic acid. An intermediate in the catabolism of phenylalanine and tyrosine, in which it is formed by isomerization of maleylacetoacetic acid and is hydrolyzed to form fumaric and acetoacetic acids.

fume   [L *fum(are)* (from *fumus* smoke, fume) to emit smoke or fumes]   1 A noxious and usually odorous gaseous emanation. 2 To give out fumes.

fumigacin   An outmoded term for HELVOLIC ACID.

fumigant   [L *fumigans*, gen. *fumigantis*, pres. part. of *fumigare* to smoke, from *fum(us)* smoke + *agere* to do]   A gas or aerosol used for disinfecting rooms or materials.

fumigate   [L *fumigat(us)*, past part. of *fumigare* (from *fum(us)* smoke + -*igare*, combining form akin to *agere* to do, drive) to smoke]   To expose to fumes, as of a disinfecting agent or pesticide, or of smoke, as from the emission of chimneys.

fumigation   [Late L *fumigatio* (from *fumigatus*, past part. of *fumigare* to smoke), a smoking, fumigating. See FUMIGANT.] The process of introducing a fumigant into an enclosed atmosphere for the purpose of disinfecting the enclosure and/or its contents.

fumigator   [*fumigat(e)* + -OR]   1 An appliance used for the fumigation of rooms or materials.   2 A person who undertakes fumigation.

fuming   Describing solutions of nitric, sulfuric, and hydrochloric acids that contain extra oxides of nitrogen, sulfur trioxide, and hydrogen chloride, respectively, dissolved in the acid or in its solution. Such acids fume in moist air. Fuming sulfuric acid is a powerful dehydrating agent, since sulfur trioxide reacts violently with water to form sulfuric acid.

Fumiron   A proprietary name for ferrous fumarate.

functio FUNCTION.

functio laesa A loss of function.

function [L *functio* (from *functus*, past part. of *fungi* to do, execute) a doing, executing] **1** The action or office performed by an organ, part, or substance of the body. Also called *functio*. **2** The characteristic action of a compound due to its composition or structure.

allomeric function The coordinated activity of the lower brainstem and spinal cord when considered as a single functioning unit.

arousal function The capacity that a sensory stimulus possesses to induce a state of vigilance, awareness, or readiness in the cerebral cortex; the induction of an activated electroencephalogram by a sensory stimulus.

Carnot's function CARNOTIC FUNCTION.

carnotic function The relationship between the amount of heat lost and the quantity of work performed as a result of the heat expended. Also called *Carnot's function*.

correlation function CORRELATION COEFFICIENT.

discriminant function An algebraic expression embodying a linear combination of variables that contribute to differentiating or discriminating two or more conditions or categories.

ego function The work of the ego in perceiving reality, mediating between it and the person and adapting the person to reality. Its tasks include perception, self-awareness, motor control, defense mechanisms, replacement of the primary process of the id with the secondary process, memory, affects, thinking, thought synthesis, and creativity.

executant ego function The task of the ego to replace the id's primary process with the secondary process.

frequency function A mathematical expression indicating the frequency attaching to each value of a random variable as a function of that value.

glottal area function The area defined by the vocal folds and the posterior laryngeal commissure plotted as a dependent variable of time.

group function The harmonious contacts of a group of teeth with their antagonists.

isomeric function The sensory, motor, or reflexive function of an isolated segment of the spinal cord.

life table function See under LIFE TABLE.

linear function A function of the general form $y = a + bx$ where a and b are constants. The graph of y against x is a straight line with slope $= b$ and intercept $= a$.

line-spread function A plot of count rate against the position of a thin "line" source of radioactivity as it is moved, at right angles to the line, across the field of vision of a collimated detector. The line source is oriented at right angles to the detector's axis, and the distance from the detector is kept constant throughout a given pass. This distance must be specified, since the spread is a function of the distance.

logistic function A function expressing the relationship between two variables, x and y, that has the general form:

$$y = \frac{k}{1 + e^{a+bx}},$$

where a and b are parameters and e is the exponential constant ($= 2.71828 \ldots$). The growth (or decline) in populations may be represented at least aproximately by the logistic function, with x as time and y as size. With suitable parameters a logistic function may also express the risk of disease (y) according to the level (x) of a risk factor.

modulation transfer function A measure of the efficiency of an imaging system in transferring the details of an object to those of the image. It is the ratio of image modulation to object modulation, plotted through some practical range of spatial frequencies in the object. In gamma imaging, the radioactivity in the object is assumed to vary sinusoidally with position from A_{max} to A_{min}, in which case the object modulation is $(A_{max} - A_{min})/(A_{max} + A_{min})$. The spatial frequency is the reciprocal of the distance between adjacent maximum peaks. The image modulation is derived in the same way, and the ratio between mod_m and mod_{ob} is then calculated for the range of spatial frequencies of practical interest. Because of imperfect system resolution, the ratio becomes smaller as the spatial frequency increases, that is, as maxima and minima crowd closer together. The modulation transfer function is the Fourier transform of the line-spread function. Abbreviation: MTF

multiple logistic function A function used in the statistical analysis of the results of epidemiologic investigations to assess the relative contribution of several independent variables to the outcome under study. An example would be the influence of blood pressure, serum cholesterol, and smoking, separately, on the occurrence of coronary heart disease.

probability density function A frequency function in which the relative frequencies are regarded as probabilities.

psychological function An ongoing behavior or mental activity that contributes to some adaptation of the organism as a whole to the conditions of its surroundings. It is analogous to the physiologic function of an organ, such as the secretion of thyroxin by the thyroid gland. Thus, learning and the operation of the sensory processes underlying distance perception are held to be psychological functions of the cerebral cortex.

functional **1** Of or relation to a function; specifically, serving to contribute to the operation of a bodily function. **2** Having no known organic cause, as *functional disorder*.

functionalism One of the early schools of psychological thought which took as the proper subject matter for psychological study those mental processes or chains of actions that demonstrate a usefulness in the adjustment of the organism to its environment. The principles of functionalism have been absorbed into the main themes of contemporary psychology.

funda A four-tailed bandage used in a slinglike fashion, as, for example, to support and limit the motion of the mandible.

fundal Of or pertaining to a fundus.

fundament [L *fundament(um)* (from *funda(re)* to lay a foundation (from *fundus* bottom) + -*mentum* -MENT) a foundation] **1** In anatomy, the anus and surrounding region; the buttocks. **2** The base of a part or structure. **3** A structure when it first begins to develop its shape or form.

fundectomy FUNDUSECTOMY.

fundi Plural of FUNDUS.

fundic Pertaining to a fundus.

fundiform Having a slinglike configuration.

fundoplasty [*fund(us)* + *o* + -PLASTY] GASTROESOPHAGOPLASTY.

fundoplication Plication of the fundus of the stomach around the lower esophagus, a surgical treatment for gastroesophageal reflux.

fundoscopy [*fund(us)* + *o* + -SCOPY] An imprecise term for OPHTHALMOSCOPY. ● *Fundoscopy* might equally well describe examination of the fundus of the uterus or of the stomach as the fundus of the eye.

Fundulus [L, dim. of *fundus* the bottom or base of a thing] A genus of small omnivorous fish of the family cyprinodontidae; the killfish. They are used extensively in research and for mosquito control.

fundus [L, the bottom or base of a thing] The base, bottom, or lowest part of an organ, often opposite the main opening, to or from, a hollow organ.

albinotic fundus The fundus of the eye of a patient with a congenital deficiency of melanin in the choroid and retina.

fundus albipunctatus   A genetic disease of the retinal pigment epithelium, characterized by the appearance of multiple, small, discrete, pale, rounded discolorations of this layer. It is generally benign. Also called *Lauber's disease.*

fundus of bladder   FUNDUS VESICAE URINARIAE.

fundus of cecum   The sacculation lateral to the tenia libera of the cecum that has grown more rapidly and larger than the sacculation on the medial side, resulting in its becoming the apex and lowest part of the cecum. The medial side of the cecum, with the appendix attached, is thus displaced to the left and superiorly. This appearance of the cecum in adults is the most common of the four variations in the shape and position of the cecum usually described. An outmoded term.

fundus of eye   FUNDUS OCULI.

fundus flavimaculatus   A genetic disease of the retinal pigment epithelium, characterized by the appearance of multiple, small, elongated, pale discolorations of this layer. It often is associated with a juvenile macular degeneration.

fundus of gallbladder   FUNDUS VESICAE BILIARIS.

fundus gastricus   [NA] The dome-shaped part of the stomach which is situated above and to the left of the cardiac orifice and is usually distended with gas. Also called *fundus of stomach, fundus ventricularis, fundus ventriculi* (outmoded), *fornix gastricus, fornix ventricularis, fornix of stomach.* • In radiologic anatomy, the term *fornix gastricus* is more common than *fundus gastricus.*

fundus of internal acoustic meatus   FUNDUS MEATUS ACUSTICI INTERNI.

leopard fundus   TESSELATED FUNDUS.

fundus meatus acustici interni   [NA] The lateral end or bottom of the internal acoustic meatus, formed by a vertical plate of bone which separates it from the internal ear and is divided by the transverse crest. Above the crest the facial nerve area is anterior to the superior vestibular area, while below the crest the tractus spiralis foraminosus is anterior to the inferior vestibular area and the foramen singulare. Also called *fundus of internal acoustic meatus.*

fundus oculi   The posterior part of the interior of the eye as viewed on ophthalmoscopy. It comprises the optic part of the retina and parts of the choroid and sclera. Also called *fundus of eye, eyeground.*

fundus of seminal vesicle   The rounded superolateral blind end of the seminal vesicle that lies below the termination of the ureter at the base of the bladder. An outmoded term.

fundus of stomach   FUNDUS GASTRICUS.

tesselated fundus   The mottled appearance of the fundus if a moderate amount of choroidal melanin contrasts with the reddish choroidal vessels, a normal variant of the fundus pattern. Also called *tigroid fundus, leopard fundus, tigroid retina, leopard retina.*

tigroid fundus   TESSELATED FUNDUS.

fundus tympani   PARIES JUGULARIS CAVITATIS TYMPANICAE.

fundus of urinary bladder   FUNDUS VESICAE URINARIAE.

fundus uteri   [NA] The domelike upper part of the body of the uterus that lies above the plane through the points of attachment of the uterine tubes. It is covered with peritoneum continuous with that on the anterior and posterior surfaces. Also called *fundus of uterus.*

fundus of uterus   FUNDUS UTERI.

fundus of vagina   FORNIX VAGINAE.

fundus vaginae   An outmoded term for FORNIX VAGINAE.

fundus ventricularis   FUNDUS GASTRICUS.

fundus ventriculi   An outmoded term for FUNDUS GASTRICUS.

fundus vesicae biliaris   [NA] The rounded, dilated end of the gallbladder that usually extends downwards and forwards beyond the inferior margin of the liver to come into contact with the anterior abdominal wall at the point where the ninth costal cartilage meets the right lateral line. It is covered by peritoneum. Also called *fundus of gallbladder, fundus vesicae felleae.*

fundus vesicae felleae   FUNDUS VESICAE BILIARIS.

fundus vesicae urinariae   [NA] The triangular base of the urinary bladder, directed posteriorly and inferiorly. In males it is separated from the rectum by the rectovesical pouch of peritoneum superiorly and by the seminal vesicles, deferent ducts, and rectovesical fascia inferiorly. In females it is related to the cervix uteri and the upper part of the anterior wall of the vagina. The internal aspect of the fundus constitutes the trigonum vesicae. Also called *fundus of urinary bladder, fundus of bladder, infundibulum of urinary bladder, base of bladder.*

funduscope   [*fundu(s)* + -SCOPE]   An imprecise term for OPHTHALMOSCOPE.

funduscopy   [*fundu(s)* + -SCOPY]   An imprecise term for OPHTHALMOSCOPY. • *Funduscopy* might equally well describe examination of the fundus of the uterus or of the stomach as the fundus of the eye.

fluorescein funduscopy   The use of intravenous fluorescein to permit more detailed examination of the circulation of the retina and choroid.

fundusectomy   [FUNDUS + -ECTOMY]   **1** A surgical removal of the base of or a broad part of an organ. Also called *fundectomy.* **2** The surgical removal of the fundus of the stomach.

fungal   Of, pertaining to, charactistic of, or caused by a fungus. Also *fungous.*

fungate   [*fung(us)* + -ATE]   To grow rapidly, like a mushroom, away from the substrate.

fungating   Descriptive of a lesion that, by virtue of its proliferative capacity, protrudes from its site of origin as a spongy growth.

fungemia   MYCETHEMIA.

fungi   Plural of FUNGUS.

fungicidal   Destructive of or deleterious to fungi.

fungicide   [L *fungi,* pl. of *fungus* fungus + -CIDE]   Any agent used to kill or inhibit fungi. Also called *mycocide* (seldom used).

fungicidin   An outmoded term for NYSTATIN.

fungiform   Resembling a mushroom.

Fungi Imperfecti   DEUTEROMYCETES.

fungimycin   An antifungal antibiotic agent obtained from *Streptomyces coelicolor* var. *aminophilus.* It is an amorphous yellow solid that is practically insoluble in water. It is an aromatic antibiotic and it contains an amino-sugar, perosamine. Also called *perimycin.*

fungistasis   [FUNGI + STASIS]   Inhibition of the growth of a fungus brought about by a chemical or physical agent.

fungistat   [L *fungi,* pl. of *fungus* fungus + -STAT]   Any agent that inhibits fungal growth without killing the fungus. Also called *mycostat.*

fungistatic   Inhibiting the growth of a fungus or fungi. Also *mycostatic.*

fungitoxic   Having the ability to kill or inhibit fungi.

fungitoxicity   The attribute of having a destructive effect on fungi.

fungivore   An animal that consumes fungi.

Fungizone   A proprietary name for amphotericin B.

fungoid   Resembling or having characteristics of a fungus. Also *fungous, mycetoid, mycoid.*

chignon fungoid   A nodular condition of human hair that is presumed to be caused by a fungal infection. An obsolete term.

fungosity   A fungus or funguslike growth.

fungous 1 FUNGOID. 2 FUNGAL.

funguria [*fung(us)* + -URIA] The presence of a fungus in the urine.

fungus [L (from or akin to Gk *spongos, sphongos* a sponge), a mushroom, toadstool, a kind of blasting or measles in a tree] (*plural* fungi) Any of a large group of achlorophyllous, spore-bearing eukaryotes having either a typically walled thallus with absorptive nutrition or an unwalled thallus with saprophytic nutrition.

aphrodisiac fungus A fungus, *Elaphomyces cervinus,* considered to increase sexual desire if ingested.

bakanae fungus The fungus *Gibberella fujikuroi,* which causes so-called foolish seedling disease of rice. A metabolic by-product of the fungus, gibberellin, causes infected rice plants to become very tall. Extracts of the fungus are sold commercially as promoters of plant growth. Also called *rice fungus.*

beefsteak fungus The fungus *Gyromitra esculenta* (sometimes classified as *Helvella esculenta*). It is generally believed that eastern North American forms of the fungus contain varying amounts of monomethylhydrazine. This fungus can cause gastrointestinal upsets, and some instances of death have been recorded. Also called *lorchel.*

biphasic fungi False yeasts, such as *Candida,* which are able to grow by budding to typical ovoid yeast cells or develop in a mycelial form.

bird's-nest fungus Any fungus of the order Nidulariales. These fungi, at maturity, resemble minute birds' nests containing eggs.

bracket fungus Any fungus that forms a shelflike or bracketlike growth, usually projecting from a tree trunk. Also called *shelf fungus, conk.*

fungus of the brain A morbid, granulating protrusion of brain tissue through an opening in the skull. Also called *cerebral fungus, fungus cerebri.*

cerebral fungus FUNGUS OF THE BRAIN.

fungus cerebri FUNGUS OF THE BRAIN.

club fungus Any fungus of the family Clavariaceae.

coral fungus Any of certain fungi which resemble coral and belong to the family Clavariaceae.

cup fungus Any ascomycetous fungus having a cuplike shape.

cutaneous fungus A seldom used term for DERMATOPHYTE.

dematiaceous fungi 1 Fungi which have dark-colored vegetative structures and/or conidia. 2 Fungi of the form-family Dematiaceae.

dimorphic fungus Any fungus that is capable of responding to environmental conditions by growing a different form for each substrate, such as a filamentous form on or in a solid substrate, and a yeastlike form in liquid media.

fission fungus An obsolete term for BACTERIUM. • This is a literal translation of *schizomycete.*

foot fungus 1 An organism that causes tinea pedis. 2 An organism that causes mycetoma of the foot. 3 An imprecise term for TINEA PEDIS. 4 See under MYCETOMA.

fungus haematodes A soft hemorrhagic tumor. An obsolete term.

imperfect fungus Any member of the form-class Deuteromyces; a fungus having no known sexual stage of reproduction. Also called *adelomycete.*

jack-o'-lantern fungus The luminescent fungus *Omphalotus olearius.*

jelly fungus Any of a group of fungi of the family Tremellaceae, that, when wet or moist, appear or feel gelatinous or jellylike. Also called *trembling fungus.*

kefir fungus A mixture of yeasts and bacteria used to produce kefir milk, a fermented milk popular in the Balkans.

mold fungus MYCELIAL FUNGUS.

mosaic fungus An incorrect term for MOSAIC ARTIFACT. • The hexagonally patterned network seen in microscopic examinations of skin scrapings that are cleaned with potassium hydroxide solution was once believed to be fungal hyphae, hence the misleading term *mosaic fungus.*

mycelial fungus Any fungus that produces a mat of intermingled hyphae, forming a mycelium. Also called *mold fungus.*

oyster-cap fungus Any fungus of the species *Pleurotus ostreatus.*

perfect fungus Any fungus whose sexual and asexual methods of reproduction are known.

pore fungus Any of the basidiomyceteous fungi of the orders Agaricales and Aphyllophorales, having pores instead of gills.

proper fungus Any fungus included in the obsolete grouping Eumycetes. An obsolete term. Also called *true fungus.*

ray fungus An outmoded term for ACTINOMYCETE.

rice fungus BAKANAE FUNGUS.

sac fungus ASCOMYCETE.

saddle fungus Any fungus of the genus *Helvella.*

shelf fungus BRACKET FUNGUS.

slime fungus Any member of the class Myxomycota.

sulfur fungus SULFUR POLYPORE.

thread fungus Any fungus having a hyphal growth which resembles a thread.

thrush fungus *CANDIDA ALBICANS.*

trembling fungus JELLY FUNGUS.

true fungus PROPER FUNGUS.

umbilical fungus GRANULOMA OF THE UMBILICUS.

yeastlike fungus Any fungus which lacks the sexual means of reproduction and which is also diphasic, one form resembling ovoid yeast cells and the other form being hyphal.

funic 1 Pertaining to a funis. 2 Pertaining to the umbilical cord. For defs. 1 and 2 also *funicular.*

funicalgia [*funic(ulus)* + -ALGIA] Pain caused by compression of a nerve root as it enters or runs through the intervertebral foramen in the spinal column. A rarely used term.

funicle FUNICULUS.

funicular 1 Pertaining to any funiculus. 2 FUNIC.

funiculate Possessing or forming a funiculus.

funiculi Plural of FUNICULUS.

funiculitis [*funicul(us)* + -ITIS] 1 Inflammation of the spermatic cord. Also called *corditis.* 2 Inflammation of a spinal nerve or of a nerve fiber tract within the spinal canal.

endemic funiculitis An acute inflammation of the spermatic cord, usually associated with orchitis, caused by filarial infections (*Wuchereria bancrofti* or *Brugia malayi*). Hydrocele may occur. A high concentration of microfilariae can usually be demonstrated in the tunica vaginalis. Abscess formation and necrosis rarely occur.

filarial funiculitis Lymphatic filariasis caused by *Wuchereria bancrofti* and *Brugia malayi* with secondary involvement of the spermatic cord.

syphilitic funiculitis SYPHILIS OF THE SPERMATIC CORD.

funiculopexy [*funicul(us)* + *o* + -PEXY] Surgical correction of undescended testes by suturing the spermatic cord to surrounding tissue.

funiculus [L (dim. of *funis* a rope, cord), a thin rope] [NA] A small cordlike or bandlike structure, as of nerve fibers. Also called *funicle.*

funiculus anterior medullae spinalis The white matter of the spinal cord lying between the anterior median fissure and the ventral root entry zone and containing longitudinal ascending and descending tracts. Also called *ventral funiculus, funiculus ventralis, anterior funiculus of spinal cord.*

anterior funiculus of spinal cord FUNICULUS ANTERIOR MEDULLAE SPINALIS.

cuneate funiculus FASCICULUS CUNEATUS MEDULLAE OBLONGATAE.

funiculus cuneatus Burdachi An outmoded term for FASCICULUS CUNEATUS MEDULLAE OBLONGATAE.

funiculus cuneatus lateralis The longitudinal tract of the medulla oblongata that is lateral to the cuneate funiculus and demarcated laterally by the rootlets of the spinal accessory nerve. It contains afferent fibers from the upper cervical dorsal roots to the external cuneate nucleus, and some fibers of the dorsolateral tract of the spinal cord.

funiculus cuneatus medullae oblongatae An outmoded term for FASCICULUS CUNEATUS MEDULLAE OBLONGATAE.

dorsal funiculus FUNICULUS POSTERIOR MEDULLAE SPINALIS.

funiculus dorsalis FUNICULUS POSTERIOR MEDULLAE SPINALIS.

funiculus gracilis An outmoded term for FASCICULUS GRACILIS MEDULLAE OBLONGATAE.

funiculus gracilis medullae oblongatae An obsolete term for FASCICULUS GRACILIS MEDULLAE OBLONGATAE.

hepatic funiculus An outmoded term for DUCTUS CHOLEDOCHUS.

hepatic funiculus of Rauber ARTERIA HEPATICA PROPRIA.

funiculus lateralis medullae oblongatae The medullary continuation of the lateral funiculus of the spinal cord, consisting principally of the anterolateral and spinocerebellar tracts. Also called *lateral funiculus of medulla oblongata*.

funiculus lateralis medullae spinalis The white matter of the spinal cord lateral to the dorsal and ventral horns, especially the ascending tracts. Also called *lateral funiculus of spinal cord, anterolateral column*.

lateral funiculus of medulla oblongata FUNICULUS LATERALIS MEDULLAE OBLONGATAE.

lateral funiculus of spinal cord FUNICULUS LATERALIS MEDULLAE SPINALIS.

ligamentous funiculus LIGAMENTUM COLLATERALE CARPI ULNARE.

funiculi medullae spinalis Longitudinally oriented segments of the white matter of the spinal cord. Dorsal, lateral, and ventral funiculi are recognized. Also called *funiculi of spinal cord*.

funiculus posterior medullae spinalis The longitudinal white matter between the posterior median sulcus and the dorsal root entry zone, consisting principally of myelinated ascending axons including a large component derived from spinal ganglion cells, most of which terminate in the cuneate and gracile nuclei of the medulla oblongata. It consists of two main components, the medial (gracile) and lateral (cuneate) fasciculi. Also called *dorsal funiculus, funiculus dorsalis, posterior funiculus of spinal cord*.

posterior funiculus of spinal cord FUNICULUS POSTERIOR MEDULLAE SPINALIS.

funiculus of Rolando FASCICULUS OF ROLANDO.

funiculus separans The oblique ridge on the caudal floor of the fourth ventricle of the medulla oblongata that separates the area postrema and the vagal trigone.

funiculus solitarius TRACTUS SOLITARIUS.

funiculus spermaticus [NA] The rounded cord extending from the deep inguinal ring and suspending the testis in the scrotum. It is composed of the testicular, cremasteric, and deferential arteries, the testicular veins and pampiniform plexus, lymph vessels, nerves, and the ductus deferens, which in their course through the inguinal canal become surrounded by the internal spermatic fascia, the cremasteric fascia, and the external spermatic fascia that extend down into the wall of the scrotum. Also called *spermatic cord, chorda spermatica* (outmoded), *testicular cord*.

funiculi of spinal cord FUNICULI MEDULLAE SPINALIS.

funiculus teres The median eminence of the floor of the fourth ventricle of the medulla. An obsolete term.

funiculus umbilicalis UMBILICAL CORD.

ventral funiculus FUNICULUS ANTERIOR MEDULLAE SPINALIS.

funiculus ventralis FUNICULUS ANTERIOR MEDULLAE SPINALIS.

funiform Ropelike; cordlike.

funis [L, a rope, cord] 1 Any ropelike structure. 2 UMBILICAL CORD.

funis argenteus An obsolete term for MEDULLA SPINALIS. • The term derives from the spinal cord's fancied resemblance to a silver rope.

funis brachii An outmoded term for VENA INTERMEDIA CEPHALICA.

funis hippocratis TENDO CALCANEUS.

Funkenstein [Daniel Hertz *Funkenstein*, U.S. psychiatrist, born 1910] See under TEST.

funnel [L *fundibulum*, also *infundibulum* (from *infundere* to pour into) a funnel] 1 A device used to transfer or filter liquids that has a wide upper orifice and tapers, often in conical shape, to a narrow neck through which effluent flows in a controllable fashion. 2 An infundibulum.

accessory müllerian funnel A supernumerary uterine tube, or female genital duct or part thereof derived anomalously from the upper end of the paramesonephric duct.

mitral funnel A funnel-shaped mitral valve seen in some cases of mitral stenosis.

muscular funnel The area bounded by the four rectus muscles of the eyeball. It resembles a funnel in shape. An outmoded term.

pial funnel The adventitial sheath surrounding blood vessels leaving and entering the central nervous system, forming a funnel-shaped channel, the Virchow-Robin space, containing cerebrospinal fluid.

Renver's funnel A conic instrument used to expand urethral strictures.

vascular funnel An outmoded term for EXCAVATIO DISCI.

FUO fever of undetermined origin.

Furacin A proprietary name for nitrofurazone.

Furadantin A proprietary name for nitrofurantoin.

furan The heterocyclic compound whose molecule consists of a ring of four —CH= groups and an oxygen atom.

furanose A sugar in the 5-membered ring form produced by reaction of the 5-hydroxyl group with the aldehyde group in an aldose, or of the 6-hydroxyl group with the 2-carbonyl group in a ulose.

furanoside Any glycoside in which the sugar is in its furanose form, i.e. as a five-membered ring. Nucleosides are in the furanoside form, and fructosyl groups, as in sucrose, are usually furanosides.

Furaspor A preparation of 5-nitrofurfuryl methyl ether. A proprietary name.

furazolidone $C_8H_7N_3O_5$. 3-[[(5-Nitro-2-furanyl)methylene]amino]-2-oxazolidinone. An antibacterial and antiprotozoal agent that is used as both a topical anti-infective and as an oral antibacterial dr ug. It is specific for many Gram-negative enteric bacterial species. It is used in the treatment of diarrhea, enteritis, and, often with nifuroxime, candidal, bacterial, and trichomonal forms of vaginitis.

furazolium $C_9H_7N_3O_3S$. 6,7-Dihydro-3-(5-nitro-2-furanyl)-5*H*-imidazo[2,1-*b*]thiazolium. An antibacterial agent. It is also prepared as the tartrate and chloride salts.

furazolium chloride $C_9H_8ClN_3O_3S$. 6,7-Dihydro-3-(5-nitro-

2-furanyl)-5*H*-imidazo[2,1-*b*]thiazol-4-ium chloride. An anti-bacterial agent.

furazosin PRAZOSIN.

furca [L (from *ferre* to bear), a fork]   In anatomy, a fork, usually referring to a two-pronged fork.

caudal furca   The two terminal processes on the last abdominal segment in certain crustaceans.

furca orbitalis ORBITAL FORK.

furcal   Forklike; forked or branched. Also *furcate.*

furcate FURCAL.

furcation [Med L *furcatio* (from *furcatus*, past part. of *furcare* to branch, from L *furca* a two-pronged fork, from *ferre* to bear) a branching, forking]   A region of a multirooted tooth where the individual roots leave the common root stock.

furcocercous [*furc(a)* + *o* + Gk *kerk(os)* tail + -OUS]   Having a bifid (forked) tail, as seen in schistosome and strigeid trematode cercariae.

furcula   A forked ridge, like an inverted U, in the ventral wall of the primitive pharynx. The groove contained between the ridges of the furcula is continued downwards on the ventral wall of the foregut as the laryngotracheal groove from which the lower part of the larynx, trachea, bronchial tree, and lungs will eventually develop.

fureur genitale   An obsolete term for HYPERSEXUALITY.

furfur [L, bran, scales on head, face, skin]   A dry, branlike scale, such as that of pityriasis capitis.

furfuraceous   Resembling furfur; scaling.

furfural   Furan-2-carbaldehyde, i.e. furan substituted with a — CHO group. It is formed by the action of sulfuric acid on pentoses, and its derivatives by the action of sulfuric acid on many sugars.

furfurous   Of or relating to furfur.

furlong [Old English *furlang*, from *furk* furrow + *lang* long]   A unit of length equal to 220 yards; 0.125 mile; 201.168 meters. An obsolete unit.

furnace / dental furnace   A furnace used by a dental technician. There are two types, one which is used for heating refractory molds and which may be heated by a gas flame, and another which is used for firing porcelain and is heated by electricity because a higher temperature is required.

inlay furnace   A dental furnace used for heating the refractory mold in preparation for the casting of inlays.

furocoumarin PSORALEN.

furoic acid   Furancarboxylic acid, either the 2- or the 3- compounds. 2-Furoic acid is obtained by oxidation of furfural.

furor [L (from *furere* to rage, rave), madness, raving, passionate love, poetic frenzy]   Anger; rage; agitation.

furor amatorius   An obsolete term for HYPERSEXUALITY.

furor epilepticus EPILEPTIC FRENZY.

furor femininus NYMPHOMANIA.

furor genitalis   An obsolete term for HYPERSEXUALITY.

paroxysmal furor EPILEPTIC FRENZY.

furor uterinus NYMPHOMANIA.

furosemide $C_{12}H_{11}ClN_2O_5S$.   5-(Aminosulfonyl)-4-chloro-2-[(2-furanylmethyl)amino]benzoic acid, a diuretic that inhibits chloride and sodium reabsorption in the ascending loop of Henle. It is used to treat hypertension and to relieve edema that stems from cardiac, hepatic, or renal disease. It is given orally, but parenteral administration may be employed. Also called *fursemide.*

Furoxone   A proprietary name for furazolidone.

furred   Having the appearance of a hairlike coating such as that acquired by the tongue in certain diseases as a result of the accumulation of debris on its surface.

furrow [Old English *furh*]   A groove or v-shaped hollow; a sulcus.

atrioventricular furrow SULCUS CORONARIUS CORDIS.

digital furrow   The flexure line on the anterior, or palmar, surface of any finger opposite the interphalangeal or metacarpophalangeal joints.

division furrow   One of the ringlike indentations on an animal cell during cytokinesis, due to infolding of the plasma membrane. The cytoplasm beneath the division furrow contains a dense ring of microfilaments (the contractile ring) encircling the cell like a purse string.

genital furrow   The groove on the caudal surface of the genital tubercle of the two month old fetus, which becomes the primary urethral groove. Also called *genital groove.*

gluteal furrow CRENA ANI.

mentolabial furrow SULCUS MENTOLABIALIS.

naso-optic furrow ORBITONASAL CLEFT.

nympholabial furrow   The groove separating the labium majus and labium minus.

primitive furrow   A longitudinal groove on the outer surface of the primitive streak.

Schmorl's furrow   A variable linear depression across the surface of the apex of the lung thought to be secondary to developmental variation of the first rib. Some observers believe the associated pulmonary tissue to be more than normally susceptible to tuberculosis.

scleral furrow SULCUS SCLERAE.

Sibson's furrow   The hollow between the lower border of the pectoralis major muscle and the thoracic wall. Also called *Sibson's groove.*

skin furrows SULCI CUTIS.

fursemide FUROSEMIDE.

Furst [William *Furst*, U.S. physician, flourished mid-20th century]   Ostrum-Furst syndrome. See under KLIPPEL-FEIL SYNDROME.

Fürstner [Carl *Fürstner*, German psychiatrist, 1848–1906]   See under DISEASE.

Furth [Jacob *Furth*, Hungarian-born pathologist active in the U.S., born 1896]   See under TUMOR.

furuncle   A deep staphylococcal folliculitis. Also called *furunculus, boil* (popular).

furuncular FURUNCULOUS.

furunculoid   Resembling a furuncle.

furunculosis [*furuncul(us)* + -OSIS]   A condition marked by the presence of furuncles. Also called *furuncular diathesis, dothienesia* (obsolete).

furunculosis blastomycetica   A systemic mycosis with furuncular lesions of the skin. It is not necessarily caused by blastomycosis. An imprecise and obsolete term.

furunculosis cryptococcica   A systemic mycosis with furunclelike skin involvement. This condition is unusual in cryptococcosis, in which fewer than 10% of the cases have skin lesions. An obsolete term.

furunculosis orientalis CUTANEOUS LEISHMANIASIS.

furunculous   Pertaining to a furuncle. Also called *furuncular.*

furunculus [L (dim. of *fur* a cheat, knave, from Gk *phōr* a thief, from *pherein* to bear, carry), a petty thief]   FURUNCLE.

furunculus orientalis CUTANEOUS LEISHMANIASIS.

furunculus vespajus   A furuncle with several small cavities that exude pus.

fury / alcoholic fury PATHOLOGIC INTOXICATION.

maniacal fury   Rage and aggression that occur as part of manic hyperirritability.

fusariotoxicosis   A toxic condition of swine, cattle, horses and poultry caused by ingestion of feed contaminated with molds of the genus *Fusarium.* Clinical signs are diarrhea, staggers, and anorexia.

Fusarium [L *fus(us)* (akin to *fustis* a stake, club, pole and to *festuca* a stalk, straw) a spindle + *-arium* -ARY] A form-genus of imperfect fungi, some of which are agents of mycotic keratitis.

Fusarium oxysporum A species which causes banana wilt. It also attacks pears, sweet potatoes, and tomatoes.

Fusarium solanae A species which causes potato wilt and has been implicated in occasional cases of mycotic keratitis.

Fusarium sporotrichiella A species of fungus that grows on cereal grains. It is implicated in mycotoxicosis of children of Siberia, northern China, and northern Korea.

fuscin The melanin pigment of the retinal pigment epithelium.

fuse [L *fus(us),* past part. of *fundere* to pour out, fuse, melt] To blend or join, either by melting together to form a combined substance or, with adjacent structures, growing into one another.

fuseau [French (from L *fusus* spindle), spindle] MACROCONIDIUM.

fusible Capable of being liquified or combined by the application of heat.

fusicellular Composed of spindle-shaped cells. Also *fusocellular.*

fusidic acid $C_{16}H_{30}O_6$. A fermentation product derived from the fungus *Fusidium coccineum* and employed as an antibiotic.

fusiform [L *fus(us)* spindle + *i* + -FORM] ° Shaped like a spindle; pointed at both ends.

fusimotor **1** Denoting specifically the γ-efferent nerve fibers which innervate the intrafusal fibers of muscle spindles, in distinction to skeletofusimotor and skeletomotor fibers. **2** Denoting any motor innervation of intrafusal fibers. **3** Denoting the contractile activity of intrafusal fibers.

fusion [L *fusio* (from *fusus,* past part. of *fundere* to pour) a pouring out] **1** In psychology, the union of the libidinal and aggressive drives. **2** Perception of a flickering light as a single, uninterrupted stimulus once the critical flicker frequency is reached. **3** The formation of an ankylosis. **4** Union of two adjacent tooth germs along their whole length or partially. This may result in a large abnormally-shaped tooth or two teeth united at crown or root level. In true fusion the dentin is confluent. Deciduous, permanent, or supernumerary teeth may be involved.

binocular fusion The cortical synthesis of the visual impulses of the same image from both eyes to form an integrated perceptual sensation.

cell fusion The merging of two cells to form one cell. When cells are grown *in vitro* the incidence of fusion is greatly increased by the presence of deactivated Sendai virus, which, by adhering strongly to cell surfaces holds cells together and thus increases the opportunity for fusion.

centric fusion A chromosome rearrangement in which the centromeres of two homologous or nonhomologous chromosomes fuse. It usually involves two acrocentric chromosomes with generation of a metacentric or submetacentric chromosome and a fragment that is composed of the satellites of the original chromosomes. The fragment is usually lost during the next mitosis.

fusion of cervical vertebrae KLIPPEL-FEIL SYNDROME.

diaphyseal-epiphyseal fusion The operative arrest of growth in the length of a bone by fusing the diaphysis and epiphysis. It is used in treating discrepancies in leg length.

flicker fusion The ability of the visual system to perceive a rapid alternation of light and dark as a steady and uniform

illumination. This normally occurs when the alternation occurs more rapidly than at 50 Hz.

gene fusion The fusion of the early part of one gene with the later part of another, producing a hybrid protein if the two regions of DNA are in phase.

nuclear fusion The coalescence of two light atomic nuclei to form a single heavier one. Some of the combined mass disappears, being converted into energy. Because of repulsion between the two positively charged nuclei, strong forces must be present to drive them together. In thermonuclear fusion this is provided by exceedingly high thermal energy.

operon fusion A process of genetic manipulation in cells, or of DNA recombination *in vitro,* that combines the early part of one operon with the later part of another, thus imposing the regulatory mechanisms of one operon on products of another. In cells it is generally achieved by a deletion between two adjacent operons.

protein fusion The hybrid product of a gene fusion.

renal fusion FUSED KIDNEY.

spinal fusion The union of two or more vertebrae, congenitally, as a result of infection, or due to a surgical procedure. Spinal fusion most often applies to a surgical operation designed to abolish motion between vertebrae.

vertebral fusion SPINAL FUSION.

Fusobacterium [*fus(us)* + *o* + BACTERIUM] A genus of Gram-negative anaerobic rods with tapered ends, often found in human cavities and in abscesses. They differ morphologically from the genus *Bacteroides* (both being in the family Bacteroidaceae), and also in forming butyric acid as a major fermentation product.

Fusobacterium fusiformis The type species of *Fusobacterium.* It is a probable cause of Vincent's angina. Also called *Fusobacterium nucleatum, Fusobacterium plantivincenti, Bacteroides fusiformis* (older term), *Bacillus fusiformis* (obsolete), *Vincent's bacillus.*

Fusobacterium nucleatum FUSOBACTERIUM FUSIFORMIS.

Fusobacterium plautivincenti FUSOBACTERIUM FUSIFORMIS.

fusocellular FUSICELLULAR.

fusospirillosis [*fus(us)* + *o* + *spirill(um)* + -OSIS] An outmoded term for FUSOSPIROCHETOSIS.

fusospirochetal Pertaining to the association of *Fusobacterium* species and spirochetes in mixed infections.

fusospirochetosis [*fus(us)* + *o* + SPIROCHETOSIS] Infection with *Fusobacterium* species and spirochetes, involving most commonly the throat, mouth, and gums. These organisms may also be implicated in lung abscesses, vulvovaginitis, and balanitis. Also called *fusospirochetal disease, fusospirillosis.* See also VINCENT'S ANGINA, NECROTIZING ULCERATIVE GINGIVITIS.

fustigation **1** A form of massage in which the body is tapped with light wooden rods. **2** A form of flagellation in which a stick or rod is used.

fusus [L (akin to *fustis* a stake, club, pole and to *festuca* a stalk, straw), a spindle] (*plural* fusi.) A minute, spindle-shaped object or part.

cortical fusi The spindle-shaped air spaces in the cortex of the hair shaft.

fracture fusi Clefts between the fibrils of the hair cortex which are produced by trauma.

fusus neuromuscularis MUSCLE SPINDLE.

fusus neurotendineus TENDON ORGAN.

-fy [from Old French *-fier,* suffix denoting to make, from L *-ficare,* from *facere* to make, do] A suffix meaning to make or form into.

G

G   **1** Symbol for giga-: used with SI units.   **2** Symbol used in physics for the unit, gauss.   **3** Symbol for glycine.   **4** Symbol for guanosine.   **5** gravitational constant.   **6** gonidial (colony).

G₁   A phase of the interphase stage of the cell cycle that precedes DNA synthesis (S phase).

G₂   A phase of the interphase stage of the cell cycle that follows DNA synthesis (S phase) and precedes mitosis.

g   **1** Symbol for the unit, gram.   **2** Symbol for the unit, grade, expressed as a superscript.

g.   gravity.

G   Symbol for the quantities (1) gravitation constant, expressed in newton square meters per kilogram squared; (2) conductance, expressed in siemens (3) Gibbs energy, expressed in joules; (4) weight, expressed in newtons.

g   Symbol for the quantity, acceleration of free fall, expressed in meters per second squared.

gₙ   Symbol for the quantity, standard acceleration of free fall.

γ   **1** The third letter of the Greek alphabet, gamma.   **2** Symbol for the obsolete unit, gamma.

γ   Symbol for the quantities (1) conductivity, expressed in siemens per meter; (2) gyromagnetic ratio, expressed in ampere square meters per joule second; (3) propagation coefficient, expressed in reciprocal meters; (4) ratio of specific heat capacities.

GA   glutaric aciduria.

Ga   Symbol for the element, gallium.

GABA   γ-aminobutyric acid.

gadfly [Middle English *gadd* (from Old Norse *gaddr* a sting) a sharp stick, rod, or tool + Middle English *flie*, from Old English *flȳge, flēoge* a housefly]   Any of various biting, blood-sucking flies of the genus *Tabanus* or of the genus *Hypoderma,* such as the heel fly and ox-warble fly, which cause myiasis in cattle, deer, horses, and occasionally in man.

gadolinium   A rare-earth metal having atomic number 64 and atomic weight 157.25. Seven isotopes occur naturally, six of them stable and the seventh, of 0.2% natural abundance, having a half-life of 1.1×10^{14} years. Ten other unstable isotopes have been described. Symbol: Gd

Gaenslen [Frederick Julius *Gaenslen,* U.S. surgeon, 1877–1937]   Gaenslen's test. See under SIGN.

Gaertner [Gustav *Gaertner,* Austrian pathologist, 1855–1937]   See under TONOMETER.

gafeira   The Portuguese word for MANGE.

Gaffky [Georg Theodor August *Gaffky,* German bacteriologist, 1850–1918]   Gaffky table. See under SCALE.

gag [Middle English *gaggen* to strangle, of imitative origin]   **1** An instrument for forcing open or holding open the mouth of the unconscious patient, particularly when under general anesthesia, and often designed to facilitate surgical access to the mouth, pharynx, and larynx.   **2** To strain involuntarily to vomit; retch.

Boyle-Davis gag   The British term for DAVIS GAG.

Davis gag   An instrument combining an incisor gag and tongue depressor, with the latter incorporating an anesthetic tube. It is used extensively in peroral surgery, particularly dissection tonsillectomy. The chief advantage lies in the manner of use. The gag is introduced and supported with the patient's head hyperextended and the shoulders raised, thereby reducing the risk of the inhalation of blood, which gravitates away from the lower air passages towards the nasopharynx. Also called *Boyle-Davis gag (British usage).*

Davis-Crowe mouth gag   A modification of the Boyle-Davis gag.

Dingman mouth gag   A complex, self-retaining surgical retractor that is used for the intraoral exposure of the palate, usually in the repair of congenital cleft palate. It holds the mouth open and the cheeks aside and keeps the tongue depressed.

Dott gag   A modification of the Boyle-Davis gag, used in operations for the repair of cleft palate.

Doyen gag   A widely used variety of incisor gag.

incisor gag   A mouth gag designed to act by application between the incisor teeth.

Kilner-Dott gag   The Dott gag modified by the inclusion of a suture frame.

Mason gag   A widely used variety of molar gag.

molar gag   A mouth gag designed to act by application between the molar teeth.

gage   GAUGE.

Gaillard [François Lucien *Gaillard,* French physician, 1805–1869]   Gaillard-Arlt suture. See under SUTURE.

gain   An increase in signal voltage or power from input to output in an electronic amplifier or system.

antigen gain   The appearance in cells of new antigenic determinants which were not normally present or expressed in the parent cell.

coarse gain   An instrument control that makes large changes in a parameter while the fine gain makes small changes.

end gain   PARANOSIC GAIN.

epinosic gain   Those advantages, of a secondary nature, that may be derived from an illness or its symptoms, such as the attentiveness and overprotection showered on an invalid by family members. Also called *secondary gain, advantage by illness.*

fine gain   An instrument control that makes small changes in a parameter while the coarse gain makes large changes.

near gain   Electronic amplification of echoes returning from structures close to the ultrasound transducer.

paranosic gain   The fundamental gain derived from an illness, such as the avoidance of anxiety in neurosis. Also called *primary gain, paranosis, end gain.*

primary gain   PARANOSIC GAIN.

secondary gain   EPINOSIC GAIN.

swept gain   Compensation for the effects of attenuation by increasing gain with time from when a pulse was emitted by an ultrasound imaging system. Also called *attenuation compensa-*

tion, electronic distance compensation, time gain compensation.

Gairdner [Sir William Tennant *Gairdner*, Scottish physician, 1824–1907] Gairdner's coin test. See under COIN SOUND.

Gaisböck [Felix *Gaisböck*, Austrian internist, 1868–1955] Gaisböck's disease, Gaisböck syndrome. See under STRESS ERYTHROCYTOSIS.

gait The way in which an individual walks.

antalgic gait A form of gait in which the patient uses a cane, crutch, or other means to avoid painful weight-bearing.

ataxic gait An unsteady gait, due as a rule either to cerebellar ataxia or to sensory ataxia. Also called *staggering gait.*

ataxospastic gait TABETOSPASTIC GAIT.

cerebellar gait A staggering, swaying, and unstable gait, like that of intoxication, seen in cases of bilateral or central cerebellar lesions. In truncal ataxia due to midbrain cerebellar lesions, the patient walks on a broad base and has difficulty in stopping and in turning. When the cerebellar syndrome is unilateral, there is a tendency to deviate to the affected side.

cerebellospastic gait Combined cerebellar ataxia and spasticity with both unsteadiness and stiffness of the legs, as seen most often in multiple sclerosis, but sometimes in the hereditary ataxias. A seldom used term.

Charcot's gait TABETOCEREBELLAR GAIT.

clowns' gait The waddling gait of pelvic girdle muscle weakness, as often seen in myopathy. A seldom used term.

double step gait A syncopated gait in which the time intervals or distances between successive steps are unequal and this uneven sequence occurs repetitively.

drag-to gait A gait in which the patient drags an impaired lower limb towards the advanced crutch.

drunken gait The ataxic gait seen in intoxication with alcohol or other drugs, such as barbiturates. Also called *staggering gait, reeling gait.*

duck gait MYOPATHIC GAIT.

dystrophic gait The waddling gait with accentuation of the lumbar lordosis which is typical of muscular dystrophy or other forms of neuromuscular disease causing weakness of pelvifemoral muscles.

equine gait STEPPAGE GAIT.

festinating gait A type of gait characteristic of some extrapyramidal syndromes and particularly of parkinsonism. It consists of involuntary acceleration of the gait, in which very small steps are taken (marche à petits pas), with the body leaning forward, as if chasing its center of gravity. Also called *festination.*

footdrop gait STEPPAGE GAIT.

four-point gait A sequential gait pattern alternating a crutch or cane with placement of the opposite foot: right crutch, left foot, left crutch, right foot.

gluteal gait The gait produced by paralysis of the gluteus medius muscle and characterized by marked tilting of the pelvis and trunk towards the affected side with every other step. This type of gait is seen particularly in patients with congenital hip dislocation. Also called *Trendelenburg gait.*

gluteus maximus gait A lurching backward movement of the trunk in order to place the center of gravity over the supporting limb, commonly used when there is weakness of the gluteus maximus on the side of that limb.

gluteus medius gait A compensatory shifting of the trunk laterally, to the weakened gluteus medius side, in order to place the center of gravity closer to the supporting limb.

heel-toe gait A normal walking pattern in which the heel strikes first and then the toes push off the surface.

helicopod gait A walk in which the feet are moved in half-circles before they touch the floor, often seen in hysteria.

hemiplegic gait The gait of a patient with hemiplegia. The

affected arm and hand are held flexed across the front of the trunk and there is extensor spasticity with circumduction of the affected leg.

hypotonic gait Myopathic gait in subjects with hypotonia and weakness of pelvifemoral muscles.

intermittent double-step gait A hemiplegic gait in which there is a prolonged pause each time after the normal foot is advanced before the hemiplegic foot is moved.

myopathic gait A type of gait in which the patient rolls from side to side in walking, with accentuation of the lumbar lordosis, as is seen in myopathy and in other neuromuscular disorders that cause weakness of the pelvic girdle musculature. Also called *duck gait, waddling gait.*

Oppenheim's gait A type of combined spastic and ataxic gait often seen in multiple sclerosis. An obsolete term.

paralytic gait Any abnormality of gait seen in patients with partial paralysis of one or both lower limbs. An imprecise and outmoded term.

paraparetic gait The spastic gait seen in patients with spastic weakness of the lower limbs.

paretic gait Any gait disorder seen in patients with weakness of the lower limbs. An imprecise and outmoded term.

Petren gait MARCHE À PETITS PAS.

reeling gait DRUNKEN GAIT.

scissor gait The type of spastic gait seen in patients with Little's disease in which with each step one leg crosses over in front of the other. Also called *scissoring, cross-legged progression.*

senile gait An uncertain gait, often with short steps and with flexion of the trunk, as seen in very elderly people.

skaters' gait Walking accomplished with abrupt flinging movements of the arms and legs and with repeated flexion and extension of the trunk, as seen in some patients with Huntington's chorea.

spastic gait The gait which results from spasticity. When both lower limbs are spastic, the patient walks stiffly, scraping the feet along the ground. With severe spasticity, as in cerebral diplegia, the legs may cross each other alternately while walking ("scissors"). In hemiplegia there may be circumduction or dragging of the affected leg. Also called *frozen attitude* (obsolete).

spastic equinus gait A gait characterized by spastic and incoordinated movements of the lower limbs, with weight borne primarily on the forefoot since the ankles are plantar flexed. There is often associated adduction and internal rotation of the hips causing the knees and feet to turn inward.

staggering gait 1 ATAXIC GAIT. 2 DRUNKEN GAIT.

stamping gait TABETIC GAIT.

star gait The star-shaped course followed by the patient with unilateral labyrinthine disease required to perform the Babinski-Weill test.

steppage gait A gait in which the advancing foot is lifted high and the toes barely clear the ground or drag along the floor. It is due to paralysis of the anterior tibial muscles as in polyneuropathy and peroneal nerve injuries. Also called *footdrop gait, equine gait.*

swaying gait The ataxic gait of cerebellar ataxia.

swing-through gait A gait in which both crutches are advanced to the same point and then the patient lifts both feet off the ground, swinging and landing ahead of the crutches.

swing-to gait A gait in which both crutches are advanced and the patient then swings both limbs so that the feet are advanced the same distance as the crutches.

tabetic gait A gait due to sensory ataxia in tabes dorsalis, in which steps are taken on a wide base with slapping of the feet heavily on descent. Often the subject watches his feet as he walks so that he will know where they are. Tabetic gait is due to posterior column disease with consequent loss of proprioception. Also called *stamping gait.*

tabetocerebellar gait A type of gait due to combined cerebellar and sensory ataxia, described in cases of hereditary spinocerebellar degeneration and especially in Friedreich's disease. Also called *Charcot's gait, Charcot sign* (outmoded).

tabetospastic gait The type of gait observed in patients with lesions of the posterior columns of the spinal cord (sensory ataxia exacerbated by covering the eyes, with impairment of deep sensitivity), and corticospinal tracts (spastic lower limbs). This combination is often seen in subacute combined degeneration of the cord (vitamin B_{12} deficiency), multiple sclerosis, some of the hereditary ataxias, and in chronic spinal cord ischemia. Also called *ataxospastic gait, spastic ataxia.*

tandem gait Heel-to-toe walking, used in neurology as a test for the presence of ataxia.

three-point gait A gait pattern in which both crutches and the impaired lower limb are advanced together and then the uninvolved lower limb is advanced by itself.

Todd's gait HELICOPODIA.

Trendelenburg gait GLUTEAL GAIT.

two-point gait A gait in which a crutch or cane is advanced together with the opposite lower limb.

waddling gait MYOPATHIC GAIT.

Gal Symbol for the unit, gal.

gal [after *Galileo* Galilei, Italian astronomer and mathematician, 1564-1642] **1** Symbol for the unit, gallon. **2** A unit of acceleration, used especially in geodesy and geophysics, equal to one centimeter per second squared, 0.01 meter per second squared. Also called *galileo* (outmoded). Symbol: Gal

galact- GALACTO-.

galactacrasia [GALACT- + Gk *a-* priv. + *kras(is)* a mixture, mixing + -IA] An abnormality of breast milk. Also called *galactocrasia.*

galactagogin HUMAN PLACENTAL LACTOGEN.

galactagogue [GALACT- + -AGOGUE] **1** Promoting the flow of breast milk. **2** Any agent that promotes the flow of breast milk. For defs. 1 and 2 also called *galactogogue, lactogogue.*

galactan A polysaccharide composed of galactose residues. Galactans are found in cell walls of algae and as a constituent of agar, but are otherwise rare.

galactapostema [GALACT- + Gk *apostēma* (from *aphistanai* to remove) an abscess] MILK ABSCESS.

galactemia The presence of milk in the blood.

galactic [Gk *galaktik(os)* (from *gala,* gen. *galaktos,* milk + *-ikos* -IC) pertaining to milk, milky] Of, pertaining to, denoting, or characteristic of breast milk.

galactin An outmoded term for PROLACTIN.

galactischia [GALACT- + Gk *isch(ein)* to suppress + -IA] Interference with or suppression of the flow of breast milk. A seldom used term. Also called *galactoschesis.*

galactitol The achiral alcohol formed by reducing the —CHO group of galactose to —CH$_2$OH. It is formed in a type of galactosemia associated with a lack of galactokinase, and its accumulation leads to cataract formation in the eye. It is found in manna and other plant products. Also called *dulcitol.*

galacto- [Gk *gala* (genitive *galaktos*) milk] A combining form meaning milk, milky. Also *galact-.*

galactocele [GALACTO- + -CELE²] **1** A mammary gland cyst containing milk, presumably caused by duct obstruction. Also called *lactocele, lacteal cyst, milk cyst, lacteal tumor, galactoma.* **2** A hydrocele in the testis containing milky fluid.

galactocerebroside A cerebroside whose hexose sugar is galactose, i.e. an *O*-galactosyl-*N*-acylsphingoid. Such compounds are the main cerebrosides of brain and myelin.

galactocrasia GALACTACRASIA.

galactogenous [GALACTO- + -GENOUS] Allowing or assisting in the production of milk.

galactoglycosuria [GALACTO- + GLYCOSURIA] Glycosuria that occurs only during the time of lactation.

galactogogue GALACTAGOGUE.

galactography [GALACTO- + -GRAPHY] Radiographic examination of the mammary ducts after the injection of a radiopaque medium into them.

galactokinase The enzyme (EC 2.7.1.6) that catalyzes the phosphorylation of galactose to yield galactose 1-phosphate at the expense of ATP. This reaction enables galactose formed by digestion of lactose to be metabolized.

galactolipid Any lipid containing galactose residues. Many glycolipids of cell surfaces do so, with galactose linked either directly to a ceramide or through glucose. Galactolipids are found in the myelin sheath of nerves and in the brain.

galactoma [GALACT- + -OMA] GALACTOCELE.

galactometastasis [GALACTO- + METASTASIS] Secretion of milk from an abnormal location. Also called *galactoplania.*

galactometer [GALACTO- + -METER] A hydrometer adapted to measure the relative density of milk. Also called *lactometer, lactodensimeter.*

galactonic acid The acid formed by oxidation of C-1 of galactose to form a carboxyl group.

galactopexic Relating to galactopexy.

galactopexy The incorporation of galactose into tissues.

galactophagous [GALACTO- + -PHAGOUS] Having a diet of milk.

galactophagy [GALACTO- + -PHAGY] The consumption of milk.

galactophlebitis [GALACTO- + PHLEBITIS] PHLEGMASIA ALBA DOLENS.

galactophlysis A vesicular eruption that is marked by the presence of a milky fluid. An obsolete term.

galactophore DUCTUS LACTIFERI.

galactophoritis [*galactophor(e)* (from GALACTO- + -PHOR) a duct carrying milk + -ITIS] Milk duct inflammation or infection.

galactophorous LACTIFEROUS.

galactophyga LACTIFUGE.

galactophygous [GALACTO- + Gk *phyg(ē)* flight, escape + -OUS] Decreasing the flow of breast milk.

galactoplania [GALACTO- + Gk *plan(ē)* a wandering + -IA] GALACTOMETASTASIS.

galactopoiesis LACTOGENESIS.

galactopoietic LACTOGENIC.

galactopyra MILK FEVER.

galactorrhea [GALACTO- + -RRHEA] Excessive or persistent flow of milk from the breasts due to a pathologic condition of either sex unrelated to the puerperium. Also called *lactorrhea.*

galactosamine 2-Amino-2-deoxygalactose. A substance found widely as a constituent of glycoproteins. Its *N*-acetylated residues occur in chondroitin. Also called *chondrosamine* (outmoded).

galactoschesis [GALACTO- + Gk *schesis* (from *schein,* 2nd aorist inf. of *echein* to have, hold) retention] GALACTISCHIA.

galactoscope [GALACTO- + -SCOPE] A device that permits estimation of the fat content of milk by measuring its translucency. Also called *lactoscope.*

galactose A 6-carbon aldose sugar, differing from glucose in its configuration at C-4. It is a constituent of lactose, which is hydrolyzed by β-galactosidase to galactose and glucose. Galactose can subsequently give rise to glucose by an epimerization at C-4, but this involves the prior formation of UDP-galactose which then forms UDP-glucose.

galactosemia [*galactos(e)* + -EMIA] A metabolic defect in the conversion of galactose, a monosaccharide derived from lactose in milk, to glucose, due to a deficiency of galactose-1-phosphate uridyltransferase, which is one of four enzymes involved. The process takes place in the liver and in red cells in which an accumulation of galactose-1-phosphate is found and is suspected of being the toxic substance giving rise to clinical symptoms including the principal tetrad of hepatomegaly, cataracts, marasmus, and mental retardation. Galactosuria and amino-aciduria may result from possible renal damage. All these symptoms, except brain damage, may regress completely if the subject is placed on a galactose-free diet. Brain damage can be prevented by early diagnosis by demonstration of excess galactose-1-phosphate in the infant's red cells. In a family with a previously affected child, subsequent children should be tested for a galactokinase deficiency in the red cells of cord blood and given lactose-free milk till the result is known. The condition isinherited as an autosomal recessive trait. Also called *galactokinase defect, congenital galactosemia in infants, hereditary galactose intolerance.*

congenital galactosemia in infants GALACTOSEMIA.

galactose-1-phosphate uridylyltransferase The enzyme (EC 2.7.7.10) that transfers a uridylyl group from UDP-glucose onto the phosphate group of galactose 1-phosphate to form UDP-galactose and glucose 1-phosphate. The step is involved in lactose synthesis and in the metabolism of galactose derived from lactose. Also called *phosphogalactose uridylyltransferase.*

galactosidase Any enzyme hydrolyzing galactosides. Thus β-galactosidases hydrolyze lactose. Study of the synthesis by bacteria of β-galatosidase and other enzymes concerned in lactose metabolism has revealed simultaneous control of transcription of related genes. Deficiency of various isomers results in the G_{m1} gangliosidoses and in mucopolysaccharidosis IVB. A combined deficiency of this activity and of neuraminidase occurs in the Goldberg syndrome.

galactoside A compound containing a galactose residue whose aldehyde group is bound as an acetal with the hydroxyl group on C-5 or C-4 and with another alcohol.

galactoside acetylase An enzyme which transfers an acetyl group from acetylcoenzyme A to β-galactoses. The production is under control of the Lac operon in *Escherichia coli.*

galactoside permease A membrane protein which is responsible for allowing galactoside to enter the cytoplasm. Production of this protein is controlled by the Lac operon in *Escherichia coli.*

galactosis [GALACTO- + -SIS] LACTATION.

galactostasia GALACTOSTASIS.

galactostasis [GALACTO- + -STASIS] **1** Cessation of breast milk secretion. **2** An abnormal accumulation of milk in the breasts. For defs. 1 and 2 also called *galactostasia.*

galactosuria [*galactos(e)* + -URIA] The excretion of galactose in the urine. This occurs only when the diet contains galactose.

galactosyl The group formed by removal of the hydroxyl group from C-1 of a ring (hemiacetal) form of galactose.

galactotherapy The administration of medicinal remedies to infants via the breast milk by treating the mother or wet nurse. The practice is obsolete, although the giving of Vitamin B_1 to thiamin-depleted lactating mothers for prevention of infantile beriberi could be regarded as prophylactic galactotherapy.

galactotoxicon GALACTOTOXIN.

galactotoxin A toxic substance of unknown composition found in decomposed milk. Also called *galactotoxicon.*

galactotoxism Poisoning from consumption of milk containing galactotoxin. Also called *galactoxism, galactoxismus.*

galactotrophic [GALACTO- + TROPHIC] Causing milk secretion.

galactotrophy [GALACTO- + TROPH- + -Y] The process of feeding on a diet of milk.

galactowaldenase An obsolete term for UDPGLUCOSE 4-EPIMERASE.

galactoxism GALACTOTOXISM.

galactoxismus GALACTOTOXISM.

galacturia [GALACT- + -URIA] An obsolete term for CHYLURIA.

galacturonic acid The acid formed by oxidation of C-6 of galactose to form a carboxyl group. It occurs combined in glycoproteins and in pectins.

galanga The dried shavings of the rhizome of *Alpinia officinarum* of the Zingiberaceae family, having aromatic and carminative properties. Also called *galangal, Chinese ginger.*

galangal GALANGA.

Galant [Ivan Borisovich *Galant*, Russian psychiatrist, born 1893] See under REFLEX.

galanthamine $C_{17}H_{21}NO_3$. A pharmaceutic compound obtained from *Galanthus waronowii*, Caucasian snowdrop; *Leucojum aestivum*, and *Ungernia victoris*. An inhibitor of cholinesterase, it has been used in Europe to treat various myopathies.

gale The French term for SCABIES.

galea [L, a helmet] **1** A structure shaped like a helmet. **2** GALEA APONEUROTICA.

galea aponeurotica [NA] The fibrous membrane that not only joins the six component parts of the epicranius muscle to each other but is also anchored posteriorly to the external occipital protuberance and supreme nuchal line, anteriorly to the skin near the eyebrows, and laterally to muscles of the ear and to the zygomatic arch, thereby covering the calvaria deep to the superficial fascia of the scalp. Also called *epicranial aponeurosis, galea, aponeurosis of occipitofrontal muscle, tendinous part of epicranius muscle.*

galeamaurosis [L *galea* (from Gk *galeē* or *gatē* a cat, polecat) helmet + *maur(oun)* to darken, become obscure + -OSIS. Helmets once were made from cat skin.] Faulty vision in which objects appear transparent.

Galeati [Domenico Gusmano *Galeati*, Italian physician, 1686–1775] Galeati's glands. See under GLANDULAE INTESTINALES.

galeatomy [GALEA + -TOMY] An incision in the galea.

galeatus [L (from *galea* helmet), wearing a helmet] Birth with the amniotic membranes lying over the skull.

Galeazzi [Riccardo *Galeazzi*, Italian orthopedic surgeon, 1866–1952] See under FRACTURE, SIGN.

Galen [Claudius *Galen*, Greek physician active in Rome, c. 130–200 A.D.] **1** See under FORAMEN. **2** Galen's pore. See under CANALIS INGUINALIS. **3** Arteria maxima galeni. See under AORTA. **4** Galen's ventricle. See under VENTRICULUS LARYNGIS. **5** Galen's veins. See under VENAE CARDIACAE ANTERIORES. **6** Galen's veins. See under VEIN. **7** Ansa of Galen, Galen's nerve, Galen's anastomosis. See under RAMUS COMMUNICANS NERVI LARYNGEI SUPERIORIS CUM NERVO LARYNGEO INFERIORE. **8** Great vein of Galen. See under VENA MAGNA CEREBRI.

galeophilia [Gk *galē*, also *gale(ē)* marten, weasel + *o* + -PHILIA] AILUROPHILIA.

galeophobia [Gk *galē*, also *gale(ē)* marten, weasel + *o* + -PHOBIA] AILUROPHOBIA.

Galeotti [Gino *Galeotti*, Italian bacteriologist, born 1867] Lustig-Galeotti vaccine. See under VACCINE.

galeropia GALEROPSIA.

galeropsia [Gk *galer(os)* cheerful + -OPSIA] A condition in which objects seem transparent. Also called *galeropia.*

galileo [after *Galileo* Galilei, Italian astronomer and mathematician, 1564–1642] An outmoded term for GAL.

gall¹ [Old English *gealla* (akin to Old English *geolu* yellow).] BILE.

ox gall OX BILE EXTRACT.

gall² [Old English *gealla* (from L *galla* a gallnut, oak apple) a skin sore.] A localized swelling of the skin of a nonspecific nature, as a *saddle gall.*

gall³ [Middle English *galle* (from L *galla* a gallnut, oak apple).] A tumorlike or cystlike excrescence on a plant that may be caused by a disease, insect damage or a physical disturbance of the plant tissue.

Aleppo gall OAK GALL.

Hungarian gall OAK GALL.

oak gall A tumorous growth in the tissues of species of oak, *Quercus,* produced by eggs and larvae of various species of gall wasps. It is a source of tannic acid. Also called *nutgall, oak apple, Aleppo gall, Hungarian gall, Smyrna gall, Syrian gall, Turkey gall, gallnut.*

Smyrna gall OAK GALL.

Syrian gall OAK GALL.

Turkey gall OAK GALL.

gallacetophenone $C_8H_8O_4$. 2′,3′,4′-Trihydroxyacetophenone. A phenolic compound which is used as an antiseptic for external use only.

gallamine triethiodide $C_{30}H_{60}I_3N_3O_3$. 2,2′,2″-[1,2,3-Benzenetriyltris(oxy)]tris(*N,N,N*-triethylethanaminium] triiodide. A synthetic muscle relaxant that inhibits neurotransmission at the myoneural junction. It is given intravenously during surgical procedures, or for endoscopic or intubation operations. It may produce respiratory paralysis that requires artificial respiration. Its actions are reversed by neostigmine. Also called *benzcurine iodide.*

Gallavardin [Louis *Gallavardin,* French physician, 1875–1957] See under PHENOMENON.

gallbladder VESICA BILIARIS.

Courvoisier's gallbladder A distended gallbladder due to biliary obstruction, often a sign of carcinoma of the head of the pancreas. See also COURVOISIER SIGN.

fish-scale gallbladder A gallbladder with multiple small mucosal cysts. The mucosal surface resembles fish scales.

floating gallbladder MOBILE GALLBLADDER.

folded fundus gallbladder A gallbladder with a kinking between the body and the fundus; phrygian cap.

hourglass gallbladder A gallbladder with an annular constriction in its mid-body. It may be either congenital or acquired.

mobile gallbladder A gallbladder that is not attached to the ventral surface of the liver but is freely movable on the cystic duct or is restrained only by a ligamentous attachment. Also called *floating gallbladder, wandering gallbladder.*

phrygian cap gallbladder See under PHRYGIAN CAP.

sandpaper gallbladder Cholesterolosis of the gallbladder.

strawberry gallbladder The appearance of the gallbladder affected by cholesterolosis, in which a strawberrylike appearance develops due to the infiltration of cholesterol into the mucosa, with accompanying inflammation.

wandering gallbladder MOBILE GALLBLADDER.

gallein A dye, poorly soluble in water or alcohol, that is used principally as a pH indicator, changing from brownish yellow to rose at a pH of 3.8 to 6.6. Also called *pyrogallolphthalein.*

gallery A space or burrow in the skin occupied by a metazoan parasite.

gallic acid 3,4,5-Trihydroxybenzoic acid. It can be liberated from tannins by hydrolysis and is used in dyeing. It is a strong reducing agent, and is oxidized to quinones.

Galli Mainini [Carlos *Galli Mainini,* Argentinian physician, 1879–1943] Galli Mainini test. See under MALE FROG TEST.

gallinaceous [L *gallinaceus* (from *gallin(a)* a hen + -*aceus* English -*aceous*) pertaining to poultry] Of or pertaining to birds of the order Galliformes, which includes chickens, turkeys, and grouse.

Gallionella A stalked bacterium that oxidizes Fe^{2+} and accumulates $Fe(OH)_3$.

gallium A rare metallic element having atomic number 31 and atomic weight 69.737. It has a low melting point (29.78°C) and can exist as a liquid at room temperature. Two stable isotopes occur in nature and 12 unstable isotopes are known. Valences are 2 and 3. Gallium often accumulates in tumors and inflammatory processes. Symbol: Ga

gallium 67 A radioactive isotope of gallium that decays by orbital electron capture. The half-life is 78.26 hours. Symbol: ^{67}Ga

gallium 68 A radioactive isotope of gallium that decays by positron emission and orbital electron capture. The half-life is 68.2 minutes. Symbol: ^{68}Ga

gallium 67 citrate Gallium citrate labeled with gallium 67. It is used for external imaging of tumors and inflammatory processes.

gallnut OAK GALL.

gallocyanin A synthetic blue dye that is used together with chrome alum as a mordant to stain both DNA and RNA within cells.

gallon [Old North French *galun, galon* (from Med L *galo* a liquid measure) a liquid measure] **1** In the United States, a unit of capacity used to measure liquids only, equal to 231 cubic inches exactly; 3.785 41 liters. Also called *Winchester gallon, liquid gallon.* Symbol: gal **2** In Great Britain and Australia, a unit of capacity equal to 4.546 09 liters exactly. Symbol: gal • *Gallon* was formerly defined in terms of the volume of 10 pounds of water under specified conditions of weighing.

liquid gallon GALLON.

Winchester gallon GALLON.

gallop See under GALLOP RHYTHM.

atrial gallop The atrial component of a gallop rhythm.

filling gallop The component of a gallop rhythm due to rapid ventricular filling.

S_3 gallop Gallop rhythm due to the presence of a third heart sound; ventricular gallop.

systolic gallop Gallop rhythm due to an extra sound during systole.

ventricular gallop Gallop rhythm due to ventricular filling; S_3 gallop.

gallotannic acid TANNIC ACID.

gallstone A concretion formed primarily of cholesterol, bile pigments, or a mixture of the two, found in the gallbladder or the biliary tree. Also called *biliary calculus, cholelith, chololith* (seldom used).

Gallus A genus of birds of the family Phasianidae. It includes the domestic chicken, *G. domesticus.*

Galton [Francis *Galton,* English anthropologist, 1822–1911] **1** Galton system of classification of fingerprints. See under SYSTEM. **2** See under DELTA, WHISTLE. **3** Galton's law. See under GALTON'S LAW OF REGRESSION.

galvanic Pertaining to galvanism.

galvanism [after Luigi *Galvani,* Italian physician and physicist, 1737–1798 + -ISM] **1** Direct current electricity as that from a chemical battery. **2** Therapeutic use of direct current electricity. **3** Electric shocks or inflammation resulting from the use of dissimilar metals such as silver and gold used in dental restorations.

dental galvanism The formation of a painful electric current in the teeth by the presence of two dissimilar metals in the saliva, which acts as an electrolyte. An amalgam restoration in intermittent contact with a gold restoration may cause this effect.

galvanization The use of galvanism in treatment or in electroplating metal.

galvanocautery ELECTRIC CAUTERY.

galvanochemical ELECTROCHEMICAL.

galvanocontractility [after Luigi *Galvan(i)* + *o* + CONTRACTILITY. See GALVANOMETER.] The ability of muscle to respond to a continuous, direct electric current.

galvanofaradic Pertaining to the simultaneous use of galvanic and faradic currents.

galvanogustometer An instrument for testing taste sensation by applying an electrical stimulus to the lingual mucosa.

galvanoionization IONTOPHORESIS.

galvanolysis ELECTROLYSIS.

galvanometer [after Luigi *Galvani*, Italian physician and physicist, 1737–1798 + *o* + -METER] An instrument for measuring a small electric current flowing through a wire or coil that moves in a magnetic field. The output is observed as the needle movement on a meter, deflection of a light beam, or deflection of a pen such as that on an electrocardiograph recorder. Also called *rheometer*.

Einthoven's galvanometer STRING GALVANOMETER.

string galvanometer A thin thread of silvered quartz or platinum stretched in a strong magnetic field. An arc lamp projected the optically magnified movements to form the first electrocardiograph in 1901. Also called *Einthoven's galvanometer, thread galvanometer*.

thread galvanometer STRING GALVANOMETER.

galvanomuscular Denoting the effect of a continuous, direct current in exciting muscle.

galvanonarcosis ELECTRONARCOSIS.

galvanonervous [*galvano-*, combining form denoting galvanic, after Luigi *Galvani*, Italian physician and physicist, 1737–1798 + NERVOUS] Describing or pertaining to the use of galvanic electrical stimulation in neurological diagnosis. An outmoded usage.

galvanopalpation An outmoded method of testing cutaneous sensibility quantitatively by applying a galvanic electrical stimulus to the skin.

galvanoprostatectomy GALVANOPROSTATOTOMY.

galvanoprostatotomy [*galvano-*, combining form denoting galvanic, after Luigi *Galvani*, Italian physician and physicist, 1737–1798 + PROSTATO- + -TOMY] Partial excision of a hypertrophic prostate by use of galvanocautery. Also called *galvanoprostatectomy*.

galvanopuncture The completion of a galvanic current circuit by insertion of needle electrodes into the body.

galvanosurgery [after Luigi *Galvan(i)*, Italian physician and physicist, 1737–1798 + *o* + SURGERY] The surgical use of an electric current to cut or cauterize tissue.

galvanotaxis ELECTROTAXIS.

galvanotherapeutics GALVANOTHERAPY.

galvanotherapy The therapeutic use of galvanic electric currents. Also called *galvanotherapeutics*.

galvanotonic Denoting a direct electric current capable of exciting muscle. An outmoded term.

galvanotonus Muscular contraction induced by direct current.

nonpermanent galvanotonus Nonsustained muscular contraction induced by direct current.

permanent galvanotonus Sustained muscular contraction in response to direct current.

galvanotropism The growth or orientation of a plant in response to an electric current.

gam- GAMO-.

gamasid HAEMOGAMASID.

Gamasidae HAEMOGAMASIDAE.

gamasoidosis [Gk *gamēs*, fut. stem of *gamein* to marry + -OID + -OSIS] A dermatitis caused by an infestation with the poultry mite, *Dermanyssus gallinae*.

gambir CATECHU.

gamblegram A bar graph representation of the electrolyte composition of body fluids in normal and diseased states.

gamboge The yellow gum resin extracted from *Garcinia hanburyi*. It is used as a cathartic and purgative. Also called *cambogia, gutti*.

Gambusia A genus of small bony fish of the family Poeciliidae; the mosquito fish. They occur in tropical and subtropical lakes and rivers and have been introduced extensively in the United States for control of mosquito larvae.

gamefar A proprietary name for pamaquine.

gametangia Plural of GAMETANGIUM.

gametangium (*plural* gametangia) A specialized cell or organ that produces gametes.

gametangy [*gamet(o)-* + *ang(i)-* + -Y] Sexual reproduction where gametangia (antheridium and oogonium) make contact prior to gametic plasmogamy and karyogamy.

gamete [Gk *gametē(s)* a husband, *gametē* a wife] A mature cell with a haploid chromosome set that participates in sexual reproduction. Two gametes of opposite sex (in humans, the male sperm and the female ovum) fuse to form a diploid zygote. Also called *gonosome* (obsolete).

gametic Referring to or of parallel function to a gamete.

gameticidal GAMETOCIDAL.

gameticide GAMETOCIDE.

gameto- [Gk *gametē* wife, *gametēs* husband] A combining form meaning gamete.

gametoblast [GAMETO- + -BLAST] An obsolete term for SPOROZOITE.

gametocidal [GAMETO- + *cid(e)* + -AL] Destructive to gametes or gametocytes. Also *gameticidal*.

gametocide [GAMETO- + -CIDE] An agent that kills gametes or gametocytes. Also called *gameticide*.

gametocyst [GAMETO- + CYST] A protective envelope in which paired gregarine sporozoan gametocytes in the gut of the invertebrate host become encysted. Ultimately, each gametocyte produces numerous isogametes within the cyst which fuse in pairs (isogamy) to form numerous zygotes in each gametocyst. A secondary cyst or oocyst forms around each zygote. Each oocyst then divides internally to produce eight sporozoites, the infective agents in the next host following ingestion of the oocyst.

gametocyte [GAMETO- + -CYTE] A cell able to produce one or more sexual (haploid) progeny, the male or female gametes which undergo fusion to complete the sexual phase of reproduction. A great many types of such cells are found in both plants and animals, and many examples can be found among the sporozoan protozoa. Also called *gamont*.

gametocytemia [*gametocyt(e)* + -EMIA] The presence of gametocytes, as, for example, of protozoan parasites, in the blood of the host.

gametogenesis The process of formation and maturation of gametes.

gametogenic 1 Of or relating to gametogenesis. 2 Capable of gametogenesis.

gametogonia GAMETOGONY.

gametogony [GAMETO- + GON-² + -Y] The gamete-producing stage in the sexual reproductive cycle, as in many protozoa, including *Plasmodium* species. In the latter, gametocytes are produced in the human blood stream. After ingestion by the mosquito vector, the gametes are released, leading to zygote formation, followed by growth of the oocyst from the zygote (ookinete) and production of great numbers of sporozoites. Also called *gametogonia, gamogony*.

gametoid Resembling gametes; having characteristics of reproductive cells.

gametologist [GAMETO- + -LOGIST] A scientist who studies gametology.

gametology [GAMETO- + -LOGY] The study of gametes.

gametophagia [GAMETO- + -PHAGIA] The elimination of the male or female element during conjugation of unicellular organisms. Also called *gamophagia*.

gametophore [GAMETO- + -PHORE] A stalk that bears or holds a gametangium. This structure is characteristic of plants classified as bryophytes.

gametophyte [GAMETO- + Gk *phyt(on)* a plant, tree] Among plants exhibiting alternation of generations, a member in the haploid, gamete-producing phase. Also called *oophyte*.

gametotropic [GAMETO- + -TROPIC¹] Attracted to gametes; having an affinity for gametes.

Gamgee [Joseph Sampson *Gamgee*, English surgeon, 1828–1886] See under TISSUE.

gamic Pertaining to a gamete (usually an ovum) that completes development only after fertilization.

gamma [third letter of the Gk alphabet] **1** The name of the third letter of the Greek alphabet. **2** A gamma ray or photon. **3** A unit of magnetic field strength equal to 10^{-5} oersted; 0.795 775 $\times 10^{-3}$ ampere per meter. An obsolete unit. Symbol: γ **4** An obsolete, informal term for MICROGRAM.

prompt gamma A gamma photon emitted at the time of nuclear fission or radioactive decay, as distinguished from gamma photons emitted by radioactive daughter products.

gammacism A defect of speech, occurring mostly in younger children, in which the sounds represented by *g* and *k* are not articulated, being replaced by other sounds, usually that represented by *d*. It results in the "baby talk" of young children.

Gammacorten A proprietary name for dexamethasone.

gamma-emitter Any nuclide that emits gamma photons.

gamma globulin See under GLOBULIN.

gammaglobulinopathy GAMMOPATHY.

gammagram A record of the photon emanations from a radioactive material, usually on photographic film.

gammagraphic Relating to a radioisotope image.

gammaloidosis An obsolete term for AMYLOIDOSIS.

gammexane LINDANE.

gammography Imaging by means of gamma radiation; scintigraphy. A rarely used term.

cerebral gammography GAMMA ENCEPHALOGRAPHY.

gammopathy [*gamm(a)* + *o* + -PATHY] Any quantitative or qualitative abnormality of plasma immunoglobulins, such as agammaglobulinemia, hyperglobulinemia, and the monoclonal hypergammaglobulinemia associated with multiple myeloma. Also called *immunoglobulinopathy, gammaglobulinopathy*.

benign monoclonal gammopathy MONOCLONAL GAMMOPATHY OF UNDETERMINED SIGNIFICANCE.

biclonal gammopathy A condition in which serum contains abnormal globulins that are derived from two separate clones of abnormally proliferating B lymphocytes.

monoclonal gammopathy An immunoproliferative disorder characterized by the abnormal proliferation of a single clone of lymphoid cells, which results in an excess of one specific class of immunoglobulins. Diseases in this category include multiple myeloma, macroglobulinemia, and heavy chain disease.

monoclonal gammopathy of undetermined significance A greater than normal serum concentration of immunoglobulin of type IgG or IgM, represented as a homogeneous single band on serum protein electrophoresis, of either kappa or lambda light chain type, but not both, in a patient who is otherwise well and without other evidence of myeloma. The monoclonal protein is usually less than 2.0 g/l. Plasma cells may be slightly increased in bone marrow, but they are not immature or myeloma cells. Bone lesions are absent. The condition is usually very indolent, but approximately 15% of patients ultimately develop myeloma or Waldenström's macroglobulinemia. Also called *benign monoclonal gammopathy*.

Gamna [Carlo *Gamna*, Italian physician, 1886–1950] **1** Gamna-Favre bodies. See under MIYAGAWA BODIES. **2** Gamna nodules, Gandy-Gamna nodules. See under GAMNA-GANDY BODIES. **3** Gandy-Gamna spleen, Gamna's disease. See under SIDEROTIC SPLENOMEGALY.

gamo- [Gk *gamos* marriage] A combining form meaning (1) united, joined; (2) sexually united. Also *gam-*.

gamobium [New L (from Gk *gamo(s)* marriage + New L *-bium*, neut. sing. of *-bius*, noun suffix denoting mode of life, from Gk *bios* life, way of life)] The sexual generation among organisms that are characterized by an alternation of generations.

gamogenesis SEXUAL REPRODUCTION.

gamogenetic Capable of or pertaining to sexual reproduction.

gamogony GAMETOGONY.

gamon Any substance produced by a gamete of one sex to facilitate fertilization by a gamete of the opposite sex.

gamont GAMETOCYTE.

gamopetalous SYMPETALOUS.

gamophagia [GAMO- + -PHAGIA] GAMETOPHAGIA.

gamophobia [Gk *gamo(s)* marriage + -PHOBIA] Pathologic fear of marriage.

gamosepalous SYNSEPALOUS.

Gamper [E. *Gamper*, Austrian neurologist, 1887–1938] See under REFLEX.

gampsodactylia CLAW FOOT.

gampsodactyly CLAW FOOT.

Gamstorp [Ingrid *Gamstorp*, Swedish pediatrician, flourished mid-20th century] Gamstorp's disease. See under PERIODIC PARALYSIS II.

Gandy [Charles *Gandy*, French physician, born 1872] **1** Gandy-Gamna nodules. See under GAMNA-GANDY BODIES. **2** Gandy-Nanta disease, Gandy-Gamna disease, Gandy-Gamna spleen. See under SIDEROTIC SPLENOMEGALY.

ganga An extract obtained from the flowers of *Cannabis sativa*, a plant indigenous to India. The material is smoked for its euphoric and mild sedative effects.

gangli- GANGLIO-.

ganglia Plural of GANGLION.

ganglial GANGLIONIC.

gangliated Possessing ganglia.

gangliectomy GANGLIONECTOMY.

gangliform GANGLIOFORM.

gangliitis GANGLIONITIS.

ganglio- [Gk *ganglion* swelling, knot] A combining form meaning ganglion. Also *gangli-*.

ganglioblast [GANGLIO- + -BLAST] One of the immature cells, similar to neuroblasts, which differentiate into the principal cells of nerve ganglia. Also called *esthesioblast*.

gangliocyte [GANGLIO- + -CYTE]   GANGLION CELL.

gangliocytoma [GANGLIO- + CYTOMA]   A tumor of ganglion cells. Non-neoplastic glial elements may be present.

ganglioform [GANGLIO- + -FORM]   Having the knotlike form of a ganglion.

ganglioglioma [GANGLIO- + GLIOMA]   A tumor of ganglion cells and neoplastic glial cells. Also called *glioneuroma, ganglionic glioma, neuroastrocytoma, neuroglioma ganglionare.*

ganglioglioneuroma [GANGLIO- + GLIONEUROMA]   A tumor of ganglion cells, glial cells, and nerve fibers.

ganglioid [GANGLI- + -OID]   Having the form or appearance of a ganglion.

gangliolytic   **1** GANGLIOPLEGIC.   **2** Denoting a substance capable of destroying ganglion cells.

ganglioma [GANGLI- + -OMA]   A tumor of a lymph node. An outmoded term.

ganglion

ganglion [Gk *ganglion* a knot, swelling]   (*plural* ganglia, ganglions)   **1** An aggregation of neuron cell bodies in the peripheral nervous system, such as the sensory root ganglia and the autonomic ganglia. Also called *neuroganglion, nerve ganglion.*   **2** A knot or mass of connective or nerve tissue, or a cystic swelling containing jellylike fluid rich in mucopolysaccharides, arising from the synovium of a tendon on the dorsum of the wrist or foot, or within a semilunar cartilage of a knee. Also called *peritendinitis serosa.*   **3** A neuronal aggregate of the central nervous system, usually associated with a grossly visible bulge. An outmoded usage.

aberrant ganglion   A small aggregate of spinal ganglion cells displaced medially in the dorsal root and distinct from the main ganglion mass.

accessory ganglia   GANGLIA INTERMEDIA.

acoustic ganglion   **1** A ganglion mass differentiated in the embryo from the cranial neural crest lying between the rhombencephalon and the developing labyrinth. It is formed from the caudal part of the larger acousticofacial ganglion and divides into two parts, the cochlear (spiral) ganglion and the vestibular ganglion. Also called *vestibulocochlear ganglion.*   **2** GANGLION SPIRALE COCHLEAE.

acousticofacial ganglion   An embryonic ganglion-mass arising from neural crest cells and initially common to the seventh and eighth cranial nerves. At the 7 mm stage in man (end of the fourth week) the cranial portion of the ganglion-mass separates to become the geniculate ganglion of the facial nerve. The caudal portion becomes the acoustic (vestibulocochlear) ganglion which divides into two parts, the vestibular and the cochlear (spiral) ganglia.

Acrel's ganglion   A cystic swelling seen on a wrist extensor tendon.

Andersch ganglion   GANGLION INFERIUS NERVI GLOSSOPHARYNGEI.

anterior ganglion of thalamus   The anterior tubercle of the thalamus, which protrudes into the third ventricle and contains the three nuclei of the anterior group, the nuclei anterodorsalis, anteroventralis, and anteromedialis. An obsolete term.

aorticorenal ganglion   GANGLIA AORTICORENALIA.

ganglia aorticorenalia   [NA] The semidetached inferior extension of the ganglia of the celiac plexus. Also called *aorticorenal ganglion, nephrolumbar ganglia* (obsolete).

Arnold's ganglion   **1** GANGLION OTICUM.   **2** GLOMUS CAROTICUM.

auditory ganglion   GANGLION SPIRALE COCHLEAE.

Auerbach's ganglion   Any of the small aggregates of parasympathetic ganglion cells of the myenteric plexus (Auerbach's plexus). Also called *Auerbach's node.*

auricular ganglion   A seldom used term for GANGLION OTICUM.

autonomic ganglia   Any of the visceral ganglia associated with the sympathetic or parasympathetic nervous system.

ganglia of autonomic plexuses   The small aggregates of postganglionic autonomic neurons of the submucosal (Meissner's) plexus and myenteric (Auerbach's) plexus. Also called *enteric ganglia.*

azygous ganglion   GANGLION IMPAR.

basal ganglia   The nuclear masses of gray matter in the cerebrum, comprising the corpus striatum (caudate, putamen, and globus pallidus) and the amygdaloid complex, sometimes including the claustrum and septal nuclei. Also called *basal nuclei.*

Bezold's ganglion   A linear aggregation of parasympathetic ganglion cells in the interatrial septum.

Bidder's ganglia   VENTRICULAR GANGLIA.

Blandin's ganglion   GANGLION SUBMANDIBULARE.

Bochdalek's ganglion   A ganglionlike structure containing no ganglion cells and located on the superior alveolar nerve. Also called *ganglion bochdalekii.*   ● The structure was described by the Czech anatomist V.A. Bochdalek in 1855, and is believed to be the plexus dentalis superior.

ganglion bochdalekii   BOCHDALEK'S GANGLION.

Bock's ganglion   INFERIOR CAROTID GANGLION.

Böttcher's ganglion   **1** GANGLION SPIRALE COCHLEAE.   **2** A ganglion lying within the cochlear nerve. An incorrect usage. ● There is no ganglion lying within the cochlear nerve.

cardiac ganglia   GANGLIA CARDIACA.

ganglia cardiaca   Parasympathetic ganglia of the cardiac plexus lying between the aortic arch and the bifurcation of the pulmonary artery. Also called *cardiac ganglia, Wrisberg's ganglion, ganglion Wrisbergi.*

carotid ganglion   **1** GLOMUS CAROTICUM.   **2** INFERIOR CAROTID GANGLION.

celiac ganglia   GANGLIA CELIACA.

ganglia celiaca   A pair of large sympathetic prevertebral ganglia within the diaphragmatic celiac plexus located on the upper part of the abdominal aorta. They innervate the stomach, spleen, liver, gallbladder, and the small and large intestines. Also called *celiac ganglia, solar ganglia, centrum nervosum of Willis.*

cephalic ganglion   Any of the parasympathetic ganglia of the head, such as the ciliary, otic, pterygopalatine, and submandibular ganglia. A seldom used term.

cerebrospinal ganglia   The ganglia associated with the afferent cranial and spinal nerve roots, containing the cell bodies of sensory neurons. They differ from other ganglia in lacking dendrites and synapses on their cell bodies.

ganglion cervicale inferius   [NA] A portion of the ganglion cervicothoracicum (stellate ganglion). Also called *inferior cervical ganglion.*

ganglion cervicale medium   [NA] The small middle cervical sympathetic ganglion at about the level of the cricoid cartilage. Its postganglionic axons innervate the cervical region, upper extremity, and heart. Also called *inferior thyroid ganglion, superior thyroid ganglion, middle cervical ganglion.*

ganglion cervicale superius   [NA] The largest and most rostral ganglion of the sympathetic trunk, lying anterior to the second and third cervical vertebrae between the internal carotid artery and the internal jugular vein. Also called *superior cervical ganglion.*

cervical ganglion of uterus   A parasympathetic ganglion near the uterine cervix. Also called *Lee's ganglion, Frankenhäuser's ganglion, cervicouterine ganglion.*

cervicothoracic ganglion GANGLION CERVICOTHORACICUM.

ganglion cervicothoracicum [NA] The sympathetic ganglion at the seventh cervical level, usually partially fused with the first thoracic ganglion. Its postganglionic axons innervate the heart, upper extremity, neck, and head. Also called *cervicothoracic ganglion, ganglion stellatum, stellate ganglion.*

cervicouterine ganglion CERVICAL GANGLION OF UTERUS.

ganglion of Chassaignac One of the submandibular lymph nodes which may become enlarged and painful in tonsillitis. An outmoded term.

ganglion ciliare [NA] A small parasympathetic ganglion lying in the posterior orbit between the optic nerve and external rectus muscle. Its postganglionic axons innervate the ciliary muscle and the pupillary sphincter. Also called *lenticular ganglion* (obsolete), *Schacher's ganglion* (seldom used), *ciliary ganglion, ophthalmic ganglion, optic ganglion, orbital ganglion.*

ciliary ganglion GANGLION CILIARE.

Cloquet's ganglion A ganglion of the nasopalatine nerve, the existence of which has been questioned.

coccygeal ganglion GANGLION IMPAR.

collateral ganglion Any of the sympathetic ganglia of the mesenteric plexus surrounding the abdominal aorta and its major branches.

compound ganglion A cystic swelling of a tendon sheath that is constricted by a ligament around the sheath.

Corti's ganglion GANGLION SPIRALE COCHLEAE.

Darkschewitsch's ganglion An obsolete term for NUCLEUS OF DARKSCHEWITSCH.

diaphragmatic ganglia GANGLIA PHRENICA.

diffuse ganglion A swelling, usually on the dorsum of the hand or wrist, composed of tendon sheath, synovium, and synovial fluid.

dorsal root ganglion GANGLION SPINALE.

ganglion of duct of Botallo NODUS LIGAMENTIS ARTERIOSI.

Ehrenritter's ganglion GANGLION SUPERIUS NERVI GLOSSOPHARYNGEI.

enteric ganglia GANGLIA OF AUTONOMIC PLEXUSES.

ganglion extracraniale GANGLION INFERIUS NERVI GLOSSOPHARYNGEI.

ganglion of facial nerve GANGLION GENICULI.

false ganglion An enlargement of a peripheral nerve not containing ganglion cells.

Frankenhäuser's ganglion CERVICAL GANGLION OF UTERUS.

Froriep's ganglion A transient embryonic dorsal root ganglion related to the metencephalon and probably to the structures of the fourth occipital somite.

Ganser's ganglion An obsolete term for NUCLEUS INTERPEDUNCULARIS.

Gasser's ganglion GANGLION TRIGEMINALE.

gasserian ganglion GANGLION TRIGEMINALE.

geniculate ganglion GANGLION GENICULI.

ganglion geniculi [NA] The intracranial sensory ganglion of the facial nerve root associated with the nervus intermedius gustatory receptors of the anterior two thirds of the tongue. Also called *ganglion of facial nerve, geniculate ganglion.*

ganglion of habenulae The habenular nuclear complex of the thalamus, derived from the embryonic epithalamus.

hepatic ganglion An autonomic ganglion located near the hepatic artery.

Huber's ganglion A cerebrospinal ganglion sometimes found at the C_1 level. There is usually no sensory ganglion at this level in man and other higher mammals. An obsolete term.

hypogastric ganglia An imprecise term for GANGLIA PELVINA.

hypoglossal ganglion A ganglion associated with sensory fibers of the twelfth cranial nerve. The ganglion is present at one stage of embryonic development but regresses and is rarely seen in the adult.

ganglion impar [NA] The unpaired, most caudal ganglion of the sympathetic trunk, lying in front of the coccyx. Also called *coccygeal ganglion, Walther's ganglion, azygous ganglion.*

inferior carotid ganglion A small ganglion on the ventral surface of the internal carotid artery in the cavernous sinus. Also called *Bock's ganglion, Laumonier's ganglion, Schmiedel's ganglion, carotid ganglion.*

inferior cervical ganglion GANGLION CERVICALE INFERIUS.

inferior ganglion of glossopharyngeal nerve GANGLION INFERIUS NERVI GLOSSOPHARYNGEI.

inferior jugular ganglion GANGLION INFERIUS NERVI GLOSSOPHARYNGEI.

inferior mesenteric ganglion GANGLION MESENTERICUM INFERIUS.

inferior petrosal ganglion GANGLION INFERIUS NERVI GLOSSOPHARYNGEI.

inferior thyroid ganglion GANGLION CERVICALE MEDIUM.

inferior vagal ganglion GANGLION INFERIUS NERVI VAGI.

inferior ganglion of vagus GANGLION INFERIUS NERVI VAGI.

ganglion inferius nervi glossopharyngei The lower of the two sensory ganglia on the glossopharyngeal nerve at the site of its entrance into the jugular foramen. Also called *ganglion petrosum, petrous ganglion, petrosal ganglion, ganglion extracraniale, Andersch ganglion, inferior ganglion of glossopharyngeal nerve, inferior jugular ganglion, inferior petrosal ganglion, lower ganglion of glossopharyngeal nerve.*

ganglion inferius nervi vagi The large inferior sensory ganglion of the vagus located below the jugular foramen at the level of the first and second cervical vertebrae. Also called *nodose ganglion, ganglion nodosum, inferior vagal ganglion, inferior ganglion of vagus, lower ganglion of vagus nerve.*

inhibitory ganglion Any autonomic ganglion the stimulation of which results in inhibition of its target organ.

intercarotid ganglion An outmoded term for GLOMUS CAROTICUM.

intercrural ganglion NUCLEUS INTERPEDUNCULARIS.

ganglia intermedia Small aggregates of sympathetic ganglion cells on the rami communicantes in the cervical, lower thoracic, and upper lumbar levels of the spinal cord. Also called *accessory ganglia, intermediate ganglia.*

intermediary ganglion An outmoded term for GANGLION VERTEBRALE.

intermediate ganglia GANGLIA INTERMEDIA.

interpeduncular ganglion NUCLEUS INTERPEDUNCULARIS.

ganglion intervertebrale GANGLION SPINALE.

intracranial ganglion GANGLION SUPERIUS NERVI GLOSSOPHARYNGEI.

ganglion isthmi An obsolete term for NUCLEUS INTERPEDUNCULARIS.

ganglion jugulare nervi vagi GANGLION SUPERIUS NERVI VAGI.

jugular ganglion of glossopharyngeal nerve GANGLION SUPERIUS NERVI GLOSSOPHARYNGEI.

jugular ganglion of vagus nerve GANGLION SUPERIUS NERVI VAGI.

Küttner's ganglion A constant, large lymph node, belonging to the superior deep cervical group, that lies on the internal jugular vein at the point where it is crossed by the posterior belly of the digastric muscle, to which a large number of marginal lymphatic vessels of the tongue converge. Also called *hauptganglion of Küttner*.

Langley's ganglion A collection of ganglion cells found in the hilus of the submandibular gland of most mammals.

Laumonier's ganglion INFERIOR CAROTID GANGLION.

Lee's ganglion CERVICAL GANGLION OF UTERUS.

lenticular ganglion An obsolete term for GANGLION CILIARE.

lesser ganglion of Meckel GANGLION SUBMANDIBULARE.

lingual ganglion An obsolete term for GANGLION SUBMANDIBULARE.

Lobstein's ganglion GANGLION SPLANCHNICUM.

Loetwig's ganglion BULBUS CORDIS.

lower ganglion of glossopharyngeal nerve GANGLION INFERIUS NERVI GLOSSOPHARYNGEI.

lower ganglion of vagus nerve GANGLION INFERIUS NERVI VAGI.

Ludwig's ganglion A small parasympathetic ganglion of the cardiac interatrial plexus innervating the right atrium.

ganglia lumbalia [NA] The four or five pairs of lumbar sympathetic ganglia on the border of the psoas muscles. Also called *lumbar ganglia*.

lumbar ganglia GANGLIA LUMBALIA.

Luschka's ganglion GLOMUS COCCYGEUM.

ganglion lymphaticum NODUS LYMPHATICUS.

maxillary ganglion An outmoded term for GANGLION SUBMANDIBULARE.

Meckel's ganglion GANGLION PTERYGOPALATINUM.

Meissner's ganglion The numerous aggregates of parasympathetic ganglion cells in the submucosal plexus (of Meissner).

ganglion mesentericum inferius [NA] The inferior ganglion of the sympathetic prevertebral chain in the inferior mesenteric plexus, innervating the descending and sigmoid colon. Also called *inferior mesenteric ganglion*.

ganglion mesentericum superius [NA] One or more paired sympathetic ganglia forming part of the celiac ganglion at the origin of the superior mesenteric artery. Also called *superior mesenteric ganglion*.

middle cervical ganglion GANGLION CERVICALE MEDIUM.

ganglion of Müller GANGLION SUPERIUS NERVI GLOSSOPHARYNGEI.

nasal ganglion GANGLION PTERYGOPALATINUM.

nephrolumbar ganglia An obsolete term for GANGLIA AORTICORENALIA.

nerve ganglion GANGLION.

ganglion nervi splanchnici GANGLION SPLANCHNICUM.

nodose ganglion GANGLION INFERIUS NERVI VAGI.

ganglion nodosum GANGLION INFERIUS NERVI VAGI.

olfactory ganglion BULBUS OLFACTORIUS.

ophthalmic ganglion GANGLION CILIARE.

optic ganglion GANGLION CILIARE.

orbital ganglion GANGLION CILIARE.

otic ganglion GANGLION OTICUM.

ganglion oticum [NA] A parasympathetic ganglion, located below the foramen ovale medial to the mandibular nerve, that innervates the parotid gland and receives preganglionic fibers from the glossopharyngeal nerve via the lesser petrosal nerve. Also called *otic ganglion*, *auricular ganglion* (seldom used), *Arnold's ganglion*, *splanchnic ganglion of Arnold*, *otoganglion* (seldom used).

ganglion of palm of hand A rarely occurring lymph nodule located toward the medial side of the middle of the thenar eminence of the hand. An outmoded term.

parasympathetic ganglia The peripheral postganglionic, cholinergic ganglia innervated by preganglionic neurons of the brainstem and middle (second to fourth) sacral segments of the spinal cord.

paravertebral ganglion One of the ganglia of the thoracolumbar sympathetic trunk.

paravertebral sympathetic ganglion Any of the sympathetic ganglia located in the sympathetic trunk that courses paravertebrally along the spinal column. Also called *ganglion sympathicum*.

pelvic ganglia GANGLIA PELVINA.

ganglia pelvina [NA] The parasympathetic and sympathetic ganglia within the pelvic plexus of both sides. Also called *pelvic ganglia*, *hypogastric ganglia* (imprecise).

periosteal ganglion A ganglion cyst occurring in a subperiosteal location.

petrosal ganglion GANGLION INFERIUS NERVI GLOSSOPHARYNGEI.

ganglion petrosum GANGLION INFERIUS NERVI GLOSSOPHARYNGEI.

petrous ganglion GANGLION INFERIUS NERVI GLOSSOPHARYNGEI.

phrenic ganglia GANGLIA PHRENICA.

ganglia phrenica [NA] The small aggregates of sympathetic ganglion cells of the phrenic plexus adjacent to the celiac plexus. Also called *diaphragmatic ganglia*, *phrenic ganglia*.

pleural ganglion One of two ganglia which innervate part of the body behind the head and the mantle in mollusks.

ganglia plexuum autonomicorum [NA] Aggregates of ganglion cells of autonomic plexuses such as the sympathetic celiac and inferior mesenteric ganglia, along with the parasympathetic ganglia of the myenteric plexus. Also called *ganglia plexuum sympathicorum* (imprecise), *ganglia of sympathetic plexuses*.

ganglia plexuum sympathicorum 1 Aggregates of sympathetic postganglionic neurons lying in plexuses of autonomic fibers. 2 An imprecise term for GANGLIA PLEXUUM AUTONOMICORUM.

posterior root ganglion GANGLION SPINALE.

prevertebral ganglia The irregular aggregates of sympathetic ganglia lying anterior to the vertebral column in the mesenteric plexuses of the thorax and abdomen surrounding the abdominal aorta and its main visceral branches.

primary ganglion A ganglion that arises primarily and does not follow injury or an episode of local inflammation.

prostatic ganglion A ganglion of the prostatic plexus lying on the prostate gland.

pterygopalatine ganglion GANGLION PTERYGOPALATINUM.

ganglion pterygopalatinum [NA] The small parasympathetic ganglion in the upper pterygopalatine fossa. Its preganglionic innervation is via the greater petrosal nerve, and its postganglionic axons innervate the lacrimal, palatine, and nasal glands. Also called *sphenopalatine ganglion*, *ganglion sphenopalatinum*, *Meckel's ganglion*, *sphenomaxillary ganglion*, *nasal ganglion*, *pterygopalatine ganglion*.

Remak's ganglion 1 SINOATRIAL GANGLION. 2 A sympathetic ganglion on the inferior vena cava at the diaphragm. 3 A ganglion of the gastric plexus.

renal ganglia GANGLIA RENALIA.

ganglia renalia [NA] Small, scattered, sympathetic ganglia in the renal plexus. Also called *renal ganglia*.

ganglion retinae The outer portion of the internal nuclear layer of the retina, containing bipolar, horizontal, and amacrine cells.

Ribes ganglion The most rostral sympathetic ganglion on the anterior communicating artery of the brain. It is rarely seen.

sacral ganglia GANGLIA SACRALIA.

ganglia sacralia The three or four ganglia of the sacral part of the sympathetic trunk. Also called *sacral ganglia*.

Scarpa's ganglion GANGLION VESTIBULARE.

Schacher's ganglion A seldom used term for GANGLION CILIARE.

Schmiedel's ganglion INFERIOR CAROTID GANGLION.

semilunar ganglion 1 GANGLION TRIGEMINALE. 2 Either of the ganglia celiaca.

ganglion semilunare gasseri GANGLION TRIGEMINALE.

sensory ganglion GANGLION SPINALE.

simple ganglion A cystic tumor in a tendon sheath that contains transparent jellylike material rich in mucopolysaccharides.

sinoatrial ganglion A sympathetic ganglion in the cardiac sinoatrial wall near the superior vena cava. Also called *Remak's ganglion.*

sinus ganglion A small collection of parasympathetic neurons found near the point of entrance of the coronary sinus into the right atrium. A seldom used term.

Soemmering's ganglion An obsolete term for SUBSTANTIA NIGRA.

solar ganglia An outmoded term for GANGLIA CELIACA.

sphenomaxillary ganglion GANGLION PTERYGOPALATINUM.

sphenopalatine ganglion GANGLION PTERYGOPALATINUM.

ganglion sphenopalatinum GANGLION PTERYGOPALATINUM.

spinal ganglion GANGLION SPINALE.

ganglion spinale [NA] The sensory ganglion of each spinal dorsal root, containing neuron cell bodies whose peripheral neurites form or contact somatosensory end organs in the skin, deep tissue, and viscera. Also called *dorsal root ganglion, posterior root ganglion, sensory ganglion, spinal ganglion, ganglion intervertebrale.*

spiral ganglion GANGLION SPIRALE COCHLEAE.

spiral ganglion of cochlear nerve GANGLION SPIRALE COCHLEAE.

ganglion spirale cochleae [NA] The olongate, spiral ganglion of the cochlear division of the eighth nerve within the temporal bone modiolus. Its peripheral axons terminate in the spiral organ (of Corti), and its central root ends in the brainstem cochlear nuclear complex. Also called *auditory ganglion, acoustic ganglion, Corti's ganglion, spiral ganglion, spiral ganglion of cochlear nerve, ganglion spirale nervi cochleae, ganglion spirale partis cochlearis nervi octavi, Böttcher's ganglion.*

ganglion spirale nervi cochleae GANGLION SPIRALE COCHLEAE.

ganglion spirale partis cochlearis nervi octavi GANGLION SPIRALE COCHLEAE.

splanchnic ganglion GANGLION SPLANCHNICUM.

splanchnic ganglion of Arnold GANGLION OTICUM.

splanchnic ganglion of Lobstein GANGLION SPLANCHNICUM.

ganglion splanchnicum [NA] The variable small sympathetic ganglion on the greater splanchnic nerve at the T_{12} vertebral level innervating portions of the gastrointestinal tract. Also called *splanchnic ganglion, splanchnic ganglion of Lobstein, ganglion nervi splanchnici, Lobstein's ganglion.*

stellate ganglion GANGLION CERVICOTHORACICUM.

ganglion stellatum GANGLION CERVICOTHORACICUM.

sublingual ganglion of Blandin GANGLION SUBLINGUALE.

ganglion sublinguale A ganglion constituted by some parasympathetic nerve cells which are occasionally found on fibers running distally from the submandibular ganglion to the lingual nerve. It is believed to be distributed to the sublingual salivary gland but its function is not yet clearly understood. Also called *sublingual ganglion of Blandin.*

submandibular ganglion GANGLION SUBMANDIBULARE.

ganglion submandibulare [NA] A small parasympathetic ganglion on the lingual nerve above the submandibular gland. It controls salivary secretion of the submandibular and sublingual glands, receiving preganglionic fibers via the chorda tympani of the facial nerve. Also called *submandibular ganglion,*

ganglion submaxillare, *Blandin's ganglion, lesser ganglion of Meckel, lingual ganglion, maxillary ganglion.*

ganglion submaxillare GANGLION SUBMANDIBULARE.

subpharyngeal ganglion A ganglion, usually bilobed, located ventral to the pharynx in arthropods and annelids. It is the most anterior of a series of ventral ganglia.

superior cardiac ganglion A small gangliform formation that is situated on the cardiac branch of the middle cervical sympathetic ganglion at the level of the inferior thyroid artery. An outmoded term.

superior carotid ganglion A sympathetic ganglion of the upper internal carotid plexus.

superior cervical ganglion GANGLION CERVICALE SUPERIUS.

superior ganglion of glossopharyngeal nerve GANGLION SUPERIUS NERVI GLOSSOPHARYNGEI.

superior mesenteric ganglion GANGLION MESENTERICUM SUPERIUS.

superior thyroid ganglion An obsolete term for GANGLION CERVICALE MEDIUM.

superior vagal ganglion GANGLION SUPERIUS NERVI VAGI.

superior ganglion of vagus nerve GANGLION SUPERIUS NERVI VAGI.

ganglion superius GANGLION SUPERIUS NERVI GLOSSOPHARYNGEI.

ganglion superius nervi glossopharyngei The upper of the two sensory ganglia on the glossopharyngeal nerve in the jugular foramen. Also called *superior ganglion of glossopharyngeal nerve, Ehrenritter's ganglion, intracranial ganglion, ganglion superius, ganglion of Müller, jugular ganglion of glossopharyngeal nerve.*

ganglion superius nervi vagi The small sensory ganglion on the vagus nerve in the jugular foramen. Its peripheral processes extend into the vagus, meningeal, and auricular nerves. Also called *jugular ganglion of vagus nerve, superior vagal ganglion, superior ganglion of vagus nerve, ganglion jugulare nervi vagi.*

suprarenal ganglion A small sympathetic ganglion of the celiac portion of the prevertebral plexus supplying the adrenal gland.

ganglia of sympathetic plexuses GANGLIA PLEXUUM AUTONOMICORUM.

ganglia of sympathetic trunk GANGLIA TRUNCI SYMPATHICI.

ganglion sympathicum PARAVERTEBRAL SYMPATHETIC GANGLION.

synovial ganglion A cystic tumor containing synovial-like fluid, usually attached to a tendon sheath and most commonly observed on the dorsum of the wrist or foot. Also called *synovial cyst, myxoid cyst, ganglion cyst.*

terminal ganglion GANGLION TERMINALE.

ganglion terminale 1 [NA] A dispersed aggregate of nerve cellson the nervus terminalis medial to the olfactory bulb. Also called *terminal ganglion.* 2 A parasympathetic ganglion in or close to the wall of a visceral organ.

ganglia thoracalia GANGLIA THORACICA.

thoracic ganglia GANGLIA THORACICA.

ganglia thoracica [NA] The eleven or twelve paired paravertebral sympathetic ganglia located at the heads of the ribs. Also called *ganglia thoracalia, thoracic ganglia.*

ganglion thoracicum primum A variable, separate thoracic component of the sympathetic cervicothoracic ganglion.

trigeminal ganglion GANGLION TRIGEMINALE.

ganglion trigeminale A large sensory ganglion on the portio major of the trigeminal nerve, containing segments for the ophthalmic, maxillary, and mandibular nerves. It lies on the anterior slope of the petrous pyramid and is partially surrounded by an extension of the subarachnoid space (cavum trigeminale). Also called *semilunar ganglion, ganglion semilunare gasseri,*

Gasser's ganglion, gasserian ganglion, trigeminal ganglion, ganglion of trigeminal nerve.

ganglion of trigeminal nerve   GANGLION TRIGEMINALE.

Troisier's ganglion   An enlarged supraclavicular lymph node associated with a mediastinal tumor.

ganglia trunci sympathici   [NA] The ganglia of the sympathetic trunk extending from the superior cervical ganglion caudally to the ganglion impar. Also called *ganglia of sympathetic trunk.*

tympanic ganglion   GANGLION TYMPANICUM.

ganglion tympanicum   [NA] A ganglion on the tympanic branch of the glossopharyngeal nerve in the petrous portion of the temporal bone. Also called *tympanic ganglion.*

tympanic ganglion of Valentin   VALENTIN'S GANGLION.

Valentin's ganglion   **1** A ganglion on the superior alveolar nerve. Also called *tympanic ganglion of Valentin.* **2** An enlargement on the tympanic branch of the glossopharyngeal nerve.

ventricular ganglia   Aggregates of parasympathetic ganglion cells in the inferior portion in the interatrial septum of the heart. Also called *Bidder's ganglia.*

vertebral ganglion   GANGLION VERTEBRALE.

ganglion vertebrale   [NA] A small, variable sympathetic ganglion between the middle cervical ganglion and the cervicothoracic ganglion. Its postganglionic fibers are distributed in the brachial plexus and in the vertebral nerve and plexus. Also called *vertebral ganglion, intermediary ganglion* (outmoded).

vestibular ganglion   GANGLION VESTIBULARE.

ganglion vestibulare   [NA] The sensory ganglion of the vestibular portion of the eighth nerve, located in the internal auditory meatus. It innervates the sensory epithelium of the saccule, utricle, and semicircular canal, and its central processes terminate in the medullary vestibular nuclei. Also called *vestibular ganglion, Scarpa's ganglion, vestibular end organ* (outmoded).

vestibulocochlear ganglion   ACOUSTIC GANGLION.

Walther's ganglion   GANGLION IMPAR.

Wrisberg's ganglion   GANGLIA CARDIACA. • This ganglion should not be confused with the geniculate ganglion associated with the nervus intermedius (nerve of Wrisberg).

ganglion Wrisbergi   GANGLIA CARDIACA.

---

ganglionated   Denoting structures, especially visceral ones, containing ganglia.

ganglionectomy   [GANGLION + -ECTOMY] Excision of a ganglion. Also called *gangliectomy.*

ganglioneure   An outmoded term for GANGLIONEURON.

ganglioneuroblastoma   [GANGLIO- + NEUROBLASTOMA] A tumor of varying degrees of malignancy composed of a mixture of neuroblasts and ganglion cells in various stages of differentiation. As in neuroblastoma, the majority occur along the thoracolumbar sympathetic chain or in the adrenal gland. They are most common in children under five years of age. In rare cases maturation into a ganglioneuroma occurs. Increased catecholamine levels may be observed. Also called *gangliosympathicoblastoma.*

ganglioneurofibroma   [GANGLIO- + NEUROFIBROMA] A neurofibroma with ganglion cells. Also called *ganglionic neuroma.*

   melanogenic ganglioneurofibroma   A ganglioneurofibroma containing melanin.

ganglioneuroma   [GANGLIO- + NEUROMA] A benign tumor composed of mature ganglion cells associated with well-differentiated neurofibromatous elements. Also called *neurofibroma gangliocellulare, neurofibroma ganglionare, ganglionic neuroma,*

neuroma verum, neuroganglioma.

   dumbbell ganglioneuroma   HOURGLASS TUMOR.

   hourglass ganglioneuroma   HOURGLASS TUMOR.

   ganglioneuroma telangiectatum cysticum   A very vascular cystic ganglioneuroma.

ganglioneuromatosis   [GANGLIO- + NEUROMATOSIS] Multiple widespread ganglioneuromas.

ganglioneuron   [GANGLIO- + NEURON] A neuron within a sensory or autonomic ganglion. A rarely used term. Also called *ganglioneure* (outmoded).

ganglionic   Pertaining to a ganglion. Also *ganglial.*

ganglionitis   [GANGLION + -ITIS] Nonspecific inflammation of an autonomic ganglion. Also called *gangliitis.*

   acute posterior ganglionitis   HERPES ZOSTER.

   gasserian ganglionitis   HERPES OPHTHALMICUS.

ganglionoplegic   GANGLIOPLEGIC.

ganglionostomy   [GANGLION + o + -STOMY] A surgical procedure that creates an opening into a cystic lesion on a tendon sheath, particularly on the dorsum of the wrist.

gangliopathy   [GANGLIO- + -PATHY] Any pathological condition affecting a ganglion. A rarely used term.

ganglioplegic   A chemical substance that blocks conduction in autonomic ganglia. Also called *gangliolytic, ganglionoplegic.*

ganglioplexus   [GANGLIO- + PLEXUS] The neural interconnections within an autonomic ganglion.

ganglioside   Any glycolipid consisting of a ceramide glycosylated with an oligosaccharide that contains at least one residue of sialic acid. Such glycolipids are important components of cell membranes.

   ganglioside GM₁   A ganglioside consisting of ceramide glycosylated by a particular oligosaccharide. This oligosaccharide contains five residues: one of glucose, two of galactose, one of N-acetylgalactosamine, and one of N-acetylneuraminic acid.

   ganglioside GM₂   A ganglioside related to ganglioside GM₁ by lacking a terminal galactose residue.

gangliosidoses   Plural of GANGLIOSIDOSIS.

gangliosidosis   [GANGLIOSIDE + -OSIS] Any of the several inborn errors of ganglioside metabolism that cause an accumulation of gangliosides in nervous tissue, primarily in lysosomes. They are due in all but one case to a deficit of a catabolic enzyme. One synthetic defect is known. Also called *ganglioside lipidosis.*

   general gangliosidosis   GM₁ GANGLIOSIDOSIS.

   GM₁ gangliosidosis   Any of several inborn errors of ganglioside GM₁ catabolism. All are autosomal recessive, result in neuronal and somatic accumulation of GM₁ gangliosides, and are associated with GM₁ β-galactosidase deficiency. Several distinct, and apparently allelic, disorders are known, which have widely variable phenotypes and ages of onset. The most severe begins in early infancy and causes severe skeletal changes and rapid neurologic deterioration. Also called *general gangliosidosis, neurovisceral lipidosis.*

   GM₂ gangliosidosis   TAY-SACHS DISEASE.

gangliospore   [GANGLIO- + SPORE] A fungal spore formed by the enlargement and pinching off of a hyphal tip.

gangliosympathectomy   [GANGLIO- + SYMPATHECTOMY] Ganglionectomy of sympathetic ganglia.

gangliosympathicoblastoma   [GANGLIO- + SYMPATHICO- + BLASTOMA] GANGLIONEUROBLASTOMA.

Gangolphe   [Louis *Gangolphe*, French surgeon, 1858–1920] See under SIGN.

gangosa   [Spanish, fem. of *gangoso* speaking with a nasal twang; of onomatopoeic origin] A form of treponematosis, tertiary yaws. Ulceration occurs in the nasal and palatal structures and nasopharynx, which it ultimately destroys. It is found in any region in which yaws is endemic, particularly Africa, South America, southeast Asia, and the Pacific. Also called *rhino-pharyngitis mutilans, ogo, kaninloma*.

gangraena oris CANCRUM ORIS.

gangrene [L *gangraena* (from Gk *gangraine* a gangrene, an eating sore, from *grainein* to gnaw) an eating sore] A form of coagulative necrosis principally due to ischemia that is modified by the liquefactive action of bacteria and polymorphonuclear leukocytes. It may affect the lower extremities, gallbladder, appendix, and intestines. • The term is commonly used in clinical surgery.

angiosclerotic gangrene ARTERIOSCLEROTIC GANGRENE.

arteriosclerotic gangrene Gangrene due to arteriosclerosis. Also called *angiosclerotic gangrene*.

carbolic gangrene Gangrene caused by the repeated application of phenol.

chemical gangrene Tissue necrosis resulting from the application or injection of various chemical agents. It is seen with extravasation of vasoactive drugs and, in drug abusers, from the inadvertent intra-arterial injection of intravenous preparations.

circumscribed gangrene Gangrene that is demarcated from the surrounding viable tissue by an inflammatory rim.

cold gangrene DRY GANGRENE.

cutaneous gangrene Necrosis of the skin. Also called *sphaceloderma* (obsolete), *pemphigus gangrenosus* (obsolete).

decubital gangrene BEDSORE.

diabetic gangrene Gangrene due to peripheral vascular insufficiency associated with diabetes mellitus. It most commonly affects the toes or feet, rarely the fingers. Also called *glycemic gangrene* (outmoded).

disseminated cutaneous gangrene GANGRENOUS DERMATITIS OF INFANTS.

dry gangrene A type of gangrene where coagulative necrosis predominates, resulting in mummification of the affected tissue. The liquefactive action of bacteria and leukocytes is minimal or absent. Also called *dry necrosis* (rarely used), *mummification necrosis, cold gangrene*.

embolic gangrene Gangrene due to embolic occlusion of the arterial supply of a tissue.

emphysematous gangrene GAS GANGRENE.

epidemic gangrene Gangrene resulting from ergotism, which formerly occurred in epidemics caused by local consumption of contaminated grain.

Fournier's gangrene FOURNIER'S DISEASE.

frost gangrene An obsolete term for FROSTBITE.

fusospirochetal gangrene Gangrene of the upper respiratory tract, oropharynx, and other tissues associated with a mixed anaerobic flora. An obsolete term.

gas gangrene Gangrene characterized by a fulminant, painful, and severely toxic infection, typically in a wound, by any of several species of the anaerobic bacterium *Clostridium*, especially *C. welchii*, with putrefaction of tissue and the formation of gas. Surgery is the usual treatment. Also called *progressive emphysematous necrosis, emphysematous gangrene, mephitic gangrene* (seldom used), *putrid degeneration* (obsolete).

glycemic gangrene An outmoded term for DIABETIC GANGRENE.

hospital gangrene **1** Infective gangrene that occurred in crowded hospital wards before the introduction of antisepsis and antiseptic techniques of wound management. Also called *phagedena nosocomialis*. **2** BEDSORE.

hot gangrene INFLAMMATORY GANGRENE.

humid gangrene WET GANGRENE.

inflammatory gangrene Gangrene that develops as a complication of inflammation. Also called *hot gangrene*.

ischemic gangrene A condition of one or more digits or the skin of the distal foot in far-advanced arterial insufficiency, where actual tissue necrosis has occurred. In dry gangrene the dead tissue has simply mummified, while in wet gangrene, secondary infection has occurred, threatening the more proximal limb.

Kaposi's bulloserpiginous gangrene A severe form of diabetic gangrene. It has virtually disappeared since the introduction of insulin.

Meleney synergistic gangrene PROGRESSIVE POSTOPERATIVE GANGRENE.

mephitic gangrene A seldom used term for GAS GANGRENE.

mixed gangrene Gangrene having both dry and wet areas. A seldom used term.

moist gangrene WET GANGRENE.

multiple gangrene Gangrene affecting several body sites.

neuropathic gangrene Secondary gangrene following severe sensory loss due to damage to a peripheral nerve or to the spinal cord. Also called *necrotic trophoneurosis* (obsolete).

oral gangrene CANCRUM ORIS.

postoperative progressive gangrene PROGRESSIVE POSTOPERATIVE GANGRENE.

presenile spontaneous gangrene Gangrene due to thromboangiitis obliterans.

pressure gangrene BEDSORE.

primary gangrene Gangrene occurring in a tissue not previously inflamed.

progressive gangrene Gangrene lacking demarcation from healthy tissue and which continues to expand.

progressive bacterial synergistic gangrene A superficial, spreading infection, often following surgery, due to synergistic multiplication of microaerophilic streptococci and *Staphylococcus aureus* and resulting in destruction of tissue. When the condition occurs postoperatively, it is called Meleney's synergistic gangrene or progressive postoperative gangrene.

progressive postoperative gangrene Cutaneous gangrene caused by a microaerophilic streptococcus in a rare complication of an abdominal surgical wound. Also called *Meleney synergistic gangrene, postoperative progressive gangrene*.

gangrene of the pulp Necrosis of the dental pulp following pulpitis or severance of the apical vessels.

Raynaud's gangrene Gangrene occurring in association with Raynaud's phenomenon.

gangrene of the scrotum A gangrenous necrosis of the scrotal skin and wall occurring commonly after urinary extravasations or diseases of the urinary tract.

secondary gangrene Gangrene developing within an inflammatory focus.

senile gangrene A form of dry gangrene of the lower extremities seen in the elderly and resulting from advanced occlusive atherosclerosis.

spirochetal gangrene A form of gangrene in which the bacterial contamination is due to spirochetes.

static gangrene Gangrene resulting from severe venous stasis. Also called *venous gangrene*.

symmetric gangrene Gangrene in similar distribution on the two sides of the body due to vasomotor disorder.

sympathetic gangrene Gangrene resulting from a preexisting disease process.

thrombotic gangrene Gangrene as a consequence of arterial thrombosis.

traumatic gangrene Gangrene resulting from traumatic injury that interferes with the blood supply to the affected region.

trophic gangrene Gangrene developing in part of an extremity which has been deprived of sensory innervation and in which trophic changes have occurred.

venous gangrene STATIC GANGRENE.

wet gangrene A form of gangrene in which the necrotic tissues are soft, edematous, and inflamed. It is commonly the result of bacterial infection. Also called *moist gangrene, humid gangrene.*

gangrenescent   Demonstrating early signs of gangrene. A seldom used term.

gangrenopsis   CANCRUM ORIS.

gangrenous   Pertaining to or characterized by gangrene.

ganja   MARIHUANA.

ganoblast   AMELOBLAST.

ganoin [Gk *gano(s)* sheen + -IN] An enamel-like substance forming an outer layer on the scales of the ganoid fish.

Ganong [William Francis *Ganong,* U.S. physiologist, born 1924] Lown-Ganong-Levine syndrome. See under SHORT PR SYNDROME.

Ganser [Sigbert Joseph Maria *Ganser,* German psychiatrist, 1853–1931] **1** Ganser's ganglion. See under NUCLEUS INTERPEDUNCULARIS. **2** Psychotic Ganser syndrome. See under SYNDROME. **3** Ganser state, Ganser symptom. See under GANSER SYNDROME. **4** Commissure of Ganser. See under DORSAL SUPRAOPTIC COMMISSURE.

Gant [Frederick James *Gant,* English surgeon, 1825–1905] See under LINE, OPERATION.

Gant [Samuel Goodwin *Gant,* U.S. surgeon, 1869–1944] See under CLAMP.

Gantrisin   A proprietary name for sulfisoxazole.

gantry   The cylindrical opening located at or near the center of an imaging scanner into which the subject is placed.

Ganz [William *Ganz,* U.S. cardiologist, born 1919] Swan-Ganz catheter. See under CATHETER.

Ganzfeld   A homogeneous visual field, evenly illuminated and devoid of all texture or microstructure, which gives rise to an impression of looking into a diffuse and three-dimensional fog.

gap   **1** An opening or space between objects; aperture. **2** An interruption in a series or sequence. **3** In cytogenetics, any euchromatic region of a chromatid or chromosome that appears unstained on cytologic preparation and that is longer than the usual unstained band. A gap resembles a discontinuity microscopically, but the proximal and distal pieces of the chromatid remain together.

air-bone gap   The difference between the impaired air-conduction auditory threshold and the better or normal bone-conduction threshold. It is indicative of middle-ear pathology.

anion gap   The excess of unmeasured anions over unmeasured cations, comprising the negative charges contributed by phosphates, sulfates, and other metabolites. It is approximated by subtracting the sum of chloride and bicarbonate anions from the sum of sodium and potassium cations. The normal range of 12 to 18 mEq/liter is exceeded in ketoacidosis, severe alcohol toxicity, lactic acidosis, renal failure, and in many toxic ingestions. Also called *cation-anion difference.*

auscultatory gap   A period of silence, in the measurement of blood pressure by sphygmomanometry, following the initial period of sounds as the pressure falls in the manometer. It is mainly encountered in hypertension and aortic stenosis. Also called *silent gap.*

Bochdalek's gap   PLEUROPERICARDIAL HIATUS.

chromatid gap   In cytogenetics, a region of a chromatid which is euchromatic and which, presumably because of less compact packing of chromatin, does not stain in usual cytologic preparations but which is more extensive than an unstained band. A gap does not disrupt the continuity of the chromatid. Gaps on human karyotypes are termed marker sites, markers, or fragile sites.

cranial gaps   Congenital fissures of the fetal skull.

interocclusal gap   INTEROCCLUSAL DISTANCE.

isochromatid gap   In cytogenetics, the occurrence of a gap at the same level of two isochromatids.

leaf gap   A region of parenchyma in a primary vascular cylinder that is located above the site of an extension from the stem to a leaf.

silent gap   AUSCULTATORY GAP.

gapes [Middle English *gapen* (from Old Norse *gapa* yawn) to gape, akin to Gk *chasma* chasm] SYNGAMIASIS.

gapeworm   A parasitic nematode worm that lodges in the air passages of birds. The most important species economically is *Syngamus trachea,* which causes gapes (syngamiasis) in domestic poultry. Worms of the related genus *Cyathostoma* infect domestic waterfowl and various wild birds. Also called *forked worm, throatworm.*

Garamycin   A proprietary name for gentamicin sulfate.

Garbe [William *Garbe,* Canadian dermatologist, born 1908] Sulzberger-Garbe syndrome. See under EXUDATIVE DISCOID LICHENOID DERMATITIS.

Gardenia   A genus of Old World tropical plants of the Rubiaceae family. The stipules of many species secrete a resinous fluid. The fruits of *G. florida, G. grandiflora,* and *G. radicans* are used as demulcents and refrigerants. Fruits of *G. lucida* yield a yellow dye, gardenin. Some species exude volatile oils that are used as scents.

Gardner [Eldon John *Gardner,* U.S. geneticist, born 1909] Fitzgerald-Gardner syndrome. See under GARDNER SYNDROME.

Garel [Jean *Garel,* French physician, 1852–1931] Garel sign. See under BROWN KELLY SIGN.

garg.   *gargarismus* (L, gargle).

gargalanesthesia   Absence of sensibility for tickle.

gargalesthesia [Gk *gargal(os)* a tickling, itching + ESTHESIA] The sense of tickle. Adjective: gargalesthetic.

gargareon   UVULA.

garget [Middle English, from Old French *gargate* throat, from echoic base] An inflammation of the mammary gland (mastitis) in cattle and sheep. An outmoded term.

gargle [Middle French *gargouiller* to gurgle, of onomatopoeic origin] **1** To rinse the throat by agitating fluid there with the head back, the soft palate being caused to vibrate against the back of the tongue by a controlled expiration. **2** A preparation, usually medicated, with which to rinse the throat.

gargoylism [English *gargoyl(e)* (from Middle English *gargule* throat, from Old French *gargouille* throat, waterspout, gargoyle, of imitative origin as Gk *gargarizein* to gargle) + -ISM] **1** An outmoded term for MUCOPOLYSACCHARIDOSIS IH. **2** Any of the severe mucopolysaccharide or mucolipid storage disorders that produce coarse facies and dysostosis multiplex. An outmoded term.

X-linked recessive gargoylism   An outmoded term for MUCOPOLYSACCHARIDOSIS II.

Garland [George Minot *Garland,* U.S. physician, 1848–1926] Curve of Ellis and Garland, Garland's curve, Ellis-Garland line. See under ELLIS LINE.

Garland [Hugh *Garland,* English neurologist, flourished mid-20th century] Marinesco-Garland syndrome, Marinesco-Sjögren-Garland syndrome. See under MARINESCO-SJÖGREN SYNDROME.

garlic [Middle English *garlek,* from Old English *garleac,* from *gar* a spear + *leac* a leek] The bulb of *Allium sativum,* used as a flavoring in foods. Garlic oil, distilled from the bulb, has been used medicinally as an anthelmintic and rubefacient.

garment / elastic garment   Any of several specially measured and fitted elastic bandages used to provide constant pressure over a healed burn in hopes of reducing hypertrophic scarring.

garnet [Old French (*pome* or *pomme*) *grenate* a deep-red apple or fruit, pomegranate, from L *granatum* a fruit containing grains or seeds] Fine particles of vitreous mineral used as an abrasive in dental procedures.

Garré [Karl *Garré*, Swiss surgeon and bacteriologist, 1857–1928] Garré's disease, Garré's osteitis. See under NONSUPPURATIVE OSTEOMYELITIS.

garrot [French (from the Germanic), a tourniquet] 1 To strangle by means of a thin wire or cord crossed behind the neck and pulled tight. 2 SPANISH WINDLASS.

garroting [Spanish *garrot(e)* a club, garrote + -ING] 1 The strangulation of an unsuspecting victim from behind with a ligature or other device used to compresss the tissues of the victim's neck. 2 The practice of judicial strangulation as a method of capital punishment. This was practiced during the centuries in Spain, Portugal, and some Latin American countries. An iron collar was applied to a criminal's neck and tightened by a screw until death occurred. These collars, known as garrotes, were often made with long, pointed screws that constricted the collar while slowly piercing the skin, cervical vertebrae, and spinal cord.

Gärtner [Gustav *Gärtner*, Austrian pathologist, 1855–1937] See under PHENOMENON.

Gartner [Hermann Treschow *Gartner*, Danish anatomist, 1785–1827] 1 Cyst. 2 Gartner's canal, Gartner's duct, canal of Malpighi-Gartner. See under LONGITUDINAL DUCT OF EPOOPHORON.

Garymicin A proprietary name for gentamicin.

gas [a term invented by Jean-Baptiste van Helmont, Belgian chemist, 1577–1644; suggested by Gk *chaos* chaos, space] A substance in the state of matter in which its molecules are widely dispersed and spend only a small fraction of time in strong interaction with each other (collision).

alveolar gas Air that has been subjected to gas exchange with pulmonary blood through the epithelium of the lung alveoli. Also called *alveolar air*.

blood gas Gas dissolved in blood.

carrier gas A gas, usually oxygen with or without nitrous oxide, used as a conveyor of liquid anesthetics that have been vaporized for inhalation.

choking gas SUFFOCATING GAS.

Clayton gas Sulfur dioxide used at one time for ridding ships of rats.

coal gas A gas produced by the distillation of coal. It is poisonous because of its carbon monoxide content.

flue gas STACK GAS.

hemolytic gas ARSINE.

ideal gas A gas that obeys Boyle's law (the product of pressure and volume is constant when the temperature is constant) and Joule's law (the internal energy is a function of temperature alone). Also called *perfect gas*.

inert gas 1 Any gas unreactive under specified experimental conditions, sometimes nitrogen, but usually one of the noble gases, as these are particularly inert. 2 Any of the exhaust gases from engines such as carbon monoxide, carbon dioxide, water vapor, or nitrogen dioxide, that are fed into empty oil tanks on tankers in order to reduce the risk of explosion.

lacrimator gas TEAR GAS.

laughing gas NITROUS OXIDE.

marsh gas See under METHANE.

mustard gas $S(-CH_2-CH_2-Cl)_2$. Dichlorodiethyl sulfide. It is a powerful alkylating agent, since it can lose chloride ion to form an unstable 3-membered ring containing positively charged sulfur. This makes it toxic, and also mutagenic and carcinogenic, since it alkylates nucleic acid as well as protein. Low exposures cause erythema of the exposed surfaces of the skin. More severe exposure causes vesication and skin ulceration, with inflammation of the respiratory tract. It was used as a war gas in World War I. Also called *yperite* (obsolete).

natural gas The mixture of gases obtained from petroleum deposits underground. It consists of lower hydrocarbons, such as methane, ethane, and propane.

nerve gas Any of a group of organophosphate compounds which interfere with the central, peripheral, and parasympathetic nervous systems by inhibiting cholinesterase.

noble gas An element of the final group of the periodic table. Such an element has a complete electron shell, so is stable as an uncombined atom. Compounds of these elements are known, but they only form with a few other elements.

olefiant gas An obsolete term for ETHYLENE.

perfect gas IDEAL GAS.

persistent war gas A war gas that persists in the atmosphere for a significant length of time, usually specified as 10 minutes or more.

premixed gas A fixed combination of gases, as oxygen and nitrous oxide, in compressed gas cylinders, used for analgesia or general anesthesia.

sewer gas The mixture of gases and vapors formed in a sewer as a result of the decomposition of organic matter in the sewage. If not properly vented, toxic amounts of hydrogen sulfide may accumulate.

sneezing gas DIPHENYLCHLORARSINE.

stack gas The mixture of gases and suspended particles discharged from an industrial stack or chimney. Also called *stack effluent, flue gas*.

suffocating gas A war gas which causes extreme damage to the lungs and respiratory tract. Also called *choking gas*.

sweet gas CARBON MONOXIDE.

tear gas A volatile fluid that is dispersed in the air to induce tearing and irritation of the eyes as a means of temporarily disabling a person or controlling a crowd. Also called *lacrimator, lacrimator gas*.

vomiting gas A gas that induces vomiting. This effect is often preceded by irritation of the nose and throat, coughing, sneezing, and headache.

war gas A chemical warfare agent, either a true gas or a finely dispersed liquid or solid, which produces a toxic or strongly irritant effect. On the basis of physiologic action there are five classes of war gas: lacrimators, lung irritants, sternutators, systemic poisons, and vesicants.

gaseous Of the nature of gas.

Gaskell [Walter Holbrook *Gaskell*, English physiologist, 1847–1914] 1 Gaskell's bridge. See under FASCICULUS ATRIOVENTRICULARIS. 2 Gaskell's nerves. See under ACCELERATOR NERVES.

gaskin [short for *galligaskins*, from Middle French *garguesques*, from Old Spanish *gregüescos*, both meaning loose, wide breeches of the 16th and 17th centuries, from *Griego* Greek, from L *Graecus* Greek] The anterior muscular part of the hind leg of a horse, between the stifle joint and the hock.

gasometer [GAS + *o* + -METER] A device that contains and measures gases, especially those evolved in analytic reactions.

Tissot gasometer TISSOT SPIROMETER.

gasometric Of or relating to a gasometer.

gasometry The measurement of gas volume, either as constituents of a gaseous mixture or as the product evolved in an analytic reaction.

gasp [Middle English *gaspen* to gasp, from Old Norse *geispa* to yawn] A short, sharp inspiration of air.

Gasser [Johann Ludwig *Gasser*, Austrian anatomist, 1723–1765] 1 Gasserian syndrome. See under GASSERIAN GANGLION SYNDROME. 2 Ganglion semilunare Gasseri, Gasser's ganglion.

See under GANGLION TRIGEMINALE.

Gasser [Konrad Johann *Gasser*, Swiss pediatrician, born 1912] Gasser syndrome. See under HEMOLYTIC UREMIC SYNDROME.

gasserectomy [*gasser(ian ganglion)* + -ECTOMY] Excision of the gasserian ganglion of the trigeminal nerve. Also called *Rose operation*.

gasseritis [*gasser(ian ganglion)* + -ITIS] Inflammation of the gasserian ganglion.

gassing Poisoning by toxic gases.

Gastaut [Henri Jean-Pascal *Gastaut*, French biologist, born 1915] Gastaut's disease. See under LENNOX-GASTAUT SYNDROME.

gaster [Gk *gaster* belly] [NA] The most dilated part of the digestive tube, situated in the upper part of the abdominal cavity and extending from the cardiac orifice at the termination of the esophagus to the pyloric orifice that opens into the duodenum. It presents two borders, namely, the greater and lesser curvatures; and two surfaces, namely, anterosuperior and posteroinferior; and its body separates the fundus at the proximal end from the pyloric antrum distally. Also called *ventriculus, stomach.*

gaster- GASTERO-.

-gaster [Gk *gastēr* belly] A combining form meaning stomach or digestive tract.

gastero- [Gk *gastēr* belly] A combining form meaning stomach or digestive tract. Also *gaster-.*

Gasteromycetes [GASTERO- + -MYCETES] A subclass of basidiomycetous fungi characterized by an inner spore-bearing area, (gleba) that is enclosed by a distinct peridium. It includes the puffballs, earthstars, stinkhorns, and bird's-nest fungi.

Gasterophilidae [*Gasterophil(us)* + -IDAE] A family of flies whose larvae, or bots, cause enteric myiasis in horses and other equids. Also called *Gastrophilidae.*

Gasterophilus [GASTERO- + Gk *philos* beloved, loving] The principal genus of horse botflies (family Gasterophilidae). The adult flies resemble honeybees. A female deposits about a thousand eggs on hairs of the horse, usually within reach of the mouth. (In one species, eggs are deposited on grass.) Eggs licked up by the horse hatch immediately in the warmth of the mouth. The larvae excavate galleries in subepithelial layers of the tongue and then migrate, usually to the lining of the stomach. They remain attached to the gastric mucosa as second and third instars until the following spring or summer. Then they detach, pass out with the feces, pupate in droppings or soil, emerge as adults, mate, and lay the eggs that begin another cycle. Also called *Gastrophilus.*

Gasterophilus haemorrhoidalis The nose bot fly, which deposits its eggs on hairs around the lips and nose of horses, a process called "strike." Gastrointestinal disturbances are rare but may occur as the larvae develop on the gastric mucosa and move to the rectal area prior to detachment and evacuation with the feces. The fly's attempt to oviposit causes considerable annoyance to horses and may prevent them from grazing.

Gasterophilus intestinalis A species of horse botfly which deposits its eggs on hairs mainly of a horse's shoulders and forelegs. Human infection also occurs, producing a form of cutaneous larva migrans. The newly hatched larvae penetrate human skin and produce visible, tortuous dermal burrows. These larvae, about 1–2 mm long, do not develop beyond the first stage and usually can easily be surgically removed from the skin. In the horse the larval bots attach to the cardiac part of the gastric mucosa but even large numbers of them are well tolerated.

Gasterophilus nasalis The equine throat botfly, which deposits its eggs on hairs in the intermandibular region causing the horse to throw its head back violently. The migrating larvae form pockets between the teeth prior to passage to the stomach where they attach to the mucosa of the pyloric portion of the stomach or anterior duodenum, after which the larvae detach and pass out with the feces.

Gasterophilus pecorum An Old World horse botfly, probably the most common as well as most pathogenic species. The eggs are deposited on the hooves of horses as well as on grass and are taken up by the feeding horse. The larval bots attach to the gastric mucosa. Heavy infestations can lead to serious injury that either kills the horse or necessitates its destruction.

gastr- GASTRO-.

gastral GASTRIC.

gastralgia [GASTR- + -ALGIA] STOMACHACHE.

gastramine BETAZOLE HYDROCHLORIDE.

gastrectasia [GASTR- + ECTASIA] Distension of the stomach. Also called *gastrectasis.*

gastrectasis GASTRECTASIA.

gastrectomy [GASTR- + -ECTOMY] A surgical procedure in which all or part of the stomach is removed.

antecolic gastrectomy A surgical procedure in which all or part of the stomach is removed and the loop of jejunum that bears the efferent loop is sutured anterior to the transverse colon.

physiologic gastrectomy A procedure in which gastric function is arrested either chemically, neurologically, or by means of a limited resection.

subtotal gastrectomy A surgical procedure in which eighty percent or more, but not all, of the stomach is resected.

transthoracic gastrectomy A gastrectomy using a transdiaphragmatic approach through the chest.

gastric [GASTR- + -IC] Affecting, originating in, or relating to the stomach. Also *gastral.*

gastricism [GASTRIC + -ISM] **1** Any disorder of the stomach associated with impaired digestion. **2** The obsolete doctrine that most illnesses are related to gastric dysfunction.

gastrin [GASTR- + -IN] A gastrointestinal hormone, the most powerful known stimulant of gastric acid secretion. It is located in G cells of the gastric antrum and proximal duodenum, less abundantly in the small and large intestinal mucosa and in delta cells of the islets of Langerhans. Gastrin release is stimulated after eating, vagus nerve activation, or insulin hypoglycemia and is secreted excessively in the Zollinger-Ellison syndrome. Also called *gastric secretin.*

gastrinoma [GASTRIN + -OMA] An endocrine tumor which produces gastrin. It occurs most frequently in the pancreas, less often in the duodenum, and rarely in the stomach. It morphologically resembles the carcinoid or the islet cell tumor. It may be malignant. Gastrin overproduction can lead to the Zollinger-Ellison syndrome. Also called *G-cell tumor, G-cell carcinoid.*

gastritic Affected by or relating to gastritis.

gastritis [GASTR- + -ITIS] Inflammation of the mucosal lining of the stomach.

acute hemorrhagic gastritis An acute inflammation of the stomach with associated hemorrhage, often related to alcohol or salicylate ingestion.

acute phlegmonous gastritis Acute gastritis with abscess formation in the gastric wall.

alcoholic gastritis Gastritis caused by alcohol ingestion.

allergic gastritis Gastritis due to allergic reaction.

antral gastritis Gastritis primarily affecting the gastric antrum.

atrophic gastritis Idiopathic, chronic gastritis characterized by diffuse atrophy of the mucosa, loss of the normal rugal folds, and diminished or absent production of gastric acid and intrinsic factor, which may lead to pernicious anemia. It is also associated with an increased risk of gastric cancer. Also called *Fenwick's disease.*

catarrhal gastritis Inflammation and hypertrophy of the mucosal lining of the stomach associated with secretion of excessive quantities of mucus and gastric juices.

chemical gastritis CORROSIVE GASTRITIS.

chronic alcoholic gastritis Gastritis induced by the chronic ingestion of alcohol.

chronic cystic gastritis Chronic gastritis with cyst formation in the gastric wall.

corrosive gastritis Acute necrotizing destructive gastritis following ingestion of highly concentrated acid or alkaline agents. Also called *chemical gastritis.*

endogenous acute gastritis Acute gastritis usually associated with very severe physical stress such as life-threatening sepsis, major traumas, extensive burns, or the like.

eosinophilic gastritis Gastritis with predominance of eosinophilic polymorphonuclear leukocytes in the inflammatory infiltrate.

erosive gastritis Gastritis with erosions or ulcerations of the gastric mucosa. Also called *exfoliative gastritis.*

exfoliative gastritis EROSIVE GASTRITIS.

exogenous acute gastritis Acute gastritis resulting from the ingestion of irritating substances.

fibrinous gastritis Gastritis characterized by the presence of a fibrinous exudate.

follicular gastritis Inflammation of the mucosal glands of the stomach.

giant hypertrophic gastritis MÉNÉTRIER'S DISEASE.

granulomatous gastritis Gastritis characterized by the presence of a granulomatous mucosal infiltrate such as may occur in patients with tuberculosis, sarcoidosis, or regional enteritis.

hemorrhagic gastritis Gastritis complicated by gastric hemorrhage.

hypertrophic gastritis MÉNÉTRIER'S DISEASE.

interstitial gastritis Inflammation of the stomach involving the lamina propria, submucosa, and muscular coats.

pellagrous gastritis Gastritis secondary to niacin deficiency.

phlegmonous gastritis SUPPURATIVE GASTRITIS.

polypous gastritis Gastritis characterized by the presence of hyperplastic inflammatory polyps of the gastric mucosa.

pseudomembranous gastritis Inflammation of the stomach characterized by formation of a pseudomembrane over the gastric mucosa.

radiation gastritis Gastritis from exposure to radiation, usually x-ray irradiation.

suppurative gastritis Severe inflammation of the stomach caused by transmural purulent infection of the gastric wall. Also called *phlegmonous gastritis.*

toxic gastritis Gastritis secondary to drug, toxin, or corrosive injury.

traumatic gastritis A disease of cattle, caused by penetration of the anterior wall of the reticulum by a sharp object, such as a nail or piece of wire that the animal has swallowed.

uremic gastritis Inflammation of the stomach occurring in association with renal failure and characterized by a variety of pathologic findings, varying from mucosal petechiae to superficial ulceration and submucosal hemorrhage, and by clinical symptoms such as anorexia, nausea, and vomiting.

gastro- [Gk *gastēr* belly] A combining form denoting the stomach. Also *gastr-.*

gastroacephalus [GASTRO- + Gk *a*- priv. + -CEPHALUS] Unequal conjoined twins in which an acephalic parasite is attached at the abdomen of the host.

gastroamorphus [GASTRO- + Gk *amorphos* misshapen] Unequal conjoined twins in which an amorphous parasite is included within the abdomen of the host.

gastroanastomosis [GASTRO- + ANASTOMOSIS] GASTROGASTROSTOMY.

gastrocamera [GASTRO- + CAMERA] A small photographic instrument which may be passed into the stomach to record the state of the gastric mucosa. It is now largely replaced by fiberoptic endoscopes.

gastrocarp The spore-bearing portion of a gastromycete.

gastrocele [GASTRO- + -CELE[1]] A hernia involving a part of the stomach.

gastrocnemius MUSCULUS GASTROCNEMIUS.

gastrocoele [GASTRO- + -COELE] ARCHENTERON.

gastrocolic Relating to or connecting the stomach and the colon.

gastrocoloptosis [GASTRO- + COLO- + -PTOSIS] Ptosis or prolapse of the stomach and colon.

gastrocolostomy [GASTRO- + COLOSTOMY] The surgical creation of an opening between the colon and the stomach. Such an opening may rarely occur spontaneously after trauma, inflammation, or formation of a neoplasm.

gastrocolotomy [GASTRO- + COLOTOMY] A surgical procedure in which an incision is made into the stomach and colon.

gastrocolpotomy [GASTRO- + COLPOTOMY] A transabdominal incision into the vagina. An older term.

gastrocutaneous [GASTRO- + CUTANEOUS] Relating to or connecting the stomach and the skin.

gastrodermis [GASTRO- + DERMIS] The layer of cells lining the gastrovascular cavity of certain invertebrates, including the Coelenterata. These cells carry out intracellular digestion of food particles.

gastrodidymus [GASTRO- + DI-[2] + -DYMUS] GASTROPAGUS.

gastrodisciasis [GASTRO- + DISC- + -IASIS] Infection with *Gastrodiscoides hominis,* a trematode that inhabits the cecum and the colon of cynomolgus monkeys, pigs, and man in India, Asia, and the Philippines. It is characterized by mild, mucoid diarrhea.

Gastrodiscoides [GASTRO- + Late L *discoides* quoit-shaped] A genus of amphistome trematodes parasitic in the intestine of humans and other mammals. The species *Gastrodiscoides hominis* (formerly called *Gastrodiscus hominis* and *Amphistomum hominis*) has been reported to occur in humans, rodents, and certain primates in southeast Asia, India, and the Philippines. It is a cone-shaped, fleshy, pink worm typical of the family Paramphistomatidae (though it is sometimes placed in a separate family, Gastrodiscidae). The planorbid snail *Helicorbus coenosus* has served in India as an experimental intermediate host. Transmission to humans is presumed to be via metacercariae encysted on aquatic plants.

Gastrodiscus hominis See under *GASTRODISCOIDES.*

gastrodisk [GASTRO- + DISK] EMBRYONIC DISK.

gastroduodenal Relating to or connecting the stomach and the duodenum.

gastroduodenectomy [GASTRO- + DUODENECTOMY] A surgical procedure in which a part or all of the duodenum and stomach are removed.

gastroduodenitis [GASTRO- + DUODENITIS] Inflammation of the stomach and duodenum, often peptic in origin.

gastroduodenoenterostomy [GASTRO- + DUODENOENTEROSTOMY] A surgical procedure that creates an opening between the stomach, the duodenum, and the small bowel following a resection or bypass procedure. Usually created surgically, it may rarely result from a spontaneous traumatic, neoplastic, or inflammatory process.

gastroduodenoscopy [GASTRO- + DUODENOSCOPY] Examination of the interior of the stomach and duodenum by means of a gastroscope.

gastroduodenostomy [GASTRO- + DUODENOSTOMY]　A surgical procedure involving a resection or bypass that creates an opening between the stomach and the duodenum. It may occur spontaneously after trauma, neoplasm, or inflammatory disease, but this is rare.

　end-to-side gastroduodenostomy　A surgical procedure involving a resection or bypass that creates an opening between the distal end of the stomach and the lateral or side wall of the duodenum. It may occur spontaneously after trauma, inflammation, or neoplasm, but this is rare.

gastrodynia [GASTR- + -ODYNIA]　STOMACHACHE.

gastroenteric　Pertaining to or connecting the stomach and small intestine.

gastroenteritis [GASTRO- + ENTERITIS]　A syndrome characterized by gastrointestinal symptoms, including nausea and vomiting, diarrhea, and abdominal discomfort, and usually viral, bacterial, or parasitic in origin. There may or may not be inflammation of the intestinal tract. Also called *enteronitis* (older term).

　acute epidemic nonbacterial gastroenteritis　Gastroenteritis frequently occurring in epidemic form and characterized by severe nausea and vomiting, and, less frequently, diarrhea. Many such outbreaks are proabably caused by viral infection, but attempts to identify a specific agent are generally unsuccessful. Chemical or bacterial food poisoning may present similar symptoms. Also called *epidemic vomiting, epidemic vomiting syndrome, nausea epidemica, Bradley's disease.*

　acute infectious gastroenteritis　Acute inflammation of the stomach and small intestine due to viral or bacterial infection. Also called *polytropous enteronitis* (older term).

　eosinophilic gastroenteritis　A form of gastroenteritis with eosinophilia of the peripheral blood, eosinophilic infiltration of the lamina propria of the stomach and small intestine, and varying amounts of abdominal pain, diarrhea, and malabsorption.

　infantile gastroenteritis　A form of gastroenteritis common in children in the first two or three years of life, and characterized by acute vomiting and diarrhea leading to dehydration. There is a high mortality rate among victims, particularly in communities with a low socioeconomic standard. The infecting agent may be bacterial or viral. Also called *summer diarrhea* (outmoded), *cholera infantum, epidemic diarrhea in children.*

　gastroenteritis paratyphosa B　Gastroenteritis due to infection with *Salmonella paratyphi* B. (*S. schottmuelleri*).

　transmissible gastroenteritis of swine　A noninflammatory disease of the small intestine of swine, caused by a coronavirus, and characterized by atrophy of the intestinal villi. Abbreviation: TGE.

　gastroenteritis typhosa　Gastroenteritis due to infection with *Salmonella typhi.*

gastroenteroanastomosis [GASTRO- + ENTERO- + ANASTOMOSIS]　GASTROENTEROSTOMY.

gastroenterocolitis [GASTRO- + ENTEROCOLITIS]　Inflammation of the stomach, the small intestine, and the colon.

gastroenterocolostomy [GASTRO- + ENTEROCOLOSTOMY]　A surgical procedure involving a bypass or resection that creates an opening between the stomach, the small bowel, and the large bowel. Rarely, it may occur spontaneously after trauma, neoplasm, or inflammatory disease.

gastroenterologic　Of or pertaining to gastroenterology.

gastroenterologist [GASTRO- + ENTERO- + -LOGIST]　A specialist in diseases of the esophagus, stomach, small and large intestine, pancreas, and liver.

gastroenterology [GASTRO- + ENTERO- + -LOGY]　The branch of medicine dealing with the function and disorders of the stomach, small and large intestines, esophagus, pancreas, liver, and biliary tract.

gastroenteropathy [GASTRO- + ENTEROPATHY]　Any disorder of the stomach or small or large bowel.

gastroenteroplasty　Any plastic operation involving the stomach and an adjacent segment of small intestine.

gastroenteroptosis [GASTRO- + ENTEROPTOSIS]　Ptosis of the stomach and small intestine.

gastroenterostomy [GASTRO- + ENTERO- + -STOMY]　A surgical procedure involving a resection or bypass that creates an opening between the stomach and the small bowel. Although it may occur spontaneously after trauma, neoplasm formation, or inflammation, such incidences are rare. Also called *gastroenteroanastomosis, gastronesteostomy.*

　Roux's gastroenterostomy　ROUX EN Y GASTROENTEROSTOMY.

　Roux en Y gastroenterostomy　A surgical procedure involving a bypass or resection, using a defunctionalized Y-shaped jejunal limb to create a connection between the stomach and the small bowel. Also called *Roux's gastroenterostomy, Roux-Y gastrojejunostomy.*

gastroenterotomy [GASTRO- + ENTEROTOMY]　A surgical incision into the stomach and the small bowel.

gastroepiploic　Pertaining to the stomach and the greater omentum.

gastroesophageal　Pertaining to the stomach and the esophagus.

gastroesophagitis [GASTRO- + ESOPHAGITIS]　Inflammation, usually peptic in origin, of the stomach and the esophagus.

gastroesophagoplasty [GASTRO- + ESOPHAGO- + -PLASTY]　Any plastic operation on the lower end of the esophagus and the cardiac end of the stomach, usually for the relief of stricture or reflux esophagitis. Also called *fundoplasty.* See also FUNDOPLICATION.

gastroesophagostomy　A surgical procedure, involving a resection or bypass, that creates an opening between the stomach and the esophagus. It may result from trauma, neoplasm, or inflammation, but this is rare. Also called *esophagogastrostomy, esophagogastroanastomosis.*

gastrofiberscope　FIBEROPTIC GASTROSCOPE.

gastrogastrostomy [GASTRO- + GASTROSTOMY]　A surgical procedure involving a partial gastric resection or biopsy, creating an opening between two parts of the stomach. Also called *gastroanastomosis.*

gastrogavage [GASTRO- + GAVAGE]　Feeding via nasogastric intubation.

gastrogenic　Originating in the stomach.

Gastrografin　A proprietary name for meglumine diatrizoate.

gastrograph [GASTRO- + -GRAPH]　An instrument for recording gastric motility. Also called *gastrokinesograph.*

gastrohepatic　Pertaining to the stomach and the liver.

gastrohydrorrhea　Gastric hypersecretion.

gastrohysterectomy [GASTRO- + HYSTERECTOMY]　An older term for ABDOMINOHYSTERECTOMY.

gastroid [GASTR- + -OID]　Similar to the stomach, in shape or in function.

gastroileac　Of or relating to the stomach and the ileum.

gastroileitis [GASTRO- + ILEITIS]　Inflammation of the stomach and the ileum.

gastroileostomy　A surgical anastomosis of the stomach to the ileum. Such a connection, which has no therapeutic use and causes death from malnutrition, has occasionally been made erroneously in place of a gastrojejunostomy.

gastrointestinal Relating to the stomach and the intestinal tract.

gastrojejunal Relating to the stomach and the jejunum.

gastrojejunitis [GASTRO- + JEJUNITIS] Inflammation of the stomach and the jejunum.

gastrojejunocolic Relating to or connecting the stomach, jejunum, and colon.

gastrojejunoesophagostomy ESOPHAGOJEJUNOGASTROSTOMOSIS.

gastrojejunostomy A surgical anastomosis creating a direct connection between the stomach and the jejunum.

Roux-Y gastrojejunostomy ROUX EN Y GASTROENTEROSTOMY.

gastrokinesograph GASTROGRAPH.

gastrolavage [GASTRO- + LAVAGE] Irrigation of the stomach via a nasogastric tube.

gastrolienal Relating to or connecting the stomach and the spleen; gastrosplenic.

gastrolith [GASTRO- + -LITH] GASTRIC CALCULUS.

gastrolithiasis [GASTRO- + LITHIASIS] A condition characterized by the tendency to form gastric calculi.

gastrologist [GASTRO- + -LOGIST] A specialist in the study and treatment of diseases of the stomach.

gastrology [GASTRO- + -LOGY] That branch of medical science devoted to the study of the stomach and its diseases.

gastrolysis [GASTRO- + LYSIS] A surgical procedure in which the adhesions that surround the stomach are lysed in preparation for a gastric resection or to expose perigastric structures.

gastromalacia A softening of the gastric wall usually involving the mucosa and submucosa, commonly an incidental autopsy finding indicating advanced autolysis. Also called *softening of the stomach.*

gastromanometry [GASTRO- + MANOMETRY] Measurement of the pressures in the stomach, esophagus, and proximal small intestine.

gastromelus [GASTRO- + Gk *melos* limb] Unequal conjoined twins in which the parasitic member is represented by a supernumerary limb attached to the abdomen of the host.

gastromenia [GASTRO- + *men(o)-* + -IA] Gastric hemorrhage as a form of vicarious menstruation or possibly secondary to endometriosis of the gastrointestinal tract.

gastromycete [GASTRO- + -*mycete(s)*] Any of various fungi, including puffballs, earthstars, stinkhorns, and bird's-nest fungi, in which sexually reproduced basidiospores are produced internally in a glebal mass enclosed by a distinct peridial layer.

gastromycosis Any fungal disease involving the stomach, as gastritis occurring in disseminated histoplasmosis or mucormycosis, or *Candida* infection of the stomach occurring in immunocompromised hosts.

gastromyeloma [GASTRO- + MYELOMA] A sarcoma of the stomach. An obsolete term.

gastromyotomy [GASTRO- + MYOTOMY] A surgical incision into the stomach wall down to but not through the mucosa.

gastromyxorrhea [GASTRO- + MYXORRHEA] Excessive production of mucus by the stomach; gastric myxorrhea.

gastronesteostomy GASTROENTEROSTOMY.

gastro-oesophagostomy A British spelling for GASTROESOPHAGOSTOMY.

gastro-omental Pertaining to the stomach and omentum.

gastropagus [GASTRO- + -PAGUS] Equal conjoined twins united at the abdominal region. Also called *gastrodidymus, celiadelphus.*

gastropagus parasiticus Unequal conjoined twins in which

the parasite is attached to the abdomen of the host. Also called *gastroparasitus.*

gastropancreatic Pertaining to the stomach and pancreas.

gastropancreatitis Inflammation involving the stomach and pancreas.

gastroparalysis [GASTRO- + PARALYSIS] Loss of smooth muscle function in the stomach; gastroparesis.

gastroparasitus [GASTRO- + L *parasitus* a guest, parasite] GASTROPAGUS PARASITICUS.

gastroparesis An incomplete gastric paralysis, seen especially in diabetic acidosis or coma. A seldom used term. Also called *gastroplegia.*

gastropathic Pathologic with respect to the stomach; pertaining to gastropathy.

gastropathy [GASTRO- + -PATHY] A pathologic condition of the stomach; a disease of the stomach.

hypertrophic gastropathy MÉNÉTRIER'S DISEASE.

gastroperiodynia [GASTRO- + PERI- + -ODYNIA] Intermittent attacks of pain in the area of the stomach.

gastroperitonitis [GASTRO- + PERITONITIS] An inflammatory process involving the stomach and peritoneum.

gastropexy [GASTRO- + -PEXY] A surgical procedure in which the stomach is fixed or resuspended to change the axis or relative position of the gastroesophageal junction.

Gastrophilidae GASTEROPHILIDAE.

Gastrophilus *GASTEROPHILUS.*

gastrophore [GASTRO- + -PHORE] A surgical device designed to support the stomach during operative procedures involving that organ.

gastrophotography Photography of the stomach. The interior of the stomach is visualized most often using a fiberoptic endoscope, and a specially adapted camera may be used for still photography, motion pictures, or videotape.

gastrophrenic Pertaining to the stomach and the respiratory diaphragm. Also *phrenogastric, phrenicogastric.*

gastrophthisis [GASTRO- + PHTHISIS] **1** Hyperplasia of the lining of the stomach producing thickening of its wall. **2** Wasting or cachexia due to disease of the stomach.

gastroplasty [GASTRO- + -PLASTY] Any plastic operation on the stomach.

gastroplegia GASTROPARESIS.

gastroplication [GASTRO- + L *plicat(us)*, past part. of *plicare* to fold + -ION] A surgical procedure in which a fold is created in a redundant gastric wall in order to reduce its size. Also called *gastroptyxis, stomach reefing.*

gastropneumonic Pertaining to the stomach and the lungs; pneumogastric. Also *gastropulmonary.*

gastropod [GASTRO- + -POD] Any mollusk of the class Gastropoda.

Gastropoda [GASTRO- + New L -*poda*, neut. pl. of -*pod*, combining form denoting foot] The largest class of the phylum Mollusca, including snails, slugs, limpets, and whelks. The head has eyes and tentacles, the foot is well developed and flattened, the body is usually asymmetrical, with a coiled visceral hump contained in a spiral shell. There are freshwater, marine, and terrestrial species.

gastropore BLASTOPORE.

gastroptosis [GASTRO- + -PTOSIS] Downward displacement of the stomach. Also called *ventroptosis, ventroptosia* (obsolete), *descensus ventriculi.*

gastroptyxis [GASTRO- + Gk *ptyxis* a fold] GASTROPLICATION.

gastropulmonary GASTROPNEUMONIC.

gastropylorectomy [GASTRO- + PYLORECTOMY] A surgical

procedure in which the pylorus and part of the stomach proximal to the pylorus are resected.

gastropyloric   Pertaining to the stomach and pylorus.

gastroradiculitis   Inflammation of the posterior nerve roots which convey afferent sensory impulses from the stomach. An imprecise and outmoded concept.

gastrorrhagia [GASTRO- + -RRHAGIA]   Hemorrhage from the mucosal surface of the stomach.

gastrorrhaphy   Closure of an incision into or laceration of the stomach.

gastrorrhea [GASTRO- + -RRHEA]   Excessive secretion of gastric juice or of mucus by the stomach.

gastrorrhexis [GASTRO- + -RRHEXIS]   Gastric rupture.

gastrosalpingotomy [GASTRO- + SALPINGOTOMY]   A transabdominal incision of a fallopian tube. A seldom used term.

gastroschisis [GASTRO- + Gk *schisis* a cleaving, division]   Failure of closure of the embryonic anterior abdominal wall at the midventral line. The viscera may protrude with or without a complete or partial covering of a membrane, variably comprised of modified skin, peritoneum, and muscle aponeuroses. The abdominal wall may be left in a deficient state. When the thorax is involved, the condition is called thoracogastroschisis. Also called *celoschisis, coeloschisis*.

gastroscope [GASTRO- + -SCOPE]   An instrument used to visualize the mucosal surface of the stomach.
  fiberoptic gastroscope   An endoscope made with flexible synthetic fibers permitting observation of the stomach. Also called *gastrofiberscope*.

gastroscopic   Relating to gastroscopy; done by means of a gastroscope.

gastroscopy [GASTRO- + -SCOPY]   Inspection of the inner surface of the stomach with an endoscope. Also called *stomachoscopy*.

gastrosia   GASTROSIS.
  gastrosia fungosa   A disease process of the stomach caused by fungi.

gastrosis [GASTRO- + -SIS]   A disease process involving the stomach. Also called *gastrosia*.

gastrospasm [GASTRO- + SPASM]   Spasm of the walls of the stomach.

gastrospiry [GASTRO- + SPIR(O)-² + -Y]   Swallowing of air into the stomach; aerophagia.

gastrosplenic   Pertaining to the stomach and the spleen.

gastrostaxis [GASTRO- + Gk *staxis* a dropping, dripping]   Oozing of blood from the mucosal surface of the stomach.

gastrostenosis [GASTRO- + STENOSIS]   A narrowing of the stomach lumen.

gastrostogavage [*gastrosto(my)* + GAVAGE]   Alimentation via a gastrostomy tube.

gastrostolavage [*gastrosto(my)* + LAVAGE]   Irrigation of the stomach via a gastrostomy tube.

gastrostoma   An opening into the stomach from the abdominal wall.

gastrostomosis   GASTROSTOMY.

gastrostomy [GASTRO- + -STOMY]   A surgical procedure creating an opening into the stomach from the abdominal wall for drainage or feeding purposes. Also called *gastrostomosis*.
  Beck's gastrostomy   A surgical procedure creating an opening between the skin and the stomach, utilizing a tube created from the greater curvature of the gastric wall. Also called *Beck's method*.
  Stamm gastrostomy   A surgical procedure for gastric decompression and/or feeding, in which a mushroom catheter is inserted through two concentric purse-string sutures into the stomach. The anterior gastric wall is then tacked securely to the peritoneal surface of the anterior abdominal wall.

gastrosuccorrhea [GASTRO- + SUCCORRHEA]   Excessive secretion of gastric juice. Also called *Reichmann's disease* (obsolete).
  digestive gastrosuccorrhea   Excessive secretion of gastric juices during digestion.

gastrotherapy   **1** Treatment of diseases of the stomach.   **2** Treatment of pernicious anemia with extract of the mucous membrane of a hog's stomach. An obsolete term.

gastrothoracic   Pertaining to the stomach and the thorax.

gastrothoracopagus   THORACOGASTROPAGUS.

gastrotome [GASTRO- + -TOME]   A surgical instrument used to incise the stomach.

gastrotomy [GASTRO- + -TOMY]   A surgical procedure in which one or more incisions are made into the stomach.

gastrotonometer [GASTRO- + TONOMETER]   An apparatus used to measure intragastric pressure.

gastrotonometry [GASTRO- + TONOMETRY]   The measurement of intragastric pressure.

gastrotoxic   Having a toxic effect on the stomach.

gastrotoxin   Any toxic substance that exerts an adverse effect on the stomach.

Gastrotricha [GASTRO- + New L -*tricha*, taxonomic suffix denoting hair, from Gk *thrix*, gen. *trichos*, the hair]   A class of small, vermiform, ciliated, aquatic organisms of the phylum Aschelminthes.

gastrotropic [GASTRO- + -TROPIC¹]   Having an effect upon the stomach.

gastrotympanites [GASTRO- + TYMPANITES]   Distention of the stomach caused by the presence of air or gas.

gastrovolumetry [GASTRO- + VOLUMETRY]   Measurement of gastric volume through use of insufflated air.

gastrula [Late L, an early embryo]   A stage in embryonic development, following that of the blastula, during which there appears for the first time, as the result of morphogenetic movements, several layers (two or three, depending on the animal group) representing the primary germ layers of ectoderm, mesoderm, and endoderm. This process of formation (gastrulation) establishes the anteroposterior axis of the body in the embryo. Also called *invaginate planula*.

gastrulation [Late L *gastrul(a)* (dim. of Gk *gastēr* the belly) an early embryo + -ATION]   The process by which the blastula is developed to the gastrula, a folding of a portion of the blastula on to the opposed part. It is during this part of embryonic development that the segmental ovum generally obtains three primary germ layers. The mechanics of gastrulation differs among animal groups.

gate [Middle English, from Old English *geat, gæt* a gate, opening, akin to Gk *chezein* to defecate]   **1** A combinational logic circuit whose output is determined by the states of its inputs.   **2** The control electrode in a field-effect transistor.   **3** An interval of time during which an electronic circuit is operative and can pass data.

AND gate   A combinational logic circuit that gives a high, or 1, output only if all inputs are high.

gating   **1** The process of selecting those portions of a wave that lie between certain times or amplitudes.   **2** The inhibition or blocking out of one set of sensations by the action of another set of sensations. Gating occurs most notably during shifts of attention, when selective focusing on the information arriving over one sensory channel tends to minimize or eliminate other sensory information, or at least to keep it at the periphery of awareness.   **3** The process by which sodium channels become opened during the electrical activity of a neuron.

gatism [French *gâtisme* (from L *vastare* to lay waste) a physical or mental deterioration] Bladder and rectal incontinence.

gatophilia [Spanish *gato* (from LateL *cattus* a cat) a cat + -PHILIA] AILUROPHILIA.

gatophobia [Spanish *gato* (from LateL *cattus* a cat) a cat + -PHOBIA] AILUROPHOBIA.

gattine [French] A disease of silkworm larvae probably caused by a mixed infection with a virus and an enterococcus similar to *Streptococcus faecalis*.

Gaucher [Philippe Charles Ernst *Gaucher*, French physician, 1854–1918] **1** Gaucher lipid. See under CEREBROSIDE. **2** See under CELL. **3** Gaucher splenomegaly. See under GAUCHER'S DISEASE.

gauge [French *jauge* (from the Germanic) gauge] **1** Any of various instruments used to measure a physical quantity, either directly or by converting one physical quantity into another giving an observable output, as a blood-pressure gauge. **2** Any arbitrarily chosen range of sizes, as of wires, generally referred to by numbers. **3** A specific size within such a range of sizes, as a 16-gauge hypodermic needle. For defs. 1, 2, and 3 also *gage*.

beta ray gauge An instrument using a source of beta radiation and a radiation detector to measure the thickness of a material, such as plastic foil, by detecting the transmission of the beta rays through it.

bite gauge A device used in prosthodontics to determine the rest position, by measurement from the nose or other fixed point. Also *bitegauge*.

Boley gauge A small linear gauge with vernier attachment, used in dentistry.

catheter gauge A plate with holes of increasing size used to measure the outside diameter of a catheter.

deposit gauge An instrument designed for measuring the amount of air-borne solid material that is deposited over a specified period of time.

directional gauge An instrument designed to measure air pollution from one or more directions.

Livingston binocular gauge A device consisting of a metric ruler, used to measure the ocular ability of an individual to accommodate and to converge.

strain gauge A thin wire transducer of metal, semiconductor, or mercury in a rubber tube. Its increase in resistance is proportional to strain, which enables measurement of stress, displacement, or pressure.

undercut gauge A device used with a surveyor for measuring the depth of undercut.

x-ray emission gauge X-RAY THICKNESS GAUGE.

x-ray thickness gauge An instrument using the transmission of x rays through a material to measure its thickness. Also called *x-ray emission gauge*.

Willis gauge A device for measuring the face.

gauntlet GAUNTLET BANDAGE.

Gause [G. F. *Gause*, German geneticist, flourished 20th century] Gause principle. See under COMPETITIVE EXCLUSION.

Gauss [Carl Friedrich *Gauss*, German mathematician, 1777–1855] Gaussian distribution. See under NORMAL DISTRIBUTION.

gauss [Karl Friedrich *Gauss,* German mathematician, 1777–1855.] A CGS electromagnetic unit of magnetic flux, equal to 10^{-4} tesla. An obsolete unit. Symbol: Gs • In physics, the symbol G is preferred.

Gaussel [Amans *Gaussel*, French physician, 1871–1937] **1** Grasset-Gaussel phenomenon. See under GRASSET'S PHENOMENON. **2** Grasset-Gaussel-Hoover sign. See under SIGN.

gauze [sixteenth-century English, from *Gaza*, Palestine, where a light, loosely woven fabric was made] A woven, usually cotton, fabric of coarse or fine mesh that is treated in various ways for use as a dressing. See also entries under BANDAGE and DRESSING.

absorbable gauze Gauze made of oxidized cellulose that can be degraded within the body.

absorbent gauze Gauze made of material that will take up serum and other liquid exudation from a wound. Also called *carbasus absorbens* (obsolete).

antiseptic gauze Gauze to which any of a number of antimicrobial agents have been added. Common among these are dyes, iodinated compounds, and sulfonamides.

aseptic gauze Gauze that has been sterilized.

fine mesh gauze A narrow woven, single-layer cotton dressing. The small interstices do not allow much adherence of the dressing to the serum and wound exudate. As a result there is less trauma to the wound or fresh graft when the dressing is removed.

medicated gauze Gauze to which any of a number of ointments or antiseptics have been added.

petrolatum gauze Gauze impregnated with petrolatum to exclude air from the wound and thus prevent drying.

ribbon gauze Gauze made in a long thin strip and used to pack a deep wound so as to keep the edges apart and allow healing from the interior outward.

tullegras gauze TULLE GRAS.

gavage [French (from Picard French *gav(e)* internal part of the neck + French *-age* -AGE), a gorging, force-feeding] **1** Alimentation via a tube placed into the stomach. **2** Superalimentation of animals.

Gavard [Hyacinthe *Gavard*, French anatomist, 1753–1802] Gavard's muscle. See under FIBRAE OBLIQUAE GASTRICAE.

Gay [Alexander H. *Gay*, Russian anatomist, 1842–1907] Glands of Gay. See under CIRCUMANAL GLANDS.

Gayet [Charles-Jules-Alphonse *Gayet*, French physician, 1833–1904] Gayet-Wernicke encephalopathy, Gayet's disease. See under WERNICKE'S DISEASE.

Gay-Lussac [Joseph Louis *Gay-Lussac*, French chemist and physicist, 1778–1850] Gay-Lussac law. See under LAW.

gaze [Middle English *gazen*, of Scandinavian origin] **1** To direct the eyes persistently. **2** The act of gazing; a stable and persistent direction of the eyes.

conjugate gaze Simultaneous movement of both eyes into a position of use.

Gb Symbol for the obsolete unit, gilbert.

GBM glomerular basement membrane.

GBq Symbol for the unit, gigabecquerel.

G + C Guanine paired with cytosine, as in DNA. See also BASE RATIO.

g-cal. Symbol for the unit, gram-calorie.

Gd Symbol for the element, gadolinium.

GDA glycidaldehyde.

GDH **1** glucose dehydrogenase. **2** glutamate dehydrogenase. **3** glycerol-3-phosphate dehydrogenase. • Because of its various meanings this abbreviation is best avoided.

GDP guanosine diphosphate.

Ge Symbol for the element, germanium.

gear / cervical gear The device used in cervical anchorage.

Geastrum A genus of fungi belonging to the order Lycoperdales; the earthstars. At maturity, the outer peridial layer splits open exposing the inner peridial layer covering the spore-bearing gleba.

Gee [Samuel Jones *Gee*, English physician, 1839–1911] **1** Gee's disease, Gee-Herter disease, Gee-Herter-Heubner disease, Gee-Herter-Heubner syndrome. See under INFANTILE CELIAC DIS-

EASE. **2** Gee-Thaysen disease. See under ADULT CELIAC DISEASE.

Gegenbaur [Carl *Gegenbaur*, German anatomist, 1826–1903] **1** Gegenbaur's muscle. See under AURICULOFRONTALIS. **2** Gegenbaur cell. See under OSTEOBLAST.

gegenhalten [German *gegen* against, counter + *halten* to hold, stop] Uneven resistance to passive movement of the limbs. Superficially it resembles in some cases the lead-pipe or cogwheel rigidity of parkinsonism and may be noted in some stuporous or demented patients. Also called *paratonia*.

Geigel [Richard *Geigel*, German physician, 1859–1930] See under REFLEX.

Geiger [Hans Wilhelm *Geiger*, German physicist, 1882–1945] **1** Geiger-Müller counter. See under COUNTER. **2** Geiger-Nuttall law. See under LAW. **3** Geiger-Müller survey meter. See under METER. **4** See under REGION, PLATEAU, THRESHOLD. **5** Halogen-quenched Geiger-Müller tube. See under TUBE. **6** Side-window Geiger-Müller tube. See under TUBE. **7** Geiger-Müller tube. See under TUBE.

Geissler [Johann Heinrich Wilhelm *Geissler*, German mechanic and glassblower, 1815–1879] Geissler-Pluecker tube. See under GEISSLER'S TUBE.

geissoschizoline $C_{19}H_{26}N_2O$. A white alkaloid obtained from the bark of *Geissospermum vellosii* and used as an antiperiodic, antipyretic, and tonic. Also called *pereirine*.

gel [short for GELATIN] A phase that is largely liquid but incapable of flow because it is held rigid by molecular chains, usually cross-linked, that pass through it.

gelasmus [New L (irreg. from Gk *gelasma* a laugh, from *gelan* to laugh)] Spasmodic, involuntary laughter sometimes seen in schizophrenia and hysteria.

gelatin [French *gélatine* (from L *gelatus*, past part. of *gelare* to cause to freeze) gelatin] A soluble protein obtained by boiling collagen with water, during which process the collagen is partly degraded.

gelatin compound phenolized A preparation with a gelatin base containing zinc oxide, glycerin, water, and phenol. It is used in bandages that are applied to the skin for the treatment of ulcers and burns.

formalin gelatin Gelatin that has been treated with an enteric coating to render it insoluble. Capsules or coverings for pills from such material are protected from the acidity of the stomach and remain intact until they reach the alkaline conditions of the small intestine.

medicated gelatin A gelatin base that contains medicinally active agents. It is most often applied topically.

zinc gelatin A medicinal preparation that is composed of 15 percent zinc oxide, gelatin, water, and glycerin. It is applied topically and serves as a protective coating.

gelatinosa Gelatinous: said of portions of the nervous system.

gelatinous **1** Having a gelatinlike consistency that varies with moisture conditions: often used of a layer or part of a fungus. **2** Pertaining to or resembling gelatin; jellylike.

gelation [GEL + -ATION] The process of gel formation.

geld [Middle English *gelden*, from Old Norse *gelda* to castrate] To castrate (a male horse).

gelding [GELD + -ING] A castrated male horse.

Gelfilm A sterilized gelatin sponge prepared as small thin sheets, and used in ear surgery. A proprietary name. See also GELFOAM.

Gelfoam A sterilized gelatin sponge used widely in ear surgery to aid hemostasis, for packing, and to support grafts. Its great advantage is its ability to be absorbed by the tissues so that it need not be removed. A proprietary name.

gelidusi An obsolete term for PELIDISI.

Gélineau [Jean Baptiste Edouard *Gélineau*, French neurologist, born 1859] Gélineau syndrome. See under NARCOLEPSY.

Gellé [Marie Ernest *Gellé*, French otologist, 1834–1923] See under SYNDROME, TEST.

Gellhorn [George *Gellhorn*, U.S. gynecologist, 1870–1936] See under PESSARY.

geloplegia [Gk *gelō(s)* laughter + -PLEGIA] Loss of muscle tone induced by laughter. Also called *gelotolepsy*.

gelosis [L *gel(are)* to freeze + -OSIS] A hard mass in a tissue, especially in a muscle. An outmoded term.

gelotherapy [Gk *gelō(to)*- (from *gelan* to laugh), combining form denoting laughter + THERAPY] The use of humor as a form of therapy in the treatment of illness. An older term. Also called *gelotoherapy*.

gelotolepsy GELOPLEGIA.

gelototherapy GELOTHERAPY.

gel. quav. *gelatina quavis* (L, in any kind of jelly).

gelsemine $C_{20}H_{22}N_2O_2$. An alkaloid obtained from the dried roots and rhizomes of *Gelsemium sempervirens* of the Loganiaceae family. It has a depressant effect on the central nervous system and has been used as an antispasmodic, a nerve sedative, and a mydriatic.

gelseminine A poisonous mixture of alkaloids, including sempervirine, that is found in the plant *Gelsemium sempervirens*, the Carolina jessamine or yellow jasmine.

gelsemism [*Gelsem(ium)* + -ISM] Poisoning caused by the ingestion of the Carolina or yellow jessamine, *Gelsemium sempervirens*. The symptoms are muscular weakness, excessive perspiration, and respiratory depression.

Gély [Jules Aristide *Gély*, French surgeon, 1806–1861] See under SUTURE.

gem- [L *geminus* twin] A prefix used in chemical names to show that the two substituents named after it are attached to the same atom.

gemästete [German, past part. of *mästen* to feed, fatten, cram] Swollen or ballooning: said of astrocytes around a lesion in the central nervous system.

gemellary [L *gemell(us)*, dim. of *geminus* double, a twin + -ARY] Pertaining to a twin gestation. An older term.

gemellipara [L (from *gemellus*, dim. of *geminus* double, a twin + *parere* to bear young), bearing twins] A mother of twins. An older term.

gemellology [L *gemell(us)*, dim. of *geminus* double, a twin + o + -LOGY] The scientific study of twin gestations. An obsolete term.

gemellus [L, dim. of *geminus* double, twin] An outmoded term for TWIN.

gemina [L, neut. pl. of *geminus* double, twin] CORPORA QUADRIGEMINA.

geminal [L *gemin(us)* double, twin + -AL] Attached to the same atom: said of two chemical groups.

geminate [L *geminat(us)*, past part. of *geminare* to double] Occurring in pairs. Also *geminous*.

gemination [L *geminatio* (from *geminatus*, past part. of *geminare* to double, be double) a doubling] The union of two teeth.

false gemination The joining together of two normal teeth by an overgrowth of cementum.

true gemination Incomplete or partial division of an embryonic primordium into two parts, as a tooth with two partially united crowns but with a single root; any incomplete duplication of a part of or an organ.

gemini Plural of GEMINUS.

geminous GEMINATE.

geminus [L, double, twin] (*plural* gemini) An outmoded term for TWIN.

gemini aequales An older term for MONOZYGOTIC TWINS.

gemistocyte PROTOPLASMIC ASTROCYTE.

gemistocytic Describing, pertaining to, or consisting of gemistocytes: used especially of certain astrocytomas.

gemistocytoma [Gk *gemisto(s)* laden, full + *cytoma*] GEMISTOCYTIC ASTROCYTOMA.

gemma [L, a bud] (*plural* gemmae) **1** A thick-walled fungal cell, sometimes irregularly shaped, similar to a chlamydospore. **2** A nonmotile, asexual spore produced by certain algae. **3** Any structure with a budlike form.

gemmae Plural of GEMMA.

gemmangioma [L *gemm(a)* a bud, jewel + ANGIOMA] An obsolete term for ANGIOSARCOMA.

gemmation [L *gemmat(us)*, past part. of *gemmare* to put forth buds or gems + -ION] Asexual cell reproduction in which part of the cell body organizes as a separate growth on the surface or within the parent body, and then differentiates as a new individual. Also called *bud fission*. See also GEMMA, GEMMULE, BUDDING.

gemmulae Hobokenii Varicosities of the umbilical cord arteries. An older term.

gemmule **1** An asexually produced bud from which an independent fungal hypha forms. **2** A nonexistent organelle said to be transferred from somatic cells to germinal tissue, thereby providing a hypothetical mechanism for the inheritance of acquired characteristics.

Gemonil A proprietary name for metharbital.

gen- GENO-.

-gen [Gk *genos* race, descent, descendant; genus as opposed to species] A combining form meaning (1) producing; (2) produced by.

gena BUCCA.

genal BUCCAL.

gender [Middle English *gendre*, from Old French *genre* kind, from L *genere*, ablative of *genus* class, kind] Sex; a categorical differentiation of organisms based on sex.

gene [Gk *gennan* (from *genna*, poetic form of *genos* race, descent, from root *genō* of *gignesthai* to become, be born) to beget (of the father), bear (of the mother)] A segment of DNA (or RNA in certain viruses) that codes for a specific polypeptide or RNA molecule. Also called *locus* (imprecise), *genetic material* (imprecise). See also CISTRON.

allelic gene ALLELE.

amorphic gene An allele that produces either no product or a nonfunctional product. The effect on phenotype is not predictable, can vary from none to extreme, and depends on the action of the companion allele in diploid organisms, among many factors. Also called *amorph*.

antimutator gene A gene whose mutation can decrease the spontaneous mutation rate.

autosomal gene Any gene located on an autosomal chromosome.

complementary genes Two or more genetic loci that interact, generally through their products, with the resulting phenotype being distinct from those of any of the loci acting independently. Also called *reciprocal genes*.

control gene REGULATOR GENE.

cumulative gene POLYGENE.

cytoplasmic gene Any gene that ordinarily exists on nucleic acid in the cytoplasm, especially one on mitochondrial or chloroplast chromosomes.

dominant gene An allele that directs the production or appearance of a mendelian dominant phenotype, regardless of

whether the allele is heterozygous or homozygous. Also called *dominant allele*.

hemizygous gene Any gene present in but one copy in a cell or organism that is diploid or polyploid: used especially of genes on either sex chromosome in the heterogametic sex.

histocompatibility gene A gene determining the specificity of tissue antigenicity and therefore the compatibility of donor and recipient in transplantation.

holandric gene **1** A gene that occurs only in the male of a species. A popular usage. **2** Y-LINKED GENE.

hologynic genes **1** Genes that determine traits limited to females. A popular usage. **2** In humans, genes that determine X-linked dominant traits lethal *in utero* to hemizygous males or autosomal traits limited to females. **3** In certain species in which the female is the heterogametic sex, genes linked to the female-determining sex chromosome, such as the W chromosome.

homoeotic gene A mutant gene whose effect on phenotype is homoeosis. Such genes, when not mutated, are thought to have roles in developmental processes.

Ir gene **1** A gene specifying an immune response function. **2** A gene in the major histocompatibility complex of the mouse.

jumping gene TRANSPOSABLE GENE.

leaky gene HYPOMORPH.

lethal gene LETHAL ALLELE.

major gene Any gene whose effect on the phenotype is evident, regardless of how this effect is modulated by the rest of the genotype.

marker gene Any gene that determines a distinct phenotype and can therefore be used in experimental genetics.

mimic gene **1** An allele that results in a phenotype similar to that of a distinct genetic locus. **2** An allele that causes a genocopy or genetic mimic.

modifying gene A gene that affects the phenotypic expression of another genetic locus. The interaction may enhance, reduce, or suppress the action of the modified locus. Also called *modifying factor, modifier, modification allele*.

mutable gene Any gene capable of undergoing mutational change. In so far as is known, all genes are mutable.

mutant gene Any allele distinct in structure or function from the wild-type allele because of mutation at that genetic locus.

mutator gene A gene whose mutation can increase the spontaneous mutation rate. In bacteria several mechanisms, affecting DNA repair or the accuracy of DNA replication, have been identified.

nonstructural genes A genetic locus whose function is other than to determine the amino acid sequence of a polypeptide chain. Compare STRUCTURAL GENE.

operator gene See under OPERATOR LOCUS.

gene pool See under POOL.

recessive gene In diploid organisms, an allele that, when homozygous, directs the production or appearance of a mendelian recessive phenotype. Also called *recessive allele*.

reciprocal genes COMPLEMENTARY GENES.

regulator gene A genetic locus that regulates expression of one or more other genes. Also called *control gene, regulator*.

repressor gene A regulator gene that directs the synthesis of a regulator protein, usually a repressor.

resistance gene Any locus that encodes a product, process, or trait capable of rendering a cell or organism less susceptible to, usually, a specific deleterious agent. An example would be a gene encoding penicillinase that results in resistance of a bacterium to penicillin.

restorer gene A gene that reverses the changes brought about by cytoplasmically induced sterility. Restorer genes have been isolated for use as fertility agents in plant genetics.

Rh genes Genes that encode the rhesus blood group antigens. They are located on the distal short arm of chromosome 1.

sex-conditioned gene SEX-INFLUENCED GENE.

sex-influenced gene A genetic locus that determines a sex-influenced phenotype. It may be either linked to a sex chromosome or autosomal. A popular usage. Also called *sex-conditioned gene.*

sex-limited gene A genetic locus, whether autosomal or linked to a sex chromosome, that determines a sex-limited phenotype. A popular usage.

sex-linked gene 1 A genetic locus located on a sex chromosome. 2 X-LINKED GENE. • This term is often used imprecisely in reference to humans.

silent gene SILENT ALLELE.

split gene A gene which consists of at least two coding sequences, separated by introns. Most genes of higher organisms are split, whereas bacterial and viral genes are rarely split.

structural gene A genetic locus that determines the amino acid sequence of a polypeptide. The gene coding for RNA molecules such as transfer RNAs or ribosomal RNAs are considered by some to be structural genes also. Compare NONSTRUCTURAL GENE.

sublethal gene SUBLETHAL ALLELE.

supplementary genes Two separate genetic loci that interact such that the dominant locus specifies its phenotype regardless of the presence or action of the second locus, whereas expression of the second locus requires the presence of the dominant locus.

suppressor gene A gene capable of blocking or otherwise modifying the effect of a mutation in a separate locus.

switch gene In developmental genetics, a regulator gene that determines the developmental sequence of an organism.

syntenic genes Genes located on the same chromosome.

taster gene PTC LOCUS.

transposable gene A transposon that contains a coding sequence. Also called *jumping gene* (popular).

tRNA gene A gene that codes for a transfer RNA molecule.

uninducible gene A gene which is present as a part of the genome, but which is not transcribed even in the presence of an inducer.

wild-type gene An allele that, when heterozygous, specifies a dominant wild-type phenotype or, when homozygous, specifies either a recessive or a dominant wild-type phenotype.

X-linked gene A genetic locus on the X chromosome in any species. Also called *sex-linked gene* (imprecise).

Y-linked gene A genetic locus on the Y chromosome in any species. Also called *holandric gene.*

geneogenous CONGENITAL.

genera Plural of GENUS.

general Affecting the whole organism rather than a local area or part.

generalization The extrapolation of conclusions or judgments about an entire group or class based on experience with a limited number of said group or class.

response generalization In operant conditioning, the tendency for an experimental subject, initially conditioned to make a specific response to a particular stimulus, to begin to make responses, when presented with the same stimulus, that are different from but recognizably similar to the original conditioned response.

stimulus generalization The elicitation of a conditioned response by a stimulus that is in some way similar to but not identical with the original stimulus.

generalize To progress from local to general: said of a disease.

generation [French *génération* (from L *generatio,* from *genera-*

tus, past part. of *generare* to beget, produce, from *genus,* gen. *generis,* class, kind, from Gk *genos* race, descent, kind) generation] 1 Reproduction. 2 One complete cycle from parents to offspring in the life of sexually reproducing organisms. 3 The group of individuals descended from a given ancestor in the same number of parent-offspring cycles. 4 In demography, a group of persons born during a given period, usually a calendar year. 5 In demography, the offspring of a group of persons born during a callendar year.

alternate generation ALTERNATION OF GENERATIONS.

asexual generation ASEXUAL REPRODUCTION.

direct generation ASEXUAL REPRODUCTION.

first filial generation All offspring resulting from the sexual reproduction of two individuals. Symbol: F_1

nonsexual generation ASEXUAL REPRODUCTION.

parental generation 1 All individuals in a population of approximately the same age as a designated set of parents. A popular usage. 2 In genetics, all sibs and first cousins of a particular set of parents. 3 In experimental genetics, the original two individuals in a breeding experiment, the mating of which produced the first filial generation. Symbol: P_1

second filial generation All offspring produced by the sexual reproduction of two individuals who were members of the first filial generation. Symbol: F_2

sexual generation SEXUAL REPRODUCTION.

spontaneous generation The theory that living organisms are created from nonliving matter. Also called *abiogenesis, autogenesis, archegony* (seldom used).

virgin generation PARTHENOGENESIS.

generative [L *generat(us),* past part. of *generare* to beget, produce + -IVE] Pertaining to the reproductive process.

generator [L (from *generatus,* past part. of *generare* to beget, produce, from *genus,* gen. *generis,* class, kind, from Gk *genos* race, descent, kind), a begetter, producer] 1 Anything that produces a particular form of matter or energy. 2 A device that produces electricity by conversion from other forms of energy, such as mechanical, nuclear, or chemical energy.

aerosol generator A device which produces an aerosol.

asynchronous pulse generator A pulse generator which is unaffected by cardiac electrical activity and generates pulses at a fixed rate. Also called *fixed-rate pulse generator.*

atrial synchronous pulse generator A pulse generator which is triggered by normal atrial activity to stimulate the ventricle. Also called *atrial triggered pulse generator.*

atrial triggered pulse generator ATRIAL SYNCHRONOUS PULSE GENERATOR.

barium-131 generator A radionuclide generator that continuously produces radioactive cesium 131 from its parent radionuclide barium 131. • This term reflects common usage, although it would be preferable to name a generator after the daughter.

character generator A unit that converts input alphanumeric codes to the signals necessary to create characters on a cathode-ray tube or dot matrix printer.

demand pulse generator VENTRICULAR INHIBITED PULSE GENERATOR.

electrostatic generator An apparatus for producing a high voltage by the separation of electric charges. Also called *static machine.*

fixed-rate pulse generator ASYNCHRONOUS PULSE GENERATOR.

pattern generator The neuronal circuitry directly involved in the production of a stereotyped form of motor activity of complex, usually repetitive pattern, such as ambulation, swimming, or chewing. The pattern generator is at once the total of distinctive interneuronal connections and the activity channeled through them which results in the pattern behavior.

pulse generator An electronic device that generates sharp pulses, usually of very short duration and either regular or random in timing.

radionuclide generator A device that contains a relatively long-lived parent radionuclide fixed to an ion exchange column from which a daughter radionuclide may be eluted. • In nuclear medicine, this is commonly termed a "cow," because it is "milked" from time to time.

standby pulse generator VENTRICULAR INHIBITED PULSE GENERATOR.

supervoltage generator An apparatus for producing voltages greater than one million volts, for use in x-ray therapy.

technetium-99m generator A radionuclide generator that produces the daughter nuclide, technetium 99m, from the parent, molybdenum 99.

Van de Graaff generator An apparatus for producing a high voltage, typically several million volts, by means of a fast-moving belt stretched between two pulleys. Electric charges are sprayed onto the belt at one pulley and taken off at the other. Also called *Van de Graaff machine.* • This apparatus was invented by R.J. Van de Graaff in 1933.

ventricular inhibited pulse generator A pulse generator whose activity is inhibited by intrinsic ventricular activity. Also called *demand pulse generator, standby pulse generator.*

ventricular synchronous pulse generator VENTRICULAR TRIGGERED PULSE GENERATOR.

ventricular triggered pulse generator A pulse generator which delivers its impulse synchronously with natural ventricular activity unless this fails, in which case it provides a pacemaking impulse. Also called *ventricular synchronous pulse generator.*

generic 1 Of or relating to a genus. 2 Nonproprietary, as a drug that can be substituted for a proprietary brand in a prescription.

genesial GENESIC.

genesic Relating to generation; generative. Also *genesial.*

genesiology [*genesi(s)* + *o* + -LOGY] The study of reproduction. An older term.

genesis [Gk *genesis* (from root *genō* of *gignesthai* to become, be, be born) origin, source, birth, race, descent] The process of being formed; origin; beginning: often used in combination, as in *spermatogenesis.*

genesistasis [*genesi(s)* + STASIS] The inhibition of cell multiplication.

gene-splicing The *in vitro* manipulation of DNA or RNA to achieve rearrangement of an organism's genes; molecular recombination. The introduction of a foreign nucleotide sequence into a specific location in the host genome, as in bacterial recombination.

genestatic [*gene(sis)* + Gk *statik(os)* (from *histanai* to make stand) causing to stand] Tending to inhibit sporulation.

genetic 1 Of or relating to the study of genetics. 2 Referring to or pertaining to anything controlled or defined by genes. Also *genic, heredobiologic* (outmoded). 3 HERITABLE.

geneticist One who specializes in the acquisition and application of knowledge about heredity and genetic processes.

genetics [Gk *gene(sis)* (from root *genō* of *gignesthai* to become, to be born) an origin, source, birth, race, descent + *t* + -ICS] That branch of the life sciences that deals with the structure and function of genes; the expression of genes in individuals, families, and populations; and the causes and extent of genetic variation. Also called *thremmatology.*

behavioral genetics A subfield of psychology concerned with investigating the influence of heredity on behavior. It combines the methods of psychology and genetics to inquire into the influence of heredity and environment on behavior, and especially into the nature of their interactions.

biochemical genetics That amalgamation of the sciences of biochemistry and genetics that focuses on the expression of normal and mutant genes in individuals and populations, usually at the level of enzymes and other proteins.

clinical genetics That branch of medicine involved with the diagnosis and treatment of human disorders caused, at least in part, by abnormal genes or chromosomes in patients and their families.

developmental genetics The study of the genetic and epigenetic control and modulation of organismal development.

human genetics That branch of genetics concerned with humans. Included are clinical genetics, medical genetics, and the study of the genetic foundations of human phenotypic variation.

medical genetics That branch of medicine concerned with clinical genetics as well as the discovery, nosology, epidemiology, and pathogenesis of hereditary disorders.

microbial genetics The branch of genetics concerned with microorganisms, especially bacteria, viruses, and phage.

molecular genetics The branch of genetics that focuses on the molecular structure of nucleic acids, the molecular organization of genetic information, and the processes through which this information is expressed.

population genetics The branch of genetics that focuses on gene and allele frequencies and their interactions in populations, as well as the forces and processes that alter gene frequencies.

statistical genetics The branch of genetics concerned with the analysis of data or the elaboration of genetic theory in quantitative terms according to the precepts of statistics.

genetotrophic Related to genetics and nutrition; relating to hereditary factors that affect the nutritional status of a person.

genetous [*genet(ics)* + -OUS] Originating in the fetal stage.

Geneva Convention An international agreement signed in Geneva, Switzerland in 1864 that established principles for the wartime treatment of prisoners, the wounded, and the dead, and that included provisions on the neutrality of hospitals.

Gengou [Octave *Gengou*, Belgian bacteriologist, 1875–1957] 1 Bordet-Gengou agar. See under AGAR. 2 Bordet-Gengou bacillus. See under *BORDETELLA PERTUSSIS.* 3 Gengou phenomenon, Bordet-Gengou phenomenon, Bordet and Gengou reaction. See under COMPLEMENT FIXATION.

genial [Gk *geny(s)* the chin + -AL] Pertaining to the chin. Also *genian.*

genian GENIAL.

genic GENETIC.

-genic [Gk *genikos* (adjective from *genos* race, descent, descendant) descended, begotten, produced] A combining form meaning producing, creating.

genicula Plural of GENICULUM.

genicular Of or pertaining to the knee, or genus.

geniculate [L *genicul(um)* the knee, a knot in a plant + -ATE] Resembling or shaped like a knee in a flexed position; bent sharply.

geniculocalcarine Denoting the visual radiation fibers projecting from the lateral geniculate body to the calcarine portion of the visual cortex.

geniculotemporal Denoting the visual radiation fibers emanating from the lateral geniculate body and coursing around the temporal horn of the lateral ventricle en route to the visual cortex.

geniculum [L (dim. of *genu* the knee, akin to Gk *gony* the knee), the knee, a knot in a plant] 1 A small acute bend or angulation, resembling a knee, in a structure or organ.   **2** A kneelike or knotlike structure.

geniculum canalis facialis   [NA] The sharp, posteriorly directed bend in the lateral part of the facial canal above the vestibular part of the internal ear and in the petrous part of the temporal bone where the canal runs from the internal acoustic meatus. The canal is dilated at this bend, where it lodges the geniculate ganglion. Also called *genu of facial canal, little knee of facial canal, knee of aquaeductus fallopii, geniculum of facial canal.*

geniculum of facial canal   GENICULUM CANALIS FACIALIS.

geniculum of facial nerve   GENICULUM NERVI FACIALIS.

geniculum nervi facialis   [NA] The portion of the facial nerve root within the facial canal that bends sharply posteriorly at the site of the geniculate ganglion. Also called *external genu of facial nerve, genu of facial nerve* (imprecise), *geniculum of facial nerve.* Compare GENU NERVI FACIALIS.

genin   Any steroid of the cardenolide or sapogenin class, found naturally as its glycoside.

geniocheiloplasty   [Gk *geneio(n)* chin + CHEILO- + -PLASTY] Any plastic operation on the lower lip and chin. Also called *genycheiloplasty, genychiloplasty.*

genioglossal   Pertaining to the chin and the tongue.

genioglossus   MUSCULUS GENIOGLOSSUS.

geniohyoglossus   MUSCULUS GENIOGLOSSUS.

geniohyoid   **1** Pertaining to the chin and the hyoid bone.   **2** Denoting the musculus geniohyoideus.

geniohyoideus   MUSCULUS GENIOHYOIDEUS.

genion   [Gk *geneion* chin, jaw, cheek] A craniometric point situated on the inner aspect of the mandible in the midline at the apex of the spine of the genial tubercles.

genioplasty   [Gk *geneio(n)* the chin + -PLASTY] Any plastic surgical procedure on the chin, usually one designed to enlarge, reduce, or change the shape of the chin. Also called *genyplasty.*

genital   [L *genital(is)* generative, begetting, leaving] **1** Of or relating to the reproductive organs (the genitals), or to reproduction.   **2** Pertaining to the final phase of psychosexual development.

genitalia   [L (neut. pl. of *genitalis* generative, begetting, bearing, from root *geno* of early L *genere* to generate and L *gignere*, past part. *genitus*, to generate and of Gk *gignesthai* to become, be born), the genitals] The organs of reproduction in both males and females, usually used in reference to external genitals. Also called *genitals, gonae, reproductive organs.*

ambiguous external genitalia   External genitalia not conforming clearly to either the male or female pattern. Causes include chromosome defects, metabolic errors of hormone synthesis, and anatomical malformations.

external genitalia   The organa genitalia masculina externa and the organa genitalia feminina externa.

indifferent genitalia   The embryonic genital organs before differentiation into the organs peculiar to either sex.

internal genitalia   Organa genitalia feminina interna and organa genitalia masculina interna.

genitality   The mature genital aspects of sexuality as opposed to the pregenital aspects.

genitaloid   [GENITAL + -OID] Relating to primary sex cells and indicating possible differentiation in the male or female genitals.

genitals   GENITALIA.

genito-   [L *genitus* (past participle of *gignere* to beget, produce) begotten, produced] A combining form meaning genital.

genitocrural   GENITOFEMORAL.

genitofemoral   Pertaining to the genitalia and the thigh. Also *genitocrural.*

genitoinfectious   VENEREAL.

genitoplasty   [GENITO- + -PLASTY] Any plastic operation on the genitalia.

genitourinary   UROGENITAL.

genitovesical   Pertaining to the genitalia and the urinary bladder.

genius   **1** A representative type; model.   **2** Extraordinary intellect, talent, or creative ability, or an individual so endowed. A popular usage.

genius epidemicus   Variations in epidemic disorders due to cosmic or atmospheric conditions. An obsolete term.

genius loci   Susceptibility of a tissue to the development of metastases.

Gennari   [Francesco *Gennari*, Italian anatomist, 1750–1795] Line of Gennari, stripe of Gennari, Gennari's layer, stria of Gennari. See under BAND.

geno-   [Gk *gennan* to beget, produce, bring forth] A combining form meaning (1) producing, bringing forth, generating; (2) genus; (3) race. Also *gen-.*

genoblast   [GENO- + -BLAST] **1** GERM CELL.   **2** ZYGOTE.

genocide   [GENO- + -CIDE] The deliberate extermination of an entire human ethnic, political, or cultural group.

genocopy   An individual whose phenotype is similar to or indistinguishable from another individual of different genotype. Also called *genetic mimic, isophene.*

genodermatology   The study of genodermatoses.

genodermatosis   Any hereditary skin disease.

genome   [German *Genom*, from *Gen* gene, factor + *(Chromos)om* chromosome] **1** The total genetic information present in a cell.   **2** In diploid cells, the genetic information contained in one chromosome set.   **3** The genetic information contained in a haploid gamete of a diploid organism.

genomic   **1** Of or pertaining to the genome.   **2** In molecular genetics, referring to DNA purified from and representative of the nuclear DNA.

genophobia   [GENO- + -PHOBIA] Pathologic fear of sex.

genophore   [GENO- + -PHORE] A prokaryotic chromosome. ● This term is used occasionally to emphasize the distinction from the more complex eukaryotic chromosome.

genotype   **1** The total genetic information in a somatic cell, or the total potential genetic information in a germ cell or an organism.   **2** The genetic constitution at one or several loci in a given cell or organism.

genotypic   **1** Of or relating to a genotype.   **2** Of or pertaining to a phenotype determined solely by the genome, with no environmental modulation. An imprecise usage.

-genous   [Gk *-gen* from *gennan* to beget, produce, bring forth + English adjectival suffix *-ous*] A combining form meaning (1) producing; (2) produced by.

Gensoul   [Joseph *Gensoul*, French surgeon, 1797–1858] Gensoul's disease. See under LUDWIG'S ANGINA.

gentamicin   A broad-spectrum, aminocyclitol antibiotic elaborated by *Micromonospora purpurea* and *M. echinospora*. It inhibits bacterial protein synthesis and is active against many Gram-negative and Gram-positive bacteria, particularly *Pseudomonas aeruginosa*. The sulfate salt is used. The major side effect is that this drug is ototoxic and may cause irreversible damage. Also *gentamycin.*

gentamycin   GENTAMICIN.

gentian   [French *gentiane* (from L *gentiana*, after the Illyrian king *Gentius*, 180–167 B.C., who discovered its properties) an aperitive and tonic plant of the temperate regions] A drug prepared from dried, fermented rhizomes and roots of *Gentiana lutea* of the Gentianaceae family. It has been used as a bitter tonic to stimulate gastric secretion and improve the appetite. Also called *bitter root*.

Indian gentian   CHIRATA.

gentiavern   GENTIAN VIOLET.

gentisic acid   2,5-Dihydroxybenzoic acid. It is formed by some molds. Like all *p*-dihydroxybenzenes it is easily oxidized to form a quinone.

Gentran   A proprietary name for dextran 75.

gentrogenin   BOTOGENIN.

genu [L, the knee]   (*plural* genua)   **1** GENUS². **2** Any of various angulated or curved anatomic structures suggestive of a bent knee.

genu capsulae internae   [NA] The angular bend formed by the anterior and posterior limbs of the internal capsule. Also called *genu of internal capsule, knee of internal capsule*.

genu corporis callosi   [NA] The ventrally directed, kneelike bend at the rostrum of the corpus callosum. Also called *genu of corpus callosum*.

genu of corpus callosum   GENU CORPORIS CALLOSI.

external genu of facial nerve   GENICULUM NERVI FACIALIS.

genu extrorsum   GENU VARUM.

genu of facial canal   GENICULUM CANALIS FACIALIS.

genu of facial nerve   **1** GENU NERVI FACIALIS. **2** An imprecise term for GENICULUM NERVI FACIALIS.

genu impressum   A deformity of the knees in which the knee is bent to one side with abnormal positioning of the patella upwards and to that side.

genu of internal capsule   GENU CAPSULAE INTERNAE.

internal genu of facial nerve   GENU NERVI FACIALIS.

genu internum radicis nervi facialis   GENU NERVI FACIALIS.

genu introrsum   GENU VALGUM.

genu nervi facialis   [NA] The bend in the motor fibers of the facial nerve at the point where they arch over the abducens nucleus, resulting in an elevation of the floor of the fourth ventricle (the facial colliculus), before coursing ventrally to emerge from the brainstem. Also called *internal genu of facial nerve, genu of facial nerve, genu internum radicis nervi facialis*. Compare GENICULUM NERVI FACIALIS.

genu recurvatum   A congenital hyperextension at the knee joint, giving a forward concavity of the lower extremity when fully extended. Also called *back knee*.

genu valgum   A congenital curvature of the lower extremity so that the knees are abnormally approximated and the ankles abnormally divergent. Also called *genu introrsum, knock-knee, gonycrotesis, in knee, tragopodia, baker leg, tibia valga*.

genu varum   A congenital curvature of the lower extremities that results in the knees being abnormally divergent and the ankles abnormally approximated. Also called *bowleg, genu extrorsum, tibia vara, gonyectyposis, bandy leg, out knee*.

genua   **1** Plural of GENU. **2** Plural of GENUS².

genual   Pertaining to or resembling a genu, or knee; genicular.

genus¹ [L (from Gk *genos* race, stock, descent), race, stock, family, species]   (*plural* genera)   A taxonomic group ranking below a family and including one or more species that have certain characteristics in common.

genus² [L, variant of *genu* knee]   (*plural* genua)   [NA] The region of the knee joint, comprising the regio genus anterior, regio genus posterior, and the fossa poplitea; the knee. Also called *genu*.

genyantralgia   An obsolete term for ANTRODYNIA.

genyantritis   An obsolete term for MAXILLARY SINUSITIS.

genyantrum   An outmoded term for SINUS MAXILLARIS.

genycheiloplasty   GENIOCHEILOPLASTY.

genychiloplasty   GENIOCHEILOPLASTY.

genyplasty   GENIOPLASTY.

geo- [Gk *gē* the earth, land]   A combining form meaning earth, soil.

geobiont [GEO- + -BIONT]   An organism that spends its entire life in the ground.

geochemistry [GEO- + CHEMISTRY]   The chemistry of the components of the earth.

geocole [GEO- + L *col(ere)* to till, inhabit]   An organism such as a fly, beetle, or moth that spends the egg or larval stage of its life in the ground. Also called *geophile, geophil*.

geode [Gk *geōdē(s)* (from *gē*, contraction of *gea* the earth + *-ōdēs* resembling) earthlike, from its similarity to a stone geode]   In anatomy, an enlarged lymphatic space or the dilatation occurring where several lymphatic capillaries join together. An outmoded term.

geoecotype   GEOTYPE.

geogen [GEO- + -GEN]   A physical or chemical feature of the earth that affects the well-being of organisms.

geomedicine [GEO- + MEDICINE]   The branch of medicine concerned with the influence of environmental, climatic, and topographic conditions on health and the prevalence of disease in different parts of the world. Also called *nosochthonography* (seldom used), *nosogeography* (seldom used).

geometry [L *geometri(a)* (from Gk *geōmetria* a land measuring, from *gē*, contraction of *gea* the earth + *o* + *metrein* to measure) geometry]   In nuclear medicine, any of the various arrangements between a radioactive source and a detector that affects the accuracy of counting or measurement. Also called *counting geometry*.

counting geometry   GEOMETRY.

good geometry   A physical relationship between a radioactive source and a detector that is favorable to the quantitative counting of the source. Two factors are usually involved: the necessity to minimize the fraction of the emitted radiation that misses the detector entirely, and the necessity to minimize the effects of scattered radiation. The latter is often beyond the experimenter's control, as when the source is buried in a patient.

poor geometry   Any relationship between a radioactive source and a detector that makes quantitative counting difficult, such as a small detector, a large source-to-detector distance, too much absorption between the two, or radiation scattering that can't be adequately duplicated for the counting of the standard source.

geopathology   The science concerned with the harmful effects on the body of environment, topography, climate, food and water supplies, and ecological factors.

geophagia [GEO- + -PHAGIA]   The eating of dirt, a form of pica. Also called *geophagy, geophagism, geotragia, chthonophagia* (obsolete), *chthonophagy* (obsolete).

geophagism   GEOPHAGIA.

geophagist   One who suffers from geophagia.

geophagy   GEOPHAGIA.

geophil [GEO- + -PHIL]   GEOCOLE.

geophile [GEO- + -PHILE]   GEOCOLE.

geophilic   Pertaining to a geocole.

Geophilus   A genus of centipedes having 47 to 67 pairs of legs. American species include *G. californius, G. rubens,* and *G. umbraticus*.

geophyte [GEO- + Gk *phyt(on)* a plant, tree]   **1** A perennial cryptophyte. **2** A land or terrestrial plant.

Georgi [Walter *Georgi*, German bacteriologist, 1880–1930]   Sachs-Georgi test. See under TEST.

Geosciurus   A genus of ground squirrels found in Africa, considered by some a subgenus of *Xerus*. Often kept as pets, they can serve as reservoirs for plague and therefore are a potential human health hazard.

geosere **1** A sere as viewed through geologic time periods. **2** A series of climax communities on a site over a long interval of time.

geotaxis [GEO- + Gk *taxis* an arranging, order] A locomotor movement by an animal in response to a gravitational stimulus.

geotragia [GEO- + Gk *trag(ein)*, 2nd aorist inf. of *trōgein* to chew, + -IA] GEOPHAGIA.

geotrichosis Infection due to the fungus *Geotrichum candidum*. It affects humans, with lesions developing in the mouth and in the digestive and respiratory systems.

Geotrichum A form-genus of fungi, one species of which is the causal agent of geotrichosis. Also called *Oospora* (obsolete).

geotropism The growth of a sessile animal or plant part relative to the gravitational attraction of the earth. Geotropism is positive when the movement is directed toward the earth and negative when directed away from the earth.

geotype A genotypic population that is isolated by physiographic barriers. Also called *geoecotype.*

geoxene [GEO- + Gk *xen(os)* a host, guest, stranger] An organism found in a soil stratum of which it is not normally a resident.

Geraghty [John Timothy *Geraghty*, U.S. physician, 1876–1924] **1** See under OPERATION. **2** Geraghty's test. See under PHENOLSULFONPHTHALEIN TEST.

geraniol $Me_2C=CH-CH_2-CH_2-C(Me)=CH-CH_2OH$. An alcohol found in plant oils in the *trans* configuration. Its molecule contains two isoprene units. Its ester with diphosphoric acid (geranyl pyrophosphate) is an important metabolic intermediate.

geranium The dried rhizome of *Geranium maculatum*. It contains tannin and gallic acid and is used as an astringent. Also called *cranesbill, alum root.*

geranyl pyrophosphate The ester of geraniol and diphosphoric acid. It is an intermediate in the synthesis of steroids and terpenes, being formed from isopentenyl pyrophosphate and dimethylallyl pyrophosphate. It reacts with a further molecule of isopentenyl pyrophosphate to form farnesyl pyrophosphate.

geratology A seldom used term for GERONTOLOGY.

gerbil [French *gerbille* (from New L *gerbillus*, dim. of *gerboa*, from Arabic *yarbū'*, a jumping rodent) gerbil] A small burrowing rodent of the genus *Gerbillus*, native to arid regions of Africa and southwest Asia, known to be an agent for the transmission of plague.

Gerdy [Pierre Nicholas, *Gerdy*, French surgeon, 1797–1856] **1** Gerdy's fontanel. See under SAGITTAL FONTANEL. **2** Gerdy's fibers. See under FIBER. **3** Gerdy's hyoid fossa. See under TRIGONUM CAROTICUM. **4** Gerdy's ligament. See under SUSPENSORY LIGAMENT OF AXILLA.

gereology GERONTOLOGY.

Gerhardt [Carl Jakob Christian Adolph *Gerhardt*, German physician, 1833–1902] **1** See under DULLNESS, TRIANGLE. **2** Gerhardt's disease. See under ERYTHROMELALGIA. **3** Gerhardt syndrome. See under BILATERAL LARYNGEAL ABDUCTOR PARALYSIS. **4** Gerhardt-Semon law. See under LAW.

geriatric [GER- + IATR- + -IC] **1** Pertaining to geriatrics. **2** Pertaining to old age.

geriatrician A physician who specializes in the practice of geriatric medicine. Also called *geriatrist.*

geriatrics [*ger(o)-* + IATR- + -ICS] A popular term for GERIATRIC MEDICINE.

    dental geriatrics GERODONTICS.

geriatrist GERIATRICIAN.

geriodontics GERODONTICS.

geriodontist GERODONTIST.

geriopsychosis SENILE DEMENTIA.

Gerlach [Andreas Christian *Gerlach*, German veterinary surgeon, 1811–1877] Gerlach's valvula. See under LIGAMENTUM PECTINATUM ANGULI IRIDOCORNEALIS.

Gerlach [Joseph von *Gerlach*, German anatomist, 1820–1896] **1** See under NETWORK, VALVE. **2** Gerlach's annular tendon, annular ring of Gerlach. See under ANNULUS FIBROCARTILAGINEUS MEMBRANAE TYMPANI. **3** Gerlach's tonsil. See under TONSILLA TUBARIA.

Gerlier [Felix *Gerlier*, Swiss physician, 1840–1914] **1** Gerlier's disease. See under VESTIBULAR NEURONITIS. **2** Gerlier syndrome. See under DISEASE. **3** Gerlier syndrome. See under PALLIDAL SYNDROME.

germ [French *germe* (from L *germen*, gen. *germinis*, sprout, fetus, seed, from root *geno* of L *gignere* to generate or from *gerere* to bear) germ] **1** The portion of an ovum which divides to give rise to the embryo, the rest of the ovum (including the yolk) being responsible for providing nourishment. **2** A precursor of certain structures in embryology, as *tooth germ, germ layer.* **3** A spore. **4** A microorganism capable of causing a disease.

dental germ TOOTH GERM.

enamel germ An epithelial bud which develops at an early stage of tooth formation.

hair germ HAIR MATRIX.

reserve tooth germ A primordium of a successional tooth.

tooth germ An embryonic precursor or dental organ of a tooth which develops at intervals along the dental lamina in the shape of a cap of ectoderm with mesenchyme on its inner aspect, forming the dental papilla which will become the dentine and the pulp. The dental organ soon becomes bell-shaped (the bell stage) and four cell layers develop: an external dental epithelium, a stellate reticulum, a stratum intermedium, and an internal dental epithelium. The latter becomes folded to determine the crown pattern of the tooth, and its cells, now called ameloblasts, lay down the enamel. Odontoblasts develop from the superficial cells of the dental papilla and lay down predentin which is the precursor of dentin. Also called *dental germ.*

wheat germ The embryo of the wheat seed. It is valuable as a source of vitamin E, thiamin, riboflavin, and other vitamins. The oil obtained from wheat germ, wheat germ oil, consists mainly of glycosides of oleic, palmitic, and linoleic acids, vitamin E, and other tocopherols.

germanium A metallic element having atomic number 32 and atomic weight 72.59. Five stable natural isotopes are known and 12 radioactive isotopes have been identified. Valences are 2 and 4. Elemental germanium is a brittle, crystalline solid with a metallic luster. The element is a semiconductor and is important in the manufacture of electronic and optical instruments. Symbol: Ge

germ-free AXENIC.

germicidal [GERM + *i* + -*cid(e)* + -AL] Able to destroy microorganisms.

germicide [GERM + *i* + -CIDE] An agent capable of destroying microorganisms.

germifuge An obsolete term for DISINFECTANT.

germinal [L *germen*, gen. *germinis*, a bud, seed + -AL] Of or relating to a germ cell or to germination.

germination [L *germinatio* (from *germinatus*, past part. of *germinare* to sprout, put forth) a sprouting, budding] The initiation of growth by a bud, seed, spore, or other structure.

germinative **1** Of or relating to a germ cell. **2** Pertaining to the process of germination.

germinoblast **1** LARGE NONCLEAVED FOLLICULAR CENTER CELL. **2** SMALL NONCLEAVED FOLLICULAR CENTER CELL.

germinocyte **1** LARGE CLEAVED FOLLICULAR CENTER CELL.

2 SMALL CLEAVED FOLLICULAR CENTER CELL.

germinoma [L *germen*, gen. *germinis*, a bud, sprout, fetus + -OMA] A malignant tumor composed of large, primitive, round cells resembling germ cells. It occurs in the pineal region, mediastinum, and retroperitoneum. It is histologically indistinguishable from testicular seminoma and ovarian dysgerminoma.

pineal germinoma A germinoma of the pineal region. It is indistinguishable from the testicular seminoma or ovarian dysgerminoma. Geminomas are the most frequent tumor of the pineal region. Also called *pineal seminoma*.

germogen [GERM + *o* + -GEN] The cytoplasmic mass from which germ cells originate.

gero- [Gk *gerōn* (genitive *gerontos*) old man] A combining form meaning old age, relating to old people. Also *geronto-, geront-*.

geroderma [GERO- + -DERMA] Atrophy of the skin, as that seen in old age. Also called *gerodermia*.

osteodysplastic geroderma GERODERMA OSTEODYSPLASTICA.

geroderma osteodysplastica A hereditary disorder, transmitted as an autosomal recessive trait and usually seen in women, that is characterized by dystrophy of the skin and genitalia, osteoporosis, and prominent bony trabeculae which are visible radiographically. Also called *osteodysplastic geroderma*.

gerodermia [GERO- + -DERM + -IA] GERODERMA.

gerodontia GERODONTICS.

gerodontics [*ger(o)-* + -ODONT + -ICS] The practice of dentistry among old people. Also called *dental geriatrics, geriodontics, gerodontia*.

gerodontist A dentist specializing in gerodontics. Also called *geriodontist*.

gerodontology [*ger(o)-* + ODONTO- + -LOGY] The study of dentistry in relation to the aging and aged.

geromarasmus The wasting of the body, as that sometimes associated with old age.

geromorphism [GERO- + MORPH- + ISM] Bodily characteristics of old age in the young; premature senility.

cutaneous geromorphism The premature aging of the skin.

geront- GERO-.

geronto- GERO-.

gerontologist [GERONTO- + -LOGIST] One who specializes in gerontology.

gerontology [GERONTO- + -LOGY] **1** The study of aging as a biologic, sociological, and psychological process. Also called *gereology, nostology* (obsolete), *geratology* (seldom used). **2** Clinical gerontology; geriatric medicine.

gerontophilia [GERONTO- + -PHILIA] Excessive love of old people.

gerontophobia [GERONTO- + -PHOBIA] Pathologic fear of aging or of old people. Also called *gerophobia*.

gerontopia [GERONT- + -OPIA] SECOND SIGHT.

gerontotherapy [GERONTO- + THERAPY] A seldom used term for GERIATRIC MEDICINE.

gerontotoxon [GERONTO- + Gk *toxon* a bow] ARCUS SENILIS.

gerontoxon [Gk *gerōn* old man + *toxon* a bow] ARCUS SENILIS.

gerophobia GERONTOPHOBIA.

geroprophylaxis An attempt to prevent the effects of biologic aging.

geropsychiatry [GERO- + PSYCHIATRY] PSYCHOGERIATRICS.

Gerota [Dimitru *Gerota*, Rumanian surgeon, 1867–1939] **1** Parammammary route of Gerota. See under ROUTE. **2** Gerota's fascia, Gerota's capsule. See under CAPSULA FIBROSA RENIS. **3** See under METHOD.

Gersh [Isidore *Gersh*, U.S. histologist, born 1907] Altmann-Gersh method. See under METHOD.

Gerstmann [Josef *Gerstmann*, Austrian neurologist, 1887–1969] See under SYNDROME.

Gersuny [Robert *Gersuny*, Austrian surgeon, 1844–1924] See under OPERATION.

gerüstmark [German *Gerüst* scaffold + *Mark* marrow, pith] The presence in scurvy of connective tissue within the bone marrow,.

Gesell [Arnold Lucius *Gesell*, U.S. psychologist, 1880–1961] Gesell developmental scales. See under SCALE.

gestagen PROGESTOGEN.

gestalt [German, form, figure, shape, vision, look] A perceptual configuration organized in such a way as to lend it properties that exceed the summation of its component parts; a pattern, a figure, or a perceptually integrated whole.

gestaltism GESTALT PSYCHOLOGY.

gestaltist An advocate of gestalt psychology.

gestation [L *gestatio* (from *gestatus*, past part. of *gestare* to bear, carry, from *gestus*, past part. of *gerere* to produce, bear, carry) a bearing, carrying in the womb] The duration of the embryo in the uterus, from fertilization of the ovum until delivery; the period of normal pregnancy.

exterior gestation The development of an infant from birth until it has the ability to use all four extremities for movement, at about nine months of age.

interior gestation The development inside the mother of a fetus from the time of fertilization of the ovum until delivery.

gestosis [L *gest(are)* (frequentative of *gerere* to bear, carry) to bear, carry + -OSIS] An abnormal or pathologic condition occurring during pregnancy. An older term.

gesture [Med L *gestura* (from L *gest(us)*, past part. of *gerere* to bear, carry + -*ura* -URE) a way of acting] An expressive movement of the body as an aspect of communication. In man, it most often involves movement of the hands or arms.

GeV Symbol for the unit, gigaelectronvolt. Also *BeV* (outmoded).

gf Symbol for the unit, gram-force.

GFR glomerular filtration rate.

GH growth hormone.

ghee [Hindi *ghī* fluid butter] The clarified butter fat that remains after the evaporation of its water. It is made from the milk of a cow, buffalo, goat, or sheep and is used in India. It does not turn rancid as quickly as butter. Also called *samna (Arabic)*.

GHIH growth hormone inhibiting hormone.

Ghilarducci [Francesco *Ghilarducci*, Italian physician, 1857–1924] See under REACTION.

Ghon [Anton *Ghon*, Czech pathologist, 1866–1936] **1** Ghon focus, Ghon's primary lesion, Küss-Ghon focus. See under GHON TUBERCLE. **2** Ghon complex. See under PRIMARY COMPLEX.

ghost [Middle English *goste*, from Old English *gast* spirit, soul, demon, akin to German *Geist* ghost] The faint and barely perceivable remains of some object, especially of an erythrocyte. Also called *shadow, phantom*.

blood ghost ERYTHROCYTE GHOST.

erythrocyte ghost The hemoglobin-free erythrocyte membrane, usually obtained by lysing erythrocytes with hypotonic solutions. Also called *ghost corpuscle, phantom corpuscle, shadow corpuscle, discoplasm, blood ghost, erythrocyte stroma, discostroma, ghost cell, phantom cell, shadow cell*.

GHRF   growth hormone releasing factor (growth hormone releasing hormone).

GHRH   growth hormone releasing hormone.

GHRIH   growth hormone release inhibiting hormone.

GHz   Symbol for the unit, gigahertz.

GI   gastrointestinal.

gi   In the United States, symbol for the unit, gill.

Giacobini [Genaro *Giacobini*, Argentinian physician, 1889–1954]   Lucherini-Giacobini syndrome. See under SYNDROME.

Giacomini [Carlo *Giacomini*, Italian anatomist, 1841–1898]   Frenulum of Giacomini. See under BAND.

Giannuzzi [Giuseppe *Giannuzzi*, Italian physiologist, 1839–1876]   **1** Giannuzzi's body, semilunar body, crescent of Giannuzzi. See under DEMILUNE OF GIANNUZZI.   **2** Cell of Giannuzzi. See under DEMILUNE CELL.

Gianotti [Ferdinando *Gianotti*, Italian dermatologist, born 1920]   Gianotti-Crosti syndrome. See under INFANTILE PAPULAR ACRODERMATITIS.

giant [L *gigas* (gen. *gigantis*; from Gk *gigas* a giant) a giant]   **1** A person or creature of great size.   **2** MEGASOME.

eunuchoid giant   An adolescent of apparently excessive height in association with delayed puberty and the concomitant delay in osseous epiphysial closure and undue growth of the long bones.

giantism [GIANT + -ISM]   GIGANTISM.

Giardia [after Alfred *Giard*, French biologist, 1846–1908 + -IA]   A genus of parasitic flagellates (order Diplomonadida, class Zoomastigophorea) found in the small intestine of many mammals, including humans. The question of which species besides *G. lamblia* may be responsible for human giardiasis remains unresolved. Also called *Lamblia*.

Giardia bovis   A species parasitic in the small intestine of cattle.

Giardia canis   A species found in the small intestine of dogs.

Giardia cati   A species found in the intestines of cats.

Giardia intestinalis   GIARDIA LAMBLIA.

Giardia lamblia   The common intestinal flagellate of humans, an abundant, cosmopolitan parasite, and probably the most common protozoan human parasite in the United States. It is spread by drinking water contaminated with human feces or feces of infected animals, such as rodents and possibly domesticated animals. Also called *Giardia intestinalis, Lamblia intestinalis*. See also GIARDIASIS.

giardiasis [*Giard(ia)* + -IASIS]   **1** Infection with protozoa of the genus *Giardia*.   **2** Specifically, human infection with *Giardia lamblia*; lambliasis. Heavy infection may cause protracted diarrhea with symptoms suggestive of malabsorption. Light infections are usually asymptomatic but are probably capable of causing disease if the host's resistance falls. Some human infections have been shown to be derived from animals via mountain streams and other sources, but most are transmitted by human sewage in public water supplies.

chinchilla giardiasis   Infection of chinchillas with flagellates of the genus *Giardia*. It is characterized by diarrhea and anorexia, often resulting in death.

gibber [L, hump]   A humplike or pouchlike enlargement or projection.

gibber inferior thalami   NUCLEUS POSTERIOR THALAMI.

gibber ulnae   An outmoded term for OLECRANON.

gibberellic acid   A plant hormone which stimulates the growth of stems and leaves. It is a C_{19} compound with five rings, derived from a diterpene, and it contains a carboxyl group, a lactone ring, two hydroxyl groups, and two double bonds. It occurs in plants, but was originally discovered in the mold *Gibberella*.

gibberellin   Any of about twenty compounds found in plants

and related chemically to gibberellic acid and possessing similar hormonal effects.

Gibbon [Q. V. *Gibbon*, U.S. surgeon, 1813–1894]   Gibbon's hydrocele. See under HERNIA.

Gibbs [Josiah Willard *Gibbs*, U.S. physicist, 1839–1903]   See under ENERGY.

gibbus [L (akin to Gk *kyphos* a hump, hunch), a hump, hunch]   An angulation of the spine due to anterior collapse of the disk space and vertebral bodies. It is usually caused by an abscess, especially a tuberculous abscess.

Gibert [Camille Melchior *Gibert*, French dermatologist, 1797–1866]   Gibert's disease, Gibert's pityriasis. See under PITYRIASIS ROSEA.

Gibney [Virgil Pendleton *Gibney*, U.S. orthopedist, 1847–1927]   **1** Gibney's disease. See under PERISPONDYLITIS.   **2** See under STRAPPING.

Gibson [George Alexander *Gibson*, Scottish physician, 1854–1913]   See under MURMUR, RULE.

Gibson [Stanley *Gibson*, U.S. pediatrician, born 1883]   Potts-Smith-Gibson operation. See under POTTS OPERATION.

gid [from *gid(dy)*, based on the swaying gait of affected animals]   A popular term for STAGGERS.

Giemsa [Berthold Gustav Carl *Giemsa*, German chemotherapeutist, 1867–1948]   See under METHOD, STAIN.

Gierke [Hans Paul Bernard *Gierke*, German anatomist, 1847–1886]   **1** Gierke cells. See under CELL.   **2** Gierke's respiratory bundle. See under TRACTUS SOLITARIUS.

Gifford [Harold *Gifford*, U.S. ophthalmologist, 1858–1929]   **1** Gifford's reflex, Gifford-Galassi reflex. See under WESTPHAL-PILTZ REFLEX.   **2** See under SIGN, OPERATION.

giga- [Gk *gigas* a giant]   A combining form denoting 10^9: used with SI units. Symbol: G.

gigabecquerel [GIGA- + BECQUEREL]   A unit of activity of a radionuclide equal to 10^9 becquerel. Symbol: GBq.

gigaelectronvolt [GIGA- + ELECTRONVOLT]   A unit of energy equal to 10^9 electronvolt; $1.602\ 19 \times 10^{-10}$ joule. Symbol: GeV.

gigahertz [GIGA- + HERTZ]   A unit of frequency equal to 10^9 hertz. Symbol: GHz.

giganewton [GIGA- + NEWTON]   A unit of force equal to 10^9 newtons. Symbol: GN.

gigantism [*gigant(o)-* + -ISM]   **1** The state or quality of having excessively large stature; abnormally large size.   **2** PITUITARY GIGANTISM.

acromegalic gigantism   Gigantism combined with changes in osseous and soft tissues characteristic of acromegaly in patients who because of an adenohypophysial tumor, began secreting growth hormone excessively before puberty and before epiphysial closure, the hormonal excess persisting into adult life. Also called *acromegalogigantism*.

cerebral gigantism   SOTOS SYNDROME.

constitutional gigantism   Excessively large stature with normal body proportions and without demonstrable endocrine or other somatic dysfunction; gigantism attributed to genetic factors. Also called *normal gigantism, primordial gigantism* (rarely used).

digital gigantism   MACRODACTYLY.

eunuchoidal gigantism   The state of being a eunuchoid giant.

fetal gigantism   A size or weight in excess of the usual range in a fetus or newborn infant, often seen in the offspring of diabetic mothers or other conditions predisposing to postmaturity.

hyperpituitary gigantism   PITUITARY GIGANTISM.

hypothalamic gigantism   Gigantism associated with excessive release of growth hormone by the adenohypophysis, presumably owing to failure or deficiency of hypothalamic somatostatin (growth hormone inhibiting hormone).

normal gigantism CONSTITUTIONAL GIGANTISM.

pituitary gigantism Gigantism owing to excessive secretion of growth hormone by an adenohypophysial tumor or hypoplasia of the adenohypophysial alpha cells. Also called *hyperpituitary gigantism, Launois syndrome, gigantism.* • When used without qualification, *gigantism* usually refers to pituitary gigantism.

primordial gigantism A rarely used term for CONSTITUTIONAL GIGANTISM.

total lipodystrophy and acromegaloid gigantism See under SEIP SYNDROME.

giganto- [Gk *gigas* (genitive *gigantos*) a giant] A combining form meaning great in size, enormously large.

Gigantobilharzia A genus of schistosome blood flukes (family Schistosomatidae) infecting birds. Some have been implicated in human cercarial dermatitis, or swimmer's itch.

Gigantobilharzia monocotylea A species of schistosome that infects gulls, grebes, and ducks in Europe and has been associated with cases of human cercarial dermatitis.

gigantoblast A very large normoblast. An obsolete term. Also called *gigantochromoblast.*

gigantochromoblast GIGANTOBLAST.

gigantomastia [GIGANTO- + MAST- + -IA] Excessive growth of the breasts.

Gigantorhynchus 1 A genus of Acanthocephala (family Gigantorhynchidae) parasitic in mammals, characterized by a single row of large hooks at the apex of the proboscis and minute hooks on the remaining portion. 2 A former name for *MACRACANTHORHYNCHUS.*

Gigantorhynchus hirudinaceus *MACRACANTHORHYNCHUS HIRUDINACEUS.*

gigantosoma [GIGANTO- + Gk *sōma* body] An older term for GIGANTISM.

gigatonne [GIGA- + TONNE] A unit of mass or weight equal to 10^9 tonnes or 10^{12} kilograms, used especially to describe the equivalent explosive power of nuclear weapons in terms of tonnes of TNT. Symbol: Gt

gigawatt [GIGA- + WATT] A unit of power equal to 10^9 watts. Symbol: GW

Gigli [Leonardo *Gigli*, Italian gynecologist, 1863–1908] See under OPERATION.

gikiyami NANUKAYAMI.

gilbert [after William *Gilbert*, English physicist, 1544–1603] The CGS unit of magnetomotive force, equal to $1/4\pi$ abampere turns. An obsolete unit. Symbol: Gb

Gilbert [Augustin-Nicholas *Gilbert*, French physician, 1858–1927] 1 See under SIGN, SYNDROME. 2 Gilbert-Behçet syndrome. See under BEHÇET SYNDROME.

Gilbert Dreyfus [*Gilbert Dreyfus*, French physician, born 1902] See under SYNDROME.

Gilchrist [Thomas Caspar *Gilchrist*, U.S. physician, 1862–1927] Gilchrist's mycosis, Gilchrist's disease. See under BLASTOMYCOSIS.

gildable [*gild* + -ABLE] Capable of combining with the gold salts that are used as stains for nerve tissue preparations.

gilding The application of gold salts or of a thin layer of gold to biologic material, especially fixed nerve tissue.

Gilford [Hastings *Gilford*, English physician, 1861–1941] Hutchinson-Gilford progeria syndrome, Hutchinson-Gilford syndrome, Hutchinson-Gilford disease. See under PROGERIA.

Gill [Arthur Bruce *Gill*, U.S. orthopedic surgeon, 1876–1965] See under OPERATION.

gill¹ [Middle English *gile*, from the Scandinavian] 1 BRAN-CHIA. 2 The platelike structure located on the underside of a basidiomycetous mushroom cap, on which basidia are developed. Also called *lamella.*

gill² [Middle English *gille*, a wine measure, from Late L *gillo* a cooling vessel] 1 In the United States, a unit of capacity equal to 1/32 (US) gallon; 1/4 liquid pint; 0.118 294 liter. Symbol: gi 2 In Great Britain, a unit of capacity equal to 1/32 (UK) gallon; 1/4 pint; 0.142 065 liter.

Gilles de la Tourette [Georges Edouard Albert Brutus *Gilles de la Tourette*, French physician, 1859–1904] Gilles de la Tourette's disease, Tourette's disease. See under SYNDROME.

Gillespie [James Donaldson *Gillespie*, Scottish physician, 1823–1891] See under OPERATION.

Gillette [Eugene Paulin *Gillette*, French surgeon, 1836–1886] Gillette suspensory ligament. See under TENDO CRICOESOPHAGEUS.

Gilliam [David Tod *Gilliam*, U.S. gynecologist, 1844–1923] See under OPERATION.

Gillies [Harold Delf *Gillies*, New Zealand surgeon, 1882–1960] 1 See under OPERATION. 2 Gillies flap, Gillies graft. See under TUBED FLAP. 3 Gillies up-and-down flap. See under FLAP. 4 Filatov-Gillies tubed pedicle. See under PEDICLE.

gill raker A bony process on the inside of the gill arches of a typical fish. It prevents passage of solid food particles.

Gilmer [Thomas Lewis *Gilmer*, U.S. oral surgeon, 1849–1931] 1 See under METHOD. 2 Gilmer wiring. See under SPLINT.

gilt [Middle English *gilte, gylte*, from Old Norse *gyltr* a young sow] A young female pig before she has had her first litter.

Gimbernat [Antonio de *Gimbernat*, Spanish surgeon and anatomist, 1734–1816] 1 Gimbernat's ligament, lacunar ligament of Gimbernat, ligamentum lacunare Gimbernati. See under LIGAMENTUM LACUNARE. 2 Reflex ligament of Gimbernat. See under LIGAMENTUM REFLEXUM.

ginger [French *gingembre* (from L *zingiber* ginger, from Gk *zingiberis* ginger) ginger] The dried rhizome of *Zingiber officinale*, which contains a volatile oil, resin, and gingerol. It is used as a flavoring in foods and beverages.

American wild ginger ASARUM.

Chinese ginger GALANGA.

wild ginger ASARUM.

gingiva [L, the gum of the mouth; pl. *gingivae* the gums] (*plural gingivae*) A combination of epithelial and connective tissues that surrounds and is attached to the tooth and alveolar bone and extends to the mucogingival junction; the gum. On the palatal side it is a rim of tissue that merges with the masticatory mucosa of the hard palate. Also called *oula* (outmoded), *ula* (outmoded).

areolar gingiva The loose areolar connective tissue overlying part of the alveolar process. This is no longer considered to be part of the gingiva. An outmoded term.

attached gingiva The major portion of the gingiva, which is firmly bound down to the underlying bone and tooth. Also called *gingival zone* (outmoded).

buccal gingiva The gingiva on the buccal aspects of the teeth.

cleft gingiva GINGIVAL CLEFT.

free gingiva The collar of gingival tissue surrounding the gingival sulcus. This sulcus may be absent in the healthy state. An outmoded term.

interdental gingiva That portion of the gingiva between adjacent teeth. It comprises the labiobuccal and lingual papillae and the interdental col. Also called *interproximal gingiva, septal gingiva.*

interproximal gingiva INTERDENTAL GINGIVA.

labial gingiva The gingiva on the labial aspects of the teeth.

lingual gingiva The gingiva on the lingual aspects of the teeth.

marginal gingiva The tissue adjacent to the gingival margin.

self-cleansing gingiva Gingiva characterized by knife-edged margins, accentuated interdental grooves, and good sluiceways, features considered to be important for gingival health.

septal gingiva INTERDENTAL GINGIVA.

gingivae Plural of GINGIVA.

gingival Of or relating to the gingivae. Also *uletic* (obsolete).

gingivalgia [*gingiv(a)* + -ALGIA] Pain in the gums. An outmoded term.

gingivally Toward the gums.

gingivectomy [*gingiv(a)* + -ECTOMY] The elimination of a gingival or periodontal pocket by excision. The bevel of raw tissue left is then covered by a surgical pack for 7–10 days while re-epithelialization is occurring. In a reverse-bevel gingivectomy, the initial incision is directed towards the apices of the roots and the gingiva remaining is sutured interdentally to bring the raw surfaces into contact with the teeth. Also called *gingivoectomy* (outmoded), *ulectomy* (outmoded).

gingivitis [*gingiv(o)-* + -ITIS] Any inflammatory condition of the gingivae, regardless of the etiology. Also called *oulitis* (outmoded), *ulitis* (outmoded).

acute gingivitis Gingivitis of sudden onset and relatively short duration but without ulceration of the gingival margin.

acute necrotizing gingivitis NECROTIZING ULCERATIVE GINGIVITIS.

acute ulcerative gingivitis The British term for NECROTIZING ULCERATIVE GINGIVITIS. Abbreviation: AUG

bismuth gingivitis Chronic gingivitis modified by the systemic influence of a bismuth compound in a medicine. A dark bluish line in the gingiva is related to plaque stagnation areas.

catarrhal gingivitis Acute exacerbation of a chronic gingivitis associated with upper respiratory infection.

chronic gingivitis Long-standing plaque-associated gingivitis.

chronic desquamative gingivitis Uncommon plaque-associated gingivitis in which the oral gingival epithelium becomes extremely thin as a result of cellular desquamation and the gingiva bright red and sharply demarcated from the normal tissue. This lesion is not to be confused with erosive lichen planus, benign mucous membrane pemphigoid, pemphigus, or foreign-body reactions. Also called *desquamative gingivitis*.

desquamative gingivitis CHRONIC DESQUAMATIVE GINGIVITIS.

diphenylhydantoin gingivitis A plaque-associated gingivitis showing marked hyperplasia caused by the systemic action of an anticoagulant drug diphenylhydantoin sodium (phenytoin sodium in British usage) used in treating epilepsy. Also called *Dilantin gingival hyperplasia (used especially in the U.S.)*.

eruptive gingivitis Gingivitis around erupting teeth. Mild trauma may produce false pockets allowing increased stagnation areas for plaque accumulation. With further eruption, these areas are reduced.

fusospirochetal gingivitis NECROTIZING ULCERATIVE GINGIVITIS.

gingivitis gravidarum PREGNANCY GINGIVITIS.

hemorrhagic gingivitis Gingivitis with marked tendency to bleeding.

herpetic gingivitis HERPETIC STOMATITIS.

hormonal gingivitis A plaque-associated gingivitis modified and aggravated by sex steroids released during phases of the menstrual cycle or pregnancy or administered in the form of contraceptives. The disease may present as a hyperplastic lesion called a pregnancy tumor (epulis). Hormonal imbalance may also be a factor in the hyperplastic gingivitis of puberty.

hyperplastic gingivitis Chronically enlarged and inflamed gingival tissues. The gingivitis is plaque-associated but may have been modified by systemic factors, such as pregnancy or ingestion of Dilantin sodium. Also called *proliferative gingivitis*.

marginal gingivitis Gingivitis limited to the gingival margins and the interdental col.

necrotizing ulcerative gingivitis A disease involving necrosis and ulceration of the surface of the gingiva with underlying inflammation. It begins in an area of gingiva in contact with plaque, often interdental, and results in the clinically pathognomonic "punched-out" papilla. The plaque is characterized by a complex flora with relative proliferation of fusiform bacilli and spirochetes. The spirochetes penetrate the apparently still vital gingival tissues. The disease is associated with a typical fetor oris. Also called *acute ulcerative gingivitis (British usage), acute necrotizing gingivitis, fusospirochetal gingivitis, ulceromembranous gingivitis, Vincent's disease, Vincent's infection, Vincent's gingivitis, trench mouth, ulcerative gingivitis, Vincent stomatitis, fusospirochetal stomatitis.* Abbreviation: NUG

phagedenic gingivitis A rapidly spreading ulcerative gingivitis.

pregnancy gingivitis A plaque-associated gingivitis that has been exacerbated by pregnancy. It is sometimes considered a form of hormonal gingivitis. It may be hemorrhagic and hyperplastic in type. Also called *gingivitis gravidarum*.

proliferative gingivitis HYPERPLASTIC GINGIVITIS.

puberty gingivitis Hyperplastic, plaque-associated chronic gingivitis in children of pubertal age or in adolescents. It is assumed to be a form of hormonal gingivitis.

scorbutic gingivitis Hemorrhagic gingivitis associated with vitamin C deficiency.

senile atrophic gingivitis Gingival inflammation in the aged, with areas of desquamation and hyperkeratinization. It is sometimes associated with oral lichen planus. An outmoded term.

simple marginal gingivitis Chronic gingivitis caused by local factors only.

streptococcal gingivitis An acute erythematous gingivitis that was once thought to be caused by streptococci.

suppurative marginal gingivitis The first stage of pyorrhea. An outmoded term.

ulcerative gingivitis NECROTIZING ULCERATIVE GINGIVITIS.

ulceromembranous gingivitis NECROTIZING ULCERATIVE GINGIVITIS.

Vincent's gingivitis NECROTIZING ULCERATIVE GINGIVITIS.

gingivo- [L *gingiva* the gum] A combining form denoting the gingivae.

gingivoectomy An outmoded term for GINGIVECTOMY.

gingivoglossitis Inflammation of the gingivae and tongue.

gingivoplasty [GINGIVO- + -PLASTY] A surgical procedure to improve the contours of the gingiva and facilitate plaque control.

gingivosis [GINGIVO- + -SIS] A noninflammatory degenerative disease of the gingiva. Chronic desquamative gingivitis has been cited as an example of the condition. An outmoded term.

gingivostomatitis Inflammation of the gingivae and the mucosa of the oral cavity.

herpetic gingivostomatitis HERPETIC STOMATITIS.

necrotizing ulcerative gingivostomatitis The extension of necrotizing ulcerative gingivitis to involve adjacent oral mucosa. The tonsillar region may be involved (Vincent's angina), and extensive gangrene may occur (cancrum oris).

primary herpetic gingivostomatitis An infection of the mouth by the herpes simplex virus, occurring usually in the first five years of life, rarely in adults. The characteristic vesicular lesions of the gingivae, but also of the tongue and lips, quickly give way to small painful ulcers. Fever and local lymphadenopathy are the rule.

white folded gingivostomatitis WHITE SPONGE NEVUS.

gingivostomatosis / white folded gingivostomatosis 1 WHITE SPONGE NEVUS. **2** ORAL FAMILIAL WHITE FOLDED DYSPLASIA.

Gingko A monotypic genus of a deciduous, resinous tree in the family Gingkoaceae. *G. biloba*, gingko, or maidenhair tree, bears a nut that is a source of gingkolic acid, which is active against *Mycobacterium tuberculosis*. The nut kernels are poisonous.

ginglyform GINGLYMOID.

ginglymal Pertaining to a ginglymus.

ginglymoarthrodial Pertaining to a joint with elements of both hinge and plane joints.

ginglymoid Pertaining to or resembling a ginglymus, or hinge joint. Also *ginglyform*.

ginglymus [New L, from Gk *ginglymos* hinge] [NA] A uniaxial synovial joint in which movement is generally limited to to-and-fro movements in one plane, like a door on a hinge. Typically, the joint has powerful collateral ligaments tending to contain the movements, such as in the humeroulnar joint. Also called *hinge joint, ginglymoid joint, hinge articulation.*

    helicoid ginglymus ARTICULATIO TROCHOIDEA.

    lateral ginglymus ARTICULATIO TROCHOIDEA.

ginseng [Chinese, ginseng] The root of *Panax ginseng*, a perennial herb of the family Araliaceae. It contains saponin, glucosidal, and bitter substances, and it has been used in Oriental medicine as a tonic and aromatic bitter. Also called *panax*.

ginsenin A glycoside obtained from the roots and leaves of *Panax quinquefolium*, American ginseng. It reduces blood sugar levels.

Giordano [Davide *Giordano*, Italian surgeon, 1864–1954] Giordano sphincter. See under MUSCULUS SPHINCTER DUCTUS CHOLEDOCHI.

Giorgi [Giovanni *Giorgi*, Italian physicist, 1871–1950] Giorgi system. See under METER-KILOGRAM-SECOND-AMPERE SYSTEM.

GIP glucose-dependent insulinotropic peptide.

Giraldès [Joaquim Pedro Casado *Giraldès*, Portuguese-born French surgeon, 1808–1875] Organ of Giraldès. See under PARAGENITAL DUCTS.

Girard [Alfred Conrad *Girard*, Swiss-born U.S. surgeon, 1841–1914] **1** See under TREATMENT. **2** Girard's method. See under TREATMENT.

girdle CINGULUM.

    firmisternal shoulder girdle A pectoral girdle, present in certain frogs, in which the margins of two coracoid plates meet ventrally, cushioning the impact of landing from a leap.

    hip girdle CINGULUM MEMBRI INFERIORIS.

    Hitzig's girdle A girdle of sensory loss around the trunk, situated at breast level, and corresponding to the region innervated by the third, fourth, fifth, and sixth dorsal nerves. This is sometimes an early manifestation of tabes dorsalis.

    girdle of inferior extremity CINGULUM MEMBRI INFERIORIS.

    limb girdle Either cingulum membri inferioris or cingulum membri superioris.

    limbus girdle WHITE LIMBAL GIRDLE OF VOGT.

    Neptune's girdle A wet pack worn around the abdomen.

    pectoral girdle CINGULUM MEMBRI SUPERIORIS.

    pelvic girdle CINGULUM MEMBRI INFERIORIS.

    girdle of resistance The bony pelvis and soft tissue that form the birth canal. An older term.

    shoulder girdle CINGULUM MEMBRI SUPERIORIS.

    girdle of superior extremity CINGULUM MEMBRI SUPERIORIS.

    thoracic girdle CINGULUM MEMBRI SUPERIORIS.

    upper limb girdle CINGULUM MEMBRI SUPERIORIS.

    white limbal girdle of Vogt A narrow fenestrated white crescent situated in the very superficial layers of the peripheral

cornea in the nasal and temporal interpalpebral space. It is a benign, asymptomatic change of no significance. Also called *limbus girdle.*

Girdner [John Harvey *Girdner*, U.S. physician, 1856–1933] Girdner's probe. See under ELECTRIC PROBE.

girth [Middle English *gerth*, from Old Norse *gjörth* a girdle, saddle girth] The measurement around the body of an animal behind the forelegs.

Gitaligin A preparation of gitalin in the form of an amorphous powder. A proprietary name.

gitalin A mixture of cardiotonic glycosides from the foxglove, once believed to be a pure compound.

gitaloxin A cardioactive glycoside that is obtained from the leaves of *Digitalis purpurea* and is a component of gitalin.

githagenin A toxic sapogenin that causes gastrointestinal irritation, found in all parts of *Agrostemma githago*, corn cockle, and in the seeds of *Saponaria officinalis*, soapwort, and *S. vaccaria*, cow cockle.

githagism [*(Agrostemma) githag(o)* + -ISM] Poisoning by seeds of corn cockle, *Agrostemma githago*. They contain the toxic substances agrostemmic acid and githagin, a glucoside. Corn cockle is a common weed whose seed is often found mixed in wheat. When ingested, it causes irritation of the digestive tract, vomiting, nausea, diarrhea, depressed respiration, and vertigo. Also called *corn cockle poisoning.*

gitogenin A sapogenin whose glycosides, e.g. gitonin, are saponins found in foxglove leaves.

gitonin A saponin found in foxglove leaves.

gitoxigenin A cardenolide whose glycosides, e.g. digitalin and gitoxin, are cardiotonic and found in foxglove.

gitoxin $C_{41}H_{64}O_{14}$. A cardioactive glycoside obtained from the leaves of *Digitalis purpurea*.

Gitterfasern [German *Gitter* lattice, trellis + *Fasern*, pl. of *Faser* thread, fiber] The reticular fibers of the dermis.

Giuffrida-Ruggieri [Vincenzo *Giuffrida-Ruggieri*, Italian anthropologist, 1872–1922] See under STIGMA.

GIX A proprietary name for DFDT.

gizzard [earlier *gysard, gysar*, from Middle English *giser*, from Old Norman French *guisier* or *gisier* liver of a fowl, gizzard, from L *gigeria* cooked entrails of poultry, from *gizeria* giblets] The muscular stomach of birds, which grinds food, with the aid of ingested foreign objects, such as stones.

Gjessing [Leiv Rolvssoen *Gjessing*, Norwegian physician, born 1918] See under SYNDROME.

GL greatest length.

gl. *glandula* (L, gland).

glabella [New L (substantive from *glabella*, fem. of *glabellus*, dim. of L *glaber* smooth), the small space in the human forehead between the eyebrows] [NA] A craniometric point situated in the midline of the frontal bone at the most prominent point between the medial ends of the superciliary arches. Also called *nasal eminence* (rarely used), *metopic point, intercilium, antinion* (outmoded), *glabellum* (outmoded), *mesophryon.*

    coccygeal glabella A small bald area in the coccygeal region.

glabellad Toward the glabella.

glabellum An outmoded term for GLABELLA.

glabrate GLABROUS.

glabrous [L *glaber*, gen. *glabris*, bald, bare + -OUS] Smooth: used especially in reference to a surface that lacks terminal hair but is not strictly hairless. Also *glabrate.*

gladiate [New L *gladiat(us)* (from L *gladi(us)* sword + -*atus* -ATE) sword-shaped] Sword-shaped; ensiform.

gladiolic acid $C_{11}H_{10}O_5$. 2,3-Diformyl-6-methoxy-5-methylbenzoic acid, a naturally occurring antibiotic substance from

Penicillium gladioli. It also has antifungal properties.

gladiolus (*plural* gladioli, gladiolus, gladioluses) **1** Any plant of the genus *Gladiolus.* **2** CORPUS STERNI.

gladiomanubrial Pertaining to the gladiolus and the manubrium of the sternum.

Glaesser [Karl *Glaesser*, German veterinarian, flourished early 20th century] See under DISEASE.

glairy Resembling glair, as in texture; viscid; glutinous.

gland

gland [L *glans* (gen. *glandis*; from early L form *galans*, akin to Gk *balanos*, Doric *galanos*, an acorn, date, akin to Gk *ballein* to throw, let fall) any kernel fruit, an acorn, chestnut, date, walnut] An organized group of epithelial cells, either tightly clustered or scattered, that produces a secretion or an excretion for discharge; glandula.

absorbent gland An outmoded term for NODUS LYMPHATICUS.

accessory adrenal glands GLANDULAE SUPRARENALES ACCESSORIAE.

accessory lacrimal glands GLANDULAE LACRIMALES ACCESSORIAE.

accessory mammary glands **1** SUPERNUMERARY MAMMAE. **2** An outmoded term for MONTGOMERY'S GLANDS.

accessory parotid gland GLANDULA PAROTIDEA ACCESSORIA.

accessory salivary glands GLANDULAE SALIVARIAE MINORES.

accessory sublingual glands Occasional small glandular lobules that are scattered irregularly about the sublingual gland. They open at the level of the sublingual caruncle of the submandibular duct. An outmoded term.

accessory suprarenal glands GLANDULAE SUPRARENALES ACCESSORIAE.

accessory thyroid glands Small remnants of thyroid tissue, residua of embryogenesis, along the course of the thyroglossal duct and in the thorax. Also called *Gley's glands, prehyoid glands, suprahyoid glands, Sandström's glands, glandulae thyroideae accessoriae, thyroidea ima* (outmoded), *thyroidea accessoria* (outmoded).

acid gland GLANDULA GASTRICA PROPRIA.

acinar gland An exocrine gland that is composed of rounded clusters of cells discharging their secretion into a central lumen.

acinotubular gland A gland made up of both tubules and acini. Also called *tubuloacinar gland.*

acinous gland A gland that is formed of cells arranged in small clusters which often encompass central lumens. Also called *alveolar gland.*

admaxillary gland An outmoded term for GLANDULA PAROTIDEA ACCESSORIA.

adrenal gland GLANDULA SUPRARENALIS.

aggregate glands FOLLICULI LYMPHATICI AGGREGATI.

agminated glands FOLLICULI LYMPHATICI AGGREGATI.

Albarrán's glands SUBCERVICAL GLANDS OF ALBARRÁN.

albuminous gland Any gland that secretes a notably proteinaceous substance.

alveolar gland ACINOUS GLAND.

anal gland Any gland associated with the anus or rectum. Such glands are found in many vertebrates and invertebrates, and their function is usually excretory or secretory.

anteprostatic gland An outmoded term for GLANDULA BULBOURETHRALIS.

anterior lingual gland GLANDULA LINGUALIS ANTERIOR.

anterior lingual gland of Blandin and Nuhn GLANDULA LINGUALIS ANTERIOR.

aortic glands CORPORA PARA-AORTICA.

apical gland of tongue GLANDULA LINGUALIS ANTERIOR.

apocrine gland A gland whose secretory discharge contains a part (the apex) of the secreting cell, as in certain sweat glands.

apocrine sweat gland A gland that opens into the hair follicle via a duct above the sebaceous duct. Such glands are small and inactive during childhood but enlarge at puberty. They are usually confined to the axillary and anogenital skin and to the areolae of the breasts.

aporic glands A seldom used term for ENDOCRINE GLANDS.

areolar glands MONTGOMERY'S GLANDS.

arterial gland A small aggregation of arteriovenous anastomoses or vascular tissue, such as the glomus coccygeum. An outmoded term.

arteriococcygeal gland An outmoded term for GLOMUS COCCYGEUM.

arytenoid gland GLANDULA ARYTENOIDEA.

Aselli's glands The nodi lymphatici mesenterici in carnivores.

atrabiliary gland An outmoded term for GLANDULA SUPRARENALIS.

Avicenna's gland An encapsulated tumor. An obsolete term.

axillary glands NODI LYMPHATICI AXILLARES.

Bartholin's gland GLANDULA VESTIBULARIS MAJOR.

Bauhin's glands GLANDULA LINGUALIS ANTERIOR.

Baumgarten's glands Convoluted tubular glands that are situated near the fornices in the medial part of the palpebral conjunctiva and open on the surface of the conjunctiva. Also called *Henle's glands.*

glands of biliary mucosa GLANDULAE MUCOSAE BILIOSAE.

Blandin's gland GLANDULA LINGUALIS ANTERIOR.

Blandin and Nuhn gland GLANDULA LINGUALIS ANTERIOR.

blood glands A seldom used term for ENDOCRINE GLANDS.

blood vessel glands A seldom used term for ENDOCRINE GLANDS.

Boerhaave's glands SWEAT GLANDS.

Bonnot's gland INTERSCAPULAR GLAND.

Bowman's gland GLANDULA OLFACTORIA.

brachial glands NODI LYMPHATICI BRACHIALES.

branching gland An exocrine gland that contains a branching pattern of secretory ducts.

bronchial glands GLANDULAE BRONCHIALES.

Bruch's glands Lymphatic follicles situated in the conjunctiva of the lower eyelid chiefly near the medial palpebral commissure.

Brunner's glands GLANDULAE DUODENALES.

buccal glands GLANDULAE BUCCALES.

bulbocavernous gland GLANDULA BULBOURETHRALIS.

bulbourethral gland GLANDULA BULBOURETHRALIS.

cardiac gland Either the glandula cardiaca esophagi or the glandula cardiaca gastricae.

carotid gland GLOMUS CAROTICUM.

glands of the caruncle The sebaceous and sweat glands within the lacrimal caruncle.

celiac glands NODI LYMPHATICI COELIACI.

ceruminous glands The wax-forming glands of the external ear, located in the external portions of the external auditory meatus. Also called *glandulae ceruminosae.*

cervical glands of uterus GLANDULAE CERVICALES UTERI.

cheek glands GLANDULAE BUCCALES.

choroid gland PLEXUS CHOROIDEUS.

Ciaccio's glands GLANDULAE LACRIMALES ACCESSORIAE.

ciliary glands GLANDULAE CILIARES PALPEBRARUM.

ciliary glands of conjunctiva An outmoded term for GLAN-

DULAE CILIARES PALPEBRARUM.

circumanal glands The large, specialized, sebaceous glands around the anus, present in most mammals. Also called *glands of Gay, perianal glands, glandulae circumanales*.

Cloquet's gland CLOQUET'S NODE.

closed glands A seldom used term for ENDOCRINE GLANDS.

Cobelli's gland GLANDULA CARDIACA ESOPHAGI.

coccygeal gland An outmoded term for GLOMUS COCCYGEUM.

coil gland CONVOLUTED GLAND.

compound gland Any exocrine gland comprising multiple units whose ducts unite to form ductules and ducts of progressively larger size. The salivary glands and the pancreas are glands of this kind. Also called *conglomerate gland* (obsolete), *glomer (British)*.

conglobate gland NODUS LYMPHATICUS.

conglomerate gland An obsolete term for COMPOUND GLAND.

conjunctival glands GLANDULAE CONJUNCTIVALES.

convoluted gland A tubular gland of the skin, as a sweat gland, whose secretory, proximal end is coiled like a glomerulus. Also called *coil gland*.

Cowper's gland GLANDULA BULBOURETHRALIS.

crop gland A gland in the crop of certain birds, such as pigeons, which secretes a milklike substance used to nourish the young.

cutaneous gland A gland of the skin. Also called *glandula cutis*.

cytogenic gland The testis or ovary. A seldom used term. Also called *genital gland*.

deep gland Any exocrine gland whose secretory element lies deep to a mucous membrane, usually in the submucosa.

ductless glands ENDOCRINE GLANDS.

duodenal glands GLANDULAE DUODENALES.

Duverney's gland GLANDULA VESTIBULARIS MAJOR.

Ebner's glands GLANDULA GUSTATORIA.

eccrine gland Any of the more numerous type of sweat glands, whose cells do not form part of its secretary discharge, thus distinguishing them from apocrine glands; a merocrine gland.

ecdysal glands Glands in the thorax of insects, originating from the ectoderm of the ventrocaudal part of the head, which secrete ecdysone. Also called *peritracheal glands, prothoracic glands, thoracic glands, ventral glands*.

Eglis glands Small mucous glands in the renal pelvis.

endocrine glands Glands that secrete gland-specific molecules, or hormones, directly into the bloodstream. The hormones influence body functions generally and at remote anatomic sites. Endocrine glands include the pituitary gland, the thyroid, parathyroids, adrenals, gonads, pancreatic islets, and specialized cells of the gastrointestinal tract and the lung. The status of the pineal and the thymus as endocrine glands is controversial. Also called *ductless glands, glandulae endocrinae, aporic glands* (seldom used), *blood glands* (seldom used), *blood vessel glands* (seldom used), *closed glands* (seldom used), *incretory glands* (rarely used), *glandulae sine ductibus* (seldom used).

endoepithelial gland A gland that is located in an epithelium. Also called *intraepithelial gland*.

endo-exocrine gland A gland that functions both as an endocrine and an exocrine gland, secreting some products into the bloodstream and others through ducts, as onto the exterior of the body either directly or indirectly.

endometrial glands GLANDULAE UTERINAE.

epithelial gland A mass of glandular cells within an epithelium.

esophageal glands GLANDULAE ESOPHAGEAE.

esophageal gland proper GLANDULA ESOPHAGEA PROPRIA.

excretory gland A gland excreting the products of metabolism from the system, as the sweat glands.

exocrine gland A gland which secretes its product to an internal or external surface through a duct or system of ducts, as the sweat glands or salivary glands.

external salivary gland An outmoded term for GLANDULA PAROTIDEA.

extraparotid lymph glands Nodi lymphatici parotidei superficiales. An outmoded term. See under NODI LYMPHATICI PAROTIDEI SUPERFICIALES ET PROFUNDI.

follicular glands of tongue An outmoded term for FOLLICULI LINGUALES.

Fraenkel's glands Minute laryngeal glands situated just below the vocal folds.

fundic gland GLANDULA GASTRICA PROPRIA.

fundus gland GLANDULA GASTRICA PROPRIA.

Galeati's glands GLANDULAE INTESTINALES.

gas gland Any of various glands which secrete a gas, such as those in the wall of the swim bladder of fishes and in the floats of certain pelagic coelenterates.

gastric glands The several groups and types of glands secreting the gastric juice, including glandula cardiaca, glandula gastrica propria, and glandula pylorica. They contain zymogenic, oxyntic, and mucous cells.

gastric gland proper GLANDULA GASTRICA PROPRIA.

gastroepiploic glands The nodi lymphatici gastrici dextri and nodi lymphatici gastrici sinistri.

glands of Gay CIRCUMANAL GLANDS.

genal glands GLANDULAE BUCCALES.

genital gland CYTOGENIC GLAND.

gingival glands SERRES GLANDS.

Gley's glands ACCESSORY THYROID GLANDS.

globate gland An outmoded term for NODUS LYMPHATICUS.

glomerate glands GLOMIFORM GLANDS.

glomiform glands Arteriovenous shunts in the skin. Also called *glomerate glands, glandulae glomiformes, glomus bodies*. • The term is inaccurate, since the bodies referred to are not glands.

glossopalatine glands Lingual mucous glands in the posterior part of the tongue behind the vallate papillae. An outmoded term.

greater vestibular gland GLANDULA VESTIBULARIS MAJOR.

green gland An excretory organ of certain crustaceans. It is located anteroventrally in the cephalothorax and the duct opens to the exterior at the base of the first antenna.

Guérin's glands 1 DUCTUS PARAURETHRALES. 2 GLANDULAE URETHRALES URETHRAE FEMININAE.

gustatory gland GLANDULA GUSTATORIA.

guttural gland Any mucous gland in the walls of the pharynx. An outmoded term.

glands of Haller GLANDULAE PREPUTIALES.

Harder's gland HARDERIAN GLAND.

harderian gland An accessory lacrimal gland near the inner corner of the eye in animals that possess nictitating membranes. It secretes an oily fluid which facilitates the movement of the third eyelid. This gland is rudimentary in humans. Also called *Harder's gland*.

haversian glands Villi synoviales or adipose tissue that is covered by a synovial lining in the joints.

hemal gland HEMAL NODE.

hemal lymph gland HEMAL NODE.

hematopoietic glands Those organs or glands that contribute to blood formation in fetal or postnatal life, including the thymus, liver, spleen, lymph glands, and bone marrow. A seldom used term.

hemolymph glands HEMOLYMPH NODE.

Henle's glands BAUMGARTEN'S GLANDS.

hepatic glands An outmoded term for GLANDULAE MUCOSAE BILIOSAE.

heterocrine gland GLANDULA SEROMUCOSA.

hibernating gland INTERSCAPULAR GLAND.

holocrine gland An exocrine gland whose secreting cells form part of its secretory discharge.

Home's gland SUBTRIGONAL GLAND.

incretory glands A rarely used term for ENDOCRINE GLANDS.

infraorbital gland A salivary gland located below the eye in certain mammals, such as the rabbit.

inguinal gland Any one of either nodi lymphatici inguinales profundi or nodi lymphatici inguinales superficiales.

intercarotid gland GLOMUS CAROTICUM.

intermaxillary gland A large mucous gland located on the anterior palate of certain amphibians.

internal salivary gland Either glandula sublingualis or glandula submandibularis. An outmoded term.

interrenal gland A variously distributed endocrine gland within the body cavity of certain fishes that secretes steroid hormones. It is homologous to the mammalian adrenal cortex. Also called *interrenal body.*

interscapular gland A lobulated deposit of brown fat in the interscapular region of some mammals, especially those that hibernate, and human fetuses. It does not have glandular structure, and is comprised of cells gorged with lipid droplets. Its specific function is unknown, but it may be involved in heat production and the regulation of body temperature due to the numerous mitochondria contained in the fat cells. Also called *Bonnot's gland, hibernating gland, brown fat, multilocular adipose tissue, primitive fat organ, brown adipose tissue, textus adiposus fuscus.*

interstitial glands An outmoded term for LEYDIG CELLS.

intestinal glands GLANDULAE INTESTINALES.

intraepithelial gland ENDOEPITHELIAL GLAND.

intramuscular gland of tongue An outmoded term for GLANDULA LINGUALIS ANTERIOR.

jugular glands NODI LYMPHATICI SUPRACLAVICULARES.

Kölliker's gland GLANDULA OLFACTORIA.

Krause glands 1 Glands in the mucous membrane of the tympanic cavity. 2 GLANDULAE CONJUNCTIVALES. 3 GLANDULAE LACRIMALES ACCESSORIAE.

labial glands of mouth GLANDULAE LABIALES ORIS.

lacrimal gland GLANDULA LACRIMALIS.

lactiferous gland An outmoded term for GLANDULA MAMMARIA.

glands of large intestine See under GLANDULAE INTESTINALES.

large sweat gland An apocrine sweat gland that has developed to full size following the onset of puberty.

laryngeal glands GLANDULAE LARYNGEALES.

lateral nasal gland of Stensen A serous-type gland situated laterally in the nasal cavity but found only in the embryo.

lenticular glands of tongue An outmoded term for FOLLICULI LINGUALES.

lesser vestibular glands GLANDULAE VESTIBULARES MINORES.

glands of Lieberkühn GLANDULAE INTESTINALES.

lingual glands GLANDULAE LINGUALES.

lingual mucous glands GLANDULAE LINGUALES.

Littre's glands 1 GLANDULAE PREPUTIALES. 2 GLANDULAE URETHRALES URETHRAE MASCULINAE.

Luschka's gland GLOMUS COCCYGEUM.

lymph gland NODUS LYMPHATICUS.

lymphatic gland NODUS LYMPHATICUS.

main salivary glands GLANDULAE SALIVARIAE MAJORES.

malar glands GLANDULAE BUCCALES.

malpighian glands FOLLICULI LYMPHATICI SPLENICI.

mammary gland GLANDULA MAMMARIA.

mandibular gland An outmoded term for GLANDULA SUBMANDIBULARIS.

Manz glands Depressions in the bulbar conjunctiva adjacent to the limbus. They were originally considered to be caused by glands but are now thought to be artifacts.

marrow-lymph gland A lymph gland that is largely composed of hematopoietic cells, and that serves as a site of blood formation, as normally occurs in embryonic and fetal life. A rarely used term.

master gland A popular term for PITUITARY GLAND.

Mehlis glands A group of unicellular glands that surround and secrete into the ootype of trematodes and cestodes. The following functions have been attributed to them, though none has been clearly established: (1) secretion of a substance that tans or hardens the egg shell, (2) production of a releaser stimulus for vitelline gland shell globules, (3) secretion of a membrane under which the shell forms around the eggs, (4) lubrication of the eggs as they pass through the ootype into the uterus, and (5) activation of spermatozoa.

meibomian glands GLANDULAE TARSALES.

merocrine gland An exocrine gland whose cells do not form part of its secretory discharge, as the commonest form of human sweat gland.

mesenteric glands NODI LYMPHATICI MESENTERICI.

mesocolic glands NODI LYMPHATICI MESOCOLICI.

metrial gland A collection of cellular elements concerned with the nutrition of the embryo. It comprises giant cells of the maternal part of the placenta, the myometrial gland, and hypertrophied epithelial cells.

minor salivary glands GLANDULAE SALIVARIAE MINORES.

mixed gland GLANDULA SEROMUCOSA.

molar glands GLANDULAE MOLARES.

Moll's glands GLANDULAE CILIARES PALPEBRARUM.

monoptychic gland An exocrine gland in which the secretory cell lining consists of a single layer of cells. A seldom used term.

Montgomery's glands The enlarged sebaceous glands seen on the areola of the nipple during pregnancy. Also called *glandulae areolares, glandulae areolares Montgomerii, glandulae sebaceae mammae, areolar gland, Montgomery's follicles, accessory mammary glands* (outmoded).

Morgagni's glands GLANDULAE URETHRALES URETHRAE MASCULINAE.

glands of mouth GLANDULAE ORIS.

mucilaginous glands SYNOVIAL VILLI.

muciparous gland GLANDULA MUCOSA.

mucous gland GLANDULA MUCOSA.

mucous glands of auditory tube GLANDULAE TUBARIAE.

mucous glands of duodenum GLANDULAE DUODENALES.

mucous glands of eustachian tube GLANDULAE TUBARIAE.

mucous gland of the urethra A mucous gland that lies in the connective tissue around the penile part of the male urethra.

musk gland Any of the glands which secrete musk, such as those located under the abdominal skin of the male musk deer or in the cloacae of alligators.

myometrial gland A collection of cells which respond to steroids and are diffusely distributed during pregnancy in the myometrium of rabbits and some rodents. The myometrial gland has been considered a possible source of a hormone.

nabothian glands NABOTHIAN CYSTS.

nasal glands GLANDULAE NASALES.

nasolabial gland A modified sweat gland in the nasolabial plane of large ruminants.

gland of neck An outmoded term for TONSILLA PHARYNGEALIS.

nidamental gland Any of four cylindrical, specialized shell glands in the mantle of a female squid. These glands secrete a jelly that covers the eggs.

Nuhn's gland GLANDULA LINGUALIS ANTERIOR.

odoriferous glands of prepuce GLANDULAE PREPUTIALES.

oil glands SEBACEOUS GLANDS.

olfactory gland GLANDULA OLFACTORIA.

optic glands A pair of endocrine structures located near the cephalopod brain that secrete a gonadotropic hormone.

oxyntic gland GLANDULA GASTRICA PROPRIA.

pacchionian glands GRANULATIONES ARACHNOIDEALES.

palatine glands GLANDULAE PALATINAE.

palpebral glands GLANDULAE TARSALES.

pancreaticosplenic glands Nodi lymphatici pancreatici and nodi lymphatici splenici considered together.

parafrenal glands Preputial glands that open alongside the frenulum of the prepuce.

parathyroid glands Yellow bodies that occur in pairs behind or in the substance of the thyroid gland. They arise embryologically from the branchial clefts, In humans they usually comprise two superior and two inferior glands. Composed of chief cells and oxyphil cells, they secrete parathyroid hormone, the principal endocrine regulator of calcium and phosphorus and of the metabolism of bone. Also called *glandulae parathyroideae, Sandström's bodies, parathyroid bodies* (obsolete), *epithelial bodies* (obsolete).

paraurethral glands 1 DUCTUS PARAURETHRALES. **2** GLANDULAE URETHRALES URETHRAE FEMININAE.

parotid gland GLANDULA PAROTIDEA.

pectoral glands NODI LYMPHATICI AXILLARES.

peptic gland GLANDULA GASTRICA PROPRIA.

perianal glands CIRCUMANAL GLANDS.

peritracheal glands ECDYSAL GLANDS.

perspiratory glands SWEAT GLANDS.

Peyer's glands FOLLICULI LYMPHATICI AGGREGATI.

pharyngeal glands GLANDULAE PHARYNGEAE.

pharyngeal pituitary gland A group of adenohypophysial cells embedded in small clusters in the sphenoid bone, richly innervated but with a blood supply lacking in hypothalamic hypophysiotropic hormones. It may play a role in the secretion of anterior pituitary hormone.

Philip's glands Lymph glands situated in the anterior triangle of the neck close to the sternoclavicular joint. They become enlarged in children suffering from pulmonary tuberculosis, by extension from a primary focus in the apex of the lung, via the bronchial and hilar lymph nodes.

pilar glands SEBACEOUS GLANDS.

pineal gland CORPUS PINEALE.

pituitary gland An unpaired, ovoid body that lies below the hypothalamus in the pituitary fossa of the sella turcica; the hypophysis. In humans it weighs 400–900 mg. It is attached to the tuber cinereum by a stalk containing the hypothalamic-hypophysial portal venous system (which conveys to the pituitary the hypothalamic hypophysiotropic hormones) and the supraopticoneurohypophysial neurosecretory tract (which acts as a conduit for the neurohypophysial peptides oxytocin and vasopressin and their carrier proteins). The gland consists of two main lobes. The anterior lobe, the adenohypophysis, arises in embryogenesis from the ectodermal roof of the stomatodeum. It has three constituent parts, the pars distalis, or main body of the adenohypophysis; the pars intermedia, which is not a separate entity in man; and the pars tuberalis, which forms a tenuous cell layer on the outer surface of the pituitary stalk. The posterior lobe, the neurohypophysis, arises in embryogenesis from an outpouching of the hypothalamic floor, and includes the pars posterior, the infundibular stem, and the median eminence. Regulated by the hypothalamic releasing hormones, the adenohypophysis periodically secretes growth hormone, prolactin, thy-

rotropin, adrenocorticotropin, gonadotropin, and lipotropin. These hormones exert a major regulatory influence through other endocrine glands upon growth, development, maturation, and reproduction. Acted upon by many stimuli, the chief being the osmolarity of the plasma, the supraoptic nuclei secrete vasopressin, which is ultimately released from the neurohypophysis. The neurohypophysis also releases oxytocin at parturition, but the physiologic role of this hormone in man is not fully understood. Also called *glandula pituitaria, hypophysis cerebri, pituitary body, master gland* (popular), *glandula basilaris, pituitarium.*

Poirier's gland A lymph node located in the base of the broad ligament of the uterus where the uterine artery crosses medially over the ureter.

polyptychic gland A gland in which the secretory cells are multilayered.

preen gland UROPYGIAL GLAND.

pregnancy glands The structures capable of secreting supporting hormones of pregnancy and comprising the ovarian follicle, corpus luteum, and placenta. A seldom used term.

prehyoid glands ACCESSORY THYROID GLANDS.

preputial glands GLANDULAE PREPUTIALES.

principal lacrimal gland PARS ORBITALIS GLANDULAE LACRIMALIS.

prostate gland PROSTATA.

prothoracic glands ECDYSAL GLANDS.

puberty glands Leydig interstitial cells in the testis and lutein cells in the ovary.

pyloric gland GLANDULA PYLORICA.

racemose glands Exocrine glands that have a ramifying duct system and attached cluster of acini. The resulting whole resembles a bunch of grapes.

rectal gland A finger-shaped gland associated with the rectum of certain vertebrates, such as sharks, which secretes a lubricating mucus.

retromolar glands GLANDULAE MOLARES.

Rivinus gland GLANDULA SUBLINGUALIS.

Rosenmüller's gland 1 CLOQUET'S NODE. **2** PARS PALPEBRALIS GLANDULAE LACRIMALIS.

saccular gland An exocrine gland that is composed of one or more sacs lined with secretory cells.

salivary gland One of either glandulae salivariae majores or glandulae salivariae minores.

Sandström's glands ACCESSORY THYROID GLANDS.

scent gland A specialized sebaceous gland that secretes an odorous substance used by territorial animals in marking or as a defense mechanism.

Schüller's glands 1 Diverticula of the ductus epoophori longitudinalis. **2** DUCTUS PARAURETHRALES.

sebaceous glands Small lobulated glands in the dermis that produce sebum by a process of holocrine secretion. Most sebaceous glands open via the sebaceous duct into a hair follicle, but in a few sites, such as the female genitalia, the glands open directly onto the skin surface. Also called *oil glands, glandulae sebaceae, sebaceous holocrine glands, pilar glands.*

sebaceous glands of conjunctiva An outmoded term for GLANDULAE SEBACEAE PALPEBRARUM.

sebaceous glands of eyelids GLANDULAE SEBACEAE PALPEBRARUM.

sebaceous holocrine glands SEBACEOUS GLANDS.

sentinel gland An enlarged regional lymph node calling attention to a nearby disease process, usually inflammatory in nature. It often refers to an enlarged lymph node adjacent to an ulcer of the stomach.

seromucous gland GLANDULA SEROMUCOSA.

serous gland An exocrine gland that secretes a wheylike or watery fluid that contains proteins such as lysozymes and digestive enzymes. The nuclei of the cells are spherical and placed near the base of the cell and the apical cytoplasm contains zymogen granules. Also called *glandula serosa*.

Serres glands Aggregations of epithelial cells situated in the gingival mucosa of the newborn infant. Also called *gingival glands*.

sexual gland The testis or ovary.

glands of Shambaugh The specialized stratified columnar epithelium of the stria vascularis on the outer wall of the cochlear duct that some investigators believe secretes endolymph. An imprecise usage.

shell gland A specialized region in the oviduct of certain fishes, reptiles, and birds which produces the egg albumin and the shell.

Sigmund's glands NODI LYMPHATICI CUBITALES.

simple gland An exocrine gland that is drained by a duct without branches.

Skene's glands 1 DUCTUS PARAURETHRALES. 2 GLANDULAE URETHRALES URETHRAE FEMININAE.

glands of small intestine See under GLANDULAE INTESTINALES.

solitary gland of small intestine SOLITARY LYMPHOID NODULE OF SMALL INTESTINE.

splenoid gland Tissue resembling that of the spleen which is stated to develop after removal of the spleen at that site. This is not generally accepted. An outmoded term.

splenolymph gland A hemal node that contains tissue resembling that of the spleen.

Stahr's gland One of the nodi lymphatici faciales, situated adjacent to the facial artery as it crosses the base of the mandible.

staphyline glands An outmoded term for GLANDULAE PALATINAE.

subauricular glands NODI LYMPHATICI MASTOIDEI.

subcervical glands of Albarrán Submucosal glands of the prostatic part of the urethra that are situated just distal to the neck of the urinary bladder where the subtrigonal glands are located. Some consider these glands to be true mucous glands. It is believed by some authorities that hyperplasia of the glands produces the so-called middle lobe hypertrophy of the prostate. Also called *Albarrán's glands, Albarrán's tubules*.

sublingual gland GLANDULA SUBLINGUALIS.

submandibular gland GLANDULA SUBMANDIBULARIS.

submaxillary gland An outmoded term for GLANDULA SUBMANDIBULARIS.

subtrigonal gland 1 One of several epithelial outgrowths of the urethra during development of the glandular tissue of the prostate which are situated beneath the mucous membrane near the apex of the trigone of the urinary bladder and constitute part of the middle lobe of the prostate, especially when they undergo hyperplasia. They lie deep to and form the uvula vesicae. Also called *Home's gland, Home's lobe*. 2 GLANDULA TRIGONI VESICAE.

sudoriferous glands SWEAT GLANDS.

sudoriparous glands SWEAT GLANDS.

suprahyoid glands ACCESSORY THYROID GLANDS.

suprahyoid accessory thyroid gland GLANDULA THYROIDEA ACCESSORIA SUPRAHYOIDEA.

suprarenal gland GLANDULA SUPRARENALIS.

Suzanne's gland A mucous gland situated in the mucous membrane of the floor of the mouth near the midline.

sweat glands Glands in the skin that produce sweat. Also called *glandulae sudoriferae, sudoriferous glands, perspiratory glands, Boerhaave's glands, sudoriparous glands*.

synovial glands SYNOVIAL VILLI.

target gland A gland whose function is affected by an external influence, as the thyroid gland, gonads, or the adrenal cortex by an anterior pituitary hormone.

tarsal glands GLANDULAE TARSALES.

tarsoconjunctival glands An outmoded term for GLANDULAE TARSALES.

Theile's glands LUSCHKA'S CRYPTS.

thoracic glands ECDYSAL GLANDS.

thymus gland THYMUS.

thyroid gland A highly vascular endocrine gland weighing 10 to 60 g in the human adult, located in the front of the neck and closely apposed to the upper part of the trachea, and consisting of two lobes joined in front by an isthmus. It arises embryologically from the pharyngeal floor. The gland is ultimately concerned with nutrition, having the capacity to concentrate iodine and forming the thyroid hormones, thyroxine and triiodothyronine, which play a major part in regulating metabolic rate, rate of cellular oxygen consumption, normal growth, and orderly somatic and mental development. It consists of follicles 200 μm in diameter, among which are interspersed parafollicular cells that secrete thyrocalcitonin, which is important in calcium metabolism. Also called *glandula thyroidea, thyroidea, thyroid body* (outmoded).

Tiedemann's gland GLANDULA VESTIBULARIS MAJOR.

glands of tongue GLANDULAE LINGUALES.

tracheal glands GLANDULAE TRACHEALES.

trachoma glands Follicular enlargements of the conjunctiva due to infection with *Chlamydia trachomatis*.

tubular gland An exocrine gland whose component cells are arranged in the form of tube about a central lumen.

tubuloacinar gland ACINOTUBULAR GLAND.

tympanic gland 1 A minute ganglionic mass situated on the tympanic nerve in its canaliculus. 2 One of the previously hypothesized mucous glands in the tympanic cavity. It has been shown that only goblet cells are present, near the entrance of the pharyngotympanic tube. An outmoded term. Also called *glandula tympanica* (outmoded).

glands of Tyson GLANDULAE PREPUTIALES.

unicellular gland A single cell that secretes directly onto a surface, as the goblet cells that line the large bowel mucosa.

urethral glands Glandulae urethrales urethrae femininae and glandulae urethrales urethrae masculinae.

urethral glands of female urethra GLANDULAE URETHRALES URETHRAE FEMININAE.

urethral glands of male urethra GLANDULAE URETHRALES URETHRAE MASCULINAE.

uropygial gland A gland at the base of the tail feathers in birds, that secretes an oily substance used to preen and waterproof the feathers. Also called *preen gland, glandula uropygialis*.

uterine glands GLANDULAE UTERINAE.

utricular glands GLANDULAE UTERINAE.

vaginal gland A mucous gland in the mucous membrane of the vagina. The gland is seldom present.

vascular gland 1 GLOMUS. 2 HEMAL NODE.

ventral glands ECDYSAL GLANDS.

vesical glands 1 Mucous follicles in the mucous membrane of the urinary bladder, especially near the neck. Also called *glandulae vesicales vesicae urinariae* (outmoded). 2 GLANDULA TRIGONI VESICAE.

vestibular glands Either glandula vestibularis major or glandulae vestibulares minores.

Virchow's gland SENTINEL NODE.

vitelline gland VITELLARIUM.

vulvovaginal gland An outmoded term for GLANDULA VESTIBULARIS MAJOR.

Waldeyer's glands Small sweat glands in the skin of the attached margin of the eyelid, especially the lower.

Wasmann's gland GLANDULA GASTRICA PROPRIA.

Weber's glands Lingual mucous glands situated in the posterior part of the tongue at its margins.

Wepfer's glands   GLANDULAE DUODENALES.

gland of Wertheimer   A gland that is stated to open on the inferior surface of the glans clitoridis. An outmoded term.

Willis gland   CORPUS ALBICANS.

gland of Wölfler   An accessory lobe of the thyroid gland which is situated above the arch of the aorta. It is commonly observed in dogs.

glands of Wolfring   GLANDULAE LACRIMALES ACCESSORIAE.

glands of Zeis   GLANDULAE SEBACEAE PALPEBRARUM.

Zuckerkandl's gland   An occasional accessory thyroid gland situated left of center on the front of the hyoid bone.

---

glandebala   An obsolete term for HIRCUS.

glanderous   Pertaining to or affected with glanders.

glanders   [Old French *glandres*, from L *glandulae* (pl. of *glandula*, dim. of *glans*, gen. *glandis*, chestnut, acorn, kernel fruit) swollen glands, esp. in the neck]   A serious, often fatal, infectious disease of horses, mules, and donkeys caused by *Pseudomonas mallei* and characterized by ulcerous nodules in the upper respiratory tract, lungs, and skin. When the lymphatic system is affected, with formation of nodules and abscesses (farcy buds), the disease is known as farcy. In the chronic form, large stellate scars in the mucosa of the nasal septum are characteristic. Formerly distributed worldwide, it has been eliminated or controlled in many countries, including the United States. Man and many other animals species are susceptible to infection. Human infection acquired from an infected animal or another human case, can be a chronic suppurative infection or acute, being localized and suppurative, pulmonary, or septicemic. The septicemic form is always fatal.

glandes   Plural of GLANS.

glandiform   Having the form or anatomic features of a gland. A seldom used term.

glandilemma   The outer covering or capsule of a gland, as the adrenal capsule. A rarely used term.

glandula

---

glandula   [L (dim. of *glans*, gen. *glandis*, any kernel fruit, an acorn, chestnut, date, walnut), any small kernel fruit, acorn, chestnut, date, walnut]   (*plural* glandulae) An organized group of epithelial cells, either tightly clustered or scattered, that produces a secretion or an excretion for discharge; gland. Either it may discharge directly onto a surface or via a duct (exocrine gland) or it may discharge into the blood and lymph streams (endocrine gland). The classification of glands is based either on structure or the nature and composition of the secretions. Also called *glandule*.

glandulae areolares   MONTGOMERY'S GLANDS.

glandulae areolares Montgomerii   MONTGOMERY'S GLANDS.

glandula arytenoidea   One of several laryngeal glands located in the triangular fovea of the arytenoid cartilage and around the cuneiform cartilage in the free edge of the aryepiglottic fold. Also called *arytenoid gland*.

glandula atrabiliaris   GLANDULA SUPRARENALIS.

glandula basilaris   PITUITARY GLAND.

glandulae bronchiales   [NA] Mixed mucoserous and mucous glands situated in the submucosa of the bronchi. Their ducts penetrate the more superficial layers to open on the surface of the mucous membrane. Also called *bronchial glands*.

glandulae buccales   [NA] Small mucous glands situated between the mucous membrane of the cheek and the buccinator muscle. Also called *buccal gland, genal glands, cheek glands, malar glands*.

glandula bulbourethralis   [NA] A small, rounded, lobulated gland situated on each side of the membranous urethra just superior to the perineal membrane and the bulb of the penis and surrounded by the sphincter urethrae. The lobules are invested with fibrous tissue and comprise acini of columnar epithelium. Its excretory duct pierces the perineal membrane and opens on the floor of the spongy part of the urethra. It is homologous to the greater vestibular gland in the female. Also called *bulbourethral gland, glandula bulbourethralis cowperi* (outmoded), *Cowper's gland, anteprostatic gland* (outmoded), *anteprostate, antiprostate, antiparastata* (outmoded), *bulbocavernous gland*.

glandula bulbourethralis cowperi   An outmoded term for GLANDULA BULBOURETHRALIS.

glandula cardiaca esophagi   Any of the small compound tubuloalveolar glands that are situated at the extremities of the esophagus. One group is at a level between the cricoid cartilage and the fifth tracheal cartilage and a lower group is near the cardiac orifice of the stomach. The glands are limited to the lamina propria mucosae, and their large ducts open on the tip of a papilla. They vary considerably or may be absent entirely. Also called *Cobelli's gland*.

glandula cardiaca gastrica   One of a small number of simple and compound tubular glands that are situated in a narrow ring-shaped area near the cardiac orifice of the stomach. Mucus-secreting cells are common, whereas zymogenic and oxyntic cells are scarce. They closely resemble the superficial mucosal glands in the esophagus adjacent to the cardiac orifice.

glandulae ceruminosae   CERUMINOUS GLANDS.

glandulae cervicales uteri   [NA] Extensively branched large glands situated in the mucosa of the cervical canal of the uterus and lined with a tall columnar epithelium that secretes a clear, alkaline mucus. Also called *cervical glands of uterus*.

glandulae ciliares conjunctivales   An outmoded term for GLANDULAE CILIARES PALPEBRARUM.

glandulae ciliares molli   An outmoded term for GLANDULAE CILIARES PALPEBRARUM.

glandulae ciliares palpebrarum   [NA] A number of large, modified sweat glands that form several rows near the free margin of each eyelid and open either into or near the follicles of the eyelashes. The nature of their secretion is uncertain. Also called *ciliary glands of conjunctiva* (outmoded), *ciliary glands, Moll's glands, glandulae ciliares conjunctivales* (outmoded), *glandulae ciliares molli* (outmoded).

glandulae circumanales   CIRCUMANAL GLANDS.

glandula clausa   Any of the endocrine glands; a ductless gland. A rarely used term.

glandulae conjunctivales   [NA] Groups of mucus-secreting goblet cells that are either scattered throughout the epithelium of the conjunctiva or are lining irregular invaginations of the epithelium, especially where it is reduced to two cell layers at the upper edge of the tarsus. Also called *conjunctival glands, Krause glands, glandulae mucosae conjunctivae krausei* (outmoded).

glandula cutis   CUTANEOUS GLAND.

glandulae duodenales   [NA] Mucous tubuloalveolar glands that are situated in the submucosa of the duodenum, most extensively in the superior part and diminishing in number towards the jejunum. Their excretory ducts pierce the muscularis mucosae and open into the intestinal glands. Also called *duodenal glands, Brunner's glands, glandulae duodenales brunneri* (outmoded), *Wepfer's glands, cryptae mucosae duodeni, mucous crypts of duodenum, mucous glands of duodenum*.

glandulae duodenales brunneri   An outmoded term for GLANDULAE DUODENALES.

glandulae endocrinae [NA] ENDOCRINE GLANDS.

glandula epiglottica One of several mucous glands located in little pits on both surfaces of the epiglottis. Also called *glandulae laryngeae anteriores.*

glandulae esophageae The glandula esophagea propria and glandula cardiaca esophagi considered together. Also called *esophageal glands.*

glandula esophagea propria One of the small compound glands with branched tubuloalveolar secretory portions that contain only mucous glands and are situated in the submucosa of the middle two thirds of the esophagus. Their long, dilated main ducts pierce the lamina muscularis mucosae to open on the mucosal surface. Also called *esophageal gland proper.*

glandula gastrica propria One of the main gastric glands that are situated in the mucosa of the body and fundus of the stomach and open into the bottom of the gastric pits. Some are compound racemose while others are simple tubular glands and they contain highly differentiated cells including chief or zymogenic cells, oxyntic or parietal cells, argentaffin cells, mucous neck cells and undifferentiated cells. Also called *gastric gland proper, fundic gland, fundus gland, Wasmann's gland, gastric follicle, oxyntic gland, acid gland, peptic gland.*

glandulae glomiformes GLOMIFORM GLANDS.

glandula gustatoria [NA] One of the specialized racemose serous or albuminous glands located in the muscle tissue of the tongue near the taste buds, the ducts of which open mostly into the sulci surrounding the vallate papillae. Also called *gustatory gland, Ebner's gland.*

glandulae hepaticae An outmoded term for GLANDULAE MUCOSAE BILIOSAE.

glandula incisiva A seldom present palatine mucous gland situated in the midline behind the upper incisors.

glandula intercarotica GLOMUS CAROTICUM.

glandulae intestinales [NA] Numerous tubular glands in the mucous membrane of the small and large intestine. They are simple tubular structures or crypts, set at right angles to the surface, that extend deeply through the thickness of the mucosa to the muscularis mucosae. In the small intestine they open by small round apertures between the bases of the villi, the epithelium of which continues into the glands and contains large zymogenic cells of Paneth at the bottom of the crypts. Scattered in their epithelium are argentaffin cells. In the large intestine their epithelium contains more goblet cells than are seen in the small intestine and there are no Paneth cells. Also called *intestinal glands, glands of Lieberkühn, crypts of Lieberkühn, Lieberkühn's follicles, intestinal follicles, Galeati's glands, cryptae mucosae* (outmoded).

glandulae labiales oris [NA] Small, rounded mucous glands, situated between the mucous membrane of the lips and the orbicularis oris muscle, the ducts of which open into the vestibule of the mouth. Also called *labial glands of mouth.*

glandulae lacrimales accessoriae [NA] Small tear-secreting glands that are situated near and in the conjunctival fornices, being more numerous in the upper eyelid than the lower. Also called *accessory lacrimal glands, Krause glands, glands of Wolfring, Ciaccio's glands.*

glandula lacrimalis [NA] The large tear-secreting gland that is situated in the anterolateral part of the orbital cavity above the lateral angle of the eye. There its fine excretory ducts open into the superior conjunctival fornix. Its anterior margin lies against the orbital septum. It is imperfectly divided into two unequal parts by the tendinous expansion of the levator palpebrae superioris muscle, namely the pars orbitalis and pars palpebralis. It is a compound tubuloalveolar gland comprising many small lobules. Also called *lacrimal gland.*

glandula lacrimalis inferior An outmoded term for PARS PALPEBRALIS GLANDULAE LACRIMALIS.

glandula lacrimalis superior An outmoded term for PARS ORBITALIS GLANDULAE LACRIMALIS.

glandulae laryngeae anteriores An outmoded term for GLANDULA EPIGLOTTICA.

glandulae laryngeae mediae Laryngeal glands grouped in the vestibular fold, the triangular fovea of the arytenoid cartilage, and the free edge of the aryepiglottic fold. An outmoded term.

glandulae laryngeae posteriores Laryngeal glands located in the mucous membrane over the transverse arytenoid muscle. An outmoded term.

glandulae laryngeales [NA] Mucous glands situated in the mucous membrane of the larynx, designated according to their location glandula epiglottica, glandula arytenoidea, glandula ventriculi laryngis, and glandula sacculi laryngis, as well as in the infraglottic cavity. They were formerly designated simply as anterior, middle, and posterior groups. Also called *laryngeal glands.*

glandulae linguales [NA] Mucous and serous glands located in the mucous membrane of the tongue. The mucous glands (glandula lingualis apicalis and glandula radicis linguae) are numerous in the posterior part but are also found along the margins and at the tip. The racemose serous glands are located near taste buds, their ducts opening into the sulci of the vallate papillae. Also called *lingual glands, lingual mucous glands, glands of tongue.*

glandula lingualis anterior [NA] One of a pair of mixed, though chiefly mucous, glands situated on the inferior surface of the apex of the tongue, on either side of the midline adjacent to the frenulum. They are covered by mucous membrane and by a few longitudinal muscle fibers. Their several small ducts open on the inferior surface between the anterior ends of the plicae fimbriatae. Also called *anterior lingual gland, anterior lingual gland of Blandin and Nuhn, apical gland of tongue, Bauhin's gland, Blandin's gland, Blandin and Nuhn gland, intramuscular gland of tongue* (outmoded), *Nuhn's gland.*

glandula mammaria [NA] The glandular element, or parenchyma, of the mamma, or breast, which undergoes growth and development after puberty in the female but remains rudimentary in the male. It is situated in the superficial fascia on each side of the front of the thorax, being separated from the ribs by the pectoral and thoracic muscles. It comprises about 15 to 20 lobes composed of lobules formed by acini and surrounded by areolar tissue, blood vessels, and lymphatics. The lobules are drained by ducts that join together so that each lobe has a single lactiferous duct opening on the surface of the nipple, or papilla. The lobes and ducts are distributed in a radial fashion around the nipple. The lobules and lobes are held together by connective tissue and surrounded by varying amounts of fat, giving the mamma its contour. The glandular structure varies with age, pregnancy, and lactation and secretes milk when functioning. Also called *mammary gland, lactiferous gland* (outmoded).

glandulae molares [NA] Several of the larger buccal glands situated external to the buccinator muscle and around the entrance of the parotid duct in the cheek. Their ducts pierce the buccinator and open into the oral cavity opposite the upper third molar tooth. Also called *molar glands, retromolar glands.*

glandula mucosa A unicellular or multicellular gland containing mucous or goblet cells that usually have small, dark nuclei flattened against the basal plasma membrane of the cell and a clear cytoplasm containing pale droplets of mucigen, a protein-polysaccharide complex. Mucigen leaves the cell to form mucin, the basic constituent of mucus. Also called *mucous gland, muciparous gland, cryptae mucosae.*

glandulae mucosae biliosae [NA] Numerous lobulated mucous glands situated in the mucous membrane of the neck of the gallbladder and groups of tubuloalveolar glands distributed throughout the mucosa of the larger bile ducts. Also called *glands of biliary mucosa, hepatic glands* (outmoded), *glandulae hepaticae* (outmoded).

glandulae mucosae conjunctivae krausei An outmoded term for GLANDULAE CONJUNCTIVALES.

glandulae mucosae tubae auditivae An outmoded term for GLANDULAE TUBARIAE.

glandulae mucosae ureteris Mucous glands of the ureter, rarely observed in humans but common in horses. An outmoded term.

glandulae nasales [NA] Groups of serous and mucous glands situated deep to the basal lamina of the respiratory epithelium of the nasal cavity. Also called *nasal glands, nasal mucous follicles* (outmoded).

glandula olfactoria One of the several branched tubuloalveolar glands deep to the olfactory epithelium of the nasal mucous membrane, on the surface of which their narrow, short ducts open. Also called *olfactory gland, Bowman's gland, Kölliker's gland.*

glandulae oris [NA] Glandulae salivariae majores and glandulae salivariae minores. Also called *glands of mouth.*

glandulae palatinae [NA] Numerous mucous glands situated between the periosteum and the mucous membrane of the posterior half of the bony palate and beneath and in the mucous membrane of both surfaces of the soft palate, especially on the inferior surface and around the uvula. Those on the superior surface are mixed glands. Also called *palatine glands, staphyline glands.*

glandulae parathyroideae PARATHYROID GLANDS.

glandula parotidea [NA] The largest of the main salivary glands, shaped like an inverted three-sided pyramid and situated below and anterior to the external acoustic meatus in the gap between the mandible and the sternocleidomastoid muscle. Superiorly it reaches the zygomatic arch and inferiorly extends beyond the angle of the mandible. It is divided into a pars superficialis and a pars profunda by the branches of the facial nerve, the superficial part extending forward over the masseter muscle and ending in the parotid duct, while the deep portion extends medially to the styloid process behind the mandible. Its investing capsule is derived from the deep cervical fascia. Within the substance of the gland are the external carotid artery and its terminal branches as well as the retromandibular vein and its tributaries and termination. Its lobules contain only serous alveoli. Also called *parotid gland, glandula parotis, parotid, external salivary gland* (outmoded), *parotis* (outmoded).

glandula parotidea accessoria [NA] The most anterior portion of the superficial part of the parotid gland, either fully or partially detached, situated between the zygomatic arch above and the parotid duct below. It is present in about 30 percent of individuals and its duct joins the parotid duct. Also called *accessory parotid gland, glandula parotis accessoria, admaxillary gland* (outmoded), *accessory part of parotid gland, masseteric part of parotid gland* (outmoded), *socia parotidis* (outmoded).

glandula parotis GLANDULA PAROTIDEA.

glandula parotis accessoria GLANDULA PAROTIDEA ACCESSORIA.

glandulae pelvis renalis Small, solid nests of epithelial cells that are situated in the epithelium of the renal pelvis and that resemble glands. No true glands are present. An outmoded term.

glandulae pharyngeae [NA] Mucous glands situated beneath the mucous membrane of the pharynx and especially numerous in the nasopharynx around the orifices of the auditory tubes. Also called *pharyngeal glands.*

glandula pituitaria PITUITARY GLAND.

glandulae preputiales [NA] A few modified sebaceous glands situated on the corona and the neck of the glans penis that secrete smegma. Also called *preputial glands, Littre's crypts,*

Littre's glands, Haller's crypts, glands of Haller, glands of Tyson, crypts of Tyson, odoriferous crypts of prepuce, odoriferous glands of prepuce, cryptae odoriferae, cryptae praeputiales.

glandula prostata An outmoded term for PROSTATA.

glandula prostata muliebris An outmoded term for GLANDULAE URETHRALES URETHRAE FEMININAE.

glandula prostatica An outmoded term for PROSTATA.

glandula pylorica One of the simple, branched tubular glands that are situated in the pyloric part of the stomach. Each comprises a few short convoluted tubules opening into the gastric pits which extend deep into the mucous membrane. The epithelial cells are mainly of the mucous type with some oxyntic cells. They may also produce gastrin. Also called *pyloric gland.*

glandula sacculi laryngis One of several laryngeal glands located in the saccule of the larynx.

glandulae salivariae majores [NA] The three pairs of main salivary glands, the ducts of which carry their secretions into the oral cavity to assist the process of digestion. They are the glandula parotidea, glandula sublingualis, and glandula submandibularis, compound racemose glands the lobules of which contain both mucous and serous alveoli, except for the parotid gland which only has serous alveoli. Also called *main salivary glands.*

glandulae salivariae minores [NA] Numerous small glands in the mucous membrane of the tongue, lips, cheeks and palate that produce either mucous or serous secretions or both so as to assist the process of digestion in the oral cavity. The groups include glandulae labiales, glandulae buccales, glandulae molares, glandulae palatinae, glandulae linguales and glandulae linguales anteriores. Also called *minor salivary glands, accessory salivary glands.*

glandulae sebaceae SEBACEOUS GLANDS.

glandulae sebaceae conjunctivales An outmoded term for GLANDULAE SEBACEAE PALPEBRARUM.

glandulae sebaceae labii majoris pudendalis Sebaceous glands situated on the medial, or inner, surface of each labium majus. An outmoded term.

glandulae sebaceae mammae MONTGOMERY'S GLANDS.

glandulae sebaceae palpebrarum [NA] Small sebaceous glands that are situated in the eyelids and open into the follicles of the eyelashes. In addition, they are also associated with the sparse, downy hairs on the skin of the eyelids. Also called *sebaceous glands of eyelids, glandulae sebaceae conjunctivales* (outmoded), *glands of Zeis, sebaceous glands of conjunctiva* (outmoded).

glandula seromucosa [NA] A mixed exocrine gland containing either mucous and serous secretory units or acini with both mucous and serous cells. In various glands one or other type of cell may predominate, affecting the constitution of the secretion produced. Also called *seromucous gland, mixed gland, heterocrine gland.*

glandula serosa SEROUS GLAND.

glandulae sine ductibus A seldom used term for ENDOCRINE GLANDS.

glandula sublingualis [NA] The smallest of the three main salivary glands situated in the floor of the mouth deep to the mucous membrane on each side of the lateral surface of the tongue, resting on the mylohyoid muscle and lying along the medial surface of the anterior part of the corpus mandibulae above the mylohyoid line. Its superior border elevates the mucous membrane to form the plica sublingualis, on the surface of which open individually up to 20 of the gland's excretory ducts. Also called *sublingual gland, Rivinus gland.*

glandula submandibularis [NA] One of the three main salivary glands, part of which is superficial to the posterior part of the mylohyoid muscle, and part deep to the muscle. It is ovoid in shape and variable in size, situated deep to the posterior part of the corpus mandibulae and extending downward into the digastric triangle of the neck. It is crossed superficially by the facial vein, while the facial artery grooves the posterosuperior part of the gland and then emerges between its lateral surface and the mandible. Its long excretory duct crosses the hyoglossus muscle and lingual nerve to open in the floor of the mouth, one on each side of the base of the frenulum of the tongue. Also called *submandibular gland, glandula submaxillaris* (outmoded), *submaxillary gland* (outmoded), *mandibular gland* (outmoded).

glandula submaxillaris   An outmoded term for GLANDULA SUBMANDIBULARIS.

glandulae sudoriferae   SWEAT GLANDS.

glandulae suprarenales accessoriae   [NA] Isolated, encapsulated nodules of either cortical tissue only (cortical bodies) or medullary and cortical tissue of the suprarenal gland. They may be located either in areolar tissue near the main gland and the celiac axis or in or near the kidney, along the ureter, in or near the ovaries, in the broad ligament of the uterus, in the spermatic cord, or in the caput epididymidis. Also called *accessory suprarenal glands, accessory adrenal capsules, accessory adrenal glands.*

glandula suprarenalis   A paired endocrine gland that is pyramidal in shape on the right and crescentic on the left, flattened anteroposteriorly, and situated on the anterosuperior aspect of each kidney. It is retroperitoneal, enclosed in the renal fascia, and composed of a mesodermal cortex and an ectodermal medulla. The embryologically fused cortex forms the greater part of the gland and comprises three layers, the zona glomerulosa, zona fasiculata, and zona reticularis, which contain no chromaffin tissue and secrete lipids. The cortex, essential to life, is regulated by two hormones. One, adenohypophysial adrenocorticotropin, maintains the glandular structure and stimulates the secretion of more than thirty C_{21} corticosteroids such as cortisol, adrenal androgens, progestins, and perhaps estrogens. The second, renin-angiotensin, controls aldosterone secretion. The medulla secretes epinephrine and norepinephrine. Its irregular chromaffin cells form either rounded masses or short cords surrounded by venules and blood capillaries. The medulla can be extirpated without lethality. Also called *adrenal gland, suprarenal gland, atrabiliary gland* (outmoded), *paranephros* (outmoded), *adrenal body, suprarenal body, adrenal capsule, suprarenal capsule, epinephros, renicapsule* (outmoded), *atrabiliary capsule, glandula atrabiliaris, suprarene* (outmoded).

glandulae tarsales   [NA] A row of about 30 modified sebaceous glands embedded transversely in a groove in the tarsus of each eyelid. They have lobulated terminal alveolar portions which are connected by short lateral branching ducts to long central excretory ducts. The long ducts are lined with stratified squamous epithelium and open on the inner free margins of the eyelids. Their oily secretion forms a barrier for the tears so that they do not overflow on to the cheeks. Also called *tarsal glands, meibomian glands, glandulae tarsales meibomi* (outmoded), *palpebral glands, palpebral follicles* (outmoded), *tarsoconjunctival glands* (outmoded).

glandulae tarsales meibomi   An outmoded term for GLANDULAE TARSALES.

glandula thyroidea   [NA] THYROID GLAND.

glandula thyroidea accessoria suprahyoidea   A small, isolated nodule of thyroid tissue occasionally located in the midline above the hyoid bone. Also called *suprahyoid accessory thyroid gland.*

glandulae thyroideae accessoriae   ACCESSORY THYROID GLANDS.

glandulae tracheales   Small tubuloacinous, mixed mucous glands situated mostly in the submucosa between the cartilaginous rings and on the posterior wall of the trachea. Their short ducts pierce the elastic fibers of the lamina propria to open on the inner surface of the trachea. Also called *tracheal glands.*

glandula trigoni vesicae   One of the glands in the mucous membrane near the internal urethral opening in the urinary bladder, considered by some authorities to be true mucous glands. Pathological enlargement may produce urinary obstruction. Also called *vesical gland, subtrigonal gland.*

glandulae tubariae   [NA] Mucous glands of the auditory tube that are located, associated with lymph nodules, in the loose, thick mucosa of the cartilaginous portion, particularly near the pharynx. Also called *mucous glands of auditory tube, mucous glands of eustachian tube, glandulae mucosae tubae auditivae.*

glandula tympanica   An outmoded term for TYMPANIC GLAND.

glandulae urethrales littrei   An outmoded term for GLANDULAE URETHRALES URETHRAE MASCULINAE.

glandulae urethrales urethrae femininae   [NA] A number of small mucous glands situated in the mucous membrane of the female urethra and opening separately on its surface. A group of glands on each side of the distal end of the urethra occasionally open into the paraurethral duct. Also called *urethral glands of female urethra, paraurethral glands, Skene's glands, Guerin's glands, cryptae urethrae muliebris, glandula prostata muliebris* (outmoded), *glandulae urethrales urethrae muliebris* (outmoded), *female prostate* (outmoded).

glandulae urethrales urethrae masculinae   [NA] Numerous small glands and follicles situated in the submucosa of the proximal two-thirds of the spongy part of the male urethra that open in the grooves between the longitudinal folds of the urethra. Also called *urethral glands of male urethra, Littre's glands, glandulae urethrales littrei* (outmoded), *crypts of Littre, Morgagni's glands.*

glandulae urethrales urethrae muliebris   An outmoded term for GLANDULAE URETHRALES URETHRAE FEMININAE.

glandula uropygialis   UROPYGIAL GLAND.

glandulae uterinae   [NA] Tubular glands found within the inner layer of the uterine wall. These glands undergo cyclical changes in the reproductive phase of life that constitute the menstrual cycle. Also called *uterine glands, endometrial glands, utricular glands.*

glandula ventriculi laryngis   One of several laryngeal glands located on the vestibular fold and in the ventricle of the larynx.

glandulae vesicales vesicae urinariae   An outmoded term for VESICAL GLANDS.

glandulae vestibulares minores   [NA] Numerous small mucous glands that open on the surface of the vestibule between the external urethral orifice and the vaginal orifice. Also called *lesser vestibular glands.*

glandula vestibularis major   [NA] A small, oval tubuloalveolar gland situated on each side of the vaginal orifice contiguous with and medial to the posterior end of the bulb of the vestibule, its duct opening between the labium minus and the vaginal orifice. It is homologous to the bulbourethral gland in the male. Also called *greater vestibular gland, Bartholin's gland, vulvovaginal gland* (outmoded), *Duverney's gland, Tiedemann's gland.*

---

glandulae   Plural of GLANDULA.

glandular   Of, resembling, or having the characteristics of a gland.

glandule   GLANDULA.

glandulous   Having many glandules. A rarely used term.

glans   [L, acorn]   An acorn-shaped, rounded body or mass of tissue, specifically the glans penis and glans clitoridis.

glans clitoridis   [NA] The small, rounded free end of the body of the clitoris, composed of erectile tissue and covered by a highly sensitive epithelium. Overhanging it superiorly is the prepuce and inferiorly the frenulum is attached to it. It is homologous to the glans penis in the male. Also called *glans of clitoris*.

glans of clitoris   GLANS CLITORIDIS.

glans penis   [NA] The conical expansion of the corpus spongiosum at the distal extremity of the penis. Its proximal end, or base, forms the corona glandis projecting over the distal ends of the corpora cavernosa, which are attached in its proximal concavity. The spongy urethra pierces it and opens on its distal end. The thin skin of the penis attaches around its neck and extends over it as a double fold forming the prepuce. Also called *head of penis, caput penis*.

Glanzmann   [Eduard *Glanzmann*, Swiss physician, 1887–1959] Glanzmann's thrombasthenia. See under GLANZMANN'S DISEASE.

glare   An irritating sensation accompanying visual perception of very bright light, either direct or reflected. It can sharply reduce perception of one's normal field of vision.

glarometer   A device used to quantitate the handicap produced by scattering of light within the ocular media.

Glasgow   [William Carr *Glasgow*, U.S. physician, 1845–1907] See under SIGN.

glass   [Old English *glæs*, akin to Old English *glær* amber and Old English *geolu* yellow]   A hard, brittle, usually transparent substance formed by fusing sand with various oxides. See also GLASSES.

cover glass   A thin disk or oblong of glass placed upon material to be examined microscopically. It is often used with a sealing material to provide permanent protection. Also called *coverslip*. Also *coverglass*.

crown glass   A type of glass used in the fabrication of optical lenses. It has a relatively low dispersion of light.

cupping glass   A glass vessel from which the air has been withdrawn and which is applied to the body to draw the blood to the surface.

flint glass   A type of glass used in the fabrication of optical lenses. It has a relatively high dispersion of light.

holvi glass   VITA GLASS.

lead glass   Transparent glass containing compounds of lead, used for viewing windows, etc., in radiation protection.

lithium glass   A lithium-containing glass used for x-ray tubes which produce photons of very low voltage, such as grenz ray tubes.

magnifying glass   A convex lens used to produce an image larger than the object being observed.

object glass   OBJECTIVE.

optical glass   Any type of fine quality glass with uniform refracting properties, suitable for the manufacture of lenses.

Pfund's gold-plated glass   A multiple-component filter that transmits only visible light. The gold plating reflects infrared rays.

protective glass   An impact-resistant type of glass fabricated in eyeglasses, masks, or shields intended to guard against injury.

quartz glass   A glass composed of the mineral, quartz, which has the property of transmitting ultraviolet rays.

safety glass   Any transparent optical material made resistant to breakage by heat treatment, lamination, plastic composition, or any other process, and therefore suitable for fabrication of protective, shatter-resistant materials.

soluble glass   A solution of potassium or sodium silicate which is applied to a dressing. As it dries it hardens and helps immobilize the wound. It has generally been replaced by newer methods. Also called *water glass*.

test glass   A small glass container, often tapering at the bottom, that is used in the examination of biologic fluids.

vita glass   Glass containing a high percentage of quartz and especially transparent to ultraviolet light. Also called *holvi glass, vitaglass*.

watch glass   A shallow concave glass vessel that is similar in shape and appearance to the crystal of a large pocket watch. It is used for evaporating small quantities of fluid or containing reagents whose interaction is to be viewed with the naked eye.

water glass   SOLUBLE GLASS.

Wood's glass   A nickel oxide filter glass used with ultraviolet light to remove the visible radiation so that any weak fluorescence may be seen. It is used to detect ringworm infection of the scalp. See also WOOD'S LIGHT.

glasses   Eyeglasses; optical spectacles.

bifocal glasses   Eyeglasses for the correction of presbyopia in which the left and right lenses are each divided into two separate segments with different focal distances, the upper portions for distant vision and the lower portions for near vision. Also called *bifocals*.

bloomed glasses   Lenses covered with an antireflective coating.

crutch glasses   Eyeglasses having a frame with an attached extension shaped to press upon the upper lid and hold it open as a corrective measure for ptosis.

franklinic glasses   [after Benjamin *Franklin*, American scientist and diplomat, 1706–1790]   Bifocal glasses in which the two segments of each lens are joined at a horizontal line. • The original invention of Benjamin Franklin was composed of separate lenses fastened together at their optical centers.

Frenzel glasses   A pair of shielded glasses fitted with +20 diopter biconvex lenses and enclosed with a source of illumination for use in the investigation of nystagmus and in caloric testing, so as to abolish optic fixation and facilitate observation of the subject's eyes.

half glasses   Spectacles for near vision purposes mounted low enough so the wearer may look above them for distance vision. The name is derived from their appearance as if only the bottom half of a spectacle frame is present. Also called *clerical spectacles, pulpit spectacles, pantoscopic spectacles*.

Hallauer's glasses   Absorptive glasses that do not transmit ultraviolet.

hyperbolic glasses   Lenses designed with an exaggerated anterior convexity.

pantoscopic glasses   HALF GLASSES.

safety glasses   Glasses designed to protect the eyes against impacts, projectiles, molten metal, chemical splash, dust, gases, and radiations.

snow glasses   Eyeglasses with protective lenses designed to shield the eyes against intense light reflected from the surface of snow. This may be accomplished by using absorptive filters or by a narrow slitlike aperture that mechanically excludes most of the incident light.

sun glasses   See under SUNGLASSES.

tinted glasses   Eyeglasses with protective lenses that transmit only selected spectral wavelengths of light.

toric glasses   Cylindrical lenses used to correct astigmatism.

trifocal glasses   Eyeglasses in which the left and right lenses are divided into three separate segments with different focal distances, the upper portions for seeing at infinity, the middle portions for seeing at arm's length, and the lower portions for near vision.

glasspox   1 An obsolete term for ALASTRIM.   2 An obsolete term for VARICELLA.

glassy   Having a semitransparent appearance, as the hyaline cartilage.

Glauber [Johann Rudolph *Glauber*, German chemist, 1604–1670] See under SALT.

glaucoma [Gk *glaukōma* (from *glauk(os)* gleaming, pale green, bluish green, gray, light-blue-eyed, gray-eyed + *-ōma*) opacity of the crystalline lens] An increase of intraocular pressure sufficient to damage the structure or function of the eye. Also called *choroiditis serosa, green cataract* (obsolete), *oculus caesius*. Adjective: glaucomatous.

absolute glaucoma The end stage of glaucoma in which the eye is completely blind. Also called *glaucoma absolutum, glaucoma consummatum*.

glaucoma absolutum ABSOLUTE GLAUCOMA.

acute congestive glaucoma Increased intraocular pressure to an angle-closure mechanism, as that of angle-closure glaucoma or narrow-angle glaucoma.

air-block glaucoma Increased intraocular pressure due to interference with aqueous flow caused by a bubble of gas within the anterior chamber.

angle-closure glaucoma Glaucoma due to obstruction of aqueous outflow by occlusion of the trabecular meshwork from mechanical contact with the peripheral iris.

angle-recession glaucoma A post-traumatic increase in intraocular pressure associated with a circumferential rupture of the portion of the ciliary body between the scleral spur and the iris base. Such an injury widens the angle of the anterior chamber.

aphakic glaucoma Increased intraocular pressure occurring in an eye without its crystalline lens.

apoplectic glaucoma Increased intraocular pressure associated with anterior chamber hemorrhage.

capsular glaucoma Increased intraocular pressure associated with exfoliation of the lens capsule.

chronic narrow-angle glaucoma Long-standing increased intraocular pressure associated with an abnormally small distance between the peripheral iris and cornea, usually resulting in adhesions between these two surfaces.

chronic simple glaucoma OPEN ANGLE GLAUCOMA.

closed-angle glaucoma Increased intraocular pressure due to obstruction of access to the trabecular meshwork from physical contact by the peripheral iris.

congenital glaucoma BUPHTHALMOS.

congestive glaucoma An increased intraocular pressure associated with obvious redness and edema of the eye. Also called *incompensated glaucoma*.

glaucoma consummatum ABSOLUTE GLAUCOMA.

Donders glaucoma Long-standing increased intraocular pressure with much visual loss.

enzyme glaucoma A transitory increased intraocular pressure following the use of alpha chymotrypsin for zonulysis in cataract extraction. The enzymatic digestants may occlude the trabecular meshwork for several weeks.

glaucoma fulminans A rapidly developing, severe, increased intraocular pressure.

hemorrhagic glaucoma Increased intraocular pressure associated with neovascularization of the iris and intraocular bleeding, usually due to diabetes or venous occlusion.

glaucoma imminens A status in which the onset of increased intraocular pressure is anticipated.

incompensated glaucoma CONGESTIVE GLAUCOMA.

infantile glaucoma BUPHTHALMOS.

inflammatory glaucoma Increased intraocular pressure due to angle obstruction by iridocyclitis or other infection.

inverse glaucoma Increased intraocular pressure due to pupil block mechanisms, as by a dislocated lens or vitreous. This is characterized by a paradoxical response to treatment in that miotics worsen and mydriatics benefit the condition.

iris block glaucoma Increased intraocular pressure due to occlusion of the trabecular meshwork by iris adhesions.

juvenile glaucoma Increased intraocular pressure occurring in young adult life due to developmental structural faults of the outflow mechanism.

lenticular glaucoma Increased intraocular pressure secondary to faulty lens position or to toxic or allergic responses of the cortex lentis.

malignant glaucoma Increased intraocular pressure resulting from a forward shift of the vitreous structure, which compresses the iris against the trabecular meshwork.

narrow-angle glaucoma Increased intraocular pressure resulting from forward displacement of the iris towards the cornea because of structural reasons in the anterior segment of the eye.

neovascular glaucoma Increased intraocular pressure caused by growth of connective tissue and new blood vessels upon the trabecular meshwork.

noncongestive glaucoma Increased intraocular pressure in an eye that appears uninflamed upon external inspection.

obstructive glaucoma Increased intraocular pressure caused by blocked access of the aqueous to the trabecular meshwork.

open-angle glaucoma Increased intraocular pressure due to an inherent loss of permeability of the trabecular meshwork itself. This is the commonest form of glaucoma. Also called *chronic simple glaucoma, simple glaucoma, glaucoma simplex*.

phakogenic glaucoma Increased intraocular pressure originating from a cellular response to lens protein.

phakolytic glaucoma Increased intraocular pressure caused by occlusion of the trabecular meshwork of macrophages entering the anterior chamber in response to the presence of liquefied lens cortex.

pigmentary glaucoma Increased intraocular pressure associated with a heavy deposit of melanin granules upon the trabecular meshwork.

postinflammatory glaucoma Increased intraocular pressure due to scarring of the angle of the anterior chamber subsequent to iridocyclitis or infection.

primary glaucoma Spontaneously occurring inherited glaucoma, the more common form of glaucoma, either open-angle or closed-angle.

pseudoexfoliative capsular glaucoma Increased intraocular pressure associated with the shedding of lens capsular material.

secondary glaucoma Increased intraocular pressure due to ocular disease rather than to an inherited tendency to glaucoma.

simple glaucoma OPEN-ANGLE GLAUCOMA.

glaucoma simplex OPEN-ANGLE GLAUCOMA.

traumatic glaucoma Increased intraocular pressure secondary to ocular injury.

vitreous-block glaucoma Increased intraocular pressure due to occlusion of the pupil by the vitreous humor, usually occurring in aphakic eyes.

wide-angle glaucoma Increased intraocular pressure due to inherent decrease in permeability of the trabecular meshwork itself, associated with a normally large distance between the peripheral cornea and iris.

glaucomatous Of or pertaining to glaucoma; associated with increased intraocular pressure.

glaucosis [Gk *glauko(s)* gleaming, pale green, bluish green, gray, light-blue-eyed, gray, gray-eyed + *-sis*] Blindness caused by increased intraocular pressure.

glaucosuria [Gk *glaukos* gleaming, pale green, bluish green, gray, light-blue-eyed, gray-eyed + *-URIA*] INDICANURIA.

GLC gas-liquid chromatography.

Glc Symbol for glucose.

GlcA **1** Symbol for glucuronic acid. **2** Symbol for gluconic acid.

GlcN   A symbol for glucosamine (systematically 2-amino-2-deoxyglucose).

GlcNAc   Symbol for *N*-acetylglucosamine.

GlcUA   Symbol for glucuronic acid.   • The preferred symbol is GlcA.

gleba [L, a clod or lump of earth, soil, a little ball]   The inner, spore-bearing portion of the fruiting body of Gasteromycetes.

gleet [Middle English *glet, glette* (from L *glittus* sticky) slime]   **1** Chronic gonococcal urethritis.   **2** The slight mucous discharge seen in the chronic stage of gonococcal urethritis.

vent gleet   CLOACITIS.

Glenn [William Wallace Lumpkin *Glenn*, U.S. cardiovascular surgeon, born 1914]   See under OPERATION.

glenohumeral   Pertaining to the glenoid cavity of the scapula and the humerus.

glenoid   Pertaining, belonging to, or resembling the glenoid cavity of the scapula.

Glenospora khartoumensis   An obsolete term for *MADURELLA MYCETOMI*.

glenosporosis [*Glenospor(a)* + -OSIS]   Any infectious condition caused by fungi earlier classified in the form-genus *Glenospora*. An obsolete term..

Gley [Emile *Gley*, French physiologist, 1857–1930]   **1** Gley cells. See under LEYDIG CELLS.   **2** Gley's glands. See under ACCESSORY THYROID GLANDS.

GLI   gastrointestinal glucagonlike immunoreactivity.

glia [Gk *glia*, also *gloia* glue]   NEUROGLIA.

ameboid glia   Microgliocytes displaying an ameboid form during degenerative processes.

cytoplasmic glia   Glial cells, usually astrocytes, containing abundant perikaryal cytoplasm.

glia of Fañanás   CELLS OF FAÑANÁS.

fibrillary glia   Astrocytes possessing numerous silver-impregnated fibrils consisting of bundles of microfilaments. They are often prominent in zones of neural degeneration in which astrocytic processes proliferate.

gliacyte [GLIA + -CYTE]   A neuroglial cell body. Also called *gliocyte, gliocytus.*

gliadin   A protein of wheat seeds, poor in lysine, which is an essential amino acid.

glial   Of or pertaining to neuroglia.

Glick [Paul Charles *Glick*, U.S. sociologist, born 1910]   See under EFFECT.

glide / mandibular glide   Lateral or protrusive movement of the mandible with teeth or other occluding surfaces in contact. Also called *gliding movement of the mandible.*

occlusal glide   An eccentric movement of the mandible during closure caused by a deflective occlusal contact.

gliding   The slow progress over a surface characteristic of myxobacteria.

glio- [Gk *glia* or *gloia* glue]   A combining form meaning (1) glue, gluelike; (2) gliomatous.

glioblast   SPONGIOBLAST.

glioblastoma [GLIO- + BLASTOMA]   A highly malignant brain tumor composed of glial tissue. It contains poorly differentiated cells and areas of necrosis, pseudopalisading, vascular endothelial proliferation, hemorrhage, and invasive growth. It usually occurs in the cerebral hemispheres of adults. Also called *gliocarcinoma, glioblastoma multiforme, spongioblastoma multiforme.*

giant cell glioblastoma   A glioblastoma with a predominance of bizarre, highly multinucleated giant cells. Also called *monstrocellular sarcoma, magnocellular glioblastoma.*

glioblastoma isomorphe   MEDULLOBLASTOMA.

magnocellular glioblastoma   GIANT CELL GLIOBLASTOMA.

glioblastoma multiforme   GLIOBLASTOMA.

gliocarcinoma [GLIO- + CARCINOMA]   GLIOBLASTOMA.

Gliocladium   A form-genus of fungi which are similar to and classified with *Aspergillus* and *Penicillium,* all of which produce metabolites which have an antibiotic effect.

gliocyte   GLIACYTE.

retinal gliocytes   MÜLLER'S FIBERS.

gliocytoma [GLIO- + CYTOMA]   GLIOMA.

gliocytus   GLIACYTE.

gliocytus radiatus   CELLS OF FAÑANÁS.

gliofibrilla   One of the cytoplasmic filaments within a glial cell. These filaments are primarily composed of glial fibrillary acid protein.

gliofibrillary   Pertaining to the silver-impregnated fibrils of neuroglial cells, consisting chiefly of microfilaments of astrocytic cytoplasmic processes.

gliofibrosarcoma [GLIO- + FIBROSARCOMA]   A glioblastoma with a fibrosarcomatous component.

gliogenous   Derived from or pertaining to glial cells. An obsolete term.

glioma [*gli(o)-* + -OMA]   A tumor of glial cells, such as astrocytoma, glioblastoma, or oligodendroglioma. Also called *gliocytoma, neurogliocytoma, neuroglioma, neurospongioma.* Adjective: gliomatous.

ameboid glioma   A glioma showing hyaline and fatty degeneration. An outmoded term.

astrocytic glioma   ASTROCYTOMA.

glioma endophytum   A glioma of the inner part of the retina. It may enter into the vitreous space.

ependymal glioma   EPENDYMOMA.

glioma exophytum   A glioma of the outer part of the retina. It may enter into the choroid.

extramedullary glioma   HETEROTOPIC GLIOMA.

ganglionic glioma   GANGLIOGLIOMA.

heterotopic glioma   A glioma formed outside the central nervous system. Also called *extramedullary glioma.*

malignant peripheral glioma   MALIGNANT SCHWANNOMA.

mixed glioma   A glioma with more than one cell type. Most commonly it is an oligoastrocytoma.

nasal glioma   An incorrect term for NASAL GLIAL HETEROTOPIA.

optic glioma   A glioma arising from the optic nerve.

perineural glioma   An outmoded term for NEURILEMMOMA.

peripheral glioma   An outmoded term for NEURILEMMOMA.

glioma retinae   A glioma arising from the retina.

glioma sarcomatoides   An obsolete term for MEDULLOBLASTOMA.

glioma sarcomatosum   A glioblastoma with a sarcomatous component.

telangiectatic glioma   A glioma rich in dilated blood vessels. An obsolete term.

gliomatosis [*gliomat(a)*, pl. of GLIOMA + -OSIS]   Diffuse gliomatous change.

gliomatosis cerebri   A rare disease in which there is diffuse involvement of the cerebral hemispheres by neoplastic glial cells. Also called *astrocytomatosis cerebri, oligodendrogliomatosis cerebri.*

meningeal gliomatosis   Glioma spreading diffusely throughout the meninges.

gliomatous [*gliomat(a)*, pl. of GLIOMA, + -OUS]   Characteristic of a glioma.

gliomyoma [GLIO- + MYOMA]   A tumor containing glial tissue and muscle.

glioneuroma [GLIO- + NEUROMA]   GANGLIOGLIOMA.

gliophagia [GLIO- + -PHAGIA] The condition in which neuroglial cells are phagocytosed by other cells.

gliopil [GLIO- + Gk *pil(os)* wool or hair wrought into felt] The matrix of glial cell processes, consisting principally of astrocytes.

gliosa [prob. neut. pl. of Gk *gloios* slippery, thick, gummy] The densely packed small cells lying on the apex of the dorsal horn and surrounding the central canal of the spinal cord. An obsolete and rarely used term.

gliosarcoma [GLIO- + SARCOMA] **1** A malignant glioma. **2** A mixed glioblastoma and sarcoma.

gliosis [GLIO- + -SIS] Proliferation of astrocytes in response to disease or injury. It is one means of scar formation in the central nervous system. Also called *astrogliosis*.

aqueductal gliosis Gliosis in or around the cerebral aqueduct, often narrowing its lumen.

basilar gliosis Gliosis in the brainstem and in basal areas of the brain roughly corresponding to the vascular territory of the basilar artery.

diffuse gliosis Gliosis occurring diffusely throughout the central nervous system.

hemispheric gliosis Gliosis limited to one cerebral hemisphere. Also called *unilateral gliosis*.

heteromorphous gliosis Gliosis giving rise to an irregular meshwork of interlacing glial fibers.

hypertrophic nodular gliosis Severe diffuse but patchy gliosis producing general as well as nodular enlargement of the cerebral hemispheres. This condition is seen particularly in tuberous sclerosis.

isomorphic gliosis Gliosis characterized by orderly arrangement of reactive glial fibers. An obsolete term.

lobar gliosis Gliosis limited to one lobe of the cerebrum or cerebellum.

perivascular gliosis Gliosis around blood vessels.

progressive subcortical gliosis BINSWANGER'S DISEASE.

spinal gliosis Gliosis in the spinal cord.

unilateral gliosis HEMISPHERIC GLIOSIS.

gliosome [GLIO- + Gk *sōma* body] A cytoplasmic organelle or inclusion seen in neuroglial cells by light microscopy. They are probably mostly mitochondria but may also include liposomes and lysosomes.

gliotic Composed of connective tissue.

gliotoxin $C_{13}H_{14}N_2O_4S_2$. A cytotoxic substance produced by certain fungi of the genus *Gliocladium*.

Gliricola A genus of chewing lice (order Mallophaga, suborder Amblycera, family Gyropidae), parasitic on mammals, chiefly rodents, in Central and South America.

Gliricola porcelli A species infesting guinea pigs, commonly found on laboratory animals and on their handlers.

glischroidia [Gk *glischr(os)* gluey, viscid, importunate + -OID + -IA] An obsolete term for EPILEPTIC CHARACTER.

glischruria [*glischr(in)* + -URIA] The presence of glischrin in the urine.

Glisson [Francis *Glisson*, English anatomist, physiologist, and pathologist, 1597–1677] **1** See under CIRRHOSIS, SLING. **2** Glisson's capsule. See under CAPSULA FIBROSA PERIVASCULARIS. **3** Glisson's capsule. See under TUNICA FIBROSA HEPATIS. **4** Glissons's disease. See under RICKETS.

glissonitis PERIHEPATITIS.

Gln Symbol for glutamine.

global **1** Of or relating to a globe, as the eye. **2** Of or involving the entire world. **3** Considered in its entirety; with attention to the broadest view of the situation.

globate GLOBOSE.

globe [L *globus*. See GLOBUS.] A spherical mass, as the eye; globus.

globefish PUFFER.

globi Plural of GLOBUS.

globidiosis BESNOITIASIS.

Globidium [New L, from L *globus* ball, globe, sphere + -IDIUM] *BESNOITIA*.

globin [*glob(us)* + -IN] The protein of hemoglobin after removal of heme.

Globocephalus A genus of hookworms of the family Ancylostomatidae, subfamily Uncinariinae, with about five species, chiefly found in pigs, and characterized by a globular buccal capsule with heavy walls and subventral lancets deep within the capsule.

Globocephalus macaci See under *TERNIDENS*.

Globocephalus urosubulatus A widespread species of hookworm common in the small intestine of domestic and wild pigs. It lacks internal and external leaf-crowns and has a well-developed buccal capsule with paired subventral teeth or lancets.

globoid Having a shape similar to that of a sphere.

globomyeloma [L *glob(us)* ball, sphere, globe + *o* + MYELOMA] A sarcoma composed of undifferentiated round cells. An obsolete term.

globose Having the shape of a globe; globular. Also *globate*.

globoside A compound, usually a glycosphingolipid, containing Gal(α1-4)Gal(β1-4)Glc(globotriaose) or GalNAc(β1-3)Gal(α1-4)Gal(β1-4)Glc(globotetraose) as its oligosaccharide.

globular **1** Characterized by a spherical shape. **2** Consisting of globules.

globule [French (from L *globulus*, dim. of *globus* a ball, sphere), a very small spherical body] **1** Any small spheroidal particle. Also called *globulus*. **2** A French term, sometimes used in English, for ERYTHROCYTE.

dentin globules Small spherical bodies of mineralized matrix seen in regions of dentin in which mineralization is incomplete.

Marchi's globule An obsolete term for MARCHI'S BALL.

milk globules In milk, the small round particles of fat that separate out as cream.

Morgagni's globules Fluid droplets within a cataractous lens.

globuli Plural of GLOBULUS.

globulicidal Causing destruction of erythrocytes; hemolytic.

globulicide Any substance that damages erythrocytes and causes their destruction. A rarely used term.

globuliferous [GLOBUL(E) + *i* + -FEROUS] Having the property of taking up erythrocytes.

globulin [*globul(e)* + -IN] A category of protein, comprising those that are soluble in dilute salt solutions and are precipitated by half saturation with ammonium sulfate, in distinction from the albumins, which require complete saturation to precipitate them. Typical globulins were once considered to be insoluble in water in the absence of salt, but the globulins have since been subdivided into the euglobulins, which possess this property, and the pseudoglobulins, which dissolve even in the absence of salt.

accelerator globulin FACTOR V. Abbreviation: AcG

alpha globulin Any of the globulins of plasma which have the greatest electrophoretic mobility of the globulins in neutral or alkaline solutions.

antihemophilic globulin The original term for FACTOR VIII. Abbreviation: AHG

antihuman globulin An antibody directed against human globulin: usually applied to the antibodies against human immunoglobulins used to detect incomplete antibodies to erythrocytes by the antiglobulin (Coombs) test.

antilymphocyte globulin An antibody directed against lymphocyte surface antigens. Such antibodies are produced by immunization of experimental animals with heterologous lymphocytes and are used as immunosuppressive agents, for example in organ transplantation. Antilymphocyte antibodies may also occur spontaneously in the presence of disease states such as systemic lupus erythematosus. Abbreviation: ALG

Bence Jones globulin BENCE JONES PROTEIN.

beta globulin Any of the globulins of blood plasma characterized by electrophoretic mobility intermediate between those of alpha (fast) and gamma (slow).

beta-1A globulin Immunoelectrophoretic designation of the major C3 conversion product found in serum after complement activation. It corresponds to the fragment properly called iC3b, but has also been used as an alternative name for the later C3 breakdown product C3c, which is difficult to distinguish from iC3b on immunoelectrophoresis. Native C3 (immunoelectrophoretic designation η1C globulin) has a slower mobility.

beta-2A globulin An obsolete term for IMMUNOGLOBULIN A.

beta-1C globulin An obsolete term for C3.

beta-1E globulin An obsolete term for C4.

beta-1F globulin An obsolete term for C5.

beta-2M globulin An obsolete term for IMMUNOGLOBULIN M.

corticosteroid-binding globulin An alpha globulin that binds and transports biologically active, unconjugated cortisol in plasma. Also called *transcortin, corticosteroid-binding protein.*

D antigen immune globulin The globulin fraction of human serum directed against the D antigens of the rhesus blood group system. It is now given within 36 hours of the birth of an Rh+ child to an Rh− mother to prevent isoimmunization of the mother.

gamma globulin **1** A group of plasma proteins characterized by very slow electrophorectic mobility in alkaline buffers. Most antibodies are gamma globulins and gamma globulins are thus usually identified with immunoglobulins. **2** IMMUNOGLOBULIN.

gamma-A globulin An obsolete term for IMMUNOGLOBULIN A.

gamma-D globulin An obsolete term for IMMUNOGLOBULIN D.

gamma-E globulin An obsolete term for IMMUNOGLOBULIN E.

gamma-G globulin An obsolete term for IMMUNOGLOBULIN G.

gamma-M globulin An obsolete term for IMMUNOGLOBULIN M.

human gamma globulin **1** The fraction of human serum that migrates most anodically on electrophoresis. **2** IMMUNOGLOBULIN G.

human immune serum globulin The globulin fraction of human serum which contains specific antibodies against various pathogenic agents.

human rabies immune globulin A preparation of human immunoglobulin based on pooled plasma from individuals who had been recently vaccinated against rabies. It is used with rabies vaccine for protection in people bitten by rabid animals or those who have been in contact with saliva from an animal suspected of being rabid.

human tetanus immune globulin An antibody fraction isolated from human serum with high specific tetanus antibody activity. It is usually obtained following deliberate immunization with tetanus toxoid.

immune globulin IMMUNOGLOBULIN.

immune serum globulin Immunoglobulin that is either from or contained in antiserum, usually with specificity for certain microorganisms or viruses.

measles immune globulin A sterile preparation from pooled human plasma of people convalescent from or immunized against measles, which contains 90% gamma globulin and 10–18 g of protein per 100 ml. It is used to prevent or modify measles in susceptible people previously exposed to a measles infection, within 6 days of that exposure.

pertussis immune globulin A sterile preparation of immunoglobulins of pooled plasma from adult human donors who previously were immunized with pertussis vaccine. It contains glycine as a stabilizing agent and some suitable preservative. It is used to confer passive protection against whooping cough to individuals exposed to that disease.

poliomyelitis immune globulin A sterile globulin solution prepared from the blood plasma of normal adult humans who have been immunized against or have recovered from poliomyelitis.

rh$_o$(D) immune globulin A sterile globulin solution prepared from human blood plasma containing immunoglobulins to the erythrocyte factor Rh$_o$(D). Intramuscular injection is used to prevent production of Rh$_o$(D) antibodies in Rh$_o$(D)-negative mothers following birth or miscarriage of an Rh$_o$(D)-positive baby or fetus, avoiding erythroblastosis fetalis in a subsequent pregnancy if the child is Rh$_o$(D)-positive.

serum globulin Any globulin in blood serum. Such proteins are divided into α, β, and γ according to their electrophoretic mobility. The γ-globulins (gamma globulins) include immunoglobulin antibodies.

T globulin A large immunoglobulin band seen in the electrophoresis of horse serum following hyperimmunization. It is postulated to be a subclass of IgG.

tetanus immune globulin A sterile gamma globulin solution used in the prophylaxis and treatment of tetanus. It is prepared from the blood plasma of normal adult human subjects who have been immunized with tetanus toxoid.

thyroid-binding globulin An imprecise term for THYROXINE-BINDING GLOBULIN.

thyroxine-binding globulin A serum globulin having a mass of about 60 000 daltons, moving electrophoretically between α_1- and α_2-globulin, which at one major binding site binds thyroxine and, less readily, triiodothyronine and acts as their carrier protein in the circulation. Serum concentration of the globulin is raised during pregnancy and estrogen administration, lowered when testosterone is given, and is deficient in one or more genetic disorders. Also called *thyroid-binding globulin* (imprecise). Abbreviation: TBG

vitamin D-binding globulin A protein synthesized in the liver, migrating in the $\alpha2$ globulin band on electrophoresis. It binds both natural D vitamins and the metabolically active hydroxylated forms. Several phenotypic variants can be identified, but no association has been found between protein variants and pathophysiologic conditions. Levels decline in severe hepatocellular diseases. Also called *Gc protein.*

globulinuria [GLOBULIN + -URIA] **1** The excretion of serum globulins in the urine, an indication of nonselective proteinuria resulting from severe glomerular damage. **2** The excretion of Bence-Jones protein in urine.

globulolysis HEMOLYSIS.

globulolytic HEMOLYTIC.

globulomaxillary Pertaining to the globular and maxillary processes of the developing embryonic face.

globulus GLOBULE.

globuli ossei A rounded area of bone tissue found within the lacunae of calcified cartilage.

globulysis HEMOLYSIS.

globus [L, ball, sphere, globe] (*plural* globi) **1** A spherical mass. **2** A lump or swelling. **3** In leprology, a macrophage swollen by its content of leprosy bacilli, as seen in lepromatous leprosy.

globus abdominalis A subjective sensation as if there were a lump in the abdomen.

globus of the heel The posterior part of the equine hoof, where the wall curves forward to form the bar.

globus hystericus The sensation of a lump in the throat that is not due to organic pathology. It may appear as the single symptom of conversion hysteria, or it may constitute a significant part of an anxiety disorder or of anorexia nervosa. Also called *anchone* (obsolete), *dysphagia globus, apopnixis* (obsolete).

globus major epididymidis An outmoded term for CAPUT EPIDIDYMIDIS.

globus minor epididymidis An outmoded term for CAUDA EPIDIDYMIDIS.

globus pallidus [NA] The smaller, medial portion of the lentiform nucleus, which is divided by the lamina medullaris medialis into a lateral or external part and a medial or internal part. The globus pallidus is separated from the more laterally located putamen by the lamina medullaris lateralis. Afferent fibers reach the globus pallidus from the putamen, subthalamic nucleus, substantia nigra, thalamus, and cerebral cortex, while efferent fibers from the globus pallidus course to the nucleus ventralis anterior of the thalamus and the subthalamic nucleus in the diencephalon, the substantia nigra and red nucleus in the midbrain, and the reticular formation and inferior olivary nucleus in the lower brain stem. Also called *pallidus, pallidum, paleostriatum*. Adjective: pallidal, paleostriatal.

Gloger [Constantine Wilhelm Lambert *Gloger*, German zoologist and ornithologist, 1803–1863] See under RULE.

glomangioma [*glom(us)* + ANGIOMA] GLOMUS TUMOR.

glomangiosis The occurrence of multiple arteriovenular anastomoses in a tissue or organ.

    pulmonary glomangiosis Arteriovenular anastomoses occurring in severe pulmonary hypertension.

glome GLOMUS.

glomectomy [*glom(us)* + -ECTOMY] Excision of a glomus, especially the glomus caroticum.

glomer A British term for COMPOUND GLAND.

glomera Plural of GLOMUS.

glomerular Of or relating to the glomerulus.

glomeruli Plural of GLOMERULUS.

glomerulitis [*glomerul(us)* + -ITIS] Inflammation of renal glomeruli with endothelial cell proliferation and often with infiltration by leukocytes. It may occur in a variety of diseases. • *Glomerulitis* usually denotes a relatively mild inflammation of the glomeruli, but is a nonspecific term.

    focal glomerulitis Glomerulitis involving only some glomeruli, usually less than half the glomeruli.

    segmental glomerulitis Glomerulitis involving only a single tuft or portion of a tuft rather than the entire glomerulus, typically seen in lupus erythematosus.

glomerulography [*glomerul(us)* + *o* + -GRAPHY] Radiographic visualization of the glomeruli of the kidney during magnification-selective renal angiography.

glomerulonephritis [*glomerul(e)* + *o* + NEPHRITIS] Any glomerular disease characterized by acute, subacute, or chronic inflammation. Also called *glomerular nephritis*. • This term has been inappropriately used at times to designate noninflammatory lesions, as in *membranous glomerulonephritis*.

    acute glomerulonephritis ACUTE DIFFUSE GLOMERULONEPHRITIS.

    acute benign hemorrhagic glomerulonephritis A syndrome of transient hematuria and proteinuria following any type of infection, rarely accompanied by hypertension, edema, or more than mild renal functional impairment. This syndrome also may represent mild poststreptococcal acute glomerulonephritis. Re-

nal biopsy may reveal the underlying lesion to be a mild, diffuse, acute, proliferative glomerulonephritis or focal glomerulitis. When the syndrome is recurrent, it usually is associated with mesangial IgG/IgA glomerulonephritis.

    acute diffuse glomerulonephritis An acute inflammatory process involving glomeruli, characterized by endothelial and mesangial proliferation, and often leukocytic infiltration. Deposition of soluble antigen-antibody complexes is the most common pathogenesis, especially after pharyngeal or skin infections due to nephritogenic strains of group A hemolytic streptococci, bacterial endocarditis, and other infections. Acute glomerulonephritis also may follow minor infections, or be associated with systemic diseases such as Henoch-Schönlein purpura, systemic lupus erythematosus, the Goodpasture syndrome, and periarteritis nodosa. Clinically the disease may be characterized by the acute nephritic syndrome, or may be so mild that it can be detected only by serial urinalysis. Also called *acute Bright's disease, acute nephritis, acute glomerulonephritis, acute hemorrhagic nephritis, Ellis type 1 glomerulonephritis* (outmoded).

    acute nonpoststreptococcal glomerulonephritis A form of acute benign hemorrhagic glomerulonephritis, not caused by group A hemolytic streptoccal infection. It sometimes occurs in epidemics and is presumably of viral etiology. Complete recovery is the rule.

    acute poststreptococcal glomerulonephritis POSTSTREPTOCOCCAL ACUTE GLOMERULONEPHRITIS.

    antiglomerular basement membrane antibody glomerulonephritis GOODPASTURE SYNDROME.

    autoimmune glomerulonephritis An experimental glomerular disease, produced in sheep by injection of a glomerular basement membrane preparation plus Freund's adjuvant, and presumably due to autoantibodies against the glomerular basement membrane. Also called *Steblay nephritis*.

    chronic glomerulonephritis Any chronic renal disease of glomerular origin. A few instances follow acute glomerulonephritis that fails to heal, but most begin with asymptomatic proteinuria, the nephrotic syndrome, hypertension, slowly developing chronic renal failure, or uremic symptoms. Even if an accurate pathologic diagnosis is established by renal biopsy, the etiology rarely is known. Also called *Ellis type 2 glomerulonephritis* (outmoded).

    circulating immune-complex glomerulonephritis Any of a group of glomerular diseases characterized by deposition of circulating antigen-antibody complexes along the glomerular capillary basement membrane in an irregular, granular pattern as revealed by immunofluorescent microscopy and by electron microscopy. The glomerular lesions may be proliferative, exudative, or both. Circulating immune-complex glomerulonephritis includes glomerulonephritis associated with group A hemolytic streptococcal infections, subacute bacterial endocarditis, malaria, lupus erythematosus, periarteritis, and other conditions. Also called *immune-complex glomerulonephritis*.

    congenital chronic glomerulonephritis CONGENITAL GLOMERULOSCLEROSIS.

    crescentic glomerulonephritis EXTRACAPILLARY GLOMERULONEPHRITIS.

    diffuse lupus glomerulonephritis A renal complication of systemic lupus erythematosus in which all glomeruli are involved, with proliferative or membranous changes. See also DIFFUSE PROLIFERATIVE GLOMERULONEPHRITIS.

    diffuse proliferative glomerulonephritis A form of glomerulonephritis that may occur during the course of systemic lupus erythematosus, characterized by proteinuria, hematuria, cylinduria, and renal functional impairment.

    Ellis type 1 glomerulonephritis An outmoded term for ACUTE DIFFUSE GLOMERULONEPHRITIS.

    Ellis type 2 glomerulonephritis An outmoded term for

CHRONIC GLOMERULONEPHRITIS.

embolic glomerulonephritis FOCAL EMBOLIC GLOMERULO-NEPHRITIS.

endocapillary acute proliferative glomerulonephritis A form of acute glomerulonephritis characterized by proliferation of glomerular endothelial cells. It is a common form of poststreptococcal acute glomerulonephritis.

extracapillary glomerulonephritis Extracapillary proliferation of epithelial cells (crescents) lining Bowman's space. Crescents may occur in a variety of glomerular diseases including poststreptococcal acute glomerulonephritis and idiopathic rapidly progressive glomerulonephritis, or may occur as part of systemic disorders such as the Goodpasture syndrome, glomerulonephritis associated with bacterial endocarditis, polyarteritis, Henoch-Schönlein purpura, systemic lupus erythematosus, and essential mixed cryoglobulinemia. Involvement of more than 50 percent of the glomeruli is usually associated with the clinical syndrome of rapidly progressive glomerulonephritis. Also called *crescentic glomerulonephritis, glomerulocapsular nephritis* (rarely used), *capsular nephritis* (rarely used), *extracapillary acute proliferative glomerulonephritis.*

extracapillary acute proliferative glomerulonephritis EXTRACAPILLARY GLOMERULONEPHRITIS.

focal glomerulonephritis Proliferation in some but not all glomeruli. Leukocytes, fibrin, and necrosis also may be present in the lesions. Such lesions occur in systemic diseases such as polyarteritis, systemic lupus erythematosus, subacute bacterial endocarditis, and Schönlein-Henoch purpura. Other cases are associated with recurrent hematuria, asymptomatic proteinuria, or the nephrotic syndrome.

focal embolic glomerulonephritis A condition characterized by proliferative, focal, and sometimes necrotizing glomerular lesions, usually associated with subacute bacterial endocarditis due to a variety of organisms but especially to *Streptococcus viridans* or staphylococci. Also called *focal proliferative glomerulonephritis, embolic nonsuppurative focal nephritis (original term), embolic nephritis, embolic glomerulonephritis, focal embolic nephritis, Löhlein's nephritis.*

focal necrotizing glomerulonephritis Necrosis of some or parts of some glomeruli, as evidenced by nuclear fragmentation and debris. Total necrosis of glomeruli results form occlusion of their blood supply.

focal proliferative glomerulonephritis FOCAL EMBOLIC GLOMERULONEPHRITIS.

focal sclerosing glomerulonephritis FOCAL GLOMERULOSCLEROSIS.

hypocomplementemic glomerulonephritis MEMBRANOPROLIFERATIVE GLOMERULONEPHRITIS.

immune-complex glomerulonephritis CIRCULATING IMMUNE-COMPLEX GLOMERULONEPHRITIS.

lobular glomerulonephritis A prominence of glomerular lobules, often associated with hyaline. This histologic feature may be associated with several different clinical states, including the nephrotic syndrome. Also called *glomerular lobulation.* • This is a nonspecific pathologic term which may be applied to lesions of chronic proliferative glomerulonephritis and rapidly progressive glomerulonephritis of various etiologies.

malignant glomerulonephritis RAPIDLY PROGRESSIVE GLOMERULONEPHRITIS.

membranoproliferative glomerulonephritis A form of chronic glomerulonephritis characterized by mesangial cell proliferation, increased mesangial matrix, and thickened glomerular capillary walls. The thickened capillary wall results from interposition of mesangial matrix and cell cytoplasm between the glomerular basement membrane and the endothelium. Two types of membranoproliferative glomerulonephritis are distinguished by electron microscopy. Type 1 is characterized by electron-dense deposits between the endothelium and the glomerular basement membrane, and type 2 by very electron-dense deposits within the basement membrane. By immunofluorescent technique C3, properdin, and to a lesser extent C3 activator are distributed as granular deposits along the capillary wall. IgG and IgM are present in approximately half the cases. The disease, which may occur at any age, is often associated with the nephrotic syndrome and is accompanied by slowly progressive renal failure over five to ten years. Spontaneous remissions sometimes occur. Type 2 is sometimes associated with partial lipodystrophy. Also called *mesangiocapillary glomerulonephritis, dense deposit disease, hypocomplementemic glomerulonephritis.*

membranous glomerulonephritis A disease characterized by heavy proteinuria and often by the nephrotic syndrome. Progressive renal failure is usual, but spontaneous remissions may occur in approximately 20 percent of the cases. Histologically, diffuse membranous lesions are characterized by protein deposits initially on the epithelial side of the glomerular capillary membrane. Basement membrane material subsequently separates the deposits, forming spikes and thickening of the membrane. The deposits contain gamma globulin and complement (C_3) in a granular distribution. Also called *membranous glomerulopathy, membranous nephropathy.*

mesangial IgA/IgG glomerulonephritis A glomerulonephritis characterized by diffuse enlargement and hypercellularity of the mesangial regions which on immunofluorescent stain contain large amounts of IgA and some IgG in most instances. Clinical features include recurrent hematuria, usually associated with respiratory infections, and persistent proteinuria only rarely great enough to result in the nephrotic syndrome. Renal failure may develop after several years and is slowly progressive. Also called *Berger's disease, mesangial IgA/IgG disease, mesangial IgA/IgG nephropathy, mesangial nephropathy, mesangial proliferative glomerulonephritis.*

mesangial proliferative glomerulonephritis MESANGIAL IGA/IGG GLOMERULONEPHRITIS.

mesangiocapillary glomerulonephritis MEMBRANOPROLIFERATIVE GLOMERULONEPHRITIS.

minimal lesion glomerulonephritis LIPOID NEPHROSIS.

nodular glomerulonephritis DIABETIC GLOMERULOSCLEROSIS.

postinfectious acute glomerulonephritis Acute glomerulonephritis following an infection. Some instances may represent a nonspecific response to infection characterized by a focal glomerulitis and asymptomatic urine abnormalities, while others may be related to circulating immune complexes as in poststreptococcal acute glomerulonephritis.

poststreptococcal acute glomerulonephritis A disorder, most common in childhood, characterized by sudden onset of proteinuria, hematuria, and cylindruria, often associated with hypertension, renal function impairment, and circulatory congestion in varying combinations. It begins 5 to 28 days after infection with a nephritogenic strain of group A hemolytic streptococci. The severity may vary from asymptomatic urine abnormalities to acute oliguric renal failure. The healing rate is high, especially in children. However, chronic glomerulonephritis follows some severe instances, usually in adults. The glomeruli are diffusely involved with endothelial cell proliferation and infiltration with polymorphonuclear leukocytes. In severe instances crescents and adhesions between the glomerular tufts and Bowman's capsule are present. By immunofluorescent techniques, IgG, complement (usually C3, sometimes C4), and properdin are deposited in a granular pattern along the epithelial side of the glomerular basement membrane. By electron microscopy characteristic electron-dense "humps" are observed up to six weeks after onset along the epithelial side of the glomerular capillary basement membrane. The latent period, glomerular deposits, and the presence of serum cryoglobulins and reduced serum complement suggest that the disorder is associated with circulating immune complexes. Also called *acute poststreptoccal glomerulonephritis, poststreptococcal nephritis.*

proliferative glomerulonephritis Any lesion characterized by proliferation of glomerular, epithelial, endothelial, or mesangial cells.

rapidly progressive glomerulonephritis A serious form of glomerulonephritis, characterized histologically by diffuse extracapillary proliferation with crescent formation, and clinically by rapidly progressive renal insufficiency, which leads to end-stage renal disease in weeks or months. The syndrome can be associated with poststreptococcal acute glomerulonephritis, mesangiocapillary glomerulonephritis, malignant hypertension, the Goodpasture syndrome, and idiopathic rapidly progressive glomerulonephritis. In the latter case, immunofluorescent study reveals deposition in a linear fashion of IgG along glomerular capillary basement membranes can be demonstrated in association with antiglomerular basement membrane antibodies in the serum. The glomerular lesions are identical to those of the Goodpasture syndrome. Also called *subacute glomerulonephritis* (outmoded), *malignant glomerulonephritis, subacute nephritis.*

segmental glomerulonephritis Glomerulonephritis limited to segments of some or all glomeruli. It is a form of focal glomerulonephritis.

subacute glomerulonephritis An outmoded term for RAPIDLY PROGRESSIVE GLOMERULONEPHRITIS.

glomerulopathy [*glomerul(e)* + *o* + -PATHY] Any lesion that involves the glomeruli.

diabetic glomerulopathy Any renal complication of diabetes mellitus involving glomeruli and including diffuse or nodular diabetic glomerulosclerosis.

membranous glomerulopathy MEMBRANOUS GLOMERULONEPHRITIS.

minimum change glomerulopathy LIPOID NEPHROSIS.

glomerulosclerosis [*glomerul(e)* + *o* + SCLEROSIS] Replacement of all or part of some or all glomeruli by collagen, mesangial matrix, or fibrillar material. This condition may be diffuse or focal and may follow proliferative glomerular lesions, or may be associated with vascular lesions, diabetes, or some instances of idiopathic nephrotic syndrome. Also called *glomerular sclerosis.*

congenital glomerulosclerosis Small and scarred glomeruli in the renal cortex of infants. If extensive, tubular atrophy and interstitial fibrosis may lead to renal failure during the first year of life. The cause is unknown. Also called *congenital chronic glomerulonephritis.*

diabetic glomerulosclerosis A common and serious complication of diabetes mellitus, characterized by diffuse but irregular thickening of the glomerular capillary basement membrane and mesangial areas. Accumulations of strongly acidophilic and PAS-positive mesangial matrix form nodules of varying size in the centers of peripheral capillary loops. Nodules may occur in association with diffuse glomerular changes. Both types of lesions may be associated with hyaline deposits ("exudative droplets"). Arteriolosclerosis involving both the afferent and efferent glomerular arterioles is characteristic of diabetes mellitus. Diabetic glomerulosclerosis is part of a generalized microangiopathy that involves arterioles of many organs, including the retina, and is characterized by proteinuria, microscopic hematuria, progressive renal failure, and sometimes the nephrotic syndrome. Also called *intercapillary glomerulosclerosis, nodular glomerulosclerosis, Kimmelstiel-Wilson syndrome, nodular glomerulonephritis, intercapillary nephrosclerosis.*

diffuse glomerulosclerosis Sclerosis of all or almost all glomeruli.

focal glomerulosclerosis 1 Sclerosis of some but not all glomeruli. 2 A renal disease characterized by the nephrotic syndrome and small hyaline foci in some glomeruli, at first involving only the juxtamedullary glomeruli. Microscopic hematuria is common, and hypertension and chronic renal failure develop within a few years. Remissions are rare, whether spontaneous or treatment-induced. The etiology is unknown. Although many features, including diffuse smudging of epithelial foot processes on electron microscopy, are similar to lipoid nephrosis, focal glomerulosclerosis probably is a separate entity. Also called *congenital nephrosclerosis, focal sclerosing glomerulonephritis.*

intercapillary glomerulosclerosis DIABETIC GLOMERULOSCLEROSIS.

nodular glomerulosclerosis DIABETIC GLOMERULOSCLEROSIS.

glomerulus [New L (dim. of L *glomus,* gen. *glomeris,* a clue, skein, ball of thread, akin to *globus* a ball, sphere, globe), a small skein, small ball of thread] (*plural* glomeruli) 1 A knot or tuft of convoluted capillary blood vessels or nerve fibers. 2 [NA] In the renal cortex and columns, a tufted network of anastomosing capillaries derived from an afferent arteriole (arteriola glomerularis afferense) and ending in an efferent arteriole (arteriola glomerularis efferens) which enter and leave at the vascular pole of a renal corpuscle. It is held together by loose connective tissue and surrounded by the glomerular capsule (capsula glomeruli). Also called *renal glomerulus, malpighian glomerulus, glomerulus renis, glomerulus renalis, renal tuft* (outmoded), *glomerular tuft* (outmoded), *malphigian tuft* (outmoded).

glomeruli arteriosi cochleae [NA] The capillary network formed by the ramification of the cochlear branch of the labyrinthine artery in the lamina spiralis and basilar membrane of the cochlea.

caudal glomeruli An outmoded term for GLOMUS COCCYGEUM.

caudal arterial glomeruli GLOMUS COCCYGEUM.

coccygeal arterial glomeruli An outmoded term for GLOMUS COCCYGEUM.

malpighian glomerulus GLOMERULUS.

glomerulus of mesonephros One of the excretory units of the mesonephros which may be functional for a short time in the embryo. Each lies medial to the mesonephric duct and is supplied by a lateral branch from the aorta.

nonencapsulated nerve glomerulus A spherical terminal cluster of nerve fibers associated with an internal organ and lacking a specialized corpuscular surrounding structure.

olfactory glomerulus One of a series of rounded areas of neuropil containing complex axodendritic and dendrodendritic synapses between olfactory afferent nerve fibers and the apical dendrites of the mitral and tufted cells and the dendrites of periglomerular cells in the glomerular layer of the main and accessory olfactory bulbs.

glomerulus of pronephros An arterial tuft covered by a thin epithelium which projects into the coelom in lower vertebrates having a functional pronephros. Waste is excreted into the coelom and removed through segmentally arranged nephrostomes to the pronephric duct.

renal glomerulus GLOMERULUS.

glomerulus renalis GLOMERULUS.

glomerulus renis GLOMERULUS.

glomic Pertaining to a glomus.

glomoid Resembling a glomus or ball.

glomus [L (gen. *glomeris*), a clue, skein, ball of thread] (*plural* glomera) [NA] A neurovascular body, generally ball-shaped, containing richly innervated small arterioles. Also called *vascular gland, glome.* Adjective: glomic.

glomera aortica CORPORA PARA-AORTICA.

glomus caroticum [NA] A small, oval neurovascular body situated at the bifurcation of each common carotid artery, containing chemoreceptors that monitor blood gas concentration and aid in the regulation of respiration by means of central connections via the glossopharyngeal nerve. Also called *carotid glomus, glomus carotideum, carotid body, intercarotid body, carotid gland, intercarotid gland, glandula intercarotica, Arnold's ganglion, carotid ganglion, intercarotid ganglion* (outmoded), *nodulus intercaroticus* (outmoded).

carotid glomus GLOMUS CAROTICUM.

glomus carotideum GLOMUS CAROTICUM.

choroid glomus GLOMUS CHOROIDEUM.

glomus choroideum [NA] The enlarged body of choroid plexus in the lateral ventricle at the junction of the main body with the inferior horn. Also called *choroid glomus.*

coccygeal glomus GLOMUS COCCYGEUM.

glomus coccygeum [NA] A small, irregularly rounded mass in front of the apex of the coccyx and at the termination of the median sacral vessels that communicate with it by efferent and afferent vessels. It is composed of a large central nodule surrounded by smaller nodules each of which is composed of spherical or polyhedral epithelial cells surrounding a sinusoidal capillary that takes part in a complex arrangement of arteriolovenular anastomoses. The cells are considered to be shortened muscle cells of the tunica media of vessels adjacent to the dilated capillaries. Its functions are not clearly understood. Similar masses are found anterior to the caudal vertebrae of many other mammals. Also called *coccygeal glomus, caudal glomeruli* (outmoded), *caudal arterial glomeruli, Luschka's body, Luschka's ganglion, Luschka's gland, corpus coccygeum, coccygeal body, arteriococcygeal gland* (outmoded), *coccygeal vascular plexus, coccygeal arterial glomeruli* (outmoded), *coccygeal gland* (outmoded).

cutaneous glomus DIGITAL GLOMUS.

digital glomus A structure that provides a short circuit of blood directly from arterioles to venules in the dermis of the fingers and toes as well as the palms and soles, face, and ears. Also called *cutaneous glomus, neuromyoarterial glomus.*

glomus intravagale One of a number of small bodies, similar in structure to that of the carotid body, situated near the arch of the aorta, ductus arteriosus, and right subclavian artery, supplied by branches of the vagus nerve and considered to contain chemoreceptor endings. An outmoded term.

glomus jugulare A microscopic neurovascular specialization in the adventitia of the jugular bulb.

glomus of Masson A special variety of arteriolovenular anastomosis that is present in the cutaneous circulation and that consists of two to six anastomoses with thick muscular walls between the afferent arteriole and the efferent venule. An outmoded term.

neuromyoarterial glomus DIGITAL GLOMUS.

glomus pulmonale A chemoreceptor similar in structure to the carotid body and associated with the left pulmonary artery near the ligamentum arteriosum. An outmoded term.

gloss- GLOSSO-.

glossa [Gk *glōssa* the tongue] LINGUA.

glossagra A seldom used term for GLOSSODYNIA.

glossal Pertaining to the tongue; lingual.

glossalgia GLOSSODYNIA.

glossauxesis Increased bulk of the tongue from whatever cause. An obsolete term.

glossectomy [GLOSS- + -ECTOMY] Surgical removal of the tongue. Also called *glossosteresis* (rarely used).

Glossina [GLOSS- + -INA] A genus of African muscoid flies, the tsetse flies, which are vectors of the various trypanosomes

that cause African trypanosomiasis of humans and domestic animals. Both sexes feed exclusively and avidly on the blood of vertebrates. Twenty-two species have been described. The feeding and breeding habits of these flies, in the so-called tsetse belts or fly belts, determine the distribution of the various trypanosomes they carry. There are three major habitat groups that are important in the epidemiology of trypanosomiasis: (1) lacustrine and riverine, including *G. palpalis, G. fuscipes,* and *G. tachinoides,* which feed largely on reptiles but also on the bushbuck, livestock, and humans; (2) forest or forest-edge thicket dwellers, including *G. tabaniformis* and *G. austeni* which feed on suids, and *G. fusca, G. pallidipes,* and *G. longipalpis,* which attack cattle and antelope, particularly the bushbuck; (3) savannah feeders, including *G. morsitans* and *G. swynnertoni,* which attack bovids and suids. Of particular adaptive importance in the survival of these flies is their pupiparous habit, the female fly possessing "milk glands" which enable a single larva to pass through its first three larval instars within the female, protected from external conditions and predation. The larvae are deposited on loose soil, into which they burrow by peristaltic movements. The integument quickly hardens to form a puparium within which the fourth larval and the pupal stage develop.

Glossina morsitans A savannah-inhabitating species that transmits *Trypanosoma brucei,* the agent of nagana in central Africa and *T. (brucei) rhodesiense,* the cause of Rhodesian, or east African, human sleeping sickness.

Glossina pallidipes The chief vector of the trypanosome that causes nagana, the rapidly fatal trypanosomiasis of cattle. It also transmits *Trypanosoma rhodesiense,* the agent of human east African sleeping sickness.

Glossina palpalis A species of tsetse fly that transmits *Trypanosoma gambiense,* an agent of Gambian, or west African, sleeping sickness. The illness is associated with riverine vegetation and villages located along water courses, in keeping with the local distribution patterns of the vector fly.

Glossinidae [*Glossin(a)* + -IDAE] A monotypic family of muscoid flies that contains the genus *Glossina,* the tsetse flies.

glossitic Having to do with glossitis.

glossitis [GLOSS- + -ITIS] Inflammation, usually superficial, of the tongue. Also called *glottitis* (seldom used).

acute aphthous glossitis A glossitis, seen mainly in children, that is characterized by the development at the sides of the tongue of vesicles which rupture to leave small erosions.

acute parenchymal glossitis Cellulitis of the tongue. Also called *parenchymatous glossitis.*

glossitis areata exfoliativa GEOGRAPHIC TONGUE.

atrophic glossitis HUNTER'S GLOSSITIS.

benign migratory glossitis GEOGRAPHIC TONGUE.

chronic superficial glossitis Red, swollen, and painful tongue, which may be smooth in its entirety or in patches, associated with many systemic diseases, including pernicious anemia, neural disturbances, and vitamin B deficiency. It is due to tissue atrophy. Also called *chronic superficial erythematous glossitis, Moeller's glossitis, pellagrous glossitis.*

chronic superficial erythematous glossitis CHRONIC SUPERFICIAL GLOSSITIS.

Clarke-Fournier glossitis INTERSTITIAL SCLEROUS GLOSSITIS.

cortical superficial sclerotic glossitis Chronic superficial glossitis characterized by red or whitish plaques and both superficial induration and atrophic furrows, an appearance seen in a number of varieties of chronic glossitis, for instance the hobnail tongue of tertiary syphilis.

deep sclerotic glossitis INTERSTITIAL SCLEROUS GLOSSITIS.

dissecting glossitis Chronic glossitis associated with painful fissures of the lingual mucous membrane.

exfoliative glossitis GEOGRAPHIC TONGUE.

Fournier's glossitis INTERSTITIAL SCLEROUS GLOSSITIS.

gummatory glossitis A rarely used term for GUMMATOUS GLOSSITIS.

gummatous glossitis 1 Gumma of the tongue. 2 Chronic, diffuse, interstitial glossitis caused by syphilis. Also called *gummatory glossitis* (rarely used).

Hunter's glossitis Glossitis associated with pernicious anemia, in which the tongue is smooth and red. Also called *atrophic glossitis.*

idiopathic glossitis Glossitis of unknown cause.

interstitial sclerous glossitis Glossitis associated with tertiary syphilis, in which there are nodules, lobulation, and induration. Also called *Clark-Fournier glossitis, Fournier's glossitis.*

leukoplakic glossitis Leukoplakia of the tongue. Also called *smokers' tongue.*

median rhomboid glossitis A rare congenital anomaly characterized by a smooth, oval, red patch in the midline of the dorsum of the tongue immediately anterior to the circumvallate papillae, due to the persistence of the tuberculum impar on the surface of the tongue. Also called *glossitis rhomboidea mediana* (seldom used).

glossitis migrans GEOGRAPHIC TONGUE.

Moeller's glossitis CHRONIC SUPERFICIAL GLOSSITIS.

monilial glossitis Thrush affecting the tongue.

parasitic glossitis An obsolete term for BLACK HAIRY TONGUE. • This term was used at a time when this condition was considered to be due to a fungus, then called a parasite.

glossitis parasitica An obsolete term for BLACK HAIRY TONGUE. • See note at PARASITIC GLOSSITIS.

parenchymatous glossitis ACUTE PARENCHYMAL GLOSSITIS.

pellagrous glossitis CHRONIC SUPERFICIAL GLOSSITIS.

glossitis rhomboidea mediana A seldom used term for MEDIAN RHOMBOID GLOSSITIS.

syphilitic glossitis Inflammation of the tongue due to syphilis. Although lesions of the tongue may occur in primary and secondary syphilis, the term is usually preserved for the hobnail tongue of the late disease. One-third of such lesions progress to carcinoma of the tongue.

ulcerative glossitis Any variety of glossitis characterized principally by ulceration.

ulceromembranous glossitis Ulceration of the tongue associated with the formation of membranes, as seen in granulocytopenia and necrotizing ulcerative gingivitis.

glosso- [Gk *glōssa* or *glōtta* tongue] A combining form meaning (1) the tongue; (2) speech, language. Also *gloss-, glotto-.*

glossodesmus A seldom used term for FRENULUM LINGUAE.

glossodynamometer An instrument for measuring the strength of the muscles of the tongue.

glossodynia [GLOSS- + -ODYNIA] 1 Pain in the tongue. 2 Paresthesia marked by a burning sensation of the tongue. A wide variety of causes have been proposed but frequently no cause can be found. For defs. 1 and 2 also called *glossalgia, glossagra* (seldom used).

glossodynia exfoliativa Painful, bald, beefy tongue, seen in certain deficiency diseases. Many varieties of glossitis, such as Hunter's glossitis, are characterized as such.

glossoepiglottic Pertaining to the tongue, usually the posterior portion, and the epiglottis. Also *glossoepiglottidean.*

glossoepiglottidean GLOSSOEPIGLOTTIC.

glossograph [GLOSSO- + -GRAPH] An instrument for recording movements of the tongue during speech.

glossohyal 1 HYOGLOSSAL. 2 The median basihyal of fishes.

glossohyoidal HYOGLOSSAL.

glossoid [GLOSS- + -OID] Resembling a tongue.

glossolabial Pertaining to the tongue and the lip or lips.

glossolabiolaryngeal Pertaining to the tongue, the lips, and the larynx.

glossolabiopharyngeal Pertaining to the tongue, the lips, and the pharynx. Also *glossopharyngeolabial.*

glossolalia [GLOSSO- + -LALIA] Speech in which neologisms are used that mimic the words, sentences, and formal structure of language.

glossology [GLOSSO- + -LOGY] 1 The study of the tongue and the conditions affecting it. 2 The definition and explanation of terms. An outmoded and seldom used term. Also called *glottology.*

glossolysis [GLOSSO- + LYSIS] GLOSSOPLEGIA.

glossomantia [GLOSSO- + Gk *manteia* a prophesying, power of divination] A prognosis of a disease on the basis of the appearance of the tongue.

glossoncus A tumor of the tongue. An obsolete term.

glossopalatine Pertaining to the tongue and the palate.

glossopalatinus MUSCULUS PALATOGLOSSUS.

glossopalatolabial Pertaining to the tongue, the palate, and the lips.

glossopathy [GLOSSO- + -PATHY] Any disease of the tongue.

glossopexy [GLOSSO- + -PEXY] The attachment of the tongue to the lower lip to prevent asphyxia in the Pierre Robin syndrome.

glossopharyngeal Pertaining to the tongue and the pharynx. Also *pharyngoglossal.*

glossopharyngeolabial GLOSSOLABIOPHARYNGEAL.

glossopharyngeum The tongue and the pharynx considered as one unit.

glossopharyngeus 1 PARS GLOSSOPHARYNGEA MUSCULI CONSTRICTORIS PHARYNGIS SUPERIORIS. 2 NERVUS GLOSSOPHARYNGEUS.

glossophytia [GLOSSO- + PHYT- + -IA] An older term for BLACK HAIRY TONGUE.

glossoplasty [GLOSSO- + -PLASTY] A plastic operation performed on the tongue.

glossoplegia [GLOSSO- + -PLEGIA] Paralysis of the tongue. This is usually unilateral, caused by damage to the hypoglossal nerve, and it brings about deviation of the tongue towards the affected side on protrusion. Also called *glossolysis.*

glossoptosis The prolapse backwards and downwards of the abnormally small tongue characteristic of the Pierre Robin syndrome.

glossopyrosis [GLOSSO- + PYROSIS] The sensation of burning in the tongue. It is a variety of glossodynia. Also called *burning tongue, pyroglossia.*

glossorrhaphy [GLOSSO- + -RRHAPHY] Suturing of the tongue. A seldom used term.

glossospasm [GLOSSO- + SPASM] A seldom used term for LINGUAL SPASM.

glossosteresis [GLOSSO- + Gk *sterēsis* privation, loss] A rarely used term for GLOSSECTOMY.

glossotomy [GLOSSO- + -TOMY] Incision of the tongue.

glossotrichia [GLOSSO- + TRICH- + -IA] Hypertrophied, filiform papillae as in black hairy tongue. A rarely used term.

glossy Forming bacterial colonies with an even more shiny surface than those designated as smooth, usually indicating the formation of a thick capsule.

glottal Of or relating to the glottis. Also *glottic, glottidean.*

glottic GLOTTAL.

glottidean GLOTTAL.

glottides   Plural of GLOTTIS.

glottidospasm   LARYNGOSPASM.

glottis   [Gk *glōttis*, also *glōssis* (from *glōtta* or *glōssa* the tongue), the glottis]   [NA] The vocal apparatus of the larynx, composed of the two vocal folds and the intermembranous part of the rima glottidis between them.

false glottis   RIMA VESTIBULI.

intercartilaginous glottis   PARS INTERCARTILAGINEA RIMAE GLOTTIDIS.

glottis respiratoria   PARS INTERCARTILAGINEA RIMAE GLOTTIDIS.

respiratory glottis   PARS INTERCARTILAGINEA RIMAE GLOTTIDIS.

glottis spuria   RIMA VESTIBULI.

true glottis   RIMA GLOTTIDIS.

glottis vera   RIMA GLOTTIDIS.

glottis vocalis   An outmoded term for PARS INTERMEMBRANACEA RIMAE GLOTTIDIS.

glottitis   A seldom used term for GLOSSITIS.

glotto-   GLOSSO-.

glottogram   [GLOTTO- + -GRAM]   ELECTROLARYNGOGRAM.

glottograph   [GLOTTO- + -GRAPH]   ELECTROLARYNGOGRAPH.

glottography   [GLOTTO- + -GRAPHY]   ELECTROLARYNGOGRAPHY.

glottology   GLOSSOLOGY.

glow   [Old English *glōwan*, akin to Old English *geolu* yellow]

cathode glow   The incandescence appearing at the surface of the cathode of a discharge tube. Also called *negative glow*.

negative glow   CATHODE GLOW.

Glu   Symbol for glutamic acid.

gluc-   GLUCO-.

glucagon   A 29-residue peptide hormone secreted by the α-cells of the pancreatic islets of Langerhans and released in response to hypoglycemia, amino-acid administration, dietary protein, and pituitary growth hormone. Its effects generally oppose those of insulin, stimulating liver cells to release glucose from stored glycogen through its activation of adenylate cyclase in the cell membrane, thus raising the intracellular concentration of cyclic AMP (adenosine 3′,5′-cyclic phosphate). The hormone appears to exert subtle effects in concert with insulin upon glucose homeostasis, and it probably plays a part in the pathogenesis of diabetes mellitus. Also called *insulin-antagonizing factor, hyperglycemic-glycogenolytic factor* (outmoded), *pancreatic hyperglycemic hormone* (obsolete), *hyperglycemic factor* (imprecise).

glucagon hydrochloride   A pharmaceutical preparation of glucagon. It has found limited clinical use in the experimental treatment of some cases of heart failure and in diagnostic tests of hypoglycemic disorders.

glucagonoma   [*glucagon* + -OMA]   An islet cell tumor of the alpha cells of the pancreas which secretes glucagon. It can occur clinically with diabetes mellitus, and may be malignant. Also called *alpha cell tumor*.

4-α-D-glucanotransferase   An enzyme (EC 2.4.1.25) which transfers a segment of a 1,4-α-D-glucan to a new 4-position in an acceptor which may be glucose or a 1,4-α-glucan. Also called *dextrin glycosyltransferase*.

glucaric acid   HOOC—[CHOH]$_4$—COOH. The acid formed from glucose by oxidizing agents that are strong enough to oxidize both C-1 and C-6 to carboxyl groups. It has little biologic significance.

gluci-   GLUCO-.

Gluck   [Themistokles *Gluck*, German surgeon, born 1853]   See under INCISION.

gluco-   [Gk *gleukos* (akin to *glykys* sweet) sweetness]   A combining form denoting glucose. Also *gluc-, gluci-*.

glucoascorbic acid   An analogue of ascorbic acid, which acts as a competitive inhibitor of the latter.

glucocerebrosidosis   GAUCHER'S DISEASE.

glucocorticoid   A C$_{21}$ adrenocortical steroid hormone which stimulates gluconeogenesis, chiefly in the liver, and opposes the hypoglycemic action of insulin. In man the major natural glucocorticoid is cortisol. In rats and mice, it is corticosterone. All the semisynthetic hormones used to treat allergic and inflammatory diseases are glucocorticoids. Also called *glucosteroid, S. hormone* (older term), *glucocorticosteroid*.

glucocorticosteroid   GLUCOCORTICOID.

Gluco-Ferrum   A proprietary name for ferrous gluconate.

glucofuranose   The 5-membered ring form of glucose, in which a hemiacetal is formed between C-1 and O-4. It is only a minor form of glucose in solution, and is rare in glycosides.

glucogenesis   The formation of glucose from the dissolution of glycogen.

glucohemia   GLYCEMIA.

glucokinase   The enzyme (EC 2.7.1.2) that catalyzes the reaction of glucose and ATP to yield glucose 6-phosphate and ADP, and has a greater specificity for glucose than does hexokinase. This enzyme has not been found in mammals, but the term is sometimes applied to the liver isoenzyme of hexokinase, because its affinity for glucose and fructose is lowered in comparison with the muscle isoenzymes, so that it may appear inactive with fructose at the concentrations used for assay. This isoenzyme is not easily saturated with glucose (K_m 10mM, compared with 0.1 mM for muscle isoenzymes), and so the rate of reaction it catalyzes increases with the blood sugar concentration. It also differs in not being inhibited by glucose 6-phosphate.

glucokinetic   Tending to ensure the maintenance and stability of glucose concentration in the blood.

Glucomannan   A fiber extracted from konjac tubers and marketed as a slimming aid. It swells when mixed with fluid in the stomach, thus giving the feeling of satiety. A proprietary name.

gluconate   The anion derived from gluconic acid, a salt containing it, or more rarely an ester.

gluconeogenesis   [GLUCO- + NEO- + GENESIS]   The formation of glucose or glucose residues of glycogen, from noncarbohydrate sources, especially from amino acids derived from proteins. Thus alanine yields pyruvate by transamination, and much but not all of the subsequent pathway is the reverse of glycolysis.

gluconic acid   The acid formed by oxidation of C-1 of glucose to form a carboxyl group. The oxidation of glucose by glucose oxidase, an enzyme found in molds, produces its lactone together with hydrogen peroxide.

gluconolactone   A lactone derived from gluconic acid, usually the 1,4- or the 1,5-lactone. 6-Phosphoglucono-1,5-lactone is the initial product of glucose-6-phosphate dehydrogenase, and glucono-1,5-lactone is likewise the initial product of glucose oxidase. In each case dehydrogenation of the —O—CHOH— group in the ring forms —O—CO—.

glucopenia   [*gluc(ose)* + -PENIA]   A condition marked by a lower-than-normal concentration of glucose in the blood and tissues.

glucophylline   THEOPHYLLINE METHYLGLUCAMINE.

glucopyranose   Glucose in its pyranose form. This form greatly predominates for free glucose, in which pyranose, furanose and chain forms equilibrate, and in natural glucosides and polysaccharides, where they do not.

glucosamine   2-Amino-2-deoxyglucose, an important component of many polysaccharides, usually acetylated on its amino group. Such polysaccharides occur, for example, in bacterial call walls. Cell membrane glycoproteins also contain glucosamine in the oligosaccharides attached to their outer portions. Symbol: GlcN

glucosaminephosphate isomerase The enzyme (EC 5.3.1.10) that catalyzes the interconversion of glucosamine 6-phosphate and water with fructose 6-phosphate and ammonia. It is so named because the first product is presumed to be the imine of fructose 6-phosphate and ammonia formed by isomerization of glucosamine phosphate. It provides a pathway for the breakdown of glucosamine. Another enzyme, present in liver and some molds, glucosaminephosphate isomerase (glutamine-forming) (EC 5.3.1.19), catalyzes a similar reaction in which glutamate replaces water, and the products are therefore fructose 6-phosphate and glutamine.

glucose [French (irreg. from Gk *gleukos*, must, sweet new wine, akin to *glykys* sweet), the sugar of grapes, of potato flour] The sugar present in blood. It is the most stable aldohexose because in its predominant pyranose form C-6 and all hydroxyl groups are equatorial substituents of the ring. It occurs widely in combined form, usually esterified with orthophosphoric acid, in metabolic pathways. Also called *starch sugar*.

liquid glucose A colorless, odorless, viscous syrup consisting of dextrose, maltose, dextrins, and water, prepared by the incomplete acid hydrolysis of starch. Also called *corn syrup*.

medicinal glucose DEXTROSE MONOHYDRATE.

glucose-glycinuria Excretion of excess amounts of glucose and glycine in the urine; a very rare condition.

glucose oxidase An enzyme (EC 1.1.3.4) that catalyzes the oxidation of glucose to gluconolactone, which in turn hydrolyzes spontaneously to gluconic acid with the concomitant reduction of oxygen to hydrogen peroxide. It is not found in mammals and it is usually derived from molds. Many methods for determining glucose concentration depend on measurement of the hydrogen peroxide that it forms. This enzyme was originally isolated from the mold *Penicillium notatum* and was mistakenly thought to be an antibiotic because of the antibacterial action of the hydrogen peroxide. Also called *notatin* (obsolete), *penicillin B* (obsolete).

glucose-6-phosphatase The enzyme (EC 3.1.3.9) that hydrolyzes glucose 6-phosphate to glucose and orthophosphate. It occurs in liver and enables liver cells to regulate blood glucose concentration. Elaborate mechanisms exist for controlling its activity.

glucose 1-phosphate An important metabolic intermediate, interconvertible with glucose 6-phosphate. It is on the route of glycogen synthesis as well as being the direct product of glycogen breakdown by phosphorylase. Unlike glucose 6-phosphate, it is a glycoside. Also called *Cori ester* (older term).

glucose 6-phosphate An important metabolic intermediate, it is the product of phosphorylation of glucose by hexokinase, glucokinase, or, in all anaerobic bacteria, phosphotransferase. It may be oxidized by glucose-6-phosphate dehydrogenase, interconverted with glucose 1-phosphate on the route to or from glycogen, or interconverted with fructose 6-phosphate in the glycolytic pathway. Also called *Embden ester* (obsolete), *Robison ester* (obsolete).

glucose-6-phosphate dehydrogenase The enzyme (EC 1.1.1.49) that catalyzes the conversion of glucose 6-phosphate into 6-phosphogluconolactone with concomitant reduction of $NADP^+$ to NADPH. This is the first step of the oxidative pentose phosphate pathway. The NADPH formed is used for reductions in fatty acid synthesis, etc. Also called *zwischenferment* (obsolete).

glucose-phosphate isomerase The enzyme (EC 5.3.1.9) that catalyzes the interconversion of glucose 6-phosphate and fructose 6-phosphate, an early step of glycolysis. Also called *oxoisomerase* (outmoded), *phosphohexoisomerase*.

glucose-1-phosphate phosphodismutase An enzyme (EC 2.7.1.41) which catalyzes the conversion of two molecules of D-glucose 1-phosphate into D-glucose and D-glucose 1,6-bisphosphate.

glucose-1-phosphate uridylyltransferase The enzyme (EC 2.7.7.9) that catalyzes the transfer of a uridylyl group from UTP onto glucose 1-phosphate to form UDPglucose and diphosphate. It is important in the formation of glycogen, because UDPglucose is the donor of glucosyl groups for the biosynthesis of glycogen and of some other polysaccharides.

glucosidase Any enzyme, such as an amylase, that catalyzes the hydrolysis of a glucoside.

glucoside A compound in which the hydroxyl group on C-1 of a ring form of glucose is substituted, i.e. the potential aldehyde group is combined as an acetal with two alcoholic hydroxyl groups, one of them already in the glucose molecule on C-4 or C-5, the other from another molecule. Polysaccharides of glucose are glucosides.

glucosinolate progoitrin A natural inhibitor of the synthesis of thyroxine, found in brassica seeds and in lesser amounts in their leaves and roots. This substance is inactive until converted to the active goitrin 5-vinyloxazolidine-2-thione by the enzyme thioglucosidase. This enzyme is destroyed by cooking, thus preventing the production of the goitrogen. Also called *cabbage factor*.

glucosteroid GLUCOCORTICOID.

glucosulfone sodium $C_{24}H_{34}N_2Na_2O_{18}S_3$. 1,1′-[Sulfonylbis(4,1-phenyleneimino)]bis[1-deoxy-1-sulfo-D-glucitol] disodium salt. An antibacterial agent with leprostatic action. It is used as an injectable solution.

glucosuria GLYCOSURIA.

glucosyl The group formed from a ring form of glucose by removing the hydroxyl group on C-1.

glucosylation The process of substituting with a glucosyl group. It is by glucosylation of O-4 of the terminal residue in a glycogen chain that the chain gains a residue during its biosynthesis.

glucuronate The anion derived from glucuronic acid.

glucuronic acid The substance formed from glucose by oxidizing C-6 from —CH_2OH to —COOH. It occurs in polysaccharides, and many substances are excreted in the urine in the form of glycosides of glucuronic acid.

glucuronidase Any enzyme that hydrolyzes the glycoside bond formed between glucuronic acid and an alcohol. The best known is β-glucuronidase (EC 3.2.1.31), which has little specificity for the alcohol, but more specific enzymes are also known. It is used in the chemical analysis of urine, as for steroid hormones, to release metabolites that are combined as glucuronides.

glucuronide A glycoside of glucuronic acid. Many substances such as steroid metabolites are converted into their glucuronides to solubilize them for excretion.

glucuronolactone A lactone of glucuronic acid, formed by esterification of the carboxyl group (C-6) with one of the hydroxyl groups, usually O-3.

glue [Low L *glus* (akin to L *gluten* glue) glue]

plasma glue PLASMA CLOT.

glumitocin [Ser⁴,Gln⁸]oxytocin. A peptide found as a hormone in certain cartilaginous fishes.

glutamate 1 A negatively charged ion derived from glutamic acid. It may bear a net charge of −1 or −2 according to pH. A glutamate residue in a protein is the deprotonated form of a glutamic residue, i.e. the form that occurs at neutral pH. 2 An ester of glutamic acid.

glutamate family   The amino acids that derive all or part of their carbon from glutamate. They include glutamine, proline, arginine, and, in many fungi and higher plants, lysine.

glutamate decarboxylase   The enzyme (EC 4.1.1.15) that catalyzes the decarboxylation of glutamic acid. The product is 4-aminobutyrate, which is important as a neurotransmitter, especially in arthropods. Also called *glutamic decarboxylase*.

glutamate dehydrogenase   An enzyme that catalyzes the reaction: glutamate $+$ NAD(P)$^+$ $\rightleftharpoons$ 2-oxoglutarate $+$ NH$_4^+$ $+$ NAD(P)H. It is probably responsible for both the biosynthesis and the catabolism of glutamate, and hence indirectly, via transamination, of other amino acids.

glutamate oxaloacetate transaminase   A previous name for ASPARTATE AMINOTRANSFERASE. Abbreviation: GOT.

glutamate pyruvate transaminase   ALANINE AMINOTRANSFERASE.

glutamic acid   HOOC—CH$_2$—CH$_2$—CH(NH$_2$)—COOH. An amino acid central to the metabolism of other amino acids, especially because it can reversibly transfer its nitrogen to many 2-oxoacids to form a new amino acid and 2-oxoglutarate. It can also form 2-oxoglutarate and ammonia with concomitant reduction of NAD$^+$ (or NADP$^+$), and the reverse of this reaction is a route of its biosythesis. Its conversion into glutamine allows some storage of ammonia. In microorganisms its formation from glutamine and 2-oxoglutarate, in which the amide nitrogen is transferred, is a key step in a major route of assimilation of ammonia nitrogen. Also called *aminoglutaric acid*.

glutamic acid hydrochloride   C$_5$H$_9$NO$_4$·HCl. A dicarboxylic amino acid which has been used as an acidifying agent in cases of achlorhydria and hypochlorhydria, and as an antiepileptic agent.

glutamic decarboxylase   GLUTAMATE DECARBOXYLASE.

glutamic semialdehyde   HCO—[CH$_2$]$_2$—CH(NH$_3^+$)—COO$^-$. An intermediate in the metabolism of glutamate, from which it can be formed by reduction of γ-glutamyl phosphate, in turn formed from glutamate and ATP. It is on the pathway of conversion of glutamate into proline, and on the pathways of glutamate formation from ornithine and proline.

glutaminase   The enzyme (EC 3.5.1.2) that catalyzes the hydrolysis of glutamine to form glutamate and ammonia.

glutamine   H$_2$N—CO—CH$_2$—CH$_2$—CH(NH$_2$)—COOH. An amide of glutamic acid. It is also one of the 20 amino acids incorporated into proteins. Many animal cells require it, although the whole organism can make it via glutamate. It is made by glutamine synthase, by a reaction that enables ammonia to be stored. Symbol: Gln

glutamine synthase   The enzyme (EC 6.3.1.2) that catalyzes the reaction: glutamate $+$ NH$_3$ $+$ ATP $\rightleftharpoons$ glutamine $+$ ADP $+$ orthophosphate. This enables ammonia to be stored. In bacteria this reaction is a key step in the assimilation of ammonia. In addition, glutamine is an intermediate in many biosyntheses, including those of amino acids, purines and pyrimidines, and the enzyme is subject to elaborate control mechanisms.

glutaminyl   The group H$_2$N—CO—CH$_2$—CH$_2$—CH(NH$_2$)—CO—, derived from glutamine.

glutamyl   The group HOOC—CH$_2$—CH$_2$—CH(NH$_2$)—CO—, derived from glutamic acid.

γ-glutamyl   The group HOOC—CH(NH$_2$)—CH$_2$—CH$_2$—CO—, derived from glutamic acid. It occurs in glutathione.

γ-glutamyl transferase   γ-GLUTAMYL TRANSPEPTIDASE.

γ-glutamyl transpeptidase   An enzyme that catalyzes the transfer of glutamyl groups among peptides or amino acids. It is derived primarily from the liver, although renal and pancreatic cells contain substantial quantities. Serum levels are markedly elevated in obstructive liver disease and hepatocellular carci-

noma, and moderately elevated with liver cell damage. It is usually measured as an indirect index of ethanol ingestion, because hepatocellular levels increase temporarily after stimulation by alcohol, barbiturates, and phenytoins. Also called *γ-glutamyl transferase*.

glutaraldehyde   OCH(CH$_2$)$_3$ CHO. A chemical having a molecular weight of 100.13 daltons, commonly used as a fixative in preservation of tissue for electron microscopy. Also called *1,5-pentanediol*.

glutaredoxin   A small protein, of molecular mass about 12 kDa, containing one disulfide bond. Its reduced form can function as the reductant for converting ribonucleotides into 2′-deoxyribonucleotides for DNA synthesis, and its oxidized form can be reduced by glutathione.

glutaric acid   HOOC—[CH$_2$]$_3$—COOH. Pentanedioic acid. It is found in some plants.

glutaryl-CoA synthetase   An enzyme (EC 6.2.1.6) that catalyzes the conversion of glutarate, adenosine triphosphate, and coenzyme A into adenosine diphosphate, orthophosphate, and glutaryl-CoA.

glutathione   The peptide γ-glutamylcysteinylglycine. In animals, it supplies reducing power to keep hemoglobin in its Fe(II) state despite spontaneous oxidation. It can also reduce ribonucleoside diphosphates to 2′-deoxyribonucleoside diphosphates. Its oxidized form, the dimeric disulfide, is reconverted into the thiol form by glutathione reductase.

   oxidized glutathione   The dimeric disulfide formed by oxidation of glutathione with formation of an —S—S— bridge.

   reduced glutathione   Glutathione in its nonoxidized form.

glutathione reductase   A flavoprotein enzyme (EC 1.6.4.2) that catalyzes the reduction of oxidized glutathione using NADPH or NADH as hydrogen donor.

gluteal   Pertaining to the buttocks or to one of its component structures.

glutelin   Any protein, according to a classification of 1908, that was insoluble in water, salt solution and aqueous ethanol, but soluble in acid and alkali. An obsolete term.

gluten [L, glue]   The part of the wheat seed consisting of protein. It causes intestinal inflammation to those who have celiac disease.

gluten-casein   A protein preparation derived from grain that has been used in gastrointestinal surgical procedures to elicit an inflammatory response and thereby cause adhesions to form.

glutenin   One of the main components of gluten.

gluteofascial   Pertaining to the fascia of the buttocks.

gluteofemoral   **1** Pertaining to the buttock and the thigh.   **2** Pertaining to a gluteal muscle and the thigh or the femoral bone.

gluteoinguinal   Pertaining to the buttock and the groin.

gluteotrochanteric   Pertaining to a gluteal muscle and the greater trochanter of the femur.

glutethimide   C$_{13}$H$_{15}$NO$_2$. 2-Ethyl-2-phenylglutarimide. A piperidinedione derivative that is used as a sedative and hypnotic. It is general central nervous system depressant, and it is used in the treatment of insomnia and as preoperative medication for its sedative properties. It is given orally.

gluteus [New L, irreg. from Gk *gloutos* the rump, bottom]   Denoting a musculus gluteus, either maximus, medius, or minimus.

glutinous   Gluelike; gummy; sticky.

glutitis [Gk *glout(os)* the rump, bottom + -ITIS]   An inflammation of the muscles of the buttocks.

Glx   A symbol for a residue that may be glutamic acid, or glutamine, or 5-oxoproline, or 4-carboxyglutamic acid. Any method of locating the residue in a protein or peptide that uses acid hydrolysis converts all the last three into glutamic acid, and hence cannot distinguish between these four residues.

Gly Symbol for glycine.

glyc- GLYCO-.

glycal An unsaturated monosaccharide derivative, which differs from the ring form of an aldose by lack of hydroxyl groups on C-1 and C-2 and by possessing a double bond between these two carbon atoms. A seldom used term.

glycanohydrolase Denoting any enzyme that catalyzes the hydrolysis of a glycan: used in systematic names.

glycemia [Gk *glyk(ys)* sweet + -EMIA] The presence of glucose in the blood. Also called *glycohemia, glucohemia, glycosemia.*

glyceral GLYCERALDEHYDE.

glyceraldehyde CH_2OH—$CHOH$—CHO. The simplest chiral sugar. Its dextrorotatory form, D-glyceraldehyde, was taken as the standard of D configuration for sugars. It is the *R* compound. Also called *glyceric aldehyde* (obsolete), *glycerose* (obsolete), *glyceral.*

glyceraldehyde 3-phosphate CHO—$CHOH$—CH_2—O—PO_3H_2. A three-carbon intermediate in glycolysis, formed when fructose 1,6-bisphosphate is cleaved under the influence of aldolase. It is interconvertible with the other triose phosphate produced with it, dihydroxyacetone phosphate. Also called *3-phosphoglyceraldehyde.*

glyceraldehyde-3-phosphate dehydrogenase Any of the enzymes (EC 1.2.1.9, 1.2.1.12, and 1.2.1.13) that catalyze the oxidation of glyceraldehyde 3-phosphate to form either 3-phosphoglycerate with concomitant reduction of $NADP^+$, or, with uptake of orthophosphate and concomitant reduction of NAD^+ or $NADP^+$, 3-phosphoglyceroyl phosphate. The term when unqualified refers to the enzyme (EC 1.2.1.12) that uses NAD^+ as hydrogen acceptor and forms 3-phosphoglyceroyl phosphate. This enzyme catalyzes an important step in the glycolytic pathway. The enzyme reacts with substrate through the thiol group of a cysteine residue, so that if the enzyme is portrayed as E—SH and the substrate as R—CHO, the hemithioacetal E—S—CHOH—R is formed and is then dehydrogenated to form an acyl enzyme, which can transfer the acyl group to orthophosphate to complete the reaction. The 3-phosphoglyceroyl phosphate formed can phosphorylate ADP to form ATP. The mammalian enzyme is a tetramer of four identical polypeptide chains, each of about 330 residues. Also called *triose phosphate dehydrogenase* (obsolete).

glycerate kinase The enzyme (EC 2.7.1.31) that catalyzes the conversion of glycerate into 3-phosphoglycerate by transfer of a phospho group from ATP. This enzyme is particularly important in microbial and plant metabolism.

glycerate phosphomutase **1** Phosphoglyceromutase, which interconverts 2- and 3-phosphoglycerates. **2** Bisphosphoglyceromutase, which interconverts 2,3-bisphosphoglycerate and 3-phosphoglyceroyl phosphate. An obsolete term.

glyceric acid CH_2OH—$CHOH$—$COOH$. A compound that is an intermediate in the metabolism of glycolate by bacteria and plants, but whose phosphates are biologically more important as glycolytic intermediates. Its 2,3-bisphosphate regulates the affinity of hemoglobin for oxygen. Symbol: Gri

glyceric aldehyde An obsolete term for GLYCERALDEHYDE.

glyceride A compound of glycerol.

glycerin GLYCEROL.

glycerin of alum A solution of potassium sulfate in water and glycerol. It is used as a topical astringent.

glycerin of belladonna An extract of belladonna in solution with water and glycerin. It has been used as a local medication on the skin to relieve pain and inflammation.

glycerin of boric acid A thick, yellow, liquid prepared by dissolving boric acid in glycerol at 140–150°C. The product

contains 31% w/w of boric acid. The weak bacteriostatic and fungistatic powers of boric acid, and the possible absorption of boric acid through abraded and broken skin areas, limit the usefulness of this medication. Also called *glyceritum boroglycerini, boroglycerin glycerite.*

compound glycerin of thymol A liquid mixture containing thymol, volatile oils, menthol, and glycerol. It has been used as a mouthwash.

glycerin of ichthammol A preparation containing 10% ichthammol in glycerin w/w which has been used as ear drops for external ear inflammatory conditions.

glycerin of lead subacetate A solution of lead subacetate ($C_4H_{10}O_8Pb_3$) in glycerin and water to a concentration of 1.48 g per ml. It has been used externally as an astringent solution for sprains and bruises.

glycerin of pepsin A suspension of pepsin in water and glycerin with hydrochloric acid as a vehicle. It is used to administer pepsin to patients with a deficiency of this proteolytic enzyme.

phenol glycerin A solution of phenol in glycerin, 16% w/w. It is further diluted with glycerin for use as a local treatment for mouth ulcers or tonsillitis. Dilute preparations in glycerin are also used as ear drops.

starch glycerin A mixture of starch, glycerin, and water. It is a translucent jelly, and has been used as a protective ointment or coating on inflamed skin. Also called *gliceritum amyli, starch glycerite.*

glycerinated Treated with glycerol: used especially of muscle fibers extracted with glycerol to remove small molecules and leave the system of actin and myosin, to which substrates and effectors can be added.

glycerine GLYCEROL.

glycerite [L *glyceritum.* See GLYCERITUM.] A solution or mixture of medicines with glylcerol as the main solvent. Also called *glyceritum.*

boroglycerin glycerite GLYCERIN OF BORIC ACID.

starch glycerite STARCH GLYCERIN.

glyceritum [L (from Gk *glykeros,* variant of *glykys* sweet), sweet] GLYCERITE.

glyceritum amyli STARCH GLYCERIN.

glyceritum boroglycerini GLYCERIN OF BORIC ACID.

glycerol (CH_2OH $CHOH$ CH_2OH). Trihydroxyproprane a clear, colorless, syrupy liquid obtained from the hydrolysis of neutral fats. It is used as a solvent, an emollient, and a suppository. Also called *glycerin, glycerine.*

glycerol kinase The enzyme (EC 2.7.1.30) that catalyzes the conversion of glycerol into *sn*-glycerol 3-phosphate by transfer of a phospho group from ATP with concomitant formation of ADP.

glycerol phosphate An ester of glycerol with phosphoric acid. The natural glycerol phosphate, formed by glycerol kinase from glycerol and ATP, or by glycerol-3-phosphate dehydrogenase by reduction of glycerone phosphate, is the *R* compound. It is known as *sn*-glycerol 3-phosphate, the prefix *sn* indicating stereospecific numbering in which the pro-*S* hydroxymethyl group is numbered 1. Glycerol phosphate is an intermediate in the metabolism of glycerol derived from fats. Also called *glycerophosphate.*

glycerol-phosphate dehydrogenase Any enzyme that dehydrogenates glycerol phosphate. The commonest of such enzymes (EC 1.1.1.8) uses NAD^+ as hydrogen acceptor, and its activity provides a means of reoxidizing NADH when glycolysis is accelerating, and the concentration of pyruvate (in plants acetaldehyde) is low, because glycerone phosphate can act as the oxidant. It may also allow glycerol phosphate derived from glycerol to enter the glycolytic pathway, although in bacteria this oxidation is effected by a glycerol-phosphate dehydrogenase

(EC 1.1.99.5) that uses a flavin as immediate hydrogen acceptor.

glycerone DIHYDROXYACETONE. Symbol: Grn

glycerophosphatase Any enzyme that hydrolyzes glycerol phosphate. Such enzymes have proven to be unspecific phosphatases, and are now designated, according to their pH optimum, as acid phosphatase or alkaline phosphatase. An obsolete term.

glycerophosphate GLYCEROL PHOSPHATE.

glycerose An obsolete term for GLYCERALDEHYDE.

glyceryl A group derived from glycerol by removal of one, two, or three hydrogen atoms from its hydroxyl groups.

glycidaldehyde A chemical which has the ability to inactivate virions, used in the preparation of virus vaccines. Abbreviation: GDA

glycidol 2,3-Epoxypropanol. Its phosphate is a powerful inhibitor of triosephosphate isomerase, being a substrate analogue that can react with a carboxyl group at the active site of the enzyme.

glycinamide ribonucleotide A substance whose molecule is composed of a ribose phosphate with the amide nitrogen of glycinamide linked to C-1 of the ribose. It is an intermediate in purine biosynthesis. Also called *N-(5-phosphoribosyl)glycineamide*.

glycinate The anion, or occasionally an ester, derived from glycine.

glycine [Gk *glyk(ys)* sweet + -IN] NH_2CH_2COOH. α-Amino acetic acid. The simplest of the amino acids and a common constituent of proteins.

glycine amidinotransferase The enzyme (EC 2.1.4.1) that catalyzes the transfer of the amidino group $-C(=NH)-NH_2$ from arginine to glycine with the formation of ornithine and guanidinoacetate, a step in the biosynthesis of creatine.

glycinemia HYPERGLYCINEMIA.

    glycinemia with ketosis HYPERGLYCINEMIA, KETOTIC FORM.

glycinol 2-AMINOETHANOL.

glycinuria [*glycin(e)* + -URIA] Excretion of excess amounts of glycine in the urine. Also called *hyperglycinuria (redundant)*.

    de Vries type renal glycinuria Excess excretion of glycine in the urine, often associated with nephrolithiasis and hypophosphatemic rickets. It is inherited as a dominant trait.

    hereditary glycinuria A rare condition, genetically transmitted as a dominant, characterized by hyperglycinuria with normoglycinemia due to decreased renal tubular reabsorption of glycine.

Glyciphagus [Gk *glyky(s)* sweet + *phagein* to eat] *GLYCYPHAGUS*.

glyco- [Gk *glykys* sweet] A combining form meaning sugar, relating to sugar. Also *glyc-*.

glycobiarsol $C_8H_9AsBiNO_6$. A pentavalent arsenical which also contains bismuth. It is used as an amebicidal drug in treating intestinal infections.

glycocalyx A thin layer of acid polysaccharides, particularly sialic acid, adherent to the outer surface of many cells. It may be the site of intense enzyme activity and also contains the surface antigens of the cell. Also called *fuzzy coat*.

glycocholic acid The conjugate of cholic acid with glycine, containing an amide bond between the carboxyl group of cholic acid and the amino group of glycine. It is present in mammalian bile.

glycocyamine Guanidinoacetic acid, an intermediate in the biosynthesis of creatine. It is made by the action of glycine amidinotransferase on glycine and arginine.

glycogen [Gk *glyk(ys)* sweet + *o* + -GEN] A storage polysaccharide, found in mammalian liver and muscle, and in microorganisms. It conists of glucose residues joined by α1-4 links, with branches formed by occasional α1-6 links.

glycogenesis **1** The formation or elaboration of glycogen. **2** The production of glucose. An older term. Also called *glycogeny*.

glycogenic [GLYCO- + -GENIC] Capable of forming carbohydrate: said of substances that can act as precursors of glycogen.

glycogenolysis The process of glycogen breakdown.

glycogenolytic Capable of causing glycogen breakdown.

glycogenosis [GLYCOGEN + -OSIS] GLYCOGEN STORAGE DISEASE.

    brancher deficiency glycogenosis GLYCOGEN STORAGE DISEASE IV.

    generalized glycogenosis GLYCOGEN STORAGE DISEASE.

    hepatic glycogenosis Any glycogenosis characterized by excessive glycogen storage within the liver.

    hepatophosphorylase deficiency glycogenosis GLYCOGEN STORAGE DISEASE VI.

    hepatorenal glycogenosis GLYCOGEN STORAGE DISEASE I.

    myophosphorylase deficiency glycogenosis GLYCOGEN STORAGE DISEASE V.

    Pompe's glycogenosis GLYCOGEN STORAGE DISEASE II.

    glycogenosis type II GLYCOGEN STORAGE DISEASE II.

    glycogenosis type III GLYCOGEN STORAGE DISEASE III.

    glycogenosis type V GLYCOGEN STORAGE DISEASE V.

    glycogenosis type VI GLYCOGEN STORAGE DISEASE VI.

glycogen phosphorylase The phosphorylase (EC 2.4.1.1) that acts on glycogen, catalyzing its reaction with orthophosphate to form glucose 1-phosphate.

glycogen synthase The enzyme (EC 2.4.1.11) responsible for the synthesis of glycogen. It acts by transferring glucosyl groups from UDPglucose onto the O-4 atom of the terminal residue of an existing glycogen chain. This enzyme is phosphorylated by the cAMP-dependent protein kinase. In its phosphorylated form it is inactive except in the presence of glucose 6-phosphate. This control allows glycogen synthesis to be shut off when glycogen breakdown is enhanced in response to hormones such as epinephrine. Also called *UDPG-glycogen transglucosidase* (outmoded).

glycogeny GLYCOGENESIS.

glycogeusia [GLYCO- + Gk *gleus(is)* taste + -IA] A spontaneous sensation of a sweet taste in the mouth.

glycohemia GLYCEMIA.

glycohistechia Abnormally high sugar content of a tissue. An obsolete term.

glycol Any 1,2-diol; especially, ethane-1,2-diol. This compound is used as an antifreeze in the cooling system of automobiles, and is toxic.

glycolacria Raised concentration of glucose in tears as a consequence of hyperglycemia.

glycolaldehyde $CH_2OH-CHO$. A highly reactive aldehyde, the simplest hydroxy aldehyde. Its adduct with thiamine pyrophosphate ("active glycolaldehyde") is an intermediate in the enzymatic transfer of C_2-units between sugar phosphates catalyzed by transketolase. Also called *glycolic aldehyde*.

glycolic acid $HO-CH_2-COOH$. 2-Hydroxyacetic acid.

glycolic aldehyde GLYCOLALDEHYDE.

glycolipid Any lipid which contains a carbohydrate group.

    blood group A glycolipid A ANTIGEN.

    blood group B glycolipid B ANTIGEN.

glycolysis [GLYCO- + LYSIS] The breakdown of carbohydrate, such as glycogen, to a simpler compound, such as pyruvate. This process does not require oxygen, but in order to regenerate NAD^+ used during glycolysis, the end-product has also to serve as a hydrogen acceptor. A variety of substances, such as lactate, ethanol and carbon dioxide, succinate, and propionate are thus formed. This overall sequence forms the basis of many industrially important fermentations. Adjective: glycolytic.

glycolytic Concerned with glycolysis, as an enzyme catalyzing one of the steps of glycolysis.

glyconeogenesis The formation of glycogen or other carbohydrate from noncarbohydrate sources, such as lactic acid or some amino acids derived from the breakdown of protein.

glycopenia [GLYCO- + -PENIA] A condition marked by a lower-than-normal concentration of sugar in the blood and tissues.

glycopeptide A compound of a peptide and a carbohydrate. Such compounds are formed by the partial hydrolysis of glycoproteins.

glycopexia The incorporation of sugars into tissues. Also called *glycopexis*.

glycopexic Of or relating to glycopexia.

glycopexis GLYCOPEXIA.

glycophorin A One of the major proteins of the erythrocyte cytoskeleton. It is a glycoprotein that contains 131 amino acids. Glycophorin spans the lipid bilayer of the membrane, with its carbohydrate-rich region on the exterior surface, its hydrophobic region with the lipid bilayer, and its interior C terminus attached to spectrin. Glycophorin is the MNSs blood group surface antigen. It is believed to constitute the anion channel.

glycopolyuria [GLYCO- + POLYURIA] Polyuria due to glycosuria. A seldom used term.

glycoprival Having to do with the removal of carbohydrates from the diet.

glycoprotein A conjugated protein containing one or more carbohydrate residues. The glycoproteins are important components of the plasma membrane, as well as of mucin and chondroitin.

alpha₁-acid glycoprotein A plasma protein conjugated with oligosaccharide elements which constitute approximately 40% of its weight. It migrates on electrophoresis with alpha globulins, and is elevated in inflammatory conditions of diverse etiologies. It is measured clinically by immunologic means and is considered an acute phase reactant, which rises within a day of inflammatory stimulus and declines within 4 or 5 days. Also called *orosomucoid glycoprotein*. Symbol: α_1 Gp

orosomucoid glycoprotein ALPHA₁-ACID GLYCOPROTEIN.

glycoptyalism GLYCOSIALIA.

glycoregulation The control of the processes associated with the metabolism of sugar.

glycoregulatory Relating to sugar regulation.

glycorrhachia [GLYCO- + Gk *rhach(is)* the back, spine, backbone + -IA] An abnormally high sugar content in the cerebrospinal fluid.

glycorrhea [GLYCO- + -RRHEA] Any sugar-containing discharge such as urine in diabetes mellitus.

glycosaminoglycan A polysaccharide that contains amino surgars or monosaccharides in which one of the —OH groups is replaced with an —NH₂ group. They occur either alone or in combination with proteins. Also called *mucopolysaccharide*.

glycosemia GLYCEMIA.

glycosialia [GLYCO- + SIAL- + -IA] The occurrence of glucose in the saliva, amounting to no more than 10–30 mg per 100 ml. Amounts occurring in excess of this almost certainly come from the diet. Also called *glycoptyalism*.

glycosialorrhea [GLYCO- + SIALO- + -RRHEA] A profuse flow of glucose-containing saliva.

glycosidase Any enzyme that catalyzes the hydrolysis of a glycoside.

glycoside Any substance consisting of an alcohol with the hydrogen of its hydroxyl group replaced by a glycosyl group. The alcohol can be released from it by acid hydrolysis, and is known as the aglycone.

cardiac glycoside Any of the glycosides of a cardenolide. They are found in plants and possess cardiotonic action.

N-glycoside A substance containing a glycosylated nitrogen atom, it is analogous with a glycoside but with nitrogen in place of oxygen. Nucleosides are *N*-glycosides.

glycostasis The maintenance of a constant sugar concentration in the body.

glycostatic Of or relating to glycostasis.

glycosuria [GLYCO- + *s* + -URIA] Excretion of abnormal amounts of glucose in urine. Normal persons may excrete up to 200 mg/24 hours of glucose and other sugars, and other substances with reducing activity, notably ascorbic acid. Glycosuria results either from excessively high plasma glucose levels or from reduced renal capacity to reabsorb glucose from normal plasma ultrafiltrate. Also called *glucosuria, saccharorrhea* (rarely used), *glycuresis, dextrosuria, saccharuria* (rarely used). Adjective: glycosuric.

alimentary glycosuria Glycosuria secondary to excess dietary sugar intake.

anxiety glycosuria Glycosuria resulting from emotional stress.

artificial glycosuria 1 The presence in the urine of sugar added inadvertently or else deliberately and surreptitiously by the patient. Also called *factitious glycosuria*. 2 The neurogenic glycosuria which results from irritation or damage to autonomic centers in the floor of the third or fourth ventricle of the brain, as in subarachnoid hemorrhage. An incorrect usage.

benign glycosuria RENAL GLYCOSURIA.

diabetic glycosuria Excessive excretion of glucose in the urine secondary to the hyperglycemia of diabetes mellitus.

epinephrine glycosuria Glycosuria secondary to secretion or administration of epinephrine, which causes hyperglycemia secondary to glycogenolysis.

factitious glycosuria ARTIFICIAL GLYCOSURIA.

hyperglycemic glycosuria Glycosuria due to hyperglycemia, as in diabetes mellitus or rapid intravenous injection of glucose.

nondiabetic glycosuria Glycosuria due to any cause other than diabetes mellitus including renal, stress, and alimentary glycosuria.

nonhyperglycemic glycosuria RENAL GLYCOSURIA.

normoglycemic glycosuria RENAL GLYCOSURIA.

phlorizin glycosuria Glycosuria produced in experimental animals by injection of phlorizin. The phlorizin decreases or abolishes renal tubular reabsorption of glucose.

pituitary glycosuria 1 Glycosuria associated with the hyperglycemia of acromegaly due to excessive growth hormone. An older term. 2 Glycosuria accompanying the hypercortisolism that occurs in the pituitary-dependent form of the Cushing syndrome.

renal glycosuria 1 The benign, usually asymptomatic presence of glucose in the urine when the blood glucose is normal, due to defective reabsorption of glucose by the proximal convoluted tubules. Familial renal glycosuria may be inherited as an autosomal recessive trait. 2 Glycosuria in the presence of normal blood glucose, due to defective reabsorption of glucose by diseased renal tubules, which may be part of the Fanconi syndrome, chronic renal failure, or due to effects on the renal tubules of toxins or poisons, such as the heavy metals, phlorizin, and carbon monoxide. Also called *benign glycosuria, nonhyperglycemic glycosuria, normoglycemic glycosuria*.

toxic glycosuria Excess amount of glucose in urine secondary to impairment of the reabsorptive ability of the proximal convoluted tubules by any toxic agent.

traumatic glycosuria Excess excretion of glucose in the urine following serious trauma. It is probably secondary to increased epinephrine secretion which causes hyperglycemia secondary to increased glycogenolysis.

glycosuric acid HOMOGENTISIC ACID.

glycosyl The group formed from a sugar, oligosaccharide, or polysaccharide by removal of its anomeric hydroxyl group.

glycosylation **1** Substitution with a glycosyl group. **2** The formation, by nonenzymatic means, of an irreversible bond between glucose and the N-terminal valine of the hemoglobin β chain to form a detectable, electrophoretically fast-moving hemoglobin, hemoglobin A_{1c}, the level of which rises in association with the raised blood glucose concentration in uncontrolled or poorly controlled diabetes mellitus.

glycosyltransferase Any of the enzymes that transfer glycosyl groups, including enzymes responsible for the synthesis of polysaccharides and those responsible for their phosphorolysis. Enzymes that hydrolyze polysaccharides are not so classed, although they transfer glycosyl groups onto water.

glycotaxis The distribution of sugars in the body by metabolic processes.

glycotropic Acting upon or influenced by the concentration of sugar.

glycuresis GLYCOSURIA.

glycyl- [GLYC- + -YL] A combining form indicating substitution with the acyl group NH_2—CH_2—CO—, derived from glycine.

glycylglycine $NH_3{}^+$—CH_2—CO—NH—CH_2—COO^-. The dipeptide formed by condensation of two molecules of glycine. It is often used as a buffer near pH 8.5.

Glycyphagus A genus of mites that infest stored food products and induce dermatitis among grocers and other food handlers. The reaction may be caused by the bites directly or may be a contact allergy. Also *Glyciphagus*.

Glycyrrhiza A genus of perennial herbs, native to Europe and North America, of the family Leguminosae (Fabaceae). The stolon and root of *Glycyrrhiza glabra* is the source of the glycyrrhiza (licorice) that is used pharmaceutically.

glycyrrhiza The dried roots of *Glycyrrhiza glabra*, used in extracts and syrups as a demulcent, expectorant, and flavoring vehicle for drugs. Also called *licorice, licorice root, liquorice, sweet root.*

glycyrrhizic acid $C_{42}H_{62}O_{16}$. A glycoside found in licorice root.

glycyrrhizin A white crystalline substance consisting of potassium and calcium salts of glycyrrhizic acid. It is the dominant constituent of licorice root. It is used as a demulcent and as an expectorant.

glyoxal CHO—CHO. A highly reactive dialdehyde.

glyoxalase The combination of two enzymes, lactoyl glutathione lyase and hydroxyacylglutathione hydrolase, whose activity interconverts methylglyoxal, CH_3—CO—CHO, and (R)-lactic acid, CH_3—CHOH—COOH, requiring glutathione as a cofactor.

glyoxalase I An obsolete term for LACTOYL-GLUTATHIONE LYASE.

glyoxalase II An obsolete term for HYDROXYACYLGLUTATHIONE HYDROLASE.

glyoxalic acid GLYOXYLIC ACID.

glyoxalin An outmoded term for IMIDAZOLE.

glyoxylate An anion, salt, or ester of glyoxylic acid.

glyoxylic acid CHO—COOH. 2-Oxoacetic acid. An intermediate in the glyoxylate pathway, by which plants and micro-

organisms, but not higher animals, can convert fat into carbohydrate. The aldehyde group is hydrated both in solution and in the solid form. Also called *glyoxalic acid.*

glyoxysome An organelle in the cells of plants and of some eukaryotic microorganisms that contains the enzymes necessary to catalyze the glyoxylate cycle.

glyphylline DYPHYLLINE.

Glyptocranium MASTOPHORA.

Glytheonate A proprietary name for theophylline sodium glycinate.

Gm See under GM ALLOTYPE.

gm Symbol for the unit, gram. An incorrect symbol.

Gmelin [Leopold *Gmelin*, German chemist, 1788–1853] Gmelin's reaction. See under TEST.

GMP guanosine monophosphate.

GN Symbol for the unit, giganewton.

gnashing Grinding or striking the teeth, usually as an accompaniment of conscious anger or other strongly felt emotion. See also BRUXISM.

gnat [Old English *gnætt*] Any of various small dipteran insects, especially pestiferous ones, such as blackflies, biting midges, or sandflies. • The term *gnat* also includes mosquitoes in British and South African usage, but not in U.S. usage.

buffalo gnat BLACKFLY.

eye gnat A fly of the genus *Hippelates*, especially *H. pusio.*

turkey gnat A blackfly of the species *Simulium meridionale* or other species that attack poultry.

gnath- GNATHO-.

gnathalgia [GNATH- + -ALGIA] GNATHODYNIA.

gnathic [GNATH- + -IC] Pertaining to the cheek or jaw, or to the alveolar process.

gnathion [New L, irreg. from Gk *gnathos* the jaw, esp. the lower jaw] A point on the surface of the mandible in the sagittal plane midway between the most anterior and the most inferior points on the chin.

gnathitis [GNATH- + -ITIS] Inflammation in the jaw. An imprecise and rarely used term.

gnatho- [Gk *gnathos* jaw, especially lower jaw] A combining form denoting the jaw. Also *gnath-.*

Gnathobdellidae A family of leeches (class Hirudinea) including the medically important genera *Hirudo* (medicinal leeches), *Haemadipsa* (terrestrial leeches), *Macrobdella* (horse leeches), *Theromyzon* (water-bird leeches), *Dinobdella* (cattle pharyngeal leeches), and *Hirudinaria* (Indian medicinal leeches).

gnathocephalus [GNATHO- + -CEPHALUS] A malformed embryo, fetus, or neonate lacking most of the head above the mandibular arch or the lower jaw.

gnathodynamics [GNATHO- + DYNAMICS] GNATHOLOGY.

gnathodynamometer [GNATHO- + DYNAMOMETER] An instrument for measuring forces exerted by the teeth. Also called *occlusometer.*

Bimeter gnathodynamometer A gnathodynamometer with a central bearing point. A proprietary name. Also called *Bimeter.*

gnathodynia [GNATH- + -ODYNIA] Pain in the jaw. Also called *gnathalgia.*

gnathography [GNATHO- + -GRAPHY] Recording with a gnathodynamometer.

gnathology [GNATHO- + -LOGY] The study of the forces exerted by the teeth, especially during mastication. Also called *gnathodynamics.*

gnathopagus parasiticus MYOGNATHUS.

gnathopalatoschisis [GNATHO- + PALATO- + Gk *schisis* a cleaving, division] A facial cleft in which the prepalate or premaxilla as well as the palate is cleft. In the usual cleft of jaw and palate, the cleft passes to either or both sides of the premaxilla.

gnathoplasty [GNATHO- + -PLASTY] Any plastic operation on either jaw.

gnathoplegia [GNATHO- + -PLEGIA] Paralysis of the muscles of the cheek.

gnathoschisis [GNATHO- + -SCHISIS] A cleft of the jaw, usually of the maxilla, thus the usual cleft of lip and jaw. Rarely the mandible and lower lip may show midline hypoplasia of sufficient degree to constitute a developmental defect.

gnathostatics [GNATHO- + Gk *statik(ē)*, fem. of *statikos* skilled in weighing; as substantive, statics, the science that treats bodies at rest; + *s*] A system of orthodontic diagnosis using cephalometry.

Gnathostoma [GNATHO- + Gk *stoma* the mouth] A genus of some 19 species of spiruroid nematodes (family Gnathostomatidae) parasitic in the stomach wall of cats, dogs, other predatory mammals, and occasionally humans. Members of the genus have heads with rows of cuticular spines, and multiple-host aquatic life cycles, involving copepods and a varied assortment of aquatic second intermediate hosts. They may also use a series of transport or paratenic hosts, leading to the final, carnivorous, mammalian host. In humans, they have been associated with a cutaneous larva migrans, especially in southeastern Asia. Also called *Cheiracanthus, Gnathostomum.*

Gnathostoma hispidum A species parasitic in the stomach of pigs, found in parts of Europe, Asia, and Africa. An incidental human parasite, it has been found in subcutaneous tissues where it causes creeping eruption, or cutaneous larva migrans. Parasites may also invade the lungs and the abdominal cavity.

Gnathostoma siamense *GNATHOSTOMA SPINIGERUM.*

Gnathostoma spinigerum A species found in cats, dogs, cattle, swine, wild carnivores, and sometimes in humans, particularly in the Far East. Transmitted by copepods and fish, human infections are usually limited to the skin but larvae have also been reported in the brain and eye. Also called *Gnathostoma siamense.*

Gnathostomata [pl. of GNATHOSTOMA] The group consisting of those vertebrates which have true jaws associated with the mouth. Compare AGNATHA.

gnathostomiasis [*Gnathostom(a)* + -IASIS] Infection with *Gnathostoma*, especially *G. spinigerum*. The larvae may affect the skin and subcutaneous tissues, and the adult worms sometimes cause intestinal infections.

Gnathostomum *GNATHOSTOMA.*

gnotobiology [Gk *gnōto(s)* known + BIOLOGY] The maintenance of laboratory animals all of whose microbiologic commensals are known, or which have been reared as germ-free. Also called *gnotobiotics.*

gnotobiosis The rearing of an organism under germ-free conditions or conditions of controlled contamination from microorganisms.

gnotobiota The microflora and microfauna of a gnotobiote.

gnotobiote [Gk *gnōto(s)* known + New L *biot(a)* (from Gk *biotos* life) the plant and animal life of a region] An animal reared so as to control the floral and faunal species found on and within its body.

gnotobiotic 1 Of or relating to gnotobiology. 2 Characteristic of a gnotobiote.

gnotobiotics GNOTOBIOLOGY.

gnotophoric Harboring a known flora and fauna on the body.

GnRF gonadotropin releasing factor.

GnRH gonadotropin releasing hormone.

goal 1 The end state toward which motivated action is directed, whether behavioral or ideational; any target for behavior or incentive for action. 2 In experimental usage, an end result, specified in advance by the experimenter, the accomplishment of which completes a behavioral sequence.

goatpox An often fatal, cutaneous pox disease of goats, caused by the goat poxvirus *Capripoxvirus*. It is characterized by widespread skin lesions that progress from round red areas to edematous plaques and finally to dry hard scabs. Lesions occur mostly on the ears and muzzle and can extend to the lungs. The disease is confined to Africa, Asia, and southeastern parts of Europe. Also called *variola caprina.*

Godélier [Charles Pierre *Godélier*, French physician, 1813–1877] See under LAW.

godet [French, a drinking cup without foot or handle] SCUTULUM.

Godman [John Davidson *Godman*, U.S. anatomist, 1794–1830] See under FASCIA.

Godtfredsen [Erik *Godtfredsen*, Danish radiologist, flourished 20th century] See under SYNDROME.

Goeckerman [William Henry *Goeckerman*, U.S. dermatologist, 1884–1954] See under TREATMENT.

Goethe [Johann Wolfgang von *Goethe*, German writer, statesman, and scientist, 1749–1832] 1 See under BONE. 2 Goethe's bone. See under OS INCISIVUM.

Goetsch [Emil *Goetsch*, U.S. physician, born 1883] Goetsch's test. See under REACTION.

Gofman [Moses *Gofman*, German physician, born 1897] See under TEST.

Goggia [Carlo Paolo *Goggia*, Italian physician, flourished 20th century] See under SIGN.

goggles Protective eyewear worn like spectacles to protect the eyes against occupational hazards such as particles flying from a lathe, molten metal, chemical splash, dust, gases, and radiation from welding or lasers.

plethysmographic goggles A device apposed to the facial contours sufficiently snugly as to permit measurement of volume changes in the eye and orbit by means of fluid linkage to a measuring system.

goiter [French *goitre* (from L *guttur* the throat) goiter] Any diffuse or nodular enlargement or swelling of the thyroid gland, often visible as a prominence in the lower anterior neck. Also called *struma, big neck* (popular), *Derbyshire neck* (popular), *Nithsdale neck* (popular), *thyroncus* (rarely used), *thyromegaly.* Adjective: strumous.

aberrant goiter Goiter affecting an ectopic or supernumerary thyroid gland, usually in the anterior and superior mediastinum.

adenomatous goiter NODULAR GOITER.

adolescent goiter Idiopathic generalized enlargement of the thyroid gland, often transient, usually seen in pubescent girls.

amyloid goiter Enlargement of the thyroid gland occurring rarely as a concomitant of amyloidosis.

Basedow's goiter A diffuse nontoxic goiter that becomes toxic or hyperfunctional after iodine administration.

cabbage goiter Diet-induced goiter caused by the goitrogenic substances contained in cabbage and related plants.

colloid goiter A diffuse enlargement of the thyroid gland caused by greatly distended, colloid-filled follicles. This is the typical form of endemic goiter seen in areas of iodine deficiency. Also called *follicular goiter, parenchymatous goiter, struma colloides, struma parenchymatosa, struma follicularis, struma gelatinosa, adenoma gelatinosum.*

congenital goiter Goiter present in the neonate or due to heritable deficiency of one of several enzymes involved in the biosynthesis of thyroid hormone. There is subnormal thyroid hormone secretion, excessive pituitary secretion of thyrotropin, and consequent hypertrophy of the thyroid gland.

cyanide goiter   Goiter experimentally induced in animals by administration of thiocyanate, which blocks the production of thyroid hormones, thus inducing the pituitary gland to increase production of thyroid stimulating hormone. If prolonged, this condition results in enlargement of the thyroid.

cystic goiter   Any enlarged thyroid gland that contains cysts, whether related to colloid or mucoid degeneration or old hemorrhage.

diet-induced goiter   Any goiter induced by the goitrogenic substances contained in foodstuffs.

diffuse goiter   Uniform and symmetrical enlargement of the thyroid gland. A seldom used term.

diving goiter   A goiter, located at the level of the sternal notch, that is freely movable and thus may change its location from above to below the sternal notch. Also called *wandering goiter.*

endemic goiter   Goiter occurring in parts of the world where the iodine content of the diet is low, as in the Alps, the Andes, the Himalayas, and the Great Lakes region of North America. In some areas dietary goitrogens may also be operative, as in Africa and South America. Also called *nontoxic diffuse goiter.*

exophthalmic goiter   Goiter associated with proptosis of the eyeballs, as seen in Graves disease. Also called *Flajani's disease* (rarely used).

familial goiter   1 Goiter associated with heritable inborn errors of thyroid hormone biosynthesis. Also called *A familial goitrous hypothyroidism.*   2 Goiter afflicting extended families in a region where goiter is endemic. A popular usage.

familial goiter with deaf-mutism   Nerve-deafness associated with familial goiter which is inherited as an autosomal recessive defect. The basic thyroid defect may be a partial failure of the incorporation of iodide into organic hormones. The subjects are euthyroid. Also called *Pendred syndrome.*

fibrous goiter   An enlargement of the thyroid gland resulting from fibrous replacement of the parenchyma. An imprecise and seldom used term.

follicular goiter   COLLOID GOITER.

iatrogenic goiter   Goiter caused by medical intervention. It may result from iodine administration, as in Basedow's goiter, or from treatment with an antithyroid drug such as propyl-thiouracil.

intrathoracic goiter   A form of goiter that extends into the thoracic cavity, usually the superior and anterior mediastinum in proximity to the thymus or thymic remnant. Also called *plunging goiter, struma endothoracica.*

lingual goiter   A mass of ectopic thyroid tissue lying at the base of the tongue in the region from which the embryonic thyroglossal duct arose. Also called *struma lingualis, struma baseos linguae, struma baseous linguae.*

lymphadenoid goiter   HASHIMOTO'S DISEASE.

malignant goiter   An enlargement of the thyroid gland caused by a malignant neoplasm. An obsolete term.

multinodular goiter   Goiter characterized by the presence of numerous localized enlargements of various sizes, most often colloid nodules.

myxedematous goiter   Any goiter associated with severe hypothyroidism, congenital or acquired.

nodular goiter   The usual form of goiter, in which the enlarged gland has a nodular pattern due to the development of multiple, discrete foci of hyperplasia with interstitial fibrosis and sometimes calcification. Also called *adenomatous goiter.*

nontoxic goiter   Any goiter not associated with hyperthyroidism or thyrotoxicosis. There are two types, diffuse (endemic goiter) and nodular (nontoxic nodular goiter).

nontoxic diffuse goiter   ENDEMIC GOITER.

nontoxic nodular goiter   Nodular goiter occurring singly or multiply and unaccompanied by hyperthyroidism.

parenchymatous goiter   COLLOID GOITER.

perivascular goiter   A goiter which surrounds a large blood vessel such as the carotid artery. A seldom used term.

plunging goiter   INTRATHORACIC GOITER.

retrovascular goiter   A form of goiter in which a portion of thyroid tissue lies behind a major blood vessel. A seldom used term.

simple goiter   Goiter with normal thyroid function.

sporadic goiter   Goiter occurring spontaneously in individuals inhabiting regions where goiter is not endemic.

substernal goiter   Goiter affecting primarily the isthmus, with downward extension into the substernal region. Also called *substernal struma, retrosternal struma.*

suffocative goiter   A goiter so large or so placed as to impinge on the trachea, causing respiratory distress.

thoracic goiter   An enlargement of accessory or ectopic thyroid tissue in the superior mediastinum. Thryoid tissue, either coextensive with or separate from the normally located thyroid gland, may develop in the upper thorax in association with the thymus. It tends to become goitrous under conditions similar to those affecting thyroid tissue generally, as in dietary iodine lack.

toxic goiter   Goiter associated with hyperthyroidism and thyrotoxicosis. There are two types, diffuse (toxic diffuse goiter) and nodular (toxic nodular goiter).

toxic diffuse goiter   Diffuse, generalized enlargement of the thyroid, accompanied by hyperthyroidism and thyrotoxicosis and often with exophthalmos.

toxic nodular goiter   Nodular goiter, more often single than multiple, accompanied by hyperthyroidism and thyrotoxicosis and not usually associated with exophthalmos. Also called *Plummer's disease.*

vascular goiter   Thyroid enlargement with prominent vascular dilatation and congestion. A seldom used term. Also called *struma vasculosa.*

wandering goiter   DIVING GOITER.

goitre   A British spelling for GOITER.

goitrin C_5H_7NOS. A goitrogenic substance that is isolated from the seeds of such *Brassica* species as rutabagas and turnips.

goitrogen   [*goit(e)r* + *o* + -GEN]   Any goiter-producing substance, as contained in peanuts, turnips and rutabagas, thiourea and its derivatives, thionamides, aminoheterocyclic compounds, substituted phenols, thicyanate and perchlorate ions.

goitrogenic   [GOITROGEN + -IC]   Tending to produce goiter. Also *goitrogenous.*

goitrogenicity   The property of being goitrogenic; tendency to produce goiter.

goitrogenous   GOITROGENIC.

gold   Element number 79, having atomic weight 196.9665. It is a soft, heavy (specific gravity, 19.32), malleable and ductile yellow metal that does not tarnish in air. The sole stable isotope, gold 197, is found free and also combined in the lithosphere and is present in sea water in concentrations as high as 2 mg/ton. Eighteen radioactive isotopes are known. Gold is used in dentistry and in some pharmaceuticals. Symbol: Au

crystal gold   MAT GOLD.

crystalline gold   MAT GOLD.

direct gold   Gold used in particulate form, such as gold foil, mat gold, or powdered gold, for the restoration of teeth, as opposed to cast gold.

fibrous gold   GOLD FOIL. See under FOIL.

inlay gold   An alloy of which the principal ingredient is gold, used in cast restorations.

mat gold   A noncohesive type of pure gold made by electrodeposition. Also called *crystal gold, crystalline gold, sponge gold.*

powdered gold Pure gold in granule form, used in combination with gold foil.

radioactive gold Any of the 25 radioactive isotopes of gold, ranging in atomic mass from 185 to 203 and having half-lives from 0.44 millisecond to 183 days. Also called *radiogold*.

sponge gold MAT GOLD.

white gold An alloy of which the principal ingredient is gold and which is given a silvery appearance by its high palladium content. It is harder than the usual (yellow) gold alloy.

gold 198 A radioactive isotope of gold, emitting beta and gamma radiation. In years past, it was used in a colloid preparation for liver imaging but has been replaced by technetium 99m agents. Intracavitary injection of a colloidal preparation of gold 198 has been used for treatment of peritoneal and pleural effusions. Interstitial implantation of gold 198 seeds or wires is used in tumor therapy. Physical half-life is 2.7 days. Symbol: ^{198}Au

Goldberg [Minnie Berelson *Goldberg*, U.S. physician, born 1900] Goldberg-Maxwell syndrome. See under TESTICULAR FEMINIZATION.

Goldberger [Joseph *Goldberger*, U.S. physician, 1874–1929] Anderson and Goldberger test. See under TEST.

Goldblatt [Harry *Goldblatt*, U.S. pathologist, 1891–1977] **1** See under KIDNEY, CLAMP. **2** Goldblatt phenomenon. See under HYPERTENSION.

Golden [William Wolfe *Golden*, U.S. physician, 1866–1929] See under SIGN.

Goldenhar [Maurice *Goldenhar*, Swiss physician, flourished mid-20th century] Goldenhar syndrome. See under OCULOAURICULOVERTEBRAL DYSPLASIA.

Goldent A type of pure gold consisting of powdered gold in small envelopes of gold foil. A proprietary name.

Goldflam [Samuel Valfovish *Goldflam*, Polish neurologist, 1852–1932] Hoppe-Goldflam syndrome, Erb-Goldflam syndrome, Erb-Oppenheim-Goldflam syndrome, Goldflam's disease, Goldflam-Erb disease, Erb-Goldflam disease. See under MYASTHENIA GRAVIS.

Goldman [Henry M. *Goldman*, U.S. periodontist, born 1911] Goldman-Fox knife. See under KNIFE.

Goldmann [Hans *Goldmann*, Swiss ophthalmologist, born 1899] See under TONOMETER.

Goldscheider [Johann Karl August Eugen Alfred *Goldscheider*, German physician, 1858–1935] Goldscheider's percussion. See under THRESHOLD PERCUSSION.

gold sodium thiomalate AUROTHIOMALATE DISODIUM.

Goldstein [Eugen *Goldstein*, German physicist, 1850–1930] See under RAYS.

Goldstein [Hyman Isaac *Goldstein*, U.S. physician, 1887–1954] **1** See under HEMATEMESIS, HEMOPTYSIS, SIGN. **2** Goldstein's disease. See under HEREDITARY HEMORRHAGIC TELANGIECTASIA.

Goldstein [Kurt *Goldstein*, German-born U.S. psychologist, 1878–1965] **1** Goldstein syndrome. See under ACQUIRED CEREBELLAR SYNDROME. **2** See under CLASSIFICATION. **3** Goldstein-Reichmann syndrome. See under ACQUIRED CEREBELLAR SYNDROME. **4** Goldstein-Scheerer tests for brain damage. See under TEST. **5** Weigl-Goldstein-Scheerer test. See under TEST.

gold thioglucose An insoluble colloidal gold compound, used in the treatment of rheumatoid arthritis.

gold thiomalate A soluble gold compound, used in the treatment of rheumatoid arthritis.

goldthread COPTIS.

Goldthwait [Joe Ernest *Goldthwait*, U.S. surgeon, 1866–1961]

Goldthwait symptom, Goldthwait's test. See under SIGN.

gold toning The optimal step in the silver impregnation techniques for reticulin, fungi, and axons, using gold chloride to provide a completely permanent preparation with a neutral black color of high density. Also called *aftergilding*.

Golé [L. *Golé*, French physician, flourished 20th century] Touraine-Solente-Golé syndrome. See under PACHYDERMOPERIOSTOSIS.

Golgi [Camillo *Golgi*, Italian histologist, 1843–1926] **1** Golgi type I neurons. See under NEURON. **2** Golgi type II neurons. See under NEURON. **3** Apparatus of Golgi-Rezzonico. See under APPARATUS. **4** See under LAW, METHOD. **5** Cox modification of Golgi's corrosive sublimate method. See under METHOD. **6** Golgi complex. See under APPARATUS. **7** Golgi body. See under DICTYOSOME. **8** Golgi-Mazzoni corpuscles. See under GOLGI-MAZZONI ENDINGS. **9** Golgi cisternae. See under CISTERNA. **10** Golgi-Rezzonico spiral. See under SPIRAL. **11** Holmgren-Golgi canals. See under ENDOPLASMIC RETICULUM. **12** Golgi cells. See under GOLGI TYPE I OR TYPE II NEURON. **13** Threads of Rezzonico-Golgi. See under THREAD. **14** See under THEORY, ZONE.

golgiokinesis [*Golgi (apparatus)* + *o* + KINESIS] The process of division of the Golgi apparatus, and its distribution to daughter cells during mitosis.

golgiosome DICTYOSOME.

Goll [Friedrich *Goll*, Swiss anatomist, 1829–1903] **1** Goll's fibers. See under FIBER. **2** Nucleus of Goll's column. See under NUCLEUS GRACILIS. **3** Column of Goll, fasciculus gracilis Golli, fasciculus of Goll, tract of Goll. See under FASCICULUS GRACILIS MEDULLAE SPINALIS. **4** Tract of Goll. See under COLUMNA POSTEROMEDIANA.

Goltz [Friedrich Leopold *Goltz*, German physiologist, 1834–1902] See under EXPERIMENT, REFLEX.

Goltz [Robert William *Goltz*, U.S. physician, born 1923] **1** Gorlin-Goltz syndrome. See under BASAL CELL NEVUS SYNDROME. **2** Goltz syndrome. See under FOCAL DERMAL HYPOPLASIA.

Gombault [François Alexis Albert *Gombault*, French neurologist, 1844–1904] **1** Tract of Philippe-Gombault, triangular tract of Philippe-Gombault, Gombault-Philippe triangle. See under FASCICULUS TRIANGULARIS. **2** Gombault's degeneration, Gombault's neuritis. See under HEREDITARY HYPERTROPHIC INTERSTITIAL NEUROPATHY.

gomitoli [Italian, pl. of *gomitolo* a coil or ball of thread] A network of specialized capillaries in the hypothalamic-hypophysial portal venous system of the infundibular stalk that envelops the terminal anteriolar branches of the superior hypophyseal arteries and empties into the hypophysial portal veins. It is often associated with the pathogenesis of the Sheehan's syndrome.

Gomori [George *Gomori*, Hungarian-born U.S. pathologist, 1904–1957] Gomori stain. See under METHOD.

Gompertz [Benjamin *Gompertz*, English mathematician, 1779–1865] **1** See under EQUATION, LAW. **2** Gompertz curve. See under GROWTH CURVE.

gomphiasis [Gk *gomphi(os)* a molar + -ASIS] **1** An outmoded term for TOOTHACHE. **2** Looseness of teeth. An outmoded term.

gomphosis [Gk *gomph(os)* nail, peg, pin + -OSIS] [NA] A type of fibrous joint in which the roots of teeth are fixed in sockets in the mandible and the maxilla by the periodontal ligament. Also called *peg-and-socket joint, socket joint of tooth, clavation, incuneation, peg-and-socket suture*.

gon The German term for GRADE.

gon-[1] [Gk *gony* (genitive *gonatos*) knee] A combining form denoting the knee. Also *gony-*.

gon-² GONO-.

gonacratia [GON-² + Gk *akrateia* (early form of *akrasia*) incontinence] SPERMATORRHEA.

gonad [New L, from Gk *gonē* (pl. *gonades*; from root *genō* of *gignesthai* to become, be born) seed, offspring, race, birth, womb] A structure capable of producing a gamete; testis or ovary. Adjective: gonadal.

female gonad OVARIUM.

indifferent gonad An undifferentiated gonad in the embryo, which has not acquired the characteristics of an ovary or a testis.

male gonad The testis.

primitive gonad An often undifferentiated anlage in an early embryo, destined to become either a testis or an ovary.

streak gonad An undeveloped gonadal structure located in the broad ligament in close proximity to the fallopian tube. It is characteristically seen in individuals with Turner syndrome, with XO genotype, in which the phenotypic development is female. It is composed of whorled connective tissue stroma with no germinal or secretory cells. The etiology is unclear, as mice with an XO genotype possess morphologically normal ovaries and may have definite, if limited, fertility.

third gonad The adrenal cortex. It has been called an additional or third gonad because it secretes sex hormones, or androstenedione, which may exert androgenic effects directly or by conversion to testosterone, and which is also peripherally converted to estrone/estradiol which exert estrogenic effects. A seldom used term.

gonadal Of or relating to a gonad. Also *gonadial.*

gonadectomize [GONAD + -*ectom(y)* + -IZE] To remove one or both gonads from surgically.

gonadectomy [GONAD + -ECTOMY] The surgical removal of one or both gonads.

gonadial GONADAL.

gonadoblastoma An ovarian or testicular tumor composed of large germ cells similar to those of seminoma and dysgerminoma and small cells resembling immature Sertoli and granulosa cells. The stroma may contain Leydig cells. The tumor almost always arises in those with dysgenetic gonads. Most subjects are phenotypic females who have a Y chromosome. Also called *dysgenetic gonadoma.*

gonadocentric Focused on the genitals, as in adolescent and adult sexuality when genital primacy is attained.

gonadogenesis [GONAD + *o* + GENESIS] Embryonic development of the ovaries or testes according to the sex of the individual.

gonadoinhibitory [GONAD + *o* + INHIBITOR + -Y] Capable of inhibiting the activity of the testis or ovary.

gonadokinetic [GONAD + *o* + Gk *kinētik(os)* putting in motion, stirring up] Capable of stimulating the actions of the testis or ovary.

gonadoma [GONAD + -OMA] A tumor of a gonad.

dysgenetic gonadoma GONADOBLASTOMA.

gonadopathy [GONAD + *o* + -PATHY] A disease of the testis or ovary. A seldom used term.

gonadopause [GONAD + *o* + PAUSE] The physiologic loss of gonadal activity through the aging process.

gonadotherapy [GONAD + *o* + THERAPY] The therapeutic use of hormones produced by the gonads. Also called *gland treatment.*

gonadotrope 1 A gonadotropin-secreting cell of the anterior pituitary. Also called *gonadotroph.* 2 A gonadotropic substance. A rarely used term. 3 One who secretes pituitary gonadotropins excessively. An outmoded term.

gonadotroph GONADOTROPE.

gonadotrophic GONADOTROPIC.

gonadotrophin GONADOTROPIN.

luteotrophic gonadotrophin An outmoded term for PROLACTIN.

gonadotrophism An outmoded term for GONADOTROPISM.

gonadotropic Acting to stimulate the gonads: used especially of the hormones of the adenohypophysis and the placenta which regulate the structure, function, and development of the gonads. Also *gonadotrophic.*

gonadotropin [GONAD + *o* + *trop(ic)* + -IN] Any hormone acting to stimulate the gonads, regulate their development, structure, or hormone-secreting functions, or contribute to gametogenesis, as the follicle-stimulating hormone or luteinizing hormone of the pituitary and the chorionic gonadotropin secreted by the placenta. Also called *gonadotrophin, gonadotropic hormone.*

chorionic gonadotropin The gonadotropin synthesized and secreted by the placenta. The hormone is a glycopeptide having an α subunit virtually identical to those of luteinizing hormone and thyroid-stimulating hormone and a specific β subunit responsible for its gonadotropic activity. Its actions resemble those of luteinizing hormone. Presence of this hormone in urine in early pregnancy is the basis for most pregnancy tests. Human chorionic gonadotropin maintains the secretory integrity of the corpus luteum of pregnancy. The urinary preparation is used pharmaceutically to treat cryptorchidism and to induce ovulation in anovulatory women. The hormone is secreted in excess in hydatidiform mole, choriocarcinoma, and certain tumors of the testis. Chorionic gonadotropin from the urine of pregnant women and pregnant mares' serum is used in the treatment of hypogonadism. Also called *pregnant mares' serum hormone, prolan* (obsolete), *anterior-pituitary-like substance.* Abbreviation: CG

equine gonadotropin PREGNANT MARE SERUM GONADOTROPIN.

human chorionic gonadotropin See under CHORIONIC GONADOTROPIN. Abbreviation: HCG

human menopausal gonadotropin The gonadotropin isolated and concentrated from the urine of postmenopausal women. The pharmaceutical preparation is used to stimulate ovulation in infertile women.

pituitary gonadotropin A gonadotropin secreted by the pituitary, as distinguished from chorionic gonadotropin; follicle-stimulating hormone or luteinizing hormone.

pregnant mare serum gonadotropin A gonadotropin obtained from the serum of pregnant mares. It has a molecular weight of about 53 000 and contains a high concentration of carbohydrate and sialic acid. Also called *equine gonadotropin.* Abbreviation: PMSG

gonadotropism [*gonadotrop(in)* + -ISM] Excessive pituitary secretion of gonadotropin. An outmoded term. Also called *gonadotrophism.*

gonaduct Oviduct or seminal duct.

gonae GENITALIA.

gonagra [GON-¹ + -AGRA] Acute pain in the knee, as in gout of the knee. An obsolete term.

gonalgia [GON-¹ + -ALGIA] Pain in the knee. An obsolete term.

gonangiectomy [GON-² + ANGI- + -ECTOMY] VASECTOMY.

gonapophysis (*plural* gonapophyses) A tubular outgrowth of the medial border of the coxite of the insect gonopod, an abdominal appendage that forms the external genitalia of insects.

gonarthritis [GON-¹ + ARTHRITIS] Arthritis of the knee. An obsolete term.

gonarthrocace [GON-¹ + ARTHRO- + Gk *kak(os)* bad] Tuberculosis of the knee. An obsolete term.

gonarthromeningitis [GON-¹ + ARTHRO- + MENINGITIS] Synovitis of the knee. An obsolete term.

gonarthrosis Arthritis of the knee.

gonarthrotomy An operative opening into the knee.

gonatocele [Gk *gonato(s)*, gen. of *gony* the knee, + -CELE¹] A tumor of the knee. An obsolete term.

Gonderia annulata THEILERIA ANNULATA.

gonecyst An obsolete term for VESICULA SEMINALIS.

gonecystis An obsolete term for VESICULA SEMINALIS.

gonecystitis [Gk *goné* seed + CYSTITIS] Inflammation of the seminal vesicles.

gonecystolith [Gk *goné* seed + CYSTO- + Gk *lith(os)* stone] A calculus or mass in a seminal vesicle.

gonecystopyosis [Gk *goné* seed + CYSTO- + PYOSIS] The formation and discharge of pus from a seminal vesicle.

goneitis GONITIS.

gonepoiesis [Gk *goné* seed + -POIESIS] The formation of semen. An obsolete term. Also called *gonopoiesis*.

gonepoietic Pertaining to gonepoiesis. An obsolete term. Also *gonopoietic*.

Gongylonema [Gk *gongylo(s)* round, spherical + *néma* thread, tissue] A genus of nematodes of the superfamily Spiruroidea, family Gongylonematidae (or the related family Spiruridae). They are characterized by possession of scattered cuticular plaques, especially over the anterior half of the worm. A number of species are known, several of which infect domestic animals and birds. Transmission is via various insects.

Gongylonema ingluvicola A species found in the esophagus, crop, and proventriculus of chickens, turkeys, and quail. Transmitted by species of infected beetles, it tunnels into the crop wall but causes little disease in the host.

Gongylonema neoplasticum A species found in the tongue, esophagus, and stomach of rodents, transmitted by cockroaches. Experimental infections have been produced in rabbits, sheep, and other mammals by using various beetles, earwigs, and fleas, as well as roaches. The lesions produced by these worms have been associated with neoplasms in the stomach and esophagus of rats. Also called *Spiroptera neoplastica*.

Gongylonema pulchrum A cosmopolitan species of gullet worm found in the esophageal mucosa and rumen of wild and domestic ruminants, and also in bears, pigs, and humans. It is transmitted by coprophagous beetles. Human infections are usually caused by immature worms. Also called *Gongylonema scutatum*.

Gongylonema scutatum GONGYLONEMA PULCHRUM.

gongylonemiasis Infection by nematode worms of the genus *Gongylonema*. It is characterized by little or no reaction by the host.

gonia Plural of GONION.

gonial Pertaining to the gonion.

gonic [GON-² + -IC] **1** Referring to reproduction. An obsolete term. **2** Referring to semen.

gonidia Plural of GONIDIUM.

gonidiospore [*gonidi(um)* + *o* + SPORE] An older term for CONIDIUM.

gonidium [GON-² + -IDIUM] (*plural* gonidia) **1** The algal component of a lichen. An older term. **2** An endospore of a fungus. **3** One of the motile reproductive cells of certain nitrogen-fixing bacteria. Adjective: gonidial.

Gonin [Jules *Gonin*, Swiss ophthalmologist, 1870–1935] See under OPERATION.

gonio- [Gk *gónia* corner, angle] A combining form meaning angle.

Goniobasis [GONIO- + Gk *basis* a stepping, walk, pedestal] A genus of freshwater operculated snails in the prosobranch family Pleuroceridae. A number of trematode flukes utilize snails of this genus as a first intermediate host. *G. livescens* is the molluscan host for the pronocephalid *Macrovestibulum obtusicaulum* of turtles, the heterophyid *Apophallus venustus* of birds, and the azygiid *Proterometra dickermani*, a most unusual neotenic digenean having this snail as its only known host. A similar array of flukes develop in *G. plicifera silicula* and *G. proxima*.

Goniobasis silicula A species of snail that serves as an intermediate host of the fluke *Nanophyetus salmincola*, a parasite of foxes, dogs, and cats in the northwestern United States. This parasite, known as the salmon-poisoning fluke, serves as a vector for *Neorickettsia helminthoeca*, which is highly toxic to canine hosts that feed on raw salmon that are host to infected flukes. The same snail species also harbors the allocreadid fluke *Plagioporus silicula*, which infects fishes, and the heterophyid *Metagonimoides oregonensis*, which infects raccoons.

goniocraniometry The measurement of cranial angles.

goniolens [GONIO- + LENS] A contact lens that modifies the corneal refraction of light so as to permit observation of the details of the peripheral angle of the anterior chamber, evaluation of which is particularly important in glaucoma.

gonioma [GON-² + *i* + -OMA] A tumor of germ cells.

goniometer [GONIO- + -METER] An instrument used to measure angles. In medicine, it is often used to test the range of flexion extension in joints.

finger goniometer An instrument for measuring flexion and extension at interphalangeal joints.

gonion [New L, irreg. from Gk *gónia* corner, angle] A craniometric point situated at the apex of the angle of the mandible formed by the body and the ramus.

goniophotography The technique of obtaining pictures of the angle of the anterior chamber of the eye.

gonioprism / Allen gonioprism A four-sided contact lens used for microscopic viewing of the internal aspect of the peripheral circumference of the anterior chamber of the eye.

goniopuncture [GONIO- + PUNCTURE] Perforation from within the trabecular meshwork and scleral structures to create a fistula leading from the anterior chamber to the subconjunctival space, particularly useful in the management of congenital glaucoma.

gonioscope [GONIO- + -SCOPE] A device for viewing the anterior chamber angle of the eye *in vivo*.

gonioscopy [GONIO- + -SCOPY] Examination of the anterior chamber angle of the eye by means of a gonioscope.

goniosynechia [GONIO- + SYNECHIA] Adhesion between the peripheral iris and the trabecular meshwork.

goniotomy [GONIO- + -TOMY] A wide incision of the trabecular meshwork, performed by approaching from within the eye via a puncture entering the opposite limbal area, useful in management of congenital glaucoma. Also called *Barkan's operation*.

gonitis [Gk *gon(y)* knee + -ITIS] An inflammation of the knee. Also called *goneitis*.

fungous gonitis An inflammation of the knee characterized by a marked thickening of the synovium.

gonitis tuberculosa A tuberculous inflammation of the knee.

gono- [Gk *goné* seed] A combining form meaning seed, semen. Also *gon-²*.

gonoblast [GONO- + -BLAST] Any cell or bud involved in reproduction.

gonoblennorrhea [GONO- + BLENNORRHEA] Gonorrheal infection of the surface of the eye.

gonocampsis A fixed flexion deformity of the knee.

gonocele [GONO- + -CELE¹] A cystic distention of the spermatic cord.

gonochorism [GONO- + Gk *chōrism(os)* a separating, dividing] The divergence of the structure of the gonads to male or female type at the time of sexual differentiation.

gonocide GONOCOCCOCIDE.

gonococcal **1** Pertaining to the presence of gonorrhea. **2** Of or relating to *Neisseria gonorrhoeae*.

gonococcemia [*gonococc(us)* + -EMIA] The presence of gonococci in the bloodstream.

gonococci Plural of GONOCOCCUS.

gonococcide GONOCOCCOCIDE.

gonococcocide [*Gonococc(us)* + *o* + -CIDE] A substance capable of killing the *Neisseria gonorrhoeae*. Also called *gonococcide, gonocide*. Adjective: gonococcocidal.

gonococcus [GONO- + L *coccus* the kermes berry, scarlet berry] (*plural* gonococci) An organism of the species *Neisseria gonorrhoeae*.

gonocyte [GONO- + -CYTE] **1** GERM CELL. **2** A secondary oocyte or secondary spermatocyte.

male gonocyte SPERMATOGONIUM.

primordial gonocyte ARCHIGONOCYTE.

gonocytoma [*gonocyt(e)* + -OMA] A tumor of germ cells.

gonoducts [GONO- + *ducts*, pl. of DUCT] The mesonephric and paramesonephric ducts considered together.

gonoid [GON-² + -OID] Resembling semen.

gonomery [GONO- + -*mer(e)* + -Y] A condition in which paternal and maternal chromosomes remain in separate groups and do not completely fuse. In birds, cross-breeding between two species renders the female hybrid offspring sterile but the males are fertile.

gononephrotome [GONO- + NEPHROTOME] The mass of secondary segmental mesoderm that in the embryo gives rise to the gonad and nephrotome.

gonophore [GONO- + -PHORE] An accessory reproductive organ utilized in addition to the gonads, such as the uterus or seminal vesicles. A seldom used term.

gonopod GONOPODIUM.

gonopodium **1** A modified anal fin which serves as a copulatory organ in fish of the family Poeciliidae, guiding spermatozoa from the vent of the male to the vent of the female for internal fertilization. **2** A clasper of a male insect or a myriapod. For defs. 1 and 2 also called *gonopod*.

gonopoiesis GONEPOIESIS.

gonopoietic GONEPOIETIC.

gonorrhea [GONO- + -RRHEA] Infection of the genitourinary organs and more rarely of the rectum, pharynx, or conjunctiva caused by *Neisseria gonorrhoeae*. The disease, detectable three to five days after sexual contact with an infected partner, is usually characterized by a purulent urethral discharge in men. Symptoms are less prominent in women. Complications include salpingitis, chronic pelvic inflammatory disease with sterility, and hematogenous dissemination producing arthritis and rash. Also called *gonococcal disease, blennorrhagia, clap* (popular), *purgación (South American Spanish)*.

gonorrheal Of or relating to gonorrhea. Also *blennorrhagic*.

gonorrhoea A British spelling for GONORRHEA.

gonoscheocele [GON-² + OSCHEO- + -CELE¹] Testicular swelling due to excessive seminal fluid.

gonosome **1** An obsolete term for GAMETE. **2** An outmoded term for SEX CHROMOSOME.

gonotokont [GONO- + Gk *tokōn*, gen. *tokōntos*, pres. part of *tokan* to be nearing childbirth] AUXOCYTE.

gonotome [GONO- + -TOME] That part of the secondary segmental mesoderm in the embryo which gives rise to the gonad.

gonotoxemia A toxic state caused by the presence in blood of substances derived from *Neisseria gonorrhoeae*.

gonotyl [GONO- + Gk *tyl(os)* knob, callus, penis] A retractile suckerlike structure that encloses the genital pore of heterophyid flukes either within or alongside the acetabulum. Possession of this structure is an important defining characteristic of the trematode family Heterophyidae.

gony- GON-¹.

-gony [Gk *gonos* or *gonē* (from *geno*, root of *gignesthai* to be, become, be born) that which is begotten, offspring, a race, family; also (*gonē*) seed] A combining form denoting reproduction.

gonyalgia paresthetica Pain and paresthesia occurring in the distribution of the infrapatellar branch of the saphenous nerve.

Gonyaulax A genus of marine dinoflagellates (order Dinoflagellida, class Phytomastigophorea) known to cause paralytic shellfish poisoning. These protozoans can synthesize and secrete a toxin that is often fatal to humans who eat filter-feeding shellfish (mussels, clams, oysters, scallops) that have filtered out the flagellates from the water. The flagellates are not destroyed by the shellfish but continue to produce their toxin in an unusual form of protective symbiosis. Species of importance in causing paralytic shellfish poisoning include *G. catenella* (Pacific coast of North America), *G. tamarensis* (North Atlantic coastlines), *G. acatenella* (Pacific coast, British Columbia), *G. polyhedra* (Pacific coast, southern California).

gonycampsis An abnormal curvature of the knee.

gonycrotesis GENU VALGUM.

gonyectyposis GENU VARUM.

gonyocele [GONY- + *o* + -CELE²] Effusion of the knee. An obsolete term.

gonyoncus A tumorous swelling of the knee.

Gooch [Frank Austin *Gooch*, U.S. chemist, 1852–1929] See under FILTER.

Good [R. A. *Good*, U.S. pediatrician, born 1922] Good syndrome. See under IMMUNODEFICIENCY WITH THYMOMA.

Goodell [William *Goodell*, U. S. gynecologist, 1829–1894] Goodell's law. See under SIGN.

Goodenough [Florence Laura *Goodenough*, U.S. psychologist, born 1886] Goodenough draw-a-man test. See under GOODENOUGH TEST.

goodness of fit The extent of agreement between a set of observed values and those predicted by a mathematical function or a statistical model. Goodness of fit is measured by some criterion involving minimizing the sum of the squared differences between the observed and the predicted values.

Goodpasture [Ernest William *Goodpasture*, U.S. pathologist, 1886–1960] **1** See under STAIN, SYNDROME. **2** Goodpasture's polychrome stain. See under GOODPASTURE STAIN FOR GRAM-NEGATIVE BACTERIA.

Goormaghtigh [Norbert *Goormaghtigh*, Belgian physicist, 1890–1960] **1** Apparatus of Goormaghtigh. See under JUXTAGLOMERULAR APPARATUS. **2** Goormaghtigh cells. **3** Goormaghtigh cells. See under JUXTAGLOMERULAR CELLS.

gooseflesh GOOSE FLESH. See under FLESH.

Gopalan [C. *Gopalan*, Indian biochemist, flourished 20th century] Gopalan syndrome. See under BURNING FEET SYNDROME.

Gordan [Gilbert S. *Gordan*, U.S. physician, born 1916] Gordan-Overstreet syndrome. See under SYNDROME.

Gordiacea NEMATOMORPHA.

Gordius A genus of the phylum Nematomorpha (or Gordiacea), the horsehair snakes, or horsehair worms. Adults are free-living, elongate, rather stiff-bodied aschelminths related to the nematodes. The larval forms undergo nearly all of their growth and development in the body cavity of an insect or other arthropod host. The fully developed larva leaves its host, usually killing it in the process, only when the host is in or near water.

Gordius aquaticus   A species sometimes found as a pseudoparasite in the human intestinal tract following ingestion of infected insects or drinking water containing infective larvae.

Gordius medinensis   DRACUNCULUS MEDINENSIS.

Gordius robustus   A species found as a pseudoparasite in human intestines and reported also in periorbital tissues and the urinary tract, probably as a result of ingesting water containing infective larvae.

Gordon [Alexander *Gordon*, Irish physician, 1818–1887]   See under SPLINT.

Gordon [Alfred *Gordon*, U.S. neurologist, 1874–1953]   **1** Gordon's test, Gordon sign. See under REFLEX.   **2** See under SIGN.

Gordon [Mervyn Henry *Gordon*, English bacteriologist, 1872–1953]   Gordon's biological test. See under TEST.

gorget [French (dim. of *gorge* throat), a plane for making hollow moldings]   A surgical instrument with a broad base that is used as a director for the insertion of a lithotome.

    probe gorget   A lithotome guide with a probe tip.

Gorgodera   A genus of trematodes of the family Gorgoderidae that are parasitic in the urinary bladder of frogs and toads. They have a complex cercarial form of the cysticercous type in which the xiphidiocercaria is enclosed in a greatly enlarged tail, and is activated by the presence of an appropriate second intermediate snail host, in which the cercaria encysts.

Gorlin [Richard *Gorlin*, U.S. cardiologist, born 1926]   See under FORMULA.

Gorlin [Robert James *Gorlin*, U.S. oral pathologist, born 1923]   **1** Gorlin-Chaudhry-Moss syndrome. See under SYNDROME.   **2** Gorlin-Goltz syndrome, Gorlin syndrome. See under BASAL CELL NEVUS SYNDROME.

gorondou   GOUNDOU.

Gosselin [Leon Athanase *Gosselin*, French surgeon, 1815–1887]   See under FRACTURE.

gossypol $C_{30}H_{30}O_8$. A sesquiterpene phenol that is a toxic principle found in cottonseed meal and cottonseed cake. It has been used in China as a male antifertility agent.

GOT   glutamate oxaloacetate transaminase (aspartate aminotransferase).

Göthlin [Gustaf *Göthlin*, Swedish physiologist, 1874–1949]   See under TEST.

Gottlieb [Bernhard *Gottlieb*, Austrian dentist, 1885–1950]   Gottlieb's cuticle. See under PRIMARY CUTICLE.

Gottron [Heinrich Adolf *Gottron*, German dermatologist, born 1890]   **1** See under SIGN.   **2** Gottron syndrome. See under PROGRESSIVE SYMMETRICAL VERRUCOUS ERYTHROKERATODERMA.

Gottschaldt [Kurt *Gottschaldt*, German psychologist, born 1902]   Gottschaldt figures. See under FIGURE.

Gottstein [Jacob *Gottstein*, German otologist, 1832–1895]   Gottstein's basal process. See under PROCESS.

gouge [Middle English *gowge*, from Old French *gouge*, from Vulgar L *gubia* for late L *gulbia* a hollow chisel]   A chisel-like surgical instrument with a handle and a blade that is U-shaped in cross section. It is designed to facilitate bone and cartilage removal.

    Kelley gouge   A surgical instrument with a handle and sharp blade designed to harvest a free graft of cartilage.

Gougerot [Henri *Gougerot*, French physician, 1881–1955]   **1** See under TRIAD.   **2** Gougerot-Carteaud syndrome. See under CONFLUENT AND RETICULATE PAPILLOMATOSIS.

Goulard [Thomas *Goulard*, French surgeon, 1720–1790]   See under LOTION.

Gould [Sir Alfred Pearce *Gould*, English surgeon, 1852–1922]   See under SUTURE.

Gould [George Milbry *Gould*, U.S. ophthalmologist and medical lexicographer, 1848–1922]   See under SIGN.

Gouley [John William Severin *Gouley*, U.S. surgeon, 1832–1920]   See under CATHETER.

goundou [French, from West African tongue]   A nasal osteoblastic periostitis, a sequel to yaws. It is characterized by purulent nasal discharge, headache, and painless symmetric nasal swellings. Orbital invasion and visual impairment may develop at a later stage. The condition occurs in West and Central Africa and in South America. A similar disease is found in the larger apes and chimpanzees. Also called *anákhré, dog nose, gorondou, gundo, henpue, henpuye.*

gourd [Middle English *gourde*, from Old French *gouorde* gourd, from L *cucurbita* gourd]   A fruit of certain plants in the Cucurbitaceae family that has a hard rind and is inedible when mature.

gout [French *goutte* (from L *gutta* a drop, akin to Gk *chytos* poured, made liquid) a drop, the gout]   Acute or chronic arthritis due to the presence of monosodium urate crystals in polymorphonuclear leukocytes within the joint space or as tophi. Also called *uratic arthritis, gouty arthritis, uarthritis, urarthritis.*

    abarticular gout   Gout involving extra-articular tissues. A seldom used term. Also called *irregular gout.*

    articular gout   Gout of a joint. Also called *regular gout.*

    calcium gout   The deposition of calcium in periarticular soft tissues. An imprecise and obsolete term.

    chalky gout   TOPHACEOUS GOUT.

    irregular gout   ABARTICULAR GOUT.

    juvenile gout   LESCH-NYHAN SYNDROME.

    latent gout   A condition, usually hyperuricemia, predisposing one to an attack of gout. Also called *masked gout.*

    lead gout   Gout associated with lead poisoning, specifically lead nephropathy. Also called *saturnine gout.*

    masked gout   LATENT GOUT.

    misplaced gout   A form of gout previously believed to consist of the disappearance of joint symptoms followed by constitutional symptoms. This concept of gout is no longer held. Also called *DaCosta's disease.*

    oxalic gout   Musculoskeletal pain associated with oxalosis.

    polyarticular gout   Gout occurring in multiple joints.

    primary gout   Gout occurring spontaneously and not induced by lead poisoning, myeloproliferative disease, or other states.

    regular gout   ARTICULAR GOUT.

    rheumatic gout   An imprecise term for POLYMYALGIA RHEUMATICA.

    saturnine gout   LEAD GOUT.

    secondary gout   Gout associated with hyperuricemia of nongenetic origin, such as a myeloproliferative disorder or diuretic therapy.

    tophaceous gout   Chronic gout associated with deposits of monosodium urate (tophi) either subcutaneously or in or near joints. Also called *chalky gout, urate thesaurismosis.*

    visceral gout   A disorder of poultry, characterized by a deposit of white material (uric acid crystals) over the surface of the abdominal viscera.

gouty [GOUT + -Y]   Pertaining to or having gout.

government / patient government   A situation, in a therapeutic community, in which the patients participate in the administration of their ward or unit in the hospital.

Gowers [Sir William Richard *Gowers*, English neurologist, 1845–1915]   **1** Gowers disease, Gowers syndrome. See under VASOVAGAL ATTACK.   **2** Panatrophy of Gowers. See under PANATROPHY.   **3** See under SIGN, PARAPLEGIA.   **4** Gowers contraction. See under FRONT TAP CONTRACTION.   **5** Fasciculus of Gowers. See under TRACTUS SPINOCEREBELLARIS VENTRALIS.

Goyrand [Jean Gaspar Blaise *Goyrand*, French surgeon, 1803–1866] **1** See under HERNIA. **2** Goyrand's injury. See under PULLED ELBOW.

GP **1** general practitioner. **2** general paresis.

G6PD glucose-6-phosphate dehydrogenase.

GPI gingival periodontal index.

gr Symbol for the unit, grain.

Grace Arthur [Mary *Grace Arthur*, U.S. psychologist, born 1883] Grace Arthur point scale. See under SCALE.

gracile [French (from L *gracilis* tall, slender), slender] Slender or lightly built.

gracilothalamic Denoting the projection from one gracile nucleus to the opposite nucleus ventralis posterolateralis of the thalamus.

grad. *gradatum* (L, by degrees).

g·rad Symbol for the unit, gram-rad.

gradatim Gradually.

grade [L *gradus* a step, degree] A unit of plane angle equal to 0.01 right angle; 0.005 π radian. Also called *gon (German usage)*. Symbol: ^{g}

Gradenigo [Giuseppe *Gradenigo*, Italian otorhinolaryngologist, 1859–1926] Gradenigo-Lannois syndrome. See under GRADENIGO SYNDROME.

gradient [L *gradiens*, gen. *gradientis*, pres. part. of *gradi* to step] The rate of change of pressure, oxygen tension, or other variable as a function of distance, time, or other continuously changing influence.

gradient of approach The changing strength of the attractiveness of a positive goal as it is approached, growing stronger as it is neared and marked by a measurable increase in effort.

atrioventricular gradient The difference, during diastole, between atrial and ventricular pressures.

gradient of avoidance The relative decrease in the attractiveness of a negative goal as it is neared; marked by a tendency to draw away from it.

axial gradient The rate of change of a variable with position along an axis.

concentration gradient The changing concentration of solute in solvent before equilibrium is reached, reflecting the effect of mass or solubility on dispersal in a confined system.

density gradient A column of liquid of gradually increasing density from top to bottom.

goal gradient The tendency for an experiemental animal to increase the vigor of responding as the goal of a task is neared, such as in maze-running, resulting in a performance that is faster and more free of error.

mitral gradient The pressure difference across the mitral valve during diastole.

physiologic gradient A regular quantitative change in a physiologic function.

proton gradient A higher concentration of protons on one side of the inner mitochondrial membrane as compared to the other side. The establishment of this gradient by transport stores free energy and the free energy of this gradient then drives the phosphorylation reaction. The proton gradient is essential to the chemiosmotic hypothesis.

gradient of response generalization In operant conditioning, in accordance with the principle of response generalization, the tendency for responses that are similar to the one originally conditioned to begin to appear when the animal is presented with the same stimulus, and the greater the degree of similarity, the more frequently will the stimulus elicit the response. The vigor or frequency of these responses may also be diminished in

a systematic way, according to the degree of their resemblance to the response originally conditioned.

gradient of stimulus generalization A variation observed after an experimental animal has learned a conditioned response and has also begun to make the conditioned response to other stimuli that resemble the conditioned stimulus: the strength or frequency of these generalized responses vary with the degree of apparent similarity to the original conditioned stimulus.

systolic gradient The pressure difference across a semilunar valve during systole.

temperature gradient Temperature difference divided by distance, expressed in kelvins per meter.

gradient of transfer In bacterial conjugation, the decreasing frequency of entry of a gene as its distance from the origin of entry increases.

triple descending gradient The normal contractile weave of the uterus during labor, consisting of an initial propagation of the contraction, the duration of the contraction, and the intensity or strength of the contraction.

venous pressure gradient The difference in pressure within the veins of the circulatory system between the capillaries and the right atrium (systemic circulation) or the left atrium (pulmonary circulation).

ventricular gradient The net difference in electrical activity between the algebraic sum of the area enclosed within the QRS complex and that within the T wave of the electrocardiogram.

vertical gradient A change in temperature or salinity or oxygen concentration from the surface of a body of water to a given depth.

graduate [Med L *graduat(us)*, past part. of *graduare* (from L *gradus* a step, degree) to graduate] A container, usually cylindrical and with a pouring lip, that is marked off in units of fluid volume and is used to contain, measure, and pour liquids.

graduated Marked with a scale by which measurements can be taken.

Graefe [Albrecht Friedrich Wilhelm Ernst von *Graefe*, German ophthalmologist, 1828–1870] **1** See under PHENOMENON, DISEASE, KNIFE, OPERATION, TEST. **2** Pseudo-Graefe sign. See under PSEUDO-GRAEFE PHENOMENON. **3** Von Graefe sign, Graefe sign. See under EYELID LAG. **4** Graefe spots. See under SPOT.

Graefenberg [Ernst *Graefenberg*, German gynecologist, active in the U.S., 1881–1957] See under RING.

Graffi [Arnold *Graffi*, German pathologist, born 1910] See under VIRUS.

graft

graft [Middle English *graffe*, from French *greffe* (from L *graphium* an iron pen or stylus) a branch or bud inserted into another plant] **1** Tissue, living or preserved, that is transferred from location to another on the same organism or from one organism to another. ● In strict usage, the term *graft* means a free graft. **2** To transfer such tissue.

accordion graft A full-thickness skin graft which is fenestrated with multiple slits to provide more extensive surface coverage.

activated graft A graft in which a nerve and blood supply have developed.

adrenal graft A procedure sometimes done experimentally after bilateral total adrenalectomy, in which a small piece of the patient's own adrenal is implanted subcutaneously in order to provide for continued secretion of adrenocorticotrophin.

allogeneic graft   ALLOGRAFT.

alloplast graft   A graft of an inert material.

animal graft   A graft from an animal to a human being. Also called *zoograft*.

anorganic bone graft   KIEL BONE GRAFT.

aortofemoral bypass graft   A conduit, usually composed of prosthetic material, that joins the aorta to the common femoral arteries in cases of aortoiliac occlusive disease. Such grafts are usually constructed to connect both common femoral arteries and thus have the configuration of an inverted Y.

aortorenal bypass graft   A conduit of autogenous vein or artery or of prosthetic material that links the aorta to the renal artery beyond a point of stenosis or occlusion. It is usually designed to correct inadequate arterial blood flow to a kidney.

arterial graft   An arterial segment that is used to replace a defect in another artery.

autochthonous graft   An older term for AUTOGRAFT.

autodermic graft   A skin autograft. An older term. Also called *autoepidermic graft* (older term).

autoepidermic graft   An older term for AUTODERMIC GRAFT.

autogenous graft   A graft from another part of the same individual, such as the implantation of bone marrow from the iliac crest to the mandible.

autologous graft   An older term for AUTOGRAFT.

autoplastic graft   An older term for AUTOGRAFT.

avascular graft   WHITE GRAFT.

axillobifemoral bypass graft   AXILLOFEMORAL BYPASS GRAFT.

axillofemoral bypass graft   An extra-anatomic bypass in which the axillary artery is used as the source for blood flow through a graft, usually of prosthetic material, to the common femoral artery. It is often used to bypass the site of aortoiliac occlusive disease in subjects who might not tolerate a direct surgical attack upon the aorta. Also called *axillobifemoral bypass graft*.

Blair-Brown graft   SPLIT-SKIN GRAFT.

blanket graft   A large sheet of split-skin graft, made by sewing several smaller sheets together edge to edge.

bone graft   A free graft composed of bone, with or without attached periosteum. Also called *bone implant, osseous graft.*

brephoplastic graft   BREPHOPLASTY.

bridge graft   INTERPOSITION GRAFT.

cable graft   A graft in which several small-caliber nerves are used to form a cable to bridge a gap in nerve anastomosis.

calibrated graft   A split-skin graft in which the thickness is measured in millimeters.

cantilever graft   A graft of bone, cartilage, or alloplastic material which is secured to the nasal bones or the frontal bone, and extends downward to support the tip of the nose.

cartilage graft   A graft of hyaline or elastic cartilage, with or without the attached perichondrium.

chessboard graft   POSTAGE STAMP GRAFT.

chondrocutaneous graft   A graft consisting of contiguous skin and cartilage, usually obtained from the ear.

chorioallantoic graft   A graft of cells, tissues, or parts of organs on the allantochorion of the chick embryo.

composite graft   Any graft, contiguous in nature, consisting of tissues of more than one type.

crossover bypass graft   An extra-anatomic vascular reconstruction, usually between the femoral vessels in both groins, performed to bypass unilateral iliac vessel occlusion.

cross-zygomaticus muscle graft   A graft used to restore animation to the angle of the mouth in unilateral facial nerve paralysis. The palmaris longus muscle and tendon are removed from the forearm, and the muscle is firmly sewn to the surface of the unparalyzed processus zygomaticus from which the pal-

maris longus muscle gains innervation. The palmaris tendon is passed through the substance of the upper lip and through a tendon sling suspended from the processus zygomaticus of the maxilla on the paralyzed side. The pull of the palmaris longus muscle is thus transmitted to the paralyzed side.

cutis graft   DERMAL GRAFT.

Davis graft   PINCH GRAFT.

delayed graft   **1** A skin graft which is elevated and then sutured back onto its donor area, where it remains for a time before being transferred.   **2** A split-skin graft which is applied to a surgically created raw surface one or more days after the excision which resulted in this recipient area.

derma-fat-fascia graft   A free graft consisting of dermis and the attached subjacent subcutaneous fat and fascia. Such a graft is sometimes inserted subcutaneously in a depressed area to fill out the contour.

dermal graft   A free graft consisting of part or all of the thickness of the dermis without any attached epidermis or subcutaneous fat. Also called *cutis graft, dermic graft, dermis graft.*

dermic graft   DERMAL GRAFT.

dermis graft   DERMAL GRAFT.

dermis-fat graft   A graft consisting of dermis and contiguous fat. Also called *dermis-fat composite graft.*

dermis-fat composite graft   DERMIS-FAT GRAFT.

diced cartilage grafts   Cartilage grafts, usually from the human rib, cut into many small pieces. Such grafts were once used by molding the pieces into the shape desired.

double-end graft   An incorrect term for TUBED FLAP.

Douglas graft   SIEVE GRAFT.

Dragstedt graft   A modified sieve graft.

epidermic graft   A very thin split-skin graft consisting of the epidermis but less than the usual amount of dermis. An old-fashioned misnomer.

Esser graft   INLAY GRAFT.

extracranial-intracranial bypass graft   The anastomosis of a branch of the external carotid artery, such as the superficial temporal artery, with an intracranial artery, such as the middle cerebral artery or one of its branches, in order to revascularize the intracranial artery. It is usually performed to relieve atherosclerotic stenoses or occlusions of the intracranial carotid artery. Such a procedure may also be performed using autogenous vein bypass grafts from the common or external carotid artery.

fascia graft   A free graft of fascia. Such a graft is sometimes used in ribbon form as a strong suture, sometimes as a pad of several thicknesses in a subcutaneous pocket to fill out defects of contour, and sometimes for other purposes.

fascia-fat graft   A graft consisting of fascia and contiguous fat.

fascicular graft   A nerve graft in which each fascicle is sutured to a corresponding fascicle in the recipient nerve.

fat graft   A free graft of fat, usually obtained from the subcutaneous tissue.

femoral-femoral graft   The connection of both common femoral arteries by a graft of autogenous or prosthetic material, usually in order to bypass a unilateral iliac artery stenosis or occlusion.

femoral-tibial bypass graft   A conduit, either autogenous vein or prosthetic material, that joins the common femoral artery at the groin and one of the tibial arteries below the popliteal trifurcation.

filler graft   A graft used to fill a cavity or defect.

free graft   A graft completely detached from the donor area and transferred to the recipient area without the use of vascular anastomoses.

free gingival graft   A graft of masticatory mucosa which is completely detached from its donor site and used to extend the area of attached gingiva.

full-thickness graft **1** A skin graft containing all the elements of the skin (epidermis and dermis) but none of the subcutaneous tissue. Such a graft will produce better cosmetic and functional results than a split-thickness graft, but its survival rate is more tenuous and the donor site must be grafted or surgically closed. Also called *Krause-Wolfe graft, Wolfe-Krause graft, Wolfe's graft.* **2** An operation utilizing a full-thickness skin graft. Also called *Krause's method, Wolfe-Krause operation.*

Gillies graft An incorrect term for TUBED FLAP.

heterodermic graft A xenograft of skin. An older term.

heterogenous graft XENOGRAFT.

heterologous graft An older term for XENOGRAFT.

heteroplastic graft An older term for XENOGRAFT.

heterotopic graft A graft of an organ or tissue to a site where it is not normally found. Also called *heterotopic transplantation.*

homogenous graft ALLOGRAFT.

homologous graft An older term for ALLOGRAFT.

homoplastic graft An older term for ALLOGRAFT.

ileal graft A graft consisting of a portion of the ileum.

iliac graft A bone graft utilizing the ilium, especially the crest of the ilium, as the donor site.

implantation graft A pinch graft, or a small bit of a split-skin graft measuring no more than three or four millimeters in any direction, which is tucked within the granulations of an open-wound recipient site. These implantation grafts are usually spaced about one centimeter apart and, if they take, grow and spread until they form a continuous cover made up mostly of scar tissue.

inlay graft A split-skin graft which is wrapped, raw side out, around a mold, usually of stent dressing, and buried just under the skin or mucosa. After the graft has taken, the overlying cover is cut through down to the mold, which is removed. The graft may remain as a pocket or trench, or it may gradually flatten to produce more laxity in the area. Also called *Esser graft, skin graft inlay, epithelial inlay, Esser's operation* (outmoded).

intermediate graft A split-skin graft of medium thickness, containing all of the epidermis and from about one third to one half of the underlying dermis. Also called *intermediate split graft.*

intermediate split graft INTERMEDIATE GRAFT.

interposition graft Tissue or prosthetic material used to bridge a gap, as to replace a missing segment of artery or reconstitute a missing segment of nerve. Also called *bridge graft.*

intramedullary graft A graft of spongy bone obtained from the medulla of the donor bone.

island graft An incorrect term for ISLAND FLAP.

isogeneic graft ISOGRAFT.

isologous graft ISOGRAFT.

isoplastic graft ISOGRAFT.

jump graft An incorrect term for JUMP FLAP.

kebab graft A graft used in the reconstruction of a segment of the mandible involving the duplication of the curve of the mandible by skewering small blocks of iliac bone on a Kirschner wire and then bending the wire into the proper curve.

Kiel graft KIEL BONE GRAFT.

Kiel bone graft A preserved, dry, deproteinized bone graft from a young calf, intended for use in human patients. It was once thought that these grafts were nonantigenic and would stimulate the growth of new bone, but the results were often disappointing and they are seldom used today. Also called *anorganic bone graft, Kiel graft.*

Krause-Wolfe graft FULL-THICKNESS GRAFT.

lamellar graft A partial-thickness corneal transplant used for the correction of a superficial corneal scar or defect.

mesh graft A split-skin graft containing multiple small slits, usually cut by machine. When tension is applied, these slits open

out into spaces and the area of the graft increases.

mesocaval H graft A mesocaval shunt constructed to relieve portal hypertension. It is most often composed of a short segment of prosthetic material and connects the superior mesenteric vein and the inferior vena cava. Also called *Drapanas shunt.*

microvascular free graft FREE FLAP.

muscle graft A free graft of muscle tissue.

nerve graft The interposition of a human or animal nerve segment to bridge a gap between the ends of a divided nerve.

Ollier graft OLLIER-THIERSCH GRAFT.

Ollier-Thiersch graft A thin split-skin graft cut with an old-fashioned straight razor or similar blade. Also called *thin-split graft, Thiersch graft, Ollier graft, razor graft, Thiersch operation.*

omental graft A free graft of a portion of the omentum, which is essentially fat. If the graft is revascularized by anastomoses of blood vessels, it is called a free omental flap. If the vascularity is continuously retained through a pedicle during the transfer, it is called an omental flap. The latter is often used to cover suture lines in gastrointestinal surgery. The free grafts and the free omental flaps are used for distant transfers, such as to the scalp or breast. Of these, the incidence of success is far greater with the free omental flap.

onlay graft Any graft, of any tissue, that is applied by laying it on a flat or convex surface. Also called *onlay, outlay.*

onlay bone graft A bone graft applied to the cortical plate at the recipient site. It is sometimes used for recontouring the jaw. Also called *bone onlay.*

orthotopic graft A graft of an organ or tissue to a site where the tissue is normally found. Also called *orthotopic transplantation, homotopic transplantation.*

osseous graft BONE GRAFT.

panel graft The construction of a large-caliber venous conduit by longitudinally incising a vein, then laterally suturing segments of the opened vein to form a panel.

parathyroid graft A procedure sometimes done experimentally after removal of more than one parathyroid for hyperparathyroidism in which a small piece of the patient's own parathyroid is implanted subcutaneously in order to provide for continued secretion of parathyroid hormone.

patch graft A graft of autologous tissue or inert prosthetic material used to enlarge the lumen of tubular structures. It is used primarily in surgery on blood vessels, ureters, or bile ducts.

pedicle graft A full-thickness graft, or a graft including subcutaneous tissues or even deeper tissues, in which the blood supply is retained, either by leaving the tissue permanently or temporarily attached to its site of origin, or by anastomosing blood vessels within the tissue to blood vessels at the recipient site. Also called *flap, pedicle flap* (incorrect).

pedicled bone graft An autograft consisting of bone, usually covered with surrounding soft tissue and transferred on a pedicle of soft tissue containing the nutrient vessels to the bone so that the bone graft remains continuously alive.

penetrating graft A full-thickness graft of cornea from an enucleated or a dead eye, used to replace an opaque cornea in a live eye, or for structural reinforcement.

periosteal graft A graft of periosteum, the purpose of which is to produce bone in the recipient area.

pinch graft A skin graft obtained by pinching up a small bit of skin with a thumb forceps and cutting it off with a knife or scissors. When many of these are placed on a wound, the epithelial cells from the edges coalesce to heal over the recipient bed.

postage stamp graft A skin graft obtained by cutting a sheet of split-skin graft into pieces about the size of an average postage stamp, usually one or two square centimeters in area. The pieces are scattered on the raw recipient site in much the same manner as a Reverdin graft, and the intervening spaces become covered by the growth of scar tissue. Also called *chessboard graft, stamp graft.*

preserved bone graft A bone graft preserved by physical or chemical means or both for a considerable period of time between removal and use. Usually these are bone homografts removed from a human patient shortly after death and preserved in a bone bank in a hospital or other institution.

prosthetic vascular graft Any of a variety of artificial blood vessel substitutes. The earliest grafts were composed of metal, but these have been superseded by Dacron, polytetrafluoroethylene, and, most recently, silicone rubber, polycarbons, and other new materials.

punch graft A full-thickness graft that is harvested with a small circular knife or trephine and most commonly used in hair transplants where hair follicles are transferred along with the skin.

razor graft OLLIER-THIERSCH GRAFT.

Reverdin graft A full-thickness graft produced by elevating a cone of skin on the point of a straight needle and cutting off the top portion of this cone. A number of these grafts are placed at intervals of about one centimeter on a raw recipient site. The separate pieces will fuse and form one whole graft. Also called *Reverdin's method, seed graft, Reverdin's operation.*

rope graft An incorrect term for TUBED FLAP.

seed graft REVERDIN GRAFT.

sequential graft A conduit that uses a bypass graft already in place as a blood flow source to other more distal arteries. It is commonly used in coronary artery bypass grafting and occasionally in tibial vessel reconstruction. Also called *snake graft.*

sheet graft A skin transplant removed from the donor site with a dermatome and placed on the recipient site as a single piece without alteration.

sieve graft A full-thickness graft in which, before removal from the donor site, multiple holes are made with a small tube with a sharpened end. Upon removal of the graft, the areas of skin within these holes are left on the donor site to spread and heal over it. The graft itself, which is moved to the recipient site, contains multiple holes, similar to a mesh graft. Also called *Douglas graft.*

skin graft A piece of skin, partial-thickness or full-thickness, completely removed from one part of the body and transferred to a raw area on another part of the same body (autograft), or transferred from one individual to another of the same species (allograft), or transferred from one individual to another of a different species (xenograft). The transfer is done without surgical vascular anastomoses.

sleeve graft A graft, often consisting of perineurium, used to connect the central and peripheral ends of a severed nerve. It is sleevelike in shape.

snake graft SEQUENTIAL GRAFT.

splenorenal bypass graft An anastomosis of the splenic artery, which is disconnected from the spleen and dissected from its bed, to the renal artery beyond a point of stenosis or occlusion.

split-rib graft A bone graft utilizing a rib or ribs that have been split along their long axes. Such a graft is useful in reconstructing the skull or facial bones.

split-skin graft A free graft of skin consisting of the entire thickness of the epidermis and part of the thickness of the dermis. The donor site regenerates skin from the remnant of dermis left on it. Such a graft can be cut in large sheets to repair large raw areas. Also called *Blair-Brown graft.*

split-thickness graft A graft of oral mucosa or skin utilizing only a portion of the thickness available at the donor site. Compare FULL-THICKNESS GRAFT.

sponge graft A graft consisting of a small piece of sponge. Such grafts were once placed at intervals on a raw area in the

hope that they would stimulate the formation of epidermis. The use of these grafts has been abandoned.

stamp graft POSTAGE STAMP GRAFT.

stent graft A skin graft held in place with a tie-over dressing. ● Formerly, the term was used only when the material in the dressing was dental wax (stent dressing), but now it is used regardless of the material.

syngeneic graft ISOGRAFT.

tendon graft A free graft consisting of a tendon.

testis graft The replacement by transplantation of all or part of a testis.

thick-split graft A split-skin graft containing half or more of the thickness of the dermis.

Thiersch graft OLLIER-THIERSCH GRAFT.

thin-split graft OLLIER-THIERSCH GRAFT.

thyroid graft A graft formerly used in the treatment for myxedema in which a piece of heterologous thyroid gland was implanted in the subcutaneous tissues.

tube graft An incorrect term for TUBED FLAP.

valise-handle graft A tubed flap from the rim of the external ear. An incorrect usage.

vascular graft A segment of artery, vein, or prosthetic conduit that is used to bypass or replace a diseased vessel.

vein graft A graft utilizing an intact segment of vein as a means of bypassing a blocked arterial segment or of replacing an arterial segment that is missing.

white graft A skin graft which has failed to become vascularized. Also called *avascular graft.*

Wolfe's graft FULL-THICKNESS GRAFT.

Wolfe-Krause graft FULL-THICKNESS GRAFT.

xenogeneic graft XENOGRAFT.

---

grafting / fascicular nerve grafting INTERFASCICULAR NERVE GRAFTING.

interfascicular nerve grafting The technique of placing individual grafts between each of the fascicles of a severed nerve to bridge the gap. Also called *fascicular nerve grafting.*

mesh grafting A method of expanding a skin transplant by running it through a special device that cuts multiple slits in the sheet of skin. Depending on the length of the slits, the graft can be expanded in ratios of up to twelve to one to cover larger areas than the original sheet.

skin grafting The implantation of skin from a different site or source in order to repair a defect. See under SKIN GRAFT. Also called *epidermization* (rarely used).

graftschizophrenia PROPFSCHIZOPHRENIA.

Graham [Evarts Ambrose *Graham*, U.S. surgeon, 1883–1957] **1** See under OPERATION. **2** Graham's test. See under CHOLECYSTOGRAPHY.

Graham [George Sellers *Graham*, U.S. pathologist, 1879–1942] Kay-Graham pasteurization test. See under TEST.

Graham [Thomas *Graham*, Scottish chemist, 1805–1869] See under LAW.

Graham Little [Sir Ernest Gordon *Graham Little*, English physician, 1867–1950] **1** See under SYNDROME. **2** Piccardi-Lassueur-Graham Little syndrome. See under LASSUEUR-LITTLE SYNDROME.

grain [Middle English *grein, greyne*, from Old French *grein* a seed, a grain, from L *granum* a seed; and from Old French *grainne* seed or grain in general, from L *grana*, pl. of L *granum*] **1** A simple, dry, one-seeded indehiscent fruit, with a pericarp firmly united around the seed coat. Also called *caryopsis, frumentum.* **2** A unit of mass or weight equal to 1/7000 pound; $64.798\ 91 \times 10^{-6}$ kilogram, 64.798 91 milligrams. The grain is the same in avoirdupois, apothecaries', and troy weight. Symbol: gr

grainage [*grain* + -AGE] Weight expressed in grains.

grains [pl. of *grain*, partly from Middle French *grain* cereal, grain, from L *granum* a grain of corn, seed, and partly from Middle French *graine* seed, from L *grana*, pl. of *granum*] Dyskeratotic, parakeratotic cells present in the epidermis in cases of keratosis follicularis.

grains of paradise CARDAMOM.

Gram [Hans Christian Joachim *Gram*, Danish physician, 1853–1938] Gram's method. See under GRAM STAIN.

gram [French *gramme* (from Gk *gramma* that which is drawn or written, a small weight) one thousandth of a kilogram] A unit of mass or weight equal to 0.001 kilogram; 15.43 grains, or 0.035 27 ounce. Symbol: g

-gram [Gk *gramma* that which is drawn or written, a letter, a small weight] A combining form meaning a record, something written.

Gram-amphophilic Staining positively in part and negatively in part with the Gram stain.

gram-atom The quantity of an element having a mass in grams numerically equal to the atomic weight. One gram-atom contains the Avogadro number of atoms. Also called *gram-atomic weight, g atom.*

gram-calorie 15°C CALORIE. Symbol: g-cal.

gram-force A unit of force equal to 10^{-3} kilogram-force; 9.806 65×10^{-3} newtons, 9.806 65 millinewtons. Also called *pond (German usage).* Symbol: gf

gramicidin A cyclic decapeptide antibiotic formed by *Bacillus brevis.* Its molecule consists of the sequence D-Phe-L-Pro-L-Val-L-Orn-L-Leu occurring twice. Peptide bond formation in its biosynthesis is accomplished by transfer of aminoacyl groups from their thioesters formed with thiol groups in the enzyme complex that makes it. It enters biologic membranes and renders them permeable to cations including Na^+ and K^+.

gramine An indolealkyl amine that acts as a vasopressor. It is found in *Hordeum vulgare,* barley, and in the blades of *Arundo donax,* giant reed.

graminivorous Subsisting on a diet of grasses or cereal grains.

gram-ion A mole, when the entity measured is an ion rather than a molecule. • This term is outmoded, since *mole* is now used for all kinds of specifiable entities.

grammeter [GRAM + METER] A unit of work equal to the work necessary to raise one gram by one meter against gravity; 9.806 65×10^{-3} joule. An obsolete unit.

gram-mole gram-molecule.

gram-molecule That quantity of substance containing the number of grams equal to its molecular weight. Also called *molugram* (obsolete). Abbreviation: gram-mole.

Gram-negative [after Hans Christian Joachim *Gram,* Danish physician, 1853–1938] Decolorized by alcohol or acetone when stained with the Gram stain. Gram-negative bacteria have an inner (cytoplasmic) membrane, a very thin murein wall, often only a single peptidoglycan layer, and a surrounding, adherent outer membrane. Compare GRAM-POSITIVE. • The lower-case form *gram-negative* is often preferred in the United States.

Gram-positive [after Hans Christian Joachim *Gram,* Danish physician, 1853–1938] Not decolorized by alcohol or acetone when stained with the Gram stain. Gram-positive bacteria have a multilayered murein wall and no outer membrane. Compare GRAM-NEGATIVE. • The lower-case form *gram-positive* is often preferred in the United States.

gram-rad A unit of absorbed dose of ionizing radiation, equal to 100 ergs; 10^{-5} joule. Symbol: g·rad

gram-roentgen In radiology, formerly the unit of integral dose, defined as the real energy conversion when one roentgen is delivered to one gram of air (83.7 ergs). This unit has been superseded by the gram-rad (100 ergs) and the kilogram-gray (1 joule).

grana [L, pl. of *granum* a grain, kernel] Structures within chloroplasts that are composed of stacked thylakoids. The grana contain chlorophylls and carotenoids and are the sites of the light reactions of photosynthesis.

Grancher [Jacques Joseph *Grancher,* French physician, 1843–1907] See under TRIAD.

grandiose Characterized by immensity, greatness, eminence, distinction, or majesty.

grand mal [French *grand* great + *mal* sickness] MAJOR EPILEPSY. • This term was once used to identify any convulsive epileptic attack with major manifestations, as opposed to petit mal.

Grandry [M. *Grandry,* Belgian anatomist, flourished 19th century] Grandry-Merkel corpuscles. See under GRANDRY'S CORPUSCLES.

Granger [Amedee *Granger,* U.S. radiologist, 1879–1939] See under SIGN, LINE.

granivore [back-formation from *granivorous,* from L *grani,* pl. of *granum* a grain of corn, seed, kernel + English *-vorous,* combining form from L *vor(are)* to swallow, devour + -OUS] An organism that makes grains and other seeds an important part of its diet.

granivorous [L *gran(um)* a grain of corn, seed, kernel + *i* + English *-vorous,* suffix denoting devouring, swallowing] Feeding on small seeds or grain.

grant / formula grant In the United States, a grant from the federal government usually, but not always, to states for specific purposes in which the amount of the grant is based on the total funds available divided by all eligible grantees.

project grant In the United States, a grant or award of federal funds to a public or private agency for specific purposes such as the development of an ambulatory care center. Grantees are usually selected on a merit basis and through a competitive process. The amount of the grant is based on the support level needed to carry out the project without regard to the number of applicants for support.

granula GRANULE.

granula iridica An irregular granular growth from the pupillary edge of the iris in horses. Also called *corpora nigra.*

granular Having a texture like grains of sand or salt. Also *granulose, granuliform.*

granulate 1 To undergo granulation; to form granulation tissue. 2 Composed of or covered with granules; granular.

granulatio [Late L *granul(um)* (dim. of *granum* grain, akin to *crescere* to grow) a little grain + *-atio* -ATION] [NA] A granular, collagenous body.

granulationes arachnoideales [NA] The numerous bulbous protrusions of the arachnoid extending chiefly into the sagittal sinus and venous lacunae, and constituting the main site of cerebrospinal fluid reabsorption into venous blood. Similar, less numerous arachnoid granulations are found in the transverse sinus and elsewhere. Those to either side of the sagittal sinus become calcified with increasing age, are visible with the naked eye, and often indent the calvaria. Also called *pacchionian bodies, pacchionian glands, pacchionian granulations, arachnoidal granulations, granulationes arachnoideales Pacchioni, granulationes cerebrales, granulationes pacchioni, meningeal granules, arachnoid villi.*

granulationes arachnoideales Pacchioni GRANULATIONES ARACHNOIDEALES.

granulationes cerebrales GRANULATIONES ARACHNOIDEALES.

granulationes pacchioni GRANULATIONES ARACHNOIDEALES.

granulation [L *granulatio.* See GRANULATIO.] The formation of a tissue composed of capillaries, fibroblasts, and inflammatory cells. It is characteristic of wounds healing by second intention.

arachnoidal granulations GRANULATIONES ARACHNOIDEALES.

Bayle's granulations Organized and fibrotic miliary tubercles of the lung. An obsolete term.

Bright's granulations The individual components of the granular scarring imparted to the renal surface by several end-stage renal diseases, mainly chronic glomerulonephritis and arteriolar nephrosclerosis. A rarely used term.

cell granulations Small particles or granules that are demonstrable by their differential staining capacity when compared with the surrounding cell cytoplasm.

exuberant granulations The overproduction of granulation tissue associated with a healing wound.

fungous granulation Exuberant development of granulation tissue in a wound or ulcer. An obsolete term.

hypertrophic granulation The process by which granulation tissue in a chronic wound, if unimpeded by wound closure, may become exuberant and rise above the edges of the wound.

Mezei granulations Brown granules seen in smears made from the lesions of actinomycosis, representing colonies of the fungus. An obsolete term.

pacchionian granulations GRANULATIONES ARACHNOIDEALES.

pyroninophlic granulations Cytoplasmic granules, which are composed of RNA, that have a particular affinity for the histologic stain pyronin.

Reilly granulations Alder-Reilly bodies. See under ALDER-REILLY ANOMALY.

Virchow's granulations Focal areas of glial proliferation in the ependymal and subependymal area around the lateral cerebral ventricles found in patients with general paresis.

granulationes Plural of GRANULATIO.

granule

granule [Late L *granulum* (dim. of *granum* grain, akin to *crescere* to grow) a little grain] **1** A small mass or particle, as a beadlike mass of tissue. **2** Any small sugar-coated or gelatin-coated pill containing a minute dose of a drug. For defs. 1 and 2 also called *granula.*

acrosomal granule A large granule formed by fusion of proacrosomal granules during spermiogenesis and enclosed within a large acrosomal vesicle. It spreads out over the nuclear membrane, flattens, and forms a cap over the nucleus in man, bull, and ram, but the form is more complicated in rodents and other mammals.

aleuronoid granules Starch granules.

alpha granules **1** Platelet granules that contain mostly platelet-derived growth factor, and also platelet factor 4, fibrinogen, β thromboglobulin, and thrombin-sensitive protein. **2** Granules of the alpha cells of the islets of the pancreas, presumed to be the source of glucagon. **3** Granules of the pituitary gland.

Altmann's granule MITOCHONDRION.

amphophil granules Granules in the cytoplasm of cells that take up both acidophilic and basophilic dyes.

argentaffin granules Cytoplasmic particles that can be stained with silver solutions without the addition of a reducing agent.

azurophil granule A granule approximately 0.1 μm in diameter, that is commonly found in the cytoplasm of normal lymphocytes, especially natural killer lymphocytes, and that stains red or violet with azure dyes. Also called *kappa granule.*

Babès-Ernst granules BABÈS-ERNST BODIES.

basal granule BASAL BODY.

basophil granules Cytoplasmic granules that stain with basic dyes.

Bensley specific granules Granules in the cytoplasm of any of the cells of the pancreatic islets of Langerhans.

beta granules Secretory or presecretory granules in the cytoplasm of the beta cells of the pancreatic islets, which contain insulin and C-peptide, and in the various beta cells or basophilic cells of the anterior pituitary, containing adrenocorticotropin, β-lipotropin, endorphins, and in other cells, the gonadotropins.

Bollinger's granules Small yellowish granular masses seen in the cutaneous lesions of botryomycosis, composed of heterogeneous aggregates of Gram-positive cocci, generally staphylococci.

Bütschli granules Enlargements or swellings located along the fibers of the mitotic spindle in an ovum.

carbohydrate granules Beadlike masses of carbohydrate found in body fluids.

chromatic granules NISSL SUBSTANCE.

chromophilic granules NISSL SUBSTANCE.

chromophobe granules Cytoplasmic granules that fail to stain with either acid or basic dyes, usually as a consequence of a relationship to secretory inactivity in the cells of the anterior lobe of the hypophysis.

cone granule The nucleus of a cone cell in the external nuclear lamina of the retina.

cortical granules Subcortically located round or elliptical membrane-bound bodies, usually 0.5 μm–0.8 μm in diameter, found in animal oocytes. These are particularly visible just before fertilization. Following sperm fusion with the egg's vitelline membrane their contents (largely mucopolysaccharides) are released into the perivitelline space (cortical reaction). This consequently modifies the properties both of the vitellus and zona pellucida (zona reaction) so that additional sperm penetration is inhibited. The cortical granules are probably derived from the coalescence of tiny vesicles produced by the Golgi apparatus.

Crooke's granules The characteristic granules of Crooke's hyaline degeneration.

cytoplasmic granule A granule in the cytoplasm of a cell. Also called *ozonophore.*

delta granules Cytoplasmic granules in delta cells of the pancreatic islets.

dense core granule NEUROSECRETORY GRANULE.

Ehrlich's granules Cell granules that are evidenced by using Ehrlich's triple stain. Also called *Ehrlich-Heinz granules.*

Ehrlich-Heinz granules EHRLICH'S GRANULES.

entomophthoramycotic granules Granules formed by growth of the fungus *Basidiobolus* and the responding eosinophilic cellular growth of the host.

eosinophil granules Cytoplasmic granules with a particular affinity for acidic dyes; especially, granules that are present in the cytoplasm of a class of polymorphonuclear leukocytes. These granules are relatively large, approximately 0.5 to 1.0 micron, round, numerous, and stain red to red-orange with Romanowsky dyes. They release a protein (eosinophil basic protein) that is toxic on contact to bacteria or living cells.

Fauvel's granules Pulmonary microabscesses found surrounding small bronchi in the early stages of bronchopneumonia. An obsolete term.

Fordyce granules FORDYCE SPOTS.

fuchsinophil granules Cytoplasmic granules that stain preferentially with acid or basic fuchsin.

glycogen granules Small particles of glycogen that can be identified within the cytoplasm of cells by electron microscopy. The granules vary between 150 and 450 Å in diameter.

Heinz granules HEINZ BODIES.

interstitial granule A fine eosinophilic particle within cell cytoplasm. It corresponds to a mitochondrion in electron microscopy.

Isaac's granules RETICULAR SUBSTANCE.

juxtaglomerular granules Granules in cells of the juxtaglomerular apparatus which represent secretion or storage of renin.

kappa granule AZUROPHIL GRANULE.

keratohyaline granule Cytoplasmic material that is identifiable by light microscopy within the cells of the granular layer of the epidermis. It is considered to be the precursor of keratin.

Kölliker's interstitial granules Small particles corresponding to mitochondria in the sarcoplasm of striated muscle cells. They are visible under light microscopy.

Kretz granules Granules found within the cirrhotic liver.

Langerhans cell granule A tennis racket-shaped cytoplasmic inclusion within a Langerhans cell of the epidermis, which is considered to be specific to this cell type.

Langley's granules Cytoplasmic granules that are visible in serous secretory cells.

lipofuscin granule A form of hyaline droplet containing lipofuscin and reflecting cellular damage. Lipofuscin granules are yellow-brown in unstained section and appear on electron microscopy as vacuoles filled with granular and membranous material. An estimate of the age of an animal can often be made based on the number of lipofuscin granules.

mast-cell granule A metachromatic particle within the cytoplasm of a mast cell. Heparin sulfate, histamine, and serotonin have been identified within such granules.

melanin granule MELANOSOME.

meningeal granules GRANULATIONES ARACHNOIDEALES.

Much's granules Cylindrical or spherical granules present in smears of tuberculous sputum. They stain with gram but not acid fast stains and are considered altered tubercle bacilli. An obsolete term. Also called *Schrön-Much granules* (obsolete).

mucinogen granules Cytoplasmic granules that are visible in mucous secretory cells.

mucous granule A cytoplasmic vesicle that contains mucin.

neurosecretory granule A small intracytoplasmic vesicle that contains an electron-dense aggregate of neurosecretory material such as oxytocin, vasopressin, or norepinephrine. Also called *dense core granule, neurosecretory sphere.*

neutrophil granules Minute granules, generally less than 0.1 μm in diameter, that are numerous in the cytoplasm of a class of polymorphonuclear leukocytes, and that stain a pale rose color with Romanowsky dyes. The granules are lysosomes that contain peroxidases and esterases.

Nissl granules NISSL SUBSTANCE.

Palade granule RIBOSOME.

Paschen's granules GUARNIERI BODIES.

perichromatin granules Particles found at the boundary between the euchromatin and heterochromatin of the nucleus. They are believed to carry messenger RNA.

pigment granules Colored or pigmented granules in a cell, generally cytoplasmic granules.

Plehn's karyochromatophil granules Basophilic granules commonly found in the conjugating form of malarial parasites. Also called *Schuegner's granules.*

polar granules VOLUTIN GRANULES.

proacrosomal granules The granular precursors of the acrosome situated inside the acroblast during spermiogenesis. Several of the cisternae in the Golgi complex accumulate these protein granules which fuse to form a single acrosomal granule containing much carbohydrate.

prosecretion granules Cytoplasmic granules containing materials that will be secreted from the cell.

protein granules Small globules or masses of proteins within the cytoplasm of a cell.

rod granule The nucleus of a rod cell in the external nuclear lamina of the retina.

Schrön's granule A small body alleged to be present in the nucleolus of an ovum.

Schrön-Much granules An obsolete term for MUCH'S GRANULES.

Schuegner's granules PLEHN'S KARYOCHROMATOPHIL GRANULES.

Schüffner's granules Numerous minute reddish granules that stipple erythrocytes infected with *Plasmodium vivax* or *P. ovale,* when stained with a Romanowsky dye. Such granules do not appear in erythrocytes infected with *P. malariae* or *P. falciparum.* Also called *Schüffner's dots, Schüffner stippling, malarial stippling.*

secondary granule SPECIFIC GRANULE.

secretory granule SECRETORY VACUOLE.

seminal granules Very small granular masses formed in seminal fluid.

specific granule The smaller type of lysosome that is found in the cytoplasm of mature neutrophil polymorphs and that contains alkaline phosphatase, collagenase, and aminopeptidase. Also called *secondary granule.*

sphere granule A large cell with granular cytoplasm found in serous exudates. An obsolete term.

sulfur granules Characteristic yellow granular bodies found in the exudate of actinomycotic lesions.

tannophil granules Cytoplasmic granules that are readily identified after mordanting with tannic acid.

toxic granules Small, basophilic, intracytoplasmic granules found in leukocytes, at one time believed to be related to infections. They probably represent aberrantly developed lysosomes.

volutin granules Metachromatic particles consisting of free nucleic acids stored in granular form in the cytoplasm of certain microorganisms such as coccidia and trypanosomes, protozoa that undergo rapid nuclear division and require substantial quantities of nucleic acids. Also called *polar granules.*

yolk granules Nutritive, nonliving material made of fatty and albuminous substance synthesized by the cytoplasm of most animal ova in the form of only a few or of many granules. The amount present enables the classification of egg types.

zymogen granules Granules in the cytoplasm of enzyme-secreting cells such as those of the salivary glands or pancreas. The granules contain the zymogenic material.

---

granuliform GRANULAR.

granulo- [Late L *granulum* little grain, dim. of L *granum* (akin to *crescere* to grow and English *grow*) grain] A combining form meaning granule, granular.

granuloblast A precursor granular cell giving rise to any adult blood cell containing granules, such as the various types of leukocyte.

granuloblastosis [GRANULO- + BLAST- + -OSIS] A neoplastic disease of poultry characterized by proliferation of malignant granulocytes in the bone marrow and granulocytic leukemia. It belongs to the leukosis-sarcoma group of the avian leukosis complex.

granulocorpuscle A small corpuscle seen in infected tissue in cases of lymphogranuloma venereum.

granulocytapheresis Leukapheresis for the collection specifically of granulocytes.

granulocyte [*granul(e)* + *o* + -CYTE] A leukocyte that characteristically contains many granules in its cytoplasm. Included among granulocytes are neutrophils, eosinophils, basophils, and the precursors of these cells. Also called *granular leukocyte.*

heterophil granulocyte NEUTROPHIL.

neutrophil granulocyte NEUTROPHIL.

polymorphonuclear granulocyte SEGMENTED NEUTROPHIL.

granulocytopenia An abnormally decreased number of granulocytes in the blood. Also called *granulopenia, hypogranulocytosis.*

granulocytopoiesis GRANULOPOIESIS.

granulocytopoietic GRANULOPOIETIC.

granulocytosis [GRANUL(E) + *o* + CYTOSIS] Increased numbers of granulocytes in blood or tissue.

granuloma

granuloma [*granul(e)* + -OMA] **1** A chronic inflammatory lesion characterized by an accumulation of macrophages which have undergone epithelioid transformation, with or without lymphocytes and multinuclear giant cells, into a discrete granule. **2** A chronic inflammatory lesion which forms microscopic or macroscopic nodules in response to multiple infectious, immunologic, neoplastic, or foreign body challenges. For defs. 1 and 2 also called *granulation tumor.*

adjuvant granuloma An inflammatory lesion that forms at the site of injection of adjuvants, particularly complete Freund's adjuvant.

alum granuloma A small inflammatory lesion that occurs at the injection site of aluminum adjuvant.

amebic granuloma A rare form of colonic amebiasis characterized by a tumorlike induration of the wall due to exuberant granulation tissue.

granuloma annulare A benign skin disorder of unknown origin characterized clinically by small dermal nodules that sometimes appear in annular configuration, and histologically by a histiocytic and granulomatous response to focal necrobiosis of collagen. Also called *heloderma simplex et annularis* (obsolete).

apical granuloma PERIAPICAL GRANULOMA.

aquarium granuloma FISH TANK GRANULOMA.

balnei granuloma SWIMMING POOL GRANULOMA.

benign granuloma of thyroid A chronic inflammatory disease of the thyroid, which enlarges and eventually becomes very firm.

beryllium granuloma The characteristic lesion of berylliosis, consisting of a usually non-caseating granuloma with multinucleated giant cells. It is most frequently seen in the lung, but the skin, liver, and spleen may also be involved.

***Candida* granuloma** **1** One of the granulomatous, crusted nodules of the scalp, face, mucous membranes, and fingers occurring in chronic, generalized candidiasis in association with impaired immune response. Also called *candidal granuloma, Monilia granuloma, monilial granuloma.* **2** Any granuloma seen in tissues infected by *Candida* oranisms.

candidal granuloma *CANDIDA* GRANULOMA.

canine venereal granuloma TRANSMISSIBLE CANINE VENEREAL TUMOR.

central giant cell reparative granuloma A giant cell reparative granuloma occurring in one of the bones of the jaw.

cholesterol granuloma A chronic granulomatous inflammatory disease involving both the tympanic and mastoid segments of the middle-ear cleft and regarded as a late stage in the progress of chronic exudative otitis media. The granulations are typified by cholesterol crystals and foreign-body giant cells. A brownish glairy exudate filling the tympanic cavity and mastoid air cells gives a characteristic bluish appearance when viewed through the tympanic membrane.

chronic granuloma PERIAPICAL GRANULOMA.

coccidioidal granuloma COCCIDIOIDOMA.

coli granuloma See under COLIGRANULOMA.

granuloma contagiosum GRANULOMA INGUINALE.

dental granuloma PERIAPICAL GRANULOMA.

Dürck's granuloma MALARIAL GRANULOMA.

granuloma endemicum An obsolete term for CUTANEOUS LEISHMANIASIS.

eosinophilic granuloma **1** A circumscribed, cystic lesion of bone most often seen in children and adolescents, consisting of histiocytes and eosinophils. See also HISTIOCYTOSIS. **2** The eosinophilic intestinal wall mass resulting from infection with the roundworm *Anisakis marina.*

eosinophilic granuloma of the skin The least severe form of histiocytosis, characterized by papular lesions and ulcerated plaques. Histologically the granulomatous lesions contain many eosinophils as well as histiocytes.

favic granuloma A chronic granulomatous ringworm infection due to *Trichophyton schoenleinii.*

fish tank granuloma A chronic, ulcerative skin lesion, usually on the forearm, caused by *Mycobacterium marinum* infection. It is the same as swimming pool granuloma, but is generally seen in persons who keep fish as a hobby and generally acquired in the process of cleaning a fish tank or aquarium. Also called *aquarium granuloma.*

granuloma fissuratum A chronic inflammatory response of the skin to repeated localized trauma, as is seen in the transversely ridged soft red nodule that forms on the skin because of the pressure of the earpiece of spectacles. Also called *fissured angioma.*

foreign body granuloma A granuloma caused by the aspiration, injection, or inoculation of foreign matter. The granuloma is usually noncaseating, and the foreign body is often visible within it.

granuloma fungoides MYCOSIS FUNGOIDES.

granuloma gangraenescens LETHAL MIDLINE GRANULOMA.

giant cell reparative granuloma A benign tumorlike lesion arising as an abnormal reaction to injury and containing numerous multinuclear giant cells. It occurs in the gingiva or in the bones of the jaw.

granuloma gluteale infantum Dull red granulomatous nodules in the diaper area of infants. Topical corticosteroids favor this development in which *Candida albicans* is believed to play a part.

granuloma inguinale A chronic, ulcerogranulomatous venereal disease of the skin and mucous membranes caused by the Gram-negative bacillus *Calymmatobacterium granulomatis* (formerly *Donovania granulomatis* or Donovan's bodies). It is characterized by ulcerating skin lesions on the genitalia which contain macrophages packed with Donovan bodies. Rectovaginal fistula is a common complication. The disease is most commonly seen in tropical and subtropical areas and is especially common in Papua New Guinea. Streptomycin is the antibiotic of choice. Also called *granuloma contagiosum, granuloma venereum, granuloma pudendi, granuloma pudente tropicum, ulcerating granuloma of the pudenda, venereal granuloma.*

intubation granuloma Laryngeal granuloma occurring at the site of minor injury caused by laryngeal intubation, usually during general anesthesia. The principal site is somewhere on the vocal cords, usually over the vocal processes of the arytenoid cartilages.

iodide granuloma   A follicular skin rash, one of many types of cutaneous reaction caused by the intake of iodides in sensitized individuals.

laryngeal granuloma   Any variety of granuloma arising within the larynx, apart from the infective granulomata. It is likely to follow trauma, particularly minor injury during laryngeal intubation.

lethal midline granuloma   A rare, progressive disease of unknown etiology, characterized by local erosive destruction of the paranasal sinuses, palate, and nose, with later extention to the orbits and other facial structures. The process involves nonspecific acute or chronic inflammation resulting in necrosis of soft tissue, bone, and cartilage with or without the formation of granulomas. Also called *midline granuloma, malignant granuloma of the face, granuloma gangraenescens.*

lipoid granuloma   A granuloma characterized by lipid-containing foamy histiocytes. It may be caused by excessive amounts of endogenous or exogenous lipid.

lipophagic granuloma   A granuloma occurring when subcutaneous fat undergoes necrosis, usually as a result of traumatic injury. This lesion is characterized by a central focus of necrotic, oily debris surrounded by lipid-laden macrophages, proliferating fibroblasts, and granulation tissue.

lycopodium granuloma   A granulomatous inflammation that used to complicate the healing of surgical wounds when they became contaminated with lycopodium spores. A rarely used term.

granuloma of Majocchi   MAJOCCHI'S GRANULOMA.

Majocchi's granuloma   An uncommon chronic infection of the hair follicles of the lower leg caused by a ringworm species, typically *Trichophyton rubrum*. It usually arises by extension of primary tinea pedis. Also called *trichophytic granuloma of Majocchi, granuloma trichophyticum, granuloma of Majocchi, hypertrophic ringworm, trichophytic granuloma, tinea profunda.*

malarial granuloma   A granulomatous lesion found in the brain in some cases of fatal cerebral malaria. Also called *Dürck's granuloma.*

malignant granuloma of the face   LETHAL MIDLINE GRANULOMA.

midline granuloma   LETHAL MIDLINE GRANULOMA.

Miescher's granuloma   CHRONIC PROGRESSIVE DISCIFORM GRANULOMATOSIS.

milkers' granuloma   Granulomatous nodules at the sides of the fingers, induced by the penetration into the skin of cow's hairs during the process of milking.

Monilia granuloma   *CANDIDA* GRANULOMA.

monilial granuloma   *CANDIDA* GRANULOMA.

granuloma multiforme   A disease of unknown origin endemic in parts of central Africa. The chronic skin lesions, often annular, show focal necrobiosis and histiocytic granuloma formation.

paracoccidioidal granuloma   SOUTH AMERICAN BLASTOMYCOSIS.

granuloma pendulum   A granuloma pyogenicum which hangs by a stalk.

periapical granuloma   Granuloma occurring adjacent to the apex of a nonvital tooth. Also called *apical granuloma, chronic granuloma, dental granuloma.*

periorificial eosinophilic granuloma   A granulomatous process in which the eosinophils are conspicuous, involving the gums and sometimes also the perianal region. An outmoded term.

peripheral giant cell reparative granuloma   A giant cell reparative granuloma occurring on the gingiva. Also called *giant cell epulis, epulis gigantocellularis.*

plasma cell granuloma   A granulomatous inflammatory response in which plasma cells predominate. At times it is not a true granuloma, but rather a nonspecific chronic inflammatory infiltrate largely composed of mature plasma cells.

granuloma of the prostate   A chronic inflammatory process of the prostate probably caused by partial obstruction of the larger ducts followed by chronic inflammation and the formation of granulomatous nodules.

granuloma pudendi   GRANULOMA INGUINALE.

granuloma pudente tropicum   GRANULOMA INGUINALE.

pyogenic granuloma   An exophytic red nodule occurring primarily in the skin and oral mucosa and composed of proliferated capillaries in an edematous stroma containing inflammatory cells. Undoubtedly benign, this lesion is believed by some to be an exaggerated response to minor trauma, i.e., exuberant granulation tissue. Others classify it as a polypoid form of capillary hemangioma. Also called *septic granuloma, granulation tumor, granuloma pyogenicum.*

granuloma pyogenicum   PYOGENIC GRANULOMA.

renal cholesterol granuloma   A granuloma in the renal cortex characterized by accumulation of nucleated giant cells in association with cholesterol clefts on histologic examination.

reticulohistiocytic granuloma   An older term for DERMATOFIBROMA.

rheumatic granulomas   Granulomas and/or subcutaneous nodules appearing in various parts of the body in certain types of inflammatory rheumatic disease, such as rheumatoid arthritis and rheumatic fever.

granuloma sarcomatodes   MYCOSIS FUNGOIDES.

septic granuloma   PYOGENIC GRANULOMA.

granuloma silica   A granulomatous reaction to the presence in the tissues of particles of silicon dioxide or magnesium silicate. Also called *silicotic granuloma.*

silicotic granuloma   GRANULOMA SILICA.

surgical-glove talc granuloma   TALC GRANULOMA.

swimming pool granuloma   A chronic skin infection caused by *Mycobacterium marinum* and acquired in nonchlorinated swimming pools or lakes. Also called *balnei granuloma.*

talc granuloma   A granulomatous reaction of the foreign-body type induced by talcum powder. This type of granuloma used to be quite frequent in the past, when surgical gloves were routinely coated with talcum powder. The introduction of starch-coated gloves solved the problem. Also called *surgical-glove talc granuloma, talcum-powder granuloma.*

talcum-powder granuloma   TALC GRANULOMA.

granuloma telangiectaticum   A granuloma composed of dilated small blood vessels.

trichophytic granuloma   MAJOCCHI'S GRANULOMA.

trichophytic granuloma of Majocchi   MAJOCCHI'S GRANULOMA.

granuloma trichophyticum   MAJOCCHI'S GRANULOMA.

granuloma tropicum   An obsolete term for YAWS.

tuberculoid granuloma   A granuloma composed of epithelioid and multinucleated giant cells in the renal cortex, usually in association with tuberculosis or sarcoidosis.

ulcerating granuloma of the pudenda   GRANULOMA INGUINALE.

umbilical granuloma   Granulation tissue that forms on the umbilical cord stump of newborn infants.

granuloma of the umbilicus   A small mass of granulation tissue formed at the site of separation of the umbilical cord, which the dermal epithelium cannot cover and which gives rise to a discharge of thin pus from the navel. It is curable by judicious application of silver nitrate. Also called *umbilical fungus.*

urate granuloma   A foreign body type of inflammatory reaction characterized by multinucleated giant cells surrounding urate crystals, as seen in gout. A rarely used term.

venereal granuloma   GRANULOMA INGUINALE.

granuloma venereum   GRANULOMA INGUINALE.

Wegener's granuloma   See under WEGENER'S GRANULOM-ATOSIS.

zirconium granuloma   A granuloma simulating sarcoidosis that is induced by the application of deodorant preparations containing zirconium lactate or zirconium oxide.

---

granulomatosis [*granulomat(a)*, pl. of GRANULOMA + -OSIS] A condition or disease characterized by multiple granulomas.

beryllium granulomatosis   A granulomatous condition of the lung resembling sarcoidosis and resulting from exposure to beryllium.

chronic familial granulomatosis   CHRONIC GRANULOMA-TOUS DISEASE.

chronic progressive disciform granulomatosis   Necrobiosis lipoidica with a granulomatous rather than a necrobiotic reaction in the dermis. Also called *Miescher's granuloma.*

chronic X-linked granulomatosis   CHRONIC GRANULOMA-TOUS DISEASE.

granulomatosis disciformis chronica et progressiva   NEC-ROBIOSIS LIPOIDICA.

lipid granulomatosis   HAND-SCHÜLLER-CHRISTIAN DIS-EASE.

lipophagic intestinal granulomatosis   WHIPPLE'S DISEASE.

lymphomatoid granulomatosis   A rare disease characterized by vasculitis and lymphoid infiltrates in nodules within the lung, subcutaneous tissue, and brain.

malignant granulomatosis   HODGKIN'S DISEASE.

necrotizing respiratory granulomatosis   Wegener's granulomatosis in the respiratory tract.

reticuloendothelial granulomatosis   HISTIOCYTOSIS.

granulomatosis siderotica   An obsolete term for GAMNA-GANDY BODIES.

Wegener's granulomatosis   An illness of unknown cause characterized by necrotizing sinusitis, other oral and ocular infiltrative granulomas, necrotizing pneumonia with nodules, systemic vasculitis, and glomerulonephritis. The disease occurs in two forms, limited Wegener's granulomatosis, which does not involve the kidneys, and generalized Wegener's granulomatosis, in which the kidneys are involved. Also called *Wegener syndrome.*

granulomatous [*granulomat(a)*, pl. of GRANULOMA, + -OUS] Describing or pertaining to a form of subacute inflammation in which there is exuberant proliferation of inflammatory cells and reactive fibrous or glial tissue.

granulomere   The central portion of a blood platelet as seen on a stained blood smear, characterized by purplish granules. Compare HYALOMERE.

granulopenia   GRANULOCYTOPENIA.

granulopexy   Fixation of granules.

granulophthisis   The wasting or inhibition of granulopoiesis.

granuloplasm [GRANULO- + -PLASM]   **1** The portion of the cytoplasm which contains granules. **2** The more centrally located cytoplasm of amebas and certain other unicellular organisms.

granuloplastic   Having the capacity to form granules.

granulopoiesis   The normal maturation and release of granulocytes by the bone marrow. Also called *granulocytopoiesis.*

granulopoietic   Pertaining to or stimulating granulopoiesis. Also *granulocytopoietic.*

granulosarcoid   An obsolete term for MYCOSIS FUNGOIDES.

granulosarcoma   An obsolete term for MYCOSIS FUNGOIDES.

granulose   GRANULAR.

granulosis [*granul(e)* + -OSIS]   The granular appearance of the surface of an organ. An imprecise usage. Also called *granulosity.*

granulosis rubra nasi   A rare childhood disease of uncertain origin, characterized by excessive sweating and the development of circumscribed erythema papulosum that gradually extends from the tip of the nose to the cheeks and upper lip. Also called *dermatitis micropapulosa erythematosa hyperidrotica nasi*, *perisyringitis chronica nasi.*

granulosity   GRANULOSIS.

granulotuberculoma   A tuberculous lesion of grossly granular appearance. An outmoded term.

laryngeal granulotuberculoma   A conspicuous tuberculous laryngeal granuloma. It is an increasingly rare occurrence.

granulovacuolar   Characterized by the presence of both granules and vacuoles in the cytoplasm, as seen in neurons in Alzheimer's disease.

granum [L, a grain]   (*plural* grana.) A grain.

graph [*graph(ic formula)*, from Gk *graphik(os)* able to draw or paint, suited for writing]   A diagrammatic representation of the relationship between two variables, such as one in which the positions of the values of the variables are determined by a system of coordinates.

graph-   GRAPHO-.

-graph [Gk *graphein* to write, draw, record]   A combining form meaning (1) an instrument that writes or records; (2) a record, something written.

graphics   The process whereby a computer generates drawings on a cathode-ray tube and an operator manipulates them with a keyboard or light pen.

graphite   The black form of the element carbon, consisting of planes of carbon atoms in fused benzene rings. The ability of the planes of atoms to slide easily over each other gives graphite its lubricant properties. The π electrons are delocalized over long distances, and this gives graphite its electrical conductivity. Also called *plumbago.*

graphitosis   GRAPHITE FIBROSIS.

grapho- [Gk *graphein* to write, draw, record]   A combining form meaning writing, a record. Also *graph-.*

graphocatharsis [GRAPHO- + CATHARSIS]   Attainment of catharsis by means of writing.

graphology [GRAPHO- + -LOGY]   The analysis of handwriting for the purpose of assessing or predicting personality type and character traits. Also called *graphopathology.*

forensic graphology   The comparative analysis of handwriting samples and handwritten documents in order to determine the authenticity of questioned documents.

graphomania [GRAPHO- + -MANIA]   A compulsive need to write, often without regard to the worth of what is being written. Also called *scribomania.*

graphomotor [GRAPHO- + MOTOR]   Describing, pertaining to, or affecting the movements used in writing.

graphopathology   GRAPHOLOGY.

graphophobia [GRAPHO- + -PHOBIA]   Pathologic fear of writing, a common form of which is severe anxiety or tremulousness if forced to sign one's name while being observed by others.

graphorrhea [GRAPHO- + -RRHEA]   Inordinate, uncontrolled, senseless writing at length, performed to fill pages rather than to record or transmit a message.

graphoscope [GRAPHO- + -SCOPE]   A device that measures surface contours of the eye.

graphospasm [GRAPHO- + SPASM]   WRITERS' CRAMP.

-graphy [Gk *graphein* to write, draw, record]   A combining form meaning (1) writing, a record; (2) a manner or means of writing or recording.

GRAS [from *generally regarded as safe*] Designating a list of food additives that were introduced before the Delaney Law was passed in 1958. They are assumed to be safe and there are no restrictions on their use. Any substance on the list found to be unsafe is immediately banned and removed from the list.

Graser [Ernst *Graser*, German surgeon, 1860–1929] See under DIVERTICULUM.

Grashey [Hubert *Grashey*, German physician, 1839–1911] See under APHASIA.

grasp / finger grasp A type of instrument grasp in which the handle is held by all the fingers flexed around it and the thumb is used to provide a finger rest.

instrument grasp The way in which an instrument is held in dentistry.

inverted pen grasp An instrument grasp similar to the pen grasp but with the wrist rotated so that the instrument tip points away from the operator.

palm-and-thumb grasp An instrument grasp in which the handle is held in the palm of the hand and gripped by all the fingers flexed around it, the thumb being used to provide a finger rest.

pen grasp An instrument grasp in which the handle is held in the same way as a pen or pencil. The finger rest is provided by the middle, third, and little fingers, separately or in combination.

grasping / forced grasping GRASP REFLEX.

grass [Middle English *gras*, from Old English *græs, gærs*; akin to Old English *grōwan* to grow and to L *gramen* herb, plant, *germen* a sprout, and *herba* grass] Any plant in the Gramineae family. The grasses are predominantly monocotyledonous herbs characterized by narrow, elongated leaves with parallel veins that grow from the stem at nodes. Small flowers which lack petals and sepals arise from the stem atop the most recent leaf growth.

Grasset [Joseph *Grasset*, French physician, 1849–1918] **1** Grasset's law. See under LANDOUZY-GRASSET LAW. **2** Grasset-Gaussel phenomenon, Grasset-Bychowski sign, Grasset sign. See under GRASSET'S PHENOMENON. **3** Grasset-Gaussel-Hoover sign. See under SIGN.

graticule [French (alteration of L *craticula* latticework, dim. of *cratis* a wicker frame or basket), a grid] A grid, usually of plastic, for measurement of quantities displayed on the cathode-ray tube of an oscilloscope.

eyepiece graticule GRADUATING DIAPHRAGM.

gratification [L *gratificatio* (from *gratificatus*, past part. of *gratificari* to gratify, from *grat(us)* pleasing + *i* + *-ficare*, combining form denoting to make) a gratifying] **1** Satisfaction of one's needs or desires. **2** The feeling of pleasure attendant upon such satisfaction.

grating A perforated frame or latticework.

diffraction grating A device that consists of closely ruled, parallel, equidistant lines on a transparent or polished plate. It is used to produce spectra of transmitted or reflected light, through interference of the waves diffracted by the individual rulings.

Gratiolet [Louis Pierre *Gratiolet*, French anatomist and physiologist, 1815–1865] **1** Peduncular ansa of Gratiolet. See under ANSA PEDUNCULARIS. **2** Fibers of Gratiolet, radiation of Gratiolet, radiatio occipitothalamica Gratioleti, Gratiolet's radiating fibers. See under RADIATIO OPTICA.

grattage [French, a scratching] The removal of surface scale by gentle scraping. The technique is used in the diagnostic examination of suspected psoriasis.

Graux [Gaston *Graux*, French physician, flourished 19th century] Féréol-Graux palsy. See under FÉRÉOL-GRAUX PARALYSIS.

grave [L *grav(is)* heavy, grave] Very serious; apt to be life-threatening.

gravel [Middle English, from Old French *gravelle*, dim. of *grave* coarse or pebbly sand] Granular urinary-tract concretions, smaller than calculi and ordinarily the size of pinheads, which can be passed through the urethra without discomfort.

graveolent An obsolete term for FETID.

Graves [Robert James *Graves*, Irish physician, 1796–1863] **1** See under DISEASE. **2** Euthyroid Graves disease. See under DISEASE. **3** Graves scapula. See under SCAPHOID SCAPULA.

grave-wax An obsolete term for ADIPOCERE.

gravid Pregnant.

gravida [L, from fem. of *gravidus* heavy, pregnant] A pregnant woman. A numerical designation is often used following the term to denote the total number of pregnancies the woman has experienced including the current one. For example, a woman who has had one prior pregnancy and is currently pregnant is designated gravida 2.

gravidic [L *gravid(us)* (from *gravis* heavy) heavy, pregnant + -IC] Relating to or occurring in pregnancy. A seldom used term.

gravidism Pregnancy, or the signs and symptoms associated with it.

graviditas [L (from *gravid(us)* heavy, pregnant, from *gravis* heavy, burdened + *-itas* -ITY), pregnancy] A condition related to pregnancy.

graviditas examnialis A pregnancy in which the amnion is retracted, leaving only the chorion to surround the fetus.

graviditas exochorialis A pregnancy in which the membranes have ruptured and retracted such that the fetus lies outside the chorion.

gravidity [L *graviditas*. See GRAVIDITAS.] PREGNANCY.

gravidocardiac [L *gravid(us)* heavy, pregnant + *o* + Gk *kardia* the heart] Referring to cardiac disease occurring during the course of pregnancy. A seldom used term.

gravidopuerperal [L *gravid(us)* heavy, pregnant + *o* + *puerpera* (from *puer* a child + *parere* to give birth) a woman giving birth] Relating to the duration of pregnancy and the postpartum period.

gravimeter An apparatus for measuring specific gravity. Also called *gravitometer*.

gravimetric [L *gravi(s)* weighty + *metric(us)* pertaining to measuring] Of or relating to measurement by weight.

gravis [L, heavy, severe, grave] A colony type of *Corynebacterium diphtheriae* found on tellurite agar. It is larger and more brittle than the intermedius or mitis strains. The presumed parallelism with the severity of the disease has not been borne out.

gravistatic Relating to the accumulation of body fluids or sedimentary material in dependent parts from the effects of gravity.

gravitation [New L *gravitatio* (from *gravitatus*, past part. of *gravitare* (a newtonian coinage) to move by force of gravity, from L *gravitas* weightiness) gravitation] The force of attraction between any two bodies. Also called *gravity*. See also NEWTON'S LAW OF GRAVITATION.

gravitometer GRAVIMETER.

gravity [L *gravitas* (from *grav(is)* weighty + *-itas* -ITY) weightiness] GRAVITATION. • Physicists tend to use *gravity* to mean the force exerted on an object near the surface of a celestial body, such as the Earth or the moon, and to use *gravitation* for the general phenomenon, but for most purposes they can be used interchangeably.

specific gravity   RELATIVE DENSITY.

standard gravity   STANDARD ACCELERATION OF FREE FALL.

Grawitz [Paul Albert *Grawitz*, German pathologist, 1850–1932] **1** Grawitz tumor. See under RENAL CELL CARINOMA. **2** Grawitz degeneration. See under BASOPHILIC STIPPLING OF ERYTHROCYTES. **3** See under CACHEXIA.

Gray [Joseph Alexander *Gray*, Australian physician, 1884–1966] Bragg-Gray principle. See under PRINCIPLE.

gray¹ [after Louis Harold *Gray*, British radiologist, 1905–1965] Special name for the SI derived unit of absorbed dose in the field of ionizing radiation, equal to one joule per kilogram. The absorbed dose is the mean energy imparted by ionizing radiation to matter per unit of mass of irradiated material at the place of interest. Symbol: Gy

gray per second   The SI derived unit of radiation absorbed dose rate. 1 gray per second = 100 rad per second. Symbol: Gy/s, Gy·s⁻¹

gray²   SUBSTANTIA GRISEA.

central gray   SUBSTANTIA GRISEA CENTRALIS CEREBRI.

periaqueductal gray   SUBSTANTIA GRISEA CENTRALIS CEREBRI.

gray-out   Mild, short-lived, or partial loss of consciousness, most commonly due to temporary anoxemia.

graze   To feed on herbaceous vegetation such as the grasses in a pasture.

grease [Middle English *grese, grees*, from Old French *craisse, graisse* grease, fat, from Vulgar L *crassia* greasiness, from L *crass(us)* coarse, fat + *-ia* -Y] A chronic, idiopathic, proliferative dermatitis of the posterior aspect of the pastern of the horse. Also called *grease heel*.

green   **1** A color of the visible spectrum falling between blue and yellow.   **2** A substance, usually a stain or dye, that is green in appearance, or that produces a cytochemical reaction resulting in green staining. For chemical names including *green*, see under the chemical name.

acid green   LIGHT GREEN S F YELLOWISH.

brilliant green   A basic arylmethane synthetic dye used sometimes as a stain for bacteria, spirochetes, fungi, and yeasts. It is used more frequently as a constituent of bacteriologic media, as in the brilliant green bile medium for the identification of *Escherichia coli*. Also called *ethyl green, new solid green*.

diamond green   MALACHITE GREEN.

fast green   A dye that is closely related to light green chemically and has been used as an alternative to it in staining techniques where greater permanency is required.

fast acid green N   LIGHT GREEN S F YELLOWISH.

fast green FCF   A dye that substitutes for light green SF yellowish but that has superior resistance to fading. It is used in various staining techniques involving bacteria, collagen fibers, and plant histology.

Hoffman green   IODINE GREEN.

Janus green B   A synthetic basic dye that contains both an azine and an azo chromophore group, and is therefore related to the safranin dyes. It is used particularly for intravital staining of mitochondria in blood leukocytes. Also called *diazin green S*.

light green N   MALACHITE GREEN.

light green S F yellowish   A synthetic acid dye derived from brilliant green. It is used as a stain for microorganisms and for collagen fibers in Masson's trichrome modification of the Mallory aniline blue method. Also called *acid green, fast acid green N*.

malachite green   A diaminotriphenylmethane dye variously used as a counterstain, as a vital stain, as an indicator at both

pH 0.0–2.0 and 11.6–14.0 ranges, and as a constituent in Löwenstein-Jensen agar for mycobacteria. It has also been used as an antiseptic and antimycotic agent. Also called *diamond green, solid green O, Victoria green, light green N*.

new solid green   BRILLIANT GREEN.

solid green O   MALACHITE GREEN.

Victoria green   MALACHITE GREEN.

Greenberg [David Morris *Greenberg*, U.S. biochemist, born 1895] See under METHOD.

Greenfield [Joseph Godwin *Greenfield*, English neuropathologist, 1844–1958] **1** Greenfield's disease. See under BALÓ'S DISEASE. **2** Greenfield syndrome, Scholz-Greenfield disease. See under METACHROMATIC LEUKODYSTROPHY.

Greenwood [Major *Greenwood*, English physician, born 1880] Greenwood-Yule method. See under METHOD.

greffotome [French *greffe* (from L *graphium* iron pen, stylus for writing on waxed tablets) a graft, grafting + *o* + -TOME] A surgical blade used for harvesting thin slices of tissue, particularly skin, for use in grafts.

gregaloid [L *gregal(is)* (from *grex*, gen. *gregis*, a herd, flock + *-alis* -AL) of the same herd or flock + -OID] Characterizing a group or colony of protozoa formed by a fusion or combining of independent cells.

Gregarina [L *gregar(ius)* (from *grex*, gen. *gregis*, a herd, flock) pertaining to a flock + -INA] A genus of septate gregarine sporozoans (suborder Septatina, subclass Gregarinia) found in the alimentary canal or reproductive system of annelids and arthropods.

gregarine [L *gregar(ius)* pertaining to a flock + -INE] **1** Belonging or pertaining to the protozoan order Eugregarinida. **2** A protozoan belonging to the order Eugregarinida.

Gregarinida   A former name for EUGREGARINIDA.

gregarinosis [*gregarin(e)* + -OSIS] The condition of harboring gregarine parasites.

gregarious [L *gregarius* (from *grex*, *gregis*, a herd, flock + *-arius* -ARY) pertaining to a herd or flock] **1** Of humans, tending to live in social groups and seek the company of and social interchange with other members of one's group. **2** Having a distinct tendency to remain together in herds or flocks: used of animals belonging to certain species.

Gregory [James *Gregory*, Scottish physician, 1753–1821] Gregory's mixture. See under COMPOUND POWDER OF RHUBARB.

Greig [David Middleton *Greig*, Scottish scientist, 1864–1936] Greig syndrome. See under ORBITAL HYPERTELORISM.

Greither [Aloys *Greither*, German dermatologist, born 1913] See under SYNDROME.

Greppi [Encrico *Greppi*, Italian hematologist, born 1896] Microelliptopoikilocytic anemia of Rietti, Greppi, and Micheli. See under ANEMIA.

gression [L *gress(us)*, past part. of *gradi* to step, + English *-ion*] Backward displacement of a tooth.

Grey Turner   See under TURNER.

gribouillist [French *gribouill(e)* a foolish, naive, disorganized person + -IST] One who accentuates the most unattractive aspects of old age, particularly in a way intended to promote guilt among other people.

grid [short for *gridiron*] In radiology, a series of very thin lead strips separated by spacers which are transparent to x rays. The strips are set on edge, parallel to the beam axis, and reduce the amount of scattered x rays reaching the film.

Amsler grid   A checkerboardlike pattern of lines used as a background for the subjective drawing of visual field defects.

baby grid   Any of various growth charts of weight and length of babies.

Bucky grid   BUCKY DIAPHRAGM.

fixed grid STATIONARY GRID.

focused grid A radiographic grid in which the lead strips are angled slightly so that they focus on a line at a specified distance, which determines the optimal placement of the x-ray tube.

moving grid A radiographic grid which moves during the x-ray exposure, in order to blur out the shadows caused by the lead strips.

parallel grid A radiographic grid in which the lead strips are parallel to each other in their longitudinal axis.

Potter-Bucky grid BUCKY DIAPHRAGM.

stationary grid A radiographic grid that does not move during the x-ray exposure. Also called *fixed grid.*

Thoms grid A grid used in pelvimetry to allow direct measurement from the radiograph of pelvic diameters.

Wetzel grid Formerly, a growth chart of heights and weights for children according to age. A second measurement of the child after a sufficient interval, when plotted on the grid, gave the growth trend of that child, whether accelerating, slowing, arrested, catching up, or normal.

Gridley [Mary F. *Gridley*, U.S. medical technologist, 1908–1954] See under STAIN.

grief Sorrow or pain secondary to bereavement; sadness or remorse.

Griesinger [Wilhelm *Griesinger*, German neurologist, 1817–1868] **1** Griesinger symptom. See under GRIESINGER SIGN. **2** Duchenne-Griesinger disease. See under PROGRESSIVE MUSCULAR ATROPHY.

Griffith [Frederick *Griffith*, English bacteriologist, died 1941] See under CLASSIFICATION.

Grifulvin A proprietary name for griseofulvin.

Grignard [François Auguste Victor *Grignard*, French chemist, 1871–1935] See under REAGENT.

grimace [French (from Old French *grimache* a grimace, from the Germanic, akin to Old English *grima* a mask, helmet), a making faces] A distortion of the face, as in choreoathetosis, facial tics, or catatonic mannerisms and stereotypies involving the face.

grindelia The leaves and flowering heads of *Grindelia camporum* or *G. cunefolia.* It is used as a mild expectorant.

grinding [Old English *grindan* (akin to L *frendere* to gnash the teeth, crush, grind), to grind]

night grinding BRUXISM.

selective grinding Alteration of the occlusal surfaces of the teeth by grinding away points or areas of contact. Also called *spot grinding.*

spot grinding SELECTIVE GRINDING.

grinding-in A method of adjusting the occlusal surfaces of the teeth by moving the jaws (or the equivalents thereof on an articulator) relative to one another with an abrasive paste in between the upper and lower occlusal surfaces. Also called *milling-in.*

grip An older term for INFLUENZA. • In this sense, the French spelling *grippe* is more usual.

Dabney's grip EPIDEMIC PLEURODYNIA.

devil's grip EPIDEMIC PLEURODYNIA.

Pawlik's grip An old-fashioned obstetrical maneuver whereby the fetus during labor is palpated transabdominally with one hand in order to determine whether the presenting part is descending into the pelvis.

grippal Pertaining to grippe or influenza.

grippe [French (from *gripper* to seize, from Low German *gripan* to clutch, seize), an epidemic catarrh, influenza] An older term for INFLUENZA.

grippe aurique Polyneuropathy resulting from the therapeutic administration of gold salts.

Balkan grippe Q fever that occurred in outbreaks in the Balkans during the Second World War.

grisein An antibiotic produced by strains of *Streptomyces griseus.* It is an amorphous red powder containing ferric iron. Acid hydrolysis yields 3-methyluracil and at least two amino acids. It is active against some Gram-positive and Gram-negative bacteria and certain fungi.

Grisel [P. *Grisel*, French physician, flourished early 20th century] Grisel's disease. See under NASOPHARYNGEAL TORTICOLLIS.

griseofulvin $C_{17}H_{17}ClO_6$. A naturally occurring antibiotic derived from *Penicillium griseofulvum.* It is used in the treatment of fungal infections of the skin. It is given orally.

Grisolle [Augustin *Grisolle*, French physician, 1811–1869] See under SIGN.

Grisonella ratellina A species of South American weasel that is a reservoir host of *Trypanosoma cruzi.*

gristle [Middle English *gristel*, from Old English *gristle*] CARTILAGE.

grit [Middle English *greet, grete*, from Old English *grēot*] Coarse particulate matter, usually referring to particles having a diameter greater than 75 μm.

Gritti [Rocco *Gritti*, Italian surgeon, 1828–1920] **1** Gritti's operation. See under GRITTI'S AMPUTATION. **2** Gritti-Stokes amputation. See under AMPUTATION.

Grocco [Pietro *Grocco*, Italian physician, 1856–1916] **1** Orsi-Grocco method. See under METHOD. **2** See under TEST, SIGN.

Groenouw [Arthur *Groenouw*, German ophthalmologist, 1862–1945] **1** Groenouw type I corneal dystrophy. See under GRANULAR CORNEAL DYSTROPHY. **2** Groenouw type II corneal dystrophy. See under MACULAR CORNEAL DYSTROPHY.

groin [early modern English rendering of *grine*, also *grinde*, from Middle English *grynde*, from Old English *grynde* abyss] The curved linear groove forming the junction between the anterior abdominal wall and the front of the thigh lateral to the perineal area. Also called *inguen.*

grommet [obsolete French *gromette* (now *gourmette*) a bridle chain for curbing animals] A popular term for VENTILATION TUBE.

Grönblad [Esther Elisabeth *Grönblad*, Swedish ophthalmologist, born 1898] Grönblad-Strandberg syndrome. See under PSEUDOXANTHOMA ELASTICUM.

groove

groove [Middle English *grofe*, from Old Norse *grof* and Middle Dutch *groeve* a pit] A linear depression or furrow found on the surfaces of teeth, bones, and other anatomical structures.

abomasal groove The third segment of the ruminant gastric groove. It extends along the lesser curvature of the abomasum.

alveolabial groove ALVEOLOLABIAL GROOVE.

alveolingual groove ALVEOLOLINGUAL GROOVE.

alveolobuccal groove The curved groove at the uppermost and lowermost margins of the vestibule of the mouth that is formed by the mucous membrane reflected from the gums to the cheeks and lips. Also called *alveolobuccal sulcus, gingivobuccal sulcus.*

alveololabial groove The groove that develops in the embryo between the lips and the jaws. It is a deepening of the labiodental lamina. Also called *alveolabial sulcus, alveolabial groove, gingi-*

vobuccal sulcus, gingivobuccal groove, gingivolabial sulcus, gingivolabial groove.

alveololingual groove   A groove that develops in the embryo between the tongue and the lower jaw. Also called *alveolingual groove, alveololingual sulcus, alveolingual sulcus, gingivolingual sulcus.*

anterior auricular groove   INCISURA ANTERIOR AURIS.

anterior interventricular groove   SULCUS INTERVENTRICULARIS ANTERIOR.

anterior palatine groove   CANALIS INCISIVUS.

anterior paramedian groove of spinal cord   SULCUS INTERMEDIUS ANTERIOR MEDULLAE SPINALIS.

anterolateral groove of medulla oblongata   SULCUS LATERALIS ANTERIOR MEDULLAE OBLONGATAE.

anterolateral groove of spinal cord   SULCUS LATERALIS ANTERIOR MEDULLAE SPINALIS.

anteromedian groove of spinal cord   FISSURA MEDIANA ANTERIOR MEDULLAE SPINALIS.

arterial grooves   SULCI ARTERIOSI.

atrioventricular groove   SULCUS CORONARIUS CORDIS.

auriculoventricular groove   SULCUS CORONARIUS CORDIS.

basilar groove   SULCUS BASILARIS PONTIS.

basilar groove of occipital bone   An outmoded term for CLIVUS OSSIS OCCIPITALIS.

basilar groove of sphenoid bone   An outmoded term for CLIVUS OSSIS SPHENOIDALIS.

bicipital groove of humerus   SULCUS INTERTUBERCULARIS HUMERI.

Blessig's groove   The future ora serrata of the retina, seen in the developing eye as a groove between the nervous part of the retina and its ciliary part.

branchial groove   A furrow on the outside of an embryo, lying between two branchial arches and having its floor made of ectoderm. Also called *visceral groove.*

buccal groove   A developmental groove on the buccal surface of a posterior tooth, running from the occlusal surface towards the cervical margin.

carotid groove of sphenoid bone   SULCUS CAROTICUS OSSIS SPHENOIDALIS.

cavernous groove of sphenoid bone   SULCUS CAROTICUS OSSIS SPHENOIDALIS.

cerebral groove   The cerebral portion of the neural groove.

chiasmatic groove   SULCUS PRECHIASMATICUS.

costal groove   SULCUS COSTAE.

deltopectoral groove   The curved vertical groove between the anterior margin of the deltoid muscle and the clavicular part of the pectoralis major muscle in which the cephalic vein and deltoid branch of the thoracoacromial artery are situated. It is continuous superiorly with the fossa infraclavicularis.

dermal groove of cubital fossa   The transverse flexure line in front of the elbow joint. An outmoded term. Also called *surface groove of cubital fossa.*

developmental groove   A groove on the surface of an anatomical structure such as a tooth or a bone, which is an intrinsically determined feature of its shape. Also called *developmental line.*

digastric groove   INCISURA MASTOIDEA OSSIS TEMPORALIS.

distobuccal groove   The distal of the two vertical grooves that are often present on the buccal surfaces of the human lower first permanent molar tooth and lower second deciduous molar tooth.

dorsal groove for subclavian vein   An outmoded term for SULCUS VENAE SUBCLAVIAE.

duodenopyloric groove   PYLORIC CONSTRICTION.

enamel grooves   Two grooves, one on each side of the enamel knot, seen in histologic sections of a developing tooth during the late cap stage.

epicondylar-olecranon groove   The vertical distal continua-

tion of the sulcus nervi ulnaris behind the medial surface of the olecranon process of the ulna in which the ulnar nerve runs with the posterior ulnar recurrent artery. It is separated from the articular capsule by the ulnar collateral ligament before the nerve passes between the two heads of the flexor carpi ulnaris muscle. A superficial fibrous expansion between the latter muscle and the medial head of the triceps muscle converts the groove into a tunnel.

esophageal groove   In ruminants, a groove which forms a direct communication between the esophagus and the abomasum, bypassing the forestomachs. Also called *reticular groove, sulcus reticuli.*

ethmoidal groove   SULCUS ETHMOIDALIS OSSIS NASALIS.

groove for eustachian tube   SULCUS TUBAE AUDITIVAE.

groove for extensor carpi ulnaris   A shallow groove on the posterior aspect of the distal end of the ulna that lies between the styloid process and the head of the ulna and contains the tendon of extensor carpi ulnaris muscle. It is converted into a tunnel by the extensor retinaculum.

groove for facial artery on mandible   A groove on the base of the mandible that is immediately anterior to the angle and is traversed by the facial artery.

free gingival groove   A groove on the surface of the gingiva at the junction between the free and attached gingiva.

frontal groove   Any of the sagittal fissures of the frontal lobe. An imprecise usage.

gastric groove   The central axis from which the four compartments of the ruminant stomach develop. It is divided into three segments.

genital groove   GENITAL FURROW.

groove for gluteal artery   An inconstant groove that is situated in the middle of the upper margin of the greater sciatic notch at its junction with the anterior gluteal line and is traversed by the superior gluteal artery. Rarely it is traversed by a nutrient branch of the artery to the gluteal surface of the ilium. An outmoded term.

groove of great superficial petrosal nerve   SULCUS NERVI PETROSI MAJORIS.

hamular groove   SULCUS HAMULI PTERYGOIDEI.

Harrison's groove   A horizontal indentation of the ribs making up the chest wall opposite the attachment of the diaphragm, produced by softening of the bones in rachitic children. Also called *Harrison's curve, Harrison sulcus.*

groove of helix   SCAPHA.

hyperbranchial groove   A mid-dorsal furrow in the pharynx of a cephalochordate.

hypobranchial groove   A ciliated groove located in the floor of the pharynx of cephalochordates.

inferior dental groove   The inferior dental (mandibular) canal during development in the embryo. At first it is not closed over by bone on its medial (lingual) aspect.

infraorbital groove of maxilla   SULCUS INFRAORBITALIS MAXILLAE.

interatrial groove   A slight sulcus extending between the left sides of the superior and inferior venae cavae on the external dorsal surface of the heart, indicating the division between the right and left atria and usually only visible if the heart is somewhat distended. Also called *interatrial sulcus.*

interdental groove   A vertical furrow on the surface of the interdental papilla.

interosseous groove of calcaneus   SULCUS CALCANEI.

intertubercular groove of humerus   SULCUS INTERTUBERCULARIS HUMERI.

labial groove   A thin ectodermal formation in the embryo which, after delamination, forms the gingivolabial furrow (alveololabial sulcus). From its internal part the dental lamina originates.

lacrimal groove   FOSSA SACCI LACRIMALIS.

groove of lacrimal bone   SULCUS LACRIMALIS OSSIS LACRIMALIS.

laryngotracheal groove   A ventrally placed gutter at the caudal end of the primitive pharyngeal floor in an embryo, marking the site of early development of the larynx and trachea.

lateral bicipital groove   SULCUS BICIPITALIS LATERALIS.

lateral groove for lateral sinus of occipital bone   An outmoded term for SULCUS SINUS TRANSVERSI.

lateral groove for lateral sinus of parietal bone   An outmoded term for SULCUS SINUS SIGMOIDEI OSSIS PARIETALIS.

lateral groove of occipital bone   SULCUS SINUS TRANSVERSI.

lateral phallic groove   A groove on each side of the developing penis in the embryo, separating it from the future scrotum.

lateral groove for sigmoidal part of lateral sinus   An outmoded term for SULCUS SINUS SIGMOIDEI OSSIS TEMPORALIS.

Liebermeister's grooves   Slight grooves on the surface of the fetal liver which may persist after birth.

lingual groove   A developmental groove on the lingual surface of a posterior tooth running from the occlusal surface towards the cervical margin.

groove of Lucas   STRIA SPINOSA.

main groove   A groove on the surface of a tooth which separates one major cusp from another.

mastoid groove   INCISURA MASTOIDEA OSSIS TEMPORALIS.

medial bicipital groove   SULCUS BICIPITALIS MEDIALIS.

median groove of patellar surface of femur   A slight median and obliquely vertical groove on the patellar surface of the femur. It separates two articular surfaces, of which the lateral is wider and more prominent. The groove articulates with the slight longitudinal ridge on the articular surface of the patella during flexion of the knee.

median groove of trochlea of humerus   A median, spiral groove that forms almost a complete circle and separates the two sloping articular surfaces of the trochlea of the humerus, articulating with a corresponding smooth ridge in the trochlear notch of the ulna.

medullary groove   NEURAL GROOVE.

meningeal grooves   Sulci arteriosi and sulci venosi.

mesiobuccal groove   The mesial of the two vertical grooves that are often present on the buccal surfaces of the human lower first permanent and second deciduous molar teeth.

mesiolingual groove   A groove between a cusp or tubercle of Carabelli and the crown of a human upper first permanent or upper second deciduous molar tooth.

groove for middle temporal artery   SULCUS ARTERIAE TEMPORALIS MEDIAE.

musculospiral groove   SULCUS NERVI RADIALIS.

mylohyoid groove   SULCUS MYLOHYOIDEUS MANDIBULAE.

mylohyoid groove of inferior maxillary bone   An outmoded term for SULCUS MYLOHYOIDEUS MANDIBULAE.

nail groove   SULCUS MATRICIS UNGUIS.

nasal groove   SULCUS ETHMOIDALIS OSSIS NASALIS.

groove for nasal nerve   SULCUS ETHMOIDALIS OSSIS NASALIS.

nasolabial groove   SULCUS NASOLABIALIS.

nasolacrimal groove   An elongated thickening that forms from ectoderm medial to the nasomaxillary groove and sinks below the surface, becomes canalized, and gives rise to the nasolacrimal duct.

nasomaxillary groove   The groove formed at the line of union of the maxillary and lateral nasal processes during the development of the cheek.

naso-optic groove   ORBITONASAL CLEFT.

nasopalatine groove   A narrow, deep channel running anteroinferiorly on each lateral surface of the vomer, lodging the nasopalatine nerve and vessels.

nasopharyngeal groove   A shallow sulcus on the lateral nasal wall extending from the body of the sphenoid bone to the junction of the hard and soft palates and separating the nasal fossa posteriorly from the nasopharynx.

neural groove   A groove, formed in an early temporary stage in the development of the central nervous system, situated in the middle of the embryo in front of Hensen's node. It follows the neural plate stage and is formed by sinking in of the neural plate to give rise to a midline groove. The margins of the groove fold over and meet centrally, at first in its middle portion, to begin the formation of the neural tube containing the neural canal. Also called *medullary groove, medullary streak.*

notochordal groove   A ventral depression in the notochordal process during early embryonic development, as seen in the Chordata.

nuchal groove   The vertical median furrow of the nape of the neck.

nutrient artery groove   A linear translucency produced on a radiograph of a bone by the canal of a nutrient artery.

obturator groove   SULCUS OBTURATORIUS OSSIS PUBIS.

occipital groove   SULCUS ARTERIAE OCCIPITALIS.

groove for occipital artery   SULCUS ARTERIAE OCCIPITALIS.

occipital groove for occipital artery   An occasional sinuous groove for the occipital artery that runs on the squamous part of the occipital bone lateral to the inferior nuchal line and the attachment of the superior oblique muscle of the head. It then crosses the superior nuchal line between the attachments of the splenius capitis and trapezius muscles. An outmoded term.

occlusal groove   A developmental groove between the cusps on the occlusal surface of a posterior tooth. Also called *occlusal sulcus.*

olfactory groove   1 SULCUS OLFACTORIUS NASI. 2 ETHMOID FOSSA.

omasal groove   In ruminants, a canal that joins the reticuloomasal orifice to the omasoabomasal orifice.

optic groove   SULCUS PRECHIASMATICUS.

oral groove   A ciliated groove or depression leading to the oral opening on the surface of certain ciliated protozoans, such as *Tetrahymena* and *Paramecium.*

palatine grooves of maxilla   SULCI PALATINI MAXILLAE.

palatine groove of palatine bone   SULCUS PALATINUS MAJOR OSSIS PALATINI.

palatomaxillary groove of palatine bone   SULCUS PALATINUS MAJOR OSSIS PALATINI.

palatovaginal groove   SULCUS PALATOVAGINALIS.

paracolic grooves   SULCI PARACOLICI.

paraglenoid groove of hip bone   An outmoded term for PREAURICULAR SULCUS.

grooves between patellar surface and condyles of femur   Two faint grooves that separate the patellar surface from the tibial surfaces of the medial and lateral condyles of the femur. The more clearly marked lateral groove extends obliquely from the front part of the medial margin of the lateral condyle to the anterior part of the lateral margin, while the medial groove extends anteroposteriorly for a short distance across the medial condyle. Both grooves rest against their corresponding menisci during full extension of the knee joint.

pharyngeal groove   A groove delineating adjacent pharyngeal or branchial arches. Pharyngeal grooves are of two varieties, endodermal and ectodermal. Endodermal grooves are found in the foregut and extend laterally to form pouches. Ectodermal grooves lie opposite the endodermal pouches.

pharyngotympanic groove   SULCUS TUBAE AUDITIVAE.

popliteal groove   A deep, smooth sulcus below and behind the lateral epicondyle of the femur, the anterior portion of which gives attachment to the tendon of the popliteus muscle, while the posterior part receives the tendon in full flexion of the knee joint.

posterior auricular groove   SULCUS AURICULAE POSTERIOR.

posterior interventricular groove   SULCUS INTERVENTRIC-ULARIS POSTERIOR.

posterior paramedian groove of spinal cord   SULCUS IN-TERMEDIUS POSTERIOR MEDULLAE SPINALIS.

posterolateral groove of spinal cord   SULCUS LATERALIS POSTERIOR MEDULLAE SPINALIS.

preauricular groove of ilium   PREAURICULAR SULCUS.

preputiolabial groove   A depression separating the two genital folds in female embryos. Also called *urogenital groove.*

primary labial groove   LABIAL LAMINA.

primary urethral groove   A median groove that develops along the caudal surface of the embryonic phallus. It is in contact with the lower margin of the urethral plate and its raised margins are the genital folds. The groove deepens and eventually becomes the greater part of the spongy urethra. Also called *urethral groove, urogenital groove.*

primitive groove   PRIMITIVE STREAK.

primitive dental groove   DENTAL LAMINA.

pterygopalatine groove of pterygoid plate   An outmoded term for SULCUS VOMEROVAGINALIS.

groove of the pulse   The anterior surface of the distal end of the radius, covered by the pronator quadratus muscle, that is crossed by the radial artery lying lateral to the tendon of the flexor carpi radialis muscle and medial to the brachioradialis muscle. The radial artery is palpated here to observe the pulse. An outmoded term.

radial groove   SULCUS NERVI RADIALIS.

groove for radial nerve   SULCUS NERVI RADIALIS.

retention groove   A groove in a tooth preparation in which a corresponding ridge of the restoration lodges for the purpose of improving the retention.

reticular groove   ESOPHAGEAL GROOVE.

rhombic groove   One of the grooves between the segments or neuromeres of the rhombencephalon.

sagittal groove   SULCUS SINUS SAGITTALIS SUPERIORIS.

second branchial groove   The U.S. term for HYOBRANCHIAL CLEFT.

groove for semimembranosus muscle   A deep transverse groove immediately below the posterior part of the articular margin of the medial condyle of the tibia. Into it is inserted the central part of the tendon of the semimembranosus muscle.

Sibson's groove   SIBSON'S FURROW.

sigmoid groove of temporal bone   SULCUS SINUS SIGMOIDEI OSSIS TEMPORALIS.

groove of small superficial petrosal nerve   SULCUS NERVI PETROSI MINORIS.

sphenobasilar groove   The shallow depression on the superior surface of the basiocciput and the dorsum sellae of the sphenoid bone to which the ventral surface of the pons is related. Also called *spheno-occipital groove.*

spheno-occipital groove   SPHENOBASILAR GROOVE.

spiral groove   SULCUS NERVI RADIALIS.

subclavian groove   GROOVE OF SUBCLAVIUS MUSCLE.

groove of subclavius muscle   A transverse groove in the middle third of the inferior surface of the clavicle for the proximal attachment of the subclavius muscle. The clavipectoral fascia is attached to the anterior and posterior margins of the groove. A nutrient foramen is located in the lateral end of the groove. Also called *subclavian groove.*

subcostal groove   SULCUS COSTAE.

groove for superior longitudinal sinus   SULCUS SINUS SAGITTALIS SUPERIORIS.

supplemental groove   A groove on the surface of the crown of a posterior tooth in addition to those which separate the major cusps.

surface groove of cubital fossa   DERMAL GROOVE OF CUBITAL FOSSA.

groove for tibialis posticus muscle   An outmoded term for SULCUS MALLEOLARIS TIBIAE.

tracheobronchial groove   A median groove that appears in the floor of the embryonic pharynx and is rapidly converted into a tubular outgrowth parallel to the foregut. It is the primordium of the larynx, trachea, bronchi, and lungs. Also called *laryngotracheal groove.*

trigeminal groove   The earliest indication in the embryo of the formation of the ganglion of the trigeminal nerve.

tympanic groove   SULCUS TYMPANICUS OSSIS TEMPORALIS.

ulnar groove   SULCUS NERVI ULNARIS.

groove of ulnar nerve   SULCUS NERVI ULNARIS.

urethral groove   PRIMARY URETHRAL GROOVE.

urogenital groove   1 PRIMARY URETHRAL GROOVE. **2** PREPUTIOLABIAL GROOVE.

venous grooves   SULCI VENOSI.

ventricular grooves   Sulcus interventricularis anterior and sulcus interventricularis posterior.

Verga's lacrimal groove   A furrow occasionally found in the lateral wall of the inferior meatus of the nose, extending downward just below the opening of the nasolacrimal duct.

vertebral groove   A marked hollow on each side of the spinous processes of the vertebral column, posterior to the laminae and the transverse processes and occupied by the deep muscles of the back.

visceral groove   BRANCHIAL GROOVE.

Gross [Ludwik *Gross*, Polish-born U.S. physician, born 1904] See under LEUKEMIA.

Gross [Samuel David *Gross*, U.S. surgeon, 1805–1884]   See under DISEASE.

gross   Visible to the naked eye; macroscopic.

Grossich [Antonio *Grossich*, Yugoslavian physician, 1849–1926] See under METHOD.

ground   1 A point in an electric circuit used as a common reference for measuring voltages.   **2** The connection between an electric circuit and the earth.   **3** A backdrop or setting on which something else, the figure, is displayed or superimposed; background. Difficulty in differentiating the figure from the ground is characteristic of some organic mental disorders.

equipment ground   A connection from earth ground to non-current-carrying metal parts of a wiring installation or of electric equipment to prevent shock and provide shielding.

ground-glass   In radiography, referring to a hazy appearance.

group   A number of mutually bonded atoms in a molecule, forming an identifiable part of that molecule.

A group   In human cytogenetics, the largest metacentric chromosomes, numbers 1, 2, and 3.

age group   A group of individuals which is determined by a range of consecutive ages, used for purposes of statistical analysis and presentation. The span of ages defining the group is chosen so as to reduce sampling variation while avoiding significant loss of information due to lack of homogeneity within the group with respect to the characteristics of interest. Also called *age class.*

alkalescens-dispar group   A group of nonpathogenic Enterobacteriaceae, classified formerly with *Shigella* (because they do not form gas) but now with *Escherichia coli.*

Arizona group   A group of microorganisms sometimes classified as *Salmonella arizonae.* They are very similar to *Salmonella* biochemically and in pathogenesis, but often lactose-positive. Reptiles seem to be the natural reservoir.

B group   In human cytogenetics, the largest submetacentric chromosomes, numbers 4 and 5.

Bethesda-Ballerup group   A group of enteric bacteria, closely related metabolically and antigenically to *Escherichia coli* and now included in *Citrobacter*.

blood group   See under BLOODGROUP.

C group   In human cytogenetics, the submetacentric chromosomes intermediate in length to those in the B and E groups, namely numbers 6 through 12 and the X.

California group   A group of eleven serologically related mosquito-borne bunyaviruses found in the United States, Europe, and Africa. Five viruses of the group are associated with human illness ranging from mild fever to encephalitis.

closed group   A therapy group to which no new patients are admitted once the series of sessions has begun.

compatibility group   INCOMPATIBILITY GROUP.

complementophil group   In side chain theory, the group on the amboceptor which attaches to complement.

continuous group   OPEN GROUP.

control group   A group used as a control in an experiment or study (control experiment). See under CONTROL. Compare EXPERIMENTAL GROUP.

cytophil group   Ehrlich's side chain theory, the group on the amboceptor serving to fix the amboceptor to the sensitive cell.

D group   In human cytogenetics, the largest acrocentric chromosomes, numbers 13, 14, and 15.

diagnosis-related group   In the United States, a group of conditions for which health-care treatment has been received and charges are to be assessed, considered to be related by diagnoses, with the object of establishing in a prospective manner a specific, reimbursable fee or range of fees for an episode of care for each such group. Thus, all diagnoses within a group are reimbursed at the same rate, regardless of length-of-stay in an inpatient facility, the severity of illness, or the specific services provided. This system was initiated primarily for prospective payment of inpatient care under the Medicare program. Abbreviation: DRG • In Japan, a similar payment system was instituted in 1983 specifically for the care of those over 70 years of age. In the United Kingdom, no comparable system exists, although the concept is reflected in the term *performance indicator*, broadly applied to various hospital services, including administrative services as well as patient management.

E group   In human cytogenetics, the smallest of the submetacentric chromosomes, numbers 16, 17, and 18.

encounter group   A therapy group in which there is an emphasis on intensive face-to-face interaction, the encouraging of interpersonal confrontation and self-disclosure, and a striving to modify behavior on the basis of increased awareness of self and of how others react to one's self. The encounter group is an outgrowth of sensitivity training. Also called *T-group, sensitivity training group*.

ethnic group   A predominantly or traditionally endogamous human group that is differentiated from other such groups by physical or cultural factors such as race, language, tribe, national origin, or religious background.

experimental group   The group in a control experiment that is exposed to the variable under study. Compare CONTROL GROUP.

F group   In human cytogenetics, the smallest of the metacentric chromosomes, numbers 19 and 20.

functional group   A chemical group to which a molecule owes some of its reactions, such as the hydroxyl group of an alcohol.

G group   In human cytogenetics, the smallest acrocentric chromosomes, numbers 21 and 22, and the Y.

high-risk group   Persons whose risk of disease or injury is higher than that of the average person in the population to which they belong or in other comparable populations. The members of the group may be defined in terms of genetic makeup, physical or chemical attributes, habits of life, socioeconomic and educational characteristics, etc., as well as the nature of the environment to which they are or have been exposed.

incompatibility group   A group of plasmids with the same specificity in the system regulating their copy number. As a result, a cell infected with two plasmids of the same group will soon yield progeny lines that contain one or the other. This feature is a fundamental criterion for classifying plasmids. Also called *compatibility group*.

leaving group   A group that leaves a molecule in the course of a chemical reaction, usually a group that takes with it both the electrons of the bond that had kept it attached. Combination with a hydrogen ion often makes a group better at leaving, e.g. $-OH_2{}^+$ can leave as OH_2, whereas $-OH$ has to leave as the more reactive OH^-, which has difficulty in getting away.

leukocyte group   White cells typed by antigenic determinants and generally recognized by their reactivity with corresponding antibodies by agglutination, cytotoxicity, or fluorescence.

leukosis-sarcoma group   One of three groups of neoplastic diseases of chickens, comprising collectively the avian leukosis complex. The leukosis-sarcoma diseases are caused by a C-type RNA oncornavirus which affects mainly the hemopoietic system. Compare MAREK'S DISEASE, RETICULOENDOTHELIOSIS GROUP.

linkage group   Two or more genes found by family, biochemical, or cytogenetic studies to be linked. Such genes do not segregate independently, in apparent violation of Mendel's second law. All genes of a given linkage group are syntenic, but all syntenic loci are not necessarily linked in the genetic sense and may show independent assortment through crossing over.

marathon group   A type of encounter group that meets for long stretches of time, sometimes for as long as 48 or 72 hours without interruption except for short sleep periods and toilet breaks.

open group   A therapy group that accepts new participants at any time. Also called *continuous group*.

prosthetic group   A group in a protein molecule not composed of amino-acid residues. The flavin of a flavoprotein is an example. The prosthetic group of an enzyme often plays a part in the reaction it catalyzes. It differs from a coenzyme in being more tightly bound so that it remains with the enzyme when this is isolated.

protecting group   A group substituted onto another in order to prevent reaction of that other during chemical synthesis. The Boc group, $(CH_3)_3C-O-CO-$, for example, may be used to acylate an amino acid for use in peptide synthesis. It renders the amino group it is on unreactive, so that the compound containing it may be made to react with another amino group, and it can then be removed after the reaction.

reporter group   A group in a molecule, often inserted artificially, that is capable of providing information about the parts of the molecule around it. It possesses some measurable characteristic, such as absorbance, fluorescence, or nuclear magnetic resonance signal, whose nature is responsive to changes in its environment. Such groups in proteins have been used to indicate conformation changes or the binding of ligands.

reticuloendotheliosis group   One of three groups of neoplastic diseases of chickens, comprising collectively the avian leukosis complex. The reticuloendotheliosis diseases are caused by an oncornavirus distinct from that causing the leukosis-sarcoma group diseases. The form of leukosis usually seen in this group is manifested by enlargement of the liver and spleen caused by neoplastic lymphoid cells. Compare LEUKOSIS-SARCOMA GROUP, MAREK'S DISEASE.

sensitivity training group   ENCOUNTER GROUP.

structured group   A therapy group whose members are chosen so that individually and as a group they will have a therapeutic effect on every other member of the group.

therapy group   Two or more patients who gather together in the presence of one or more therapists in order to participate in treatment of their emotional disorders or social maladjustments.

transitional group   A therapy group for children in the latency period or puberty, which emphasizes the acquiring of social skills.

ventral thalamic group   The several nuclei lying ventrolateral to the internal medullary lamina, constituting the thalamic centers for somatosensory and motor integration.

grouping / blood grouping   Typing of blood cell antigenic determinants by their specific reactivity with corresponding antibodies and generally determined *in vitro* by cell agglutination. (For specific blood groups, see under BLOOD GROUP.).

group-specific   Specific for a particular group.

growth [Middle English *grouth*, from Old Norse *grōa* to grow]   **1** The process by which an organism increases in size as part of its normal development.   **2** Any increase in size of an organism or part.   **3** A tumor.   **4** An increase in the number of units making up a whole, as, for example, population growth, or growth of a tissue or organ by cellular multiplication.

absolute growth   An actual increase in size, in whole or in part.

accretionary growth   Any growth process involving an increase in the amount of intercellular, nonliving substances.

allometric growth   The growth of a part of the body as an exponential function of the growth of the body as a whole.

appositional growth   A growth process which occurs by increase at the edges or on the outside of a structure, thus adding new material or tissue at the periphery.

auxetic growth   AUXESIS.

balanced growth   The part of the exponential phase in a bacterial culture when the population has not yet altered the medium enough to begin to influence the growth rate and therefore cell composition remains constant.

condylar growth   An increase in size of the condylar process of the mandible accompanied by the growth of cartilage and its replacement by bone.

confluent growth   The growth of animal cells to form a sheet in which the cells are brought into intimate contact. Normally this results in cessation of DNA synthesis and of further growth (contact inhibition), but many types of cancer cell continue to grow.

differential growth   The difference in growth rates as exhibited by the several parts of a structure or an organism.

histiotypic growth   Profuse uncontrolled growth of cells.

interstitial growth   Growth occurring inside a structure or organ by increase in number and size of the elements or components contained within them.

intussusceptive growth   AUXESIS.

isometric growth   The growth of various body parts at the same rate.

multiplicative growth   Growth which results from an increase in number of cells.

new growth   NEOPLASM.

organotypic growth   A growth process ordained to produce the cellular structure and organization which will result in the formation of a particular organ.

population growth   The change in size of a population with the passage of time, being the balance between the increments (live births and immigration) and the decrements (deaths and emigration) that have occurred during the period in question.

synchronous growth   Simultaneous division of all the cells in a culture. Inocula of bacteria that yield such growth for a few generations may be obtained by various procedures, such as collecting in the cold the cells that have just been released from

mother cells wedged in the pores of a membrane filter.

grub [Middle English *grobbe, grubbe*]   A larva or maggot, thick and wormlike in form, characteristic of insects in the orders Coleoptera, Hymenoptera, and Diptera.

cattle grub   A larva of *Hypoderma bovis* or *H. lineatum*. Also called *ox bot*.

grübelsucht [German *grübel(n)* to ponder, brood + *Sucht* illness]   Brooding over trifles, a frequent symptom in obsessive-compulsive neurosis and depressive psychosis.

Gruber [Georg Benno Otto *Gruber*, German pathologist, born 1884]   Gruber syndrome, Meckel-Gruber syndrome. See under MECKEL SYNDROME.

Gruber [Josef *Gruber*, Austrian otologist, 1827–1900]   See under SPECULUM, TEST, METHOD.

Gruber [Maximilian Franz Maria von *Gruber*, Austrian bacteriologist, 1853–1927]   Gruber-Widal reaction, Gruber's reaction, Gruber-Widal test. See under WIDAL TEST.

Gruber [Wenzel Leopold *Gruber*, Russian anatomist, 1814–1890]   **1** Petrospheno-occipital suture of Gruber. See under FISSURA PETRO-OCCIPITALIS.   **2** Gruber's fossa, sac of Gruber. See under GRUBER'S CUL-DE-SAC.   **3** Sac of Gruber. See under BURSA OF SINUS TARSI.   **4** See under MUSCLE.   **5** Gruber-Landzert fossa. See under RECESSUS PARADUODENALIS.   **6** Gruber-Landzert fossa. See under FOSSA.

gruel [Middle English *gruel, grewel*, from Old French *gruel* (from Med L *grutellum*, dim. of *grutum* meal) coarse meal]   A thin watery porridge made from cereal grain.

grumose   GRUMOUS.

grumous   Any semisolid material containing small, lumpy concretions. It is often used to describe the gross appearance of the contents of advanced atheromatous plaques. Also called *grumose*.

grundplatte [German *Grund* ground + *Platte* plate]   BASAL LAMINA.

grunt / expiratory grunt   A low-pitched, harsh sound resulting from brief, rapid expiration through partially closed, tense vocal ligaments. It is a vocal expression indicative of respiratory distress, or a response to noxious stimuli in general anesthesia.

Grünwald [Ludwig *Grünwald*, German rhinologist, born 1863]   May-Grünwald stain. See under STAIN.

grutum [Med L, meal, akin to English *groats*]   An obsolete term for MILIUM.

Grütz [Otto *Grütz*, German dermatologist, born 1886]   Bürger-Grütz syndrome. See under FAMILIAL HYPERLIPOPROTEINEMIA TYPE I.

Grynfelt [Joseph Casimir *Grynfelt*, French surgeon, 1840–1913]   Grynfelt's triangle, triangle of Grynfelt and Lesshaft. See under SUPERIOR LUMBAR TRIANGLE.

gryochrome   Designating any nerve cell or neuronal perikaryon containing stainable granules in its cytoplasm, such as the anterior horn cells of the spinal cord.

gryphosis   ONYCHOGRYPOSIS.

gryposis [Gk *gryp(os)* curved, esp. hook-nosed + -OSIS]   ONYCHOGRYPOSIS.

gryposis penis   CHORDEE.

gryposis unguium   ONYCHOGRYPOSIS.

Gs   Symbol for the obsolete unit, gauss.

GSH   Symbol for reduced glutathione.

GSR   galvanic skin response (psychogalvanic response).

GSSG   Symbol for oxidized glutathione.

Gt   Symbol for the unit, gigatonne.

gt.   *gutta* (L, drop).

GTH   gonadotropic hormone (gonadotropin).

GTO   Golgi tendon organ (tendon organ).

GTP   guanosine triphosphate.

gtt.   *guttae* (L, drops).

GU   **1** genitourinary.   **2** gastric ulcer.

Gua   Symbol for guanine.

guaiacol $C_7H_8O_2$. 2-Methoxyphenol, a phenolic compound of creosote produced primarily by destructive distillation of beechwood. It has antiseptic, disinfectant, deodorant, expectorant, and mucolytic properties. It may be synthesized from catechol and may be used to synthesize vanillin. Also called *catechol methyl ether, methylcatechol.*

guaiacol carbonate $C_{15}H_{14}O_5$. Carbonic acid bis(2-methoxyphenyl)ester, a white, crystalline powder used as an expectorant medication.

guaiacum   GUAIACUM WOOD.

guaiaci lignum   GUAIACUM WOOD.

guaiacum resin   A resin obtained from guaiacum wood. It has mild laxative and diuretic actions and it has been used to treat rheumatism. The resin is also used in a test for occult blood in feces that also employs acetic acid and hydrogen peroxide.

guaifenesin $C_{10}H_{14}O_4$. 3-(2-Methoxyphenoxy)-1,2-propanediol, a compound that is believed to reduce the viscosity of sputum. It is used as an expectorant in cough medicine.

guanase   GUANINE DEAMINASE.

guanazolo   AZAGUANINE.

guanethidine $C_{10}H_{22}N_4$. A potent synthetic agent that is used in the treatment of hypertension by reducing the epinephrine level in the body.

guanethidine sulfate $C_{20}H_{46}N_8O_4S$. 2-(1′-Azacyclooctyl)ethylguanidine sulfate, a compound that is used in the management of moderate to severe hypertension, and for hypertension secondary to renal disease, amyloidosis, and renal artery stenosis. It is given orally.

guanidine $(NH_2)_2C{=}NH$. A strong base (pK 13.6), which forms a highly symmetrical cation. Strong solutions of its hydrochloride are used to denature and dissolve proteins.

guanidine phosphate   **1** A salt between guanidine and phosphoric acid.   **2** An incorrect term for PHOSPHOGUANIDINE.

guanidino   The group $NH_2{-}C({=}NH){-}NH{-}$, derived from guanidine. It is strongly basic and is an important feature of the arginine molecule.

guanidinoacetic acid $NH_2{-}C({=}NH_2{}^+){-}NH{-}CH_2{-}COO^-$. An intermediate in the biosynthesis of creatine, it is formed by transfer of an amidino group from arginine onto glycine by glycine amidinotransferase.

γ-guanidinobutyramide $H_2N{-}C({=}NH){-}NH{-}[CH_2]_3{-}CO{-}NH_2$. A compound related in structure to both arginine and γ-aminobutyric acid, found to lower urea and influence autonomic neuropathy in diabetes.

guanidinosuccinic acid   A complex of guanidine and succinic acid, having a molecular weight of approximately 158, that accumulates in the blood of uremic patients and inhibits platelet aggregation. The hemorrhagic diathesis of uremia has been attributed to this substance.

guanine   One of the two purines found in all nucleic acids; 2-amino-6-hydroxypurine and its tautomers, predominantly 2-amino-6-oxo-1,6-dihydropurine. Its nucleotides are important in a number of biologic processes, such as the decarboxylation of oxaloacetate, the oxidation of 2-oxoglutarate, and, in bacteria, the integration of the biosynthesis of proteins and nucleic acids.

guanine deaminase   The enzyme (EC 3.5.4.3) that catalyzes the hydrolysis of guanine to xanthine and ammonia, a step in the catabolism of guanine. Also called *guanase.*

guanine deoxyriboside   A nucleoside, composed of the purine base guanine and the pentose deoxyribose. It is one of the four nucleosides present in DNA, and it base-pairs with cytosine deoxyriboside.

guano   [Spanish (from Quechua *huanu* dung), seabirds' droppings]   The accumulated excrement of marine birds or cave-dwelling bats. It is a valuable source of phosphates and is used as a fertilizer.

guanophores   [Spanish *guano* (from Quechua *huanu* excrement) dung + -PHORE]   Epidermal cells, found in some poikilotherms, which contain granules rich in guanine. The granules give the animal a metallic luster, usually gold or silver.

guanosine   The nucleoside formed by condensation of guanine and ribose. It is a constituent of nucleic acids and of many biologically important nucleotides. Also called *ribofuranosylguanine.*

guanosine diphosphate   The nucleotide formed by esterification of O-5′ of guanosine with diphosphoric (pyrophosphoric) acid. Symbol: GDP

guanosine 3′-diphosphate-5′-diphosphate   A purine riboside bearing diphosphate groups on two oxygen atoms of the ribose. It accumulates in bacteria when they are starved of a required amino acid, and inhibits the synthesis of some but not all types of RNA in those bacteria.

guanosine triphosphate   The nucleotide formed by esterification of O-5′ of guanosine with triphosphoric acid. It is the precursor of guanosine-phosphate residues in RNA, and also acts as an intermediate in biologically important energy-transfer and biosynthetic processes. Symbol: GTP

guanyl   An obsolete term for AMIDINO.

guanyl cyclase   GUANYLATE CYCLASE.

guanylate cyclase   The enzyme (EC 4.6.1.2) responsible for the breakdown of GTP into cGMP and diphosphate. Guanylate cyclase is an important metabolic regulator in bacteria and in higher cells. Some enterotoxins act by activating this enzyme. Also called *guanyl cyclase, guanylyl cyclase.*

guanylic acid   A guanosine phosphate, usually guanosine 5′-phosphate. Its residues occur in RNA and in several nucleotides.

guanyloribonuclease   RIBONUCLEASE T$_1$.

guanylyl cyclase   GUANYLATE CYCLASE.

guanylyl methylene diphosphonate   The anhydride between GMP and methylenebis(phosphonic acid), i.e., the analogue of GTP in which the oxygen atom between P-β and P-γ is replaced by CH_2. It is a competitive inhibitor of guanosine triphosphate reactions in protein synthesis.

guarana   A dried paste of the crushed seeds of *Paullinia cupana* which contains nearly three times the amount of caffeine as coffee.

guard   A device that protects or shields.

bite guard   A removable appliance that covers the occlusal surfaces of the teeth in one jaw. It is used to protect teeth from occlusal stress and in the treatment of temporomandibular joint pain. Also called *occlusal overlay appliance.*

mouth guard   A device for protecting the teeth from injury during sporting activities. It covers the teeth occlusally, labially, and buccally, and extends into the labial and buccal vestibules. It is made in one piece of resilient material, such as rubber, on casts of the teeth and gums.

night guard   A bite guard worn only during sleep.

guarding   A reflex or voluntary reaction of a subject during physical examination that firmly contracts the abdominal wall, thereby making deep palpation difficult. It is usually associated with an underlying inflammatory process. Also called *muscle guarding, muscular defense.*

muscle guarding   GUARDING.

Guarnieri   [Giuseppe *Guarnieri*, Italian pathologist, 1856–1918]

Guarnieri's corpuscles, Guarnieri's inclusions. See under GUAR-
NIERI BODIES.

guaza   MARIHUANA.

gubernacular   Of or relating to a gubernaculum.

gubernaculum [L (from *guberna(re)* to steer, govern, from Gk
kybernan to steer + L *-culum* English *-cle*), the helm or rudder
of a ship]   A fibrous cord directing the course of a structure
attached to it during development.

   gubernaculum dentis   An epithelial tract that for some time
   attaches the apex of unerupted deciduous and permanent teeth
   to the gum epithelium. It is a remnant of the dental lamina and
   eventually disappears completely.

Hunter's gubernaculum   GUBERNACULUM TESTIS.

   gubernaculum testis   A fibromuscular cord which, in the male
   embryo, connects the lower pole of the wolffian body (mesonephros) to the part of the inguinal peritoneum that sends out,
   through the abdominal wall, a diverticulum called the processus
   vaginalis. The gubernaculum is crossed on its ventral aspect by
   the urogenital cord. The gubernaculum then becomes adherent
   to the lower pole of the testis, as it starts to descend and connects
   it through the cord and the processus vaginalis to the coverings
   of the genital swelling. There is thus formed a pathway for the
   descent of the testis: intra-abdominal within the inguinal fold of
   peritoneum, then intraparietal within the bulk of the abdominal
   muscles (internal oblique and transversus where the inguinal
   canal will form), and finally extra-abdominal within the scrotum.
   The testis normally descends along this pathway to reach the
   scrotum where it projects into the distal end of the processus
   vaginalis which later becomes the tunica vaginalis testis. The
   gubernaculum in adult males contributes to the fascial coverings
   of the testis and spermatic cord. In adult females the homologous
   structure is retained as the round ligament of the uterus and the
   ligament of the ovary. Also called *Hunter's gubernaculum, scrotal ligament of testis.*

Gubler [Adolphe Marie *Gubler*, French physician, 1821–1879]
   1 See under SIGN, LINE, TUMOR. **2** Gubler's hemiplegia, Gubler's paralysis, Millard-Gubler paralysis, Gubler-Millard paralysis. See under MILLARD-GUBLER SYNDROME. **3** Gubler's icterus. See under HEMOLYTIC JAUNDICE.

Gudden [Johann Bernhard Aloys von *Gudden*, German psychiatrist, 1824–1886]   **1** See under LAW, ATROPHY. **2** Tegmental nuclei of Gudden. See under NUCLEI TEGMENTI MESENCE-
   PHALICI. **3** Commissura inferior guddeni. See under GUD-
   DEN'S COMMISSURE.

Guedel [Arthur Ernest *Guedel*, U.S. anesthesiologist, 1883–
   1956]   Guedel stages of general anesthesia. See under STAGE.

Guenther [Carl Oskar *Guenther*, German physician, 1854–1929]
   See under STAIN.

Guérin [Alphonse François Marie *Guérin*, French surgeon,
   1816–1895]   **1** Guérin's glands. See under DUCTUS PARAURE-
   THRALES. **2** Guérin's glands. See under GLANDULAE URE-
   THRALES URETHRAE FEMININAE. **3** Guérin's fold, valvule of
   Guérin, Guérin's valve. See under VALVULA FOSSAE NAVICU-
   LARIS. **4** Guérin's fracture. See under LEFORT I FRACTURE.
   5 Guérin sinus. See under LACUNA MAGNA.

Guérin [Camille *Guérin*, French bacteriologist, 1872–1961]   Bacille Calmette-Guérin. See under CALMETTE-GUÉRIN BACIL-
   LUS.

guidance   **1** Counseling and supportive psychotherapy that en-
   courages the subject to set specific goals and to avoid anxiety-
   provoking situations. **2** The act or process of guiding.

   child guidance   Measures taken to enhance familial and social
   supports available during a child's developmental years as a
   means of preventing or minimizing the chances of the development of mental illness.

   condylar guidance   The guidance supplied by a condylar
   guide on an articulator.

   contact guidance   The condition in which the direction of
   growth of a cellular process or the direction of cellular movement is dependent upon the contour of the solid substratum
   with which the cell is in physical contact. The influence of
   nonuniform surfaces on cell growth or movement is seen during
   embryogenesis or in tissue culture.

   incisal guidance   **1** The guidance supplied by an incisal guide
   on an articulator. **2** The effects on mandibular movement of
   sliding contacts of upper and lower incisor teeth.

   vocational guidance   Professional counseling applied to an
   individual's choice of and preparation for a vocation or career.
   Although a comparative evaluation of the client's abilities and
   talents is essential, the selection of an appropriate career goes
   well beyond purely cognitive factors to include questions of
   temperament, motivation, planning ability, and the like.

guide   **1** A device that directs the course of something else, as
   by preceding it or confining its motion, or that indicates by
   pointing. **2** To serve as a guide for.

   anterior guide   INCISAL GUIDE.

   condylar guide   That part of an articulator which controls the
   path of the simulated condyle.

   incisal guide   That part of an articulator which simulates the
   natural incisal guidance angle. Also called *anterior guide.*

   light guide   Fiberoptics used for illumination only and not for
   transmitting images.

   mold guide   A series of samples, photographs, or diagrams
   showing the various shapes and sizes of artificial teeth available
   from a manufacturer.

guideline   **1** A line used as a guide or indicator. **2** A statement or rule that serves to guide conduct in accordance with
   policy.

   clasp guideline   SURVEY LINE.

   Cummer's guideline   A survey line on teeth for insertion of
   partial dentures.

Guidi [Guido *Guidi* (Vidius), Italian-born anatomist active in
   France, 1500–1569]   Canal of Guidi, canalis pterygoideus Vi-
   dii. See under CANALIS PTERYGOIDEUS.

Guillain [Georges *Guillain*, French neurologist, 1876–1961]   **1**
   Barré-Guillain syndrome, Guillain-Barré polyneuritis, Guillain-
   Barré-Strohl syndrome, Landry-Guillain-Barré syndrome. See
   under GUILLAIN-BARRÉ SYNDROME. **2** Guillain-Barré reflex.
   See under SOLE-TAP REFLEX.

guillotine [French, originally a machine for beheading with a
   sharp blade sliding down vertical guides, after Joseph Ignace
   Guillotin, French physician, 1738–1814]   A sharp surgical instrument designed to excise the tonsils or the uvula.

   tonsil guillotine   One of a family of instruments for performing tonsillectomy, all descended from the Physick tonsillotome.
   Modern instruments do not cut off the tonsils, as the name
   suggests, but enucleate them. Also called *tonsillotome* (obsolete),
   tonsillectome (obsolete), *amygdalotome* (obsolete).

guilt [Middle English *gilt*, from Old English *gylt* an offense, sin]
   Anxiety stemming from knowledge or belief of one's own wrong-
   doing and anticipation of punishment for it.

Guinard [Aimé *Guinard*, French surgeon, 1856–1911]   See under TREATMENT.

guinea pig   A small rodent of the genus *Cavia* used extensively
   in biologic research.

Guinon [Georges *Guinon*, French physician, 1859–1929]   Guinon's disease, tic de Guinon. See under GILLES DE LA TOUR-
   ETTE SYNDROME.

gula   GULLET.

gulf / **Lecat's gulf**   A dilatation of the lumen of the bulb of the urethra just beyond the membranous portion where the ducts of the bulbourethral glands open.

Gull [Sir William Withey *Gull*, English physician, 1816–1890] Arteriocapillary fibrosis of Gull and Sutton. See under GULL-SUTTON DISEASE.

gullet [Middle English *golet*, from Middle French *goulet*, dim. of Old French *gole, goule* throat, from L *gula* gullet, windpipe, neck]   The hollow muscular canal extending from the mouth to the stomach, comprising the pharynx and the esophagus. Also called *gula*.

Gullstrand [Allvar *Gullstrand*, Swedish ophthalmologist, 1862–1934]   See under LAMP, LAW.

gulose   An aldohexose isomeric with glucose, from which it differs in configuration at both C-3 and C-4. It has little biochemical importance.

guluronic acid   The acid related to gulose by oxidation of C-6 to a carboxyl group. L-Guluronic acid is a precursor in the biosynthesis of ascorbic acid.

gum¹ [L *gummi*. See GUMMI.]   A diverse group of complex carbohydrate derivatives that are amorphous, translucent, and water-soluble, and that are produced by plants following mechanical injury. Also called *gummi*.

acacia gum   ACACIA.

gum arabic   ACACIA.

Australian gum   WATTLE GUM.

Bassora gum   STERCULIA GUM.

gum benjamin   BENZOIN.

gum benzoin   BENZOIN.

gum dragon   GUM TRAGACANTH.

eucalyptus gum   An exudation obtained primarily from the bark of *Eucalyptus longirostris* that is used as an astringent in treating throat ailments and as an antidiarrheal. Also called *red gum, eucalyptus kino*.

ghatti gum   STERCULIA GUM.

gum guaiac   A resin obtained from the heartwood of *Guiacum officinale* and *Guiacum sanctum*. It is a hard, glossy, reddish brown substance that takes on a green color on long exposure to the air. It has a balsamic odor and a slightly acrid taste. The powder made from the resin is yellow-brown becoming olive-brown on exposure to air. It dissolves incompletely but readily in alcohol, ether, chloroform, and alkalis, and dissolves slightly in carbon disulfide and benzene. It is used as a preservative or antioxidant in foods. It can be detected by adding one drop of freshly prepared $FeCl_3 6H_2O$ (5 g in 50 ml absolute alcohol) to 5 ml of alcoholic solution (1 in 100) of the gum guaiac. If present, blue color is produced that turns green and then yellowish green.

guar gum   A gum obtained from the guar plant, *Cyamopsis tetragonolobus*, that is used as a stabilizer and thickener in processed foods.

Indian gum   STERCULIA GUM.

gum juniper   SANDARAC.

karaya gum   STERCULIA GUM.

Kordofan gum   ACACIA.

mesquite gum   A gum obtained principally from *Prosopis juliflora*, mesquite. It has been used as a substitute for acacia gum.

gum opium   OPIUM.

red gum   EUCALYPTUS GUM.

gum senegal   ACACIA.

sterculia gum   An exudate obtained from several species of *Sterculia*, the most important being *S. urens*. It is used as a bulk cathartic. Also called *Bassora gum, karaya gum, Indian gum, ghatti gum, karaya, Indian tragacanth*.

gum tragacanth   The gummy exudate obtained from several species of *Astragalus*, the most important commercially being

A. gummifer. It is used pharmaceutically as an emulsifying agent, adhesive, and emollient. Also called *gum dragon, tragacanth, mucilago tragacanthae*.

wattle gum   A gum obtained from *Acacia decurrens* and several other Australian species of the genus. It is used as a substitute for gum arabic. Also called *Australian gum*.

gum² [Old English *gōma* (akin to German *Gaumen* palate and to Gk *chaunos* gaping) palate, in pl., jaws]   The gingiva or the mucosa covering edentulous ridges; usually used in the plural.

blue gum   The appearance of gingiva with a lead line.

gumboil [GUM¹ + BOIL]   **1** See under ALVEOLAR ABSCESS.   **2** The external end of the draining tract from a chronic alveolar abscess.

gumma [L *gummi*. See GUMMI.]   The characteristic but inconstant lesion of tertiary syphilis. It may be solitary or multiple, range from microscopic to several centimeters in diameter, and is most commonly found in the liver, testis, bone, skin, and mucosal areas. Gummas have a rubbery consistency and are often surrounded by a fibrous capsule. Microscopically, the center consists of necrotic debris with faint outlines of preexisting structures. Epithelioid cells, occasional multinucleated giant cells, and plasma cells surround the necrotic center. Gummas are clinically important because of local tissue destruction. The large ones must be differentiated from neoplasms. Therapy shrinks the gumma, which becomes a fibrotic scar. Also called *gummy tumor*.

scrofulous gumma   TUBERCULOUS GUMMA.

tuberculous gumma   A granulomatous nodule of tuberculous origin. Also called *scrofuloderma gummosa, scrofulous gumma*.

gummata   Plural of GUMMA.

gummatous   Having the gross appearance of a gumma.

gummi [L (from Gk *kommi* gum, gummy substance), gum, gummy substance]   GUM.

gummy   Resembling the consistency of gum.

gun / balling gun   A metal, syringelike device used in veterinary medicine for dosing animals, mainly sheep, cattle, and horses, with medicaments in the form of tablets or capsules.

electron gun   A device for producing a beam of electrons from a thermionic source.

gundo   GOUNDOU.

Gunn   See under MARCUS GUNN.

Gunn [Moses *Gunn*, U.S. surgeon, 1822–1887]   See under LAW.

Gunning [Jan Willem *Gunning*, Dutch chemist, 1827–1901]   See under MIXTURE.

Gunning [Thomas Brian *Gunning*, U.S. dentist, 1813–1889]   See under SPLINT.

Günther [Hans *Günther*, German physician, 1884–1956]   Günther's disease. See under CONGENITAL ERYTHROPOIETIC PORPHYRIA.

Günz [Justus *Günz*, German anatomist, 1714–1789]   See under LIGAMENT.

Günzberg [Alfred *Günzberg*, German physician, born 1861]   See under SIGN.

Guo   Symbol for guanosine.

gurney   A wheeled stretcher or cart for the transport of patients, usually within a hospital.

Gussenbauer [Carl Ignatz *Gussenbauer*, Austrian surgeon, 1842–1903]   See under SUTURE, OPERATION.

gustation [L *gustatio* (from *gustatus*, past part. of *gustare* to taste) a tasting]   DEGUSTATION.

gustatory [L *gustat(us)*, past part. of *gustare* to taste + -ORY]   Having to do with the sense of taste.

gustometry [L *gust(us)* a tasting + *o* + -METRY]   The measurement of taste thresholds either by applying the appropriate stimulus (salt, sweet, sour, or bitter) to the dorsum of the tongue or by the technique of electrogustometry.

gut [Old English *guttas* (pl.) viscera, akin to *geotan* to pour] **1** In embryology, the foregut, midgut, or hindgut. **2** INTESTINE. **3** The digestive or alimentary tract, or a part of it.

blind gut CAECUM.

head gut FOREGUT.

postanal gut The extension tailwards of the posterior part of the embryonic intestine (the hindgut) beyond the cloacal membrane. It becomes obliterated and disappears early in development. Also called *tailgut.*

preoral gut SEESSEL'S POUCH.

primitive gut ARCHENTERON.

ribbon gut A broad band of animal intestine that has been heated and processed and is used to reinforce surgical suture lines where the natural tissues are weakened.

silkworm gut A strand of treated and processed suture material drawn from a silkworm. It is fairly stiff and nonabsorbable.

surgical gut CATGUT.

Guthrie [Clyde Graeme *Guthrie*, U.S. physician, 1880–1931] See under FORMULA.

Guthrie [George James *Guthrie*, English surgeon, 1785–1856] Guthrie's muscle. See under MUSCULUS SPHINCTER URETHRAE.

Guthrie [Robert *Guthrie*, U.S. pediatrician and microbiologist, born 1916] See under TEST.

Gutmann [Carl *Gutmann*, German physician, born 1872] Michaelis-Gutmann bodies. See under BODY.

gutta [Malay *getah* the gum of the percha tree]   (*plural* guttae.) A drop.

guttae ophthalmicae HASSALL-HENLE BODIES.

gutta serena An obsolete term for AMAUROSIS.

guttae Plural of GUTTA.

gutta-percha [Malay *getah* gum + *percha* the tree yielding the juice] A thermoplastic material made from the latex of certain sapotaceous trees which has been used as a temporary filling in dentistry.

baseplate gutta-percha Gutta-percha that has been mixed with filler and coloring and made into sheets. It is no longer used for baseplates.

temporary stopping gutta-percha Gutta-percha that has been mixed with filler and coloring and made into rods. It is made plastic by heating and is used for sealing dressings into tooth cavities.

guttat. *guttatum* (L, drop by drop).

guttate Denoting a lesion of the skin having the shape of a drop.

guttation [L *gutt(a)* a drop + -ATION] The exudation of water from leaves.

gutter **1** A shallow furrow. **2** One of the sulci paracolici.

hepatic gutter HEPATIC DIVERTICULUM.

left lateral paracolic gutter The longitudinal intraperitoneal channel that lies between the descending colon and the left lateral abdominal wall and is formed by the visceral peritoneum of the colon, dipping posteriorly to become continuous with the parietal peritoneum of the posterolateral abdominal wall.

paracolic gutters SULCI PARACOLICI.

pleuroperitoneal gutters Paired gutters between somatopleure and splanchnopleure which at one stage constitute the posterior parts on each side of the primitive coelomic cavity (becoming closed off as the coelomic duct). Each pleuroperitoneal communication is subsequently obliterated, between the fifth and eighth weeks of gestation, by the formation of a pleuroperitoneal membrane and by the enlargement of neighboring

organs such as the liver on the right and the suprarenal gland on the left.

right lateral paracolic gutter The longitudinal intraperitoneal channel that lies between the ascending colon and the right lateral abdominal wall. It is formed by the visceral peritoneum of the colon dipping posteriorly to become continuous with the parietal peritoneum of the posterolateral abdominal wall. Superiorly it is continuous with the hepatorenal pouch and with the superior omental recess, and inferiorly it is continuous over the brim of the pelvis with the rectovesical or rectouterine pouch.

synaptic gutter SYNAPTIC TROUGH.

guttering An operation in which the surface of a bone is grooved deeply.

gutti GAMBOGE.

Guttmann [E. *Guttmann*, German physician, flourished 20th century] Bodechtel-Guttmann disease. See under SUBACUTE SCLEROSING PANENCEPHALITIS.

Guttmann [Paul *Guttmann*, German physician, 1834–1893] See under SIGN.

gutt. quibusd. *guttis quibusdam* (L, with a few drops).

guttur [L, the throat] The throat.

guttural [L *guttur* the throat + -AL] **1** Concerned with or relating to the throat. **2** The quality of an individual's speech and of certain spoken languages in which there is a greater proportion of sounds produced with the posterior part of the tongue in the velar or pharyngeal regions of the vocal tract.

gutturophony An unduly throaty quality of speech.

gutturotetany A hypertonic state of the pharyngeal and related musculature resulting in a tense, thin, throaty speech quality.

Guy [E. F. *Guy*, U.S. physiologist, flourished early 20th century] Leake and Guy method. See under METHOD.

Guye [Ambroise Arnold Guillaume *Guye*, Dutch laryngologist, 1839–1904] Guye sign. See under GUYE'S APROSEXIA.

Guyon [Jean Casimir Felix *Guyon*, French surgeon, 1831–1920] **1** See under SIGN. **2** Guyon's operation. See under AMPUTATION. **3** Guyon's isthmus. See under ISTHMUS UTERI.

GVH graft-versus-host (reaction).

GVHD graft-versus-host disease.

GW Symbol for the unit, gigawatt.

Gwathmey [James Taylor *Gwathmey*, U.S. surgeon, 1863–1944] See under ANESTHESIA.

Gy Symbol for the unit, gray.

Gymnamoebia [*gymn(o)-* + *amoeb(a)* + *-IA*] A subclass of nontestate amebas (class Lobosea, superclass Rhizopoda, subphylum Sarcodina) which includes the familiar amebas of the order Amoebida, such as *Amoeba, Entamoeba, Platyamoeba, Flabellula, Paramoeba, Naegleria, Tetramitis,* and *Pelomyxa.*

gymnastics [L *gymnasticus* (from Gk *gymnastikos* fond of athletics, from *gymnos* naked, lightly clad) gymnastic] Systematic exercise patterns and procedures, often of a complex or athletic nature.

antagonistic gymnastics Gymnastic exercises involving at least two participants who resist one another's movements. Also called *resistance-antagonistic gymnastics.*

medical gymnastics Gymnastic exercises performed for medical reasons, including the improvement of trunk and limb physical disabilities.

ocular gymnastics Exercises consisting of movement of the eyes into various positions.

resistance-antagonistic gymnastics ANTAGONISTIC GYMNASTICS.

Swedish gymnastics A system of exercises developed by a

Swedish fencing master in 1813, originally for use in the military but later proposed as a means of attaining physical fitness for the general population. It involves detailed directions classifying starting positions and specific degrees of activity, and regulating dosage and progress. As a result of royal backing and the founding of the Central Institute of Gymnastics in Stockholm, this program, to which massage was added, became known as Swedish gymnastics and massage. Also called *Swedish movement, Ling's method, lingism.*

gymnemic acid $C_{32}H_{55}O_{12}$. A bitter powder obtained from the leaves of *Gymnema sylvestre*, a shrub native to southern Asia. When placed in the mouth, it temporarily blocks the capacity to distinguish between bitter and sweet tastes.

gymno- [Gk *gymnos* naked, lightly clad] A combining form meaning naked, bare, exposed.

Gymnoascus   A genus of fungi which includes several common saprobic species.

gymnocarpous [GYMNO- + *carp(o)-*² + -OUS] Not protected or covered during basidiocarp development: used of the gill layer of a mushroom.

gymnocyte [GYMNO- + -CYTE] A cell without a limiting membrane or a cell wall. Also called *gymnoplast.*

gymnophobia [GYMNO- + -PHOBIA] Pathologic fear of nudity.

gymnoplast [GYMNO- + -PLAST] GYMNOCYTE.

gymnoscopic   Referring to a desire to see naked bodies.

Gymnosomata [GYMNO- + Gk *sōmata*, pl. of *sōma* body] A suborder of Mollusca lacking shells.

gymnosperm [GYMNO- + SPERM] A seed plant with seeds that are not enclosed in an ovary. The conifers are the most familiar group of gymnosperms. Compare ANGIOSPERM.

gymnospore [GYMNO- + SPORE] A spore without a protective envelope.

gymnothecium [GYMNO- + *thec(a)* + 1 *-ium*, neut. noun suffix] A cluster of ascocarps covered by a thin veil of hyphae which leave the asci essentially unprotected.

Gymnothorax   A genus of marine eels of the family Muraenidae; the moray eels. They occur on tropical reefs and have caused cases of poisoning when eaten.

gyn-   GYNECO-.

gynaeco-   A British spelling for GYNECO-.

gynaecology   A British spelling for GYNECOLOGY.

gynaecomastia   A British spelling for GYNECOMASTIA.

Gynaecophorus   A former name for *SCHISTOSOMA*.

gynander [GYN- + Gk *anēr*, gen. *andros*, a man] An older term for GYNANDROMORPH.

gynandria   **1** An imprecise term for HERMAPHRODITISM. **2** An older term for FEMALE PSEUDOHERMAPHRODITISM.

gynandrism   **1** An imprecise term for HERMAPHRODITISM. **2** An older term for FEMALE PSEUDOHERMAPHRODITISM.

gynandroblastoma [GYN- + ANDRO- + BLASTOMA] A very rare ovarian tumor in which collections of granulosa cells with typical Call-Exner bodies coexist with hollow tubules lined by Sertoli cells. Used morphologically, the term does not imply a specific type of hormone production. Also called *sex cord-stromal tumor of mixed cell types.*

gynandroid [GYN- + ANDROID] FEMALE PSEUDOHERMAPHRODITE.

gynandromorph [GYN- + ANDRO- + -MORPH] An individual having both male and female external genitalia and/or secondary sexual features. Also called *gynander* (older term).

gynandromorphism [GYN- + ANDRO- + MORPH- + -ISM] HERMAPHRODITISM.

gynandromorphous   Possessing both male and female anatomic characteristics. Also *hermaphroditic.*

gynandry   **1** An imprecise term for HERMAPHRODITISM. **2** An older term for FEMALE PSEUDOHERMAPHRODITISM.

gynanthropia   **1** An imprecise term for HERMAPHRODITISM. **2** An older term for FEMALE PSEUDOHERMAPHRODITISM.

gynanthropism   **1** An imprecise term for HERMAPHRODITISM. **2** An older term for FEMALE PSEUDOHERMAPHRODITISM.

gynatresia [GYN- + ATRESIA] An occlusion of any part of the female genital tract, particularly an occlusion of the vagina by a residual urogenital membrane.

gyne-   GYNECO-.

gynec-   GYNECO-.

gynecic [GYNEC- + -IC] GYNOPATHIC.

gyneco- [Gk *gynē* (genitive *gynaikos*) a woman] A combining form meaning woman or female. Also *gyn-, gyne-, gyno-, gynaeco- (British spelling).*

gynecogen [GYNECO- + -GEN] Any agent, as female sex hormones, which induces the development of or stimulates female somatic or behavioral characteristics.

gynecogenic [GYNECO- + -GENIC] Producing or tending to produce female characteristics.

gynecography [GYNECO- + -GRAPHY] Radiography of the female genital organs using air or other gas injected intraperitoneally as a contrast medium. Also called *gynography.*

gynecoid [GYNEC- + -OID] Pertaining to or resembling women.

gynecologist [GYNECO- + -LOGIST] A physician who specializes in the diseases of women's reproductive organs and associated diseases.

gynecology [GYNECO- + -LOGY] The branch of medicine which devotes itself to the care and prevention of genital tract disorders in women and which for the most part is not concerned with pregnancy. Gynecology is also associated with public-health functions, and includes family planning, preconception counseling, genetic counseling, and sexual therapy. Also called *gyniatry.* Adjective: gynecologic, gynecological.

gynecomania [GYNECO- + -MANIA] SATYRIASIS.

gynecomastia [GYNECO- + Gk *mast(os)* (from earlier *mazos* a woman's breast) a woman's breast + -IA] Enlargement of the male breast, occurring sometimes in mild form as a normal phenomenon of male puberty, and as a sequela of various pathologic conditions, such as the Klinefelter syndrome, or hepatic cirrhosis, or thyrotoxicosis. The bulk of the overgrowth is fibrous, regardless of cause. Galactorrhea occurs uncommonly. Also called *mammary feminism* (older term), *gynecomasty* (seldom used), *gynecomastism* (rarely used), *gynecomazia* (rarely used).

nutritional gynecomastia   REFEEDING GYNECOMASTIA.

refeeding gynecomastia   Transient gynecomastia appearing during nutritional rehabilitation after a period of severe undernutrition. Also called *nutritional gynecomastia, rehabilitation gynecomastia.*

rehabilitation gynecomastia   REFEEDING GYNECOMASTIA.

gynecomastism   A rarely used term for GYNECOMASTIA.

gynecomasty   A seldom used term for GYNECOMASTIA.

gynecomazia   A rarely used term for GYNECOMASTIA.

gynecopathy [GYNECO- + -PATHY] Any disease of women, especially of the female reproductive system. Also called *gynopathy.*

gynecophoral [GYNECO- + PHOR- + -AL] See under GYNECOPHORIC CANAL.

gynecotelic [GYNECO- + *tel(e)-*² + -IC] Characterizing social insects which become functional females (queens) if given special care and feeding during their larval development, otherwise becoming infertile, neuter adults (workers).

gynecotokology [GYNECO- + TOKO- + -LOGY] The measurement of uterine contractions, usually during labor. An older term.

gyneduct [GYNE- + DUCT] PARAMESONEPHRIC DUCT.

gynephilia [GYNE- + -PHILIA] SATYRIASIS.

gynephobia [GYNE- + -PHOBIA] Aversion to or fear of women. Also called *gynophobia*.

gyneplasty GYNOPLASTY.

Gynergen A proprietary name for ergotamine tartrate.

gyniatrics [GYN- + -IATRICS] The treatment of diseases of women.

gyniatry [GYN- + -IATRY] GYNECOLOGY.

gyno- GYNECO-.

gynoecium [GYN- + New L *oecium* (from *oec-*, combining form denoting house, from Gk *oikos* a house + L *-ium*, neut. noun suffix) an ovicell] The aggregate carpels in a flower.

gynogamon A gamon produced by a female gamete to attract or stimulate fertilization by the male gamete.

gynogenesis [GYNO- + GENESIS] Development of an embryo from an egg that has been stimulated by a male gamete, but where the spermatozoon does not contribute any genetic material to the conceptus.

gynography GYNECOGRAPHY.

gynoid GYNECOID.

gynomerogon [GYNO- + MERO-¹ + Gk *gon(os)* offspring, procreation] An organism derived from an ovum possessing solely a female pronucleus and thus with maternal chromosomes only. Also called *gynomerogone*.

gynomerogone GYNOMEROGON.

gynomerogony [GYNO- + MERO-¹ + -GONY] Development of the part of a fertilized ovum having only the female pronucleus with its maternal chromosomes.

gynopathic [GYNO- + -PATH + -IC] Pertaining to diseases peculiar to women. Also *gynecic*.

gynopathy GYNECOPATHY.

gynophobia GYNEPHOBIA.

gynoplastic Pertaining to gynoplasty.

gynoplasty [GYNO- + -PLASTY] Reconstructive surgery of the female reproductive organs. Also called *gyneplasty*.

gypsum $CaSO_4 \cdot 2H_2O$. A mineral, the dihydrate of calcium sulfate. With heat treatment and rehydration it forms plaster of Paris which in the past was much used as a dental impression material.

gyr- GYRO-.

gyral Pertaining to a gyrus.

gyrase A name for the ATP-hydrolyzing DNA topoisomerase (EC 5.99.1.3), the enzyme that unwinds the DNA helix, introducing a region of positive supercoiling into the duplex ahead of the replication fork. Also called *helicase*.

gyrate Twisted or coiled; convoluted.

Gyraulus [New L (from Gk *gyr(os)* a ring, circle + *aulos* a tube, flute, wind instrument)] A large genus of freshwater pulmonate snails in the family Planorbidae. It is worldwide in distribution.

Gyraulus convexiusculus A planorbid snail common in southeastern Asia, Indonesia, and the Philippines, which serves as the first intermediate host of an echinostome of rats and humans, *Echinostoma ilocanum*.

Gyraulus parvus A species that serves as the intermediate

host of the schistosome *Gigantobilharzia gyrauli*, a parasite of birds, and of the plagiorchid fluke *Haematoloechus parviplexus*, a common fluke in the lungs of North American frogs.

gyre An obsolete term for GYRUS.

gyrectomy [GYR- + -ECTOMY] Excision of a convolution, or gyrus, of the cerebrum.
  frontal gyrectomy Gyrectomy of the frontal lobe.

Gyrencephala [GYR- + New L *encephala*, pl. of *encephalon* (alteration of Gk *enkephalos* the brain) the brain] The group composed of mammals having a convoluted cerebral cortex, including anthropoid primates and cetaceans.

gyrencephalic [GYR- + ENCEPHAL- + -IC] Denoting the presence of convolutions in the cerebral cortex.

gyri Plural of GYRUS.

gyro- [Gk *gyros* ring, circle] A combining form meaning (1) ring, ringlike; (2) rotating, rotatory. Also *gyr-*.

gyrochrome [GYRO- + Gk *chrōm(a)* color] A neuron containing a ring-shaped perikaryal array of basophilic granules (Nissl bodies). An obsolete term.

gyromele [GYRO- + Gk *mēlē* a probe] A flexible rod passed through a stomach tube and rotated with any of several attachments affixed to the end. It was formerly used for stomach cleansing or other treatment and for taking specimens for culture.

gyrometer [*gyr(us)* + *o* + -METER] A device for measuring cerebral gyri.

gyromitrin Monomethylhydrazine, a hemolytic toxin produced in varying quantities by all species of *Gyromitra* fungi.

Gyropus A genus of biting lice (order Mallophaga, suborder Amblycera, family Gyropidae) which includes several important ectoparasites of mammals.
  Gyropus ovalis A species commonly found on guinea pigs and a troublesome pest in laboratory colonies.

gyrosa [Gk *gyros* a ring, circle + *a*] ROTATORY VERTIGO.

gyrospasm [GYRO- + SPASM] Rotatory spasm of the head.

gyrotrope RHEOTROPE.

gyrus

gyrus [L (from Gk *gyros* a ring, circle), a circle, circuit, ring] (*plural* gyri) [NA] An elevation of the cerebral cortex resulting from the infolding of adjacent sulci or fissures; convolution. Also called *gyre* (obsolete).

angular gyrus GYRUS ANGULARIS.

gyrus angularis [NA] The gyrus of the inferior parietal lobule formed by the caudal union of the superior and middle temporal gyri. Also called *angular gyrus*.

annectant gyri GYRI ANNECTENTES.

gyri annectentes The small gyri (convolutions) within the sulcal depths formed by inconstant, small indentations or furrows. Also called *annectant gyri, gyri transitivi cerebri, transitional gyri, transitional convolutions*.

anterior central gyrus GYRUS PRECENTRALIS.

anterior sigmoid gyrus The cerebral gyrus rostral to the cruciate sulcus of carnivores, the principal site of primary motor cortex.

anterior sylvian gyrus In the carnivore brain, the gyrus along the anterior border of the sylvian fissure.

ascending frontal gyrus GYRUS PRECENTRALIS.

ascending parietal gyrus GYRUS POSTCENTRALIS.

gyri breves insulae [NA] The short, rostral gyri on the insular surface, within the lateral sulcus. Also called *preinsular gyri, short gyri of insula, gyri operti* (obsolete).

Broca's gyrus BROCA'S MOTOR SPEECH AREA.

callosal gyrus GYRUS CINGULI.

gyrus callosus GYRUS CINGULI.

gyrus centralis anterior GYRUS PRECENTRALIS.

gyrus centralis posterior GYRUS POSTCENTRALIS.

gyri cerebelli The folia of the cerebellar cortex.

gyri cerebri [NA] The convolutions of the cerebral cortex, separated by sulci, or fissures. Also called *convolutions of cerebrum, gyri of cerebrum.*

gyri of cerebrum GYRI CEREBRI.

cingulate gyrus GYRUS CINGULI.

gyrus cinguli [NA] The convolution on the medial surface of the cerebrum surrounding the corpus callosum, consisting of a transitional cortex (principally Brodmann's areas 24 and 23) and the retrosplenial fields. Also called *callosal convolution, mesocortex, limbic cortex, gyrus callosus, callosal gyrus, rhinencephalic arch, cingulum hemispherii, cingulate gyrus, cingulate cortex.*

coronal gyrus An outwardly-bowed gyrus in the frontoparietal region of the carnivore brain joining the anterior and posterior sigmoid gyri. Medially it embraces the end of the cruciate sulcus, and laterally it is limited by the coronal sulcus.

gyrus cunei CUNEUS.

cuneolingual gyri The gyri on the medial surface of the human cerebral hemisphere surrounding the calcarine sulcus and containing portions of the visual areas.

deep gyri GYRI PROFUNDI CEREBRI.

deep transitional gyrus The central, transverse zone of cortex in the fetal human cerebrum that forms the buried portion of the sulcus centralis in later development.

dentate gyrus GYRUS DENTATUS.

gyrus dentatus [NA] The innermost cortex of the hippocampal gyrus capping the hippocampal fissure. It consists of a zonal lamina, a densely packed granular layer, and a loose pyramidal or polymorphic layer bounded on its ventricular surface by a myelinated tract, the alveus hippocampi. Also called *fascia dentata hippocampi, dentate gyrus, dentate band, dentate fascia, fascia of Tarin, fascia tarini, fasciola dentata, denticulate body* (obsolete).

gyrus descendens POSTERIOR OCCIPITAL GYRUS.

ectosylvian gyrus On the carnivore brain, the inverted U-shaped convolution surrounding the anterior and posterior sylvian gyri, from which it is separated by anterior and posterior ectosylvian sulci. Anterior, middle, and posterior ectosylvian gyri are distinguished.

gyrus epicallosus INDUSIUM GRISEUM.

external orbital gyrus GYRUS ORBITALIS LATERALIS.

gyrus fasciolaris [NA] The band of cortex surrounding the splenium of the corpus callosum, contiguous with the underlying induseum griseum rostrally and with the hippocampal formation ventrocaudally. Also called *fasciola cinerea cinguli, fascia cinerea, splenial gyrus.*

gyrus fornicatus LIMBIC LOBE.

gyrus frontalis inferior [NA] The inferior convolution below the inferior frontal sulcus of the anthropoid cerebral cortex, divided into triangular, orbital, and opercular sectors by branches of the lateral sulcus. Also called *Broca's convolution, inferior frontal gyrus, Broca's region.*

gyrus frontalis medialis [NA] A convolution on the medial surface of the frontal lobe, lying above the sulcus cinguli and extending dorsally to meet the superior frontal gyrus. Also called *medial frontal gyrus, lateral gyrus (used of carnivores), gyrus marginalis, marginal gyrus of Turner.*

gyrus frontalis medius [NA] The middle convolution of the

frontal lobe, extending rostrally from the precentral gyrus and bordered by the superior and inferior frontal sulci. Also called *middle frontal gyrus.*

gyrus frontalis superior [NA] A frontal lobe convolution extending forward from the precentral gyrus above the sulcus frontalis superior. Also called *superior frontal gyrus.*

fusiform gyrus GYRUS FUSIFORMIS.

gyrus fusiformis A convolution on the ventral surface of the temporal lobe, bounded laterally by the inferior temporal gyrus and limited medially by the collateral and rhinal sulci. It comprises medial and lateral lobules, the gyri occipitotemporalis medialis and lateralis. Also called *fusiform gyrus, fusiform lobule.*

gyrus geniculi GYRUS SUBCALLOSUS.

Heschl's gyri The obliquely oriented transverse temporal gyri lying on the temporal operculum of the lateral sulcus. They are the site of the primary auditory cortex (Brodmann's area 41 and probably a portion of area 42). Also called *Heschl's convolutions.*

hippocampal gyrus 1 GYRUS HIPPOCAMPI. 2 An imprecise term for GYRUS PARAHIPPOCAMPALIS.

gyrus hippocampi 1 [NA] The hippocampal cortical fields (of Ammon's horn), sometimes including the fascia dentata and the subiculum. Also called *hippocampal gyrus.* 2 An imprecise term for HIPPOCAMPAL FORMATION.

inferior frontal gyrus GYRUS FRONTALIS INFERIOR.

inferior occipital gyrus The more ventral of the two gyri on the lateral surface of the occipital lobe, limited anteriorly by the occipital lateral sulcus.

inferior temporal gyrus GYRUS TEMPORALIS INFERIOR.

gyrus infracalcarinus GYRUS LINGUALIS.

gyri insulae The gyri forming the surface of the insula, deep within the lateral sulcus, comprising the gyrus longus insulae and the gyri breves insulae.

internal orbital gyrus GYRUS ORBITALIS MEDIALIS.

gyrus intralimbicus The caudal bulge of the uncus at its junction with the hippocampus.

lateral gyrus the equivalent in carnivores of GYRUS FRONTALIS MEDIALIS.

lateral occipital gyri The two gyri (superior and inferior) on the lateral surface of the occipital lobe, delimited by the lateral occipital sulcus.

lateral occipitotemporal gyrus GYRUS OCCIPITOTEMPORALIS LATERALIS.

gyrus limbicus LIMBIC LOBE.

lingual gyrus GYRUS LINGUALIS.

gyrus lingualis [NA] A rostrally oriented, tongue-shaped gyrus on the medial and ventral surfaces of the occipital and temporal lobes, separated from the cuneus by the calcarine sulcus and from the fusiform gyrus by the collateral sulcus. It is the site of contralateral, upper quadrant visual field representation. Also called *gyrus infracalcarinus, lingual gyrus.*

long gyrus of insula GYRUS LONGUS INSULAE.

gyrus longus insulae [NA] The largest and most caudal of the longitudinally oriented gyri of the insula. It lies within the lateral sulcus. Also called *long gyrus of insula.*

gyrus marginalis GYRUS FRONTALIS MEDIALIS.

marginal gyrus of Turner GYRUS FRONTALIS MEDIALIS.

medial frontal gyrus GYRUS FRONTALIS MEDIALIS.

medial occipitotemporal gyrus GYRUS OCCIPITOTEMPORALIS MEDIALIS.

middle frontal gyrus GYRUS FRONTALIS MEDIUS.

middle temporal gyrus GYRUS TEMPORALIS MEDIUS.

gyrus occipitotemporalis lateralis [NA] The lateral portion of the fusiform gyrus. It is continuous with the inferior temporal gyrus laterally and is separated from the medial portion of the fusiform gyrus by the occipitotemporal sulcus. Also called *lat-*

eral occipitotemporal gyrus, occipitotemporal convolution.

gyrus occipitotemporalis medialis   [NA] The medial portion of the fusiform gyrus. It lies on the ventral surface of the temporal lobe and extends between the collateral sulcus and the occipitotemporal sulcus. Also called *medial occipitotemporal gyrus.*

gyrus olfactorius lateralis of Retzius   A rarely used term for LIMEN INSULAE. • The term is misleading because this gyrus apparently lacks an olfactory role.

gyrus olfactorius medialis of Retzius   A seldom used term for AREA SUBCALLOSA. • The term is misleading because the region has no direct role in olfaction.

gyri operti   An obsolete term for GYRI BREVES INSULAE.

orbital gyri   GYRI ORBITALES.

gyri orbitales   The several irregular convolutions on the basal surface of the frontal lobe overlying the orbit and lateral to the olfactory sulcus. Also called *orbital gyri.*

gyrus orbitalis lateralis   The most lateral of the contiguous convoluted orbital gyri on the base of the human frontal lobe. Also called *external orbital gyrus.*

gyrus orbitalis medialis   The most medial of the contiguous convoluted orbital gyri on the base of the human frontal lobe cortex. Also called *internal orbital gyrus.*

paracentral gyrus   GYRUS PARACENTRALIS.

gyrus paracentralis   A convolution on the medial surface of the cerebral hemisphere continuous with the precentral and postcentral gyri at the termination of the central sulcus, bounded ventrally by the cingulate sulcus. It is the site of sensory and motor representation of the lower extremities and of a separate, supplementary representation of the entire body (called the supplementary motor cortex). Also called *paracentral gyrus.*

parahippocampal gyrus   GYRUS PARAHIPPOCAMPALIS.

gyrus parahippocampalis   [NA] A convolution on the ventral and medial surface of the temporal lobe, lying between the hippocampal sulcus medially and the collateral (rhinal) sulcus laterally. It contains the subicular and entorhinal cortical fields. Also called *parahippocampal gyrus, hippocampal gyrus* (imprecise).

parahippocaudal gyrus   The cerebral cortex between the rhinal fissure marking the neocortical boundary and the hippocampal fissure marking the site of contact with the hippocampus proper.

parasplenial gyrus   A convolution on the medial surface of the carnivore brain adjacent to the splenium. It is bordered superiorly by the parasplenial sulcus, and inferiorly by the corpus callosum.

paraterminal gyrus   GYRUS SUBCALLOSUS.

gyrus paraterminalis   [NA] GYRUS SUBCALLOSUS.

postcentral gyrus   GYRUS POSTCENTRALIS.

gyrus postcentralis   [NA] The rostral convolution of the parietal lobe, lying behind the central sulcus and anterior to the postcentral sulcus. It is the primary area of somatosensory cortex, corresponding approximately to Brodmann's areas 3, 1, and 2. Also called *posterior central gyrus, postrolandic gyrus, ascending parietal gyrus, gyrus centralis posterior, postcentral gyrus.*

posterior central gyrus   GYRUS POSTCENTRALIS.

posterior occipital gyrus   The inferior portion of the gyrus occipitalis lateralis. Also called *gyrus descendens.*

posterior sylvian gyrus   In the carnivore brain, the gyrus immediately posterior to the sylvian fissure.

postrolandic gyrus   GYRUS POSTCENTRALIS.

precentral gyrus   GYRUS PRECENTRALIS.

gyrus precentralis   [NA] The caudal convolution of the frontal lobe anterior to the central sulcus. It is the thickest cortical area, the principal site of origin of the corticospinal tract, and the principal motor area, corresponding approximately to Brod-

mann's area 4 and a portion of area 6. Also called *anterior central gyrus, precentral gyrus, prerolandic gyrus, ascending frontal gyrus, gyrus centralis anterior.*

preinsular gyri   GYRI BREVES INSULAE.

prerolandic gyrus   GYRUS PRECENTRALIS.

gyri profundi   Deep or hidden gyri.

gyri profundi cerebri   Gyri of cerebral cortex, formed within the depths of sulci, that reach the surface. Also called *deep gyri.*

gyrus proreus   On the carnivore brain, the cortical area occupying the tip of the frontal pole and extending caudally to the anterior sigmoid gyrus. It is homologous to the premotor frontal cortex in man.

quadrate gyrus   A seldom used term for PRECUNEUS.

gyrus rectus   [NA] The medial convolution on the orbital surface of the frontal lobe, bordered laterally by the olfactory sulcus. Also called *straight gyrus.*

retrosplenial gyrus   The posterior continuation of the cingulate gyrus, extending behind the splenium of the corpus callosum. See also RETROSPLENIAL CORTEX.

gyrus of Retzius   **1** GYRUS INTRALIMBICUS. **2** LIMEN INSULAE.

gyrus rolandicus   A rarely found gyrus of the human cerebral cortex in the anomalous condition in which two central sulci are present.

short gyri of insula   GYRI BREVES INSULAE.

sigmoid gyrus   The area of sensorimotor cortex on a carnivore brain. The U-shaped gyrus embraces the cruciate sulcus, and on its other side is bounded by the ansate, coronal, and presylvian sulci.

splenial gyrus   GYRUS FASCIOLARIS.

straight gyrus   GYRUS RECTUS.

subcalcarine gyrus   The gyrus forming the inferior lip of the calcarine sulcus.

subcallosal gyrus   GYRUS SUBCALLOSUS.

gyrus subcallosus   [NA] A thin, paramedian gyrus rostral and ventral to the genu of the corpus callosum. Also called *gyrus paraterminalis, Zuckerkandl's convolution, subcallosal gyrus, gyrus geniculi, external marginal arc of Zuckerkandl, area paraterminalis, septal area, paraterminal body, paraterminal gyrus, corpus paraterminalis, penduculus corporis callosi* (obsolete).

subcollateral gyrus   Either of the occipitotemporal gyri. An obsolete term.

superior frontal gyrus   GYRUS FRONTALIS SUPERIOR.

superior occipital gyrus   The uppermost of the gyri on the lateral surface of the occipital lobe, lying above the lateral occipital sulcus.

superior temporal gyrus   GYRUS TEMPORALIS SUPERIOR.

supracallosal gyrus   GYRUS SUPRACALLOSUS.

gyrus supracallosus   The thin horizontal band lying between the cingulate gyrus and the corpus callosum containing the indusium griseum (hippocampal rudiment). Also called *supracallosal gyrus.*

supramarginal gyrus   GYRUS SUPRAMARGINALIS.

gyrus supramarginalis   [NA] The convolution of the inferior portion of the parietal lobe surrounding the caudal end of the lateral sulcus and continuous anteriorly with the superior temporal gyrus. Also called *supramarginal gyrus.*

suprasylvian gyrus   On the carnivore brain, the large arc of cortex laterally embracing the ectosylvian gyri.

gyri temporales transversi   The transverse convolutions of the superior temporal gyrus lying within the lateral sulcus. It is the site of the primary auditory cortex. The anterior transverse temporal gyrus is called Heschl's gyrus or convolution. Also called *transverse temporal gyri.*

gyrus temporalis inferior   [NA] The longitudinal inferolateral gyrus of the temporal lobe, below the inferior temporal sulcus and continuous caudally with the lateral occipitotemporal gyrus. Also called *inferior temporal gyrus.*

gyrus temporalis medius [NA] The middle longitudinal gyrus of the temporal lobe, bounded by the superior and inferior temporal sulci. Also called *second temporal convolution, middle temporal gyrus.*

gyrus temporalis superior [NA] The horizontal, dorsal sulcus of the temporal lobe lying above the superior temporal sulcus and below the lateral sulcus, merging caudally with the supramarginal gyrus. Also called *first temporal convolution, superior temporal gyrus.*

transitional gyri   GYRI ANNECTENTES.

gyri transitivi cerebri   GYRI ANNECTENTES.

transverse gyri of Heschl   AUDITORY CORTEX.

transverse temporal gyri   GYRI TEMPORALES TRANSVERSI.

uncinate gyrus   UNCUS.

gyrus uncinatus   UNCUS.

Gy/s   Symbol for the unit, gray per second.

Gy·s⁻¹   Symbol for the unit, gray per second.

H

H **1** Symbol for the unit, henry. **2** Symbol for the element, hydrogen. **3** Symbol for histidine.

H. **1** horizontal. **2** hyperopia.

¹H Symbol for protium.

²H Symbol for deuterium.

³H Symbol for tritium.

h **1** Symbol for hecto-: used with SI units. **2** Symbol for the unit, hour.

H **1** A symbol for the quantity, enthalpy, measured in joules. **2** Symbol for the quantity, magnetic field strength, expressed in amperes per meter. **3** Symbol for the quantity, magnetization, expressed in amperes per meter.

h Symbol for the quantities (1) height, expressed in meters; (2) Planck's constant, expressed in joule seconds; (3) coefficient of heat transfer, expressed in watts per square meter; (4) specific enthalpy, expressed in joules per kilogram.

ha Symbol for the unit, hectare.

HAA hospital activity analysis.

Haab [Otto *Haab*, Swiss ophthalmologist, 1850–1931] **1** See under MAGNET, REFLEX. **2** Biber-Haab-Dimmer dystrophy. See under DYSTROPHY.

Haagensen [Cushman Davis *Haagensen*, U.S. surgeon, born 1900] See under TEST.

haarscheibe [German *Haar* + *Scheibe* disk] HAIR DISK.

Habel [Karl *Habel*, U.S. virologist, born 1908] See under METHOD.

habena [L (from *habere* to have, hold), a thong, strap] Any straplike fibrous structure, resembling a bridle; frenum.

habenal Pertaining to the habena. Also *habenar*.

habenar HABENAL.

habenula [dim. of HABENA. See HABENA.] (*plural* habenulae) **1** A small, straplike fibrous structure; frenulum. **2** [NA] A caudal, dorsal thalamic nuclear group derived from the embryonic epithalamus bordering the third ventricle. Its association with the overlying pineal gland is evident in some species. The habenular complex consists of a medial nucleus with neurosecretory cells, and a lateral nucleus from which the main efferent tract, the habenulointerpeduncular tract, arises. Also called *habenula conarii, habenular body*.

habenula arcuata An outmoded term for ZONA ARCUATA.

habenula conarii HABENULA. ● The term is derived from the relation of the habenula to the conarium (pineal gland).

Haller's habenula RUDIMENT OF VAGINAL PROCESS.

habenula pectinata An outmoded term for ZONA PECTINATA.

habenula perforata FORAMINA NERVOSA LIMBUS LAMINAE SPIRALIS OSSEAE.

pineal habenula The stalk of the pineal gland extending to the habenular nuclear complex of the thalamus, a prominent feature of certain reptiles.

Scarpa's habenula An outmoded term for RUDIMENT OF VAGINAL PROCESS.

habenula urethralis Either of the two whitish lines extending from the external urethral orifice to the glans clitoridis in young females, considered by some to be related to the two slender bands of erectile tissue connecting the anterior ends of the bulbs of the vestibule to the glans. An outmoded term.

habenular Denoting the habenula.

habenulopeduncular Denoting the habenulo-interpeduncular tract. An outmoded term.

Haber [Henry *Haber*, English dermatologist, flourished mid-20th century] See under SYNDROME.

Habermann [Rudolf *Habermann*, German dermatologist, 1884–1941] Habermann's disease, Mucha-Habermann disease, Mucha-Habermann syndrome. See under PITYRIASIS LICHENOIDES.

habilitation [Med L *habilitatio* (from Late L *habilitatus*, past part. of *habilitare* to make suitable) a making suitable or fit] Training given to develop skills not previously possessed, as in compensation for early-acquired handicaps or congenital defects. Also called *compensatory education*.

habit [L *habitus*. See HABITUS.] A learned response, practiced often enough to have become relatively permanent and virtually automatic, requiring very little conscious attention for an efficient execution. Habitual responses are notable for their invariance and ease of evocation.

clamping habit CLENCHING.

glaucomatous habit A predisposition to spontaneous development of increased intraocular pressure.

oral habit An abnormal habit involving the mouth, such as thumb sucking, that often persists from childhood.

position habit The tendency for an experimental subject to go to a specific place in the test apparatus, or to select one side consistently in making a discrimination response.

tongue habit Habitual malposition of the tongue, as in the forward malposition of lisping.

habitat [L (3rd person sing. of *habitare* to inhabit), it inhabits] The site or area where an organism normally lives.

habituation [Med L *habituatio* (from Late L *habituatus*, past part. of *habituare* to bring into a bodily condition, from L *habitus* condition, habit) habituation] **1** The process of gradual adaptation to a stimulus or an environment. **2** ADDICTION.

habitus [L (from *habitus*, past. part. of *habere* to have, hold), habit, condition, fashion, state of health, attire] **1** Physical appearance; physique or attitude. **2** The physical appearance of one who is particularly subject to a specific disease or condition.

acromegaloid habitus A body form and physique like that of patients with acromegaly but found in the absence of growth hormone hypersecretion, reported in familial cases in Europe.

Buddhalike habitus The normal posture of the fetus, with folded upper and lower extremities. A seldom used term.

habitus enteroptoticus The appearance of the body in persons said to have enteroptosis, characterized by a long and narrow chest and abdomen. An obsolete term.

habitus phthisicus A general bodily appearance, characterized by pallor, thinness, and limited muscular and osseous development, formerly thought to indicate a predisposition to tuberculosis.

ptotic habitus A drooping of the upper eyelids.

Habronema [Gk *habro(s)* delicate, dainty, soft + *nēma* that which is spun, thread, yarn, tissue] A genus of parasitic nematodes (family Spiruridae, subfamily Habronematinae) found in the stomach of horses. Maggots of houseflies and stable flies serve as intermediate hosts. The nematode larvae are ingested by the fly maggots and become infective to horses when the fly maggots pupate and carry the parasites to open wounds of horses. The nematode larvae collect in the fly proboscis and escape when the fly probes around the mouth, lips, or sores in the skin. The nematode larvae in skin wounds cause cutaneous habronemiasis. The horse is infected as a definitive host by ingesting flies, either with its feed or by licking infected wounds.

Habronema majus A species similar to *H. muscae* in life cycle, distribution, and hosts. The stable fly (*Stomoxys calcitrans*) is the chief intermediate host, though other fly larvae can also serve. The nematodes interfere with the fly's ability to suck blood, forcing it to probe around sores as the housefly does, allowing escape of the nematode larvae in an appropriate site, with far greater likelihood of being licked up by the horse to initiate the final stage of infection. The adult worms may penetrate the stomach glands or lie in the paramucosal lumen. Also called *Habronema microstoma*.

Habronema microstoma *HABRONEMA MAJUS.*

Habronema muscae A species widely distributed and commonly found in the stomach of horses, mules, zebras, and asses. The common housefly (*Musca domestica*) serves as the usual intermediate host, though other muscids can also serve. The mature larvae collect in the fly's mouthparts and exit when the fly contacts the horse's lips, nose, eyes, or cutaneous sores. The larvae induce nonhealing summer sores, which the horse licks and bites, allowing ingestion of the larvae. Occasionally granular conjunctivitis also develops if the conjunctival sac is invaded. In rare instances *H. muscae* larvae may also be found in the lungs of the equid host, where they induce nodule formation. The usual site, however, is the gastric mucosa.

habronemiasis [*Habronem(a)* + -IASIS] Infection with nematodes of the genus *Habronema*, chiefly in horses but also in zebras, asses, and other equids. The adult nematodes occur in nodules in the gastric mucosa whereas their larvae often are deposited in skin wounds where they cause granulomatous dermatitis.

cutaneous habronemiasis A skin disease of horses characterized by chronic granulomatous sores caused by larvae of gastric nematodes which are species of *Habronema* and *Draschia*. Persisting for long periods, pulpy lesions with a large raw surface develop, causing the horse to lick and bite them and in the process swallow some of the larvae. The sores regress spontaneously in the winter. Also called *bursatti, summer sores, summer wounds, bursautee.*

gastric habronemiasis The condition caused in the glandular gastric mucosa of the horse by adult worms of the genera *Habronema* and *Draschia*. *Draschia* causes rounded mucosal swellings in which it resides. Several swellings may become confluent to form lesions several centimeters in diameter. *Habronema* adults reside on the mucosal surface where they cause irritation and a chronic inflammatory thickening of the mucosa. The intermediate hosts for these worms are the house fly (*Musca*) and stable fly (*Stomoxys*).

habronemic Pertaining to or caused by nematodes of the genus *Habronema.*

habu The highly venomous snake *Trimeresurus flavoviridis*, found on the Ryukyu Islands.

hachement [French (from *hache(r)* to cut into small pieces + -*ment* -MENT), a cutting into small pieces] A form of massage in which the therapist uses chopping or hacking strokes to improve circulation and muscle tone.

Hacker [Viktor von *Hacker*, Austrian surgeon, 1852–1933] See under OPERATION.

HACS hyperactive child syndrome.

hadal [French, from *Had(ès)* (Gk *Haidēs*) Hades + French -*al* -AL] Of or pertaining to an oceanic zone below 5000 m.

hadephobia [Gk *Haidē(s)* the god of the lower world, home of the dead + -PHOBIA] Pathologic fear of hell or damnation. Also called *stygiophobia.*

Hadfield [Geoffrey *Hadfield*, English pathologist, born 1889] Hadfield-Clarke syndrome. See under CLARKE-HADFIELD SYNDROME.

Hadrurus A genus of scorpions characterized by having many setae on the stinger. The most common species is *H. arizonensis,* the large hairy scorpion, found in the southwestern United States. It has a very painful sting but there is very little systemic reaction to it.

Haeckel [Ernst Heinrich *Haeckel*, German biologist, 1834–1919] **1** Haeckel's law, Müller-Haeckel law. See under RECAPITULATION THEORY. **2** Haeckel's gastrea theory. See under GASTREA THEORY.

haem A British spelling for HEME.

haem- A British spelling for HEM-. See under HEMO-.

Haemadipsa [HAEM- + *a* + Gk *dipsa* thirst] A genus of terrestrial leeches of the family Gnathobdellidae, found in the Far East and South America, especially in tropical forests. The leeches, 2–3 cm long when not engorged, are found on leaves and under stones in damp places and quickly drop onto or attach to human or animal skin, adhere with their posterior sucker, lacerate a wound that bleeds freely, and engorge large amounts of blood, usually exceeding their body weight and more than doubling their volume.

Haemadipsa ceylonica *HAEMADIPSA ZEYLANDICA.*

Haemadipsa chiliani A land leech, common in tropical areas of South America, that attacks horses and cattle and other animals, causing severe blood loss or even death in cases of particularly heavy infestations.

Haemadipsa japonica The Japanese land leech, an infamous and abundant species found in wet forested regions of Japan.

Haemadipsa zeylandica A species found in Sri Lanka and the humid tropics of Asia, the Philippines, Australia, and the Chilean Andes. It attaches itself to the skin of humans and other mammals, biting painfully and taking a large volume of blood. Multiple bites may result in anemia or even death. The bites continue bleeding because of an anticoagulant in the saliva of the leech, and often become sites of infection. Also called *Haemadipsa ceylonica.*

Haemagogus A genus of tree-hole-breeding treetop mosquitoes, many species of which are vectors of jungle yellow fever in Central and South America. They are closely related to *Aedes*, with brilliantly metallic colors. Some of the important species in the transmission of jungle yellow fever, such as *H. spegazzinii falco* and *H. splendens*, have become adapted to breeding in waterfilled hollows, tree stumps, cut bamboo stalks, or even old tires and water tanks at the forest fringe.

Haemamoeba A former genus of hematozoan parasites that included *Plasmodium* species. Also *Hemameba.*

haemangioma A British spelling for HEMANGIOMA.

Haemaphysalis [HAEM- + *a* Gk *physalis*, also *physallis*, a bladder, bubble, wind instrument, from *physan* to blow, puff, snort] A genus of mostly small inornate ticks characterized by a lack of eyes, the presence of festoons, and a distinctive basis capituli. The sexes are usually similar. The larvae and nymphs parasitize small mammals and birds, and the adults are found on larger animals and some birds. Among the approximately 150 species described, several are medically important as vectors of infectious agents, particularly viruses.

Haemaphysalis chordeilis A species commonly found on turkeys and game birds in North America. It is an economically important pest of turkeys and may be a vector of several diseases of wildlife.

Haemaphysalis cinnabarina A species, found principally in the drier regions of British Columbia, containing strains which can cause tick paralysis, or ascending paraplegia, in humans and various animals.

Haemaphysalis cinnabarina punctata A subspecies found in Europe, Japan, and North Africa. Immature forms feed on terrestrial reptiles, and adults are parasites of various domestic herbivores and of hedgehogs and rabbits. It is of veterinary importance as a vector of anaplasmosis and bovine babesiosis.

Haemaphysalis concinna A vector of *Rickettsia sibirica,* the agent of Siberian tick typhus. It is also a vector of a form of Russian spring-summer encephalitis virus found in China and the eastern USSR.

Haemaphysalis humerosa The bandicoot tick, a vector of *Coxiella burnetii.*

Haemaphysalis leachi A species common on dogs in South Africa, Asia, and Australia, and found also on other domestic and wild carnivores, small rodents, and rarely, on cattle. It is of veterinary importance as a vector of canine babesiosis.

Haemaphysalis leporispalustris The rabbit tick, widely distributed in the western hemisphere. It is a vector of Colorado tick fever virus, rickettsias including the agent of Rocky Mountain spotted fever, and *Francisella tularensis,* the agent of tularemia. It is medically important only in maintaining infection in wild animal reservoir hosts.

Haemaphysalis punctata A species that transmits a benign form of bovine babesiosis in southern Europe and may cause tick paralysis in chickens in southern Europe and in sheep, dogs, and cats in Crete. It also may rarely transmit tick-borne encephalitis virus, and it has been implicated as a vector of Tribec virus and Bhanja virus in Italy.

Haemaphysalis spinigera A species that transmits Kyasanur Forest disease among tropical forest workers in India.

haemato- A British spelling for HEMATO-. See under HEMO-.

Haematobia A genus of muscid flies, including highly irritating and economically costly horn flies such as *H. irritans* and *H. minuta.*

Haematobia irritans The horn fly of cattle, a small fly that is very annoying to cattle and causes economically significant weight loss or unthriftiness. The subspecies *H. i. irritans,* the true horn fly, is a particular pest of dairy and beef cattle. *H. i. exigua,* the buffalo fly, is found in Australia and the Oriental region, where it attacks water buffalo, cattle, horses, dogs, and man. Also called *Siphona irritans, Lyperosia irritans, Haematobia stimulans.*

Haematobia minuta A horn fly that attacks cattle and water buffalo in Africa and may become a serious pest of humans if present in large numbers.

Haematobia stimulans *HAEMATOBIA IRRITANS.*

haematocrit A British spelling for HEMATOCRIT.

haematology A British spelling for HEMATOLOGY.

haematoma A British spelling for HEMATOMA.

Haematopinus [HAEMATO- + Gk *pinein* to drink] A genus

of sucking lice (order Anoplura), the single genus in the family Haematopinidae. Several species are abundant and widespread parasites of swine, cattle, horses, and some wild animals. Each host or group of related hosts has its characteristic species of louse.

Haematopinus asini A species found on horses, asses, and mules. It is a common and cosmopolitan parasite.

Haematopinus eurysternus The short-nosed louse of cattle, the most important anopluran infesting domestic cattle. It is universally distributed but is especially common in cold and temperate areas.

Haematopinus quadripertusus A sucking louse of cattle, found around the eyes and in the ears as well as in the long hair around the tail. It is normally found on zebu (*Bos indicus*) and hybrids of zebu and *Bos taurus.* Its distribution is chiefly tropical or subtropical.

Haematopinus suis A large (5–6 mm) louse of swine, the so-called blue louse or common pig louse. It is the only louse infesting pigs and it is cosmopolitan in distribution. It is a serious pest of hogs and also feeds readily on humans.

Haematopota A genus of horseflies, related to *Tabanus,* with characteristic densely mottled wings. *H. americana* is a species found from Alaska to New Mexico. Other species are common in the Oriental zoogeographic region, though they are absent from Australia. *H. pluvialis* is a vector of *Trypanosoma theileri,* a relatively nonpathogenic widespread parasite of cattle, oxen, and antelopes.

Haematosiphon A genus of bedbugs similar to *Cimex,* but with longer legs and an unusually elongated sucking proboscis and beak.

Haematosiphon inodorus The poultry bug or Mexican chicken bug; a bedbug that attacks chickens, owls, eagles, and condors in southwestern United States and Mexico. It rarely attacks humans though it may be severe among poultry handlers.

haematuria A British spelling for HEMATURIA.

Haementeria A genus of leeches in the family Rhynchobdellidae. It includes *H. officinalis,* the medicinal leech of South and Central America. Also *Hementaria.*

-haemia A British spelling for -HEMIA.

haemo- A British spelling for HEMO-.

Haemobartonella [HAEMO- + *bartonella,* after Alberto L. *Barton,* Peruvian physician, 1871–1950 + L *-ella,* fem. diminishing suffix] A genus of spherical or rod-shaped microorganisms (family Bartonellaceae, order Rickettsiales) parasitic on the surface of red cells of many animals. Disease rarely ensues except after splenectomy or other interference with the host's resistance. Also *Hemobartonella.*

Haemobartonella bovis A species widely distributed in cattle. Its pathogenicity is low.

Haemobartonella canis A cosmopolitan blood parasite of dogs, transmitted by fleas of the genus *Ctenocephalides.*

Haemobartonella felis A blood parasite of cats that causes feline infectious anemia. The method of spread is unknown.

Haemobartonella muris A very common rodent-infecting species transmitted by the rat lice *Haematopinus* and *Polyplax,* the bedbug *Cimex lectularius,* and the rat flea *Xenopsylla cheopis.* The infection is found in most laboratory rats in a latent form, but acute disease may develop after splenectomy, resulting in large numbers of the microorganisms appearing in the circulating blood.

Haemobartonella peromysci A bacillus-shaped microorganism found in erythrocytes of the North American deer mouse *Peromyscus leucopus novaboracensis.*

Haemobartonella sciuri A bacillus-shaped microorganism invading the erythrocytes of the gray squirrels (*Sciurus caroli-*

enensis leucotis). It can cause mild disease in the squirrel but is not pathogenic for laboratory white mice.

Haemococcidium A former genus of blood parasites that included *Plasmodium* species.

Haemocytozoa [HAEMO- + CYTO- + Gk *zōa*, pl. of *zōon* a living being, animal] An obsolete term for HAEMOSPORIDIA.

haemodialysis A British spelling for HEMODIALYSIS.

Haemodipsus A genus of sucking lice found on rodents and lagomorphs.

Haemodipsus ventricosus A louse commonly infesting rabbits and one of many insects that transmit the agent of tularemia.

haemogamasid [HAEMO- + GAMASID] **1** Of or belonging to the family Haemogamasidae. **2** A member of the family Haemogamasidae. For defs. 1 and 2 also called *gamasid*.

Haemogamasidae [HAEMO- + GAMASIDAE] A family of bloodsucking mites in the suborder Mesostigmata, superfamily Parasitoidea, which are thought to transmit tularemia and probably other infections among rodents. Also called *Gamasidae*.

haemoglobin A British spelling for HEMOGLOBIN.

haemoglobinuria A British spelling for HEMOGLOBINURIA.

Haemogregarina A genus of sporozoans (family Haemogregarinidae, suborder Adeleina, order Eucoccidiida) parasitic in the blood cells of cold-blooded animals and found in the digestive system of the initial invertebrate host. Aquatic hosts such as the European turtle *Emys orbicularis* infected with *Haemogregarina stepanowi* are infected by the leech, in which sporogony takes place, schizogony occurring in the turtle. Haemogregarines of terrestrial reptiles apparently are transmitted chiefly by mites.

haemolysis A British spelling for HEMOLYSIS.

haemolytic A British spelling for HEMOLYTIC.

Haemonchus [HAEM- + New L *-onchus* (combining form irreg. from Gk *onkos* a barb, sharp hook) pertaining to a barb or sharp hook] An economically important genus of bloodsucking nematodes (family Trichostrongylidae) found in the abomasum of ruminants. Infection by large numbers of worms results in severe anemia and death, particularly in previously uninfected or young animals.

Haemonchus contortus The large stomach worm of cattle, sheep, goats, and other ruminants and the most economically important member of the genus. The female is characterized by white filamentous ovaries that spiral around a straight, blood-filled gut. This species causes a serious anemia and even death, particularly in sheep and infrequently in man. The infective stage is the nonfeeding third-stage larva, which retains the cuticle of the second stage as a protective sheath. The larvae undergo the final two molts and mature in the abomasum, the usual site of the adult worms.

Haemonchus placei The large stomach worm of cattle and other ruminants. It is distinguished from *H. contortus* by differences in genitalia and larval size. There is also a difference in the size of the X chromosome in the two species, though the question of separate species status of *H. placei* remains unsettled. In heavy infections, particularly in young animals, severe anemia and even death can ensue.

Haemonchus similis A species found in the abomasum of cattle and sheep. It resembles *H. contortus* but is smaller.

haemophilia A British spelling for HEMOPHILIA.

Haemophilus [HAEMO- + Gk *philos* beloved, loving] A genus of small, Gram-negative, nonmotile facultatively anaerobic coccobacilli with complex growth requirements provided by blood. These requirements include the heat-stable factor X (hemin) and the heat-labile factor V (nicotinamide adenine dinucleotide). They are generally grown on chocolate agar, in which mild heating has released the factors and destroyed an inhibitor of

factor V. Growth is often enhanced by elevated carbon dioxide concentrations. The major species is *H. influenzae*. Also *Hemophilus*.

Haemophilus aegyptius A species, very similar to *H. influenzae*, that produces purulent conjunctivitis. Also called *Koch-Weeks bacillus*.

Haemophilus ducreyi A hemophilus that causes chancroid. Also called *Ducrey's bacillus*.

Haemophilus haemolyticus A nonpathogenic hemophilus often present in the upper respiratory tract. It forms β-hemolytic colonies, especially with rabbit blood, that are easily mistaken for those of *Streptococcus pyogenes*.

Haemophilus influenzae A hemophilus found normally in the human nasopharynx; the influenza bacillus. Strains with polysaccharide capsules, of six types (designated *a* to *f*), may cause disease. Type *b* is the most frequent. The organism is the commonest cause of meningitis in children. It also causes sinusitis, otitis media, pneumonia, arthritis, and a fulminating epiglottitis and obstructive laryngitis. The organism was once considered, mistakenly, the cause of pandemic influenza. Also called *Pfeiffer's bacillus*.

Haemophilus parainfluenzae An organism closely related to *H. influenzae*, often found as a commensal in the human respiratory tract.

Haemophilus pertussis An obsolete term for BORDETELLA PERTUSSIS.

Haemophilus suis A hemophilus that causes various diseases in swine, including a pneumonia that depends on its association with swine influenza virus.

Haemophoructus A genus of bloodsucking midges or gnats (family Ceratopogonidae).

Haemopis A genus of horse leeches (family Gnathobdellidae) found in the pharynx and nasal passages, rarely in the urethra, where they may remain for some days or even weeks.

Haemoproteidae [HAEMO- + *Prote(us)* Roman and Gk sea god of changeable shape + -IDAE] A family of protozoa in the suborder Haemosporina, order Eucoccidiida, class Sporozoea, parasitic in various cells of vertebrates. It includes the genera *Haemoproteus* and *Leucocytozoon*. The life cycle is metoxenous, requiring both an invertebrate and a vertebrate host.

Haemoproteus The type genus of sporozoans in the family Haemoproteidae, parasitic in visceral endothelial cells and erythrocytes of birds and reptiles. Pupiparous insects generally are the vectors in most known life cycles, although a species parasitic in ducks utilizes biting midges as vectors. Also called *Halteridium*. Also *Hemoproteus*.

haemorrhage A British spelling for HEMORRHAGE.

haemorrhoids A British spelling for HEMORRHOIDS.

haemosiderosis A British spelling for HEMOSIDEROSIS.

Haemosporidia [pl. of HAEMOSPORIDIUM.] A former order of sporozoans in the class Telosporidia, equivalent to the present suborder Haemosporina in the order Eucoccidiida, class Sporozoea. Many of the most important pathogens of humans, domestic animals, and birds are included, notably the malarial parasites of the genus *Plasmodium* and various bird pathogens included in the genus *Leucocytozoon*. Also called *Acystosporidia*, *Haemocytozoa* (obsolete). Also *Hemosporidia*.

haemosporidian **1** Pertaining to or belonging to the former sporozoan order Haemosporidia (now replaced by the suborder Haemosporina). **2** A member of the Haemosporidia (Haemosporina).

haemosporidium [HAEMO- + SPORIDIUM] (*plural* haemosporidia) Any of the sporozoan blood parasites formerly classified as members of the order Haemosporidia and now as members of the suborder Haemosporina. Also called *hematospori-dium*. Also *hemosporidium*.

Haemosporina A suborder of sporozoans in the order Eucoccidiida, equivalent to the former order Haemosporidia. It includes the genera *Haemoproteus, Hepatocystis, Leucocytozoon,* and *Plasmodium*.

haemostasis A British spelling for HEMOSTASIS.

haemostatic A British spelling for HEMOSTATIC.

Haemostrongylus vasorum ANGIOSTRONGYLUS VASORUM.

haemothorax A British spelling for HEMOTHORAX.

haemozoin A British spelling for HEMOZOIN.

Haenel [Heinrich G. *Haenel*, German neurologist, 1874–1942] Haenel's variant. See under SYMPTOM.

Haffkine [Waldemar Mordecai Wolff *Haffkine*, Russian bacteriologist, 1860–1930] See under VACCINE.

Hafnia alvei An enterobacterium found in feces and in nature. It is an opportunistic pathogen. Also called *Enterobacter hafniae, Enterobacter alvei*.

hafnium Element number 72, having atomic weight 178.49. It is found combined in minerals containing zirconium, which it resembles chemically. One of its six natural isotopes, hafnium 74, is radioactive, having a half-life of 2×10^{15} years and emitting alpha particles. Many additional radioactive isotopes have been identified, with mass numbers ranging from 168 to 183 and half-lives from 5 seconds to 9×10^6 years. The metal absorbs neutrons and is used to make control rods for nuclear reactors. Symbol: Hf

Hagedorn [Hans Christian *Hagedorn*, Danish physician, born 1888] Hagedorn and Jensen method. See under METHOD.

Hagedorn [Werner *Hagedorn*, German surgeon, 1831–1894] See under NEEDLE.

Haglund [Sims Emil Patrik *Haglund*, Swedish physician, 1870–1937] Haglund's disease, Haglund's deformity. See under ACHILLES BURSITIS.

Hagner [Francis Randall *Hagner*, U.S. surgeon, 1873–1940] See under OPERATION, BAG.

Hagner [Karl *Hagner*, 19th-century German hospital patient] See under DISEASE.

Hahn [Eugen *Hahn*, German surgeon, 1841–1902] See under OPERATION.

Hahn [Friedrich Lazarus *Hahn*, German chemist, born 1888] See under REAGENT.

hahnemannism [after Samuel C. F. *Hahnemann*, German physician, 1755–1843 + -ISM] HOMEOPATHY.

Haidinger [Wilhelm Karl von *Haidinger*, Austrian mineralogist, 1795–1871] Haidinger's brushes. See under BRUSH.

Haig Ferguson [James *Haig Ferguson*, Scottish obstetrician, born 1862] See under FORCEPS.

Hailey [Hugh E. *Hailey*, U.S. dermatologist, born 1909] Hailey-Hailey disease. See under BENIGN FAMILIAL PEMPHIGUS.

Hailey [William Howard *Hailey*, U.S. dermatologist, 1898–1967] Hailey-Hailey disease. See under BENIGN FAMILIAL PEMPHIGUS.

Haines [Walter Stanley *Haines*, U.S. toxicologist, 1850–1923] See under COEFFICIENT.

hair [Old English *hær*] **1** A keratinized threadlike skin appendage consisting of cornified epidermal cells that is formed in specialized follicles and is a characteristic feature of mammals; pilus. Also called *capillus* (rarely used), *crinis* (obsolete), *thrix* (obsolete). **2** The entire coat of a mammal.

auditory hairs The stereocilia and kinocilia of each cellula sensoria pilosa located on the inner surface of the utricle, saccule, and semicircular ducts and in the auditory portion of the inner

ear. The cells communicate with afferent vestibular fibers. An imprecise usage.

bamboo hair TRICHORRHEXIS INVAGINATA.

bayonet hair A structural defect of the hair shaft in which the shaft tapers to a fine point above a spindle-shaped thickening of the cortex immediately below the tip of the hair. The origin of the defect is uncertain.

beaded hair Hair characterized by regular elliptical nodes separated by internodes. It is a shaft defect characteristic of monilethrix. Also called *moniliform hair*.

burrowing hair A hair that fails to emerge from the follicle and grows into its wall. Also called *pilus cuniculatus*.

club hair A hair in the telogen phase of the hair cycle. It is the state in which it is shed in all physiologic and in some pathologic circumstances. Also called *resting hair*.

exclamation mark hair The British term for EXCLAMATION POINT HAIR.

exclamation point hair A broken hair shaft of normal caliber and 5–10 mm in length, tapering to an atrophic or shrunken bulb or to a more or less normal club. Such hairs are characteristic of the periphery of extending patches of alopecia areata. Also called *exclamation mark hair (British)*.

Frey's hairs A device composed of stiff hairs mounted at right angles to the end of a wooden handle. It is used to measure skin touch sensitivity. The hairs are graded in tensile strength and can be flexed according to the degree of pressure exerted, thus enabling the examiner to measure sensory tactile acuity.

guard hairs The long coarse hairs that form an outer protective covering over the underfur in the coat of a mammal.

gustatory hairs The hairlike protrusions of taste cells, consisting of microvilli. Also called *taste hairs*.

ingrown hair The penetration of the surface epidermis or the wall of a follicle by the tip of a tightly coiled hair. It commonly occurs on the neck, when the resulting inflammatory changes give rise to pseudofolliculitis. Also called *pilus incarnatus*.

kinky hair Short, brittle, lightly colored hair marked by pili torti and other structural defects. It is characteristic of the Menkes syndrome.

knotted hair TRICHONODOSIS.

lanugo hair The fine hair that grows on the body of a fetus.

moniliform hair BEADED HAIR.

pubic hair The terminal hair of the mons pubis. Also called *crinis pubis* (obsolete).

resting hair CLUB HAIR.

ringed hair A hereditary defect of the hair shaft in which light bands on the shaft mark areas containing an increased number of air spaces within the cortex. Also called *thrix annulata, trichonosus versicolor* (obsolete), *leukotrichia annularis* (obsolete), *pili annulati* (obsolete).

root hair A tubular outgrowth of epidermal cells on young roots in the zone of maturation, or zone of differentiation, that absorb water and dissolved mineral salts from the soil.

Schridde cancer hairs Coarse black hairs on the temples and the beard area that are alleged to be associated with cancer of the internal organs.

sensory hairs The hairlike cilia, stereocilia, and microvilli of the sensory cells of the olfactory epithelium, the hair cells of the organ of Corti, the ampullary crests and the maculae of the utricle and saccule, and the cells of the taste buds.

stellate hair A hair that shows terminal splitting, the divergent parts of the hair assuming a starlike pattern.

stinging hairs Rigid, glandular hairlike structures found on certain plants and urticating insects, such as the tussock moths, browntail moths, and other caterpillars that secrete an irritating or acrid fluid at the base of the stinging hair or spine.

taste hairs GUSTATORY HAIRS.

terminal hair The long, strong hair of the scalp, eyebrows, eyelashes, male beard, axillae, and pubic region of the adult human.

vellus hair   VELLUS.

hairball   TRICHOBEZOAR.

haircast   A trichobezoar which has filled and acquired the shape of a segment of the alimentary canal, usually the stomach.

hairworm [HAIR + WORM]   **1** A nematode worm of the genus *Trichostrongylus.*   **2** A nematode worm of the genus *Capillaria.* **3** HORSEHAIR WORM.

Hajek [M. *Hajek,* Austrian otolaryngologist, 1861–1941] See under OPERATION.

halation [*hal(o)* + -ATION]   A scattering of light to the sides of its primary focus.

Halban [Josef Van *Halban,* Austrian gynecologist, 1870–1937] See under SIGN.

Halberstraedter [Ludwig *Halberstraedter,* German physician, 1876–1949]   Halberstraedter-Prowazek bodies. See under TRACHOMA BODIES.

halcinonide $C_{24}H_{32}ClFO_5$. 21-Chloro-9α-fluoro-11β-hydroxy-16α,17α-isopropylidenedioxypregn-4-ene-3,20-dione, a synthetic steroidal agent that is used topically as an anti-inflammatory medication.

Haldane [John Burdon Sanderson *Haldane,* Scottish geneticist, 1892–1964]   See under LAW, SCALE.

Haldane [John Scott *Haldane,* Scottish physiologist, 1860–1936] **1** Haldane's chamber. See under HALDANE APPARATUS. **2** Haldane-Priestley sampling. See under SAMPLING. **3** See under EFFECT, TUBE.

Haldol   A proprietary name for haloperidol.

Haldrone   A proprietary name for paramethasone acetate.

Hales [Stephen *Hales,* English physiologist, 1677–1761]   See under PIESIMETER.

half-center   See under HALF-CENTER HYPOTHESIS.

half-cycle   Half of a sequential movement or period.

half-layer   HALF-VALUE LAYER.

half-life   **1** See under RADIOACTIVE HALF-LIFE.   **2** The time taken for the concentration of a substance to fall to half its initial value. This time is independent of the initial concentration in many processes, as for example in radioactive decay, and approximately so for others, as in the elimination of many foreign substances from the body.

antibody half-life   A measurement of the mean lifetime of antibodies after synthesis, most often referring to the time required to eliminate 50 percent of a known quantity of immunoglobulin from the circulation.

biologic half-life   The time required for a biologic system to eliminate half of some specified constituent if this constituent is nonradioactive. If it is radioactive, the biologic half-life is the effective half-life back-corrected for the physical decay.

effective half-life   The time required for half of the original amount of a constituent to disappear from a biological or other system, whether because of radioactive decay or any other process such as diffusion or chemical change. Symbol: $t_{1/2}$.

environmental half-life   The half-life of a chemical such as DDT when exposed to natural environmental conditions.

physical half-life   RADIOACTIVE HALF-LIFE.

radioactive half-life   The time required for the radioactivity of a sample of a radionuclide to decrease to half of its initial value, and thus the time when half of its atoms have disintegrated. The half-life of a radionuclide is a physical constant which is equal to 0.693 divided by the disintegration constant. Also called *physical half-life.* Symbol: $T_{1/2}$

half-moon   A crescent-shaped structure or marking; a lunula or demilune.

red half-moon   The suffused lunula characteristic of cardiac failure.

half-retinal   Pertaining to approximately fifty percent of the ocular retina.

half-thickness   HALF-VALUE LAYER.

half-time   The time after which half remains of the amount originally present of a given substance. This time will be constant for any substance being destroyed by a first-order reaction, e.g. radioactive decay. See also HALF-LIFE.

halide   Any of the ions, or the salts that contain them, derived from a halogen atom by addition of an electron.

halimetry [Gk *hals,* gen. *halos,* salt + *i* + -METRY]   The measurement of salts or of electrolytes in a solution.

haliphagia [*hal(o)-* + *i* + -PHAGIA]   The ingestion of an abnormally large amount of salts, especially sodium chloride, sodium bicarbonate, and the salts of calcium, magnesium, and potassium.

halisteresis   An obsolete term for OSTEOMALACIA.

halisteresis cerea   A waxlike softening of bone.

halitosis [L *halit(us)* breath, exhalation + -OSIS]   FETOR ORIS.

halitus [L, breath, vapor, exhalation]   Breath; exhalation.

halitus saturninus   LEAD BREATH.

Hall [Josiah Newhall *Hall,* U.S. physician, 1859–1939]   See under SIGN.

hallachrome   A quinonoid pigment found in the annelid worm *Halla.*

Hallauer [Otto *Hallauer,* Swiss ophthalmologist, born 1866] See under GLASSES.

Hallé [Adrien Joseph Marie Noel *Hallé,* French physician, 1859–1947]   See under POINT.

Haller [Albrecht von *Haller,* Swiss physiologist, 1708–1777] **1** See under CHANNEL, CRESCENT, ANSA. **2** Haller's line. See under FISSURA MEDIANA ANTERIOR MEDULLAE SPINALIS. **3** Haller's unguis. See under CALCAR AVIS. **4** Haller's habenula. See under RUDIMENT OF VAGINAL PROCESS. **5** Rete halleri, rete testis halleri, rete of Haller. See under RETE TESTIS. **6** Arcus lumbocostalis lateralis halleri, lateral lumbocostal arch of haller. See under LIGAMENTUM ARCUATUM LATERALE. **7** Haller's arches. See under ARCH. **8** Circulus vasculosus nervi optici halleri, circle of Haller. See under CIRCULUS VASCULOSUS NERVI OPTICI. **9** Haller's crypts. See under GLANDULAE PREPUTIALES. **10** Thoracic branch of Haller. See under BRANCH. **11** Arcus lumbocostalis medialis halleri, medial lumbocostal arch of Haller. See under LIGAMENTUM ARCUATUM MEDIALE. **12** Circle of Haller, venous ring of Haller. See under PLEXUS VENOSUS AREOLARIS. **13** Haller's cones. See under LOBULI EPIDIDYMIDIS. **14** Haller's layer, Haller's membrane. See under LAMINA VASCULOSA CHOROIDEAE. **15** Vas aberrans of Haller. See under DUCTULUS ABERRANS SUPERIOR. **16** Haller's aberrant duct. See under DUCTULUS ABERRANS INFERIOR. **17** Haller's tripod. See under TRUNCUS COELIACUS. **18** Haller's tunica vasculosa. See under TUNICA VASCULOSA BULBI.

Hallermann [Wilhelm *Hallermann,* German physician, born 1901]   Hallermann-Streiff-François syndrome. See under HALLERMANN-STREIFF SYNDROME.

Hallervorden [Julius *Hallervorden,* German neurologist, 1882–1965]   Hallervorden-Spatz syndrome. See under HALLERVORDEN-SPATZ DISEASE.

hallex   HALLUX.

Hallgren [Bertil *Hallgren,* Swedish geneticist, flourished mid-20th century]   See under SYNDROME.

Hallion [Louis *Hallion,* French physiologist, 1862–1940] **1** Hallion's test. See under TUFFIER'S TEST. **2** See under LAW.

Hallopeau [François Henri *Hallopeau,* French dermatologist,

1842–1919] **1** Adenoma sebaceum of Hallopeau. See under ADENOMA. **2** Hallopeau's acrodermatitis. See under ACRODERMATITIS CONTINUA. **3** Hallopeau-Siemens syndrome. See under EPIDERMOLYSIS BULLOSA DYSTROPHICA (RECESSIVE).

hallucal   Pertaining to the hallux.

halluces   Plural of HALLUX.

hallucination [L *hallucinatio* or *alucinatio* (from past parts. of *hallucinari* or *alucinari* to talk idly, dote, prob. from Gk *alyein* to wander in the mind, be ill at ease) carelessness, blundering] A false sensory perception unrelated to any external stimulus, such as hearing voices when one is alone in a forest, or seeing people coming out of the fireplace when one is in an empty room.

auditory hallucination   A hallucination of hearing, including audible thoughts, music, mumbled voices, or entire conversations between different voices.

autoscopic hallucination   AUTOSCOPY.

blank hallucination   A hallucination in which there is a disorder of one's sense of equilibrium and space. It may be typified by the rhythmic approaching and receding of objects. Also called *Isakower phenomenon, dream screen, abstract perception.*

elementary hallucination   A hallucination of unformed perceptions such as sparks or tapping.

epileptic hallucination   A somatosensory, visual, or auditory hallucination, occurring either as one manifestation or as the entire evidence of an attack of epilepsy, and usually resulting from neuronal discharge arising in the sensory association areas. Epileptic hallucinations can be differentiated from epileptic illusions and from attacks of primary sensory epilepsy. Also called *hallucinatory aura* (incorrect).

gustatory hallucination   A hallucination of taste, as of burned meat even though the subject is not eating.

haptic hallucination   A hallucination of touch, as of electrical impulses being applied to various parts of the body. Also called *tactile hallucination.*

hypnagogic hallucination   A hallucination, usually visual, that occurs during the transitional phase from being awake to sleeping.

hypnopompic hallucination   A hallucination, usually visual, that occurs in the half-awake state between sleeping and full arousal.

induced hallucination   A hallucination prompted or suggested by another person, such as a hypnotist.

lilliputian hallucination   MICROPSIA.

microptic hallucination   MICROPSIA.

olfactory hallucination   A hallucination of smell, such as the odor of burning rubber. Also called *phantosmia* (seldom used).

hallucination of perception   An auditory hallucination involving a voice whose origin is outside the body of the subject.

psychomotor hallucination   A hallucination that parts of one's body are being transferred to different regions of the body.

reflex hallucination   A hallucination aroused by stimulation of a different sensory area, such as the sight of people scrambling about when one receives an intramuscular injection.

sexual hallucination   A sensation of sexual excitement in a nonsexual part of the body, often occurring as a somatic delusion.

stump hallucination   PHANTOM LIMB.

tactile hallucination   HAPTIC HALLUCINATION.

visual hallucination   A hallucination of sight, as of faces leering or grimacing. Also called *parablepsia, pseudoblepsia, pseudoblepsis, pseudopsia, subjective vision.*

hallucinatory   **1** Pertaining to or characterized by hallucinations. **2** Having the quality of a hallucination.

hallucinogen   A drug that is capable of producing hallucinations, such as mescaline or LSD. Also called *psychotomimetic, psychotogen.*

hallucinogenic   Giving rise to hallucinations, such as occurs with certain drugs. Also *psychotogenic, psychotomimetic.*

hallucinosis [L *hallucin(atio)* or *alucin(atio)* (see HALLUCINATION) + -OSIS]   The occurrence of hallucinations, usually visual or auditory, without disorientation or intellectual impairment.

acute alcoholic hallucinosis   An acute hallucinatory state occurring in a clear intellectual state and without other features of delirium, sometimes observed in alcoholics following an unusual excess of alcohol intake or, less commonly, as a part of alcohol withdrawal. Most often the hallucinations are auditory and derogatory or critical in content, and sometimes they are accompanied by paranoid delusions of a persecutory nature.

alcoholic hallucinosis   Hallucinosis in which auditory hallucinations are often accompanied by paranoid delusions of a persecutory or derogatory nature. It occurs in alcoholics following an excessive intake of alcohol or as a symptom of alcohol withdrawal. Also called *alcoholic withdrawal hallucinosis, alcoholic paranoia* (seldom used).

alcoholic withdrawal hallucinosis   ALCOHOLIC HALLUCINOSIS.

hallucinotic   Of or pertaining to hallucinosis.

hallux [L, the big toe]   [NA] The big toe; the first digit of the foot. Also called *pollex pedis, hallex, great toe, digitus primus, digitus I.*

hallux dolorosa   A painful condition of the big toe that is seen in flatfoot deformity.

hallux flexus   A hammer toe deformity characterized by acute flexion of the interphalangeal joint. Also called *hallux malleus.*

hallux malleus   HALLUX FLEXUS.

hallux rigidus   A painful limitation of motion in the metatarsophalangeal joint of the big toe in flexion. Also called *stiff toe.*

hallux valgus   A displacement of the big toe away from the midline at the metatarsophalangeal joint. When the joint is covered with an adventitious bursa, it is called a bunion.

hallux varus   A displacement of the big toe towards the midline and away from the other toes.

Hallwachs [Wilhelm Ludwig Franz *Hallwachs*, German physicist, 1859–1922]   See under EFFECT.

halmatogenesis   SALTATORY VARIATION.

halo [L (from Gk *alōs* a threshing floor, the disk of the sun or moon), a halo, circle around the sun or moon]   **1** A circumferential scattering of light around its focus or origin. **2** A type of cranial skeletal traction used to immobilize the neck or keep pressure off the scalp.

anemic halo   A pale area surrounding a skin lesion.

Fick's halo   Dispersion of light into its spectral components by fluid droplets in the cornea, occurring because of the prolonged wearing of a contact lens. This is recognized by the patient because of a circular rainbow seen around lights.

halo glaucomatosus   GLAUCOMATOUS HALO.

glaucomatous halo   A rainbow-colored ring seen around lights when the cornea is edematous due to increased intraocular pressure. Also called *halo glaucomatosus.*

peripapillary senile halo   CIRCUMPAPILLARY CHORIORETINAL ATROPHY.

halo saturninus   LEAD LINE.

senile halo   CIRCUMPAPILLARY CHORIORETINAL ATROPHY.

halo- [Gk *hals* (gen. *halos*) grain of salt; pl. *haloi* salt in general]   **1** A combining form designating a salt. **2** A combining form designating replacement of a hydrogen atom by an atom of any halogen.

Halobacterium   A genus of Gram-negative aerobic rods that require a high salt concentration, found in salt-preserved meats and in salt-evaporating ponds. They lack a peptidoglycan wall.

halocline [HALO- + Gk *klin(ein)* to make slope or slant, to incline] A salinity concentration gradient of the ocean marked by lowered salinity nearer the surface as a result of precipitation.

halodermia [*halo(gen)* + DERM- + -IA] A skin condition caused by exposure to certain halogens, such as bromine, chlorine, and iodine, either by inhalation, ingestion, or skin absorption.

halogen [HALO- + -GEN] An element of group VII of the periodic table, including fluorine, chlorine, bromine, iodine, and astatine. All form stable anions on addition of an electron to an atom of the element.

halogenation [HALOGEN + -ATION] The chemical reaction of adding halogen to a molecule. This may be by an addition of the element to a double bond, or it may be by a substitution reaction. Such reactions are common in organic synthesis. Tyrosine is halogenated to form diiodotyrosine in the biosynthesis of thyroxin.

halogeton A grayish brown annual herb indigenous to the southwestern United States and other arid regions of the world. The major species is *Halogeton glomeratus*. Ingestion by cattle and sheep has caused poisoning because of soluble oxalates in the plant.

halometer A device for measuring the scattering of light to the side of the object or focus.

halometry [HALO + -METRY] Measurement of the scattering of light to the side of the object or focus by a halometer.

haloperidol $C_{21}H_{23}ClFNO_2$. A neuroleptic drug of the butyrophenone class.

halophile [HALO- + -PHILE] A microorganism that tolerates or even requires a high concentration of sodium chloride for growth. Such organisms, e.g. *Halobacterium*, are found in the sea and in salted foods. Adjective: halophilic.

halophyte [Gk *hals*, gen. *halos*, salt + *phyt(on)* a plant, tree] A plant that is normally found growing in a saline habitat.

haloscope [Gk *hals*, gen. *halos*, salt + -SCOPE] Any device used to measure a salt concentration. An outmoded term.

halosteresis OSTEOMALACIA.

Halotestin A proprietary name for fluoxymesterone.

halothane CHBrCl—CF₃. Bromochlorotrifluoroethane. A nonflammable general anesthetic which occurs in liquid form but which can be converted into a vapor for inhalation. It consists of a halogenated trifluoride amide and will produce all stages of general anesthesia.

Halsted [William Stewart *Halsted*, U.S. surgeon, 1852–1922] **1** Halsted radical mastectomy, Halsted's operation. See under RADICAL MASTECTOMY. **2** See under HERNIORRHAPHY, SUTURE, OPERATION.

Halteridium HAEMOPROTEUS.

halzoun [Arabic *ḥalzūn* snail] An acute parasitic pharyngitis causing respiratory distress or blockage, nasal and lacrimal discharges, episodic sneezing and coughing, hemolysis, dyspnea, dysphonia, dysphagia, and frontal headache, associated with the eating of raw liver or other viscera of sheep, goat, camel, or ox infected with *Fasciola hepatica*. It is prevalent in parts of the Near and Middle East, north Africa, and south Asia. Nymphs of the pentastome worm *Linguatula serrata* have also been recovered from the nasal passages and throats of a number of persons suffering from this syndrome in Lebanon. Other trematodes have also been held responsible for it.

Ham [Thomas Hale *Ham*, U.S. physician, born 1905] See under TEST.

ham [Middle English *hamme*, from Old English *hamm*, akin to Gk *knēmē* the part of the leg between knee and ankle] **1** FOSSA POPLITEA. **2** The buttock and the back of the thigh, or the

back of the thigh below the buttock. **3** The hindleg of a quadrupedal animal.

hamadryad [Gk *Hamadryas* (from *hama* at the same time with + *Dryas*, gen. *Dryados*, a wood nymph, from *drys* the oak, any timber tree) a wood nymph whose life was entwined with that of the tree in which she dwelt] KING COBRA.

hamamelis The dried leaves of *Hamamelis virginiana*, which have been used as an astringent. An extract made from them has been used in making suppositories and in treating hemorrhoids. Also called *witch hazel*.

hamamelose The sugar 2-*C*-(hydroxymethyl)-D-ribose, found combined in plant tannins. It is one of the rare branched-chain sugars.

hamarthritis An obsolete term for POLYARTHRITIS.

hamartia [Gk *hamartia* error, failure, sin] A localized disturbance of the normal arrangement, organization, or patterning of tissues during development. A rarely used term.

hamartoblastoma [*hamarto(ma)* + BLASTOMA] A neoplasm developing from a hamartoma. A rarely used term.

hamartoblastoma of the kidney An outmoded term for NEPHROBLASTOMA.

hamartochondromatosis [HAMARTO- + CHONDROMATOSIS] Multiple cartilaginous hamartomas.

hamartoma [Gk *hamart(ia)*, also *hamart(ēma)* a failure, error, sin + -OMA] A benign tumor or tumorlike lesion composed of one or more tissues normal to the organ but abnormally mixed and overgrown. For example, a hamartoma of the lung may contain a mixture of cartilage, connective tissue, and bronchial epithelium. Compare CHORISTOMA.

chondromatous hamartoma CHONDROMA OF LUNG.

fetal hamartoma MESOBLASTIC NEPHROMA.

infantile mesenchymal hamartoma MESOBLASTIC NEPHROMA.

hamartoma of the kidney RENAL ANGIOMYOLIPOMA.

leiomyomatous hamartoma MESOBLASTIC NEPHROMA.

neuromuscular hamartoma A tumorlike lesion containing differentiated skeletal muscle admixed with nerves. It is multinodular, separated by fibrous tissue bonds, and associated with major nerves. It typically occurs in infancy. Also called *benign Triton tumor*.

renal hamartoma RENAL ANGIOMYOLIPOMA.

temporal hamartoma A malformation of developmental origin situated in the temporal lobe of the brain.

hamartomatosis [*hamartomat(a)*, pl. of HAMARTOMA + -OSIS] The presence of multiple hamartomas.

hamartomatous [*hamartomat(a)*, pl. of HAMARTOMA + -OUS] Of the nature of or resembling a hamartoma.

hamartophobia [Gk *hamart(ia)*, also *hamart(ēma)* a failure, error, sin + *o* + -PHOBIA] Fear that one will commit or has committed some grievous error or unpardonable sin.

hamartoplasia Overgrowth of a tissue as a consequence of an excessive repair process. An obsolete term.

hamate **1** OS HAMATUM. **2** Hook-shaped at the tip. Also *hamose*.

hamatum OS HAMATUM.

hamaxophobia AMAXOPHOBIA.

Hamberger [Georg Erhard *Hamberger*, German physician, 1697–1755] See under SCHEMA.

Hamburger [Franz *Hamburger*, German physician, born 1874] See under TEST.

Hamburger [Hartog Jakob *Hamburger*, Dutch physiologist, 1859–1924] **1** Hamburger phenomenon, shift of Hamburger. See under CHLORIDE SHIFT. **2** See under LAW.

Hamilton [David James *Hamilton*, Scottish pathologist, 1849–1909] See under METHOD.

Hamilton [Frank Hastings *Hamilton*, U.S. surgeon, 1813–1886] See under PSEUDOPHLEGMON, TEST.

Hamman [Louis *Hamman*, U.S. physician, 1877–1946] **1** Hamman syndrome. See under DISEASE. **2** Hamman-Rich disease. See under HAMMAN-RICH SYNDROME. **3** Hamman sign. See under HAMMAN'S MURMUR.

hammer MALLEUS.

Neef's hammer WAGNER'S HAMMER.

percussion hammer REFLEX HAMMER.

reflex hammer An instrument for testing tendon reflexes, usually consisting of a rubber-headed mallet. Also called *percussion hammer.*

Wagner's hammer A switch for the rapid opening and closing of an electric circuit. Also called *Neef's hammer.*

Hammerschlag [Albert *Hammerschlag*, Austrian physician, 1863–1935] See under METHOD, TEST.

hammock / pelvic hammock A suspensory support for a fractured pelvis.

Hammond [William Alexander *Hammond*, U.S. neurologist, 1823–1900] Hammond syndrome, Hammond's disease. See under DOUBLE ATHETOSIS.

hamose HAMATE.

Hampton [Aubrey Otis *Hampton*, U.S. radiologist, 1900–1955] See under MANEUVER, HUMP.

Hamspon [William *Hampson*, English inventor, 1854–1926] See under UNIT.

hamstring [Old English *hamm* (akin to Gk *knēmē* the leg between knee and ankle) + Old English *streng* (akin to L *stringere* to tie, bind, and to Gk *strangein* to draw tight) string] **1** See under HAMSTRING TENDON. **2** See under HAMSTRING MUSCLE.

inner hamstrings MEDIAL HAMSTRINGS.

lateral hamstring The tendon of insertion of the biceps femoris muscle. Also called *outer hamstring.*

medial hamstrings The tendon of insertion of the semimembranosus and semitendinosus muscles. Also called *inner hamstrings.*

outer hamstring LATERAL HAMSTRING.

hamular Hook-shaped; unciform.

hamulate Shaped like or possessing a small hook. Also *hamulose.*

hamulose HAMULATE.

hamulus [L (dim. of *hamus* a hook, thorn), a little hook] A small, hooklike structure.

hamulus cochleae HAMULUS LAMINAE SPIRALIS.

hamulus of ethmoid bone PROCESSUS UNCINATUS OSSIS ETHMOIDALIS.

frontal hamulus ALA CRISTAE GALLI.

hamulus frontalis ALA CRISTAE GALLI.

hamulus of hamate bone HAMULUS OSSIS HAMATI.

lacrimal hamulus HAMULUS LACRIMALIS.

hamulus lacrimalis [NA] The hooklike process, situated at the lower end of the vertical posterior lacrimal crest on the orbital surface of the lacrimal bone, that turns anteriorly to articulate with the orbital surface of the maxilla, forming the upper bony opening of the nasolacrimal canal. Also called *lacrimal hamulus, hamular process of lacrimal bone, uncinate process of lacrimal bone* (outmoded).

hamulus laminae spiralis [NA] The hooklike termination of the osseous spiral lamina at its apex after it has wound around the modiolus of the cochlea. Also called *hamulus cochleae, rostrum of spiral lamina* (outmoded).

hamulus ossis hamati [NA] The hooklike projection, flat-tened from side to side, on the palmar surface of the hamate bone to which the flexor retinaculum, pisohamate ligament, and two hypothenar muscles are attached. Also called *hamulus of hamate bone, hook of hamate bone, hamular process of unciform bone* (outmoded), *uncus of hamate bone* (outmoded), *uncinate process of unciform bone* (outmoded).

pterygoid hamulus HAMULUS PTERYGOIDEUS.

hamulus pterygoideus [NA] The narrow, curved, fingerlike projection from the inferior end of the medial pterygoid plate of the sphenoid bone on the lateral side of which there is a groove for the tendon of the tensor veli palatini muscle that hooks around it to the soft palate. Also called *pterygoid hamulus, hamular process of sphenoid bone.*

trochlear hamulus SPINA TROCHLEARIS.

hamycin A polyene, antifungal antibiotic obtained from *Streptomyces pimprina.* It is very similar to trichomycin and candicidin. Also called *primamycin.*

Hancock [Henry *Hancock*, English surgeon, 1809–1880] Hancock's operation. See under AMPUTATION.

Hand [Alfred *Hand*, Jr., U.S. pediatrician, 1868–1949] Hand-Schüller-Christian syndrome, Hand syndrome. See under HAND-SCHÜLLER-CHRISTIAN DISEASE.

hand The extremity of the upper limb distal to the forearm; manus.

accoucheur's hand The position of the hand in tetany, as in hypocalcemia of hypoparathyroidism, the hand being flexed at the wrist, the fingers flexed at the metacarpophalangeal joints but extended at the interphangeal joints, with the thumb tightly flexed over and into the palm. Also called *obstetrician's hand, main d'accoucheur.*

ape hand A developmental defect in which the thumb extends almost at right angles to the longitudinal axis of the hand, resembling the nonapposed position of the thumb of the great apes.

apostolic hand PREACHER'S HAND.

beat hand Cellulitis of the hand occurring among miners and caused by friction and pressure.

benediction hand PREACHER'S HAND.

Charcot's hand PREACHER'S HAND.

claw hand A hand which superficially resembles a claw and which usually results from an ulnar nerve lesion or from some other process causing diffuse atrophy and weakness of the interosseous and lumbrical muscles. The digits are hyperextended at the metacarpophalangeal joints, and flexed at the interphalangeal joints. Also called *griffin-claw hand, griffin claw, main en griffe.* Also *clawhand.*

cleft hand **1** LOBSTER CLAW HAND. **2** A congenital defect in which separation between any two adjacent fingers extends into the metacarpal region. More often than not, this defect involves lobster-claw deformity, with the partial or total absence of one or more of the middle digits. Also called *split hand, main en pince, main fourchée.* See also LOBSTER-CLAW DEFORMITY.

club hand TALIPOMANUS.

corpse hand A hand in which the interosseous muscles and those of the thenar and hypothenar eminences are severely atrophic, giving the hand an emaciated appearance, like that of a skeleton. A seldom used term. Also called *skeleton hand, main de squelette.*

crab hand Erysipeloid of the hand that is usually a result of a scratch from a crab shell.

cubital club hand TALIPOMANUS.

dead hand See under VIBRATION DISEASE.

drop hand WRISTDROP.

fakir's hand A hand with fingers maximally and firmly flexed into the palm. This is almost invariably due to hysterical contracture, much less often to organic contracture. An older term.

flat hand   MANUS PLANA.

flipper hand   1 A hand that lacks spontaneous motion due to destruction of most of the wrist and interphalangeal joints by inflammatory arthritis.   2 A hand affected by a severe form of syndactyly.

ghoul hand   A yellowish-white hand with blotchy pigmentation, attributed to tertiary yaws.

griffin-claw hand   CLAW HAND.

hypotonic hollow hand   PARETIC HOLLOW HAND.

Krukenberg's hand   KRUKENBERG'S ARM.

lobster claw hand   1 An attitude of the hand, sometimes seen in syringomyelia, in which the thumb is held away from the index finger, which is semiflexed, giving a pincerlike appearance. The three other fingers are strongly flexed. Also called *cleft hand*.   2 LOBSTER-CLAW DEFORMITY.

Marinesco's hand   A seldom used term for SUCCULENT HAND.

mitten hand   Multiple syndactyl deformities of the fingers.

monkey's hand   A hand showing severe atrophy of the muscles of the thenar and hypothenar eminences so that opposition of the thumb and fingers becomes impossible, seen in many lesions of the cervical spinal cord, of the inner cord of the brachial plexus, and in combined lesions of the ulnar and median nerves, but most often occurring in motor neuron disease. An imprecise and seldom used term. Also called *simian hand, main de singe, monkey-paw*.

obstetrician's hand   ACCOUCHEUR'S HAND.

opera-glass hand   A hand in which the joints are severely damaged by inflammatory arthritis resulting in telescoped fingers. Also called *main en lorgnette*.

paretic hollow hand   A hand exhibiting wasting of the small hand muscles. An outmoded term. Also called *hypotonic hollow hand*.

phantom hand   A sensation, following amputation, as if the hand were still present. See under PHANTOM LIMB.

preacher's hand   A position of the hand marked by flexion of the two terminal phalanges of all the fingers and extension of the first, with extension of the hand at the wrist. This may be caused by paralysis of the ulnar and median nerves, precluding any action antagonistic to that of the long extensor muscles or by a lesion of the first thoracic spinal nerve or inner cord of the brachial plexus. Often the flexion of the little and ring fingers is more striking than that of the others. Also called *Charcot's hand, benediction hand, apostolic hand*.

simian hand   MONKEY'S HAND.

skeleton hand   CORPSE HAND.

spade hand   The characteristic thick, massive hand of patients who have acromegaly, with heavy, spadelike fingers, bulky overgrowth of soft tissue, and strikingly prominent superficial veins.

split hand   CLEFT HAND.

stiff hand   Restricted movement of the hand and fingers, whether resulting from joint disease or from organic or hysterical contracture of muscles and tendons. An imprecise and outmoded term.

succulent hand   A hand that is swollen and plump, with dimpling over the knuckles. It is sometimes caused by edema resulting from immobility and dependency but more often due to brawny swelling and induration of the soft tissues. It is most often seen in syringomyelia but can develop in other conditions such as shoulder-hand syndrome or reflex dystrophy of the upper extremity. It has been attributed at least in part to the effects of loss of pain and temperature sensation and repeated minor trauma. Also called *main succulente, Marinesco's hand* (seldom used).

swan-neck hand   A drooping hand or wristdrop, caused by paralysis of the extensor muscles of the carpus and fingers, and

giving an appearance like the neck of a swan. A seldom used term.

thalamic hand   A characteristic posture of the hand seen in cases of the thalamic syndrome. In such cases bizarre mobile posturing of the hand, especially when the eyes are closed, is attributable to severe loss of position and joint sense in the affected member (pseudoathetosis). Contractures of the hands and fingers in such cases may be due to an associated hemiparesis but are not a consequence of the thalamic lesion. An outmoded and imprecise term.

trailing hand   The hand which lags behind the other in bimanual activity when both hands are carrying out comparable movements, as in dysdiadochokinesia. Also called *trailer*.

trench hand   Frostbite of the hand, resulting in a loss of soft tissue and skin, which produces stiffness and atrophy. Also called *main des tranchées*.

trident hand   The hand characteristically seen in achondroplasia in which all digits tend to be of equal length, with fingers somewhat splayed at the first interphalangeal joint.

ulnar hand   The posture of the hand following paralysis of the ulnar nerve, combining the characteristics of the so-called claw and corpse hands.

useless hand   A hand which cannot be used for any useful motor activity because of severe loss of position and joint sense.

Warner's hand   The posture of the outstretched hand seen in rheumatic chorea, with flexion of the wrist and hyperextension of the fingers at the metacarpophalangeal joints.

writing hand   The "pill-rolling" tremor with opposition of the thumb and fingers, as seen in Parkinson's disease. An imprecise usage.

handedness   The use of one hand in preference to the other in the performance of motor acts.

handicap   [obsolete English, a game in which forfeits were drawn from a cap, alteration of *hand in cap*]   A physical or mental limitation, which may be correctable, in the ability to function normally.

handicapped   Limited in a physical or mental capacity, such that the ability to function normally is impaired. Legal definitions in some jurisdictions have been determined to fix standards of eligibility for specific programs and services.

perceptually handicapped   Having limitations of activity and ability related to sensory difficulties, frequently, resulting from birth defects or subsequent injury or illness.

handle / handle of malleus   MANUBRIUM MALLEI.

Handley   [William Sampson *Handley*, English surgeon, 1872–1962]   Handley's method. See under LYMPHANGIOPLASTY.

Handovsky   [Hans *Handovsky*, Czech pharmacologist, born 1888]   Wiechowski and Handovsky method. See under METHOD.

handpiece   1 A device, held in the hand, that holds the bur and either transmits rotational power from a dental engine to the bur or has within it a small engine.   2 A similar device for producing vibratory movements of a tip, which replaces the bur.

air turbine handpiece   A contra-angle handpiece containing a turbine that is driven by compressed air and that drives the bur directly. Because of its high speed, over 100 000 rpm, special ball bearings or air-cushion bearings and cooling water sprays are incorporated in the handpiece.

high-speed handpiece   A handpiece for use with a high-speed dental engine, speed 60 000–100 000 rpm, It incorporates a cooling water jet and special bearings.

right-angle handpiece   A handpiece in which the long axis of the bur is at right angles to the long axis of the handle.

straight handpiece   A handpiece in which the long axis of the bur is in line with the long axis of the handle.

ultrasonic handpiece   A handpiece using ultrasonic vibrations and an abrasive slurry as the cutting mechanism.

water-turbine handpiece An experimental handpiece containing a water turbine which drives the bur.

handprint 1 The patterned impression of the epidermal ridges and skin creases of the fingers, thumb, and palm, made by chance contact of an individual's hand with a surface capable of retaining the impression. 2 The impression made by applying ink or some other substance to the hand and pressing the hand on paper or another suitable medium. Handprints of newborns are often made for the purpose of identification, and occasionally they are required for biologic investigations and in cases of disputed paternity.

handshaking The exchange of a certain sequence of control signals by two communication devices such as modems to synchronize transmission of data.

Hanfmann [Eugenia *Hanfmann*, U.S. psychologist, flourished 20th century] Hanfmann-Kasanin test. See under TEST.

hanging Subjecting to asphyxial injury or death by ligature strangulation in which the weight of the victim's suspended body produces the force to tighten the ligature. Death results from compression of the upper airway and cervical blood vessels, except in a judicial hanging in which the sudden snap of the laterally placed knot when the victim is dropped is designed to fracture the upper cervical vertebrae and cause transection of the spinal cord.

hangnail [alteration of English and Middle English *agnail* (from Old English *angnægl* a corn, from *ang(e)* pain (akin to English *anger*) + Old English *nægl* a metal nail) a sore around a toenail or fingernail] A hard spicule at the edge of the nail. It is common among nail biters. Also called *agnail*.

hangover A syndrome that follows ingestion of alcohol and/or other sedations. Symptoms include a bad taste in one's mouth, nausea, pallor, sweating, and conjunctival infection. A popular usage. Also called *katzenjammer (German)*.

Hanhart [Ernst *Hanhart*, Swiss internist, flourished mid-20th century] 1 Hanhart syndrome. See under PITUITARY DWARFISM III. 2 See under DWARF. 3 Hanhart syndrome. See under AGLOSSIA-ADACTYLIA SYNDROME.

Hanlon [C. Rollins *Hanlon*, U.S. surgeon, born 1915] Blalock-Hanlon operation. See under OPERATION.

Hann [F. von *Hann*, Hungarian physician, flourished early 20th century] See under DISEASE.

Hannover [Adolph *Hannover*, Danish anatomist, 1814–1894] 1 Hannover's intermediate membrane. See under NASMYTH'S MEMBRANE. 2 Hannover's canal. See under SPATIUM ZONULARE.

Hanot [Victor Charles *Hanot*, French physician, 1844–1896] 1 Hanot-Chauffard syndrome. See under SYNDROME. 2 Hanot cirrhosis, Hanot's disease, Hanot syndrome. See under PRIMARY BILIARY CIRRHOSIS.

Hansen [Gerhard Henrik Armauer *Hansen*, Norwegian bacteriologist, 1841–1912] 1 Hansen's disease. See under LEPROSY. 2 Hansen's bacillus. See under LEPROSY BACILLUS.

hanseniasis [after Gerhard Henrik Armauer *Hansen*, Norwegian bacteriologist and physician, 1841–1912 + -IASIS] A rarely used term for LEPROSY. • In Brazil the Portuguese translation of the term, hanseníase, is the official name for the disease.

hansenid [after Gerhard Henrik Armauer *Hansen*, Norwegian bacteriologist and physician, 1841–1912 + -ID²] TUBERCULOID LEPROSY.

Hansenula anomala A nonpathogenic species of yeast fungus sometimes found as normal flora of the throat and digestive tract of humans.

hapalonychia [Gk *hapal(os)* soft, tender + ONYCH- + -IA]

The presence of very soft nails, which may be thinner than usual and bend and split easily. The affected nail may be eggshell in color. The condition is seen in chronic arthritis, myxedema, leprosy, and cachexia.

haphalgesia [Gk *haph(e)* a touching, sense of touch + ALGESIA] Cutaneous pain caused by the faintest contact, occurring in hysterical states and in diseases such as tabes. Also called *aphalgesia*.

haphephobia HAPTEPHOBIA.

hapl- HAPLO-.

haplo- [Gk *haploos* or *haplous* single, simple] 1 A combining form meaning single or simple. 2 A combining form meaning haploid. For defs. 1 and 2 also *hapl-*. Compare DIPLO-.

haplodermatitis Dermatitis with no complications, such as a secondary infection. A seldom used term. Also called *haplodermitis*.

haplodermitis HAPLODERMATITIS.

haplodiploidy [HAPLO- + DIPLOIDY] A state in which males develop from unfertilized ova and are haploid, and females develop from fertilized ova and are diploid, as in honeybees. Compare HAPLOID-DIPLOID MOSAICISM.

haplodont [HAPL- + -ODONT] Denoting molar teeth with simple crowns and no tubercles.

Haplographiaceae [HAPLO- + Gk *graphei(on)*, pencil, brush + -ACEAE] An obsolete form-family of fungi, presently included in the form-subclass Blastomycetidae.

haploid [HAPL- + -OID] 1 Having a chromosome complement composed either of a single chromosome (as in bacteria and viruses) or multiple nonhomologous chromosomes (as in the gametes of eukaryotes). In humans, the haploid number of chromosomes is 23, and it is the normal situation in ova and sperm. Also *monoploid*. Compare DIPLOID. 2 A cell or organism having such a chromosome complement. Also called *haplont*.

haploidy The condition of having a single set of nonhomologous chromosomes. Also called *haploid state*.

haplomycosis ADIASPIROMYCOSIS.

haplont HAPLOID.

haplopathy [HAPLO- + -PATHY] A disease that lacks complications.

haplophase The phase of the cell cycle of gametes or of the life cycle of some organisms during which nuclei contain a haploid chromosome set. Compare DIPLOPHASE.

haplopia [HAPL- + -OPIA] The normal condition of binocular vision without diplopia.

Haplorchis [HAPL- + Gk *orchis* testicle] A genus of heterophyid flukes having only one testis. They are found in a variety of birds and mammals throughout the Middle East and in Taiwan. Operculated snails of the genus *Melania* serve as the first intermediate hosts, and a variety of fishes serve as the vertebrate transport hosts, conveying the metacercariae to fish-eating birds or mammals. Also called *Monorchotrema*.

Haplorchis taichui A species found in Taiwan in the intestine of birds and mammals, and infrequently in humans. Various species of fish serve as the intermediate host to the vertebrate, and cercariae develop in the snail *Melania obliquegranosa*.

haploscope [HAPLO- + -SCOPE] A device presenting a separate picture to each eye. Adjective: haploscopic.

mirror haploscope A device that uses mirrors in order to show a different view to each eye, used in the study of binocular vision and in treatment of its disorders.

haploscopic Pertaining to a haploscope.

haplosporangin An antigen prepared from the fungus *Chrysosporium parva* and used in serologic testing for coccidioidomycosis.

Haplosporidia [HAPLO- + *sporidia*, pl. of SPORIDIUM] A group of unusual sporozoans in which reproduction is by schizogony and production of simple spores without polar capsules or polar filaments. Flagella are absent and pseudopodia present in some forms. It was formerly considered a class, Haplosporea, which was combined with the class Microsporea in the subphylum Microspora. A more recent classification raises both to separate phyla of protozoa, Microspora and Ascetospora, the latter including the haplosporidians in the class Stellatosporea. Representative genera, parasitic in cells, tissues, and body cavities of invertebrates, include *Bertramia* (in the coelom of rotifers and worms), *Anurosporidium* (hyperparasitic in sporocysts of digenetic trematodes), *Urosporidium* (coelom of polychaete worms), *Coelosporidium* (coelom and Malpighian tubules of cockroaches), *Haplosporidium* (aquatic annelid worms and mollusks).

haplotype 1 In linked genes, the alleles contributed from one or the other parent. 2 A linear combination of specific linked alleles or nucleotide sequences, such as restriction enzyme site polymorphisms, that are inherited in coupling (as the alleles of the Rh locus) and may be subject to linkage disequilibrium (as the alleles of the major histocompatibility complex).

hapt- HAPTO-.

hapte- HAPTO-.

hapten [HAPT- + *-ene*, suffix from Gk *-ēnē*, fem. patronymic suffix] A substance that is unable to induce antibody formation but that can react with antibody: applied especially to organic chemicals of low molecular weight. To raise antibodies to haptens it is necessary to couple them to an immunogenic "carrier" molecule which can recruit a helper T cell response. Also called *partial antigen, incomplete antigen, proantigen.* Also *haptin, haptene.* Adjective: haptenic.

haptene HAPTEN.

haptenic Produced by or having the qualities of a hapten.

haptephobia [HAPTE- + -PHOBIA] Pathologic fear of being touched. Also called *haphephobia, aphephobia.*

hapteron [New L (from Gk *haptein* to cling to)] A mass of highly adhesive fungal hyphae that forms an attachment organ at the base of the funicular cord in bird's-nest fungi.

haptics [HAPT- + -ICS] The science of touch, pertaining not only to passively perceived cutaneous sensations of touch and pressure, but including also the active component of exploration via these senses.

haptin HAPTEN.

hapto- [Gk *haptein* to touch, handle, fasten to or on, perceive] A combining form meaning touching or bound together. Also *hapt-, hapte-.*

haptocyst [HAPTO- + CYST] A surface organelle of suctorian protozoa found in the tentacular swellings. They are extremely small, 0.3–0.4 μm, yet are complex tripartite swollen structures used to penetrate the pellicle of the prey upon contact.

haptoglobin An α_2 globulin, normally present in plasma, that specifically binds hemoglobin released from erythrocytes lysed within the circulating blood.

haptometer [HAPTO- + -METER] An instrument for measuring tactile sensitivity, usually consisting of calibrated hairs or filaments.

haptophil [HAPTO- + -PHIL] Having a marked affinity for a haptophore. Also *haptophile.*

haptophile HAPTOPHIL.

haptophore [HAPTO- + -PHORE] In Ehrlich's side chain theory of the nature of antibodies, the group that gave the antibody its specific activity. It thus corresponds to the antigen-binding site. An obsolete term. Adjective: haptophorous, haptophoric.

Harada [Einosuke *Harada*, Japanese surgeon, 1892–1947]

Harada's disease. See under SYNDROME.

harara [Arabic *ḥarāra* heat, rash] A form of papular urticaria caused by the bites of the sand fly, *Phlebotomus papatasii*. It occurs on the posterior aspects of the hands as urticaria or inflammatory papules, often seen in travelers in the Middle East, particularly in the Nile valley. Also called *urticaria multiformis endemica.*

Harden [Sir Arthur *Harden*, English biochemist, 1865–1940] Harden-Young ester. See under FRUCTOSE 1,6-BISPHOSPHATE.

hardening 1 The process of making or becoming firm. 2 In microscopy, the process of making a tissue firmer, usually by chemical fixation or by quick-freezing, so as to facilitate sectioning.

hardening of the arteries ARTERIOSCLEROSIS.

Harder [Johann Jacob *Harder*, Swiss anatomist, 1656–1711] 1 Harder's gland. See under HARDERIAN GLAND. 2 Harderian fossa. See under FOSSA.

hardness 1 HARDNESS OF WATER. 2 The property of a solid that characterizes its resistance to scratching or indentation.

indentation hardness The measure of a material's resistance to being dented by a standard load applied to a measured surface area.

permanent hardness Hardness of water that cannot removed by boiling. It is caused by the presence of the sulfates, chlorides, and nitrates of calcium and magnesium.

temporary hardness Hardness of water that can be removed by boiling. It is caused by the soluble carbonates and hydroxides of calcium and magnesium, which lose carbon dioxide on boiling and precipitate as carbonates.

hardness of water A characteristic of water that reflects the total concentration of calcium and magnesium ions. Also called *hardness.*

hardware The physical components, circuits, and mechanical equipment that make up a computer, as distinguished from software.

hardwood ANGIOSPERM.

Hardy [Godfrey Harold *Hardy*, English mathematician, 1877–1947] 1 Hardy-Weinberg law. See under LAW. 2 Hardy-Weinberg equilibrium. See under EQUILIBRIUM.

Hare [Edward Selleck *Hare*, English physician, 1812–1838] Hare syndrome. See under PANCOAST SYNDROME.

harelip [HARE + LIP] CLEFT LIP.

acquired harelip A cleft of the upper lip caused by an injury.

bilateral harelip A harelip with the upper lip cleft on both sides of the philtrum and premaxilla. Also called *double harelip.*

double harelip BILATERAL HARELIP.

lateral harelip A harelip consisting of a unilateral cleft of the upper lip on one side or the other of the philtrum and premaxilla, with or without an associated cleft of the maxilla. Also called *single harelip, unilateral harelip.*

median harelip A harelip consisting of a cleft of the upper lip and maxilla at the midline. It results from failed development of the embryonic medial nasal processes. It is analogous to the midline cleft normally seen in a hare.

single harelip LATERAL HARELIP.

unilateral harelip LATERAL HARELIP.

harmaline $C_{13}H_{14}ON_2$. A cardioactive alkaloid obtained from the seeds and roots of *Peganum harmala.*

Harmer [William Douglas *Harmer*, English otolaryngologist, born 1873] Finzi-Harmer operation. See under OPERATION.

harmine $C_{13}H_{12}N_2O$. A β-carboline alkaloid found in a variety of plants, including *Peganum harmala* and *Banisteria caapi*. A central nervous system stimulant and inhibitor of monoamine oxidase, it is used to treat paralysis agitans. Its sedative and depressive effect is usually more pronounced than its hallucinogenic effect.

harmonia   SUTURA PLANA.

harmonic   A sinusoidal component of a periodic wave having a frequency that is an integral multiple of the fundamental frequency. Twice the fundamental frequency is the second harmonic.

harmony [Gk *harmonia* (from *harmozein* to fit together, set in order) a fitting together, harmony (in music), intonation of the voice (in rhetoric)]

functional occlusal harmony   A state of occlusal balance providing maximum masticatory efficiency.

occlusal harmony   A dental occlusion compatible with complete health of teeth, periodontium, temporomandibular joints, and neuromuscular mechanisms.

Harmonyl   A proprietary name for deserpidine.

harness / shoulder harness   A restraint attached to the frame of a motor vehicle, passing diagonally from behind a shoulder and fastening next to the opposite hip of a seated passenger or the driver. It prevents forward motion of the upper torso during sudden deceleration and is more effective in preventing injury than a lap belt alone.

Harpirhynchus   A genus of mites, parasitic on birds, usually found as colonies in feather follicles and which often induce tumors and cysts.

harpoon [Dutch *harpoen* harpoon, from Middle French *harpon* harpoon, from Middle French *harper* to claw, from the Scandinavian]   An elongated, thin, barbed surgical instrument designed to obtain a small sample of tissue for diagnostic testing.

Harrington [David O. *Harrington*, U.S. ophthalmologist, born 1904]   Harrington-Flocks test. See under TEST.

Harrington [S. W. *Harrington*, U.S. surgeon, born 1889]   See under OPERATION.

Harris [Downey Lamar *Harris*, U.S. pathologist, 1875–1956]   See under METHOD.

Harris [Franklin I. *Harris*, U.S. surgeon, born 1895]   See under TUBE.

Harris [Henry Albert *Harris*, English anatomist, 1886–1968]   Harris line. See under GROWTH ARREST LINE.

Harris [Henry Fauntleroy *Harris*, U.S. physician, 1867–1926]   See under HEMATOXYLIN.

Harris [James Arthur *Harris*, U.S. scientist, born 1880]   Harris and Benedict standard. See under STANDARD.

Harris [Malcolm LaSalle *Harris*, U.S. surgeon, 1862–1936]   Harris separator. See under SEGREGATOR.

Harris [Seale *Harris*, U.S. physician, 1870–1957]   See under SYNDROME.

Harris [Wilfred John *Harris*, English physician, 1869–1960]   Harris migrainous neuralgia. See under MIGRAINOUS NEURALGIA.

Harrison [Edward *Harrison*, English physician, 1766–1838]   Harrison's curve, Harrison sulcus. See under GROOVE.

Harrison [Harold Edward *Harrison*, U.S. physician, born 1908]   See under TEST.

Harrison Antinarcotic Act   An act regulating the importation, sale, and use of all substances defined in the act as narcotics. It was originally passed by the U.S. Congress in 1914, and amended several times subsequently.

Harrower [Henry Robert *Harrower*, U.S. physician, born 1883]   See under HYPOTHESIS.

Harrower-Erickson [Molly R. *Harrower-Erickson*, U.S. psychologist, born 1906]   See under TEST.

harrowing [Middle English *harwe*, prob. akin to Gk *keirein* to clip, cut out, hew off, + -ING]   HERSAGE.

Hart [Theodore Stuart *Hart*, U.S. physician, born 1869]   See under METHOD.

Hartel [Fritz *Hartel*, German surgeon, flourished early 20th century]   See under TREATMENT, METHOD.

Hartley [Frank *Hartley*, U.S. surgeon, 1857–1913]   Hartley-Krause operation. See under OPERATION.

Hartman [Le Roy Leo *Hartman*, U.S. dentist, 1893–1951]   See under SOLUTION.

Hartmann [Arthus *Hartmann*, German laryngologist, 1849–1931]   See under SPECULUM.

Hartmann [Henri *Hartmann*, French surgeon, 1860–1952]   **1** Hartmann's point, Hartmann's critical point. See under POINT OF SUDECK. **2** See under POUCH.

Hartmann [Robert *Hartmann*, German anatomist, 1831–1893]   Hartmann's fossa. See under RECESSUS ILEOCECALIS INFERIOR.

Hartmannella   A genus of amebas (order Amoebida) normally free-living, although some species are facultative parasites in the respiratory passages and central nervous system of mammals, including humans.

Hartmannella castellanii   ACANTHAMOEBA CASTELLANII.

Hartmannella hyalina   A coprozoic species found in human feces.

Hartnup [Edward *Hartnup*, English hospital patient of 20th century]   **1** Hartnup's disorder. See under DISEASE. **2** See under SYNDROME.

harvest   To obtain (tissue or an organ) from a donor for use in another site in the same subject or as a transplant into another subject.

hasamiyami [Japanese, after *Hasami*, a place name + *-yami*, combining form denoting illness]   HASAMI FEVER.

Hashimoto [Hakaru *Hashimoto*, Japanese surgeon, 1881–1934]   Hashimoto struma, Hashimoto's thyroiditis. See under HASHIMOTO DISEASE.

hashish [Arabic *ḥashīsh* dried hemp, hashish]   A resin obtained from the Indian hemp plant, *Cannabis sativa*, ingested for its intoxicating qualities.

Hasner [Joseph Ritter von Artha *Hasner*, Czech physician, 1819–1892]   Hasner's fold, Hasner's valve. See under PLICA LACRIMALIS.

Hassall [Arthur Hill *Hassall*, English physician, 1817–1894]   **1** Virchow-Hassall body, Hassall's body. See under HASSALL'S CORPUSCLE. **2** Hassall-Henle warts. See under HASSALL-HENLE BODIES.

Hasselbalch [Karl Albert *Hasselbalch*, Danish biochemist and physician, 1874–1962]   Henderson-Hasselbalch equation. See under EQUATION.

Hassin [George Boris *Hassin*, U.S. neurologist, 1873–1951]   See under SYNDROME.

Hata [Sahachiro *Hata*, Japanese physician, 1873–1938]   **1** See under PHENOMENON. **2** Ehrlich-Hata treatment. See under TREATMENT.

hatchet [Middle French *hachette* (from *hache* battle-axe + dim. suffix *-ette*) a small axe]   A manual dental instrument, the tip of which is a very small, angled chisel. Also called *enamel hatchet*.

enamel hatchet   HATCHET.

Haudek [Martin *Haudek*, Austrian roentgenologist, 1880–1931]   Haudek sign. See under NICHE.

haunch   The hips and buttocks considered as a single unit.

hauptganglion of Küttner   KÜTTNER'S GANGLION.

haust.   *haustus* (L, a draft).

haustoria   Plural of HAUSTORIUM.

haustorium [L *haust(us)* a drinking, drawing of water + *-orium* -ORY]   (*plural* haustoria) An absorbent organ originating on a fungal hypha of a parasite and penetrating into a cell of the host. It is most often associated with obligate parasites but is produced also by some facultative parasites.

haustra   **1** Plural of HAUSTRUM.   **2** HAUSTRA COLI.

haustral   **1** Pertaining to a haustrum.   **2** Of or relating to the haustra coli.

haustrations [*haustr(um)* + -ATION + English pl. *s*]   HAUS-TRA COLI.

haustrum [L (from *haustus*, past part. of *haurire* to draw forth or out, drink off, from Gk *aryein* to draw water), a machine for drawing water]   (*plural* haustra) Any one of the pouches, or sacculations, in the wall of the colon.

cecal haustra   Haustra coli located on the cecum.

haustra coli   [NA] The sacculations of the colon that are formed because of the shortness of the taeniae coli relative to the circular muscle coat and the length of the large intestine. The number and distribution of the sacculations are modified according to the physiologic status of the colon, and they disappear in the vicinity of the rectum. In the newborn and infants they are fewer and shallower than in adults. Also called *haustra of colon, haustrations, haustra, cellulae coli* (outmoded), *colic sacculations, cecal sacculations, colic haustra.*

colic haustra   HAUSTRA COLI.

haustra of colon   HAUSTRA COLI.

haustus [L (from *haustus*, past part. of *haurire* to draw forth or out, drink off), a drawing, drinking, the right of drawing water]   **1** A potion.   **2** A measure of a liquid drug or medicinal preparation.

haustus niger   COMPOUND MIXTURE OF SENNA.

haut mal [French *haut* high + *mal* sickness]   MAJOR EPILEPSY.

HAV   HEPATITIS A VIRUS.

Haven [Hale *Haven*, U.S. neurologist, born 1902]   Haven syndrome. See under SCALENUS ANTERIOR SYNDROME.

Haverhillia multiformis   *STREPTOBACILLUS MONILIFORMIS.*

Hawes [Sir Richard Brunel *Hawes*, English physician, flourished 20th century]   Hawes-Pallister-Landor syndrome. See under STRACHAN-SCOTT SYNDROME.

hawthorn   CRATAEGUS.

Hayem [Georges *Hayem*, French physician, 1841–1933]   **1** See under DISEASE, SOLUTION.   **2** Hayem's encephalitis. See under HYPERPLASTIC ENCEPHALITIS.   **3** Hayem's elementary corpuscle. See under PLATELET.   **4** Hayem's hematoblast. See under HEMOCYTOBLAST.

hay fever   See under FEVER.

Hayflick [Leonard *Hayflick*, U.S. microbiologist, born 1928]   See under PHENOMENON.

Haygarth [John *Haygarth*, English physician, 1740–1827]   Haygarth nodes. See under NODE.

Haynes [Irving Samuel *Haynes*, U.S. surgeon, 1861–1946]   See under OPERATION.

hayrake   HAYRAKE SPLINT.

hazard [Middle English, from Old French *hazard* a dice game, from Arabic *az-zahr* the dice, dice game]   **1** A circumstance or agent that increases the probability of loss or damage.   **2** The chance that injury will result from exposure to a substance under specified conditions of use.

haze   An atmospheric suspension of tiny dry particles that are invisible to the naked eye, but that reduce visibility or give the sky an opalescent appearance. The particles may become the nuclei of water droplets that produce a mist.

Hazen [Allen *Hazen*, U.S. civil engineer, 1869–1930]   See under THEOREM.

Hb   hemoglobin (or hemoglobin concentration).

HB$_c$Ag   hepatitis B core antigen.

HBeAg   hepatitis B e antigen.

HB$_s$Ag   hepatitis B surface antigen.

HbO$_2$ oxyhemoglobin (oxygenated hemoglobin).

HBV   hepatitis B virus.

HCG   Human chorionic gonadotropin.

HCT   hematocrit.

HD$_{50}$ [from *hemolyzing dose*]   The amount of complement which will cause hemolysis of 50 percent of a population of sensitized red blood cells.

h.d.   *hora decubitus* (L, at bedtime).

HDCV   human diploid cell vaccine.

HDL   high-density lipoprotein.

HDN   hemolytic disease of the newborn.

H and E   hematoxylin and eosin stain.

He   Symbol for the element, helium.

Head [Sir Henry *Head*, English neurologist, 1861–1940]   **1** See under CLASSIFICATION, ZONE.   **2** Head-Holmes syndrome. See under SYNDROME.

head

head [Old English *hēafod*, akin to L *caput* head]   **1** The upper extremity of the human body; caput. It comprises the cranium and the face.   **2** The proximal or superior extremity of any organ or structure.

angular head of quadratus labii superioris muscle   An outmoded term for MUSCULUS LEVATOR LABII SUPERIORIS ALAE-QUE NASI.

articular head   The cartilage-covered rounded extremity of a bone that articulates with another bone.

head of astragalus   CAPUT TALI.

head of blind colon   An outmoded term for CAECUM.

box head   The characteristically flattened head which results from rickets.

bulldog head   The head of an achondroplastic individual, marked by a high vault and relatively of a large size.

head of condyloid process of mandible   CAPUT MANDIBU-LAE.

coronoid head of pronator teres muscle   CAPUT ULNARE MUSCULI PRONATORIS TERETIS.

deep head of triceps brachii muscle   An outmoded term for CAPUT MEDIALE MUSCULI TRICIPITIS BRACHII.

deep head of triceps extensor cubiti muscle   An outmoded term for CAPUT MEDIALE MUSCULI TRICIPITIS BRACHII.

drum head   MEMBRANA TYMPANI.

engaged head   A fetal head which as the presenting part has descended to a level such that the biparietal plane of the fetal head is below that of the pelvic inlet.

head of epididymis   CAPUT EPIDIDYMIDIS.

head of femur   CAPUT OSSIS FEMORIS.

head of fibula   CAPUT FIBULAE.

first head of triceps brachii muscle   An outmoded term for CAPUT LONGUM MUSCULI TRICIPITIS BRACHII.

first head of triceps extensor cubiti muscle   An outmoded term for CAPUT LONGUM MUSCULI TRICIPITIS BRACHII.

floating head   A condition in which the fetal head as the presenting part lies well above the plane of the pelvic inlet.

great head of adductor hallucis muscle   An outmoded term for CAPUT OBLIQUUM MUSCULI ADDUCTORIS HALLUCIS.

great head of triceps brachii muscle   An outmoded term for CAPUT LATERALE MUSCULI TRICIPITIS BRACHII.

great head of triceps extensor cubiti muscle   An outmoded term for CAPUT LATERALE MUSCULI TRICIPITIS BRACHII.

great head of triceps femoris muscle   An outmoded term for MUSCULUS ADDUCTOR MAGNUS.

hot cross bun head   **1** A head in which depressions trace the lines of the cranial sutures; the condition is seen in infants and children with rickets or syphilitic osteitis.   **2** CAPUT QUADRATUM.

hourglass head   A head having a transverse depression on the skull at the coronal suture. It can be a manifestation of congenital syphilis.

humeral head of biceps brachii muscle   An occasional accessory head of the biceps brachii muscle that arises from the medial margin of the humerus just below the insertion of the coracobrachialis muscle and inserts into the posterior surface of the fleshy belly of the biceps brachii. It is innervated by the musculocutaneous nerve.

humeral head of flexor carpi ulnaris muscle   CAPUT HUMERALE MUSCULI FLEXORIS CARPI ULNARIS.

humeral head of flexor digitorum sublimis muscle   CAPUT HUMEROULNARE MUSCULI FLEXORIS DIGITORUM SUPERFICIALIS.

humeral head of pronator teres muscle   CAPUT HUMERALE MUSCULI PRONATORIS TERETIS.

humeroulnar head of flexor digitorum superficialis   CAPUT HUMEROULNARE MUSCULI FLEXORIS DIGITORUM SUPERFICIALIS.

head of humerus   CAPUT HUMERI.

infraorbital head of quadratus labii superioris muscle   An outmoded term for MUSCULUS LEVATOR LABII SUPERIORIS.

lateral head of gastrocnemius muscle   CAPUT LATERALE MUSCULI GASTROCNEMII.

lateral head of triceps brachii muscle   CAPUT LATERALE MUSCULI TRICIPITIS BRACHII.

lateral head of triceps extensor cubiti muscle   CAPUT LATERALE MUSCULI TRICIPITIS BRACHII.

lateral head of triceps muscle   CAPUT LATERALE MUSCULI TRICIPITIS BRACHII.

little head of humerus   CAPITULUM HUMERI.

little head of mandible   An outmoded term for PROCESSUS CONDYLARIS MANDIBULAE.

little head of metatarsal bone   An outmoded term for CAPUT METATARSALE.

long head of adductor hallucis muscle   An outmoded term for CAPUT OBLIQUUM MUSCULI ADDUCTORIS H ALLUCIS.

long head of adductor triceps muscle   An outmoded term for MUSCULUS ADDUCTOR LONGUS.

long head of biceps brachii muscle   CAPUT LONGUM MUSCULI BICIPITIS BRACHII.

long head of biceps femoris muscle   CAPUT LONGUM MUSCULI BICIPITIS FEMORIS.

long head of biceps flexor cruris muscle   An outmoded term for CAPUT LONGUM MUSCULI BICIPITIS FEMORIS.

long head of biceps flexor cubiti muscle   CAPUT LONGUM MUSCULI BICIPITIS BRACHII.

long head of triceps brachii muscle   CAPUT LONGUM MUSCULI TRICIPITIS BRACHII.

long head of triceps extensor cubiti muscle   CAPUT LONGUM MUSCULI TRICIPITIS BRACHII.

long head of triceps femoris muscle   An outmoded term for MUSCULUS ADDUCTOR LONGUS.

long head of triceps muscle   CAPUT LONGUM MUSCULI TRICIPITIS BRACHII.

head of malleus   CAPUT MALLEI.

head of mandible   **1** CAPUT MANDIBULAE.   **2** PROCESSUS CONDYLARIS MANDIBULAE.

medial head of biceps brachii muscle   CAPUT BREVE MUSCULI BICIPITIS BRACHII.

medial head of biceps flexor cubiti muscle   An outmoded term for CAPUT BREVE MUSCULI BICIPITIS BRACHII.

medial head of gastrocnemius muscle   CAPUT MEDIALE MUSCULI GASTROCNEMII.

medial head of triceps brachii muscle   CAPUT MEDIALE MUSCULI TRICIPITIS BRACHII.

medial head of triceps extensor cubiti muscle   An outmoded term for CAPUT MEDIALE MUSCULI TRICIPITIS BRACHII.

medial head of triceps muscle   CAPUT MEDIALE MUSCULI TRICIPITIS BRACHII.

medusa head   CAPUT MEDUSAE.

head of metacarpal bone   CAPUT METACARPALIS.

head of metatarsal bone   CAPUT METATARSALE.

middle head of triceps brachii muscle   An outmoded term for CAPUT LONGUM MUSCULI TRICIPITIS BRACHII.

middle head of triceps extensor cubiti muscle   An outmoded term for CAPUT LONGUM MUSCULI TRICIPITIS BRACHII.

head of muscle   CAPUT MUSCULI.

nasal head of levator labii superioris alaeque nasi muscle   MUSCULUS LEVATOR LABII SUPERIORIS ALAEQUE NASI.

nerve head   DISCUS NERVI OPTICI.

oblique head of adductor hallucis muscle   CAPUT OBLIQUUM MUSCULI ADDUCTORIS HALLU CIS.

oblique head of adductor pollicis muscle   CAPUT OBLIQUUM MUSCULI ADDUCTORIS POLLICIS.

head of optic nerve   DISCUS NERVI OPTICI.

overriding head   An unengaged fetal head which as the presenting part lies over the symphysis pubis.

head of pancreas   CAPUT PANCREATIS.

head of penis   GLANS PENIS.

head of phalanx   Either caput phalangis digitorum manus or caput phalangis digitorum pedis.

head of phalanx of fingers   CAPUT PHALANGIS DIGITORUM MANUS.

head of phalanx of toes   CAPUT PHALANGIS DIGITORUM PEDIS.

plantar head of flexor digitorum pedis longus muscle   An outmoded term for MUSCULUS QUADRATUS PLANTAE.

quadrate head of flexor digitorum pedis longus muscle   An outmoded term for MUSCULUS QUADRATUS PLANTAE.

radial head of flexor digitorum sublimis muscle   CAPUT RADIALE MUSCULI FLEXORIS DIGITORUM SUPERFICIALIS.

radial head of flexor digitorum superficialis muscle   CAPUT RADIALE MUSCULI FLEXORIS DIGITORUM SUPERFICIALIS.

radial head of humerus   An outmoded term for CAPITULUM HUMERI.

head of radius   CAPUT RADII.

head of rib   CAPUT COSTAE.

saddle head   CLINOCEPHALY.

scapular head of triceps brachii muscle   An outmoded term for CAPUT LONGUM MUSCULI TRICIPITIS BRACHII.

scapular head of triceps extensor cubiti muscle   An outmoded term for CAPUT LONGUM MUSCULI TRICIPITIS BRACHII.

second head of triceps brachii muscle   An outmoded term for CAPUT LATERALE MUSCULI TRICIPITIS BRACHII.

short head of biceps brachii muscle   CAPUT BREVE MUSCULI BICIPITIS BRACHII.

short head of biceps femoris muscle   CAPUT BREVE MUSCULI BICIPITIS FEMORIS.

short head of biceps flexor cruris muscle   An outmoded term for CAPUT BREVE MUSCULI BICIPITIS FEMORIS.

short head of biceps flexor cubiti muscle   An outmoded term for CAPUT BREVE MUSCULI BICIPITIS BRACHII.

short head of coracoradialis muscle   An outmoded term for CAPUT BREVE MUSCULI BICIPITIS BRACHII.

short head of triceps brachii muscle   An outmoded term for CAPUT MEDIALE MUSCULI TRICIPITIS BRACHII.

short head of triceps extensor cubiti muscle   An outmoded term for CAPUT MEDIALE MUSCULI TRICIPITIS BRACHII.

short head of triceps femoris muscle   An outmoded term for MUSCULUS ADDUCTOR BREVIS.

head of spermatozoon   The ovoid head of a male germ cell or spermatozoon. It is somewhat pear-shaped in man because the tip is flattened. It is nearly 4 μm long and consists of a nucleus enclosed by a nuclear membrane with its front half covered by a two-layered cap (the acrosome).

head of spleen   An outmoded term for EXTREMITAS POSTERIOR SPLENIS.

head of stapes   CAPUT STAPEDIS.

steeple head   OXYCEPHALY.

swell head   LECHUGUILLA POISONING.

head of talus   CAPUT TALI.

head of thigh bone   CAPUT OSSIS FEMORIS.

tower head   OXYCEPHALY.

transverse head of adductor hallucis muscle   CAPUT TRANSVERSUM MUSCULI ADDUCTORIS HALLUCIS.

transverse head of adductor pollicis muscle   CAPUT TRANSVERSUM MUSCULI ADDUCTORIS POLLICIS.

head of ulna   CAPUT ULNAE.

ulnar head of flexor carpi ulnaris muscle   CAPUT ULNARE MUSCULI FLEXORIS CARPI ULNARIS.

ulnar head of pronator teres muscle   CAPUT ULNARE MUSCULI PRONATORIS TERETIS.

white head   FAVUS.

zygomatic head of quadratus labii superioris muscle   An outmoded term for MUSCULUS ZYGOMATICUS MINOR.

---

headache [HEAD + Old English *æce*]   Pain in the head. Also called *angina capitis, dolor capitis*.

anemic headache   Headache occurring in a patient with anemia and not due to any other cause.

anoxic headache   Headache due to lowered partial oxygen pressure in the blood. It may occur at high altitudes or as a result of carbon monoxide poisoning at blood saturations of more than 20 percent.

bilious headache   MIGRAINE HEADACHE.

blind headache   MIGRAINE HEADACHE.

caffeine-withdrawal headache   Headache following the withdrawal of caffeine taken as a drug or following heavy consumption of caffeine-containing beverages such as coffee or tea.

cervical myalgic headache   A feeling of tightness or pressure in the head, most often in the suboccipital area, associated with tonic contraction of the head or neck muscles, and usually resulting from stress or nervous tension. Also called *muscle-contraction headache, rheumatic headache*.

cluster headache   MIGRAINOUS NEURALGIA.

congestive headache   Headache resulting either from vascular dilatation or from raised intracranial pressure. An imprecise and outmoded term.

cough headache   A syndrome in which attacks of severe headache are precipitated by coughing. This may be a benign syndrome for which no cause is discovered but cough headache sometimes occurs in patients with raised intracranial pressure.

cyclic headache   Any periodic headache, such as that of migraine.

drainage headache   LUMBAR PUNCTURE HEADACHE.

dynamite headache   Headache due to the hypotensive effects of the nitroglycerin component of dynamite. It is accompanied by arterial dilatation, increased heart rate, and a reduced blood pressure. Workers usually acclimatize rapidly to this hypoten-

sive action. Headache is a common symptom on first exposure and on Monday mornings after loss of acclimatization. Also called *nitroglycerin headache*.

epinephrine headache   Headache following the administration of epinephrine.

fibrositic headache   A headache involving the occipital region of the skull. There is often pain and tenderness associated with the presence of small nodules in the scalp. It is often evoked by atmospheric cold.

functional headache   Headache produced by conflict or tension and not based upon demonstrable organic pathology.

helmet headache   Headache limited to the upper part of the head which would be covered by a helmet.

histamine headache   MIGRAINOUS NEURALGIA.

Horton's vascular headache   MIGRAINOUS NEURALGIA.

hyperemic headache   Any vascular headache resulting from, or associated with, dilatation of extracranial or intracranial arteries.

hypertensive headache   Headache resulting from essential hypertension.

jolt headache   Headache induced by sudden head movement.

lumbar puncture headache   Headache due to reduced intracranial pressure after lumbar puncture resulting from leakage of cerebrospinal fluid through the hole in the dura mater left by the exploring needle. Also called *drainage headache, postspinal headache, puncture headache, spinal headache, spinal-fluid loss headache*.

meningeal headache   Headache due to inflammation or irritation of the meninges, usually accompanied by neck stiffness.

migraine headache   The typical paroxysmal throbbing headache occurring in attacks of migraine. Also called *bilious headache, blind headache, sick headache*.

muscle-contraction headache   CERVICAL MYALGIC HEADACHE.

neuralgic headache   Any headache involving the head and neck in which pain radiates or shoots along the course of a sensory nerve or is sharp, intermittent, and transient in character.

nitroglycerin headache   DYNAMITE HEADACHE.

nodular headache   Headache arising in the tissues of the scalp and sometimes associated with nodular or tender areas. This may have been an early description of cranial arteritis. An imprecise usage.

ocular headache   Headache related to the use of the eyes or to their disorders.

organic headache   Any headache due to physical as distinct from mental disease.

paraplegic headache   Transient pressor headache occurring in paraplegic patients in whom a sudden sharp rise in systemic blood pressure may be reflexly induced by stimuli originating below the level of the spinal cord lesion, such as distension of the bladder or rectum.

pheochromocytoma headache   An acute headache usually of great intensity resulting from a transient hypertensive episode in patients with a pheochromocytoma.

postconcussional headache   Recurrent headache following a closed head injury giving rise to concussion. This headache usually declines in frequency and severity with the passage of time and ultimately resolves.

postspinal headache   LUMBAR PUNCTURE HEADACHE.

pressor headache   Headache due to transient or persistent arterial hypotension or to pharmacologic pressor agents.

puncture headache   LUMBAR PUNCTURE HEADACHE.

pyrexial headache   Headache developing in the context of fever.

reflex headache   A form of headache resulting from a disease or abnormality outside the brain. Also called *symptomatic head-ache.*

rheumatic headache   CERVICAL MYALGIC HEADACHE.

rhinogenous headache   Headache caused by disease of the nose.

sick headache   MIGRAINE HEADACHE.

spinal headache   LUMBAR PUNCTURE HEADACHE.

spinal-fluid loss headache   LUMBAR PUNCTURE HEADACHE.

symptomatic headache   REFLEX HEADACHE.

tension headache   A headache, typically occipital in location, resulting from emotional stress or conflict.

toxemic headache   A headache marking the onset of an acute infectious disease such as typhoid fever.

toxic headache   A headache resulting from systemic poisoning.

traction headache   Headache resulting from traction upon pain-sensitive intracranial or extracranial structures such as the dura mater, arteries, veins, and muscles.

traumatic headache   Headache following head injury.

vacuum headache   Frontal headache apparently due to obstruction of the ostia of the anterior group of paranasal sinuses. The obstruction is said to be caused by swelling of the mucosa beneath the middle nasal concha leading to absorption of air in the sinuses and the establishment of a partial vacuum.

vascular headache   A headache resulting from disease or dysfunction of extracranial or intracranial arteries.

vasomotor headache   Headache resulting from constriction or, alternatively, from vasodilatation, of extracranial or intracranial arteries.

head-banging   The hitting of the head against a wall, crib, or other object, generally as a part of a child's temper tantrum and more rarely as a manifestation of a stereotypy. Also called *head-knocking.*

headcap   A cap-shaped device, fitting closely to the skull and used in occipital anchorage.

plaster headcap   A headcap, made of plaster of Paris and gauze to fit the individual patient, used as a base for fixation and traction in the treatment of jaw fractures.

headdress   A cover placed over a patient's hair during operations.

headgear   The headcap or neck device used as the base for external anchorage in orthodontic treatment.

headgut   FOREGUT.

head-knocking   HEAD-BANGING.

headlight   An electric light incorporated into a head mirror worn on a headband, enabling the wearer, as a surgeon, to observe deeply situated structures under good illumination while leaving his hands free.

headlock   A condition whereby the chins of twins *in utero* catch on each other. Usually the first twin presents as a breech while the second twin is in the vertex presentation.

head-nodding   SPASMUS NUTANS.

headpiece   A bandage or splint support for the head.

head-rolling   Rhythmical head movements of a rotatory nature, occurring usually just before the child falls asleep. If frequent in occurrence, it is considered a stereotypy.

head wrapping   A method once used to treat hydrocephalus by constricting the infant's head in tight bandages. An obsolete term.

Heaf [Frederick R. G. *Heaf,* English physician, born 1894]   See under TEST.

heal [Middle English *helen,* from Old English *hælan*]   **1** To make or become whole or well.   **2** To bring about the recovery of (a lesion).

healer   One who heals, as a physician.

healing [Old English *hælan*]   The act of making or the process of becoming whole or healthy; restoration to health.

healing by first intention   The normal, uncomplicated healing of a wound. It is seen in small, smooth lacerations and sutured surgical wounds when continuity is reestablished without infection or granulation tissue. Also called *primary adhesion, primary union, immediate union.*

healing by granulation   HEALING BY SECOND INTENTION.

healing by second intention   A type of healing of a surface wound, usually large and irregular or infected, which is characterized by development of granulation tissue from the depth and margins of the wound. Eventually, the epithelium grows over and covers the defect. It often results in a prominent scar. Also called *secondary adhesion, healing by granulation.*

faith healing   Treatment of disease through prayer, often invoking faith in God's power to heal or in the healing power of faith itself.

mental healing   PSYCHOTHERAPY.

health [Old English *hælth* (from *hāl* whole)]   **1** A state of well-being of an organism or part of one, characterized by normal function and unattended by disease.   • *Health* is defined in the constitution of the World Health Organization as "a state of complete physical, mental, and social well-being and not merely the absence of disease and infirmity." ⟨"This definition emphasizes that our attitude towards health should be a positive one but, for practical purposes, heavy reliance is placed on negative indices—mortality, morbidity, and disability—in measuring the health status of communities." —M. J. Goldacre and M. P. Vessey, *Oxford Textbook of Medicine,* Vol. 1, p. 2.3⟩   **2** The relative condition of an individual, either physiologic or psychologic, as in *ill health.*

emotional health   MENTAL HEALTH.

environmental health   **1** ENVIRONMENTAL HYGIENE.   **2** The quality of an environment and the state of its ecology considered in relation to health.

mental health   A state of psychologic well-being and absence of mental illness. Its characteristics include ability to work and accept responsibility, to relax and enjoy oneself both alone and in the company of others, to make friends and tolerate people, to show love and devotion beyond caring for oneself, and a reasonable degree of independence, persistence, creativity, and humor. Also called *emotional health.*

occupational health   A professional discipline designed to promote and protect the health of workers by identifying and controlling health hazards in the workplace. Occupational health comprises mainly occupational medicine and occupational hygiene but also includes ergonomics and occupational psychology.

public health   **1** Services designed to promote the health of populations, especially those provided on a community rather than individual basis.   **2** The publicly organized system through which members of the health professions and others work to reduce morbidity and mortality.   **3** The health status of a population as measured by morbidity and mortality indices and other relevant information.

radiological health   That discipline concerned with the protection of people from the harmful effects of ionizing radiation. Also called *radiation hygiene.*

healthy [HEALTH + -Y]   Characterized by a state of well-being; functioning normally and free from disease.

hearing [Middle English *hering(e),* from *her(en)* to hear, from Old English *hieran* to hear, + *-inge* -ING]   A primary sensory and perceptual function. Extremely small rapidly recurring variations of air pressure originating from a sound source often some distance away are converted first into vibrations of the tympanic membrane and ossicular chain, so matching variations in air pressure to variations in fluid pressure within the inner ear, and subsequently initiating neural activity through the organ of Corti. Hearing does not only refer to middle-ear or end-organ activity but includes all that takes place from the periphery to the higher auditory and related centers until the sound enters consciousness and is located and identified. Also called *acouesthesia* (obsolete), *acuesthesia* (obsolete).

double hearing   DIPLACUSIS.

double disharmonic hearing   DISHARMONIC DIPLACUSIS.

monaural hearing   Hearing by one ear only, because the other ear is purposefully occluded or there is a unilateral hearing loss.

residual hearing   The hearing remaining available to an individual with a hearing loss. In audiometric terms this lies between the sometimes greatly increased auditory threshold and the upper limit of hearing when discomfort is experienced on exposure to very loud sounds.

hearing aid   See under AID.

hearing loss   See under LOSS.

heart [Old English *heorte*, akin to L *cor*, gen. *cordis*, heart, and Gk *kardia* heart]   The hollow, chambered organ that serves as the muscular pump for the circulation of the blood; cor.

addisonian heart   The small, ptotic heart of untreated Addison's disease. At necropsy, there is a characteristic brown degeneration of myocardium, now rarely encountered since most patients are treated.

amyloid heart   A heart infiltrated by amyloid, as is usually the case in senile amyloidosis.

armor heart   ARMORED HEART.

armored heart   Chronic adhesive pericarditis with calcification. Also called *armor heart, panzerherz.*

artificial heart   Any of various extracorporeal or intracorporeal circulatory devices used as a substitute for the heart or a part of it. An implanted device consisting of two separate ventricles for perfusion of both systemic and pulmonary circulations, as the Jarvik heart, is powered by an external air-driven system. Also called *mechanical heart.*

athlete's heart   Hypertrophy of the heart due to athletic activity. It is not thought that this type of hypertrophy is ever pathologic. Also called *athletic heart.*

athletic heart   ATHLETE'S HEART.

atrophic heart   CARDIAC ATROPHY.

beer heart   BEER-DRINKER'S CARDIOMYOPATHY.

beriberi heart   The enlarged heart and associated cardiac disorders resulting from thiamin deficiency. The heart becomes enlarged with the right side becoming very prominent. The pulmonary second sound is accentuated. Tachycardia occurs at the slightest physical exertion, and heart failure of the right side, precipitated by physiologic stress, is the end result.

boat-shaped heart   The shape of the heart seen radiologically, suggestive of a boat, in some cases of aortic regurgitation as a result of combined dilatation and hypertrophy.

bony heart   A heart affected by calcareous deposits in the myocardium or pericardium.

booster heart   AUXILIARY VENTRICLE.

bovine heart   COR BOVINUM.

chaotic heart   A heart characterized by frequent ectopic beats.

drop heart   A condition in which the heart appears long and thin, usually in tall asthenic individuals but also occurring in conditions where the diaphragm is unusually low, as in asthma or emphysema. Also called *hanging heart, pendulous heart, suspended heart, cardioptosis, cardioptosia.*

dynamite heart   A heart disorder in individuals industrially exposed to nitroglycerine in which coronary spasm develops on withdrawal from exposure to the chemical.

encased heart   A heart affected with constrictive pericarditis.

extracorporeal heart   An artificial heart device located outside the body as in a heart-lung machine.

fat heart   FATTY HEART.

fatty heart   A non-specific accumulation of fat within the myocardium, usually the consequence either of chronic mild hypoxia as seen in anemia, or ischemia associated with coronary atherosclerosis. Other causes include toxic injury, myocarditis, and cardiomyopathy. The microscopic distribution of fat tends to be in the form of small cytoplasmic droplets. Also called *Quain's fatty heart* (obsolete), *steatosis cordis, steatosis cardiaca, adipositas cordis, fat heart.*

fibroid heart   A heart characterized by much fibrotic tissue, as in chronic myocarditis.

flask-shaped heart   The radiological appearance of the heart in pericardial effusion.

frosted heart   A condition in which the pericardium becomes hyalinized, opaque, and glistening. Also called *icing heart.*

goiter heart   HYPERTHYROID HEART.

hairy heart   PERICARDITIS VILLOSA.

hanging heart   DROP HEART.

horizontal heart   The electrical position of the heart in which the QRS deflection is predominantly positive in aVL and negative in aVF.

hypertensive heart   A hypertrophied heart as a consequence of hypertension.

hyperthyroid heart   An overactive heart due to hyperthyroidism and characterized by tachycardia and a tendency to atrial arrhythmias and cardiac failure of the high output type. Also called *goiter heart, thyroid heart, thyrotoxic heart.*

hypoplastic heart   An abnormally small heart as seen, for example, in Addison's disease.

icing heart   FROSTED HEART.

intermediate heart   An electrical position of the heart intermediate between the horizontal and vertical heart.

intracorporeal heart   An artificial heart implanted in the body.

irritable heart   NEUROCIRCULATORY ASTHENIA.

Jarvik heart   See under ARTIFICIAL HEART.

kyphoscoliotic heart   A form of cor pulmonale secondary to kyphoscoliosis.

left heart   The left atrium and the left ventricle considered together. Also called *cor sinistrum, cor arteriosum* (outmoded).

luxus heart   Hypertrophy of the heart.

lymph heart   A small, two-chambered organ which aids in distributing lymph back into the venous circulation. It occurs in teleost fishes, amphibians, reptiles, and some birds. This structure is generally paired and is located in the pelvic or tail region.

mechanical heart   ARTIFICIAL HEART.

myxedema heart   The enlarged, flabby heart of severe hypothyroidism. Pericardial effusion is sometimes present. Coronary artery atherosclerosis, interstitial edema, and swelling of muscle fibers are usual findings. Clinical characteristics are slow rate, distant heart sounds, some tendency to heart failure, and low amplitude on the electrocardiogram.

ox heart   COR BOVINUM.

paracorporeal heart   An artificial heart placed beside the body.

parchment heart   HYPOPLASIA OF THE RIGHT VENTRICLE.

pear-shaped heart   The radiological appearance of the heart seen in combined aortic and mitral valve disease.

pectoral heart   Bulging of the anterior chest wall as a result of cardiac enlargement.

pendulous heart   DROP HEART.

porpoise heart   A heart with right ventricular preponderance.

pulmonary heart   The right side of the heart, which serves the pulmonary circulation.

Quain's fatty heart   An obsolete term for FATTY HEART.

rheumatic heart A heart affected by rheumatic fever and its sequelae.

right heart The right atrium and the right ventricle considered together. Also called *cor dextrum, cor venosum* (outmoded).

round heart The circular appearance of the heart seen radiologically in gross mitral stenosis and regurgitation.

sabot heart COEUR EN SABOT.

scleroderma heart The structural and functional changes seen in the heart in progressive systemic sclerosis. These changes are nonspecific and include interstitial myocardial fibrosis, thickening of small vessels, and possibly vasospasm.

semihorizontal heart The electrical position of the heart when it is between the horizontal and intermediate positions, with a QRS axis of approximately 0°.

semivertical heart The electrical position of the heart when it is situated between the intermediate and vertical positions with an electrical axis of approximately 60°.

soldier's heart NEUROCIRCULATORY ASTHENIA.

stony heart ISCHEMIC CONTRACTURE OF THE LEFT VENTRICLE.

suspended heart DROP HEART.

systemic heart The left side of the heart, which serves the systemic circulation.

tabby cat heart The appearance of heart muscle affected by pale areas of fatty degeneration; tigering. Also called *tiger heart, tiger lily heart.*

three-chambered heart COR TRILOCULARE.

thrush breast heart Patchy fatty change of the myocardium that appears streaked due to alternating lipid-laden and normal myofibers.

thyroid heart HYPERTHYROID HEART.

thyrotoxic heart HYPERTHYROID HEART.

tiger heart TABBY CAT HEART.

tiger lily heart TABBY CAT HEART.

Traube's heart Heart disease as a consequence of renal disease.

triatrial heart COR TRIATRIUM.

trilocular heart COR TRILOCULARE.

vertical heart The electrical position of the heart in which there is a dominant R wave in aVF and an S wave and negative T wave in aVL, the electrical axis of the QRS being approximately +90°.

wooden shoe heart COEUR EN SABOT.

heartbeat A contraction of the heart; a complete cardiac cycle. Also called *ictus cordis.*

heartburn A substernal burning sensation usually due to the reflux of gastric acid into the esophagus. Also called *pyrosis, phagopyrosis, ardor ventriculi* (obsolete), *brash.*

heartmobile [HEART + *(auto)mobile*] An ambulance specially equipped for the emergency transport to a hospital of persons with heart attacks; a mobile coronary care unit pending transfer to a hospital.

heartwater A fatal disease of domestic ruminants, caused by a rickettsial organism, *Cowdria ruminantium,* transmitted by the bont tick, *Amblyomma hebraeum* and marked by fluid accumulation in the pleural cavity and pericardium. Also called *veld disease, heartwater disease, veldt sickness, cowdriosis.*

heartwood The innermost, oldest, nonliving wood of a tree trunk. It is usually dark in color and devoid of water transport. It is surrounded by sapwood.

heartworm A filarial worm of the species *Dirofilaria immitis.*

heat **1** A form of energy that is caused by motion of molecules. **2** A sensation resulting from exposure of the body to high temperatures. **3** ESTRUS.

animal heat The heat resulting from biologic processes in living animals.

blood heat BODY TEMPERATURE.

heat of combustion The heat evolved when a substance is burnt. Measurement of this quantity for the products and reactants of a reaction can be part of determination of the change in Gibbs energy of the reaction and hence of its equilibrium position.

heat of compression The heat produced by simple compression of a body or substance.

conductive heat The heat transmitted from a body of higher temperature to one of lower temperature by flow of heat through a material body.

convective heat The heat transmitted by material currents driven by temperature gradients in gases or liquids.

conversive heat The heat produced from the absorption of radiation.

delayed heat RECOVERY HEAT.

dry heat The heat of a moistureless environment.

heat of fusion The heat required to convert a substance from a solid to a liquid state without a temperature change.

initial heat The heat produced at the beginning of muscular contraction. Compare RECOVERY HEAT.

latent heat The heat lost or gained by a body or system undergoing a change in state but without a change in temperature.

prickly heat MILIARIA RUBRA.

radiant heat Heat transferred from one point to another without an intervening conductive medium, such as heat from the sun or a heating lamp; a form of electromagnetic radiation.

recovery heat The heat produced as a result of a muscular contraction. Also called *delayed heat.* Compare INITIAL HEAT.

sensible heat The heat that produces an elevation in temperature in a body that absorbs it.

specific heat The amount of heat required to change the temperature of a known mass of a substance 1°C divided by the amount of heat required to change the temperature of an equal mass of water by the same number of degrees. The specific heat of water is 1.0.

heat of vaporization The heat required to convert a substance from a liquid to a gaseous state without a temperature change.

Heath [Christopher *Heath*, English surgeon, 1835–1905] See under OPERATION.

heating / conductive heating Transfer of heat by direct contact with a warm object such as a hot pack or hot water bottle.

convective heating Application of heat by means of an intermediary fluid substance such as warmed air or water.

conversive heating Application of heat by conversion of energy from a form other than heat, as in diathermy or ultrasound therapy.

deep heating Application of heat to relatively deep parts of the body by conversive heating, utilizing short wave, microwave, or ultrasound.

radiant heating Application of heat radiating directly as electromagnetic waves, either luminous or nonluminous, and from a natural source such as the sun or from special devices such as a heat lamp or other radiator.

reflex heating Heating of one portion of the body by reflex vasodilation secondary to heat application at a distance.

superficial heating Application of heat to the surface of the body, by means of radiation, conduction, or convection.

ultrasonic heating Heating by absorption of ultrasound.

heat-labile Having the property of being destroyed by a rise in temperature. This property is often used in biochemistry as evidence that a process involves the action of proteins, often enzymes.

Heaton [George *Heaton*, U.S. surgeon, 1808–1879] See under OPERATION.

heatstroke [HEAT + STROKE] A condition caused by environmental temperatures too high for the body's compensatory mechanism. It is characterized by dry skin, high body temperature, nausea, headache, thirst, and confusion. If untreated, it can lead to coma and death. Also called *heat apoplexy, thermoplegia, thermic fever, heat hyperpyrexia, heat pyrexia, anhidrotic heat exhaustion.*

heave / parasternal heave Palpable elevation of the ribs adjacent to the sternum with heartbeat, usually due to enlargement of the right ventricle.

heaves A clinical state in horses characterized by a double expiratory effort resulting from chronic obstructive lung disease. It is seen in chronic alveolar emphysema and chronic bronchiolitis. Also called *broken wind* (popular).

hebdom. *hebdomada* (L, a week).

hebeosteotomy [Gk *hēbē* manhood, youth + OSTEO- + -TOMY] PUBIOTOMY.

hebephrenia [Gk *hēbē* manhood, freshness of youth, time just before manhood + -PHRENIA] A subtype of schizophrenia characterized by marked disorganization of speech and behavior, inappropriate affect, and unsystematized and bizarre delusions that are often concerned with ideas of omnipotence, sex change, cosmic identification, and rebirth.

grafted hebephrenia PROPFHEBEPHRENIA.

hebephrenic 1 Having the characteristics of hebephrenia. Also *heboid* (outmoded). 2 An individual afflicted with hebephrenia.

Heberden [William *Heberden*, Sr., English physician, 1710–1801] 1 Heberden's asthma, Rougnon-Heberden disease. See under ANGINA PECTORIS. 2 See under DISEASE. 3 Heberden's arthropathy, Heberden sign. See under HEBERDEN'S NODES. 4 Heberdin's rheumatism. See under OSTEOARTHRITIS.

hebetic [Gk *hēbētik(os)* (from *hēbē* youth, manhood + *t* + -*ikos* -IC) pertaining to youth, youthful] Of or relating to puberty.

hebetomy [Gk *hēbē* manhood, youth + -TOMY] PUBIOTOMY.

hebetude [Late L *hebetud(o)* (from L *hebe(s)* dull, slow + Late L *-tudo* English *-tude*) mental dullness, lethargy] An outmoded term for EMOTIONAL DETERIORATION.

hebiatrics [Gk *hēb(ē)* manhood, youth + -IATRICS] ADOLESCENT MEDICINE.

heboid An outmoded term for HEBEPHRENIC.

heboidophrenia [L *heb(es)* dull, slow + -OID + *o* + -PHRENIA] An outmoded term for SIMPLE SCHIZOPHRENIA.

heboid-paranoid Having some of the characteristics of both the hebephrenic and paranoid forms of schizophrenia.

hebosteotomy [Gk *hēb(ē)* manhood, youth + OSTEO- + -TOMY] PUBIOTOMY.

hebotomy [Gk *hēb(ē)* manhood, youth + *o* + -TOMY] PUBIOTOMY.

Hebra [Ferdinand Ritter von *Hebra*, Austrian dermatologist, 1816–1880] 1 Hebra's pityriasis. See under ERYTHRODERMA. 2 See under PRURIGO.

hecatomeral HECATOMERIC.

hecatomeric Denoting a neuron sending axonal processes to both sides of the spinal cord. Also *hecatomeral.*

Hecht [Selig *Hecht*, U.S. physiologist, born 1892] Hecht-Schlaer adaptometer. See under ADAPTOMETER.

Hecht [Victor *Hecht*, Austrian pathologist, flourished early 20th century] Hecht's pneumonia. See under GIANT CELL PNEUMONIA.

Hecker [Karl von *Hecker*, German obstetrician, 1827–1882] See under LAW.

hectare [French (from Gk *hekaton* one hundred + French *are*

an area of one hundred square meters, from L *area* a piece of ground, field), ten thousand square meters] A unit of area equal to 100 are; 101^4 square meters; 2.47 acres: used especially for the measurement of land. Symbol: ha

hectic [Middle English *etik, etyk*, from Old French *étique* hectic, from Late L *hecticus* habitual, from Gk *hektikos* habitual, consumptive, from *hexis* a habit of body, from root of *exō*, fut. of *echein* to have] Characterized by wide swings in temperature which recur daily: said of a fever or of a condition involving such a fever.

hecto- [Gk *hekaton* one hundred] A combining form denoting 10^2, one hundred: used with SI units. Symbol: h

hectogram [HECTO- + GRAM] A unit of mass or weight equal to 100 grams or 0.1 kilogram; 3.527 ounces. Symbol: hg

hectoliter [HECTO- + LITER] A unit of volume or capacity equal to 100 liters or 0.1 cubic meter; 26.417 (US) gallons or 21.997 (UK) gallons. Symbol: hl

hectometer [HECTO- + METER] A unit of length equal to 100 meters, 328.08 feet, or 109.36 yards. Symbol: hm

Hectopsyllidae [*hecto-*, combining form from Gk *hekaton* a hundred, + *psyll(a)* a flea + -IDAE] A family of fleas that parasitize rodents.

hedeoma PENNYROYAL.

hederagenin $C_{30}H_{48}O_4$. A hemolytic saponin found in *Hedera helix*, English ivy.

hederiform Denoting the ivy-shaped appearance of certain silver-impregnated sensory endings in the stratum germinativum of the epidermis. An obsolete term.

Hedinger [Christoph Ernst *Hedinger*, Swiss pathologist, born 1917] Hedinger syndrome. See under CARCINOID SYNDROME.

hedonia [Gk *hēdon(ē)* pleasure + -IA] Enjoyment, pleasure, happiness; especially self-centered pleasure with a disregard of others' wants and needs.

hedonic Characterized by or productive of hedonia.

hedonism [Gk *hēdon(ē)* delight, pleasure sensation + -ISM] Devotion to pleasure as the supreme good. Compare HORMISM.

hedonophobia [Gk *hēdon(ē)* pleasure + *o* + -PHOBIA] Pathologic fear of pleasure or enjoyment.

hedratresia [Gk *hedr(a)* the fundament + *a*- priv. + *trēs(is)* a perforation + -IA] IMPERFORATE ANUS.

hedrocele [Gk *hedr(a)* the fundament + *o* + -CELE²] RECTAL PROLAPSE.

hedrosyrinx [Gk *hedr(a)* the fundament + *o* + *syrinx* a pipe, tube, fistula] ANAL FISTULA.

Hedström [Erik Gustav *Hedström*, Swedish dental scientist, born 1869] See under FILE.

Hedulin A proprietary name for phenindione.

heel 1 The distal end of a part. 2 The rounded protuberance forming the posterior end of the foot; calx.

anterior heel A bar of leather placed behind the weight-bearing line of the metatarsal heads on the sole of a shoe. It is designed to redistribute the weight-bearing forces of the foot.

basketball heels BLACK HEEL.

black heel Bluish black specks occurring just above the hyperkeratotic edge of the heel, due to rupture of superficial capillaries and accumulation of blood in the dermis and epidermis. It usually occurs in athletic adolescent girls. Also called *talon noir pseudochromidrose plantaire, basketball heels.*

cracked heels Hyperkeratotic heels marked by fissures.

heel of denture One of the ends of a full lower or free end of an extension of a partial denture.

gonorrheal heel Plantar fasciitis with osteophytic invasion of the fascia at its attachment to the os calcis. It is a manifestation of the Reiter syndrome. An incorrect and out-of-date term.

grease heel   GREASE.

painful heel   Pain or local tenderness on the plantar surface of the heel when bearing weight. Also called *calcodynia*.

prominent heel   A painful swelling around the posterior aspect of the os calcis at the attachment of the Achilles tendon.

Thomas heel   A 4.7 mm rise of leather that is placed along the inner side of the shoe heel and extended forward onto the longitudinal arch area. It is used as an additional support and to force the foot into a more inverted position to correct flatfoot deformities.

HEENT   head, eyes, ears, nose, throat.

Heerfordt [Christian Frederik *Heerfordt*, Danish oculist, born 1871]   Heerfordt's disease. See under SYNDROME.

Hefke [H. W. *Hefke*, U.S. radiologist, born 1871]   Hefke-Turner sign. See under OBTURATOR SIGN.

Hegar [Alfred *Hegar*, German gynecologist, 1830–1914]   **1** Hegar's dilators. See under DILATOR.   **2** See under SIGN.

Hegglin [Robert Marquand *Hegglin*, Swiss internist, born 1907]   Hegglin's anomaly. See under MAY-HEGGLIN ANOMALY.

Heidenhain [Rudolf Peter Heinrich *Heidenhain*, German physiologist, 1834–1897]   **1** See under POUCH, LAW.   **2** Heidenhain's iron hematoxylin stain. See under HEIDENHAIN'S IRON HEMATOXYLIN.   **3** Heidenhain's liquid. See under SUSA FIXATIVE.

height   A distance or a corresponding measurement from the lowest part to the top of an object or part.

alveolonasal height   A craniometric distance measured between the prosthion and the nasal spine.

anterior facial height   A craniometric distance measured between the nasion and the menton.

apex height   The peak magnitude of several interacting muscular contractions.

height of contour   The points of greatest convexity of a tooth, relative to a more or less vertical reference line through the crown. The height of contour may change when the reference line is inclined to different angles. Also called *surveyed height of contour*.

cusp height   The average height of the cusps of a tooth measured perpendicularly from the central fossa.

effective chimney height   EFFECTIVE STACK HEIGHT.

effective stack height   The height of a chimney stack plus the additional height to which the plume initially rises above the top of the stack as a result of its efflux velocity and its buoyancy. Also called *effective chimney height*.

gnathion-nasion height   A craniometric distance measured between the gnathion and the nasion.

posterior facial height   **1** The length of the perpendicular from the sella-nasion plane intersecting the mandibular plane.   **2** The height of the ramus of the mandible from gonion to condylare.

sitting height   The height of the vertex of a child above a table he is sitting on, when the external auditory meatus and the lower edge of the orbit are in a horizontal plane, (the Frankfort plane), the back is held straight with no sagging or rounding, and the weight is taken by the ischial tuberosities on the table, to ensure which the thighs should be kept just clear of the surface of the table by placing the feet on a stool of suitable height. Also called *sitting vertex height*.

sitting suprasternal height   The length of the trunk, as measured by the vertical distance between the notch of the manubrium sterni and the surface on which the subject is sitting.

sitting vertex height   SITTING HEIGHT.

standing height   A measurement of a child's height taken with the child standing upright against a wall or fixed ruler. It is the distance between the horizontal plane of the vertex, when the external auditory meatus and the lower edge of the orbit are in

a horizontal plane (the Frankfort plane) and the floor. The heels of the subject must be together, knees straight, and buttocks and upper back touching the measuring rod or wall.

surveyed height of contour   HEIGHT OF CONTOUR.

Heilbronner [Karl *Heilbronner*, Dutch physician, 1869–1914]   Heilbronner sign. See under THIGH.

Heim [Ernst Ludwig *Heim*, German physician, 1747–1834]   Heim-Kreysig sign. See under SIGN.

Heimlich [Henry Jay *Heimlich*, U.S. surgeon, born 1920]   See under MANEUVER.

Heine [Jakob von *Heine*, German orthopedist, 1800–1879]   Heine-Medin disease. See under ACUTE ANTERIOR POLIOMYELITIS.

Heine [Leopold *Heine*, German ophthalmologist, 1870–1940]   See under OPERATION.

Heineke [Walter Hermann *Heineke*, German surgeon, 1834–1901]   **1** See under OPERATION.   **2** Heineke-Mikulicz operation. See under HEINEKE-MIKULICZ PYLOROPLASTY.

Heiner [D. C. *Heiner*, U.S. pediatrician, born 1925]   See under SYNDROME.

Heinz [Robert *Heinz*, German pathologist, 1865–1924]   **1** Heinz body test. See under TEST.   **2** Ehrlich-Heinz granules. See under EHRLICH'S GRANULES.   **3** Heinz granules. See under HEINZ BODIES.   **4** Heinz-body anemia. See under ANEMIA.   **5** Heinz-body anemia, congenital Heinz-body anemia. See under UNSTABLE HEMOGLOBIN HEMOLYTIC ANEMIA.

Heisrath [Friedrich *Heisrath*, German ophthalmologist, 1850–1904]   See under OPERATION.

Heister [Lorenz *Heister*, German anatomist, 1683–1758]   **1** Heister's fold, valvula spiralis Heisteri, spiral valve of Heister, Heister's valve. See under PLICA SPIRALIS.   **2** Heister's diverticulum. See under BULBUS SUPERIOR VENAE JUGULARIS.

hekistotherm [Gk *hēkisto(s)* worst, least + *therm(ē)* heat]   An organism that lives in extremely cold areas.

helcodermatosis   An ulcerated skin lesion. An obsolete term.

helcoid   Resembling an ulcer.

helcology [Gk *helko(s)* a sore, ulcer + -LOGY]   The study of ulcers.

helcoma [Gk *helk(os)* a wound, later a sore, ulcer, abscess + -OMA]   An ulcer of the cornea.

helcomenia [Gk *helk(os)* a wound, later a sore, ulcer, abscess + *o* + *mēn* a month + -IA]   Vicarious menstruation from a peptic ulcer.

helcoplasty [Gk *helko(s)* a sore, ulcer + -PLASTY]   An operation performed in the treatment of skin ulcers. A rarely used term.

helcosis   ULCERATION.

Helcosoma tropicum   LEISHMANIA TROPICA.

helcotic   Relating to helcosis; ulcerous.

Held [Hans *Held*, German anatomist, 1866–1942]   **1** End feet of Held. See under FOOT.   **2** Striae of Held. See under STRIAE MEDULLARES VENTRICULI QUARTI.   **3** End bulb of Held. See under END BULB.   **4** See under DECUSSATION.   **5** His-Held space. See under PERIVASCULAR SPACE.

Heleidae   CERATOPOGONIDAE.

helenalin $C_{15}H_{18}O_4$. An extremely toxic substance, derived from *Helenium autumnale*, that is used in cancer chemotherapy.

heli-   HELIO-.

helianthin   METHYL ORANGE.

heliation   HELIOTHERAPY.

helic-   HELICO-.

helical   Referring to or having the shape of a helix.

helicase   GYRASE.

Helicella A genus of land snails (family Helicellidae) that serves in Europe as an intermediate host of the little liver fluke of sheep, *Dicrocoelium dentriticum* and of a parasitic fluke of birds, *Brachylaema nicolli.*

Helicellidae [HELIC- + -*ell(a)* + -IDAE] A family of land snails in the suborder Stylommatophora, order Pulmonata, that serve as intermediate hosts of various trematodes infecting humans.

helices Plural of HELIX.

helicine Having a helical or spiral form; coiled.

helico- [Gk *helix* (genitive *helikos*) coil, spiral, whirl] A combining form meaning helical, spiral. Also *helic-.*

helicoconidium [HELICO- + CONIDIUM] (*plural* helicoconidia) A spirally curved fungal conidium. Also called *helicospore.*

helicoid Having the shape of a helix, a coil, or a spiral.

helicopodia [HELICO- + -POD + -IA] A sweeping type of gait observed in spastic hemiplegia, resulting from the inability of the leg to be moved forward without describing an arc, the radius of which is external to the body, with the foot scraping the ground. This is due to a combination of extensor spasticity, causing difficulty in flexing the knee, together with spastic footdrop. Also called *Todd's gait.* Adjective: helicopod.

helicospore [HELICO- + SPORE] HELICOCONIDIUM.

helicotrema [NA] The narrow opening connecting the scala tympani to the scala vestibuli at the apex of the modiolus of the cochlea where the cochlear duct ends. It is bounded by the hamulus of the spiral lamina. Also called *Breschet's hiatus, Scarpa's hiatus.*

heliencephalitis [HELI- + ENCEPHALITIS] Encephalitis formerly thought to be due to sunstroke. An outmoded term.

helio- [Gk *hēlios* the sun] A combining form denoting the sun. Also *heli-.*

helioaerotherapy Therapeutic use of the sun's rays and fresh air.

heliopathia [HELIO- + -PATHIA] Any pathological changes induced by light. A seldom used term. Also called *heliopathy.*

heliopathy HELIOPATHIA.

heliosis [HELIO- + -SIS] SUNSTROKE.

heliotaxis [HELIO- + Gk *taxis* an arranging] Movement, as of a plant, in response to sunlight; heliotropism.

heliotherapy The use of the sun's rays for therapeutic purposes. Also called *heliation, solar therapy, solar treatment.*

Heliotiales [Gk *hēlioti(s)* pertaining to dawn or to the sun + L -*ales,* pl. of -*alis* -AL] An order of fungi belonging to the class Ascomycetes. Most of the fungi of this group are saprobic but some are very important plant pathogens, such as brown rot of stone fruits, lettuce drop, and various leaf spots.

heliotropism [HELIO- + TROPISM] The tendency in a plant to turn toward the sun; phototropism. Compare APHELIOTROPISM.

Heliozoa [HELIO- + Gk *zōa,* pl. of *zōon* living being, animal] A class of amebas (superclass Actinopoda, subphylum Sarcodina, phylum Sarcomastigophora) which lack a central capsule and are characterized by stiff radiating filaments on all sides, usually clear. Members commonly form colonies and most live in fresh water. Representative genera include *Actinophrys, Actinosphaerium,* and *Gymnosphaera.*

Helisoma [HELI- + Gk *sōma* body] A large genus of North American freshwater planorbid snails in the subfamily Helisomatinae, none of which transmits parasites to humans but many of which harbor trematodes that infect various vertebrate hosts. A number of trematode parasites of birds and mammals have been found in *H. anceps,* and of birds, mammals, reptiles, frogs, and fishes in *H. trivolvulus.* The heart of *H. trivolvulus* and *H. companulatum,* furthermore, is parasitized by the nematode

Daubaylia potomaca. H. duryi is a common subtropical species that has been used in laboratory studies of immune responses in snails.

helium Element number 2, having atomic weight 4.0026. It is a chemically inert gas, the second most abundant element (after hydrogen) in the universe, though it is present in the earth's atmosphere in a concentration of only about five parts per million. It tends to escape from the earth, but it is constantly replenished as a radioactive decay product, since alpha particles, emitted from many of the natural radioactive minerals, are the nuclei of helium atoms. Natural helium consists of two stable isotopes, helium 3 (comprising only about 0.00013%) and helium 4 (virtually 100%). The boiling point of helium is close to absolute zero, and the liquid displays unique properties that are of great interest in physics research. Being much less soluble in blood than nitrogen, helium is used in place of nitrogen in artificial atmospheres for divers, caisson workers, and the like. Symbol: He

Helix [See HELIX.] A genus of land snails (family Helicidae) that includes the common garden snails *H. pomatia* and *H. aspersa.*

helix (*plural* helices, helixes) **1** A circular pattern in which each successive loop is a constant distance from the last, in the manner of a spring, and every point of the pattern is equidistant from its central axis, such that any two lines drawn through corresponding points of successive loops would be parallel. Adjective: helical. **2** [NA] The prominent curved outer rim of the auricle of the external ear. It is separated from the antihelix by the scapha.

alpha helix One of the regular arrangements of amino-acid residues in proteins. It is a helix of 3.6 residues per turn, with each carbonyl group hydrogen-bonded to the fourth NH group towards the C terminus of the chain. Many proteins have regions of such helix, with side chains pointing out from the helix axis. Also called *Pauling-Corey helix.*

double helix The molecular arrangement of double-stranded DNA. Each of the two polynucleotide chains forms a right-handed coil. Bases of the nucleotides project toward the axis of the helix. The chains are complementary with the C-5′ end of one chain pairing with the C-3′ end of the second chain. The coil makes one turn each 3.4 nm, with 10 nucleotides per turn. The polynucleotide chains are held together by hydrogen bonds between bases, adenine bonding to thymine and cytosine to guanine. Also called *Watson-Crick helix, twin helix.*

Pauling-Corey helix ALPHA HELIX.

twin helix DOUBLE HELIX.

Watson-Crick helix DOUBLE HELIX.

Helkesimastix A genus of coprozoic flagellates.

Hellat [Peter *Hellat,* Russian otologist, 1857–1912] See under SIGN.

hellebore [L *helleborus,* also *helleborum* (from Gk *helleboros* hellebore, possibly from *hellos* a fawn + *boros* gluttonous) hellebore] Any of the members of the genus *Veratrum* of the Liliaceae family.

American hellebore VERATRUM VIRIDE.

green hellebore VERATRUM VIRIDE.

helleborism [*Hellebor(us)* + -ISM] Poisoning from the consumption of the toxic substance in a common garden perennial, *Helleborus niger,* Christmas rose.

Hellebrand Hering-Hellebrand deviation. See under DEVIATION.

hellebrin $C_{36}H_{52}O_{15}$. A cardiac glycoside obtained from the rhizome of *Helleborus niger.*

Hellendall [Hugo *Hellendall,* German gynecologist, born 1872] Hellendall's sign. See under CULLEN SIGN.

Hellenopolypus   A genus of sea anemones which are poisonous upon contact.

Heller [Arnold Ludwig Gotthilf *Heller*, German pathologist, 1840–1913]   **1** Heller-Döhle disease. See under SYPHILITIC AORTITIS.   **2** See under PLEXUS.

Heller [Carl George *Heller*, U.S. physiologist, born 1913]   Heller-Nelson syndrome. See under SYNDROME.

Heller [Ernst *Heller*, German surgeon, 1877–1964]   Heller's operation, Heller esophagomyotomy. See under CARDIOMYOTOMY.

Heller [Theodor O. *Heller*, German neuropsychiatrist, born 1869]   Heller's disease. See under DEMENTIA INFANTILIS.

Hellin [Dyonizy *Hellin*, Polish pathologist, 1867–1935]   See under LAW.

Helly [Konrad *Helly*, Swiss pathologist, born 1875]   Helly's fixative. See under FLUID.

Helmholtz [Hermann Ludwig Ferdinand von *Helmholtz*, German physicist and physiologist, 1821–1894]   **1** Helmholtz line. See under ATROPIC LINE.   **2** Wheel rotation of Helmholtz. See under ROTATION.   **3** Young-Helmholtz theory. See under HELMHOLTZ THEORY OF COLOR VISION.   **4** See under ENERGY, RESONATOR, LIGAMENT.   **5** Helmholtz theory of hearing. See under THEORY.

helminth [Gk *helmins*, gen. *helminthos*, a worm]   A parasitic worm, especially a cestode, trematode, or nematode parasite of vertebrates.

helminthagogue   ANTHELMINTIC.

helminthemesis [HELMINTH + EMESIS]   The vomiting of intestinal worms.

helminthiasis [Gk *helmins*, gen. *helminthos*, a worm + -IASIS]   Any infection with helminths.

    cutaneous helminthiasis   CUTANEOUS LARVA MIGRANS.

helminthic   HELMINTIC.

helminthicide [HELMINTH + *i* + -CIDE]   A compound lethal to helminths; an anthelmintic.

helminthism [HELMINTH + -ISM]   The presence of worms; helminthiasis.

helminthoid   Resembling a worm; wormlike.

helminthologist [HELMINTH + *o* + -LOGIST]   A biologist who specializes in the study of parasitic worms.

helminthology [HELMINTH + *o* + -LOGY]   The scientific study of parasitic worms. Also called *scolecology*.

helminthoma [HELMINTH + -OMA]   A tumor caused by a helminth. A seldom used term.

helminthous   HELMINTIC.

helmintic [*helmint(h)* + -IC]   Relating to or infected with parasitic worms or helminths. Also *helminthic, helminthous*.

helo- [Gk *hēlos* nail, wart, callus, corn]   A combining form meaning (1) nail or callus; (2) wart, warty.

Heloderma   A genus of poisonous lizards of the family Helodermatidae, containing two extant species, *H. suspectum*, the gila monster, and *H. horridum*, the Mexican beaded lizard. They are found in the southwestern United States and Mexico, and are the only lizards known to be poisonous.

heloderma [HELO- + -DERMA]   A warty or nodulated condition of the skin. An obsolete term.

    heloderma simplex et annularis   An obsolete term for GRANULOMA ANNULARE.

helodes [Gk *helōdēs* (from *hel(os)* marsh + *eidos* like) marshy]   MALARIA.

heloma [Gk *hēl(os)* a nail, stud (more for ornament than use) + -OMA]   CORN[2].

    heloma durum   An obsolete term for CORN[2].

    heloma molle   SOFT CORN.

helophilous [Gk *helo(s)* marshland + -PHIL + -OUS]   Dwelling in or attracted to low, wet areas such as marshes or swamps.

Helophilus   A genus of flies (family Syrphidae) known as hover flies. The larvae (rat-tail maggots) may cause myiasis in nasal cavities or intestines of man or domestic animals. See also RAT-TAIL MAGGOT.

helosis [HELO- + -SIS]   The state of being marked by corns. A seldom used term.

helotic   Marked by corns. A seldom used term.

helotomy [HELO- + -TOMY]   The cutting of a corn or callus as a method of surgical treatment.

helplessness / learned helplessness   **1** The condition of passivity or apathy that can be created by subjecting an experimental animal to unavoidable noxious stimulation, such as electric shock. Following a prolonged exposure to aversive stimuli which he can neither avoid nor escape, the experimental animal demonstrates difficulty in learning an avoidance response when it is made available. Because humans faced with stressful and uncontrollable events may also exhibit apathy which can then generalize to other situations, this animal model has been proposed as a key for understanding states of depression.   **2** In geriatric medicine, a condition of dependency greater than the accompanying physical or mental disability would suggest as appropriate. It is caused, at least in part, by environmental circumstances, such as overprotective attendants in a nursing home.

Helvella   A genus of ascomycetous fungi; the saddle fungi. One or more species of this group contain monomethylhydrazine, a toxin which causes gastrointestinal distress and, in some instances, death.

helvellic acid $C_{12}H_{20}O_7$. An extremely toxic hemolytic constituent of the fungus *Helvella infula*.

Helvetius [Johannis Claudius Adrian *Helvetius*, French anatomist, born 1685]   Ligaments of Helvetius. See under LIGAMENTA PYLORI.

helvolic acid $C_{33}H_{44}O_8$. An antibiotic chemical derived from cultures of *Aspergillus fumigatus*. Also called *fumigacin* (outmoded).

Helweg [Hans Kristian Saxtorph *Helweg*, Danish physician, 1847–1901]   **1** Bundle of Helweg. See under BUNDLE.   **2** Helweg's tract. See under TRACTUS OLIVOSPINALIS.

hem-   HEMO-.

hema-   HEMO-.

hemabarometer   An instrument which determines specific gravity of blood. An imprecise usage.

hemachromatosis   HEMOCHROMATOSIS.

hemachrome   HEMOCHROME.

hemachrosis   Abnormally increased redness of the blood, as seen in carbon monoxide poisoning or in the presence of cyanhemoglobin.

hemacyte   HEMOCYTE.

hemacytometer   HEMOCYTOMETER.

hemacytopoiesis   HEMATOPOIESIS.

hemacytozoon   HEMOCYTOZOON.

hemaden [HEM- + -ADEN]   An endocrine gland. A rarely used term.

hemadenology [HEMADEN + *o* + -LOGY]   A rarely used term for ENDOCRINOLOGY.

hemadostenosis [Gk *haimas*, gen. *haimados*, a stream of blood + STENOSIS]   Stenosis or narrowing of a blood vessel.

hemadsorbent   **1** Causing or characterized by hemadsorption.   **2** A substance causing hemadsorption.

hemadsorption [HEM- + ADSORPTION]   **1** The adherence of red cells to mammalian cells or viruses whose surfaces possess receptors. **2** A technique in which antiglobulin antibodies are coupled to erythrocytes and used to detect antibodies bound on tissue cells.

mixed hemadsorption   MIXED ANTIGLOBULIN REACTION.

hemadynometry   HEMOMANOMETRY.

hemafacient   Promoting hematopoiesis.

hemafecia [HEMA- + Middle English *fex, feces,* from L *faex,* gen. *faecis,* dregs or lees of wine or any liquid, sediment + -IA] The presence of blood in feces.

hemagglutination [HEM- + AGGLUTINATION]   HEMOAGGLU-TINATION.

passive hemagglutination   Passive agglutination in which red blood cells are the indicator particles to which an antigen has been adsorbed.

tanned cell hemagglutination   Any hemagglutination procedure in which the indicator particles are red cells treated with tannic acid, a process that increases their capacity to adsorb immunologically active materials.

viral hemagglutination   Agglutination of erythrocytes brought about by a virus, such as the mumps virus or an influenza virus.

hemagglutinative   Capable of agglutinating erythrocytes.

hemagglutinin   A substance capable of causing agglutination of erythrocytes: used especially of the surface components of myxoviruses and paramyxoviruses that have this activity, but also applicable to antierythrocyte antibodies. Also *hemoagglutinin.*

cold hemagglutinin   An erythrocyte-agglutinating antibody, usually of anti-I specificity and IgM class, which is active only at temperatures below 37°C. This reflects the low affinity of the antibodies. Cold hemagglutinins are found in man following infections with *Mycoplasma pneumoniae,* but more usually as a result of a lymphoproliferative process. In this case they are monoclonal.

warm hemagglutinin   An erythrocyte-agglutinating antibody which is active at normal body temperature (37°C). These antibodies are usually characterized by high affinity and are often IgG.

hemagogic   Any substance which stimulates flow of blood.

hemagonium   HEMOCYTOBLAST.

hemal   **1** Of, pertaining to, or characteristic of blood or blood vessels. **2** Designating the area ventral to the spine, which contains the heart and great vessels.

hemalum   ALUM HEMATOXYLIN.

Mayer's hemalum   An alum hematoxylin solution containing sodium iodate as an oxidant. It is often used where acid-alcohol differentiation would be inappropriate. Also called *Mayer solution.*

Hemameba   HAEMAMOEBA.

hemamebiasis [HEM- + AMEBIASIS]   An infection of red blood cells with ameboid parasites, as is seen in malaria.

hemanalysis   Examination or analysis of the blood.

hemangiectasia   ANGIECTASIA.

hemangio- [HEM- + ANGIO-]   A combining form denoting blood and blood vessels.

hemangioameloblastoma [HEMANGIO- + AMELOBLASTOMA] A very vascular amelobastoma. Also called *ameloblastic hemangioma.*

hemangioblast [HEMANGIO- + -BLAST]   One of the precursor cells which give rise in an embryo to both blood cells and blood vessels.

hemangioblastoma [HEMANGIO- + BLASTOMA]   A vascular tumor of the central nervous system composed of capillary type blood cells separated by stromal cells. Histologically it resembles the hemangioblastic meningioma, but it arises mainly in the

cerebellum, medulla, or spinal cord. It may be part of the Lindau syndrome or of Von Hippel-Lindau disease. Also called *angioblastoma.*

hemangioblastoma retinae   HEMANGIOMATOSIS RETINAE.

hemangioblastomatosis [HEMANGIO- + *blastomat(a),* pl. of BLASTOMA + -OSIS]   The presence of multiple hemangioblastomas.

hemangioelastomyxoma [HEMANGIO- + ELASTOMYXOMA] A benign tumor of blood vessels and mucinous elastic tissue.

hemangioendothelioblastoma [HEMANGIO- + ENDOTHE-LIOBLASTOMA]   HEMANGIOENDOTHELIOMA.

hemangioendothelioma [HEM- + ANGIOENDOTHELIOMA]   A tumor of blood vessels, mainly capillaries, with prominent endothelial cells. It may occur in benign or malignant forms. Also called *hemangioendothelioblastoma, hemendothelioma.*

benign hemangioendothelioma   ANGIOENDOTHELIOMA.

infantile hemangioendothelioma   A hemangioendothelioma of infants, typically in the liver. It may be locally aggressive and replace large portions of the organ.

malignant hemangioendothelioma   ANGIOSARCOMA.

hemangioendothelioma tuberosum multiplex   Multiple vascular nodules caused by hyperplasia of the endothelium of dermal blood vessels.

hemangioendotheliosarcoma [HEMANGIO- + ENDOTHELIO-SARCOMA]   ANGIOSARCOMA.

hemangiofibroma [HEMANGIO- + FIBROMA]   ANGIOFI-BROMA.

hemangiogliomatosis retinae   HEMANGIOMATOSIS RETI-NAE.

hemangiolipoma [HEMANGIO- + LIPOMA]   A benign tumor of vascular and fatty tissue.

hemangiolymphangioma [HEMANGIO- + LYMPHANGIOMA] HEMOLYMPHANGIOMA.

hemangioma [HEM- + ANGIOMA]   A benign lesion composed of proliferated blood vessels. It may occur in various forms, such as capillary, venous or cavernous, and is subtyped accordingly. In many of the lesions of this group, the distinction between malformations and neoplasms is difficult and in some cases unresolved. Also called *hemartoma* (obsolete). • *Angioma* is often used synonymously but can also apply to lymphangioma.

ameloblastic hemangioma   HEMANGIOAMELOBLASTOMA.

arterial hemangioma   CAPILLARY HEMANGIOMA.

capillary hemangioma   A nevoid vascular defect consisting of a dense cluster of capillaries of various size separated by a sparse network of reticular tissue. The endothelial cells making up the walls of the capillaries are large and tend to protrude into the lumina so as to reduce the internal diameter. Also called *hemangioma congenitale, arterial hemangioma, hemangioma simplex, capillary angioma, capillary nevus.*

hemangioma cavernosum   CAVERNOUS HEMANGIOMA.

cavernous hemangioma   A hemangioma composed of large channels lined by a single layer of endothelial cells. Also called *hemangioma cavernosum, erectile tumor, cavernous tumor, angiocavernoma, nevus cavernosus, cavernoma, cavernous angioma, angioma cavernosum.*

cirsoid hemangioma   RACEMOSE HEMANGIOMA.

hemangioma congenitale   CAPILLARY HEMANGIOMA.

hemangioma hypertrophicum cutis   ANGIOMA CUTIS.

hemangioma of the kidney   A benign vascular tumor of the kidney parenchyma that causes all degrees of hematuria from microscopic bleeding to massive hemorrhage.

multiple hemorrhagic hemangioma of Kaposi   KAPOSI SAR-COMA.

hemangioma planum extensum   A large cutaneous hemangioma which is not noticeably elevated above the general level of the skin.

racemose hemangioma   A lesion resembling a malformation composed of tortuous, thick-walled blood vessels of the venous and arterial type. Also called *cirsoid hemangioma*.

renal hemangioma   A hemangioma usually arising in the medulla. Intermittent hematuria is the most common symptom, often associated with renal colic due to clots in the ureter. Differential diagnosis includes malignant tumors and calculi. When the diagnosis is not clear nephrectomy is indicated.

sclerosing hemangioma   DERMATOFIBROMA.

hemangioma simplex   CAPILLARY HEMANGIOMA.

venous hemangioma   A benign lesion composed of irregular medium-to-large-sized vessels, predominantly of the venous type.

verrucous hemangioma   VERRUCOUS KERATOTIC HEMANGIOMA.

verrucous keratotic hemangioma   A lesion in which the epidermis shows verruciform projections with dilated capillaries in close apposition to the basal layer and simulating angiokeratoma, but with vascular changes extending into the underlying dermis and subcutis, usually in the form of a capillary angioma. Also called *verrucous hemangioma*.

hemangiomatosis [HEM- + ANGIOMATOSIS]   Regional or diffuse proliferation of capillaries or thin-walled vascular structures with or without a congenital arteriovenous fistula. Sometimes this lesion is accompanied by overgrowth of fat and/or bone. Also called *angiomatosis*.

hemangiomatosis retinae   A vascular tumor of the retina, as in von Hippel-Lindau syndrome. Also called *hemangioblastoma retinae, hemangiogliomatosis retinae*.

systemic hemangiomatosis   A condition involving one or more organs or tissues which is characterized by multicentric or diffuse hemangiomatous lesions. Rendu-Osler-Weber disease, Sturge-Weber disease, the Mafucci syndrome, the Bourneville syndrome, and Hippel-Lindau disease are forms of systemic hemangiomatosis.

hemangiomyolipoma [HEMANGIO- + MYOLIPOMA]   ANGIOMYOLIPOMA.

hemangiopericyte   PERICYTE.

hemangiopericytoma [HEMANGIO- + PERI- + CYT- + -OMA]   A vascular tumor in which the pericytic cells of vessel walls proliferate. Microscopically the tumor cells surround vascular channels which are lined by a single layer of endothelial cells. The tumor may be benign or malignant. Also called *perithelioma, perithelial endothelioma, periangioma, pericytoma*.

renal hemangiopericytoma   JUXTAGLOMERULAR CELL TUMOR.

hemangiosarcoma [HEMANGIO- + SARCOMA]   ANGIOSARCOMA.

hemaphein   A derivative of hemoglobin that imparts a brown color to serum or urine. Adjective: hemapheic.

hemaphersis   The process of separating freshly drawn blood into various constituents, retaining the desired portions, and returning the remaining portions to the donor. Erythrocytes are virtually always one of the components returned. Components retained may be plasma, leukocytes, or platelets, or some combination of these. The restoration of erythrocytes and replacement of lost fluids prevent the donor from experiencing untoward effects from repeated donations, so the process can be repeated more than once, at intervals as short as 48 hours. Also called *apheresis, pheresis (widely used but incorrect)*.

hemaphotograph   HEMOPHOTOGRAPH.

hemapoiesis   HEMATOPOIESIS.

hemapoietic   HEMATOPOIETIC.

hemapophysis [HEM- + APOPHYSIS]   The anterior segment of the hemal arch. A costal cartilage can be regarded as an apophysis of the hemal spine.

hemarthros   HEMARTHROSIS.

hemarthrosis   A hemorrhage into a joint. Also called *hemarthros*.

hemartoma   An obsolete term for HEMANGIOMA.

hemastrontium   A histologic staining solution containing hematein with strontium chloride and aluminium chloride in alcohol and citric acid.

hemat-   HEMO-.

hematal [HEMAT- + -AL]   Relating to blood or blood vessels; hemal.

hemateikon   The microscopic appearance of the blood. A rarely used term.

hematemesis [HEMAT- + EMESIS]   The vomiting of blood, which may be clearly recognizable as such or may be in an altered state as dark-colored or blackish material.

   Goldstein's hematemesis   Hematemesis resulting from bleeding telangiectases in the gastric mucosa.

hematencephalon [HEMAT- + ENCEPHALON]   The brain suffused with blood.

hematherapy   The administration of blood or blood components such as packed erythrocytes, plasma, platelets, granulocytes, or cryoprecipitate.

hemathermal [HEMA- + THERMAL]   HOMEOTHERMIC.

hemathermous [HEMA- + THERM- + -OUS]   HOMEOTHERMIC.

hemathidrosis   HEMATIDROSIS.

hemathorax   HEMOTHORAX.

hematic   Pertaining to blood.

hematid   A skin eruption due to hypersensitivity to a component of blood.

hematidrosis   The perspiring of blood-tinged sweat. Also called *hemathidrosis, hemtohidrosis, dermorrhagia, sudor cruentus* (obsolete), *sudor sanguineus* (obsolete), *bloody sweat*.

hematimeter   HEMOCYTOMETER.

hematimetry   The enumeration of blood cells.

hematin [HEMAT- + -IN]   A complex of prophyrin and hydroxide ion with iron(III). It may be isolated from hemoglobin as the dimer formed by dehydration, in which the two iron atoms are linked by an oxygen bridge.

   acid hematin   A brown pigment released from hemoglobin upon treatment with hydrochloric acid. It is apparently identical with heme.

hematinemia   The presence of heme in blood, usually bound to hemopexin.

hematinic   Any substance that promotes blood formation, such as iron, vitamin B_{12}, or folic acid. Also called *hematinogen, hematonic*.

hematinogen   HEMATINIC.

hematinometer   HEMOGLOBINOMETER.

hematinuria   The presence in the urine either of oxidized heme pigment or hematin, the dark brown, granular microcrystalline pigment formed from heme by malarial or schistosomal parasites.

hemato-   HEMO-.

hematobia   Plural of HEMATOBIUM.

hematobilia [HEMATO- + *bil(i)*- + -IA]   The presence of blood within the biliary system. Also called *hemobilia*.

hematobium [HEMATO- + New L *-bium*, neut. of *-bius*, combining form from Gk *bios* life]   (*plural* hematobia) Any microorganism, particularly an animal form or hematozoon, which is parasitic in the blood.

hematoblast HEMOCYTOBLAST.

Hayem's hematoblast HEMOCYTOBLAST.

hematoblastosis HEMOBLASTOSIS.

hematocele [HEMATO- + -CELE¹] A collection of extravasated blood in a cavity or part, often forming a tumorlike or cystlike swelling, especially in the tunica vaginalis testis.

parametric hematocele RECTOUTERINE HEMATOCELE.

pelvic hematocele A collection of effused blood within the peritoneal cavity; usually, a rectouterine hematocele.

pudendal hematocele A hematocele in a labium of the pudenda.

rectouterine hematocele A collection of blood in the rectouterine excavation (pouch of Douglas). Also called *parametric hematocele.*

scrotal hematocele A hematocele of the scrotum, either in the subcutaneous tissue or within the cavity of the tunica vaginalis.

vaginal hematocele A hematocele of the tunica vaginalis testis.

hematocelia HEMATOCOELIA.

hematochezia [HEMATO- + Gk *chez(ein)* to defecate + -IA] The passage of bright red, easily identifiable blood from the anus, usually a sign of fresh bleeding distal to the ileocecal valve. Also called *hemochezia.* Compare MELENA.

hematochlorin A green hemoglobin degradation product obtained from placentas. It may be a mixture of verdohemoglobin and related pigments.

hematochromatosis HEMOCHROMATOSIS.

hematochylocele A localized collection of both blood and chyle, as seen in the tunica vaginalis of the testis in filariasis.

hematochyluria [HEMATO- + CHYLURIA] HEMATOLYMPHURIA.

hematocoelia Bleeding into the peritoneal cavity. Also *hematocelia.*

hematocolpometra [HEMATO- + COLPO- + Gk *mētra* uterus] A collection of blood in the uterus and vagina, usually because of an imperforate hymen or vaginal atresia.

hematocolpos [HEMATO- + Gk *kolpos* bosom, womb, fold] Retention of blood in the vagina usually because of an imperforate hymen. Also *hematokolpos, retained menstruation.*

hematocrit [HEMATO- + Gk *krit(ēs)* a discerner, judge, arbiter] **1** The proportion of erythrocytes in blood, as determined by centrifugation of anticoagulated blood and the calculation:

$$100 \times \frac{\text{volume of packed erythrocytes}}{\text{volume of specimen}}.$$

Also called *packed cell volume.* **2** With some automated particle counters, the product $0.1 \times$ mean corpuscular volume $\times$ erythrocyte count. **3** Originally, the centrifuge used to determine the ratio of the volume of packed erythrocytes per unit volume of blood. An obsolete usage. For defs. 1, 2, and 3 also *hematokrit (German spelling).*

large vessel hematocrit The volume of erythrocytes ($\times 100$) per unit volume of blood in an artery or vein. Due to passage of fluid out of the blood in the capillaries, venous hematocrit is slightly higher than arterial hematocrit. The hematocrit of capillary blood, as from a finger prick, more nearly resembles the arterial hematocrit. For most clinical studies, either venous or capillary hematocrits are employed.

whole body hematocrit The volume of erythrocytes ($\times 100$) per unit volume of blood for all the blood in circulation. Usually this is determined by measuring, for example with radiolabeled albumen, the plasma volume and the total erythrocyte volume of blood, and then calculating:

$$\frac{\text{whole body}}{\text{hematocrit}} = \frac{100 \times \text{total erythrocyte volume}}{\text{plasma volume} + \text{total erythrocyte volume}}$$

Wintrobe's hematocrit **1** The proportion of packed erythrocytes in a column of blood following centrifugation for 30 minutes at relative centrifugal force 2260. **2** A graduated glass tube, 10 cm in length with a uniform internal diameter, used for making this measurement.

hematocyst **1** A cyst that contains blood. **2** The presence of blood in the urinary bladder. For defs. 1 and 2 also called *hematocystis.*

hematocystis HEMATOCYST.

hematocyte HEMOCYTE.

hematocytoblast HEMOCYTOBLAST.

hematocytolysis HEMOLYSIS.

hematocytometer HEMOCYTOMETER.

hematocytopenia A less than normal number of cells in blood, as in erythrocytopenia, leukopenia, neutropenia, lymphocytopenia, thrombocytopenia, and pancytopenia.

hematocytosis POLYCYTHEMIA.

hematocytozoon HEMOCYTOZOON.

hematocyturia HEMATURIA.

hematodyscrasia BLOOD DYSCRASIA.

hematodystrophy NUTRITIONAL ANEMIA.

hematoencephalic Pertaining to a suffusion of blood in the intracranial cavity.

hematoencephalon [HEMATO- + ENCEPHALON] Hemorrhage in or about the brain. An imprecise and outmoded term.

hematogenesis HEMATOPOIESIS.

hematogenic **1** A rarely used term for HEMATOPOIETIC. **2** A rarely used term for HEMATOGENOUS.

hematogenous Arising from the blood or disseminated by the bloodstream. Also *hematogenic* (rarely used).

hematogone A lymphocytelike cell, normally present in bone marrow, that is approximately 7 μm in diameter, has very condensed nuclear chromatin without nucleoli, and contains very little cytoplasm. The relationship of hematogones to other blood cells is unclear. They have been considered to be the common hematopoietic stem cells. Also called *lymphoid hemoblast of Pappenheim, myelogone.*

hematohidrosis HEMATIDROSIS.

hematohistioblast HEMOHISTIOBLAST.

hematohyaloid Describing the hyaline thrombi resulting from degenerative agglutination of erythrocytes and/or platelets.

hematoid Bloodlike.

hematoidin An iron-free derivative of hemoglobin that resembles bilirubin.

hematokolpos HEMATOCOLPOS.

hematokrit The German spelling of HEMATOCRIT. • This spelling occasionally appears in English-language texts.

hematolith HEMOLITH.

hematologist [HEMATO- + -LOGIST] A medical scientist concentrating on the study of blood and blood-forming tissues, and/or specializing in diagnosis and treatment of disorders of same.

hematology [HEMATO- + -LOGY] The science of blood and blood-forming tissues, including disorders thereof. Also called *hemology.*

hematolymphangioma [HEMATO- + LYMPHANGIOMA] HEMOLYMPHANGIOMA.

hematolymphuria [HEMATO- + LYMPH + -URIA] The presence of red blood cells and lymph in the urine, usually due to bladder infection with *Wuchereria bancrofti.* Also called *hematochyluria.*

hematolysis HEMOLYSIS.

hematolytic   HEMOLYTIC.

hematoma [HEMAT- + -OMA]   A localized accumulation of blood in a tissue or space. It is usually composed of clotted blood in various stages of organization depending on the length of time it is present. Among the most common causes are trauma, erosion of a blood vessel by pathologic processes such as cancer or abscess, and disorders of blood coagulation.

aneurysmal hematoma   FALSE ANEURYSM.

hematoma auris   A condition usually resulting from injury to the external ear in which blood is extravasated between the perichondrium and the cartilage, producing a characteristic unsightly swelling of the pinna. Boxers and rugby football players are particularly at risk. Cases of spontaneous hematoma have sometimes been reported. Failure to evacuate the hematoma promptly may lead to cauliflower ear. Also called *othematoma* (rarely used).

cystic hematoma   A hematoma which, in the the process of organization, has developed a wall and whose contents have undergone liquefaction.

dissecting hematoma   ARTERIAL DISSECTION.

dural hematoma   EPIDURAL HEMATOMA.

epidural hematoma   A collection of blood external to the dura, usually found within the skull following fracture. Also called *dural hematoma, extradural hematoma.*

extradural hematoma   EPIDURAL HEMATOMA.

intracerebral hematoma   An accumulation of blood within the substance of the brain, a common cause of death, dependent on the size and location of the accumulation.

intracranial hematoma   A hematoma anywhere within the cranial cavity.

intramural hematoma   A hematoma located in the wall of a hollow organ.

nasal septum hematoma   Hematoma located beneath the mucoperichondrium and mucoperiosteum of the nasal septum. It can occur either postoperatively, for instance following submucous resection of the septum, or as a result of accidental trauma. The latter is particularly liable to infection with the formation of a nasal septum abscess.

pelvic hematoma   A hematoma in the soft tissues of the pelvis.

perianal hematoma   A painful hematoma developed under the perianal skin.

perinephric hematoma   A collection of blood anywhere around the kidney, caused by trauma, surgery, or rupture of a blood vessel.

puerperal hematoma   A hematoma that occurs during the postpartum period.

retroperitoneal hematoma   Hemorrhage into the retroperitoneal or perirenal areas caused by injury, including a renal biopsy: It may produce severe pain, hematuria, and swelling.

retrouterine hematoma   A hematoma occurring in connective tissue located behind the uterus.

subchorial tuberous hematoma of the placenta   TUBEROUS MOLE.

subdural hematoma   A collection of blood between the dura and arachnoid. Intracranially, the hematoma usually comes from torn veins near the longitudinal venous sinus. Also called *hemorrhagic internal pachymeningitis* (obsolete), *hemorrhagic pachymeningitis* (obsolete).

subungual hematoma   A localized collection of blood beneath a digital nail.

tuberous subchorial hematoma   TUBEROUS MOLE.

hematomancy   HEMODIAGNOSIS.

hematomanometer   SPHYGMOMANOMETER.

hematomatous   Resembling or resulting from a hematoma.

hematomediastinum   HEMOMEDIASTINUM.

hematometakinesis   The redistribution of blood from one part of the body to another. Also called *borrowing-lending hemodynamic phenomenon, hemometakinesia, hemometakinesis.*

hematometer   HEMOGLOBINOMETER.

hematometra [HEMATO- + Gk *mētra* the uterus]   An accumulation of blood in the uterus usually due to obstruction either at the level of the uterine cervix or occasionally due to an imperforate hymen. Also called *hemometra.*

hematometry   Quantitative analysis of the formed elements of blood.

hematomole [HEMATO- + MOLE[2]]   TUBEROUS MOLE.

hematomphalocele   The presence of frank blood within an omphalocele.

hematomphalus [HEMAT- + Gk *omphalos* the navel]   CULLEN SIGN.

hematomyelia [HEMATO- + MYEL- + -IA]   Hemorrhage within the spinal cord occurring spontaneously or as a result of trauma. Also called *hematorrhachis interna.*

central hematomyelia   MINOR'S DISEASE.

obstetric hematomyelia   MINOR'S DISEASE.

hematomyelitis   Acute myelitis complicated by areas of hemorrhage within the spinal cord. Also called *hemorrhagic myelitis.*

hematomyelopore [HEMATO- + MYELO- + PORE]   Posthemorrhagic cavitation or softening of the spinal cord.

hematoncometry   The measurement of total blood volume.

hematonephrosis   The presence of blood within the renal pelvis.

hematonic   HEMATINIC.

hematopathology   The pathology of blood and of blood-forming and lymphoid tissues.

hematopedesis   HEMODIAPEDESIS.

hematopenia   An imprecise and seldom used term for CYTOPENIA.

hematopericardium   HEMOPERICARDIUM.

hematoperitoneum   HEMOPERITONEUM.

hematophage   ERYTHROPHAGOCYTE.

hematophagia [HEMATO- + -PHAGIA]   Ingestion of blood or subsistence on blood, especially by parasites. Also called *hematophagy, hemophagia.*

parasitic hematophagia   Blood parasitism, as in the erythrocytic cycle of malaria parasites.

hematophagocyte   ERYTHROPHAGOCYTE.

hematophagous [HEMATO- + -PHAGOUS]   Bloodsucking; subsisting on blood: said primarily of parasites. Also *sanguivorous.*

hematophagus [HEMATO- + -PHAGUS]   A hematophagous parasite, especially an insect.

hematophagy   HEMATOPHAGIA.

hematophilia   HEMOPHILIA.

hematophobia   HEMOPHOBIA.

hematophyte [HEMATO- + Gk *phyt(on)* a plant, tree]   Any plantlike microorganism found living in the blood, for example, a fungus or bacterium.

hematophytic   Relating to or caused by hematophytes.

hematopiesis [HEMATO- + Gk *piesis* a pressing, squeezing]   An outmoded term for BLOOD PRESSURE.

hematoplasmopathy   HEMOPLASMOPATHY.

hematoplast   HEMOCYTOBLAST.

hematoplastic   HEMATOPOIETIC.

hematopneic   Promoting, relating to, or characteristic of the oxygenation of blood.

hematopoiesis [HEMATO- + -POIESIS]   The growth and maturation of the formed elements of the blood. Also called *hemapoiesis, hemacytopoiesis, hematogenesis, hemogenesis, hemo-*

cytogenesis, hemocytopoiesis, hemopoiesis, sanguification (rarely used), *sanguinification* (rarely used). Adjective: hematopoietic.

extramedullary hematopoiesis The production of formed elements of the blood in tissues outside of the bone marrow.

hematopoietic **1** Relating to hematopoiesis. Also *hemapoietic, hematogenic, hemogenic, hematoplastic, hemopoietic, hemopoiesic, sanguinopoietic.* **2** Any agent that promotes hematopoiesis.

hematoporphyria An obsolete term for PORPHYRIA.

hematoporphyrin **1** A porphyrin two of whose pyrrole rings have methyl and 1-hydroxyethyl substituents, and two have methyl and 2-carboxyethyl substituents. Hematoporphyrins are not found in nature, but can be prepared from the protoporphyrin of hemoglobin by addition of the elements of water to its vinyl groups. **2** Any of several naturally occurring porphyrins. An older usage.

hematoporphyrinemia The presence of hematoporphyrin in plasma or serum. A seldom used term.

hematoporphyrinism A clinical syndrome of hematoporphyrinemia and cutaneous sensitivity to sunlight.

hematoporphyrinuria [HEMATOPORPHYRIN + -URIA] The excretion of hematoporphyrin, a degradation product of hemoglobin, in the urine.

hematopsia [HEMAT- + -OPSIA] The subjective perception of blood suspended in the vitreous cavity, recognized by the sudden onset of many floating spots, usually black but sometimes reddish or other colors.

hematorrhachis [HEMATO- + Gk *rhachis* the back, spine, backbone] The effusion of blood into the spinal canal. Also called *hemorrhachis.*

hematorrhachis externa The effusion of blood into the spinal canal, sparing the spinal cord itself. Also called *intramedullary hemorrhage.*

hematorrhachis interna HEMATOMYELIA.

hematosalpinx [HEMATO- + Gk *salpinx* a tube] An accumulation of blood in a fallopian tube often in association with a tubal ectopic pregnancy. Also called *hemosalpinx.*

hematosarcoma A rarely used term for LYMPHOMA.

hematoscheocele [HEMAT- + OSCHEO- + -CELE¹] An accumulation of blood in the scrotum.

hematoscopy Examination of the blood. A rarely used term.

hematosepsis SEPTICEMIA.

hematosiphoniasis An infestation with the Central American chicken bug, *Haematosiphon inodorus.*

hematospectroscope A device for examining the optical spectrum of light that has passed through a thin layer of blood. Dark bands that are seen in certain regions of the spectrum indicate the presence of specific pigments, such as oxyhemoglobin, methemoglobin, or sulfhemoglobin.

hematospectroscopy Examination of the optical spectrum of light that has passed through a thin layer of blood.

hematospermatocele [HEMATO- + SPERMATOCELE] A spermatocele that contains blood.

hematospermia HEMOSPERMIA.

hematosporidium HAEMOSPORIDIUM.

hematostatic **1** Characterized by or resulting from stagnation of the blood. **2** HEMOSTATIC.

hematosteon Hemorrhage into the medullary cavity of a bone.

hematotherapy HEMOTHERAPY.

hematothermal [HEMATO- + THERMAL] HOMEOTHERMIC.

hematothorax HEMOTHORAX.

hematotoxic HEMOTOXIC.

hematotoxin Any substance that damages blood or blood cells or blood-forming organs.

hematotrachelos [HEMATO- + Gk *trachēlos* the throat, neck] Distension of the uterine cervix due to an accumulation of blood, usually secondary to obstruction at that level.

hematotropic HEMOTROPIC.

hematotympanum HEMOTYMPANUM.

hematoxic HEMOTOXIC.

hematoxylin An extract from the heartwood of the tree *Haematoxylon campechianum* that is extensively used as a stain for nuclear chromatin. Hematoxylin itself is colorless and needs to be oxidized to the dye hematin, either by natural oxidation by exposure to light and air or by chemical oxidation using sodium iodate or mercuric oxide. Hematin on its own has a poor affinity for tissue and requires a mordant which is usually a salt of a heavy metal.

Delafield's hematoxylin An alum hematoxylin that is oxidized to its active form by exposing to light and air for about five days.

Ehrlich's hematoxylin An alum hematoxylin that naturally oxidizes to its active form, hematin, over a period of about two months. Also called *Ehrlich's acid hematoxylin.*

Ehrlich's acid hematoxylin EHRLICH'S HEMATOXYLIN.

Harris hematoxylin An alum hematoxylin in which mercuric oxide is used as an oxidant. It provides particularly clear nuclear staining.

Heidenhain's iron hematoxylin A form of iron hematoxylin in which ferric ammonium sulfate is used as a combined oxidizing agent and mordant on tissue specimens, staining nuclei a deep purple. Also called *Heidenhain's iron hematoxylin stain.*

Kulchitsky's hematoxylin A solution of hematoxylin in alcohol that is mixed with acetic acid and used to stain lipids and phospholipids a blue-black color.

Weigert's iron hematoxylin A nuclear stain using alcoholic hematoxylin and ferric chloride. It is the standard iron hematoxylin solution used for staining nuclei. Also called *Weigert solution, Weigert's iron hematoxylin stain.*

hematoxylinophilic Characterized by a staining affinity to hematoxylin.

hematozoa Plural of HEMATOZOON.

hematozoic [HEMATO- + zo(o)- + -IC] Parasitic in the blood of vertebrates: said principally of protozoa. Also *hemozoic.*

hematozoon [HEMATO- + Gk *zōon* living being, animal] (*plural* hematozoa) A protozoon that is parasitic in the blood of vertebrates. Also called *hemozoon.*

hematrophe HEMOTROPH.

hematuria [HEMAT- + -URIA] Excretion of urine containing blood, either gross (visible) or microscopic (seen only by microscopic examination). The source of bleeding may be the kidney, ureter, bladder, urethra, or prostate. Also called *erythrocyturia, erythruria, hematocyturia, hemuresis* (rarely used).

angioneurotic hematuria Hematuria without demonstrable cause. An imprecise usage.

Egyptian hematuria SCHISTOSOMIASIS HAEMATOBIA.

endemic hematuria SCHISTOSOMIASIS HAEMATOBIA.

enzootic bovine hematuria A disease of cattle, resulting from ingestion of bracken fern which induces tumors of the urinary bladder and the subsequent passage of blood in the urine. The disease is endemic in various parts of the world.

essential hematuria Hematuria of unknown cause.

false hematuria Red blood cells in the urine from sources other than the urinary tract, as in contamination from feces or vaginal secretions.

hereditary hematuria HEREDITARY NEPHRITIS.

initial hematuria Hematuria only at the beginning of urination, a sign of a urethral lesion.

microscopic hematuria Hematuria detectable only through microscopic examination.

recurrent hematuria A form of glomerulonephritis characterized by recurrent gross or microscopic hematuria in association with infections. Edema, hypertension, and renal functional impairment are uncommon. The most common histologic finding is focal glomerulonephritis, sometimes with IgA deposition in the mesangium. The prognosis usually is excellent.

renal hematuria Red blood cells in the urine due to lesions in the kidneys rather than other urinary tract sources. Red blood cell casts signify glomerular origin of hematuria.

Sydenham's hematuria Hematuria due to a renal calculus. A seldom used term.

terminal hematuria Hematuria at the end of micturition, reflecting a hemorrhagic lesion in the posterior urethra or base of the bladder.

total hematuria Hematuria throughout micturition, reflecting a hemorrhagic lesion in the kidneys or ureter.

urethral hematuria The passing of blood in the urine due to a urethral hemorrhage.

vesical hematuria Blood in the urine from a hemorrhage in the bladder.

hemautography The recording of hemautographs.

hembra A form of ulcerative cutaneous leishmaniasis.

heme [contraction of HEMATIN] Any iron-porphyrin coordination complex. Porphyrins bind iron(II) and iron(III) very tightly. Also called *oxyhematin, oxyheme, oxyhemochromogen, ferriheme.*

hemelytrometra [HEM- + ELYTRO- + Gk *mētra* the uterus] An accumulation of blood in the uterus and vagina secondary to an imperforate hymen.

hemendothelioma [HEM- + ENDOTHELIOMA] HEMANGIOENDOTHELIOMA.

Hementaria HAEMENTARIA.

hemeralope An individual with hemeralopia.

hemeralopia [Gk *hēmeralōp(s)* (from *hēmer(a)* the day, daylight + *al(aos)* blind + *ōps* the eye) blind by day + -IA] Inability to see well in bright illumination. Also called *day blindness.* ● This term is commonly used incorrectly to designate night blindness (nyctalopia).

Hemerocampa A genus of moths.

Hemerocampa leukostigma The white-marked tussock moth, whose larvae bear urticating venomous white hairs that can cause a severe dermatitis.

hemerythrin An oxygen-carrying red protein found in the blood of certain annelid worms.

hemi- [Gk prefix *hēmi-* half] A prefix meaning half.

-hemia [New L suffix from Gk suffix *-aimia* from Gk *haima* (genitive *haimatos*) blood] A combining form denoting blood. Also *-haemia* (British spelling).

hemiablepsia [HEMI- + ABLEPSIA] HEMIAMBLYOPIA.

hemiacardius [HEMI- + ACARDIUS] Conjoined twins in which circulation of both is effected partially or wholly by the heart of only one member.

hemiacephalus [HEMI- + Gk *a-* priv. + -CEPHALUS] ANENCEPHALUS.

hemiacetal 1 A compound containing the grouping —C(OH)(OR)—. It is formed reversibly by combination of the carbonyl group —CO— with the alcohol R—OH. A second molecule of alcohol could convert it into the acetal —C(OR)$_2$—, which would not revert so easily to the free carbonyl compound. The ring forms of sugars are hemiacetals, formed by combination of a carbonyl group with a hydroxyl group within the same molecule. **2** Such a substance having the carbonyl group contributed only by an aldehyde rather than by a ketone. In the

latter case, the term *hemiketal* was once used. An obsolete usage.

hemiachromatopsia [HEMI- + ACHROMATOPSIA] Faulty color perception in a portion of the visual field, due to neurologic disease rather than to the inherited forms of color blindness. Also called *hemichromatopsia, color hemianopia.*

hemiacrosomia [HEMI- + ACRO- + Gk *sōm(a)* body + -IA] CONGENITAL HEMIHYPERTROPHY.

hemiagenesis [HEMI- + AGENESIS] Agenesis of only one of a pair of organs or unilateral agenesis of an organ normally displaying prominent bilaterality, such as the cerebrum or the cerebellum of the brain.

hemiageusia [HEMI- + AGEUSIA] Lack or partial loss of the sense of taste on one side of the tongue. Also called *hemiageustia.*

hemiageustia HEMIAGEUSIA.

hemiagnosia [HEMI- + AGNOSIA] Agnosia restricted to half of the body, with regard to the sense of touch, or to half the visual field of each eye, with regard to visual perception.

hemiagnosia for pain Hemiasomatognosia giving rise to lack of reaction to painful stimuli restricted to one half of the body.

hemialbumin A polypeptide sometimes found in the urine of patients with osteomalacia or diphtheria. An outmoded term. Also called *hemialbumose.*

hemialbumose HEMIALBUMIN.

hemialbumosuria [*hemialbumos(e)* + -URIA] Urinary excretion of hemialbuminose, a degradation product of protein normally present in the bone marrow. It may be associated with osteomalacia or with infections. Also called *propeptonuria.*

hemialgia [HEMI- + -ALGIA] Neuralgic pain on one side of the head or body.

hemiamaurosis [HEMI- + AMAUROSIS] HEMIAMBLYOPIA.

hemiamblyopia [HEMI- + AMBLYOPIA] Inability to see in all or part of one half of the visual field, usually affecting both eyes. Also called *hemiablepsia, hemiamaurosis.*

hemiamyosthenia [HEMI- + AMYOSTHENIA] Unilateral muscular weakness.

hemianacusia Severe hearing loss restricted to one ear only.

hemianalgesia [HEMI- + ANALGESIA] Analgesia on one side of the body.

hemianencephaly [HEMI- + ANENCEPHALY] Anencephaly affecting one side or primarily one side of the brain and related cranial structures.

hemianesthesia [HEMI- + ANESTHESIA] Loss of sensation on one side of the body.

alternate hemianesthesia Loss of feeling on one side of the face due to a lesion of the trigeminal nucleus or tract which also involves ascending sensory pathways resulting in loss of sensation over the contralateral trunk and limbs. The most typical picture is that seen in the Wallenberg syndrome.

bulbar hemianesthesia Loss of sensation on one half of the body due to a contralateral brainstem lesion, sometimes associated with hemiplegia, such as that occurring in the paramedian syndrome and in the syndromes of Schmidt and Avellis, in Jackson's lateral bulbar syndrome, and in the Wallenberg syndrome.

cerebral hemianesthesia Hemianesthesia resulting from a cerebral lesion.

cheiro-oral hemianesthesia Impaired sensation on one side of the peribuccal region and on the radial edge of the hand on the same side of the body. This is most often seen in patients with thalamic lesions and less often in postrolandic cortical lesions.

crossed hemianesthesia Hemianesthesia due to a contralateral lesion in the central nervous system. Also called *hemianesthesia cruciata.*

hemianesthesia cruciata CROSSED HEMIANESTHESIA.

hysterical hemianesthesia Hemianesthesia, usually involving all sensory modalities, including vibration sense on one half of the skull, resulting from hysteria and not from organic disease of the nervous system.

mesocephalic hemianesthesia Hemianesthesia resulting from a midbrain lesion.

peduncular hemianesthesia Hemianesthesia due to a lesion of the opposite cerebral peduncle. This may involve all forms of sensation or may affect only pain and temperature sense, touch, or deep sensibility, depending upon the situation and extent of the lesion. Sometimes there is an associated hemiplegia on the side of the impaired sensation and/or a third nerve palsy with signs of cerebellar dysfunction on the side of the lesion.

pontile hemianesthesia PONTINE HEMIANESTHESIA.

pontine hemianesthesia Hemianesthesia due to a contralateral pontine lesion, often associated with signs of cranial nerve dysfunction on the side of the lesion. Also called *pontile hemianesthesia.*

spinal hemianesthesia Hemianesthesia due to a spinal cord lesion.

hemianopia [HEMI- + ANOPIA] Inability to see in half of the visual field. Also called *hemianopsia, visus dimidiatus, half vision.* Adjective: hemianopic.

absolute hemianopia The complete loss of sight in the affected part of an eye that has lost all or part of half of its visual field.

altitudinal hemianopia The loss of the upper or lower half of the field of vision.

bilateral hemianopia BINOCULAR HEMIANOPIA.

binasal hemianopia Loss of the medial half of the visual field in both eyes.

binocular hemianopia Loss of half of the visual field in both eyes. Also called *bilateral hemianopia.*

bitemporal hemianopia Loss of the lateral half of the field of vision in both eyes.

hemianopia bitemporalis fugax Transitory loss of the lateral half of the field of vision in both eyes.

color hemianopia HEMIACHROMATOPSIA.

complete hemianopia Loss of a complete half of the visual field, extending to the midline.

congruous hemianopia A loss of part or all of half of the visual field that has exactly identical borders in both eyes.

crossed hemianopia Loss of opposite vertical halves of the visual fields in the two eyes, top loss on one side, bottom on the other.

equilateral hemianopia A symmetrical loss of half of the visual field in each eye.

heteronymous hemianopia Loss of different (crossed) halves of the visual field for each eye, as loss of the right field in one eye and of the left field in the other.

homonymous hemianopia Loss of the same (uncrossed) halves of the visual field for each eye, as loss of the right field for each eye.

horizontal hemianopia LATERAL HEMIANOPIA.

incomplete hemianopia Loss of less than half of a visual field.

incongruous hemianopia Losses of half of the visual field that are of different extent in each eye.

lateral hemianopia Loss of all or part of the upper or lower half of the visual field. Also called *horizontal hemianopia.*

lower hemianopia Loss of all or part of the bottom half of the visual field.

nasal hemianopia Loss of all or part of the medial half of the visual field.

quadrantic hemianopia Loss of all or part of a fourth of the visual field, bounded by the vertical and horizontal midlines.

relative hemianopia Loss of all or part of half of the visual field that is demonstrable only when the test objects are simultaneously presented on both sides of the visual field.

temporal hemianopia Loss of all or part of the lateral half of the visual field.

true hemianopia Loss of vision of half of the visual field, affecting both eyes, and limited to one side of the vertical midline, as would result from a visual pathway lesion at or posterior to the optic chiasm.

unilateral hemianopia UNIOCULAR HEMIANOPIA.

uniocular hemianopia Loss of all or part of half of the visual field in only one eye. Also called *unilateral hemianopia.*

upper hemianopia VERTICAL HEMIANOPIA.

vertical hemianopia Loss of all or part of the upper half of the visual field. Also called *upper hemianopia.*

hemianopic [HEMI- + Gk *an-* priv. + *ōp(ē)* vision + -IC] Characterized by or relating to hemianopia; being unable to see in all or part of half of the visual field. Also *hemianoptic.*

hemianopsia HEMIANOPIA. Adjective: hemianoptic.

hemianoptic HEMIANOPIC.

hemianosmia Anosmia affecting only one side of the nose.

hemiapraxia [HEMI- + APRAXIA] Unilateral apraxia.

Hemiascomycetidae [HEMI- + *asc(us)* + *o* + MYCET- + -IDAE] A subclass of ascomycetous fungi that develop directly from zygotes or single cells, without ascogenous hyphae or ascocarps.

hemiasomatognosia [HEMI- + Gk *a-* priv. + SOMATO- + Gk *-gnōsia,* combining form from *gnōs(is)* knowledge + -IA] Inability to appreciate and interpret somatic sensation upon one side of the body.

hemiasynergia HEMIASYNERGY.

hemiasynergy [HEMI- + ASYNERGY] Unilateral asynergy. Also called *hemiasynergia, hemisynergia.*

hemiataxia [HEMI- + ATAXIA] Unilateral ataxia. Also called *hemiataxy.*

hemiataxy HEMIATAXIA.

hemiathetosis [HEMI- + ATHETOSIS] Unilateral athetosis.

hemiatonia [HEMI- + ATONIA] Unilateral muscular atonia (flaccid paralysis) or hypotonia.

hemiatonia apoplectica Flaccid hemiplegia resulting from apoplexy.

hemiatrophy [HEMI- + ATROPHY] Atrophy of tissues involving one side of the body or one half of a structure, organ, or part. Also called *hemihypoplasia.*

cranial hemiatrophy Hemiatrophy of the face and cranium.

facial hemiatrophy ROMBERG'S PROGRESSIVE FACIAL HEMIATROPHY.

progressive lingual hemiatrophy A progressive, unilateral paralysis of the tongue, accompanied by atrophy.

Romberg's progressive facial hemiatrophy A rare condition characterized by unilateral facial atrophy, involving especially the subcutaneous tissues. The condition, of unknown cause, occurs more frequently in women, first appears in adolescence, and is slowly progressive. Also called *Romberg's disease, facial trophoneurosis, Parry-Romberg syndrome, facial hemiatrophy, trophoneurosis of Romberg.*

hemiautotrophic Synthesizing proteins from inorganic nitrogen in the presence of organic compounds: said of partially self-nourishing microorganisms.

hemiazygos Partially paired. Also *hemiazygous.*

hemiazygous HEMIAZYGOS.

hemiballism HEMIBALLISMUS.

hemiballismus [HEMI- + Gk *ballismos* a throwing oneself about] A syndrome, usually of sudden onset, in elderly patients, giving rise to violent, writhing, involuntary movements, often of wide excursion, and confined to one half of the body. The movements are continuous and often exhausting but cease during sleep. It results from cerebral vascular disease and is usually due to infarction of one subthalamic nucleus (corpus Luysii) or of the pathway connecting this nucleus to the midbrain. The condition was often fatal in the past, due to exhaustion, but can now sometimes be controlled by phenothiazine drugs or abolished by stereotaxic surgery. Milder forms of the condition may be identified as hemichorea. Also called *syndrome of the corpus Luysii, subthalamic syndrome, hemiballism, body of Luys syndrome.*

hemibranch [HEMI- + BRANCH]   A gill which has a layer of gill filaments on one side of the gill arch.

hemic   Related to blood or blood flow.

hemicanities   The occurrence of gray hair that is confined to one side of the body.

hemicardia [HEMI- + CARDIA]   A developmentally defective heart with only two chambers, a single atrium and a single ventricle. These chambers have structural features common to the respective right and left chambers, therefore efforts to identify them with the normal right and left chambers are meaningless. Also called *cor biloculare.*

hemicardius   An embryo, fetus, or neonate with hemicardia, that is only half of the usual four-chambered heart.

hemicellulose   Any of several alkali-soluble polysaccharides found in the walls of plant cells. They include polymers of xylose, mannose, L-arabinose, glucuronic acid, and galacturonic acid.

hemicentrum   Either of the two lateral halves of a body of a vertebra.

hemicephalalgia [HEMI- + CEPHAL- + -ALGIA]   HEMICRANIA.

hemicephalia   HEMICEPHALY.

hemicephalus [HEMI- + -CEPHALUS]   An embryo, fetus, or infant with hemicephaly. Also called *hemiencephalus.*

hemicephaly [HEMI- + CEPHAL- + -Y]   Agenesis or partial agenesis of the cerebral hemispheres. The basal ganglia may be present to a variable degree but the brainstem and cerebellum tend to be normally formed. Also called *hemicephalia.*

hemicerebrum   The cerebral hemisphere of one side. Also called *hemiencephalon.*

Hemichorda   HEMICHORDATA.

Hemichordata [HEMI- + CHORDATA]   A phylum of primitive prechordate marine organisms, characterized by gill-slits that enter the pharynx, by a conical proboscis, and by a wormlike appearance. The ciliated larval stage (a dipleurula) is similar to that of echinoderms, giving the group an important phylogenetic position between the echinoderms and the other protochordates. Also called *Hemichorda.*

hemichorea [HEMI- + CHOREA]   Chorea in which the choreic movements affect only one half of the body. Also called *hemiplegic chorea, hemilateral chorea, chorea dimidiata, unilateral chorea, one-sided chorea.*

paralytic hemichorea   Hemichorea giving such a degree of weakness and hypotonia in the affected limbs that hemiplegia is simulated.

posthemiplegic hemichorea   Hemichorea developing as a sequel of hemiplegia.

preparalytic hemichorea   A condition in which choreiform movements in the affected limbs precede the development of hemiplegia.

rheumatic hemichorea   Hemichorea occurring as a result of rheumatic fever.

syphilitic hemichorea   Hemichorea developing as a manifestation of neurosyphilis.

hemichromatopsia   HEMIACHROMATOPSIA.

hemichromosome   **1** An isolated fragment of a chromosome. **2** An isochromosome arm.   **3** A chromatid with half of a centromere. A seldom used term.

hemiclonus [HEMI- + CLONUS]   Myoclonus restricted to one half of the body.

hemicolectomy [HEMI- + COLECTOMY]   The surgical removal of approximately half of the large bowel.

left hemicolectomy   The surgical removal of the large bowel from the midtransverse colon to the rectum.

right hemicolectomy   The surgical removal of a few distal centimeters of the small bowel and the large bowel from the cecum to the midtransverse colon.

hemiconvulsion [HEMI- + CONVULSION]   Jacksonian epilepsy involving one side of the body.

hemicorporectomy   The surgical removal of the lower half of the body, including all of the pelvic contents and the pelvic bones.

hemicrania [HEMI- + *cran(i)-* + -IA]   **1** Pain or neuralgia on one side of the head. Also called *hemicephalalgia.*   **2** MIGRAINE.

hemicrania cerebellaris   BÁRÁNY SYNDROME.

hemicraniectomy [HEMI- + CRANIECTOMY]   Removal of one side of the cranium, as for extensive decompression of the brain. Also called *hemicraniotomy.*

hemicraniosis   An enlargement of one side of the cranium and/or face.

hemicraniotomy [HEMI- + CRANIOTOMY]   HEMICRANIECTOMY.

hemicryptophyte   A plant whose buds or shoot apices are located at or just below the soil surface.

hemidecerebration   The experimental separation of the brainstem from or destruction of one cerebral hemisphere. Also called *semidecerebration* (outmoded).

hemidecortication [HEMI- + DECORTICATION]   Excision of the cortex of the cerebrum on one side.

hemidesmosome   An attachment point between an epidermal cell and the underlying basement membrane, seen by electron microscopy to correspond to one-half of a desmosome.

hemidiaphoresis [HEMI- + DIA- + -PHORESIS]   HEMIHYPERHIDROSIS.

hemidiaphragm   One half of the diaphragm (right or left).

hemidrosis   HEMIHIDROSIS.

hemidysergia [HEMI- + DYS- + Gk *erg(on)* work + -IA]   Dyssynergia on one side of the body.

hemidysesthesia   Spontaneous abnormal sensation occurring over one half of the body.

hemidystrophy   A developmental defect characterized by underdevelopment of one side of the body.

hemiectromelia [HEMI- + ECTRO- + MEL-[1] + -IA]   A reduction deformity of the limbs on one side of the body.

hemiencephalon   HEMICEREBRUM.

hemiencephalus   HEMICEPHALUS.

hemiepilepsy [HEMI- + EPILEPSY]   Any of the clinical manifestations of epilepsy, such as convulsive movements, restricted to one half of the body.

hemifacial [HEMI- + FACIAL]   Describing, pertaining to, or affecting one side of the face only.

hemigastrectomy   The surgical removal of approximately half of the stomach.

hemigeusia [HEMI- + Gk *geus(is)* taste + -IA]   Taste sensation on one side of the tongue only.

hemigigantism   Extreme hypertrophy of a lateral half of the body or of one or more parts on one side of the body.

hemiglossal   HEMILINGUAL.

hemiglossectomy   The excision of half the tongue.

hemiglossitis   Glossitis confined to one side of the tongue.

hemiglossoplegia [HEMI- + GLOSSOPLEGIA]   Paralysis of one side of the tongue.

hemignathia [HEMI- + GNATH- + -IA]   Defective development of the mandibular region on one side.

hemihepatectomy   The surgical removal of approximately half of the liver.

hemihidrosis [HEMI- + HIDROSIS]   Sweating confined to one side of the body. Also called *hemidrosis.*

hemihydranencephaly [HEMI- + HYDRANENCEPHALY]   Hydranencephaly affecting only one side of the head.

hemihypalgesia   A reduction in pain sensibility on one half of the body.

hemihyperesthesia [HEMI- + HYPERESTHESIA]   An apparent heightening of acuteness of perception of touch on one side of the body.

hemihyperhidrosis [HEMI- + HYPERHIDROSIS]   Excessive sweating on one side of the body. Also called *hemidiaphoresis, hyperhidrosis unilateralis.*

hemihypermetria [HEMI- + HYPERMETRIA]   Hypermetria on one side of the body.

hemihyperplasia [HEMI- + HYPERPLASIA]   Hyperplasia of tissues on one side of the body or on one side of an organ or part.

hemihypertonia [HEMI- + HYPERTONIA]   Hypertonia restricted to one half of the body. Also called *hemitonia.*

hemihypertrophy [HEMI- + HYPERTROPHY]   Hypertrophy of tissues, organs, or parts on one side of the body.

   congenital hemihypertrophy   Hemihypertrophy that is apparent at birth. Also called *hemiacrosomia.*

   facial hemihypertrophy   Hemihypertrophy affecting structures on only one side of the face.

hemihypesthesia [HEMI- + HYP- + -ESTHESIA]   Impairment of the sense of touch over one half of the body. Also called *hemihypoesthesia.*

hemihypoesthesia   HEMIHYPESTHESIA.

hemihypogeusia [HEMI- + HYPOGEUSIA]   Reduced perception of taste on one side of the tongue.

hemihypometria [HEMI- + HYPOMETRIA]   Hypometria on one side of the body.

hemihypoplasia [HEMI- + HYPOPLASIA]   HEMIATROPHY.

hemihypothermia   A condition in which the temperature upon one side of the body is lower than on the other.

hemihypotonia [HEMI- + HYPOTONIA]   Hypotonia restricted to one half of the body.

hemikaryon   The nucleus of a cell which contains the haploid number of chromosomes.

hemiketal   A hemiacetal derived from a ketone rather than from an aldehyde. An obsolete term.

hemilaminectomy   Excision of a vertebral lamina on one side. Also called *hemilaminotomy.*

hemilaminotomy   HEMILAMINECTOMY.

hemilaryngectomy [HEMI- + LARYNGECTOMY]   An operation to remove half the larynx for malignant disease localized strictly within the part removed. See also HEMILARYNX.

   horizontal hemilaryngectomy   Hemilaryngectomy in which the part of the larynx removed is that situated above the level of the vocal folds, including the hyoid bone, epiglottis, and ventricular bands. Also called *supraglottic laryngectomy.*

   vertical hemilaryngectomy   A partial laryngectomy in which the greater part of the hemilarynx situated to one side of the anteroposterior midline vertical plane is removed.

hemilarynx   Half the larynx; particularly a half that is surgically removed. It can be either the half to one side of the midline vertical plane through the laryngeal eminence or the half above the horizontal plane transecting the larynx immediately above the true vocal cords.

hemilateral   Pertaining to or involving the outer half of one side.

hemilesion [HEMI- + LESION]   A lesion involving one side of the spinal cord or brain. An outmoded term.

hemilingual   Pertaining to either lateral half of the tongue. Also *hemiglossal.*

hemimacrocephaly [HEMI- + MACRO- + CEPHAL- + -Y]   Hemihypertrophy affecting the head.

hemimacroglossia   Enlargement of the tongue confined to one side.

hemimandible   Either half of the mandible situated on one side or the other of the midline vertical plane passing through the symphysis menti.

hemimandibulectomy   Surgical excision of half the mandible, from close to the symphysis menti to, and including, the mandibular condyle. It is undertaken chiefly for the removal of various tumors confined to this part. Reconstruction may make use of a bone graft or of a metal implant splint.

hemimandibuloglossectomy   Hemimandibulectomy combined with excision of part of the tongue. It is undertaken for malignant disease involving both mandible and tongue. Reconstruction presents formidable problems.

hemimelia [HEMI- + MEL-¹ + -IA]   A developmental defect involving major reduction in the distal portion of a limb. It is one of the conditions that can result when a pregnant woman takes thalidomide. Compare PHOCOMELIA.

   axial hemimelia   The agenesis of one of the distal long bones of a limb.

   fibular hemimelia   The agenesis of the fibula, with or without associated reduction defects of the foot and toes.

   radial hemimelia   The agenesis of the radius with or without associated reduction defects of the hand and fingers.

   tibial hemimelia   The agenesis of the tibia with or without associated reduction defects of the foot and toes.

   transverse hemimelia   The natural developmental amputation of a limb at the elbow or wrist in an upper extremity or at the knee or ankle in a lower extremity.

   ulnar hemimelia   The agenesis of the ulna with or without associated reduction defects of the hand and fingers.

hemimelus [HEMI- + MEL-¹ + L -us, masc. noun suffix]   Any embryo, fetus, or postnatal individual with hemimelia.

Hemimetabola [HEMI- + Gk *metabola,* neut. pl. of *metabolos* (from *metaballein* to turn about, change) changeable]   A taxonomic category, the series within the class Insecta, which includes those insect orders that develop by simple or hemimetabolous metamorphosis, characterized by development of the imago through a number of gradual nymphal changes rather than by a single pupation step as found in the more advanced, holometabolous orders. The hemimetabolous stages include egg, nymph (through a succession of instars), and imago or sexual, flying adult. Examples of hemimetabolous insect orders include: Orthoptera (grasshoppers and crickets), Dictyoptera (cockroaches), Mallophaga (chewing lice), Ephemeroptera (mayflies), Thysanoptera (thrips), Anoplura (sucking lice), Hemiptera (true bugs), Homoptera (cicadas, aphids, scale insects, leafhoppers, and others), and Isoptera (termites). Compare HOLOMETABOLA.

hemimetabolous   Characterized by gradual or simple metamorphosis, involving a series of preadult nymphal stages: said primarily of insects. See also HEMIMETABOLA.

hemimyasthenia [HEMI- + MYASTHENIA]   Unilateral muscular weakness. An imprecise and outmoded term. Also called *hemineurasthenia.*

hemimyoclonus [HEMI- + MYOCLONUS] Myoclonus occurring on one side of the body only.

hemin The complex of a porphyrin and chloride with iron(III). It may be isolated from hemoglobin. Also called *ferriprotoporphyrin* (incorrect).

heminephrectomy [HEMI- + NEPHRECTOMY] Surgical removal of a portion of a kidney.

heminephroureterectomy [HEMI- + NEPHRO- + URETER- + -ECTOMY] Surgical removal of a portion of a kidney with its ureter.

hemineurasthenia [HEMI- + NEURASTHENIA] HEMIMYASTHENIA.

hemiobesity Obesity localized to one side of the body.

hemiopalgia [HEMI- + Gk *ōp(s)* eye + -ALGIA] Pain on one side of the head and in the eye on the same side.

hemiopia [HEMI- + -OPIA] The loss of all or part of half of the visual field. Also called *hemiscotosis*. Adjective: hemiopic.

hemipagus [HEMI- + -PAGUS] THORACOPAGUS.

hemipalatectomy Surgical excision of one half of the palate, usually one half of the hard palate along with the corresponding alveolar process. An ambiguous usage.

hemipalatolaryngoplegia Paralysis of the muscles of the palate and larynx, confined to one side.

hemiparalysis [HEMI- + PARALYSIS] HEMIPLEGIA.

hemiparanesthesia [HEMI- + *par(a)* + ANESTHESIA] Anesthesia on one side of the lower half of the body. An outmoded and inaccurate term.

hemiparaplegia [HEMI- + PARAPLEGIA] Paralysis of one side of the lower half of the body. • This usage is incorrect as *paraplegia* by definition means paralysis of both lower limbs.

  spinal hemiparaplegia BROWN-SÉQUARD SYNDROME.

hemiparesis [HEMI- + PARESIS] Slight or incomplete motor weakness affecting one side of the body.

hemiparesthesia [HEMI- + PARESTHESIA] Paresthesia restricted to one half of the body.

hemiparkinsonism [HEMI- + PARKINSONISM] Parkinsonism in which the abnormal physical signs are restricted to one half of the body.

hemipelvectomy The surgical removal of half of the bony pelvis.

hemipelvis Either of the two lateral halves of a pelvis.

hemipelvisectomy HINDQUARTER AMPUTATION.

hemipenis [HEMI- + PENIS] One of a pair of copulatory structures present in most male snakes and lizards.

hemiphalangectomy An excision of part of a digit.

hemiphonia [HEMI- + PHON- + -IA] An uneven quality of voice resulting from involuntary alternation between normally voiced speech and whispering.

hemipinta Pinta involving only one half of the body.

hemiplegia [HEMI- + -PLEGIA] Paralysis of one half of the body. The paralysis may be total, involving face, limbs, and trunk, or partial (hemiparesis). Bilateral hemiplegia may occur, giving a clinical picture which is difficult to distinguish from tetraplegia. Also called *hemiparalysis, semiplegia, semisideratio*. Adjective: hemiplegic.

  acute infantile hemiplegia An acute cerebral disorder affecting infants and children up to about two years, characterized by hemiplegia, lateralized seizures, and severe neurologic residual defects. Fever and coma are common. The etiology is manifold and includes thrombosis of the internal carotid artery and cortical thrombophlebitis secondary to severe dehydration. Also called *Marie-Strümpell disease, polioencephalitis of Marie-Strümpell, hemiconvulsive-hemiplegic syndrome, Strümpell's disease, polioencephalitis acuta infantum (imprecise and outmoded),* *Strümpell-Leichtenstern disease, H.H.E. syndrome, Strümpell-Marie disease.*

  hemiplegia alternans hypoglossica MEDIAN MEDULLARY SYNDROME.

  alternate hemiplegia CROSSED HEMIPLEGIA.

  alternating oculomotor hemiplegia WEBER SYNDROME.

  ascending hemiplegia Hemiplegia in which paralysis begins in the foot and leg and spreads upwards to the trunk and upper limb.

  Avellis hemiplegia AVELLIS PARALYSIS.

  bulbar hemiplegia Any type of hemiplegia caused by damage to the medulla oblongata.

  capsular hemiplegia Hemiplegia resulting from a lesion of the contralateral internal capsule.

  cerebellar hemiplegia Severe unilateral ataxia due to a lesion of the ipsilateral cerebellum or of cerebellar pathways in the brainstem on the same side. Strictly, although the affected limbs may be grossly ataxic and also weak, this is not a true hemiplegia. Also called *cerebellar hemisyndrome*.

  cerebral hemiplegia Hemiplegia due to any cerebral lesion.

  chronic ascending spinal hemiplegia A rare form of hemiplegia beginning in the lower limb and spreading to the upper limb after one or two years. It is doubtful whether this can be accepted as a specific syndrome.

  collateral hemiplegia Hemiplegia occurring on the same side as the cerebral lesion. This may be due, among other causes, to pressure upon the contralateral crus cerebri against the free edge of the tentorium cerebelli, produced by a space-occupying lesion.

  congenital hemiplegia Hemiplegia present at birth and attributable to impaired cerebral development or to birth trauma. A form of cerebral palsy, it is rarely discernible before the age of two or three months.

  contralateral hemiplegia The usual form of hemiplegia, occurring on the side opposite to the cerebral lesion.

  cortical hemiplegia Hemiplegia due to a lesion of the contralateral motor cortex. The weakness is often incomplete and involves distal muscle groups in the limbs more severely than proximal. Associated features may include jacksonian epilepsy, impairment of fine sensibility in the affected limbs, if the sensory as well as the motor cortex is involved, and expressive dysphasia when the lesion also involves Broca's area and the lesion is in the dominant hemisphere.

  crossed hemiplegia 1 Hemiplegia due to a contralateral brainstem lesion which may have produced signs of cranial nerve dysfunction or cerebellar signs on the side of the lesion (the side opposite to the hemiplegia). Also called *hemiplegia cruciata, alternate hemiplegia, stauroplegia*. 2 A very rare situation in which a lesion of the pyramidal decussation in the medulla oblongata results in paralysis of the upper limb on one side and of the lower limb on the other. An incorrect usage.

  hemiplegia cruciata CROSSED HEMIPLEGIA.

  epileptic hemiplegia Transient or persistent hemiplegia following an epileptic attack or status epilepticus. Also called *postepileptic hemiplegia*. • This term is incorrect when used to designate transient hemiplegia, which is occasionally the manifestation of a unilateral atonic epileptic attack.

  facial hemiplegia Unilateral facial paralysis. Also called *hemiprosoplegia*.

  facial hemiplegia alternans Crossed paralysis, with facial weakness on one side of the body and hemiplegia on the other.

  faciobrachial hemiplegia Paralysis of one side of the face and of the arm on the same side.

  faciolingual hemiplegia Paralysis of one side of the face and of half the tongue on the same side.

  flaccid hemiplegia Hemiplegia with atonia or severe hypotonia and absent or depressed tendon reflexes in the affected limbs. This may be an initial manifestation of an acute lesion, such as an infarct, in the opposite cerebral hemisphere, seen in the phase of "shock", in which case spasticity often develops subsequently in the affected limbs. But when there is extensive involvement of the parietal sensory cortex as well as motor cortex, flaccidity may persist in the paralyzed limbs.

functional hemiplegia HYSTERICAL HEMIPLEGIA.

Gubler's hemiplegia MILLARD-GUBLER SYNDROME.

hereditary hemiplegia Familial hemiplegic migraine.

hysterical hemiplegia Hemiplegia due to subconscious mental motivation and not to any physical cause, usually developing as a means of escape from a stressful situation. Often there is also total loss of all forms of sensation in the affected limbs. Also called *functional hemiplegia*.

infantile hemiplegia Hemiplegia which may be present from birth, normally due to perinatal brain damage, or which develops during infancy. It may develop acutely and is often associated with seizures occurring at the onset. It is usually due to infarction resulting from arterial or, less often, cerebral venous occlusion, but may in rare cases be due to encephalitis or encephalopathy. A hemiplegia developing gradually in infancy or early childhood may be a manifestation of the Sturge-Weber syndrome.

infantile acquired hemiplegia Infantile hemiplegia resulting from a postnatal, as distinct from a prenatal, lesion.

laryngeal hemiplegia **1** Unilateral paralysis of the intrinsic muscles of the larynx, usually caused by damage to the recurrent laryngeal nerve. **2** Paralysis and atrophy of the laryngeal muscles of a horse, usually on the left side. This condition causes a loud inspiratory noise, especially after strenuous exercise. Also called *roaring*.

middle alternating hemiplegia Recurrent hemiplegia due to ischemia in the area of the middle cerebral artery occurring first on one side of the body, then on the other. A seldom used term.

organic hemiplegia Any form of hemiplegia due to a physical lesion of the nervous system.

peduncular hemiplegia Hemiplegia due to a lesion of the contralateral cerebral peduncle.

pontine hemiplegia Hemiplegia due to a contralateral pontine lesion. In most cases, this is associated with signs of cranial nerve or cerebellar dysfunction on the side of the lesion.

postepileptic hemiplegia EPILEPTIC HEMIPLEGIA.

proportional hemiplegia Hemiplegia which affects the face and the upper and the lower limb with equal intensity. A seldom used term.

puerperal hemiplegia Hemiplegia due to cerebral vascular disease developing in the puerperium.

spastic hemiplegia Hemiplegia with spasticity, as distinct from flaccidity, of the affected limbs.

spinal hemiplegia Hemiplegia resulting from a unilateral lesion of the pyramidal (corticospinal) tract in the spinal cord. The face is spared. Depending upon the extent of the lesion, sensory pathways may also be affected.

superior alternate hemiplegia WEBER SYNDROME.

Wernicke-Mann hemiplegia Partial or incomplete hemiplegia. An outmoded term.

hemiplegic Pertaining to hemiplegia.

hemiprosoplegia [HEMI- + *proso(p)* + -PLEGIA] FACIAL HEMIPLEGIA.

hemiprostatectomy [HEMI- + PROSTATECTOMY] The surgical removal of one of the lateral halves of the prostate.

Hemiptera [HEMI- + Gk *ptera* (pl. of *pteron* feather) feathers, wings] An order of hemimetabolous insects, the true bugs, which includes many species of varied habits and structures, but all equipped with piercing and sucking mouthparts. A few are of medical importance, being adapted for bloodsucking, enabling them to be disease vectors. The triatomine or cone-nosed bugs

serve to transmit the flagellate *Trypanosoma cruzi*, the agent of Chagas disease. *Cimex lectularius*, the common bedbug, is a member of the order. Though a notorious pest and bloodsucker, it appears not to serve as an efficient vector of human parasites.

hemipterous Of or belonging to the order Hemiptera.

hemipylorectomy The surgical removal of half of the gastric pylorus.

hemipyonephrosis [HEMI- + PYONEPHROSIS] Unilateral pyonephrosis.

hemirachischisis Spina bifida with more severe involvement of one-half of the spinal cord. An imprecise and outmoded term.

hemisacralization The unilateral fusion of the transverse process of the fifth lumbar vertebra to the wing of the sacrum.

hemiscotosis [HEMI- + *scot(o)* + -OSIS] HEMIOPIA.

hemisection BISECTION.

hemisection of the spinal cord A longitudinal incision dividing the spinal cord in the midline.

hemiseptum Half of a septum, especially one side of the septum pellucidum of the telencephalon.

hemiseptum cerebri The septum pellucidum of one side of the telencephalon.

hemisotonic Having the same osmolarity as the blood.

hemispasm [HEMI- + SPASM] Unilateral spasm.

alternate facial hemispasm A rare syndrome due to lesions of the lower pons, and giving rise to homolateral facial spasm with paralysis of the limbs on the opposite side. Also called *Brissaud-Sicard syndrome, Brissaud-Lereboullet syndrome*.

facial hemispasm Spasmodic unilateral contraction of facial muscles, usually due to an irritative lesion of the facial nerve in its canal, less often to a lesion of the facial nucleus in the brainstem. This is a not infrequent sequel of facial paralysis (Bell's palsy). Also called *clonic facial spasm, facial myoclonus, facial myospasm*.

glossolabial hemispasm Unilateral recurrent contraction of tongue and lip muscles, which may extend to the orbicularis oculi or be associated with blepharospasm. This may be hysterical, but similar manifestations can occur in facial dyskinesia due to phenothiazine drugs.

hemisphaerium HEMISPHERIUM.

hemisphere [L *hemisphaerium*. See HEMISPHERIUM.] HEMISPHERIUM.

animal hemisphere In a cleaving telolecithal ovum, the hemisphere where the yolk material does not accumulate. Compare VEGETAL HEMISPHERE.

cerebellar hemisphere HEMISPHERIUM CEREBELLI.

cerebral hemisphere HEMISPHERIUM CEREBRI.

dominant hemisphere The cerebral hemisphere which controls speech and executive and cognitive skills. This is almost invariably the left hemisphere in right-handed individuals. In the left-handed, it is usually the right, but sometimes it may be the left. Also called *talking hemisphere*.

mute hemisphere NONDOMINANT HEMISPHERE.

nondominant hemisphere The cerebral hemisphere other than the dominant one, such that ablation results in a less severe deficit. Also called *mute hemisphere*.

talking hemisphere DOMINANT HEMISPHERE.

vegetal hemisphere The hemisphere of a cleaving ovum of the telolecithal type where the yolk becomes concentrated. Compare ANIMAL HEMISPHERE.

hemispherectomy [*hemispher(e)* + -ECTOMY] Excision or extensive resection of one cerebral hemisphere.

hemispheria Plural of HEMISPHERIUM.

hemispherium [L *hemisphaerium* (from Gk *hēmisphairion* a small hemisphere, from *hēmi-* half + *sphairion* a little ball or sphere) hemisphere] Half of a spherical structure or organ such as the cerebrum or cerebellum. Also called *hemisphere, hemisphaerium.*

hemispherium bulbi urethrae   Each lateral half of the bulbus penis (occasionally called bulbus urethrae), on each side of the commencement of the spongy part of the urethra.

hemispherium cerebelli   [NA] The cerebellar hemisphere of one side, lateral to the midline vermis and consisting of the lobuli centralis, quadrangularis, simplex, semilunaris, biventer, and tonsil. Also called *cerebellar hemisphere.*

hemispherium cerebri   [NA] The largest mass of the brain on either side, derived from the embryonic telencephalon and consisting principally of the cerebral cortex and the underlying basal ganglia and their associated fiber systems. Also called *cerebral hemisphere.*

hemisphygmia   A condition in which there are twice as many pulse beats as heart beats, such as pulsus bisferiens.

Hemispora stellata   An obsolete form-species of fungus at one time considered to be the etiologic agent of various granulomas.

hemispore [HEMI- + SPORE]   A type of fungal conidium which is formed at the terminus of a hypha and undergoes division to form two or more secondary conidia.

hemistrumectomy   A seldom used term for HEMITHYROIDEC-TOMY.

hemisyndrome [HEMI- + SYNDROME]   Any syndrome in which the symptoms and signs of disease or dysfunction are confined to one side of the body.

cerebellar hemisyndrome   CEREBELLAR HEMIPLEGIA.

hemisynergia   HEMIASYNERGY.

hemiterpene   A terpene formed from a single isoprene unit and of formula C_5H_8.

hemitetany [HEMI- + TETANY]   Tetany on only one side of the body.

hemithermoanesthesia [HEMI- + THERMO- + ANESTHESIA]   Loss or impairment of temperature sensation on one side of the body.

hemithorax   One of the two lateral halves of the chest.

hemithyroidectomy   Removal of half the mass of the thyroid gland, as for a localized goiter or relatively benign tumor. Also called *hemistrumectomy* (seldom used).

hemitomias [HEMI- + Gk *tomias* (from *temnein* to cut) a eunuch]   An individual having only one testis.

hemitonia   HEMIHYPERTONIA.

hemitoxin   A toxin that has half of its original toxicity.

hemitremor [HEMI- + TREMOR]   Tremor on only one side of the body.

hemivagotonia   Unilateral hyperactivity of the vagus nerve. Also called *hemivagotony.*

hemivagotony   HEMIVAGOTONIA.

hemivertebra   A failure in the development of a lateral half, or major part thereof, of a vertebra. It is usually accompanied by agenesis of the rib ordinarily associated with the missing vertebral part.

hemizygosity   The state of being hemizygous.

hemizygote   A cell, tissue, organism, or sex having but one copy of a specific gene, genes, chromosome segment, or entire chromosome in its otherwise diploid genome. The human male is a hemizygote with reference to the X and Y chromosomes.

hemizygotic   HEMIZYGOUS.

hemizygous   **1** Of or pertaining to a specific gene, group of genes, chromosome segment, or entire chromosome that is present only once in an otherwise diploid genome. **2** Referring to a cell, tissue, organism, or sex that is in some way a hemizygote. The heterogametic sex of a species is hemizygous for genes on both sex chromosomes. For defs. 1 and 2 also *hemizygotic.*

hemlock [Old English *hemlic*, prob. from Finno-Ugrian *humala* hop plant]   **1** A plant of the species *Conium maculatum*; poison hemlock. **2** A tree of the genus *Tsuga*; hemlock spruce.

poison hemlock   CONIUM.

hemo- [Gk *haima* (genitive *haimatos*) blood]   A combining form meaning blood. Also *haemo- (British spelling), hem-, hema-, haem- (British spelling), hemat-, hemato-, haemato- (British spelling).*

hemoagglutination   A phenomenon characterized by the clumping of blood cells and induced by an antibody reacting with the corresponding antigen present on the cell surface. Also called *hemagglutination.*

hemoagglutinin   HEMAGGLUTININ.

hemoantitoxin   An antibody that counteracts the effects of a hemolytic toxin.

Hemobartonella   *HAEMOBARTONELLA.*

hemobilia   HEMATOBILIA.

hemoblast   HEMOCYTOBLAST.

lymphoid hemoblast of Pappenheim   HEMATOGONE.

hemoblastosis   Any neoplastic disorder of the hematopoietic system, such as leukemias of all types, malignant lymphomas, myeloma, polycythemia vera, and essential thrombocythemia. A rarely used term. Also called *hematoblastosis, hemolymphadenosis, hemomyelosis.*

hemocatharsis   HEMODIALYSIS.

hemocatheresis   A seldom used term for HEMOLYSIS.

hemocele   HEMOCOEL.

hemochezia   HEMATOCHEZIA.

hemocholecyst   A hollow structure, usually the gallbladder, containing both blood and bile and resulting from nontraumatic hemorrhage.

hemocholecystitis   Inflammation of the gallbladder accompanied by bleeding into the gallbladder.

hemochorial   Pertaining to a type of placentation containing only trophoblast, connective tissue, and endothelium, occurring in lower rodents, bats, and anthropoids. The endothelium of uterine vessels is lost and blood circulates in channels in the fetal syncytium.

hemochromatosis [HEMO- + CHROMATOSIS]   A chronic, progressive disease of unclear pathogenesis that is associated with iron overload and iron deposition in many tissues. The idiopathic form is an autosomal recessive condition. A similar phenotype, hemosiderosis, can result from multiple transfusions or a diet very high in iron. Clinical sequelae include a bronze hue to the skin, hepatic failure with cirrhosis, diabetes, heart failure, pituitary insufficiency, and arthropathy. Also called *hemachromatosis, hematochromatosis, Recklinghausen-Applebaum disease, iron storage disease.*

exogenous hemochromatosis   Hemochromatosis caused by an excess of iron taken into the body, as through repeated blood transfusions or prolonged and excessive ingestion of iron.

hemochromatotic   Characterized by hemochromatosis.

hemochrome   Any oxygen-carrying pigment of blood. The hemochrome of vertebrates is hemoglobin. A variety of hemochromes occur in invertebrate species, such as hemocyanin, erythrocruorin, chlorocruorin, and hemoerythrin. Also *hemachrome.*

hemochromogen   Any substance that contains heme in combination with protein or other constituents.

hemoglobin hemochromogen   Denatured hemoglobin.

hemochromometer   HEMOGLOBINOMETER.

hemochromometry   HEMOGLOBINOMETRY.

hemocidal   Having the capability of destroying blood.

hemoclasia   The destruction of blood or blood cells. A seldom used term. Also called *hemoclasis*. Adjective: hemoclastic.

hemoclasis HEMOCLASIA.

hemoclip [HEMO- + *clip*, from Middle English *clippen* to embrace, from Old English *clyppan* to clasp] A malleable metal clip used to occlude small vessels during a surgical operation or to mark structures for radiographic study or postoperative irradiation.

hemocoagulation The clotting of blood.

hemocoagulin A substance in the venom of certain snakes, especially vipers, that induces the clotting of blood.

hemocoel [HEMO- + *coel(om)*] **1** A body cavity in which blood circulates freely without being confined to vessels, as in arthropods. **2** In vertebrates, the part of the coelomic body cavity involved in the development of the heart. For defs. 1 and 2 also called *hemocoelom, hemocoeloma*. Also *hemocele*.

hemocoelom HEMOCOEL.

hemocoeloma HEMOCOEL.

hemoconcentration A relative increase in the proportion of cellular components of blood due to reduction in the fluid component. Hemoconcentration may result from dehydration, from severe or extensive burns, or transiently in an extremity from prolonged application of a tourniquet prior to drawing a blood specimen.

hemocrine [HEMO- + *(endo)crine*] Capable of producing a hormonal influence in the blood.

hemocrinia The occurrence of hormones in the blood. A seldom used term.

hemoculture Culture of the blood to isolate microbial agents, usually bacteria.

hemocyanin An oxygen-carrying, copper-containing blood pigment found in arthopods and mollusks. It is often used as an experimental antigen in immunologic studies.

hemocyte [HEMO- + -CYTE] Any formed element of the blood. Also called *hematocyte*. Also *hemacyte*.

hemocytoblast The totipotential precursor of mesenchymal origin, probably of lymphoid appearance, which can develop into any of the formed blood elements. It is the keystone of the monophyletic theory of hematopoiesis. Also called *hematoblast, Hayem's hematoblast, hematocytoblast, hematoplast, hemoblast, hemagonium, lymphoidocyte*.

hemocytoblastoma LEUKEMIA.

hemocytocatheresis HEMOLYSIS.

hemocytogenesis HEMATOPOIESIS.

hemocytology The study of blood cells.

hemocytolysis The destruction of formed elements of the blood. The term includes hemolysis, leukocytolysis, and thrombocytolysis.

hemocytolytic HEMOLYTIC.

hemocytoma [HEMO- + CYTOMA] A tumor of hematopoietic cells.

hemocytometer A device used in the microscopic enumeration of blood cells. It consists of a thin glass tablet on which are scored grids of precise dimensions, so that when a 0.1 mm thick film of diluted blood is placed above the grids, the number of cells in a volume of blood may be determined by microscopic examination. Also called *counting chamber, hemacytometer, hematocytometer, hematimeter, Zappert's chamber*.

hemocytophagia The ingestion of blood cells by phagocytes.

hemocytophagic **1** Relating to hemocytophagia. **2** Capable of ingesting blood cells: used of phagocytes.

hemocytopoiesis HEMATOPOIESIS.

hemocytotripsis The mechanical destruction of blood cells.

hemocytozoa Plural of HEMOCYTOZOON.

hemocytozoon [HEMO- + CYTO- + Gk *zōon* living being, animal] (*plural* hemocytozoa) A parasitic protozoan found in blood cells; a haemosporidium. A seldom used term. Also called *hemacytozoon, hematocytozoon*.

hemodia [Gk *haimōdia(ein)* to set the teeth on edge] The condition of having abnormally sensitive teeth.

hemodiafiltration [HEMO- + DIA- + FILTRATION] SIMULTANEOUS HEMODIALYSIS AND HEMOFILTRATION. See under HEMOFILTRATION.

hemodiagnosis A diagnosis resulting from examination of the blood. Also called *hematomancy*.

hemodialysis [HEMO- + DIALYSIS] A process by which certain molecules are removed from circulating blood of uremic patients by diffusion through a semipermeable membrane. Access to blood is achieved through an external arteriovenous shunt, or more commonly, an arteriovenous fistula produced surgically. Also called *hemocatharsis*.

sequential ultrafiltration-hemodialysis A process by which fluid, electrolytes, and substances of relatively small molecular weight are removed from whole blood by convective transport through a conventional hemodialysis membrane combined with ultrafiltration. The ultrafiltration may be performed before or after the hemodialysis.

simultaneous hemodialysis and hemofiltration See under HEMOFILTRATION.

hemodialyzer An apparatus by which hemodialysis may be carried out, blood being separated by a semipermeable membrane from a solution of such composition as to cause diffusion of certain unwanted molecules out of the blood. A variety of different hemodialysis machines and semipermeable membranes are available. Treatments are given two or three times weekly in endstage renal disease, with repeated access to the vascular system usually through an internal, surgically produced arteriovenous shunt. Also called *artificial kidney* (popular).

ultrafiltration hemodialyzer A hemodialyzer in which fluid pressure causes filtration of a protein-free fluid out of the blood, used in the management of fluid overload in the presence of acute or chronic renal failure, or in intractable congestive heart failure.

hemodiapedesis The passage of red cells through capillary walls into the tissues. Also called *hematopedesis*.

hemodilution The reduction of hematocrit, or the lowering of hemoglobin or erythrocyte concentration of blood, resulting from augmentation of plasma volume.

hemodromogram [HEMO- + DROMO- + -GRAM] A graphic record of blood flow velocity.

hemodromograph An instrument for recording speed of blood flow. Also called *hemodromometer*.

hemodromography [HEMO- + DROMO- + -GRAPHY] The procedure of recording blood flow velocity. Also called *hemodromometry*.

hemodromometer HEMODROMOGRAPH.

hemodromometry HEMODROMOGRAPHY.

hemodynamic [HEMO- + DYNAMIC] Of or relating to the process of blood circulation.

hemodynamics The science concerned with the study of blood circulation. Also called *hemohydraulics*.

hemodynamometer HEMOMANOMETER.

hemodynamometry HEMOMANOMETRY.

hemodyscrasia Any disorder of the blood or blood-forming tissues, especially diseases of the formed elements. Also called *hemodystrophy* (incorrect).

hemodystrophy An incorrect term for HEMODYSCRASIA. ● Usage excludes temporary disorders although the term implies remediable nutritional causes.

hemoendothelial Describing a type of placentation in which maternal blood comes in contact with the endothelium of the placenta, occurring in rats, guinea pigs, and rabbits. The endothelium alone, of fetal vessels, separates fetal blood from the maternal blood sinuses. See also HEMOENDOTHELIAL PLACENTA.

Hemofil A proprietary name for factor VIII.

hemofiltration [HEMO- + FILTRATION] An extracorporeal process by which the fluid and solute composition of blood and body fluids can be corrected by a combination of ultrafiltration and convective solute loss and dilution with physiologic saline solution. Dilution may occur before or after the ultrafiltration. This treatment requires an apparatus similar to a hemodialyzer. The membrane has a high ultrafiltration capability. Usually rates of blood flow of 250–350 ml/min are required to maintain ultrafiltration rates in the range of 50–150 ml/min. The process removes 25–30 liters of ultrafiltrate during a period of five or six hours. During therapy, simultaneous reinfusion of a physiologic saline solution is required. Equipment which can balance fluid removal and replacement, preventing marked intravascular shifts, is necessary for the performance of hemofiltration. Although the technique is less efficient than hemodialysis for removing substances of small molecular weight, such as urea nitrogen and creatinine, it has the advantage of efficient removal of excess fluid without cardiovascular instability. The technique also allows for the removal of substances of larger molecular weight. Increased protein loss could mean retrogression if repeated therapy is necessary.

simultaneous hemodialysis and hemofiltration A system of extracorporeal treatment which utilizes convective and diffusive transport simultaneously. Membranes must have high permeability for fluid and be satisfactory for hemodialysis, such as polyacrylonitrile or cellulose acetate. The patient may be simultaneously hemodialyzed while up to 100 ml of ultrafiltrate is removed each minute. A replacement solution is reinfused at the rate of 60–90 ml/min. The combined and additive effectiveness of diffusion and convective transport results in a reduction of treatment time. Also, the combined therapy results in a lower incidence of cardiovascular instability during treatment. A major advantage of this form of therapy is a shortened treatment time. However, it does require more complicated and expensive equipment. Also called *hemodiafiltration.*

hemoflagellate [HEMO- + FLAGELLATE] Any flagellate protozoan of the family Trypanosomatidae that is parasitic in the blood. Found in many species of birds and animals, including man, hemoflagellates include the genera *Trypanosoma* and *Leishmania,* which contain species that are important human and animal pathogens, causing a wide spectrum of diseases.

hemofuscin A yellow-brown nonferrous pigment present in the tissues in hemochromatosis.

hemogenesis HEMATOPOIESIS.

hemogenic HEMATOPOIETIC.

hemoglobin [HEMO- + GLOBIN (for GLOBULIN)] A heme protein of approximately 64 000 MW that transports oxygen and carbon dioxide and constitutes approximately 99% of the protein content of mammalian erythrocytes. It also occurs also in other animal phyla and in plants, as in root nodules o f legumes (leghemoglobin). Hemoglobin is a tetramer of four subunits, each consisting of a globin chain of amino acids and a heme group.

hemoglobin A The predominant form of human hemoglobin, the molecule of which consists of two α and two β chains.

hemoglobin A_2 A normally present component of hemoglobin that is a tetramer of α and δ globin chains, i.e. $\alpha_2\delta_2$. Hemoglobin A_2 normally makes up 1.5–3% of the hemoglobin in adults or children of age greater than six months. An elevated proportion of hemoglobin A_2 is usually indicative of β-thalassemia trait.

hemoglobin A_{1c} A minor form of hemoglobin in normal blood. It contains carbohydrate linked to the N-terminal valine of the β chains, probably in the form of the Amadori rearrangement product of glucosylated protein, i.e. the furanose form of fructose in which O-1 is replaced by the amino group of the valine residue. Its concentration is raised in diabetes. See also GLYCOSYLATED HEMOGLOBIN.

abnormal hemoglobin Any hemoglobin found in only a minority of individuals. Such hemoglobins often contain a single change in amino-acid sequence.

hemoglobin Bart's A hemoglobin variant that is a tetramer of γ chains (γ_4) and which, when present in blood, is evidence of α-thalassemia.

hemoglobin C An abnormal human hemoglobin in which lysine occurs instead of glutamate at position 6 of the beta chain, i.e. $\beta6(A2)$Glu→Lys. This is due to a mutation at the beta locus, allelic to the mutation for hemoglobin S. The presence of hemoglobin C causes a mild hemolytic anemia in the heterozygote and a more severe disorder when homozygous. Hemoglobin C is common in West Africa and among a small proportion of black Americans.

hemoglobin Constant Spring A hemoglobin variant in which the α chain is extended by addition of 31 amino acids to the C-terminal end as a result of mutation of a nonsense (termination) codon of DNA. When present in blood, it usually comprises 1–3% of the total hemoglobin, and has the effect of a mild α-thalassemia trait. Although described from the village of Constant Spring, Jamaica, hemoglobin Constant Spring is found only in Asians. It is a common hemoglobin variant in Chinese and in Southeast Asians.

hemoglobin D Any of a group of hemoglobin variants due to amino acid substitutions in the β-globin chain that confer abnormal electrophoretic mobility. The most common of these is hemoglobin D-Punjab (or hemoglobin D-Los Angeles), which differs from normal adult hemoglobin A by having glutamine rather than glutamic acid as the 121st amino acid of the β-globin chain, i.e. $\beta121(GH4)$Glu→Gln.

hemoglobin E A hemoglobin variant that differs from the normal hemoglobin A by having lysine rather than glutamic acid as the 26th amino acid of the β-globin chain, i.e. $\beta26(B8)$Glu→Lys. Hemoglobin E is very common in persons of Southeast Asian ancestry.

hemoglobin F The predominant hemoglobin of fetal life. It is a tetramer of α and γ globin chains, $\alpha_2\gamma_2$, and has a higher affinity for oxygen than does adult hemoglobin. At birth, hemoglobin F is 50–70% of the total hemoglobin, but the proportion of hemoglobin F declines rapidly. In adults and children of age greater than one year, hemoglobin F normally is not more than 1% of total hemoglobin. Elevated proportions of hemoglobin F occur in thalassemias and other chronic anemias. Also called *fetal hemoglobin.*

fast hemoglobins Those variant hemoglobins that, upon electrophoresis at pH 8.6–9.0, run ahead of the normal hemoglobin A. They are more negatively charged than hemoglobin A. Glycosylated hemoglobin is the fast hemoglobin component that is in the first fraction eluted from certain ion-exchange resin chromatography columns.

fetal hemoglobin HEMOGLOBIN F.

hemoglobin G Any of several hemoglobin variants that exhibit mobility identical with, or just slightly greater than hemoglobin S upon electrophoresis in alkaline media. The most commonly encountered is hemoglobin G-Philadelphia [$\alpha68(E17)$ Asn→Lys], a hemoglobin variant that is found commonly in the blood of black people. Other G-hemoglobins are rare.

glycosylated hemoglobin Any complex of hemoglobin with glucose or related monosaccharides, in which the monosaccharide binds to the N-terminal end of the β globin chain. Among glycosylated hemoglobins are hemoglobin A_{Ic}, a complex of hemoglobin A with glucose; A_{Ia1}, a complex of hemoglobin A with fructose diphosphate; and A_{Ia2}, a complex of hemoglobin A with glucose 6-phosphate.

hemoglobin Gower Either of two human hemoglobins normally present in blood during the first three months of embryonic life. They contain the prefetal globin chains ζ (a prefetal α chain) and ϵ (a prefetal non-α chain). Hemoglobin Gower-1 is $\zeta_2\epsilon_2$ and hemoglobin Gower-2 is $\alpha_2\epsilon_2$. • The term is never used without specifying it as Gower-1 or Gower-2.

hemoglobin H A hemoglobin variant that is a tetramer of β-globin chains, (β_4). Hemoglobin H is an expression of α-thalassemia. Rarely it occurs as an epiphenomenon of erythroleukemia.

homozygous hemoglobin C A disorder that results from inheritance of a gene for hemoglobin C from both parents. The condition is associated with mild anemia, erythrocytic hypochromia, and numerous target erythrocytes. Also called *called hemoglobin C disease.*

homozygous hemoglobin D A minor disorder that results from inheritance of a gene for hemoglobin D from both parents. Homozygous hemoglobin D-Punjab has been associated with mild erythrocytic microcytosis. It is very rare except in northwest India. Also called *hemoglobin D disease.*

homozygous hemoglobin E A minor condition due to inheritance of a gene for hemoglobin E from both parents. The condition is associated with moderate erythrocytic microcytosis and hypochromia, and occasionally with minimal anemia. Also called *hemoglobin E disease* (incorrect).

hemoglobin J Any of several hemoglobin variants that exhibit more rapid anodal mobility than hemoglobin A upon electrophoresis in alkaline media. In such media, the position of hemoglobin J is as far ahead of (anodal to) hemoglobin A as hemoglobin S is behind (cathodal to)hemoglobin A. Hemoglobins J-Baltimore $[\beta15(A12)Gly \rightarrow Asp]$ and J-Oxford $[\alpha15(A13) Gly \rightarrow Asp]$ are found occasionally in blood specimens of blacks and Caucasians respectively. All other J-hemoglobins are very rare.

hemoglobin K Any of three hemoglobin variants, with amino acid substitutions in the β chain, that exhibit slightly faster anodal mobility than hemoglobin A, but less than hemoglobin J, upon electrophoresis in alkaline media. Of the three K-hemoglobins, (K-Woolwich, K-Ibadan, and K-Cameroon), all were reported in blood specimens from black persons, and all appear to be quite rare.

hemoglobin Köln An unstable hemoglobin variant that causes continual mild hemolytic anemia, jaundice, and splenomegaly. Although rare, it is the unstable hemoglobin most commonly encountered in people of north European origin. Hemoglobin Köln is $\beta98(FG5) Val \rightarrow Met.$

hemoglobin Lepore An abnormal human hemoglobin in which two normal α chains pair with two abnormal globin chains, the latter being 146 amino acids long and composed of the N-terminal portion of normal δ-globin chains and the C-terminal portion of normal β-globin chains. It is thought to arise from unequal recombination between the closely linked delta and beta globin genes. • This hemoglobin is named for the family in which the variant was first discovered.

hemoglobin M Any of a group of hemoglobin variants in which the heme iron of one pair of globin chains is in the Fe(III) state because of an amino acid substitution.

mean corpuscular hemoglobin The average amount of hemoglobin per erythrocyte in a sample of blood, expressed in picograms. It is calculated by dividing hemoglobin (in grams per liter) by erythrocyte count. Also called *blood quotient.* Abbreviation: MCH, MCHg

muscle hemoglobin An outmoded term for MYOGLOBIN.

hemoglobin N Any of three hemoglobin variants, with amino acid substitutions in the β chain, that exhibit a slightly more rapid anodal mobility than hemoglobin J upon electrophoresis in alkaline media. Hemoglobin N-Baltimore $[\beta95(FG2) Lys \rightarrow Glu]$ is found occasionally in blood specimens of black persons. The other N-hemoglobins are very rare.

hemoglobin O Any of three hemoglobin variants that exhibit mobility identical with that of hemoglobin C upon electrophoresis in alkaline media. The most commonly encountered is hemoglobin O-Arab $[\beta121(GH4)Glu \rightarrow Lys]$, a hemoglobin variant that is found occasionally in the blood of black people or of Bulgarians.

oxidized hemoglobin **1** METHEMOGLOBIN. **2** OXYHEMOGLOBIN. • Because of the ambiguity of this term, it is best avoided.

reduced hemoglobin The deoxygenated form of hemoglobin. Also called *deoxyhemoglobin.*

hemoglobin S An abnormal human hemoglobin due to the presence of a valine residue instead of glutamate at position 6 of the β-globin chain, i.e. $\beta6(A2)Glu \rightarrow Val$. This mutation results in a conformational alteration in the hemoglobin molecule when deoxygenation occurs, with the result that the erythrocyte assumes a "sickle" shape. When both alleles at the beta locus have this mutation, sickle cell disease results. Heterozygosity for the mutant allele and the normal allele results in sickle cell trait. Hemoglobin S occurs in approximately 8% of black people in North America. Also called *sickle hemoglobin.* Abbreviation: HbS

sickle hemoglobin HEMOGLOBIN S.

slow hemoglobins Hemoglobin variants which, on electrophoresis at pH 8.6–9.0, migrate more slowly toward the anode than does the normal hemoglobin A. The reason for their slow electrophoretic mobility is that they contain more positively charged amino acids than does hemoglobin A.

unstable hemoglobin A hemoglobin variant that precipitates more readily than does normal adult hemoglobin A upon mild heating or chemical or mechanical stress.

hemoglobin Zürich An unstable hemoglobin variant that predisposes a person having it to hemolytic anemia when sulfonamides are ingested. Hemoglobin Zürich is $\beta63(E7) His \rightarrow Arg.$ The condition is very rare.

hemoglobinated Containing or mixed with hemoglobin.

hemoglobinemia [HEMOGLOBIN + -EMIA] A greater than normal concentration of hemoglobin in plasma. Also called *hyperhemoglobinemia.*

hemoglobinemia paralytica An incorrect term for PARALYTIC MYOGLOBINURIA.

puerperal hemoglobinemia A hemolytic disease of cattle, sometimes fatal, characteristically seen in stabled cows 14 to 28 days after calving. Also called *puerperal hemoglobinuria.*

hemoglobiniferous **1** Bearing hemoglobin. **2** Of or pertaining to hemoglobin. For defs. 1 and 2 also *hemoglobinous.*

hemoglobinocholia The presence of free hemoglobin in bile.

hemoglobinolysis Splitting or fractionation of the hemoglobin molecule by chemical means. Also called *hemoglobinopepsia.*

hemoglobinometer An instrument for determining hemoglobin concentration of blood, plasma, or other fluids. Also called *hematinometer, hematometer, hemochromoneter, hemometer.*

hemoglobinometry The determination of hemoglobin concentration of blood, plasma, or other fluids. Also called *hemochromometry, hemometry.*

Sahli's hemoglobinometry Measurement of blood hemoglobin concentration by conversion of hemoglobin to acid hematin, and estimating its concentration by comparison with a calibrated tinted glass wedge. An obsolete procedure.

hemoglobinopathy   Any abnormality of the hemoglobin molecule, whether inherited or acquired, quantitative or qualitative, including unbalanced globin chain production, amino acid substitutions, deletions, and additions within globin chains, and abnormalities of the heme group. Most hemoglobinopathies do not result in clinical disease.

hemoglobinopepsia   HEMOGLOBINOLYSIS.

hemoglobinous   HEMOGLOBINIFEROUS.

hemoglobinuria [HEMOGLOBIN + -URIA]   The presence of free hemoglobin or its derivatives in urine, whenever its concentration in plasma exceeds the maximum saturation of plasma haptoglobin. The urine is dark brown in color. Hemoglobinuria should be differentiated from lysis of erythrocytes during hematuria by dilute or alkaline urine. Hemoglobinuria may result from toxins, some infections, incompatible blood transfusions, extensive burns, excessive physical exertion, and as a feature of paroxysmal nocturnal hypoglobinuria, or paroxysmal cold hemoglobinuria. Sudden hemoglobinuria may be a primary cause of or a contributing factor to acute renal failure. Also called *methemoglobinuria*.

epidemic hemoglobinuria   WINCKEL'S DISEASE.

intermittent hemoglobinuria   Recurrent attacks of hemoglobinuria characteristic of paroxysmal nocturnal hemoglobinuria or paroxysmal cold hemoglobinuria.

malarial hemoglobinuria   BLACKWATER FEVER.

march hemoglobinuria   An episodic form of hemolysis, caused by unusually intense or prolonged physical activity (such as running or marching) sufficient to cause mechanical injury to circulating erythrocytes.

paroxysmal cold hemoglobinuria   A rare disorder characterized by acute severe hemolytic anemia following exposure to cold. There is usually hemoglobinuria, and a serum test for Donath-Landsteiner antibody is positive. Also called *Donath-Landsteiner syndrome*.

paroxysmal nocturnal hemoglobinuria   A rare disorder, reflecting acquired erythrocyte hypersensitivity to the lytic effect of complement, that is manifested by intravascular hemolysis, hemoglobinuria, hemosiderinuria, positive Ham test, Crosby test, and sucrose lysis test, and is often accompanied by other cytopenias. Also called *Marchiafava-Micheli syndrome* (rarely used), *Marchiafava-Micheli disease* (rarely used). • The name implies increased nocturnal hemolysis, because the first morning urine is most concentrated and pigments from hemolysis more noticeable. In fact, hemolysis is not greater at night.

puerperal hemoglobinuria   PUERPERAL HEMOGLOBINEMIA.

toxic hemoglobinuria   The presence of free hemoglobin in the urine following exposure to various toxic substances, or as a result of infection.

hemoglobinuric   Of or pertaining to hemoglobinuria.

hemogram   COMPLETE BLOOD COUNT.

hemohistioblast   A mesenchymal progenitor capable of differentiating into any normal cellular element of blood. Also called *hematohistioblast, Ferrata cell*.

hemohydraulics   HEMODYNAMICS.

hemohydrosalpinx [HEMO- + HYDROSALPINX]   An accumulation of blood and fluid in a fallopian tube.

hemokinesis   The movement of blood.

hemokinetic   Pertaining to blood flow.

hemolith [HEMO- + -LITH]   A concretion in the wall of a blood vessel; an angiolith. An obsolete term. Also called *hematolith*.

hemology   HEMATOLOGY.

hemolymph   **1** The circulating body fluids, including blood and lymph, taken as a whole.   **2** A type of body fluid in certain invertebrates, analogous to both blood and lymph. It may be found free in the body cavity, or in restricted parts of the coelom, or within the vascular bed, as in insects.

hemolymphadenosis   HEMOBLASTOSIS.

hemolymphangioma [HEMO- + LYMPHANGIOMA]   A tumor composed of blood vessels and lymphatics. Also called *hematolymphangioma, hemangiolymphangioma*.

hemolymphocytotoxin   A factor found in the hemolymph of invertebrates which has the ability to kill mammalian cells. Such factors are quite frequent but seem to have no close relationship to the antibodies or complement components found in vertebrates.

hemolysate   The fluid that is formed upon lysis of blood cells. Also called *blood cytolysate*.

hemolysin [HEMO- + LYSIN]   An antibody capable of inducing red cell destruction in the presence of complement. Also called *erythrolysin, erythrocytolysin, erythrocyto-opsonin*.

α-hemolysin   The most common of the four cytolytic toxins produced by *Staphylococcus aureus*. It lyses rabbit but not human erythrocytes. When injected into experimental animals it causes aggregation and lysis of platelets of man and rabbits, and causes local necrosis of skin and tissue.

β-hemolysin   One of the four cytolytic toxins produced by *Staphylococcus aureus*, found most often in bovine strains and in about 20 percent of human strains. A hot-cold lysin, it lyses sheep, beef, and human erythrocytes only when incubation at 37°C is followed by refrigeration.

γ-hemolysin   One of the four cytolytic toxins produced by *Staphylococcus aureus*. It consists of two components that synergistically induce hemolysis of rabbit, sheep, and human erythrocytes. Its action is inhibited by sulfated polymers, including agar.

δ-hemolysin   One of the four cytolytic toxins produced by *Staphylococcus aureus*. It has a broad range of lytic and cytotoxic activity, but serum phospholipids inhibit its action and it therefore may not exert an effect *in vivo*.

acid hemolysin   A hemolytic antibody with a pH optimum below 7.0.

bacterial hemolysin   Any hemolysin produced by bacteria.

cold hemolysin   DONATH-LANDSTEINER ANTIBODY.

hot-cold hemolysin   A hemolytic antibody with biphasic activity such that the temperature at which it attaches to its specific antigen is different from that at which the antibody-coated cells hemolyze.

immune hemolysin   A hemolytic antibody produced in the host animal or individual after immunizing exposure to blood cells carrying the antigen for which the antibody is specific. It may be a human antibody against an alloantigen or an antibody raised in animals against a heterogenous antigen.

natural hemolysin   A naturally occurring antibody capable of inducing red cell destruction in the presence of complement.

specific hemolysin   Antibody capable of inducing red cell destruction by its specific reactivity with the corresponding antigen on the red cell surface and complement fixation.

hemolysis [HEMO- + LYSIS]   The destruction or dissolution of erythrocytes. Also called *erythrocytolysis, erythrolysis, cythemolysis, globulysis, globulolysis, hemocatheresis* (seldom used), *hematocytolysis, hemolyzation* (seldom used), *hematolysis, hemocytocatheresis, hemoclastic reaction*. Adjective: hemolytic.

α hemolysis   The partial decomposition of hemoglobin characteristic of certain strains of streptococci and pneumococci. It appears as a greenish color surrounding a bacterial colony in blood agar. Also called *viridans hemolysis*.

β hemolysis   Hemolysis in which a transparent area is apparent surrounding a colony of certain pathogenic bacteria in blood agar.

biologic hemolysis   Hemolysis by substances produced by animals or plants.

contact hemolysis   Accelerated destruction of erythrocytes as a result of mechanical stress during or following contact with a foreign surface.

immune hemolysis   The lysis by complement of antibody-sensitized erythrocytes.

osmotic hemolysis   Disruption of erythrocytes, and loss of their cytosol, as a consequence of swelling and bursting in hypotonic solution.

passive hemolysis   Hemolysis occurring in the presence of complement and antibody directed to an antigen adsorbed or chemically coupled onto the surface of erythrocytes. It is used as a test for antibodies to various antigens that can be bound to erythrocytes.

siderogenous hemolysis   Any condition in which accelerated destruction of blood (hemolysis) is associated with increased body iron stores, as in thalassemia major.

venom hemolysis   The lysis of erythrocytes by toxins produced by animals such as snakes and arachnids.

viridans hemolysis   α HEMOLYSIS.

hemolytic   Relating to, characterized by, or producing hemolysis. Also *hematolytic, hyperhemolytic, hemocytolytic, globulolytic.*

hemolyzable   Subject to hemolysis.

hemolyzation   A seldom used term for HEMOLYSIS.

hemolyze   To subject to or undergo hemolysis. Also *lake.*

hemomanometer   An instrument for measuring the blood pressure. Also called *hemopiezometer.*

hemomanometry   The process of blood pressure measurement. Also called *hemodynamometry, hemadynometry.*

hemomediastinum   A hematoma in the mediastinum. Also called *hematomediastinum.*

hemometakinesia   HEMATOMETAKINESIS.

hemometakinesis   HEMATOMETAKINESIS.

hemometer   HEMOGLOBINOMETER.

hemometra   HEMATOMETRA.

hemometry   HEMOGLOBINOMETRY.

hemomyelogram   A differential cell count, or tabulation by cell type, of the cells identified in a specimen aspirated from the bone marrow.

hemomyelosis   HEMOBLASTOSIS.

hemonchosis [*Hemonch(us)*, var. of *Haemonchus* + -OSIS]   A disease mainly of sheep and cattle, characterized by anemia, due to bloodsucking of the stomach worm, *Haemonchus contortus.*

hemonephrosis [HEMO- + NEPHROSIS]   The presence of blood in the renal pelvis.

hemonormoblast   NORMOBLAST.

hemopathology   1 Disease of the blood or blood-forming organs or lymphatic tissues.   2 The study, especially by histologic technique, of diseases of the blood or blood-forming organs or lymphatic tissues.

hemopathy [HEMO- + -PATHY]   Any disease primarily involving the blood or blood-forming organs. Adjective: hemopathic.

hemoperfusion [HEMO- + PERFUSION]   The removal of substances from blood by passage through a column containing a substance over the surface of which the blood passes and comes into contact before leaving the column and returning to the patient. In contradistinction to hemodialysis, there is no semipermeable dialysis membrane and no dialysate. Blood comes directly into contact with the sorbent contained within the column, or the sorbent may be coated with a material preventing direct contact between the blood and the active ingredient of the column, if such contact would be detrimental, as by damaging or trapping formed elements of the blood, or by permitting embolization of the active ingredient of the column into the

blood. A variety of substances may be used as the active ingredient in the column over which blood is perfused. Selection of the active ingredient is determined by its affinity for the substance or substances whose removal from blood is desired.

charcoal hemoperfusion   Hemoperfusion performed through a column containing charcoal, usually activated charcoal. The charcoal may be uncoated or it may be coated with a protective substance to prevent direct contact between blood and charcoal.

resin hemoperfusion   Hemoperfusion performed through a column containing a resin as absorbent. A large variety of resins are available. Selection of the right resin depends upon its affinity for the substance whose removal from blood is desired. The resin may be uncoated, permitting direct contact between blood and resin, or it may be coated with a substance to prevent direct contact between blood and resin.

hemopericardium   Blood in the pericardial space. Also called *hematopericardium.*

hemoperitoneum   The presence of frank blood within the peritoneal cavity. Also called *hematoperitoneum.*

hemopexin   A plasma beta-globulin, produced by the liver, that binds heme when heme appears in plasma. The heme-hemopexin complex is removed from plasma by macrophages.

hemophage   ERYTHROPHAGOCYTE.

hemophagia [HEMO- + -PHAGIA]   HEMATOPHAGIA.

hemophagocyte   ERYTHROPHAGOCYTE.

hemophagocytosis   ERYTHROPHAGOCYTOSIS.

hemophil [HEMO- + -PHIL]   1 Any of the microorganisms which culture most successfully on media containing blood.   2 Any organism which prefers, or thrives on, blood.

hemophilia [HEMO- + -PHILIA]   A serious inherited hemorrhagic disease. Hemophilias A and B are X-linked while factor XI deficiency (hemophilia C) is autosomal. Also called *bleeders' disease, thromboplastinopenia* (obsolete), *hematophilia.* Adjective: hemophilic.

hemophilia A   An X-linked recessive disorder of blood coagulation due to deficiency of the coagulation moiety of factor VIII. The gene for factor VIII is located near the telomere of the long arm of the X chromosome, closely linked to the gene encoding glucose-6-phosphate dehydrogenase. Morbidity and mortality can be improved considerably by infusion of concentrates of human coagulation factors enriched for factor VIII. Also called *classical hemophilia.* See also VON WILLEBRAND'S DISEASE.

hemophilia B   An X-linked hereditary bleeding disease caused by a deficiency of factor IX. Also called *factor IX deficiency, Christmas disease, deuterohemophilia* (outmoded).

hemophilia C   An autosomally inherited bleeding disease resulting from a deficiency of factor XI. Also called *Rosenthal syndrome, plasma thromboplastin antecedent deficiency.*

classical hemophilia   HEMOPHILIA A.

hemophilia neonatorum   An incorrect term for HEMORRHAGIC DISEASE OF THE NEWBORN.

vascular hemophilia   The association of a prolonged bleeding time with a reduction of plasmatic factor VIII. Most, if not all, patients with vascular hemophilia have von Willebrand's disease.

hemophiliac   A person or animal with hemophilia.

hemophilic   Relating to hemophilia or hemophiliacs.

hemophilioid   Describing any bleeding tendency, usually of unknown origin, resembling one or another hemophilia.

Hemophilus [HEMO- + Gk *philos* beloved, loving]   *HAEMOPHILUS.* • This spelling is preferred by many microbiologists in the United States.

hemophilus   Any microorganism of the genus *Haemophilus.*

hemophobia [HEMO- + -PHOBIA] Pathologic fear of blood. Also called *hematophobia*.

hemophoresis [HEMO- + -PHORESIS] The movement of blood.

hemophoric [HEMO- + -*phor(e)* + -IC] Concerning the movement of blood.

hemophotograph A photograph of formed elements of the blood. An imprecise usage. Also *hemaphotograph*.

hemophotometer An instrument for determining hemoglobin concentration of blood by photometric or colorimetric means.

hemophthalmia [HEM- + OPHTHALMIA] Hemorrhage within the eye. Also called *hemophthalmos, hemophthalmus*.

hemophthalmos HEMOPHTHALMIA.

hemophthalmus HEMOPHTHALMIA.

hemophthisis Anemia due to impaired formation of erythrocytes.

hemopiezometer HEMOMANOMETER.

hemoplasmopathy Any disease characterized by quantitative or qualitative disturbance of plasma proteins. Also called *hematoplasmopathy*.

hemoplastic Relating to the growth and maturation of formed elements of the blood.

hemoplasty The formation of formed elements of the blood.

hemopleura HEMOTHORAX.

hemopneumopericardium The presence of both blood and gas in the pericardial space.

hemopneumothorax The presence of blood and air in the pleural cavity.

hemopoiesic HEMATOPOIETIC.

hemopoiesis HEMATOPOIESIS.

hemopoietic HEMATOPOIETIC.

hemoposia [HEMO- + Gk *pos(is)* a drinking + -IA] The drinking of blood, as by vampire bats, insects, or other metazoan parasites, or by humans for nutrition, therapy, or ritual purposes.

hemoproctia [HEMO- + PROCT- + -IA] Rectal bleeding.

hemoprotein Any protein containing a heme group, such as hemoglobin or cytochrome c.

Hemoproteus HAEMOPROTEUS.

hemoprotozoa [HEMO- + PROTOZOA] (*singular* hemoprotozoon) Protozoan parasites that circulate in the bloodstream during some stage in their development, for example, plasmodia and trypanosomes.

hemoptic HEMOPTYSIC.

hemoptoic HEMOPTYSIC.

hemoptysic Relating to or characterized by hemoptysis. Also *hemoptoic, hemoptic*.

hemoptysis [HEMO- + Gk *ptysis* a spitting] The expectoration of blood. Also called *emptysis*.

  cardiac hemoptysis Hemoptysis secondary to a cardiac disorder, particularly mitral stenosis.

  endemic hemoptysis PARAGONIMIASIS.

  Goldstein's hemoptysis Hemoptysis due to telangiectasia of the tracheobronchial tree.

  Manson's hemoptysis Hemoptysis as a result of pulmonary infection with *Paragonimus westermani*.

  oriental hemoptysis PARAGONIMIASIS.

  parasitic hemoptysis PARAGONIMIASIS.

  vicarious hemoptysis The coughing up of blood at the time of menstruation, usually caused by endometriosis of the lung or bronchial passages.

hemopyelectasis [HEMO- + PYELECTASIS] The presence of blood in a dilated renal pelvis. A rarely used term. Also called *hydrohematonephrosis*.

hemorepellant 1 Resistant to wetting by blood: said of a surface or substance. 2 A hemorepellant surface or substance.

hemorheology The study of the effect of blood flow on the constituents of the blood, especially the cellular components, and upon the vessel walls.

hemorrhachis HEMATORRHACHIS.

hemorrhage [HEMO- + -RRHAGE] 1 The escape of blood from blood vessels. Such bleeding continues until external pressure exceeds that within the blood vessel. 2 An accumulation of extravasated blood. See also PETECHIA, PURPURA, ECCHYMOSIS, HEMATOMA.

  accidental hemorrhage ABRUPTIO PLACENTAE.

  accidental antepartum hemorrhage ABRUPTIO PLACENTAE.

  arterial hemorrhage Hemorrhage from a ruptured artery. Also called *arteriorrhagia* (seldom used).

  capillary hemorrhage Hemorrhage from damaged capillary vessels.

  capsular hemorrhage Cerebral hemorrhage occurring in the internal capsule.

  capsuloganglionic hemorrhage Cerebral hemorrhage involving the internal capsule and basal ganglia.

  cerebellar hemorrhage Hemorrhage arising in or extending into the cerebellum.

  cerebral hemorrhage Hemorrhage occurring in one cerebral hemisphere or, less often, in both. The many causes include arteriosclerosis, hypertension, aneurysm, angioma, cerebral tumor, head injury, arteritis, and blood diseases. Also called *ictus sanguinis*.

  choroidal hemorrhage Hemorrhage within the posterior part of the uveal tract.

  concealed hemorrhage Hemorrhage that is not apparent on the surface.

  concealed antepartum hemorrhage The occurrence of abruptio placentae with accumulation of blood behind the placenta but without concomitant vaginal bleeding.

  consecutive hemorrhage RECURRING HEMORRHAGE.

  critical hemorrhage Hemorrhage that threatens either life or the function of the organ into which the bleeding occurs.

  cyclic hemorrhage MENORRHAGIA.

  dot hemorrhage A small hemorrhage, as may occur in the retina from diabetes.

  epidural hemorrhage EXTRADURAL HEMORRHAGE.

  essential hemorrhage Hemorrhage of unknown cause.

  essential uterine hemorrhage Hemorrhage into the cavity of the uterus which occurs in connection with pelvic, uterine, or cervical diseases.

  expulsive hemorrhage A severe choroidal hemorrhage occurring at the time of cataract extraction, usually forcing a large portion of the intraocular contents out of the incision.

  external hemorrhage Blood escaping through a wound in the skin. Unless issuing from deep-seated blood vessels, it can usually be controlled by direct pressure.

  extradural hemorrhage Hemorrhage occurring between the dura mater and the skull, usually caused by head injury with skull fracture and division of the middle meningeal artery or one of its branches. Also called *epidural hemorrhage*.

  fetomaternal hemorrhage Leakage of fetal blood cells into the maternal circulation. This usually occurs at the time of placental separation.

  fibrinolytic hemorrhage Hemorrhage due to a disorder of the fibrinolytic system.

  flame-shaped hemorrhages Bleeding into the nerve fiber layer of the retina, recognizable by its linear configuration. Also called *flame spots*.

  glomerular hemorrhage The presence of blood in the glomerular capsular space. This is a feature of glomerulonephritis.

gravitating hemorrhage   Hemorrhage within the spinal subarachnoid space with accumulation of blood, under the influence of gravity, in the lowest part of the spinal canal.

intermediary hemorrhage   A minor or moderate episode of bleeding preceding a catastrophic hemorrhage.

intermediate hemorrhage   Bleeding of moderate severity.

internal hemorrhage   Bleeding that is confined within the body cavity. It is usually not readily apparent on physical examination, but may be suspected from systemic reactions to blood loss.

intracerebral hemorrhage   Hemorrhage arising within the cerebrum. Also called *encephalorrhagia*.

intracranial hemorrhage   Hemorrhage occurring anywhere within the cranial cavity. Also called *sanguineous apoplexy* (outmoded).

intradural hemorrhage   SUBDURAL HEMORRHAGE.

intramedullary hemorrhage   HEMATOMYELIA.

intrapartum hemorrhage   The occurrence of hemorrhage usually due to abruptio placentae or placenta previa during labor.

intraventricular hemorrhage   Hemorrhage arising within the cerebral ventricles.

massive hemorrhage   Hemorrhage severe enough to cause shock. In otherwise healthy individuals this amounts to 15 to 20 percent of the blood volume, or about 1.2 liters in a person weighing 70 kg.

meningeal hemorrhage   SUBARACHNOID HEMORRHAGE.

nasal hemorrhage   EPISTAXIS.

neonatal subdural hemorrhage   Subdural hemorrhage occurring in neonates.

nuclear hemorrhage   Cerebral hemorrhage involving the central grey nuclei of the cerebral hemisphere, and most often involving the external portion of the lenticular nucleus (putamen).

parenchymatous hemorrhage   Hemorrhage into the parenchyma of an organ.

hemorrhage per rhexin   Hemorrhage due to rupture of a vessel.

petechial hemorrhage   Punctate hemorrhage under the skin, producing petechiae.

plasma hemorrhage   The loss of blood plasma from the vascular system.

pontine hemorrhage   Hemorrhage arising in or extending into the pons.

postpartum hemorrhage   The occurrence of hemorrhage during the postpartum period. The most frequent causes are uterine atony, retained placental tissue, or an unrecognized laceration of the birth canal.

primary hemorrhage   1 Hemorrhage immediately following injury.   2 SPONTANEOUS HEMORRHAGE.

pulmonary hemorrhage in newborn   Hemorrhage into the pulmonary alveoli, and to a lesser degree into the interstitial tissue of the lung, a complication of the respiratory distress syndrome, pneumonia, or severe anoxia, and a common autopsy finding in neonatal deaths from varied causes. Symptoms are respiratory distress and oozing of frothy blood from nose and mouth, with death ensuing in 48 hours.

punctate hemorrhage   Hemorrhage at minute points in the skin or other organs.

recurring hemorrhage   Recurrent episodes of capillary hemorrhage. Also called *consecutive hemorrhage*.

renal hemorrhage   Hemorrhage from or into a kidney. An imprecise usage. Also called *renal apoplexy* (rarely used).

retinal hemorrhage   Bleeding within the retina of the eye.

revealed antepartum hemorrhage   Hemorrhage due to abruptio placentae with concomitant vaginal bleeding.

secondary hemorrhage   1 Hemorrhage that is delayed fol-lowing injury. It usually occurs when a vessel is damaged but is able to withstand the internal pressure for a time. It also occurs when an expanding hematoma finally ruptures the capsule of an organ such as the liver, spleen, or kidney.   2 Bleeding that is delayed following surgery. It may be caused by slippage of a ligature by or elevation of the patient's blood pressure enough to overcome pressure external to the blood vessel.

slit hemorrhage   A linear extension of intracerebral hemorrhage usually found in the white matter, separating fiber bundles or tracts.

splinter hemorrhage   A linear hemorrhage found at the base of or under the nail bed. It is diagnostically important in bacterial endocarditis, microembolic disease, and some forms of vasculitis. It may also occur as a result of minor trauma to the fingers.

spontaneous hemorrhage   Hemorrhage occurring without evident provocation. Also called *primary hemorrhage*.

subarachnoid hemorrhage   Hemorrhage occurring in the subarachnoid space. The many causes include intracranial aneurysm, angioma, head injury, neoplasia, and blood disease. Also called *meningeal hemorrhage*.

subconjunctival hemorrhage   Hemorrhage beneath the conjunctiva, arising spontaneously or resulting from trauma.

subdural hemorrhage   Hemorrhage occurring in the subdural space, between the dura and the arachnoid. This usually results from head injury with rupture of veins which traverse the space, and it can be acute, subacute, or chronic. In rare cases it results from blood or liver disease or occurs as a complication of anticoagulant therapy. Also called *intradural hemorrhage*.

subgaleal hemorrhage   Hemorrhage arising beneath the galea aponeurotica.

subhyaloid hemorrhage   Hemorrhage occurring between the retina and the hyaloid membrane of the eye which separates the retina from the vitreous. It is usually brick-red in color, extending outwards from the optic disk and is diagnostic of subarachnoid hemorrhage.

thalamic hemorrhage   A fairly common form of cerebral hemorrhage which normally involves the posterior part of the internal capsule as well as the thalamus.

toxemic accidental hemorrhage   Abruptio placentae associated with the manifestations of toxemia of pregnancy. Also called *toxemic antepartum hemorrhage*.

toxemic antepartum hemorrhage   TOXEMIC ACCIDENTAL HEMORRHAGE.

unavoidable hemorrhage   Hemorrhage in association with placenta previa.

venous hemorrhage   Loss of blood from a vein.

vicarious hemorrhage   The occurrence of hemorrhage in one area as a result of suppression of bleeding in another area.

hemorrhagic   Causing, resulting from, or characterized by hemorrhage.

hemorrhagin   A toxic substance present in certain venoms and plant seeds, such as snake venom and castor beans (*Ricinus communis*). It causes extensive destruction of the endothelial cells in blood vessels.

hemorrheology   The study of the flow of blood. Adjective: hemorrheologic.

hemorrhoid [Gk *haimorrhoos* (from *haima* blood + *rhoos* a stream, from *rheein* to flow, stream) a streaming with blood] A varicosity of one of the veins comprising the hemorrhoidal venous plexus (plexus venosus rectalis).

acute hemorrhoid   A newly formed hemorrhoid.

combined hemorrhoid   MIXED HEMORRHOID.

cutaneous hemorrhoid   EXTERNAL HEMORRHOID.

external hemorrhoid   A hemorrhoid below the pectinate line, covered by anal skin, and involving only the inferior venous plexus. Also called *cutaneous hemorrhoid*.

internal hemorrhoid   A hemorrhoid above the pectinate line, covered by mucous membrane, and involving the superior venous plexus.

mixed hemorrhoid   A hemorrhoid extending above and below the pectinate line, usually representing a connection between the superior and inferior rectal venous plexuses. Also called *combined hemorrhoid, mucocutaneous hemorrhoid*.

mucocutaneous hemorrhoid   MIXED HEMORRHOID.

prolapsed hemorrhoid   An internal hemorrhoid which protrudes from the anus.

strangulated hemorrhoid   A prolapsed internal hemorrhoid which has been cut off from its blood supply.

thrombosed hemorrhoid   A strangulated hemorrhoid which, because of compromised blood flow, has become thrombosed. The hemorrhoid becomes hard, tender, and nonreducible and results in perianal pain.

hemorrhoidal   **1** Of or relating to hemorrhoids.   **2** Rectal: designating arteries, veins, and nerves of the rectum.

hemorrhoidectomy [HEMORRHOID + -ECTOMY]   Surgical excision or removal of hemorrhoids.

hemorrhoidolysis   The destruction of hemorrhoids by means other than direct surgical removal, as by diathermy or chemical treatment.

hemorrhoids   A condition in which there are varicosities in veins of the hemorrhoidal plexus, often associated with hematochezia, pruritus ani, or anorectal pain. Although often associated with constipation, its cause is not known. Also called *piles, St. Fiacre's disease* (obsolete).

hemosalpinx   HEMATOSALPINX.

hemosarcoma   An obsolete term for LEUKEMIA.

hemosialemesis [HEMO- + SIAL- + EMESIS]   The production of saliva containing traces of blood.

hemosiderin [HEMO- + *sider(o)*- + -IN]   An iron-rich protein found in the liver and some other organs. It is probably a form of ferritin.

hemosiderinuria   The presence of hemosiderin in the urine, associated with hemosiderosis.

hemosiderosis [*hemosider(in)* + -OSIS]   The deposition of iron within tissues, either diffusely or focally, not associated with injury or fibrosis of the affected organs.

hepatic hemosiderosis   Deposition of large quantities of iron in hepatic tissue, generally seen within sinusoidal Kupffer cells and not resulting in hepatic cirrhosis or fibrosis.

nutritional hemosiderosis   The presence of excess iron in the body arising from an excessive dietary intake and demonstrated by the presence of hemosiderin in the tissues. When slight overloading occurs, the iron is deposited in the liver's parenchymal cells but no clinical manifestations are apparent. With increasing iron intake, the Kupffer cells become loaded and eventually their portals contract. This may result in fibrosis and be a contributing cause to cirrhosis. Alcoholics who drink inexpensive wines rich in iron (10–350 mg/l) are especially subject to the condition. Hemosiderosis is also common among those peoples who traditionally cook in iron pots. Also called *nutritional siderosis*.

pulmonary hemosiderosis   The presence of hemosiderin-laden macrophages within alveoli and interstitium of the lung. In addition to an idiopathic form occurring in children and young adults, it may result from severe left-sided heart failure and the Goodpasture syndrome.

transfusional hemosiderosis   Chronic iron overload that results from repeated blood transfusions.

hemosite [HEMO- + *(para)site*]   A blood parasite. An obsolete term.

hemospermia [HEMO- + SPERM + -IA]   The occurrence of blood in the semen. Also called *hematospermia*.

Hemosporidia   HAEMOSPORIDIA.

hemosporidium   HAEMOSPORIDIUM.

hemosporine [HEMO- + *spor(e)* + -INE]   **1** Pertaining or belonging to the suborder Haemosporina of the sporozoan order Eucoccidiida; haemosporidian.   **2** A sporozoan blood parasite belonging to the suborder Haemosporina; a haemosporidium.

hemostasia   HEMOSTASIS.

hemostasis [HEMO- + -STASIS]   The arrest of hemorrhage. Also called *hemostasia*.

hemostat   A device or material designed to occlude or compress tissues or vessels in order to control bleeding, as during surgery or following trauma. Also called *angioclast* (obsolete).

hemostatic [HEMO- + -STAT + -IC]   **1** Tending to cause hemostasis. Also *hematostatic*.   **2** An agent that causes hemostasis. For defs 1 and 2 also *hemostyptic*.

capillary hemostatic   An agent which arrests capillary hemorrhage.

hemostix   A styletlike instrument used to pierce skin and obtain a small amount of blood for diagnostic testing.

hemostyptic   HEMOSTATIC.

hemotherapeutics   A rarely used term for HEMOTHERAPY.

hemotherapy   The administration of blood or such blood components as packed erythrocytes, platelets, leukocytes, plasma, or serum. Also called *hematotherapy, hemotherapeutics* (rarely used).

hemothorax   A collection of blood within the pleural cavity. It may be either internal or external to the pleura but not within the mediastinum. Also called *hematothorax, hemathorax, hemopleura*.

hemotoxic   Having the property of damaging blood cells. Also *hematotoxic, hematoxic*.

hemotoxicity   Injury to blood or blood-forming tissues by drugs, chemicals, or other substances.

hemotoxin   Any substance that is injurious to blood cells, causing them to be destroyed or removed from circulation at a greater than normal rate.

cobra hemotoxin   A toxic substance in cobra venom which is capable of hemolyzing red blood cells in man and animals.

hemotroph [HEMO- + Gk *troph(ē)* nourishment]   The nutrients supplied to an embryo by maternal blood either as carried by the bloodstream or from blood cells. Also *hematrophe*. Adjective: hemotrophic.

hemotrophe   HEMOTROPH.

hemotropic   **1** Having an affinity for blood or blood cells.   **2** Influencing phagocytic cells to migrate toward blood. For defs. 1 and 2 also *hematotropic*.

hemotympanum   Hemorrhage into the tympanic cavity. It often occurs after head injury and indicates a skull fracture involving the middle ear. Also called *hematotympanum*.

hemovolumetry   The measurement of blood volume.

hemozoic   HEMATOZOIC.

hemozoin   The pigment product of malarial breakdown of hemoglobin in the infected red blood cell.

hemozoon   HEMATOZOON.

hemp [Old English *hænep*, prob. from non-Indo-European source of Gk *kannabis* hemp]   CANNABIS.   • The word *hemp* is applied chiefly to varieties of cannabis that are cultivated for their fiber. The word also enters into the names of various other plants or their products that are similar in some respect, such as *Manila hemp, Canada hemp*.

American hemp   CANNABIS.

black Indian hemp   See under *APOCYNUM*.

Indian hemp 1 CANNABIS. 2 A plant of the species *Apocynum cannabinum*; Canada hemp. ● This ambiguous term is derived either by reference to India, where much cannabis has been grown, or to North American Indians, who have used *A. cannabinum* in various ways.

hemuresis [HEM- + -URESIS] A rarely used term for HEMATURIA.

HEMPAS hereditary erythroblastic multinuclearity with positive acid serum test. See under CONGENITAL DYSERYTHROPOIETIC ANEMIA.

henbane HYOSCYAMUS.

black henbane HYOSCYAMUS.

Hench [Philip Showalter *Hench*, U.S. physician, 1896–1965] Hench-Rosenberg syndrome. See under PALINDROMIC RHEUMATISM.

Henderson [Lawrence Joseph *Henderson*, U.S. biochemist, 1878–1942] Henderson-Hasselbalch equation. See under EQUATION.

Henderson [Melvin Starkey *Henderson*, U.S. orthopedic surgeon, 1883–1954] Henderson-Jones disease. See under OSTEOCHONDROMATOSIS.

Hendersonula A genus of black or grey molds found on vegetation in tropical regions of Africa, India, and the West Indies. It is capable of causing skin and nail disease in man in a form that closely resembles *Trichophyton rubrum* ringworm. The usual species are *Hendersonula toruloidea* and *Scytalidium hyalinum*.

hendersonulosis An infection of the skin or nails with the saprophytic mold *Hendersonula toruloidea*.

Henke [Wilhelm *Henke*, German anatomist, 1834–1896] 1 Henke's triangle, Henke's trigone. See under TRIGONUM INGUINALE. 2 Henke space. See under SPATIUM RETROPHARYNGEUM.

Henle [Adolf Richard *Henle*, German surgeon, born 1864] Henle-Coenen test. See under TEST.

Henle [Friedrich Gustav Jacob *Henle*, German anatomist and pathologist, 1809–1885] 1 See under LIGAMENT, BAND, SPHINCTER. 2 Henle's reaction. See under CHROMAFFIN REACTION. 3 See under LAYER. 4 Henle's nervous layer. See under ENTORETINA. 5 Henle's elastic membrane. See under EXTERNAL ELASTIC LAMINA. 6 Internal cremaster of Henle. See under CREMASTER. 7 Henle's ansa, Henle's canal. See under LOOP OF HENLE. 8 Hassall-Henle warts. See under HASSALL-HENLE BODIES. 9 Henle's membrane. See under COMPLEXUS BASALIS CHOROIDEAE. 10 Henle's glands. See under GLAND. 11 Henle's fissures. See under FISSURE. 12 Henle's ampulla. See under AMPULLA DUCTUS DEFERENTIS. 13 Crural canal of Henle. See under CANALIS ADDUCTORIUS. 14 Medial accessory ligament of Henle. See under LIGAMENTUM SPHENOMANDIBULARE. 15 Lumbocostal ligament of Henle. See under LIGAMENTUM LUMBOCOSTALE. 16 Henle's fiber layer. See under LAYER. 17 Inferior ligament of neck of rib of Henle. See under LIGAMENTUM COSTOTRANSVERSARIUM. 18 Lateral accessory ligament of Henle. See under LIGAMENTUM LATERALE ARTICULATIONIS TEMPOROMANDIBULARIS. 19 Transverse ligament of pelvis of Henle. See under LIGAMENTUM TRANSVERSUM PERINEI. 20 Sheath of Henle. See under ENDONEURIUM. 21 Henle's tubules. See under TUBULE. 22 Spine of Henle. See under SPINA SUPRAMEATUM. 23 Muscle of Henle. See under MUSCULUS AURICULARIS ANTERIOR. 24 Henle's fenestrated membrane. See under MEMBRANE. 25 External tuber of Henle. See under TUBERCULUM MENTALE MANDIBULAE. 26 Scapular tuberosity of Henle. See under PROCESSUS CORACOIDEUS SCAPULAE. 27 Superior tubercle of Henle. See under TUBERCULUM OBTURATORIUM POSTERIUS.

28 Thick limb of the loop of Henle. See under THICK ASCENDING LIMB. 29 Thin limb of the loop of Henle. See under LIMB.

henna A natural coloring from the dried leaves of *Lawsonia inermis* and other *Lawsonia* species. When combined with any of a number of acids it is a relatively permanent dye, imparting a red color to the hair, nails, and other protein compounds.

Henneberg [Richard *Henneberg*, German physician, born 1868] 1 Henneberg's disease. See under PSEUDOBULBAR PARALYSIS. 2 Scholz-Bielschowsky-Henneberg diffuse cerebral sclerosis. See under METACHROMATIC LEUKODYSTROPHY.

Hennebert [Camille *Hennebert*, Belgian otologist, born 1867] See under TEST, SIGN.

Henoch [Eduard Heinrich *Henoch*, German pediatrician, 1820–1910] 1 Henoch's chorea, Henoch-Bergeron electric chorea. See under HENOCH-BERGERON CHOREA. 2 Schönlein-Henoch purpura nephritis. See under NEPHRITIS. 3 Schönlein-Henoch disease, Henoch's disease, Henoch's purpura, Schönlein-Henoch purpura, Schönlein-Henoch syndrome, Henoch-Schönlein syndrome. See under HENOCH-SCHÖNLEIN PURPURA.

henogenesis ONTOGENY.

henpue [West African] GOUNDOU.

henpuye [West African] GOUNDOU.

Henry [Sir Edward Richard *Henry*, English goverment official, 1850–1931] Henry system of classification of fingerprints. See under SYSTEM.

Henry [William *Henry*, English chemist, 1775–1836] See under LAW.

henry [after Joseph *Henry*, US physicist, 1797–1878] (*plural* henrys, henries) The SI derived unit of inductance; the inductance of a closed circuit in which an electromotive force of one volt is produced when the electric current in the circuit varies uniformly at the rate of one ampere per second; 1 henry = 1 volt $\times$ 1 second/1 ampere. Symbol: H

Henseleit [Kurt *Henseleit*, German biochemist, born 1907] Krebs-Henseleit cycle. See under UREA CYCLE.

Hensen [Viktor *Hensen*, German physiologist, 1835–1924] 1 See under NODE, KNOT, BODY, STRIPE. 2 Hensen's disk, Hensen's line, Hensen's plane. See under H BAND. 3 Hensen's canal. See under DUCTUS REUNIENS. 4 Hensen cells. See under CELL. 5 Hensen's duct. See under DUCTUS REUNIENS.

Hensing [Friedrich W. *Hensing*, German anatomist, 1719–1745] Hensing's fold, Hensing's ligament. See under LIGAMENTUM PHRENICOCOLICUM.

HEP high egg passage (a form of Flury vaccine for rabies).

hepar [NA] A wedge-shaped, reddish brown gland that is situated in the upper right portion of the abdominal cavity immediately beneath the diaphragm; liver. It is the largest organ in the body and weighs an average of 1500 g in adults. Its diaphragmatic surface is in contact with the diaphragm and adjacent body walls, and its visceral surface is related to abdominal organs. It is divided into right and left lobes, and on its visceral surface its caudate and quadrate lobes are demarcated by various fissures and the porta hepatis. The internal substance is divided into segments on the basis of the ramification of the bile ducts and the hepatic vessels. It is almost totally invested by peritoneum, on the inner aspect of which is a connective tissue capsule. It has a dual blood supply from the hepatic artery and the portal vein and drains through multiple hepatic veins into the inferior vena cava. For information on the physiologic function of the organ, see LIVER. Also called *jecur* (obsolete).

hepar adiposum FATTY LIVER.

hepar lobatum The grossly misshapen and scarred liver that develops after congenital syphilis. It is characterized by multiple lobes of variable size separated by deep fissures resulting from the scars of healed syphilitic gummas.

heparan sulfate A polysaccharide derived from a sequence of alternating residues of D-glucuronic acid and N-acetylglucosamine by partial deacetylation and sulfation of amino groups. As the process proceeds, inversion at C-5 of the D-glucuronic residues forms L-iduronic residues, which also become sulfated at O-2, and the glucosamine residues are sulfated at O-6. As these processes advance, the heparan sulfate becomes heparin.

heparin A polysaccharide, consisting typically of alternate residues of L-iduronic acid 2-sulfate and 2-deoxy-2-sulfoaminoglucose 6-sulfate. The processes that form it from heparan sulfate may, however, not be complete, so less sulfated residues and glucuronic residues may be present. Its anticoagulant properties are probably due to its binding to thrombin and antithrombin in plasma and assisting their combination. It may also affect lipid metabolism by binding lipoprotein lipase to cell surfaces.

heparinase 1 An outmoded term for HEPARIN LYASE. 2 Any enzyme that degrades heparin, whether by hydrolytic or elimination reactions.

heparinemia Active heparin circulating in the blood. Normally, negligible amounts are found in the blood, and demonstrable amounts reflect a very rare state in man unless exogenous heparin has been administered.

heparinize To administer heparin in order to achieve some degree of anticoagulation.

heparin lyase The enzyme (EC 4.2.2.7) that degrades heparin by an elimination reaction in which a hexosamine residue is liberated as a new reducing end by cleavage of the oxygen it glycosylates from a glucuronate residue, with the introduction of a 4,5-double bond in the latter. Also called *heparinase* (outmoded).

heparitinuria The presence of heparan sulfate in the urine, as may occur in mucopolysaccharidoses, notably the Hurler syndrome.

hepat- HEPATO-.

hepatalgia Pain in the liver, most often related to capsular distension.

hepatalgic Pertaining to pain in the liver.

hepatatrophia HEPATATROPHY.

hepatatrophy Atrophy of the liver. Also called *hepatatrophia*. See also ACUTE YELLOW ATROPHY OF THE LIVER.

hepatauxe [HEPAT- + Gk *auxē* growth, increase] HEPATOMEGALY.

hepatectomize To remove all or a major part of the liver tissue.

hepatectomy [HEPAT- + -ECTOMY] The surgical removal of all or a part of the liver.

hepatic [Gk *hēpatik(os)* (from *hēpar*, gen. *hēpatos*, the liver + -*ikos* -IC) pertaining to the liver] Of or relating to the liver.

hepatico- HEPATO-.

hepaticocholangiojejunostomy The surgical creation of an opening between the common hepatic bile duct and a proximal loop of small intestine in order to bypass obstructed or damaged distal bilary ducts. It may also involve a second communication with another bile duct.

hepaticocholedochostomy The surgical creation of an opening between the common hepatic duct and the common bile duct.

hepaticodochotomy A surgical procedure in which an incision is made into the hepatic and common bile ducts.

hepaticoduodenostomy A surgically created opening between the common hepatic duct and the duodenum. It is performed to alleviate damage to or an obstruction of the distal biliary tree.

hepaticoenterostomy The surgical creation of an opening between a hepatic bile duct and the small bowel. It is usually performed to bypass the distal biliary tree after resection, because of an obstruction, or because of trauma.

hepaticogastrostomy A surgical procedure creating an opening between a hepatic bile duct and the stomach.

hepaticojejunostomy The surgical creation of an opening between a hepatic bile duct and the proximal small intestine. It is frequently performed following biliary duct resection or for damage or obstruction of the distal biliary tree.

Hepaticola *CAPILLARIA*.

hepaticoliasis CAPILLARIASIS.

hepaticolithotomy A surgical procedure in which an incision is made into a hepatic bile duct for the purpose of stone removal.

hepaticolithotripsy A surgical procedure in which hepatic duct stones are crushed to facilitate their passage or removal.

hepaticopancreatic Pertaining to the liver and the pancreas.

hepaticopulmonary Pertaining to the liver and the lung or lungs.

hepaticostomy [HEPATICO- + -STOMY] A surgical procedure in which an incision is made into a hepatic bile duct to permit drainage, usually through a tube.

hepaticotomy [HEPATICO- + -TOMY] A surgical incision into a hepatic bile duct.

hepatism [HEPAT- + -ISM] Illness due to liver disease or malfunction.

hepatitic Of or relating to hepatitis.

hepatitides Plural of HEPATITIS.

hepatitis [HEPAT- + -ITIS] 1 Inflammation of the liver, involving alteration of hepatocytes, either degenerative or necrotic. 2 Any of various diseases characterized primarily by liver inflammation.

hepatitis A An acute illness of global distribution caused by hepatitis virus A, a picornavirus. After an incubation period of two to six weeks, the disease begins with fever, nonspecific gastrointestinal symptoms, and malaise. Subsequently, hepatosplenomegaly, jaundice, dark urine, and pruritis usually develop, with convalescence marked by persistent malaise, fatigue, and slight liver function abnormalities. The disease is usually acquired by oral consumption of contaminated material or by close person-to-person contact, especially via the fecal-oral route. It is rarely transmitted by blood transfusion. Hepatitis A occurs most frequently in children and young adults. Also called *infectious hepatitis, viral hepatitis type A, epidemic hepatitis, epidemic catarrhal jaundice.*

active chronic hepatitis See under CHRONIC ACTIVE HEPATITIS.

acute hepatitis Hepatitis of relatively short duration and recent onset.

alcoholic hepatitis An inflammatory process in the liver caused by alcohol ingestion.

amebic hepatitis Invasion of the liver by trophozoites of *Entamoeba histolytica*.

anicteric hepatitis An inflammatory process in the liver not accompanied by jaundice.

anicteric viral hepatitis Inflammation of the liver induced by a virus which is unaccompanied by clinically detectable jaundice.

avian hepatitis AVIAN VIBRIONIC HEPATITIS.

avian vibrionic hepatitis A disease of chickens, marked by necrosis and hemorrhage in the liver, and caused by infection with an organism of the genus *Vibrio*. Also called *avian hepatitis*.

hepatitis B Inflammation of the liver caused by hepatitis B virus. The infectious agent may circulate in the blood for long periods of time (months or years) and is characteristically transmitted by parenteral, percutaneous, or permucosal inoculation of even minute amounts of blood, blood products, or bodily secretions. The disease may be acute or chronic, symptomatic or asymptomatic. Also called *viral hepatitis type B, homologous serum hepatitis, human serum jaundice, homologous serum jaundice.*

canine viral hepatitis   INFECTIOUS CANINE HEPATITIS.

cholangiolitic hepatitis   CHOLESTATIC HEPATITIS.

cholestatic hepatitis   An inflammatory process in the liver accompanied by manifestations of cholestasis. Also called *cholangiolitic hepatitis.*

chronic active hepatitis   A chronic inflammatory disease of the liver characterized by progressive destruction of the hepatic lobule, progressing to scarring and cirrhosis. Known etiologies are hepatitis virus, drugs, and certain autoimmune phenomena. The morphologic lesion of chronic active hepatitis can also be seen as part of the spectra of Wilson's disease and primary biliary cirrhosis. Also called *chronic aggressive hepatitis, subacute hepatitis, relapsing epidemic jaundice* (outmoded).

chronic aggressive hepatitis   CHRONIC ACTIVE HEPATITIS.

chronic interstitial hepatitis   Cirrhosis of the liver.

chronic persistent hepatitis   A chronic hepatitis manifested histologically by an infiltrate of inflammatory cells in the portal areas without disruption of the limiting plate, with minimal piecemeal necrosis and without fibrosis. Known causative agents include hepatitis B virus and a virus of non-A, non-B hepatitis. Clinical manifestations include mild fatigue and malaise, but most patients are asymptomatic.

hepatitis contagiosa canis   INFECTIOUS CANINE HEPATITIS.

delta hepatitis   DELTA AGENT HEPATITIS.

delta agent hepatitis   Infection with delta agent, an RNA virus, occurring as a coinfection with hepatitis B or as a superinfection in a hepatitis B carrier and manifested as a fulminant, acute, or chronic exacerbation of hepatitis B infection. The agent is transmissible person-to-person via percutaneous or permucosal exposure to infected blood, serous fluid, or bodily secretions, but the presence in the host of hepatitis B surface antigen (HBsAg) is necessary for its replication. There is an unusually high incidence of cirrhosis in persons with chronic hepatitis due to delta agent superinfection. Delta agent infection probably occurs worldwide and is endemic in Italy. Incidence in the United States is low except among users of intravenous drugs. Also called *delta hepatitis.*

drug-induced hepatitis   Hepatitis caused by administration of any of various pharmacologic agents or by their metabolites.

duck virus hepatitis   A severe, acute hepatitis of ducklings, caused by a picornavirus.

enzootic hepatitis   RIFT VALLEY FEVER.

epidemic hepatitis   HEPATITIS A.

hepatitis externa   PERIHEPATITIS.

familial hepatitis   WILSON'S DISEASE.

fulminant hepatitis   A rare form of hepatitis which rapidly develops massive liver damage characterized by acute yellow atrophy, commonly ending in coma and death. In most cases it is the result of viral or toxic liver injury.

giant cell hepatitis   A histologic pattern of liver damage where multinucleate giant cells are conspicuous. It occurs particularly in newborn infants as a response to a variety of noxious agents.

gonococcal hepatitis   A hepatitis caused by *Neisseria gonorrhoeae.* See also FITZ-HUGH AND CURTIS SYNDROME.

halothane hepatitis   Liver damage that has occurred in some patients following administration of the anesthetic halothane.

homologous serum hepatitis   HEPATITIS B.

infectious hepatitis   HEPATITIS A.

infectious canine hepatitis   A common, worldwide disease of dogs caused by canine adenovirus type 1 and characterized by

liver damage. Intranuclear inclusion bodies occur in liver and endothelial cells. Fever, leukopenia, severe depression, abdominal pain, anorexia, and edema of the head and neck are common signs. Transient corneal opacity of one or both eyes may occur during recovery. Mortality may be high. Also called *canine viral hepatitis, hepatitis contagiosa canis, Rubarth's disease* (outmoded).

infectious necrotic hepatitis   An acute, infectious, and usually fatal disease of sheep and occasionally cattle, caused by *Clostridium novyi* which proliferates in necrotic foci in the liver. Also called *black disease.*

ischemic hepatitis   Inflammtory change in the liver, most prominent in the centrolobular zone, caused by acute hepatic ischemia and characterized by dramatic elevations of serum transaminase concentrations.

leptospiral hepatitis   Hepatitis as a feature of leptospirosis.

long-incubation hepatitis   SERUM HEPATITIS.

lupoid hepatitis   Chronic active hepatitis characterized by LE cells in the circulating blood. Despite the immunologic abnormalities, the illness is not thought to be related to systemic lupus erythematosus. Also called *plasma cell hepatitis.*

mouse hepatitis   A disease, mainly of neonatal mice, caused by any of several strains of a coronavirus. The virus usually is latent, and resistance to it increases with age. Also called *murine hepatitis.*

murine hepatitis   MOUSE HEPATITIS.

neonatal hepatitis   A giant cell hepatitis of unknown cause although possibly due to maternal-infant transmission of hepatitis B. It is one of the main causes of an obstructive type of jaundice in the newborn infant. Recovery is sometimes complete, but the condition may develop into hepatic cirrhosis.

non-A, non-B hepatitis   Hepatitis in humans apparently caused by an as-yet uncharacterized retrovirus or retroviruslike agent. Diagnosis continues to depend on serological exclusion of hepatitis A and B viruses, cytomegalovirus, and Epstein-Barr virus. The clinical picture is indistinguishable from that produced by hepatitis B virus, it may be acquired by transfusion of blood and blood products, and infection may lead to chronic active or chronic persistent hepatitis.

plasma cell hepatitis   LUPOID HEPATITIS.

post-transfusion hepatitis   Hepatitis occurring following a blood transfusion. The vast majority of cases are caused by either hepatitis B or non-A, non-B virus. Also called *transfusion hepatitis.*

postvaccinal hepatitis   Hepatitis following either the administration of human serum or following vaccination, usually for yellow fever.

serum hepatitis   **1** Viral hepatitis transmitted parenterally (by contaminated needles or the administration of infective blood products) or by oral ingestion of contaminated material. This general category of hepatitis is now usually specified according to the types of virus responsible: either hapatitis B, non-A, or non-B hepatitis, or delta agent hepatitis. Also called *long-incubation hepatitis, syringe jaundice, transfusion jaundice.* Abbreviation: SH **2** THEILER'S DISEASE.

subacute hepatitis   Chronic active hepatitis.

suppurative hepatitis   An inflammatory process in the liver accompanied by abscess formation. Also called *purohepatitis.*

toxic hepatitis   Hepatitis caused by the administration of or exposure to a toxic compound. Also called *toxipathic hepatitis.*

toxipathic hepatitis   TOXIC HEPATITIS.

transfusion hepatitis   POST-TRANSFUSION HEPATITIS.

trophopathic hepatitis   An inflammatory process of the liver caused by nutritional deficiency.

tuberculous hepatitis   A hepatitis, usually granulomatous, caused by the tubercle bacillus, *Mycobacterium tuberculosis.*

viral hepatitis   Any inflammation of the liver caused by a virus, including hepatitis A, hepatitis B, non-A, non-B hepatitis, delta agent hepatitis, and hepatitis due to Epstein-Barr virus, cytomegalovirus, or yellow fever virus. The clinical manifestations range from asymptomatic to fulminant disease resulting in coma and early death. Common symptoms are malaise, weakness, and nausea, and icterus occurs in approximately 25% of cases. Recovery is usually complete, but chronic hepatitis may occur after hepatitis B, non-A, non-B hepatitis, or delta agent hepatitis.

viral hepatitis of turkeys An acute adenoviral infection of turkeys, marked by focal necrosis of the liver.

viral hepatitis type A HEPATITIS A.

viral hepatitis type B HEPATITIS B.

hepatization The transformation of a loose tissue into a dense, homogenous mass with the texture and consistency of liver. It usually denotes the conversion of normal lung to the consolidated inflammatory infiltrate of lobar pneumonia.

gray hepatization The gross appearance of the second stage in the evolution of lobar pneumonia in which the lung parenchyma is firm rather than spongy, and has a grayish discoloration. This color is due to the degradation of leukocytes, red blood cells, and fibrin that fill the alveoli.

red hepatization Hepatization in which the affected portion of lung is firm and red as a result of hyperemia and extravasation of blood in the early stages of pneumonia.

hepatized Denoting an organ or structure that has been altered by disease so as to have the consistency of liver.

hepatizon [Gk *hepatizon* (pres. part. of *hepatizein* to be like the liver, from *hepar*, gen. *hepatos*, the liver) liver-colored] A patchy pigmentation of the skin. An obsolete term.

hepato- [Gk *hepar* (genitive *hepatos*) the liver; Gk *hepatikos* pertaining to the liver] A combining form denoting the liver. Also *hepat-*, *hepatico-*. • The use of *hepato-* is often confined to terms pertaining to the liver itself, whereas *hepatico-* usually refers to the liver ducts.

hepatobiliary Pertaining to the liver and biliary system.

hepatoblast [HEPATO- + -BLAST] The precursor in the fetus of the parenchymatous hepatic cell of the liver.

hepatoblastoma [HEPATO- + BLASTOMA] A malignant tumor of the liver, composed of cells resembling embryonal and fetal hepatic parenchyma with or without mesenchymal elements, such as cartilage and bone. It occurs mainly in early childhood and is not associated with cirrhosis. Also called *embryonal carcinoma of the liver, embryonal mixed tumor.*

hepatobronchial Pertaining to the liver and the bronchial tree.

hepatocarcinogen [HEPATO- + CARCINOGEN] An agent that is the cause of a cancer of the liver.

hepatocarcinogenesis [HEPATO- + CARCINOGENESIS] The establishment of cancer of the liver.

hepatocarcinogenic [HEPATO- + CARCINOGENIC] Capable of causing cancer of the liver.

hepatocarcinoma [HEPATO- + CARCINOMA] HEPATOCELLULAR CARCINOMA.

hepatocele [HEPATO- + -CELE[1]] A herniation of part of the liver.

hepatocellular Pertaining to liver cells.

hepatocerebral [HEPATO- + CEREBRAL] Describing, pertaining to, or affecting the liver and brain.

hepatocholangeitis HEPATOCHOLANGITIS.

hepatocholangioduodenostomy A surgical procedure creating an opening between the hepatic biliary tree and the duodenum in order to treat distal biliary tract disease.

hepatocholangioenterostomy The surgical formation of an opening between the hepatic bile ducts and the small bowel in order to treat distal biliary tract disease.

hepatocholangiogastrostomy A surgical procedure that creates an opening between the hepatic ducts and the stomach. It is performed to bypass diseased areas of the distal biliary tract.

hepatocholangiojejunostomy The surgical creation of an opening between the hepatic ducts and the proximal part of the small bowel. It is performed to bypass a diseased biliary tract.

hepatocholangiostomy A surgical procedure creating an opening between the hepatic ducts and the skin, usually through a tube, for the purpose of drainage.

hepatocholangitis Inflammation of the liver and biliary ducts. Also called *hepatocholangeitis.*

hepatocirrhosis CIRRHOSIS OF THE LIVER.

hepatocolic Referring to the liver and the colon.

hepatocystic Referring to the liver and the gallbladder. Also *hepatovesicular.*

Hepatocystis A genus of sporozoans (family Plasmodiidae), parasitic in the blood of lower primates and other arboreal animals, rodents, bats, and hippopotamuses. Gametocytes are found in red blood cells and cystlike schizonts occur in parenchymal cells of the liver. Vectors are biting midges of the genus *Culicoides.*

Hepatocystis kochi A species commonly found in baboons and other African monkeys, transmitted by bloodsucking midges of the genus *Culicoides.* Also called *Plasmodium kochi.*

hepatocyte LIVER CELL.

hepatoduodenal Referring to the liver and duodenum.

hepatoduodenostomy A surgical procedure creating an opening between the liver and the duodenum for the purpose of bile drainage.

hepatodynia [HEPAT- + -ODYNIA] Pain emanating from the liver.

hepatodystrophy ACUTE YELLOW ATROPHY OF THE LIVER.

hepatoenteric Referring to the liver and intestine.

hepatoenterostomy A surgical procedure creating an opening between the liver and small bowel for the purpose of biliary decompression and drainage.

hepatofugal Tending to move or flow away from the liver.

hepatogastric Referring to the liver and stomach.

hepatogenic HEPATOGENOUS.

hepatogenous Originating in or from the liver. Also *hepatogenic.*

hepatogram A radiograph of the liver.

emission hepatogram LIVER SCAN.

isotope hepatogram An incorrect term for LIVER SCAN.

radionuclide hepatogram LIVER SCAN.

hepatography [HEPATO- + -GRAPHY] Radiography of the liver usually after the injection of a contrast agent into the hepatic artery or retrogradely into hepatic veins. The liver can also be made radiopaque as a result of picking up special contrast agents, such as thorotrast or iodinated fat preparations, by the reticuloendothelial system. This method has experimental use only.

isotope hepatography Scintigraphic study of the liver. An incorrect usage.

hepatohemia [HEPATO- + HEM- + -IA] Congestion of the sinusoids of the liver.

hepatoid Resembling the liver or liver tissue.

hepatojejunal Referring to the liver and jejunum.

hepatojugular Referring to the liver and jugular vein, as in *hepatojuglar reflux.*

hepatojugularometer An instrument used to measure the amount of hepatojugular reflux.

hepatolenticular Involving the liver and the lenticular nucleus, as in *hepatolenticular degeneration.*

hepatolienal   Referring to the liver and the spleen.

hepatolienography   HEPATOSPLENOGRAPHY.

hepatolienomegaly   HEPATOSPLENOMEGALY.

hepatolith   A calculus in an intrahepatic bile duct.

hepatolithectomy [HEPATO- + LITH- + -ECTOMY]   The surgical removal of one or more stones from the liver.

hepatolithiasis   A pathologic condition characterized by the presence of calculi within the intrahepatic bile ducts.

hepatologist [HEPATO- + -LOGIST]   A specialist in diseases of the liver.

hepatology [HEPATO- + -LOGY]   The study of the liver and its diseases.

hepatolysis   Necrosis of liver cells. A seldom used term.

hepatolytic   Capable of causing liver necrosis.

hepatoma [HEPAT- + -OMA]   **1** A primary tumor of the liver parenchymal cells. **2** HEPATOCELLULAR CARCINOMA. **3** A benign or malignant experimental tumor of liver parenchymal cells.

    malignant hepatoma   HEPATOCELLULAR CARCINOMA.

hepatomalacia   A condition marked by the softening of the liver.

hepatomegalia   HEPATOMEGALY.

    hepatomegalia glycogenica   GLYCOGENIC HEPATOMEGALY.

hepatomegaly [HEPATO- + -MEGALY]   Enlargement of the liver. Also called *hepatomegalia, hepatauxe, megalohepatia.*

    glycogenic hepatomegaly   Enlargement of the liver caused by a glycogen storage disease. Also called *hepatomegalia glycogenica.*

hepatomelanosis   A condition characterized by an abnormal dark pigmentation of the liver.

hepatometry [HEPATO- + -METRY]   Measurement of the size of the liver.

hepatomphalocele   An omphalocele which contains part of the liver within the membranous sac.

hepatomyeloma [HEPATO- + MYELOMA]   A soft cancer of the liver.An obsolete term.

hepatonecrosis   Massive necrosis of hepatocytes, as in acute fulminant viral hepatitis. A seldom used term.

hepatonephric   Relating to or connecting the liver and the kidney; hepatorenal.

hepatonephritis   Simultaneous inflammation of the liver and kidneys, as in leptospirosis.

hepatopathic   Causing or relating to liver disease.

hepatopathy [HEPATO- + -PATHY]   Disease of the liver.

hepatoperitonitis   Inflammation of the hepatic peritoneum.

hepatopetal   Flowing or tending toward the liver: said, for example, of blood in the portal vein or anything carried along in it.

hepatopexy [HEPATO- + -PEXY]   A surgical procedure in which the liver is resuspended to prevent ptosis.

hepatophlebitis   Inflammation of veins in the liver.

hepatophlebography   Radiologic visualization of the hepatic venous outflow tracts.

hepatopleural   Relating to or connecting the liver and the pleura or pleural cavity.

hepatopneumonic   HEPATOPULMONARY.

hepatoportal   Relating to the portal venous system of the liver.

hepatoptosis   Ptosis of the liver.

hepatopulmonary   Relating to, connecting, or affecting the liver and the lungs. Also *hepatopneumonic.*

hepatorenal   Relating to liver and kidneys.

hepatorrhagia [HEPATO- + -RRHAGIA]   Bleeding from the liver.

hepatorrhaphy [HEPATO- + -RRHAPHY]   A surgical procedure in which sutures are placed in the liver substance either for repair of a defect or for fixation.

hepatorrhexia [HEPATO- + -*rrhex(is)* + -IA]   Rupture of the liver.

hepatoscan   A scintiscan depicting the liver.

hepatoscirrhus [HEPATO- + Gk *skiros* or *skirrhos* gypsum, stucco, hard tumor]   A scirrhous carcinoma of the liver. An outmoded term.

hepatosis [HEPAT- + -OSIS]

    hepatosis dietetica   A nutritional disease of swine, associated with deficiencies of vitamin E and selenium. Massive necrosis of the liver is the main feature.

hepatosplenic   Relating to or connecting the liver and the spleen; hepatolienal.

hepatosplenitis   Inflammation of the liver and the spleen.

hepatosplenography [HEPATO- + SPLENO- + -GRAPHY]   Radiography of the liver and spleen, usually after opacification of these organs by injecting contrast medium into feeding vessels, such as the celiac axis, or by intravenous administration of radiopaque preparations which are picked up by the cells of the reticuloendothelial system. Also called *hepatolienography.*

hepatosplenomegaly   Simultaneous enlargement of the liver and spleen. Also called *hepatolienomegaly, splenohepatomegaly, splenohepatomegalia.*

hepatosplenopathy   A disorder of the liver and the spleen.

hepatostomy [HEPATO- + -STOMY]   A surgical procedure creating an opening between the liver and the skin, usually through a tube, in order to establish drainage.

hepatothrombin   Hepatic component of thrombin. An outmoded term.

hepatotomy [HEPATO- + -TOMY]   A surgical incision into the liver.

    transthoracic hepatotomy   A surgical incision into the liver using a transdiaphragmatic approach through the chest.

hepatotoxic   Toxic to the liver.

hepatotoxicity   Toxicity with respect to the liver; the property of being toxic to the liver.

hepatotoxin [HEPATO- + TOXIN]   A drug, chemical, or other substance toxic to the liver.

hepatotropic   Having an affinity for the liver; specifically affecting the liver.

hepatovesicular   HEPATOCYSTIC.

Hepatozoon [HEPATO- + Gk *zōon* living being, animal]   A genus of heteroxenous sporozoans (order Coccidia, family Haemogregarinidae), parasitic in blood cells of birds and mammals. Schizogony takes place in the viscera, gametes are formed in erythrocytes or leukocytes, and sporogony occurs in certain ticks and other arthropods. Examples are *H. canis* of dogs, cats, jackals and hyenas, transmitted by *Rhipicephalus appendiculatus,* and *H. perniciosum* of dogs, transmitted by the mite *Echinolaelops echidninus.*

HEPES   *N*-2-hydroxyethylpiperazine-*N'*-propanesulfonic acid. It is used as a buffer, all of whose forms are impermeable to biologic membranes due to the presence of the sulfo group. The p*K* values of piperazine are greatly depressed in this compound, and the p*K* of 7.5 normally used is that between its zwitterionic and anionic forms.

hephephilia   HYPHEPHILIA.

hept-   HEPTA-.

hepta- [Gk *hepta* seven]   A combining form meaning seven.

heptabarbital $C_{13}H_{18}N_2O_3$.   5-(1-Cyclohepten-1-yl)-5-ethylbarbituric acid, a barbiturate with sedative and hypnotic properties. It is a short-acting agent, is given orally, and may lead to habituation or addiction.

heptachromic [HEPTA- + CHROM- + -IC] Being able to recognize normally the various spectral hues.

heptadactylia HEPTADACTYLY.

heptadactyly [HEPTA- + DACTYL- + -Y] The presence of seven digits on a hand or foot. Also called *heptadactylia*.

heptylpenicillin PENICILLIN K.

heptyne Any of the acetylenic hydrocarbons of general formula C_7H_{12}. Some of them are used in perfumery.

herb [L *herba* (akin to Gk *phorbē* pasture, forage, from *pherbein* to feed) an herb, herbage] **1** Any nonwoody seed-bearing plant that dies completely at the end of the growing season or passes through dormancy following a growing season, when its life is sustained by means of underground structures such as bulbs, corms, or rhizomes. **2** A prepared drug that consists of plants or plant parts.

death's herb BELLADONNA.

herbaceous Of or relating to an herb.

herbal A manuscript or book of information, usually illustrated, that contained the names, descriptions, and properties of plants. It focused primarily on those of pharmacologic significance.

herbalist **1** A person who collects, identifies, and studies herbs. **2** One who writes herbals.

herbarium [L *herb(a)* grass, herbage, an herb + *-arium* -ARY] A collection of dried plant specimens that is maintained and preserved for the purpose of scientific study.

Herbert [Herbert *Herbert*, English ophthalmic surgeon, 1865–1942] **1** See under OPERATION. **2** Herbert's pits. See under PIT.

herbicide An agent that kills plants.

herbivore [from New L *herbivor(a)*, neut. pl. of *herbivorus* feeding on grass or herbs, from L *herb(a)* grass, herb + *i* + *vor(are)* to swallow, devour + L *-us*, masc. suffix] An animal that is a member of the second trophic level in the food chain and that feeds primarily on vegetation. Also called *primary consumer*.

herbivorous [HERB + *i* + L *vor(are)* to devour, swallow + -OUS] Characterized by a plant-eating diet. Also *phytophagous*.

herbology [HERB + *o* + -LOGY] The study of herbs and their uses.

hereditable HERITABLE.

hereditary Transmitted or transmissable from parent to child through the genes. Also *inborn*.

heredity [L *hereditas* (from *heres* or *haeres* an heir, heiress, akin to *herus* the master of a family or of slaves and to German *Herr* master) inheritance] **1** The genetic endowment an offspring receives from the parents. **2** The transmission of genetic information from parents to offspring.

autosomal heredity AUTOSOMAL INHERITANCE.

dominant heredity DOMINANT INHERITANCE.

infectious heredity The alteration of the genome of a cell by the addition of a plasmid, the integration of a virus, or the incorporation of transforming or transfecting DNA.

sex-linked heredity An imprecise term for X-LINKED INHERITANCE.

X-linked heredity X-LINKED INHERITANCE.

heredo- [L *heres* (genitive *heredis*) heir] A combining form meaning heredity, hereditary.

heredoakinesia [HEREDO- + AKINESIA] A familial syndrome characterized by episodes of limb pain, paralysis, and exhaustion. No such specific syndrome is now recognized.

heredoataxia Any of the group of hereditary ataxias.

Pierre Marie cerebellar heredoataxia MARIE'S HEREDITARY CEREBELLAR ATAXIA.

heredobiologic An outmoded term for GENETIC.

heredodegeneration [HEREDO- + DEGENERATION] Any hereditary degeneration of the nervous system.

neuroradicular heredodegeneration Any of a group of hereditary neuropathies, including hereditary sensory neuropathy, progressive hypertrophic interstitial polyneuropathy and peroneal muscular atrophy.

spinocerebellar heredodegeneration Any of a group of hereditary ataxias including Friedreich's disease, Marie's cerebellar ataxia, the Roussy-Lévy syndrome, olivopontocerebellar degeneration, and many other inherited degenerative diseases of the nervous system.

heredodiathesis Proneness to one or more diseases based upon genetic transmission.

heredoimmunity Inherited immunity. A seldom used term.

heredoinfection [HEREDO- + INFECTION] Infection transmitted to offspring as a result of infection of the sperm or ovum of a parent. Also called *germinal infection*.

heredolues CONGENITAL SYPHILIS.

heredoluetic HEREDOSYPHILITIC.

heredomacular Pertaining to inherited diseases of the central portion of the retina.

heredopathia An outmoded term for HEREDITARY DISORDER.

heredopathia atactica polyneuritiformis An older term for REFSUM'S DISEASE.

heredosyphilis CONGENITAL SYPHILIS.

heredosyphilitic Of or relating to congenital syphilis. Also *heredoluetic*.

heredotrophedema HEREDITARY LYMPHEDEMA.

Herellea A former genus of aerobic, Gram-negative diplobacilli, now included in *Acinetobacter*.

herelleosis An infection caused by bacteria of the genus *Herellea*.

Hering [Heinrich Ewald *Hering*, German physiologist, 1866–1948] **1** See under PHENOMENON, EFFECT. **2** Hering's nerve. See under RAMUS SINUS CAROTICI NERVI GLOSSOPHARYNGEI. **3** Hering-Breuer reflex. See under REFLEX.

Hering [Karl Ewald Constantin *Hering*, German physiologist, 1834–1918] **1** See under TEST, THEORY, AFTERIMAGE. **2** Hering-Hellebrand deviation. See under DEVIATION. **3** Traube-Hering waves. See under WAVE. **4** Semon-Hering hypothesis. See under MNEMIC HYPOTHESIS. **5** Canal of Hering. See under CHOLANGIOLE.

heritability Any measure of capability of being inherited.

broad sense heritability The proportion of the phenotypic variance that is due to genetic factors. It can be calculated from the analysis of twins:

$$H = \frac{V_{DZ} - V_{MZ}}{V_{DZ}},$$

where H is broad sense heritability and V_{DZ} and V_{MZ} are the means of the squares of the differences between members of dizygotic and monozygotic twin pairs, respectively.

$$H' = \frac{r_{MZ} - r_{DZ}}{1 - r_{DZ}},$$

where r_{DZ} and r_{MZ} are the intraclass correlations for dizygotic and monozygotic twin pairs. H and H' are approximately equal provided the total variance for dizygotic twins does not differ too greatly from that for monozygotic twins.

narrow sense heritability The proportion of the phenotypic variance that is due to additive genetic variation.

$$h^2 = \frac{V_A}{V_A + V_D + V_E},$$

where h^2 is narrow sense heritability, V_A is the additive genetic variance, V_D is the dominance variance, and V_E is the environmental variance.

heritable **1** Capable of being inherited. **2** Referring to a phenotype determined by a gene. For defs. 1 and 2 also *hereditable, genetic.*

heritage **1** All characteristics passed from one generation to the next, irrespective of genetic considerations. A popular usage. **2** All characteristics, due in part to genes, that are transmitted from one generation to the next.

Herlitz [Carl Gillis *Herlitz*, Swedish pediatrician, born 1902] Herlitz syndrome. See under EPIDERMOLYSIS BULLOSA LETALIS.

Hermansky [F. *Hermansky*, Czech internist, flourished 20th century] Hermansky-Pudlak syndrome. See under SYNDROME.

hermaphrodism [See HERMAPHRODITISM.] HERMAPHRODITISM.

hermaphrodite [after *Hermaphroditos*, mythological son of *Hermes* (Mercury) and *Aphrodite* (Venus)] An individual with some anatomic attributes of both sexes.

true hermaphrodite A person who has both ovarian and testicular tissue and a highly variable clinical syndrome ranging from external genitalia which simulate normal male or female structures through any degree of ambiguity. Gonads are of three types: testis on one side, ovary on the other; ovotestes on each side; ovotestis on one side, testis or ovary on the other. Internal genitalia are variable. Chromosomal constitution is normal male or female or XX/XY chimerism or XY/XXY mosaicism. Also called *true intersex.*

hermaphroditic [*hermaphrodit(e)* + -IC] GYNANDROMORPHOUS.

hermaphroditism [*hermaphrodit(e)* + -ISM] The condition of having both male and female anatomic characteristics. Also called *hermaphrodism, hermaphroditismus, gynadromorphism, gynandrism* (imprecise), *gynandria* (imprecise), *gynandry* (imprecise), *gynanthropism* (imprecise), *gynanthropia* (imprecise).

adrenal hermaphroditism Female pseudohermaphroditism of the female fetus and infant, in congenital adrenocortical hyperplasia. A seldom used term.

bilateral hermaphroditism True hermaphroditism in which ovarian and testicular tissue is present on both sides. Also called *hermaphroditismus verus bilateralis.*

dimidiate hermaphroditism LATERAL HERMAPHRODITISM.

false hermaphroditism PSEUDOHERMAPHRODITISM.

lateral hermaphroditism True hermaphroditism in which an ovary is present on one side and a testis on the other, without admixture of gonadal tissue. Also called *dimidiate hermaphroditism, hermaphroditismus verus lateralis.*

male hermaphroditism **1** An incorrect term for MALE PSEUDOHERMAPHRODITISM. **2** True hermaphroditism with predominately male somatotype. An imprecise usage.

ovotesticular hermaphroditism TRUE HERMAPHRODITISM.

protandrous hermaphroditism The condition in a hermaphroditic organism in which the male reproductive organs develop earlier than the female organs.

protogynous hermaphroditism Hermaphroditism in which the female reproductive organs develop earlier than the male organs.

spurious hermaphroditism PSEUDOHERMAPHRODITISM.

synchronous hermaphroditism Hermaphroditism in which female and male generative functions occur concurrently, or sometimes alternately.

transverse hermaphroditism Pseudohermaphroditism in which the gonads are characteristic of one sex and the external genitalia are characteristic of the other.

true hermaphroditism The condition of being a true hermaphrodite. Also called *hermaphroditismus verus.*

unilateral hermaphroditism The presence of both ovarian and testicular tissue on one side of the body and of either an ovary or a testis on the other side. Also called *hermaphroditismus verus unilateralis.*

hermaphroditismus [See HERMAPHRODITISM.] HERMAPHRODITISM.

hermaphroditismus verus TRUE HERMAPHRODITISM.

hermaphroditismus verus bilateralis BILATERAL HERMAPHRODITISM.

hermaphroditismus verus lateralis LATERAL HERMAPHRODITISM.

hermaphroditismus verus unilateralis UNILATERAL HERMAPHRODITISM.

Hermetia A genus of flies (family Stratiomyidae), one species of which, *H. illucens,* the black soldier fly, has been implicated as causing human enteric myiasis. The larvae develop in overripe fruit, vegetables, and organic matter, and apparently are accidentally ingested.

hermetic Sealed by fusion to ensure a very low rate of gas or water-vapor leakage.

hernia

hernia [L, hernia, rupture] Protrusion of an organ or tissue through an abnormal opening. Also called *rupture* (popular).

abdominal hernia A hernia in the abdominal wall, usually of small intestine.

acquired hernia A hernia that develops after birth, commonly one brought on by lifting or straining.

adipose hernia FAT HERNIA.

annular hernia INDIRECT INGUINAL HERNIA.

Barth's hernia An abdominal hernia at the site of a persistant vitelline duct.

Birkett's hernia A hernia of the stratum synoviale through the stratum fibrosum of a joint capsule. Also called *synovial hernia.*

hernia of the bladder **1** A projection of a portion of the urinary bladder through any opening. Also called *cystic hernia, vesical hernia, vesicocele.* **2** EXSTROPHY OF THE BLADDER.

hernia of the brain Protrusion of the brain through a defect in the skull, the falx cerebri, or the tentorium cerebelli, or through anatomical openings such as the incisura of the tentorium or the foramen magnum. Also called *hernia cerebri, cerebral hernia.*

broad-ligament hernia HERNIA OF THE BROAD LIGAMENT OF THE UTERUS.

hernia of the broad ligament of the uterus A protrusion of a loop of intestine into the substance of the broad ligament of the uterus. Also called *broad-ligament hernia.*

cerebral hernia HERNIA OF THE BRAIN.

hernia cerebri HERNIA OF THE BRAIN.

Cloquet's hernia PECTINEAL HERNIA.

complete hernia A hernia which has passed entirely through the orifice: applied especially to an indirect inguinal hernia that has passed into the scrotum or the labium majus.

Cooper's hernia   RETROPERITONEAL HERNIA.

crural hernia   FEMORAL HERNIA.

cystic hernia   HERNIA OF THE BLADDER.

diaphragmatic hernia   A hernia of abdominal viscera into the thorax at any of several areas of the diaphragm, most commonly in one of the less supported areas such as the pleuroperitoneal membrane, Morgagni's foramen, or the esophageal hiatus. It may also occur at other points owing to congenital underdevelopment of the usual muscular and tendinous supports. In the newborn, it most commonly occurs through the pleuroperitoneal canal (foramen of Bochdalek).

direct hernia   DIRECT INGUINAL HERNIA.

direct inguinal hernia   An inguinal hernia which leaves the abdomen between the inferior epigastric artery and the rectus muscle. Also called *direct hernia, internal hernia.*

diverticular hernia   A hernia of a congenital intestinal diverticulum.

exomphalos hernia   OMPHALOCELE.

fat hernia   Hernia of fatty tissue, either from the mesentery or the properitoneal fat, through the abdominal wall. Also called *adipose hernia, pannicular hernia.*

femoral hernia   A hernia of intestine into the femoral canal. Also called *femorcele, enteromerocele, crural hernia.*

funicular hernia   A hernia involving either the spermatic or the umbilical cord.

gastroesophageal hernia   A hiatal hernia involving a portion of stomach and esophagus.

Gibbon's hernia   An inguinal hernia occurring together with a hydrocele. Also called *Gibbon's hydrocele.*

Goyrand's hernia   An inguinal hernia in which the protrusion does not reach the scrotum.

Hesselbach's hernia   A hernia that has a diverticulum through the fascia cribrosa.

hiatal hernia   Hernia through the diaphragmatic hiatus, usually of a portion of the stomach and lower esophagus. It may be a sliding hernia or a paraesophageal hernia. Also called *hiatus hernia, parahiatal diaphragmatic hernia.*

hiatus hernia   HIATAL HERNIA.

incarcerated hernia   A hernia which cannot be reduced. Also called *irreducible hernia.*

incisional hernia   A hernia occurring at the site of a surgical incision, usually in the abdomen.

incomplete hernia   A hernia which has not passed entirely through the orifice.

indirect hernia   INDIRECT INGUINAL HERNIA.

indirect inguinal hernia   An inguinal hernia in which the internal orifice is the deep inguinal ring. Also called *indirect hernia, annular hernia, oblique hernia.*

infantile hernia   A congenital inguinal hernia.

inguinal hernia   Hernia into the inguinal canal. See also DIRECT INGUINAL HERNIA, INDIRECT INGUINAL HERNIA.

inguinofemoral hernia   Hernia into both the inguinal and the femoral canal.

internal hernia   1 A hernia not involving the abdominal wall. 2 DIRECT INGUINAL HERNIA.

interstitial hernia   A hernia contained between muscular layers of the abdominal wall.

hernia of the iris   Extrusion to the surface, through a wound, of the anterior portion of the uveal tract.

irreducible hernia   INCARCERATED HERNIA.

labial hernia   Protrusion of a loop of intestine into the labia majora, usually through the canal of Nuck.

Laugier's hernia   A femoral hernia passing through the lacunar ligament.

hernia of the lung   Protrusion of the lung through a defect in the chest wall or diaphragm. Also called *pneumatocele, pneumocele, pneumonocele.*

Malgaigne's hernia   A temporary fetal structure consisting of a small empty pocket of peritoneum attached to the gubernaculum testis and protruding into the inguinal canal. It is later occupied by the descending testis.

mesenteric hernia   Hernia through the mesentery.

mesocolic hernia   Hernia through the mesocolon.

hernia of the nucleus pulposus   INTERVERTEBRAL DISK PROTRUSION.

oblique hernia   INDIRECT INGUINAL HERNIA.

obturator hernia   A hernia through the obturator canal.

omental hernia   Hernia of a portion of omentum.

ovarian hernia   Protrusion of an ovary as part of a hernia.

pannicular hernia   FAT HERNIA.

paraesophageal hernia   A form of hiatal hernia in which the gastroesophageal junction remains in its infradiaphragmatic position and the fundus and body of the stomach herniate into the thorax.

parahiatal diaphragmatic hernia   HIATAL HERNIA.

para-umbilical hernia   Protrusion of an infant's viscera, through a weakness in the rectus fascia just above the umbilical scar. This hernia, which is uncommon, has no tendency to disappear spontaneously. Also called *parumbilical hernia.*

parumbilical hernia   PARA-UMBILICAL HERNIA.

pectineal hernia   A femoral hernia that enters the femoral canal and perforates the pectineus fascia rather than the fascia cribrosa, simulating an obturator hernia. Also called *pectineal crural hernia, Cloquet's hernia.*

pectineal crural hernia   PECTINEAL HERNIA.

pleuroperitoneal hiatus hernia   A congenital diaphragmatic hernia through the pleuroperitoneal membrane. It usually occurs on the left side.

posterior labial hernia   Protrusion of a loop of intestine into both the labial and vaginal areas. The hernia usually involves the posterior portion of the labia majora. Also called *vaginolabial hernia.*

posterior vaginal hernia   Downward displacement of the pouch of Douglas (excavatio rectouterina). Also called *enterocele.*

properitoneal hernia   Hernia between the parietal peritoneum and the fascia transversalis.

pudendal hernia   Hernia in the pudendum via the levator muscle.

hernia of pulp   CHRONIC OPEN HYPERPLASTIC PULPITIS.

pulsion hernia   Hernia produced by a sudden force such as an increase in intra-abdominal pressure.

rectal hernia   Hernia of a loop of small intestine into the wall of the rectum.

rectovaginal hernia   RECTOCELE.

reducible hernia   Hernia in which the protruding portion of bowel may be manipulated back into its normal position.

retroperitoneal hernia   Hernia of intestine into the retroperitoneum, usually in the region of the retroperitoneal duodenum. Also called *Cooper's hernia.*

sciatic hernia   Hernia through the greater sciatic foramen. Also called *ischiocele.*

scrotal hernia   An inguinal hernia that extends into the scrotum. Also called *orchiocele, oscheocele, scrotocele.*

sliding hernia   A hernia either of the cecum or of the sigmoid colon into the parietal peritoneum.

strangulated hernia   An incarcerated hernia which may become ischemic and gangrenous.

synovial hernia   BIRKETT'S HERNIA.

tentorial hernia   TENTORIAL HERNIATION.

tonsillar hernia   TONSILLAR HERNIATION.

transmesenteric hernia   A herniation of a loop or larger segment of intestine through a defect of a mesentery, which is often of developmental origin.

hernia of the tunica albuginea A minute hernia in which seminiferous epithelium penetrates through the tunica albuginea of the testis.

umbilical hernia A protrusion of a segment of the gastrointestinal tract and/or the great omentum through a defect in the abdominal wall at the umbilicus, the herniated mass being circumscribed and covered by normal skin. It is almost universal in children in tropical countries, sometimes to a late age, but it is a self-curing condition. Compare OMPHALOCELE.

uterine hernia Protrusion of the uterus as part of a hernia.

vaginal hernia Protrusion of a loop of intestine into the vagina.

vaginolabial hernia POSTERIOR LABIAL HERNIA.

ventral hernia The herniation of peritoneal contents through the abdominal wall, often associated with a defect resulting from an incompletely closed surgical incision. Also called *laparocele*.

vesical hernia HERNIA OF THE BLADDER.

---

hernial Of or referring to a hernia. Also *herniary*.

herniary HERNIAL.

herniated Having undergone herniation; protruding through a hernial opening.

herniation [*herni(a)* + -ATION] The formation of a hernia; rupture.

caudal transtentorial herniation Herniation of the brain caudally through the hiatus of the tentorium.

cingulate herniation Hernia of the cingulate gyrus beneath the falx cerebri.

disk herniation The protrusion of nucleus pulposus material through the annulus fibrosus of an intervertebral disk. Also called *herniation of intervertebral disk, intravertebral disk herniation*.

foraminal herniation Herniation through an anatomic opening, usually of the cerebellar tonsils through the foramen magnum or the rostral displacement of the cerebral peduncles through the tentorial incisura.

herniation of intervertebral disk DISK HERNIATION.

intravertebral disk herniation DISK HERNIATION.

herniation of nucleus pulposus A protrusion of the nucleus puposus of the intervertebral disk through a tear in the anulus fibrosus.

rostral transtentorial herniation Partial protrusion of the temporal lobe through the incisura of the tentorium, the result of supratentorial pressure at birth.

subfalcial herniation Herniation of the medial aspects of a cerebral hemisphere beneath the inferior edge of the falx cerebri.

tentorial herniation Herniation of the brain through the tentorial hiatus, usually involving the inferomedial portion of one or both temporal lobes (the uncus), due to supratentorial pressure. Also called *tentorial hernia, uncal herniation*.

tonsillar herniation Herniation of one or both cerebellar tonsils through the foramen magnum due to intracranial pressure. Also called *tonsillar hernia*.

transtentorial herniation Herniation of the brain through the tentorial hiatus.

uncal herniation TENTORIAL HERNIATION.

hernio- [L *hernia* rupture] A combining form meaning hernia.

hernioappendectomy [HERNIO- + APPENDECTOMY] A combined hernioplasty and appendectomy.

hernioceliotomy [HERNIO- + CELIOTOMY] A surgical procedure that combines a hernia repair with an exploratory incision into the peritoneal cavity.

hernioenterotomy [HERNIO- + ENTEROTOMY] A surgical procedure that combines a hernia repair with an incision into the small bowel.

hernioid [*herni(o)-* + -OID] Resembling a hernia.

herniolaparotomy [HERNIO- + LAPAROTOMY] A surgical procedure in which an incision into the abdominal cavity is combined with a hernia repair.

herniology [HERNIO- + -LOGY] The study of hernias.

hernioplasty [HERNIO- + -PLASTY] Any surgical procedure for repairing a hernia.

Cooper's ligament hernioplasty MCVAY'S OPERATION.

herniopuncture [HERNIO- + PUNCTURE] A surgical procedure in which a hole is made in a hernia sac.

herniorrhaphy [HERNIO- + -RRHAPHY] A sutural procedure designed to repair a hernia.

Halsted's inguinal herniorrhaphy One of two variants of a surgical procedure for repairing a groin hernia.

herniotome [HERNIO- + -TOME] HERNIA KNIFE.

Cooper's herniotome A surgical instrument used to incise a hernia sac.

herniotomy [HERNIO- + -TOMY] Any surgical procedure that involves an incision into a hernia, usually to effect a repair. Also called *celotomy, kelotomy*.

heroic Involving extreme risk to a patient but resorted to in an effort to save life: said of a procedure.

heroin $C_{21}H_{23}O_5N$. A derivative of morphine that is formed by acetylation. It produces intense euphoria and excitation, and its use is likely to result in dependence and addiction. Also called *diamorphine, diacetylmorphine, acetomorphine*.

herpangina [*herp(es)* + ANGINA] An infectious disease caused by group A coxsackieviruses and characterized by fever, dysplasia, severe sore throat, anorexia, malaise, and typical gray-white vesicles in the tonsillar region. The disease occurs most frequently in children under seven years of age. Also called *benign croupous angina, pharyngitis herpetica*.

herpes [Gk *herpēs* (from *herpein* to creep, crawl, akin to L *serpere* to creep, crawl) a skin eruption] **1** Either of two diseases caused by a herpesvirus and characterized by a vesicular eruption: herpes simplex or herpes zoster. • When not followed by *zoster* or by *virus*, the word *herpes* now usually refers specifically to herpes simplex. **2** Any of various serpiginous skin diseases. An obsolete usage.

buccal herpes Herpes simplex appearing on the buccal mucous membrane.

herpes catarrhalis Herpes simplex manifested as a cold sore.

herpes circinatus An obsolete term for DERMATITIS HERPETIFORMIS.

herpes corneae Infection of the ocular cornea with either herpes simplex or herpes zoster virus.

herpes desquamans TINEA IMBRICATA.

herpes digitalis Herpes simplex that involves one or more fingers or toes.

herpes disseminatus The presence of scattered varicelliform vesicles in a subject with herpes zoster.

herpes facialis Herpes simplex on the face.

herpes febrilis Herpes simplex manifested as a fever blister (cold sore) or accompanying fever. See also HERPES LABIALIS.

herpes generalisatus Herpes zoster occurring as a generalized vesicular eruption, usually in the presence of an immune defect.

herpes of the geniculate ganglion An incorrect term for HERPES ZOSTER AURICULARIS.

genital herpes Genital infection with *Herpesvirus hominis*, the herpes simplex virus (HSV), usually HSV-2. Most often transmitted by sexual contact and affecting both males and females, the infection is characterized clinically by itching, hyperemia, and the formation of closely grouped vesicles filled with clear fluid at the site of the infection. These rupture and develop into superficial ulcerations which heal after several weeks but recur in most patients and become active and infective again. Primary infection is frequently associated with systemic manifestations such as fever, malaise, anorexia, and bilateral inguinal lymphadenopathy. Also called *herpes genitalis, herpes progenitalis.*

herpes genitalis   GENITAL HERPES.

herpes gestationis   A rare disease characterized by an itchy erythematous eruption which later blisters. Clinically it resembles pemphigoid but occurs only in late pregnancy and the puerperium. It recurs in successive pregnancies and can be reactivated by the oral contraceptive. Histologically there are foci of epidermal basal cell necrosis over the tips of dermal papillae and subepidermal blister formation. Patients have an IgG (herpes gestationis factor) circulating which fixes complement to the basement membrane zone. Symptomatic treatment is often sufficient although occasionally corticosteroids may be necessary to control blistering. Also called *hydroa gestationis* (obsolete), *hydroa gravidarum* (obsolete), *dermatitis gestationis.*

herpes gladiatorum   TRAUMATIC HERPES.

herpes iris   An obsolete term for ERYTHEMA MULTIFORME.

labial herpes   HERPES LABIALIS.

herpes labialis   Herpes simplex manifested as an acute vesicular eruption on the lip or lips; a labial cold sore. The infection is usually acquired in childhood, and exacerbations may occur throughout life, especially during febrile illnesses such as pneumonia and malaria. Also called *labial herpes.*

lingual herpes   Herpes simplex on the tongue.

menstrual herpes   Herpes simplex recurring in the premenstrual or menstrual phase of the menstrual cycle. Also called *herpes menstrualis, mensual herpes.*

herpes menstrualis   MENSTRUAL HERPES.

mensual herpes   MENSTRUAL HERPES.

herpes mentalis   Herpex simplex below the chin.

nasal herpes   An eruption on or in the nose due either to the herpes simplex virus or to the virus of herpes zoster.

nasal herpes simplex   The characteristic eruption around the anterior nares caused by the herpes simplex virus. In many individuals such sores are liable to recur whenever the patient has a cold or is overexposed to the sun, as the virus resides in the cells of the skin and becomes active in response to local irritation.

nasal herpes zoster   A painful vesicular eruption which may occur on the skin of the external nose, in the nasal vestibule or, rarely, within the nasal cavity, due to herpes zoster of the maxillary division of the trigeminal nerve. Postherpetic pain may persist after the eruption has healed. The diagnosis may be more apparent if vesicles appear elsewhere in the distribution of the second division of the affected nerve, for instance on the ipsilateral cheek, but not across the midline.

neuralgic herpes   Genital herpes marked by painful straining of the bladder and rectum.

ocular herpes   Infection of any part of the eye with either herpes simplex or herpes zoster virus.

herpes ophthalmicus   Herpes zoster involving the trigeminal ganglion and giving rise to pain and vesiculation in the distribution of the first division of the trigeminus, often including the cornea. Also called *herpes zoster ophthalmicus, zoster ophthalmicus, zona ophthalmica, gasserian ganglionitis.*

orofacial herpes simplex   An eruption around the mouth or nose or, less often, elsewhere on the face, due to infection with the virus of herpes simplex.

herpes phlyctaenodes   An obsolete term for DERMATITIS HERPETIFORMIS.

herpes praeputialis   Genital herpes affecting the prepuce.

herpes progenitalis   GENITAL HERPES.

herpes pyaemicus   PUSTULAR PSORIASIS.

herpes recurrens   HERPES SIMPLEX RECURRENS.

recurrent herpes   HERPES SIMPLEX RECURRENS.

herpes simplex   A disease caused by infection with *Herpesvirus hominis* (herpes simplex virus), types 1 and 2, usually characterized by vesicles 3–6 mm in diameter developing around the lips or nostrils (usually type 1) or in the genital area (usually type 2). Infection may also involve the eye, the brain, or the meninges. The principal mode of spread is direct contact, usually by means of infected secretions. Once acquired, infection may be recurrent, and recurrences may be precipitated by physical illness or emotional stress. Neonatal infection may occur in offspring of mothers with active cervical herpes. Also called *hydroa febrile* (obsolete).

herpes simplex recurrens   Herpes simplex that tends to recur at or near the same site. Also called *herpes recurrens, recurrent herpes.*

herpes tonsurans   An inflammatory form of tinea capitis. An obsolete term.

herpes tonsurans barbae   An obsolete term for TINEA BARBAE.

herpes tonsurans capillitii   An obsolete term for TINEA CAPITIS.

traumatic herpes   Herpes simplex developing at the site of recent trauma, as may occur in wrestling and other body-contact sports. Also called *wrestlers' herpes, herpes gladiatorum.*

herpes vegetans   An obsolete term for PEMPHIGUS VEGETANS.

wrestlers' herpes   TRAUMATIC HERPES.

herpes zoster   An acute viral disease resulting from the activation of a latent herpesvirus (varicella-zoster virus) and characterized by inflammation of sensory ganglia, radicular neuralgic pain, and the usually unilateral eruption of groups of varicellalike vesicular lesions in a dermatomic distribution. Vesicles at sites distant from the primary infection occur in 2–5% of cases and more often in immunocompromised persons. The frequency of disseminated infection increases with age and with immunosuppression. Also called *shingles, zoster, zona, zona ignea* (older term), *zona serpiginosa, zona volatica* (obsolete), *erysipelas zoster* (obsolete), *acute posterior ganglionitis.*

herpes zoster auricularis   A painful eruption of vesicles in the concha of the ear or elsewhere in or around the ear, due to infection with the virus of herpes zoster. Some cases are complicated by facial paralysis, deafness, and vertigo. Postherpetic neuralgia may occur particularly in the elderly. Also called *zoster auricularis, herpes zoster oticus, zoster oticus, herpes of the geniculate ganglion* (incorrect), *geniculate zoster* (incorrect). See also RAMSAY HUNT SYNDROME.

herpes zoster ophthalmicus   HERPES OPHTHALMICUS.

herpes zoster oticus   HERPES ZOSTER AURICULARIS.

herpes zoster varicellosus   Disseminated herpes zoster characterized by a varicelliform eruption.

Herpesvirus   A generic designation used to include various herpes viruses, including herpes simplex viruses, varicella-zoster virus, and Epstein-Barr virus.

Herpesvirus hominis   A genus-species designation for herpes simplex virus.

Herpesvirus papio   A herpesvirus of baboons which is related to Epstein-Barr virus of humans.

Herpesvirus simiae   A genus-species designation for herpes B virus.

Herpesvirus suis   A genus-species designation for pseudorabies virus.

herpesvirus   **1** A virus belonging to the genus *Herpesvirus*. **2** Any herpes virus; a virus belonging to the family Herpetoviridae.

herpesvirus B   HERPES B VIRUS.

equine herpesvirus 1   The herpesvirus that causes equine viral rhinopneumonitis and equine viral abortion. Also called *equine rhinopneumonitis virus, equine abortion virus.*

herpesvirus simian B   HERPES B VIRUS.

herpesvirus T A virus that causes mild herpetic lesions in the mouth of its natural host, the squirrel monkey, *Saimiri sciureus.*

herpetic [Gk *herpet(on)* a creeping thing, reptile + -IC] **1** Pertaining to herpes. **2** Of or relating to the herpesvirus.

herpetiform Resembling a cutaneous herpesvirus infection: said of grouped vesicles.

herpetology [Gk *herpeto(n)* a creeping thing, reptile + -LOGY] The branch of zoology concerned with the study of reptiles and amphibians.

Herpetomonas [Gk *herpeto(n)* (from *herpein* to creep, crawl) a creeping thing + *monas* single, alone (as adj.), a unit (as substantive)] A genus of monogenetic insect-parasitizing flagellates of the family Trypanosomatidae. Transmission occurs via infective forms passed in feces of the host. The type species is *H. muscaedomesticae,* found in the common housefly. *H. sarcophagae* is a parasite of the flesh fly *Sarcophaga haemorrhoidalis.*

herpetomoniasis [*Herpetomon(as)* + -IASIS] Infection with any member of the genus *Herpetomonas.*

herpetophobia [Gk *herpeto(n)* a creeping thing, reptile + -PHOBIA] **1** Pathologic fear of snakes, lizards, or any creeping animal. **2** Pathologic fear of herpesvirus infection and, in particular, exaggerated fear of contracting genital herpes.

Herpetoviridae [Gk *herpeto(n)* a reptile, esp. snake + *vir(us)* + -IDAE] A family of large, enveloped, DNA-containing viruses. Those causing human disease belong to two genera: *Herpesvirus,* which includes herpes simplex virus, varicella-zoster virus, and Epstein-Barr virus, and *Cytomegalovirus,* which includes the agent of cytomegalic inclusion disease.

Herrick [James Bryan *Herrick,* U.S. physician, 1861–1954] Herrick's anemia. See under SICKLE CELL ANEMIA.

Herring [Percy Theodore *Herring,* English physiologist, 1872–1967] Herring bodies. See under HYALINE BODIES OF THE PITUITARY.

hersage [French (from L *irpex* or *hirpex* a harrow), a harrowing] The separation of fibers of a scarred nerve. Also called *combing, harrowing, endoneurolysis.*

Herter [Christian Archibald *Herter,* U.S. physician, 1865–1910] Herter's disease, Gee-Herter disease, Herter-Heubner disease, Gee-Herter-Heubner syndrome, Herter's infantilism. See under INFANTILE CELIAC DISEASE.

Hertig [Arthur T. *Hertig,* U.S. pathologist, born 1904] Hertig-Rock ova. See under OVUM.

Hertwig [Richard Carl Wilhelm Theodor von *Hertwig,* German zoologist, 1850–1937] Hertwig-Magendie phenomenon, Magendie-Hertwig sign, Hertwig-Magendie sign, Hertwig-Magendie syndrome. See under SKEW DEVIATION.

Hertwig [Wilhelm August Oskar *Hertwig,* German physiologist, 1849–1922] See under SHEATH.

hertz [after Heinrich Rudolph *Hertz,* German physicist, 1857–1894] (*plural* hertz) Special name for the SI derived unit of frequency, the frequency of a periodic phenomenon having a periodic time of one second; one cycle per second. Symbol: Hz

Herxheimer [Karl *Herxheimer,* German dermatologist, 1861–1944] **1** Jarisch-Herxheimer reaction, Herxheimer's fever. See under HERXHEIMER REACTION. **2** Herxheimer's fibers. See under HERXHEIMER SPIRALS.

Heryng [Theodor *Heryng,* Polish laryngologist, 1847–1925] See under SIGN.

Herz [Max *Herz,* German physician, born 1865] Triad of Herz. See under NEUROCIRCULATORY ASTHENIA.

herzstoss [German *Herz* heart + *Stoss* a thrust, push, shock] A diffuse precordial cardiac impulse.

Heschl [Richard L. *Heschl,* Austrian pathologist, 1824–1881] Transverse gyri of Heschl. See under AUDITORY CORTEX.

hesperanopia [K *hesper(a)* the evening + *an-* priv. + -OPIA] Inability of the eye to adapt for scotopic vision.

hesperidin $C_{28}H_{34}O_{15}$. A bioflavonoid present in citrus fruits, especially lemons and sweet oranges.

Hess [Alfred Fabian *Hess,* U.S. physician, 1875–1933] Hess capillary test. See under TEST.

Hess [Walter Rudolf *Hess,* Swiss physiologist, 1881–1973] Trophotropic zone of Hess. See under ZONE.

Hesselbach [Franz Kaspar *Hesselbach,* German surgeon, 1759–1816] **1** Hesselbach's fascia. See under FASCIA CRIBROSA. **2** Ligamentum interfoveolare hesselbachi, Hesselbach's ligament. See under LIGAMENTUM INTERFOVEOLARE. **3** Hesselbach's triangle. See under TRIGONUM INGUINALE.

heter- HETERO-.

heteradelphus [HETER- + Gk *adelphos* a twin, brother] CONJOINED UNEQUAL TWINS.

heteradenia Any abnormality of a gland or glands. A rarely used term. Adjective: heteradenic.

heterakid [*Heterak(is)* + -ID[1]] A member of the genus *Heterakis.*

Heterakis A genus of nematodes (family Heterakidae, order Ascaridida), parasitic in poultry. *H. gallinae,* the cecal worm of domestic fowl and other gallinaceous birds, is involved in transmission of *Histomonas meleagridis,* the agent of histomoniasis.
Heterakis gallinae An extremely common nematode worm that inhabits the cecum of numerous avian species. It is the carrier of *Histomonas meleagridis,* the cause of histomoniasis.

heteralius [HETER- + Gk *halios* fruitless] CRYPTODIDYMUS.

heterauxesis [HETER- + AUXESIS] The disproportionate growth of a part in relation to another part of the same organism.

heteraxial Having perpendicular axes of unequal length.

heterecious [Gk *heter(a),* fem. of *heteros* the other of two + *oiki(a)* a dwelling + -OUS] Requiring more than one host to complete the life cycle: a characteristic of many parasites. Also *heteroecious, metecious, metoecious, heteroxenous, metoxenous.* Compare AUTECIOUS.

heterecism [Gk *heter(a),* fem. of *heteros* the other of two + *oik(ia)* a dwelling + -ISM] A life cycle pattern, characteristic of many parasites, in which more than one host is required for the organism to complete its life cycle. Also called *heteroxeny, metoxeny, metaxeny.* Also *heteroecism.*

heterergic Capable of producing varying pharmacologic effects: said of drugs or pharmaceutical agents.

heteresthesia [HETER- + -ESTHESIA] Alternate hypesthesia and hyperesthesia in adjoining areas of the skin, occurring in spinal cord lesions.

hetero- [Gk *heteros* (adjective) other, one of two] **1** A combining form meaning other, different. **2** In organic chemistry, a combining form specifically meaning containing elements other than carbon. Also *heter-.* Compare HOMO-.

heteroagglutinin An antibody that agglutinates xenogeneic erythrocytes. Also called *heterohemoagglutinin.*

heteroallele In diploid cells, a mutant allele whose paired allele on the homologous chromosome also carries a mutation but in a different codon. Compare EUALLELE.

heteroallelic Pertaining to mutant alleles that differ from the wild type because of mutations in different codons. Compare EUALLELIC.

heteroatom An atom other than carbon, especially such an atom in a chain of carbon atoms.

heteroauxin An obsolete term for INDOLE-3-ACETIC ACID. ● This name was given when it was thought to be only one of the auxins, and that other substances were the main plant growth hormones.

Heterobasidiomycetes HETEROBASIDIOMYCETIDAE.

Heterobasidiomycetidae [HETERO- + BASIDIO- + MYCET- + -IDAE]   A former subclass of rust and smut fungi (plant pathogens), now contained in the subclass Teliomycetidae. Also called *Heterobasidiomycetes.*

heterobasidium [HETERO- + BASIDIUM]   (*plural* heterobasidia) Any type of fungal basidium other than a single-celled, club-shaped basidium.

Heterobilharzia   A genus of schistosomes parasitic in various mammals, and rarely reported from man.

Heterobilharzia americana   A species found in mesenteric veins of the lynx and other mammals. The cercariae may be responsible for a form of dermatitis common among oil workers in Louisiana.

heteroblastic   Derived from different kinds of precursor or from various embryonic cell types.

heterocaryon HETEROKARYON.

heterocellular [HETERO- + CELLULAR]   Formed of two or more kinds of cells.

heterocephalic   Having heads of unequal size: said of conjoined twins.

heterocephalus [HETERO- + -CEPHALUS]   Conjoined twins with heads of unequal size.

heterocercal   Curving upward at the caudal end of the vertebral column, resulting in a caudal fin that has a dorsal lobe larger than the ventral lobe, as in sharks.

heterochiral   Relating to the other hand.

heterochromatin   Regions of chromosomes characterized by condensation during interphase, late replication of DNA, transcriptional inactivity, and enrichment for highly repititious DNA. Compare EUCHROMATIN.

constitutive heterochromatin   Heterochromatin such as that at the centromere which is relatively invariant in an organism, regardless of cell type, state of differentiation, or transcriptional acitivity of the cell or of the surrounding euchromatin.

facultative heterochromatin   Heterochromatin that may become euchromatin, depending on the cell type, developmental stage, or sex. The inactive X chromosome in mammalian females is largely facultative heterochromatin.

paracentric heterochromatin   Heterochromatin that surrounds the centromere of a chromosome.

heterochromatinization   The process during which the euchromatin of a chromosome, or a part of a chromosome is changed to heterochromatin.

heterochromatosis HETEROCHROMIA.

heterochromia [HETERO- + CHROM- + -IA]   The presence of more than one color where uniformity of color is normal. Also called *heterochromatosis.*

binocular heterochromia   Variations in the color of the iris affecting both eyes, with or without associated pigmentation defects elsewhere in the body.

heterochromia iridis CHROMATIC ASYMMETRY.

monocular heterochromia   Loss of part of the melanin pigmentation of one iris.

heterochromic   Manifesting heterochromia. Also *heterochromous.*

heterochromosome ALLOSOME.

heterochromous HETEROCHROMIC.

heterochron [HETERO- + Gk *chron(os)* time]   Denoting excitable tissue displaying more than one chronaxy value. An obsolete term.

heterochronia   The development of tissues, organs, or other parts of an organism out of normal temporal sequence. Compare SYNCHRONIA.

heterochronic HETEROCHRONOUS.

heterochronous   Pertaining to or exhibiting heterochronia. Also *heterochronic.*

heterochthonous [HETERO- + Gk *chthōn* the earth, ground + -OUS]   ALLOCHTHONOUS.

heterocladic   Relating to or characterized by anastomosis between branches of different arterial trunks.

heterocoelous [HETERO- + COEL- + -OUS]   Having saddle-shaped articular faces between centra: said of vertebrae, as in the neck of birds.

heterocrine [HETERO- + Gk *krin(ein)* to separate, put apart]   Secreting more than one kind of substance: used of both endocrine and exocrine glands. Also called *allocrine.*

heterocrisis   A crisis marked by unusual symptoms or occurring at an unusual time.

heterocycle   A closed chain (ring) in an organic molecule in which at least one of the ring atoms is replaced by an atom other than carbon, such as O, N, S, P, Se, As, and B. Heterocyclic compounds are extremely numerous, and some, like pyrroles, furans, oxazines, thiazines, pyrimidines, and purines, play important parts in biologic chemistry and the dyestuffs industry.

heterocyclic [HETERO- + CYCLIC]   Designating a compound whose molecule contains a ring of atoms of which one or more is not carbon.

heterocyst   A large, transparent cell with a thickened wall that forms in filaments of certain species of cyanobacteria.

heterocytolysin HETEROLYSIN.

heterocytotoxin   A cytotoxin effective in a species other than that which produced it.

heterocytotropic   Having an affinity for cells of another species.

heterodactyl [HETERO- + Gk *daktyl(os)* finger]   Having two toes pointing forward and two toes pointing backward, as in certain birds.

Heterodera radicicola   A nematode parasite of root vegetables including carrots, radishes, potatoes, turnips, and others. Ova may be found in stools of humans and are often confused with true human parasites. Also called *Oxyuris incognita.*

heterodesmotic   Pertaining to fascicles or tracts of nerve fibers that interconnect neural centers of differing function.

heterodisperse   Exhibiting variation in some characteristic as in the particle sizes of an aerosol.

Heterodon   A common genus of harmless snakes, the hognose snakes, or puff adders, of the eastern and central United States, noted for their distinctive manner of flattening the head and neck region and hissing loudly when alarmed, and of feigning death or thrashing about wildly in response to threat.

heterodont [*heter(o)*- + -ODONT]   Denoting a dentition in which the teeth are specialized into different types, such as the incisors, canines, premolars, and molars of mammals.

Heterodoxus   A genus of biting lice (order Mallophaga, family Boopidae) that attack mammals. Examples include the Australian louse, *H. longitarsus,* found on kangaroos, wallabies, and occasionally dogs, and *H. spiniger,* a parasite of coyotes and wolves in North America which may also infest dogs.

heteroduplex   **1** Any double-stranded nucleic acid, either totally or partially base paired, in which the two strands are derived from different sources, such as different species.   **2** A completely or partially base paired nucleic acid in which one strand is DNA and the other is RNA.

heteroecious HETERECIOUS.

heteroecism HETERECISM.

heteroerotism [HETERO- + EROTISM] Investment of energy of the libido onto others, and specifically onto persons of the opposite sex, a normal phase of development.

heterofermentative Carrying out heterolactic fermentation. Also *heterolactic*. Compare HOMOFERMENTATIVE.

heterogamete Any gamete that differs in structure or size from the one that is usually joined in fertilization with it, as in the human ovum and sperm.

heterogametic **1** Referring to or characterized by the production of different kinds of gametes, usually in reference to the sex chromosome present. In humans, males are heterogametic. **2** Referring to or characterized by the production of gametes that differ in size or structure. Humans are heterogametic in this regard.

heterogamety An individual organism, a specific sex, or a species that gives rise to different kinds of gametes, usually used in reference to the sex chromosome present, and occasionally used with respect to size or structure.

heterogamous Pertaining to or characterized by heterogamy.

heterogamy [HETERO- + *gam(o)-* + -Y] **1** A mating preference for individuals of unlike characteristics. **2** ALTERNATION OF GENERATIONS. **3** The property of bearing different types of flowers. **4** The reproduction of plants by indirect pollination. Compare HOMOGAMY.

heteroganglionic Denoting the interconnecting ganglia of the sympathetic chain.

heterogeneic HETEROGENIC.

heterogeneity GENETIC HETEROGENEITY.

genetic heterogeneity The occurrence of different mutations, either at a single locus or at distinct loci, that determine the same phenotype. Also called *heterogenicity, heterogeneity*.

heterogeneous HETEROGENIC.

heterogenesis **1** ALTERNATION OF GENERATIONS. **2** XENOGENESIS. **3** Origination or development by asexual multiplication, sport, or bud variation.

heterogenetic HETEROGENIC.

heterogenic Characterized by heterogeneity. Also *heterogenetic, heterogeneous, heterogenous, heterogeneic*.

heterogenicity GENETIC HETEROGENEITY.

heterogenote A bacterium which is heterozygous for a region of a chromosome owing to the presence of an F-prime factor or a transducing phage.

heterogenous HETEROGENIC.

heterogeusia [HETERO- + Gk *geus(is)* taste + -IA] A variety of dysgeusia characterized by a persistent, consistent change in the taste of all food and drink, for example everything may taste sweet.

heterogonic [HETERO- + GON-² + -IC] Characterizing an alternative cycle in which larvae, under appropriate circumstances, develop into free-living male and female adults instead of developing directly into the infective parasitic form. Alternative heterogonic and homogonic cycles are seen in rhabditoid nematode worms. See also *STRONGYLOIDES*.

heterograft XENOGRAFT.

bovine heterograft A prosthetic vascular graft composed of preserved calf carotid artery.

heterogynous [HETERO- + GYN- + -OUS] Having two different types of females in a species, such as queen and worker bees.

heterohemagglutination Hemagglutination induced by hemagglutinins from a different species.

heterohemagglutinin HETEROAGGLUTININ.

heterohemolysin An antibody occurring naturally or raised by immunization which is effective in producing a complement-mediated lysis of xenogeneic erythrocytes.

heteroimmune Having or inducing heteroimmunity.

heteroimmunity Immunity induced in an animal by introducing immunizing cells derived from an animal of a different species.

heteroinfection [HETERO- + INFECTION] An infection contracted from a source outside the host; an exogenous infection. Compare AUTOINFECTION.

heteroinoculable Susceptible to heteroinoculation.

heteroinoculation [HETERO- + INOCULATION] Inoculation of one individual with a microorganism from another.

heterointoxication Poisoning resulting from the introduction of an exogenous substance into the body. Also called *heterotoxis*.

heterokaryon A cell that contains two or more genetically different nuclei in a common cytoplasm, as somatic cell hybrids, or cells of some ascomycetes or basidiomycetes. Also *heterocaryon*. Compare HOMOKARYON.

heterokaryosis The condition of a heterokaryon.

heterokeratoplasty [HETERO- + KERATOPLASTY] The transplantation of a cornea to an individual of a different species of animal.

heterokinesia [HETERO- + KINESIA] Difficulty in performing a movement, due to the fact that one limb is moved spontaneously when one attempts to move the other (allokinesia or mirror movement), or that a movement contrary to the one desired is made. Also called *heterokinesis*.

heterokinesis **1** The segregation of the sex chromosomes during meiosis in a heterogametic organism. **2** HETEROKINESIA.

heterolactic HETEROFERMENTATIVE.

heterolalia [HETERO- + -LALIA] A form of partial aphasia in which the patient says a word which is not the one he intended. A seldom used term. Also called *allophemia, heterophasia, heterophasis, heterophemia*.

heterolateral CONTRALATERAL.

heterolecithal [HETERO- + LECITH- + -AL] Describing an ovum in which yolk substances are unequally distributed.

heterolith [HETERO- + -LITH] A nonmineral intraintestinal concretion. An obsolete term.

heterologous **1** Different: said of a graft between divergent species. Also *xenogenic, xenogeneic*. **2** Noncorresponding, as two nonhomologous chromosomes, or an antigen and an antibody that do not interact. For defs. 1 and 2 also *heterospecific*. Compare HOMOLOGOUS.

heterolysin An antibody occurring naturally or raised by immunization which is effective in producing complement-mediated lysis of xenogeneic cells. Also called *heterocytolysin*.

heterolysis Lysis occurring in an animal of a species other than that which produced the lysin.

heterolysosome [HETERO- + LYSOSOME] A membrane-limited organelle in the cytoplasm of the cell which is formed by fusion of a phagosome and a lysosome.

heterolytic Of or characterized by heterolysis.

heteromastigote A flagellate characterized by dissimilar flagella, one or several extended anteriorly, the other posteriorly.

heteromeral HETEROMERIC.

heteromeric [HETERO- + *mer(o)-¹* + -IC] **1** Possessing a different chemical composition. **2** Denoting neurons of the spinal cord emitting axons that cross to the opposite side. Also *heteromeral, heteromerous*.

heteromerous HETEROMERIC.

heterometaplasia Metaplasia in which the transformed tissue is not normally present at the site.

heterometric [HETERO- + METR- + -IC] Concerning changes in dimension.

heterometropia [HETERO- + Gk *metr(on)* measure + -OPIA]

A difference in the refractive errors of the two eyes.

heteromorphic HETEROMORPHOUS.

heteromorphosis The regeneration of a structure, part, or organ different from that lost or removed.

heteromorphous [HETERO- + -MORPHOUS] **1** Departing from the norm in shape or structure. **2** Exhibiting variation in form: anisomorphous. **3** Of or relating to heteromorphosis. For defs. 1, 2, and 3 also *heteromorphic.*

heteronymous Of or relating to another muscle: said of the response in one muscle, motoneuron, or nerve upon stimulation of the nerve to a second muscle, which is usually a synergist.

hetero-osteoplasty The xenografting of bone.

heteropagus [HETERO- + -PAGUS] DUPLICITAS ASYMMETROS.

heterophagous [HETERO- + -PHAGOUS] Eating a variety of food types.

heterophany [HETERO- + Gk *-phan(ēs)*, combining form denoting making to appear, shining + -Y] Variation in the manifestations of a certain disease or condition.

heterophasia HETEROLALIA.

heterophasis HETEROLALIA.

heterophemia HETEROLALIA.

heterophil [HETERO- + -PHIL] Having the property of reacting or combining with more than one substance, as an antiserum that reacts with both human and sheep erythrocytes or a cell that is stainable by both acidic and basic dyes.

heterophonia [HETERO- + PHON- + -IA] Disordered voice production resulting from inflammatory, structural, neurologic, or psychogenic factors. Also called *heterophony.*

heterophony HETEROPHONIA.

heterophoralgia [HETERO- + PHOR- + ALGIA] Ocular symptoms attributable to heterophoria.

heterophoria [HETERO- + -PHORIA] A latent tendency to misalignment of the eyes in any direction, recognizable only when fusion is interrupted, as by covering one eye. Adjective: heterophoric.

heterophoric Of or relating to heterophoria.

heterophthalmia [HETER- + OPHTHALMIA] A difference in the structure of the two eyes. Also called *heterophthalmos, allophthalmia.*

heterophthalmos HETEROPHTHALMIA.

heterophydiasis HETEROPHYIASIS.

Heterophyes [HETERO- + Gk *phyē* (from *phyein* to bring forth, make to grow) growth, stature, one's natural powers] A genus of small fish-borne trematodes of the family Heterophyidae, parasitic in the small intestine of humans, dogs, cats, other mammals, and fish-eating birds. Infection of the final host occurs through ingestion of raw or undercooked infected fish, which are in turn infected from cercariae from infected first intermediate snail hosts. Also called *Cotylogonimus.*

Heterophyes heterophyes A species parasitic in the cecum and small intestine of man and other fish-eating mammals; the Egyptian or small intestinal fluke. It is widely distributed in Egypt and the Far East. Also called *Distoma heterophyes* (obsolete), *Fasciola heterophyes, Mesogonimus heterophyes.*

Heterophyes katsuradai A species of trematode, smaller in size than *H. heterophyes,* which occurs in Japan. Infections resulting from ingestion of raw, smoked, pickled, or undercooked fresh- or brackish-water fish are common.

heterophyiasis [*Heterophy(es)* + -IASIS] Infection with flukes of the genus *Heterophyes.* Also called *heterophydiasis.*

Heterophyidae [*Heterophy(es)* + -IDAE] A family of small trematodes which are freshwater-fish-borne parasites of fish-eating birds, humans, and other mammals. It includes the genus

Heterophyes, species of which are common human parasites. Some members of the family are thought to cause blockage of coronary vessels by the extremely small eggs of the parasites that enter the submucosa and the mesenteric circulation. These cases, reported chiefly in the Philippines, involved bird heterophyids not well adapted to humans.

heteroplasia [HETERO- + -PLASIA] **1** The development of cells or tissues of a distinctive type in a location where they do not normally occur. Also called *alloplasia.* **2** An abnormal position, termination, or origin of an organ or part that is otherwise normal, as an ectopic termination of the ureter.

heteroplasm [HETERO- + -PLASM] A tissue found in an abnormal location.

heteroplastic Exhibiting heteroplasia; ectopic.

heteroplastid XENOGRAFT.

heteroplasty [HETERO- + -PLASTY] An obsolete term for HETEROTRANSPLANTATION.

heteroploid Characterized by heteroploidy.

heteroploidy [HETERO- + -PLOID + -Y] The condition of a cell or an individual organism that has a number of chromosomes different from the usual haploid or diploid complement, as the states of aneuploidy and polyploidy.

Heteropoda A genus of large tarantulalike spiders, capable of inflicting a painful but nonvenomous bite to humans.

Heteropoda venatoria A large spider, confused with tarantulas, often found in shipments of tropical fruit, particularly bananas. The bite of this spider is painful but not serious.

heteropodal Possessing branches, such as the dendrites of neurons, having different morphologic and functional characteristics.

heteroprosopus [HETERO- + Gk *prosōp(on)* a face + L *-us,* noun suffix] JANICEPS.

heteropsia [HETER- + -OPSIA] A difference in the visual acuity of the two eyes.

heteropsychology ABNORMAL PSYCHOLOGY.

Heteroptera [HETERO- + Gk *ptera* feathers, wings (pl. of *pteron* feather)] A suborder of bugs in the order Hemiptera. Most possess two pairs of wings, one coriaceous or horny, the other membranous. The medically important families Reduviidae and Cimicidae are included in the suborder.

heteroptics [HETER- + OPT- + -ICS] Variations from normal visual perceptions, such as hallucinations.

heteropyknosis [HETERO- + PYKN- + -OSIS] The condition in which a substance appears to have different densities, as the different degrees of staining intensity of different chromosomes. Increased capacity to stain or increased density is called positive heterpyknosis, and decreased capacity or density negative. Adjective: heteropyknotic.

heteropyknotic Referring to or demonstrating heteropyknosis, as heterochromatin.

heteroscope [HETERO- + -SCOPE] A device that can present to the two eyes separate images that may be varied with respect to the angular alignment of the two eyes with each other.

heteroscopy [HETERO- + -SCOPY] The use of a heteroscope to present images at different angles to the two eyes.

heterosexual [HETERO- + SEXUAL] **1** Characterized by heterosexuality. **2** A heterosexual individual.

heterosexuality [HETERO- + SEXUALITY] Sexuality directed toward the opposite sex.

heterosis [HETERO- + -SIS] The vitality of a hybrid that exceeds the vitality of either parent. Also called *hybrid vigor.*

monohybrid heterosis OVERDOMINANCE.

heterosmia [HETER- + *osm(o)*-² + -IA] A disorder of the sense of smell in which the odor perceived is at variance with the stimulus producing it. Also called *allotriosmia* (seldom used).

heterosome A rarely used term for SEX CHROMOSOME.

heterospecific HETEROLOGOUS.

heterosporous Having spores of two kinds, each of which reproduces asexually.

heterotaxia ECTOPIA.

heterotaxic [New L *heterotax(is)* (from Gk *hetero(s)* other, one of two + *taxis* an arranging) an abnormal ordering + -IC] ECTOPIC.

heterotaxis ECTOPIA.

heterotaxy ECTOPIA.

heterothallic Having hyphae that are observably similar in form, but sexually segregated, therefore requiring two opposite mating types for sexual reproduction: used especially of certain fungi. Compare HOMOTHALLIC.

heterotherapy Treatment directed at the chief symptoms of a disorder.

heterotherm POIKILOTHERM.

heterothermic POIKILOTHERMIC.

heterothermy POIKILOTHERMY.

heterotonia A condition characterized by variations in muscle tone.

heterotonic Concerning heterotonia.

heterotopia [HETERO- + Gk *top(os)* place + -IA] ECTOPIA.

nasal glial heterotopia A tumorlike mass of mature glial tissue occurring intranasally or at the base of the nose. Astrocytes may simulate nerve cells. Also called *nasal glioma* (incorrect).

neuronal heterotopia A pathologic state in which neurons are found in parts of the brain (as in the white matter) where they are not normally present.

heterotopic 1 ECTOPIC. 2 Describing or relating to heterotopia.

heterotopy ECTOPIA.

heterotoxic Producing toxic effects in individuals of a different species from the originating individual. Compare HOMEOTOXIC.

heterotoxin [HETERO- + TOXIN] A toxin which produces adverse effects in individuals of a different species from the originating individual.

heterotoxis HETEROINTOXICATION.

heterotransplant XENOGRAFT.

heterotransplantation An operation involving the transplantation of tissue or an organ from an unrelated species (xenograft) to replace lost or damaged tissue. Also called *heteroplasty* (obsolete), *xenoplasty*.

heterotrichia [HETERO- + TRICH- + -IA] The growth of hair of more than one color.

heterotrichosis The growth of one or more sites of hair differing in color from the scalp hair.

heterotrichosis superciliorum A state of having eyebrows that differ in color from the scalp hair.

heterotrichous [HETERO- + TRICH- + -OUS] Having hair of more than one color.

heterotroph [HETERO- + Gk *troph(ē)* nourishment] An organism unable to synthesize nutrients from inorganic compounds and therefore dependent on complex organic molecules from external sources for growth. Also called *metatroph*. Compare AUTOTROPH.

heterotrophic 1 Of or relating to a heterotroph. 2 Denoting the mode of nutrition characterizing heterotrophs; requiring complex organic molecules as sources of carbon and other nutrients. For defs 1 and 2 also *metatrophic*.

heterotropia STRABISMUS.

comitant heterotropia CONCOMITANT HETEROTROPIA.

concomitant heterotropia A manifest deviation of the two eyes that is the same in all directions of gaze. Also called *comitant heterotropia*.

noncomitant heterotropia A manifest deviation of the two eyes that is not the same in all directions of gaze.

paralytic heterotropia A manifest deviation of an eye due to nonfunction of one or more of the extraocular muscles.

heterotropy [HETERO- + Gk *trop(ē)* a turn, turning around + -Y] STRABISMUS.

heterotype A representative of a population whose characters are widely divergent from the mean for that population. Compare HOMOTYPE.

heterotypic 1 Differing from what is normal or commonly found. 2 Designating the first meiotic division of germ cells. An outmoded usage.

heterovaccination Vaccination with a vaccine produced from a microorganism different from the agent causing the disease for which the vaccine is used. The use of BCG to attempt to increase resistance to leprosy is an example. An outmoded term.

heterovaccine A vaccine manufactured from a microorganism different from the causative agent of the disease for which the vaccine is used.

heteroxenous HETERECIOUS.

heteroxeny HETERECISM.

heterozygosis The union of gametes of unlike genetic constitution to form a zygote.

heterozygosity A condition of a diploid or polyploid organism in which different alleles are found at one or more loci.

heterozygote An individual having different alleles at one or more genetic loci in homologous chromosome segments. This situation provides a much greater potential store of genetic diversity than is possible in a population of homozygotes with identical alleles at these loci.

compound heterozygote GENETIC COMPOUND.

double heterozygote A cell or organism that is heterozygous at two separate genetic loci. In experimental genetics, it is usually the offspring of parents who were homozygous for different alleles at two loci. Also called *dihybrid, diheterozygote*.

inversion heterozygote A cell or organism that contains an inverted region of chromosome or detectable DNA sequence at one allele at one or more loci.

triple heterozygote An individual cell or organism that is heterozygous at three separate genetic loci. In experimental genetics, it is usually the offspring of parents who were homozygous for different alleles at the three loci. Also called *triheterozygote, trihybrid*.

heterozygotic HETEROZYGOUS.

heterozygous Characterized by different alleles at a given locus: used especially of diploid or polyploid cells or organisms. Also *heterozygotic*.

Hetherington [D. C. *Hetherington*, U.S. anatomist, born 1895] See under STAIN.

Hetrazan A proprietary name for diethylcarbamazine.

Heublein [Arthur Carl *Heublein*, U.S. radiologist, 1879–1932] See under METHOD.

Heubner [Johann Otto Leonhard *Heubner*, German pediatrician, 1843–1926] 1 Heubner's specific endarteritis. See under SYPHILITIC CEREBRAL ENDARTERITIS. 2 Herter-Heubner disease, Gee-Herter-Heubner disease, Gee-Herter-Heubner syndrome. See under INFANTILE CELIAC DISEASE. 3 See under ARTERY.

Heuser [Chester *Heuser*, U.S. embryologist, 1885–1965] Heuser's membrane. See under EXOCOELOMIC MEMBRANE.

hex- HEXA-.

hexa- [Gk *hex* six] A combining form meaning six. Also *hex-*.

Hexa-Betalin A proprietary name for pyridoxine hydrochloride.

hexacanth [HEX- + -ACANTH] ONCOSPHERE.

hexachlorane HEXACHLOROCYCLOHEXANE.

hexachlorobenzene C_6Cl_6. A white crystalline solid used as a fungicidal dressing on seed grains. It is not known to cause poisoning to workers manufacturing it or using it in the field. Poisoning has occurred among persons who have eaten wheat treated with this fungicide.

hexachlorocyclohexane $C_6H_6Cl_6$. A halogenated hydrocarbon that is an effective agent in the treatment of scabies and pediculosis. It is used in creams, ointments, and shampoos. The gamma isomer is lindane, which is used as an insecticide. Poisoning may occur from ingestion or prolonged inhalation. Also called *hexachlorane, benzene hexachloride*.

hexachlorophane HEXACHLOROPHENE.

hexachlorophene $C_{13}H_6Cl_6O_2$. 2,2'-Methylenebis-[3,4,6-trichlorophenol]. A mild detergent that is used as a topical antiseptic agent and as a component of some soaps and scrubbing preparations. It is contraindicated for burn or skin dressings, the skin of infants, or other situations in which absorption of the chemical might occur and lead to toxic reactions. Also called *compound G-11, hexachlorophane*.

hexachromic [HEXA- + CHROM- + -IC] Descriptive of the ability to perceive six of the major spectral hues, the faulty discrimination usually being in the short wavelength end of the visible spectrum.

hexacontane $C_{60}H_{122}$. The saturated hydrocarbon whose molecules have unbranched chains of sixty carbon atoms.

hexacosane $C_{26}H_{54}$. The saturated hydrocarbon whose molecules have unbranched chains of 26 carbon atoms.

hexadactylia HEXADACTYLY.

hexadactylism HEXADACTYLY.

hexadactyly [HEXA- + DACTYL- + -Y] Polydactyly in which there are six digits on a hand or foot. Also called *hexadactylia, hexadactylism*.

hexadimethrine bromide $(C_{13}H_{30}Br_2N_2)_x$. *N,N,N',N'*-Tetramethyl-1,6-hexanediamine polymer with 1,3-dibromopropane. A polymer with basic properties that has the capacity to combine with and neutralize the effects of heparin and prevent its anticoagulant action.

Hexadrol A proprietary name for dexamethasone.

Hexagenia bilineata A mayfly that is abundant on the shores of Lake Erie. Cast skins of this species are associated with asthma in the susceptible local population.

hexamethonium $(CH_3)_3N^+$—$[CH_2]_6$—$N^+(CH_3)_3$. A ganglion-blocking agent, available as its chloride or bromide, used for the treatment of hypertension.

hexamethylenaminesalicylsulfonic acid METHENAMINE.

hexamethylendiamine NH_2—$[CH_2]_6$—NH_2. An amine used in the manufacture of nylon.

hexamethyl violet CRYSTAL VIOLET.

hexamine METHENAMINE.

hexamine hippurate METHENAMINE HIPPURATE.

hexamine mandelate METHENAMINE MANDELATE.

Hexamita A genus of protozoan flagellates (order Diplomonadida, class Zoomastigophorea), members of which are characterized by two anterior nuclei, and six anterior and two posterior flagella. Some species are found as parasites in the small intestine of certain mammals and gallinaceous birds, but many other species are strictly free-living. The genus is related to the common human parasitic flagellate *Giardia*. Also called *Octomitus*.

Hexamita meleagridis A species that causes acute enteritis, or hexamitiasis, in turkeys, pheasant, quail, chickens, chukkar partridges and other gallinaceous birds. The most severe form of disease occurs in young turkeys.

hexamitiasis [*Hexamit(a)* + -IASIS] An enteric disease of turkeys and other avian species, caused by infection with the flagellate protozoan parasite *Hexamita meleagridis*, which causes a severe enteritis in wild and domestic fowl.

hexane CH_3—$[CH_2]_4$—CH_3. The saturated hydrocarbon whose molecules have unbranched chains of six carbon atoms.

Hexanicotol A proprietary name for inositol niacinate.

hexanoic acid CH_3—$[CH_2]_4$—$COOH$. One of the lower fatty acids. Its residues occur in milk fat. Also called *caproic acid* (outmoded).

hexaploid [HEXA- + -PLOID] Having six sets of chromosomes in the cell nucleus.

hexaploidy [HEXA- + -PLOID + -Y] The state of having six sets of chromosomes in the nuclei of somatic cells.

Hexapoda [HEXA- + New L -*poda*, neut. pl. of -*pod*, combining form from Gk *pous*, gen. *podos*, foot] INSECTA.

hexavaccine A vaccine composed of six different antigens.

Hexavibex A proprietary name for pyridoxine hydrochloride.

hexavitamin A combination of vitamins containing six components: Vitamins A, C, and D, and thiamine hydrochloride, riboflavin, and nicotinamide. It is formed into a tablet or capsule for oral administration.

hexaxial Having or pertaining to six axes, as in the hexaxial reference system, used for determining the electrical axis of the heart.

hexenmilch [German, witches' milk] WITCH'S MILK.

hexestrol $C_{18}H_{22}O_2$. 4,4'-(1,2-Diethyl-1,2-ethanediyl) bisphenol, a synthetic derivative of diethylstilbestrol, used orally and parenterally in substitutive and pharmacologic estrogen therapy.

hexetidine $C_{21}H_{45}N_3$. 1,3-Bis(2-ethylhexyl)hexahydro-5-methyl-5-pyrimidinamine. An oil used as a 0.1% solution in mouth and throat infections. The agent has antibacterial and antiprotozoal activity, and it is effective against *Candida* infections as well as mixed bacterial infections.

hexobarbital $C_{12}H_{16}N_2O_3$. 5-(1-Cyclohexen-1-yl)-1,5-dimethylbarbituric acid, a barbiturate used therapeutically as a sedative and short-acting hypnotic. It is given orally. Also called *enhexymal, methexenyl*.

hexocyclium methylsulfate $C_{21}H_{36}N_2O_5S$. 4-(β-Cyclohexyl-β-hydroxy-β-phenethyl)-1,1-dimethylpiperazinium methylsulfate. A quarternary anticholinergic agent that is used to decrease gastric motility and gastric secretory activity. In larger doses it is also used to produce parasympathetic blockade. It is given orally.

hexokinase The enzyme (EC 2.7.1.1) that catalyzes the transfer of a phosphate group from ATP to glucose to yield glucose 6-phosphate. Most of its forms, such as those of muscle, have a low Michaelis constant for glucose and are normally saturated by it. The main liver isoenzyme, however, has a Michaelis constant comparable with the glucose concentration in the blood, and therefore phosphorylates more glucose when this concentration is raised.

hexonate The anion or salt of a hexonic acid, i.e. the acid formed by oxidation of C-1 of an aldohexose to yield a carboxyl group.

hexonic acid The acid formed by oxidation of C-1 of an aldohexose to yield a carboxyl group.

hexosamine The derivative of an aldohexose in which one hydroxyl group, normally on C-2, is replaced by an amino group.

hexosaminidase Any enzyme that catalyzes the hydrolysis of glycosides formed by hexosamines or *N*-acylated hexosamines. The removal of *N*-acetylglucosamine and *N*-acetylgalactosamine residues from glycolipids is a function of hexosaminidases.

hexosaminidase A The more negatively charged (pI = 5) of two hexosaminidases found in tissues. It catalyzes the hydrolytic cleavage of *N*-acetylglucosamine residues from glycolipids. If the enzyme is absent as in Tay-Sachs disease, a ganglioside accumulates.

hexosaminidase B The less negatively charged of two hexosaminidases found in tissues. It has an isoelectric point of 7. Unlike hexosaminidase A, it is not deficient in Tay-Sachs disease.

hexose [HEX- + -OSE²] A sugar whose molecule consists of a chain of six carbon atoms, such as glucose or fructose.

hexose diphosphate Any of the bisphosphates of hexoses. Biologically these are mainly fructose 1,6-bisphosphate and, to a lesser extent, glucose 1,6-bisphosphate. An obsolete term.

hexose monophosphate Any or several of the phosphates of various hexoses, including glucose 6-phosphate, glucose 1-phosphate and fructose 6-phosphate: used to indicate that the particular compounds are not distinguished.

hexosephosphoric esters Phosphate esters of hexose sugars. They are important intermediates in carbohydrate metabolism.

hexylcaine hydrochloride $C_{16}H_{24}ClNO_2$. 1-(Cyclohexylamino)-2-propanol benzoate (ester) hydrochloride, a local anesthetic used primarily for topical anesthesia of intact membranes of the respiratory tract, the upper gastrointestinal tract, and the urinary tract.

hexylresorcinol $C_{12}H_{18}O_2$. 4-Hexyl-1,3-benzenediol, an antiseptic used in a solution which usually contains glycerin in water, as a wash, or for application to topical wounds or membranes. It is also administered internally as an antihelminthic against roundworms and hookworms.

Hey [William *Hey*, English surgeon, 1736–1819] **1** See under SAW. **2** Hey's internal derangement. See under DERANGEMENT. **3** Hey's operation. See under AMPUTATION. **4** Hey's ligament. See under MARGO FALCIFORMIS HIATUS SAPHENUS.

Heyer [W. T. *Heyer*, U.S. scientist, born 1902] Pudenz-Heyer valve. See under VALVE.

Heyman [James *Heyman*, Swedish gynecologist, born 1882] See under TECHNIQUE.

Heymans [Corneille Jean François *Heymans*, Belgian physiologist, 1892–1968] See under LAW.

Heyns [O. S. *Heyns*, South African obstetrician, flourished 20th century] See under DECOMPRESSION.

Hf Symbol for the element, hafnium.

Hfr Denoting a strain of *Escherichia coli* capable of high-frequency gene transfer to a recipient because its F plasmid has integrated into the host chromosome. The site of integration determines the locus of entry of the chromosome.

HFT high-frequency transduction (denoting certain strains of bacteriophage).

Hft high-frequency transduction (denoting certain strains of bacteriophage).

Hg Symbol for the element, mercury.

hg Symbol for the unit, hectogram.

Hgb hemoglobin.

HGH human growth hormone.

HGPRT hypoxanthine-guanine-phosphoribosyl transferase.

HHA health hazard appraisal (health risk appraisal).

H. + Hm. compound hypermetropic astigmatism.

HHS Department of Health and Human Services.

hiatal Of or referring to a hiatus, especially the esophageal hiatus of the diaphragm.

hiation [L *hiat(us)*, past part. of *hiare* to gape, yawn + -ION] YAWNING.

hiatopexia HIATOPEXY.

hiatopexy [L *hiat(us)* an opening, a gaping + *o* + -PEXY] A surgical procedure to repair a space, gap, or widened opening, usually employing suture plication. Also called *hiatopexia*.

hiatus [L, a cleft, opening] Any large opening, gap, or cleft; a foramen.

adductor hiatus HIATUS TENDINEUS.

hiatus adductorius HIATUS TENDINEUS.

aortic hiatus HIATUS AORTICUS.

hiatus aorticus [NA] The osseoaponeurotic opening in, or behind, the diaphragm, bounded by the median arcuate ligament anteriorly, the right and left crura of the diaphragm on either side, and the lower border of the body of twelfth thoracic vertebra posteriorly, transmitting the aorta, the thoracic duct and, occasionally, the azygos vein. Also called *aortic opening, aortic foramen, aortic hiatus, inferior left foramen* (outmoded), *aortic opening in diaphragm, aortic orifice.*

Breschet's hiatus HELICOTREMA.

buccal hiatus A cleft at the angle of the mouth in the embryo, which, if it persists, gives rise to macrostomia. Also called *transverse facial cleft.*

hiatus of canal for greater petrosal nerve HIATUS CANALIS NERVI PETROSI MAJORIS.

hiatus canalis facialis HIATUS CANALIS NERVI PETROSI MAJORIS.

hiatus canalis nervi petrosi majoris [NA] The opening in the anterior petrous portion of the temporal bone that leads to the facial canal and contains the greater petrosal nerve and a branch of the middle meningeal artery. Also called *hiatus of canal for greater petrosal nerve, hiatus canalis facialis, hiatus of facial canal, hiatus for greater superficial petrosal nerve, superficial petrosal fissure, foramen of Fallopio, hiatus of Fallopius, hiatus of fallopian canal, hiatus fallopii, false hiatus of fallopian canal, spurious aperture of fallopian canal* (outmoded), *spurious aperture of facial canal* (outmoded), *foramen of Tarin* (outmoded), *Ferrein's foramen.*

hiatus canalis nervi petrosi minoris [NA] The small lateral opening in the petrous portion of the temporal bone through which the lesser petrosal nerve passes. Also called *hiatus of canal for lesser petrosal nerve, opening for lesser superficial petrosal nerve, opening for smaller superficial petrosal nerve.*

hiatus of canal for lesser petrosal nerve HIATUS CANALIS NERVI PETROSI MINORIS.

esophageal hiatus HIATUS ESOPHAGEUS.

hiatus esophageus [NA] The oval opening formed by the separation of the medial muscular fibers of the right crus of the diaphragm at the level of the tenth thoracic vertebra, transmitting the esophagus, the anterior and posterior vagal trunks, and esophageal branches of the left gastric vessels. Also called *esophageal hiatus, esophageal foramen, superior left foramen* (outmoded), *hiatus oesophageus, esophageal opening in diaphragm, opening of esophagus.*

ethmoidal hiatus HIATUS SEMILUNARIS.

hiatus of facial canal HIATUS CANALIS NERVI PETROSI MAJORIS.

hiatus of fallopian canal HIATUS CANALIS NERVI PETROSI MAJORIS.

hiatus fallopii HIATUS CANALIS NERVI PETROSI MAJORIS.

hiatus of Fallopius HIATUS CANALIS NERVI PETROSI MAJORIS.

false hiatus of fallopian canal HIATUS CANALIS NERVI PETROSI MAJORIS.

hiatus femoralis FEMORAL FOSSA.

hiatus finalis sacralis The portion of the hiatus sacralis involving the fifth, or last, sacral vertebra. An outmoded term.

genital hiatus A so-called deficient area of the urogenital region in the female, bounded in front of the vagina by the medial margins of the two levator ani muscles, the pubic bones, and the symphysis pubis. It corresponds to the space between the arcuate pubic ligament and the anterior or upper margin of the perineal membrane. An outmoded term.

hiatus for greater superficial petrosal nerve HIATUS CANALIS NERVI PETROSI MAJORIS.

hiatus intermedius lumbosacralis A fissure resulting from delayed normal ossification occasionally observed in the first sacral vertebra in young individuals.

hiatus interosseus The gap proximal to the interosseous membrane between the radius and the ulna and distal to the oblique ligament through which the posterior interosseous vessels pass.

hiatus leukemicus A maturation gap in the granulocytic series that is often seen in acute granulocytic leukemia. For example, there may be myeloblasts, progranulocytes, and mature neutrophils, without any cells of the normally intermediate stages of maturation.

hiatus lumbosacralis The large space between the vertebral arches of the fifth lumbar and the first sacral vertebrae.

hiatus maxillaris [NA] The large, irregular aperture opening into the maxillary sinus on the posterosuperior aspect of the nasal surface of the maxilla, partly closed by the perpendicular plate of palatine bone, the maxillary process of inferior nasal concha, the uncinate process of ethmoid, and part of the lacrimal bone. Also called *maxillary hiatus, hiatus of maxillary sinus, maxillary foramen, ostium maxillare, orifice of maxillary sinus.*

maxillary hiatus HIATUS MAXILLARIS.

hiatus of maxillary sinus HIATUS MAXILLARIS.

neural hiatus An opening in the neural tube of early embryos during the closure process which eventually results in a complete neural tube with anterior and posterior neuropores.

hiatus oesophageus HIATUS ESOPHAGEUS.

pleuropericardial hiatus An opening by which the early pericardial cavity communicates with each pleural canal. Subsequently each hiatus is closed off by the corresponding pleuropericardial fold, and contributes to the definitive diaphragm. If not closed, each opening is a potential site of a diaphragmatic hernia. Also called *pleuroperitoneal sinus, sinus of Bochdalek, foramen of Bochdalek* (seldom used), *hiatus pleuroperitonealis, Bochdalek's gap.*

hiatus pleuroperitonealis PLEUROPERICARDIAL HIATUS.

sacral hiatus HIATUS SACRALIS.

hiatus sacralis [NA] An inverted U-shaped opening at the apex of the dorsal surface of the sacrum, produced by the failure of the laminae of the fifth, and often the fourth, sacral vertebra to meet in the midline. This opening into the sacral canal is roofed over by the superficial dorsal sacrococcygeal ligament. Also called *sacral hiatus, inferior opening of sacral canal.*

saphenous hiatus HIATUS SAPHENUS.

hiatus saphenus [NA] The opening in the fascia lata of the thigh just below and lateral to the pubic tubercle, closed by the cribriform fascia through which pass the great saphenous vein to join the femoral vein, as well as small arteries, veins, and lymphatics. Also called *saphenous hiatus, saphenous opening, fossa ovalis femoris, oval fossa of thigh, fossa ovalis, foramen of saphenous vein, subinguinal triangle* (outmoded).

Scarpa's hiatus HELICOTREMA.

hiatus of Schwalbe The gap between the obturator fascia and the origin of the levator ani muscle when the latter occasionally arises by a tendinous sling attached only to bone anteriorly and posteriorly. The gap is a potential communication between the pelvic cavity and the ischioanal fossa.

semilunar hiatus HIATUS SEMILUNARIS.

hiatus semilunaris [NA] A curved, long and narrow fissure between the free, posterior border of the uncinate process of the ethmoid bone inferiorly and the rounded ethmoidal bulla superiorly. It is continuous anteriorly with the ethmoidal infundibulum in the lateral wall of the middle meatus of the nasal cavity, and often receives the opening of the maxillary sinus. Also called *semilunar hiatus, ethmoidal hiatus, semilunar opening of ethmoid bone.*

subarcuate hiatus FOSSA SUBARCUATA OSSIS TEMPORALIS.

hiatus tendineus [NA] The large osseoaponeurotic opening in the tendon of the adductor magnus muscle at the medial supracondylar line about the junction of the middle and lower thirds of the thigh through which the femoral vessels pass from the adductor canal into the popliteal fossa. Also called *hiatus adductorius, tendinous opening, femoral opening, adductor hiatus, opening in adductor magnus muscle, inferior opening of Hunter's canal* (outmoded).

tentorial hiatus INCISURA TENTORII.

hiatus totalis sacralis A gap extending along the whole dorsal wall of the sacral canal due to failure of the laminae to meet in the midline.

vena caval hiatus FORAMEN VENAE CAVAE.

hiatus of Winslow FORAMEN OMENTALE.

Hibbs [Russell Aubra *Hibbs,* U.S. surgeon, 1869–1932] See under OPERATION.

hibernaculum [L, winter quarters] The wintertime nest chamber of a hibernator.

hibernal Indicating the season of the year extending from mid-November to late winter. Also *heimal.*

hibernation [L *hibernatus,* past part. of *hibernare* (akin to *hiems* winter) to winter] A period of dormant inactivity, marked by hypothermia, that occurs in winter among many rodents, bats, and some large carnivores, such as the bear. Also called *winter torpor.* Compare ESTIVATION.

artificial hibernation A drug-induced state of narcosis and reduced metabolic activity resembling the natural state of hibernation exhibited by certain animal species.

hibernoma [L *hibern(us)* pertaining to winter + -OMA; so called because the tumor suggests a fad pad of some hibernating animals] A benign, lobulated and encapsulated tumor made up of granular or vacuolated, round, acidophilic cells having the appearance of brown fat. It usually involves the shoulder and neck region of young adults. Also called *fetal fat cell lipoma, lipoma fetalocellulare, brown fat tumor.*

hiccough HICCUP.

hiccup [earlier *hikop,* of imitative origin] **1** An involuntary, spasmodic diaphragmatic contraction interrupted by a sudden closure of the glottis which results in a characteristic sound. Also called *singultus, singultation, spasmolygmus.* Also *hiccough.* **2** To produce a hiccup or hiccups.

epidemic hiccup An uncommon disorder, thought to be a monosymptomatic manifestation of encephalitis lethargica, in which strong recurrent diaphragmatic contractions occur and are often accompanied by glottal spasm, possibly for several hours or even for days. Also called *diaphragmatic myoclonus.*

Hicks See under BRAXTON HICKS.

hidebound Adhering tightly to the subcutaneous tissues, as of the skin in scleroderma.

hidr- HIDRO-.

hidradenitis [HIDR- + ADENITIS] An inflammation of the sweat glands. It most often affects the apocrine sweat glands. Also called *hidrosadenitis, spiradenitis.* Also *hydradenitis.*

hidradenitis axillaris Hidradenitis suppurativa of the axillary region. Also called *hidrosadenitis axillaris.*

hidradenitis suppurativa A chronic infective disorder that involves apocrine gland follicles of the axilla and anogenital region producing indolent discharging sinuses. Some cases are associated with acne conglobata. Also called *apocrine acne, spiradenitis suppurativa, hidrosadenitis suppurativa.*

hidradenocarcinoma [HIDR- + ADENOCARCINOMA] SWEAT GLAND CARCINOMA.

hidradenocyte The epithelial cell that characterizes apocrine metaplasia of the breast in fibrocystic disease. It resembles apocrine sweat gland epithelium.

hidradenoid Resembling sweat glands.

hidradenoma [HIDR- + ADENOMA] A sweat gland adenoma. Also called *hidroadenoma.* Also *hydradenoma.*

clear cell hidradenoma ECCRINE ACROSPIROMA.

eruptive hidradenoma SYRINGOMA.

hidradenoma eruptivum SYRINGOMA.

nodular hidradenoma A nodular sweat gland adenoma.

papillary hidradenoma A benign sweat gland tumor composed of papillae arranged in a lacelike pattern with superficial apocrine-type cells. It occurs in women in the anogenital region. Also called *papilliferous hidradenoma, apocrine adenoma.*

papilliferous hidradenoma PAPILLARY HIDRADENOMA.

verrucous hidradenoma A sweat gland adenoma with a verrucous appearance.

hidro- [Gk *hidrōs* sweat] A combining form denoting sweat or sweat glands. Also *hidr-.*

hidroa [HIDRO- + -(i)a] **1** Any skin condition occurring with associated abnormal sweating. A seldom used term. **2** HYDROA.

hidroadenoma HIDRADENOMA.

hidrocystoma A benign sweat gland tumor with single or multiple cysts that are lined by apocrine cells and occasional papillary structures. Also called *hydrocystadenoma.* Also *hydrocystoma.*

hidrocystomatosis [*hidrocystomat(a)*, pl. of HIDROCYSTOMA, + -OSIS] A skin eruption of multiple hidrocystomas.

hidroid [HIDR- + -OID] Pertaining to sweating or to a sweat gland.

hidropoiesis [HIDRO- + -POIESIS] The formation of sweat. Adjective: hidropoietic.

hidrorrhea HYPERHIDROSIS.

hidrosadenitis [Gk *hidros* sweat + ADENITIS] HIDRADENITIS.

hidrosadenitis axillaris HIDRADENITIS AXILLARIS.

hidrosadenitis destruens suppurativa An obsolete term for PAPULONECROTIC TUBERCULID.

hidrosadenitis suppurativa HIDRADENITIS SUPPURATIVA.

hidroschesis HYPOHIDROSIS.

hidrosis [HIDR- + -OSIS] HYPERHIDROSIS.

hidrotic Of, relating to, or inducing sweating or increased sweating; sudorific or hyperhydrotic.

hidrotopathic Relating to any disorder of sweating. A seldom used term.

hiemal HIBERNAL.

hieralgia [Gk *hier(on)* (L *sacrum* a sacred or secret thing) a temple, a sacred place + ALGIA] Pain in the sacrum.

hierarchy / anxiety hierarchy The ranking of stimuli or situations to which a phobic patient responds with anxiety, ranging from those least fear-provoking to those most anxiety-provoking. This gradual series can then be used to gradually reduce crippling anxiety-laden responses by means of behavior modification techniques, such as systematic desensitization.

Maslow's motivational hierarchy The theory that human motivations can best be understood as a hierarchical arrangement ascending in five stages from the most basic and potent to the least, beginning with insistent biologic needs, as for water,

food, or sleep; to safety needs (order, security, and predictability); to affiliative needs (belongingness and love); to social needs (competence, prestige, and power); and finally to the highest and most weakly impelling of human needs, that is, knowing, understanding, esthetics, and self-fulfillment. See also MASLOW'S THEORY OF HUMAN MOTIVATION.

hierarchy of needs An ordering of human needs according to their urgency and potency, ranging from the most basic of physiologic drives to the most highly evolved motive for self-actualization. Each need must be satisfied, at least partially, before the next highest can emerge. Thus, the primary needs, such as food and water, are the most urgent and must be satisfied first, followed by successive levels of needs categorized as those for safety and security, affiliation, love and belongingness, esteem needs, and, finally, the need for self-actualization.

hieric SACRAL.

hierolisthesis A displacement of the sacrum which results in an abnormal angulation at the lumbosacral junction.

hierotherapy [Gk *hiero(s)* pertaining to the gods, holy + THERAPY] The use of prayer or other religious practices to treat illness.

Higashi [Ototaka *Higashi*, Japanese physician, flourished mid-20th century] Chédiak-Higashi disease, Chédiak-Steinbrinck-Higashi disease. See under CHÉDIAK-HIGASHI ANOMALY.

high-energy ENERGY-RICH.

Highmore [Nathaniel *Highmore*, English anatomist, 1613–1685] **1** Antrum highmori, antrum of Highmore. See under SINUS MAXILLARIS. **2** Body of Highmore. See under MEDIASTINUM TESTIS.

highmoritis [after Nathaniel *Highmore* English anatomist, 1613–1685 + -ITIS] A seldom used term for MAXILLARY SINUSITIS.

high-risk **1** More liable to develop a disease or sustain an injury than others in the population at large or in some other defined group. 〈"babies classified as 'high risk' have distinctly different cry patterns from 'normals.' High risk was determined by the prevalence among mothers during pregnancy of factors such as toxemia, narrow birth canal, infection and poor nutrition. . . . many high risk babies displayed these traits: Took longer to respond to the cry stimulus [;] sustained their cry for less time but took an average of 11 seconds longer to start crying after being snapped with a rubber band; had a pitch twice as high as normals." —*Science News*, 19 Nov. 1983, 327.〉 **2** More hazardous for the patient than an alternative procedure. **3** Having a poor prognosis.

high-spin Denoting the state of a transition metal ion in which the electrons have as few paired spins as possible and are therefore spread among different orbitals. This state is energetically favored when different orbitals differ little in energy, usually because no strong interactions with electrons of ligands are provided in particular directions. This form of iron(II) is just favored in hemoglobin, and the iron in its high-spin state is larger than in its low-spin state and is further out of the plane of the porphyrin, whereas the low-spin state is favored in oxyhemoglobin.

high-spinal With reference to spinal preparations, denoting the highest cervical levels of the spinal cord, above the outflow of the phrenic nerve.

hila Plural of HILUM.

hilar Pertaining to a hilum.

Hildenbrand [Johann Valentin Edler von *Hildenbrand*, Austrian physician, 1763–1818] Hildenbrand's disease. See under TYPHUS.

hili Plural of HILUS.

hilifuge [L *hili*, gen. of *hilum* the black spot on top of a bean, a trifle (*hilus*, often used, is erroneous) + -FUGE] Extending from the pulmonary hilus: said of the configuration of a density seen on a chest radiograph, as in pulmonary edema.

hilitis [*hil(us)* + -ITIS] Inflammation of the hilus of the lung or of any hilus. An imprecise and seldom used term.

Hill [Archibald Vivian *Hill*, English physiologist, 1886–1977] See under COEFFICIENT, EQUATION.

Hill [Sir Leonard Erskine *Hill*, English physiologist, born 1866] See under SIGN.

Hill [Robin *Hill*, English chemist, flourished early 20th century] See under REACTION.

Hillis [David S. *Hillis*, U.S. obstetrician and gynecologist, 1873–1942] **1** DeLee-Hillis obstetric stethoscope. See under STETHOSCOPE. **2** Müller-Hillis maneuver. See under MANEUVER.

hillock A small prominence or elevated part.

anal hillock ANAL TUBERCLE.

auricular hillocks EAR HILLOCKS.

axon hillock The conical portion of the axon as it emerges from a neuron soma, distinguished by a relative paucity of Nissl bodies and a specialized plasmalemma. It is believed to be the site of initiation of the conducted action potential. Also called *nerve hillock, basis axonis* (rarely used).

cloacal hillock GENITAL TUBERCLE.

Doyère's hillock MOTOR ENDPLATE.

ear hillocks Small mounds on the side of the head of an embryo which are destined to form the external ear. Also called *auricular hillocks.*

facial hillock COLLICULUS FACIALIS.

germ hillock CUMULUS OOPHORUS.

germ-bearing hillock CUMULUS OOPHORUS.

nerve hillock AXON HILLOCK.

seminal hillock COLLICULUS SEMINALIS.

Hilton [John *Hilton*, English surgeon, 1804–1878] **1** See under METHOD, LAW. **2** Hilton's white line. See under LINE. **3** Hilton sac. See under SACCULUS LARYNGIS. **4** Hilton's muscle. See under MUSCULUS ARYEPIGLOTTICUS.

hilum [L akin to Gk *kēlis* a stain, spot), the black spot on the top of a bean, a trifle] **1** A small gap or hollow in an organ where vessels, nerves, and ducts enter or leave it. Also called *hilus* (outmoded). **2** A scar on the seed where the seed was attached to the funiculus.

hilum of broad ligament An outmoded term for LIGAMENTUM SUSPENSORIUM OVARII.

hilum of caudal olivary nucleus HILUM NUCLEI OLIVARIS CAUDALIS.

hilum glandulae suprarenalis A short groove for the passage of the corresponding suprarenal vein, which is situated on the anterior surface of each suprarenal gland. Also called *hilum of suprarenal gland.*

glomerular hilum The vascular pole, or polus vascularis, of a renal corpuscle. An outmoded term.

hilum hepatis An outmoded term for PORTA HEPATIS.

hilum of inferior olivary nucleus HILUM NUCLEI OLIVARIS CAUDALIS.

hilum of kidney HILUM RENALE.

hilum lienis An outmoded term for HILUM SPLENICUM.

hilum of lung HILUM PULMONIS.

hilum of lymph node HILUM NODI LYMPHATICI.

hilum lymphoglandulae An outmoded term for HILUM NODI LYMPHATICI.

hilum nodi lymphatici A depression on one side of a lymph node through which the efferent lymph vessel emerges and its blood vessels enter and leave. Dense fibrous tissue extends from it into the medulla. Also called *hilum of lymph node, hilum lymphoglandulae.*

hilum nuclei dentati The axonal core of the dentate nucleus

of the cerebellum, giving rise to fibers of the superior cerebellar peduncle.

hilum nuclei olivaris caudalis The medial axonal core of the inferior olivary nucleus of the medulla oblongata. Also called *hilum of olivary nucleus, hilum of inferior olivary nucleus, hilum of caudal olivary nucleus.*

hilum of olivary nucleus HILUM NUCLEI OLIVARIS CAUDALIS.

hilum ovarii [NA] A slit in the mesovarian border of the ovary through which its arteries, veins, and lymphatics enter or leave. Also called *hilum of ovary.*

hilum of ovary HILUM OVARII.

pulmonary hilum HILUM PULMONIS.

hilum pulmonis [NA] The depression on the mediastinal surface of each lung through which the structures of the root of the lung enter or leave the lung. Also called *hilum of lung, porta of lung* (outmoded), *porta pulmonis* (outmoded), *pulmonary lung.*

renal hilum HILUM RENALE.

hilum renale [NA] A deep vertical fissure in the medial margin of each kidney that contains the renal artery, vein, and nerves and the renal pelvis. The vein usually lies anterior to the artery and the pelvis is often posterior to both. Also called *hilum of kidney, hilum renalis* (outmoded), *porta renis, renal hilum.*

hilum renalis An outmoded term for HILUM RENALE.

hilum of spleen HILUM SPLENICUM.

hilum splenicum [NA] A fissure in the lower part of the gastric surface of the spleen for the passage of the splenic vessels and nerves. Also called *hilum of spleen, porta of spleen* (outmoded), *hilum lienis* (outmoded), *porta lienis* (outmoded).

hilum of suprarenal gland HILUM GLANDULAE SUPRARENALIS.

hilus An outmoded term for HILUM.

himantosis [Gk *himas*, gen. *himantos*, a leather thong + -OSIS] Elongation of the uvula. A rarely used term.

hinchazón [Spanish, swelling (referring to the edema of wet beriberi)] A Cuban term for BERIBERI.

hindbrain RHOMBENCEPHALON.

hindfoot The foot structure posterior to the midtarsal joint.

hindgut [*hind* + GUT] **1** The posterior segment of the embryonic intestine, precursor of the sigmoid colon and the rectum. It is extended by the cloaca, the partitioning of which separates the anal canal from the urogenital sinus. It is temporarily extended in the tail bud by a diverticulum, the postanal gut, which usually disappears before the end of the fifth week in human development. Also called *epigaster.* **2** The posterior ectodermal segment of the digestive tract of arthropods.

hind-kidney METANEPHROS.

hindwater [*hind* + *water*] That portion of the amniotic fluid that lies behind the presenting fetal part.

Hines [Edgar Alphonso *Hines*, Jr. U.S., physician, born 1906] **1** Hines and Brown test. See under COLD PRESSOR TEST. **2** Hines-Bannick syndrome. See under SYNDROME.

hinge-bow A face-bow used in locating the external projection of the hinge axis on the face.

hinny [irreg. from L *hinnus* mule, from Gk *hinnos, innos, ginnos* (and other variants) mule, prob. imitative of equine whinney] The offspring of a male horse and a female ass.

Hinton [William Augustus *Hinton*, U.S. physician, 1883–1959] See under TEST.

hip[1] [Old English *hype*, akin to L *cubitus* or *cubitum* the elbow, the arm below the elbow, a curvature, and to Gk *kybos* a cube, vertebra] **1** ARTICULATIO COXAE. **2** The lateral bulge of the body below the waist and lateral to the hip joint.

snapping hip The crepitus and associated audible snapping noise that occurs when the fascia lata tendon rides over an enlarged posterior margin of the greater trochanter of the femur. Also called *Perrin-Ferraton disease*.

hip² [Middle English *hepe, hipe*, from Old English *heope*]   The fruit of the rose, a plant of the genus *Rosa*. It contains high quantities of vitamin C.

Hippel   See under VON HIPPEL.

Hippelates   A genus of acalyptrate flies of the western hemisphere (family Chloropidae, order Diptera) known as eye gnats. Attracted to eye secretions and fluids of man and animals, some species are believed to transmit conjunctivitis, bovine mastitis, and yaws.

Hippelates flavipes   A tropical species thought to be involved in mechanical transmission of yaws in Haiti and Jamaica.

Hippelates pallipes   A member of the *H. pusio* group, and an annoying eye fly of New World temperate regions. Also called *Oscinis pallipes*.

Hippelates pusio   The black-bodied, shining eye gnat of California and Florida. Also found in other southern states, it is a mechanical vector of a form of epidemic conjunctivitis and a particularly troublesome pest.

Hippeutis   A genus of freshwater pulmonate snails in the subfamily Segmentininae, family Planorbidae. *H. cantori,* found in China, is the intermediate host of the trematode *Fasciolopsis buski.*

hippiatria   HIPPIATRICS.

hippiatrics   [HIPP(O)- + -IATRICS]   A branch of veterinary medicine that deals with diseases of the horse. Also called *hippiatria.*

hippo-   [Gk *hippos* horse]   A combining form meaning horse.

Hippobosca   A genus of primarily Old World louse flies of the family Hippoboscidae, ectoparasitic on mammals and ostriches. Species reported to attack humans include *H. equina,* the forest fly of England, which is normally parasitic on horses, mules, and sometimes cattle and other mammals, *H. variegata,* a widespread parasite of cattle and equines, *H. camelina* of camels, and *H. longipennis,* parasitic on dogs in the Mediterranean region. The bite of the last-mentioned fly is reported to be as painful as the sting of a yellow jacket. *H. rufipes* is a vector of *Trypanosoma theileri* in South America.

Hippoboscidae   [HIPPO- + Gk *bosk(ein)* to feed + -IDAE]   A family of pupiparous flies parasitic on birds and mammals. Both winged and wingless species are contained in the three genera, *Hippobosca, Melophagus,* and *Psuedolynchia.* Adult flies are flattened and leathery, with wings fully developed, short, or absent. They also have short, well-clawed, widely separated legs for rapid movement between feathers or hair. The sheep ked, *Melophagus ovinus* is the most important pest in the family, though a number of pathogenic agents can be transmitted by other members of the family as well.

hippocampal   Pertaining to the hippocampus of the cerebral hemispheres.

hippocampus   [New L (from Gk *hippokampos* seahorse, from *hippos* horse + *kampos* sea monster), a seahorse]   [NA] An infolded region of the cerebral cortex forming an arched elevation in the floor of the lateral ventricle bordering the choroid fissure. It is composed of two sectors: Ammon's horn, or hippocampus proper, and the dentate gyrus, both of which together are sometimes called the hippocampal formation. The laminar structure constitutes a unique form of allocortex, with white matter (the alveus) on the surface. The main afferent connections derive from the entorhinal cortex of the parahippocampal gyrus. It gives rise to a large efferent bundle, the fornix, partially originating in the subiculum and projecting to the mamillary nuclei, septal nuclei, and anterior nuclei of the thalamus. Also called *hippocampus major, cornu Ammonis, horn of Ammon, pes*

hippocampi major. Adjective: hippocampal.

hippocampus major   HIPPOCAMPUS.

hippocampus minor   **1** An ambiguous and obsolete term for CALCAR AVIS. **2** An obsolete term for INDUSIUM GRISEUM.

hippocampus nudus   The portion of the hippocampus exposed at the splenial bend where the fascia dentata is sometimes separated. An obsolete term.

Hippocrates   **1** A physician of ancient Greece (460 B.C.–377 B.C.), customarily described as the "Father of Medicine" in recognition of his contribution to the scientific foundation of medicine through his and his followers' writings and practice. His name is also associated with the fundamental principles of medical ethics through the Hippocratic Oath, an ancient oath of uncertain origin still sworn by new physicians. Adjective: hippocratic. **2** Cord of Hippocrates. See under TENDO CALCANEUS. **3** Hippocratic maneuver. See under MANEUVER.

hippocratic   Associated with or attributed to Hippocrates.

hippomanes   [Gk *hippomanes* (from *hippo(s)* a horse + *maō,* aorist root of *mainesthai* to rage) a humor that falls from mares]   Flattened oval bodies found in the allantoic fluid of Equidae.

Hippuran   A proprietary name for iodohippurate sodium.

hippurate   A compound, often the sodium salt, of hippuric acid, used in studies of kidney function. To provide a gamma emitter for scintillation detection, radioiodine may be attached to the benzene ring, usually in the *ortho* position, thus making possible gamma images of the kidney (scintigrams) and time-activity graphs of excretory function (renograms).

hippuric acid C_6H_5—CO—NH—CH$_2$—COOH. *N*-Benzoylglycine, the form in which benzoic acid is mainly excreted in the urine.

hippus   [New L (from Gk *hippos* a horse, an eye ailment causing winking]   A spasmodic alternation of large and small pupil size occurring spontaneously or associated with light or accommodation reflexes. Also called *pupillary athetosis, bounding pupil.*

Hiprex   A proprietary name for methenamine hippurate.

hirci   [See HIRCUS.]   (*singular* hircus) [NA] Axillary hair.

hircism   [L *hirc(us)* the smell of the armpits + -ISM]   The odor of axillary sweat. Also called *hircismus.*

hircismus   HIRCISM.

hircus   [L, he-goat, goatlike smell, smell of the armpits]   (*plural* hirci) An axillary hair. Also called *glandebala* (obsolete).

Hirschberg   [Julius *Hirschberg,* German ophthalmologist, 1843–1925]   **1** See under METHOD, MAGNET. **2** Hirschberg's test for strabismus. See under TEST.

Hirschberg   [Leonard Keene *Hirschberg,* U.S. physician, born 1877]   Hirschberg's reflex, Hirschberg sign. See under ADDUCTOR REFLEX OF FOOT.

Hirschfeld   [Felix *Hirschfeld,* German physician, born 1863]   See under DISEASE.

Hirschfeld   [Isador *Hirschfeld,* U.S. dentist, 1881–1965]   **1** See under METHOD. **2** Hirschfeld's canals. See under INTERDENTAL CANALS.

Hirschfeld   [Ludwig Moritz *Hirschfeld,* Polish anatomist, 1816–1896]   See under NERVE.

Hirschfelder   [Joseph Oakland *Hirschfelder,* U.S. pathologist, 1854–1920]   Hirschfelder's tuberculin. See under OXYTUBERCULIN.

Hirschsprung   [Harald *Hirschsprung,* Danish pediatrician, 1830–1916]   Hirschsprung's disease. See under CONGENITAL MEGACOLON.

hirsute   [L *hīrsut(us)* hairy, shaggy]   **1** Characterized by hirsutism. **2** Having a hairy appearance: said of a mushroom cap.

hirsuties   HIRSUTISM.

hirsuties papillaris penis HIRSUTOID PAPILLOMAS OF THE PENIS.

hirsutism [L *hirsutus* hairy, shaggy + -ISM] The growth of hair in women in the male sexual pattern, either in part or wholly. Also called *trichosis hirsuties, hirsuties.* Compare HYPERTRICHOSIS.

constitutional hirsutism Hirsutism in women due to hereditary factors and not to excessive androgen secretion. Also called *idiopathic hirsutism.*

idiopathic hirsutism CONSTITUTIONAL HIRSUTISM.

hirudicidal [*hirudicid(e)* + -AL] Capable of killing leeches.

hirudicide [*Hirud(o)* + *i* + -CIDE] An agent that destroys leeches.

hirudin A substance secreted by the salivary glands of leeches. It acts as an antithrombin, preventing the coagulation of blood.

Hirudinaria [*Hirudin(is)*, gen. of HIRUDO, + -ARIA] A genus of parasitic leeches in the family Gnathobdellidae.

Hirudinea [L *hirudo*, gen. *hirudinis* a leech + *-ea* (neut. pl. of *-eus* English *-eous*), suffix denoting a class] The leeches, a class of worms of the phylum Annelida that includes the genera *Haementeria, Helobdella, Hirudo, Hirudinaria, Haemadipsa, Haemopis, Limnatis, Macrobdella,* and *Pontobdella,* characterized by an extremely branched alimentary system for food storage, flat, segmented bodies, and a sucker at the posterior and often the anterior end. Most feed on the tissues of soft-bodied invertebrates, such as snails, but a number take the blood and exudates of vertebrates. Fish are frequently attacked, as are amphibians and other aquatic organisms. Human infestation often occurs while bathing or drinking hastily from contaminated pools. The worms enter rapidly and attach deep within the nostrils, pharynx, throat, ears, urethra, or vagina. The land leeches of the Far East (*Haemadipsa*) and South America, especially in humid or tropical rainforests, are notorious for mass attacks on horses, cattle or humans, often causing death.

hirudiniasis [*Hirudin(aria)* + -IASIS] A condition caused by an attack by leeches, generally resulting in blockage of channels such as the urethra, or bleeding caused by a temporary attachment in the nares, pharynx, or ears.

external hirudiniasis Hirudiniasis resulting from attachment of aquatic or land leeches to the skin, resulting in blood loss, possible secondary infection, and transmission of parasites.

internal hirudiniasis Hirudiniasis resulting from accidental ingestion through drinking, or invasion of the mouth, nose, pharynx, larynx or genitalia.

hirudinization The injection of hirudin in order to prevent coagulation of blood.

hirudinize To render (blood) incoagulable by the addition of hirudin. This may be *in vitro* or done by the leech (*Hirudo*) during blood sucking.

Hirudo [L (akin to *haerere* to hold, stick, adhere), a leech, bloodsucker] A genus of leeches (family Gnathobdellidae, class Hirudinea), used traditionally for blood-letting or hirudinization. Also called *Iatrobdella, Sanguisuga.*

Hirudo aegyptiaca LIMNATIS NILOTICA.

Hirudo japonica The medicinal leech used for therapy in Japan.

Hirudo javanica A species found in Java and Burma, reported to cause internal hirudiniasis.

Hirudo medicinalis The medicinal leech, formerly a species of great importance in medicine as a therapeutic agent for hemorrhoids and many other conditions, and still in use by some local practitioners, especially in the Orient. Aquatic leeches serve as intermediate hosts for trypanosomes and sporozoan parasites of fish, amphibians, and turtles.

Hirudo quinquestriata A species found in Australia that is an economic pest in sheep raising areas.

Hirudo troctina A species of leeches common in Europe, marked with a troutlike pattern of green, orange, and black spots.

His [Wilhelm *His*, Jr., Swiss-born anatomist active in Germany, 1863–1934] **1** See under ELECTROGRAPHY. **2** His disease, His-Werner disease, Werner-His disease. See under TRENCH FEVER. **3** Ventriculoseptal artery to bundle of His. See under ARTERY. **4** Kent-His bundle, His band, bundle of His. See under FASCICULUS ATRIOVENTRICULARIS. **5** Bifurcation of bundle of His. See under BIFURCATION. **6** His-Tawara node. See under NODUS ATRIOVENTRICULARIS. **7** Left branch of bundle of His. See under CRUS SINISTRUM FASCICULI ATRIOVENTRICULARIS. **8** Right branch of bundle of His. See under CRUS DEXTRUM FASCICULI ATRIOVENTRICULARIS. **9** Trunk of bundle of His. See under TRUNCUS FASCICULI ATRIOVENTRICULARIS. **10** His spindle. See under AORTIC SPINDLE.

His [Wilhelm *His*, Sr., Swiss-born anatomist active in Germany, 1831–1904] **1** See under RULE, BURSA, PLANE. **2** Duct of His, His canal. See under THYROGLOSSAL DUCT. **3** His zones. See under ZONE. **4** Isthmus of His. See under ISTHMUS RHOMBENCEPHALI. **5** Copula of His. See under LINGUAL COPULA. **6** His perivascular space, His-Held space. See under PERIVASCULAR SPACE. **7** Germinal cell of His. See under MEDULLOEPITHELIAL CELL. **8** His tubercle. See under TUBERCULUM AURICULAE.

His Symbol for histidine.

hispid [L *hispid(us)* hairy, shaggy] Having a rough surface because of stiff or bristly hairs.

Hiss [Philip Hanson *Hiss*, U.S. bacteriologist, 1868–1913] Hiss capsule stain. See under STAIN.

hist- HISTO-.

Histadyl A proprietary name for methapyrilene.

Histalog A proprietary name for betazole.

histaminase A copper-containing amine oxidase. An outmoded term. • This term is misleading because it suggests that the reaction is a hydrolysis rather than an oxidation.

histamine Imidazolylethylamine. The substance formed by decarboxylation of histidine. It is released from mast cells during the allergic response. It stimulates the contraction of smooth muscle and increases vascular permeability.

histamine acid phosphate HISTAMINE PHOSPHATE.

histamine dihydrochloride $C_5H_9N_3 \cdot 2HCl$. A compound with the same general properties and actions as histamine.

histamine-fast Not responsive to histamine.

histaminemia The presence of histamine in the blood.

histamine phosphate $C_5H_9N_3 \cdot 2H_3PO_4$. The diphosphate salt of histamine, which is used as a diagnostic tool for the study of gastric secretions and in the treatment of some allergic conditions. Also called *histamine acid phosphate.*

histaminia A state of shock caused by an excess of histamine.

histic HISTOID.

histidase An outmoded term for HISTIDINE AMMONIA-LYASE.

histidinase An outmoded term for HISTIDINE AMMONIA-LYASE.

histidine One of the amino acids incorporated into proteins. Its molecule consists of alanine substituted on C-3 by imidazole (at C-4 of the imidazole). The imidazole ring is weakly basic, so histidine residues in proteins are partly, but not overwhelmingly, protonated at neutral pH. They are involved in the catalytic mechanism of several enzymes.

histidine ammonia-lyase The enzyme (EC 4.3.1.3) that catalyzes the interconversion of histidine with ammonia and urocanate, the *trans* isomer of 3-(imidazol-4-yl)propenoic acid. This is a step in the catabolism of histidine. Also called *histidase* (outmoded), *histidinase* (outmoded).

histidine decarboxylase   The enzyme (EC 4.1.1.22) that catalyzes the conversion of histidine into histamine and carbon dioxide.

histidinemia   A rare inborn error of amino acid metabolism characterized by an elevated level of plasma histidine, excessive urinary excretion of histidine and imidazole metabolites, mental retardation, and defective speech. It is caused by a deficiency of histidine α-deaminase that is inherited as an autosomal recessive trait.

histidinuria   The excessive urinary excretion of histidine. The condition is a feature of histidinemia.

histio-   [Gk *histion* web, cloth, sheet]   A combining form denoting tissue.

histioblast   [HISTIO- + -BLAST]   A histiocyte precursor.

histiocyte   [HISTIO- + -CYTE]   A connective-tissue macrophage. Also called *histocyte, reticulum cell, reticuloendothelial cell, reticular cell.*

   cardiac histiocyte   A multinucleate cell found in the inflammatory nodules of rheumatic carditis. Such cells may represent a fusion of macrophages or alternatively a damaged and degenerating cardiac muscle cell. Also called *Anichkov cell, Anichkov's myocyte.*

   sea-blue histiocyte   A histiocyte that contains an excess of ceroid pigment within the cytoplasm.

histiocytoid   Having the morphologic features of a histiocyte.

histiocytoma   [HISTIO- + CYT- + -OMA]   **1** DERMATOFIBROMA.   • This term is not recommended because of its possible confusion with fibrous histiocytoma.   **2** A cutaneous tumor peculiar to the dog and especially common in dogs less than two years old.

   fibrous histiocytoma   A benign tumor of histiocytes and fibroblasts which typically grow in a storiform pattern. Lipid-laden macrophages, as foam cells and giant cells, are also present. It is most commonly found in the dermis. Also called *fibroxanthoma, lipoid histiocytoma, fibroma xanthoma, xanthofibroma.*

   juvenile histiocytoma   JUVENILE XANTHOMA.

   lipoid histiocytoma   FIBROUS HISTIOCYTOMA.

   malignant fibrous histiocytoma   The malignant counterpart of a fibrous histiocytoma. Also called *malignant fibroxanthoma, xanthosarcoma.*

histiocytomatosis   A generalized disorder of the reticuloendothelial system. An imprecise and obsolete term.

histiocytosis   [HISTIO- + CYTOSIS]   Any of several disorders in which there is proliferation of histiocytes without any known underlying cause, such as infection, or disorder of lipid metabolism. Histiocytosis may be solitary or multiple, and may be restricted to bone or may be generalized. It is seen in eosinophilic granuloma, Hand-Schüller-Christian disease, and Letterer-Siwe disease, but although these disorders may be neoplastic in nature they are to be distinguished from malignant histiocytosis, which is a separate entity. Also called *histocytosis, histiocytosis X, reticuloendothelial granulomatosis.*

   kerasin histiocytosis   An incorrect and obsolete term for GAUCHER'S DISEASE.

   lipid histiocytosis   An incorrect and obsolete term for NIEMANN-PICK DISEASE.

   malignant histiocytosis   A rapidly progressive neoplastic proliferation of histiocytes, especially those of bone marrow, liver, and spleen. The disorder is characterized by fever, enlargement of spleen and liver, pancytopenia, and infiltration of bone marrow by large, bizarre histiocytes that typically exhibit much

erythrophagocytosis. Also called *histiocytic medullary reticulosis, bony reticulosis.*

   nonlipid histiocytosis   LETTERER-SIWE DISEASE.

   pulmonary histiocytosis   An uncommon condition of unknown cause characterized by proliferation of histiocytes and granulomas in the lungs, often with subsequent fibrosis.

   sinus histiocytosis   A nonspecific, benign reactive change of lymph nodes characterized by proliferation of histiocytes within peripheral and medullary sinuses. It may be seen in lymph nodes draining certain carcinomas.

histiocytosis X   HISTIOCYTOSIS.

histiogenic   HISTOGENOUS.

histioid   HISTOID.

histioirritative   An agent capable of irritating tissues, particularly connective tissue. A seldom used term.

histioma   [*histi(o)-* + -OMA]   An obsolete term for NEOPLASM.

histionic   Of or relating to connective tissue.

histiotrophe   HISTOTROPH.

histo-   [Gk *histos* loom, web of loom, warp]   A combining form denoting tissue. Also *hist-*.

histoangic   Pertaining to the character of blood vessels.

histoautoradiography   The process or technique of producing autoradiographs from histologic sections of tissue.

histoblast   [HISTO- + -BLAST]   One of the precursor cells that give rise to the tissues of the body, usually in the embryo and fetus but also later in life.

histochemistry   The chemistry of tissues, especially in the sense of the characterization of the distribution of specific chemical compounds within cells. Also called *histologic chemistry.*

histochemotherapy   CHEMOTHERAPY.

histochromatosis   Any of several diseases involving the reticuloendothelial system. An obsolete and imprecise term.

histoclastic   Pertaining to the breakdown or resorption of tissue by cells.

histocompatibility   A compatibility between the genotypes of donor and host such that a graft generally will not be rejected. Genetically determined alloantigens, present on the surface of nucleated cells of many tissues and easily detected on blood leukocytes, determine histocompatibility. The best studied antigens are those of the H-2 histocompatibility system in mice and the HLA histocompatibility system in man.

histocompatible   Marked by histocompatibility; not likely to induce an immune response leading to rejection: said especially of a tissue graft or organ transplant.

histocyte   HISTIOCYTE.

histocytosis   HISTIOCYTOSIS.

histodiagnosis   The diagnosis of disease processes by means of microscopic examination of the affected tissues and cells.

histodialysis   HISTORRHEXIS.

histodifferentiation   The development of the characteristics peculiar to a particular tissue type from less organized groups of cells.

histofluorescence   [HISTO- + FLUORESCENCE]   Fluorescence produced in tissue by the administration of some substance, such as one that had been previously irradiated.

histogenesis   [HISTO- + GENESIS]   The creation and development of tissues arising from undifferentiated embryonic cells. Also called *histogeny, morphologic synthesis.* Adjective: histogenetic.

histogenous   Of or relating to histogenesis. Also *histiogenic.*

histogeny   HISTOGENESIS.

histogram   [HISTO- + -GRAM]   A graphic representation of a frequency distribution by means of a set of rectangles, the base of each representing a class-interval and the area being proportional to the frequency of that class.

histography [HISTO- + -GRAPHY]   A written account of tissue structure.

histohematogenous   Developed from blood and some tissue type.

histohydria   An obsolete term for EDEMA.

histohypoxia   An abnormally decreased oxygen pressure in the tissues. A seldom used term.

histoid [HIST- + -OID]   Possessing a weblike structure of normal connective tissue. Also *histioid, histic.*

histoincompatibility   An incompatibility between the genotypes of donor and host such that a graft will almost invariably be rejected.

histoincompatible   Marked by histoincompatibility; likely to induce an immune response leading to rejection: said especially of a tissue graft or organ transplant.

histokinesis   Fundamental tissue movement, such as is seen in peristalsis.

histologic   Of or relating to histology.

histologist [HISTO- + -LOGIST]   A scientist who studies tissues and cells by using microscopic techniques. Also called *microanatomist.*

histology [HISTO- + -LOGY]   An integral subspecialty of anatomy wherein the tissues and cells of an organism's structures are treated with special chemicals and studied with the light microscope. Also called *microscopic anatomy, micranatomy, micranatomy, microhistology, histomorphology, histologic anatomy, minute anatomy.*

   normal histology   The study of normal tissues and cells using microscopic techniques.

   pathologic histology   HISTOPATHOLOGY.

   topographic histology   The study of cell and tissue specialization according to the anatomic site in which they occur.

histolysate   Any substance formed by the lysis of tissue cells.

histolysis   Dissolution of tissue. Also called *physiolysis.* Adjective: histolytic.

histolytic   Characterized by or inducing histolysis.

histoma [HIST- + -OMA]   An obsolete term for NEOPLASM.

histometaplastic   Pertaining to or causing tissue metaplasia. A seldom used term.

Histomonas   A genus of protozoa (order Trichomonadida, class Zoomastigophorea) parasitic in the liver, cecum, and other tissues of turkeys, chickens, geese, and ducks. It possesses ameboid and flagellated stages, and lives on intestinal mucosal cells of the host.

Histomonas meleagridis   A species that parasitizes the liver and intestine of many gallinaceous birds, including turkeys and chickens. It is highly pathogenic in turkey poults, causing histomoniasis or blackhead disease. Although common in chickens, it rarely causes disease in these hosts. Consequently, in order to avoid passing the parasites to young turkeys, chickens and turkeys are ordinarily not raised together. Also called *Amoeba meleagridis.*

histomoniasis [*Histomon(as)* + -IASIS]   A serious avian disease caused by an ameboflagellate protozoan, *Histomonas meleagridis.* Young turkeys up to three months old are most susceptible, but chickens and other poultry may be affected. Focal necrosis of cecal mucosa and liver is the main lesion. Common signs are depression, anorexia, loss of condition, and cyanosis of skin of the head (blackhead). However, death may be sudden without clinical signs. Also called *blackhead, avian blackhead, enterohepatitis, infectious enterohepatitis, avian enterohepatitis.*

histomorphology   HISTOLOGY.

histomycosis [HISTO- + MYCOSIS]   A deep dermatomycosis.

histone   One of the strongly basic proteins usually associated with DNA in eukaryotic nuclei. There are five main types, and they show very little variation in sequence from one species to another.

histoneurology   An obsolete term for NEUROHISTOLOGY.

histonomy [HISTO- + *nom(o)-* + -Y]   The use of quantitative techniques in the analysis of histologic observations.

histonuria [*histon(e)* + -URIA]   The presence of histone in the urine, associated with dissolution of cells, as occurs in leukemias and in febrile and wasting illnesses.

histopathogenesis   Abnormal embryonic development of cells or tissues; abnormal histogenesis.

histopathology [HISTO- + PATHOLOGY]   The study of the structural alterations of cells and tissues caused by disease. Also called *micropathology* (rarely used), *pathologic histology.*

histophysiology   The relationship between the microscopic structure and the function of living things.

Histoplasma [HISTO- + PLASMA]   A genus of dimorphic fungi that includes the agent of histoplasmosis, *Histoplasma capsulatum.* The perfect state is *Emmonsiella.*

Histoplasma capsulatum   The species of yeastlike dimorphic fungus known to cause histoplasmosis. Also called *Cryptococcus capsulatus* (obsolete).

Histoplasma capsulatum var. duboisii   The form-species and variety of the false yeast found to cause African histoplasmosis.

Histoplasma farciminosum   The form-species of fungi found to be the contagious etiologic agent of epizootic lymphangitis of horses and mules. Also called *Blastomyces farciminosus* (obsolete), *Cryptococcus farciminosus* (obsolete).

histoplasmin   A sterile liquid preparation containing soluble antigenic material that is derived from cultures of *Histoplasma capsulatum.* It is injected intradermally as a skin test for the presence of cell-mediated immunity to *H. capsulatum.*

histoplasmoma [*Histoplasm(a)* + -OMA]   A tissue response to *Histoplasma capsulatum* consisting of a small tumorlike nodule, often located in the lung or in a lymph node. The nodule may contain calcifications in a caseous center or concentric rings of calcification.

histoplasmosis   A systemic fungal disease contracted by inhalation of spores of *Histoplasma capsulatum.* It may vary in severity from an asymptomatic infection to an acute influenza-like respiratory illness to a progressive disseminated disease, usually fatal if untreated, marked by hepatosplenomegaly, lymphadenopathy, fever, and organ or system involvement such as endocarditis or hypoadrenalism. The disease may also occur as a chronic cavitary pulmonary infection. Healing lesions frequently undergo calcification. Histoplasmosis occurs worldwide but is endemic in some areas, such as the Ohio and lower Mississippi river valleys of the south central United States. Also called *Darling's disease.*

African histoplasmosis   A systemic fungal disease reported in Africa (especially west Africa) and caused by *Histoplasma duboisii,* which although producing a separate disease is identical in culture to *H. capsulatum.* There are characteristic cutaneous nodules, papules, or ulcers, bony lesions, and lymphadenopathy with liquefaction necrosis. The portal of entry is thought to be respiratory. Diagnosis is from biopsy or smears from skin or bone lesions.

historadiograph   A microradiograph of a tissue section.

historadiography   Microradiography of tissue sections.

historetention   The retention of substances by tissues. An obsolete term.

historrhexis [HISTO- + -RRHEXIS]   Disintegration of a tissue caused by conditions other than infection. An obsolete term. Also called *histodialysis.*

history / **case history**   A recording of information relating to a particular case, as in medicine, social work, or the like.

client history   The medical and administrative background on an enrollee in a medical plan or insurance program, usually maintained in written form.

life history   A description of the various phases through which an individual organism passes, from the formation of the zygote until the death of the organism.

medical history   A recording, often in written form as part of the medical record, of a patient's prior medical and health care status, illnesses, treatments, and problems.

natural history   **1** The study of a group of organisms with respect to their classification, distribution, ecology, and life cycles, usually in their unaltered environment.   **2** The observation and study of natural phenomena, as animals, plants, and minerals.   • In this sense the term is now outmoded, embracing the body of knowledge which, though often based on acute and careful observation, lacked the systematic rigor of modern zoology, botany, or mineralogy.

histospectroscopy   The application of spectroscopy to tissue sections.

emission histospectroscopy   The identification of compounds within tissue sections according to the specific wavelengths of radiant energy they may be caused to emit.

roentgen absorption histospectroscopy   Spectroscopy that is applied to tissue sections using x rays.

ultraviolet absorption histospectroscopy   Spectroscopy that is applied to tissue sections using ultraviolet light.

histotome [HISTO- + -TOME]   MICROTOME.

histotomy [HISTO- + -TOMY]   The sectioning of tissues for histological study. An obsolete term.

histotoxic   Toxic to or destructive of tissue: used especially in reference to infection by bacteria such as *Clostridium perfringens*, which form tissue-destroying enzymes.

histotroph [HISTO- + Gk *trophē* nourishment]   The nutrients supplied to the mammalian embryo from the maternal tissues as distinct from that derived from the maternal blood and bloodstream, which is called hemotroph. Also called *histiotrophe*. Adjective: histotrophic, histiotrophic.

histotropic   Having an affinity for tissue cells: said of certain chemicals, stains, and parasites.

histozoic [HISTO- + *zo(o)-* + -IC]   Living within host tissues: used especially of protozoan parasites.

hit-and-run   Describing an accident in which a pedestrian is unintentionally struck by a vehicle which immediately leaves the scene of the accident.

Hittorf [Johann Wilhelm *Hittorf*, German physicist, 1824–1914]   See under TUBE.

Hitzig [Eduard *Hitzig*, German neurologist and psychiatrist, 1838–1907]   See under GIRDLE, SYNDROME, TEST.

hives [Scots dialect]   URTICARIA.

Hjärre [Albert *Hjärre*, Swedish veterinarian, 1897–1958]   Hjärre's disease. See under COLIGRANULOMA.

Hl   **1** latent hyperopia.   **2** half-life.   **3** hearing loss.

hl   Symbol for the unit, hectoliter.

HLA   **1** human leukocyte antigen.   **2** human leukocyte, locus A.   • *HL-A* or *HLA* referred originally to locus A, but subsequently various loci have been identified and are designated as *HLA-A, HLA-B, HLA-C*, and *HLA-D*.

HL-A   human leukocyte, locus A. See under HLA.

Hm   manifest hyperopia.

hm   Symbol for the unit, hectometer.

HMG   human menopausal gonadotropin.

HMO   health maintenance organization.

hnRNA   heterogeneous nuclear RNA.

Ho   Symbol for the element, holmium.

hoarhound   HOREHOUND.

hoarse [Middle English *hors*, from Old English *has*]   **1** Husky, croaking, rough: said of the sound of the voice.   **2** Suffering from such a change of voice.

hoarseness   The condition of being hoarse. Also called *trachyphonia*.

Hoboken [Nicolaas *Hoboken*, Dutch anatomist and physician, 1632–1678]   **1** Valvulae Hobokenii. See under VALVULA.   **2** Hoboken's valves. See under VALVE.

Hoche [Alfred Erich *Hoche*, German psychiatrist, 1865–1945]   Hoche's tract. See under FASCICULUS SEPTOMARGINALIS.

Hochenegg [Julius von *Hochenegg*, Austrian surgeon, 1859–1940]   See under OPERATION.

Hochsinger [Karl *Hochsinger*, Austrian pediatrician, born 1860]   See under PHENOMENON, SIGN.

hock [Middle and Old English *hōh* heel]   The tarsus, which comprises several small bones between the tibia and the metatarsal bone of horses, cattle, and swine.

capped hock   A hock with swelling over the tuber calcis. The swelling results from inflammation of the subcutaneous bursa in that area.

curby hock   CURB.

Hodara [Menahem *Hodara*, Turkish physician, died 1926]   Hodara's disease. See under TRICHORRHEXIS NODOSA.

Hodge [Hugh Lenox *Hodge*, U.S. gynecologist, 1796–1873]   **1** See under PESSARY, MANEUVER, FORCEPS.   **2** Hodge's planes. See under PLANE.

Hodgen [John Thompson *Hodgen*, U.S. surgeon, 1826–1882]   Hodgen's apparatus. See under SPLINT.

Hodgkin [Alan Lloyd *Hodgkin*, British physiologist, born 1914]   See under CYCLE.

Hodgkin [Thomas *Hodgkin*, English physician, 1798–1866]   **1** Reed-Hodgkin disease. See under HODGKIN'S DISEASE.   **2** See under PRURIGO.   **3** Hodgkin-Key murmur. See under MURMUR.   **4** Hodgkin's disease of lung. See under DISEASE.   **5** Hodgkin cells. See under STERNBERG-REED CELLS.   **6** Non-Hodgkin's lymphoma. See under LYMPHOMA.

Hodgson [Joseph *Hodgson*, English physician, 1788–1869]   See under DISEASE.

hodograph   An instrument that records the movements of locomotion.

hodology [Gk *hodo(s)* path, road, way + -LOGY]   The scientific study of tracts or pathways in the central nervous system.

hodoneuromere [Gk *hodo(s)* a way, path + NEURO- + -MERE]   An embryonic body segment together with the segmental nerves that supply it.

hodophobia [Gk *hodo(s)* a traveling, path, road + =PHOBIA]   Pathologic fear of traveling.

hoe [Middle English *howe*, from Old French *houe* axe, hoe, of Germanic origin]   HOE SCALER.

Hoehne [Ottomar *Hoehne*, German gynecologist, 1871–1932]   See under SIGN.

Hoeppli [Reinhard J. C. *Hoeppli*, German parasitologist, born 1893]   See under PHENOMENON.

hof [German *Hof* courtyard]   A pale or lucent area in the cytoplasm of cells stained with Romanowsky stains (such as the Wright stain), corresponding to the Golgi zone. A hof is characteristically seen in plasma cells and osteoblasts, toward the center of the cell from the eccentrically located nuclei.

nuclear hof   A deep nuclear indentation that is often situated opposite the Golgi apparatus. Also called *nuclear pocket*.

Hofacker [Johann Daniel *Hofacker*, German obstetrician, 1788–

1828]　Hofacker-Sadler laws. See under LAW.

Hofbauer [J. Isfred Isidore *Hofbauer*, U.S. gynecologist, 1878–1961]　Hofbauer cells. See under CELL.

Hoff [Jacobus Hendricus van't *Hoff*, Dutch chemist, 1852–1911] Hoff's law. See under VAN'T HOFF'S PRINCIPLE OF MOBILE EQUILIBRIUM.

Hoffa [Albert *Hoffa*, German surgeon, 1859–1907]　**1** Hoffa's operation, Hoffa-Lorenz operation. See under LORENZ OPERATION.　**2** Hoffa-Kastert disease. See under HOFFA'S DISEASE.

Hoffmann [Friedrich *Hoffmann*, German physician and chemist, 1660–1742]　**3** Hoffmann's drops. See under ETHER SPIRIT.

Hoffmann [Johann *Hoffmann*, German neurologist, 1857–1919]　**1** See under REFLEX, SYNDROME, SIGN, PHENOMENON.　**2** Werdnig-Hoffmann paralysis, Hoffmann's atrophy, Werdnig-Hoffmann atrophy, Hoffmann-Werdnig syndrome, Werdnig-Hoffmann syndrome. See under WERDNIG-HOFFMANN DISEASE.

Hoffmann [Moritz *Hoffmann*, German anatomist, 1622–1698] Hoffmann's duct. See under DUCTUS PANCREATICUS.

Hofmann [August Wilhelm von *Hofmann*, German chemist, 1818–1892]　See under VIOLET.

Hofmann [Georg von *Hofmann* Wellenhof, Austrian bacteriologist, 1843–1890]　Hofmann's bacillus. See under *CORYNEBACTERIUM PSEUDODIPHTHERITICUM*.

Hofmeister [Franz von *Hofmeister*, German surgeon, 1867–1926]　See under OPERATION.

hogg HOGGET.

hogget [Middle English *hogg(e)* hog, from Old English *hogg*, + *-et*, diminishing suffix]　A young sheep of either sex, usually over ten months old, whose central incisor teeth have not erupted. Also called *hogg*.

Hoguet [Joseph Pierre *Hoguet*, U.S. surgeon, 1882–1946]　See under MANEUVER.

hogweed SCOPARIUS.

Högyes [Endre *Högyes*, Hungarian physician, 1847–1906]　See under TREATMENT.

Hoke [Michael *Hoke*, U.S. surgeon, 1872–1944]　See under OPERATION.

hol- HOLO-.

holagogue PANACEA.

holandric　Pertaining to traits, usually heritable ones, that only occur in the males of a species.

holarthritis　An obsolete term for POLYARTHRITIS.

hold / inspiratory hold　A device used to delay the onset of expiration during mechanical ventilation.

Holden [Luther *Holden*, English anatomist, 1815–1905]　See under LINE.

holder / broach holder　A manual dental instrument with a chuck for holding broaches securely during endodontic treatment.

　clamp holder　RUBBER DAM CLAMP FORCEPS.

　foil holder　A manual dental instrument used for holding foil pellets in place in the cavity during condensing.

　matrix holder　MATRIX RETAINER.

　needle holder　A surgical device somewhat resembling scissors that is designed to hold a needle near the points of the blades and thus facilitate the placement of surgical sutures. Also called *suture forceps*.

　rubber dam holder　A device for holding a rubber dam in place. It may be a wire frame with lugs on which the rubber is stretched, or an arrangement of clips attached to elastics that encircle the head.

　rubber dam clamp holder　RUBBER DAM CLAMP FORCEPS.

sponge holder　A surgical instrument with two blades and two handles that is designed to hold small absorbent pads. It is used for blunt dissection and hemostasis. Also called *sponge-holding forceps*.

holdfast　An organ found on certain parasites used for adherence, such as the scolex of tapeworms, highly modified for sucking and attachment to the intestinal wall of a vertebrate host, or the special basal structure by which Trichomycetes fungi attach to their insect hosts. The spiny rostellum of acanthocephalans or spiny head of some nematodes, such as *Gnathostoma spinigerum* serve a similar purpose.

hole / beam hole　A hole through a reactor shield and reflector which enables a beam of radiation or elementary particles to escape for use outside the reactor. Also called *glory hole*.

　burr hole　An opening in the skull made with a burr.

　glory hole　BEAM HOLE.

　shot hole　**1** The appearance of plant leaves as if riddled by shot, due to loss of necrotic tissue from infection by microorganisms, particularly fungi.　**2** Any plant disease characterized by perforated leaves. A popular usage.

holergasia [HOL- + Gk *ergasia* work, occupation]　Any syndrome involving disorganization of the entire personality, such as schizophrenia or a major affective disorder.

Holger Nielsen [*Holger Nielsen*, Danish army officer, 1866–1955]　Holger Nielsen method. See under COPENHAGEN METHOD.

holiday / drug holiday　A period during which maintenance drugs used in the treatment or suppression of mental illnesses, are discontinued, to assess the level of activity of the underlying disorder and to prevent or minimize undesirable side effects.

holism [HOL- + -ISM]　HOLISTIC PSYCHOLOGY.

holistic [HOL- + -IST + -IC]　Pertaining to or considering the whole rather than just individual parts or aspects. See also HOLISTIC MEDICINE, HOLISTIC PSYCHOLOGY.

Holl [Moritz *Holl*, Austrian surgeon, 1852–1920]　See under LIGAMENT.

Hollander [Franklin *Hollander*, U.S. physiologist, 1899–1966] See under TEST.

Hollenhorst [Robert William *Hollenhorst*, U.S. ophthalmologist, born 1913]　Hollenhorst bodies. See under PLAQUE.

hollow　In anatomy, a depression or concavity in a surface.

　Sebileau's hollow　A depression on the floor of the mouth between the sublingual fold and the inferior surface of the tongue. An outmoded term.

hollow-back LORDOSIS.

Holmes [Eric Gordon *Holmes*, English neurologist, born 1897] Stewart-Holmes sign. See under SIGN.

Holmes [Gordon Morgan *Holmes*, English neurologist, 1876–1965]　**1** Holmes-Adie syndrome. See under ADIE SYNDROME.　**2** Holmes phenomenon, Holmes-Stewart phenomenon, Holmes sign. See under HOLMES REBOUND PHENOMENON.　**3** Holmes ataxia, Holmes type cerebellar ataxia, Holmes degeneration, Holmes familial cerebellar degeneration. See under PRIMARY PROGRESSIVE CEREBELLAR DEGENERATION.　**4** Head-Holmes syndrome. See under SYNDROME.　**5** Holmes rebound sign phenomenon. See under PHENOMENON.

Holmes [Timothy *Holmes*, English surgeon, 1825–1907]　See under OPERATION.

Holmgren [Alarik Frithiof *Holmgren*, Swedish physiologist, 1831–1897]　**1** Holmgren skeins. See under SKEIN.　**2** See under TEST.

Holmgren [Emil Algot *Holmgren*, Swedish histologist, 1866–1922]　Holmgren-Golgi canals. See under ENDOPLASMIC RETICULUM.

holmium Element number 67, having atomic weight 164.93. Holmium is a somewhat toxic rare-earth metal. One stable isotope occurs in nature and many synthetic radioisotopes have been identified. Symbol: Ho

holo- [Gk *holos* whole, complete] A combining form meaning whole, complete, integral, undivided. Also *hol-*.

holoacardius [HOLO- + ACARDIUS] A monozygotic twin that lacks a heart and depends for circulation of blood upon the heart of the more nearly normal twin via the placenta and umbilical cord.

 holoacardius acephalus A holoacardius lacking a head.

 holoacardius acormus A holoacardius lacking the entire caudal part of the body.

 holoacardius amorphus A holoacardius consisting wholly or in large part of a shapeless mass of tissue attached to the placenta by an umbilical cord.

holoanencephalic [HOLO- + ANENCEPHALIC] Completely lacking a brain and a cranium.

holoanencephalus [HOLO- + ANENCEPHALUS] An embryo, fetus, or newborn infant lacking a brain and a cranium.

holoanencephaly [HOLO- + ANENCEPHALY] The total absence of the brain and cranium.

holoantigen A complete antigen, as distinguished from a hapten.

Holobasidiomycetidae A subclass of basidiomycetous fungi (mushrooms). This subclass is characterized by a basidiocarp or other hymenial mass within which or upon which numerous single-celled basidia are formed.

holobasidium [HOLO- + BASIDIUM] (*plural* holobasidia) A single-celled basidium. Although typically club-shaped, holobasidia may resemble tuning forks in some taxa, and in others the basidium may become divided by adventitious septa.

holobenthic [HOLO- + BENTHIC] Referring to an organism which lives on the deep sea bottom throughout its life.

holoblast [HOLO- + -BLAST] An early embryo in which cleavage is total. Adjective: holoblastic.

holoblastic [HOLO- + -BLAST + -IC] See under HOLOBLASTIC CLEAVAGE.

Holocaine A proprietary name for phenacaine hydrochloride.

holocarpic Having the entire thallus converted into one or more reproductive structures.

holocephalic [HOLO- + CEPHAL- + -IC] Pertaining to or exhibiting holocephaly.

holocephaly [HOLO- + CEPHAL- + -Y] A condition in which the head is normal in the presence of demonstrable malformation elsewhere in the body.

holocoenotic [HOLO- + COENO- + *t* + -IC] Pertaining to the interaction of multiple environmental factors affecting an organism.

holocortex [HOLO- + CORTEX] The cerebral cortex, conceived as formed by a continuous and contiguous migration. It includes the isocortex, cingulate region, and Ammon's formation.

holocrine [HOLO- + Gk *krin(ein)* to separate] Denoting or characterized by secretion in which the secreting cells form part of the secretory product. Compare MEROCRINE.

holodiastolic Occupying the whole of diastole.

holoendemic [HOLO- + ENDEMIC] HYPERENDEMIC.

holoenzyme An enzyme including its removable prosthetic group, in distinction from the apoenzyme formed when the prosthetic group is removed.

hologamy A characteristic by which the gametes of an organism are indistinguishable from somatic cells. Reproduction involves the fusion of two gametes, as is seen in unicellular organisms.

hologastroschisis [HOLO- + GASTRO- + -SCHISIS] A developmental defect in the body wall caused by the failure of the anterior (or ventral, in quadrupeds) abdominal wall to close about the umbilicus. It represents an extreme degree of omphalocele.

hologenesis Worldwide genesis; a theory proposing that the human species did not originate in any one place, but evolved at the same time from many ancestral populations in many different parts of the world.

hologram [HOLO- + -GRAM] An interference pattern recorded on photographic film by using a split beam of coherent light. When the film is illuminated from behind by coherent light, the viewer sees a three-dimensional image.

holography [HOLO- + -GRAPHY] The process of recording or viewing a hologram.

 acoustic holography An imaging technique whereby a diffraction pattern is first generated from the original object and an image is subsequently reconstructed by coherent radiation.

hologynic Pertaining to traits, usually heritable ones, that occur in the females of a species.

holomastigote [HOLO- + MASTIGOTE] Having many flagella on the surface of the body, as in the termite-gut mutualist flagellate *Holomastigotes elongatum* (order Hypermastigida).

Holometabola [HOLO- + Gk *metabola*, neut. pl. of *metabolos* changeable] The group of insect orders characterized by holometabolous or complete metamorphosis, with development in four very distinct stages: egg, larva (through successive molts), pupa, and imago or adult. Examples of biomedical interest include the Diptera (flies, mosquitoes, gnats), Hymenoptera (bees, hornets, wasps), Coleoptera (beetles), Lepidoptera (moths, butterflies), Strepsiptera (twisted-wing insect parasites), and Siphonaptera (fleas). Compare HEMIMETABOLA.

holometabolous Characterized by complete metamorphosis, with fully distinct larval, pupal, and imago stages: said of insects. See also HOLOMETOBOLA.

holomicrography The use of microscopic equipment to generate and record three-dimensional holographic images.

holomorphosis The reattainment of physical wholeness through development or regeneration of a part that has been lost.

holonephros [HOLO- + Gk *nephros* kidney] All of the embryonic renal tubular systems considered as an all-embracing, continuous series. Also called *segmental organ*. • There are anatomic and other attributes to indicate resemblances between the tubules of the pronephros, mesonephros, and metanephros, and so the term *holonephros* would include all three of these tubular excretory systems.

holoparasite [HOLO- + PARASITE] An organism that is parasitic throughout its life cycle.

holopelagic Pertaining to a marine organism that spends its entire life in the open ocean.

Holophyra coli BALANTIDIUM COLI.

holophytic Capable of manufacturing food from inorganic sources, like a green plant: said of certain protozoa.

holoplankton Organisms that remain in the plankton stage throughout their lives.

holoplexia [HOLO- + Gk *plēx(is)* (from *plēssein* to strike) a stroke + -IA] GENERAL PARESIS.

holoprosencephaly The failure of the embryonic prosencephalon, or forebrain, to differentiate into two cerebral hemispheres and the diencephalon. It is seen in severe degrees of cyclopia.

 familial alobar holoprosencephaly The autosomal recessive inheritance of malformations of the cranium (orbital hypotelorism), the face (median cleft lip and palate), and the brain (absence of the corpus callosum and/or a single ventricle).

holorachischisis   RACHISCHISIS TOTALIS.

holoschisis [HOLO- + -SCHISIS]   AMITOSIS.

holosymphysis   A complete continuity: said of bones.

holosystolic   Occupying the whole of systole; pansystolic.

holotelencephaly [HOLO- + TELENCEPHALY]   The persistence of a single cerebral lobe and a single cerebral ventricle because of the failure of the embryonic telencephalon to differentiate into two hemispheres. It is seen in arrhinencephaly and severe degrees of cyclopia.

holotetanus [HOLO- + TETANUS]   Generalized tetanus or generalized tetanic spasms. An outmoded term. Also called *holotonia*.

Holothuroidea [L *holothur(ion)*, Gk *holothour(ion)* an unidentified sea monster + New L *-oidea*, from L *-oid(es)* -OID + *-ea*, neut. pl. of *-eus* English *-eous*]   A class of invertebrates in the phylum Echinodermata; the sea cucumbers. Its members are elongated along an oral-aboral axis, and the skeleton is reduced to microscopic ossicles embedded in the body wall. It is found in all marine environments.

Holothyrus   A genus of mites parasitic in poultry and other domestic animals. A species from Mauritius, *H. coccinella* has poisoned ducks, geese, and chickens that ingested it. In humans this species may cause a painful swelling of the tongue and throat.

holotomy [HOLO- + -TOMY]   Any surgical procedure in which a whole organ is excised, usually intact.

holotonia [HOLO- + *ton(o)*- + -IA]   HOLOTETANUS.

holotonic [HOLO- + TONIC]   Of or relating to holotetanus.

holotopic   Pertaining to the relationship between a specific portion of an organ and the whole organ.

holotopy   The position of a part or an organ with respect to the whole body or organism.

Holotricha   HOLOTRICHIDIA.

Holotrichidia [HOLO- + TRICH- + -ID¹ + -IA]   A subclass of Ciliata in which the cilia cover the body surface of the protozoan in a complex network of cilia and kinetodesmal fibrils. It includes the widespread and well-known genera *Paramecium* and *Tetrahymena*. A newer classification system places these genera in the subclass Hymenostomatia and the phylum Ciliophora. Also called *Holotricha*.

holotrichous [HOLO- + TRICH- + -OUS]   Having cilia of approximately equal length over the entire body surface: said of microorganisms.

holotype   A seldom used term for TYPE SPECIMEN. Adjective: holotypic.

holozoic   Concerning the ingestion and metabolism of food in a manner common to most animals, involving heterotrophic nutrition, in which the energy source or food is derived directly from the cells or cell products of other organisms, as distinguished from saprozoic organisms.

Holt [Mary Clayton *Holt*, English pediatrician, flourished 20th century]   Holt-Oram syndrome. See under SYNDROME.

Holth [Soren *Holth*, Norwegian ophthalmologist, 1863–1937]   See under OPERATION.

Holtz [Wilhelm *Holtz*, German physicist, 1836–1913]   See under MACHINE.

Holzknecht [Guido *Holzknecht*, Austrian roentgenologist, 1872–1931]   **1** See under UNIT, CHROMORADIOMETER, STOMACH. **2** Lambert-Holzknecht law. See under LAW. **3** Holzknecht space. See under RETROCARDIAC SPACE.

Holzmann [Walter *Holzmann*, German physician, born 1878]   Much-Holzmann reaction. See under REACTION.

homalocephalus   An individual possessing a flat head.

homalographic   Pertaining to homalography.

homalography   The study of the structural organization of a body by plane sections of parts or regions, or by drawings of such sections.

Homalomyia   A genus of flies of which the larvae may cause accidental intestinal myiasis in animals or humans.

homaluria [Gk *homal(os)* even, level + -URIA]   Excretion in the urine of any substance at a constant rate, or production of urine itself at a constant rate.

Homans [John *Homans*, U.S. surgeon, 1877–1954]   See under SIGN.

Homaridae [New L *homar(us)* (from French *homard* a lobster, akin to Old Norse *humarr* a lobster) a genus of decapod crustaceans + -IDAE]   A family of crustaceans in the order Decapoda, including the American and European lobsters.

homarine   *N*-Methylpyridinium-2-carboxylate. A zwitterionic substance found in lobster (*Homarus*) muscle.

homatropine $C_{16}H_{21}NO_3$. An alkaloid medication made by combining in ester form tropine and mandelic acid. It is used as an antispasmodic because of its anticholinergic action as a parasympathetic blocking agent like atropine. Its salts are used as mydriatics.

homatropine hydrobromide $C_{16}H_{21}NO_3 \cdot HBr$. A white, crystalline powder that is used as a cycloplegic and mydriatic agent. It is given topically in the conjunctiva.

homatropine methylbromide $C_{17}H_{24}BrNO_3$. The methylbromide salt of homatropine, which has the same properties as the parent drug. It is a parasympatholytic agent and used in the treatment of spasms in the gastrointestinal tract. It is given orally.

homaxial   Possessing axes of equal length, as in a sphere.

Home [Sir Everard *Home*, English surgeon, 1756–1832]   Home's lobe, Home's gland. See under SUBTRIGONAL GLAND.

home / home for the aged   A residence provided for a group of old people to live in together. Generally, services such as meals are provided on the assumption that the aged residents can no longer provide these for themselves. Also called *old age home*.

adult foster home   A private household which accepts an adult, usually an elderly person, into the household to live as a member of the family.

boarding home   A custodial care facility that provides room and board.

maternity home   A residential facility providing for the needs of pregnant women, usually young women, and often from home environments considered unsupportive or unwholesome.

nursing home   A health care institution which provides various levels of long-term care for people who usually have medical disabilities or limitations in activity or mobility. • The term is used in this sense in many countries (except Japan), but in some (such as the United Kingdom and South Africa) it may apply also to some institutions providing short-term acute care.

old age home   HOME FOR THE AGED.

residential home   A residence provided for any of various groups requiring special care, such as the old or the handicapped. Such a home typically provides room and board and limited personal assistance in a group or family setting within the community.

homebound   HOUSEBOUND.

homecious   AUTECIOUS.

Homén [Ernst Alexander *Homén*, Finnish physician, 1851–1926]   See under SYNDROME.

homeo- [Gk *homoios* like, resembling]   A combining form meaning like, similar, same. Also *homoeo- (variant British spelling), homoio-*.

homeograft ALLOGRAFT.

homeokinesis Mitotic division in which each daughter cell nucleus contains the same number of chromosomes as the mother cell nucleus.

homeometric Maintaining like size.

homeomorphous Of like form and shape.

homeo-osteoplasty The allografting of bone.

homeopath A practitioner of homeopathy.

homeopathic Of or relating to homeopathy.

homeopathy [HOMEO- + -PATHY] A system of medicine in which the treatment of disease depends upon the administration of minute doses of drugs that would in larger doses produce symptoms of the disease being treated. Homeopathy was originally propounded by Samuel C. F. Hahnemann (1755–1843), a German physician. Also called *hahnemannism*. Compare ALLOPATHY.

homeoplasia [HOMEO- + -PLASIA] The growth of new tissue similar to the tissue present in the region. Also called *homoioplasia*.

homeoplastic Of or relating to homeoplasia.

homeorrhesis [HOMEO- + -*rrhe(a)* + -SIS] The continuation of a biological process along an unchanged course that remains unaffected by potentially diverting influences.

homeosis A change or substitution in one structure or organ of the body to or by a related or homologous structure from another body segment.

homeostasis [HOMEO- + -STASIS] **1** The relative stability of the internal environment of a normal organism which is preserved through feedback mechanisms despite the presence of influences capable of causing profound changes. For example, when oxygen level decreases, sensors cause respiration to increase to preserve a level within a limited variability consistent with normal functioning. Also called *homeostatic equilibrium*. **2** Those processes considered collectively by which homeostasis is maintained by normal organisms. For defs. 1 and 2 also called *homoiostasis*.

genetic homeostasis In a breeding population, the combination of forces and processes that stabilize the genotype.

immunologic homeostasis The immunologic condition of a normal animal, in which an immune response is produced by the introduction of foreign antigens but not by the animal's own antigens.

homeostatic Of or relating to homeostasis.

homeotherapeutic Relating to homeotherapy or to homeopathy.

homeotherapy Therapy or prevention of a disease using a material similar to, but not identical with, the pathogenic agent of that disease. See also HOMEOPATHY.

homeotherm [HOMEO- + Gk *therm(ē)* heat] An animal that can maintain a more or less constant body temperature by metabolic activity and by modifications that carefully regulate the rate of heat exchange with the environment. Also called *homotherm, warm-blooded animal*. Compare POIKILOTHERM.

homeothermal HOMEOTHERMIC.

homeothermic [HOMEO- + THERM- + -IC] Exhibiting or characterized by homeothermy. Also *homeothermal, hemathermal, hematothermal, hemathermous, homoiothermal, homoiothermic, homothermal, homothermic, endothermic, warm-blooded*.

homeothermy [HOMEO- + THERM- + -Y] The maintenance of a constant body temperature independent of ambient temperatures. Homeothermy is typical only of birds and mammals. Also called *endothermy*.

homeotoxic Producing toxic effects in individuals of the same species as the originating individual; characteristic of or pertaining to a homeotoxin. Also *isotoxic*. Compare HETEROTOXIC.

homeotoxin [HOMEO- + TOXIN] A toxin from an individual which is toxic to other individuals of the same species. Also called *isotoxin*. Also *homoeotoxin, homoiotoxin*.

homeotransplant ALLOGRAFT.

homeotransplantation ALLOTRANSPLANTATION.

homeotypic Pertaining to or resembling the normal or usual cell type: used especially of products of the second meiotic division of the male germ cells.

homergic Characterizing drugs or pharmacologic agents that produce the same type of pharmacologic effects, even though they may not accomplish this by the same mechanism or by the same receptors.

homicide [L *homocid(ium)* (from *homo* a human being + *caedere* to kill) homicide] **1** The killing of a human being by the act, by omission, or by negligence under circumstances which may be justifiable, excusable, or felonious. **2** One who commits homicide.

homicidomania [*homicid(e)* + *o* + -MANIA] The compulsion to kill, or repeated executions of the compulsion. Also called *homicidal insanity, phonomania* (older term).

homiculture A seldom used term for POSITIVE EUGENICS.

hominid **1** Belonging to the primate family Hominidae. **2** A member of the primate family Hominidae.

Hominidae The primate family comprising humans and the ancestral and collateral forms most closely related to them. There is only one extant genus, *Homo*, but numerous earlier forms are known from the fossil record. Some zoologists include the anthropoid apes in this family.

Hominoidea [L *homo*, gen. *hominis*, man + New L -*oidea*, neut. pl. combining form from L -*oïd(es)* -OID + -*ea*, neut. pl. of -*eus* English -*eous*] A superfamily of the mammalian order Primates. It comprises the anthropoid families Hominidae and Pongidae and includes fossil apes, early man, and other fossil species having characteristics of both ("ape-men"), as well as modern great apes and modern man.

homme [French, man]

homme rouge [French, lit., red man] A patient with mycosis fungoides having red plaquelike lesions on the skin. • An ambiguous and outmoded term. The great majority of these cases are now recognized as suffering not from mycosis fungoides but from other lymphomas.

Homo [L, a human being, man] A genus of the family Hominidae of which *H. sapiens* is the only living species. Extinct species such as *H. habilis* and *H. erectus* are known from fossil remains, as are *H. neanderthalensis* and others which are now often considered subspecies of *H. sapiens*.

Homo heidelbergensis See under HEIDELBERG MAN.

Homo neanderthalensis A fossil human species represented by the type specimen from La Chapelle-aux-Saints, France. Many other examples are known from Europe and the Middle East. The skeleton of this species is typically of short stature and robust structure, with large joints and a large cranial capacity. The face is large and projects forward from heavy brow ridges. Sites yielding Neandertal remains are mostly dated to between 50 000 and 100 000 years before the present. Some authorities regard Neandertal man as belonging to the species *Homo sapiens*, designating it as the subspecies *H. sapiens neanderthalensis*.

Homo sapiens The species that includes all the living races of mankind. It is characterized by striding, upright bipedalism, brain size in the order of 1350 cm^3, and an orthognathic face with a chin. These characters, as well as several others, serve to distinguish modern human anatomy from that of other species such as *H. habilis* and *H. erectus.* Early examples of *H. sapiens* are known from Swanscombe, England and Omo, Ethiopia, dated to between 100 000 and 250 000 years before the present. Some authorities recognize fossil subspecies such as *H. sapiens neanderthalensis, H. sapiens rhodesiensis, H. sapiens steinheimensis,* and others.

homo- [Gk *homos* one and the same] **1** A combining form meaning same, alike. **2** In organic chemistry, a combining form indicating the addition of a methylene group to a compound. Compare HETERO-.

homoallele   EUALLELE.

homoallelic   EUALLELIC.

homobiotin   A compound homologous to biotin but having an additional CH_2 grouping in its side-chain. It acts as a biotin antagonist.

homoblastic   Derived from one particular type of tissue.

homocercal [HOMO- + Gk *kerk(os)* a tail + -AL]   Designating a tail in which the dorsal and ventral portions are similar and the vertebral column ends at the middle of its base, as in most bony fishes.

homochromous [HOMO- + CHROM- + -OUS]   Being of only one color; monochromatic.

homochronous [HOMO- + CHRON- + -OUS]   Occurring at the same age in succeeding generations.

homocladic   Relating to or characterized by anastomosis between small branches of the same artery.

homocysteine $HS—CH_2—CH_2—CH(NH_3{}^+)—COO^-$.   An amino acid not incorporated into proteins but important as an intermediate in the metabolism of cysteine and methionine. In the breakdown of methionine it reacts with serine to form cystathionine, and it can alternatively by methylated to yield methionine. Symbol: Hcy

homocysteine desulfhydrase   A pyridoxal-containing enzyme (EC 4.4.1.2) that catalyzes the reaction of homocysteine and water to yield 2-oxobutyrate, ammonia, and hydrogen sulfide. This is not the main route of homocysteine degradation in mammals.

homocysteine methyltransferase   **1** The enzyme (EC 2.1.1.10) present in plants and microorganisms that is responsible for the methylation of homocysteine to yield methionine. It uses *S*-adenosylmethionine or *S*-methylmethionine as methyl donor.   **2** The cobamide-containing enzyme that uses methyltetrahydrofolate as methyl donor.

homocystine $[S·CH_2·CH_2·CH(NH_2)COOH]_2$.   A substance made by the demethylation of methionine. It provides a source of sulfur for the body and is homologous to cystine.

homocystinemia   The presence of homocystine in blood, a rare finding in patients with homocystinuria.

homocystinuria   **1** The abnormal excretion of homocysteine or homocystine in the urine. It is usually due to one of several inborn errors of transsulfuration, but it can also be caused by drugs or bacterial contamination of the urine.   **2** A clinical condition caused by a deficiency of cystathionine β-synthase. The condition is of widely variable severity and is characterized by overgrowth of tubular bones, osteoporosis, ectopia lentis, thrombosis, and mental retardation. In one of at least two biochemical (and perhaps allelic) variants, the administration of pyridoxine increases enzyme activity, corrects biochemical abnormalities, and reduces the likelihood of further clinical deterioration. Also called *cystathionine β-synthase deficiency.*

homocytotropic   Capable of binding to cells of the same animal species: said of antibodies.

homodesmotic [HOMO- + DESMO- + *t* + -IC]   Describing or pertaining to nerve tracts or fascicles of nerve fibers which interconnect neural centers of similar function.

homodont [*hom(o)-* + -ODONT]   Having all teeth of the same general form. This dentition is characteristic of all toothed vertebrates except mammals, and it was exhibited in some early mammals. It has been secondarily developed in some cetaceans. Also *isodont.*

homodromous   Moving in the same direction, or directing activity toward the same end.

homodynamic   Of or relating to drugs or pharmacological agents that interact specifically with the same receptor and thus produce the same type of pharmacological response.

homodynamy   Similarity in structure and development of parts or organs arranged in series along the main axis of the body. Also called *metameric homology, serial homology.*

homoecious   AUTECIOUS.

homoeo-   A British spelling for HOMEO-.

homoeopathy   A British spelling for HOMEOPATHY.

homoeosis   A British spelling for HOMEOSIS.

homoeostasis   A British spelling for HOMEOSTASIS.

homoeotoxin   HOMEOTOXIN.

homoerotic [HOMO- + EROTIC]   Characterized by homoeroticism. Also *isophilic* (seldom used).

homoeroticism [HOMO- + EROTICISM]   Libidinal attraction to others of the same sex, a normal phase in the development of object relationships, but considered deviant by many authorities if it remains the preferred way of relating sexually in adult life. Homoeroticism implies that the attraction remains sublimated. Also called *homoerotism.*

homoerotism   HOMOEROTICISM.

homofermentative   Carrying out homolactic fermentation. Also *homolactic.* Compare HETEROFERMENTATIVE.

homogamete   A germ cell produced by the homogametic parent.

homogametic   **1** Referring to or characterized by the production of the same kinds of gametes, usually in reference to the sex chromosome present. In humans, females are homogametic. **2** Referring to or characterized by the production of gametes that are of the same size or structure.

homogamous   Having male and female sex organs functional at the same time. Compare DICHOGAMOUS.

homogamy   **1** A mating preference between organisms that share certain aspects of phenotype or are of similar genotype. It is a contributing factor to assortative mating.   **2** Simultaneous maturation of the sexual elements of flowers. Compare HETEROGAMY.

homogenate [HOMO- + -GEN + -ATE]   Material that has been reduced to a uniform consistency by homogenization.

homogeneity [Med L *homogeneitas* (from *homogene(us)* of the same kind, from Gk *homogenios* of the same race or blood, from *homo(s)* one and the same + *genos* race, descent; + -*itas* -ITY) the state of being homogeneous]   The property of having all its parts the same. Of chemical substances it signifies purity, because all the molecules are identical.

homogeneization   HOMOGENIZATION.

homogeneous   Possessing homogeneity.

homogenesis   The continuity of characteristics over successive generations of organisms. Also called *homogeny.* Adjective: homogenetic.

homogenetic   Characterized by homogenesis.

homogenic   Pertaining to a gamete that has but one allele of a given gene or of all genes. All haploid gametes are homogenic.

homogenitality [HOMO- + GENITAL + -ITY]   The expression of homoeroticism in overt sexual activity.

homogenization   The process whereby material is reduced to a uniform consistency. Also called *homogeneization.*

homogenize   To reduce to uniform consistency or composition; to render homogeneous.

homogenous [HOMO- + -GENOUS]   Marked by similar form and structure resulting from common ancestry.

homogentisic acid   (2,5-Dihydroxyphenyl)acetic acid. An intermediate in the catabolism of tyrosine, it appears in the urine in alkaptonuria, in which its oxidation to maleylacetoacetate is deficient. Also called *alkapton* (obsolete), *alcapton* (obsolete), *glycosuric acid.*

homogentisuria   The presence of homogentisic acid in the urine.

homogeny   HOMOGENESIS.

homoglandular   Of or relating to the same gland. Estrogen and progesterone, for example, have a *homoglandular* source (the ovary) in the female mammal.

homogonic [HOMO- + GON-² + -IC]   Characterizing an alternative cycle in which larvae develop directly into infective parasitic forms instead of developing into free-living adults. Alternative homogonic and heterogonic cycles are seen in rhabditoid nematode worms. See also *STRONGYLOIDES.*

homograft [HOMO- + GRAFT]   ALLOGRAFT.
  isogeneic homograft   ISOGRAFT.

homoio-   HOMEO-.

homoioplasia   HOMEOPLASIA.

homoiopodal   Describing or relating to neurons which have branches of one type only.

homoiosmotic   Describing an aquatic animal that maintains an internal concentration of body fluids unlike that of the environment.

homoiostasis   HOMEOSTASIS.

homoiothermal   HOMEOTHERMIC.

homoiothermic   HOMEOTHERMIC.

homoiotoxin   HOMEOTOXIN.

homokaryon   A cell that contains two or more genetically identical nuclei in a common cytoplasm. Compare HETEROKARYON.

homokeratoplasty [HOMO- + HERATO- + -PLASTY]   Surgical exchange of a cornea from one individual to another of the same species.

homolactic   HOMOFERMENTATIVE.

homolalia [HOMO- + -LALIA]   Similarity or identity of speech.

homolateral   IPSILATERAL.

homologic   Pertaining to homology.

homologous   **1** Resembling in structure and origin. In biology, of organs or structures having the same evolutionary history but divergent adaptation, such as the skeleton in the forelimb of a land vertebrate and that in the wing of a bat. Compare ANALOGOUS.   **2** Obtained from an animal of the same species but not from the same individual as that providing the other constituents of the experiment or study: said especially of serum, tissue, cells, etc., under immunologic study. Also *isologous.* Compare AUTOLOGOUS, HETEROLOGOUS.

homologue   **1** Any organ or structure similar in structure and origin to that in another organism or series of organisms. Compare ANALOGUE.   **2** HOMOLOGOUS CHROMOSOME.

homology [HOMO- + -LOGY]   Similarity in structure and evolutionary development of organs or structures either in one individual or in two or a series of organisms; the state of being homologous. Compare ANALOGY.
  metameric homology   HOMODYNAMY.
  serial homology   HOMODYNAMY.

homolysin   A lysin produced in an animal in response to an antigen obtained from another animal of the same species.

homolysis   ISOHEMOLYSIS.

homomorphic   **1** In cytogenetics, of or relating to the synapsis of two chromosomes that are similar in shape and size, and are usually homologues, during meiosis.   **2** Having a superficial resemblance: used especially of organisms of different taxa. For defs. 1 and 2 also *homomorphous.*

homomorphosis [HOMO- + MORPH- + -OSIS]   Replacement of a part of an organism with a similar part through regeneration.

homomorphous   HOMOMORPHIC.

homonomous   Belonging to a set of similar structures: used especially of those structures that occur in series, such as ribs and fingers.

homonymous [Gk *homōnymos* (from *hom(os)* one and the same + Gk *onyma,* also *onoma* name) having the same name]   **1** Being in the same relation, as *homonymous diplopia* (uncrossed diplopia).   **2** Designating or of the nature of an interrelated sequence of a muscle's nerve and motor response, as a muscle's reflex response elicited upon stimulating the nerve to that muscle.

homophene   One of two or more spoken words that are indistinguishable to the deaf lip-reader but that may sound different to a hearer and have different meanings.

homophile [HOMO- + -PHILE]   HOMOSEXUAL.

homoplasmy   HOMOPLASY.

homoplastic   Referring to homoplasty.

homoplasty [HOMO- + -PLASTY]   **1** An operation utilizing allografting.   **2** The similarity in function and form of the anatomic units of dissimilar species.

homoplasy [HOMO- + Gk *plas(is)* a shaping, molding + -Y]   The possession by two or more species of a similar trait or characteristic that was not derived from an ancestor common to both species. Also called *homoplasmy.*

homopolymer [HOMO- + POLYMER]   A polymer which is composed of only one type of monomer.

homorganic [*hom(o)-* + ORGANIC]   **1** Arising from the same organ.   **2** Stemming from homologous organs.

homoserine $HOCH_2—CH_2—CH(NH_3{}^+)—COO^-$. 2-Amino-4-hydroxybutyric acid. An intermediate in the biosynthesis of threonine from aspartate in those organisms (not including man) that can make threonine. Symbol: Hse

homoserine lactone   The cyclic compound formed from homoserine by ester formation between its carboxyl and hydroxyl groups. This formation occurs spontaneously in acid. A residue of homoserine lactone is found at the C terminus of a peptide formed by scission of polypeptide chains at methionine by the action of cyanogen bromide.

homosexual [HOMO- + SEXUAL]   **1** Characterized by homosexuality. Also *isosexual* (seldom used).   **2** A homosexual individual. Also called *homophile, invert* (older term).

homosexuality [HOMO- + SEXUALITY]   Preferential sexual attraction to members of one's own sex, considered a disorder only if such attraction is ego-dystonic and the subject desires to increase heterosexual responsivity. Also called *sexual inversion* (obsolete), *uranism* (outmoded).
  ego-dystonic homosexuality   Homosexuality in which the sexual attraction is unwanted and a source of distress. In addition, the subject seeks to acquire or increase heterosexual responsivity so that heterosexual relations can be initiated or maintained and homosexual inclinations forsaken.
  female homosexuality   A female's preferential sexual attraction to other females. Also called *lesbianism, sapphism, amor lesbicus* (obsolete).
  latent homosexuality   Homosexuality that is not expressed in overt sexual activity or even, in some cases, fully recognized as such by the subject.

male homosexuality A male's preferential sexual attraction to other males. Also called *commasculation* (outmoded), *Dorian love* (obsolete).

overt homosexuality Attraction to members of one's own sex and willful indulgence in sexual relations with them.

unconscious homosexuality An extreme form of latent homosexuality in which the subject is attracted to members of his own sex but is not aware of it.

homosporous Having only one kind of spore.

D-homosteroid A steroid having an extra methylene group in ring D, which therefore becomes a six-membered ring like the other rings in the molecule.

homostimulant 1 Effecting the stimulation of the same or a homologous organ. 2 A stimulant prepared from the same organ or from an organ homologous to that being stimulated.

homostimulation The stimulation of an organ by a material from the same organ or from a homologous organ.

homothallic Having hyphae that are sexually integrated such that reproduction can take place within one individual: used especially of certain fungi. Compare HETEROTHALLIC.

homotherm HOMEOTHERM.

homothermal HOMEOTHERMIC.

homothermic HOMEOTHERMIC.

homotonia ISOTONIA.

homotonic ISOTONIC.

homotopic In or involving the same or corresponding sites or parts of the body.

homotransplant ALLOGRAFT.

homotransplantation ALLOTRANSPLANTATION.

homotropism [HOMO- + TROPISM] The property of a cell which causes similar cells to move toward or away from it.

homotype 1 Any part or organ with the same structure and function as another, especially in reversed symmetry, such as the hand. 2 A representative of a population whose characters most nearly approach the mean for that population. Compare HETEROTYPE.

homotypic Pertaining to or exhibiting the characteristics of a homotype. Also *homotypical*.

homotypical HOMOTYPIC.

homovanillic acid 3-Methoxy-4-hydroxymandelic acid. A metabolite of dopa, dopamine, and norepinephrine, found in urine.

homozygosis 1 HOMOZYGOSITY. 2 The generation of an offspring that is homozygous at one or more specific loci by union of gametes having identical alleles at those loci.

homozygosity In genetics, a condition in which one or more specific loci are homozygous. Also called *homozygosis*.

homozygote A nonhaploid cell or organism that has identical alleles at a given locus.

homozygous Characterized by identical alleles at a given locus or loci: said of nonhaploid cells or organisms.

homunculus [L (dim. of *homo* man), a little man, mannikin] A dwarf characterized by proportions that are typical of most normal-sized people.

honeycomb RETICULUM.

hood 1 A covering used in laboratories to provide a protected space. 2 In soft or argasid ticks, the anterior extension of the dorsal, leathery or wrinkled integument that covers the ventrally positioned mouthparts. A ventral groove or camerostome in the hood encloses the mouthparts.

tooth hood DENTAL OPERCULUM.

hoof [Old English *hōf*] The horn-covered foot of certain animals such as the large domestic animals.

cloven hoof A hoof which is divided into two parts, as the bovine hoof.

hook [Middle English *hoc*, hook, from Old English *hōc*] 1 A long, thin surgical instrument with a curved, sharpened end. It is often used for retraction or fixation of tissues. 2 A double curved terminal device for an upper-limb prosthesis. One part is opened by the amputee using a steel cable, allowing grasping when it is closed.

blunt hook An obstetric instrument formerly used to exert traction on a fetus in the breech presentation. Also *blunthook*.

Braun's hook An obsolete obstetric instrument formerly used to decapitate a fetus.

hook of cartilaginous auditory tube The superior part of the cartilaginous part of the auditory tube that is bent laterally and downwards to form a broad medial lamina and a narrow, short lateral lamina. On transverse section the cartilage has a hooklike appearance. An outmoded term.

dural hook A small, sharp, hooked instrument for picking up the dura mater.

embrasure hook A type of rest for a partial denture, occupying the occlusal part of an embrasure.

fixation hook A surgical instrument used to retract or immobilize tissues during an operation.

hook of hamate bone HAMULUS OSSIS HAMATI.

Loughnane's hook A surgical instrument that has two curved prongs and is designed for postresectional transurethral prostate gland removal.

Malgaigne's hooks A surgical instrument with two bone-holding hooks that is used to produce apposition of the fragments in a fractured patella.

muscle hook A surgical instrument with a right angled tip that may be positioned beneath an extraocular muscle to isolate and identify its insertion, for use in strabismus surgery. Also called *squint hook*.

nerve hook A dull, right-angled hook for lifting a nerve.

Pajot's hook An obstetric instrument formerly used to decapitate a fetus.

posterior palate hook PALATE RETRACTOR.

retraction hook A surgical instrument with a blunt, curved tip for retraction of tissue.

squint hook MUSCLE HOOK.

tracheostomy hook An instrument used in tracheostomy to hook forward and steady the trachea prior to incising it. It has a straight handle approximately 14 cm long, terminating in a fine sharp hook.

Tyrrell's hook A very small angulated metal rod for use in eye surgery.

hooklet A small, clawlike rostellar structure of tapeworms, especially of the larval forms. The hooklets are arranged in various patterns that characterize families and genera. The hexacanth cestode embryo uses its six hooklets to claw out of its membrane sheath and to penetrate the gut wall of the host. • The larger, more robust holdfast structures of adult *Taenia* tapeworms are usually termed hooks rather than hooklets.

hook-up 1 The circuit arrangement of electrical equipment, cables, and electrodes for diagnosis or therapy. 2 A connection to a source of electricity, water, oxygen, suction, etc.

hookworm Any of various bloodsucking worms of the family Ancylostomatidae, which are parasitic in the intestine of humans and other vertebrates. Medically and veterinarily important genera include *Ancylostoma*, *Necator*, and *Uncinaria*.

American hookworm NEW WORLD HOOKWORM.

dog hookworm Any hookworm that primarily or commonly infects dogs, such as *Ancylostoma caninum* or *Uncinaria stenocephala*.

European hookworm OLD WORLD HOOKWORM.

New World hookworm A hookworm of the species *Necator Americanus.* Also called *American hookworm.*

Old World hookworm A hookworm of the species *Ancylostoma duodenale.* Also called *European hookworm.*

rat hookworm A hookworm of the genus *Nippostrongylus.*

hookworm of ruminants Any of various hookworms that parasitize ruminants. Important genera are in the subfamily Uncinariinae and include *Bunostomum* and *Gaigeria.*

Hoorweg [Jan Leendert *Hoorweg*, Dutch biophysicist, born 1841] See under LAW.

hoose [possibly variant of *wheeze*] PARASITIC BRONCHITIS.

Hoover [Charles Franklin *Hoover*, U.S. physician, 1865–1927] **1** See under SIGN. **2** Grasset-Gaussel-Hoover sign. See under SIGN.

Hopkins [Andrew Delmar *Hopkins*, U.S. entomologist, born 1857] Hopkins rule. See under HOPKINS BIOCLIMATIC LAW.

Hopkins [Sir Frederick Gowland *Hopkins*, English biochemist, 1861–1947] Benedict-Hopkins-Cole reagent. See under REAGENT.

Hoplonemertini [Gk *hoplo(n)* a weapon + New L *Nemertini* (from Gk *Nēmērt(ēs)* a Nereid + *-ini* -INA)] An order of ribbon worms or nemertine worms in the phylum Rhynchocoela, class Enopla. These worms are nonsegmented, and possess a proboscis armed with a stylet apparatus. The intestine has lateral diverticula and a cecum. They are found in terrestrial, fresh water or marine habitats.

Hoplopsyllus anomalus A species of flea found as an ectoparasite of ground squirrels in the western United States and serving as a vector of sylvatic plague.

Hopmann [Carl Melchior *Hopmann*, German rhinologist, 1844–1925] See under POLYP.

Hoppe [Hermann Henry *Hoppe*, U.S. neurologist, 1867–1929] Hoppe-Goldflam syndrome. See under MYASTHENIA GRAVIS.

hora somni At bedtime, used in prescription writing.

hor. decub. *hora decubitus* (L, at bedtime).

hordein A prolamin that is insoluble in water but soluble in 80% alcohol. Hordein is found in barley.

hordenine $C_{10}H_{15}NO$. 4-[2-(Dimethylamino)ethyl]phenol. A natural substance, present in malted barley, that is very similar to adrenaline in its pharmacologic activity. It is a sympathomimetic agent and it is used as a stimulant for the heart, a vasoconstrictor, and a bronchodilator.

hordeolum [New L, variant of Late L *hordeolus*, dim. of L *hordeum* barley, barleycorn] STYE.

horehound *Marrubium vulgare* of the Labiatae family. It is used as an expectorant in lozenges. Also *hoarhound.*

Horgan [Edmund J. *Horgan*, U.S. surgeon, born 1884] Horgan's operation. See under TRANSANTRAL ETHMOIDECTOMY.

hor. interm. *horis intermediis* (L, in the intermediate hours).

horizocardia A horizontal position of the heart.

horizon / retinal horizon The line of retinal loci centered upon the fovea and extending directly medial and lateral.

horizontalis Denoting a flat plane at right angles to a vertical plane, either the median or the coronal, with respect to the anatomical position of the body; horizontal.

hormesis [Gk *hormēsis* (from *horm(an)* to set in motion + *-ēsis* -ESIS) rapid motion] The stimulating effect of small doses of any substance which in larger doses is inhibitory.

hormic [Gk *horm(ē)* an assault, onset, impulse, impetus + -IC] Denoting a theory that all behavior is purposeful in nature and largely determined by instinctive impulses or their derivatives. A rarely used term.

hormion [New L, irreg. from Gk *hormos* a cord, collar, necklace] A craniometric point situated at the posterior border of the vomer in the midline at its junction with the sphenoid.

hormism [Gk *horm(ē)* onrush, impulse, setting oneself in motion + -ISM] The philosophy that goals are sought for their own sake and value, rather than because of pleasure at their attainment. Compare HEDONISM.

hormogonium A short segment of a filament of a cyanobacterium that is capable of developing into an independent organism.

hormonagogue An agent that stimulates the secretion of hormone or hormones.

hormonal Of or relating to a hormone or hormones. Also *hormonic.*

hormone

hormone [Gk *hormōn*, pres. part. of *horman* to set in motion, rouse, urge on] Any substance secreted by specialized cells in the endocrine glands or in clusters or diffusely spread through the brain, lungs, and gastrointestinal tract. These substances act upon specific target tissues more or less remote from the site of secretion or upon the regulation of metabolic processes throughout the organism. Also called *internal secretion, incretion* (obsolete).

adaptive hormone A hormone secreted during adaptation to stressful changes as epinephrine, cortisol, or vasopressin. A popular usage.

adenohypophysial hormone A hormone secreted by the adenohypophysis (anterior pituitary), as growth hormone, prolactin, the gonadotropins, thyrotropin, adrenocorticotropin, or lipotropin. Also called *anterior pituitary hormone.*

adipokinetic hormone **1** ADIPOKININ. **2** An older term for LIPOTROPIN.

adrenocortical hormone Any of several steroid hormones synthesized in and secreted by the adrenal cortex, suggested as comprising four classes. They are C_{19} androgens, C_{21} progestogens, C_{21} corticosteroids, and perhaps C_{18} estrogens. Also called *cortical hormone.*

adrenocorticotropic hormone The adenohypophysial polypeptide hormone that regulates the structure and function of the adrenal cortex. A single chain of 39 amino acids, of 4567 daltons, it is controlled by the hypophysiotropic hormone, corticotropin-releasing hormone, and by the level of plasma cortisol, is secreted in a free-running circadian cycle, and is highly labile to external stimuli, increasing during stress. The hormone primarily stimulates the secretion of corticosteroids and androgens, having a lesser influence upon aldosterone. Adrenocorticotropic hormone is subnormally secreted in hypopituitarism and when corticosteroids are given medicinally, and excessively secreted in pituitary-dependent Cushing syndrome. As a pharmaceutical, most of its uses in inflammatory and allergic disease have been superseded by the introduction of the semisynthetic corticosteroids. Also called *adrenocorticotropin, corticoptropin, corticotrophin, adrenocorticotrophin, adrenotropin, adrenotrophin, adrenotropic hormone* (seldom used), *acortan (seldom used in the U.S.), adrenotropic hormone, adrenocorticotropic peptide* (outmoded). Abbreviation: ACTH

adrenomedullary hormone Epinephrine or norepinephrine of the adrenal medulla.

adrenotropic hormone A seldom used term for ADRENOCORTICOTROPIC HORMONE.

androgenic hormone ANDROGEN.

anterior pituitary hormone ADENOHYPOPHYSIAL HORMONE.

antidiabetic hormone An obsolete term for INSULIN.

antidiuretic hormone VASOPRESSIN.

antigonadotropic hormone Antibody or antibodies formed in response to administered gonadotropic hormone derived from another species.

Aschheim-Zondek hormone An outmoded term for LUTEINIZING HORMONE.

brain hormone Any of a group of insect hormones secreted in the brain that control development and maturation. See also ECDYSIOTROPIN.

chondrotropic hormone An outmoded term for GROWTH HORMONE.

chorionic growth hormone-prolactin HUMAN PLACENTAL LACTOGEN.

chromaffin hormone An older term for EPINEPHRINE.

chromatophorotropic hormone MELANOCYTE STIMULATING HORMONE.

circulatory hormone A hormonal substance that exerts its effects at a distant site via the bloodstream. This is in contrast to the products of enterochromaffin cells, which can only exert direct local effects on adjacent structures because they do not enter the circulatory system.

conjugated estrogen hormones CONJUGATED ESTROGENS.

corpus luteum hormone PROGESTERONE.

cortical hormone ADRENOCORTICAL HORMONE.

corticotropin releasing hormone A presumably peptide hormone of the hypothalamus that stimulates the release of adrenocorticotropin (ACTH) by adenohypophysial cells, whose own secretory rate is regulated by diurnal fluctuations in plasma cortisol values, plasma ACTH concentration, and stress. Also called *corticoliberin, corticotropin releasing factor* (older term). Abbreviation: CRH

diabetogenic hormone A heterogenous substance identified in crude extracts of anterior pituitary tissue and found to induce hyperglycemia and act as an insulin antagonist. Most of the diabetogenic activity is probably due to growth hormone, some to adrenocorticotropin.

environmental hormone Any substance derived from biologic materials that has an effect on the growth of other organisms. Some of these hormones can be produced from the combination of decomposition products and minerals. The effect may be inhibitory, as from antibiotics, or stimulatory, as from vitamins. Also called *external diffusion hormone, ecomone.*

estrogenic hormone ESTROGEN.

external diffusion hormone ENVIRONMENTAL HORMONE.

fat-mobilizing hormone LIPOLYTIC HORMONE.

female hormone Estrogen or progesterone. A popular usage.

follicle hormone FOLLICULAR HORMONE.

follicle-ripening hormone An older term for FOLLICLE STIMULATING HORMONE.

follicle stimulating hormone An anterior pituitary polypeptide hormone of 24 000–35 000 daltons, a sialic acid-containing gonadotropin which regulates the growth and maturation of the ovarian or graafian follicle and stimulates testicular spermatogenesis. For maximal effect on the male or female gonad this hormone requires also the presence of luteinizing hormone, the two hormones having a subunit in common. Pharmaceutical preparations from human pituitary extracts and postmenopausal urine are used in treatment of infertility in women. Also called *gametogenic hormone* (seldom used), *gametokinetic hormone* (seldom used), *follicle-ripening hormone* (older term), *follicle stimulating principle* (older term), *thylakentrin* (older term). Abbreviation: FSH

follicle stimulating hormone releasing hormone A hypothalamic hormone specifically regulating the adenohypophysial release of follicle stimulating hormone (FSH). It is probably identical to gonadotropin releasing hormone which controls the release of both FSH and luteinizing hormone. Also called *follicle stimulating hormone releasing factor.* Abbreviation: FSHRH

follicular hormone A hormone secreted by the ovarian or graafian follicle; estrogen. Also called *follicle hormone.*

galactopoietic hormone An outmoded term for PROLACTIN.

gametogenic hormone A seldom used term for FOLLICLE STIMULATING HORMONE.

gametokinetic hormone A seldom used term for FOLLICLE STIMULATING HORMONE.

gastrointestinal hormone Any of the hormones arising from specialized cells in the mucosa of the stomach and intestine and acting to control the motility and secretory activity of the gastrointestinal tract. The hormones include cholecystokinin, gastrin, secretin, vasoactive intestinal polypeptide, gastric inhibitory polypeptide, motilin, and bombesin. Also called *gut hormone* (popular).

glycoprotein hormone Any polypeptide hormone containing sialic acid, as the anterior pituitary gonadotropins, thyrotropin, and chorionic gonadotropin.

gonadotropic hormone GONADOTROPIN. Abbreviation: GTH

gonadotropin releasing hormone A decapeptide, hypophysiotropic hormone which stimulates the release of follicle stimulating hormone (FSH) and luteinizing hormone from the anterior pituitary. It may also act on both gonadotropins, there being no separate releasing hormone for FSH. Also called *gonadotropin releasing factor, luteinizing hormone releasing factor, luteinizing hormone releasing hormone, luliberin.* Abbreviation: GnRH

growth hormone 1 An adenohypophysial hormone that promotes and regulates somatic and skeletal growth and influences carbohydrate, fat, and protein metabolism. Human growth hormone is a polypeptide of about 21 500 daltons and containing 191 amino acids. It is secreted by specialized acidophil cells under the control of the hypothalamus, undergoing a periodic sleep-wake secretory cycle and responding briskly to many stimuli, being increased by stress and exercise, inhibited by obesity and glucocorticoids. Deprivation leads to dwarfism, excess to gigantism, acromegaly, and glucose intolerance. The pharmaceutical preparation from human or monkey but not other animal pituitary glands is used to treat human hypopituitary dwarfism. Also called *somatotropin, somatotrophin, somatropin, chondrotropic hormone* (outmoded), *somatotropic hormone.* Abbreviation: GH **2** Any hormone that promotes growth.

growth hormone inhibiting hormone SOMATOSTATIN. Abbreviation: GHIH

growth hormone release inhibiting hormone SOMATOSTATIN. Abbreviation: GHRIH

growth hormone releasing hormone A hypothalamic releasing hormone which stimulates the secretion of growth hormone into the circulation by the adenohypophysis. Its chemical structure is not yet known. Also called *growth hormone releasing factor, somatotropin releasing hormone, somatotropin releasing factor.* Abbreviation: GHRH

gut hormone A popular term for GASTROINTESTINAL HORMONE.

human growth hormone See under GROWTH HORMONE. Abbreviation: HGH

hypophysial hormone Any adenohypophysial or neurohypophysial hormone, as growth hormone or vasopressin; any pituitary hormone.

hypophysiotropic hormone Any of the hormones that act to regulate the hormone secretion of the hypophysis by stimulating or inhibiting secretion, such as thyrotropin releasing hormone, gonadotropin releasing hormone, and somatostatin.

hypothalamic inhibitory hormone Any of several peptide hormones of the hypothalamus which inhibit release of anterior pituitary hormones, such as somatostatin (inhibiting growth hormone) and prolactin inhibitory hormone. It is conveyed to the adenohypophysis via the hypothalamic-hypophysial portal venous system.

hypothalamic releasing hormone Any of several peptide hormones of the hypothalamus which stimulate release of anterior pituitary hormones. In general there is a specific releasing hormone for each adenohypophysial hormone. It is conveyed to the adenohypophysis via the hypothalamic-hypophysial portal venous system.

inhibitory hormone Any hormone that exerts an inhibitory action on the secretion or function of its target tissue, as the inhibition of gonadotropin secretion by estrogen or of growth hormone release by somatostatin.

interstitial cell-stimulating hormone An outmoded term for LUTEINIZING HORMONE. ● The name is derived from the property of stimulating the Leydig or interstitial cells of the testis as well as the corpus luteum of the ovary. Abbreviation: ICSH

intestinal hormone Any of the hormones secreted by specialized cells in the mucosa of the intestinal tract. They act mainly to regulate the motility and secretory functions of the gut itself.

intracellular hormone A hormone located or acting inside a cell.

juvenile hormone A secretion of the corpora allata and other tissues of insects, also found in certain plants. Acting in conjunction with ecdysone, juvenile hormones in insects ensure the normal preadult development. During the final nymphal or larval stage, the corpora allata are inactivated and ecdysone becomes dominant, leading to metamorphosis into the adult stage. Juvenile hormones are terpenoids, related esters of tridecadienoic acid. Also called *neotenin*.

ketogenic hormone LIPOLYTIC HORMONE.

lactation hormone A seldom used term for PROLACTIN.

lactogenic hormone PROLACTIN.

langerhansian hormone Any hormone of the pancreatic islets of Langerhans, including insulin or glucagon. A seldom used term.

lipolytic hormone Any hormone that stimulates the release of free fatty acids and glycerol from adipose tissue triglyceride by augmenting the formation of cyclic AMP which stimulates a protein kinase activating a hormone-sensitive lipase. These hormones include epinephrine, norepinephrine, adrenocorticotropin, glucagon, β-lipotropin, and arginine vasopressin. Growth hormone and cortisol stimulate delayed lipopysis. Also called *ketogenic hormone, fat-mobilizing hormone*.

lipotropic hormone LIPOTROPIN.

local hormone A chemical transmitter other than a neurotransmitter that exerts its effect in a restricted area near its site of production.

luteal hormone PROGESTERONE.

luteinizing hormone An adenohypophysial gonadotropic hormone that stimulates ovulation, maintains progesterone secretion by the corpus luteum, and regulates secretion of testicular Leydig cells. It is a glycoprotein of 28 000 daltons, has an α unit in common with other glycopeptides, and a specific β subunit. Under the control of hypothalamic gonadotropin releasing hormone, it undergoes the cyclic secretory variations of the menstrual cycle and more rapid diurnal oscillations. Also called *interstitial cell-stimulating hormone* (outmoded), *Aschheim-Zondek hormone* (outmoded), *metakentrin* (older term), *luteinizing principle* (older term). Abbreviation: LH

luteinizing hormone releasing hormone GONADOTROPIN RELEASING HORMONE. Abbreviation: LHRH

luteotropic hormone PROLACTIN.

mammary stimulating hormone PROLACTIN.

mammogenic hormone PROLACTIN.

mammotropic hormone An outmoded term for PROLACTIN.

melanocyte stimulating hormone A specific pigmentary hormone secreted by the hypophysial intermediate lobe of lower forms, as amphibians, and stimulating the rearrangement of dermal melanin granules so as to produce darkening of the skin. In man, lacking a separate intermediate lobe, the adenohypophysis contains the β form, a peptide of 2734 daltons and 22 amino acids which can also be radioimmunologically detected in plasma. β-melanocyte stimulating hormone in man is thought to be an extraction artifact of anterior pituitary β-lipotropin, not a distinct hormone. Also called *melanophore stimulating hormone, chromatophorotropic hormone, intermedin, melanophore dilating principle*. Abbreviation: MSH

melanocyte stimulating hormone inhibitory hormone A hypothalamic hypophysiotropic hormone that inhibits the release of melanocyte stimulating hormone from the anterior pituitary. Such hormonal activity has been demonstrated but the hormone has not been identified chemically. Also called *melanocyte stimulating hormone release inhibiting factor, melanocyte stimulating hormone inhibiting factor, intermediate lobe inhibiting factor*.

melanocyte stimulating hormone regulatory hormone MELANOCYTE STIMULATING HORMONE RELEASING HORMONE.

melanocyte stimulating hormone releasing hormone A hypothalamic releasing hormone which causes the release of melanocyte stimulating hormone from the anterior pituitary. Such hormonal activity has been demonstrated but the hormone has not been identified chemically. Also called *melanocyte stimulating hormone releasing factor, melanocyte stimulating hormone regulatory hormone*. Abbreviation: MSHRH

melanophore stimulating hormone MELANOCYTE STIMULATING HORMONE.

molting hormone ECDYSONE.

morphogenetic hormone EVOCATOR.

morphogenic hormone A substance capable of bringing about changes in shape, form and structure of parts or the whole of a developing organism. Steroids exert a morphogenetic effect when they modify the course of development of the genital ducts and genitalia.

N. hormone Androgen, specifically adrenocortical androgen which stimulates nitrogen or nitrogen retention, as distinct from s. (sugar) hormone or glucocorticoid. An outmoded and seldom used term. Also called *nitrogen hormone*.

natriuretic hormone A postulated hormone of the adrenal cortex which is supposed to act on the renal tubule to promote sodium excretion, especially such a steroid hormone secreted in the salt-losing form of congenital adrenocortical hyperplasia.

nitrogen hormone N. HORMONE.

orchidic hormone A rarely used term for TESTOSTERONE.

ovarian hormone A hormone secreted by the ovary; any estrogen or progestogen.

oxytocic hormone OXYTOCIN.

pancreatic hyperglycemic hormone An obsolete term for GLUCAGON.

parathyroid hormone PARATHYRIN.

placental hormone Any hormone secreted or released by the placenta in pregnancy, including many estrogens, chorionic gonadotropin, and human placental lactogen.

placental growth hormone HUMAN PLACENTAL LACTOGEN.

plant hormone PHYTOHORMONE.

posterior pituitary hormone Either of the hormones oxytocin and vasopressin, which come from the neurohypophysis (posterior part of the pituitary gland).

pregnant mares' serum hormone   CHORIONIC GONADOTRO-PIN.

preproparathyroid hormone   The initial hormonal substance synthesized in the cells of the parathyroid gland, the precursor of proparathyroid hormone and of parathyroid hormone. It contains 115 amino acids.

progestational hormone   PROGESTERONE.

prolactin inhibitory hormone   A hypothalamic hypophysiotropic hormone that inhibits the release of prolactin from the adenohypophysis. The principal component is dopamine. Also called *prolactin inhibiting factor*. Abbreviation: PIH

prolactin releasing hormone   A hypothalamic hypophysiotropic hormone that stimulates the release of prolactin from the anterior pituitary. It is a peptide but has not been identified chemically. Also called *prolactin releasing factor*. Abbreviation: PRH

proparathyroid hormone   An intermediate product in the biosynthesis of parathyroid hormone in the parathyroid gland. It contains 90 amino acids.

prothoracic gland hormone   ECDYSONE.

prothoracotropic hormone   ECDYSIOTROPIN.

PU hormone   Pregnancy urine hormone, chorionic gonadotropin in the urine of pregnant women. A seldom used term.

releasing hormone   Any of the hormones that stimulate release of the pituitary hormones and thus regulate secretion; a hypophysiotropic hormone. Also called *releasing factor*. Abbreviation: RH.

S. hormone   An older term for GLUCOCORTICOID.

salivary gland hormone   PAROTIN.

sex hormone   Any hormone affecting structure or function of a sexual organ or sexual behavior, especially testosterone and estrogen.

somatotropic hormone   GROWTH HORMONE.

somatotropin releasing hormone   GROWTH HORMONE RELEASING HORMONE.

steroid hormone   A group of biologically and pharmaceutically important hormones secreted by the testis, ovary, adrenal cortex, and placenta, as the androgens, estrogens, glucocorticoids, and mineralocorticoid.

sympathetic hormone   SYMPATHIN.

testicular hormone   Any hormone secreted by the testis, specifically testosterone. Also called *testis hormone*.

testis hormone   TESTICULAR HORMONE.

thyroid hormone   Any of the active hormonal principles secreted by the thyroid gland, comprising thyroxine, triiodothyronine, and thyrocalcitonin. ● In ordinary use the term refers to thyroxine or to thyroxine and triiodothyronine.

thyroid stimulating hormone   THYROTROPIC HORMONE. Abbreviation: TSH

thyrotropic hormone   The adenohypophysial glycopeptide that regulates the growth, development, and secretory activity of the thyroid gland. It is a polypeptide having a molecular mass of about 28 000 daltons. It contains an α subunit structurally almost identical with those of follicle stimulating hormone, luteinizing hormone, and chorionic gonadotropin, and a specific β subunit. The hormone stimulates many metabolic processes in the thyroid, including release of thyroxine and triiodothyronine from the thyroid follicles. Excessive thyrotropic hormone produces thyroid hyperplasia. The hormone is chiefly regulated by hypothalamic thyrotropin releasing hormone. Also called *thyrotropin, thyrotrophin, thyroid stimulating hormone*. ● *TSH* (from *thyroid stimulating hormone*) is often used as the abbreviation for *thyrotropic hormone*, since *TH* could be taken to refer to thyroid hormone.

thyrotropin releasing hormone   The hypothalamic hypophysiotropic hormone that regulates the secretion of thyrotropic hormone. Its chemical structure is that of a tripeptide amide, 5-oxoprolylhistidyl prolineamide. Also called *thyrotropin releasing factor, thyroid stimulating hormone releasing factor*. Abbreviation: TRH

trophic hormones   An older term for TROPIC HORMONES.

tropic hormones   Hormones that stimulate or regulate the function of other endocrine glands. Examples include the gonadotropic, thyrotropic, and adrenocorticotrophic hormones of the anterior pituitary. Also called *trophic hormones* (older term).

---

hormonic   HORMONAL.

hormonogen [*hormon(e)* + *o* + -GEN]   Any hormone or agent that fosters the production of another hormone.

hormonogenesis [*hormon(e)* + *o* + GENESIS]   The synthesis, production, or elaboration of a hormone or hormones. Also called *hormonopoiesis, hormopoiesis* (rarely used).

hormonogenic   Producing or stimulating the production of hormones; characterized by hormonogenesis.

hormonology [*hormon(e)* + *o* + -LOGY]   The study of the chemistry and biology of hormones.

hormonopexic   Having the property of fixing hormones, as to tissue, naturally or artificially.

hormonopoiesis [*hormon(e)* + *o* + -POIESIS]   HORMONOGENESIS. Adjective: hormonopoietic.

hormonopoietic   Of or relating to hormonogenesis or hormonopoiesis.

hormonoprivia   Deprivation of hormones or of a specific hormone, or the somatic, clinical, or cellular condition resulting from it.

hormonotherapeutic   Of or relating to hormonotherapy.

hormonotherapy   Treatment by the administration of hormones. Also called *endocrinotherapy, incretotherapy* (outmoded).

hormopoiesis   A rarely used term for HORMONOGENESIS. Adjective: hormopoietic.

horn [Middle English, from Old English, akin to L *cornu* horn]   **1** One of the pointed projections from the skull of certain artiodactyls, such as the American antelope, the giraffe, and the rhinoceros. The number, position, and structure of these projections vary among major groups.   **2** Any comparable projection from the head of other animals, such as the tentacles in snails or the horn of rhinoceros beetles.   **3** CORNU.

horn of Ammon   HIPPOCAMPUS.

anterior gray horn of spinal cord   CORNU ANTERIUS MEDULLAE SPINALIS.

anterior horn of lateral ventricle   CORNU ANTERIUS VENTRICULI LATERALIS.

anterior horn of spinal cord   CORNU ANTERIUS MEDULLAE SPINALIS.

cicatricial horn   The elevated edge of a scar resulting from proliferation of fibrous tissue.

coccygeal horn   CORNU COCCYGEUM.

cutaneous horn   A benign warty excrescence of the skin that may develop on a solar keratosis or other epidermal lesion. Also called *warty horn, cornu cutaneum, dermatokeras* (obsolete).

dorsal horn of spinal cord   CORNU DORSALE MEDULLAE SPINALIS.

frontal horn of lateral ventricle   CORNU ANTERIUS VENTRICULI LATERALIS.

greater horn of hyoid bone   CORNU MAJUS OSSIS HYOIDEI.

iliac horn   A pointed bony projection arising from the back of the leaf of the iliac bones that is seen in the nail-patella syndrome.

inferior horn of cerebrum   CORNU INFERIUS VENTRICULI LATERALIS.

inferior horn of falciform margin CORNU INFERIUS MARGINIS FALCIFORMIS.

inferior horn of Haller The lowest point of the line of reflection of serous pericardium on the ascending aorta and pulmonary trunk. It is situated slightly below the bifurcation of the pulmonary trunk at the level of the space between the aorta and pulmonary trunk into which the pericardium extends. An outmoded term.

inferior horn of lateral ventricle CORNU INFERIUS VENTRICULI LATERALIS.

inferior horn of saphenous opening CORNU INFERIUS MARGINIS FALCIFORMIS.

inferior horns of thymus The distal extremities, or apices, of the two lobes of the thymus that extend into the lower part of the neck or the thorax. An outmoded term.

inferior horn of thyroid cartilage CORNU INFERIUS CARTILAGINIS THYROIDEAE.

lateral horn of coccyx Either of two transverse projections from the base of the coccyx. They represent rudimentary transverse processes of the first coccygeal vertebra and may articulate or fuse with the inferior lateral angle of the sacrum.

lateral gray horn of spinal cord CORNU LATERALE MEDULLAE SPINALIS.

lateral horn of hyoid bone An outmoded term for CORNU MAJUS OSSIS HYOIDEI.

lateral horn of spinal cord CORNU LATERALE MEDULLAE SPINALIS.

lateral horn of uterus 1 CORNU UTERI (DEXTRUM/SINISTRUM). **2** Either horn of a uterus bicornis.

lesser horn of hyoid bone CORNU MINUS OSSIS HYOIDEI.

Libby horn A horn-shaped connection between a postaural hearing aid and the ear mold, designed to enhance and extend high-frequency response and fitted in some cases of high-frequency hearing loss.

motor horn CORNU ANTERIUS MEDULLAE SPINALIS.

occipital horn of lateral ventricle CORNU POSTERIUS VENTRICULI LATERALIS.

posterior gray horn of spinal cord CORNU DORSALE MEDULLAE SPINALIS.

posterior horn of lateral ventricle CORNU POSTERIUS VENTRICULI LATERALIS.

posterior horn of spinal cord CORNU DORSALE MEDULLAE SPINALIS.

pulp horn A diverticulum of the pulp chamber beneath a cusp or mamelon of a tooth.

sacral horn CORNU SACRALE.

sebaceous horn A horny outgrowth from a sebaceous cyst.

superior horn of falciform margin CORNU SUPERIUS MARGINIS FALCIFORMIS.

superior horn of Haller The highest point of the line of reflection of the serous pericardium on the ascending aorta and pulmonary trunk. It is situated on the commencement of the arch of the aorta about 1 cm from the origin of the brachiocephalic trunk. An outmoded term.

superior horn of hyoid bone An outmoded term for CORNU MINUS OSSIS HYOIDEI.

superior horn of saphenous opening CORNU SUPERIUS MARGINIS FALCIFORMIS.

superior horn of thymus The conical proximal extremity of each of the two lobes of the thymus.

superior horn of thyroid cartilage CORNU SUPERIUS CARTILAGINIS THYROIDEAE.

temporal horn of lateral ventricle CORNU INFERIUS VENTRICULI LATERALIS.

uterine horn CORNU UTERI (DEXTRUM/SINISTRUM).

ventral horn of spinal cord CORNU ANTERIUS MEDULLAE SPINALIS.

warty horn CUTANEOUS HORN.

Horner [Johann Friedrich *Horner*, Swiss ophthalmologist, 1831–1886] **1** See under PTOSIS, PUPIL, LAW. **2** Claude Bernard-Horner syndrome, Bernard-Horner syndrome, Horner-Bernard syndrome. See under HORNER SYNDROME.

Horner [William Edmonds *Horner*, U.S. anatomist, 1793–1853] **1** Horner's teeth. See under TOOTH. **2** Horner's muscle. See under PARS LACRIMALIS MUSCULI ORBICULARIS OCULI.

hornification KERATINIZATION.

hornskin Thickening of the skin keratin in response to abnormal pressures or stresses.

horny Resembling horn, especially in having a hard, rigid consistency. Also *keratic, corneous*.

horopter [Gk *hor(os)* a boundary + *optēr* one who looks or spies] The projection of corresponding retinal points into visual space; a concept of importance in explaining the perception of distance. Adjective: horopteric.

Vieth-Müller horopter A conceptual spherical surface in space defined as the locus of spatial projection from the corresponding retinal points of the two eyes.

horrida cutis [L *horrida* (substantive, from *horrida*, neut. pl. of *horridus* horrid, rough) + *cutis*, gen. of *cutis* skin] GOOSE FLESH.

horripilation PILOERECTION.

horror [L, a shuddering, terror, horror] Intense fear, dismay, or alarm.

horror autotoxicus SELF-TOLERANCE.

horror feminae Fear or revulsion at the thought of intercourse with a woman or at the sight of female genitalia. An outmoded term.

horror fusionis A pathologic change in binocular vision in which simultaneous macular alignment by the two eyes is impossible.

horrors The hallucinations of delirium tremens. A popular usage.

horsefly A large-bodied avidly bloodsucking fly of the genus *Tabanus* or other genus of the family Tabanidae. Also *horse fly*.

horsepower A unit of power equal to 550 foot pounds-force per second; 745.700 watts. Symbol: hp

metric horsepower A unit of power equal to 75 kilogramforce meters per second; 735.499 watts. Also called *cheval vapeur (French usage), pferdestärke (German usage)*.

horsepower-hour A unit of work equal to the work done by a power of one horsepower in one hour; 1.98×10^6 foot pounds-force; $2.684\ 52 \times 10^6$ joules. Symbol: hp·h

horsepox A rare disease of horses caused by a poxvirus and characterized by skin lesions that progress from macules to pustules which dry and form scabs. Also called *equine variola, equine smallpox* (seldom used), *equine contagious pustular stomatitis* (seldom used).

horseshoe An orthopedic surgical device that acts as a suspending support following the placement of Steinmann's pins or threaded wires.

Horsfall [Frank L. *Horsfall*, Jr., U.S. physician, 1906–1971] Tamm-Horsfall mucoprotein. See under MUCOPROTEIN.

Horsley [Sir Victor Alexander Haden *Horsley*, English surgeon and physiologist, 1857–1916] **1** See under OPERATION, TREPHINE, SIGN, PUTTY. **2** Horsley's bone wax. See under PUTTY.

Hortega [Pío del Río *Hortega*, Spanish-born anatomist active in Argentina, 1882–1945] **1** See under TUMOR, METHOD. **2** Hortega cells. See under MICROGLIA.

hortobezoar [L *hort(us)* herbs, vegetables + *o* + English *bezoar*, from Persian *bādzahr, pādzahr* antidote against poison, from *pād* protection against + *zahr* poison] PHYTOBEZOAR.

Horton [Bayard Taylor *Horton*, U.S. physician, born 1895] **1** Horton's vascular headache, Bing-Horton syndrome, Horton's disease. See under MIGRAINOUS NEURALGIA. **2** Horton's arteritis. See under TEMPORAL ARTERITIS.

hortungskörper [German *Hortung* accumulation + *Körper* body] Senile amyloid or other material found upon pathologic examinations of body organs in aged individuals.

hor. un. spatio *horae unius spatio* (L, at the end of one hour).

hospice [L *hospitium* a chamber for guests, lodging, hospitality. Compare HOSPITAL.] **1** A program or facility which provides palliative and supportive care for terminally ill patients and their families. **2** Originally, a shelter or short-term care facility for homeless or destitute people.

hospital [L *hospitalis* (from *hospes*, gen. *hospitis*, a host, guest, visitor, stranger, akin to *hostis* a stranger and *gustare* to taste, enjoy, from Gk *geuein* to taste, eat) relating to a guest] An institution equipped with inpatient facilities for the 24-hour care, diagnosis, and treatment of the sick and injured, usually for both medical and surgical conditions, and staffed with professionally trained medical practitioners.
affiliated hospital A hospital that is associated with a medical school or with a larger organizational entity such as a chain of hospitals.
camp hospital A hospital used in military activity to service the needs of a troop encampment.
closed hospital A hospital whose medical staff membership is not open to all physicians in the community.
cottage hospital A general hospital, usually maintained by a municipality but sometimes privately owned, originally designed to provide general practitioners with bed privileges for treating their own patients in hospital. An old-fashioned term used in the United Kingdom, South Africa, and in Newfoundland, Canada.
county hospital A hospital which is owned by and operated by or for a county unit of government. A term used only in the U.S.
day hospital A hospital that serves patients on an ambulatory basis without overnight stays, as for example in mental health day care.
district hospital A hospital serving a geographic area defined as a district. A term used chiefly in the U.S., Canada, Australia, and New Zealand.
district general hospital A hospital which provides general inpatient care for a health district in the United Kingdom.
evacuation hospital A hospital, often established on a temporary basis, for treating individuals who have been moved from a casualty area such as combat or a natural disaster.
field hospital A military hospital located in an area of troop activity such as a battle zone.
for-profit hospital See under PROPRIETARY HOSPITAL.
general hospital A hospital that provides a wide range of health care services rather than only one type of specialty care.
geriatric day hospital A facility attended by old people which provides some of the functions of a hospital but which does not provide overnight or weekend accommodation. ● A term used in the United Kingdom, Australia, and New Zealand. Similar services exist in the United States, but are usually called simply "day care for the elderly.".
government hospital A hospital that is owned, operated, and funded by a governmental authority.
isolation hospital A hospital utilized for the removal, often on a temporary basis and sometimes for a specific disease, of individuals from society for purposes of treatment and of protecting society from communicable disease.
long-term care hospital A hospital designed to care for people who need continuing care, often over one month, as the disabled elderly or psychiatric patients.
lying-in hospital MATERNITY HOSPITAL.
maternity hospital A hospital that primarily provides obstetrical services. Also called *lying-in hospital.*
mental hospital An inpatient facility for the care of patients with psychiatric disorders or developmental disabilities, or both. ● Before the development of somatic treatments such as insulin coma and electroconvulsive treatment in the 1930s and neuroleptics, lithium, antidepressants, and other psychopharmacologic agents in the 1950s, mental hospitals were generally institutions for long-term care and protection. At the present time, most are oriented toward short-term, intensive treatment of acute episodes, in addition to longer-term custodial care for refractory patients who continue to be dangerous to themselves or others.
mobile army surgical hospital An easily transportable, usually temporary, hospital designed for use in military battlefield situations to treat injured soldiers.
municipal hospital An inpatient facility for medical and surgical care, in the United States usually for short-term care, operated by a municipal government.
open hospital A hospital whose medical staff membership is open to any physician in the community subject to meeting specified training and experience criteria.
philanthropic hospital A hospital that is supported or sponsored by a charitable organization. A rarely used term.
private hospital A hospital that serves only private patients, thus excluding patients who do not have their own private physician and source of funding.
proprietary hospital A hospital owned by individuals or a corporation and operated for profit. A term used chiefly in the United States. ● In the United Kingdom, India, and New Zealand, such a hospital is called a private hospital operated for profit. In the U.S., *for-profit hospital* is sometimes used as a variant of *proprietary hospital.*
psychogeriatric hospital A hospital designed to treat and care for people suffering from mental illnesses associated with old age. A term not used in the U.S.
public hospital An inpatient facility for medical and surgical care, in the United States usually short-term care, owned or operated by a governmental authority.
special hospital A hospital that limits its services to certain specialties or to special categories of patients.
state hospital **1** In the United States, an inpatient facility, either short-term or long-term, owned and often also operated by a state government. **2** In the United Kingdom, a special hospital for the custodial care of subnormal, severely subnormal, or psychopathic patients of dangerous, violent, or criminal propensities.
surgical hospital A hospital that primarily provides surgical and surgery-related services.
teaching hospital Any hospital that operates one or more teaching programs for medical, dental, or osteopathic students, interns, or residents.
Veterans Administration hospital A hospital operated by the United States Veterans Administration for the care of war veterans and retired members of the armed forces.
voluntary hospital A nongovernmental, nonprofit hospital.

hospitalism Anaclitic depression in infants associated with prolonged institutionalization, as in a hospital.

hospitalitis [HOSPITAL + -ITIS] A condition in which a patient is psychologically dependent on a hospital in which he has been admitted. Attempts at discharge result in a surge of symptoms. Also called *sanatorium disease.*

hospitalization The admission or stay of a patient in a hospital.

hospitalize To admit (a person) to inpatient status at a hospital.

host [L *hospes*, gen. *hospitis*, a host, guest, visitor, stranger, akin to *hostis* a stranger] **1** An organism that harbors or provides nourishment, a habitat, or transport to another organism, whether symbiont, commensal, or parasite. **2** The recipient of any transplant from another organism.

accidental host A host not normally associated with a particular parasite. Also called *incidental host.*

alternate host A facultative intermediate host.

biological intermediate host An intermediate host in which biologic or cyclic development takes place. Also called *cyclic intermediate host.* Compare MECHANICAL INTERMEDIATE HOST.

cyclic intermediate host BIOLOGICAL INTERMEDIATE HOST.

dead-end host A human host infected by a parasite that is unable to complete its life cycle unless the human is consumed by another host in the transmission chain. Examples would be a human infected with *Trichinella, Echinococcus,* or tissue cysts of *Sarcocystis.*

definitive host The host in which a parasite or symbiont reaches adulthood, completes its development, or becomes sexually mature. Also called *final host, primary host* (incorrect).

final host DEFINITIVE HOST.

incidental host ACCIDENTAL HOST.

intermediary host INTERMEDIATE HOST.

intermediate host A host in which the symbiont or parasite undergoes larval or developmental stages or asexual multiplication. Also called *intermediary host.*

maintaining host RESERVOIR.

maintenance host RESERVOIR.

mechanical intermediate host An intermediate host in which the parasite or symbiont does not undergo development or reproduction, and transmission is by mechanical means. Tabanid flies, for example, can transmit many species of trypanosomes by direct inoculation from one host to another, with no intervening development. Compare BIOLOGICAL INTERMEDIATE HOST.

overwintering host An intermediate host or vector or a final host in which a parasite survives over the winter and can be transmitted to a new host the following spring.

paratenic host TRANSPORT HOST.

host of predilection The preferred or normal host of a parasite.

primary host **1** The first intermediate host, such as the snail host of digentic trematodes. **2** An incorrect term for DEFINITIVE HOST.

reservoir host RESERVOIR.

secondary host **1** A second intermediate host. **2** A host of secondary importance. **3** RESERVOIR. AN AMBIGUOUS USAGE.

transfer host TRANSPORT HOST.

transport host An intermediate host in which maturation or cyclic development does not occur, but which carries the parasite to another host in which it does occur. It may be one of a succession of transport hosts, as exemplified in the second intermediate hosts of pseudophyllidean cestodes such as *Diphyllobothrium latum.* Also called *paratenic host, transfer host.* See also PHORESIS.

HOT human old tuberculin.

hot-box An appliance usually of metal or wood designed to enclose a limb or the entire body excluding the head and equipped with an electrical system to produce dry heat. Temperatures for local treatment are 60–70°C. and for general heat treatment, 50–70°C. Also called *hot air box, heat cabinet, light cabinet, fever cabinet* (outmoded), *Japanese hot-box* (outmoded).

Japanese hot-box An outmoded term for HOT-BOX.

Hotchkiss [Lucius Wales *Hotchkiss*, U.S. surgeon, 1859–1926] See under OPERATION.

hot line A telephone counseling service for people in crisis situations. A service will specialize in a particular condition, as in suicide or child abuse. See also CRISIS CONSULTATION.

Hottentot bustle STEATOPYGIA.

hour [L *hora* (from Gk *hōra* a fixed, limited time; akin to L *heri* yesterday, *cras* tomorrow) an hour, season] A unit of time equal to 60 minutes. Symbol: h

house / halfway house Any facility that provides care designed to facilitate the transition between inpatient institutional care, such as for mental health, and outpatient community-based care. Also called *interim accommodation center.* • The term is used chiefly in the U.S., Canada, and New Zealand. It is known but less commonly used in the United Kingdom and Australia.

housebound Characterizing an individual who is confined to his home or residence due to physical or mental illness. Also *homebound.*

housefly A fly of the species *Musca domestica* (common housefly), or *Fannia canicularis* (lesser housefly). Also called *typhoid-fly* (obsolete). Also *house fly.*

household A social unit of complex socioeconomic nature comprising a group of individuals habitually residing together in the same dwelling. • The way this concept is defined for statistical purposes varies from country to country and according to the investigator. So as to enable international comparisons to be made it has been recommended that a household be defined as a group living together in the same dwelling and taking their meals together.

multiperson household Any household consisting of more than one person.

housekeeping In a computer, that portion of the hardware or software that performs routine tasks such as saving addresses during subroutines or setting up constants.

housing / adapted housing Residential quarters that have been specially altered or reconstructed for the benefit of disabled or handicapped persons.

diagnostic-type protective tube housing An x-ray tube housing so constructed that the leakage radiation measured at one meter from the source cannot exceed 1 mR in one hour when operated at maximum ratings.

satellite housing One of the settings used in long-term care, consisting of apartments or single-family houses for patients. There is no live-in staff, but some professional supervision is ordinarily provided as well as easy access to more intensive care in emergencies.

sheltered housing Dwellings for the elderly, provided with an employee whose responsibility is to initiate daily contact with each resident and summon assistance if it is required. A British usage.

therapeutic-type protective tube housing An x-ray tube housing so constructed that the leakage radiation, averaged over any 100 cm² area at one meter from the source, does not exceed either one roentgen in one hour or 0.1 percent of the useful beam rate, whichever is greater.

Houssay [Bernardo Alberto *Houssay*, Argentinian physiologist, 1887–1971] **1** See under PHENOMENON, ANIMAL. **2** Houssay-Biasotti syndrome. See under SYNDROME.

Houston [John *Houston*, Irish physician, 1802–1845] **1** Houston's valves. See under PLICAE TRANSVERSALES RECTI. **2** See under MUSCLE, VALVE.

hoven [early past part. of *heave*] BLOAT.

Hovius [Jacob *Hovius*, Dutch anatomist, 1710–1786] **1** See under CANAL, PLEXUS. **2** Hovius membrane. See under COM-

PLEXUS BASALIS CHOROIDEAE. **3** Circulus venosus hovii. See under CIRCLE OF HOVIUS.

Howard [Benjamin Douglas *Howard*, U.S. physician, 1840–1900] See under METHOD.

Howard [John Eager *Howard*, U.S. physician, born 1902] Ellsworth-Howard test. See under HOWARD TEST.

Howe [Percy *Howe*, U.S. dentist, 1864–1950] **1** Howe's silver nitrate. See under AMMONIACAL SILVER NITRATE SOLUTION. **2** Howe silver precipitation method. See under METHOD.

Howell [William Henry *Howell*, U.S. physiologist, 1860–1945] **1** Howell's bodies. See under HOWELL-JOLLY BODIES. **2** See under METHOD.

Howship [John *Howship*, English anatomist, 1781–1841] **1** Romberg-Howship symptom. See under SYMPTOM. **2** See under LACUNA.

Hoyer [Heinrich F. *Hoyer*, Polish anatomist and histologist, 1834–1907] Sucquet-Hoyer anastomosis. See under SUCQUET-HOYER CANAL.

HP   House Physician.

Hp   haptoglobin.

hp   Symbol for the unit, horsepower.

HPFH   hereditary persistence of high fetal hemoglobin.

HPG   human pituitary gonadotropin.

HPI   history of present illness.

HPL   human placental lactogen.

HPLC   high-pressure liquid chromatography.

hr   Symbol for the unit, hour. An incorrect symbol.

HRA   **1** health risk appraisal. **2** Human Resources Administration.

h.s.   *hora somni* (L, at bedtime).

HSA   human serum albumin.

5-HT   5-hydroxytryptamine (serotonin).

Ht   total hyperopia.

HTLV   human T cell leukemia/lymphoma virus; human T cell lymphotrophic virus; human T cell leukemia virus; human lymphotrophic retrovirus.

htone na [Burmese] A peripheral neuropathy found in Burma. It has been attributed, probably wrongly, to malaria.

Hua   A genus of freshwater snails of China. The species *H. ningpoensis*, found in central and southern China, serves as an initial intermediate host of the Chinese liver fluke *Clonorchis sinensis*. The eggs hatch in the body of the snail which ingests them, and development of the fluke continues through sporocyst, redial, and cercarial stages. *H. toucheana* serves as a first intermediate host of the lung fluke *Paragonimus westermani*.

Hubbard [Leroy Watkins *Hubbard*, U.S. orthopedic surgeon, 1857–1938] See under TANK.

Huber [Johann Jacob *Huber*, Swiss anatomist, 1707–1778] See under GANGLION.

Hubrecht [Ambrosius *Hubrecht*, Dutch anatomist, 1858–1915] Hubrecht's protochordal knot. See under HENSEN'S KNOT.

Huchard [Henri *Huchard*, French physician, 1844–1910] See under DISEASE.

hucklebone   TALUS.

Hudson [Arthur Cyril *Hudson*, English ophthalmologist, 1875–1962] Hudson's line. See under HUDSON-STÄHLI LINE.

Hudson [William E. *Hudson*, U.S. surgeon, 1862–1915] See under DRILL.

hue   The particular attribute of a color that distinguishes it as red, green, or blue, or as any other color.

Hueck [Alexander Friedrich *Hueck*, German anatomist, 1802–1842] Hueck's ligament. See under LIGAMENTUM PECTINATUM ANGULI IRIDOCORNEALIS.

Huët [G. J. *Huët*, Dutch physician, born 1879] Pelger-Huët nuclear anomaly. See under PELGER-HUËT ANOMALY.

Hueter [Karl *Hueter*, German surgeon, 1838–1882] **1** Vogt-Hueter point. See under POINT. **2** See under SIGN, LINE.

Huggins [Charles Brenton *Huggins*, Canadian-born U.S. surgeon, born 1901] See under OPERATION.

Hughes [Charles Hamilton *Hughes*, U.S. neurologist, 1839–1916] See under REFLEX.

Huguenin [Gustave *Huguenin*, Swiss physician, 1841–1920] See under EDEMA.

Huguier [Pierre Charles *Huguier*, French surgeon, 1804–1874] **1** Huguier's disease. See under LEIOMYOMA. **2** Huguier's canal. See under ITER CHORDAE ANTERIUS. **3** See under CIRCLE, SINUS.

Huhner [Max *Huhner*, U.S. urologist, 1873–1947] See under TEST.

hum   A dull, continuous sound, usually of unvarying tone.

venous hum   A continuous murmur heard to the right of the sternum and over the right jugular vein, especially in children. It may also be heard sometimes in adults, especially those who are anemic or pregnant. It is abolished by compression on the jugular vein or on assuming a recumbent posture. Also called *humming-top murmur, bruit de diable, nun's murmur*.

human [Middle English *humayne*, from Old French *humaine* human, from L *human(us)* (akin to *homo* man) pertaining to human beings, human] **1** Of or belonging to mankind, humanity, or the genus *Homo*. **2** A human being; a member of the genus *Homo*.

humanol   A liquefied human fat placed about a nerve or tendon to minimize adhesions.

humanoscope   An early form of anatomical atlas wherein a series of overlapping anatomical diagrams were arranged so that flipping the pages resulted in an appreciation of the relative sizes, shapes and relationships of regions of the body.

Human Tissue Act   See under UNIFORM ANATOMICAL GIFT ACT.

Humatin   A proprietary name for paromomycin sulfate.

Humber [John Davis *Humber*, U.S. physician, born 1895] Coffey-Humber treatment. See under TREATMENT.

humectant   **1** An agent that brings about a moistening effect. **2** Moist or damp.

humectation   The process or act of moistening.

humeral   Pertaining to the humerus.

humeri   Plural of HUMERUS.

humeroradial   Pertaining to the humerus and the radius.

humeroscapular   Pertaining to the humerus and the scapula.

humeroulnar   Pertaining to the humerus and the ulna.

humerus [L (akin to Gk *ōmos* the shoulder with upper arm), the shoulder of man and animal] [NA] The long bone of the arm, presenting an upper extremity carrying a rounded head for articulation with the scapula, a shaft, and a lower extremity with a condyle adapted to articulate with the radius and the ulna. Also called *humeral bone*.

humerus varus   An abnormally angulated humerus that curves toward the midline.

humicolin   An antifungal metabolite produced by *Aspergillus humicola*.

humidification   The process of making humid or more humid.

humidifier   A device that increases the moisture content of the air. Its use may be to increase the general ambient humidity or localized to a small area for purposes of breathing supersaturated air.

nebulizing humidifier   A heated water container used to permit entrainment of water vapor in a dry gas, as in the case of oxygen given for inhalation therapy, or in the application of a general inhalation anesthetic. Also called *vaporizing humidifier*.

vaporizing humidifier   NEBULIZING HUMIDIFIER.

humidistat [L *humid(us)* moist + *i* + -STAT] An appliance for maintaining the vapor pressure in the air of a room or other enclosed space within set limits.

humidity [L *humiditas* (from *humidus* moist, wet, humid, from *humere* to be wet or moist, akin to *hiems* rainy weather, winter and to Gk *cheimōn* winter) humidity] The amount of moisture in an atmosphere.

absolute humidity   The mass of water vapor in the air per unit volume of air or gas.

relative humidity   The ratio of the amount of water vapor in the air to the amount it would contain if saturated at the same temperature and pressure.

specific humidity   The ratio of the mass of water vapor in the air to the mass of the air plus the water vapor.

humification   The formation of humus from particulate organic matter.

humin   Insoluble material formed during acid hydrolysis of proteins, largely by reaction between tryptophan and carbohydrates.

humor [Med L (from L *humor*, also *umor* dampness, moisture, a liquid), humor of the body] Any of the four elemental body fluids believed by the ancients to be the physiologic and pathologic basis of health and disease. The humors are blood, phlegm, yellow bile, and black bile.

aqueous humor   HUMOR AQUOSUS.

humor aquosus   [NA] A nutritive watery fluid that is formed by the ciliary processes and diffuses through the posterior and anterior chambers of the eye. It is reabsorbed into the venous system by filtering through the spaces of the iridocorneal angle into the sinus venosus sclerae, which communicates with the anterior ciliary veins. Besides serving as a refractive medium, it maintains the intraocular pressure and provides glucose, amino acids, and ascorbic acid to the avascular lens and cornea. Also called *aqueous humor, aqueous, hydatoid, aqua oculi, intraocular fluid*.

humor cristallinus   An outmoded term for LENS.

crystalline humor   An outmoded term for LENS.

ocular humor   Either humor aquosus or humor vitreus.

plasmoid humor   See under PLASMOID AQUEOUS HUMOR.

plasmoid aqueous humor   The aqueous humor modified by damage to the blood-eye barrier, which permits entry of blood proteins into the anterior chamber.

vitreous humor   HUMOR VITREUS.

humor vitreus   [NA] The structureless gel within the loose network of collagen fibrils of the vitreous body of the eyeball. It is often equated with corpus vitreum. Also called *vitreous humor, vitreous*.

humoral   Pertaining to the humors, or certain fluids, of the body.

humoralism   The ancient doctrine that elemental body fluids (humors: blood, phlegm, yellow bile, and black bile) are the physiologic and pathologic basis of health and disease. Also called *humorism, fluidism, humoral theory*.

humorism   HUMORALISM.

Humorsol   A proprietary name for demecarium bromide.

humour   A British spelling for HUMOR.

hump / buffalo hump   A nuchal and upper dorsal prominence seen in subjects with severe spontaneous or iatrogenic Cushing syndrome, caused by deposition of fat and upper dorsal kyphosis. Also called *buffalo neck, buffalo obesity, bison neck*.

dromedary hump   A normal radiologic finding characterized by a bulging of the lateral border of the left kidney, often due to pressure from the spleen.

Hampton hump   A convex opacity seen adjacent to the chest wall or diaphragm on the chest radiograph following pulmonary infarction.

humpback   KYPHOSIS.

Humphry [George Murray *Humphry*, English surgeon, 1820–1896] **1** See under OPERATION. **2** Humphry's ligament. See under LIGAMENTUM MENISCOFEMORALE ANTERIUS.

humulene   2,6,10,10-Tetramethylcycloundeca-1,4,8-triene, a sequiterpene found in clove oil.

humulin   LUPULIN.

humus [L, the ground, earth, soil] Organic matter that is decomposing in the soil.

hunchback   KYPHOSIS.

hunchbacked   KYPHOTIC.

hundredweight   **1** In the United States, a unit of mass or weight equal to 100 pounds; 45.3592 kilograms. Also called *short hundredweight*. Symbol: cwt **2** In Great Britain, a unit of mass or weight equal to 112 pounds; 50.8023 kilograms. Symbol: cwt • In the United States, *long hundredweight* is used to distinguish the British hundredweight of 112 pounds from the *short hundredweight* of 100 pounds used in the United States.

long hundredweight   See under HUNDREDWEIGHT. Symbol: long cwt

short hundredweight   HUNDREDWEIGHT. Symbol: sh cwt

Hünermann [Carl *Hünermann*, German physician, flourished mid-20th century] Hünermann's disease, Conradi-Hünermann syndrome. See under CHONDRODYSPLASIA PUNCTATA.

Hung [See-Lu *Hung*, U.S. scientist, flourished 20th century] Hung's method. See under FÜLLEBORN'S METHOD.

hunger [Old English *hungor*] A craving, usually for food. Also called *fames*.

affect hunger   Insatiable demand for attention and affection, which may take the form of provocative antisocial behavior. It occurs in children who have suffered emotional deprivation.

air hunger   KUSSMAUL RESPIRATION.

calcium hunger   An irrational desire to eat substances rich in calcium, such as calcium salts. It is a form of pica. Also called *calcifames, status calcifames*.

periodic morbid hunger with somnolence   KLEINE-LEVIN SYNDROME.

Hunner [Guy Leroy *Hunner*, U.S. surgeon, 1868–1957] **1** See under STRICTURE. **2** Fenwick-Hunner ulcer. See under HUNNER'S ULCER.

Hunt [James Ramsay *Hunt*, U.S. neurologist, 1872–1937] **1** See under TREMOR, ATROPHY. **2** Ramsay Hunt neuralgia, Hunt's neuralgia. See under GENICULATE GANGLION NEURALGIA. **3** Hunt syndrome. See under RAMSAY HUNT SYNDROME. **4** Hunt striatal syndrome, Ramsay Hunt's parkinsonian syndrome, Hunt's disease, Ramsay Hunt paralysis. See under JUVENILE PARALYSIS AGITANS. **5** Hunt's disease. See under DYSSYNERGIA CEREBELLARIS MYOCLONICA. **6** Hunt's paradoxical phenomenon. See under PHENOMENON.

Hunt [Reed *Hunt*, U.S. pharmacologist, 1870–1948] See under METHOD.

Hunt [William Edward *Hunt*, U.S. neuro surgeon, born 1921] Tolosa-Hunt syndrome. See under SYNDROME.

Hunter [Charles *Hunter*, Canadian physician, flourished 20th century] Hunter syndrome. See under MUCOPOLYSACCHARIDOSIS II.

Hunter [John *Hunter*, Scottish surgeon, 1728–1793] **1** Hunter's gubernaculum. See under GUBERNACULUM TESTIS. **2** Hunter's canal. See under CANALIS ADDUCTORIUS. **3** Fascia of Hunter's canal. See under FASCIA. **4** Inferior opening of Hunter's canal. See under HIATUS TENDINEUS.

Hunter [William *Hunter*, English botanist active in India, 1755–1812] See under GLOSSITIS.

Hunter [William *Hunter*, English anatomist, 1718–1783] **1** Bands of Hunter-Schreger. See under SCHREGER'S LINES. **2** Hunter's line. See under LINEA ALBA. **3** Hunter's ligament. See under LIGAMENTUM TERES UTERI.

Huntington [George *Huntington*, U.S. physician, 1850–1916] **1** See under SIGN. **2** Huntington's disease. See under CHOREA.

huratoxin A toxic, carcinogenic diterpene found in the plant exudate and seeds of *Hura crepitans*, the sandbox tree.

Hurler [Gertrud *Hurler*, Austrian pediatrician, flourished early 20th century] **1** Hurler-Pfaundler syndrome, Hurler syndrome. See under MUCOPOLYSACCHARIDOSIS IH. **2** Hurler-Scheie syndrome. See under MUCOPOLYSACCHARIDOSIS IH/S. **3** Pseudo-Hurler's disease, pseudo-Hurler polydystrophy. See under MUCOLIPIDOSIS III. **4** Hurler-Scheie compound. See under COMPOUND.

Hurst [Edward Weston *Hurst*, English physician active in Australia, flourished 20th century] Hurst's disease. See under ACUTE HEMORRHAGIC LEUKOENCEPHALITIS.

Hürthle [Karl *Hürthle*, German histologist, 1860–1945] **1** See under CARCINOMA, TUMOR. **2** Hürthle cell adenoma. See under ONCOCYTIC ADENOMA.

Huschke [Emil *Huschke*, German anatomist, 1797–1858] **1** Auditory teeth of Huschke. See under DENTES ACUSTICI. **2** Vomerian cartilage of Huschke. See under CARTILAGO VOMERONASALIS. **3** See under CANAL. **4** Gastropancreatic folds of Huschke. See under FOLD. **5** Huschke's valve. See under PLICA LACRIMALIS. **6** Gastropancreatic ligaments of Huschke, Huschke's ligaments. See under PLICAE GASTROPANCREATICAE. **7** Stria vascularis of Huschke. See under STRIA VASCULARIS DUCTUS COCHLEARIS.

husk [from obsolete English *husk* to have a dry cough] PARASITIC BRONCHITIS.

Hutchinson [Sir Jonathan *Hutchinson*, English surgeon, 1828–1913] **1** Hutchinson's patch. See under SALMON PATCH. **2** Hutchinson's incisors. See under INCISOR. **3** Hutchinson's malignant lentigo. See under FRECKLE. **4** Hutchinson's mask. See under TABETIC MASK. **5** See under FACIES, NOTCH, PUPIL, PRURIGO, SIGN. **6** Hutchinson's tooth, hutchinsonian tooth. See under SYPHILITIC TOOTH. **7** Hutchinson-Gilford progeria syndrome, Hutchinson-Gilford syndrome, Hutchinson-Gilford disease. See under PROGERIA. **8** Summer prurigo of Hutchinson, Hutchinson's disease. See under HUTCHINSON SUMMER PRURIGO. **9** Hutchinson syndrome. See under TRIAD. **10** Hutchinson-Boeck syndrome, Hutchinson-Boeck disease. See under SARCOIDOSIS.

Hutchison [Sir Robert *Hutchison*, English pediatrician, 1871–1960] See under NEUROBLASTOMA.

Huxley [Thomas Henry *Huxley*, English biologist, 1825–1895] Huxley's membrane, Huxley sheath. See under LAYER.

Huygens [Christiaan *Huygens*, Dutch physicist, 1629–1695] **1** See under PRINCIPLE. **2** Huygen's ocular. See under HUYGENIAN EYEPIECE.

HV **1** hyperventilation. **2** herpes virus.

HVL half-value layer.

Hy. hyperopia.

hyal HYOID.

hyal- HYALO-.

hyalin [Gk *hyal(os)* or *hyel(os)*, a clear, transparent stone, oriental alabaster, crystal, glass + -IN] A clear homogeneous tissue formed as an eosinophilic product of amyloid degeneration.

hematogenous hyalin The glassy, translucent material formed following platelet aggregation. An older term.

hyaline Nearly transparent, glasslike in appearance. Also *hyaloid*.

hyalinization The process by which a tissue or structure becomes dense, homogeneous, and glassy. It is usually associated with atrophy of cellular elements. Also called *hyalinosis*.

tympanic hyalinization TYMPANOSCLEROSIS.

hyalinogen A precursor of hyalin material.

hyalinosis [HYALIN + -OSIS] HYALINIZATION.

hyalinosis cutis LIPOID PROTEINOSIS.

hyalinosis cutis et mucosae LIPOID PROTEINOSIS.

tympanic hyalinosis TYMPANOSCLEROSIS.

hyalitis [HYAL- + -ITIS] Inflammation within the vitreous humor. Also called *hyaloiditis*.

asteroid hyalitis ASTEROID HYALOSIS.

hyalitis punctata PUNCTATE HYALOSIS.

hyalitis suppurativa Purulent inflammation of the vitreous humor.

hyalo- [Gk *hyalos* glass] A combining form denoting glass. Also *hyal-*.

hyalocapsulitis The hyalinization of the capsule of an organ, usually the spleen or liver. A seldom used term.

hyaloid HYALINE.

hyaloideocapsular [HYALO- + IDEO- + CAPSUL- + -AR] Related to the junction of the vitreous humor and the lens capsule.

hyaloiditis HYALITIS.

hyaloidopathy [HYAL- + -OID + *o* + -PATHY] Any disease or deterioration of the vitreous humor.

asteroid hyaloidopathy ASTEROID HYALOSIS.

hyalomere The granule-free, pale, clear peripheral zone of platelet cytoplasm. Compare GRANULOMERE.

hyalomitome HYALOPLASM.

Hyalomma A genus of large, extremely hardy ixodid ticks of Asia and Africa, characterized by submarginal eyes, lack of body ornamentation, a long rostrum, and coalesced festoons. Adults of the approximately 21 species are ectoparasites of all domestic and many wild animals. Larval forms parasitize birds and reptiles as well as small mammals. Life cycles are variable, with one, two, or three hosts, sometimes even variable within the same species. Members of this genus transmit many microorganisms pathogenic in humans and other animals, and they can also cause significant mechanical damage to hosts. Crimean-congo hemorrhagic fever (CCHF), boutonneuse fever, canine and equine babesioses, and ehrlichioses are carried by various *Hyalomma* ticks. *H. anatolicum anatolicum* is a vector of Siberian tick typhus, Thogoto virus, a swine pox virus, CCHF, *Nocardia* fungal infections, and *Theileria annulata*; *H. a. excavatum* carries animal leptospirosis; *H. asiaticum* carries Siberian tick typhus, Q fever, and *Nocardia* infections; *H. dromedarii* carries viruses of the Dera Ghazi Kahn group; *H. marginatum issaci* carries Wad Medani virus; *H. m. marginatum* carries CCHF and Absettarov virus; *H. M. rufipes* carries CCHF and Dugbe virus; and *H. truncatum*, CCHF.

hyalomucoid HYALURONIC ACID.

hyalonyxis [HYALO- + Gk *nyxis* a pricking, piercing, stabbing] Incision of the vitreous body.

hyaloplasm [HYALO- + -PLASM] The clear fluid portion of the protoplasm generally supported by the cytoreticulum. Also called *cytohyaloplasm, cytolymph, cytosol, enchylema, endochylema, hyalomitome, hyalotome, hydroplasm, cell sap, cytochylema, interfilar substance, interspongioplastic substance, paraplasm*.

nuclear hyaloplasm KARYOLYMPH.

hyaloserositis Hyalinization and fibrosis of the capsule of an organ such as the spleen or liver. An obsolete term.

progressive multiple hyaloserositis Progressive inflammation of the serous membranes, including the pericardium, pleura, and peritoneum, in which a fibrinous exudate gradually hyalinizes so that the inflamed areas acquire a thick, opaque, shiny, white or off-white coating.

hyalosis [HYAL- + -OSIS] Degenerative change of the vitreous body.

asteroid hyalosis The presence of numerous tiny white spheres composed of calcium soaps deposited upon the collagen framework of the vitreous humor as a result of a benign degenerative change. It is unassociated with systemic disease. Also called *asteroid hyalitis, asteroid hyaloidopathy, Benson's disease.*

punctate hyalosis A condition of the vitreous humor in which multiple localized opacities exist. Also called *hyalitis punctata.*

hyalosome A spherical or oval body in the cell which stains weakly, and shows little internal structure.

hyalotome HYALOPLASM.

hyaluronate lyase The enzyme (EC 4.2.2.1) that catalyzes the breakdown of hyaluronic acid by an elimination reaction in which the *N*-acetylglucosamine residue is liberated as a new reducing end by cleavage of the oxygen it glycosylates from a glucuronate residue with the introduction of a double bond between C-4 and C-5 of the latter.

hyaluronic acid A major polysaccharide of connective tissue, consisting of alternate residues of D-glucuronic acid (glycosylated on O-4) and of *N*-acetylglucosamine (glycosylated on O-3). Also called *hyalomucoid.*

hyaluronidase An enzyme, produced by some strains of streptococci, that hydrolyzes hyaluronic acid. This reaction, in the ground substance of connective tissue, may promote spread of the microorganisms. Its presence in pathologic amounts in the joint fluid results in a reduced viscosity of the joint fluid. Also called *spreading factor, Duran-Reynals factor, Reynals factor.*

hyaluronidase for injection A sterile enzyme powder derived from mammalian testes that is used to promote enzymatic hydrolysis of mucopolysaccharides and thus facilitate the rate of absorption of medical agents that are administered parenterally. It is suitable for either subcutaneous or intramuscular injection.

Hyazyme A preparation of hyaluronidase for injection. A proprietary name.

hybaroxia HYPERBARIC OXYGEN THERAPY.

hybrid [L *hybrida* or *hibrida* (perhaps akin to *geminus* a twin and to German *Kebse* a concubine) a mongrel animal begotten by animals of different species, a person whose parent was a slave] **1** Any offspring of two parents with different genotypes. In this sense, all humans are hybrids. **2** An organism produced by the union of two parents of different species. Also called *crossbreed.* **3** In experimental genetics, a cell formed by the fusion of two genetically distinct cells. **4** In molecular biology, a duplex nucleic acid formed *in vitro* between complementary DNA and RNA chains or DNA chains. **5** In population genetics, a group of organisms that results from the mating of genetically distinct populations.

cell hybrid CYBRID.

F₁ hybrid The offspring of a parental cross; a member of the first filial generation.

graft hybrid A hybrid produced by grafting one genetically distinct strain of plant to another.

somatic hybrid A cell formed by fusion of two cells from different organisms in tissue culture; heterokaryon. The inactivated Sendai virus increases the incidence of fusion in culture.

hybridism The condition of being a hybrid. A seldom used term. Also called *hybridity* (seldom used).

hybridity A seldom used term for HYBRIDISM.

hybridization **1** The production of a hybrid cell, organism, or population through any of the numerous processes of fusing or mating genetically distinct parents or precursors. Also called *crossbreeding.* **2** In molecular biology, the process of forming a double helix between DNA chains or DNA and RNA chains that are at least partially complementary.

cell hybridization The process of the fusion of two somatic cells of different genotypes to produce a hybrid cell.

colony hybridization In work with recombinant DNA, a method of detection of a desired sequence of DNA in a colony. The cells are made permeable and their DNA hybridized with radioactively labeled homologous DNA or RNA.

cross hybridization In molecular biology, the hybridization of polynucleotide chains that are not perfectly complementary, as between species or strains.

in situ **hybridization** A technique by which a known nucleic acid is applied to a cytologic preparation in which the DNA has been partially denatured. The conditions are then altered to promote annealing of the test nucleic acid to complementary sequences in the cell. The location of hybridization is usually detected by autoradiography.

introgressive hybridization The phenomenon, associated with the hybridization of two populations, of the back-cross of the hybrids and the stabilization of a back-cross progeny.

molecular hybridization A procedure used to compare the similarities of base sequences between two polynucleotide chains from different sources. The polynucleotide chains are heated to separate the single strands (melting). Recombination or annealing occurs upon slow cooling.

hybridoma [HYBRID + -OMA] A cell type formed by fusion of two or more different types of cells.

hybrimycin A hybrid aminoglycoside antibiotic, with the streptamine ring derived from streptomycin and the other rings from neomycin.

hycanthone $C_{20}H_{24}N_2O_2S$. 1-[[2-(Dimethylamino)ethyl] amino]-4-(hydroxymethyl)-9*H*-thioxanthen-9-one. An antischistosomal drug that is given by parenteral injection, usually as the mesylate salt.

Hycodan A preparation of hydrocodone bitartrate. A proprietary name.

hydantoic acid *N*-Carbamoylglycine. It is an intermediate in the chemical synthesis of hydantoin, which it forms on treatment with acid.

hydantoin A compound, occurring in plants, whose molecule is the five-membered ring formed by the —CO—NH—CO—NH— group and a methylene group. Its derivative may be formed from amino acids.

hydathode [Gk *hydōr*, gen. *hydatos*, water + *hod(os)* a path, way, channel] A glandular structure on a leaf that exudes water during guttation.

hydatid [Gk *hydatis* (from *hydōr*, gen. *hydatos*, water) a drop of water, watery vesicle] **1** HYDATID CYST. **2** Any vesicle or cystlike structure that contains clear watery fluid. It may be a remnant of an embryonic structure or produced by larval parasites.

alveolar hydatid ALVEOLAR HYDATID CYST.

hydatid of Morgagni **1** APPENDIX MORGAGNII. **2** APPENDIX TESTIS.

nonpedunculated hydatid APPENDIX TESTIS.

pedunculated hydatid APPENDIX OF THE EPIDIDYMIS.

pedunculated hydatid of Morgagni **1** Any of the appendices vesiculosae epoöphori. **2** APPENDIX OF THE EPIDIDYMIS.

sessile hydatid APPENDIX TESTIS.

sessile hydatid of Morgagni APPENDIX TESTIS.

Virchow's hydatid ALVEOLAR HYDATID CYST.

hydatidiform Having the appearance of watery drops or a watery cyst.

hydatidosis [HYDATID + -OSIS] ECHINOCOCCOSIS.

hydatidostomy [HYDATID + *o* + -STOMY] A surgical procedure in which an opening is created in a hydatid cyst for the purpose of drainage. Such an opening may occur spontaneously, but it is rare.

Hydatigena *TAENIA.*

Hydatigera A genus of cestodes of the family Taeniidae, characterized by a columnar rostellum, a double row of hooks, large suckers, and gravid segments longer than wide. Adult worms are found in the small intestine of carnivores, strobilocercus larvae in rodents.

Hydatigera taeniaeformis *TAENIA TAENIAEFORMIS.*

hydatism [Gk *hydat(is)* a drop of water, watery vesicle + -ISM] The sound caused by fluid movement in a body cavity.

hydatoid 1 An outmoded term for HUMOR AQUOSUS. 2 An outmoded term for MEMBRANA VITREA. 3 Pertaining to the aqueous humor. An outmoded term.

hydatorrhea HYDRORRHEA.

Hydeltra A proprietary name for prednisolone.

Hydergine A mixture of dihydrogenated ergot alkaloids used to treat cerebrovascular deficiency and mental impairment in the elderly. A proprietary name.

hydr- HYDRO-.

hydracetin ACETYLPHENYLHYDRAZINE.

Hydrachnoidea [New L (from *hydr-*, suffix denoting water + Gk *achn(ē)* foam, froth + New L *-oidea*, suffix denoting characterized by] A large superfamily of mites of the order Acariformes, consisting of the single family Hydrachnidae. They are typically bright red in color, and are found in standing water and sluggish streams throughout much of the world. The aquatic nymphs and adults are predaceous, the semiaquatic larvae are parasitic in larvae of aquatic beetles and hemipterans, living with them for long periods, including overwintering in some examples.

hydracrylic acid $HO-CH_2-CH_2-COOH$. 3-Hydroxypropionic acid. It can be formed by hydration of acrylic acid. Unlike its isomer, lactic acid, it is not of biologic importance.

hydradenitis HIDRADENITIS.

hydradenoma HIDRADENOMA.

hydraemia A British spelling for HYDREMIA.

hydragogue 1 Promoting or causing the expulsion of water, as from the gastrointestinal tract. 2 A cathartic that brings about a watery purgation.

hydralazine $C_8H_8N_4$. An antihypertensive agent that is administered orally or parenterally.

hydramnion HYDRAMNIOS.

hydramnios [HYDR- + New L *amnios*, irreg. from Gk *amnion* the membrane around a fetus] The presence of an abnormally large amount of amniotic fluid for a particular stage of pregnancy. It is commonly associated with fetal abnormality, maternal illnesses, such as diabetes mellitus, or with interference in normal fetal physiology by toxic or other substances. Also called *hydramnion, hydrops amnii, dropsy of amnion, polyhydramnios.*

hydranencephaly [HYDR- + + Gk *an-* priv. + ENCEPHALY] An extreme degree of hydrocephaly in which the lateral and third ventricles form essentially a single cerebral cavity enclosed within the three layers of meninges, the skull, and the skin. Cerebral hemispheres are largely reduced to basal ganglia and remnants of the choroid plexus, other nervous tissue presumably having succumbed to pressure atrophy from long-continued internal hydrocephalus. Other parts of the brain may appear to be developmentally normal but signs of pressure may be evident.

hydrangin UMBELLIFERONE.

hydrangiography [HYDR- + ANGIOGRAPHY] LYMPHANGIOGRAPHY.

hydrangiology LYMPHANGIOLOGY.

hydrargyria [HYDR- + ARGYRIA] MERCURY POISONING.

hydrargyrism [HYDR- + ARGYRISM] MERCURY POISONING.

hydrargyromania ERETHISM.

hydrargyrophthalmia Ophthalmia due to chronic mercury poisoning.

hydrargyrosis [HYDR- + ARGYROSIS] MERCURY POISONING.

hydrargyrum [L from Gk *hydrargyros* liquid silver, from *hydōr* water + *argyros* silver), liquid silver] MERCURY.

hydrargyrum ammoniatum AMMONIATED MERCURY.

hydrargyrum oleatum MERCURY OLEATE.

hydrargyri oxycyanidum MERCURIC OXYCYANIDE.

hydrargyri perchloridum MERCURIC CHLORIDE.

hydrargyri salicylas MERCURIC SALICYLATE.

hydrargyri subchloridum CALOMEL.

hydrarthrodial Of or relating to hydrarthrosis.

hydrarthrosis [HYDR- + ARTHROSIS] The presence of excessive synovial fluid within a joint. Also called *hydrops articuli, articular dropsy.*

intermittent hydrarthrosis A periodic swelling of a joint due to excessive synovial fluid.

hydrastine $C_{21}H_{21}O_6N$. An alkaloid obtained from *Hydrastis candensis.* It has been used as a uterine hemostat.

hydrastis *Hydrastis canadensis*, an herb of the family Ranunculaceae. The rhizome and roots, which contain hydrastine, berberine, and canadine, have been used to prepare a uterine hemostatic drug. Also called *yellow root, golden seal.*

hydratase Any enzyme catalyzing the reaction of a carbon-carbon double bond with water to add —OH to one carbon atom and —H to another, such as fumarate hydratase.

hydrate A compound with water combined, usually reversibly.

hydrated Having water added, usually by reversible chemical reaction.

hydration 1 The addition of water, as by intravenous fluids to replace water lost from the body as a result of dehydration. 2 The binding of water molecules to ions or molecules in solution.

hydraulicity [*hydraulic* + -ITY] The ability to set when in contact with moisture: said of cement.

hydraulics The branch of science and technology dealing with the mechanics of fluids, especially liquids, comprised of hydrostatics and hydrodynamics.

hydrazide Any of the compounds, R—CO—NH—NH₂, derived from hydrazine by acylation, such as the hydrazides of α-amino acids (NH₂—CHR—CO—NH—NH₂).

hydrazine NH_2-NH_2. A toxic, weakly basic ($pK = 8.2$) substance, normally liquid, used as a reagent for carbonyl compounds, for which it has high affinity. It is a mild reducing agent.

hydrazinolysis Treatment of a protein at high temperature with hydrazine to break its peptide bonds and form hydrazides of its amino acids. Since the free carboxyl group of the C-terminal residue is less reactive than the peptide bonds, this residue remains as a free amino acid and can thereby be identified.

hydrazoic acid HN_3. A toxic, highly explosive, colorless liquid of boiling point 37°C and pK 4.6. Many of its salts, the azides, are also explosive, but sodium azide is stable.

hydrazone The imine formed between hydrazine and a carbonyl compound, often used for the characterization of carbonyl compounds. Such imines are usually very stable.

hydrelatic Of or relating to any stimulation that brings about a watery secretion. A seldom used term.

hydremia An increase in the plasma volume of blood without a corresponding increase in the number of erythrocytes or hemoglobin concentration.

hydrencephalitis [HYDR- + ENCEPHALITIS] Hydrocephalus and encephalitis occurring together. An outmoded term.

hydrencephalocele HYDROENCEPHALOCELE.

hydrencephalomeningocele [HYDR- + ENCEPHALO- + MENINGOCELE] A hydrencephalocele specifically demonstrated to contain meninges. Also called *hydroencephalomeningocele.*

hydrencephalus HYDROCEPHALUS.

hydrencephaly HYDROCEPHALUS.

hydriatric Relating to hydriatrics.

hydriatrics [HYDR- + -IATRICS] The use of water for medical purposes, especially its outmoded internal use as in water cures. See also HYDROTHERAPY.

hydriatrist A practitioner of hydriatrics.

hydric Relating to hydroxyl groups, as *dihydric alcohol,* which has two such groups in its molecule.

hydride [HYDR- + -ID] **1** Any compound of hydrogen with an element, particularly if the hydrogen is the more electronegative element. **2** The ion H^-.

hydrindantin A derivative of ninhydrin in which two molecules of ninhydrin are joined by formation of a C-C bond between a carbonyl group in each, with concomitant hydrogenation.

hydrindicuria The presence in urine of indoles related to phenylalanine and tryptophane.

hydriodic acid HI. A strong acid, easily oxidized to iodine. It is used as a reducing agent. Also called *hydrogen iodide.*

hydriodide The salt formed by reaction of a base with hydriodic acid.

hydrion An outmoded term for HYDRON.

hydro- [Gk *hydōr* (genitive *hydatos*) water] **1** A combining form denoting water. **2** In chemistry, a combining form denoting the presence of hydrogen or water in a compound. For defs. 1 and 2 also *hydr-.*

hydroa [HYDR- + Gk *ōa,* pl. of *ōon* egg] Any condition characterized by vesicle formation. An older term. Also *hidroa.*

hydroa aestivale An older term for HUTCHINSON SUMMER PRURIGO.

hydroa febrile An obsolete term for HERPES SIMPLEX.

hydroa gestationis An obsolete term for HERPES GESTATIONIS.

hydroa gravidarum An obsolete term for HERPES GESTATIONIS.

hydroa herpetiforme An obsolete term for DERMATITIS HERPETIFORMIS.

hydroa puerorum An obsolete term for HUTCHINSON SUMMER PRURIGO.

hydroa vacciniforme A rare photodermatosis of early childhood in which deep-seated umbilicated vesicles appear on exposed sites. After healing they leave large varioliform scars. In most subjects it persists into adult life. Also called *recurrent summer eruption.*

vesicular hydroa An obsolete term for ERYTHEMA MULTIFORME.

hydroadipsia Absence of thirst for water.

hydroangiography An anatomic and physiologic description of the lymphatic system. Also called *angiohydrography.* Compare HYDRANGIOGRAPHY.

Hydrobiidae [HYDRO- + bi(o)- + -IDAE] A family of prosobranch (operculated) snails found in freshwater, brackish, and marine habitats. Those of the type genus, *Hydrobis,* live in marine or brackish water in Europe and eastern North America.

The family formerly included the important host snails of *Schistosoma japonicum* (the *Oncomelania hupensis* complex) and of the lung fluke *Paragonimus* (in *Pomatiopsis* and related host species), as well as the genus *Amnicola,* host of a number of North American trematode species. These medically important snails are now placed in a separate family, Pomatiopsidae. Also called *Amniocolidae.*

hydroblepharon [HYDRO- + Gk *blepharon* an eyelid] A watery swelling of the eyelid.

hydrobromic acid An aqueous solution of hydrogen bromide.

hydrobromide The salt formed from an organic base with hydrogen bromide.

Hydrocal A proprietary name for a brand of artificial stone used in dentistry.

hydrocalycosis [HYDRO- + L *calyx,* gen. *calycis,* a bud, covering, shell of fruit + -OSIS] A dilatation of a single renal calix, usually due to a congenital stricture or to an abnormal narrowing of the caliceal cup stalk.

congenital hydrocalycosis A rare congenital anomaly consisting of dilatation of a single renal calix due to stricture or abnormal narrowing of the stalk of a calyceal cup.

hydrocalyx [HYDRO- + L *calyx* a bud, covering, shell of fruit] Dilatation of a renal calix.

hydrocarbarism HYDROCARBONISM.

hydrocarbon [HYDRO- + CARBON] A compound consisting only of the elements carbon and hydrogen. Squalene is the only important hydrocarbon metabolite in mammals.

carcinogenic hydrocarbon A hydrocarbon, usually aromatic polycyclic in type, that acts on living tissue to cause cancer.

chlorinated hydrocarbon A hydrocarbon containing a chlorine grouping in its molecular structure. Such compounds have many uses, particularly in pesticides or insecticides. Many are environmentally harmful because of their stability and undesirable ecological effects.

Diels hydrocarbon A hydrocarbon, obtained from sterols by selenium-catalyzed dehydrogenation, whose molecules consist of phenanthrene carrying a methylated cyclopentane ring. Its discovery was important in elucidation of the structure of steroids.

fluorinated hydrocarbon FLUOROCARBON.

halogenated hydrocarbon Any hydrocarbon molecule with one or more halogen atoms attached. Some such compounds are toxic and are used for the control of certain pest species. They are fat soluble and may accumulate in the food chain.

hydrocarbonism Poisoning produced by hydrocarbons. An imprecise usage. Also called *hydrocarbarism.*

hydrocardia HYDROPERICARDIUM.

hydrocele [HYDRO- + -CELE¹] An accumulation of serous fluid in a body cavity, especially between the visceral and parietal layers of the tunica vaginalis in the scrotum. It may be congenital.

bilocular hydrocele A collection of serous fluid in the tunica vaginalis testis or persistent processus vaginalis testis in the scrotum and/or inguinal regions of both sides.

cervical hydrocele BRANCHIAL CYST.

chylous hydrocele A type of hydrocele in which the liquid contents are milky white.

hydrocele colli BRANCHIAL CYST.

communicating hydrocele A hydrocele that communicates with the peritoneal cavity.

congenital hydrocele A hydrocele of the tunica vaginalis present at birth and due to failure of closure of the processus vaginalis, leaving a communication with the abdominal cavity. Also called *infantile hydrocele.*

diffused hydrocele　A collection of fluid diffused in spermatic cord tissue.

Dupuytren's hydrocele　A bilocular hydrocele in which all or major parts of the processus vaginalis testis of both sides persist.

encysted hydrocele　A small, localized hydrocele of the testis or epididymis situated at the point of reflection of the tunica vaginalis testis.

hydrocele feminae　A collection of fluid in the canal of Nuck along the round ligament sometimes extending into the labia majora. Also called *hydrocele muliebris, Nuck's hydrocele.*

filarial hydrocele　A hydrocele due to the presence, in the tunica vaginalis of the testicle, of microfilariae, usually of *Wuchereria bancrofti.*

funicular hydrocele　A persistence of the embryonic saccus vaginalis testis in its upper extent but not continuously with the tunica vaginalis testis. It may be either a blind cyst beside the spermatic cord or an elongated sac continuous with the peritoneal cavity.

Gibbon's hydrocele　GIBBON'S HERNIA.

infantile hydrocele　CONGENITAL HYDROCELE.

inguinal hydrocele　A hydrocele accompanying an undescendedtesticle. It may be found in the inguinal canal or the pubic area.

Maunoir's hydrocele　BRANCHIAL CYST.

hydrocele muliebris　HYDROCELE FEMINAE.

Nuck's hydrocele　HYDROCELE FEMINAE.

scrotal hydrocele　A hydrocele in the tunica vaginalis testis in the scrotum. Also called *oscheohydrocele.*

spermatic hydrocele　The collection of spermatic fluid along the spermatic cord.

hydrocele of the spermatic cord　An encysted hydrocele in that portion of the peritoneum surrounding the spermatic cord. It usually lies in the upper part of the scrotum or the inguinal canal.

hydrocele spinalis　SPINA BIFIDA.

hydrocele of the testis　A hydrocele of the testicular part of the tunica vaginalis. It is the commonest type of hydrocele. Also called *hydrorchis.*

hydrocelectomy　The surgical process of removing a hydrocele.

hydrocenosis　A procedure by which an abnormal serous fluid accumulation is drained from the body.

hydrocephalic　Describing, pertaining to, or affected by hydrocephalus.

hydrocephalocele　HYDROENCEPHALOCELE.

hydrocephaloid　Resembling hydrocephalus in having an apparently enlarged cranium, as is seen in some cases of starvation, but without any abnormal accumulation of cerebrospinal fluid.

hydrocephalus　[HYDRO- + L -*cephalus* (from Gk -*kephalos* combining form of *kephalē* the head) combining form meaning in relation to the head]　Any condition in which there is an abnormally large volume of cerebrospinal fluid within the skull. Also called *hydrencephalus, hydrencephaly, dropsy of head* (obsolete), *dropsy of brain* (obsolete), *hydrocephaly, hydrocrania, hydrops capitis* (obsolete).

acute acquired hydrocephalus　Hydrocephalus developing acutely as the result of an acquired pathologic process as distinct from a developmental anomaly.

communicating hydrocephalus　Hydrocephalus in which there is obstruction to the flow of cerebrospinal fluid within the subarachnoid space. Also called *external hydrocephalus, serous internal pachymeningitis.*

compensating hydrocephalus　HYDROCEPHALUS EX VACUO.

compensatory hydrocephalus　HYDROCEPHALUS EX VACUO.

congenital hydrocephalus　Primary hydrocephalus due to developmental obstruction or stenosis of any of the passages through which cerebrospinal fluid normally passes. Also called *primary hydrocephalus.*

external hydrocephalus　COMMUNICATING HYDROCEPHALUS.

hydrocephalus ex vacuo　The replacement of lost or atrophic brain tissue by cerebrospinal fluid, occurring as a compensatory mechanism to restore intracranial volume. Also called *compensating hydrocephalus, compensatory hydrocephalus.*

hypertonic hydrocephalus　Hydrocephalus with increased intracranial pressure.

internal hydrocephalus　OBSTRUCTIVE HYDROCEPHALUS.

low-pressure hydrocephalus　A form of communicating hydrocephalus identified as a cause of dementia, intermittent confusion, and gait disturbance, in which the cerebrospinal fluid pressure as measured by lumbar puncture is often low or normal.

noncommunicating hydrocephalus　OBSTRUCTIVE HYDROCEPHALUS.

normal-pressure hydrocephalus　LOW-PRESSURE HYDROCEPHALUS.

obstructive hydrocephalus　Hydrocephalus due to a disease process or to a developmental or acquired lesion which causes obstruction to the normal flow of cerebrospinal fluid through the cerebral ventricular system. Also called *internal hydrocephalus, noncommunicating hydrocephalus.*

occult hydrocephalus　Hydrocephalus which is asymptomatic and produces no abnormal physical signs.

otitic hydrocephalus　Benign intercranial hypertension occurring in association with otitis media and with thrombosis of one or more intercranial venous sinuses.

postmeningitic hydrocephalus　Communicating hydrocephalus following meningitis.

post-traumatic hydrocephalus　Hydrocephalus, usually of the communicating variety, developing as a sequel to head injury.

primary hydrocephalus　CONGENITAL HYDROCEPHALUS.

secondary hydrocephalus　Hydrocephalus resulting from any acquired disease process or lesion.

thrombotic hydrocephalus　Hydrocephalus resulting from intracranial venous sinus thrombosis.

toxic hydrocephalus　Benign intracranial hypertension due to an exogenous or endogenous toxin.

hydrocephaly　[French *hydrocéphalie* hydrocephalus]　HYDROCEPHALUS.

hydrochloric acid　HCl. The aqueous solution of hydrogen chloride. Also called *muriatic acid, spirit of salt* (obsolete).

diluted hydrochloric acid　A diluted medicinal preparation of hydrochloric acid that contains 9.5 to 10.5 g of HCl in 100 ml of water. It is used as an acidifying medium in formulations.

hydrochloride　The salt formed from a base by combination with hydrogen chloride.

hydrochlorothiazide　$C_7H_8ClN_3O_4S_2$. 6-Chloro-3,4-dihydro-2H-1,2,4-benzothiadiazine-7-sulfonamide 1,1-dioxide, an important antihypertensive, diuretic agent that inhibits the reabsorption of sodium by the renal tubular cells. It is administered orally.

hydrocholeretic　Inducing or provoking increased bile flow, especially of more dilute bile.

hydrochory　[HYDRO- + Gk *chōr(ein)* to spread abroad + -Y]　Distribution of fungal propagules via water.

hydrocinnamic acid　3-Phenylpropionic acid, which may be prepared by hydrogenation of cinnamic acid. An obsolete term.

hydrocirsocele　[HYDRO- + CIRSO- + -CELE[1]]　A hydrocele and a varicocele occurring simultaneously.

hydroclimatology　The study and therapeutic utilization of waterfront climates. An outmoded term. See also MARINOTHERAPY.

hydrocodone $C_{18}H_{21}NO_3$. 4,5-Epoxy-3-methoxy-17-methylmorphinan-6-one, a semisynthetic analgesic derived from codeine. It is a stronger analgesic than codeine with antitussive properties. It is usually administered as its bitartrate salt, and chronic use can lead to addiction.

hydrocodone resin complex A combination of hydrocodone and a cationic resin for oral administration with slow release and absorption of the drug. The antitussive agent should act for about 12 hours after one dose in this formulation.

hydrocole [HYDRO- + L col(ere) to cultivate, inhabit] An animal that lives in a swamp, marsh, or other wet terrestrial habitat.

hydrocolloid [HYDRO- + COLLOID] An elastic water-based impression material.

irreversible hydrocolloid A hydrocolloid, prepared by adding a powder to water, which can be used only once.

reversible hydrocolloid A thermoplastic hydrocolloid.

hydrocolpocele [HYDRO- + COLPO- + -CELE²] An accumulation of fluid other than blood or pus in the vagina. Such accumulation is usually dependent upon an imperforate hymen or atresia of the lower vaginal canal and is usually seen in the neonatal period. Also called hydrocolpos.

hydrocolpos HYDROCOLPOCELE.

hydroconion ATOMIZER.

hydrocortamate $C_{27}H_{41}NO_6$. An ester derivative of hydrocortisone that is used as a 0.5 percent ointment in the treatment of dermatologic conditions that respond to corticosteroids.

hydrocortisone CORTISOL.

hydrocortisone acetate The acetate ester of hydrocortisone (cortisol) at the C-21 position. It has the same uses as cortisol, the parent compound, and is given intra-articularly by soft-tissue injection and applied topically to the skin or conjunctiva.

hydrocortisone sodium phosphate The phosphate ester of hydrocortisone (cortisol). It has the same uses as the parent compound but has greater solubility in water. It is given intravenously and by intramuscular injection.

hydrocortisone sodium succinate The hemisuccinate ester sodium salt derivative of hydrocortisone. It has greater water solubility but is used for the same purposes as hydrocortisone. It is administered intravenously or intramuscularly.

hydrocortisone tebutate HYDROCORTISONE TERTIARY-BUTYLACETATE.

hydrocortisone tertiary-butylacetate The tertiary butylacetate ester of hydrocortisone. It has the same uses as hydrocortisone. Also called hydrocortisone tebutate.

Hydrocortone A proprietary name for hydrocortisone.

hydrocrania [HYDRO- + cran(i)- + -IA] HYDROCEPHALUS.

hydrocyanic acid HYDROGEN CYANIDE.

hydrocyanism [hydro(gen) + cyan(ide) + -ISM] Poisoning due to hydrogen cyanide. Toxic symptoms depend upon the dose, the form in which it is administered, and the route. With high concentrations, respiration ceases immediately. At lower concentrations, symptoms of muscular incoordination and decreased respiration develop more slowly, and may be fatal if left untreated.

hydrocyst Any cystic structure that has watery or serous contents. An obsolete term.

hydrocystadenoma HIDROCYSTOMA.

hydrocystoma HIDROCYSTOMA.

hydrodiascope A refracting device linked to the cornea with fluid, with the intent of subtracting the optical characteristics of the cornea from the refractive findings.

hydrodictiotomy [HYDRO- + Gk diktyo(n) a net + -TOMY] Correction of retinal detachment.

hydrodiffusion 1 The diffusion of a substance through water. 2 The diffusion of one liquid through another liquid.

hydrodipsia [HYDRO- + DIPSIA] A craving for water. An outmoded term.

hydrodipsomania PSYCHOGENIC POLYDIPSIA.

Hydrodiuril A proprietary name for hydrochlorothiazide.

hydrodynamics The science and technology dealing with the motion of fluids and the forces they exert on solids within them.

hydroelectric 1 Relating to the conversion of water power into electric power. 2 An outmoded term for HYDROGALVANIC.

hydroelectrization Galvanic stimulation of a portion of the body immersed in water. An outmoded term.

hydroencephalocele [HYDRO- + ENCEPHALOCELE] An encephalocele in which cerebrospinal fluid has accumulated either in meningeal spaces or in the ventricles of herniated brain, causing dilatation of the herniated mass. Also called encephalocystocele, encephalocystomeningocele, hydrencephalocele, hydrocephalocele.

hydroencephalomeningocele HYDRENCEPHALOMENINGOCELE.

hydrofluoric acid HF. Hydrogen fluoride and its solutions. It is strongly corrosive and a moderately strong acid.

hydrofugous Shedding water, as the cuticle of many insects.

hydrogalvanic Relating to galvanic stimulation to a portion of the body immersed in water. Also hydroelectric (outmoded).

hydrogen Element number 1, having atomic weight 1.0019. Hydrogen is the most abundant element in the universe but constitutes less than 0.22% of the total atoms on earth. It is a fuel sustaining the thermonuclear reactions in the sun and stars. It is the lightest of all gases, and only traces (less than 1 ppm) occur free in the atmosphere. It occurs chiefly in combination with oxygen in water. There are three isotopes. Hydrogen 1 (protium) has a natural abundance of 99.985%. The remaining .015% consists mostly of hydrogen 2 (deuterium). The one unstable isotope, hydrogen 3 (tritium) occurs naturally in minute traces. Hydrogen combines with other elements, often explosively. The valence is 1. As a constituent of water and of most organic compounds, hydrogen is essential to life. See also DEUTERIUM, TRITIUM. Symbol: H

arseniuretted hydrogen ARSINE.

heavy hydrogen DEUTERIUM.

hydrogen ion The positively charged nucleus of the hydrogen atom; a proton. Acids have the ability to liberate hydrogen ions. Symbol: H^+

nascent hydrogen Hydrogen being formed by reaction of a metal with an acid. It has greater reducing properties than hydrogen gas.

radioactive hydrogen TRITIUM.

sulfuretted hydrogen An obsolete term for HYDROGEN SULFIDE.

hydrogen 2 DEUTERIUM.

hydrogen 3 TRITIUM.

hydrogen arsenide ARSINE.

hydrogenase 1 The enzyme (EC 1.18.3.1) that catalyzes the reduction of ferredoxin by hydrogen gas. It is an iron-sulfur protein. 2 Any of various other enzymes that catalyze reductions by hydrogen gas. An outmoded usage.

hydrogenate To add hydrogen to a molecule, usually by reaction with the atoms at either end of a double bond. It may be performed catalytically with hydrogen gas, or with numerous other reagents.

hydrogenation The process of adding hydrogen atoms to a compound, often using hydrogen gas. In nonbiological systems, it is frequently catalyzed by a noble metal or by one of its salts.

hydrogen bromide A colorless gas that browns on prolonged exposure to light, is dangerous to breathe, and is obtained by hydrolysis of phosphorus tribromide. Its saturated aqueous solution contains 66% HBr at 25°C. It is a strong acid and reducing agent, used for preparing bromides.

hydrogen chloride HCl. A gas, soluble in water and organic solvents. Its aqueous solution is hydrochloric acid. The commercial product is a concentrated solution about 12 M or 38% HCl, of density 1.19. It is a colorless liquid, which fumes in air and is highly corrosive with an irritant smell. When heated it loses hydrogen chloride until "constant boiling" hydrochloric acid is formed, of concentration about 6 M. Dilute solutions are used for preparing certain medicaments, especially hydrochlorides of alkaloids and other bases.

hydrogen cyanide HCN. A very volatile liquid in the anhydrous state, with, for some persons, a penetrating smell. It is miscible with water, ether, and alcohol in all proportions. Its melting point is −14°C and its boiling point 26°C. It is a very weak acid (pK 9). It is very toxic because of the high affinity of the cyanide ion for the iron of cytochrome oxidase. Also called *hydrocyanic acid, prussic acid*.

hydrogen fluoride HF. A colorless, corrosive gas, very irritating and toxic. It is soluble in water and alcohol in all proportions and in ether. $d^{20} = 0.699$. The freezing point is −14°C, and the boiling point 26°C. The commercial product is a solution of 47–53% HF. In dilute solution it is a weak acid (pK 3.2) but the associated forms present in concentrated solution are much stronger acids. The anhydrous liquid is a powerful solvent with hydrogen-bonding properties like water. It is used for etching glass. It may cause severe burns to skin, eyes, and mucous membranes. Inhalation of the vapor may cause pulmonary edema.

hydrogen iodide HYDRIODIC ACID.

hydrogenlyase An outmoded term for DEHYDROGENASE.

hydrogenolysis A reaction in which the molecules of one reactant are broken into two parts, each containing one atom of hydrogen derived from the the other reactant, hydrogen gas.

hydrogen peroxide H_2O_2. A compound available in aqueous solution, but unstable when the solution is concentrated. It is both an oxidizing agent (being reduced to water) and a reducing agent (being oxidized to oxygen). It is produced when oxygen oxidizes the reduced form of many enzymes, particularly flavoproteins. The enzyme catalase converts it into water and oxygen, and peroxidases catalyze oxidations in which it is reduced to water. Also called *peroxide*.

hydrogen sulfate ACID SULFATE.

hydrogen sulfide H_2S. A colorless, flammable, highly poisonous gas (boiling point −60°C) with a sweetish taste and an odor of rotten eggs. It owes its toxicity to its high affinity for iron compounds, such as cytochrome oxidase. It is used in the identification of metal ions, since many form insoluble sulfides. It is a reducing agent, being easily oxidized to sulfur, sulfur dioxide, and sulfuric acid. Colorless and photosynthetic sulfur bacteria use biologic and light energy respectively to decompose it to sulfur and to form a reducing agent of its hydrogen. Other bacteria, particularly those living in marine muds, form it from decomposing organic matter and sulfate. It can also be formed bacterially from cysteine derived from proteins. In low concentrations it causes irritation of mucous membranes, particularly of the eyes, leading to keratitis. In high concentrations it causes death from paralysis of the respiratory center. Also called *sul-*

furetted hydrogen (obsolete), *hydrosulfuric acid, sulfur hydride, sulfhydric acid*.

hydroglossa An obsolete term for RANULA.

hydrogymnasium A therapeutic pool or hydrotherapy tank. A British term.

hydrogymnastic Relating to hydrogymnastics.

hydrogymnastics Exercises performed while immersed in water.

hydrohemarthrosis [HYDRO- + HEM- + ARTHROSIS] Hemorrhagic effusion of the joint.

hydrohematonephrosis [HYDRO- + HEMATO- + NEPHROSIS] HEMOPYELECTASIS.

hydrohematosalpinx [HYDRO- + HEMATO- + Gk *salpinx* tube] A collection of fluid and blood in an oviduct, usually due to damage by chronic salpingitis.

hydrohymenitis Inflammation of a serosal membrane such as the pleura. An obsolete term.

hydrohystera [HYDRO- + Gk *hystera* the uterus] HYDROMETRA.

hydroid [HYDR- + -OID] **1** Any of the hydrozoan coelenterates, characterized by having a polyp stage during their life cycle. They may be solitary or colonial and are usually attached. Members of colonial species may be specialized, as for defense. **2** HYDROZOAN.

hydrokinesitherapy The therapeutic use of exercises performed while the patient is immersed in water.

hydrokinetic Pertaining to the use of moving water or other fluid for therapeutic purposes, as in hydromassage.

hydrokinetics The study of water in motion and its therapeutic applications.

hydrokollag A graphite suspension that is used to study ciliary and lymphatic activity.

hydrolabile [HYDRO- + LABILE] Marked by a tendency to experience alterations in water content. Compare HYDROSTABILE.

hydrolabyrinth A rarely used term for MENIÈRE'S DISEASE. ● See note at LABYRINTHINE HYDROPS.

hydrolase Any enzyme that catalyzes the hydrolysis of its substrate.

hydrology [HYDRO- + -LOGY] The scientific study of water. ● When unmodified, *hydrology* most commonly refers to the study of water as a large-scale component of the earth's surface, crust, and atmosphere.
medical hydrology The study of medical properties and uses of water.

Hydrolose A proprietary name for methylcellulose.

hydrolyase Any enzyme that catalyzes the elimination of water from a molecule, usually with formation of a double bond, such as enolase.

hydrolysate The product or products of hydrolysis of a substance.

hydrolysis [HYDRO- + LYSIS] A reaction in which bonds in the reactant are broken by reaction with water, with addition of a hydroxyl group and a hydrogen atom to the two atoms previously joined. Adjective: hydrolytic.
papain hydrolysis The hydrolysis of proteins using the protease obtained from the papaya plant. This enzyme is commonly used in immunologic research to split the IgG molecule into three parts (two Fab fragments and one Fc fragment).

hydrolytic Pertaining to or bringing about hydrolysis.

hydrolyze To split a substance into component parts with addition of the elements of water: to bring about the process of hydrolysis.

hydroma HYGROMA.

hydromassage Therapeutic manipulation of soft tissues by means of agitated water, as in a whirlpool bath.

hydromeningitis [HYDRO- + MENINGITIS] **1** Hydrocephalus resulting from meningitis. **2** An obsolete term for BENIGN INTRACRANIAL HYPERTENSION.

hydromeningocele A herniation of a fluid-filled sac of spinal or cranial meninges through a defect in the bony structures that normally prevent such protrusion.

   cranial hydromeningocele A hydromeningocele through the skull.

hydrometer [HYDRO- + -METER] A meter used to determine a fluid's specific gravity. Also called *aerometer*.

hydrometra [HYDRO- + Gk *mētra* the uterus] A collection of watery fluid or mucus in the uterus. Also called *hydrohystera*.

hydrometric **1** Of or pertaining to hydrometry. **2** Relating to a hydrometer. For defs. 1 and 2 also *areometric*.

hydrometrocolpos [HYDRO- + METRO- + Gk *kolpos* bosom, womb, fold] An accumulation of fluid other than blood or pus in the uterus and vagina. Such accumulation is usually contingent on an imperforate hymen or atresia of the lower vaginal canal.

hydrometry [HYDRO- + -METRY] The determination of a fluid's specific gravity by using a hydrometer. Also called *areometry*.

hydromicrocephaly [HYDRO- + MICROCEPHALY] Microcephaly associated with a disproportionately large volume of cerebrospinal fluid.

hydromorphone hydrochloride $C_{17}H_{20}ClNO_3$. 4,5α-Epoxy-3-hydroxy-17-methylmorphinan-6-one hydrochloride, a chemically produced derivative of morphine with about 10 times the analgesic potency of morphine. It is given orally or by subcutaneous injection. Chronic use may lead to addiction.

hydromphalus A cystic mass containing watery fluid associated with the umbilicus. The cyst is most likely a remnant of the embryonic vitelline duct or sac, or of the embryonic allantoic stalk.

hydromyelia [HYDRO- + MYEL- + -IA] **1** A dilatation of the central canal of the spinal cord containing cerebrospinal fluid. **2** Any fluid-containing cavity within the spinal cord except those of syringomyelia. Also called *hydrorachis*.

   acquired hydromyelia Hydromyelia due to an acquired lesion or process as distinct from a developmental anomaly.

hydromyelocele [HYDRO- + MYELOCELE] The protrusion through a spina bifida of a fluid-filled sac enclosed by attenuated spinal cord tissue and associated meninges. The presence of cord tissue in the sac may be difficult to demonstrate, but its former presence may be inferred from the intact meninges.

hydromyelomeningocele A hydromyelocele with demonstrable spinal cord tissue in the wall of the fluid-filled sac protruding from a spina bifida.

hydromyoma [HYDRO- + MYOMA] A myoma containing fluid-filled cystic areas.

hydron H$^+$. The cation formed from hydrogen, irrespective of isotope. Thus a hydron may be a proton, a deuteron, or a triton. Also called *hydrion* (outmoded).

hydronephrectasia [HYDRO- + NEPHR- + ECTASIA] Enlargement of a kidney due to accumulation of fluid in the pelvis or in kidney substance.

hydronephrosis [HYDRO- + NEPHROSIS] Dilatation of the renal pelvis and calices, and sometimes collecting ducts, secondary to obstruction of urine flow by calculi, tumors, neurologic disorders, or any of various congenital anomalies. Also called *nephrydrosis, uronephrosis*. Adjective: hydronephrotic.

   closed hydronephrosis Permanent hydronephrosis due to total obstruction of the ureter.

   congenital hydronephrosis Hydronephrosis present at birth, sometimes due to atresia of ureters or the urethra or to hypertonicity of sphincters within the tract.

   external hydronephrosis URINOMA.

   infected hydronephrosis Hydronephrosis and an associated infection, usually caused by *E. coli*, with symptoms resembling those of severe pyelonephritis. Also called *pyonephrosis, pyopyelectasis*.

   intermittent hydronephrosis Dilatation of the pelvis and calices due to intermittent, incomplete obstruction of ureters by an aberrant renal artery, movable kidney, calculi, etc.

   open hydronephrosis Distention of the pelvis and calices of the kidney caused by occasional obstruction of the ureter.

   perirenal hydronephrosis URINOMA.

   subcapsular hydronephrosis URINOMA.

hydronephrotic Pertaining to or having the characteristics of hydronephrosis.

hydronium An outmoded term for OXONIUM.

Hydronol A proprietary name for isosorbide.

hydroparasalpinx The accumulation of serous fluid in any of the embryonic mesonephric duct or tube remnants associated with the oviduct.

hydroparotitis Swelling of the parotid gland due to distension of the duct system with secretions, usually from acute obstruction to salivary flow as in sialolithiasis. A seldom used term.

hydropathic Relating to hydropathy.

hydropathy [HYDRO- + -PATHY] An obsolete form of therapy based on the supposed universal curative properties of ingested water.

hydropedesis HYPERHIDROSIS.

hydropelvis [HYDRO- + PELVIS] Dilatation of the renal pelvis by urine.

hydropenia [HYDRO- + -PENIA] A condition marked by an inadequate amount of water.

hydropenic Of or relating to hydropenia.

hydropericarditic Pertaining to or characterized by hydropericarditis.

hydropericarditis Pericarditis with liquid effusion into the pericardial sac.

hydropericardium The presence of an abnormally large volume of fluid in the pericardial sac. Also called *hydrocardia, hydrops pericardii*.

hydroperinephrosis [HYDRO- + PERI- + NEPHROSIS] The accumulation of fluid in the retroperitoneal connective tissue communicating with the renal pelvis.

hydroperion [HYDRO- + PERI- + Gk *ōon* egg] Fluid lying between the capsular and parietal portions of the decidua.

hydroperitoneum ASCITES.

hydroperitonia ASCITES.

hydropexia [HYDRO- + -*pex(y)* + -IA] The incorporation of water into tissues. Also called *hydropexis*.

hydropexic [HYDRO- + -*pex(y)* + -IC] Of or relating to the incorporation of water into tissues.

hydropexis HYDROPEXIA.

hydrophagocytosis The internalization by phagocytes of surrounding liquid. Also called *Lewis phenomenon*.

hydrophallus [HYDRO- + PHALLUS] Dilatation of the penis by accumulated fluid in its tissues.

Hydrophiidae [HYDR- + OPHI- + -IDAE] The family of marine reptiles which includes the true sea snakes. Members have a proteroglyphic jaw, a ventrally compressed body, and a dorsally flattened tail. They produce a strongly neurotoxic venom, but their behavior is nonaggressive.

hydrophilic [HYDRO- + -PHILIC]   Having an affinity for water: used of substances that are soluble in water or of chemical groups that raise the solubility in water of substances that contain them. Also *hydrophilous*.

hydrophilous   HYDROPHILIC.

hydrophobia [HYDRO- + -PHOBIA]   **1** A clinical manifestation, usually of rabies, involving glottal spasm and paralysis of the muscles of deglutition and provoked by attempts to drink fluids or by the sight of fluids.   **2** A popular term for RABIES. **3** Morbid aversion to water.

paralytic hydrophobia   PARALYTIC RABIES.

hydrophobic   **1** Having low affinity for water. Hydrophobic groups have affinity for each other when they are in an aqueous environment, because of the tendency of their interface with water to diminish. Hydrocarbons are typically hydrophobic.   **2** Relating to or characterized by hydrophobia.

hydrophone [HYDRO- + Gk *phōnē* sound, voice]   A liquid-filled tube for conveying sound to the ear in auscultatory percussion.

hydrophorograph [HYDRO- + PHORO- + -GRAPH]   An apparatus for measuring the pressure or flow of a fluid.

hydrophthalmia [HYDR- + OPHTHALMIA]   BUPHTHALMOS.

hydrophthalmos [HYDR- + Gk *ophthalmos* the eye]   BUPHTHALMOS.

hydrophthalmos anterior   Congenital glaucoma that preferentially enlarges the front portion of the eye.

hydrophthalmos posterior   Congenital glaucoma that preferentially enlarges the back part of the eye.

hydrophthalmos totalis   Congenital glaucoma that symmetrically enlarges the entire eye.

hydrophthalmoscope [HYDR- + OPHTHALMOSCOPE]   A contact lens used in viewing the ocular fundus.

hydrophthalmus [See HYDROPHTHALMOS.]   BUPHTHALMOS.

hydrophysometra [HYDRO- + PHYSO- + Gk *mētra* the uterus]   PNEUMOHYDROMETRA.

hydrophyte [HYDRO- + Gk *phyt(on)* a plant, tree]   A plant that grows partly or completely underwater.

hydropic   A rarely used term for EDEMATOUS.

hydropigenous [Gk *hydrōps*, gen. *hydropos*, also *hydropos* (from *hydōr* water, without further significant combination) dropsy, any watery humor, a dropsical person + *i* + -GENOUS]   Causing edema.

hydroplasm   HYALOPLASM.

hydroplasmia   A reduction in the osmolarity of blood plasma, due either to an increase in the water content or a decrease in the concentration of electrolytes and colloids. Also called *hydroplasmy*.

hydroplasmy   HYDROPLASMIA.

hydropleura   HYDROTHORAX.

hydropneumatosis   A condition characterized by the presence of fluid and gas within a tissue.

hydropneumogony   An obsolete term for ARTHROGRAPHY.

hydropneumopericardium   The presence of fluid and gas within the pericardial sac.

hydropneumoperitoneum [HYDRO- + PNEUMO- + PERITONEUM]   An intraperitoneal accumulation of air and fluid.

hydropneumothorax   The presence of air and watery fluid in the pleural cavity. Also called *pneumohydrothorax, seropneumothorax*.

hydroponics [HYDRO- + Gk *pon(os)* labor + -ICS]   The culture of plants by immersing the roots in an inert aqueous or particulate substratum to which nutrient salts have been added.

hydrops [L (from Gk *hydrōps* dropsy, a dropsical person, from *hydōr* water), dropsy]   An excessive accumulation of serous fluid in interstitial tissues or body cavities.

hydrops abdominis   An obsolete term for ASCITES.

hydrops amnii   HYDRAMNIOS.

hydrops antri   An accumulation of serous fluid within the maxillary sinus. The fluid, often straw-colored, usually proves to be the contents of a retention cyst within the antrum.

hydrops articuli   HYDRARTHROSIS.

Bart's hemoglobin hydrops fetalis   A form of α-thalassemia due to homozygosity for α-thalassemia-1 that is lethal during fetal life. Only hemoglobin Bart's is present in the blood of such a fetus.

hydrops capitis   An obsolete term for HYDROCEPHALUS.

hydrops of the cornea   Gross entry of aqueous humor into the cornea as a result of a rupture of the endothelium and Descemet's membrane, as may occur in keratoconus.

endolymphatic hydrops   **1** MENIÈRE'S DISEASE.   **2** A distended state of the membranous labyrinth found in Menière's disease.

fetal hydrops   The abnormal accumulation of fluid in the tissues of a fetus or newborn infant, as in erythroblastosis fetalis. Also called *hydrops fetalis*.

hydrops fetalis   FETAL HYDROPS.

hydrops folliculi   Accumulation of fluid in the graafian follicle of the ovary.

hydrops gravidarum   Edema occurring during pregnancy.

hypertensive meningeal hydrops   BENIGN INTRACRANIAL HYPERTENSION.

hydrops hypostrophos   An obsolete term for ANGIONEUROTIC EDEMA.

hydrops labyrinthi   MENIÈRE'S DISEASE.   ● See note at LABYRINTHINE HYDROPS.

labyrinthine hydrops   An incorrect term for MENIÈRE'S DISEASE.   ● The term is misleading as it implies involvement of the entire labyrinth when in fact only the endolymphatic compartment is involved.

hydrops pericardii   HYDROPERICARDIUM.

hydrops spurius   PSEUDOMYXOMA PERITONEI.

hydrops tubae   HYDROSALPINX.

hydrops tubae profluens   Vaginal secretion of profuse amounts of serous fluid originating in the fallopian tube. It may be a sign of a tubal carcinoma.

tympanic hydrops   SECRETORY OTITIS MEDIA.

hydropyonephrosis [HYDRO- + PYO- + NEPHROSIS]   Dilatation of the renal pelvis and calyces with pus, secondary to obstructive uropathy.

hydroquinol   HYDROQUINONE.   ● This term was produced by confusion of the two terms *hydroquinone* and *quinol*.

hydroquinone $C_6H_4(OH)_2$. The compound benzene-1,2-diol, which is easily oxidized to a quinone. It occurs as the glucoside arbutin in leaves of *Arctostaphylos uva-ursi*, the bearberry, and in all parts of *Kalmia latifolia*, the mountain laurel. Hydroquinone has been associated with poisoning, and it has been used as an antiseptic, astrigent, diuretic, and tonic. Also called *hydroquinol*.

hydrorachis [HYDRO- + Gk *rhachis* the back, spine, backbone]   HYDROMYELIA.

hydrorachitis [HYDRO- + RACHITIS]   Spinal meningitis with marked exudation of fluid. An outmoded term.

hydrorchis [HYDR- + Gk *orchis* testicle]   HYDROCELE OF THE TESTIS.

hydrorheostat   A rheostat in which the resistance varies by varying the distance between electrodes in an electrolyte.

hydrorrhea [HYDRO- + -RRHEA]   An excessive or copious discharge of water or other fluid. Also called *hydatorrhea*.

hydrorrhea gravidarum Intermittent vaginal drainage of fluid during pregnancy. The fluid may come from the extra-amniotic space or may be amniotic fluid.

nasal hydrorrhea Watery rhinorrhea. A seldom used term.

hydrosalpinx [HYDRO- + Gk *salpinx* tube] Distension of the fallopian tube by clear fluid, usually occurring as a result of closure of the fimbricated end of the tube by inflammation. Also called *tubal dropsy, salpingian dropsy, hydrops tubae, sactosalpinx.*

hydrosalpinx follicularis A loculated accumulation of fluid in the oviduct.

intermittent hydrosalpinx An accumulation of watery, serous fluid which periodically discharges itself from the oviduct.

hydrosalpinx simplex A single cavity of fluid within the oviduct.

hydrosarcocele [*hydro(cele)* + SARCOCELE] Hydrocele and sarcocele combined.

hydrosaturnism [HYDRO- + Med L *saturnus* (after 1 *Saturnus* the planet) alchemists' term for lead + -ISM] Poisoning from the ingestion of water containing lead.

hydroscheocele [HYDR- + OSCHEO- + -CELE[1]] A scrotal hernia in which the hernial sac contains serous fluid.

hydroscope [HYDRO- + -SCOPE] An instrument used for detecting water. Adjective: hydroscopic.

hydrospermatocele [HYDRO- + SPERMATOCELE] SPERMATOCELE.

hydrospermatocyst [HYDRO- + SPERMATO- + CYST] A hydrocele with spermatozoa in its fluid.

hydrosphere [HYDRO- + *(bio)sphere*] The aquatic portion of the biosphere.

hydrosphygmograph A sphygmograph that utilizes a water manometer.

hydrospirometer A spirometer which uses displacement of water to measure gas volumes.

hydrostabile [HYDRO- + STABILE] Having the quality of maintaining a constant water content. Compare HYDROLABILE.

hydrostat [HYDRO- + -STAT] A device that regulates the level of fluid in a column or other container.

hydrostatics [HYDRO- + -STAT + -ICS] The science of pressures and levels in water and hence in liquids generally.

hydrostomia A rarely used term for PTYALISM.

hydrosudopathy HYDROSUDOTHERAPY.

hydrosudotherapy The combination of induced sweating and hydrotherapy, such as may be utilized in a Turkish bath setting. Also called *hydrosudopathy.*

hydrosulfite An obsolete term for DITHIONITE.

hydrosulfuric acid HYDROGEN SULFIDE.

hydrosyringomyelia Syringomyelia.

Hydrotaea A genus of muscid flies that includes bloodsuckers and pests of ruminants and humans. *H. meteorica* may cause summer mastitis in heifers and dry cows in Asia and the United States and also attacks man. *H. pandella* rasps the skin to stimulate blood flow. *H. irritans,* the sheep head fly, will also attack man and may cause serious damage to lambs.

hydrotaxis [HYDRO- + Gk *taxis* an arranging, ordering] A movement or orientation directed by the presence of water.

hydrotherapeutic Relating to hydrotherapy or hydrotherapeutics.

hydrotherapeutics The study of the therapeutic properties of water in all of its applications, including both internal and external.

hydrotherapist A specialist in or practitioner of hydrotherapy.

hydrotherapy 1 Utilization of water by external application or by immersion as a primary therapeutic measure or adjunctive

technique. 2 Therapeutic use of water by ingestion as in spa therapy. Also called *water cure.*

hydrothermal Relating to hot water, especially to naturally occurring hot water as in thermal springs. Also *hydrothermic.*

hydrothermic HYDROTHERMAL.

hydrothermostat A thermostat for regulating the temperature of water.

hydrothermotherapy Hydrotherapy in which heated water is utilized.

hydrothionemia The presence of hydrogen sulfide in blood, as in a person who has inhaled hydrogen sulfide gas.

hydrothoracic Pertaining to hydrothorax.

hydrothorax [HYDRO- + THORAX] Watery fluid in the pleural cavity, usually due to heart failure or a state of generalized edema. Also called *dropsy of chest, hydropleura.*

chylous hydrothorax CHYLOTHORAX.

pseudochylous hydrothorax The presence of opalescent fluid in the pleural cavity whose appearance is due to substances other than fat, usually cholesterol.

hydrotimeter [HYDRO- + -METER] An apparatus for testing the hardness of water.

hydrotimetry [HYDRO- + -METRY] The measurement of the hardness of water.

hydrotis A seldom used term for SECRETORY OTITIS MEDIA.

hydrotomy [HYDRO- + -TOMY] A procedure in which tissues are separated or dissected free by injecting water or other fluid under high pressure.

hydrotoxicity WATER INTOXICATION.

hydrotropism [HYDRO- + TROPISM] The growth or directional response of an organism toward or away from water or moisture.

hydrotympanum SECRETORY OTITIS MEDIA.

hydroureter [HYDRO- + URETER] Acquired dilatation of the ureter by fluid, usually due to obstruction of the urinary outflow tract or to vesicoureteral reflux. Also called *hydroureterosis.*

hydroureteronephrosis [HYDRO- + URETERO- + NEPHROSIS] Dilatation of kidney and ureter by fluid, usually due to obstruction of urinary outflow or to vesicoureteral reflux.

hydroureterosis HYDROURETER.

hydrouria [HYDRO- + -URIA] Excretion of dilute urine.

hydrovarium [HYDR- + New L *ovarium* (from L *ov(um)* egg + New L suffix -*arium*) ovary] Edema or cyst of the ovary.

hydrox- HYDROXY-.

hydroxamic acids Derivatives of carboxylic acids, such as fatty acids or amino acids, in which a hydroxylamine bonds to the carbon of the carboxyl group, to give the structure R—CO—NH—OH. They are easily detected, and their spontaneous formation from thioesters allows these to be detected as metabolic intermediates.

hydroxide The ion HO^- or a compound containing it.

hydroxo- [*hydrox(yl)* + *o*] A combining form used in inorganic chemistry to show that a hydroxide ion, OH^-, is a ligand in a complex.

hydroxocobalamin The cobalamin in which the sixth ligand of the cobalt is a hydroxide ion. It is an important form of vitamin B_{12}.

hydroxy- [Gk *hydōr* water + *oxys* sharp] A combining form designating the presence of a hydroxyl group, —OH, as a substituent in a molecule. Also *hydrox-.*

3-hydroxyacyl-CoA dehydrogenase The enzyme (EC 1.1.1.35) of fatty-acid catabolism responsible for the oxidation of a 3-hydroxyacyl-CoA to a 3-oxoacyl-CoA with transfer of hydrogen to NAD^+.

hydroxyacylglutathione hydrolase An enzyme that catalyzes the hydrolysis of an *S*-(2-hydroxyacylglutathione) to glutathione and a 2-hydroxy acid. Also called *glyoxalase II* (obsolete).

hydroxyamphetamine $C_9H_{13}NO$. *p*-(2-Aminopropyl)phenol, an adrenergic agent that is applied topically to the conjunctiva as a mydriatic. The hydrochloride and hydrobromide salts are commonly used.

hydroxyamphetamine hydrobromide $C_9H_{13}NO \cdot HBr$. 4-(2-Aminopropyl)phenol hydrobromide, an adrenergic agent that is used as a mydriatic medication to the conjunctiva. It also acts as a nasal decongestant and, when given orally, is an effective pressor agent for the treatment of the carotid sinus syndrome, postural hypotension, and some types of heart block.

11β-hydroxyandrostenedione 11β-hydroxy-4-androstene-3,17-dione. A C_{19} adrenal steroid, a weak androgen, and a major source with cortisol of the 11-oxygenated 17-ketosteroids in the urine.

hydroxyapatite $[Ca_3(PO_4)_2]_3 \cdot Ca(OH)_2$. A compound whose crystals form a lattice that is embedded in the protein matrix of bones and teeth and contribute the major portion of rigid mineral structure to these structures. Also called *bone-salt*.

hydroxybenzene PHENOL.

3-hydroxybutyrate dehydrogenase The enzyme (EC 1.1.1.30) that interconverts 3-hydroxybutyrate and acetoacetate, which uses NAD^+ as hydrogen acceptor.

3-hydroxybutyric acid $CH_3-CHOH-CH_2-COOH$. An acid found in blood during ketosis, along with acetoacetic acid, from which it is formed by hydrogenation, and with acetone. Also called *β-hydroxybutyric acid*. See also KETONE BODY.

β-hydroxybutyric acid 3-HYDROXYBUTYRIC ACID.

hydroxychloroquine sulfate $C_{18}H_{26}ClN_3O \cdot H_2SO_4$. 7-Chloro-4-{4-[ethyl(2-hydroxyethyl)amino]-1-methylbutylamino}-quinoline sulfate, the sulfate salt of a quinoline analog that is used as an antimalarial agent and as a suppressant drug for lupus erythematosus. It is also used in the treatment of rheumatoid arthritis and giardiasis. It is given orally.

25-hydroxycholecalciferol A precursor of 1,25-dihydroxycholecalciferol, which can act directly on intestine and kidney to enhance calcium absorption and retention. It is formed in the liver by hydroxylation of cholecalciferol (the main form of vitamin D).

11-hydroxycorticosteroid A steroid of the adrenal cortex containing an 11-hydroxyl group. Most corticosteroids contain such a group. This group is very unreactive, being axial and having access to it hindered by the neighboring methyl groups (C-18 and C-19).

17-hydroxycorticosteroid A steroid of the adrenal cortex containing a 17-hydroxyl group. The addition of this group converts corticosterone, the main adrenocortical hormone in the rat, into cortisol, the main such hormone in man.

17-hydroxycorticosterone CORTISOL.

25-hydroxydihydrotachysterol One of the most potent compounds synthesized from vitamin D_2 (ergocalciferol). It is used in the treatment of hypoparathyroidism and is often found to be more effective for this purpose than is vitamin D_2, as it causes a greater mobilization of bone.

hydroxydione sodium A compound related to adrenal steroids and once injected intravenously for the induction of general or basal anesthesia.

25-hydroxyergocalciferol A compound formed by hydroxylation of ergocalciferol, a minor form of vitamin D, in the same way as 25-hydroxycholecalciferol is formed from cholecalciferol.

hydroxyestradiols A large class of estradiol metabolites, comprising compounds with a hydroxyl group at the 2,6,15 and

2,6,16 positions. Some of these are further metabolized in the periphery to methoxyestrones.

hydroxyestrin benzoate ESTRADIOL BENZOATE.

hydroxyethylapocupreine A derivative of quinine that was formerly used in the treatment of pneumonia.

5-hydroxyindoleacetic acid A metabolite of tryptophan found in urine.

11-hydroxy-17-ketosteroid A steroid likely to be androgenic, because of the carbonyl group at C-17 and the removal of the two-carbon side chain of adrenocortical hormones. It is also likely to be of adrenal origin, since the 11-hydroxyl group is present.

hydroxyl [HYDR- + *ox(y)-*[1] + Gk *(h)yl(ē)* wood, material, stuff] The group formed from one hydrogen atom and one oxygen atom.

hydroxylamine 1 Any compound of general formula $R-NH-OH$ where R is an alkyl radical. 2 NH_2-OH. An unstable compound forming colorless crystals, soluble in water and various organic solvents. It is a weak base (pK 7.97). Because of its instability its salts (hydrochloride, sulfate) are used as reducing agents or as reagents in organic chemistry. It is a nucleophile, and liberates thiols and alcohols from their esters. Sensitive tests exist for the hydroxamic acids formed, and this is used for assaying thioesters.

hydroxylase Any enzyme that replaces a hydrogen atom with a hydroxyl group, usually using molecular oxygen as oxidant. Such enzymes are monooxygenases if the second atom of oxygen is reduced to water, and they are dioxygenases if it is incorporated into the same substrate or into a second substrate. An outmoded term.

hydroxylation The process of replacing a hydrogen atom with a hydroxyl group.

5-hydroxylysine An amino acid present in collagen and some other proteins. It is produced by hydroxylation of lysine residues already incorporated into the protein. In some proteins the hydroxyl group is glycosylated.

hydroxymethylglutaryl-CoA synthase The enzyme (EC 4.1.3.5) that forms 3-hydroxy-3-methylglutaryl-CoA and coenzyme A from acetyl-CoA, acetoacetyl-CoA, and water. This reaction is a step both in the formation of isoprenoid compounds, including steroids and terpenses, and in the liberation of free acetoacetate.

5-hydroxymethyl cytosine Cytosine with a hydroxymethyl substituent on C-5. It occurs in certain forms of DNA, especially those of bacteriophages. It is made as part of the 2'-deoxycytidine 5'-phosphate molecule by transfer of the hydroxymethyl group from methylene-tetrahydrofolate.

hydroxymethylglutaryl-CoA lyase The enzyme (EC 4.1.3.4) that cleaves 3-hydroxy-3-methylglutaryl-CoA into acetoacetate and acetyl-CoA. This is the main reaction that forms free acetoacetate during ketosis.

hydroxymethylglutaryl-CoA reductase One of the enzymes responsible for the conversion of 3-hydroxy-3-methylglutaryl-CoA into mevalonate and coenzyme A. Two molecules of NADH are required by one such enzyme (EC 1.1.1.88), and two of NADPH by another (EC 1.1.1.34). The reaction is involved in the synthesis of isoprenoid compounds such as steroids.

β-hydroxy-β-methylglutaryl-coenzyme A $HOOC-CH_2-C(OH)(CH_3)-CH_2-CO-$coenzyme-A. A thioester formed by the action of hydroxymethylglutaryl-CoA synthase in the pathway of conversion of acetyl-CoA derived from fats into steroids and other isoprenoid compounds.

hydroxymethyltransferase Any enzyme that catalyzes the transfer of a hydroxymethyl group, $HO-CH_2-$, in exchange for a hydrogen atom. Such enzymes often use 5,10-methylene-tetrahydrofolate as the donor of the hydroxymethyl group. The reaction is equivalent to the addition of formaldehyde.

β-hydroxymyristic acid   A C_{14} saturated fatty acid found attached to the amino groups of glucosamine in lipid A of lipopolysaccharide.

hydroxyphenamate   2-Hydroxy-2-phenylbutyl carbamate. A carbamate with properties like those of meprobamate. It has been used as a minor tranquilizer for anxiety and tension states.

p-hydroxyphenylpyruvic acid   The 2-oxoacid formed from tyrosine by transamination. It is an intermediate in the pathway of tyrosine catabolism, in which it is degraded to homogentisic acid and carbon dioxide by reaction with oxygen catalyzed by 4-hydroxyphenylpyruvate dioxygenase.

hydroxyphenyluria   Urinary excretion of phenylalanine and tyrosine. It occurs in premature infants deficient in ascorbic acid.

17α-hydroxyprogesterone   17α-Hydroxy-pregn-4-ene-3,20-dione, a C_{21} steroid hormone, of great importance as an intermediate step between pregnenolone and cortisol in adrenocortical hormone biosynthesis. Also called *α-progesterone*.

hydroxyprogesterone caproate   3,20-Dioxopregn-4-en-17α-yl hexanoate. It is used to treat functional uterine bleeding, dysmenorrhea, endometriosis, and threatened abortion. It is given intramuscularly and has a slow onset and prolonged effect for 7 to 17 days. Also called *hypoprogesterone hexanoate*.

hydroxyproline   An amino acid found in collagen, formed by hydroxylation of proline residues after they have been incorporated into the protein. Most of the hydroxyproline present is 4-hydroxyproline, but some is 3-hydroxyproline.

hydroxyproline epimerase   The bacterial enzyme (EC 5.1.1.8) that catalyzes the inversion of configuration at C-2 of 4-hydroxyproline, irrespective of the configuration at C-4.

hydroxyprolinemia   An excess quantity of hydroxyproline in the blood, as in conditions of collagen degradation.

hydroxyprolinuria   An excess quantity of hydroxyproline in the urine, as in conditions of collagen degradation.

15-α-hydroxy prostaglandin dehydrogenase   An enzyme that inactivates prostaglandins by converting the 15-α-hydroxy groups to a ketone.

hydroxypyridine   Each of the three isomeric phenols derived from pyridine, $C_5H_4N(OH)$. The o- and p- compounds exist largely in their quinonoid tautomers with —NH— and =O groups.

8-hydroxyquinoline sulfate   A yellow powder, soluble in water, that is used in very low concentrations as a preservative in syrups, and in skin medications as an antibacterial and antifungal agent. Also called *oxyquinoline sulfate*.

hydroxystearin sulfate   A hydrophilic ointment base prepared by sulfating hydrogenated castor oil.

12-hydroxystearyl alcohol CH_3—$[CH_2]_5$—CHOH—$[CH_2]_{10}$—CH_2OH. Octadecan-1,12-diol, made by hydrogenating ricin oil, and having a melting point of 69°C. It is used to make plastics, surface-active agents, and pharmaceutical products.

11-hydroxysteroid   A steroid hydroxylated at C-11, usually a product of the adrenal cortex.

hydroxystilbamidine isethionate $C_{16}H_{16}N_4O \cdot 2C_2H_6O_4S$. 2-Hydroxy-4,4'-diquanylstilbene diisethionate. A yellow powder used in the treatment of fungal and protozoan diseases. It is effective against leishmanial infections and North American blastomycosis.

hydroxytetracycline   OXYTETRACYCLINE.

hydroxytoluic acid   Each of the phenolic acids of formula CH_3—$C_6H_3(OH)$—CO_2H, derived from a cresol by substituting a carboxyl group for a hydrogen atom. Ten isomers exist.

5-hydroxytryptamine   See under SEROTONIN.

5-hydroxytryptophan   The product of hydroxylation of tryptophan at C-5. It is an intermediate in the formation of serotonin (5-hydroxytryptamine), which is formed by its decarboxylation.

hydroxyurea $CH_4N_2O_2$. A white powder used to treat chronic granulocytic leukemia, melanoma, and inoperable tumors of the ovary. It inhibits DNA synthesis.

hydroxyzine $C_{21}H_{27}ClN_2O_2$. N-(4-Chlorobenzhydryl)-N'-(hydroxyethyloxyethyl)-piperazine. An antihistaminic drug with sedative properties. It is used as an antiemetic agent, for pre- and postoperative sedation, and for the treatment of anxiety and tension.

Hydrozoa   [HYDRO- + Gk *zōa*, pl. of *zōon* living being, animal] A class of invertebrates of the phylum Cnidaria; the hydroids and velum-bearing medusae. They are characterized by radial symmetry, gastric tentacles or septa in the gastrovascular cavity, and a horny or calcareous exoskeleton. They are chiefly marine and may be either colonial or solitary.

hydrozoan   [HYDRO- + Gk *zō(on)* living being, animal + English *-an*, suffix denoting belonging to] Any member of the class Hydrozoa. Also called *hydroid*.

hyenanchin $C_{15}H_{18}O_7$. A poisonous substance isolated from the fruit of *Toxicodendron capense (Hyaenache globosa)*.

Hyflo supercel   A purified form of kieselguhr. A trade name.

hygeiolatry   1 A preoccupation with one's health. An obsolete term. 2 An obsolete term for HYPOCHONDRIASIS.

hygeiophrontis   [after *Hygei(a)* goddess of health in ancient Greece + *o* + Gk *phrontis* care, heed, thought] HYPOCHONDRIASIS.

hygieiology   [Gk *hygiei(a)* health + *o* + -LOGY] The science of hygiene and sanitation. Also *hygieology, hygiology*.

hygiene   [Gk *hygieinē*, fem. of *hygieinos* wholesome, healthy, healthful, sound] The principles governing healthy development and the maintenance of health, and the practice of those principles. Also called *hygienics*.

criminal hygiene   A branch of mental hygiene concerned with the causes, prevention, and treatment of antisocial behavior.

environmental hygiene   The science concerned with environmental influences in promoting or preserving health and preventing disease or infirmity. Also called *environmental health, environmental medicine* (imprecise).

industrial hygiene   OCCUPATIONAL HYGIENE. ● See note at OCCUPATIONAL HYGIENE.

mental hygiene   The totality of measures undertaken to deal with mental disorders through prevention, early detection, and treatment, and to improve the adaptation of patients to their social and occupational milieu. Also called *psychophylaxis*.

occupational hygiene   A branch of occupational health which deals with the measurement, evaluation, and control of these environmental factors in the workplace to which exposure may be hazardous to health. Also called *industrial hygiene*. ● The term is used chiefly in the United Kingdom, Australia, and India. In New Zealand and Japan, *industrial hygiene* is the preferred term, and is also used in Britain. Neither term is used in the U.S. or South Africa.

radiation hygiene   RADIOLOGICAL HEALTH.

sex hygiene   Those aspects of hygiene relating to the sex organs and to sexual behavior.

social hygiene   The prevention and treatment of venereal disease. An obsolete term.

hygienic   1 Of or relating to hygiene. 2 Conducive to health; sanitary.

hygienics   HYGIENE.

hygienist One who specializes in hygiene, or in a specific branch of hygiene, as a dental hygienist.

dental hygienist A skilled and sometimes licensed ancillary worker who assists a dentist and performs certain therapeutic and preventive services under the dentist's supervision.

hygieology HYGIEIOLOGY.

hygiology HYGIEIOLOGY.

hygr- HYGRO-.

hygrechema [HYGR- + Gk *ēchēma* a sound] The sound heard on auscultation of the lungs over a fluid-containing cavity. A seldom used term.

hygremometry Estimation of hemoglobin concentration of blood by drying and weighing a measured volume of blood. An obsolete procedure.

hygric [HYGR- + -IC] **1** Concerning moisture. **2** Moist.

hygric acid *N*-methylproline, which can be formed from hygrine by oxidation. An outmoded term. Also called *hygrinic acid.*

hygrine 2-(2-Oxopropyl)-*N*-methylpyrrolidine. An alkaloid derived from ornithine.

hygrinic acid HYGRIC ACID.

hygro- [Gk *hygros* moist, wet, liquid] A combining form meaning moist, moisture. Also *hygr-.*

hygroblepharic [HYGRO- + BLEPHAR- + -IC] Having a condition resulting in wet eyelids.

hygrocole [HYGRO- + L *col(ere)* to cultivate, inhabit] An animal that lives in a moist habitat.

hygrograph [HYGRO- + -GRAPH] An instrument for recording changes in atmospheric humidity.

hygroma [HYGR- + -OMA] **1** A cystic lymphangioma. **2** A fluid-filled tumor. Also called *hydroma.*

acute traumatic subdural hygroma A subdural hygroma forming over one or both cerebral hemispheres following head injury.

hygroma axillare A hygroma of the axilla.

hygroma colli A hygroma or cystic hygroma of the neck.

cystic hygroma A congenital cystic lymphangioma of the neck. Also called *hygroma cysticum, hygroma cysticum colli.*

hygroma cysticum CYSTIC HYGROMA.

hygroma cysticum colli CYSTIC HYGROMA.

Fleischmann's hygroma An accumulation of fluid in the bursa found occasionally between the genioglossus muscle and the septum linguae.

multiloculated hygroma A hygroma with multiple cystic cavities.

hygroma praepatellare Fluid collection in the prepatellar bursa.

subdural hygroma A collection of cerebrospinal fluid in the subdural space.

hygromatous Pertaining to a hygroma.

hygrometer [HYGRO- + -METER] An instrument used to measure the moisture of the atmosphere. Also called *psychrometer.*

dew point hygrometer DEW POINT INDICATOR.

hair hygrometer A hygrometer that indicates changes in atmospheric moisture by measuring the extension and contraction in length of a human hair. Also called *Saussure's hygrometer.*

Saussure's hygrometer HAIR HYGROMETER.

wet and dry bulb hygrometer A hygrometer consisting of two identical thermometers. The bulb of one is dry and the other is covered by a thin film of water or ice. Evaporation results in a depressed reading on the wet bulb thermometer, the degree of which will vary according to the amount of atmospheric moisture. The humidity percentage is determined by reference to tables. Also called *wet and dry bulb psychrometer, Mason psychrometer.*

hygrometric [HYGRO- + *metr(e)* + -IC] Pertaining to the measurement of atmospheric humidity.

hygrometry [HYGRO- + -METRY] The science of measuring the moisture in the atmosphere. Adjective: hygrometric.

hygrophanous [HYGRO- + Gk *-phan(ēs)*, combining form from *phainein* to bring to light, make appear + -OUS] Having the property of changing color as conditions change from moist to dry.

hygroscopic Capable of absorbing water from moist air.

hygrothermograph [HYGRO- + THERMO- + -GRAPH] A visual record of temperature and relative humidity readings taken over a period of several days.

hygrothermometer [HYGRO- + THERMOMETER] An instrument that measures temperature and relative humidity.

Hygroton A proprietary name for chlorthalidone.

Hyl Symbol for hydroxylysine.

hyl- HYLO-.

hyla [Gk *hyl(ē)* wood, material, stuff, forest] A lateral evagination of the cerebral aqueduct (of Sylvius). Also called *paraqueduct.*

hyle- HYLO-.

Hylemyia A genus of flies that breed in vegetables, and whose larvae may be ingested by humans causing accidental or false parasitism.

hylergography The recording of the activity of cells as they respond to environmental influences.

hylo- [Gk *hylē* wood, material, stuff] A combining form denoting matter, substance. Also *hyl-, hyle-.*

hyloma [HYL- + -OMA] A tumor of embryonic tissue. An obsolete term. Also called *hylic tumor.* ● Tumors of specific embryonic tissues have been described with this term, such as *mesenchymal hyloma* and *mesothelial hyloma.* These too are obsolete.

hylophobia [Gk *hyl(ē)* wood, a wood, forest + *o* + -PHOBIA] Pathologic fear of being in a forest.

hymen [Gk *hymēn* a skin, membrane] A thin crescentic or annular fold of mucous membrane that partially or completely occludes the vaginal orifice. It varies considerably in shape and extent and may be absent. Also called *claustrum virginale* (outmoded), *virginal membrane* (outmoded), *hymenal membrane, maidenhead* (obsolete).

annular hymen CIRCULAR HYMEN.

hymen bifenestratus A hymen in which there are two openings separated by a wide band of tissue. Also called *hymen biforis, bilobate hymen.*

hymen biforis HYMEN BIFENESTRATUS.

bilobate hymen HYMEN BIFENESTRATUS.

circular hymen A hymen that has a circular opening. Also called *annular hymen.*

crescentic hymen A crescent-shaped hymen that partially closes the ostium vaginae posteriorly, as is normal in many virgins. Also called *falciform hymen, lunar hymen.*

cribriform hymen A hymen with a number of small perforations. Also called *fenestrated hymen.*

denticular hymen A hymen with an opening that has serrated edges resembling teeth.

embryonic hymen A plug of epithelial tissue at the lower end of the paramesonephric ducts. It is the anlage of the hymen.

falciform hymen CRESCENTIC HYMEN.

fenestrated hymen CRIBRIFORM HYMEN.

fimbriate hymen A hymen with ragged edges.

imperforate hymen A hymen without an opening.

infundibuliform hymen A funnel-shaped hymen.

lunar hymen CRESCENTIC HYMEN.

septate hymen A hymen with two openings separated by a

narrow band of tissue. Also called *hymen septus*.

hymen septus   SEPTATE HYMEN.

hymen subseptus   A hymen that is partially closed by a band of adventitious tissue.

hymenal   Pertaining to the hymen.

hymenectomy [HYMEN + -ECTOMY]   Excision of the hymen.

hymenia   Plural of HYMENIUM.

hymenitis [HYMEN + -ITIS]   Inflammation of the hymen.

hymenium [Gk *hymēn* skin, membrane + L -*ium*, noun suffix] (*plural* hymenia)   A fertile layer of a fungus, consisting of asci or basidia. Also called *thecium*.

hymenography   HYMENOLOGY.

hymenolepiasis   An infection or disease due to worms of the cestode genus *Hymenolepis*.

hymenolepidid [from *Hymenolepidid(ae)*]   **1** Pertaining or belonging to the cestode family Hymenolepididae.   **2** Any cestode of the family Hymenolepididae.

Hymenolepididae   A large family of small to medium-sized tapeworms (order Cyclophyllidea, subclass Cestoda) parasitic in a variety of vertebrates, including humans. *Hymenolepis* is the medically important genus, *H. nana* being one of the most common tapeworms of humans.

Hymenolepis [*hymeno-*, combining form of HYMEN + Gk *lepis* a scale, husk, shell, flake]   The largest genus of tapeworms in the order Cyclophyllidea and the type genus of the family Hymenolepididae, containing over 300 species, parasitic chiefly in aquatic birds and rodents. The genus has been subdivided by various taxonomists into a number of genera, placing the human parasite *H. nana* for example, in the genus *Vampirolepis*, while retaining unarmed species, including *H. diminuta*, in the type genus.

Hymenolepis diminuta   The rat tapeworm, a common species found in rats and mice, and rarely in humans. The cysticercoid larvae occur in fleas, beetles, caterpillars, and other insects. Also called *Taenia diminuta*.

Hymenolepis fraterna   A non-human-adapted form of the dwarf mouse tapeworm. It is regarded by some as conspecific with the dwarf tapeworm of man, *H. nana*.

Hymenolepis lanceolata   *DREPANIDOTAENIA LANCEOLATA.*

Hymenolepis microstoma   A species found in the biliary passages of rodents. Also called *Rodentolepis microstoma*.

Hymenolepis nana   A species common in humans as well as in mice and rats; the dwarf mouse tapeworm. It is 7–80 mm long and is sometimes found in large numbers in the intestines, especially in children. The cysticercoid larvae can develop through all stages in a single host, or they may pass through a two-host cycle, with flour beetles or other insects as intermediate hosts. Human infections are usually asymptomatic, but in very heavy infections abdominal pain, diarrhea, insomnia, and other symptoms may occur. Rodent and human strains of the parasite appear to have developed. The rodent strain has been called *H. nana* var. *fraterna* or given the species designation *H. fraterna*. Also called *Taenia minima*, *Taenia nana*.

Hymenolepis nana var. fraterna   A variety of the dwarf mouse tapeworm that is not adapted to the human intestine. It is regarded by some as a separate species, *H. fraterna*.

hymenology   The study of the structural organization and functions of the membranes of the body. Also called *hymenography*.

Hymenoptera [HYMEN + o + Gk *ptera* (pl. of *pteron* feather) feathers, wings]   An order of holometabolous insects having locked pairs of membranous wings. It includes wasps, hornets, bees, and ants. They are considered among the most advanced and remarkable of insects owing to their high degree of social development, in which all individuals are members of one or another highly specialized caste.

hymenopteran   **1** Of or belonging to the insect order Hymenoptera.   **2** A member of the order Hymenoptera.

hymenopterism [*Hymenopter(a)* + -ISM]   Poisoning by stings of bees, hornets, or other insects of the order Hymenoptera. Symptoms are local inflammation and various hypersensitivity reactions, sometimes resulting in death due to anaphylactic shock.

hymenorrhaphy [HYMEN + o + -RRHAPHY]   A plastic operation on the hymen to produce partial or complete closure of the vagina.

hymenotome   A surgical instrument used to incise the hymen.

hymenotomy [HYMEN + o + -TOMY]   Surgical incision in the hymen.

hyo- [Gk prefix *hyo-* denoting υ-shaped (upsilon-shaped)]   A combining form meaning (1) U-shaped, υ-shaped; (2) relating to the hyoid.

hyobasioglossus   The posteroinferior part of musculus hyoglossus. A rarely used term.

hyodeoxycholic acid   3,6-Dihydroxycholanic acid. A bile acid whose conjugates are found in pig bile.

hyoepiglottic   Pertaining to the hyoid bone and the epiglottis, specifically their connecting ligament. Also *hyoepiglottidean*.

hyoepiglottidean   HYOEPIGLOTTIC.

hyoglossal   Pertaining to the hyoid bone and the tongue. Also *glossohyal, glossohyoidal*.

hyoid [*hy(o)-* + -OID]   **1** Shaped like the Greek letter upsilon or the Roman letter U, as the hyoid bone.   **2** Pertaining to either the hyoid bone or, in comparative anatomy, the series of bones at the base of the tongue developed from the embryonic hyoid arch. Also *hyal*.   **3** OS HYOIDEUM.

hyolaryngeal   Pertaining to the hyoid bone and the larynx.

hyomandibular   Pertaining to the first and second branchial arches and the groove or pouches lying between them.

hyomental   Pertaining to the hyoid bone and the chin.

hyoscine   SCOPOLAMINE.

hyoscyamine $C_{17}H_{23}NO_3$. 3α-Tropanyl *S*-(-)-tropate. An alkaloid obtained from *Hyoscyamus niger*, *Atropa belladonna*, and other sources. It is the levorotatory isomer of atropine, which is a racemic mixture. Its actions are like those of atropine, but its central and peripheral effects are more pronounced. It is an anticholinergic drug, can be given orally or parenterally, and is used in the treatment of asthma, bronchitis, and mental illness.

hyoscyamine hydrobromide   The hydrobromide salt of hyoscyamine. It has the same properties and uses as atropine.

hyoscyamine sulfate   The sulfate salt of hyoscyamine. It has the same properties and uses as atropine.

hyoscyamus   *Hyoscyamus niger*, an herb of the family Solanaceae. It contains the alkaloids hyoscyamine and scopolamine and has been cultivated for its narcotic properties, but is used medicinally as an antispasmodic. Also called *insane root, henbane, black henbane, poison tobacco*.

hyostapedial   Pertaining to the second branchial arch and its derivatives.

hyosternal   Pertaining to the hyoid bone and the sternum.

Hyostrongylus   A genus of trichostrongyle nematodes. One species, *H. rubidus*, is found in the stomach of swine.

Hyostrongylus rubidus   The red stomach worm of swine; a small, reddish, bloodsucking trichostrongyle nematode found in the mucosa of the stomach of the pig. It causes little damage unless present in very large numbers or the animal is in a general state of poor health, with low resistance to infection.

hyothyroid   THYROHYOID.

hyovertebrotomy [HYO- + VERTEBRO- + -TOMY]   A surgical

opening of the guttural pouch in the horse.

hyp- HYPO-.

hypacusia HYPERACUSIS.

hypadrenia An outmoded term for HYPOADRENALISM.

hypalbuminemia HYPOALBUMINEMIA.

hypalbuminosis HYPOALBUMINEMIA.

hypalgesia [HYP- + ALGESIA] Reduction in sensitivity to pain. Also called *hypalgia, hypoalgesia.* Adjective: hypalgesic, hypalgetic.

hypalgesic Relating to hypalgesia. Also *hypalgetic.*

hypalgetic HYPALGESIC.

hypalgia HYPALGESIA.

hypamnion HYPAMNIOS.

hypamnios [HYP- + Gk *amnion* (from *amnos* a lamb) the membrane around the fetus] Insufficiency of amniotic fluid. Also called *hypamnion.*

hypanakinesia HYPOKINESIA.

hypanakinesis HYPOKINESIA.

hypanisognathism [HYP- + Gk *aniso(s)* unequal + GNATH- + -ISM] A form of malocclusion in which the upper dental arch is too wide to occlude normally with the lower dental arch.

hypaphorine $C_{14}H_{18}N_2O_2$. A poisonous alkaloid obtained from the seeds of *Erythrina americana* and other *Erythrina* species. It causes central nervous system stimulation and convulsions.

hypaphrodisia [HYP- + APHRODISIA] SEXUAL ANESTHESIA.

hyparterial Situated below an artery. Also *hypoarterial.* Compare EPARTERIAL. • The term was first suggested and used with reference to the branches of the bronchi as related to the pulmonary artery.

hypasthenia [HYP- + ASTHENIA] A state of reduced strength. Compare HYPERSTHENIA.

hypatonia HYPOTONIA.

hypaxial 1 Below the axis of the vertebral column, usually with reference to quadrupedal forms, fish, etc.; ventral. 2 Below any axis.

hypemia An obsolete term for ANEMIA.

hypencephalon [HYP- + ENCEPHALON] The midbrain, pons, and medulla oblongata. An obsolete term.

hypenchyme [HYP- + *enchym(a)* + *e*] Primitive cells formed in the archenteron of an embryo.

hypengyophobia [Gk *hypengyo(s)* (from *hyp(o)* under + *engyos* surety) responsible + -PHOBIA] Pathologic fear of responsibility.

hypeosinophil A cell of the granulocyte series that shows only weak staining of the granules with eosin.

hyper- [Gk *hyper* over, above] A prefix meaning (1) over, above; (2) increased, excessive, too much or too many, above the normal. Compare HYPO-.

hyperabduction Excessive abduction. Also called *superabduction.*

hyperacanthosis ACANTHOSIS.

hyperacidaminuria HYPERAMINOACIDURIA.

hyperacidity [HYPER- + ACIDITY] Any condition characterized by a higher than normal concentration or quantity of acid. Also called *peracidity.*

   gastric hyperacidity The secretion of increased amounts of acid by the stomach. See also HYPERCHLORHYDRIA.

hyperacousia HYPERACUSIS.

hyperactive [HYPER- + ACTIVE] Demonstrating an excess of motor activity. Also called *hyperdynamic.*

hyperactivity Excessive activity especially as a part of minimal

brain dysfunction. Also called *hyperdynamia, hyperenergia, hyperergasia, hyperfunction.*

   purposeless hyperactivity Random excess activity that fulfills no purpose. In organic brain disease stimulation sufficient to produce any response typically provokes purposeless hyperactivity in addition to the appropriate response.

hyperacuity [HYPER- + ACUITY] Increased sharpness of sense perception.

hyperacusia HYPERACUSIS.

hyperacusis [HYPER- + ACU-² + -SIS] A condition in which sounds are perceived as unduly loud. Also called *hyperacousia, hypacusia, hyperacusia, oxyacoia, macracusia, paracusia acris.* Also *hyperakusis.*

hyperacute Exceptionally acute or of explosive onset.

hyperadenosis Enlargement of lymph nodes. An obsolete term.

hyperadiposis OBESITY.

hyperadiposity OBESITY.

hyperadrenal [HYPER- + ADRENAL] Marked by excessive function or secretion of the adrenal, especially of the adrenal cortex; hyperadrenocortical. Also *hyperinterrenal.*

hyperadrenalemia HYPEREPINEPHRINEMIA.

hyperadrenalism [HYPERADRENAL + -ISM] Any excessive function of the adrenal gland, especially hyperadrenocorticism. An imprecise usage. Also called *hyperadrenia* (outmoded), *hyperinterrenopathy* (rarely used), *hypersuprarenalism* (outmoded).

hyperadrenia An outmoded term for HYPERADRENALISM.

hyperadrenocortical Of, caused by, or relating to hyperadrenocorticism.

hyperadrenocorticalism HYPERADRENOCORTICISM.

hyperadrenocorticism The clinical condition induced by excessive amounts of glucocorticoids, either due to oversecretion of cortisol by the adrenal cortex in Cushing syndrome (hypercortisolism) or to long-term administration of any corticosteroid during treatment, as for an allergic or inflammatory disease. Also called *hyperadrenocorticalism, hypercorticalism, hypercorticism.*

hyperaemia A British spelling for HYPEREMIA.

hyperaeration [HYPER- + AERATION] HYPERVENTILATION.

hyperaesthesia A British spelling for HYPERESTHESIA.

hyperaffectivity Emotional overreaction to mild stimuli.

hyperakusis HYPERACUSIS.

hyperalbuminemia A greater than normal concentration of albumin in plasma. Also called *hyperalbuminosis, polyemia hyperalbuminosa, albuminosis* (rarely used).

hyperalbuminosis HYPERALBUMINEMIA.

hyperalcoholemia ALCOHOLEMIA.

hyperaldosteronemia A greater than normal concentration of aldosterone in plasma.

hyperaldosteronism ALDOSTERONISM.

hyperaldosteronuria [HYPER- + *aldosteron(e)* + -URIA] Excess excretion of aldosterone in the urine, associated with any condition that increases aldosterone secretion by the adrenal cortex.

hyperalgesia [HYPER- + ALGESIA] Excessive sensitivity to painful stimuli. Also called *hyperalgia.* Adjective: hyperalgesic, hyperalgetic.

   auditory hyperalgesia A condition of the ear in which pain is experienced in response to auditory stimuli insufficiently intense to cause pain in the normal subject.

   muscular hyperalgesia Pain induced by movement in fatigued muscles.

   olfactory hyperalgesia Pain in the nose induced by specific olfactory stimuli.

hyperalgesic Pertaining to hyperalgesia. Also *hyperalgetic*.

hyperalgetic HYPERALGESIC.

hyperalgia [HYPER- + -ALGIA] HYPERALGESIA.

hyperalimentation Administration of nutritive substances in quantities exceeding the normal requirements of the individual; superalimentation. • *Hyperalimentation* is usually used to refer specifically to parenteral hyperalimentation or total parenteral nutrition.

 parenteral hyperalimentation The intravenous administration of greater than the normally optimal amounts of essential nutrients. See also TOTAL PARENTERAL NUTRITION.

hyperalimented Having received total parenteral nutrition.

hyperalimentosis [HYPER- + ALIMENT + -OSIS] Disease arising from the consumption of too much food.

hyperallantoinuria [HYPER- + ALLANTOIN + -URIA] An increased urinary content of allantoin. An end product of purine metabolism, it is not normally produced by humans because they lack the enzyme uricase.

hyperalonemia A greater than normal concentration of anions and cations in plasma.

hyperaminoacidemia The presence of amino acids in the blood in greater than normal concentration.

hyperaminoaciduria [HYPER- + AMINOACIDURIA] Excess urinary excretion of amino acids, either specific or general. It is usually related to chronic nephritis or to specific defects in tubular reabsorption, as in the Fanconi syndrome. Also called *hyperacidaminuria*.

hyperammonemia A greater than normal concentration of ammonium in plasma, commonly observed in patients with decompensation of liver function. Also called *hyperammoniemia, ammonemia, ammoniemia*.

hyperammoniemia HYPERAMMONEMIA.

hyperammonuria [HYPER- + AMMONURIA] Excess urinary excretion of ammonia, usually as a compensatory response to systemic acidosis.

hyperamylasemia A greater than normal activity of amylase in plasma, as is commonly observed in acute pancreatitis. Also called *diastemia*.

hyperanabolism Excessive retention of nitrogen, as in excessive growth hormone secretion.

hyperandrogenism [HYPER- + ANDROGEN + -ISM] Any condition caused by oversecretion of androgenic hormones, as virilism in the female.

hyperaphia [HYPER- + Gk *(h)aph(ē)* a touching, touch + -IA] Increased sensitivity to touch. Also called *hyperaphy, tactile hyperesthesia, hyperselaphesia, oxyaphia*. Adjective: hyperaphic.

hyperaphy HYPERAPHIA.

hyperazotemia AZOTEMIA.

hyperbaric [HYPER- + BAR-² + -IC] At greater than atmospheric pressure.

hyperbarism [HYPER- + BAR-² + -ISM] Any condition caused by exposure of the body to excessive ambient pressures, including adverse effects on body fluids, tissues, and cavities. An example is oxygen toxicity.

hyperbasophilic Characterized by a strong affinity for basic dyes.

hyperbetaalaninemia A rare, severe, inborn error of alanine metabolism presumably due to a deficiency of β-alanine-α-ketoglutarate aminotransferase. The condition's profound mental retardation and seizures are accompanied by an abnormal accumulation of alanine and γ-aminobutyric acid in the plasma and the urine.

hyperbetalipoproteinemia Elevated concentration of β-lipoproteins in the blood.

familial hyperbetalipoproteinemia FAMILIAL HYPERCHOLESTEROLEMIA.

hyperbicarbonatemia An elevated concentration of bicarbonate in the blood or blood serum. Also called *bicarbonatemia*.

hyperbilirubinemia [HYPER- + BILIRUBINEMIA] An increased concentration of bilirubin in the blood or blood serum, causing jaundice when sufficiently increased.

 hyperbilirubinemia I GILBERT SYNDROME.

 anicteric hyperbilirubinemia Hyperbilirubinemia without clinically evident jaundice.

 congenital hyperbilirubinemia CRIGLER-NAJJAR SYNDROME.

 constitutional hyperbilirubinemia GILBERT SYNDROME.

 hereditary nonhemolytic hyperbilirubinemia GILBERT SYNDROME.

hyperblastosis HYPERPLASIA.

hyperbrachycephalic Exhibiting hyperbrachycephaly. Also *hyperbrachycranial*.

hyperbrachycephaly An abnormally great degree of brachycephaly, with a cephalic index exceeding 85.

hyperbrachycranial HYPERBRACHYCEPHALIC.

hyperbulia [HYPER- + Gk *boul(ē)* determination, task + -IA] Bizarre or inappropriate application and assiduousness in trivial tasks.

hypercalcemia [HYPER- + CALCEMIA] An elevated concentration of calcium in the blood or blood serum. Also called *hypercalcinemia*.

 idiopathic hypercalcemia A rare disease of infants, with symptoms of failure to thrive, constipation, thirst, and dehydration. A characteristic elfin facies is described. Serum calcium is raised and blood urea is high. Cardiac lesions such as aortic and pulmonary stenosis are often present. The disorder is thought to be due to an abnormal sensitivity to vitamin D. Few cases have been seen since about 1960.

hypercalcinemia HYPERCALCEMIA.

hypercalcinuria [HYPER- + CALCINE + -URIA] HYPERCALCIURIA.

hypercalcipexy An excessive fixation of calcium salts.

hypercalcitoninemia The presence of excessive calcitonin in the blood, as in the Sipple syndrome or multiple endocrine neoplasia type II. Detection of this abnormality is used as early evidence of dysfunction of the thyroidal parafollicular cells before a definite medullary carcinoma develops. Blood calcitonin concentrations are also raised, that is, above 100–200 pg/ml, in hypercalcemic states, oat cell carcinoma of the lung, carcinoma of the breast, and chronic renal disease.

hypercalciuria [HYPER- + CALCIURIA] Excretion in the urine of more than 200 mg calcium per day on a diet containing 400 mg calcium per day. Nephrolithiasis is a common complication while nephrocalcinosis also may occur. Hypercalciuria may occur whenever hypercalcemia due to any cause is present. It may occur without hypercalcemia in renal tubular acidosis, normocalcemic hyperparathyroidism, or in an idiopathic form. Mechanisms for hypercalciuria include resorptive, absorptive, and renal hypercalciuria. Also called *hypercalcinuria*.

 absorptive hypercalciuria Hypercalciuria in which the primary mechanism is excessive absorption of calcium from the intestines, most commonly in primary or idiopathic hyperabsorption of calcium, but also in sarcoidosis and hypervitaminosis D.

 idiopathic hypercalciuria Hypercalciuria either from idiopathic hyperabsorption of calcium for the intestines or idiopathic decreased renal tubular absorption of calcium.

 renal hypercalciuria Hypercalciuria in which the primary mechanism is reduction of renal tubular reabsorption of calcium.

The idiopathic form is the most common. Renal hypercalciuria also occurs in untreated renal tubular acidosis and in treated hyperparathyroidism.

resorptive hypercalciuria Hypercalciuria in which the primary mechanism is excess mobilization of skeletal calcium, as in primary hyperparathyroidism, malignancy of the bone, or in the active phases of degenerative bone diseases.

secondary hypercalciuria Hypercalciuria due to known causes such as primary hyperparathyroidism, renal tubular acidosis, bone malignancy, sarcoidosis, or hypervitaminosis D.

hypercapnia An elevated concentration of carbon dioxide in the blood. Also called *hypercarbia*.

hypercapnic Relating to or characterized by hypercapnia.

hypercarbia HYPERCAPNIA.

hypercardia [HYPER- + -CARDIA] HYPERCARDIOTROPHY.

hypercardiotrophy Cardiac hypertrophy; enlargement of the heart. Also called *hypercardia*.

hypercarotenemia An elevated concentration of carotene in the blood or blood serum. The condition arises when one regularly eats very large amounts of foods rich in carotenoids, such as carrots. The plasma becomes orange-yellow and the skin can become tinged with the same color. It can be distinguished from jaundice as the eyes do not become yellow. The condition is benign, since vitamin A is not formed in toxic amounts in the body, and the skin reverts to its normal color on reducing the in take of carotenoids. Also called *hypercarotenosis, aurantiasis, carotenemia* (imprecise), *carotinemia* (imprecise), *carotenosis, carotinosis, xanthemia*.

hypercarotenosis HYPERCAROTENEMIA.

hypercatabolic Relating to hypercatabolism.

hypercatabolism A state of abnormally excessive breakdown of complex compounds into simpler substances.

hypercathexis Excessive investment of psychic force in an object or person, including parts of one's self.

hypercedemonia Excessive grief or anxiety. An outmoded term.

hypercellularity An increase in the number of cells within a structure such as the bone marrow or the renal glomeruli. Adjective: hypercellular.

    glomerular hypercellularity An increase in the number of cells of the renal glomerulus caused by proliferation of intrinsic cells as well as infiltration by inflammatory cells. It is characteristic of certain forms of glomerulonephritis.

hypercementosis [HYPER- + CEMENTOSIS] CEMENTOSIS.

hypercenesthesia A feeling of exaggerated well-being, euphoria, or elation.

hyperchloremia An elevated concentration of chloride in the blood or blood serum. Also called *chloridemia, chloruremia* (obsolete).

hyperchloremic Relating to or characterized by hyperchloremia. Also called *chloruremic* (obsolete).

hyperchlorhydria Excessive gastric secretion of hydrochloric acid, seen particularly in duodenal ulcer disease and the Zollinger-Ellison syndrome. Also called *Rossbach's disease, hyperhydrochloria*.

hyperchloridation The creation of a state of excessive blood chloride content by the administration of sodium chloride.

hyperchloruria [HYPER- + *chlor(ide)* + -URIA] Excretion of greater than normal amounts of chloride in the urine. In general, chloride excretion approximates its intake, and parallels that of sodium. Hyperchloruria may be associated with excess chloride intake, diuretics, or spontaneous diuresis.

hypercholesteremia HYPERCHOLESTEROLEMIA.

hypercholesteremic HYPERCHOLESTEROLEMIC.

hypercholesterinemia HYPERCHOLESTEROLEMIA.

hypercholesterolemia [HYPER- + CHOLESTEROLEMIA] An elevated concentration of cholesterol in the blood or blood serum. Also called *hypercholesterinemia, hypercholesteremia, cholesteremia, cholesterinemia*.

    essential hypercholesterolemia FAMILIAL HYPERLIPOPROTEINEMIA TYPE III.

    familial hypercholesterolemia A hereditary disorder of lipid metabolism of autosomal dominant transmittance, characterized by cutaneous and tendon xanthomas, premature arcus corneae, recurrent polyarthritis, accelerated atherosclerosis, and myocardial infarction in the fourth or fifth decade of life. Heterozygotes are relatively common, with a frequency of 1 in 500. The rare homozygotes have a qualitatively similar, but much more severe, condition, and often die in their teens. There is a marked increase in cholesterol of the low density lipoprotein (LDL) fraction. Serum concentration of high density lipoprotein is reduced. The disorder is due to a mutation in the LDL receptor of cell membranes, resulting in a functional deficiency of LDL receptors. Also called *familial hyperlipoproteinemia type IIa, familial hyperbetalipoproteinemia, LDL-receptor disorder*.

hypercholesterolemic 1 Having a greater than normal cholesterol concentration: said of a blood specimen. 2 Denoting a person who has hypercholesterolemic blood. For defs. 1 and 2 also *hypercholesteremic*.

hypercholesterolia Excessive cholesterol in bile.

hypercholia [HYPER- + CHOL- + -IA] Excessive bile secretion.

hyperchondroplasia The excessive formation of cartilage.

hyperchromaffinism A disorder characterized by excessive secretion of chromaffin substances (sympathicomimetic agents) and associated with paroxysmal hypertension.

hyperchromasia HYPERCHROMATISM.

hyperchromatic Characterized by intense coloration, either from natural pigments or from strong affinity for colored dyes. Also *hyperchromic*.

hyperchromatin Chromatin which stains with a blue aniline dye.

hyperchromatism The increased or excessive staining capacity of a structure such as the nuclei of cancer cells, which stain excessively with hematoxylin owing to their increased nucleic acid (chromosomal) content. Also called *hyperchromasia, hyperchromia*.

hyperchromatopsia [HYPER- + CHROMAT- + -OPSIA] A disorder of visual perception in which everything the individual sees is colored or abnormally colored.

hyperchromatosis Increased avidity for a stain. A seldom used term.

hyperchromia 1 HYPERCHROMATISM. 2 The more intense staining, in blood films, of macrocytes when compared with normal erythrocytes. Also called *macrocytic hyperchromia*. • The term in this latter sense has been used on analogy with *hypochromia*, but seldom.

    macrocytic hyperchromia HYPERCHROMIA.

hyperchromic HYPERCHROMATIC.

hyperchromicity An increase in the absorption of ultraviolet light by solutions of polynucleotides due to a loss of the secondary structure. The secondary structure can be lost as the nucleotide "melts" due to heating.

hyperchylia [HYPER- + CHYL- + -IA] GASTRIC HYPERSECRETION.

hyperchylomicronemia [HYPER- + CHYLOMICRONEMIA] CHYLOMICRONEMIA.

    familial hyperchylomicronemia FAMILIAL HYPERLIPOPROTEINEMIA TYPE I.

hypercitruria [HYPER- + citr(ate) + -URIA] Increased urinary excretion of citrate in alkalosis. The increased citrate enhances calcium solubility and thus may decrease or prevent calcium precipitation in urine and renal parenchyma.

hypercoagulability **1** A thrombotic tendency. **2** Elevation of one or more coagulation factors. **3** Reduction of coagulation inhibitors. **4** Accelerated clotting in vitro. A vague term.

hypercoagulable Characterized by hypercoagulability.

hypercompensation OVERCOMPENSATION.

hypercoria HYPERKORIA.

hypercorticalism HYPERADRENOCORTICISM.

hypercorticism HYPERADRENOCORTICISM.

hypercorticotropism [HYPER- + CORTICO- + TROPISM] A condition resulting from excessive production of adrenocorticotropic hormone, as by the anterior pituitary in Cushing's disease or by a hormone-producing carcinoma.

hypercortisolism The condition resulting from excessive endogenous production of cortisol or administration of exogenous cortisol or its congeners; hyperadrenocorticism.

hypercreatinemia Excessive creatine in the blood, evidence of excessively rapid breakdown of muscle tissue, as in thyrotoxicosis.

hypercrine [HYPER- + Gk krin(ein) to separate, put apart] Resulting from an excess of a hormone or hormones. A seldom used term.

hypercrinism The somatic condition resulting from excessive secretion of a hormone or hormones. An obsolete term.

hypercryalgesia HYPERCRYESTHESIA.

hypercryesthesia [HYPER- + CRY- + -ESTHESIA] Extreme sensitivity to cold. Also called hypercryalgesia.

hypercupremia A greater than normal concentration of copper in blood.

hypercupriuria Excretion of greater than usual amounts of copper in the urine. Hypercupriuria is a characteristic of hepatolenticular disease, and reflects the excess accumulation of copper in the body in this disease.

hypercyanotic Characterized by extreme cyanosis.

hypercyesis SUPERFETATION.

hypercythemia ERYTHROCYTOSIS.

hypercytochromia [HYPER- + CYTO- + CHROM- + -IA] A heightened affinity of a cell, especially a blood cell, for stains.

hypercytosis An abnormally elevated number of cells in blood. An obsolete term.

hyperdacryosis [HYPER- + DACRYO- + -SIS] A condition of excessive tearing of the eyes.

hyperdactylia POLYDACTYLY.

hyperdactylism POLYDACTYLY.

hyperdactyly POLYDACTYLY.

hyperdiadochokinesia [HYPER- + DIADOCHOKINESIA] Diadochokinesia in which the rotatory movements of the hand are of greater excursion than usual, thus constituting a particular type of hypermetria. It is usually associated with dysdiadochokinesia in cerebellar lesions.

hyperdiastole Extreme dilatation of the heart during diastole. Also hyperdiastoly.

hyperdiastoly HYPERDIASTOLE.

hyperdicrotic Characterized by exaggerated dicrotism.

hyperdicrotism A state of exaggerated dicrotism.

hyperdiemorrhysis Increased blood flow through the veins.

hyperdiploid Having a chromosome complement slightly in excess of that found in the usual diploid state of a cell or an organism.

hyperdiploidy The state of being hyperdiploid.

hyperdipsia Increased thirst and consequently an increased consumption of fluids.

hyperdolichocranial Having an extremely long and narrow head, with a breadth considerably less than 70 percent of its length.

hyperdontia [HYPER- + -(o)dontia] POLYDONTIA.

hyperdontogeny [HYPER- + (o)donto- + -GEN + -Y] The replacement of the permanent dentition by a third series of teeth.

hyperdynamia HYPERACTIVITY.

hyperdynamia uteri Hypertonic uterine contractions during labor.

hyperdynamic HYPERACTIVE.

hypereccrisia A state marked by excessive excretion. Also called hypereccrisis.

hypereccrisis HYPERECCRISIA.

hypereccritic Of or relating to hypereccrisia.

hyperechoic [HYPER- + ECHOIC] Producing echoes of higher amplitude or density than the surrounding medium.

hyperelastic Characterized by an unusually increased state of elasticity.

hyperelectrolytemia A greater than normal concentration of anions and cations in blood, as may occur due to dehydration. A seldom used term.

hyperemesis [HYPER- + EMESIS] Excessive or severe, protracted vomiting.

hyperemesis gravidarum Excessive and persistent vomiting associated with pregnancy, usually experienced during the first trimester.

hyperemetic Relating to or characterized by hyperemesis.

hyperemia [HYPER- + -EMIA] An increase in the volume of blood in an affected part or tissue due to arterial or arteriolar dilatation.

active hyperemia Increase of blood flow to a segment of the body through vascular dilatation. Also called fluxionary hyperemia.

arterial hyperemia Increase in blood flow due to arterial dilatation.

Bier's passive hyperemia BIER'S TREATMENT.

collateral hyperemia A compensatory increase in arterial blood flow through preexisting collateral vessels as a consequence of the interruption of blood flow through the main artery supplying a part.

constriction hyperemia Passive hyperemia induced by a constriction, as by application of a tourniquet. Also called stauungs hyperemia. See also BIER'S TREATMENT.

fluxionary hyperemia ACTIVE HYPEREMIA.

leptomeningeal hyperemia Congestion of the meninges.

passive hyperemia An increase of blood in an area or part resulting from an obstruction to the blood's outflow path. Also called venous hyperemia.

pulpal hyperemia A mild reversible pulpitis, characterized by sensitivity to heat. There is no spontaneous pain or tenderness of the tooth to pressure. It is caused by chemical injury, trauma, heat, or bacterial infection. If caused by the last, it usually progresses to acute or chronic pulpitis.

reactive hyperemia An increase of blood in a region following the restoration of the blood supply after a period of temporary arrest.

stauungs hyperemia CONSTRICTION HYPEREMIA.

venous hyperemia PASSIVE HYPEREMIA.

hyperemization Induced hyperemia for therapeutic purposes.

hyperemotivity Excessive display of feelings; overreaction to emotionally laden stimuli.

hyperencephalic [HYPER- + ENCEPHAL- + -IC] An incorrect term for ANENCEPHALIC.

hyperencephalus [HYPER- + Gk *enkephalos* the brain] ANEN-CEPHALUS.

hyperencephaly An incorrect term for ANENCEPHALY.

hyperendemic [HYPER- + ENDEMIC] Endemic to a high degree; so prevalent and persistent in an area that the inhabitants are in effect exposed from birth, as can occur, for example, with malaria in certain regions or with yellow fever in some of the foci of that disease. Also called *holoendemic*.

hyperendemicity The characteristic of being hyperendemic.

hyperendocrinism Excessive secretion of a hormone by an endocrine gland, or the condition resulting from it. Also called *hyperhormonism,*.

hyperenergia HYPERACTIVITY.

hyperenzymemia A greater than normal activity of any of several enzymes normally present in plasma.

hypereosinophilia A marked increase in the number of eosinophils in the blood, often to 1×10^9 per liter or more.

hyperephidrosis HYPERHIDROSIS.

hyperepinephrinemia A greater than normal concentration of epinephrine in blood. Also called *suprarenalemia* (obsolete), *hyperadrenalemia*, *hypersuprarenalemia* (obsolete).

hyperepinephry Excessive production of epinephrine by the adrenal medulla. A seldom used term.

hyperequilibrium A state in which a susceptible individual is more than usually liable to lose balance or experience vertigo.

hypererethism HYPERSENSITIVITY.

hyperergasia HYPERACTIVITY.

hyperergia [HYPER- + *(all)erg(en)* + -IA] Extreme sensitivity to allergens; hypersensitivity. Also called *hyperergy*. Adjective: hyperergic.

hyperergy HYPERERGIA.

hypererythrocythemia ERYTHROCYTOSIS.

hyperesophoria [HYPER- + ESOPHORIA] A combination of vertical and inward latent deviations of the eyes with respect to each other.

hyperesthesia [HYPER- + ESTHESIA] Exaggerated sensibility. According to the organ or sensory pathway affected, hyperesthesia may be acoustic (auditory), gustatory, olfactory, optic, sexual, or tactile. Also called *oxyesthesia*. Adjective: hyperesthesic.

    acoustic hyperesthesia DYSACUSIS.

    auditory hyperesthesia DYSACUSIS.

    cervical hyperesthesia Hypersensitivity of the necks of the teeth.

    gustatory hyperesthesia HYPERGEUSIA.

    muscular hyperesthesia Increased pain sensitivity of muscle. Also called *hypermyesthesia*.

    olfactory hyperesthesia HYPEROSMIA.

    optic hyperesthesia A heightened sensitivity of the eye to brightness.

    sexual hyperesthesia Inordinate sensitivity to tactile stimulation of the genitals, or to any kind of erotic stimulation.

    tactile hyperesthesia HYPERAPHIA.

    hyperesthesia unguium ONYCHALGIA.

hyperesthesic Pertaining to, or affected by, hyperesthesia.

hyperestrinemia HYPERESTROGENEMIA.

hyperestrinism HYPERESTROGENISM.

hyperestrogenemia An increased concentration of estrogens in the blood or blood serum. Also called *hyperestrinemia, hyperfolliculinemia* (older term).

hyperestrogenism [HYPER- + ESTROGEN + -ISM] A condition resulting from excessive estrogen secretion or exogenous administration of estrogens. Also called *hyperestrinism, hyperfolliculinism*.

hyperestrogenosis Raised concentrations of estrogens in body fluids or tissues. A rarely used term.

hyperestrogenuria [HYPER- + ESTROGEN + -URIA] Increased excretion of estrogens in the urine. Also called *hyperfolliculinuria* (rarely used).

hypereuryopia [HYPER- + EURYOPIA] Very large palpebral apertures, both in width and height.

hyperexcretory Of or characterized by excessive excretion.

hyperexophoria [HYPER- + EXOPHORIA] A combination of vertical and outward latent deviations of the eyes with respect to each other.

hyperexplexia Excessive jerking or jumping of the limbs and trunk on being startled. Also called *essential startle disease*.

hyperextensible Capable of excessive extension: said of a limb or part.

hyperextension The excessive extension of a limb or a joint. Also called *superextension*.

hyperferremia An increased concentration of iron in the blood or blood serum. Also called *hyperferricemia*.

hyperferremic Relating to or characterized by hyperferremia.

hyperferricemia HYPERFERREMIA.

hyperfibrinogenemia Increase in the concentration of plasma fibrinogen above normal. Also called *hyperinosemia* (obsolete), *superfibrination* (outmoded), *hyperinosis* (outmoded).

hyperfibrinolysis Excessive fibrinolysis.

    systemic hyperfibrinolysis A coagulation disorder characterized by poor clot formation, rapid clot dissolution, and low plasma fibrinogen. It is the result of enhanced activity of plasma fibrinolysins and is considered part of the disorder of disseminated intravascular coagulation.

hyperflexion An excessive flexion of a limb or a joint. Also called *superflexion, overflexion*.

hyperfolliculinemia An older term for HYPERESTROGENEMIA.

hyperfolliculinism [HYPER- + *folliculin* + -ISM] HYPERESTROGENISM.

hyperfolliculinuria [HYPER- + FOLLICULIN + -URIA] A rarely used term for HYPERESTROGENURIA.

hyperfunction HYPERACTIVITY.

hypergalactia [HYPER- + GALACT- + -IA] Excessive secretion of breast milk. Also called *hypergalactosis*. Adjective: hypergalactous.

hypergalactosis HYPERGALACTIA.

hypergalactous Pertaining to hypergalactia.

hypergammaglobulinemia [HYPER- + GAMMA + GLOBULIN-EMIA] A greater than normal concentration of IgG immunoglobulin in blood, plasma, or serum.

    M-component hypergammaglobulinemia Hypergammaglobulinemia due to an excess of monoclonal immunoglobulin.

hypergasia The manic form of bipolar or manic-depressive psychosis. An outmoded term.

hypergenesis Excessive or exaggerated development of a tissue, organ, or part, usually in an unnatural or unwanted manner. Adjective: hypergenetic.

hypergenitalism Excessive growth or activity of the sexual organs: used especially in reference to precocious puberty.

hypergeusesthesia HYPERGEUSIA.

hypergeusia [HYPER- + Gk *geus(is)* taste + -IA] Heightened taste perception. Also called *gustatory hyperesthesia, hypergeusesthesia*.

hypergigantosoma [HYPER- + GIGANTO- + Gk *sōma* body] An older term for GIGANTISM.

hyperglandular Of or characterized by excessive glandular secretion or size.

hyperglobulia POLYCYTHEMIA VERA.

hyperglobulinemia An elevated concentration of globulin in the blood or blood serum.

hyperglobulism POLYCYTHEMIA VERA.

hypergluconeogenesis Excessive formation of carbohydrate from amino acids or fatty acids, a characteristic of hyperadrenocorticism. A seldom used term. Also called *hyperglyconeogenesis.*

hyperglycaemia A British spelling for HYPERGLYCEMIA.

hyperglycemia [HYPER- + GLYCEMIA] A greater than normal concentration of glucose in blood. Also called *hyperglycosemia, hyperglycoplasmia.*

anacidotic hyperglycemia NONKETOTIC HYPERGLYCEMIA.

nonketotic hyperglycemia Marked hyperglycemia with plasma hyperosmolality, dehydration, and risk of seizures, but without ketoacidosis. Also called *anacidotic hyperglycemia.*

hyperglycemic 1 Pertaining to, characterized by, or resulting from hyperglycemia. 2 Capable of increasing blood glucose concentration.

hyperglyceridemia [HYPER- + GLYCERIDEMIA] An increased concentration of glycerides, especially triglycerides, in the blood or serum.

hyperglyceridemic 1 Pertaining to, characterized by, or resulting from hyperglyceridemia. 2 Capable of increasing blood glyceride concentration.

hyperglycinemia A congenital metabolic disorder marked by high blood levels of glycine and occurring in two forms, the ketotic form and the nonketotic form. The ketotic form is secondary to a number of organic acidemias, such as methylmalonic acidemia. The nonketotic form is due to a specific enzyme deficit. Patients show mental retardation, failure to thrive, and seizures but do not have episodic ketosis with neutropenia and thrombocytopenia, as in the ketotic form. Also called *glycinemia.*

ketotic hyperglycinemia The association of an elevated concentration of glycine in the plasma and urine with a presence of organic acids in the plasma. It occurs in several inborn errors of organic acid metabolism, especially the proprionic acidemias. Also called *glycinemia with ketosis.*

nonketotic hyperglycinemia An autosomal recessive inborn error of glycine metabolism characterized by mental retardation, seizures, hypotonia, and lethargy, with onset and often death in infancy. The presumed basic defect is in glycine decarboxylation, perhaps in the enzyme glycine formiminotransferase.

hyperglycinuria [HYPER- + GLYCINURIA] A redundant term for GLYCINURIA.

hyperglycistia An increased content of sugar in the tissues. An obsolete term. Also *hyperglycystia.*

hyperglycodermia Excessive levels of glycose in the skin.

hyperglyconeogenesis HYPERGLUCONEOGENESIS.

hyperglycoplasmia HYPERGLYCEMIA.

hyperglycorrhachia [HYPER- + GLYCO- + *rrhach(i)*- + -IA] An abnormally high glucose content of the cerebrospinal fluid.

hyperglycosemia HYPERGLYCEMIA.

hyperglycystia HYPERGLYCISTIA.

hyperglyoxylemia Greater than normal concentration of glyoxylate in plasma, as may occur in thiamine deficiency.

hypergnosis Excessive elaboration of a single concept or percept.

hypergonadism [HYPER- + GONAD + -ISM] A condition resulting from untimely or excessive secretion of sex hormones by the gonads, and characterized by abnormally great somatic growth and precocious puberty.

hypergonadotrophic HYPERGONADOTROPIC.

hypergonadotropic Having or characterized by excessive secretion of gonadotropic hormone or hormones, as in the hypergonadotropic eunuchoidism of the Klinefelter syndrome. Also *hypergonadotrophic.*

hypergonia The increased gonial angle of the mandible.

hypergranulation / juxtaglomerular cell hypergranulation Abnormal increase in granules in juxtaglomerular cells reflecting renin hypersecretion and storage, often associated with hyperplasia and hypertrophy of the cells, and with large distorted nuclei.

hyperguanidinemia Greater than normal concentration of guanidine in plasma.

hypergynecosmia [HYPER- + Gk *gynē* a woman + *kosm(os)* good order + -IA] 1 Premature or precocious development of female secondary sex characters in girls. 2 Excessive development in women of secondary sex characters.

hyperhedonia Excessive craving for pleasure.

hyperhemoglobinemia HEMOGLOBINEMIA.

hyperhemolytic HEMOLYTIC.

hyperheparinemia Greater than normal concentration of heparin in plasma, as occurs during therapeutic administration of heparin to prevent or retard formation of clots in blood vessels.

hyperhidrosis [HYPER- + HIDROSIS] A state of increased sweating. Also called *hidrorrhea, hyperephidrosis, idrosis, hyperidrosis, hydropedesis, ephidrosis, hidrosis, sudoresis, polyhidria, polyhidrosis, polyidrosis, diaphoresis, sudorrhea.*

gustatory hyperhidrosis AURICULOTEMPORAL SYNDROME.

hyperhidrosis nudorum Axillary hyperhidrosis provoked by the contact of the underarm area with cold air, as is experienced when undressing.

hyperhidrosis unilateralis HEMIHYPERHIDROSIS.

hyperhidrotic Characterized by increased sweating.

hyperhistaminemia Very high concentration of histamine in blood or serum.

hyperhormonal [HYPER- + HORMONAL] Of, characterized by, or resulting from excessive hormone or hormones. A seldom used term. Also *hyperhormonic.*

hyperhormonic HYPERHORMONAL.

hyperhormonism HYPERENDOCRINISM.

hyperhydration [HYPER- + HYDRATION] A greater than normal amount of water in the body or any tissue.

hyperhydrochloria HYPERCHLORHYDRIA.

hyperhypnosis [HYPER- + HYPNOSIS] HYPERSOMNIA.

hyperhypophysism [HYPER- + *hypophys(is)* + -ISM] A rarely used term for HYPERPITUITARISM.

hypericin A polyhydroxypolycyclic hydrocarbon present in *Hypericum* species (St. John's wort). Cattle eating this plant develop photosensitization.

hyperidrosis HYPERHIDROSIS.

hyperimmune Having a high degree of immunity: usually said of an animal that has been repeatedly immunized.

hyperimmunity The state of being highly immune.

hyperimmunization The induction of a high level of antibodies in the serum, especially by the administration of successive booster doses of antigen for the production of therapeutic antisera, as in horses and other animals. Also called *hypervaccination.*

maternal hyperimmunization Hyperimmunization in a pregnant or postpartum mammalian female marked by increasing levels of circulating antibody and having the effect of ensuring that sufficient protection is passed from mother to offspring *in utero* via the placenta or to her nursing young via colostrum.

hyperimmunoglobulinemia   An increase in immunoglobulin concentration of serum.

hyperindicanemia   A very high concentration of indican in the blood.

hyperinflation   An abnormal degree of distension of the lungs with air.

hyperingestion [HYPER- + INGESTION]   The intake of more nutrients than are required for good health.

hyperinnervation   Abnormal, functionally effective connection of more than one axon with a given extrafusal muscle fiber, i.e., inclusion of the fiber in two or more motor units.

hyperinosemia   An obsolete term for HYPERFIBRINOGENE-MIA.

hyperinosis   An outmoded term for HYPERFIBRINOGENEMIA.

hyperinsulinemia   A very high concentration of insulin in the blood.

hyperinsulinism [HYPER- + INSULIN + -ISM]   Abnormally increased secretion of insulin by the pancreatic islets, leading to hypoglycemia. Also called *insulism* (older term).

  alimentary hyperinsulinism   Excess release of insulin following food ingestion, a postulated cause of reactive or functional hypoglycemia.

  functional hyperinsulinism   Hyperinsulinism characterized by hypoglycemic attacks provoked by carbohydrate ingestion, not by the fasting state. Pancreatic islet cell adenoma is absent.

  iatrogenic hyperinsulinism   Insulin overdosage resulting in hypoglycemia. The relative overdose may be due to error in insulin administration, failure to ingest a meal at the proper time, faulty timing of insulin dosage, brittle diabetes, or from unknown cause. The deliberate induction of hypoglycemic coma for treatment of schizophrenia is now obsolete.

  organic hyperinsulinism   HARRIS SYNDROME.

hyperinterrenal [HYPER- + INTER- + RENAL]   An outmoded term for HYPERADRENAL.

hyperinterrenopathy [*hyperinterren(al)* + *o* + -PATHY]   A rarely used term for HYPERADRENALISM.

hyperinvolution [HYPER- + INVOLUTION]   Excessive postpartum involution of the uterus of a nursing mother, resulting in a very small uterus. Also called *superinvolution.*

hyperiodemia   A high concentration of iodide in blood or plasma or serum, for example a serum protein-bound iodine concentration in excess of 8 mg/100 ml.

hyperirritability   A state of excessive reactivity or responsiveness to stimuli either from the internal or the external environments.

hyperisotonic   HYPERTONIC.

hyperisotonicity   HYPERTONICITY.

hyperkalemia   A high concentration of potassium in plasma, such as a concentration greater than 5 mEq/l. Also called *hyperpotassemia, potassemia*. Also *hyperkaliemia.*

hyperkaliemia   HYPERKALEMIA.

hyperkaluresis [HYPER- + KALURESIS]   A redundant term for KALURESIS.

hyperkaluria [HYPER- + New L *kal(ium)* (from Arabic *kali* or *qali* potash) potassium + -URIA]   KALURESIS.

hyperkeratinization   HYPERKERATOSIS.

hyperkeratomycosis   Any fungus infection of the skin that causes thickening of the stratum corneum. An imprecise and outmoded term.

hyperkeratosic   HYPERKERATOTIC.

hyperkeratosis [HYPER- + KERATOSIS]   An excessive thickening of the horny layer of the epidermis. Also called *acanthokeratodermia, hyperkeratinization.*

  bovine hyperkeratosis   A disease of cattle, caused by contact with or ingestion of chlorinated naphthalene compounds which were formerly used as wood preservatives and lubricants. The disease is of historic interest only. It is characterized by a thickening of the horny layers of the skin and proliferation of the mucous membranes.

  bullous ichthyosiform hyperkeratosis   BULLOUS ICHTHYO-SIFORM ERYTHRODERMA.

  hyperkeratosis congenitalis palmaris et plantaris   PALMOPLANTAR KERATODERMA.

  diffuse congenital hyperkeratosis   ICHTHYOSIS CONGENITA.

  hyperkeratosis eccentrica   An obsolete term for POROKERATOSIS OF MIBELLI.

  epidermolytic hyperkeratosis   Any of several forms of bullous ichthyotic skin disorders sharing onset prenatally or in early infancy and autosomal dominant inheritance. They include a generalized form (bullous ichthyosiform erythroderma) and a localized form (ichthyosis hystrix).

  follicular hyperkeratosis   KERATOSIS PILARIS.

  hyperkeratosis follicularis et parafollicularis in cutem penetrans   A rare disease of the skin in which large horny follicular plugs develop, particularly on the lower legs. Also called *Kyrle's disease, hyperkeratosis follicularis in cutem penetrans, hyperkeratosis penetrans, hyperkeratosis in cutem penetrans.*

  hyperkeratosis follicularis in cutem penetrans   HYPERKERATOSIS FOLLICULARIS ET PARAFOLLICULARIS IN CUTEM PENETRANS.

  hyperkeratosis follicularis vegetans   Keratosis follicularis accompanied by hypertrophic lesions.

  generalized ichthyosiform hyperkeratosis   ICHTHYOSIS CONGENITA.

  hyperkeratosis in cutem penetrans   HYPERKERATOSIS FOLLICULARIS ET PARAFOLLICULARIS IN CUTEM PENETRANS.

  hyperkeratosis lacunaris   KERATOSIS PHARYNGIS.

  hyperkeratosis lacunaris pharyngis   KERATOSIS PHARYNGIS.

  hyperkeratosis lenticularis perstans   Warty keratosis of a distinctive type that is seen on the trunk and limbs.

  hyperkeratosis penetrans   HYPERKERATOSIS FOLLICULARIS ET PARAFOLLICULARIS IN CUTEM PENETRANS.

  perifollicular hyperkeratosis   Hyperkeratosis surrounding the ostium of a pilosebaceous follicle.

  precancerous hyperkeratosis   A persistent keratosis in which malignant change may occur, such as happens in solar keratosis and arsenical keratosis.

  hyperkeratosis subungualis   Epithelial hyperplasia of the tissues beneath the nail plate. It is commonly seen in psoriasis and local chronic inflammatory conditions.

hyperkeratotic   Manifesting hyperkeratosis. Also *hyperkeratosic.*

hyperketonemia   Very high concentration of ketones in plasma or serum, as in uncontrolled severe diabetes mellitus.

hyperketonuria   KETONURIA.

hyperketosis   A state of excessive ketone formation.

hyperkinemia   A condition in which there is abnormally high blood flow.

hyperkinemic   1 Characterized by or causing an abnormally high volume of blood flow.   2 An agent that increases the volume of blood flow.

hyperkinesia [HYPER- + KINESIA]   1 Abnormally intense motor activity, often associated with agitation.   2 Certain recurring or continuous involuntary movements seen in disease of the central nervous system, such as chorea and athetosis. For defs. 1 and 2 also called *hyperkinesis, hyperpraxia.* Adjective: hyperkinetic.

  essential hyperkinesia   Excessive and often purposeless activity shown by a child, of unknown cause.

reflex hyperkinesia Reflex movements of the paralyzed limbs of a hemiplegic patient, brought about by an external stimulus.

hyperkinesis HYPERKINESIA.

hyperkinetic **1** Characterized by abnormally intense motor activity, often associated with agitation; overactive. **2** Able to stimulate movements.

hyperkoria A feeling of satiety occurring before sufficient food has been consumed to meet the immediate needs of the body. A seldom used term. Also *hypercoria.*

hyperlactation [HYPER- + LACTATION] Puerperal lactation that persists for a longer than usual time and is thought to be excessive in quantity. Also called *superlactation.*

hyperlacticacidemia Very high concentration of lactic acid in plasma.

hyperlecithinemia A greater than normal concentration of lecithin in blood.

hyperlethal Exceeding the minimum required for a lethal effect: said of a dosage of a drug or other agent.

hyperleukocytosis A very marked increase in the white blood count; leukocytosis.

hyperleydigism [HYPER- + *Leydig (cells)* + -ISM] Excessive increase in the activity of the Leydig cells of the testes; excessive secretion of testosterone.

hyperlipaemia A British spelling for HYPERLIPEMIA.

hyperlipemia [HYPER- + LIPEMIA] HYPERLIPIDEMIA.

carbohydrate-induced hyperlipemia CARBOHYDRATE-INDUCED HYPERLIPIDEMIA.

essential familial hyperlipemia FAMILIAL HYPERLIPOPROTEINEMIA.

retention hyperlipemia An obsolete term for FAMILIAL HYPERLIPOPROTEINEMIA TYPE I.

hyperlipidemia [HYPER- + LIPIDEMIA] A greater than normal concentration of lipids in blood plasma. Also called *hyperlipemia, hyperlipoidemia, hyperliposis, lipidemia* (imprecise), *lipemia* (imprecise), *lipohemia* (imprecise), *lipoidemia* (imprecise), *pionemia* (obsolete).

carbohydrate-induced hyperlipidemia A greater than normal concentration of lipids in the blood, especially of triglycerides, following ingestion of carbohydrates. The phenomenon is characteristic of familial hyperlipoproteinemia types IV and V. Also called *carbohydrate-induced hyperlipemia, carbohydrate-induced hypertriglyceridemia.*

combined fat- and carbohydrate-induced hyperlipidemia A form of hyperlipoproteinemia in which ingestion of fat or carbohydrates results in greater than normal plasma concentration of very low density lipoproteins and persistent chylomicronemia during fasting.

fat-induced hyperlipidemia Greater than normal concentration of plasma lipids following ingestion of food containing fat. See also FAMILIAL HYPERLIPOPROTEINEMIA TYPE I.

mixed hyperlipidemia A subtype of familial hyperlipoproteinemia type II, characterized by increased concentrations of serum low density lipoproteins and very low density lipoproteins during fasting. Also called *familial hyperlipoproteinemia type IIb.*

hyperlipoidemia HYPERLIPIDEMIA.

hyperlipoproteinemia [HYPER- + LIPOPROTEINEMIA] Greater than normal concentration of lipoprotein in blood, plasma, or serum.

acquired hyperlipoproteinemia Persistently greater than normal plasma concentration of lipoproteins that is nonhereditary in cause, secondary to some other disorder such as myxedema.

familial hyperlipoproteinemia Any of several genetic disorders of lipid metabolism characterized by increase in concentration of one or more types of serum lipoprotein. These disorders are classified as hyperlipoproteinemia types I, II, III, IV, and V. Also called *essential familial hyperlipemia.*

familial mixed hyperlipoproteinemia A disorder of lipid metabolism that is of autosomal dominant transmittance in which affected members of a kindred may exhibit different serum lipid abnormalities like those of hyperlipoproteinemia types IIa, IIb, or V.

familial hyperlipoproteinemia type I A rare hereditary disorder of lipid metabolism, characterized by onset in childhood of xanthomas of skin, abdominal pain and pancreatitis, enlargement of liver and spleen, lipemic retinopathy, accelerated atherosclerosis, lipemic plasma, and marked increase in serum chylomicrons, extreme increase in serum triglycerides, and low concentration of serum cholesterol. Inheritance is autosomal recessive. Two different metabolic defects are responsible: in some families there is a deficiency of the enzyme lipoprotein lipase; in others there is a deficiency of apolipoprotein C-II, a cofactor of lipoprotein lipase, causing a functional deficiency of lipoprotein lipase. Also called *familial hyperchylomicronemia, familial hypertriglyceridemia, endogenous hypertriglyceridemia, familial fat-induced hypertriglyceridemia, Bürger-Grütz syndrome, retention hyperlipemia* (obsolete).

familial hyperlipoproteinemia type II Any of a number of disorders of lipid metabolism characterized by elevated serum cholesterol and low density lipoprotein, including familial hypercholesterolemia (type IIa) and mixed hyperlipidemia (type IIb).

familial hyperlipoproteinemia type IIa FAMILIAL HYPERCHOLESTEROLEMIA.

familial hyperlipoproteinemia type IIb MIXED HYPERLIPIDEMIA.

familial hyperlipoproteinemia type III A hereditary disorder of lipid metabolism of autosomal recessive transmittance, characterized by adult onset of cutaneous xanthomas, accelerated atherosclerosis, increase in serum very low density lipoprotein, marked increase in serum cholesterol and triglyceride. The metabolic defect is a deficiency of apoprotein E-3. Also called *essential hypercholesterolemia* (outmoded), *xanthoma tuberosum* (outmoded), *xanthoma tuberosum multiplex, dysbetalipoproteinemia, broad-beta disease, floating beta disease.*

familial hyperlipoproteinemia type IV A disorder of lipid metabolism characterized by elevation of both plasma cholesterol and triglyceride levels secondary to an increase in the very-low density lipoprotein fraction. It occurs in response to a high carbohydrate diet in persons who are sensitive to this form of dietary induction. The genetics and metabolic defect are unknown. Also called *familial hyperprebetalipoproteinemia, endogenous hypertriglyceridemia, familial hypertriglyceridemia.* See also CARBOHYDRATE-INDUCED HYPERLIPIDEMIA.

familial hyperlipoproteinemia type V A disorder of lipid metabolism characterized by adult onset of cutaneous xanthomas, sometimes by pancreatitis, peripheral neuropathy, hyperglycemia or abnormal glucose tolerance, increase in serum chylomicrons and triglycerides and very low density lipoproteins, but decrease in low density and high density lipoproteins. The disorder appears to have autosomal dominant transmittance, but penetrance is often incomplete. defect is unknown. Affected relatives in a family may exhibit either type IV or type V hyperlipoproteinemia. A similar acquired lipoprotein abnormality may be seen in diabetes mellitus, alcoholism, nephrotic syndrome, or hypothyroidism.

hyperliposis HYPERLIPIDEMIA.

hyperlithemia A high concentration of lithium in the blood.

hyperlithuria HYPERURICURIA.

hyperlogia HYPERPHRASIA.

hyperlordosis An increase in the natural degree of lordosis.

hyperlucency [HYPER- + (radio)lucency] An extreme radiolucency.

hyperluteinization **1** A condition in which an excessive number of graafian follicles of the ovary are luteinized, that is, are corpora lutea. **2** Abnormally long persistence of the luteal phase of the ovarian cycle.

hyperlutemia [HYPER- + lutemia, from lut- (from the corpus luteum hormone, progesterone) + -EMIA] HYPERPROGESTERONEMIA.

hyperlysinuria [HYPER- + lysin(e) + -URIA] Increased urinary excretion of lysine, a feature of persistent hyperlysinemia.

hypermagnesemia An elevated concentration of magnesium in the blood or blood serum. Also called magnesemia.

hypermania DELIRIOUS MANIA.

hypermastia [HYPER- + MAST- + -IA] Excessive enlargement of the breasts.

hypermature [HYPER- + MATURE] **1** Beyond the mature state. **2** Overripe.

hypermedication Excessive administration or use of therapeutic agents, either in the number of drugs taken, or in the amounts given.

hypermegasoma [HYPER- + MEGA- + Gk sōma body] An outmoded term for GIGANTISM.

hypermegasthenic Of or relating to excessive strength.

hypermelanosis An excess of melanin pigmentation.

hypermelanotic Showing excessive melanin pigmentation.

hypermenorrhea [HYPER- + MENORRHEA] Frequent menstrual periods or an abnormal increase in the duration and/or amount of menstrual flow. Also called epimenorrhagia, epimenorrhea.

hypermery [HYPER- + -mer(e) + -Y] In embryology, an abnormal increase in the number of body segments. It is seen as a developmental variant in most vertebrates and is most often expressed in mammals, including man, in the presence of supernumerary vertebrae.

hypermesosoma Stature somewhat greater than normal. A rarely used term.

hypermetabolism A state of excessive metabolic activity; an excessively high metabolic rate.

extrathyroidal hypermetabolism A state of excessive metabolic activity not attributable to hyperthyroidism.

hypermetamorphosis Overreactivity to visual stimuli, suggestive of temporal lobe pathology.

hypermetamorphosis of Wernicke Excessive automatic behavior, including the repeated handling of any object placed within the field of vision, seen as a part of the Klüver-Bucy syndrome in monkeys after bilateral temporal lobe ablation.

hypermetaplasia Exuberant metaplasia. An obsolete term.

hypermetria [HYPER- + -metr(y) + -IA] Motor incoordination such that movements overreach their target, as seen in cerebellar dysfunction. This can be noted in spontaneous movements but is often more obvious in actions rapidly executed on command, as in the finger-nose test or the heel-knee test.

hypermetric Of or relating to hypermetria.

hypermetrope [HYPER- + Gk metr(on) a measure + -OPE] HYPEROPE.

hypermetropia [HYPER- + Gk metron a measure, rule, standard + -OPIA] HYPEROPIA.

hypermetropic HYPEROPIC.

hypermicrosoma Extreme generalized dwarfism.

hypermimia ECHOPRAXIA.

hypermineralization Excessive deposit of minerals in the body.

hypermnesia [HYPER- + Gk mnēs(is) remembrance + -IA] Ability to recall material to a greater degree than is usual.

hypermodal [HYPER- + MODAL] Describing or pertaining to the measured values greater than or, when represented graphically, to the right of the mode in a data distribution.

hypermorph [HYPER- + -MORPH] A long-limbed individual with a disproportionally small sitting height due to a small, slender trunk and an asthenic musculature.

hypermotility The capability of moving excessively.

hypermyesthesia [HYPER- + MYESTHESIA] MUSCULAR HYPERESTHESIA.

hypermyotonia A seldom used term for HYPERTONIA.

hypermyotrophy A state of excessive muscular development.

hypernanosoma An extremely short stature.

hypernasality The nasal quality imparted to speech when an undue proportion of the airflow passes through the nasal cavity, as may happen in cleft palate, following palatal paralysis, or as a result of surgery. Also called rhinolalia aperta, open rhinolalia, hyperrhinolalia.

hypernatremia An elevated concentration of sodium in the blood or blood serum. Also called hypernatronemia.

hypernatremic Characteristic of, resulting from, or causing hypernatremia.

hypernatronemia Hypernatremia.

hypernea [HYPER- + nea, irreg. from Gk noos mind, thought] HYPERPRAGIA.

hyperneocytosis **1** RETICULOCYTOSIS. **2** Leukocytosis with an increased proportion of immature forms. Also called hyperskeocytosis.

hypernephritis [HYPER- + NEPHRITIS] Inflammation of the adrenal gland. An obsolete term.

hypernephroid Like the adrenal gland. A rarely used term.

hypernephroma [HYPER- + NEPHROMA] RENAL CELL CARCINOMA.

adrenal hypernephroma malignum ADRENAL CORTICAL CARCINOMA.

hypernephrotrophy [HYPER- + NEPHRO- + Gk trophē nourishment] A rarely used term for RENAL HYPERTROPHY.

hyperneuroma [HYPER- + NEUROMA] A rapidly growing nerve tumor. An obsolete term.

hyperneurotization [HYPER- + NEURO- + t + -IZE + -ATION] Implantation of a motor nerve into a muscle already possessing motor nerve innervation.

hypernidation [HYPER- + L nid(us) nest + -ATION] More than one implantation, as in a multiple pregnancy.

hypernitremia An elevated concentration of nitrogen in the blood or blood serum.

hypernormal [HYPER- + NORMAL] In excess of the normal.

hypernutrition [HYPER- + NUTRITION] Overeating or consuming more food than is required to meet the metabolic needs of the body, as a form of therapy. Hypernutrition is sometimes used in treating anorexic conditions by having the subject consume high-protein milk. Also called supernutrition.

hyperocclusion [HYPER- + OCCLUSION] A tooth extrusion which causes premature contact.

hyperoic A rarely used term for PALATINE.

hyperoitis [Gk hyperō(ē) the palate + -ITIS] A rarely used term for PALATITIS.

hyperoncosis [HYPER- + ONCO-¹ + -SIS] A state of excessive swelling.

hyperoncotic **1** Marked by oncotic pressure that is greater than normal. **2** Of or relating to excessive swelling.

hyperontomorph [HYPER- + Gk onto(s), gen. of ōn, pres. part.

of *einai* to be + -MORPH] A person subject to hyperthyroidism. A rarely used term.

hyperonychia [HYPER- + ONYCH- + -IA] The presence of thickened or hypertrophic nails. Also called *hyperonychosis.*

hyperonychosis HYPERONYCHIA.

hyperope [HYPER- + -OPE] A person with hyperopia; a far-sighted person. Also called *hypermetrope.*

hyperopia [HYPER- + -OPIA] The refractive error in which additional dioptric power obtained by accommodation or by wearing a convex spectacle lens is needed in order to see clearly in the distance. Also called *hypermetropia, farsightedness, far sight, long sight, longsightedness.* Adjective: hyperopic.

absolute hyperopia That portion of hyperopia in excess of the amount of available accommodation and therefore uncorrectible by accommodative effort.

axial hyperopia Hyperopia caused by a relative shortness of the anteroposterior length of the eye.

curvature hyperopia Hyperopia caused by an increased convexity of the surfaces of the cornea or lens. Also called *hyperopia of curvature.*

facultative hyperopia That portion of hyperopia that can be corrected by accommodative effort.

high hyperopia Presence of an unusually large amount of hyperopia; extreme farsightedness.

index hyperopia Hyperopia due to an increased refractive strength of the lens substance.

latent hyperopia The portion of hyperopia that cannot be measured without use of a cycloplegic drug for refraction.

manifest hyperopia The portion of hyperopia that may be readily measured by a noncycloplegic refraction.

physiologic hyperopia A relatively minor degree of hyperopia, as commonly exists asymptomatically.

relative hyperopia Hyperopia that induces excessive convergence, resulting in muscle imbalance.

total hyperopia The entire amount of hyperopia, as disclosed by cycloplegic refraction.

hyperopic Of or characterized by hyperopia. Also *hypermetropic, farsighted.*

hyperorchidism [HYPER- + *orchid(o)-* + -ISM] An abnormal increase in testicular function.

hyperorexia [HYPER- + Gk *orex(is)* (from stem of *orexō*, fut. of *oregein* to reach) a longing for + -IA] BULIMIA.

hyperornithemia [HYPER- + *ornith(ine)* + -EMIA] A metabolic fault in which an excess of ornithine accumulates within the body. This results in gyrate atrophy of the choroid.

hyperorthocytosis Leukocytosis with a normal differential distribution.

hyperosmia [HYPER- + *osm(o)-*² + -IA] Abnormally heightened olfactory perception. Also called *hyperosphresis, olfactory hyperesthesia.*

hyperosmolality Having an osmolality greater than normal for body fluids.

hyperosmolarity A state of high molecular density within a solution such that it will absorb water across a semipermeable membrane from a less dense solution.

hyperosmotic 1 Having a higher concentration of osmotically active solutes than a comparative solution. 2 Characterized by excessive osmotic activity.

hyperosphresia HYPEROSMIA.

hyperostatic HYPEROSTOTIC.

hyperosteogenesis HYPEROSTOSIS.

hyperosteogeny Excessive bone development.

hyperosteopathy An abnormal bone formation and/or development.

hyperostosis [HYPER- + OSTOSIS] A hypertrophy of bone, either in the form of a local increase in size, such as an exostosis, or a generalized increase that involves a whole bone. Also called *hyperosteogenesis.*

calvarial hyperostosis A generalized irregular thickening of the cortex of the skull. It can take the form of the van Buchem syndrome or hyperostosis frontalis interna.

hyperostosis corticalis generalisata VAN BUCHEM SYNDROME.

disseminated cortical hyperostosis VAN BUCHEM SYNDROME.

flowing hyperostosis MELORHEOSTOSIS.

hyperostosis frontalis interna Calvarial hyperostosis that affects only the inner wall of the frontal bone. It may be associated with obesity and hypertrichosis in middle-aged women. Also called *Stewart-Morel syndrome, endocraniosis, Morel syndrome, Morgagni's hyperostosis, Morgagni-Stewart-Morel syndrome, Morgagni's disease, Morgagni syndrome.*

infantile hyperostosis An intermittent inflammatory process characterized by multiple subperiosteal new bone formation points in the long bones, the mandible, and the clavicles, and resulting in swelling of the soft tissues. It is seen in young infants with pyrexia. Also called *infantile cortical hyperostosis syndrome, Caffey's disease, Caffey syndrome, Caffey-Silverman syndrome, infantile cortical hyperostosis.*

infantile cortical hyperostosis INFANTILE HYPEROSTOSIS.

Morgagni's hyperostosis HYPEROSTOSIS FRONTALIS INTERNA.

senile ankylosing hyperostosis of spine The generalized formation of new bone, with osteophytes most often bridging and forming within the interligamentous structures of the thoracic and upper lumbar vertebrae to produce a marked loss of movement and kyphosis. It is seen primarily in the elderly. Also called *senile vertebral ankylosing hyperostosis.*

senile vertebral ankylosing hyperostosis SENILE ANKYLOSING HYPEROSTOSIS OF SPINE.

hyperostotic Of or relating to hyperostosis. Also *hyperostatic.*

hyperovaria An outmoded term for HYPEROVARIANISM.

hyperovarianism 1 Precocious puberty in girls, due to untimely secretion of estrogen by the ovaries. Also called *hyperovaria, hyperovarism.* 2 Excessive ovarian secretion of estrogen at any age. A rarely used term.

hyperovarism An outmoded term for HYPEROVARIANISM.

hyperoxaluria [HYPER- + OXALURIA] Increased excretion of oxalate in the urine, often a cause of calcium oxalate nephrolithiasis or nephrocalcinosis, or of chronic interstitial nephritis leading to renal failure. Hyperoxaluria may be genetic (primary), or secondary to ingestion or administration of excess amounts of oxalate precursors, or to intestinal diseases.

primary hyperoxaluria The progressive deposition of calcium oxalate in the kidneys and other tissues (oxalosis) due to either of two inborn errors of oxalic acid metabolism, oxalosis I or oxalosis II.

primary hyperoxaluria type I OXALOSIS I.

primary hyperoxaluria type II OXALOSIS II.

secondary hyperoxaluria Increased oxalate in the urine, associated with intestinal disorders such as Crohn's disease or following ileal bypass surgery for obesity.

hyperoxemia Increased or excessive acidity of the blood or blood serum; acidosis.

hyperoxemic 1 Having excess acid in blood. An obsolete usage. 2 Characterized by hyperoxia.

hyperoxia 1 Increased or excessive oxygen concentration. 2 Elevated oxygen tension in blood.

hyperoxic Characteristic of, resulting from, or causing hyperoxia.

hyperpallesthesia [HYPER- + PALLESTHESIA] Abnormally acute pallesthesia. Also called *pallhyperesthesia* (seldom used).

hyperparasite A parasite whose host is itself a parasite.

second degree hyperparasite A parasite that exists within or preys on a hyperparasite. Complex interactions such as this sometimes occur in connection with biological control efforts involving hyperparasitic or parasitoid wasps, some of which parasitize one another while they are in a primary host, such as a scale insect.

hyperparasitic [HYPER- + PARASITIC] Parasitic upon a parasite. Also *biparasitic, paraneoexenous.*

hyperparasitism [HYPER- + PARASITISM] Parasitism in which the host is itself parasitic upon yet another organism. Also called *biparasitism, superparasitism.*

hyperparasitoidism The phenomenon of a parasitoid preying upon another species of parasitoid.

hyperparathyroid Of or relating to hyperparathyroidism.

hyperparathyroidism [HYPER- + PARATHYROID + -ISM] A condition resulting from excessive secretion of parathyroid hormone by the parathyroid glands, accompanied by hypercalcemia, hypophosphatemia, loss of calcium from bones, renal calculi, and gastrointestinal and mental disturbances. It is caused by hyperplasia, adenoma, and occasionally by a hormone-secreting cancer, as squamous cell carcinoma of the lung. Rarely, it is caused by carcinoma of the parathyroids.

acute hyperparathyroidism Sudden exacerbation of systemic symptoms of hypercalcemia occurring in the course of hyperparathyroidism, as constipation becoming ileus and lethargy coma.

nutritional hyperparathyroidism A nutritional disease associated with consumption of a diet with a low calcium to phosphorus ratio. All mammals are susceptible. It is characterized by hyperplasia of the parathyroid glands and by fibrous osteodystrophy.

primary hyperparathyroidism Hyperparathyroidism resulting from intrinsic disease of the parathyroid glands.

secondary hyperparathyroidism Excessive secretion of parathyroid hormone by the parathyroid glands in chronic renal insufficiency characterized by high serum phosphate concentration and low, normal, or subnormal calcium value. The cause is assumed to be failure of the diseased kidney to synthesize 1-α-25-dihydroxycholecalciferol, the most active form of vitamin D, absence or deficiency of which leads to subnormal absorption of calcium from the gut and relative hypocalcemia, which stimulates parathyroid hormone oversecretion.

tertiary hyperparathyroidism A condition developing in the course of secondary hyperparathyroidism in which, after protracted oversecretion of parathyroid hormone in response to renal failure, the parathyroids become autonomous, and a state virtually identical to primary hyperparathyroidism develops, accompanied by high normal or excessive concentration of serum calcium. Treatment by parathyroidectomy is required.

hyperparotidism [HYPER- + *parotid (gland)* + -ISM] Excessive secretion by the parotid gland.

hyperpathia [HYPER- + PATH- + -IA] Abnormally enhanced sensitivity to pain, seen particularly in the thalamic syndrome and sometimes in lesions of peripheral nerves or of the spinothalamic tract. The sensation evoked by the painful stimulus is excessive and may persist after removal of the stimulus. Also called *oxypathia, oxypathy.* Adjective: hyperpathic.

thalamic hyperpathia THALAMIC PAIN.

hyperpathic Relating to hyperpathia. Also *oxypathic.*

hyperpepsia GASTRIC HYPERSECRETION.

hyperpepsinemia An elevated concentration of pepsin in the blood.

hyperpepsinia Excessive production of pepsin by the stomach. See also GASTRIC HYPERSECRETION.

hyperpeptic Relating to or characterized by gastric hypersecretion.

hyperperistalsis Excessively active intestinal peristalsis.

hyperperistaltic Relating to or characterized by hyperperistalsis.

hyperpermeability A state of excessive permeability.

hyperpexia [HYPER- + -*pex(y)* + -IA] The incorporation of an excessive quantity of substance into tissues. Also called *hyperpexy.*

hyperpexy HYPERPEXIA.

hyperphagia [HYPER- + -PHAGIA] BULIMIA.

hyperphagic Characterized by eating to excess: said of animals whose satiety centers in the ventromedial nucleus of the hypothalamus have been damaged for experimental purposes.

hyperphalangia [HYPER- + Gk *phalanx*, gen. *phalangos*, a round piece of wood, log, a bone of a finger or toe, spider + -IA] POLYPHALANGIA.

hyperphalangism [*hyperphalang(ia)* + -ISM] POLYPHALANGIA.

hyperphalangy [See HYPERPHALANGIA.] POLYPHALANGIA.

hyperphenylalaninemia An elevated concentration of phenylalanine in the blood.

hyperphoria [HYPER- + -PHORIA] A latent misalignment of the eyes in which the visual axis of an eye is higher than its fellow eye. This may be observed only when fusion is interrupted, as by covering one eye.

hyperphosphatasemia An increase in concentration of phosphatase in blood to above a normal level.

hyperphosphatasia A hereditary, autosomal recessive, chronic osteopathy characterized by an increased serum phosphatase concentration in the presence of normal serum calcium and phosphate concentrations. Also called *juvenile Paget's disease.*

hyperphosphatemia An elevated concentration of phosphate or phosphorus in the blood or blood serum.

hyperphosphaturia Increased excretion of inorganic phosphates in the urine, secondary to excess phosphate intake, to excess amounts of parathyroid or thyroid hormone, or to proximal tubular defects. It is sometimes associated with osteomalacia, defective growth in children, and a variety of other conditions.

hyperphosphoremia An elevated concentration of phosphorus compounds in the blood or blood serum.

hyperphrasia Pathologic verbosity or loquacity. Also called *hyperlogia.*

hyperpiesia [HYPER- + Gk *pies(is)* pressure, a squeezing + -IA] HYPERTENSION.

hyperpiesis [HYPER- + Gk *piesis* pressure, a squeezing] HYPERTENSION.

hyperpietic HYPERTENSIVE.

hyperpigmentation Excessive pigmentation of any origin. Also called *superpigmentation.*

periocular hyperpigmentation Hypermelanosis of the periorbital skin. It is determined by an autosomal dominant gene. Also called *melanosis of the eyelids.*

hyperpinealism [HYPER- + PINEAL + -ISM] Excessive secretion of a postulated hormone or hormones by the pineal gland: used especially in reference to the precocious puberty sometimes observed in association with pineal tumors.

hyperpituitarism [HYPER- + PITUITARISM] Any condition characterized by excessive secretion of pituitary hormones, particularly those of the anterior pituitary, as acromegaly, Cushing's disease, or nonpuerperal galactorrhea associated with a prolactin-secreting microadenoma. Also called *hyperhypophysism* (rarely used), *antuitarism* (obsolete).

basophilic hyperpituitarism Cushing's disease associated with basophil adenoma of the adenohypophysis, or more specifically, of the anterior pituitary corticotrophs.

eosinophilic hyperpituitarism Pathologic overactivity of the eosinophil cells of the anterior pituitary (adenoma or hyperplasia), causing acromegaly or gigantism due to excessive secretion of growth hormone. A seldom used term.

hyperplasia [HYPER- + -PLASIA] Increase in the number of cells in a tissue or organ with a concomitant increase in the size of the structure involved. It is a controlled, finite change, caused by known stimuli, and one that ceases when the causative stimulus stops. Also called *hyperblastosis, quantitative hypertrophy* (obsolete), *numeric hypertrophy (incorrect and obsolete), merisis*.

angiofollicular mediastinal lymph node hyperplasia BENIGN MEDIASTINAL LYMPH NODE HYPERPLASIA.

basal cell hyperplasia An increase in the proportion of basal-type cells in a stratified, usually squamous epithelium. It is characteristic of the early stages of epithelial dysplasia.

benign mediastinal lymph node hyperplasia A condition characterized by benign, solid, lymphoid masses occurring in the mediastinum of young adults. Histologically they are characterized by concentric perivascular aggregations of lymphocytes. Although usually asymptomatic, they may cause mechanical compression of vital structures. Surgical removal is the treatment of choice to prevent obstructive sequelae or neoplastic transformation. Also called *angiofollicular mediastinal lymph node hyperplasia*.

benign hyperplasia of the prostate Noncancerous enlargement of the prostate, common after the age of 50 and characterized by obstruction of the bladder outlet, impeding the outflow of urine and leading to obstruction with back pressure.

cementum hyperplasia CEMENTOSIS.

chronic perforating hyperplasia of pulp CHRONIC OPEN HYPERPLASTIC PULPITIS.

condylar hyperplasia The overgrowth of one or both condyles of the mandible.

congenital adrenal hyperplasia CONGENITAL ADRENOCORTICAL HYPERPLASIA.

congenital adrenocortical hyperplasia An inherited metabolic disorder due to partial or complete lack of an enzyme, most commonly steroid 21-hydroxylase, in the synthesis of cortisol by the adrenal cotex. A reduced concentration of cortisol in plasma allows overproduction of adrenocorticotropic hormone by the anterior pituitary, leading to hypertrophy and hyperplasia of the adrenal cortex, and to excessive secretion of androgenic steroids. The affected male is born with enlarged penis, the female with enlarged clitoris and varying degrees of masculinization of the genitalia. Salt loss is an additional feature in some cases. Treatment is with cortisol or its analogs, together with salt replacement. Inheritance is autosomal recessive. Also called *adrenogenital syndrome, androgenital syndrome* (seldom used), *Wilkins disease, adrenal struma* (older term), *Cooke-Apert-Gallais syndrome, adrenal virilism* (imprecise), *congenital adrenal virilism, congenital adrenal hyperplasia*.

congenital sebaceous gland hyperplasia SEBACEOUS NEVUS.

cystic hyperplasia Hyperplasia of glandular epithelium accompanied by cysts, resulting from a combination of retention of secretions and obstruction by the proliferated epithelium. It is most commonly seen in endometrium, breast, and prostate. Also called *Swiss-cheese hyperplasia*.

cystic hyperplasia of the breasts CYSTIC MASTOPATHY.

cystic-glandular hyperplasia of the endometrium A form of endometrial hyperplasia characterized by proliferation of endometrial and stromal cells and cyst formation. It is most frequently seen at the time of the menopause or later and results from unremitting estrogenic stimulation. Also called *Swiss-cheese endometrium*.

denture hyperplasia Hyperplasia of the oral mucous membrane caused by repeated irritation from an ill-fitting denture. Also called *inflammatory fibrous hyperplasia, denture hypertrophy*.

Dilantin gingival hyperplasia A term used chiefly in the U.S. for DIPHENYLHYDANTOIN GINGIVITIS.

endometrial hyperplasia An abnormal growth response in the endometrium due to excessive, unremitting or noncyclic, unopposed estrogenic stimulus. Also called *hyperplasia endometrii*.

hyperplasia endometrii ENDOMETRIAL HYPERPLASIA.

epiphyseal hyperplasia DYSPLASIA EPIPHYSIALIS HEMIMELICA.

fibromuscular hyperplasia See under FIBROMUSCULAR DISEASE.

focal adenomyomatous hyperplasia of the gallbladder A focal lesion in the fundus of the gallbladder in which diverticuli are surrounded by fibrous and muscular tissue to form a tumorlike nodule. Also called *adenomyoma* (incorrect).

focal nodular hyperplasia of the liver A reactive or hamartomatous lesion of the liver characterized by the presence of one or several nodular, well circumscribed but not encapsulated hepatic nodules ranging in size from 1–15 cm. The lesion usually occurs in women of childbearing age and is generally asymptomatic and has a benign prognosis.

follicular hyperplasia Increased numbers of secondary follicles with active germinal centers, detectable on microscopic examination of a lymph node. There may or may not be accompanying enlargement of the lymph node.

giant follicular hyperplasia A peculiar form of lymph node hyperplasia characteristically involving the mediastinum but also found in the neck, axilla, and other sites. Large follicles are present within a mass of lymphoid tissue that may show prominent vascular proliferation and hyalinization, and sometimes plasma cells.

gingival hyperplasia Enlargement of the gingiva produced by an increase in the number of its elements. Usually gingival hyperplasia is a plaque-associated gingivitis, more common in the young. A severe form may be found in patients on long-term diphenylhydantoin sodium therapy. Also called *gingival hypertrophy* (incorrect), *macrogingiva, gingival proliferation*.

hemifacial hyperplasia The overgrowth of one side of the face.

inflammatory hyperplasia Hyperplasia of a tissue resulting from an inflammatory reaction.

inflammatory fibrous hyperplasia DENTURE HYPERPLASIA.

inflammatory papillary hyperplasia Red papillary projections from the hard palate, developing under a denture. Also called *papillary hyperplasia, inflammatory papillomatosis, multiple papillomatosis*.

islet cell hyperplasia A ribbonlike overgrowth, associated with excessive insulin secretion, of the β-cells of the pancreatic islets of Langerhans, and sometimes occurring as a part of multiple endocrine neoplasia Type I.

juxtaglomerular cell hyperplasia Hyperplasia and hypertrophy of the juxtaglomerular cells of the kidney with consequent excessive secretion of renin, hyperangiotensinemia, aldosteronism, hypokalemia, alkalosis, insensitivity to the hypertensive action of angiotensin, and absence of hypertension.

juxtaglomerular hyperplasia with hyperaldosteronism See under BARTTER SYNDROME.

lipoid hyperplasia Hyperplasia of lipid-containing cells. A rarely used term.

lipomelanotic reticular hyperplasia   An enlargement of the lymph glands secondary to chronic skin disease.

ovarian stromal hyperplasia   THECOMATOSIS.

papillary hyperplasia   INFLAMMATORY PAPILLARY HYPERPLASIA.

polar hyperplasia   Overdevelopment of the cranial or caudal end of an embryo, resulting in an abnormal fetus with two heads or three or four hind limbs.

polypoid hyperplasia   Focal hyperplasia of a tissue in which the affected area has the shape of a polyp.

pseudocarcinomatous hyperplasia   PSEUDOEPITHELIOMATOUS HYPERPLASIA.

pseudoepitheliomatous hyperplasia   Abundant proliferation of squamous epithelium simulating carcinoma. The lesion occurs over areas of chronic inflammation. Also called *pseudocarcinomatous hyperplasia*.

Schwann hyperplasia   HEREDITARY HYPERTROPHIC INTERSTITIAL NEUROPATHY.

Swiss-cheese hyperplasia   CYSTIC HYPERPLASIA.

thymic medullary hyperplasia   A condition in which hyperplastic germinal centers are present in the medulla of the thymus. It is particularly common in myasthenia gravis.

hyperplasmia   Increase in volume of blood plasma.

hyperplasminemia   The abnormal emergence of the fibrinolytic enzyme plasmin in the blood, characteristic of disseminated intravascular coagulation.

hyperplastic   Pertaining to or characterized by hyperplasia.

hyperplexia   A state of apparent muscular rigidity or increased tone occurring in states of excitement or ecstasy. A seldom used term.

hyperploid [HYPER- + -PLOID]   Having a chromosome complement slightly in excess of that found in a complement having any integral multiple of the haploid set.

hyperploidy   The state of being hyperploid.

hyperpnea   Excessively rapid or deep breathing. Adjective: hyperpneic.

hyperpnoea   A British spelling for HYPERPNEA.

hyperpolarization   An increase in the transmembrane potential across nerve or muscle cells that occurs with an increased net difference in charge between the interior and exterior surfaces.

early hyperpolarization   POSITIVE AFTERPOTENTIAL.

hyperpolypeptidemia   An elevated concentration of polypeptides in the blood.

hyperponesis [HYPER- + Gk *pon(os)* toil + -ESIS]   Dysponesis with enhanced action potential discharge from the motor and premotor parts of the cerebral cortex. Adjective: hyperponetic.

hyperposia [HYPER- + Gk *pos(is)* a drinking, drink + -IA]   The consumption of abnormally large volumes of liquids over short periods of time.

hyperpostpituitary [HYPER- + POST- + PITUITARY]   Characterized by excessive neurohypophysial hormone secretion, as in the Schwartz-Bartter syndrome.

hyperpotassemia   HYPERKALEMIA.

hyperpragia [HYPER- + Gk *prag*, a root of *prassein* to achieve, manage + -IA]   Excessive mental activity. Also called *hypernea, hyperpsychosis* (obsolete).

hyperpraxia   HYPERKINESIA.

hyperprebetalipoproteinemia   An elevated concentration of prebetalipoproteins (very low density lipoproteins) in the blood or blood serum. Also called *prebetalipoproteinemia*.

familial hyperprebetalipoproteinemia   FAMILIAL HYPERLIPOPROTEINEMIA TYPE IV.

hyperpresbyopia [HYPER- + PRESBYOPIA]   The complete loss of accommodation due to aging.

hyperprogesteronemia   An abnormally high concentration of progesterone in the blood. Also called *hyperlutemia*.

hyperprolactinemia   Raised concentration of prolactin in the blood, normal in pregnancy, lactation and response to stress, pathologic in pituitary adenomas, nonpuerperal galactorrhea, amenorrhea, and renal failure.

hyperprolactinism   The presence of excessive levels of circulating prolactin, usually due either to an adenoma of the anterior pituitary gland or to stimulation with any of a number of drugs or conditions of physiologic stress. Normal levels are below 25 ng/ml.

hyperprolinemia   1 An elevated concentration of proline in the blood.   2 A genetically determined metabolic disorder characterized by elevated plasma proline and increased urinary excretion of proline, hydroxyproline, and glycine, due to impairment of oxidation of proline. Clinical manifestations include mental retardation and renal dysfunction. For defs. 1 and 2 also called *prolinemia*.

familial hyperprolinemia   ENCEPHALOPATHY WITH PROLINEMIA.

hyperprosessis [HYPER- + Gk *prosessis* for *prosexis* (from *prosexō*, fut. of *prosechein* to turn one's attention to) attention]   Exaggerated attentiveness. Also called *hyperprosexia*.

hyperprosexia   HYPERPROSESSIS.

hyperproteinemia   An elevated concentration of protein in the blood or blood serum.

hyperproteosis [HYPER- + *prote(in)* + -OSIS]   A condition caused by excessive dietary intake of protein.

hyperpselaphesia [HYPER- + Gk *psēlaphēs(is)* a touching, groping + -IA]   HYPERAPHIA.

hyperpsychosis   An obsolete term for HYPERPRAGIA.

hyperptyalism   An incorrect term for PTYALISM.

hyperpyretic   HYPERPYREXIAL.

hyperpyrexia [HYPER- + PYREXIA]   An excessively high body temperature, usually over 40.5°C (105°F).

fulminant hyperpyrexia   MALIGNANT HYPERPYREXIA.

heat hyperpyrexia   HEATSTROKE.

malignant hyperpyrexia   A familial disorder in which severe muscular pain and rigidity with hyperpyrexia, leading sometimes to a fatal termination, may be induced in susceptible individuals by various inhalational anesthetic agents, especially halothane, or by a muscular relaxant such as succinylcholine. Also called *fulminant hyperpyrexia*.

hyperpyrexial   Suffering from or relating to hyperpyrexia. Also *hyperpyretic*.

hyperreactive   Exhibiting or pertaining to an excessive reaction to a stimulus.

hyperreflectivity   A seldom used term for HYPERREFLEXIA.

hyperreflexia [HYPER- + REFLEX + -IA]   Exaggeration of reflexes. Also called *hyperreflectivity* (seldom used), *surreflectivity (more correct, but obsolete)*.

autonomic hyperreflexia   A condition in which there is an excessive autonomic response to visceral or somatic afferent stimuli.

hyperresonance   A greater than normal resonance.

hyper-rhinencephalia   RHINOCEPHALY.

hyperrhinolalia   HYPERNASALITY.

hyperrhinoplaty [HYPER- + RHINO- + Gk *platy(s)* flat, broad]   A facial deformity resulting from undue widening of the nose.

hypersalemia   An elevated concentration of salt in the blood or blood serum.

hypersaline   Characterized by increased or excessive salinity: used of treatment involving the administration of large doses of sodium chloride.

hypersalivation PTYALISM.

hypersecretion [HYPER- + SECRETION] Excessive secretion, as of a gland. Also called *supersecretion*.

gastric hypersecretion Excessive production of mucus, acid, and/or pepsin by the gastric secretory cells. It occurs in the Zollinger-Ellison syndrome. Also called *hyperchylia, hyperpepsia*.

intestinal hypersecretion Pathologically increased secretion of mucus by the intestine.

hypersegmentation The state of having many segments or lobes.

hereditary hypersegmentation of neutrophils UNDRITZ ANOMALY.

hypersensibility Abnormally sharp sensory perception.

hypersensitive Exhibiting hypersensitivity. Also *supersensitive*.

hypersensitivity [HYPER- + SENSITIVITY] 1 A state of reactivity where a subsequent exposure to an antigen produces a greater effect than that produced on the initial exposure. 2 Excessive reactivity to any stimulus. Also called *hypererethism*.

atopic hypersensitivity ATOPY.

carotid sinus hypersensitivity Abnormal sensitivity of the carotid sinus, causing bradycardia or transient asystole and/or hypotension, which may result in syncope.

contact hypersensitivity Delayed (type 4) hypersensitivity reaction occurring in the skin at sites which have been in contact with agents that can bind to the skin to give rise to antigenic stimulation. Examples of substances that can induce contact hypersensitivity reactions are poison ivy (to which almost all exposed subjects react), and various drugs and cosmetics (to which comparatiely few react). Induction of contact hypersensitivy to dinitrochlorobenzene is used as a test of immune competence.

cutaneous basophil hypersensitivity JONES-MOTE REACTION.

delayed hypersensitivity An increased sensitivity to a foreign agent which is cell-mediated. The lesions in which lymphocytes and macrophages are prominent do not appear before 24 hours after contact or injection of the foreign substance. This reactivity can be transferred by lymphocytes from the sensitized individual to an unsensitized individual. Also called *type 4 hypersensitivity*. See also IMMUNOLOGICAL MECHANISMS OF TISSUE DAMAGE.

immediate hypersensitivity An increased sensitivity to a foreign agent, clinically manifest within minutes, characterized by the release of histamine and other pharmacologic mediators following the reaction of antigen with IgE antibody bound to mast cells. Serum of an affected individual that is introduced in another individual will allow immediate hypersensitivity to be produced in the second individual when challenged with the appropriate antigen. Also called *immediate allergy, type 1 hypersensitivity*. See also IMMUNOLOGICAL MECHANISMS OF TISSUE DAMAGE.

Jones-Mote hypersensitivity JONES-MOTE REACTION.

type 1 hypersensitivity IMMEDIATE HYPERSENSITIVITY.

type 2 hypersensitivity Type 2 hypersensitivity reaction. See under IMMUNOLOGICAL MECHANISMS OF TISSUE DAMAGE.

type 3 hypersensitivity Type 3 hypersensitivity reaction. See under IMMUNOLOGICAL MECHANISMS OF TISSUE DAMAGE.

type 4 hypersensitivity DELAYED HYPERSENSITIVITY.

hypersensitization The induction of a state of hypersensitivity. Also called *supersensitization*.

hyperserotonemia An elevated concentration of serotonin in the blood or blood serum.

hypersexuality [HYPER- + SEXUALITY] Pathologically increased sexual activity, as in the compulsive masturbator who masturbates seven times a day, the satyriasist whose quest for sexual conquests is insatiable, or the nymphomaniac whose search for sexual partners dominates her life. Also called *acolasia* (obsolete), *eroticomania, erotomania, fureur genitale* (obsolete), *furor amatorius* (obsolete), *furor genitalis* (obsolete).

hypersialosis An outmoded term for PTYALISM.

hyperskeocytosis HYPERNEOCYTOSIS.

hypersomatotropism [HYPER- + SOMATO- + TROPISM] 1 Excessive secretion of the anterior pituitary growth hormone. 2 ACROMEGALY.

hypersomia [HYPER- + Gk *sōma* body + -IA] GIGANTISM.

hypersomnia [HYPER- + L *somnia*, pl. of *somnium* (from *somnus* a sleep, sleepiness) a dream] A pathologic state of prolonged sleep, from which the patient can be roused only partly and very briefly. Also called *hyperhypnosis, lethargy*.

continuous hypersomnia A pathologic state of prolonged and uninterrupted sleep. This may be the principal symptom of such diseases as epidemic encephalitis or sleeping sickness, and can occur in patients with cerebral tumors, especially those situated in the third ventricular region or hypothalamus.

episodic hypersomnia PAROXYSMAL HYPERSOMNIA.

paroxysmal hypersomnia Hypersomnia occurring in bouts which may last for several minutes or for several hours. Hypersomnia differs from narcolepsy in that the cause may be an identifiable organic disorder of cerebral structure and function. Also called *episodic hypersomnia*.

periodic hypersomnia KLEINE-LEVIN SYNDROME.

hypersphyxia [HYPER- + Gk *sphyx(is)* for *sphygmos*, in earliest medical writers, the throbbing pulse in inflamed parts, later the beating of the heart, and finally the common pulse + -IA] A disorder characterized by a high blood pressure and increased circulatory activity.

hypersplenia HYPERSPLENISM.

hypersplenism A pathologic increase in the normal splenic functions of sequestration and destruction of aged or damaged formed blood elements, often associated with enlargement of the organ. It is manifested as varying combinations of anemia, leukopenia, thrombocytopenia, and hyperplasia of corresponding precursors in the bone marrow. Also called *hypersplenia, sissorexia*.

hypersplenotrophy SPLENOMEGALY.

hyperspongiosis An increase in the amount of substantia spongiosa ossium.

hypersteatosis SEBORRHEA.

hyperstereoroentgenography [HYPER- + STEREOROENTGEN-OGRAPHY] Stereoroentgenography in which the homologous points are separated by a greater distance than usual. Also called *hyperstereoskiagraphy*.

hyperstereoskiagraphy HYPERSTEREOROENTGENOGRAPHY.

hypersthenia [HYPER- + STHEN- + -IA] A state of excessive strength. Compare HYPASTHENIA.

hypersthenic [HYPER- + STHENIC] Concerning excessive strength.

hypersthenuria A condition characterized by a highly concentrated urine.

hypersuprarenalemia An obsolete term for HYPEREPINEPHRINEMIA.

hypersuprarenalism [HYPER- + SUPRA- + RENAL + -ISM] An outmoded term for HYPERADRENALISM.

hypersusceptibility Higher than normal susceptibility to a toxin or infectious agent.

hypersympathicotonus Abnormally great activity in the sympathetic nervous system.

hypersynchronism The sequence of electrical events that accompany the simultaneous repetitive discharge of large numbers of neurons, producing discharge patterns of high amplitude and sinusoidal in form. In the electroencephalogram this is observed as slow waves of abnormally high voltage. An incorrect usage. Also called *hypersynchrony.*

hypersynchrony HYPERSYNCHRONISM.

hypersystole Abnormally forceful or prolonged cardiac systole.

hypersystolic Pertaining to or characterized by hypersystole.

hypertarachia [HYPER- + Gk *tarach(ē)* trouble, complaint + -IA] Abnormal irritability of the nervous system.

hypertelorism [HYPER- + TELORISM] **1** Abnormally increased distance between paired organs or parts. **2** ORBITAL HYPERTELORISM.

canthal hypertelorism TELECANTHUS.

ocular hypertelorism ORBITAL HYPERTELORISM.

orbital hypertelorism The abnormally great interorbital distance associated with an enlarged sphenoid bone and sometimes with mental retardation and other developmental disorders such as craniofacial and cleidocranial dysostosis. Also called *Greig syndrome, ocular hypertelorism, hypertelorism.*

hypertensin Angiotensin II amide 5-valine.

hypertensinase ANGIOTENSINASE.

hypertensinogen ANGIOTENSINOGEN.

hypertension [HYPER- + TENSION] Abnormally high tension or pressure: applied especially to systemic arterial or pulmonary arterial blood pressure. Also called *hyperpiesis, hyperpiesia.*

accelerated hypertension A form of hypertension characterized by extremely high arterial pressures and usually by papilledema, fundic hemorrhages and exudates, and rapidly progressing renal failure. It is associated with a very poor prognosis if no treatment is given. Also called *malignant hypertension.*

adrenal hypertension Hypertension as a consequence of adrenal disease. Also called *suprarenal hypertension.*

arterial hypertension Hypertension in the systemic arterial circuit.

benign hypertension Hypertension in which the blood pressure is only modestly elevated in the absence of any secondary effects of the high blood pressure. Also called *red hypertension.*
• The term *benign* here is a misnomer, in that such cases often progress later to develop the serious complications of hypertension.

benign intracranial hypertension A syndrome of high intracranial pressure associated with cerebral edema, sometimes resulting from intracranial venous sinus thrombosis but more often of undetermined cause. The cerebral ventricles are normal or smaller than normal in size and the course is benign unless papilledema damages vision. Also called *pseudotumor cerebri, hypertensive meningeal hydrops, hydromeningitis* (obsolete), *pseudoabscess.*

diastolic hypertension Increased diastolic pressure in the systemic arteries, usually considered to be present in adults if 90 mmHg or greater when determined by the fifth phase of the Korotkoff sounds.

episodic hypertension PAROXYSMAL HYPERTENSION.

essential hypertension Hypertension for which no causative factor can be determined. Also called *idiopathic hypertension, primary hypertension.*

gestational hypertension Elevated blood pressure associated with pregnancy.

Goldblatt hypertension **1** An experimental hypertension in animals caused by constriction of one or both renal arteries. **2** Hypertension in man secondary to renal artery stenosis. For defs. 1 and 2 also called *Goldblatt phenomenon.*

idiopathic hypertension ESSENTIAL HYPERTENSION.

intracranial hypertension Increased intracranial pressure caused by a space-occupying lesion, cerebral edema, by obstruc-

tive or communicating hydrocephalus or by any process which increases the brain volume or pressure of the cerebrospinal fluid. The principal symptoms and signs are headache, vomiting, and papilledema.

malignant hypertension ACCELERATED HYPERTENSION.

neuromuscular hypertension Excessive muscular tension, including spasticity and rigidity of the musculature.

ocular hypertension The presence of an intraocular pressure level higher than usually considered normal, but which has not yet resulted in any demonstrable visual field defects. Ocular hypertension is not necessarily benign, inasmuch as some cases progress to overt glaucomatous damage. The distribution of intraocular pressure levels in the normal population extends through a considerable range and overlaps with the range of pressures found in glaucoma. Classification of a given pressure (for example, greater than 22 mmHg) as representing glaucoma on the one hand or a normal value on the other is not possible without careful medical evaluation of both ocular function and structure. Also called *hypertonia oculi.*

pale hypertension Hypertension associated with skin pallor due to constriction of superficial blood vessels. An outmoded term.

paroxysmal hypertension A form of hypertension in which the blood pressure rises in paroxysms, characteristically associated with pheochromocytoma. Also called *episodic hypertension.*

pituitary hypertension Associated with disorders of the adenohypophysis, such as Cushing's disease and acromegaly. An older term.

portal hypertension Elevation of portal vein pressure due to intrahepatic or extrahepatic cause, resulting in collateral circulation giving rise to esophageal and gastric varices or hemorrhoids, and in ascites, splenomegaly, and other manifestations.

primary hypertension ESSENTIAL HYPERTENSION.

pulmonary hypertension Increase in the pressure in the pulmonary circulation. Also called *pulmonary artery hypertension.*

pulmonary artery hypertension PULMONARY HYPERTENSION.

red hypertension BENIGN HYPERTENSION.

renal hypertension Hypertension secondary to renal disease, renal artery stenosis, or obstruction of the urinary tract. Renin often is increased in renal veins of affected kidneys.

renin-dependent hypertension Hypertension due to increased renin production in renal artery stenosis, renal parencyhmal disease, or in urinary tract obstruction.

renoprival hypertension Hypertension in an anephric patient or in a patient whose kidneys do not function. Renoprival hypertension may result from fluid overload, absence of vasodepressor factors produced by the kidneys, or both.

renovascular hypertension Hypertension secondary to stenosis of the main renal artery or its primary branches, or of an aberrant artery, usually due to atherosclerosis or fibromuscular hyperplasia. The renal artery rarely may be narrowed by extrinsic pressure, aneurysm, thrombosis, embolism, or arteritis. Renin is increased in renal venous blood from affected kidneys. The hypertension may be cured by surgical reconstruction of the affected artery, or by nephrectomy if the condition is unilateral.

saturnine hypertension Hypertension associated with lead encephalopathy.

secondary hypertension Hypertension which is secondary to another disorder, such as renal disease, adrenal tumors, or coarctation of the aorta. Also called *symptomatic hypertension.*

suprarenal hypertension ADRENAL HYPERTENSION.

symptomatic hypertension SECONDARY HYPERTENSION.

systolic hypertension Increased systolic pressure in the systemic arteries, usually considered to be present if the systolic pressure is greater than 140 mmHg in adults. It is commonly accompanied by diastolic hypertension, but may be isolated in hyperthyroidism and in the elderly with rigid arteries due to arteriosclerosis.

transient hypertension Hypertension that is evident only intermittently.

vascular hypertension Abnormally high pressure in the blood vessels; hypertension.

venous hypertension Increased venous pressure.

hypertensive Affected by or pertaining to hypertension. Also *hyperpietic.*

hypertensor Any agent that raises blood pressure; a pressor substance.

hypertestosteronism Excessive secretion of testosterone from any source, as in Leydig cell tumor of the testis in prepubertal boys.

hyperthecosis [HYPER- + *thec(a)* + -OSIS] The development of stromal hyperplasia and foci of luteinization in the ovary. Most patients are of age 20–30.

testoid hyperthecosis Diffuse hyperplasia and often focal luteinization of ovarian stromal cells associated with testosterone secretion, virilization, obesity, and sometimes diabetes.

hyperthelia [HYPER- + THEL- + -IA] POLYTHELIA.

hyperthermal [HYPER- + THERMAL] Concerning excessively high temperatures.

hyperthermalgesia [HYPER- + THERMALGESIA] Excessive sensitivity to heat. Also called *hyperthermesthesia, hyperthermoesthesia.*

hyperthermesthesia HYPERTHERMALGESIA.

hyperthermia [HYPER- + Gk *thermē* heat, feverish heat + -IA] Fever, especially therapeutic fever. Also called *hyperthermy.*

malignant hyperthermia See under MALIGNANT HYPERTHERMIA SYNDROME.

whole-body hyperthermia The deliberate raising of body temperature for the treatment of disease. It may be used to enhance the effect of other therapeutic agents.

hyperthermoesthesia HYPERTHERMALGESIA.

hyperthermy HYPERTHERMIA.

hyperthrombinemia An elevated concentration or activity of thrombin in the blood.

hyperthymergasia The manic form of manic-depressive psychosis. A seldom used term.

hyperthymia A state of overactivity as a manifestation of cyclothymia.

hyperthymism An abnormal increase in activity of the thymus.

hyperthyrea A rarely used term for HYPERTHYROIDISM.

hyperthyreosis A seldom used term for HYPERTHYROIDISM.

hyperthyroid [HYPER- + THYROID] Of, characterized by, or resulting from hyperthyroidism.

hyperthyroidism [HYPER- + THYROID + -ISM] **1** Excessive secretion by the thyroid gland of thyroxine or triiodothyronine or both, accompanied by increased rate of oxygen consumption, accelerated basal metabolic rate, thyroid enlargement, and systemic disturbances, the most prominent symptoms being weakness, weight loss, and nervousness. Also called *hyperthyreosis* (seldom used), *hyperthyrea* (rarely used), *hyperthyroidosis* (seldom used), *thyroidism.* **2** An ambiguous term for GRAVES DISEASE.

apathetic hyperthyroidism MASKED HYPERTHYROIDISM.

factitious hyperthyroidism Hyperthyroidism produced by self-medication with thyroid hormone.

iatrogenic hyperthyroidism Hyperthyroidism resulting from the administration of too much thyroid hormone in the course of medical treatment.

iodine-induced hyperthyroidism Unexplained induction of true hyperthyroidism by ingestion of excessive iodine. Also called *Jod-Basedow, Jod-Basedow phenomenon, iod-Basedow.*

latent hyperthyroidism A condition clinically resembling Graves disease but in which the secretion of thyroid hormone appears normal. ● The term is misleading since it does not refer to a single entity.

masked hyperthyroidism Excessive secretion of thyroid hormone by the thyroid gland, usually in middle-aged or elderly persons, but without the typical signs and symptoms of hyperthyroidism. It is characterized by weakness, lethargy, and often by cardiac arrhythmia or congestive heart failure. Also called *apathetic hyperthyroidism.*

primary hyperthyroidism Hyperthyroidism due to intrinsic disease of the thyroid gland.

secondary hyperthyroidism Hyperthyroidism due to stimulation of the thyroid gland by adenohypophysial oversecretion of thyrotropic hormone. The condition is very rare. Also called *hyperthyrotropinism.*

hyperthyroidosis A seldom used term for HYPERTHYROIDISM.

hyperthyrotropinism SECONDARY HYPERTHYROIDISM.

hyperthyroxinemia An elevated concentration of thyroxine in the blood or blood serum.

hypertonia [HYPER- + Gk *tonos* (from *teinein* to stretch, strain, draw tight) a tightening, rope, sinew, force + -IA] **1** Increased muscle tone. Also called *hypertonus, hypermyotonia* (seldom used). Adjective: hypertonic. **2** A seldom used term for HYPERTENSION.

hypertonia oculi OCULAR HYPERTENSION.

hypertonia polycythaemica The combination of polycythemia and arterial hypertension.

hypertonic **1** More than normally tonic, as the state of a muscle. **2** Having a greater tonicity than the solution with which it is compared. **3** Having an osmotic pressure higher than that of an isotonic solution or more concentrated than isotonic. Sodium chloride solutions are said to be hypertonic at concentrations of more than 0.45%, the point at which red blood cells undergo crenation. Also *hyperisotonic.*

hypertonicity The property of being hypertonic. Also called *hyperisotonicity.*

hypertonus HYPERTONIA.

hypertoxic [HYPER- + TOXIC] Extremely or excessively toxic.

hypertoxicity [HYPER- + TOXICITY] Excessive or extreme toxicity.

hypertrichiasis HYPERTRICHOSIS.

hypertrichophobia Pathologic fear or intense dislike of excess hair, as on a hairy chest or hairy back.

hypertrichophrydia [HYPER- + TRICH- + Gk *ophry(s)* the eyebrow + *d* + -IA] An excessive growth of the eyebrows.

hypertrichosis [HYPER- + TRICHOSIS] The growth of hair in any pattern which is excessive for the age, sex, and race of the subject. Also called *hypertrichiasis.* Compare HIRSUTISM.

familial hypertrichosis Hypertrichosis as a family trait, suggesting some type of hereditary transmission.

fetal hypertrichosis An excessive growth of lanugo *in utero.*

hypertrichosis pinnae auris The growth of coarse hair on the rim of the helix that occurs between the ages of 17 and 45 in many Bengali and Sinhalese males. A Y-linked inheritance is probable. Also called *hairy ears.*

hypertrichosis universalis lanuginosa The presence at birth and persistence throughout life of long, fine lanugo in all follicles.

hypertriglyceridemia [HYPER- + TRIGLYCERIDE + -EMIA]

An elevated concentration of triglycerides in the blood or blood serum. See also HYPERLIPOPROTEINEMIA.

alimentary hypertriglyceridemia EXOGENOUS HYPERTRIGLYCERIDEMIA.

carbohydrate-induced hypertriglyceridemia CARBOHYDRATE-INDUCED HYPERLIPIDEMIA.

endogenous hypertriglyceridemia 1 FAMILIAL HYPERLIPOPROTEINEMIA TYPE I. **2** FAMILIAL HYPERLIPOPROTEINEMIA TYPE IV.

exogenous hypertriglyceridemia A greater than normal concentration of triglycerides in plasma as a consequence of high triglyceride content of the diet or parenteral administration of large amounts of triglycerides. Also called *alimentary hypertriglyceridemia.*

familial hypertriglyceridemia 1 FAMILIAL HYPERLIPOPROTEINEMIA TYPE I. **2** FAMILIAL HYPERLIPOPROTEINEMIA TYPE IV.

familial fat-induced hypertriglyceridemia FAMILIAL HYPERLIPOPROTEINEMIA TYPE I.

hypertrophia A seldom used term for HYPERTROPHY.

hypertrophia musculorum vera A syndrome of generalized hypertrophy of the skeletal muscles. It is of multiple etiology, the causes including myotonia congenita and hypothyroidism.

hypertrophic Pertaining to or characterized by hypertrophy.

hypertrophied Characterized by hypertrophy.

hypertrophy [HYPER- + Gk *trophē* nourishment, food] Increase in size of an organ or part due to an increase in the size of its individual cells. A common example is hypertrophy of the left ventricular myocardium as a result of systemic arterial hypertension. Also called *hypertrophia* (seldom used), *simple hypertrophy.*

adaptive hypertrophy Hypertrophy of the walls of a hollow organ as a result of increased resistance to the emptying function, as occurs in the left ventricle of the heart in aortic valve stenosis and in the urinary bladder in outflow obstruction due to prostatic gland enlargement.

adult hypertrophy of the pylorus Acquired hypertrophy of the pylorus which presents in adults as partial or complete gastric outlet obstruction. It may be related in some cases to underlying peptic ulcer disease. Also called *Billroth hypertrophy.* See also ADULT PYLORIC STENOSIS.

benign masseteric hypertrophy The enlargement of one or both masseter muscles. Also called *hypertrophy of masseter muscle.*

benign hypertrophy of the pons Enlargement of the pons resulting from the presence of a slowly growing pontine glioma.

bilateral hypertrophy of masseters A benign syndrome of unknown cause in which there is marked enlargement of both masseter muscles.

Billroth hypertrophy ADULT HYPERTROPHY OF THE PYLORUS.

biventricular hypertrophy Hypertrophy affecting both cardiac ventricles.

breast hypertrophy of the newborn The enlargement of breast tissue common in infants of both sexes during the first week of life. It is sometimes associated with the secretion of a few drops of milk that may be released during this period.

cardiac concentric hypertrophy Uniform hypertrophy of the ventricles.

cicatricial hypertrophy The overproduction of fibrous connective tissue in a scar.

compensatory hypertrophy Hypertrophy of a tissue or organ following damage or loss of a portion of such tissue. It is seen, for example, in the viable myocardium adjacent to an infarct, and in the remaining kidney following unilateral nephrectomy. Also called *complementary hypertrophy, vicarious hypertrophy.*

compensatory hypertrophy of the heart Hypertrophy of the heart as a response to increased work load as imposed by valvular heart disease or hypertension.

complementary hypertrophy COMPENSATORY HYPERTROPHY.

concentric hypertrophy Hypertrophy, especially of a cardiac chamber, characterized by increased thickness of the walls but without dilatation.

congenital hypertrophy of the bladder neck MARION'S DISEASE.

denture hypertrophy DENTURE HYPERPLASIA.

eccentric hypertrophy Hypertrophy, especially of a cardiac chamber, characterized by normal or increased thickness of the walls and dilatation of the lumen.

false hypertrophy PSEUDOHYPERTROPHY.

functional hypertrophy An increase in the size of an organ due to an increase in functional load or activity. Also called *physiologic hypertrophy.*

gingival hypertrophy An incorrect term for GINGIVAL HYPERPLASIA.

hemangiectatic hypertrophy KLIPPEL-TRENAUNAY-WEBER SYNDROME.

hemifacial hypertrophy Asymmetrical hypertrophy involving one side of the face.

juxtaglomerular cell hypertrophy Enlargement of the renal juxtaglomerular cells secondary to decreased blood flow. Associated degranulation reflects greater secretion than storage of renin.

hypertrophy of the kidney RENAL HYPERTROPHY.

mammary hypertrophy Hypertrophy of one or both breasts, so excessive as to constitute a cosmetic or mechanical burden and require surgical correction. Also called *barymazia.*

Marie's hypertrophy Swelling of an extremity due to periostitis.

hypertrophy of masseter muscle BENIGN MASSETERIC HYPERTROPHY.

mulberry hypertrophy See under HYPERTROPHIC RHINITIS.

numeric hypertrophy an incorrect and obsolete term for HYPERPLASIA.

physiologic hypertrophy FUNCTIONAL HYPERTROPHY.

pseudomuscular hypertrophy MUSCULAR PSEUDOHYPERTROPHY.

quantitative hypertrophy An obsolete term for HYPERPLASIA.

renal hypertrophy Compensatory increase in mass and function of one kidney in response to absence or marked impairment of function of the contralateral kidney. This may be congenital or acquired, and occurs in transplanted kidneys. Also called *hypernephrotrophy* (rarely used), *nephrohypertrophy, hypertrophy of the kidney.*

simple hypertrophy HYPERTROPHY.

true hypertrophy Hypertrophy due to an increase in the size of all structural elements of an organ or part.

unilateral hypertrophy Hypertrophy involving only one side of the body or of a portion of it, or one of a paired organ such as the kidney.

ventricular hypertrophy Myocardial hypertrophy of a cardiac ventricle.

vicarious hypertrophy COMPENSATORY HYPERTROPHY.

work hypertrophy Muscle hypertrophy resulting from increased workload.

hypertropia [HYPER- + TROPIA] A constant deviation of alignment of the eyes in which the visual axis of one eye points in a direction higher than the other. The designation is applied to the higher of the two eyes, irrespective of which eye is used in fixation. Thus, in right hypertropia, the right eye is higher; in left hypertropia, the left.

alternating hypertropia   Hypertropia in which the visual axis of each eye is higher from time to time.

hypertyrosinemia   A greater than normal concentration of tyrosine in blood.

hyperuresis [HYPER- + -URESIS]   POLYURIA.

hyperuricacidemia   HYPERURICEMIA.

hyperuricaciduria   HYPERURICURIA.

hyperuricemia   A greater than normal concentration of uric acid or urates in blood. Also called *hyperuricacidemia, agremia* (older term), *uricemia, uratemia, uricacidemia, lithemia.* Adjective: hyperuricemic.

congenital hyperuricemia   LESCH-NYHAN SYNDROME.

X-linked hyperuricemia   HYPOXANTHINE PHOSPHORIBOSYL-TRANSFERASE DEFICIENCY.

hyperuricemia-oligophrenia   LESCH-NYHAN SYNDROME.

hyperuricosuria   HYPERURICURIA.

hyperuricuria [HYPER- + -URIC + -URIA]   Urinary excretion of more than 600 mg uric acid per day while on a low purine diet. It is associated with uric acid overproduction and hyperuricemia in some gouty patients, the Lesch-Nyhan syndrome, myeloproliferative disorders, polycythemia, hemolytic and certain other anemias, and some carcinomas, and may occur during treatment of gout with a uricosuric agent. Chronic hyperuricuria may result in uric acid calculi and gouty nephropathy, while acute hyperuricuria secondary to rapidly effective treatment of myeloproliferative disorders or large tumors may lead to precipitation of uric acid in the urinary tract with resultant acute renal failure. Also called *hyperuricosuria, hyperlithuria, hyperuricaciduria.*

hypervaccination   HYPERIMMUNIZATION.

hypervalinemia   A metabolic disorder, of which a single case has been described, characterized by retardation and vomiting, and by increased valine in both plasma and urine.

hypervascular   Having increased vascularity; very highly vascular.

hypervenosity   An abnormal increase in venous circulation.

hyperventilation [HYPER- + VENTILATION]   Pulmonary ventilation beyond that necessary for metabolism, causing excessive alveolar ventilation. Hyperventilation, often a reaction to anxiety or fear, results in progressive hypocapnia, producing symptoms of palpitations, dizziness or faintness, paresthesiae, and tetany. Also called *overventilation, hyperaeration, overbreathing* (popular).

central neurogenic hyperventilation   Hyperventilation resulting from a lesion in the central nervous system.

hysterical hyperventilation   A syndrome of voluntary hyperventilation resulting from hysteria and usually occurring in young women, in which tetany and even syncope may occur.

hyperviscosity   The quality of being extremely viscous.

hypervitaminosis [HYPER- + VITAMIN + -OSIS]   Adverse effects resulting from the consumption of excessive quantities of one or more vitamins. Also called *supervitaminosis.*

hypervitaminosis A   A condition resulting from the ingestion of excessive amounts of vitamin A. It is characterized by loss of weight, soreness of the eyes, loss of hair, demineralization of the skeleton, and hemorrhages. The doses necessary to produce these effects are approximately 10 000 times the daily requirement and are therefore rarely encountered.

hypervitaminosis D   A condition resulting from the daily ingestion of excessive amounts of vitamin D. It increases excretion of blood phosphorus by the kidney, extracts calcium and phosphorus from bone, produces osteoporosis and causes deposition of calcium salts in the soft tissues.

hypervitaminotic   Relating to the excessive consumption of one or more vitamins.

hypervolaemia   A British spelling for HYPERVOLEMIA.

hypervolemia   Greater than normal blood volume.

hypervolemic   Having or pertaining to greater than normal blood volume.

hypervolia [HYPER- + *vol(ume)* + -IA]   Increased water content in a given compartment, such as a cell.

hypervolume   The total niches of all community members.

hypervolumic   Of or relating to excessive volume or bulk.

hypesthesia   HYPOESTHESIA.

hypesthetic   HYPOESTHETIC.

hypha [Gk *hyphē* or *hyphos* a weaving, web]   (*plural* hyphae) The unit of structure of most fungi, consisting of a tubular filament, combined into a complex network that makes up the thallus or body of a fungus. Also called *mycelial thread.*

apical hypha   The growing tip of a fungal hypha and the region immediately behind it upon which it depends metabolically.

nonseptate hypha   A hypha without crosswalls, so that nuclei lie in the common cytoplasmic matrix. Such hyphae are seen in fungal subdivisions Haplomastigomycotina, Diplomastigomycotina, and Zygomycotina.

racquet hypha   A specialized form of hypha consisting of a series of small paddleshaped units with the narrow end of each attached to the larger end of the preceding segment.

receptive hypha   A female reproductive structure of certain fungi.

septate hypha   A hypha with crosswalls which divide the filamentous tube into compartments or cells, as in the fungal subdivisions Ascomycotina, Basidiomycotina, and Deuteromycotina.

hyphae   Plural of HYPHA.

hyphaema   A British spelling for HYPHEMA.

hyphal   Of or pertaining to a hypha or hyphae.

hyphedonia [*hyp(o)-* + *hēdon(ē)* pleasure + -IA]   A state in which there is an inability to experience pleasure to a normal degree.

hyphema [See HYPHEMIA.]   The presence of free blood in the inferior portion of the anterior chamber of the eye. Being heavier than the aqueous humor, blood cells settle to the bottom, becoming oriented with a characteristic horizontal flat top as determined by gravity. This readily observable sign signifies the presence of serious intraocular pathology requiring prompt ophthalmological evaluation. Also called *hyphemia.*

hyphemia [HYP- + -HEMIA]   **1** HYPHEMA.   **2** An obsolete term for ANEMIA.

hyphephilia [Gk *hyphē* a weaving, web + -PHILIA]   A paraphilia in which sexual gratification depends upon contact with a specific fabric, such as silk or velvet. Also called *hephephilia, stuff erotism.*

hyphidrosis   HYPOHIDROSIS.

hyphology   The study of fungal hyphae. An obsolete term.

Hyphomyces destruens   A species of fungus which is one among several agents of phycomycotic lesions on the head and lower legs of horses and mules.

hyphomycete [*hyph(a)* + *o* + -MYCETE]   An imperfect fungus of the form-subclass Hyphomycetidae, which produces neither acervuli nor pycnidia.

hyphomycetoma [*hyphomycet(e)* + -OMA]   The swelling accompanying any form of disease caused by any member of the fungal form-class Deuteromycetes. An obsolete term.

hyphomycosis   **1** Any infection with a *Hyphomyces* fungus.   **2** HYPHOMYCOSIS DESTRUENS EQUI.

hyphomycosis destruens equi   A fungal infection of horses, caused by *Hyphomyces destruens* and characterized by subcutaneous abscesses and cutaneous necrosis. Also called *hypomycosis.*

hyphylline   DYPHYLLINE.

hypinosis   An obsolete term for HYPOFIBRINOGENEMIA.

hypinotic   Characterized by hypinosis (hypofibrinogenemia). An obsolete term.

hypn-   HYPNO-.

hypnagogic   **1** Sleep-producing;   hypnotic. **2** Preceding sleep: used of images or dreams perceived during the transition between the waking state and sleep.

hypnagogue   [HYPN- + -AGOGUE]   **1** A hypnotic agent. **2** An agent causing sleepiness or drowsiness.

hypnenergia   An obsolete term for SOMNAMBULISM.

hypnic   Describing, pertaining to, or inducing sleep.

hypno-   [Gk *hypnos* sleep]   A combining form meaning sleep. Also *hypn-.*

hypnoanalysis   The use of hypnosis to open paths to memories that are not available to the subject during sessions when he is fully conscious. Also called *hypnonarcoanalysis.*

hypnoanesthesia   A trancelike state produced by hypnosis and sometimes suitable for performance of minor surgery.

hypnobatia   [HYPNO- + Gk *bat(os)*, verbal of *bainein* to go, walk + -IA]   An obsolete term for SOMNAMBULISM.

hypnocatharsis   The reliving of repressed material and its affective associations that have been brought forth during hypnoanalysis.

hypnocinematograph   An instrument for recording movements made during sleep.

hypnocyst   A dormant or quiescent cyst. An obsolete term.

hypnodontia   [HYPN- + -ODONTIA]   The study of hypnosis in dentistry.

hypnodontics   [HYPN- + -ODONT + -ICS]   The practice of hypnosis in dentistry.

hypnogenetic   HYPNOGENIC.

hypnogenic   [HYPNO- + -GENIC]   Productive of hypnosis or sleep, as a spot which, upon being touched by a subject, puts him into a hypnotic state. Also *hypnogenetic.*

hypnogenous   [HYPNO- + -GENOUS]   Arising from a state of hypnosis, such as unconscious material uncovered during the course of hypnoanalysis.

hypnoid   Resembling a state of hypnosis or sleep.

hypnolepsy   NARCOLEPSY.

hypnology   [HYPNO- + -LOGY]   The study of the phenomena of sleep and hypnosis.

hypnonarcoanalysis   HYPNOANALYSIS.

hypnonarcosis   A hypnotic trance.

hypnophobia   [HYPNO- + -PHOBIA]   Pathologic fear of falling asleep.

hypnopompic   [HYPNO- + Gk *pomp(ē)* an escorting, procession + -IC]   Denoting imagery characteristic of the drowsy state following wakening from a deep sleep but before becoming fully awake.

hypnosia   Excessive or uncontrollable drowsiness.

hypnosigenesis   [*hypnosi(s)* + GENESIS]   The induction of hypnosis. A seldom used term.

hypnosis   [HYPN- + -OSIS]   **1** A state of decreased general awareness but increased attention to a constricted area of rhythmic or repetitive stimulation, usually induced by another person, and distinguishable from sleep by the presence of catatonia and increased suggestibility. Also called *braidism* (obsolete), *hypnotic sleep, teleotherapeutics.* **2** The induction of a hypnotic state. Adjective: hypnotic.

lethargic hypnosis   **1** A hypnotic trance. **2** Sleep following a period of hypnosis.

hypnosophy   The study of sleep and of associated phenomena.

hypnotherapy   The use of hypnosis as the major or sole modality of treatment. Also called *hypnotic psychotherapy, Bernheim's therapy* (older term).

hypnotic   **1** A sleep-producing or sedative agent. **2** Inducing sleep or having an anodyne effect. **3** Of, relating to, or resulting from hypnotism.   ● In modern usage, *hypnotics* is applied more often to sedative agents and *narcotics* to pain-relieving agents.

hypnotism   [Gk *hypnōt(ikos)* (from *hypnoein* to lull to sleep, from *hypnos* sleep) inclined to sleep + -ISM]   The theory and applications of hypnosis. Also called *donatism, pathetism* (obsolete), *somnolism* (obsolete), *mesmerism* (obsolete).

hypnotoxin   **1** A toxin which depresses the activity of the central nervous system and which is released from the tentacles of *Physalia* (the Portuguese man-of-war). **2** A toxic substance which, according to a discredited hypothesis, accumulates in the bloodstream during drowsiness and ultimately induces sleep.

hypo-   [Gk *hypo* under, from under]   **1** A prefix meaning (1) under, beneath; (2) diminished, deficient, too little or too few, below the normal. **2** In chemistry, a prefix designating an oxyacid or its salt with less oxygen than in the unprefixed compound. Compare HYPER-.

hypoactive   [HYPO- + ACTIVE]   Less than normally active.

hypoactivity   [HYPO- + ACTIVITY]   A state of less than normal activity.

hypoacusis   [HYPO- + ACU-² + -SIS]   Partial hearing loss. Also called *acoustic hypoesthesia, auditory hypoesthesia.*

hypoadenia   Subnormal function of a gland or glands. A rarely used term.

hypoadrenalemia   Less than normal concentration of adrenal hormones and epinephrine in blood.

hypoadrenalism   [HYPO- + ADRENAL + -ISM]   Any deficient function of the adrenal gland, especially hypoadrenocorticism. An imprecise usage. Also called *hypadrenia* (outmoded), *hypoadrenia* (rarely used), *hyposuprarenalism* (seldom used).

hypoadrenia   A rarely used term for HYPOADRENALISM.

hypoadrenocortical   Of, caused by, or relating to hypoadrenocorticism.

hypoadrenocorticalism   HYPOADRENOCORTICISM.

hypoadrenocorticism   The clinical condition induced by deficient secretion of hormones by the adrenal cortex, as in Addison's disease or panhypopituitarism. Also called *hypoadrenocorticalism, hypocorticalism, hypocorticism.*

pituitary hypoadrenocorticism   SECONDARY HYPOADRENOCORTICISM.

secondary hypoadrenocorticism   Deficient secretion of adrenocortical hormones, particularly cortisol, due either to pituitary failure and subnormal secretion of adrenocorticotropin, suppression of the pituitary adrenocortical axis by exogenous corticosteroids, or, rarely, systemic disease, as Laennec cirrhosis of the liver. Also called *pituitary hypoadrenocorticism.*

hypoaesthesia   A British spelling for HYPOESTHESIA.

hypoaffective   Lacking in emotional responsivity, with a blunted or flattened affect.

hypoagnathus   An individual with a much reduced or with no lower jaw.

hypoalbuminemia   Less than normal concentration of albumen in blood, plasma, or serum. Also called *hypoalbuminosis, hypalbuminemia, hypalbuminosis.*

hypoalbuminosis   HYPOALBUMINEMIA.

hypoaldosteronemia   Less than normal concentration of aldosterone in blood, plasma, or serum.

hypoaldosteronism [HYPO- + ALDOSTERONISM] Deficient adrenocortical secretion of aldosterone, usually accompanying primary adrenocortical insufficiency or Addison's disease, and causing excessive renal salt wasting with depletion of blood volume, hyponatremia and hypotension. Also called *aldosteronopenia*.

hyporeninemic hypoaldosteronism A disorder seen in elderly subjects and characterized by selective aldosterone deficiency and low plasma renin levels, hyperkalemia, and frequently hypertension. Possible causes are chronic renal disease, diabetes mellitus with autonomic neuropathy, and chronic overexpansion of blood volume.

isolated hypoaldosteronism A very rare form of primary adrenocortical insufficiency in which aldosterone secretion is subnormal or absent with normal secretion of other adrenocortical steroids, as cortisol.

hypoaldosteronuria An abnormally low concentration of aldosterone in the urine.

hypoalgesia HYPALGESIA.

hypoalimentation [HYPO- + ALIMENTATION] Insufficient ingestion or administration of the essential nutrients needed to satisfy the metabolic needs of the body.

hypoallergenic Not likely to induce an allergic reaction.

hypoalonemia A less than normal concentration of cations and anions in blood. A rarely used term.

hypoalphalipoproteinemia ANALPHALIPOPROTEINEMIA.

hypoaminoacidemia Less than normal concentration of amino acids in blood, plasma, or serum.

hypoamphotonia Simultaneous reduction of parasympathetic and of sympathetic activity.

hypoandrogenism [HYPO- + ANDROGEN + -ISM] A deficiency of androgenic hormone or hormones, or the condition resulting from it.

hypoarterial HYPARTERIAL.

hypoazoturia [HYPO- + AZOTURIA] Decreased urinary excretion of nitrogenous substances in advanced renal failure. A rarely used term.

hypobaric [HYPO- + BAR-² + -IC] At less than normal atmospheric pressure.

hypobarism [HYPO- + BAR-² + -ISM] Any condition which results from a decrease in ambient pressure to a level below that in body fluids, tissues, and cavities. Also called *hypobaropathy*.

hypobaropathy HYPOBARISM.

hypobasophilism Deficient function of the basophil cells of the anterior pituitary, specifically in a rare form of isolated adrenocorticotropin deficiency associated with a subnormal number of pituitary corticotrophs. A seldom used term.

hypobetalipoproteinemia **1** Any reduction in β-lipoproteins in plasma. **2** A syndrome heritable as an autosomal dominant trait and characterized by reduced serum cholesterol and β-lipoprotein. Atherosclerosis is not a feature and longevity is either unaffected or increased. Other clinical features, including acanthocytosis, are inconsistent. Heterozygosity for the defect that causes abetalipoproteinemia has not been substantiated as the cause for hypobetalipoproteinemia. Also called *familial hypobetalipoproteinemia*.

familial hypobetalipoproteinemia HYPOBETALIPOPROTEINEMIA.

hypobilirubinemia Less than normal concentration of bilirubin in blood, plasma, or serum.

hypoblast [HYPO- + -BLAST] A deeply placed germ layer, either in the general sense of endoderm or more often in primitive Amniota in the sense of entophyll. At the start of gastru-

lation the chick blastoderm consists of two layers, the epiblast above, the hypoblast beneath. The hypoblast arises at the posterior end of the area pellucida. It extends anteriorly until it lies beneath the whole of the area pellucida. Later the definitive endoblast invaginates through the anterior end of the primitive streak and becomes inserted into the sheet of hypoblast. Adjective: hypoblastic.

hypoblepharon [HYPO- + Gk *blepharon* an eyelid] Outward displacement of the eyelid by the presence of an underlying mass. A seldom used term.

hypoboulia [HYPO- + Gk *boul(ē)* will, determination, task + -IA] Lacking in volition, willpower, or drive. Also *hypobulia*.

hypobranchial Situated beneath the branchial arches.

hypobromite The ion BrO⁻ and any salt containing it.

hypobromous acid HBrO. An acid that has not been isolated but is known in solution. Its salts are formed, together with bromides, when bromine is dissolved in alkali. It is a powerful oxidizing agent.

hypobulia HYPOBOULIA.

hypocalcemia Less than normal concentration of calcium in blood or serum. Adjective: hypocalcemic.

neonatal hypocalcemia The decrease in serum calcium level which occurs during the first week of life. It is associated with an increase in the serum phosphorous level. Signs of tetany may become apparent in some infants where the calcium level falls below 2 mmol/l. This may occur with or without brief convulsive episodes. The hypocalcemia is considered to be secondary to a renal failure to clear phosphate. Since cow's milk contains more phosphorous than does human milk clinical symptoms are largely confined to artificially fed infants.

hypocalcia A state of reduced calcium content.

hypocalcification [HYPO- + CALCIFICATION] A decrease in the calcification process.

enamel hypocalcification An abnormality in which the enamel is of normal thickness but is chalky and weak. It may be caused by fluorosis, or it may be hereditary.

hereditary enamel hypocalcification Enamel hypocalcification affecting all the teeth as a genetic defect.

hypocalcipectic HYPOCALCIPEXIC.

hypocalcipexic Of or relating to hypocalcipexy. Also *hypocalcipectic*.

hypocalcipexy A state of reduced fixation of calcium.

hypocalcitonemia HYPOCALCITONINEMIA.

hypocalcitoninemia A concentration of calcitonin in the blood below the normal value of 5–100 pg/ml. Also called *hypocalcitonemia*.

hypocalciuria Decreased urinary excretion of calcium. It is an inconstant sign of low dietary calcium intake, but is common during growth, pregnancy, and lactation, and in the intestinal malabsorption syndrome. The condition may be a sign of deficiency of parathyroid or thyroid hormones, or vitamin D. It also may occur during salt depletion or diuretic therapy.

hypocapnia [HYPO- + Gk *kapn(os)* smoke, vapor + -IA] An abnormally low concentration of carbon dioxide in the blood. Also called *hypocarbia*.

hypocapnic Characterized by hypocapnia.

hypocarbia HYPOCAPNIA.

hypocatalasemia Less than normal activity of catalase in blood cells, especially in erythrocytes.

hypocellularity A state characterized by an abnormally low number of cells, as seen in the bone marrow in aplastic anemia or following cancer chemotherapy. Adjective: hypocellular.

hypocelom HYPOCOELOM.

hypocenter That point on the surface of the earth that is directly at the center of a nuclear bomb explosion.

hypoceruloplasminemia A reduced concentration of plasma ceruloplasmin, as is usually found in Wilson's disease and Menkes disease and normally in the newborn.

hypochloremia Less than normal concentration of chloride in blood, plasma, or serum. Also called *hypochloridemia, chloropenia.* Adjective: hypochloremic.

hypochlorhydria Diminished gastric secretion of hydrochloric acid. Also called *hypohydrochloria.*

hypochlorhydric Relating to or characterized by hypochlorhydria.

hypochloridation A level of chloride insufficient to accomplish the purpose for which it is intended.

hypochloridemia HYPOCHLOREMIA.

hypochlorite The ion ClO⁻ and salts containing it.

hypochlorization A limitation placed on the dietary intake of salt.

hypochlorous acid HClO. An acid that has not been isolated. It is formed by the action of water on Cl_2O. Its solution is used for making hypochlorites almost free from chlorides.

hypochloruria Decreased urinary excretion of chloride, as in dietary salt restriction or accumulating edema. It may be secondary to excess chloride loss in gastric secretions or to secretion or administration of salt-retaining mineralocorticoid hormones.

hypocholesteremia HYPOCHOLESTEROLEMIA.

hypocholesterinemia HYPOCHOLESTEROLEMIA.

hypocholesterolemia A less than normal concentration of cholesterol in blood, plasma, or serum. Also called *hypocholesteremia, hypocholesterinemia.* Adjective: hypocholesterolemic, hypocholesteremic.

hypocholia [HYPO- + CHOL- + -IA] Diminished secretion of bile.

hypochondria HYPOCHONDRIASIS.

hypochondriac A person who suffers from hypochondriasis.

hypochondriacal Pertaining to or suffering from hypochondriasis.

hypochondriasis A somatoform disorder characterized by a misinterpretation of physical signs that leads to the belief of having a serious disease even though repeated evaluations can elicit no indications of physical disorder. Also called *hypochondria, hypochondriacal neurosis, nosomania* (obsolete), *nosophilia* (obsolete), *hygeiophrontis, hygeiolatry* (obsolete), *somatophrenia, vapors* (obsolete).

hypochondrium REGIO HYPOCHONDRIACA (DEXTRA ET SINISTRA).

hypochondroplasia A less severe form or variant of achondroplasia, with dwarfism that is not apparent until mid-childhood. It may be inherited as an autosomal dominant trait. Also called *chondrohypoplasia* (obsolete).

hypochordal [HYPO- + Gk *chord(ē)* a cord, string of gut + -AL] Lying below or ventral to the notochord.

hypochromasia Hypochromia.

hypochromatic In genetics, referring to a cell or organism with fewer than normal chromosomes. An obsolete term.

hypochromatism 1 A less than usual intensity of color in any structure. 2 A fading of the chromatin of the cell nucleus.

hypochromatosis 1 The condition of having less than the usual amount of color intensity. 2 A less than normal amount of chromatin in the cell nucleus.

hypochromemia HYPOCHROMIA.

hypochromia A paler than normal appearance of erythrocytes when stained by a Romanowsky type stain and examined microscopically. The reduction in color intensity of such erythrocytes is due to diminution in their hemoglobin content. Also

called *hypochromemia, hypochromasia, oligochromasia.*

hypochromic Exhibiting hypochromia. Hypochromic erythrocytes are characteristic of thalassemias, severe iron deficiency anemia, anemia of chronic disease, and sideroblastic anemias.

hypochromicity A decrease in the absorption of ultraviolet light by a solution of polypeptide polynucleotide chains as the secondary structure is established.

hypochromotrichia A reduced pigmentation of the hair, as is seen in protein malnutrition.

hypochylia [HYPO- + CHYL- + -IA] Diminished gastric secretion; insufficiency of chyle.

hypocinesia HYPOKINESIA.

hypocinesis HYPOKINESIA.

hypocitremia Less than normal concentration of citrate in blood.

hypocitruria [HYPO- + *citr(ate)* + -URIA] Decreased urinary excretion of citrate and increased potassium excretion during acidosis.

hypocleidium [HYPO- + CLEID- + L *-ium,* noun suffix] The median projection from the wishbone of birds, representing the interclavicle fused to the ends of the paired clavicle bones.

hypocoagulability Retardation of the clotting process because of either a deficiency of one or more clotting factors or platelets, or the presence of coagulation inhibitors.

hypocoagulable Less able than normal to clot.

hypocoelom [HYPO- + COELOM] The ventral part of coelomic cavity. Also called *hypocelom.*

hypocomplementemia A condition in which there is less than normal activity of complement or any of the complement components of blood. The condition may be hereditary or acquired. Various immune complex diseases result in acquired deficiency of complement components. Also called *acomplementemia.* Adjective: hypocomplementemic.

hypocone [HYPO- + Gk *kōn(os)* pine cone, cone] 1 The cusp of the talon; the distolingual cusp of a mammalian upper molar tooth. 2 In dinoflagellates, that part posterior to the equatorial groove.

hypoconid The buccal cusp of the talonid; the distobuccal cusp of a mammalian lower molar tooth.

hypoconulid The distal cusp of the talonid; the distal cusp of a mammalian lower molar tooth.

hypocorticalism A seldom used term for HYPOADRENOCORTICISM.

hypocorticism A seldom used term for HYPOADRENOCORTICISM.

hypocotyl The part on the axis of a plant embryo that is located between the attachment of the radicle and the cotyledons. It develops into the stem.

Hypocreales [HYPO- + Gk *kre(as)* flesh + L *-ales,* pl. of -ALIS -AL] A family of ascomycetous fungi known for their fleshy texture and bright colors. Some of them are insect parasites.

hypocrine Of, relating to, or characterized by hypoendocrinism.

hypocrinia A rarely used term for HYPOENDOCRINISM.

hypocrinism A rarely used term for HYPOENDOCRINISM.

hypocupremia An abnormally low concentration of copper in the blood or blood serum.

hypocyclosis [HYPO- + CYCLO- + -SIS] A deficient functioning of the ciliary muscle, resulting in an inadequacy of the accommodation of the eye. ● *Hypocyclosis* connotes a departure from normal and is not synonymous with *presbyopia,* which refers to the normal loss of accommodation that accompanies aging.

hypocystotomy [HYPO- + CYSTOTOMY]   Cystotomy by way of the perineum.

hypocythemia   **1** An abnormally low concentration of erythrocytes in the blood.   **2** A rarely used term for HYPOCYTOSIS.

hypocytosis   Any cytopenia involving formed elements of the blood, including oligocythemia, oligocytosis, and pancytopenia. Also called *hypocythemia* (rarely used).

hypodactylia   ECTRODACTYLY.

hypodactylism   ECTRODACTYLY.

hypodactyly   ECTRODACTYLY.

hypoderm   TELA SUBCUTANEA.

Hypoderma [HYPO- + DERMA]   A genus of heel flies, or ox warble flies, (family Oestridae, sometimes placed in a separate family Hypodermatidae). The larvae (cattle grubs) migrate through the body of the host for about four months, reach the spinal cord, and eventually burrow to the skin. The larva cuts a hole in the skin for its spiracles and completes larval development in a furuncular boil, or warble. After a period of 5 to 12 weeks, it drops out of the warble to the ground, pupates, and emerges in four or five weeks as an adult fly. Eggs are laid on the hair of cattle or other host (deer, horse, or, rarely human) and hatch in a week. The larvae then burrow through the skin or via a hair follicle and begin their long and destructive visceral migration. The adult flies, which do not feed, attack cattle to lay eggs on their hairs, often terrorizing and stampeding them in a process known as "gadding." Parasitization of humans by various species has been reported, involving extensive visceral and dermal migration with severe pain or discomfort, and sometimes temporary paralysis.

Hypoderma bovis   The northern cattle grub or ox warble fly. It attacks cattle and Old World deer, rarely horses and humans. The adult fly is 15 mm in length with light and dark bands that make it resemble a bumblebee. The full-grown larva measures about 27–28 mm. It causes extensive damage to hides, retards growth, and opens cutaneous wounds to infection and to other myiasis agents such as screwworms.

Hypoderma lineatum   The common cattle grub, a species widely distributed in the United States. Adults are slightly smaller than those of *H. bovis*, but the pattern of attacking cattle and other hosts is similar. Human infections have been reported, which result in a painful visceral larva migrans, sometimes reaching the eye and requiring surgical removal.

hypodermatic   SUBCUTANEOUS.

hypodermatoclysis   A seldom used term for HYPODERMOCLYSIS.

hypodermatomy [HYPO- + DERMA- + -TOMY]   An incision into the tela subcutanea.

hypodermiasis   Infestation of cattle by larvae of the genus *Hypoderma*. The larvae develop from eggs deposited on hairs by certain flies of the family Oestridae and burrow into the subcutaneous tissue. They wander about the body for months and may be found more or less anywhere in connective tissue. *H. lineatum* usually resides in the submucosa of the esophagus and *H. bovis* in the epidural fat. Eventually the larvae migrate to the subcutis of the back where they make holes through the skin above them. The cycle is completed when encysted larvae fall to the ground and pupate to form adult flies. Rarely, other animals and man may be affected.

hypodermic [HYPO- + -DERM + -IC]   **1** SUBCUTANEOUS.   **2** Applied or used beneath the skin: said especially of an injection or an instrument.

hypodermis   TELA SUBCUTANEA.

hypodermoclysis [HYPO- + DERMO- + Gk *klysis* a washing out, esp. by a clyster]   Subcutaneous administration of fluids, most frequently used as an alternative to intravenous administration of replacement for body fluid loss or dehydration. Also called *hypodermatoclysis* (seldom used).

hypodermolithiasis   The formation of calcified nodules in the dermis.

hypodermomycosis [HYPO- + DERMO- + MYCOSIS]   A subcutaneous fungal infection.

hypodiaphragmatic   SUBPHRENIC.

hypodiploid   Deficient in one or more chromosomes or chromosome segments compared to the diploid state: said of a cell or an individual.

hypodiploidy [HYPO- + DIPLOIDY]   The condition in which an organism or cell is hypodiploid.

hypodipsia [HYPO- + DIPSIA]   Diminished thirst with consequential reduction of fluid intake. Also called *oligodipsia*.

hypodontia [HYP- + -ODONTIA]   The congenital condition of having fewer teeth than normal.

hypodynamia   A reduced force or power.

hypodynamia cordis   Reduced force of cardiac contraction.

hypodynamic   Reduced in power or force; pertaining especially to reduced contractility of the heart.

hypodynia [HYP- + -ODYNIA]   Slight pain. An obsolete term.

hypoeccrisia   The state of decreased secretion. Also called *hypoeccrisis*. Adjective: hypoeccritic.

hypoeccrisis   HYPOECCRISIA.

hypoeccritic [HYPO- + ECCRITIC]   Relating to or pertaining to decreased secretion.

hypoechoic [HYPO- + ECHOIC]   Producing echoes of lower amplitude or density than the surrounding medium.

hypoelectrolytemia   An abnormally low electrolyte concentration in the blood.

renal hypoelectrolytemia   Decreased blood electrolyte content secondary to renal tubular dysfunction.

hypoemia   An obsolete term for ANEMIA.

hypoendocrinia   A rarely used term for HYPOENDOCRINISM.

hypoendocrinism [HYPO- + *endocrin(e)* + -ISM]   Subnormal or deficient secretion of an endocrine hormone or hormones, or the condition resulting it. Also called *hypocrinia* (rarely used), *hypocrinism* (rarely used), *hypoendocrisia* (rarely used), *hypoendocrinia* (rarely used), *hypohormonism* (seldom used).

hypoendocrisia   A rarely used term for HYPOENDOCRINISM.

hypoeosinophilia   EOSINOPENIA.

hypoepinephrinemia   An abnormally low concentration of epinephrine in the blood.

hypoequilibrium   Lack of sensitivity to stimuli normally inducing vertigo.

hypoergasia [HYPO- + Gk *ergasia* work, toil]   The depressive form of bipolar or manic-depressive psychosis. An outmoded term.

hypoergia [HYPO- + *(all)erg(en)* + -IA]   Reduced sensitivity to allergens; hyposensitivity. Also called *hypoergy*. Adjective: hypoergic.

hypoergy   HYPOERGIA.

hypoesophoria [HYPO- + ESOPHORIA]   A latent deviation of ocular alignment characterized by the lower eye turning inward, toward the nose.   • Precise usage specifies the separate presence of *hypophoria* and *esophoria*, including the accurate measurement of each individual deviation. The combined prefix *hypoeso* does not permit accurate evaluation of the status of the extraocular muscle functions and is not good clinical usage.

hypoesthesia [HYPO- + ESTHESIA]   Reduction in sensitivity. Also called *hypesthesia*. Adjective: hypoesthetic, hypesthetic.

acoustic hypoesthesia   HYPOACUSIS.

auditory hypoesthesia   HYPOACUSIS.

gustatory hypoesthesia   HYPOGEUSIA.

olfactory hypoesthesia HYPOSMIA.

tactile hypoesthesia A reduced perception of touch. Also called *amblyaphia*.

hypoesthetic Relating to hypoesthesia. Also *hypesthetic*.

hypoestrinemia An older term for HYPOESTROGENEMIA.

hypoestrinism An older term for HYPOESTROGENISM.

hypoestrogenemia Abnormally low concentrations of estrogens, as estrone or estradiol or both, in the blood. Also called *hypoestrinemia* (older term).

hypoestrogenism [HYPO- + ESTROGEN + -ISM] Subnormal or deficient ovarian secretion of estrogens, or the condition resulting from it. Also called *hypoestrinism* (older term).

hypoexcitability A state of reduced excitability, either of the whole person, or of neurons or other nervous structures and pathways.

hypoexcitable Inadequately or subnormally reactive to normally exciting stimuli.

hypoexophoria [HYPO- + EXOPHORIA] A latent deviation of ocular alignment characterized by the lower eye turning outward, toward the ear. • Precise usage specifies the separate presence of *hypohoria* and of *exophoria,* including the accurate measurement of each individual deviation. The combined prefix *hyopexo* does not permit accurate evaluation of the status of the extraocular muscle functions and is not good clinical usage.

hypoferremia An abnormally low concentration of iron in the blood or blood serum. Also called *oligosideremia*.

hypoferrism IRON DEFICIENCY.

hypofibrinogenemia Reduced concentration of plasma fibrinogen. Also called *fibrinogenopenia, fibrinopenia, hypinosis* (obsolete).

hypofunction [HYPO- + FUNCTION] Reduced function of an organ, tissue, or system, often signifying function at a subnormal level, as of an endocrine gland.

convergence hypofunction Deficient amplitude of ocular convergence. Also called *insufficiency of the interni*.

divergence hypofunction Deficient amplitude of ocular divergence. Also called *insufficiency of the externi*.

hypogalactia [HYPO- + GALACT- + -IA] Reduced milk formation.

hypogalactous In a state of reduced milk formation.

hypogammaglobulinemia [HYPO- + GAMMAGLOBULIN + -EMIA] A condition of immunologic deficiency marked by abnormally low levels or the virtual absence of immunoglobulins in the blood, causing increased vulnerability to infectious diseases. Also called *agammaglobulinemia*. Adjective: hypogammaglobulinemic.

acquired hypogammaglobulinemia Hypogammaglobulinemia which is due to causes other than genetic defects in antibody formation and which becomes manifest after early childhood.

Bruton hypogammaglobulinemia INFANTILE SEX-LINKED HYPOGAMMAGLOBULINEMIA.

congenital hypogammaglobulinemia INFANTILE SEX-LINKED HYPOGAMMAGLOBULINEMIA.

infantile sex-linked hypogammaglobulinemia A congenital disorder affecting male infants, in which all classes of immunoglobulins may be deficient, with subnormal plasma concentrations. The affected infant is prone to infections, particularly respiratory, due to bacterial pathogens and especially *Pneumocystis carinii*. Replacement therapy with regular injections of plasma protein derivatives rich in immunoglobulin G is partially effective. Also called *Bruton's disease, congenital hypogammaglobulinemia, Bruton hypogammaglobulinemia, X-linked hypogammaglobulinemia, Bruton type agammaglobulinemia*.

lymphopenic hypogammaglobulinemia SEVERE COMBINED IMMUNODEFICIENCY.

physiologic hypogammaglobulinemia The normal fall in plasma concentration of immunoglobulin which occurs during the first three to six months after birth. It is due to a delay before the start of synthesizing immunoglobulin G (IgG).

primary hypogammaglobulinemia Hypogammaglobulinemia resulting from defects in or diseases of the normal antibody-forming mechanism.

secondary hypogammaglobulinemia Hypogammaglobulinemia resulting from nonimmunologic disease, as from conditions causing protein loss into the gut or urine, certain drugs, infections, or malnutrition.

Swiss type hypogammaglobulinemia SEVERE COMBINED IMMUNODEFICIENCY.

transient hypogammaglobulinemia of infancy The low plasma level of immunoglobulin, particularly IgG, that normally occurs at about three months of life because in early infancy the amount of immunoglobulin received through the placenta before birth is catabolized more rapidly than new immunoglobulin is formed.

X-linked hypogammaglobulinemia INFANTILE SEX-LINKED HYPOGAMMAGLOBULINEMIA.

hypogastralgia Pain in the hypochondrium of gastric origin.

hypogastric [HYPO- + GASTRIC] **1** Pertaining to the hypogastrium. **2** Below the stomach.

hypogastrium REGIO PUBICA.

hypogastropagus [HYPO- + GASTRO- + -PAGUS] Equal conjoined twins joined in the hypogastric regions.

hypogastroschisis [HYPO- + GASTRO- + -SCHISIS] The developmental failure of the abdominal wall to close in the region below the umbilicus and above the pubis.

hypogean [Gk *hypoge(ios)* (from *hypo-* under + *gē* the earth, land) underground + English *-an,* adjectival suffix] Living or growing below the surface of the ground, as do burrowing animals and certain fungi. Also *hypogeous*.

hypogenesis [HYPO- + GENESIS] Failure of development or growth of an embryo, fetus, or a part of it. Adjective: hypogenetic.

polar hypogenesis Specific underdevelopment at the cephalic or caudal ends of the body, or both.

hypogenitalism [HYPO- + GENITAL + -ISM] Underdevelopment of the genitalia owing to hypogonadism.

hypogeous HYPOGEAN.

hypogeusesthesia HYPOGEUSIA.

hypogeusia [HYPO- + Gk *geus(is)* taste + -IA] Diminished acuity of taste perception. Because of the close association of the senses of taste and smell, patients with anosmia will usually complain of hypogeusia although the sense of taste may be shown to be unaffected. Also called *gustatory hypoesthesia, hypogeusesthesia*.

hypoglandular [HYPO- + GLANDULAR] Characterized by subnormal or deficient glandular secretion.

hypoglobulia An abnormally low concentration of erythrocytes in the blood, or of erythrocyte precursors in the bone marrow.

hypoglossal Below the tongue.

hypoglossis HYPOGLOTTIS.

hypoglossus NERVUS HYPOGLOSSUS.

hypoglottis The inferior surface of the tongue. Also called *hypoglossis*.

hypoglycaemia A British spelling for HYPOGLYCEMIA.

hypoglycemia [HYPO- + GLYCEMIA] Subnormal concentration of glucose in the blood. It may be caused by pancreatic islet cell overactivity, overdosage of insulin, intestinal malabsorption, or hepatic or endocrine disease. It produces symptoms of headache, tremor, sweating, blanching, mental and emotional disturbances (faintness, impaired concentration and memory), convulsions, and coma. Adjective: hypoglycemic.

fasting hypoglycemia Pathologically low blood glucose concentration in the fasting state, that is, after a 48 to 72 hour fast. It is characteristic of the hypoglycemia of organic as opposed to functional disease, and is found in insulinoma, very severe hepatic disease, sprue, advanced malnutrition, Addison's disease, and panhypopituitarism.

functional hypoglycemia REACTIVE HYPOGLYCEMIA.

leucine-induced hypoglycemia Hypoglycemia of infants, induced by most proteins, which contain leucine. A familial disease, it is transmitted as an autosomal recessive.

mixed hypoglycemia Hypoglycemia with the characteristics of both fasting and reactive hypoglycemia, marked by low blood sugar when fasting and after a carbohydrate feeding. It is found in some patients with infantile hypoglycemia, Addison's disease, panhypopituitarism, and insulinoma.

reactive hypoglycemia Hypoglycemia occurring in response to a carbohydrate feeding, due to abnormally increased insulin secretion. It is found in functional hypoglycemia, sometimes in the postgastrectomy syndrome, and after the excessively rapid absorption of carbohydrate in thyrotoxicosis. Also called *functional hypoglycemia*.

hypoglycemic 1 Of, relating to, or characterized by hypoglycemia. 2 Acting to lower the level of glucose in the blood, as *hypoglycemic agent*.

hypoglycemosis Subnormal concentration of glucose in the blood and in the cells; hypoglycemia.

hypoglycin 2-Amino-3-(2-methylenecyclopropyl)propionic acid. A toxic amino acid present in unripe ackee fruits. It lowers the blood sugar and inhibits the catabolism of branched-chain amino acids.

hypoglycogenolysis [HYPO- + GLYCOGENOLYSIS] A reduced level of glycogenolysis.

hypoglycorrhachia [HYPO- + GLYCO- + Gk *rhach(is)* the back, spine, backbone + -IA] An abnormally small glucose content of the cerebrospinal fluid.

hypognathous [HYPO- + GNATH- + -OUS] Having a protruding mandible.

hypognathus [HYPO- + Gk *gnathos* jaw, esp. lower jaw] An incorrect term for MYOGNATHUS.

hypogonadal Having or pertaining to hypogonadism.

hypogonadia An older term for HYPOGONADISM.

hypogonadism [HYPO- + GONAD + -ISM] The condition resulting from subnormal secretion of sex hormones by the gonads, with consequent retardation of growth, eunuchoidism, and failure of the secondary sex characters to develop. Also called *hypogonadia* (older term).

hypogonadism with anosmia KALLMANN SYNDROME.

familial hypogonadotropic hypogonadism Failure of secondary sexual characters to develop owing to isolated deficiency of anterior pituitary secretion of gonadotropin. It appears to be inherited as an autosomal recessive trait.

hypogonadotropic hypogonadism Hypogonadism owing to deficient anterior pituitary secretion of gonadotropic hormones. Also called *secondary hypogonadism*.

pituitary hypogonadism Hypogonadism resulting from disease of the anterior pituitary with deficient secretion of gonadotropic hormones.

primary hypogonadism Insufficient development, hormone secretion, and gamete production by the gonads due to intrinsic gonadal disease, as contrasted to hypergonadotropic hypogo-

nadism (secondary hypogonadism).

secondary hypogonadism HYPOGONADOTROPIC HYPOGONADISM.

hypogonadotrophic HYPOGONADOTROPIC.

hypogonadotrophism HYPOGONADOTROPISM.

hypogonadotropic Of or characterized by hypogonadotropism. Also *hypogonadotrophic*.

hypogonadotropism [HYPO- + GONAD + *o* + TROPISM] Subnormal or deficient secretion of the gonadotropic hormones of the anterior pituitary, or the condition resulting from it. Also called *hypogonadotrophism*.

hypogranulocytosis GRANULOCYTOPENIA.

hypogyny [HYPO- + GYN- + -Y] A condition of having the calyx, corolla, and stamens located at the base of or below the free ovary. Adjective: hypogenous.

hypohemia An obsolete term for ANEMIA.

hypohidrosis [HYPO- + HIDROSIS] Diminished sweating. Also called *hidroschesis, hyphidrosis, olighidria, oligidria, olighydria, oligohidrosis, hypoidrosis*.

hypohidrotic 1 Characterized by diminished sweating. 2 A substance that inhibits sweating.

hypohormonal [HYPO- + HORMONAL] Marked by insufficient secretion of a hormone or hormones. Also *hypohormonic* (seldom used).

hypohormonic A seldom used term for HYPOHORMONAL.

hypohormonism [HYPO- + *hormon(e)* + -ISM] A seldom used term for HYPOENDOCRINISM.

hypohyal The hyoid element that lies between the ceratohyal and basihyal of the hyoid apparatus. It is derived from the anterior end of the distal part of the cartilage of the second branchial arch, and it forms the lesser horn of the hyoid bone in the human adult.

hypohyals [HYPO- + *hy(o)-* + -AL + s] The bones or cartilages serving for the attachment of the hyoid apparatus in fishes.

hypohydration [HYPO- + HYDRATION] A state of decreased water content.

hypohydrochloria HYPOCHLORHYDRIA.

hypohyloma [HYPO- + HYLOMA] A tumor of endodermal origin. An obsolete term.

hypohypnotic 1 Relating to light sleep. 2 Concerning partial hypnosis.

hypohypophysism [HYPO- + *hypophys(is)* + -ISM] A rarely used term for HYPOPITUITARISM.

hypoidrosis HYPOHIDROSIS.

hypoinsulinemia [HYPO- + INSULIN + -EMIA] The condition of having a subnormal concentration of insulin in the blood relative to the blood glucose concentration. A degree of hypoinsulinemia is present in all patients with diabetes mellitus.

hypoinsulinism [HYPO- + INSULIN + -ISM] The incapacity to secrete normal amounts of insulin, as in diabetes mellitus.

hypoiodidism A deficiency of iodide in the body which occurs after prolonged dietary intake of less than 35–45 μg of iodine in infants and less than 50 μg in adults, leading to goiter in the latter. In children, hypoiodidism is believed to induce myxedematous cretinism.

hypoisotonic HYPOTONIC.

hypokalemia An abnormally low concentration of potassium in the blood or blood serum. It may be congenital, as in familial periodic paralysis, or acquired through intestinal or renal loss. Manifestations may include muscle weakness or paralysis, electrocardiographic abnormalities, and impairment of renal tubular function. Also called *hypopotassemia*. Also *hypokaliemia*.

hypokalemic 1 Pertaining to or resulting from hypokalemia. Also *hypopotassemic*. 2 Any substance which lowers potassium content of blood or tissue.

hypokaliemia   HYPOKALEMIA.

hypokeratosis   Deficient keratinization.

hypokinemia   Reduced cardiac output.

hypokinesia   A reduction in motor activity or in the range of movement of the body or limbs. Also called *hypanakinesia, hypanakinesis, hypokinesis, hypocinesis*. Also *hypocinesia*. Adjective: hypokinetic.

hypokinesis   HYPOKINESIA.

hypokinetic   Pertaining to or affected by hypokinesia.

hypokolasia [HYPO- + Gk *kolas(is)* a checking, pruning, correcting + -IA]   Impairment of inhibitory mechanisms in the central nervous system.

hypolarynx   The lower part of the laryngeal cavity, extending from the vocal folds to the level of the lower border of the cricoid cartilage.

hypolemma [HYPO- + Gk *lemma*, a peel, rind, husk]   The space beneath a sheath, such as muscle sheath.

hypolemmal   Pertaining to hypolemma.

hypolepidoma [HYPO- + LEPIDOMA]   A tumor of endodermal origin. An obsolete term.

hypolethal   Describing a mutant allele that may reduce fitness of the organism without totally eliminating the possibility of reproduction.

hypoleukemia   Either aleukemic or subleukemic leukemia. An obsolete and imprecise term.

hypoleukocytic   LEUKOPENIC.

hypoleydigism   Deficient secretion of androgen (testosterone) by the testicular interstitial cells of Leydig.

hypolipemia   An abnormally low concentration of fat in the blood or blood serum.

hypolipoproteinemia   An abnormally low concentration of lipoprotein in the blood or blood serum. See also HYPOBETA-LIPOPROTEINEMIA, ABETALIPROTEINEMIA, ANALPHALIPOPRO-TEINEMIA.

hypoliposis   An abnormally low concentration of lipids in the blood or tissues.

hypolutemia   An abnormally low concentration of progesterone in the blood or blood serum.

hypolymphemia   LYMPHOCYTOPENIA.

hypomagnesemia   An abnormally low concentration of magnesium in the blood or blood serum, manifested chiefly by muscular hyperirritability.

hypomania [HYPO- + -MANIA]   A relatively mild form of mania characterized by elated mood, restlessness and irritability, overproductivity, distractibility and an increase in ideas and the rate of speech. Also called *submania*.

hypomanic   Characterized by hypomania.

hypomastia [HYPO- + MAST- + -IA]   Congenital underdevelopment of the female breast. Also called *hypomazia*.

hypomazia   HYPOMASTIA.

hypomelancholia   A mild degree of the depressed form of bipolar disorder.

hypomelanism   A state of reduced skin pigmentation.

  dominant oculocutaneous hypomelanism   An autosomal dominant hereditary disorder, similar to albinism, in which the iris is translucent when light is passed through it and the skin is hypersensitive to ultraviolet radiation.

hypomelanosis [HYPO- + MELANOSIS]   A reduced melanin pigmentation of the skin.

  hereditary hypomelanosis   A reduced melanin pigmentation that is of hereditary origin.

  idiopathic guttate hypomelanosis   The development of small macules of hypomelanosis. It is a common but inconspicuous condition that begins in late childhood.

hypomenorrhea [HYPO- + MENORRHEA]   Diminution in the amount of flow or a shortening of the duration of menstruation.

hypomere [HYPO- + -MERE]   The part of the mesoderm in an embryo that gives rise to the mesothelial lining of the serous cavities. It is derived from lateral plate mesoderm.

hypomery [HYPO- + -mer(e) + -Y]   Diminution in the number of the primitive embryonic segments.

hypomesosoma   A stature that is shorter than the median percentile.

hypometabolism   A state of reduced metabolic activity; a reduced rate of metabolism.

  euthyroid hypometabolism   A state of reduced metabolic activity in the presence of normal thyroid function.

hypometria [HYPO- + Gk *metr(on)* a measure + -IA]   A form of dysmetria in which movement of a limb falls short of the intended target.

hypometropia [HYPO- + METROPIA]   A seldom used term for MYOPIA.

hypomicron   SUBMICRON.

hypomicrosoma   The smallest stature within the normal percentiles.

hypomineralization   A state marked by a deficiency of minerals in the body.

hypomnesis [HYPO- + Gk *mnēsis* memory]   A state characterized by deficient memory.

hypomodal   Describing or pertaining to the measured values less than or, when represented graphically, to the left of the mode in a data distribution.

hypomorph [HYPO- + -MORPH]   **1** An individual who is short in standing height in proportion to sitting height. This results from a lower limb length that is proportionally shorter than trunk length. Adjective: hypomorphic.   **2** An allele of reduced effect compared to the wild-type allele. The protein product, for example, would have reduced—but not absent—enzymatic activity. Also called *leaky gene, leaky allele*.

hypomotility   A condition marked by levels of movement that are less than normal.

hypomyosthenia [HYPO- + MYO- + -STHEN + -IA]   Muscular weakness. A seldom used term.

hypomyotonia   A seldom used term for HYPOTONIA.

hypomyxia [HYPO- + MYX- + -IA]   Diminished mucus secretion.

hyponanosoma   An extreme degree of dwarfism.

hyponasality   The nasal quality of speech when there is an obstruction to normal airflow through the nose, particularly for the nasal consonants such as m or n. Also called *rhinolalia clausa, denasality*.

hyponatremia   An abnormally low concentration of sodium in the blood serum. Adjective: hyponatremic.

hyponatruria   Decreased urinary excretion of sodium, as in dietary salt restriction or accumulating edema, or secondary to increased secretion or to administration of salt-retaining mineralocorticoid hormones.

hyponeocytosis   Fewer than normal young erythrocytes in blood.

hyponeuria [HYPO- + NEUR- + -IA]   Reduction in sensitivity; numbness. A seldom used term.

hyponoderma   An obsolete term for CUTANEOUS LARVA MIGRANS.

hyponoetic   Pertaining to or under voluntary control.

hyponomoderma   An obsolete term for CUTANEOUS LARVA MIGRANS.

hyponychial　Of or relating to the hyponychium.

hyponychium　[NA] The part of the fingertip that extends from the distal end of the nail bed to the distal crease on the palmar aspect of the finger. It corresponds to the pulp of the finger.

hyponychon　[irreg. from HYP- + Gk *onyx*, gen. *onychos*, talon, claw, nail] An ecchymosis that lies beneath a fingernail or toenail.

hyponym　[HYP- + Aeolian Gk *onym(a)* a name] A generic name of an organism, often used provisionally, which is not based on a type species.

hypo-oncotic　Marked by oncotic pressure that is less than the normal.

hypo-orchidia　An older term for HYPO-ORCHIDISM.

hypo-orchidism　Subnormal spermatogenic or hormone-secreting function of the testis. Also called *hypo-orchidia* (older term).

hypo-orthocytosis　Leukopenia with normal proportions of granulocytes, lymphocytes, and monocytes. A rarely used term.

hypo-osmosis　The reduced movement of a solvent as a result of a diminished difference in osmotic activity between two solutions.

hypo-osmotic　1 Having a lower concentration of osmotically active solutes than a comparative solution.　2 Of or relating to hypo-osmosis.

hypo-ovaria　An older term for HYPOVARIANISM.

hypo-ovarianism　HYPOVARIANISM.

hypopallesthesia　[HYPO- + PALLESTHESIA] Abnormal reduction in sensitivity to applied vibration. Also called *pallhypesthesia* (seldom used).

hypopancreatism　Pancreatic hyposecretion of insufficiency.

hypoparathyreosis　A rarely used term for HYPOPARATHYROIDISM.

hypoparathyroid　Of, relating to, or characteristic of hypoparathyroidism.

hypoparathyroidism　[HYPO- + PARATHYROID + -ISM] The condition resulting from subnormal or absent secretion of parathyroid hormone by the parathyroid glands, most often due to inadvertent parathyroidectomy or injury to the glands during thyroid surgery. The idiopathic form is rare and may have an autoimmune basis. It is sometimes associated with pernicious anemia, Addison's disease, or ovarian failure. Hypoparathyroidism is characterized by hypocalcemia, high serum phosphorous, low levels of plasma, immunoreactive parathyroid hormone, increased bone density, cataracts, tetany, convulsions, ectopic calcifications, and mental disturbances. There may be associated abnormalities of skin, nails, hair, and teeth. Also called *parathyroid insufficiency, hypoparathyreosis* (rarely used), *hypoparathyrosis* (rarely used).

familial hypoparathyroidism　Any of three forms of hereditary hypoparathyroidism, comprising neonatal hypoparathyroidism, an X-linked recessive disorder occurring only in males; the familial disorder without Addison's disease and moniliasis, an autosomal recessive disorder often associated with consanguinity; and the familial disorder with Addison's disease and mucocutaneous moniliasis, an autosomal recessive disorder sometimes associated with other autoimmune disorders, as pernicious anemia, thyroiditis or ovarian failure. Familial hypoparathyroidism constitutes about 25 percent of cases of hypoparathyroidism.

hypoparathyrosis　A rarely used term for HYPOPARATHYROIDISM.

hypopepsia　Diminished gastric secretion.

hypopepsinia　Diminished gastric secretion of pepsin.

hypopeptic　Relating to or characterized by hypopepsia.

hypoperistalsis　Diminished or inadequate peristalsis.

hypoperistaltic　Relating to or characterized by hypoperistalsis.

hypopermeability　A condition in which the permeability of a membrane is less than normal.

hypopexia　[HYPO- + *-pex(y)* + -IA] The reduced fixation of a substance into tissues. Also called *hypopexy*.

hypopexy　HYPOPEXIA.

hypophalangism　[HYPO- + *phalang(es)*, pl. of PHALANX + -ISM] A condition of having fewer than the normal number of phalanges.

hypophamine　A substance formerly believed to be the active hormone of the neurohypophysis. An obsolete term.

α-hypophamine　A seldom used term for OXYTOCIN.

β-hypophamine　A seldom used term for VASOPRESSIN.

hypopharyngitis　Pharyngitis in which the hypopharynx or laryngopharynx is the main site of the inflammation.

hypopharyngoscope　ESOPHAGEAL SPECULUM.

hypopharyngoscopy　The examination of the interior of the hypopharynx, often combined with the examination of the cricopharyngeal region and the upper esophagus.

hypopharynx　PARS LARYNGEA PHARYNGIS.

hypophonia　[HYPO- + PHON- + -IA] The weak or thin voice, or whisper, resulting from impaired respiratory or vocal fold activity. Also called *subenergetic phonation*.

hypophoria　[HYPO- + -PHORIA] A latent, downward deviation of one eye, spontaneously corrected by the fusion mechanisms. The specified eye is the deviating lower eye. Thus, in right hypophoria, the right eye tends to deviate downward and the left to fix; in left hypophoria, the left eye tends to deviate downward and the right eye to fix.

hypophosphatasia　An inherited deficiency of alkaline phosphatase. Severe forms occur in infancy and childhood and are inherited as autosomal recessive traits. Features include severe undermineralization of the skeleton and stillbirth in the most severe cases, irritability, seizures, rachitic skeletal changes, premature loss of teeth, and susceptibility to bleeding and infection. The adult-onset form is inherited as an autosomal dominant trait and features bone fragility, osteoporosis, and premature loss of teeth.

hypophosphate　An anion, salt, or ester of hypophosphoric acid.

hypophosphatemia　[HYPO- + PHOSPHATEMIA] Less than normal concentration of phosphate in blood, plasma, or serum. Also called *hypophosphoremia*.

familial hypophosphatemia　FAMILIAL HYPOPHOSPHATEMIC RICKETS.

hereditary hypophosphatemia　X-LINKED HYPOPHOSPHATEMIA.

renal hypophosphatemia　FAMILIAL HYPOPHOSPHATEMIC RICKETS.

X-linked hypophosphatemia　The most common form of familial hypophosphatemic rickets, inherited as an X-linked dominant trait, and characterized by radiologic rickets and osteomalacia, slow growth, bowed legs, hypophosphatemia, decreased renal tubular phosphate reabsorption, and normal plasma calcium and parathyroid hormone. The biochemical defect is unclear. Also called *familial vitamin D-resistant rickets, hereditary hypophosphatemia, phosphate diabetes* (obsolete).

hypophosphaturia　Decreased urinary excretion of inorganic phosphates when dietary phosphate intake is low, but more commonly when phosphates are bound in the gastrointestinal tract by nonabsorbable antacids. It is also caused by normal somatic growth, pregnancy, lactation, hypoparathyroidism, Addison's disease, and sodium depletion.

hypophosphite An anion, salt, or ester of hypophosphorous acid.

hypophosphoremia HYPOPHOSPHATEMIA.

hypophosphoric acid $(HO)_2P(O)—P(O)(OH)_2$. 'The tetrabasic acid formed by two phospho groups joined by a phosphorus-phosphorus bond. It is a crystalline solid.

hypophosphorous acid An outmoded term for PHOSPHINIC ACID.

hypophrenia [HYPO- + -PHRENIA] MENTAL RETARDATION.

hypophrenic SUBPHRENIC.

hypophrenium The part of the peritoneal cavity between the diaphragm above and the transverse colon and mesocolon below. It comprises all the subphrenic and subhepatic recesses and the omental bursa. An outmoded term. Also called *supracolic space, supraomental region, subphrenic region*.

hypophrenosis [HYPO- + PHRENO- + -SIS] Mental retardation or handicap. An obsolete term.

hypophyseal HYPOPHYSIAL.

hypophysectomize [*hypophys(is)* + -ECTOMIZE] To excise or destroy the hypophysis.

hypophysectomy [*hypophys(is cerebri)* + -ECTOMY] The excision or destruction of the hypophysis cerebri. Among the indications are certain pituitary tumors, particularly chromaphobe adenomas, and certain endocrine disorders, particularly acromegaly and Cushing's disease. The operation as a means of relieving advanced breast cancer and carcinoma of the prostate has been largely superseded by chemotherapy and hormone therapy. The surgical approach may be transcranial or extracranial (as in transeptal and transethmoidal hypophysectomy). Also called *hypophysiectomy*.

trans-sphenoidal hypophysectomy An operation for removal of the pituitary by traversing the sphenoid sinus and removing the floor of the sella turcica. It is now performed with the aid of a surgical microscope. To prevent cerebrospinal-fluid leakage the operation attempts to preserve the diaphragma sellae, uses material to pack the cavity of the sella turcica, and employs a substituting material for replacing the defect in the floor of the sella.

hypophyseoportal HYPOPHYSIOPORTAL.

hypophysial Of or relating to the pituitary gland (hypophysis). Also *hypophyseal*.

hypophysiectomy HYPOPHYSECTOMY.

hypophysin 1 The hormone of the posterior pituitary gland. Rarely used in this sense. 2 An extract of bovine pituitary gland containing oxytocin and vasopressin.

hypophysioportal Pertaining to the portal vascular system supplying the hypophysis. Also *hypophyseoportal*.

hypophysioprivic Characterized by subnormal secretion of a hormone or hormones of the pituitary gland. Also *hypophysoprivic* (seldom used).

hypophysiotrophic HYPOPHYSIOTROPIC.

hypophysiotropic Acting upon the pituitary gland (hypophysis cerebri), as the hypothalamic hypophysiotropic hormones. Also *hypophysiotrophic*.

hypophysis [HYPO- + PHYSIS] [NA] An unpaired, ovoid body that lies below the hypothalamus in the pituitary fossa of the sella turcica; the pituitary gland.

accessory hypophysis One or more rests of adenohypophyseal tissue up to 5 mm in diameter found near the junction of the sphenoid and the vomer in relation to the site of the embryologic craniopharyngeal canal. In man they often merge with the mucous glands in the nasopharynx. They may hypertrophy and become functional if the hypophysis is destroyed. Also called *pharyngeal hypophysis*.

hypophysis cerebri PITUITARY GLAND.

pharyngeal hypophysis ACCESSORY HYPOPHYSIS.

hypophysis sicca An outmoded term for NEUROHYPOPHYSIS.

hypophysitis [*hypophys(is cerebri)* + -ITIS] Inflammation of the pituitary gland.

hypophysoma [*hypophys(is)* + -OMA] A tumor of the hypophysis. An outmoded term.

hypophysomegaly A seldom used term for ACROMEGALY.

hypophysoprivic A seldom used term for HYPOPHYSIOPRIVIC.

hypopiesia HYPOTENSION.

hypopiesis HYPOTENSION.

hypopietic HYPOTENSIVE.

hypopigmentation Pigmentation that is lighter than normal.

hypopigmenter An individual whose pigmentary response to light exposure is less than normal.

hypopinealism Postulated hyposecretion of pineal hormones.

hypopituitarism [HYPO- + PITUITARISM] Deficient secretion of anterior pituitary hormones. Hypopituitarism may result from postpartum necrosis of the pituitary gland as in the Sheehan syndrome, to tumors, to surgical hypophysectomy, or to sudden infarction of the gland (pituitary apoplexy). It is associated with varying degrees of stunted growth and with gonadal, thyroidal, and adrenocortical deficiency. Also called *anterior pituitary insufficiency, hypophysial dystrophy, hypohypophysism* (rarely used), *pituitary insufficiency, subpituitarism*.

postpartum hemorrhagic hypopituitarism SHEEHAN SYNDROME.

hypopituitary Of or characteristic of hypopituitarism.

hypoplasia [HYPO- + -PLASIA] An underdevelopment of a tissue, organ, or region of the body. It implies fewer than the usual number of cells. Also called *hypoplasty, microgenesis*. Compare AGENESIS, APLASIA, DYSPLASIA.

hypoplasia of the aortic tract complexes See under HYPOPLASTIC LEFT HEART SYNDROME.

cartilage-hair hypoplasia METAPHYSEAL CHONDRODYSPLASIA, MCKUSICK TYPE.

chronologic enamel hypoplasia Enamel hypoplasia caused by a short-lived, specific interference with amelogenesis.

condylar hypoplasia The underdevelopment of one or both condyles of the mandible.

congenital adrenal hypoplasia 1 Congenital aplasia of the zona fasciculata and zona reticularis in children with miniature adrenal cortices comprising zona glomerulosa cells only, and secreting only aldosterone. 2 A familial disease, confined to boys and young men, including diffuse leukodystrophy of the central nervous system and primary adrenocortical insufficiency.

congenital generalized muscular hypoplasia A syndrome marked by generalized muscle hypoplasia, with onset at birth with generalized muscular weakness, hypotonia, and delay in walking and in reaching other physical milestones. There are no other constitutional abnormalities, and the deep tendon reflexes are usually normal. It is now known that this is a syndrome of multiple etiology and not a specific disease. The condition often tends to improve spontaneously. Also called *Krabbe syndrome, Krabbe's disease, congenital universal muscular hypoplasia*.

congenital universal muscular hypoplasia CONGENITAL GENERALIZED MUSCULAR HYPOPLASIA.

craniofacial hypoplasia Congenital underdevelopment of the cranial and facial bones frequently associated with other malformations.

hypoplasia cutis congenita 1 Developmental ectodermal dysplasia involving absence or deficiency of hair, nails, and glands of the skin. 2 Any developmental dysplasia or hypoplasia of the skin.

enamel hypoplasia A hereditary abnormality in which the enamel is defective in thickness or structure. What enamel is present may be of normal structure and calcification. The condition is most often seen as pits on what are normally smooth surfaces. The pits may become carious. Also called *hereditary enamel hypoplasia.*

focal dermal hypoplasia An X-linked, dominant, congenital syndrome of asymmetric scarlike regions and hyperpigmented streaks on the skin, isolated herniations of subcutaneous fat, papillomas of the lips, mouth, and anogenital area; sparse hair, dysplastic nails, digital anomalies, ear malformations with conductive deafness, and osteopathia striata. Mental retardation and dental, palatal, and cardiac anomalies also occur. The syndrome is usually lethal *in utero* in males, producing an increased miscarriage rate in affected women. Also called *Goltz syndrome.*

granulocytic hypoplasia Reduction in the rate of formation of granulocytes by bone marrow.

hereditary brown hypoplasia of enamel AMELOGENESIS IMPERFECTA.

hereditary enamel hypoplasia ENAMEL HYPOPLASIA.

lobular hypoplasia LOBULAR APLASIA.

nasomaxillary hypoplasia The underdevelopment of the structures forming the nose and the upper jaw.

oligonephronic hypoplasia Renal underdevelopment characterized by reduced numbers of nephrons.

pluricystic hypoplasia Renal underdevelopment associated with numerous cysts, as is seen in polycystic kidney.

hypoplasia of the right ventricle A congenital abnormality of the right ventricular wall, which may be so underdeveloped that it has no muscular tissue and is paper thin. Also called *right ventricular hypoplasia, parchment heart.* See also UHL'S ANOMALY.

right ventricular hypoplasia HYPOPLASIA OF THE RIGHT VENTRICLE.

thymic hypoplasia Incomplete development of the thymus.

hypoplasia of tooth Defective formation of a tooth, most often of the enamel, but occasionally of the dentin.

Turner's hypoplasia Hypoplasia of a permanent tooth caused by infection of, or trauma affecting, its deciduous predecessor.

hypoplastic Characterized by or exhibiting hypoplasia.

hypoplasty HYPOPLASIA.

hypoploid [HYPO- + -PLOID] Having a chromosome complement which is aneuploid through loss of chromosomes from the usual integral number of sets: usually said of a complement slightly less than an integral multiple, as in hypodiploid.

hypoploidy The condition or state of being hypoploid.

hypopnea [HYPO- + -PNEA] Slow and shallow breathing. Also called *oligopnea.*

hypopnoea A British spelling for HYPOPNEA.

hyponesis [HYPO- + Gk *ponēsis* work, action] Functional insufficiency of the motor cortex in inducing motor activity. A seldom used term.

hypoporosis [HYPO- + POROSIS] Inadequate callus formation during the healing of a fracture.

hypoposia [HYPO- + Gk *pos(is)* a drinking, drink + -IA] The drinking of abnormally small amounts of liquids.

hypopotassemia HYPOKALEMIA.

hypopotassemic HYPOKALEMIC.

hypopotentia 1 Reduced electrical activity of the cerebral cortex. 2 Weakness. An outmoded term.

hypopraxia A diminished or reduced motor activity. An imprecise and seldom used term.

hypoproaccelerinemia Factor V deficiency in plasma.

hypoproconvertinemia A condition marked by low plasma factor VII activity, which may result from administration of coumarin anticoagulants, from severe liver disease, or from a genetic disorder.

hereditary hypoproconvertinemia FACTOR VII DEFICIENCY.

hypoprogesterone hexanoate HYDROXYPROGESTERONE CAPROATE.

hypoprosessis [HYPO- + Gk *prosessis* for *prosexis* (from *prosexō*, fut. of *prosechein* to turn one's attention to) attention] Inattentiveness; distractiblity. Also called *hypoprosexia.*

hypoprosexia HYPOPROSESSIS.

hypoprosody A state in which a lack of the normal variations in pitch or rhythm results in monotonous speech.

hypoproteinemia [HYPO- + PROTEINEMIA] Less than normal concentration of protein in blood, plasma, or serum.

chronic idiopathic hypoproteinemia in the child Unexplained hypoproteinemia in a young child, often presenting as edema. Investigation usually reveals a chronic gastrointestinal disorder, such as celiac disease, lymphangiectasis, or ulcerative colitis.

hypoproteinemic Marked by a less-than-normal protein concentration in the plasma.

hypoproteinia An abnormally low level of protein in the blood plasma due to a very low intake from the diet or arising from a disease state such as nephrosis, or liver disease.

hypoproteinic Of or relating to hypoproteinia.

hypoproteinosis Protein deficiency due to the chronic ingestion of a diet low in protein.

hypoprothrombinemia A less than normal activity or concentration of prothrombin in blood. Also called *prothrombinopenia.*

hypopselaphesia [HYPO- + Gk *psēlaphēs(is)* a touching, groping + -IA] Impairment of the sensation of touch.

hypopsychosis Diminished or inadequate mental functioning. An obsolete term.

hypopteronosis cystica An avian disease, particularly of canaries, in which the feather follicles develop one or more cysts and feathers do not form.

hypopus [Gk *hypopous* furnished with feet] (*plural* hypopi) An unusual transport stage in the life cycle of certain grain mites (order Acariformes, suborder Astigmata), in which a distinctive body form develops between the first and second nymphal stages. In some species phoretic or active hypopi occur, adapted for clinging to arthropods or mammals. Another type is a passive form, the dauernymph, which is able to use air currents for dispersal or which is simply a waiting stage.

hypopyon [HYPO + Gk *pyon* pus] The sedimentation of white blood cells into the inferior portion of the anterior chamber of the eye, where a flat-topped gravity line is formed. This inferior white deposit is an easily observed sign of serious intraocular inflammation. Also called *lunella* (outmoded).

hypopyon recidivans BEHÇET SYNDROME.

hyporeactive Exhibiting a reduced responsiveness to stimulation.

hyporeflectivity HYPOREFLEXIA.

hyporeflexia Reduction or weakening of reflexes. Also called *hyporeflectivity.*

hyporiboflavinosis RIBOFLAVIN DEFICIENCY.

hyposalemia Less than normal concentration of cations and anions in the blood or serum. A seldom used term.

hyposalivation Reduced flow of saliva, causing a dry mouth. Also called *hyposialosis, oligosialia, asialorrhea.*

hyposarca ANASARCA.

hyposcheotomy [HYP- + OSCHEO- + -TOMY] Incision of a hydrocele at the inferior portion of the tunica vaginalis testis.

hyposcleral [HYPO- + SCLERAL] Situated between the sclera and the choroid.

hyposecretion [HYPO- + SECRETION] Subnormal secretion, as of a substance or hormone by a gland.

hyposensitive Showing subnormal sensitivity.

hyposensitivity [HYPO- + SENSITIVITY] A state in which an immune individual reacts with diminished response on subsequent exposure to a specific antigen to which he has been previously sensitized.

hyposensitization The induction of a state of hyposensitivity.

hyposensitize To subject to repeated and gradually increasing doses of a sensitizing allergen to induce a state hyposensitivity for that specific allergen.

hyposexuality Diminished sexual desire or responsivity.

hyposiagonarthritis [HYPO- + Gk *siagōn* jawbone, jaw + ARTHRITIS] Arthritis of the temperomandibular joint. An obsolete term.

hyposialadenitis Inflammation of the submaxillary salivary gland or glands.

hyposialosis HYPOSALIVATION.

hyposmia [HYP- + *osm(o)*-² + -IA] Subnormal olfactory perception. Also called *hyposphresia, olfactory hypoesthesia*.

hyposomatotropism [HYPO- + SOMATO- + TROPISM] **1** Deficient or absent adenohypophysial secretion of growth hormone, or the condition resulting from it. **2** Hypopituitary dwarfism of children. See under HYPOPHYSIAL DWARF.

hyposomia [HYPO- + *som(a)* + -IA] A condition marked by an underdeveloped body.

hyposomnia INSOMNIA.

hyposomniac INSOMNIAC.

hypospadia HYPOSPADIAS.

hypospadiac [HYPO- + Gk *span* to draw, draw out or forth, tear] **1** An individual exhibiting hypospadias. **2** Characterized by or exhibiting hypospadias.

hypospadias [HYPO- + Gk *span* to draw, draw out or forth, tear] A developmental defect of the urethra in which the urethral folds have failed to unite to complete the ventral wall of the urethra. The defect may involve only localized segments of a major portion of the urethra. Urine is discharged at the most proximal point of the defect. Also called *hypospadia*.
  balanic hypospadias Hypospadias on or near the glans penis. Also called *coronal hypospadias, glandular hypospadias, balanitic hypospadias*.
  balanitic hypospadias BALANIC HYPOSPADIAS.
  coronal hypospadias BALANIC HYPOSPADIAS.
  female hypospadias Hypospadias in the female, allowing leakage or discharge of urine into the lower vagina.
  glandular hypospadias BALANIC HYPOSPADIAS.
  male hypospadias PENILE HYPOSPADIAS.
  penile hypospadias Hypospadias in the male at any point in or throughout the length of the penile urethra. Also called *male hypospadias*.
  penoscrotal hypospadias Hypospadias occurring either separately or continuously on both the ventral aspect of the penis and at the midline of the scrotum.
  perineal hypospadias Hypospadias in which the entire scrotum is cleft by an extensive defect in the base of the penile urethra and in more or less of the urethra on the shaft of the penis. The testes often do not descend and the penis may be rudimentary, with a chordee.

hypospermatogenesis A diminishing of male germ cell production due to testicular disease.

hyposphresia HYPOSMIA.

hypostasis [Gk *hypostasis* (from *hypo-* under + *stasis* a standing)

deposited matter, sediment] **1** The settling or pooling of a fluid or suspended solid due to gravity; especially, stasis of the circulation in a dependent part or organ. **2** The failure of the usual phenotypic expression of a gene when in the presence of another gene that is epistatic toward it.

hypostatic **1** Of or characterized by hypostasis. **2** Failing to be expressed phenotypically when in the presence of an epistatic gene: said of a gene.

hyposteatolysis A reduced capacity to hydrolyze fats during digestion.

hyposteatosis OLIGOSTEATOSIS.

hyposthenia A state of reduced strength; weakness.

hyposthenia nt **1** Characterized by hyposthenia. Also *hyposthenic*. **2** Any substance that brings about hyposthenia.

hyposthenic HYPOSTHENIANT.

hyposthenuria [HYPO- + STHEN- + -URIA] Impaired ability of the kidneys to concentrate urine appropriately in response to fluid deprivation or administration of antidiuretic hormone. It may be measured by the relative density of urine under conditions of known fluid deficit or by the urine-to-plasma osmolality ratio.
  tubular hyposthenuria Impaired urinary concentrating ability secondary to injury or disease of the renal tubular epithelium. This may occur in any parenchymal renal disease, especially interstitial nephritis.

hypostome [HYPO- + Gk *stom(a)* mouth] **1** An organ of attachment in the tick capitulum. Centrally located and covered with spines, it allows the tick to anchor itself while feeding. **2** In Diptera, the anterior region of the head between the eyes and above the mouth. **3** In coelenterate polyps, a raised conical area surrounding the proctostome.

hypostomia [HYPO- + STOM- + -IA] Microstomia in which the oral orifice tends to be a small sagittal slit rather than a transverse one.

hypostosis [HYP- + OSTOSIS] A decreased development of bone.

hyposulfite An outmoded term for DITHIONITE.

hyposulfurous acid An obsolete term for THIOSULFURIC ACID.

hyposuprarenalemia Less than normal concentration of epinephrine (adrenaline) in blood.

hyposuprarenalism [HYPO- + SUPRA- + RENAL + -ISM] A seldom used term for HYPOADRENALISM.

hyposympathicotonus [HYPO- + SYMPATHICO- + TONUS] A reduction from the normal level of tonic activity induced by the sympathetic nervous system.

hyposynergia [HYPO- + Gk *synergia* (from *syn-* with + *erg(on)* work + -*ia* -IA) cooperation] Defective coordination.

hyposystole Diminished cardiac systole.

hypotelorism [HYPO- + TELORISM] Abnormal closeness of paired organs or parts.
  orbital hypotelorism An abnormally short interorbital or interocular distance. It is seen in trigonocephaly, and in some instances may represent a minimal expression of cyclopia.

hypotension [HYPO- + TENSION] Abnormally low tension or pressure, especially blood pressure. Also called *hypopiesis, hypopiesia*.
  arterial hypotension Abnormally low systemic arterial pressure.
  chronic orthostatic hypotension SHY-DRAGER SYNDROME.
  controlled hypotension INDUCED HYPOTENSION.
  familial orthostatic hypotension The Shy-Drager syndrome involving more than one member of a family.
  idiopathic hypotension Hypotension of undetermined cause.

induced hypotension Hypotension intentionally produced, either by mechanical or by pharmacological means, usually for the purpose of reducing blood loss in surgery. Also called *controlled hypotension*.

intracranial hypotension Reduced intracranial pressure.

orthostatic hypotension Hypotension on assuming the upright posture, commonly manifested by faintness or syncope. It is a feature of certain disorders of the autonomic nervous system and also of treatment with certain antihypertensive agents. Also called *postural hypotension*.

postural hypotension ORTHOSTATIC HYPOTENSION.

spinal hypotension Hypotension resulting from the block of sympathetic nerve fibers during spinal anesthesia or spinal cord trauma.

vascular hypotension Hypotension as a consequence of vascular dilatation.

ventricular hypotension Reduction in the pressure of the cerebrospinal fluid in the cerebral ventricles following cranial surgery or head injury or occurring in states of dehydration, but most often following lumbar puncture or occurring in conditions causing extracranial leakage of cerebrospinal fluid. The principal symptoms are headache, which is worse when the patient stands or sits up, vomiting, and stiffness of the neck.

hypotensive Characterized by or causing abnormally low tension or pressure, especially blood pressure. Also *hypopietic*.

hypothalamic Describing, pertaining to, or affecting the hypothalamus.

hypothalamotomy [*hypothalam(us)* + *o* + -TOMY] Incision into the hypothalamus or into the floor of the third ventricle.

hypothalamus [HYPO- + THALAMUS] A subdivision of the diencephalon that extends from the lamina terminalis to the mamillary bodies and comprises the ventrolateral wall and floor of the third ventricle below the hypothalamic sulcus. It can be divided into three zones (supraoptic, infundibulotuberal, and mamillary) and contains various groups of nuclei which exert control over autonomic functions, water balance, regulation of body temperature, appetite and food intake, sleep, and certain endocrine functions, including the neurosecretory control of the adenohypophysis and neurohypophsysis.

hypothecium [HYPO- + *thec(a)* + L -*ium*, noun suffix] A thin layer of interwoven fungal hyphae immediately below the hymenium of an apothecium.

hypothenar [NA] The elongated eminence along the ulnar border of the palm of the hand, produced mainly by the three intrinsic muscles that abduct, flex and oppose the fifth digit. Also called *hypothenar eminence, antithenar, antithenar eminence*.

hypothermal Descriptive of a body temperature below the normal.

hypothermesthesia Subnormal temperature sensibility.

hypothermia [HYPO- + Gk *therm(ē)* heat, feverish heat + -IA] A body temperature below the normal value of 98.6°F or 37°C. Clinically, hypothermia is not important unless the body temperature declines to 91°–92°F or about 33°C. Also called *cold stroke, hypothermy, frozen sleep*.

accidental hypothermia Hypothermia caused by exposure to a cold environment and characterized by a dangerous fall in body temperature. It occurs most often in infants and in the elderly.

hypothermia by extracorporeal methods Cooling of all or part of the body by refrigeration or by perfusion with cold blood.

hypothermia by surface cooling Induction of a subnormal body temperature by cooling of the body surface, which may be accidental or intentional. When done for therapeutic purposes appropriate medications are given to prevent or diminish the normal physiological responses to cold.

endogenous hypothermia Hypothermia caused by bodily disease or dysfunction rather than exogenous causes.

induced hypothermia Reduction in body temperature intentionally produced, for therapeutic purposes or as an adjunct to surgical techniques in which a reduction in body metabolism is helpful.

moderate hypothermia Hypothermia in which the body temperature is reduced to a range of 23–32°C.

profound hypothermia Body temperature of 12–20° C.

regional hypothermia Local cooling of an ischemic organ by refrigeration or perfusion with cold blood to reduce its metabolic requirements.

total body hypothermia Hypothermia of the entire body, as opposed to regional hypothermia, which may be limited to an extremity or organ.

hypothermy HYPOTHERMIA.

hypothesis [Gk *hypothesis* (from *hypotithenai* to place under, lay down, presuppose) a groundwork, assumption, principle] An assumption advanced to explain phenomena subject to tests that confirm, modify, or disprove it, or to serve as a basis for further experimentation or argument.

anniversary hypothesis A hypothesis stating that if a person who loses a parent during childhood, who later marries and has children, who still later is hospitalized for a first episode of mental illness, is likely to have that first episode at the time that his eldest child is within a year of his own age when he lost his parent.

biogenic amine hypothesis The theory that the biogenic amines are significant and perhaps even etiologic factors in the development of the major affective disorders and schizophrenia. The catecholamine hypothesis of affect disorders states that depressions are associated with a relative or absolute deficiency of catecholamines in functionally important sites in the brain. The permissive hypothesis of affect disorders states that a defect in central indolaminergic transmission permits affect disorder but is not enough to cause it. When superimposed on the indolamine defect, excess catecholamine produces mania while deficiency produces depression. The dopamine hypothesis of schizophrenia states that excess dopaminergic activity in the brain causes, precipitates, provokes, or exaggerates schizophrenic symptoms.

Buergi's hypothesis A theory that if two drugs have identical pharmacologic effects, their combined activity will be more than additive, when given simultaneously, if they have different mechanisms of pharmacologic action. Also called *Buergi's theory*.

cardionector hypothesis The hypothesis that two pacemaker regions in the heart, the sinoatrial node (atrionector) and the atrioventricular node (ventriculonector), control the heart rhythm. An obsolete term.

cascade hypothesis of coagulation An explanation of the sequence of events in coagulation in which the product of each step is a protease that activates the ensuing step by converting an inactive plasma protein to an active protease that in turn activates the next step. Thus, activation of factor XII by contact with glass or platelet phospholipids results in formation of factor XIIa, which converts factor XI to factor XIa, which in the presence of factor VIII converts factor IX to factor XIa, which converts factor X to factor Xa in the presence of factor V. Then factor Xa converts prothrombin to thrombin, which converts fibrinogen to fibrin, thus forming a blood clot. The above sequence is for the intrinsic coagulation cascade, which involves only plasma coagulation factors. The extrinsic coagulation cascade includes activation of factor VII to factor VIIa by a tissue factor (phospholipid). Factor VIIa activates factor IX and factor X to factors IXa and Xa, which then convert prothrombin to thrombin, etc.

catecholamine hypothesis See under BIOGENIC AMINE HYPOTHESIS.

chemiosmotic hypothesis The hypothesis that the action of the respiratory chain leads to the formation of a gradient in chemical potential of hydrogen ions across the membrane containing that respiratory chain, e.g. the mitochondrial membrane of eukaryotes, and that the passage of hydrogen ions down this gradient is used to drive chemical reactions, such as the condensation of ADP and orthophosphate to form ATP. The difference in chemical potential of the hydrogen ions consists of two parts, the pH difference and the difference in electrical potential across the membrane. The hypothesis was formulated to explain the coupling of oxidation to ATP formation by mitochondria, but it has also been extended to ATP formation in photosynthesis and to membrane transport by bacteria.

disuse hypothesis A theory that changes similar to those of aging may be brought about in a part of the body which is constantly neglected or disused.

dopamine hypothesis See under BIOGENIC AMINE HYPOTHESIS.

frustration-aggression hypothesis The hypothesis that frustration always leads to aggressive reactions of either an explicit or implicit nature and, conversely, that any observed aggressive behavior is always the result of frustration of one kind or another.

Gad's hypothesis The unsubstantiated theory that a wedge-shaped valve is formed by the acute angle at the junction of the branches of the hepatic artery and the portal vein in the portal canal of the liver.

Haldane-Oparin hypothesis The hypothesis that life arose on earth from dilute solutions of organic compounds formed by inorganic forces and able to accumulate because lack of atmospheric oxygen, and absence of microbial degradation, made them much more stable than they would be today.

half-center hypothesis An outmoded hypothesis to explain stepping in the spinal animal. The circuitry of the cord that provides excitation to extensor muscles (one half-center) was said to be in delicate, mutually inhibitory balance with another portion (the other half-center) excitatory to flexor activity. Crossed influences from the two comparable half-centers on the opposite side of the spinal cord were also proposed.

Harrower's hypothesis The proposal that certain organ abnormalities may be ascribed to the defective supply of hormones on which the proper functioning of the organ depends.

inactive X hypothesis LYON PHENOMENON.

insular hypothesis The idea that malfunction of the pancreatic islets of Langerhans is the cause of diabetes mellitus.

intact nephron hypothesis The hypothesis that chronic renal failure is characterized by a progressive decrease in the number of functioning nephrons rather than from separate impairment of the function of glomeruli and tubules. As nephrons decrease in number those remaining are thought to undergo structural and functional hypertrophy.

Lyon hypothesis LYON PHENOMENON.

Lyon-Russell hypothesis LYON PHENOMENON.

Makeham's hypothesis The proposal that death is due to both chance, which is constant, and the inability to prevent destruction, a factor that increases geometrically with age.

master-slave hypothesis The concept, now largely disproven, that structural genes are present in multiple, tandemly repeated copies in the genome. One copy is the master and serves as a corrective template for the other copies (the slaves) during each replication of the chromosome, a process termed rectification. The hypothesis was advanced by H.G. Callan in the 1960s and sought to account for the immense variation in nuclear DNA content among closely related organisms.

mnemic hypothesis The hypothesis that a stimulus or irritant

produces a change, or engram, in the protoplasm of a cell which persists after cessation of the stimulus. An obsolete portion of the hypothesis states further that germ cells as well as nerve cells form engrams, and thus acquired responses to stimuli may be passed on to descendants. Also called *Semon-Hering hypothesis*.

multiple factor hypothesis QUANTITATIVE INHERITANCE.

null hypothesis In statistics, the assumption that a measured difference between two samples of the same population is purely accidental, rather than being the result of some systematic variation.

one gene-one enzyme hypothesis The concept that each gene specifies a single enzyme. Although of historical importance, this hypothesis has been superseded by the one gene-one polypeptide hypothesis.

one gene-one polypeptide hypothesis The concept that each gene specifies a sequence in mRNA that directs the translation of one functional polypeptide.

Orgel's hypothesis ERROR CATASTROPHE.

permissive hypothesis of affective disorders See under BIOGENIC AMINE HYPOTHESIS.

polarization hypothesis The hypothesis that blastomeres at the 8-cell stage "recognize" an asymmetry of cell contacts by developing a polarized phenotype with an axis normal to the points of contact. The polarity is stable throughout division to the 16-cell stage yielding distinguishable superficial and deep subpopulations of cells. Continuing interactions between these cell subpopulations cause increasingly divergent differentiation to generate trophectoderm and inner cell mass tissues at the 32-cell stage.

polyneme hypothesis The hypothesis that a chromatid consists of more than one molecule of DNA. This concept has now been generally supplanted by the unineme hypothesis.

Rubner's hypothesis Within a given gene pool, longevity is inversely related to the intensity of living.

self-marker hypothesis A hypothesis to explain self/nonself discrimination by proposing that the body's own antigens carry markers which are recognized as self by immunologically competent cells. The latter cells are then inhibited from responding against those antigens which carry the self-marker. No molecular basis for the theory was proposed.

Semon-Hering hypothesis MNEMIC HYPOTHESIS.

sliding-filament hypothesis The hypothesis that the basic mechanism responsible for the contractile force and shortening of muscle tissue depends upon longitudinally arranged and interdigitating actin and myosin filaments which, through activation of cross-bridges, increase the overlap along their lengths and so shorten the sarcomere.

statistical hypothesis A hypothesis stating the value of parameters or the form of a probability function of a given population. See also STATISTICAL TEST, STATISTICAL SIGNIFICANCE.

structural hypothesis The hypothesis that the psyche has three divisions, id, ego, and superego. Also called *structural theory*.

topographic hypothesis The hypothesis that the psyche has three divisions, conscious, preconscious, and unconscious.

trade-off hypothesis The hypothesis that as renal function declines various compensatory changes tend to maintain the concentration of solutes in body fluids at near normal levels, at the expense of some other organs or organ systems. This is based on the retention of phosphate as glomerular filtration rate decreases, which in turn causes an increase in the secretion of parathyroid hormone. The increased parathyroid hormone inhibits proximal reabsorption of phosphate, thus returning the plasma phosphate level to normal. However, the persistent increase in parathyroid hormone mobilizes calcium from the bones and thus leads to the osteodystrophy of chronic renal failure. In this manner, maintainence of a normal plasma phosphate level is "traded-off" for secondary hyperparathyroidism and renal osteodystrophy.

triplet hypothesis   The hypothesis that a sequence of three nucleotides in the deoxyribonucleic acid molecule (a codon), carries the genetic information needed to place a specific amino acid in a polypeptide chain.

unineme hypothesis   The concept, generally accepted for all eukaryotes, that one double helix of DNA extends from one end of a chromatid to the other.

unitarian hypothesis   The theory, now obsolete, that antibody is a single species of immunoglobulin regardless of the types of reaction seen with various antigens. Also called *unitarian theory of antibodies.*

wobble hypothesis   The hypothesis which states that the terminal nucleotide (3′) in a codon may be either of the two purines without altering the amino acid incorporated into the polypeptide chain, or in other codons either of two pyrimidines without altering specificity. The specificity of the codon is dependent on the first two nucleotides, with some freedom in the third nucleotide. The wobble is dependent on the geometry of the ribosome.

hypothrepsia   MALNUTRITION.

hypothromboplastinemia   A deficiency of one of the hemophilic factors, VIII, IX, or XI.

hypothymia [HYPO- + -THYMIA]   Reduced intensity of affect or emotion; emotional blandness.

hypothymism   Subnormal function of the thymus.

hypothyrea   An older term for HYPOTHYROIDISM.

hypothyreosis   A seldom used term for HYPOTHYROIDISM.

hypothyroid [HYPO- + THYROID]   Of, relating to, or characteristic of hypothyroidism. Also *athyreotic* (seldom used).

hypothyroidation   The process of inducing or contributing to hypothyroidism.

hypothyroidea   A rarely used term for HYPOTHYROIDISM.

hypothyroidism [HYPOTHYROID + -ISM]   Deficient hormone secretion by the thyroid gland, or the condition resulting from it. In infants, hypothyroidism leads to cretinism. In adults, it is characterized by lowered oxygen consumption, a slowed basal metabolic rate, sluggishness, lethargy, pallor, menstrual disorders, and disturbances in mentation. In advanced stages, myxedema ensues and coma may follow. The commonest form of thyroid gland failure may have an autoimmune basis. Also called *thyroid insufficiency, subthyroidism, thyroprivia, athyreosis* (seldom used), *hypothyreosis* (seldom used), *hypothyrosis* (seldom used), *hypothyroidea* (rarely used), *hypothyrea* (older term), *athyroidism* (seldom used), *athyrosis* (obsolete), *athyria* (obsolete), *athyroidosis* (obsolete), *athyrea* (obsolete).

familial goitrous hypothyroidism   FAMILIAL GOITER.

hypothalamic hypothyroidism   Hypothyroidism due to failure of hypothalamic thyrotropin releasing hormone secretion, which leads to hyposecretion of adenohypophysial thyrotropin, causing atrophy and diminished elaboration of thyroid hormones by the thyroid gland. Also called *tertiary hypothyroidism, hypothalamic myxedema, tertiary myxedema.*

infantile hypothyroidism   CRETINISM.

postablative hypothyroidism   POSTOPERATIVE HYPOTHYROIDISM.

postoperative hypothyroidism   Hypothyroidism following surgical removal of all or part of the thyroid gland. Also called *postablative hypothyroidism.*

primary hypothyroidism   Hypothyroidism due to disease of the thyroid gland itself, as in idiopathic atrophy of the gland (Gull's disease).

secondary hypothyroidism   TROPHOPRIVIC HYPOTHYROIDISM.

tertiary hypothyroidism   HYPOTHALAMIC HYPOTHYROIDISM.

thyroprivic hypothyroidism   Hypothyroidism due to loss or atrophy of thyroid gland tissue with hyposecretion of thyroid hormone; primary hypothyroidism.

trophoprivic hypothyroidism   Hypothyroidism due to deficient secretion of the anterior pituitary hormone, thyrotropin. Also called *secondary hypothyroidism.*

hypothyrosis   A seldom used term for HYPOTHYROIDISM.

hypotonia [HYPO- + Gk *ton(os)* (from *teinein* to stretch, strain, draw tight) a tightening, rope, sinew, force + -IA]   Reduction in muscle tone. Also called *hypotony, hypomyotonia* (seldom used), *hypatonia.*

benign congenital hypotonia   Diffuse hypotonia of the skeletal musculature present from birth accompanied by delayed physical development and showing a tendency to spontaneous improvement and sometimes complete recovery. This is now known to be a syndrome of multiple etiology and not a single disease entity. Also called *benign infantile hypotonia.*

benign infantile hypotonia   BENIGN CONGENITAL HYPOTONIA.

infantile hypotonia   FLOPPY INFANT SYNDROME.

hypotonia oculi   OCULAR HYPOTONY.

hypotonic   **1** Less than normally tonic, as the state of a muscle. **2** Having an osmotic pressure less than that of an isotonic solution or less concentrated than isotonic. Also *hypoisotonic.*

hypotonicity   A condition in which the effective osmotic pressure of a body fluid is lower than that in surrounding tissues.

hypotonus [HYPO- + TONUS]   A reduced force or tension exerted by a muscle while the muscle is in the relaxed state.

hypotony   HYPOTONIA.

ocular hypotony   Abnormally soft intraocular pressure, as may occur in the presence of a perforating wound or a diminished rate of formation of the aqueous humor. Also called *hypotonia oculi.*

hypotoxicity [HYPO- + TOXICITY]   Low or moderate toxicity.

hypotransferrinemia   Less than normal concentration of transferrin in plasma or serum, as occurs in many chronic disorders, malignancies, infectious diseases, rheumatoid arthritis, and chronic renal disease.

hypotrichiasis   HYPOTRICHOSIS.

Hypotrichida [HYPO- + TRICH- + New L -*ida*, neut. pl. in form, from L -*ides*, patronymic suffix]   An order of ciliates in the protozoan subclass Spirotrichia. They are usually large, free-living, and free-swimming, and are found in a great variety of habitats. Genera include *Urostyla, Holosticha, Euplotes,* and *Stylonychia.*

hypotrichosis [HYPO- + TRICHOSIS]   Any condition marked by a partial lack of hair. Also called *hypotrichiasis, oligotrichy.*

hypotrichous [HYPO- + TRICH- + -OUS]   Marked by an absence of cilia on the dorsal surface: said of certain ciliates.

hypotriploid   Designating a cell or an organism in which the chromosome number is one less than the triploid number.

hypotrophy [HYPO- + TROPH- + -Y]   Wasting or reduction in size.

hypotropia [HYPO- + TROPIA]   A vertical misalignment of the eyes. The specified eye is the deviating lower eye. Thus, in right hypotropia, the right eye is the nonfixing, downward-directed eye; in left hypotropia, the left.

hypotryptophanic   Due to a dietary deficiency of tryptophan.

hypotympanic   Pertaining to the hypotympanum.

hypotympanum   The part of the tympanic cavity below the level of the tympanic membrane, bounded inferiorly by the paries jugularis. An outmoded term.

hypotype [HYPO- + TYPE] A specimen whose description aids in amplifying or correcting the identification and classification of a species.

hypouremia Less than normal concentration of blood urea.

hypouresis [HYPO- + URESIS] Deficient urine excretion. A seldom used term.

hypouricosuria HYPOURICURIA.

hypouricuria [HYPO- + -URIC + -URIA] Decreased urinary excretion of uric acid. The hyperuricemia of most patients with gout results from increased reabsorption of uric acid from the glomerular filtrate by the renal tubule cells, often due to inherited enzyme defects. Secondary causes of hypouricuria include increased plasma organic acids which inhibit tubular reabsorption of uric acid, as in starvation, ketosis, of lactic acid acidosis. Volume depletion due to any cause, including diuretics, and renal failure also are common causes of hypouricuria. Also called *hypouricosuria*.

hypovaria A rarely used term for HYPOVARIANISM.

hypovarianism Deficient hormone secretion by the ovary. Also called *hypo-ovarianism, hypovaria* (rarely used), *hypo-ovaria* (older term).

hypovasopressinemia Less than normal concentration of vasopressin in blood, as in pituitary insufficiency or diabetes insipidus.

hypovenosity The deficient development of veins in a region or part.

hypoventilation [HYPO- + VENTILATION] Insufficient ventilation of the alveoli of the lungs to maintain normal levels of oxygen and/or carbon dioxide in arterial blood.

   central hypoventilation Hypoventilation due to disease or dysfunction of the brainstem.

   chronic alveolar hypoventilation Hypoventilation often resulting from chronic neuromuscular disease giving rise to weakness of the respiratory muscles and carbon dioxide retention, with consequential headache, drowsiness, and confusion.

   primary alveolar hypoventilation Hypoventilation occurring in a patient with normal ventilatory function, due to a deficiency in the brainstem regulation of breathing. Also called *Ondine's curse.*

hypovigility Diminished responsivity to or awareness of external stimuli.

hypovitaminosis [HYPO- + VITAMIN + -OSIS] A disorder due to a deficiency of one or more vitamins. Also called *avitaminosis* (imprecise).

hypovolaemia A British spelling for HYPOVOLEMIA.

hypovolemia [HYPO- + VOL(UME) + -EMIA] Abnormal reduction in the circulating blood volume.

hypovolemic Related to or characterized by hypovolemia.

hypovolia A reduced volume or diminished water content.

hypovolumic Characterized by reduced or subnormal volume.

hypoxaemia A British spelling for HYPOXEMIA.

hypoxanthine 4-Hydroxypurine and its keto tautomer. It is produced by the hydrolysis of adenine when this is catabolized. Xanthine oxidase converts it, via xanthine, into uric acid, which is excreted in man, although most other mammals break it down further. Also called *adenine hypoxanthine.*

hypoxanthine-guanine-phosphoribosyl-transferase The enzyme responsible for purine salvage, whereby guanine and hypoxanthine are converted to guanilic acid and inosinic acid. The absence of this enzyme results in an accumulation of uncombined phosphoribosyl-l-pyrophosphate, which causes an acceleration in purine production and an excess in uric acid production.

hypoxanthine oxidase An outmoded term for XANTHINE OXIDASE. • The name was given because this enzyme not only oxidizes xanthine to uric acid, but also hypoxanthine to xanthine.

hypoxemia [*hyp(o)-* + *ox(ygen)* + -EMIA] Reduced oxygen concentration in arterial blood.

hypoxia [HYP- + *ox(ygen)* + -IA] Inadequate oxygen concentration in body tissues. Also called *suboxidation* (rarely used).

   anemic hypoxia Less than normal oxygen content of blood due to decreased hemoglobin concentration of blood. Also called *anemic anoxia* (imprecise).

   circulatory hypoxia Impaired oxygen delivery to tissues due to decreased blood flow.

   diffusion hypoxia Hypoxia that may result at termination of nitrous oxide-oxygen anesthesia, believed to be the result of outward diffusion of nitrous oxide reducing the concentration of oxygen in alveoli.

   histotoxic hypoxia A condition marked by a reduced ability of a tissue to utilize oxygen.

   hypoxic hypoxia A reduced supply of oxygen to tissues due to a reduced partial pressure of oxygen in the blood.

hypoxic [*hyp-* + *ox(y)-*[1] + -IC] Marked by a reduced oxygen supply. Also *anoxic* (incorrect).

hypoxidosis [HYP- + OXIDOSIS] A reduction of cell function or activity due to an inadequate oxygen supply.

hypsarhythmia HYPSARRHYTHMIA.

hypsarrhythmia [*hyps(o)-* + ARRHYTHMIA] In electroencephalography, a pattern of continuous generalized irregular wave and spike activity occurring in children. This pattern is not specific. It may be seen in various forms of cerebral lipidosis, in some other neuronal storage diseases and in tuberous sclerosis, but most often occurs in infants suffering from infantile massive spasm. These attacks are often very frequent. They may be partially responsive to ACTH treatment, but most affected infants become severely mentally retarded. Similar appearances in the EEG may occur in adults with Creutzfeldt-Jakob disease. Also *hypsarhythmia.*

hypsarrhythmoid Exhibiting or pertaining to electroencephalographic waveforms resembling but not identical with those of hypsarrhythmia.

hypsi- HYPSO-.

hypsibrachycephalic [HYPSI- + BRACHYCEPHALIC] Having a tall yet broad cranial vault.

hypsicephalic [HYPSI- + CEPHALIC] Having a skull in which the cranial height-length index is equal to or greater than 75. Also *hypsocephalous.*

hypsicephaly [HYPSI- + CEPHAL- + -Y] The conformation of a skull with a cranial height-length index equal to or greater than 75. Also called *hypsocephaly.*

hypsiconchous [HYPSI- + *conch(a)* + -OUS] Characterizing a skull in which the orbital index is relatively high.

hypsiloid UPSILOID.

hypsistaphylia [HYPSI- + STAPHYL- + -IA] A narrow, highly-arched palate. An obsolete term.

hypsistenocephalic [HYPSI- + STENO- + CEPHALIC] Characterizing a skull in which the cranial vault is high and narrow.

hypsithermal Pertaining to the geologic time period, 5000–7000 years ago, during which the mean temperature of the earth was 2°–3°C above normal. This resulted in the loss of plants and animals adjusted to cooler climate conditions and is believed to have led to the extinction of some forms of life.

hypso- [Gk *hypsos* height; Gk *hypsi* on high, aloft] A combining form meaning height, high. Also *hypsi-.*

hypsocephalous HYPSICEPHALIC.

hypsocephaly [HYPSO- + CEPHAL- + -Y] HYPSICEPHALY.

hypsochromic Denoting a shifting to a shorter wavelength, usually of an absorption band in a spectrum. Compare BATHOCHROMIC.

hypsochromy The shift of a band in the light absorption spectrum of a chemical compound to shorter wavelengths as the result of a modification in the structure of the compound.

hypsodont [*hyps(o)*- + -ODONT] Denoting teeth in which the crowns are very high in relation to the length of the roots.

hypsokinesis [HYPSO- + KINESIS] An abnormality of gait in which there is displacement of the center of gravity, as in parkinsonism, so that the patient may move more and more quickly, usually forwards, but occasionally backwards, and may ultimately fall.

hypsometer [HYPSO- + -METER] An instrument for measuring the boiling point of water under reduced atmospheric pressure. The value of the atmospheric pressure, and hence the altitude of the measurement point, are derived from tables. Also called *boiling-point barometer.*

hypsonosus [HYPSO- + Gk *nosos* disease, illness] Hypoxemia due to reduced oxygen pressure at high altitudes.

hypsotherapy [HYPSO- + THERAPY] The therapeutic use of either a permanent or temporary residence at a high elevation.

hypurals [HYP- + Gk *our(a)* tail + -AL + *s*] The enlarged hemal spines of the caudal vertebrae of teleost fish. These spines fuse to form the base of the homocercal tail fin.

Hyrtl [Joseph *Hyrtl*, Austrian anatomist, 1811–1894] **1** Hyrtl's foramen. See under PORUS CROTAPHITICOBUCCINATORIUS. **2** Hyrtl's anastomosis. See under LOOP. **3** Hyrtl sphincter. See under SPHINCTER ANI TERTIUS. **4** Hyrtl's recess. See under RECESSUS EPITYMPANICUS. **5** Ophthalmomeningeal vein of Hyrtl. See under VEIN.

hyster- HYSTERO-.

hystera UTERUS.

hysteralgia [HYSTER- + -ALGIA] UTERALGIA.

hysteratresia Atresia of the uterine lumen. It is usually a result of inflammation. Developmental atresia occurs when a paramesonephric duct fails to join with the urogenital sinus, thereby leaving an oviduct and part of the uterus isolated from the rest of the female genital tract.

hysterauxesis [HYSTER- + AUXESIS] An enlargement of the uterus, either pathologic or associated with pregnancy

hysterectomy [HYSTER- + -ECTOMY] Surgical removal of the uterus. Also called *metrectomy, myohysterectomy.*

abdominal hysterectomy Removal of the uterus through an incision in the abdominal wall. Also called *supravaginal hysterectomy, celiohysterectomy.*

abdominovaginal hysterectomy Surgical removal of the uterus from a combined abdominal and vaginal approach.

cesarean hysterectomy Removal of the uterus at the time of cesarean section. Also called *radical caesarian section, Porro hysterectomy.*

complete hysterectomy Removal of the uterine fundus and cervix. Also called *panhysterectomy, total hysterectomy.*

partial hysterectomy SUBTOTAL HYSTERECTOMY.

Porro hysterectomy CESAREAN HYSTERECTOMY.

radical hysterectomy Removal of the uterus, upper vagina, and parametrium for cancer.

subtotal hysterectomy Removal of the uterus at or above the level of the internal os. Also called *partial hysterectomy, supracervical hysterectomy.*

supracervical hysterectomy SUBTOTAL HYSTERECTOMY.

supravaginal hysterectomy ABDOMINAL HYSTERECTOMY.

total hysterectomy COMPLETE HYSTERECTOMY.

vaginal hysterectomy Surgical removal of the uterus through the vagina. Also called *colpohysterectomy.*

hysteremphysema [HYSTER- + EMPHYSEMA] Gas in the uterus.

hysteresis [Gk *hysterēsis* (from *hysterein* to be behind, come later, from *hysteros* coming after) a coming short, want, need] The dependence of a system output on the history and direction of the input. The mechanical hysteresis of the lung causes different transpulmonary pressures after inspiration and expiration. The thermal hysteresis of a reversible colloid causes differing temperatures of gelation and liquefaction. The magnetization of a magnetic material differs for increasing and decreasing magnetic forces.

protoplasmic hysteresis A condition in which the protoplasm becomes less dispersed due to a loss of water and a reduction of electrical charge, postulated as a cause of cell senescence.

hystereurynter [HYSTER- + Gk *eurynein* to widen] METREURYNTER.

hystereurysis [HYSTER- + EURY- + -SIS] Dilatation of the cervix.

hysteria [Gk *hyster(a)* (mostly in pl. *hysterai*) the uterus + -IA] **1** See under CONVERSION HYSTERIA. **2** See under ANXIETY HYSTERIA. **3** HISTRIONIC PERSONALITY DISORDER. **4** Any of various disorders characterized by conversion symptoms, such as paralysis, tremor, anesthesia, vomiting, amnesia, somnambulism, fugue, or other dissociation manifestations. An outmoded term. Also called *hysterical neurosis.* • *Hysteria* is no longer recognized as a separate clinical entity without qualification.

anxiety hysteria A phobic disorder, consisting of a specific, persistent, and irrational fear that leads to avoidance of all situations in which the feared object may be encountered and significant constriction of usual activities. The fear comes to dominate the patient's entire life. In time, if often spreads to include more than the original object as well as anticipatory fear that the anxiety or panic associated with exposure to the object may recur spontaneously. Also called *phobic neurosis, phobism* (outmoded), *phobic reaction.*

Arctic hysteria PIBLOKTO.

conversion hysteria A disorder, without detectable organic basis, characterized by a motor, sensory, or visceral physical manifestation, such as paralysis, tic, paresthesia, or vomiting, or a mental manifestation such as amnesia, fugue, depersonalization, or multiple personality. The subject displays a surprisingly calm mental attitude concerning his symptoms. Also called *somatic conversion, hysteroneurosis, conversion neurosis.*

convulsive hysteria Conversion hysteria in which epileptiform seizures constitute the major somatic manifestation.

fixation hysteria Conversion hysteria in which the affected somatic area is one that is, or has been, the site of some organic disorder, such as the development of paralysis in a hand that had been injured months previously in an accident. Also called *pathergasia, pathergasis, pathoneurosis, pathopsychosis.*

grand hysteria MAJOR HYSTERIA.

hysteria major MAJOR HYSTERIA.

major hysteria A rare type of conversion hysteria in which attacks occur in stages: (1) aura; (2) epileptoid convulsions; (3) tonic spasms followed by clonic spasms; (4) dramatic emotional display; and (5) delirium. A seldom used term. Also called *hysteroepilepsy, grand hysteria, hysteria major, hysteroepilepsy.*

hysteria minor A form of conversion hysteria in which consciousness is maintained during mild convulsions.

monosymptomatic hysteria Conversion hysteria manifested as a single symptom, such as torticollis without the accompanying mental state of dissociation.

traumatic hysteria Conversion hysteria that develops after an injury. It is a traumatic neurosis that ordinarily does not become manifest until some time after the injury.

hysteric 1 A person suffering from hysteria. 2 HYSTERICAL.

hysterical Characterized by hysteria. Also *hysteric*.

hystericoneuralgia Conversion hysteria in which neuralgic-like pain is the major somatic manifestation.

hysterics Emotional outburst, similar to a child's temper tantrums. A seldom used term.

hysteriform HYSTEROID.

hysteritis [HYSTER- + -ITIS] Inflammation of the uterus.

hystero- [Gk *hystera* uterus] A combining form meaning (1) the uterus; (2) hysteria. Also *hyster-*.

hysterobubonocele [HYSTERO- + Gk *boubōn*, gen. *boubōno(s)*, the groin + -CELE¹] A groin hernia containing the uterus. The condition is extremely rare.

hysterocarcinoma [HYSTERO- + CARCINOMA] Carcinoma of the uterus. An outmoded term.

hysterocatalepsy Conversion hysteria with posturing and waxy flexibility or rigidity as the major manifestation. A seldom used term.

hysterocele [HYSTERO- + -CELE¹] A hernia containing the uterus. Also called *metrocele*.

hysterocleisis [HYSTERO- + -CLEISIS] A surgical procedure in which the uterine cervix is sutured closed.

hysterocolpectomy [HYSTERO- + COLPECTOMY] Removal of the uterus and vagina. Also called *panhysterocolpectomy*.

hysterocolposcope [HYSTERO- + COLPOSCOPE] An instrument for viewing the vagina, cervix, and uterine cavity.

hysterocystic [HYSTERO- + CYSTIC] Referring to the uterus and bladder.

hysterocystocleisis [HYSTERO- + CYSTO- + -CLEISIS] An operation in which the uterus is used to aid the closure of a vesicovaginal fistula. Also called *Bozeman's operation*.

hysterocystopexy [HYSTERO- + CYSTO- + -PEXY] A surgical procedure in which the uterus is sutured to the urinary bladder, which is then sutured to the anterior abdominal wall, for purposes of fixation. Also called *ventrovesicofixation*.

hysterodynia [HYSTER- + -ODYNIA] UTERALGIA.

hysteroedema [HYSTERO- + EDEMA] Swelling of the uterus from edema.

hysteroepilepsy MAJOR HYSTERIA.

hysteroepileptogenic Giving rise to or precipitating an attack of major hysteria.

hysterofrenic [HYSTERO- + *fren(um)* + -IC] Arresting or tending to arrest hysterical attacks: said especially of points on the body where pressure may have this effect, or to the pressure applied.

hysterogenic [HYSTERO- + -GENIC] Causing or predisposing to symptoms of hysteria.

hysterogram [HYSTERO- + -GRAM] A roentgenogram obtained during hysterography.

hysterograph [HYSTERO- + -GRAPH] A device which measures the strength of uterine contractions.

hysterography [HYSTERO- + -GRAPHY] Radiographic examination of the uterine canal after the instillation of an opaque contrast medium through the cervical os. Also called *uterography, metrography* (obsolete).

hysteroid Resembling hysteria. Also called *hysteriform*.

hysterolith [HYSTERO- + -LITH] A stone or calcification in the uterus.

hysterology [HYSTERO- + -LOGY] The body of scientific knowledge concerning the uterus.

hysteromania [HYSTERO- + -MANIA] 1 NYMPHOMANIA. 2

A state of hyperactivity and agitation, occurring in hysteria. An obsolete term.

hysterometer [HYSTERO- + -METER] UTERINE SOUND.

hysterometry [HYSTERO- + -METRY] The process of measuring uterine size. Also called *uterometry*.

hysteromucography [HYSTERO- + MUCO- + -GRAPHY] HYSTEROSALPINGOGRAPHY.

hysteromyoma [HYSTERO- + MYOMA] Myoma of the uterus.

hysteromyomectomy [HYSTERO- + MYOMECTOMY] Excision of uterine leiomyomas.

hysteromyotomy [HYSTERO- + MYOTOMY] Uterine incision for removal of a solid tumor.

hysteroneurosis CONVERSION HYSTERIA.

hystero-oophorectomy [HYSTERO- + OOPHORECTOMY] Removal of the uterus and one or both ovaries. Also called *panhystero-oophorectomy*.

hysteropathy [HYSTERO- + -PATHY] METROPATHY.

hysterope [HYSTER- + -OPE] A person with visual symptoms due to the functional disorder of hysteria.

hysteropexy [HYSTERO- + -PEXY] The operative fixation of an abnormally positioned uterus. Also called *uterofixation, uteropexy, metropexy*.

hysteropia [HYSTER- + -OPIA] The presence of visual symptoms caused by hysteria. Characteristically, these are variable even within a very short time of examination and are readily influenced by suggestion. Bizarre, nonphysiologic visual field constrictions of tunnel configuration are common. Inability to see during stressful situations is the typical complaint. The affected person shows little concern over this visual loss, in contrast to the apprehension that most patients show when suffering from an organic loss of sight.

hysteroplasty [HYSTERO- + -PLASTY] UTEROPLASTY.

hysteropsychosis HYSTERICAL PSYCHOSIS.

hysteroptosia [HYSTERO- + Gk *ptōs(is)* a fall, falling + -IA] PROLAPSE OF UTERUS.

hysteroptosis [HYSTERO- + -PTOSIS] PROLAPSE OF UTERUS.

hysterorrhaphy [HYSTERO- + -RRHAPHY] Suture of the uterus.

hysterorrhea [HYSTERO- + -RRHEA] A uterine discharge.

hysterorrhexis [HYSTERO- + -RRHEXIS] METRORRHEXIS.

hysterosalpingectomy [HYSTERO- + SALPINGECTOMY] Removal of the uterus and an oviduct. Also called *panhysterosalpingectomy*.

hysterosalpingography [HYSTERO- + SALPINGO- + -GRAPHY] Radiographic examination of the uterus and fallopian tubes following the instillation of opaque contrast medium via the cervical os. Also called *hysteromucography, hysterotubography, uterosalpingography, uterotubography, metrosalpingography* (rarely used), *metrotubography* (rarely used).

hysterosalpingo-oophorectomy [HYSTERO- + SALPINGO- + OOPHORECTOMY] Surgical removal of the uterus, fallopian tubes, and ovaries. Also called *hysterosalpingo-oothectomy, panhysterosalpingo-oophorectomy*.

hysterosalpingo-oothecectomy HYSTEROSALPINGO-OOPHORECTOMY.

hysterosalpingostomy [HYSTERO- + SALPINGO- + -STOMY] A reimplantation of a partially occluded oviduct for the purpose of establishing fertility.

hysterosalpinx TUBA UTERINA.

hysteroscope [HYSTERO- + -SCOPE] A transcervical instrument for examining the uterine cavity. Also called *metroscope, uteroscope*.

hysteroscopy [HYSTERO- + -SCOPY] Inspection of the uterine cavity.

hysterospasm A spasm of the uterus. An obsolete term.

hysterostat [HYSTERO- + -STAT] A device in which are placed sealed sources of radioactive substances, such as radium, for intrauterine insertion. It is used in radiation therapy for cancer of the uterus.

hysterostomatocleisis An operation for vesicovaginal fistula in which the uterus is sutured over the defect.

hysterostomatome [HYSTERO- + *stoma(t)-* + -TOME] A knife used in hysterostomatomy or cervical incisions.

hysterostomatomy [HYSTERO- + *stoma(t)-* + -TOMY] Surgical enlargement of the os uteri by an incision.

hysterotabetism [HYSTERO- + *tabe(s)* + *t* + -ISM] Concomitant hysteria and tabes dorsalis.

hysterothermometry [HYSTERO- + THERMOMETRY] UTEROTHERMOMETRY.

hysterotome [HYSTERO- + -TOME] An instrument for making an incision into the uterus.

hysterotomotocia [HYSTERO- + *-tom(e)* + *o* + *toc(o)-* + -IA] An older term for CESAREAN SECTION.

hysterotomy [HYSTERO- + -TOMY] Incision into the uterus extending into the uterine cavity. It may be performed vaginally or transabdominally. Also called *uterotomy, metrotomy, metratomy.*

abdominal hysterotomy Hysterotomy carried out through an abdominal incision.

vaginal hysterotomy Hysterotomy carried out through a vaginal incision.

hysterotrachelectasia Surgical dilatation of the uterine cervix. A seldom used term.

hysterotrachelectomy [HYSTERO- + TRACHEL- + -ECTOMY] Removal of uterus and cervix; hysterectomy.

hysterotracheloplasty TRACHELOPLASTY.

hysterotrachelorrhaphy [HYSTERO- + TRACHELO- + -RRHAPHY] Plastic surgery of a lacerated cervix by paring the edges and suturing them together.

hysterotrachelotomy [HYSTERO- + TRACHELO- + -TOMY] Surgical incision of the neck of the uterus.

hysterotraumatic Pertaining to or exhibiting hysterotraumatism.

hysterotraumatism Symptoms of hysteria following trauma.

hysterotrismus [HYSTERO- + Gk *trismos* a creaking] Conversion hysteria in which the major symptom is a locking of the jaw.

hysterotubography [HYSTERO- + TUBO- + -GRAPHY] HYSTEROSALPINGOGRAPHY.

hysterovaginoenterocele Prolapse of the uterus and small intestine into the vagina.

hysterythrine An outmoded term for ESTROGEN.

hystrichiasis [Gk *hystrix*, gen. *hystrichos*, porcupine + -IASIS] Abnormal piloerection.

hystrix [Gk *hystrix* porcupine] Warty and spiny: said of some forms of nevi and ichthyosis.

Hytakerol A proprietary name for dihydrotachysterol.

hyther [Gk *hy(dōr)* water + *ther(mē)* heat] The combined effect of the atmospheric temperature and humidity on an organism.

Hz Symbol for the unit, hertz.

I

I **1** Symbol for the element, iodine. **2** Symbol for isoleucine. **3** Symbol for inosine.

I Symbol for the quantities (1) electric current, expressed in amperes; (2) moment of inertia, expressed in kilogram meters squared; (3) radiant intensity, expressed in watts per steradian; (4) luminous intensity, expressed in candelas; (5) sound intensity, expressed in watts per square meter.

i Symbol for the quantities (1) frequency interval, expresssed in octaves; (2) specific enthalpy, expressed in joules per kilogram; (3) van't Hoff's factor.

i- iso-.

-ia [L and Gk feminine-noun termination *-ia* denoting state or condition] **1** A suffix meaning state or condition: used especially in the names of diseases or pathologic conditions. **2** A suffix used in taxonomic names.

IAA indole-3-acetic acid.

iamatology [Gk *iama*, gen. *iamatos*, a means of healing + *o* + -LOGY] The science of medical cures and remedies.

IANC International Anatomical Nomenclature Committee. (The Committee which prepares the *Nomina Anatomica*).

ianthinopsia [Gk *ianthin(os)* violet-colored + -OPSIA] A distortion of color vision in which a violet discoloration is falsely perceived.

-iasis [Gk suffix *-sis* denoting state or condition] A suffix meaning (1) diseased or abnormal condition; (2) formation, production, or increase.

iathergy [Gk *iath(ēnai)* (aorist inf. passive of *iasthai* to heal, cure) to have been cured + *erg(on)* work + -Y] An immune state following specific desensitization by a given antigen. An obsolete term.

iatr- IATRO-.

iatraliptic [Gk *iatraleiptik(ē)* (from *iatr(os)* surgeon + *aleiptik(os)* pertaining to an anointer, from *aleiphein* to anoint with oil) the practice of surgery by anointing, friction, or exercise] Relating to the administration of medicinal substances by surface application to the skin.

iatraliptics [*iatralipt(ic)* + -ICS] The methods and practice of surface application of medicinal substances.

iatreusiology [Gk *iatreusi(s)* a means of healing + *o* + -LOGY] The science of therapeutics.

iatreusis [Gk *iatreusis*, also *iatreia* a healing, means of healing] Medical treatment.

iatric Of or pertaining to a physician or to medicine.

-iatrics [Gk *iatr(os)* physician, surgeon, leech + -ICS] A combining form meaning medical care or treatment.

iatro- [Gk *iatros* physician, surgeon, leech] A combining form meaning physician or medicine. Also *iatr-*.

Iatrobdella HIRUDO.

iatrochemistry The study of the relation between chemistry and medicine, especially in connection with the 17th-century doctrine that attributed to chemical substances a key role in physiologic processes and disease. Also called *chemiatry*.

iatrogenesis The production, by medical treatment, of complications, injuries, unfavorable results, or other problems in addition to those already present in a patient. Adjective: iatrogenic.

iatrogenic [IATRO- + -GENIC] **1** Pertaining to or describing a complication, injury, unfavorable result, or other problem which can be directly attributed to medical care. **2** Pertaining to or describing any effect upon a patient resulting from the action of a physician.

iatrology [IATRO- + -LOGY] Medical science.

iatrotechnical Pertaining to the techniques of medical practice.

iatrotechnics IATROTECHNIQUE.

iatrotechnique The technique of medical practice; the practical application of the art of medicine. Also called *iatrotechnics*.

-iatry [Gk *iatreia* the practice of healing] A combining form meaning medical treatment.

IB **1** immune body (antibody). **2** inclusion body.

IBC iron-binding capacity.

-ible -ABLE.

ibogaine $C_{20}H_{26}N_2O$. An alkaloid obtained from the root of the African plant *Tabernanthe iboga* and species of *Peschiera* and *Voacanga*. It is said to prevent fatigue and has been used as a possible antidepressant drug, but it may produce serious psychological disturbances.

ibufenac $C_{12}H_{16}O_2$. 4-(2-Methylpropyl)benzeneacetic acid. An analgesic drug formerly used in the treatment of rheumatoid arthritis. It was found to cause jaundice.

ibuprofen $C_{13}H_{18}O_2$. α-Methyl-4-(2-methylpropyl)benzeneacetic acid. A nonsteroidal anti-inflammatory agent with antipyretic and analgesic properties. It is employed in the treatment of rheumatoid and osteoarthritis by oral administration.

IC **1** internal conversion. **2** intermittent claudication.

-ic [L suffix *-icus* or Gk suffix *-ikos*] **1** A suffix meaning (1) being related to, derived from, or consisting of; (2) causing or being caused by. **2** In chemistry, a suffix applied to names of elements to indicate that they are in their higher oxidation state. It is also used in forming names of acids.

ICC intensive coronary care.

ICD **1** International Classification of Diseases (of the World Health Organization). **2** ischemic coronary disease. **3** intra-uterine contraceptive disease.

ICDA International Classification of Diseases Adapted (for use in the United States).

ice The solid state of water.

dry ice SOLID CARBON DIOXIDE.

ich [*Ich(thyophthirius)*, genus of the causative organism] A disease of the skin of marine and fresh-water fish caused by the protozoan parasite *Ichthyophthirius multifilis*. Also called *white spot disease*.

ichnogram [Gk *ichno(s)* footstep, track + -GRAM] FOOT-PRINT.

ichor [Gk *ichōr* the watery part of blood or of milk, serum, lymph, impure discharge] A thin, serous discharge from a wound or an ulcer. An obsolete term. Adjective: ichorous.

ichoremia SEPTICEMIA.

ichoroid Resembling a serous fluid. An obsolete term.

ichorrhea A copious and persistent discharge of watery serous fluid. A rarely used term.

ichorrhemia SEPTICEMIA.

ichthammol A darkly colored, viscous fluid obtained from the distillation of particular bituminous schists, sulfonation of the distillate, and subsequent neutralization of the product with ammonia. It is used as a topical anti-infective medication for skin diseases. Also called *ammonium ichthyosulfonate*.

ichthyo- [Gk *ichthys* fish] A combining form meaning fish.

ichthyocolla A gelatinous substance obtained from the swim-bladder of the fish, *Acipenser huso*. It is used as an adhesive as well as a clarifying agent. Also called *isinglass*.

ichthyoid Fishlike; fish-shaped.

Ichthyol A proprietary name for ichthammol.

ichthyology [ICHTHYO- + -LOGY] The study of fishes.

ichthyolsulfonate An ichthammol derivative, a salt form of ichthyolsulfonic acid. It was formerly used as a dermatologic medication due to its demulcent and emollient properties.

ichthyophagia [ICHTHYO- + -PHAGIA] The consumption of fish in the diet. Adjective: ichthyophagous.

Ichthyophthirius multifilis A ciliate protozoan fish parasite (subclass Hymenostomatia, suborder Ophryoglenina). It is an ectoparasite that causes lesions in the skin of marine and fresh-water fish, often with fatal consequences. The disease is commonly known as ich or white spot disease.

ichthyosarcotoxin A substance that occurs in the flesh of certain fishes, which causes it to be poisonous upon ingestion.

ichthyosarcotoxism A pathological condition caused by ingestion of the flesh of fishes that contains ichthyosarcotoxin. Clinical signs of poisoning are numbness of the lips, tongue, and throat, followed shortly by nausea, vomiting, abdominal pain, and diarrhea. Later symptoms are nervousness, muscle pain, sore teeth, visual disturbances, and convulsions. Some deaths have been reported due to respiratory paralysis.

ichthyosic ICHTHYOTIC.

ichthyosiform Resembling ichthyosis.

ichthyosis [*ichthy(o)-* + -OSIS] Any of a group of disorders of keratinization that are characterized by dryness and fine scaling. Also called *fish-skin disease*.

  acquired ichthyosis Nonhereditary ichthyosis, often occurring as a manifestation of systemic disease, particularly neoplastic disease.

  autosomal dominant ichthyosis ICHTHYOSIS VULGARIS.

  ichthyosis congenita A rare, severe form of ichthyosis in which grossly hyperkeratotic lesions are present at birth. Also called *ichthyosis congenita neonatorum, diffuse congenital hyperkeratosis, ichthyosis intrauterina, keratosis universalis congenita, generalized ichthyosiform hyperkeratosis.*

  ichthyosis congenitalis palmare et plantare A diffuse keratoderma of the palms and soles, seen in young infants.

  ichthyosis congenita neonatorum ICHTHYOSIS CONGENITA.

  ichthyosis cornea ICHTHYOSIS HYSTRIX.

  ichthyosis fetalis 1 Gross ichthyosis present at birth. **2** Any ichthyosis present in the fetus.

  follicular ichthyosis An obsolete term for KERATOSIS PILARIS.

  ichthyosis hystrix Autosomal dominant dermatoses that share congenital or perinatal onset of hyperkeratotic quill-like projections. In the Lambert type, only rudimentary tonofilaments occur. In the Curth-Macklin type, concentric unbroken shells of abnormal tonofilaments cluster around the nucleus. Also called *sauriosis, nevus keratoticus papillomatosus, ichthyosis cornea, porcupine skin, ichthyosis spinosa.*

  ichthyosis hystrix, Curth-Macklin type See under ICHTHYOSIS HYSTRIX.

  ichthyosis hystrix, Lambert type See under ICHTHYOSIS HYSTRIX.

  ichthyosis intrauterina ICHTHYOSIS CONGENITA.

  lamellar ichthyosis A hereditary disorder of keratinization characterized by diffuse erythema and large lamellar scales.

  lamellar ichthyosis of the newborn The lamellar scaling and erythema seen at birth in a collodion baby. Also called *collodion dermatitis*.

  ichthyosis lethalis The most severe form of ichthyosis vulgaris. It is seen in the harlequin fetus.

  linear ichthyosis A linearly arranged wartlike nevus that involves only the epidermis.

  ichthyosis linearis circumflexa A rare form of hereditary icthyosis, presenting at or soon after birth, and characterized by a generalized erythema and scaling, with some lesions having a thickened horny serpiginous border.

  ichthyosis linguae Leukoplakia of the tongue. A rarely used term.

  nacreous ichthyosis Ichthyosis with pearly scales.

  ichthyosis palmaris PALMAR KERATODERMA.

  ichthyosis palmaris et plantaris PALMOPLANTAR KERATODERMA.

  ichthyosis plantaris PLANTAR KERATODERMA.

  ichthyosis sauroderma Persistent ichthyosis congenita. An obsolete term.

  ichthyosis scutulata Ichthyosis with lozenge-shaped lesions. An obsolete term.

  ichthyosis sebacea cornea Ichthyosis accompanied by abundant vernix caseosa and occurring in the newborn. An obsolete term.

  senile ichthyosis The dryness and scaling of the skin associated with old age.

  sex-linked recessive ichthyosis An inherited ichthyosis determined by a sex-linked recessive gene. Unlike ichthyosis vulgaris, it does not spare the flexures. Also called *X-linked ichthyosis*.

  ichthyosis simplex ICHTHYOSIS VULGARIS.

  ichthyosis spinosa ICHTHYOSIS HYSTRIX.

  ichthyosis vulgaris The common form of ichthyosis. It is of autosomal dominant inheritance. Also called *ichthyosis simplex, autosomal dominant ichthyosis, fish skin.*

  X-linked ichthyosis SEX-LINKED RECESSIVE ICHTHYOSIS.

ichthyotic 1 Pertaining to ichthyosis. **2** Affected by ichthyosis. Also *ichthyosic*.

ichthyotoxicology [ICHTHYO- + TOXICOLOGY] The study of the natural toxins present in fish.

ichthyotoxin [ICHTHYO- + TOXIN] Any natural toxin present in fish.

iconotype [Gk *eikōn*, gen. *eikonos*, image, likeness + TYPE] A representation, drawing, or photograph of a type specimen.

icosa- [Gk *eikos(i)* (*eikosin* before a vowel) twenty + *a-*] A combining form meaning twenty. Also *eicosa-*.

icosahedron [Gk *eikosaedron*, substantive from neut. sing. of *eikosaedros* having twenty sides or surfaces, from *eikos(i)* twenty + *a* + *(h)edra* seat, base] The regular solid figure with 20 faces, which are equilateral triangles. It is the most complex of the five regular solids in that it has the largest number of faces. Many viruses have this form.

icosane $CH_3—[CH_2]_{18}—CH_3$. The parent linear C_{20} saturated hydrocarbon. Also *eicosane (obsolescent spelling).*

icosanoid   Any of a large number of fatty acids that are 20 carbons in length, including arachidonic acid, prostaglandins, thromboxanes, and related compounds.

icosapentaenoic acid   An unsaturated fatty acid, twenty carbons in length, that contains five double bonds. It is a precursor of some prostaglandins, such as PGI_2.

icosatrienoic acid   An unsaturated fatty acid twenty carbons in length that contains three double bonds. It is a precursor of some prostaglandins.

-ics [L suffix *-icus* and Gk suffix *-ikos*] A suffix (forming nouns from words originally adjectives) meaning (1) a study or discipline, as a science or branch of science; (2) practice, method, manner.

ICSH   interstitial cell-stimulating hormone (luteinizing hormone).

ICT   **1** insulin coma therapy.   **2** inflammation of connective tissue.

ictal   Describing or pertaining to an ictus.

icteric   Relating to or characterized by the presence of icterus, or jaundice.

ictero- [Gk *ikteros* jaundice] A combining form denoting jaundice.

icteroanemia   Anemia associated with jaundice.

swine icteroanemia   An acute febrile disease of swine caused by *Eperythrozoon suis,* characterized by icterus, anemia, and emaciation. It occurs mainly in young animals. Morbidity and mortality are usually low. *E. parvum,* which is of much lower virulence than *E. suis,* is rarely, if ever, pathogenic.

icterogenic [ICTERO- + -GENIC] Causing or contributing to the development of jaundice.

icterogenicity [ICTERO- + -GENIC + -ITY] The quality of being icterogenic, or the degree to which something is icterogenic.

icterohematuria   Hematuria associated with jaundice.

icterohematuric   Characterized by jaundice and hematuria; relating to icterohematuria.

icterohemoglobinuria   The combination of jaundice and hemoglobinuria.

icterohepatitis [ICTERO- + HEPATITIS] Inflammation of the liver with associated jaundice.

icteroid [*icter(us)* + -OID] Jaundicelike; characterized by a yellow color.

icterus [New L, from Gk *ikteros* jaundice] JAUNDICE.

benign familial icterus   GILBERT SYNDROME.

icterus castrensis gravis   Icteric leptospirosis occurring among troops in camp.

icterus castrensis levis   Mild jaundice of apparently infectious but not leptospiral origin, occurring among troops in camp. An obsolete term.

icterus catarrhalis   Hepatitis of infectious origin; catarrhal jaundice. An outmoded term.

chronic familial icterus   HEREDITARY SPHEROCYTOSIS.

congenital familial icterus   HEREDITARY SPHEROCYTOSIS.

congenital hemolytic icterus   HEREDITARY SPHEROCYTOSIS.

cythemolytic icterus   Jaundice caused by increased bile formation due to hemolysis.

enzootic icterus   A disease of sheep, that occurs in areas where they graze on plants that contain pyrrolizidine alkaloids. Affected sheep eventually have jaundice and a hemolytic crisis.

epidemic catarrhal icterus   Mild icteric leptospirosis.

familial hemolytic icterus   HEREDITARY SPHEROCYTOSIS.

febrile icterus   Severe jaundice caused by an infectious agent. Also called *icterus febrilis.*

icterus febrilis   FEBRILE ICTERUS.

icterus gravis   An acute destructive disease of the liver; massive liver necrosis.

icterus gravis neonatorum   ERYTHROBLASTOSIS FETALIS.

Gubler's icterus   An obsolete term for HEMOLYTIC JAUNDICE.

icterus infectiosus   ICTERIC LEPTOSPIROSIS.

icterus melas   WINCKEL'S DISEASE.

icterus neonatorum   **1** PHYSIOLOGIC JAUNDICE.   **2** A rare, congenitally induced jaundice due to occlusion of the common bile duct or to congenital malformation of the liver. Also called *jaundice of the newborn.*

nuclear icterus   KERNICTERUS.

physiologic icterus   PHYSIOLOGIC JAUNDICE.

icterus praecox   Mild jaundice that occurs during a newborn's first 24 hours, due to ABO blood group incompatibility of mother and fetus.

icterus simplex   Any jaundice caused by hepatitis of infectious etiology. An outmoded term.

spirochetal icterus   ICTERIC LEPTOSPIROSIS.

icterus typhoides   The jaundice accompanying fulminant hepatitis and acute yellow atrophy.

ictometer [L *ict(us)* a stroke, beat + *o* + -METER] An instrument for measuring the force of the cardiac apex beat.

Ictotest   A tablet containing sulfosalicylic acid and *p*-nitrobenzene diazonium *p*-toluene sulfonate that is used to detect bilirubin in urine. A purple discoloration constitutes a positive result. A proprietary name.

ictus [L (from *ictus,* past part. of *icere* to beat, stab, strike), a stroke, blow, stab, hit] An event of sudden onset, such as a stroke or cerebrovascular accident. Adjective: ictal.

ictus cordis   HEARTBEAT.

epileptic ictus   An epileptic attack of explosive onset. A seldom used term. Also called *epileptic stroke* (obsolete), *epileptic apoplexy* (obsolete), *ictus epilepticus.*

ictus epilepticus   EPILEPTIC ICTUS.

ictus paralyticus   A stroke causing paralysis.

ictus sanguinis   CEREBRAL HEMORRHAGE.

ictus solis   A seldom used term for SUNSTROKE.

ICU   intensive care unit.

ID   **1** infective dose.   **2** intradermal.   **3** infectious disease(s).   **4** inside diameter.

ID$_{50}$ **1** minimal infecting dose.   **2** median infective dose.

id [L (neut. sing. of *is* he), it] That portion of the psychic apparatus which precedes the ego and superego and contains the psychic representatives of the drives and all the phylogenetic acquisitions. The processes of the id are completely unconscious and its operation is governed by the pleasure principle and the primary process.

id.   *idem* (L, the same).

-id[1] [French suffix *-ide* from Gk suffix *-idos* from *eidos* form, shape] A suffix designating a member of a group, as a taxonomic class.

-id[2] [from L *-id-,* stem of *-is,* fem. patronymic suffix; denoting a skin rash] A suffix signifying that a skin eruption is an allergic manifestation of an underlying infection, as *tuberculid.* Also *-ide[2].*

-idae [pl. of L *-ides* denoting son of, from Gk *-idēs* denoting son of] A taxonomic suffix used in forming the names of families.

IDDM   insulin-dependent diabetes mellitus.

-ide[1] [French (ox)ide oxide]   **1** A combining form used in chemistry for a binary compound to signify the more electronegative of the two elements. It replaces the ending of the name of one of them, e.g. sodium and chlorine give sodium chloride. **2** A combining form used in chemistry to signify negative ions formed from an atom by the gain of one or more electrons, e.g. chloride for Cl^-. By extension it signifies other anions formed by loss of hydrogen ions, e.g. amide for NH_2^-, acetylide for $HC{\equiv}C^-$, methanide for CH_3^-. Amines are also considered to become amides when acylated. ● When *-ide* replaces *-e* at the end of the name of a sugar ending in *-ose*, it signifies glycoside formation. Several other words contain the ending, e.g. *nucleoside*, *lactide*, and here the relationship to the original meaning is more distant.

-ide² -ID².

idea [L (from Gk *idea*, from *idein* to see), a form or image present to the mind, idea, form] Any mental image or thought.

autochthonous idea A delusion, characteristic of schizophrenia, that appears without external cause or explanation, within the subject's mind. It has an imperative quality and since it seems so convincing the subject frequently believes that it has been implanted in his mind by a malevolent external agent.

dominant idea Abnormal thought that occupies the forefront of consciousness and to which other thoughts and actions are subordinated. Also called *hyperquantivalent idea* (obsolete).

fixed idea IDÉE FIXE. See under IDÉE.

hyperquantivalent idea An obsolete term for DOMINANT IDEA.

imperative idea OBSESSION.

obtrusive idea An obsessive idea that repeatedly forces itself into the subject's thoughts even though the subject recognizes it as ego-alien and undesirable.

idea of reference A delusion in which the subject believes that anything that happens in the world has a specific meaning for him or has been done only because of him. A clap of thunder or a drop of rain is taken personally, the subject feeling it has special significance. Most commonly, an idea of reference accompanies a delusion of persecution and the subject misinterprets anything that happens in reality as a sign that imagined persecutors are about to succeed in destroying or disgracing him. Also called *delusion of reference, self-referential delusion, referential idea.*

referential idea IDEA OF REFERENCE.

ruminative idea OBSESSION.

ideal [Late L *ideal(is)* (from L *ide(a)* idea + *-alis* -AL) ideal. See IDEA.] An abstraction or standard of perfection that is strongly desired and which serves as a goal for the guidance of behavior.

ego ideal The image of perfection that one constructs for oneself, typically on the basis of identification with the parents. It is a precipitation of the superego but, unlike the latter, it is not confined to the earliest parental images but continues to be added to during life by identification with heroes, mentors, etc.

idealization Overestimation of the attributes of another individual, usually the love object. The subject is not only blind to defects, but also regards the loved one as being perfect.

ideation The process of forming ideas or mental images and examining their relationships. Adjective: ideational.

idée The French word for idea.

idée fixe A delusion that tends to have a dominating impact on behavior. Also called *fixed idea.*

identification [Middle French *identité* (irreg. from L *idem* the same, the same one, from *is* he) identity + French *-fication* -FICATION] **1** The act of identifying or the means by which an identity is established. **2** In psychoanalytic psychology, an unconscious, intrapsychic process in which a part of the self is transformed into a facsimile of one or more external objects, and the subject then begins to think, feel, or act as he imagines

the external object would do. Identification is a primitive method of recognizing reality that provides a means of rendering the frightening unknown into the tolerable familiar. **3** In developmental psychology, the assimilation of parental values in the child, assisting the gradual formation of a sense of self.

anthropometric identification An inaccurate, obsolete system of criminal identification based on the measurement of a subject's height, weight, thoracic diameter, seated height, maximal head length and width, auriculobregmatic distance, bizygomatic width, and other body measurements and physical traits. The system was devised in approximately 1880 but was superseded by the emergence of fingerprinting in the 20th century. Also called *Bertillon system.*

cosmic identification A state in which the various phenomena of the external world, such as sunsets or moonglow, become part of the subject and reflect his thoughts and desires. Thus there is a loss of the boundary between the self and the external world.

firearms identification FORENSIC BALLISTICS.

hostile identification Incorporation or assimilation of the aggressive, negative, intimidating, or otherwise socially undesirable characteristics of another, as is seen in identification with the aggressor.

projective identification A dual process of attributing one's own impulses to another and then fearing that the other will turn that impulse, often aggression, against oneself.

identity [French *identité* (from L *idem* the same one, the same, from *is* he) identity] The image, concept, or inner conviction that one has of oneself, whether as a whole or in relation to particular functions or roles, as in *body indentity, gender identity, mental* or *psychological identity, social identity*, etc.

body identity BODY IMAGE.

core gender identity The inner conviction that one is male, female, ambivalent, or neutral. It is established in accordance with the sex of assignment and of rearing and becomes evident by 18 months of age. By the age of 30 months, it is generally irreversible. Also called *gender identity.*

ego identity Delineation of the physical and mental self as distinct from the external world; the existence of a persistent and coordinate system that distinguishes between the self and the environment and situates the self in relation to the environment.

gender identity CORE GENDER IDENTITY.

sexual identity The biologically determined sex of a person, no matter what form that same person's core gender identity and gender role may take.

ideo- [Gk *idea* idea, form] A combining form meaning idea, mental.

ideodynamism The excitation of a cerebral neuron by a mental act or idea.

ideogenetic Relating to mental processes that involve sense impressions and images rather than formed ideas that are ready for verbal expression.

ideokinetic IDEOMOTOR.

ideology [IDEO- + -LOGY] A sociopolitical belief system concerning the way human interchanges, especially those involving power, should be governed.

ideomotion [IDEO- + MOTION] Muscular activity aroused by an idea or thought; involuntary movement associated with mental activity, as moving the lips while reading. Also called *ideomotor phenomenon.*

ideomotor Initiated directly by an idea: said of a motor response or action, usually those involuntary, tentative, and diminished body movements that are evoked by thought processes rather than by sensory stimulation. Also *ideomuscular, ideokinetic.*

ideomuscular IDEOMOTOR.

ideophobia [IDEO- + -PHOBIA] Pathologic fear of ideas or of letting one's mind wander freely.

ideophrenia [IDEO- + -PHRENIA] An obsolete term for DELIRIUM.

ideosynchysia [IDEO- + SYN- + Gk *chys(is)* a pouring, squandering, a heap + -IA] An obsolete term for DELIRIUM.

ideovascular Vascular changes stemming from mental activity.

idio- [Gk *idios* one's own, personal] A combining form meaning applying to or originating within oneself, personal, individual.

idioblast [IDIO- + -BLAST] BIOPHORE.

idiochromatin An outmoded term for BARR BODY.

idiochromidia The extranuclear chromatin component that plays a role in the reproduction of the cell.

idiochromosome SEX CHROMOSOME.

idiocrasy IDIOSYNCRASY.

idiocratic IDIOSYNCRATIC.

idiocy [See IDIOT.] Profound mental retardation, with an IQ below 25. An outmoded term.

absolute idiocy PROFOUND IDIOCY.

adult amaurotic familial idiocy KUFS DISEASE.

amaurotic familial idiocy Any of various neurodegenerative disorders. An ambiguous, obsolete, and regrettable term. See under TAY-SACHS DISEASE, JANSKY-BIELSCHOWSKY DISEASE, BATTEN DISEASE, KUFS DISEASE.

athetosic idiocy Any degenerative disease of the brain involving both athetosis and mental retardation. An outmoded term.

Bielschowsky's amaurotic idiocy BIELSCHOWSKY-DOLLINGER SYNDROME.

cretinoid idiocy An older term for CRETINISM.

developmental idiocy Mental retardation due to any disorder of brain development. An outmoded term.

eclamptic idiocy Mental retardation in a child born to a mother who suffered from eclampsia during the relevant pregnancy.

epileptic idiocy Severe mental retardation occurring in epileptic patients. • This was once thought to result from repeated attacks, whereas in fact the epilepsy is but one manifestation of the underlying brain disease which also causes the mental retardation. The term should be discarded.

genetous idiocy IDIOPATHIC CONGENITAL IDIOCY.

hydrocephalic idiocy Mental retardation in a child with hydrocephalus. An outmoded term.

idiopathic congenital idiocy Severe or profound mental retardation of developmental but otherwise obscure origin. An outmoded term. Also called *genetous idiocy*.

infantile amaurotic familial idiocy An obsolete term for TAY-SACHS DISEASE.

intrasocial idiocy Profound mental retardation but with the ability to carry out one or more specific, routine tasks.

juvenile amaurotic familial idiocy BATTEN DISEASE.

Kalmuk idiocy An outmoded term for DOWN SYNDROME.

Kufs type amaurotic familial idiocy KUFS DISEASE.

late infantile amaurotic familial idiocy JANSKY-BIELSCHOWSKY DISEASE.

microcephalic idiocy Severe or profound mental retardation associated with an abnormally small cranium and without indication of a focal lesion. An outmoded term.

mongolian idiocy An outmoded term for DOWN SYNDROME.

plagiocephalic idiocy Severe or profound mental retardation associated with marked deformity of the cranium, as in asymmetric craniostenosis. An outmoded term.

porencephalic idiocy Mental retardation associated with congenital cavities in the brain substance.

profound idiocy Mental retardation of a severe degree. An outmoded term. Also called *absolute idiocy*.

scaphocephalic idiocy Severe or profound mental retardation associated with scaphocephaly.

sensorial idiocy Mental retardation of severe degree associated with loss or impairment of any of the special senses. An outmoded term.

spastic amaurotic axonal idiocy An obsolete term for INFANTILE NEUROAXONAL DYSTROPHY.

torpid idiocy Profound mental retardation associated with inactivity and anergy.

traumatic idiocy Severe mental retardation due to injury at birth or in early childhood. An outmoded term.

xerodermic idiocy An outmoded term for DE SANCTIS-CACCHIONE SYNDROME.

idiogamist [IDIO- + GAM- + -IST] A man who can perform sexually only with his wife or a limited number of partners, being impotent with other women.

idiogenesis Origin without apparent or evident cause, as in idiopathic disease. A rarely used term.

idiogenic Pertaining to or characterized by idiogenesis.

idioglossia 1 The speech of a deaf child which may be intelligible to its parents but not to others. 2 A form of developmental dysarthria characterized by frequent consonant substitutions and showing a tendency to spontaneous improvement. Adjective: idioglottic.

idioglottic Of, pertaining to, or suffering from idioglossia.

idiogram A diagram, drawn to scale, that represents a single chromosome or the entire karyotype. Ordinarily, chromosome bands (according to standard conventions and stage of mitosis or meiosis), the centromere, and any secondary constrictions and satellites are included.

idiographic [IDIO- + -GRAPH + -IC] 1 Denoting the search for an understanding of the behavior of one individual through an exhaustive examination of the behavior of that person alone, without specific reference to others as in the in-depth, single-case study. 2 Referring to the value of a variable, such as pulse rate or blood pressure, for an individual at a given time as compared with the personal norm or baseline value of that variable for that individual.

idiohypnotism An obsolete term for AUTOHYPNOSIS.

idiolalia [IDIO- + -LALIA] A condition characterized by the development of one's own private language, sometimes developed by children with Wernicke's aphasia. An obsolete and imprecise term.

idiomere A structural unit of a chromosome. Each idiomere contains one gene. An outmoded term.

idiometritis [IDIO- + METRITIS] MYOMETRITIS.

idiomiasma A self-produced offensive odor.

idiomuscular Pertaining to muscular activity that results from an idea or some other thought process.

idioneurosis [IDIO- + NEUROSIS] Idiopathic or unexplained neurosis. An obsolete term.

idionodal Arising in the atrioventricular node itself; junctional: applied particularly to cardiac rhythms.

idiopathetic IDIOPATHIC.

idiopathic [IDIO- + -PATH + -IC] Having no known cause: said of a disease or other pathologic condition. ⟨"Originally, when it first came into the language of medicine, the term had a different, highly theoretical meaning. It was assumed that most human diseases were intrinsic, due to inbuilt failures of one sort or another, things gone wrong with various internal humors. The word 'idiopathic' was intended to mean, literally, a disease having its own origin, a primary disease without any external cause." —Lewis Thomas, *The Medusa and the Snail*, 1979⟩ Also called *idiopathetic, autopathic* (seldom used).

idiopathy [IDIO- + -PATHY]   A disease of spontaneous origin or without apparent external cause.

idiophase   The phase of metabolism, after growth has ceased, that yields secondary metabolites. Compare TROPHOPHASE.

idioplasm   The total of the hereditary determinants of an organism. An outmoded term.

idioreflex   A self-induced reflex.

idioretinal [IDIO- + RETINAL]   Distinctively characteristic of the retina.

idiosome [IDIO- + Gk *sōma* body]   **1** The centriole with its associated Golgi apparatus and mitochondria in a spermatocyte or an oocyte.   **2** A hypothetical smallest unit of living matter. Also called *idiozome, centrotheca.*

idiospasm   Any localized spasm. An outmoded term.

idiospastic   Describing or pertaining to idiospasm.

idiosthenia [IDIO- + STHEN- + -IA]   Inherent strength.

idiosyncrasy   **1** A property or characteristic peculiar to an individual's physical or mental constitution. Also called *idiocrasy.*   **2** An unusual or exaggerated reaction to a drug or food that is due to some inherent characteristic of the responder's metabolism and not to allergy (or immunologic response to the drug or food). Idiosyncratic reactions occur on first exposure to the drug or food in contrast to the requirement of immunologic reactions for presensitization.

idiosyncratic   Of the nature of an idiosyncrasy; peculiar to an individual's physical or mental constitution. Also *idiocratic.*

idiot [L *idiota* (from Gk *idiōtēs* a private person, individual, layman, unskilled or commonplace person, from *idios* one's own, personal, peculiar) an ignorant, unskilled person]   A person with idiocy. An outmoded term.

idiot savant   A mentally retarded person of any grade who has a special but limited talent of some sort, most often a memory for the details of music or an ability to make rapid arithmetic calculations.

idiotope [IDIO- + Gk *top(os)* a place]   An epitope on the variable region of an antibody molecule that can be recognized by the combining site of other antibodies in the same animal species.

idiotopy   The interrelationships of the positions of parts of an organ.

idiotype   The antigenic determinants, associated with the hypervariable regions in the variable domains of antibody molecules, which characterize individual antibodies; the set of idiotopes of the antibody produced by a given clone of cells. Similar antigenic determinants have been described on T cells and presumably occur in the T cell receptor. It is a central tenet of the network theory of immune regulation that all antibodies are anti-idiotypes in addition to reacting with other antigens.

idiovariation   A mutation or alteration in the hereditary units of an organism.

idioventricular   Arising in the ventricles themselves, or pertaining to or affecting the cardiac ventricles alone. See also IDIOVENTRICULAR RHYTHM.

idiozome   IDIOSOME.

iditol   The alcohol formed by reduction of idose at C-1.

-idium [New L (from Gk *-idion* diminishing suffix), suffix denoting smaller or lesser]   A suffix meaning a smaller or lesser one.

idolomania [*idol(um)* + *o* + -MANIA]   FETISHISM.

idolum [L (from Gk *eidōlon* image, phantasm, idol), image]   An obsolete term for FETISH.

idonic acid   The acid formed by the oxidation of idose at C-1.

idose   The aldohexose with the opposite configuration to glu-

cose at C-2, C-3, and C-4. Thus the inversion of configuration at these three carbon atoms of D-glucose would yield D-idose, whereas inversion at C-5 of D-glucose yields L-idose. Residues of L-iduronic acid are produced in heparin by this latter route from glucuronic residues.

idoxuridine $C_9H_{11}IN_2O_5$. A pyrimidine analogue of the structure 2-deoxy-5-iodo-uridine. It is a white powder used as an antiviral agent in the treatment of herpes simplex keratitis. It inhibits viral DNA synthesis, and is applied topically to the conjunctiva. Also called *5-iododeoxyuridine.* Abbreviation: IDU

idrosis   HYPERHIDROSIS.

IDS   inhibitor of DNA synthesis.

IDU   idoxuridine.

iduronate   The anion, salt, or ester of iduronic acid, formed by the oxidation of C-6 of idose to —COOH.

iduronic acid   The substance produced by oxidation of C-6 of idose to form a carboxyl group. Residues of L-iduronic acid occur in heparin, where they are produced from D-glucuronic residues by inversion at C-5.

IE   immunoelectrophoresis.

IEM   **1** immune electron microscopy.   **2** inborn error of metabolism.

IEP   **1** isoelectric point.   **2** isoelectric precipitation.

IF   **1** intrinsic factor.   **2** interferon.   **3** interstitial fluid.   **4** initiation factor (in protein synthesis).

IFN   interferon.

Ig   immunoglobulin.

IgA   immunoglobulin A.

IgD   immunoglobulin D.

IgE   immunoglobulin E.

IgG   immunoglobulin G.

IgM   immunoglobulin M.

ignatia   The dried and ripened seeds of *Strychnos ignatii*, containing alkaloids such as strychnine and brucine, as well as igasuric acid and loganin. It is used in the preparation of certain bitter tonics.

igniextirpation [L *igni(s)* fire + EXTIRPATION]   A surgical procedure in which one or more organs are removed by use of a cautery.

ignioperation   Any surgical procedure in which a hot cautery is used to perform all or part of the operation.

ignipedites [L *ignipes*, gen. *ignipedis* (from *ignis* five + *pes* foot) + Gk *-ites*, a pl. of -ITIS]   BURNING FEET.

ignis [L, fire]   Fire.

ignis infernalis   ERGOTISM.

ignisation [L *ignis* fire, heat + -ATION]   HEAT EXHAUSTION.

IH   infectious hepatitis.

IK   Immune Körper (German, immune bodies).

IL   interleukin.

Il   Symbol for the element, illinium, now called promethium.

il-   **1** IN-¹.   **2** IN-².

ILA   insulinlike activity.

Ile   Symbol for isoleucine.

-ile [L *-ilis*, suffix denoting relating to, proper to, of]   A suffix meaning of, like, relating to, or capable of.

ileac   **1** Relating to or characterized by ileus.   **2** Relating to the ileum; ileal.

ileadelphus [*ile(o)-* + Gk *adelphos* twin, brother]   DUPLICITAS POSTERIOR.

ileal   Pertaining to the ileum.

ileectomy [*ile(o)-* + -ECTOMY]   A surgical procedure in which all or a part of the distal small bowel is removed.

ileitis [*ile(o)-* + -ITIS]   Inflammation of the ileum.

backwash ileitis Mucosal changes in the ileum consisting of colonic metaplasia and also inflammatory changes typical of ulcerative colitis. This condition is found in patients with ulcerative colitis.

distal ileitis TERMINAL ILEITIS.

regional ileitis Crohn's disease involving the ileum.

terminal ileitis Crohn's disease involving the terminal ileum. Also called *distal ileitis.*

ileo- [New L *ileum* (from L *ile, ileum,* or *ilium,* pl. *ilia,* groin, flank, lower part of body, gut, bowels, abdomen, loins, from Gk *eileos,* verbal of *eilein* to roll or twist tight up; early used interchangeably with *ilium,* but later referred to the entire intestine) last division of the small intestine. Compare ILIO-.] A combining form denoting the ileum.

ileocecal Pertaining to the ileum and the cecum.

ileocecostomy [ILEO- + CECOSTOMY] A surgical procedure creating an opening between the distal small bowel and the cecum. Such an opening may rarely result spontaneously from inflammatory, neoplastic, or traumatic causes.

ileocecum The ileum and the cecum considered as a single entity.

ileocolic Pertaining to the ileum and the colon, usually the ascending colon. Also *ileocolonic, coloileal.*

ileocolitis [ILEO- + COLITIS] **1** Mucous membrane inflammation of the ileum and colon. **2** Crohn's disease involving both the ileum and the colon.

tuberculous ileocolitis Inflammation of the mucous membranes of the colon and small intestine caused by tuberculosis.

ileocolitis ulcerosa chronica A form of ileocolitis characterized by anemia, right ileac pain, tachycardia, fever, and a chronic course.

ileocolonic ILEOCOLIC.

ileocolostomy [ILEO- + COLOSTOMY] A surgical procedure creating an opening between the distal small bowel and the large bowel, following resection or bypass. Such an opening may rarely occur spontaneously following neoplastic, inflammatory, or traumatic disease.

ileocolotomy [ILEO- + COLOTOMY] A surgical procedure in which an incision is made into the distal small bowel and large bowel. A similar result may rarely be produced by trauma.

ileocutaneous Pertaining to or communicating between the ileum and the skin.

ileocystoplasty A surgical procedure in which a defect in the urinary bladder wall is repaired with a small defunctionalized loop of distal small bowel.

ileocystostomy A surgical procedure creating an opening between the distal small bowel and the urinary bladder.

ileoentectropy [ILEO- + ENT- + Gk *ektrop(ē)* a turning off or out + -Y] The turning of a segment of ileum inside out.

ileoileal Pertaining to or connecting different segments of ileum.

ileoileostomy [ILEO- + ILEOSTOMY] A surgical procedure creating an opening between two sections of distal small bowel following resection or bypass. Such an opening may rarely result from neoplastic, inflammatory, or traumatic causes.

ileojejunitis The involvement of the ileum, in part or totally, and the jejunum with a chronic inflammatory condition.

ileoparietal Situated on the wall of the ileum.

ileopathy [ILEO- + -PATHY] Disease of the ileum.

ileopexy [ILEO- + -PEXY] A surgical procedure in which the distal small bowel is suspended and fixed to prevent ptosis or torsion.

ileoproctostomy [ILEO- + PROCTOSTOMY] A surgical procedure creating an opening between the distal small bowel and

the rectum following a colonic resection or bypass. Such an opening may rarely result spontaneously from neoplastic, inflammatory, or traumatic causes. Also called *ileorectostomy.*

ileorectal Pertaining to or communicating between the ileum and the rectum.

ileorectostomy [ILEO- + RECTOSTOMY] ILEOPROCTOSTOMY.

ileorrhaphia ILEORRHAPHY.

ileorrhaphy [ILEO- + -RRHAPHY] A surgical procedure in which sutures are placed into the distal small bowel for purposes of plication or repair. Also called *ileorrhaphia.*

ileosigmoid Concerning both the ileum and the sigmoid colon.

ileosigmoidostomy [ILEO- + SIGMOIDOSTOMY] A surgical procedure creating an opening between the distal small bowel and the sigmoid colon following bypass or resection of the colon. Such an opening may rarely result from neoplastic, traumatic, or inflammatory causes.

ileostomy [ILEO- + -STOMY] A surgical procedure in which a loop or end of the distal small bowel is brought out through an opening in the abdominal wall following colonic bypass or resection. Such a protrusion may rarely result spontaneously from an inflammatory, neoplastic, or traumatic process.

end ileostomy An exteriorization on the abdominal wall of the divided proximal ileum.

ileotomy [ILEO- + -TOMY] A surgical procedure in which an incision is made into the distal small bowel.

ileotransverse Relating to the ileum and the transverse colon.

ileotransversostomy [ILEO- + *transvers(e)* + *o* + -STOMY] ILEOTRANSVERSE COLOSTOMY.

ileotyphlitis [ILEO- + TYPHL-[1] + -ITIS] Inflammation of the ileum and the cecum.

ileovesical Concerning or communicating with both the ileum and the urinary bladder.

Iletin A proprietary name for insulin injection.

ileum [See ILEO-.] [NA] The distal three-fifths of the small intestine, continuous with the jejunum proximally and ending at the junction of the cecum and the ascending colon. It is attached to the posterior abdominal wall by the mesentery and most of it is situated in the hypogastric and pelvic regions. Its wall is thinner than that of the jejunum, and it contains characteristic aggregated lymph follicles. Also called *intestinum ileum* (outmoded).

ileus [L (from Gk *eileos* rolled up tight, from *eilein* to roll or twist tight up), twisted gut, colic, renal colic] **1** Slowing or stoppage of the transit of intestinal contents due to diminished or absent bowel motility. **2** Any intestinal obstruction.

acute duodenal ileus Acute obstruction of the duodenum often as a result of compression by the superior mesenteric artery. See also SUPERIOR MESENTERIC ARTERY SYNDROME.

adynamic ileus Intestinal obstruction due to a lack of intestinal motility.

angiomesenteric ileus SUPERIOR MESENTERIC ARTERY SYNDROME.

chronic duodenal ileus Chronic obstruction of the duodenum in the superior mesenteric artery syndrome.

dynamic ileus Intestinal obstruction due to spasm of some part of the intestinal musculature. Also called *hyperdynamic ileus, spastic ileus.*

foreign-body ileus Intestinal obstruction as the result of the presence of a foreign body in the intestine.

hyperdynamic ileus DYNAMIC ILEUS.

mechanical ileus Intestinal obstruction from a mechanical cause such as a gallstone, hernia, adhesion, volvulus, or foreign body. Also called *occlusive ileus.*

meconium ileus Intestinal obstruction in neonates as the result of a mass of thickened meconium. It is commonly due to cystic fibrosis.

metabolic ileus　Ileus as the result of a systemic metabolic abnormality such as severe acidosis.

occlusive ileus　MECHANICAL ILEUS.

paralytic ileus　Ileus as the result of inhibition of bowel motility. Also called *ileus paralyticus.*

ileus paralyticus　PARALYTIC ILEUS.

parasitic ileus　Intestinal obstruction as the result of masses of parasites in the intestine. Also called *verminous ileus.*

postoperative ileus　Adynamic ileus following surgery.

spastic ileus　DYNAMIC ILEUS.

ileus subparta　Intestinal obstruction due to the pressure of a pregnant uterus on the colon.

terminal ileus　Obstruction of the terminal part of the small intestine.

verminous ileus　PARASITIC ILEUS.

ilia　Plural of ILIUM.

iliac　Pertaining to the ilium.

iliadelphus [*ili(o)-* + Gk *adelphos* twin, brother]　DUPLICITAS POSTERIOR.

ilicin　A bitter principle isolated from the leaves of *Ilex aquifolium,* the European holly.

Ilidar　A preparation of azapetine phosphate. A proprietary name.

ilio- [New L *ilium* (from L *ile, ileum,* or *ilium,* pl. *ilia,* groin, flank, lower part of the body, gut, bowels, abdomen, loins, from Gk *eileos,* verbal of *eilein* to roll or twist tight up; early used interchangeably with *ileum,* but later used with *os* bone *(os ilium)* to denote the bone of the soft parts) hip bone. Compare ILEO-.]　A combining form denoting the ilium.

iliocapsularis　MUSCULUS ILIACUS MINOR.

iliococcygeal　Pertaining to the ilium and the coccyx.

iliococcygeus　MUSCULUS ILIOCOCCYGEUS.

iliocolotomy [ILIO- + COLOTOMY]　An incision into the colon in the iliac region.

iliocostal　Pertaining to the ilium and the ribs, specifically the muscles between them.

iliocostocervicalis　Denoting the iliocostalis cervicis and iliocostalis thoracis muscles. An outmoded term.

iliodorsal　Of or pertaining to the posterior, or gluteal, surface of the ilium.

iliofemoral　Pertaining to the ilium and the femur, or to the iliac region and the thigh.

iliofemoroplasty　A surgical procedure in which a reconstruction of the iliac and femoral arteries is performed.

iliohypogastric　Pertaining to the iliac and hypogastric regions.

ilioinguinal　Pertaining to the iliac and inguinal regions.

iliolumbar　**1** Pertaining to the iliac and the lumbar regions. **2** Pertaining to the flank and the loin.

iliolumbocostoabdominal　Pertaining to the iliac, lumbar, costal, and abdominal regions.

iliometer [ILIO- + -METER]　An instrument that is used to measure the relative positions of the iliac spines and the center of the vertebral column.

iliopagus [ILIO- + -PAGUS]　Equal conjoined twins with union restricted to the iliac region.

iliopagus parasiticus　ILIOPARASITUS.

ilioparasitus [ILIO- + L *parasitus* a guest, parasite]　Unequal conjoined twins with the parasitic member attached at the iliac region of the host. Also called *iliopagus parasiticus.*

iliopectineal　Pertaining to the ilium and the pecten of the pubic bone.

iliopelvic　Pertaining to the iliac region and the pelvis, or to the iliacus muscle and the pelvic cavity.

ilioperoneal　Pertaining to the ilium and the fibula, or to the inguinal region and the lateral compartment of the leg.

iliopsoas　MUSCULUS ILIOPSOAS.

iliopubic　Pertaining to the ilium and the pubis or pubes; iliopectineal.

iliosacral　Pertaining to the ilium and the sacrum.

iliosacralis　An occasional separate muscle bundle of the coccygeus muscle that runs anterior to it from the iliopectineal line to the anterolateral border of the sacrum.

iliosciatic　Pertaining to the ilium and the ischium.

ilioscrotal　Of or pertaining to the ilium and the scrotum.

iliospinal　Pertaining to the ilium and the vertebral column.

iliospinale [IDIO- + Late L *spinale,* neut. sing. of *spinalis* (from L *spin(a)* spine + *-alis* -AL) pertaining to the spinal column]　An anthropometric point situated at the apex of the anterior superior iliac spine.

iliothoracopagus [ILIO- + THORACO- + -PAGUS]　Equal conjoined twins with union extending from the thoracic to the iliac regions.

iliotibial　Pertaining to or connecting the ilium and the tibia.

iliotrochanteric　Pertaining to the ilium and a trochanter, usually the greater trochanter of femur.

ilioxiphopagus [ILIO- + *xipho(id)* + -PAGUS]　Equal conjoined twins with union extending from the xiphoid to the iliac regions.

-ility [L *-ilitas* a noun-forming suffix denoting quality or condition]　A suffix denoting a quality or condition.

ilium [See ILIO-.]　[NA] OS ILII.

ill [Middle English, from Old Norse *illr* ill]　**1** Not well; sick. **2** A disorder or disease: used especially in veterinary medicine.

colt ill　STRANGLES.

joint ill　A common disease of young animals, in which infectious bacteria gain systemic circulation and localize in one or more joints. Also *joint-ill.*

louping ill　OVINE ENCEPHALOMYELITIS.

navel ill　Any of various disorders of young animals (lambs, calves, and foals) involving a serious systemic infection that is acquired through the umbilical vessels. The specific disease that results depends on the infecting organism. Streptococci and staphylococci usually cause a local umbilical abscess and often abscesses in the lungs, heart, liver, and kidney. Other organisms, such as those of *Pasteurella,* may cause an acute febrile septicemia leading to death in a few days. Limb joints and joints of the vertebral column often become involved by the suppurative infections with resultant lameness and swelling of the affected joints (joint-ill).

quarter ill　A popular term for EMPHYSEMATOUS ANTHRAX.

thorter ill　A popular term for STAGGERS.

trembling ill　OVINE ENCEPHALOMYELITIS.

illaqueate [L *illaqueat(us),* past part. of *illaqueare* to ensnare + e]　To correct the position of an inwardly misdirected eyelash; correct trichiasis. A rarely used term.

illaqueation [*illaqueat(e)* + -ION]　The correction of an inwardly misdirected eyelash position. A rarely used term.

illinition [L *illinitus,* past part. of *illinere* to smear, daub, lay on]　Friction of the skin to facilitate absorption of a medicinal substance; inunction.

illness [ILL + -NESS]　**1** The state of being ill. **2** A disorder producing such a state; a disease.

catastrophic illness　An unusually severe illness that is expensive to treat.

emotional illness　An imprecise term for MENTAL DISORDER.

functional illness Disturbance or variation in the way in which an organ or body system functions, with no evidence of alteration of that organ's structure. Psychogenic illnesses are functional, but not all functional illnesses are psychogenic.

mental illness An imprecise term for MENTAL DISORDER.

psychosomatic illness PSYCHOSOMATIC DISORDER.

radiation illness RADIATION SICKNESS.

terminal illness An illness from which the patient is not expected to recover and which is expected to be the proximate cause of death.

illumination [Late L *illuminatio* (from L *illuminatus*, past part. of *illuminare* to make light or bright, from *lumen*, gen. *luminis*, light, akin to Gk *lampros* radiant) light, illumination] The act or process of casting light on an object, as that seen under a microscope, or in an enclosed space, as within a body cavity, to render it visible for examination.

axial illumination The transmission or reflection of light along the optical axis of the objective and eyepiece of a microscope. Also called *central illumination.*

central illumination AXIAL ILLUMINATION.

contact illumination A method of inspecting the interior of the eye by means of light transmitted from a source touching the eye. This is most useful as a method of producing retroillumination, or backlighting, of the area under observation.

critical illumination In microscopy, the focusing of light from the source precisely upon the object to be observed. The image of the light source falls at the plane and location of the object observed.

dark-field illumination The illumination of an object by light rays striking it only from the periphery. The central or vertically oriented light is obstructed, causing the field to appear dark and the object to appear bright as it scatters or reflects the peripherally incident light. Also called *dark-ground illumination.*

dark-ground illumination DARK-FIELD ILLUMINATION.

direct illumination In microscopy, illumination by a light source situated above the object being observed, with the light reflected upward through the optical system. Also called *surface illumination.*

focal illumination The concentration of light upon an object by focusing from a lens or mirror.

Köhler illumination A means to obtain optimum microscopic illumination by focusing light from the source first upon the lower focal plane of the condensing lens and then focusing the image from the condensing lens upon the object.

lateral illumination Illumination by light from a source whose axis is diagonal to the optical axis of the microscope. Also called *oblique illumination.*

oblique illumination LATERAL ILLUMINATION.

orthogonal illumination Illumination for microscopic examination using light rays that are perpendicular to the axis of observation.

stroboscopic illumination Illumination by means of a rapidly and regularly intermittent light source. When the rate of light flashing is the same as the rotation of a wheel or the rate of presentation of similar features, the illusion of stopping the movement occurs. This phenomenon may be used to calibrate a desired rate of movement or to measure an unknown rate.

surface illumination DIRECT ILLUMINATION.

through illumination TRANSILLUMINATION.

illuminator A light source for observing an object.

Abbé's illuminator ABBÉ'S CONDENSER.

illusion [L *illusio* (from *illusus*, past part. of *illudere* to divert oneself with, jest with, pollute) a bantering, jeering, sneering] **1** A false perception of the actual appearance or character of an object. **2** Any perception based on erroneous interpretation of sensory stimuli.

autokinetic illusion The apparent movement of a pinpoint of light when regarded continuously in a darkened room.

illusions of doubles CAPGRAS SYNDROME.

epileptic illusion A perceptual disorder which is the basis, often the initial, and sometimes the only, symptom of an attack of focal epilepsy, and which is caused by epileptic discharge arising in part of the temporal cortex. According to the exact area involved, one can distinguish between perceptual illusions, in which the object in question is perceived in a distorted manner, and agnosic illusions, in which the object in question is perceived correctly but not recognized, thus giving rise either to déjà vu or jamais vu. Perceptual illusions can be classified, according to the sense involved, into somatosensory, visual, auditory, vertiginous, olfactory, and gustatory epileptic illusions. The dreamlike epileptic state is a prolonged epileptic illusional condition. Also called *illusional aura.*

epileptic dreamlike illusion See under EPILEPTIC ILLUSION.

Fregoli's illusion The belief that a persecutor has assumed the guise of various people whom the subject encounters routinely. Also called *Fregoli's phenomenon, illusion of negative double.*

illusion of negative double FREGOLI'S ILLUSION.

optical illusion A false visual interpretation. The cerebral perception of patterns and designs is subject to variable interpretations, depending upon associated forms and perspectives. Thus, a given line may seem spontaneously to change from the background to the foreground of a drawing, causing the shape to turn inside out. In other examples, perceptions of distance and shape may be changed. Alternatively, optical devices may be used to produce distortions of space, as with anisokonic lenses.

illutation [IL- + L *lut(um)* (substantive from neut. sing. of *lutus*, past part. of *luere* to wash) mud + -ATION] Therapeutic application of moist earth, usually heated, as in mud baths at thermal spas.

Ilosone A preparation of erythromycin estolate. A proprietary name.

Ilotycin A preparation of erythromycin. A proprietary name.

IM 1 intramuscularly (injection site). **2** internal medicine. **3** infectious mononucleosis.

im intramuscularly (injection site).

im- **1** IN-[1]. **2** IN-[2].

image [L *imago* (pl. *imagines*; akin to *imitari* to copy, and to *similis* like, similar) an image, likeness, conception] The physical reproduction or mental picture of an object.

accidental image AFTERIMAGE.

acoustic image AUDITORY IMAGE.

aerial image An image formed in air rather than upon a surface. It may be seen if positioned conjugate with the retina of the observing eye. For example, in the process of indirect ophthalmoscopy, the hand-held 20 diopter lens produces a real aerial image between the observer and the patient. The observer sees the aerial image of the object (the patient's fundus).

auditory image A conception of something previously heard. Also called *acoustic image.*

body image The image or concept that one holds of one's self and one's body as an object in space. Also called *body identity.*

direct image VIRTUAL IMAGE.

double image DIPLOPIA.

eidetic image See under EIDETIC.

erect image VIRTUAL IMAGE.

false image The incorrectly localized double image originating from the nonfixing eye in strabismus. There is no real object in space corresponding to the apparent location of the false image.

flood field image The image produced when a gamma camera is exposed to a uniform field of gamma radiation.

gamma image   SCINTISCAN.

heteronymous image   A false image projected to the opposite side from the corresponding eye, as occurs in physiologic diplopia when the fixation point is more distant than the object of diplopia, thereby causing stimulation of the temporal side of both retinas.

homonymous image   A false image projected to the same side as the corresponding eye, as occurs in physiologic diplopia when the fixation point is closer than the object of diplopia, thereby causing stimulation of the nasal side of both retinas.

hypnagogic image   The especially vivid imagery sometimes experienced during the drowsy state just before sleep. It may occur in any sense mode but is most often visual and of near hallucinatory quality. Also called *hypnagogic phenomenon.*

hypnopompic image   The imagery that occurs in the state following termination of sleep and before complete wakefulness.

idealized image   A false picture of one's self and worth developed as a characterological defense.

incidental image   AFTERIMAGE.

inverted image   REAL IMAGE.

memory image   A mental reconstruction of an event or object experienced in the past, often only partial in its detail and including an active effort to revive, by association, other missing elements from the memory store.

mental image   The ideational representation in consciousness of an experience originally sensory or perceptual in nature but not at the moment present to the senses.

mirror image   The reflection of an object in a mirror, with particular reference to its side to side reversal from the original object. Also called *lateral inversion.*

motor image   Self-awareness of the entire body with regard to motor function.

negative image   See under NEGATIVE AFTERIMAGE.

optical image   An image formed by the projection of light rays through a lens system which reassembles them at a point of focus where they may be perceived as a visual replica of an object.

primordial image   An imprint or engram that develops from a condensation of innumerable similar processes and is a basic form of some frequently recurring psychic experience. Also called *archetype.*

pulse echo image   A two-dimensional image achieved by sending pulses of ultrasound into the body and processing and displaying reflected echoes from tissue interfaces and parenchyma as an anatomic image.

Purkinje images   The four images resulting from reflection of light by the front and back surfaces of the cornea and the lens of the eye. Also called *Purkinje-Sanson mirror images, Sanson's images.*

Purkinje-Sanson mirror images   PURKINJE IMAGES.

real image   An image formed at the intersection of convergent light rays and which may be visibly displayed on a surface. Also called *inverted image.*

retinal image   The real image projected upon the retina. The quality of this image is dependent upon such components of the object-image relationship as the refractive status of the eye, accommodation, corrective lenses, and clarity of the ocular media.

Sanson's images   PURKINJE IMAGES.

specular image   1 An image caused by a reflecting surface. 2 The fine detail of a surface that may be perceived by observation of light reflected from the surface. The endothelial cells of the living cornea, for example, may be studied in microscopic detail by the technique of specular reflection.

tactile image   The three dimensional concept elicited by palpation of an object.

true image   The correctly localized image of the double images in strabismus. It originates from the fixing eye. The real object in space corresponds to the apparent location of the true image.

virtual image   An image situated at the theoretical point of intersection of light rays but which cannot be displayed on a surface, as that seen in a plane mirror. Also called *direct image, erect image.*

imagery   An inner evocation of some prior perceptual experience that retains many of the sensory qualities of the external stimuli giving rise to the original experience.

imaging   The process of obtaining or producing an image.

dynamic imaging   Imaging in which a rapid sequence of static images is used for real-time display of moving structures.

magnetic resonance imaging   NUCLEAR MAGNETIC RESONANCE. Abbreviation: MRI

pulse echo imaging   Imaging of normally nonvisible tissues and tissue interfaces by ultrasonic pulse echo technique. See also PULSE ECHO IMAGE.

static imaging   Imaging in which a single still image is produced.

stop-action imaging   Imaging of cyclical motion in such a way as to produce a stationary representation. This is accomplished by repetitively imaging at the same point in time of the repetitive cycle, for example with a stroboscope.

through-transmission imaging   Imaging by transmission of an interrogating beam through the specimen and receiving on a far surface.

imago [L, an image, likeness, conception]   1 The adult, sexually mature stage in the life cycle of an insect.   2 In psychoanalysis, the likeness of another that is stored in the unconscious, such as the image or internal representation of a parent.

imagocide   A chemical agent that destroys the adult stage of the insect, most often adult malarial parasites.

imbalance [IM- + BALANCE]   Lack of balance, whether in motor activities or in the activities of various organs, glands, viscera, or systems.

autonomic imbalance   Any disorder of the autonomic nervous system in which there is unequal activity of the sympathetic and parasympathetic systems. Also called *vasomotor imbalance.*

gene imbalance   Any situation in which the number of alleles being expressed at one or more loci has deleterious consequences on phenotype, and in aneuploidy. It is a potential complication of abnormal gene dosage.

sex chromosome imbalance   Any karyotype in which an abnormal number of entire or partial sex chromosomes is present. The most common examples in humans are 47,XXX; 47,XXY; and 47,XYY.

vasomotor imbalance   AUTONOMIC IMBALANCE.

imbecile [French *imbécile* (from L *imbecillis* or *imbecillus* weak, weak-headed, from *im-* not + *bacillum* a little stick) stupid, deprived of intellect]   A person with severe to moderate mental retardation with an IQ between 25 and 54. An outmoded term.

imbecility [IMBECILE + -ITY]   The state of being an imbecile.

imbed   EMBED.

imbibition [L *imbibitus,* past part. of *imbibere* (from *im-* -IN + *bibere* to drink) to drink in]   The absorption of a liquid by a gel, solid, or organized body.

imbricate [Late L *imbricat(us),* past part. of *imbricare* (from L *imbrex,* gen. *imbricis* a gutter tile) to furnish with gutter tiles]   1 To cause to overlap, as tissue: used in surgery to denote the intentional overlapping of adjacent tissues in order to improve contour or tensile strength.   2 IMBRICATED.

imbricated   Overlapped or layered, as tissue in a surgical procedure, in the manner of roof shingles or the elements of a pine cone. Also *imbricate.*

imbrication **1** A surgical technique in which tissues are imbricated. **2** The overcrowding of incisor teeth in the same arch.

ImD$_{50}$ The dose of an antigen sufficient to immunize 50 percent of a test group of animals.

Imerslund [Olga *Imerslund*, Scandinavian physician, flourished 20th century] Imerslund-Najman-Gräsbeck syndrome. See under IMERSLUND SYNDROME.

Imhoff [Karl *Imhoff*, German engineer, 1876–1965] Imhoff tank. See under EMSHER TANK.

imidamine ANTAZOLINE.

imidazole $C_3H_4N_2$. The heterocyclic aromatic base whose molecules contain a five-membered ring consisting of two nitrogen atoms at positions 1 and 3, one of them carrying a hydrogen atom, and three CH groups. It is a weak base (pK 7.2) and a very weak acid (pK 14.2). It is used as a buffer and as a basic catalyst, and it is the functional component of histidine residues in proteins. Also called *glyoxalin* (outmoded), *iminazole* (outmoded).

imidazoline Any of the isomeric dihydroimidazoles.

imidazolylethylamine The systematic name for histamine.

imide A compound containing the NH group joined to two CO groups. Such a compound is stable only if the grouping is part of a ring.

imido- [variant of *amido-*] A combining form denoting imide. ● Since an imide is ammonia doubly acylated by a bivalent acyl group, words in *imido-* will normally take also a suffix indicating the compound substituted, e.g., *succinimidoacetic acid*. It is also used in the word *imidoester* to indicate a compound of the type R—C(=NH)—O—R'.

imidocarb hydrochloride $C_{19}H_{20}N_6O \cdot 2HCl$. 3,3'-Di(2-imidazolin-2-yl)carbanilide dihydrochloride. An antiprotozoal agent specifically effective as a babesicide in veterinary medicine.

iminazole An outmoded term for IMIDAZOLE.

imine Any compound formed by condensation of a primary amine (or ammonia), R—NH$_2$, with a carbonyl compound, R'—CO—R", to give the structure R—N=CR'R". Several enzymes, such as aldolase, combine with their substrates by reversible imine formation. Also called *Schiff base, azomethine.*

imino- [variant of AMINO-] A prefix indicating the bivalent = NH group, as in iminodiacetic acid, HN(—CH$_2$—COOH)$_2$.

imino acids Organic acids containing the =NH group. Proline and hydroxyproline are examples of imino acids. Also called *secondary amino acids.*

iminodipeptidase An outmoded term for PROLYLDIPEPTIDASE. ● The name was given because proline contains an imino group.

iminoglycinuria The urinary excretion of the imino acids, proline and hydroxyproline, and the amino acid glycine. It occurs normally in newborns until renal transport mechanisms mature, and abnormally in the Fanconi syndrome, in hyperprolinemia, in hyperhydroxyprolinemia, and in benign familial iminoglycinuria. Also called *proline-hydroxyproline-glycinuria.*

familial iminoglycinuria A benign, autosomal, recessive phenotype characterized by iminoglycinuria.

familial renal iminoglycinuria A familial defect in renal tubular transport that leads to increased excretion of L-proline, glycine, and the imino acids. Transmitted as an autosomal recessive trait, the condition usually is benign, but may be associated with decreased intestinal absorption of the same imino acids, seizures, and mental retardation.

iminoquinone A derivative of a quinone in which one or both =O groups are replaced by =NH. They are more stable than the imines of simple ketones.

imipramine hydrochloride $C_{19}H_{24}N_2 \cdot HCl$. 10,11-Dihydro-$N,N$-dimethyl-5$H$ dibenz[b,f]azepine-5-propanamine monohydrochloride. A member of the class of tricyclic antidepressant drugs. It is used in the treatment of depression and in enuresis, and is given orally.

imitation An action initiated or guided by the actions of another person; copying behavior.

hysterical imitation A mimicry of symptoms that are observed in others, based on identification with those persons.

Imlach [Francis *Imlach*, Scottish anatomist and surgeon, 1819–1891] Imlach's fat plug. See under PLUG.

immature Not mature; not fully developed.

immaturity The state of being immature.

immedicable Not subject to being cured by medical practice.

immersion [L *immersio* (from *immersus*, past part. of *immergere* to plunge into, immerse, sink, from *im-* in, into + *mergere* to put under water, dip) a plunging into] **1** The placing of a body or part entirely in water or another liquid. **2** In microscopy, the interposition of a liquid between the objective lens and the object under examination so that the liquid bathes both surfaces.

Abbé homogeneous immersion The use of cedarwood oil as the immersion fluid for microscopic examination.

cold immersion A syndrome consisting of hypothermia and sometimes frostbite resulting from prolonged contact of a part or the whole of the body with a cold liquid.

homogeneous immersion In microscopy, the use of an immersion liquid with virtually the same refractive index as that of glass.

oil immersion The use of oil as the immersion fluid in microscopy between the objective lens and the object examined.

water immersion The use of water as the immersion fluid in microscopy between the objective lens and the object examined.

immigration In population genetics, the introduction of genes through reproduction by individuals foreign to a breeding population.

immiscible Possessing qualities that prevent mixing; unmixable.

immobilization The act of making immovable, as a fractured part with a splint.

immobilize To make immovable, as a fractured limb with a splint; fix in place.

immune [L *immun(is)* (from *im-* IM-² + *mun(us)* a person's work or function) exempt from public duty or taxes, free from] **1** Characterized by a high degree of resistance to a specific foreign substance, either antibody-mediated resistance or resistance manifested as delayed hypersensitivity (T cell-mediated). **2** Incapable of being affected by a pathogen or other foreign substance.

immunifacient Causing immunity: said of an infection that subsequently produces immunity against infections with the same infective agent.

immunifaction IMMUNIZATION.

immunisin A rarely used term for ANTIBODY.

immunity [L *immunitas* (from *immunis* exempt from a public duty, from *im-* not + *munus* one's work, function, akin to *manus* hand, labor) exemption from a public duty, immunity] A state of increased resistance against the harmful effects of a noxious agent, as an infectious agent or toxin. Immunity can be innate or acquired. Acquired immunity may be humoral or cellular in origin and may be achieved as a result of a host's response to a prior disease or infection, or it may be produced in a host by means of immunization.

acquired immunity Immunity to infectious disease gained during one's lifetime, not inherited. It may be active or passive, with active immunity the result when antibody (or specifically reactive lymphocytes) is produced by the individual's immune system in response to a naturally acquired infection or to vaccination, and passive immunity the result when antibody is transferred to the individuals from another, immune human or animal host. Passive immunity can also be transferred with lymphocytes from an immune syngeneic animal.

active immunity Acquired immunity in which specific antibody (or specifically reactive lymphocytes) is produced by the individual's own immune system in response to a naturally acquired infection or to vaccination.

adoptive immunity Passive immunity of the cell-mediated type following the administration of sensitized lymphocytes from an immune donor.

artificial immunity Active or passive immunity, produced artificially, as distinguished from naturally acquired immunity. The administration of an antitoxin is an example of artificial immunity.

cell-mediated immunity Those manifestations of the immune response that are brought about by cells, in particular by T lymphocytes and macrophages. Also called *cellular immunity*. Abbreviation: CMI

cellular immunity CELL-MEDIATED IMMUNITY.

charitable immunity The doctrine in medical malpractice that nonprofit or charitable hospitals and other health care facilities are not subject to litigation for malpractice.

community immunity HERD IMMUNITY.

congenital immunity The immunity an individual has at birth.

cross immunity Immunity to a disease occurring subsequent to either natural infection or immunization with a different, but usually closely related, organism or toxin.

familial immunity NATURAL IMMUNITY.

functional immunity PROTECTIVE IMMUNITY.

genetic immunity NATURAL IMMUNITY.

governmental immunity The doctrine in medical malpractice that a government cannot be sued for the negligent acts of its employees unless it consents to such a suit.

herd immunity The epidemiologic concept that a population can be more resistant to the spread of a disease than would be suggested by the immunities of its members. Also called *community immunity*.

heterologous immunity Passive immunity conferred by the administration of serum from a different species.

homologous immunity A state of immunity conferred as a result of administration of antibodies from members of the same species. A seldom used term.

humoral immunity Those manifestations of the immune response that are brought about by components of plasma, in particular antibodies and complement, and do not require the presence of cells. Humoral immunity does, however, recruit cells secondarily in a number of situations.

induced immunity Immunity acquired as a result of either active or passive immunization.

inherent immunity NATURAL IMMUNITY.

inherited immunity NATURAL IMMUNITY.

innate immunity NATURAL IMMUNITY.

intrauterine immunity Fetal immunity acquired by the passage of maternal immunoglobulins across the placenta and into the fetal circulation. Also called *placental immunity*.

local immunity Immunity confined chiefly to a particular organ, part, or kind of tissue.

maternal immunity Passive immunity transferred humorally from mother to offspring before or after birth. In man and other primates, maternal immunoglobulins pass into the fetal circulation by crossing the placenta. In cows, colostrum is the vehicle of transport of immunity to the young. In birds, antibodies in the egg yolk provide immunity. Also called *natural immunity*.

native immunity NATURAL IMMUNITY.

natural immunity 1 Immunity to a microorganism that does not require prior experience of the organism and does not depend on the generation of specific lymphocytes or the formation of specific antibody. Also called *innate immunity, native immunity, inherited immunity, inherent immunity, natural resistance, genetic immunity, familial immunity, autarcesis, occult immunization* (rarely used). 2 MATERNAL IMMUNITY.

naturally acquired immunity Immunity acquired by fortuitous exposure to an antigen and not by deliberate immunization.

nonspecific immunity Resistance to infection resulting from any mechanism other than the formation of antibodies and the generation of antigen-reactive lymphocytes.

passive immunity Acquired immunity in which specific antibody is transferred to the individual from another, already immune human or animal host (as from mother to fetus) or by injection with serum. In inbred strains of animals or in identical twins, passive immunity can also be conferred by transfer of lymphocytes from an immune donor. Also called *passive protection*.

phagocytic immunity An inherent defense system that is based on the ability of macrophages and neutrophil polymorphs to ingest and destroy infective agents.

placental immunity INTRAUTERINE IMMUNITY.

postoncolytic immunity Immunity that follows destruction of tumor cells.

preemptive immunity Immunity conferred by the interference phenomenon: cells infected with one virus may be insusceptible to superinfection with another.

Profeta's immunity Supposed immunity to syphilis in offspring of syphilitic parents.

protective immunity Immunity following administration of an antigen which stimulates antibodies or cellular immunity protective against a disease or an allergic state. Also called *functional immunity*.

racial immunity Immunity or resistance manifested particularly by members of one human race rather than another towards a particular infection or antigenic stimulus.

residual immunity Immunity of indeterminate duration following the disappearance of an infection.

species immunity Immunity or resistance to a given antigen shown by members of a particular species.

specific immunity Immunity resulting from the formation of antibodies or the generation of specifically reactive lymphocytes against a particular antigen. It may occur following natural infection or as a result of immunization.

superinfection immunity In bacteriophage-infected cells, an alteration in the cell surface that prevents superinfection with another bacteriophage strain.

toxin-antitoxin immunity Acquired immunity brought about by subcutaneous inoculation with a toxin combined with its specific antitoxin. This method was developed as a form of diphtheria prophylaxis in the late nineteenth century.

transplantation immunity The development of an immune response on the part of the host to transplanted allogenic tissue.

immunization [*immun(o)-* + *-iz(e)* + *-ATION*] The act or process of making a subject immune, as to decrease susceptibility to infection. Also called *immunifaction*.

active immunization The induction of active immunity by the administration of antigen. Also called *active sensitization, isopathic immunization*.

collateral immunization Immunization with an organism different from the one that is the cause of the existing infection.

isopathic immunization ACTIVE IMMUNIZATION.

occult immunization A rarely used term for NATURAL IMMUNITY.

passive immunization The conferring of passive immunity by the administration of antibody or, less frequently, of syngeneic, specifically reactive lymphocytes. Also called *passive sensitization*.

prophylactic immunization   Immunization that prevents disease.

immunizator   Any agent producing immunity.

immunize [*immun(e)* + -IZE]   To make immune.

immuno- [L *immunis* (from *in-* not + *munus* one's work, function) exempt from a public duty]   A combining form meaning immune, immunity.

immunoadsorbent   IMMUNOSORBENT.

immunoadsorption   A technique for the separation or quantification of an antibody from a serum or mixture, or of an antigen from a solution. The material sought is brought into contact with a solid phase that has the specific antigen or antibody on its surface. The specific antigen-antibody reaction attaches the material to the solid phase, resulting in physical separation from the original fluid medium. The adsorbed material can then be measured, eluted, purified, or otherwise manipulated in relatively pure form.

immunoagglutination   Clumping of blood cells or other antigen-bearing particulate matter induced by their reactivity with a corresponding antibody.

immunoassay [IMMUNO- + ASSAY]   The measurement of a material by means of an antigen-antibody reaction that can be precisely quantified. Radioimmunoassay, enzyme-multiplied procedures, and rocket immunoelectrophoresis are frequently used techniques. Also called *immune assay*.

enzyme-multiplied immunoassay   A competitive binding technique employing an antibody specific for the substance being measured and a readily detectible enzyme that is coupled to a known quantity of the analyte in reagent form. The reaction of the antibody with the analyte inactivates the attached enzyme. The quantity of analyte in the unknown is calculated from the proportion of inactivated enzyme in the aliquot of indicator material.

immunobiology   The study of the immunologic factors that affect the growth, development, and health of biological organisms.

immunoblast   A transformed B lymphocyte or T lymphocyte with pyroninophilic cytoplasm and a centrally placed nucleolus. Such cells are capable of differentiating further to form either plasma cells or committed T lymphocytes. Also called *pyroninophilic blast cell*.

immunochemical [IMMUNO- + CHEMICAL]   Of or relating to immunochemistry; involving the chemical aspects of immunologic phenomena.

immunochemistry   The study of the chemical basis of the antigen-antibody reaction and other immunologic responses. Also called *chemoimmunology*.

immunocompetence   The property of being immunocompetent; the capacity to respond immunologically to an antigen. Also called *immunologic competence*.

immunocompetent   Capable of responding immunologically to an antigen, as by producing antibodies or by developing cell-mediated immunity.

immunocompromised   In a state of diminished or impaired immunity, such as may be brought on by cytotoxic chemotherapy or irradiation or by certain disease processes.

immunoconglutinin   An anticomplement antibody produced in the body which binds the individual's own complement components, usually when bound at a complement fixation site. These antibodies react with bound C3 and bound C4. Also called *autoanticomplement*.

immunocyte   A lymphoid cell capable of reacting with antigen

to induce antibody synthesis or cell-mediated immunity. Also called *immunologically competent cell, immunocompetent cell, I cell*.

immunocytoadherence   A means of determining cell surface properties, in which receptors or immunoglobulins on the surface of one cell population cause cells with corresponding molecular configurations on their surface to adhere in rosettes around the indicator cells.

immunocytochemistry   A histologic and cytologic process in which antigens can be identified using specific antibodies labeled with fluorescein or enzymes that can give a colored reaction product. Also called *immunohistochemistry*.

immunocytology   The branch of histology that employs immunologic probes in studying cells and their origins, structure, function, and pathology.

immunodeficiency [IMMUNO- + DEFICIENCY]   Any deficiency in the capacity to respond immunologically, as by defective production of humoral or cell-mediated immunity. Also called *immunologic deficiency*.

acquired primary immunodeficiency   Abnormal lack of resistance to infection due to disorder of the immunological apparatus and first appearing after early childhood.

combined immunodeficiency   Immunodeficiency involving both humoral and cell-mediated immunity. See also SEVERE COMBINED IMMUNODEFICIENCY.

common variable immunodeficiency   The most frequent form of primary immunodeficiency which includes sporadic cases of congenital immunodeficiency not falling into a recognized category and most cases of acquired primary immunodeficiency. Antibody deficiency disease is the most common manifestation, but abnormalities of T cells as well as of B cells can be found. It is likely to represent a mixture of different diseases which have not so far been clearly delineated.

severe combined immunodeficiency   A group of disorders in which both antibody formation and cellular immunity are highly deficient, usually occurring in infants. The disease is associated with a propensity to overwhelming infections in early life, often due to *Pneumocystis carinii* or other organisms of low pathogenicity, and unless corrected by bone marrow grafting is fatal. The primary defect in most cases is unknown, but a proportion is due to homozygous deficiency of adenine deaminase. Also called *severe combined immunodeficiency disease, combined immunodeficiency disease, combined immunodeficiency syndrome, Swiss type agammaglobulinemia, Swiss type hypogammaglobulinemia, Swiss type immunodeficiency, lymphopenic agammaglobulinemia, lymphopenic hypogammaglobulinemia*. Abbreviation: SCID

Swiss type immunodeficiency   SEVERE COMBINED IMMUNODEFICIENCY.

immunodeficiency with thymoma   A primary immunodeficiency which develops in older adults in association with benign tumors of the thymus and is characterized by agammaglobulinemia and defective antibody formation. Persons with this disorder have little or no resistance to bacterial, viral, and fungal infections and are subject to frequent, recurrent infections. Also called *Good syndrome* (outmoded).

thymus-dependent immunodeficiency   Those immunity deficiency states that arise from a failure of thymus function. Congenital absence of the thymus, as occurs in nude mice or in DiGeorge syndrome in man, is associated with absence or serious deficiency of peripheral T cells and a consequent failure of cell-mediated immunity. Homozygous deficiency of purine nucleotide phosphorylase also produces selective T cell defects in man. Clinically, thymus-dependent immunodeficiency is associated particularly with unusually severe or persistent viral exanthematous disease and infection with *Candida*. Removal or destruction of the thymus after infancy produces no obvious immunodeficiency. Also called *thymus-dependent deficiency*.

X-linked immunodeficiency with undue susceptibility to Epstein-Barr virus A rare disease of apparently immunologically normal males who, upon first infection with the Epstein-Barr virus, develop fulminating infectious mononucleosis, agammaglobulinemia, or B-cell lymphoma, or bone-marrow aplasia. It shows the inheritance characteristic of X chromosome genetic defects. Also called *X-linked lymphoproliferative syndrome, X-linked progressive combined variable immunodeficiency*.

X-linked progressive combined variable immunodeficiency X-LINKED IMMUNODEFICIENCY WITH UNDUE SUSCEPTIBILITY TO EPSTEIN-BARR VIRUS.

immunodeficient Deficient in the capacity to respond immunologically; characterized by an immunodeficiency.

immunodepressant IMMUNOSUPPRESSANT.

immunodepression IMMUNOSUPPRESSION.

immunodepressive IMMUNOSUPPRESSIVE.

immunodepressor IMMUNOSUPPRESSANT.

immunodiagnosis The diagnosis, usually of infectious conditions but increasingly of other altered tissue conditions, by detecting and quantifying antibodies or antigenic material in serum or other body materials.

immunodiffusion [IMMUNO- + DIFFUSION] A precipitin technique in which an antigen and an antibody diffuse through a gel medium, producing precipitin lines at those sites where the antigen and antibody concentrations are optimal for precipitation of insoluble complexes. This basic principle is used, either alone or in combination with electrophoretic principles, in a variety of qualitative, semiquantitative, and quantitative techniques such as radial diffusion and immunoelectrophoresis. Also called *diffusion test, immunodiffusion test*.

double immunodiffusion A qualitative technique to demonstrate the presence of an antigen and an antibody by allowing both reactants to diffuse toward one another from wells in immunologically inert agar. A precipitin line forms where the antigen and antibody concentrations are optimal for immune complex deposition. The location, shape, and intensity of the line depend on the relative concentrations of the reactants and the geometrical relationship of the wells.

radial immunodiffusion A technique for quantifying antigen in a solution. A measured quantity of the antigen is placed in a well in an agar plate containing a uniformly distributed antibody. As the antigen diffuses outward, a precipitin ring forms where antigen and antibody concentrations are optimal. The radius of the ring is proportional to the antigen concentration. Absolute figures can be derived by comparison with ring sizes observed when using standards of known concentration. Abbreviation: RID

reverse radial immunodiffusion A procedure for quantifying antibodies in which an antigen is uniformly distributed in a gel and the antibody-containing material is placed in a well from which it diffuses into the antigen-containing medium. The radius of the precipitin ring formed is proportional to the amount of antibody in the original material.

single immunodiffusion A precipitin technique in which one reactant, either an antigen or antibody, diffuses through the inert supporting medium while the other is fixed in location and concentration.

immunodominance The property of being immunodominant.

immunodominant 1 Describing those antigenic determinants in a molecule, or those components in an antigenic mixture, to which an immune response is produced preferentially. 2 Contributing a disproportionately large amount of binding energy in an antigen-antibody reaction. For example, the monosaccharide unit determining the antigenic specificity of a polysac-

charide is immunodominant, as is the action of haptens.

immunoelectroadsorption Immunoadsorption in which the reaction of the antibody with the adsorbing antigen is enhanced by passage of electric current. To quantify the antibody, a layer of antigen is applied to an inert surface, and the thickness of the antibody layer adsorbed after application of the current is measured.

immunoelectrophoresis [IMMUNO- + ELECTROPHORESIS] A semiquantitative analytic technique in which electrically charged molecules, usually proteins, are separated by electrophoresis in an agar gel and then further characterized by the precipitin lines developing after suitable antibodies are introduced into the gel. Also called *immunophoresis*. Abbreviation: IE

counter immunoelectrophoresis See under COUNTERIMMUNOELECTROPHORESIS.

crossed immunoelectrophoresis TWO-DIMENSIONAL IMMUNOELECTROPHORESIS.

Laurell crossed immunoelectrophoresis ROCKET IMMUNOELECTROPHORESIS.

reverse immunoelectrophoresis Counterimmunoelectrophoresis in which the starting positions for the antigen and antibody are reversed.

rocket immunoelectrophoresis A technique for quantifying proteins that employs both the immunodiffusion of an antigen into an antibody-containing gel and the electrophoretic stimulation of protein migration. Test samples and standards of known concentration are placed in wells and then current is applied to speed and direct the migration into agarose that contains a uniformly distributed antibody to the protein being measured. Convex precipitin arcs, which resemble the shape of a rocket, form at a distance from the origin that is determined by the concentration of protein present. Also called *Laurell rocket test, Laurell crossed immunoelectrophoresis*.

two-dimensional immunoelectrophoresis Crossed electrophoresis in which the antiserum to the migrating proteins is introduced with the second application of current, producing precipitin arcs that move perpendicularly to the initial direction of protein migration. Also called *crossed immunoelectrophoresis*.

immunoenhancement Any means by which the strength of an immune response is augmented.

immunoferritin Any antibody to which ferritin has been conjugated. The use of a ferritin-labeled antibody allows electron microscopic visualization of the antigen-antibody combining site.

immunofiltration [IMMUNO- + FILTRATION] Immunoadsorption in which the fluid material is filtered through a column containing the immunosorbent. Also called *electrosyneresis*.

analytical immunofiltration ANTIBODY AFFINITY CHROMATOGRAPHY.

immunofluorescence [IMMUNO- + FLUORESCENCE] A technique in which antigen or antibody is coupled with a fluorochrome dye (i.e., fluorescein isothiocyanate or rhodamine) and used to localize the site of an immune reaction. It is used in tissue sections, cell or bacterial smears, and flow cytometry.

direct immunofluorescence Immunofluorescence in which antigens in tissue sections or cell surfaces are localized with a fluorochrome-conjugated antibody specific for that tissue constituent. Also called *single-layer immunofluorescence technique*.

indirect immunofluorescence A two-step technique for detecting antibodies reactive against cellular antigens. The unmodified serum is incubated with fixed cells containing the antigen. The specific antibody, if present, attaches to antigen sites. The presence of attached antibody is detected by adding fluorochrome-labeled antiglobulin serum, which attaches to the previously fixed antibody and produces a marker visible by fluorescent microscopic examination. Also called *double layer fluorescent antibody technique*.

membrane immunofluorescence The use of a fluorochrome-labeled antibody to the antigens on the outer membrane surface of living cells. The viable membrane prevents the antibody from entering the cell and staining intracellular constituents. It is useful in studying cell surface topography, especially those configurations that change when antigen-antibody reactions occur.

immunogen [IMMUNO- + -GEN] ANTIGEN.

immunogenetic Pertaining to or characterized by the interplay between immunology and genetics.

immunogenetics **1** The study of genetic mechanisms of immunologic control, expression, and disease. **2** The application of immunologic methods, such as monoclonal antibodies, to genetic investigations.

immunogenic [IMMUNO- + -GENIC] Capable of inducing an immune response: often said of antigens.

immunogenicity The capacity of an antigen to induce an immune response. Also called *antigenicity*.

immunoglobulin A family of proteins having antibody activity. Immunoglobulins are composed of a basic structural unit comprising two identical heavy and two identical light chains linked together by disulfide bonds. There are five distinct kinds of heavy chains which form the basis for the five classes of immunoglobulins (IgA, IgD, IgE, IgG, IgM). Subclasses of IgG, IgA, and IgM with related but different heavy chains also occur. In addition, there are two different light chains designated κ and λ which are found in all classes. Also called *immune globulin, immunoprotein, gamma globulin*.

immunoglobulin A The class of immunoglobulin which is secreted in saliva, mucus, and other external secretions and reacts with viruses, bacteria, and other antigens to protect epithelial cells. IgA monomer has a molecular weight of 170 000. Molecules of IgA are commonly linked by an additional J chain to form IgA dimers. Prior to secretion, a secretory piece, formed in epithelial cells, is attached to each IgA monomer, and the secretory immunoglobulin so formed then has a molecular weight of about 400 000. In serum, IgA is a monomer with a normal concentration of 150–400 mg/dl. IgA does not pass the placenta into the fetal circulation. It usually does not fix complement. In humans there are at least two subclasses of IgA. Also called *gamma-A globulin* (obsolete), *secretory immunoglobulin, exocrine immunoglobulin, beta-2a globulin* (obsolete). Abbreviation: IgA

Bence-Jones monoclonal immunoglobulin BENCE JONES PROTEIN.

immunoglobulin D The class of immunoglobulin which is found on the surface of B lymphocytes. It occurs in human plasma at low concentrations (0.3–40 mg/100 ml), primarily in the intravascular space. It has a molecular weight of 150 000. Also called *gamma-D globulin* (obsolete). Abbreviation: IgD

immunoglobulin E The class of immunoglobulin which has reaginic or homocytotropic antibody activity. It occurs in normal human plasma at very low concentrations (300 ng/ml). The concentration is greater in the presence of atopic allergy. It has a molecular weight of 196 000 and a high carbohydrate content. Also called *gamma-E globulin* (obsolete). Abbreviation: IgE

exocrine immunoglobulin IMMUNOGLOBULIN A.

immunoglobulin G The class of immunoglobulin present in largest amount in plasma and which fixes complement and crosses the placenta. It occurs in normal human plasma at concentrations of 800–1600 mg/100 ml. It has a molecular weight of 150 000. Four subclasses, called IgG1, IgG2, IgG3, and IgG4, have been identified. Also called *gamma-G globulin* (obsolete), *human gamma globulin*. Abbreviation: IgG

immunoglobulin M The class of immunoglobulin which is active against bacteria or erythrocytes and in certain pathologic states may be active against autologous antibody. It occurs in normal human plasma at concentrations of 50–200 mg/ml. It is composed of a cyclic pentamer of five basic units of heavy and light chains linked by disulfide bonds. Its heavy chain is larger than that of other immunoglobulins. Because of its size, it does not cross the placental barrier in man. It has a molecular weight of 900 000 daltons. Also called *gamma-M globulin* (obsolete), *beta-2M globulin* (obsolete), *γ macroglobulin* (obsolete). Abbreviation: IgM

monoclonal immunoglobulin Immunoglobulin derived from a single cell or clone. It may be present in the serum of patients with multiple myeloma, in which case antibody specificity is rarely identifiable, or it may be an antibody deliberately produced and harvested by hybridoma techniques.

secretory immunoglobulin IMMUNOGLOBULIN A.

surface immunoglobulin Immunoglobulin present on the cell membrane, an important characteristic of a β-lymphocyte.

immunoglobulinopathy GAMMOPATHY.

immunohematology The study of the humoral and cellular immune mechanisms as these relate to the pathogenesis, diagnosis, or treatment of diseases of blood and hematopoietic tissues. Blood banking is part of the field of immunohematology.

immunohistochemistry IMMUNOCYTOCHEMISTRY.

immunologic Of or relating to immunology. Also *immunological*.

immunological IMMUNOLOGIC.

immunologist [IMMUNO- + -LOGIST] A specialist in immunology.

immunology [IMMUNO- + -LOGY] The science concerned with the phenomena that allow an animal to respond to a subsequent exposure to a foreign substance in a way that is distinct from the way it responds to the initial exposure to that same substance. The modified response is specific for the particular foreign substance and can be elicited after long intervals (months or years) from the initial exposure. Immunology may be considered the study of the phenomena that enable organisms to distinguish self from nonself macromolecules and to respond specifically to foreign macromolecules. The formation of antibodies and the generation of antigen-reactive lymphocytes are the two principal phenomena studied. All aspects of these two phenomena and the effector mechanisms that they can recruit are included in the science of immunology.

immuno-osmophoresis COUNTERIMMUNOELECTROPHORESIS.

immunopathologic Of or relating to immunopathology.

immunopathology That part of the science of immunology that is concerned with the role of immune reactions in the pathogenesis, diagnosis, and treatment of disease.

immunophoresis IMMUNOELECTROPHORESIS.

immunoprecipitation Precipitation produced by the introduction of a specific antibody to a soluble antigen. Also called *precipitation*.

immunoprecipitin An older term for PRECIPITIN.

immunoproliferative Marked by an increase in the number of cells that play a role in antibody formation, i.e. lymphocytes and plasma cells. Immunoproliferative disorders include malignant lymphomas, lymphocytic leukemias, and multiple myeloma.

immunoprophylaxis Disease prevention by immunologic means. Active immunoprophylaxis involves the administration of antigens to stimulate the host's own immune system. Passive immunoprophylaxis involves the administration of antibody (or, in inbred species or identical twins, of lymphocytes) from an immune donor.

immunoprotein IMMUNOGLOBULIN.

immunoreaction IMMUNE RESPONSE.

immunoreactive Having the capacity to participate in an antigen-antibody reaction: often applied to hormones where assays of the immunoreactive material may not always parallel assay of the functional hormone.

immunoreactivity The capability for or degree of interaction between antigen and antibody or antigen and lymphocyte or plasma cell.

gastrointestinal glucagonlike immunoreactivity Extrapancreatic material detected by immunoassays for glucagon. It is of incompletely known structure and function, produced by mucosal cells of the postduodenal bowel, as in the dog. It is distinct from gastric glucagon. Abbreviation: GLI

immunoselection The survival of certain cell lines based on their ability to escape the cytotoxic actions of antibody or immune lymphoid cells.

immunosenescence The decline in immune function that occurs with advancing age. This decline has been held as the cause of many manifestations of aging, but on the basis of little substantive evidence.

immunosmoelectrophoresis COUNTERIMMUNOELECTROPHORESIS.

immunosorbent The insoluble or solid form of an antigen or antibody that is used in immunoadsorption. Also called *immunoadsorbent*.

immunosuppressant Any substance capable of inhibiting or depressing the immune response to an antigen, an immunosuppressive substance. Also called *immunodepressant, immunodepressor*.

immunosuppression The inhibition or suppression of the immune response, as by antimetabolites or irradiation, or by the administration of antilymphocytic sera or cyclosporin A to prevent the rejection of grafts or organ transplants; or by infection, as in acquired immune deficiency syndrome (AIDS). Also called *immunodepression*.

immunosuppressive Causing or contributing to immunosuppression. Also *immunodepressive*.

immunosurveillance IMMUNOLOGIC SURVEILLANCE.

immunosympathectomy An experimental procedure performed on embryonal or newborn laboratory animals in which certain sympathetic ganglia are destroyed by the injection of an extract containing antibodies that prevent production of a protein necessary for the development of the sympathetic nervous system.

immunotherapy [IMMUNO- + THERAPY] **1** The treatment of disease by the administration to the patient of antibody raised in another individual or another species (passive immunotherapy) or by immunizing the patient with antigens appropriate to the disease (active immunotherapy). **2** Therapy, used especially in the treatment of cancer, intended to stimulate the effector mechanisms of the immune response nonspecifically.

immunotolerance IMMUNOLOGIC TOLERANCE.

immunotolerant [IMMUNO- + TOLERANT] Characterized by immunologic tolerance.

immunotransfusion The use of blood or blood components from a donor who has developed an appropriate immune response to a particular pathogen. This is a form of adoptive immunotherapy. Also called *phylactotransfusion*.

IMP inosine monophosphate (inosinic acid).

IMPA incisal mandibular plane angle.

impact [L *impact(us)*, past part. of *impingere* to hit, throw against, fasten] **1** To press firmly into a space, as food between the teeth. **2** To jam forcibly together as a result of trauma, as

the ends of bones. **3** The force that a moving body imparts to another upon colliding with it.

impacted [L *impact(us)*, past part. of *impingere* to thrust, drive against + English *-ed*, suffix denoting past participle] **1** Pressed firmly into a space, as food between two teeth. **2** Prevented from erupting by some obstacle: said of a tooth. **3** Forcibly jammed together as a result of trauma, as the fractured ends of bones: said of a fracture.

impaction [L *impactio*, from *impactus*, past part. of *impingere* to thrust, drive against] The condition of being impacted.

cecal impaction A concretion in the cecum causing obstruction.

ceruminal impaction IMPACTED CERUMEN.

dental impaction A condition in which a tooth is prevented from erupting by an obstacle such as another tooth.

fecal impaction A mass of compressed, often inspissated and hard feces found in the sigmoid colon or rectum.

food impaction A condition in which food is firmly fixed in some location as between teeth or between an appliance and teeth.

mucoid impaction Obstruction of a bronchus by mucuslike material.

impactor [L *impact(us)*, past part. of *impingere* to thrust, drive against + -OR] A device for removing suspended material from a gas. A stream of the gas, emitted under pressure through a nozzle, is directed against a solid surface on which the suspended material is deposited. It is commonly used for measuring the concentrations of suspended particulate matter. Also called *impinger*.

cascade impactor A device for determining particle size distribution in an aerosol by passage of the aerosol through a series of nozzles of different apertures to produce a fractional deposition of the particles according to size.

impaired Acting under a handicap, as that arising from drug or alcohol abuse, that is likely to diminish significantly the effectiveness or competence of performance with respect to the medical service rendered, as *impaired physician*. • The term is used in this sense in India and New Zealand as well as the United States. In the United Kingdom, *sick*, as in *sick doctor*, is sometimes used with this sense, but *impaired* is not used.

impairment [Old French *empeirier* (from Vulgar L *impejorare*, from L *im-* intensive + *pejorare* to make worse, from *pejor* worse) to diminish, lessen + -MENT] **1** A partial disability or loss of function; a functional deficit. **2** Diminution or reduction below normal, as applied, for example, to resonance on percussion or to loudness of breath or voice sounds on auscultation of the chest.

conductive hearing impairment CONDUCTIVE HEARING LOSS.

hearing impairment HEARING LOSS.

impalpable Impossible to perceive by touch.

impaludation [IM- + L *palus*, gen. *paludis*, swamp, marsh + -ATION] The use of malarial therapy.

impaludism [IM- + L *palus*, gen. *paludis*, a marsh, swamp + -ISM] CHRONIC MALARIA.

impar [L (from *im-* IM-² + *par* equal, a pair), unequal] Unpaired; azygous.

imparidigitate [L *impar* unequal, uneven + *i* + DIGIT + -ATE] PERISSODACTYLOUS.

impatency The state of being closed or blocked.

impatent Closed or blocked; not patent.

impedance [L *imped(ire)* (from *im-* in, into + *pes*, gen. *pedis*, foot) to entangle, hinder, impede + -ANCE] **1** The opposition to flow from an alternating source at a given frequency. **2** In electricity, the sum, in quadrature, of the resistance and the reactance, which is composed of capacitance and inductance. **3** In fluid flow, the sum, in quadrature, of the viscous resistance and the reactance, which is composed of compliance and inertance. **4** In acoustics, the product of the velocity of sound and the density.

acoustic impedance　The opposition to the flow of sound energy in a mechanical system such as the tympanic membrane and ossicular chain, its measurement being related to the wavelength of the sound and the inertia, stiffness, and mass of the system. Also called *ear impedance.*

characteristic acoustic impedance　Density multiplied by the sound speed of a medium.

ear impedance　ACOUSTIC IMPEDANCE.

specific acoustic impedance　The ratio of sound pressure to particle velocity.

imperative [L *imperat(us)* (past part. of *imperare* to order, command) ordered + -IVE]　Something obligatory or compelling.

authoritative imperative　A directive, parental or social, emanating unconsciously through the superego.

categorical imperative　In psychiatry, a blanket demand for total obedience, with anything less being unacceptable.

ethical imperative　The guidance of behavior by the moral principles that are part of the superego.

immoral imperative　A compulsion to act against the rules of society.

imperception [IM-(IN-²) + PERCEPTION]　Impaired perception in any sensory modality.

auditory imperception　ANACHROASIA.

imperforate [IM-² + L *perforat(us)*, past part. of *perforare* to pierce, form by boring]　Lacking a normal orifice.

imperforation [IM- + PERFORATION]　A failure of a normal opening to occur in an organ during embryonic development.

otic imperforation　ATRESIA OF THE EXTERNAL AUDITORY CANAL.

impermeable　Not permeable; incapable of being penetrated by a fluid, as a gas.

impersistence / motor impersistence　Inability to sustain any motor act or movement.

impervious　Not permitting passage, as of fluids or light; blocking penetration.

impetiginization　The secondary development of impetigo as a complication of another skin disorder.

impetiginoid　Resembling impetigo.

impetiginous　Of or relating to impetigo.

impetigo [L (from *impetere* to attack, assault), a skin infection]　A contagious bullous, crusted, or pustular eruption of the skin that is caused by streptococci and/or staphylococci. Also called *impetigo vulgaris, impetigo contagiosa, pyoderma superficialis, crusted tetter* (obsolete).

Bockhart's impetigo　A staphylococcal infection of the skin characterized by superficial follicular pustules. Also called *superficial pustular perifolliculitis.*

impetigo bullosa　BULLOUS IMPETIGO.

bullous impetigo　Impetigo of the newborn characterized by predominantly bullous lesions. Also called *pemphigus neonatorum* (older term), *pyosis of Corlett, impetigo contagiosa bullosa, impetigo bullosa, impetigo neonatorum, epidemic pemphigus of the newborn.*

chronic symmetric impetigo　Extensive impetigo that affects the trunk. Also called *impetigo pityroides.*

impetigo circinata　CIRCINATE IMPETIGO.

circinate impetigo　Impetigo in which the lesions are grouped in a coiled configuration. Also called *impetigo circinata.*

impetigo contagiosa　IMPETIGO.

impetigo contagiosa bullosa　BULLOUS IMPETIGO.

impetigo contagiosa gyrata　Impetigo in which the lesions are in a convoluted configuration.

impetigo follicularis　Impetigo that involves the pilosebaceous follicles.

impetigo herpetiformis　An outmoded term for PUSTULAR PSORIASIS.

miliary impetigo　PUSTULAR MILIARIA.

impetigo neonatorum　BULLOUS IMPETIGO.

impetigo parasitica　Impetigo complicating a parasitic infection, particularly pediculosis capitis.

impetigo pityroides　**1** PITYRIASIS ALBA. **2** CHRONIC SYMMETRIC IMPETIGO.

impetigo sicca　An incorrect term for PITYRIASIS ALBA.

impetigo simplex　STAPHYLOCOCCAL IMPETIGO.

staphylococcal impetigo　Impetigo caused by staphylococci, which are common secondary invaders of streptococcal impetigo. Also called *impetigo simplex, staphylococcic impetigo.*

staphylococcic impetigo　STAPHYLOCOCCAL IMPETIGO.

impetigo streptogenes　Impetigo of streptococcal origin.

impetigo of Tilbury Fox　Impetigo characterized by thin-walled bullae that soon rupture to form yellow-brown crusts.

impetigo varicellosa　Varicella with bullae or pustular lesions.

impetigo vulgaris　IMPETIGO.

impetus [L, an attack, onset, impulse]　The thrust or force of a drive.

impf-malaria　A German term for MALARIOTHERAPY.

impilation　The formation of rouleaux.

impinger　IMPACTOR.

implant [L *im-* in + PLANT]　**1** ORAL IMPLANT. **2** To insert into the body, usually at operation, as to preserve or restore function or to maintain configuration or for other therapeutic purposes. **3** An object so inserted.

anchor endosteal implant　An endosteal implant with wedges shaped, when viewed from the side, like nautical anchors.

basket implant　A fenestrated globe that is buried in the muscle cone following enucleation of an eye in order to enhance shape and motility of the socket.

blade endosteal implant　An endosteal implant of which the wedges are perforated to allow the tissues to grow through.

bone implant　BONE GRAFT.

carcinomatous implants　The growth of carcinoma from cells transferred from another site, as on peritoneal surfaces from an ovarian primary tumor.

cartilaginous implant　Cartilage, usually autogenous tragal cartilage, implanted into the middle ear for a variety of tympanoplastic and other therapeutic procedures.

ceramic endosteal implant　An endosteal implant the infrastructure of which is made of porcelainlike material.

cochlear implant　An electrode, usually a multichannel electrode, implanted into the inner ear, less often into the middle ear, in an attempt to restore a modicum of hearing to someone deafened as the result of the total loss of cochlear function.

complete-arch blade endosteal implant　A blade endosteal implant inserted in an edentulous jaw and carrying multiple abutments.

complete subperiosteal implant　A subperiosteal implant inserted in an edentulous jaw and carrying multiple abutments.

dental implant　ORAL IMPLANT.

deoxycortone acetate implant　A formulation as a cylinder or tablet of deoxycortone acetate suitable for subcutaneous administration to provide slow, sustained release of the drug.

diodontic implant　ENDODONTIC IMPLANT.

dynamic implant　A significant idea that is introduced into the subject's consciousness with the expectation that he will assimilate the idea and reorganize his thinking and behavior accordingly.

endodontic implant　An endosteal implant inserted through the root canal of a tooth for the purpose of splinting the tooth. Also called *diodontic implant*.

endometrial implants ENDOMETRIOSIS.

endosseous implant ENDOSTEAL IMPLANT.

endosteal implant An oral implant entering, and surrounded by, bone. The infrastructure may consist of wedge-shaped blades which fit into longitudinal grooves cut into the bone. In the case of single tooth implants, it may be a simple spiral or perforated structure which fits into a tooth socket or prepared substitute. Also called *endosseous implant*.

fabricated implant An implant made individually to fit a particular site.

frame type of ramus endosteal implant A complete arch endosteal implant consisting of two ramus endosteal implants connected to an anterior endosteal implant by a connector bar.

helicoid endosteal implant An oral implant, commonly to support a single artificial tooth, having a spiral of wire which is placed in a tooth socket. Also called *spiral endosteal implant*.

hormone implant A fused or compressed hormone formulation in the shape of a cylinder or tablet suitable for subcutaneous or intramuscular placement. Slow release of the hormone is provided by this route of administration.

intraosseous implant A metal implant for intraosseous fixation of fractures.

intraperiosteal implant An oral implant inserted beneath the fibrous outer layer of the periosteum.

magnetic implant An oral implant completely buried in the bone. Its function is to improve the retention of a denture by the mutual attraction between it and another magnet attached to the denture.

mesostructure implant An oral implant supporting an intermediate structure which itself supports the denture.

needle endosteal implant PIN ENDOSTEAL IMPLANT.

oral implant An insert of biologic or alloplastic material in the hard or soft oral tissues for cosmetic purposes or to support or retain a denture, bridge, or crown. Also called *dental implant*, *ventplant*.

orbital implant A form buried in the orbital tissues after enucleation of the eye. Its purpose is to restore partially the volume of the orbit so as to permit a better fit and movement of the artificial eye.

pin implant PIN ENDOSTEAL IMPLANT.

pin endosteal implant An oral implant of which the infrastructure is a number of pins driven into the bone at various angles. Also called *needle endosteal implant, pin implant*.

ramus endosteal implant A blade endosteal implant placed in the anterior part of the ramus, with an abutment at its lower end, in the retromolar area.

self-tapping implant A helicoid endosteal implant which is screwed into place.

spiral endosteal implant HELICOID ENDOSTEAL IMPLANT.

stock implant A manufactured implant made in various shapes and sizes.

subperiosteal implant An oral implant made to fit the surface of the bone and covered, apart from the necks of the abutments, with mucoperiosteum.

transosteal implant An anterior mandibular implant of which the infrastructure passes through the whole of the body of the mandible. It is usually inserted through an extraoral opening.

two-piece implant An implant made in two parts so that the infrastructure may be inserted first and the abutments or mesostructure attached by screws after initial healing has taken place.

universal subperiosteal implant An implant for a partially edentulous jaw, which enters the edentulous spaces but does not touch the natural teeth.

implantation [IMPLANT + -ATION] **1** The attachment of the fertilized ovum to, or penetration into, an organ where it develops during gestation. Implantation almost always takes place in the uterus on the receptive mucous lining or endometrium. Penetration is accompanied by destruction of endometrial tissue. Exceptionally (about 0.1%), it occurs outside the uterus (ectopic pregnancy) in the lining of the uterine tube or even in some other intra-abdominal organ, such as the ovary. Implantation generally occurs when the fertilized ovum has reached the blastocyst stage, or at the start of gastrulation after the appearance of secondary mesoderm. Also called *nidation*. **2** The surgical fixation or insertion of a tissue such as muscle, tendon, nerve, or bone to establish a new union. **3** The act or process of placing a surgical implant. **4** In radiotherapy, the insertion of needles or other emitters of ionizing radiation such as radium.

implantation of the bile ducts A surgical procedure in which some part of the intrahepatic or extrahepatic biliary tree is connected to the intestinal tract to bypass an absolute or relative distal obstruction of the biliary tree.

central implantation SUPERFICIAL IMPLANTATION.

circumferential implantation SUPERFICIAL IMPLANTATION.

delayed implantation A pause in development of the blastocyst, which in many mammalian species remains unimplanted inside the uterine horn for varying periods. One type of delayed implantation is short and related to lactation, as in rodents. Another type is continued long after lactation has ceased, as in some of the Carnivora, and can last for several months or even longer in the European badger, with the result that parturition occurs at the same time of each year.

eccentric implantation Implantation of the ovum in which the chorionic sac lies for a time in a fold or pocket of the uterine mucosa where it eventually implants by destruction of some tissue and becomes closed off from the main uterine cavity, as in the mouse and rat.

endometrial implantation The process whereby the blastocyst penetrates and becomes fixed in the endometrium.

filigree implantation A surgical procedure in which a mesh of fine steel wire or other material is used to close a large defect where primary closure is not suitable. Also called *filigree repair*.

hypodermic implantation The insertion of a medication into the tissue under the skin.

interstitial implantation Implantation of the ovum in which the ovum penetrates into the substance of the uterine mucosa, as in the hedgehog, guinea pig, and some primates, including man.

intrafollicular implantation Ectopic implantation of an embryo within an ovarian (graafian) follicle which occurs following spontaneous (parthenogenetic) activation and intrafollicular development of an ovarian oocyte. This phenomenon has been reported in various mammalian species, but most commonly in the LT/SV strain of mice, and is the likely origin of most ovarian teratocarcinomas where development becomes disorganized shortly after the blastocyst stage.

juxtafollicular implantation The ectopic embedding of the blastocyst near to or adjoining an ovarian (graafian) follicle.

nerve implantation Grafting by insertion of a nerve into muscle.

periosteal implantation A surgical procedure in which the tendon from one or more functional muscles is inserted into the periosteum to take the place of a nonfunctional muscle.

silk implantation A surgical procedure in which silk sutures are placed along the course of a nonfunctional tendon for the purpose of inducing fibrosis in the same region and thereby strengthen or replace the defective tendon.

superficial implantation Implantation of the ovum in which the chorionic sac (the outer surface of the expanding blastocyst) makes a simple contact with the uterine mucosa, as in the pig, sheep, cow, horse, dog, cat, and some primates. Also called *central implantation, circumferential implantation*.

teratic implantation   FETAL INCLUSION.

tooth implantation   The surgical insertion of a structure or material into or on the bone of the jaw to support a dental restoration, for cosmetic correction, or for the immobilization of a fracture.

implantation of the ureters   A surgical procedure in which the distal ureters are either reinserted into the bladder or inserted into a loop of bowel following a cystectomy.

implantodontics   [IMPLANT + ODONT- + -ICS]   The practice of oral implantology.

implantodontist   ORAL IMPLANTOLOGIST.

implantodontology   ORAL IMPLANTOLOGY.

implantologist / oral implantologist   A dentist specializing in oral implantology. Also called *implantodontist*.

implantology / oral implantology   The study of the implantation of teeth or implants. Also called *implantodontology*.

impletion   [Late L *impletio* (from L *impletus*, past part. of *implere* to fill in, fill up) a filling in or up]   The phenomenon that one is normally unaware of the existence of the blind spot of the eye.

implosion   [IM-¹ + *plos(us)* for *plausus*, past part. of *plaudere* to clap, beat + -ION]   A therapeutic technique in which the phobic patient imagines the object or situation he fears.

importation   The introduction of an infectious disease into an area from which it is absent at the time.

impotence   [L *im-* not + *potentia* (from *potens*, gen. *potentis*, pres. part. of *posse* to be able) power, might, ability]   A dysfunction in which the male is unable to perform the sexual act. It may be of psychosexual or organic origin. Also called *impotency, impotentia* (obsolete), *improcreance, invirility* (obsolete).

anal impotence   Constipation resulting from anxiety over the injurious or dirty aspect of the fecal mass.

atonic impotence   Impotence due to a lesion of the nervi erigentes.

erectile impotence   Impotence due to an inability to achieve or maintain erection. Also called *astyphia* (obsolete), *astysia* (obsolete).

functional impotence   PSYCHIC IMPOTENCE.

organic impotence   Impotence resulting from any organic disorder of the sexual apparatus, its innervation, or its blood supply. Also called *secondary impotence*.

orgastic impotence   Failure of either the male or female to achieve orgasm, despite adequacy of response in earlier phases of the sexual act. Also called *anorgasmy*.

paretic impotence   Impotence due to a lesion of the spinal cord or any other part of the central nervous system.

primary impotence   PSYCHIC IMPOTENCE.

psychic impotence   A psychosexual dysfunction consisting of inability of the male to perform sexual intercourse despite sexual desire and despite the lack of any organic condition that affects genital structure or function. Also called *functional impotence, primary impotence, psychogenic impotence*.

psychogenic impotence   PSYCHIC IMPOTENCE.

relative impotence   A male's inability to perform the sex act under certain conditions or with certain partners.

secondary impotence   ORGANIC IMPOTENCE.

symptomatic impotence   Impotence due to a lesion of the afferent (perineal nerve) components of the reflex arcs concerned with erection and ejaculation.

impotency   IMPOTENCE.

impotentia   An obsolete term for IMPOTENCE.

impotentia coeundi   Sexual impotence in the male.

impotentia generandi   Inability to produce offspring.

impregnate   **1** To make pregnant; fertilize.   **2** To permeate; saturate.

impregnation   **1** The act of impregnating or making pregnant; fertilization. Also called *ingravidation*.   **2** The process of saturating a substance or the condition resulting from it.

artificial impregnation   ARTIFICIAL INSEMINATION.

impressio   [L (from *impressus*, past part. of *imprimere* to press into, stamp into, from *im-* into + *premere* to press), a pressing in or into, stamping into]   (*plural* impressiones)   A concave depression or indentation in the surface of an organ or structure produced by the contact of another, as of the surface of the liver in contact with the stomach. Also called *impression*.

impressio cardiaca hepatis   [NA]   A shallow depression on the superior portion of the diaphragmatic surface of the liver, related to the heart through the diaphragm. Also called *cardiac impression of liver*.

impressio cardiaca pulmonis   [NA]   A deep concavity on the mediastinal part of the medial surface of each lung, more pronounced on the left, for accommodation of the heart and pericardium. Also called *cardiac impression of lung*.

impressio colica hepatis   [NA]   A variable hollow on the visceral surface of the right lobe of the liver, adjacent to the inferior border and to the right of the gallbladder, and related to the right flexure of the colon. Also called *colic impression of liver*.

impressiones digitatae   [NA]   Faint hollow markings on the inner surface of the cranium produced by the cerebral gyri. Also called *digitate impressions, digital impressions*.

impressio duodenalis hepatis   [NA]   A small, shallow depression on the visceral surface of the right lobe of the liver, wedged between the colic and the renal impressions to the right of the neck and adjacent part of the gallbladder and produced by the junction of the superior and descending parts of the duodenum. Also called *duodenal impression of liver*.

impressio esophagealis hepatis   [NA]   A small, shallow depression on the posterior aspect of the left lobe of the liver to the left of the upper end of the fissure for ligamentum venosum and related to the abdominal part of the esophagus. Also called *esophageal impression of the liver, impressio oesophagea hepatis*.

impressio gastrica hepatis   [NA]   A large concavity, occupying most of the visceral surface of the left lobe and continuing on to the anterior part of the quadrate lobe of the liver, related to the anterior surface and pyloric part of the stomach respectively. Also called *gastric impression of liver*.

impressio gastrica renis   A variable small triangular area wedged between the left suprarenal gland medially, the splenic area laterally, and the pancreatic area inferiorly on the anterior surface of the left kidney, and related to the posteroinferior surface of the stomach separated by the omental bursa.   • This term is a misnomer since it is not a true impression, but an area of relationship.

impressio hepatica renis   A large area occupying most of the anterior surface of the right kidney, below the suprarenal gland, related to the renal impression on the visceral surface of the right lobe of the liver and covered by peritoneum.   • This term is a misnomer since it is not a true impression, but an area of relationship.

impressio ligamenti costoclavicularis   [NA]   A rough raised area on the inferior surface of the medial, or sternal, end of the clavicle for the attachment of the costoclavicular ligament. Also called *impression of costoclavicular ligament, rhomboid impression of clavicle, tuberositas costalis claviculae, costal tuberosity of clavicle, tuberosity of clavicle* (outmoded).

impressio meningealis   FOVEOLAE GRANULARES.

impressio muscularis renis   A longitudinal area on the lower part of the posterior surface of each kidney, adjacent to the medial border, that is related to the psoas major muscle.

impressio oesophagea hepatis IMPRESSIO ESOPHAGEALIS HEPATIS.

impressio petrosa cerebri IMPRESSIO PETROSA PALLII.

impressio petrosa pallii A shallow indentation on the inferior surface of the temporal lobe made by the superior ridge of the petrous portion of the temporal bone. Also called *impressio petrosa cerebri, petrous impression.*

impressio renalis hepatis [NA] A large hollow on the posterior part of the visceral surface of the right lobe of the liver, bounded posteriorly by the inferior layer of the coronary ligament, medially by the duodenal impression, and anteriorly by the colic impression, and related to most of the anterior surface of the right kidney below the suprarenal gland. Also called *renal impression of liver.*

impressio suprarenalis hepatis [NA] A small depression on the "bare area" of the posterior surface of the right lobe of the liver, to the right of the lower end of the groove for inferior vena cava and superomedial to the renal impression. It is related to the right suprarenal gland. Also called *suprarenal impression of liver.*

impressio trigeminalis ossis temporalis [NA] A small, oval hollow on the anterior surface of the petrous part of the temporal bone, just behind its apex, on which rests the trigeminal ganglion. Also called *trigeminal impression of temporal bone, angular impression for gasserian ganglion* (outmoded), *fossa of gasserian ganglion* (outmoded), *trigeminal impression for gasserian ganglion.*

impression [L *impressio.* See IMPRESSIO.] **1** IMPRESSIO. **2** An imprint of a shape resulting from pressure applied against a plastic surface, often for the purpose of making a mold that can be cast, as a *dental impression.* **3** The immediate, unanalyzed effect of sensory information received.

anatomic impression A dental impression made without distorting the tissues.

angular impression for gasserian ganglion An outmoded term for IMPRESSIO TRIGEMINALIS OSSIS TEMPORALIS.

aortic impression of the trachea The close contact of the arch of the aorta with the left side of the trachea just above its bifurcation. No impression is produced on the trachea. An outmoded term.

basilar impression PLATYBASIA.

cardiac impression Either impressio cardiaca hepatis or impressio cardiaca pulmonis.

cardiac impression of liver IMPRESSIO CARDIACA HEPATIS.

cardiac impression of lung IMPRESSIO CARDIACA PULMONIS.

cleft palate impression A negative mold of a cleft palate from which an exact model can be cast in order to assist in the fabrication of a prosthetic device.

closed mouth impression A dental impression made with the mouth closed so that the margins of the impression can be molded by the orofacial muscles.

colic impression of liver IMPRESSIO COLICA HEPATIS.

colic impression of pancreas The occasional close contact of the transverse colon with the inferior surface of the body of the pancreas. In actuality, no impression is produced on the pancreas. An outmoded term.

colic impression of spleen FACIES COLICA SPLENIS.

composite impression SECTIONAL IMPRESSION.

copper-ring impression An impression of a prepared tooth taken in a fitted copper ring.

impression of coracobrachialis muscle A rough impression near the middle of the medial margin of the shaft of the humerus for the insertion of the coracobrachialis muscle.

costal impressions Transverse and oblique grooves on the surface of the hardened lungs of cadavers that are produced by the pressure of the ribs. They are not present in living persons.

impression of costoclavicular ligament IMPRESSIO LIGAMENTI COSTOCLAVICULARIS.

deltoid impression of humerus TUBEROSITAS DELTOIDEA HUMERI.

dental impression A mold made from the teeth and associated structures by surrounding them with a plastic material which sets in position. The impression, which is held in an impression tray, is then withdrawn from the mouth and plaster of paris is poured into it to form a model or cast of the teeth and contiguous structures.

digastric impression FOSSA DIGASTRICA.

digital impressions IMPRESSIONES DIGITATAE.

digitate impressions IMPRESSIONES DIGITATAE.

direct bone impression A dental impression, for a subperiosteal implant, taken of the bone after it has been exposed.

dual impression A dental impression made, for a partial denture, as a combination of two types. An anatomically correct impression is made of the teeth, while the denture-bearing soft tissue is compressed.

duodenal impression of liver IMPRESSIO DUODENALIS HEPATIS.

duodenojejunal impression of pancreas The close contact of the duodenojejunal flexure with the medial part of the inferior surface of the body of the pancreas. No impression is actually produced on the pancreas. An outmoded term.

elastic impression A dental impression made with a material which when set yields enough to permit its removal from undercuts and which then returns to its original set shape.

esophageal impression of the heart A faint impression on the posterior wall of the left atrium of the heart that is produced by the esophagus behind it. An outmoded term.

esophageal impression of liver IMPRESSIO ESOPHAGEALIS HEPATIS.

final impression A dental impression used to make the cast which will be used in making the denture or restoration.

fluid wax impression A dental impression which has been corrected by the addition of wax in a fluid state and then returned to the mouth.

functional impression A dental impression taken with the supporting tissues compressed and the orofacial muscles active. Also called *registration of functional form, mucodisplacement impression.*

gastric impression Either impressio gastrica hepatis or impressio gastrica renis.

gastric impression of liver IMPRESSIO GASTRICA HEPATIS.

gastric impression of pancreas The close contact of the posterior surface of the stomach with the anterior surface of the body of the pancreas. An outmoded term.

gastric impression of spleen FACIES GASTRICA SPLENIS.

hydrocolloid impression A dental impression made with hydrocolloid.

meningeal impression FOVEOLAE GRANULARES.

mercaptan impression A dental impression made with mercaptan, an elastic material containing polysulfide.

mucodisplacement impression FUNCTIONAL IMPRESSION.

mucostatic impression A dental impression causing minimal mucosal displacement.

petrous impression IMPRESSIO PETROSA PALLII.

pickup impression A dental impression made with an implant superstructure in place on the abutments. The impression material flows under the superstructure. When set and withdrawn, it holds the superstructure within it.

preliminary impression A dental impression taken for the purpose of making a study cast or impression tray. Also called *primary impression, snap impression.*

presurgical impression   A dental impression taken before oral surgery is carried out.

primary impression   PRELIMINARY IMPRESSION.

impression of pronator teres muscle   A rough, low ridge near the middle of the lateral surface of the radius for the insertion of the pronator teres muscle.

renal impression of liver   IMPRESSIO RENALIS HEPATIS.

rhomboid impression of clavicle   IMPRESSIO LIGAMENTI COSTOCLAVICULARIS.

secondary impression   A second, more accurate, and usually final impression, in the making of a denture.

sectional impression   A dental impression, usually for a partial denture, made in sections so that a material which is rigid when set can be withdrawn from undercuts and reassembled in the impression tray for casting. Also called *composite impression.*

small intestinal impression of pancreas   The close contact of the coils of the jejunum with the left side of the inferior surface of the pancreas, lateral to the duodenojejunal flexure. In fact, no impression is produced on the pancreas. An outmoded term.

snap impression   PRELIMINARY IMPRESSION.

suprarenal impression of liver   IMPRESSIO SUPRARENALIS HEPATIS.

thyroid impression of trachea   The close contact of the left lobe of the thyroid gland with the upper third of the left side of the trachea. No impression is produced on the trachea, however. An outmoded term.

trigeminal impression for gasserian ganglion   IMPRESSIO TRIGEMINALIS OSSIS TEMPORALIS.

trigeminal impression of temporal bone   IMPRESSIO TRIGEMINALIS OSSIS TEMPORALIS.

impressiones   Plural of IMPRESSIO.

impressorium [L *impress(io)* (from *impressus,* past part. of *imprimere* to press into, impress) a pressing into, impressing + *-orium* -ORY]   SENSORIUM.

imprinting   A mode of rapid learning by some animals depending on very brief and very early exposure to adults, usually parents, such as the following behavior of birds soon after hatching.

improcreance   IMPOTENCE.

improcreant [IM- + PROCREANT]   A seldom used term for INFERTILE.

impulse [L *impulsus* (from *impulsus,* past part. of *impellere* to push, drive, impel, from *im-* into, toward + *pellere* to set in motion, from Gk *pelein* to be in motion, go) a setting in motion, moving, impulse]   **1** A sudden urge to act in response to subjective or external stimuli: used especially of behavior viewed as powerfully motivated, compulsive, or irrational.   **2** Any driving force.   **3** A nerve impulse.

apex impulse   APEX BEAT.

apical impulse   APEX BEAT.

cardiac impulse   The visible or palpable thrust of the heart against the chest wall; apex beat. Also called *pulsus cordis.*

component impulse   Any of the pregenital manifestations of a drive. They usually manifest themselves as foreplay in the adult and remain subservient to genital primacy.

ectopic impulse   An electrical impulse arising in any part of the heart other than the sinuatrial node.

enteroceptive impulses   Nerve impulses derived from the viscera.

episternal impulse   An impulse from aortic pulsation in the suprasternal notch.

exteroceptive impulses   Nerve impulses derived from sense organs of the skin and distance receptors.

involuntary impulse   **1** REFLEX ACT.   **2** Autonomic neural activity. An outmoded term.

irresistible impulse   Inability to restrain or ignore the desire to perform an action due to mental illness, used in some jurisdictions as a means of evaluating criminal responsibility.

left parasternal impulses   Impulses felt along the left sternal border due to pulsation of the pulmonary artery, right ventricle, or left atrium.

morbid impulse   **1** Any socially unacceptable action.   **2** An uncontrollable action that may represent a compulsion or be based upon a delusional idea. An imprecise and old-fashioned term.

nerve impulse   A rapid, electrochemical, conducted event propagated in nerve fibers. Also called *neural impulse.*

neural impulse   NERVE IMPULSE.

noise impulse   Noise in which the onset is abrupt, as when a hammer strikes a metal plate or when a gun is fired. The sound is usually transient and its intensity considerable so that it cannot be measured accurately with conventional sound level meters.

proprioceptive impulses   Nerve impulses derived from receptors in muscles, tendons, and joints.

right parasternal impulses   Abnormal impulses felt along the right border of the sternum.

voluntary impulse   Excitation of nerve impulses in the corticospinal tract, volitionally initiated to evoke movement. An outmoded term.

impulsion [L *impulsio* (from *impulsus,* past part. of *impellere* to push, drive, impel) impulse, external impression]   In psychology, indiscriminate gratification of every wish, typical of children before the superego has become firmly established.

im-pyeng   COLLAPSING TYPHUS.

imu [Ainu]   A culture-specific syndrome of the Ainu of Japan consisting of hyperkinesia, catalepsy, echolalia, echopraxia, and command automatism. It appears almost exclusively in adult females.

Imuran   A proprietary name for azathioprine.

imus   Lowest.

IMViC   A set of tests used to distinguish various Enterobacteriaceae, and especially to distinguish coliforms of fecal origin from *Enterobacter* species. The tests are for indole production, methyl red color change with pH, Voges-Proskauer reaction for acetoin, and citrate utilization.

In   Symbol for the element, indium.

in   Symbol for the unit, inch.

in²   Symbol for the unit, square inch.

in-¹ [L preposition *in* (in all combinations with L words *in-* becomes *im-* before *b, m, p; il-* before *l, ir-* before *r;* with English words *in-* may remain unchanged regardless of following letter) in, on, into]   A prefix meaning in, into, toward, inward. Also *il-, im-, ir-.*

in-² [L prefix *in-* (regularly *im-* before *b, m, p; il-* before *l; ir-* before *r*) not]   **1** A prefix meaning not, negative.   **2** A prefix used as an intensive. Also *il-, im-, ir-.*

-in [noun suffix from French *-ine,* from L *-ina,* fem. of *-inus* of or belonging to]   A suffix meaning of or belonging to.

-ina [fem. sing. or neut. pl. of L *-inus* combining form denoting belonging to]   A suffix meaning one related or belonging to.

inacidity [IN-² + ACIDITY]   The lack of acidity; anacidity.

inaction   **1** Lack of action.   **2** Sluggish response to a stimulus.

inactivate   To make biologically inactive, as viruses or bacteria, toxins, or serum complement, by any of various means, such as by physical means (exposure to x rays, ultraviolet irradiation, or heating), or by exposure to chemical agents or to immunologic antagonists.

inactivation   The process by which a substance or agent, as a virus, a toxin, or enzyme, is rendered biologically inactive, or the condition thus effected by such a process.

paternal-X inactivation The nonrandom inactivation of the X chromosome that is derived from the father in the somatic cells of females of some species, including marsupials.

random-X inactivation The inactivation of most of one of the two X chromosomes present in the homogametic sex, such as human females, as a mechanism of dosage compensation. The selection of which X chromosome becomes inactive occurs randomly in normal cells.

inactivator / C3b inactivator An outmoded term for FACTOR I. • The reference is to factor I (the letter, not the roman numeral).

inagglutinable Not capable of being agglutinated.

inalimental **1** Not nourishing. **2** Not suitable for food.

inanagenesis [IN-¹ + Gk *anagennēsis* (from *ana*- up + *genn(an)* to beget + *-ēsis* -ESIS) regeneration] Muscle regeneration. A rarely used term. Also called *inanaphysis*.

inanaphysis INANAGENESIS.

inangulate Without angles.

inanimate Lacking life; not animate.

inanition [Middle English *in-anisioun*, from late L *inanitio*, from L *inanitus*, past part. of *inanire* to empty, from *inanis* empty] Any disorder of the body due to the insufficient intake of one or more essential nutrients including water, as vitamin deficiency diseases, starvation, kwashiorkor, marasmus, goiter, and anemia.

inapparent Not apparent; specifically, present but undetectable clinically, as an infection.

inappetence Lack of desire or appetite.

Inapsine A proprietary name for droperidol.

inarticulate **1** Incapable of producing the sounds of intelligible speech. **2** Unable to speak easily or well; uncommunicative. **3** Lacking articulations or joints.

in articulo mortis [L *in* in + *articulo*, ablative of *articulus* juncture, fit moment + *mortis*, gen. of *mors* death] At the exact moment of death.

inassimilable Not capable of being assimilated, as ingested nutrients.

inattention [L *in*- not + ATTENTION] Lack of attention.

selective inattention The ignoring or disregard of events, attitudes, values, etc., because they are given no value by the significant people in the subject's environment.

sensory inattention INATTENTION PHENOMENON.

inaxon INTERNAL MESAXON.

inborn **1** HEREDITARY. **2** CONGENITAL.

inbred **1** Pertaining to inbreeding. **2** Describing a population in which the occurrence of consanguineous matings is relatively high.

inbreeding **1** The selective crossing of related plants or animals. Compare OUTBREEDING. **2** A mating system, whether directed or occurring in nature, in which mates are on average more closely related than expected on the basis of random selection. Also called *intermarriage* (popular), *linebreeding*. **3** In human populations, the occurrence of consanguineous matings that are productive of offspring.

incallosal Describing or pertaining to agenesis of the corpus callosum. A seldom used term.

incanate An obsolete term for INCANOUS.

incandescent Producing light caused by heating.

incanous [L *incanus* gray-white] Having a grayish white hue. Also *incanate* (obsolete).

incaparina [*I(nstitute of) N(utrition of) C(entral) A(merica and) P(anama)* + L *(f)arina* flour] A dietary supplement containing 27.5% protein used in the prevention and treatment of protein-calorie malnutrition, including kwashiorkor. Different

formulas exist but all have the same protein content. A typical product consists of 38% cottonseed flour, 29% ground corn, 39% sorghum, 3% Torula yeast, 1% calcium carbonate and 1350 μg vitamin A per 100 g. Many versions contain maize or soya flour.

incarcerated Abnormally enclosed or confined; trapped.

incarceration [Late L *incarceratio* imprisonment, from L *in* IN + *carcer* prison + *-atio* -ATION] Abnormal enclosure or confinement of a part.

incarnatio [Late L, from *incarnatus*, past part. of *incarnare* to clothe with flesh, from L *-in* -IN¹ + *caro*, gen. *carnis*, flesh] INGROWING NAIL.

incarnatio unguis INGROWING NAIL.

incarnative **1** Promoting formation of granulation tissue. **2** Any agent that increases the formation of granulation tissue.

incasement [IN-¹ + *case* (from Old Norman French *casse* a box, from L *capsa* a box, chest, from *capere* to take) + -MENT] PREFORMATION.

inceal INCUDAL.

incendiarism [L *incendiar(ius)* (from *incendium* fire, heat) an incendiary + -ISM] PYROMANIA.

incentive An external stimulus that increases an already existing internal motivational state to produce some action or to maintain a behavioral sequence necessary for the achievement of a distant goal. If an ultimate goal is remote, the partial reinforcement offered by extrinsic incentives along the path to that goal may be absolutely necessary for the maintenance of the behavior sequence.

inceptus [L, from *inceptus*, past part. of *incipere* to begin, undertake] ANLAGE.

incertae sedis Of uncertain affiliation: used in taxonomy.

incest [L *incest(um)* (from neut. of *incestus* unchaste, polluted, from *in*- not + *castus* chaste, pure) impurity, incest] Sexual intercourse between two persons who are close blood relatives.

inch [Old English *ince*, from L *uncia* the twelfth part of any whole] A unit of length equal to 1/36 yard; 1/12 foot; 2.54 centimeters exactly. Symbol: in

conventional inch of mercury A unit of pressure equal to 25.4 conventional millimeters of mercury; 13.5951 conventional inches of water; $3.386\,39 \times 10^3$ pascals. Symbol: inHg

conventional inch of water A unit of pressure equal to 25.4 conventional millimeters of water; 249.089 pascals. Symbol: inH₂O

cubic inch A unit of volume equal to a cube of one inch side; 16.3871 cubic centimeters. An obsolescent unit. Symbol: in³

inch of mercury See under CONVENTIONAL INCH OF MERCURY.

square inch A unit of area equal to 6.4516 square centimeters approximately; 645.16 square milllimeters approximately. Symbol: in²

inch of water See under CONVENTIONAL INCH OF WATER.

inchação [Portuguese, a swelling (referring to the edema of wet beriberi)] A Brazilian term for BERIBERI.

incidence [Late L *incidentia* (from L *incidens*, gen. *incidentis*, pres. part. of *incidere* to happen, befall) a happening, befalling, incidence] The number of cases of a disease, abnormality, accident, etc., arising in a defined population during a stated period, expressed as a proportion, such as *x* cases per 1000 population per year. Also called *incidence rate, attack rate*.

incident Falling upon, or impinging on, as *incident light*.

incinerate [Med L *incinerat(us)*, past part. of *incinerare* to burn to ashes, from L *in*- IN¹ + *cinis*, gen. *cineris*, ashes, cinders] To subject to incineration; to burn (a substance) or to oxidize (it) completely in some other way. Organic materials are frequently incinerated by heating in sulfuric acid in the presence of catalysts to convert all their carbon into carbon dioxide. This permits analysis for various elements in the residue, e.g. nitrogen as ammonium ions.

incineration [Med L *incineratio* (from L *incineratus*, past part. of *incinerare* to incinerate, from *in-* IN-¹ + *cinis*, gen. *cineris*, cinders, ashes) incineration]   The process of complete oxidation of an organic substance, often performed in order to allow its content of certain elements to be measured. It may be carried out by heating the substance in air, or it may be performed by heating the substance in sulfuric acid containing catalysts.

incipient [L *incipiens*, gen. *incipientis*, pres. part. of *incipere* to begin]   About to appear or come into existence; initial, as a stage of illness.

incisal   **1** Relating to an incisor tooth.   **2** Relating to the cutting edge of an incisor tooth.

incise [L *incis(us)*, past part. of *incidere* to cut into, from *in-* into + *caedere* to cut]   To cut into or divide with a knife, scissors, or other sharp instrument during a surgical procedure. Adjective: incised.

incision [*incis(e)* + *-ION*]   A surgical cut with a sharp instrument into the body that results in a division of tissue and creation of a wound.

Agnew-Verhoeff incision   An obsolete method of surgical drainage of an abscess of the lacrimal sac by means of a stab cut through the overlying tissues.

Auvray incision   A surgical incision, usually made during a splenectomy, into the skin and abdominal wall parallel to the lateral border of the left rectus muscle.

Bar's incision   An incision in the midline of the upper abdomen used in an obsolete method of performing a cesarean section.

Battle's incision   A vertical incision through the paramedian part of the anterior abdominal wall in which the anterior and posterior parts of the rectus sheaths are longitudinally divided and the muscles are retracted. Also called *Battle-Jalaguier-Kammerer incision, lateral rectus incision.*

Battle-Jalaguier-Kammerer incision   BATTLE'S INCISION.

Bergmann's incision   A surgical incision in the abdominal wall for purposes of exposing the kidney. The line of incision extends from the twelfth rib to the midportion of Poupart's ligament.

Bevan's incision   A sigmoid-shaped right paramedian incision for exposure of the biliary tree through the anterior abdominal wall.

buttonhole incision   A small, linear surgical incision into an organ or body cavity.

Cherney incision   A transverse suprasymphyseal incision in the anterior abdominal wall. After the rectus muscles are exposed, the tendinous insertions are transected at the symphysis.

collar incision   A surgical incision of one of the natural transverse creases of the skin of the front of the neck, particularly such an incision based on the midline low in the neck. The object of such an incision is to ensure that the scar, by coinciding with a natural crease, will be inconspicuous.

confirmatory incision   An incision into an organ, tissue, or mass for diagnostic purposes.

cruciate incision   A surgical incision in the shape of a cross, frequently employed for drainage procedures.

Deaver's incision   A paramedian incision in the right lower abdominal wall in which the rectus muscle is retracted rather than divided. It is used in appendectomy procedures.

decompression incision   An incision to relieve pressure within a tight body compartment. In the case of burns this may be made through the skin, and in other forms of trauma or vascular compromise it may be made through the investing muscle fascia.

double-Y incision   HAYES MARTIN INCISION.

Dührssen's incisions   Longitudinal incisions in the uterine cervix utilized to facilitate vaginal delivery of a fetus.

endaural incision   **1** A surgical incision, used in middle-ear surgery, made within the confines of the external ear in contrast to the classic postauricular incision.   **2** An extracartilaginous incision which consists of a curved incision down to bone at the entrance to the external auditory meatus posteriorly, in front of the anterior edge of the conchal cartilage. The incision continues with an extension upwards and forwards between the tragus and the ascending portion of the helix, this part remaining superficial to the temporalis fascia.

eyebrow incision   A surgical approach through the eyebrow with the intent of concealment of the scar.

Fergusson's incision   WEBER-FERGUSSON INCISION.

incision of food   The penetration of food by incisor teeth, as in biting an apple.

Fowler's angular incision   A surgical incision in the anterolateral part of the abdominal wall for abdominal exploration.

Gluck incision   A skin incision in the front of the neck performed for total laryngectomy. It consists of three parts: a gently curved transverse incision convex downward at the level of the hyoid bone, a second shorter curved transverse incision convex upward at the level of the second tracheal ring, and a vertical incision in or to one side of the midline joining the transverse incisions. Though still employed, the incision has been modified.

Hayes Martin incision   A composite skin incision on one side of the neck, utilized for total laryngectomy combined with radical neck dissection. It consists of three parts: a shallow V-shaped incision convex downward extending from the tip of the mastoid process to a point beneath the tip of the chin, a second incision in the form of an inverted V based on the clavicle and, the third, a vertical incision joining the nearest points of the other two. Also called *double-Y incision.*

hockey stick incision   An incision consisting of two joined straight incisions that form an obtuse angle. It is usually made to extend an otherwise inadequate incision.

Howarth's incision   A curved incision approximately 3.5 cm in length carried down to bone, approximately 1 cm medial to the inner canthus of the eye, and extending downward from a point just below the inner end of the eyebrow. It originated as the first step in frontoethmoidectomy but has since been used in a number of other surgical procedures including transsphenoidal hypophysectomy. Also called *Lynch incision.*

Kehr's incision   A long midline incision through the abdominal wall, beginning at the xiphoid cartilage, passing around the umbilicus, and continuing to the pubis.

Kocher's incision   A right subcostal incision in the abdominal wall two finger breadths below and parallel to the costal margin.

Küstner's incision   A transverse incision in the lower abdomen above the symphysis pubica that follows the natural semilunar curve of the skin. The upper flap of skin and subcutaneous tissue is elevated to expose the aponeurosis of the external oblique muscle, and then an incision is made parallel to the rectus muscle.

Langenbeck's incision   A surgical incision in the anterior abdominal wall that extends through the semilunar line, parallel to the fibers of the rectus muscle.

lateral rectus incision   BATTLE'S INCISION.

Longuet's incision   LONGUET'S OPERATION.

Lynch incision   HOWARTH'S INCISION.

MacFee incisions   Two parallel transverse incisions, one at the base of the neck and the other just below the jaw line, utilized during radical neck dissection.

Mason's incision   A vertical incision into the anterior abdominal wall designed to preserve the nerve supply of the rectus abdominis muscles.

mastoid incision   POSTAURICULAR INCISION.

Maylard incision A transverse suprasymphyseal incision into the anterior abdominal wall. The rectus muscles are transected transversely.

McArthur's incision A vertical incision through the paramedian region of the anterior abdominal skin and anterior paramedian sheath. The posterior sheath and peritoneum are then incised transversely.

McBurney's incision A surgical incision for appendectomy in the right lower quadrant of the anterior abdominal wall parallel to the fibers of the external oblique muscle through a point one third the distance between the umbilicus and the anterior superior iliac spine. All of the underlying muscles are split rather than incised. This was originally developed as a drainage incision for acute appendicitis.

median incision An incision along all or part of the midline of the anterior abdominal wall.

Meyer's hockey stick incision A lower abdominal L-shaped surgical incision that in part splits and in part divides the muscles.

muscle-splitting incision Any surgical incision in which the muscle groups are split or separated in the direction of the fibers without cutting into them.

Owens incision A modification of Ruddy's incision. The deep U-shaped incision, convex forward is made just within the alveolar margin to preserve the blood supply and nerve supply of the large palatal mucoperiosteal flap.

paramedian incision A surgical incision in the anterior abdominal wall parallel to the rectus muscle and away from the midline.

paravaginal incision A surgical incision made into the vagina and perineum designed to increase the diameter of the vaginal outlet.

Perthes incision A surgical incision into the right upper quadrant of the abdomen. It has a vertical paramedian component from the xiphoid to the umbilicus and a transverse component from the umbilicus to the costal margin.

Pfannenstiel's incision A lower abdominal curvilinear transverse incision through the skin, followed by a midline fascial and peritoneal incision.

postaural incision POSTAURICULAR INCISION.

postauricular incision An incision made behind the ear to provide surgical access to the interior of the mastoid process and, frequently, thereby to the tympanic cavity and its contents. At one time, the skin incision was carried through the periosteum down to bone, but increasingly surgeons have incised the periosteum separately backward of the skin incision to create a separate periosteal flap. Also called *postaural incision, mastoid incision, Schwartze incision.*

preauricular incision Any incision made anterior to the ear.

rectus incision Any surgical incision into the abdominal wall that passes through the rectus muscle on one or both sides of the midline.

relief incision An incision, usually made into fascia, that releases tension on a suture line or within a tissue. Also called *relieving incision.*

relieving incision RELIEF INCISION.

Risdon's incision An incision at the angle of the mandible, used to gain access to the ramus.

Robertson incision A surgical procedure for treating hypertrophic pyloric stenosis, in which a transverse incision is made opposite the eighth costal cartilage. The underlying muscles are split according to fiber direction, and a transverse peritoneal incision is made.

Rodman's incision An incision across the axilla, through which the axillary lymph nodes are removed before it is extended around the breast for the completion of a radical mastectomy. The procedure is obsolete.

Ruddy's incision A curved surgical incision, through the mucoperiosteum of the hard palate, used as an approach for the correction of congenital choanal atresia.

Schuchardt's incision A large paravaginal incision used in preparation for a radical vaginal hysterectomy.

Schwartze incision POSTAURICULAR INCISION.

Singleton's incision An incision in the abdominal wall that is used for upper abdominal procedures.

Sloan's incision An incision in the abdominal wall used for upper abdominal surgery.

Smith incision An incision once used to facilitate skin closure following a radical mastectomy. An obsolete term.

Sorensen incision A skin incision in the front of the neck frequently used for laryngectomy. It is a symmetrical U-shaped incision centered on the midline, following the anterior border of the sternomastoid muscle on either side from the level of the hyoid bone above to the level of the third ring of the trachea below where the lateral limbs of the incision are united by a short transverse incision convex downwards.

stab incision A small surgical incision, similar to a knife wound, that is usually used to provide an egress for open or closed drainage.

Stewart's incision A transverse incision frequently used in the performance of modified radical mastectomy. An obsolete term.

transfixion incision In rhinoplasty, an incision that traverses the membranous septum from one side of the nose to the other, thus separating the columella from the nasal septum.

Vischer's lumboiliac incision A lateral abdominal wall incision in which the fibers of the lumboiliac muscles are split immediately above the central portion of the iliac crest. Care is taken to spare these muscles and the local nerves from any injury.

Weber-Fergusson incision An incision that courses through the upper lip, along the side of the nose, and then along the inferior orbital rim. The cheek and lip can then be reflected to the side permitting wide exposure of the maxilla, as is needed during total maxillectomy. Also called *Fergusson's incision.*

Wilde's incision An obsolete procedure involving an incision into the swelling behind the ear carried down to the mastoid bone, for the relief of mastoiditis. It has been replaced by mastoidectomy.

incisive **1** Cutting; penetrating. **2** Relating to an incisor tooth.

incisolabial [L *incis(us)*, past part. of *incidere* to cut into + *o* + *labi(a)* a lip + *-alis* -AL] Relating to both an incisor tooth and the lip.

incisolingual [L *incis(us)*, past part. of *incidere* to cut into + *o* + *lingu(a)* the tongue + *-alis* -AL] Relating to both an incisor tooth and the tongue.

incisoproximal [L *incis(us)*, past part. of *incidere* to cut into + *o* + *proxim(us)* very near, next, nearest + *-alis* -AL] Describing the angle between the incisal edge and the mesial or distal surface of an incisor tooth.

incisor [L *incis(us)* (past part. of *incidere* to cut into, from *in-* into + *caedere* to cut) cut into, made by cutting + *-or*] A tooth situated in front of the canines. In human dentition, one of the four most anterior teeth in either jaw. Also called *cutting tooth, incisor tooth.*

central incisor The incisor nearest to the midsagittal plane in each quadrant. Also called *first incisor, medial incisor.*

first incisor CENTRAL INCISOR.

Hutchinson's incisors Hypoplastic incisors caused by congenital syphilis. They are barrel-shaped when viewed from the front and have a crescentic notch in the center of the incisal edge. The upper central incisors are the most commonly affected.

lateral incisor   The incisor situated distal to the first incisor and mesial to the canine. Also called *second incisor*.

medial incisor   CENTRAL INCISOR.

scalpriform incisor   One of the chisel-shaped incisors of a rodent.

second incisor   LATERAL INCISOR.

shovel-shaped incisors   Upper central incisor teeth with large crowns concave lingually.

winged incisor   A rotated maxillary incisor tooth with the distal edge protruding labially.

incisura [L (from *incisus*, past part. of *incidere* to cut into, from *in-* into + *caedere* to cut, + *-ura* -URE), cut into] (*plural* incisurae) A notch, depression, or indentation, often on the edge of a structure. Also called *incisure, notch.*

incisura acetabuli [NA] A gap between the inferior ends of the lunate surface of the acetabulum of the hip bone which is bridged by the transverse ligament to form the cotyloid foramen. Also called *incisure of acetabulum, acetabular notch, cotyloid notch, cotyloid incisure.*

anacrotic incisura   ANACROTIC NOTCH.

incisura angularis gastrica [NA] A depression at the most dependent point of the lesser curvature of the stomach, usually at the junction of its upper two thirds and lower one third. It separates the body of the stomach on the left from the pyloric antrum on the right. Its position varies with the degree of distension of the stomach and with the inherent shape of the stomach. Also called *incisura angularis ventriculi, gastric notch, sulcus angularis, angulus of stomach, angular notch, angular sulcus, angular incisure.*

incisura angularis ventriculi   INCISURA ANGULARIS GASTRICA.

incisura anterior auris [NA] A marked notch separating the crus of the helix from the tragus of the external ear, occasionally surmounted by the supertragic tubercle. Also called *anterior incisure of ear, anterior auricular groove, anterior notch of ear, sulcus auriculae anterior* (outmoded).

incisura apicis cordis [NA] A small notch on the right margin of the heart just to the right of the apex where the anterior interventricular sulcus on the sternocostal surface becomes continuous with posterior interventricular sulcus on the diaphragmatic surface. Also called *incisure of apex of heart, notch of apex of heart.*

incisura cardiaca pulmonis sinistri [NA] A wide notch in the anterior margin of the superior lobe of the left lung, just above the lingula and anterior to the cardiac fossa occupied by the heart and pericardium. Also called *cardiac incisure of left lung, cardiac notch of left lung, fovea cardiaca.*

incisura cardiaca gastrica [NA] The acute-angled notch at the junction of the left margin of the esophagus and the greater curvature of the stomach, above the level of which the fundus is located. Also called *cardiac incisure of stomach, cardiac notch of stomach, cardiac incisura of stomach.*

cardiac incisura of stomach   INCISURA CARDIACA GASTRICA.

incisurae cartilaginis meatus acustici [NA] Two or three fissures in the anterior wall of the cartilaginous part of the external acoustic meatus providing mobility of the ear. Also called *Santorini's clefts, Santorini's fissures, Duverney's fissures, incisures of Duverney, incisurae santorinii.*

incisura cerebelli anterior   The broad indentation on the anterior surface of the cerebellum, overlying the inferior colliculus and the superior cerebellar peduncle. Also called *anterior cerebellar notch.*

incisura cerebelli posterior   The narrow indentation behind the cerebellar hemispheres containing the falx cerebelli. Also called *posterior cerebellar notch, marsupial notch* (obsolete).

incisura clavicularis sterni [NA] The oval, concave articular surface on either side of the jugular notch on the superior margin of the manubrium sterni for receiving the medial end of the clavicle and the intervening articular disk. Also called *clavicular incisure of sternum, clavicular notch of sternum, lateral incisure of sternum* (outmoded), *semilunar incisure of sternum* (outmoded), *clavicular facet.*

incisurae costales sterni [NA] Notches on the lateral borders of the sternum, seven on each side, for articulation with the first seven costal cartilages. Also called *costal incisures of sternum, costal foveae of sternum, costal notches of sternum, articular foveae for rib cartilages, lateral facets of sternum, costal facets of sternum, articular facets for rib cartilages, costal sinuses of sternum* (outmoded).

incisura ethmoidalis ossis frontalis [NA] A wide, quadrangular space between the orbital parts of the frontal bone occupied by the cribriform plate of the ethmoid bone articulating in the frontoethmoidal suture. Also called *ethmoidal incisure of frontal bone, ethmoidal notch of frontal bone, ethmoidal notch, notch of ethmoid, incisure of ethmoid.*

incisura fastigii   A transverse notch seen on the ventricular surface during fetal development of the cerebellar lamina.

incisura fibularis tibiae [NA] A triangular notch on the lateral surface of the distal end of the tibia, the rough upper part of which receives the attachment of the lower end of the interosseous membrane while the lower part may be covered with articular cartilage for articulation with the lower end of the fibula. Also called *fibular incisure of tibia, fibular notch, incisura peronea tibiae* (outmoded), *incisura semilunaris tibiae* (outmoded), *peroneal incisure of tibia, semilunar incisure of tibia* (outmoded), *peroneal sinus of tibia* (outmoded), *semilunar sinus of tibia* (outmoded), *fibular notch of tibia.*

incisura frontalis [NA] A minute notch occasionally present medial to the supraorbital notch or foramen and transmitting a diploic branch of the supraorbital artery and a frontal branch of supraorbital nerve to the frontal sinus. The notch may be bridged over by bone, converting it into foramen frontale. Also called *frontal incisure, frontal notch, supraciliary canal, supraorbital notch, notch of frontal bone.*

incisura glenoidalis   A notch in the anterosuperior rim of the glenoid fossa of the scapula that indicates the junction of the coracoid and scapular parts of the articular surface. The part above the notch has a separate center of ossification. The notch is more apparent in young individuals than in older person. An outmoded term. Also called *notch of glenoid cavity.*

incisura interarytenoidea laryngis [NA] A small notchlike prolongation of the aditus laryngis posteriorly between the corniculate cartilages and the apices of the arytenoid cartilages on each side as far back as the interarytenoid fold of mucosa. Also called *interarytenoid incisure of larynx, interarytenoid notch.*

incisura interlobaris hepatis   An outmoded term for INCISURA LIGAMENTI TERETIS.

incisura interlobaris pulmonis   Either fissura obliqua pulmonis or fissura horizontalis pulmonis dextri.

incisura intertragica [NA] A deep notch between the tragus and the antitragus just above the lobe of the ear pinna. Also called *intertragic incisure, intertragic notch, incisura tragica, intertragic incisure of ear.*

incisura ischiadica major [NA] A wide, deep notch in the posterior border of the ilium, above, and the ischium, below, extending from the posterior inferior iliac spine to the sciatic, or ischial, spine, and converted into a foramen by the sacrotuberous and sacrospinous ligaments. Also called *greater ischiadic incisure, greater ischiatic notch, greater sciatic notch, greater sacrosciatic notch* (outmoded), *iliosciatic notch* (outmoded).

incisura ischiadica minor [NA] A shallow notch on the posterior margin of the ischium, limited by the sciatic, or ischial, spine above and the upper end of the ischial tuberosity below, and converted into a foramen by the sacrotuberous and sacrospinous ligaments. Also called *lesser ischiadic incisure, lesser ischiadic notch, lesser sciatic notch, lesser iliac incisure* (outmoded), *lesser sacrosciatic notch* (outmoded).

incisura jugularis ossis occipitalis [NA] An indentation on the front of the jugular process of the occipital bone, forming the posterior part of the jugular foramen. The notch is subdivided by the intrajugular process. Also called *jugular incisure of occipital bone, jugular notch of occipital bone.*

incisura jugularis ossis temporalis [NA] A large, ellipsoid notch on the inferior surface of the petrous part of the temporal bone, posterior to the external carotid foramen, forming the anterior and lateral parts of the jugular foramen and containing the superior bulb of the internal jugular vein. Also called *jugular incisure of temporal bone, jugular notch of temporal bone.*

incisura jugularis sterni [NA] A concavity in the center of the superior border of the manubrium sterni, bounded by the clavicular notch on each side. Also called *jugular incisure of sternum, jugular notch of sternum, suprasternal notch, sternal notch, sternal incisure, superior semilunar incisure of sternum* (outmoded), *interclavicular incisure, interclavicular notch, presternal notch.*

incisura lacrimalis maxillae [NA] A narrow, vertical depression located anteriorly on the medial border of the orbital surface of the maxilla where the lacrimomaxillary suture is in the fossa for the lacrimal sac adjacent to the orbital orifice of the nasolacrimal duct. Also called *lacrimal incisure of maxilla, lacrimal notch of maxilla, lacrimal notch.*

incisura ligamenti teretis [NA] A notch of varying size and depth in the inferior border of the liver slightly to the right of the median plane, continuous posteriorly with the fissure for ligamentum teres and containing the ligamentum teres. Also called *incisura umbilicalis, umbilical incisure, umbilical notch, notch of ligamentum teres, incisura interlobaris hepatis* (outmoded), *interlobar notch.*

incisura mandibulae [NA] A deep concavity in the superior border of the ramus of the mandible, between the coronoid and condylar processes, through which the masseteric nerve and vessels pass. Also called *incisure of mandible, mandibular notch, semilunar notch of mandible* (outmoded), *sigmoid incisure of mandible, sigmoid notch* (outmoded), *semilunar incisure of mandible* (outmoded).

incisura mastoidea INCISURA MASTOIDEA OSSIS TEMPORALIS.

incisura mastoidea ossis temporalis [NA] A deep longitudinal furrow, medial to the base of the mastoid process of the temporal bone and lateral to the groove for occipital artery, to which the posterior belly of the digastric muscle is attached. Also called *mastoid incisure of temporal bone, mastoid notch, mastoid groove, digastric groove, digastric notch, digastric incisure of temporal bone, digastric fossa, incisura mastoidea.*

incisura nasalis maxillae [NA] A large concavity on the medial border of the anterior surface of the body of the maxilla, forming the lateral and inferior margin of the piriform aperture, the lower end of which continues anteriorly to meet the opposite side at the anterior nasal spine. Also called *nasal incisure of maxilla, nasal notch of maxilla, nasal notch.*

incisura pancreatis [NA] A groove between the head and the neck of the pancreas inferiorly where the uncinate process hooks posterior to the superior mesenteric vessels. Also called *pancreatic notch, inferior notch of neck of pancreas.*

incisura parietalis ossis temporalis [NA] The angle, or notch, formed by the posterior part of the superior border of the squamous part of the temporal bone meeting the mastoid part. It is located at the posterior end of the petrosquamous suture internally and the squamomastoid suture externally. Also

called *parietal incisure of temporal bone, parietal notch of temporal bone, parietosphenoid fissure, parietal notch.*

incisura peronea tibiae An outmoded term for INCISURA FIBULARIS TIBIAE.

incisura preoccipitalis [NA] The ventrolateral notch demarcating the caudal limit of the temporal lobe and the rostral boundary of the occipital lobe. Also called *preoccipital notch, preoccipital incisure.*

incisura pterygoidea [NA] The angular fissure separating the lower parts of the medial and lateral plates of the pterygoid process of the sphenoid bone, the margins of which articulate with the pyramidal process of the palatine bone. Also called *pterygoid fissure, pterygoid notch, fissura pterygoidea, palatine incisure, pterygoid incisure, palatine notch.*

incisura radialis ulnae [NA] A shallow concavity on the lateral surface of the coronoid process of the ulna for articulation with the circumference of the head of radius, while the anterior and posterior edges of the notch provide attachment for the annular ligament. Also called *radial incisure of ulna, radial notch of ulna, lesser semilunar incisure of ulna* (outmoded), *lesser sigmoid fossa of ulna, lesser sigmoid cavity of ulna, radial fossa of ulna* (outmoded), *lunate sinus of ulna* (outmoded).

incisura rivini INCISURA TYMPANICA.

incisurae santorinii INCISURAE CARTILAGINIS MEATUS ACUSTICI.

incisura scapulae [NA] A deep notch on the superior margin of the scapula at its junction with the coracoid process. The notch is bridged over by the superior transverse scapular ligament, over which the suprascapular vessels pass and deep to which the suprascapular nerve runs. Also called *incisure of scapula, scapular notch, suprascapular notch, semilunar incisure* (outmoded), *suprascapular incisure, coracoid notch, semilunar incisure of scapula* (outmoded), *semilunar notch of scapula* (outmoded), *lunula of scapula* (outmoded).

incisura semilunaris tibiae An outmoded term for INCISURA FIBULARIS TIBIAE.

incisura semilunaris ulnae INCISURA TROCHLEARIS ULNAE.

incisura sphenopalatina INCISURA SPHENOPALATINA OSSIS PALATINI.

incisura sphenopalatina ossis palatini [NA] A narrow gap between the orbital and the sphenoidal processes at the top of the perpendicular plate of the palatine bone which is converted into a foramen by the body of the sphenoid bone coming into contact with the processes superiorly. The gap lies between the pterygopalatine fossa laterally and the posterior part of the nasal cavity near its roof medially. Also called *sphenopalatine incisure of palatine bone, sphenopalatine notch of palatine bone, palatine incisure of Henle, palatine notch of palatine bone, sphenopalatine notch, incisura sphenopalatina.*

incisura supraorbitalis [NA] A small notch, often converted to a bony foramen, at the junction of the rounded medial one third and the sharp lateral two thirds of the supraorbital margin of the frontal bone for the transmission of the supraorbital nerve and vessels. Also called *supraorbital incisure, supraorbital notch, supraorbital fissure* (outmoded).

incisura temporalis The notch between the uncus and the tip of the temporal lobe. Also called *temporal incisure.*

incisura tentorii [NA] The large, oval opening that contains the midbrain and the anterior part of the superior surface of the vermis of the cerebellum. It is bounded anteriorly by the dorsum sellae of the sphenoid bone and laterally and posteriorly by the concave, free margin of the tentorium cerebelli. Also called *tentorial notch, incisure of tentorium of cerebellum, incisure of cerebellum, tentorial hiatus, foramen ovale of Pacchioni.*

incisura terminalis auris [NA] A deep notch almost completely separating the cartilage of the auricle from that of the external acoustic meatus. Also called *terminal incisure of ear, terminal notch of auricle.*

incisura thyroidea inferior [NA] A shallow notch in the inferior margin of the thyroid cartilage at the junction of the laminae in the midline, where the median cricothyroid ligament is attached. Also called *inferior thyroid incisure, inferior thyroid notch.*

incisura thyroidea superior [NA] A deep V-shaped notch situated anteriorly in the midline between the superior margins of the laminae of the thyroid cartilage and just above the laryngeal prominence. Also called *superior thyroid incisure, superior thyroid notch.*

incisura tragica INCISURA INTERTRAGICA.

incisura trochlearis ulnae [NA] A deep concave notch at the upper end of the ulna formed by the superior surface of the coronoid process and the anterior surface of olecranon for articulation with the trochlea of the humerus. It is unevenly divided by a longitudinal ridge fitting the groove on the trochlea. Also called *trochlear notch of ulna, incisura semilunaris ulnae, humeral incisure of ulna* (outmoded), *semilunar incisure of ulna, sigmoid incisure of ulna* (outmoded), *greater semilunar incisure of ulna* (outmoded), *trochlear incisure of ulna, semilunar fossa of ulna, sigmoid fossa of ulna, greater sigmoid cavity of ulna.*

incisura tympanica [NA] A gap in the superior part of the tympanic sulcus of the temporal bone occupied by the pars flaccida of the tympanic membrane above the malleolar folds. Also called *tympanic notch, Rivinus incisure, notch of Rivinus, incisura rivini, Rivinus foramen* (outmoded), *rivinian foramen* (outmoded), *rivinian notch, tympanic incisure, rivinian segment, segment of Rivinus.*

incisura ulnaris radii [NA] A concavity on the medial surface of the lower end of radius for articulation with the circumference of the head of ulna in the inferior radioulnar joint. Also called *ulnar incisure of radius, ulnar notch of radius, semilunar incisure of radius* (outmoded), *sigmoid cavity of radius, lunate sinus of radius* (outmoded), *semilunar sulcus of radius* (outmoded).

incisura umbilicalis INCISURA LIGAMENTI TERETIS.

incisura vertebralis inferior [NA] A notch on the inferior border of the pedicle of a vertebra, forming the upper part of an intervertebral foramen. Also called *inferior vertebral incisure, inferior vertebral notch, greater vertebral incisure.*

incisura vertebralis superior [NA] A notch on the superior border of the pedicle of a vertebra, forming the lower part of an intervertebral foramen. Also called *superior vertebral incisure, superior vertebral notch, lesser vertebral incisure.*

incisurae Plural of INCISURA.

incisural Pertaining to an incisura.

incisure

incisure [L *incisura.* See INCISURA.] INCISURA.

incisure of acetabulum INCISURA ACETABULI.

angular incisure INCISURA ANGULARIS GASTRICA.

anterior incisure of ear INCISURA ANTERIOR AURIS.

incisure of apex of heart INCISURA APICIS CORDIS.

incisure of calcaneus SULCUS TENDINIS MUSCULI FLEXORIS HALLUCIS LONGI CALCANEI.

cardiac incisure of left lung INCISURA CARDIACA PULMONIS SINISTRI.

cardiac incisure of stomach INCISURA CARDIACA GASTRICA.

incisure of cerebellum INCISURA TENTORII.

clavicular incisure of sternum INCISURA CLAVICULARIS STERNI.

costal incisures of sternum INCISURAE COSTALES STERNI.

cotyloid incisure INCISURA ACETABULI.

digastric incisure of temporal bone INCISURA MASTOIDEA OSSIS TEMPORALIS.

incisures of Duverney INCISURAE CARTILAGINIS MEATUS ACUSTICI.

incisure of ethmoid INCISURA ETHMOIDALIS OSSIS FRONTALIS.

ethmoidal incisure of frontal bone INCISURA ETHMOIDALIS OSSIS FRONTALIS.

falciform incisure of fascia lata MARGO FALCIFORMIS HIATUS SAPHENUS.

fibular incisure of tibia INCISURA FIBULARIS TIBIAE.

frontal incisure INCISURA FRONTALIS.

incisure of gallbladder FOSSA VESICAE BILIARIS.

greater ischiadic incisure INCISURA ISCHIADICA MAJOR.

greater semilunar incisure of ulna An outmoded term for INCISURA TROCHLEARIS ULNAE.

greater vertebral incisure INCISURA VERTEBRALIS INFERIOR.

humeral incisure of ulna An outmoded term for INCISURA TROCHLEARIS ULNAE.

inferior maxillary incisure An outmoded term for MARGO LACRIMALIS MAXILLAE.

inferior thyroid incisure INCISURA THYROIDEA INFERIOR.

inferior vertebral incisure INCISURA VERTEBRALIS INFERIOR.

interarytenoid incisure of larynx INCISURA INTERARYTENOIDEA LARYNGIS.

interclavicular incisure INCISURA JUGULARIS STERNI.

intertragic incisure INCISURA INTERTRAGICA.

intertragic incisure of ear INCISURA INTERTRAGICA.

jugular incisure of occipital bone INCISURA JUGULARIS OSSIS OCCIPITALIS.

jugular incisure of sternum INCISURA JUGULARIS STERNI.

jugular incisure of temporal bone INCISURA JUGULARIS OSSIS TEMPORALIS.

lacrimal incisure of maxilla INCISURA LACRIMALIS MAXILLAE.

incisures of Lanterman-Schmidt SCHMIDT-LANTERMAN INCISURES.

lateral incisure of sternum An outmoded term for INCISURA CLAVICULARIS STERNI.

lesser iliac incisure An outmoded term for INCISURA ISCHIADICA MINOR.

lesser ischiadic incisure INCISURA ISCHIADICA MINOR.

lesser semilunar incisure of ulna An outmoded term for INCISURA RADIALIS ULNAE.

lesser vertebral incisure INCISURA VERTEBRALIS SUPERIOR.

incisure of mandible INCISURA MANDIBULAE.

mastoid incisure of temporal bone INCISURA MASTOIDEA OSSIS TEMPORALIS.

nasal incisure of frontal bone MARGO NASALIS OSSIS FRONTALIS.

nasal incisure of maxilla INCISURA NASALIS MAXILLAE.

obturator incisure of pubic bone An outmoded term for SULCUS OBTURATORIUS OSSIS PUBIS.

palatine incisure INCISURA PTERYGOIDEA.

palatine incisure of Henle INCISURA SPHENOPALATINA OSSIS PALATINI.

parietal incisure of temporal bone INCISURA PARIETALIS OSSIS TEMPORALIS.

patellar incisure of femur An outmoded term for FACIES PATELLARIS FEMORIS.

peroneal incisure of tibia INCISURA FIBULARIS TIBIAE.

popliteal incisure An outmoded term for FOSSA INTERCON-DYLARIS FEMORIS.

preoccipital incisure INCISURA PREOCCIPITALIS.

pterygoid incisure INCISURA PTERYGOIDEA.

radial incisure of ulna INCISURA RADIALIS ULNAE.

Rivinus incisure INCISURA TYMPANICA.

incisure of scapula INCISURA SCAPULAE.

Schmidt-Lanterman incisures Oblique channels of Schwann cell cytoplasm extending across the myelin sheaths of peripheral nerves. Also called *incisures of Lanterman-Schmidt, Schmidt-Lanterman clefts, Lanterman's clefts.*

semilunar incisure An outmoded term for INCISURA SCAP-ULAE.

semilunar incisure of mandible An outmoded term for IN-CISURA MANDIBULAE.

semilunar incisure of radius An outmoded term for INCI-SURA ULNARIS RADII.

semilunar incisure of scapula An outmoded term for IN-CISURA SCAPULAE.

semilunar incisure of sternum An outmoded term for IN-CISURA CLAVICULARIS STERNI.

semilunar incisure of tibia An outmoded term for INCISURA FIBULARIS TIBIAE.

semilunar incisure of ulna INCISURA TROCHLEARIS ULNAE.

sigmoid incisure of mandible INCISURA MANDIBULAE.

sigmoid incisure of ulna An outmoded term for INCISURA TROCHLEARIS ULNAE.

sphenopalatine incisure of palatine bone INCISURA SPHE-NOPALATINA OSSIS PALATINI.

sternal incisure INCISURA JUGULARIS STERNI.

superior semilunar incisure of sternum An outmoded term for INCISURA JUGULARIS STERNI.

superior thyroid incisure INCISURA THYROIDEA SUPERIOR.

superior vertebral incisure INCISURA VERTEBRALIS SUPE-RIOR.

supraorbital incisure INCISURA SUPRAORBITALIS.

suprascapular incisure INCISURA SCAPULAE.

incisure of talus SULCUS TENDINIS MUSCULI FLEXORIS HAL-LUCIS LONGI TALI.

temporal incisure INCISURA TEMPORALIS.

incisure of tentorium of cerebellum INCISURA TENTORII.

terminal incisure of ear INCISURA TERMINALIS AURIS.

trochlear incisure of ulna INCISURA TROCHLEARIS ULNAE.

tympanic incisure INCISURA TYMPANICA.

ulnar incisure of radius INCISURA ULNARIS RADII.

umbilical incisure INCISURA LIGAMENTI TERETIS.

---

incitant The causative agent of a disorder or condition, such as the agent that triggers an allergic response.

incitogram [irreg. from L *incit(atus)*, past part. of *incitare* to set in rapid motion + *o* + -GRAM] The events within the central nervous system that initiate efferent nervous impulses.

inclinatio [L (from *inclinatus*, past part. of *inclinare* to incline, bend), an inclining, leaning, bending] A leaning, bending, or sloping with respect to a particular plane. Also called *inclination, incline.*

inclinatio pelvis [NA] The angle between the plane of the superior aperture of the pelvis and the horizontal plane, which, in the standing anatomical position, varies in individuals from 50° to 60°. Also called *inclination of pelvis, pelvic inclination, pelvic incline, incline of pelvis, angle of inclination, angle of pelvis, pelvivertebral angle.*

inclination [INCLINE + -ATION] INCLINATIO.

axial inclination The inclination of a tooth relative to the vertical. The inclination is usually described as mesial, distal, lingual, labial or buccal. Also called *inclination of tooth.*

enamel rod inclination The angle between an enamel prism and a line or plane such as the surface of a tooth.

lateral condylar inclination The direction of movement of the head of the condyle on the balancing side when the mandible is swung laterally.

pelvic inclination INCLINATIO PELVIS.

inclination of pelvis INCLINATIO PELVIS.

inclination of tooth AXIAL INCLINATION.

inclinationes Plural of INCLINATIO.

incline [L *inclinare* (*in-* in + obsolete *clinare* to bend, lean, from Gk *klinein* to make a thing slope or slant, to make recline) to incline, bend, curve] INCLINATIO.

pelvic incline INCLINATIO PELVIS.

incline of pelvis INCLINATIO PELVIS.

inclinometer A device to measure the axis of astigmatism.

inclusion [L *inclusio* (from *inclusus*, past part. of *includere* to shut up, confine, from *in-* in + *claudere* to close, shut, from Gk *kleiein* to shut) a shutting up, confinement] **1** The state of being included or enclosed. **2** Something included or enclosed. **3** CELL INCLUSION.

cell inclusion **1** A foreign body contained within a cell. Also called *inclusion.* **2** A storage substance, a pigment, or a metabolic product found as a granule or vesicle in a cell.

dental inclusion The presence of an unerupted tooth completely surrounded by bone after the time when it should have erupted.

fetal inclusion A parasitic and usually incomplete member of a pair of unequal conjoined twins enclosed within the body of the host twin. Also called *fetus in fetu, intrafetation, teratic implantation.*

Guarnieri's inclusions GUARNIERI BODIES.

intranuclear inclusions Foreign matter found within the nucleus, usually representing viral material.

leukocyte inclusions Small, round or oval, gray-blue bodies found in the cytoplasm of neutrophils in severe infections, burns, septicemia, and toxic conditions. They are common in scarlet fever, but contrary to earlier beliefs are not specific for this disease. They are comprised of RNA fibrils in an area free of specific granules. They are also seen occasionally in thrombo-cytopenic purpura, myeloproliferative syndromes, chronic mye-logenous leukemia, pernicious anemia, and hemolytic anemia. They are a permanent morphologic feature of the May-Hegglin anomaly of platelets.

Walthard's inclusions WALTHARD'S CELL NESTS.

incoagulability A state characterized by the inability of blood or plasma to clot. Absolute incoagulability is rare.

incoagulable Exhibiting incoagulability.

incomitance [IN-² + L *comitans*, pres. part. of *comitari* to go along with] The characteristic of strabismus whereby the amount of ocular misalignment changes with different positions of gaze. Adjective: incomitant.

incomitant Pertaining to incomitance.

incompatibility [French *incompatibilité* (from L *in-* not + COM- + L *pati* to bear, suffer, from Gk *paschein* to suffer, be affected by) antipathy] The quality of being incompatible, as drugs whose interaction renders them ineffective or harmful, or blood types which in combination induce an undesirable immunologic reaction in the host.

ABO incompatibility Lack of compatibility of cells bearing the ABO blood group when mixed with serum containing the corresponding, naturally occurring isoantibodies. The lack of compatibility is manifested *in vivo* by hemolysis.

chemical incompatibility Chemical unmixability, e.g., of oil and water.

physiologic incompatibility Unsuitability for being administered together because of antagonistic pharmacologic actions.

therapeutic incompatibility Unsuitability for combination, as of drugs administered at the same time.

incompatible Having an adverse or unwanted effect if combined or used together, as drugs, blood types, or other substances.

incompetence [L *in-* not + COMPETENCE] **1** Failure of an organ, part, or system to meet an accepted standard for quality of function, often of a specific physiologic function; substandard function; insufficiency. **2** Inability to understand adequately a particular transaction or to conduct one's own affairs responsibly. A legal term. Also called *incompetency.*

aortic incompetence AORTIC REGURGITATION.

ileocecal incompetence The lack of function of the ileocecal valve allowing for cephalad flow of fecal material into the small bowel. Also called *ileocolic incompetence, ileocecal insufficiency.*

ileocolic incompetence ILEOCECAL INCOMPETENCE.

valvular incompetence Incompetence of a cardiac valve due to inadequate closure, resulting in valvular regurgitation.

velopharyngeal incompetence VELOPHARYNGEAL INSUFFICIENCY.

incompetency INCOMPETENCE.

incompetent **1** Characterized by incompetence; substandard in function; insufficient. **2** Held to be unable to enter into certain contractual relationships or to make certain kinds of decisions independently. A legal term.

incongruence [L *in-* not + *congruentia* (from *congruens,* gen. *congruentis,* agreeing + *-ia* -IA) conformity, symmetry] A characteristic of binocular visual field defects in which the defects are dissimilar in the two eyes. Adjective: incongruent.

incongruity / retinal incongruity Noncorrespondence of retinal visual elements serving comparable portions of the binocular field.

incontinence [L *incontinentia.* See INCONTINENTIA.] **1** Absence of voluntary control of an excretory function, especially defecation or urination. **2** Willing or unwilling lack of restraint of one's appetites or impulses. Also called *incontinentia.*

active incontinence Defecation or urination which is normal and regular but not subject to voluntary control.

emotional incontinence EMOTIONAL LABILITY.

fecal incontinence The inability to voluntarily control the anal sphincters, resulting in involuntary release of flatus and stool. Also called *incontinence of the feces, rectal incontinence, incontinentia alvi, copracrasia, scatacratia, scoracratia.*

incontinence of the feces FECAL INCONTINENCE.

intermittent incontinence Urinary incontinence which is not continuous but is characterized by lack of voluntary inhibitory response to stress on the bladder or to sudden movement. It is one manifestation of the neurogenic bladder.

incontinence of milk Inability to control the secretion of breast milk.

overflow incontinence Dribbling of urine due to pressure in a full, overdistended bladder. Also called *paradoxical incontinence.*

paradoxical incontinence OVERFLOW INCONTINENCE.

paralytic incontinence Incontinence due to an inoperative or paralyzed sphincter, resulting from disease or dysfunction of the central nervous system. Also called *sphincteric incontinence.*

passive incontinence Urinary incontinence in which, because emptying cannot occur normally or voluntarily, urine dribbles out under the pressure of a full bladder.

rectal incontinence FECAL INCONTINENCE.

sphincteric incontinence PARALYTIC INCONTINENCE.

stress incontinence Discharge of urine or feces due to in-

creased intra-abdominal pressure, as in coughing, straining, or sudden movement.

urgency incontinence Urinary incontinence due to excessive feelings of urgency.

urinary incontinence Inability to control urination, with resultant repeated or continuous involuntary passage of urine. Also called *incontinentia urinae.*

incontinent Exhibiting or characterized by incontinence.

incontinentia [L (from *incontinens,* gen. *incontinentis,* intemperate, immoderate, incontinent, from *in-* not + *continens,* pres. part. of *continere* to hold or keep together, hold), inability to restrain one's desires, incontinence] INCONTINENCE.

incontinentia alvi FECAL INCONTINENCE.

incontinentia pigmenti An X-linked dominant syndrome of neonatal onset characterized by progressive skin lesions leading to swirling patterns of hyperpigmentation, alopecia of the crown of the head, ocular changes including optic atrophy, absent or malformed teeth, mental retardation, and seizures. A paucity of affected males and an increased miscarriage rate among affected women are consistent with this disorder's being lethal *in utero* in hemizygous males. Also called *Bloch-Sulzberger syndrome.*

incontinentia urinae URINARY INCONTINENCE.

incoordination [L *in-* not + COORDINATION] Lack of coordination, whether in motor activities (ataxia) or in the activities of various organs, glands, or viscera.

first-degree uterine incoordination PRIMARY UTERINE INERTIA.

second-degree uterine incoordination SECONDARY UTERINE INERTIA.

incorporation [Late L *incorporatio* (from *incorporatus,* past part. of *incorporare* to incorporate, from L *in-* IN¹ + *corpus,* gen. *corporis,* body) an incorporating or being incorporated] In psychoanalytic psychology, assimilation of external objects into the self, usually applied to the earliest phase of object recognition when everything pleasurable is something to swallow. Less commonly, incorporation is equated with identification or introjection, or both.

incostapedial INCUDOSTAPEDIAL.

incrassate [Late L *incrassat(us),* past part. of *incrassare* to thicken, from L *in-* IN¹ + *crassare* to thicken] Thickened or swollen. An obsolete term.

increase / natural increase An increase during a given period in the size of a population which is attributable to an excess of births over deaths.

increment [L *incrementum* (from *increscere* to increase, grow, grow upon + *-mentum* -MENT) growth, increase] A small increase in the value of a variable. If the value of a variable changes from x to $x + \Delta x$, the increment Δx is taken to be small relative to x and in the limit approaches zero. Adjective: incremental.

absolute increment An increment Δx expressed as the difference between $x + \Delta x$ and x.

relative increment An increment Δx expressed as a proportion of the initial value of the variable, i.e. Δx divided by x.

incretin A seldom used term for SECRETIN.

incretion An obsolete term for HORMONE.

incretology [IN-¹ + L *(se)cret(us),* past part. of *secernere* to separate, sever + *o* + -LOGY] An older term for ENDOCRINOLOGY.

incretopathy [IN-¹ + L *(se)cret(us),* past part. of *secernere* to separate, sever + *o* + -PATHY] An outmoded term for ENDOCRINOPATHY.

incretory An outmoded term for ENDOCRINE.

incretotherapy An outmoded term for HORMONOTHERAPY.

incross In experimental genetics, the mating of two organisms that are both homozygous at a given locus for the same allele.

incrustation 1 The formation of a crust. 2 CRUST.

incubate [L *incubat(us)*, past part. of *incubare* to lie in or on a thing, brood, hatch] To maintain a microbiologic culture or a preparation of biological or chemical materials at a fixed temperature.

incubation 1 The maintenance of microbiologic cultures or of preparations of biologic or chemical material at a fixed temperature for a prescribed period of time. 2 The development of an infectious disease in a host from the time the infecting agent is introduced into the body until the first clinical features manifest themselves. 3 The maintenance of a newborn infant in an environment controlled for temperature and atmospheric conditions, used especially for premature or sick newborns.

incubator A device in which fixed temperature and atmospheric conditions can be maintained, used for incubation of biologic or chemical materials and in pediatrics to provide a controlled environment for the care of premature or sick newborns. Also called *couveuse* (obsolete).

incubus [Middle English, from Late L *incubus* (from L *incubare* to lie in or upon a thing) an evil being believed to lie upon persons in their sleep, esp. in sexual intercourse with women] A nightmare, especially one in which a woman dreams that a man or devil has entered her bed to have intercourse with her. An obsolete term.

epileptic incubus An obsolete term for EPILEPTIC NIGHT-MARE.

incudal Pertaining to the incus. Also *inceal*.

incudectomy Excision of the incus or, more often, of the remains thereof as in a radical mastoidectomy.

incudiform In the shape of an anvil.

incudius LIGAMENTUM MALLEI ANTERIUS.

incudomalleal MALLEOINCUDAL.

incudostapedial Pertaining to the incus and the stapes. Also *incostapedial*.

incuneation GOMPHOSIS.

incurable Admitting of no cure; not curable.

incurvation The bending inwards of a structure, such as a limb bone.

incus [L (from *incudere* to stamp, strike), anvil] [NA] The middle of the three auditory ossicles of the middle ear. It has a cuboid body that articulates anteriorly with the head of the malleus, a long crus that terminates in the lentiform process for articulation with the head of the stapes, and a short crus which is attached to the fossa incudis. Also called *anvil, stithe* (outmoded).

incyclodeviation [IN-¹ + CYCLO- + DEVIATION] Torsional displacement of an eye on its anteroposterior axis so that its upper (12 o'clock) part is rotated inward in the direction of the nose. Also called *positive torsion*.

incyclophoria [IN-¹ + CYCLO- + -PHORIA] A latent tendency to torsion of the eye, the superior portion turning nasalward.

incyclotropia [IN-¹ + CYCLO- + TROPIA] A manifest tendency to torsion of the eye, the superior portion turning nasalward.

incyclovergence [IN-¹ + CYCLO- + VERGENCE] Inward torsion of the top of both eyes.

in d. *in dies* (L, meaning daily), used in prescription writing.

indehiscent [IN-² + L *dehiscens*, gen. *dehiscentis*, pres. part. of *dehiscere* to break open] Remaining closed at maturity: used especially of a seed pod or fruit.

indemnity [L *indemnitas* (from *indemn(is)* suffering no financial loss, from -*in* not + *damnum* damage, harm, + -*itas* -ITY) security from loss] The agreement of an insurer to provide health insurance benefits in the form of cash payments to, or on behalf of, a beneficiary for services provided, rather than the provision of the services themselves.

aggregate indemnity The maximum amount, specified in currency, payable for any disability, period of disability, or covered service under an insurance policy.

indenization COLONIZATION.

indentation [L *in-* into + *dens*, gen. *dentis*, tooth + -ATION] 1 The formation of notches in an edge or pits in a surface. 2 A notch or pit.

aortic indentation of esophagus AORTIC NARROWING OF ESOPHAGUS.

indentation of Hahn An anterior defect of the vertebral body seen on the lateral radiograph of the vertebral column of the young child, giving to the vertebra a "turtle head" appearance. It may persist in the adult as a fine medial vertebral canal in one or more vertebrae.

indentation of the tongue The impression made on the surface of the tongue by the occlusal surfaces of the teeth. It is caused by the development of rigor mortis in the muscles of mastication.

independence / statistical independence A lack of statistical bearing of the outcome of one eventuality on that of the outcome of another. Two events are statistically independent if the probability of both occurring is equal to the product of the separate probabilities of the occurrence of each. For example, let the probability of a patient having a given disease be P(A) and the probability of a random individual being of a certain blood group be P(B); the occurrence of the disease and the presence of the blood group are statistically independent if P(A and B), that is, the probability of a diseased patient having that blood group, is equal to the product of P(A) and P(B).

index

index (*plural* indices, indexes) 1 The second finger of the hand. Also called *indicator, index finger, digitus secundus, digitus demonstrativus, forefinger, digitus II.* 2 Anything used to indicate or point out. 3 Any numerical characteristic developed for use in the analysis of quantitative information; specifically, a number expressing the magnitude of a given quantity as a ratio of that of another quantity of similar kind, or of itself at some other period, these latter in each case being given by convention the value 100 (or other power of ten) in the scale of relative values.

absolute refractive index The ratio between the velocity of light in a vacuum and the velocity of light in the designated medium.

ACH index An index of a child's nutritional state based on measurement of the arm, chest, and hip.

air pollution index A measurement or aggregate of several measurements of one or more air contaminants. It is used to compare the pollution of different areas or the same area at different times.

air velocity index The ratio of the maximum breathing capacity to the vital capacity. An obsolete term.

alpha index The proportion of time during which alpha rhythms are recorded by an electroencephalograph during any single recording.

altitudinal index A measure of the relationship between cranial height and length: (height × 100)/length. Also called *height-length index, length-height index, vertical index*.

alveolar index   A measure of the degree of prognathism of a skull: (basion-nasion length × 100)/basion–alveolar point length.

anesthetic index   **1** A measure of the potency of a local or general anesthetic.   **2** An indication of the depth of general anesthesia as it is administered to an individual.

antitryptic index   A numerical indicator of the degree of effectiveness of antagonism to digestion by trypsin. It was used in diagnosing cancer. Also called *antitryptic efficiency.*

Arneth index   A numerical expression of neutrophilic segmentation, derived by adding the percentage of one-lobed and two-lobed cells to one half of the percentage of three-lobed cells. The normal value is 60%. See also ARNETH FORMULA.

auricular index   The relation between the width of the pinna and its height.

auricular-height index of the skull   A measure of the relationship between the height of the head and its length: (bregma–auricular point × 100)/glabella-opisthocranion.

auriculoparietal index   A measure of the relationship between the breadth of the skull between the auricular points to its maximum breadth: (biauricular breadth × 100)/maximum biparietal breadth.

auriculovertical index   A measure of the relationship between the height of the skull vertically above the auricular point to its maximum height from the same point: (vertical height from auricular point × 100)/maximum height from auricular point.

Ayala's index   AYALA'S QUOTIENT.

baric index   A formula, no longer in use, that was designed to relate body weight to height. The body weight was multiplied by 100 and divided by the cube of the height.

basilar index   A measure of the relationship between the basion and the auricular point to the maximum length of the skull: (basion–alveolar point × 100)/maximum length.

Becker-Lennhoff index   LENNHOFF'S INDEX.

body build index   A formerly used index relating body weight to height in which the body weight was divided by the square of the height.

Boedecker's index   The ratio of the number of carious tooth surfaces in a mouth to the number of tooth surfaces at risk.

Bouchard's index   A formerly used index of adiposity derived by dividing the weight by height.

brachial index   A measure of the relationship between the length of the upper arm and the forearm: (length of forearm × 100)/length of upper arm.

breadth-height index   A measure of the relationship between the maximum breadth and the maximum height of the head: (breadth × 100)/height.

Broders index   BRODERS CLASSIFICATION.

Brugsch index   The chest circumference × 100 divided by the length of the body.

calcification index   CALCIUM INDEX.

calcium index   A formula relating the amount of calcium in the blood with a standard solution of calcium oxide. Also called *calcification index.*

cardiac index   The cardiac output of blood per unit of time divided by the body surface area.

cardiothoracic index   The ratio between the greatest transverse diameter of the heart and the greatest transverse diameter of the chest as measured on a PA chest x ray. This is normally less than 1:2 in the adult and children over four years.

centromeric index   In cytogenetics, a measure of relative centromere position, C. If p is the length of the short chromosome arm and q the length of the long arm, C equals p divided by the sum of p and q, multiplied by 100.

cephalic index   A measure of the relationship between the maximum breadth of the head and and the maximum length of the head: (maximum head breadth × 100)/maximum head length.

cephalic height index   A measure of the relationship between the height of the head and its length: (vertex–auricular point × 100)/glabella-opisthocranion.

cephalo-orbital index   A measure of the relationship between the volume of the cranium and the combined volume of the two orbits: (cranial volume × 100)/combined orbital volume.

cephalospinal index   A measure of the relationship between the area of the foramen magnum in square meters and the cranial volume in cubic centimeters.

cerebral index   A measure of the relationship between the maximum transverse diameter to the maximum anteroposterior length of the cranial cavity: (maximum internal breadth × 100)/maximum anteroposterior internal length.

chemotherapeutic index   THERAPEUTIC INDEX.

coliform index   COLIFORM TEST.

color index   An index of the hemoglobin concentration of erythrocytes that was once widely used, but is now obsolete. The color index was obtained by dividing hemoglobin concentration by the erythrocyte count and multiplying the quotient by 0.345. The factor was used to make the color index of normal blood approximately 1.0. The color index has been supplanted by measurement of mean corpuscular hemoglobin. Also called *cell color ratio.*

Colour Index   A joint publication of the English Society of Dyers and Colourists and the American Association of Textile Chemists and Colorists that lists and characterizes dyes and stains and assigns to each a number (CI number). The index permits appropriate classification and allows accurate identification. Abbreviation: CI

combined thyroid hormone index   A calculated value that reflects overall biologic effects of thyroid gland secretion, achieved by combining the values of free thyroxine index, free triiodothyronine index, and thyroid-binding globulin activity expressed by percentage of resin uptake. Because it corrects for hormonal or drug-induced alterations of thyroid-binding globulin activity, it appears to give more precise distinction among hypothyroid, euthyroid, and hyperthyroid states than the free hormone index for either thyroxine or triiodothyronine.

community periodontal index of treatment needs   A method of assessing the requirement for periodontal treatment based on bleeding, calculus formation, and depth of pockets, utilizing the WHO periodontal probe. The mouth is divided into sextants and the worst condition in each is coded as follows: a pocket of 6 mm or more is code 4; a pocket of 4–5 mm is code 3; supragingival or subgingival calculus is code 2, bleeding after probing is code 1; and no symptoms is code 0.

comparative mortality index   **1** An index for use in comparisons of mortality usually employed to express changes over time in the experience of the population of a given area. Formally, the index is the ratio of the weighted sums of age-specific death rates in the initial or base year to those of subsequent years, the weights being the average of the proportions of the population in each age group in the years in question. Abbreviation: CMI   **2** STANDARDIZED MORTALITY RATIO.

Cooke's index   COOKE'S FORMULA.

coronofrontal index   A measure of the relationship between the maximum frontal breadth of the skull to the maximum coronal breadth: (maximum frontal breadth × 100)/maximum coronal breadth.

corpuscular thickness index   THICKNESS INDEX.

cranial index   A measure of the relationship between the maximum breadth to the maximum length of the skull: (maximum breadth × 100)/maximum length. Also called *length-breadth index.*

creatine index   A test formerly used to measure the capacity of the organism to retain administered creatine under standard conditions of diet. It is low in hyperthyroidism and high in hypothyroidism. Also called *creatine tolerance test.*

crural index A measure of the relationship between the length of the lower leg and the length of the thigh: (length of lower leg × 100)/length of thigh.

def index An index of the effects of caries on the deciduous dentition. A tooth has a postive score if it is decayed (d), extraction is indicated (e), or it contains a filling (f). Missing teeth, not known to have been extracted, are ignored because of normal exfoliation. Also called *def rate, def.*

degenerative index The proportion of granulocytes containing toxic cytoplasmic granules. An obsolete term.

dental index A measure of the relationship between the length of the tooth row and the basion-nasion length: (length of tooth row × 100)/basion-nasion length. Also called *Flower's index.*

dilution index A numerical statement of air quality expressed as the concentration of an air pollutant emitted by a specified source divided by the rate of emission.

diversity index The numerical expression of species diversity within a community that can be expressed by dividing the number of species by the total number of individuals. The number of individuals is usually expressed as a logarithm or square root.

DMF index An index of the effects of caries on the permanent dentition. Decayed, missing and filled teeth are counted as equals. A tooth is given a positive score if is decayed, has been extracted because of caries, or is filled. Also called *DMF rate, DMF.* • This index is also called DMFT to distinguish it from a related, more refined index, DMFS, in which the surfaces involved are counted.

dynamic index A measure of the dynamic response of a muscle spindle afferent. It is the difference between the peak frequency of spike discharge during the dynamic phase of muscle stretch and the discharge frequency at the new steady length. The second frequency is commonly measured at 0.5 second following the change in muscle length.

effective temperature index An index of apparent warmth relating the temperature, movement, and humidity of air.

endemic index A measure of the prevalence of an endemic disease, such as the proportion of the population suffering from it at a given time.

erythrocyte indices A set of calculated figures for cell size, hemoglobin content, and hemoglobin concentration of individual red blood cells. They include mean cell volume, mean cell hemoglobin, and mean cell hemoglobin concentration.

facial index Either of two measures of the relationship between the length of the face to its width: (nasion–alveolar point × 100)/maximum bizygomatic width = superior facial index, or (nasion–mental tubercle × 100)/maximum bizygomatic width = total facial index.

fatigue index The ratio between the muscle tension remaining after a test period of tetanic stimulation to the value present initially. Generally the stimulus consists of repeated brief trains of pulses.

femorohumeral index A measure of the relationship between the length of the upper arm and the length of the thigh: (length of humerus × 100)/length of femur. Also called *humerofemoral index.*

firing index A Measure of the responsiveness of a single nerve cell, usually a motoneuron, to successive stimulation of a reflex or motor pathway. The index is calculated as the number of trials eliciting a discharge divided by the total number of trials, expressed as a percent.

Flower's index DENTAL INDEX.

forearm-hand index A relationship between the length of the hand and the length of the forearm: (total hand length × 100)/forearm length.

Fourmentin's thoracic index A relationship between the transverse and anteroposterior diameters of the thorax: (total transverse width × 100)/anteroposterior depth.

free thyroxine index The product of the serum total thyroxine concentration and the triiodothyronine resin uptake. Since this product is proportional to the serum free thyroxine concentration over a wide range of values, the derived figure provides a valid index of free thyroxine concentration. Abbreviation: FTI

free triiodothyronine index An indicator of the serum concentration of free triiodothyronine based on calculations similar to those used for determining the free thyroxine index. The tests in common use correct for abnormalities in thyroxine-binding globulin.

gingiva-bone count index A method of assessing periodontal disease that includes gingival condition and bone loss.

gingival periodontal index An index of periodontal disease based on the worst condition in each of the six segments of the mouth. A score of up to 3 is given for gingivitis and 4–6 for the depth of pocketing from the cementoenamel junction. Abbreviation: GPI

gnathic index The ratio between the distance from the basion to the prosthion multiplied by 100 and the distance between the basion and the nasion, an index of prominence of the maxilla.

habitus index A relationship between the girth of the trunk and stature: (maximum thoracic girth + maximum abdominal girth × 100)/height.

hair index A mathematical expression of the shape of the hair, obtained by dividing the least diameter of a hair by the greatest diameter and multiplying by 100.

hand index A relationship between the breadth and length of the hand: maximum hand breadth × 100)/maximum hand length.

height-breath index of the nose NASAL INDEX.

height-length index ALTITUDINAL INDEX.

hematopneic index A measure of blood oxygenation.

hemophagocytic index PHAGOCYTIC INDEX.

humerofemoral index FEMOROHUMERAL INDEX.

icteric index ICTERUS INDEX.

icterus index An approximation of bilirubin concentration in serum, obtained by comparing the intensity of color in the specimen against that of an aqueous solution of potassium dichromate with added sulfuric acid. It has been rendered obsolete by the widespread availability of chemical determination of bilirubin. Also called *icteric index.*

inhibition index The ratio of the weight of an antimetabolite required to inhibit the biological effect of a unit weight of metabolite.

intermembral index The relationship between total arm length and total leg length: (total arm length × 100)/total leg length.

iron index An obsolete expression of the iron content of erythrocytes, obtained by dividing the iron content of blood by the erythrocyte count. The normal value was 8–9.

juxtaglomerular index A morphologic estimation of the degree of cytoplasmic granularity of the juxtaglomerular cells, and therefore an indirect assessment of renin content.

Kaup index An expression of the relationship between body weight and stature: body weight divided by the square of the body length.

Langelier's index The hydrogen ion concentration of a water when in equilibrium with its calcium carbonate content.

length-breadth index CRANIAL INDEX.

length-height index ALTITUDINAL INDEX.

Lennhoff's index Sternal notch to pubic symphysis length × 100, divided by the maximum circumference of abdomen. Also called *Becker-Lennhoff index.*

leukopenic index The ratio of a decrease in the number of leukocytes compared to the normal total leukocyte count following administration of a drug or ingestion of foods, useful in testing for allergy.

lower leg–foot index   The relationship between the length of the foot and the lower leg: (foot length $\times$ 100)/lower leg length.

lymphocyte-monocyte index   The ratio of lymphocytes to monocytes in the blood, expressed using a monocyte denominator of one.

Macdonald index   The proportion of a population of children with enlarged spleen in which malarial parasites are also found on microscopic examination of blood.

malocclusion index   An index of the severity of a malocclusion using values assigned to various observations.

maturation index   A cytologic evaluation of vaginal cells in which there is a calculated ratio of parabasal, intermediate, and superficial cells.

maxilloalveolar index   The relationship between the length and the breadth of the dental arcade: (maximum alveolar breadth $\times$ 100)/maxilloalveolar length.

index of mental deterioration   A measure of the degree of psychologic or intellectual deficit produced by the condition under study, often expressed as a deterioration quotient or ratio obtained by comparing relatively stable functions such as vocabulary retention with relatively unstable functions, such as digit symbol or arithmetic abilities.

metacarpal index   A relationship between the length and breadth of the second through fifth metacarpal bones of the right hand taken as an average: (length M_2/breadth M_2 + length M_3/breadth M_3 + length M_4/breadth M_4 + length M_5/breadth M_5)/4.

mitotic index   The proportion of a population of cells that are in mitosis at a given point in time.

monocyte-leukocyte index   The ratio of monocytes to total leukocytes in the blood, expressed using a monocyte numerator of one.

morphologic face index   The relationship between the length and breadth of the facial skeleton: (nasion-gnathion $\times$ 100)/maximum bizygomatic breadth.

nasal index   The relationship between the height and breadth of the nasal aperture: (maximum breadth $\times$ 100)/nasion-nasospinale height. Also called *height-breadth index of the nose.*

nucleoplasmic index   The ratio obtained by dividing the volume of the nucleus of a cell by the cytoplasmic volume.

obesity index   A method of estimating the degree of overweight in which body weight is divided by body volume.

odor intensity index   The number of times an odorant must be diluted by a factor of two in order to reach the threshold of detectability by the human subject.

opsonic index   A measure of the opsonizing antibodies to a given microorganism, obtained by comparing the number of bacteria phagocytized by leukocytes in the presence of the test serum with that of serum from a normal individual. Also called *opsonocytophagic index.*

opsonocytophagic index   OPSONIC INDEX.

optical index   An index of microscope objectives. It reflects both the magnification and the numerical aperture of the lenses involved.

orbital index   The relationship between the height and breadth of the orbit: (maximum orbital height $\times$ 100)/maximum orbital breadth.

palatal index   The relationship between the length and breadth of the palate: (maximum palatal breadth $\times$ 100)/maximum palatal length in the midline. Also called *palatine index, palatomaxillary index.*

palatine index   PALATAL INDEX.

palatomaxillary index   PALATAL INDEX.

parasite index   The proportion of individuals in a population

in which malarial parasites are found on examination of blood smears.

pelvic index   A value based on comparative measurements of the conjugate and transverse diameters of the maternal pelvis as a means of estimating whether or not cephalopelvic disproportion is likely. Also called *pelvic inlet index.*

pelvic inlet index   PELVIC INDEX.

periodontal index   A weighted index of periodontal disease used extensively for epidemiological surveys. Scores are recorded for gingivitis, the presence of pockets, and mobility with loss of function. Also called *Russell index.* Abbreviation: PI

periodontal disease index   An index based on a clinical examination around six teeth: the upper right first molar, upper left central incisor and first bicuspid, lower left first molar, lower right central incisor and first bicuspid. Also called *Ramfjord index.* Abbreviation: PDI

phagocytic index   The mean number of bacteria in leukocyte cytoplasm after incubation of washed leukocytes and serum with the bacteria to be tested. The index reflects the presence of antibodies to the bacteria in the serum and the ability of leukocytes to ingest the bacteria. Also called *hemophagocytic index.*

physiognomonic upper face index   The relationship between the height and breadth of the upper face: (nasion-stomion $\times$ 100)/maximum bizygomatic breadth.

Pignet index   The categorization of strength potential based on Pignet's formula.

Pirquet's index   An estimate of nutritional status in infants and children based on measurement of weight and sitting height. A value below 94 pelidisi indicates the child is undernourished, between 95 and 100, the nutritional status is good, and over 101, overnutrition is apparent.

PMA index   An index of gingivitis: scores are recorded for inflammation of the papilla (P), the labial gingival margin (M) and the attached gingiva (A).

polymorphonuclear lymphocyte index   The ratio of polymorphonuclear leukocytes to lymphocytes in the blood, expressed using a lymphocyte denominator of one.

ponderal index   The ratio of height, measured in inches, to the cube root of body weight in pounds.

Pont's index   An index relating the inclusive width of the four incisors, the distance between the left and right first premolars, and the distance between the left and right first molars.

profunda-popliteal collateral index   A determination of the adequacy of profunda collaterals when the superficial femoral artery is occluded. It is suggested as a means for determining whether lower extremity revascularization can be accomplished with an inflow procedure alone, or whether outflow must be augmented as well.

prothrombin index   An index devised to simplify the correlation of prothrombin time and clotting activity: normal prothrombin time $\times$ 100 divided by patient's prothrombin time. The prothrombin time and concentrations of plasma coagulation factors are correlated in a rectangular hyperbolic fashion.

pulsatile index   An objective measure of the effect of a proximal stenosis upon an arterial waveform. It is the quotient peak-to-peak waveform excursion divided by mean velocity.

radiohumeral index   The relationship between the lengths of the radius and the humerus: (maximum length of radius $\times$ 100)/maximum length of humerus.

Ramfjord index   PERIODONTAL DISEASE INDEX.

recession index   An assessment of chronic periodontal disease obtained by counting the number of teeth where gingival recession has exposed the cementoenamel junction. It is expressed as a percentage of the total teeth in the mouth. Abbreviation: RI

refractive index   The ratio between the velocity of light in air and the velocity of light in a designated medium.

index of relative refraction   A ratio between the refractive index of the designated material or object and the refractive index of the material surrounding it. Also called *relative refractive index.*

relative refractive index   INDEX OF RELATIVE REFRACTION.

risk index   A numerical determination or estimation of the probability of the occurrence of harmful effects resulting from a risk.

Röhrer's index   An estimate of nutritional status based on body weight in grams multiplied by 100 and the product divided by the height, in centimeters, cubed.

Russell index   PERIODONTAL INDEX.

sacral index   The relationship between the length and breadth of the sacrum: (maximum sacral breadth $\times$ 100)/maximum sacral length.

salivary lactobacillus index   A caries potential index based on the incubation of a sample of saliva, founded on the belief that *Lactobacillus acidophilus* is the causative organism. This index was used in the 1930s but is now discredited.

saturation index   An obsolete expression of hemoglobin concentration within erythrocytes, obtained by dividing the percentage of standard of hemoglobin by the percentage of standard of hematocrit. The normal value was 0.97–1.02.

Schneider index   A test of physical fitness comprising observations on pulse rate and blood pressure under standard conditions of rest and exercise.

index of similarity   In ecology, any numerical index that compares two communities.

simplified oral hygiene index   The combination of a debris index and calculus index obtained by the examination of six selected tooth surfaces. Twelve surfaces were examined for the original oral hygiene index.

smog index   An index of photochemical smog based on the relationship of this type of smog and the meteorological conditions conducive to its formation.

soiling index   A numerical expression of the concentration of smoke in the atmosphere. It is measured by assessing the stain produced by an air sample passed through white filter paper.

spleen index   The proportion of individuals in a population that have enlarged spleens, as used in malaria surveys. This index is generally based on the examination of children, which has been found to be a useful indicator of malaria in the entire population.

splenometric index   An index indicating the amount of malarial infection in a particular district, equal to the product of the spleen rate by a standard measure of spleen enlargement.

superior facial index   See under FACIAL INDEX.

tension-time index   The product of heart rate and the time interval of ventricular systolic pressure.

therapeutic index   A measure of drug safety, given by the ratio of the median lethal dose (LD_{50}) divided by the median effective dose (ED_{50}). The larger the ratio, the safer the drug. This ratio, however, does not include allowance for the differences in distribution of the population about these median values, and may not show the differences between the doses required for effectiveness in most of the population and the dose required for toxicity in a few individuals. Also called *chemotherapeutic index, therapeutic ratio, curative ratio.*

thickness index   The ratio of the observed mean erythrocyte thickness to the normal value (2.1 μm). Also called *corpuscular thickness index.*

thoracic index   The relationship between the width and depth of the thorax: (maximum thoracic depth $\times$ 100)/maximum thoracic breadth.

tibiofemoral index   The relationship between the length of the tibia and the length of the femur: (maximum tibial length $\times$ 100)/maximum femoral length.

tibioradial index   The relationship between the length of the

tibia and the length of the radius: (maximum radial length $\times$ 100)/maximum tibial length.

trunk index   The relationship between the length and breadth of the trunk: (biacromial breadth $\times$ 100)/maximum sitting height at suprasternale.

urea index   AMBARD'S FORMULA.

ureosecretory index   AMBARD'S FORMULA.

uricolytic index   The ratio, expressed as a percentage, of urinary nitrogen derived from allantoin to that derived from allantoin plus uric acid. It reflects the capacity to metabolize uric acid into allantoin, a reaction determined by the enzyme uricase. Because they have virtually no uricase, humans have a uricolytic index near zero.

Vaughan's leukopenic index   An obsolete test for the presence of a food allergy in which a drop in the circulating total leukocyte count that occurs after ingestion of a foodstuff indicates the presence of hypersensitivity to that food.

ventilation index   A ratio of pulmonary ventilation per minute divided by the vital capacity. An outmoded term.

vertical index   ALTITUDINAL INDEX.

vital index   A measure of the extent to which a population reproduces itself, being the number of births during a specified period expressed as a percentage of the number of deaths. An obsolete term. Also called *birth-death ratio.*

volume index   A numerical expression of erythrocyte size, calculated by dividing percent of normal hematocrit by percent of normal erythrocyte count. The normal value is 1.0.

wet-bulb globe temperature index   An index for measuring outdoor thermal environments. It is calculated from the formula 0.2(globethermometer temperature) + 0.1(dry-bulb thermometer temperature) + 0.7(natural wet-bulb thermometer temperature). The latter temperature is measured with the wet-bulb thermometer exposed to natural air movements and unprotected from radiation. A modified formula, 0.7(natural wet-bulb thermometer temperature) + 0.3(globe thermometer temperature) is used for measuring indoor thermal environments. Abbreviation: WBGT

xanthoproteic index   XANTHOPROTEIC REACTION.

Youden's index   An index for rating the accuracy of diagnostic tests. The index is the figure obtained by subtracting one from the sum of the specificity and the sensitivity.

zygomaticoauricular index   The relationship between the biauricular and bizygomatic breadths of the skull: (maximum biauricular breadth $\times$ 100)/maximum bizygomatic breadth.

---

indican   The plant glucoside whose aglycon, indoxyl, is oxidized by air to yield the dye indigo.

indicanemia   The presence of indican of animal origin in the blood.

indicanorachia   Indican in the cerebrospinal fluid.

indicant   1 Providing an indication. 2 Something that serves as an indication, as a symptom that indicates a diagnosis.

indicanuria   [INDICAN + -URIA] The presence of excessive amounts of indican in the urine. Also called *glaucosuria, urocyanosis* (obsolete).

indicarmine   SODIUM INDIGOTINDISULFONATE.

indicarminum   SODIUM INDIGOTINDISULFONATE.

indicatio   [L, an indicating, valuing. See INDEX.]   INDICATION.

indication   [L *indicatio.* See INDICATIO.]   1 A symptom, sign, or circumstance that points to a specific treatment for an illness. Also called *indicatio.* 2 A mode of treatment indicated as appropriate or necessary based on an evaluation of the condition and history of the patient and the nature of his illness.

indicator   [L (from *indicatus,* past part. of *indicare* to show, reveal, + -*or* -OR), that which or one who indicates or values. See INDEX.] **1** INDEX. **2** MUSCULUS EXTENSOR INDICIS. **3** A substance used to produce color in response to a specific metabolic activity such as fermentation or acid production. **4** A strain of microorganisms used to test for the presence of a substance, as in bioautography. **5** A phage-sensitive strain used to test for release of a phage by a lysogenic strain.

anaerobic indicator   A solution whose appearance reflects the oxygen status of its environment.

biologic indicator   A plant or animal species characteristic of a certain state of pollution of surface waters. Three pollution "zones" have been described in terms of biologic indicators, the polysaprobic zone, the mesosaprobic zone, and the oligosaprobic zone.

complex indicator   Any stimulus arousing emotion because it has touched upon an unconscious conflict area of the subject.

dew point indicator   A device that measures the moisture content of a gas by recording the temperature at which condensation occurs as the vapor is cooled. Also called *dew point hygrometer.*

fluorescent indicator   An indicator that is labeled with fluorescein or some other fluorescent substance. It is used to localize materials in fluorescence microscopy or to permit titrimetric examination, under ultraviolet light, of materials that are turbid or highly pigmented in ordinary light.

health indicator   A statistical index or combination of indices intended to reflect the health status of a population. An indicator is usually concerned with morbidity and mortality rather than with the positive aspects of health.

oxidation-reduction indicator   A substance whose color changes with differences in oxidation potential. Also called *redox indicator.*

pH indicator   A substance that undergoes a color change with a change in pH. It is used in titration and as a means for visual estimation of the pH of solutions or substances.

proportional mortality indicator   The percentage of all deaths in a population during a given period that occur at age 50 years or over, proposed by WHO in 1957 as a simple but effective index to distinguish countries of differing levels of health.

radioactive indicator   RADIOACTIVE TRACER.

redox indicator   OXIDATION-REDUCTION INDICATOR.

universal indicator   A mixture of indicator substances compounded so that distinct colors will develop at different points along a range of pH values.

indices   Plural of INDEX.

indicophose [L *Indic(um)* a blue pigment from India, indigo + *o* + Gk *phōs* light, daylight]   A blue subjective light sensation.

indictment [L *indict(us),* past part. of *indicere* to denounce, enjoin + -MENT]   A written accusation presented to a court of law by a grand jury.

indifférence [French, indifference]

    belle indifférence   LA BELLE INDIFFÉRENCE.

    la belle indifférence   A situation seen in patients with conversion hysteria, where the patient exhibits an apparent lack of concern about the accompanying disabling symptoms. Also called *belle indifférence.*

indigency / medical indigency   The state of being medically indigent.

indigenous [L *indigen(a)* (masc. and fem.) inborn, native + -OUS]   Native to an area and not introduced by man.

indigent / medically indigent   Having inadequate financial resources to pay for or otherwise obtain medical care without depriving oneself or one's family of the other basic necessities of life.

indigestible   Not easily digested.

indigestion [L *indigestio* (from *in-* not + *digestio* a putting in order, digestion, from *digerere* to distribute, dispose) a nondisposing of things in order, indigestion]   **1** Inadequate or disordered digestion of food in the alimentary canal. **2** Gastric or abdominal discomfort experienced after eating. A popular usage.

acid indigestion   Indigestion attributed to excessive gastric acid secretion.

fat indigestion   Malabsorption or inadequate digestion of fats. See also STEATORRHEA.

gastric indigestion   The lack of proper digestion of food as a result of an abnormality or disorder of the stomach.

intestinal indigestion   The lack of proper digestion as a result of intestinal dysfunction.

sugar indigestion   Inadequate or ineffective digestion of sugars, often resulting in diarrhea.

indigitation [From L *indigitatus,* past part. of *indigitare* (origin unknown) to call upon, invoke (a deity), utter, declare. Erroneously associated in the sixteenth century with L *digitus* finger.]   An invagination, especially an intussusception.

indigo   A blue dye that was originally derived from plants of the genera *Isatis* and *Indigofera* by fermentation of the plant glucoside indican. It is now commercially obtained and is used in both histological and cytologic techniques as a counterstain. Also called *indigo blue.*

false indigo   BAPTISIA.

wild indigo   BAPTISIA.

indigo carmine   SODIUM INDIGOTINDISULFONATE.

indigodisulfonic acid   A dye used in some measurements of renal function, usually as the sodium salt known as indigo carmine.

indigopurpurine   A purple coloration present in the urine due to the presence of indoxyl sulphate, the conjugate of indoxyl derived from tryptophane.

indigotin $C_{16}H_{10}N_2O_2$. The main component of indigo.

indigotindisulfonate sodium   SODIUM INDIGOTINDISULFONATE.

indirubin   A red pigment sometimes seen in urine as a result of oxidation of indoxyl to isatin which then combines with unaltered indoxyl.

indirubinuria   The presence of indirubin in the urine, producing red urine.

indisposition [Middle English *indisposicioun* unfitness, prob. from *indisposes* unfitted, from *in-* not + *disposed* fitted]   A slight illness or feeling of being unwell. A popular usage.

indium [L *indicum* indigo]   A soft metallic element having atomic number 49 and atomic weight 114.82. It is found in ores of zinc and other metals. There are two naturally occurring stable isotopes. Some 20 radioactive isotopes are known. Indium has various technologic applications. Symbol: In

indium 111   The radioactive isotope of indium of atomic mass 111, having a half-life of 2.83 days and gamma ray energies of 171 and 245 keV. Symbol: ^{111}In

indium 113m   A radioactive form of indium, with a half-life of 1.7 hours, which decays by isomeric transition, emitting gamma rays of 391.7 keV. Indium 113m is generator-produced from the parent tin 113. When labeled to appropriate substances, it can be used for blood-pool, liver-spleen, lung, and brain scanning.

individualization [INDIVIDUAL + -*iz(e)* + -ATION]   The process of becoming an independent organism separated from the support of mother or surrogate or from a similar organism, as in the separation of conjoined twins.

individuation   **1** In embryology, an inductive process which results in the formation of complete or entire organic structures. **2** The behavioral principle that wholes emerge prior to partial patterns distinguishable as subunits of the total pattern; in popular usage, the gradual definition of an individual, as growth and experience combine to produce a unique person.   **3** Jung's treatment procedure which moves through successive layers of psychologic conflict to reach the inner core, the self.

Indocin   A proprietary name for indomethacin.

indocyanine green   A nontoxic, nonirritating dye used to measure hepatic excretory function. When injected intravenously, it is bound to plasma proteins. It is removed and excreted solely by hepatocellular action, with no enterohepatic recirculation. Plasma levels are measured spectrophotometrically at an absorbance peak of 805 nm. The normal plasma decay curve has a half-life of 3.8 minutes.

Indoklon   A proprietary name for flurothyl.

indolaceturia   The occurrence of indoleacetic acid in urine.

indole   The heterocyclic compound whose molecules contain a benzene ring fused to C-2 and C-3 of a pyrrole ring. It is not very basic, and when protonated by strong acids it loses its aromatic character and is then easily oxidized. Tryptophan and many alkaloids are substituted indoles.

indole-3-acetic acid   A plant hormone, or auxin, which evokes the faster lengthening of growing tips on the side away from light, and hence the phototropic response. It is derived from tryptophan. Also called *heteroauxin* (obsolete).

indolent   Characterized by slow progression, as of a disease process or a tumor of low malignancy.

indoline   2,3-Dihydroindole, the compound formed by reduction of the pyrrole ring of indole.

indoloemia   [Gk *Indo(s)* Indian + *loim(os)* plague, pestilence + -IA]   CHOLERA.

indoluria   [*indol(e)* + -URIA]   The presence of indoles in the urine. This is of uncertain clinical significance.

indolylacryloylglycine   A conjugate of indolyacrylic acid and glycine formed as a product of the colonic fermentation of tryptophan. It is found in abnormal quantities in the urine of patients with Hartnup disease following the ingestion of large doses of tryptophan.

indomethacin $C_{19}H_{16}ClNO_4$.   1-(4-Chlorobenzoyl)-5-methoxy-2-methyl-1H-indole-3-acetic acid. An agent with anti-inflammatory, antipyretic, and analgesic properties. It is used in the treatment of several types of arthritis, including rheumatoid arthritis, osteoarthritis of the hip, and gouty arthritis. It is given orally.

indophenol   **1** Any of a series of colored compounds of the quinone-imine group that do not readily form salts with mineral acids and whose halogenated substitution products are used as pH indicators, losing color in the reduced state.   **2** The specific compound consisting of the imine formed between *p*-benzoquinone and *p*-hydroxyaniline, the simplest of the indophenol series.

indophenol blue   *N*-(*p*-Dimethylaminophenyl)naphthoquinone monoimine. A blue compound formed by condensing *p*-nitroso-*N*,*N*-dimethylaniline with 1-naphthol.

indophenol oxidase   The enzyme responsible for forming an indophenol from a phenol and a *p*-diamine, now known to be cytochrome oxidase.

Indoplanorbis   A genus of freshwater pulmonate snails of the family Planorbidae, common in east Asia.

Indoplanorbis exustus   A widespread freshwater snail in Asia that serves as the first intermediate host of a number of parasites, such as *Schistosoma indicum* of horses, sheep, goats, dogs, and camels in India, *S. spindale* of cattle and buffalo in India, Sumatra, and Malaysia, *S. nasale* of cattle in India, as well as various echinostome flukes, including *Echinostoma malayanum,* reportedly found in man in Malaysia and Indonesia.

indoxole $C_{22}H_{19}NO_2$.   2,3-Bis(4-methoxyphenyl)-1-*H*-indole.

A substituted indole compound with anti-inflammatory and antipyretic properties.

indoxyl   2-Hydroxyindole. It is released from the plant glucoside indican by hydrolysis. It is oxidized by the air to the dye indigo. Some indoxyl is formed from tryptophan by intestinal bacteria and is excreted in the urine as its sulfate.

indoxylemia   The presence of indole oxidation products in the blood.

indoxyluria   [INDOXYL + -URIA]   Excessive indoxyl in the urine.

induced   Brought about, especially by intervention, as *induced labor.*

inducer   A small molecule that accelerates the transcription of particular genes by binding to a regulatory protein.

inductance   [See INDUCTION.]   The property of an electric circuit by which a changing current induces in the same or a neighboring circuit an electromotive force proportional to the rate of change of the current, expressed in henrys.

induction   [L *inductio* (from *inductus*, past part. of *inducere* to lead in, introduce, induce) a bringing or leading in or into, intention, induction]   **1** In embryology, the production of a specific morphogenetic effect, or the determination of the developmental fate of a cell or tissue, in the developing embryo through the influence of chemical substances (evocators) produced within and released by another cell or tissue.   **2** In microbiology, the process by which a foodstuff or metabolite stimulates the formation of a protein related to its metabolism. This is a major mechanism in enzyme adaptation.   **3** Any change in the composition or behavior of a cell in response to an environmental stimulus, such as lysis by ultraviolet activation of a potentially lytic prophage.   **4** That phase of inhalation anesthesia from the start to attainment of a surgical plane of anesthesia.   **5** The production of electric charge in a body by moving a second charged body near it.   **6** The production of magnetism in a body by moving a magnet near it.   **7** The voltage produced in a coil when the magnetic flux through it is varied.

induction of abortion   The stimulation of expulsive uterine contractions by artificial means to bring about abortion.

aerosol induction of sputum   Stimulation of sputum production by inhalation of an aerosol.

autonomous induction   Induction in which the cells which produce the inducing substance do not themselves become incorporated into the resultant tissue or organ so formed. Compare COMPLEMENTARY INDUCTION.

complementary induction   A particular type of induction in which the cells which produce the inducing substance become incorporated into the resultant tissue or organ so formed. Compare AUTONOMOUS INDUCTION.

enzyme induction   The increase in the rate of biosynthesis of an enzyme in response to a stimulus. It differs from, but is physiologically complementary to, the increase of activity of preexisting enzyme as a control mechanism.

induction of labor   The use of artificial means to bring about the onset of labor, as by artificial rupture of the fetal membranes or through the administration of oxytocic drugs.

magnetic induction   A quantity used as measure of the strength of a magnetic field, expressed in teslas. Also called *magnetic flux density, magnetoinduction.* Symbol: B

medical induction of labor   Induction of labor through the use of oxytocic drugs.

persistent induction   The induction of an active transport system that concentrates the inducer, thus permitting bacteria to maintain induced enzymes at inducer concentrations too low to initiate induction.

somatic induction   The production of new characters in succeeding generations through the influence of the cellular tissues of the parent on its own germ cells.

Spemann's induction The original demonstration of the controlling influence of localized parts of the early embryo on the morphohgenetic development of neighboring tissues or parts. This effect was later shown to be due to the production and diffusion of chemical substances (inductors) from these parts.

spinal induction The process in the spinal cord by which activity in one nerve cell or group of cells lowers the threshold of activity in other nerve cells.

surgical induction of labor Induction of labor by artificial rupture of the fetal membranes.

zygotic induction Conversion of prophage into vegetatively multiplying phage, induced by transfer from the repressive cytoplasm of a lysogenic donor to the nonrepressive cytoplasm of a recipient.

inductive Able to procure embryologic induction, as a group of cells or tissue.

inductogram [L *induct(us)*, past part. of *inducere* to lead or bring in + *o* + -GRAM] A rarely used term for RADIOGRAPH.

inductometer An instrument that measures the voltage induced in a conductor.

inductopyrexia ELECTROPYREXIA.

inductor [L (from *inductus*, past part. of *inducere* to lead in, introduce, induce, + -*or* -OR), one who persuades or induces] **1** A tissue which elaborates a chemical substance during embryonic development that determines the developmental fate of another cell or tissue. The ability of a cell or tissue to respond in this way is a demonstration of its competence. Also called *evocator, organizer.* **2** ORGANIZER. **3** A coil of wire, with or without a magnetic core, for introducing inductance into an electrical circuit.

gene inductor A substance, such as a nutrient, in the cell's environment which allows an operon to be transcribed. The inductor may function by the inactivation of a repressor protein.

inductorium A coil designed to produce high-voltage electrical discharges by induction for physiologic experiments.

inductotherm An instrument for elevating body temperature by using high-frequency current.

inductothermy The process of elevating body temperature by using an inductotherm.

indulin INDULIN BLACK.

indulin black A synthetic dye with a black guinone-imine chromatophore used as a background stain in the study of bacteria and in the staining of tissue of the central nervous system. Also called *indulin.*

indulinophil INDULINOPHILIC.

indulinophilic Having the property to be stained by the synthetic dye indulin black. Also *indulinophil.*

indurated Hardened, or characterized by an increase in consistency.

induration [Late L *induratio* (from L *induratus*, past part. of *indurare* to make hard, make shameless, from *in-* in, within + *durare* to harden, remain, last) a hardening] The hardening of normally soft tissues or organs due to inflammation or infiltration.

black induration Dark pigmentation and fibrosis of the lung due to anthracosis.

brawny induration Hardening of soft tissues caused by chronic inflammation.

brown induration Induration of the lung seen in chronic venous congestion.

fibroid induration CIRRHOSIS.

Froriep's induration A seldom used term for MYOSITIS FIBROSA.

granular induration Cirrhosis.

gray induration Induration of the lung due to fibrosis after pneumonia.

laminate induration A pallisade of lymphocytes and plasma cells in the corium, seen histologically in cases of syphilitic chancre. Also called *parchment induration.*

parchment induration LAMINATE INDURATION.

penile induration PEYRONIE'S DISEASE.

phlebitic induration Induration of the skin of the leg as a consequence of chronic phlebitis, occurring initially around phlebitic veins of the lower leg, but sometimes extending to form large plaques on legs with chronic venous insufficiency.

plastic induration PEYRONIE'S DISEASE.

plastic induration of penis PEYRONIE'S DISEASE.

red induration Induration of the lung seen in persisting pneumonia with vascular congestion.

rigid induration of the bladder neck MARION'S DISEASE.

indurative Characterized by or pertaining to induration.

indurescent Becoming hardened and thickened.

indusium INDUSIUM GRISEUM.

indusium griseum [NA] The dorsal continuation of the hippocampus, lying above the corpus callosum and continuous with the lower margin of the cingulate gyrus. Also called *hippocampal rudiment, hippocampus minor* (obsolete), *gyrus epicallosus, indusium.*

indwelling Remaining in place in the body, as to provide drainage or to allow administration of nutrients or drugs: said especially of a catheter or similar tubular implement.

-ine [noun suffix from French *-ine*, from L *-ina*, fem. of *-inus* of or belonging to] An ending of the names of many chemical substances, including amino acids and amines, but with no precise definition. It may also be part of some more complex suffixes, e.g. *-olidine*, which signifies a 5-membered saturated ring containing nitrogen.

inebriant Producing inebriation; intoxicating.

inebriation [Late L *inebriatio*, from L *inebriatus*, past part. of *inebriare* (from *in-* -IN[1] + *ebrius* one who has drunk up a vat) to make drunk] A stuporous state induced by ingesting an intoxicating substance, especially alcohol, characterized by motor incoordination and slurred speech; drunkenness.

inebriety [IN-[1] + English *ebriety*, from L *ebriet(as)* drunkenness + -Y] Repeated and pathologic abuse of intoxicants; habitual drunkenness.

inelastic Not elastic; inflexible.

Inermicapsifer A genus of tapeworms (family Linstowiidae), found in rodents and hyraxes in Africa. A few cases of human infection have been reported from *I. madagascariensis,* normally a parasite of rats.

inert Having little or no tendency to react chemically.

inertance [L *iners*, gen. *inertis* (from *in-* IN-[2] + *ars*, gen. *artis*, art, skill) without art, unskilled, inactive + -ANCE] In a fluid, the pressure difference divided by the rate of change of flow. It is also equal to the mass divided by the square of the cross-sectional area.

inertia [L (from *iners*, gen. *inertis*, without art, without skill, weak, insipid, from *in-* not + *ars*, gen. *artis*, the method, way, an art, faculty, from Gk *arō*, root of *arariskein* to join, fasten, fit), unskillfulness, sloth] **1** The property of matter that causes it to continue in a state of rest or uniform motion in a straight line unless acted upon by an external force. **2** A state of little or no action or movement.

chemical inertia The absence of reaction in a chemical system of substances that should theoretically react. It can result from imperfect contact, the presence of a gaseous film on an insulating solid, etc.

colonic inertia   The lack of strong colonic muscular activity, often resulting in colonic distention and subsequent constipation.

primary uterine inertia   Abnormal uterine contractions probably synonymous with the latent phase of labor or false labor but characterized by failure to progress in labor. Inherent musculature weakness or faulty innervation is felt to be etiologic if such contractions persist for prolonged periods of time. Also called *first-degree uterine incoordination*.

psychic inertia   FIXATION.

secondary uterine inertia   Abnormal uterine contractions characterized by poor intensity attributed to exhaustion of the uterine musculature due to protracted uterine activity. Also called *second-degree uterine incoordination*.

inertia uteri   UTERINE INERTIA.

uterine inertia   Abnormal contraction of the uterus during or just preceding labor. Also called *inertia uteri*.

inexcitability   The inability to respond to stimulation.

temporary postreflex inexcitability   Exhaustion Leading to abolition of the knee or ankle jerks after these reflexes have been elicited repetitively. This phenomenon may occur unduly rapidly in Parkinson's disease.

inexcitable   Incapable of responding to stimulation. Also *unirritable*.

in extremis [L *in* in + *extremis*, ablative pl. of *extremus* (superl. of *exter* outward, external) outermost, final]   At the point of death.

inf.   *infunde* (L, pour in).

infancy [L *infantia* inability to speak, infancy. See INFANT.]   The period from birth to about one year of age.

infant [L *infans*, gen. *infantis* (pres. part. of assumed *infari*, from *in*- not + *fari* to say, speak), speechless, young, little, childish; as substantive, a little child, infant]   A child from birth to about one year of age.

floppy infant   See under FLOPPY INFANT SYNDROME.

infant Hercules   A young male child exhibiting marked hypertrophy or pseudohypertrophy of skeletal muscles and therefore having the superficial and deceptive appearance of extraordinary muscular development. It is most often seen in Duchenne type muscular dystrophy, less often in myotonia congenita.

immature infant   A premature infant born before 27 weeks of gestational age measured from the first day of the last menstrual period.

liveborn infant   A fetus that is born alive.

mature infant   TERM INFANT.

newborn infant   NEONATE.

postmature infant   An infant born after 42 weeks of gestation measured from the first day of the last menstrual period. The fetus may show a normal growth rate or may be of a reduced birth weight with loss of soft tissue mass. Also called *post-term infant*.

post-term infant   POSTMATURE INFANT.

premature infant   An infant having a birth weight less than 2500 grams and born after a gestation period of less than 38 weeks from the first day of the last menstrual period. The low birth weight is a result of normal fetal growth for an abnormally short period of time. Also called *preterm infant*.

preterm infant   PREMATURE INFANT.

stillborn infant   An infant born without evidence of life.

term infant   An infant born between 38 and 42 weeks of gestational age measured from the first day of the last menstrual period and having a weight greater than 2500 grams. Also called *mature infant*.

infanticide [INFANT + *i* + -CIDE]   **1** The killing of an infant. The period of infancy as defined in such cases is usually designated as the time from birth through the first year of life, but varies slightly from jurisdiction to jurisdiction.   **2** One who commits infanticide.

infantile [L *infantilis* (from *infans*, gen. *infantis*, pres. part. of assumed *infari*, from *in*- not + *fari* to say, speak + -*ilis* -ILE[1])   pertaining to children, young]   **1** Of or characteristic of infants or infancy.   **2** Relating to behavioral or developmental characteristics like those of infancy.

infantilism [*infantil(e)* + -ISM]   The persistence of physical and/or mental characteristics of childhood into adult life.   ● In endocrinologic contexts, the term *infantilism* is outmoded.

Brissaud's infantilism   An outmoded term for INFANTILE MYXEDEMA.

celiac infantilism   INFANTILE CELIAC DISEASE.

dysthyroidal infantilism   Failure of growth and development in early life due to hypothyroidism, as in cretinism. An outmoded term.

hepatic infantilism   Infantilism associated with cirrhosis of the liver.

Herter's infantilism   INFANTILE CELIAC DISEASE.

hypophysial infantilism   An older term for HYPOPHYSIAL DWARFISM.

idiopathic infantilism   An older term for HYPOPHYSIAL DWARFISM.

intestinal infantilism   INFANTILE CELIAC DISEASE.

Lévi-Lorain infantilism   An outmoded term for HYPOPHYSIAL DWARFISM.

Lorain's infantilism   An outmoded term for HYPOPHYSIAL DWARFISM.

myxedematous infantilism   An older term for CRETINISM.

pancreatic infantilism   Growth failure due to deficient endocrine function of the pancreas, as uncontrolled diabetes mellitus in children, or subnormal exocrine activity, as in cystic fibrosis of the pancreas. An older term.

partial infantilism   A block in the development of an organ or part. A seldom used term.

pituitary infantilism   An older term for HYPOPHYSIAL DWARFISM.

proportionate infantilism   An older term for HYPOPHYSIAL DWARFISM.

pulmonary infantilism   The failure of a child to grow and develop as a result of chronic lung disease.

renal infantilism   Stunted growth due to renal osteodystrophy in the early years of life.

sexual infantilism   Failure of the secondary sex characters to develop, as in hypophysial dwarfism.

symptomatic infantilism   Infantilism due to any general or systemic developmental failure. A seldom used term.

thyroid infantilism   A seldom used term for CRETINISM.

toxemic infantilism   An obsolete term for INFANTILE CELIAC DISEASE.

universal infantilism   Dwarfism accompanied by failure of the secondary sex characters to develop, as in hypophysial dwarfism.   ● The term is applicable to many forms of dwarfism.

infantorium [English *infant* + L -*orium* -ORY]   A hospital for infants or the newborn. An outmoded term.

infarct [L *infarctus* (pref. *infartus*; past part. of *infarcire* or *infercire* to stuff or cram into, from *in*- into + *farcire* to fill up, stuff, cram; Gk *phrassein* to fence, defend, block up, fill) filled, filled up]   A discrete, usually wedge-shaped area of ischemic coagulative necrosis caused by interruption of blood flow. The apex of the wedge usually points toward the point of vascular occlusion.

anemic infarct   An infarct caused by arterial occlusion. They are distinctly pale in gross appearance because they result from ischemic coagulative necrosis affecting an organ with a single arterial blood supply. Also called *pale infarct, white infarct*.

aseptic infarct   BLAND INFARCT.

bilirubin infarct   An infarct containing bilirubin crystals found in the renal pyramids, usually in the newborn.

bland infarct   An infarct that is not contaminated by infectious microorganisms. Also called *aseptic infarct.*

Brewer's infarcts   Conical dark red areas seen on section of the kidney in pyelonephritis. They are not considered true infarcts.

calcareous infarct   An infarct that has undergone dystrophic calcification. An obsolete term.

cerebral infarct   An infarct of cerebral tissues. It may be either anemic or hemorrhagic. The cause is usually atherosclerotic occlusion with or without thrombosis or thromboembolism from a remote source. In their evolution, cerebral infarcts undergo liquefaction and cystic transformation with permanent loss of brain parenchyma.

cicatrized infarct   A healed infarct. A rarely used term.

cystic infarct   An infarct that has undergone liquefaction and cystic transformation as, for example, in old cerebral infarcts.

embolic infarct   An infarct caused by embolic occlusion of an artery.

hemorrhagic infarct   An infarct that appears red due to interstitial hemorrhage throughout the necrotic area. This is usually the result of venous occlusion or arterial occlusion in organs that have a double blood supply. It may also follow the reestablishment of blood flow after the ischemic tissue has undergone necrosis. Also called *red infarct, red softening.*

hepatic infarct   An infarct in the liver resulting from an inadequate blood supply, usually following the blockage of an artery or arteriole.

infected infarct   SEPTIC INFARCT.

inflammatory infarct   an incorrect and seldom used term for SEPTIC INFARCT.

kidney infarct   RENAL INFARCT.

mesenteric infarct   Necrosis of the intestine and mesentery resulting from the impairment of the intestinal blood supply within the mesentery.

pale infarct   ANEMIC INFARCT.

placental infarct   An area of ischemic necrosis located in the substance of a placenta.

pulmonary infarct   Dead lung tissue resulting from obstruction of its blood supply.

red infarct   HEMORRHAGIC INFARCT.

renal infarct   Necrosis secondary to ischemia due to interruption of arterial or venous circulation of the kidneys. Arterial obstruction usually is secondary to arteriosclerotic narrowing of a renal artery or to emboli. Obstruction of arcuate or larger arteries may cause infarction. Vasculitis, aneurysm, compression by tumors, or trauma also may precipitate renal infarcts. Venous thrombosis secondary to hypercoagulable states, dehydration, or some kidney diseases such as membranous glomerulonephritis also, on rare occasions, may contribute to renal infarction. Clinically, renal infarction is characterized by lumbar pain, transient proteinuria and hematuria, and renal function impairment. Renal infarction leads to scarring and contracted depressions. Also called *kidney infarct, renal apoplexy, infarcted kidney, renal infarction.*

septic infarct   An infarct that is contaminated by infectious microorganisms. Such infarcts may result from necrosis of a previously infected area, or by the seeding of a developing infarct with microorganisms contained in emboli of vegetations from infected heart valves. These infarcts commonly progress to abscess formation. Also called *infected infarct, inflammatory infarct (an incorrect and seldom used term).*

thrombotic infarct   An infarct that is due to vascular occlusion by a thrombus.

uric acid infarct   The presence of yellow streaks in the tips of the renal papillae of newborn infants. The streaks are caused by uric acid crystals in the terminal collecting ducts, but infarction is not present. This appears to be a normal physiologic condition of unknown explanation. • This term is inappropriate but nevertheless accepted.

white infarct   ANEMIC INFARCT.

infarctectomy [INFARCT + -ECTOMY]   A surgical procedure in which a localized area of necrotic or hypoperfused tissue is excised.

infarction [INFARCT + -ION]   The process of infarct formation.

acute myocardial infarction   The acute phase of a myocardial infarction.

anterior myocardial infarction   Myocardial infarction involving the anterior wall of the heart, revealed in the electrocardiogram by involving most of the leads from V_1 to V_6.

anterolateral myocardial infarction   Infarction affecting the lateral wall of the heart, revealed on the electrocardiogram by changes in V_5 and V_6 and in leads I and aVL.

anteroseptal myocardial infarction   Infarction involving the anterior wall and septum of the heart and revealed in the electrocardiogram by changes in V_1 to V_4.

apical myocardial infarction   Infarction involving the apex of the heart.

atrial myocardial infarction   Myocardial infarction involving one or both of the atria.

cardiac infarction   MYOCARDIAL INFARCTION.

diaphragmatic myocardial infarction   INFERIOR MYOCARDIAL INFARCTION.

high lateral myocardial infarction   Myocardial infarction involving the high lateral wall of the ventricle and sometimes only revealed in the electrocardiogram in leads such as aVL and the high lateral leads. Also called *lateral myocardial infarction.*

inferior myocardial infarction   Infarction involving the inferior surface of the myocardium and usually revealed on the electrocardiogram best in leads II, III, and aVF. It is usually due to occlusion of the right coronary artery, but may result from circumflex artery occlusion. Also called *diaphragmatic myocardial infarction, posterior myocardial infarction (incorrect and outmoded).*

inferolateral myocardial infarction   Infarction affecting both the inferior and lateral surfaces of the heart and revealed on the electrocardiogram by changes in leads II, III, aVF, V_5 and V_6.

lateral myocardial infarction   HIGH LATERAL MYOCARDIAL INFARCTION.

myocardial infarction   An acute necrotic process of the myocardium resulting from sudden loss of blood supply to the affected tissue. It is usually associated with thrombosis, but embolism, rupture of a plaque, and coronary arterial spasm may all be factors in its genesis. Also called *cardiac infarction.*

pituitary infarction   An acute vascular accident accompanying thrombus, embolus, or vasospasm of the blood vessels of the hypothalamic-adenohypophysial portal venous system, leading to ischemic necrosis with or without hemorrhage into the adenohypophysis, and sometimes also involving the neurohypophysis. The lesion characterizes the Sheehan syndrome. It may occur in five to ten percent of cases of pituitary tumor and in a small number of cases of diabetes mellitus. Other precipitating causes are anticoagulation therapy, radiotherapy of the pituitary fossa, and basilar fractures of the skull. Impairment of pituitary function is variable. The lesion may figure in the pathogenesis of empty-sella syndrome. The clinical syndrome associated with pituitary infarction is sometimes called pituitary apoplexy.

posterior myocardial infarction   **1** Infarction involving the posterior wall of the left ventricle. It is not readily visualized on the electrocardiogram but is often associated with lateral and inferior changes and also with the development of a dominant R wave in V_1. **2** An incorrect and outmoded term for INFERIOR MYOCARDIAL INFARCTION.

posterolateral myocardial infarction Infarction affecting posterior and lateral walls of the heart.

pulmonary infarction Infarction in a lung, commonly resulting from obstruction of the blood supply by an embolus.

renal infarction RENAL INFARCT.

right ventricular infarction Infarction involving the wall of the right ventricle. It is virtually always associated with an inferior myocardial infarction. Transient ST segment elevation may be seen in the right precordial leads.

septal myocardial infarction Infarction involving the interventricular septum. It usually produces changes in leads V_1 to V_4.

silent myocardial infarction Myocardial infarction occurring in the absence of the characteristic symptoms.

subendocardial infarction Infarction involving only that part of the myocardium which is adjacent to the endocardium.

through-and-through myocardial infarction TRANSMURAL MYOCARDIAL INFARCTION.

transmural myocardial infarction Infarction involving the full thickness of the myocardium. Also called *through-and-through myocardial infarction.* • The term *transmural* is sometimes used inaccurately to describe any infarction associated with pathological Q waves, which were at one time thought to indicate infarction through the full thickness, though it is now known that this is not necessarily the case.

infarctoid Resembling an infarct.

infaust [L *infaust(us)* (from *in-* IN-² + *faustus* auspicious, akin to *favere* to favor) unfortunate, unpropitious] Unfavorable; not propitious.

infect [L *infect(us),* past part. of *inficere* to infect. See INFECTION.] **1** To invade and become established in or on (the body of a host): said of pathogenic microorganisms and internal parasites, such as bacteria, viruses, fungi, protozoa, helminths, and sometimes arthropods. **2** To transmit an infection to; contaminate with an infectious agent.

infectible [INFECT + -IBLE] Capable of becoming infected.

infection [Late L *infectio* (from *infectus,* past part. of *inficere* to put into, mix, dye, color, tinge, spoil, infect, taint, from *in-* in, into + *facere* to make, do) an injurious affecting or infecting] **1** The process whereby pathogenic organisms become established and multiply in or on the body of a host. **2** The state resulting from this process, which often includes local or systemic disease with cellular or systemic injury.

abortive infection An infection which terminates before it has run its usual course.

aerial infection AIR-BORNE INFECTION.

agonal infection TERMINAL INFECTION.

air-borne infection Infection caused by microorganisms carried on droplets of moisture or particles suspended in the air and which usually gain access to the host through inhalation. Also called *aerial infection.*

apical infection Infection from the apex of a tooth. It may be acute (acute apical periodontal abscess or alveolar abscess), or it may be chronic (periapical granuloma or chronic apical abscess). The last may have a draining sinus. Apical infection was once thought to be a source of danger to the whole body but it is now considered that this danger is of importance only in persons with certain pathologic conditions, particularly conditions of the heart following rheumatic fever or heart surgery.

autochthonous infection Infection by organisms indigenous or native to the environment.

canine herpesvirus infection A severe viral disease with high mortality that particularly affects puppies from one to three weeks old.

***Capillaria philippinensis* infection** A nematode infection of the small intestine, occurring in humans in central Luzon in the northern Philippines and in Thailand. Infection can be massive, resulting in morphological jejunal mucosal changes which are associated with malabsorption, sometimes severe, and intestinal protein loss. Treatment is with thiabendazole or mebendazole. Untreated, there is significant mortality. Fish and rodents can be alternative hosts to man.

complex infection CONCURRENT INFECTION.

concurrent infection Simultaneous infections by two or more causative agents. Also called *complex infection.*

contact infection An infection resulting from direct contact with an infected person or animal. Also called *direct infection.* Compare INDIRECT INFECTION.

covert infection Any clinically inapparent infection, which may be either dormant or latent. Also called *inapparent infection, silent infection, subclinical infection.*

cross infection An infection spread from one person or animal to another person or animal. • The term is sometimes reserved for infections contracted in hospital.

cryptogenic infection An infection in which the origin or entry point of the causative agent is unknown.

cytomegalovirus infection CYTOMEGALIC INCLUSION DISEASE.

diaplacental infection Infection transmitted to the embryo or fetus through the placenta.

direct infection CONTACT INFECTION.

dormant infection An infection in which a pathogenic microorganism can be recovered from the host but is not at that time causing symptomatic disease in that individual. If the organism is shed the individual is called a carrier.

droplet infection An infection caused by the inhalation of liquid particles containing infective organisms.

dust-borne infection An infection caused by the inhalation of dust particles carrying pathogenic microorganisms.

ectogenous infection EXOGENOUS INFECTION.

***Ehrlichia* infection** CANINE EHRLICHIOSIS.

endogenous infection Infection by organisms already present in or on the host as components of its normal flora and fauna or as pathogens in a dormant state. Compare EXOGENOUS INFECTION.

exogenous infection An infection due to a pathogen which originated outside the body of the host. Also called *ectogenous infection.* Compare ENDOGENOUS INFECTION.

focal infection An infection which is confined to a single site, such as the prostatic bed or sinuses. • In the past certain systemic diseases were often erroneously attributed to focal infections.

germinal infection HEREDOINFECTION.

hand-borne infection Infection transmitted by contaminated hands.

herd infection Infection in a large group, either animal or human.

inapparent infection COVERT INFECTION.

indirect infection An infection transmitted by an intermediary such as food, water, air or fomes rather than transmitted directly from host to host. Compare CONTACT INFECTION.

intercurrent infection An infection occurring during the course of another infection.

invasive burn infection A bacterial or fungal infection of a burn wound that has invaded the living tissue under the area of necrotic skin. It is a harbinger of systemic sepsis.

latent infection **1** An infection in which the causative agent (the tubercle bacillus, for example) cannot be recovered from a patient although its continued presence can be inferred from continuing immunologic reactivity or, retrospectively, from the later emergence of overt illness. **2** An infection with certain viruses where the viral genome becomes integrated into the cellular DNA of host cells and is replicated at cell division but where no virions are formed. Such latent infections (for example, with herpes simplex virus) may become reactivated to give a productive infection.

local infection An infection confined to a definite area or tissue.

mass infection An infection caused by the introduction of a large number of pathogenic microorganisms into the circulation or tissues.

metastatic infection An infection which is transferred from an original focus to another part or parts of the body by conveyance of the pathogen in the blood or lymph.

mixed infection Concurrent infection at the same site by different kinds of pathogen, such as occurs commonly in open wounds.

nonspecific infection An infection in which a specific causative organism has not been identified.

nosocomial infection An infection acquired in a hospital or other health-care facility.

opportunistic infection An infection in a patient with diminished resistance by an organism that is ordinarily a harmless commensal.

phycomycotic infection MUCORMYCOSIS.

puerperal infection An infection of the birth canal occurring during the postpartum period.

pyogenic infection An infection due to pus-producing organisms, especially *Staphylococcus aureus* and *Streptococcus pyogenes*.

retrograde infection An infection that spreads up a tube or duct in a direction contrary to the flow of secretions or excretions.

secondary infection **1** An infection complicating a prior infection. **2** An infection complicating another underlying disease, as, for example, bacterial pneumonia occurring in a patient with bronchial carcinoma.

silent infection COVERT INFECTION.

slow infection An infection in which there is a lengthy period of incubation and/or latency (months or years) followed by the appearance of illness which may be severe and associated with life-threatening signs and symptoms. Such infections are usually of viral origin and include kuru, subacute sclerosing panencephalitis, progressive multifocal leukoencephalopathy, and scrapie in sheep.

subclinical infection COVERT INFECTION.

terminal infection An infection preceding and often causing death, typically as a complication of a chronic disease or of a debilitated or immunocompromised state. Also called *agonal infection.*

Vincent's infection NECROTIZING ULCERATIVE GINGIVITIS.

water-borne infection An infection in which the pathogenic organisms are transmitted by water used for drinking, bathing, or other purposes.

zoogenic infection **1** An infection of humans for which there is an animal reservoir. **2** Infection by an animal organism, as, for example, by a parasite helminth.

infectiosity The relative capacity of a microorganism to cause infection.

infectious **1** Caused by infection with pathogenic organisms: said of diseases. **2** Capable of causing an infection; infective. **3** Capable of being spread from one host to another, with or without direct contact.

infectiousness The state or quality of being able to cause or to communicate infection. Also called *infectivity.*

infective Capable of causing infection.

infectivity INFECTIOUSNESS.

infecundity [IN-² + FECUNDITY] Inability to become pregnant.

inference / statistical inference A generalization about a population or universe based on observations of one or more samples thought to be derived therefrom. For example, the recovery rate observed in a series of patients following therapy for a given disease might be inferred as applicable to all patients with that disease similarly treated.

inferent AFFERENT.

inferior [NA] Lower; near or toward the bottom: used in human anatomy with reference to the upright posture and designating structures or parts relatively near the caudal end of the body as compared with others nearer the cranial (cephalic) end.

inferiority Inadequacy; any type of adaptation of lower than the expected degree.

inferocostal INFRACOSTAL.

inferofrontal Denoting the inferior portion of the frontal lobe.

inferolateral Situated below and at or toward the side.

inferomedial Situated below and at or toward the median plane.

inferomedian Situated below and in the middle.

inferoparietal Denoting the inferior parietal lobule of the cerebrum, including the angular and supramarginal gyri.

inferoposterior Situated below and behind.

infertile [IN-² + FERTILE] Unable to conceive; unable to become pregnant; unable to sire offspring. Also *improcreant* (seldom used).

infertilitas [L, infertility. See INFERTILITY.] INFERTILITY.

infertility [L *in*- not + FERTILITY] **1** Inability to conceive; inability to become pregnant. **2** Inability to impregnate. Also called *infertilitas.*

primary infertility Infertility of a couple in which the woman has never conceived.

secondary infertility Current infertility of a couple although the woman has previously had at least one pregnancy.

infest [L *infest(are)* to attack, damage, infest] **1** To dwell in or invade (a habitat or locality): said of populations of disease vectors or other pestiferous organisms. **2** To dwell on or in (a host): said of populations of metazoan parasites, especially ectoparasites.

infestation [Late L *infestatio* (from L *infestatus*, past part. of *infestare* to molest) a molesting, infestation] The invasion or inhabitation of a place, or of a host organism, by a population of pests or parasites. • The term *infection*, rather than *infestation*, is normally used for the invasion or inhabitation of a host by noxious microorganisms, and many consider *infection* the only correct term to use in reference to larger internal parasites as well, limiting *infestation* of a host to surface-dwelling parasites such as lice, fleas, or ticks.

infestive Likely or apt to cause an infestation.

infibulation The practice of fastening by stitches or clasps the labia majora in girls or the prepuce in boys in order to prevent copulation.

infiltrate [L *in*- into + FILTRATE] The extracellular accumulation of fluids, cells, or other materials as a result of a pathologic process.

Assmann's tuberculous infiltrate ASSMANN FOCUS.

infraclavicular infiltrate A pulmonary infiltrate seen as an abnormal shadowing below the clavicles on the chest radiograph. It is typically of tuberculous origin.

leukemic infiltrate The accumulation of leukemic cells within any organ other than the bone marrow. Common sites include the liver, spleen, lymph nodes, and meninges.

infiltration [L *in-* into + FILTRATION] The extracellular accumulation within a tissue or organ of any material or cell type that is not a normal component of that tissue.

adipose infiltration FATTY INFILTRATION.

calcareous infiltration CALCIFICATION.

calcium infiltration CALCIFICATION.

cellular infiltration The permeation or accumulation of cells within tissues that are distant from their point of origin.

diffuse pulmonary infiltration Widespread accumulation of abnormal material in the lungs.

epituberculous infiltration Infiltration of lung tissue related to large tuberculous lymph nodes, seen in children with tuberculosis.

fatty infiltration The permeation or accumulation of fat in cells or tissues. Also called *adipose infiltration, lipolipoidosis* (obsolete).

gelatinous infiltration A type of lung infiltration characterized by a grayish appearance, seen in severe tuberculosis.

glycogen infiltration The vacuolated or empty appearance of the nucleus and/or cytoplasm of cells due to excessive accumulation of glycogen, as may occur in diabetes mellitus, glycogen-storage disease, or in patients receiving glucose-rich intravenous infusions.

inflammatory infiltration An accumulation of the effector cells of inflammation, mostly granulocytes, macrophages, and lymphocytes.

lymphocytic infiltration of skin A benign disorder of unknown origin that is characterized by the development of reddish brown plaques. Histologically it appears as an intense lymphocytic infiltration of the dermis. The condition affects men primarily. Also called *Jessner-Kanof disease.*

mineral infiltration The deposition of mineral salts in the tissues, such as calcium in dystrophic calcification.

paraneural infiltration PERINEURAL ANESTHESIA.

pulmonary infiltration with eosinophilia LÖFFLER SYNDROME.

round-cell infiltration The accumulation of mononuclear cells such as monocytes and lymphocytes, usually associated with viral infections and chronic inflammation.

sanguineous infiltration An infiltration of blood.

serous infiltration EDEMA.

urinous infiltration An infiltration of urine resulting from a break in the continuity of the wall of the ureter or bladder. It may be caused by cancer, trauma, or inflammation.

waxy infiltration An obsolete term for AMYLOIDOSIS.

infirm [L *infirm(us)* weak, feeble] Weak or enfeebled, as by a chronic condition: used especially of the old.

infirmary [Med L *infirmar(ium)* (from L *infirm(us)* not strong, infirm + *-arium* -ARY) infirmary + -Y] A primary or short-term medical care facility, usually serving a larger institution. • The term was originally applied to that part of a monastery or other institution where the sick or infirm were cared for, and is still used in this sense, as in *school infirmary,* but is now also used more broadly of much larger health-care facilities, even of large hospitals.

infirmity [L *infirm(itas)* weakness, feebleness + -ITY] **1** A condition that produces prolonged weakness or enfeeblement, especially in the aged. **2** Weakness; feebleness.

inflame To cause or to undergo inflammation.

inflamed Affected by inflammation.

inflammation [L *inflammatio* (from *inflammatus,* past part. of *inflammare* to set on fire, excite, rouse, from *in-* in + *flamma* flame, fire, ardor) an inflaming, kindling, inflammation] The localized response of vascularized tissues to injury caused by chemical, physical, or biological agents. Clinically, the cardinal

signs of inflammation include redness, swelling, heat, pain, loss of function, and fever. Events that follow injury include vasodilation, stasis, leukocytic margination and emigration, and exudation of leukocytes and plasma. The purpose of inflammation is to dilute, contain and destroy the injurious agent. The exact nature of this response, and the healing that follows it, depend on several factors, including the nature and extent of the injury, the tissue injured, and the responsiveness of the organism.

acute inflammation Inflammation of sudden onset, usually characterized by the cardinal signs (swelling, heat, redness, pain, and fever) clinically, and by predominately vascular and exudative responses pathologically.

adhesive inflammation Inflammation in which the amount of fibrin in the exudate is sufficient to stimulate, in the healing stage, the formation of fibrous adhesions between adjacent structures such as the pleural or pericardial surfaces.

allergic inflammation Inflammation resulting from a hypersensitivity reaction.

alterative inflammation DEGENERATIVE INFLAMMATION.

atrophic inflammation A form of chronic inflammation that results in excessive fibrous tissue formation that retracts and atrophies and compresses the intervening parenchymal tissue. Also called *fibroid inflammation* (seldom used), *sclerosing inflammation.*

bacterial inflammation Inflammation caused by bacterial infection.

catarrhal inflammation Inflammation of a mucous membrane characterized by excess mucin production, resulting in a copious mucous discharge, as in the common cold. A seldom used term.

chemical inflammation Inflammation due to a chemical injury to tissues.

chronic inflammation Inflammation that is persistent over time, due to the continuation of an acute stimulus, repeated bouts of acute inflammation, or the continuation over time of a low-grade, subclinical focus. It is characterized by mononuclear cell infiltration and the proliferation of fibroblasts, and frequently leads to scarring.

cirrhotic inflammation Atrophy of an organ or part as a result of chronic inflammation. An obsolete term.

croupous inflammation Pseudomembranous inflammation of the larynx, which may extend into the trachea and bronchi. A seldom used term.

degenerative inflammation A form of inflammation characterized by degenerative cellular changes in parenchymal cells, including frank necrosis, and by little or no exudation. It is seen in response to intracellular injury by agents such as viruses and chemicals. A seldom used term. Also called *alterative inflammation.*

diffuse inflammation Inflammation that involves most of an organ or tissue in a homogeneous manner.

disseminated inflammation Inflammation affecting several distinct foci throughout the body.

exudative inflammation Inflammation that is characterized principally by an exudate, which may be serous, serofibrinous, fibrinous, or mucous.

fibrinopurulent inflammation A form of acute inflammation whose exudate is mainly composed of fibrin and pus.

fibrinous inflammation Inflammation characterized by an exudate containing large amounts of fibrin.

fibroid inflammation A seldom used term for ATROPHIC INFLAMMATION.

focal inflammation Inflammation that is localized in a discrete area.

granulomatous inflammation Chronic inflammation characterized by granuloma formation and the presence of giant cells, as in tuberculosis.

hyperplastic inflammation A form of chronic inflammation associated with an exaggerated repair process that often results in abundant fibrovascular scar tissue. Also called *plastic inflammation* (obsolete), *productive inflammation*, *proliferous inflammation*.

hypertrophic inflammation Inflammation characterized by an increase in size of the cellular elements of the affected tissue.

immune inflammation Inflammation resulting from an immune response.

interstitial inflammation Inflammation of the stroma, or interstitium, of an organ with relative sparing of the parenchymatous elements.

metastatic inflammation Inflammation that is spread to distant sites via hematogenous or lymphatic routes. A rarely used term.

necrotic inflammation Inflammation characterized by extensive necrosis of the affected tissue.

obliterative inflammation Inflammation that results in the obliteration or replacement of a structure with scar tissue.

parenchymatous inflammation Inflammation of the parenchymal cells of an organ, with relative sparing of its stromal connective tissue framework.

plastic inflammation An obsolete term for HYPERPLASTIC INFLAMMATION.

productive inflammation HYPERPLASTIC INFLAMMATION.

proliferous inflammation HYPERPLASTIC INFLAMMATION.

pseudomembranous inflammation Acute inflammation of a mucosal surface that is characterized by the formation of a friable membrane on the affected mucosa. The membrane is composed of precipitated fibrin, polymorphonuclear leukocytes, and necrotic epithelial cells. This response is the result of powerful necrotizing toxins, such as diphtheria toxin.

purulent inflammation SUPPURATIVE INFLAMMATION.

sclerosing inflammation ATROPHIC INFLAMMATION.

serofibrinous inflammation Inflammation characterized by a serous exudate containing a relatively large amount of fibrin.

seroplastic inflammation Inflammation characterized by both a hyperplastic response of the affected tissue, and a serous exudate. An obsolete term.

serous inflammation Inflammation characterized by an exudate comprised mostly of serum and lacking significant cellular infiltration.

simple inflammation Inflammation devoid of distinguishing features such as pus formation.

specific inflammation Inflammation that is caused by a single, identified agent, usually a microorganism.

subacute inflammation Inflammation that is intermediate between acute and chronic in the duration and characteristics of the response.

suppurative inflammation Inflammation that is characterized by pus formation, such as that caused by pyogenic bacteria. Also called *purulent inflammation*.

toxic inflammation Inflammation caused by a poison, which may be bacterial products, such as exotoxins, or chemical compounds, such as chlorinated hydrocarbons.

traumatic inflammation Inflammation caused by a mechanical injury to tissues.

ulcerative inflammation Inflammation accompanied by sloughing of the inflamed necrotic tissue, resulting in a local defect, or ulceration, in the surface of the affected area.

inflammatory Characterized by or resulting from inflammation.

inflation [L *inflatio* (from *inflatus*, past part. of *inflare* to inflate, cause to swell) an inflating] **1** The condition of being distended, as with a gas or fluid. **2** The process of becoming distended.

inflator A device for injecting air, gases, or fumes into a tissue or organ. It is used with formalin fumes to fix tissue for macroscopic examination.

inflected INFLEXED.

inflection The act of bending inward or the state of being bent inward. Also called *inflexion*.

inflexed Bent or curved inward. Also *inflected*.

inflexion INFLECTION.

inflorescence [New L *inflorentia* (from Late L *inflorescens*, gen. *inflorentis*, pres. part. of *inflorescere* to begin blossoming, from *in-* IN- + *flos*, gen. *floris*, a flower; + *-ia* -Y) a flowering] **1** A flower cluster. **2** The definite arrangement of flowers on the stalk that is characteristic of a given species.

inflow The adequacy of arterial perfusion into an arterial segment.

nervous inflow Afferent neural activity. Also called *nervous influx*.

influents [L *influens*, gen. *influentis*, pres. part. of *influere* to flow or run into, + *s*] The animals present in an ecological community and which exert an influence on the dominant species in the community.

influenza [Italian (from Med L *influentia* influence, from *influens*, gen. *influentis*, pres. part. of L *influere* to flow or run into), influence, influenza, epidemic] An acute respiratory disease of viral origin which is distributed worldwide and often occurs in widespread epidemics. It is characterized by fever, headache, myalgia, and prostration and occurs with rapid onset. Complications such as bronchitis and bacterial pneumonia are common. Two serologically distinct viruses cause the disease, influenza virus A and influenza virus B. These viruses, particularly A, periodically undergo changes in antigenic composition and as a result, world populations become newly susceptible to the disease. New serologic types and the illnesses they cause are designated according to where they are first identified, for example, Hong Kong influenza, Asian influenza and Russian influenza. Also called *flu* (popular), *epidemic catarrhal fever* (outmoded), *epidemic rheuma* (outmoded), *grippe* (older term), *grip* (older term), *la grippe (French)*.

influenza A Influenza caused by a serotype of the type A influenza virus. It is the most widespread and frequently occurring influenza type.

avian influenza A worldwide disease of many avian species, caused by one of the type A avian influenza viruses. The disease varies greatly in severity, from mild to one with sudden onset and high mortality. Main signs are respiratory, with dyspnea, oral and nasal mucoid discharge, and edema of the head and neck. In mild forms, decreased egg production and fertility are observed. Also called *fowl plague* (obsolete), *avian plague* (obsolete), *chicken pest* (obsolete), *fowl pest* (obsolete).

influenza B Influenza caused by the type B influenza virus. Although less frequently a cause of epidemics than influenza A, it produces illness indistinguishable from that produced by influenza A and it contributes to excess mortality. It is also associated as an antecedent infection with the Reye syndrome.

influenza C A mild respiratory infection caused by the type C influenza virus and resembling the common cold. This illness is not influenza in the clinical or epidemiological sense of the term.

clinical influenza An infection which clinically resembles influenza but for which the specific pathogen has not been identified. It is characterized by the abrupt onset of fever, headache, muscle ache, and cough in winter months.

endemic influenza Influenza occurring in localized, usually seasonal, outbreaks. It tends to be less severe than the epidemic disease. Also called *influenza nostras*.

epidemic influenza Influenza occurring in large numbers of people in a given region or area over a period of a few weeks or months.

equine influenza An acute, typical mild influenzal pneumonia of horses caused by either of two subtypes of influenza virus type A.

influenza lymphatica INFECTIOUS MONONUCLEOSIS.

influenza nostras ENDEMIC INFLUENZA.

pandemic influenza Influenza that spreads in waves worldwide, for example, the influenza pandemic of 1918 in Europe and America.

Spanish influenza SWINE INFLUENZA.

summer influenza of Italy An outmoded term for SANDFLY FEVER.

swine influenza An acute influenzal illness caused by influenza A virus, subtype Hsw1N1. It affects swine, is transmissible to man, and is often highly contagious among members of these two populations. This particular type of influenza was responsible for the great pandemic of 1918–1919, which killed 21 000 000 persons worldwide in three waves of disease. Reports of isolated cases of human infection and a small outbreak among recruits at a U.S. military base in 1975–1976 prompted development of a vaccine and a national immunization program. However, the infection did not spread and no epidemics occurred. Also called *Spanish influenza.*

influenzal Pertaining to influenza.

influx / nervous influx NERVOUS INFLOW.

infold [IN-¹ + *fold*] To fold inward so as to be self-enclosing, either surgically (as for a lesion) or developmentally (as an embryonic structure).

information [L *informatio* (from *informatus*, past part. of *informare* to shape, describe) an idea, first draft]

genetic information GENETIC CODE.

sensory information Afferent input to the central nervous system, essential for sensory experience.

infra- [L *infra* (for *infera*) below, beneath, under] A prefix meaning below, beneath.

infra-alveolar 1 Below an alveolus. 2 Below the alveolar part of the mandible.

infra-auricular Below the ear pinna.

infra-axillary Below the axilla.

infrabulge [INFRA- + *bulge*] The undercut part of an axial tooth surface, i.e. the part apical to the height of contour.

infracardiac Below the heart or the level of the heart.

infracerebral Beneath the cerebrum.

infraclass [INFRA- + *class*] A taxonomic subdivision of a subclass.

infraclavicular Below the clavicle. Also *subclavicular.*

infraclavicularis A rare variant of the pectoralis major muscle in which an upper slip of the clavicular portion is fused with the deltoid muscle or its fascia.

infraclinoid Below any clinoid process of the sphenoid bone.

infraclusion [INFRA- + *(oc)clusion*] The failure of a tooth to erupt fully to the height of its neighbors. Also called *infraocclusion, infraversion.*

infracommissure One or several commissures of the ventral portion of the hypothalamus. An outmoded term.

infracondylism [INFRA- + *condyl(e)* + -ISM] Deviation downwards of the condyles of the mandible.

infraconstrictor An outmoded term for MUSCULUS CONSTRICTOR PHARYNGIS INFERIOR.

infracortical Beneath the cortex of an organ; subcortical.

infracostal Below a rib or the ribs. Also *inferocostal.*

infracotyloid Below the acetabulum.

infraction [L *infractio* (from *infractus*, past part. of *infringere*

to break, break into pieces, dishearten, interrupt) a breaking into pieces, weakening, dejection] INCOMPLETE FRACTURE.

Freiberg's infraction KÖHLER SECOND DISEASE.

infracture INCOMPLETE FRACTURE.

infradentale [INFRA- + L *dentale*, neut. sing. of *dentalis* pertaining to teeth, from *dens*, gen. *dentis*, tooth + *-alis* -AL] A cephalometric point situated at the highest point on the gingiva between the two lower central incisor teeth. Also called *symphysion.*

infradiaphragmatic SUBPHRENIC.

infraduction [INFRA- + L *ductus*, past part. of *ducere* to lead, draw, carry along] The rotation of one eye downward.

infrageniculate 1 Below the knee. 2 Below the geniculum of the facial nerve.

infragenual INFRAPATELLAR.

infraglenoid Below the glenoid cavity of the scapula. Also *subglenoid.*

infraglottic Below the glottis. Also *subglottic.*

infrahyoid Below the hyoid bone. Also *subhyoid, subhyoidean.*

infrainguinal Below the inguinal region.

inframamillary Below the nipple of the breast.

inframammary Below the mammary gland or the breast, submammary.

inframandibular Below the mandible; submandibular.

inframarginal Below any margin or border.

inframaxillary Below the maxilla; submaxillary. • The term was formerly used to refer to either the mandibular or the inframandibular area.

infranatant [INFRA- + L *natans*, gen. *natantis*, pres. part. of *natare* to swim, float, be overflowed with water] 1 Denoting a fluid that, because of its greater density, settles below a layer of solids or other fluid after the mixture is subjected to centrifugation or sedimentation by gravity. 2 An infranatant fluid. For defs. 1 and 2 also *subnatant.* Compare SUPERNATANT.

infranuclear Denoting an axonal process originating in a nuclear neuronal aggregate, especially with respect to the functional changes resulting from interruption of motor nerves, in contrast to damage to the cell bodies and the descending axons impinging upon them.

infraoccipital Below the occipital bone or the occipital region of the head; suboccipital.

infraocclusion INFRACLUSION.

infraorbital Located below the orbit. Also *suborbital.*

infrapatellar Below the patella, referring particularly to the infrapatellar synovial fold and its contained pad of fat. Also *infragenual, subpatellar.*

infraphysiologic Of or relating to reduced functional activity. A seldom used term.

infraplacement [INFRA- + PLACEMENT] Displacement of a tooth downwards.

infrapsychic [INFRA- + PSYCHIC] Below the level of consciousness.

infrapubic SUBPUBIC.

infrared [INFRA- + RED] That portion of the electromagnetic spectrum having wavelengths longer than the red part of the visible spectrum and shorter than microwaves, from 0.77 to 300 micrometers.

long-wave infrared Infrared radiation having wavelengths farthest from the visible spectrum, 1.5 to 300 micrometers.

short-wave infrared Infrared radiation having wavelengths closest to those of the visible spectrum, from 0.77 to 1.5 micrometers.

infrascapular Below the scapula.

infrasonic Relating to infrasound; having a frequency below 20 hertz.

infrasound [INFRA- + SOUND] Wave motion with a frequency too low (below about 20 hertz) to be perceived as sound. Adjective: infrasonic.

infraspecific [INFRA- + SPECIFIC] Pertaining to a category of organisms within a species, as a variety or subspecies.

infraspinous Below any spinous process or spine, such as of the scapula or of a vertebra. Also *subspinous*.

infrasplenic Below the spleen.

infrastapedial Below the stapes.

infrasternal Below the sternum.

infrastructure / implant infrastructure The part of an oral implant which is embedded in the bone or covered with mucoperiosteum. Also called *implant substructure*.

infratemporal Below the temporal fossa of the skull.

infratemporale [INFRA- + Late L *temporale*, neut. sing. of *temporalis* (from L *tempus*, gen. *temporis*, the temple of the head + *-alis* -AL) pertaining to the temple of the head] A craniometric point situated on the base of the skull at the point of maximum medial convexity on the sutural line between the temporal bone and the greater wing of the sphenoid. The distance between the two points gives a minimum breadth of the skull base.

infratentorial Situated below the tentorium cerebelli in the posterior cranial fossa.

infrathoracic Below the thorax.

infratonsillar Below the palatine tonsil.

infratracheal Below the trachea.

infratrochlear Below a trochlea, particularly that of the superior oblique muscle of the eye.

infratubal Below a tube.

infraturbinal CONCHA NASALIS INFERIOR.

infraumbilical Below the umbilicus.

infravaginal Below the vagina.

infraversion [INFRA- + VERSION] 1 The downward turning of both eyes simultaneously. 2 INFRACLUSION.

infravesical Below the urinary bladder.

infrazygomatic Below the zygomatic, or cheek, bone.

infriction An obsolete term for INUNCTION.

infundibula Plural of INFUNDIBULUM.

infundibular 1 Pertaining to, resembling, or having the characteristics of an infundibulum. 2 Denoting the infundibulum hypothalami.

infundibulectomy [*infundibul(um)* + -ECTOMY] Excision of the infundibular region of the right ventricle in subvalvar pulmonary stenosis, especially in the tetralogy of Fallot.
Brock's infundibulectomy TRANSVENTRICULAR CLOSED VALVOTOMY.

infundibuliferous Bearing an infundibulum.

infundibuliform Funnel-shaped; cone-shaped.

infundibuloma [*infundibul(um)* + -OMA] A tumor of the infundibulum of the pituitary.

infundibulo-ovarian Pertaining to the infundibulum of the uterine tube and the ovary.

infundibulopelvic Pertaining to an infundibulum and a pelvis, such as the expanded calix of the kidney and the renal pelvis, or the infundibulum of the uterine tube and the lateral wall of the pelvis.

infundibulum [L, a funnel] 1 Any funnel-shaped structure or passage. 2 INFUNDIBULUM HYPOTHALAMI. 3 CONUS ARTERIOSUS.
cardiac infundibulum CONUS ARTERIOSUS.

crural infundibulum An outmoded term for CANALIS FEMORALIS.

infundibulum crurale An outmoded term for CANALIS FEMORALIS.

ethmoidal infundibulum INFUNDIBULUM ETHMOIDALE.

ethmoidal infundibulum of cavity of nose INFUNDIBULUM ETHMOIDALE.

infundibulum ethmoidale [NA] A deep, crescentic groove in the lateral wall of the middle nasal meatus, formed by the medial surface of the ethmoidal labyrinth. The groove lies anterior to hiatus semilunaris, below bulla ethmoidalis, and above the uncinate process. At its middle it receives the ostium of the maxillary sinus, while anteriorly are the openings of the anterior ethmoidal cells and the opening of either the frontal sinus or the frontonasal duct. It may end blindly in the anterior ethmoidal cells. Also called *ethmoidal infundibulum of cavity of nose, ethmoidal infundibulum of ethmoid bone, infundibulum of frontal air sinus, infundibulum of frontal sinus, infundibulum of nose, infundibulum nasi, ethmoidal infundibulum.*

ethmoidal infundibulum of ethmoid bone INFUNDIBULUM ETHMOIDALE.

infundibulum of fallopian tube INFUNDIBULUM TUBAE UTERINAE.

infundibulum of frontal sinus 1 FRONTONASAL DUCT. 2 Infundibulum ethmoidale, when the frontonasal duct is absent.

infundibulum of frontal air sinus INFUNDIBULUM ETHMOIDALE.

infundibulum of heart CONUS ARTERIOSUS.

infundibulum of hypophysis INFUNDIBULUM HYPOTHALAMI.

infundibulum hypothalami [NA] The funnel-shaped, hollow stalk of the posterior lobe of the pituitary gland, extending forward from the rostral tuber cinereum of the hypothalamus. Also called *hypophysial stalk, neural stalk, infundibulum of hypophysis, infundibulum of hypothalamus, infundibulum, peduncle of hypophysis* (obsolete), *pituitary stalk, infundibular nucleus, infundibular process.*

infundibulum of hypothalamus INFUNDIBULUM HYPOTHALAMI.

infundibula of kidney CALICES RENALES MINORES.

infundibulum of lacrimal duct The initial vertical segment of each lacrimal canaliculus that ends at an ampulla at the angle before continuing in a somewhat sloping horizontal section. An outmoded term.

infundibulum of lung INFUNDIBULUM PULMONIS.

infundibulum nasi INFUNDIBULUM ETHMOIDALE.

infundibulum of nose INFUNDIBULUM ETHMOIDALE.

infundibulum pulmonis Any of the ductuli alveolares in the substance of the lung. Also called *infundibulum pulmonum, infundibulum of lung.*

infundibulum pulmonum INFUNDIBULUM PULMONIS.

infundibula renum An outmoded term for CALICES RENALES MINORES.

infundibulum of Scarpa The cavity formed at the lowest part of an artificial anus by progressive contraction of the septum between the two intestinal orifices. It is created to stabilize the evacuation of the intestinal contents. An outmoded term.

infundibulum tubae uterinae [NA] The funnel-shaped dilatation at the lateral, or abdominal, end of the uterine tube, from the margins of which the fimbriae diverge. Also called *infundibulum of uterine tube, infundibulum of fallopian tube.*

infundibulum of urinary bladder FUNDUS VESICAE URINARIAE.

infundibulum of uterine tube INFUNDIBULUM TUBAE UTERINAE.

infused Placed in an aqueous or other suitable solution, as a substance, to extract the soluble portion.

infusible 1 Incapable of being melted or fused. 2 Capable of being infused.

infusion [L *infusio* (from *infusus*, past part. of *infundere* to pour in or into, impart, instill) a pouring in or into, imparting] 1 The addition of water or other suitable liquid to a substance to obtain an extract of its soluble components. 2 The steeping of a therapeutic agent in order to extract its medicinally active ingredients. 3 The administration of a fluid other than blood into a vein for therapeutic purposes, e.g., the intravenous administration of saline. 4 A solution containing the water-soluble principles of a vegetable drug. Also called *infusum*. 5 A solution to be administered intravenously by infusion for therapeutic purposes.
　amniotic fluid infusion AMNIOTIC FLUID EMBOLISM.
　cold infusion The extraction of a drug or drug source with cold water to obtain the active material.
　drop infusion Administration of a medication, such as an intravenous fluid, by slow, drop-by-drop injection.
　saline infusion The procedure of introducing saline solution into the body parenterally.

infusodecoction A preparation containing both a decoction and an infusion of a source of a medicinal material.

infusor [L *infus(us)*, past part. of *infundere* to pour in or into + -OR] A device that slowly infuses liquids into a vein or the parenchyma.

Infusoria [New L (from *infusoria*, neut. pl. of *infusorius*, pertaining to infusions, from L *infus(us)*, past part. of *infundere* to pour into, + -*orius* -ORY)] An outmoded term for CILIATA.

infusum INFUSION.

-ing [Middle English *-ing*, *-inge*, irreg. from Old English *-ende*, suffix indicating pres. part. of verbs; also Old English *-ing*, *-ung*, suffix forming nouns and gerunds from verbs] A suffix used to indicate the present participle in verbs and to form nouns and gerunds from verbs with the meaning of an act or result of doing (the action expressed in the verb).

ingesta [L, neut. pl. of *ingestus*, past part. of *ingerere* to carry] Material that has been swallowed or is intended for swallowing. Also called *ingestant*.

ingestant INGESTA.

ingestion [Late L *ingestio* (from L *ingestus*, past part. of *ingerere* to carry) a carrying or pouring in] The process of taking materials into the gastrointestinal tract through the mouth.

ingestive Of or relating to ingestion.

ingluvies [L, the maw, crop, or gorge of a bird] 1 The crop of a bird. 2 A seldom used term for RUMEN.

Ingrassia [Giovanni Filippo *Ingrassia*, Italian anatomist, 1510–1580] 1 Ingrassia's process, processus of Ingrassia, apophysis of Ingrassia. See under ALA MINOR OSSIS SPHENOIDALIS. 2 Wings of Ingrassia. See under WINGS OF SPHENOID BONE.

ingravescent Becoming more severe.

ingravidation IMPREGNATION.

ingrowth A process progressing inward from the surface.
　epithelial ingrowth Invasion of the interior of the eye by surface tissue cells that enter at the site of a wound or incision.

inguen GROIN.

inguina Plural of INGUEN.

inguinal Pertaining to the groin, or inguen.

inguinoabdominal Pertaining to or located in the groin and the abdomen.

inguinocele A pathologic swelling found in the groin or inguinal region.

inguinocrural Pertaining to or located in the groin and the thigh.

inguinodynia [L *inguen*, gen. *inguinis*, the groin, a swelling in the groin + -ODYNIA] Pain in the groin.

inguinointerstitial Located or occurring in the tissues of the groin.

inguinolabial Pertaining to or located in the groin and the labium majus.

inguinoscrotal Pertaining to or located in the groin and the scrotum.

INH A proprietary name for isoniazid.

inhalant An agent or medicinal substance that is administered in a vaporous form into the upper respiratory passages. Also *inhalent*.
　antifoaming inhalant A medicinal agent administered in the form of a vapor for the purpose of preventing the accumulation of foam in the respiratory passages of patients suffering from pulmonary edema.

inhalation 1 The process of drawing materials into the lungs through the respiratory passages. 2 An agent suitable for administration through the respiratory passages into the lungs; inhalant.
　smoke inhalation A syndrome that occurs following inhalation of the by-products of combustion. These by-products, besides carbon monoxide are tissue-toxic, and can produce severe respiratory distress and pulmonary damage. Diagnosis can be made from history of closed space fire and elevated carbon monoxide levels. The syndrome is particularly lethal in combination with cutaneous burns, approximately doubling the mortality for burns of any size.

inhale [L *in-* in + *halare* to breath, exhale] To draw materials into the lungs through the mouth or nasal passages. Also *inspire*.

inhalent INHALANT.

inhaler [*inhal(e)* + -ER] 1 A device to administer medicinal agents in a vapor phase into the respiratory system by inhalation. 2 A mask or face covering that prevents smoke or other particulate matter from entering the respiratory tract by inhalation. It may also be used to protect against breathing cold or damp air.
　Clover's inhaler CLOVER'S CHLOROFORM VAPORIZER.
　EMO inhaler An EMO ether vaporizer with attachments for inhalation anesthesia. Also called *Oxford inhaler*.
　ether inhaler A device used to vaporize ether for inhalation anesthesia.
　Junker inhaler A device once used to vaporize chloroform for inhalation anesthesia. Also called *Junker apparatus, Junker bottle*.
　Morton's inhaler The original ether inhaler. It was first demonstrated in general anesthesia in Boston on October 16, 1846.
　Oxford inhaler EMO INHALER.
　Snow's inhaler An ether inhaler formerly used with an ether or chloroform vaporizer, where a constant vapor pressure was assured by a water jacket encircling the anesthetic being vaporized, thus maintaining constant temperature. This inhaler and similar ones were pioneering devices used originally in Britain.

inheritance [L *in-* in + *hereditans*, pres. part. of *hereditare* to inherit] Those characters which are transmitted from parent to offspring through the genes. Also called *transmission*.
　inheritance of acquired characteristics HOMOTROPIC INHERITANCE.
　alternative inheritance The transmission to offspring of phenotypes found in only one of the parents. An obsolete term.
　amphigonous inheritance A seldom used term for BIPARENTAL INHERITANCE.
　autosomal inheritance The transmission of a phenotype determined by a gene located on an autosome. Also called *autosomal heredity*.

biparental inheritance Transmission to offspring of phenotypes present in both parents. A seldom used term. Also called *amphigonous inheritance* (seldom used) duplex inheritance (seldom used).

blending inheritance The appearance in offspring of phenotypes that appear intermediate in qualitative or quantitative characteristics to those of the parents. Compare MENDELIAN INHERITANCE.

collateral inheritance The appearance of a phenotype in second or higher degree relatives. An example is multifactorial inheritance. A seldom used term.

complemental inheritance The appearance in offspring of a phenotype, the expression of which is determined by two (complementary) loci.

criss-cross inheritance The transmission to offspring of one sex a phenotype present in the parent of the opposite sex.

cytoplasmic inheritance The transmission of phenotypes, usually found in the mother, that are controlled or determined by genes not part of the nuclear chromosome set. Such phenotypes are characterized by nonsegregation and constancy of the phenotype in backcrosses to the parents. It is due to mitochondrial DNA (in most animals), non-nuclear DNA-containing plasmids, or chloroplast DNA. Also called *mitochondrial inheritance, maternal inheritance, extranuclear inheritance, extrachromosomal inheritance, matrilinear inheritance.*

dominant inheritance The appearance of a phenotype in relatives who are heterozygous for a mutant allele. Characteristics of this form of transmission of traits are a vertical pattern in a pedigree, with multiple affected generations; an equality of frequency and severity of effect between males and females; a 50 percent chance of transmitting the phenotype from an affected parent to each offspring; and a possibility of cases arising from a sporadic germinal mutation in a parent. A paternal age effect is often demonstrated in sporadic cases. Also called *dominant heredity.*

duplex inheritance A seldom used term for BIPARENTAL INHERITANCE.

extrachromosomal inheritance CYTOPLASMIC INHERITANCE.

extranuclear inheritance CYTOPLASMIC INHERITANCE.

galtonian inheritance QUANTITATIVE INHERITANCE.

holandric inheritance The appearance of a trait, determined at least in part by a gene or genes, that arises only in males. In humans, it is usually due to a locus on the Y chromosome.

hologynic inheritance The appearance of a trait, determined at least in part by a gene or genes, that arises only in females. In humans, examples are X-linked dominant traits that are lethal *in utero* in males, traits such as hydrometrocolpos which are sex-limited, and structural abnormalities of the X chromosome that result in defective segregation.

homochronous inheritance The transmission of phenotypes that appear in offspring at the same age or stage of development as in the parents.

homotropic inheritance The alleged transmission to offspring of traits acquired by the parent by design or environmental influences. Also called *inheritance of acquired characteristics.*

maternal inheritance CYTOPLASMIC INHERITANCE.

matrilinear inheritance CYTOPLASMIC INHERITANCE.

mendelian inheritance The transmission of phenotypes from parent to offspring in accordance with mendelian theory. Also called *monogenic inheritance, unit inheritance, monofactorial inheritance, particulate inheritance.* Compare BLENDING INHERITANCE.

mitochondrial inheritance CYTOPLASMIC INHERITANCE.

monofactorial inheritance MENDELIAN INHERITANCE.

monogenic inheritance MENDELIAN INHERITANCE.

mosaic inheritance In an individual, with respect to a given trait, the transmission of some proportion of the cells with a phenotype determined by a paternal allele and the rest of the cells with a phenotype determined by a maternal allele. This is seen with X-linked traits in mammalian females.

multifactorial inheritance 1 The transmission of a phenotype, the presence and nature of which are determined by multiple genes and environmental factors. 2 The transmission of a phenotype that is determined by multiple genes and environmental factors, but that holds to the following empiric rules: the appearance or severity often differs between the sexes; the occurrence is greater in first-degree relatives than in second-degree relatives, which, in turn, is greater than in third-degree relatives; the risk of recurrence in offspring is greater if the affected parent is of the less commonly affected sex; and the average risk of recurrence in offspring approximates the square root of the population prevalence.

particulate inheritance MENDELIAN INHERITANCE.

polygenic inheritance The transmission of a phenotype that is determined by several, often many, genes. It is an essential component of multifactorial inheritance.

quantitative inheritance The transmission of a metrical phenotype, usually one that exhibits continuous variation in the population, such as height. The phenotype is determined by the cumulative and inseparable action of many genes. Also called *galtonian inheritance, multiple factor hypothesis.*

quasidominant inheritance The transmission of a phenotype through multiple generations of a family in a pattern that is consistent with autosomal dominant inheritance but is in fact due to mating of a homozygous affected individual with a heterozygous carrier of a recessive trait. Such inheritance is rare except when the mutant allele frequency is high or consanguinity is common.

recessive inheritance The transmission of a phenotype, determined by a single genetic locus in diploid organisms, that is present only when that locus is homozygous for the responsible allele.

sex-linked inheritance 1 The transmission of a phenotype that is determined by one or more loci on one of the sex chromosomes. 2 An imprecise term for X-LINKED INHERITANCE.

supplemental inheritance The transmission of a phenotype that is determined by two genes, with the alleles at one locus affecting those of the second locus.

unit inheritance 1 The transmission of a phenotype that is apparently unaltered through successive generations. 2 MENDELIAN INHERITANCE.

X-linked inheritance The transmission of a phenotype that is determined by a gene located on the X chromosome. Characteristics of this form of inheritance are: males are more severely or obviously affected than females; a heterozygous (carrier) female transmits the mutant X-chromosome, on average, to one half of her daughters (who are also carriers) and one half of her sons (who are hemizygous); and hemizygous fathers cannot have affected sons, but all of their daughters are heterozygous. Also called *X-linked heredity, sex-linked inheritance* (imprecise), *sex-linked heredity* (imprecise).

inherited 1 Acquired through the genotype. 2 Of, referring to, or pertaining to a trait present in organisms of successive generations because of descent of the genotype.

inHg Symbol for the unit, conventional inch of mercury.

inhibin A peptide hormone apparently secreted by the Sertoli cells of the seminiferous tubules of the testis and acting to suppress or inhibit the release of anterior pituitary follicle-stimulating hormone (FSH). Loss of inhibin secretion presumably accounts for the raised FSH secretion observed in disorders of the testis associated with tubular destruction, such as the Klinefelter syndrome and myotonic muscular dystrophy.

inhibit To restrain or suppress.

inhibiter INHIBITOR.

inhibition [L *inhibitio* (from *inhibitus*, past part. of *inhibere* to hold in, hold back, restrain, from *in-* in + *habere* to have, hold) a restraining] **1** The diminishing or total suppression of a function or activity of the nervous system. **2** In chemistry, the phenomenon whereby certain substances can slow or stop a reaction. **3** Unconscious restriction of an impulse or its manifestations. **4** A restriction or suppression of thought or behavior not dependent on any known neural mechanism.

allogeneic inhibition A phenomenon in which the interaction of lymphocytes differing at the major histocompatibility locus depresses the reactivity of the lymphocytes to other antigens.

allosteric inhibition Inhibition of an enzyme by an allosteric effector. The flux through many reaction pathways is controlled by allosteric inhibition of an enzyme early in the pathway by the final product of the pathway.

antidromic inhibition RECURRENT INHIBITION.

associative inhibition **1** The blocking or weakening of an established association by the formation of a newly learned association for one of the elements in the original associative bond. **2** A resistance offered to the forming of new associative bonds because of strong existing associations between preexisting associative elements.

autogenous inhibition A reflex inhibition taking place at the point of stimulation.

central inhibition The suppression of excitation of the neurons within the central nervous system.

competitive inhibition Enzyme inhibition in which the inhibitor raises the Michaelis constant (K^m) without affecting the limiting rate (V) of the catalyzed reaction that is approached at high substrate concentration. The inhibition is said to have a competitive component if the inhibitor diminishes V/K^m. The simplest mechanism proposed for competitive inhibition is that the inhibitor and substrate compete for the same site on the enzyme, which cannot bind both at once.

contact inhibition **1** A cessation of the increase in cell numbers when the population density allows physical contact between cells. Also called *density-dependent inhibition*. **2** A cessation of movement of cells and inhibition of the undulatory behavior of the lamellipodia when two cells in a culture come into contact.

density-dependent inhibition CONTACT INHIBITION.

end-product inhibition Inhibition of a process by the final product that it forms. In metabolic sequences, end-product inhibition is usually exerted on the first step of the sequence.

enzyme inhibition The suppression of enzyme activity by the reversible, and usually noncovalent, binding of a substance to the enzyme.

feedback inhibition Inhibition of a step in a pathway by a product of that pathway. This provides a mechanism for controling the rate of a metabolic pathway.

fertility inhibition Decreased formation of sex pili by cells carrying the F factor, when superinfected with an R factor forming a repressor with the same specificity. R factors are thus classified into fi$^+$ and fi$^-$.

hemagglutination inhibition An immunologic procedure capable of demonstrating the presence of either an antigen or antibody, employing as its end point the inhibition of previously established hemagglutination. It can be used to demonstrate the presence of an antibody against a hemagglutinating virus, or the presence of soluble antigen that combines with and inhibits action of an antibody directed against antigens on the red cell surface.

mixed inhibition Inhibition of an enzyme-catalyzed reaction by an inhibitor that has both a competitive and an uncompetitive component. • *Mixed inhibition* has sometimes been called *noncompetitive inhibition*, although the latter term has usually been reserved for the particular case of mixed inhibition in which the specificity constant and the limiting velocity are lowered by the same factor.

motor inhibition A suppression of motor activity; a state of persistent reduction in motor activity resulting in immobility, weakness, or diminished speed of execution of movements and actions. This must be differentiated from fading, in which there is progressive diminution followed by total cessation of the movement, and from bradykinesia, which is simply an abnormal slowness of movement.

noncompetitive inhibition **1** See under MIXED INHIBITION. **2** Inhibition of an enzyme-catalyzed reaction in which the inhibitor diminishes the limiting rate (V) that the reaction approaches at high substrate concentration without affecting the Michaelis constant (K_m). This type of inhibition is rare.

potassium inhibition Cardiac arrest as a result of potassium infusion.

proactive inhibition The inhibiting effect of prior learning on material to be learned later. This effect is found especially in studies of verbal learning. The rate of learning is faster for elements appearing early in a sequence to be mastered than for those coming later.

reciprocal inhibition Suppression of excitability of the motor neurons or reflex responses of one muscle or synergist group when an antagonist muscle is reflexly facilitated. The classic example is the inhibition of activity in a flexor when a stretch reflex is elicited in an antagonist extensor muscle.

recurrent inhibition The reduction of neuron discharge via a feedback circuit involving axon collaterals that excite interneurons, e.g., Renshaw cells, which provide inhibitory control. Also called *Renshaw inhibition, antidromic inhibition.*

reflex inhibition A consistent negative response to a stimulus involving two or more neurons, especially muscle relaxation or a reduction of impulse discharge.

Renshaw inhibition RECURRENT INHIBITION.

retroactive inhibition The inhibition of recall of something once learned by the action of something learned later, especially if there is a degree of similarity between the learned elements.

substrate inhibition The phenomenon of decrease in the rate of an enzyme-catalyzed reaction with increasing concentration of substrate. Such a decrease may occur at high substrate concentrations after the usual increase of rate with concentration at lower values of the concentration.

uncompetitive inhibition Enzyme inhibition in which the inhibitor diminishes to the same degree both the limiting rate (V) of the catalyzed reaction that is approached at high substrate concentration and the Michaelis constant (K^m) for the substrate. Inhibition is said to have an uncompetitive component when the inhibitor diminishes V.

Wedensky inhibition A nerve conduction block resulting from previous high frequency electrical stimulation.

inhibitive INHIBITORY.

inhibitor [L *inhibit(us)*, past part. of *inhibere* to hold in, hold back, restrain, from *in-* in + *habere* to have, hold + *-OR*] **1** Anything that causes inhibition. **2** Denoting a neuron which inhibits the activity of the organ or structure which it innervates. **3** In biochemistry, any substance that diminishes the rate of an enzymatic reaction, such as competitive inhibitors, noncompetitive inhibitors, or allosteric inhibitors. Also *inhibiter.*

active-site-directed irreversible inhibitor An inhibitor of an enzyme-catalyzed reaction that binds to the active site of the enzyme, usually because it is similar in properties to the natural substrate, and there reacts with the enzyme irreversibly.

aldosterone inhibitor A drug or medicinal agent capable of inhibiting or antagonizing the effects of aldosterone on the renal tubules of the nephron.

C1-inhibitor   A stoichiometric inhibitor of C1 and of a number of other serine proteases, including plasmin, kallikrein, and factors XIIa and XIa of the clotting system. It is the only inhibitor of C1 in plasma. Heterozygous deficiency of C1-inhibitor is associated with hereditary angioedema.

cholesterol inhibitor   A drug or agent capable of inhibiting the synthesis of cholesterol and reducing its concentration in the blood.

competitive inhibitor   A substance that inhibits an enzyme reversibly by binding to it in competition with the substrate, since the enzyme cannot bind both substrate and inhibitor simultaneously. The degree of inhibition is therefore diminished as the substrate concentration is increased. Such inhibitors are usually substrate analogues that bind to the enzyme at the substrate-binding site.

complement inhibitor   Any natural protein inhibitor of complement components, serving to regulate the sequence of enzymes of complement.

irreversible inhibitor   An inhibitor of an enzyme-catalyzed reaction whose effect is not reversed by removing unreacted inhibitor from the enzyme. Although this may sometimes be due to very tight binding, so that no dissociation can normally be observed, it is more often due to an irreversible reaction that leads to a covalent compound between enzyme and inhibitor.

mitotic inhibitor   A chemical that slows or stops mitotic activity, e.g. colchicine, which arrests mitosis in metaphase.

noncompetitive inhibitor   A substance that inhibits an enzyme reversibly in such a way that the degree of inhibition is independent of the concentration of substrate.

reversible inhibitor   An inhibitor of an enzyme-catalyzed reaction whose action is reversed by removing the inhibitor. It acts by binding to the enzyme, but the binding is reversible, so that lowering the concentration of free inhibitor allows dissociation to regenerate unligated, active enzyme.

inhibitory   Tending to inhibit; acting to restrain or suppress. Also *inhibitive.*

inH₂O   Symbol for the unit, conventional inch of water.

inhomogeneity   **1** The property of being inhomogeneous.   **2** The difference between one part of inhomogeneous material and others.   **3** A part that so differs.

inhomogeneous   Possessing differences between its different parts. In an inhomogeneous substance, the molecules differ, so that the substance is not a pure compound.

iniac   Relating to the inion. A seldom used term.

iniad   Toward the inion.

inial   Pertaining to the inion.

iniencephalus   An embryo, fetus, or newborn infant with iniencephaly.

iniencephaly   [Gk *ini(on)* back of the head, nape of the neck + ENCEPHAL- + -Y]   A developmental defect in which the occipital part of the cranium and upper spinal regions fail to close about the neural tube, thus permitting exposure of brain and cord tissue. The condition often involves extreme retroflection of the head combined with variable degrees of cervical rachischisis.

iniodymus   [Gk *inio(n)* the back of the head + -DYMUS]   IN-IOPAGUS.

inion   [Gk *inion* (dim. of *is*, gen. *inos*, strength, a nerve, sinew, muscle) the sinews between occiput and back, the back of the head, nape of the neck]   [NA]   The most prominent point of the external occipital protuberance in the midline, used in craniometry.

iniopagus   [Gk *inio(n)* the back of the head + -PAGUS]   A pair of equal conjoined twins with union at the occipital region. Also called *craniopagus posterior, iniodymus.*

iniops   [Gk *ini(on)* the back of the head + *-ōps* eye]   JANICEPS ASYMMETRUS.

initial   [L *initialis* (from *initium* a going in, entrance, beginning, from *initus,* past part. of *inire* to go into, + *-alis* -AL) entering, beginning]   First, as of a series or set of stages; being a beginning or opening part.

fusiform initials   Long, flattened cells of the vascular cambium that form axial or vertical phloem and xylem elements.

initiation   [L *initiatus,* past part. of *initiare* to initiate]   The initial carcinogenic event in a tissue or cell caused by a tumor-producing substance.

initis   Inflammation involving the interstitium of muscle. A rarely used term.

inject   To instill or infuse (a fluid) into an artery, vein, organ, body cavity, or tissue region.

injectable   **1** Suitable for injection.   **2** A preparation of a drug or agent designed to be given by injection.

disposable injectable   A packaging system in which a standard dose of an agent is contained in a disposable syringe for injection. The syringe is not to be reused.

injectio   INJECTION.

injection   **1** The administration of a medicinal or nutritional substance into the subcutaneous tissue, muscular tissue, the veins, or one of the body canals or orifices, such as the vagina, rectum, or urethra. Also called *injectio.*   **2** A condition of visible hyperemia, as *conjunctival injection.*

adrenal cortex injection   An aqueous solution containing the active principles of the adrenal cortex steroids. It was formerly used for the treatment of Addison's disease, but it has been superseded by hydrocortisone and other preparations of adrenal steroids.

anatomical injection   The injection of one of several formulae of special fluids, and occasionally dyes, into vessels, cavities, or organs of a cadaver so as to preserve the body for dissection or to facilitate demonstration.

booster injection   A booster dose administered by injection. See under BOOSTER DOSE.

capillary injection   Capillary dilatation, evident especially in the face or conjuctiva.

circumcorneal injection   Capillary dilatation causing redness at the limbal area. Such a red halo encircling the cornea is often associated with iridocyclitis.

coarse injection   An anatomic injection that involves only the large vessels.

depot injection   An injection of a medical agent in a vehicle that causes slow release of the substance from the injection site over a prolonged interval.

dextrose injection   A sterile solution of dextrose in water suitable for parenteral administration of dextrose as a nutrient or as fluid replacement.

endermic injection   INTRADERMAL INJECTION.

epidural injection   An injection of material into the extradural space.

epifascial injection   A procedure in which liquid is forced through a needle into a fascial plane.

exciting injection   SENSITIZING INJECTION.

fine injection   An anatomic injection that reaches the smallest vessels.

fructose injection   A sterile solution of fructose in water given parenterally for nutritional needs or fluid replacement.

gelatin injection   An anatomic injection in which gelatin forms the basic ingredient in order to prevent the tissues from becoming too hard.

hypodermic injection   SUBCUTANEOUS INJECTION.

insulin injection A sterile, neutralized solution of the active principle of the pancreatic islet cells that affects the metabolism of glucose. It acts promptly as a hypoglycemic agent in the treatment of diabetes mellitus. Also called *neutral insulin, regular insulin.*

intracutaneous injection INTRADERMAL INJECTION.

intradermal injection An injection into the corium, or substance of the skin. Also called *endermic injection, intracutaneous injection, intradermic injection.*

intradermic injection INTRADERMAL INJECTION.

intramuscular injection An injection made into the body of a muscle.

intrathecal injection An injection into the subarachnoid space, as of gas, contrast material, anesthetic agent, or medication.

intravascular injection An injection made directly into a blood vessel.

intravenous injection An injection made directly into a vein.

iron-dextran injection A sterile, colloidal solution of ferric hydroxide and low molecular weight dextrans suitable for parenteral administration of iron. Also called *iron dextran complex.*

iron sorbitex injection A sterile, brown, colloidal solution composed of a complex of ferric iron, sorbitol, and citric acid. It is stabilized with dextran and sorbitol. It is used as a parenteral form of iron for the treatment of iron deficiency anemia where oral treatment is not possible or is ineffective.

jet injection The injection of a drug through the skin by a very fine jet of solution under high pressure.

lactated Ringer's injection A sterile solution containing calcium chloride, potassium chloride, sodium chloride, and sodium lactate in water for parenteral infusion to replenish fluid and electrolyte loss. Also called *Ringer's lactate.*

molding injection The injection of a plastic material into the hollow space of a mold.

nerve injection The injection of a substance into or close to a nerve for temporary or permanent anesthesia or nerve block.

opacifying injection An injection of a radiopaque contrast medium into a lumen or into tissue as part of a roentgenographic examination. Also called *opaque injection.*

opaque injection OPACIFYING INJECTION.

oxytocin injection A clear, sterile, aqueous solution containing the active principle of the posterior pituitary, which may be prepared from domestic animals or by synthesis. It is used to stimulate uterine contractions and for the control of postpartum hemorrhage.

parathyroid injection A sterile aqueous solution containing the water-soluble principles obtained from bovine parathyroid glands. It is administered parenterally to maintain normal levels of calcium in the blood. Also called *parathyroid extract, parathyroid solution.*

parenchymatous injection An injection made into the substance of an organ.

plaster injection An anatomic injection in which a gypsum and water paste fills the vessels for special demonstration purposes.

posterior pituitary injection A sterile aqueous solution containing the water-soluble principles of the posterior lobe of the pituitary gland from domestic animals. It is administered parenterally for its oxytocic properties and the treatment of diabetes insipidus. Also called *pituitary solution, posterior pituitary solution, liquor pituitarii posterii.*

preparatory injection SENSITIZING INJECTION.

preservative injection An anatomic injection that preserves the cadaver or any specimen and prevents decomposition.

protamine sulfate injection A sterile solution of protamine sulfate in sodium chloride injection. It is used to neutralize the anticoagulant effect of heparin and prevent hemorrhage from heparin overdosage.

protein hydrolysate injection A sterile solution of amino acids and small peptides derived by hydrolysis of casein, lactalbumin, or other suitable protein sources. It is used as a parenteral nutrient replacement for oral protein intake.

repository injection The injection of a medication in a formulation that permits slow absorption and a prolonged drug effect.

Ringer's injection A sterile solution containing sodium chloride, potassium chloride, and calcium chloride in water. It is used parenterally to replace fluid and electrolyte loss.

Schlösser's injection Injection of alcohol into major branches of the trigeminal nerve in cases of intractable facial neuralgia. An obsolete term.

sclerosing injection The injection into a blood vessel, usually a varicose vein, of a substance which causes obliteration of the vessel. See also INJECTION SCLEROTHERAPY.

sensitizing injection The initial injection of any substance which induces allergic hypersensitivity to itself. Also called *exciting injection, preparatory injection.*

sodium chloride injection A sterile, isotonic aqueous solution of sodium chloride. It is used as a parenteral injection to replace the loss of fluid and electrolytes, and as a vehicle for the administration of other therapeutic agents.

subcutaneous injection An injection into the loose connective tissue beneath the skin using a needle or syringe. Also called *hypodermic injection.*

Teflon injection of vocal cord The injection of a measured amount of Teflon paste lateral to the conus elasticus in cases of unilateral abduction of the vocal cord and imperfect glottic closure, the object being to compel the affected cord towards the midline.

trigger point injection Infiltration of trigger points with local anesthetics and/or cortisone to relieve muscle spasm.

vasopressin injection A sterile, aqueous solution containing the pressor principle of the posterior pituitary. It is prepared from the glands of domestic animals or from synthetic material. It is used as a diuretic medication.

injector [L *inject(us)*, past part. of *inicere* to throw in or into, put in or into + -OR] An instrument, such as a syringe, used to inject solutions into body organs or tissues.

jet injector A high-pressure syringelike apparatus used to instill doses of drugs hypodermically without using a needle to puncture the skin.

Sanders injector A device utilizing the Venturi principle to entrain oxygen and insure adequate ventilation during a bronchoscopy.

injure [back-formation from *injury* (from L *injuri(a)* injury, injustice, from fem. sing. of *injurius* wrongful, from *in-* IN-² + *jus*, gen. *juris*, justice, right, law)] To harm or hurt; disrupt the integrity or function of a tissue or organ by external, usually mechanical, means.

injury [L *injuria* (from *in-* not + *jus*, gen. *juris*, justice, right, law) a thing done unjustly, injury] A disruption of the integrity or function of a tissue or organ by external means, which are usually mechanical but can also be chemical, electrical, thermal, or radiant.

air-blast injury An injury caused by the rapid expansion of air. Common examples include explosions and direct injection of compressed air into the body in industrial accidents.

atmospheric blast injury An injury resulting from rapid changes in pressure of the ambient air, as in an explosion. It may also result from sudden decompression, as in high altitude aircraft accidents.

birth injury Bodily damage suffered by an infant as a result of the birth process.

blunt injury A mechanical injury produced by the impact of a blunt instrument that tears, shears, or crushes tissue in contrast to an incision injury. The three basic forms are lacerations, contusions, and abrasions.

bucket-handle injury BUCKET-HANDLE TEAR.

bumper injury An injury to a pedestrian, marked by wedge-shaped fractures of the tibial shafts produced by automobile bumper impact with the legs. The fractures are often bilateral, and the fibulae are commonly involved. The apex of the triangular fragment of fractured bone often, but not invariably, points in the direction in which the vehicle was moving.

closed head injury An injury to the brain without an associated skull fracture.

cold injury An injury resulting when the circulation of a part is insufficient to protect the cells from damage by a cold environment. The severity of the injury is proportional to the adequacy of the circulation in relation to the temperature of the environment. If the environment is wet, trench foot results, or if dry, frostbite results.

compression injury CRUSH INJURY.

contrecoup injury An injury caused by a blow to the brain but found on the side opposite the blow. The blow starts the brain in motion and momentum is stopped by the opposite side of the skull, creating damage to the brain at that opposite point. Although such lesions can occur in a fluid-filled organ, a contrecoup other than to the brain is quite rare. Also called *counterstroke, contrecoup contusion.*

contrecoup injury of brain Localized contusion or laceration of the brain substance on the side opposite to the point of the impact causing a head injury due to the brain substance being driven forcibly against the inner table of the skull.

coup injury of brain Contusion or laceration of the brain substance underlying the point of impact upon the skull.

coup-contrecoup injury Contusion or laceration of the brain substance both on the side of the impact and on the opposite side.

crush injury A tissue or organ injury caused by severe squeezing or pressure. The squeezing may be purely mechanical or it may be due to sudden expansion of liquid or gas, as in an explosion or the passage of a high-velocity missile. The damage is not usually evident immediately or at the time of initial examination. Intense swelling occurs in the crushed part, and unless compartments are decompressed, further tissue damage may occur from vascular compromise. Also called *compression injury.*

deceleration injury An injury that occurs when there is a sudden deceleration and stopping of a moving vehicle, as in an automobile or aircraft crash. The magnitude of the injury is related to the deceleration force to which the individual is subjected. The force is directly proportional to the square of the vehicle speed and inversely proportional to the stopping distance. The most serious of these is traumatic rupture of the thoracic aorta at the point where the arch meets the descending aorta.

egg-white injury An obsolete term for EGG-WHITE SYNDROME.

Goyrand's injury An obsolete term for PULLED ELBOW.

high-explosive injury An injury caused by the sudden change in atmospheric pressure resulting from the instantaneous reaction of unstable compounds. The injuries result both from the blast and from flying debris. Also called *shell injury.*

hyperextension-hyperflexion injury An injury to a joint caused by forcibly moving the joint beyond its normal range. See also WHIPLASH INJURY.

immersion blast injury A blast injury caused by an under-water explosion from a mine or depth charge to anyone in the water near the explosion. Because water is not compressible the shock wave is transmitted over long distances with almost undiminished force. Such injuries may be more severe than those caused by comparable explosions transmitted through the atmosphere.

inhalation injury Injury to the lung resulting from inhalation of smoke or of any of various damaging chemical gases.

internal injury Injury to organs or tissues within body cavities.

injury of intervertebral disk A tearing or fissuring of the annulus fibrosus that permits movement of the nucleus pulposus.

minimal brain injury MINIMAL BRAIN DYSFUNCTION.

minimal cerebral injury MINIMAL BRAIN DYSFUNCTION.

neonatal cold injury The effect of hypothermia in the newborn infant. There is gradually increasing lethargy and failure to feed. The body temperature falls below 32°C (89.6°F), leading to hardening of the subcutaneous tissue of the buttocks and thighs (sclerema), although the face remains misleadingly rosy. The blood sugar is low. Treatment requires slow rewarming, but the mortality is high.

occupational injury An injury which arises out of and in the course of work. In some countries, injuries received traveling to and from work or occurring at the place of work outside working hours are also classified as occupational for purposes of claiming compensation.

open head injury An injury to the brain associated with a fracture of the skull, especially with compound or depressed fractures or with in-driven fragments of bone, hair, or foreign material.

patterned injury A wound, most commonly resulting from blunt force, in which an impression of the wound-producing instrument's surface remains on the skin.

radiation injury Tissue or intracellular damage or death caused by absorbed radiation, which may operate through atomic excitation, ion production, free radicals, circulatory disturbances, etc. Cells, tissues, and species vary widely in their susceptibility to radiation injury.

shell injury HIGH-EXPLOSIVE INJURY.

soft tissue injury Any injury to muscle, fascia, tendon, ligament, skin, fat, or other nonosseous, noncartilaginous tissue of the body.

steering wheel injury An injury to the anterior chest wall and/or the mediastinal contents resulting from forcible contact with the steering wheel of a motor vehicle during sudden deceleration.

straddle injury An injury to the perineum and/or the pelvis caused by a fall directly onto the perineum. Injury results because the force of the fall is not dispersed through the lower extremities.

thermal injury A burn.

vital injury In forensic medicine, an antemortem injury occurring at a sufficient interval prior to death to initiate tissue and organ reactions such as hemorrhage, coagulation, inflammation, swelling, and initial or partial healing of the injured tissue.

whiplash injury Injury to the soft tissues (muscles and ligaments) supporting the cervical spine, usually in the area of the third and fourth cervical vertebrae (C-3 and C-4). It is usually caused by sudden hyperextension of the neck in a rear-end motor vehicle collision as the supported body is accelerated and the unsupported head initially remains stationary. The head reaches the end of its travel and then snaps forward, doing further damage. Objective assessment of injury is difficult, and such injuries are a frequent cause of legitimate as well as spurious claims for damages following such accidents.

wringer injury **1** Any injury, usually to an extremity, caused when the extremity is drawn between spring-loaded rollers. In the process, the skin and subcutaneous tissues are avulsed from their underlying blood supply, causing them to slough and necessitating skin grafts or other methods to replace the lost skin. **2** Any similar injury causing avulsion of the skin from its blood supply.

inky cap A fungus of the deliquescent *Coprinus* species, so-called because at maturity the pileus "melts away" thus distributing the spores.

inlay [IN-¹ + *lay*] A restoration, made out of the mouth to fit in a prepared tooth cavity and fixed in place by a thin layer of dental cement. An inlay is usually made of cast gold alloy, but fused porcelain has also been used.

bone inlay The grafting of bone into a slot or gutter.

epithelial inlay INLAY GRAFT.

gold-shell inlay Gold inlay cast in the form of a hollow shell.

skin graft inlay INLAY GRAFT.

inlet A space or passage leading into a cavity.

pelvic inlet APERTURA PELVIS SUPERIOR.

inlet of pelvis APERTURA PELVIS SUPERIOR.

thoracic inlet The superior mediastinum and the base of the neck, through which pass the great brachiocephalic vessels.

inlet of thorax APERTURA THORACIS SUPERIOR.

INN International Nonproprietary Names.

innate [L *innat(us)* (past part. of *innasci* to be born or spring up in a place) inborn, innate] Inborn; hereditary.

innervate To supply with nerve fibers or a nerve stimulus, as to a neuron, muscle, or gland.

innervation [L *in-* in + NERVE + -ATION] The distribution of nerve fibers or a neural stimulus to a neuron, muscle, or gland.

crossed innervation The experimental condition wherein innervation to two structures is interchanged surgically by cutting the nerves and anastomosing the stubs.

double innervation Nerve fiber distribution from two distinct sources, such as autonomic innervation by sympathetic and parasympathetic axons or a muscle by two nerves of differing origin.

multiple innervation The presence of more than one motor endplate on a given muscle fiber.

plurisegmental innervation Innervation of a single structure, such as a muscle, by two or more consecutive segments of the spinal cord.

polyneuronal innervation Innervation by more than one neuron, as is characteristic of ordinary muscle fibers at one stage in the development of a mammal, and of intrafusal muscle fibers in the adult.

reciprocal innervation Innervation of muscle antagonist pairs whereby the agonist is excited and its antagonist inhibited to achieve synchronized contraction and relaxation. Also called *Sherrington's law*.

innidiation [IN-¹ + L *nid(us)* nest + *i* + -ATION] The growth and proliferation of cells in a region of the body to which they have been transported in a metastatic process.

innocent Not inherently harmful; benign.

innominata Plural of INNOMINATUM.

innominatal Pertaining to truncus brachiocephalicus or to the innominate bone.

innominate [Late L *innominat(us)* (from L *in-* IN-² + *nominatus*, past part. of *nominare* to name, from *nomen* a name) unnamed, nameless] Nameless or unnamed: applied to certain anatomic structures.

innominatum (*plural* innominata.) OS COXAE.

Innovar A fixed combination of fentanyl citrate, a narcotic analgesic, and droperidol, a neuroleptic agent. A proprietary

name. • While listed in many references, such combinations are of limited value and not encouraged. The mixture is appropriate only when this particular dose of each drug is required. Otherwise, the two should each be given in the proper amount.

innoxious Safe; harmless.

innutrition A lack of nourishment.

Ino Symbol for the nucleoside inosine.

ino- [Gk *is* (genitive *inos*, plural nominative *ines*) nerve, thew, sinew; in plural, fibrous vessels] A combining form meaning fiber, fibrous. • In oncology *ino-* has been combined with a variety of terms to indicate combinations of fibrous tissue with the other tumor elements, as in *inomycoma, inomyxoma, inoneuroma, inoleiomyoma, inoglioma,* and *inochondroma.* All are obsolete.

inoblast [INO- + -BLAST] An undifferentiated connective tissue cell.

inoccipitia [IN-² + L *occipit(ium)* the back part of the head + -IA] Agenesis of one or both occipital lobes. A rarely used term.

inochondritis An inflammatory reaction affecting fibrocartilage. A seldom used term.

inocula Plural of INOCULUM.

inoculability The fact or property of being inoculable.

inoculable **1** Capable of being transmitted by inoculation. **2** Subject to a disease transmitted by inoculation.

inoculate [See INOCULATION.] **1** To introduce microorganisms into (culture media, tissue culture, on animal, soil, etc.) for the purposes of growth and identification of the organism. **2** To introduce infectious material or noninfectious antigenic material parenterally into (the body) in order to stimulate a protective immune response.

inoculation [L *in-* into + *oculus* eye, bud + -atio -ATION] Introduction of a microorganism or other antigenic material into an organism or a culture medium, usually in order to stimulate a protective immune response or to study the cultured substance.

inoculative Pertaining to or done by inoculation: said especially of the mode of transmission of an infective agent or a venom, as by the sting or bite of an animal.

inoculator A scarifying device used to inoculate.

inoculum [New L (from L *in-* in + *oculum,* accus. of *oculus* eye, bud)] The substance inoculated into culture or into an experimental animal.

inocyte FIBROBLAST.

inogen A substance once believed to be present in muscles that breaks down to form lactic acid and carbon dioxide and releases energy for contraction. A recombination of the lactic acid with other carbon molecules reforms the inogen. An obsolete term.

inogenesis Fibrous tissue formation.

inogenous Derived from or producing fibrous tissue.

inoglia [INO- + GLIA] The matrix, or ground substance, of fibrous connective tissue.

inohymenitis An inflammatory reaction involving a fibrous membrane. An obsolete term.

inolith A calcified fibrous nodule. A rarely used term.

inoma [*in(o)-* + -OMA] An obsolete term for FIBROMA.

inomyositis An obsolete term for FIBROMYOSITIS.

inopectic Characterized by inopexia; hypercoagulable. A seldom used term.

inoperable [IN-² + OPERABLE] Describing a disease or condition, or a stage thereof, that would not be improved by surgical intervention.

inopexia A tendency to accelerated coagulation; a hypercoagulable state. A seldom used term. Adjective: inopectic.

inorganic **1** Denoting compounds that do not contain carbon-carbon and carbon-hydrogen bonds. **2** Denoting the chemistry of inorganic compounds.

inosclerosis Induration of a tissue as a result of an increase in fibrous tissue. An obsolete term.

inoscopy [INO- + -SCOPY] An arcane diagnostic method based on the examination of the fibrous or fibrinous elements of specimens such as sputum, tissues, effusion fluids, and clotted blood. An obsolete term.

inosculate [IN-¹ + L *osculat(us)*, past part. of *osculari* to kiss, from *osculum* a little mouth, kiss, dim. of *os*, gen. *oris*, mouth] To link by small openings; anastomose.

inosculation [English *in* + L *osculatio* (from *asculatus*, past part. of *osculari* to kiss, from *osculum*, dim. of *os* mouth) a kissing] ANASTOMOSIS.

inose INOSITOL.

inosemia The presence of inositol in blood.

inosine A nucleoside resulting from the deamination of adenosine.

inosinic acid Inosine 5′-phosphate. It can be formed from adenylic acid by biologic deamination with release of ammonia, or by deamination *in vitro* with nitrous acid.

inosite INOSITOL.

inositide Any of various compounds of inositol, usually a lipid such as phosphatidylinositol.

inositis [Gk *is* (gen. *inos*) nerve, in pl., fibrous vessels + -ITIS] An inflammatory process involving fibrous tissue. A rarely used term.

inositol $C_6H_{12}O_6$. The compound formed by a ring of six — CHOH— groups. It is found combined in phospholipids, e.g. as phosphatidylinositol. The main isomer found naturally is *myo*-inositol, which has the two hydroxyl groups on C-4 and C-6 on the opposite side of the plane of the ring from the other four. Its biosynthesis is as its 1-phosphate, which is formed by cyclization of glucose 6-phosphate with inversion at C-5 of the glucose residue (C-2 of the inositol residue). Its hexaphosphate is phytic acid. Also called *inose, inosite, antialopecia factor, mouse antialopecia factor*.

inositol niacinate $C_{42}H_{30}N_6O_{12}$. *myo*-Inositol hexa-3-pyrimidinecarboxylate. A polyester of inositol and nicotinic acid. It has been used therapeutically as a peripheral vasodilator in the treatment of peripheral vascular disease. It is given orally.

inositoluria INOSITURIA.

inosituria [Gk *inos*, gen. of *is* nerve, fiber + -it(e) + -URIA] The appearance of inosinic acid in the urine of a subject in shock. Also called *Mosler's diabetes, inosuria, inositoluria, melituria inosita*.

inostosis [IN-¹ + OST- + -OSIS] The re-formation of bone in an area of damage.

inosuria [Gk *inos*, gen. of *is* nerve, fiber + -URIA] **1** An abundance of fibrin present in urine. **2** INOSITURIA.

inotagma [INO- + Gk *tagma* anything arranged] The ordered, linear arrangement of contractile elements in a striated muscle fiber.

inotropic [INO- + -TROPIC¹] Affecting the force or speed of muscular contraction either by enhancing or inhibiting it.

in ovo [L *in* in + *ovo*, ablative of *ovum* egg] Describing a laboratory procedure that uses duck or chick embryos.

inpatient [IN-¹ + PATIENT] **1** An individual admitted to a health care institution, usually for a period including at least one overnight stay. **2** Pertaining to or serving inpatients. Compare OUTPATIENT.

input **1** Anything that is put into a system, such as data into a computer, a signal into an amplifier, or a stimulus into an animal. **2** The place where an input is made, such as the terminals of a computer or amplifier. **3** The process of entering data or a signal.

input/output The peripheral equipment, such as a video terminal or a printer, that communicates with a computer, usually through special circuits called ports. Symbol: I/O

inquest [Late L *inquesta* (from *inquesta*, past part. of *inquirere* to search into, from L *in* into + *quaerere* to search) a searching into] CORONER'S INQUEST.

coroner's inquest A judicial inquiry, convened by a coroner and usually conducted before a jury, into the manner of death of an individual whose death occurred suddenly under suspicious, unusual, or violent circumstances. The performance of forensic autopsies has greatly reduced the need for inquests. In many jurisdictions, however, it remains a legal requirement that all deaths in penal institutions, foster homes, mental institutions, etc. be subjected to an inquest. Also called *inquest*.

inquiline [L *inquilin(us)* (for *incolinus* inhabitant of a place, from *incolere* to dwell in a place) an inhabitant of a place that is not his own] An animal that habitually resides in another species' abode without causing inconvenience to the host. The clownfish *Amphiprion*, living among the tentacles of its anenome host, is one of many examples. Also called *inquiline parasite*.

inquisition [L *inquisitio* (from *inquisitus*, past part. of *inquirere* to seek for, examine) an inquiry] Any judicial inquiry, particularly one made to determine mental competence.

inructation [L *irructatus* (for *inructatus*), past part. of *irructare* (from *ir-* -IN¹ + *ructare* to bring up wind noisily, belch) a noisy swallowing of air] A kind of noisy aerophagy.

insaccation The condition of being surrounded by a sac.

insalivation [IN-¹ + SALIVATION] The mixing of food with saliva during mastication. Also called *inviscation*.

insalubrious Not healthful, as a climate.

insane [L *insan(us)* (from *in-* not + *sanus* sound, sane) not well, diseased in mind, insane] Of or pertaining to unsoundness of mind or insanity. Also *mad* (imprecise). • The term is no longer used in psychiatry except in legal contexts.

insane on arraignment Designating an individual found incompetent to stand trial by reason of mental disorder or legal insanity. A term used only in the U.S. Also called *unfit to plead (British and New Zealand usage)*.

criminally insane Describing a person who has committed a crime and who suffers or did at the time suffer mental illness of enough severity to reduce or abolish responsibility for his action: a legal or judicial finding.

insanitary [IN-² + SANITARY] Not sanitary; unclean; not conducive to good health.

insanity [L *insanitas* (from *insan(us)* insane + -*itas* -ITY) insanity] As determined by a court of law, a mental disorder of such a nature or degree as to interfere with the subject's capacity to discharge his legal responsibilities. Also called *lunacy* (obsolete), *madness* (imprecise).

acute confusional insanity Delirium characterized by a sudden onset of short-term memory defects and disorientation.

affective insanity An obsolete term for AFFECTIVE PSYCHOSIS.

alcoholic insanity An outmoded term for ALCOHOLIC PSYCHOSIS.

alternating insanity An outmoded term for ALTERNATING MANIC-DEPRESSIVE DISORDER.

anticipatory insanity Psychosis appearing in a patient at an earlier age than it previously occurred in the patient's parent.

basedowian insanity Psychosis associated with hyperthyroidism as may occur in Grave disease (Basedow's disease). A seldom used term.

circular insanity An outmoded term for ALTERNATING MANIC-DEPRESSIVE DISORDER.

climacteric insanity An obsolete term for INVOLUTIONAL MELANCHOLIA.

collective insanity SHARED DELUSION.

communicated insanity SHARED DELUSION.

compound insanity More than one type of psychosis simultaneously developing in the same subject.

compulsive insanity OBSESSIVE-COMPULSIVE NEUROSIS.

confusional insanity EXHAUSTION PSYCHOSIS.

consecutive insanity Psychosis developing subsequent to other disease. A seldom used term.

criminal insanity The state of mind resulting from a mental defect or disorder and which was present when an individual committed a crime and rendered him unable to understand the wrongfulness of his conduct or to conform his conduct to the requirements of the law.

cyclic insanity An outmoded term for ALTERNATING MANIC-DEPRESSIVE DISORDER.

degenerative insanity **1** An obsolete term for INVOLUTIONAL MELANCHOLIA. **2** An obsolete term for SENILE DEMENTIA.

delusional insanity PARANOIDISM.

double insanity FOLIE À DEUX.

doubting insanity FOLIE DU DOUTE.

homicidal insanity HOMICIDOMANIA.

homochronous insanity Psychosis developing in a patient at the same age as it previously occurred in the patient's parent.

idiophrenic insanity ENDOGENOUS PSYCHOSIS.

imposed insanity SHARED DELUSION.

induced insanity SHARED DELUSION.

intermittent insanity An obsolete term for MANIC-DEPRESSIVE PSYCHOSIS.

manic-depressive insanity An obsolete term for MANIC-DEPRESSIVE PSYCHOSIS.

moral insanity A pattern of behavior that characterizes the antisocial personality. An obsolete term. Also called *Ray's mania* (seldom used).

insanity of negation Psychosis accompanied by nihilistic delusions, for example, the patient may believe that he has no body. Also called *Cotard syndrome*.

partial insanity In the legal system, a mental disorder that limits the subject's responsibility for his actions but which is not severe enough to render him totally free of responsibility.

perceptional insanity Psychosis accompanied by prominent hallucinations or illusions. An obsolete term.

periodic insanity An obsolete term for MANIC-DEPRESSIVE PSYCHOSIS.

primary insanity A seldom used term for ENDOGENOUS PSYCHOSIS.

pubescent insanity An obsolete term for HEBEPHRENIC SCHIZOPHRENIA.

puerperal insanity POSTPARTUM PSYCHOSIS.

recurrent insanity An obsolete term for MANIC-DEPRESSIVE PSYCHOSIS.

religious insanity A psychosis, usually schizophrenic, with prominent delusions concerning religious beliefs or figures. An obsolete term.

senile insanity SENILE DEMENTIA.

simultaneous insanity FOLIE À DEUX.

toxic insanity A state of mental confusion due to the ingestion of an animal poison or plant poison, alcohol, opium, heroin, cocaine, or other hallucinogenic agent. It may also be precipitated by drug withdrawal or certain metabolic disorders.

inscriptio [L (from *inscriptus*, past part. of *inscribere* to write in

or on, inscribe), a writing in or on, inscription] (*plural* inscriptiones) INSCRIPTION.

inscriptio tendinea INTERSECTIO TENDINEA.

inscriptiones tendineae musculi recti abdominis INTERSECTIONES TENDINEAE MUSCULI RECTI ABDOMINIS.

inscription [L *inscriptio*. See INSCRIPTIO.] **1** The main section of a prescription, in which are listed the drug ingredients and the amounts of each to be compounded . **2** A mark or line. For defs. 1 and 2 also called *inscriptio*.

tendinous inscription INTERSECTIO TENDINEA.

tendinous inscriptions of rectus abdominis muscle INTERSECTIONES TENDINEAE MUSCULI RECTI ABDOMINIS.

inscriptiones Plural of INSCRIPTIO.

insect [L *insect(um)*, neut. sing. of *insectus*, past part. of *insecare* to make an incision in, cut] A member of the class Insecta.

social insects Colonial members of the insect orders Hymenoptera (wasps, bees, ants) and Insoptera (termites), which form highly organized communities within a single colony and are controlled by a single fertile queen. Infertile members are organized into classes or castes of workers and soldiers, sometimes with striking morphologic specializations, as seen among certain ants and termites.

Insecta [pl. of L *insectum*. See INSECT.] A class of arthropods, the largest group of animals known, whose members have three pairs of jointed legs and are characteristically divided into three anatomical portions: head, thorax, and abdomen. Many members are parasitic and others serve as intermediate hosts for human and animal pathogens. Also called *Hexapoda*.

insectarium INSECTARY.

insectary [INSECT + -ARY] A place in which insects are bred and raised. Also called *insectarium*.

insecticide [INSECT + *i* + -CIDE] Any substance that kills insects. Insecticides are widely used in agriculture to increase crop production and in disease control. Many are highly toxic and can give rise to hazardous exposures in both occupational and nonoccupational situations. The toxic dose and clinical picture vary with the compound. • By U.S. statute, an *insecticide* is "any substance or mixture of substances intended for preventing, destroying, repelling, or mitigating any insects which may be present in the environment whatsoever." It thus embraces a broader range of effect than that employed in ordinary usage.

insectiform [INSECT + *i* + -FORM] Resembling an insect; insectlike in shape.

insectifuge An insect repellent.

Insectivora [INSECT + *i* + New L -*vora*, neut. pl. of -*vorus*, combining form from L *vorare* to swallow, devour] An order of mammals. They are usually small animals with long narrow snouts. They are plantigrade and pentadactyl with claws on each digit. The diet consists characteristically of insects and other invertebrates. All members are primitive in some respects. The distribution is cosmopolitan. Echolocation has been observed in many members of this order.

insectivore [INSECT + *i* + English -*vore*, combining form from L *vorare* to swallow, devour] **1** Any organism that feeds on insects. **2** Any member of the order Insectivora.

insectivorous [*insectivor(e)* + -OUS] Characterized by a diet of insects.

insectology [INSECT + *o* + -LOGY] ENTOMOLOGY.

insemination [L *in-* in + SEMINATION] The deposit of semen in the female genital tract. Also called *semination*.

artificial insemination Introduction of semen into the female genital tract by means of a suitably designed instrument. Also called *artificial fecundation, artificial impregnation*.

donor insemination Artificial insemination utilizing semen from a male other than the female's husband. Also called *heterologous insemination*. Abbreviation: A.I.D.

heterologous insemination   DONOR INSEMINATION.

homologous insemination   Artificial insemination utilizing the husband's sperm. Abbreviation: A.I.H.

insenescence   The condition of growing old without the usual signs of aging. Adjective: insenescent.

insenescent   Growing old without the usual signs of aging.

insensible   **1** UNCONSCIOUS.   **2** Without the awareness of the senses.

insensitivity   A lack of sensitivity.

congenital insensitivity to pain   ASYMBOLIA FOR PAIN.

insert [L *insertus* (past part. of *inserere* to put, bring, or introduce into, insert, mix, connect) put, brought, or introduced into]   **1** To put in or implant.   **2** Something that is put in or implanted.   **3** To attach, as a tendon to a bone.

intramucosal insert   A mushroom-shaped addition to the fitting surface of a denture, extending into a preformed pouch in the mucosa, and serving to increase retention of the denture.

package insert   The labeling included with a prescription drug shipped to the pharmacist by the manufacturer and which may be required by law in certain jurisdictions to contain specific types of information.

insertio [L, from *insertus*. See INSERT.]   INSERTION.

insertio velamentosa   VELAMENTOUS INSERTION.

insertion [L *insertio*. See INSERTIO.]   The more movable attachment of a muscle during the principal action of that muscle, usually the distal end of a muscle's attachment to a bone and the point on which the force of a muscle is applied. Also called *insertio*.

parasol insertion   Separation of the umbilical vessel some distance from the center of the placenta so that they spread out like the ribs of an umbrella or parasol.

velamentous insertion   The attachment of the umbilical cord to the placenta so that the umbilical vessels ramify some distance from the placental margin and diverge on the chorion before reaching the substance of the placenta. Also called *insertio velamentosa*.

insheathed   Enveloped by a sheath.

insidious   Denoting the progression of a disease process that gives little or no symptomatic indication of its severity.

insight   In psychiatry, awareness and acknowledgment that one's symptoms or complaints represent some disorder or abnormality, and some degree of understanding of the relationship between probable causes or predisposing factors and the ensuing dysfunction.

in situ   **1** In its original or normal position.   **2** Not invasive: applied especially to carcinomas which have not invaded beyond their original epithelial confines.

insolation [L *insolatio* (from *insolatus*, past part. of *insolare* to place in the sun, from *in-* IN-¹ + *sol* the sun) a placing in the sun]   **1** Exposure to the sun; treatment by exposure to sunlight. A rarely used term.   **2** SUNSTROKE.

asphyxial insolation   Sunstroke so severe as to be fatal, marked by cold skin, hypothermia, and feeble pulse. An obsolete term.

hyperpyrexial insolation   An obsolete term for SUNSTROKE.

insoluble   Not capable of being dissolved in the solvent medium under consideration.

insomnia [L (from *insomnis* sleepless, from *in-* not + *somnus* sleep, akin to Gk *hypnos* sleep), sleeplessness]   A sleep disorder in which the individual is unable to initiate or to maintain sleep. Also called *agrypnia* (seldom used), *anhypnia* (obsolete), *asomnia* (obsolete), *hyposomnia*, *pernoctation* (obsolete), *sleeplessness*.

insomniac [*insomni(a)* + -AC]   One who suffers from insomnia. Also called *hyposomniac*.

inspection   Careful visual examination, as of the body or a part.

inspersion   The sprinkling around of a liquid or the scattering about of a powder.

inspiration   The act or process of breathing in; in humans, the taking in of air into the lungs as part of the process of respiration.

crowing inspiration   INSPIRATORY STRIDOR.

inspirator   A respirator or inhaler.

inspiratory   Of or relating to inspiration.

inspire   INHALE.

inspirometer   An instrument for measuring the volume of inspired air.

inspissant [Late L *inspissans*, gen. *inspissantis*, pres. part. of *inspissare* (from L *in-* IN¹ + *spissare* to thicken) to make thicker]   **1** Causing an increased thickness of a body fluid by extracting water.   **2** Any agent that decreases the liquidity of a body fluid by extracting water.

inspissate [Late L *inspissat(us)*, past part. of *inspissare* (from L *in-* -IN¹ + *spissare* to thicken, from *spissus* dense, thick) to thicken]   To bring about a decreased liquidity in (a body fluid) by the extraction of water.

inspissated   Of or relating to inspissation.

inspissation [Med L *inspissatio* (from Late L *inspissatus*, past part. of *inspissare* to thicken) a thickening. See INSPISSATE.]   The process of lessening the water content of a body fluid.

inspissator [New L *inspissat(us)*, past part. of *inspissare* to thicken, from L *in* into + *spissare* to thicken, condense, + -OR]   A device for evaporating a fluid in order to render the residual material thicker or more concentrated.

instability   The condition of being unstable; lack of stability.

instar [L, image, form, likeness]   A single growth stage of an insect or other arthropod which occurs between molts.

instauration [L *instauratio* (from *instauratus*, past part. of *instaurare* to renew) a renewing]   Restoration; repair.

instep   The highest part of the medial longitudinal arch on the dorsum of the foot.

instillation   The delivery of a liquid, drop-by-drop, into some body cavity or part.

instillator   A medicine dropper.

instinct [L *instinctus* (from *instinctus*, past part. of *instinguere* to incite, instigate, from *in-* in, into + *stinguere* to sting, extinguish, annihilate; Gk *stizein* to prick, puncture, burn a mark in, brand) instigation, impulse, incitement, instinct]   A complex unlearned response that is usually genetically determined and species-specific.

aggressive instinct   DEATH INSTINCT.

death instinct   In psychoanalytic psychology, a biologic tendency, under the control of the repetition-compulsion principle, toward self-destruction and the destruction of anything, whether arising from outside or inside the organism, that threatens to disturb the status quo. Also called *ego instinct, aggressive instinct, Thanatos.*

ego instinct   DEATH INSTINCT.

herd instinct   The tendency to be a group member and to conform to the behavior of the group.

homing instinct   An ability of an animal to return to its home territory when released at a remote site, as found especially in certain birds.

life instinct   SEXUAL INSTINCT.

sexual instinct   In psychoanalytic psychology, an instinct hypothesized to be under the control of the pleasure principle and its primary function being the preservation of life. Also called *eros, life instinct.*

instinctive [INSTINCT + -IVE] Pertaining to a behavioral act performed without the use of reason or past learning.

institutionalization 1 Commitment of an individual to a custodial or health care facility. 2 A syndrome of dehumanization and depersonalization described in some patients who have been in a mental hospital for an extended period. It consists of loss of individuality and self-esteem, apathy, depression, and decreasing involvement with others.

instruction A code that tells a computer to perform arithmetic and logic functions, control peripheral devices, or indicate succeeding instructions.

instrument [L *instrumentum* (from *instruere* to put together, set in order, erect, build in or into + *-mentum* -MENT) a tool, implement, furniture, utensils] An implement or tool.

Cawthorne's instrument An instrument designed for emergency laryngotomy, combining a retractable scalpel with a curved trocar and a cannula of oval cross-section.

double-plane instrument A binangled dental hand instrument with the angles in different planes.

Feleky's instrument An instrument used to massage the prostate gland.

gnathologic instrument ARTICULATOR.

hand instrument An instrument held in and worked by the hand as opposed to a rotary instrument which is held in a handpiece and is driven by an external power source.

McCall's instrument A dental hand instrument for scaling and root planing. It has a curette-shaped tip and is made with various different angles of shank.

nib instrument PLUGGING INSTRUMENT.

plastic instrument A dental hand instrument used for placing a plastic restorative material such as dental amalgam or cement.

plugging instrument A dental instrument used for condensing. It may be worked by hand or by engine. Also called *nib instrument*.

screwdriver instrument A screwdriver, used in oral surgery, made of the same metal as the screws used, thus avoiding the electrolytic problems caused by small deposits of alien metal on the screw heads.

single-plane instrument A dental hand instrument with bends in the shaft which are all in one plane.

stereotaxic instrument STEREOTAXIC APPARATUS.

stitching instrument A surgical device with two blades and handles that is used to facilitate the placement of stitches during the course of an operative procedure.

test handle instrument A root canal instrument in the form of a mandrel for adjusting the effective length of a reamer or file.

instrumentarium [Med L (from L *instrument(um)* tool, instrument + *-arium* -ARY), a case for carrying or storing papers] The instruments or other equipment required for a given surgical or medical procedure.

instrumentation [INSTRUMENT + -ATION] 1 The set of instruments that measure, monitor, record, control, and treat subject variables. 2 The use of instruments.

insuccation The process of soaking, as in the treatment of a crude drug source to obtain an extract for further purification of the active principle.

insufficiency [L *insufficientia* (from *in-* not + *sufficientia* sufficiency, from *sufficiens*, gen. *sufficientis*, pres. part. of *sufficere*, to afford, supply, be sufficient, from SUB- + L *facere* to do, make) insufficiency] A failure of an organ, part, or system to perform at a normal or adequate level of function; relative ineffectuality of function. Also called *insufficientia*.

active insufficiency A limitation of the contraction of a muscle stemming from the approximation of its origin and insertion.

acute adrenocortical insufficiency ADDISONIAN CRISIS.

acute coronary insufficiency UNSTABLE ANGINA.

adrenocortical insufficiency 1 Failure of adrenocortical secretion of steroid hormones due to any cause, such as bilateral total adrenalectomy, primary disease of the adrenal cortex (as autoimmune or tuberculous infiltration of the gland), or hypopituitarism. Also called *capsular insufficiency* (older term). 2 ADDISON'S DISEASE.

anterior pituitary insufficiency HYPOPITUITARISM.

aortic insufficiency AORTIC REGURGITATION.

basilar insufficiency Vertebrobasilar syndrome.

capsular insufficiency An older term for ADRENOCORTICAL INSUFFICIENCY.

cardiac insufficiency HEART FAILURE.

chronic adrenocortical insufficiency ADDISON'S DISEASE.

chronic mesenteric arterial insufficiency A chronic obstructive syndrome of the mesenteric arterial circulation presenting with abdominal pain, diarrhea, malabsorption, and anorexia. This may be the result of a variety of perivascular or intravascular lesions such as atherosclerosis, aneurysms, or vasculitis.

chronic renal insufficiency A disorder characterized by progressive decrease in renal function, including the glomerular filtration rate, over months or years. Urea and other nonprotein nitrogenous substances increase in the blood. A large number of other biochemical abnormalities gradually develop along with anemia, osteodystrophy, hypertension, anorexia, and many other signs and symptoms of the uremic syndrome.

coronary insufficiency Inadequate coronary blood flow.

insufficiency of the externi DIVERGENCE HYPOFUNCTION.

insufficiency of the eyelids Inadequate closure of the eyelids.

functional pyloric insufficiency Inadequate functioning of the pyloric valve which allows duodenal-gastric reflux, causing gastric mucosal irritation from bile salts. It has been suggested as a mechanism in the production of gastric ulcer.

gastric insufficiency Deficient ability of the stomach to empty itself, resulting in dilatation. Also called *gastromotor insufficiency*.

gastromotor insufficiency GASTRIC INSUFFICIENCY.

hepatic insufficiency Inability of the liver to perform its function properly. See also HEPATIC FAILURE.

ileocecal insufficiency ILEOCECAL INCOMPETENCE.

insufficiency of the interni CONVERGENCE HYPOFUNCTION.

left ventricular insufficiency LEFT VENTRICULAR HEART FAILURE.

mitral insufficiency See under MITRAL REGURGITATION.

muscular insufficiency Muscle weakness.

pancreatic insufficiency Inadequate production or release of pancreatic enzymes, resulting in inadequate digestion of nutrients and in abdominal symptoms.

parathyroid insufficiency HYPOPARATHYROIDISM.

pineal insufficiency A condition postulated as resulting from a nonparenchymal tumor of the pineal body which destroys its endocrine function. As a result, the pituitary-inhibiting hormone, perhaps melatonin, is not elaborated, the pituitary releases gonadotropin prematurely, and precocious puberty follows.

pituitary insufficiency HYPOPITUITARISM.

placental insufficiency Abnormal growth or function of the placenta due to inadequate oxygenation or nutrition, so that it is often unable to sustain adequately the developing fetus.

post-traumatic pulmonary insufficiency ADULT RESPIRATORY DISTRESS SYNDROME.

primary adrenocortical insufficiency ADDISON'S DISEASE.

proteopexic insufficiency Severe neutropenia that follows the entry into the bloodstream of a foreign protein that results in immunologic sensitization or anaphylaxis.

pulmonary insufficiency 1 Failure of the lungs to maintain normal levels of oxygen and/or carbon dioxide in arterial blood. **2** Regurgitation of the pulmonic valve.

pulmonic insufficiency See under PULMONARY REGURGITATION.

pyloric insufficiency A condition characterized by inadequate closure of the pyloric valve, resulting in too rapid emptying of the stomach.

renal insufficiency Impairment of renal function, whether acute or chronic.

right ventricular insufficiency RIGHT VENTRICULAR HEART FAILURE.

secondary adrenocortical insufficiency Adrenocortical insufficiency resulting from hypopituitarism. Also called *secondary adrenocortical failure.*

thyroid insufficiency HYPOTHYROIDISM.

total renal insufficiency A decrease in all renal function.

tricuspid insufficiency See under TRICUSPID REGURGITATION.

uterine insufficiency Abnormal or inadequate uterine contractions during labor which do not effectively dilate the cervix.

insufficiency of the valves See under VALVULAR REGURGITATION.

valvular insufficiency See under VALVULAR REGURGITATION.

velopharyngeal insufficiency Imperfect closure of the palatopharyngeal sphincter on swallowing or while speaking. Important causes include a variety of neurologic diseases producing paralysis of the palate or of the palate and pharynx, and cleft palate. Also called *velopharyngeal incompetence.* Compare VELOPHARYNGEAL ADEQUACY.

venous insufficiency Impairment of venous return as a result of incompetence of the venous valves.

vertebral insufficiency VERTEBROBASILAR SYNDROME.

vertebrobasilar insufficiency VERTEBROBASILAR SYNDROME.

insufficientia INSUFFICIENCY.

insufflate [See INSUFFLATION.] To blow, or deliver under pressure (air, gas, vapor, or particulate matter) into (a chamber or body cavity).

insufflation [L *insufflatio* (from *insufflatus,* past part. of *insufflare* to blow on or into, from *in-* in + *sufflare* to blow at or against, inflate, from SUB- + L *flare* to blow, breathe) a blowing into] **1** The delivery under pressure of air, gas, vapor, or particulate matter into a chamber or cavity of the body, as, for example, the delivery of air to the lungs in artificial respiration. **2** An inhalant or other substance to be insufflated.

cranial insufflation The blowing of air or a gas into the intracranial spaces.

endopharyngeal insufflation INSUFFLATION ANESTHESIA.

endotracheal insufflation The insufflation of air or gas into the lungs through an endotracheal tube.

perirenal insufflation An outmoded radiologic procedure entailing the percutaneous injection of air into the perirenal space to visualize the borders of the adrenal gland and kidney.

presacral insufflation An outmoded radiographic technique characterized by injection of gas, usually carbon dioxide, through a needle placed into retrorectal space for radiologic visualization of the kidneys, adrenal glands, and other retroperitoneal structures.

tubal insufflation The transcervical instillation of carbon dioxide gas in order to allow distension and subsequent passage of the gas from the fimbriae of the fallopian tubes into the peritoneal cavity. The procedure is most commonly utilized to determine patency of the fallopian tubes.

insufflator An instrument used for insufflation.

insula [L, an island] [NA] The expanded area of cerebral cortex at the depth of the lateral sulcus, delimited below by the underlying claustrum. Also called *insula Reilii, insula of Reil, island of Reil, caudate lobe of cerebrum* (obsolete).

insulae of Peyer FOLLICULI LYMPHATICI AGGREGATI.

insula of Reil INSULA.

insula Reilii INSULA.

insulae Plural of INSULA.

insular **1** Of or relating to the insula. **2** Of or relating to the islets of Langerhans.

insular-pancreatotropic Tending to affect the secretory functions of the pancreatic islets of Langerhans.

insulate To separate conductors by a material of poor conductivity to minimize the passage of electricity, heat, or sound.

insulation [L *insulat(us)* (from *insul(a)* island + *-atus* -ATE) made into an island + -ION] **1** Material of poor conductivity used to insulate. **2** The act of insulating. **3** The state of being insulated.

insulator A material that insulates or a device made of such material. Compare CONDUCTOR.

insulin [*insul(a)* + -IN] A peptide hormone synthesized and secreted by the beta cells of the pancreatic islets of Langerhans, the principal fuel-metabolizing hormone of mammals. It is a polypeptide having two chains (the A chain of 21 amino acids and the B chain of 30 amino acids) linked by two disulfide bonds, and having a molecular weight of 5734. The hormone accelerates the transport of glucose, amino acids, and potassium across cell membranes, and elicits the release of one or more intracellular second messengers, with consequent changes in the levels of enzyme action and other activities, thereby regulating carbohydrate, lipid, and amino acid metabolism. Diabetes mellitus is the result of insulin deficiency. Preparations of the crystalline or chemically modified or bound hormone derived from hog or beef pancreas are used in treating the human disease. Also called *insuline* (obsolete), *antidiabetic hormone* (obsolete).

dealinated insulin A derivative of porcine insulin prepared by the removal of the alanine residue at the C-terminal end of the B chain. Replacement by phenylalanine yields human insulin. Porcine insulin so treated is biologically active and useful in instances where antibodies to porcine or bovine insulin have reduced the effectiveness of those preparations.

depot insulin A preparation of insulin that is slowly absorbed from the site of injection.

globin insulin GLOBIN ZINC INSULIN.

globin zinc insulin A combination of insulin, globin, and zinc, with an intermediate time of onset of action and a duration of activity between regular insulin and protamine zinc insulin. Also called *globin insulin.*

hexamine insulin A combination of hexamethylenetetramine and insulin that is no longer used.

histone insulin A complex of thymus histone and insulin that is no longer used.

histone zinc insulin A combination of thymus histone, insulin, and zinc that is no longer used.

immunoreactive insulin The insulin measured by immunoassay rather than by its hormonal activity. Immunoassays detect both insulin and proinsulin, but not the various nonsuppressible insulinlike activities of human plasma.

insulin lente INSULIN ZINC SUSPENSION.

neutral insulin INSULIN INJECTION. ● The terms are now equivalent, but previously insulin injection was not neutralized, and this distinction was of importance because of the greater stability of the neutralized preparation.

pectin insulin A combination of insulin and pectin that is no longer used.

plant insulin Any substance obtained from plant material that produces a hypoglycemic effect in experimental animals. Also called *vegetable insulin.*

protamine insulin   A combination of insulin with protamine but without zinc, no longer used clinically. Also called *insulin protaminate.* Abbreviation: PI

protamine zinc insulin   A sterile suspension of insulin in buffered water to which zinc chloride and protamine sulfate have been added. It is administered by injection. Also called *zinc protamine insulin, protamine zinc insulin suspension.*

regular insulin   INSULIN INJECTION.

synalbumin insulin   A postulated antagonist of insulin that is present in the blood of some diabetics and is believed to be a polypeptide related to the B chain of insulin associated with serum albumin.

three-to-one insulin   A combination of regular insulin and protamine zinc insulin in a ratio of these two activities of 3:1. Such combinations have been largely replaced by combinations of amorphous and crystalline insulins and limited concentrations of zinc, to obtain both rapid onset and prolonged duration of insulin activity.

vegetable insulin   PLANT INSULIN.

zinc protamine insulin   PROTAMINE ZINC INSULIN.

insuline   An obsolete term for INSULIN.

insulinemia   The presence of insulin in the blood. A seldom used term.

insulinization [INSULIN + -iz(e) + -ATION]   Treatment with exogenous insulin. A seldom used term.

insulinlipodystrophy   Atrophy of fat at the sites of insulin injection.

insulinogenesis   Synthesis or synthesis and release into the bloodstream of insulin by the beta cells of the pancreatic islets.

insulinogenic   Pertaining or promoting insulinogenesis. Also *insulogenic.*

insulinoid   Having hypoglycemic properties like insulin.

insulinoma [INSULIN + -OMA]   A tumor of the beta cells of the pancreatic islets. Such tumors are usually benign and are characterized by excessive secretion of insulin with consequent severe hypoglycemia. Also called *insuloma.*

insulinopenia [INSULIN + o + Gk *penia,* poverty, need]   Relative or absolute lack of insulin, as in diabetes mellitus or following pancreatectomy. Adjective: insulinopenic.

insulinoprivic [insulin + o + L *priv(us)* deprived of + -IC]   Lacking insulin; marked by insulinopenia.

insulin protaminate   PROTAMINE INSULIN.

insulism   An older term for HYPERINSULINISM.

insulitis [L *insul(a)* an island + -ITIS]   Cellular infiltration of the pancreatic islets, presumably a result of inflammation or infection. A seldom used term.

insulogenic   INSULINOGENIC.

insuloma   INSULINOMA.

insulopathic   Of or characterized by abnormal secretion of insulin. A seldom used term.

insult [French *insult(er)* (from L *insultare* to leap upon or against, scoff at, insult, from -*in* -IN¹ + *saltare* to leap; frequentative form of *insilire* to leap into or upon, from -*in* -IN¹ + *salire* to leap) to offend by hurtful words]   **1** To abuse or attack.   **2** Any injury to the body or to tissue, as that resulting from an attack. Also called *insultus.*

insultus [Late L, from L *in-* IN-¹ + *saltus* a leap]   INSULT.

insurance   A contractual relationship between an insurer and another party under which the insurer agrees to reimburse or otherwise provide compensation for a loss, should one occur, in exchange for the payment of a fee. Also called *assurance.*

catastrophic health insurance   Health insurance which pro-

vides protection against the high cost of treating severe or lengthy illness or disability; major medical.

contributory insurance   Group insurance in which all or part of the premium is paid by the employee and the remainder, if any, by the employer or other party.

disability income insurance   A form of health insurance that provides periodic payments to replace income when the insured is unable to work as the result of injury or illness.

dread disease insurance   An insurance policy that provides benefits against specified and feared disease.

group insurance   Any insurance whereby members of a group, such as employees of an employer, along with their dependents, are insured under a single policy covering all members of the group.

health insurance   Insurance against loss by disease, bodily injury, or illness, and related health care needs.

individual health insurance   Health insurance covering an individual, and sometimes the individual's dependents, rather than a group.

malpractice insurance   PROFESSIONAL LIABILITY INSURANCE.

professional liability insurance   Insurance purchased by a health care provider to protect against the risk of or actual financial loss on the part of the provider due to damages awarded as a result of the provider's negligent acts. Also called *malpractice insurance.*

sponsored malpractice insurance   Medical malpractice insurance under which a professional society sponsors a specific insurer's insurance program and cooperates in the administration of the program.

supplemental health insurance   Health insurance which covers medical expenses not covered by separate health insurance already held by the insured.

insured   The individual or organization protected in the event of loss under the terms of an insurance policy.

insurer   The party to an insurance policy who contracts to pay losses or render services in the event of a loss.

intake   The entry into the body of a solid, liquid, or gaseous substance.

acceptable daily intake   **1** The amounts of the various nutrients that need to be consumed to satisfy a person's metabolic needs.   **2** The maximum amount of a substance added to food that can be consumed without causing a health hazard. Abbreviation: ADI

caloric intake   The caloric value of substances taken into the body.

conditional daily intake   The amount of a given food absorbed per day by the body.

daily intake   The amount of any given food substance consumed per day. Also called *unconditional daily intake.*

fluid intake   The volume of fluid taken into the body.

food intake   The amount of food consumed by a person or animal in a given period of time.

provisional total weekly intake   The amount of food expected to be consumed by a person given an itemized dietary regimen.

total daily intake   The absolute amount of all nutrients consumed per day.

unconditional daily intake   DAILY INTAKE.

Intal   A proprietary name for disodium chromoglycate.

integration [L *integratio* (from *integratus,* past part. of *integrare* to make whole, renew, heal, from *integer* whole, complete, intact, from *in-* in + *tangere* to touch, affect) a renewing, restoration]   **1** The amalgamation of different parts into a coordinated whole.   **2** In microbiology or cell biology, the incorporation of a piece of DNA, often a viral genome or a plasmid, into a chromosome.   **3** In psychology, the process of making integral the several contributing elements or characteristics of a subject.

nervous integration   The process by which a neuron or set of neurons provides an output or behavior in response to the synaptic interactions of inputs.

personality integration   The dynamic organization of all of the traits, motives, and moral acquisitions of an individual into a coherent whole that will permit a consistent and harmonious adjustment to the constantly changing circumstances of life, especially to those of the social milieu.

structural integration   ROLFING.

integrity   Wholeness; intactness; unimpaired condition.

integument   INTEGUMENTUM.

common integument   INTEGUMENTUM COMMUNE.

spore integument   The envelope of a bacterial spore, consisting of the core membrane, cortex, coat, and exosporium.

integumentary   **1** Pertaining to the integumentum commune. **2** Providing a covering.

integumentum   [L (from *in-* IN-¹ + *tegumentum*, also *tegmentum* a covering, protection, from *teg(ere)* to cover + *-mentum* -MENT), a covering, integument]   A covering or investing layer of a part or the body. Also called *integument*.   • The term is often used instead of *integumentum commune*.

integumentum commune   [NA] The layer enveloping the whole body, i.e., the skin, comprising epidermis, dermis, and all appendages such as hairs, nails, sweat and sebaceous glands, and mammary glands. Also called *common integument, cutaneous system, integumentary system, dermoid system* (seldom used), *dermal system* (seldom used), *skin.*

in tela   [L *in* in + *telā*, ablative of TELA]   Within membranous connective tissue: said especially of preparations for the light microscope.

intellect   [L *intellect(us)* (from *intellectus*, past part. of *intelligere*, also *intellegere* to understand, perceive, know) an understanding, intellect. See INTELLIGENCE.]   That grasp of cognitive mental processes by means of which humans think, especially those processes permitting the discovery of relationships, and of judging, conceiving, and reasoning.

intellectualization   An attempt to analyze a personal problem in purely intellectual terms, to the neglect or exclusion of affective considerations that would be normal under the circumstances. It is often a defensive measure by which the individual can achieve some degree of insulation against the feelings of emotional hurt that would otherwise be experienced.

intelligence   [L *intelligentia* or *intellegentia* (from *intelligens, intellegens*, gen. *intelligentis, intellegentis*, pres. part. of *intelligere, intellegere* to understand, perceive, know, from INTER- + L *legere* to collect, pick up, read) perception, understanding, intellect]   **1** A quality of behavior demonstrating the degree to which an organism is able to learn quickly and to adopt responses rapidly and effectively when faced with novel situations. **2** The ability to manipulate symbols and to grasp abstract relationships in problem-solving and to respond flexibly to changing demands within a given context. Human intelligence would encompass the collective repertory of cognitive powers possessed by an individual which can be brought to bear on the solution of difficult and complex problems, such as reason, insight, foresight, judgment, or imagination.

abstract intelligence   The ability to understand and to deal effectively with abstract concepts or relationships, typically by the use of symbols, either verbal or numerical.

artificial intelligence   The programing of a computer to perform functions that are normally associated with human intelligence, such as learning, reasoning, and decision-making.

mechanical intelligence   A demonstrated native ability to quickly grasp mechanical interrelationships among concrete objects, and a quick comprehension of the operation of mechanical devices.

social intelligence   The ability of an individual to deal effectively with other persons, and to adapt to novel situations involving other members of one's social group. A rarely used term.

intensification   An increase in intensity.

image intensification   In radiology, the method of increasing the brightness of fluoroscopic image by means of an image intensifier tube.

intensimeter   [*intensi(ty)* + -METER]   An apparatus, no longer used, to measure x-ray intensity, based on the ability of irradiation to vary the electric resistance of a selenium cell.

intensity   [*intens(e)* + -ITY]   The magnitude or strength of a variable, such as brightness, ionizing radiation, sound, electric field, or magnetic field.

compensation intensity   The degree of light intensity at which a plant produces just enough oxygen by photosynthesis to carry on respiration.

intensity of electric field   The force on a stationary positive charge per unit charge at a point in an electric field. Also called *electric field vector, electric field strength, electric vector.*

intrauterine intensity   The strength of intrauterine pressure that occurs with a uterine contraction during labor.

light intensity   LUMINOUS INTENSITY.

luminous intensity   The luminous flux incident on a small surface which lies in a specified direction from a light source and is normal to this direction, divided by the solid angle (in steradians) which the surface subtends at the source of light. Also called *light intensity.*

pulse average intensity   Intensity averaged over the pulse duration.

intensity of roentgen rays   The radiation energy passing per unit time through a unit area perpendicular to the beam of radiation.

intensity of service   A measure of the quantity and sophistication of services provided in a hospital or other health care facility.

spatial average intensity   Intensity averaged over the transducer area or the ultrasound beam cross-sectional area.

spatial average temporal average intensity   Intensity averaged over the cross-sectional area of an ultrasound transducer beam and over the pulse repetition period.

spatial peak intensity   Intensity at the point in an ultrasound beam where it is maximum.

spatial peak temporal average intensity   Intensity averaged over the ultrasound pulse repetition period at the point in the beam where it is maximum.

temporal average intensity   Intensity averaged over an ultrasound pulse repetition period.

temporal peak intensity   The maximum intensity reached in an ultrasound pulse repetition period.

threshold intensity   The stimulus magnitude necessary for tissue excitation or sensory detection.

intensive   Marked by intensity; specifically, requiring special attention or strong measures, as *intensive care.*

intent / criminal intent   The intent to do harm, as evidenced by the commission of a criminal act, or the mental ability to form such an intention, or both, frequently an important consideration in establishing responsibility of a person accused of having committed such an act. Also called *mens rea.*

intention   A manner of healing of wounds and incisions, such as healing by first intention.

inter-   [L *inter* between, among]   A prefix meaning (1) between or among; (2) mutual, shared, combined.

interaccessory Denoting structures connecting accessory processes of vertebrae.

interacinar Between acini. Also *interacinous.*

interacinous [INTER- + *acin(us)* + -OUS] INTERACINAR.

interaction [INTER- + ACTION] In statistics, the relationship obtaining between two independent variables when their joint effect on the dependent variable is greater than that of the sum of the effects of both acting separately. For example, if respiratory function (dependent variable) is affected both by occupational exposure to dust and by cigarette smoking (independent variables) but their effect when acting jointly exceeds the sum of their separate effects, occupational exposure and smoking are said to show interaction with respect to respiratory function.

complementary interaction Nonallelic gene interaction in which the phenotype produced is distinct from that of either gene separately.

coulombic interactions Interactions between particles or bodies that are due to the attraction of unlike or repulsion of like electrical charges.

heme-heme interaction Interaction between two heme groups. Such interactions occur in hemoglobin, where oxygenation (or deoxygenation) of one heme facilitates the oxygenation (or deoxygenation) of others. The interactions are indirect, since they are effected by alterations in the structural configuration of the globin chains rather than of their heme components.

ion-dipole interaction An interaction or attraction between a neutral molecule and an ion. The ion-dipole interactions are weak and the forces decrease rapidly as the interacting groups are moved apart.

primary interaction The binding of antibody to antigen, regardless of whether it can be detected serologically.

interalveolar Between alveoli, particularly those of the lung.

interamnios [INTER- + New L *amnios,* variant of AMNION] A cavity between the amnion and the embryophore in the eggs of mammals showing inversion of germ layers.

interangular Between angles.

interannular Between two ringlike structures or constrictions.

interapophyseal Between two bony processes or projections.

interarticular Between the articular surfaces of a joint or between two joints.

interarytenoid Between the two arytenoid cartilages of the larynx. Also *interarytenoidal.*

interarytenoidal INTERARYTENOID.

interasteric Between the right and left asterion of the skull, a distance occasionally measured in craniometry.

interatrial Between the atria of the heart. Also *interauricular.*

interauricular 1 INTERATRIAL. 2 Between the auricles of the external ears. 3 Between the auricles of the atria.

interaxonal Between axons, with reference to the Schwann cell processes and endoneurial collagen in peripheral nerves.

interbands The regions of a polytene chromosome between the cytologic bands.

interbrain [INTER- + BRAIN] DIENCEPHALON.

intercadent [INTER- + L *cadens,* gen. *cadentis,* pres. part. of *cadere* to fall, drop] 1 Interpolated, as an extra beat in cardiac rhythm. 2 Characterized by interpolated beats.

intercalary Inserted between; additional, interposed, as intercalary ducts of compound exocrine glands and intercalated disks of cardiac muscle. Also *intercalated, intercalate.*

intercalate INTERCALARY.

intercalated INTERCALARY.

intercalatum [L (substantive from neut. sing. of *intercalatus,* past part. of *intercalare* to interpose, place between, from *inter-*

INTER- + *calare* to call), an inserting between] An obsolete term for SUBSTANTIA NIGRA.

intercanalicular Between canaliculi.

intercapillary Between or among capillary vessels.

intercarotic INTERCAROTID.

intercarotid Between the external and internal carotid arteries. Also *intercarotic.*

intercarpal Between carpal bones.

intercartilaginous Located between, or connecting, cartilages. Also *interchondral.*

intercavernous 1 Between two cavities. 2 Between or connecting the two cavernous sinuses.

intercellular Between and among cells.

intercentra A series of small crescent shaped bones wedged between the centra of vertebrae of reptiles and of the tails of mammals.

intercentral Connecting or situated between two centers of the brain and/or spinal cord.

intercept [L *intercept(us),* past part. of *intercipere* (from *inter-* between + *capere* to seize, take) to catch up, intercept] The point at which the graph of a linear function cuts the abscissa; the value of y in a linear function when $x = 0$.

intercerebral Situated between or connecting the cerebral hemispheres. Also *interhemicerebral.*

interchange In cytogenetics, any redistribution of chromatin, which is detectable microscopically, between or among chromosomes or between chromatids, such as translocations and sister chromatid exchanges.

interchondral INTERCARTILAGINOUS.

intercilium 1 GLABELLA. 2 The gap between the eyebrows.

interclavicle A small, diamond-shaped bone located between the tips of the clavicular bones in the pectoral girdle of reptiles.

interclavicular Between the clavicles.

interclinoid Between the clinoid processes of the sphenoid bone, either between anterior and posterior or across the midline. Also *interclinoidal.*

interclinoidal INTERCLINOID.

intercoccygeal Between segments of the coccyx.

intercolumnar Between any two columnlike or pillarlike structures.

intercondylar Between any two condyles. Also *intercondylous, intercondyloid.*

intercondyloid INTERCONDYLAR.

intercondylous INTERCONDYLAR.

intercornual Lying between paired horn-shaped structures of the nervous system.

intercoronary Between coronary arteries.

intercoronoideal Between the right and the left coronoid processes of the mandible.

intercostal Between the ribs.

intercostohumeral Pertaining to an intercostal space and the humerus or the arm.

intercoupler An electrical device that connects together the anesthesia machine, the operating table, the patient, and the anesthetist to keep them at the same electrical potential. This minimizes static-electricity sparks which might ignite a flammable anesthetic. The device is now obsolete.

intercourse Exchange or communication between people.
sexual intercourse COITUS.

intercoxal Between the hips or the hip bones.

intercricothyrotomy CRICOTHYROTOMY.

intercristal Between two crests, particularly those of the ilia of the hip bones: applied to measurement of the distance between them or to the level of the plane between their highest points.

intercross The mating of diploid individuals who are both heterozygous for one or more of the same alleles at given loci.

intercrural **1** Between any two crura. **2** Between the legs.

intercurrent Denoting a disease process affecting a patient already suffering from a preexisting illness.

intercuspal Pertaining to the relationship, or fit, of the cusps of the teeth of the upper or lower jaw against those on the teeth of the opposite jaw.

intercuspation [INTER- + CUSP + -ATION] The fitting of the cusps of the teeth of one arch into the fossae and occlusal embrasures of the opposing arch. Also called *intercusping, interdigitation.*

intercusping INTERCUSPATION.

intercutaneomucous Between the skin and the mucous membrane.

interdeferential Between the two ductus deferentes.

interdental Describing the space or position between adjacent teeth in the same jaw. Also *interproximal.*

interdentium [INTER- + L *dens* tooth + -*ium*, New L noun suffix] The space between two adjacent teeth.

interdigit The part of the hand or foot between any two adjacent fingers or toes.

interdigital Between any two adjacent fingers or toes.

interdigitate To interlock or interweave in elongated or fingerlike processes.

interdigitation **1** The state of being interlocked or interwoven in elongated or fingerlike processes. **2** INTERCUSPATION.

interductal Between ducts.

interface [INTER- + FACE] **1** In a biological system, the junctional layer between two different materials. **2** The point in a process where independent systems interact.

dermoepidermal interface DERMOEPIDERMAL JUNCTION.

gamma camera interface The electronic equipment that functionally connects a gamma camera to a computer and serves to convert the analog signals generated by the camera to digital signals compatible with the computer format.

interfacial Of or relating to an interface.

interfascicular Between fasciculi.

interfeminium The space between the thighs, or the inner side of the thighs. An obsolete term. Also called *interfemus.*

interfemoral Between the thighs.

interfemus INTERFEMINIUM.

interference [*interfer(e)* + -ENCE] **1** The combination of two or more wave disturbances, differing in frequency or in direction of propagation, acting at the same point, to produce a net disturbance. **2** In the presence of atrioventricular dissociation, the interruption of the regular rhythm of one pair of chambers by activation deriving from the other, most often of the ventricles (ventricular capture) by an impulse deriving from the atria. **3** In genetics, any statistically significant alteration in cross-over frequency from randomness. Chromosome interference may be either positive or negative, depending on whether a given cross-over decreases or increases, respectively, the frequency of another cross-over. Also called *chiasma interference.* **4** See under OCCLUSAL INTERFERENCE.

chiasma interference INTERFERENCE.

chromatid interference Any statistically significant alteration from random in successive cross-over frequencies between any two chromatids of the four present in paired homologues.

cuspal interference The presence of tooth contacts which prevent a normal path of closure or cause instability of a denture.

electromagnetic interference Interference to a circuit from

an outside source, such as power line, radio, or radar. Abbreviation: EMI

initial interference PREMATURE INTERFERENCE.

interceptive occlusal interference PREMATURE INTERFERENCE.

interchromosomal interference Balancing of negative interference in one pair of homologues by positive interference in another such that the overall cross-over frequency is less altered than in either situation alone.

occlusal interference A contact between antagonistic teeth which prevents proper closure or function.

premature interference Occlusal interference during closure in centric position. Also called *initial interference, interceptive occlusal interference.*

working interference Occlusal interference on the working side.

interferometer [*interfer(ence)* + *o* + -METER] An instrument that measures extremely small displacements by counting maxima and minima of interference patterns of light.

acoustic interferometer An interferometer that examines sound waves rather than light waves.

electron interferometer An interferometer that examines electron beams rather than light waves.

interferometry The process of measuring very small distances or movements by use of an interferometer.

interferon A protein produced in organisms infected by viruses, and effective at protecting those organisms from other virus infections. In the presence of a double-stranded RNA, such as viral RNA, it stimulates the synthesis of 2′,5′-linked oligonucleotides of adenylate, carrying a 5′-triphosphate group, and these stimulate a ribonuclease that degrades messenger RNA. Also, in the presence of double-stranded RNA, it stimulates a kinase that phosphorylates an initiation factor and thereby inactivates it. Interferon therefore suppresses protein biosynthesis by two mechanisms.

α interferon Any of a number of closely related antiviral proteins synthesized by many types of cell in response to viral infections or to a variety of inducers (e.g. double-stranded DNA). Lymphoblastoid cells are a good source of α interferon, which has been purified from them. All α interferons show a characteristic resistance to acid pH. Also called *lymphoblastoid cell interferon.*

β interferon A particular molecular species of interferon that shares most of its properties, including acid stability, with α interferons. It is synthesized by many types of cell in response to virus infection, but was first isolated from fibroblast cells. Also called *fibroblast interferon.*

γ interferon The variety of interferon that is produced by sensitized T lymphocytes on stimulation by specific antigens. Besides its action in preventing viral replication, it is a macrophage-activating factor. It is structurally quite distinct from the classical interferons (α interferon and β interferon). Also called *immune interferon.*

antigenic interferon Interferon measured by reaction with specific antibody rather than by its biologic activity. Also called *immunoreactive interferon.*

fibroblast interferon β INTERFERON.

immune interferon γ INTERFERON.

immunoreactive interferon ANTIGENIC INTERFERON.

lymphoblastoid cell interferon α INTERFERON.

interfibrillar Between and among fine fibers. Also *interfibrillary.*

interfibrillary INTERFIBRILLAR.

interfibrous Between and among fibers.

interfilamentous Located between filaments.

interfilar Located between the filaments of a reticulum.

interfollicular   Situated between and around follicles.

interfrontal   Between the two unfused frontal bones, with reference to the frontal, or metopic, suture.

interfurca [INTER- + FURCA]   The area between the roots of a multirooted tooth.

interfurcae   Plural of INTERFURCA.

interganglial   Denoting connections between autonomic ganglia. Also called *interganglionic*.

interganglionic   **1** Denoting connections, which have been shown to be nonexistent, between sensory ganglion cells. An outmoded term.   **2** INTERGANGLIAL.

intergemmal   Between two or more bulblike bodies or structures, such as taste buds.

intergenic   **1** Pertaining to a region of DNA or chromosome that is located between two genetic loci, but not necessarily involving either.   **2** Of or relating to a mutation that is located between two genetic loci, but not necessarily involving either.   **3** Designating a mutation which affects the expression of two juxtaposed loci.

interglandular   Between glands.

interglobular   Situated between globules: said especially of microscopic spaces between globules of calcified dentin in teeth.

intergluteal   Between the buttocks; internatal.

intergonial   Between the gonia, or angles of the mandible.

intergrade   A stage of transition between two other stages.
sex intergrade   INTERSEX.

intergranular   Situated within the granule cell layers of the cerebrum or cerebellum.

intergyral   Connecting or situated between cerebral gyri.

interhemal   Between the hemal arches.

interhemicerebral   INTERCEREBRAL.

interhemispheric   Situated or occurring between, or connecting, the cerebral hemispheres.

interictal [INTER- + ICTAL]   Present or occurring between attacks. Also *interparoxysmal*.

interinhibitive   Mutually inhibiting: said of drugs or other agents.

interior   Located on or toward the inside.

interischiadic   Between the two ischia, particularly their tuberosities. Also *intersciatic*.

interjacent   Being or lying between or among.

interjugal   **1** Between the zygomatic processes.   **2** Between right and left jugale, a measurement used in craniometry.

interkinesis [INTER- + KINESIS]   The interval between cell divisions, especially the first and second meiotic divisions.

interlabial   **1** Between the lips.   **2** Between the labia.

interlamellar   Situated between lamellae.

interlaminar   Situated between laminae.

interleukin-1   A mediator produced by macrophages which acts upon lymphocytes enhancing their capacity to respond to antigens. Interleukin-1 is also believed to be the same as endogenous pyrogen and as catabolin and to be responsible for inducing the increased synthesis of many acute phase proteins during an inflammatory response *in vivo*. Also called *lymphocyte-activating factor*. Abbreviation: IL-1

interleukin-2   A lymphokine that supports growth and differentiation of thymus-derived cells and plaque-forming cells. Also called *T-cell growth factor*. Abbreviation: IL-2

interligamentary   INTERLIGAMENTOUS.

interligamentous   Between or among ligaments. Also *interligamentary*.

interlobar   Between the lobes of any structure or organ.

interlobular   Between the lobules of a structure or organ.

interlock   A device that prevents the operation of any piece of equipment until various components or specific preliminary conditions have been brought to a predetermined operational state.

interlocking   The locking together of twins by the chins where the first twin presents as a breech and the second one presents as a vertex. Also called *compaction, head locking*.

intermalar   Between the zygomatic bones.

intermalleolar   Between the medial and the lateral malleolus.

intermamillary   **1** Between the nipples of the breasts, with reference to an imaginary line between them.   **2** INTERMAMMARY.

intermammary   Between the breasts. Also *intermamillary*.

intermarginal   Between two margins or borders.

intermarriage   **1** A popular term for INBREEDING.   **2** The marriage of individuals of different races, cultures, religions, or other groups.

intermastoid   Between the mastoid processes of the temporal bone, a distance measured in craniometry.

intermaxilla   OS INCISIVUM.

intermaxillary   Between the two maxillae.

intermediary   Situated or coming between.
fiscal intermediary   A contractor who processes or pays provider claims under a health insurance policy on behalf of the insurer. Also called *fiscal agent*.

intermediate   **1** Occurring at or representing a middle position between others more extreme; halfway.   **2** INTERMEDIUS.   **3** A substance formed from the reactant in a chemical reaction and then transformed into the product.

intermedin [after *pars intermedia*, the intermediate lobe of the pituitary gland, the site of the hormone in amphibia, reptiles, and other forms]   MELANOCYTE STIMULATING HORMONE.

intermediolateral   Intermediate and on the lateral side.

intermediomedial   Intermediate and on the medial side.

intermedius   Denoting the middle of three structures, the other two being on either side of it, the one being nearest and the other furthest from the median plane; intervening; between two extremes. Also *intermediate*.

intermembral   Located or occurring between the limbs of an organism.

intermembranous   Located between two membranes.

intermeningeal   Situated or occurring between the layers of meninges surrounding the brain or spinal cord.

intermenstrual [INTER- + MENSTRUAL]   Between the menses or menstrual periods.

intermenstruum [INTER- + L *menstruum*, neut. of *menstruus* monthly]   The time from one menstrual period to the next.

interment [Middle English *enterren*, from Middle French *interrer* to inter, from assumed Vulgar L *interrare* (from *in-* IN-[1] + *terra* earth) to place into a grave + English *-ment*]   The act of burial, especially of a human body.

intermesenteric   Occurring between any mesenteries.

intermesoblastic   Lying between the layers of the mesoderm or the lateral plates thereof.

intermetacarpal   Between metacarpal bones.

intermetameric   Placed between two metameres.

intermetatarsal   Between metatarsal bones.

intermission [L *intermissio* (from *intermissus*, past part. of *intermittere* to leave off, discontinue) a ceasing, intermission]   Any interval, such as a quiet period between attacks or episodes of any form of disease or dysfunction.

intermit [L *intermit(tere)* (from *inter-* INTER- + *mittere* to send, let go) to leave off, discontinue]   To cease temporarily.

intermitotic Pertaining to the period and the events occurring between mitotic divisions.

intermittence Occurrence at intervals rather than continuously; interruptedness: commonly used with reference to the occasional dropping of heart beats or pulses. Also called *intermittency*.

glomerular intermittence Intermittent function of glomeruli, as demonstrated by *in vivo* dissecting microscope studies of frog kidneys. Glomerular intermittence has not been demonstrated in mammals.

intermittency INTERMITTENCE.

intermittent Occurring at intervals rather than continuously.

intermolecular Located or occurring between the molecules of a substance.

intermural Between the walls of an organ or organs of the body. Also *interparietal*.

intermuscular Between muscles, as of a septum.

intern [French *interne* (from L *internus* internal) one who is inside] An individual in professional training in a health care field, usually immediately after the awarding of the degree but before independent practice. Also *interne*.

internal Situated or occurring on the inside of a part, organ, or body; interior. Also *internus*. • Occasionally used, incorrectly, to describe a medial position.

internalization The process hypothesized to account for an individual's incorporation of the mores and standards of conduct of his society. Moral values, attitudes, and opinions are learned from others, primarily from parents, and these internalized principles then substitute for outer controls in the guidance of behavior.

internarial Between the nostrils. Also *internasal*.

internasal 1 Between the nasal bones or cartilages. 2 INTERNARIAL.

internatal Between the buttocks, or nates; intergluteal.

internation [INTERN (v.) + -ATION] The confinement of an individual, ordered by law, in a specified institution such as a prison or psychiatric hospital.

International Classification of Diseases A list of diseases, injuries, and causes of death, arranged under numbered categories according to etiology and anatomic localization and intended to ensure by international agreement comparability of mortality and morbidity statistics. Although every morbid condition can be assigned to a category, each does not necessarily have a category of itself. Contrary, therefore, to what is often assumed, the list does not constitute a nomenclature of diseases and injuries but a classification intended primarily for statistical use. Originally produced at the International Statistical Congress of Paris, in 1855, with various subsequent modifications, the Classification now undergoes a decennial revision under the auspices of the World Health Organization. The most recent edition, ICD-9, became effective in January 1979. Abbreviation: ICD

International Health Regulations A set of regulations introduced by the World Health Organization in 1969, with subsequent amendments, to replace the International Sanitary Regulations. They are binding on member states of WHO, unless specific reservations have been formally entered, and lay down the maximum measures that may be imposed on international traffic when there is a risk of transmission of a disease subject to be dealt with under the regulations. The regulations also deal with preventive arrangements at ports and airports and provide for the international surveillance of other diseases such as influenza and salmonellosis.

International Nonproprietary Names The nonproprietary names recommended by the World Health Organization for any drug. Lists of such names are published regularly. Abbreviation: INN

International Organization for Standardization An international body, founded in 1946, that promotes the development of standards in the areas of intellectual, scientific, technical, and economic activities in order to facilitate the international exchange of goods and services and to develop cooperation in those areas. Abbreviation: ISO

International Pharmacopeia A collection of specifications prepared by the World Health Organization for the quality control of pharmaceutical products which would enable all countries to establish standards in common. It differs from national pharmacopeias in that it lacks legal force. Each member state of the World Health Organization is, however, authorized to incorporate any part of the International Pharmacopeia in its own national pharmacopeia or to adopt it *in toto* as its national pharmacopeia.

International Red Cross Society An international philanthropic nongovernmental organization founded in 1864 with headquarters in Geneva, Switzerland, and having national affiliated societies in many countries. Its objectives are humanitarian and include disaster relief, the welfare of prisoners of war, public education, and training in first aid. It is known popularly as the Red Cross. In predominantly Muslim countries a comparable organization is known as the Red Crescent.

International Sanitary Regulations A set of regulations established by the World Health Organization for preventing the dissemination across international boundaries of the quarantinable diseases and superseded in 1969 by the International Health Regulations.

International System of Units See under SYSTÈME INTERNATIONAL D'UNITÉS.

interne INTERN.

interneural Between the vertebral, or neural, arches.

interneuron [INTER- + NEURON] Any neuron in a neural chain other than a primary afferent ganglion cell or a motor fiber innervating muscle. Also called *internuncial cell, connector neuron, intercalary neuron, intercalated neuron, internuncial neuron*.

inhibitory interneuron A short-axon neuron whose excitation produces an inhibitory postsynaptic potential on a nearby neuron, such as the Renshaw cells of the spinal cord.

interneuronal Pertaining to interneurons and their action.

internist A physician specializing in internal medicine.

internodal Situated between nodes. Also *internodular*.

internode INTERNODAL SEGMENT.

internode of Ranvier INTERNODAL SEGMENT.

internodular 1 Between two nodules. 2 INTERNODAL.

internship [INTERN + -ship, from Middle English -ship, scipe, from Old English -scipe, all noun suffixes denoting nature, position, quality; of Germanic origin] A period of training in a health care field such as medicine, usually following the awarding of a professional degree but preceding residency or independent practice.

internuclear Situated between nuclei: used especially of nuclear groups in the central nervous system.

internuncial Denoting an intermediary neural effect mediated between nerve cells or centers through the action of interneurons.

internus INTERNAL.

interocclusal Located between the occlusal surfaces of the opposing dental arches.

interoception [*inter-* as in *interior* + *o* + *(re)ception*] VISCERAL SENSE.

interoceptive Denoting the internal receptive apparatus associated with viscera and mediating internal sensation.

interoceptor A sense organ located in the viscera.

interofection [*inter(ior)* + *o* + *-fection* as in *affection*] The organismal response to internal changes.

interofective Denoting the autonomic nervous system and its influence on the interior of the body.

interogestate [INTER- + *o* + L *gestatus*, past part. of *gestare* to carry, bear] An embryo or fetus in the period of interior gestation. Compare EXTEROGESTATE.

interoinferiorly Inward and below or downward.

interolivary Situated between the paired inferior olivary bodies of the medulla oblongata.

interorbital Between the orbits.

interosculate ANASTOMOSE.

interosseal 1 Denoting the interosseous muscles. 2 INTEROSSEOUS.

interosseous Connecting or located between bones, particularly with reference to muscles, nerves, and vessels. Also *interosseal*.

interpalatine Between the palatine bones.

interpalpebral Situated between the upper and lower eyelid. The interpalpebral aperture is the opening for the eye.

interpandemic [INTER- + PANDEMIC] Existing or occurring between pandemics.

interpapillary Located between papillae.

interparietal 1 Between the parietal bones. 2 INTERMURAL. 3 Between certain gyri of the parietal lobe of the cerebrum.

interparoxysmal [INTER- + PAROXYSMAL] INTERICTAL.

interpediculate Between pedicles of a vertebra or vertebrae.

interpeduncular Situated between paired peduncles, like the fossa separating the cerebral peduncles from the nucleus interpeduncularis.

interpenetration 1 A disorder in which the subject inserts irrelevant material into his verbal productions. The material may consist of references to his complexes or conflicts but is unrelated to the topic of the moment. 2 A disorder in which the subject states only parts of an answer to a question he has been asked. The subject's ramblings or preoccupation with other material do not permit a direct, full, organized, or relevant answer.

interphalangeal Between contiguous phalanges of a finger or toe.

interphase The phase of the cell cycle between cell divisions, during which much of the synthesis of cellular constituents occurs. Interphase is divided into the following stages: G_1, a period immediately after mitosis or meiosis, during which no DNA synthesis is occurring; S, during which DNA synthesis occurs; and G_2, after DNA synthesis and before the onset of division.

interpial Located between the layers of the pia mater.

interplant [INTER- + PLANT[1]] The insertion of a part or piece of one embryo into a reasonably indifferent environment of another, such as the coelom or the chorioallantoic membrane.

interpleural Between the pleurae, or between two layers of a pleural sac.

interpleuricostal Between a pleural sac and the surrounding ribs.

interpolar Positioned between two poles.

interpolate [L *interpolatus*, past part. of *interpolare* (from *interpolis* altered in appearance, painted, dressed) to give a new appearance, polish, furbish] To perform the act of interpolation.

interpolated 1 Obtained or implanted by interpolation. 2 Inserted; intercalated.

interpolation [*interpolat(e)* + -ION] 1 Estimation of the value taken by a function at points intermediate between two known values. In the simplest form of interpolation it is assumed that the dependent variable is directly proportional to the independent variable, and in this case the interpolation is said to be linear. 2 In surgery, the insertion of a flap between two or more structures.

interposition A putting between; the condition of being interposed.

interpositum [L, neut. sing. of *interpositus*, past part. of *interponere* to interpose] An interposed structure, such as the veli of the central nervous system. A rarely used term.

interpretation [L *interpretatio* (from *interpretatus*, past part. of *interpretari* to interpret, explain, from *interpres*, gen. *interpretis*, an agent, mediator, negotiator, from INTER- + L *pres*, root of *pretium* worth, value, price, akin to Gk *priasthai* to buy) interpretation] The therapist's description or formulation of the significance of a patient's productions during psychoanalytic treatment, often presented as a hypothesis to explain contradictions or inconsistencies in the patient's behavior or feelings.

mutative interpretation An interpretation that produces change in the subject's attitude or behavior, in particular one that makes the subject realize that his transference reaction to the analyst is based on his inner conflicts and not on accurate evaluation of current reality.

psychoanalytic interpretation Interpretation, by the analyst, of the patient's symbols, resistances, and defenses into a form that is meaningful to the patient.

serial interpretation Interpretation, by an analyst, of a consecutive number of dreams considered as a group centering on the same conflict.

interpreter A specialized computer program that translates each line of a high-level language such as BASIC into machine language and executes the specified instruction before going on to the next instruction.

interprotometamere [INTER- + PROTO- + META- + -MERE] That which lies between the initial segmental divisions of an embryo.

interproximal INTERDENTAL.

interpterion Between the two pteria of the skull, a distance sometimes measured in craniometry.

interpterygoid Between the pterygoid processes of the sphenoid bone.

interpubic Between the pubic bones.

interpupillary Pertaining to the space between the pupils of the two eyes.

interpyramidal 1 Situated within the pyramidal tract. 2 Situated between the paired pyramids of the medulla oblongata.

interrenal Between the kidneys.

interreticular Located between the elements of a reticulum, as the cytoplasmic material between the elements of the endoplasmic reticulum.

interrupted Broken in continuity; characterized by intervals of discontinuity; irregular.

interrupter / ground fault circuit interrupter A special circuit breaker that disconnects the source of electric power when a ground fault (leakage path) greater than about six milliamperes occurs. Safety codes require their use in wet areas such as bathrooms, swimming pools, and hydrotherapy areas to prevent electrocution.

interscapilium INTERSCAPULUM.

interscapular Between the two scapulae.

interscapulothoracic   INTERTHORACICOSCAPULAR.

interscapulum   The area between the scapulae. Also called *interscapilium.*

intersciatic   INTERISCHIADIC.

intersectio [INTER- + SECTIO]   (*plural* intersectiones) A site of meeting or crossing of two structures; a division or separation. Also called *intersection.*

  intersectio tendinea   [NA] A fibrous band that extends transversely or obliquely across a muscle belly, dividing it, wholly or partly, into segments. Also called *inscriptio tendinea, tendinous intersection, tendinous inscription, aponeurotic intersection.*

  intersectiones tendineae musculi recti abdominis   [NA] Fibrous bands, usually three in number, that pass transversely or obliquely across the rectus abdominis muscle, one being at the level of the umbilicus, a second opposite the tip of the xiphoid process, and a third being midway between the former two. They extend partly or totally through the substance of the muscle and are fixed to the anterior lamina of the rectus sheath. Also called *tendinous intersections of rectus abdominis muscle, inscriptiones tendineae musculi recti abdominis, tendinous inscriptions of rectus abdominis muscle.*

intersection [L *intersectio.* See INTERSECTIO.]   INTERSECTIO.

  aponeurotic intersection   INTERSECTIO TENDINEA.

  tendinous intersection   INTERSECTIO TENDINEA.

  tendinous intersections of rectus abdominis muscle   INTERSECTIONES TENDINEAE MUSCULI RECTI ABDOMINIS.

intersectiones   Plural of INTERSECTIO.

intersegment [INTER- + SEGMENT]   A metamere or any one of a series of similar segments. An older term.

intersegmental   **1** Placed between two segments.   **2** In embryology, lying between two metameres.

interseptal   Between septa, or partitions.

interseptum   DIAPHRAGMA.

intersex [INTER- + SEX]   An individual exhibiting ambiguous sexual characteristics, largely with respect to anatomical or behavioral traits. Also called *sex intergrade.*   ● The term is used in a more general sense than hermaphrodite or gynandromorph.

  female intersex   FEMALE PSEUDOHERMAPHRODITE.

  male intersex   MALE PSEUDOHERMAPHRODITE.

  true intersex   TRUE HERMAPHRODITE.

intersexual   Pertaining to or having the characteristics of intersexuality.

intersexuality [INTER- + SEXUALITY]   Any combination of male and female genetic, chromosomal, morphologic, hormonal, gonadal, and behavioral characteristics within the same individual; sexual ambiguity due to any cause. A popular usage.

  female genital intersexuality   Ambiguity of internal or external genitalia due to any cause in a genotypic female.

  gonadal intersexuality   TRUE HERMAPHRODITISM.

  male genital intersexuality   Ambiguity of internal or external genitalia due to any cause in a genotypic male.

intersigmoid   Between two parts of the sigmoid colon.

interspace [INTER- + SPACE]   A gap or area between two similar structures, such as the space between two ribs, or between two lobules of an organ.

  dineric interspace   The region of contact between two liquids.

interspinal   Between two spines or spinous processes. Also *interspinous.*

interspinous   INTERSPINAL.

intersternal   Between segments of the sternum.

interstice   **1** Any small gap or space in the structure of a tissue or organ.   **2** A crevice or interval between parts of the body. Also called *interstitium.*

interstitial   Pertaining or belonging to interstices or interspaces of a tissue or organ.

interstitialoma [*interstitial (cell tumor)* + -OMA]   LEYDIG CELL TUMOR.

interstitioma [*interstiti(al cell tumor)* + -OMA]   LEYDIG CELL TUMOR.

interstitium   **1** INTERSTICE.   **2** INTERSTITIAL TISSUE.

intersuperciliary   Between the superciliary arches of the frontal bone.

intertarsal   Between tarsal bones.

intertendinous   Between tendons.

interthoracicoscapular   Between the thorax and the scapula. Also *interscapulothoracic.*

intertragic   Between the tragus and the antitragus of the pinna.

intertransversalis   Any one of the musculi intertransversarii. Also called *intertransversarius.*

intertransversarius   INTERTRANSVERSALIS.

intertransverse   Between transverse processes of the vertebrae.

intertriginous   Pertaining to intertrigo, or to sites anatomically susceptible to intertrigo.

intertrigo [L (from *inter-* between + *tri(tus)*, past part. of *terere* to rub + -(i)go, suffix forming nouns from verbs, often indicating diseased condition), a sore place caused by chafing]   Erythema or eczema that affects apposed skin surfaces, as in flexurae or beneath a pendulous breast. Also called *intertriginous eczema, eczema intertrigo, paratrimma.*

  intertrigo labialis   An obsolete term for ANGULAR CHEILITIS.

intertrochanteric   Between the greater and lesser trochanters of the femur.

intertuberal   Between tubers or tuberosities.

intertubercular   Between tubercles.

intertubular   Between or among tubules or tubes.

interureteral   INTERURETERIC.

interureteric   Between the ureters. Also *interureteral.*

interuteroplacental [INTER- + UTERO- + PLACENTAL]   Located or occurring between the uterus and placenta.

intervaginal   Between sheaths.

interval [L *intervallum* (from INTER- + L *vallum* a palisade made from stakes and set up on a rampart) a space between two palisades, an intervening space, interval]   A gap between two parts or structures; a period between two points in time.

  a-c interval   The interval between the onset of the a wave and that of the c wave of the jugular pulse.

  A-H interval   The time between the onset of the atrial deflection and the His bundle deflection. This is normally between 50 and 150 milliseconds.

  atrioventricular interval   The interval between the onset of atrial systole and that of ventricular systole. Also called *A-V interval, auriculoventricular interval.*

  auriculoventricular interval   ATRIOVENTRICULAR INTERVAL.

  A-V interval   ATRIOVENTRICULAR INTERVAL.

  BH interval   The duration of His bundle deflection.

  birth interval   The time interval between births, sometimes including the protogenetic interval.

  cardioarterial interval   The interval between the onset of the apex beat and that of the radial pulse.

  closed birth interval   The time interval between consecutive births to a woman.

  confidence interval   In statistics, the interval, as calculated from observations on a random sample, within which will lie, with a degree of probability specified in advance, the true value of a given population parameter. The complement of the probability is an index of the risk of being in error when regarding the interval so defined as containing the true value. A commonly observed convention is to accept a risk of error of 5% or 1%. The boundary values of the interval are termed confidence limits.

coupling interval The interval between the onset of a QRS complex in sinus rhythm and that of a succeeding premature beat, usually expressed in hundredths of a second or milliseconds.

first birth interval PROTOGENETIC INTERVAL.

first pregnancy interval The interval between marriage and the first pregnancy within that marriage.

focal interval The distance between the principal foci of an optical system.

H-V interval The time from the onset of the earliest His bundle deflection to the earliest component of ventricular depolarization.

induction-delivery interval The period of time between starting an induction of labor and the delivery of the infant.

interectopic interval The interval between two successive ectopic beats.

interpregnancy interval The interval between pregnancies measured from the termination of one to the commencement of the next. Also called *pregnancy interval*.

interstimulus interval In classical conditioning, the time elapsing between the onset of a conditioned stimulus and the onset of the paired unconditioned stimulus.

intertrial interval The interval between successive presentations of any kind of stimuli, such as words in a list of nonsense syllables.

isometric interval ISOVOLUMETRIC INTERVAL.

isovolumetric interval The period during which the cardiac ventricle is contracting but its volume remains the same; the period between the onset of mechanical systole and the opening of the semilunar valves. Also called *isometric interval, presphygmic interval*.

lucid interval 1 A period of relative freedom from confusion, hallucinations, delusions, and other grossly psychotic symptoms, as may occur during organic deliria as well as acute schizophrenic episodes. 2 In forensic medicine, a sufficient restoration of reason so that the subject is able to comprehend and perform an action with such memory, perception, and judgment as to be held legally responsible for the action.

open birth interval The time interval between the last birth to a woman and the point when that information was obtained, as in a census or during an ad hoc survey.

open pregnancy interval The time interval between the end of a woman's last pregnancy and the point when that information is recorded, as in a census or during an ad hoc survey.

P-A interval The time between the earliest deflection of the P wave and the deflection caused by depolarization of the lower atrial septum in intracardiac electrography.

P-J interval The interval between the onset of the P wave of the electrocardiogram and the junction (J) between the terminal part of the S wave and the ST segment.

postmortem interval In forensic medicine, the amount of time between a person's death and the discovery of the body. The determination of this period is never exact except under circumstances in which death is witnessed. In unwitnessed deaths, the estimate is made by an assessment of the development of algor, rigor, and livor mortis and by vitreous humor analysis and other tests and examinations.

postsphygmic interval The period of isovolumetric relaxation.

P-P interval The interval between two successive P waves.

P-R interval The interval between the onset of the P wave and the beginning of the QRS complex, whether this be a Q wave or an R wave. It is usually between 0.12 and 0.20 seconds.

pregnancy interval INTERPREGNANCY INTERVAL.

presphygmic interval ISOVOLUMETRIC INTERVAL.

protogenetic interval In demography, the interval between marriage and the first birth. Also called *first birth interval*.

Q-R interval The interval between the onset of the QRS complex and the peak of the R wave.

QRS interval The interval between the onset of the Q wave and the termination of the S wave.

QRST interval Q-T INTERVAL.

Q-T interval The interval between the onset of the Q wave and the termination of the T wave, representing the duration of ventricular depolarization and repolarization. Also called *QRST interval*.

S₂-OS interval The interval between the second heart sound and the opening snap in mitral stenosis. The shorter the interval, the more severe the stenosis is apt to be.

Sturm's interval The distance between the two linear foci of a cylindrical lens.

temperature interval The value assigned to a unit of temperature on any particular temperature scale.

turnover interval The average time a hospital bed remains unoccupied between patients. It is a measure of the extent to which available beds in a ward, a hospital, or group of hospitals are being used to capacity. It is the ratio of the average daily number of unoccupied beds during a given period to the number of discharges and deaths during the period, times the number of days in the period.

intervalvular Between valves.

intervascular Between blood vessels.

intervention [Late L *interventio* (from *interventus*, past part. of *intervenire* to come between) an intervening] 1 Any procedure implemented to assist or educate a patient in preserving or improving his health or well-being. 2 In psychiatry, any therapeutic maneuver in which the therapist enters into the disequilibrium between subject and environment so as to help the patient regain a satisfactory level of adaptation.

interventricular Between ventricles.

intervertebral [INTER- + VERTEBRAL] Between two adjacent vertebrae.

interview / depth interview An interview that probes nonconscious attitudes or motivations which may contribute to observable behavior. To be effective, the depth interview must be conducted in a permissive atmosphere in which the subject can feel free to express inner feelings without disapproval or admonition.

stress interview A psychiatric evaluation session in which the interviewer deliberately avoids the usual ways of reducing the subject's anxiety in order to heighten pressure and have it released within the controlled environment of the interview.

intervillous Among or between villi.

interzonal Between zones, as the interzonal fibers connecting chromatids during anaphase of mitosis.

intestinal Concerning the intestine.

intestine [L *intestinum*. See INTESTINUM.] The tubular portion of the digestive apparatus which extends from the pylorus of the stomach to the anus. It is divided into the small intestine and the large intestine. Also called *bowel, gut, intestinum*.

blind intestine CAECUM.

empty intestine JEJUNUM.

iced intestine PERITONITIS CHRONICA FIBROSA ENCAPSULANS.

jejunoileal intestine The jejunum and ileum considered together.

large intestine INTESTINUM CRASSUM.

mesenterial intestine INTESTINUM TENUE MESENTERIALE.

preoral intestine The part of the embryonic intestine in front of the buccopharyngeal membrane and forming the deep part of the stomadeum.

primitive intestine   The hollow embryonic precursor of the adult intestine.

segmented intestine   An outmoded term for COLON.

small intestine   INTESTINUM TENUE.

straight intestine   An outmoded term for RECTUM.

intestinointestinal   Involving or relating two or more segments of the intestine; enteroenteric.

intestinum [L, neut. of *intestinus* inward, internal; as substantive, a gut; in pl. *intestina*, the guts, bowels, intestines]   INTESTINE.

intestinum caecum   An outmoded term for CAECUM.

intestinum crassum   [NA] The distal portion of the intestine which extends from the termination of the ileum to the anus. It is divided into the cecum with the vermiform appendix, the colon, the rectum, and the anal canal. It is arranged to surround the small intestine and functions mainly in the absorption of fluid and solutes. It differs from the small intestine in several ways including its wider caliber and the presence of taeniae coli, haustrations, plicae semilunares coli, and appendices epiploicae. Also called *large intestine*.

intestinum ileum   An outmoded term for ILEUM.

intestinum jejunum   An outmoded term for JEJUNUM.

intestinum rectum   An outmoded term for RECTUM.

intestinum tenue   [NA] The convoluted proximal portion of the intestine which extends from the pyloric orifice to the ileocecal valve. It is divided into duodenum, jejunum, and ileum, of which the latter two are suspended from the posterior abdominal wall by the mesentery. It is situated in the central and lower portions of the abdominal cavity and is surrounded by the large intestine. Its major functions include the continued digestion of food by intestinal juices and the absorption of nutrients into the blood and lymph vessels, for which the mucosal surface is considerably increased by the formation of the plicae circulares and the villi. Also called *small intestine, enteron*.

intestinum tenue mesenteriale   The portion of the small intestine that is suspended from the posterior abdominal wall by the mesentery, namely, jejunum and ileum. Also called *mesenterial intestine*.

intima [L, fem. sing. of *intimus* innermost, superl. of assumed *interus* inward (the comparative is *interior* inner, interior)]   **1** Denoting an innermost layer.   **2** TUNICA INTERNA VASORUM.

intimal   Pertaining to the tunica intima of a blood vessel.

intimectomy [*intim(a)* + -ECTOMY]   Removal of a portion of the intima of an artery.

intimitis [*intim(a)* + -ITIS]   Inflammation of the intima of an artery or vein; endangiitis.

intine [L *int(us)* within + -INE]   The inner layer of the wall of a bryophyte spore or a pollen grain.

Intocostrin   A proprietary name for tubocurarine chloride.

intoe   A deformity of the foot in which, when walking or standing, the foot turns inward. It can arise from metatarsus varus, tibial torsion, or persistence of the fetal alignment.

intolerance [L *intolerantia* (from *in-* not + *tolerantia* a bearing, enduring, from *tolerans*, gen. *tolerantis*, a pres. part. of *olerare* to bear, endure, abide, akin to *tollere* to bear, endure and to Gk *tlan* to bear, undergo) insolence, insufferable pride]   **1** Inability or unwillingness to accept or withstand.   **2** A tendency to react hypersensitively, as to a drug.

congenital lactose intolerance   A condition of diarrhea and a failure to thrive due to the malabsorption of lactose. In some it is due to congenital deficiency of lactase, which is inherited as an autosomal recessive trait. In others it is due to an autosomal dominant, more severe disorder associated with lactosuria.

disaccharide intolerance   An inability to digest one or more disaccharides, leading to symptoms of bloating, abdominal discomfort, nausea, vomiting, and explosive, acidic diarrhea when the offending sugar is ingested. This arises as a result of a deficiency in the disaccharidases present in the brush border membrane of the intestinal villi. Human jejunal mucosa contains five maltases, two sucrases, two lactases and an α-dextrinase. Such a deficiency can arise as a primary, inherited enzyme defect or an acquired defect secondary to another disease such as kwashiorkor, celiac disease, giardiasis, sprue, acute enteric infections, and cystic fibrosis.

fructose intolerance   HEREDITARY FRUCTOSE INTOLERANCE.

hereditary fructose intolerance   A rare, inherited, metabolic disorder due to an absence of the enzyme 1-phosphate aldolase from the liver. This leads to interference with several aspects of carbohydrate metabolism, including that of glycogen breakdown, with consequent hypoglycemia which may be severe. Symptoms consisting of vomiting, sweating, and convulsions occur after sucrose or fructose are introduced into an infant's diet. These disappear if glucose is given. Older children and adults may have epigastric pain, bloating, diarrhea, and hepatomegaly. Symptoms are brought on acutely by eating fruit or food sweetened with cane sugar (sucrose). Symptoms are reversible and competely preventable by excluding fructose from the diet. The inheritance is autosomal recessive. Also called *fructose intolerance, fructokinase deficiency, fructose-1,6-diphosphatase deficiency*. Abbreviation: HFI.

hereditary galactose intolerance   GALACTOSEMIA.

lactose intolerance   Inadequate capacity of the intestine to hydrolyze lactose, resulting in a syndrome of abdominal discomfort, cramps, and watery diarrhea, mostly occurring within thirty minutes to a few hours after ingesting milk or milk products. It may be genetic or occur in association with other gastrointestinal disorders. Also called *milk intolerance*.

leucine intolerance   Intolerance of the branched-chain amino acid leucine, one of the causes of hypoglycemia in early infancy. Ingestion of leucine causes a rapid fall in blood sugar. It also occurs in maple sugar urine disease, the dietetic control of which requires regulating the amounts of the three branched-chain amino acids, leucine, valine, and isoleucine.

lysine intolerance   An autosomal recessive disorder that is caused by a deficiency of L-lysine:NAD-oxido-reductase. It is evident in infancy, and it is characterized by vomiting, coma, and hyperammonemia. A low-protein diet to restrict lysine constitutes treatment.

milk intolerance   LACTOSE INTOLERANCE.

intonation [Med L *intonatio* (from *intonatus*, past part. of *intonare* to utter in a singing tone, to intone, from L *in-* IN-¹ + *tonus* a sound) an intoning]   The variations in voice pitch characteristic of the natural speaker of a language. Patterns of intonation are specific to particular languages.

nasal intonation   NASAL RESONANCE.

intorsion   Rotation of the eye upon its anteroposterior axis so that the upper part of the eye approaches the midline of the body. Also called *conclination*.

intort   To rotate the eye upon its anteroposterior axis so that the upper part of the eye approaches the midline of the body.

intorter [L *intort(us)*, past part. of *intorquere* to turn around, twist + -ER]   An extraocular muscle that turns the eye on its anteroposterior axis so that the upper part of the eye moves nasalward.

intoxation   A seldom used term for INTOXICATION.

intoxicant   A substance that produces intoxication or drunkenness.

intoxication [L *in-* intensive + *toxicum* poison for arrows, poison, from Gk *toxikon* poison for arrows, + -ATION] **1** The action of an absorbed and diffused toxic substance upon an organism, or the resultant pathological state of the organism; poisoning. Also called *toxication, intoxation* (seldom used). **2** Drunkenness; acute alcoholism or a clinically similar condition.

acid intoxication Severe acidosis. A seldom used term.

alkaline intoxication Severe alkalosis. A seldom used term.

anaphylactic intoxication ANAPHYLACTIC SHOCK.

bromide intoxication BROMIDE POISONING.

citrate intoxication A condition that may develop from blood transfusions in which citrate has been used as an anticoagulant. Tetany may result from the citrate combining with the blood calcium, thereby reducing the concentration of ionized calcium.

digitalis intoxication Poisoning with one of the digitalis alkaloids. Overdosage causes increased cardiac irritability and irregularities, gastrointestinal and visual disturbances, and occasionally, bizarre neurologic symptoms and psychoses in later stages of intoxication.

intestinal intoxication Intoxication from the production and accumulation of toxins formed in the intestine. Also called *autointoxication, intestinal autointoxication.*

manganese intoxication A syndrome resembling parkinsonism which results from chronic exposure to the dust of manganese ores and which is seen almost exclusively in miners of the metal and those handling the ores in factories.

pathologic intoxication Idiosyncratic hypersensitivity to alcohol, a small amount of which precipitates extreme excitement with persecutory ideas and aggressive, destructive, and sometimes homicidal outbursts. The reaction lasts several hours and ends with the subject falling into a deep sleep from which he wakes with total amnesia for the episode. Also called *alcoholic fury, mania à potu, mania à poter, alcoholic mania.*

roentgen intoxication RADIATION SICKNESS.

serum intoxication SERUM SICKNESS.

water intoxication An excessive water content in the body. Also called *hydrotoxicity.*

intra- [L *intra* (for *intera*) within, inside] A prefix meaning within, inside.

intra-abdominal Situated or occurring within the abdomen.

intra-acinous Within an acinus or acini.

intra-alveolar Within an alveolus or alveoli.

intra-appendicular Situated or occurring within the appendix.

intra-arachnoid Situated within the trabeculae of the arachnoid in the subarachnoid space.

intra-arterial Within an artery or arteries.

intra-articular Within a joint cavity.

intra-atomic Existing or occurring within an atom.

intra-atrial Within an atrium or the atria of the heart. Also *intra-auricular* (outmoded).

intra-aural Within the ear.

intra-auricular **1** Within an auricle of the ear or the atrium of the heart. **2** An outmoded term for INTRA-ATRIAL.

intrabronchial Within a bronchus or the bronchi. Also *endobronchial.*

intrabronchiolar Within a bronchiole or the bronchioles.

intrabuccal **1** Within the mouth. **2** Within the mass of the cheek.

intracaliceal Within a renal calix.

intracanalicular Within a canaliculus or canaliculi.

intracapsular Within a capsule, particularly of a joint.

intracardiac Within the heart. Also *intracordal.*

intracarpal Within the wrist or among wrist bones.

intracartilaginous Located or formed within cartilage or cartilaginous tissue. Also *endochondral, enchondral, intrachondral, intrachondrial, endchondral.*

intracatheter [INTRA- + CATHETER] A plastic tube introduced through a metal needle into a vein or artery and used for fluid infusion, drug injection, sampling blood, or keeping track of pressures.

intracavernous Within a cavernous sinus of the skull.

intracavitary Within the cavity of an organ or part.

intracelial Within any of the body cavities; endoceliac.

intracellular Within a cell. Also *endocellular.*

intracephalic Within the cranium or within the brain.

intracerebellar Within the cerebellum.

intracerebral Within the cerebrum.

intracervical Within any cervical canal, particularly that of the cervix uteri.

intrachange HOMOSOMAL ABERRATION.

intrachondral INTRACARTILAGINOUS.

intrachondrial INTRACARTILAGINOUS.

intrachordal [INTRA- + CHORDAL] Situated or occurring inside the notochord.

intrachorionic [INTRA- + CHORIONIC] Situated or occurring within the chorion.

intracisternal Within a cistern, usually with reference to a subarachnoid cistern, especially the cisterna magna (cisterna cerebellomedullaris).

intracolic Situated or occurring within the colon.

intracordal INTRACARDIAC.

intracorneal Within the cornea.

intracoronal Situated within the crown of a tooth: used especially of an attachment placed in a prepared cavity.

intracorporal INTRACORPOREAL.

intracorporeal Located or occurring within a body. Also *intracorporal.*

intracorpuscular Located inside a corpuscle, especially inside an erythrocyte. Hemolytic disorders may be divided into those of intracorpuscular and those of extracorpuscular cause. Also *endocorpuscular, endoglobular, endoglobar.*

intracostal On the internal surface of a rib or ribs.

intracranial Within the skull or cranium.

intracrureus The medial part of musculus vastus intermedius. An outmoded term.

intractable Resistant to therapy.

intracutaneous Situated within the skin.

intracuticular Situated within the cuticle.

intracystic Occurring within a cyst or within the urinary bladder.

intracytoplasmic Located in the cytoplasm of a cell.

intrad Inward; entad. An obsolete term.

intradermal Situated within the dermis. Also *intradermic.*

intradermic INTRADERMAL.

intradermoreaction INTRACUTANEOUS REACTION.

intraduct Within a duct or ducts. Also *intraductal.*

intraductal INTRADUCT.

intraduodenal Within the duodenum.

intradural Situated within or below the dura mater of the brain or spinal cord.

intraembryonic [INTRA- + EMBRYONIC] Situated or occurring within the embryo.

intraepidermal Situated within the epidermis. Also *intraepidermic.*

intraepidermic INTRAEPIDERMAL.

intraepiphyseal Within an epiphysis.

intraepithelial   Situated within the epithelium.

intraerythrocytic   Located within the cytoplasm of erythrocytes.

intraesophageal   Within the esophagus.

intrafascicular   Within a fascicle or the fasciculi of a tissue.

intrafebrile   Occurring during the febrile phase of a disease. Also *intrapyretic*.

intrafetation   [INTRA- + FETATION]   FETAL INCLUSION.

intrafilar   Located within a network or reticulum.

intrafissural   Within a fissure of the cerebral cortex.

intrafistular   Within a fistula.

intrafollicular   Within a follicle.

intrafusal   Denoting the striated muscle fibers situated within the fusiform capsule of a muscle spindle.

intragastric   Found or occurring within the stomach.

intragemmal   Within any bulblike structure or body, such as a taste bud.

intragenic   1 Pertaining to a region of DNA or chromosome entirely within a genetic locus.   2 Referring to a mutation, particularly a deletion or an insertion, that is located entirely within a given locus.

intraglandular   Within a gland or glandular tissue.

intraglobular   Located within a globule.

intragluteal   Within the buttock or the gluteal region.

intragyral   Within a gyrus of the cerebral cortex.

intrahepatic   Within the liver.

intrahyoid   Occurring within the hyoid bone, as accessory thyroid glands.

intraictal   [INTRA- + ICTAL]   Present or occurring during an attack.

intraintestinal   Situated or occurring within the intestine.

intrajugular   Within the jugular fossa, notch, process, foramen, or vein.

intralamellar   Within lamellae.

intralaryngeal   Within the larynx.

intralesional   Present within a lesion.

intraleukocytic   Located within the cytoplasm of leukocytes.

intraligamentous   Within any ligament.

intralingual   Within the tongue.

intralobar   Within a lobe.

intralobular   Within a lobule.

intralocular   Within the loculi of a tissue.

intralumbar   Situated within the lumbar segments of the spinal cord.

intraluminal   Within the lumen of any tubular structure, such as an artery or the intestine.

intramammary   Within the mammary gland or breast.

intramarginal   Within the margin or edge of any structure or organ.

intramatrical   Situated within a matrix.

intramedullary   1 Lying within the spinal cord.   2 Lying within the medulla oblongata.   3 Lying within the bone marrow.   4 Lying within the myelin sheath.

intramembranous   Within the layers of a membrane.

intrameningeal   Situated within the meninges surrounding the brain and spinal cord.

intramenstrual   [INTRA- + MENSTRUAL]   Occurring within the menstrual period.

intramolecular   Located or occurring within a molecule.

intramucosal   Within the layers of a mucous membrane.

intramural   Within the substance or the boundary of the wall of any organ or cavity. Also *intraparietal*.

intramuscular   Within the substance of a muscle.

intramyocardial   Within the myocardium.

intramyometrial   Being within the myometrium of the uterus.

intranarial   Within the naris or nares.

intranasal   Within the nose.

intranatal   Occurring during the process of birth.

intraneural   1 Within or extending into a nerve.   2 Within or extending into the central nervous system.   3 Within or extending into the cytoplasm of a neuron or one of its processes. Also *intraneuronal*.

intraneuronal   INTRANEURAL.

intranidal   [INTRA- + L *nid(us)* nest + -AL]   Taking place within the uterus before birth.

intranuclear   Situated or occurring within the nucleus.

intraocular   [INTRA- + OCULAR]   Located or occurring within the eyeball.

intraoperative   [INTRA- + OPERATIVE]   Pertaining to the period of time between the beginning and the completion of a surgical procedure.

intraoptic   [INTRA- + OPTIC]   Within the eye.

intraoral   Within the mouth.

intraorbital   Within the orbit.

intraosseous   Within a bone or bony tissue. Also *intraosteal*.

intraosteal   INTRAOSSEOUS.

intraovarian   Being within the substance of the ovary.

intraovular   [INTRA- + OVULAR]   Being within an ovum.

intrapancreatic   Situated or occurring within the pancreas.

intraparenchymatous   Within the parenchyma of a gland or an organ.

intraparietal   1 INTRAMURAL.   2 Within the parietal lobe of the cerebrum, specifically denoting the intraparietal sulcus.

intrapartum   [INTRA- + *partum*, accusative of *partus* a birth, begetting]   Occurring during labor or delivery.

intrapelvic   Within the pelvis.

intrapericardial   Within the pericardium or the pericardial cavity.

intraperineal   Within the structures of the perineum.

intraperitoneal   Within the cavity of the peritoneum.

intraphalangeal   Within a phalanx or phalanges.

intrapial   Lying within or covered by the pia mater.

intraplacental   [INTRA- + PLACENTAL]   Being within the substance of the placenta.

intrapleural   Within the pleura or pleural cavity.

intrapontine   Within the metencephalic pons.

intraprostatic   Within the prostate gland.

intraprotoplasmic   Within the cell cytoplasm.

intrapulmonary   Within the lung or lungs.

intrapyretic   INTRAFEBRILE.

intrarachidian   INTRASPINAL.

intrarectal   Within the rectum.

intrarenal   Within the kidney.

intraretinal   Located within the retina.

intrascapular   Within the scapula.

intrascleral   Located within the sclera.

intrascrotal   Within the scrotum.

intrasegmental   Within a segment, such as of the spinal cord.

intrasellar   Within the sella turcica of the sphenoid bone.

intraspinal   Within the vertebral column, the vertebral canal, or the spinal cord. Also *intrarachidian*.

intraspinous   Within a spinous process, as of a vertebra.

intrasplenic   Within the spleen.

intrasternal   Within the sternum.

intrastitial   Situated within the fibers or cells of a tissue.

intrastromal   Within the stroma, or framework, of an organ.

intrasynovial   Within the synovial membrane of a joint cavity or the synovial sheath of a tendon.

intratarsal   Within the tarsus.

intratesticular   Within a testis.

intrathecal   1 Within a sheath.   2 Within the subarachnoid space; intradural.

intrathenar   Pertaining to the shallow sulcus between the thenar and the hypothenar eminences in the palm of the hand.

intrathoracic   ENDOTHORACIC.

intratonsillar   Within a tonsil.

intratrabecular   Within a trabecula or trabeculae.

intratracheal   Within the trachea.

intratrochanteric   Within a trochanter.

intratubal   Within a tube or tubular structure, particularly the uterine tube.

intratubular   Within a tubule or tubules of an organ.

intratympanic   Within the tympanic cavity.

intraumbilical   Within the umbilicus.

intraureteral   Within the ureter.

intraurethral   Within the urethra. Also *endourethral*.

intrauterine   Within the uterus. Also *endouterine*.

intravaginal   Within the vagina.

intravasation   [INTRA- + VAS + -ATION]   The entry or introduction of foreign matter into a vein or artery.

intravascular   Within a vessel or vessels, particularly blood and lymphatic vessels.

intravenous   Within a vein or veins. Also *endovenous*.

intraventricular   Within a ventricle.

intraversion   [INTRA- + VERSION]   The position of a tooth or other oral structure which is nearer the median plane than is normal.

intravertebral   Within the vertebral column or canal.

intravesical   Within the bladder, particularly the urinary bladder.

intravillous   Within a villus.

intravital   1 Found or occurring during life.   2 Used, or capable of being used, on the cells or tissues of living organisms: said of a stain. Also *intra vitam*. Compare SUPRAVITAL.

intra vitam   [L *intra*, for *intera* within, inside + *vitam*, accus. sing. of *vita* life]   1 During life.   2 INTRAVITAL.

intravitelline   [INTRA- + VITALLINE]   Situated inside the vitellus.

intravitreal   INTRAVITREOUS.

intravitreous   Located or occurring within the vitreous cavity. Also *intravitreal*.

intrinsic   Belonging or inherent to and located entirely within a part or organ.

intro-   [L *intro* (for *intero*) inward, within]   A prefix meaning into, inward, being directed within.

introcession   An indentation or depression distorting the regular contour of a surface.

introcision   [INTRO- + -*cision* (from L *caesus*, past part. of *caedere* to cut) as in INCISION]   Intentional rupture of the hymen.

introducer   Any instrument designed to facilitate the introduction of some other instrument or appliance. For example, the introducer of a tracheostomy tube converts the blunt open end of the tube into a smooth, rounded tip and provides a handle.

Sise introducer   An awl used to puncture skin and deeper tissues, especially tough interspinous ligaments, thus facilitating the insertion of a lumbar-puncture needle in spinal anesthesia and the introduction of a fine lumbar-puncture needle without its touching the skin.

introflexion   A bending or flexing inward.

introgastric   Moved or transported into the stomach.

introgression   [INTRO- + (*di*)*gression*]   A theory of evolution by hybridization in which genes of one isolated species population infiltrate the genes of another isolated species population.

introitus   [L (from INTRO- + L *itus* past part. of *ire* to go) a going in, entrance]   The opening into a cavity, canal, or hollow organ.

introitus esophagi   The entrance to the esophagus at the lower end of the pharynx.

introitus pelvis   APERTURA PELVIS SUPERIOR.

introitus vaginae   OSTIUM VAGINAE.

introjection   [INTRO- + (*pro*)*jection*]   An unconscious defense mechanism of the ego consisting of incorporation or assimilation of an external object into one's ego, a part of which is thereby transformed into the representation of that object so that what originally occurred between the real object and self now occurs between the introjected object and self.

intromission   [L *intromissus*, past part. of *intromittere* (from *intro*- inward, within + *mittere* to send, cause to go) to send into or to]   1 The act of inserting the penis into the vagina in coitus.   2 Introduction or insertion of an object or part within something else.

intromittent   Inserted or capable of being inserted into a cavity.

intron   A region of a gene that lies between exons and is transcribed into RNA, but later is spliced out and does not code for translated gene product. Also called *intervening sequence*. Compare EXON.

intropunitive   [INTRO- + PUNITIVE]   Denoting a self-punishing reaction to frustration characterized by self-blame and feelings of shame, guilt, or humiliation. Compare EXTRAPUNITIVE.

introrsus   Turned inward or toward the center.

introspection   [L *introspect(us)*, past part. of *introspicere* to look into, examine + -ION]   Self-examination, particularly of one's thoughts and feelings.

introsusception   INTUSSUSCEPTION.

introversion   [New L *introversio* (from L *intro*- INTRO- + -*versio*, from *versus*, past part. of *vertere* to turn, as in *conversio* revolution) introversion]   The dynamic process in personality development by which the psychic energy of the individual is directed inwardly toward the self.

introversion-extroversion   A hypothetical bipolar dimension of the personality which attempts to classify individuals along a continuum varying from complete absorption in the self, to a complete outer-directedness towards external objects and other people.

introvert   [INTRO- + L *vert(ere)* to turn]   One whose personality is turned primarily inward, whose interests are vested more in personal thoughts, feelings, and experiences than in the world of external objects, other people, or social concerns.

intrude   [L *intrud(ere)* to thrust in, obtrude oneself]   To move a tooth into the bone in the direction of its root.

intrusion   Inward protrusion, thrusting, or penetration.

intubate   [IN-¹ + *tub(e)* + -ATE]   To introduce a tube into.

intubation   [L *in*- in + TUBE + -ATION]   The introduction of a tube, as into a vessel or orifice.

altercursive intubation   The surgical placement of a drainage tube for intermittent drainage or diversion of a secretion such as bile or urine.

aqueductal intubation   The introduction of a catheter

through the aqueduct of Sylvius.

blind nasal intubation   Nasal intubation in which the physician uses tactile and visual senses and the breathing sounds made by the patient as a guide, thus obviating the use of a laryngoscope. A topical or general anesthetic is applied prior to this procedure.

blind nasotracheal intubation   Nasotracheal intubation in which the physician does not have direct vision of the trachea.

esophageal intubation   The introduction of a tube or bougie into the esophagus for purposes of diagnosis or treatment.

nasal intubation   The passage of a tube, via the nose, into the trachea or stomach.

nasotracheal intubation   The passage of a tube into the trachea via the nose, either blindly or under direct vision.

oral intubation   The passage of a tube into the stomach or trachea via the mouth, done under direct vision.

orotracheal intubation   The passage of a tube, via the mouth, into the trachea done under direct vision.

intubationist [INTUBATION + -IST] One who passes a tube through a patient's nose or mouth into the trachea or stomach.

intubator   One who performs intubation.

intuition [Late L *intuitio* (from L *intuitus*, past part. of *intueri* to look at or upon) a beholding, contemplation] Judgment, perception, or knowledge that arrives in consciousness without prior, conscious, systematic thinking or reflection. The meaning of the data that are directly apprehended often contains an emotional component and is notable for its immediacy and the absence of any need for cogitation.

intuitive   Characterized by intuition.

intumesce   TUMEFY.

intumescence [L *intumescens*, pres. part. of *intumescere* to swell, grow angry] **1** INTUMESCENTIA. **2** The process of swelling.

intumescent [L *intumescens* (gen. *intumescentis*, pres. part. of *intumescere* to swell, grow angry) swelling, growing angry] Swelling up; swollen up.

intumescentia [INTUMESCENT + -IA] [NA] A swelling or enlargement.

intumescentia cervicalis   [NA] The cervical enlargement of the spinal cord, reaching its maximum thickness at the level of the fifth and sixth cervical vertebrae. It contains the motoneurons, interneurons, and fiber connections for C_5–T_1 spinal roots. Also called *cervical enlargement*.

intumescentia ganglioformis   A swelling in the shape of a ganglion.

intumescentia lumbalis   [NA] The lumbar enlargement of the spinal cord beginning at the level of the tenth thoracic vertebra, reaching its maximum thickness at the level of the first lumbar vertebra and tapering caudally. It includes central neurons and connects for L_4–S_3 spinal roots. Also called *lumbar enlargement*.

intumescentia tympanica   A swelling of the tympanic branch of the glossopharyngeal nerve lacking ganglion cells. Also called *Valentin pseudoganglion*.

intussusception [L *intus* within, inside + *susceptio* (from *susceptus*, past part. of *suscipere* to take or lift up, undertake, from SUB- + L *capere* to hold, seize) an undertaking] The invagination or telescoping of one segment of the intestine within a neighboring segment, most commonly the ileum into the colon. Also called *introsusception*.

acute intussusception   The invagination of one part of intestine into another resulting in paroxysms of pain, vomiting, and the development of an abdominal mass.

agonic intussusception   POSTMORTEM INTUSSUSCEPTION.

appendicular intussusception   The intussusception of the vermiform appendix upon itself. This mostly occurs in infancy and early childhood.

colocolic intussusception   The intussusception of one segment of colon into another.

compound intussusception   The combination of appendicular and ileocecal intussusception.

double intussusception   The occurrence of a second intussusception proximal to the first so that the mass formed by the first intussusception is enveloped by the second.

enterocolic intussusception   An intussusception of both the terminal ileum and the right colon such that the terminal ileum passes distally through the ileocecal valve into the cecum or colon.

gastric intussusception   The intussusception of the stomach on itself.

gastroduodenal intussusception   The invagination of the duodenum into the stomach.

ileal intussusception   An intussusception involving two segments of the ileum.

ileocecal intussusception   An enterocolic intussusception with the passage of the ileum into the cecum.

ileocolic intussusception   An enterocolic intussusception with the passage of the ileum into the ascending colon.

jejunogastric intussusception   A post-gastrojejunostomy complication involving the intussusception of either an efferent or afferent loop of bowel into the stomach.

postmortem intussusception   The development of an intestinal intussusception during the early postmortem interval. Also called *agonic intussusception*.

retrograde intussusception   Intussusception of distal bowel into a proximal segment.

secondary intussusception   A telescoping of one segment of the gastrointestinal tract into a more distal segment in which the leading point or intussusceptor is a tumor or mass lesion.

intussusceptum   A segment of intestine which has prolapsed into an immediately adjacent portion of intestine.

intussuscipiens   A segment of intestine into which an immediately adjacent portion of intestine has prolapsed.

inulase   An outmoded term for INULINASE.

inulase II   An enzyme that breaks down inulin by removing two fructose residues at a time from the nonreducing end in the form of a cyclic disaccharide.

inulin   A vegetable polysaccharide composed of fructofuranose units in a polymer form. It is used as a test substance to evaluate renal excretory function.

inulinase   The enzyme (EC 3.2.1.7) that catalyzes endohydrolysis of $2,1$-β-D-fructoside linkages in inulin. Also called *inulase* (outmoded).

inunction [L *inunctio* (from *inunctus*, past part. of *inungere* to anoint, besmear) an applying of an ointment] **1** Surface application of an ointment with friction to facilitate penetration into the skin. Also called *perfrication, infriction* (obsolete), *entripisis* (obsolete). **2** An ointment or other medication to be applied with friction. Also called *inunctum*.

inunctum   INUNCTION.

inunctum mentholis compositum   COMPOUND MENTHOL OINTMENT.

in utero [L *in* in + *utero*, ablative of UTERUS] Situated within the uterine cavity.

invaccination [IN-² + VACCINATION] Vaccination that inadvertently includes pathogenic organisms.

in vacuo [L *in* in + *vacuo*, ablative of *vacuum* (substantive from neut. sing. of *vacuus* empty, void) a vacuum] **1** Taking place in a vacuum. **2** Designating events or actions that occur seemingly without causal relationship to any other event.

invade   To penetrate or spread into injuriously, as infectious organisms or diseased tissue.

invaginate [IN-¹ + L *vagin(a)* sheath + -ATE] To infold (one portion of a structure) so that it becomes ensheathed within the structure.

invagination [L *in-* in + VAGINA + -ATION] **1** A type of gastrulation in which part of the blastoderm of an early embryo folds inward so that the hollow sphere becomes a double-walled cup. **2** The portion of the structure so ensheathed.

basilar invagination PLATYBASIA.

invagination of enamel DENS INVAGINATUS.

epithelial invagination The growth of oral epithelium over the surface of an implant so that it becomes entirely covered.

mammary invagination The primitive epithelial invagination, which during the eighth week in human development develops internally from the surface of the skin to form the galactiferous ducts.

invaginator [See INVAGINATION.] A surgical instrument that is used to fold in one portion of a structure onto another portion of the same structure.

invalid [L *invalidus* (from *in-* IN-² + *validus* strong, from *valere* to be strong, have force) weak, powerless] **1** Suffering from a disabling condition. **2** A person whose condition is disabling, as from chronic illness, infirmity, or injury.

invalidism [INVALID + -ISM] The condition of being an invalid, especially when of long duration.

invalidity [INVALID + -ITY] The state of being an invalid or incapacitated and unable to work.

invasion The infiltration of adjacent tissues by a disease process, usually cancer.

invasive [Med L *invasiv(us)* (from L *invas(us)*, past part. of *invadere* to enter upon, invade + *-ivus* -IVE) invasive] **1** Marked by invasiveness; tending to spread to other tissues. **2** Involving the penetration of a body cavity or the skin; used especially of a therapeutic or diagnostic procedure.

invasiveness **1** The aspect of pathogenicity involving penetration into a tissue or stable attachment to an epithelial surface, thus promoting spread in the body. **2** The quality of being invasive, as a therapeutic or diagnostic procedure.

inventory [Med L *inventor(ium)* (irreg. from Late L *inventarium* a finding out, from *invent(us)*, past part. of *invenire* to find, obtain information on + *-arium* -ARY) a finding information on + -Y] A list of questions to be answered to determine the presence or absence of certain interests, behaviors, or attitudes.

Bernreuter personality inventory A questionnaire appraising six personality traits: neurotic tendency, self-sufficiency, introversion, dominance, confidence, and sociability. Its main use has been as a screening device, to identify those individuals falling at the extremes of maladjustment on the self-descriptive scale.

California personality inventory A paper-and-pencil questionnaire designed to measure personality traits among normal individuals for age levels varying from preschool children to the adult. Subscales of the inventory reflect such traits as dominance, sociability, self-acceptance, and responsibility.

emission inventory SOURCE EMISSION DATA.

Maudsley personality inventory A questionnaire consisting of a variety of items about characteristic personal behaviors and interpersonal reactions. It is designed to measure two dimensions of personality held to be basic: neuroticism and introversion-extroversion.

Minnesota multiphasic personality inventory A widely used paper-and-pencil personality test in which the subject marks 550 items, concerning behavior, feelings, abnormal symptoms, social attitudes, or reactions, as "agree," "disagree," or "cannot say." Also called *Minnesota multiphasic personality test.*

source inventory SOURCE EMISSION DATA.

invermination [IN-¹ + VERMIN + -ATION] Infestation by vermin.

Inversine A proprietary name for mecamylamine hydrochloride.

inversion [L *inversio* (from *inversus*, past part. of *invertere* to turn over, transpose, alter, from *in-* in + *vertere* to turn) irony, a transposition, allegory] **1** The condition of being inside out, upside down, or out of place or usual position. **2** Any developmental reversal of the usual position, sidedness, or relationship of organs or parts. It occurs most commonly in the viscera, as in situs inversus viscerum. **3** The conversion of a chiral center in a molecule into its enantiomeric configuration. **4** An alteration in a section of DNA that reverses the direction of transcription. Inversion plays a key role in the regulation of a number of bacterial genes, such as those involved in phase variation in *Salmonella.*

atmospheric inversion TEMPERATURE INVERSION.

inversion of the bladder A partial or complete inversion of the urinary bladder through the urethral meatus due to relaxation of the vesical outlet. It is in many cases a result of straining during urination. Also called *cystanastrophe.*

chromosome inversion A chromosome aberration in which one portion of the chromatid is rotated 180° about its longitudinal midpoint. The phenotype may or may not be affected.

inversion of the foot TALIPES VARUS.

forced inversion Iatrogenic inversion of the uterus caused by undue traction on the umbilical cord or excessive fundal pressure in an effort to deliver a placenta following delivery of an infant.

inversion of germ layers A reversal in the relative position of germ layers. Complete inversion of the germ layers occurs in rat, mouse, and rabbit embryos, with the disappearance of the bilaminar omphalopleure so that the trilaminar omphalopleure is directly exposed to the uterine tissues during pregnancy. In incomplete inversion, the vascular embryonic segment of the yolk sac is invaginated into the nonvascular abembryonic segment and, as in primitive rodents, the yolk sac cavity is reduced or absent.

inversion of gradient Abnormal uterine contractions during labor which start in the lower uterine segment and spread toward the fundus. Normally contractions start in the fundus and spread toward the lower uterine segment.

lateral inversion MIRROR IMAGE.

paracentric inversion A chromosome aberration in which a portion of one chromosome arm, not including the centromere, is inverted.

pericentric inversion A chromosome aberration in which a portion of both chromosome arms and the centromere is inverted.

inversion of the polar formula An obsolete term for ERB'S REACTION.

sexoesthetic inversion An obsolete term for TRANSVESTISM.

sexual inversion An obsolete term for HOMOSEXUALITY.

inversion of sleep rhythm A sleep disorder consisting of somnolence by day and wakefulness at night.

sound inversion SONOINVERSION.

spontaneous inversion The turning inside out of the uterus as a natural occurrence during or following placental delivery as opposed to its occurrence as a complication of too vigorous traction on the umbilical cord to speed placental delivery (forced inversion).

temperature inversion An atmospheric condition in which the temperature of the air in the troposphere increases with altitude rather than decreases with distance from the earth. Such a situation is likely to interfere with the dispersion of fog, haze, and atmospheric pollutants. Also called *atmospheric inversion.*

thermic inversion A reversal of the normal circadian rhythm of body temperature that results in the temperature being at its highest in the morning. Also called *typhus inversus.*

inversion of uterus Abnormal turning of the uterus inside out so that the internal surface of the corpus uteri lies in or outside of the vagina. Also called *metranastrophe.*

visceral inversion SITUS INVERSUS VISCERUM.

inversus [L, past part. of *invertere* to turn about, change, invert] Denoting a reversal of the normal position or relations of a structure or an organ, from right side to left side, or vice versa, or upside down; transposition of viscera.

invert An older term for HOMOSEXUAL.

invertase β-D-Fructofuranosidase, an enzyme especially important for its hydrolysis of sucrose to glucose and fructose. The mixture produced was once known as invert sugar, owing to its possessing an optical rotation of opposite sign to that of the sucrose substrate. An outmoded term. Also called *invertin.*

invertebral Lacking a vertebral column. A seldom used term.

Invertebrata [New L (neut. pl. of *invertebratus,* lacking a backbone, from L *in-* not + New L *vertebratus* vertebrate, from L *vertebr(a)* a turning point in the body, a joint in the backbone + *-atus* -ATE)] **1** The group of all animals that lack a nerve cord, or in which the nerve cord is not enclosed by bony segments. **2** All members of the animal kingdom not classified in the chordate subphylum Vertebrata. The division of the animal kingdom into Vertebrata and Invertebrata is artificial. An obsolete term.

invertebrate [See INVERTEBRATA.] **1** Any animal that lacks a nerve cord, or in which the nerve cord is not enclosed in a skeletal backbone. **2** Any animal that is not classified as a member of the chordate subphylum Vertebrata.

invertin INVERTASE.

invertor A muscle responsible for turning a part, such as the foot, inward.

invest To surround, envelop, or ensheath with a particular material.

investing The act of surrounding a wax pattern or any solid form with a setting material so as to make a mold.

vacuum investing The subjecting of a dental investment mixture to a vacuum in order to remove air bubbles.

investiture INVESTMENT.

investment [L *invest(ire)* (from *in-* in + *vestire* to cover, clothe, from *vestis* a garment, clothing, akin to Gk *esthēs* a garment) to clothe + -MENT] **1** An outer covering, enveloping material, or sheath. **2** The setting material used to surround a wax pattern in the making of a mold, especially refractory material used in casting. For defs. 1 and 2 also called *investiture.*

emotional investment CATHEXIS.

fibrous investment A fibrous connective tissue layer surrounding a structure but separate from its capsule.

hygroscopic investment An investment using the property of hygroscopic expansion to compensate for the contraction of the cast on cooling.

myelin investment MYELIN SHEATH.

soldering investment An investment partly surrounding and supporting metal dentures and bridge units during soldering.

inveterate [L *inveterat(us),* past part. of *inveterare* (from *in-* IN-¹ + *vetus,* gen. *veteris,* old, of long standing) to become old, last a long time] Long-standing, chronic, and resistant to cure or correction.

invirility An obsolete term for IMPOTENCE.

inviscation [IN¹ + L *visc(us),* also *visc(um)* mistletoe, birdlime made from mistletoe berries + -ATION] INSALIVATION.

in vitro [L *in* in + *vitro,* ablative of *vitrum* glass] Describing a biological event that occurs in a laboratory in an artificial environment. Compare IN VIVO.

in vivo [L *in* in + *vivo,* ablative of *vivum* that which is living, from neut. sing. of *vivus* living] Describing a biological event that occurs in an intact animal or in the natural environment. Compare IN VITRO.

involucre INVOLUCRUM.

involucrum [L (from *involvere* to wrap up, envelop, cover), a wrapper, covering] **1** A surrounding sheath or membrane. Also called *involucre.* **2** The growth of new bone that forms around necrosed bone (sequestrum).

involuntary **1** Not voluntary. **2** In psychiatry, not consciously desired.

involute **1** CATABOLIZE. **2** To infold within another structure.

involution [L *involutio* (from *involutus,* past part. of *involvere* to roll in, envelop, from *in-* in + *volvere* to roll, turn) an enveloping] **1** An infolding. **2** A return to a former state. **3** Retrogression or decay. **4** CATABOLISM.

buccal involution The turning inward of ectoderm as the primitive oral cavity is formed in the embryo.

pituitary involution The first sign of Rathke's pouch as an upgrowth from the roof of the buccal cavity which will form the anterior lobe of the pituitary gland.

senile involution **1** An impairment of function due to aging, as of an organ. **2** A wasting of tissues due to aging.

involution of the uterus The gradual restoration to normal size of the uterus following a pregnancy.

involutional Relating to or characterized by involution.

involvement [L *involvere* to to roll in, envelop, cover, from *in-* in + *volvere* to roll, turn + -MENT] The inclusion in a disease process of a part not previously affected.

bifurcation involvement The extension of a periodontal pocket between the roots of a two-rooted tooth.

interradicular involvement The extension of a periodontal pocket between the roots of a multirooted tooth.

pulp involvement Presence in the pulp of a noxious agent likely to cause pulpitis; in particular, the spread of dental caries into the pulp.

trifurcation involvement The extension of a periodontal pocket between the roots of a three-rooted tooth.

iobenzamic acid $C_{16}H_{13}I_3N_2O_3.$ *N*-(3-Amino-2,4,6-triiodobenzoyl)-*N*-phenyl-β-alanine, a compound used in radiology as a radiopaque contrast agent for cholecystography.

iocetamic acid $C_{12}H_{13}I_3N_2O_3.$ *N*-Acetyl-*N*-(3-amino-2,4,6-triiodophenyl)-2-methyl-β-alanine, a compound used in radiology as radiopaque contrast medium.

iodalbumin Albumin containing covalently linked iodine in tyrosyl residues. It is a source of iodine and has properties like those of thyroglobulin, although it is much less active.

iodamide α,5-Diacetamide-2,4,6-triiodo-*m*-toluic acid. It is a radiopaque contrast medium.

Iodamoeba [French *iode* (from Gk *ioeides* violet-colored, from *ion* the violet + *eidos* form, shape) iodine + AMOEBA] A genus of amebas (order Amoebida, superclass Rhizopoda) which occur in the intestinal tract of humans and other mammals. The trophozoites have a large endosome, surrounded by granules of a globular form, and the cysts generally are uninucleate and have a large glycogen vacuole.

Iodamoeba buetschlii A species parasitic in the large intestine of humans. The trophozoites range from 5 to 20 μm in diameter and are infrequently found in feces. Cysts, ranging from 5 to 14 μm in diameter, are of irregular shape, uninucleate, and thick-walled, with a compact mass of glycogen that stains deeply with iodine solution. Cysts are the infective forms passed in feces. The organism is normally not pathogenic in man. Also called *Iodamoeba williamsi, Entamoeba buetschlii.*

Iodamoeba suis A species found in the intestine of pigs which is morphologically indistinguishable from *I. buetschlii.*

Iodamoeba williamsi IODAMOEBA BUETSCHLII.

iodate **1** The ion IO_3^- and its salts. This ion is a mild oxidizing agent. It is formed by the reduction of periodate when this acts as an oxidizing agent. **2** Any polyatomic anion with a central iodine atom.

iod-Basedow [*iod(ine-induced)* + *Basedow('s disease)*] IODINE-INDUCED HYPERTHYROIDISM.

iodemia The presence of iodine or iodide in blood, plasma, or serum.

iodeosin The analogue of eosin in which four iodine atoms replace the four bromine atoms of eosin. The term is used especially of the free acid, its salt being known as erythrosin.

iodic acid HIO_3. An oxoacid of iodine which exists as a white solid but is known mostly in solution or as its salts, the iodates.

iodide **1** The ion I^- or a salt that contains it. **2** Iodine in covalent combination, e.g. iodomethane, CH_3-I, may be called methyl iodide.

iodidoderma [*iodid(e)* + *o* + -DERMA] A cutaneous lesion resulting from adverse reaction to ingested iodides. Also called *iodide acne.*

iodimetry A measurement of iodine, usually by titration. It is used either to measure the amount of iodine in a material or liberated from a material, or to measure the amount of iodine consumed or displaced by some other material in an analytic reaction.

iodinate To add iodine to a compound, usually in substitution for hydrogen, but sometimes by simple addition.

iodination The process of treating a substance with, or causing it to combine with, iodine or with an iodine compound.

iodine A nonmetallic element of the halogen group, having atomic number 53 and atomic weight 126.9045. It consists of lustrous blackish crystalline flakes that volatilize at room temperature, forming a violet vapor with a strong odor. Iodine occurs in salt deposits and in sea water, where it is concentrated in the fronds of seaweeds. Inland areas are often deficient in iodine. The only isotope found in nature is the stable iodine 127. Valences are 1, 3, 5, and 7. Iodine is insoluble in water but soluble in an aqueous solution of potassium or sodium iodide. Its characteristic reaction with starch, the formation of a dark blue compound, provides a simple test for either starch or iodine. Iodine is an essential constituent of thyroid hormones and small amounts of iodine are essential in the diet. Symbol: I

butanol-extractable iodine Iodine, largely deriving from thyroid hormones, that is separated from serum by extraction with butanol, a step that eliminates some but not all of the interfering compounds that render the protein-bound iodine level inaccurate as a measurement of circulating thyroxine. This test is now supplanted by direct measurement of thyroxine. Abbreviation: BEI

protein-bound iodine Iodine present in serum and precipitated with serum proteins. Although largely derived from thyroid hormones, protein-bound iodine values also include inorganic iodides, abnormal iodinated proteins, and exogenous iodine-containing materials. It was formerly measured to indicate circulating thyroxine levels, but is now supplanted by direct measurement of thyroxine. Abbreviation: PBI

radioactive iodine Any iodine isotope other than iodine 127, which is stable. Three of these have been useful as diagnostic and therapeutic tools in diseases of the thyroid gland. The one in longest use is eight-day iodine 131, but it has been replaced to some extent by three-hour iodine 123 and iodine 125. Also called *radioiodine.*

iodine 123 An unstable isotope of iodine having atomic mass

123 and a half-life of 13.1 hours, with a major gamma photon emission of 159 keV. Symbol: ^{123}I

iodine 125 The radioactive isotope of iodine having atomic mass 125 and a half-life of 59.7 days, with a gamma photon emission of 35.5 keV. Symbol: ^{125}I

iodine 131 A radioactive isotope of iodine emitting beta and gamma radiation. As the radioactive element itself, it is used for thyroid imaging and function tests. It can also be used as a marker for renal imaging (sodium iodohippurate I-131), hepatobiliary imaging (rose bengal I-131), and for many other labeled agents. In therapeutic doses, it is used in the treatment of hyperthyroidism and thyroid carcinoma. Physical half-life is 8.04 days. Symbol: ^{131}I

iodine 132 A radioactive isotope of iodine having atomic mass 132 and a half-life of 2.285 hours, with beta emissions ranging from 0.72 to 2.12 MeV and gamma emissions from 147 to 2395 keV. Symbol: ^{132}I

iodine-fast Describing hyperthyroidism unresponsive to treatment with iodine.

iodine green A chromatin stain containing triphenylmethane. Also called *Hoffman green.*

iodine pentoxide I_2O_5. A crystalline white substance used as an oxidizing agent in carbon monoxide analysis to convert carbon monoxide to the dioxide form.

iodine violet HOFMANN'S VIOLET.

iodinin $C_{12}H_8N_2O_4$. 1,6-phenazinediol 5,10-dioxide, a purple chemical isolated from *Chromobacterium iodinum*. It has antibiotic activity against staphy lococci, streptococci, and some Gram- negative bacteria.

iodinometry The quantitative measurement of iodine, either as a constituent of a mixture or compound or as released from an iodide after oxidation. Also called *iodometry.*

iodinophil **1** Readily combining with or staining with iodine. Also *iodinophilous.* **2** An iodinophil cell or other tissue constituent. Also called *iodophil.*

iodinophilous IODINOPHIL.

iodipamide $C_{20}H_{14}I_6N_2O_6$. 3,3'-[1,6-Dioxo-1,6-hexanediyl)diimino]bis[2,4,6-triiodobenzoic acid]. A contrast substance for radiographic visualization of the biliary system.

iodism Poisoning from the chronic ingestion of iodine or its compounds, or from intensive, repeated therapy. Symptoms are coryza, ptyalism, headache, and skin eruptions.

iodize To treat with iodine and incorporate or attach (iodine) to a product; iodinate.

iodo- [French *iod(e)* iodine + *o*] A combining form indicating substitution of iodine for hydrogen in a chemical compound.

iodoacetamide $I-CH_2-CO-NH_2$. A reagent often used for alkylating thiol groups in proteins. Their ionized form, $R-S^-$, attacks its methylene group, expelling I^- to form $R-S-CH_2-CO-NH_2$.

iodoacetic acid $I-CH_2-COOH$. An acid forming colorless crystals, soluble in alcohol and ether, which darken on keeping, especially in the light, with release of iodine, so that pure samples need to be freshly recrystallized. It is a moderately strong acid (pK 3.1). It carboxymethylates nucleophiles, especially the thiol group, and inhibits thiol enzymes by the reaction: $R-SH + I-CH_2-COO^- \rightarrow R-S-CH_2-COO^- + H^+ + I^-$.

iodoalphionic acid $C_{15}H_{12}I_2O_3$. 3-(4-Hydroxy-3,5-diiodophenyl)-2-phenylproprionic acid. A radiopaque contrast agent used for cholecystography.

iodoantipyrine A freely diffusible radioisotope-labeled tracer used to measure the blood flow in skin and other tissues.

iodobrassid $C_{24}H_{44}I_2O_2$. 13,14-Diiodo-13-docosenic acid ethyl ester. A source of iodine for iodide therapy and a radiopaque contrast medium.

iodocasein An iodinated casein preparation containing 5.7% iodine, attached to the tyrosine residues. It has thyroxinelike activity.

iodochlorhydroxyquin C_9H_5ClINO. 5-Chloro-7-iodo-8-quinolinol. A brownish yellow powder, prepared as a powder, cream, or ointment, in suppositories, or as enteric-coated tablets. It has a direct amebicidal action and is used to treat acute and chronic intestinal amebiasis. It has also been used to treat *Trichomonas, Candida*, and various dermatitis infections by local or tropical application. It has also been used in dusting powders on wounds, ulcers, and burns of the skin. Also called *clioquinol*.

iodocholesterol Cholesterol that has been labeled with one or more iodine atoms. The iodine may be radioactive (radioiodinated cholesterol).

5-iododeoxyuridine IDOXURIDINE.

iododerma A cutaneous lesion resulting from an adverse reaction to ingested iodine.

iodoform CHI_3. A compound containing approximately 96% iodine. It is a yellow, crystalline powder and it is used topically as an anti-infective agent. Also called *triiodomethane*.

iodoformism Poisoning from iodoform. Topical application of large quantities has produced inflammation of the brain or cord and fatty degeneration of internal organs. It has been replaced by more desirable and effective drugs.

iodogorgonine An iodinated protein from corals which produces diiodotyrosine upon hydrolysis.

iodogorgoic acid A term seldom used in the U.S. for DIIODOTYROSINE.

iodohippurate sodium A compound used for studying renal function when labeled with an appropriate radionuclide. It has also been used as a radiopaque compound for urography.

iodolography [English *iodol* (from French *iode* iodine, from Gk *ioeid(ēs)* violet-colored, + L *ol(eum)* oil) + *o* + -GRAPHY] Roentgenography of an organ or body part after its being injected with an iodized oil.

iodometry IODINOMETRY.

iodonium The unstable ion I^+.

iodopanoic acid IOPANOIC ACID.

iodophendylate IOPHENDYLATE.

iodophil IODINOPHIL.

iodophilia An affinity for iodine or iodide, characteristic of starch and amyloid. Although iodophilia is said to be characteristic of neutrophil leukocytes in certain pathologic states, such as toxemia, it is not currently considered of diagnostic value. A rarely used term.

iodophor A high molecular weight carrier, such as polyvinylpyrrolidone, which holds iodine and can be used as a disinfectant on the skin. It is applied to skin surfaces before operations in veterinary medicine.

iodophthalein sodium The disodium salt of tetraiodophenolphthalein, a compound which has been used as a radiopaque contrast medium in cholecystography.

iodoprotein [IODO- + PROTEIN] An endogenous protein of the serum in which iodine is covalently bound within the peptide sequence. It is measured by the difference between protein-bound iodine and serum thyroxine. Its concentration is often raised in Hashimoto's disease and subacute thyroiditis, and sometimes in thyroid cancers and nontoxic goiter.

iodopsin The retinal visual pigment of the cone photoreceptors, responsible for day vision. Also called *visual violet*. Compare RHODOPSIN.

iodopyracet $C_{11}H_{16}I_2N_2O_5$. Diethanolammonium-3,5-diiodo-

4-pyridone-*N*-acetate. A compound which is radiopaque due to its iodine content. It is used in urographic procedures.

iodoquinol DIIODOHYDROXYQUIN.

iodosobenzoic acid 2-Iodosylbenzoic acid. It is used as a reagent for oxidizing thiol groups in proteins to disulfides, when it is concomitantly reduced to 2-iodobenzoate.

iodostick An applicator composed of iodine and potassium iodide. It is used topically as an antiseptic.

iodosulfate A combination of iodine and sulfuric acid with a basic compound to yield a complex salt of these two acidic components.

iodosyl The chemical group —IO.

iodotherapy [*iodo*- (from French *iode* iodine) combining form denoting iodine + THERAPY] Treatment with iodine or iodides. An older term.

iodothiouracil 5-Iodo-2-thiouracil. An iodine-containing derivative of thiouracil which has an advantage over the latter because preoperative iodine administration is no longer necessary. It is given orally as the sodium salt.

iodothyroglobulin A seldom used term for THYROGLOBULIN.

iodothyronine A compound formed by the oxidative coupling of two iodotyrosines through an ether linkage in the *para* configuration. Compounds of this class comprise the thyroid hormones, thyroxine, triiodothyronine, and their metabolites.

iodotyrosine Tyrosine iodinated *ortho* to its hydroxyl group. The term is sometimes used to include the tyrosine doubly iodinated. These two compounds are precursors of thyroxine and triiodithyronine, the thryoid hormones.

iodoventriculography [*iod(ine)* + *o* + VENTRICULO- + -GRAPHY] Roentgenography of the head in various positions after the placement of an iodine-containing oily contrast medium in the cerebral ventricular system.

iodovolatilization The release of free iodine by certain cells of brown algae or kelp.

iodoxyquinolinesulfonic acid An amebicidal agent given in a mixture with sodium bicarbonate as chiniofon, or as chiniofon sodium.

ioduria [*iod(ide)* + -URIA] The presence of iodides in the urine.

ioglycamic acid $C_{18}H_{10}I_6N_2O_7$. 3,3-(Diglycoloyldiimino) bis [2,4,6 triiodobenzoic acid], the meglumine and sodium salts of which are used in radiology as radiopaque contrast media for cholecystography.

iometer [*io(n)* + -METER] A chamber for measuring radiation. A seldom used term.

ion [Gk *iōn*, pres. part. neut. of *ienai* to go] An atom or radical that is electrically charged as a result of having lost or gained one or more electrons.

dipolar ion A molecular entity carrying charges of opposite sign.

-ion [L *-io*, gen. *-ionis*, suffix denoting an act or process, the result thereof, a condition or state, or thing acted upon] A noun suffix denoting action, process, or result.

ionium An obsolete term for THORIUM 230.

ionization [ION + -*iz(e)* + -ATION] **1** Dissociation into charged atoms or groups of atoms by electrolytes in aqueous solution. **2** Production of charged atoms or molecules in a gas by electric discharge or by irradiation.

avalanche ionization A process occurring among gaseous ions in an ionization chamber radiation detector. Given an adequate mean free path, a primary ion caused by the incident radiation can be accelerated by the applied voltage to the point where its collisions produce several other ions, whereupon each secondary ion does the same thing, and so on, causing an "avalanche." The multiplication of ions can be millionfold or more.

Also called *Townsend avalanche, avalanche, Townsend ionization.*

primary ionization The initial ionization produced by incident radiation.

secondary ionization Ions produced by collisions between primary ions or electrons and other atoms in an absorber.

Townsend ionization AVALANCHE IONIZATION.

ionize To undergo or cause to undergo ionization.

ionocolorimeter A device for determining the pH of a solution by the color it imparts to a suitably selected indicator.

ionogram [ION + *o* + -GRAM] ELECTROPHORETOGRAM.

ionometer [ION + *o* + -METER] Any apparatus which measures the intensity or quantity of radiation by measuring the ionization it produces. Also called *iontoquantimeter, iontoradeometer.*

ionometry [ION + *o* + -METRY] Measurement of ionizing radiation.

ionone Either of two isomeric compounds that smell of violets and are found in plant oils. Both are based on a cyclohexene ring, which carries on three adjacent carbon atoms the substituents dimethyl, 3-oxobut-1-enyl, and methyl. The α and β isomers differ in the position of the double bond in the ring. The synthetic material has largely displaced violets themselves from the perfumery trade.

ionopherogram ELECTROPHORETOGRAM.

ionophore [ION + *o* + -PHORE] An antibiotic that carries specific ions across a membrane, such as the plasma membrane of bacterial or animal cells or the mitochondrial membrane. Examples of ionophores are valinomycin and alamethicin.

ionophoresis The electrophoresis of small molecules.

ionophose [Gk *ion* the violet + *o* + *phōs*, contraction of *phaos* light] A violet-colored subjective light sensation.

ionosphere [ION + *o* + SPHERE] The stratum of the earth's atmosphere in which the atmospheric gases are highly ionized by the action of the solar ultraviolet rays and particle radiation. It extends from about 50 km to perhaps 600 km in altitude, overlapping the thermosphere.

ionotherapy [ION + *o* + THERAPY] **1** A seldom used term for IONTOPHORESIS. **2** An obsolete term for ULTRAVIOLET THERAPY.

iontherapy A seldom used term for IONTOPHORESIS.

iontophoresis [Gk *ionto(s)*, gen. of *iōn*, pres. part. of *ienai* to go + -PHORESIS] The tranference of ions into the body by an electromotive force for purposes of local or systemic medicinal effect. Also called *galvanoionization, iontotherapy, ionic medication, ionotherapy* (seldom used), *iontherapy* (seldom used).

iontophoretic Relating to iontophoresis.

iontoquantimeter IONOMETER.

iontoradeometer IONOMETER.

iontotherapy IONTOPHORESIS.

IOP intraocular pressure.

iopanoic acid $C_{11}H_{12}I_3NO_2$. 3-Amino-α-ethyl-2,4,6-triiodohydrocinnamic acid, a radiopaque contrast agent for cholecystography. Also called *iodopanoic acid.*

iophendylate $C_{19}H_{29}IO_2$. An iodine-containing, oily radiopaque medium that has been used diagnostically for both the examination of the biliary tract and for myelography. Also called *ethyl iodophenylundecylate, iodophendylate.*

iophenoxic acid $C_{11}H_{11}I_3O_3$. α-Ethyl-3-hydroxy-2,4,6-triiodohydrocinnamic acid, a compound used as a radiopaque contrast agent for cholecystography. Also called *triiodoethionic acid.*

iopydol $C_8H_9I_2NO_3$. 1-(2,3-Dihydroxypropyl)-3,5-diiodo-4(1*H*)-pyridinone. A radiopaque material used diagnostically in bronchoscopy to visualize the bronchial structures.

iopydone $C_5H_3I_2NO$. 3,5-Diiodo-4(1*H*)-pyridinone. A radiopaque agent used diagnostically in bronchography.

iosefamic acid $C_{28}H_{28}I_6N_4O_8$. 5,5'-(Sebacoyldiimino) bis [2,4,6-triiodo-*N*-methylesophthalamic acid]. An acid used in radiology as a radiopaque contrast agent.

iothalamate A salt of iothalamic acid. The meglumine and sodium salts are the main forms used diagnostically as radiopaque agents.

iothalamic acid $C_{11}H_9I_3N_2O_4$. 5-Acetamido-2,4,6-triiodo-*N*-methylisophthalamic acid, the meglumine and sodium salts of which are used in radiology as water-soluble contrast media, such as in intravenous urography.

iothiouracil $C_4H_3IN_2OS$. 5-Iodo-2-thiouracil. An agent used in the treatment of hyperthyroidism. It acts as a thyroid inhibitor, and it is used when a surgical thyroidectomy is contraindicated.

IP intraperitoneally (injection site).

ipecac [shortened form of *ipecacuanha*, Portuguese form of Tupi *ipekaaguéne* (from *pe* flat + *kaa* an herb + *guéne* vomit) a small creeping plant that induces sickness] The dried roots and rhizome of *Cephaelis ipecacuanha* or *C. acuminata*, which is used as an emetic and amebicidal drug. Also called *ipecacuanha.*

powdered ipecac Ipecac that is reduced to a fine powder to make a syrup.

ipecacuanha IPECAC.

ipodate sodium An iodinated compound used for radiologic cholangiography and cholecystography. It is thought to increase T_3 uptake. Also called *sodium ipodate.*

ipomea A cathartic medication obtained from the dried root of *Ipomoea orizabensis*. Also called *orizaba jalap root.*

ipomoea [Gk *ips*, gen. *ipos*, a worm + *homoios* similar to] *Ipomoea orizabensis*, a plant of the Convolvulaceae family. Its roots, when dried, yield a resin that is used as a cathartic. Also called *Mexican scammony, wild jalap, jalapa, ololiuqui.*

IPPB intermittent positive pressure breathing.

Ipral A proprietary name for probarbital.

iprindole $C_{19}H_{28}N_2$. 6,7,8,9,10,11-Hexahydro-*N,N*-dimethyl-5*H*-cyclooct[*b*]indole-5-propanamine. An agent with pharmacologic actions like those of imipramine. It is used as an antidepressant drug in the form of the hydrochloride.

iproniazid $C_9H_{13}N_3O$. 4-Pyridinecarboxylic acid 2-(1-methylethyl)hydrazide. An antidepressant agent chemically related to isoniazid. It is an inhibitor of monoamine oxidase and it has antituberculosis activity. It is not regularly used to treat tuberculosis, however, because its toxicity is greater than that of other agents now available.

ipronidazole $C_7H_{11}N_3O_2$. 1-Methyl-2-(1-methylethyl)-5-nitro-1*H*-imidazole. An imidazole derivative that is used as an antihistomonal agent in domestic fowl.

ips impulses per second (used to express the rate of spiking discharge in a muscle or nerve cell).

ipsation [L *ips(e)* self + -ATION] A seldom used term for MASTURBATION.

ipsefact [L *ipse* self + *fact(um)* a thing made, from neut. sing. of *factus*, past part. of *facere* to make] Any portion or aspect of an animal's habitat or environment created by its own behavior, such as nests, beehives, and prairie dog villages.

ipselateral An outmoded spelling of IPSILATERAL.

ipsilateral Located on or affecting the same side. Also *ipselateral (outmoded spelling), homolateral, isolateral.* Compare CONTRALATERAL.

ipsiversive [L *ipsi*, dative of *ipse* self + *vers(us)*, past part. of *vertere* to turn + -IVE] Tending to turn or twist to the side of the body on which a brain structure has been damaged or stimulated.

IPSP inhibitory postsynaptic potential.

IPTG isopropyl thiogalactoside.

IQ intelligence quotient.

deviation IQ An intelligence quotient expressed as a standard score, with the average preset at 100 and with a standard deviation of approximately 15–16, depending on the test used. The statistical conversion of scores to a common base facilitates comparison between performances at different ages.

Ir Symbol for the element, iridium.

ir- 1 IN-[1]. **2** IN-[2].

iralgia IRIDALGIA.

-irane [*ir-* (prob. alteration of TRI-) + *-ane*, variant of -INE] A suffix that signifies a saturated three-membered ring, as in *oxirane* the systematic name for epoxide.

IRC inspiratory reserve capacity (inspiratory reserve volume).

Ircon A proprietary name for ferrous fumarate.

IRI immunoreactive insulin.

irid- IRIDO-.

iridadenosis [IRID- + ADENOSIS] Infiltration of the iris by lymphoid cells.

iridal IRIDIC.

iridalgia [IRID- + -ALGIA] Pain referred to the iris. Also called *iralgia.*

iridauxesis [IRID- + AUXESIS] Thickening of the iris.

iridavulsion [IRID- + AVULSION] IRIDODIALYSIS.

iridectasis [IRID- + ECTASIS] Prolapse of the iris through a wound or incision.

iridectome [IRID- + Gk *ectom(ē)* a cutting out] A surgical instrument for cutting the iris.

iridectomesodialysis [IRID- + ECTO- + MESO- + DIALYSIS] A combination of excision of a portion of the iris and freeing of pupillary adhesions.

iridectomize [IRID- + *-ectom(y)* + -IZE] To excise a portion of iris.

iridectomy [IRID- + -ECTOMY] The surgical removal of a portion of the iris.

basal iridectomy An excision of a portion of iris that includes its peripheral base.

broad iridectomy Excision of a wide section of iris.

buttonhole iridectomy PERIPHERAL IRIDECTOMY.

complete iridectomy Excision of a sector of the iris, including the pupil margin.

optical iridectomy Excision of a central portion of the iris with the intent of enhancing the entry of light into the eye. Also called *iridocystectomy.*

peripheral iridectomy Excision of a very small portion of the peripheral iris, with preservation of the pupil. Also called *coretomedialysis, buttonhole iridectomy, stenopeic iridectomy.*

preliminary iridectomy A sector iridectomy performed as a separate operation, to be followed later by cataract extraction. Also called *preparatory iridectomy.*

preparatory iridectomy PRELIMINARY IRIDECTOMY.

sector iridectomy Excision of a portion of iris extending from its base to the pupil margin.

stenopeic iridectomy PERIPHERAL IRIDECTOMY.

therapeutic iridectomy Removal of a portion of iris with the intent of treating an ocular disorder.

iridectopia [IRID- + Gk *ektop(os)* displaced + -IA] Displacement of the pupil.

iridectropium [IRID- + *ectrop(ion)* + L *-ium*, noun suffix] Outward turning of a portion of the margin of the pupil.

iridemia [IRID- + -EMIA] Hemorrhage from the iris.

iridencleisis [IRID- + EN- + -CLEISIS] Incarceration of a tongue of iris in a limbal wound with the intention of creating an artificial channel for drainage of aqueous from the eye, in management of glaucoma.

iridentropium [IRID- + *entrop(ion)* + L *-ium*, noun suffix] Posterior inturning of a portion of the margin of the iris.

irideremia [IRID- + Gk *erēmia* want of, absence] ANIRIDIA.

irides Plural of IRIS.

iridescence [IRID- + L *-escentia*, combining form denoting becoming] A condition of color marked by changing hue and metallic sheen. It is produced by the reflection and refraction of different lengths of light waves at the apparently colored surface. The effect is seen in certain birds, fishes, and reptiles. Adjective: iridescent.

iridesis [IRID- + -ESIS] Iris inclusion surgery for glaucoma, in which the iris is interposed in a corneoscleral incision to block its closure.

iridiagnosis IRIDODIAGNOSIS.

iridial IRIDIC.

iridian IRIDIC.

iridic [IRID- + -IC] Of or relating to the iris. Also *iritic, iridal, iridial, iridian.*

iridis rhizoma ORRIS.

iridium A metallic element having atomic number 77 and atomic weight 192.22. It occurs uncombined in nature along with platinum and other metals. It is heavier than any other known element except osmium, and is the most corrosion-resistant metal. Symbol: Ir

iridium 192 An artificial radioactive isotope of iridium, emitting beta and gamma rays. Physical half-life is 75 days. Symbol: ^{192}Ir

iridization The dispersion of light by corneal edema, resulting in the perception of colored halos around lights.

irido- [Gk *iris* (genitive *iridos*) rainbow, iris] A combining form denoting the iris. Also *irid-.*

iridoavulsion [IRIDO- + AVULSION] IRIDODIALYSIS.

iridocapsulitis [IRIDO- + CAPSULITIS] Inflammation of the iris and lens capsule.

iridocapsulotomy [IRIDO- + CAPSULOTOMY] Surgical excision of a portion of the iris and adherent lens capsule.

iridocele [IRIDO- + -CELE[1]] Prolapse of the iris through a wound in cornea or limbus. Also called *myiocephalon* (outmoded), *myiocephalum* (outmoded).

iridochoroiditis [IRIDO- + CHOROIDITIS] UVEITIS.

iridocoloboma [IRIDO- + COLOBOMA] COLOBOMA IRIDIS.

iridoconstrictor [IRIDO- + CONSTRICTOR] The sphincter muscle of the iris or any autonomic stimulus that activates it.

iridocorneosclerectomy [IRIDO- + *corne(a)* + *o* + SCLER- + -ECTOMY] A glaucoma operation consisting of excision of a portion of the limbus and underlying iris.

iridocyclectomy [IRIDO- + CYCL- + -ECTOMY] Excision of a portion of iris and ciliary body, as for a neoplasm.

iridocyclitis [IRIDO- + CYCLITIS] Inflammation of the iris and ciliary body. Also called *anterior uveitis.*

heterochromic iridocyclitis A mild, persistent anterior uveitis associated with a developmental melanin deficiency of the affected eye.

iridocyclitis septica BEHÇET SYNDROME.

iridocyclochoroiditis [IRIDO- + CYCLO- + CHOROIDITIS] UVEITIS.

iridocystectomy [IRIDO- + CYSTECTOMY] OPTICAL IRIDECTOMY.

iridocyte [IRIDO- + -CYTE] A specialized cell occurring in fish scales. It contains crystalline guanin which breaks light into a spectrum of colors.

iridodesis [IRIDO- + -DESIS] A filtering operation for glaucoma in which an iris wick is utilized.

iridodiagnosis The purported recognition of systemic disease by observation of the iris, having no scientific validity. Also called *iridiagnosis, iridology.*

iridodialysis [IRIDO- + DIALYSIS] A tearing of the iris from its base upon the ciliary body. Also called *iridoavulsion, iridavulsion.*

    congenital iridodialysis A separation of the base of the iris from the ciliary body, present at birth.

iridodiastasis [IRIDO- + DIASTASIS] Absence of a portion of the iris at its peripheral base.

iridodilator 1 MUSCULUS DILATOR PUPILLAE. 2 A neurochemical acting to innervate this muscle.

iridodonesis [IRIDO- + Gk *don(ein)* to shake + -ESIS] Tremulousness of the iris, which results when the physical support of the lens is lost, as following dislocation of the lens or cataract extraction.

iridokeratitis [IRIDO- + KERATITIS] Inflammation of the iris and cornea.

iridokinesia Movement of the iris. Also called *iridokinesis.*

iridokinesis IRIDOKINESIA.

iridokinetic Pertaining to movement of the iris.

iridoleptynsis [IRIDO- + Gk *leptynsis* a making thin, growing thin] Atrophy of the iris.

iridology IRIDODIAGNOSIS.

iridolysis [IRIDO- + LYSIS] A freeing of the iris from synechiae.

iridomalacia A softening and deterioration of the iris.

iridomesodialysis [IRIDO- + MESO- + DIALYSIS] A freeing of the iris from adhesions affecting the pupil margin.

iridomotor Pertaining to or causing movement of the iris.

iridoncosis [IRID- + ONCO- + -SIS] Edema of the iris.

iridoncus [IRID- + -ONCUS] A tumor of the iris.

iridoparalysis [IRIDO- + PARALYSIS] IRIDOPLEGIA.

iridoparelkysis [IRIDO- + Gk *parelky(sō)*, fut. of *parelkein* to draw aside + -SIS] A displacement of the pupil for optical purposes, achieved by prolapsing the peripheral iris into a limbal incision.

iridoparesis [IRIDO- + PARESIS] Incomplete loss of motor function of the iris.

iridopathy [IRIDO- + -PATHY] Any disorder of the iris.

iridoperiphakitis [IRIDO- + PERI- + PHAKITIS] Inflammation of the iris and the lens capsule.

iridophore [IRIDO- + -PHORE] An iridescent chromatophore.

iridoplania [IRIDO- + L *plan(us)* flat + -IA] Flattening of the iris due to loss of posterior support by the lens.

iridoplegia [IRIDO- + -PLEGIA] Loss of motor function of the iris. Also called *iridoparalysis, pupilloplegia.*

    accommodation iridoplegia Loss of the pupillary reaction component of the accommodation-convergence reflex.

    complete iridoplegia Paralysis of the iris musculature that renders the pupil immobile on both neural and chemical stimulation.

    reflex iridoplegia Failure of the pupil to constrict in response to light or accommodation-convergence.

    sympathetic iridoplegia Failure of the pupil to dilate in response to a painful stimulus.

iridoptosis [IRIDO- + PTOSIS] Prolapse of the iris through a wound.

iridopupillary [IRIDO- + PUPILLARY] Pertaining to both iris and pupil.

iridorhexis [IRIDO- + -RHEXIS] Tearing or rupture of the iris.

iridoschisis [IRIDO- + -SCHISIS] A splitting of the frontal plane of mesodermal layers of the iris, usually as a spontaneous degenerative change.

iridosclerotomy [IRIDO- + -SCLEROTOMY] An incision through sclera and iris, as for acute angle-closure glaucoma.

iridosis IRIDOTASIS.

iridosteresis [IRIDO- + Gk *sterēsis* loss] Absence of all or most of the iris owing to trauma, disease, or developmental cause.

iridotasis [IRIDO- + Gk *tasis* a stretching, straining] Incarceration of iris in a corneoscleral incision. Also called *iridosis.*

iridotome [IRIDO- + -TOME] A surgical instrument designed for incising the iris.

iridotomy [IRIDO- + -TOMY] A cut into the iris without removal of tissue. This is performed during cataract extraction as a prophylactic measure against possible pupillary blockage by the vitreous humor.

iris [Gk, rainbow] (*plural* irides) [NA] The visible, colored portion of the vascular tunic of the eye, in front of the lens, functioning as a diaphragm and encompassing a central orifice (pupil) whose size is regulated by sphincter and dilator muscles to control the passage of light. It is lined posteriorly by a double layer of pigmented epithelial cells and is attached at the margins to the ciliary body. Adjective: iridic, iridal, iridial, iridian.

    iris bombé Forward displacement of the midportion of the iris due to a pupillary block that occludes aqueous flow into the anterior chamber. Also called *umbrella iris.*

    tremulous iris An iris that has lost its posterior support by the lens and therefore moves within the eye whenever eye movement occurs.

    umbrella iris IRIS BOMBÉ.

irisopsia [IRIS + -OPSIA] The dispersion of light by corneal edema that causes spectral colors to be seen around lights.

iritic Pertaining to or characterized by iritis.

iritis [*ir(is)* + -ITIS] Inflammation of the iris.

    iritis catamenialis Inflammation of the iris associated with menstruation.

    diabetic iritis Neovascularization of the iris due to diabetes mellitus.

    endogenous iritis NONGRANULOMATOUS IRITIS.

    follicular iritis Iritis associated with lymphoid infiltration.

    gouty iritis Iritis occurring during acute arthritis, such as Reiter's disease or ankylosing spondylitis. It was formerly and incorrectly thought to be gout. An obsolete term. Also called *uratic iritis.*

    granulomatous iritis Iritis characterized by formation of inflammatory nodules.

    nongranulomatous iritis Inflammation of the iris due to immunologic factors. Also called *endogenous iritis.*

    iritis papulosa Iritis that produces localized nodules.

    plastic iritis Iritis that results in fibrinous outpouring into the aqueous.

    purulent iritis Iritis that results in leukocytic outpouring into the aqueous.

    quiet iritis Very mild inflammation of the iris.

    rheumatoid iritis Iritis associated with rheumatoid arthritis.

    iritis septica BEHÇET SYNDROME.

    serous iritis Iritis associated with leakage of plasma proteins into the aqueous.

    spongy iritis Iritis associated with fibrin clots in the anterior chamber.

sympathetic iritis Iritis consequent upon injury to the opposite eye.

uratic iritis GOUTY IRITIS.

iritoectomy [IRITO- (irreg. for IRIDO-) + -ECTOMY] Excision of secondary cataract and adherent iris.

iritomy [*iri(d)-* + -TOMY] Incision of the iris. Also called *irotomy*.

irium A hard, white, metallic element having atomic number 77, and atomic weight 192.2. Symbol: Ir

iron Element number 26, having atomic weight 55.847. By weight, iron is the fourth most abundant element in the lithosphere, where it is found combined with oxygen. The core of the earth is believed to be largely molten iron. Ordinary iron is a mixture of four stable isotopes. Valences are 2, 3, 4, and 6. The metal has been central to technology from prehistoric times. Its compounds figure in such plant and animal life processes as photosynthesis, oxygen transport, and the action of many enzymes. Symbol: Fe Adjective: ferric, ferrous.

iron and ammonium acetate A combination of ferric citrate and ammonium acetate, used as a solution as an iron tonic.

iron and ammonium citrate A combination of ferric citrate and ammonium citrate, soluble in water and often used to treat iron deficiency anemia. Also called *ferric ammonium citrate*.

iron and ammonium sulfate A combination of ferric iron and ammonium sulfate as a complex salt, $FeNH_4(SO_4)_2 \cdot 12H_2O$. It is used as an astringent and styptic medication. Also called *ferric ammonium sulfate*.

iron and ammonium tartrate Reddish-brown scales composed of ferric ammonium tartrate. It is used as a convenient source of iron for the treatment of iron deficiency anemia.

available iron The component of dietary iron which can be absorbed from the gastrointestinal tract.

nonheme iron Iron that is not part of the heme group: describing particularly the iron-sulfur proteins. These contain iron bound, often in a complex with S^{2-} ions, to cysteine residues of the protein in their deprotonated form.

Quevenne's iron REDUCED IRON.

iron and quinine citrate A complex ammonium quinine ferric citrate containing 14.5–15.5% anhydrous quinine and 12–14% iron. It has been used as a tonic.

radioactive iron RADIOIRON.

reduced iron A fine, black powder of metallic iron prepared from iron salts by reduction with hydrogen under standard conditions. It is insoluble in water, but dissolves in dilute mineral acids. It has the same uses as iron salts, but its bioavailability is limited and variable. Also called *Quevenne's iron*.

iron 52 A radioactive isotope of iron, having a half-life 8.3 hours, and producing beta emissions of 0.8 MeV and gamma emissions of 169 and 378 keV. Symbol: ^{52}Fe

iron 55 A radioisotope of iron. It decays by electron capture, emitting characteristic x rays of 5.9 keV. Physical half-life is 2.7 years. Symbol: ^{55}Fe

iron 59 A radioisotope of iron, emitting beta and gamma rays. Physical half-life is 45 days. Symbol: ^{59}Fe

iron acetate $Fe(O_2CCH_3)_3$. An iron salt of limited value as an astringent agent.

iron adenylate A form of iron used for parenteral (intramuscular) administration.

iron arsenate A preparation of iron formerly used in the treatment of skin diseases. Also called *ferrous arsenate*.

iron arsenite A yellow powder preparation of iron formerly used in the treatment of iron deficiency anemia.

iron ascorbate A soluble complex of reduced iron and ascorbic acid that is used for the treatment of iron deficiency anemia. Also called *iron cevitaminate*.

Ironate A proprietary name for ferrous sulfate.

iron cevitaminate IRON ASCORBATE.

iron choline citrate FERROCHOLINATE.

iron citrate FERRIC CITRATE.

iron citrate green GREEN FERRIC AMMONIUM CITRATE.

iron dextrin A sterile, clear, dark brown solution containing a complex of ferric hydroxide and partially hydrolyzed dextrin in water suitable for intravenous administration.

iron gluconate FERROUS GLUCONATE.

iron glycerophosphate FERRIC GLYCEROPHOSPHATE.

iron hematoxylin A hematoxylin solution containing an iron salt that acts as both an oxidizing agent and a mordant.

iron hypophosphite FERRIC HYPOPHOSPHITE.

iron iodide FERROUS IODIDE.

iron iodobehanate An amorphous, reddish brown powder, formerly used in the treatment of rickets, tuberculosis, and iron deficiency anemia.

iron lactate FERROUS LACTATE.

iron magnesium sulfate A mixture of ferrous sulfate and magnesium sulfate used in the treatment of iron-deficiency anemia.

iron malate A preparation of iron in apple juice used as an oral form of iron treatment for anemia.

iron oleate An iron salt of oleic acid that is a waxy, solid preparation. It is used as an astringent.

iron phosphate A mixture of ferric and ferrous phosphates that has been used to treat iron-deficiency anemias.

soluble iron phosphate Ferric phosphate made soluble by the addition of sodium citrate. It has been used in the treatment of iron-deficiency anemia.

iron protosulfate FERROUS SULFATE.

iron pyrophosphate $Fe_4(P_2O_7)_3 \cdot 9H_2O$. A salt of iron, insoluble in water, that has been used as a nutrient source of iron to prevent anemia.

iron sorbitex A sterile, brown, colloidal solution containing ferric iron, sorbitol, and citric acid, stabilized with dextrin and sorbitol. It can be used intramuscularly in the treatment of iron-deficiency anemia, but should not be given intravenously.

iron subcarbonate An amorphous powder consisting mostly of iron hydroxide.

iron sulfate FERROUS SULFATE.

iron valerianate $FeC_5H_9O_2(OH)_2$. A ferric salt of valeric acid, insoluble in water, that has been used in the treatment of iron deficiency anemia.

Irosul A proprietary name for ferrous sulfate.

irotomy IRITOMY.

irradiate [IR- + RADIATE] To expose to ionizing radiation, as for diagnosis, treatment, or sterilization, or by accident.

irradiation [L -*ir* in + *radiatus*, past part. of *radiare* to emit rays, radiate, from *radi(us)* a sunbeam, ray of light + -ATION] **1** In radiology, treatment by ionizing radiations. **2** LUMINESCENCE.

heterogeneous irradiation Radiotherapy by means of ionizing radiation unequally distributed in the body tissues.

homogeneous irradiation Radiotherapy by means of ionizing radiation equally distributed in the tissues.

interstitial irradiation Therapeutic irradiation by the insertion, in the tissue, of an encapsulated radioactive nuclide such as radium, cobalt 60, etc.

intracavitary irradiation INTRACAVITARY RADIOTHERAPY.

Medinger-Craver irradiation A seldom used term for WHOLE-BODY IRRADIATION.

painful irradiation The propagation or extension of pain into a region which may be near to, or less often far from, its origin, as in propagation of the chest pain of angina pectoris, which is usually retrosternal, into the left or both shoulders and arms or into the neck and jaw.

palliative irradiation Radiation therapy to slow down the progress of a lesion, especially cancer, or to alleviate pain, without hope of curing the disease.

surface irradiation Radiation from a radioactive ionizing source applied to the surface of the body.

ultraviolet blood irradiation A method of irradiation consisting of the extracorporeal exposure of blood to ultraviolet light.

whole-body irradiation Irradiation of the entire body by an external source of radiation. Also called *Medinger-Craver irradiation* (seldom used).

irrational In psychiatry, characterized by behavior or thinking that is unreasonable, such as harming oneself without an adequate reason, or wanting to suffer evil or be harmed.

irreducible 1 Impossible to be lowered by the application of current knowledge or techniques, as an irreducible infection rate. 2 Not able to be corrected further.

irregular 1 Not regular, orderly, or proper. 2 Occurring at uneven intervals, as *irregular heartbeat*.

irremediable Not capable of being remedied; lacking a remedy.

irrespirable Unsuitable for breathing: said of air or gas that will not support the respiratory processes, or is toxic, or of aerosols in which the particle size is too large.

irresponsibility / criminal irresponsibility Exemption from responsibility for criminal conduct due to mental illness or defect which can be demonstrated to have been present in an individual at the time a criminal act was committed. Compare CRIMINAL RESPONSIBILITY.

irresuscitable [IR- + L *resuscit(are)* to revive + -ABLE] Denoting a shock state or injury so severe that currently known treatment cannot restore enough vital function to prevent death.

irreversibility The quality of being unable to return to its original form or state.

irreversibility of conduction The theory that conduction can occur in one direction only in a reflex arc. This principle is physiologically unsound with respect to nerve fibers which are capable of antidromic conduction, but holds for transmission through the synapse which occurs in one direction only.

irrigant A fluid used to flush out or irrigate a cavity or surface.

irrigate [L *irrigat(us)*, past part. of *irrigare* to conduct water, irrigate] To flush thoroughly, especially a cavity or wound, with a fluid to rid of unwanted substances.

irrigation [L *irrigatio* (from *irrigatus*, past part. of *irrigare* to conduct water to, irrigate, from *in-* in + *rigare* to water, akin to Gk *rheein* to flow and to English *rain*) a watering, irrigating] The process of flushing a cavity or wound thoroughly with water, salt solution, or medicated fluid, as to wash out debris, foreign material, or dead tissues.

continuous irrigation Irrigation performed with an uninterrupted stream of fluid.

irrigator Any of a number of devices used for irrigation. Examples are syringes, tubing connected to a bottle elevated for gravity flow, and pumps that provide continuous or pulsatile flow.

irrigoradioscopy [L *irrig(are)* to water, conduct water to + *o* + RADIOSCOPY] Fluoroscopy of the large bowel during the administration of a contrast enema. Also called *irrigoscopy*.

irrigoscopy IRRIGORADIOSCOPY.

irritability [L *irritabilitas* (from *irritabil(is)* irritable + -*itas* -ITY) irritability] 1 EXCITABILITY. 2 Excessive sensitivity.

chemical irritability Responsiveness to chemical stimuli.

electric irritability Responsiveness to electric current.

faradic irritability The responsiveness of tissue to repetitive electric currents. An outmoded term.

galvanic irritability Responsiveness of nerve and muscle to direct (continuous) current.

mechanical irritability Responsiveness to mechanical force or displacement.

muscular irritability The contractile response of muscle to a stimulus.

myotatic irritability Responsiveness of muscle to transient muscle stretch.

nervous irritability The property of nervous tissue of being excited by a stimulus.

specific irritability LAW OF SPECIFIC IRRITABILITY.

irritability of the stomach A condition in which abdominal pain, nausea, or vomiting results after ingestion of normal amounts and types of foods.

uterine irritability An increased propensity for uterine contractions following any type of stimulus.

irritable 1 Capable of reacting to a stimulus. 2 Hypersensitive to stimulation.

irritant An agent that causes irritation or inflammation.

primary irritant An agent or substance capable of producing inflammation on first contact with a tissue, especially the skin.

irritation [L *irritatio* (from *irritatus*, past part. of *irritare* to stir up, incite, excite) a stirring up, provoking, incitement] 1 The response of excitable tissue to a stimulus. 2 The incipient inflammatory response of tissue to a noxious stimulus. 3 The application of a stimulus or excitation.

cerebral irritation 1 The state produced by any lesion or disease which irritates brain cells. 2 The clinical state of irritability or intolerance of interference which may result from brain injury or disease.

direct irritation Irritation resulting from direct action on the affected part.

functional irritation Irritation associated with abnormal function of the affected organ or part.

meningeal irritation Irritation of the meninges due to meningitis or hemorrhage and giving rise to headache and neck stiffness.

spinal irritation Spinal rigidity and pain due to a lesion or disease in the spinal column or canal.

sympathetic irritation Inflammation of an organ as a consequence of inflammation of a related organ. Typically seen in one eye following trauma or surgery to the other.

irritative 1 Causing irritation. 2 An obsolete term for EXCITATORY.

irrumation [L *irrumat(us)*, past part. of *irrumare* (from IR-¹ + *ruma* woman's breast, teat) to give suck, perform fellatio + -*io* -ION] FELLATIO.

Irvine [A. Ray *Irvine*, Jr., U.S. ophthalmologist, born 1917] See under SYNDROME.

Irving [Frederick Carpenter *Irving*, U.S. obstetrician, born 1883] See under OPERATION.

IS 1 intercostal space. 2 intraspinal. 3 immune serum.

Isaacs [Charles Edward *Isaacs*, U.S. physiologist, 1811–1860] Isaacs-Ludwig arteriole. See under ARTERIOLE.

Isambert [Emile *Isambert*, French physician, 1827–1876] See under DISEASE.

isatin The indole derivative formed by oxidizing indoxyl. Its molecules consist of the group —CO—CO—NH— substituting the hydrogen atoms on adjacent carbons of benzene. It reacts with amino acids in a manner similar to that of ninhydrin. It has a bright orange color.

isauxesis [*is(o)-* + AUXESIS] A proportionate equality of growth between parts and the whole.

ischaemia A British spelling for ISCHEMIA.

ischemia [Gk *ischaimos* (from *ischein* to hold, check, a form of *echein* to have, hold + -EMIA) stanching blood; as substantive, a styptic] Inadequate blood flow to a part or organ.

  coronary ischemia Myocardial ischemia resulting from coronary artery disease.

  intestinal ischemia Deficiency of blood flow to the intestine.

  mesenteric ischemia The impairment of blood supply to a part of the small or large bowel leading to impairment of cellular function but not to cell death.

  myocardial ischemia Deficient blood flow to the myocardium.

  postural ischemia Reduction of the blood flow in a limb or part thereof during a surgical procedure, by elevating it above the level of the heart.

  renal ischemia Decreased blood perfusion of the kidney, either from organic causes, such as stenosis of the main renal artery or its primary branches due to atherosclerosis or fibromuscular disease, to arteriolar nephrosclerosis, or to functional prerenal situations such as heart failure, hypovolemia, or shock.

  ischemia retinae Inadequate retinal circulation due to shock following profuse blood loss.

  subendocardial ischemia Inadequate blood flow to a part of the myocardium adjacent to the endocardium.

  subepicardial ischemia Inadequate blood flow to the myocardium subjacent to the pericardium.

  transient cerebral ischemia Temporary reduction of arterial blood supply to the cerebrum. Transient cerebral ischemic attacks can present with many different clinical features including weakness, paresthesia, amblyopia, vertigo, and many others, depending upon the area of the brain or brainstem to which blood supply is temporarily reduced. Microembolism due to atherosclerosis is the commonest cause. Abbreviation: TCI

  vasospasm cerebral ischemia A temporary reduction of cerebral blood supply as a result of spasm of nutrient arteries.

ischemic Characterized by or affected with ischemia.

ischesis [Gk *isch(ein)* (variant of *echein* to have, hold) to check, hold back + -ESIS] The prevention or suppression of a discharge, applied especially to a condition affecting a normal secretion. A seldom used term.

ischi- ISCHIO-.

ischia Plural of ISCHIUM.

ischiac ISCHIAL.

ischiadelphus [ISCHI- + Gk *adelphos* twin, brother] ISCHIOPAGUS.

ischiadic ISCHIAL.

ischial Of or relating to the ischium or the hip joint; sciatic. Also *ischiadic, ischiatic, ischiac.*

ischialgia [ISCHI- + -ALGIA] Pelvic pain in the region of the ischium. Also called *ischias, ischiodynia, ischioneuralgia.* Adjective: ischialgic.

ischias ISCHIALGIA.

ischiatic ISCHIAL.

ischiatitis An obsolete term for SCIATICA.

ischidrosis ANHIDROSIS.

ischiectomy [ISCHI- + -ECTOMY] The surgical removal of all or part of one or both hips.

ischigalactic ISCHOGALACTIC.

ischio- [Gk *ischion* (plural *ischia*) hip joint; in plural, hips or loins] A combining form denoting the ischium. Also *ischi-.*

ischioanal Pertaining to the ischium and the anus.

ischiobulbar Pertaining to the ischium and the bulb of the penis.

ischiocapsular Pertaining to the ischium and the capsule of the hip joint.

ischiocavernous Pertaining to the ischium and the corpus cavernosum penis or clitoridis.

ischiocele SCIATIC HERNIA.

ischiococcygeal Pertaining to the ischium and the coccyx.

ischiococcygeus MUSCULUS COCCYGEUS.

ischiodidymus [ISCHIO- + Gk *didymos* double, a twin] ISCHIOPAGUS.

ischiodymia [ISCHIO- + -*dym(us)* + -IA] ISCHIOPAGIA.

ischiodynia ISCHIALGIA.

ischiofemoral Pertaining to the ischium and the femur.

ischiofemoralis An occasional fasciculus of the gluteus maximus muscle that extends from the ischial tuberosity to the lower border of the muscle near the greater trochanter.

ischiofibular Pertaining to the ischium and the fibula.

ischiohebotomy A surgical procedure in which the two pubic rami, the ischiopubic and the ascending, are divided.

ischiomelus [ISCHIO- + Gk *melos* a limb] Unequal conjoined twins in which the parasitic member is represented mainly by an extra arm or leg attached to the host in the pelvic region.

ischiomyelitis [ISCHIO- + MYELITIS] Myelitis of the lumbar part of the spinal cord. An outmoded term.

ischioneuralgia ISCHIALGIA.

ischionitis An inflammation of the ischium.

ischiopagia [ISCHIO- + -*pag(us)* + -IA] The condition displayed by an ischiopagus. Also called *ischiodymia.*

ischiopagus [ISCHIO- + -PAGUS] Equal conjoined twins united in the ischial region. Also called *ischiodidymus, ischiadelphus.*

  ischiopagus parasiticus Unequal conjoined twins with the parasitic member attached at the ischial region of the host.

  ischiopagus tetrapus An ischiopagus parasiticus with four feet, the parasitic member being represented largely by an extra pair of lower extremities.

  ischiopagus tripus An ischiopagus parasiticus with three feet, the parasitic member being represented by a single lower extremity with or without variable other parts.

ischioperineal Pertaining to the ischium and the perineum.

ischioprostatic Pertaining to the ischium and the prostate gland.

ischiopubic Pertaining to the ischium and the pubis.

ischiopubis 1 The ischium and the pubis considered as a single unit. 2 The junction of the ischium and the pubis.

ischiorectal Pertaining to the ischium and the rectum. Also *rectischiac.*

ischiosacral Pertaining to the ischium and the sacrum.

ischiothoracopagus [ISCHIO- + THORACO- + -PAGUS] Equal conjoined twins united from the thorax to the pelvis. The pelvic union more often involves the ilium than the ischium.

ischiotibial Pertaining to the ischium and the tibia.

ischiovaginal Pertaining to the ischium and the vagina.

ischiovertebral Pertaining to the ischium and the vertebral column.

ischium [L (from Gk *ischion* the hip joint), the hip joint] OS ISCHII.

ischnophonia A rarely used term for STUTTERING.

ischocholia [Gk *isch(ein)* for *echein* to have, hold + *o* + CHOL- + -IA] The suppression of bile flow. A seldom used term.

ischochymia [Gk *isch(ein)* for *echein* to have, hold + *o* + Gk *chym(os)* juice + -IA] The suppression of gastric digestive processes. A seldom used term.

ischogalactia [Gk *isch(ein)* to check, restrain + *o* + GALACT-

+ -IA] Suppression of secretion of breast milk. Adjective: ischogalactic.

ischogalactic Tending to suppress the secretion of breast milk. Also *ischigalactic*.

ischogyria [Gk *isch(ein)* to check, hold back, stop + *o* + *gyr(us)* + -IA] A jagged or nodular appearance of cerebral gyri as seen sometimes in tuberous sclerosis.

ischolochia [Gk *isch(ein)* + *o* + LOCHIA] Stoppage of the lochial flow.

ischomenia [Gk *isch(ein)* to check, restrain + *o* + *mēn* month + IA] The stopping of the menstrual flow. An ambiguous and rarely used term.

ischospermia [Gk *isch(ein)* to hold, check + *o* + SPERM- + -IA] The retention of semen, or the suppression of semen excretion.

ischuretic Referring to ischuria.

ischuria [*isch(i)-* + -URIA] URINARY RETENTION.

ischuria paradoxa Excessive dilatation of the bladder from urine, although the passing of urine continues.

ischuria spastica Retention of urine due to spasm of the bladder sphincter.

-ise A British spelling for -IZE.

iseiconia ISEIKONIA.

iseiconic ISEIKONIC.

iseikonia [*is(o)-* + Gk *eikōn* image, likeness + -IA] Equality of image size perceived by the two eyes. Also called *iso-iconia*. Also *iseiconia*. Adjective: iseikonic.

iseikonic [*is(o)-* + Gk *eikōn* image, likeness + -IC] Characterized by or pertaining to iseikonia; relating to equal size of the images perceived by the two eyes. Also *iso-iconic, iseiconic*.

Ishihara [Shinobu *Ishihara*, Japanese ophthalmologist, 1879–1963] See under TEST.

isinglass ICHTHYOCOLLA.

Japanese isinglass AGAR.

island [Old English *īgland*] ISLET.

blood island An aggregate of mesenchymal cells in the embryo that give rise to primitive blood vessels and the first blood cells. Collectively, blood islands are known as angioblastema. Also called *Wolff's island, Pander's island*.

bone island Isolated piece of bone found with either normal cortical or cancellous bone.

islands of Calleja Dense clusters of granular and polymorphic neurons in the cortex of the anterior perforated space within the tuberculum olfactorium. Also called *Calleja's islets, olfactory islands*.

cartilage island A residual area of cartilaginous tissue that remains within bony tissue following endochondral ossification.

heat island An area of slightly higher environmental temperatures observed in and around urban areas as a result of spatially concentrated fuel combustion.

islands of Langerhans ISLETS OF LANGERHANS.

Life Island A trademark for a controlled environment system.

olfactory islands ISLANDS OF CALLEJA.

Pander's island BLOOD ISLAND.

island of Reil INSULA.

skin island EPITHELIAL BUD.

tonal islands Regions of residual hearing in the severely deafened subject, in whom hearing is restricted to certain frequencies, usually in the low frequency range of the tonal spectrum.

Wolff's island BLOOD ISLAND.

islet [Middle French *islette* (from *isle* island, from L *insuale* island, + *-ette* French diminishing suffix) a small island] A small cluster of cells with a similar or related function. Also called *island*.

Calleja's islets ISLANDS OF CALLEJA.

islets of Langerhans Localized clusters of endocrine cells scattered through the acinar substance of the pancreas. They contain alpha, beta, and delta cells that secrete, respectively, glucagon, insulin, and gastrin. Also called *islands of Langerhans*.

Walthard's islets Small, glistening nodules found on the surface of the fallopian tubes. They are composed of serosal cells that have become hyperplastic or metaplastic. They are benign, and must be distinguished from tumor implants.

-ism [Gk suffix *-ismos* from verb termination *-izein* denoting to perform an act + *-mos* termination converting verb to noun] A suffix meaning (1) act or process; (2) state or condition; (3) abnormal condition, anomaly; (4) doctrine of belief or system of practice.

Ismelin A proprietary name for guanethidine sulfate.

ISO International Organization for Standardization.

iso- [Gk *isos* equal to] **1** A combining form meaning equal, equivalent. **2** A combining form used in chemical nomenclature to indicate a slight difference, most commonly to indicate chain branching. Thus, whereas the propyl group is CH_3—CH_2—CH_2—, the isopropyl group is $(CH_3$—$)_2CH$—. Abbreviation: *i*-

isoacceptor One of two or more tRNA molecules capable of accepting the same amino acid and transferring it to a nascent polypeptide.

isoadrenocorticism EUADRENOCORTICISM.

isoallele An allele that is distinguishable from another, which is usually the wild type, only by its effect on the phenotype when it is present with certain mutant alleles in heterozygotes or by its DNA sequence.

isoalloxazine The compound whose molecule provides the basic ring system of flavins. It consists of three rings. The central one is pyrazine, with a benzene ring fused to one of its C-C bonds, and a uracil ring to the other. In flavins, the benzene ring carries two methyl substituents, and one nitrogen atom of the central ring is substituted with ribitol. This ring system can undergo reversible hydrogenation.

isoalloxazine mononucleotide FLAVIN MONONUCLEOTIDE.

isoamyl An outmoded term for 3-METHYLBUTYL.

isoamylase The enzyme (EC 3.2.1.68) that catalyzes the hydrolysis of the 1,6-α-glucosidic branch linkages in glycogen, amylopectin, and related polysaccharides.

isoamylene $(CH_3)_2C$—$CHCH_3$. Trimethylethylene. A chemical at one time used as an anesthetic but discarded because it was too toxic.

isoamylethylbarbituric acid AMOBARBITAL.

isoamyl nitrite AMYL NITRITE.

isoandrosterone EPIANDROSTERONE.

isoantibody An outmoded term for ALLOANTIBODY.

isoantigen An outmoded term for ALLOANTIGEN.

H isoantigen One of the antigens of the ABH blood groups, expressed predominantly in type O individuals and to a lesser degree in type B, A, and AB individuals.

isoascorbic acid The epimer of ascorbic acid with inverted configuration at C-5. It is related to D-sugars.

isobar Any of two or more nuclides having the same mass number but different atomic numbers, such as uranium 235 and neptunium 235.

isobarbituric acid An isomer of barbituric acid. It is 2,4,5-trihydroxypyrimidine and its tautomers (i.e. 5-hydroxyuracil), whereas barbituric acid is 2,4,6,-trihydroxypyrimidine and its tautomers.

isobaric [ISO- + BAR- + -IC] Of equal pressure.

isobody An outmoded term for ALLOANTIBODY.

isobucaine hydrochloride $C_{15}H_{23}NO_2 \cdot HCl$. 2-Isobutylamino-2-methylpropylbenzoate hydrochloride. A white, crystalline powder which is used as a local anesthetic for dental anesthesia.

isobutanol $(CH_3)_2CH$—CH_2OH. 2-Methyl propan-1-ol. A colorless liquid arising by fermentation of carbohydrates. It is inflammable and slightly soluble in water. It is used as a solvent and for preparing essences. It is irritant to skin and mucous membranes.

isobutylallylbarbituric acid   BUTALBITAL.

isocaloric   EQUICALORIC.

isocarboxazid $C_{12}H_{13}N_3O_2$. 5-Methyl-3-isoxazolecarboxylic acid 2-benzylhydrazide. It is a monoamine oxidase inhibitor and used in the treatment of depressed patients who are refractory to tricyclic antidepressant drugs, or in patients in which the tricyclic antidepressants are contraindicated.

isocellular   Composed of identical or closely similar cells.

isocercal   Ending in the median line of the caudal fin: said of the vertebral column of certain fish.

isocholesterol   LANOSTEROL.

isochoric   Of or relating to the effect upon pressure that occurs when a substance whose volume remains constant undergoes a change in temperature.

isochromatic   1 Being of uniform color throughout. 2 Having exactly the same color as something else. For defs. 1 and 2 also *isochroous*.

isochromatophil   ORTHOCHROMOPHIL.

isochromosome   A mediocentric chromosome with homologous arms, probably resulting from an abnormal transverse division of the centromere during meiosis.

isochron   Possessing equal time or chronaxy in excitable tissues.

isochronal   ISOCHRONIC.

isochronia [ISO- + CHRON- + -IA] 1 ISOCHRONISM. 2 A correspondence in time, rate, or frequency, as between biological processes.

isochronic   Occurring or performed at the same time. Also *isochronal*.

isochronism   The condition of nerve and muscle possessing the same chronaxy (i.e. excitability). Also called *isochronia, law of isochronism, Lapicque's law*.

isochronous [ISO- + CHRON- + -OUS] Occurring simultaneously; at the same time.

isochroous   ISOCHROMATIC.

isocitratase   An outmoded term for ISOCITRATE LYASE. ● The name is misleading because it implies that the reaction catalyzed by this enzyme is a hydrolysis.

isocitrate dehydrogenase   The enzyme (EC 1.1.1.41), of the citric acid cycle, that converts the CHOH group of isocitrate into a carbonyl group with concomitant reduction of NAD^+. The initial product undergoes decarboxylation to form 2-oxoglutarate before it dissociates from the enzyme. There is also an NADP-linked enzyme (EC 1.1.1.42), which is cytosolic.

isocitrate lyase   The enzyme (EC 4.1.3.1) that converts isocitrate into succinate and glyoxylate. It is found in microorganisms, some worms, and plants, but not in mammals, and is part of the glyoxylate cycle, which effects the net conversion of fat into carbohydrate. Also called *isocitratase* (outmoded).

isocitric acid   HOOC—CH_2—CH(COOH)—CHOH—COOH. 1-Hydroxypropane-1,2,3-tricarboxylic acid. The natural compound is the $1R,2S$ isomer. It is an intermediate in the citric acid cycle, being produced from citrate by the enzyme aconitase, and being converted into 2-oxoglutarate by the enzyme isocitrate dehydrogenase. It is also an intermediate in the glyoxylate cycle in plants, where it is split by isocitrate lyase to form glyoxylate and succinate.

isocomplement   Complement derived from serum of a member of the same species or the same individual that also was a source of antibody.

isocoria [ISO- + *cor(e)*- + -IA] Equality of pupil size.

isocortex   The portion of the cerebral cortex that is most complex in structure and considered phylogenetically most recent. It is characteristically six-layered, and covers the lateral cerebral hemispheres. All other cortical areas contain fewer layers and are located medially. Also called *neopallium, neocortex, homogenetic cortex, homotypic cortex, eulaminate cortex* (older term), *nonolfactory cortex* (outmoded). ● According to the schema of O. Vogt, who devised the term, the cerebral cortex was seven-layered, but the conventionally accepted scheme of Brodmann recognizes six layers.

Isocrin   A proprietary name for oxyphenisatin acetate.

isocyanate   The group —N═C═O or a compound that contains it. Such compounds are hydrolyzed slowly by water, and they react with amines to form urea derivatives.

isocyanide   The group —NC or a compound that contains it. Such compounds are formed by the action of alkali and trichloromethane on primary amines, and this reaction was once widely used as a test for such amines, since the isocyanide formed could be detected by its distinctive smell. Also called *carbylamine* (obsolete).

isocytosis   Uniformity of cell size, especially of erythrocytes. Also called *anisocytosis*.

isocytotoxin [ISO- + CYTO- + TOXIN] A toxin active against cells of the animal species from which it is derived.

isodactylism   A trait of equal-length digits.

isodactylous   Of or relating to isodactylism.

isodiagnosis   The diagnosis of a subclinical or inapparent infection by inoculation of a susceptible laboratory animal with blood from the patient suspected of having the condition.

isodialuric acid   2,4,5,6-Tetrahydroxypyrimidine and its tautomers. It is one of the acidic pyrimidines.

isodiametric   Having all diameters of equal length.

isodont [*is(o)*- + -ODONT] HOMODONT.

isodose [ISO- + DOSE] In radiotherapy, designating a curve or surface in which all the points receive the same dose of radiation.

isodynamic [ISO- + DYNAMIC] Possessing the same force or power. Also *isoenergetic, isodynamogenic*.

isodynamogenic   ISODYNAMIC.

isoeffect [ISO- + EFFECT] An equal effect.

isoelectric   Possessing the same electric potential, as ions having the same electric charge; isopotential.

isoelectronic   Having the same number and arrangement of electrons. The ammonium ion is, for example, isoelectronic with the methane molecule.

isoenergetic [ISO- + ENERGETIC] ISODYNAMIC.

isoenzyme   One of different forms of an enzyme, all judged to be the same enzyme by the fact that they catalyze the same reaction. The term was originally used for enzymes that differed in any way, usually because they were separable by electrophoresis or isoelectric focusing, but it has since become restricted to forms that differ by genetically determined differences in amino-acid sequence, rather than those that differ by modification of the same sequence, as by loss of amide nitrogen. Also called *isozyme*.

isoephedrine   PSEUDOEPHEDRINE.

isoerythrolysis   The destruction of red cells by alloantibodies. **neonatal isoerythrolysis**   Destruction of neonate red cells by alloantibodies, generally of maternal origin, as in hemolytic disease of the newborn.

isoetharine $C_{13}H_{21}NO_3$. 3,4-Dihydroxy-α-[1-(isopropylamino)propyl]benzyl alcohol. An adrenergic drug used for the treatment of bronchial asthma and as a bronchiolar dilator.

isoflurophate   DIISOPROPYL FLUOROPHOSPHATE.

isogame   ISOGAMY.

isogamete [ISO- + GAMETE]   A gamete similar in size and form to the cell with which it unites.

isogametic   Producing similar gametes that fuse in syngamy. Some protozoa and algae are isogametic.

isogamety   The production of gametes by a homogametic individual, with all gametes having the same sex chromosome. It is the situation found in the normal human female.

isogamous   Reproducing by fusion of gametes which are similar in size and form.

isogamy [ISO- + GAM- + -Y]   Reproduction in which the two uniting gametes are similar in size, shape, and motility. Also called *microgamy*. Also *isogame*.

isogeneic   Of or relating to transplantation of tissues in which the donor and the host are genetically identical, as in grafts between monozygous twins. Also *isologous, isoplastic*.

isogeneric [ISO- + GENERIC]   Of or pertaining to members of the same genus.

isogenesis   Development occurring by the same processes.

isogenic   **1** Of or relating to two or more cells, clones, tissues, or individuals that have the same genotypes. Also *syngeneic*.   **2** Pertaining to two or more cells, clones, tissues, or individuals that have the same genotype at specific loci. For defs. 1 and 2 also *isologous*.

isogenous   Originating from one cell.

isoglutamine $^-OOC—CH_2—CH_2—CH(NH_3{}^+)—CO—NH_2$. The 1-amide of glutamic acid, in distinction from glutamine, its 5-amide.

isograft [ISO- + GRAFT]   A graft transferred from one individual to another individual who is genetically identical, as in identical twins or animals so highly inbred that they have complete compatibility of genes. Also called *isogeneic homograft, syngraft, isogeneic graft, isologous graft, isoplastic graft, syngeneic graft, isotransplant*.

isohemolysin   Antibody directed against an antigen found in the same species and capable of inducing red cell destruction.

isohemolysis   Hemolysis caused by antierythrocyte antibodies formed in response to stimulation by antigens of another member of the same species. Also called *homolysis*. Adjective: isohemolytic.

isohydruria   The excretion of urine at a fixed pH.

isohypercytosis   ISOLEUKOCYTOSIS.

isohypocytosis   Leukopenia with normal proportions of different classes, especially granulocytes.

iso-iconia   ISEIKONIA.

iso-iconic   ISEIKONIC.

isoimmunization   Immunization following exposure to antigens originating in a genetically different member of the same species.

Rh isoimmunization   Isoimmunization resulting from exposure to an Rh antigen, formerly the most common cause of hemolytic disease of the newborn. See also RH ANTIGEN.

isoindicial   Within a medium of progressively changing refractive index, such as the crystalline lens, referring to a zone or region within which the index of refraction is the same.

isolabeling   The appearance of radioactive precursors of DNA synthesis (usually tritiated thymidine) in both daughter chromatids at the second metaphase after the labelled precursor is administered. It is the consequence of sister chromatid exchange.

isolate [French *isolé* (from Italian *isolato* like an island, from *isola* an island, from L *insula* island) separated, little frequented, insulated + -ATE]   **1** To separate from other chemicals, ma-

terials, objects, persons or other living organisms a population or group of one kind.   **2** Any isolated substance, organism, population, etc.

geographic isolate   A population that must breed within itself because of geographic restriction, the result of which is assortative mating and inbreeding.

mating isolate   A population that is genetically isolated from other members of its species.

isolateral   **1** Having sides that are equal or identical.   **2** IPSILATERAL.

isolation [*isolat(e)* + -ATION]   The condition of being set apart from others, as to minimize the risk of spreading infection.

behavioral isolation   The prevention of breeding between two or more populations of animals due to behavioral differences. Also called *psychosexual isolation, ecobiotic isolation*.

ecobiotic isolation   BEHAVIORAL ISOLATION.

ethologic isolation   **1** The inability of members of a population to reproduce because of profound differences in mating behavior.   **2** The inability of related species to produce hybrids due to different mating behavior.

genetic isolation   The prevention of interbreeding between two populations by differences in genotype or chromosome complement.

psychosexual isolation   BEHAVIORAL ISOLATION.

reproductive isolation   The inability of two sexually reproducing populations to interbreed freely in their natural environment.

reverse isolation   Isolation to prevent contamination or infection from spreading into the environment from an infected source.

seasonal isolation   The inability of two sexually reproducing populations to interbreed because they are reproductively active at different seasons of the year.

sensory isolation   SENSORY DEPRIVATION.

isolator   **1** A surgical instrument that functions to separate one region of tissue from another.   **2** A person whose function is to preserve separation of one region of tissue from another during operative procedures.

surgical isolator   A large plastic bag in which the patient and operative team are placed during a surgical procedure in order to prevent infective contamination of the patient.

isolecithal [ISO- + LECITHAL]   MIOLECITHAL.

isoleucine $CH_3—CH_2—CH(CH_3)—CH(NH_3{}^+)—COO^-$. One of the 20 amino acids that are incorporated in proteins. It is essential in the human diet. The name is restricted to the 2*S*,3*S* compound (L-isoleucine) and its enantiomer, the 2*R*,3*R* compound, the other two diastereoisomers being known as alloisoleucine. Symbol: Ile

[8-isoleucine] oxytocin   See under MESOTOCIN.

isoleukocytosis   Leukocytosis with normal proportions of different classes, especially granulocytes. Also called *isohypercytosis*.

isologous   **1** ISOGENIC.   **2** ISOGENEIC.   **3** HOMOLOGOUS.

isomaltase   Oligo-1,6-glucosidase. An enzyme that hydrolyzes 1,6-α-glucoside bonds in isomaltose and related oligosaccharides.

isomaltose   6-*O*-(α-D-Glucosyl)glucose. An isomer of maltose, from which it differs in that the reducing residue is glucosylated on O-6 rather than on O-4. It is derived from partial hydrolysates of glycogen and amylopectin, in which it represents the points where their chains branch.

isomastigote   A protozoan with two or four flagella that are equal in size and at one extremity.

isomer [Gk *iso(s)* equal to + *mer(os)* a part]   **1** One of two or more substances whose molecules possess equal numbers of each type of atom they contain, such as $CH_3—CH_2—OH$ and $CH_3—O—CH_3$, both C_2H_6O but having very different properties. The term is applied especially to closely related substances, such as citric acid and isocitric acid, that differ in the locations of — OH and an —H in their molecules. **2** Any of two or more atomic nuclei which have the same number of protons and neutrons but different energy states, such as technetium 99 and technetium 99m.

cis-trans isomer   Either of two stereoisomers that differ only in having certain atoms located on different sides of a specified plane. The plane is usually that of a double bond or a ring. Also called *geometric isomer*.

conformational isomer   Any of two or more isomers that can be interconverted without bond breakage, but which nevertheless are in conformations to which their atoms return spontaneously after small displacements. Conformational isomers often interconvert fairly rapidly. Also called *conformer*.

geometric isomer   CIS-TRANS ISOMER.

metastable isomer   A radioactive nuclide belonging to the same nuclear species as some nuclide of interest, i.e., it has the same proton and neutron numbers, but exists at a higher level of nuclear excitation. It discharges its excess energy by gamma emission, with a measurable half-life. See also ISOMERIC TRANSITION.

optical isomer   ENANTIOMER.

positional isomer   One of two or more isomers that differ in the position of a substituent.

isomerase   Any enzyme which converts a substrate to its isomer.

isomeric   **1** Being in the relation of isomers: said of substances. **2** Having the same atomic number and same mass number, but different internal energy states. For defs. 1 and 2 also called *isomerous*.

isomerism [ISOMER + -ISM]   The phenomenon that molecules can differ when they contain the same numbers of the same atoms.

optical isomerism   The phenomenon of molecules differing by being the mirror images of each other (enantiomers). Such isomers rotate the plane of polarized light in opposite directions.

isomerization   The conversion of one isomer into another.

isomerous   ISOMERIC.

isomethadone $C_{21}H_{27}NO$. 6-(Dimethylamino)-5-methyl-4,4-diphenyl-3-hexanone. A compound similar to methadone in structure and in pharmacologic properties. It is an analgesic with addicting properties if taken chronically.

isometheptene $C_9H_{19}N$. *N*,1,5-Trimethyl-4-hexenylamine. An adrenergic drug used as an antispasmodic for intestinal, biliary, or ureteral spasm or colic.

isometheptene mucate $C_{24}H_{48}N_2O_8$. The mucate derivative of isometheptene. It has the same adrenergic properties and uses as the parent drug.

isometric [ISO- + METRIC]   Possessing the same length or dimensions, as a muscle contraction in which the force is increased without a change in length.

isometrics   Movements or exercises in which the muscles are tensed without motion at the joints they bridge.

isometropia [ISO- + METROPIA]   A similar refraction state in each eye.

isometry [ISO- + -METRY]   An equality of dimensions.

isomicrogamete [ISO- + MICRO- + GAMETE]   A small gamete that is equal in size to the cell with which it conjugates. Such gametes are produced by some protozoa.

isomorph   An outmoded term for ALLELE.

isomorphic   ISOMORPHOUS.

isomorphism   The property of being morphologically similar.

isomorphous [ISO- + MORPH- + -OUS]   Occurring in the same form. Also *isomorphic*.

isonephrotoxin   A nephrotoxin derived from the same species as that on which it acts.

isoniazid $C_6H_7N_3O$. 4-Pyridinecarboxylic acid hydrazide. A

crystalline solid, soluble in water and alcohol, practically insoluble in ether and benzene, used in the treatment of tuberculosis. Also called *isonicotinic acid hydrazide, isonicotinoylhydrazine*.

isonicotinic acid   Pyridine-4-carboxylic acid, an isomer of nicotinic acid. Its hydrazide inhibits pyridoxal-containing enzymes, particularly in some bacteria. Its consequent toxicity to them is the basis of the use of the hydrazide in treating tuberculosis.

isonicotinic acid hydrazide   ISONIAZID.

isonicotinoylhydrazine   ISONIAZID.

isonipecaine   MEPERIDINE HYDROCHLORIDE.

isonormocytosis   Having a normal total leukocyte count and normal proportions of different classes of leukocytes.

isonymous   Having the same surname. Such a characteristic is an indicator, but not proof, of the consanguinity of spouses in pedigree analysis.

iso-oncotic   Possessing the same oncotic pressure.

iso-osmotic   ISOSMOTIC.

Isoparorchidae [ISO- + *par(asite)*- + *orch(i)*- + -IDAE]   A small family of trematode parasites of fishes in the superfamily Hemiuroidea which contains the genus *Isoparorchis*. The species *I. hypselobagri* from the swine bladder of siluroid fishes in India and the Far East has occasionally been found in humans, probably from the ingestion of raw fish.

isopentenyl diphosphate $CH_2=C(CH_3)-CH_2-CH_2-O-PO(OH)-O-PO(OH)_2$. 3-Methylbut-3-enyl diphosphate. This substance is formed from diphosphomevalonic acid by a decarboxylation and elimination linked with the hydrolysis of ATP, in an early step of the pathway by which steroids and other terpenes are made. Also called *isopentenyl pyrophosphate*.

isopentenyldiphosphate isomerase   The enzyme (EC 5.3.3.2) that catalyzes the interconversion of isopentenyl diphosphate (3-methylbut-3-enyl diphosphate) and dimethylallyl diphosphate (3-methylbut-2-enyl phosphate). In a further reaction of the pathway of terpene and steroid biosynthesis, isopentenyl and dimethylallyl diphosphates condense with the formation of the C_{10}-compound, geranyl diphosphate, and the release of inorganic diphosphate.

isopentenyl pyrophosphate   ISOPENTENYL DIPHOSPHATE.

isophagy   An obsolete term for AUTOLYSIS.

isophan   **1** PHENOCOPY.   **2** In plant breeding, a hybrid of similar phenotype but different germ lines from other hybrids.

isophene   GENOCOPY.

isophenolization   The technique of injecting nerves with isophenol in order to destroy neurons, such as during a sympathectomy.

isophilic   A seldom used term for HOMOEROTIC.

isophoria [ISO- + -PHORIA]   **1** A constant balance of ocular muscles regardless of the position of the eyes. **2** The visual axes of the two eyes are on the same horizontal plane so that there is no hyperphoria or hypophoria.

isophotometer [ISO- + PHOTOMETER]   A device for locating points of equal density on a radiograph or another type of film.

Isophrin   A proprietary name for phenylephrine hydrochloride.

isopia [*is(o)*- + -OPIA]   Similar visual acuity in each eye.

isoplastic   ISOGENEIC.

isopleural   Symmetrical in appearance on both sides, particularly in reference to the thorax.

isopotential   Possessing the same potential force or energy; having the same ability to do work.

isopregnenone   DYDROGESTERONE.

isoprenaline   ISOPROTERENOL.

isoprene $CH_2=CH-C(CH_3)=CH_2$. 2-Methylbuta-1,3-diene. A hydrocarbon that is the fundamental unit from which many natural products, including steroids, are built.

isoprenoid Any substance biosynthesized from C_5-units with the isoprene skeleton. Such compounds include squalene, the precursor of steroids, and terpenes. Isopentenyl diphosphate and dimethylallyl diphosphate are the two precursors of the C_5-units present in more complex molecules.

Isoprinosine $C_{52}H_{78}N_{10}O_{17}$. A drug which stimulates T cells and lymphocytes *in vitro* and *in vivo*, and has been reported to have some antiviral activity *in vitro*. A proprietary name.

isopropamide iodide $C_{23}H_{33}IN_2O$. γ-(Aminocarboxyl)-*N*-methyl-*N*-*N*-bis(1-methylethyl)-γ-phenylbenzene propanaminium iodide. An anticholinergic agent used to treat peptic ulcer. It is given orally.

isopropanol CH_3—CHOH—CH_3. Propan-2-ol. A colorless liquid having a smell like ethanol. It is present in wine alcohols and can be made from propene, from cracking petroleum. Its toxicity is comparable to that of ethanol. It is used as solvent, to denature ethanol, in preparing cosmetics, and as a surgical antiseptic. Also called *isopropyl alcohol*.

isopropenyl The univalent group CH_2=C(—CH_3)—.

isopropyl $(CH_3—)_2CH$—. The group formed by removing a hydrogen atom from C-2 of propane. Also called *propyl*.

isopropyl alcohol ISOPROPANOL.

isopropylarterenol ISOPROTERENOL.

isopropylepinephrine ISOPROTERENOL.

isopropyl meprobamate CARISOPRODOL.

isopropyl myristate $C_{17}H_{34}O_2$. An ester used in topical medicinal preparations because of its ability to promote absorption of externally applied drugs through the skin.

isopropyl thiogalactoside A synthetic galactoside derivative containing sulfur instead of oxygen as the glycosylated atom. It is used as an inducer of the formation of bacterial enzymes of galactoside metabolism, specifically those controlled by the *lac* operon.

isoproterenol $C_{11}H_{17}NO_3$.   3,4-Dihydroxy-α-[(isopropylamino)methyl]benzyl alcohol. A synthetic adrenergic agent similar to epinephrine, with a propyl group replacing the methyl group. It is a potent cardiac stimulant and bronchodilator. As the hydrochloride, it is given by inhalation, sublingually, or parenterally for treatment of bronchial asthma. It is used also for some cardiac conditions responding to these drugs. Also called *isoprenaline, isopropylarterenol, isopropylepinephrine*.

isopter [*is(o)-* + Gk *optēr* one who looks or spies] A line on a visual field chart passing through points of equal visual acuity.

isopycnotic ISOPYKNOTIC.

isopyknic [ISO- + PYKN- + -IC] Having equal density: said especially of a substance and a suspending medium in centrifugation.

isopyknosis [ISO- + PYKN- + -OSIS] A state of equivalent condensation of chromatin, as applied particularly to comparisons between and within chromosomes.

isopyknotic Of or relating to isopyknosis. Also *isopycnotic*.

isoquinoline C_9H_7N. 3,4-Benzpyridine. A heterocyclic amine of p*K* 5.1, it is a colorless liquid of repulsive smell and is soluble in organic liquids. The melting point is 24–25°C and the boiling point is 243°C. The isoquinoline ring occurs in the molecules of some alkaloids and some antimalarial drugs.

Isordil A proprietary name for isosorbide dinitrate.

isorhythmic Having a constant, invariable rhythm.

isoriboflavin $C_{17}H_{20}N_4O_6$.   8-Demethyl-6-methylriboflavin. An antimetabolite of riboflavin which has methyl groups on the 6 and 5 positions, rather than 6 and 7 positions, of the isoalloxazine nucleus. It has been used to produce a riboflavin deficiency in experimental animals.

isorrhea [ISO- + -RRHEA] A homeostasis of body fluid volume and composition.

isorrheic Of or relating to isorrhea.

isosaccharic acid 2,5-Anhydromannaric acid, a product of chemical breakdown of glucosamine. An obsolete term.

isoscope A device for evaluating cyclotorsion.

isosensitize AUTOSENSITIZE.

isoserine 3-Amino-2-hydroxypropionic acid; i.e. serine with its amino and hydroxyl groups interchanged.

isoserotherapy Therapy involving injections of isoserum.

isoserum Serum taken from a person who is convalescing from the same disease as that of the patient to be treated with such serum.

isosexual [ISO- + SEXUAL] A seldom used term for HOMOSEXUAL.

isosmotic Having equal osmotic pressure: used of two fluids. Also *iso-osmotic*.

isosmoticity The quality of being isosmotic.

isosorbide $C_6H_{10}O_4$. 1,4:3,6-Dianhydro-D-glucitol. A derivative of sorbitol used as an osmotic diuretic agent. It also reduces the intraocular pressure and is used to lower the tension quickly in glaucoma.

isosorbide dinitrate $C_6H_8N_2O_8$. 1,4:3,6-Dianhydro-D-glucitol dinitrate. A form of nitrate used to dilate the coronary vessels of the heart. It is given in tablets for sublingual absorption and in sustained-release oral tablets, the latter being considerably less effective.

isospermotoxin An antibody which is cytotoxic to spermatozoa of the same species.

Isospora A genus of monoxenous coccidian parasites in the suborder Eimeriina, found chiefly in mammals, but also in birds, amphibians, and reptiles. The mature oocysts, found in feces, contain two sporocysts, each with four sporozoites.

Isospora belli A species found in the small intestine of humans in the tropics, and probably throughout the world. The infection, known as coccidiosis, is usually asymptomatic and self-limiting, but has been associated with mucous diarrhea or steatorrhea, anorexia, nausea, and, in some cases, colicky abdominal pain and malabsorption.

Isospora bigemina A species found in the small intestine of dogs, cats, minks, foxes, and probably other carnivores. It is the cause of diarrhea and enteritis in dogs and cats. The oocysts are extremely similar to those of *Toxoplasma* and *I. hominis*. Also called *Coccidium bigeminum*.

Isospora canis A worldwide species that causes a mild diarrheal disease in dogs.

Isospora felis A worldwide species found in cats, lions, and other felids. Its effects usually are mild but occasionally it causes severe enteritis and even death.

Isospora hominis SARCOCYSTIS HOMINIS.

Isospora rivolta A worldwide species found in dogs, cats, and other carnivores. It causes a mild intestinal coccidiosis. Separate strains or species of dog and cat forms may exist.

Isospora suis A species common in swine, producing a catarrhal enteritis and mild diarrhea which lasts three to four days.

isosporiasis [*Isospor(a)* + -IASIS] Infection by sporozoans of the genus *Isospora*, which are found in the intestines of a wide variety of animals and which occasionally infect man. Also called *isosporosis*. See also COCCIDIOSIS.

isosporosis ISOSPORIASIS.

isostere A compound similar to another compound in the shape of its molecule but differing from it in chemical structure. Isosteres of natural compounds are often useful as research tools, since they may bind to enzymes and other receptors for the natural compounds.

isosthenuria [ISO- + STHEN- + -URIA] Excretion of urine with a fixed relative density (± 1.010) under all circumstances. It is a sign of advanced renal failure.

isotachophoresis [ISO- + TACHO- + -PHORESIS] An electrophoretic separation technique in which the substances being separated move at the same speed, but form separate zones, at the boundary between two electrolyte solutions. These solutions have ions chosen to have higher and lower mobilities, respectively, than the ions of the sample.

isotel [ISO- + Gk *tel(os)* end, completeness, fulfillment] A dietary factor which can effectively replace another essential nutrient.

isotherm [ISO- + Gk *therm(ē)* heat] A line drawn on a chart that connects points of the same temperature.

isothermagnosia [ISO- + *therm-* + Gk *agnōsia* a not knowing, ignorance] **1** Inability to distinguish between heat and cold. **2** An abnormality of sensation in which the patient perceives pain, heat, and cold as a feeling of heat. Also called *isothermognosis*.

isothermal ISOTHERMIC.

isothermic [ISO- + THERM- + -IC] Possessing the same temperature. Also *isothermal, synthermal*.

isothermognosis ISOTHERMAGNOSIA.

isothermy The process of maintaining a constant temperature.

isothiazine hydrochloride ETHOPROPAZINE HYDROCHLORIDE.

isothipendyl $C_{16}H_{19}N_3S$. 10-(2-Dimethylamino-2-methylethyl)-10*H*-pyrido[3,2-*b*][1,4]benzothiazine. An antihistamic agent often given in the hydrochloride salt form. It is a potent, but short acting antihistaminic medication, given by oral or parenteral routes for severe allergies.

isotocin A pituitary hormone of fishes. It differs from mammalian oxytocin in replacing glutamine at locus 4 with serine, and leucine at locus 8 with isoleucine.

isotomin A substance found in *Isotoma longiflora*, longflower shrubharebell, that paralyzes the heart.

isotone Any of two or more atomic nuclei which have the same number of neutrons but different atomic numbers and different mass numbers such as $^{30}_{14}Si$, $^{31}_{15}P$, and $^{32}_{16}S$. .

isotonia Equality of osmotic pressure in two solutions that are being compared. Also called *homotonia*.

isotonic **1** Denoting a fluid exerting the same osmotic pressure as another fluid with which it is being compared and in which cells can be immersed without changing their size and shape. **2** Maintaining a uniform muscle tone. For defs. 1 and 2 also *homotonic*.

isotonicity The quality of being isotonic.

isotope [Gk *iso(s)* equal to, the same as + *topos* a place] Any of several atoms which have the same number of protons, and thus are members of the same element, but have different numbers of neutrons. Thus ^{129}I and ^{131}I are isotopes of iodine. • At one time *isotope* was widely but incorrectly used to refer to any radioactive atom, for which the preferred term is now *radioactive nuclide* or *radionuclide*, unless reference is made specifically to two nuclides of the same element. Adjective: isotopic.

heavy isotope An isotope of greater nuclear mass than that of the naturally most abundant isotope of the element concerned, or the more massive of two naturally occurring isotopes. Although many radioactive isotopes are heavier than their naturally most abundant forms, e.g. ^3H or ^{14}C compared with ^1H or ^{12}C, the term is often used specifically for isotopes that do not emit radiation, e.g. ^2H, ^{13}C, ^{15}N, or ^{18}O.

radioactive isotope An incorrect term for RADIONUCLIDE.

stable isotope An isotope that does not transmute into another element; a nonradioactive isotope.

isotopic Of or pertaining to isotopes.

isotoxic HOMEOTOXIC.

isotoxin [ISO- + TOXIN] HOMEOTOXIN.

isotransplant ISOGRAFT.

Isotricha A genus of endocommensal ciliates of ruminants. *I. prostoma* is abundant in the rumen and reticulum of cattle, *I. intestinalis* is common in those of cattle, sheep, and goats.

isotron [ISO- + Gk *-tron*, suffix denoting an instrument] An electromagnetic instrument that separates isotopes of ions into groups relative to their masses. It has a strong direct field and weak fields that vary at radio frequency.

isotropic [ISO- + -TROPIC¹] Having physical properties that are independent of direction in the material.

isotropy The state or quality of being isotropic.

isotypical Of the same type.

isovaleric acid $(CH_3)_2CH-CH_2-COOH$. 3-Methylbutyric acid. It contains the carbon chain of the amino acid valine.

isovalericacidemia An inborn error of metabolism of the branched-chain amino acid leucine. The basic defect is thought to be a deficiency of the enzyme isovaleryl-CoA dehydrogenase. Serum isovaleric acid levels are markedly elevated, with clinical consequences appearing as psychomotor retardation, an objectionable body odor that resembles sweaty feet, and a tendency for developing dehydration, acidosis, and coma. The condition is inherited as an autosomal recessive trait. Also called *Sidbury syndrome, odor-of-sweaty-feet syndrome, sweaty feet syndrome*.

isoxazolyl penicillin A group of semisynthetic penicillins that are resistant to penicillinase and to acid hydrolysis. They include cloxacillin, dicloxacillin, flucloxacillin, and oxacillin.

isoxsuprine hydrochloride $C_{18}H_{23}NO_3 \cdot HCl$. *p*-Hydroxy-α-[1-[(1-methyl-2-phenoxyethylamino]ethyl]benzyl alcohol hydrochloride. A white, crystalline powder, sparingly soluble in water, used as a vasodilator in the treatment of peripheral vascular disease associated with arteriosclerosis.

isozyme ISOENZYME.

issue [French, from Old French *issue, eissue* an issue, end, event, fem. of *issu*, past part. of *issir* to go out, from L *exire* to go out, from *ex-* EX-¹ + *ire* to go] **1** A purulent or bloody discharge, sometimes associated with the presence of a foreign body. A seldom used term. **2** Offspring; progeny.

-ist [Gk suffix *-istēs* from verb termination *-izein* denoting to perform an act + *-tēs* forming agent nouns] A suffix denoting a person engaged in a profession or activity.

isthmectomy [*isthm(us)* + -ECTOMY] A surgical procedure in which a narrow bridge of tissue connecting two larger tissue masses is excised, as removal of the thyroid isthmus. Also called *median strumectomy*.

isthmi Plural of ISTHMUS.

isthmian Pertaining to any anatomical isthmus. Also *isthmic*.

isthmic ISTHMIAN.

isthmitis [*isthm(us)* + -ITIS] Inflammation of the isthmus faucium. An ambiguous and obsolete term.

isthmoid Resembling an anatomical isthmus.

isthmoparalysis Paralysis of the musculature of the isthmus faucium. An obsolete term. Also called *isthmoplegia*.

isthmoplegia ISTHMOPARALYSIS.

isthmus [Gk *isthmos* a neck, narrow passage, isthmus] **1** A narrow strip of tissue connecting the larger structures or parts of an organ. **2** A short narrow passage or constriction connecting two cavities or canals.

anterior isthmus of fauces ISTHMUS FAUCIUM.

isthmus of aorta ISTHMUS AORTAE.

isthmus aortae [NA] A narrowing of the lumen of the aorta, especially marked in the fetus, between the final site of origin of the left subclavian artery and the attachment of the ductus arteriosus, which becomes the ligamentum arteriosum after birth. The constriction occasionally persists in the adult. Also called *isthmus of aorta, aortic isthmus.*

aortic isthmus   ISTHMUS AORTAE.

isthmus of auditory tube   ISTHMUS TUBAE AUDITIVAE.

isthmus of auricle   ISTHMUS CARTILAGINIS AURIS.

isthmus of cartilage of auricle   ISTHMUS CARTILAGINIS AURIS.

isthmus cartilaginis auris   [NA] A narrow strip of cartilage joining the cartilage of the auricle of the external ear to that of the external acoustic meatus. Also called *isthmus of cartilage of auricle, isthmus of auricle, isthmus of cartilaginous part of ear.*

isthmus of cartilaginous part of ear   ISTHMUS CARTILAGINIS AURIS.

isthmus of cingulate gyrus   ISTHMUS GYRI CINGULI.

isthmus of eustachian tube   ISTHMUS TUBAE AUDITIVAE.

isthmus of external auditory meatus   A very narrow segment of the osseous part of the external acoustic meatus that is situated at the junction of the outer three fourths and the inner one fourth of the meatus.

isthmus of fallopian tube   ISTHMUS TUBAE UTERINAE.

isthmus of fauces   ISTHMUS FAUCIUM.

isthmus faucium   [NA] The slightly narrowed opening between the oral cavity and the oral pharynx, bounded superiorly by the free border of the palatal velum and the uvula, laterally by the palatoglossal arches, and inferiorly by the dorsum of the tongue. Also called *isthmus of fauces, oropharyngeal isthmus, pharyngo-oral isthmus, anterior isthmus of fauces, velopharyngeal portal* (outmoded).

isthmus glandulae thyroideae   [NA] A horizontal strip of thyroid tissue, of varying size, anterior to the upper part of the trachea, connecting the lower parts of the lateral lobes of the thyroid gland. Occasionally the pyramidal lobe is attached to it. Also called *isthmus of thyroid gland.*

Guyon's isthmus   ISTHMUS UTERI.

gyral isthmus   A narrow bridge interposed between two gyri of the cerebral cortex.

isthmus gyri cinguli   The constriction of the cingulate gyrus behind and below the splenium of the corpus callosum at its transition to the parahippocampal gyrus. Also called *isthmus gyri fornicati, isthmus of limbic lobe, isthmus of cingulate gyrus.*

isthmus gyri fornicati   ISTHMUS GYRI CINGULI.

isthmus hippocampi   The narrow retrosplenial cortex bridging the cingulate gyrus and the parahippocampal gyrus.

isthmus of His   ISTHMUS RHOMBENCEPHALI.

Krönig's isthmus   KRÖNIG'S AREA.

isthmus of limbic lobe   ISTHMUS GYRI CINGULI.

isthmus meatus acustici externi   A constriction in the osseous part of the external acoustic meatus less than one inch from the porus acusticus externus. An outmoded term.

oropharyngeal isthmus   ISTHMUS FAUCIUM.

isthmus pharyngonasalis   CHOANA.

pharyngo-oral isthmus   ISTHMUS FAUCIUM.

isthmus prostatae   [NA] A band of fibromuscular tissue that joins the right to the left lobe of the prostate in front of the urethra. Also called *isthmus of prostate.*

isthmus of prostate   ISTHMUS PROSTATAE.

isthmus rhombencephali   The constriction formed in fetal development by a bend in the neural tube at the juncture of the rhombencephalon and mesencephalon. Also called *isthmus of His.*

isthmus of thyroid gland   ISTHMUS GLANDULAE THYROIDEAE.

isthmus tubae auditivae   [NA] The narrowest part of the auditory tube, occurring at the junction of the osseous and cartilaginous portions. Also called *isthmus of auditory tube, isthmus of eustachian tube.*

isthmus tubae uterinae   [NA] The narrow, cordlike medial one third of the uterine tube, lying between its ampulla and the wall of the uterus. Also called *isthmus of fallopian tube, isthmus of uterine tube.*

isthmus urethrae   An outmoded term for PARS MEMBRANACEA URETHRAE MASCULINAE.

isthmus uteri   [NA] The transverse constriction between the cervix and the body of the uterus. Also called *isthmus of uterus, Guyon's isthmus.*

isthmus of uterine tube   ISTHMUS TUBAE UTERINAE.

isthmus of uterus   ISTHMUS UTERI.

isthmus of Vieussens   LIMBUS FOSSAE OVALIS.

Isuprel   A proprietary name for isoproterenol.

isuria   The excretion of urine at a rate that remains constant over time.

itaconic acid $CH_2{=}C(COOH){-}CH_2{-}COOH$. An acid originally obtained by heating citric acid, but also excreted by some fungi as a fermentation product. It is an intermediate in chemical syntheses.

itch   [(substantive) Middle English *icche*, from Old English *gicce*; (verb) Middle English *icchen*, from Old English *giccan*]   **1** A sensation that elicits the desire to scratch; pruritus.   **2** A skin disorder characterized by an itch.   **3** A popular term for SCABIES.

alkali itch   Dermatitis caused by contact with alkalis.

Aujeszky's itch   PSEUDORABIES.

azo itch   Contact dermatitis caused by sensitization and exposure to azo dyes.

bakers' itch   BAKERS' ECZEMA.

barbers' itch   Infections and other disorders of the skin of the beard area in men, including ringworm, bacterial folliculitis, and pseudofolliculitis. An imprecise usage.

barley itch   An infestation by the mite *Pyemotes tritici* associated with grains, cause of a common human dermatitis.

bath itch   Pruritus caused by soap.

bedouin itch   MILIARIA RUBRA.

bricklayers' itch   A form of occupational dermatitis that occurs among bricklayers. Trauma and a sensitivity to compounds such as cement are causative factors. A popular usage.

Caripito itch   Dermatitis caused by airborne scales from the wings of various species of moth.   ● It was initially described following a massive flight of *Hylesia canitia* on a tank ship on the Orinoco river at Caripito, Venezuela.

cavalryman's itch   Scabies caused by the equine form of the scabies mite, *Sarcoptes scabiei* var. *equi.*

cheese itch   A contact dermatitis caused by mites associated with mold on cheese or other food products, caused by *Tyrophagus putrescentiae* (*Tyroglyphus longior* var. *castellani*) in the family Acaridae. It often affects workers who handle cheese.

clam diggers' itch   SCHISTOSOME DERMATITIS.

coolie itch   **1** GROUND ITCH.   **2** An eruption among tea plantation workers that is caused by the mite *Rhizoglyphus parasiticus.*

copra itch   An irritable papular eruption among those handling copra that is caused by the itch mite, *Tyrophagus Putrescentiae* (*Tyroglyphus longior* var. *Castellani*) of the family Acaridae.

Cuban itch   ALASTRIM.

dew itch   A seldom used term for GROUND ITCH.

dhobie itch   An outmoded term for TINEA CRURIS.

Dogger Bank itch   Contact dermatitis due to a sensitization to the marine animal *Alcyonidium gelatinosum.*

drysalters' itch   An occupational dermatitis occurring in drysalters from contact with rock salt in mines, brine, or sea salt which has been dried.

farmers' itch An eruption caused by contact with mites that infest stored grain, such as *Acorus siro* (*Tyrophagus farinae*) of the family Acaridae.

filarial itch ONCHOCERCAL DERMATITIS.

foot itch GROUND ITCH.

frost itch WINTER PRURIGO.

grain itch ACARODERMATITIS URTICARIOIDES.

grocers' itch An irritable eruption of the hands and forearms that is sometimes attributable to the house mite *Glycophagus domesticus* (family Glycophagidae).

ground itch An irritable eruption of the skin of the feet that is caused by penetration by hookworm or *Strongyloides* larvae. Also called *miners' itch, water itch, water pox, toe itch, foot itch, swamp itch, dew itch* (seldom used), *water sore, uncinarial dermatitis, waterpox* (obsolete), *coolie itch.*

gym itch TINEA CRURIS.

Haberswein itch An itching eruption caused by the hairs of certain species of moth in the Haberswein region of Kenya.

harvest itch An eruption caused by the harvest mite.

jock itch A popular term for TINEA CRURIS.

kabure itch SCHISTOSOMIASIS.

laundryman's itch An incorrect term for TINEA CRURIS. • It was once widely held that the condition resulted from the contamination of clothing during laundering.

lumberman's itch WINTER PRURIGO.

mad itch PSEUDORABIES.

Malabar itch TINEA IMBRICATA.

mattress itch ACARODERMATITIS URTICARIOIDES.

millers' itch ACARODERMATITIS URTICARIOIDES.

miners' itch GROUND ITCH.

Norway itch NORWEGIAN SCABIES.

Philippine itch ALASTRIM.

poultryman's itch A dermatitis caused by the chicken mite, *Dermanyssus gallinae.*

psoroptic itch PSOROPTIC MANGE.

rank itch SCABIES.

Saint Ignatius itch PELLAGRA.

sandhogs' itch The itching and mottling of the skin that occurs in decompression sickness, particularly if the skin is chilled during decompression.

sarcoptic itch SARCOPTIC SCABIES.

Sawah itch An East Indian term for SCHISTOSOMIASIS.

scrub itch An eruption caused by the harvest mite, which in some regions may carry scrub typhus.

seven-year itch SCABIES.

straw itch ACARODERMATITIS URTICARIOIDES.

straw-bed itch ACARODERMATITIS URTICARIOIDES.

sugar itch An occupational dermatitis that occurs in those who frequently handle large quantities of sugar, such as bakers.

summer itch HUTCHINSON SUMMER PRURIGO.

swamp itch GROUND ITCH.

swimmers' itch SCHISTOSOME DERMATITIS.

tar itch An irritable dermatosis caused by exposure to tar. A popular usage.

toe itch GROUND ITCH.

vanilla-workers' itch VANILLISM.

warehouseman's itch Dermatitis caused by exposure to mites that infest food. Warehouse workers are most at risk, but other wholesale and retail food handlers may also be affected.

washerwoman's itch Skin irritation that is brought on by repeated and prolonged exposure to water and/or laundry products.

water itch GROUND ITCH.

wheat pollard itch A dermatitis caused by handling grain infested with the scaly grain mite, *Suidasia nesbitti*, of the family Acaridae.

winter itch WINTER PRURIGO.

itching [ITCH + -ING] PRURITUS.

-ite [Gk-*itēs* (feminine -*itis*) suffix denoting resembling, of the nature of; also L -*itus* general past participle ending; also arbitrary variant of -*ate* from L -*atus* past participle ending] **1** A suffix meaning (1) substance of or derived from (something specified); (2) constituent or division, especially an early developmental stage of an anatomic part. **2** A suffix designating an anion, salt, or ester containing less oxygen than that contained in another anion, salt, or ester based on the same element, as nitrite, NO_2^- in contrast with nitrate, NO_3^-.

iter [L (gen. *itineris*; from *itus*, past part. of *ire* to go), a going along, walk, road, way, path] A tubular passage or channel between two structures or parts.

iter ad infundibulum The median tubular passage of the infundibular stalk connecting the hypothalamic third ventricle with the pituitary.

iter a tertio ad quartum ventriculum AQUEDUCTUS CEREBRI.

iter chordae anterius A foramen situated at the inner end of the petrotympanic fissure that transmits the chorda tympani from the cavity of the middle ear to the deep face. Also called *Huguier's canal, Civinini's canal.*

iter chordae posterius CANALICULUS CHORDAE TYMPANI.

iter dentium The channel through which a permanent tooth emerges into the oral cavity.

iter of Sylvius AQUAEDUCTUS CEREBRI.

iteral Pertaining to an iter.

iterative [Late L *iterativus* (from L *iterat(us)*, past part. of *iterare* to repeat + -*ivus* -IVE) repetitive] Repeatedly executing a series of operations or instructions until some condition is satisfied: said of a procedure or computer program.

iteroparity [L *iter(um)* again + *o* + *par(ere)* to bring forth young, procreate + -ITY] The state of having reproduced more than one time.

iteroparous [L *iter(um)* + *o* + *par(erere)* to bring forth young, procreate + -OUS] Having reproduced more than once.

ithycyphos An obsolete term for ITHYOKYPHOSIS.

ithylordosis Lordosis without accompanying lateral deviation of the spine. An obsolete term.

ithyokyphosis A backward projection of the spine with no accompanying lateral deviation. Also called *ithycyphos* (obsolete).

-itides Plural of -ITIS.

-itis [Gk -*itis* (feminine of -*ites*) noun suffix denoting disease, especially inflammatory] (*plural* -itides) A suffix meaning inflammation or disease associated with inflammation.

Ito [Hayazo *Ito*, Japanese pathologist, born 1865] Ito-Reenstierna reaction. See under ITO-REENSTIERNA TEST.

Ito [Minor *Ito*, Japanese dermatologist, flourished 20th century] See under NEVUS.

ITP idiopathic thrombocytopenic purpura.

Itrumil A proprietary name for iothiouracil.

Itsenko [N. N. *Itsenko*, Russian physician, flourished mid-20th century] Itsenko's disease. See under CUSHING SYNDROME.

-ity [L -*itas*, suffix forming nouns from adjectives and denoting state or condition] A suffix denoting state or condition.

IU **1** international unit. **2** immunizing unit. **3** intrauterine.

IUCD intrauterine contraceptive device.

IUD intrauterine device.

IV **1** intravenous(ly). **2** intravertebral.

Ivalon A proprietary name for polyvinyl alcohol.

IVC inferior vena cava.

-ive [L -*ivus*, suffix usually adjectival, sometimes substantive, denoting possession of a quality or nature] A suffix meaning having the nature or quality of.

ivermectin One of a class of potent antiparasitic drugs, the avermectins, used against a wide variety of nematodes and arthropods. It is the 22,23-dihydro derivative of avermectin B1, which is a macrocyclic lactone produced by *Actinomyces avermitilis*. The antiparasitic activity apparently is associated with blocking neuromuscular transmission mediated by γ-aminobutyric acid. It is used currently to control parasites of domestic animals, but its use may be extended to man.

ivory [Old French *yvoire* (from L *eboreus* made of ivory, from *ebur*, gen. *eboris*, ivory, akin to Sanskrit *ibhas* elephant) ivory] Dentin, especially of very large teeth such as the tusks of the elephant, walrus, hippopotamus, and narwhal. Also called *ebur*.

IVP **1** intravenous pyelogram. **2** intraventricular pressure.

IVT intravenous transfusion.

Ivy [Andrew Conway *Ivy*, U.S. physiologist, 1893–1978] Ivy's method. See under IVY BLEEDING TIME TEST.

Ivy [Robert H. *Ivy*, U.S. oral and plastic surgeon, 1881–1974] Ivy loop wiring. See under EYELET WIRING.

ivy **1** Any of various members of the genus *Hedera*, which is composed primarily of climbing plants. **2** See under POISON IVY.

poison ivy **1** Any of several plants of the genus *Toxicodendron* (especially *T. radicans*) widely distributed in North America and occurring also in South Africa, producing contact dermatitis with itching and in severe cases blistering. Smoke from the burning plant is also toxic. **2** Dermatitis resulting from contact or exposure to the toxin of the poison ivy plant.

Iwanoff [Wladimir *Iwanoff*, Russian ophthalmologist, born 1861] Iwanoff cysts. See under CYST.

Ixodes [Gk *ixōdēs* (from *ix(os)* mistletoe, birdlime prepared from the mistletoe berry + *eidos* form, shape or from *-ōdēs* suffix denoting resemblance, from *ozein* to smell, have a smell; akin to L *viscum* mistletoe, birdlime) like birdlime] The largest genus of ixodid or hard ticks, consisting of about 250 species, 40 from North America. They are all three-host ticks. Many are ectoparasites of man and domestic and wild mammals, causing severe reactions by their bites, and transmitting a number of disease agents.

Ixodes canisuga A common species, the British dog tick, found on dogs in Britain, western Europe, and North America.

Ixodes cavipalpus A tick infesting monkeys as well as children in Africa.

Ixodes cookei A species of tick that transmits Powassan virus in Canada.

Ixodes frequens A species found in Japan that infests cattle and horses, and will also attack humans.

Ixodes hexagonus A species found on domestic and wild carnivores in Africa and Europe, and implicated in transmission of tick-borne encephalitis virus and several human cases of tick paralysis in Europe.

Ixodes holocyclus An Australian species, the scrub tick, commonly found on wild rodents, but which often infests dogs, cats, other domestic animals, birds, and humans. It secretes a toxin that causes ascending flaccid paralysis and death from respiratory failure. One tick can cause death of a dog. Larger animals are unlikely to be affected. It is also the probable vector of Queensland tick typhus.

Ixodes pacificus The California black-legged tick, a species common on cattle and deer in California. It readily attacks man. It is considered a possible vector of tularemia in humans, and is a cause of tick paralysis.

Ixodes persulcatus A low-temperature-tolerant Eurasian species, the taiga tick, which is a vector of Russian spring-summer encephalitis, Omsk hemorrhagic fever virus, Absettarov virus, and Kemerovo virus in western Siberia. It plays an important role in the transmission of viruses to man and of bovine babesiosis in cattle. It is associated with a wide variety of small forest mammals and birds in its larval stages, and with larger domestic and wild animals as an adult tick.

Ixodes pilosus A species found on sheep in South Africa and thought to cause tick paralysis.

Ixodes putus A species found in the nests of a variety of marine birds.

Ixodes rasus A species found on insectivores, carnivores, ungulates, and occasionally man and other primates in Africa.

Ixodes ricinus The European castor bean tick, one of the most important viral and babesiosis vectors in this large genus. It is parasitic on sheep, cattle, and many wild animals. Larvae are found on a great range of small mammals and birds. It transmits a variety of disease agents including the virus of louping ill, Omsk hemorrhagic fever virus (the Bukovinian agent), Absettarov virus, Tribec virus, central European tick-borne encephalitis virus, and the Uukuniemi group viruses. It is also the vector of *Babesia bovis*, possibly of the Japanese B encephalitis virus, and is the etiologic agent of tularemia.

Ixodes rubicundus The Karoo paralysis tick, found on wild lagomorphs, carnivores, sheep, cattle, and goats in southern and southwestern Africa, and which causes flaccid paralysis. One human case has been reported.

Ixodes scapularis An American species, the black-legged or shoulder tick closely related to *I. ricinus* and *I. persulcatus* of Europe. This species is found in the eastern United States and frequently attacks man, inflicting a painful bite. It is closely related to the recently described vector of human babesiosis caused by *Babesia microti* and occurring in Massachusetts.

Ixodes spinipalpis A tick vector of the Powassan encephalitis virus, which was isolated from white-footed mice (*Peromyscus*) in Connecticut and South Dakota.

ixodiasis [*Ixod(es)* + -IASIS] **1** Any disease caused by tick bites. **2** Infestation with ticks. Also called *ixodism*.

ixodic Pertaining to or caused by ticks of the genus *Ixodes* or the family Ixodidae.

ixodid **1** Pertaining or belonging to the family Ixodidae. **2** A tick of the family Ixodidae.

Ixodidae [*Ixod(es)* + -IDAE] A family of ticks (order Acarina, suborder Ixodides) comprising some 660 species in 14 genera; the hard ticks. They are characterized by a rigid body form and the presence of a scutum. Many have a three-host life cycle with larvae on rodents or small birds, nymphs on intermediate-sized mammals, and adults on larger mammals, especially ruminants. It includes the genera *Amblyomma, Anocentor, Aponomma, Boophilus, Demacentor, Haemaphysalis, Hyalomma, Ixodes, Margaropus, Nosomma,* and *Rhipicephalus*.

Ixodides [*Ixod(es)* + L *-ides*, patronymic suffix] A suborder of Acarina which includes the superfamily Ixodoidea, comprising the families Ixodidae (hard ticks) and Argasidae (soft ticks).

Ixodiphagus A genus of hymenopteran parasitoids that attack ixodid ticks. An example is the species *I. caucurtei*.

ixodism IXODIASIS.

Ixodoidea [*Ixod(es)* + New L *-oidea*, neut. pl. suffix, from L *-oid(es)* -OID + *-ea*, neut. pl. of *-eus* English *-eous*] A superfamily of the order Acarina, suborder Ixodides, that includes the soft and hard ticks all of which are contained in the families Argasidae and Ixodidae, respectively.

-ize [Gk *-izein* infinitive verb termination meaning to perform an act] A suffix meaning to subject to. Also *-ise (British spelling).*

J

J **1** Symbol for the unit, joule. **2** Symbol for Joule's equivalent.

J Symbol for the quantities (1) electric current density, expressed in amperes per square meter; (2) magnetic polarization, expressed in teslas; (3) dynamic moment of inertia, expressed in kilogram meters squared; (4) sound intensity, expressed in watts per square meter.

jaagziekte [See JAGZIEKTE.] PULMONARY ADENOMATOSIS OF SHEEP.

jaborandi PILOCARPUS.

Jaboulay [Mathieu *Jaboulay*, French surgeon, 1860–1913] **1** See under BUTTON, PYLOROPLASTY, METHOD. **2** Jaboulay's amputation. See under INTERPELVIABDOMINAL AMPUTATION. **3** Jaboulay's operation. See under INTERPELVIABDOMINAL AMPUTATION.

Jaccoud [François-Sigismond *Jaccoud*, French physician, 1830–1913] See under FEVER, SIGN.

jacket [French *jaquette*, dim. of *jaque* a medieval short cloak, after *Jaques* an appellation for a peasant] **1** A popular term for COMPLETE VENEER CROWN. **2** A device that surrounds the torso and provides support and/or immobilizes the body.

leather jacket A leather appliance used to support the spine.

Minerva jacket A closely molded plaster-of-Paris jacket that extends from the iliac crest to the external occiput. • The term is named after *Minerva*, the Roman goddess of wisdom.

plaster-of-Paris jacket A Minerva jacket that does not encompass the neck and occiput. It is used for spinal fractures and for correcting deformities. Also called *Sayre's jacket*.

polyethylene jacket A jacket similar in shape and molding to the plaster-of-Paris jacket and made from polyethylene.

Sayre's jacket PLASTER-OF-PARIS JACKET.

strait jacket CAMISOLE.

jackscrew [*jack* + *screw*] A screw used in oral surgery to move segments of bone.

Jackson [Chevalier Q. *Jackson*, U.S. otolaryngologist, 1865–1958] **1** Jackson's safety triangle. See under TRIANGLE. **2** Chevalier Jackson's operation. See under VENTRICULOCORDECTOMY.

Jackson [Jabez North *Jackson*, U.S. surgeon, 1868–1935] Jackson's membrane, Jackson's veil. See under PERICOLIC MEMBRANE.

Jackson [John Hughlings *Jackson*, English neurologist, 1835–1911] **1** Bravais-Jacksonian epilepsy. See under JACKSONIAN EPILEPSY. **2** Jacksonian fit. See under FIT. **3** See under THEORY, SIGN. **4** Jackson's rule. See under LAW. **5** Hughlings Jackson syndrome, Jackson's lateral bulbar syndrome, Jackson syndrome, Jackson-Mackenzie syndrome. See under JACKSON'S PARALYSIS.

Jackson [Victor Hugo *Jackson*, U.S. dentist, 1850–1929] See under CRIB.

jacksonism [after John Hughlings *Jackson*, English neurologist, 1835–1911 + -ISM] **1** A seldom used term for JACKSONIAN MARCH. **2** A seldom used term for JACKSON'S THEORY.

Jacob [Arthur *Jacob*, Irish ophthalmologist, 1790–1874] **1** See under ULCER. **2** Jacob's membrane. See under STRATUM NEUROEPITHELIALE RETINAE.

Jacobaeus [Hans Christian *Jacobaeus*, Swedish physician, 1879–1937] See under OPERATION.

jacobine $C_{18}H_{25}NO_6$. A toxic alkaloid isolated from ragwort, *Senecio jacobaea*. It causes hepatic toxicosis of sheep and cattle. In cattle it may be either acute or chronic depending on the amount of ragwort ingested.

Jacobsohn [Ludvig Levin *Jacobsohn*, Danish anatomist, 1783–1843] Nucleus supraspinalis of Jacobsohn. See under SUPRASPINAL NUCLEUS.

Jacobson [Julius *Jacobson*, German ophthalmologist, 1828–1889] Jacobson's retinitis. See under RETINITIS SYPHILITICA.

Jacobson [Ludvig Levin *Jacobson*, Danish anatomist, 1783–1843] **1** Jacobson's plexus, plexus tympanicus Jacobsoni, Jacobson's anastomosis. See under PLEXUS TYMPANICUS. **2** Jacobson's nerve, tympanic nerve of Jacobson. See under NERVUS TYMPANICUS. **3** Ramus tubae plexus tympanici Jacobsoni. See under RAMUS TUBARIUS PLEXUS TYMPANICI. **4** See under REFLEX. **5** Organ of Jacobson. See under VOMERONASAL ORGAN. **6** Jacobson's canal, canal for Jacobson's nerve, tympanic canaliculus of Jacobson's nerve. See under CANALICULUS TYMPANICUS. **7** Cartilago vomeronasalis jacobsoni, cartilago jacobsoni, Jacobson's cartilage. See under CARTILAGO VOMERONASALIS. **8** Jacobson sulcus. See under SULCUS PROMONTORII CAVITATIS TYMPANICAE.

Jacod [Maurice *Jacod*, French physician, born 1880] Jacod syndrome, Jacod-Negri syndrome. See under PETROSPHENOID SYNDROME.

Jacquart [Henri *Jacquart*, French physician, born 1881] Jacquart's angle. See under OPHRYOSPINAL ANGLE.

Jacquemet [Marcel *Jacquemet*, French anatomist, 1872–1908] See under RECESS.

Jacquemier [Jean Marie *Jacquemier*, French obstetrician, 1806–1879] See under SIGN.

Jacquemin [Emile *Jacquemin*, French chemist, flourished late 19th century] See under TEST.

Jacques [Paul *Jacques*, French physician, flourished late 19th century] See under PLEXUS.

Jacquet [Leonard Marie Lucien *Jacquet*, French dermatologist, 1860–1914] **1** Jacquet's dermatitis. See under DIAPER DERMATITIS. **2** See under ERYTHEMA.

jactatio [L (from *jactatus*, past part. of *jactare* to throw), a tossing, shaking] JACTITATION.

jactation JACTITATION.

jactitation [Late L *jactitatio* (from L *jactitatus*, past part. of *jactitare* to throw out, display) a making a show, displaying] **1** The tossing, restless, to-and-fro movements of a delirious subject. **2** Any irregular jerking, twitching, and repetitive movements of the trunk and limbs, such as the movements of focal motor epilepsy. Also called *jactatio, jactation*.

periodic jactitation   CHOREA.

jaculiferous   Bearing sharp spines or prickles.

Jadassohn [Josef *Jadassohn*, German dermatologist, 1863–1936] **1** Jadassohn-Lewandowsky syndrome. See under PACHYONYCHIA CONGENITA. **2** Jadassohn-Lewandowsky syndrome. See under PALMOPLANTAR KERATODERMA. **3** Sebaceous nevus of Jadassohn. See under NEVUS. **4** Jadassohn's macular atrophy. See under ATROPHY. **5** Franceschetti-Jadassohn syndrome. See under NAEGELI SYNDROME. **6** Jadassohn's test. See under IRRIGATION TEST.

Jadelot [Jean François Nicolas *Jadelot*, French physician, 1791–1830] Jadelot lines. See under LINE.

Jaeger [Eduard *Jaeger* von Jaxtthal, Austrian oculist, 1818–1884] See under TYPE.

Jaesche [George Emanuel *Jaesche*, German surgeon, born 1815] Arlt-Jaesche operation. See under OPERATION.

Jaffe [Henry Lewis *Jaffe*, U.S. pathologist, born 1907] Jaffe's disease, Jaffe-Lichtenstein disease, Jaffe-Lichtenstein syndrome. See under FIBROUS DYSPLASIA.

Jaffé [Max *Jaffé*, Russian physician, 1841–1911] Jaffé reaction. See under TEST.

jag / naphtha jag   Intoxication from inhaling any of various organic solvents. The acute response consists of a brief euphoria, excitement and giddiness, followed by central nervous system depression.

jagziekte [Afrikaans *jagsiekte* (from *jag(en)* to drive, hunt, hurry + *siekte* disease) an infectious disease of sheep] PULMONARY ADENOMATOSIS OF SHEEP.

Jakob [Alfons *Jakob*, German physician, 1884–1931] Jakob-Creutzfeldt disease, Jakob's disease, Jakob spastic pseudosclerosis, Creutzfeldt-Jakob presenile encephalopathy, Creutzfeldt-Jakob syndrome. See under CREUTZFELDT-JAKOB DISEASE.

Jaksch   See under VON JAKSCH.

Jalaguier [Adolphe *Jalaguier*, French surgeon, 1853–1924] Battle-Jalaguier-Kammerer incision. See under BATTLE'S INCISION.

jalap [Spanish *jalapa*, from *Jalapa* or *Xalapa*, a town in Mexico named from Mayan *xalapa* the sand beside the water] The resinous material present in the dried roots of *Exogonium purga* and various *Ipomocu* species. The powdered material or a tincture derived from the resin have been used as a cathartic. Also called *jalap resin*.

Tampico jalap   The root of *Ipomoea simulans*, containing a resin like that from jalap. The resin has been used as a purgative.

wild jalap   IPOMOEA.

jalapa   IPOMOEA.

jamais vu [French *jamais* never + *vu*, past part. of *voir* to see] A form of paramnesia consisting of a powerful sense of unreality or depersonalization and a feeling that one has never before seen what is being perceived, even though the visual experience, as of a domestic scene, is one that ought to be familiar to the subject. It often occurs as a manifestation of temporal lobe epilepsy, but sometimes in states of emotional disturbance or anxiety (the phobic anxiety-depersonalization syndrome) in which the patient feels curiously detached from his environment as if in a dream or unreal world. Hence this is sometimes an epileptic illusion which, if prolonged, gives a so-called epileptic dreamy state.

jambul   The bark and seeds of *Syzygium jambolana*. Along with the fruit of the plant, it is used as an antidiarrheal, deriving its effectiveness from its volatile oils, resins, and tannin.

James [G. C. W. *James*, U.S. physician, flourished 20th century]

Swyer-James-Macleod syndrome, Swyer-James syndrome. See under MACLEOD SYNDROME.

James [T. N. *James*, U.S. cardiologist and physiologist, born 1925] See under FIBER.

James [William *James*, U.S. psychologist and philosopher, 1842–1910] James-Lange-Sutherland theory. See under JAMES-LANGE THEORY.

Jampel [Robert Steven *Jampel*, U.S. ophthalmologist, born 1926] Schwartz-Jampel syndrome. See under CHONDRODYSTROPHIC MYOTONIA.

Janet [Pierre Marie Felix *Janet*, French psychologist and neurologist, 1859–1947] **1** Janet's disease. See under PSYCHASTHENIA. **2** See under TEST, PSYCHOLOGY.

Janeway [Edward Gamaliel *Janeway*, U.S. physician, 1841–1911] Janeway spots. See under JANEWAY LESIONS.

janiceps [after *Jan(us)* a two-faced Roman god + *i* + L *-ceps*, combining form from *caput* head] Equal conjoined twins united at the head, with two faces oriented in different directions. Also called *heteroprosopus, janus*.

janiceps asymmetros   JANICEPS ASYMMETRUS.

janiceps asymmetrus   Janiceps with one of the two faces imperfectly formed. Also called *syncephalus asymmetros, iniops, janiceps asymmetros, janus asymmetros*.

janiceps parasiticus   Unequal conjoined twins in which the parasitic member consists primarily of a head with recognizable facial features.

Janin [Joseph *Janin*, French physician, born 1864] Janin's tetanus. See under CEPHALIC TETANUS.

Jansen [Albert *Jansen*, German otologist, 1859–1933] See under FORCEPS, OPERATION.

Jansen [Murk *Jansen*, Dutch orthopedic surgeon, 1867–1935] See under TEST, DISEASE.

Jansky [Jan *Jansky*, Czech physician, 1873–1921] **1** Bielschowsky-Jansky disease. See under BIELSCHOWSKY-DOLLINGER SYNDROME. **2** See under CLASSIFICATION. **3** Jansky-Bielschowsky disease. See under DISEASE.

Janthinosoma [L *ianthinus* (from Gk *ianthinos* violet-colored, from *ion* the violet + *anthos* a bud, sprout, flower, bloom) violet-colored + Gk *sōma* the body] A genus of mosquitoes, considered by some workers to be a subgenus of *Psorophora*. Some species are used by the common botfly, *Dermatobia hominis*, for egg transport. The fly captures the mosquito, adheres its eggs to the body or legs, and allows the mosquito to transport the eggs, which hatch on contact, to a human or animal host. Examples include *J. lutzi* and *J. posticata* in tropical South America.

janus [See JANICEPS.]   JANICEPS.

janus asymmetros   JANICEPS ASYMMETRUS.

jar¹ [French *jarre* a large stoneware vessel for holding liquids, from Old Provençal *jarra* jar, from Arabic *jarrah* an earthen water vessel] A vessel with a wide mouth, usually of glass or earthenware.

anaerobic jar   A closed container with a device for eliminating molecular oxygen. It is used for incubating plates inoculated with anaerobic bacteria.

bell jar   A bell-shaped enclosure that is usually made of glass and is placed over or around a substance or device. It is used most often in procedures that involve gases or vacuums.

candle jar   A convenient means of providing an atmosphere of elevated carbon dioxide content when required for the growth of certain bacteria: a candle is lit in a jar containing the inoculated plates, the jar is sealed, and the candle extinguishes itself when part of the oxygen present is converted to carbon dioxide.

Coplin jar   A wide-mouthed glass container with a rectangular internal cross-section and vertically oriented grooves on two sides. It is used to immerse microscope slides in staining solutions.

Leyden jar A glass vessel with metal foil on the inner and outer surfaces of its lower portion. It was once used as a capacitor in early work with electricity.

jar² [onomatopoeic] A jolt or wrenching movement.

heel jar A sudden jolting of the heels to the ground, which will produce pain in cases of tuberculosis of the spine, other infective conditions of the spinal column, or a protrusion of an intervertebral disk.

jararaca [Brazilian Portuguese, from the Tupi and Guarani] The venomous snake *Bothrops jararaca.*

Jarcho [Julius *Jarcho*, U.S. obstetrician, 1882–1963] See under PRESSOMETER.

jargon [Middle English *jargoun*, from Middle French *jargon* (of imitative origin) a chattering, as of birds] In aphasia, the combination of syllables or segments of speech into fluent but meaningless gibberish.

organ jargon The symbolic meaning of somatoform symptoms.

jargonagraphia JARGON AGRAPHIA.

jargonaphasia JARGON APHASIA.

jargonapraxia [*jargon* + APRAXIA] A type of apraxia in which aimless and inappropriate movements are made. A seldom used term.

jargonomimia [*jargon* + Gk *min(os)* imitator, mime + -IA] An attempt to express meaning by clownlike or inappropriate gestures. A seldom used term.

jargonorrhea [JARGON + *o* + -RRHEA] JARGON APHASIA.

Jarisch [Adolf *Jarisch*, Austrian dermatologist, 1850–1902] **1** Jarisch-Herxheimer reaction. See under HERXHEIMER REACTION. **2** Bezold-Jarisch effect, Bezold-Jarisch reflex. See under BEZOLD REFLEX.

Jarjavay [Jean François *Jarjavay*, French physician, 1815–1868] **1** Jarjavay's ligaments. See under LIGAMENT. **2** See under MUSCLE.

Jarvik [Robert Koffler *Jarvik*, U.S. biomedical engineer and physician, born 1946] Jarvik heart. See under ARTIFICIAL HEART.

Jarvis [William Chapman *Jarvis*, U.S. laryngologist, 1855–1895] See under OPERATION, SNARE.

jaundice [Middle English *jaundis*, from Old French *jaunisse* jaundice, from *jaune* yellow, from L *galbinus* greenish yellow] Yellow discoloration of the skin and mucous membranes resulting from hyperbilirubinemia and subsequent deposition of bile pigment in the involved structure. Also called *icterus.*

acholuric jaundice HEMOLYTIC JAUNDICE.

acholuric familial jaundice An obsolete term for HEREDITARY SPHEROCYTOSIS.

acute febrile jaundice CATARRHAL JAUNDICE.

acute infectious jaundice CATARRHAL JAUNDICE.

anhepatic jaundice ANHEPATOGENOUS JAUNDICE.

anhepatogenous jaundice Jaundice that is not due to impaired liver function. Also called *anhepatic jaundice.*

black jaundice WINCKEL'S DISEASE.

breast-milk jaundice Severe hyperbilirubinemia due to raised concentration of unconjugated bilirubin in nursing infants two to four weeks postpartum. The cause appears to be a steroidal agent in breast milk that interferes with the action of hepatic glucuronyl transferase in the infant.

Budd's jaundice An obsolete term for MALIGNANT JAUNDICE.

catarrhal jaundice Hepatitis of infectious origin. An outmoded term. Also called *febrile jaundice, acute febrile jaundice, acute infectious jaundice.*

cholestatic jaundice Jaundice due to a reduction in bile flow, either because of hepatocyte necrosis with reduction of all liver cell functions, or because of interference with the excretory function of the liver cell only, with preservation of other functions.

chronic intermittent juvenile jaundice A rarely used term for GILBERT SYNDROME.

congenital hemolytic jaundice HEREDITARY SPHEROCYTOSIS.

congenital nonhemolytic jaundice **1** Any condition in which neonatal jaundice occurs in the absence of hemolysis. **2** CRIGLER-NAJJAR SYNDROME.

congenital obliterative jaundice Obstructive jaundice of the newborn associated with the absence or nonpatency of the hepatic bile duct system. It is uncertain whether the condition is genetic or caused by intrauterine infection.

constitutional jaundice GILBERT SYNDROME.

Crigler-Najjar jaundice CRIGLER-NAJJAR SYNDROME.

epidemic catarrhal jaundice An outmoded term for HEPATITIS A.

familial acholuric jaundice An obsolete term for HEREDITARY SPHEROCYTOSIS.

febrile jaundice CATARRHAL JAUNDICE.

hematohepatogenous jaundice Jaundice that is due to both hemolysis and impaired liver function, as in malaria. A rarely used term.

hemolytic jaundice Jaundice due to increased destruction of erythrocytes and characterized by the absence of bilirubin in the urine and increase in the indirect-reacting bilirubin concentration in blood. Also called *acholuric jaundice, Gubler's icterus* (obsolete).

hemorrhagic jaundice ICTERIC LEPTOSPIROSIS.

hepatic jaundice HEPATOGENOUS JAUNDICE.

hepatocanalicular jaundice HEPATOCELLULAR JAUNDICE.

hepatocellular jaundice Jaundice resulting from intrinsic disease of the liver cells rather than hemolysis or obstruction of the biliary drainage system. Also called *parenchymatous jaundice, intralobular jaundice* (rarely used), *hepatocanalicular jaundice.*

hepatogenic jaundice HEPATOGENOUS JAUNDICE.

hepatogenous jaundice Jaundice due to the inability of hepatocytes to conjugate and/or to secrete a bilirubin load. This condition may be the result of a congenital abnormality of bilirubin secretion or an acquired hepatic parenchymal or intrahepatic biliary tract lesion. Also called *hepatogenic jaundice, hepatic jaundice.*

homologous serum jaundice HEPATITIS B.

human serum jaundice HEPATITIS B.

infectious jaundice Viral or leptospiral hepatitis. An ambiguous term. Also called *infective jaundice.*

infective jaundice INFECTIOUS JAUNDICE.

intralobular jaundice A rarely used term for HEPATOCELLULAR JAUNDICE.

latent jaundice Hyperbilirubinemia without visible yellow staining of skin or mucous membranes. Also called *occult jaundice.*

leptospiral jaundice ICTERIC LEPTOSPIROSIS.

malignant jaundice Jaundice associated with the fulminant form of acute viral hepatitis. A rarely used term. Also called *Budd's jaundice* (obsolete).

malignant jaundice of dogs CANINE BABESIOSIS.

mechanical jaundice OBSTRUCTIVE JAUNDICE.

medical jaundice Jaundice due to hepatocyte dysfunction and not amenable to surgical therapy.

jaundice of the newborn **1** PHYSIOLOGIC JAUNDICE. **2** ICTERUS NEONATORUM.

nonhemolytic jaundice Jaundice due to liver disease rather than hemolysis.

nonobstructive jaundice Jaundice that is due to any cause other than stoppage of the flow of bile from the liver to the small intestine.

nuclear jaundice KERNICTERUS.

obstructive jaundice Jaundice due to anatomic obstruction of the biliary drainage system at any level. Also called *mechanical jaundice*.

occult jaundice LATENT JAUNDICE.

parenchymatous jaundice HEPATOCELLULAR JAUNDICE.

physiologic jaundice The mild jaundice common in newborn infants from the second or third day and which usually disappears within a week. The main cause is the low activity of the liver enzyme glucuronyl transferase at birth. Thus, bilirubin released by red cell breakdown is only slowly changed to a conjugated form which enables it to be excreted. Also called *icterus neonatorum, physiologic icterus, jaundice of the newborn, Ritter's disease*.

picric acid jaundice Local yellow discoloration of the skin, simulating jaundice, which may occur following ingestion or inhalation of picric acid dust.

pleiochromic jaundice POSTARSPHENAMINE JAUNDICE.

polychromic jaundice POSTARSPHENAMINE JAUNDICE.

postarsphenamine jaundice Jaundice following the administration of arsphenamine. Also called *pleiochromic jaundice, polychromic jaundice*.

prehepatic jaundice Jaundice resulting from an overproduction of bile pigments, especially by hemolysis, in the absence of disease of the liver or biliary drainage system.

regurgitation jaundice Jaundice due to reflux of conjugated bilirubin from the bile canuliculi into the blood with resulting high levels of urinary urobilinogen. Also called *resorptive jaundice*.

relapsing epidemic jaundice An outmoded term for CHRONIC ACTIVE HEPATITIS.

resorptive jaundice REGURGITATION JAUNDICE.

retention jaundice Jaundice resulting from production of bilirubin in excess of the liver's ability to excrete it, as from hemolysis.

spirochetal jaundice ICTERIC LEPTOSPIROSIS.

Sumatra jaundice A leptospiral liver infection endemic in Sumatra and caused by *Leptospira interrogans* serovar *pyrogenes*.

surgical jaundice Jaundice due to an obstruction of the biliary tract which can be treated by surgical intervention, such as a gallstone in the common bile duct.

syringe jaundice SERUM HEPATITIS.

toxemic jaundice TOXIC JAUNDICE.

toxic jaundice Jaundice due to acute or chronic exposure to toxic chemical agents. Also called *toxemic jaundice*.

transfusion jaundice SERUM HEPATITIS.

urobilin jaundice Jaundice caused by the presence of urobilin in the blood.

xanthochromic jaundice Jaundice accompanied by yellowish discoloration of palms, soles, and sclerae without bile pigment in urine, as in chronic hemolytic jaundice. A rarely used term.

jaw [Middle English *jowe, jawe*; spelling perhaps influenced by Middle French *joue* cheek] Either of two bony or cartilaginous structures of the face supporting the teeth and forming the framework of the mouth in most vertebrates. In humans, they are entirely bony in adults and used in opening and closing the mouth, chewing, and adjusting the size and shape of the oral cavity for speech. The upper jaw comprises the two maxillae, and the lower jaw, the mandible. • The term is commonly used for the mouth region.

bird-beak jaw A facial deformity produced by forward pro-

trusion of the upper jaw and teeth.

cleft jaw A midline cleft or hypoplastic groove involving the chin or the entire lower jaw. The mandible is variably affected, from minimal notching to complete separation at the midline.

crackling jaw Crepitus arising from a diseased meniscus of the temporomandibular joint when the jaw is opened or closed. Also called *snapping jaw*.

Hapsburg jaw 1 MANDIBULAR PROGNATHISM. 2 A prominence of the jaw that is transmitted as an autosomal dominant trait, as seen in the Hapsburg royal house of Europe.

inferior jaw MANDIBULA.

lock jaw See under LOCKJAW.

locked jaw TRISMUS.

lower jaw MANDIBULA.

lumpy jaw See under ACTINOMYCOSIS.

parrot jaw A facial deformity produced by the forward projection of the incisor teeth.

phossy jaw A condition caused by chronic yellow phosphorous poisoning and characterized by periostitis with suppuration, ulceration, necrosis, and severe deformity of the mandible. It is a most distressing disease because it is painful and accompanied by a foul, fetid discharge which makes its victim unendurable to others. It occurred among workers making matches before the use of yellow phosphorous was prohibited, and the condition is now mainly of historical interest. Also called *phosphonecrosis, phosphorus necrosis, mandibular necrosis*.

snapping jaw CRACKLING JAW.

upper jaw MAXILLA.

jawbone 1 MANDIBULA. 2 A bone of the upper or lower jaw, usually the mandible. Also *jaw bone*.

jaw chattering Repetitive clonic contraction or spasm of the masseters occurring as a tic or in a rigor.

jaw-limb In tonic torsion of the head to one side, the arm or forelimb toward which the jaw is rotated.

Jaworski [Walery *Jaworski*, Polish physician, 1849–1924] 1 Jaworski bodies. See under BODY. 2 Jaworski's corpuscles. See under CORPUSCLE.

jaw winking MARCUS GUNN SYNDROME.

Jeanselme [Edouard *Jeanselme*, French dermatologist, 1858–1935] Jeanselme's nodules. See under LUTZ-JEANSELME NODULES.

jecorize [L *jecur*, gen. *jecoris*, the liver + -IZE] To give a food the same antirachitic properties as cod liver oil by increasing its vitamin D content. This is often done by exposing it to ultraviolet light, as in the case of milk.

jecur An obsolete term for HEPAR.

Jefferson [Sir Geoffrey *Jefferson*, English neurosurgeon, born 1886] 1 See under SYNDROME. 2 Jefferson syndrome. See under INFRACLINOID SYNDROME.

Jeffersonia A small disjunct genus of herbs of the Berberidaceae family, found in Asia and North America. *J. diphylla*, American twinleaf, has roots which are used as a stimulant and a tonic.

Jeghers [Harold *Jeghers*, U.S. physician, born 1904] Peutz-Jeghers syndrome. See under SYNDROME.

jejunal Pertaining to the jejunum.

jejunectomy [*jejun(o)-* + -ECTOMY] A surgical procedure in which the proximal part of the small intestine is resected, usually in association with a reanastomosis.

jejunitis [*jejun(o)-* + -ITIS] An inflammatory process involving the jejunum.

jejuno- [L *jejunus* empty, hungry] A combining form denoting the jejunum.

jejunocecostomy A surgical procedure creating an opening between the proximal part of the small bowel and the cecum after a bypass or resection of the intervening bowel. Such an opening may rarely occur spontaneously following trauma or inflammatory or neoplastic disease.

jejunocolostomy A surgical procedure creating an opening between the proximal small intestine and the large intestine following a resection or bypass. Such an opening may rarely result from trauma or inflammatory or neoplastic disease.

jejunogastric Relating to the jejunum and the stomach; gastrojenunal.

jejunoileitis An inflammatory process involving both the jejunum and the ileum.

jejunoileostomy A surgical procedure that creates an opening between the proximal and distal parts of the small bowel following a resection or bypass of the intervening bowel. Such an opening may rarely result spontaneously from traumatic, neoplastic, or inflammatory causes.

jejunoileum The jejunum and ileum considered as a unit.

jejunojejunostomy A surgical procedure to create an opening between two loops of the proximal small bowel following resection or bypass. Such an opening may rarely result spontaneously from traumatic, neoplastic, or inflammatory causes.

jejunoplasty [JEJUNO- + -PLASTY] A surgical procedure in which the proximal part of the small bowel is repaired or plicated.

jejunorrhaphy [JEJUNO- + -RRHAPHY] A surgical procedure in which the proximal part of the small bowel is sutured.

jejunostomy [JEJUNO- + -STOMY] A surgical procedure creating an opening in the proximal part of the small bowel that communicates with the skin. Such an opening may rarely result from traumatic, neoplastic, or inflammatory causes. Also called *nesteostomy, nestiostomy.*

jejunotomy [JEJUNO- + -TOMY] A surgical procedure in which an incision is made into the proximal part of the small bowel.

jejunum [L *(intestinum) jejunum* empty intestine, a translation of Gk *nēstis* fasting, empty, from the belief that this portion of the intestine was always found empty after death] [NA] The proximal two-fifths of the small intestine, extending from the duodenojejunal flexure to its junction with the ileum, and arranged in coils or loops suspended from the posterior abdominal wall by the mesentery. Typically, it has larger villi and is thicker and more vascular than the ileum. Also called *intestinum jejunum* (outmoded), *empty intestine.*

Jelks [John Lemuel *Jelks*, U.S. surgeon, 1870–1945] See under OPERATION.

Jellinek [Stefan *Jellinek*, Austrian physician, born 1871] Jellinek symptom. See under SIGN.

jelly [French *gelée* (past part. of *geler* to freeze into ice, from L *gelare* to freeze) jelly, frost] A semisolid, colloidal gelatinous substance that is often clear or nearly translucent.

cardiac jelly A gelatinous material, probably of mucopolysaccharide nature, occupying the space between endocardium and myocardium in the early embryonic heart tube. It is thought to be responsible for preventing regurgitation of blood before identifiable valves are present. Subsequently, it accumulates as subendocardial cushions in restricted parts of the heart such as the atrioventricular canal and the truncus arteriosus and eventually is invaded by fibrous connective tissue to contribute to definitive cardiac valves and septa. Elsewhere it disappears in step with the differentiation of the muscle fibers.

contraceptive jelly A spermicidal medication of jellylike consistency used alone or in conjunction with a mechanical barrier as a means of preventing sperm from reaching an ovum. Similar preparations are formulated as medicated creams and foams.

electrode jelly Jelly used in electrocardiography, electroen-

cephalography, and surface electromyography to improve contact between the electrode and the skin.

enamel jelly STELLATE RETICULUM.

interlaminar jelly A jellylike substance appearing between the embryonic ectoderm and endoderm. It is said to aid movements of developing mesoderm.

mineral jelly PETROLATUM.

petroleum jelly PETROLATUM.

royal jelly A highly nutritious substance produced by the pharyngeal glands of worker bees, which when fed to a female bee larva results in her development into a queen.

Wharton's jelly Mucous tissue peculiar to the umbilical cord. It has few fibers but is rich in mucoid (mucopolysaccharide) jelly and differentiates from the primitive extraembryonic mesenchyme included in the cord at the time of its formation. It is the only part that remains of the primitive extraembryonic mesenchyme itself representing the magma rectulare of the blastocoel.

jellyfish 1 A planktonic, mushroom-shaped medusa stage of scyphozoan coelenerates, having gastric filaments and marginal tentacles. 2 A free-swimming or floating hydrozoan that is often implicated in stings suffered by swimmers. A popular usage.

Jena Nomina Anatomica A revision of the 1933 Birmingham Revision (BR) of the Basle Nomina Anatomica (1895), prepared and adopted by German anatomists at Jena in 1936 and now superseded by several revisions of Nomina Anatomica.

Jendrassik [Ernö *Jendrassik*, Hungarian physician, 1858–1936] See under MANEUVER.

Jenner [Edward *Jenner*, English physician, 1749–1823] 1 Jennerian vaccination. See under VACCINATION. 2 Jennerian vaccine. See under SMALLPOX VACCINE.

Jenner [Sir William *Jenner*, English physician, 1815–1898] Jenner's emphysema. See under SENILE EMPHYSEMA.

jennerian [after Edward *Jenner*, English physician, 1749–1823] Pertaining to the smallpox vaccine or vaccination developed by Edward Jenner.

jennerization [after Edward *Jenner*, English physician, 1749–1823 + -iz(e) + -ATION] The induction of immunity to a disease by vaccination with the attenuated form of the virus producing the disease. An obsolete term.

Jensen [B. Norman *Jensen*, Danish biochemist, flourished early 20th century] Hagedorn and Jensen method. See under METHOD.

Jensen [Carl Oluf *Jensen*, Danish veterinarian and pathologist, 1864–1934] See under TUMOR.

Jensen [Edmund *Jensen*, Danish ophthalmologist, 1861–1950] See under CHOROIDITIS, DISEASE, RETINITIS.

Jensen [Sigurd Orla *Jensen*, Danish bacteriologist, born 1870] Löwenstein-Jensen agar, Löwenstein-Jensen medium. See under AGAR.

jerk A momentary, involuntary movement, usually of an extremity or the head.

Achilles jerk ACHILLES TENDON REFLEX.

ankle jerk ACHILLES TENDON REFLEX.

biceps jerk BICEPS REFLEX.

crossed adductor knee jerk Adduction of the thigh in response to elicitation of the patellar reflex in the contralateral limb.

crossed knee jerk Contraction of the quadriceps in response to tapping the patellar tendon on the contralateral leg.

elbow jerk TRICEPS REFLEX.

epileptic jerk INFANTILE MASSIVE SPASM.

finger jerk HOFFMAN'S REFLEX.

jaw jerk Brisk contraction of the muscles of mastication when the chin of the partially opened and lax jaw is tapped. It is mediated by the trigeminal nerve. Also called *jaw reflex, mandibular reflex, jaw jerk reflex, chin reflex, chin-jerk reflex*.

knee jerk   PATELLAR REFLEX.

massive myoclonic jerk   INFANTILE MASSIVE SPASM.

myoclonic jerk   MYOCLONUS.

nystagmoid jerks   Transient, lateral, jerking movements of the eyes, which are not sustained and may be seen on extreme lateral gaze. They are neither as regular nor as repetitive as true nystagmus and are of no pathologic significance. Also called *deviational nystagmus, end-point nystagmus, end-position nystagmus.*

pendular knee jerk   The type of knee jerk seen in patients with chorea in which there is hypotonia and impaired inhibition in that the leg swings backwards and forwards several times like a pendulum after a single blow on the patellar tendon. Also called *pendulousness of the legs test.*

quadriceps jerk   PATELLAR REFLEX.

supinator jerk   BRACHIORADIALIS REFLEX.

tendon jerk   TENDON REFLEX.

triceps surae jerk   ACHILLES TENDON REFLEX.

Jervell [Anton *Jervell*, Norwegian cardiologist, born 1901]   Jervell and Lange-Nielsen syndrome. See under SYNDROME.

Jesionek [Albert *Jesionek*, German dermatologist, 1870–1935]   See under LAMP.

Jeune [Mathis *Jeune*, French pediatrician, born 1910]   Jeune syndrome. See under ASPHYXIATING THORACIC DYSTROPHY.

Jewett [Eugene Lyon *Jewett*, U.S. surgeon, born 1900]   See under OPERATION, NAIL.

jhin jhinia   A hysterical mimicking of organic disease described as occurring in epidemic form in India.

jigger   CHIGOE.

jitter   Small, rapid irregularities in echo location on an ultrasound display due to electronic noise, mechanical disturbances, and other variables.

JNA   Jena Nomina Anatomica.

Jobert de Lamballe [Antoine Joseph *Jobert de Lamballe*, French surgeon, 1799–1867]   **1** See under SUTURE.   **2** Jobert's fossa. See under FOSSA.

Jobling [James Wesley *Jobling*, U.S. pathologist, 1876–1961]   Flexner-Jobling carcinosarcoma. See under CARCINOSARCOMA.

Jod-Basedow [German *Jod* iodine + Karl Adolph von *Basedow*, German physician, 1799–1854]   IODINE-INDUCED HYPERTHYROIDISM.

Joest [Ernst *Joest*, German veterinary pathologist, 1873–1926]   Joest's bodies. See under BODY.

Joffroy [Alex *Joffroy*, French physician, 1844–1908]   See under SIGN, REFLEX.

jogging   Slow or moderately paced running, often done on a regular basis as an exercise for cardiovascular or general fitness.

Johansson [Sven Christian *Johansson*, Swedish surgeon, born 1880]   Sinding-Larsen-Johansson disease. See under LARSEN-JOHANSSON DISEASE.

Johne [Heinrich Albert *Johne*, German veterinarian, 1839–1910]   **1** Johne's disease. See under PARATUBERCULOSIS.   **2** Johne's bacillus. See under *MYCOBACTERIUM PARATUBERCULOSIS*.

johnin   A substance prepared from cultures of *Mycobacterium paratuberculosis*, and used in the skin test for detecting paratuberculosis (Johne's disease) in cattle. Also called *paratuberculin*.

Johnson [Frank B. *Johnson*, U.S. pathologist, born 1919]   Dubin-Johnson syndrome. See under SYNDROME.

Johnson [Frank Chambliss *Johnson*, U.S. pediatrician, 1894–1934]   Johnson-Stevens disease, Stevens-Johnson disease. See under STEVENS-JOHNSON SYNDROME.

Johnson [Treat Baldwin *Johnson*, U.S. chemist, 1875–1947]   Wheeler and Johnson test. See under TEST.

joint

joint [Old French *joint* (from L *junct(us)*, past part. of *jungere* to join, unite) a joining of two things]   ARTICULATIO.

acromioclavicular joint   ARTICULATIO ACROMIOCLAVICULARIS.

amphidiarthrodial joint   AMPHIDIARTHROSIS.

ankle joint   ARTICULATIO TALOCRURALIS.

anterior talocalcanean joint   ARTICULATIO TALOCALCANEONAVICULARIS.

arthrodial joint   ARTICULATIO PLANA.

arycorniculate joint   The cartilaginous, sometimes synovial, joint between the apex of each arytenoid cartilage and the corresponding corniculate cartilage.

atlantoaxial joint   Either articulatio atlantoaxialis lateralis or articulatio atlantoaxialis mediana.

atlanto-occipital joint   ARTICULATIO ATLANTO-OCCIPITALIS.

ball-and-socket joint   ARTICULATIO SPHEROIDEA.

biaxial joint   A variety of joint that permits totally independent movements around two axes at right angles to each other and possesses two degrees of freedom, such as condyloid and saddle-shaped joints.

bilocular joint   A variety of synovial joint in which the intra-articular disk divides the joint into two distinct cavities, such as the temporomandibular joint.

bleeders' joint   Repeated hemorrhages into a joint of a person with a disorder of the blood clotting system, such as hemophilia.

Brodie's joint   HYSTERIC JOINT.

Budin's joint   SYNCHONDROSIS INTRAOCCIPITALIS POSTERIOR.

calcaneocuboid joint   ARTICULATIO CALCANEOCUBOIDEA.

capitular joint   ARTICULATIO CAPITIS COSTAE.

carpometacarpal joints   ARTICULATIONES CARPOMETACARPALES.

cartilaginous joint   ARTICULATIO CARTILAGINEA.

Charcot's joint   NEUROGENIC ARTHROPATHY.

Chopart's joint   ARTICULATIO TARSI TRANSVERSA.

Clutton's joint   Painless joint effusions seen in congenital syphilis.

coccygeal joint   ARTICULATIO SACROCOCCYGEA.

cochlear joint   A variety of hinge joint that also allows some rotation or lateral deviation because the cylindrical axis of the condyle tends to be spiral in section rather than a simple arc of a circle. Also called *spiral joint, screw joint, cochlear articulation, screw articulation* (rarely used).

coffin joint   The third phalangeal joint within the hoof of the horse.

composite joint   ARTICULATIO COMPOSITA.

compound joint   ARTICULATIO COMPOSITA.

condylar joint   ARTICULATIO BICONDYLARIS.

condyloid joint   An imprecise term for ARTICULATIO BICONDYLARIS.

coracoclavicular joint   An occasional joint formed between the medial end of the horizontal part of the coracoid process and the lateral end of the groove for the subclavius muscle on the inferior surface of the clavicle. Often there is a bursa between these bony parts, which are joined by the conoid and trapezoid ligaments, and occasionally these bony parts are closely apposed and covered with synovial cartilage, forming a joint.

costochondral joints ARTICULATIONES COSTOCHONDRALES.

costotransverse joint ARTICULATIO COSTOTRANSVERSARIA.

costovertebral joints ARTICULATIONES COSTOVERTE-BRALES.

cotyloid joint Either articulatio spheroidea or articulatio coxae. The latter use is outmoded.

cricoarytenoid joint ARTICULATIO CRICOARYTENOIDEA.

cricothyroid joint ARTICULATIO CRICOTHYROIDEA.

Cruveilhier's joint 1 ARTICULATIO ATLANTOAXIALIS MEDIANA. 2 ARTICULATIO ATLANTO-OCCIPITALIS.

cubital joint ARTICULATIO CUBITI.

cuboideonavicular joint A fibrous joint connecting the navicular and cuboid bones by dorsal, plantar, and interosseous ligaments, the movements being limited to gliding.

cuneocuboid joint ARTICULATIO CUNEOCUBOIDEA.

cuneometatarsal joints ARTICULATIONES TARSOMETATARSALES.

cuneonavicular joint ARTICULATIO CUNEONAVICULARIS.

diarthrodial joint ARTICULATIO SYNOVIALIS.

digital joints Articulationes interphalangeales manus and articulationes interphalangeales pedis.

dry joint 1 A joint lacking normal synovial fluid. 2 In chronic arthritis, a joint characterized predominantly by fibrosis rather than proliferative synovitis with joint effusion.

elbow joint ARTICULATIO CUBITI.

ellipsoidal joint ARTICULATIO ELLIPSOIDEA.

enarthrodial joint ARTICULATIO SPHEROIDEA.

false joint PSEUDARTHROSIS.

femoropatellar joint That portion of the knee joint in which the articular facets on the posterior surface of the patella articulate with the patellar surface of the femur, sharing the same articular cavity with the tibiofemoral portion. Also called *patellofemoral articulation, articulatio femoropatellaris (used of quadrupeds).*

femorotibial joint That portion of the knee joint in which the two condyles of the femur articulate with the superior articular surface of the tibia, sharing the same articular cavity with the femoropatellar portion. Also called *articulatio femorotibialis (used of quadrupeds).*

fibrocartilaginous joint SYMPHYSIS.

fibrous joint ARTICULATIO FIBROSA.

flail joint A joint in which there is pathological mobility and instability that is caused by a loss of motor power in the surrounding muscles.

freely movable joint ARTICULATIO SYNOVIALIS.

ginglymoid joint GINGLYMUS.

glenohumeral joint An outmoded term for ARTICULATIO HUMERI.

gliding joint ARTICULATIO PLANA.

hemophilic joint Painful hemarthrosis progressing to degenerative changes and limited motion, characteristic of inadequately treated hemophilias.

hinge joint GINGLYMUS.

hip joint ARTICULATIO COXAE.

humeroradial joint ARTICULATIO HUMERORADIALIS.

humeroulnar joint ARTICULATIO HUMEROULNARIS.

hysteric joint Abnormal posturing of a joint caused by hysteria rather than by organic abnormality at the joint. Also called *Brodie's joint.*

immovable joint ARTICULATIO FIBROSA.

incudomalleolar joint ARTICULATIO INCUDOMALLEARIS.

incudostapedial joint ARTICULATIO INCUDOSTAPEDIA.

inferior radioulnar joint ARTICULATIO RADIOULNARIS DISTALIS.

inferior sternal joint SYNCHONDROSIS XIPHOSTERNALIS.

inferior tibiofibular joint SYNDESMOSIS TIBIOFIBULARIS.

interarticular joints ARTICULATIONES ZYGAPOPHYSIALES.

intercarpal joints ARTICULATIONES INTERCARPALES.

interchondral joints ARTICULATIONES INTERCHONDRALES.

intercoccygeal joints Symphyseal joints between the coccygeal vertebrae which are present in young people but become ossified at varying times in adult life. Occasionally the joint between the first and second coccygeal vertebrae is synovial in type.

intercuneiform joints ARTICULATIONES INTERCUNEIFORMES.

intermetacarpal joints ARTICULATIONES INTERMETACARPALES.

interphalangeal joints Either articulationes interphalangeales manus or articulationes interphalangeales pedis.

irritable joint A joint subject to repeated episodes of inflammation without discernible cause.

jaw joint ARTICULATIO TEMPOROMANDIBULARIS.

knee joint ARTICULATIO GENUS.

ligamentous joint SYNDESMOSIS.

Lisfranc's joints ARTICULATIONES TARSOMETATARSALES.

lumbosacral joint ARTICULATIO LUMBOSACRALIS.

lunate-triquetrum joint One of the intercarpal joints of the proximal row between the lunate and the triquetrum bones which are held together by dorsal, palmar, and interosseous ligaments and by a thin fibrous capsule.

joints of Luschka A series of small synovial joints between the raised bony lips on the lateral sides of the bodies of contiguous cervical vertebrae, i.e., between the lips on the lower surface of one vertebra and those on the upper surface of the subjacent vertebra. They develop in childhood at the age of about ten years. Medial to each is the intervertebral disk and laterally is a capsular ligament. Some authorities believe that they are not synovial joints but merely clefts in the intervertebral disks. See also PROCESSUS UNCINATUS OF CERVICAL VERTEBRAE.

mandibular joint ARTICULATIO TEMPOROMANDIBULARIS.

manubriosternal joint SYNCHONDROSIS MANUBRIOSTERNALIS.

mediocarpal joint ARTICULATIO MEDIOCARPALIS.

metacarpophalangeal joints ARTICULATIONES METACARPOPHALANGEALES.

metatarsophalangeal joints ARTICULATIONES METATARSOPHALANGEALES.

midcarpal joint ARTICULATIO MEDIOCARPALIS.

midcoccygeal joint The intercoccygeal symphyseal joint between the first and second coccygeal vertebrae which generally ossifies in the fourth or fifth decade of life. Occasionally it is synovial in type. An outmoded term.

midtarsal joint ARTICULATIO TARSI TRANSVERSA.

mixed joint A type of joint in which characteristics of different varieties of joints are found.

mortise joint ARTICULATIO TALOCRURALIS.

movable joint Articulatio synovialis, or, to a lesser extent, articulatio cartilaginea.

multiaxial joint ARTICULATIO SPHEROIDEA.

naviculocuneiform joint An outmoded term for ARTICULATIO CUNEONAVICULARIS.

neurocentral joint One of the cartilaginous joints which during the first two years of life connects the vertebral body to each half of the vertebral arch.

open joint A joint, especially of an equine or bovine animal, that has become open to the skin surface, usually through infection.

pastern joint The joint, especially in the horse, between a metacarpal or metatarsal bone and the first phalanx.

Pavy's joint Arthritis occurring with typhoid fever. A rarely used term.

peg-and-socket joint GOMPHOSIS.

pisotriquetral joint ARTICULATIO OSSIS PISIFORMIS.

pivot joint ARTICULATIO TROCHOIDEA.

plane joint ARTICULATIO PLANA.

polyaxial joint ARTICULATIO SPHEROIDEA.

posterior talocalcanean joint ARTICULATIO SUBTALARIS.

radiocarpal joint ARTICULATIO RADIOCARPALIS.

rotary joint ARTICULATIO TROCHOIDEA.

sacrococcygeal joint ARTICULATIO SACROCOCCYGEA.

sacroiliac joint ARTICULATIO SACROILIACA.

saddle joint ARTICULATIO SELLARIS.

saddle-shaped joint ARTICULATIO SELLARIS.

scapholunate joint One of the intercarpal joints of the proximal row between the superior articular facet on the medial surface of the scaphoid and the lateral surface of the lunate bone, which are connected by dorsal, palmar, and interosseous ligaments and by a thin fibrous capsule.

scapuloclavicular joint An outmoded term for ARTICULATIO ACROMIOCLAVICULARIS.

screw joint COCHLEAR JOINT.

sellar joint ARTICULATIO SELLARIS.

shoulder joint ARTICULATIO HUMERI.

simple joint ARTICULATIO SIMPLEX.

skin joint FLEXURE LINE.

slightly movable joint ARTICULATIO CARTILAGINEA.

slip joint A connector fitted into the proximal end of an endotracheal tube for attachment to a breathing circuit.

socket joint of tooth GOMPHOSIS.

spheno-occipital joint SYNCHONDROSIS SPHENO-OCCIPITALIS.

spheroidal joint ARTICULATIO SPHEROIDEA.

spiral joint COCHLEAR JOINT.

sternoclavicular joint ARTICULATIO STERNOCLAVICULARIS.

sternocostal joints ARTICULATIONES STERNOCOSTALES.

stifle joint In animals, especially larger animals such as horses and cattle, the joint formed by the femur, patella, and tibia. It corresponds to the human knee joint. Also called *stifle.*

subtalar joint ARTICULATIO SUBTALARIS.

superior radioulnar joint ARTICULATIO RADIOULNARIS PROXIMALIS.

superior sternal joint SYNCHONDROSIS MANUBRIOSTERNALIS.

superior tibiofibular joint ARTICULATIO TIBIOFIBULARIS.

suture joint SUTURA.

synarthrodial joint ARTICULATIO FIBROSA.

synovial joint ARTICULATIO SYNOVIALIS.

talocalcaneal joint Either the posteroinferior part of the articulatio talocalcaneonavicularis or the articulatio subtalaris.

talocalcaneonavicular joint ARTICULATIO TALOCALCANEONAVICULARIS.

talocrural joint ARTICULATIO TALOCRURALIS.

talonavicular joint The portion of the talocalcaneonavicular joint that combines with the calcaneocuboid articulation to form the transverse tarsal joint.

talotibiofibular joint ARTICULATIO TALOCRURALIS.

tarsal joints ARTICULATIONES INTERTARSEAE.

tarsometatarsal joints ARTICULATIONES TARSOMETATAR-SALES.

temporomandibular joint ARTICULATIO TEMPOROMANDIBULARIS.

thigh joint An outmoded term for ARTICULATIO COXAE.

joints of thorax ARTICULATIONES THORACIS.

through joint An outmoded term for ARTICULATIO SYNOVIALIS.

thyroepiglottic joint An outmoded term for LIGAMENTUM THYROEPIGLOTTICUM.

tibiofibular joint 1 ARTICULATIO TIBIOFIBULARIS. 2 SYNDESMOSIS TIBIOFIBULARIS.

transverse tarsal joint ARTICULATIO TARSI TRANSVERSA.

trochoid joint ARTICULATIO TROCHOIDEA.

uniaxial joint A joint in which movement of a bone is limited to rotation about one axis only, possessing one degree of freedom, as in a hinge joint.

unilocular joint A synovial joint having a single cavity, even when an articular disk may be present.

joints of the vertebral column ARTICULATIONES VERTEBRALES.

von Gies joint Chronic syphilitic arthritis.

wedge-and-groove joint SCHINDYLESIS.

wrist joint ARTICULATIO RADIOCARPALIS.

xiphisternal joint SYNCHONDROSIS XIPHOSTERNALIS.

zygapophysial joints ARTICULATIONES ZYGAPOPHYSIALES.

---

jointed Provided with or forming a joint.

joint-ill JOINT ILL.

Jolly [Friedrich *Jolly,* German neurologist, 1844–1904] 1 Jolly's reaction. See under MYASTHENIC REACTION. 2 See under SIGN.

Jolly [Justin *Jolly,* French histologist, 1870–1953] Jolly's bodies. See under HOWELL-JOLLY BODIES.

Jonas [Siegfried *Jonas,* Austrian physician, born 1874] See under SYMPTOM.

Jones See under BENCE JONES.

Jones [Hugh T. *Jones,* U.S. orthopedic surgeon, born 1892] Henderson-Jones disease. See under OSTEOCHONDROMATOSIS.

Jones [Sir Robert *Jones,* English orthopedic surgeon, 1858–1933] See under POSITION.

Jones [T. D. *Jones,* U.S. physician, 1899–1954] Jones criteria. See under CRITERION.

Jonnesco [Thoma *Jonnesco,* Rumanian physician, 1860–1926] 1 See under OPERATION, FOSSA. 2 Jonnesco's fold. See under PARIETOPERITONEAL FOLD. 3 Fossa of Jonnesco. See under RECESSUS DUODENALIS SUPERIOR.

Jordan [David Starr *Jordan,* U.S. zoologist, 1851–1931] See under RULE.

Joseph [Jacques *Joseph,* German surgeon, 1865–1934] See under CLAMP, KNIFE, OPERATION.

Joseph [Rene *Joseph,* French pediatrician, born 1907] Joseph's disease. See under ENCEPHALOPATHY WITH PROLINEMIA.

Joule [James Prescott *Joule,* English physicist, 1818–1889] See under EQUIVALENT, LAW.

joule [after James Prescott *Joule,* English physicist, 1818–1889] Special name for the SI derived unit of energy, work, or quantity of heat; the work done when the point of application of a force of one newton is displaced through a distance of one meter in the direction of the force; equal to one newton meter. It is also equal to the work done when a power of one watt is dissipated for one second; equal to one watt second. Symbol: J

joule per kilogram-second WATT PER KILOGRAM.

joule per second The SI derived unit of power, generally known by the special name watt. Symbol: J/s, J·s⁻¹

Jourdain [Anselme-Louis-Bernard-Berchillet *Jourdain,* French surgeon, 1734–1816] Jourdain's disease. See under CHRONIC PERIDONTITIS.

joystick A hand-operated lever in which fore-and-aft motion and side-to-side motion send analogous voltages to a device or computer, usually for control of motion.

J/s Symbol for the unit, joule per second.

J·s⁻¹ Symbol for the unit, joule per second.

juccuya A zoonotic infection of gerbils and marmots transmitted by *Phlebotomus papatasii* (sandfly) to man, in whom it produces a form of cutaneous leishmaniasis.

judgment / time judgment An apprehension of the duration of a stimulus or experience that is accomplished purely subjectively, without external aids such as clocks or a view of the sun's position, and without reliance on internal physiologic factors such as pulse rate or respiration.

juga Plural of JUGUM.

jugal **1** Pertaining to the zygomatic bone. **2** Uniting; yoked together.

jugale [L, neut. sing. of *jugalis* (from *jug(um)* a yoke + *-alis* -AL) yoked together] A craniometric point situated at the apex of the angle of the posterior border of the zygomatic bone. Also called *jugal point.*

jugate **1** Possessing a jugum; ridged. **2** Paired. **3** Joined together.

juglandic acid NUCIN.

juglone $C_{10}H_6O_3$. 5-hydroxy-1,4-naphthoquinone. An antibiotic substance obtained from the leaves of *Juglans* species. It has antibiotic activity against some fungi.

jugomaxillary Pertaining to the zygomatic bone and the maxilla.

jugular [Late L *jugular(is)* (from L *jugul(um)* the collarbone, neck, throat, dim. of *jugum* a yoke, collar + *-aris* -AR) pertaining to the neck or throat] **1** Pertaining to the neck or throat. **2** JUGULAR VEIN.

jugulocephalic Pertaining to the neck and the head.

jugulum [L, collarbone, neck, throat] The neck or throat.

jugum [L (root of *jungere* to join, connect, yoke, akin to Gk *zeugos* a yoke or team of horses), a yoke or collar on the necks of oxen, a team or yoke of oxen or horses] (*plural* juga) [NA] A ridge or depression connecting two structures or two points. Also called *yoke.*

juga alveolaria [NA] The eminences produced by the roots of the incisors and canines on the anterior surface of the alveolar part of the mandible and the alveolar process of the maxilla. Between them are depressions corresponding to the interalveolar septa. Also called *alveolar eminences, alveolar yokes.*

juga alveolaria maxillae [NA] Vertical furrows on the anterior surface of the maxilla between the ridges produced by the roots of the incisor teeth.

juga cerebralia ossium cranii Faint ridges corresponding to the sulci of the brain that outline the digitate impressions on the internal surface of the cranium. Also called *cerebral ridges of cranial bones, cerebral crests of cranial bones.*

jugum penis A double-bladed instrument designed to compress the penis.

jugum petrosum An outmoded term for EMINENTIA ARCUATA.

jugum sphenoidale [NA] The smooth anterior part of the cerebral surface of the body of the sphenoid bone, grooved on each side of the midline by the olfactory tracts and limited posteriorly by the anterior border of sulcus prechiasmatis, and separating the anterior cranial fossa from the sphenoidal sinus. Also called *sphenoidal yoke.*

juice [L *jus* broth, soup] **1** Any fluid of plant or animal tissues. **2** SUCCUS.

appetite juice Gastric juice secreted upon the sight or smell of food as a vagally mediated conditioned reflex.

cancer juice A yellow-white fluid that can be expressed from some cancers. It is comprised of plasma, neoplastic cells, and debris, and results from liquefaction of the necrotic centers of large, rapidly growing tumors.

gastric juice The clear, colorless fluid secretion of the glands and mucosal epithelium of the stomach which contains mainly water, mucus, hydrochloric acid, and enzymes, such as pepsin, rennin, and lipase, and which functions in the digestion of food. Also called *succus gastricus, liquor gastricus.*

intestinal juice The colorless, alkaline fluid secretion of the mucosal epithelium and glands of the small intestine which contains mucus and several enzymes used in the digestion of food, including peptidases, lipase, amylase, and enzymes for breaking down disaccharides to monosaccharides. Also called *succus entericus, liquor entericus.*

pancreatic juice The clear, colorless, alkaline fluid secreted by the exocrine glands of the pancreas and discharged through the pancreatic ducts into the duodenum for digestion of food. It contains several enzymes including trypsin, chymotrypsin, carboxypeptidase, amylase, lipase, DNAase, RNAase, and phospholipase A. Also called *succus pancreaticus, liquor pancreaticus.*

jumper A person with myoclonic epilepsy.

jumping the bite **1** The forcible movement forward of a retruded mandible to obtain a normal occlusion. **2** The changing of cuspal relationships in centric occlusion, as when moving a lingually placed upper incisor buccally without disoccluding it, causing a temporary premature contact and occlusion of convenience until it is in place.

jumping Frenchmen of Maine A syndrome resembling Gilles de la Tourette syndrome. Some consider it a culture-specific syndrome, such as lata, as it was originally described in a group of inhabitants of the state of Maine who were of French Canadian descent. Also called *jumper disease of Maine.*

jumps **1** Jerking, twitching, or choreiform movements. **2** The premonitory muscular twitching and jerking which may occur in alcoholic subjects on the verge of delirium tremens. An imprecise usage.

junction [L *junctio* (from *junctus*, past part. of *jungere* to join, connect, akin to Gk *zeugos* a yoke or team of horses) a joining, connection, union] The place where two organs, structures, or parts meet; an interface. Also called *junctura.*

amelodentinal junction The interface between the enamel and dentin of a tooth. Also called *dentinoenamel junction, dentoenamel junction.*

anorectal junction The lower end of the perineal flexure at the level of the urogenital diaphragm, where the rectal ampulla narrows and continues posteriorly as the anal canal. The puborectalis muscle forms a palpable sling at the sides and back of this region, while the circular muscle coat of the rectum thickens here to form the sphincter ani internus which surrounds the anal canal. Also called *linea sinuosa analis* (outmoded). ● This term is occasionally used synonymously with *anorectal line (linea anorectalis)* and even with *pectinate line.*

cell junction Any modification of a cell surface that provides cohesion between adjacent cells.

cementodentinal junction The interface between the cementum and dentin of a tooth. Also called *dentinocemental junction.*

cementoenamel junction The boundary between the cementum and enamel of a tooth. In animals which do not have coronal cementum, it forms the cervical line demarcating the anatomical crown from the root.

cervicomedullary junction That part of the neuraxis where the cervical spinal cord becomes medulla oblongata; the zone of transition between the rostral part of the spinal cord and the caudal part of the brain stem.

choledochoduodenal junction The site, just below the middle of the descending part of the duodenum, where the bile and the main pancreatic ducts join to form the hepatopancreatic ampulla before it narrows to open on the major duodenal papilla. However, the ducts may open separately on the papilla.

dentinocemental junction CEMENTODENTINAL JUNCTION.

dentinoenamel junction   AMELODENTINAL JUNCTION.

dentoenamel junction   AMELODENTINAL JUNCTION.

dentogingival junction   The interface between a tooth and its surrounding gingiva.

dermoepidermal junction   The interdigitating interface between the epidermis and the papillary layer of the corium, or dermis, where the perpendicular papillae fit into corresponding pits on the deep surface of the epidermis. Also called *dermoepidermal interface.*

esophagogastric junction   The interface, about 2.5 cm below the diaphragm, where the abdominal part of the esophagus becomes confluent with the stomach, marked internally by an abrupt transition from the stratified squamous epithelium of the esophagus to the simple columnar epithelium of the stomach, and externally, on the left, by the cardiac notch. Internally the junction is visible as a notched line, the esophagus being smooth and pinkish-grey in comparison with the pitted, honeycomblike, red gastric mucosa.

fibromuscular junction   The site of the blending of the thick smooth muscle layer of the wall of the body of the uterus with the dense fibrous tissue of the cervix uteri.

gap junction   A type of intercellular junction which allows communication between cells by affording passage to small molecules and ions. At gap junctions the space between plasma membranes of adjacent cells is about 30 Å, and cylinders with an inside diameter of 20 Å run as a pipeline between the cytoplasm of the two cells. The cylinders are each composed of 12 protein subunits, six associated with each plasma membrane. Also called *nexus.*

intercellular junction   A junction or membrane specialization exhibited by neighboring cells in a tissue playing roles in cell-to-cell adhesion and intercellular transport. Types of intercellular junctions include tight junctions, desmosomes, gap junctions, and plasmodesmata.

intermediate junction   ZONULA ADHERENS.

intermembrane junction   ZONE OF ADHESION.

iridociliary junction   MARGO CILIARIS IRIDIS.

junction of the lips   1 COMMISSURA LABIORUM ORIS.   2 ANGULUS ORIS.

manubriogladiolar junction   An outmoded term for SYNCHONDROSIS MANUBRIOSTERNALIS.

mucocutaneous junction   The site where the skin becomes confluent with a mucous membrane, such as the lips of the mouth and the anus.

mucogingival junction   A scalloped linear boundary between the attached gingiva and the nonkeratinized lining mucosa of the sulcus. Also called *health line* (popular).

myoneural junction   MOTOR ENDPLATE.

myotendinal junction   MUSCLE-TENDON ATTACHMENT.

neuromuscular junction   MOTOR ENDPLATE.

osseous junction   ARTICULATIO.

pentilaminar junction   TIGHT JUNCTION.

rectosigmoid junction   The site of union of the lower end of the sigmoid colon with the rectum which is situated in the median plane at the level of the third sacral vertebra.

root-cord junction   The site of junction of the spinal roots with the substance of the spinal cord. Also called *cornuradicular zone.*

sclerocorneal junction   LIMBUS CORNEAE.

ST junction   J POINT.

tendinous junctions   CONNEXUS INTERTENDINEUS.

tight junction   A region where the plasma membranes of two adjacent cells are closely apposed, preventing the movement of materials between the cells. When observed by electron microscopy, the outer dark layer of the plasma membranes of the adjacent cells form a common layer. The junction may be a zone around the cell (zonula occludens) or only a point (macula

occludens). Also called *pentilaminar junction.*

tympanostapedial junction   SYNDESMOSIS TYMPANOSTAPEDIA.

ureteropelvic junction   The site at which the renal pelvis becomes continuous with the ureter, often marked by a slight constriction outside the hilum.

ureterovesical junction   The site of the oblique passage of the ureter through the wall of the urinary bladder, into which it opens by a slitlike ostium. Also called *ureterotrigonal complex.*

junctional   Pertaining to a junction.

junctura [L (from *junct(us)*, past part. of *jungere* to join, connect, akin to Gk *zeugos* a yoke or team of horses + *-ura* -URE), a joining, uniting, joint, seam]   1 [NA] JUNCTION.   2 An outmoded term for ARTICULATIO.

junctura cartilaginea   ARTICULATIO CARTILAGINEA.

juncturae cinguli membri inferioris   ARTICULATIONES CINGULI MEMBRI INFERIORIS.

juncturae cinguli membri superioris   ARTICULATIONES CINGULI MEMBRI SUPERIORIS.

junctura fibrosa   ARTICULATIO FIBROSA.

junctura lumbosacralis   ARTICULATIO LUMBOSACRALIS.

juncturae membri inferioris liberi   ARTICULATIONES MEMBRI INFERIORIS LIBERI.

juncturae membri superioris liberi   ARTICULATIONES MEMBRI SUPERIORIS LIBERI.

junctura ossium   ARTICULATIO.

juncturae ossium   Articulations; joints.

juncturae ossium cinguli extremitatis pelvinae   An outmoded term for ARTICULATIONES CINGULI MEMBRI INFERIORIS.

juncturae ossium cinguli extremitatis thoracicae   An outmoded term for ARTICULATIONES CINGULI MEMBRI SUPERIORIS.

junctura sacrococcygea   ARTICULATIO SACROCOCCYGEA.

junctura synovialis   ARTICULATIO SYNOVIALIS.

juncturae tendinum   CONNEXUS INTERTENDINEUS.

juncturae zygapophyseales   ARTICULATIONES ZYGAPOPHYSIALES.

juncturae   Plural of JUNCTURA.

Junet [Robert Maurice *Junet*, Swiss internist, born 1907]   Troell-Junet syndrome. See under SYNDROME.

Jung [Karl Gustav *Jung*, Swiss anatomist, 1793–1864]   Jung's muscle. See under MUSCULUS PYRAMIDALIS AURICULAE.

Jungbluth [Hermann *Jungbluth*, German physician, flourished 20th century]   Jungbluth's vessels, vasa propria of Jungbluth. See under VASA.

jungian [Carl Gustav *Jung*, Swiss psychologist and psychiatrist, 1875–1961]   Pertaining to the theories proposed by or associated with Carl Jung.

Jüngling [Otto *Jüngling*, German physician, 1888–1944]   See under DISEASE.

juniper   The dried, ripe fruit of the evergreen shrub *Juniperus communis* of the Coniferae family. An infusion of the berries is diuretic. Its volatile oil is used as a diuretic, urinary antiseptic, and carminative.

Junius [Paul *Junius*, German ophthalmologist, born 1871]   Kuhnt-Junius disease, Kuhnt-Junius degeneration. See under DISCIFORM MACULAR DEGENERATION.

Junker [Ferdinand Ethelbert *Junker*, English physician, flourished 1868]   Junker apparatus, Junker bottle. See under INHALER.

jurisprudence [Late L *jurisprudentia* (from L *jus*, gen. *juris*, law + *prudentia*, a foreseeing, prudence, from *prudens*, gen. *prudentis*, for *providens*, pres. part. of *providere* to look forward, make provision) jurisprudence]   The science of law, or a particular system or division of law.

dental jurisprudence 1 The philosophy, principles, doctrines, and statutes of law and justice as they apply to all aspects of dental practice. Of particular concern are issues such as malpractice, negligence, causation, and product liability and their effect upon the relationship between society and the practice of dentistry and between dental practitioners. **2** FORENSIC DENTISTRY.

medical jurisprudence 1 The philosophy, principles, doctrines, and statutes of law and justice as they apply to and govern various aspects of medical practice, particularly the relationships between patients and medical practitioners as well as the relationship of medical practitioners to each other. **2** FORENSIC MEDICINE.

jury / coroner's jury A jury that inquires into the cause and manner of sudden, unusual, unattended, or violent deaths to determine whether unlawful activity was involved in the death and, if so, to issue appropriate indictments. It is assembled at the request of a coroner. Also called *inquest jury.*

inquest jury CORONER'S JURY.

jury-mast A single bar neck brace formerly utilized to support the head in cases of spinal tuberculosis.

jusculum [L, dim. of *jus* broth, soup, liquid] A broth, soup, juice, or gravy.

Juster [Emile *Juster*, French neurologist, flourished 20th century] See under REFLEX.

justo major [L (from *justo,* ablative of *justum* what is right + *major* larger), larger than right] GIANT PELVIS.

justo minor [L (from *justo,* ablative of *justum* what is right + *minor* less, smaller), smaller than is right] PELVIS JUSTO MINOR.

juvantia [L, neut. pl. of *juvans,* pres. part. of *juvare* to help] Adjuvant substances and appliances.

juvenile [L *juvenil(is)* (from *junven(is)* young; as substantive, young man, young people + *ilis* -ILE) youthful, juvenile] **1** Of or relating to youth or to an early period of development. **2** A juvenile specimen or individual.

juxta-articular Near or adjacent to a joint.

juxtacortical Near or adjacent to the cortex of an organ or a structure.

juxtaepiphyseal Close to or adjoining an epiphysis.

juxtaglomerular Near or adjacent to a renal glomerulus.

juxtallocortex [L *juxt(a)* next to + ALLO- + CORTEX] The cerebral cortex transitional between typical allocortex and isocortex.

juxtapapillary [L *juxta* + *papill(a)* + -ARY] Adjacent to the optic disk.

juxtaposition A side by side position; apposition.

juxtapyloric Near or adjacent to the pylorus or the pyloric portion of the stomach.

juxtaspinal Near or adjacent to the vertebral column.

K

K **1** Symbol for the element, potassium. **2** Symbol for the unit, kelvin. **3** Symbol for lysine.

K. cathode.

°K Symbol for the unit, kelvin. An obsolete and incorrect symbol.

k Symbol for kilo-: used with SI units.

K Symbol for the quantities (1) bulk modulus, or modulus of compression, expressed in pascals; (2) kerma, expressed in joules per kilogram; (3) coefficient of heat transfer, expressed in watts per square meter kelvin; (4) kinetic energy, expressed in joules.

K_m Symbol for the quantity, Michaelis constant.

κ **1** Symbol for the quantity, compressibility, expressed in reciprocal pascals. **2** Symbol for the quantity, magnetic susceptibility.

kA Symbol for the unit, kiloampere.

kabure [Japanese, a rash, skin eruption] A Japanese term for SCHISTOSOME DERMATITIS.

Kader [Bronislaw *Kader*, Polish surgeon, 1863–1937] Kader's operation. See under KADER-SENN OPERATION.

Kaes [Theodor *Kaes*, German neurologist, 1852–1913] Band of Kaes-Bekhterev, Kaes feltwork, line of Kaes, layer of Kaes-Bekhterev, stripe of Kaes-Bekhterev. See under BEKHTEREV'S LAYER.

kafindo ONYALAI.

Kahlbaum [Karl Ludwig *Kahlbaum*, German physician, 1828–1899] **1** Kahlbaum syndrome, Kahlbaum's disease. See under CATATONIC STUPOR. **2** Kahlbaum-Wernicke syndrome. See under PRESBYOPHRENIA.

Kahlden [Clemens von *Kahlden*, German pathologist, 1809–1903] See under TUMOR.

Kahler [Otto *Kahler*, German physician, 1849–1893] **1** Kahler's disease. See under MYELOMA. **2** See under LAW.

Kahn [Friedel *Kahn*, German physician, flourished early 20th century] Kahn-Falta sign. See under SIGN.

Kahn [Reuben Leon *Kahn*, U.S. bacteriologist, born 1887] See under TEST.

kaino-¹ CENO-¹.

kaino-² CENO-².

kainophobia CAINOPHOBIA.

kainotophobia CAINOPHOBIA.

Kaiserling [Carl *Kaiserling*, German pathologist, 1869–1942] Kaiserling's fixative, Kaiserling solutions, Kaiserling's method. See under FLUID.

kak- CACO-.

kakergasia [KAK- + Gk *ergasia* work, occupation] MERERGASIA.

kakesthesia CACESTHESIA.

kakidrosis BROMHIDROSIS.

kakke A Japanese term for BERIBERI.

kako- CACO-.

kakodyl CACODYL.

kakosmia CACOSMIA.

kakotrophy [KAKO- + *troph(o)*- + -Y] MALNUTRITION.

kala-azar [Hindi (from *kālā* black + Persian *āzār* disease, poison, or fever), black disease, black poison, or black fever] An acute, infectious, systemic disease characterized by irregular fever of long duration, splenomegaly, hepatomegaly, hyperglobulinemia, and progressive emaciation. Leukopenia and anemia result from bone-marrow infiltration, and lymphadenopathy, malaise, and secondary infections are frequent accompaniments. If untreated, death may occur. The disease is caused by the protozoan parasite *Leishmania donovani* and transmitted by sandfly bites (*Phlebotomus* species and related genera). The organism lives and multiplies throughout the reticuloendothelial system. Kala-azar is widespread and occurs with local differences in India, Kenya, the Sudan, China, Brazil, and the USSR. Also called *visceral leishmaniasis, Assam fever, Dumdum fever, febrile tropical splenomegaly, old world leishmaniasis, black sickness*.

canine kala-azar Kala-azar occurring in dogs. It is probably identical to the human disease. The causative organisms are morphologically and serologically identical. Also called *canine leishmaniasis*.

Mediterranean kala-azar A variant of kala-azar which occurs on the Mediterranean littoral, especially in Greece and Portugal, and usually affects infants and children. It is caused by *Leishmania infantum* which is antigenically identical to *L. donovani*. Also called *infantile leishmaniasis, ponos (local Greek)*.

kalafungin An antibiotic from *Streptomyces tanashiensis* var. *kala*. It has antifungal properties.

kaliopenic Deficient in potassium.

kaliuresis KALURESIS.

Kalischer [Siegfried *Kalischer*, German physician, born 1862] Kalischer's disease, Sturge-Kalischer-Weber syndrome. See under STURGE-WEBER SYNDROME.

kallak [Eskimo, a North American Indian language] A pustular dermatitis commonly seen among Eskimos.

kallidin Either of two peptides, bradykinin and lysyl-bradykinin, released by the action of the enzyme kallikrein from a plasma protein. The 9-residue peptide bradykinin is sometimes known as kallidin-9 or kallidin I, whereas the 10-residue peptide lysyl-bradykinin is sometimes known as kallidin-10 or kallidin II.

kallikrein The enzyme (EC 3.4.21.8) that releases bradykinin or lysyl-bradykinin from the plasma protein kininogen. At least three types, characteristic of plasma, pancreas, and kidney, are physiologically important. They are proteinases with a preference for splitting on the C-terminal side of arginine and lysine residues. Also called *kininogenase*. Also *callicrein*.

kallikreinogen PREKALLIKREIN.

Kallmann [Franz Josef *Kallmann*, German-born U.S. geneticist and psychiatrist, 1897–1965] See under SYNDROME.

kalmegh The dried plant or the dried leaves and shoots of *Andrographis paniculata* (Acanthaceae), containing not less than 1% of a bitter principle, andrographolide. It has been used in Asia as a bitter in the form of a liquid extract.

kaluresis [L *kal(ium)* potassium + -URESIS] Increased urinary excretion of potassium secondary to hyperkalemia, adrenocortical hyperfunction, or administration of adrenocortical hormones or any of many diuretic agents. Also called *hyperkaluria, hyperkaluresis (redundant), kaliuresis, kaluria.*

kaluretic **1** Pertaining to or causing kaluresis. **2** Any agent or condition that increases renal excretion of potassium.

kaluria [New L *kal(ium)* (from *kal(i)* alkali, from Arabic *qali* saltwort + L -*ium*, neut. sing. noun suffix) potassium + -URIA] KALURESIS.

kamala The glands and hairs of the capsules of *Mallotus philippinensis*, the kamala tree. They are used to prepare an anthelmintic. Also called *rottlera.*

Kammerer [Frederic *Kammerer*, U.S. surgeon, 1856–1928] Battle-Jalaguier-Kammerer incision. See under BATTLE'S INCISION.

kanamycin $C_{18}H_{36}N_4O_{11}$. An antibiotic produced by *Streptomyces kanamyceticus* which is active against many Gram-positive and Gram-negative bacteria. Excessive or prolonged use may cause irreversible damage to the eighth cranial nerve. The sulfate salt has been most commonly used, but resistant organisms, hypersensitivity, and ototoxicity have limited its usefulness.

Kanavel [Allen Buckner *Kanavel*, U.S. surgeon, 1874–1938] **1** See under OPERATION, SIGN, TRIANGLE. **2** Lumbrical canals of Kanavel. See under CANAL. **3** Kanavel's cockup splint. See under SPLINT.

Kandinsky [Victor Chrisanfovic *Kandinsky*, Russian psychiatrist, 1825–1890] Clérambault-Kandinsky syndrome. See under CLÉRAMBAULT-KANDINSKY COMPLEX.

Kandori [Fumio *Kandori*, Japanese ophthalmologist, born 1904] Kandori's flock retina. See under RETINA.

kaninloma GANGOSA.

Kanner [Leo *Kanner*, Austrian-born U.S. child psychiatrist, born 1894] Kanner syndrome. See under EARLY INFANTILE AUTISM.

kansasiin A tuberculinlike preparation made from *Mycobacterium kansasii* that is used in skin tests.

Kanter [Aaron Elias *Kanter*, U.S. gynecologist, born 1893] See under SIGN.

Kantor [John Leonard *Kantor*, U.S. physician, 1890–1947] Kantor sign. See under STRING SIGN.

Kantrex A proprietary name for kanamycin.

kanyemba [native language of southern Africa] A severe necrotic inflammatory disorder of the colon and rectum seen in mountain regions of Malawi, Zambia, and South America.

kaodzera [Bantu] RHODESIAN TRYPANOSOMIASIS.

kaolin [Chinese *Kao-ling* (High Ridge), in Kiangsi province, southeast China, where kaolin was first obtained] $Al_2O_3 \cdot 2SiO_2 \cdot 2H_2O$. Hydrated aluminum silicate, found in natural deposits. It is used as an absorbent, in filters to clarify liquids, and as a constituent of dusting powders. Also called *bolus alba, terra alba.*

kaolinosis Pneumoconiosis resulting from inhalation of kaolin dust.

Kaposi [Moritz *Kaposi*, Hungarian-born Austrian dermatologist, 1837–1902] **1** Kaposi's disease, multiple hemorrhagic hemangioma of Kaposi. See under KAPOSI SARCOMA. **2** Xeroderma of Kaposi. See under XERODERMA PIGMENTOSUM. **3**

Kaposi's varicelliform eruption. See under ERUPTION.

Kappadione A proprietary name for menadiol sodium diphosphate.

kaps- CAPS-.

karakurt [*Turki*, from *kara* black + *kurt* wolf] A spider of the species *Latrodectus lugubris*, a central Asian variant of the venomous black widow.

karaya STERCULIA GUM.

Karell [Philip Jakob *Karell*, Russian physician, 1806–1886] See under DIET, TREATMENT.

Karl Fischer [*Karl Fischer*, German chemist, flourished 20th century] See under REAGENT.

Karr [Walter Gerald *Karr*, U.S. biochemist, born 1892] See under METHOD.

Kartagener [Manes *Kartagener*, Swiss physician, born 1897] Kartagener's triad. See under SYNDROME.

Karyamoebina falcata *ENTAMOEBA HISTOLYTICA.*

karyapsis [*kary(o)-* + Ionic Gk *apsis* a juncture, knot, arch] The fusion of nuclei following cell conjugation.

karyenchyma [*kary(o)-* + ENCHYMA] KARYOLYMPH.

karyo- [Gk *karyon* nut, nucleus] A combining form meaning nucleus. Also *caryo-.*

karyochromatophil Having a nucleus which has a high affinity for stains: said of a cell.

karyochrome A neuron in which the nucleus stains very deeply and in which there are few Nissl bodies or none. Also called *karyochrome cell.* Also *caryochrome.*

karyochylema [KARYO- + CHYLE + -*ma* as in -OMA] KARYOLYMPH.

karyoclasis [KARYO- + -CLASIS] NUCLEORRHEXIS. Adjective: karyoclastic.

karyoclastic **1** Pertaining to karyoclasis. **2** Able to reversibly suppress mitosis without being lethal to the cell. Also *karyoklastic.*

karyocyte [KARYO- + -CYTE] Any nucleated cell. A rarely used term.

karyogamic Pertaining to karyogamy.

karyogamy [KARYO- + GAM- + -Y] The fusion of nuclei, the ultimate event of fertilization. The result of karyogamy is the reestablishment of the diploid number of chromosomes in the zygote. Adjective: karyogamic.

karyogenesis [KARYO- + GENESIS] The formation of the cell nucleus.

karyogenic [KARYO- + -GENIC] Pertaining to or effecting karyogenesis.

karyogonad [KARYO- + GONAD] MICRONUCLEUS.

karyokinesis [KARYO- + Gk *kinēsis* movement] Division of the cell nucleus by mitosis. Adjective: karyokinetic.

asymmetric karyokinesis A mitotic division in which the chromosome complement is unequally distributed to the two daughter cells.

hyperchromatic karyokinesis A nuclear division in which the number of chromosomes involved is greater than the normal number.

hypochromatic karyokinesis A nuclear division in which the number of chromosomes involved is lower than the normal number.

karyokinetic Pertaining to karyokinesis.

karyoklastic KARYOCLASTIC.

karyolobic Having a lobate nucleus: said of a cell.

karyolobism The condition in which the cell nucleus has a number of lobes, as the nucleus of a neutrophil leukocyte.

karyology The study of the cell nucleus, its organelles, structures, and functions. Also called *nuclear cytology*.

karyolymph [KARYO- + LYMPH] The fluid content of the cell nucleus. Also called *karyenchyma, karyochlema, nuclear hyaloplasm, nuclear sap, nucleolymph, nucleochylema*.

karyolysis [KARYO- + LYSIS] **1** Dissolution of the nucleus so that it no longer takes a basic stain. **2** The disappearance of the interphase nucleus during the early prophase of mitosis. Adjective: karyolytic.

Karyolysus lacertarum A coccidian parasite in the family Haemogregarinidae, found in the blood of lizards.

karyolytic Pertaining to or causing karyolysis.

karyomegaly [KARYO- + -MEGALY] A slight, uniform increase in nuclear size in the cells of a tissue.

karyomere Any of a series of small nuclei resulting when chromosomes which are widely spaced on the spindle diverge at anaphase. This condition occurs commonly during cleavage in some animal cells and can be induced chemically in others.

karyometry [KARYO- + -METRY] The measurement of the nuclei of cells.

karyomicrosome [KARYO- + MICROSOME] A small granule or particle occurring within the cell nucleus.

karyomit [KARYO- + Gk *mit(os)* a thread] A thread of chromatin which is part of the nuclear reticulum.

karyomitome The fibrillar network in the nucleus.

karyomitosis MITOSIS.

karyomitotic [KARYO- + MITOTIC] MITOTIC.

karyomorphism The shape of the cell nucleus.

karyon [Gk *karyon* a nut] The nucleus of a cell. Also called *karyoplast*.

karyonide Any of the nuclei in a clone, all nuclei being derived from a single nucleus.

karyophage [KARYO- + Gk *phagein* to eat, feed on] An intracellular protozoan parasite that feeds on the nucleus of the host cell.

karyoplasm NUCLEOPLASM.

karyoplasmic Pertaining to karyoplasm.

karyoplast [KARYO- + -PLAST] KARYON.

karyoplastin [KARYO- + -PLAST + -IN] The achromatic nuclear material which forms the spindle apparatus.

karyopyknosis Shrinkage of nuclei and condensation of the chromatin into structureless masses, as in squamous epithelium when it forms cornified epithelium. Adjective: karyopyknotic.

karyopyknotic Pertaining to, undergoing, or causing karyopyknosis.

karyoreticulum [KARYO- + RETICULUM] The reticular network within the cell nucleus.

karyorrhexis [KARYO- + -RRHEXIS] NUCLEORRHEXIS. Adjective: karyorrhectic.

karyosome [KARYO- + Gk *sōm(a)* body] A mass of aggregated chromatin material in an interphase nucleus. It is often confused with the nucleolus. Also called *net knot, chromatin nucleolus, false nucleolus, pseudonucleolus, chromatin reservoir, chromocenter*.

karyospherical Having a spherical cell nucleus.

karyostasis [KARYO- + STASIS] The nondividing condition of the cell nucleus during interphase.

karyotheca NUCLEAR ENVELOPE.

karyotype The particular chromosome complement of an individual as defined by the number, size, and centromere position of the chromosomes, usually in mitotic metaphase. See also IDIOGRAM. Adjective: karyotypic.

karyotypic Pertaining to a karyotype.

karyotyping Examination of the chromosomes to determine the karyotype.

karyozoic Parasitic in the nuclei of cells: said of certain protozoa.

Kasabach [Haig Haigouni *Kasabach*, U.S. physician, 1898–1943] Kasabach-Merritt syndrome. See under SYNDROME.

kasai [Bantu] A syndrome marked by anemia, edema, and dermal depigmentation and associated with protein-calorie malnutrition or kwashiorkor. It has been described in Zaire. Also called *Belgian Congo anemia*.

Kasanin [Jacob Sergi *Kasanin*, U.S. psychologist, 1897–1946] Hanfmann-Kasanin test. See under TEST.

Kashin [Nikolai Ivanovich *Kashin*, Russian physician, 1825–1872] Kashin-Beck disease. See under DISEASE.

Kast [Alfred *Kast*, German internist, 1856–1903] Kast syndrome. See under MAFUCCI SYNDROME.

Kastert [Josef *Kastert*, German orthopedic surgeon, born 1910] Hoffa-Kastert disease. See under HOFFA'S DISEASE.

Kastle [Joseph Hoeing *Kastle*, U.S. chemist, 1864–1916] See under TEST.

kasugamycin An antibiotic, containing an aminosugar and a cyclohexitol, that interferes with the initiation step in protein synthesis. It has had little use in medicine, against *Pseudomonas*, but it is widely used against a fungal disease of rice plants.

kat Symbol for the unit, katal.

kat- CATA-.

kata- CATA-.

katabolism CATABOLISM.

katachromasis [KATA- + GK *chrōma* color + -SIS] The formation of daughter nuclei during the telophase of mitosis. The chromatin is dispersed in the daughter nuclei. An obsolete term.

katadidymus CATADIDYMUS.

katal The special name for the unit of catalytic activity equal to one mole per second. With reference to the concentration of enzymatic activity, a katal is the amount of enzyme that catalyzes the transformation of substrate at a rate of one mole per second. Symbol: kat

katal per liter The unit of catalytic concentration or concentration of enzymatic activity. Symbol: kat/l, kat·l^{-1}

kataphrasis [Gk *kataphrasis* (from *kata* down, down from above + a root *phrax* of *phrassein* to secure) a stopping up] A surgical procedure in which metallic support is provided for a ptotic, or floating, organ.

kataphylaxis CATAPHYLAXIS.

katathermometer [KATA- + *thermometer*] An instrument used for measuring air velocity, particularly where air movements are turbulent or multidirectional. It consists of a thermometer which is heated, the cooling time between two temperature marks being measured and converted into wind speed. It was originally designed to measure the cooling power of the atmosphere but was unsatisfactory owing to its sensitivity to air movements.

Katayama [Kunika *Katayama*, Japanese physician, 1856–1931] Katayama disease. See under KATAYAMA SYNDROME.

Katayama ONCOMELANIA.

kath- CATA-.

katharometer [Gk *katharo(s)* pure, clean + -METER] An instrument for gas analysis, using the principle of thermal conductivity.

katharophore [Gk *katharo(s)* clear, pure + -PHORE] A device by which the urethra is washed.

kathisophobia [Gk *kathis(is)* a sitting down + *o* + PHOBIA] A syndrome resembling akathisia, possibly of psychogenic origin. A seldom used term.

katholysis [Gk *katho(dos)* a going down + English *(electro)lysis*] Electrolysis in which a cathode needle is used. An obsolete term.

katine $C_9H_{13}NO$. *d*-norpseudoephedrine. An alkaloid isolated from *Catha edulis*. It has an effect on the central nervous system like that of cocaine, but no local anesthetic properties, and it has been used as an anorectic agent. The leaves (catha) are used for tea and chewed in several regions of Africa.

kation CATION.

katipo [Maori, an eastern Polynesian language spoken in New Zealand] A venomous spider of the black widow genus, *Latrodectus hasselti,* found in New Zealand.

kat/l Symbol for the unit, katal per liter.

kat·l⁻¹ Symbol for the unit, katal per liter.

Kato [Kan *Kato*, Japanese scientist, born 1879] See under TEST.

katolysis [Gk *katō* below + LYSIS] A partial digestion or breakdown.

katophoria [KAT- + *o* + -PHORIA] A tendency to downward deviation of the eyes.

katotropia [KAT- + *o* + -TROPIA] A downward deviation of the eyes.

Katz [Johann Rudolf *Katz*, German chemist, 1880–1938] See under FORMULA.

katzenjammer A German word for HANGOVER.

kava 1 An intoxicating, addictive beverage prepared from the roots of *Piper methysticum*. 2 The dried roots and rhizome of *P. methysticum*, which contain kawain. Also called *kava-kava, ava-kava, ava.*

kavaism A condition resulting from the abuse of kava, or ava, a beverage prepared from the dried rhizome and roots of *Piper methysticum* in Polynesia. Symptoms are muscular weakness and mental confusion, progressing to convulsions or paralysis. Also called *avaism.*

kava-kava KAVA.

Kawasaki [T. *Kawasaki*, Japanese pediatrician, flourished 20th century] Kawasaki disease. See under SYNDROME.

Kay [Herbert Davenport *Kay*, Canadian biochemist, born 1893] Kay-Graham pasteurization test. See under TEST.

Kayser [Bernhard *Kayser*, German ophthalmologist, 1869–1954] 1 Kayser-Fleischer ring. See under RING. 2 Kayser's disease. See under WILSON'S DISEASE.

Kayser [Heinrich *Kayser*, German physician, 1876–1940] Brion-Kayser disease. See under PARATYPHOID FEVER.

Kazanjian [Varaztad Hovhannes *Kazanjian*, Armenian-born U.S. otorhinolaryngologist, born 1879] 1 Kazanjian procedure. See under RIDGE EXTENSION. 2 See under FORCEPS, OPERATION.

kBq Symbol for the unit, kilobecquerel.

kC Symbol for the unit, kilocoulomb.

kc Symbol for the obsolete unit, kilocycle per second. An incorrect symbol.

kcal Symbol for the unit, kilocalorie.

kCi Symbol for the unit, kilocurie.

kc.p.s. Symbol for the unit, kilocycle per second. An incorrect symbol.

kc/s Symbol for the unit, kilocycle per second.

KCT kathodal (cathodal) closure tetanus.

kDa Symbol for kilodalton.

KDO ketodeoxyoctonate.

kdyn Symbol for the unit, kilodyne.

Keating-Hart [Walter-Valentin *Keating-Hart*, French physician, 1870–1922] 1 Keating-Hart fulguration. See under METHOD. 2 See under TREATMENT.

kebocephaly CEBOCEPHALY.

ked [origin unknown] A wingless fly of the species *Melophagus ovinus*. Also called *sheep tick, tick fly.*

kedani A Japanese term for CHIGGER.

Keegan [Denis Francis *Keegan*, English surgeon, 1840–1920] See under OPERATION.

keel Something suggesting the shape or function of the keel of a ship (the ridged, bottommost, lengthwise part of a vessel's framework), as a ridged or protuberant process or a device used to divide parts lengthwise. Adjective: keeled.

McNaught keel A small, flanged, metal plate inserted between the anterior parts of the vocal cords at the conclusion of certain laryngeal operations and removed only when it is judged that there is no longer a risk of cicatricial stenosis.

Keeler [Leonard *Keeler*, U.S. criminologist, 1903–1949] Keeler's lie polygraph. See under POLYGRAPH.

Keen [W. W. *Keen*, U.S. surgeon, 1837–1932] See under POINT, SIGN.

Kehr [Hans *Kehr*, German surgeon, 1862–1916] See under SIGN, INCISION.

Kehrer [Ferdinand Adalbert *Kehrer*, German physician, born 1883] 1 See under SIGN. 2 Kehrer-Adie syndrome. See under ADIE SYNDROME. 3 Kehrer's reflex. See under EXTERNAL AUDITORY MEATUS REFLEX.

keirospasm [Gk *keir(ein)* to clip, cut short, esp. the hair + *o* + SPASM] An occupational cramp occurring among barbers and hairdressers and characterized by muscle spasms in the hands and forearms. It results from continued use of the same muscles. Also called *shaving cramp.*

Keith [Sir Arthur *Keith*, Scottish anatomist, 1866–1955] Keith's node, sinuatrial node of Keith and Flack, Keith-Flack node, Keith's bundle. See under NODUS SINUATRIALIS.

Keith [Norman MacDonnell *Keith*, U.S. physician, born 1885] See under DIET.

kelectome [Gk *kēl(ē)* a tumor + *ektomē* a cutting out] A surgical instrument that is used to obtain a piece of tissue for pathologic examination.

Kelene A proprietary name for ethyl chloride.

kelis 1 An obsolete term for KELOID. 2 An obsolete term for MORPHEA.

Kellie [George *Kellie*, Scottish anatomist, flourished late 18th century] Monro-Kellie doctrine. See under DOCTRINE.

Kelly See under BROWN KELLY.

Kelly [Howard Atwood *Kelly*, U.S. gynecologist, 1858–1943] See under CYSTOSCOPE, OPERATION, SIGN, SPECULUM, SPHINCTEROSCOPE.

keloid [Gk *kēlē* a rupture, hernia + -OID or from Gk *kēlis* a stain, spot, or blemish + -OID.] A firm, scarlike nodule of the skin, composed of fibrous tissue with broad bands of homogeneous acidophilic collagen. It develops as a response to trauma that may be trivial and far exceeds the physiologic needs appropriate to the site and the degree of injury. It is usually found in heavily pigmented people, and, unlike a hyperplastic scar, it tends to recur. Also called *cheloid, cheloma* (obsolete), *kelis* (obsolete), *keloma.*

acne keloid A keloid that forms at the nape of the neck as a result of keloid acne.

Addison's keloid MORPHEA.

Alibert's keloid A keloid formed by the hypertrophy of a scar rather than as a response to trauma. Also called *cicatricial keloid, false keloid.*

cicatricial keloid ALIBERT'S KELOID.

false keloid ALIBERT'S KELOID.

keloid of gums An outmoded term for GINGIVAL FIBROMATOSIS.

keloidal Of or relating to a keloid.

keloma KELOID.

kelosomia CELOSOMIA.

kelosomus CELOSOMUS.

kelotomy [Gk *kēl(ē)* a rupture, hernia + *o* + -TOMY] HERNIOTOMY.

kelp [Middle English *culp*] Any of the large brown marine algae.

Kelser [Raymond Alexander *Kelser*, U.S. pathologist, born 1892] See under VACCINE.

Kelvin [William Thomson (Lord *Kelvin*), English physicist, 1824–1907] See under SCALE, THERMOMETER.

kelvin [after William Thomson, Lord *Kelvin*, British physicist, 1824–1907] **1** The SI base unit of thermodynamic temperature, defined as the fraction 1/273.16 of the thermodynamic temperature of the triple point of water. Also called *degree absolute, degree kelvin* (outmoded). Symbol: K **2** A unit of electrical energy equal to the kilowatt-hour. An obsolete unit.

Kemadrin A proprietary name for procyclidine hydrochloride.

Kempner [Walter *Kempner*, U.S. physician, born 1903] See under DIET.

Kenacort A proprietary name for triamcinolone.

Kenalog A proprietary name for triamcinolone acetonide.

Kendall [Edward Calvin *Kendall*, U.S. biochemist, 1886–1972] **1** Kendall's compound A. See under 11-DEHYDROCORTICOSTERONE. **2** Kendall's compound B. See under CORTICOSTERONE. **3** Kendall's compound D. See under COMPOUND. **4** Kendall's compound E. See under CORTISONE. **5** Kendall's compound F. See under CORTISOL.

Kennedy [Edward *Kennedy*, U.S. dentist, born 1883] **1** Kennedy bar. See under CONTINUOUS BAR RETAINER. **2** See under CLASSIFICATION.

Kennedy [Robert Foster *Kennedy*, U.S. neurologist, 1884–1952] Kennedy syndrome. See under FOSTER KENNEDY SYNDROME.

Kenny [Elizabeth *Kenny*, Australian nurse, 1886–1952] Kenny's treatment. See under METHOD.

keno- CENO-³.

kenophobia [KENO- + -PHOBIA] Pathologic fear of open or barren space; a type of agoraphobia. Also called *cenophobia*.

kenotoxin [KENO- + TOXIN] FATIGUE TOXIN.

Kent [Albert Frank Stanley *Kent*, English physiologist, 1863–1958] **1** See under BUNDLE. **2** Kent-His bundle, bundle of Stanley Kent. See under FASCICULUS ATRIOVENTRICULARIS.

Kent [Grace Helen *Kent*, U.S. psychologist, born 1875] **1** See under SCALE. **2** Kent EGY test. See under KENT EMERGENCY SCALE.

Kepler [Edwin John *Kepler*, U.S. physician, born 1894] Robinson-Kepler test, Robinson-Kepler-Power water test. See under TEST.

Kepone A proprietary name for chloredecone.

Keq Symbol for equilibrium constant.

Kerandel [Jean François *Kerandel*, French physician, 1873–1934] Kerandel sign. See under SYMPTOM.

keraphyllocele KERATOMA.

kerat- KERATO-.

keratalgia [KERAT- + -ALGIA] Pain referred to the cornea.

keratectasia [KERAT- + ECTASIA] A localized thinning and protrusion of the cornea; a forward bulging of part of the corneal curvature. Also called *corneal ectasia*.

keratectomy [KERAT- + -ECTOMY] Excision of a portion of the cornea. Also *ceratectomy*.

keratein The protein formed by the reduction of the disulfide bonds of keratin to thiol groups.

keratiasis [*kerat(oma)* + -IASIS] The presence of keratomas on the skin. An obsolete term.

keratic HORNY.

keratin [KERAT- + -IN] A scleroprotein or albuminoid found in horny tissues such as hair, nails, feathers, and scales. Keratins are insoluble in water, in dilute acids, and in dilute alkalis, and are generally not digested by proteolytic enzymes. Keratins have a high sulfur content. The amino acids cystine and arginine generally predominate. Also *ceratin*.

false keratin PSEUDOKERATIN.

keratinase A keratin-hydrolyzing enzyme that catalyzes the breakdown of keratin.

keratinization The formation of keratin, as in the development of a horny layer of tissue. Also called *cornification, hornification*.

keratinize To turn into horny tissue.

keratinocyte A cell of the epidermis that produces keratin.

keratinoid **1** Resembling keratin. **2** A pill or tablet having keratin as an enteric coating.

Keratinomyces A form-genus of dermatophytic and keratinophilic fungi.

keratitic Pertaining to the cornea; corneal.

keratitis [KERAT- + -ITIS] Inflammation of the cornea. Also called *corneitis, keratoiditis*. Also *ceratitis*.

acne rosacea keratitis ROSACEA KERATITIS.

actinic keratitis Corneal epithelial damage from the ultraviolet rays of the sun.

aerosol keratitis Corneal damage due to the propellant vehicle in a pressurized aerosol can.

alphabet keratitis STRIATE KERATOPATHY.

keratitis arborescens DENDRITIC KERATITIS.

artificial silk keratitis Keratoconjunctivitis occurring as a result of exposure to low concentrations of hydrogen sulfide used in the manufacture of viscose rayon fibers. Also called *artificial silk keratoconjunctivitis*.

band keratitis BAND KERATOPATHY.

keratitis bandelette BAND KERATOPATHY.

band-shaped keratitis BAND KERATOPATHY.

keratitis bullosa A condition characterized by the formation of blebs and vesicles on the corneal epithelium.

deep keratitis Inflammation of the posterior stromal and Descemet's layers of the cornea. Also called *keratitis profunda*.

dendriform keratitis DENDRITIC KERATITIS.

dendritic keratitis Linear and branching corneal ulceration due to herpes simplex or herpes zoster. Also called *dendriform keratitis, keratitis arborescens*.

desiccation keratitis Corneal damage due to local exposure and dehydration of the tissue.

Dimmer's keratitis KERATITIS NUMMULARIS.

disciform keratitis Stromal scarring and infiltration from herpes. Also called *keratitis disciformis*.

keratitis disciformis DISCIFORM KERATITIS.

exfoliative keratitis Loss of the corneal epithelium due to inflammation of the cornea.

exposure keratitis EXPOSURE KERATOPATHY.

fascicular keratitis Progressive, ulcerative corneal damage associated with localized vascularization.

keratitis filamentosa Corneal irritation, usually from inadequate lubrication, that causes strands of epithelial cells to hang from the corneal surface.

furrow keratitis Linear ulceration of the cornea due to herpes.

herpetic keratitis Corneal infection with herpes simplex or herpes zoster.

hypopyon keratitis Severe corneal inflammation associated with leukocytic sedimentation in the anterior chamber.

infectious bovine keratitis INFECTIOUS BOVINE KERATO-CONJUNCTIVITIS.

interstitial keratitis Inflammation of the deep corneal stroma, often due to congenital syphilis.

lagophthalmic keratitis EXPOSURE KERATOPATHY.

lattice keratitis A familial corneal dystrophy that forms linear intrastromal opacities.

marginal keratitis Superficial defects of the peripheral corneal epithelium.

metaherpetic keratitis Chronic, corneal stromal infection with herpes simplex or herpes zoster. Also called *metaherpes*.

mycotic keratitis Corneal infection with a fungus, commonly *Aspergillus, Fusarium,* or *Candida.*

necrogranulomatous keratitis A severe corneal disorder in which focal infiltrates of inflammatory cells break down and ulcerate.

neuroparalytic keratitis Corneal damage resulting from loss of sensitivity due to trigeminal nerve damage. Infrared lacrimation may be a contributing factor. Also called *neurotrophic keratitis, neuropathic keratitis, neuroparalytic ophthalmia.*

neuropathic keratitis NEUROPARALYTIC KERATITIS.

neurotrophic keratitis NEUROPARALYTIC KERATITIS.

keratitis nummularis A mild inflammation of the cornea in which small superficial disk-shaped opacities exist. Also called *Dimmer's keratitis.*

parenchymatous anaphylactic keratitis Immunologic inflammation of the corneal stroma.

keratitis petrificans Calcification of the corneal surface.

phlyctenular keratitis Superficial sector allergic response of the cornea.

keratitis profunda DEEP KERATITIS.

keratitis punctata PUNCTATE KERATITIS.

keratitis punctata leprosa The most common form of leprotic keratitis, in which there are minute white spots on the cornea.

keratitis punctata subepithelialis The presence of multiple, small, deep infiltrates of the corneal epithelium.

punctate keratitis The presence of multiple small erosions of the corneal epithelium. Also called *keratitis punctata, superficial punctate keratitis.*

purulent keratitis Leukocytic invasion of the cornea. Also called *keratitis purulenta, suppurative keratitis.*

keratitis purulenta PURULENT KERATITIS.

keratitis pustuliformis profunda A deep purulent infection of the cornea.

keratitis ramificata superficialis The loss of the superficial corneal epithelium resulting from exposure to tropical conditions. A rarely used term.

reapers' keratitis Traumatic keratitis sustained while harvesting grain, such as barley.

reticular keratitis A familial corneal dystrophy causing netlike patterns of intrastromal opacity.

ribbonlike keratitis A familial corneal dystrophy causing linear intrastromal opacities.

rosacea keratitis Corneal inflammation associated with the dermatologic disease, acne rosacea. Also called *acne rosacea keratitis.*

sclerosing keratitis Opacification of the cornea continuous with the white sclera, due to inflammation.

scrofulous keratitis TUBERCULOUS KERATITIS.

secondary keratitis Keratitis due to disorder of an adjacent ocular tissue.

senile guttate keratitis Endothelial dystrophy, with Hassall-Henle bodies on Descemet's membrane.

serpiginous keratitis A chronic, ulcerative corneal inflammation occurring in older persons.

keratitis sicca Corneal damage secondary to deficient lacrimal secretion.

striate keratitis STRIATE KERATOPATHY.

superficial linear keratitis Erosion or folding of the superficial layers of the cornea.

superficial punctate keratitis PUNCTATE KERATITIS.

suppurative keratitis PURULENT KERATITIS.

syphilitic keratitis Corneal infection with *Treponema pallidum.*

trachomatous keratitis Corneal infection with *Chlamydia trachomatis.*

traumatic keratitis Corneal damage from injury.

trophic keratitis Corneal damage from nutritional or innervational defect.

tuberculous keratitis Corneal infection with *Mycobacterium tuberculosis.* Also called *scrofulous keratitis.*

vascular keratitis Keratitis characterized by the invasion of blood vessels in the cornea.

vasculonebulous keratitis Keratitis characterized by scarring and the invasion of blood vessels in the cornea.

vernal keratitis Keratitis due to allergic response of the cornea to spring pollens.

vesicular keratitis Keratitis characterized by the presence of multiple, localized, fluid spaces between the corneal epithelium and Bowman's membrane.

xerotic keratitis Corneal damage due to pathologic dryness, as in vitamin A deficiency.

zonular keratitis BAND KERATOPATHY.

kerato- [Gk *keras* (genitive *keratos*) horn, cornea] A combining form denoting (1) the cornea; (2) horny tissue. Also *kerat-, cerat-, cerato-.*

keratoacanthoma A rapidly growing benign squamous cell, tumorlike lesion occurring predominantly in exposed skin and forming a nodule with a central crater filled with keratin. It occurs especially in individuals exposed to sunlight, tar, and other environmental carcinogens. The crateriform nodule enlarges for 3–4 weeks after which it decreases in size and is eventually shed, to be followed by a distinctive scar. This spontaneous recovery takes place in the vast majority of keratoacanthomas, but occasional transformation to squamous cell carcinoma occurs, notably with lesions of the pinna and lower lip and more particularly in the very elderly. Also called *Ackerman's tumor.*

keratoangioma ANGIOKERATOMA.

keratocele [KERATO- + -CELE¹] DESCEMETOCELE.

keratocentesis [KERATO- + CENTESIS] Incision of the cornea.

keratochromatosis [KERATO- + CHROMATOSIS] Discolored opacification of the cornea.

keratochromomycosis [KERATO- + CHROMO- + MYCOSIS] Corneal infection with pigment-producing fungi.

keratoconjunctivitis [KERATO- + CONJUNCTIVITIS] Inflammation of both the cornea and conjunctiva.

actinic keratoconjunctivitis Superficial damage to the cornea and conjunctiva by the ultraviolet rays of the sun.

adenoviral keratoconjunctivitis An infection of the cornea and conjunctiva of adenoviral etiology. It has occurred in epidemic form among shipyard workers. Also called *Sander's disease.*

artificial silk keratoconjunctivitis ARTIFICIAL SILK KERATITIS.

epidemic keratoconjunctivitis An acute infectious conjunctivitis usually caused by adenovirus types 8 and 19 and characterized by scanty exudate and development of corneal subepithelial infiltrations 7–10 days after the onset of inflammation. Epidemic outbreaks have occurred, with one of the first large-scale epidemics involving shipyard workers. Also called *shipyard* *keratoconjunctivitis, shipyard eye, shipyard conjunctivitis.*

flash keratoconjunctivitis   Irritation of the cornea and conjunctiva by ultraviolet radiation from welding, particularly electric-arc welding.

infectious bovine keratoconjunctivitis   An acute contagious keratoconjunctivitis of cattle, caused by *Moraxella bovis.* Also called *infectious bovine keratitis.*

phlyctenular keratoconjunctivitis   Superficial sector allergic response of the cornea and conjunctiva.

shipyard keratoconjunctivitis   EPIDEMIC KERATOCONJUNCTIVITIS.

keratoconjunctivitis sicca   XEROPHTHALMIA.

superior limbic keratoconjunctivitis   Inflammation of the superior cornea and adjacent conjunctiva of unknown etiology.

vernal keratoconjunctivitis   An allergic response of the conjunctiva and cornea occurring primarily in children, with a tendency to be more severe in the spring. It is characterized by giant papillary formation on the palpebral conjunctiva. Also called *spring ophthalmia.*

viral keratoconjunctivitis   Any keratoconjunctivitis caused by adenoviruses or other viruses. The epidemic form is usually caused by adenoviruses types 1–3, 7–9, 19.

keratoconometer   A device for measuring or identifying keratoconus.

keratoconus [KERATO- + L *conus* a cone]   A dystrophy in which the central cornea becomes thin and ectatic, to form a symmetrical, conical protrusion. Also called *conical cornea, sugar-loaf cornea.*

congenital keratoconus   A developmental anomaly of corneal curvature in which the central cornea is thinned and conical in shape.

keratocricoid   CERATOCRICOID.

keratocyst [KERATO- + CYST]   A dental cyst lined by keratinizing epithelium. The probable origin is from the dental lamina and there is a risk of recurrence unless enucleation is thorough.

keratocyte   **1** An abnormally shaped erythrocyte that has two hornlike projections on the same side. Keratocytes may be found in blood films from persons who have been exposed to drugs or toxins that cause oxidative injury to erythrocytes, such as dapsone. Also called *bite cell.*   **2** A stromal cell of the cornea.

keratoderma [KERATO- + DERMA]   The thickening of the horny layer of the epidermis. Also called *keratodermia.*

keratoderma blennorrhagicum   The distinctive warty lesions of the skin that are symptomatic of the Reiter syndrome, occurring typically on the soles of the feet and the nail beds and palms of the hand, and often elsewhere. Also called *keratosis blennorrhagica, keratodermia blennorrhagica, gonorrheal keratosis* (incorrect).

keratoderma climactericum   A circumscribed palmoplantar keratoderma that occurs among women of middle age. It has been ascribed without evidence to menopausal hormonal changes. Also called *endocrine keratoderma.*

endocrine keratoderma   KERATODERMA CLIMACTERICUM.

gonorrheal keratoderma   Warty lesions of the palms and soles that have been falsely attributed to gonorrhea. They are part of the Reiter syndrome.

palmar keratoderma   An increased thickness in the palmar skin. It may be diffuse, striated, or papular, or it may be confined to areas of pressure. Also called *ichthyosis palmaris.*

keratoderma palmare et plantare   PALMOPLANTAR KERATODERMA.

palmoplantar keratoderma   A thickening of the horny layer of the palms and soles. Also called *keratoderma palmare et plantare, dermatitis exsiccans palmaris* (obsolete), *keratodermia palmaris et plantaris, keratoma palmare et plantare, keratosis palmaris et plantaris, ichthyosis palmaris et plantaris, symmetric*

keratoderma, symmetrical keratoderma of adults, Jadassohn-Lewandowsky syndrome, tylosis palmaris et plantaris, hyperkeratosis congenitalis palmaris et plantaris.

plantar keratoderma   Increased thickness of the plantar skin. The increase may be diffuse, striate, or papular, or confined to areas of pressure. Also called *ichthyosis plantaris.*

punctate keratoderma   A form of hereditary palmoplantar keratoderma in which the lesions are circumscribed keratoses. Also called *keratosis punctata.*

symmetric keratoderma   PALMOPLANTAR KERATODERMA.

symmetrical keratoderma of adults   PALMOPLANTAR KERATODERMA.

syphilitic keratoderma   Warty lesions of the palms and soles that occur in syphilis.

keratodermatocele [KERATO- + DERMATOCELE]   DESCEMETOCELE.

keratodermatosis [KERATO- + DERMATOSIS]   Any skin disorder in which the horny layer is thickened or abnormal. An obsolete term.

keratodermia [KERATO- + -DERM + -IA]   KERATODERMA.

keratodermia blennorrhagica   KERATODERMA BLENNORRHAGICUM.

keratodermia excentrica   An obsolete term for POROKERATOSIS OF MIBELLI.

keratodermia palmaris et plantaris   PALMOPLANTAR KERATODERMA.

keratodermia plantaris sulcata   PITTED KERATOLYSIS.

keratoectasia [KERATO- + ECTASIA]   A forward bulging of thinned cornea without the iris being adherent posteriorly.

keratogenesis   The formation of keratin.

keratogenetic   Of or relating to keratogenesis.

keratogenous   Giving rise to keratin.

keratoglobus [KERATO- + GLOBUS]   MEGALOCORNEA.

keratohelcosis [KERATO- + HELCOSIS]   An ulceration of the cornea.

keratohemia [KERATO- + -HEMIA]   Hemorrhage within the cornea.

keratohyal   CERATOHYAL.

keratohyalin   The hyaline material found in the granular layer of the epidermis.

keratohyaline   Resembling keratohyalin.

keratoid [KERAT- + -OID]   Resembling or pertaining to the cornea.

keratoiditis   KERATITIS.

keratoiridocyclitis [KERATO- + IRIDO- + CYCLITIS]   Inflammation of the cornea and anterior uveal tract.

keratoiridoscope   BIOMICROSCOPE.

keratoiritis [KERATO- + IRITIS]   Inflammation of the cornea and iris.

hypopyon keratoiritis   Inflammation of the cornea and iris with leukocytic sediment in the anterior chamber.

keratoleptynsis [KERATO- + Gk *leptynsis* a making thin]   Surgical placement of a conjunctival flap overlying the cornea.

keratoleukoma [KERATO- + LEUKOMA]   A white scarring of the cornea.

keratolysis [KERATO- + LYSIS]   The separation of the horny layer from the rest of the epidermis.

keratolysis neonatorum   TOXIC EPIDERMAL NECROLYSIS.

pitted keratolysis   A superficial infection of the skin of the soles by species of *Corynebacterium* or of *Actinomyces.* Also called *keratolysis plantare sulcatum, chaluni, keratoma plantare sulcatum* (obsolete), *keratodermia plantaris sulcata.*

keratolysis plantare sulcatum   PITTED KERATOLYSIS.

keratolytic **1** Of or relating to keratolysis. **2** Any agent used to soften or break up keratin.

keratoma [KERAT- + -OMA] **1** KERATOSIS. **2** A condition of the equine foot in which there is overgrowth of horn, usually at the toe on the inner surface of the wall. It usually is a sequel to chronic inflammation of the sensitive laminae of the hoof and can cause pressure atrophy of the phalangeal bone. Also called *keraphyllocele*.

keratoma auriculare Nodular chondrodermatitis of the ear.

congenital diffuse malignant keratoma KERATOSIS DIFFUSA FETALIS.

keratoma diffusum KERATOSIS DIFFUSA FETALIS.

keratoma palmare et plantare PALMOPLANTAR KERATODERMA.

keratoma plantare sulcatum An obsolete term for PITTED KERATOLYSIS.

senile keratoma ACTINIC KERATOSIS.

keratomalacia [KERATO- + MALACIA] A wasting and opacification of the cornea classically associated with vitamin A deficiency, but also occurring with other nutritional or metabolic defects.

keratomata Plural of KERATOMA.

keratome KERATOTOME.

keratometer A device for measuring the anterior curvatures of the cornea, of particular use in evaluating astigmatism and in fitting contact lenses. Also called *ophthalmometer*.

keratometric Pertaining to keratometry.

keratometry [KERATO- + -METRY] The measurement of corneal curvature. Also called *ophthalmometry*. Adjective: keratometric.

keratomileusis [KERATO- + Gk *(s)mileusis* the act of carving] A surgical modification of the corneal curvature in order to change refractive error; refractive keratoplasty.

keratomycosis [KERATO- + MYCOSIS] A fungus infection of the cornea.

keratomycosis linguae An old-fashioned and incorrect term for BLACK HAIRY TONGUE.

keratonosis [KERATO- + *n* + -OSIS] Any abnormality of the horny layer of the epidermis. An obsolete term.

keratonosus [KERATO- + Gk *nosos* disease, illness] Degeneration of the cornea.

keratonyxis [KERATO- + Gk *nyxis* a pricking] Surgical perforation of the cornea.

keratopathy [KERATO- + -PATHY] A noninflammatory corneal disease.

band keratopathy A superficial, interpalpebral, corneal calcification usually associated with severe general degeneration of an eye. Also called *band-shaped keratopathy, band keratitis, band-shaped keratitis, keratitis bandelette, zonular keratitis*.

band-shaped keratopathy BAND KERATOPATHY.

exposure keratopathy Keratopathy due to faulty lid closure. Also called *exposure keratitis, lagophthalmic keratitis*.

striate keratopathy A deep linear folding of the inner corneal layers caused by ocular hypotony and corneal edema. Also called *alphabet keratitis, striate keratitis*.

keratoplasia [KERATO- + -PLASIA] The formation or renewal of a horny layer.

keratoplasty [KERATO- + -PLASTY] The replacement of a faulty cornea by a portion of a normal cornea obtained from another eye. Also called *corneal transplantation*.

lamellar keratoplasty Transplantation of only partial thickness of the cornea.

optic keratoplasty Corneal transplantation to improve eyesight.

penetrating keratoplasty Transplantation of full-thickness cornea.

tectonic keratoplasty Corneal transplantation for structural reasons, as in infections or traumatic loss of tissue.

keratoprosthesis [KERATO- + PROSTHESIS] Implantation of a transparent foreign substance into the cornea.

keratorhexis [KERATO- + -RHEXIS] Rupture of the cornea.

keratoscleritis [KERATO- + SCLERITIS] Inflammation of the cornea and sclera.

keratoscope A device to observe or measure corneal curvature.

keratoscopy [KERATO- + -SCOPY] Observation or measurement of corneal curvature.

keratosis [KERAT- + -OSIS] A benign horny lesion. It is usually actinic or seborrheic in origin. Also called *keratoma*.

acneform keratosis follicularis Follicular keratosis associated with inflammatory changes that resemble acne vulgaris.

actinic keratosis An erythematous scaly lesion of the skin that is provoked by prolonged exposure to sunlight. Also called *solar keratosis, senile keratosis, keratosis senilis, senile keratoma, verruca plana senilis*.

arsenical keratosis Warty keratosis, particularly on the palms and soles, caused by the ingestion of inorganic arsenic.

aural keratosis CHOLESTEATOMA.

keratosis blennorrhagica KERATODERMA BLENNORRHAGICUM.

contagious keratosis follicularis Acneform keratosis follicularis that occurs in epidemic proportions within a population. It was once believed to be contagious. Also called *keratosis follicularis contagiosa, epidemic keratosis follicularis*.

keratosis diffusa fetalis A very severe form of congenital ichthyosiform erythroderma. An obsolete term. Also called *congenital diffuse malignant keratoma, keratoma diffusum*.

epidemic keratosis follicularis CONTAGIOUS KERATOSIS FOLLICULARIS.

keratosis follicularis A hereditary disorder of keratinization characterized by the widespread development of dyskeratotic follicular papules. Also called *Darier's disease, keratosis vegetans* (obsolete), *psorospermosis*.

keratosis follicularis contagiosa CONTAGIOUS KERATOSIS FOLLICULARIS.

keratosis follicularis decalvans Keratosis follicularis that results in the destruction of the follicles and subsequent alopecia.

gonorrheal keratosis An incorrect term for KERATODERMA BLENNORRHAGICUM.

inverted follicular keratosis A hyperkeratotic papule arising as a result of an abnormality in growth of hair follicle epithelium. It is a benign lesion.

keratosis labialis Actinic keratosis occurring on the mucous membrane of the lip.

keratosis linguae Leukoplakia of the tongue.

keratosis nigricans ACANTHOSIS NIGRICANS.

keratosis obliterans KERATOSIS OBTURANS.

keratosis obturans A disease of the external ear in which the canal becomes obstructed and sometimes expanded by a firm mass of keratin, epidermic scales, and cerumen. Also called *keratosis obliterans, wax keratosis, otitis desquamativa* (older term).

keratosis palmaris et plantaris PALMOPLANTAR KERATODERMA.

keratosis pharyngis A disease of unknown pathogenesis, affecting the epithelial covering of the lymphoid tissue of the fauces and pharynx. It is characterized by grayish white horny spicules scattered over the palatine or lingual tonsils or the adenoids or pharyngeal lymphoid nodules, but most often over the palatine tonsils. The disease causes few if any symptoms and eventually resolves spontaneously. Also called *hyperkeratosis* *lacunaris, hyperkeratosis lacunaris pharyngis, pharyngitis keratosa.*

keratosis pilaris Hyperkeratosis of the hair follicles which gives rise to small horny papules, visible most often on the extensor aspect of the limbs. Also called *follicular hyperkeratosis, keratosis pilaris rubra, pityriasis pilaris* (obsolete), *follicular xeroderma* (obsolete), *keratosis suprafollicularis* (obsolete), *follicular ichthyosis* (obsolete).

keratosis pilaris atrophicans Follicular keratosis in which the horny plugs are succeeded by atrophic scars.

keratosis pilaris rubra KERATOSIS PILARIS.

keratosis pilaris rubra atrophicans of the face Keratosis pilaris atrophicans that is primarily confined to the face.

keratosis punctata PUNCTATE KERATODERMA.

roentgen keratosis A keratosis, possibly premalignant, occurring in skin that has been damaged by ionizing radiation. Also called *x-ray keratosis.*

keratosis rubra figurata ERYTHROKERATODERMA VARIABILIS.

seborrheic keratosis A benign tumor, common among the elderly, that is formed of immature epidermal cells. Also called *basalcell papilloma, acanthosis verrucosa, acanthosis seborrheica, verruca seborrheica, verruca senilis, senile wart, seborrheica wart, pigmented wart, keratosis seborrheica, seborrheic nevus.*

keratosis seborrheica SEBORRHEIC KERATOSIS.

senile keratosis ACTINIC KERATOSIS.

keratosis senilis ACTINIC KERATOSIS.

solar keratosis ACTINIC KERATOSIS.

stucco keratosis A small warty papule most commonly seen on the feet and ankles of elderly men.

keratosis suprafollicularis An obsolete term for KERATOSIS PILARIS.

tar keratosis A keratosis induced by exposure to tar.

keratosis universalis congenita ICHTHYOSIS CONGENITA.

keratosis vegetans An obsolete term for KERATOSIS FOLLICULARIS.

wax keratosis KERATOSIS OBTURANS.

x-ray keratosis ROENTGEN KERATOSIS.

keratosulfate A polysaccharide of connective tissue. It consists of alternate residues of β-D-galactose, glycosylated on O-3, and β-D-*N*-acetylglucosamine 6-sulfate, glycosylated on O-4.

keratosulfaturia The excretion of excessive keratosulfates in the urine. It is symptomatic of mucopolysaccharidosis IV.

keratotic Warty or horny, as in keratosis.

keratotome [KERATO- + -TOME] A triangular surgical knife designed to cut through the cornea to enter the anterior chamber. Also called *keratome.*

keratotomy [KERATO- + -TOMY] An incision in the cornea.

delimiting keratotomy Incision of the cornea with the hope of preventing progression of an ulcer.

radial keratotomy A technique of refractive keratoplasty in which a series of radial incisions are made in the peripheral cornea in order to flatten the corneal curvature, thereby reducing myopia. The procedure gives inconstant and variable results and leaves permanent corneal scars, and is therefore considered controversial.

keratotorus [KERATO- + TORUS] An ectasia of the cornea, producing irregular astigmatism.

Kerckring [Thomas Theodor *Kerckring,* Dutch anatomist, 1640–1693] **1** See under CENTER, OSSICLE. **2** Circular folds of Kerckring, Kerckring's folds of small intestine, Kerckring's valves. See under PLICAE CIRCULARES. **3** Nodules of Kerckring. See under NODULI VALVULARUM SEMILUNARIUM VALVAE AORTAE.

kerectasis [*ker(at)-* + ECTASIS] A forward bulging of a thin or weakened cornea.

kerectomy KERATECTOMY.

kerion [Gk *kērion* a honeycomb, a waxen tablet, from *kēros* beeswax, wax; L *cera* wax] A highly inflammatory, purulent ringworm infection usually occurring on the scalp, beard area, or limb where there are coarse follicles. It is typically caused by a dermatophyte contracted from an animal or from the soil. Also called *tinea kerion, conglomerate folliculitis, conglomerative pustular folliculitis, kerion celsi* (outmoded), *conglomerative pustular perifolliculitis, honeycomb ringworm.*

kerion celsi An outmoded term for KERION.

keritherapy [Gk *kēr(os)* beeswax, wax + *i* + THERAPY] Treatment by paraffin baths. A seldom used term. Also called *kerotherapy.*

Kerley [Peter James *Kerley,* English radiologist, born 1900] Kerley's lines. See under LINE.

kerma [from *k(inetic) e(nergy) r(eleased in) ma(tter)*] The kinetic energy transferred to charged particles by uncharged particles in unit mass of material, expressed in rads or joules per kilogram.

kermes ALKERMES.

kernel [Old English *cyrnel,* akin to Old Norse *korn* grain] **1** That part of the atom existing when the charged sheath is removed. **2** A seed, especially a seed contained within a fruit or the body of a seed within its husk.

kernicterus [German *Kernikterus* (from *Kern* a kernel, nucleus, core + *Ikterus* jaundice; in botany, chlorosis) nuclear jaundice] Damage to the globus pallidus, putamen, and caudate nucleus and to the cerebral cortical gray matter and cerebellar and brainstem nuclei, with deep yellow staining of the affected areas resulting from high levels of serum bilirubin. Clinical manifestations include deafness, mental retardation, and athetosis. The condition has usually but not invariably been the result of hemolytic jaundice due to Rh incompatibility. Also called *bilirubin encephalopathy, nuclear icterus, nuclear jaundice.*

Kernig [Vladimir Michailovich *Kernig,* Russian physician, 1840–1917] See under SIGN.

kernschwund [German *Kern* kernel, nucleus + *Schwund* disappearance, decline, decay] A congenital faulty development of cellular nuclei in the central nervous system, as in congenital ophthalmoplegia.

keroid Like the cornea.

kerosene [Gk *kēros* wax + *-ene,* adjectival suffix, from Gk *-en(os)* adjectival suffix] A mixture of hydrocarbons derived from petroleum, with boiling points of about 150–200°C.

kerosis [Gk *kērōsis* the formation of wax] A condition of the skin, seen in seborrhea, in which the follicular orifices are patent and conspicuous.

kerotherapy KERITHERAPY.

Kerr See under MUNRO KERR.

Kerr [Harry Hyland *Kerr,* U.S. surgeon, born 1881] Parker-Kerr suture. See under SUTURE.

Ketaject A proprietary name for ketamine hydrochloride.

ketal Any acetal that is derived from a ketone. An outmoded term.

Ketalar A proprietary name for ketamine hydrochloride.

ketamine hydrochloride $C_{13}H_{16}ClNO$. A fast-acting general anesthetic administered intravenously or intramuscularly. It is related to the hallucinogen phencyclidine. It produces dissociation in the central nervous system with a lack of awareness. It is a competent analgesic but reflexes and strong sympathetic response are retained.

ketazolam $C_{20}H_{17}ClN_2O_3$. A benzodiazepine tranquilizer with properties much like diazepam.

keten $O{=}C{=}CH_2$. The parent compound indicated in the formula or any of its substituted derivatives. Ketens are highly reactive with nucleophiles; the parent compound reacts with water to form acetic acid and with ammonia to form acetamide. Ketens are useful in organic synthesis.

ketimine   An imine formed between a ketone and an amine, as between enzyme-bound pyridoxamine phosphate and a 2-oxoacid in an aminotransferase. Compare ALDIMINE.

keto-   [German *Keton* ketone, from French *acétone* ketone, from L *acetum* vinegar + Gk suffix *-ōnē* denoting female descendant] A combining form indicating the presence of a carbonyl group. ● Although *keto-* was once used in systematic nomenclature, the form *oxo-* is now used in its place to signify replacement of CH_2 by CO, but the word *keto* is still used to designate a class of substance. Thus, 2-oxoglutaric acid is a keto acid. It is sometimes used in carbohydrate nomenclature to signify replacement of CHOH by CO.

keto acid   A substance containing both a carbonyl group and an acidic group. 2-Oxoacids, formed by oxidation of carbohydrates and of branched-chain amino acids, as well as by transamination of amino acids, are the most biologically important keto acids.

ketoacidosis   A metabolic acidosis associated with an accumulation of ketone bodies that are characteristic of uncontrolled diabetes mellitus.

   diabetic ketoacidosis   Ketoacidosis resulting from uncontrolled diabetes mellitus. The precipitating cause may be failure to take insulin, infection, or acute stressful illness. The clinical picture is one of severe dehydration, prostration, fever, hypotension, hyperpnea, and, if untreated, shock and death. Also called *diabetic acidosis*.

ketoaciduria   KETONURIA.

   branched chain ketoaciduria   MAPLE SYRUP URINE DISEASE.

β-ketoacyl-ACP reductase   3-OXOACYL-ACP REDUCTASE.

3-ketoacyl-CoA thiolase   An outmoded term for ACE-TYL-COA ACETYLTRANSFERASE.

ketoaminoacidemia   MAPLE SYRUP URINE DISEASE.

ketodeoxyoctonate   Usually 2-keto-3-deoxyoctonate. It is an octose sugar, oxidized to the carboxylic acid at C-1, and to the ketone at C-2, and reduced to CH_2 at C-3. It is alternatively described as a 3-deoxyoctulosonic acid, or more strictly as a 2-dehydro-3-deoxyoctonic acid. It occurs in the pyranose form, with O-6 bound to C-2. The compound with the mannose configuration at C-4 to C-7 is important in the linking of the antigenic branched polysaccharides of bacterial cell walls to the core lipopolysaccharide structure. Abbreviation: KDO

ketogenesis   The formation of the ketones acetoacetate, acetone, and β-hydroxybutyrate.

ketogenetic   KETOGENIC.

ketogenic   Of or relating to ketogenesis. Also *ketogenetic*.

2-ketogluconate   The compound formed when the hydroxyl group on the number 2 carbon of gluconic acid is oxidized to a ketone group.

α-ketoglutarate dehydrogenase   An outmoded term for OX-OGLUTARATE DEHYDROGENASE.

α-ketoglutaric acid   An outmoded term for 2-OXOGLUTARIC ACID.

ketol   A ketone that carries a hydroxyl group on one of the carbon atoms next to the carbonyl group. A seldom used term.

ketolytic   Capable of destroying ketones, particularly of lowering the blood concentration of ketone bodies.

ketonaemia   A British spelling for KETONEMIA.

ketone   A compound containing a carbonyl group, CO, bonded to two other carbon atoms. Ketones are typically less reactive than aldehydes, because the two alkyl groups are usually elec-

tron-donating and diminish the electrophilic reactivity of the carbonyl group.

ketonemia   ACETONEMIA.

ketonic   Related to a ketone. A ketonic substance contains the carbonyl group, but often contains other functional groups.

ketonuria   The excretion of ketone bodies in the urine, as seen in starvation, fever, and diabetes mellitus. Also called *ketoaciduria*, *ketosuria*, *hyperketonuria*, *acetonuria* (seldom used), *oxonuria* (seldom used).

ketopantoic acid $CH_2OH—C(CH_3)_2—CO—COOH$. 4-Hydroxy-3,3-dimethyl-2-oxobutyric acid, i.e. 2-dehydropantoic acid. A precursor of pantoic acid in its biosynthesis from valine. This reaction does not occur in mammals, which require pantothenic acid in their diet.

ketoplasia   [*keto-*, combining form from *ketone*, arbitrary variant of French *acétone* acetone + -PLASIA]   The formation of ketone bodies.

ketoplastic   Causing ketone body production.

ketopregnene   A progestational steroid isolated from human corpus luteum and placenta in two isomeric forms, 20α- and 20β-hydroxy-pregn-4-ene-3-one.

ketose   A sugar that is a ketone, in distinction from an aldose, which is a sugar that is an aldehyde. All monosaccharide molecules consist of a chain of carbon atoms. One of these carbon atoms is in a carbonyl group, and each of the others carries a hydroxyl group. Hence the carbonyl group of a ketose is not at the end of the chain. All natural ketoses known are uloses, i.e. the second atom in the chain is in the carbonyl group.

ketoside   The glycoside formed by a ketose, e.g. a fructoside.

ketosis   [*keto(ne bodies)* + -SIS]   A disordered metabolic state occurring in starvation, acute alcoholism, and uncontrolled diabetes mellitus, characterized by the accumulation of ketone bodies in cells, extracellular fluid, and plasma. The biochemical basis is incomplete combustion of long-chain fatty acids to carbon dioxide and water. Adjective: ketotic.

   bovine ketosis   A disease of cows, characterized by ketonemia and ketonuria. It is most prevalent in high-producing dairy cows, occurring within a few weeks after parturition. It is associated with a disturbance of carbohydrate metabolism. Also called *bovine acetonemia*.

ketosteroid   A steroid that is a ketone.

17-ketosteroid   A steroid with a carbonyl group at C-17. Measurements of neutral 17-ketosteroids are taken to indicate metabolites of androgens, because C-21 steroids derived from progesterone and corticosteroids cannot possess the 17-carbonyl group, and estrogens are phenolic and so are not neutral, i.e. they are extracted from an organic solvent by alkali before the test is made.

ketosuria   KETONURIA.

β-ketothiolase   An outmoded term for ACETYL-COA ACYL-TRANSFERASE.

ketotic   Of, relating to, or characteristic of ketosis.

ketourine   [*keto(ne)*, arbitrary variant of *acetone*, from L *acetum* vinegar, + URINE]   Urine produced while the patient is on a ketogenic diet. A seldom used term.

ketoxime   An oxime formed from a ketone, in distinction from an aldoxime, which is formed from an aldehyde.

kettle / bronchitis kettle   A kettle used to humidify air with steam in treatment of bronchitis.

keV   Symbol for the unit, kiloelectronvolt.

Key   [Charles Aston *Key*, English surgeon, 1793–1849]   **1** See under OPERATION.   **2** Hodgkin-Key murmur. See under MURMUR.

Key   [Ernst Axel Henrik *Key*, Swedish anatomist, 1832–1901]

1 Foramen of Key and Retzius. See under APERTURA LATERALIS VENTRICULI QUARTI. **2** Key-Retzius sheath, connective tissue sheath of Key and Retzius. See under ENDONEURIUM.

key / coding key A listing of data groupings and the various letters, numbers, or symbols assigned to each, such as might be used in a double-blind clinical trial.

dental key TOOTH KEY.

determinative key A diagram of the properties of various bacteria which enables one to identify a species by tracing its properties through successive forks in a branching tree.

tetanizing key A reed that vibrates a copper contact in and out of mercury to interrupt current.

tooth key An instrument used for the extraction of teeth before the introduction of dental forceps. It consisted of a shaft with a double right-angled handle, like a corkscrew handle. At the distal end of the shaft was a hinged claw which gripped the tooth on the lingual side when the shaft was laid horizontally on the buccal side. A rotary movement of the shaft extracted the tooth. Also called *dental key.*

torquing key An orthodontic instrument for fitting rectangular arch wires into edgewise brackets.

keypunch A machine with a keyboard which enables an operator to punch holes in punch cards for entering data into a computer. Also called *card punch.*

keyway [*key* + *way*] **1** The dovetailed part of a prepared cavity in a tooth, designed to improve retention of the restoration. **2** The dovetailed groove in the female part of a precision attachment.

kg Symbol for the unit, kilogram.

kgf Symbol for the unit, kilogram-force.

kgm **1** Symbol for the unit, kilogram-meter. **2** Symbol for the unit, kilogram. An incorrect symbol.

khat CATHA.

KHN Knoop hardness number.

Khoisan A human racial and linguistic group including the Bushmen and Hottentots of Southern Africa, characterized by short stature, gracile body form, a light brown skin, reduced body hair and peppercorn scalp hair. Another characteristic feature of the group is the presence of steatopygia.

kHz Symbol for the unit, kilohertz.

kibe [Middle English *kybe*] Mild frostbite; chilblain. An obsolete term.

kibisitome [Gk *kibisi(s)* a pocket, pouch + -TOME] A surgical device for cutting the capsule of the crystalline lens.

kick / atrial kick Forceful contraction of the atrium which leads to distension and rise in pressure in the ventricle, especially in the presence of ventricular hypertrophy as in aortic stenosis or hypertension. It is associated with a marked a wave in the apexcardiogram and a fourth heart sound.

kidingapopo [Swahili, dengue fever] A viral disease that may be dengue. It has been described in Zanzibar.

kidney

kidney [Middle English *kidenei,* prob. from the Scandinavian] Either of a pair of organs in the dorsal area of the abdominal cavity of vertebrates which function to excrete waste products and to maintain fluid, electrolyte, and acid-base homeostasis; ren.

aglomerular kidney A kidney which contains no glomeruli, such as that found in elasmobranchs.

amyloid kidney RENAL AMYLOIDOSIS.

arteriolosclerotic kidney ARTERIOLONEPHROSCLEROSIS.

artificial kidney A popular term for HEMODIALYZER.

atrophic kidney RENAL ATROPHY.

blue kidney Renal hemosiderosis with a blue tinge to the kidney, secondary to considerable intravascular hemolysis.

branny kidney A kidney on whose surface are seen opaque granules representing fatty degeneration.

cake kidney A form of fused kidney characterized by a lobular anterior renal surface, from which the ureters arise, and a smooth concave posterior surface. It is usually situated in the pelvis. Also called *clump kidney, L-shaped kidney.*

cicatricial kidney CONTRACTED KIDNEY.

clump kidney CAKE KIDNEY.

coarsely granular kidney A kidney with large, depressed, irregular scars on its surface, with irregular elevations between the scars, usually associated with arterionephrosclerosis.

confluent kidney FUSED KIDNEY.

congenital double kidney Reduplication of the ureter, renal pelvis and kidney occurring to a varying degree (usually incomplete), resulting from a reduplication of the embryologic ureteric bud. It may be associated with other urogenital anomalies. Although usually asymptomatic, the congenital duplication of these structures may make them prone to infection, obstruction, and calculus formation.

congested kidney Excess blood in the kidney, usually secondary to congestive heart failure or obstruction of the vena cava or renal veins. Renal function may be moderately decreased, but it returns to normal when the heart failure or obstruction responds to treatment. Also called *cyanotic kidney* (seldom used).

contracted kidney A small, shrunken kidney with a finely and coarsely granular surface and a thick adherent capsule. Scattered elevations 0.5 to 2 cm long separated by deep, wedge-shaped scars may be present, while small cysts are common. Many chronic glomerular, vascular, or interstitial diseases may lead to contracted kidneys and uremia. Also called *cicatricial kidney.*

crush kidney Acute tubular necrosis secondary to shock resulting from severe crushing injuries.

cyanotic kidney A seldom used term for CONGESTED KIDNEY.

cystic kidney A kidney marked by the presence of one or more cysts.

definitive kidney METANEPHROS.

disk kidney A disk-shaped excretory organ formed by fusion of both poles of the renal anlagen. Also called *doughnut kidney.* See also RENAL FUSION.

double kidney An incorrect term for DOUBLE URETER.

doughnut kidney DISK KIDNEY.

dystopic kidney A congenital anomaly in which one or both kidneys are in an abnormal position, held in place by anomalous blood vessels which persisted from early fetal life. The abnormally placed kidney usually is deformed and small. It may be located in the pelvis, sacroiliac area, thorax or elsewhere. It is more common in males, and may be associated with other congenital anomalies. Also called *ectopia of the kidney, renal ectopia, ectopia renis, ectopic kidney.*

ectopic kidney DYSTOPIC KIDNEY.

embryonic kidney The pronephros, mesonephros, and metanephros.

fatty kidney A large, white kidney with increased lipid content, usually associated with the nephrotic syndrome. The medulla is darker than the cortex. Also called *large white kidney, putty kidney, renal lipoidosis* (rarely used).

finely granular kidney A kidney sometimes seen when the capsule is stripped off at autopsy. Small, pale, surface elevations of approximately 0.2 cm or less are separated by darker, shallow depressions. The elevations represent dilated tubules, the depressions atrophy and scarring.

flea-bitten kidney A kidney with pinhead-sized red spots scattered irregularly over the surface, sometimes seen in the focal glomerulonephritis of subacute bacterial endocarditis.

floating kidney A popular term for NEPHROPTOSIS.

Formad's kidney An enlarged, deformed kidney alleged to occur in chronic alcoholism. There is no documentation for this condition. An obsolete term.

fused kidney A congenital anomaly characterized by fusion of both kidneys at the upper or lower pole (horseshoe kidney), at both poles (disk or doughnut kidney), along the entire length (cake kidney), or at the contralateral upper and lower poles (sigmoid kidney), or location of both kidneys on one side, with fusion between the lower and upper poles (tandem kidney). Fused kidneys are usually in the pelvis or at level of the fifth lumbar vertebra. The vascular supply and course of the ureters also usually are anomolous. It is caused by adherence during embryogenesis of the metanephric organs after they have passed through the crotch between the embryonic umbilical arteries in ascending from their pelvic site of origin. Fused kidneys are susceptible to calculi, hydronephrosis, and infection. Also called *confluent kidney, renal fusion.*

Goldblatt kidney A kidney in which, in experimental animals, the renal artery has been constricted, producing hypertension.

gouty kidney URATE NEPHROPATHY.

granular kidney A kidney characterized by elevations separated by depressed scars and distributed over the renal surface, which may be fine or coarse.

head kidney PRONEPHROS.

horseshoe kidney A form of fused kidney in which the kidneys are fused at either the upper or, more commonly, the lower poles. There may also be some caudal ectopia and hyporotation. This condition is associated with an increased risk of calculi, hydronephrosis, and infection. Also called *ren unguliformis.*

infarcted kidney RENAL INFARCT.

intrathoracic kidney A very rare congenital anomaly in which the kidneys are located in the thorax.

lardaceous kidney RENAL AMYLOIDOSIS.

large red kidney A kidney congested because of inflammation, impaired venous drainage, or urinary tract obstruction. A rarely used term.

large white kidney FATTY KIDNEY.

L-shaped kidney CAKE KIDNEY.

lump kidney SIGMOID KIDNEY.

medullary cystic kidney MEDULLARY CYSTIC DISEASE.

medullary sponge kidney A congenital anomaly affecting one or, much more commonly, both kidneys, in which a large number of small cysts arise from the calices or collection ducts in the pyramids. The condition usually is asymptomatic, the diagnosis being made on characteristic changes in the intravenous pyelogram. In a few patients calculi, recurrent infections, or recurrent hematuria may complicate the condition. However, prognosis is good and life expectancy is normal. Also called *sponge kidney, Cacchi-Ricci disease.*

middle kidney MESONEPHROS.

monopyramidal kidney UNILOBAR KIDNEY.

mortar kidney A rarely used term for RENAL TUBERCULOSIS.

movable kidney NEPHROPTOSIS.

multicystic kidney POLYCYSTIC RENAL DISEASE.

multilobar kidney A kidney consisting of more than one lobe, up to 18 having been reported in humans.

mural kidney An uncommon anomalous condition in which the kidney is situated in a peritoneal pouch in the abdominal wall.

myelin kidney A gray and mottled kidney with yellow flecks on gross examination, usually in patients who have had nephrotic syndrome. An outmoded term.

myeloma kidney A complication of multiple myeloma characterized by diffuse atrophy of tubules associated with dense casts and multinucleated giant cells, and by an interstitial nephritis often leading to uremia. Myeloma kidney is almost always associated with Bence Jones proteinuria. Bence Jones protein has been demonstrated to have a toxic effect on renal tubule cells. Excretion of other proteins is usual, and may be great enough to lead to the nephrotic syndrome.

palpable kidney A kidney that can be palpated in a flank. In adults a palpable kidney usually indicates an enlarged kidney.

pelvic kidney A kidney abnormally located in the pelvic cavity, often a fused kidney.

polycystic kidney POLYCYSTIC RENAL DISEASE.

polypyramidal kidney A kidney with more than the usual five to seven pyramids.

primitive kidney PRONEPHROS.

primordial kidney PRONEPHROS.

putty kidney FATTY KIDNEY.

sacciform kidney NEPHRECTASIA.

sclerotic kidney NEPHROSCLEROSIS.

sigmoid kidney A type of fused kidney in which the two kidneys are fused at their upper and lower contralateral poles. Also called *lump kidney, tandem kidney.*

single kidney Fused kidneys in which there is little external indication of their original duality and in which a single irregular mass at any of several locations serves the functional role of the two normal organs. Two ureters usually emerge from separate sites on the surface.

soapy kidney An outmoded term for RENAL AMYLOIDOSIS.

solitary kidney A single kidney, either congenital or due to surgical removal.

sponge kidney MEDULLARY SPONGE KIDNEY.

sulfa kidney SULFONAMIDE TOXICITY.

tandem kidney SIGMOID KIDNEY.

unilateral kidney 1 UNILATERAL FUSED KIDNEY. 2 The one existing kidney in unilateral renal agenesis, usually located at the approximate normal level of the kidney of that side.

unilateral fused kidney A fused kidney lying on one or the other side of the vertebral column, usually at or near the vertebral level of the normal kidney of that side. Also called *unilateral kidney.*

unilobar kidney A kidney containing a single lobe; a rare, abnormal condition in a human kidney, which normally contains 5 to 11 lobes each comprising a pyramid, protruding into the calyx region, and associated cortex. In some species, such as the beaver and the pig, a single lobe is the typical appearance. Also called *monopyramidal kidney.*

wandering kidney A popular term for NEPHROPTOSIS.

waxy kidney A rarely used term for RENAL AMYLOIDOSIS.

Kielland [Christian *Kielland*, Norwegian gynecologist, 1871–1941] See under FORCEPS.

Kien [Alphonse-Marie-Joseph *Kien*, German physician, flourished 19th century] Kussmaul-Kien respiration. See under KUSSMAUL RESPIRATION.

Kienböck [Robert *Kienböck*, Austrian physician, 1871–1953] **1** See under UNIT, DISEASE, DISLOCATION, PHENOMENON. **2** Kienböck-Adamson points. See under POINT.

Kiernan [Francis *Kiernan*, Irish-born British physician, 1800–1874] Kiernan spaces. See under PORTAL CANAL.

kieselguhr [German *Kiesel* quartz, hard stone, flint + *Guhr* loose earth deposited in cavities by water] DIATOMACEOUS EARTH.

Kieser [Willibald *Kieser*, German physician, flourished mid-20th century] Turner-Kieser syndrome. See under NAIL-PATELLA SYNDROME.

Kiesselbach [Wilhelm *Kiesselbach*, German laryngologist, 1839–1902] Kiesselbach space. See under AREA.

kiestein KYESTEIN.

kil A white clay found near the Black Sea that was once used as a vehicle (ointment) for dermatotherapy.

Kilian [Hermann Friedrich *Kilian*, German gynecologist, 1800–1863] See under LINE.

killeen CARRAGEEN.

Killian [Gustav *Killian*, German laryngologist, 1860–1921] **1** Killian's tubes. See under TUBE. **2** Killian's operation. See under KILLIAN FRONTAL SINUS OPERATION. **3** See under DEHISCENCE. **4** Killian nasal speculum. See under SPECULUM.

killing / mercy killing See under EUTHANASIA.

kilo- [Gk *chilioi* one thousand] A combining form denoting 10^3, one thousand: used with SI units. Symbol: k

kiloampere [KILO- + AMPERE] A unit of electric current equal to 10^3 amperes. Symbol: kA

kilobecquerel [KILO- + BECQUEREL] A unit of activity of a radionuclide equal to 10^3 becquerel. Symbol: kBq

kilocalorie [KILO- + CALORIE] A unit of quantity of heat equal to 10^3 calories; 4.2 kilojoules approximately. Symbol: kcal

kilocoulomb [KILO- + COULOMB] A unit of quantity of electricity, electric charge, or electric flux, equal to 10^3 coulombs. Symbol: kC

kilocurie [KILO- + CURIE] A unit of activity of a radionuclide or of a radioactive source equal to 10^3 curies; 3.7×10^{13} becquerels, exactly. Symbol: kCi

kilocycle [KILO- + CYCLE] See under KILOCYCLE PER SECOND.

kilocycle per second A unit of frequency equal to 10^3 cycles per second; 10^3 hertz. Symbol: kc/s • The term *kilohertz,* a unit with the same meaning, is more commonly used than *kilocycle per second. Kilocycle* is often but incorrectly used for *kilocycle per second.*

kilodalton A unit of mass equal to 1000 daltons. It is used to describe a molecule with a molar mass of 1 kg/mol, and a relative molecular mass of 1000. This unit is widely used in biochemistry. Symbol: kDa

kilodyne [KILO- + DYNE] A unit of force equal to 10^3 dynes; 10^{-2} newton. Symbol: kdyn

kiloelectronvolt A unit of energy equal to 10^3 electronvolts. Symbol: keV

kilogram [KILO- + GRAM] The SI base unit of mass, equal to 10^3 grams; 2.2046 pounds. It is equal to the mass of the international prototype of the kilogram, a solid cylinder of platinum-iridium in the custody of the Bureau International des Poids et Mesures, Sèvres, France. The kilogram is also the unit of weight used in commercial trading. Symbol: kg

kilogram-calorie CALORIE.

kilogram-force The technical unit of force in the metric gravitational system of units, being that force which, acting on a mass of one kilogram, gives to it an acceleration equal to the internationally agreed acceleration of free fall, 9.806 65 meters per second squared; 9.806 65 newtons. Also called *kilopond (German usage).* Symbol: kgf

kilogram-force meter A unit of moment of force, the product of one kilogram-force and one meter, equal to 9.806 65 newton-meters. Also called *kilopond-meter (German usage), kilogram-meter (incorrect but often used).* Symbol: kgf·m

kilogram-meter An incorrect but commonly used term for KILOGRAM-FORCE METER. See under KILOGRAM-FORCE.

Kiloh [Leslie Gordon *Kiloh*, Australian physician, flourished 20th century] Kiloh-Nevin syndrome. See under OCULAR MYOPATHY.

kilohertz A unit of frequency equal to 10^3 hertz. Symbol: kHz

kilohm A unit of electrical resistance equal to 10^3 ohms. Also called *kiloohm.* Symbol: kΩ

kilojoule [KILO- + JOULE] A unit of energy, work, or quantity of heat equal to 10^3 joules. Symbol: kJ

kilokatal [KILO- + KATAL] A unit of catalytic activity equal to 10^3 katal; 10^3 mole per second. Symbol: kkat

kiloliter [KILO- + LITER] A unit of volume or capacity equal to 10^3 liters or one cubic meter. A rarely used term. Symbol: kl

kilomegacycle [KILO- + MEGACYCLE] See under KILOMEGACYCLE PER SECOND.

kilomegacycle per second A unit of frequency equal to 10^9 cycles per second; 10^9 hertz; 1 gigahertz. An obsolete unit. Symbol: kMc/s

kilometer [KILO- + METER] A unit of length equal to 10^3 meters; 0.6214 mile or 1093.6 yards or 3280.8 feet. Symbol: km

square kilometer A unit of area equal to 10^6 square meters; 100 hectares; 0.386 square mile or 247.105 acres. Symbol: km²

kilonem [KILO- + NEM] A nutritional milk unit, equal to 10^3 nem.

kilonewton [KILO- + NEWTON] A unit of force equal to 10^3 newtons. Symbol: kN

kiloohm KILOHM.

kilopascal [KILO- + PASCAL] A unit of pressure or stress equal to 10^3 pascals. Symbol: kPa

kilopascal second per liter The SI derived unit of vascular resistance to flow (and resistance to flow in airways), equal to 10.204 conventional centimeters of water second per liter; 10 dyne second per centimeter to the fifth power; 0.125 conventional millimeter of mercury minute per liter. Symbol: kPa·s/l, kPa·s·l^{-1}

kilopond [KILO- + POND] The German term for KILOGRAM-FORCE. Symbol: kp

kilopond-meter The German term for KILOGRAM-FORCE METER.

kiloroentgen [KILO- + ROENTGEN] A unit of ionization exposure equal to 10^3 roentgen; 0.258 coulomb per kilogram. Symbol: kR

kilosecond [KILO- + SECOND] A unit of time equal to 10^3 seconds. Symbol: ks

kilotonne [KILO- + TONNE] A unit of mass or weight equal to 10^3 tonnes, or 10^6 kilograms. It is used especially to describe the equivalent explosive power of nuclear weapons in terms of tonnes of TNT. Symbol: kt

kilounit [KILO- + UNIT] A quantity equal to 10^3 units.

kilovar [KILO- + VAR] A unit of electrical power equal to 10^3 var. Symbol: kvar

kilovolt [KILO- + VOLT] A unit of electrical potential, potential difference, or electromotive force, equal to 10^3 volts. Symbol: kV

kilovolt-ampere A unit of electric power equal to 10^3 volt-amperes. Symbol: kV·A

kilowatt [KILO- + WATT] A unit of power equal to 10^3 watts. Symbol: kW

kilowatt-hour A unit of energy, especially electric energy, equal to the work done by a power of one kilowatt in one hour; 3.6×10^6 joules. Symbol: kW·h

kilurane [*kil(o)* + *uran(ium)* + *e*] A unit of radioactivity equal to 10^3 uranium units. An obsolete unit.

Kimmelstiel [Paul *Kimmelstiel*, German-born physician, 1900–1970] **1** Kimmelstiel-Wilson syndrome. See under DIABETIC GLOMERULOSCLEROSIS. **2** Kimmelstiel-Wilson lesion. See under LESION.

kimputu An African term for RELAPSING FEVER.

kin- KINE-.

kinaesthesia A British spelling for KINESTHESIA.

kinaesthesiometer A British spelling for KINESTHESIOMETER.

kinanaesthesia A British spelling for KINANESTHESIA.

kinanesthesia [KIN- + ANESTHESIA] Loss of position and joint sense and of deep pressure sensation, resulting in the inability to perceive movement at joints, especially in the limbs. Also *cinanesthesia*.

kinase Any enzyme that transfers a phospho group from ATP or from another nucleoside triphosphate onto a hydroxyl group to form a phosphate or onto an amino group to form a phosphoramidate.

kindling A neurological phenomenon characterized by the relatively enduring reduction in threshold of a function or of neuronal activity by a brain structure following a period of sustained activation of a distant locus with which the structure has neuronal connections. Often the distant locus is the contralateral homologue of the affected structure. Activation of the distant site may occur through pathologic change or may be induced experimentally by electrical or chemical stimuli.

kine- [Gk *kinein* to move] A combining form meaning movement, motion. Also *cine-, kin-, cin-*.

kinemadiagraphy [*kinema* for *cinema* + DIA- + -GRAPHY] An obsolete term for CINERADIOGRAPHY.

kinematics [French *cinématique* (from Gk *kinēma*, gen. *kinēmatos*, motion + French *-ique* -ICS) the part of mechanics that studies motion] The science of motion without reference to force or mass. Also called *cinematics*.

kinemia [KIN- + -EMIA] An outmoded term for CARDIAC OUTPUT.

kinemic Relating to cardiac output.

kineplastics KINEPLASTY.

kineplasty [KINE- + -PLASTY] A method of amputation, usually of the upper extremity of man, in which the muscles and tendons in the stump are arranged so that they can transmit movements through a mechanical prosthesis. Skin grafts or flaps are often used to isolate the tendons or muscles. Also called *cinematic amputation, cineplastic amputation, cinematization* (outmoded), *cineplastics, cineplasty, kineplastics, cineplastic surgery*.

kinesalgia Pain evoked by movement. Also called *kinesialgia, cinesalgia*.

kinescope [KINE- + -SCOPE] A device for refraction based upon the principle of subjective movement of an object positioned in front of the pupil.

kinesi- KINESIO-.

kinesia [*kines(i)-* + -IA] MOTION SICKNESS.

   kinesia paradoxa PARADOXICAL KINESIA.

   paradoxical kinesia Transient disappearance of akinesia, chiefly in parkinsonism, with the concomitant appearance of rapid movements, such as running, boxing, etc. Also called *kinesia paradoxa*.

kinesialgia KINESALGIA.

kinesiatrics KINESITHERAPY.

kinesic **1** KINETIC. **2** Pertaining to kinesics.

kinesics [*kines(o)-* + -ICS] The study of motion and action as a communications vehicle.

kinesiesthesiometer KINESTHESIOMETER.

kinesigenic Produced by movement. Also *kinesogenic*.

kinesimeter An instrument used for measuring bodily movements. Also called *cinometer*.

kinesio- [Gk *kinēsis* movement] A combining form meaning movement, motion. Also *cinesio-, kinesi-, cinesi-, kineso-, cineso-*.

kinesiodic KINESODIC.

kinesiology The study of muscular movements of the body and of its parts, especially with reference to therapy. Also called *kinology, cinology*.

kinesiometer KINESTHESIOMETER.

kinesioneurosis [KINESIO- + NEUROSIS] Any neurosis in which tics or other movements are seen. An older term.

   vascular kinesioneurosis A neurosis associated with vasomotor manifestations.

kinesiotherapy KINESITHERAPY.

kinesipathist A practitioner of kinesitherapy.

kinesis [Gk *kinēsis* movement] (*plural* kineses) **1** Generalized movements of an organism or population of organisms, especially in response to an environmental stimulus, such as light. **2** MOTION SICKNESS.

kinesitherapy [KINESI- + THERAPY] The therapeutic use of muscle or body movements administered as a course of exercises. Also called *kinesiotherapy, kinetotherapy, kinesotherapy, kinesiatrics*.

kineso- KINESIO-.

kinesodic Concerning the conduction of impulses in motor nerves. Also *kinesiodic*.

kinesogenic **1** KINETOGENIC. **2** KINESIGENIC.

kinesophobia Pathologic fear of motion or motion sickness.

kinesotherapy KINESITHERAPY.

kinesthesia [KIN- + ESTHESIA] The sensation or perception of movement of the body or its parts. Also called *kinesthesis, kinesthetic sense, kinesthetic sensation, kinesthetic sensibility*. Compare PROPRIOCEPTION. • The term is often imprecisely used to include sensations of static position, loading, or resistance to movement.

kinesthesiometer An instrument for testing joint sense. Also called *kinesiometer, kinesiesthesiometer*.

kinesthesis KINESTHESIA.

kinesthetic Of or related to kinesthesia.

kinetia MOTION SICKNESS.

kinetic [See KINETICS.] Relating to or characterized by motion. Also *kinesic*.

kineticist One who studies kinetics.

kinetics [Gk *kinētikos* putting in motion, stirring up, from *kinēsis* a moving, motion, from *kinein* to move, set in motion] The branch of science dealing with the production of movement and the rate of change, acceleration, and deceleration of bodies in motion in relation to the forces acting on them.

   chemical kinetics The study of the rates of chemical reactions and the factors that affect them.

   first-order kinetics The kinetics characteristic of first-order reactions. In these reactions the rate is proportional to the concentration of reactant, and the logarithm of this concentration falls linearly with time. In a given interval a constant fraction of reactant disappears.

   Michaelis kinetics The relationship between the rate of an enzyme-catalyzed reaction and the concentration of free substrate that is expressed by the Michaelis-Menten equation. Also called *Michaelis-Menten kinetics*.

   Michaelis-Menten kinetics MICHAELIS KINETICS.

   pre-steady-state kinetics The study of the rates of enzyme-catalyzed reactions under conditions when it cannot be assumed that the concentration of enzyme-substrate complex is constant.

For much of the course of the reaction this constancy may be assumed, but at early stages after mixing enzyme and substrate the concentration of this complex must rise, and the study of the rate it does so can reveal some rate constants that cannot be determined from measurements made once the steady state has been reached. Also called *transient kinetics*.

transient kinetics   PRE-STEADY-STATE KINETICS.

kinetin   6-Furfurylaminopurine, a purine that acts as a growth factor in plants which at low concentrations increases the mitotic rate in meristems, generally by reducing the duration of the interphase. It may not occur in nature.

kinetism   The ability to produce muscular activity.

kineto-   [Gk *kinētikos* (from *kinein* to move) putting in motion] A combining form meaning movement, motion. Also *cineto-*.

kinetocardiogram   A record of the low-frequency vibrations of the anterior chest wall over the cardiac region. Also called *precordial cardiogram*.

kinetocardiograph   The instrument used to detect and display the kinetocardiogram.

kinetocardiography   The process of recording the low frequency vibrations of the anterior chest wall over the cardiac region.

kinetochore   CENTROMERE.

kinetogenic   Causing movement. Also *kinesogenic*.

kinetographic   Of or relating to kinetography. Also called *motorgraphic*.

kinetography   The process of recording movement. Also called *kinetoscopy*.

kinetoplasm   1 The highly contractile portion of the cell cytoplasm.   2 A region of the cytoplasm of a neuron which contains chromophilic material.

kinetoplast [KINETO- + -PLAST]   A DNA-rich organelle forming part of the cytoplasmic kinetic complex of certain protozoans, such as the flagellates (order Kinetoplastida, subphylum Mastigophora). The kinetoplast is included within a single large mitochondrion extending the length of the body. It is associated with the basal granule (kinetosome) from which the flagellum arises. It is also closely associated with the parabasal body, which appears to be related to nuclear division. The exact function of each of these entities is uncertain, and some authorities consider the entire complex to form a single kinetoplast. Also called *motion nucleus*.

Kinetoplastida   [Gk *kinēto(s)* moving, movable + -PLAST + New L *-ida*, neut. pl. in form from L *-ides*, patronymic suffix] An order of flagellate protozoa in the class Zoomastigophorea, subphylum Mastigophora, characterized by one or two anterior flagella and a single mitochondrion extending the length of the body, with a conspicuous DNA-containing kinetoplast near the flagellar kinetosomes. The order contains the suborders Bodonina (typical genera: *Bodo, Cryptobia, Rhynchomonas)* and Trypanosomatina (genera *Leishmania, Trypanosoma)*. Most species are parasitic. Also called *Protomastigida (former name)*.

kinetoscope   An instrument for making serial photographs of movements.

kinetoscopy   KINETOGRAPHY.

kinetoses   Plural of KINETOSIS.

kinetosis   MOTION SICKNESS.

kinetosome   BASAL BODY.

kinetotherapeutic   Relating to kinesitherapy.

kinetotherapy   KINESITHERAPY.

King   [Brien Thaxton *King*, U.S. surgeon, born 1886]   See under OPERATION.

King   [Earl Judson *King*, Canadian biochemist, 1901–1962] King-Armstrong unit. See under UNIT.

kingdom   [Middle English, from Old English *cyningdom*, from *cyning* king + *dom* a condition, state, judgment] A taxonomic group, the primary category in the classification of organisms. For various methods of classifying kingdoms see under TWO-KINGDOM SYSTEM, THREE-KINGDOM SYSTEM, etc.

Kingsley   [Norman William *Kingsley*, U.S. dentist, 1829–1913] See under SPLINT.

kinin   A basic peptide released from a plasma protein by proteolysis in the allergic response, and capable of causing vasodilatation and contraction of smooth muscle.

venom kinin   A peptide in the venom of certain insects that acts on blood vessels, smooth muscles, and certain nerve endings.

wasp kinin   A peptide in wasp venom which induces rapid and intense pain.

kininogen   A protein that, upon cleavage by a kininogenase such as kallikrein, forms kinins. Two kininogens are recognized: high molecular weight kininogen, which yields bradykinin following kallikrein cleavage, and low molecular weight kininogen, which yields kallidin following cleavage.

high molecular weight kininogen   A plasma protein of 110 000 MW that normally exists in plasma in a 1:1 complex with prekallikrein. The complex is a cofactor in the activation of coagulation factor XII. The product of this reaction, factor XIIa, in turn activates prekallikrein to kallikrein, which cleaves high molecular weight kininogen to form bradykinin, a vasodilator, and two other fragments that accelerate coagulation.

low molecular weight kininogen   A protein of 50 000 MW that occurs in various normal tissues and which, upon cleavage by kallikrein or other kininogenase, forms kallidin. Kallidin, in turn, is converted to bradykinin.

kininogenase   KALLIKREIN.

kink   A sharp twist or bend.

ileal kink   Obstruction of the terminal ileum due to kinking of Lane's band, an anomalous membrane connecting the ileum and mesentery to the cecum. Also called *Lane's kink*.

Lane's kink   ILEAL KINK.

Kinnier Wilson   [Samuel Alexander *Kinnier Wilson*, English neurologist, 1877–1937]   1 Kinnier Wilson sign. See under WILSON SIGN.   2 Kinnier Wilson disease. See under WILSON'S DISEASE.

kino   The dried juice from the trunk of *Pterocarpus marsupium*, a powerful astringent. It was used often in combination with opium to treat diarrhea and dysentery. Depending upon its origin, it is called East Indian kino, Malabar kino, Madras kino, or Cochino kino.

eucalyptus kino   EUCALYPTUS GUM.

kino-   [Gk *kinein* to move]   A combining form meaning movement, motion. Also *cino-*.

kinocentrum   [KINO- + CENTRUM]   CENTROSOME.

kinocilium   [KINO- + CILIUM]   (*plural* kinocilia) A cytoplasmic filament that is motile and extends out from the plasma membrane or free surface of a cell.

kinohapt   [KINO- + Gk *hapt(ein)* to touch]   An instrument for making a number of tactile stimuli at established intervals of time or space.

kinology   KINESIOLOGY.

kinomere   CENTROMERE.

kinomometer   An instrument that measures the range of motion.

kinosphere   [KINO- + SPHERE]   ASTER.

kinotoxin   [KINO- + TOXIN]   FATIGUE TOXIN.

kinship   1 Relatedness among individuals or groups based on consanguinity or on connect ion through marriage.   2 A group of individuals whose relatedness is based on consanguinity.

kiono- CIONO-.

kiotome [Gk *kiō(n)* a pillar, the uvula + -TOME] An obsolete term for UVULATOME.

kiotomy [Gk *kiō(n)* a column, the uvula + -TOMY] An obsolete term for UVULOTOMY.

kip [*ki(lo)-* + *p(ound)*] In the United States, a unit of force equal to 10^3 pounds-force; 4.448 22 kilonewtons. A popular unit. Symbol: kip

Kirk [Norman Thomas *Kirk*, U.S. surgeon, 1888–1960] See under AMPUTATION.

Kirkland [Olin *Kirkland*, U.S. periodontist, 1876–1969] See under KNIFE.

kirromycin An antibiotic that blocks release of EFTu·GDP from the ribosome, thus preventing completion of the initiation step in protein synthesis in bacteria.

Kirschner [Martin *Kirschner*, German surgeon, 1879–1942] 1 See under WIRE, APPARATUS. 2 Kirschner wire splint. See under SPLINT.

Kisch [Bruno *Kisch*, German physiologist, 1890–1966] Kisch reflex. See under EXTERNAL AUDITORY MEATUS REFLEX.

kitasamycin An antibiotic compound from *Streptomyces kitasatoensis*, with properties much like those of erythromycin.

kiting Falsification of a prescription by increasing the quantity of the drug prescribed.

kitol A vitamin A precursor from whale oil.

kJ Symbol for the unit, kilojoule.

Kjeldahl [Johan Gustav Christoffer *Kjeldahl*, Danish chemist, 1849–1900] Kjeldahl's method, macro-Kjeldahl method. See under TEST.

kkat Symbol for the unit, kilokatal.

kl Symbol for the unit, kiloliter.

Klapp [Rudolph *Klapp*, German surgeon, 1873–1949] 1 Klapp's suction cups. See under CUP. 2 Klapp's method. See under KLAPP'S CREEPING TREATMENT.

Klauder [Joseph Victor *Klauder*, U.S. dermatologist, 1888–1962] See under SYNDROME.

Klebs [Theodor Albrecht Edwin *Klebs*, German pathologist, 1834–1913] Klebs Löffler bacillus. See under *CORYNEBACTERIUM DIPHTHERIAE*.

Klebsiella A genus of Enterobacteriaceae closely related metabolically to *Enterobacter*, but differing in its range of surface antigens and in often being a primary pathogen.

Klebsiella ozaenae A species that causes a progressive fetid atrophy of the nasal mucosa.

Klebsiella pneumoniae The most important human pathogen of the *Klebsiella* group. It forms an unusually large capsule of various serologic types. It is an occasional component of the normal throat flora, a secondary invader in chronic pulmonary infection, and a primary cause of severe pneumonia and of urinary-tract infection. Also called *Friedlaender's bacillus* (older term).

Klebsiella rhinoscleromatis A species that causes a destructive granuloma of the nose and pharynx.

Klein [David *Klein*, Swiss geneticist, born 1908] Franceschetti-Zwahlen-Klein syndrome, Franceschetti-Klein syndrome. See under MANDIBULOFACIAL DYSOSTOSIS.

Klein [Edward Emanuel *Klein*, Hungarian bacteriologist active in England, 1844–1925] Klein's muscle. See under AEBY'S MUSCLE.

Kleine [Willi *Kleine*, German psychiatrist, flourished 20th century] Kleine-Levin syndrome. See under SYNDROME.

-kleisis -CLEISIS.

Kleist [Karl *Kleist*, German neurologist and physician, born 1879] 1 See under CLASSIFICATION, SIGN. 2 Kleist's oppo-

sition motor phenomenon. See under MAYER-REISCH PHENOMENON.

Klemm [Paul *Klemm*, Russian physician, 1861–1921] Klemm's tetanus. See under CEPHALIC TETANUS.

Klemperer [Felix *Klemperer*, German physician, 1866–1931] See under TUBERCULIN.

Klemperer [Georg *Klemperer*, German physician, 1865–1946] 1 Klemperer's disease. See under BANTI'S DISEASE. 2 See under TUBERCULIN.

kleptolagnia [Gk *klept(ein)* to steal + *o* + *lagneia* lust, desire] Sexual excitement induced by stealing.

kleptomania [Gk *klept(ein)* + *o* + -MANIA] A disorder of impulse control consisting of stealing. It is senseless in that the objects are not taken for use or for their value. Also *cleptomania*.

kleptomaniac A person exhibiting kleptomania.

Kleyn [Adrianus Paulus Huibertus Antoine de *Kleyn*, Dutch otorhinolaryngologist, flourished mid-20th century] Van der Hoeve-Kleyn syndrome. See under SYNDROME.

KLHC keyhole-limpet hemocyanin.

Klieg [after John H *Kliegl*, German-born U.S. lighting equipment manufacturer, 1869–1959] See under EYE.

Kligler [Israel J. *Kligler*, U.S. bacteriologist, 1889–1943] See under AGAR.

Kline [Benjamin Schoenbrun *Kline*, U.S. pathologist, 1886–1968] Kline-Young test. See under KLINE TEST.

Klinefelter [Harry Fitch *Klinefelter*, Jr., U.S. physician, born 1912] See under SYNDROME.

Klippel [Maurice *Klippel*, French neurologist, 1858–1942] 1 Kippel's disease. See under ARTHRITIC GENERAL PSEUDOPARALYSIS. 2 Klippel-Feil sign. See under SIGN. 3 Klippel-Feil syndrome. See under SYNDROME. 4 Klippel-Feil malformation. See under MALFORMATION. 5 Klippel and Weil sign. See under THUMB SIGN. 6 Klippel-Trenaunay syndrome. See under KLIPPEL-TRENAUNAY-WEBER SYNDROME.

kliseometer CLISEOMETER.

Kloeckera A form-genus of yeastlike fungi of the form-class Blastomycetidae.

Kloeckera apiculatus A form-species of fungi which ferment glucose sugar in fruit. Also called *Saccharomyces apiculatus* (incorrect).

Klossiella A worldwide genus of sporozoan parasites of the family Klossiellidae which infect endothelial cells of renal capillaries and arterioles after ingestion by the host of infective sporocysts, which then release sporozoites. Sexual stages occur in the epithelial cells of renal tubules, after which sporocysts are passed in the urine. *K. equi* is a usually nonpathogenic species in equids. *K. muris* is a fairly common parasite of laboratory mice, ordinarily nonpathogenic except in very heavy infections.

Klotz [Henri Pierre *Klotz*, French endocrinologist, born 1910] See under SYNDROME.

Kluge [Karl Alexander Ferdinand *Kluge*, German obstetrician, 1782–1844] Kluge sign. See under CHADWICK SIGN.

Klumpke [Augusta Dejerine-*Klumpke*, French neurologist, 1859–1927] Dejerine-Klumpke paralysis, Klumpke's paralysis, Klumpke-Dejerine syndrome, Klumpke-Dejerine paralysis. See under DEJERINE-KLUMPKE SYNDROME.

Klüver [Heinrich *Klüver*, German-born U.S. neurologist, born 1897] Klüver-Bucy syndrome. See under SYNDROME.

km Symbol for the unit, kilometer.

km² Symbol for the unit, square kilometer.

kMc kilomegacycle.

kMc.p.s. Symbol for the obsolete unit, kilomegacycle per second. An incorrect symbol.

kMc/s Symbol for the obsolete unit, kilomegacycle per second.

kN Symbol for the unit, kilonewton.

Knapp [Herman Jakob *Knapp*, U.S. ophthalmologist, 1832–1911] **1** Knapp streak, Knapp stria. See under ANGIOID STREAK,. **2** See under OPERATION. **3** Knapp's forceps. See under TRACHOMA FORCEPS.

Knaus [Hermann Hubert *Knaus*, Austrian physiologist, born 1892] **1** See under REACTION, RULE. **2** Ogino-Knaus method. See under METHOD.

kneading A massage technique in which the muscles are grasped and pressed in a manner similar to kneading dough. Also called *pétrissage.*

knee [Old English *cnēow*; akin to L *genu* knee and Gk *gony* knee] The articulation of the lower limb that joins the femur, patella, and tibia, along with the region surrounding this articulation; genus; articulatio genus.

knee of aquaeductus fallopii GENICULUM CANALIS FACI-ALIS.

back knee GENU RECURVATUM.

beat knee Bursitis and/or cellulitis due to prolonged pressure and friction on the knee. It occurs in miners who are obliged to work in a kneeling position. A similar condition may affect the elbow.

Brodie's knee BRODIE'S DISEASE.

conventional single axis knee A simple low-cost prosthetic knee mechanism that provides for a constant friction or braking action during the swing phase of locomotion.

housemaids' knee A prepatellar bursitis caused by excessive kneeling on a hard surface, as found among housemaids who regularly scrub floors. A similar condition may affect clergymen and nuns.

hydraulic knee A complex prosthetic knee that allows for variations in swing more closely duplicating the normal movement of the lower extremity than does the conventional single axis knee.

in knee GENU VALGUM.

knee of internal capsule GENU CAPSULAE INTERNAE.

jumpers' knee Chondromalacia of the patella occurring in basketball players and long-distance runners. It is probably caused by repeated minor trauma. Also called *runners' knee.*

little knee of facial canal GENICULUM CANALIS FACIALIS.

locked knee The inability to extend fully the knee because of the presence of a loose body in the joint, a tear of a meniscus, or patellofemoral derangement.

out knee GENU VARUM.

rugby knee OSGOOD-SCHLATTER DISEASE.

runners' knee JUMPERS' KNEE.

snapping knee Crepitus within the knee.

kneecap PATELLA.

kneippism A therapeutic regimen utilizing applications of cold water and particularly walking barefoot in snow or dewy grass. The practice is primarily restricted to Germany and carried out at specialized Kneipp health resorts.

Knemidokoptes [Gk *knēmis*, gen. *knēmidos*, a greave, leg armor, from *knēmē* the leg between the knee and ankle + *koptein* to strike, cut, knock down, slay] A genus of bird mange mites in the family Knemidokoptidae. Also *Cnemidocoptes.*

Knemidokoptes gallinae The depluming mite, a species that causes irritation at the base of the feathers, principally of the wings and tail, of fowl. Feather loss often results from the itching which causes the birds to pluck their feathers.

Knemidokoptes mutans The scalyleg mite, a species of microscopic mite found under the scales of the legs of domestic fowl and cage birds, and which causes thickening, crusting, and deformity.

Knemidokoptes pilae A species that causes mange among caged parakeets *(Melopsittacus)* in the United States. It princi-

pally affects the face and the base of beak and the legs.

Knies [Max *Knies*, German ophthalmologist, 1851–1917] See under SIGN.

knife [Old English *cnīf*] Any surgical instrument with one or more sharp blades, designed in many shapes and configurations and used to incise tissues.

amputating knife Any surgical blade used for performing limb amputations.

Ballenger swivel knife An instrument for removing large portions of the quadrilateral cartilage in submucous resection of the nasal septum. The small knife blade, set at right angles at the end of the divided shaft, swivels so as to remain in line with the direction of thrust.

Beer's knife A rather broad, pointed knife designed to make corneal incisions.

Blair knife A long, straight-edged knife used for the free-hand harvesting of split-thickness skin grafts.

buck knife A spear-shaped gingivectomy knife.

button knife A small-bladed knife used for cutting cartilage.

cataract knife A slim knife designed for making an incision across the superior one-third of the limbus during the procedure for extraction of an opaque crystalline lens.

cautery knife A modified scalpel that utilizes current from an electric cautery. Also called *electric knife, electrosurgical knife, endotherm knife.*

electric knife CAUTERY KNIFE.

electrosurgical knife CAUTERY KNIFE.

endotherm knife CAUTERY KNIFE.

gold knife **1** A dental hand instrument used for trimming gold foil restorations. **2** A large knife used to cut gold foil into small pieces for insertion into a tooth cavity.

Goldman-Fox knife One of a set of gingivectomy knives.

Graefe's knife A type of cataract knife.

hernia knife A small, sharp surgical blade designed to incise a hernial sac. Also called *herniotome.*

Humby knife A knife for harvesting split-thickness skin grafts or excising burned tissue, having a roller guide for adjusting the thickness of the graft.

Joseph knife A pointed, double-edged scalpel used in the performance of a rhinoplasty.

Kirkland knife A heart-shaped gingivectomy knife.

lenticular knife A knife designed for surgical procedures on or about the lens of the eye.

Liston's knife A long surgical blade used in limb amputations.

meniscectomy knife A knife with a short, sharp cutting edge that is used to excise the peripheral attachment of a torn meniscus.

Merrifield's knife A gingivectomy knife with a triangular blade.

Ramsbotham sickle knife A seldom-used, sickle-shaped instrument designed to decapitate a fetus in order to facilitate vaginal delivery.

Thiersch knife A specially designed knife for cutting partial-thickness skin grafts.

Knight [James *Knight*, U.S. physician, born 1810] **1** See under BRACE. **2** Knight-Taylor brace. See under BRACE.

knismogenic [Gk *knismo(s)* a tickling, itching + -GENIC] Giving rise to a sensation of tickling.

knismolagnia [Gk *knismo(s)* a tickling + *lagneia* lust, desire] A paraphilia in which sexual gratification depends upon being tickled by the sexual partner.

knitting The repair process of a bone fracture. A popular usage.

knob [Middle English *knobbe* knob, bud] A rounded protuberance or mass.

aortic knob The prominence caused by the aortic arch in a chest radiograph.

basal knob A node or swelling at the cell surface from which the cilium projects.

double aortic knob Persistence of two aortic arches, resulting from a variation in development of the primitive vascular arches.

embryonic knob The part of the inner cell mass consisting of the primary ectoderm and endoderm after the migration of the parietal endodermal cells, which are involved in the formation of the yolk sac, has occurred. In some mammals, notably the rodents, this represents the earliest stage of egg cylinder formation.

surfers' knobs SURFERS' KNOTS.

synaptic knob END FOOT.

terminal knob END FOOT.

knock / pericardial knock A clicking sound occasionally heard on auscultation of the heart after penetrating trauma to the pericardium.

knock-knee GENU VALGUM.

Knoepfelmacher [Wilhelm *Knoepfelmacher*, Austrian pediatrician, born 1866] See under MEAL.

knokkelkoorts [Dutch *knokkel* knuckle + *koorts* fever] A Dutch term for DENGUE, used in Indonesia.

Knoop [Frederick *Knoop*, U.S. metallurgist, flourished 20th century] Knoop hardness number. See under NUMBER.

knot [Old English *cnotta*] **1** An interlacing or looping of a string, thread, rope, or strip of material such as may be used in attaching or securing it to another structure. **2** A knoblike mass, such as a node; a clump of cells, vessels, or nerves suggestive of a knot.

clove-hitch knot A knot in which two contiguous loops are applied around the end of a limb to permit traction on the part for reduction of a dislocation or for immobilizing fractures.

double knot FRICTION KNOT.

enamel knot A cluster of epithelial cells associated with a small protuberance at the center of the enamel organ. It appears during the cap stage of tooth development. Also called *enamel node*.

false knot A varicosity of umbilical cord vessels, giving the appearance of a knot.

friction knot A knot used in surgical procedures that is made by twisting the ends of the suture twice rather than once before the knot is tied. Also called *double knot, surgeons' knot, surgical knot*.

granny knot A surgical knot consisting of two separate knots placed in such a way that the two knots may slide on the suture when pressure is applied.

Hensen's knot A primitive node at the cephalic end of the primitive streak. Also called *Hubrecht's protochordal knot, protochordal knot*.

Hubrecht's protochordal knot HENSEN'S KNOT.

net knot KARYOSOME.

primitive knot HENSEN'S NODE.

protochordal knot HENSEN'S KNOT.

reef knot SQUARE KNOT.

sailor's knot SQUARE KNOT.

square knot A surgical double knot in which the two throws of the knot lie in the same plane, thus preventing slippage. Also called *sailor's knot, reef knot*.

stay knot A surgical knot made with two or more square-knotted sutures.

surfers' knots A conditon characterized by fibrotic hyperplastic nodules approximately 3 cm or less in diameter that appear over the bony prominences of the feet and legs of surfers as a result of repeated trauma from kneeling on surfboards. Also called *Malibu disease, surfers' knobs, surfers' nodules*.

surgeons' knot FRICTION KNOT.

surgical knot FRICTION KNOT.

syncytial knot A multinucleated mass on the outer aspect of the chorionic trophoblast in the established placenta.

true knot An actual knot in the umbilical cord that occurs as a result of intrauterine movement of the fetus. Also called *knot of umbilical cord*.

knot of umbilical cord TRUE KNOT.

knowledge of results Information given a learner about the correctness or error of responses made, thus providing a system of feedback. A hypothesis of the learning theory proposes that learning is much facilitated when the learner is informed promptly about the occurrence of error, and its direction. Abbreviation: KR.

knuckle [Middle English *knokel*, akin to Old English *cnotta* knot] **1** A prominence produced by the posterior aspect of any interphalangeal or metacarpophalangeal joint when the finger is flexed or the hand is clenched. **2** Any of various anatomical structures resembling such a flexed, knoblike prominence.

aortic knuckle The terminal part of the arch of the aorta seen above the heart as a rounded shadow, usually to the left of the vertebral column, in anteroposterior radiographs.

cervical aortic knuckle An anomaly of the aortic arch when it extends into the neck, forming an anteroposterior arch, for varying distances as high as the hyoid bone.

kΩ Symbol for the unit, kilohm.

Kobelt [George Ludwig *Kobelt*, German physician, 1804–1857] **1** See under CYST. **2** Kobelt's tubes. See under TUBE. **3** Kobelt's tubules. See under TUBULE.

Köbner [Heinrich *Köbner*, German dermatologist, 1838–1904] Köbner's phenomenon. See under ISOMORPHIC EFFECT.

KOC kathodal (cathodal) opening contraction.

Koch [Heinrich Herman Robert *Koch*, German bacteriologist, 1843–1910] **1** Koch's postulates. See under LAW. **2** Koch-Weeks conjunctivitis. See under ACUTE CONTAGIOUS CONJUNCTIVITIS. **3** Koch-Weeks bacillus. See under *HAEMOPHILUS AEGYPTIUS*. **4** Koch's phenomenon. See under REACTION. **5** Koch's lymph. See under OLD TUBERCULIN.

Koch [Walter *Koch*, German surgeon, born 1880] Koch's node. See under NODUS ATRIOVENTRICULARIS.

Kocher [Emil Theodor *Kocher*, Swiss surgeon, 1841–1917] **1** Kocher's sign, Kocher symptom. See under GLOBE LAG. **2** See under INCISION, POINT, FORCEPS, MANEUVER, OPERATION, SYNDROME. **3** Kocher's reflex. See under TESTICULAR COMPRESSION REFLEX. **4** Kocher-Debré-Semelaigne syndrome. See under DEBRÉ-SEMELAIGNE SYNDROME.

kocherization [after Emil Theodor *Kocher*, Swiss surgeon, 1841–1917 + *-iz(e)* + -ATION] The surgical technique of reflecting the second portion of the duodenum and head of the pancreas, commonly used to facilitate the transduodenal exposure of the ampulla of Vater.

Kocks [Joseph *Kocks*, German surgeon, 1846–1916] See under OPERATION.

Koeppe [Leonhard *Koeppe*, German physician, born 1884] Koeppe nodules. See under NODULE.

Koerber [Hermann *Koerber*, German ophthalmologist, born 1878] Koerber-Salus-Elschnig syndrome. See under AQUEDUCT OF SYLVIUS SYNDROME.

Koester [Karl *Koester*, German pathologist, 1843–1904] See under NODULE.

Koga [Kensai *Koga*, Japanese physician, flourished 20th century] See under TREATMENT.

Kogoj [Franjo *Kogoj*, Yugoslavian dermatologist, born 1894] Spongiform pustule of Kogoj. See under PUSTULE.

Köhler [Alban *Köhler*, German roentgenologist, 1874–1947] **1** See under DISEASE. **2** Köhler's second disease. See under DISEASE. **3** Köhler-Pellegrini-Stieda disease. See under PELLEGRINI-STIEDA DISEASE.

Köhler [August Karl Johann Valentin *Köhler*, German microscopist, 1866–1948] See under ILLUMINATION.

Köhlmeier [W. *Köhlmeier*, German dermatologist, flourished mid-20th century] Köhlmeier-Degos disease, progressive arterial occlusive disease (Köhlmeier-Degos). See under MALIGNANT ATROPHIC PAPULOSIS OF DEGOS.

Kohlrausch [Otto Ludwig Bernhard *Kohlrausch*, German physician, 1811–1854] **1** Kohlrausch folds, Kohlrausch valves. See under PLICAE TRANSVERSALES RECTI. **2** Kohlrausch veins. See under VEIN.

Kohn [Hans N. *Kohn*, German pathologist, born 1866] See under PORE.

Kohnstamm [Oskar *Kohnstamm*, German physician, 1871–1917] See under PHENOMENON.

koilo- [Gk *koilos* (adjective) hollow] A combining form meaning hollow in shape, concave.

koilocytosis A cell conformation that is characterized by concavity of the cell membrane, as seen in the normal mature red blood cell.

koilonychia [*koil(o)*- + *onych*- + -IA] The presence of spoon-shaped nails, with a concave surface. Also called *spoon nail*.

koilorrhachic [KOILO- + *rrach(i)*- + -IC] Exhibiting a reversal of normal lumbar lordosis such that the spine appears concave in the lumbar region when viewed anteriorly.

koilosternia PECTUS EXCAVATUM.

koilosternum PECTUS EXCAVATUM.

koino- CENO-².

kojic acid 2-Hydroxymethyl-5-hydroxypyran-4-one. A compound formed by bacterial action on any of several sugars, including glucose. It retains the pyran ring of the sugar, being the product of dehydration and dehydrogenation of aldopyranoses.

koktigen A vaccine prepared by boiling a suspension of bacteria in isotonic saline for 30 minutes.

Kolle [Wilhelm *Kolle*, German bacteriologist, 1868–1935] See under SERUM.

Kölliker [Rudolf Albert von *Kölliker*, Swiss anatomist and physiologist, 1817–1905] **1** Kölliker's nucleus. See under SUBSTANTIA INTERMEDIA CENTRALIS MEDULLAE SPINALIS. **2** Kölliker's interstitial granules. See under GRANULE. **3** Kölliker's reticulum. See under NEUROGLIA. **4** Kölliker's layer. See under STROMA IRIDIS. **5** Kölliker's gland. See under GLANDULA OLFACTORIA. **6** Kölliker's membrane. See under MEMBRANA RETICULARIS DUCTUS COCHLEARIS. **7** Column of Kölliker. See under SARCOSTYLE.

Kollmann [Arthur *Kollmann*, German urologist, born 1858] See under DILATOR.

Kolmer [John A. *Kolmer*, U.S. pathologist, 1886–1962] See under TEST.

kolp- COLPO-.

kolpo- COLPO-.

kolypeptic [Gk *kōly(ein)* to hinder + *peptik(os)* (from *pept(ein)*, also *pessein* to cook, digest + *-ikos* -IC) promoting digestion, able to digest] Inhibiting or interfering with digestion. Also *colypeptic*.

kolyphrenia [Gk *kōly(ein)* to hinder + -PHRENIA] A state characterized by inhibition of thinking. Also *colyphrenia*.

kombé [Swahili, a climbing plant yielding poison for arrows] An African arrow poison derived from the ripe seeds of *Strophathnus kombé*. It contains the glycosides cymarin and stro-

phanthin. The latter, in large doses, is a muscle poison, but in small doses is a cardiac stimulant.

kombic acid An acid occurring as a glucoside in the ripe seeds of *Strophanthus kombé*. It is a powerful cardiac stimulant.

Konakion A proprietary name for vitamin K₁.

Kondoleon [Emmanuel *Kondoleon*, Greek surgeon, 1879–1939] See under OPERATION.

kongo [Kongo, a native language of Zaire] An epidemic disease of unknown etiology, found in Zaire and marked by painful paresthesiae in the legs, leading rapidly to paraplegia.

König [Charles Joseph *König*, French otologist, born 1868] König's rods. See under KÖNIG CYLINDERS.

König [Franz *König*, German surgeon, 1832–1910] **1** König's disease. See under OSTEOCHONDRITIS DISSECANS. **2** See under OPERATION.

konimeter [Gk *koni(s)* dust + -METER] A portable instrument for making a rough and rapid evaluation of airborne dust concentrations. It consists of a hand-primed pump that draws a known volume of air through a jet on to a plate on which particles are counted under magnification. Also called *coniometer, jet dust counter, konometer*.

koniocortex [Gk *koni(a)* dust + *o* + CORTEX] The areas of the cerebral cortex, especially the sensory areas, containing a thick granular layer. Also called *coniocortex*.

koniology CONIOLOGY.

koniosis CONIOSIS.

konjac [Japanese *konjak(u)* a large aroid] The poisonous corm of *Amorphophallus rivieri*. It has been used medicinally in Asia to treat snake bite, insect bites, and as a febrifuge.

konometer KONIMETER.

kopf-tetanus [German *Kopf* head + TETANUS] CEPHALIC TETANUS.

kopiopia COPIOPIA.

Koplik [Henry *Koplik*, U.S. pediatrician, 1858–1927] **1** Koplik sign, Koplik's spots. See under SPOT. **2** Koplik stigma of degeneration. See under STIGMA.

Kopp [Johann Heinrich *Kopp*, German physician, 1777–1858] Kopp's asthma. See under LARYNGISMUS STRIDULUS.

kopr- COPRO-.

kopro- COPRO-.

Korányi [Friedrich von *Korányi*, Hungarian physician, 1828–1913] See under TREATMENT.

Korff [Karl von *Korff*, German anatomist and histologist, flourished 20th century] Korff's fibers. See under FIBER.

Kornberg [Arthur *Kornberg*, U.S. physician and biochemist, born 1918] See under ENZYME.

Kornzweig [Abraham Leon *Kornzweig*, U.S. physician, born 1900] Bassen-Kornzweig disease, Bassen-Kornzweig syndrome. See under ABETALIPOPROTEINEMIA.

koro [Malayan] An acute delusional syndrome seen in Malaya and Southern China and characterized by depersonalization and the delusion that the subject's penis is shrinking into his abdomen.

koronion CORONION.

koroscopy [Gk *kor(ē)* the pupil of the eye + *o* + -SCOPY] Retinoscopic measurement of the refractive error.

Korotkoff [Nikolai Sergeivich *Korotkoff*, Russian physician, 1874–1920] **1** See under METHOD, TEST. **2** Korotkoff sounds. See under SOUND.

Korsakoff [Sergei Sergeivich *Korsakoff*, Russian psychiatrist, 1854–1900] **1** Korsakoff's disease, Korsakoff syndrome. See under PSYCHOSIS. **2** Wernicke-Korsakoff syndrome. See under WERNICKE-KORSAKOFF PSYCHOSIS.

Körte [Werner *Körte*, German surgeon, 1853–1937] Körte-Ballance operation. See under OPERATION.

Kostmann [Rolf *Kostmann*, Swedish physician, born 1909] **1** Kostmann's disease. See under FANCONI'S ANEMIA. **2** Kostmann's disease. See under CONGENITAL NEUTROPENIA.

koumiss [Tatar *kumyz*] **1** Originally, a fermented alcoholic drink made from mare's milk by Tatars. **2** A powder preparation containing yeast and lactic-acid producing organisms, used to make fermented milk drinks for dietary purposes from cow's milk, or a beverage so made. Also called *lac fermentum.*

kousso BRAYERA.

Kovalevsky [Aleksandr Onufrievich *Kovalevsky*, Russian embryologist, 1840–1901] Kovalevsky's canal. See under NEURENTERIC CANAL.

Koyanagi [Yoshizo *Koyanagi*, Japanese ophthalmologist, 1880–1954] Vogt-Koyanagi syndrome. See under SYNDROME.

Kozhevnikov [Aleksei Yakovlevich *Kozhevnikov*, Russian neurologist, 1836–1902] Kozhenvnikov's disease, Kozhevnikov's epilepsy, Kozhevnikov syndrome. See under CONTINUOUS PARTIAL EPILEPSY.

KP **1** keratitic precipitates. **2** keratitis punctata.

kp Symbol for the unit, kilopond.

kPa Symbol for the unit, kilopascal.

kPa·s/l Symbol for the unit, kilopascal second per liter.

kPa·s·l⁻¹ Symbol for the unit, kilopascal second per liter.

Kr Symbol for the element, krypton.

kR Symbol for the unit, kiloroentgen.

Krabbe [Knud H. *Krabbe*, Danish neurologist, 1885–1961] **1** Krabbe syndrome. See under CONGENITAL GENERALIZED MUSCULAR HYPOPLASIA. **2** Krabbe's leukodystrophy, Krabbe type diffuse sclerosis. See under DISEASE. **3** Christensen-Krabbe disease, Christensen-Krabbe progressive infantile cerebral poliodystrophy. See under KRABBE'S DISEASE.

Kraepelin [Emil *Kraepelin*, German psychiatrist, 1856–1926] **1** See under CLASSIFICATION. **2** Morel-Kraepelin disease. See under SCHIZOPHRENIA.

krait [Hindi *karait*] Any venomous snake of the elapid genus *Bungarus.*

banded krait A poisonous elapid snake of southeastern Asia belonging to the species *Bungarus fasciatus.* These snakes have highly colored rings around their bodies.

kra-kra [prob. from Dutch *krauw(en)* to scratch] A west African term for DERMATITIS NODOSA.

krameric acid A tannic acid from *Krameria*, a South American shrub. It is an astringent compound that has been used in mouthwashes and in the treatment of diarrhea.

Kraske [Paul *Kraske*, German surgeon, 1851–1930] See under POSITION, OPERATION.

kratom [Thai (also called Siamese)] The leaf of *Mitragyna speciosa.* It is chewed for its opiumlike effect.

kratometer [Gk *krato(s)* strength + -METER] An orthoptic device for strabismus measurement and training.

krauomania A form of tic exhibiting rhythmic movements such as nodding or intermittent rotation of the head.

kraurosis / kraurosis penis BALANITIS XEROTICA OBLITERANS.

kraurosis vulvae Primary atrophy of the vulva.

Krause [Fedor *Krause*, German surgeon, 1857–1937] **1** Krause-Wolfe graft, Wolfe-Krause graft, Krause's method, Wolfe-Krause operation. See under FULL-THICKNESS GRAFT. **2** Hartley-Krause operation. See under OPERATION.

Krause [Karl Friedrich Theodor *Krause*, German anatomist, 1797–1868] **1** Krause glands. See under GLAND. **2** Krause glands. See under GLANDULAE LACRIMALES ACCESSORIAE. **3**

Krause glands, glandulae mucosae conjunctivae krausei. See under GLANDULAE CONJUNCTIVALES. **4** Krause ligament. See under LIGAMENTUM TRANSVERSUM PERINEI. **5** Posterior costotransverse ligament of Krause. See under LIGAMENTUM COSTOTRANSVERSARIUM LATERALE. **6** Krause valve. See under BÉRAUD'S VALVE.

Krause [Wilhelm *Krause*, German anatomist, 1833–1910] **1** Krause respiratory bundle. See under TRACTUS SOLITARIUS. **2** Krause line, Krause membrane. See under Z BAND. **3** Krause bone. See under OS ACETABULI. **4** Ulnar collateral nerve of Krause. See under NERVE. **5** Bulbs of Krause. **6** Bulbs of Krause. See under CORPUSCULA BULBOIDEA. **7** Posterior jugular process of occipital bone of Krause. See under PROCESSUS PARAMASTOIDEUS OSSIS OCCIPITALIS.

kreat CREAT.

krebiozen A substance, isolated from the blood of horses previously injected with *Actinomyces bovis*, that was claimed to cure cancer. The major component in the preparations was identified as creatine. Its use has been prohibited in the United States by the Food and Drug Administration.

Krebs [Carl *Krebs*, Danish pathologist, born 1892] See under TUMOR.

Krebs [Sir Hans Adolf *Krebs*, German-born English biochemist, born 1900] **1** Krebs cycle. See under TRICARBOXYLIC ACID CYCLE. **2** Krebs-Henseleit cycle. See under UREA CYCLE. **3** Krebs-Ringer solution. See under SOLUTION.

kreotoxicon [Gk *kre(as)* meat + *o* + *toxicon* a poison for arrows] The substance present in contaminated meat that causes toxic symptoms. Also *creatoxicon, creotoxicon.*

kreotoxin [Gk *kre(as)* meat + *o* + TOXIN] A toxin in meat produced by microorganisms. Also *creatoxin, creotoxin.*

kreotoxism [Gk *kre(as)* meat + *o* + TOX- + -ISM] Meat poisoning. Also *creatoxism, creotoxism.*

Kretschmann [Friederick *Kretschmann*, German otologist, 1858–1934] See under SPACE.

Kretz [Richard *Kretz*, German pathologist, 1865–1920] Kretz granules. See under GRANULE.

Kreysig [Fridrich Ludwig *Kreysig*, German physician, 1770–1839] Kreysig sign. See under HEIM-KREYSIG SIGN.

krinin CRININ.

Krishaber [Maurice *Krishaber*, Hungarian physician active in France, 1836–1883] See under DISEASE.

Kristeller [Samuel *Kristeller*, German gynecologist, 1820–1900] **1** Kristeller technique. See under KRISTELLER'S METHOD. **2** Kristeller expression. See under EXPRESSION OF FETUS. **3** See under MANEUVER.

Krogh [Schack August Steenberg *Krogh*, Danish physiologist, 1874–1949] See under APPARATUS.

Kromayer [Ernst L. F. *Kromayer*, German dermatologist, 1862–1933] See under TREATMENT, LAMP.

Krompecher [Edmund *Krompecher*, Hungarian pathologist, 1870–1926] Krompecher's tumor, Krompecher's carcinoma. See under BASAL CELL CARCINOMA.

Kronecker [Karl Hugo *Kronecker*, Swiss pathologist, 1839–1914] **1** See under PUNCTURE. **2** Kronecker center. See under CARDIOINHIBITORY CENTER.

Krönig [Georg *Krönig*, German physician, 1856–1911] **1** See under PERCUSSION. **2** Krönig's field, Krönig's isthmus. See under AREA.

Krönlein [Rudolf U. *Krönlein*, Swiss surgeon, 1847–1910] See under OPERATION.

Krukenberg [Adolph *Krukenberg*, German anatomist, 1816–1877] Krukenberg's veins. See under VENAE CENTRALES HEPATIS.

Krukenberg [Friedrich Ernst *Krukenberg*, German pathologist, 1871–1946] **1** See under TUMOR. **2** Axenfeld-Krukenberg spindle. See under KRUKENBERG SPINDLE.

Krukenberg [Herman *Krukenberg*, German surgeon, born 1863] **1** Krukenberg's hand. See under ARM. **2** See under AMPUTATION.

Krumwiede [Charles *Krumwiede*, U.S. physician, 1879–1930] Krumwiede triple sugar agar. See under AGAR.

krymotherapy CRYOTHERAPY.

kryolith CRYOLITE.

krypto- CRYPTO-.

krypton A rare gas having atomic number 36, atomic weight 83.80. It is present in the atmosphere in a concentration of about one part per million. Six stable isotopes occur in nature and 15 unstable isotopes have been reported. Long believed to be inert chemically, krypton forms a few compounds with fluorine. The most notable of the few uses of krypton is based on the wavelength of the orange-red line in the spectrum of krypton 86, which has been adopted as the basic standard of length in defining the meter. Symbol: Kr

krypton 85 A radioactive isotope of krypton, emitting beta and gamma radiation. It has been used in the study of respiratory exchange, cardiac output, and peripheral blood flow. Physical half-life is 10.6 years. Symbol: ^{85}Kr

17-KS 17-ketosteroid.

ks Symbol for the unit, kilosecond.

KSC kathodal (cathodal) closing contraction.

KST kathodal (cathodal) closing tetanus.

kt Symbol for the unit, kilotonne.

KUB A roentgenogram of the abdomen designed to reveal abnormalities of the kidneys, ureters, or bladder; a scout film of the abdomen.

kubisagari [Japanese *kubi* head, neck + *sagaru* to hang down] A Japanese term for VESTIBULAR NEURONITIS.

Kufs [H. *Kufs*, German psychiatrist, 1871–1955] Kufs type amaurotic familial idiocy. See under KUFS DISEASE.

Kugelberg [Eric Klas Henrik *Kugelberg*, Swedish neurologist, born 1913] Kugelberg-Welander disease, Kugelberg-Welander syndrome. See under JUVENILE FAMILIAL MUSCULAR ATROPHY.

Kuhn [Ernst *Kuhn*, German physician, 1873–1920] See under MASK.

Kuhn [Franz *Kuhn*, German surgeon, 1866–1929] See under TUBE.

Kühne [Wilhelm Friedrich *Kühne*, German physiologist and histologist, 1837–1900] **1** Kühne's terminal plates. See under PLATE. **2** Kühne's muscular phenomenon. See under PHENOMENON. **3** Kühne's fiber. See under MUSCLE SPINDLE.

Kuhnt [Hermann *Kuhnt*, German ophthalmologist, 1850–1925] **1** Kuhnt-Szymanowski procedure. See under KUHNT-SZYMANOWSKI OPERATION. **2** See under MENISCUS, TISSUE. **3** Kuhnt-Junius disease, Kuhnt-Junius degeneration. See under DISCIFORM MACULAR DEGENERATION. **4** Kuhnt spaces. See under SPACE. **5** Kuhnt's postcentral vein. See under VEIN.

kukuruku [Hausa] A Nigerian disease of unknown origin characterized by jaundice and fever. Although it resembles yellow fever, it is probably caused by a virus of the viral hepatitis group.

Kulchitsky [Nicholas *Kulchitsky*, Russian histologist, 1856–1925] **1** Kulchitsky cell carcinoma. See under CARCINOID. **2** Kulchitsky cell. See under ARGENTAFFIN CELL. **3** See under HEMATOXYLIN.

Kulenkampff [Dietrich *Kulenkampff*, German surgeon, born 1880] See under ANESTHESIA.

Kümmell [Hermann *Kümmell*, German surgeon, 1852–1937]

Kümmell-Verneuil disease, Kümmell spondylitis. See under KÜMMELL'S DISEASE.

Kunkel [Henry George *Kunkel*, U.S. physician, born 1916] See under SYNDROME.

Küntscher [Gerhard *Küntscher*, German surgeon, 1902–1972] See under NAIL.

Kupffer [Karl Wilhelm von *Kupffer*, German anatomist, 1829–1902] **1** Kupffer cell sarcoma. See under SARCOMA. **2** Von Kupffer cell. See under KUPFFER CELL.

Kupressoff [J. *Kupressoff*, Russian physician, flourished latter 19th century] Kupressoff center. See under MICTURITION CENTER.

Kurie [Franz Newell Devereux *Kurie*, U.S. physicist, born 1907] See under PLOT.

Kurloff [Mikhail Georgievich *Kurloff*, Russian physician, 1859–1932] **1** Kurloff bodies. See under BODY. **2** See under CELL.

kurtosis [Gk *kyrtōsis* (from *kyrt(os)* curved, convex + -*ōsis* -OSIS) convexity] The relative height at the mode of the curve of a unimodal frequency distribution.

kuru [Malayo-Polynesian] A transmissible spongiform encephalopathy due to a slow infection believed to be caused by a prion, found only among the Fore people in the eastern highlands of Papua New Guinea. After a very long incubation period (10–20 years), the disease presents as progressive cerebellar ataxia with tremor of the head, trunk, and limbs, dysarthria, and dementia. Death usually ensues in 3–9 months. At autopsy, the vermis cerebelli and its afferent and efferent connections show marked degenerative changes. Kuru was seen principally in Fore women and children, the traditional participants in a cannibalistic mourning rite involving consumption of a dead kinsman, with infection resulting from autoinoculation from ingestion of infected brain tissue. As cannibalism among the Fore has ceased, the disease is now rare. Little is known about the agent, which is extremely small, highly resistant to activation, and similar to the agents of other slow infections such as scrapie and Creutzfeldt-Jakob disease. The agent is transmissible by peripheral or intracerebral inoculation to chimpanzees, some monkeys, ferrets, and mink. Also called *smiling corpse disease, laughing disease*.

Küss [Emil *Küss*, German physiologist, 1815–1871] See under EXPERIMENT.

Küss [Georges *Küss*, French physician, 1867–1936] Küss-Ghon focus. See under GHON TUBERCLE.

Kussmaul [Adolf *Kussmaul*, German physician, 1822–1902] **1** See under COMA. **2** Kussmaul's aphasia. See under HYSTERICAL MUTISM. **3** Kussmaul breathing, Kussmaul symptom, Kussmaul-Kien respiration, Kussmaul respiration. See under KUSSMAUL RESPIRATION. **4** Kussmaul-Maier disease, Kussmaul disease. See under POLYARTERITIS NODOSA. **5** Kussmaul's pulse. See under SIGN. **6** Kussmaul paralysis, Kussmaul-Landry paralysis, Landry-Kussmaul syndrome. See under LANDRY'S PARALYSIS.

Küster [Hermann *Küster*, German gynecologist, flourished early 20th century] Rokitansky-Küster syndrome. See under ROKITANSKY-KÜSTER-HAUSER SYNDROME.

Küstner [Heinz *Küstner*, German gynecologist, born 1897] **1** Prausnitz-Küstner antibody. See under ANTIBODY. **2** Prausnitz-Küstner test. See under PRAUSNITZ-KÜSTNER REACTION. **3** Reversed Prausnitz-Küstner test. See under TEST.

Küstner [Otto Ernst *Küstner*, German gynecologist, 1849–1931] See under SIGN.

Kutrol A proprietary name for urogastrone.

kuttarosome [Gk *kyttaro(s)* a hollow, cell of a honeycomb, pinecone + *sōm(a)* body] A multilayered structure, at the outer segments of the retinal rods and cones, that acts as a receptor of light energy. Also called *photoreceptor lamella.*

kV Symbol for the unit, kilovolt.

kV·A Symbol for the unit, kilovolt-ampere.

kvar Symbol for the unit, kilovar.

Kveim [Morton Ansgar *Kveim*, Norwegian physician, born 1892] Kveim antigen. See under KVEIM-SILTZBACH TEST.

kvp kilovolt peak.

kW Symbol for the unit, kilowatt.

kwashiorkor [native word in Ghana, prob. meaning "displaced child" or "red boy"] A severe form of malnutrition characterized by edema, anemia, impaired growth, diarrhea, a crazy-paving dermatosis, and brittle, red hair. The pancreas and the liver are particularly involved, the liver is infiltrated to an excessive degree with fat, and serum albumin is severely depressed. Secondary infections are common and can cause the patient to go into negative nitrogen balance if the protein intake is borderline. Untreated, there is a very high death rate. Kwashiorkor is found especially in children (peak age one to four years) in tropical countries where children are weaned onto food with a very low protein content. It is particularly common where maize, rice, yams, cassava, and plantain are staple foods. Secondary forms of the disease exist in both children and adults and are usually superimposed on a disease associated with gross catabolism, such as tuberculosis. Also called *malignant malnutrition, plurideficiency syndrome, fatty liver of Brahmin children (used in India), protein malnutrition, deposed child syndrome.*

marasmic kwashiorkor A clinical condition midway between the two extreme forms of protein-calorie malnutrition, kwashiorkor and marasmus. It frequently develops in a child who is subject to a severe caloric restriction and marginal protein intake, and who develops a systemic or intestinal infection. Acute protein deficiency results. The child characteristically shows loss of subcutaneous fat, muscle wasting, and severe dehydration. Following treatment, the characteristics of kwashiorkor disappear but the child is still grossly emaciated.

kwaski See under KWASKI SHAKES.

Kwell A proprietary name for lindane.

kW·h Symbol for the unit, kilowatt-hour.

kw.-hr. Symbol for the unit, kilowatt-hour. An incorrect symbol.

kyan- CYANO-.

kyano- CYANO-.

kyanophane [KYANO- + -phane, combining form from Gk -phanēs, combining form denoting appearing, shining, from *phainein* to make to appear, shine] A photosensitive pigment that is associated with the retinal cones.

kyestein [Gk *ky(ein)* to be pregnant + *est(h)ein* to clothe] A film that may appear on putrefactive urine, formerly regarded as an indication of pregnancy. Also called *kiestein.*

kyllosis [Gk *kyllo(s)* crippled, halt + -SIS] Any deformity of the foot, but particularly talipes.

kymatism [Gk *kyma*, gen. *kymatos*, anything swollen + -ISM] MYOKYMIA.

kymbocephaly CYMBOCEPHALY.

kymocyclograph KYMOGRAPH.

kymogram [Gk *kym(a)* anything swollen + *o* + -GRAM. See KYMOGRAPH.] The image obtained by kymography.

kymograph [Gk *kym(a)* (from *kyein* to hold, contain, carry in the womb) anything swollen, the swell of the sea, a wave, billow + *o* + -GRAPH] An instrument that records oscillating motion or pressure. Also called *cymograph, kymocyclograph.*

multiple slit kymograph X-RAY KYMOGRAPH.

x-ray kymograph A device for recording the movement of

the heart or other types of motion on a single x-ray film. It contains a lead sheet with multiple parallel slits 1 mm wide and 1 cm apart. The lead sheet, placed on an x-ray cassette, moves 1 cm in its logitudinal direction during x-ray exposure to the heart in order to record on x-ray film pulsation amplitude and direction from many points of the cardiac border. Also called *multiple slit kymograph.*

kymography The use of a kymograph to record oscillating motion.

roentgen kymography A roentgenographic technique for recording on a single x-ray film the extent and rate of movements of the borders of an organ or structure. Abbreviation: RKY

kymotrichous [Gk *kym(a)* a wave + *o* + TRICH- + -OUS] Having wavy hair, as an anthropological characteristic. Compare LEIOTRICHOUS.

Kynex A proprietary name for sulfamethoxypyridazine.

kynocephalus CYNOCEPHALUS.

kynurenic acid 4-Hydroxyquinoline-2-carboxylic acid. It is an intermediate in one pathway of tryptophan catabolism. Transamination of kynurenine gives a 2-oxoacid that cyclizes spontaneously to form kynurenic acid. This loses its hydroxyl group to form quinoline-2-carboxylic acid (quinaldic acid), which is found in urine. Kynurenic acid may be present in the urine in increased quantities in certain hereditary disorders of metabolism.

kynureninase The enzyme (EC 3.7.1.3) that hydrolyzes kynurenine to form anthranilate, i.e. *o*-aminobenzoate, and alanine. It contains pyridoxal phosphate, and is on one of the pathways of tryptophan catabolism.

kynurenine 2-Amino-4-(2-aminophenyl)-4-oxobutyric acid. It is an intermediate in the catabolism of tryptophan. It is broken down in various ways, partly by hydroxylation at C-3 of its phenyl group followed by hydrolysis to alanine and 2-amino-3-hydroxybenzoate.

kynurenine formamidase The enzyme (EC 3.5.1.9) that catalyzes the hydrolysis of *N*-formylkynurenine to formate and kynurenine, a step in the catabolism of tryptophan. Also called *formamidase.*

kyphorachitis A curvature of the vertebral column and thorax to create an exaggerated anterior concavity or posterior hump as a result of rickets. The pelvis may also be involved in the abnormal anterior curvature.

kyphos [Gk *kyphos* crookedness, esp. a hump] **1** An Abnormal spinal curvature with anterior concavity. **2** A hump.

kyphoscoliosis The combined deformity of kyphosis and scoliosis in the thoracic spine. Adjective: kyphoscoliotic.

kyphosis [Gk *kyphōsis* (from *kyphos* bent or bowed forward, stooping, from *kekypha*, perf. of *kyptein* to bend forward, stoop) a humpback] An excessive flexion of the thoracic spine that results in marked convexity when viewed from the side. Also called *cyrtosis, round back deformity, rachiocyphosis, rachiokyphosis, thoracic kyphosis, hunchback, humpback, anterior curvature.*

angular kyphosis A sharp, anterior flexion of several segments of the thoracic spine that have been diseased by tumor or infection or deformed by trauma.

kyphosis dorsalis juvenilis SCHEUERMANN'S KYPHOSIS.

juvenile kyphosis SCHEUERMANN'S KYPHOSIS.

post-traumatic kyphosis An angular flexion deformity of the spine that follows a crush injury of one or more vertebral bodies.

Scheuermann's kyphosis Osteochondritis of the epiphyses of the vertebral bodies. Also called *juvenile kyphosis, kyphosis dorsalis juvenilis, Scheuermann's disease, vertebral epiphysitis, osteochondritis deformans juvenilis dorsi.*

senile kyphosis Abnormally increased convexity in the curvature of the thoracic spine when viewed from the side, resulting in hunchback deformity.

thoracic kyphosis KYPHOSIS.

kyphotic **1** Of or relating to kyphosis. **2** Exhibiting kyphosis. Also *hunchbacked.*

kyphotone [Gk *kypho(s)* crookedness, hump + *ton(os)* a stretching, brace] An obsolete device for reducing kyphotic deformity secondary to tuberculosis of the spine.

Kyrle [Josef *Kyrle*, Austrian dermatologist, 1880–1926]

Kyrle's disease. See under HYPERKERATOSIS FOLLICULARIS ET PARAFOLLICULARIS IN CUTEM PENETRANS.

kyrtorrhachic [Gk *kyrto(s)* curved, bent, humped + *rrhach(i)-* + -IC] Exhibiting lumbar lordosis such that the spine appears convex in the lumbar region when viewed from the side.

kysth- KYSTHO-.

kystho- [Gk *kysthos* a hollow] A combining form designating the vagina. An obsolete form. Also *kysth-.*

kyto- CYTO-.

L

L **1** Symbol for the unit, lambert. **2** Alternative symbol for the unit, liter. **3** Symbol for leucine. **4** lethal.

L_0 Symbol for limes zero.

L_{EPN} Symbol for effective perceived noise level.

l- A prefix denoting a certain configuration of atoms around a chiral carbon atom. The enantiomeric configuration is designated D-. A subscript "s" is sometimes used to show that the center is named by relation to serine, or a subscript "g" to show relation to glyceraldehyde, to clarify the configuration.

l Symbol for the unit, liter.

L Symbol for the quantities (1) diffusion length, expressed in meters; (2) latent heat, expressed in joules per kilogram; (3) radiance, expressed in watts per steradian square meter; (4) self-inductance, expressed in henrys; (5) luminance, expressed in candelas per square meter.

L_P Symbol for the quantities, sound pressure level, or sound power level.

L_v Symbol for the quantity, brightness or luminance, expressed in candelas per square meter.

l Symbol for the quantities (1) length, expressed in meters; (2) specific latent heat, expressed in joules per kilogram; (3) mean free path, expressed in meters.

l- levo-. • This abbreviation has been abandoned because of ambiguity, as it was sometimes used to refer to optical rotation of a compound, now designated $(-)$, and sometimes to configuration, now designated L.

λ **1** The eleventh letter of the greek alphabet, lambda. **2** Symbol for the unit, microliter. An outmoded symbol.

λ Symbol for the quantities (1) decay constant, disintegration constant, expressed in reciprocal seconds; (2) mean free path, expressed in meters; (3) thermal conductivity, expressed in watts per meter kelvin; (4) wavelength, expressed in meters.

L & A light and accomodation (used with reference to pupil response).

LA50 [from *lethal area*.] The total body surface size of a burn that will kill 50 percent of the patients (or experimental animals). It is used in statistical analyses of mortality figures for burn patients.

La **1** Symbol for the element, lanthanum. **2** Symbol for the unit, lambert.

la Symbol for the unit, lambert.

Labarraque [Antoine Germaine *Labarraque*, French apothecary, 1777–1850] See under SOLUTION.

Labbé [Ernest Marcel *Labbé*, French physician, 1870–1939] Labbé's neurocirculatory syndrome. See under SYNDROME.

Labbé [Leon *Labbé*, French surgeon, 1832–1916] **1** See under TRIANGLE. **2** Labbé's vein. See under VENA ANASTOMOTICA INFERIOR.

label [Old French, a ribbon, rag, from the Germanic] **1** A chemical or radioactive marker that can be attached to some pharmaceutical or other material of interest, the vector, to show what the vector is doing. The label must be detectable in amounts so small that the behavior of the vector is not significantly altered, which is why radioactive labels are useful. The label may be an isotope, not necessarily radioactive, of one of the elements in the vector. Also called *tracer.* **2** To add such a marker to (a substance). For defs. 1 and 2 also *tag.*

radioactive label RADIOACTIVE TRACER.

labeling **1** The process or procedure followed in using chemical or radioactive labels as an aid in diagnosis or in experimental study. Also called *tagging.* **2** The appending or accompaniment of written, printed, or graphic information to a food, drug, medical device, equipment or cosmetic, the content of which may be specified by law.

affinity labeling A method of identifying functional groups, such as enzymes, in macromolecules by allowing them to react with synthetic compounds that resemble the substance with which they bind biologically, such as substrate or allosteric effector, but which also contains a reactive grouping capable of rapidly forming a covalent bond with a group at or near the binding site of the macromolecule.

ferritin labeling The technique of identifying substances in electron micrographs by treating the specimen with antibodies specific to the substances to be identified after attaching these antibodies to ferritin. The ferritin may be identified by its high electron density, which is due to its high content of iron.

isotope labeling The technique of using a labeled compound in an experiment so that the products made from it may be identified. The labeled compound is a mixture of the ordinary compound with the substance in which an unusual isotope replaces one or more of its atoms. For example, ethanol might be mixed with (^{18}O)ethanol (the parentheses indicating isotope substitution) to give [^{18}O]ethanol (the square brackets indicating isotope labeling). Appearance of ^{18}O in another compound would then indicate that it originated from the ethanol added.

peroxidase labeling A technique for iodinating tyrosine residues in proteins with ^{131}I-labeled iodine. Since it is inconvenient and dangerous to handle the radioactive isotope in the form of volatile di-iodine, in this technique it is added as the iodide ion, which is not volatile. A low concentration of the I_2 species is then produced in solution by oxidizing the iodide with hydrogen peroxide in the presence of the enzyme iodide peroxidase, which is found in milk. The di-iodine then reacts with tyrosine residues.

pulse labeling An experimental technique in which cells are exposed for a short time to a compound labeled with a radioactive nuclide, followed by a "chaser" (a large quantity of the same compound without the label). The emitted radiation can then be followed as the compound is metabolized.

spin labeling The insertion into a molecule of a stable radical. The radical possesses an unpaired electron, and hence net spin. This can be observed by electron paramagnetic resonance, so that the radical acts as a reporter group, because the environment of the molecule interacts with the spin of the radical.

Labhart [A. *Labhart*, Swiss physician, flourished mid-20th century] Prader-Labhart-Willi syndrome. See under PRADER-WILLI SYNDROME.

labia Plural of LABIUM.

labial 1 Pertaining to the lip or lips or any labium. **2** Toward or facing the lips.

labialism [LABIAL + -ISM] Undue use of bilabial consonants, that is /b/, /p/, sometimes /w/, and the /β/ and /φ/ sounds which are not used in English, usually as substitutions for sounds involving the tongue, such as /d/, /z/ or /g/, which the speaker cannot produce.

labichorea LABIOCHOREA.

labidometer [Gk *labis*, gen. *labidos*, a forceps + -METER] An instrument capable of measuring the size of a fetal head which formerly was used by obstetricians as an attachment to obstetric forceps. Also called *labimeter*.

labile [L *lab(ilis)* (from *labi* to glide, slip, fall + -*ilis* -ILE¹) a slipping down, falling] **1** Easily or spontaneously changed; responding readily to conditions inducing change; unstable. **2** In psychiatry, referring to emotions that are inordinately changeable.

lability [*labil(e)* + -ITY] The property of being easily changed or destroyed, often by some specified agent, such as heat.

emotional lability Laughing or weeping in an uncontrolled manner, constituting an exaggerated or inappropriate response to a stimulus. It occurs often in schizophrenic persons and in patients with disease of the cerebral cortex, usually bilateral, and most commonly secondary to vascular disease. Also called *emotional incontinence*.

labimeter LABIDOMETER.

labio- [L *labia* (fem.) and *labium* (neuter) lip] A combining form denoting the lips.

labioalveolar 1 Pertaining to the lip and the dental alveoli. **2** Relating to the labial aspect of a dental alveolus.

labiocervical Pertaining to the labial aspect of the neck of a tooth.

labiochorea Jerky or grimacing movements of the lips, associated with stuttering, and seen in some neurologic conditions. Also called *labichorea*.

labioclination [LABIO- + *(in)clination*] The inclination of a tooth in a labial direction.

labioglossolaryngeal Concerning the lips, tongue, and larynx.

labioglossopharyngeal Pertaining to the lips, tongue, and pharynx.

labiograph An instrument used to record lip movement during speech.

labiologic Having to do with labiology.

labiology [LABIO- + -LOGY] The study of lip movements in speech and singing.

labiomental Pertaining to the lip or lips and the chin; mentolabial.

labiomycosis Any fungal infection of the lips.

labionasal Pertaining to the lip or lips and the nose.

labiopalatine Pertaining to the lip or lips and the palate.

labioplacement [LABIO- + PLACEMENT] LABIOVERSION.

labioplasty [LABIO- + -PLASTY] **1** Any plastic operation on the labium majus or the labium minus. **2** CHEILOPLASTY.

labiotenaculum [LABIO- + Late L *tenaculum* a tool for holding a thing] An instrument used for holding a lip or lips, as the labia majora.

labioversion [LABIO- + VERSION] The deviation of tooth from the arch towards the lip. Also called *labioplacement*.

Labitome [Gk *labi(s)* forceps + -TOME] A surgical forceps with two sharp cutting blades.

labium [L, a lip] (*plural* labia) **1** [NA] A lip or lip-shaped structure; a fleshy margin or fold. **2** A posterior mouthpart of certain insects, analogous to a lower lip. Compare LABRUM.

labium anterius orificii externi uteri An outmoded term for LABIUM ANTERIUS OSTII UTERI.

labium anterius ostii pharyngei tubae auditivae The anterior lip of ostium pharyngeum tubae auditivae, or pharyngeal opening of auditory tube. An outmoded term.

labium anterius ostii uteri [NA] The anterior lip of the external os of the uterus, thicker and shorter than the posterior lip, both being more obvious in multiparous women in whom the os has become a transverse slit and is no longer rounded as in nulliparous women. It is closely related to the posterior wall of the vagina. Also called *anterior lip of ostium of uterus, anterior lip of cervix of uterus, labium anterius orificii externi uteri* (outmoded).

labium cerebri The outer lip of any deep cerebral sulcus.

labium externum cristae iliacae [NA] The outer margin or lip of the iliac crest that provides attachment along its whole length for fascia lata as well as for the tensor fasciae latae muscle from the anterior third, the lower fibers of the external oblique muscle of abdomen along the anterior two thirds, and the lowest fibers of the latissimus dorsi muscle from the posterior one-third. At the junction of the anterior and middle thirds the prominent tubercle of the crest is located. Also called *external lip of iliac crest*.

labium inferius oris [NA] The fleshy lower margin or fold of the oral fissure, formed internally of mucous membrane and externally of skin, which surround the orbicularis oris muscle, vessels, nerves, areolar tissue, and small salivary glands. Externally it extends to the mentolabial sulcus which separates it from the chin. Also called *lower lip, inferior lip, labium mandibulare* (outmoded).

labium inferius valvulae coli The lower margin of the ileocecal valve, which varies considerably in shape. Only in about 50 percent of them are lips obvious. An outmoded term. Also called *inferior lip of ileocecal valve*.

labium internum cristae iliacae [NA] The inner margin, or lip, of the iliac crest that provides attachment for the fascia iliaca and lower fibers of the transversus abdominis muscle along its anterior two thirds, for the lumbodorsal fascia and quadratus lumborum muscle just posterior to them, and for part of the erector spinae muscle posteriorly. Also called *internal lip of iliac crest*.

labium laterale lineae asperae femoris [NA] The outer lip of linea aspera of femur, continuous with the gluteal tuberosity superiorly and with the lateral supracondylar line bounding the popliteal surface inferiorly, and providing attachment, from medial to lateral side, to the short head of the biceps femoris muscle, the lateral intermuscular septum, and the fused vastus lateralis and vastus intermedius muscles. Also called *lateral lip of linea aspera of femur, external lip of linea aspera of femur, greater trochanteric spine* (outmoded).

labium limbi tympanicum laminae spiralis [NA] The extended and tapering lower part of the C-shaped, periosteal-formed sulcus spiralis internus, within the duct of the cochlea, which is perforated by foramina for branches of the cochlear nerve and by means of which the basilar membrane is attached to the tympanic lip of the osseous spiral lamina. Also called *tympanic lip of limb of spiral lamina, labium tympanicum laminae spiralis, zona perforata* (outmoded).

labium limbi vestibulare laminae spiralis [NA] The upper part of the C-shaped, periosteal-formed sulcus spiralis internus, within the duct of the cochlea, produced by the projecting edge of the limbus laminae spiralis to which the inner, thin part of the membrana tectoria is attached. The upper surface of the lip has furrows separated by projections, forming the auditory teeth.

Also called *vestibular lip of limb of spiral lamina, labium vestibulare laminae spiralis, crista spiralis, spiral crest, lamina dentata.*

labia majora   The greater lips of the pudendum. See under LABIUM MAJUS PUDENDI.

labium majus pudendi   [NA] One of two prominent, elongated and rounded cutaneous folds, one on either side of the rima pudendi of the vulva, extending from the mons pubis anteriorly, where they meet to form the anterior commissure, to a short distance in front of the anus posteriorly where they form the posterior commissure. Each is separated from the medial surface of the thigh by a deep cleft, and the external surface of each is covered with hairs while the internal surface is smooth, bearing numerous openings of sebaceous glands. Between the two surfaces is a varying amount of fat, areolar tissue and dartos muscle fibers. Also called *greater lip of pudendum.*

labium mandibulare   An outmoded term for LABIUM INFERIUS ORIS.

labium maxillare   An outmoded term for LABIUM SUPERIUS ORIS.

labium mediale lineae asperae femoris   [NA] The inner lip of the linea aspera of femur, continuous superiorly with the spiral line and then the intertrochanteric line, and inferiorly with the medial supracondylar line, and having the medial intermuscular septum attached to it. Lateral to the septum the adductor longus muscle and medially the the vastus medialis muscle are attached. Also called *medial lip of linea aspera of femur, lesser trochanteric spine* (outmoded).

labia minora   The lesser lips of the pudendum. See under LABIUM MINUS PUDENDI.

labium minus pudendi   [NA] One of two thin cutaneous folds located on either side of the external openings of the vagina and urethra and between the labia majora. Anteriorly each one splits into two folds to meet those of the opposite side anterior and posterior to the free end of the clitoris. Posteriorly each either blends with the corresponding labium majus or, in the virginal state, becomes joined to the other by a fold of skin, frenulum labiorum pudendi. The labium is smooth and pigmented, devoid of hair and fat, and contains areolar tissue, blood vessels, and small sebaceous and sweat glands. Also called *lesser lip of pudendum, nympha.*

labia oris   [NA] The fleshy upper and lower borders of the rima oris that form the front wall of the oral cavity and are continuous laterally with the cheeks; the lips. Internally they are separated from the teeth and gums by the vestibule.

labium posterius orificii externi uteri   An outmoded term for LABIUM POSTERIUS OSTII UTERI.

labium posterius ostii pharyngei tubae auditivae   The posterior lip of ostium pharyngeum tubae auditivae, or pharyngeal opening of auditory tube. An outmoded term.

labium posterius ostii uteri   [NA] The posterior lip of the external os of the uterus, thinner and longer than the anterior lip, both being more obvious in multiparous women in whom the os has become a transverse slit and is no longer rounded as in nulliparous women. It is closely related to the posterior wall of the vagina. Also called *posterior lip of ostium of uterus, posterior lip of cervix of uterus, labium posterius orificii externi uteri.* (outmoded).

labia pudendi   Labium majus pudendi and labium minus pudendi considered together. An outmoded term.

labium superius oris   [NA] The fleshy upper border of the oral fissure, formed internally of mucous membrane and externally of skin which surround orbicularis oris muscle, vessels, nerves, areolar tissue and small salivary glands. Superiorly it extends as far as the nose, and laterally it is separated from the cheek by the nasiolabial sulcus. Internally it is separated from the teeth and gums by the vestibule. Also called *upper lip,*

superior lip, labium maxillare (outmoded).

labium superius valvulae coli   The upper margin of the ileocecal valve, which varies considerably in shape. Only in about 50 percent of them are lips obvious. An outmoded term. Also called *superior lip of ileocecal valve.*

labium tympanicum laminae spiralis   LABIUM LIMBI TYMPANICUM LAMINAE SPIRALIS.

labium urethrae   One of the two lateral margins of the slightly elevated and irregular external ostium of the urethra.

labium uteri   Either labium anterius ostii uteri or labium posterius ostii uteri.

labium vestibulare laminae spiralis   LABIUM LIMBI VESTIBULARE LAMINAE SPIRALIS.

labium vocale   PLICA VOCALIS.

labor   [L (earlier *labos,* gen. *laboris;* akin to Irish *labhar* a day's work), labor, fatigue, drudgery, industry, sickness, pain]   The process which, by the utilization of uterine musculature contractions as a force, results in the delivery of the products of conception of a pregnancy from the uterus and through the vaginal outlet. Customarily, labor is divided into three stages: the first, from onset of purposeful uterine contractions until full dilatation of the cervix; the second, from full cervical dilatation until vaginal delivery of the fetus; and the third, from delivery of the fetus through delivery of the placenta. Also called *confinement, travail* (older term), *tocus* (older term), *accouchement* (old-fashioned and seldom used).

active labor   ACTIVE PHASE.

arrested labor   Labor that has failed to progress at an expected rate given the particular characteristics of fetus and mother.

artificial labor   INDUCED LABOR.

atonic labor   Labor that is prolonged due to hypotonic uterine dysfunction.

complicated labor   Abnormal labor resulting from cephalopelvic disproportion, fetal distress, third trimester hemorrhage, or some other untoward complication.

delayed labor   POSTMATURE LABOR.

dry labor   Labor that occurs following premature rupture of the fetal membranes with subsequent escape of amniotic fluid from the uterine cavity. Also called *xerotocia, partus siccus.*

false labor   Uterine contractions that mimic those of labor but do not result in any measurable progress. Also called *dolores praesagientes, mimetic labor, spurious labor.*

habitual premature labor   Premature labor occurring in at least three successive pregnancies.

immature labor   Labor occurring in a pregnancy between 20 and 27 weeks after the first day of the last menstrual period.

induced labor   Labor that is initiated by artificial means, as by the artificial rupture of the fetal membranes or through the administration of oxytocic drugs. Also called *artificial labor.*

inert labor   Ineffective labor due to uncoordinated uterine contractions.

instrumental labor   Labor that is assisted with instruments to facilitate vaginal delivery of the fetus.

mimetic labor   FALSE LABOR.

missed labor   Uterine contractions occurring at or near term, followed by fetal death and cessation of all uterine contractions. The fetus may be retained *in utero* for months in some instances.

multiple labor   Labor in the presence of more than one fetus.

normal labor   Labor that results in cervical effacement, cervical dilatation, and descent of the fetus such that vaginal delivery occurs. For primiparas the duration is about 14 hours, while for multiparas the duration is about 8 hours.

obstructed labor   Labor that fails to progress due to cephalopelvic disproportion.

onset of labor   The start of uterine contractions which are purposeful and result in progress in labor, as cervical dilatation or descent of the fetus.

postmature labor   Labor occurring after a gestation of more than 42 weeks measured from the first day of the last menstrual period. Also called *delayed labor, postponed labor, partus serotinus.*

postponed labor   POSTMATURE LABOR.

precipitate labor   Labor that proceeds so rapidly that there is some danger of maternal or fetal harm due to inability to control delivery. Also called *artus precipitatus.*

premature labor   Labor occurring less than 38 weeks after the first day of the last menstrual period. Also called *partus immaturus, partus prematurus.*

prolonged labor   Labor of duration longer than expected. Labor is said to be prolonged if the latent phase continues more than 20 hours in a nullipara or 14 hours in a multipara. In the active phase, labor is said to be prolonged if cervical dilatation occurs at a rate of less than 1.2 cm per hour in a nullipara or 1.5 cm per hour in a multipara. Also called *protracted labor.*

protracted labor   PROLONGED LABOR.

spontaneous labor   Labor that occurs naturally without the use of instruments or oxytocic drugs.

spurious labor   FALSE LABOR.

stages of labor   See under STAGE.

stimulation of labor   See under STIMULATION.

trial of labor   See under TRIAL.

laboratorian   An individual whose professional concerns lie in the laboratory rather than in clinical areas. The title applies to professional workers across a spectrum of educational levels.

laboratory [Med L *laborat(orium)* (from L *laborat(us),* past part. of *laborare* to labor + *-orium* -ORY) a room for scientific research or experiment]   **1** The space and the equipment used to perform experimental and analytical tests.   **2** A group of persons engaged in testing, especially those associated with a discrete organizational entity.

hot laboratory   A laboratory equipped for the safe manipulation of highly radioactive materials.

Laborde [Jean-Baptiste-Vincent *Laborde,* French physician, 1831–1903]   **1** See under FORCEPS, METHOD.   **2** Laborde's test. See under CLOQUET'S NEEDLE SIGN.

labour   A British spelling for LABOR.

labra   Plural of LABRUM.

labrale [*labr(um)* + L *-ale,* neut. sing. of *-alis* -AL]   A cephalometric point situated on the red margin of the lip.

labrale inferius   A cephalometric point situated at the lowest point in the midline on the red margin of the lower lip.

labrale superius   A cephalometric point situated at the highest point in the midline on the red margin of the upper lip.

labrocyte   MAST CELL.

labrum [L (from *lambere* to lick, wash gently), a lip, edge, rim] (*plural* labra)   **1** A brim or liplike structure.   **2** An anterior mouthpart of certain insects, analogous to an upper lip. Compare LABIUM.

acetabular labrum   LABRUM ACETABULARE.

labrum acetabulare   [NA] A triangular rim of fibrocartilage, the base of which is fixed to the margin of the acetabulum, deepening its cavity. Inferiorly it stretches across the acetabular notch as the transverse ligament. The free edge of the labrum grips the head of the femur. Also called *acetabular lip, labrum glenoidale articulationis coxae, circumferential cartilage, border of acetabulum, cotyloid fibrocartilage, cotyloid ligament, fibrocartilaginous lip of acetabulum, cartilaginous margin of acetabulum* (outmoded), *glenoid lip of articulation of hip* (outmoded), *acetabular labrum.*

glenoid labrum   LABRUM GLENOIDALE.

labrum glenoidale   [NA] A triangular rim of fibrocartilage,

the base of which is fixed to the circumference of the glenoid cavity of the scapula, deepening it. Superiorly it is continuous with the tendon of the long head of the biceps brachii muscle. Also called *glenoid lip, labrum glenoidale articulationis humeri, glenoid lip of articulation of humerus* (outmoded), *circumferential cartilage, ligamentum glenoidale* (outmoded), *glenoid ligament of humerus* (outmoded), *glenoid ligament of Macalister* (outmoded), *glenoid labrum.*

labrum glenoidale articulationis coxae   LABRUM ACETABULARE.

labrum glenoidale articulationis humeri   LABRUM GLENOIDALE.

laburinine   CYTISINE.

labyrinth [L *labyrinthus.* See LABYRINTHUS.]   A complex of interconnecting cavities or canals; labyrinthus.

acoustic labyrinth   COCHLEA.

bony labyrinth   LABYRINTHUS OSSEUS.

cortical labyrinth   PARS CONVOLUTA LOBULI CORTICALIS RENALIS.

labyrinth of ethmoid   LABYRINTHUS ETHMOIDALIS.

ethmoidal labyrinth   LABYRINTHUS ETHMOIDALIS.

Ludwig's labyrinths   Spaces between the renal columns and the cortical arches.

membranous labyrinth   LABYRINTHUS MEMBRANACEUS.

nasal labyrinth   The series of interconnecting spaces in the nasal cavity between the nasal conchae. An outmoded term.

nonacoustic labyrinth   An outmoded term for LABYRINTHUS VESTIBULARIS.

olfactory labyrinth   An outmoded term for LABYRINTHUS ETHMOIDALIS.

osseous labyrinth   LABYRINTHUS OSSEUS.

renal labyrinth   PARS CONVOLUTA LOBULI CORTICALIS RENALIS.

Santorini's labyrinth   PLEXUS VENOSUS PROSTATICUS.

statokinetic labyrinth   An outmoded term for LABYRINTHUS VESTIBULARIS.

labyrinth of vestibule   LABYRINTHUS VESTIBULARIS.

labyrinthectomy [LABYRINTH + -ECTOMY]   Surgical destruction, either partial or complete, of the sensory elements of the labyrinth, chiefly for the relief of Menière's disease. Techniques used include the injection of absolute alcohol into the labyrinth, membranous labyrinthectomy, and the use of diathermy, ultrasound, and cryosurgery. Also called *vestibulectomy* (seldom used).

membranous labyrinthectomy   Labyrinthectomy effected by avulsing the membranous lateral semicircular canal. The osseous lateral semicircular canal is exposed by mastoidectomy and opened to reveal the contained membranous canal which is avulsed together with the ampulla.

transtympanic labyrinthectomy   Labyrinthectomy effected by transtympanic avulsion of the utricle. The stapes is exposed by tympanotomy and either removed or turned aside. The utricle, drawn into view with a small hook, is then avulsed using fine forceps.

ultrasonic labyrinthectomy   Selective destruction of the vestibular labyrinth by means of ultrasound, used for relief of Menière's disease. The object is to conserve hearing while destroying the source of the vertigo.

labyrinthi   Plural of LABYRINTHUS.

labyrinthine   Relating to a labyrinth, especially to that of the inner ear.

labyrinthitis [LABYRINTH + -ITIS]   Inflammation of the inner ear. Also called *otitis interna* (rarely used), *otitis labyrinthica* (obsolete), *otitis intima* (outmoded).

circumscribed labyrinthitis   A disorder in which transient vertigo is associated with a fistula between the middle and inner ears. The fistula may be caused by cholesteatoma or may occur accidentally during mastoid surgery or deliberately as in stapedectomy or fenestration. The true cause of vertigo will often be perilymph leakage rather than inflammation of the labyrinth. Also called *perilabyrinthitis* (imprecise).

primary labyrinthitis VOLTOLINI'S DISEASE.

serous labyrinthitis Nonsuppurative labyrinthitis, occurring especially in the presence of a fistula between the middle-ear cleft and the periotic labyrinth, characteristically at the site of the lateral semicircular canal. Also called *toxic labyrinthitis*.

suppurative labyrinthitis An infection of the inner ear caused by pus-forming organisms and usually resulting in a dead ear. In most cases the labyrinthitis is a complication of chronic suppurative otitis media, the infection reaching the inner ear by one of a number of routes. Also called *pyolabyrinthitis, empyema of the labyrinth*.

toxic labyrinthitis SEROUS LABYRINTHITIS.

traumatic labyrinthitis Labyrinthitis complicating head injury, where a fracture line passes through the inner ear, or complicating aural surgery. Most cases result in a dead ear.

labyrinthotomy [LABYRINTH + *o* + -TOMY] A double vestibulotomy once used in the treatment of suppurative labyrinthitis. Access to the inner ear was gained both through the foramen vestibuli and by an opening in the osseous lateral semicircular canal.

labyrinthus [L (from Gk *labyrinthos* labyrinth, maze, anything of spiral or twisted shape), a labyrinth, esp. the one in Crete built by Daedalus] (*plural* labyrinthi) [NA] A complex of interconnecting cavities or canals; a labyrinth.

labyrinthus ethmoidalis [NA] A roughly oblong mass of thin-walled air cells between two parallel vertical plates of bone, suspended from the lateral part of the cribriform plate and situated on each side of the perpendicular plate of the ethmoid bone. The lateral or orbital plate forms part of the medial wall of the orbit while the vertical medial plate is part of the lateral wall of the nasal cavity and has the superior and middle nasal conchae projecting medially into the cavity. Also called *ethmoidal labyrinth, labyrinth of ethmoid, olfactory labyrinth* (outmoded), *lateral mass of ethmoid bone, massa lateralis ossis ethmoidalis* (outmoded).

labyrinthus membranaceus [NA] A closed system of communicating membranous sacs and ducts situated within the bony labyrinth of the internal ear, containing endolymph, surrounded by perilymph, and having the branches of the vestibulocochlear nerve distributed in its walls. It comprises the labyrinthus vestibularis formed by the utricle, saccule, and three semicircular ducts, and the labyrinthus cochlearis, formed by the duct of the cochlea. Also called *membranous labyrinth, auditory bulb* (outmoded).

labyrinthus osseus [NA] The system of bony cavities of the internal ear lodged in the petrous part of the temporal bone and connected to the middle ear by the fenestra vestibuli and fenestra cochleae in the intervening wall. It is divided into the vestibulum, the canales semicirculares ossei, and the cochlea and it communicates with the cranial cavity by the meatus acusticus internus, which transmits the vestibulocochlear nerve to it. It is lined by periosteum and houses the membranous labyrinth, from which it is separated by the perilymph in the perilymphatic space. Also called *bony labyrinth, osseous labyrinth, bony canals of ear*.

labyrinthus vestibularis [NA] The portion of the membranous labyrinth of the internal ear comprising the sacculus and utriculus and their connections and the three semicircular canals. It is the component of the inner ear concerned with the direction of linear and rotational acceleration. Also called *nonacoustic labyrinth* (outmoded), *statokinetic labyrinth* (out-

moded), *labyrinth of vestibule, vestibular system, labyrinthine system, vestibular organ, endovestibular system*.

lac¹ [L (gen. *lactis*; from Gk *gala*, gen. *galaktos*, milk), milk, the juice of herbs, a milky color] Natural milk or any medication resembling milk.

lac coactum Curdled milk.

lac defloratum Skimmed milk.

lac femininum Human milk.

lac fermentum KOUMISS.

lac sulfuris PRECIPITATED SULFUR.

lac vaccinum Cow's milk.

lac² [Persian *lak* and Hindi *lākh* lac, from Sanskrit *lākṣā*, variant of *rākṣā* a resin, secreted on trees by various scale insects, from which a crimson dye is obtained.] The reddish, resinous secretion of the scale insect *Laccifer (Tachardia) lacca*, produced after the insects suck the sap of various resiniferous trees, chiefly in India. Varying in color and occasionally bleached or dewaxed, it is the basis of lacquer, has a great many industrial uses, and is used for the enteric coating of pills and tablets. A variety produced by *Coccus lactis* in India is used in dentistry and surgery. Also called *shellac, lacca*.

Lacassgne [Antoine Marcelin *Lacassagne*, French physician, born 1884] Regaud and Lacassagne technique. See under PARIS TECHNIQUE.

lacca [Italian and New Latin, from Persian *lak*, lac².] LAC².

laccase Any of a group of copper-containing enzymes (EC 1.10.3.2) of low specificity that catalyze the reaction: 4 benzenediol + O_2 → 4 benzosemiquinone + $2H_2O$. The semiquinone formed may spontaneously dismute to form reactant and quinone. The enzymes act on both 1,2-diols and 1,4-diols. The enzyme was first found in the Japanese lac tree. Also called *polyphenol oxidase* (outmoded).

laccate [Italian *lacc(a)* lacquer + -ATE] Having a surface that appears waxed, varnished, or otherwise shiny.

lacer / thigh lacer A thigh corset that is a component of a below-knee prosthesis or orthosis, used for suspension and reduction of weight-bearing by the patellar tendon.

lacerable Susceptible to laceration.

lacerate [See LACERATION.] To tear by blunt force and produce a torn, irregular, ragged wound.

lacerated [See LACERATION.] Wounded by the tearing, crushing, and shearing action of blunt force.

laceration [L *laceratio* (from *laceratus*, past part. of *lacerare* to hew, tear to pieces, mangle, from *lacer* hewn, mangled, torn in pieces, akin to *ligo* a hoe and to Gk *lakis* a rent, tearing) a hewing, tearing, mangling] **1** An injury produced by a blunt instrument in which the skin and/or soft tissues are torn by the crushing and shearing forces produced at impact. Lacerations are characterized by ragged, irregular margins, surrounding contusion, marginal abrasion, tissue bridging in the wound depths, and undermining of the sound in the direction of the blunt force. **2** The act of producing a laceration.

brain laceration Laceration of any part of the brain due to head injury.

dicing lacerations DICING ABRASIONS.

first-degree obstetric laceration An obstetric laceration of the perineum involving the fourchette, the vaginal mucosa, and adjacent skin but not the underlying fascia and muscle.

fourth-degree obstetric laceration An obstetric laceration of the perineum which extends from the vaginal canal to and through the rectal canal and involves underlying fascia and musculature.

obstetric laceration LACERATION OF THE PERINEUM.

laceration of the perineum A laceration that occurs during vaginal delivery and involves the perineum of the mother. Also called *obstetric laceration.*

second-degree obstetric laceration An obstetric laceration of the perineum which involves the skin, vaginal mucosa, and underlying fascia and musculature but does not involve the anal sphincter or extend into the rectal canal.

stellate laceration A star-shaped laceration.

third-degree obstetric laceration An obstetric laceration of the perineum which involves the skin, vaginal mucosa, underlying fascia and musculature, including the anal sphincter, but does not extend into the anal canal.

lacerocondylar Pertaining to the foramen lacerum and the occipital condyle.

lacertus [L, the upper part of the arm] (*plural* lacerti) A fibrous band or bundle.

lacertus cordis Any one of the trabeculae carneae cordis.

lacertus fibrosus musculi bicipitis brachii APONEUROSIS MUSCULI BICIPITIS BRACHII.

lacertus medius weitbrechtii LIGAMENTUM LONGITUDINALE ANTERIUS.

lacertus medius wrisbergii LIGAMENTUM LONGITUDINALE ANTERIUS.

lacertus musculi recti lateralis bulbi [NA] A fascial band extending from the sheath of the lateral rectus muscle of the orbit to a small tubercle on the orbital surface of the zygomatic bone, and considered to check excessive movement of the muscle. Also called *lateral check ligament of eyeball.*

Lachesis A genus of venomous snakes of the family Crotalidae, distributed in South America. It includes *L. mutus*, the bushmaster.

lacinia An outmoded term for FIMBRIA.

lacmoid A synthetic indicator prepared from resorcinol. It changes from red at a pH of 4.4 to blue at a pH of 6.4.

lacmus LITMUS.

lacrima [L, a tear] The fluid of tears which is an isotonic sodium chloride solution of low protein content with a pH of about 7.4. It contains lysozyme, a bactericidal enzyme. Adjective: lacrimal.

lacrimae Plural of LACRIMA.

lacrimal Relating to the tears or to their secretory and drainage apparatus.

lacrimale [Med L, neut. sing. of *lacrimalis* (from L *lacrim(a)* a tear + *-alis* -AL) pertaining to tears] A craniometric point situated at the junction of the crest of the lacrimal bone and the frontolacrimal suture.

lacrimation [L *lacrima* a tear + -ATION] The production of tears.

lacrimator [L *lacrim(a)* a tear + -ATOR] TEAR GAS.

lacrimatory Producing tears or associated with lacrimation.

lacrimonasal Pertaining to the lacrimal apparatus and the nose; nasolacrimal.

lacrimotome [L *lacrim(a)* a tear + *o* + -TOME] A surgical device for cutting the lacrimal ducts or sacs.

lacrimotomy [L *lacrim(a)* a tear + *o* + -TOMY] Incision into the lacrimal duct or sac.

lact- LACTO-.

lactacidemia LACTICACIDEMIA.

lactaciduria The presence of lactic acid in the urine.

lactagogue [LACT- + -AGOGUE] GALACTAGOGUE.

lactalbumin Any of a group of proteins found in milk that are not precipitated by half-saturation with ammonium sulfate. One such is α-lactalbumin, which is a component of the enzyme lactose synthase. In its absence the other component of the enzyme catalyzes transfer of a β-galactosyl group from UDPga-

lactose onto O-4 of *N*-acetylglucosamine. In its presence, the recipient is glucose and the product is lactose.

lactam 1 A cyclic amide. 2 The tautomer containing the group $-NH-CO-$, which may be written $-NH^+=C(-O^-)-$, as opposed to the tautomer containing the group $-N=C(-OH)-$, in heterocyclic bases such as uracil and cytosine.

β-lactam See under β-LACTAM ANTIBIOTIC.

β-lactamase Any bacterial enzyme that hydrolyzes the β-lactam bond in β-lactam antibiotics, resulting in the loss of antimicrobial activity. Specificities for various penicillins and cephalosporins vary. The enzyme may be membrane-bound, excreted, or periplasmic, and it may be coded for by a chromosomal gene or by a plasmid.

lactamide $CH_3-CHOH-CO-NH_2$. The amide of lactic acid.

Lactarius A genus of basidiomycetous agaric (mushroom) fungi which characteristically exude white or colored latex when cut.

lactaroviolin $C_{15}H_{14}O$. 7-Isopropenyl-4-methyl-1-azulenecarboxaldehyde. An antibiotic purple pigment obtained from the fungus *Lactarius deliciosus*.

lactase β-D-Galactosidase. Lactose is one of its most important natural substrates. An outmoded term.

lactate 1 To produce breast milk. 2 The anion, or a salt, or an ester, of lactic acid.

Ringer's lactate LACTATED RINGER'S INJECTION.

lactate dehydrogenase An enzyme (EC 1.1.1.27) that catalyzes the reaction: lactate + NAD^+ ⇌ pyruvate + NADH + H^+. The equilibrium of the reaction greatly favors lactate and NAD^+ at neutral pH. In this direction the reaction allows muscle glycolysis to occur under anaerobic conditions, the lactate passing into the blood as it is formed. The enzyme is a tetramer consisting of two types of chain. The first (type 1, or α, or H) is predominant in the enzyme from heart muscle, and the other (type 2, or β, or M) is predominant in the enzyme from skeletal muscle. The five tetrameric forms, H_4, H_3M, H_2M_2, HM_3, and M_4, may be separated by electrophoresis. The different forms have different kinetic characteristics. Thus forms with M chains predominating are less inhibited by high pyruvate concentrations, which may occur in anaerobic skeletal muscle but are unlikely to be present in heart muscle. The enzyme acts on (S)-lactate. Dehydrogenases acting on (R)-lactate also exist.

lactate racemase An enzyme (EC 5.1.2.1) that interconverts (S)-lactate and (R)-lactate. It enables animals to metabolize (R)-lactate, which is mainly of bacterial origin.

lactation [LACT- + -ATION] 1 The secretion of milk. Also called *galactosis.* 2 The period during which secretion of milk occurs. Adjective: lactational.

lactational Pertaining to lactation.

lacteal [L *lacte(us)* (from *lac*, gen. *lactis*, milk) milky, pertaining to milk + English -AL] 1 Of or relating to milk. 2 A lacteal vessel; one of the chyliferous lymphatic capillaries of the small intestine. Also called *chyliferous vessel* (outmoded).

central lacteal The central lymphatic capillary of an intestinal villus, important in the absorption of chyle.

lactein [*lacte(us)* made of milk, milky + -IN] CONDENSED MILK.

lactescent Describing blood serum that displays a milky or opalescent character.

lacti- LACTO-.

lactic [LACT- + -IC] 1 Pertaining to milk. 2 Producing lactic acid, as in fermentations.

lactic acid $CH_3-CHOH-COOH$. The product of anaerobic glycolysis by milk-souring bacteria and in animal tissues. It is formed when muscles are strenuously exercised. It is formed by the action of lactate dehydrogenase on pyruvate, and this reaction reoxidizes NADH to supply the NAD^+ needed in glycolysis. The same reaction occurs in the reverse direction, particularly in liver, reconverting lactate into pyruvate at the start of its reconversion into carbohydrate. (S)-Lactate is the isomer involved in animal tissues. (R)-Lactate is formed by many species of bacteria. Also called *sarcolactic acid*.

D-lactic acid   The form of lactic acid produced from methylglyoxal and NADPH by some microorganisms.

L-lactic acid   The form of lactic acid produced from pyruvate by the action of lactate dehydrogenase and NADH. It has the *S* configuration at C-2.

lacticacidemia   Greater than normal concentration of lactic acid in blood, plasma, or serum. Also called *lactacidemia, lacticemia*.

lacticemia   LACTICACIDEMIA.

lactide   A cyclic dimeric derivative of lactic acid, formed by esterification of the hydroxyl group of one molecule with the carboxyl group of the other.

lactiferous   Capable of producing, transporting, or secreting milk. Also *lactigenous, lactigerous, galactophorus*.

lactifuge   1 Inhibiting the secretion of milk.   2 An agent that inhibits or stops lactation. Also called *galactophyga*.

lactigenous   LACTIFEROUS.

lactigerous   LACTIFEROUS.

lactim   The tautomer of a cyclic amide (lactam), in which the amide group —NH—C(=O)— or —NH$^+$=C(—O$^-$)— has become —N=C(—OH)—. In purines and pyrimidines it is usually a minor form.

lactimorbus   [LACTI- + MORBUS]   MILK SICKNESS.

lactinated   Made with lactose.

lactiphagous   [LACTI- + -PHAGOUS]   LACTIVOROUS.

lactisugium   [LACTI- + New L *sugium* a pump, from L *sugere* to suck]   A type of breast pump.

lactivorous   [LACTI- + L *vor(are)* to swallow, devour + -OUS]   Consuming a diet composed entirely of milk. Also *lactiphagous*.

lacto-   [L *lac* (genitive *lactis*) milk]   A combining form denoting milk. Also *lact-, lacti-*.

lactobacilli   Plural of LACTOBACILLUS.

Lactobacillus   [LACTO- + BACILLUS]   A genus of Gram-positive, nonsporulating, anaerobic or facultative rods of the family Lactobacillaceae. Growth requirements are complex. Various species are homofermentative or heterofermentative, producing D- or L- or DL-lactic acid. Major species include *L. delbrueckii, L. leichmannii, L. lactis, L. bulgaricus, L. helveticus, L. casei*, and *L. plantarum*. Some species are found in the human mouth, intestine, and vagina. In metabolism and distribution, lactobacilli are very much like the Gram-positive cocci of the family Streptococcaceae.

Lactobacillus acidophilus   1 A homofermentative lactobacillus that is prominent in infants' feces and has also been isolated from the human mouth and vagina.   2 A mixture of lactobacilli of dental origin. An obsolete usage.

Lactobacillus bifidus   An obsolete term for *BIFIDOBACTERIUM*.

Lactobacillus bulgaricus   An organism prominent in the fermentation of yogurt.

Lactobacillus casei   An organism isolated from the human mouth, intestine, and vagina, as well as from dairy products.

Lactobacillus salivarius   An organism isolated from the mouth of humans and of some lower animals.

lactobacillus   (*plural* lactobacilli)   A microorganism of the genus *Lactobacillus*.

lactobutyrometer   LACTOCRIT.

lactocele   GALACTOCELE.

lactocrit   [LACTO- + Gk *krit(ēs)* (from *krinein* to separate, divide, judge) a decider, judge]   A device used to measure the total fat content of milk. Also called *lactobutyrometer*.

lactodensimeter   [LACTO- + DENSIMETER]   GALACTOMETER.

lactofarinaceous   [LACTO- + FARINACEOUS]   Made up of foods containing milk and flour.

lactoferrin   An iron-binding protein of milk, other tissue fluids, and neutrophils that chelates iron, thereby retarding bacterial proliferation.

lactoflavin   The original name for RIBOFLAVIN.

lactogen   [LACTO- + -GEN]   Any agent that stimulates lactation, such as prolactin.

human placental lactogen   A polypeptide hormone, structurally related to human growth hormone and prolactin, secreted by the placenta and disappearing from maternal circulation within 48 hours after parturition. The hormone has several effects, growth-stimulating, lactogenic, and luteotropic, and it may be important in the maintenance and growth of the fetus. The concentration in plasma is raised in molar pregnancy and choriocarcinoma. Also called *human chorionic somatomammotropin, placental growth hormone, chorionic growth hormone-prolactin, galactagogin, somatomammotropin, human chorionic somatomammotropin*. Abbreviation: HPL.

lactogenesis   The production of milk by the mammary glands. Also called *galactopoiesis*.

lactogenic   Stimulating lactation; enhancing the production of milk. Also *galactopoietic*.

lactoglobulin   A protein present in milk. It has a subunit molecular mass of 18 kDa, and in most species forms dimers, which may associate further. In cow's milk it has a concentration of about 3 g/l, second only to casein among the milk proteins. Also called *β-lactoglobulin*.

β-lactoglobulin   LACTOGLOBULIN.

lactolin   [LACTO- + *l* + -IN]   CONDENSED MILK.

lactometer   [LACTO- + -METER]   GALACTOMETER.

lactone   An internal cyclic ester within an organic molecule, formed by the elimination of water from a carboxyl group and combination with an alcoholic hydroxyl nearby.

γ-lactone   A compound that contains a five-membered ring of atoms including the —CO—O— group. It is the lactone formed between a carboxyl group and the γ-hydroxyl group of an acid.

lacto-ovovegetarian   [LACTO- + OVO- + VEGETARIAN]   One whose diet is composed of vegetables, fruit, milk, and eggs.

lactoperoxidase   The iodide peroxidase found in milk. It is a hemoprotein.

lactophenin $C_{11}H_{15}NO_3$. A product derived from the combination of phenetidin and lactic acid. It was used in the past as an analgesic and antipyretic agent.

lactophosphate   A salt of both lactic acid and phosphonic acid, using the same base component.

lactoprecipitin   A precipitin that precipitates the casein of milk. It is produced in the serum of an animal by injecting milk of another species.

lactorrhea   [LACTO- + -RRHEA]   GALACTORRHEA.

lactoscope   [LACTO- + -SCOPE]   GALACTOSCOPE.

lactose   [*lact(o)-* + -OSE^2]   4-*O*-β-D-Galactosyl-D-glucose. It is the main sugar of milk. It is hydrolyzed by β-galactosidase to galactose and glucose. A genetic inability to continue production of this enzyme into adult life is common in many parts of the world, especially in hot countries where milk has not normally been in the adult diet. People with this inability suffer discomfort after drinking milk, as the lactose is not hydrolyzed and absorbed but instead provides nutrient for gas-forming intestinal flora. Also called *saccharum lactis, milk sugar* (outmoded).

lactoserum　The serum of an animal previously injected with milk from another species. The serum contains lactoprecipitin, which precipitates milk casein.

lactose synthase　The enzyme (EC 2.4.1.22) that catalyzes the synthesis of lactose by galactosylating glucose using UDPgalactose as donor. It is found in milk and in mammary glands. It consists of two proteins, one of which is by itself capable of galactosylating *N*-acetylglucosamine to form *N*-acetyllactosamine, but not glucose, and the other, from which it dissociates fairly easily, modifies its specificity so that it galactosylates glucose. The modifying protein has proved identical with that previously described as α-lactalbumin.

lactosuria　The presence of lactose in the urine.

lactotherapy　Any treatment involving the use of a milk-based diet.

lactotoxin [LACTO- + TOXIN]　Any toxic substance formed in milk.

lactotroph　MAMMOTROPIC CELL.

lactovegetarian [LACTO- + VEGETARIAN]　One whose diet consists of vegetables, fruit, and milk.

lactoyl　The acyl group CH₃—CHOH—CO—, derived from lactic acid.

lactoyl-glutathione lyase　An enzyme (EC 4.4.1.5) that catalyzes the interconversion of *S*-lactoylglutathione with methylglyoxal (CH₃—CO—CHO) and glutathione. Since there is another enzyme that hydrolyzes *S*-lactoylglutathione, the two enzymes together act to interconvert lactate and methylglyoxal. The function of this interconversion, which involves the less common isomer *R*-lactate, is unknown. Also called *glyoxalase I* (obsolete).

lactucarium　The dried milky juice of *Lactuca virosa* (wild lettuce), which has mild sedative properties. It has been used for the treatment of coughs. Also called *lettuce opium, thridacium.*

lactucic acid　An acid in the juice from *Lactuca virosa* (wild lettuce), reported to have sedative properties. It has been used to treat coughs.

lactucin　C₁₅H₁₆O₅. An active principle isolated from various *Lactuca* species. It is one of several bitter chemicals present in lettuce of several species which are said to have properties as a sedative.

lactucism　Poisoning from overdose of preparations containing lactucin, a crystallizable extractive of the wild lettuce *Lactuca virosa*. Symptoms are headache, dizziness, ataxia, and dyspnea.

lactulose　4-O-β-D-Galactopyranosyl-D-fructose. A synthetic disaccharide of galactose and fructose. It has been used as a cathartic and in the treatment of hepatic coma to increase the rate of ammonia formation.

lactulum unguis　MATRIX UNGUIS.

lacuna [L (from *lacus* a lake, cistern, basin, akin to *liquere* to be liquid, be clear; also to *lacrima* a tear; Gk *lakkos*, erroneously *lakos*, a hollow, pit, cistern, pond), a ditch, pool, cleft, opening, loss, want] (*plural* lacunae)　**1** A space or cavity between cells or structures or within a structure; a small depression or pit in a surface. **2** An abnormal gap or discontinuity. For defs. 1 and 2 also called *lacune.*

absorption lacuna　HOWSHIP'S LACUNA.

air lacuna　A small air-filled space, such as the cortical fusi of the hair shaft.

Blessig's lacuna　Cysts in the peripheral retina due to physiologic degenerative changes.

blood lacunae　TROPHOBLASTIC LACUNAE.

cartilage lacuna　One of the spaces within cartilaginous tissue which house the formative cells or chondrocytes. Also called *cartilage space.*

cerebral lacunae　Tiny cavities, often measuring no more than a millimeter or two in diameter, found within the gray or white matter of the cerebrum and almost invariably resulting from minute areas of infarction due to occlusion of one or more small cerebral arteries. Hypertension is the most common cause, and several specific syndromes of so-called lacunar strokes have been defined.

great lacuna of urethra　LACUNA MAGNA.

Howship's lacuna　A rounded pit or defect on the surface of bony tissue that is usually occupied by one or more osteoclasts. It is believed to be a site of bone resorption. Also called *absorption lacuna.*

intervillous lacuna　INTERVILLOUS SPACE.

lacunae laterales [NA]　The venous network within the dura mater through which arachnoid villi project into the superior sagittal sinus. Also called *parasinoidal lacunae, parasinoidal sinus.*

lacuna magna　A pitlike recess in the roof of the fossa navicularis urethrae from which it is separated by the valvula fossae navicularis. Also called *great lacuna of urethra, Guérin sinus.*

lacunae of Morgagni　Lacunae urethrales in the male urethra. Also called *urethral lacunae of Morgagni, mucous sinuses of male urethra.*

lacunae morgagnii urethrae muliebris　Lacunae urethrales in the female urethra. An outmoded term.

lacuna of muscles　LACUNA MUSCULORUM.

lacuna musculorum [NA]　The space between the inguinal ligament and the hip bone, lateral to the iliopectineal arch and transmitting the iliopsoas muscle and femoral nerve into the thigh. Also called *lacuna of muscles, muscular compartment, iliac canal.*

osseous lacunae　Small spaces within bony tissue that contain the osteocytes and are connected to each other by fine radiating channels or canaliculae.

parasinoidal lacunae　LACUNAE LATERALES.

lacuna pharyngis　An insignificant depression in the auditory tube near its orifice in the nasopharynx. An outmoded term.

superego lacunae　Superego defects that engender antisocial behavior. They are believed to represent unconscious wishes of the parents.

trophoblastic lacunae　Small spaces that develop in the syncytial trophoblast of the developing human placenta and fuse to form the intervillous space. Also called *blood lacunae, lacunae trophoblasticae.*

lacunae trophoblasticae　TROPHOBLASTIC LACUNAE.

lacunae of urethra　LACUNAE URETHRALES.

urethral lacunae　LACUNAE URETHRALES.

lacunae urethrales [NA]　Pitlike recesses of varying size in the mucous membrane of the spongy part of the urethra in the male and the entire urethra in the female. It is considered that some are the wide ostia of the urethral glands. Also called *urethral lacunae, foramina of urethra* (outmoded), *lacunae of urethra.*

urethral lacunae of Morgagni　LACUNAE OF MORGAGNI.

lacuna vasorum [NA]　The space between the inguinal ligament and the hip bone, medial to the iliopectineal arch and lateral to the lacunar ligament, transmitting the femoral sheath and its contents. Also called *lacuna of vessels, vascular compartment, venous lacuna.*

lacuna venosa durae matris　One of the lacunae laterales.

venous lacuna　LACUNA VASORUM.

lacuna of vessels　LACUNA VASORUM.

lacunae　Plural of LACUNA.

lacunar　Relating to a lacuna or characterized by lacunae.

lacune LACUNA.

lacunose Pitted; having many cavities or depressions.

lacunula A very small lacuna. Also called *lacunule*.

lacunule LACUNULA.

lacus [L, a lake, cistern, basin. See LACUNA.] (*plural* lacus) A space in which fluid collects; lake.

lacus lacrimalis LACRIMAL LAKE.

lacus seminalis The vagina following intercourse and insemination. An older term. Also called *seminal lake*.

Ladd [William Edwards *Ladd*, U.S. pediatric surgeon, 1880–1967] **1** Ladd's bands. See under BAND. **2** See under PROCEDURE.

Ladd-Franklin [Christine *Ladd-Franklin*, U.S. psychologist and logician, 1847–1930] Ladd-Franklin theory. See under THEORY.

Ladin [Louis Julius *Ladin*, U.S. obstetrician, born 1862] Ladin sign. See under HEGAR SIGN.

lady's slipper CYPRIPEDIUM.

Laelaps *ECHINOLAELAPS*.

Laennec [René Theophile Hyacinthe *Laennec*, French physician, 1781–1826] **1** See under CATARRH. **2** Laennec's disease. See under CIRRHOSIS.

laetrile [*lae(vorotaryni)trile*, from LAEVO- + *rotary* + *nitrile*] A preparation of amygdalin, a cyanide-containing substance obtained from the pits of apricots, peaches, and bitter almonds. Though sometimes promoted as a cancer treatment, no responsible scientist has been able to find any valid basis to the theory that it has an antineoplastic effect. Also called *vitamin B₁₇*.

laeve [L, neut. sing. of *laevis*, also *levis* smooth, bald] Bald, as *chorion laeve*.

laevo- A British spelling for LEVO-.

laevocardia A British spelling for LEVOCARDIA.

LAF lymphocyte-activating factor.

Lafora [Gonzalo Rodriguez *Lafora*, Spanish neurologist, 1887–1971] **1** See under SIGN. **2** Lafora's bodies. See under BODY. **3** Myoclonic epilepsy with Lafora bodies, Lafora's disease, Lafora body disease. See under PROGRESSIVE MYOCLONIC EPILEPSY.

lag **1** A slowness to act or react. **2** The interval between an expected action or reaction and its occurrence.

anaphase lag A retarded movement of chromosomes during mitosis. If homologous chromosomes do not separate far enough or fast enough, the daughter cells will be aneuploid for the involved chromosomes. Also called *lagging*.

eyelid lag Failure of the upper eyelid to descend promptly and steadily when the gaze is directed downward. Instead the eyelid moves belatedly and jerkily, a sign of Graves disease. Also called *lid lag, Graefe sign, von Graefe sign, Boston sign*.

globe lag An ocular sign of Graves disease. In the act of looking upward, the patient's upper eyelid pulls back faster than the eyeball is raised, thus exposing the sclera above the iris. Also called *Kocher sign, Kocher symptom*.

jet lag An alteration in biologic rhythm due to rapid transport, as by jet aircraft, from one time zone to another. Patterns of sleep and wakefulness and of hunger and satiety are often temporarily disrupted, producing disorientation and fatigue. Also called *flying fatigue*.

lid lag EYELID LAG.

nitrogen lag The interval between the ingestion of protein and the appearance of an equivalent amount of nitrogen in urine.

phenomic lag A period of multiplication in a mutated cell in which the premutational phenome is diluted and is replaced by a phenome corresponding to the mutated genome. Several generations are required before an auxotrophic mutation is phenotypically expressed.

phenotypic lag An interval between the occurrence of a mutation and its phenotypic expression in bacteria. Its components are stabilization of the mutation by its replication on a complementary strand, nuclear segregation, and phenomic lag.

segregation lag The lag in expression of a mutation in bacteria until cell division has segregated it from the nonmutant allele in other copies of the chromosome.

lagena [L, a flagon, flask, bottle] (*plural* lagenae) **1** CAECUM CUPULARE DUCTUS COCHLEARIS. **2** A more or less distinct portion of the cochlear duct of the membranous labyrinth in nonmammalian vertebrates, especially in reptiles. In a few lizards and nearly all snakes the lagena occupies the major portion of the cochlear duct. It contains a sensory end-organ, the lagenar macula, possessing hair cells and often regarded as a possible auditory receptor, but the evidence is scanty. ⟨Wever, E.G., *The Reptile Ear*, 1978.⟩

lageniform Flask-shaped.

lagging **1** Reduced or retarded movement of one side of the chest, as might be seen in a patient with pulmonary tuberculosis. **2** ANAPHASE LAG.

lagnosis [Gk *lagno(s)* lustful + -SIS] SATYRIASIS.

Lagochilascaris minor A small nematode (male 9 mm; female 15 mm) of the family Ascarididae, found in subcutaneous, tonsillar, and mastoid abscesses of humans in Trinidad and Suriname. It probably occurs normally in the intestines of South American felids, including leopards. Treatment is with diethylcarbamazine.

lagochiline A substance presumed to be psychoactive that is found in the leaves of *Lagochilus inebrians* of the family Lamiaceae. In Turkestan a narcotic and intoxicating tea is prepared from the roasted leaves.

lagophthalmos [Gk *lag(ōs)* a hare + *ophthalmos* the eye] Inability to close the eyelids completely, as in facial nerve paralysis. Also called *oculus leporinus, hare's eye*. Also *lagophthalmus*.

lagophthalmus LAGOPHTHALMOS.

Lagrange [Pierre-Felix *Lagrange*, French ophthalmologist, 1857–1928] See under OPERATION.

la grippe A French term for INFLUENZA.

laity The lay public; the nonprofessional population in respect to any particular profession.

lake¹ [L *lacus*. See LACUS.] A small collection of fluid or the space in which it collects; lacus.

capillary lake The total volume of blood contained in the capillary beds.

lacrimal lake The pool of tears normally existing in the medial portion of the lower cul-de-sac. Also called *lacus lacrimalis*.

marginal lakes Dilated regions of the peripheral part of the intervillous space of the human placenta which merge medially with the subchorial space.

seminal lake LACUS SEMINALIS.

lake² [Persian *lak* lac. See LAC².] **1** Any of a class of pigments, originally red or purplish red but now including various colors, produced by precipitation of a soluble natural or synthetic dye with a metallic compound. Some lakes are used as coloring agents in foods and in medicinal tablets and capsules. **2** A seldom used term for HEMOLIZE.

Laki [Koloman *Laki*, Hungarian-born U.S. physiologist, born 1909] Laki-Lorand factor. See under FACTOR XIII.

laky Denoting the reddish hue of serum or plasma, which results from hemoglobin released from hemolyzed erythrocytes.

-lalia [Gk *lalia* (from *lalein* to prate, chatter, speak) talking, chattering] A combining form designating a disorder involving speech.

Lallemand [Claude François *Lallemand*, French surgeon, 1790–1854] Lallemand's bodies, Lallemand-Trousseau bodies,

Trousseau-Lallemand bodies. See under BENCE JONES CYLIN-DERS.

lalo- [Gk *lalein* to prate, chatter, speak] A combining form denoting speech.

lalochezia A seldom used term for COPROLALIA.

lalognosis [LALO- + Gk *gnōsis* knowledge] Knowledge and understanding of speech.

laloneurosis Any psychogenic speech disorder.

lalophobia Pathologic fear of speaking in public.

lalorrhea [LALO- + -RRHEA] LOGOMANIA.

Lalouette [Pierre *Lalouette*, French physician, 1711–1742] Lalouette's pyramid. See under LOBUS PYRAMIDALIS GLANDULAE THYROIDEAE.

Lamarck [Jean Baptiste Pierre Antoine de Monet *Lamarck*, French naturalist, 1744–1829] See under THEORY.

lamarckism [after Jean Baptiste Pierre Antoine de Monet *Lamarck*, French naturalist, 1744–1829 + -ISM] LAMARCK'S THEORY.

Lamaze [Fernand *Lamaze*, French obstetrician, 1890–1957] See under METHOD.

lambda 1 The name of the eleventh letter of the Greek alphabet. Symbol: λ 2 A craniometric point marking the position of the occipital fontanel situated at the junction of the sagittal and lambdoid sutures.

lambdoid Shaped like or relating to the Greek letter lambda (λ). Also *lambdoidal*.

lambdoidal LAMBDOID.

Lambert [Alexander *Lambert*, U.S. physician, 1861–1939] See under TREATMENT.

Lambert [Edward Howard *Lambert*, U.S. physiologist, born 1915] Eaton-Lambert syndrome. See under LAMBERT-EATON SYNDROME.

Lambert [Johann Heinrich *Lambert*, German mathematician, 1728–1777] 1 Lambert law, Lambert-Holzknecht law. See under LAW. 2 Beer-Lambert law. See under BEER'S LAW.

lambert [after Johann Heinrich *Lambert*, German mathematician and physicist, 1728–1777] The CGS unit of illuminance equal to one lumen per square centimeter; 10^4 lumen per square meter; 10^4 lux. Symbol: La

Lamblia GIARDIA.

Lamblia intestinalis GIARDIA LAMBLIA.

lambliasis Infection caused by *Giardia lamblia*. Also called *lambliosis*. See also GIARDIASIS.

lambliosis LAMBLIASIS.

lambo lambo A local name for TROPICAL PYOMYOSITIS.

Lambotte [Albin *Lambotte*, Belgian surgeon, 1866–1912] See under TREATMENT.

lame [Old English *lama*] Unable to walk with a normal gait because of pain or impairment.

lame foliacée FOLIATE LAMINA.

lamel LAMELLA.

lamella [L (dim. of *lamina*, *lammina*, or *lamna* a plate or thin piece of wood, metal, marble, a saw blade, the thin shell of fruit; akin to *liber* the inner bark of a tree, paper made of bark, a book), a small metal plate, disk, wafer] (*plural* lamellae) 1 A thin plate, layer, or sheet, as of compact bone. 2 GILL. 3 A medicated disk to be inserted under the eyelid, consisting of an alkaloid drug, contained in a mixture of gelatin, glycerine, and distilled water. Also called *lamel*.

annulate lamellae Flattened lamellar stacks, having fenestrae (windows) similar to nuclear pores located in the cytoplasm of some cells. The annulate lamellae are believed to arise as blebs from the nuclear envelope.

articular lamella A layer of smooth compact bone to which articular cartilage is firmly attached.

basic lamella CIRCUMFERENTIAL LAMELLA.

lamella of bone OSSEOUS LAMELLA.

circumferential lamella One of a varying number of layers of bone encircling either the external surface of compact bone (lamella circumferentialis externa) or the internal surface lining the wall of the marrow cavity (lamella circumferentialis interna). Also called *basic lamella, primary lamella*.

lamella circumferentialis externa See under CIRCUMFERENTIAL LAMELLA.

lamella circumferentialis interna See under CIRCUMFERENTIAL LAMELLA.

concentric lamella One of a number of concentric layers (4 to 20) of bony tissue surrounding a central Haversian canal, or canalis centralis osteoni, and its contained neurovascular bundle. Also called *haversian lamella, lamella osteoni*.

cornoid lamella A parakeratotic horny structure histologically characteristic of porokeratosis of Mibelli.

elastic lamella One of the layers of elastic tissue that form part of the tunica media of an artery. The elastic lamellae are particularly prominent in the larger arteries. Also called *elastic lamina, elastic membrane*.

enamel lamella One of the microscopic layers of organic material that run through tooth enamel to reach the dentine layer.

endosteal lamella One of the circumferential lamellae under the endosteum lining the wall of the marrow cavity.

ground lamella INTERSTITIAL LAMELLA.

haversian lamella CONCENTRIC LAMELLA.

intermediate lamella INTERSTITIAL LAMELLA.

interstitial lamella One of the curved bony layers occupying the irregular intervals between the haversian systems or osteons. These bony layers are the remains of older osteons partly resorbed during bone remodeling. Also called *ground lamella, intermediate lamella, lamella interstitialis*.

lamella interstitialis INTERSTITIAL LAMELLA.

lamella ossea OSSEOUS LAMELLA.

osseous lamella One of a series of contiguous thin layers of bone matrix that comprises the basic structural unit of bone, such as a concentric or circumferential lamella. Also called *lamella of bone, lamella ossea*.

lamella osteoni CONCENTRIC LAMELLA.

periosteal lamella A bony layer at the external surface of a bone adjacent to the periosteum. Also called *peripheral lamella*.

peripheral lamella PERIOSTEAL LAMELLA.

photoreceptor lamella KUTTAROSOME.

posterior border lamella of Fuchs COMPLEXUS BASALIS CHOROIDEAE.

primary lamella CIRCUMFERENTIAL LAMELLA.

triangular lamella TELA CHOROIDEA VENTRICULI TERTII.

vitreous lamella COMPLEXUS BASALIS CHOROIDEAE.

lamellae Plural of LAMELLA.

lamellar Pertaining to, composed of, or characterized by lamellae.

lamellasome [LAMELLA + Gk *sōm(a)* body] A membranous cytoplasmic inclusion, unique to the blue-green algae, consisting of a series of lamellae within a common membrane.

lamelliform Resembling lamellae.

lamellipodia (*singular* lamellipodium) Broad flattened projections from the leading edge of a cell, such as fibroblast, when growing in tissue culture. The lamellipodia are ruffled in appearance and have an undulating motion. Microfilaments are abundant, especially at points of adhesion to the substrate.

lameness / fescue lameness A lameness in cattle, associated with the ingestion of an unidentified toxin in tall fescue grass (*Festuca arundinacea*). Symptoms are gangrene of the hind feet. In severe cases, the front feet, tip of the tail, and ears may also be involved. Animals are distressed by extremes of hot and cold weather with cold intensifying the severity of the gangrenous attacks. Also called *fescue foot, fescue.*

lamina

lamina [L, a plate or thin piece of wood, metal, marble, a saw blade, the thin shell of fruit; akin to *liber* the inner bark of a tree, paper made of bark, a book] (*plural* laminae) A thin, flat layer or plate; a scale.

lamina affixa [NA] The tela choroidea of the medial wall of the lateral ventricle that fuses during development in the midline, attaches to the dorsal surface of the thalamus overlying the stria terminalis, and covers the thalamostriate and choroid veins.

alar lamina That part of the lateral wall of the neural tube of the embryo lying between the sulcus limitans and the roof plate of the tube. Formed by proliferation of the germinal cells of the ependymal zone, the neuroblasts of each alar lamina become the receptor cells of the posterior horns of the spinal cord and sensory cells in the medulla. Also called *lamina alaris, flügelplatte, dorsolateral plate, wing plate, encephalic region, epencephalic region, dorsal zone of His.*

lamina alaris   ALAR LAMINA.

laminae albae cerebelli [NA] The myelinated fiber bundles underlying the cerebellar cortex. Also called *laminae medullares cerebelli, white laminae of cerebellum, white layers of cerebellum.*

anterior limiting lamina   LAMINA LIMITANS ANTERIOR CORNEAE.

lamina anterior vaginae musculi recti abdominis [NA] The anterior layer of the sheath of the rectus abdominis muscle, extending from the costal margin to the symphysis pubis and formed in its entirety by the aponeurosis of the external oblique muscle which is strengthened by the anterior lamina of the internal oblique muscle in its upper two thirds and by the aponeuroses of the internal oblique and transversus abdominis muscles in its lower one third. Also called *anterior layer of the rectus abdominis sheath.*

lamina arcus vertebrae [NA] One of two broad symmetrical plates of bone that fuse at their junction with the spinous process to form the posterior wall of the vertebral arch, each extending laterally to the base of the transverse process where each fuses with the corresponding pedicle. Also called *lamina of vertebral arch, lamina of vertebra, neural lamina.*

basal lamina That part of the lateral wall of the neural tube of the embryo lying between the sulcus limitans and the floor plate of the tube. Formed by proliferation of the germinal cells of the ependymal zone, the neuroblasts of each basal lamina become the motor cells of the anterior horns of gray matter of the spinal cord and the motor cells in the medulla. Also called *ventrolateral plate, hypencephalic region, ventral zone of His, lamina basalis, grundplatte.*

basal lamina of choroid   COMPLEXUS BASALIS CHOROIDEAE.
basal lamina of ciliary body   LAMINA BASALIS CORPORIS CILIARIS.
lamina basalis   BASAL LAMINA.
lamina basalis chorioideae An outmoded term for COMPLEXUS BASALIS CHOROIDEAE.
lamina basalis choroideae   COMPLEXUS BASALIS CHOROIDEAE.
lamina basalis corporis ciliaris The anterior extension of lamina basalis choroideae into the ciliary body. An outmoded term. Also called *basal lamina of ciliary body.*

basement lamina   BASEMENT MEMBRANE.
lamina basilaris ductus cochlearis [NA] The fibrous membrane of the floor of the cochlear duct extending from the tympanic lip of the osseous spiral lamina to the crista basilaris of the spiral ligament of the lateral wall, supporting the spiral organ of Corti within the duct and completing the roof of the scala tympani. Also called *basilar membrane of cochlear duct, basilar membrane, membrana basilaris ductus cochlearis* (outmoded), *cochlear zone* (outmoded), *Valsalva zone* (outmoded), *zona Valsalvae* (outmoded), *basilar membrane envelope.*

bony spiral lamina   LAMINA SPIRALIS OSSEA.
Bowman's lamina   LAMINA LIMITANS ANTERIOR CORNEAE.
buccal lamina   LATERAL ENAMEL STRAND.
buccogingival lamina   VESTIBULAR LAMINA.

lamina cartilaginis cricoideae [NA] The flat, quadrate posterior expansion of the signet-ring-shaped cricoid cartilage, its anterior surface forming much of the posterior wall of the larynx, and its posterior surface providing attachment to the posterior cricoarytenoid muscles and ligaments. The arytenoid cartilages articulate with the superior border of the lamina. Also called *lamina of cricoid cartilage, cricoid lamina.*

lamina cartilaginis lateralis tubae auditivae [NA] The narrow lateral plate of the troughlike, bent superior part of the cartilaginous portion of the auditory tube. Also called *lamina lateralis cartilaginis tubae auditivae, lateral cartilaginous layer, lateral lamina of cartilage of auditory tube.*

lamina cartilaginis medialis tubae auditivae [NA] The broad medial plate of the troughlike, bent superior part of the cartilaginous portion of the auditory tube. Also called *lamina medialis cartilaginis tubae auditivae, medial cartilaginous layer, medial lamina of cartilage of auditory tube.*

lamina cartilaginis thyroideae dextra/sinistra [NA] One of a pair (right and left) of quadrate-shaped plates of the thyroid cartilage, widely separated posteriorly and fused in the midline anteriorly to form the laryngeal prominence surmounted by the thyroid notch. The posterior border has two slender projections, the superior and inferior cornua. The smooth internal surface, lined by mucous membrane, encloses the specialized vocal apparatus while the external surface provides attachment for muscles. Also called *lamina of thyroid cartilage.*

lamina choriocapillaris An outmoded term for LAMINA CHOROIDOCAPILLARIS.
lamina choroidea epithelialis thalami The lamina epithelialis of the superior and medial surface of the thalamus.
lamina choroidea epithelialis ventriculi lateralis The ependymal cell layer of the choroid plexus lining the lateral cerebral ventricles.
lamina choroidea epithelialis ventriculi quarti The ependymal cell lining of the roof of the fourth ventricle overlying the rostral medulla oblongata.
lamina choroidocapillaris [NA] A layer of capillaries forming a network in the choroid in which the choroidal arteries end and which is separated from the retina by Bruch's membrane. The spaces in the network are very small posteriorly but become larger anteriorly and contain elastic and collagenous fibers. Near the ciliary body the capillaries join those of the ciliary processes. Also called *lamina choriocapillaris* (outmoded), *membrana choriocapillaris, Ruysch membrane, Ruysch tunic, ruyschian membrane, tunica ruyschiana* (outmoded), *mesochoroidea* (outmoded), *choriocapillary layer, membrana ruyschiana* (outmoded).

lamina cinerea terminalis An obsolete term for LAMINA TERMINALIS.

cribriform lamina An outmoded term for FASCIA CRIBROSA.
cribriform lamina of ethmoid bone   LAMINA CRIBROSA OSSIS ETHMOIDALIS.

cribriform lamina of transverse fascia   An outmoded term for SEPTUM FEMORALE.

lamina cribrosa   Either lamina cribrosa ossis ethmoidalis or lamina cribrosa sclerae.

lamina cribrosa ossis ethmoidalis   [NA] The perforated horizontal plate of the ethmoid bone, forming part of the roof of the nasal cavity and occupying the ethmoidal notch of the frontal bone. Attached inferiorly are the labyrinth on each side and the perpendicular plate in the center, above which the crista galli projects superiorly. The plate is perforated by numerous branches of the olfactory nerves, which are connected to the olfactory bulbs superior to it. The gyrus rectus is also above the plate. Also called *cribriform lamina of ethmoid bone, cribriform plate of ethmoid bone, cribrum, cribriform plate, sieve bone.*

lamina cribrosa sclerae   [NA] The posterior circular, sievelike area of the sclera which is pierced by the nerve bundles of the optic nerve. At its periphery the sclera is continuous with the fibrous sheath of the nerve. At the center of the area there is a large opening for the central artery and vein of the retina. This is the weakest part of the sclera which may bulge outward if the intraocular pressure becomes raised. Also called *optic foramen of sclera, perforated layer of sclera, optic foramen* (outmoded), *porus opticus* (outmoded).

cricoid lamina   LAMINA CARTILAGINIS CRICOIDEAE.

lamina of cricoid cartilage   LAMINA CARTILAGINIS CRICOIDEAE.

lamina densa   An outmoded term for GLOMERULAR BASEMENT MEMBRANE.

dental lamina   A flat band of epithelial cells that develops in embryos as a medially placed strip from the primary dental band of the mandibular arch and opposed surface of the maxillary process. The dental organs (tooth germs) develop at intervals along the dental lamina to give rise to the primary and secondary dentition. Also called *primitive dental groove, lamina dentalis, dentogingival lamina, dental ledge, enamel ledge, maxillary ridge.*

lamina dentalis   DENTAL LAMINA.

lamina dentata   LABIUM LIMBI VESTIBULARE LAMINAE SPIRALIS.

dentogingival lamina   DENTAL LAMINA.

descending lamina of sphenoid bone   An outmoded term for PROCESSUS PTERYGOIDEUS OSSIS SPHENOIDALIS.

lamina dura   A dense linear radiographic image of the bone which lines the socket of a tooth.

elastic lamina   ELASTIC LAMELLA.

lamina elastica anterior bowmani   An outmoded term for LAMINA LIMITANS ANTERIOR CORNEAE.

lamina elastica posterior demoursi   An outmoded term for LAMINA LIMITANS POSTERIOR CORNEAE.

lamina elastica posterior descemeti   An outmoded term for LAMINA LIMITANS POSTERIOR CORNEAE.

episcleral lamina   LAMINA EPISCLERALIS.

lamina episcleralis   [NA] The loose fibroelastic tissue which forms the outermost layer of the sclera and is continuous externally with the dense connective tissue of the vagina bulbi, while its inner surface blends with the substantia propria sclerae. Also called *episcleral lamina.*

lamina epithelialis   [NA] The modified layer of ependymal cells forming the ventricular surface of the tela choroidea.

lamina externa   LAMINA EXTERNA CRANII.

lamina externa cranii   [NA] The dense outer layer of compact bone of the flat cranial bones. It encloses the diploë and certain paranasal sinuses between it and the inner layer. Also called *outer plate of cranial bones, outer table of bones of skull, tabula externa ossis cranii* (outmoded), *lamina externa.*

external elastic lamina   A fenestrated layer of elastic tissue that represents the boundary between the tunica media and the tunica adventitia of an artery. Also called *membrana elastica externa, external elastic membrane, Henle's elastic membrane.*

external medullary lamina of thalamus   See under LAMINAE MEDULLARES THALAMI.

external lamina of peritoneum   An outmoded term for PERITONEUM PARIETALE.

external plexiform lamina   STRATUM PLEXIFORME EXTERNUM.

external lamina of pterygoid process   LAMINA LATERALIS PROCESSUS PTERYGOIDEI.

lamina fibrocartilaginea interpubica   An outmoded term for DISCUS INTERPUBICUS.

fibrocartilaginous interpubic lamina   DISCUS INTERPUBICUS.

foliate lamina   A laminated connective tissue sheath present in some melanocytic nevi. Also called *lame foliacée.*

lamina fusca sclerae   [NA] The thin, pigmented innermost layer of the sclera, composed of small bundles of collagen fibers and many elastic fibers between which are branching chromatophores containing melanin. Its inner surface has grooves for the ciliary vessels and nerves. Also called *membrana fusca.*

hepatic lamina   A sheet or layer of liver cells that lies between adjacent sinusoids.

lamina horizontalis ossis palatini   [NA] The quadrilateral horizontal plate of the palatine bone which articulates anteriorly with the palatine process of the maxilla so that its palatal surface forms the posterior part of the hard palate and its nasal surface forms the back of the floor of the nasal cavity on each side. Also called *horizontal plate of palatine bone, pars horizontalis ossis palatini* (outmoded), *palate plate* (outmoded).

inferior lamina of sphenoid bone   An outmoded term for PROCESSUS PTERYGOIDEUS OSSIS SPHENOIDALIS.

lamina interna   LAMINA INTERNA CRANII.

lamina interna cranii   [NA] The dense internal layer of compact bone of the flat cranial bones. It lies on the inner aspect of the diploë and, in certain parts, of the paranasal sinuses. Also called *inner plate of cranial bones, inner table of bones of skull, vitreous table* (outmoded), *tabula vitrea* (outmoded), *tabula interna ossis cranii* (outmoded), *lamina interna, inner table.*

internal elastic lamina   The innermost layer of elastic tissue in the wall of an artery. It forms the boundary between the tunica interna and the tunica media. Also called *internal elastic membrane, membrana elastica interna, internal elastic coat of artery.*

internal medullary lamina of thalamus   See under LAMINAE MEDULLARES THALAMI.

internal plexiform lamina   STRATUM PLEXIFORME INTERNUM.

internal lamina of pterygoid process   LAMINA MEDIALIS PROCESSUS PTERYGOIDEI.

labial lamina   The ectodermal precursor demarcating the lips from the gums, at first in the form of a semicircular band along the upper and lower jaws of a developing embryo. The lateral portion of the labial lamina, sometimes called the vestibular lamina, becomes grooved (vestibular groove), and the grooves deepen to give rise to the vestibule of the mouth. Also called *primary labial groove, labiogingival lamina, lip furrow band, tenia labiogingivalis.*

labiodental lamina   One of the ectodermal ingrowths that give rise to the dental and labiogingival laminae.

labiogingival lamina   LABIAL LAMINA.

lateral lamina of cartilage of auditory tube   LAMINA CARTILAGINIS LATERALIS TUBAE AUDITIVAE.

lateral dental lamina   A band of cells extending from the dental lamina to a tooth germ.

lamina lateralis cartilaginis tubae auditivae   LAMINA CARTILAGINIS LATERALIS TUBAE AUDITIVAE.

lamina lateralis processus pterygoidei　[NA] The broad, short and everted lateral plate of each of the two pterygoid processes projecting down from the junctions of the body and greater wings of the sphenoid bone. The outer surface is part of the medial wall of the infratemporal fossa and gives attachment to the lateral pterygoid muscle, while the inner surface is separated from the medial plate by the pterygoid fossa and gives attachment to the medial pterygoid muscle. The upper portion of the anterior border forms the posterior margin of the pterygomaxillary fissure. Also called *lateral plate of pterygoid process, external lamina of pterygoid process, lateral lamina of pterygoid process, lateral pterygoid plate, lateral pterygoid lamina, external pterygoid plate* (outmoded).

lateral medullary lamina　LAMINA MEDULLARIS LATERALIS CORPORIS STRIATI.

lateral medullary lamina of lentiform nucleus　LAMINA MEDULLARIS LATERALIS NUCLEI LENTIFORMIS.

lateral pterygoid lamina　LAMINA LATERALIS PROCESSUS PTERYGOIDEI.

lateral lamina of pterygoid process　LAMINA LATERALIS PROCESSUS PTERYGOIDEI.

lamina limitans anterior corneae　[NA] The layer of tightly interwoven fibrils which is situated directly underneath the corneal epithelium and is considered to be a modified layer of the underlying substantia propria but without fibroblasts. Also called *anterior limiting lamina, lamina elastica anterior bowmani* (outmoded), *Bowman's membrane, Bowman's layer, anterior elastic layer, Reichert's membrane, ectocornea.*

lamina limitans posterior corneae　[NA] The thin, homogeneous, transparent membrane separating the substantia propria from the epithelium posterius of the cornea, of the latter of which it is considered to be the basement membrane. At the circumference of the cornea it breaks up into the trabecular meshwork on the inner wall of sinus venosus sclerae. Also called *posterior limiting lamina, Descemet's membrane, Demours membrane, lamina elastica posterior demoursi* (outmoded), *lamina elastica posterior descemeti* (outmoded), *posterior elastic layer, Duddell's membrane, vitreous membrane.*

lamina limitans tubuli seminiferi convoluti　The limiting membrane that surrounds the cellular wall of a convoluted seminiferous tubule. It comprises a basement membrane surrounded by an envelope of loose connective tissue containing a single continuous layer of myoid cells, the stratum myoideum. Also called *tunica propria tubuli testis* (outmoded), *tunica propria tubuli seminiferi* (outmoded).

medial lamina of cartilage of auditory tube　LAMINA CARTILAGINIS MEDIALIS TUBAE AUDITIVAE.

lamina medialis cartilaginis tubae auditivae　LAMINA CARTILAGINIS MEDIALIS TUBAE AUDITIVAE.

lamina medialis processus pterygoidei　[NA] The long, narrow inner plate of each of the two pterygoid processes projecting down from the junctions of the body and greater wings of the sphenoid bone. It fuses anteriorly with the lateral plate to form the pterygoid fossa between them. Its medial surface helps to form the corresponding posterior aperture of the nose. Extending inferiorly from the plate is a hooklike process, or hamulus, around which the tendon of the tensor veli palatini muscle passes, while superiorly the plate is prolonged along the inferior surface of the body of the sphenoid as the vaginal process. The posterior border provides attachment for part of the superior constrictor muscle of the pharynx. Also called *medial lamina of pterygoid process, medial plate of pterygoid process, internal lamina of pterygoid process, medial pterygoid plate, medial pterygoid lamina, internal pterygoid plate* (outmoded).

medial medullary lamina　LAMINA MEDULLARIS MEDIALIS CORPORIS STRIATI.

medial pterygoid lamina　LAMINA MEDIALIS PROCESSUS PTERYGOIDEI.

medial lamina of pterygoid process　LAMINA MEDIALIS PROCESSUS PTERYGOIDEI.

laminae mediastinales　The reflections of the mediastinal pleura at the right and left sides of the mediastinum. They extend over the pericardium, to which they adhere, and over the other structures of the mediastinum.

laminae medullares cerebelli　LAMINAE ALBAE CEREBELLI.

laminae medullares thalami　Two bands of myelinated fibers associated with the thalamus. The outer or external medullary lamina surrounds the lateral and ventral surfaces, and the inner or internal medullary lamina separates the medial from the ventrolateral tier of nuclei. Also called *medullary laminae of thalamus.*

lamina medullaris lateralis corporis striati　The band of myelinated fibers coursing between the medial and lateral segments of the globus pallidus. Also called *lateral medullary lamina.*

lamina medullaris lateralis nuclei lentiformis　The nerve bundle lateral to the nucleus lentiformis. Also called *lateral medullary lamina of lentiform nucleus.*

lamina medullaris medialis corporis striati　The layer of myelinated fibers coursing between the globus pallidus and the putamen. Also called *medial medullary lamina.*

lamina medullaris transversa corporis quadrigemini　STRATUM ALBUM PROFUNDUM CORPORIS QUADRIGEMINI.

medullary laminae of lentiform nucleus　Lamina medullaris lateralis nuclei lentiformis and lamina medullaris medialis nuclei lentiformis.

medullary laminae of thalamus　LAMINAE MEDULLARES THALAMI.

lamina membranacea tubae auditivae　[NA] A membranous connective tissue layer extending between the free edges of the medial and lateral plates of the troughlike cartilaginous portion of the auditory tube, completing it inferiorly and laterally. Also called *membranous layer of auditory tube.*

membranous lamina of auditory tube　LAMINA MEMBRANACEA TUBAE AUDITIVAE.

lamina mesenterii propria　An outmoded term for COMMON DORSAL MESENTERY.

lamina modioli　[NA] The upper part of lamina spiralis ossea.

lamina muscularis mucosae　A thin layer of smooth muscle in the wall of most parts of the digestive tube, located between the lamina propria mucosae and the loose connective tissue of the tela submucosa.

lamina muscularis mucosae coli　Lamina muscularis mucosae intestini crassi as observed in the colon.

lamina muscularis mucosae esophagi　[NA] The thin layer of longitudinal muscle fibers and some elastic fibers located external to the lamina propria mucosae of the esophagus. This muscular lamina and the tela submucosa form longitudinal folds in the lumen which flatten out during the swallowing of food.

lamina muscularis mucosae gastricae　[NA] The thin layer of smooth muscle, consisting of an inner circular and an outer longitudinal layer and, in some areas, of an additional outer circular layer, located in the wall of the stomach between the lamina propria mucosae and the tela submucosa. The inner circular layer may send fibers between the glands to the mucosal surface, the contraction of which flattens the longitudinal folds of the mucosa in the presence of food.

lamina muscularis mucosae intestini crassi　[NA] A well-developed layer of smooth muscle in the mucous membrane of the large intestine, composed of outer longitudinal and inner circular fibers. It is situated between the lamina propria mucosae and the tela submucosa. It may be irregular or lacking at the sites of lymphatic nodules. Occasionally thin bundles of muscle cells extend toward the surface epithelium.

lamina muscularis mucosae intestini recti LAMINA MUSCULARIS MUCOSAE RECTI.

lamina muscularis mucosae intestini tenuis [NA] The regular and well-developed layer of smooth muscle of the wall of the small intestine located between the lamina propria mucosae and the tela submucosa.

lamina muscularis mucosae recti [NA] The well-developed layer of smooth muscle deep in the tunica mucosa of the rectum, which has the same characteristics as the lamina muscularis mucosae coli, except that the rectal mucosa presents folds in the lumen. Also called *lamina muscularis mucosae intestini recti.*

neural lamina LAMINA ARCUS VERTEBRAE.

nuclear fibrous lamina A fibrillar layer that is applied to the internal aspect of the inner nuclear membrane.

orbital lamina LAMINA ORBITALIS OSSIS ETHMOIDALIS.

lamina orbitalis ossis ethmoidalis [NA] A vertical, oblong bony plate which forms the lateral surface of the ethmoidal labyrinth and a large part of the medial wall of the orbit. It articulates with the lacrimal bone anteriorly, the sphenoid bone posteriorly, the orbital part of the frontal bone superiorly and the maxilla and palatine bone inferiorly. Also called *orbital lamina, orbital plate of ethmoid bone, lamina papyracea* (outmoded), *paper plate* (outmoded), *os planum.*

osseous spiral lamina LAMINA SPIRALIS OSSEA.

palatine lamina of maxilla PROCESSUS PALATINUS MAXILLAE.

lamina papyracea An outmoded term for LAMINA ORBITALIS OSSIS ETHMOIDALIS.

lamina parietalis pericardii [NA] The outer layer of serous pericardium that is reflected off the great vessels and heart to line the fibrous pericardium of the cavity in which the heart lies. Also called *parietal layer of serous pericardium, parietal pericardium, parietal layer of pericardium.*

lamina parietalis tunicae vaginalis propriae testis LAMINA PARIETALIS TUNICAE VAGINALIS TESTIS.

lamina parietalis tunicae vaginalis testis [NA] The outer layer of tunica vaginalis testis. It is reflected from the testis and from a short way up the front and medial side of the spermatic cord on to the internal surface of the scrotum, where it adheres to the internal spermatic fascia. Also called *perietal layer of tunica vaginalis of testis, lamina parietalis tunicae vaginalis propriae testis, tunica adnata testis* (outmoded), *periorchium* (outmoded).

periclaustral lamina CAPSULA EXTERNA.

perpendicular lamina of ethmoid bone LAMINA PERPENDICULARIS OSSIS ETHMOIDALIS.

lamina perpendicularis ossis ethmoidalis [NA] The thin quadrilateral plate of the ethmoid bone, descending vertically from the crista galli at its junction with the cribriform plate to form the upper part of the nasal septum and join the septal cartilage below. The posterior margin articulates with the vomer inferiorly and with the sphenoidal crest superiorly. Also called *perpendicular lamina of ethmoid bone, perpendicular plate of ethmoid bone, perpendicular layer of ethmoid bone, vertical layer of ethmoid bone* (outmoded).

lamina perpendicularis ossis palatini [NA] The thin quadrangular vertical part of the palatine bone, the anterior border of which articulates with the maxilla and the inferior nasal concha so that its nasal surface forms part of the lateral wall of the nasal cavity, while its lateral, or maxillary, surface forms part of the posterior wall of maxillary sinus and the medial wall of the pterygopalatine fossa and has a deep vertical groove, the greater palatine groove, posteriorly. The superior border has the orbital process in front, the sphenoidal process posteriorly and the sphenopalatine notch between them. Also called *perpendicular plate of palatine bone, pars perpendicularis ossis palatini*

(outmoded), *vertical plate of palatine bone.*

posterior limiting lamina LAMINA LIMITANS POSTERIOR CORNEAE.

posterior membranous lamina of trachea PARIES MEMBRANACEUS TRACHEAE.

lamina posterior vaginae musculi recti abdominis [NA] The posterior layer of the sheath of the rectus abdominis muscle. It is formed by the posterior lamina of the aponeurosis of the internal oblique muscle blending with the aponeurosis of the transversus abdominis muscle, extending from the costal margin to the arcuate line about halfway between the umbilicus and symphysis pubis. Also called *posterior layer of rectus sheath.*

lamina pretrachealis fasciae cervicalis [NA] A layer of deep cervical fascia continuous with the investing layer behind the sternocleidomastoid muscle. It passes in front of the trachea and larynx, ensheathing the infrahyoid muscles and forming a sheath around the thyroid gland. Superiorly it is attached to the hyoid bone and laterally it forms the carotid sheath and blends with the buccopharyngeal fascia. Inferiorly it extends to the back of the manubrium sterni becoming continuous with the fibrous covering of the aorta and of the pericardium. Also called *middle layer of cervical fascia, pretracheal fascia, pretracheal layer, thyrolaryngeal fascia* (outmoded), *cervical visceral fascia.*

lamina prevertebralis fasciae cervicalis [NA] The circular layer of deep cervical fascia that covers the prevertebral and scalene muscles, forming a fascial floor for the posterior triangle of the neck. Posteriorly it is continuous with the ligamentum nuchae, attaching to the external occipital protuberance and the spine of the seventh cervical vertebra. Anteriorly it lies behind the pharynx, the esophagus, and the carotid sheath, to which it is attached by fibroareolar tissue. Inferiorly it extends into the superior mediastinum to blend with the anterior longitudinal ligament. Also called *prevertebral fascia, fascia prevertebralis.*

lamina profunda fasciae temporalis [NA] The inner, or deep, layer of the aponeurotic fascia over the temporalis muscle that is attached to the medial surface of the zygomatic arch, just above which it is connected to the superficial layer by dense, fibrous tissue and separated by fat and vessels. It provides origin to fibers of the temporalis muscle.

lamina profunda musculi levatoris palpebrae superioris MUSCULUS TARSALIS SUPERIOR.

proper lamina of mesentery An outmoded term for COMMON DORSAL MESENTERY.

lamina propria LAMINA PROPRIA MUCOSAE.

lamina propria membranae tympani The middle, or fibrous, layer of the tympanic membrane separating the external acoustic meatus from the tympanic cavity. The layer comprises two united layers, namely, stratum radiatum and stratum circulare, which are not found in the pars flaccida. An outmoded term.

lamina propria mucosae [NA] A layer of connective tissue between the superficial epithelium and the underlying lamina muscularis mucosae of the alimentary tract. Also called *lamina propria, membrana propria* (outmoded), *mucoderm.*

lamina quadrigemina LAMINA TECTI MESENCEPHALI.

reticular lamina MEMBRANA RETICULARIS DUCTUS COCHLEARIS.

reticular lamina of the cochlea In the organ of Corti, a delicate layer of cytoplasmic processes that extend from the cells of Deiters and the outer rod or pillar cells. This membrane is perforated by the stereocilia of the hair cells. Also called *lamina reticularis, reticular lamina of the spiral organ.*

lamina reticularis RETICULAR LAMINA OF THE COCHLEA.

reticular lamina of the spiral organ RETICULAR LAMINA OF THE COCHLEA.

laminae of Rexed A group of cytoarchitectural layers and zones of the spinal gray matter which have provided an anatomically consistent and physiologically meaningful way of grouping spinal neurons. These consist of laminae I–IX arranged in the dorsoventral direction and a centrally situated lamina X.

rostral lamina   LAMINA ROSTRALIS.

lamina rostralis   The thin median bridge extending from the rostrum of the corpus callosum down to the lamina terminalis. It comprises the median reflection of pia mater, and contrary to some earlier beliefs does not contain commissural fibers. Also called *rostral lamina, taeniola corporis callosi of Reil.*

secondary spiral lamina   LAMINA SPIRALIS SECUNDARIA.

lamina septi pellucidi   [NA] The vertical neural laminae separated by a space, the cavum septi pellucidi. The lamina contains the medial and lateral nuclei of the septum pellucidum and fibers of the fornix. Also called *lamina of septum pellucidum.*

lamina of septum pellucidum   LAMINA SEPTI PELLUCIDI.

lamina spiralis ossea   [NA] The ledge of bone projecting from the modiolus of the cochlea and winding screwlike around it, partially dividing the cochlear canal into an upper passage, or scala vestibuli, and a lower one, or scala tympani. It ends at the apex in the hooklike hamulus. It comprises an upper and a lower lamella between which minute canals transmit fibers of the cochlear nerve to its edge and the organ of Corti. Also called *bony spiral lamina, spiral plate, osseous spiral lamina.*

lamina spiralis secundaria   [NA] A bony ridge projecting inwards from the outer wall of the lower part of the first turn of the cochlea, opposite the osseous spiral lamina but not reaching it. Also called *secondary spiral lamina, secondary spiral plate.*

submucous lamina of stomach   A layer of loose connective tissue that contains vessels and autonomic nerves. It is situated between the main muscle layer externally and the mucosal layer internally. Also called *vascular lamina of stomach.*

superficial lamina of cervical fascia   LAMINA SUPERFICIALIS FASCIAE CERVICALIS.

lamina superficialis fasciae cervicalis   [NA] The superficial, or investing, layer of deep fascia of the neck, fused posteriorly with the ligamentum nuchae, surrounding the trapezius muscle and covering the posterior triangle of the neck, then investing the sternocleidomastoid muscle, anterior to which it covers the anterior triangle of the neck and becomes continuous with the corresponding layer of the opposite side at the midline. Inferiorly it is attached to the clavicle and manubrium sterni while superiorly it attaches to the superior nuchal line and the body of the mandible and extends over the parotid gland to the masseteric fascia, as well as attaching to the symphysis menti and the hyoid bone. Also called *external cervical fascia, superficial lamina of cervical fascia, investing layer of cervical fascia.*

lamina superficialis fasciae temporalis   [NA] The superficial layer of the aponeurotic fascia covering the temporalis muscle that is attached to the outer surface of the zygomatic arch, above which it is connected to the deep layer by dense, fibrous tissue. The superficial temporal vessels and the auriculotemporal nerve cross it superficially while deep to it the middle temporal artery and fatty and areolar tissue may be found.

lamina superficialis musculi levatoris palpebrae superioris [NA] The fibrous, aponeurotic superior layer of the levator palpebrae superioris muscle of the orbit that is inserted partly into the anterior surface of the superior tarsus, and partly into the skin of the upper eyelid after passing through fibers of the orbicularis oculi muscle.

lamina suprachorioidea   An outmoded term for LAMINA SUPRACHOROIDEA.

suprachoroid lamina   LAMINA SUPRACHOROIDEA.

lamina suprachoroidea   [NA] A thin layer of pigmented, nonvascular, obliquely directed lamellae which is situated on the external surface of the choroid and connected to the lamina fusca sclerae. Each lamella consists of a meshwork of delicate collagen and elastic fibers within which are branching melanocytes, ganglionic neurons and nerve fibers. Also called *supra-*

choroid lamina, suprachorioid layer (outmoded), *lamina suprachorioidea* (outmoded), *cellulosa chorioideae* (outmoded), *suprachoroidea, stratum perichorioideum* (outmoded).

lamina supraneuroporica   That part of the lamina terminalis located caudal to the anterior neuropore in an embryo. It is virtually indiscernible in human embryos.

tectal lamina of mesencephalon   LAMINA TECTI MESENCEPHALI.

lamina tecti mesencephali   The roof of the mesencephalon, consisting of laminae of fibers and nerve cells. In submammalian forms, it forms the roof of the optocoele. In mammals it refers to the superior and inferior colliculi (corpora quadrigemina). Also called *quadrigeminal plate, lamina quadrigemina, tectal lamina of mesencephalon.*

terminal lamina of hypothalamus   LAMINA TERMINALIS.

lamina terminalis   [NA] A membrane formed in the developing embryo by the closure of the anterior neuropore at the cephalic end of the early neural tube. In the adult brain the lamina terminalis remains as a thin layer of gray matter, derived from the telencephalon, that extends from the superior surface of the optic chiasma to the rostrum of the corpus callosum. It forms part of the anterior wall of the third ventricle. Also called *lamina terminalis hypothalami, terminal lamina of hypothalamus, terminal plate, velum terminale, lamina cinerea terminalis* (obsolete), *gray plate* (obsolete).

lamina terminalis hypothalami   LAMINA TERMINALIS.

lamina of thyroid cartilage   LAMINA CARTILAGINIS THYROIDEAE DEXTRA/SINISTRA.

lamina tragi   [NA] The arched longitudinal lamina of cartilage of the tragus of the auricle, quite separate from the cartilage of the auricle and attached to the outer margin of the cartilage of the external auditory meatus. Also called *lamina tragica.*

lamina tragica   LAMINA TRAGI.

ungual laminae   CRISTAE MATRICIS UNGUIS.

vascular lamina of choroid   LAMINA VASCULOSA CHOROIDEAE.

vascular lamina of stomach   SUBMUCOUS LAMINA OF STOMACH.

lamina vasculosa chorioideae   An outmoded term for LAMINA VASCULOSA CHOROIDEAE.

lamina vasculosa choroideae   [NA] The outermost layer of the choroid proper which consists of the branches of the short posterior ciliary arteries extending anteriorly, a venous plexus which converges in whorls on the vorticose veins, and a loose connective tissue containing melanocytes. It is situated between the lamina suprachoroideae externally and the lamina choroidocapillaris deep to it. The vessels tend to diminish in size from the outer to the inner aspects of this layer. Also called *vascular lamina of choroid, vascular layer of choroid, Haller's layer, Haller's membrane, lamina vasculosa chorioideae* (outmoded), *secundina oculi* (outmoded).

lamina vasculosa testis   TUNICA VASCULOSA TESTIS.

lamina of vertebra   LAMINA ARCUS VERTEBRAE.

lamina of vertebral arch   LAMINA ARCUS VERTEBRAE.

vestibular lamina   That part of the labial lamina, extending backwards between the developing cheek and gums, that will split to form the vestibule of the mouth. Also called *buccogingival lamina.*

lamina visceralis pericardii   [NA] The layer of the serous pericardium that closely invests the heart and the beginning of the aorta and pulmonary trunk. Also called *epicardium, visceral layer of pericardium, visceral pericardium, cardiac pericardium* (outmoded).

lamina visceralis tunicae vaginalis propriae testis   LAMINA VISCERALIS TUNICAE VAGINALIS TESTIS.

lamina visceralis tunicae vaginalis testis   [NA] The layer of the tunica vaginalis testis that closely invests the testis on its medial and lateral surfaces and anterior border and also covers the lateral and medial aspects of the epididymis as well as the upper surface of its head. Also called *visceral layer of tunica vaginalis of testis, lamina visceralis tunicae vaginalis propriae testis, eporchium* (outmoded), *tunica serosa testis* (outmoded).

lamina vitrea   An outmoded term for COMPLEXUS BASALIS CHOROIDEAE.

vitreal lamina   An outmoded term for COMPLEXUS BASALIS CHOROIDEAE.

vitreous lamina   An outmoded term for COMPLEXUS BASALIS CHOROIDEAE.

white laminae of cerebellum   LAMINAE ALBAE CEREBELLI.

zonal lamina   STRATUM MOLECULARE.

lamina zonalis   STRATUM MOLECULARE.

lamina zonalis of cerebellum   STRATUM MOLECULARE CEREBELLI.

---

laminae   Plural of LAMINA.

laminagram [LAMINA + -GRAM]   A roentgenogram obtained during laminagraphy. Also called *laminogram.*

laminagraph [LAMINA + -GRAPH]   X-ray equipment for doing body section roentgenography. Also called *laminograph.*

stroboscopic laminagraph   An x-ray machine for doing body section roentgenography, equipped with a stroboscopic system to allow clear unblurred images of a moving structure by causing the motion to appear slowed or stopped.

laminagraphy [LAMINA + -GRAPHY]   BODY SECTION ROENTGENOGRAPHY.

laminar   Consisting of, arranged in, or pertaining to laminae; laminated.

laminaran   LAMINARIN SULFATE.

Laminaria   A genus of brown algae in the division Phaeophycophyta. Species of this genus have been used to gradually dilate the cervix in induced abortions. Algin from *L. digitata* is used as a thickening agent in pharmaceuticals, cosmetics, and dentrifices. Kelp, a common name for many genera of brown algae, has served as a source of iodine and bromine.

laminarin   A polysaccharide obtained from brown algae of the *Laminaria* genus. It is chiefly composed of β-D-glucose residues. When the glucose units are sulfated, resulting in two sulfate groups per glucose unit, the molecule attains maximum stability and has anticoagulant properties. With fewer sulfate groups, the molecule has antilipemic activity only.

laminarin sulfate   The sulfated form of a polysaccharide from a seaweed, *Laminaria*, having anticoagulant properties, like heparin. Also called *laminaran.*

laminate   LAMINATED.

laminated   Consisting of or arranged in layers or laminae. Also *laminate.*

lamination   A layered arrangement or formation.

laminectomy [lamin(a) + -ECTOMY]   Excision of the posterior arches and spinous processes of a vertebra. Also called *rachiotomy, spondylotomy, rachitomy.*

laminester   A naturally occurring polyester found in beehives as a waterproofing coat to protect the brood cells.

laminitis [lamin(a) + -ITIS]   An inflammatory condition of the hoof, especially of horses, that often results from excessive intake of grain. It may become chronic with considerable malformation of the foot. Also called *founder.*

laminogram   LAMINAGRAM.

laminograph   LAMINAGRAPH.

laminography [lamin(a) + o + -GRAPHY]   BODY SECTION ROENTGENOGRAPHY.

laminotomy [lamin(a) + o + -TOMY]   The division or partial removal of vertebral laminae.

lamp   A device for producing light artificially for illumination.

arc lamp   A lamp in which an electric arc passes through a gas between two electrodes, heating the gas and electrodes to incandescence. Also called *arc light.*

Birch-Hirschfeld lamp   An intense source of visible radiation intended for use in treatment of eye disease.

carbon arc lamp   A lamp that produces intense white light by electric discharge between carbon rod electrodes.

cold quartz mercury vapor lamp   A quartz mercury arc lamp that generates ultraviolet rays with the resonance emission of mercury vapor (254 mμ) and operates at low vapor pressure and low intensity. It was formerly used for bactericidal effect.

Eldridge-Green lamp   A color-vision testing device using spectral filters.

Finsen lamp   A carbon arc lamp producing concentrated ultraviolet radiation at 50 volts and 50 amperes and utilized for dermatological treatment, particularly lupus vulgaris.

Finsen-Reya lamp   A modified Finsen lamp in which the electrodes are placed at right angles.

Gullstrand slit lamp   One of the earliest models of a biomicroscope, the combination of a microscope and a narrow beam of collimated light.

infrared lamp   A device that produces radiation in the lower range of the visible spectrum and below, utilized therapeutically as a source of radiant heat in the near infrared (760–1500 mμ) and far infrared (1500–15 000 mμ) ranges.

Jesionek lamp   An early type of sun lamp.

Kromayer lamp   A hand-held, water- or air-cooled mercury quartz ultraviolet lamp for localized application of intense bactericidal wave length, utilized in the treatment of skin ulcers.

mercury vapor lamp   A carbon arc lamp in which the electric arc is enclosed in a quartz burner containing mercury vapor, producing ultraviolet radiation that may be used therapeutically for general irradiation of large body areas, artificially duplicating the effect of sunlight, or adapted for focal application as a Kromayer lamp.

mignon lamp   A tiny surgical instrument with a light at the end, used during endoscopic procedures.

mouth lamp   A light source placed in the mouth.

quartz lamp   A mercury vapor lamp emitting ultraviolet light. Two types exist, cold quartz, operating at low vapor pressure and low intensity, producing shorter wave lengths (Kromayer lamp), and hot quartz, operating under high vapor pressure and high intensity at a relatively high temperature, producing longer wave lengths (sun lamp).

Simpson lamp   An electric arc lamp emitting heat rays and visible and ultraviolet light. One electrode is made from tungstenate of iron and the other from manganese. Also called *Simpson light.*

slit lamp   A combination of a microscope and a narrow beam of collimated light, used to observe the eye. Also called *corneal microscope, slit lamp microscope.*

sun lamp   Any lamp used for irradiation or sunbathing purposes that emits radiation which simulates that of the sun in some respect, especially in the ultraviolet range.

tungsten arc lamp   A lamp having compressed tungsten electrodes.

ultraviolet lamp   Any lamp that principally emits ultraviolet rays.

uviol lamp   An electric lamp with special glass to emit violet rays.

Wood's lamp   A device for producing ultraviolet rays (Wood's light) filtered through nickel glass and peaking at 365 nm, which gives a characteristic fluorescence in the presence of some microbial agents. It is commonly used to demonstrate *Microsporum* species in the hair of children. Infected hair has a bright green fluorescence. A pink fluorescence appears in skin lesions of erythrasma, a gold fluorescence in areas of pityriasis versicolor, and a bright green in wounds, lesions, and toe webs of *Pseudomonas*. Wood's light is invaluable in controlling outbreaks of *Microsporum* infection. However, some fungi causing tinea capitis (ringworm of the scalp), such as *Trichophyton tonsurans*, produce no fluorescence when subjected to ultraviolet light.

lampas [French (from *lamper* to guzzle, nasalized form of *laper*, onomatopoeic word meaning to lap liquids), a swelling of the roof of the mouth in young horses]   A painful swelling of the hard palate of a horse, immediately behind the upper incisor teeth, especially the central incisors.

Lamus   A former genus of reduviid bugs now included in the genera *Panstrongylus* and *Triatoma*.

Lamy [Maurice Emile Joseph *Lamy*, French physician, born 1895]   **1** Maroteaux-Lamy disease. See under DISEASE.   **2** Maroteaux-Lamy syndrome. See under MUCOPOLYSACCHARIDOSIS VI.

lana [L, wool]   Wool.

Lancaster [Walter Brackett *Lancaster*, U.S. ophthalmologist, born 1863]   See under ADVANCEMENT.

lance   **1** To incise tissue with a lancet for purposes of drainage.   **2** LANCET.

Mauriceau's lance   An obstetric knife formerly used to carry out embryotomy.

Lancefield [Rebecca Craighill *Lancefield*, U.S. bacteriologist, born 1895]   **1** See under CLASSIFICATION.   **2** Lancefield precipitation test. See under TEST.

lancelet [*lance* + *-let*, diminishing suffix]   CEPHALOCHORDATE.

lanceolate   Tapering to a point and broad at the base or in the middle; lance-shaped.

Lancereaux [Étienne *Lancereaux*, French physician, 1829–1910]   **1** See under NEPHRITIS.   **2** Lancereaux-Mathieu disease. See under ICTERIC LEPTOSPIROSIS.

lancet [French *lancette*, dim. of *lance* a spear, from L *lance(a)* a lance, spear]   A small surgical blade, usually with two honed edges, used for making small drainage incisions. Also called *lance*.

abscess lancet   A surgical knife with one convex and one concave cutting edge that is used for drainage of an abscess.

acne lancet   A narrow-bladed lancet for piercing acne pustules and abscesses.

gingival lancet   A knife for incising the gum. Also called *gum lancet*.

gum lancet   GINGIVAL LANCET.

spring lancet   A surgical blade, usually concealed in a case, that is released and activated by a spring.

thumb lancet   A short surgical knife that has a blade which folds back into a metallic sheath.

lancinate [L *lancinat(us)*, past part. of *lancinare* (akin to *lacerare* to hew, tear to pieces) to lacerate, mangle, tear to pieces]   **1** To cut sharply, tear, or make sharp darting movements such as would be made with a lancet.   **2** Pertaining to a lancet.

lancinating [L *lancinat(us)*, past part. of *lancinare* (akin to *lacer* hewn, mangled) to tear in pieces, lacerate + -ING. *Lancinare* is not related in meaning to L *lancea* a lance, which Latin borrowed from the Celtic of Gaul.]   Describing a sudden sharp and transient pain, supposedly like the pain of being pierced with the point of a lance.

Lancisi [Giovanni Maria *Lancisi*, Italian physician, 1654–1720]   **1** See under SIGN.   **2** Longitudinal nerves of Lancisi. See under NERVES OF LANCISI.

Landau [Leopold *Landau*, German gynecologist and obstetrician, 1848–1920]   See under REFLEX.

landfill   A depression that is set aside for the deposition of waste material.

sanitary landfill   A landfill formed by controlled tipping, in which the solid waste is spread in thin layers, compacted, and covered with soil at the end of each working day. Compare DUMP.

landmark   A specified and recognized anatomical marking or structure that is used in locating other structures or as a reference point in making measurements.

Landolt [Edmund *Landolt*, French ophthalmologist, 1846–1926]   **1** See under OPERATION, RING.   **2** Landolt's bodies. See under BODY.   **3** Landolt ring chart. See under CHART.

Landor [J. V. *Landor*, English physician, flourished 20th century]   Hawes-Pallister-Landor syndrome. See under STRACHAN-SCOTT SYNDROME.

Landouzy [Louis Theophil Joseph *Landouzy*, French physician, 1845–1917]   **1** Landouzy-Grasset law. See under LAW.   **2** Landouzy-Dejerine atrophy, Landouzy-Dejerine myopathy, Duchenne-Landouzy dystrophy, Dejerine-Landouzy dystrophy, Landouzy's dystrophy, Landouzy-Dejerine dystrophy. See under FACIOSCAPULOHUMERAL MUSCULAR DYSTROPHY.   **3** Landouzy's disease. See under ICTERIC LEPTOSPIROSIS.

Landry [Jean Baptiste Octave *Landry*, French physician, 1826–1865]   **1** Landry-Guillain-Barré syndrome. See under GUILLAIN-BARRÉ SYNDROME.   **2** Landry's disease, Landry's palsy, Kussmaul-Landry paralysis, Landry-Kussmaul syndrome, Landry syndrome. See under LANDRY'S PARALYSIS.

Landsberg [J. W. *Landsberg*, U.S. hematologist, born 1907]   Wintrobe and Landsberg method. See under METHOD.

Landschutz [Christoph *Landschutz*, German medical researcher, flourished 20th century]   See under TUMOR.

Landsteiner [Karl *Landsteiner*, Austrian-born U.S. pathologist, 1868–1943]   **1** Donath-Landsteiner cold autoantibody. See under DONATH-LANDSTEINER ANTIBODY.   **2** Donath-Landsteiner syndrome. See under PAROXYSMAL COLD HEMOGLOBINURIA.   **3** Donath-Landsteiner test. See under TEST.   **4** See under CLASSIFICATION.

Landström [John *Landström*, Swedish surgeon, 1869–1910]   See under MUSCLE.

Landzert [Theodor *Landzert*, German anatomist, died 1889]   **1** Landzert's fossa, Gruber-Landzert fossa. See under RECESSUS PARADUODENALIS.   **2** Gruber-Landzert fossa. See under FOSSA.

Lane [Clayton Arbuthnot *Lane*, British parasitologist active in India, born 1868]   Lane method. See under DIRECT CENTRIFUGAL FLOTATION METHOD.

Lane [John Edward *Lane*, U.S. dermatologist, 1872–1933]   Lane's disease. See under ERYTHEMA PALMARE HEREDITARIUM.

Lane [Sir William Arbuthnot *Lane*, English surgeon, 1856–1943]   **1** Lane's kink. See under ILEAL KINK.   **2** Lane's band. See under GENITOMESENTERIC BAND.   **3** Lane plates. See under PLATE.

Lang [Basil Thorn *Lang*, English ophthalmologist, 1880–1928]   Frost-Lang operation. See under OPERATION.

Langdon-Down [John *Langdon* (Haydon) *Down*, English physician, 1828–1896]   Langdon-Down disease. See under DOWN SYNDROME.

Lange [Carl *Lange*, German physician, born 1883]   **1** Lange's reaction, Lange's test. See under COLLOIDAL GOLD TEST.   **2** See under SOLUTION.

Lange [Carl Georg *Lange*, Danish psychologist, 1834–1900]

James-Lange-Sutherland theory. See under JAMES-LANGE THEORY.

Lange [Fritz *Lange*, German orthopedic surgeon, 1864–1952] See under OPERATION.

Langenbeck [Bernhard Rudolph Konrad von *Langenbeck*, German surgeon, 1810–1887] **1** See under INCISION, TRIANGLE. **2** Langenbeck flap. See under VON LANGENBECK'S BIPEDICLED MUCOPERIOSTEAL FLAP.

Langendorff [Oscar *Langendorff*, German physiologist, 1853–1908] Langendorff's method. See under PREPARATION.

Lange-Nielsen [Fredrik *Lange-Nielsen*, Norwegian cardiologist, flourished mid-20th century] Jervell and Lange-Nielsen syndrome. See under SYNDROME.

Langer [Karl Ritter von *Langer*, Austrian anatomist, 1819–1887] **1** Langer's axillary arch. See under PECTORODORSALIS MUSCLE. **2** Langer's lines. See under CLEAVAGE LINES. **3** See under MUSCLE.

Langerhans [Paul *Langerhans*, German pathological anatomist, 1847–1888] **1** Langerhansian adenoma. See under ISLET CELL ADENOMA. **2** Langerhansian hormone. See under HORMONE. **3** Islands of Langerhans. See under ISLETS OF LANGERHANS. **4** Langerhans stellate corpuscle. See under CELL. **5** Langerhans cell granule. See under GRANULE. **6** Langerhans layer. See under GRANULAR LAYER OF EPIDERMIS.

Langhans [Theodor *Langhans*, German anatomist, 1839–1915] **1** Langhans layer. See under CYTOTROPHOBLAST. **2** See under STRIA, CELL. **3** Langhans cell. See under LANGHANS GIANT CELL.

Langley [John Newport *Langley*, English physiologist, 1852–1925] **1** Langley's nerve. See under PILOMOTOR NERVES. **2** Langley's granules. See under GRANULE. **3** See under GANGLION.

Langmuir [Irving *Langmuir*, U.S. chemist, 1881–1957] See under TROUGH.

language [L *lingua* (from *lingare* to lick, lap; Gk *leichein* to lick) the tongue, language, speech, voice] **1** Any system making use of word symbols to convey meaning to other individuals and, possibly, to influence their behavior. The signals of any language system, whether they are spoken, written, or conveyed by gesture, are learned, and they permit an exchange of information with any other individual who has also learned the rules of that system. **2** The means for communicating with a computer.

assembly language A computer language in which mnemonically grouped sets of letters represent machine-language instructions, e.g. LDA for load accumulator.

body language The communication of the emotions, feelings, or motives of an individual to others by means of gesture, posture, facial expression, or other nonverbal signs.

higher level language A computer language such as FORTRAN, BASIC, or COBOL that enables easy solution of users' problems but is less efficient than assembly language.

irrelevant language Speech with words that have meaning only to the speaker, and which is thus unintelligible to others.

machine language The set of binary codes that control the logic gating of the internal circuits of a computer. All other programing languages must be translated into these codes.

metaphoric language Speech with metaphoric substitutions that are known only to the speaker, and which is thus incomprehensible to others.

laniary [L *laniar(ius)* (from *lani(us)* a butcher, from the Etruscan + *-arius* -ARY) pertaining to a butcher + -Y] Shaped like a dagger, as some canine teeth.

Lankesterella ranarum A small, unpigmented, nucleophilic, intracellular, coccidian parasite found in frogs. Its structure is similar to that of *Isospora*. Schizogony, gametogony, and spo-

rogony take place in macrophage cells of spleen, liver, lungs, or kidneys. Endodyogeny and endopolygeny occur, and multiple sporozoites develop from oocysts directly without forming sporocysts. They enter red cells and are taken up in blood meals by the vector, probably one of the common leeches attacking frogs.

Lankesteria culicis A gregarine sporozoon parasitic in the gut of *Aedes aegypti* and possibly other mosquitoes.

Lannelongue [Odilon Marc *Lannelongue*, French surgeon, 1840–1911] **1** Foramina of Lannelongue. See under FORAMEN. **2** Foraminula of Lannelongue. See under FORAMINA VENARUM MINIMARUM CORDIS.

Lannois [Maurice *Lannois*, French otorhinolaryngologist, born 1856] Gradenigo-Lannois syndrome. See under GRADENIGO SYNDROME.

lanolin A waxy, fatty secretion of the sebaceous glands of the sheep, which is deposited on the wool fibers. It contains about 25–30% water and is used as an ointment base. Also called *wool fat*.

anhydrous lanolin A yellowish, semisolid fat, obtained from sheep's wool, that is practically insoluble in water but can be mixed with water to form a stable emulsion. It is used as an ointment base. Also called *adeps lanae*.

lanosterol A sterol originally found in wool fat. It differs from cholesterol by possessing two methyl groups on C-4 and one on C-14, by the absence of a double bond at C-5, and by the presence of two at C-8 and C-24. It is the first steroid made in the pathway by which squalene is converted into sterols in animals. Cycloartenol plays a similar role in plants. It is made by the action of lanosterol synthase on squalene 2,3-epoxide. Also called *isocholesterol*.

lanosterol synthase The enzyme (EC 5.4.99.7) responsible for the biosynthesis of the steroid ring in animals. It isomerizes squalene 2,3-epoxide with formation of four rings.

Lanoxin A proprietary name for digoxin.

Lanterman [A. J. *Lanterman*, U.S. anatomist active in France, flourished late 19th century] **1** Schmidt-Lanterman segment. See under MEDULLARY SEGMENT. **2** Lanterman's clefts, Schmidt-Lanterman clefts, incisures of Lanterman-Schmidt. See under SCHMIDT-LANTERMAN INCISURES.

lanthanic Denoting a disease or condition that produces no symptoms and is discovered by chance. The patient may have other, nonrelated complaints. A rarely used term.

lanthanides The chemical elements having atomic numbers from 58 (cerium) to 71 (lutetium) inclusive. Lanthanum, just before cerium in the periodic table, is sometimes included in the lanthanide series. Also called *rare earth elements, rare earths*.

lanthanum Element number 57, having atomic weight 138.9055. It is a soft, silvery white metal, the first member of the lanthanide series of elements. The valence is 3. Lanthanum and its compounds are somewhat toxic. Symbol: La

lanthopine A minor alkaloid of opium.

lanugo [L, soft, tender hair or down] The fine downy hairs, devoid of a medulla, that cover the skin of a human fetus, except for the palms and soles, at about midterm. They are mostly shed before birth and are replaced on the trunk and limbs by the fine secondary hairs of the vellus during the first few months after birth, and by longer and coarser terminal hair on the scalp. Also called *down, pappus* (obsolete). Adjective: lanuginous. ● The term *lanugo* is often misused for the vellus hair.

lanulous [L *lanul(a)* (from *lan(a)* wool + *-ula*, fem. diminishing suffix) a small piece of wool + -OUS] Covered with fine, downy hair.

Lanum A proprietary name for lanolin.

Lanz [Otto *Lanz*, Swiss-born surgeon active in the Netherlands,

1865–1935] **1** See under OPERATION, POINT. **2** Lanz line. See under INTERSPINAL LINE.

LAP leukocyte alkaline phosphatase.

lapactic PURGATIVE.

lapar- LAPARO-.

laparacolpotomy LAPAROCOLPOTOMY.

laparectomy [LAPAR- + -ECTOMY] A surgical procedure in which part or all of the abdominal wall is excised and then reconstructed. It is usually performed to correct laxity but may be done because of a neoplasm, inflammation, or trauma.

laparo- [Gk *lapara* the soft part of the body between ribs and hip, flank, loin] A combining form denoting (1) the flank or loin; (2) the abdominal wall. Also *lapar-*.

laparocele VENTRAL HERNIA.

laparocholecystotomy [LAPARO- + CHOLECYSTOTOMY] CHOLECYSTOTOMY.

laparoclysis A British term for PERITONEAL DIALYSIS.

laparocolectomy COLECTOMY.

laparocolostomy A colostomy with the opening on the lateral or anterolateral wall of the abdomen.

laparocolotomy COLOTOMY.

laparocolpotomy [LAPARO- + COLPOTOMY] A transvaginal incision into the peritoneal cavity, usually made through the pouch of Douglas. Also called *laparacolpotomy*.

laparocystectomy A surgical procedure in which an intra-abdominal cyst is removed by way of an abdominal wall incision.

laparocystidotomy An incision into the urinary bladder made by a suprapubic approach.

laparocystotomy [LAPARO- + CYSTOTOMY] **1** SUPRAPUBIC CYSTOTOMY. **2** Evacuation of a cyst following an abdominal incision.

laparocystovariohysterotomy [LAPARO- + CYST- + OVARIO- + HYSTEROTOMY] Hysterotomy and removal of an ovarian cyst through an incision in the abdominal wall.

laparoenterostomy An enterostomy through the abdominal wall.

laparoenterotomy A surgical incision through the abdominal wall and into the small bowel. Also called *celioenterotomy*.

laparogastroscopy An exploratory operation in which the interior of the stomach is inspected after laparogastrotomy.

laparogastrotomy A surgical incision through the abdominal wall and into the stomach. Also called *celiogastrotomy*.

laparohepatotomy Incision of the liver through a laparotomy.

laparohysterectomy Hysterectomy performed through an abdominal incision.

laparohystero-oophorectomy Removal of the uterus and ovary through an incision in the abdominal wall. Also called *celiohystero-oothecectomy*.

laparohysterosalpingo-oophorectomy Removal of the uterus, uterine tube, and ovaries through an abdominal incision. Also called *celiohysterosalpingo-oothecectomy*.

laparohysterotomy [LAPARO- + HYSTEROTOMY] ABDOMINOHYSTEROTOMY.

laparoileotomy Incision of the ileum through a laparotomy.

laparomonodidymus [LAPARO- + MONO- + Gk *didymos* brother, twin] An imprecise term for DUPLICITAS ANTERIOR.

laparomyitis LAPAROMYOSITIS.

laparomyomectomy ABDOMINAL MYOMECTOMY.

laparomyomotomy [LAPARO- + MYOMOTOMY] CELIOMYOMOTOMY.

laparomyositis An inflammatory process of the lateral abdominal muscles. Also called *laparomyitis*.

laparonephrectomy A nephrectomy done via either an abdominal or a lumbar incision.

laparorrhaphia LAPARORRHAPHY.

laparorrhaphy The repair or strengthening of the abdominal wall by means of sutures. Also called *celiorrhaphy, laparorrhaphia*.

laparosalpingectomy Removal of a uterine tube through an abdominal incision. Also called *celiosalpingectomy*.

laparosalpingo-oophorectomy Removal of a uterine tube and ovary through an abdominal incision. Also called *celiosalpingo-oothecectomy*.

laparosalpingotomy An opening into an oviduct mode through an abdominal incision.

laparoscope [LAPARO- + -SCOPE] An endoscope designed for examination of the peritoneal cavity, especially the surface of the liver. Also called *peritoneoscope*.

laparoscopy [LAPARO- + -SCOPY] Endoscopic examination of the peritoneal cavity and surface of accessible abdominal organs by means of a laparoscope. Also called *peritoneoscopy ventroscopy* (rarely used).

laparosplenotomy A surgical procedure resecting all or part of the spleen through an abdominal incision. Also called *splenolaparotomy*.

laparotome [LAPARO- + -TOME] A surgical knife used to make an incision into the abdominal wall.

laparotomy [LAPARO- + -TOMY] **1** A surgical incision through the abdominal flank. **2** An imprecise term for CELIOTOMY.

laparotyphlotomy Incision of the cecum through a laparotomy.

laparouterotomy [LAPARO- + UTEROTOMY] ABDOMINOHYSTEROTOMY.

laparovaginal ABDOMINOVAGINAL.

lapathin CHRYSOPHANIC ACID.

Lapham [Maxwell Edward *Lapham*, U.S. obstetrician, born 1899] Friedman-Lapham test. See under FRIEDMAN TEST.

Lapicque [Louis *Lapicque*, French physiologist, 1866–1952] Lapicque's law. See under ISOCHRONISM.

lapilliform Having a form suggestive of small stones.

lapis [L, a stone] A stone: used in alchemy for any nonvolatile material.
  lapis albus Native calcium silicofluoride, or the precipitated compound.
  lapis calaminaris CALAMINE.
  lapis imperialis SILVER NITRATE.
  lapis infernalis SILVER NITRATE.
  lapis lunaris SILVER NITRATE.

Laplace [Pierre-Simon *Laplace*, French mathematician, astronomer, and physicist, 1749–1827] **1** See under LAW. **2** Laplace-Gauss distribution. See under NORMAL DISTRIBUTION.

lappa A decoction made from the root or whole plant of burdock, *Arctium lappa*. It has been used as a diuretic and diaphoretic.

lapsus [L, a fall, slip] A lapse or slip, as of memory.
  lapsus calami Slip of the pen.
  lapsus linguae Slip of the tongue.
  lapsus memoriae Slip of the memory.

larbish [West African] A form of cutaneous larva migrans found in Senegal.

lard [L *lardum*, also *laridum* the fat of bacon, fat] Purified fat from the omentum of the hog. It has been used in the compounding of ointments, but has been superseded by more stable vehicles. Also called *adeps, adeps praeparatus*.
  benzoinated lard ADEPS BENZOINATUS.

leaf lard   Lard prepared from the perirenal fat.

lard oil   An oil obtained from lard that is used for some pharmaceutical purposes.

lardacein   An outmoded term for AMYLOID.

lardaceous   Resembling lard in gross appearance, as the spleen in amyloidosis.

Lardennois [Henri *Lardennois*, French surgeon, born 1872] See under BUTTON.

lariat   A structure that forms during processing of mRNA in which one end of the molecule forms a covalent bond with a nucleotide at a consensus sequence within a transcribed intron, forming a loop with a tail, to resemble a rope lariat. The structure is important in proper splicing of mRNA to the mature molecule that directs translation.

laricic acid   AGARIC ACID.

larithmics [Gk *la(os)* the people at large + *(a)rithm(os)* number + -ICS]   Quantitative demography.

larkspur   The poisonous seed of *Delphinium ajacis*. Its toxicity may result from cutaneous absorption. It is used as a pediculiside. Also called *delphinium*.

Larmor [Sir Joseph *Larmor*, Irish mathematician and physicist, 1857–1942]   See under FREQUENCY, EQUATION.

Laron [Zvi *Laron*, Israeli pediatric endocrinologist, born 1927] See under DWARF.

Larrey [Baron Dominique Jean *Larrey*, French surgeon, 1766–1842]   **1** Larrey space, Larrey's cleft. See under MORGAGNI'S FORAMEN.   **2** See under LIGATION.   **3** Larrey's operation. See under AMPUTATION.   **4** Larrey-Weil disease. See under ICTERIC LEPTOSPIROSIS.

Larsen [Christian Magnus Falsen Sinding-*Larsen*, Norwegian physician, 1866–1930]   Larsen's disease, Sinding-Larsen-Johansson disease. See under LARSEN-JOHANSSON DISEASE.

Larsen [Loren Joseph *Larsen*, U.S. orthopedic surgeon, born 1914]   See under SYNDROME.

Larsson [Tage Konrad Leopold *Larsson*, Swedish scientist, born 1905]   Sjögren-Larsson syndrome. See under SYNDROME.

larva [L (akin to *lar* to a tutelary god), a ghost, specter, mask] (*plural* larvae)   **1** A usually motile feeding and developing stage in the life cycle of holometabolous insects which follows the egg stage and precedes the pupa. Larvae of some kinds of insects are known as caterpillars, maggots, grubs, and worms.   **2** An early nymphal stage of various hemimetabolous insects and other arthropods, or a morphologically distinct early stage of certain other invertebrates such as helminths, or of vertebrates such as some amphibians and fishes, which in an immature stage of development do not resemble the adult form but which will undergo a metamorphic transformation to assume it.

filariform larva   The infective or third-stage larva of certain parasitic nematodes such as *Strongyloides, Ascaris,* hookworms, and others that have larvae that penetrate or migrate through the body of the host to reach the intestine where the final molt, maturation, and completion of the life cycle occur.

rat-tailed larva   RAT-TAIL MAGGOT.

Larvacea [L *larv(a)*, evil spirit, ghost, mask + -ACEA]   A class of invertebrates in the subphylum Urochordata. Members are pelagic and free-swimming, and are considered to be neotenous in that sexually mature forms have larval organization.

larvaceous   LARVATE.

larva currens   A rapidly spreading skin infestation by the larva of *Strongyloides stercoralis*, which produces a rapidly progressing linear urticarial trail in the skin, usually starting at or near the anus. It may be caused by zoonotic species of *Stronglyoides*, such as *S. fuelleborni* in Southeast Asia (from primates) or *S. procyonis* in the United States (from racoons).

larvae   Plural of LARVA.

larval [*larv(a)* + -AL]   Pertaining to or resembling larvae.

larva migrans   A migratory phase of the life cycle of helminths, warble flies, and other parasites. It usually applies to parasites in an abnormal host or site where the wandering is random. Examples are seen in human cutaneous larva migrans by dog or cat hookworm larvae and human visceral larva migrans by dog or cat ascarid larvae.

cutaneous larva migrans   Larva migrans in the skin, as for example the linear eruption caused by hookworm larvae. Also called *creeping eruption, dermatitis linearis migrans*.

gnathostomatid larva migrans   The migration into the skin and other tissues by larvae of gnathostomatid nematodes such as *Gnathostoma spinigerum*, agent of gnathostomiasis.

spiruroid larva migrans   The migration into the skin and other tissues by larvae of spiruroid nematodes such as species of *Gongylonema* of the super family Spiruroidea.

visceral larva migrans   A disorder caused by visceral migration of the larva of *Toxocara, Toxascaris,* and other nematodes not adapted to man, so the normal migratory pathway from the intestine to liver, heart, lungs, trachea, mouth and back to the intestine is not completed. The worms leave the bloodstream and wander to the viscera until they are encapsulated usually within a few weeks to several months. Dog and cat ascarids are frequently responsible, such as *Toxacara canis, T. cati, Toxascaris leonina*. Clincal features are hypereosinophilia, hepatomegaly, and pneumonitis. Also called *nonpatent nematodiasis*.

larvate   Masked, concealed or hidden. Also *larvaceous*. • Used in describing a symptom, disease, or condition with atypical features.

larvicide   A medication effective against the larval forms of insects.

Panama larvicide   A larvicidal mixture against mosquito larvae, containing carbolic acid, rosin, and caustic soda.

larviparous [*larv(a)* + *i* + L *par(ere)* to bear or beget young + -OUS]   Depositing hatched larvae rather than eggs: a characteristic of insects such as certain myiasis flies. See also PUPIPAROUS.

larviphagic [*larv(a)* + *i* + *phag(o)-* + -IC]   LARVIVOROUS.

larviposition [*larv(a)* + *i* + *(de)position*]   The deposition of larvae, particularly in the tissues of a host.

larvivorous [*larv(a)* + *i* + L *vor(are)* to swallow, devour + -OUS]   Consuming a diet consisting of larvae. Also *larviphagic*.

laryng-   LARYNGO-.

laryngalgia [LARYNG- + -ALGIA]   Pain in the larynx. A seldom used term.

laryngeal   Pertaining to the larynx.

laryngectomy [LARYNG- + -ECTOMY]   Excision of part or all of the larynx. • When not qualified, the term is widely used to mean total laryngectomy.

frontolateral partial laryngectomy   An operation similar to lateral partial laryngectomy employed when the tumor to be excised spreads across the anterior laryngeal commissure to involve the front end of the contralateral vocal cord.

lateral partial laryngectomy   Partial laryngectomy for small tumors localized to the membranous part of one vocal cord. The larynx is opened by the laryngofissure approach and the tumor removed with a surrounding margin of healthy tissue. The procedure may also involve the excision of part of the cartilaginous thyroid ala adjacent to the tumor. Also called *laryngofissure, laryngofission*.

partial laryngectomy   One of a number of varieties of laryngectomy in which a large part of the larynx is spared and the laryngeal airway and, thus, laryngeal voice preserved.

supraglottic laryngectomy HORIZONTAL HEMILARYNGEC-TOMY.

total laryngectomy Laryngectomy of the most radical kind, necessitating removal of the whole larynx along with a variable amount of the upper trachea and, usually, the hyoid bone and preepiglottic tissues. The establishment of a permanent end tracheostome is an inevitable consequence. The indication in all but the exceptional case is malignant disease of the larynx or laryngopharynx too extensive for more limited procedures. Technical variations, for instance the excision of the homolateral thyroid lobe, may be required by the extent of the disease, which may also determine the need for removal of part of the pharynx (pharyngolaryngectomy) or radical neck dissection for lymph node metastasis.

laryngemphraxis Laryngeal obstruction. An obsolete term.

laryngendoscope An endoscope for viewing the interior of the larynx.

laryngismal Resembling or pertaining to laryngismus (laryngospasm).

laryngismus [New L, from LARYNG- + L -ismus -ISM] LARYNGOSPASM.

laryngismus stridulus Brief, nocturnal attacks of laryngospasm, usually in children, often waking the patient from sleep. There is neither evidence of other laryngeal abnormality nor, characteristically, of intercurrent disease. Also called *false croup, pseudocroup, Kopp's asthma* (obsolete), *Millar's asthma* (obsolete), *Wichmann's asthma* (obsolete).

laryngitic Having to do with laryngitis.

laryngitis [LARYNG- + -ITIS] Inflammation of the lining of the larynx. The principal symptom is hoarseness. Adjective: laryngitic.

acute catarrhal laryngitis SIMPLE LARYNGITIS.

acute spasmodic laryngitis LARYNGITIS STRIDULOSA.

atrophic laryngitis Laryngitis in which the lining of the larynx is dry and crusted and sometimes atrophic. It is a rare disease today, although once common, usually occurring as a complication of atrophic rhinitis or, occasionally, chronic suppurative sinusitis. Also called *laryngitis sicca.*

bacterial laryngitis Any variety of laryngitis due to or complicated by pathogenic bacteria.

catarrhal laryngitis Laryngitis characterized by a catarrhal reaction of the mucosa in the absence of other specific features. Also called *laryngocatarrh* (seldom used).

chemical laryngitis Laryngitis caused by irritant chemicals reaching the larynx not only by being inhaled, but sometimes through the bloodstream or through ingestion. For example swallowed caustics may spill over and damage the larynx.

chronic catarrhal laryngitis Catarrhal laryngitis running a protracted course, sometimes becoming indistinguishable from atrophic laryngitis.

chronic hyperplastic laryngitis A variety of chronic non-specific laryngitis in which the nonkeratinized squamous epithelium of the vocal cords and often the respiratory epithelium of the vestibular folds have undergone hyperplastic changes often with metaplasia and keratinization. The well-established condition is regarded as precancerous.

chronic nonspecific laryngitis Laryngitis of a chronic nature which cannot be easily ascribed to a specific cause, such as tuberculosis or syphilis, nor can the manifestations be easily circumscribed, as in the case of polyps or contact pachydermia. Metaplasia and hyperplasia of the laryngeal lining are characteristic and may possibly be caused by vocal abuse or abuse of alcohol and tobacco. Chronic infection elsewhere in the respiratory tract is present in more than half the cases.

croupous laryngitis Any of the varieties of laryngitis that cause croup, for instance membranous laryngitis and laryngitis stridulosa.

diphtheric laryngitis A seldom used term for LARYNGEAL DIPHTHERIA.

diphtheritic laryngitis LARYNGEAL DIPHTHERIA.

edematous laryngitis Edema of the larynx which presents as a feature of various types of laryngitis, both infective and non-infective, as well as a complication of major surgery of the floor of the mouth, radiotherapy to the larynx and pharynx, and adjacent severe infection such as Ludwig's angina and peritonsillar abscess. It was once regarded as a separate disease entity. Also called *phlegmonous laryngitis* (older term).

membranous laryngitis Laryngitis, usually acute, characterized by pseudomembrane formation and presenting with hoarseness, stridor, and obstruction to the laryngeal airway. The most common cause is laryngeal diphtheria but infection with β-hemolytic streptococcus or *Pseudomonas aeruginosa* may be responsible. Noninfective causes include inhalation of hot gases by the victims of fires, and of certain poisonous gases. Also called *membranous croup, fibrinous croup.*

phlegmonous laryngitis An older term for EDEMATOUS LARYNGITIS.

laryngitis sicca ATROPHIC LARYNGITIS.

simple laryngitis Acute infective laryngitis complicating the common upper respiratory tract infections, in particular the common cold. Also called *acute catarrhal laryngitis.*

laryngitis stridulosa Acute laryngitis occurring in children, characterized by brief attacks of laryngospasm that are usually nocturnal. The attacks resolve spontaneously over a short period of time. Also called *acute spasmodic laryngitis, spasmodic croup, false croup, pseudocroup.* See also LARYNGISMUS STRIDULUS.

subglottic laryngitis Laryngitis affecting especially the subglottic larynx, seen particularly in children. Subglottic edema occurs frequently and is responsible for the characteristic respiratory obstruction.

supraglottic laryngitis Inflammation of the supraglottic larynx, particularly that due to *Haemophilus influenzae* type B. It can occur at any age, complicating *H. influenzae* bacteremia, but it usually and characteristically occurs in childhood. The epiglottis, aryepiglottic folds, and other parts above the vocal cords become greatly swollen and quickly threaten the patient with asphyxia. It responds well to correct antibiotic therapy but intubation or tracheostomy may be urgently required. Also called *epiglottitis, epiglottiditis* (seldom used), *angina epiglottidea* (obsolete), *chorditis vocalis inferior.*

syphilitic laryngitis Laryngitis occurring sometimes during the secondary stage of syphilis and, rarely, during the tertiary stage. In secondary syphilis the typical mucous patches may be observed on the vocal cords, epiglottis, or ventricular bands.

tuberculous laryngitis Laryngitis caused by infection with *Mycobacterium tuberculosis*, still seen as a complication of pulmonary tuberculosis in the many parts of the world where the latter disease remains a major problem. The protean clinical features may cause confusion with other laryngeal granulomata and even carcinoma of the larynx. Also called *tuberculosis of the larynx, laryngeal tuberculosis, laryngophthisis* (seldom used), *laryngeal phthisis.*

vestibular laryngitis Supraglottic laryngitis in which *Haemophilus influenzae* cannot be identified.

viral laryngitis Acute infective laryngitis caused by one of a number of viruses, for example the rhinoviruses and the viruses of influenza and measles.

laryngo- [Gk *larynx* (genitive *laryngos*) larynx] A combining form denoting the larynx. Also *laryng-.*

laryngocatarrh CATARRHAL LARYNGITIS.

laryngocele [LARYNGO- + -CELE[1]] An air-containing pouch, usually bilateral, formed by the ballooning of a sacklike expansion of the ventricular saccule of the larynx. It is normally present in many higher apes which are able to distend them at will by an expiratory effort. In man, it occurs rarely and as an occupational hazard, particularly in glassblowers and wind-instrument players.

external laryngocele The commoner variety of laryngocele that presents intermittently as a swelling in the subhyoid region of the neck as the result of the herniation of the distended ventricular saccule through the thyrohyoid membrane.

internal laryngocele A rare variety of laryngocele presenting as a cystlike swelling at the entrance to the larynx above the vocal cord, diagnosed by demonstrating on x ray an air-containing sac distensible by the Valsalva maneuver. Also called *ventricular laryngocele, laryngocele ventricularis* (seldom used).

ventricular laryngocele INTERNAL LARYNGOCELE.

laryngocele ventricularis A seldom used term for INTERNAL LARYNGOCELE.

laryngocentesis [LARYNGO- + -CENTESIS] Surgical puncture of the larynx, as in percutaneous injection through the cricothyroid membrane. This is a rarely practiced procedure.

laryngofission 1 LARYNGOFISSURE. 2 LATERAL PARTIAL LARYNGECTOMY.

laryngofissure 1 LATERAL PARTIAL LARYNGECTOMY. 2 A surgical approach to the interior of the larynx by a midline incision carried through the cricothyroid membrane and the angle of the thyroid cartilage. Also called *laryngofission, median laryngotomy, thyrochondrotomy, thyrofissure.*

laryngogram 1 Any x-ray film showing details of the larynx, particularly films using contrast techniques. Also called *laryngograph.* See also LARYNGOGRAPHY. 2 ELECTROLARYNGOGRAM.

laryngograph 1 LARYNGOGRAM. 2 ELECTROLARYNGOGRAPH.

laryngography 1 Radiography, usually contrast radiography, of the larynx. The structures are outlined not only by the air in the larynx and pharynx but also by a radiopaque medium such as Dionosil aqueous injected over the back of the tongue. The larynx may be screened or various films taken at rest or during the Valsalva maneuver. It is of particular value in demonstrating the presence of laryngeal tumors, paralysis, and stenosis. 2 ELECTROLARYNGOGRAPHY.

laryngohypopharynx The walls of the pars laryngea pharyngis and the aditus laryngis considered together. An outmoded term.

laryngologist [LARYNGO- + -LOGIST] An otorhinolaryngologist especially interested and experienced in laryngology and, therefore, everything concerned with the voice.

laryngology [LARYNGO- + -LOGY] The branch of otorhinolaryngology concerned particularly with the larynx.

laryngomalacia [LARYNGO- + MALACIA] A flaccid condition of the supraglottic larynx found in a small proportion of newborn infants and responsible for inspiratory stridor. It tends to improve spontaneously as the child grows. Also called *chondromalacia of the larynx.*

laryngometry Measurement of the larynx.

laryngoparalysis LARYNGEAL PARALYSIS.

laryngopathy [LARYNGO- + -PATHY] Any disease of the larynx.

laryngopharyngeal Pertaining to the laryngopharynx or laryngeal part of the pharynx.

laryngopharyngectomy PHARYNGOLARYNGECTOMY.

laryngopharyngeus MUSCULUS CONSTRICTOR PHARYNGIS INFERIOR.

laryngopharyngitis Inflammation involving both the larynx and pharynx. The laryngitis occurs as a complication of the pharyngitis. Also called *pharyngolaryngitis.*

laryngopharynx PARS LARYNGEA PHARYNGIS.

laryngophony Auscultation of the larynx during phonation, usually with the stethoscope.

laryngophthisis A seldom used term for TUBERCULOUS LARYNGITIS.

laryngoplasty [LARYNGO- + -PLASTY] Any operation designed to reconstruct the larynx. It is usually done to improve the airway, as in cases of bilateral laryngeal abductor paralysis.

laryngoplegia [LARYNGO- + -PLEGIA] LARYNGEAL PARALYSIS.

laryngoptosis [LARYNGO- + -PTOSIS] The condition in which the larynx is found to have shifted to an unusually low level in the neck and may be abnormally mobile. It is regarded by some as an occasional feature of old age.

laryngopyocele An inflamed external laryngocele containing pus, caused when the narrow isthmus through the thyrohyoid membrane becomes obstructed by infection.

laryngorhinology RHINOLARYNGOLOGY.

laryngorrhagia [LARYNGO- + -RRHAGIA] Bleeding from the larynx. It is a rare occurrence, presenting as hemoptysis. Subsequent laryngoscopy reveals the cause which may be, for instance, laryngeal telangiectasia. A seldom used term.

laryngorrhaphy [LARYNGO- + -RRHAPHY] Suturing of the larynx.

laryngorrhea [LARYNGO- + -RRHEA] An excessive collection of fluid in the subglottis and larynx proper. The primary lesion may be respiratory, in which case the fluid is mostly mucoid, or it may be an obstructive upper esophageal mass, usually neoplastic, causing pooling and spillover of fluid into the larynx. The condition results in lending a gurgling quality to speech.

laryngoscleroma Scleroma of the larynx. It occurs rarely secondary to rhinoscleroma with pharyngeal involvement. Induration rather than ulceration occurs and obstruction to the airway has been reported. Healing with marked scarring and distortions is characteristic as is the case in other granulomatous diseases.

laryngoscope [LARYNGO- + -SCOPE] An instrument for inspecting the interior of the larynx.

Macintosh laryngoscope A laryngoscope for tracheal intubation. The curved tongue blade is designed so that the tip comes to rest between the base of the tongue and the epiglottis and is cut away on one side to afford the optimum view of the vocal cords. A lightbulb powered by a battery is located just beyond the midpoint of the blade.

laryngoscopic Of or relating to laryngoscopy.

laryngoscopy [LARYNGO- + -SCOPY] The inspection of the interior of the larynx.

direct laryngoscopy Laryngoscopy using a rigid instrument that permits a direct view of the interior of the larynx. Compare INDIRECT LARYNGOSCOPY.

fiberoptic laryngoscopy Laryngoscopy using a flexible fiberoptic nasopharyngoscope. This technique is particularly suitable for use on outpatients as an adjunct to indirect laryngoscopy or when the indirect method has proven unsuccessful.

indirect laryngoscopy Laryngoscopy using a special mirror held at the back of the mouth so as to reflect light into the interior of the larynx and reflect the image back to the examiner. Also called *mirror laryngoscopy.* Compare DIRECT LARYNGOSCOPY.

mirror laryngoscopy INDIRECT LARYNGOSCOPY.

suspension laryngoscopy A kind of direct laryngoscopy, usually carried out on the anesthetized patient, in which the laryngoscope is held in place mechanically so as to free both hands of the surgeon for any required operative procedure on the interior of the larynx thus exposed.

laryngospasm   Reflex spasm of the laryngeal sphincter, particularly the glottic sphincter, initiated typically by the threat of inhalation of foreign material into the lower air passages. Thus, secretions, blood, or a foreign body reaching the laryngeal inlet or, especially, the vocal cords will precipitate such spasm. The reflex is particularly brisk in children. It also occurs as a symptom of a number of other diseases, such as tabes dorsalis and tetanus. While the spasm persists the inspiration of air is impossible or very difficult and then accompanied by marked stridor. Also called *glottic spasm, glottidospasm, laryngismus, spasmus glottidis* (rarely used), *Schrötter's chorea, laryngeal chorea.*

laryngostenosis   LARYNGEAL STENOSIS.

laryngostomy [LARYNGO- + -STOMY]   The surgical establishment of an opening into the subglottic larynx maintained by the presence of an oval-section laryngotomy tube for the relief of upper airway obstruction. Although indicated occasionally in an emergency, for the most part laryngostomy has been superseded by tracheostomy or endotracheal intubation.

laryngostroboscope   A stroboscope adapted for use in laryngoscopy. In particular, it enables the movements of the vocal cords to be studied in detail by showing them in slow motion or arrested in the desired phase.

laryngostroboscopy   Study of the vocal cord in action by indirect laryngoscopy using the laryngostroboscope.

laryngotome [LARYNGO- + -TOME]   An instrument for performing laryngotomy, usually comprising a curved trocar and a cannula of oval cross section.

dilating laryngotome   A laryngotome formerly used for dividing laryngeal webs. It was passed through the mouth under indirect laryngoscopic control. It consisted of an olive-shaped dilator from within which a sharp blade could be made to protrude either forward or backward. It proved ineffective because the web would re-form.

laryngotomy [LARYNGO- + -TOMY]   **1** Surgical incision of the larynx.   **2** CRICOTHYROTOMY.

complete laryngotomy   An outmoded procedure involving opening the larynx by dividing the thyroid and cricoid cartilages vertically in the midline. Also called *cricothyreotomy* (seldom used).

inferior laryngotomy   CRICOTHYROTOMY.

median laryngotomy   LARYNGOFISSURE.

subhyoid laryngotomy   SUPERIOR LARYNGOTOMY.

superior laryngotomy   Opening of the larynx through the thyrohyoid membrane. This procedure should be properly regarded as a pharyngotomy. Also called *subhyoid laryngotomy, thyrohyoid laryngotomy.*

thyrohyoid laryngotomy   SUPERIOR LARYNGOTOMY.

laryngotracheal   Pertaining to both the larynx and trachea.

laryngotracheitis [LARYNGO- + TRACHEITIS]   **1** LARYNGOTRACHEOBRONCHITIS.   **2** Inflammation of the larynx and trachea.

avian infectious laryngotracheitis   INFECTIOUS LARYNGOTRACHEITIS.

infectious laryngotracheitis   **1** A worldwide, viral, respiratory disease, mainly of adult poultry, that affects the laryngeal and tracheal mucosa. The disease may be mild or severe. Also called *avian infectious laryngotracheitis.*   **2** LARYNGOTRACHEOBRONCHITIS.

laryngotracheobronchitis   Inflammation of the larynx, trachea, and bronchial tree but particularly such inflammation occurring in the very young as an acute illness due to one of a number of viruses, especially the parainfluenza virus type 1 and the measles virus. The characteristic slowly progressive respiratory obstruction is due chiefly to subglottic swelling and the

tenacious secretions occupying the airways. Also called *laryngotracheitis, infectious laryngotracheitis, bronchial croup.*

laryngotracheobronchoscopy   The endoscopic examination of the interior of the larynx and of the tracheobronchial tree.

laryngotracheoscopy   The examination of the interior of the larynx and trachea, usually by endoscopic means.

laryngotracheotomy   CRICOTRACHEOTOMY.

laryngovestibulitis   Inflammation of the laryngeal vestibule. A seldom used term.

laryngoxerosis   Any condition of the larynx characterized by diminished secretions resulting in a dryness of the larynx. A seldom used term.

larynx [Gk *larynx,* gen. *laryngos,* the larynx or upper part of the windpipe, the gullet, throat]   [NA]   A tubular organ which extends vertically from the root of the tongue opposite the hyoid bone to the trachea and is composed of a framework of cartilages held together by ligaments and membranes which are acted on by both extrinsic and intrinsic muscles. It is covered by skin and fasciae and is situated posteromedial to the infrahyoid muscles and is lined internally by mucous membrane which forms the true and false vocal folds. It lies anterior to the pharynx with which it is continuous through its inlet or aditus. It forms the organ of phonation and serves as an air passage to the lungs and a sphincteric mechanism to guard the trachea. Also called *voice box.*

artificial larynx   One of a number of mechanical or electronic devices designed to assist with the production of voice after total laryngectomy.

lasanum [L from Gk *lasanon* a trivet, night stool), a chamberpot]   An outmoded term for BIRTHING CHAIR.

lascivia [L, lustfulness]   An obsolete term for NYMPHOMANIA.

Lasègue [Ernest C. *Lasègue,* French physician, 1816–1883]   **1** See under SYNDROME, LAW.   **2** Lasègue's arm sign. See under SIGN.   **3** Lasègue's test. See under LASÈGUE SIGN.   **4** Lasègue's maneuver. See under NERI SIGN.   **5** Lasègue's disease. See under SCIATICA.

laser [*l(ight) a(mplification by) s(timulated) e(mission of) r(adiation)*]   A device that produces an intense, small, nondiverging beam of coherent electromagnetic radiation in the ultraviolet, visible, or infrared regions of the spectrum. It is used in retinal welding, microsurgery, cauterization, tumor therapy, and diagnosis of deep pathologic lesions. Exposure of any part of the body surface to a laser beam can cause injury. The eye is especially vulnerable to its thermal and photochemical effects.

carbon dioxide laser   A laser used to remove lesions of the skin or other superficial organs by burning them away. It operates at a wavelength of 10.6 μm and provides a very high output of 50–500 watts.

argon laser   A laser using the coherent emission spectrum of light emitted by argon. This light is blue-green and is readily absorbed by red hemoglobin, thus allowing the use of the argon laser in coagulation of bleeding sites in surgery.

Lasiohelea   A subgenus of small bloodsucking gnats in the genus *Forcipomyia,* family Ceratopogonidae, including pests that attack humans and domestic animals, especially in the tropics.

Lassar [Oskar *Lassar,* German dermatologist, 1849–1907]   **1** See under PASTE.   **2** Lassar's betanaphthol paste. See under PASTE.   **3** Lassar's plain zinc paste. See under ZINC OXIDE PASTE.

lassitude   **1** A languid state.   **2** A state of weariness.

Lassueur [Auguste *Lassueur,* Swiss physician, 1874–1949]   Piccardi-Lassueur-Graham Little syndrome. See under LASSUEUR-LITTLE SYNDROME.

lata [Malay]   An acute catatonoid reaction seen in Malay, consisting of echopraxia, automatic obedience, and coprolalia. It is most frequent in women below the age of 20 years. Also *latah*.

latah   LATA.

Latarjet [André *Latarjet*, French anatomist, born 1877]   **1** Hypogastric nerve of Latarjet. See under NERVUS HYPOGASTRICUS DEXTER ET SINISTER.   **2** Latarjet's vein. See under VENA PREPYLORICA.

lat. dol.   *lateri dolenti* (L, to the painful side).

latebra [L (from *latere* to be hidden), a hiding place]   A strand of white yolk in the eggs of birds stretching from the blastodisk to the center of the ovum.

latency [L *latens*, pres. part. of *latere* (akin to Gk *lanthanein* to escape or elude notice), to lie hidden, be unknown to + *-cy*, English noun suffix denoting state or quality, action, practice]   **1** The period between stimulus application and response onset.   **2** In psychoanalytic psychology, the developmental period extending from the end of the infantile period (normally about age 5) to the onset of adolescence. Also called *latency phase*.

absolute latency   The shortest interval between stimulus and response, elicited by increasing stimulus strength.

reducible latency   The interval between stimulus and response that can be shortened by increasing stimulus magnitude.

total reflex latency   The time period between an afferent stimulus and the reflex response.

latent [L *latens*, gen. *latentis*, pres. part. of *latere* to be low, lie hidden]   Existing but not apparent; hidden; dormant, as an infection.

latentiation   The process of modifying an active drug to a chemical derivative that then requires absorption, distribution, or metabolism to restore the active form of the drug. The modification permits the slow release or gradual formation of the active drug *in vivo*.

laterad   Toward a side; sidewards; laterally.

lateral [L *lătus* (gen. *lateris*; substantive, akin to Gaelic *leathad* flat (adj.) from L *lātus* flat, broad and to Gk *platos* breadth, width) side, width]   **1** Of, at, or toward the side.   **2** Farther toward the right or left, as compared with other structures or parts that are nearer the midline or median plane of the body. Compare MEDIAL.

left lateral   In roentgenography, describing a lateral projection with the patient's left side closest to the film.

right lateral   In roentgenography, describing a lateral projection with the patient's right side closest to the film.

lateralis   Lateral. Also *externus (outmoded and incorrect)*.

laterality [LATERAL + -ITY]   A relationship or tendency towards one side.

crossed laterality   **1** The predominant control of motor acts by the contralateral cerebral hemisphere.   **2** Paired interactions between right and left sides, as associated mirror movements.

dominant laterality   Preferential use of right or left for any structure.

mixed laterality   Preferential use of opposite sides in various paired structures in a given individual.

lateralization   **1** The tendency to perform an act predominantly on the left or right side of the body.   **2** Laterally asymmetrical functional localization in the central nervous system.

sound lateralization   The ability of the listener to determine the side on which a sound stimulus has occurred. The neurophysiology is complex and different processes are involved for low and high frequency tones, partly as a result of the relation of the wavelength of the sound to the diameter of the head.

latericeous   LATERITIOUS.

latericumbent   In a lateral recumbent position; lying on one's side.

laterigrade   LATEROGRADE.

lateritious [L *lateritius* (from *later* clay stone, brick) made of bricks]   Similar to brick dust. Also *latericeous*.

latero- [L *latus* (genitive *lateris*) side, flank]   A combining form meaning lateral.

lateroabdominal   Situated on or relating to the lateral aspect of the abdomen.

laterocele [LATERO- + -CELE¹]   A herniation through the lateral abdominal wall.

laterodetrusion [LATERO- + *detrusion*, from L *detrusus*, past part. of *detrudere* to push downward or outward]   The lateral and opening movement of the mandible at the beginning of the masticatory cycle.

laterodeviation   Displacement to the side.

laterodorsal   DORSOLATERAL.

lateroduction   Lateral movement, especially of an eye.

lateroflexion [LATERO- + FLEXION]   A bending to one side of the body.

laterognathism   The deviation of the chin to one side or the other due to underdevelopment or overdevelopment of one side of the mandible.

laterograde   Indicating a sideward movement. Also *laterigrade*.

lateromarginal   Situated on the outer edge or border.

lateroposition   A position that is farther to one side than is normal; laterodeviation.

lateroprotrusive   Pertaining to lateral protrusion.

lateropulsion   Involuntary deviation to one side when walking.

lateroretrusive   Describing movement of the mandible involving lateral and backward components.

laterosellar   At or to the side of the sella turcica.

laterotorsion   A twisting to one side, especially rotation of an eye in a lateral direction from the twelve o'clock meridian.

laterotrusion [LATERO- + TRUSION]   Outward transtrusion. Also called *side-shift*.

lateroversion   A turning or deflection to one side, as of the uterus.

latex [L, water, fluid]   An emulsion, or suspension, produced in special cells or vessels of tissues in certain plants. It can exude when the tissue is wounded.

Latham [Peter Mere *Latham*, English physician, 1789–1875]   See under CIRCLE.

lathe [Middle English *lath* a supporting stand]   An electric motor used by dental technicians for grinding and polishing. An outmoded term.

lathyrism [*Lathyr(us)* + -ISM]   Spastic paraparesis with sensory impairment in the lower limbs, resulting from the ingestion of peas of the genus *Lathyrus*. The condition is seen especially in parts of India. Turkeys fed a diet containing seeds of *L. odoratus* died of hemorrhage because of rupture of the aorta. The active principle is β-aminoproprionitrile. Adjective: lathyritic.

lathyritic   Describing, pertaining to, or suffering from lathyrism.

lathyrogen   Any substance that produces lathyrism.

lathyrogenic   Capable of producing lathyrism.

Lathyrus   A genus of annual and perennial herbs of the Leguminosae family. Many species are grown as forage or food crops. When consumed in large quantities, some species cause lathyrism in both humans and livestock. Toxic species include *L. hirsutus*, caley pea, *L. incanus*, wild pea, *L. odoratus*, sweet pea, *L. pulsillus*, singletary pea, and *L. sylvestris*, everlasting pea.

latissimocondylaris   An uncommon variation of the latissimus dorsi muscle, of which a tendinous slip may be inserted into the brachial fascia, triceps muscle, lateral epicondyle of humerus, or other neighboring structures. Often present in some lower animals, the tendinous slip in humans is usually inserted into the brachial fascia or long head of triceps muscle. Also called *latissimocondyloideus, dorsoepitrochlearis*.

latissimocondyloideus   LATISSIMOCONDYLARIS.

latissimus   Widest; usually used in reference to wide, flat muscles.

l·atm   Symbol for the unit, liter-atmosphere.

latrodectism [*Latrodect(us)* + *-ISM*]   Poisoning by the venom of spiders of the genus *Latrodectus*. The most dangerous is the black widow. The bite produces localized pain, muscle spasms, and paresthesia. Severe poisoning may result in coma, respiratory paralysis, and cardiovascular collapse.

Latrodectus   A genus of poisonous spiders of the family Theridiidae, the comb-footed spiders, of cosmopolitan distribution.

Latrodectus mactans   The black widow spider, a highly venomous species found in the southern U.S., and in warmer parts of the Americas and in similar climatic zones of other continents. The fully-grown female has a bright red hourglass-shaped mark on the ventral side of the abdomen. The male lacks this mark and is not venomous. The toxic fraction of the venom of the female is a neurotoxic labile protein which causes ascending motor paralysis and destruction of peripheral nerve endings.

LATS   long-acting thyroid stimulator.

lattice   SPACE LATTICE.

  space lattice   A three-dimensional grid or other orderly structure, as that which characterizes the arrangement of atoms in a crystal. Also called *lattice.*

latus [L, the flank]   (*plural* latera.) The side of the trunk between the lowest rib and the iliac crest; the flank.

Latzko [Wilhelm *Latzko*, Austrian gynecologist and obstetrician, 1863–1945]   See under OPERATION, SECTION.

Lauber [Hans *Lauber*, Swiss-born ophthalmologist active in Austria, born 1876]   Lauber's disease. See under FUNDUS ALBIOPUNCTATUS.

laudable   Beneficial because indicative of healing, as in *laudable pus*. An outmoded term.

laudanidine   The *l*-isomer of laudanine, an alkaloid from opium.

laudanine $C_{20}H_{25}NO_4$. The *dl*-forms of a minor alkaloid from opium that remain in solution in the usual process for extracting morphine from opium.

laudanum   OPIUM TINCTURE.

laugh [Middle English *laughen*, from Old English *hlæhhan, hleahhan, hliehhan*, akin to German *lachen* to laugh]   **1** To produce laughter.   **2** LAUGHTER.

  canine laugh   RISUS SARDONICUS.

  sardonic laugh   RISUS SARDONICUS.

laughing / spasmodic laughing   Episodic, unnatural, and violent laughing, a form of emotional lability. This can occur in rare cases of temporal lobe epilepsy (gelastic epilepsy), but periodic and inappropriate laughter is also seen in patients with lesions of the midbrain and hypothalamus, as in encephalitis lethargica or pseudobulbar palsy, as well as in schizophrenic disorders.

laughter [Middle English, from Old English *hleahtor*, akin to German *Gelächter* laughter]   The sound and accompanying facial and other movements that express amusement, exultation, or scorn. It is prompted by amusement, exultation, scorn, or nervous stimulation such as occurs in tickling. Also called *laugh, risus.*

  compulsive laughter   Inappropriate laughing without feeling, occurring in some hebephrenic schizophrenics. Also called *obsessive laughter, forced laughter.*

  forced laughter   COMPULSIVE LAUGHTER.

  obsessive laughter   COMPULSIVE LAUGHTER.

Laugier [Stanislas *Laugier*, French surgeon, 1799–1872]   See under SIGN.

Laumonier [Jean-Baptiste-Philippe-Nicolas-René *Laumonier*, French surgeon, 1749–1818]   Laumonier's ganglion. See under INFERIOR CAROTID GANGLION.

Launois [Pierre Emile *Launois*, French physician, 1856–1914]   **1** Launois syndrome. See under PITUITARY GIGANTISM.   **2** Launois-Cléret syndrome. See under FRÖHLICH SYNDROME.

laurel   Any plant of the genus *Laurus* in the family Lauraceae.

Laurence [John Zacharias *Laurence*, English physician, 1830–1874]   Laurence-Moon syndrome. See under SYNDROME.

Laurens [Georges *Laurens*, French surgeon, flourished 20th century]   See under OPERATION.

Laurer [Johann Friedrich *Laurer*, German pharmacologist, 1798–1873]   See under CANAL.

laureth 9   A mixture of polyethylene glycol monododecyl ethers with an average value of nine ethylene oxide groups per molecule. The compound is used as a pharmaceutical aid and as a spermicide.

lauric acid CH_3—$[CH_2]_{10}$—COOH. Dodecanoic acid. It is one of the fatty acids commonly found in natural fats such as butter.

Lauron   A proprietary name for aurothioglycanide.

lauryl   DODECYL.

Lauth [Ernest Alexandre *Lauth*, French anatomist and physiologist, 1803–1837]   Lauth's canal. See under SINUS VENOSUS SCLERAE.

Lauth [Thomas *Lauth*, German anatomist and surgeon, 1758–1826]   **1** See under LIGAMENT.   **2** Lauth's ligament. See under LIGAMENTUM ARCUATUM PUBIS.

LAV   lymphadenopathy-associated virus.

lavage [French *laver* (from L *lavare* to wash, bathe; Gk *louein* to wash oneself) to wash + *-age* -AGE]   **1** The washing out, especially by irrigation, of a hollow organ, or cavity, such as the stomach, bowel, or bladder. Also called *lavation, lavement* (obsolete).   **2** The purification of a solid, liquid, or gas by means of a substance or solution that is not itself contaminated and will not dissolve or decompose the substance to be purified.

  lavage of the blood   The introduction of serum to the blood based on the outmoded belief that it would dilute noxious substances.

  bronchoalveolar lavage   A technique for obtaining cells from bronchioles and alveoli of the lungs by instillation of sterile fluid through a fiberoptic bronchoscope into a lobe and subsequent removal by suction. The technique may be of diagnostic value or be used to evaluate the effectiveness of treatment.

  ether lavage   The obsolete practice of lavage of the peritoneal cavity with ether as treatment of acute intra-abdominal or pelvic infections. Also called *Souligoux-Morestin method.*

  gastric lavage   A procedure used to remove the contents of the stomach, as for example after ingestion of a toxic substance.

  intestinal lavage   A form of dialysis in which fluids are instilled and withdrawn in the small intestine in order to remove waste products from the blood across the intestinal mucosa.

  peritoneal lavage   The instillation and retrieval of a physiologic solution in the peritoneal cavity in order to examine the effluent for abnormal cells, bacteria, or evidence of internal bleeding following trauma.

  pleural lavage   Lavage of the pleural cavity.

  tracheal lavage   Irrigation of the trachea with fluid.

lavation   **1** An act of washing or cleansing.   **2** LAVAGE.

lavement   An obsolete term for LAVAGE.

lavender   *Lavandula officinalis*, a perennial shrub of the Labiatae family. The flowers are the source of lavender oil, a volatile oil that contains linalyl acetate, geraniol, linalool, limonene, pinene, and cineol. It is used in perfumes, as a flavoring, as a carminative and aromatic, and as an insect repellent.

Laveran [Charles Louis Alphonse *Laveran*, French army surgeon, 1845–1922] Laveran bodies. See under BODY.

Laverania A former genus, now considered a subgenus, that includes *Plasmodium falciparum* as opposed to the other human plasmodia.

Lavernia falcipara PLASMODIUM FALCIPARUM.

laveur [French (from L *lav(are)* to wash + French -*eur* -OR), a person or machine that washes] A device used in performing lavage. A seldom used term.

law

law [Old English *lagu*] A description of phenomena so thoroughly tested and accepted that it can be relied on as a principle governing like phenomena. See also entries under PRINCIPLE and RULE.

Adrian-Bronk law ALL-OR-NONE LAW.

Alexander's law Vestibular nystagmus is enhanced if the gaze is turned in the direction of the fast component.

Allen's paradoxic law In normal persons the more sugar taken the more is utilized, whereas in diabetes mellitus the more sugar taken the less is utilized.

all-or-none law The response of muscle and nerve cells to stimuli at or above threshold is maximal, but to stimuli below threshold is nil, i.e., no response of intermediate level is obtainable by subthreshold stimuli. The law is applicable to individual neurons or muscle cells, but not to the aggregate comprising a nerve or muscle. Also called *all-or-nothing law of excitation, Adrian-Bronk law, Bowditch's law.*

all-or-nothing law of excitation ALL-OR-NONE LAW.

law of anticipation The tendency for genetic disorders to appear at an earlier age in each succeeding generation.

antisubstitution laws Regulations concerning the substitution of generic, alternative drugs for proprietary or brand name drugs by the pharmacist. If the physician specifies a proprietary drug and adds "DAW" (Dispense as Written) in writing on the prescription, the pharmacist is forbidden in most jurisdictions to substitute a generic drug.

Aran's law Blows to the dome of the skull result in basilar skull fractures that radiate along lines of stress.

Arndt's law The doctrine that physiological activity is excited by weak stimuli, optimal with moderate stimuli, and curtailed by strong stimuli. Also called *Arndt-Schultz law.*

Arndt-Schultz law ARNDT'S LAW.

laws of articulation Rules for setting up teeth in dentures to ensure occlusal balance.

law of avalanche The hypothesis that a peripheral stimulus can be elaborated in neural pathways to produce complex sensations.

law of average localization A basic clinical principle for the localization of abdominal pain. Pain of visceral origin is localized most accurately in the least mobile organ.

Avogadro's law Equal volumes of different gases, observed at the same temperature and pressure, contain the same number of molecules.

Babinski's law A law defining the response to the galvanic test of normal subjects compared with those with labyrinthine disease. The normal subject inclines to the side of the positive pole, whereas someone with labyrinthine disease, tending to fall to one side, will incline that way on galvanic stimulation. Where the disease has destroyed the labyrinth, there will be no response. An outmoded term.

Baer's law LAW OF VON BAER.

Barfurth's law The primary axis of healing or regenerating tissue at the site of a surgical wound is perpendicular to the incision.

Baruch's law A once-held maxim that bath water at a temperature equal to that of the skin will produce a sedative effect, whereas bath water at a temperature higher or lower than that of the skin will produce a stimulating effect.

Bastian's law BASTIAN-BRUNS LAW.

Bastian-Bruns law The tendon reflexes in the legs are abolished after total section of the spinal cord above the lumbar enlargement. A seldom used term. Also called *Bastian-Bruns sign, Bastian's law.*

Baumès law COLLES LAW.

Beer's law The law relating the intensity, I, of light or other electromagnetic radiation to the length l of absorbing solution through which the radiation has passed and the concentration, c, of absorbing solute. It states that $\log(I/I_o) = \epsilon \cdot l \cdot c$, where I_o is the incident intensity, and ϵ is an empirical constant, the molar absorption coefficient. The law only holds for monochromatic radiation. Also called *Beer-Lambert law.*

Beer-Lambert law BEER'S LAW.

Behring's law Immunity may be passively transferred to a nonimmune person by injection of transfusion of serum or blood from an immunized person.

Bell's law BELL-MAGENDIE LAW.

Bell-Magendie law The concept that the dorsal spinal roots conduct sensory activity toward the spinal cord and the ventral roots conduct to muscle. Also called *Bell's law, Magendie's law.*

Bergonié-Tribondeau law A law expressing the mode of variation of tissue sensitivity to x rays: the sensitivity of a cell to x rays is directly proportional to its ability to reproduce and inversely proportional to its degree of differentiation.

biogenetic law RECAPITULATION THEORY.

Boudin's law The proposition that tuberculosis and malaria are mutually antagonistic.

Bowditch's law ALL-OR-NONE LAW.

Boyle's law The volume of a fixed mass of gas is inversely proportional to the pressure on it, provided that the temperature remains constant. Also called *Mariotte's law.*

Brenner's law The law defining the reaction of the normal auditory nerve to galvanic stimulation: with the cathode in the external auditory meatus, a sensation of sound is produced on closing the circuit which is interrupted when the circuit is opened again. With the anode in the meatus, no reaction is experienced on closing the circuit but a weak sensation of sound is experienced when the circuit is opened again.

Breton's law The psychophysical relationship between a given stimulus and the minimum discriminable increment in intensity.

Briggs law A Massachusetts state law establishing compulsory and impartial psychiatric examination of all those defendants either accused of capital crimes, previously convicted of more than one other offense, or previously convicted of a felony. The examination is conducted by a panel of experts who make determinations regarding mental status and the presence or absence of mental disorders which could exempt defendants from criminal responsibility.

Broadbent's law Lesions of the corticospinal tract in the cerebral hemisphere produce less marked paralysis of contralateral muscles (such as those of the face) which are usually involved in simultaneous bilateral movements than of muscles which are more often unilateral (those of the limbs).

Buhl-Dittrich law The assumption that in every instance of acute miliary tuberculosis there is a pre-existing caseous focus.

Bunge's law   The secretory cells of the mammary gland take minerals from the plasma in the exact proportion necessary for the optimum development of the offspring.

Camerer's law   The food requirements of children are a function of their weight and are independent of their ages.

Cannon's law of denervation   When an efferent neuron is destroyed, hypersensitivity to the neurotransmitter substance which it normally releases develops in the denervated target organ; the hypersensitivity of denervation.

Charles law   The volume of a fixed weight of a gas at constant pressure is directly proportional to its absolute temperature.

Colles law   A child with congenital syphilis does not infect its mother. It became clear later that the reason for the apparent paradox is that the mother was already infected and passed the disease to the child. Also called *Baumès law, Colles-Baumès law.*

Colles-Baumès law   COLLES LAW.

Collin's law   After removal of a tumor in infancy or childhood, if metastasis or recurrence does not develop within a period equal to the age of the patient plus nine months, the risk of such a development is small.

law of constant energy consumption   The rate of growth is proportional to the rate of metabolic activity. Also called *Rubner's law.*

law of constant growth quotient   A standard fraction of energy produced, the growth quotient, is diverted to the process of growth. Also called *Rubner's law.*

law of contiguity   One of Aristotle's primary laws of learning by association, which holds that two experiences occurring together in time or in space tend to become associated so that the reoccurrence of one of these elements at a later moment will tend to evoke the other.

law of contrary innervation   Living functions are maintained by the constant opposing forces of activation and inhibition; the concept of dualistic innervation. Also called *Meltzer's law.*

Cope's law   A less specialized genus may originate a greater number of forms than one that is more specialized.

Coulomb's law   The repulsive force between two electric charges is proportional to their product, and is therefore negative (i.e., attractive) if they have unlike sign, and the force is inversely proportional to the square of the distance between the charges and to the dielectric constant of the medium in which they reside.

Courvoisier's law   A principle differentiating physical findings in benign and malignant causes of obstructive jaundice: obstruction of the common bile duct by a gallstone rarely results in dilatation of the gallbladder, whereas obstruction due to cancer or other causes commonly results in gallbladder dilatation. See also COURVOISIER SIGN.

Cramer's law   The hypothesis that when, in a given population, the incidence of cancer of one particular organ is increased markedly, there is a compensatory decrease in the incidence of cancer in a number of other organs. First enunciated in 1942, the hypothesis is now regarded as disproved by most epidemiologists.

Cushing's law   A formerly accepted belief that an increase of intracranial pressure causes a rise of blood pressure to a value slightly greater than the pressure of cerebrospinal fluid on the medulla.

Dale-Feldberg law   Each neuron releases only a single neurotransmitter from all its terminals. This law has been challenged in the light of recent data.

Dalton's law   In a mixture of gases, the total pressure is equal to the sum of the partial pressures of the constituents.

Dastre-Morat law   The constriction of skin blood vessels is associated with dilatation of blood vessels in the splanchnic circulation, and, conversely, such dilatation of blood vessels in the splanchnic circulation is associated with the constriction of skin blood vessels.

Deiter's law   The doctrine, first enunciated in 1865, that all nerve fibers are long processes of nerve cells.

law of denervation   See under CANNON'S LAW OF DENERVATION.

Desmarres law   The diplopia of esotropia is uncrossed; that of exotropia is crossed.

law of diffusion   **1** The principle that the diffusion rate of a substance is a function of the difference in concentration between two given points.   **2** The principle that a central neural process can be broadly distributed in its effects.

law of dissolution   JACKSON'S LAW.

Dollo's law   When a structure or adaptation is lost during evolution, subsequent generations cannot regain it in the original form.

Donders law   The amount of cyclotorsion of the eye at any given line of fixation of the eyes with respect to the head is always the same regardless of the manner of adoption of that line of fixation.

DuBois-Reymond's law   The principle that the rate of change rather than the absolute magnitude of an electrical stimulus determines the excitability threshold of a muscle or nerve. Also called *law of excitation.*

Dulong-Petit law   The molar heat capacity, i.e., the specific heat multiplied by the molar mass, is approximately the same for almost all elements in solid form.

Edinger's law   Neuronal functioning enhances growth, but if not sustained or excessive can lead to atrophy and degeneration.

law of effect   The empirical generalization that a behavioral response which leads to a successful outcome is associated more rapidly to the stimuli which accompany or immediately precede it, and that learning is slow or does not occur at all if the response to such stimuli is followed by an annoying or unsuccessful outcome.

Einthoven's law   The potential in lead II of the electrocardiogram is equal to the arithmetic sum of the potentials from leads I and III. Lead I is measured between the left arm and the right arm, lead II between the left leg and the right arm, and lead III between the left leg and the left arm. See also STANDARD LEAD.

Elliott's law   The principle that stimulation of sympathetic nerves results in epinephrine release.

Emmert's law   The generalization that the size of a projected image, most often an afterimage but including eidetic images as well, will tend to increase in size in a manner proportional to the linear distance between the eye and the ground on which it is projected.

equipotentiality law   The hypothesis that any part of a cerebral cortical region acting as a nerve center can, with proper training, carry out the function of any other part of that center which may have been lost by damage to the tissue.

Ewald's Laws   Two laws defining the effect of endolymph flow in the semicircular canals of the inner ear on reflex movements of the head and eyes. The first is that the movement of the endolymph in the horizontal semicircular canal causes a slow movement of the eyes or head in the direction of the endolymph current, and the second is that in the horizontal canal the current towards the ampulla is a stronger stimulus than the current away from the ampulla.

law of excitation   DuBois-REYMOND'S LAW.

law of exponential decay   A law expressing the relationship of radioactive decay to time: for any radioactive nuclide, the change in activity can be expressed by the relation $A_t = A_o e^{-\lambda t}$ where A_t is the activity remaining from an initial activity A_o after a time t, and λ is the fractional decay per unit time, known as the decay constant.

law of facilitation Impulse activity over a synaptic pathway by repetition.

Faget's law Lack of correlation between body temperature and heart rate in yellow fever. There is either a bradycardia associated with a constant temperature, or a normal heart rate with a rising temperature. A similar dissociation may occur in *Salmonella typhi* infections. Also called *Faget sign*.

Faraday's laws Two relationships concerning electrolysis: (1) the amount of any substance deposited or dissolved by electrolysis is proportional to the quantity of electricity passed, and (2) the amounts of different substances deposited or dissolved by the same quantity of electricity are proportional to their molar masses divided by the number of electrons taken up or released per mole.

Farr's law The statement that "subsidence is a property of all zymotic diseases," meaning that a curve representing the incidence of an epidemic disease rises steeply at first, levels off somewhat as it nears its peak, and falls more steeply than it rose.

Fechner's law The principle that the magnitude of sensation increases logarithmically with stimulus intensity. Also called *range of sensibility*.

Ferry-Porter law The critical frequency of a flickering light, above which the flickering is no longer perceptible, is directly proportional to the logarithm of the light intensity.

Fick's first law of diffusion The flux of material by diffusion, which has the dimensions mass · area^{-1} · time^{-1}, is equal to a constant (the diffusion coefficient) multiplied by the concentration gradient.

Fildes law A syphilitic reagin in the blood of a newborn infant is diagnostic of syphilis in the mother.

law of filial regression GALTON'S LAW OF REGRESSION.

first law of thermodynamics Energy exchanges between systems are balanced, and no energy in either of two exchanging systems is created or destroyed.

Fitz law A clinical principle for diagnosis of acute pancreatitis: acute pancreatitis should be strongly suspected when a previously healthy person experiences sudden onset of severe epigastric pain, vomiting, and prostration which is followed within a day by abdominal distension, tympany, and guarding, in the presence of a slight fever.

Flatau's law The principle that the longer ascending and descending tracts of the spinal cord tend to be displaced peripherally by shorter axons arriving or terminating at other levels.

Flechsig's myelogenetic law MYELOGENETIC LAW.

Flint's law In embryology, a theoretical supposition that the development of the parts of an individual organism (ontogeny) is influenced by the phylogenetic significance of the heart and/or the blood supply to those parts.

Froriep's law A law that states that skull size has increased, at least in the amniotes, by the annexation of true vertebrae corresponding to occipital segments of which the hypoglossal represents the nerve.

Fuerbringer's law The developmental origin of a muscle can be determined from its nerve supply based on the fundamental pattern of innervation of muscles established in the embryo.

Galton's law GALTON'S LAW OF REGRESSION.

Galton's law of regression A principle of quantitative genetics that holds the average value of a given multifactorial trait in offspring approaches the mean of the trait in the parents. Also called *Galton's law, law of filial regression, law of regression*.

Gay-Lussac's law At constant pressure the volume of a fixed mass of gas increases by the same fraction for each degree rise in temperature.

Geiger-Nuttall law A rule referring to radioactive disintegration by alpha emission: in any radioactive series, the logs of the ranges of the alpha particles are linearly related to the logs of the decay constants.

Gerhardt-Semon law In certain disease processes affecting the motor nerve supply of the larynx, acting either centrally or peripherally, a position of the vocal cords intermediate between abduction and adduction indicates a partial lesion.

Giraud-Teulon law The perceived location of a binocularly-seen image is at the intersection of the projection of the visual axes from the corresponding retinal points that are stimulated.

Godélier's law The proposition that tuberculosis of the peritoneum always occurs in conjunction with tuberculosis of the pleural membranes.

Golgi's law The law that the severity of an attack of malaria is related directly to the number of malarial parasites in the erythrocytes.

Gompertz law The principle that there is a positive correlation that can be quantified between the probability of death from a disease and increasing age.

Goodell's law GOODELL SIGN.

Good Samaritan law Any law designed to shield from subsequent legal action those who voluntarily try to help a victim of an accident or illness in an emergency. The legislation is intended to encourage citizens to help strangers in distress. Most states of the United States have enacted such legislation. A term used chiefly in the U.S.

Graham's law The rate of diffusion of a gas is inversely proportional to the square root of its density.

Grasset's law LANDOUZY-GRASSET LAW.

law of gravitation See under NEWTON'S LAW OF GRAVITATION.

Gudden's law Upon division of an axon, some degeneration of the nerve fiber spreads centripetally towards the neuronal cell body.

Gullstrand's law Observation of the corneal light reflex as a person with strabismus turns his head will disclose that the reflex moves toward the paralyzed muscle.

Gull-Toynbee law In mastoiditis, intracranial spread of infection usually involves the cerebellum, whereas in otitis media, which particularly involves the tympanic antrum, upward spread into the temporal lobe is more common. Also called *Toynbee's law*.

Gunn's law To reduce a dislocation, the joint must be placed as at the time of the injury. A force can then be applied in the direction opposite to that of the dislocating force.

Haeckel's law RECAPITULATION THEORY.

Haldane's law A principle of genetics that pertains to hybrid offspring of two species. If one sex of the hybrids is sterile or absent, then that sex is heterogametic.

Hallion's law A law, no longer accepted, that the extract of an organ or tissue stimulates that organ or tissue.

Hamburger's law In alkaline blood, chloride tends to concentrate in plasma and phosphate in erythrocytes. Acid reverses this tendency.

Hanau's laws of articulation Laws for the formation of occlusal surfaces of dentures or in natural dentitions to provide balanced articulation.

Hardy-Weinberg law A mathematical formulation of the relationship between allele frequency and genotype frequency at genetic equilibrium in a large, randomly breeding population not subject to such influences as mutation, drift, and migration that disturb equilibrium. If the frequencies of alleles A and a are p and q, respectively, and if $p + q = 1$ at equilibrium, the frequencies of genotypes AA, Aa, and aa are p^2, $2pq$, and q^2, respectively.

law of the heart STARLING'S LAW.

Hecker's law With each successive delivery of a multipara, the infant's weight tends to exceed that of its immediate predecessor by about 200 grams.

Heidenhain's law   Secretion by a gland always entails alteration in the structure of its secretory cells.

Hellin's law   A statement of the statistical probability of multiple pregnancies: about one in 89 pregnancies results in twins. For triplets, the ratio is one in 89^2, and for each higher order the probability decreases by a factor of 89. Also called *Hellin-Zeleny law.*

Hellin-Zeleny law   HELLIN'S LAW.

Henry's law   The weight of a gas dissolved in a liquid is directly proportional to the pressure of that gas.

Heymans law   A simultaneous stimulus of vision will proportionately increase the threshold of a visual stimulus.

Hilton's law   The principle that a nerve trunk supplying a joint also contains axons innervating the muscles acting upon that joint and the skin overlying the articular insertions of those muscles.

Hofacker-Sadler laws   Different ratios of the sex of offspring purported to be statistically related to the seniority of one parent over the other or to their equivalence in age.

Hoff's law   VAN'T HOFF'S PRINCIPLE OF MOBILE EQUILIBRIUM.

Hoorweg's law   The principle that a critical duration of neural discharge is required for muscular contraction.

Hopkins bioclimatic law   Periodic biologic events occur four days earlier for each degree latitude toward the equator, or each five degrees longitude westward, or for each elevation decrease of 400 feet (about 122 meters). The law applies to the United States from the eastern states to the Rocky Mountains. Also called *bioclimatic rule, Hopkins rule.*

Horner's law   Color blindness is transmitted as a sex-linked recessive trait.

Houghton's law of fatigue   When muscles are contracted to fatigue, the work performed times the rate of work is constant.

law of independent assortment   See under MENDEL'S LAWS.

law of initial value   The more closely an organ or tissue is working to its maximum the less easily it can be stimulated to increase its work load, but it may be readily inhibited. Also called *Wilder's law of initial work.*

law of the intestines   The physiologic principle that explains the coordinated caudad progression of intestinal contents: the presence of a bolus in the intestine induces contraction cephalad and relaxation caudad to it.

law of inverse square   A rule expressing the effect of distance on x-ray or gamma ray intensity: the intensity of radiation emitted from a point source varies inversely as the square of the distance from that source.

law of isochronism   ISOCHRONISM.

isodynamic law   The body heat produced by a food is interchangeable with that of another food of the same caloric value.

law of isolated conduction   The transmission of nerve impulses between neurons occurs only through synapses.

Jackson's law   Those cerebral functions which are the last to be acquired in the course of evolution are the first to be lost when the cerebral cortex is damaged, and they are last to reappear during recovery. Also called *law of dissolution, Jackson's rule.*

Jost's law   The generalization that when two mental associations are of the same manifest strength, but unequal age, the older will benefit more from repetition, and the younger will lose strength more rapidly with the passage of time.

Joule's law   Heat is generated in an electric circuit at a rate proportional to the product of the resistance of the conductor and the square of the current.

Kahler's law   The successive addition of dorsal root fibers in the dorsal column results in a somatotopic pattern wherein each successive rostral spinal input forms a mediolateral sequence by adding to the lateral surface of the tract.

Knapp's law   The image seen by a person with a corrected refractive error is the same size as the image seen by an emmetrope if the anterior focal point of the eye and the principal plane of the correcting lens coincide.

Koch's law   The rule that four conditions must be satisfied to establish the causative organism of a specific disease: the organism must be present in every case of the disease; the organism must be isolated and grown in pure culture; the pure culture must produce the disease when it is inoculated into a susceptible animal; and the organism must be recovered from the infected animal and grown again in pure culture. Also called *Koch's postulates, law of specificity of bacteria.*

Lambert's cosine law   A law expressing the mode of variation of radiation intensity for parallel rays on an absorbing surface: the intensity varies as the cosine of the angle of incidence.

Lambert-Holzknecht law   The basic principle of superficial radiotherapy: in order to obtain a homogeneous dose on the surface of an entire area of irradiated field, the source-skin distance must be at least equal to if not greater than twice the greatest diameter of the field.

Landouzy-Grasset law   Where there is a unilateral cerebral lesion, the head turns towards the side of the lesion in a case of flaccid hemiplegia, and towards the side of the affected limbs in a case of spastic hemiplegia. A seldom used term. Also called *Grasset's law.*

Lapicque's law   ISOCHRONISM.

Laplace's law   The transmural pressure in a free sphere or cylinder is directly proportional to the circumferential tension in the wall and inversely proportional to the radius, the factor of proportionality for tension being 2 for a sphere and unity for a cylinder.

Lasègue's law   The tendon reflexes are increased in nervous or functional disorders, and more often reduced in organic nervous disease. An obsolete term.

Le Chatelier's law   Any external stresses, such as temperature or pressure, that disturb a system in equilibrium displace the equilibrium in a direction that tends to undo the effect of the stress. Also called *Le Chatelier's principle.*

Leopold's law   A law expressing a relation between the configuration of the oviducts and implantation: with posterior uterine wall implantation of the placenta, the oviducts curve anteriorly, while with anterior wall implantation the oviducts turn backwards and are parallel to the body axis when the mother is recumbent.

Levret's law   In cases of placenta previa, the umbilical cord is usually inserted marginally.

Liebig's law of the minimum   The growth of an organism is dependent on the amount of the essential nutrient that is least available to the organism. Also called *law of limiting factors, law of the minimum.*

law of limiting factors   LIEBIG'S LAW OF THE MINIMUM.

Listing's law   When the fixation of the eye changes, the angle of rotation in the new position is the same as if the eye had arrived at this position by turning on a fixed axis perpendicular to the original and new positions of the line of fixation.

Louis' law   The propositions that pulmonary tuberculosis usually originates in the left lung, and that tuberculosis in any part of the body is accompanied by localization in the lung.

Magendie's law   BELL-MAGENDIE LAW.

malthusian law   Because population increases geometrically whereas food production increases arithmetically, populations tend to outstrip their means of subsistence. See also MALTHUSIANISM.

Marey's law   The pulse rate is inversely related to the arterial blood pressure.

Mariotte's law BOYLE'S LAW.

law of mass action The rate of a chemical reaction is proportional to the concentrations of the reactants.

Meltzer's law LAW OF CONTRARY INNERVATION.

Mendel's laws A set of three principles of genetics. The first law, known as the principle of uniformity in F_1, holds that, in a mating between one parent having a dominant phenotype due to homozygosity for an allele and the other parent having a recessive phenotype controlled by a different allele at the same locus, all offspring will be heterozygotes and express the dominant phenotype. This uniformity is independent of which parent was dominant and which recessive. The second law, the principle of segregation, holds that alleles separate, or segregate, at meiosis and are carried in different gametes. The third law, the principle (or law) of independent assortment, holds that the allele pairs of unlinked loci are transmitted to gametes, or assorted, independently. Also called *mendelian law*.

mendelian law MENDEL'S LAWS.

Meyer's law The internal structure of a mature bone provides the greatest resistance with the least possible amount of material.

law of microscopic reversibility The law stating that the pathway and transition states are the same for forward and reverse reactions.

law of the minimum LIEBIG'S LAW OF THE MINIMUM.

Minot's law The most accelerated rate of aging occurs in the young.

Müller's law LAW OF SPECIFIC IRRITABILITY.

Müller-Haeckel law RECAPITULATION THEORY.

law of multiple variants Any variation in the number or general conformation of bones of the hands or feet is multiple, that is, it affects more than one bone.

myelogenetic law The order in which nerve fibers become myelinated is determined by the order in which they appear phylogenetically and become functional. The earliest to myelinate are ventral nerve root fibers, then dorsal root fibers, and central nervous system tract fibers later on. Pyramidal tract fibers myelinate late, about the first or second year after birth in man. Also called *Flechsig's mylogenetic law*.

Naegeli's law The proposition that a disease with eosinophilic leukocytes present in half-normal, normal, or increased numbers cannot be typhoid fever. The presence of even a small number of eosinophils makes a diagnosis of typhoid questionable.

Nernst's law The threshold for electrical excitation of muscle varies in proportion to the square root of stimulus frequency.

Newton's law of gravitation The principle that two bodies of matter attract each other with a force proportional to the product of thair masses and inversely proportional to the square of the distance between them.

Nysten's law Rigor mortis develops first in the masticatory muscles and then sequentially in the musculature of the neck, upper extremities, trunk, and finally the lower extremities.

Ohm's law The voltage across a resistor is equal to the product of the magnitude of the current flowing through it and a property of the resistor called resistance.

Ollier's law In children, when two longitudinal bones are joined proximally and distally, the arrest of growth in one of the bones will result in abnormal growth in the other bone.

Pajot's law A law explaining the manner of presentation of the fetus during labor: the shape of a cavity governs to some extent the position of an object within it, especially if the contained object is of a sizable mass. The law explains why a vertex presentation of a fetus is the usual one.

law of parsimony OCCAM'S RAZOR.

Pflüger's laws Rules of electrical excitation of nerve specifying that impulse initiation occurs at the cathode with stimulus onset and at the anode with stimulus removal.

Poiseuille's law The rate of flow of liquid in a tube is directly proportional to the pressure drop along the tube and to the fourth power of the radius of the tube, and is inversely proportional to the length of the tube and to the viscosity of the fluid. Also called *Poiseuille's equation*.

power function law A psychophysical hypothesis for relating the amount of physical energy required to evoke a sensory experience, in certain systems, to the subjective intensity of the sense impression: The intensity of a subjective sensory experience is equal to a constant multiplied by the magnitude of the physical stimulus energy raised to a power.

Prentice law The prism diopters of deviation caused by a spherical lens are the same as the dioptric power of the lens for each centimeter of decentralization.

Prévost's law In a unilateral cerebral lesion, the head and eyes are often turned to the affected side.

Profeta's law A clinically syphilis-free baby born of a syphilitic mother is immune to the disease. This was later refuted when it was found that the child had been infected from birth but the infection was in a latent or unrecognized form.

psychophysical law 1 WEBER-FECHNER LAW. 2 The subjective magnitude of each sensation is a specific power (i.e., an exponential) function of stimulus magnitude.

Raoult's law The proposition that the vapor pressure exerted by a component in a liquid is directly proportional to its mole fraction in that liquid. It is approximately followed for many liquids when their molecules do not interact strongly.

law of reciprocal proportions The law stating that if an element A combines separately with two other elements B and C that also combine with each other, then the ratio by mass of B and C that combine with a fixed mass of A is simply related to the ratio by mass with which they combine with each other. Observations that this law was obeyed provided early evidence for the existence of atoms.

law of referred pain The doctrine that referred pain can only arise from excitation of nociceptor axons.

law of refraction A law stating the mathematical relationship between the angle of incidence and the angle of transmission resulting from refraction of optical or acoustic waves. It can be expressed as $n_2\sin\theta_2 = n_1\sin\theta_1$ where n_2 and n_1 are the indices of refraction of two media, θ_2 is the angle between the normal to the surface and the direction of propagation, and θ_1 is the angle of refraction, i.e., the angle between the normal to the surface and the direction of the outgoing ray. Also called *Snell's law*.

law of refreshment The doctrine that the nutrient supply to muscle is a function of the rate of arterial blood supply.

law of regression GALTON'S LAW OF REGRESSION.

law of relativity The relationship of altering subjective sensation magnitude by comparing simultaneous versus successive stimuli of the same magnitude.

Ritter's law The principle that both onset and offset of an electrical current can excite nerve.

Ritter-Valli law After interruption of a peripheral nerve there is a gradual distal spread of a transient increase in excitability followed by a loss of excitability. Also called *Valli-Ritter law*.

Rosenbach's law Extensor muscles of the limbs are involved before the flexor muscles in disorders of spinal anterior horn cells or peripheral nerves.

Rubner's law 1 LAW OF CONSTANT ENERGY CONSUMPTION. 2 LAW OF CONSTANT GROWTH QUOTIENT.

Schroeder van der Kolk's law In a mixed peripheral nerve, sensory fibers are distributed to regions moved by motor fibers of the same nerve. Also called *van der Kolk's law*.

second law of thermodynamics Processes in nature are accompanied by dispersal of energy and an increase in the unavailability of heat.

law of segregation See under MENDEL'S LAWS.

Semon's law   A law purporting to explain the inconstant position assumed by the vocal cords when their motor nerve supply is affected by disease or injury: in progressive organic lesions of the motor nerve supply of the intrinsic laryngeal muscles, the function of abduction is lost before that of adduction. Also called *Semon-Rosenbach law.*

Semon-Rosenbach law   SEMON'S LAW.

Shelford's law of tolerance   Organisms have both upper and lower limits of tolerance to environmental factors. Also called *law of tolerance.*

Sherrington's law   RECIPROCAL INNERVATION.

Snell's law   LAW OF REFRACTION.

Spallanzani's law   Regeneration in the young approaches totality more so than in the old.

law of specific energies   LAW OF SPECIFIC IRRITABILITY.

law of specific irritability   The doctrine proposed by Johannes Müller that each nerve is excited via sense organs responsive to a specific form of energy, and that its excitation, because of its connections, can only give rise to one modality of sensation regardless of whether the nerve is electrically or mechanically excited, e.g., excitation of the optic nerve by any means can only lead to visual sensory impressions. Also called *doctrine of specific nerve energies, Müller's law, specific irritability, specific nerve energy, law of specific energies.*

law of specificity of bacteria   KOCH'S LAW.

Starling's law   As a general rule, the energy of contraction of cardiac muscle fibers is proportional to their length at the start of contraction. Also called *law of the heart.*

Stokes law   A muscle lying over an inflamed membrane (such as the peritoneum or pleura) often becomes paralyzed.

Talbot's law   Equal apparent brightness is perceived whether the total light energy is delivered as a constant intensity or as a light blinking at a frequency higher than can be recognized as a flickering sensation.

Teevan's law   Fractures of bones occur in lines of extension and in the line of compression.

third law of thermodynamics   Absolute zero temperature is unattainable in any finite sequence of operations, no matter how idealized.

law of tolerance   SHELFORD'S LAW OF TOLERANCE.

Toynbee's law   GULL-TOYNBEE LAW.

Valli-Ritter law   RITTER-VALLI LAW.

van der Kolk's law   SCHROEDER VAN DER KOLK'S LAW.

van't Hoff-Arrhenius law   The law that the variation of rate of reaction with temperature can be expressed as a linear decrease of the logarithm of the rate of reaction as the reciprocal of the absolute temperature rises.

Virchow's law   Tumor cells are derived from preexisting normal cells.

law of von Baer   **1** A law concerning the orientation of the embryo in a bird's egg: the axis of the embryo is perpendicular to the long axis of the egg and its head is directed to the opposite of the observer having the egg in front of him with the pointed end to the right. This orientation depends on mechanical factors. **2** The concept of embryogenic recapitulation according to which the forms of higher animals pass during their development through stages recalling those of lower forms. This concept was taken up again by Haeckel in his recapitulation theory. • K. E. von Baer (1792-1876) was the father of modern embryology. He discovered the mammalian ovum in 1827 and described many embryologic structures, including the germ layers. Also called *Baer's law.*

Vulpian's law   When a part of the brain is destroyed, its functions may be adopted by the surviving parts.

Waller's law   If sensory fibers are divided in a spinal root proximal to the ganglion, the fibers between the lesion and the ganglion remain intact while those between the lesion and the spinal cord degenerate. Also called *wallerian law.*

wallerian law   WALLER'S LAW.

Weber's law   The smallest discriminable intensity increment is a fixed fraction of the comparison stimulus magnitude for all sensory systems, i.e., $\Delta I/I$-constant.

Weber-Fechner law   For any sensory system the incremental threshold changes in relation to the background intensity in such a way that the ratio of increment (ΔI) to the background intensity (I) is always constant. Also called *psychophysical law.*

Weigert's law   The principle that the biological processes of regeneration and repair are always accompanied by overproduction of tissue, such as callus formation during bone fracture repair. A rarely used term.

Wien's displacement law   A law expressing the relationship of the wavelength of maximal intensity to the temperature of an object capable of absorbing and emitting radiations of all wavelengths: the wavelength of maximal intensity becomes shorter as the temperature increases. Wavelength times temperature equals a constant: 0.2898 cm-deg.

Wilder's law of initial value   LAW OF INITIAL VALUE.

Wolff's law   The internal structure and external shape of a bone develop in response to the change in function and to the forces acting upon it.

Zeune's law   A theory, now obsolete, that purported to link the incidence of blindness with residence in the temperate, frigid, or tropical zones. Blindness was said to be more prevalent nearer the equator, and proportionately less prevalent in the temperate than in the frigid zone.

Lawrence [Robert Daniel *Lawrence, English physician, flourished 20th century*] **1** Lawrence-Seip syndrome, Seip-Lawrence syndrome. See under SEIP SYNDROME. **2** Lawrence syndrome. See under ACQUIRED GENERALIZED LIPODYSTROPHY.

lawrencium   A synthetic element of the actinide series, having atomic number 103 and mass number 257. Several isotopes have been reported, the maximum half-life being 35 seconds. Symbol: Lr

lawsone $C_{10}H_6O_3$. 2-hydroxy-1,4-naphthoquinone. An agent isolated from the leaves of *Lawsonia inermis* that has the ability to act as a sunscreen.

laxation [L *laxatio* (from *laxatus*, past part. of *laxare* to loosen, disengage, deliver) a loosening, relaxing] DEFECATION.

laxative [Med L *laxativus* (from L *laxatus*, past part. of *laxare* to loosen + -*ivus* -IVE) loosening, lessening. See also LAXATOR.] **1** Tending to promote the onset of defecation; stimulating a bowel movement. **2** A laxative agent; a mild cathartic.

bulk laxative   A laxative that works by increasing stool volume, usually by retaining a greater proportion of water in the stool.

laxator [L *laxat(us)* (past part. of *laxare* to enlarge, widen, loosen, slacken, relax; Gk *lagaroun* to become slack, loose) enlarged, widened, loosened, freed + -OR] Something that loosens or relaxes. An outmoded term in anatomy.

laxator tympani major   An outmoded term for LIGAMENTUM MALLEI ANTERIUS.

laxator tympani minor   An outmoded term for LIGAMENTUM MALLEI LATERALE.

laxitas [L (from *lax(us)* slack, loosened, lax + -*itas* -ITY), spaciousness, looseness]

laxitas gingivarum   Spongy gums.

laxity [L *laxit(as)* (from *lax(us)* slack, loose, spacious + -*itas* -ITY) spaciousness, wideness, looseness + -Y] The capability of either normal free motion or greater than normal motion, as of a joint; looseness.

congenital laxity of ligaments   A familial disorder, often observed in families of contortionists in whom a remarkable range of movement at many joints is possible, which is believed to be due to ligamentous laxity present from birth.

lay [Middle English, *lay, lai,* from Old French *lai* lay, from Late L *lai(cus)* lay, not of the priesthood, from Gk *laikos* pertaining to the people, from *laos* the people + *-ikos* -IC] Not belonging to a given profession or group of professions; of or pertaining to laymen.

layer

layer [Middle English *leyer,* from *leyen* to lay] A sheet of tissue of more or less uniform thickness, commonly one of several superimposed sheets; a lamina or a stratum.

layer I STRATUM MOLECULARE.

layer II EXTERNAL GRANULAR LAYER OF CEREBRUM.

layer III LAYER OF SMALL PYRAMIDAL CELLS.

layer IV INTERNAL GRANULAR LAYER.

layer V INTERNAL PYRAMIDAL LAYER.

layer VI MULTIFORM LAYER.

abscission layer ABSCISSION.

adamantine layer ENAMEL.

ameloblastic layer A layer of cells which are derived from the inner enamel epithelium and which produce the enamel of a tooth. Also called *enamel layer.*

anterior elastic layer LAMINA LIMITANS ANTERIOR CORNEAE.

anterior fascial layer of transversus abdominis muscle The aponeurosis of the transversus abdominis muscle which passes transversely to the median plane to end in the linea alba, the upper three fourths lying behind the rectus abdominis muscle and blending with the posterior lamina of the rectus sheath, while the lower one fourth passes anterior to the rectus abdominis. The lowest fibers turn downward to help form the conjoint tendon. An outmoded term.

anterior limiting layer of iris FACIES ANTERIOR IRIDIS.

anterior layer of the rectus abdominis sheath LAMINA ANTERIOR VAGINAE MUSCULI RECTI ABDOMINIS.

bacillary layer STRATUM NEUROEPITHELIALE RETINAE.

Baillarger's layer A horizontal band of myelinated fibers in the internal granular layer of the cerebral neocortex, often called the inner line of Baillarger. See also BAILLARGER'S LINES.

basal layer 1 COMPLEXUS BASALIS CHOROIDEAE. 2 STRATUM BASALE ENDOMETRII.

basal layer of epidermis A single layer of columnar cells that form the deepest layer of the germinative part of the epidermis. The cells are perpendicular to a basement membrane and contain mitoses and occasional pigment cells or chromatocytes. Also called *rete malpighii, epidermal rete* (outmoded), *stratum basale epidermidis, stratum cylindricum epidermidis, palisade layer.*

basement layer BASEMENT MEMBRANE.

Bekhterev's layer A narrow band or plexus of horizontal myelinated fibers at the margin of the external granular and external pyramidal layers (layers II and III) of the cerebral cortex. Also called *line of Kaes* (outmoded), *Bekhterev's band* (outmoded), *band of Kaes-Bekhterev* (outmoded), *Kaes feltwork, layer of Kaes-Bekhterev, supraradial plexus, stria kaesbekhterevi, stripe of Kaes-Bekhterev.*

blastodermic layer GERM LAYER.

Bowman's layer LAMINA LIMITANS ANTERIOR CORNEAE.

Bruch's layer COMPLEXUS BASALIS CHOROIDEAE.

buffy layer A layer of white blood cells and platelets that forms on the top of a column of centrifuged red blood cells.

cambium layer 1 A condensation of loose connective tissue at its interface with a different layer or structure. 2 STRATUM OSTEOGENETICUM.

layers of cerebellar cortex The laminar pattern found in the superficial part of the cerebellum, comprising an outer molecular layer, a Purkinje cell layer, and a broad granule cell layer containing a variety of cell types. These layers overlie the white matter, which is devoid of neuron cell bodies.

cerebral layer An outmoded term for STRATUM NERVOSUM RETINAE.

Chievitz layer A layer of fibers temporarily situated between the inner and outer neuroblastic layers in the developing optic cup.

choriocapillary layer LAMINA CHOROIDOCAPILLARIS.

circular layer of eardrum STRATUM CIRCULARE MEMBRANAE TYMPANI.

circular layer of muscular tunic of colon STRATUM CIRCULARE TUNICAE MUSCULARIS COLI.

circular layer of muscular tunic of rectum STRATUM CIRCULARE TUNICAE MUSCULARIS RECTI.

circular layer of muscular tunic of small intestine STRATUM CIRCULARE TUNICAE MUSCULARIS INTESTINI TENUIS.

circular layer of muscular tunic of stomach STRATUM CIRCULARE TUNICAE MUSCULARIS GASTRICAE.

circular layer of tympanic membrane STRATUM CIRCULARE MEMBRANAE TYMPANI.

claustral layer An outmoded term for CLAUSTRUM. ● It is so named because the claustrum was once believed to constitute a separate layer of cortex.

clear layer of skin STRATUM LUCIDUM EPIDERMIDIS.

columnar layer 1 STRATUM NEUROEPITHELIALE RETINAE. 2 MANTLE LAYER.

compact layer STRATUM COMPACTUM ENDOMETRII.

cortical layer CORTEX.

cremasteric layer CREMASTERIC COAT OF TESTIS.

cutaneous layer of tympanic membrane STRATUM CUTANEUM MEMBRANAE TYMPANI.

cuticular layer In the skin, a single layer of scaly cells with atrophic nuclei that is closely applied to the outside of the hair root. Also called *epidermicula.*

deep layer of triangular ligament FASCIA DIAPHRAGMATIS UROGENITALIS SUPERIOR.

deep layer of urogenital diaphragm FASCIA DIPHRAGMATIS UROGENITALIS SUPERIOR.

dense layer GLOMERULAR BASEMENT MEMBRANE.

dermic layer STRATUM CUTANEUM MEMBRANAE TYMPANI.

Dobie's layer Z BAND.

electron layer The layer of electrons constituting the space charge (the region containing excess electrons) around the cathode in a vacuum tube.

enamel layer AMELOBLASTIC LAYER.

ependymal layer An internal layer of cells of the primitive neural tube bounding the central canal. The ependymal cells abut against an internal limiting membrane next to the canal while their processes extend peripherally. The thick pseudostratified epithelium present in the recently closed neural tube is known as the neuroepithelial layer. Later on the mantle and marginal layers or zones will appear, to give rise to the grey and white matter. Also called *ependymal zone.*

epitrichial layer The outermost layer of the embryonic epidermis which, after the sixth month of intrauterine life, is loosened by the growth of lanugo and contributes to the vernix caseosa as the epitrichium.

external granular layer of cerebrum The most superficial neuronal layer of cerebral neocortex, containing numerous densely packed small neurons (granule cells) and few myelinated fibers. Also called *layer II.*

external pyramidal layer LAYER OF SMALL PYRAMIDAL CELLS.

fatty layer of perineum SUPERFICIAL LAYER OF FASCIA OF PERINEUM.

fibrous layer of articular capsule MEMBRANA FIBROSA CAPSULAE ARTICULARIS.

Floegel's layer A granular layer of cytoplasm in a skeletal muscle cell adjacent to a motor endplate and containing numerous mitochondria and nuclei.

fruiting layer The spore-bearing or fertile hymenial layer of ascomycetous and basidiomycetous fungi. Also called *sporogenous layer.*

functional layer of endometrium STRATUM FUNCTIONALE ENDOMETRII.

fusiform layer MULTIFORM LAYER.

layer of fusiform cells MULTIFORM LAYER.

ganglionic layer of cerebellum STRATUM GANGLIOSUM CEREBELLI.

ganglionic layer of optic nerve STRATUM GANGLIONARE RETINAE.

ganglionic layer of retina STRATUM GANGLIONARE RETINAE.

Gennari's layer GENNARI'S BAND.

germ layer One of the three basic layers or laminae of cells of the early embryo: ectoderm (outer skin), mesoderm (middle skin), and endoderm (inner skin). The tissues of the body are derived from the germ layers and the fate of each layer is fairly well defined, though not as specifically as formerly believed. The layers may be considered assembly areas from where the parts of the embryo will emerge at the right position and in the right order. Also called *blastodermic layer.*

germinative layer A layer of cells within which new cells are formed.

germinative layer of epidermis The zone of the epidermis in which the generation of new epidermal cells occurs. It is the stratum basale epidermidis and stratum spinosum epidermidis combined. Also called *corpus mucosum, mucous layer, stratum germinativum epidermidis malpighii* (outmoded), *stratum dentatum epidermidis* (outmoded), *stratum malpighii* (outmoded), *stratum mucosum* (outmoded), *rete mucosum.*

germinative layer of nail STRATUM GERMINATIVUM UNGUIS.

granular layer INTERNAL GRANULAR LAYER.

granular-cell layer GRANULE LAYER.

granular layer of cerebellum STRATUM GRANULOSUM CEREBELLI.

granular layer of epidermis The deeper of the keratinizing layers of the epidermis, lying between the stratum spinosum of the germinative layers and the more superficial stratum lucidum. The cells derive from the stratum spinosum, become flattened, contain pyknotic nuclei, and synthesize keratohyalin granules. Also called *keratohyaline layer, Langerhans layer, Unna's layer, stratum granulosum epidermidis.*

granular layer of follicle of ovary STRATUM GRANULOSUM FOLLICULI OVARICI SECUNDARII.

granular layer of Tomes A narrow zone in the peripheral region of the dentin of a root which has a granular appearance in ground sections of teeth.

granule layer The layer of densely packed small neurons (granule cells) of the cerebral and cerebellar cortex. They constitute the principal zone of termination of afferent fibers. Also called *granular-cell layer.*

gray layer of superior colliculus STRATUM GRISEUM COLLICULI SUPERIORIS.

half-thickness layer HALF-VALUE LAYER.

half-value layer An index of photon beam radiation quality. It is the thickness of appropriate attenuating material which, when inserted in a narrow beam, reduces its intensity in half. Also called *half-value thickness, half-thickness, half-layer, half-thickness layer.* Abbreviation: Hvl

Haller's layer LAMINA VASCULOSA CHOROIDEAE.

Henle's layer A darkly staining layer that forms the outer portion of the inner root sheath of a hair.

Henle's fiber layer An outer sublayer of the external plexiform lamina around the fovea centralis. It is formed by horizontally stretched inner rod and cone fibers and corresponding parts of Müller's fibers.

Henle's nervous layer ENTORETINA.

horny layer of epidermis STRATUM CORNEUM EPIDERMIDIS.

horny layer of nail STRATUM CORNEUM UNGUIS.

Huxley's layer The two layers of cells that are immediately external to the inner root sheath cuticle of a hair. Also called *Huxley sheath, Huxley's membrane.*

inferior layer of pelvic diaphragm FASCIA DIAPHRAGMATIS PELVIS INFERIOR.

inferior layer of urogenital diaphragm MEMBRANA PERINEI.

infragranular layer A cell layer of the human fetal cerebral cortex that appears about the sixth month deep to the inner granular layer and gives rise to the ganglionic layer.

inner molecular layer An outmoded term for STRATUM PLEXIFORME INTERNUM.

inner muscular layer of stomach STRATUM CIRCULARE TUNICAE MUSCULARIS GASTRICAE.

inner neuroblastic layer The layer of the embryonic retina giving rise to ganglion cells, amacrine, and sustentacular cells.

inner nuclear layer STRATUM NUCLEARE INTERNUM.

inner plexiform layer of the retina STRATUM PLEXIFORME INTERNUM.

internal granular layer The layer of cerebral neocortex consisting of densely packed, small stellate neurons (granule cells). It is the main recipient zone of specific thalamocortical afferent terminals, and is consequently best developed in the sensory areas. Also called *granular layer, layer IV.*

internal medullary layers of optic thalamus The two bands (fused in part) of myelinated axons separating the medial from the lateral and ventral thalamic nuclear groups and containing the intralaminar nuclei.

internal pyramidal layer The lamina of cerebral neocortex containing the largest pyramidal neurons, which are especially large and conspicuous in the motor areas. Also called *layer V, Meynert's layer.*

investing layer of cervical fascia LAMINA SUPERFICIALIS FASCIAE CERVICALIS.

layer of Kaes-Bekhterev BEKHTEREV'S LAYER.

keratohyaline layer GRANULAR LAYER OF EPIDERMIS.

Kölliker's layer STROMA IRIDIS.

Langerhans layer GRANULAR LAYER OF EPIDERMIS.

Langhans layer CYTOTROPHOBLAST.

lateral cartilaginous layer LAMINA CARTILAGINIS LATERALIS TUBAE AUDITIVAE.

longitudinal layer of muscular tunic of colon STRATUM LONGITUDINALE TUNICAE MUSCULARIS COLI.

longitudinal layer of muscular tunic of rectum STRATUM LONGITUDINALE TUNICAE MUSCULARIS RECTI.

longitudinal layer of muscular tunic of small intestine STRATUM LONGITUDINALE TUNICAE MUSCULARIS INTESTINI TENUIS.

longitudinal layer of muscular tunic of stomach STRATUM LONGITUDINALE TUNICAE MUSCULARIS GASTRICAE.

malpighian layer The main portion of the epidermis, which is composed of squamous cells that are connected by numerous intercellular bridges, or desmosomes. Also called *Renaut's layer*.

mantle layer The middle layer of the neural tube, lying between the germinal layer inside it and the marginal layer outside. As the neural tube differentiates, the cell derivatives of the original neuroepithelial layer settle in different zones of the wall. All the neuroblasts, supported by numerous but not all glial precursors, occupy the mantle layer. Also called *mantle zone, columnar layer*.

marginal layer The outermost of layer of the neural tube at the start of its development, which includes few cell bodies, but mostly nerve fibers and prolongations of the interlacing neuroglia. Separated by an external limiting membrane from a dense mesenchymatous layer (future leptomeninges), it surrounds the mantle layer (future gray matter) and itself will develop into the white matter of the spinal cord. Also called *marginal zone*.

matching layer Material placed in front of the face of an ultrasound transducer element to reduce the reflection of sound at the transducer surface.

medial cartilaginous layer LAMINA CARTILAGINIS MEDIALIS TUBAE AUDITIVAE.

membranous layer of the perineum The thin, but strong, aponeurotic deep layer of the superficial fascia of the perineum, continuous with the membranous, or Scarpa's, layer of superficial fascia of the lower abdominal wall, the tunica dartos and the fascia of the penis. It is attached to the ischiopubic rami laterally, and to the posterior, or inferior, border of the perineal membrane and the perineal body posteriorly. Deep to it is the superficial perineal pouch.

Meynert's layer INTERNAL PYRAMIDAL LAYER.

middle layer of cervical fascia LAMINA PRETRACHEALIS FASCIAE CERVICALIS.

mixing layer The lower part of the atmosphere where pollutants are mixed and dispersed by atmospheric turbulence.

molecular layer STRATUM MOLECULARE.

molecular layer of cerebellar cortex STRATUM MOLECULARE CEREBELLI.

molecular layer of cerebellum STRATUM MOLECULARE CEREBELLI.

molecular layer of olfactory bulb The ill-defined external plexiform layer of the olfactory bulb. It lies between the layer of synaptic glomeruli and interglomerular spaces externally and the mitral cell layer centrally, and contains tufted cells which diminish in size throughout the layer towards the glomeruli. Some authorities include the mitral cells, which are analogous to but larger than the tufted cells, in this layer.

monomolecular layer MONOLAYER.

mucous layer GERMINATIVE LAYER OF EPIDERMIS.

mucous layer of tympanic membrane STRATUM MUCOSUM MEMBRANAE TYMPANI.

multiform layer The deepest neuronal layer of the cerebral neocortex, containing predominantly spindle-shaped (fusiform) cells. It is bordered below by the white matter and above by the internal pyramidal layer. It is distinctively pierced by bundles of radial axons, and gives rise to many short association fibers. In some earlier schemes it was subdivided into layers VI and VII (Vogt) to distinguish the cells scattered at the border of the white matter. Also called *fusiform layer, spindle-celled layer, layer of fusiform cells, layer VI*.

muscular layer of fallopian tube TUNICA MUSCULARIS TUBAE UTERINAE.

muscular layers of Renaut Strands of smooth muscle of the inner circular layer of the muscularis mucosae of the stomach which extend between the glands towards the epithelial surface. An outmoded term.

nervous layer STRATUM NERVOSUM RETINAE.

neurodermal layer ECTODERM.

neuroepidermal layer ECTODERM.

neuroepithelial layer The single layer of cells that comprises the neural plate and its derivative, the early neural tube. Subsequently, as the neural tube thickens, the cells of the neuroepithelial layer proliferate and give rise to precursors of neurons, ependyma, and glial cells.

neuroepithelial layer of retina STRATUM NEUROEPITHELIALE RETINAE.

layer of Nitabuch MEMBRANE OF NITABUCH.

odontoblastic layer The pseudostratified layer of large, elongated and radially arranged cells that line a tooth's pulp cavity adjacent to the dentin and send protoplasmic processes, or fibers of Tomes, into the dentinal tubules. The cells contain mitochondria and a Golgi net.

Oehl's layer STRATUM LUCIDUM EPIDERMIDIS.

Ollier's layer STRATUM OSTEOGENETICUM.

osteoblastic layer STRATUM OSTEOGENETICUM.

osteogenetic layer STRATUM OSTEOGENETICUM.

outer molecular layer An outmoded term for STRATUM PLEXIFORME EXTERNUM.

outer neuroblastic layer The layer of the embryonic retina giving origin to the photoreceptive elements, the rods and cones, and the bipolar neurons.

outer nuclear layer STRATUM NUCLEARE EXTERNUM.

outer plexiform layer of the retina STRATUM PLEXIFORME EXTERNUM.

ozone layer An atmospheric zone at about 10 to 50 km above the earth's surface that has a relatively high percentage of ozone. It is believed to reduce the amount of solar ultraviolet radiation reaching the earth's surface. Also called *ozonosphere*.

palisade layer BASAL LAYER OF EPIDERMIS.

Pander's layer SPLANCHNOPLEURE.

papillary layer of corium STRATUM PAPILLARE CORII.

parietal layer of pelvic fascia FASCIA PELVIS PARIETALIS.

parietal layer of pericardium LAMINA PARIETALIS PERICARDII.

parietal layer of serous pericardium LAMINA PARIETALIS PERICARDII.

parietal layer of tunica vaginalis of testis LAMINA PARIETALIS TUNICAE VAGINALIS TESTIS.

Parrot's layer A layer of calcifying cartilage within the growing region of a bone, situated between the growth cartilage and the epiphysis. This is associated with the process of epiphyseal endochondral ossification.

perforated layer of sclera LAMINA CRIBROSA SCLERAE.

pericyte layer PERITHELIUM.

peripheral layer STRATUM MOLECULARE.

perpendicular layer of ethmoid bone LAMINA PERPENDICULARIS OSSIS ETHMOIDALIS.

pigmented layer of ciliary body EPITHELIUM PIGMENTOSUM PARTIS CILIARIS RETINAE.

pigmented layer of ciliary part of retina EPITHELIUM PIGMENTOSUM PARTIS CILIARIS RETINAE.

pigmented layer of eyeball The continuous layer of pigmented epithelium which lines the inside of the eyeball from the entrance of the optic nerve to the pupillary margin of the iris and comprises the pigmented layers of the retina, ciliary body, and iris. An outmoded term. Also called *stratum pigmenti bulbi oculi*.

pigmented layer of iris EPITHELIUM POSTERIUS PIGMENTOSUM PARTIS IRIDICAE RETINAE.

pigmented layer of optic part of retina STRATUM PIGMENTOSUM PARTIS OPTICAE RETINAE.

pigmented layer of retina STRATUM PIGMENTOSUM PARTIS OPTICAE RETINAE.

plexiform layer 1 Either stratum plexiforme externum or stratum plexiforme internum. 2 STRATUM MOLECULARE.

Polyak layer The horizontal cell layer of the retina.

posterior elastic layer LAMINA LIMITANS POSTERIOR COR-
NEAE.

posterior layer of rectus sheath LAMINA POSTERIOR VA-
GINAE MUSCULI RECTI ABDOMINIS.

pretracheal layer LAMINA PRETRACHEALIS FASCIAE CER-
VICALIS.

prickle-cell layer STRATUM SPINOSUM EPIDERMIDIS.

primary blastodermic layer The single-layered embryonic
disk before the germ layers have appeared.

primitive layer The internal layer of the neuroepithelium of
the optic cup, which gives rise to the outer and inner neuroblastic
layers.

primordial layers Endoblast and ectoblast before gastrulation.

Purkinje layer STRATUM GANGLIOSUM CEREBELLI.

layer of pyramidal cells A lamina of large, pyramidal neurons in the cerebral cortex, especially the internal pyramidal
layer (layer V) of neocortex or the main neuronal lamina of the
hippocampal and dentate gyri.

radiate layer of tympanic membrane STRATUM RADIATUM
MEMBRANAE TYMPANI.

Rauber's layer PRIMITIVE ECTODERM.

Renaut's layer MALPIGHIAN LAYER.

reticular layer of corium STRATUM RETICULARE CORII.

layer of rods and cones STRATUM NEUROEPITHELIALE RET-
INAE.

Rohr's layer Fibrinoid stria in the juxtaintervillous portion
of the basal plate of a human placenta, often closely related to
Nitabuch's membrane.

Sattler's layer The part of the lamina vasculosa choroideae
which is close to the lamina choroidocapillaris and contains the
smaller caliber blood vessels.

sclerotogenous layer SKELETOGENOUS LAYER.

second half-value layer That thickness of absorbing medium
required to reduce the intensity of penetrating radiation by one
half, subsequent to a reduction by one half of the original radiation intensity by the primary absorbing medium.

skeletogenous layer The mesoderm around the notochord
that gives rise to the axial skeleton. Also called *sclerotogenous
layer.*

slime layer **1** A loosely adherent bacterial capsule. **2** A
layer of dextran or levan which promotes adherence of some
bacteria. **3** A layer, characteristic of the myxobacteria, that
holds together chains of cells.

sluggish layer STILL LAYER.

layer of small pyramidal cells The lamina of supragranular
pyramidal cells in the cerebral neocortex containing numerous
granule and Martinotti neurons intermingled in a gradient of
pyramidal neurons decreasing in size towards the surface. In
myelin-stained preparations this layer displays the horizontal
band of Kaes-Bechterev. Also called *external pyramidal layer,
layer III.*

somatic layer SOMATOPLEURE.

spindle-celled layer MULTIFORM LAYER.

spinous layer of epidermis STRATUM SPINOSUM EPIDER-
MIDIS.

splanchnic layer SPLANCHNOPLEURE.

spongy layer STRATUM SPONGIOSUM ENDOMETRII.

sporogenous layer FRUITING LAYER.

still layer The relatively slow moving layer of blood adjacent
to the wall of a capillary. Also called *sluggish layer.*

subcallosal layer A layer of myelinated axons on the inferior
surface of the corpus callosum.

subcutaneous layer TELA SUBCUTANEA.

subendocardial layer A layer of loose connective tissue that
binds the endocardium to the myocardium, is continuous with
the myocardial interstitial tissue, and contains blood vessels,

nerves, and conducting fibers of the heart. It lies deep to the
subendothelial layer.

subendothelial layer A thin collagenous layer deep to the
lining endothelium of the endocardium and of the large and
medium caliber vessels, containing a few fibroblasts and elastic
fibers.

subepicardial layer A thin collagenous layer with elastic fibers, blood vessels, and nervous elements between the mesothelial layer of the epicardium and the underlying myocardium.

submantle layer A fine layer of dentin with interglobular
spaces just deep to the peripheral layer of cover dentin at its
junction with the circumpulpar dentin. It is analagous to the
granular layer of Tomes in the root of the tooth.

submucous layer TELA SUBMUCOSA.

submucous layer of bladder TELA SUBMUCOSA VESICAE URI-
NARIAE.

submucous layer of colon TELA SUBMUCOSA COLI.

submucous layer of esophagus TELA SUBMUCOSA ESO-
PHAGI.

submucous layer of pharynx TELA SUBMUCOSA PHARYNGIS.

submucous layer of small intestine TELA SUBMUCOSA IN-
TESTINI TENUIS.

submucous layer of stomach TELA SUBMUCOSA GASTRICA.

subodontoblastic layer A layer of the peripheral pulp of the
tooth, deep to the odontoblasts and best seen in older teeth. It
is characterized by absence of cells, the fibrous tissue and cell
processes forming a clear cell-free zone. In a young tooth, a
capillary plexus is found in this zone, as well as branches from
longitudinal myelinated fibers in the pulp forming a plexus (of
Raschkow) here. Also called *Weil's basal layer.*

subpapillary layer A vascular layer deep to the papillary
layer at its junction with the reticular layer of the dermis where
the rete subpapillare is found.

subserosal layer TELA SUBSEROSA.

subserous layer TELA SUBSEROSA.

subserous layer of peritoneum TELA SUBSEROSA PERITONEI.

superficial layer of fascia of perineum The fatty, or superficial, layer of the superficial fascia of the perineum, continuous
anteriorly either with the fat-free tunica dartos and fascia of the
penis or with the labia majora where it contains a lot of fat,
laterally with superficial fascia on the medial side of the thighs,
and posteriorly with the perianal superficial fascia. Also called
fatty layer of perineum.

superficial gray layer STRATUM GRISEUM COLLICULI SU-
PERIORIS.

superficial layer of triangular ligament MEMBRANA PERI-
NEI.

superficial layer of urogenital diaphragm MEMBRANA PE-
RINEI.

superior layer of pelvic diaphragm FASCIA DIAPHRAG-
MATIS PELVIS SUPERIOR.

superior layer of urogenital diaphragm See under SPATIUM
PERINEI PROFUNDUM.

suprachorioid layer An outmoded term for LAMINA SUPRA-
CHOROIDEA.

supragranular layer The neuronal lamina above the internal
granular layer of the cerebral neocortex. It is the zone above
the principal zone of specific afferent fiber termination, and
generally recognized as comprising layers II and III, which are
difficult to separate in some cortical areas (e.g., the limbic cortex).

synovial layer of articular capsule MEMBRANA SYNOVIALIS
CAPSULAE ARTICULARIS.

trophic layer ENDODERM.

Unna's layer GRANULAR LAYER OF EPIDERMIS.

vascular layer of choroid LAMINA VASCULOSA CHOROI-
DEAE.

vascular layer of testis　TUNICA VASCULOSA TESTIS.

vegetative layer　ENDODERM.

vertical layer of ethmoid bone　An outmoded term for LAMINA PERPENDICULARIS OSSIS ETHMOIDALIS.

vessel layer of the iris　STRATUM VASCULOSUM IRIDIS.

visceral layer of pelvic fascia　FASCIA PELVIS VISCERALIS.

visceral layer of pericardium　LAMINA VISCERALIS PERICARDII.

visceral layer of tunica vaginalis of testis　LAMINA VISCERALIS TUNICAE VAGINALIS TESTIS.

Waldeyer's layer　1 GERMINAL EPITHELIUM.　2 EPITHELIUM SUPERFICIALE OVARII.

Weil's basal layer　SUBODONTOBLASTIC LAYER.

white layers of cerebellum　LAMINAE ALBAE CEREBELLI.

yellow layer　BUFFY COAT.

Zeissl's layer　A layer observed between the tela submucosa and tunica muscularis mucosae in the stomach wall of the cat.

zonal layer of cerebellum　STRATUM MOLECULARE CEREBELLI.

zonal layer of quadrigeminal body　STRATUM ZONALE CORPORIS QUADRIGEMINI.

zonal layer of thalamus　STRATUM ZONALE THALAMI.

---

layman　A nonmember of a given profession; a person who has not worked or been trained in any field of the given profession or type of profession.

lazar　[from *Lazarus*, the biblical beggar described as "full of sores"]　A medieval term for LEPER.

lazaretto　[alteration (because of *Lazarus*, the New Testament person afflicted with sores) of Italian *Nazareto* Nazareth, from Santa Maria di *Nazaret*, an important hospital in Venice]　1 A hospital for isolating cases of infectious disease.　2 A building used for housing persons being kept in quarantine.

Lb　Symbol for the unit, pound-force. An outmoded symbol.

lb　Symbol for the unit, pound.

LBF　*Lactobacillus bulgaricus* factor (folic acid).

lbf　Symbol for the unit, pound-force.

lbf·ft　Symbol for the unit, pound-force foot.

lb tr　Symbol for the unit, pound troy.

LCM　lymphocytic choriomeningitis.

l/cmH₂O　Symbol for the unit, liter per centimeter of water.

LD　1 lethal dose.　2 light difference (eye examination).

LD₅₀　median lethal dose.

LD₁₀₀　The dose of biologically active material, usually a drug, a toxin, or a microorganism, that causes death in all exposed subjects. Also called *invariably lethal dose*.

LDH　lactate dehydrogenase.

LDL　1 low-density lipoprotein.　2 loudness discomfort level.

LDV　laser Doppler velocimetry.

LE　lupus erythematosus.

leach　[prob. Old English *leccan* to wet, irrigate]　1 To separate constituents of (a mixture) by contact with a solvent in which only some of the constituents are soluble, often used to harvest the soluble material.　2 To remove (the soluble portion) of a mixture.

leachate　An aqueous liquid that contains soluble or suspended matter acquired as the water percolates through solid waste, soil, underlying mineral strata, or other materials.

leaching　[LEACH + -ING]　The process of dissolving soluble material from its combined form in an insoluble matrix. It is used to separate and collect soluble material that is otherwise inaccessible. Also called *lixiviation*.

lead¹　[Old English *lēad*]　Element number 82, having atomic weight 207.2. Lead is a soft, bluish white metal with specific gravity 11.35, easily separated from its ores and sometimes found in elemental form. Four stable isotopes are found in nature, the end products of the uranium, thorium, and actinium disintegration series. Seventeen unstable isotopes are known. Lead is corrosion resistant and it is an effective absorber of sound and a wide range of electromagnetic radiation. It is universally used as a shield against x rays and other hazardous radiation. Its compounds have many applications in technology, in storage batteries, gasoline, paints, etc. It is a cumulative poison, and lead pollution becomes an endemic health hazard in some environments. Symbol: Pb

radioactive lead　Any of the radioactive isotopes of lead that either occur in nature as intermediates in the uranium, neptunium, thorium, or actinium series or are artificially produced. The naturally occurring radioactive isotopes are lead 204, 206, 207, and 208. Also called *radiolead*.

uranium lead　LEAD 206.

lead 206　A stable isotope of lead. It is the last member of the radioactive series which starts with uranium and includes radium. Also called *uranium lead, radium G*. Symbol: ^{206}Pb

lead 207　One of the four stable isotopes of lead (about 22% abundant), this one being the end product of the actinium series of radioactive elements that starts with uranium 235.

lead 208　One of the four stable isotopes of lead, comprising 52.3% of naturally occurring lead. It is the end product of radioactive decay in the thorium 232 series. Symbol: ^{208}Pb

lead 210　A radioactive isotope of lead, atomic number 82, having a half-life of 22.3 years. It occurs naturally in the uranium series through alpha decay of polonium 214. Also called *radium D*. Symbol: ^{210}Pb

lead 214　A radioactive isotope of lead, atomic number 82, having a half-life of 26.8 minutes. It occurs naturally in the uranium series through alpha decay of polonium 218. Also called *radium B*. Symbol: ^{214}Pb

lead²　[Middle English *lede* a leading, from *leden* to lead, from Old English *lǣden* to cause to go]　1 Any of the electrical connections used for recording a biopotential, such as an electrocardiogram.　2 Any of the records made from specific sites or pair of connections.

bipolar lead　A lead in which each of two sites of location of the electrodes contributes significantly to the record, as in the standard leads I, II, and III.

CF lead　A chest lead with the indifferent electrode attached to the left leg.

chest lead　An electrocardiographic lead in which the exploring electrode is placed on the chest. See also V LEAD. Also called *precordial lead, Wilson's lead*.

CL lead　A chest lead with the indifferent electrode attached to the left arm.

CM lead　A chest lead with the indifferent electrode placed on the manubrium sterni.

CR lead　A chest lead with the indifferent electrode attached to the right arm.

electroencephalographic lead　An electrical connection of two wires to two electrodes on the scalp that measures the cerebral activity between them. Normally many leads simultaneously record from many pairs of electrodes.

esophageal lead　An electrocardiographic lead in which the electrode is placed in the esophagus.

limb lead　Any of the electrocardiographic leads in which the exploring electrode or both electrodes are placed on the limbs: leads I, II, or III, or aVR, aVL, or aVF.

precordial lead　CHEST LEAD.

standard lead　One of the three bipolar leads that were regarded as standard in the early days of electrocardiography: lead

I (right arm–left arm), lead II (left leg–right arm), and lead III (left leg–left arm). Also called *standard limb lead, standard extremity lead.*

standard extremity lead   STANDARD LEAD.

standard limb lead   STANDARD LEAD.

unipolar lead   A lead in which one electrode is an exploring electrode and the other is an indifferent electrode with effective zero input, such as the Wilson central terminal.

unipolar limb lead   A unipolar lead in which the exploring electrode is attached to one of the limbs, as aVR (right arm), aVL (left arm), or aVF (left leg).

V lead   A unipolar electrocardiographic lead in which the exploring electrode is on the chest. The locations of the most commonly used V leads are as follows: V_1 and V_2 are in the fourth intercostal space, to the right and left of the sternum, respectively. V_3 is midway between V_2 and V_4, the latter being in the fifth intercostal space on the midclavicular line. V_5, on the left anterior axillary line, and V_6, on the midaxillary line, are both on the same horizontal level as V_4.

Wilson's lead   CHEST LEAD.

Leadbetter [Guy Whitman *Leadbetter*, U.S. orthopedic surgeon, 1893–1945]   See under MANEUVER.

leading   A British term among smelters for LEAD POISONING.

lead zirconate titanate   A piezoelectric ceramic material used in ultrasonic transducers. Symbol: PZT

leaf [Old English *lēaf*, akin to L *liber* inner bark of a tree]   A plant stem appendage that functions in transpiration and photosynthesis.

anterior mesodermal leaf   The more anterior half of the portion of the iris of mesodermal origin. This portion of the iris does not extend to the pupil, but stops at an irregular border midway between the pupil edge and the iris base.

digitalis leaf   The dried leaf of *Digitalis purpurea*, the purple foxglove. This the common form of digitalis, which was prescribed for many years as powdered digitalis leaf. It has been standarized as a reference of activity for other crude digitalis preparations. The availability of the purified digitalis glycosides has gradually replaced the use of the crude leaf preparations in most countries.

***Digitalis lantana* leaf**   The dried leaf of *Digitalis lantana*, which contains cardioactive glycosides and is more potent than digitalis leaf. Also called *woolly foxglove, Austrian foxglove.*

liver leaf   AMERICAN LIVERWORT.

leaflet   **1** A small structure resembling a leaf, such as a cusp of a valvule of a heart valve. **2** A small leaf, especially one forming a part of a compound leaf.

Leake [Chauncey Depew *Leake*, U.S. physiologist, 1896–1978]   Leake and Guy method. See under METHOD.

leans   A condition in which members of an air crew, in an attempt to compensate for an illusory tilting of the aircraft, lean in the opposite direction. The illusion is caused by a labyrinthine reaction uncorrected by being able to see land. A popular usage.

Leão [A. A. P. *Leão*, Brazilian physiologist, born 1914]   Leão spreading depression. See under DEPRESSION.

learning [Old English *leornung*, from *leornian* to learn + *-ung* -ING]   The acquired responses of an organism that are the result of experience, especially of repeated experience or practice, and of such deliberate modification procedures as classical or operant conditioning. Temporary behavioral changes that are the consequence of physiologic fluctuations, such as sensory adaptation, disease, fatigue, or drug effects are not regarded as instances of learning, nor are those maturational changes rooted directly in genetic influences.

associative learning   The establishment of a functional connection between two events such that the occurrence of one tends to reinstate the other. Bonds are formed between words, ideas, or other stimulus-response units, with no causal relation implied.

avoidance learning   That type of training in which an experimental animal learns to make a particular instrumental response to prevent the occurrence of a noxious stimulus. The response is usually to some warning signal that just precedes the delivery of a painful or punishing stimulus.

computer-assisted learning   An application of the computer to individualized learning, similar to but more complex and sophisticated than that of programed learning by means of a teaching machine. Not only can the material to be learned be presented in small steps, and the student's mastery of each unit tested before advancing to the next, but the nature of any errors made can be analyzed instantaneously and remedial instruction supplied, in much the same fashion that would be followed by a human tutor. Abbreviation: C.A.L.

conditioning learning   CONDITIONING.

discriminative learning   The learning of responses to selected stimuli through the application of differential reinforcement.

escape learning   Learning which is reinforced by subjecting the experimental animal to noxious or painful stimuli which the animal can escape by making a particular response.

imitative learning   Learning based on consciously copying the behavior of another. See also MODELING.

immunologic learning   The progressive changes in the nature of the antibodies formed (including increased avidity) following antigenic stimulation.

incidental learning   Learning or remembering that takes place without any obvious intent or particular purpose, and without any formal instruction to learn or remember, or any evident motive to learn.

instrumental learning   OPERANT LEARNING.

latent learning   Learning which has taken place, but which is not exhibited at the time that it is acquired but only at some later moment when the conditions of motive or reward are appropriate.

motor learning   Learning of tasks that involve the processes of skeletomuscular action rather than ideation. Motor and ideational learning are not, however, mutually exclusive processes.

operant learning   That form of learning, based on operant conditioning, in which the reinforcement of a given response increases the likelihood of the same response being made again. By selecting a species-compatible behavior, any by reinforcing any responses made that fall in the general direction desired by the experimenter, quite specific and often complicated behavioral sequences can be shaped. Also called *instrumental learning.*

passive avoidance learning   Avoidance learning in which the experimental animal learns to inhibit responses in order to avoid receiving a punishing stimulus.

perceptual learning   Learning in which the principal task or feature is a modification in the way things are perceived.

programed learning   Self-instruction using a set of materials specially selected to allow the learner to determine the pace. Whether the content is presented by means of a teaching machine or in a printed workbook, the essence of the method is to guide learning forward in small steps, questioning the student's mastery of what has been learned in each unit before proceeding to the next.

serial order learning   The learning of a series of responses, such as those made by an animal in running a maze or by a human subject in learning a list of nonsense syllables, in which the items to be mastered must appear in a prescribed order. Serial order learning is also basic for the acquisition of any complex skill, such as typewriting.

social learning   The shaping of the behavior of an individual during the years of growth so that it will be appropriate to the social standards or mores, folkways, attitudes, habits, values, and customs to which the individual is exposed.

state-dependent learning Learning which takes place while the person is in a particular physiologic state and can' most readily be recalled when the person is once again in the same state, such as a state induced by a dissociative drug or alcohol.

trial-and-error learning Learning in which the learner, faced with a task for which the appropriate response is not known, responds either randomly, or only to the most general features of the situation, until those actions which prove unsatisfactory are abandoned and there is a gradual, rather than an insightful, focusing on those responses that are successful.

learning-to-learn Acquiring skill in learning by practice in solving problems. The learner, usually a human or one of the higher primates, approaches problems in a way that suggests that they require an instrumental behavior for solution, as if operating on an implicit hypothesis that a means to the end, or goal, is there to be discovered. See also MENTAL SET.

leash A cordlike group of nerves, blood vessels, fibers, or similar structures.

Leber [Theodor *Leber*, German ophthalmologist, 1840–1917] **1** Leber's optic atrophy. See under ATROPHY. **2** See under DISEASE. **3** Leber's corpuscle. See under HASSALL'S CORPUSCLE. **4** Amaurosis congenita of Leber. See under AMAUROSIS. **5** Leber's plexus. See under HOVIUS PLEXUS.

Lebistes reticulatus A species of top-feeding minnows that consume mosquito larvae, found in warm water ponds of South America.

lecanopagus [Gk *lekan(e)* a dish + *o* + -PAGUS] Equal conjoined twins united at the pelvis. An ambiguous usage. • A preferred term to designate such a union would include the name of the particular bone involved, if any, such as *iliopagus*.

lecanosomatopagus [Gk *lecan(e)* a dish + *o* + SOMATO- + -PAGUS] Equal conjoined twins united throughout all or most of the trunk, including the pelvis. This condition is a form of dicephaly, the head being duplicated fully and the trunk only partially.

Lecat [Claude Nicolas *Lecat*, French surgeon, 1700–1768] See under GULF.

Le Chatelier [Henry Louis *Le Chatelier*, French chemist, 1850–1936] Le Chatelier's principle. See under LAW.

leche de higuerón [Spanish *leche* milk + *de* of + *higuerón* a large Latin American fig tree] The crude latex, sap, or milk obtained from the wild fig trees *Ficus doliara* and *F. glabrata* of Central and South America. It has been used as an anthelmintic, especially in treating trichuriasis.

lechopyra [Gk *lechō* a woman in childbirth + *pyra*, pl. of *pyr* fever] PUERPERAL FEVER.

lecith- [Gk *lekithos* pulse porridge, yolk of an egg] A combining form denoting the yolk of an egg.

lecithal [LECITH- + -AL] Possessing yolk. Eggs are classified according to the amount of yolk present, and range from microlecithal (having little yolk) to megalethical (having much yolk).

lecithin PHOSPHATIDYLCHOLINE.

lecithinase **1** An obsolete term for PHOSPHOLIPASE. **2** An obsolete term for LYSOPHOSPHOLIPASE.

lecithin:cholesterol acyl transferase A normally occurring plasma enzyme that esterifies cholesterol in the reaction: lecithin + cholesterol $\underset{\longrightarrow}{\text{LCAT}}$ lysolecithin + cholesteryl ester. Abbreviation: LCAT

lecithinemia The presence of lecithin in blood.

lecitho- LECITH-.

lecithoblast [LECITHO- + -BLAST] The early endoderm of the embryonic disk.

lecithocoele [LECITHO- + -COELE] A cavity surrounded by endoblast at a late blastocyst stage. Its dorsal part will give rise to the primitive intestine while its ventral part will become the yolk sac. • The term is derived from the fact that in sauropsid embryos this formation corresponds to the part of the endoblast containing the nutritious yolk.

Leclanché [Georges *Leclanché*, French chemist, 1839–1882] See under CELL.

lectin A hemagglutinating protein substance present in the saline extracts of the seeds of certain plants. Lectins bind specifically to certain sugars and oligopolysaccharides, including certain glycoproteins present on the surface of many mammalian cells. Some lectins have specific binding properties for certain lymphocyte subsets and are thus extensively used as mitogens in immunologic experiments. Their reaction usually requires divalent cations. Adjective: lectinic.

lectotype [Gk *lekto(s)*, verbal of *legein* to choose + TYPE] The syntype designated as the type specimen subsequent to the original description of a taxon for which no holotype was originally designated.

lectual [L *lectu(s)* (from *lectus*, past part. of *legere* to lie together) a bed + English -AL] Relating to or requiring confinement to bed.

ledbänder BÜNGNER'S BANDS.

Le Dentu [Jean-François-Auguste *Le Dentu*, French surgeon, 1841–1926] See under SUTURE.

Ledercillin A proprietary name for procaine penicillin G.

Lederer [Max *Lederer*, U.S. pathologist, 1885–1952] **1** See under SYNDROME. **2** Lederer-Brill anemia. See under LEDERER'S ANEMIA.

ledge A ridgelike or shelflike projection.

dental ledge DENTAL LAMINA.
enamel ledge DENTAL LAMINA.

Leduc [Stephane A. N. *Leduc*, French physician, 1853–1939] See under CURRENT.

Lee [Robert *Lee*, English gynecologist and obstetrician, 1793–1877] Lee's ganglion. See under CERVICAL GANGLION OF UTERUS.

leech [Old English *læce* a healer, physician] **1** An annelid worm of the class Hirudinea, especially an aquatic, blood-sucking member of such genera as *Hirudo, Limnatis, Dinobdella*, or *Haemopis*. Most leeches are aquatic scavengers or predators of snails, insects, annelids, or other soft-bodied aquatic animals. Land leeches, *Haemadipsa* species, are notorious pests in southeast Asian rainforests. Also called *sanguisuga*. **2** To apply leeches to (the body of a patient) for bloodletting, reduction of hematomas or varicosities, or other therapeutic purposes. See also LEECHING. **3** A practitioner of leeching; formerly, a physician.

American leech A leech of the species *Macrobdella decora*.
horse leech A leech that is parasitic upon horses, especially one of the kinds that lodge in the nasal passages and pharynx, such as *Limnatis nilotica* or *Haemopis* species.
land leech A leech that lives in a terrestrial habitat, especially one of the genus *Haemadipsa*.
medicinal leech A leech of the species *Hirudo medicinalis*.

leeching The former practice of applying leeches to the body to draw blood as a therapeutic measure.

Leede [Carl Stockbridge *Leede*, U.S. physician, born 1882] Rumpel-Leede sign, Rumpel-Leede test, Leede-Rumpel phenomenon. See under RUMPEL-LEEDE PHENOMENON.

leet [prob. a variant of *leat* (from Middle English *leet*, from Old English *(ge)lǣt* a road junction, conduit) a water trench going to or from a mill] To exude: said of eczema. An obsolete term.

leeting The serous exudate of eczema. An obsolete term.

Leeuwenhoekia australiensis An Australian mite thought to cause severe irritation by burrowing in the skin.

Leeuwenkoek [Antony van *Leeuwenkoek*, Dutch microscopist, 1632–1723] Leeuwenkoek's canal. See under HAVERSIAN CANAL.

Lefèvre [Paul *Lefèvre*, French dermatologist, flourished 20th century] Papillon-Lefèvre syndrome. See under SYNDROME.

Le Fort [Leon Clement *Le Fort*, French surgeon, 1829–1893] **1** Operation, fracture, amputation, suture. **2** Le Fort I osteotomy, Le Fort II osteotomy, Le Fort III osteotomy. See under OSTEOTOMY.

left-eyed Having the left eye dominant.

left-footed Characterized by preferential or dominant use of the left foot. Also *sinistropedal.*

left-handed Characterized by preferential or dominant use of the left hand. Also *sinistromanual.*

left-handedness Preferential use of the left hand in motor activities.

leg [Middle English, from Old Norse *leggr* leg, hollow bone of arm or leg] **1** In human anatomy, the portion of the lower limb between the knee and the ankle joint; crus. **2** In common usage, the whole lower limb including or excluding the foot.

> **badger leg** An inequality in leg length.
>
> **baker leg** GENU VALGUM.
>
> **bandy leg** GENU VARUM.
>
> **Barbados leg** ELEPHANT LEG.
>
> **bayonet leg** Genu recurvatum combined with ankylosis.
>
> **cross leg** SCISSOR LEG.
>
> **deck legs** Edema of the legs, especially the ankles, in passengers traveling on ships in the tropics, usually for the first time and before acclimatization to the physical environment. The edema may range from a slight swelling, noticeable in the tightness of footwear, to an incapacitating swelling of the legs. The condition, which particularly affects young women, is reversible immediately after acclimatization or return to a temperate climate. An older term. Also called *Colombo flop* (obsolete), *tropical legs.*
>
> **elephant leg** Elephantiasis of the leg. Also called *Barbados leg.*
>
> **jimmy legs** RESTLESS LEGS SYNDROME.
>
> **jitter legs** RESTLESS LEGS SYNDROME.
>
> **milk leg** PHLEGMASIA ALBA DOLENS.
>
> **red leg** An acute systemic disease of amphibians, caused by infection with *Aeromonas hydrophila.*
>
> **riders' leg** Stiffness or strain of the adductor muscles of the legs in horseback riders.
>
> **scaly leg** A parasitic skin disease of the legs of poultry. It is caused by the mite *Knemidokoptes mutans.*
>
> **scissor leg** A pattern of weight bearing and walking in which the legs cross over each other. It is seen in spasticity, particularly of the adductor muscles, and in cerebral palsy. Also called *cross leg.*
>
> **tennis leg** A condition resulting from tearing the musculotendinous portion of the medial belly of the gastrocnemius muscle. It usually occurs in poorly conditioned individuals required to make sudden weight-bearing leg movements, as in playing tennis. Also called *tennis calf.*
>
> **tropical legs** DECK LEGS.
>
> **white leg** PHLEGMASIA ALBA DOLENS.

Legal [Emmo *Legal*, German physician, 1859–1922] See under TEST. See under GLOSSOPHARYNGEAL NEURALGIA.

Legendre [Gaston-Lucien-Joseph *Legendre*, French physician, born 1887. The spelling *Le Gendre* is erroneous.] Le Gendre sign. See under SIGN.

Legg [Arthur Thornton *Legg*, U.S. surgeon, 1874–1939] Legg's disease, Legg-Calvé-Perthes disease, Legg-Calvé-Waldenström's disease, Legg-Calvé-Perthes syndrome. See under PERTHES DISEASE.

leghemoglobin An oxygen-binding heme protein found in the root nodules of legumes. Soybean leghemoglobin is 142 amino acids in length and approximately 17 000 MW. Leghemoglobins are similar in structure and function to vertebrate myoglobins. They facilitate nitrogen fixation by root nodule bacteria. Also called *legoglobin.*

Legionella pneumophila A thin, nonmotile, nonspore-forming, Gram-negative rod, unrelated to other bacterial groups, causing epidemics and sporadic cases of pneumonia (legionnaire's disease). Its growth *in vitro* requires a medium rich in cysteine, methionine, and other amino acids and is enhanced by the presence of iron. In some epidemics the organism has apparently been spread from soil or from the cooling water in air-conditioning systems.

legoglobin LEGHEMOGLOBIN.

legume [French *légume* (from L *legum(en)* pulse, beans, peas, a leguminous plant) legume] **1** Any member of the Leguminosae family of which peas and beans are typical. Some legumes are capable of fixing nitrogen in the soil by way of the bacterium that inhabits nodules on the plant roots. **2** A dry fruit developed from one carpel that opens along two sides.

legumelin An albumin present in lentils, beans, and other leguminous seeds.

legumin A globulin protein that is heat-coagulable and insoluble in water. It is found in the seeds of such leguminous plants as beans, peas, lentils, and vetches.

leguminivorous Pertaining to or consuming a diet of legumes.

Lehmann [Orla J. O. L. *Lehmann*, Swedish physician, born 1927] Börjeson-Forsman-Lehmann syndrome. See under BÖRJESON SYNDROME.

leiasthenia [*lei(o)* + -ASTHENIA] Weakness of smooth muscle.

Leichtenstern [Otto Michael Ludwig *Leichtenstern*, German physician, 1845–1900] **1** Leichtenstern's encephalitis, Strümpell-Leichtenstern encephalitis. See under ACUTE HEMORRHAGIC LEUKOENCEPHALITIS. **2** Strümpell-Leichtenstern disease. See under ACUTE INFANTILE HEMIPLEGIA. **3** Leichtenstern's phenomenon. See under SIGN.

Leifson [Einar *Leifson*, U.S. bacteriologist, born 1902] Leifson's flagella stain. See under STAIN.

Leigh [Archibald Denis *Leigh*, English neuropathologist, born 1915] Leigh's necrotizing encephalomyelopathy, Leigh's disease, Leigh's encephalopathy. See under SUBACUTE NECROTIZING ENCEPHALOPATHY.

Leiner [Karl *Leiner*, Austrian pediatrician, 1871–1930] See under SYNDROME, DISEASE.

leio- [Gk *leios* smooth] A combining form meaning smooth. Also *lio-*.

leiodermatous Having a smooth and glossy skin.

leiodermia [LEIO- + -DERMIA] A smoothness and glossiness of the skin.

leiodystonia [LEIO- + DYSTONIA] Dystonia of smooth muscle.

Leiognathus bacoti *ORNITHONYSSUS BACOTI.*

leiomyoblastoma A smooth muscle tumor with polygonal cells having pale or clear cytoplasm. It is usually benign. It is most frequently found in the stomach and intestines. Also called *epithelioid leiomyoma.*

leiomyofibroma [LEIO- + MYO- + FIBROMA] A rarely used term for LEIOMYOMA.

leiomyoma [LEIO- + MYOMA] A benign tumor of smooth-muscle cells typically showing little variation in their appearance. Mitotic activity is very low. Collagen formation may be excessive, obscuring the muscular nature of the tumor. It can be found in a variety of sites but is most frequent in the uterus. Also called *fibroid, fibromyoma, myofibroma, leiomyofibroma* (rarely used), *Huguier's disease, myoma levicellulare.*

bizarre leiomyoma A leiomyoma with large, bizarrely shaped cells. Mitoses are rare.

leiomyoma cutis A cutaneous nodule containing smooth muscle tissue. Also called *dermatomyoma.*

epithelioid leiomyoma LEIOMYOBLASTOMA.

multiple cutaneous leiomyoma Multiple cutaneous nodules containing smooth muscle tissue.

parasitic leiomyoma A leiomyoma, usually uterine, which detaches from the uterine serosa and grows on the peritoneum at another site.

leiomyoma of the seminal vesicles A rare, benign, smooth-muscle tumor of the seminal vesicle. It may clinicaly resemble a vesicular cyst.

leiomyoma uteri Leiomyoma of the uterus, the most frequent site of this tumor. Also called *fibromyoma uteri.*

vascular leiomyoma ANGIOMYOMA.

Zenker's leiomyoma LEIOMYOSARCOMA.

leiomyomatosis [*leiomyomat(a)*, pl. of LEIOMYOMA, + -OSIS] Multiple widespread leiomyomas.

leiomyosarcoma [LEIO- + MYO- + SARCOMA] A malignant tumor of smooth-muscle cells, which, in its well-differentiated forms, closely simulates leiomyoma. The most important distinguishing feature is the presence of mitotic figures. It may occur at a number of body sites such as the uterus and the stomach. Also called *Zenker's leiomyoma.*

leiotrichous Having straight hair, as an anthropological characteristic. Compare KYMOTRICHOUS.

leiotrichy [LEIO- + TRICH- + -Y] A straightness of the hair.

leipo- [Gk *leip(ein)* to leave, lack] A combining form meaning lack, loss.

leipotrichia LIPSOTRICHIA.

leipyria [Gk *leipyria* malignant intermittent fever] The sensation of coldness in the limbs that is sometimes experienced during febrile attacks.

Leishman [Sir William Boog *Leishman*, British surgeon, 1865–1926] **1** Leishman's nodules. See under NODULE. **2** Leishman-Donovan body. See under AMASTIGOTE. **3** Leishman's chrome cells. See under CELL. **4** See under STAIN, ANEMIA.

Leishmania [after Sir William B. *Leishman*, British surgeon, 1865–1926 + -IA] A genus of flagellate protozoa (family Trypanosomatidae, order Kinetoplastida) found in the macrophages of vertebrate hosts in the amastigote form, and in invertebrate hosts (or cultures) in the promastigote form. Most species are morphologically indistinguishable. They may be differentiated on the basis of developmental pattern in the sandflies that are their intermediate hosts, clinical manifestations, geographic distribution, and biochemical or physicochemical characteristics, such as enzyme electrophoretic patterns, kinetoplast DNA analysis, and DNA buoyant density measurements.

Leishmania aethiopica A species responsible for cutaneous leishmaniasis in the Ethiopian highlands and on the slopes of Mt. Elgon in Kenya. It is frequently seen as blind swellings of the nose and upper lip without ulceration and with few parasites. A diffuse form is occasionally seen among anergic patients. Reservoir hosts are rock hyraxes (*Procavia* spp.) and the vector sandflies are *Phlebotomus longipes* and *P. pedifer.*

Leishmania brasiliensis A species or complex of species that includes the causative agents of mucocutaneous leishmaniasis. Also *Leishmania braziliensis.*

Leishmania brasiliensis pifanoi See under *LEISHMANIA PIFANOI.*

Leishmania braziliensis LEISHMANIA BRASILIENSIS.

Leishmania chagasi The South American agent of kala-azar, formerly thought to be a variant of the Asian *L. donovani*, but now considered likely to be an endemic form originally from the Amazon basin and subsequently spread through much of South America. Reservoirs are wild and domestic canids, and vectors are various species of the sandflies *Lutzomyia* and *Psychodopygus.*

Leishmania donovani The agent of the Old World visceral leishmaniasis, or kala azar, found in the Mediterranean region the south-central Soviet Union, India, northern China, and central and eastern Africa. In each region the disease has its own clinical characteristics, sandfly vectors, and animal reservoirs, if any. It has been proposed that the agents in each area be recognized as distinct subspecies.

Leishmania enrietti A species infecting guinea pigs in Brazil and now widely used in research into immunity in leishmaniasis. This is the only species of *Leishmania* that is readily distinguishable from those species infecting man.

Leishmania farciminosa An obsolete term for *HISTOPLASMA FARCIMINOSUM.*

Leishmania furunculosa LEISHMANIA TROPICA.

Leishmania guyanensis A species of the *L. brasiliensis* complex (sometimes treated as a subspecies, *L. brasiliensis guyanensis*) that causes a form of New World cutaneous leishmaniasis called pian bois, forest yaws, bay sore, or buba, found in forest regions of Guyana, and in northern Pará and Amazonas states and Roraima territory in Brazil. Moderate ulceration is produced, sometimes with metastatic spread over the body via the lymphatics. Espundia is rare. Reservoir hosts are arboreal rodents, and the vector is *Lutzomyia umbratilis.*

Leishmania infantum A species, sometimes treated as a subspecies of *L. donovani*, that causes visceral leishmaniasis primarily in infants in regions of the Mediterranean. Sandflies of the *Phlebotomus major* group are the vectors and the reservoir host is the dog and, in some areas, other canids. Infection is usually limited to children under two years old.

Leishmania major See under LEISHMANIA TROPICA.

Leishmania mexicana A species, or species group, that includes the causative agent of chiclero ulcer, a form of New World cutaneous leishmaniasis found among workers in chicle gum and mahogany forests in southeastern Mexico and Guatemala. The vector is the sandfly *Lutzomyia flaviscutellata*, and reservoir hosts include various marsupials, primates, and rodents, especially the arboreal spiny rat *Proechimys guyanensis.* Besides the agent of chiclero ulcer (*Leishmania mexicana mexicana*), the *L. mexicana* complex is commonly considered to include *L. m. amazonensis, L. m. pifanoi* (also called *L. pifanoi* as a separate species), *L. m. aristedesi*, and an undescribed form from Trinidad.

Leishmania nilotica LEISHMANIA TROPICA.

Leishmania peruviana A species, sometimes regarded as a subspecies of *L. brasiliensis*, that causes uta, the only form of New World cutaneous leishmaniasis that is not characteristically restricted to forest regions. It occurs in the high arid valleys of the Andes in Peru, Bolivia, and Argentina. The sandfly vectors are probably *Lutzomyia verrucarum* and/or *L. peruensis*, and dogs are reservoir hosts.

Leishmania pifanoi A species that causes diffuse cutaneous leishmaniasis, first described in Venezuela and also known in the Amazon basin and in Mato Grosso in Brazil. The vector is the sandfly *Lutzomyia flaviscutellata* and the reservoir hosts are arboreal rodents. Now considered a distinct species by many workers, it is also commonly classified as a subspecies of *Leishmania mexicana* (*L. m. pifanoi*), and formerly as a subspecies of *L. brasiliensis* (*L. b. pifanoi*).

Leishmania tropica The causative agent of Old World cutaneous leishmaniasis, or oriental sore. It is found in the Mediterranean littoral, the Middle East, India, Pakistan, and the southern USSR. It has also been reported in western Africa. Two forms of *L. tropica* have been described. *L. major* (formerly *L. t. major*) is the agent of moist, or rural, oriental sore, a zoonosis. *L. tropica* (formerly *L. t. minor*) is the agent of dry, urban, or classical oriental sore (variously known as Aleppo, Baghdad, or Delhi boil, bouton d'orient, bouton de Biskra, and by many other names), an anthroponotic disease. Various sandflies of the genus *Phlebotomus* serve as vectors, chiefly *P. papatasi* and *P. sergenti*. Various rodents serve as reservoirs of *L. major*, whereas *L. tropica* is largely dependent on human-sandfly-human or dog-sandfly-human transmission. Also called *Leishmania furunculosa, Leishmania nilotica, Helcosoma tropicum.*

leishmania (*plural* leishmaniae)   **1** An older term for AMASTIGOTE.   **2** A member of the genus *Leishmania.*

leishmanial   **1** Pertaining to or caused by organisms of the genus *Leishmania.*   **2** Pertaining to the amastigote or "leishmania" stage of certain other flagellate protozoans such as *Trypanosoma cruzi.*

leishmaniasis [LEISHMANIA + -SIS]   A group of infectious diseases caused by flagellate protozoan parasites of the genus *Leishmania* and transmitted to man by the sandfly species of the genera *Phlebotomus* and *Lutzomyia.* This group includes a visceral form of the disease (kala-azar), several cutaneous forms, and a mucocutaneous form. Also called *leishmaniosis.*

American leishmaniasis   MUCOCUTANEOUS LEISHMANIASIS.
leishmaniasis americana   MUCOCUTANEOUS LEISHMANIASIS.
American mucocutaneous leishmaniasis   MUCOCUTANEOUS LEISHMANIASIS.
anergic leishmaniasis   DIFFUSE CUTANEOUS LEISHMANIASIS.
Brazilian leishmaniasis   MUCOCUTANEOUS LEISHMANIASIS.
canine leishmaniasis   CANINE KALA-AZAR.
leishmaniasis cutanea diffusa   DIFFUSE CUTANEOUS LEISHMANIASIS.
cutaneous leishmaniasis   An infection with *Leishmania tropica, L. mexicana, L. braziliensis* and other species, transmitted to man by sandfly bites. It is characterized by localized, cutaneous ulcers most frequently found on exposed areas of the skin. Both dry, moist, and cartilaginous forms have been described. There is no visceral involvement. Following the sandfly bite, there is invasion of cutaneous reticuloendothelial cells with production of a small red papule which may become scaly and is surrounded by an erythematous margin. It may ulcerate and slowly heal, leaving a characteristic scar, and a strong, specific, permanent immunity usually follows. Satellite ulcers may also develop. Untreated, these lesions may last from months to a year or more. The disease has a wide distribution in the Mediterranean region, the Middle East, Asia, Africa, Central and South America, tropical Australia, and the USSR. Also called *dermal leishmaniasis, leishmaniasis tropica, Aleppo boil, Baghdad boil, Biskra boil, Delhi boil, Gafsa boil, godovnik boil, Jericho boil, Natal boil, oriental boil, Penjdeh boil, tropical boil, Aleppo button, Baghdad button, Biskra button, oriental button, bouton de Biskra, bouton d'orient, larcotica* (rarely used), *Cochin sore* (obsolete), *date sore, Delasoa sore, Delhi sore, Kandahar sore, Lahore sore, Madagascar sore, Moultan sore, Natal sore, Old World tropical sore, oriental sore, Penjdeh sore, tropical sore, bosch yaws, bush yaws, furunculosis orientalis, granuloma endemicum* (obsolete), *gwaliar ulcer, Jeddah ulcer, Lahore ulcer, Pendinski ulcer, Penjdeh ulcer, Persian ulcer, furunculus orientalis, tropical ulcer, Old World leishmaniasis, Syrian ulcer, Syriac ulcer, frina, lupus endemicus, Annam ulcer, annamite ulcer, Gaboon ulcer, Tashkent ulcer, Turkestan ulcer, Mozambique ulcer, Cochin-China ulcer.* See also TROPICAL ULCER. • The

local names for cutaneous leishmaniasis are in the main old descriptive terms coined before more sophisticated methods of diagnosis of this etiology were devised. Therefore, no one can say with certainty that all of these terms have historically described the same condition, but all are believed to have been used to describe the ulcers of cutaneous leishmaniasis and, by extension, the disease itself.

dermal leishmaniasis   CUTANEOUS LEISHMANIASIS.
diffuse cutaneous leishmaniasis   Cutaneous leishmaniasis caused by *Leishmania* species in Africa and Central and South America and occurring in the equatorial forests of Africa, Bolivia, Venezuela, and Brazil. Following formation of a localized, nonulcerating, nodular lesion, satellite lesions (macules, plaques, and papules) develop and spread until most of the dermis is involved. The disease is usually associated with an impaired immune response. Histologically, numerous *Leishmania* amastigotes are found in macrophages in the dermis. Also called *leishmaniasis tegumentaria diffusa, pseudolepromatous leishmaniasis, anergic leishmaniasis, leishmaniasis cutanea diffusa.*
infantile leishmaniasis   MEDITERRANEAN KALA-AZAR.
mucocutaneous leishmaniasis   Leishmaniasis caused by forms of *Leishmania braziliensis* or rarely, by strains of *L. mexicana,* and characterized by highly destructive ulcerative granulomas of the skin and mucous membranes, especially of the mucocutaneous junctions of the mouth, nasopharynx, genitalia, and rectum. It begins with a superficial skin lesion at the site of a sandfly bite, and spreads by hematogenous routes, usually after a period of several years, to a mucocutaneous location. Distribution involves much of South and Central America, though it is most prevalent in the Amazon basin. Also called *American leishmaniasis, Brazilian leishmaniasis, espundia, leishmaniasis americana, naso-oral leishmaniasis, nasopharyngeal leishmaniasis, New World leishmaniasis, American mucocutaneous leishmaniasis, Breda's disease, bubas braziliana, buba (South American Spanish), bouba (Portuguese), bouba braziliana (Portuguese), Bahia ulcer.*
naso-oral leishmaniasis   MUCOCUTANEOUS LEISHMANIASIS.
nasopharyngeal leishmaniasis   MUCOCUTANEOUS LEISHMANIASIS.
New World leishmaniasis   MUCOCUTANEOUS LEISHMANIASIS.
leishmaniasis nodosus   Cutaneous leishmaniasis of the moist, nodular, early-ulcerating variety. It is considered by some authorities, especially in the USSR, to be caused by a distinct species, *Leishmania major,* different from that which causes the dry form of the disease, *L. tropica.* Others consider them to be subspecies of *L. tropica: L.t. major* and *L.t. minor.*
Old World leishmaniasis   **1** CUTANEOUS LEISHMANIASIS. **2** KALA-AZAR.
post-kala-azar dermal leishmaniasis   A sequel to kala-azar (visceral leishmaniasis), characterized by nodular and nonulcerating hypopigmented lesions, with a scanty amount of parasites, which appear especially on the face, neck, extensor surfaces of the forearms, and inner thighs. These lesions are relatively resistant to treatment but may respond, after a period of time, to antimonial agents. The disease occurs months to several years after the original disease has remitted or been cured. It is found in up to twenty percent of persons in India and two percent of Africans who have had kala-azar.
pseudolepromatous leishmaniasis   DIFFUSE CUTANEOUS LEISHMANIASIS.
leishmaniasis recidivans   Cutaneous leishmaniasis of the dry, chronic type, marked by continuous spread by satellite lesions which may or may not ulcerate, intense granulomata, and resistance to treatment, often continuing for many years. This form of leishmaniasis, caused by *Leishmania tropica,* is thought to be sustained by an extreme granulomatous host response. It

is especially common in the southern Soviet Union, Iran, Iraq, and Turkey. Also called *leishmaniasis recidivus*.

leishmaniasis recidivus LEISHMANIASIS RECIDIVANS.

leishmaniasis tegumentaria diffusa DIFFUSE CUTANEOUS LEISHMANIASIS.

leishmaniasis tropica CUTANEOUS LEISHMANIASIS.

visceral leishmaniasis KALA-AZAR.

leishmanicidal **1** Effective against *Leishmania*. **2** A leishmanicidal drug.

leishmaniosis LEISHMANIASIS.

leishmanoid [*leishman(ia)* + -OID] POST-KALA-AZAR DERMAL LEISHMANOID.

dermal leishmanoid POST-KALA-AZAR DERMAL LEISHMANOID.

post-kala-azar dermal leishmanoid A cutaneous lesion, usually on the face, in which leishmaniae are present. It is evidence of post-kala-azar dermal leishmaniasis, and has been reported in India, Kenya, and the Sudan. It is usually cured by antimony therapy. Also called *leishmanoid, dermal leishmanoid*.

Leitner [Stefan J. *Leitner*, Swiss physician, born 1903] See under SYNDROME.

Lelaps ECHINOLAELAPS.

Leloir [Henri Camille C. *Leloir*, French dermatologist, 1855–1896] Leloir's disease. See under LUPUS VULGARIS ERYTHEMATODES.

lema [Gk *lēmē* a humor in the corners of the eye, gum, rheum] Secretions of the tarsal glands.

Lembert [Antoine *Lembert*, French surgeon, 1802–1851] Czerny-Lembert suture. See under SUTURE.

lememia [Gk *loim(os)* plague, deadly infection + -EMIA] The presence of plague bacilli *(Yersinia pestis)* in the blood. Also *loemaemia (British spellings)*.

lemic [Gk *loim(os)* plague, pestilence + -IC] Pertaining to plague or other epidemic diseases. An obsolete term. Also *loemic (British spelling)*.

Lemli [Luc *Lemli*, U.S. pediatrician, flourished 20th century] Smith-Lemli-Opitz syndrome. See under SYNDROME.

lemma [Gk *lemma* a stripped-off peel, husk, rind, skin, or scale] A layer or covering: used especially to describe cell membranes, as a sarcolemma.

lemmoblast A cell derived from the embryonic neural crest cells which gives rise to a neurilemma cell. Also called *lemnoblast*.

lemmocyte A cellular derivative of the neural crest and precursor of a neurilemma cell. Also called *lemnocyte*.

lemmocytoma [Gk *lemm(a)* a peel, husk, skin + *o* + CYTOMA] NEURILEMMOMA.

lemnisci Plural of LEMNISCUS.

lemniscus [L (from Gk *lēmniskos* a ribbon, fillet), a ribbon hanging from a victor's wreath, crown, or garland] *(plural* lemnisci) A ribbon, band, fillet, or bundle of axons. Also called *fillet*.

acoustic lemniscus LEMNISCUS LATERALIS.

lemniscus acusticus LEMNISCUS LATERALIS.

lateral lemniscus LEMNISCUS LATERALIS.

lemniscus lateralis [NA] A longitudinal tract of auditory system axons, originating in the cochlear nuclei and trapezoid body, that crosses and ascends in the lateral pontine tegmentum and terminates in the inferior colliculus and the thalamic medial geniculate body. Also called *lateral lemniscus, acoustic lemniscus, lemniscus acusticus*.

medial lemniscus LEMNISCUS MEDIALIS.

lemniscus medialis [NA] A large, myelinated tract emerging from the nuclei gracilis and cuneatus, descending in an arc as the internal arcuate fibers, and crossing above the pyramidal

tracts in the medulla oblongata. It ascends as a compact bundle terminating principally in the opposite ventrobasal thalamic nucleus. Each axon conveys impulses activated by a specific type of mechanoreceptor and from a restricted contralateral receptive field, chiefly cutaneous. It is the largest somatosensory tract in the brain and subserves tactile sensibility and position sense. Also called *sensory lemniscus, lemniscus sensitivus, medial lemniscus, lemniscus*.

optic lemniscus An obsolete term for TRACTUS OPTICUS.

lemniscus sensitivus LEMNISCUS MEDIALIS.

sensory lemniscus LEMNISCUS MEDIALIS.

spinal lemniscus A seldom used term for SPINOTHALAMIC TRACT.

lemniscus spinalis A seldom used term for SPINOTHALAMIC TRACT.

trigeminal lemniscus LEMNISCUS TRIGEMINALIS.

lemniscus trigeminalis [NA] A large band of myelinated axons originating mainly from the principal trigeminal sensory nucleus and with contributions from all sectors of the spinal trigeminal nucleus. Its fibers cross in the pons and join the lemniscus medialis, terminating in the medial sector of the thalamic ventrobasal nucleus. This large tract conveys tactile sensory information from facial skin and the oral cavity, and is considered the trigeminal homologue of the lemniscus medialis. A separate, uncrossed component conveying tactile activity from the oral and perioral regions to the ipsilateral ventral thalamus via a dorsal course is called the dorsal trigeminal lemniscus or tract, the homolateral trigeminal tract, and Wallenberg's bundle or tract. Also called *trigeminal lemniscus, tractus trigeminothalamicus, trigeminothalamic tract, central tract of cranial nerves, central tract of trigeminal nerve*.

lemnoblast LEMMOBLAST.

lemnocyte LEMMOCYTE.

lemography [Gk *loimo(s)* plague + -GRAPHY] A treatise on an epidemic disease, especially plague. An obsolete term.

lemology [Gk *loimo(s)* plague + -LOGY] The study of plague and other contagious diseases occurring in epidemic form. An obsolete term.

lemoparalysis [Gk *laimo(s)* the throat, gullet + PARALYSIS] ESOPHAGEAL PARALYSIS.

lemostenosis [Gk *laimo(s)* the throat, gullet + STENOSIS] Stenosis of the esophagus. An obsolete term.

Lenard [Philipp *Lenard*, German physicist, 1862–1947] See under RAYS.

Lendrum [A. C. *Lendrum*, Scottish pathologist, flourished 20th century] Lendrum's inclusion body stain. See under STAIN.

Lenetran A proprietary name for mephenoxalone.

length Linear extent from one point to another.

arch length The distance between the most posterior teeth in either the upper or lower jaw, measured around the periphery of the dental arch.

basialveolar length The distance between the basion and the alveolare.

basinasal length The distance between the basion and the nasion.

cranial length The length of the skull between the glabella and the inion.

crown-heel length The length of an embryo, fetus, or infant, stretched out and measured from the top of the head to the heel of the foot.

crown-rump length The distance from the top of the head to the buttocks, used in describing an embryo, fetus, or infant.

dental length The overall length of a dental quadrant.

focal length The distance at which a lens converges or appears to diverge parallel light.

foot length   The heel-to-toe measurement taken of a fetus to estimate its age. This measurement at times has an advantage in that distortion of the fetus can cause inaccuracy in other measurements.

length of generation   The average age in a cohort of mothers at which one first bears a daughter.

length of gestation   The duration of a pregnancy as measured, usually in weeks, from the first day of the last normal menstrual cycle.

greatest length   The overall length of an embryo or fetus. It is taken when the crown-rump length cannot be measured as from lack of development of the appropriate curvature, or because it is not applicable to the particular species, as in the porpoise embryo.

mean length of life   The average length of life given certain defined rates of mortality. Also called *expectation of life at birth.*

pulse length   PULSE DURATION.

sitting length   The distance between the vertex of the head and the coccyx. It is approximately equivalent to the crown-rump length used in measurement of embryos, fetuses, and infants.

length of stay   The time period, usually expressed in days, from admission to discharge of a patient in an inpatient health care facility.

stem length   The distance between the vertex of the head and the midpoint of a line joining the ischial tuberosities.

wave length   See under WAVELENGTH.

Lenhossek [Joseph von *Lenhossek*, Hungarian anatomist, 1818–1888] Lenhossek's fibers. See under STILLING'S FIBERS.

Lenhossék [Michael von *Lenhossék*, Hungarian anatomist, 1863–1937] Lenhossék's processes. See under PROCESS.

leniceps [L *leni(s)* soft, gentle + *-ceps*, combining form from *capere* to hold, seize] Short obstetric forceps. An older term.

leniquinsin $C_{20}H_{20}N_2O_4$.   *N*-[(3,4-Dimethoxyphenyl) methylene]6,7-dimethoxy-4-quinolinamine. A compound with antihypertensive properties.

lenitive   1 Soothing.   2 A lenitive agent.

Lennhoff [Rudolf *Lennhoff*, German physician, 1866–1933]   1 See under SIGN.   2 Becker-Lennhoff index. See under LENNHOFF'S INDEX.

Lennox [William Gordon *Lennox*, U.S. physician, 1884–1960] Lennox syndrome. See under LENNOX-GASTAUT SYNDROME.

Lenoir [Camille-Alexandre-Henri *Lenoir*, French anatomist, born 1867]   See under FACET.

lens [L, gen. *lentis*, a lentil]   1 A medium bound by two surfaces that refracts light rays.   2 [NA] A transparent, biconvex disk situated between the iris anteriorly and the vitreous body behind. It is encased in a capsule and held in position at its equator by the ciliary zonule. Almost spherical at birth, it becomes fairly convex in the adult, the anterior surface being less convex than the posterior surface, and it flattens in old age. The shape also changes during near and far accommodation. As a refractive medium, it focuses rays of light on the retina. Its substance comprises a soft cortex and a firm, central nucleus. Also called *crystalline lens, lens crystallina, humor cristallinus* (outmoded), *crystalline humor* (outmoded), *phacoid.* Adjective: lenticular.

Abbé apochromatic lens   APOCHROMATIC LENS.

absorption lens   A lens that does not transmit certain wavelengths.

achromatic lens   A lens corrected for chromatic aberration. Also called *achromat.*

acoustic lens   A device that focuses sound, analogous to an optical lens that focuses light.

acrylic lens   A lens fabricated from plastic, such as methyl methacrylate.

adherent lens   CONTACT LENS.

anamorphote lens   A lens that alters the size of an image without changing the focal length.

aniseikonic lens   A lens that changes the size of an image without altering the focal distance.

aplanatic lens   A lens corrected for spherical aberration.

apochromatic lens   A lens corrected for chromatic and spherical aberration. Also called *Abbé apochromatic lens.*

biconcave lens   A lens with negative power on both surfaces. Also called *concavoconcave lens.*

biconvex lens   A lens with positive power on both surfaces. Also called *bispherical lens.*

bicylindrical lens   A lens with toric power on both surfaces.

bifocal lens   A lens with two focal distances.

bispherical lens   BICONVEX LENS.

bullet lens   The very small lens of spherophakia.

cataract lens   A lens for the correction of aphakia.

compound lens   A lens system fabricated with multiple lenses.

concave lens   A lens having a concave surface and minus dioptric power.

concavoconcave lens   BICONCAVE LENS.

concavoconvex lens   A lens with negative dioptric power on a concave surface, and plus dioptric power on the other, convex surface.

condensing lens   A lens that focuses light or electron beam upon the object of microscopic observation.

contact lens   A lens that fits directly upon the cornea. Also called *adherent lens.*

converging lens   PLUS LENS.

convex lens   A lens having a convex surface and plus dioptric power.

convexoconcave lens   A lens with plus dioptric power on a convex surface, and minus dioptric power on the other, concave surface.

coquille plano lens   A blown glass lens with no dioptric power.

Crookes lens   Absorptive lenses that minimize transmission of infrared and ultraviolet especially and prevent glare.

crossed lens   A convergent lens corrected for distant spherical aberration by choice of surfaces.

lens crystallina   LENS.

lens crystallina   LENS.

crystalline lens   LENS.

cylindrical lens   An optical lens having its greatest strength along one meridian, designed to correct astigmatism. Also called *cylinder.*

decentered lens   A lens positioned with its optical center off the axis of the optical system to cause a prismatic effect and correct for muscle imbalance.

diverging lens   MINUS LENS.

electron lens   An electromagnetic device that is used to focus a beam of electrons within an electron microscope.

eye lens   The upper of the two lenses in a huygenian eyepiece.

fenestrated lens   A contact lens with small apertures to allow gaseous exchange and prevent corneal haze.

field lens   The lower of the pair of lenses in a huygenian eyepiece.

flat lens   A lens with one plane surface or with opposite surfaces both equally concave or convex.

Hruby lens   A minus 55 diopter lens designed to permit biomicroscopic viewing of the ocular fundus.

immersion lens   An objective lens intended for direct contact with an immersion fluid.

iseikonic lens   A lens that changes the size of an object to correct for aniseikonia.

lenticular lens   A strong spectacle lens with power only in its central portion, in order to reduce thickness and weight.

magnifying lens   A lens with plus power, used to increase the apparent size of objects.

meniscus lens   A deeply curved concavoconvex lens.

meter lens   A lens with a power of one diopter plus.

minus lens   A lens that diverges rays of light; a lens having minus dioptric power. Also called *negative lens, diverging lens*.

negative lens   MINUS LENS.

omnifocal lens   A bifocal lens in which the curvature of the lens is such that dioptric power increases gradually toward the lens periphery, thereby providing a continuous range of focal distances from which the user can select the one best suited for a chosen working distance at any given time. Also called *progressive lens*.

orthoscopic lens   A lens corrected for spherical aberrations.

periscopic lens   A corrected curve lens with deep curvature.

photochromic lens   A lens that darkens upon exposure to ultraviolet and is used in sunglasses.

plane lens   A lens with no dioptric strength.

planoconcave lens   A concave (negative) lens that is flat on one surface.

planoconvex lens   A convex (positive) lens that is flat on one surface.

plus lens   A lens that converges rays of light; a lens having plus dioptric power. Also called *positive lens, converging lens*.

positive lens   PLUS LENS.

progressive lens   OMNIFOCAL LENS.

rectilinear lens   A magnifying lens corrected for peripheral aberration.

retroscopic lens   A lens positioned so that its upper part is closer to the eye than the lower part.

spectacle lens   An optical lens worn in front of an eye by an individual for the purpose of correction of errors of refraction, filtering out of excessive light, or mechanical protection of the eye.

spherical lens   A lens with plus or minus dioptric power, but no cylindrical power.

spherical afocal lens   A plano lens with surfaces of constant radius of curvature.

spherocylindrical lens   A lens combining plus power with toric curvature.

telescopic lens   A corrective lens for reduced vision that permits viewing at a distance.

toric lens   A concavoconvex of or convexoconcave lens with a cylinder ground on its outer surface for the correction of astigmatism.

trial lens   A lens used to measure refractive error.

trifocal lens   A lens with three separate dioptric powers, used for presbyopia.

lensometer   A device for measurement of lens strength.

lentectomize [LENS + -*ectom(y)* + -IZE]   To extract the crystalline lens surgically.

lentectomy [LENS + -ECTOMY]   Surgical removal of the crystalline lens.

Lente Iletin   A proprietary name for insulin zinc suspension.

lentic [L *lent(us)* slow, sluggish, calm + -IC]   Pertaining to or living in a standing water habitat, such as a lake.

lenticel   A lens-shaped or lentil-shaped gland, particularly one found at the root of the tongue.

lenticonus [LENS + L *conus* a cone]   LENTIGLOBUS.

lenticula [L, dim. of *lens*, gen. *lentis*, a lentil, freckle]   NUCLEUS LENTIFORMIS.

lenticular [L *lenticular(is)* (from *lenticul(a)*, dim. of *lens* a lentil + -*aris* -AR) lenticular]   Pertaining to a lens.

lenticuli   Plural of LENTICULUS.

lenticulo-optic   Pertaining to the lenticular nucleus and the

optic thalamus. An obsolete term.

lenticulostriate   **1** Pertaining to the lenticular nucleus and the corpus striatum.   **2** Denoting the largest of the striate branches of the middle cerebral artery, one of the most frequent sites of cerebral arterial occlusion.

lenticulothalamic   Pertaining to the lenticular nucleus and the thalamus.

lenticulus [L (dim. of *lens*, gen. *lentis*, a lentil), a little lentil]   A small lens.

lentiform   **1** Shaped like a lentil or the lens of an eye.   **2** NUCLEUS LENTIFORMIS.

lentigines   Plural of LENTIGO.

lentiginosis [LENTIGO + -OSIS]   The presence of lentigines in exceptionally large numbers or in a distinctive distribution.

cardiomyopathic lentiginosis   MULTIPLE LENTIGINES SYNDROME.

centrofacial lentiginosis   A rare hereditary syndrome is which multiple lentigines develop from childhood in the central area of the face.

generalized lentiginosis   The widespread development of multiple lentigines.

lentiginous   Pertaining to or of the nature of a lentigo.

lentiglobus [L *lens*, gen. *lentis*, a lentil + GLOBUS]   An anomalous conical or spheroidal elevation on the surface of the crystalline lens. Also called *lenticonus*.

lentigo [L (gen. *lentiginis*; from LENS), a lentil-shaped spot] (*plural* lentigines.)   A small brown macule that results from an increased number of melanocytes at the dermoepidermal junction.

lentigo aestiva   FRECKLE.

Hutchinson's malignant lentigo   HUTCHINSON'S MELANOTIC FRECKLE.

lentigo maligna   HUTCHINSON'S MELANOTIC FRECKLE.

malignant lentigo   HUTCHINSON'S MELANOTIC FRECKLE.

lentigomelanoma [LENTIGO + MELANOMA]   A malignant melanoma arising in a lentigo.

lentigomelanosis [LENTIGO + MELANOSIS]   A localized, irregular, brownish black pigmentation produced by a senile lentigo.

lentitis [L *lens*, gen. *lentis*, a lentil + -ITIS]   Inflammation of the ocular lens.

lentivirus   A slow virus belonging to the *Lentivirus* genus and Lentivirinae subfamily of the Retroviridae. Maedi and visna viruses are members of this genus.

lentoptosis [L *lens*, gen. *lentis*, a lentil + *o* + -PTOSIS]   Downward displacement of the ocular lens.

lentula [possibly L, fem. of *lentulus* (dim. of *lentus* pliant, flexible) somewhat pliant, flexible]   PASTE FILLER.

Leonardo [*Leonardo* da Vinci, Italian scientist, artist, engineer, and inventor 1452–1519]   Leonardo's band. See under TRABECULA SEPTOMARGINALIS.

leontiasis [Gk *leōn*, gen. *leontos*, a lion + -IASIS]   An obsolete term for LEONINE FACIES.

leontiasis ossea   LEONTIASIS OSSIUM.

leontiasis ossea generalisata   VAN BUCHEM SYNDROME.

leontiasis ossium   A bilateral, symmetric hypertrophy of the bones of the face and cranium of unknown etiology. It results in a lion-like facial expression which must be differentiated from the leonine face of lepromatous leprosy. Also called *leontiasis ossea*.

Leopold [Christian Gerhard *Leopold*, German physician, 1846–1911]   **1** See under LAW.   **2** Leopold's maneuvers. See under MANEUVER.

Leopold Lévi   See under LÉVI.

leotropic [Gk *laio(s)* left + -TROPIC[1]] Denoting a spiral ascending from right to left, as that of a shell. Compare DEXIOTROPIC.

LEP low egg passage (a form of Flury vaccine for rabies).

leper [French *lèpre* (from Gk *lepra* leprosy, from *lepra*, fem. of *lepros* scaly) leprosy. English *leper* formerly meant the disease itself, afflicting a leprous person] A person suffering from leprosy. • The term is rarely used by the medical profession because of its alternative definition as a tainted or objectionable person. Also called *lazar*.

lepido- [Gk *lepis* (genitive *lepidos*) scale, husk, shell] A combining form meaning scale, flake.

lepidoid [*lepid(o)-* + -OID] SQUAMOUS.

lepidoma [*lepid(o)-* + -OMA] 1 A tumor of embryonal membranes. 2 A scaly tumor. An obsolete term. Also called *lepidic tumor, rind tumor*.

    endothelial lepidoma An obsolete term for ENDOTHELIOMA.

Lepidoptera [LEPIDO- + Gk *ptera* (pl. of *pteron* a feather) feathers, wings] An order of holometabolous insects characterized by wings covered with scales; the moths and butterflies.

lepidosarcoma [LEPIDO- + SARCOMA] 1 A sarcoma of embryonal membranes. 2 A scaly sarcoma. An obsolete term.

lepidosis [LEPIDO- + -SIS] A scaly eruption. An obsolete term.

Lépine [Jean *Lépine*, French physician, born 1876] Lépine-Froin syndrome. See under FROIN SYNDROME.

lepiota / poisonous lepiota A green-spored mushroom of the species *Chlorophyllum molybdites*. It causes a rather strong gastrointestinal irritation when ingested. • The name is derived from *Lepiota morganii*, an earlier name for this species.

lepocyte A nucleated cell having a distinct cell wall.

leporipoxvirus [L *lepus*, gen. *leporis*, a hare + POX + VIRUS] Any virus of the genus *Leporipoxvirus* in the family Poxviridae. They cause myxomas and fibromas in leporids and squirrels. The virions are enveloped, brick-shaped, 218–270 nm, contain double-stranded DNA, and are inactivated by ether. Serological cross-reactivity among species is common. Mechanical transmission by mosquitoes frequently occurs. Myxoma virus is the type species.

lepothrix [Gk *lepo(s)* husk, rind, scale + *thrix* hair] A superficial *Corynebacterium* infection of the axillary or pubic hair in which red, yellow, or black nodules or sheaths form on the hair shafts. Also called *trichomycosis chromatica, trichomycosis nodosa, trichomycosis palmellina* (obsolete). • This condition was originally thought to be a fungal infection, giving rise to the *trichomycosis* misnomers.

lepra [Gk *lepra* (from *lepros* rough, leprous, mangy) leprosy] 1 LEPROSY. 2 An obsolete term for PSORIASIS.

    lepra alba Macular leprosy that is characterized by hypopigmented lesions.

    lepra alphos PSORIASIS.

    lepra cutanea Leprosy that involves the skin. An obsolete term.

    lepra graecorum LEPROSY.

    lepra manchada [Spanish, spotted leprosy] LUCIO PHENOMENON.

    lepra minor Tuberculoid leprosy manifested by small, discrete lesions.

    lepra mutilans An obsolete term for TROPHONEUROTIC LEPROSY.

    lepra nervorum Leprosy that involves the nervous system. An obsolete term.

    lepra tuberculosa An obsolete term for LEPROMATOUS LEPROSY.

    lepra tuberosa An obsolete term for LEPROMATOUS LEPROSY.

    Willan's lepra PSORIASIS CIRCINATA.

lepraphobia LEPROPHOBIA.

leprechaunism [Irish Gaelic, from *lupracán*, also *luprachán*, *leipreachán* (from Middle Irish *lúchorpán* a little body, from *lú* little + *corpán*, dim. of *corp* body, from L *corpus* body] a mischievous elf who can reveal hidden treasure if caught + -ISM] A rare, lethal syndrome of infancy characterized by wide-set eyes, low-set ears, lanugo, and several metabolic-endocrine features including complete absence of subcutaneous fat like that in lipoatrophic diabetes mellitus, hyperplasia of the pancreatic islets, clitoral and breast enlargement in females and phallomegaly in males. Also called *Donohue's disease, Donohue syndrome*.

lepride [*lepr(a)* + -IDE[2]] The raised and thickened skin lesion (plaque) of tuberculoid leprosy. A rarely used term.

    major lepride The markedly raised and thickened skin lesion of tuberculoid leprosy. A rarely used term.

    minor lepride A slightly raised and thickened skin lesion of tuberculoid leprosy. A rarely used term.

leprolin A preparation of tissue containing *Mycobacterium leprae* used in the early twentieth century in attempts to induce immunity to leprosy.

leprologist [*lepro(sy)* + -LOGIST] A specialist in the diagnosis and treatment of leprosy.

leprology [*lepro(sy)* + -LOGY] The study of leprosy.

leproma [*lepr(a)* + -OMA] A histiocytic cellular reaction characteristic of lepromatous leprosy. A diagnostic feature is the demonstration of leprosy bacilli following suitable staining.

lepromatosis [Gk *lepr(os)* scaly, leprous + -*omata*, pl. of -*oma* -OMA, + -OSIS] See under LUCIO PHENOMENON.

    pure and primitive diffuse lepromatosis A rarely used and obsolete term for LUCIO LEPROSY.

lepromatous Pertaining to a leproma.

lepromin [*leprom(a)* + -IN] The material used in the lepromin test, of which there are two preparations in common use: leprominum integrale (Nitsuda-type) and Dharmendra lepromin. Also called *Mitsuda antigen*.

    Dharmendra lepromin Material used in the lepromin test consisting of a purified chloroform-ether-extracted suspension of leprosy bacilli that is practically devoid of tissue protein. It is also used in immunologic research as a source of *Mycobacterium leprae* antigen.

    integral lepromin A popular term for LEPROMINUM INTEGRALE (MITSUDA TYPE).

    Mitsuda lepromin A popular term for LEPROMINUM INTEGRALE (MITSUDA TYPE).

    lepromium integrale (Mitsuda type) A saline suspension of heat-killed leprosy bacilli, numbering between 4.0×10^7 and 1.6×10^8 bacilli/ml, together with tissue protein. It is used in the lepromin test. Also called *Mitsuda lepromin* (popular), *integral lepromin* (popular).

leprophobia Pathologic fear of leprosy, of lepers, or of contracting leprosy. Also called *lepraphobia*.

leprophthalmia Any ophthalmic complication of leprosy.

leprosarium [Med L, from Late L *lepros(us)* leprous + -*arium* -ARY] (*plural* leprosaria) A hospital or similar institution for the treatment of leprosy inpatients. Leprosaria play no part in leprosy control programs and are becoming obsolete. Also called *leprosary* (rarely used).

leprosary A rarely used term for LEPROSARIUM.

leprostatic Inhibitory to the growth of *Mycobacterium leprae*, the organism that causes leprosy.

leprosy [LEPROUS + -Y] A chronic mycobacterial disease that is sometimes infectious. It primarily affects the peripheral nervous system and secondarily involves the skin and certain other tissues. Also called *Hansen's disease, hanseniasis* (rarely used), *lepra graecorum, elephantiasis graecorum, lepra.*

anesthetic leprosy Leprosy characterized by skin insensitivity. Because a loss of feeling may complicate all types of leprosy at some stage, it is not classified as a specific form of the disease. A rarely used term.

articular leprosy Leprosy marked by joint involvement. This may take a number of different forms. An imprecise and rarely used term.

benign leprosy Leprosy in which the disease is localized, as in tuberculoid leprosy. An obsolete term.

borderline leprosy Leprosy affecting persons possessing a moderate degree of cell-mediated immunity to *Mycobacterium leprae*. Because immunity is unstable the leprosy is able to upgrade to the tuberculoid pole or downgrade to the lepromatous pole. Also called *dimorphous leprosy* (rarely used), *intermediate leprosy* (rarely used).

cat leprosy A disease of cats caused by *Mycobacterium lepraemurium*, which is the causative organism of rat leprosy. The formation of cutaneous and subcutaneous granulomas is the characteristic feature.

closed leprosy Leprosy that is noninfectious.

conjugal leprosy Leprosy acquired by contact with a marriage partner.

cutaneous leprosy Leprosy manifested by one or more skin lesions in the absence of clinical evidence of involvement of other tissues. A rarely used term. • The term is a misnomer because nerve involvement occurs in all cases of leprosy even though clinical evidence of nerve damage is lacking.

diffuse leprosy of Lucio and Latapí LUCIO LEPROSY.

dimorphous leprosy A rarely used term for BORDERLINE LEPROSY.

histoid leprosy Leprosy characterized by skin nodules that are firm, shiny, glistening, and sometimes erythematous, as in hyperactive lepromatous leprosy. These skin nodules may be seen in new patients or in relapsed cases, and the classical histological finding is of spindle-shaped histiocytes containing large numbers of leprosy bacilli.

indeterminate leprosy An early, transitory stage of leprosy, seen most often in children, in which one or more macules appear on the skin, but the immunological status of the subject has not been determined.

intermediate leprosy A rarely used term for BORDERLINE LEPROSY.

lazarine leprosy An obsolete term for LUCIO PHENOMENON.

lepromatoid leprosy Leprosy that has been successfully transmitted to a laboratory animal and is similar to lepromatous leprosy in the human.

lepromatous leprosy Leprosy affecting persons with depressed cell-mediated immunity to *Mycobacterium leprae*. As a result leprosy bacilli are widely disseminated in the tissues. Also called *nodular leprosy* (obsolete), *lepra tuberculosa* (obsolete), *lepra tuberosa* (obsolete), *virchowian leprosy*. Abbreviation: LL

Lucio leprosy A diffuse, non-nodular variant of lepromatous leprosy rarely encountered outside Mexico and Central America. Also called *diffuse leprosy of Lucio and Latapí, pure and primitive diffuse lepromatosis (rare and obsolete).* • See note at LUCIO PHENOMENON.

macular leprosy Leprosy characterized by skin lesions that are entirely composed of macules. These flat lesions cannot be felt by the examiner's finger.

maculoanesthetic leprosy Leprosy in which the only skin lesions are macules that are insensitive.

malignant leprosy Leprosy in which the disease is generalized, as in lepromatous leprosy. An obsolete term.

midborderline leprosy Borderline leprosy in which cell-mediated immunity to *Mycobacterium leprae* is in an intermediate range.

murine leprosy RAT LEPROSY.

neural leprosy Leprosy with manifestations of nerve damage. An obsolete term.

nodular leprosy An obsolete term for LEPROMATOUS LEPROSY.

polar lepromatous leprosy Lepromatous leprosy which is immunologically stable. There is no evolution to a different type, hence the leprosy is termed polar. Abbreviation: LLp

pure neural leprosy Leprosy characterized by one or more palpably thickened nerves, with or without signs of nerve dysfunction, that occur in the absence of skin lesions.

rat leprosy A spontaneous disease of rats and mice caused by *Mycobacterium lepraemurium*. Characteristic granulomas occur in the skin and subcutis, and in most abdominal viscera except the kidneys. Also called *murine leprosy.*

reactional leprosy LEPRA REACTION.

spotted leprosy LUCIO PHENOMENON.

subclinical leprosy Infection with *Mycobacterium leprae* that is apparent only by immunologic testing and is acquired by contact with infectious leprosy. There are no clinical manifestations and only a very small proportion of infected persons develop clinical disease, confirming that the rate of transmission of *Mycobacterium leprae* is very significantly higher than the disease attack rate.

subpolar lepromatous leprosy Lepromatous leprosy that has previously undergone a borderline phase. It is immunologically unstable and may upgrade to the borderline type. Abbreviation: LLs

trophoneurotic leprosy Leprosy characterized by deformity, such as the shortening of digits, or muscle paralysis. A rarely used term. Also called *lepra mutilans* (obsolete).

tuberculoid leprosy Leprosy that affects persons possessing good cell-mediated immunity to *Mycobacterium leprae*. Clinical manifestations are few and leprosy bacilli are scanty or absent in the tissues. Also called *hansenid.*

virchowian leprosy LEPROMATOUS LEPROSY. • In the new leprosy terminology officially approved in Brazil, the term *virchowian* has replaced *lepromatous*, but the change has received little general acceptance in the English-speaking world.

leprotic Of or relating to leprosy. Also *leprous.*

leprous [*lepr(a)* + L *-osus* -OUS] LEPROTIC.

-lepsia -LEPSIS.

-lepsis [Gk *lēpsis* (from *lēpsomai,* fut. of *lambanein* to take hold of, seize) a taking, seizing] A combining form meaning a seizure.

-lepsy -LEPSIS.

lept- LEPTO-.

leptandra The dried root and rhizome of *Veronica virginica*, which has been used as a cathartic. Also called *Culver's root.*

leptazol PENTYLENETETRAZOLE.

lepthymenia The condition of thinness of a membrane. An obsolete term.

lepto- [Gk *leptos* thin, fine, slender, delicate] A combining form meaning fine, slender, delicate, weak. Also *lept-.*

leptocephalic [LEPTO- + CEPHALIC] MICROCEPHALOUS.

leptocephalous [LEPTO- + CEPHAL- + -OUS] MICROCEPHALOUS.

leptocephalus [LEPTO- + -CEPHALUS] MICROCEPHALUS.

leptocephaly [LEPTO- + CEPHAL- + -Y] MICROCEPHALY.

leptochroa [LEPTO- + Ionic Gk *chroa* the skin] Abnormally delicate or sensitive skin. An obsolete term.

leptochromatic [LEPTO- + CHROMATIC] Having a delicate network of chromatin.

Leptocimex A genus of bedbugs that usually parasitize bats.

One species, *L. boueti*, is also a parasite of humans in tropical Africa.

Leptoconops A genus of bloodsucking midges of the family Certatopogonidae that is widely distributed in warm temperate and tropical areas. Many are extremely annoying pests of humans and domestic animals. *L. kerteszi* causes a dermatitis around the eyes of sheep known as leptoconops mange. *L. torrens* and *L. carteri* are seriously annoying pests in the western United States, as are *L. irritans* in Europe and *L. spinosifrons* in eastern Africa.

leptocyte An erythrocyte that is thinner than normal and hence appears hypochromic. It is commonly observed in iron deficiency anemia, thalassemias, chronic inflammatory disorders, and other conditions.

leptocytic Pertaining to leptocytes.

leptocytosis The presence of numerous leptocytes in blood.

leptodactylous [LEPTO- + DACTYL- + -OUS] Having slender fingers and toes.

leptodactyly [LEPTO- + DACTYL- + -Y] An unusual slenderness or elongation of the fingers and toes.

Leptodera pellio *RHABDITIS PELIO.*

leptodermic Marked by abnormally thin skin. An obsolete term.

leptodontous [LEPT- + -ODONT + -OUS] Having abnormally narrow teeth.

leptokurtic Describing the curve of a frequency distribution that has a sharper peak at the mode than a normal curve.

leptomeninges (*singular* leptomeninx) The arachnoidea and pia mater together. Also called *arachnopia* (obsolete), *pia-arachnoid, meningina* (obsolete), *meninx tenuis* (obsolete), *piarachnoid.*

leptomeningioma [*leptomening(es)* + *i* + -OMA] A tumor of the leptomeninges.

leptomeningitis [LEPTO- + MENINGITIS] Inflammation of the leptomeninges. Also called *meninginitis, subarachnoiditis, pia-arachnitis, piarachnitis.* See also MENINGITIS.

    leptomeningitis interna Inflammation largely confined to the pia mater.

    sarcomatous leptomeningitis Diffuse sarcomatous infiltration in the meninges and subarachnoid space.

leptomeningopathy [LEPTO- + MENINGO- + -PATHY] Any disease of the leptomeninges.

leptomeninx Singular of LEPTOMENINGES.

Leptomicrurus A genus of venomous coral snakes of the family Elapidae.

leptomonad [LEPTO- + MONAD] **1** Pertaining to the genus *Leptomonas.* **2** A member of the genus *Leptomonas.* **3** An older term for PROMASTIGOTE.

Leptomonas A genus of flagellate protozoa in the family Trypanosomatidae, order Kinetoplastida, found in the gut of various insects.

lepton Any of a group of low-mass elementary particles (of mass less than 1 amu) that includes electrons, positrons, neutrinos, antineutrinos, muons, and antimuons.

leptonema A very thin, threadlike form, as taken by the chromosomes during the leptotene stage of meiosis.

leptopellic Having an unusually narrow pelvis.

leptophonia [LEPTO- + PHON- + -IA] A weak, thin quality to the voice, resulting from general debility or certain myopathic or neurologic conditions. Also called *microphonia.* Adjective: leptophonic.

leptopodal [LEPTO- + -POD + -AL] Having slender, elongate legs or tarsals: said primarily of certain insects.

leptoprosope An individual displaying leptoprosopia.

leptoprosopia [LEPTO- + PROSOP- + -IA] An extreme narrowness of the face.

leptoprosopic Exhibiting leptoprosopia.

Leptopsylla [LEPTO- + Gk *psylla* a flea] A genus of rodent fleas in the family Leptopsyllidae. Also called *Ctenopsyllus.*

Leptopsylla musculi *LEPTOPSYLLA SEGNIS.*

Leptopsylla segnis The cosmopolitan European mouse flea, also commonly found on rats. It is able to transmit plague, but is a poor vector as it bites humans rarely. Also called *Ctenopsyllus segnis, Leptopsylla musculi.*

leptorrhine [LEPTO- + Gk *rhis*, gen. *rhinos*, nose] Having a tall, narrow nasal opening of the skull, with a nasal index of below 48.

leptoscope An optical instrument used to measure the thickness of a thin film, such as the plasma membrane.

leptosomatic Characterized by a slight, narrow bodily framework; having a small, slender physique.

leptosome A person with a narrow, slight physique.

Leptospira [LEPTO- + Gk *speira* anything wound or wrapped around a thing; pl. *speirai* the twisted folds or coils of a serpent, twists or coils of a net] A genus of coiled, aerobic spirochetes. See under *LEPTOSPIRA INTERROGANS.*

Leptospira biflexa A saprobic leptospire found in streams. It carries a genus-specific antigen used in the diagnosis of leptospiral infection.

Leptospira interrogans A species of spirochete with a very tight coil, the body often being bent at the ends in the form of a hook. It can be grown aerobically in complex media containing fatty acids. Wild rodents and domestic animals are the reservoir, often shedding the organisms in the urine during a mild, chronic illness. The human illness varies from subclinical to a severe disease with jaundice, albuminuria, and hemorrhages (Weil's disease). Many strains may be differentiated, whether antigenically, by G + C content of the DNA, or by origin. All the pathogens are classified in the one species, with serotypes such as interohaemorrhagiae from rats, canicola from dogs, etc. ● The epithet *interrogans* derives from the resemblance of the organism to a question mark.

Leptospira interrogans serotype **autumnalis** A leptospire originally isolated in Japan and shown serologically to have been the cause of an epidemic of pretibial fever at Fort Bragg.

leptospire An organism of the genus *Leptospira.* Adjective: leptospiral.

leptospirosis [*Leptospir(a)* + -OSIS] Infection by spirochetes of the genus *Leptospira*, of which there are more than 170 serotypes. The major diseases in man are caused by *L. icterohaemorrhagiae* and *L. canicola.* Many kinds of mammals serve as reservoirs of infection, especially rats and dogs. The bacteria are excreted in the animals' urine, and infection is acquired through cuts and abrasions in the skin. The disease has multiple clinical presentations.

    anicteric leptospirosis A common, relatively mild form of leptospirosis characterized by fever, headache, myalgia, nausea, malaise, and, rarely, circulatory collapse. Jaundice is absent and hepatomegaly is rare. The disease may be biphasic, with the first stage lasting three to seven days and the second, or immune, stage lasting one to three days. Fever may not be present in the second stage. Also called *benign leptospirosis.*

    benign leptospirosis ANICTERIC LEPTOSPIROSIS.

    canine leptospirosis CANICOLA FEVER.

    leptospirosis hebdomadis NANUKAYAMI.

    icteric leptospirosis The severe form of leptospirosis, characterized by biphasic fever, muscle pain, bleeding tendencies, gastrointestinal symptoms, and commonly also jaundice, azotemia, anemia, and disturbances of consciousness resulting from liver and kidney impairment. It may be caused by almost any serotype of *Leptospira interrogans*. Once common among sewer and abattoir workers and laborers in rice paddies, it now occurs primarily in young people exposed to contaminated water during outdoor recreation. Also called *Weil's disease, leptospirosis icterohemorrhagica, leptospiral jaundice, icterohemorrhagic fever, spirochetal jaundice, spirochetal icterus, icterus infectiosus, hemorrhagic jaundice, icterogenic spirochetosis* (obsolete), *spirochetosis icterohemorrhagica, Fiedler's disease, Larrey-Weil disease, Landouzy's disease, Lancereaux-Mathieu disease, Mathieu's disease, Wassilieff's disease, bilious typhoid* (outmoded), *Mediterranean yellow fever* (outmoded).

leptospirosis icterohemorrhagica   ICTERIC LEPTOSPIROSIS.

leptospiruria   Excretion of *Leptospira* in the urine.

leptostaphyline   Having a narrow palate, with a palatal index of 80 or less.

leptotene   The first stage in the first prophase of meiosis, in which chromosomes first become visible as thin threads.

leptothricosis   LEPTOTRICHOSIS.

Leptotrichia buccalis   A nonpathogenic bacterium of the Bacteroidaceae family, characterized by lactic fermentation.

leptotrichosis   Any disease attributed to species of *Leptotrichia* (or *Leptothrix*). In fact, *Leptotrichia* is considered a doubtful pathogen and this is not a useful term. Also *leptothricosis.*

leptotrichosis conjunctivae   An imprecise term for PARINAUD'S CONJUNCTIVITIS.

Leptotrombidium   A genus of chigger mites in the family Trombiculidae, formerly considered a subgenus of *Trombicula*. It probably includes all known vectors of *Rickettsia tsutsugamushi*, the causative agent of scrub typhus. The principal species that transmit this disease include *L. akamushi (Trombicula akamushi, Microtrombidium akamushi)*, which is the vector of classical Japanese scrub typhus in northern Honshu, *L. deliense (T. deliensis)*, the key vector in the Philippines, coastal Australia, and China west through southeast Asia to Pakistan, and *L. fletcheri (T. fletcheri)*, an important vector in Malaysia, New Guinea, and the Philippines. Among other important vectors are *L. scutellare (T. scutellaris)* and *L. pallidum (T. pallida)*.

Leptus   A pseudogenus of chiggers, or larval trombiculid mites. *L. autumnalis,* for example, is the larva of *Trombicula autumnalis* and *L. akamushi* is the larva of *Leptotrombidium akamushi*. It also includes some larval forms of which the adult stage has not been identified and which are therefore not yet assigned to a true genus and species.

Leq   loudness equivalent: the equivalent continuous sound level of noise, measured on the dB(A) scale, used in the investigation of noise levels as these affect the community and place of work, and in the experimental investigation of noise-induced hearing loss.

Lerch   [Otto *Lerch*, U.S. physician, born 1894]   Lerch's percussion. See under DROP PERCUSSION.

Lereboullet   [Pierre *Lereboullet*, French physician, 1874–1944]   Brissaud-Lereboullet syndrome. See under ALTERNATE FACIAL HEMISPASM.

leresis   [Gk *lērēsis* (from *lēr(os)* idle talk + *-ēsis* -ESIS) a speaking foolishly]   Childish garrulity, as seen in senile dementia.

Léri   [Andre *Léri*, French physician, 1875–1930]   **1** See under SIGN.   **2** Léri's disease. See under MELORHEOSTOSIS.   **3** Léri's pleonosteosis, Léri-Weill syndrome. See under DYSCHONDROSTEOSIS.

Leriche   [René *Leriche*, French surgeon, 1879–1955]   **1** Leriche costoclavicular outlet syndrome. See under SCALENUS ANTERIOR SYNDROME.   **2** See under TREATMENT.   **3** Leriche's disease. See under POST-TRAUMATIC OSTEOPOROSIS.

Leritine   A proprietary name for anileridine.

Lerman   [J. *Lerman*, U.S. physician, born 1902]   Lerman-

Means scratch. See under SCRATCH.

Lermoyez   [Marcel *Lermoyez*, French otolaryngologist, 1858–1929]   See under SYNDROME.

Leroy   [Emile *Leroy*, French physician, born 1873]   Fiessinger-Leroy-Reiter syndrome. See under REITER SYNDROME.

les   **1** local excitatory state.   **2** lower esophageal sphincter (cardiac sphincter).

lesbian   [Gk *Lesbi(os)* pertaining to the Gk island of Lesbos and to its people + English *-an*, adjectival suffix]   **1** A female homosexual.   **2** Characterized by female homosexuality.

lesbianism   [Gk *Lesbi(os)* Lesbian, of the Gk island of Lesbos + English *-an*, adjectival suffix denoting belonging to + -ISM]   FEMALE HOMOSEXUALITY.

Lesch   [Michael *Lesch*, U.S. pediatrician, born 1939]   Lesch-Nyhan disease. See under LESCH-NYHAN SYNDROME.

lese   To irritate or damage; produce a lesion. An outmoded term.

Leser   [Edmund *Leser*, German surgeon, 1853–1916]   Leser-Trélat sign. See under SIGN.

lesion   [L *laesio* (from *laesus*, past part. of *laedere* to strike, injure, akin to Gk *lēizesthai* to plunder, ravage) a hurting, harming]   A pathologic alteration in the structure or function of a tissue or organ.

Armanni-Ebstein lesion   A morphologic change occasionally seen in the kidney of diabetes mellitus patients. The tubule cells appear markedly vacuolated due to the accumulation of glycogen. Also called *Ebstein's lesion.*

Baehr-Löhlein lesion   LÖHLEIN-BAEHR LESION.

Blumenthal lesion   A proliferative disorder of small arteries in diabetics.

Bracht-Wächter lesions   Microscopic foci of myocardial necrosis, seen in bacterial endocarditis and resulting from either coronary embolization or endarteritis.

capsular drop lesion   HYALINE LESION.

caviar lesion   Venous ectasia of the undersurface of the tongue.

central lesion   Any lesion of the central nervous system.

cheek-chewing lesion   An ulcerated or hyperkeratotic lesion on the inside of the cheek opposite the occlusal plane when the teeth are together. It is caused by habitual chewing of the mucosa.

coin lesion   A lesion in the lung which appears radiographically as a discrete disk of opacity.

complement lesion   The consequence of the insertion of the membrane complex of complement into a membrane. It is characterized functionally by the formation of a transmembrane channel and morphologically by a characteristic ring-shaped appearance on electron microscopy.

compressive lesion of the lumbosacral region   A mass lesion within the lumbar or sacral spinal canal, as that found in herniated nucleus pulposus or in tumor. It is usually identified by symptoms of pain or weakness attributable to injury to the lumbar or sacral nerve roots.

Councilman lesion   COUNCILMAN BODIES.

degenerative lesion   A lesion resulting in degeneration or loss of function.

depressive lesion   A lesion that results in reduced function of the affected part. A rarely used term.

destructive lesion   A lesion which results in the death of the affected tissue or organ.

diffuse lesion   A poorly localized lesion.

discharging lesion   Any brain lesion which gives rise to focal electrical discharge in the electroencephalogram or to focal epilepsy.

Duret's lesion   Bleeding into the fourth ventricle of the brain as a result of head injury.

Ebstein's lesion   ARMANNI-EBSTEIN LESION.

focal lesion   A circumscribed, well-localized lesion.

functional lesion   A lesion characterized by an alteration of function of the affected part.

Ghon's primary lesion   GHON TUBERCLE.

gross lesion   A lesion visible to the naked eye. Also called *macroscopic lesion.*

hepatic veno-occlusive lesion   Occlusion of the hepatic veins, a rare condition usually caused by tumor or thrombus arising locally or by extension from the inferior vena cava. Other reported causes are thrombophlebitis migrans and clotting diseases such as polycythemia rubra vera. Membranous obliteration of the hepatic segment of the vena cava has also been described.

herpetic lesion   A vesicular lesion caused by the herpesvirus. The vesicle soon bursts, leaving an ulcer.

herpetiform lesion of Cole   The initial cutaneous or mucosal vesicular lesion of lymphogranuloma venereum.

histologic lesion   A lesion too small to be seen with the naked eye.

hyaline lesion   Hyaline accumulations in the lumina of one or more capillary peripheral loops in the glomerular capsule, or in the glomerular space, often found in but not specific for diabetic glomerulopathy. Also called *fibrin cap, fibrinoid cap, capsular drop lesion.* See also GLOMERULAR DEPOSITS, DIABETIC GLOMERULOSCLEROSIS.

indiscriminate lesion   A lesion affecting multiple organs, regions, or tissues.

initial syphilitic lesion   HARD CHANCRE.

irritative lesion   A lesion that results in stimulation of the affected part.

Janeway lesions   Hemorrhagic macules that appear usually on the palms or soles in some cases of infective endocarditis. Also called *Janeway spots.*

jet lesion   A focus of endocardial fibrosis caused by the trauma of repeated jet-like streams of blood directed at the focus, due to incompetence or stenosis of a cardiac valve.

Kimmelstiel-Wilson lesion   Round hyaline deposits in glomerular mesangial areas, characteristic of but not specific for diabetic glomerulosclerosis.

local lesion   Any lesion of the central nervous system restricted to a particular area and giving rise to focal neurologic signs.

local glomerular lesion   SEGMENTAL GLOMERULAR LESION.

Löhlein-Baehr lesion   A focal glomerular lesion in infective endocarditis. Also called *Baehr-Löhlein lesion.*

lower motor neuron lesion   Any lesion involving lower as distinct from upper motor neurons.

macroscopic lesion   GROSS LESION.

mass lesion   Any large space-occupying lesion, particularly in the central nervous system, such as a tumor, hematoma, or abscess.

molecular lesion   A lesion demonstrable at the molecular level. The lesion itself is thus not visible, although its effects on the tissue may be apparent.

onion scale lesions   Replication of the arterial laminae, specifically of the splenic arterioles, giving the histologic appearance in cross-section of concentric circles resembling a sliced onion. These lesions are characteristic of systemic lupus erythematosus, but may be seen in vasculitis and hypertension.

organic lesion   A lesion that produces an alteration in the structure of the affected organ or tissue. Also called *structural lesion.*

partial lesion   A lesion that is present in only a part of the affected tissue or organ.   • Frequently used to describe lesions that affect only part of a conducting tract in neurological disorders.

peripheral lesion   Any lesion of the terminal part of nerve fibers.

precancerous lesion   A morphologically altered tissue that has a greater risk of becoming a cancer than its normal counterpart, as in epithelial dysplasia, Barrett's esophagus, or adenoma of the colon.

primary lesion   The earliest lesion of a disease or condition: used especially of syphilis.

retrocochlear lesion   A lesion behind the cochlea, that is, central to the cochlea on the vestibular pathway. In patients with vertigo and/or sensorineural deafness it is critically important to differentiate between cochlear and retrocochlear lesions if, for instance, cases of Menière's disease, a cochlear lesion, are to be separated from cases of acoustic neuroma, a retrocochlear lesion.

ring-wall lesion   A small area of organized perivascular hemorrhage in the brain, surrounded by glial proliferation.

Scheibe lesion   A lesion of the cochlea and saccule suspected of being the most common cause of congenital genetic deafness. The sensory epithelium of the organ of Corti and the saccular macula is represented simply by a mass of entirely undifferentiated cells.

secondary lesion   **1** A lesion of secondary syphilis.   **2** A lesion that occurs as a superinfection or complication of an existing lesion, such as impetigo that arises in cases of pediculosis.

segmental glomerular lesion   Any lesion involving part of a glomerulus. Also called *local glomerular lesion.*

structural lesion   ORGANIC LESION.

swan-neck tubular lesion   A distortion of the proximal convoluted tubule caused by thinning and shortening of the first portion of the proximal tubule, often present in congenital nephrosis. It may be suspected by histologic study but can be definitively demonstrated by microdissection.

systemic lesion   A lesion that may involve multiple organ systems, such as fibrin thrombi occluding multiple capillary beds in disseminated intravascular coagulation.

total lesion   A lesion involving an entire organ or tissue. A seldom used term.

traumatic lesion   A lesion caused by trauma such as a bone fracture.

trophic lesion   A lesion that results from altered nutrition of the affected part.

tumorlike lesion   A non-neoplastic lesion resembling a neoplasm. Also called *pseudotumor, false tumor.*

upper motor neuron lesion   PYRAMIDAL SYNDROME.

wire-loop lesion   Thickened glomerular capillary walls that look like stiff wire loops in histologic sections, frequently seen in but not specific for lupus nephropathy.

Lesshaft [Pyotr Frantsovich *Lesshaft*, Russian anatomist, 1836–1909]   Triangle of Grynfelt and Lesshaft, Lesshaft's triangle, Lesshaft space. See under SUPERIOR LUMBAR TRIANGLE.

LET   linear energy transfer.

let-down   The movement of newly formed milk from the alveoli to the ducts of the mammary gland.

lethal [L *letalis* or *lethalis* (from *let(um)* death, ruin, akin to *delere* to destroy, blot out + *-alis* -AL) deadly, mortal]   Causing or capable of causing death; deadly.

polyphasic lethal   Of or relating to a mutant gene whose deleterious action or effect occurs during certain developmental stages that are separated by periods when the mutant is not harmful.

lethality [*lethal* + *-ITY*]   FATALITY RATE.

lethargogenic   **1** Producing lethargy.   **2** A drug or agent that produces lethargy.

lethargus [L, lethargy, morbid drowsiness]   **1** GAMBIAN TRYPANOSOMIASIS.   **2** RHODESIAN TRYPANOSOMIASIS.

lethargy [Late L *lethargia* (from L *lethargus* drowsiness, morbid sleepiness, from Gk *lēthargos* forgetful, lethargis, from *lēthē* forgetfulness) lethargy, forgetfulness] **1** A state of excessive fatigue or retardation, with diminished physical or mental activity. This can be due to organic disease or dysfunction of the nervous system or to mental illness, such as depression. **2** HYPERSOMNIA.

African lethargy 1 GAMBIAN TRYPANOSOMIASIS. **2** RHODESIAN TRYPANOSOMIASIS.

hypnotic lethargy A state of apparent sleep or stupor induced by hypnosis. Also called *hypnotic trance, hysteric lethargy, induced lethargy, induced trance.*

hysteric lethargy HYPNOTIC LETHARGY.

induced lethargy HYPNOTIC LETHARGY.

lucid lethargy Retention of consciousness and of the power of speech with inability to move as in sleep paralysis or, less commonly, in hysteric dissociation states.

Negro lethargy 1 GAMBIAN TRYPANOSOMIASIS. **2** RHODESIAN TRYPANOSOMIASIS.

letheral [Gk *lēthē* forgetfulness + *r* + -AL] AMNESIC.

lethologic [Gk *lēth(ē)* a forgetting + *o* + LOG- + -IC] Characterized by loss of memory for words. A seldom used term.

lethologica [Gk *lēth(ē)* forgetfulness + *o* + *logika*, neut. pl. of *logikos* pertaining to speech or reason] NOMINAL APHASIA.

letimide $C_{14}H_{18}N_2O_3$. 3-[2-(Diethylamino)ethyl]-2*H*-1,3-benzoxazine-2,4(3*H*)dione. An analgesic compound, usually administered in the hydrochloride form.

letter / confusion letters Additional letters in a visual acuity chart, intended to make memorization more difficult.

intermediary letter In the United States, a letter from the Federal Government to Medicare intermediaries providing administrative directions or setting policy.

test letter A letter or symbol printed in type of various sizes used in tests to measure visual acuity.

Letterer [Erich *Letterer*, German pathologist, born 1895] Letterer-Siwe disease. See under DISEASE.

Leu Symbol for leucine.

leuc- A British spelling for LEUK-. See under LEUKO-.

leucemia LEUKEMIA.

leucine $(CH_3)_2CH—CH_2—CH(NH_2)COOH$. One of the nutritionally essential amino acids for man and other higher animals. Also called *aminoisocaproic acid* (obsolete).

Leucine aminopeptidase The cytosolic aminopeptidase found in mammals. It is a zinc-containing enzyme that hydrolyzes peptides, removing the N-terminal residue, provided that this is not arginine or lysine. It is often used for determining the sequences of peptides.

[4-leucine] oxytocin A synthetic neurohypophysial peptide, an analog of oxytocin. It induces renal excretion of sodium, potassium and chloride, and also opposes the antidiuretic action of arginine vasopressin.

leucinosis A condition marked by the passage of leucine in the urine.

leucinuria The presence of leucine in the urine.

leucismus [Gk *leuk(os)* white + *-ismos* -ISM] Whiteness.

leucismus pilorum Whiteness of the hair, especially of a forelock.

leucitis [LEUC- + -ITIS] SCLERITIS.

leuco- LEUKO-.

leucocidin A British spelling for LEUKOCIDIN.

leucocyte A British spelling for LEUKOCYTE.

leucocytosis A British spelling for LEUKOCYTOSIS.

Leucocytozoon [LEUCO- + CYTO- + Gk *zōon* living being, animal] A genus of blood-infecting sporozoans (family Hae-

moproteidae, suborder Haemosporina), parasitic chiefly in birds and transmitted by biting flies and midges of the genera *Simulium* and *Culicoides*. The parasites are found primarily in the immature red blood cells and lymphocytes, where the gametocytes are also found. Schizogony occurs in the endothelial cells of the liver, spleen, and kidney. Acute outbreaks of disease are common, especially in ducks and turkeys. Also *Leukocytozoon.*

Leucocytozoon marchouxi A worldwide species common in wild pigeons and doves and of unknown life cycle and pathogenicity. Though gamonts are found in white blood cells, signs of illness have not been described.

Leucocytozoon sabrazesi A species that causes leucocytozoonis of chickens in Malaysia, India, Sumatra, and Java. Gamonts are found in leukocytes and erythrocytes.

Leucocytozoon simondi An important blood parasite of wild and domestic ducks, geese and other waterfowl in the northern United States and Canada. Grouse, pheasants, or chickens that are associated with sick ducks are not affected. It causes severe anemia, particularly in young ducks and geese. Gamonts are found in white and red cells, schizogony in cells of a number of organs. The onset of an outbreak is extremely rapid with death sometimes occurring the day after onset of symptoms. Black flies, such as *Simulium ruggelsi,* are the vectors.

Leucocytozoon smithi A species that occurs in domestic and wild turkeys. Gamonts develop in leukocytes, schizogony in liver cells. It is a highly pathogenic species, sometimes killing 75 percent or more of a flock. The parasite is found in North America and Europe. Vectors are various species of *Simulium* (black flies).

leucocytozoonosis [LEUCO- + CYTO- + ZOONOSIS] The infection of various species of wild and domestic water fowl, turkeys, chickens, pigeons, and doves with sporozoan parasites of the genus *Leucocytozoon.* Severe disease is produced with heavy infections particularly in young birds, often resulting in death. Otherwise infection tends to be subacute or chronic. Anemia is the main effect. Also *leukocytozoonosis.*

leucoderma A British spelling for LEUKODERMA.

leucofluorescein The product of fluorescein after reduction with zinc powder in acidic solution. It is used in solution as a diagnostic aid to detect corneal damage or injury. Also called *fluorecin.*

leucoma A British spelling for LEUKOMA.

leuconic acid C_5O_5. The substance whose molecule is a ring of five carbonyl groups. These carbonyl groups are largely hydrated, and the acidity of the compound is due to the dissociation of a hydrogen ion from a hydrated carbonyl group.

Leuconostoc A genus of Gram-positive cocci of the family Streptococcaceae that carries out a heterofermentative lactic fermentation. Various species are found in milk and on fermenting fruits and vegetables. Some form slimy dextrans from sucrose.

leuconychia A British spelling for LEUKONYCHIA.

leucopenia A British spelling for LEUKOPENIA.

leucoplakia A British spelling for LEUKOPLAKIA.

leucoplast [LEUCO- + -PLAST] A colorless plastid in the cytoplasm of plant cells. Leucoplasts can accumulate and store oils, fats, starches, or proteins. Also called *leucoplastid, leukoplastid.* Also *leukoplast.*

leucoplastid LEUCOPLAST.

leucopoiesis A British spelling for LEUKOPOIESIS.

leucopterin A white pigment found in butterfly wings. It was one of the early pterins to be discovered.

leucoriboflavin Riboflavin in its reduced (i.e., hydrogenated) and colorless form.

leucorrhoea A British spelling for LEUKORRHEA.

leucotomy   A British spelling for LEUKOTOMY.

leucovorin   FOLINIC ACID.

leucovorin calcium   The calcium salt of folinic acid (leuco-verin). It is used to counteract the toxic effects of folic acid antagonists. It is also used in the treatment of megaloblastic anemias and as an adjunct to cyanocobalamin in the treatment of pernicious anemia.

Leudet   [Theodor-Emil *Leudet*, French physician, 1825–1887]   **1** Leudet's bruit. See under TINNITUS.   **2** See under SIGN.

leuk-   LEUKO-.

leukaemia   A British spelling for LEUKEMIA.

leukagglutinin   LEUKOAGGLUTININ.

leukanemia   PROLEUKEMIA.

leukapheresis   Selective removal of leukocytes by hemapher-esis. It may be performed to obtain leukocyte donation or as a therapeutic measure in patients with elevated peripheral blood white cells where the cells are likely to cause cerebral white cell infarcts as in the acute "blast crisis" phase of chronic granulo-cytic leukemia.

leukemia   [LEUK- + -EMIA]   A malignant proliferation of blood leukocytes, usually characterized by leukocytosis and infiltration of other organs by the leukemic cells, ultimately causing death. Several distinct types of leukemia are recognized, including acute lymphocytic, acute myelogenous, acute monocytic, acute myelomonocytic, acute promyelocytic, erythroleukemia, chronic myelogenous, and chronic lymphocytic. Also called *Bennett's disease, hemosarcoma* (obsolete), *medullosis* (obsolete), *hemocytoblastoma, leukocytic sarcoma*. Also *leucemia*.

acute leukemia   Any of several acute forms of leukemia, such as acute lymphocytic leukemia, acute granulocytic leukemia, acute monocytic leukemia, acute myelomonocytic leukemia, acute erythroleukemia, or acute promyelocytic leukemia. Also called *blast cell leukemia, Bennet syndrome*. See also FRENCH-AMERICAN-BRITISH CLASSIFICATION.

acute basophilic leukemia   A very rare form of acute gran-ulocytic leukemia in which the myeloblasts or other granulocyte precursors show signs of differentiation into basophils, such as the presence of a few very large basophilic granules in the cytoplasm of cells beyond the progranulocyte stage.

acute eosinophilic leukemia   A rare form of acute granulo-cytic leukemia in which the myeloblasts or other granulocyte precursors exhibit signs of differentiation into eosinophils, such as the presence of a few large eosinophilic granules in the cy-toplasm.

acute granulocytic leukemia   An acute leukemia character-ized by a predominance of myeloblasts in the peripheral blood and bone marrow. Also called *myeloblastic leukemia, acute myeloid leukemia, myeloblastic leukosis* (rarely used), *acute mye-locytic leukemia*.

acute lymphoblastic leukemia   ACUTE LYMPHOCYTIC LEUKEMIA.

acute lymphocytic leukemia   An acute leukemia that is dis-tinguished by the presence of large numbers of lymphoblasts in the blood and bone marrow. Also called *acute lymphoid leuke-mia, acute lymphoblastic leukemia, acute lymphogenous leuke-mia, lymphoblastic leukemia*. See also FRENCH-AMERICAN-BRITISH CLASSIFICATION.

acute lymphogenous leukemia   ACUTE LYMPHOCYTIC LEUKEMIA.

acute lymphoid leukemia   ACUTE LYMPHOCYTIC LEUKEMIA.

acute myelocytic leukemia   ACUTE GRANULOCYTIC LEUKE-MIA.

acute myeloid leukemia   ACUTE GRANULOCYTIC LEUKEMIA.

acute nonlymphocytic leukemia   Any acute leukemia that is distinguished by the presence of large numbers of immature cells (usually blasts) other than lymphoblasts in the blood. Included are acute granulocytic leukemia, progranulocytic leukemia, myelomonocytic leukemia, acute monocytic leukemia, and acute erythroleukemia. See also FRENCH-AMERICAN-BRITISH CLAS-SIFICATION.

acute promyelocytic leukemia   An uncommon type of acute granulocytic leukemia in which atypical promyelocytes are the predominant leukocytes. The atypical promyelocytes have fewer of the prominent dense primary cytoplasmic granules that char-acterize promyelocytes, and they often have large numbers (5–20) of Auer rods that may be arranged in sheaves or "faggots." This leukemia is typically associated with deficiencies of clotting factors due to intravascular coagulation and with a cytogenetic abnormality in the leukemic cells that is a 15;17 translocation, i.e. t(15;17)(q26;q22).

aleukemic leukemia   Acute leukemia in which leukemic cells ("blasts") are not present in blood, nor is there leukocytosis. Often there is pancytopenia. Diagnosis is made by examination of bone marrow. A rarely used term. Also called *aleukocythmic leukemia, leukopenic leukemia, cryptoleukemia*.

aleukocythemic leukemia   ALEUKEMIC LEUKEMIA.

basophilic leukemia   A rare form of leukemia in which there is a very marked increase in basophils in blood and bone marrow. It is considered a variant of chronic granulocytic leukemia.

blast cell leukemia   ACUTE LEUKEMIA.

chronic granulocytic leukemia   A neoplastic disorder of the blood granulocytes that usually occurs in persons of age 30–50 years, and is characterized by splenomegaly, increase in the number of granulocytes in blood and bone marrow to values as high as 500 x 10⁹/l, thrombocytosis that may be very marked, absent or nearly absent leukocyte alkaline phosphatase, and a distinctive cytogenetic abnormality of granulocytes, the Phila-delphia (Ph¹) chromosome: t(9;22)(p34;q11). Approximately 10% of cases that have the other features of chronic granulocytic leukemia lack the chromosomal anomaly; the taxonomic status of "Philadelphia chromosome negative chronic granulocytic leu-kemia" is unresolved. Also called *chronic myeloid leukemia, chronic myelocytic leukemia, chronic myelogenous leukemia, chronic myelosis, myelemia* (rarely used), *splenomyelogenous leu-kemia, myelocytic leukosis* (rarely used), *mature cell leukemia, medullary leukemia, lienomyelogenous leukemia*.

chronic lymphatic leukemia   CHRONIC LYMPHOCYTIC LEUKEMIA.

chronic lymphocytic leukemia   A neoplastic disorder of adults characterized by marked increase in mature lymphocytes in blood, often by enlargement of lymph nodes and spleen, and by duration of months to years. Also called *lymphocytic leuke-mia, chronic lymphatic leukemia, chronic lymphoid leukemia, leukemic lymphadenosis* (rarely used), *lymphemia* (rarely used), *lymphosis* (incorrect).

chronic lymphoid leukemia   CHRONIC LYMPHOCYTIC LEUKEMIA.

chronic myelocytic leukemia   CHRONIC GRANULOCYTIC LEUKEMIA.

chronic myelogenous leukemia   CHRONIC GRANULOCYTIC LEUKEMIA.

chronic myeloid leukemia   CHRONIC GRANULOCYTIC LEUKEMIA.

leukemia cutis   Involvement of the skin, particularly the der-mis, by leukemia. This condition is seen particularly in the Sézary syndrome, but also in chronic lymphocytic and acute leukemias. Also called *lymphodermia perniciosa* (obsolete).

embryonal leukemia   STEM CELL LEUKEMIA.

eosinophilic leukemia   A very rare form of leukemia in which eosinophilia of peripheral blood and bone marrow is associated with an excessive number of myeloblasts (e.g. 10% or more of the granulocytic cells) in bone marrow or blood or both.

feline leukemia   An acute lymphocytic leukemia that occurs in cats infected with the feline leukemia virus. In addition to leukemia, this virus infection of cats may cause thymoma, lymphosarcoma, fibrosarcoma, hypoplastic anemia, or an immunodeficiency syndrome that mimics in many of its features the human acquired immunodeficiency syndrome (AIDS), including the propensity to fatal infections with opportunistic microorganisms.

leukemia of fowls AVIAN LEUKOSIS.

granulocytic leukemia A leukemia in which the predominant cells are of the granulocyte cell line, i.e. polymorphonuclear leukocytes and their precursors. The term includes chronic granulocytic leukemia, in which granulocytes of all stages of maturation are present in blood, and acute granulocytic leukemia, in which myeloblasts are markedly increased in blood and bone marrow. Also called *myelogenous leukemia, myeloid leukemia, myeloleukemia, myeloid granulocytic leukemia, myelocytic leukemia, neutrophilic leukemia, polymorphocytic leukemia.*

Gross leukemia A murine leukemia of experimental importance, for which the causative virus can be transmitted by inoculation from one species to another.

hairy cell leukemia LEUKEMIC RETICULOENDOTHELIOSIS.

hemoblastic leukemia STEM CELL LEUKEMIA.

hemocytoblastic leukemia STEM CELL LEUKEMIA.

histiocytic leukemia 1 The leukemic phase of histiocytic medullary reticulosis. 2 SCHILLING'S LEUKEMIA. See under MONOCYTIC LEUKEMIA.

leukopenic leukemia ALEUKEMIC LEUKEMIA.

lienomyelogenous leukemia CHRONIC GRANULOCYTIC LEUKEMIA.

lymphoblastic leukemia ACUTE LYMPHOCYTIC LEUKEMIA.

lymphocytic leukemia CHRONIC LYMPHOCYTIC LEUKEMIA.

lymphogenous leukemia LYMPHOID LEUKEMIA.

lymphoid leukemia Any neoplastic proliferation of lymphoid cells in the blood and marrow, including acute lymphocytic leukemia and chronic lymphocytic leukemia. Also called *lymphogenous leukemia.*

lymphosarcoma cell leukemia A type of lymphatic leukemia characterized by numerous large lymphocytes with prominent, usually single, nucleoli. It is often considered a variant of chronic lymphocytic leukemia. Also called *lymphosarcoleukemia.*

Mallory leukemia Leukemia, usually acute granulocytic, attributed to exposure to hydrocarbons.

mast cell leukemia A malignant proliferation of mast cells; a leukemic phase of systemic mastocytosis. Also called *malignant mastocytosis.*

mature cell leukemia CHRONIC GRANULOCYTIC LEUKEMIA.

medullary leukemia CHRONIC GRANULOCYTIC LEUKEMIA.

megakaryocytic leukemia 1 A variant of chronic granulocytic leukemia in which megakaryocytic proliferation and thrombocytosis predominate. 2 ESSENTIAL THROMBOCYTHEMIA.

micromyeloblastic leukemia A variety of acute granulocytic leukemia in which the predominant cell is a small myeloblast, resembling a lymphocyte and best distinguished by histochemistry.

mixed leukemia Chronic granulocytic leukemia, with emphasis on the different types of cells characteristically seen in the disease. Also called *mixed cell leukemia.*

mixed cell leukemia MIXED LEUKEMIA.

monocytic leukemia Neoplastic proliferation of monocytes, a broad category which combines two varieties: Naegeli type acute myelomonocytic leukemia, in which cells are relatively smaller and exhibit some myeloblastic characteristics, and Schilling's leukemia, in which cells are larger and more typically monocytoid or even histiocytic. Also called *monocytoma, monoblastoma.*

myeloblastic leukemia ACUTE GRANULOCYTIC LEUKEMIA.

myelocytic leukemia GRANULOCYTIC LEUKEMIA.

myelogenous leukemia GRANULOCYTIC LEUKEMIA.

myeloid leukemia GRANULOCYTIC LEUKEMIA.

myeloid granulocytic leukemia GRANULOCYTIC LEUKEMIA.

myelomonocytic leukemia A leukemia that is commonly subacute, but may be acute, and which is characterized by the presence in blood and bone marrow of numerous cells that have features both of myeloblasts and monocytes. These cells give positive reactions with nonspecific esterase stain (a monocyte stain) and with chloroacetate esterase stain (a granulocyte stain), and they may be peroxidase positive. In the French-American-British classification this condition is acute nonlymphocytic leukemia M4.

Naegeli leukemia NAEGELI TYPE ACUTE MYELOMONOCYTIC LEUKEMIA.

Naegeli type acute myelomonocytic leukemia An acute monocytic leukemia in which many of the leukemic cells resemble myeloblasts. It is type M-4 in the French-American-British classification. Also called *Naegeli leukemia.*

neutrophilic leukemia GRANULOCYTIC LEUKEMIA.

paramyeloblastic leukemia A seldom used term for RIEDER CELL LEUKEMIA.

plasma cell leukemia A malignant disorder of plasma cells characterized by large numbers of plasma cells in blood as well as in bone marrow. Plasma cells exceed $1 \times 10^9/l$ in blood of persons with this disorder. Also called *plasmacytic leukemia.*

plasmacytic leukemia PLASMA CELL LEUKEMIA.

polymorphocytic leukemia GRANULOCYTIC LEUKEMIA.

progranulocytic leukemia PROMYELOCYTIC LEUKEMIA.

promyelocytic leukemia A variety of myeloblastic leukemia in which promyelocytes predominate. It is often complicated by coagulation abnormalities. It is type M-3 in the French-American-British classification. Also called *progranulocytic leukemia.*

Rieder cell leukemia A variety of acute granulocytic leukemia in which the myeloblasts have indented nuclei (Rieder cells). Also called *paramyeloblastic leukemia* (seldom used).

Schilling's leukemia The acute form of monocytic leukemia. It is type M-5 in the French-American-British classification. Also called *histiocytic leukemia.*

splenic leukemia Any instance of leukemia accompanied by significant splenomegaly. An imprecise usage.

splenomyelogenous leukemia An obsolete term for CHRONIC GRANULOCYTIC LEUKEMIA.

stem cell leukemia An acute leukemia in which the primitive blast cells cannot be classified as lymphoblasts, myeloblasts, or monoblasts, but may be presumed to represent the common precursor of all three cell lines. Also called *embryonal leukemia, undifferentiated cell leukemia, hemoblastic leukemia, hemocytoblastic leukemia.*

subleukemic leukemia An acute leukemia in which primitive blast cells are present in the blood but the total leukocyte count is normal. An obsolete term. Also called *leukopenic myelosis.*

undifferentiated cell leukemia STEM CELL LEUKEMIA.

leukemic Having or pertaining to leukemia.

leukemid A nonspecific cutaneous lesion containing infiltrates of leukemia cells, seen in patients with leukemia.

leukemogen Any substance or condition that promotes the development of leukemia, including chemicals such as benzene, all forms of ionizing radiation, and some viruses.

leukemogenesis The process or mechanism of the development of leukemia.

leukemogenic Having the property of promoting the occurrence of leukemia.

leukemoid Having features resembling those of leukemia, such as marked leukocytosis or the appearance of immature leukocytes in blood or bone marrow. Leukemoid reactions may occur in the course of some infections, as in miliary tuberculosis.

leukencephalitis LEUKOENCEPHALITIS.

leukeran A proprietary name for chlorambucil.

leukexosis A collection of dead leukocytes within a vessel. An obsolete term.

leukin LEUKOCYTIC ENDOLYSIN.

leuko- [Gk *leukos* light, bright, white] A combining form meaning (1) white or colorless; (2) leukocyte. Also *leuco- (British spelling), leuk-, leuc- (British spelling).*

leukoagglutinin Any antibody that causes clumping of leukocytes. Also called *leukagglutinin.*

leukobilin An outmoded term for WHITE BILE.

leukoblast See under LEUKOBLAST OF PAPPENHEIM.

granular leukoblast An obsolete term for PROMYELOCYTE.

leukoblast of Pappenheim A leukocyte precursor with morphologic features differing slightly from a myeloblast. The cell so described may have been a lymphoblast. An obsolete term.

leukoblastosis Any malignant proliferative disorder of white blood cells, including leukemias and lymphomas.

leukocidin [LEUKO- + L *caedere* (akin to Sanskrit *chid* to cut) to cut + -IN] A complement-fixing antileukocyte antibody that, in the presence of complement, will cause the leukocytes to be killed. An older term.

leukocoria LEUKOKORIA.

leukocytal A seldom used term for LEUKOCYTIC.

leukocyte [LEUKO- + -CYTE] Any of several nucleated cells that occur in blood or tissue fluid, exclusive of erythrocytes and erythrocyte precursors. Major classes of leukocytes are lymphocytes, monocytes, neutrophils, eosinophils, and basophils. Also called *white cell, white blood cell, white corpuscle, white blood corpuscle, amebocyte* (rarely used), *amoebocyte* (rarely used).

acidophilic leukocyte See under EOSINOPHIL.

agranular leukocytes Leukocytes that do not have cytoplasmic granules. Included are, principally, lymphocytes and monocytes, but also plasma cells, lymphoblasts, myeloblasts, and monoblasts. Also called *nongranular leukocytes.*

alpha leukocyte Any leukocyte that lyses during coagulation. A rarely used term for .

beta leukocyte Any leukocyte that does not lyse during coagulation. A rarely used term.

cystinotic leukocyte A monocyte or neutrophil that contains cystine in prominent lysosomes as a manifestation of the hereditary metabolic disorder cystinosis.

endothelial leukocyte MACROPHAGE.

eosinophilic leukocyte See under EOSINOPHIL.

filament polymorphonuclear leukocyte A mature leukocyte, of the polymorphonuclear group, that has at least two nuclear lobes separated by a fine thread, or filament, of nuclear chromatin.

globular leukocyte A small lymphocyte observed in the subepithelial layers of the crypts of the intestinal mucosa. It has cytoplasmic globules which are eosinophilic. Also called *globule leukocyte.*

globule leukocyte GLOBULAR LEUKOCYTE.

granular leukocyte GRANULOCYTE.

heterophil leukocyte NEUTROPHIL.

hyaline leukocyte An obsolete term for MONOCYTE.

lymphoid leukocyte LYMPHOCYTE.

motile leukocyte Any leukocyte that shows pseudopodia and ameboid movement in supravital, or wet, nonfixed preparations. All viable leukocytes are motile or potentially motile.

neutrophil leukocyte NEUTROPHIL.

nonfilament polymorphonuclear leukocyte Any leukocyte of the polymorphonuclear class that does not have two or more nuclear lobes connected by fine strands of chromatin. Included are band neutrophils, metamyelocytes, myelocytes, promyelocytes, and myeloblasts.

nongranular leukocytes AGRANULAR LEUKOCYTES.

nonmotile leukocyte A leukocyte lacking ameboid movement capability.

polymorphonuclear leukocyte A blood leukocyte that has a distinctly segmented or lobulated nucleus, the lobules being separated by a thin strand of chromatin. Included are segmented neutrophils, eosinophils, and basophils. Also called *lobocyte, polymorphocyte, segmented leukocyte.*

segmented leukocyte POLYMORPHONUCLEAR LEUKOCYTE.

transitional leukocyte An obsolete term for MONOCYTE.

Türk's irritation leukocyte TÜRK CELL.

leukocythemia LEUKOCYTOSIS.

leukocytic Pertaining to or characteristic of leukocytes. Also *leukocytal* (seldom used).

leukocytoblast The earliest recognizable leukocyte precursor. It may be a lymphoblast, monoblast, or myeloblast.

leukocytogenesis LEUKOPOIESIS.

leukocytoid Resembling, or characteristic of, leukocytes.

leukocytology The study of leukocytes and disorders thereof.

leukocytolysis LEUKOLYSIS.

leukocytolytic LEUKOLYTIC.

leukocytoma Any of various tumorous accumulations of leukocytes, including chloroma, granulocytic sarcoma, and lymphoma.

leukocytometer A finely calibrated glass chamber which, used with a microscope, permits enumeration of leukocytes in accurately diluted samples of blood or other body fluids.

leukocytopenia LEUKOPENIA.

leukocytophagy The phagocytosis of leukocytes by cells of the monocyte-macrophage system.

leukocytoplania LEUKOPEDESIS.

leukocytopoiesis LEUKOPOIESIS.

leukocytosis [*leukocyt(e)* + -OSIS] Any condition marked by increased concentration of leukocytes in the blood, including absolute lymphocytosis and absolute neutrophilia. Also called *absolute leukocytosis, leukocythemia.*

absolute leukocytosis LEUKOCYTOSIS.

agonal leukocytosis Terminal leukocytosis.

basophilic leukocytosis Leukocytosis due to increased basophilic granulocytes. Also called *basocytosis.*

digestive leukocytosis A mild, transient leukocytosis which normally follows ingestion of food.

distribution leukocytosis Leukocytosis due to an increase in one or more specific types of leukocytes, resulting in an abnormal differential count.

emotional leukocytosis Leukocytosis attributed to emotional disturbance, usually stress.

eosinophilic leukocytosis An increase in eosinophilic leukocytes in the peripheral blood.

lymphocytic leukocytosis Leukocytosis due to an increase of lymphocytes in the peripheral blood.

mononuclear leukocytosis Leukocytosis due to an increase of monocytes in the peripheral blood.

neutrophilic leukocytosis Leukocytosis due to an increase of neutrophils in the peripheral blood. Also called *pure leukocytosis.*

leukocytosis of the newborn The normal leukocytosis observed during the first four days of life, reflecting transient increases in neutrophil numbers up to 30 000 per mm^3.

pathologic leukocytosis Leukocytosis due to infection, inflammation, or other disease.

physiologic leukocytosis Leukocytosis due to normal physiologic stimuli, including exercise or other nonpathologic factors.

pure leukocytosis NEUTROPHILIC LEUKOCYTOSIS.

relative leukocytosis An increased number of any specific leukocyte, not sufficient to cause an abnormal increase in total leukocyte numbers.

terminal leukocytosis An elevation in the number of leukocytes in blood that occurs as a person dies. Also called *agonal leukocytosis.*

toxic leukocytosis An increase in the number of leukocytes in blood in response to severe infection.

leukocytotactic Having the property of attracting the migration of leukocytes.

leukocytotaxia LEUKOCYTOTAXIS.

leukocytotaxis The migration of leukocytes to a site of inflammation or injury. Also called *leukocytotaxia.*

leukocytotherapy Treatment by injection of leukocytes, for example, transfusion of granulocytes.

leukocytotoxin Any substance that selectively damages leukocytes. Also called *leukotoxin.*

leukocytotropic Having an affinity for leukocytes.

Leukocytozoon LEUCOCYTOZOON.

leukocytozoonosis LEUCOCYTOZOONOSIS.

leukocyturia The presence of a greater than normal number of leukocytes in the urine, as in pyelonephritis.

leukoderma [LEUKO- + DERMA] Lack of normal pigmentation of the skin. Also called *leukopathia, leukopathy, leukodermia.*

acquired leukoderma **1** Any leukoderma that is not congenital. **2** VITILIGO.

leukoderma acquisitum centrifugum LEUKODERMA CENTRIFUGUM ACQUISITUM.

leukoderma centrifugum acquisitum A halo of hypomelanosis acquired around a cutaneous tumor, which is usually a melanocytic nevus but is sometimes a blue nevus or a melanoma. Also called *circumnevic vitiligo, perinevic vitiligo, leukoderma acquisitum centrifugum, circumscribed vitiligo.*

leukoderma colli VENEREAL COLLAR.

congenital leukoderma The presence of patchy areas of skin depigmentation that are noticeable at or shortly after birth, as is seen in the Waardenburg syndrome. The condition is phenotypically similar to vitiligo, an acquired phenomenon.

occupational leukoderma A depigmentation of the skin that is caused by exposure to chemicals used in the workplace. It is seen, for example, among those manufacturing rubber goods who use hydroquinone derivatives as antioxidants.

psoriatic leukoderma A temporary loss of pigment that may follow the resolution of a plaque of psoriasis.

leukoderma punctatum The presence of very small macules of white skin within melanotic areas that are symptomatic of arsenic pigmentation.

syphilitic leukoderma An area of mottled pigmentation and depigmentation that forms on the skin as a result of syphilis.

leukodermatous Of or relating to leukoderma. Also *leukodermic.*

leukodermia LEUKODERMA.

leukodermic LEUKODERMATOUS.

leukodont [LEUK- + -ODONT] A person with leukodontia.

leukodontia [LEUK- + -ODONTIA] The characteristic of having white teeth.

leukodystrophia cerebri progressiva PROGRESSIVE CEREBRAL LEUKODYSTROPHY.

leukodystrophy [LEUKO- + DYSTROPHY] A group of diseases of the central nervous system, marked anatomically by lesions of the white matter of the cerebral hemispheres and sometimes involving myelin within the cerebellum and peripheral nerves. These diseases result in progressive demyelination, and most are due to inborn errors of lipid metabolism. Among the leukodystrophies are metachromatic leukodystrophy, Krabbe's disease, and Pelizaeus-Merzbacher disease.

cerebral leukodystrophy ADRENOLEUKODYSTROPHY.

dysmyelinogenic leukodystrophy ALEXANDER'S DISEASE.

globoid leukodystrophy KRABBE'S DISEASE.

globoid cell leukodystrophy KRABBE'S DISEASE.

hereditary cerebral leukodystrophy Any cerebral leukodystrophy which is genetically determined and not acquired.

Krabbe's leukodystrophy KRABBE'S DISEASE.

melanodermic leukodystrophy ADRENOLEUKODYSTROPHY.

metachromatic leukodystrophy A form of progressive cerebral leukodystrophy, of autosomal recessive inheritance, usually beginning in childhood and marked clinically by progressive dementia and progressive spastic tetraplegia with contractures. Morphologically, there is diffuse degeneration of the white matter of the brain, with degeneration of the oligodendroglia and accumulation of degenerate myelin products which stain metachromatically with toluidine blue. The condition is now known to be due to sulfatide accumulation due to an inherited deficiency of aryl sulfatase which can be demonstrated in the leukocytes. The peripheral nerves are generally affected, showing signs of a polyneuropathy. A form of late onset producing a fatuous euphoric dementia and polyneuropathy has been described in adults. Also called *Scholz-Bielschowsky-Henneberg diffuse cerebral sclerosis, Scholz disease, Scholz cerebral sclerosis, Scholz-Greenfield disease, Scholz metachromatic leukoencephalitis, Greenfield syndrome, van Bogaert-Nyssen-Pfeiffer disease, metachromatic leukoencephalopathy, sulfatide lipidosis, cerebroside sulfatase deficiency.*

progressive cerebral leukodystrophy Any of the progressive demyelinating or dysmyelinating leukodystrophies involving the cerebral hemispheres. Also called *leukodystrophia cerebri progressiva.*

progressive familial leukodystrophy Any of a group of inherited disorders, many of autosomal recessive inheritance, which give rise to progressive demyelination in the cerebral and cerebellar hemispheres and sometimes of peripheral nerves. Most of these conditions give rise to progressive dementia and spasticity and often to epilepsy, and many are now known to be due to specific abnormalities of lipid metabolism, though some are still of unknown cause. An imprecise and outmoded term.

spongiform leukodystrophy CANAVAN'S DISEASE.

sudanophilic leukodystrophy Any of a group of demyelinating leukodystrophies, including Schilder's disease, in which the degenerating lipid is sudanophilic.

leukoedema [LEUKO- + EDEMA] An opalescent appearance of the buccal mucous membrane, noted particularly in Negroid subjects. It is debated whether it represents a normal variation or an early form of leukoplakia. ⟨Sanstead, H.R. and Lowe, J.W., *Journal of the National Cancer Institute* 14:423–438, 1953.⟩

leukoencephalitis [LEUKO- + ENCEPHALITIS] Any form of encephalitis involving predominantly the cerebral white matter rather than the gray. • The term, though outmoded, is still sometimes used to embrace the various forms of postinfective encephalomyelitis. Also called *leukoencephalitis.*

acute hemorrhagic leukoencephalitis An exceptionally acute form of acute disseminated encephalomyelitis characterized clinically by rapidly advancing coma, occasionally convulsions, and sometimes focal neurologic signs, including hemiplegia. Pathologically, there is widespread perivascular demyelination with areas of hemorrhage and cellular infiltration around blood vessels largely in the cerebral white matter. Sometimes the lesions are more severe in one cerebral hemisphere than the other, thus accounting for unilateral neurologic signs. Many cases are fatal, and in those who recover there may be significant neurologic residua. Also called *acute hemorrhagic leukoencephalopathy, acute necrotizing hemorrhagic leukoencephalopathy, Leichtenstern's encephalitis, Strümpell-Leichtenstern encephalitis, Hurst's disease*. See also BRAIN PURPURA.

concentric pariaxial leukoencephalitis BALÓ'S DISEASE.

leukoencephalitis periaxialis concentrica BALÓ'S DISEASE.

Scholz metachromatic leukoencephalitis METACHROMATIC LEUKODYSTROPHY.

subacute sclerosing leukoencephalitis SUBACUTE SCLEROSING PANENCEPHALITIS.

van Bogaert sclerosing leukoencephalitis SUBACUTE SCLEROSING PANENCEPHALITIS.

leukoencephalopathy [LEUKO- + ENCEPHALOPATHY] Any disease of the white matter of the brain. Also called *leukoencephaly*.

acute hemorrhagic leukoencephalopathy ACUTE HEMORRHAGIC LEUKOENCEPHALITIS.

acute necrotizing hemorrhagic leukoencephalopathy ACUTE HEMORRHAGIC LEUKOENCEPHALITIS.

metachromatic leukoencephalopathy METACHROMATIC LEUKODYSTROPHY.

multifocal leukoencephalopathy PROGRESSIVE MULTIFOCAL LEUKOENCEPHALOPATHY.

progressive multifocal leukoencephalopathy Progressive multifocal demyelination in cerebral white matter giving rise to dementia, spastic paralysis, and sometimes blindness and resulting from opportunistic infection with papova viruses (e.g., polyoma viruses) in patients suffering from immune deficiency states associated with systemic diseases, particularly malignant lymphomas. Also called *multifocal leukoencephalopathy, progressive multifocal encephalopathy*. Abbreviation: PML

subacute sclerosing leukoencephalopathy SUBACUTE SCLEROSING PANENCEPHALITIS.

leukoencephaly LEUKOENCEPHALOPATHY.

leukoerythroblastosis The presence in blood of numerous normoblasts together with immature cells of the granulocytic series. See also MYELOPHTHISIC ANEMIA.

leukokeratosis LEUKOPLAKIA.

congenital leukokeratosis mucosae oris ORAL FAMILIAL WHITE FOLDED DYSPLASIA.

congenital oral leukokeratosis ORAL FAMILIAL WHITE FOLDED DYSPLASIA.

leukokinesis [LEUKO- + Gk *kinēsis* movement] The movement of leukocytes through the body.

leukokinetic Of or relating to leukokinesis.

leukokinetics The study of the formation, circulation, and fate of leukocytes, usually by use of a radioactive tracer.

leukokoria [LEUKO- + Gk *kor(ē)* the pupil of the eye + -IA] A disorder causing a white reflex of the pupil, as in retinopathy of prematurity. Leukokoria does not include cataract, but only conditions posterior to the crystalline lens. Also *leukocoria*.

leukokraurosis [LEUKO- + Gk *kraur(os)* hard, dry, brittle + -OSIS] LICHEN SCLEROSUS ET ATROPHICUS.

leukolymphosarcoma A malignant lymphoma with a leukemic phase, i.e. in which lymphoblasts are present in the blood. Also called *leukosarcoma*. See also RICHTER SYNDROME.

leukolysis The destruction of leukocytes. Also called *leukocytolysis*.

leukolytic Relating to, characteristic of, or resulting from leukolysis. Also *leukocytolytic*.

leukoma [LEUK- + -OMA] A dense white scar of the cornea.

leukoma adhaerens A dense white corneal scar associated with an anterior synechia.

leukomaine Any of the nitrogenous bases formed during metabolism by living organisms.

leukomainic Concerning a leukomaine.

leukomatous Having or pertaining to leukoma.

leukomelanoderma MELANOLEUKODERMA.

leukomethylene blue The colorless derivative produced by the reduction of the dye methylene blue. Early methods of detecting dehydrogenases were based on the decolorization of methylene blue.

leukomyelitis Inflammation of the spinal cord white matter.

leukomyelopathy Any disease of the spinal cord white matter.

leukon The aggregate of all leukocytes and all leukocyte-producing cells of the body. A rarely used term.

leukonecrosis Gangrene with sloughing of whitened necrotic tissue. A seldom used term.

leukonychia [LEUK- + ONYCHIA] White nails that are attributable to a whitening of the nail plate. Also called *onychopacity, gift spots*.

leukonychia striata Transverse white lines of the nail plate.

leukonychia totalis A rare autosomal dominant abnormality that produces whitening of the entire nail plate. The nails are also brittle and easily broken.

leukopathia [*leukopathy*. See LEUKOPATHY.] LEUKODERMA.

acquired leukopathia VITILIGO.

congenital leukopathia ALBINISM.

leukopathia punctata et reticularis symmetrica A genetically determined pigmentary defect, reported in Japan, in which leukoderma develops in childhood more or less symmetrically on the backs of hands and feet and on the forearms and lower legs, and extends proximally. Also called *safu (Japanese)*.

leukopathia unguium A pallor of the nails.

leukopathy [LEUKO- + -PATHY] LEUKODERMA.

symmetric progressive leukopathy Punctate leukoderma that develops in young adults on the shins and the extensor aspects of the arms.

leukopedesis [LEUKO- + Gk *pēdēsis* a leaping] The migration of leukocytes through the walls of blood vessels or through other tissues. It is a form of diapedesis. Also called *leukocytoplania*.

leukopenia [LEUKO- + -PENIA] An abnormal decrease in the number of leukocytes in the blood. Also called *leukocytopenia, oligoleukocythemia, oligoleukocytosis*.

basophilic leukopenia An abnormal decrease in the number of basophils in the circulating blood.

congenital leukopenia CONGENITAL NEUTROPENIA.

eosinophilic leukopenia An abnormal decrease in the number of eosinophiles in the circulating blood.

lymphocytic leukopenia LYMPHOCYTOPENIA.

malignant pernicious leukopenia AGRANULOCYTOSIS.

monocytic leukopenia MONOCYTOPENIA.

neutrophilic leukopenia NEUTROPENIA.

leukopenic Pertaining to, characterized by, or resulting from leukopenia. Also *hypoleukocytic*.

leukophagocytosis The ingestion of leukocytes by phagocytes.

leukophthalmous [LEUK- + OPHTHALM- + -OUS] Characterized by unusual whiteness of the eye.

leukoplakia [LEUKO- + Gk *plax*, gen. *plakos*, anything flat and broad, a flat stone, plate + -IA] A lesion of the mucous membrane characterized by white patches due to epithelial hyperplasia with keratosis. It chiefly affects the tongue, cheeks, and gums but also the mucosa of the upper respiratory tract, particularly the larynx, the urinary bladder, and the female genitalia. It is a macroscopic and clinical diagnosis. Many sources of chronic irritation, including smoking, alcohol, and syphilis, have been blamed. Many such lesions are premalignant while others are examples of carcinoma *in situ*. Some are completely innocuous. This assessment must be made microscopically. Also called *leukoplasia, leukokeratosis, alphelasma* (obsolete), *pachymucosa alba* (seldom used), *smokers' patch, tylosis linguae*.

balanopreputial leukoplakia   LEUKOPLAKIA PENIS.

hyperkeratotic leukoplakia   VERRUCOUS LEUKOPLAKIA.

leukoplakia of the larynx   Leukoplakia involving the lining of the larynx. It is frequently a feature of chronic hyperplastic laryngitis. The vocal cords are most often the site but areas normally lined by respiratory epithelium, such as the vestibular folds, may be affected when epithelial metaplasia into squamous epithelium precedes keratinization.

leukoplakia penis   Leukoplakia of the penile skin. It is commonly secondary to lichen sclerosus et atrophicus. Also called *balanopreputial leukoplakia*.

simple leukoplakia   Leukoplakia that is not marked by verrucous thickening, fissuring, or neoplastic change. An imprecise usage.

verrucous leukoplakia   Leukoplakia characterized by well-marked, horny thickening of the epithelium. Also called *hyperkeratotic leukoplakia*.

leukoplakia vesicae   Leukoplakia affecting the mucosa of the base of the urinary bladder.

leukoplakia of the vulva   White, hypertrophic, potentially malignant plaques of the mucous membrane of the vulva. Also called *leukoplakia vulvae, Breisky's disease, leukoplakic vulvitis*.

leukoplakia vulvae   LEUKOPLAKIA OF THE VULVA.

leukoplakic   Affected by, resembling, or due to leukoplakia.

leukoplasia   LEUKOPLAKIA.

leukoplast   A colorless plastid found in the cytoplasm of plant cells. The leukoplast can accumulate and store oils, fats, starches, or proteins. Also called *leukoplastid*.

leukoplastid   LEUCOPLAST.

leukopoiesis [LEUKO- + -POIESIS]   The formation, growth, and maturation of leukocytes. Also called *leukocytogenesis, leukocytopoiesis*.

leukopoietic   1 Concerning or characterized by leukopoiesis. 2 An agent capable of stimulating leukopoiesis.

leukoprophylaxis   Augmenting of the number of leukocytes in the blood by granulocyte transfusion before surgery to reduce the risk of infection. A seldom used term.

leukopsin   The colorless product of bleaching of rhodopsin.

leukorrhagia [LEUKO- + -RRHAGIA]   Profuse leukorrhea.

leukorrhea [LEUKO- + -RRHEA]   A gynecologic disorder characterized by an abnormal, whitish, nonbloody discharge from the genital tract. Also called *fluor albus*.

menstrual leukorrhea   A white discharge associated with menstruation.

periodic leukorrhea   Intermittent vaginal discharge, which may occur at regular or irregular intervals.

leukorrheal   Pertaining to or associated with leukorrhea.

leukosarcoma   LEUKOLYMPHOSARCOMA.

leukosarcomatosis   The presence of multiple tumor masses consisting of leukemic cells. A seldom used term.

leukoscope [LEUKO- + -SCOPE]   A color-vision testing instrument that mixes spectral colors to form white.

leukosis [LEUK- + -OSIS]   Excess proliferation, usually malignant, of one or more leukocyte varieties. It includes lymphoproliferation and myeloproliferation.

avian leukosis   Any of a number of neoplastic diseases of poultry caused by a retrovirus and now identified as belonging to the avian leukosis complex. An outmoded term. Also called

fowl leukosis, avian lymphomatosis, lymphomatosis of fowl, leukemia of fowls.

avian leukosis complex   See under COMPLEX.

bovine leukosis   A neoplastic disease of cattle, caused by the bovine leukemia virus. There are numerous forms of this disease.

fowl leukosis   AVIAN LEUKOSIS.

lymphoid leukosis   A transmissible avian lymphocytic neoplasm belonging to the leukosis-sarcoma group of the avian leukosis complex. The cause is an RNA C-type oncornavirus. Lymphocytes, which are transformed within the bursa of Fabricius, spread to the liver, spleen, and other organs to cause focal or diffuse enlargement. Also called *big liver disease* (outmoded), *visceral lymphomatosis* (outmoded).

myeloblastic leukosis   A rarely used term for ACUTE GRANULOCYTIC LEUKEMIA.

myelocytic leukosis   A rarely used term for CHRONIC GRANULOCYTIC LEUKEMIA.

leukotactic   Capable of attracting leukocytes, usually to an inflammatory focus.

leukotaxin   LEUKOTAXINE.

leukotaxine   A cell-free nitrogenous material prepared from inflammatory exudates and inflamed tissues that increases capillary permeability and attracts leukocytes. Also called *leukotaxin*. • Greater definition of chemoattractants in recent years has made this term obsolete.

leukotaxis   The active, ameboid, unidirectional migration of leukocytes toward an attractant, as in an inflammatory focus.

leukotherapy   The administration by transfusion of leukocytes obtained from donor blood. Also called *granulocyte transfusion*.

preventive leukotherapy   Transfusion of leukocytes obtained from donor blood to prevent bacterial infection, as when the recipient's blood neutrophil count is less than $0.5 \times 10^9/l$.

leukothrombopenia   Combined leukopenia and thrombocytopenia. A seldom used term.

leukotic   Pertaining to or affected by leukosis.

leukotome [LEUKO- + -TOME]   An instrument for dividing the white fibers of the cerebrum in performing a lobotomy.

leukotomy [LEUKO- + -TOMY]   A chiefly British term for FRONTAL LOBOTOMY.

transorbital leukotomy   A chiefly British term for TRANSORBITAL LOBOTOMY.

leukotoxic   Toxic to leukocytes, as a serum.

leukotoxin   LEUKOCYTOTOXIN.

leukotrichia [LEUKO- + TRICH- + -IA]   A state of possessing white hair.

leukotrichia annularis   An obsolete term for RINGED HAIR.

leukotrichous [LEUKO- + TRICH- + -OUS]   White-haired.

leukotrienes   A group of icosanoid compounds derived from 5-hydroperoxy-6,8,11,14-icosatetraenoic acid, and thus ultimately from arachidonic acid, that are mediators of the inflammatory reaction. Leukotriene A_4 is an unstable intermediate that is converted to leukotriene B_4, which is a chemoattractant for and an aggregator of neutrophils. Leukotrienes C_4, D_4, and E_4 play roles in anaphylaxis (and were formerly called the slow reacting substance of anaphylaxis).

leukourobilin   A colorless product of urobilin catabolism.

Leunbach [Jonathan Hugh *Leunbach*, Danish physician, born 1884]   See under PASTE.

Levaditi [Constantin *Levaditi*, Rumanian bacteriologist, 1874–1928]   See under METHOD.

levallorphan tartrate $C_{19}H_{25}NO \cdot C_4H_6O_6$.   9a-Allylmorphinan-3-ol-hydrogen tartrate, the tartrate salt form of levallorphan, a white crystalline powder. It is used as a narcotic antagonist, particularly to treat respiratory depression caused by narcotic administration. It is given parenterally.

levamfetamine $C_9H_{13}N$. *l*-α-methylbenzeneethanamine. This form has actions similar to racemic amphetamine, but is less potent than either the racemic or dextrorototory forms of amphetamine. Also *levamphetamine*.

levamfetamine succinate $C_9H_{13}N·C_4H_6O_4$. The succinate salt of levamfetamine (or amphetamine). It is employed therapeutically in the treatment of narcolepsy and hyperkinesis. It is also used as an anorexic agent in the treatment of obesity. It is given orally.

levamisole hydrochloride $C_{11}H_{12}N_2S·HCl$. (*S*)-2,3,5,6-Tetrahydro-6-phenylimidazo[2,1-*b*]thiazole monohydrochloride. The *l*- form of tetramisole, with anthelmintic properties. It is used orally to treat roundworm, hookworm, and *Strongyloides* infections, and is also employed as an investigational drug in the treatment of cancer as an immunopotentiator agent.

levamphetamine LEVAMFETAMINE.

levan A polysaccharide formed from fructose residues, especially the polysaccharide with 2,6-linkage, as opposed to inulin, which has 1,2-linkage. An older term.

levarterenol NOREPINEPHRINE.

levator [L *levat(us)* (past part. of *levare* to lift, raise, elevate, from *levis* light in weight) + *-or* -OR] (*plural* levatores) **1** A muscle that raises or lifts up the part into which it is inserted. **2** A surgical instrument used to elevate fragments of bone, especially of the skull.

levator claviculae An occasional detached slip of musculus levator scapulae that arises from the transverse processes of the upper two or the lower cervical vertebrae and is inserted on the lateral end of the clavicle. It is commonly found in many nonhuman vertebrates. Also called *omocervicalis*.

levatores Plural of LEVATOR.

LeVeen [Harry H. *LeVeen*, U.S. surgeon, born 1914] See under VALVE.

level [L *libella* (dim. of *libra* a level, pair of scales, balance) a level, plumb line] **1** A position or value relative to others in a scale; extent or degree. **2** In neuroanatomy, a plane or stage of complexity in the cerebrospinal axis, usually referring to geographic position as well as operational complexity.

action level A threshold concentration of a pollutant or contaminant that indicates a need for taking immediate preventive or remedial action. Also called *alert level*.

alert level **1** A threshold concentration of a pollutant or contaminant above which it is considered advisable to issue warnings to the population regarding potential hazards. In cases of air pollution, for example, it may involve the issuance of advice for persons suffering from heart or respiratory disease to stay indoors. **2** ACTION LEVEL.

level of anesthesia **1** The relative depth of narcosis in general anesthesia. **2** The segmental height of spinal or epidural anesthesia.

level of aspiration The standard, set by an individual, concerning expected success or failure at a given task. It is set before the activity has actually begun. It reflects an internally felt degree of confidence and varies over time as the result of objective success or failure in performance.

A-weighted sound level The response, expressed in dB(A), of a sound level meter, the electronic filtering of which approximates to the auditory sensitivity of the human ear. See also WEIGHTING NETWORK.

bone conduction hearing level The auditory threshold of a subject as measured by bone conduction. Also called *sensorineural acuity level*.

levels of brightness A range of illuminance levels recommended for various tasks or work areas. The levels recom-

mended by the Illuminating Engineering Society of Great Britain range from 3000 lux for minute work to 150 lux for an area with no continuous work. For routine work which is not fine the value is 500 lux. Individual needs have to be considered when choosing levels for particular tasks.

B-weighted sound level The sound pressure level of sounds measured using the B-weighting network which lies between the response curves of the A- and C-weighting networks of a sound level meter.

compensation level The level in an underwater vertical light gradient at which plant photosynthesis equals community respiration. Also called *compensation point, compensation depth, zone of effective light penetration*.

complement level The serum quantity of either a specified complement component, such as C3, or of the total functional sequence of complement proteins, specified by the function tested, as whole hemolytic complement.

continuous noise level The average or the minimum level of noise measured by a sound level meter during a specified period, such as during working hours. It is important for hearing conservation programs in those locations where there are high levels of ambient noise.

C-weighted sound level The sound pressure level of sounds, in decibels, measured using the C-weighting network of a sound level meter. The network gives a virtually linear response across the frequency spectrum.

derived working level A maximum acceptable level of a pollutant in specified media other than the target. It is determined to ensure that under specified circumstances a primary protection standard is not exceeded. Also called *ambient quality standard, derived standard, environmental standard, maximum permissible limit*.

developmental level The division of the life-span according to chronologic age, corresponding with major advancements in biopsychosocial organization. One system, for example, recognizes the neonatal period, from birth to one month; infancy, from one month to one year; childhood, from one year to puberty; adolescence, from puberty to 18 or 21 years; adulthood, from 21 to 65 years; senium, after 65 years of age.

effective perceived noise level A complex rating for airborne aircraft noise which includes correction factors for pure tone frequencies and noise duration. Symbol: L_{EPN}

environmental level The concentration of a substance, frequently a contaminant, in some specified part of the environment.

hearing level The level of intensity at which sounds are heard, as during pure tone audiometry. The acoustic energy of the sound stimulus is compared with an internationally accepted standard and expressed in dB HL. This measure is not identical with the A-weighted sound level, there being a nonlinear relationship between them. Abbreviation: HL

instinctual level The stage of development of a drive, usually described in terms of object relations or libidinal changes. The stages in the development of object relationships are the autoerotic or somatogenic, narcissistic, homoerotic, heteroerotic, and alloerotic. The libidinal stages are oral, anal, phallic, latency, and genitality.

isoelectric level BASELINE.

loudness discomfort level The level of loudness at which the subject complains of discomfort as the intensity of the sound is increasing. It is usually estimated on the pure tone audiometer and expressed in dB HL. Also called *threshold of discomfort*.

masking zero reference level The reference intensity for a noise, wide or narrow band, used for masking in audiometric investigations. See also MASKING LEVEL DIFFERENCE.

neurologic level The concept that the nervous system is organized in hierarchic levels, with the cerebral cortex representing the highest level.

no adverse effect level The dose level at and below which a substance or mixture of substances produces no harmful effect in a biologic system.

no detectable effect level NO OBSERVABLE EFFECT LEVEL.

no effect level NO OBSERVABLE EFFECT LEVEL.

noise level The intensity of ambient noise or of a particular noise. The conditions under which the noise is being measured need to be specified. Important features of noise measurement are its minimum continuous level, the duration and temporal pattern of the maxima, and the spectral distribution of acoustic energy.

noise emission level The level of noise measured at a specified distance from a noise-producing source such as an engine or machine.

no observable effect level The subthreshold dose level at and below which no adverse effects from the given substance can be observed. Also called *no detectable effect level, no effect level.*

perceived noise level See under EFFECTIVE PERCEIVED NOISE LEVEL.

sensation level The magnitude of acoustic energy required for sensory detection.

sensorineural acuity level BONE CONDUCTION HEARING LEVEL.

serum transaminase level The serum quantity of either glutamic oxalacetic transaminase or glutamic pyruvate transaminase, used as a measure of tissue damage.

level of significance The probability of rejecting a test hypothesis when it is in fact true; the likelihood of a type I error. See also STATISTICAL SIGNIFICANCE.

sound pressure level The acoustic force applied to the unit area of a sound-sensitive instrument such as a microphone. Its measure is a ratio of this force to the reference sound pressure of 20 μPa and recorded in dB SPL. Abbreviation: SPL

threshold level The lowest dose level of a test substance required to elicit a response.

tonal level The auditory threshold for pitch discrimination.

trophic levels The hierarchic levels in a food chain. At the first basic level is the green plant, or producer, above that the level of herbivore, and then various levels of carnivores.

leveling The tendency, in recall, to simplify the events and to leave out details, remembering the content of experience as being more balanced and regular than actually was the case.

Leventhal [Michael Leo *Leventhal*, U.S. obstetrician and gynecologist, 1901–1971] Stein-Leventhal syndrome. See under SYNDROME.

lever / dental lever DENTAL ELEVATOR.

leverage [Middle English *lever*, from Old French *leveour, levier* lever, from *lever* to lift, raise, from L *levare* to raise] The lift provided by a lever or elevator, or the mechanical advantage gained by it.

Lévi [Leopold *Lévi*, French endocrinologist, 1868–1933] **1** Lévi syndrome. See under LEOPOLD LÉVI SYNDROME. **2** Lévi-Lorain infantilism, Lorain-Lévi syndrome, Lévi-Lorain type. See under HYPOPHYSIAL DWARFISM. **3** Lévi-Lorain dwarf, Lorain-Lévi dwarf. See under HYPOPHYSIAL DWARF.

levicellular Composed of smooth muscle.

levigate To grind finely and obtain a smooth, uniform powder, usually with a mortar and pestle.

Levin [Max *Levin*, Russian-born U.S. neurologist, born 1901] Kleine-Levin syndrome. See under SYNDROME.

Levine [Max *Levine*, Polish-born U.S. bacteriologist, born 1889] Levine's EMB agar, Levine's eosin-methylene blue agar. See under EOSIN-METHYLENE BLUE AGAR.

Levine [Samuel A. *Levine*, U.S. physician and cardiologist, 1891–1966] **1** Levine's clenched-fist sign. See under CLENCHED FIST SIGN. **2** Lown-Ganong-Levine syndrome. See under SHORT PR SYNDROME.

levitation [English *levit(y)* (lightness) (from L *levit(as)* lightness, from *lev(is)* light + *-itas* -ITY; + -Y) + -ATION] **1** A sensation of floating; a sensation of being lighter than air. **2** Any of various systems for relieving pressure on the bed-ridden patient, as one suffering severe burns, by providing a cushion of air or by using air-filled or water-filled chambers to support the patient. A seldom used term.

levo- [L *laevus* (from Gk *laios* left) left, to the left] **1** A combining form meaning left, to or on the left. **2** In stereochemistry, a combining form designating the levorotatory enantiomer of a substance. Also *laevo- (British spelling).* Compare DEXTRO-. Symbol: (−)

levoangiocardiogram A radiograph obtained by levoangiocardiography.

levoangiocardiography Angiographic examination of the chambers of the left side of the heart.

levocardia [LEVO- + -CARDIA] The presence of a normally positioned heart on the left side in an individual with situs inversus of other asymmetrical viscera. Associated malformations are often found in the heart and aortic arch.

isolated levocardia Levocardia in the absence of associated cardiac or major arterial malformations.

mixed levocardia A congenital malformation in which the heart, located in the left chest, has discordant atrial and ventricular chambers, that is, either normally arranged atria and mirror-image ventricles, or mirror-image atria and normally arranged ventricles. Most frequently it is found also with ventriculoarterial discordance and is then known as "congenitally corrected transposition."

levocardiogram The part of the electrocardiogram which represents activity of the left ventricle. An outmoded term. Also called *levogram.*

levoclination [LEVO- + (in)clination] LEVOCYCLODUCTION.

levocondylism [LEVO- + condyl(e) + -ISM] Leftward deviation of the mandibular condyles.

levocycloduction [LEVO- + CYCLODUCTION] Cyclotorsion of the eye to the left (with respect to 12 o'clock). Also called *levoclination.*

levocycloversion [LEVO- + CYCLOVERSION] Simultaneous cyclotorsion of both eyes to the left (with respect to twelve o'clock).

levodopa $C_9H_{11}NO_4$. 3-Hydroxyl-L-tyrosine. The levorotatory isomeric form of dopa. It is administered orally in the treatment of Parkinson's disease.

Levo-Dromoran A proprietary name for levorphanol tartrate.

levoduction [LEVO- + L *duct(us)*, past part. of *ducere* to lead + -ION] The turning of an eye to the left side.

levogram LEVOCARDIOGRAM.

levonordefrin *l*-3,4-Dihydroxynorephedrine. A white, odorless, crystalline powder, practically insoluble in water, usually used as the hydrochloride salt. It is used as a vasoconstrictor in dentistry in a concentration of 1:20 000 in solutions of local anesthetic agents.

Levophed A proprietary name for *l*-norepinephrine acid tartrate.

levophobia Pathologic fear of the left or of objects on the left. Also called *sinistrophobia* (seldom used).

levorotatory [LEVO- + *rotatory*, from L *rotat(us)*, past part. of *rotare* to turn around + -ORY] Capable of rotating the plane of polarized light counterclockwise, when viewed towards the light source. Compare DEXTROROTATORY. Symbol: *l*-, ($-$)

levorphanol L-3-Hydroxy-*N*-methylmorphinan. It is used as a narcotic analgesic similarly to morphine, and is usually given as the tartrate salt.

levorphanol tartrate $C_{17}H_{23}NO \cdot C_4H_6O_6 \cdot 2H_2O$. 9a-Methyl-morphinan-3-ol hydrogen tartrate dihydrate, a synthetic narcotic possessing analgesic properties. It is a white crystalline powder and is administered subcutaneously or orally.

levothyroxine sodium $C_{15}H_{10}I_4NNa_4 \cdot H_2O$. The sodium salt of L-thyroxine hydrate. It is used as replacement therapy in patients with reduced or nonexistent thyroid function. It is a yellow, hygroscopic powder which is given orally.

levotorsion [LEVO- + TORSION] Cyclorotation of the eye to the left (with respect to twelve o'clock).

levoversion [LEVO- + VERSION] Conjugate rotation of both eyes to the left.

levoxadrol hydrochloride $C_{20}H_{24}ClNO_2$. 2,2-Diphenyl-4-(2-piperidyl)-1,3-dioxolane. It is the L-isomer of dioxadiol hydrochloride. It is used as a local anesthetic and smooth muscle relaxant drug.

Levoxan [NA] Levoxadrol hydrochloride.

Levret [André *Levret*, French obstetrician, 1703–1780] See under FORCEPS, MANEUVER, LAW.

Levugen A proprietary name for fructose.

levulinate A salt or ester derivative of levulinic acid.

levulinic acid $CH_3 — CO — CH_2 — CH_2 — COOH$. 4-Oxopentanoic acid. It is formed by heating hexoses in concentrated hydrochloric acid. Its identification as a product of the ozonolysis of rubber provided a vital clue to the head-to-tail nature of the isoprene units in that polymer. It is best known as its derivative aminolevulinic acid, an intermediate in the biosynthesis of porphyrins.

levulose An outmoded term for FRUCTOSE. • This name was originally given because, in contrast to glucose, it is levorotatory.

levulosemia FRUCTOSEMIA.

levurid An obsolete term for CANDIDIDE.

levuride An obsolete term for CANDIDIDE.

Levy [Robert Louis *Levy*, U.S. physician, 1888–1974] Levy, Rowntree, and Marriott method. See under METHOD.

Lévy [Gabrielle *Lévy*, French neurologist, 1886–1935] Lévy-Roussy syndrome, Roussy-Lévy disease. See under ROUSSY-LÉVY SYNDROME.

Lewandowsky [Felix *Lewandowsky*, German dermatologist, 1879–1921] 1 Nevus elasticus of Lewandowsky. See under NEVUS. 2 Lewandowsky syndrome. See under EPIDERMODYSPLASIA VERRUCIFORMIS. 3 Jadassohn-Lewandowsky syndrome. See under PACHYONYCHIA CONGENITA. 4 Jadassohn-Lewandowsky syndrome. See under PALMOPLANTAR KERATODERMA. 5 Miliary rosaceal tuberculide of Lewandowsky. See under ROSACEALIKE TUBERCULID. 6 Lewandowsky-Lutz disease. See under EPIDERMODYSPLASIA VERRUCIFORMIS.

Lewis [Gilbert Newton *Lewis*, U.S. chemist, 1875–1946] See under BASE, ACID.

Lewis [Mrs. H. D. G. *Lewis*, 20th-century English hospital patient] Lewis antibodies. See under ANTIBODY.

Lewis [Sir Thomas *Lewis*, English cardiologist 1881–1945] 1 Lewis and Pickering test. See under TEST. 2 H factor of Lewis. See under FACTOR. 3 Lewis reaction, triple response of Lewis. See under WHEAL-FLARE REACTION.

lewisite CHLOROVINYLDICHLOROARSINE.

Lewisohn [Richard *Lewisohn*, U.S. surgeon, 1875–1961] See under METHOD.

Lewy [Frederic H. *Lewy*, German-born neurologist active in the U.S., 1885–1950] Lewy bodies. See under BODY.

Lexis [Wilhelm Hector Richard Albrecht *Lexis*, German mathematician, 1837–1914] See under DIAGRAM.

Leyden [Ernst Victor von *Leyden*, German physician, 1832–1910] 1 Leyden's ataxia. See under DIABETIC PSEUDOTABES. 2 See under DISEASE, NEURITIS. 3 Duchenne-von Leyden syndrome. See under SYNDROME. 4 Leyden-Westphal ataxia. See under ATAXIA. 5 Leyden's crystals. See under CHARCOT-LEYDEN CRYSTALS. 6 Leyden-Moebius syndrome. See under SYNDROME. 7 Leyden-Moebius muscular dystrophy. See under LEYDEN-MOEBIUS MYOPATHY. 8 Leyden-Moebius dystrophy. See under LIMB-GIRDLE MUSCULAR DYSTROPHY.

Leydenia gemmipara A protozoan parasite presumed but never proved to be present in ascitic fluid of certain cancer patients.

Leydig [Franz von *Leydig*, German anatomist, 1821–1908] 1 Leydig's duct. See under MESONEPHRIC DUCT. 2 Sertoli-Leydig cell tumor. See under TUMOR. 3 Interstitial cells of Leydig. See under LEYDIG CELLS.

leydigarche [*Leydig (cells)* + Gk *archē* a beginning] The onset of gonadal function in the male. A seldom used term.

Lf [abbreviated from Latin *limes* limit, and *flocculation*] See under LF DOSE.

LFA left frontoanterior position (of a fetus). See under BROW ANTERIOR POSITION.

LFD least fatal dose.

L-forms Slowly growing, spherical cells of certain bacterial species that have lost the rigid murein layer. They are formed either spontaneously or after exposure to an agent that impairs wall synthesis. Some are due to mutations and revert slowly if at all. Others are due to undefined phenotypic changes, and their reversion is promoted by Mg^{2+} and by a high concentration of agar. Their relation to disease is uncertain. Also called *L-phase variants*. • *L* is derived from Lister Institute.

LFP left frontoposterior position (of a fetus). See under BROW POSTERIOR POSITION.

LFT left frontotransverse position (of a fetus). See under BROW TRANSVERSE POSITION.

LGH lactogenic hormone (prolactin).

LH luteinizing hormone.

Lhermitte [Jean *Lhermitte*, French physician, 1877–1959] 1 Claude and Lhermitte syndrome. See under HYPOTHALAMIC SYNDROME. 2 See under SIGN. 3 Lhermitte-McAlpine syndrome. See under SYNDROME.

LHRF luteinizing hormone releasing factor (gonadotropin releasing hormone).

LHRH luteinizing hormone releasing hormone.

Li Symbol for the element, lithium.

liability / professional liability 1 The obligation of professional practitioners such as physicians to assume responsibility for payment of damages resulting from their negligent acts in the care of patients. 2 The obligation of professional practitioners such as physicians to provide health care that adequately meets recognized standards of quality.

Lian [Camille Constant *Lian*, French physician, born 1882] See under POINT.

liana [Norman French *liane* (from French *lierne*, *liorne*, alterations (because of *lier* to bind) of *viorne*, a shrub of the family *caprifoliaceae*, from L *viburnum* the wayfaring tree) liana] A large, epiphytic, woody vine, common in the tropics, that relies on another plant for structural support.

liberomotor Describing or pertaining to voluntary movement. An outmoded term.

libidinal Relating to libido.

libidinous Possessing, exhibiting, or originating in libido.

libido [L, desire, appetite, passion for the opposite sex] The energy of the sexual drive in Freud's psychoanalytic psychology. It is often used to include the energy of the aggressive drive as well.

bisexual libido Libidinal or erotic cathexis of both female and male love objects as seen in one individual.

ego libido Libidinal energy that cathects the ego itself, as in narcissism.

object libido Libidinal energy that cathects objects other than the self.

Libman [Emanuel *Libman*, U.S. physician, 1872–1946] Libman-Sacks disease, Libman-Sacks syndrome. See under LIBMAN-SACKS ENDOCARDITIS.

libra [L, a pound of 12 ounces, a scale, balance] **1** A Spanish unit of mass or weight equal to 1.01 pound approximately; 0.46 kilogram. An obsolete unit. **2** An ancient Roman unit of mass or weight, a pound of 12 ounces, equal to 0.72 pound approximately; 0.33 kilogram approximately.

library [Middle English *librarie*, from Old French *libraire* a copyist, from L *librarius* a transcriber of books (noun), pertaining to books (adj.), from *liber* the inner bark of a tree, which was written on] An ordered collection of complete programs or subroutines written for a particular computer.

gene library A number of independently cloned DNA fragments which theoretically contain at least one copy of each gene of the organism from which the DNA was obtained.

Librium A proprietary name for chlordiazepoxide hydrochloride.

lice Plural of LOUSE.

license [L *licentia* (from *licens*, gen. *licentis*, pres. part. of *licere* to be permitted + *-ia* -IA) freedom, liberty] Permission or franchise granted by public authority for an individual to practice a profession or for an organization to provide certain specified services which are illegal to perform or provide in the absence of such approval.

licensure [*licens(e)* + -URE] The process or administrative function, usually based on a governmental authority, of issuing an exclusive franchise to individuals or organizations who have met certain standards to provide services or practice a profession.

institutional licensure **1** Permission or granting of authority, usually by a public agency, for a health care organization to provide specified services. **2** A proposed system in which institutions rather than individuals would be licensed to allow the practice of the health care professions and under the provisions of which professionals would function under the organization's authority.

licentiate [Middle English *licentiat*, from Med L *licentiat(us)*, past part. of *licentiare* to license, from L *licentia* freedom, liberty] The holder of a license.

lichen [Gk *leichēn*, also *lichēn* a tree moss, lichen, lichenlike eruption on the skin, scurvy, blight, canker] **1** A mutualistic form of plantlike life that is composed of a union of an alga and a fungus. **2** LICHEN PLANUS. **3** Any skin lesion that resembles lichen planus.

lichen acuminatus An obsolete term for LICHEN PLANUS.

acute bullous lichen planus A rare variant of lichen planus in which some of the lesions are surmounted by bullae.

lichen agrius Severe papular prurigo. An obsolete term.

lichen albus LICHEN SCLEROSUS ET ATROPHICUS.

lichen amyloidosus The most common form of cutaneous amyloidosis, consisting of discrete, firm, hemispherical papules. The papules are brown or yellow in color, smooth, and shining. In some cases, scaling may exist. The condition most often involves the lower legs. Also called *lichenoid amyloidosis*.

lichen annularis LICHEN PLANUS ANNULARIS.

lichen aureus A rare skin condition characterized by the development of a cluster of reddish brown lichenoid papules. Its etiology is unknown.

lichen axillaris FOX-FORDYCE DISEASE.

lichen chronicus simplex LICHEN SIMPLEX.

lichen corneus hypertrophicus Hyperkeratotic lichen planus.

erythematous lichen planus **1** Lichen planus in which the lesions are red rather than violaceous, but are otherwise typical. **2** Lichenoid eruptions that are not lichen planus, but they may include a distinct entity. An imprecise usage.

lichen fibromucinoidosus LICHEN MYXEDEMATOSUS.

follicular lichen planus LICHEN PLANOPILARIS.

lichen framboesianus A papular eruption that takes place during the secondary stage of yaws.

lichen hemorrhagicus Purpura that is characterized by hemorrhaging into the follicles. An obsolete term.

hypertrophic lichen planus Chronic hyperkeratotic lesions of lichen planus that are most frequently seen on the lower leg. Also called *lichen planus hypertrophicus, lichen ruber verrucosus, lichen planus verrucosus*.

lichen infantum An obsolete term for MILIARIA RUBRA.

lichen iris Ringworm with concentric annular lesions. An obsolete term.

lichen myxedematosus The widespread proliferation of fibroblasts and the deposition of acid mucopolysaccarides in the skin. It is a rare disorder. Also called *scleromyxedema, papular myxedema, lichen fibromucinoidosus, papular mucinosis*.

lichen nitidus A rare skin disease believed to be a variant of lichen planus in which very small shiny papules develop particularly on the arms, trunk, and penis. Also called *Pinkus disease*.

lichen obtusus PRURIGO NODULARIS.

lichen obtusus corneus PRURIGO NODULARIS.

oral erosive lichen planus Lichen planus of the oral mucous membrane presenting as multiple superficial erosions.

oral nonerosive lichen planus Lichen planus of the oral mucous membrane presenting as the characteristic fine bluish white network and in the absence of superficial ulceration.

lichen pilaris LICHEN PLANOPILARIS.

lichen planopilaris Lichen planus in which the typical lesions are associated with follicular lesions that cause follicular destruction and cicatricial alopecia. Also called *lichen pilaris, follicular lichen planus*.

lichen planus A common skin disease of unknown cause, characterized by an eruption of violaceous papules, which are of variable morphology and extent. Also called *lichen ruber planus, Wilson's lichen, lichen acuminatus* (obsolete), *lichen*.

lichen planus annularis Lichen planus in which the papules are in an annular configuration. Also called *lichen annularis*.

lichen planus atrophicus Lichen planus that is followed by atrophy of the characteristic papules.

lichen planus et acuminatus atrophicans Follicular lichen planus leading to atrophy of the characteristic papules and subsequently to cicatricial alopecia. It occurs on the scalp and other areas.

lichen planus hypertrophicus HYPERTROPHIC LICHEN PLANUS.

lichen planus linearis Lichen planus in a linear configuration, which usually occurs as an isomorphic effect at the site of a scratch.

lichen planus morpheicus LICHEN SCLEROSUS ET ATROPHICUS.

lichen planus obtusus PRURIGO NODULARIS.

lichen planus verrucosus HYPERTROPHIC LICHEN PLANUS.

lichen ruber acuminatus PITYRIASIS RUBRA PILARIS.

lichen ruber moniliformis A rare skin disorder, in which red beaded papules arranged in lines affect the skin extensively. Also called *morbus moniliformis lichenoides.*

lichen ruber planus LICHEN PLANUS.

lichen ruber verrucosus HYPERTROPHIC LICHEN PLANUS.

lichen sclerosus et atrophicans LICHEN SCLEROSUS ET ATROPHICUS.

lichen sclerosus et atrophicus A superficial form of scleroderma which may be widely distributed, but affects most frequently the penis or the vulva. Also called *lichen sclerosus et atrophicans, dermatitis lichenoides chronica atrophicans, Csillag's disease, white-spot disease, lichen albus, leukokraurosis, lichen planus morpheicus.*

lichen scorbuticus A follicular purpura sometimes seen in scurvy. Slight hemorrhage into the lesions is often seen.

lichen scrofulosorum A tuberculid consisting of grouped lichenoid follicular papules. Also called *papular scrofuloderma, tuberculosis cutis lichenoides, acne scrofulosorum* (outmoded), *tuberculosis lichenoides, lichen scrofulosus.*

lichen scrofulosus LICHEN SCROFULOSORUM.

lichen simplex A response in some predisposed skins to rubbing. It is seen as isolated lesions, mainly on the nape of the neck and the lateral aspects of the lower leg in men. It often complicates eczema of any origin. In many cases no history of any preceeding disease is known, but some cause must have brought on the irritation that led to the scratching or rubbing. Also called *circumscribed neurodermatitis, Vidal's disease, lichen simplex chronicus, lichen chronicus simplex, lichen Vidal.*

lichen simplex chronicus LICHEN SIMPLEX.

lichen spinulosus A rare disease in which follicular horny papules arise in groups, each surmounted by a horny spine.

lichen striatus A linear inflammatory dermatosis of unknown origin, occurring principally on a limb and in childhood. It resolves spontaneously after weeks or months. Also called *linear dermatitis.*

lichen strophulosus An obsolete term for MILIARIA RUBRA.

lichen tropicus MILIARIA RUBRA.

lichen urticatus An outmoded term for PAPULAR URTICARIA.

lichen Vidal LICHEN SIMPLEX.

Wilson's lichen LICHEN PLANUS.

lichenase An enzyme (EC 3.2.1.73) that catalyzes hydrolysis of 1,4-β-glucosidic linkages in polysaccharides that contain both 1,3- and 1,4-glucosidic linkages, but not in those that contain only one of these types. One susceptible polysaccharide is lichenin.

licheniasis [LICHEN + -IASIS] The presence of a lichenoid eruption. An obsolete term.

lichenification [LICHEN + i + -FICATION] Thickening of the epidermis with increased prominence of the surface markings of the skin that is produced by repeated rubbing. Also called *eczema hypertrophicum, lichenization.*

licheniformin Any of a group of antibiotics isolated from *Bacillus subtilis.* Their properties resemble those of subtilin.

lichenin A polysaccharide from lichens which contains both 1,3- and 1,4-linked glucose residues.

lichenization LICHENIFICATION.

lichenoid Resembling lichen planus. Also *lichenous.*

lichenous LICHENOID.

Lichtheim [Ludwig *Lichtheim*, German physician, 1845–1928] **1** See under APHASIA, TEST. **2** Lichtheim syndrome. See under SUBACUTE COMBINED DEGENERATION OF THE SPINAL CORD. **3** Proust-Lichtheim maneuver. See under MANEUVER. **4** Lichtheim plaques. See under PLAQUE. **5** Dejerine-Lichtheim phenomenon, Lichtheim's phenomenon. See under LICHTHEIM SIGN.

licorice GLYCYRRHIZA.

lid [Old English *hlid* lid, gate] EYELID.

granular lids MARGINAL BLEPHARITIS.

tucked lid of Collier Retraction of the upper eyelid in ophthalmoplegia due to a supranuclear midbrain lesion.

Liddell [Edward George Tandy *Liddell*, English physiologist, born 1895] Liddell-Sherrington reflex. See under REFLEX.

Lidex A proprietary name for fluocinonide.

lidocaine $C_{14}H_{22}N_2O.$ 2-(Diethylamino)-N-(2,6-dimethylphenyl)acetamide. A white, crystalline powder, practically insoluble in water, very soluble in alcohol and chloroform, very soluble in ether and in oils. It is a local anesthetic applied in sprays and creams to skin and mucous membranes. Also called *lignocaine.*

lidocaine hydrochloride $C_{14}H_{22}N_2O \cdot HCl \cdot H_2O.$ A monohydrate, white, crystalline powder, soluble in water and alcohol and insoluble in ether. Injectable as a water-soluble local anesthetic, it is more potent than procaine, and has antiarrhythmic and anticonvulsant properties as well.

lidoflazine 4-[4,4-Bis(p-fluorophenyl)butyl]-1-piperazine aceto-2′,6′-xylidide. An agent with coronary vasodilator and cardiac stimulant properties.

lie [Old English *licgan* to lie, akin to L *lectus* a bed, Gk *lechos* a bed] The relationship of the long axis of the fetus to that of the mother.

life lie The neurotic defense of blaming fate or other people for one's own failures.

longitudinal lie A lie in which the long axis of both mother and fetus are in the same plane during labor.

oblique lie A lie in which the long axes of mother and fetus cross each other at an angle of 45° during labor.

transverse lie A lie in which the long axes or mother and fetus cross at an angle of 90° during labor. Except in very special circumstances, the fetus cannot be delivered vaginally in this situation. Also called *cross birth, torso presentation, transverse presentation, trunk presentation.*

Lieberkühn [Johannes Nathanael *Lieberkühn*, German anatomist, 1711–1756] **1** Lieberkühn's follicles, glands of Lieberkühn, crypts of Lieberkühn. See under GLANDULAE INTESTINALES. **2** See under AMPULLA.

Liebermann [Carl Theodore *Liebermann*, German chemist, 1842–1914] Burchardt-Liebermann test, Burchard-Liebermann reaction, Liebermann-Burchardt reaction. See under LIEBERMANN-BURCHARDT TEST.

Liebermeister [Carl von *Liebermeister*, German physician, 1833–1901] **1** Liebermeister's grooves. See under GROOVE. **2** See under RULE.

Liebig [Baron Justus von *Liebig*, German chemist, 1803–1873] See under LAW.

Liebreich [Richard *Liebreich*, Russian ophthalmologist, 1830–1917] See under SYMPTOM.

lien [L (akin to Gk *splēn* the spleen), the spleen] SPLEN.

lien accessorius SPLEN ACCESSORIUS.

lien mobilis FLOATING SPLEEN.

lien succenturiatus SPLEN ACCESSORIUS.

lien- LIENO-.

lienal Pertaining to the spleen; splenic.

lienculus SPLEN ACCESSORIUS.

lienectomy [LIEN- + -ECTOMY] SPLENECTOMY.

lienitis SPLENITIS.

lieno- [L *lien* and *lienis* (Gk *splēn*) spleen] A combining form denoting the spleen. Also *lien-.*

lienocele Hernia of the spleen; splenocele.

lienography [LIENO- + -GRAPHY] SPLENOGRAPHY.

lienointestinal Pertaining to the spleen and the intestine.

lienomalacia   SPLENOMALACIA.

lienomedullary   SPLENOMEDULLARY.

lienomyelogenous   SPLENOMEDULLARY.

lienomyelomalacia   SPLENOMYELOMALACIA.

lienopancreatic   Pertaining to the spleen and the pancreas; splenopancreatic.

lienopathy   SPLENOPATHY.

lienorenal   Pertaining to the spleen and the kidney; splenonephric; splenorenal.

lienotoxin   SPLENOTOXIN.

lienteric   Related to or characterized by lientery.

lientery [Gk *leienter(ia)* (from *lei(os)* smooth + *enter(on)* a piece of gut + *-ia* -Y) a passing of one's food undigested]   Diarrhea in which the feces contain undigested food.

lienunculus   SPLEN ACCESSORIUS.

Liesegang [Raphael Eduard *Liesegang*, German chemist, 1869–1947]   **1** Liesegang rings. See under RING.   **2** Liesegang's waves. See under LIESEGANG'S PHENOMENON.

Lieutaud [Joseph *Lieutaud*, French physician, 1703–1780]   **1** Lieutaud's triangle, Lieutaud's trigone, trigonum vesicae lieutaudi. See under TRIGONUM VESICAE.   **2** Lieutaud's uvula, Lieutaud's luette. See under UVULA VESICAE.

LIF   **1** leukocyte migration inhibition factor.   **2** left iliac fossa.

life [Old English *líf*]   The condition that distinguishes organisms from inorganic substances, characterized especially by metabolism and the capacity to grow and reproduce.
  antenatal life   Existence before birth, especially of the conceptus in viviparous animals in the intrauterine period.
  average life   MEAN EFFECTIVE LIFE.
  embryonic life   The functional activity or the period of functional activity at the embryo stage of development. In humans it is usually restricted to the first eight weeks of intrauterine life.
  fetal life   The functional activity or the period of functional activity at the fetal stage of development. In humans it is usually restricted to the period of intrauterine life that follows the first eight weeks.
  intellectual life   MENTAL LIFE.
  intrauterine life   The functional activity or the period of functional activity associated with development of an animal *in utero*. Also called *uterine life*.
  mean life   MEAN EFFECTIVE LIFE.
  mean effective life   The mean duration of existence of molecules, particles, or constituents of specified decaying nuclides, chemical substances, or biologic systems, the rate of decay often decreasing as an exponential curve. Also called *mean life, average life, mean time*.
  mental life   The functional activity associated with sensation, reasoning, and voluntary action. An outmoded term. Also called *psychic life, intellectual life*.
  potential years of life lost   A measure of the estimated effect that early deaths from a specified cause have on a given population compared to that population's normal life expectancy. Abbreviation: PYLL
  psychic life   MENTAL LIFE.
  sexual life   The directions and manifestations of the sexual drive that contribute to a person's life-style, sometimes confined to genital activity and sometimes referring to all of the manifestations of libidinal energy in the subject's personality and relationships. An imprecise usage.
  uterine life   INTRAUTERINE LIFE.
  vegetative life   **1** The level of functional activity attributable to plants.   **2** The automatic functional activity associated with mechanisms, such as metabolism and reproduction, that are essential for continued existence.

life-span   The period of time between birth and death.

life-style   The unique mode of living that characterizes an individual and lends consistency to the general patterning of his behavior, including all of the assumptions, motives, cognitive styles, and patterns of coping employed by that person in pursuit of the basic goals of life.

lig.   ligament; ligamentum.

ligament

ligament [L *ligamentum*. See LIGAMENTUM.]   LIGAMENTUM.

accessory ligament   A fibrous band that strengthens the capsule of a joint, either external or internal to it.

accessory atlantoaxial ligament   A fibrous band extending between the lateral mass of the atlas near the lower attachment of the transverse ligament and the body of the axis adjacent to the base of the dens, thereby strengthening each of the lateral atlantoaxial joints posteromedially.

accessory ligaments of digits of hand   LIGAMENTA PALMARIA ARTICULATIONUM METACARPOPHALANGEALIUM.

accessory ligament of humerus   An outmoded term for LIGAMENTUM CORACOHUMERALE.

accessory ligaments of metacarpophalangeal joints   LIGAMENTA COLLATERALIA ARTICULATIONUM METACARPOPHALANGEARUM.

accessory patellar ligaments   Ligamentum meniscofemorale anterius and ligamentum meniscofemorale posterius.

accessory plantar ligaments   LIGAMENTA PLANTARIA ARTICULATIONUM METATARSOPHALANGEALIUM.

accessory transverse ligament of scapula   An inconstant small fibrous band situated above and parallel to the superior transverse ligament of the scapula and deep to the suprascapular artery.

accessory volar ligaments   LIGAMENTA PALMARIA ARTICULATIONUM METACARPOPHALANGEALIUM.

acromioclavicular ligament   LIGAMENTUM ACROMIOCLAVICULARE.

acromiocoracoid ligament   An outmoded term for LIGAMENTUM CORACOACROMIALE.

adipose ligament of knee of Cruveilhier   An outmoded term for PLICA SYNOVIALIS INFRAPATELLARIS.

alar ligaments   **1** LIGAMENTA ALARIA.   **2** An outmoded term for PLICAE ALARES.

alar ligaments of knee   An outmoded term for PLICAE ALARES.

alveolodental ligament   PERIODONTIUM.

annular ligament of base of stapes   LIGAMENTUM ANNULARE STAPEDIS.

annular ligaments of digits of foot   PARS ANNULARIS VAGINAE FIBROSAE DIGITORUM PEDIS.

annular ligaments of digits of hand   PARS ANNULARIS VAGINAE FIBROSAE DIGITORUM MANUS.

annular ligament of femur   ZONA ORBICULARIS ARTICULATIONIS COXAE.

annular ligaments of fingers   PARS ANNULARIS VAGINAE FIBROSAE DIGITORUM MANUS.

annular ligament of radius   LIGAMENTUM ANNULARE RADII.

annular ligament of stapes   LIGAMENTUM ANNULARE STAPEDIS.

annular ligaments of tendon sheaths of fingers   PARS ANNULARIS VAGINAE FIBROSAE DIGITORUM MANUS.

annular ligament of Weber　An outmoded term for ZONA ORBICULARIS ARTICULATIONIS COXAE.

anococcygeal ligament　LIGAMENTUM ANOCOCCYGEUM.

anterior ligament of the ankle joint　The thin anterior part of the capsule of the talocrural joint attached to the articular margins of the tibia and malleoli superiorly and to the talus inferiorly.

anterior annular ligament of tarsus　An outmoded term for RETINACULUM MUSCULORUM EXTENSORUM PEDIS INFERIUS.

anterior atlantoaxial ligament　A ligament between the anterior arch of the atlas and the anterior surface of the axis and lying behind the anterior longitudinal ligament. It reinforces the capsule of the lateral atlantoaxial joint. An outmoded term.

anterior atlanto-occipital ligament　MEMBRANA ATLANTO-OCCIPITALIS ANTERIOR.

anterior auricular ligament　LIGAMENTUM AURICULARE ANTERIUS.

anterior ligament of bladder　Either ligamentum puboprostaticum or ligamentum pubovesicale.

anterior carpometacarpal ligaments　LIGAMENTA CARPOMETACARPALIA PALMARIA.

anterior cervical ligament　An outmoded term for MEMBRANA TECTORIA.

anterior ligament of colon　An outmoded term for TAENIA OMENTALIS.

anterior costocentral ligament　LIGAMENTUM CAPITIS COSTAE RADIATUM.

anterior costotransverse ligament　LIGAMENTUM COSTOTRANSVERSARIUM ANTERIUS.

anterior cruciate ligament　LIGAMENTUM CRUCIATUM ANTERIUS GENUS.

anterior cruciate ligament of knee　LIGAMENTUM CRUCIATUM ANTERIUS GENUS.

anterior fibrous ligament　An outmoded term for LIGAMENTUM STERNOCLAVICULARE ANTERIUS.

anterior ligament of head of fibula　LIGAMENTUM CAPITIS FIBULAE ANTERIUS.

anterior ligament of head of rib　LIGAMENTUM CAPITIS COSTAE RADIATUM.

anterior iliosacral ligaments　An outmoded term for LIGAMENTA SACROILIACA ANTERIORA.

anterior inguinal ligament　An outmoded term for CRUS MEDIALE ANNULI INGUINALIS SUPERFICIALIS.

anterior intermetacarpal ligament　An outmoded term for LIGAMENTUM METACARPEUM TRANSVERSUM PROFUNDUM.

anterior longitudinal ligament　LIGAMENTUM LONGITUDINALE ANTERIUS.

anterior ligament of malleus　LIGAMENTUM MALLEI ANTERIUS.

anterior meniscofemoral ligament　LIGAMENTUM MENISCOFEMORALE ANTERIUS.

anterior metacarpophalangeal ligaments　An outmoded term for LIGAMENTA PALMARIA ARTICULATIONUM METACARPOPHALANGEALIUM.

anterior metatarsal ligament　An outmoded term for LIGAMENTUM METATARSALE TRANSVERSUM PROFUNDUM.

anterior ligament of neck of rib　LIGAMENTUM COSTOTRANSVERSARIUM ANTERIUS.

anterior petrosphenoid ligament　SYNCHONDROSIS SPHENOPETROSA.

anterior phrenicopericardiac ligament　A fibrous band connecting the base of the fibrous pericardium to the anterior part of the central tendon of the diaphragm. An outmoded term.

anterior plantar metatarsal ligament　An outmoded term for LIGAMENTUM METATARSALE TRANSVERSUM PROFUNDUM.

anterior pubic ligament of Cruveilhier　An outmoded term for DISCUS INTERPUBICUS.

anterior radiate ligament of head of rib　An outmoded term for LIGAMENTUM CAPITIS COSTAE RADIATUM.

anterior radiocarpal ligament　LIGAMENTUM RADIOCARPALE PALMARE.

anterior ligament of radiocarpal joint　LIGAMENTUM RADIOCARPALE PALMARE.

anterior radioulnar ligament　A slight thickening of the anterior aspect of the fibrous capsule of the distal radioulnar joint. An outmoded term.

anterior sacrococcygeal ligament　LIGAMENTUM SACROCOCCYGEUM ANTERIUS.

anterior sacroiliac ligaments　LIGAMENTA SACROILIACA ANTERIORA.

anterior sacrosciatic ligament　LIGAMENTUM SACROSPINALE.

anterior scaphotrapezium ligament　A short bundle of the palmar ligaments of the midcarpal joint which extends between the base of the tubercle of the scaphoid and the anterior surface of the trapezium. An outmoded term.

anterior stellate ligament　An outmoded term for LIGAMENTUM CAPITIS COSTAE RADIATUM.

anterior sternoclavicular ligament　LIGAMENTUM STERNOCLAVICULARE ANTERIUS.

anterior superior ligament of neck of rib　LIGAMENTUM COSTOTRANSVERSARIUM ANTERIUS.

anterior talocalcaneal ligament　LIGAMENTUM TALOCALCANEUM ANTERIUS.

anterior talofibular ligament　LIGAMENTUM TALOFIBULARE ANTERIUS.

anterior talotibial ligament　PARS TIBIOTALARIS ANTERIOR LIGAMENTI MEDIALIS.

anterior tarsal ligament　An outmoded term for RETINACULUM MUSCULORUM EXTENSORUM PEDIS INFERIUS.

anterior tibiofibular ligament　LIGAMENTUM TIBIOFIBULARE ANTERIUS.

anterior triangular ligament of pubis　An outmoded term for LIGAMENTUM ARCUATUM PUBIS.

anterior true ligament of bladder　**1** LIGAMENTUM PUBOPROSTATICUM. **2** LIGAMENTUM PUBOVESICALE.

anterior volar ligament of wrist　An outmoded term for RETINACULUM FLEXORUM MANUS.

anteroinferior sacroiliac ligament　The strong inferior part of the anterior sacroiliac ligament, one part of which connects the third piece of the sacrum with the lateral margin of the preauricular sulcus, while the other part is attached along the superior margin of the greater sciatic notch adjacent to the posterior inferior iliac spine. An outmoded term.

anterosuperior sacroiliac ligament　The superior part of the anterior sacroiliac ligament which connects the superior surface of the ala of the sacrum with the ilium on either side of the arcuate line. An outmoded term.

ligament of antibrachium of Weitbrecht　An outmoded term for CHORDA OBLIQUA.

apical ligament of dens　LIGAMENTUM APICIS DENTIS AXIS.

apical dental ligament　LIGAMENTUM APICIS DENTIS AXIS.

apical odontoid ligament　LIGAMENTUM APICIS DENTIS AXIS.

appendiculo-ovarian ligament　A secondary peritoneal fold occasionally found between the mesoappendix and the broad ligament of the uterus.

Arantius ligament　LIGAMENTUM VENOSUM.

arcuate ligaments　An outmoded term for LIGAMENTA FLAVA.

arcuate ligament of knee　LIGAMENTUM POPLITEUM ARCUATUM.

arcuate popliteal ligament　LIGAMENTUM POPLITEUM ARCUATUM.

arcuate pubic ligament　LIGAMENTUM ARCUATUM PUBIS.

Arnold's ligament LIGAMENTUM INCUDIS SUPERIUS.

articular ligament of vertebrae An outmoded term for CAPSULA ARTICULARIS ARTICULATIONUM VERTEBRARUM.

arytenoepiglottic ligament PLICA ARYEPIGLOTTICA.

atlanto-occipital obturator ligament An outmoded term for MEMBRANA ATLANTO-OCCIPITALIS ANTERIOR.

ligaments of auditory ossicles LIGAMENTA OSSICULORUM AUDITUS.

ligaments of auricle LIGAMENTA AURICULARIA.

axis ligament of malleus An outmoded term for LIGAMENTUM MALLEI LATERALE.

Barkow's ligament 1 Vertical fibers of the part of the capsule of the elbow joint that pass through the pad of fat in the olecranon fossa of the humerus. **2** The anterior and posterior portions of the fibrous capsule of the elbow joint.

basal pelviprostatic ligament An outmoded term for FASCIA PROSTATAE.

Bellini's ligament The fibrous bandlike extension of the ischiofemoral ligament to the greater trochanter of the femur.

Béraud's ligament A fibrous band connecting the upper part of the pericardium to the front of the third thoracic vertebra and the disk below it and occasionally to the prevertebral cervical fascia. Also called *pericardiovertebral ligament.*

Berry's ligament LIGAMENTUM THYROHYOIDEUM LATERALE.

Bertin's ligament LIGAMENTUM ILIOFEMORALE.

Bichat's ligament LONG POSTERIOR SACROILIAC LIGAMENT.

bifurcate ligament LIGAMENTUM BIFURCATUM.

bifurcated ligament LIGAMENTUM BIFURCATUM.

Bigelow's ligament LIGAMENTUM ILIOFEMORALE.

bigeminate ligaments of Arnold LIGAMENTA TARSOMETATARSALIA DORSALIA.

ligament of Botallo LIGAMENTUM ARTERIOSUM.

Bourgery's ligament LIGAMENTUM POPLITEUM OBLIQUUM.

brachiocubital ligament An outmoded term for LIGAMENTUM COLLATERALE ULNARE.

brachioradial ligament An outmoded term for LIGAMENTUM COLLATERALE RADIALE.

broad ligament of liver LIGAMENTUM FALCIFORME HEPATIS.

broad ligament of lung An outmoded term for LIGAMENTUM PULMONALE.

broad ligament of uterus LIGAMENTUM LATUM UTERI.

Brodie's ligament TRANSVERSE HUMERAL LIGAMENT.

Burns ligament MARGO FALCIFORMIS HIATUS SAPHENUS.

calcaneocuboid ligament LIGAMENTUM CALCANEOCUBOIDEUM.

calcaneofibular ligament LIGAMENTUM CALCANEOFIBULARE.

calcaneonavicular ligament LIGAMENTUM CALCANEONAVICULARE.

calcaneotibial ligament PARS TIBIOCALCANEUS LIGAMENTI MEDIALIS.

ligament between calcaneus and fifth metatarsal A strong band of the lateral part of the plantar aponeurosis which extends between the lateral process of the calcaneal tuberosity and the base of the fifth metatarsal bone. Occasionally it contains muscle fibers.

Caldani's ligament LIGAMENTUM CORACOCLAVICULARE.

Campbell's ligament SUSPENSORY LIGAMENT OF AXILLA.

Camper's ligament DIAPHRAGMA UROGENITALE.

canthal ligament Any of three ligaments: (1) ligamentum palpebrale laterale; (2) ligamentum palpebrale mediale; (3) raphe palpebralis lateralis. An outmoded term.

capsular ligaments 1 LIGAMENTA CAPSULARIA. **2** Articular capsules. See under CAPSULA ARTICULARIS.

capsular ligament of atlanto-occipital joint CAPSULA ARTICULARIS ATLANTO-OCCIPITALIS.

capsular ligament of hip joint CAPSULA ARTICULARIS COXAE.

capsular ligament of sternocostal joint CAPSULA ARTICULARIS STERNOCOSTALIS.

capsular ligament of temporomandibular joint CAPSULA ARTICULARIS ARTICULATIONIS TEMPOROMANDIBULARIS.

Carcassonne's ligament MEMBRANA PERINEI.

cardinal ligament LATERAL CERVICAL LIGAMENT.

caroticoclinoid ligament An intraclinoid ligament between the anterior and the middle clinoid processes on either side of the body of the sphenoid bone, often ossified and converted into a foramen transmitting the internal carotid artery.

carpal ligaments The ligaments of the wrist, including retinaculum extensorum, retinaculum flexorum, and ligamentum carpi radiatum. An outmoded term.

carpal dorsal ligaments LIGAMENTA INTERCARPALIA DORSALIA.

Casser's ligament LIGAMENTUM MALLEI LATERALE.

casserian ligament LIGAMENTUM MALLEI LATERALE.

caudal ligament of common integument RETINACULUM CAUDALE.

cemental ligament PERIODONTIUM.

central ligament of spinal cord An obsolete term for FILUM TERMINALE.

ceratocricoid ligament LIGAMENTUM CERATOCRICOIDEUM.

cervical ligament of sinus tarsi An oblique fibrous band situated behind the attachment of the bifurcated ligament lateral to the sinus tarsi, extending upwards and medially from the superolateral aspect of the calcaneus to the inferolateral aspect of the neck of the talus. It helps to limit extensive inversion of the foot.

cervical ligament of uterus LATERAL CERVICAL LIGAMENT.

cervicobasilar ligament An outmoded term for MEMBRANA TECTORIA.

check ligament A ligament that checks or limits the movement of a muscle or joint; specifically, one of the check ligaments of the axis (ligamenta alaria), or of the eyeball, medial and lateral (lacertus musculi recti lateralis bulbi).

check ligaments of axis LIGAMENTA ALARIA.

chondroxiphoid ligaments LIGAMENTA COSTOXIPHOIDEA.

ligament of Chopart LIGAMENTUM BIFURCATUM.

ciliary ligament An outmoded term for MUSCULUS CILIARIS.

circular ligament PERIODONTIUM.

ligament of Civinini LIGAMENTUM PTERYGOSPINALE.

Clado's ligament An occasional secondary peritoneal band or fold between the mesoappendix and the infundibulopelvic ligament.

Cloquet's ligament RUDIMENT OF VAGINAL PROCESS.

collateral ligaments LIGAMENTA COLLATERALIA.

collateral ligaments of interphalangeal articulations of foot LIGAMENTA COLLATERALIA ARTICULATIONUM INTERPHALANGEARUM PEDIS.

collateral ligaments of interphalangeal articulations of hand LIGAMENTA COLLATERALIA ARTICULATIONUM INTERPHALANGEARUM MANUS.

collateral ligaments of interphalangeal joints of foot LIGAMENTA COLLATERALIA ARTICULATIONUM INTERPHALANGEARUM PEDIS.

collateral ligaments of interphalangeal joints of hand LIGAMENTA COLLATERALIA ARTICULATIONUM INTERPHALANGEARUM MANUS.

collateral ligaments of joints of fingers LIGAMENTA COLLATERALIA ARTICULATIONUM INTERPHALANGEARUM MANUS.

collateral ligaments of joints of toes LIGAMENTA COLLATERALIA ARTICULATIONUM INTERPHALANGEARUM PEDIS.

collateral ligaments of metacarpophalangeal articulations LIGAMENTA COLLATERALIA ARTICULATIONUM METACARPOPHALANGEARUM.

collateral ligaments of metatarsophalangeal articulations LIGAMENTA COLLATERALIA ARTICULATIONUM METATARSOPHALANGEARUM.

collateral ligaments of midcarpal joint Short ligaments on the radial and ulnar sides of the midcarpal joint. The radial ligament is the stronger and more distinct of the two and runs between the scaphoid and trapezium while the ulnar ligament connects the triquetrum and the hamate. They are continuous with the corresponding collateral ligaments of the wrist joint.

Colles ligament LIGAMENTUM REFLEXUM.

ligaments of colon An outmoded term for TAENIAE COLI.

common ligament of knee of Weber LIGAMENTUM TRANSVERSUM GENUS.

conjugate ligament A ligament found in the costovertebral joints of some mammals which is homologous to the intra-articular ligament in humans.

conoid ligament LIGAMENTUM CONOIDEUM.

Cooper's ligament 1 LIGAMENTUM PECTINEALE. 2 CHORDA OBLIQUA. 3 One of the ligamenta suspensoria mammaria.

Cooper suspensory ligaments LIGAMENTA SUSPENSORIA MAMMARIA.

coracoacromial ligament LIGAMENTUM CORACOACROMIALE.

coracocapsular ligaments LIGAMENTA CINGULI EXTREMITATIS SUPERIORIS.

coracoclavicular ligament LIGAMENTUM CORACOCLAVICULARE.

coracohumeral ligament LIGAMENTUM CORACOHUMERALE.

coracoid ligament of scapula LIGAMENTUM TRANSVERSUM SCAPULAE SUPERIUS.

cordiform ligament of diaphragm An outmoded term for CENTRUM TENDINEUM.

corniculopharyngeal ligament A fibroelastic band extending from the corniculate cartilage inferiorly toward the midline, where it joins the pharyngeal mucosa and the corresponding opposite ligament behind the transverse and oblique arytenoid muscles to form the cricopharyngeal ligament which descends centrally. Also called *cricosantorinian ligament, ligamentum jugale* (outmoded).

coronary ligament of the knee Fibers of the deep surface of the fibrous capsule of the knee joint that are attached to the peripheral margins of the medial and lateral menisci and to the corresponding margins of the condyles of the tibia, to which each meniscus is firmly held by each ligament.

coronary ligament of liver LIGAMENTUM CORONARIUM.

coronary ligament of radius An outmoded term for LIGAMENTUM ANNULARE RADII.

costoclavicular ligament LIGAMENTUM COSTOCLAVICULARE.

costocolic ligament LIGAMENTUM PHRENICOCOLICUM.

costocoracoid ligament An outmoded term for LIGAMENTUM TRANSVERSUM SCAPULAE SUPERIUS.

costolaminar ligament of Trolard A costovertebral ligament which extends between the superior border of the neck of a rib and the inferior border of the lamina of the adjacent vertebra above it.

costopericardiac ligament An extension of one of the bands of the sternopericardiac ligaments to the posterior aspect of the first sternocostal joint. Also called *Lannelongue's ligament.*

costotransverse ligament LIGAMENTUM COSTOTRANSVERSARIUM.

costovertebral ligament LIGAMENTUM CAPITIS COSTAE RADIATUM.

costovertebral interosseous ligament of Cruveilhier An outmoded term for LIGAMENTUM CAPITIS COSTAE INTRA-ARTICULARE.

costoxiphoid ligaments LIGAMENTA COSTOXIPHOIDEA.

cotyloid ligament LABRUM ACETABULARE.

Cowper's ligament FASCIA PECTINEA.

cricopharyngeal ligament LIGAMENTUM CRICOPHARYNGEUM.

cricopharyngeal ligament of Luschka LIGAMENTUM CRICOPHARYNGEUM.

cricosantorinian ligament 1 LIGAMENTUM CRICOPHARYNGEUM. 2 CORNICULOPHARYNGEAL LIGAMENT.

cricothyroarytenoid ligament An outmoded term for CONUS ELASTICUS LARYNGIS.

cricothyroid ligament LIGAMENTUM CRICOTHYROIDEUM MEDIANUM.

cricotracheal ligament LIGAMENTUM CRICOTRACHEALE.

cricotracheal ligament of Luschka A median thickening of the ligamentum cricotracheale. An outmoded term.

crucial ligaments of fingers PARS CRUCIFORMIS VAGINAE FIBROSAE DIGITORUM MANUS.

crucial ligament of foot RETINACULUM MUSCULORUM EXTENSORUM PEDIS INFERIUS.

cruciate ligaments LIGAMENTA CRUCIATA GENUS.

cruciate ligament of atlas LIGAMENTUM CRUCIFORME ATLANTIS.

cruciate ligaments of fingers PARS CRUCIFORMIS VAGINAE FIBROSAE DIGITORUM MANUS.

cruciate ligaments of knee LIGAMENTA CRUCIATA GENUS.

cruciate ligament of leg RETINACULUM MUSCULORUM EXTENSORUM PEDIS INFERIUS.

cruciate ligaments of toes PARS CRUCIFORMIS VAGINAE FIBROSAE DIGITORUM PEDIS.

cruciform ligament of atlas LIGAMENTUM CRUCIFORME ATLANTIS.

crural ligament LIGAMENTUM INGUINALE.

Cruveilhier's ligaments LIGAMENTA PLANTARIA ARTICULATIONUM METATARSOPHALANGEALIUM.

cubitoradial ligament An outmoded term for CHORDA OBLIQUA.

cubitoulnar ligament An outmoded term for LIGAMENTUM COLLATERALE ULNARE.

cubonavicular ligament Either ligamentum cuboideonaviculare plantare or ligamentum cuboideonaviculare dorsale.

cutaneophalangeal ligaments Fibrous strands extending from the sides of phalanges near the joints to the skin.

cysticoduodenal ligament An occasionally persisting remnant of the embryonic ventral mesentery extending between the gallbladder and the first or second portion of the duodenum or the pylorus. Also called *cystoduodenal ligament, cholecystoduodenal band, cholecystoduodenocolic fold.*

cystoduodenal ligament CYSTICODUODENAL LIGAMENT.

deep atlanto-occipital ligament MEMBRANA ATLANTO-OCCIPITALIS ANTERIOR.

deep bifurcate ligaments An outmoded term for LIGAMENTA TARSOMETATARSALIA PLANTARIA.

deep bifurcate ligaments of Arnold An outmoded term for LIGAMENTA TARSOMETATARSALIA PLANTARIA.

deep common ligament of wrist joint An outmoded term for LIGAMENTUM COLLATERALE CARPI RADIALE.

deep dorsal sacrococcygeal ligament LIGAMENTUM SACROCOCCYGEUM POSTERIUS PROFUNDUM.

deep radioscapholunate ligament One or more deep bundles of the palmar radiocarpal ligament which extend obliquely between the anterior surface of the distal end of the radius and the scaphoid and lunate bones. An outmoded term.

deep ligaments of tarsus LIGAMENTA TARSI PROFUNDA.

deep transverse metacarpal ligament LIGAMENTUM METACARPEUM TRANSVERSUM PROFUNDUM.

deep transverse metatarsal ligament LIGAMENTUM METATARSALE TRANSVERSUM PROFUNDUM.

deep transverse palmar ligament LIGAMENTUM METACARPEUM TRANSVERSUM PROFUNDUM.

deep transverse volar ligaments of carpus An outmoded term for LIGAMENTA METACARPALIA PALMARIA.

deltoid ligament Either ligamentum mediale articulationis talocruralis or ligamentum collaterale ulnare.

deltoid ligament of ankle LIGAMENTUM MEDIALE ARTICULATIONIS TALOCRURALIS.

deltoid ligament of elbow LIGAMENTUM COLLATERALE ULNARE.

deltoid ligament of talocrural joint LIGAMENTUM MEDIALE ARTICULATIONIS TALOCRURALIS.

Denonvilliers ligament SEPTUM RECTOVESICALE.

dental ligament The horizontal group of fibers of the periodontium attached to the neck of a tooth.

dentate ligament of spinal cord LIGAMENTUM DENTICULATUM.

denticulate ligament LIGAMENTUM DENTICULATUM.

Denucé's ligament LIGAMENTUM QUADRATUM.

diaphragmatic ligament An involuted remnant of the cranial genital fold in the embryo. In the female it becomes the suspensory ligament of the ovary.

digital vaginal ligaments Vaginae fibrosae digitorum manus and vaginae fibrosae digitorum pedis.

distal intermetacarpal ligament LIGAMENTUM METACARPEUM TRANSVERSUM PROFUNDUM.

distal plantar intermetatarsal ligament LIGAMENTUM METATARSALE TRANSVERSUM PROFUNDUM.

dorsal ligaments of bases of metacarpal bones LIGAMENTA METACARPALIA DORSALIA.

dorsal ligaments of bases of metatarsal bones LIGAMENTA METATARSALIA DORSALIA.

dorsal calcaneocuboid ligament A thin, wide band in the dorsal part of the capsule of the calcaneocuboid joint which is attached some distance from the articular margins and lies lateral to the calcaneocuboid ligament of the bifurcate ligament.

dorsal calcaneonavicular ligament LIGAMENTUM CALCANEONAVICULARE DORSALE.

dorsal carpal ligament RETINACULUM EXTENSORUM MANUS.

dorsal carpometacarpal ligaments LIGAMENTA CARPOMETACARPALIA DORSALIA.

dorsal common annular ligament An outmoded term for RETINACULUM EXTENSORUM MANUS.

dorsal cuboideonavicular ligament LIGAMENTUM CUBOIDEONAVICULARE DORSALE.

dorsal cuneocuboid ligament LIGAMENTUM CUNEOCUBOIDEUM DORSALE.

dorsal cuneonavicular ligaments LIGAMENTA CUNEONAVICULARIA DORSALIA.

dorsal intercarpal ligaments LIGAMENTA INTERCARPALIA DORSALIA.

dorsal intercuneiform ligaments LIGAMENTA INTERCUNEIFORMIA DORSALIA.

dorsal intermetacarpal ligaments LIGAMENTA METACARPALIA DORSALIA.

dorsal intermetatarsal ligaments LIGAMENTA METATARSALIA DORSALIA.

dorsal intertarsal ligaments LIGAMENTA TARSI DORSALIA.

dorsal metacarpal ligaments LIGAMENTA METACARPALIA DORSALIA.

dorsal metatarsal ligaments LIGAMENTA METATARSALIA DORSALIA.

dorsal posterior annular ligament of wrist An outmoded term for RETINACULUM EXTENSORUM MANUS.

dorsal proximal intermetatarsal ligaments An outmoded term for LIGAMENTA METATARSALIA DORSALIA.

dorsal radiocarpal ligament LIGAMENTUM RADIOCARPALE DORSALE.

dorsal ligament of radiocarpal joint LIGAMENTUM RADIOCARPALE DORSALE.

dorsal radioscaphoid ligament An accessory bundle of ligamentum radiocarpale dorsale which extends from the styloid process of the radius to the posterior surface of the scaphoid. An outmoded term.

dorsal radioulnar ligament A thickening of the dorsal aspect of the capsule of the distal radioulnar articulation. An outmoded term.

dorsal sacroiliac ligaments LIGAMENTA SACROILIACA DORSALIA.

dorsal scaphotriquetral ligament The superior fasciculus of the ligamenta intercarpalia dorsalia which extends between the dorsal surfaces of the scaphoid and the triquetrum. An outmoded term.

dorsal talonavicular ligament LIGAMENTUM TALONAVICULARE.

dorsal tarsometatarsal ligaments LIGAMENTA TARSOMETATARSALIA DORSALIA.

dorsal ligaments of tarsus LIGAMENTA TARSI DORSALIA.

dorsal transverse intermetacarpal ligaments An outmoded term for LIGAMENTA METACARPALIA DORSALIA.

dorsal transverse intermetatarsal ligaments An outmoded term for LIGAMENTA METATARSALIA DORSALIA.

dorsal transverse ligaments of wrist An outmoded term for LIGAMENTA INTERCARPALIA DORSALIA.

dorsal ligament of wrist RETINACULUM EXTENSORUM MANUS.

Douglas ligament PLICA RECTOUTERINA.

ligament of ductus venosus LIGAMENTUM VENOSUM.

duodenohepatic ligament LIGAMENTUM HEPATODUODENALE.

duodenorenal ligament LIGAMENTUM DUODENORENALE.

epididymal ligament Either ligamentum epididymidis superius or ligamentum epididymidis inferius.

epihyal ligament LIGAMENTUM STYLOHYOIDEUM.

external annular ligament of ankle RETINACULUM MUSCULORUM PERONEORUM SUPERIUS.

external annular ligament of malleolus An outmoded term for RETINACULUM MUSCULORUM EXTENSORUM PEDIS INFERIUS.

external arcuate ligament of diaphragm An outmoded term for LIGAMENTUM ARCUATUM LATERALE.

external capsular clavicular ligament An outmoded term for LIGAMENTUM ACROMIOCLAVICULARE.

external coracoclavicular ligament An outmoded term for LIGAMENTUM TRAPEZOIDEUM.

external inguinal ligament An outmoded term for LIGAMENTUM INGUINALE.

external intercostal ligament MEMBRANA INTERCOSTALIS EXTERNA.

external intermuscular ligament of arm An outmoded term for SEPTUM INTERMUSCULARE BRACHII LATERALE.

external intermuscular ligament of thigh An outmoded term for SEPTUM INTERMUSCULARE FEMORIS LATERALE.

external laciniate ligament RETINACULUM MUSCULORUM PERONEORUM SUPERIUS.

external lateral ligament of knee LIGAMENTUM COLLATERALE FIBULARE.

external lateral ligament of temporomandibular joint LIG-

AMENTUM LATERALE ARTICULATIONIS TEMPOROMANDIBULARIS.

external lateral ligament of wrist joint   LIGAMENTUM COLLATERALE CARPI RADIALE.

external ligament of mandibular articulation   An outmoded term for LIGAMENTUM LATERALE ARTICULATIONIS TEMPOROMANDIBULARIS.

external ligament of neck of rib   An outmoded term for LIGAMENTUM COSTOTRANSVERSARIUM POSTERIUS.

external popliteal ligament   RETINACULUM LIGAMENTI ARCUATI.

external sphenoidal ligament   **1** LIGAMENTUM INTERFOVEOLARE.   **2** One of the ligamenta intercuneiformia plantaria. An outmoded usage.

external superior ligament of neck of rib   An outmoded term for LIGAMENTUM COSTOTRANSVERSARIUM POSTERIUS.

extracapsular accessory ligaments   Any supplementary supportive ligaments distinct from and external to an articular capsule which are additional to its usual extracapsular ligaments.

fabellofibular ligament   An occasional fibrous band extending between the fabella of the lateral head of the gastrocnemius muscle and the apex of the head of the fibula.

falciform ligament   PROCESSUS FALCIFORMIS LIGAMENTI SACROTUBERALIS.

falciform ligament of liver   LIGAMENTUM FALCIFORME HEPATIS.

fallopian ligament   An outmoded term for LIGAMENTUM INGUINALE.

ligament of Fallopius   An outmoded term for LIGAMENTUM INGUINALE.

false ligament   **1** The peritoneum reflected from the superior surface and apex of the urinary bladder to either the anterior abdominal wall or the walls of the pelvis. Occasionally this is divided into superior, lateral, and posterior false ligaments.   **2** Any ligament that is actually a peritoneal fold and not truly ligamentous in structure.

Ferrein's ligament   LIGAMENTUM LATERALE ARTICULATIONIS TEMPOROMANDIBULARIS.

fibrous ligaments of breast   LIGAMENTA SUSPENSORIA MAMMARIA.

fibular collateral ligament   LIGAMENTUM COLLATERALE FIBULARE.

fibular collateral ligament of knee joint   LIGAMENTUM COLLATERALE FIBULARE.

fibular intermuscular ligament   An outmoded term for SEPTUM INTERMUSCULARE CRURIS ANTERIUS.

flaval ligaments   LIGAMENTA FLAVA.

Flood's ligament   The superior glenohumeral ligament of the shoulder joint. See also LIGAMENTA GLENOHUMERALIA.

fundiform ligament of penis   LIGAMENTUM FUNDIFORME PENIS.

gastrocolic ligament   **1** LIGAMENTUM GASTROCOLICUM.   **2** A segment of the dorsal mesogastrium in the embryo which is attached along the inferior border (greater curvature) of the stomach and forms the anterior peritoneal sheet, doubled, of the omental bursa, and is finally included within the greater omentum.

gastrohepatic ligament   LIGAMENTUM HEPATOGASTRICUM.

gastrolienal ligament   LIGAMENTUM GASTROSPLENICUM.

gastropancreatic ligaments of Huschke   PLICAE GASTROPANCREATICAE.

gastrophrenic ligament   LIGAMENTUM GASTROPHRENICUM.

gastrosplenic ligament   LIGAMENTUM GASTROSPLENICUM.

genitoinguinal ligament   The ridge extending from the caudal pole of the gonad to the inguinal region of the embryo, through which it passes to the ipsilateral labioscrotal fold. The guber-

naculum differentiates within the ridge and constitutes a potential pathway for the descent of the gonad. In the male, descent is complete so that the ridge disappears, but in the female, descent of the ovary is only partial, and the lower part of the ridge persists as the round ligaments of the ovary and uterus. Also called *ligamentum genitoinguinale, plica gubernatrix, inguinal fold, caudal genital fold, plica inguinalis.*

Gerdy's ligament   SUSPENSORY LIGAMENT OF AXILLA.

Gillette suspensory ligament   TENDO CRICOESOPHAGEUS.

Gimbernat's ligament   LIGAMENTUM LACUNARE.

gingivodental ligament   The dentogingival fibers of the periodontal membrane.

ligaments of girdle of inferior extremity   LIGAMENTA CINGULI EXTREMITATIS INFERIORIS.

ligaments of girdle of superior extremity   LIGAMENTA CINGULI EXTREMITATIS SUPERIORIS.

glenohumeral ligaments   LIGAMENTA GLENOHUMERALIA.

glenoid ligaments of Cruveilhier   LIGAMENTA PLANTARIA ARTICULATIONUM METATARSOPHALANGEALIUM.

glenoid ligament of humerus   An outmoded term for LABRUM GLENOIDALE.

glenoid ligament of Macalister   An outmoded term for LABRUM GLENOIDALE.

glenoid ligament of mandibular fossa   An outmoded and inappropriate term for DISCUS ARTICULARIS ARTICULATIONIS TEMPOROMANDIBULARIS.   ● It was probably so called because it is both thin and, occasionally, perforated, in the center and attached posteriorly, where it is thick, to the posterior wall of the articular capsule. Although the articular surface of the mandibular fossa is linked by thick fibrous tissue containing few cartilage cells, there is no specific rim of fibrocartilage attached to the periphery of the fossa.

great posterior pelvic ligament   An outmoded term for LIGAMENTUM SACROTUBERALE.

great sacrosciatic ligament   LIGAMENTUM SACROTUBERALE.

Gruber's ligament   PETROSPHENOID LIGAMENT.

ligament of Gunther   Dense connective tissue which may connect the anterior parts of the adherent fascial sheets investing the gluteus medius and minimus muscles so as to form an intermuscular septum that gives the appearance of a common tendon. Occasionally the connective tissue and fascial sheets may be so poorly developed that the muscles are fused.

Günz ligament   A layer of the obturator membrane.

hamatometacarpal ligament   An outmoded term for LIGAMENTUM PISOMETACARPEUM.

hammock ligament   A slinglike arrangement of collagen fibers that separate the apex of the developing root of a tooth from the fundus of its socket. Although original descriptions suggested otherwise, it is not attached to bone.

ligament of head of femur   LIGAMENTUM CAPITIS FEMORIS.

Helmholtz ligament   **1** A band of fibers of the anterior ligament of the malleus attached to the greater tympanic spine of the tympanic notch.   **2** The posterior part of the lateral ligament of the malleus.

ligaments of Helvetius   LIGAMENTA PYLORI.

Henle's ligament   A fascial expansion of the lowermost part of the rectus abdominis muscle tendon or sheath, or of part of the aponeurosis of the transversus abdominis muscle that reinforces the deep surface of the conjoined tendon, or falx inguinalis. Originally Henle included this expansion and Hesselbach's ligament in the description of the falx inguinalis. See also HENLE'S BAND.

Hensing's ligament   LIGAMENTUM PHRENICOCOLICUM.

hepatic ligaments   Peritoneal folds between the liver and surrounding structures.

hepatocolic ligament   LIGAMENTUM HEPATOCOLICUM.

hepatocystocolic ligament An occasional extension of the hepatocolic ligament to the gallbladder.

hepatoduodenal ligament LIGAMENTUM HEPATODUODENALE.

hepatoesophageal ligament LIGAMENTUM HEPATOESOPHAGEUM.

hepatogastric ligament LIGAMENTUM HEPATOGASTRICUM.

hepatogastroduodenal ligament OMENTUM MINUS.

hepatorenal ligament LIGAMENTUM HEPATORENALE.

hepatoumbilical ligament An outmoded term for LIGAMENTUM TERES HEPATIS.

Hesselbach's ligament LIGAMENTUM INTERFOVEOLARE.

Hey's ligament MARGO FALCIFORMIS HIATUS SAPHENUS.

Holl's ligament A ligamentous band joining the two corpora cavernosa clitoridis anterior to the external urethral ostium.

Hueck's ligament RETICULUM TRABECULARE SCLERAE.

Humphry's ligament LIGAMENTUM MENISCOFEMORALE ANTERIUS.

Hunter's ligament LIGAMENTUM TERES UTERI.

Huschke's ligaments PLICAE GASTROPANCREATICAE.

hyaloideocapsular ligament Circular fibers adhering the posterior surface of the capsule of the lens of the eye to the vitreous body.

hyoepiglottic ligament LIGAMENTUM HYOEPIGLOTTICUM.

hyothyroid ligaments Ligamentum thyrohyoideum laterale and ligamentum thyrohyoideum medianum. An outmoded term.

hypsiloid ligament LIGAMENTUM ILIOFEMORALE.

iliocostal ligament An outmoded term for LIGAMENTUM LUMBOCOSTALE.

iliofemoral ligament LIGAMENTUM ILIOFEMORALE.

iliolumbar ligament LIGAMENTUM ILIOLUMBALE.

iliopectineal ligament ARCUS ILIOPECTINEUS.

iliopubic ligament An outmoded term for LIGAMENTUM INGUINALE.

iliotibial ligament of Maissiat TRACTUS ILIOTIBIALIS.

iliotrochanteric ligament The lateral band of the iliofemoral ligament, extending between the anterior superior iliac spine and the greater trochanter and adjacent upper end of the intertrochanteric line of the femur.

ligament of the incus Ligamentum incudis posterius or ligamentum incudis superius.

inferior acromioclavicular ligament An inconstant ligament connecting the inferior surface of the acromion to the inferior surface of the lateral extremity of the clavicle. An outmoded term.

inferior annular ligament An outmoded term for LIGAMENTUM ARCUATUM PUBIS.

inferior arcuate ligament of pubis LIGAMENTUM ARCUATUM PUBIS.

inferior calcaneonavicular ligament LIGAMENTUM CALCANEONAVICULARE PLANTARE.

inferior ligament of epididymis LIGAMENTUM EPIDIDYMIDIS INFERIUS.

inferior glenohumeral ligament The lowest of the three bands of the glenohumeral ligaments, which extends from the upper part of the medial margin of the glenoid cavity and the adjacent glenoid labrum to the lower part of the anatomical neck of the humerus. See also LIGAMENTA GLENOHUMERALIA.

inferior metatarsophalangeal ligaments LIGAMENTA PLANTARIA ARTICULATIONUM METATARSOPHALANGEALIUM.

inferior ligament of neck of rib The posterior portion of ligamentum costotransversarium superius. An outmoded term.

inferior ligament of neck of rib of Henle LIGAMENTUM COSTOTRANSVERSARIUM.

inferior pubic ligament LIGAMENTUM ARCUATUM PUBIS.

inferior sternopericardial ligament The lower of the two ligamenta sternopericardiaca, which extends from the anteroin-

ferior part of the fibrous pericardium to the posterior surface of the lower end of the sternum and the xiphisternum.

inferior thyroarytenoid ligament An outmoded term for LIGAMENTUM VOCALE.

inferior transverse ligament of scapula LIGAMENTUM TRANSVERSUM SCAPULAE INFERIUS.

inferior ligament of tubercle of rib LIGAMENTUM COSTOTRANSVERSARIUM LATERALE.

infundibulo-ovarian ligament FIMBRIA OVARICA.

infundibulopelvic ligament LIGAMENTUM SUSPENSORIUM OVARII.

inguinal ligament LIGAMENTUM INGUINALE.

inguinal ligament of Blumberg An outmoded term for LIGAMENTUM INTERFOVEOLARE.

inguinal ligament of Cooper LIGAMENTUM PECTINEALE.

inguinal ligament of the kidney The caudal portion of the mesonephros in the inguinal region. An outmoded term.

interarticular ligaments An outmoded term for LIGAMENTA INTRACAPSULARIA.

interarticular ligament of articulation of humerus An outmoded term for CAPUT LONGUM MUSCULI BICIPITIS BRACHII.

interarticular chondrosternal ligament LIGAMENTUM STERNOCOSTALE INTRA-ARTICULARE.

interarticular costocentral ligament An outmoded term for LIGAMENTUM CAPITIS COSTAE INTRA-ARTICULARE.

interarticular ligament of head of rib An outmoded term for LIGAMENTUM CAPITIS COSTAE INTRA-ARTICULARE.

interarticular ligament of hip joint An outmoded term for LIGAMENTUM CAPITIS FEMORIS.

interarticular sternocostal ligament An outmoded term for LIGAMENTUM STERNOCOSTALE INTRA-ARTICULARE.

interchondral ligament 1 Either the medial or the lateral ligament which strengthens the thin fibrous capsule of each interchondral joint. 2 An outmoded term for MEMBRANA INTERCOSTALIS EXTERNA.

interclavicular ligament LIGAMENTUM INTERCLAVICULARE.

interclinoid ligament A band of dura mater extending between any two clinoid processes on either side of the body of the sphenoid bone. The caroticoclinoid ligament is an example.

intercornual ligament LIGAMENTUM SACROCOCCYGEUM LATERALE.

interfoveolar ligament LIGAMENTUM INTERFOVEOLARE.

interlaminar ligaments LIGAMENTA FLAVA.

intermaxillary ligament An outmoded term for RAPHE PTERYGOMANDIBULARIS.

internal annular ligament An outmoded term for RETINACULUM MUSCULORUM FLEXORUM PEDIS.

internal annular ligament of ankle An outmoded term for RETINACULUM MUSCULORUM FLEXORUM PEDIS.

internal annular ligament of malleolus An outmoded term for RETINACULUM MUSCULORUM FLEXORUM PEDIS.

internal arcuate ligament of diaphragm An outmoded term for LIGAMENTUM ARCUATUM MEDIALE.

internal calcaneocuboid ligament An outmoded term for LIGAMENTUM CALCANEOCUBOIDEUM.

internal capsular ligament An outmoded term for LIGAMENTUM CAPITIS FEMORIS.

internal coracoclavicular ligament An outmoded term for LIGAMENTUM CONOIDEUM.

internal inguinal ligament 1 An outmoded term for LIGAMENTUM REFLEXUM. 2 An outmoded term for CRUS MEDIALE ANNULI INGUINALIS SUPERFICIALIS.

internal intercostal ligament MEMBRANA INTERCOSTALIS INTERNA.

internal intermuscular ligament of arm An outmoded term for SEPTUM INTERMUSCULARE BRACHII MEDIALE.

internal interosseous ligaments of Barkow An outmoded term for LIGAMENTA INTERCUNEIFORMIA PLANTARIA.

internal lateral ligament of knee LIGAMENTUM COLLATERALE TIBIALE.

internal lateral ligament of temporomandibular joint An outmoded term for LIGAMENTUM SPHENOMANDIBULARE.

internal lateral ligament of wrist joint An outmoded term for LIGAMENTUM COLLATERALE CARPI ULNARE.

internal ligament of neck of rib An outmoded term for LIGAMENTUM COSTOTRANSVERSARIUM SUPERIUS.

internal patellar ligament An outmoded term for RETINACULUM PATELLAE MEDIALE.

internal sacrosciatic ligament An outmoded term for LIGAMENTUM SACROSPINALE.

interosseous ligaments of bases of metacarpal bones LIGAMENTA METACARPALIA INTEROSSEA.

interosseous ligaments of bases of metatarsal bones LIGAMENTA METATARSALIA INTEROSSEA.

interosseous ligaments of carpal bones LIGAMENTA INTERCARPALIA INTEROSSEA.

interosseous carpometacarpal ligaments Two more or less fused fibrous bands which are extensions of the palmar carpometacarpal ligament and connect the contiguous surfaces of the distal margins of the capitate and hamate bones with the adjacent surfaces of the third and fourth metacarpal bones.

interosseous cuboideonavicular ligament A ligament composed of strong transverse fibers which connects the nonarticular parts of the adjacent surfaces of the cuboid and navicular bones. It may also be continuous with the dorsal and plantar cuboideonavicular ligaments.

interosseous cuneometatarsal ligaments LIGAMENTA CUNEOMETATARSALIA INTEROSSEA.

interosseous iliosacral ligaments An outmoded term for LIGAMENTA SACROILIACA INTEROSSEA.

interosseous intercarpal ligaments LIGAMENTA INTERCARPALIA INTEROSSEA.

interosseous intercuneiform ligaments LIGAMENTA INTERCUNEIFORMIA INTEROSSEA.

interosseous intermetacarpal ligaments LIGAMENTA METACARPALIA INTEROSSEA.

interosseous intermetatarsal ligaments LIGAMENTA METATARSALIA INTEROSSEA.

interosseous intertarsal ligaments LIGAMENTA TARSI INTEROSSEA.

interosseous ligaments of knee An outmoded term for LIGAMENTA CRUCIATA GENUS.

interosseous ligament of leg An outmoded term for MEMBRANA INTEROSSEA CRURIS.

interosseous metacarpal ligaments LIGAMENTA METACARPALIA INTEROSSEA.

interosseous metatarsal ligaments LIGAMENTA METATARSALIA INTEROSSEA.

interosseous ligament of pubis **1** An outmoded term for DISCUS INTERPUBICUS. **2** An outmoded term for LIGAMENTUM TRANSVERSUM PERINEI.

interosseous ligament of pubis of Winslow An outmoded term for LIGAMENTUM TRANSVERSUM PERINEI.

interosseous sacroiliac ligaments LIGAMENTA SACROILIACA INTEROSSEA.

interosseous talocalcaneal ligament LIGAMENTUM TALOCALCANEUM INTEROSSEUM.

interosseous ligaments of tarsus LIGAMENTA TARSI INTEROSSEA.

interosseous ligament of tibiofibular syndesmosis A series of short, thick fibrous bands which connect the adjacent rough surfaces of the inferior tibiofibular joint or synchondrosis and

are continuous superiorly with the crural interosseous membrane.

interosseous transverse metatarsal ligament An outmoded term for LIGAMENTA METATARSALIA INTEROSSEA.

interprocess ligament A fibrous band between two processes on a bone.

interpubic ligament An outmoded term for DISCUS INTERPUBICUS.

interspinal ligaments LIGAMENTA INTERSPINALIA.

interspinous ligaments LIGAMENTA INTERSPINALIA.

intertransverse ligaments LIGAMENTA INTERTRANSVERSARIA.

intertransverse ligaments of vertebral arch LIGAMENTA INTERTRANSVERSARIA.

interureteral ligament An outmoded term for PLICA INTERURETERICA.

intervertebral ligaments An outmoded term for DISCI INTERVERTEBRALES.

intra-articular ligaments LIGAMENTA INTRACAPSULARIA.

intra-articular costovertebral ligament LIGAMENTUM CAPITIS COSTAE INTRA-ARTICULARE.

intra-articular ligament of head of rib LIGAMENTUM CAPITIS COSTAE INTRA-ARTICULARE.

intra-articular sternocostal ligament LIGAMENTUM STERNOCOSTALE INTRA-ARTICULARE.

intrinsic ligament A taut ligament between two points on the same bone or on another anatomical structure.

intrinsic ligaments of the auricle A number of short fibrous bands connecting some projections of the cartilage of the auricle of the ear, the main ones being between the tragus and the helix, thereby completing the meatus anteriorly and bounding the concha, and between the tail of the helix and the anthelix. There are also a few less conspicuous bands on the cranial surface of the auricle.

ischiocapsular ligament An outmoded term for LIGAMENTUM ISCHIOFEMORALE.

ischiofemoral ligament LIGAMENTUM ISCHIOFEMORALE.

ischioprostatic ligament An outmoded term for DIAPHRAGMA UROGENITALE.

ischiosacral ligaments Ligamentum sacrotuberale and ligamentum sacrospinale. An outmoded term.

Jarjavay's ligaments The uterosacral ligament and the rectovaginal fold.

Krause's ligament LIGAMENTUM TRANSVERSUM PERINEI.

labial ligament The terminal fibrous strands of the round ligament of the uterus where it attaches to the connective tissue of the upper part of the labium majus.

laciniate ligament RETINACULUM MUSCULORUM FLEXORUM PEDIS.

lacunar ligament LIGAMENTUM LACUNARE.

lacunar ligament of Gimbernat LIGAMENTUM LACUNARE.

lambdoid ligament An outmoded term for RETINACULUM MUSCULORUM EXTENSORUM PEDIS INFERIUS.

Lannelongue's ligament COSTOPERICARDIAC LIGAMENT.

lateral accessory ligament of Henle An outmoded term for LIGAMENTUM LATERALE ARTICULATIONIS TEMPOROMANDIBULARIS.

lateral ligament of the ankle LATERAL LIGAMENT OF THE ANKLE JOINT.

lateral ligament of the ankle joint A strengthening capsular ligament on the lateral side of the talocrural joint comprising three fascicles attached to the lateral malleolus and described as separate ligaments, namely, ligamentum talofibulare anterius, ligamentum talofibulare posterius, and ligamentum calcaneofibulare between them. Also called *lateral ligament of the ankle*.

lateral arcuate ligament LIGAMENTUM ARCUATUM LATERALE.

lateral atlanto-occipital ligament LIGAMENTUM ATLANTO-OCCIPITALE LATERALE.

lateral ligaments of the bladder Thickenings of fibroareolar tissue connecting the sides of the urinary bladder to the tendinous arch of the pelvic fascia on each side.

lateral cervical ligament A bandlike condensation of pelvic fascia at the base of the broad ligament of the uterus, extending from the side of the cervix and the upper end and lateral fornix of the vagina to the fibroareolar tissue around the blood vessels on the lateral wall of the pelvis. It is one of the important supporting ligaments of the uterus. Also called *cervical ligament of uterus, cardinal ligament, Mackenrodt's ligament, transverse cervical ligament of Mackenrodt.*

lateral check ligament of eyeball LACERTUS MUSCULI RECTI LATERALIS BULBI.

lateral ligament of colon An outmoded term for TAENIA OMENTALIS.

lateral costotransverse ligament LIGAMENTUM COSTO-TRANSVERSARIUM LATERALE.

lateral ligament of elbow LIGAMENTUM COLLATERALE RADIALE.

lateral intermuscular ligament of arm An outmoded term for SEPTUM INTERMUSCULARE BRACHII LATERALE.

lateral intermuscular ligament of thigh An outmoded term for SEPTUM INTERMUSCULARE FEMORIS LATERALE.

lateral ligaments of joints of fingers LIGAMENTA COLLATERALIA ARTICULATIONUM INTERPHALANGEARUM MANUS.

lateral ligaments of joints of toes LIGAMENTA COLLATERALIA ARTICULATIONUM INTERPHALANGEARUM PEDIS.

lateral ligament of knee LIGAMENTUM COLLATERALE FIBULARE.

lateral ligaments of liver Ligamentum triangulare dextrum hepatis and ligamentum triangulare sinistrum hepatis. An outmoded term.

lateral ligament of malleus LIGAMENTUM MALLEI LATERALE.

lateral maxillary ligament An outmoded term for LIGAMENTUM LATERALE ARTICULATIONIS TEMPOROMANDIBULARIS.

lateral meniscofemoral ligament An outmoded term for LIGAMENTUM MENISCOFEMORALE POSTERIUS.

lateral metacarpophalangeal ligaments LIGAMENTA COLLATERALIA ARTICULATIONUM METACARPOPHALANGEARUM.

lateral ligaments of metacarpophalangeal joints LIGAMENTA COLLATERALIA ARTICULATIONUM METACARPOPHALANGEARUM.

lateral metatarsal ligaments An outmoded term for LIGAMENTA METATARSALIA INTEROSSEA.

lateral metatarsal ligaments of Weitbrecht An outmoded term for LIGAMENTA METATARSALIA INTEROSSEA.

lateral metatarsophalangeal ligaments LIGAMENTA COLLATERALIA ARTICULATIONUM METATARSOPHALANGEARUM.

lateral ligaments of metatarsophalangeal joints LIGAMENTA COLLATERALIA ARTICULATIONUM METATARSOPHALANGEARUM.

lateral occipitoaxial ligaments LIGAMENTA ALARIA.

lateral palpebral ligament LIGAMENTUM PALPEBRALE LATERALE.

lateral patellar ligament An outmoded term for RETINACULUM PATELLAE LATERALE.

lateral proper metatarsal ligaments of Weber An outmoded term for LIGAMENTA METATARSALIA INTEROSSEA.

lateral puboprostatic ligament The lateral extension of ligamentum puboprostaticum.

lateral radial ligament An outmoded term for LIGAMENTUM COLLATERALE CARPI RADIALE.

lateral radiate ligament An outer band of the radiate carpal ligament extending from the capitate bone to the styloid process of the ulna. An outmoded term.

lateral ligament of rectum The fascia around the middle rectal vessels which passes from the posterolateral wall of the true pelvis to each side of the rectum at the level of the third sacral vertebra.

lateral sacrococcygeal ligament LIGAMENTUM SACROCOCCYGEUM LATERALE.

lateral talocalcaneal ligament LIGAMENTUM TALOCALCANEARE LATERALE.

lateral ligament of talocrural joint The complex ligament lateral to the talocrural joint which comprises three separate ligaments: ligamentum talofibulare anterius, ligamentum talofibulare posterius, and ligamentum calcaneofibulare.

lateral ligament of temporomandibular articulation LIGAMENTUM LATERALE ARTICULATIONIS TEMPOROMANDIBULARIS.

lateral ligament of temporomandibular joint LIGAMENTUM LATERALE ARTICULATIONIS TEMPOROMANDIBULARIS.

lateral thyrohyoid ligament LIGAMENTUM THYROHYOIDEUM LATERALE.

lateral true ligament of bladder LIGAMENTUM PUBOPROSTATICUM.

lateral ulnar ligament An outmoded term for LIGAMENTUM COLLATERALE CARPI ULNARE.

lateral umbilical ligament An outmoded term for LIGAMENTUM UMBILICALE MEDIALE.

lateral vesical ligament An outmoded term for LIGAMENTUM UMBILICALE MEDIALE.

Lauth's ligament 1 Some fibers of the alar ligaments of the axis that form a transverse band behind the dens and above the transverse ligament of the atlas, extending from one edge of the foramen magnum to the other. 2 LIGAMENTUM ARCUATUM PUBIS.

least sacrosciatic ligament An outmoded term for LIGAMENTUM SACROSPINALE.

ligament of left anterior vena cava PLICA VENAE CAVAE SINISTRAE.

left lateral phrenicopericardiac ligament Occasional connective-tissue fibers connecting the fibrous pericardium with the left side of the central tendon and the adjacent muscle of the diaphragm. An outmoded term.

left phrenicocolic ligament LIGAMENTUM PHRENICOCOLICUM.

ligament of left superior vena cava PLICA VENAE CAVAE SINISTRAE.

left triangular ligament of liver LIGAMENTUM TRIANGULARE SINISTRUM HEPATIS.

lienophrenic ligament LIGAMENTUM SPLENORENALE.

lienorenal ligament LIGAMENTUM SPLENORENALE.

Lisfranc's ligament One of the ligamenta cuneometatarsea interossea, namely, the strong band between the lateral surface of the medial cuneiform bone and the medial aspect of the base of the second metatarsal bone, which separates the medial from the intermediate tarsometatarsal articulation.

Lockwood's ligament SUSPENSORY LIGAMENT OF EYEBALL.

Lockwood suspensory ligament SUSPENSORY LIGAMENT OF EYEBALL.

long iliosacral ligament LONG POSTERIOR SACROILIAC LIGAMENT.

longitudinal ligament of abdomen An outmoded term for LINEA ALBA.

long occipitoaxial ligament MEMBRANA TECTORIA.

long plantar ligament LIGAMENTUM PLANTARE LONGUM.

long posterior sacroiliac ligament The lower part of ligamenta sacroiliaca dorsalia, extending from the third and/or fourth transverse tubercles of the dorsum of the sacrum to the posterior superior iliac spine and merging laterally with the upper part of the sacrotuberous ligament and medially with the posterior lamella of the thoracolumbar fascia. Also called *Bichat's ligament, ligamentum sacroiliacum posterius longum* (outmoded), *long iliosacral ligament, sacrospinous ligament of Bichat* (outmoded).

lumbocostal ligament LIGAMENTUM LUMBOCOSTALE.

lumbocostal ligament of Henle LIGAMENTUM LUMBOCOSTALE.

lumbosacral ligament The lower part of the iliolumbar ligament that extends from the inferior surface of the transverse process of the fifth lumbar vertebra to the anterosuperior surface of the lateral part of the sacrum, fusing with the ventral sacroiliac ligament.

ligaments of Luschka LIGAMENTA STERNOPERICARDIACA.

Mackenrodt's ligament LATERAL CERVICAL LIGAMENT.

ligament of Maissiat TRACTUS ILIOTIBIALIS.

ligaments of malleus The ligaments attaching the malleus to the walls of the middle ear, namely, ligamentum mallei anterius, ligamentum mallei laterale, and ligamentum malleus superius.

marsupial suspensory ligament An outmoded term for PLICA SYNOVIALIS INFRAPATELLARIS.

Mauchart's ligaments LIGAMENTA ALARIA.

ligament of Mayer LIGAMENTUM CARPI RADIATUM.

Meckel's ligament MECKEL'S BAND.

medial ligament LIGAMENTUM MEDIALE ARTICULATIONIS TALOCRURALIS.

medial accessory ligament of Henle An outmoded term for LIGAMENTUM SPHENOMANDIBULARE.

medial arcuate ligament LIGAMENTUM ARCUATUM MEDIALE.

medial calcaneocuboid ligament An outmoded term for LIGAMENTUM BIFURCATUM.

medial check ligament of eyeball A strong, triangular expansion extending medially from the junction of the bulbar sheath and the tubular sheath of the medial rectus muscle of the bulb to the lacrimal bone. It checks the action of the muscle.

medial cuneonavicular ligament A small fibrous band connecting the tuberosity of the navicular to the medial surface of the medial cuneiform bone of the foot. It is an extension of a dorsal cuneonavicular ligament to the plantar ligament. An outmoded term.

medial ligament of elbow joint LIGAMENTUM COLLATERALE ULNARE.

medial intermuscular ligament of arm An outmoded term for SEPTUM INTERMUSCULARE BRACHII MEDIALE.

medial intermuscular ligament of thigh An outmoded term for SEPTUM INTERMUSCULARE FEMORIS MEDIALE.

medial palpebral ligament LIGAMENTUM PALPEBRALE MEDIALE.

medial puboprostatic ligament The medial extension of ligamentum puboprostaticum.

medial talocalcaneal ligament LIGAMENTUM TALOCALCANEARE MEDIALE.

medial ligament of temporomandibular joint LIGAMENTUM MEDIALE ARTICULATIONIS TEMPOROMANDIBULARIS.

medial umbilical ligament LIGAMENTUM UMBILICALE MEDIALE.

medial ligament of wrist LIGAMENTUM COLLATERALE CARPI ULNARE.

median arcuate ligament LIGAMENTUM ARCUATUM MEDIANUM.

median hyothyroid ligament LIGAMENTUM THYROHYOIDEUM MEDIANUM.

median occipitoaxial ligament LIGAMENTUM APICIS DENTIS AXIS.

median thyrohyoid ligament LIGAMENTUM THYROHYOIDEUM MEDIANUM.

median umbilical ligament LIGAMENTUM UMBILICALE MEDIANUM.

mesentericomesocolic ligament A peritoneal fold bounding the rarely found paraduodenal recess inferiorly, which is continuous with the duodenomesocolic or inferior duodenal fold.

mesocolic ligament of colon An outmoded term for TAENIA MESOCOLICA.

metacarpal interosseous ligaments LIGAMENTA METACARPALIA INTEROSSEA.

middle cricothyroid ligament LIGAMENTUM CRICOTHYROIDEUM MEDIANUM.

middle glenohumeral ligament The middle of the three bands of the glenohumeral ligaments, which extends from the upper part of the medial margin of the glenoid cavity and the labrum glenoidale to the lower part of the lesser tubercle of the humerus. See also LIGAMENTA GLENOHUMERALIA.

middle interosseous cuneometatarsal ligament One of the interosseous cuneometatarsal ligaments which connects the lateral cuneiform bone with the adjacent angle of the second metatarsal bone. An outmoded term.

middle maxillary ligament An outmoded term for LIGAMENTUM SPHENOMANDIBULARE.

middle ligament of neck of rib LIGAMENTUM COSTOTRANSVERSARIUM.

middle odontoid ligament An outmoded term for LIGAMENTUM APICIS DENTIS AXIS.

middle pharyngeal ligament An outmoded term for RAPHE PHARYNGIS.

middle thyrohyoid ligament LIGAMENTUM THYROHYOIDEUM MEDIANUM.

middle umbilical ligament LIGAMENTUM UMBILICALE MEDIANUM.

mucous ligament PLICA SYNOVIALIS.

ligament of nape An outmoded term for LIGAMENTUM NUCHAE.

ligament of neck of rib LIGAMENTUM COSTOTRANSVERSARIUM.

nephrocolic ligament Fibrous strands of areolar tissue between the perirenal fascia anterior to the lower pole of each kidney and areolar tissue on the posterior aspect of the ascending and the descending colon related to corresponding kidneys.

nuchal ligament LIGAMENTUM NUCHAE.

oblique ligament CHORDA OBLIQUA.

oblique accessory carpal ligament An outmoded term for LIGAMENTUM RADIOCARPALE PALMARE.

oblique ligament of Cooper CHORDA OBLIQUA.

oblique cuboideonavicular ligament An outmoded term for LIGAMENTUM CUBOIDEONAVICULARE PLANTARE.

oblique ligament of elbow joint CHORDA OBLIQUA.

oblique ligament of forearm CHORDA OBLIQUA.

oblique ligaments of knee An outmoded term for LIGAMENTA CRUCIATA GENUS.

oblique palmar carpometacarpal ligaments An outmoded term for LIGAMENTA CARPOMETACARPALIA PALMARIA.

oblique popliteal ligament LIGAMENTUM POPLITEUM OBLIQUUM.

oblique ligament of scapula An outmoded term for LIGAMENTUM TRANSVERSUM SCAPULAE SUPERIUS.

oblique ligament of superior radioulnar joint CHORDA OBLIQUA.

obturator ligament of atlas An outmoded term for MEMBRANA ATLANTO-OCCIPITALIS ANTERIOR.

obturator ligament of pelvis An outmoded term for MEMBRANA OBTURATORIA.

occipitoaxial ligament MEMBRANA TECTORIA.

occipito-odontoid ligaments LIGAMENTA ALARIA.

odontoid ligaments of axis LIGAMENTA ALARIA.

orbicular ligament of radius LIGAMENTUM ANNULARE RADII.

ovarian ligament LIGAMENTUM OVARII PROPRIUM.

ligament of ovary LIGAMENTUM OVARII PROPRIUM.

palmar ligaments LIGAMENTA PALMARIA ARTICULATIONUM METACARPOPHALANGEALIUM.

palmar carpometacarpal ligaments LIGAMENTA CARPOMETACARPALIA PALMARIA.

palmar ligament of carpus An outmoded term for LIGAMENTUM CARPI RADIATUM.

palmar intercarpal ligaments LIGAMENTA INTERCARPALIA PALMARIA.

palmar intermetacarpal ligaments LIGAMENTA METACARPALIA PALMARIA.

palmar metacarpal ligaments LIGAMENTA METACARPALIA PALMARIA.

palmar metacarpophalangeal ligaments LIGAMENTA PALMARIA ARTICULATIONUM METACARPOPHALANGEALIUM.

palmar radiocarpal ligament LIGAMENTUM RADIOCARPALE PALMARE.

palmar ligament of radiocarpal joint LIGAMENTUM RADIOCARPALE PALMARE.

palmar scaphotriquetral ligament One of the palmar intercarpal ligaments which connects the scaphoid and triquetrum bones and bridges across the lunate. An outmoded term.

palmar ulnocarpal ligament LIGAMENTUM ULNOCARPALE PALMARE.

patellar ligament LIGAMENTUM PATELLAE.

pectinate ligament of iridocorneal angle RETICULUM TRABECULARE SCLERAE.

pectineal ligament LIGAMENTUM PECTINEALE.

pectineal ligament of Cooper LIGAMENTUM PECTINEALE.

ligaments of pelvic girdle LIGAMENTA CINGULI EXTREMITATIS INFERIORIS.

pelviprostatic capsular ligament An outmoded term for FASCIA PROSTATAE.

pericardiovertebral ligament BÉRAUD'S LIGAMENT.

perineal ligament of Carcassonne MEMBRANA PERINEI.

periodontal ligament PERIODONTIUM.

peritoneal ligament A fold or double layer of peritoneum which connects an organ either to another organ or to the abdominal or pelvic walls. It may contain extraperitoneal connective tissue, vessels, or nerves.

Petit's ligament UTEROSACRAL LIGAMENT.

Pétrequin's ligament A small tract of intercrural fibers that are attached to the inguinal ligament.

petroclinoid ligament PETROSPHENOID LIGAMENT.

petrosphenoid ligament A fibrous band between the lateral edge of the dorsum sellae at the posterior clinoid process and the superior margin of the petrous part of the temporal bone near its medial end, deep to which the abducent nerve passes into the cavernous sinus. Also called *petroclinoid ligament, Gruber's ligament.*

pharyngeal ligament RAPHE PHARYNGIS.

phrenicocolic ligament LIGAMENTUM PHRENICOCOLICUM.

phrenicolienal ligament LIGAMENTUM SPLENORENALE.

phrenicosplenic ligament LIGAMENTUM SPLENORENALE.

phrenocolic ligament LIGAMENTUM PHRENICOCOLICUM.

pisohamate ligament LIGAMENTUM PISOHAMATUM.

pisometacarpal ligament LIGAMENTUM PISOMETACARPEUM.

pisounciform ligament An outmoded term for LIGAMENTUM PISOHAMATUM.

pisouncinate ligament An outmoded term for LIGAMENTUM PISOHAMATUM.

plantar ligaments LIGAMENTA PLANTARIA ARTICULATIONUM METATARSOPHALANGEALIUM.

plantar ligaments of bases of metatarsal bones LIGAMENTA METATARSALIA PLANTARIA.

plantar calcaneocuboid ligament LIGAMENTUM CALCANEOCUBOIDEUM PLANTARE.

plantar calcaneonavicular ligament LIGAMENTUM CALCANEONAVICULARE PLANTARE.

plantar cuboideonavicular ligament LIGAMENTUM CUBOIDEONAVICULARE PLANTARE.

plantar cuboscaphoid ligament An outmoded term for LIGAMENTUM CUBOIDEONAVICULARE PLANTARE.

plantar cuneocuboid ligament LIGAMENTUM CUNEOCUBOIDEUM PLANTARE.

plantar cuneonavicular ligaments LIGAMENTA CUNEONAVICULARIA PLANTARIA.

plantar external ligaments of Barkow An outmoded term for LIGAMENTA INTERCUNEIFORMIA PLANTARIA.

plantar intercuneiform ligaments LIGAMENTA INTERCUNEIFORMIA PLANTARIA.

plantar intermetatarsal ligaments LIGAMENTA METATARSALIA PLANTARIA.

plantar intertarsal ligaments LIGAMENTA TARSI PLANTARIA.

plantar ligaments of little heads of metacarpal bones An outmoded term for LIGAMENTUM METACARPEUM TRANSVERSUM PROFUNDUM.

plantar metatarsal ligaments LIGAMENTA METATARSALIA PLANTARIA.

plantar metatarsophalangeal ligaments LIGAMENTA PLANTARIA ARTICULATIONUM METATARSOPHALANGEALIUM.

plantar navicularicuneiform ligaments An outmoded term for LIGAMENTA CUNEONAVICULARIA PLANTARIA.

plantar proximal intermetatarsal ligaments An outmoded term for LIGAMENTA METATARSALIA PLANTARIA.

plantar scaphocuneiform ligaments An outmoded term for LIGAMENTA CUNEONAVICULARIA PLANTARIA.

plantar ligament of second metatarsal bone One of ligamenta tarsometatarsalia plantaria. An outmoded term.

plantar tarsometatarsal ligaments LIGAMENTA TARSOMETATARSALIA PLANTARIA.

plantar ligaments of tarsus LIGAMENTA TARSI PLANTARIA.

plantar transverse intermetatarsal ligaments An outmoded term for LIGAMENTA METATARSALIA PLANTARIA.

popliteal arcuate ligament LIGAMENTUM POPLITEUM ARCUATUM.

posterior ligament of the ankle joint The thin posterior part of the capsule of the ankle joint, consisting mostly of transverse fibers and blending with the deep part of posterior tibiofibular ligament. An outmoded term.

posterior annular ligament of carpus RETINACULUM EXTENSORUM MANUS.

posterior atlantoaxial ligament A broad, thin membrane which extends between the lower border of the posterior arch of the atlas and the upper margin of the laminae of the axis and is in series with the ligamenta flava. It has a thickened median bundle in line with the interspinous ligaments. It stretches as far as the capsule of the lateral atlantoaxial joint and is pierced laterally by the second cervical nerve. An outmoded term.

posterior atlanto-occipital ligament MEMBRANA ATLANTO-OCCIPITALIS POSTERIOR.

posterior auricular ligament LIGAMENTUM AURICULARE POSTERIUS.

posterior ligaments of bladder of Morris SACROGENITAL FOLD.

posterior carpometacarpal ligaments LIGAMENTA CARPOMETACARPALIA DORSALIA.

posterior cervical ligament An outmoded term for LIGA-MENTUM NUCHAE.

posterior costotransverse ligament LIGAMENTUM COSTO-TRANSVERSARIUM POSTERIUS.

posterior costotransverse ligament of Krause An out-moded term for LIGAMENTUM COSTOTRANSVERSARIUM LAT-ERALE.

posterior costovertebral ligament The posterior part of the fibrous capsule of the joint of the head of the rib which is continuous with the costovertebral ligament and attached to the bones adjacent to the articular surfaces and the intervening articular disk. An outmoded term. Also called *posterior radiate ligament of head of rib* (incorrect).

posterior cricoarytenoid ligament LIGAMENTUM CRICO-ARYTENOIDEUM POSTERIUS.

posterior cruciate ligament LIGAMENTUM CRUCIATUM POS-TERIUS GENUS.

posterior cruciate ligament of knee LIGAMENTUM CRUCIA-TUM POSTERIUS GENUS.

posterior ligament of elbow joint The posterior portion of the capsule of the elbow joint which consists of fibers extending from the periphery of the olecranon fossa and the medial and lateral epicondyles of the humerus to the superior and lateral surfaces of the olecranon process, the ulna just distal to the radial notch and the annular ligament of the radius. Most fibers run straight or obliquely downward but some pass transversely at the summit of the olecranon fossa. An outmoded term.

posterior false ligaments of bladder SACROGENITAL FOLD.

posterior fibrous ligament LIGAMENTUM STERNOCLAVICU-LARE POSTERIUS.

posterior ligament of head of fibula LIGAMENTUM CAPITIS FIBULAE POSTERIUS.

posterior ligament of incus LIGAMENTUM INCUDIS POSTER-IUS.

posterior inguinal ligament An outmoded term for LIGA-MENTUM INTERFOVEOLARE.

posterior ligament of knee The posterior portion of the fi-brous capsule of the knee joint which is attached proximally to the margins of the femoral condyles and the posterior margin of the intercondylar fossa and distally to the posterior margins of the tibial condyles and the posterior edge of the intercondylar area. It is strengthened by the oblique popliteal and arcuate popliteal ligaments. An outmoded term.

posterior longitudinal ligament LIGAMENTUM LONGITU-DINALE POSTERIUS.

posterior ligament of malleus An outmoded term for PLICA MALLEARIS POSTERIOR MEMBRANAE TYMPANI.

posterior meniscofemoral ligament LIGAMENTUM MENIS-COFEMORALE POSTERIUS.

posterior meniscofemoral ligament of Wrisberg LIGAMEN-TUM MENISCOFEMORALE POSTERIUS.

posterior oblique ligament of knee LIGAMENTUM POPLI-TEUM OBLIQUUM.

posterior occipitoaxial ligament MEMBRANA TECTORIA.

posterior ligament of pinna LIGAMENTUM AURICULARE POSTERIUS.

posterior proximal intermetacarpal ligaments An out-moded term for LIGAMENTA METACARPALIA DORSALIA.

posterior radiate ligament of head of rib An incorrect term for POSTERIOR COSTOVERTEBRAL LIGAMENT.

posterior ligament of radiocarpal joint LIGAMENTUM RA-DIOCARPALE DORSALE.

posterior radioulnar ligament A slight thickening of the posterior aspect of the fibrous capsule of the distal radioulnar joint. An outmoded term.

posterior sacrococcygeal ligament Either ligamentum sac-

rococcygeum posterius profundum or ligamentum sacrococcy-geum posterius superficiale.

posterior sternoclavicular ligament LIGAMENTUM STER-NOCLAVICULARE POSTERIUS.

posterior talocalcaneal ligament LIGAMENTUM TALOCAL-CANEUM POSTERIUS.

posterior talofibular ligament LIGAMENTUM TALOFIBU-LARE POSTERIUS.

posterior talotibial ligament PARS TIBIOTALARIS POSTE-RIOR LIGAMENTI MEDIALIS.

posterior tibiofibular ligament LIGAMENTUM TIBIOFIBU-LARE POSTERIUS.

posterior ligament of uterus RECTOVAGINAL FOLD.

Poupart's ligament LIGAMENTUM INGUINALE.

preurethral ligament of Waldeyer LIGAMENTUM TRANS-VERSUM PERINEI.

prismatic ligament of Weitbrecht LIGAMENTUM CAPITIS FEMORIS.

proper ligament of costal cartilage An outmoded term for MEMBRANA INTERCOSTALIS EXTERNA.

proper ligament of the ovary LIGAMENTUM OVARII PRO-PRIUM.

proper volar ligament of carpus An outmoded term for RETINACULUM FLEXORUM MANUS.

proximal intermetacarpal ligaments Any of three groups of ligaments: (1) ligamenta metacarpalia dorsalia; (2) ligamenta metacarpalia palmaria; (3) ligamenta metacarpalia interossea.

proximal posterior intermetatarsal ligaments LIGAMENTA METATARSALIA DORSALIA.

pterygomandibular ligament RAPHE PTERYGOMANDIBU-LARIS.

pterygomaxillary ligament An outmoded term for RAPHE PTERYGOMANDIBULARIS.

pterygospinal ligament LIGAMENTUM PTERYGOSPINALE.

pterygospinous ligament LIGAMENTUM PTERYGOSPINALE.

pubic arcuate ligament LIGAMENTUM ARCUATUM PUBIS.

pubic ligament of Cowper An outmoded term for LIGAMEN-TUM INGUINALE.

pubocapsular ligament LIGAMENTUM PUBOFEMORALE.

pubofemoral ligament LIGAMENTUM PUBOFEMORALE.

puboischiadic ligament of prostate gland An outmoded term for FASCIA DIAPHRAGMATIS UROGENITALIS SUPERIOR.

puboprostatic ligament LIGAMENTUM PUBOPROSTATICUM.

puborectal ligament 1 LIGAMENTUM PUBOPROSTATICUM. 2 LIGAMENTUM PUBOVESICALE.

pubovesical ligament LIGAMENTUM PUBOVESICALE.

pulmonary ligament LIGAMENTUM PULMONALE.

quadrate ligament LIGAMENTUM QUADRATUM.

quadrate ligament of Denucé LIGAMENTUM QUADRATUM.

radial carpal collateral ligament LIGAMENTUM COLLA-TERALE CARPI RADIALE.

radial collateral ligament LIGAMENTUM COLLATERALE RA-DIALE.

radial collateral ligament of carpus LIGAMENTUM COL-LATERALE CARPI RADIALE.

radial collateral ligament of elbow joint LIGAMENTUM COLLATERALE RADIALE.

radial collateral ligament of wrist LIGAMENTUM COLLA-TERALE CARPI RADIALE.

radial ligament of cubitocarpal articulation An outmoded term for LIGAMENTUM COLLATERALE CARPI RADIALE.

radial lateral ligament of carpus An outmoded term for LIGAMENTUM COLLATERALE CARPI RADIALE.

radiate ligament LIGAMENTUM CAPITIS COSTAE RADIATUM.

radiate carpal ligament LIGAMENTUM CARPI RADIATUM.

radiate ligament of carpus LIGAMENTUM CARPI RADIATUM.

radiate costosternal ligaments An outmoded term for LIG-

AMENTA STERNOCOSTALIA RADIATA.

radiate ligament of head of rib LIGAMENTUM CAPITIS COSTAE RADIATUM.

radiate ligament of Mayer LIGAMENTUM CARPI RADIATUM.

radiate sternocostal ligaments LIGAMENTA STERNOCOSTALIA RADIATA.

radiate ligament of wrist LIGAMENTUM CARPI RADIATUM.

radioulnar interosseous ligament An outmoded term for MEMBRANA INTEROSSEA ANTEBRACHII.

rectouterine ligament Musculus rectouterinus within the plica rectouterina.

reflected ligament LIGAMENTUM REFLEXUM.

reflex ligament of Gimbernat LIGAMENTUM REFLEXUM.

reflex inguinal ligament LIGAMENTUM REFLEXUM.

reinforcing ligament Any ligament that strengthens the capsule of a joint.

Retzius ligament The stem portion of the Y-shaped inferior extensor retinaculum, attached laterally to the proximal surface of the calcaneus and surrounding the tendons of the peroneus tertius and extensor digitorum longus muscles as it passes medially to separate into its two medial portions.

rhomboid ligament of clavicle LIGAMENTUM COSTOCLAVICULARE.

rhomboid ligament of wrist An outmoded term for LIGAMENTUM RADIOCARPALE DORSALE.

right lateral phrenicopericardiac ligament Connective tissue fibers connecting the inferior surface of the fibrous pericardium with the right anterior part of the central tendon of the diaphragm and the anterolateral surface of the inferior vena cava. An outmoded term.

right phrenicocolic ligament An occasional peritoneal fold extending from the right flexure of the colon to the adjacent lateral abdominal wall. Sometimes it extends from the latter to any part of the ascending colon. An outmoded term.

right triangular ligament of liver LIGAMENTUM TRIANGULARE DEXTRUM HEPATIS.

ring ligament of hip joint ZONA ORBICULARIS ARTICULATIONIS COXAE.

Robert's ligament LIGAMENTUM MENISCOFEMORALE POSTERIUS.

round ligament of acetabulum An outmoded term for LIGAMENTUM CAPITIS FEMORIS.

round ligament of Cloquet An outmoded term for LIGAMENTUM CAPITIS COSTAE INTRA-ARTICULARE.

round ligament of elbow joint CHORDA OBLIQUA.

round ligament of femur LIGAMENTUM CAPITIS FEMORIS.

round ligament of forearm An outmoded term for CHORDA OBLIQUA.

round ligament of liver LIGAMENTUM TERES HEPATIS.

round ligament of uterus LIGAMENTUM TERES UTERI.

sacciform ligament An outmoded term for CAPSULA ARTICULARIS RADIOULNARIS DISTALIS.

sacrospinal ligament LIGAMENTUM SACROSPINALE.

sacrospinous ligament LIGAMENTUM SACROSPINALE.

sacrospinous ligament of Bichat An outmoded term for LONG POSTERIOR SACROILIAC LIGAMENT.

sacrotuberal ligament LIGAMENTUM SACROTUBERALE.

sacrotuberous ligament LIGAMENTUM SACROTUBERALE.

salpingopharyngeal ligament An outmoded term for PLICA SALPINGOPHARYNGEA.

Santorini's ligament LIGAMENTUM CRICOPHARYNGEUM.

Sappey's ligament A thickening of the posterior wall of the articular capsule of the temporomandibular joint, formed by a thick layer of loose and vascularized connective tissue fusing the articular disk to the capsule. Also called *retrodiscal pad*.

scaphocapitate ligament That part of the radiate carpal ligament which connects the head of the capitate with the anterior surface of the scaphoid. An outmoded term.

ligament of Scarpa CORNU SUPERIUS MARGINIS FALCIFORMIS.

Schlemm's ligaments Two ligamentous thickenings in the capsule of the shoulder joint in the position of the inferior glenohumeral ligament.

scrotal ligament of testis GUBERNACULUM TESTIS.

Sebileau suspensory ligaments SUSPENSORY APPARATUS OF THE PLEURA.

serous ligament LIGAMENTUM SEROSUM.

short cuboideometatarsal ligaments An outmoded term for LIGAMENTA TARSOMETATARSALIA PLANTARIA.

short lateral ligament An inconstant bundle of fibers posterior to the fibular collateral ligament of the knee joint, extending from the lowest part of the lateral condyle of the femur to the apex of the head of the fibula. Deep to it are the tendon of the popliteus muscle and the inferior lateral genicular nerve and vessels. It may be replaced by the fabellofibular ligament.

short plantar ligament LIGAMENTUM CALCANEOCUBOIDEUM PLANTARE.

short posterior pelvic ligament An outmoded term for LIGAMENTUM SACROSPINALE.

short posterior sacroiliac ligament The superior, almost horizontal, portion of ligamenta sacroiliaca dorsalia extending from the first two transverse tubercles and lateral crests of the dorsum of the sacrum to the tuberosity of the ilium. Some authorities consider this ligament to be the separated superior part of the superficial sheet of ligamenta sacroiliaca interossea lying deep to the dorsal sacroiliac ligaments. Also called *ligamentum sacroiliacum posterius breve* (outmoded).

ligaments of shoulder girdle LIGAMENTA CINGULI EXTREMITATIS SUPERIORIS.

ligaments of the skull Fibrous bands linking bones of the cranial base to each other or to bones below it, for example, the stylohyoid, stylomandibular, pterygospinous and sphenomandibular ligaments.

Soemmering's ligament Fibrous tissue connecting the convex border of the orbital part of the lacrimal gland to the orbital periosteum.

sphenoideotarsal ligaments An outmoded term for LIGAMENTA TARSOMETATARSALIA PLANTARIA.

sphenomandibular ligament LIGAMENTUM SPHENOMANDIBULARE.

sphenomandibular ligament proper The portion of the sphenomandibular ligament that is attached to the spine of the sphenoid.

spinoglenoid ligament LIGAMENTUM TRANSVERSUM SCAPULAE INFERIUS.

spinosacral ligament An outmoded term for LIGAMENTUM SACROSPINALE.

spiral ligament of cochlea LIGAMENTUM SPIRALE COCHLEAE.

splenogastric ligament An outmoded term for LIGAMENTUM GASTROSPLENICUM.

splenophrenic ligament An outmoded term for LIGAMENTUM SPLENORENALE.

spring ligament LIGAMENTUM CALCANEONAVICULARE PLANTARE.

Stanley's cervical ligament RETINACULUM CAPSULAE ARTICULARIS COXAE.

stapedial ligament LIGAMENTUM ANNULARE STAPEDIS.

sternocostal ligaments LIGAMENTA STERNOCOSTALIA RADIATA.

sternopericardiac ligaments LIGAMENTA STERNOPERICARDIACA.

sternopericardial ligaments LIGAMENTA STERNOPERICARDIACA.

stylohyoid ligament LIGAMENTUM STYLOHYOIDEUM.

stylomandibular ligament LIGAMENTUM STYLOMANDIBULARE.

stylomaxillary ligament An outmoded term for LIGAMENTUM STYLOMANDIBULARE.

stylomylohyoid ligament An outmoded term for LIGAMENTUM STYLOMANDIBULARE.

subflaval ligaments LIGAMENTA FLAVA.

subpubic ligament LIGAMENTUM ARCUATUM PUBIS.

superficial ligament of carpus 1 An outmoded term for LIGAMENTUM RADIOCARPALE DORSALE. 2 An outmoded term for LIGAMENTUM RADIOCARPALE PALMARE.

superficial dorsal sacrococcygeal ligament LIGAMENTUM SACROCOCCYGEUM POSTERIUS SUPERFICIALE.

superficial transverse metacarpal ligament LIGAMENTUM METACARPALE TRANSVERSUM SUPERFICIALE.

superficial transverse metatarsal ligament LIGAMENTUM METATARSALE TRANSVERSUM SUPERFICIALE.

superior acromioclavicular ligament An outmoded term for LIGAMENTUM ACROMIOCLAVICULARE.

superior auricular ligament LIGAMENTUM AURICULARE SUPERIUS.

superior coccygeal ligament An outmoded term for LIGAMENTUM ILIOFEMORALE.

superior costotransverse ligament LIGAMENTUM COSTOTRANSVERSARIUM SUPERIUS.

superior ligament of epididymis LIGAMENTUM EPIDIDYMIDIS SUPERIUS.

superior glenohumeral ligament The highest of the three glenohumeral ligaments, which extends from the uppermost part of the medial margin of the glenoid cavity and the adjacent labrum glenoidale to a small fossa above the lesser tubercle of the humerus. It runs along the medial margin of the tendon of the long head of the biceps brachii muscle. See also LIGAMENTA GLENOHUMERALIA.

superior ligament of hip An outmoded term for LIGAMENTUM ILIOFEMORALE.

superior ligament of incus LIGAMENTUM INCUDIS SUPERIUS.

superior ligament of malleus LIGAMENTUM MALLEI SUPERIUS.

superior ligament of pinna LIGAMENTUM AURICULARE SUPERIUS.

superior pubic ligament LIGAMENTUM PUBICUM SUPERIUS.

superior sternoclavicular ligament The weak superior part of the fibrous capsule of the sternoclavicular joint which extends between the superior margin of the medial end of the clavicle and the lateral part of the suprasternal notch. An outmoded term.

superior sternopericardial ligament The upper of the two sternopericardial ligaments which extends from the anterosuperior surface of the fibrous pericardium to the inner surface of the upper end of the sternum and the manubrium sterni.

superior transverse ligament of scapula LIGAMENTUM TRANSVERSUM SCAPULAE SUPERIUS.

superior transversocostal ligament An outmoded term for LIGAMENTUM COSTOTRANSVERSARIUM SUPERIUS.

suprascapular ligament LIGAMENTUM TRANSVERSUM SCAPULAE SUPERIUS.

supraspinal ligament LIGAMENTUM SUPRASPINALE.

supraspinous ligament LIGAMENTUM SUPRASPINALE.

suspensory ligament of axilla The fused laminae of the clavipectoral fascia extending between the lower border of the pectoralis minor muscle and the axillary fascia covering the floor of the axilla. During abduction of the arm it elevates the axillary

fascia and underlying skin to produce the hollow of the armpit. Also called *Campbell's ligament, Gerdy's ligament.*

suspensory ligament of axis An outmoded term for LIGAMENTUM APICIS DENTIS AXIS.

suspensory ligament of bladder An outmoded term for PLICA UMBILICALIS MEDIANA.

suspensory ligaments of breast LIGAMENTA SUSPENSORIA MAMMARIA.

suspensory ligament of clitoris LIGAMENTUM SUSPENSORIUM CLITORIDIS.

suspensory ligament of duodenum MUSCULUS SUSPENSORIUS DUODENI.

suspensory ligament of eyeball A thickening of the lower part of the bulbar sheath which is formed by the medial and lateral check ligaments of the eyeball fusing with the margins of the sheath of the inferior rectus muscle of the bulb, forming a broad sling below the eyeball and limiting certain of its movements. Also called *Lockwood's ligament, Lockwood suspensory ligament.*

suspensory ligament of humerus An outmoded term for LIGAMENTUM CORACOHUMERALE.

suspensory ligament of lens ZONULA CILIARIS.

suspensory ligament of liver An outmoded term for LIGAMENTUM FALCIFORME HEPATIS.

suspensory ligaments of mammary gland LIGAMENTA SUSPENSORIA MAMMARIA.

suspensory ligament of ovary LIGAMENTUM SUSPENSORIUM OVARII.

suspensory ligament of penis LIGAMENTUM SUSPENSORIUM PENIS.

suspensory ligament of spleen An outmoded term for LIGAMENTUM SPLENORENALE.

sutural ligament A layer of connective tissue in the sutural gap between any two skull bones, continuous at the margins with periosteum both outside and inside the skull. It contains thin-walled veins that communicate with diploic veins and with veins inside and outside the skull. Also called *sutural membrane, intersutural membrane.*

synovial ligament A large fold of synovial membrane inside the capsule of a joint.

synovial ligament of hip An outmoded term for LIGAMENTUM CAPITIS FEMORIS.

talonavicular ligament LIGAMENTUM TALONAVICULARE.

temporomandibular ligament LIGAMENTUM LATERALE ARTICULATIONIS TEMPOROMANDIBULARIS.

tendinotrochanteric ligament The part of the capsule of the hip joint that is attached to the greater trochanter and intertrochanteric line of the femur. An outmoded term.

tensor ligament An outmoded term for MUSCULUS TENSOR TYMPANI.

Teutleben's ligament LIGAMENTUM PULMONALE.

Thompson's ligament DEEP CRURAL ARCH.

thyroepiglottic ligament LIGAMENTUM THYROEPIGLOTTICUM.

thyrohyoid ligament LIGAMENTUM THYROHYOIDEUM LATERALE.

tibial collateral ligament LIGAMENTUM COLLATERALE TIBIALE.

tibial collateral ligament of knee joint LIGAMENTUM COLLATERALE TIBIALE.

tibiofibular ligament SYNDESMOSIS TIBIOFIBULARIS.

tibionavicular ligament PARS TIBIONAVICULARIS LIGAMENTI MEDIALIS.

Toynbee's ligament LIGAMENTUM MALLEI ANTERIUS.

tracheal annular ligaments LIGAMENTA ANNULARIA TRACHEALIA.

transverse ligament of acetabulum LIGAMENTUM TRANS-VERSUM ACETABULI.

transverse ligament of atlas LIGAMENTUM TRANSVERSUM ATLANTIS.

transverse ligament of carpus An outmoded term for RETINACULUM FLEXORUM MANUS.

transverse cervical ligament of Mackenrodt LATERAL CERVICAL LIGAMENT.

transverse ligament of elbow An oblique fibrous band of the ulnar collateral ligament that connects the margin of the coronoid process to that of the olecranon process.

transverse humeral ligament A ligamentous thickening of the capsule of the shoulder joint extending between the greater and the lesser tubercles of the humerus, converting the intertubercular sulcus into a canal for the tendon of the long head of biceps brachii as it emerges from the capsule. Also called *Brodie's ligament.*

transverse ligament of knee LIGAMENTUM TRANSVERSUM GENUS.

transverse ligament of knee joint LIGAMENTUM TRANSVERSUM GENUS.

transverse ligament of leg RETINACULUM MUSCULORUM EXTENSORUM PEDIS SUPERIUS.

transverse ligament of little head of rib An outmoded term for LIGAMENTUM CAPITIS COSTAE INTRA-ARTICULARE.

transverse ligaments of little heads of metacarpal bones An outmoded term for LIGAMENTUM METACARPEUM TRANSVERSUM PROFUNDUM.

transverse ligaments of little heads of metatarsal bones An outmoded term for LIGAMENTUM METATARSALE TRANSVERSUM PROFUNDUM.

transverse metacarpal interosseous ligaments An outmoded term for LIGAMENTA METACARPALIA INTEROSSEA.

transverse pelvic ligament LIGAMENTUM TRANSVERSUM PERINEI.

transverse ligament of pelvis LIGAMENTUM TRANSVERSUM PERINEI.

transverse ligament of pelvis of Henle LIGAMENTUM TRANSVERSUM PERINEI.

transverse perineal ligament LIGAMENTUM TRANSVERSUM PERINEI.

transverse ligament of tibia An outmoded term for RETINACULUM MUSCULORUM EXTENSORUM PEDIS SUPERIUS.

transverse tibiofibular ligament The lower, deep part of the posterior tibiofibular ligament, extending from the lateral malleolar fossa to the posterior articular margin of the medial malleolus and articulating anteriorly with the talus.

transverse ligament of wrist RETINACULUM FLEXORUM MANUS.

transversocostal interosseous ligament of Cruveilhier An outmoded term for LIGAMENTUM COSTOTRANSVERSARIUM.

trapezoid ligament LIGAMENTUM TRAPEZOIDEUM.

ligament of Treitz MUSCULUS SUSPENSORIUS DUODENI.

triangular ligament of abdomen An outmoded term for LIGAMENTUM REFLEXUM.

triangular ligament of Colles MEMBRANA PERINEI.

triangular ligament of linea alba An outmoded term for ADMINICULUM LINEAE ALBAE.

triangular ligament of scapula An outmoded term for LIGAMENTUM TRANSVERSUM SCAPULAE INFERIUS.

triangular ligament of thigh An outmoded term for LIGAMENTUM REFLEXUM.

triangular ligament of urethra An outmoded term for LIGAMENTUM PUBOPROSTATICUM.

trigeminate ligaments of Arnold An outmoded term for LIGAMENTA TARSOMETATARSALIA DORSALIA.

triquetral ligament **1** An outmoded term for LIGAMENTUM CRICOARYTENOIDEUM POSTERIUS. **2** An outmoded term for LIGAMENTUM CORACOACROMIALE.

triquetral ligament of foot An outmoded term for LIGAMENTUM CALCANEOFIBULARE.

triquetral ligament of scapula An outmoded term for LIGAMENTUM TRANSVERSUM SCAPULAE INFERIUS.

triquetrocapitate ligament The part of the radiate carpal ligament which connects the head of the capitate with the anterior surface of the triquetrum.

triquetrotrapezium-trapezoid ligament The part of the ligamenta intercarpalia dorsalia that extends between the rough posterior surface of the triquetrum and the posterior surfaces of the trapezium and trapezoid bones. An outmoded term.

trochlear ligament An outmoded term for LIGAMENTUM METACARPEUM TRANSVERSUM PROFUNDUM.

trochlear ligaments of foot An outmoded term for LIGAMENTA PLANTARIA ARTICULATIONUM METATARSOPHALANGEALIUM.

trochlear ligaments of hand An outmoded term for LIGAMENTA PALMARIA ARTICULATIONUM METACARPOPHALANGEALIUM.

trochlear ligaments of little heads of metacarpal bones An outmoded term for LIGAMENTUM METACARPEUM TRANSVERSUM PROFUNDUM.

tuberososacral ligament An outmoded term for LIGAMENTUM SACROTUBERALE.

tubopharyngeal ligament of Rauber PLICA SALPINGOPHARYNGEA.

Tuffier's inferior ligament The distal part of the mesentery extending into the iliac fossa.

ulnar carpal ligament LIGAMENTUM COLLATERALE CARPI ULNARE.

ulnar carpal collateral ligament LIGAMENTUM COLLATERALE CARPI ULNARE.

ulnar ligament of carpus LIGAMENTUM COLLATERALE CARPI ULNARE.

ulnar collateral ligament LIGAMENTUM COLLATERALE ULNARE.

ulnar collateral ligament of carpus LIGAMENTUM COLLATERALE CARPI ULNARE.

ulnar collateral ligament of elbow joint LIGAMENTUM COLLATERALE ULNARE.

ulnar collateral ligament of wrist LIGAMENTUM COLLATERALE CARPI ULNARE.

ulnar lateral ligament of carpus An outmoded term for LIGAMENTUM COLLATERALE CARPI ULNARE.

utero-ovarian ligament An outmoded term for LIGAMENTUM OVARII PROPRIUM.

uteropelvic ligaments Fibromuscular bands at the base of the broad ligament of the uterus extending from each side of the uterus and the vagina to the fascia on the obturator internus and levator ani muscles on the lateral pelvic wall. They include, for example, the lateral cervical ligament.

uterosacral ligament A band of fibrous tissue and smooth muscle fibers within the rectouterine fold, extending backward on each side from the cervix uteri to the front of the sacrum. Also called *Petit's ligament.*

uterovesical ligament A peritoneal fold extending from the junction of the cervix and the body of the uterus anteriorly to the the upper surface of the urinary bladder. Also called *vesicouterine ligament.*

vaginal ligaments An outmoded term for VINCULA TENDINUM.

vaginal ligaments of fingers VINCULA TENDINUM DIGITORUM MANUS.

ligaments of vaginal sheaths An outmoded term for VINCULA TENDINUM.

vaginal ligaments of toes VINCULA TENDINUM DIGITORUM PEDIS.

ligaments of Valsalva LIGAMENTA AURICULARIA.

venous ligament of liver LIGAMENTUM VENOSUM.

ventral sacrococcygeal ligament LIGAMENTUM SACROCOCCYGEUM ANTERIUS.

ventral sacroiliac ligaments LIGAMENTA SACROILIACA ANTERIORA.

ventricular ligament of larynx LIGAMENTUM VESTIBULARE.

vertebropelvic ligament Any of three ligaments: (1) ligamentum iliolumbale; (2) ligamentum sacrospinale; (3) ligamentum sacrotuberale.

vertebropericardial ligament Fibrous tissue intervening between the posterior surface of the fibrous pericardium and the vertebral column from the sixth cervical vertebra to the fourth thoracic vertebra.

vertebropleural ligament An outmoded term for MEMBRANA SUPRAPLEURALIS.

ligament of Vesalius LIGAMENTUM INGUINALE.

vesicopubic ligament LIGAMENTUM PUBOVESICALE.

vesicoumbilical ligament LIGAMENTUM UMBILICALE MEDIANUM.

vesicouterine ligament UTEROVESICAL LIGAMENT.

vestibular ligament LIGAMENTUM VESTIBULARE.

vocal ligament LIGAMENTUM VOCALE.

volar ligaments of bases of metacarpal bones LIGAMENTA METACARPALIA PALMARIA.

volar capitular ligament LIGAMENTUM METACARPEUM TRANSVERSUM PROFUNDUM.

volar carpal ligament The superficial part of the flexor retinaculum which overlies the ulnar nerve and vessels. An outmoded term.

volar carpometacarpal ligaments LIGAMENTA CARPOMETACARPALIA PALMARIA.

volar intercarpal ligaments LIGAMENTA INTERCARPALIA PALMARIA.

volar ligaments of little heads of metacarpal bones An outmoded term for LIGAMENTUM METACARPEUM TRANSVERSUM PROFUNDUM.

volar radiocarpal ligament LIGAMENTUM RADIOCARPALE PALMARE.

volar transverse intermetacarpal ligaments An outmoded term for LIGAMENTA METACARPALIA PALMARIA.

Walther's oblique ligament An outmoded term for LIGAMENTUM TALOFIBULARE POSTERIUS.

Weitbrecht's ligament CHORDA OBLIQUA.

Winslow's ligament LIGAMENTUM POPLITEUM OBLIQUUM.

Wrisberg's ligament LIGAMENTUM MENISCOFEMORALE POSTERIUS.

xiphicostal ligaments of Macalister LIGAMENTA COSTOXIPHOIDEA.

xiphoid ligaments An outmoded term for LIGAMENTA COSTOXIPHOIDEA.

yellow ligaments LIGAMENTA FLAVA.

ligament of Zaglas Part of the posterior sacroiliac ligament extending from the posterior superior iliac spine to the lateral crest of the second sacral vertebra.

Zinn's ligament ANNULUS TENDINEUS COMMUNIS.

zonal ligament of thigh An outmoded term for ZONA ORBICULARIS ARTICULATIONIS COXAE.

zonular ligament ANNULUS TENDINEUS COMMUNIS.

---

ligamenta Plural of LIGAMENTUM.

ligamentopexis LIGAMENTOPEXY.

ligamentopexy [LIGAMENT + *o* + -PEXY] A surgical procedure in which one or more ligaments are shortened, plicated, or strengthened. This operation, performed on the uterine round ligaments, is now rarely undertaken. Also called *ligamentopexis.*

ligamentous Pertaining to, resembling, or having the characteristics of a ligament.

ligamentum

ligamentum [L (from *liga(re)* to bind, tie, akin to *licium* a thread, string and to *laqueus* a noose, snare; + -*mentum* -MENT), a band, bandage] (*plural* ligamenta) **1** [NA] A band, sheet, or local thickening of fibrous connective tissue in which the predominantly collagenous, as well as elastic, fibers are regularly oriented in thick bundles. It may occur inside a joint capsule, outside a capsule, or replacing a capsule, and is attached to two or more bones of a joint, strengthening, supporting, and limiting its movements. **2** [NA] A fibrous band, a fascial condensation, or a fold of peritoneum attached to an organ or organs, supporting it or them. **3** A fibrous remnant of an embryological or fetal tissue or organ. For defs. 1, 2, and 3 also called *ligament.*

ligamenta accessoria plantaria An outmoded term for LIGAMENTA PLANTARIA ARTICULATIONUM METATARSOPHALANGEALIUM.

ligamenta accessoria volaria An outmoded term for LIGAMENTA PALMARIA ARTICULATIONUM METACARPOPHALANGEALIUM.

ligamentum acromioclaviculare [NA] A broad fibrous band covering the superior part of the capsule of the acromioclavicular joint, extending from the acromial end of the clavicle to the superior surface of the acromion and strengthened by the aponeuroses of the trapezius and deltoid muscles. Also called *acromioclavicular ligament, external capsular clavicular ligament, superior acromioclavicular ligament* (outmoded).

ligamenta alaria [NA] Two rounded cords extending from the sides of the dens of the axis to rough surfaces medial to the condyles of the occipital bone. They are relaxed when the head is extended, but tighten on flexion so as to limit the movement. Also called *alar ligaments, check ligaments of axis, check ligaments of odontoid, Mauchart's ligaments, occipito-odontoid ligaments, lateral occipitoaxial ligaments.*

ligamentum annulare baseos stapedis An outmoded term for LIGAMENTUM ANNULARE STAPEDIS.

ligamentum annulare bulbi RETICULUM TRABECULARE SCLERAE.

ligamentum annulare radii [NA] A thick band encircling the head of the radius and forming three-fourths of an osseofibrous ring by its attachment to the anterior and posterior margins of the radial notch. Its inner surface is lined with cartilage for articulation with the circumference of the head of the radius. Its fibers blend with the capsule of the elbow joint and with some surrounding ligaments and muscles. Also called *orbicular ligament of radius, annular ligament of radius, coronary ligament of radius* (outmoded), *ligamentum orbiculare radii* (outmoded).

ligamentum annulare stapedis [NA] A ring of elastic fibers encircling the base of the stapes and holding it to the margin of the fenestra vestibuli as well as serving as a hinge on which the base moves during contraction of the stapedius muscle. Also called *annular ligament of stapes, annular ligament of base of stapes, stapedial ligament, ligamentum annulare baseos stapedis* (outmoded).

ligamenta annularia digitorum manus An outmoded term

for PARS ANNULARIS VAGINAE FIBROSAE DIGITORUM MANUS.

ligamenta annularia digitorum pedis An outmoded term for PARS ANNULARIS VAGINAE FIBROSAE DIGITORUM PEDIS.

ligamenta annularia trachealia [NA] Fibrous membranes, composed of collagen and intermingled elastin fibers, continuous with the perichondrium of adjacent tracheal rings, linking them and connecting the ends of the incomplete rings posteriorly. Also called *tracheal annular ligaments*.

ligamentum anococcygeum [NA] A fibromuscular band, comprising fibers of the subcutaneous part of the external anal sphincter and of connective tissue, attached to the posterior aspect of the dermis of the anus and to the tip of the coccyx. Also called *anococcygeal ligament, anococcygeal body, anococcygeal raphe* (outmoded), *raphe anococcygea* (outmoded), *Symington's body, white anococcygeal line* (outmoded), *white line of ischiococcygeal muscle* (outmoded).

ligamentum apicis dentis axis [NA] A narrow fibrous band extending from the tip of the dens of the axis to the anterior border of the foramen magnum and located between the alar ligaments. It is tightened by extension of the head. Also called *apical dental ligament, ligamentum apicis dentis epistrophei* (outmoded), *apical odontoid ligament, suspensory ligament of axis* (outmoded), *apical ligament of dens, middle odontoid ligament* (outmoded), *median occipitoaxial ligament*.

ligamentum apicis dentis epistrophei An outmoded term for LIGAMENTUM APICIS DENTIS AXIS.

ligamentum arcuatum laterale [NA] A thickened transverse band in the fascia of the quadratus lumborum muscle, or anterior lamella of thoracolumbar fascia, attached laterally to the lower border of the twelfth rib and medially to the front of the transverse process of the first lumbar vertebra, serving as an origin of the diaphragm. Also called *lateral arcuate ligament, lateral lumbocostal arch, lateral lumbocostal arch of Haller, arcus lumbocostalis lateralis, arcus lumbocostalis lateralis halleri* (outmoded), *external diaphragmatic arch* (outmoded), *external lumbocostal arch of diaphragm* (outmoded), *external tendinous arch of diaphragm* (outmoded), *external arcuate ligament of diaphragm* (outmoded).

ligamentum arcuatum mediale [NA] A horizontal ligamentous band in the psoas fascia attached laterally to the front of the transverse process of the first lumbar vertebra and medially to the body of the first or second lumbar vertebra where it is continuous with the outer side of the corresponding crus of the diaphragm, serving as an origin of the diaphragm. Deep to it the sympathetic trunk enters the abdominal cavity. Also called *medial arcuate ligament, medial lumbocostal arch, medial lumbocostal arch of Haller, arcus lumbocostalis medialis, arcus lumbocostalis medialis halleri* (outmoded), *internal diaphragmatic arch* (outmoded), *internal lumbocostal arch of diaphragm* (outmoded), *internal tendinous arch of diaphragm* (outmoded), *internal arcuate ligament of diaphragm* (outmoded).

ligamentum arcuatum medianum [NA] The tendinous arch joining the crura of the diaphragm in the median plane in front of the aorta. Also called *median arcuate ligament*.

ligamentum arcuatum pubis [NA] A thick fibrous arch across the inferior surface of the body of the pubis on each side, attached to the interpubic disk superiorly and to the inferior pubic rami laterally. It forms the apex of the pubic arch, deep to which the deep dorsal vein of clitoris or penis enters the pelvis above the anterior margin of the perineal membrane. Also called *arcuate pubic ligament, inferior pubic ligament, subpubic ligament, anterior triangular ligament of pubis* (outmoded), *inferior arcuate ligament of pubis, inferior annular ligament* (outmoded), *pubic arcuate ligament, Lauth's ligament*.

ligamentum arteriosum [NA] The thick cordlike remnant of the closed ductus arteriosus, extending from the left pulmonary artery, near its origin, to the concavity of the arch of the aorta.

The left recurrent laryngeal nerve hooks around its left side while to the right is the superficial part of the cardiac plexus of nerves. Also called *ligament of Botallo, ligamentum arteriosum arteriae pulmonalis* (outmoded).

ligamentum arteriosum arteriae pulmonalis An outmoded term for LIGAMENTUM ARTERIOSUM.

ligamentum atlanto-occipitale laterale [NA] A ligament lateral to and strengthening the capsule of the atlanto-occipital joint which extends craniomedially from the transverse process of the atlas, lateral to the foramen transversarium, to the inferior surface of the jugular process of the occipital bone. It corresponds in position to an intertransverse ligament of a vertebra. Also called *lateral atlanto-occipital ligament*.

ligamentum auriculare anterius [NA] An extrinsic ligament of the ear attaching the helix and the tragus of the auricle to the root of the zygoma. Also called *anterior auricular ligament, ligamentum auriculare anterius valsalvae* (outmoded).

ligamentum auriculare anterius valsalvae An outmoded term for LIGAMENTUM AURICULARE ANTERIUS.

ligamentum auriculare posterius [NA] An extrinsic ligament of the ear extending between the posterior aspect of the concha of the auricle and the mastoid process of the temporal bone. Also called *posterior auricular ligament, ligamentum auriculare posterius valsalvae* (outmoded), *posterior ligament of pinna*.

ligamentum auriculare posterius valsalvae An outmoded term for LIGAMENTUM AURICULARE POSTERIUS.

ligamentum auriculare superius [NA] An extrinsic ligament of the ear extending between the spine of the helix and the upper margin of the bony external acoustic meatus. Also called *superior auricular ligament, superior ligament of pinna, ligamentum auriculare superius valsalvae* (outmoded).

ligamentum auriculare superius valsalvae An outmoded term for LIGAMENTUM AURICULARE SUPERIUS.

ligamenta auricularia [NA] The three extrinsic ligaments, namely, anterior, posterior, and superior, that attach the auricle to the side of the head. Also called *ligaments of auricle, ligaments of Valsalva, ligamenta auricularia valsalvae* (outmoded).

ligamenta auricularia valsalvae An outmoded term for LIGAMENTA AURICULARIA.

ligamenta basium Ligaments connecting the bases of the metacarpal bones in the intermetacarpal articulations, and of the metatarsals in the intermetatarsal articulations: ligamenta metacarpalia (dorsalia, palmaria, and interossea) and ligamenta metatarsalia (dorsalia, plantaria, and interossea).

ligamenta basium ossium metacarpalium dorsalia An outmoded term for LIGAMENTA METACARPALIA DORSALIA.

ligamenta basium ossium metacarpalium interossea An outmoded term for LIGAMENTA METACARPALIA INTEROSSEA.

ligamenta basium ossium metacarpalium volaria An outmoded term for LIGAMENTA METACARPALIA PALMARIA.

ligamenta basium ossium metatarsalium dorsalia An outmoded term for LIGAMENTA METATARSALIA DORSALIA.

ligamenta basium ossium metatarsalium interossea An outmoded term for LIGAMENTA METATARSALIA INTEROSSEA.

ligamenta basium ossium metatarsalium plantaria An outmoded term for LIGAMENTA METATARSALIA PLANTARIA.

ligamentum bifurcatum [NA] A strong short band, the stem of which is attached posteriorly to the anterior part of the superior surface of the calcaneus while anteriorly it bifurcates into two, namely, the calcaneocuboid and calcaneonavicular ligaments. Also called *bifurcate ligament, bifurcated ligament, medial calcaneocuboid ligament* (outmoded), *ligament of Chopart*.

ligamentum calcaneocuboideum [NA] The anterolateral portion of the bifurcated ligament that is attached distally to the dorsal part of the medial aspect of the cuboid bone, helping to secure the first to the second row of tarsal bones. Also called *calcaneocuboid ligament, pars calcaneocuboidea ligamenti bifurcati* (outmoded), *internal calcaneocuboid ligament* (outmoded).

ligamentum calcaneocuboideum plantare [NA] A short broad band extending from the anterior tubercle and adjacent anterior area of the calcaneus to the contiguous plantar surface of the cuboid bone. This powerful ligament tends to prevent flattening of the lateral longitudinal arch of the foot. Also called *plantar calcaneocuboid ligament, short plantar ligament.*

ligamentum calcaneofibulare [NA] A long, cordlike band extending posteriorly from the hollow anterior to the apex of the lateral malleolus of the fibula down to the tubercle near the middle of the lateral surface of the calcaneus. It is crossed by the tendons of the peroneus longus and brevis muscles and, with the anterior and posterior talofibular ligaments, forms the lateral ligament of the talocrural joint. Also called *calcaneofibular ligament, triquetral ligament of foot.*

ligamentum calcaneonaviculare [NA] The anteromedial portion of the bifurcated ligament that is attached distally to the dorsolateral part of the navicular bone. Also called *calcaneonavicular ligament, pars calcaneonaviculare ligamenti bifurcati* (outmoded), *calcaneonavicular part of bifurcated ligament.*

ligamentum calcaneonaviculare dorsale The dorsal fibers of the ligamentum calcaneonaviculare, no longer considered separately from the main ligament. An outmoded term. Also called *dorsal calcaneonavicular ligament.*

ligamentum calcaneonaviculare plantare [NA] A broad, thick, and strong band extending between the anterior margin of the sustentaculum tali of the calcaneus and the plantar aspect of the navicular bone, supporting the head of talus on the fibrocartilaginous facet on its dorsal surface while its plantar surface is supported by the tendons of the tibialis posterior, flexor hallucis longus, and flexor digitorum longus muscles. Also called *plantar calcaneonavicular ligament, spring ligament, inferior calcaneonavicular ligament.*

ligamentum calcaneotibiale An outmoded term for PARS TIBIOCALCANEUS LIGAMENTI MEDIALIS.

ligamentum capitis costae intra-articulare [NA] A short, flat band stretching transversely from the crest separating the two articular facets on the head of a rib to the adjacent intervertebral disk, dividing the joint cavity into two compartments. It is absent in the joints of the first, tenth, eleventh, and twelfth ribs. Also called *intra-articular ligament of head of rib, interarticular ligament of head of rib* (outmoded), *costovertebral interosseous ligament of Cruveilhier* (outmoded), *interarticular costocentral ligament* (outmoded), *round ligament of Cloquet* (outmoded), *ligamentum capituli costae interarticulare* (outmoded), *interarticular cartilage of little head of rib* (outmoded), *transverse ligament of little head of rib* (outmoded), *intra-articular costovertebral ligament.*

ligamentum capitis costae radiatum [NA] Fibers attached to the anterior surface of the head of a rib and radiating medially to the body of the vertebra above, to that of the vertebra below, and to the intervertebral disk in between. Also called *radiate ligament of head of rib, anterior ligament of head of rib, ligamentum capituli costae radiatum* (outmoded), *anterior stellate ligament* (outmoded), *anterior costocentral ligament, costovertebral ligament, radiate ligament, ligamentum radiatum* (outmoded), *anterior radiate ligament of head of rib* (outmoded).

ligamentum capitis femoris [NA] A flat triangular intracapsular band attached by its apex to the anterosuperior part of the fovea on the head of the femur and by its base to each side of the acetabular notch and the inferior border of the transverse ligament in between. It is surrounded by synovial membrane and it tightens when the hip joint is semiflexed or adducted. Also called *ligament of head of femur, ligamentum teres femoris* (outmoded), *round ligament of femur, round ligament of acetabulum* (outmoded), *prismatic ligament of Weitbrecht, internal capsular ligament* (outmoded), *synovial ligament of hip* (outmoded), *synovial fold of hip, interarticular fold of hip, interarticular ligament of hip joint* (outmoded).

ligamentum capitis fibulae anterius [NA] A broad band extending upwards and obliquely from the front of the head of the fibula to the lateral condyle of the tibia and fused on its deep surface with the capsule of the superior tibiofibular joint. Also called *anterior ligament of head of fibula.*

ligamentum capitis fibulae posterius [NA] A thick band extending upwards and obliquely from the back of the head of the fibula to the lateral condyle of the tibia deep to the tendon of the popliteus muscle. Its deep surface is fused with the capsule of the superior tibiofibular joint. Also called *posterior ligament of head of fibula.*

ligamentum capituli costae interarticulare An outmoded term for LIGAMENTUM CAPITIS COSTAE INTRA-ARTICULARE.

ligamentum capituli costae radiatum An outmoded term for LIGAMENTUM CAPITIS COSTAE RADIATUM.

ligamenta capituli fibulae Ligamentum capitis fibulae anterius and ligamentum capitis fibulae posterius.

ligamenta capitulorum ossium metacarpalium transversa An outmoded term for LIGAMENTUM METACARPEUM TRANSVERSUM PROFUNDUM.

ligamenta capitulorum ossium metatarsalium transversa An outmoded term for LIGAMENTUM METATARSALE TRANSVERSUM PROFUNDUM.

ligamenta capsularia [NA] Ligamentous thickenings in the fibrous layer of articular capsules. Also called *capsular ligaments.* See also MEMBRANA FIBROSA CAPSULAE ARTICULARIS.

ligamentum carpi dorsale An outmoded term for RETINACULUM EXTENSORUM MANUS.

ligamentum carpi radiatum [NA] A group of ligamentous fascicles on the palmar aspect of the carpus radiating from the head of the capitate bone to surrounding bones of the midcarpal joint. Also called *radiate carpal ligament, radiate ligament of carpus, radiate ligament of Mayer, palmar ligament of carpus* (outmoded), *radiate ligament of wrist, ligament of Mayer.*

ligamentum carpi transversum An outmoded term for RETINACULUM FLEXORUM MANUS.

ligamentum carpi volare The superficial part of the retinaculum flexorum manus.

ligamenta carpometacarpalia dorsalia [NA] A group of fibrous bands strengthening the articular capsules between the distal row of carpal bones and the bases of the metacarpal bones on their posterior surfaces, the first metacarpal receiving a single band from the trapezium and the fifth metacarpal one from the hamate, while the other metacarpals each receive two fasciculi from adjacent carpal bones. Also called *dorsal carpometacarpal ligaments, posterior carpometacarpal ligaments.*

ligamenta carpometacarpalia palmaria [NA] A group of fibrous bands strengthening the articular capsules between the distal row of carpal bones and the bases of the metacarpal bones on their anterior, or palmar, surfaces, the first metacarpal receiving a single band from the trapezium and the fifth metacarpal one from the hamate, while the third receives three fasciculi, and the second and fourth receive two from adjoining carpal bones. Also called *palmar carpometacarpal ligaments, anterior carpometacarpal ligaments, ligamenta carpometacarpea volaria* (outmoded), *volar carpometacarpal ligaments, oblique palmar carpometacarpal ligaments* (outmoded).

ligamenta carpometacarpea volaria An outmoded term for LIGAMENTA CARPOMETACARPALIA PALMARIA.

ligamentum caudale integumenti communis An outmoded term for RETINACULUM CAUDALE.

ligamenta ceratocricoidea lateralia See under LIGAMENTUM CERATOCRICOIDEUM.

ligamenta ceratocricoidea posteriora See under LIGAMEN-TUM CERATOCRICOIDEUM.

ligamentum ceratocricoideum [NA] An external accessory ligament which strengthens the fibrous capsule of the cricothyroid joint. It radiates anteriorly and downward as the ligamentum ceratocricoideum anterius, laterally and downward as the ligamenta ceratocricoidea lateralia, and posteromedially and upward as the ligamenta ceratocricoidea posteriora from the inferior cornu of the thyroid cartilage to the cricoid cartilage. Also called *ceratocricoid ligament.*

ligamentum ceratocricoideum anterius See under LIGA-MENTUM CERATOCRICOIDEUM.

ligamenta cinguli extremitatis inferioris All the ligaments of the pelvic girdle, including those of the symphysis pubis and the sacroiliac and hip joints as well as the iliolumbar, sacrotuberous, and sacrospinous ligaments. An outmoded term. Also called *ligaments of girdle of inferior extremity, ligaments of pelvic girdle.*

ligamenta cinguli extremitatis superioris The ligaments of the shoulder girdle, including the superior and inferior transverse scapular and the coracoacromial ligaments as well as the ligaments of the acromioclavicular and sternoclavicular joints. An outmoded term. Also called *coracocapsular ligaments, ligaments of girdle of superior extremity, ligaments of shoulder girdle.*

ligamentum collaterale carpi radiale [NA] A short, rather weak band lying deep to the radial artery and extending between the tip of the styloid process of the radius and the lateral side of the scaphoid and trapezium bones. Also called *radial carpal collateral ligament, radial collateral ligament of carpus, radial collateral ligament of wrist, radial lateral ligament of carpus* (outmoded), *radial ligament of cubitocarpal articulation* (outmoded), *external lateral ligament of wrist joint, deep common ligament of wrist joint* (outmoded), *lateral radial ligament* (outmoded).

ligamentum collaterale carpi ulnare [NA] A strong short band attached proximally to the tip of the styloid process of the ulna and distally by two fasciculi, one to the pisiform bone and one to the medial aspect of triquetrum. Also called *ulnar carpal collateral ligament, lateral ulnar ligament* (outmoded), *ulnar carpal ligament, ulnar collateral ligament of carpus, ligamentous funiculus, ulnar collateral ligament of wrist, ulnar ligament of carpus, ulnar lateral ligament of carpus* (outmoded), *medial ligament of wrist, internal lateral ligament of wrist joint* (outmoded).

ligamentum collaterale fibulare [NA] A strong fibrous band extending from the lateral epicondyle of the femur to the head of the fibula anterior to its apex, separated from the capsule of the knee joint by the tendon of the popliteus muscle and inferior lateral genicular vessels, while superficial to it is the tendon of the biceps femoris muscle splitting around it. Also called *fibular collateral ligament, lateral ligament of knee, external lateral ligament of knee, fibular collateral ligament of knee joint.*

ligamentum collaterale radiale [NA] A strong triangular band attached proximally by its apex to the lower part of the lateral epicondyle of the humerus and distally by its base to the annular ligament of the radius and the supinator crest of the ulna, serving as a partial origin for the supinator and extensor carpi radialis brevis muscles. Also called *radial collateral ligament, lateralligament of elbow, brachioradial ligament* (outmoded), *radial collateral ligament of elbow joint.*

ligamentum collaterale tibiale [NA] A broad fibrous band, posteromedial to the knee joint, extending from the medial epicondyle of the femur, below the adductor tubercle, to the medial condyle and adjacent shaft of the tibia, and having its deep surface firmly attached to the medial meniscus and capsule of the knee joint. Superficially there is a bursa separating it from the tendons of the sartorius, gracilis and semitendinosus mus-

cles. Also called *tibial collateral ligament, internal lateral ligament of knee, tibial collateral ligament of knee joint.*

ligamentum collaterale ulnare [NA] A strong triangular band on the medial side of the elbow joint, attached proximally at its apex to the anterior and inferior surfaces of the medial epicondyle and divisible distally into three parts: an anterior part attached to the upper end of the medial edge of the coronoid process of the ulna, a posterior part attached to the medial surface of the olecranon, and an intermediate part between these two parts attached to the oblique band between the coronoid and olecranon processes. Also called *ulnar collateral ligament, ulnar collateral ligament of elbow joint, medial ligament of elbow joint, deltoid ligament of elbow, brachiocubital ligament* (outmoded), *cubitoulnar ligament* (outmoded).

ligamenta collateralia [NA] Thick fibrous bands that are located on the sides of uniaxial hinge joints such as the interphalangeal, humeroulnar, and knee joints. They help strengthen the joint capsules and control movement. Also called *collateral ligaments.*

ligamenta collateralia articulationum digitorum manus An outmoded term for LIGAMENTA COLLATERALIA ARTICULATIONUM INTERPHALANGEARUM MANUS.

ligamenta collateralia articulationum digitorum pedis An outmoded term for LIGAMENTA COLLATERALIA ARTICULATIONUM INTERPHALANGEARUM PEDIS.

ligamenta collateralia articulationum interphalangearum manus [NA] Strong, thick cords placed obliquely on the sides of the interphalangeal joints of the fingers, extending from the posterolateral surface of the distal end of the proximal bone to the anterolateral aspect of the base of the distal bone. Posteriorly the fibers join the expansion of the extensor tendon of each finger. The ligaments are always tense, preventing lateral movements. Also called *collateral ligaments of interphalangeal articulations of hand, ligamenta collateralia articulationum digitorum manus* (outmoded), *collateral ligaments of joints of fingers, lateral ligaments of joints of fingers, collateral ligaments of interphalangeal joints of hand.*

ligamenta collateralia articulationum interphalangearum pedis [NA] Strong fibrous cords placed obliquely on the sides of the interphalangeal joints of the toes, extending from a small depression on the side of the head of the more proximal bone to a rough edge on the side of the base of the distal bone. Also called *collateral ligaments of interphalangeal articulations of foot, ligamenta collateralia articulationum digitorum pedis* (outmoded), *collateral ligaments of joints of toes, lateral ligaments of joints of toes, collateral ligaments of interphalangeal joints of foot.*

ligamenta collateralia articulationum metacarpophalangearum [NA] Strong fibrous cords placed obliquely on the sides of the metacarpophalangeal joints, extending from a posterior tubercle and depression on each side of the head of the metacarpal bone to the corresponding anterolateral side of the base of the proximal phalanx. The fibers connect posteriorly with the extensor expansion and anteriorly with the palmar ligament of each finger. In the thumb, the ligaments also attach to the sesamoid bones. Also called *collateral ligaments of metacarpophalangeal articulations, lateral ligaments of metacarpophalangeal joints, accessory ligaments of metacarpophalangeal joints, lateral metacarpophalangeal ligaments.*

ligamenta collateralia articulationum metatarsophalangearum [NA] Strong fibrous cords placed obliquely on the sides of the metatarsophalangeal joints, extending from a tubercle on each side of the posterior aspect of the head of the metatarsal bone to the corresponding anterolateral side of the base of the proximal phalanx. Also called *collateral ligaments of metatarsophalangeal articulations, lateral ligaments of metatarsophalangeal joints, lateral metatarsophalangeal ligaments.*

ligamentum colli costae An outmoded term for LIGAMEN-TUM COSTOTRANSVERSARIUM.

ligamenta columnae vertebralis et cranii Ligaments of the vertebral column and the cranium.

ligamentum conoideum [NA] The triangular, posteromedial part of the coracoclavicular ligament, attached superiorly by its base to the conoid tubercle and an adjoining line medial to it on the inferior surface of the clavicle and inferiorly by its apex to the posteromedial edge of the root of the coracoid process at the scapular notch. Also called *conoid ligament, internal cora-coclavicular ligament* (outmoded).

ligamentum coracoacromiale [NA] A strong triangular band attached at its apex near the tip of the acromion anterior to the articular surface for the clavicle and by its base to the lateral margin of the coracoid process, forming an arch over the shoulder joint and deep to the deltoid muscle. Also called *cor-acoacromial ligament, acromiocoracoid ligament* (outmoded), *triquetral ligament* (outmoded).

ligamentum coracoclaviculare [NA] A strong band holding the lateral end of the clavicle to the underlying coracoid process of the scapula and consisting of two parts, the conoid and the trapezoid ligaments, separated from each other by fat or a bursa. Also called *coracoclavicular ligament, Caldani's ligament.*

ligamentum coracohumerale [NA] A broad band, partly fused with the capsule of the shoulder joint, extending infero-laterally from the lateral side of the root of the coronoid process of the scapula to the anterior aspect of the greater tubercle of the humerus. Also called *coracohumeral ligament, accessory lig-ament of humerus* (outmoded), *suspensory ligament of humerus* (outmoded).

ligamentum coronarium [NA] The peritoneal reflection from the diaphragm to the superior and posterior surfaces of the liver, comprising an upper and a lower layer that are separated by part of the right lobe devoid of peritoneum, the bare area, and continuous with the right triangular ligament. To the left, the upper layer is continuous with the right layer of the falciform ligament while the lower layer becomes continuous with the posterior layer of the hepatogastric ligament. Also called *coro-nary ligament of liver.*

ligamentum costoclaviculare [NA] A strong V-shaped band extending inferomedially from the inferior surface of the sternal end of the clavicle to the superior surface of the first rib and adjacent cartilage, and comprising two laminae, anterior and posterior, that fuse laterally and are continuous medially with the capsule of the sternoclavicular joint. Also called *costoclavic-ular ligament, rhomboid ligament of clavicle, costoclavicular syn-chondrosis.*

ligamentum costotransversarium [NA] A short, wide band of fibers that is attached anteriorly to the posterior aspect of the neck of a rib and posteriorly to the anterior surface of the adjacent transverse process. It occupies the costotransverse for-amen. It may be weak or absent on the eleventh and twelfth ribs. Also called *costotransverse ligament, transversocostal inter-osseous ligament of Cruveilhier* (outmoded), *ligamentum colli costae* (outmoded), *inferior ligament of neck of rib of Henle, middle ligament of neck of rib, ligament of neck of rib.*

ligamentum costotransversarium anterius The anterior layer of ligamentum costotransversarium superius, attached be-low to the crest of the neck of a rib and above the lower surface of the transverse process of a vertebra. Also called *anterior costotransverse ligament, anterior ligament of neck of rib, anterior superior ligament of neck of rib.*

ligamentum costotransversarium laterale [NA] A power-ful, short fibrous band extending upward and laterally from the tip of the transverse process of a vertebra to the nonarticular part of the tubercle of the adjacent rib. It is absent on the eleventh and twelfth ribs. Also called *lateral costotransverse*

ligament, ligamentum tuberculi costae (outmoded), *posterior cos-totransverse ligament of Krause* (outmoded), *inferior ligament of tubercle of rib.*

ligamentum costotransversarium posterius The posterior layer of the ligamentum costotransversarium superius. Also called *posterior costotransverse ligament, external ligament of neck of rib* (outmoded), *external superior ligament of neck of rib* (outmoded).

ligamentum costotransversarium superius [NA] A strong, broad fibrous band consisting of two layers. The anterior layer extends from the crest on the superior margin of the neck of a rib to the inferior margin of the transverse process above it, being continuous with the medial margin of the internal inter-costal membrane. The posterior layer extends medially from the posterior surface of the neck of a rib to the transverse process above it. The ligament is absent on the first rib. Anterior to the ligament are the posterior intercostal vessels and the intercostal nerve. Also called *superior costotransverse ligament, superior transversocostal ligament* (outmoded), *internal ligament of neck of rib* (outmoded).

ligamenta costoxiphoidea [NA] Inconstant fibrous bands, varying in length and breadth, that connect the front and back of the xiphoid process to corresponding surfaces of the seventh, and occasionally the sixth, costal cartilages. Also called *costo-xiphoid ligaments, xiphicostal ligaments of Macalister, xiphoid ligaments* (outmoded), *chondroxiphoid ligaments.*

ligamentum cricoarytenoideum posterius [NA] A strong, short band reinforcing the cricoarytenoid joint and extending from the upper border of the lamina of the cricoid cartilage to the medial surface of the base and muscular process of the arytenoid cartilage, fixing and limiting the forward movements of the latter. Also called *posterior cricoarytenoid ligament, tri-quetral ligament* (outmoded), *posterior cricoarytenoid cartilage* (outmoded).

ligamentum cricopharyngeum [NA] A single band extend-ing downward in the median plane from the junction of the right and left corniculopharyngeal ligaments and the pharyngeal mucosa to the cricoid lamina and the pharyngeal mucosa. Also called *cricopharyngeal ligament, cricosantorinian ligament, San-torini's ligament, cricopharyngeal ligament of Luschka.*

ligamentum cricothyreoideum medium An outmoded term for LIGAMENTUM CRICOTHYROIDEUM MEDIANUM.

ligamentum cricothyroideum LIGAMENTUM CRICOTHYRO-IDEUM MEDIANUM.

ligamentum cricothyroideum medianum [NA] The midline band of yellow elastic tissue connecting the cricoid cartilage to the lower margin of the thyroid cartilage. Laterally it is contin-uous with the conus elasticus (cricovocal membrane), the upper edge of which is the ligamentum vocale. Also called *ligamentum cricothyroideum, cricothyroid ligament, middle cricothyroid lig-ament, ligamentum cricothyreoideum medium* (outmoded).

ligamentum cricotracheale [NA] A fibrous ring linking the lower border of the cricoid cartilage to the first cartilaginous ring of the trachea and continuous inferiorly with the tracheal annular ligaments. Also called *cricotracheal ligament, cricotra-cheal membrane.*

ligamenta cruciata digitorum manus An outmoded term for PARS CRUCIFORMIS VAGINAE FIBROSAE DIGITORUM MANUS.

ligamenta cruciata digitorum pedis An outmoded term for PARS CRUCIFORMIS VAGINAE FIBROSAE DIGITORUM PEDIS.

ligamenta cruciata genu An outmoded term for LIGAMENTA CRUCIATA GENUS.

ligamenta cruciata genus [NA] Strong intracapsular liga-ments that cross each other in the intercondylar region of the knee joint posterior to its center, and called ligamentum crucia-tum anterius genus and ligamentum cruciatum posterius genus. They represent collateral ligaments of ancestral, separate medial and lateral femorotibial joints. Also called *cruciate ligaments of knee, ligamenta cruciata genu* (outmoded), *interosseous ligaments of knee* (outmoded), *oblique ligaments of knee* (outmoded), *cruciate ligaments*.

ligamentum cruciatum anterius   LIGAMENTUM CRUCIATUM ANTERIUS GENUS.

ligamentum cruciatum anterius genu   An outmoded term for LIGAMENTUM CRUCIATUM ANTERIUS GENUS.

ligamentum cruciatum anterius genus   [NA] A thick cord-like band within the knee joint extending from the anterior intercondylar area of the tibia to the posterior part of the medial aspect of the lateral condyle of the femur. Although taut in all positions, it prevents forward gliding of the tibia on the femur. Also called *anterior cruciate ligament of knee, ligamentum cruciatum anterius genu* (outmoded), *ligamentum cruciatum anterius, anterior cruciate ligament*.

ligamentum cruciatum atlantis   An outmoded term for LIGAMENTUM CRUCIFORME ATLANTIS.

ligamentum cruciatum cruris   An outmoded term for RETINACULUM MUSCULORUM EXTENSORUM PEDIS INFERIUS.

ligamentum cruciatum posterius   LIGAMENTUM CRUCIATUM POSTERIUS GENUS.

ligamentum cruciatum posterius genu   An outmoded term for LIGAMENTUM CRUCIATUM POSTERIUS GENUS.

ligamentum cruciatum posterius genus   [NA] A strong band, shorter than the anterior cruciate ligament, extending from the posterior intercondylar area of the tibia to the front of the lateral aspect of the medial condyle of the femur. It is taut in all positions and prevents backward gliding of the tibia on the femur. Also called *posterior cruciate ligament of knee, ligamentum cruciatum posterius genu* (outmoded), *ligamentum cruciatum posterius, posterior cruciate ligament*.

ligamentum cruciforme atlantis   [NA] A cross-shaped fibrous band in which the transverse ligament of atlas forms a horizontal bar posterior to the dens where it sends ascending and descending longitudinal bundles to be attached superiorly on the internal aspect of the anterior margin of the foramen magnum, between the apical ligament of dens and the membrana tectoria, and inferiorly to the posterior surface of the body of the axis, respectively. Also called *cruciform ligament of atlas, cruciate ligament of atlas, ligamentum cruciatum atlantis* (outmoded).

ligamentum cuboideonaviculare dorsale   [NA] A fibrous band strengthening the transverse articulation of the tarsus and extending laterally and distally from the dorsal surface of the navicular to the medial side of the cuboid bone. Also called *dorsal cuboideonavicular ligament*.

ligamentum cuboideonaviculare plantare   [NA] A strong band strengthening the transverse articulation of the tarsus and extending transversely from the medial side of the plantar surface of the cuboid to the plantar surface of the navicular bone. It is often joined to the dorsal ligament by an interosseous ligament passing between the nonarticular surfaces of the two bones. Also called *plantar cuboideonavicular ligament, oblique cuboideonavicular ligament* (outmoded), *plantar cuboscaphoid ligament* (outmoded).

ligamentum cuneocuboideum dorsale   [NA] A fibrous band between the dorsal surfaces of the lateral cuneiform and the cuboid bones. Proximally it may blend with the dorsal cuboideonavicular and cuneonavicular ligaments. Also called *dorsal cuneocuboid ligament*.

ligamentum cuneocuboideum interosseum   [NA] Strong fibers connecting the adjacent nonarticular surfaces of the lateral cuneiform and cuboid bones. Also called *interosseous cuneocuboid ligament*.

ligamentum cuneocuboideum plantare   [NA] A fibrous band connecting the plantar surfaces of the lateral cuneiform and

cuboid bones, reinforced by slips from the tendon of the tibialis posterior muscle. Also called *plantar cuneocuboid ligament*.

ligamenta cuneometatarsalia interossea   [NA] Fibrous bands, usually three in number, connecting the cuneiform bones to the bases of adjoining metatarsal bones. The strongest is the one between the lateral surface of medial cuneiform and the medial surface of the base of the second metatarsal bone. The second band joins the lateral cuneiform to the second metatarsal, and the third band connects the lateral cuneiform with the bases of the third and fourth metatarsal bones. Also called *interosseous cuneometatarsal ligaments*.

ligamenta cuneonavicularia dorsalia   [NA] Strong bands, usually fusing into a continuous band, connecting each of the dorsal surfaces of the three cuneiform bones to the navicular bone. The band to the medial cuneiform sends fasciculi medially to join the plantar cuneonavicular ligaments. Also called *dorsal cuneonavicular ligaments, ligamenta navicularicuneiformia dorsalia* (outmoded).

ligamenta cuneonavicularia plantaria   [NA] Strong bands, usually fusing into a continuous band, connecting each of the plantar surfaces of the three cuneiform bones to the navicular bone, and reinforced by slips of the tendon of tibialis posterior muscle. Also called *plantar cuneonavicular ligaments, ligamenta navicularicuneiformia plantaria* (outmoded), *plantar navicularicuneiform ligaments* (outmoded), *plantar scaphocuneiform ligaments* (outmoded).

ligamentum deltoideum   LIGAMENTUM MEDIALE ARTICULATIONIS TALOCRURALIS.

ligamentum denticulatum   [NA] One of a series of flattened triangular bands of epipial tissue attached medially to the lateral surface of the spinal cord midway between the dorsal and ventral roots and lateral to the dural sheath. 18 to 24 ligaments anchor the spinal cord to the dura and alternate with the dural evaginations marking the exit of the cervical, thoracic, and first lumbar spinal nerves. Also called *denticulate ligament, dentate ligament of spinal cord*.

ligamentum duodenorenale   An occasional peritoneal fold passing from the duodenum to the front of the right kidney. Also called *duodenorenal ligament*.

ligamentum epididymidis inferius   [NA] A fold of the visceral layer of the tunica vaginalis at the lower end of the sinus epididymidis passing from the testis over the tail of the epididymis to become continuous with the parietal layer. Also called *inferior ligament of epididymis*.

ligamentum epididymidis superius   [NA] A fold of the visceral layer of the tunica vaginalis at the upper end of the sinus epididymidis passing from the testis over the head of the epididymis to become continuous with the parietal layer. Also called *superior ligament of epididymis*.

ligamenta extracapsularia   [NA] Ligaments that are outside the capsule of a synovial joint and sometimes separated from it.

ligamentum falciforme hepatis   [NA] A midline crescentic fold of peritoneum, the ventral part of the primitive ventral mesogastrium, connecting the liver to the diaphragm and the anterior abdominal wall above the umbilicus, and containing the ligamentum teres and paraumbilical veins in its free edge which is attached to the inferior border of the liver. On the superior surface of the liver the two layers separate and the right layer becomes continuous with the upper layer of the coronary ligament while the left layer is continuous with the anterior layer of the left triangular ligament of liver. Also called *falciform ligament of liver, broad ligament of liver, suspensory ligament of liver* (outmoded).

ligamenta flava   [NA] A series of plates of yellow elastic tissue forming elastic syndesmoses between the laminae of adjacent vertebrae and extending from the posterior arch of the atlas to the first sacral vertebra. The almost perpendicular fibers of each plate are attached superiorly to the medial edge of the inferior articular process and a ridge on the lower part of the anterior surface of a lamina, while inferiorly they are attached to the medial edge of the superior articular process and the superior margin of the lamina of the vertebra below. Thus they also partake in the structure of the capsules of the articular processes. They are thinnest in the neck and thickest in the lumbar region. They facilitate flexion and steady the vertebrae during regaining the erect position from a flexed one. Also called *arcuate ligaments* (outmoded), *flaval ligaments, yellow ligaments, interlaminar ligaments, subflaval ligaments.*

ligamentum flavum   Any one of the ligamenta flava.

ligamentum fundiforme penis   [NA] A thickened elastic band of the membranous layer of the superficial fascia adherent to the lower part of the linea alba and the top of the symphysis pubis that extends to the dorsum of the penis and splits around it, reuniting below it to attach to the septum of the scrotum. Also called *fundiform ligament of penis.*

ligamentum gastrocolicum   [NA] The portion of the greater omentum that extends from the greater curvature of the stomach to the transverse colon, fusing with its anterior surface. It is continuous superiorly with the gastrosplenic ligament and to the left with the phrenicocolic ligament. Also called *gastrocolic ligament.*

ligamentum gastrolienale   LIGAMENTUM GASTROSPLENICUM.

ligamentum gastrophrenicum   [NA] A short fold, formed by the merging of the splenorenal and gastrosplenic ligaments, which passes forward from the diaphragm to the posterior surface of the fundus of the stomach, the two layers separating around the esophagus. It is essentially an upper portion of the greater omentum. Also called *gastrophrenic ligament.*

ligamentum gastrosplenicum   [NA] The part of the greater omentum that extends from the greater curvature on the left side of the fundus and adjoining part of the body of the stomach to the hilum of the spleen. Also called *ligamentum gastrolienale, gastrosplenic ligament, gastrolienal ligament, splenogastric ligament* (outmoded), *gastrosplenic omentum* (outmoded), *splenogastric omentum* (outmoded).

ligamentum genitoinguinale   GENITOINGUINAL LIGAMENT.

ligamenta glenohumeralia   [NA] Three variable fibrous bands, superior, middle, and inferior, projecting on the inner aspect of the front of the capsule of the shoulder joint and extending from the edge of the glenoid cavity and labrum glenoidale to the lesser tubercle and adjoining inferior part of the neck of the humerus. Also called *glenohumeral ligaments.*

ligamentum glenoidale   An outmoded term for LABRUM GLENOIDALE.

ligamentum hepatocolicum   [NA] An occasional prolongation inferiorly of the hepatoduodenal ligament to the transverse colon and right colic flexure. Also called *hepatocolic ligament.*

ligamentum hepatoduodenale   [NA] The right portion of the lesser omentum, extending from the porta hepatis to the first part of the duodenum, forming the anterior boundary of the epiploic foramen and containing in its free edge the hepatic artery proper, the bile duct and the portal vein, as well as some lymph nodes and vessels, and a plexus of nerves. Also called *hepatoduodenal ligament, duodenohepatic ligament.*

ligamentum hepatoesophageum   The left margin of the lesser omentum extending between the liver and the abdominal part of the esophagus. Also called *hepatoesophageal ligament.*

ligamentum hepatogastricum   [NA] The upper, major part of the lesser omentum, extending between the lesser curvature of the stomach and the fissure for ligamentum venosum of the liver. Also called *hepatogastric ligament, gastrohepatic ligament.*

ligamentum hepatorenale   [NA] An occasional prolongation inferiorly of the lower layer of the coronary ligament of the liver on to the right kidney just to the right of the epiploic foramen. Also called *hepatorenal ligament.*

ligamentum hyoepiglotticum   [NA] A broad elastic sheet connecting the anterior surface of the upper part of the epiglottis to the superior margin of the body of the hyoid bone and to its greater horn. Inferiorly it is separated from the thyrohyoid membrane by a fat pad. Also called *hyoepiglottic ligament, hyoepiglottic membrane.*

ligamentum hyothyreoideum laterale   An outmoded term for LIGAMENTUM THYROHYOIDEUM LATERALE.

ligamentum hyothyreoideum medium   An outmoded term for LIGAMENTUM THYROHYOIDEUM MEDIANUM.

ligamentum iliofemorale   [NA] A strong inverted Y-shaped band attached proximally to the lower part of the anterior inferior iliac spine and distally to the anterior surface of the greater trochanter and the intertrochanteric line of the femur. The central portion is weak and the medial band is strong. The lateral band is often called the iliotrochanteric ligament. The ligament is fused with the capsule of the hip joint anteriorly, supporting the weight of the body in the erect posture, with minimal muscular action, and limiting hyperextension and lateral rotation. Also called *iliofemoral ligament, hypsiloid ligament, superior ligament of hip* (outmoded), *Bigelow's ligament, Bertin's ligament, superior coccygeal ligament* (outmoded).

ligamentum iliolumbale   [NA] A strong triangular band extending from a long attachment on the internal aspect of the iliac crest to the anteroinferior part of the transverse process of the fifth, and often the fourth, lumbar vertebra. The superior margin provides partial origin for the quadratus lumborum muscle. Also called *iliolumbar ligament.*

ligamentum iliopectineale   ARCUS ILIOPECTINEUS.

ligamentum incudis posterius   [NA] A short fibrous band connecting the tip of the short process of the incus to the fossa incudis on the posterior wall of the tympanic cavity. Also called *posterior ligament of incus.*

ligamentum incudis superius   [NA] A fold of mucous membrane extending upward from the body of the incus to the roof of the epitympanic recess of the middle ear. Also called *superior ligament of incus, Arnold's ligament.*

ligamentum inguinale   [NA] The free and upturned, hammocklike, lower edge of the aponeurosis of the external oblique muscle extending from the anterior superior iliac spine to the pubic tubercle and pecten pubis, curved convex downward and attached to the fascia lata. The lateral part is strengthened by iliac fascia while the medial part forms the inguinal canal. Also called *inguinal ligament, arcus inguinalis, crural ligament, Poupart's ligament, pubic ligament of Cowper* (outmoded), *crural arch, superficial femoral arch, ligament of Vesalius, ligament of Fallopius* (outmoded), *fallopian ligament* (outmoded), *iliopubic ligament* (outmoded), *external inguinal ligament* (outmoded), *ligamentum inguinale pouparti* (outmoded).

ligamentum inguinale pouparti   An outmoded term for LIGAMENTUM INGUINALE.

ligamentum inguinale reflexum   LIGAMENTUM REFLEXUM.

ligamentum inguinale reflexum collesi   An outmoded term for LIGAMENTUM REFLEXUM.

ligamenta intercarpalia dorsalia   [NA] Transverse bands connecting the dorsal surfaces of the carpal bones in the proximal row and of those in the distal row, as well as short, irregular bundles between the proximal and distal rows. Also called *dorsal intercarpal ligaments, carpal dorsal ligaments, dorsal transverse ligaments of wrist* (outmoded).

ligamenta intercarpalia interossea   [NA] Short, variable bands connecting the adjacent surfaces of the proximal and of the distal carpal bones. Also called *interosseous intercarpal ligaments, interosseous ligaments of carpal bones.*

ligamenta intercarpalia palmaria   [NA] Transverse bands connecting the palmar surfaces of the proximal row and of the distal row of carpal bones, as well as short, irregular bundles between the bones of the proximal and those of the distal row. Also called *palmar intercarpal ligaments, volar intercarpal ligaments, ligamenta intercarpea volaria* (outmoded).

ligamenta intercarpea volaria　An outmoded term for LIGAMENTA INTERCARPALIA PALMARIA.

ligamentum interclaviculare　[NA] A strong, flat, curved fibrous band connecting the posterosuperior parts of the sternal ends of the two clavicles, some fibers being attached to the back of the superior margin of the manubrium sterni and to the capsules of both sternoclavicular joints. Superiorly it is continuous with the deep cervical fascia. Also called *interclavicular ligament.*

ligamenta intercostalia externa　An outmoded term for MEMBRANA INTERCOSTALIS EXTERNA.

ligamenta intercostalia interna　An outmoded term for MEMBRANA INTERCOSTALIS INTERNA.

ligamenta intercuneiformia dorsalia　[NA] Transverse fibrous bands connecting the dorsal surfaces of the three cuneiform bones. Also called *dorsal intercuneiform ligaments.*

ligamenta intercuneiformia interossea　[NA] Strong, deep fibrous ligaments which connect the intermediate cuneiform with the lateral and medial cuneiform bones, occupying the total vertical depth between the nonarticular surfaces of the adjoining bones and blending with the plantar and dorsal cuneonavicular ligaments. Also called *interosseous intercuneiform ligaments.*

ligamenta intercuneiformia plantaria　[NA] Transverse fibrous bands connecting the plantar surfaces of the three cuneiform bones and reinforced by slips from the tendon of the tibialis posterior muscle. Also called *plantar intercuneiform ligaments, plantar external ligaments of Barkow* (outmoded), *internal interosseous ligaments of Barkow* (outmoded).

ligamentum interfoveolare　[NA] A thickened band of the transversalis fascia, occasionally containing muscle fibers, extending from the lower margin of the transversus abdominis muscle to the superior ramus of the pubis, or, occasionally to blend with the femoral sheath. The band passes medial to the deep inguinal ring and in front of the inferior epigastric artery. Sometimes its medial side blends with the conjoint tendon. Also called *interfoveolar ligament, Hesselbach's ligament, ligamentum interfoveolare hesselbachi* (outmoded), *interfoveolar muscle, semilunar fold of transversalis fascia, external sphenoidal ligament, posterior inguinal ligament* (outmoded), *inguinal ligament of Blumberg* (outmoded), *pubicoperitoneal muscle* (outmoded).

ligamentum interfoveolare hesselbachi　An outmoded term for LIGAMENTUM INTERFOVEOLARE.

ligamentum interspinale　Any one of the ligamenta interspinalia.

ligamenta interspinalia　[NA] Fibrous membranes located between the spines of the vertebrae, extending obliquely from the root of one spine to the tip of the adjacent spine and continuous with the ligamenta flava anteriorly and the supraspinous ligaments posteriorly. They are best developed in the lumbar region and least in the neck. Also called *interspinal ligaments, interspinous ligaments, interspinal membranes* (outmoded).

ligamenta intertransversaria　[NA] Weak fibrous bands or bundles extending between the tips of adjacent transverse processes of vertebrae, best developed in the lumbar region and replaced by the intertransverse muscles in the neck. Also called *intertransverse ligaments, intertransverse ligaments of vertebral arch.*

ligamentum intertransversarium　Any one of the ligamenta intertransversaria.

ligamenta intracapsularia　[NA] Ligaments situated inside the capsule of a joint but excluded from the joint cavity by folds of synovial membrane, such as the cruciate ligaments of the knee. Also called *intra-articular ligaments, interarticular ligaments* (outmoded).

ligamentum ischiocapsulare　An outmoded term for LIGAMENTUM ISCHIOFEMORALE.

ligamentum ischiofemorale　[NA] A strong triangular band posterior to the capsule of the hip joint, spiraling superolaterally behind the neck of the femur from its attachment on the body of the ischium, behind and below the acetabulum, to the greater trochanter and trochanteric fossa, while some of the lateral and deeper fibers are continuous with the zona orbicularis. It helps to prevent excessive medial rotation. Also called *ischiofemoral ligament, ischiocapsular ligament* (outmoded), *ligamentum ischiocapsulare* (outmoded).

ligamentum jugale　An outmoded term for CORNICULOPHARYNGEAL LIGAMENT.

ligamentum laciniatum　An outmoded term for RETINACULUM MUSCULORUM FLEXORUM PEDIS.

ligamentum lacunare　[NA] The triangular extension of the medial end of the inguinal ligament to the medial part of the pecten pubis along which it extends laterally to blend with the pectineal fascia. The apex is attached to the pubic tubercle and its laterally directed concave base forms the medial border of the femoral ring. Its superior, abdominal surface forms the floor of the inguinal canal medially. Also called *lacunar ligament, Gimbernat's ligament, lacunar ligament of Gimbernat, ligamentum lacunare Gimbernati* (outmoded), *pectineal part of inguinal ligament.*

ligamentum lacunare Gimbernati　An outmoded term for LIGAMENTUM LACUNARE.

ligamentum laterale articulationis temporomandibularis　[NA] A strong, oblique fibrous band, closely related to the lateral surface of the capsule of the temporomandibular joint, extending downward and posteriorly from its attachment on the lateral surface and crest of the tubercle on the root of the zygoma to the lateral surface and back of the mandibular neck while the deeper, medial fibers attach to the articular disk and lateral aspect of the mandibular condyle. Also called *lateral ligament of temporomandibular articulation, ligamentum temporomandibulare* (outmoded), *temporomandibular ligament, lateral accessory ligament of Henle* (outmoded), *lateral maxillary ligament* (outmoded), *Ferrein's ligament, external lateral ligament of temporomandibular joint, external ligament of mandibular articulation* (outmoded), *lateral ligament of temporomandibular joint.*

ligamentum latum pulmonis　An outmoded term for LIGAMENTUM PULMONALE.

ligamentum latum uteri　[NA] A transverse fold of peritoneum extending from each lateral surface of the uterus and supravaginal cervix to the lateral walls of the pelvic cavity. The two layers are continuous at the superior, free border which contains the uterine tube, while they diverge near the superior surface of levator ani muscle. Between the layers are the uterine and ovarian vessels, ovarian ligaments, round ligaments, epoophoron, paroophoron, some smooth muscle and fibroareolar tissue. The ligament is divided into mesosalpinx, mesovarium and mesometrium. Also called *broad ligament of uterus, ala vespertilionis* (outmoded).

ligamentum lienorenale　LIGAMENTUM SPLENORENALE.

ligamentum longitudinale anterius　[NA] A strong band, of variable width and composed of several layers of longitudinal fibers, extending down the front of the bodies of the vertebrae from the basilar part of the occipital bone to the front of the first sacral segment. It is fixed to the intervertebral disks and the upper and lower margins of the vertebral bodies, the superficial fibers extending over several vertebrae while the deep ones pass from one vertebra to the next. Also called *anterior longitudinal ligament, anterior longitudinal fascia, lacertus medius weitbrechtii, lacertus medius wrisbergii.*

ligamentum longitudinale posterius [NA] A strong band, of variable width and composed of several layers of longitudinal fibers, extending down the posterior surfaces of the bodies of the vertebrae inside the vertebral canal from the axis, where it is continuous superiorly with the membrana tectoria, to the first two segments of the sacrum. It is fixed to the intervertebral disks and the upper and lower margins of the vertebral bodies, narrowing over the center of the bodies from which it is separated by veins. Its superficial fibers span several vertebrae while the deep fibers attach to contiguous vertebrae. Also called *posterior longitudinal ligament, posterior longitudinal fascia, interarticular cartilage* (outmoded).

ligamentum lumbocostale [NA] A strong band of fibers connecting the neck of the twelfth rib to the base of the transverse process of the first lumbar vertebra, in series with the superior costotransverse ligaments. Also called *lumbocostal ligament, iliocostal ligament* (outmoded), *tendinous arch of lumbodorsal fascia, retinaculum costae ultimae* (outmoded), *lumbocostal ligament of Henle.*

ligamentum mallei anterius [NA] A band extending from the neck of the malleus near the anterior, or long, process to the anterior tympanic wall, some fibers (Meckel's band) continuing through the adjacent petrotympanic fissure to the angular spine of the sphenoid bone. A few fibers may reach the sphenomandibular ligament. Also called *anterior ligament of malleus, Toynbee's ligament, laxator tympani major* (outmoded), *incudius, Casser's muscle, casserian muscle.*

ligamentum mallei laterale [NA] A short, triangular band extending from the head of the malleus to the posterior margin of the tympanic notch. Also called *lateral ligament of malleus, axis ligament of malleus* (outmoded), *Casser's ligament, casserian ligament, Folius muscle* (outmoded), *laxator tympani minor* (outmoded).

ligamentum mallei superius [NA] A fine, round band that ascends from the head of the malleus to the roof of the epitympanic recess of the middle ear. Also called *superior ligament of malleus.*

ligamentum malleoli lateralis anterius An outmoded term for LIGAMENTUM TIBIOFIBULARE ANTERIUS.

ligamentum malleoli lateralis posterius An outmoded term for LIGAMENTUM TIBIOFIBULARE POSTERIUS.

ligamentum mediale articulationis talocruralis [NA] A strong triangular band on the medial side of the talocrural joint, attached proximally to the tip and anterior and posterior margins of the medial malleolus and passing inferiorly in four bands, namely, pars tibionavicularis, pars tibiocalcanea, pars tibiotalaris anterior, and pars tibiotalaris posterior, the names of which indicate their distal attachments to the tarsal bones. Superficial to the ligament are the tendons of the tibialis posterior and flexor digitorum longus muscles. Also called *medial ligament, deltoid ligament of ankle, deltoid ligament of talocrural joint, ligamentum deltoideum.*

ligamentum mediale articulationis temporomandibularis [NA] A horizontal fibrous band that strengthens the capsule on the medial side of the temporomandibular joint and prevents backward displacement of the mandibular condyle. Also called *medial ligament of temporomandibular joint.*

ligamentum menisci lateralis An outmoded term for LIGAMENTUM MENISCOFEMORALE POSTERIUS.

ligamentum meniscofemorale anterius [NA] An oblique fasciculus extending from the posterior part of the lateral meniscus to the medial condyle of the femur and passing anterior to and blending with the posterior cruciate ligament. Also called *anterior meniscofemoral ligament, Humphry's ligament.*

ligamentum meniscofemorale posterius [NA] A strong fasciculus extending from the posterior extremity of the lateral meniscus to the medial condyle of the femur and passing pos-

terior to and blending with the posterior cruciate ligament. Also called *posterior meniscofemoral ligament, Robert's ligament, Wrisberg's ligament, lateral meniscofemoral ligament* (outmoded), *ligamentum menisci lateralis* (outmoded), *posterior meniscofemoral ligament of Wrisberg.*

ligamentum metacarpale transversum superficiale [NA] A transverse band of fibers in the superficial fascia across the webs of the fingers, attached to the skin of the webs as well as to the fifth metacarpal bone. Also called *superficial transverse metacarpal ligament, ligamentum natatorium* (outmoded).

ligamenta metacarpalia dorsalia [NA] Short transverse bands connecting the dorsal surfaces of the bases of the second to fifth metacarpal bones to each other. Also called *dorsal metacarpal ligaments, ligamenta basium ossium metacarpalium dorsalia* (outmoded), *dorsal ligaments of bases of metacarpal bones, dorsal transverse intermetacarpal ligaments* (outmoded), *dorsal intermetacarpal ligaments, posterior proximal intermetacarpal ligaments* (outmoded).

ligamenta metacarpalia interossea [NA] Short fibrous bands connecting the apposed surfaces, distal to the articular facets, of the bases of the medial four metacarpal bones. Also called *interosseous metacarpal ligaments, interosseous intermetacarpal ligaments, ligamenta basium ossium metacarpalium interossea* (outmoded), *interosseous ligaments of bases of metacarpal bones, transverse metacarpal interosseous ligaments* (outmoded), *metacarpal interosseous ligaments.*

ligamenta metacarpalia palmaria [NA] Short transverse bands connecting the palmar surfaces of the bases of the second to fifth metacarpal bones to each other. Also called *palmar metacarpal ligaments, ligamenta basium ossium metacarpalium volaria* (outmoded), *palmar intermetacarpal ligaments, deep transverse volar ligaments of carpus* (outmoded), *volar ligaments of bases of metacarpal bones, volar transverse intermetacarpal ligaments* (outmoded).

ligamentum metacarpeum transversum profundum [NA] A series of short fibrous bands connecting the palmar ligaments of the second to fifth metacarpophalangeal joints, forming a continuous transverse band fused proximally to fascia of the interosseous muscles and to digital slips of the palmar aponeurosis and, on the sides of the joints, joining the transverse band of the dorsal digital expansion. Also called *deep transverse metacarpal ligament, ligamenta capitulorum ossium metacarpalium transversa* (outmoded), *deep transverse palmar ligament, trochlear ligament* (outmoded), *distal intermetacarpal ligament, anterior intermetacarpal ligament* (outmoded), *volar capitular ligament* (outmoded), *volar ligaments of little heads of metacarpal bones* (outmoded), *trochlear ligaments of little heads of metacarpal bones* (outmoded), *transverse ligaments of little heads of metacarpal bones* (outmoded), *plantar ligaments of little heads of metacarpal bones* (outmoded).

ligamentum metatarsale transversum profundum [NA] A series of short fibrous bands connecting the plantar ligaments of the metatarsophalangeal joints, forming a continuous transverse band that fuses with the sheaths of the flexor tendons and receives slips from digital bands of the plantar aponeurosis. The interosseous muscles pass deep to it. Also called *deep transverse metatarsal ligament, ligamenta capitulorum ossium metatarsalium transversa* (outmoded), *anterior plantar metatarsal ligament* (outmoded), *anterior metatarsal ligament* (outmoded), *distal plantar intermetatarsal ligament, transverse ligaments of little heads of metatarsal bones* (outmoded).

ligamentum metatarsale transversum superficiale [NA] Transverse bands in the superficial fascia of the sole of the foot linking the webs of the toes and attached to the skin of the webs. Also called *superficial transverse metatarsal ligament.*

ligamenta metatarsalia dorsalia [NA] Transverse membranous bands connecting the dorsal surfaces of the bases of the four lateral metatarsal bones, strengthening the capsules of the intermetatarsal joints. Also called *dorsal metatarsal ligaments, ligamenta basium ossium metatarsalium dorsalia* (outmoded), *dorsal ligaments of bases of metatarsal bones, dorsal proximal intermetatarsal ligaments* (outmoded), *proximal posterior intermetatarsal ligaments, dorsal transverse intermetatarsal ligaments* (outmoded), *dorsal intermetatarsal ligaments.*

ligamenta metatarsalia interossea [NA] Strong transverse bands connecting the nonarticular parts of the adjacent surfaces of the bases of the lateral four metatarsal bones. Also called *interosseous metatarsal ligaments, ligamenta basium ossium metatarsalium interossea* (outmoded), *interosseous ligaments of bases of metatarsal bones, interosseous intermetatarsal ligaments, interosseous transverse metatarsal ligament* (outmoded), *lateral metatarsal ligaments* (outmoded), *lateral metatarsal ligaments of Weitbrecht* (outmoded), *lateral proper metatarsal ligaments of Weber* (outmoded).

ligamenta metatarsalia plantaria [NA] Transverse membranous bands connecting the plantar surfaces of the bases of the four lateral metatarsal bones, strengthening the capsules of the intermetatarsal joints. Also called *plantar metatarsal ligaments, ligamenta basium ossium metatarsalium plantaria* (outmoded), *plantar ligaments of bases of metatarsal bones, plantar proximal intermetatarsal ligaments* (outmoded), *plantar transverse intermetatarsal ligaments* (outmoded), *plantar intermetatarsal ligaments.*

ligamentum natatorium An outmoded term for LIGAMENTUM METACARPALE TRANSVERSUM SUPERFICIALE.

ligamenta navicularicuneiformia dorsalia An outmoded term for LIGAMENTA CUNEONAVICULARIA DORSALIA.

ligamenta navicularicuneiformia plantaria An outmoded term for LIGAMENTA CUNEONAVICULARIA PLANTARIA.

ligamentum nuchae [NA] A midline fibroelastic band extending from the external occipital protuberance and crest to the spine of the seventh cervical vertebra, its deep surface being attached to the occipital bone, posterior tubercle of atlas, and the tips of the spines of the cervical vertebrae, thereby forming a septum between the posterior right and left neck muscles and providing origin to these muscles. It is homologous with the supraspinous and interspinous ligaments with which it is continuous inferiorly. Also called *nuchal ligament, apparatus ligamentosus colli, ligament of nape* (outmoded), *posterior cervical ligament* (outmoded), *posterior median raphe of neck* (outmoded).

ligamentum orbiculare radii An outmoded term for LIGAMENTUM ANNULARE RADII.

ligamenta ossiculorum auditus [NA] Either bands of collagen fibers or vascularized folds of mucous membrane that connect the malleus, incus, and stapes to the walls of the tympanic cavity. Also called *ligaments of auditory ossicles.*

ligamentum ovarii proprium [NA] A fibromuscular cord located between the layers of the broad ligament of the uterus and connecting the uterine, or inferior, extremity of the ovary to the lateral angle of the uterus below and posterior to the attachment of the uterine tube. Also called *ovarian ligament, utero-ovarian ligament* (outmoded), *proper ligament of the ovary, ligament of ovary.*

ligamenta palmaria articulationum interphalangealium manus [NA] Fibrocartilaginous bands anterior to the interphalangeal joints of the hand, similar to, but thinner than, those of the metacarpophalangeal joints. They are joined laterally to the collateral ligaments and are grooved by the flexor tendons.

ligamenta palmaria articulationum metacarpophalangealium [NA] Thick fibrocartilaginous bands anterior to the metacarpophalangeal joints, firmly attached to the margins of the bases of the phalanges but only united by areolar tissue to the metacarpals, and joined laterally to the collateral ligaments

and deep transverse metacarpal ligament. Anteriorly they are grooved by the flexor tendons which are held in the grooves by their fibrous sheaths. Also called *palmar ligaments, ligamenta accessoria volaria* (outmoded), *accessory volar ligaments, accessory ligaments of digits of hand, palmar metacarpophalangeal ligaments, anterior metacarpophalangeal ligaments* (outmoded), *trochlear ligaments of hand* (outmoded).

ligamentum palpebrale laterale [NA] A thick fibrous band lying deep to a muscular raphe and fixing the lateral ends of the tarsal plates of the eyelids to a tubercle on the zygomatic bone just within the orbital margin. Also called *lateral palpebral ligament.*

ligamentum palpebrale mediale [NA] A strong fibrous band, formed by a slip from the medial end of each tarsus, that passes medially in front of the lacrimal sac to become attached to the frontal process of the maxilla and its anterior lacrimal crest. Some deep fibers attach to the posterior lacrimal crest of the lacrimal bone. Also called *medial palpebral ligament, tendo palpebrarum* (outmoded), *tendo oculi* (outmoded).

ligamentum patellae [NA] The flattened continuation of the common tendon of the quadriceps femoris muscle extending from the apex and inferior margins of the patella to the upper part of the tuberosity of the tibia. Its deep surface is fused to the capsule of the knee joint, being separated from the synovial membrane by the infrapatellar pad of fat. Also called *patellar ligament, anterior patellar tendon* (outmoded), *inferior patellar tendon* (outmoded).

ligamentum pectinatum anguli iridocornealis RETICULUM TRABECULARE SCLERAE.

ligamentum pectinatum iridis An outmoded term for RETICULUM TRABECULARE SCLERAE.

ligamentum pectineale [NA] A strong fibrous band extending laterally from the base of the lacunar ligament along the pecten pubis where it fuses with the pectineal fascia and periosteum, as well as with the lateral extensions of the conjoint tendon and adminiculum lineae albae. Also called *pectineal ligament, Cooper's ligament, inguinal ligament of Cooper, pectineal ligament of Cooper.*

ligamentum phrenicocolicum A triangular fold of peritoneum extending from the left colic flexure to the diaphragm opposite the left tenth and eleventh ribs, against which the lower pole of the spleen may rest. Also called *phrenicocolic ligament, phrenocolic ligament, costocolic ligament, sustentaculum lienis, Hensing's ligament, Hensing's fold, costocolic fold, parietocolic fold* (outmoded), *left phrenicocolic ligament.*

ligamentum phrenicolienale LIGAMENTUM SPLENORENALE.

ligamentum phrenicosplenicum LIGAMENTUM SPLENORENALE.

ligamentum pisohamatum [NA] One of the prolongations of the tendon of insertion of the flexor carpi ulnaris muscle, extending from the pisiform bone to the hook of the hamate bone. Also called *pisohamate ligament, pisouncinate ligament* (outmoded), *pisounciform ligament* (outmoded).

ligamentum pisometacarpeum [NA] One of the prolongations of the tendon of insertion of the flexor carpi ulnaris muscle, extending from the pisiform bone to the base of the fifth metacarpal bone. Also called *pisometacarpal ligament, hamatometacarpal ligament* (outmoded).

ligamentum plantare longum [NA] A long, broad band attached proximally to the inferior surface of calcaneus anterior to the medial and lateral processes of the tuberosity, while distally the deep fibers attach to the plantar surface of the cuboid bone and the superficial fibers attach to the bases of the second through fifth metatarsal bones. Also called *long plantar ligament.*

ligamenta plantaria articulationum interphalangealium pedis [NA] Fibrocartilaginous bands anterior to the interphalangeal joints of the toes, similar to, but thinner than, those of the metatarsophalangeal joints. They are joined laterally to the collateral ligaments and are grooved by the flexor tendons.

ligamenta plantaria articulationum metatarsophalangealium [NA] Thick fibrous, sometimes fibrocartilaginous, pads on the plantar surfaces of the metatarsophalangeal joints, firmly attached to the margins of the bases of the phalanges, deepening the articular surfaces, but only loosely joined to the metatarsals, and united laterally to the collateral ligaments and the deep transverse metatarsal ligaments. Their plantar aspects are grooved by the flexor tendons which are held in the grooves by their fibrous flexor sheaths. Also called *plantar ligaments, ligamenta accessoria plantaria* (outmoded), *accessory plantar ligaments, Cruveilhier's ligaments, inferior metatarsophalangeal ligaments, glenoid ligaments of Cruveilhier, plantar metatarsophalangeal ligaments, trochlear ligaments of foot* (outmoded).

ligamentum popliteum arcuatum [NA] A broad band of fibers attached to the apex of the head of the fibula from which it arches upwards superficial to the popliteus tendon and divides into two bands: one passes medially to blend with the oblique popliteal ligament and attach to the intercondylar area of the tibia, while the other band becomes the short lateral ligament. Also called *arcuate popliteal ligament, popliteal arch, arcuate ligament of knee, popliteal arcuate ligament.*

ligamentum popliteum obliquum [NA] An oblique expansion of the tendon of the semimembranosus muscle near its insertion, extending upwards and laterally to blend with the joint capsule and to attach to the lateral epicondyle of the femur where it unites with the lateral head of the gastrocnemius muscle. Its fasciculi are separated by openings for vessels and nerves. Also called *oblique popliteal ligament, posterior oblique ligament of knee, Bourgery's ligament, Winslow's ligament.*

ligamentum pterygospinale [NA] A fibrous band, occasionally replaced by muscle fibers, extending between the posterior margin of the lateral pterygoid lamina and the spine of the sphenoid. Occasionally it ossifies to form a bony foramen through which muscular branches of the mandibular nerve pass. Also called *pterygospinal ligament, pterygospinous ligament, ligamentum pterygospinosum* (outmoded), *ligament of Civinini.*

ligamentum pterygospinosum An outmoded term for LIGAMENTUM PTERYGOSPINALE.

ligamentum pubicum superius [NA] A transverse band of yellow fibers above the symphysis pubis extending along the pubic crest on either side as far as the pubic tubercle, and fusing in the midline with the interpubic disk. Also called *superior pubic ligament.*

ligamentum pubocapsulare An outmoded term for LIGAMENTUM PUBOFEMORALE.

ligamentum pubofemorale [NA] A triangular band, the base of which is attached to the obturator crest, the iliopubic eminence, and the superior pubic ramus, while distally it unites with the capsule of the hip joint anteriorly and with the deep aspect of the medial band of the iliofemoral ligament. Also called *pubofemoral ligament, ligamentum pubocapsulare* (outmoded), *pubocapsular ligament.*

ligamentum puboprostaticum [NA] A thickened sheet of endopelvic fascia in the male that extends from the base of the prostate and the neck of the bladder anteriorly to the parietal fascia on the back of the pubis (formerly called ligamentum puboprostaticum medium) and laterally to the arcus tendineus fasciae pelvis (formerly called ligamentum puboprostaticum laterale). It is equivalent to ligamentum pubovesicale in the female. Also called *puboprostatic ligament, anterior true ligament of bladder, lateral true ligament of bladder, triangular ligament of urethra* (outmoded), *puborectal ligament.*

ligamentum puboprostaticum laterale The lateral pubo-

prostatic ligament; the lateral extension of ligamentum puboprostaticum. An outmoded term.

ligamentum puboprostaticum medium The medial puboprostatic ligament; the medial portion of ligamentum puboprostaticum. An outmoded term.

ligamentum pubovesicale [NA] A thickened sheet of endopelvic fascia in the female that extends from the neck of the bladder anteriorly to the parietal fascia on the back of the pubis (formerly called ligamentum pubovesicale medium) and laterally to the arcus tendineus fasciae pelvis (formerly called ligamentum pubovesicale laterale). It is equivalent to ligamentum puboprostaticum in the male. Also called *pubovesical ligament, vesicopubic ligament, puborectal ligament, anterior true ligament of bladder.*

ligamentum pubovesicale laterale The lateral portion of ligamentum pubovesicale. An outmoded term.

ligamentum pubovesicale medium The medial portion of ligamentum pubovesicale. An outmoded term.

ligamentum pulmonale [NA] A reflected fold of mediastinal pleura extending from the anterior and posterior surfaces of the structures in the root of the lung down along the mediastinal surface of the lung behind the cardiac impression to the diaphragm where it ends in a free falciform border. It helps to hold the lung in position. Also called *pulmonary ligament, broad ligament of lung* (outmoded), *ligamentum latum pulmonis* (outmoded), *Teutleben's ligament.*

ligamenta pylori Thickened longitudinal muscle bands along the anterior and posterior walls of the pyloric antrum, most of the muscle fibers passing deep to end in the pyloric sphincter. An outmoded term. Also called *ligaments of Helvetius, taeniae pylori.*

ligamentum quadratum [NA] A thin fibrous membrane extending from the distal margin of the radial notch of the ulna to the neck of the radius and closing the synovial membrane over the inferomedial aspect of the proximal radioulnar joint. Also called *quadrate ligament, Denucé's ligament, quadrate ligament of Denucé.*

ligamentum radiatum An outmoded term for LIGAMENTUM CAPITIS COSTAE RADIATUM.

ligamentum radiocarpale dorsale [NA] A thin fibrous sheet extending over the back of the radiocarpal joint from the posterior margin of the distal end of the radius and the edge of the articular disk to the proximal row of carpal bones and blending with the dorsal intercarpal ligaments. Also called *dorsal radiocarpal ligament, dorsal ligament of radiocarpal joint, posterior ligament of radiocarpal joint, superficial ligament of carpus* (outmoded), *rhomboid ligament of wrist* (outmoded).

ligamentum radiocarpale palmare [NA] A thick membranous band in front of the radiocarpal joint extending from the anterior margin of the styloid process and distal end of the radius to the anterior surfaces of the proximal row of carpal bones, blending with the anterior intercarpal ligaments. Also called *palmar radiocarpal ligament, ligamentum radiocarpeum volare* (outmoded), *volar radiocarpal ligament, palmar ligament of radiocarpal joint, superficial ligament of carpus* (outmoded), *anterior ligament of radiocarpal joint, anterior radiocarpal ligament, oblique accessory carpal ligament* (outmoded).

ligamentum radiocarpeum volare An outmoded term for LIGAMENTUM RADIOCARPALE PALMARE.

ligamentum reflexum [NA] According to some authorities, a poorly developed expansion of the lateral crus of the inguinal ligament, passing medially and upward behind the medial end of the superficial inguinal ring in front of the conjoint tendon, feebly reinforcing the posterior wall of the inguinal canal, and interweaving with like fibers of the opposite side in the linea alba. Others describe it as a poorly developed triangular band of the external oblique aponeurosis of one side that crosses the midline, passing behind the superficial inguinal ring of the opposite side to be attached to the pectineal line. It is seldom independent, usually being fused with the external oblique aponeurosis or with the conjoint tendon. Also called *reflex inguinal ligament, ligamentum inguinale reflexum, ligamentum inguinale reflexum collesi* (outmoded), *Colles ligament, reflex ligament of Gimbernat, reflected ligament, internal inguinal ligament* (outmoded), *triangular fascia of abdomen, triangular fascia of Quain, triangular ligament of abdomen* (outmoded), *triangular ligament of thigh* (outmoded), *medial crus of external inguinal ring.*

ligamentum sacrococcygeum anterius [NA] A series of fibers, considered to be the termination of the anterior longitudinal ligament, extending anterior to the sacrococcygeal joint from the lowest segment of the sacrum to the coccyx. Also called *ligamentum sacrococcygeum ventrale, anterior sacrococcygeal ligament, ventral sacrococcygeal ligament.*

ligamentum sacrococcygeum dorsale profundum LIGAMENTUM SACROCOCCYGEUM POSTERIUS PROFUNDUM.

ligamentum sacrococcygeum dorsale superficiale LIGAMENTUM SACROCOCCYGEUM POSTERIUS SUPERFICIALE.

ligamentum sacrococcygeum laterale [NA] A broad band, similar to an intertransverse ligament, that extends from the lateral inferior margin of the sacrum to the transverse process of the first coccygeal vertebra, forming a foramen for the ventral branch of the fifth sacral nerve. Also called *lateral sacrococcygeal ligament, intercornual ligament.*

ligamentum sacrococcygeum posterius profundum [NA] A fibrous band extending from the dorsal surface of the fifth sacral vertebra to the back of the coccyx, representing the posterior longitudinal ligament with which it may be continuous superiorly. Also called *ligamentum sacrococcygeum dorsale profundum, deep dorsal sacrococcygeal ligament.*

ligamentum sacrococcygeum posterius superficiale [NA] A flat band continuous with the supraspinous ligament and extending downward from the margin of the sacral hiatus to the dorsal surface of the coccyx covering the lower part of the sacral canal. Also called *ligamentum sacrococcygeum dorsale superficiale, superficial dorsal sacrococcygeal ligament.*

ligamentum sacrococcygeum ventrale LIGAMENTUM SACROCOCCYGEUM ANTERIUS.

ligamentum sacrodurale Filamentous fibers extending from the spinal dura to the posterior longitudinal ligament in the sacral canal. An outmoded term.

ligamenta sacroiliaca anteriora [NA] Fibrous thickenings of the anterior and inferior parts of the capsule of the sacroiliac joint, especially strong opposite the arcuate line. Also called *ligamenta sacroiliaca ventralia, anterior sacroiliac ligaments, ventral sacroiliac ligaments, anterior iliosacral ligaments* (outmoded).

ligamenta sacroiliaca dorsalia [NA] A series of thick fibrous bands posterior to the sacroiliac joint extending from the lateral sacral crest to the tuberosity of the ilium, the iliac crest, and the posterior iliac spines. The direction of different bands is irregular and the series is often divided into an upper, deep group (the short posterior sacroiliac ligament) and the lower, more superficial group (the long posterior sacroiliac ligament) which is continuous with the sacrotuberous ligament. Also called *dorsal sacroiliac ligaments.*

ligamenta sacroiliaca interossea [NA] Short, strong fibrous bands, deep to the posterior sacroiliac ligaments, extending from the iliac tuberosity to the sacral tuberosity just posterior to the auricular surface. Also called *interosseous sacroiliac ligaments, interosseous iliosacral ligaments* (outmoded).

ligamenta sacroiliaca ventralia LIGAMENTA SACROILIACA ANTERIORA.

ligamentum sacroiliacum posterius breve An outmoded term for SHORT POSTERIOR SACROILIAC LIGAMENT.

ligamentum sacroiliacum posterius longum An outmoded term for LONG POSTERIOR SACROILIAC LIGAMENT.

ligamentum sacrospinale [NA] A thin triangular fibrous band attached by its apex to the margins and pelvic surface of the ischial spine and by its base to the lateral margin and pelvic surface of the lower part of the sacrum and the coccyx. Anteriorly it gives partial attachment to the coccygeus muscle while posteriorly it is covered by the sacrotuberous ligament with which it converts the greater and the lesser sciatic notches into foramina. Also called *sacrospinal ligament, sacrospinous ligament, spinosacral ligament* (outmoded), *ligamentum sacrospinosum* (outmoded), *anterior sacrosciatic ligament, internal sacrosciatic ligament* (outmoded), *least sacrosciatic ligament* (outmoded), *short posterior pelvic ligament* (outmoded).

ligamentum sacrospinosum An outmoded term for LIGAMENTUM SACROSPINALE.

ligamentum sacrotuberale [NA] A long, strong, somewhat triangular-shaped fibrous band extending from the posterior superior and inferior iliac spines and the lateral margins and dorsal surfaces of the last three sacral and first two coccygeal vertebrae to the medial margin of the ischial tuberosity and of the ischial ramus. Superomedially its fibers mix with those of the posterior sacroiliac ligaments and its posterior surface gives partial origin to the gluteus maximus muscle. Its free anterior margin helps to convert the greater and the lesser sciatic notches into foramina. Also called *sacrotuberal ligament, sacrotuberous ligament, tuberososacral ligament* (outmoded), *ligamentum sacrotuberosum* (outmoded), *great sacrosciatic ligament, great posterior pelvic ligament* (outmoded).

ligamentum sacrotuberosum An outmoded term for LIGAMENTUM SACROTUBERALE.

ligamentum serosum Any fold of a serous membrane, particularly peritoneum, that supports or connects an organ or part and transmits blood vessels and nerves. An outmoded term. Also called *serous ligament.*

ligamentum sphenomandibulare [NA] A thin fibrous remnant of Meckel's cartilage lying medial to the capsule of the temporomandibular joint and extending from the spine of the sphenoid bone and the area adjacent to the petrotympanic fissure to the lingula and the back of the mylohyoid groove of the mandible. Also called *sphenomandibular ligament, middle maxillary ligament* (outmoded), *medial accessory ligament of Henle* (outmoded), *internal lateral ligament of temporomandibular joint* (outmoded).

ligamentum spirale cochleae [NA] A ridge of thickened and altered periosteum supporting the lateral wall of the cochlear duct and having the basilar membrane attached to it. It contains many blood vessels in its upper part. Also called *spiral ligament of cochlea.*

ligamentum splenorenale [NA] A peritoneal fold, comprising a left layer (parietal layer of greater sac) passing from the abdominal wall to the front of the left kidney, where it meets the right layer (from the lesser sac) from the front of the pancreas, extending to the hilum of the spleen and containing the splenic vessels and the tail of the pancreas, and then becoming continuous with the gastrosplenic ligament and merging into the gastrophrenic ligament. Also called *ligamentum lienorenale, lienorenal ligament, lienophrenic ligament, phrenicolienal ligament, ligamentum phrenicolienale, phrenicosplenic ligament, ligamentum phrenicosplenicum, splenophrenic ligament* (outmoded), *suspensory ligament of spleen* (outmoded).

ligamentum sternoclaviculare Ligamentum sternoclaviculare anterius or ligamentum sternoclaviculare posterius.

ligamentum sternoclaviculare anterius [NA] A broad band blending with the anterior surface of the capsule of the sternoclavicular joint and extending from the anterior and superior margins of the medial end of the clavicle to the front of the upper border of the manubrium sterni and the adjacent costal cartilage. Also called *anterior sternoclavicular ligament, anterior fibrous ligament* (outmoded).

ligamentum sternoclaviculare posterius [NA] A fibrous band blending with the posterior surface of the capsule of the sternoclavicular joint and extending from the posterior margin of the medial end of the clavicle to the posterior surface of the adjacent upper margin of the manubrium sterni. Also called *posterior sternoclavicular ligament, posterior fibrous ligament* (outmoded).

ligamentum sternocostale interarticulare An outmoded term for LIGAMENTUM STERNOCOSTALE INTRA-ARTICULARE.

ligamentum sternocostale intra-articulare [NA] An inconstant fibrocartilaginous band connecting the cartilage of the second rib to the fibrocartilage joining the manubrium to the body of the sternum, and dividing the joint into two compartments. Occasionally fibrocartilaginous filaments are found in the third and lower articular cavities between the costal cartilages and the sternum. Also called *intra-articular sternocostal ligament, ligamentum sternocostale interarticulare* (outmoded), *interarticular sternocostal ligament* (outmoded), *interarticular chondrosternal ligament, interarticular costal cartilage.*

ligamenta sternocostalia radiata [NA] Thin, triangular bands radiating from the anterior and the posterior surfaces of the medial ends of the costal cartilages of the true ribs to corresponding adjacent surfaces of the sternum. The anterior fibers interweave with those of ligaments above and below, with those of the opposite side, and with fibers of origin of the pectoralis major muscle. Also called *radiate sternocostal ligaments, sternocostal ligaments, radiate costosternal ligaments* (outmoded), *radiating fibers of anterior chondrosternal ligaments.*

ligamenta sternopericardiaca [NA] Two variable bands of dense fibrous tissue fixing the fibrous pericardium to the upper and lower parts of the posterior surface of the sternum. Also called *sternopericardiac ligaments, sternopericardial ligaments, ligaments of Luschka.*

ligamentum stylohyoideum [NA] A slender fibrous cord extending from the tip of the styloid process of the temporal bone to the lesser cornu of the hyoid bone and providing partial origin for the middle constrictor of the pharynx. Also called *stylohyoid ligament, epihyal ligament.*

ligamentum stylomandibulare [NA] A thin process of the deep cervical fascia attached proximally to the tip of the styloid process of the temporal bone and distally to the angle and posterior margin of the ramus of the mandible between the masseter and medial pterygoid muscles. It separates the parotid gland from the submandibular gland. Also called *stylomandibular ligament, stylomaxillary ligament* (outmoded), *stylomylohyoid ligament* (outmoded).

ligamentum supraspinale A longitudinal band of variable thickness connecting the tips of the spines of the vertebrae and extending from the second cervical vertebra to the median sacral crest where it is continuous with the superficial dorsal sacrococcygeal ligament. Superiorly it is continuous with ligamentum nuchae. Also called *supraspinal ligament, supraspinous ligament.*

ligamenta suspensoria mammae LIGAMENTA SUSPENSORIA MAMMARIA.

ligamenta suspensoria mammaria [NA] The coarse connective tissue strands connecting the glandular tissue of the upper part of the mammary gland to both the dermis of the overlying skin and the underlying pectoral fascia, resembling retinacula cutis. Also called *ligamenta suspensoria mammae, suspensory ligaments of mammary gland, suspensory ligaments of breast, fibrous ligaments of breast, Cooper suspensory ligaments.*

ligamentum suspensorium clitoridis [NA] A fibrous band connecting the dorsum of the body of the clitoris to the arcuate pubic ligament and symphysis pubis. Also called *suspensory ligament of clitoris.*

ligamentum suspensorium ovarii [NA] The part of the broad ligament of uterus that extends from the tubal end of the ovary and the infundibulum of the uterine tube to the lateral wall of the pelvis, transmitting the ovarian blood vessels, nerves, and lymph vessels. The fold continues superiorly over the external iliac vessels to become continuous with the parietal peritoneum over the psoas muscle either in the subcecal fossa or behind the descending colon. Also called *suspensory ligament of ovary, infundibulopelvic ligament, Clado's band, hilum of broad ligament* (outmoded).

ligamentum suspensorium penis [NA] A triangular fibroelastic band, deep to the fundiform ligament, attached above to the front of symphysis pubis and below to the fascia around the penis. Also called *suspensory ligament of penis.*

ligamentum talocalcaneare laterale [NA] A short band extending downward and posteriorly, from the talus just anteroinferior to the lateral malleolar surface, to the lateral surface of the calcaneus anterior to the attachment of the calcaneofibular ligament. Also called *lateral talocalcaneal ligament.*

ligamentum talocalcaneare mediale [NA] A narrow band extending obliquely downward from the medial tubercle of the talus to the calcaneus behind the sustentaculum tali and blending with the medial ligament of the talocrural joint. Also called *medial talocalcaneal ligament.*

ligamentum talocalcaneum anterius A fibrous band extending from the anterolateral aspect of the neck of the talus to the superior surface of the calcaneus. Also called *anterior talocalcaneal ligament.*

ligamentum talocalcaneum interosseum [NA] A broad band occupying the sinus tarsi and running obliquely and laterally from the roof of sulcus tali to sulcus calcanei. It strengthens the capsules of both the talocalcaneonavicular joint and the subtalar joint. Also called *interosseous talocalcaneal ligament.*

ligamentum talocalcaneum posterius A short band radiating from the lateral tubercle of the talus to the proximal medial aspect of the calcaneus. Also called *posterior talocalcaneal ligament.*

ligamentum talofibulare anterius [NA] A narrow band extending from the anterior margin of the lateral malleolus to the lateral aspect of the talus anterior to the malleolar surface. Also called *anterior talofibular ligament.*

ligamentum talofibulare posterius [NA] A thick horizontal band extending from the posterior border and fossa of the lateral malleolus to the lateral tubercle of the posterior process of the talus. Also called *posterior talofibular ligament, Walther's oblique ligament* (outmoded).

ligamentum talonaviculare [NA] A broad, thin band extending from the dorsolateral surface of the neck of the talus to the dorsal surface of the navicular bone. Also called *talonavicular ligament, ligamentum talonaviculare dorsale* (outmoded), *dorsal talonavicular ligament.*

ligamentum talonaviculare dorsale An outmoded term for LIGAMENTUM TALONAVICULARE.

ligamentum talotibiale anterius An outmoded term for PARS TIBIOTALARIS ANTERIOR LIGAMENTI MEDIALIS.

ligamentum talotibiale posterius An outmoded term for PARS TIBIOTALARIS POSTERIOR LIGAMENTI MEDIALIS.

ligamenta tarsi dorsalia [NA] The ligaments that connect the tarsal bones on their dorsal surfaces, including the talonavicular, intercuneiform, cuneocuboid, cuboideonavicular, and bifurcate ligaments. Also called *dorsal ligaments of tarsus, dorsal intertarsal ligaments.*

ligamenta tarsi interossea [NA] The ligaments connecting the adjoining surfaces of the tarsal bones, including the interosseous cuneocuboid, talocalcaneal, and intercuneiform ligaments. Also called *interosseous ligaments of tarsus, interosseous intertarsal ligaments.*

ligamenta tarsi plantaria [NA] The ligaments that bind the tarsal bones on their plantar surfaces, including the long plantar, calcaneocuboid, calcaneonavicular, cuneonavicular, cuboideonavicular, cuneocuboid, and intercuneiform ligaments. Also called *plantar ligaments of tarsus, plantar intertarsal ligaments.*

ligamenta tarsi profunda The deeply placed plantar ligaments of the tarsus. Also called *deep ligaments of tarsus.*

ligamenta tarsometatarsalia dorsalia [NA] Short fibrous bundles extending distally from the cuboid and the three cuneiform bones to the bases of the metatarsal bones on their dorsal surfaces. Also called *dorsal tarsometatarsal ligaments, bigeminate ligaments of Arnold, trigeminate ligaments of Arnold* (outmoded).

ligamenta tarsometatarsalia plantaria [NA] Longitudinal and oblique bands binding the plantar surfaces of the cuboid and the three cuneiform bones to the bases of the metatarsal bones. Also called *plantar tarsometatarsal ligaments, deep bifurcate ligaments* (outmoded), *deep bifurcate ligaments of Arnold* (outmoded), *short cuboideometatarsal ligaments* (outmoded), *sphenoideotarsal ligaments* (outmoded).

ligamentum temporomandibulare An outmoded term for LIGAMENTUM LATERALE ARTICULATIONIS TEMPOROMANDIBULARIS.

ligamentum teres femoris An outmoded term for LIGAMENTUM CAPITIS FEMORIS.

ligamentum teres hepatis [NA] A fibrous cord, the remnant of the obliterated umbilical vein, extending from the umbilicus to the anterior border of the liver in the free margin of the falciform ligament and ending in the left branch of the portal vein at the left side of the porta hepatis. Also called *round ligament of liver, hepatoumbilical ligament* (outmoded).

ligamentum teres uteri [NA] A narrow fibrous band attached proximally to the lateral angle of the uterus on each side, passing between the two layers of the broad ligament anteroinferior to the uterine tube to enter the deep inguinal ring and leave the inguinal canal through the superficial ring, ending in the labium majus by becoming continuous with the connective tissue. Near the uterus it also contains muscle fibers. It is homologous with part of the gubernaculum testis. Also called *round ligament of uterus, Hunter's ligament, plica cordae uteroinguinalis* (outmoded).

ligamentum testis A ligament in the embryo developing within the caudal genital ridge to form the cranial portion of the gubernaculum.

ligamentum thyreoepiglotticum An outmoded term for LIGAMENTUM THYROEPIGLOTTICUM.

ligamentum thyroepiglotticum [NA] An elastic band firmly connecting the stalk, or petiole, of the lower end of the epiglottis to the back of the thyroid cartilage in the midline just below the superior notch. Also called *thyroepiglottic ligament, ligamentum thyreoepiglotticum* (outmoded), *thyroepiglottic joint* (outmoded).

ligamentum thyrohyoideum An outmoded term for LIGAMENTUM THYROHYOIDEUM LATERALE.

ligamentum thyrohyoideum laterale [NA] The elastic, cordlike posterior edge of the thyrohyoid membrane extending from the superior cornu of the thyroid cartilage to the greater cornu of the hyoid bone. Also called *lateral thyrohyoid ligament, ligamentum hyothyreoideum laterale* (outmoded), *Berry's ligament, ligamentum thyrohyoideum* (outmoded), *thyrohyoid ligament.*

ligamentum thyrohyoideum medianum [NA] The median elastic thickening of the thyrohyoid membrane extending upward behind the body of the hyoid bone from the superior notch of the thyroid cartilage to the superior margin of the hyoid bone, a bursa interposing between the latter and the band. Also called

median thyrohyoid ligament, ligamentum hyothyreoideum medium (outmoded), *median hyothyroid ligament, middle thyrohyoid ligament.*

ligamentum tibiofibulare anterius [NA] A strong triangular band in front of the tibiofibular syndesmosis extending downward and laterally from the distal end of the tibia at the anterior margin of the fibular notch to the adjacent margin of the lateral malleolus. Also called *anterior tibiofibular ligament, ligamentum malleoli lateralis anterius* (outmoded).

ligamentum tibiofibulare medium An outmoded term for MEMBRANA INTEROSSEA CRURIS.

ligamentum tibiofibulare posterius [NA] A fibrous band situated diagonally behind the tibiofibular syndesmosis and extending from the posterior margin of the fibular notch at the distal end of the tibia to the adjacent posterior margin of the lateral malleolus. Also called *posterior tibiofibular ligament, ligamentum malleoli lateralis posterius* (outmoded).

ligamentum tibionaviculare An outmoded term for PARS TIBIONAVICULARIS LIGAMENTI MEDIALIS.

ligamentum transversum acetabuli [NA] A fibrous band of decussating fibers spanning the acetabular notch, converting it into a foramen, and attached to the margin of the acetabulum on each side of the notch and continuous with the acetabular labrum. It is also attached to the ligament of the head of femur and the capsule of the hip joint. Also called *transverse ligament of acetabulum.*

ligamentum transversum atlantis [NA] A powerful, thick fibrous band, attached at each end to a tubercle on the medial surface of the lateral mass of the atlas, converting the ring of the atlas into a small anterior portion for the dens of the axis with which it articulates and a larger posterior portion for the spinal cord and its membranes. It forms the horizontal bar of the cruciform ligament of the atlas. Also called *transverse ligament of atlas.*

ligamentum transversum cruris An outmoded term for RETINACULUM MUSCULORUM EXTENSORUM PEDIS SUPERIUS.

ligamentum transversum genu An outmoded term for LIGAMENTUM TRANSVERSUM GENUS.

ligamentum transversum genus [NA] A fibrous cord of variable thickness connecting the anterior convex margin of the lateral meniscus of the knee joint to the anterior extremity of the medial meniscus. It is occasionally absent. Also called *transverse ligament of knee, ligamentum transversum genu* (outmoded), *common ligament of knee of Weber, transverse ligament of knee joint.*

ligamentum transversum pelvis An outmoded term for LIGAMENTUM TRANSVERSUM PERINEI.

ligamentum transversum perinei [NA] A thickening at the line of fusion of the anterior margin of the perineal membrane and the endopelvic fascia deep to it, extending transversely between the inferior pubic rami and lying below the dorsal vein and nerves of penis or clitoris. Also called *transverse perineal ligament, ligamentum transversum pelvis* (outmoded), *transverse pelvic ligament, interosseous ligament of pubis, interosseous ligament of pubis of Winslow* (outmoded), *Krause's ligament, transverse ligament of pelvis, preurethral ligament of Waldeyer, transverse ligament of pelvis of Henle.*

ligamentum transversum scapulae inferius [NA] A thin membranous band extending, when present, from the lateral margin of the spine of the scapula to the margin of the glenoid cavity, forming a fibro-osseous canal through which the suprascapular vessels and nerve enter the infraspinous fossa. Also called *inferior transverse ligament of scapula, spinoglenoid ligament, triquetral ligament of scapula* (outmoded), *triangular ligament of scapula* (outmoded).

ligamentum transversum scapulae superius [NA] A fibrous band bridging the scapular notch, converting it into a foramen for the suprascapular nerve and extending from the lateral end of the superior margin to the base of the coracoid process. Superior to it are the suprascapular vessels and the fibers of attachment of the omohyoid muscle. Also called *superior transverse ligament of scapula, suprascapular ligament, costocoracoid ligament* (outmoded), *coracoid ligament of scapula, oblique ligament of scapula* (outmoded).

ligamentum trapezoideum [NA] The broad anterolateral part of the coracoclavicular ligament, extending from a ridge on the medial margin of the coracoid process to an oblique ridge running anterolaterally from the conoid tubercle on the inferior surface of the lateral end of the clavicle. It is separated from the conoid ligament by fat or a bursa. It limits anterior movement of the scapula. Also called *trapezoid ligament, external coracoclavicular ligament* (outmoded).

ligamentum triangulare An outmoded term for MEMBRANA PERINEI.

ligamentum triangulare dextrum hepatis [NA] A triangular fold of peritoneum connecting the right lobe at the apex of the bare area of the liver to the diaphragm and formed by the fusion of the superior and the inferior layers of the coronary ligament. Also called *right triangular ligament of liver.*

ligamentum triangulare sinistrum hepatis [NA] A long fold of peritoneum connecting the superior surface of the left lobe of the liver to the diaphragm, its anterior layer being continuous with the left layer of the falciform ligament while the posterior layer continues as the anterior layer of the lesser omentum. The two layers are in close contact and become continuous with each other at the left free border. Also called *left triangular ligament of liver.*

ligamentum tuberculi costae An outmoded term for LIGAMENTUM COSTOTRANSVERSARIUM LATERALE.

ligamentum ulnocarpale palmare [NA] A rounded fibrous bundle extending from the styloid process of the ulna and the front of the articular disk to the palmar surfaces of the carpal bones, particularly the lunate and triquetrum. Also called *palmar ulnocarpal ligament.*

ligamentum umbilicale laterale An outmoded term for LIGAMENTUM UMBILICALE MEDIALE.

ligamentum umbilicale mediale [NA] A fibrous cord, the remnant of the obliterated umbilical artery beyond the origin of the superior vesical artery from the internal iliac artery, lying within a fold of peritoneum, the medial umbilical fold, extending from the pelvis along the lateral wall of the bladder and the posterior surface of the anterior abdominal wall to the umbilicus. Also called *medial umbilical ligament, obliterated hypogastric artery, lateral umbilical ligament* (outmoded), *ligamentum umbilicale laterale* (outmoded), *lateral vesical ligament* (outmoded).

ligamentum umbilicale medianum [NA] The fibrous remnant of the urachus between the apex of the bladder and the umbilicus that raises up a fold of peritoneum, the median umbilical fold, on the posterior surface of the anterior abdominal wall. Also called *median umbilical ligament, ligamentum umbilicale medium* (outmoded), *middle umbilical ligament, vesicoumbilical ligament.*

ligamentum umbilicale medium An outmoded term for LIGAMENTUM UMBILICALE MEDIANUM.

ligamentum vaginale **1** An outmoded term for RUDIMENT OF VAGINAL PROCESS. **2** An outmoded term for FRENULUM SYNOVIALE.

ligamenta vaginalia digitorum manus An outmoded term for VINCULA TENDINUM DIGITORUM MANUS.

ligamenta vaginalia digitorum pedis An outmoded term for VINCULA TENDINUM DIGITORUM PEDIS.

ligamentum venae cavae sinistrae An outmoded term for PLICA VENAE CAVAE SINISTRAE.

ligamentum venosum [NA] The fibrous remnant of the ob-

literated ductus venosus connecting the left branch of the portal vein to the inferior vena cava or the left hepatic vein and occupying a fissure on the posterior aspect of the liver. Also called *venous ligament of liver, Arantius ligament, ligamentum venosum arantii* (outmoded), *ligament of ductus venosus.*

ligamentum venosum arantii An outmoded term for LIGAMENTUM VENOSUM.

ligamentum ventriculare An outmoded term for LIGAMENTUM VESTIBULARE.

ligamentum vestibulare [NA] A narrow fibrous band within the vestibular fold and extending posteriorly from the angle of the thyroid cartilage to the anterolateral surface of the arytenoid cartilage just above the vocal process. Also called *vestibular ligament, ligamentum ventriculare* (outmoded), *ventricular ligament of larynx, glandular crest of larynx* (outmoded).

ligamentum vocale [NA] The thickened free upper edge of the lateral part of the cricothyroid ligament, extending from the thyroid angle to the tip of the vocal process of the arytenoid cartilage, and lying alongside the vocalis muscle within the vocal fold. It is composed of yellow elastic tissue. Also called *vocal ligament, inferior thyroarytenoid ligament* (outmoded).

---

ligand [L *ligand(us)*, gerundive of *ligare* to bind] Any one of several molecules or ions, identical or different, that bind to the same central entity. For example, the nitrogen atoms and the oxygen molecule bind to the iron of hemoglobin. The hydrogen ions that bind to the same protein molecule are another example.

cell ligands Molecules associated with cell surfaces which interact and link the cells together. Ligands are found on surfaces of embryonic cells and are responsible for the adhesiveness of specific cells.

ligase SYNTHETASE.

ligate [L *ligat(us)*, past part. of *ligare* to bind, tie] **1** To tie or compress with a suture, as a vessel or other tissue. **2** To bind together, as one molecule (the ligand), which is considered peripheral, to another (such as a metal ion or a protein) which is considered central.

ligation [L *ligatio* (from *ligatus*, past part. of *ligare* to bind, tie, akin to *licium* a thread, string and to *laqueus* a noose, snare) a binding, tieing] A surgical procedure in which a suture is placed around a tissue, usually a vessel, in order to tie off or obliterate the lumen.

immediate ligation A surgical procedure in which a ligature is tied directly on a vessel without incorporating any surrounding tissue. An outmoded term.

Larrey's ligation A surgical procedure in which the femoral artery is ligated immediately below the inguinal ligament.

mediate ligation A surgical procedure in which a ligature is tied around a vessel along with a small amount of surrounding tissue. An obsolete term.

pole ligation The placement of a suture about one or more poles of the thyroid gland in order to impede the vascular supply, an obsolete surgical procedure for treating Graves disease.

proximal ligation A surgical procedure in which a suture is used to tie off or obliterate the proximal or near end of a vessel, duct, or other hollow organ; ligature of the upstream end of a vessel or duct.

quadruple ligation A method for controlling an arteriovenous fistula by which the two arterial and two venous components of the fistula are ligated. It is a less favored approach, because distal perfusion is dependent upon collateral flow around the operative site.

saphenous ligation A surgical procedure in which one or more sutures are passed around the saphenous vein, usually at the saphenofemoral junction, as a treatment for venous incompetence of the leg.

surgical ligation   The fixing of a ligature around the neck of an unerupted tooth so that traction can be applied to it.

tooth ligation   The tying together of two or more teeth with fine wire or thread either for splinting or for orthodontic movement.

tubal ligation   A surgical procedure in which one or both fallopian tubes are tied and cut or crushed for the purpose of sterilization.

ligator [*ligat(e)* + -OR]   A surgical instrument used to facilitate the ligation of deep, small, and otherwise inaccessible structures.

ligature [L *ligatura* (from *ligatus*, past part. of *ligare* to bind + *-ura* -URE) a band, tie]   A suture that is tied around a tissue or vessel in order to obliterate the lumen. It may be made of any naturally occurring or synthetic material.

absorbable ligature   A suture designed to decompose and be absorbed by the body. Also called *soluble ligature.*

chain ligature   An over-and-over suture used to secure hemostasis.

Desault's ligature   A ligature of the femoral artery placed immediately above the popliteal space. It is used to treat a popliteal aneurysm. An obsolete term.

distal ligature   A ligature that ties off or obliterates the lumen at the distal end of a vessel, duct, or other hollow organ; ligature of the downstream end of a vessel or duct.

double ligature   A pair of ligatures tied around the same structure, usually in close approximation, to ensure against leakage.

elastic ligature   A ligament used to tie around tissues and capable of stretching a predetermined amount.

grass-line ligature   A ligature, used in tooth ligation, which has the property of shrinking when wetted and so tightening.

immediate ligature   A ligature used to establish hemostasis by closing off the main feeding vessel. An outmoded term.

ligature in continuity   Placement and tying of ligatures on tissue prior to incising between the ligatures.

interlacing ligature   INTERLOCKING LIGATURE.

interlocking ligature   A ligature in which the loops of successive stitches interlock. Also called *interlacing ligature.*

kangaroo ligature   A surgical suture material prepared from preserved tail of a species of kangaroo. Also called *kangaroo tendon.*

lateral ligature   A surgical suture that is placed on or about a vessel in such a way that distal blood flow is controlled but not obliterated. An obsolete term.

nonabsorbable ligature   A ligature made of material that will not be degraded or absorbed by the body.

occluding ligature   A suture that is tied about a vessel to obliterate the blood flow distally.

provisional ligature   A ligature that is placed during the initial stages of a surgical procedure and may or may not be left in place at the completion of the operation.

soluble ligature   ABSORBABLE LIGATURE.

Stannius ligature   A thread tied around the heart of cold-blooded animals either at the sinoatrial junction (first Stannius ligature) or in the atrioventricular groove (second Stannius ligature). It is used in experiments demonstrating the different degrees of inherent rhythmicity in sinus, atrial, and ventricular tissues.

steel ligature   A fine stainless steel wire used in tooth ligation.

suboccluding ligature   A surgical suture that, when applied and tied, obliterates all or most of the main blood supply to an organ or tissue. It does, however, leave smaller vessels capable of dilatation and use in anastomoses. An obsolete term.

terminal ligature   A surgical tie that occludes the distal end

of a transected vessel. An obsolete term.

thread-elastic ligature   Elastic thread for orthodontic tooth movement.

light [Old English *lēoht*, akin to L *lux*, gen. *lucis*, daylight, light, brightness and to Gk *lykē*, root of Gk *lykabas* the path of light and *lykaphōs* twilight]   **1** Electromagnetic radiation to which the human eye is sensitive, comprising the wavelength range from 400 to 700 nm. Both limits are poorly defined.   **2** Electromagnetic radiation with wavelengths outside the visible limits, but excited by similar means. The portion with wavelengths longer than the visible is called infrared light, that with shorter, ultraviolet.

actinic light   Sunlight capable of producing chemical changes in the skin.

arc light   ARC LAMP.

axial light   Light whose rays are parallel to the optical axis. Also called *central light.*

central light   AXIAL LIGHT.

light chaos   INTRINSIC LIGHT.

coherent light   Light from a laser, which has a single frequency, whose waves are in phase in space and time, and which travels in intense parallel beams with very small divergence.

diffused light   Light that has been made diffuse, having its brightness at any wavelength nearly independent of the direction of observation, either by reflection from a rough surface or by transmission through a medium containing suitably distributed scatterers.

fiberoptic light   Light transmitted by fiberoptics.

Finsen light   The type of light produced by a Finsen lamp.

idioretinal light   INTRINSIC LIGHT.

intrinsic light   The variable phosphenes spontaneously seen in darkness. Also called *idioretinal light, light chaos.*

Landeker-Steinberg light   An artificial sunlight from which the ultraviolet waves have been filtered out.

Minin light   A form of ultraviolet lamp.

reflected light   Light that has returned from an illuminated surface.

refracted light   Light whose rays are deflected from a straight line by passing obliquely from one medium such as air to another such as glass.

Simpson light   SIMPSON LAMP.

stray light   Light of a wavelength other than the desired band that enters the cuvette and photocell of a photometric device.

Tyndall light   Light scattered at an angle to the incident beam by colloidal particles in solution.

white light   Light that contains substantially equal energy at all wavelengths of the visible range.

Wood's light   Ultraviolet light produced by Wood's lamp, used to detect the presence of certain microbial agents in the hair, especially of children. See also WOOD'S LAMP.

light-adapted   Adapted to daylight intensities of light; seeing with photopic vision.

lightening   The descent of the fetus deeper into the pelvis, resulting in a decrease in the fundal height. Lightening occurs a few days or weeks before labor, due to physiologic changes of the uterus.

light-headed   Having a feeling of slight dizziness, as if about to faint.

Lightwood [Reginald *Lightwood*, English pediatrician, flourished 20th century]   **1** See under SYNDROME.   **2** Lightwood-Albright syndrome. See under PROXIMAL RENAL TUBULAR ACIDOSIS.

Lignac [Georges Otto Emile *Lignac*, Dutch pediatrician, 1891–1954]   **1** Lignac syndrome, Lignac-Fanconi disease, Lignac's disease. See under CYSTINOSIS.   **2** Lignac-Fanconi syndrome. See under NEPHROGENIC CYSTINOSIS.

ligneous [L *ligneus* (from *lign(um)* wood + -*eus* English -*eous*) wooden, woody] Woody; consisting of or resembling wood.

lignification The process of lignin deposition in the secondary cell walls of a plant, thereby making the plant more rigid.

lignin A polymer of phenylpropanoid units. It is one of the most important constituents of the secondary cell wall of plants, although not all secondary cell walls contain lignin. Also called *xylogen*.

lignocaine LIDOCAINE.

lignocellulose A heterohexosan of lignin and cellulose. The compound is a constituent of the cell walls of woody plants.

lignoceric acid $CH_3—[CH_2]_{22}—COOH$. One of the higher fatty acids, having a melting point of 84°C. It occurs in natural fats such as peanut oil and in phospholipids.

ligroin A light petroleum product of boiling range about 90–120°C.

ligula [L (dim. of *lingua* tongue), a little tongue or strap] A narrow band of white matter in the brainstem connecting the nucleus gracilis to the inferior cerebellar peduncle and closely related to the most lateral part of the floor of the fourth ventricle. Also called *ligule*.

ligule LIGULA.

Lilienthal [Howard *Lilienthal*, U.S. surgeon, 1861–1946] See under PROBE.

Lillie [Ralph D. *Lillie*, U.S. pathologist, 1896–1979] **1** Lillie's allochrome stain. See under STAIN. **2** Lillie's azure-eosin stain. See under STAIN.

Limax A genus of common shell-less gastropods or land slugs in the family Limacidae which serve as the intermediate hosts for various helminth parasites, such as the nematode *Angiostrongylus*. Several species have become established in the United States, and are now widespread garden pests, for example, *L. maximus* and *L. flavus*.

limb [Old English *lim*] **1** An arm, leg, or appendage projecting from the trunk of a body; membrum. **2** Any of various internal anatomical structures resembling or suggestive of such an appendage; crus.

anacrotic limb The ascending limb of the arterial pressure pulse wave.

aneurogenic limb A limb bud of an early embryo into which no nerve has yet grown. When a limb bud appears, the nerves of the segments opposite to where it is formed grow out into its mesenchyme to innervate muscles and the skin segments forming the limb.

anterior limb of internal capsule The most anterior part of the internal capsule, separating the head of the caudate nucleus from the lentiform nucleus.

anterior limb of stapes CRUS ANTERIUS STAPEDIS.

limbs of anthelix CRURA ANTHELICIS.

artificial limb A prosthetic appliance that replaces a portion or the entirety of an arm or a leg.

ascending limb See under LOOP OF HENLE.

catacrotic limb The descending limb of the arterial pressure pulse wave.

descending limb See under LOOP OF HENLE.

inferior limb MEMBRUM INFERIUS.

inverted champagne-bottle limb The appearance produced by gross atrophy of all lower limb muscles below the knee with sparing of the thigh muscles, resembling the shape of an inverted champagne bottle, as seen in peroneal muscular atrophy.

long limb of incus CRUS LONGUM INCUDIS.

lower limb MEMBRUM INFERIUS.

pelvic limb MEMBRUM INFERIUS.

phantom limb The perception by an amputee of sensations, often interpreted as pain, that appear to issue from a limb when

in fact the limb has been amputated. It is a neurologic phenomenon originating in the transected peripheral nerve endings. Also called *stump hallucination, pseudomelia*.

posterior limb of internal capsule The most posterior part of the internal capsule lying lateral to the thalamus and lentiform nucleus.

posterior limb of stapes CRUS POSTERIUS STAPEDIS.

short limb of incus CRUS BREVE INCUDIS.

superior limb MEMBRUM SUPERIUS.

thick ascending limb The ascending limb of a Henle's loop of a subcapsular nephron, which is much shorter and thicker than that of a juxtaglomerular nephron. It forms the U-turn and the descending limb may be thin and very short. Such a loop only extends into the outer part of the medulla and produces the zonation of the medulla.

thick descending limb A descending limb of Henle's loop which develops thick squamous cells in a short loop from a subcapsular nephron.

thick limb of the loop of Henle See under THICK ASCENDING LIMB.

thin limb of the loop of Henle The descending limb of a loop of Henle. See under LOOP OF HENLE.

thoracic limb MEMBRUM SUPERIUS.

upper limb MEMBRUM SUPERIUS.

limbal [L *limb(us)* border, edge + -AL] Pertaining to the junction of cornea and sclera. Also *corneoscleral, pericorneal, perikeratic*.

limbi Plural of LIMBUS.

limbic **1** Denoting a limbus. **2** In the brain, denoting anatomically the limbic lobe (of P. Broca) constituting the cerebral cortex forming the hilus of each hemisphere.

limbous Overlapping.

limbus [L (akin to LEMNISCUS, L *limen* threshold, *labium* lip, *libella* dim. of *libra* a level), the hem, welt, border of a garment] An edge, border, or fringe. Adjective: limbal.

limbus alveolaris mandibulae An outmoded term for ARCUS ALVEOLARIS MANDIBULAE.

limbus alveolaris maxillae An outmoded term for ARCUS ALVEOLARIS MAXILLAE.

alveolar limbus of mandible An outmoded term for ARCUS ALVEOLARIS MANDIBULAE.

alveolar limbus of maxilla An outmoded term for ARCUS ALVEOLARIS MAXILLAE.

limbus angulosus An outmoded term for LINEA OBLIQUA CARTILAGINIS THYROIDEAE.

limbus chorioideus The infolded part of the ependyma in the developing medial wall of the archipallium. Between the infolded lips of this double-layered ependymal fold vascular mesodermal tissue grows to form the choroid plexus of the lateral ventricle. An outmoded term.

limbus conjunctivae An outmoded term for ANNULUS CONJUNCTIVAE.

limbus of cornea LIMBUS CORNEAE.

limbus corneae [NA] The line of junction between the cornea and the sclera which is marked on the surface of the eyeball by the sulcus sclerae. It also marks the junction of the cornea and the conjunctiva. Also called *limbus of cornea, sclerocorneal junction*.

limbus corticalis A region of the medial wall of the developing telencephalon covered by a layer of cortical cells that eventually forms the subiculum, dentate gyrus, induseum griseum, and striae Lancisii. An outmoded term.

limbus foraminis ovalis The border of the foramen ovale in the embryonic heart. An outmoded term.

limbus fossae ovalis [NA] The well-marked crescentic edge of the fossa ovalis on the interatrial septum in the right atrium of the heart, representing the margin of the septum secundum of the embryonic heart. Its anterior part is continuous with the valve of the inferior vena cava. Also called *limbus fossae ovalis vieussenii* (outmoded), *annulus ovalis, Vieussens annulus, border of oval fossa, limbus of Vieussens, isthmus of Vieussens, ring of Vieussens, interauricular valve* (outmoded).

limbus fossae ovalis vieussenii   An outmoded term for LIMBUS FOSSAE OVALIS.

limbus laminae spiralis osseae   [NA] Thickened periosteum on the upper plate of the osseous spiral lamina, projecting into the duct of the cochlea and ending laterally as the sulcus spiralis internus. Also called *zona cartilaginea*.

limbus luteus retinae   An outmoded term for MACULA RETINAE.

limbus medullaris   That part of the developing medial wall of the telencephalon that is not covered by cortical cells and eventually develops into the fimbria hippocampi. An outmoded term.

limbus membranae tympani   The thickened margin of the tympanic membrane attached by the annulus fibrocartilagineus to the tympanic sulcus of the temporal bone.

limbi palpebrales anteriores   [NA] The rounded anterior edges of the free margin of the upper and lower eyelids. They bear the eyelashes, or cilia.

limbi palpebrales posteriores   [NA] The sharp posterior edges of the free margin of the upper and lower eyelids. They rest on the surface of the eyeball and mark the junction of the skin and palpebral conjunctiva. Along them are the single rows of minute openings of the tarsal glands.

limbus sphenoidalis   LIMBUS OF THE SPHENOID BONE.

limbus of the sphenoid bone   The sharp anterior edge of the sulcus prechiasmaticus on the superior surface of the body of the sphenoid bone. Also called *limbus sphenoidalis*.

limbus of Vieussens   LIMBUS FOSSAE OVALIS.

lime   [Old English *līm* cement, akin to Old Norse *līm* lime, Old High German *līm* birdlime, L *lima* a polishing, polish, *levis* smooth, Gk *leios* smooth, level]   Either calcium oxide or calcium hydroxide.

lime arsenate   A solution of arsenic trioxide and sodium carbonate in water that was once widely used as an insecticide.

slaked lime   CALCIUM HYDROXIDE.

sulfurated lime   A mixture of calcium sulfide and calcium sulfate that is used topically as a keratolytic. At one time it was taken internally for boils and carbuncles.

limen   [L (akin to LIMBUS and to *limes* a limit, boundary), a threshold, lintel, entrance]   A threshold or boundary.

difference limen   DIFFERENCE THRESHOLD.

limen insulae   [NA] The zone of junction, on the inferior surface of the cerebral hemisphere, between the cortex of the insula and that of the frontal lobe. Also called *gyrus of Retzius, gyrus olfactorius lateralis of Retzius* (rarely used).

limen nasi   [NA] A curved ridge demarcating the junction of the skin of the vestibule and the mucous membrane of the nasal cavity proper. It corresponds to the superior margin of the lower nasal cartilage. Also called *threshold of nose*.

limen of twoness   The threshold distance for cutaneous two-point discrimination.

limes zero   The largest amount of toxin which, when mixed with one standard unit of the corresponding antitoxin and administered by subcutaneous injection to a 250-gram guinea pig, will produce no observable reaction. Also called *limes nul dose*. Symbol: L_0.

limic   [Gk *lim(os)* hunger + -IC]   Pertaining to hunger.

limina   Plural of LIMEN.

liminal   [L *limen*, gen. *liminis*, threshold + -AL]   Pertaining to the threshold of sensation.

liminometer   [L *limen*, gen. *liminis*, threshold + *o* + -METER]   An instrument capable of measuring the intensity of a stimulus applied to a tendon in order to evoke a reflex as well as the threshold intensity which will just evoke a reflex.

liminoscope   [L *limen*, gen. *liminis*, threshold + *o* + -SCOPE]   An instrument for measuring the threshold intensity at which visual stimuli can be perceived. An outmoded term.

limit   [L *limes*, gen. *limitis* boundary path, boundary]   A value or condition regarded as an end point or boundary.

Anstie's limit   The amount of absolute alcohol that may be taken without injury, as interpreted by the life insurance industry. This is equivalent to about 1.5 oz per day for adults, or approximately 3 oz of whiskey, brandy, rum, or gin. Also called *Anstie's rule*.

assimilation limit   The amount of carbohydrate an animal can metabolize without spillage into the urine resulting in glycosuria. Also called *saturation limit*.

audibility limit   The upper and lower limits of the range of hearing.

confidence limits   The boundary values of a confidence interval.

elastic limit   The greatest degree to which a pliable material may be stretched without impairing its ability to return to its original dimensions.

emergency exposure limit   The maximum concentration of a highly dangerous toxic material to which a volunteer can be exposed following a disaster or accident, on the assumption that any health impairment incurred would be reversible and that the possibility of such impairment would be justifiable on the grounds of saving human life.

exposure limit   The airborne concentration of a dust, gas, or fume in the workplace to which an individual may be safely exposed for a specified period of time. Exposure limits vary in the degree of protection offered.

genetic dose limit   A recommendation that the dose equivalent of radiation to the gonads for the population of the United States as a whole from all sources other than natural radiation and radiation from the healing arts not exceed a yearly average of 0.17 rem (1.7 mSv) per person. The recommendation was made in 1971 by the National Council of Radiation Protection.

maximum permissible limit   DERIVED WORKING LEVEL.

limit of perception   The smallest visible detail which normally subtends a visual angle of one minute and a retinal image of just greater than one cone diameter.

quantum limit   MINIMUM WAVELENGTH.

release limit   The limit imposed by a controlling authority on the amount or concentration of a toxic, harmful, or otherwise undesirable substance that may be discharged into an environmental medium such as a river.

saturation limit   ASSIMILATION LIMIT.

limitation   The state of being limited or restricted.

birth limitation   BIRTH CONTROL.

eccentric limitation   Irregular constriction of the visual field.

limitrophic   Having control over food intake and metabolism.

Limnatis   A genus of horse leeches in the order Gnathobdellida, class Hirudinea.

Limnatis nilotica   A large horse leech (8–12 cm) common in central and southern Europe, northern Africa and the Middle East. It enters the nostrils, larynx, pharynx, and gullet of mammals drinking contaminated water, where it can cause hemorrhages and anemia by attaching itself to the mucous membranes. It has also been commonly employed for therapeutic bloodletting in these areas. Also called *Hirudo aegyptiaca*.

limnemia   [Gk *limn(ē)* a lake, esp. a marshy lake + -EMIA]   A rarely used term for CHRONIC MALARIA.

limnemic   [Gk *limnē* a marshy or freshwater lake + *m* + -IC]

Suffering from chronic malaria.

limnetic [Gk *limnē* a marshy or freshwater lake + *t* + -IC] Of or relating to fresh water.

limnology [Gk *limn(ē)* a pool, lake + *o* + -LOGY] The scientific study of bodies of fresh water and their biota.

limonene $C_{10}H_{16}$. A volatile oil, a monocyclic terpene, extracted from the oils in the peels of lemons and oranges and from caraway and dill. Also called *dipentene*.

limophthisis Wasting due to a diminished food intake or fasting.

limosis [Gk *limo(s)* hunger, famine + -SIS] An abnormally large appetite.

limotherapy [Gk *limo(s)* hunger, want of food + THERAPY] The treatment of disease by restricting food intake. It is used in obesity to force the body to metabolize some of its own adipose tissue. At one time it was used in cancer treatment as it was believed that deprivation of food led to starvation of the tumor. This belief has now disappeared from modern medical practice. Also called *hunger cure, nestiatria, nestitherapy, nestotherapy, peinotherapy, pinotherapy, hunger therapy.*

limp [Middle English *lympen*, from Old English *limpan* to happen] An abnormality of gait such that full weight bearing is not applied to one of the lower extremities; commonly, a type of walking produced by pain or sensitivity in the leg or foot.

Limulus A genus of arthropods of the class Merostomata; the horseshoe crab. Amebocytes from the organism are used in a highly sensitive test for endotoxin.

linalool $C_{10}H_{17}OH$. An acyclic alcohol found in essential oils of various plants, especially *Citrus aurantium*, Seville orange; *Citrus bergamia*, bergamot orange; and *Cinnamomum pedatinervum*, wild cinnamon.

linamarin $C_{10}H_{17}NO_6$. A cyanogenic glycoside extracted from the seed chaff or embryos of *Linum usitatissimum*, flax, and *Phaseolus lunatus*, lima bean. Also called *phaseolunatin*.

Lincoln [Robert Stanley *Lincoln*, U.S. psychologist, born 1923] Lincoln-Oseretsky Motor Development Scale. See under SCALE.

lincomycin $C_{18}H_{34}N_2O_6S$. An antibiotic from a variant strain of *Streptomyces lincolnesis*. It acts primarily on Gram-positive bacteria.

lincomycin hydrochloride $C_{18}H_{34}N_2O_6S \cdot HCl \cdot H_2O$. The monohydrate, monohydrochloride salt of lincomycin. It is used as an antibiotic against susceptible strains of streptococci, pneumococci, and staphylococci. It can be administered intramuscularly and intravenously.

lincture ELECTUARY.

linctus ELECTUARY.

lindane $C_6H_6Cl_6$. The gamma isomer of hexachlorocyclohexane. A white, crystalline powder with a slightly musty odor, widely used as an insecticide. Serious poisoning and fatalities have occurred from its improper use. It acts as a systemic poison, causing lassitude, headache, limb pains, intestinal colic, and diarrhea. Convulsions and other disorders of the central nervous system may follow. Also called *gammexane, gamma benzene hexachloride.*

Lindau [Arvid Vilhelm *Lindau*, Swedish pathologist, 1892–1958] Lindau-von Hippel syndrome, Hippel-Lindau disease, Lindau's disease, von Hippel-Lindau disease, Lindau-von Hippel disease. See under VON HIPPEL-LINDAU SYNDROME.

Lindbergh [Charles Augustus *Lindbergh*, U.S. aviator, 1902–1974] **1** Carrel-Lindbergh pump. See under PUMP. **2** Lindbergh pump. See under PUMP.

Lindemann [August *Lindemann*, German surgeon, born 1880] See under METHOD, CANNULA.

Lindner [Karl David *Lindner*, Austrian ophthalmologist, 1883–

1961] Lindner's initial bodies. See under MIYAGAWA BODIES.

Lindqvist [Johan Torsten *Lindqvist*, Swedish physician, born 1906] Fahraeus-Lindqvist effect. See under EFFECT.

line

line [L *linea*. See LINEA.] **1** A connection between two points or a boundary between two areas. **2** A long thin mark, ridge, or crease on the surface of a structure; linea. **3** A measure formerly used in mensuration of objects viewed under a microscope. See also PARIS LINE.

abdominal line Any crease on the surface of the abdomen, such as one outlining the edge of a muscle, or any marking drawn to divide the surface into regions.

absorption lines Sharp bands, perceived as lines, in an absorption spectrum.

accretion lines INCREMENTAL LINES.

adrenal line SERGENT'S WHITE ADRENAL LINE.

ala-tragal line CAMPER'S LINE.

alveolar line A line from nasion to prosthion.

alveolobasilar line A line from prosthion to basion.

alveolonasal line A line from prosthion to nasion.

Amberg's line A line bisecting the angle between the anterior margin of the mastoid process and the temporal line. It indicates the location of the transverse sinus for certain surgical procedures. Also called *lateral sinus line.*

line of Amici An obsolete term for Z BAND.

angular line The zigzag line on the iris along the inner aspect of the anterior mesodermal leaf.

anocutaneous line The line of junction of the perianal skin and the stratified squamous epithelium of the lower part of the anal canal, a level where the hair follicles cease. Also called *linea anocutanea*. See also PECTINATE LINE.

anorectal line LINEA ANORECTALIS.

anterior axillary line LINEA AXILLARIS ANTERIOR.

anterior gluteal line LINEA GLUTEA ANTERIOR.

anterior intertrochanteric line An outmoded term for LINEA INTERTROCHANTERICA.

anterior median line LINEA MEDIANA ANTERIOR.

arcuate line Either linea arcuata vaginae musculi recti abdominis or linea arcuata ossis ilii.

arcuate line of ilium LINEA ARCUATA OSSIS ILII.

arcuate line of innominate bone LINEA ARCUATA OSSIS ILII.

arcuate line of pelvis LINEA TERMINALIS PELVIS.

arcuate line of sheath of rectus abdominus muscle LINEA ARCUATA VAGINAE MUSCULI RECTI ABDOMINIS.

arcuate line of Vogt The circular line sometimes found on the posterior lens capsule, corresponding to the end of the hyaloid canal.

Arlt's line A horizontal scar of the upper palpebral conjunctiva that is almost pathognomic of chronic trachoma.

atropic line Any line perpendicular to the plane defined by the axes of rotation of the two eyes (presuming that the eyes are normally aligned, without a vertical muscle imbalance). Also called *Helmholtz line*.

auriculobregmatic line A line extending from the auricular point to the bregma.

axial lines In the limbs, the dorsal and ventral lines that represent contact between nonconsecutive dermatome areas.

axillary line LINEA AXILLARIS.

Baillarger's lines Two myelinated, horizontal laminae visible in vertical sections through the cerebral cortex as pale bands running parallel to the pial surface and composed of an inner and an outer band. They lie in the fifth and fourth cortical layers, respectively, and apparently reflect the profusion of corticipetal arborizations in these areas. These laminar bands vary in conspicuousness in different cortical areas. In the area striata of visual cortex, the outer band (Gennari's band) is unusually prominent. In agranular cortex, both lines are usually absent. Also called *Baillarger's bands, Baillarger stripes, Baillarger striations, striae of Baillarger, interradial plexus.*

base line A line connecting the orbitale and the superior border of the external auditory meatus and extending to the median line of the occipital bone. It is used as the basis of the Frankfort horizontal plane in craniometric studies, and approximates the base of the skull. Also called *Reid's base line, Reid's baseline.*

base-apex line A line that is perpendicular to the base of a prism and bisects the prism's refracting angle.

basinasal line A line joining basion to nasion. Also called *nasobasilar line.*

basiobregmatic line A line joining basion to bregma, used in craniometry to measure the height of the cranium.

Baudelocque's line EXTERNAL CONJUGATE.

Beau's lines Superficial transverse depressions in the nail plates that appear several weeks after an acute illness.

biauricular line A line connecting the two external auditory meatuses across the vertex of the skull.

bi-iliac line A line joining the widest points between the two iliac crests.

bikini line Surgical incision in the lower abdomen or around the breast that approximates the outline of a bikini bathing suit.

bismuth line A black line at the gingival margin caused by the deposition of bismuth sulfide from the ingestion of bismuth salts and their reaction with sulfur-containing products of dental plaque.

blood line The line of descent of an individual in a pedigree. Also called *lineage.*

blue line LEAD LINE.

Borsieri's line A white line that quickly turns red, produced by drawing the finger across the skin: supposedly an early sign of scarlet fever. Also called *Borsieri sign.*

Bridgett's line The surface marking of the facial nerve on the mastoid process, considered at one time by some surgeons as an important means of avoiding injury to the facial nerve during mastoid operations.

Brödel's line A longitudinal line just posterior to the outer convex border of the kidney, considered to be a bloodless zone between the areas of distribution of the anterior and the posterior branches of the renal artery. However, in fact, the areas supplied by the vessels overlap and the linear zone is only relatively avascular.

Brödel's white line A longitudinal pale zone located along the anterior aspect of the outer convex border of the kidney.

Brücke's line A BAND.

Bryant's line A horizontal line drawn, with the subject in the supine position, from the greater trochanter of the femur to a vertical line, which it meets at right angles, from the anterior superior iliac spine to the table underneath the person. It is the base of Bryant's triangle.

Burton's line BURTON SIGN.

burtonian line BURTON SIGN.

calcification lines INCREMENTAL LINES.

Camper's line A line drawn from the base of the anterior nasal spine, or subnasale, to the upper border of the tragus of the ear, or tragion. Also called *ala-tragal line.*

cell line A population of cells established as a primary culture and propagated in tissue culture.

cement line In bony tissue, a line of reversal of bone growth.

It marks the junction between adjacent osteons. The increased basophilia of the line is due to a high inorganic matrix content.

cementing line The thin layer of cement exposed at the margin of any restoration which has been cemented in position.

central pupillary line An imaginary line perpendicular to the iris and centered in the pupil.

cervical line A line around the neck of a tooth where enamel and cementum meet, demarcating the anatomical crown from the root.

Chamberlain's line A line drawn on a lateral radiograph of the skull joining the posterior end of the hard palate to the posterior margin of the foramen magnum. In the normal individual the odontoid process of the axis should not extend above this line.

Chaussier's line The median line of the corpus callosum. An obsolete term.

Chiene's lines A set of reference lines established to aid in localizing cerebral centers. An obsolete term.

chorionic plate line The dense ultrasound echo line between the placental echo pattern and the uterine cavity along the placental border.

Clapton's line COPPER LINE.

clavicular line A line along the clavicles.

cleavage lines Fine linear clefts in the skin, produced by the parallel bundles of connective tissue in the reticular layer, along which the skin more easily splits especially when incised. The direction of the bundles varies in different parts of the body, generally paralleling lines of tension and compression due to ordinary movements. Also called *Langer's lines, tension lines.*

Conradi's line A line drawn between the base of the xiphisternum and the apex of the heart, to indicate the normal upper margin of the left lobe of the liver.

contour lines LINES OF OWEN.

copper line A dirty green to bluish black line between the teeth and gingiva due to ingestion of large amounts of copper sulfate. It is caused by inhalation of mist and dust of copper salts and usually marked by discoloration of the teeth and tongue as well as the gingival margin. Also called *Corrigan's line, Corrigan sign, Clapton's line.*

Corrigan's line COPPER LINE.

costoarticular line A line drawn between the sternoclavicular joint and the tip of the eleventh rib.

costoclavicular line An outmoded term for LINEA PARASTERNALIS.

costophrenic septal lines Fine horizontal lines seen mainly in the costophrenic region on the chest radiograph in pulmonary edema and several other conditions.

Crampton's line A line of incision drawn from the tip of the twelfth costal cartilage to a point just above the iliac crest and then anteriorly to a point just inferomedial to the anterior superior iliac spine. It is used for an extraperitoneal approach to ligate the common iliac artery.

crease lines Lines of tension in the skin. Maximum tension is along the crease lines rather than across them.

cricoclavicular line A line from the point of intersection of the anterior axillary line and the clavicle to the cricoid cartilage.

cruciate line EMINENTIA CRUCIFORMIS.

curved line of ilium An outmoded term for LINEA ARCUATA OSSIS ILII.

Czermak's lines Lines visible in histologic sections of dentin produced by rows of interglobular spaces.

Daubenton's line A line extending from the opisthion to the basion. An obsolete term.

deadly mesenteric line MESENTERIC TRIANGLE.

delay line A device for delaying input signals for precise periods of time.

line of demarcation An ill-defined, irregular line that separates infarcted or gangrenous tissue from healthy tissue. The line becomes more distinct with time as granulation tissue develops. Also called *surface demarcation.*

dentate line PECTINATE LINE.

developmental line DEVELOPMENTAL GROOVE.

Dobie's line An obsolete term for Z BAND.

line of Douglas LINEA ARCUATA VAGINAE MUSCULI RECTI ABDOMINIS.

line of draw The direction of withdrawal or insertion of an appliance or restoration. It is not necessarily perpendicular to the occlusal plane.

Duhot's line A line connecting the anterior superior iliac spine to the apex of the sacrum.

dynamic lines Lines on the face appearing in middle or old age as the result of lifelong repetitive use of the muscles of expression.

ectental line The line of junction between ectoderm and entoderm.

Egger's line The circular attachment of the hyaloideocapsular ligament to the posterior periphery of the crystalline lens capsule.

Ellis line An S-shaped line detected by percussion of the chest in the presence of a pleural effusion. Also called *Ellis-Garland line, Garland's curve, curve of Ellis and Garland, Damoiseau's curve.*

Ellis-Garland line ELLIS LINE.

embryonic line PRIMITIVE STREAK.

epiphyseal line 1 LINEA EPIPHYSIALIS. 2 A radiolucent line seen on a radiograph at the growing end of the diaphysis of a long bone representing a zone of cartilage next to a layer of new bone of the metaphysis.

established cell line A group of cells, cultured *in vitro*, which can be subcultured indefinitely in tissue culture.

external oblique line A ridge on the lateral surface of the mandible which extends downwards and forwards from the anterior edge of the coronoid process and becomes indistinct in the region of the first permanent molar tooth.

external superior arcuate line of occipital bone An outmoded term for LINEA NUCHAE SUPERIOR.

facial line 1 A line connecting the nasion to the pogonion. 2 A straight line tangential to the glabella and the pogonion.

Farre's white line A pale straight line along the mesovarian border of the ovary where the mesovarium meets the germinal epithelium of the ovary.

Feiss line A line drawn from the distal tip of the medial malleolus to the plantar aspect of the first metatarsophalangeal joint.

finish line The line made by the meeting of a bevel with the surface of the tooth. It indicates the margin of a restoration to the technician making a wax pattern.

fissural line A fine linear density seen on a chest x ray representing the pleura seen tangentially within the fissures separating pulmonary lobes. It is usually made up of two layers of pleura.

line of fixation An imaginary line from the fovea to the object of regard.

Fleischner line Linear density seen on a chest x ray representing atelectasis of a small area of lung. It is usually associated with decreased diaphragmatic motion, thoracic trauma, subphrenic disease, or pulmonary embolus, but can be seen also in normal people with high diaphragms. Also called *platelike atelectasis, discoid atelectasis.*

Fleischner lines Linear opacities seen just above the diaphragm on the chest radiograph, probably representing small areas of pulmonary atelectasis.

flexure line Any one of several furrows in the skin produced by folds in the dermis resulting from compression by constant joint movements, and indicative of planes of anchorage to the underlying deep fascia. During joint movements the skin on each side of a line is folded passively, making the line more prominent. These lines are conspicuous anterior to the wrist joint, on the palms, the soles, and the digits. In the palm there are usually two curved horizontal and at least two longitudinal lines. Also called *skin joint, flexion crease.*

fracture line A sharp line of radiolucency representing a fracture as seen on a roentgenogram of a bone.

Fränkel's line WHITE LINE OF FRÄNKEL.

Fraunhofer Lines Lines in the solar spectrum formed by the absorption of particular wavelengths by elements in the outer layers of the sun.

Frommann's lines STRIATIONS OF FROMMANN.

frown lines Permanent lines in the skin of the forehead, caused by habitual frowning.

fulcrum line One of the hypothetical lines about which a partial denture tends to rotate during mastication. The principle fulcrum lines are vertical, horizontal fore and aft, and horizontal cross-arch.

Gant's line A demarcation on the proximal femoral shaft just below the greater trochanter. It serves as a landmark during surgical exploration.

line of Gennari GENNARI'S BAND.

germ line 1 In an individual, all cells derived from the embryonic cells that have the potential for forming gametes. 2 In a species, the linkage of related individuals through germ cells. Also called *germ track.*

gingival line 1 The level of gingival margin on a tooth. 2 Any line on the gingiva, such as a lead line. Also called *gum line.*

Gottinger's line A line parallel to the superior margin of the zygomatic arch.

Granger's line A curved line on a specially angled posteroanterior roentgenogram of the skull, representing the superior surface of the sphenoid bone. It is used to localize and demonstrate the optic groove.

growth arrest line On radiography of a long bone, a metaphyseal transverse line of increased radiodensity. It represents a zone of increased calcification resulting usually from growth arrest due to malnutrition or disease. Also called *Harris line.*

Gubler's line A line connecting the apparent origins of the roots of the trigeminal nerve. An obsolete term.

gum line GINGIVAL LINE.

Haller's line An obsolete term for FISSURA MEDIANA ANTERIOR MEDULLAE SPINALIS.

Harris line GROWTH ARREST LINE.

health line A popular term for MUCOGINGIVAL JUNCTION.

Helmholtz line ATROPIC LINE.

Hensen's line H BAND.

highest arcuate line of occipital bone An outmoded term for LINEA NUCHAE SUPREMA.

highest curved line of occipital bone An outmoded term for LINEA NUCHAE SUPREMA.

highest nuchal line LINEA NUCHAE SUPREMA.

highest semicircular line of occipital bone An outmoded term for LINEA NUCHAE SUPREMA.

high lip line The highest level reached by the upper lip on the teeth or gingiva.

Hilton's white line The mucocutaneous junction between the upper border of the stratified squamous epithelium of the anal canal and the stratified columnar or cuboidal epithelium, slightly below the pectinate line. Common clinical usage, however, equates this with the pectinate line, that is, the clinical anorectal junction. Some consider this line to lie at the level of an intermuscular septum between the internal sphincter and the subcutaneous part of the external sphincter of the anus. See also PECTINATE LINE.

Holden's line   A flexure line in the inguinal region between the anterior superior iliac spine and the greater trochanter of the femur, crossing the position of the capsule of the hip joint.

Hudson's line   HUDSON-STÄHLI LINE.

Hudson-Stähli line   A linear, subepithelial corneal deposit of hemosiderin, occurring as a normal aging process. Also called *Hudson's line, pigmented line of the cornea, Stähli's pigment line, Stähli's line, superficial line of the cornea, linea corneae senilis.*

Hueter's line   The line drawn between the medial epicondyle of the humerus and the top of the olecranon when the elbow is extended.

Hunter's line   LINEA ALBA.

iliopectineal line   **1** The posterior continuation of pecten pubis as far as the iliopubic eminence or beyond, being part of the terminal line. Also called *linea iliopectinea* (outmoded).   **2** LINEA ARCUATA OSSIS ILII.

imbrication lines   See under PICKERILL'S IMBRICATION LINES.

incremental lines   The lines visible in histologic sections of teeth and bone which reflect the rhythmic formation of mineralized tissues. Also called *accretion lines, calcification lines, recessional lines.*

inferior arcuate line of occipital bone   An outmoded term for LINEA NUCHAE INFERIOR.

inferior curved line of ilium   An outmoded term for LINEA GLUTEA INFERIOR.

inferior curved line of occipital bone   An outmoded term for LINEA NUCHAE INFERIOR.

inferior gluteal line   LINEA GLUTEA INFERIOR.

inferior nuchal line   LINEA NUCHAE INFERIOR.

inferior semicircular line of parietal bone   An outmoded term for LINEA TEMPORALIS INFERIOR OSSIS PARIETALIS.

inferior temporal line   LINEA TEMPORALIS INFERIOR OSSIS PARIETALIS.

inferior temporal line of parietal bone   LINEA TEMPORALIS INFERIOR OSSIS PARIETALIS.

inflating line   A tube used to inflate a pilot balloon on a tracheal or tracheostomy tube.

infracostal line   SUBCOSTAL LINE.

infrascapular line   A line drawn horizontally through the tips of the inferior angles of the two scapulae.

intercondylar line   LINEA INTERCONDYLARIS FEMORIS.

intercondyloid line   LINEA INTERCONDYLARIS FEMORIS.

intermediate line of iliac crest   LINEA INTERMEDIA CRISTAE ILIACAE.

internal oblique line of mandible   An outmoded term for LINEA MYLOHYOIDEA MANDIBULAE.

interspinal line   A line drawn across the abdomen between the two anterior superior iliac spines, to help demarcate the interspinal plane. Also called *Lanz line.*

intertrochanteric line   LINEA INTERTROCHANTERICA.

intertuberal line   A line drawn between the most prominent points on the two frontal tuberosities of the cranium.

intertubercular line   A line drawn across the surface of the abdomen between the tubercles of the iliac crests, helping to demarcate the transtubercular plane.

isoeffect lines   In radiotherapy, lines on a chart showing the location of doses producing equal effects on the tissues.

isoelectric line   BASELINE.

Jadelot's lines   Lines of the face in young children, supposed to indicate specific types of disease.

line of Kaes   An outmoded term for BEKHTEREV'S LAYER.

Kerley's lines   Thin linear soft-tissue densities, a few centimeters long, of the lungs, seen on roentgenograms of the chest and thought to represent thickened interlobular septa. Kerley's

B lines are located peripherally, especially at the costophrenic sulci, often arranged horizontally in stepladder fashion. Kerley's A lines are located centrally and run obliquely. Kerley's C lines are tiny lacelike densities in the midzones of the lungs. Kerley's lines are seen with interstitial pulmonary edema and pulmonary fibrosis.

Kilian's line   A transverse line through the promontory of the sacrum.

Krause line   Z BAND.

Langer's lines   CLEAVAGE LINES.

Lanz line   INTERSPINAL LINE.

lateral line   **1** A zone, usually visible because less pigmented, extending along the sides from the head to the tail in most aquatic vertebrates. In the cyclostomes, sense organs are arranged in pores in this region, the arrangement being collectively called the lateral line system.   **2** LINEA MEDIOCLAVICULARIS.

lateral sinus line   AMBERG'S LINE.

lateral sternal line   LINEA STERNALIS.

lead line   A blue or blue-black pigmentation within the marginal gingiva caused by lead intoxication. It is found around teeth with heavy deposits of dental plaque, and precipitation within the soft tissues of dark metallic salts (probably sulfides) from reaction with absorbed products of plaque metabolism as the likely mechanism. Also called *blue line, halo saturninus.* See also BURTON SIGN.

lip line   The level on the teeth of either jaw of the margin of the lip at rest.

lower lung line   A horizontal line seen on a roentgenogram of the upper abdomen, extending from the lateral wall of the chest to the upper lumbar spine and representing the posterior costophrenic sulcus seen *en face.*

low lip line   The lowest level reached by the lower lip on the lower teeth.

magnetic line of force   A line (generally curved) in a magnetic field such that its tangent at any point is in the direction of the magnetic force exerted by the field at that point. The intensity of the field is conventionally represented by the density of the lines, i.e., the number passing normally through unit area.

mamillary line   LINEA MAMILLARIS.

mammary line   **1** MAMMARY RIDGE.   **2** A horizontal line drawn between the nipples of the breasts.

McKee's line   A line of incision drawn from the tip of the eleventh costal cartilage to a point one and a half inches medial to the anterior superior iliac spine and then across to a point just above the position of the superficial inguinal ring. It is used for an extraperitoneal approach for ligation of the common iliac artery.

median line   Either linea mediana anterior or linea mediana posterior.

median nuchal line   CRISTA OCCIPITALIS EXTERNA.

Mees lines   The transverse white striations that appear in nails as a result of arsenic poisoning. Also called *Mees stripes, bands of Mees.*

mercurial line   A dark line of variable color at the gingival margin caused by the ingestion of mercurial salts. It sometimes used to be seen in patients being treated for syphilis with mercury.

mesenteric line   MESENTERIC TRIANGLE.

Meyer's line   An axial line through the big toe that, when projected backwards, will pass through the center of the heel in a normal foot.

midaxillary line   LINEA AXILLARIS MEDIA.

midclavicular line   LINEA MEDIOCLAVICULARIS.

middle curved line of ilium   An outmoded term for LINEA GLUTEA ANTERIOR.

middle nuchal line   CRISTA OCCIPITALIS EXTERNA.

middle line of scrotum   RAPHE SCROTI.

middle semicircular line of occipital bone An outmoded term for LINEA NUCHAE SUPERIOR.

midspinal line A vertical line drawn down the center of the vertebral column in the median plane.

midsternal line A vertical line drawn down the center of the sternum.

milk line MAMMARY RIDGE.

Monro's line MONRO-RICHTER LINE.

Monro-Richter line A line drawn between the umbilicus and the left anterior superior iliac spine. Also called *Monro's line*.

Morgan's line A crease below the lower eyelids in atopic dermatitis. Also called *Dennie sign*.

Moyer's line A line drawn between the midpoint of the body of the third sacral vertebra and a point midway between the two anterior superior iliac spines.

muscular lines of scapula LINEAE MUSCULARES SCAPULAE.

mylohyoid line LINEA MYLOHYOIDEA MANDIBULAE.

mylohyoidean line LINEA MYLOHYOIDEA MANDIBULAE.

mylohyoid line of mandible LINEA MYLOHYOIDEA MANDIBULAE.

nasobasilar line BASINASAL LINE.

nasolabial line A line drawn between the ala of the nose and the angle of the mouth on the same side.

nasosubnasal line A line drawn between the nasion and the subnasal point.

Nélaton's line A line drawn from the anterior superior iliac spine to the most prominent part of the ischial tuberosity, passing through the top of the greater trochanter of the femur normally when the thigh is partly flexed. Also called *Roser's line*.

neonatal line A prominent incremental line found in enamel and in dentin. It is caused by a retardation in the formation of these tissues during the postpartum period. Also called *neonatal ring*.

nigra line LINEA NIGRA.

nipple line LINEA MAMILLARIS.

Obersteiner-Redlich line OBERSTEINER-REDLICH SPACE.

oblique line A line placed obliquely on a structure in the anatomical position.

oblique line of femur An outmoded term for LINEA INTERTROCHANTERICA.

oblique line of fibula **1** An incorrect term for CRISTA MEDIALIS FIBULAE. **2** An outmoded term for MARGO ANTERIOR FIBULAE.

oblique line of mandible LINEA OBLIQUA MANDIBULAE.

oblique line of radius The proximal part of the anterior margin of the radius extending from the anterolateral part of the radial tuberosity to the middle of the junction of the anterior and lateral surfaces just above the rough tuberosity for the insertion of the pronator teres muscle.

oblique line of thyroid cartilage LINEA OBLIQUA CARTILAGINIS THYROIDEAE.

oblique line of tibia An outmoded term for LINEA MUSCULI SOLEI.

obturator line A line normally crossing the obturator fascia internal to the acetabulum, as seen on an anteroposterior radiograph.

line of occlusion PLANE OF OCCLUSION.

Ogston's line A line drawn from the adductor tubercle to the intercondylar fossa of the femur.

omphalospinous line A line drawn between the umbilicus and the anterior superior iliac spine. Also called *umbilicoiliac line*.

orthostatic lines Flexure lines in the neck accommodating flexion and extension movements.

Ouchterlony line The precipitin line formed when antigen and antibody combine in optimal proportions in immunodiffusion in agar gel.

lines of Owen The incremental lines in dentin caused by minor bends in the dentinal tubules. Also called *contour lines*.

papillary line An outmoded term for LINEA MAMILLARIS.

parasternal line LINEA PARASTERNALIS.

Paris line A measure approximately equivalent to one-eleventh inch (0.23 cm), formerly used in mensuration of objects viewed under a microscope. An obsolete term.

Pastia's lines Transverse red lines which appear in skin creases at the inside of the elbow, wrists, and inguinal areas in the early stages of scarlet fever. They persist throughout the disease and may be of some late diagnostic value. Also called *Pastia sign, Thomson sign*.

pectinate line An uneven horizontal line formed by the continuity between the anal valves and the bases of the rectal columns about 2 cm above the anal opening. Clinicians consider this to be the upper boundary of the anal canal at the clinical anorectal junction; however, anatomists view the line as being in the middle of the anal canal. The line has commonly been considered to lie at the junction of the endodermal part of the anal canal and the ectodermal proctodeum, but there is evidence that this union is situated lower down. Various authors have also considered the anocutaneous and anorectal lines to be the same as the pectinate line, producing confusion. Also called *dentate line, dentate margin*.

pectineal line **1** PECTEN OSSIS PUBIS. **2** LINEA PECTINEA FEMORIS.

pelvic pain line An imaginary line on the abdominal wall along or beneath which it was once believed that painful stimuli from the bladder, prostate, or uterus, and other pelvic organs were perceived or conducted. An obsolete term.

Pickerill's imbrication lines Transverse grooves on the surface of enamel. They are especially numerous towards the neck of a tooth.

pigmented line of the cornea HUDSON-STÄHLI LINE.

pleuroesophageal line On an anteroposterior or posteroanterior chest roentgenogram, a vertical line of soft-tissue density to the left of the thoracic spine, representing the zone of contact of the left lung with the esophagus.

Poirier's line A line drawn from the nasion to the lambda, passing 5 mm above the external auditory meatus.

popliteal line of femur LINEA INTERCONDYLARIS FEMORIS.

popliteal line of tibia LINEA MUSCULI SOLEI.

posterior axillary line LINEA AXILLARIS POSTERIOR.

posterior gluteal line LINEA GLUTEA POSTERIOR.

posterior intertrochanteric line An outmoded term for CRISTA INTERTROCHANTERICA.

posterior median line LINEA MEDIANA POSTERIOR.

Poupart's line A line drawn on the surface of the abdomen passing vertically through the midpoint of the inguinal ligament and parallel to the median plane. Used to help demarcate regions of the abdomen, it approximates the lower extension of the midclavicular, or lateral, line (linea medioclavicularis).

precentral line An oblique line drawn on the surface of the head extending anteroinferiorly from the median plane at an angle of about 70° from the midpoint between glabella and inion. It approximates the position of the precentral sulcus.

primitive line PRIMITIVE STREAK.

profile line CAMPER'S LINE.

protrusive line A central line on a pantographic tracing.

pupillary line See under CENTRAL PUPILLARY LINE.

pure line A strain of organisms that is produced by self-fertilization of apomixic plants or by continual inbreeding of a sexual species. It is genetically pure, except for random, sporadic mutation. Each individual is homozygous at each locus and has the same genotype as every other individual of the strain.

quadrate line   A linear ridge occasionally found extending down from the quadrate tubercle of the intertrochanteric crest of the femur produced by the insertion of the quadratus femoris muscle.

radial longitudinal line   LINEA VITALIS.

recessional lines   INCREMENTAL LINES.

line of reflection of parietal layer of pericardium   An inverted J-shaped line formed by the parietal layer on the fibrous pericardium, enclosing the superior and inferior venae cavae and the four pulmonary veins and forming the cul-de-sac of the oblique sinus within the curve.

line of reflection of pleura   The line of junction of the visceral pleura and the mediastinal pleura.

regression line   A geometric representation of a regression equation in the limiting case in which only one independent variable is involved. It is a straight line when the equation is a first-degree polynomial. When there are two or more independent variables there will be a corresponding regression surface.

Reid's base line   BASE LINE.

retentive fulcrum line   A line through retentive clasps around which a partial denture tends to rotate when subjected to a pull from sticky food.

Retzius lines   STRIAE OF RETZIUS.

Robson's line   A line drawn from either nipple to the umbilicus.

Rolando's line   A line on the surface of the head marking the position of the underlying fissure of Rolando.

Roser's line   NÉLATON'S LINE.

rough line of femur   A seldom used term for LINEA ASPERA FEMORIS.

Salter's lines   Incremental lines visible in histologic sections of cementum.

scan line   A line produced on a cathode ray tube by moving an electron beam spot at constant speed.

scapular line   LINEA SCAPULARIS.

Schoemaker's line   A line drawn between the greater trochanter of the femur and the anterior superior iliac spine, the projection of which normally passes above the umbilicus.

Schreger's lines   Lines seen in longitudinal sections of human enamel when viewed by reflected light. Also called *bands of Schreger, bands of Hunter-Schreger, Schreger striae.*

Schwalbe's line   The peripheral edge of Descemet's membrane, as observed by gonioscopy. See also SCHWALBE'S RING.

semicircular line of Douglas   LINEA ARCUATA VAGINAE MUSCULI RECTI ABDOMINIS.

semicircular line of frontal bone   An outmoded term for LINEA TEMPORALIS OSSIS FRONTALIS.

semilunar line   LINEA SEMILUNARIS.

semilunar line of Spieghel   LINEA SEMILUNARIS.

septal lines   Lines on a chest roentgenogram representing thickened interlobular septa, such as Kerley B lines.

Sergent's white adrenal line   A white line that briefly persists after the fingernail is drawn across the hyperpigmented skin of the abdomen of a patient with Addison's disease. Also called *adrenal line, white adrenal line.*

Shenton's line   A smooth curve drawn on an anteroposterior roentgenogram of the normal hip, extending from the upper border of the obturator foramen to the medial cortex of the neck of the femur. Also called *Shenton's arch, Skinner's line.*

line of sight   An imaginary line from the fixation point to the center of the pupil.

simian line   A major flexion crease that completely traverses the human palm. It is found as a normal variant as well as with increased frequency in some syndromes, especially the Down syndrome. Also called *simian crease.*

Skinner's line   SHENTON'S LINE.

soleal line of tibia   LINEA MUSCULI SOLEI.

Spieghel's line   LINEA SEMILUNARIS.

spigelian line   LINEA SEMILUNARIS.

Spigelius line   LINEA SEMILUNARIS.

spiral line of femur   A curved line continuous above with the lower end of the intertrochanteric line and below with the medial lip of linea aspera femoris. It forms the medial boundary of the insertion of the iliacus muscle. Also called *linea spiralis* (outmoded).

stabilizing fulcrum line   A line through occlusal rests around which a partial denture tends to rotate during mastication.

Stähli's line   HUDSON-STÄHLI LINE.

Stähli's pigment line   HUDSON-STÄHLI LINE.

sternal line   LINEA STERNALIS.

sternomastoid line   A line along the anterior margin of the sternocleidomastoid muscle from the medial end of the clavicle to the mastoid process of the temporal bone.

subcostal line   A line drawn across the lowest points on the tenth costal cartilages on the anterior surface of the trunk. It is the level of the subcostal plane. Also called *infracostal line.*

subscapular lines   LINEAE MUSCULARES SCAPULAE.

superficial line of the cornea   HUDSON-STÄHLI LINE.

superior arcuate line of occipital bone   An outmoded term for LINEA NUCHAE SUPERIOR.

superior curved line of ilium   An outmoded term for LINEA GLUTEA POSTERIOR.

superior curved line of occipital bone   An outmoded term for LINEA NUCHAE SUPERIOR.

superior nuchal line   LINEA NUCHAE SUPERIOR.

superior semicircular line of occipital bone   An outmoded term for LINEA NUCHAE SUPERIOR.

superior semicircular line of parietal bone   An outmoded term for LINEA TEMPORALIS SUPERIOR OSSIS PARIETALIS.

superior temporal line   LINEA TEMPORALIS SUPERIOR OSSIS PARIETALIS.

superior temporal line of parietal bone   LINEA TEMPORALIS SUPERIOR OSSIS PARIETALIS.

supracondylar lines   Two diverging lines, medial and lateral, on the posterior surface of the lower third of the shaft of the femur, bounding the popliteal surface and continuous above with the medial and lateral lips of the linea aspera while ending inferiorly at the adductor tubercle and lateral epicondyle, respectively. They serve as the partial attachments of muscles and intermuscular septa.

supraorbital line   A faint horizontal line above the zygomatic process of the frontal bone continuous medially with the superciliary ridge. A rarely used term.

supreme arcuate line of occipital bone   An outmoded term for LINEA NUCHAE SUPREMA.

supreme curved line of occipital bone   An outmoded term for LINEA NUCHAE SUPREMA.

supreme nuchal line   LINEA NUCHAE SUPREMA.

supreme semicircular line   An outmoded term for LINEA NUCHAE SUPREMA.

survey line   A line joining the points of height of contour on the teeth. Also called *clasp guideline.*

suture line   **1** The site of anastomosis of two luminal structures, as the juncture of two blood vessels. **2** Any site where two tissue edges have been brought together by sutures.

Sydney line   The proximal transverse flexure line in the palm that reaches the ulnar border of the hand. Also called *Sydney crease.*

sylvian line   A line on the surface of the head extending from the external angular process of the frontal bone to a point 3/4 inch(about 20 mm) below the most prominent point of the parietal bone. It overlies the fissure of Sylvius.

temporal line of frontal bone   LINEA TEMPORALIS OSSIS FRONTALIS.

tension lines CLEAVAGE LINES.

terminal line of pelvis LINEA TERMINALIS PELVIS.

Thompson's line A red line occasionally seen on the gums of patients with pulmonary tuberculosis.

thyroid red line An erythematous streak caused by irritation of the skin on the anterior neck and upper thorax in hyperthyroid patients.

Topinard's line A line connecting the glabella and the gnathion.

tram lines Thin parallel lines on a chest radiograph, representing peribronchial interstitial thickening best seen in the central aspects of the lower lung fields, due to chronic inflammation.

transverse lines of sacral bone LINEAE TRANSVERSAE OSSIS SACRI.

transverse lines of sacrum LINEAE TRANSVERSAE OSSIS SACRI.

trapezoid line LINEA TRAPEZOIDEA.

tree line The elevational or latitudinal limit of the occurrence of forests. Beyond this limit only stunted forms of tree growth and other vegetation occur.

triradiate lines Linear sutures that develop in the embryonic lens because of the less than interpolar length of lens fibers. They give rise to complex lens stars with from three to as many as nine rays.

Trümmerfeld line The zone of rarefaction at the growing end of the shaft of a long bone, seen in infantile scurvy. It sometimes leads to fracture and displacement of the epiphysis.

type line Either of two diverging epidermal ridges seen in fingerprints.

Ullmann's line In the displacement of spondylolisthesis, a vertical line that, when drawn upward from the anterior edge of the first sacral segment, will pass through the body of the fifth lumbar vertebra.

umbilicoiliac line OMPHALOSPINOUS LINE.

line of Venus The main flexure line across the anterior aspect of the wrist.

Veslingius line RAPHE SCROTI.

vibrating line An imaginary line demarcating the hard palate from the movable tissues of the soft palate.

Virchow's line A line from nasion to lambda.

visual line VISUAL AXIS.

Wagner's line A curved, pale line at the junction of the epiphysis and the diaphysis of a long bone produced by provisional calcification in the cartilaginous plate.

Wallace's line A zoogeographic line on the map of southeastern Asia which marks a boundary of species differences between the Australian and Oriental faunal regions.

Weiger's line The circular line of attachment of the vitreous body to the posterior surface of the lens, which is located towards the lens periphery.

white line LINEA ALBA.

white adrenal line SERGENT'S WHITE ADRENAL LINE.

white anococcygeal line An outmoded term for LIGAMENTUM ANOCOCCYGEUM.

white line of Fränkel A roentgenographic sign of scurvy, consisting of a line of increased radiodensity in the metaphysis at the provisional zone of calcification. Also called *Fränkel's line.*

white line of ischiococcygeal muscle An outmoded term for LIGAMENTUM ANOCOCCYGEUM.

white line of pelvic fascia ARCUS TENDINEUS FASCIAE PELVIS.

white line of pelvis An outmoded term for ARCUS TENDINEUS MUSCULI LEVATORIS ANI.

white line of pharynx RAPHE PHARYNGIS.

Wimberger's line A zone of increased radiodensity at the periphery of the epiphysis, seen typically in scurvy.

working line A lateral line on a pantographic tracing.

Wrisberg's lines A group of filaments connecting the motor and sensory roots of the trigeminal nerve. An obsolete term.

Y line A horizontal line drawn through the Y cartilages of the hips on an anteroposterior radiograph of the pelvis to assess acetabular angles.

Z line Z BAND.

lines of Zahn Striations on the surface of a blood clot due to the layering of platelet aggregates. Also called *Zahn's ribs.*

Zöllner's lines An optical illusion of converging and diverging lines.

---

linea [L (akin to *linum* flax, lint, a fishing line, thread, a net for hunting or fishing; Gk *linon* anything made of flax, a net, fishing net, linen, lampwick), a thread made of flax, line, cord, string] (*plural* lineae) A long thin mark, ridge, or crease on the surface of a structure; a line.

linea alba [NA] A midline tendinous band extending from the xiphoid process to the symphysis pubis and formed by the aponeuroses of the external oblique, internal oblique and transversus muscles of the abdomen fusing and decussating with each other and with corresponding aponeuroses of the opposite side. It is interrupted by the umbilicus. Also called *white line, linea alba abdominis, Hunter's line, abdominal raphe* (outmoded), *longitudinal ligament of abdomen* (outmoded).

linea alba abdominis LINEA ALBA.

linea alba cervicalis The fusion of the fascial sheaths of the sternohyoid and sternothyroid muscles in the anterior midline of the neck. An outmoded term.

lineae albicantes STRIAE ATROPHICAE.

linea anocutanea ANOCUTANEOUS LINE.

linea anorectalis [NA] A vague annular region of the lumen of the large intestine usually at or below the level of the anorectal junction. It is commonly considered to be about 4 cm above the anocutaneous line and about 1.5 cm above the pectinate line, approximating the upper end of the anal columns. In this region the intestinal glands shorten and disappear and the circular muscle coat of the rectum thickens to form the upper end on the sphincter ani internus. Also called *anorectal line.* • Originally this term referred to the lower limit of the simple columnar epithelium of the rectal mucosa, which is usually lower than the level of the anorectal junction. Nevertheless, it is occasionally used synonymously with *anorectal junction.*

linea arcuata ossis ilii [NA] The thick, rounded continuation anteriorly of the anteroinferior end of the medial border of the ilium, where the latter meets the anterior angulation of the auricular surface, extending to the iliopubic eminence as the iliac portion of the terminal line and separating the iliac fossa from the internal surface of the body of the ilium in the true pelvis. It forms part of the lateral wall of the inlet of the minor pelvis, and transmits compression forces from the trunk to the lower limb. Also called *arcuate line of ilium, iliopectineal crest of iliac bone, curved line of ilium* (outmoded), *iliopectineal line, pars iliaca lineae terminalis* (outmoded), *arcuate line of innominate bone.*

linea arcuata vaginae musculi recti abdominis [NA] The concave lower margin of the posterior wall of the rectus sheath, located about midway between the umbilicus and the pubic symphysis, below which all three aponeuroses of the abdominal muscles pass anterior to the rectus abdominis muscle. The inferior epigastric vessels pass anterior to the line. Also called *arcuate line of sheath of rectus abdominis muscle, linea semicircularis douglasi* (outmoded), *semicircular line of Douglas, line of Douglas, Douglas fold.*

linea aspera femoris [NA] A rough, crestlike ridge buttressing the middle third of the posterior surface of the shaft of the femur, comprising medial and lateral lips and resisting compression forces produced by the anterior curvature of the femur. It provides attachment for muscles and intermuscular septa of the thigh. Also called *rough line of femur* (seldom used), *rough crest of femur* (outmoded), *linea aspera of femur, rough ridge of femur* (outmoded), *pilaster of Broca* (outmoded), *femoral crest, crista femoris.*

linea aspera of femur   LINEA ASPERA FEMORIS.

lineae atrophicae   STRIAE ATROPHICAE.

linea axillaris   Any one of the three parallel vertical lines related to the axillary folds: (1) linea axillaris anterior; (2) linea axillaris media; (3) linea axillaris posterior. An outmoded term. Also called *axillary line.*

linea axillaris anterior   [NA] A vertical line, parallel to the median plane, extending downward from the medial end of the anterior fold of the axilla along the side of the trunk. Also called *anterior axillary line.*

linea axillaris media   [NA] A vertical line, parallel to the anterior and the posterior axillary lines and midway between them, usually passing through the apex of the axilla. Also called *midaxillary line, linea medio-axillaris.*

linea axillaris posterior   [NA] A vertical line, parallel to the median plane, extending downward from the medial end of the posterior fold of the axilla along the side of the thorax. Also called *posterior axillary line.*

linea corneae senilis   HUDSON-STÄHLI LINE.

lineae distensae   STRIAE ATROPHICAE.

linea epiphysialis   [NA] A line seen on the surface in a mature bone at the junction between the epiphysis and the metaphyseal end of the diaphysis. It corresponds to the level of the perichondrial ring around the epiphyseal plate in an immature bone. Also called *epiphyseal line.*

linea fusca   A band of pigmentation along the frontal hair margin. It may be associated with cerebral inflammatory or neoplastic lesions.

linea glutea anterior   [NA] The middle of three curved ridges on the gluteal surface of the ala of the ilium extending from a point on the iliac crest 2–3 cm behind the anterior superior iliac spine to the middle of the superior margin of the greater sciatic notch. Between this line and the crest, the gluteus medius muscle arises. Also called *anterior gluteal line, middle curved line of ilium* (outmoded).

linea glutea inferior   [NA] The most anterior, and least distinct, of three curved ridges on the gluteal surface of the ala of the ilium, extending backwards from the notched margin below the anterior inferior iliac spine to the front angulation of the greater sciatic notch. Most of the area between the anterior and the inferior lines gives rise to the gluteus minimus muscle. Also called *inferior gluteal line, inferior curved line of ilium* (outmoded).

linea glutea posterior   [NA] The posterior, and shortest, of three curved ridges on the gluteal surface of the ala of the ilium, extending downwards from a point on the iliac crest about 5 cm in front of the posterior superior iliac spine to the superior margin of the greater sciatic notch just in front of the posterior inferior iliac spine. A small portion of gluteus maximus muscle arises behind this line. Also called *posterior gluteal line, superior curved line of ilium* (outmoded).

linea iliopectinea   An outmoded term for ILIOPECTINEAL LINE.

linea innominata   An outmoded term for LINEA TERMINALIS PELVIS.

linea intercondylaris femoris   [NA] A faint transverse ridge separating the posterior part of the intercondylar fossa of the femur from the popliteal surface and providing attachment for the capsule of the knee joint. Also called *intercondylar line, linea*

intercondyloidea femoris (outmoded), *intercondyloid line, popliteal line of femur.*

linea intercondyloidea femoris   An outmoded term for LINEA INTERCONDYLARIS FEMORIS.

linea intermedia cristae iliacae   [NA] A narrow strip between the outer and the inner lips of the iliac crest, the anterior two-thirds of which provides partial origin for the internal oblique muscle of the abdomen. Also called *intermediate line of iliac crest.*

linea intertrochanterica   [NA] A prominent oblique ridge separating the anterior surface of the neck of the femur from the shaft, extending inferomedially from a tubercle at the anterosuperior part of the greater trochanter to a point anterior to the lesser trochanter, where it becomes continuous with the spiral line. The iliofemoral ligament and the capsule of the hip joint are attached to it. Also called *intertrochanteric line, anterior intertrochanteric line* (outmoded), *oblique line of femur* (outmoded), *anterior intertrochanteric crest.*

linea intertrochanterica posterior   An outmoded term for CRISTA INTERTROCHANTERICA.

linea mamillaris   [NA] A vertical line, parallel to the median plane, passing through the nipple of either breast. Because of the variable position of the nipple, it is untenable to equate it with the linea medioclavicularis, with which it occasionally overlaps. Also called *mamillary line, nipple line, papillary line* (outmoded).

linea mediana anterior   [NA] A vertical line on the anterior surface of the body along the median plane, dividing the body into equal right and left halves. Also called *anterior median line.*

linea mediana posterior   [NA] A vertical line on the posterior surface of the body along the median plane, dividing the body into equal right and left halves. Also called *posterior median line.*

linea medio-axillaris   LINEA AXILLARIS MEDIA.

linea medioclavicularis   [NA] A vertical line, parallel to the median plane, passing through the midpoint between the jugular notch and the tip of the acromion and extending down the trunk on each side to cross the inguinal ligament midway between the anterior superior iliac spine and the symphysis pubis. Occasionally it may coincide with the mamillary line but by definition it is not the same. Also called *midclavicular line, lateral line.* See also POUPART'S LINE.

linea mensalis   Any one of the flexure lines on the palm of the hand produced by flexion of the fingers; palm crease. An outmoded term.

lineae musculares scapulae   Several ridges on the costal surface of the scapula extending superolaterally from the medial margin and providing attachment for the tendinous intersections of the subscapularis muscle. An outmoded term. Also called *muscular lines of scapula, subscapular lines, oblique ridges of scapula.*

linea musculi solei   [NA] An oblique ridge on the posterior surface of the tibia extending downward and medially from the fibular facet to the medial border about one-third of the distance from the upper end. Attached to it are the soleus muscle and its fascia, the popliteal fascia and the fascia covering the deep muscles of the leg. Also called *soleal line of tibia, linea poplitea tibiae* (outmoded), *popliteal line of tibia, oblique line of tibia* (outmoded), *linea obliqua tibiae* (outmoded).

linea mylohyoidea mandibulae   [NA] An oblique ridge on the medial surface of the body of the mandible extending from a point behind the third molar tooth just below the alveolar margin to the lower end of the symphysis menti below the mental spine. It provides attachment for the mylohyoid muscle, helping to form the floor of the mouth, and posteriorly for part of the superior constrictor muscle of the pharynx and for the pterygomandibular raphe. Also called *mylohyoid line of mandible,* *internal oblique line of mandible* (outmoded), *mylohyoidean line, mylohyoid ridge, mylohyoid line.*

linea nigra The linea alba of the abdomen during pregnancy, when it becomes pigmented. Also called *nigra line.*

linea nuchae inferior [NA] A curved bony ridge on the external surface of the squamous part of the occipital bone extending laterally from the midpoint of the external occipital crest to the jugular process and providing attachment for the upper margins of the rectus capitis posterior major and minor muscles. Also called *inferior nuchal line, inferior arcuate line of occipital bone* (outmoded), *inferior curved line of occipital bone* (outmoded).

linea nuchae superior [NA] A curved bony ridge on the external surface of the squamous part of the occipital bone extending laterally from the external occipital protuberance towards the lateral angle and providing attachment for the trapezius muscle medially and the sternocleidomastoid muscle laterally. Also called *superior nuchal line, superior semicircular line of occipital bone* (outmoded), *middle semicircular line of occipital bone* (outmoded), *superior arcuate line of occipital bone* (outmoded), *superior curved line of occipital bone* (outmoded), *external superior arcuate line of occipital bone* (outmoded).

linea nuchae suprema [NA] A faint curved bony ridge on the external surface of the squamous part of the occipital bone extending laterally from the external occipital protuberance above the superior nuchal line and providing attachment for the galea aponeurotica. Also called *highest nuchal line, supreme nuchal line, highest semicircular line of occipital bone* (outmoded), *highest curved line of occipital bone* (outmoded), *highest arcuate line of occipital bone* (outmoded), *supreme arcuate line of occipital bone* (outmoded), *supreme curved line of occipital bone* (outmoded), *supreme semicircular line* (outmoded).

linea obliqua cartilaginis thyroideae [NA] A curved line on the external surface of the lamina of the thyroid cartilage extending anteroinferiorly between the superior and the inferior tubercles and providing attachment to the sternothyroid and thyrohyoid muscles and the inferior constrictor muscle of the pharynx. Also called *oblique line of thyroid cartilage, limbus angulosus* (outmoded), *oblique crest of thyroid cartilage.*

linea obliqua fibulae An outmoded term for CRISTA MEDIALIS FIBULAE.

linea obliqua mandibulae [NA] An indefinite ridge on the outer surface of the body of the mandible extending backwards and upwards from the mental tubercle to the lower end of the anterior margin of the ramus, and providing attachment, anteriorly, for the depressor muscles of the mouth. Also called *oblique line of mandible.*

linea obliqua tibiae An outmoded term for LINEA MUSCULI SOLEI.

linea parasternalis [NA] A vertical line drawn on the anterior surface of the trunk midway between and parallel to the sternal and midclavicular lines. Also called *parasternal line, costoclavicular line* (outmoded).

linea pectinea femoris [NA] A slight ridge on the posteromedial aspect of the upper part of the shaft of the femur, descending from the base of the lesser trochanter to the top of the linea aspera and lying between the spiral line medially and the gluteal tuberosity laterally. The pectineus muscle is attached to it. Also called *pectineal line, pectineal crest of femur, middle ridge of femur* (outmoded).

linea poplitea tibiae An outmoded term for LINEA MUSCULI SOLEI.

linea scapularis [NA] A vertical line drawn through the inferior angle of the scapula and parallel to the median plane. Also called *scapular line.*

linea semicircularis douglasi An outmoded term for LINEA ARCUATA VAGINAE MUSCULI RECTI ABDOMINIS.

linea semilunaris An irregularly curved groove on the abdominal surface outlining the lateral margin of each rectus abdominis muscle and extending from the tip of the ninth costal cartilage to the pubic tubercle. It is best seen in lean, muscular individuals. Also called *semilunar line, linea semilunaris spigeli* (outmoded), *Spieghel's line, Spigelius line, spigelian line, semilunar line of Spieghel.*

linea semilunaris spigeli An outmoded term for LINEA SEMILUNARIS.

linea sinuosa analis An outmoded term for ANORECTAL JUNCTION.

linea spiralis An outmoded term for SPIRAL LINE OF FEMUR.

linea splendens A reduplication of pia mater in the fissura mediana anterior medullae spinalis forming a sheath for the anterior spinal artery. A seldom used term.

linea sternalis [NA] A vertical line corresponding to the lateral sternal margin on the anterior surface of the thorax. Also called *sternal line, lateral sternal line.*

linea temporalis inferior ossis parietalis [NA] The lower of two curved transverse lines, convex upwards, crossing the middle of the external surface of the parietal bone, to which the temporalis muscle is attached. Also called *inferior temporal line of parietal bone, inferior semicircular line of parietal bone* (outmoded), *inferior semicircular ridge of parietal bone* (outmoded), *inferior temporal line.*

linea temporalis ossis frontalis [NA] A prominent line curving back from the zygomatic process of the frontal bone and soon dividing into superior and inferior lines that are continuous with the two lines traversing the parietal bone. Also called *temporal line of frontal bone, semicircular line of frontal bone* (outmoded), *temporal crest of frontal bone, crista temporalis, external frontal crest, temporal ridge.*

linea temporalis superior ossis parietalis [NA] The upper of two curved transverse lines, convex upwards, crossing the middle of the external surface of the parietal bone and providing attachment for the temporal fascia. Also called *superior temporal line of parietal bone, superior temporal line, superior semicircular line of parietal bone* (outmoded), *superior semicircular ridge of parietal bone* (outmoded).

linea terminalis pelvis [NA] A ridge on the inner surface of the side walls of the bony pelvis, comprising the arcuate line posteriorly, the iliopectineal line and pecten pubis laterally, and crest of pubis anteriorly on each side, continuous with the promontory of the sacrum posteriorly and dividing the false, or major, pelvis above from the true, or minor, pelvis below. It forms most of the boundary of the superior aperture, or inlet, of the minor pelvis. Also called *terminal line of pelvis, iliopectineal crest of pelvis, linea innominata* (outmoded), *arcuate line of pelvis.*

lineae transversae ossis sacri [NA] Four transverse ridges on the pelvic surface of the sacrum extending between the paired pelvic sacral foramina as lines of fusion between the bodies and representing the positions of the former intervertebral disks. Also called *transverse lines of sacrum, transverse lines of sacral bone, transverse ridges of sacrum.*

linea trapezoidea [NA] A narrow ridge running anterolaterally from the conoid tubercle on the posterior border of the inferior surface of the lateral third of the clavicle and providing attachment for the trapezoid ligament, a part of the coracoclavicular ligament. Also called *trapezoid line, trapezoid ridge.*

linea visus VISUAL AXIS.

linea vitalis A flexure line encircling the thenar eminence on the palm of the hand. Also called *radial longitudinal line.*

lineae Plural of LINEA.

lineage [French *lignage* (from *ligne* line, from LINEA) race, lineage] **1** The direct descendants of an individual. **2** BLOOD

LINE. **3** The line of descent of a strain of cells cultured *in vitro*.

sympathetic cell lineage Categories of cells derived from the neural crest epithelium and including the following types: sympathogonia, unipolar sympathoblasts, multipolar sympathetic neurons, paraganglionic cells.

lineal **1** Of or relating to direct descent, as in a pedigree. **2** LINEAR.

linear Relating to or having the properties of a line. Also *lineal*.

linebreeding INBREEDING.

liner A protective or insulating layer applied to a surface, especially to the inside of a container or cavity.

asbestos liner In dentistry, a layer of asbestos placed between the investment and the casting ring to allow for expansion of the investment.

cavity liner A thin layer of varnish placed in a prepared dental cavity before placing the cement base. Also called *cavity primer, cavity varnish*.

soft liner A soft material for application to the fitting surfaces of dentures. It may be a synthetic elastomer or a plasticized acrylic polymer. Also called *soft lining*.

Lineweaver [Hans *Lineweaver*, U.S chemist, born 1907] Lineweaver-Burk equation. See under LINEWEAVER-BURK PLOT.

Ling [Per Henrik *Ling*, Swedish hygienist, 1776–1839] Ling's method. See under SWEDISH GYMNASTICS.

lingism SWEDISH GYMNASTICS.

lingua [L, the tongue, language, speech] [NA] A muscular organ covered with mucous membrane on its upper and lower surfaces, situated in the floor of the mouth and the anterior wall of the pharynx, and involved in mastication, swallowing, taste, and speech; the tongue. It is composed of three layers of intrinsic muscles which alter its shape, and it is connected to the mandible, hyoid bone, styloid process, and palate by four pairs of extrinsic muscles which can move it in all directions. The motor nerve is the hypoglossal nerve, while sensory and taste innervation come from the fifth, seventh, and ninth cranial nerves. Also called *glossa*.

lingua cerebelli The most anteroventral portion of the cerebellar vermis, bounded inferiorly by the superior medullary velum and superiorly by the lobus centralis.

lingua fisturata FISSURED TONGUE.

lingua frenata TONGUE-TIE.

lingua geographica GEOGRAPHIC TONGUE.

lingua nigra BLACK HAIRY TONGUE.

lingua plicata FISSURED TONGUE.

lingua scrotalis FISSURED TONGUE.

lingua villosa nigra BLACK HAIRY TONGUE.

lingua- LINGUO-.

linguae Plural of LINGUA.

lingual **1** Relating to the tongue; lingualis. **2** Resembling or suggestive of a tongue; linguiform. **3** Next to or in the direction of the tongue.

linguale In craniometry, the highest point on the lingual surface of symphysis menti.

Linguatula [Late L *linguatus* tongued + -ULA -*ule*] A genus of bloodsucking parasites, the tongue worms, of the phylum Pentastomida (family Linguatulidae, order Porocephalida), which are endoparasitic as adults in the lungs, sinuses, and other air passages of various animals, including man. Larvae are found in the digestive organs and lungs of a wide variety of hosts. Also called *Pentastoma*.

Linguatula rhinaria *LINGUATULA SERRATA*.

Linguatula serrata A species of which the adult is found in the nasal passages and sinuses of dogs and other canids, and rarely in felines. Larvae develop in the lymph nodes and liver of sheep, swine, cattle, rodents, rabbits, and occasionally man and other primates, eventually becoming encysted in the viscera. The parasite is widespread in Europe, and also found in the United States and South America. Infection usually causes a mild and insignificant rhinitis and sinusitis. Also called *Linguatula rhinaria*. See also HALZOUN.

linguatuliasis [*Linguatul(a)* + -IASIS] Infection with pentastome parasites of the genus *Linguatula*. Also called *linguatulosis*.

linguatulid [*Linguatul(ida)* + -ID[1]] **1** Pertaining or belonging to the family Linguatulidae. **2** A pentastome worm of the family Linguatulidae.

Linguatulida [Late L *linguat(a)* (from L *lingu(a)* tongue + -*ata*, neut. pl. of -*atus* -ATE) tongued + -*ula* -ULE + -*ida*, neut. pl. of L -*ides*, patronymic suffix] POROCEPHALIDA.

Linguatulidae A family of parasites in the order Porocephalida, class or phylum Pentostomida. Having a flattened body resembling acanthocephalan worms, they are parasitic in the nasal cavities of dogs, cats, and other carnivores in the adult form, and in the tissues of rodents, herbivores, and many other animals in the larval (or nymphal) form. Both forms have been reported from humans, the larval form from ingestion of eggs, the adult from ingestion of raw or undercooked liver or other organs. See also HALZOUN.

linguatulosis LINGUATULIASIS.

linguiform Tongue-shaped; lingulate.

lingula [L, dim. of LINGUA] A small structure or process shaped like or suggestive of a tongue. • When used without modifiers the term commonly refers to lingula cerebelli.

lingula cerebelli [NA] The most anterior and ventral portion of the vermis of the cerebellum. It is the medial component of the anterior lobe, and receives the attachment of the superior medullary velum. Also called *lingula of cerebellum*.

lingula of cerebellum LINGULA CEREBELLI.

lingula of left lung LINGULA PULMONIS SINISTRI.

lingula of lower jaw An outmoded term for LINGULA MANDIBULAE.

lingula of mandible LINGULA MANDIBULAE.

lingula mandibulae [NA] A small projection of bone anteromedial to the mandibular foramen on the medial surface of the ramus of the mandible, providing attachment to the sphenomandibular ligament. Also called *lingula of mandible, lingula of lower jaw* (outmoded), *spine of Spix*.

lingula pulmonis sinistri [NA] An occasional projection of the lower end of the anterior border of the superior lobe of the left lung, just below the cardiac notch and above the oblique fissure. Also called *lingula of left lung*.

lingula of sphenoid LINGULA SPHENOIDALIS.

sphenoidal lingula LINGULA SPHENOIDALIS.

lingula sphenoidalis [NA] A narrow bony projection between the posterior part of the lateral surface of the body of the sphenoid bone and the greater wing of the sphenoid, forming the lateral margin of the back of the carotid sulcus and roofing the posterior opening of the pterygoid canal. Also called *lingula of sphenoid, sphenoidal lingula, anterior petrosal process* (outmoded), *tongue of sphenoid bone*.

lingulae Plural of LINGULA.

lingular Pertaining to a lingula or lingulalike process.

lingulate Like a tongue or a lingula; linguiform.

lingulectomy [*lingul(a)* + -ECTOMY] Removal of the lingula of the left upper lobe of the lung.

linguo- [L *lingua* tongue, language] A combining form denoting the tongue or relationship to the tongue. Also *lingua-*.

linguocervical Pertaining to the lingual aspect of the neck of a tooth. Also *cervicolingual*.

linguoclination [LINGUO- + *(in)clination*] The inclination of a tooth in the lingual direction.

linguoclusion [LINGUO- + *(oc)clusion*] Linguoversion of a group of teeth.

linguodental [LINGUO- + DENTAL] Relating to both the tongue and the teeth.

linguopapillitis Inflammation of the lingual papillae, particularly along the edges of the tongue. An unspecific and seldom used term.

linguoplacement LINGUOVERSION.

linguoplate [LINGUO- + PLATE] A major connector in a partial denture which covers the gingivae and the cingula of the anterior teeth.

linguotrite [LINGUO- + L *trit(us)*, past part. of *terere* to rub] An obsolete term for TONGUE FORCEPS.

linguoversion [LINGUO- + VERSION] The deviation of a tooth from the arch towards the tongue. Also called *linguoplacement, lingual placement.*

liniment [L *linimentum*. See LINIMENTUM.] An oily liquid preparation, applied externally or to the gums. It may be a solution, suspension, or emulsion; and used as a counterirritant, anodyne, or cleansing agent.

   ammoniated liniment of camphor A liniment containing 12% camphor, strong ammonia solution, and lavender oil in alcohol.

   liniment of belladonna A liniment prepared by percolating belladonna root with 80% alcohol, followed by the addition of camphor.

   camphor liniment A liniment containing 20% camphor in arachis oil. Also called *camphorated oil.*

   medicinal soft soap liniment GREEN SOAP TINCTURE.

linimentum [L (from *lin(ere)* to smear + *i* + *-mentum* -MENT), an ointment, anointing] Liniment.

   linimentum saponis mollis GREEN SOAP TINCTURE.

linin A substance that forms fine threadlike structures to which nuclear chromatin granules appear to be attached. An obsolete term.

lining 1 A cement base under a dental restoration. A British usage. **2** An extra layer on the fitting surface of a denture.

   soft lining SOFT LINER.

linitis [Gk *lin(on)* a thing made of flax, thread, fishing net, linen + -ITIS] Inflammation of the stomach. An older term.

   linitis plastica A thickening and stiffening of the wall of the stomach due to diffuse mural infiltration by a poorly differentiated scirrhous carcinoma. Also called *leather bottle stomach, sclerotic stomach, gastric sclerosis, Brinton's disease* (seldom used), *cirrhosis of the stomach* (seldom used), *fibromatosis ventriculi.*

   salt link The attraction between two ions of opposite charge, i.e. the same type of bond as between the ions of a salt crystal. The term often applies to this attraction between two amino-acid side chains of a protein.

linkage The tendency for genes, during breeding, not to segregate entirely at random but in daughter cells to remain associated in their original combinations. In eukaryotic cells, linkage usually indicates that the linked genes are carried on the same chromosome. Linkage analysis is the experimental determination of the degree to which genetic markers tend to remain together during recombination. This is inversely proportional to the distance that separates these genes from each other. That is, the greater the degree of random segregation of two genes, the less the linkage, and the more recombination between them. When the chance of recombination between two genes is 50 percent, segregation is random, and the genes are unlinked, although they might still be syntenic.

medical record linkage The process of identifying and relating different medical records or sources of information through a common code, name, number, or other unique item of identification.

record linkage The systematic linking of all relevant items of information relating to each individual in a population or group so as to provide a cumulative and up-to-date record of the significant health events, such as hospitalizations and immunization and vaccination procedures, affecting the individual. • Record linkage is practiced chiefly in the U.S., United Kingdom, and Canada, although it is known and sometimes made use of in New Zealand and India.

sex linkage 1 An inheritance in which a phenotype is determined by a genetic locus on a sex chromosome. In humans, nearly all such phenotypes are X-linked. **2** A genetic locus that occurs on a sex chromosome. It is designated by specifying the chromosome on which the linkage occurs.

Y linkage Linkage associated with loci on the Y chromosome.

Linodil A proprietary name for inositol niacinate.

Linognathus [New L, from Gk *lino(n)* anything made of flax, a net, fishing net, linen, lampwick + *gnathos* jaw, esp. lower jaw] A genus of blood-sucking lice of the family Linognathidae.

   Linognathus africanus The African blue louse, a parasite of goats and sheep.

   Linognathus ovillus The sheep body louse, often found with other species of lice on the same animal, but in different preferred sites of infection.

   Linognathus pedalis The foot louse of sheep, occurring on the legs and feet where there is an absence of wool. It is found in the Americas, Australia, New Zealand, and South Africa.

   Linognathus setulosus The sucking louse of dogs, also found on other canids. It is a possible host of the filarial worm of dogs, *Dipetolonema reconditum.*

   Linognathus vituli A species of sucking louse that infects cattle; the long-nosed cattle louse.

linoleic acid $CH_3—[CH_2]_4—CH=CH—CH_2—CH=CH—[CH_2]_7—COOH$. An essential fatty acid. It is produced in plants as its coenzyme-A derivative by insertion of the 12-13 double bond in the *cis* configuration. It (or other polyunsaturated fatty acids with which it is interconvertible, such as linolenic acid and arachidonic acid) is required in the mammalian diet, especially as a precursor of prostaglandins.

linolenic acid $CH_3—[CH_2—CH=CH—]_3—[CH_2]_7—COOH$. An essential fatty acid, interconvertible with arachidonic acid and linoleic acid, required for prostaglandin synthesis.

linseed The dried ripe seed of *Linum usitatissium*, flax. It contains mucilage, protein, and a fixed oil—linseed, or flaxseed, oil—which constitutes 30 to 40 percent of the seed. If taken internally, the oil acts as a demulcent and laxative. Also called *flaxseed, linum.*

Linser [Paul *Linser*, German dermatologist, born 1871] See under METHOD.

Linstowiidae A family of small to medium-sized tapeworms (order Cyclophyllidea, subclass Cestoda) that are parasitic in reptiles, birds, and mammals, including humans. Genera of medical importance as rarely reported parasites of man include *Oochoristica* and *Inermicapsifer.* They inhabit the intestine but their effects, if any, are unknown.

lint A surgical dressing material originally made of scrapings from linen cloth but now made of a specially finished fabric. Also called *charpie.*

lintin Loosely woven absorbent cotton cloth used as a dressing for a wound.

lintine Cotton lint from which the oil has been removed. It is used as a dressing for a wound.

Linton [Robert Ritchie *Linton*, U.S. surgeon, born 1900]   See under PROCEDURE.

linum   LINSEED.

Linzenmeier [Georg *Linzenmeier*, German physician, born 1882]   See under TEST.

lio-   LEIO-.

lip [Old English *lippa*, prob. akin to L *labium* and *labia* lip and to *labrum* lip, edge, rim]   **1** Either the upper or the lower fleshy fold forming the movable anterior wall of the mouth cavity and surrounding the oral fissure; labium oris.   **2** Any projecting liplike margin or edge; labium; labrum.

acetabular lip   LABRUM ACETABULARE.

anterior lip of cervix of uterus   LABIUM ANTERIUS OSTII UTERI.

anterior lip of ostium of uterus   LABIUM ANTERIUS OSTII UTERI.

anterior lip of pharyngeal opening of auditory tube   See under LABIUM ANTERIUS OSTII PHARYNGEI TUBAE AUDITIVAE.

cleft lip   A developmental defect consisting of a notch, furrow, or open fissure of the upper lip with or without associated cleft of the maxilla. The cleavage is usually on one side of the philtrum and premaxilla. It is sometimes bilateral, in which case a segment of lip and associated premaxilla are relatively set apart on the midline. Rarely, the midline segments are absent, and then the midline cleft bears some resemblance to that of a hare. It results from the failure of the embryonic medial nasal and maxillary processes to unite in normal embryogenesis. It is often associated with cleft palate, and infrequently with genal or oblique facial cleft. Also called *harelip, cheiloschisis, chiloschisis, stomatoschisis.*

dorsal lip of blastopore   In amphibians, the dorsal edge of the blastopore, formed by invagination. It appears precociously at the start of the invagination process at gastrulation and in essence marks the appearance of the notochord. The cells of the dorsal lip have been shown to possess organizing powers.

double lip   A fold of tissue on the inner side of the lip resembling a second lip. Habitual sucking between the teeth may be a factor in its development.

external lip of iliac crest   LABIUM EXTERNUM CRISTAE ILIACAE.

external lip of linea aspera of femur   LABIUM LATERALE LINEAE ASPERAE FEMORIS.

fibrocartilaginous lip of acetabulum   LABRUM ACETABULARE.

glenoid lip   LABRUM GLENOIDALE.

glenoid lip of articulation of hip   An outmoded term for LABRUM ACETABULARE.

glenoid lip of articulation of humerus   An outmoded term for LABRUM GLENOIDALE.

greater lip of pudendum   LABIUM MAJUS PUDENDI.

inferior lip   LABIUM INFERIUS ORIS.

inferior lip of ileocecal valve   LABIUM INFERIUS VALVULAE COLI.

internal lip of iliac crest   LABIUM INTERNUM CRISTAE ILIACAE.

lateral lip of bicipital groove   CRISTA TUBERCULI MAJORIS.

lateral lips of blastopore   The two lateral edges of the blastopore which extend from the dorsal lip to the ventral lip.

lateral lip of linea aspera of femur   LABIUM LATERALE LINEAE ASPERAE FEMORIS.

lesser lip of pudendum   LABIUM MINUS PUDENDI.

lower lip   LABIUM INFERIUS ORIS.

medial lip of bicipital groove   CRISTA TUBERCULI MINORIS.

medial lip of linea aspera of femur   LABIUM MEDIALE LINEAE ASPERAE FEMORIS.

posterior lip of cervix of uterus   LABIUM POSTERIUS OSTII UTERI.

posterior lip of ostium of uterus   LABIUM POSTERIUS OSTII UTERI.

posterior lip of pharyngeal opening of auditory tube   See under LABIUM POSTERIUS OSTII PHARYNGEI TUBAE AUDITIVAE.

rhombic lip   The lateral edge of the embryonic rhombencephalon.

superior lip   LABIUM SUPERIUS ORIS.

superior lip of ileocecal valve   LABIUM SUPERIUS VALVULAE COLI.

tapir lips   TAPIR MOUTH.

tympanic lip of limb of spiral lamina   LABIUM LIMBI TYMPANICUM LAMINAE SPIRALIS.

upper lip   LABIUM SUPERIUS ORIS.

ventral lip of blastopore   The ventral edge of the blastopore, appearing after the dorsal lip and to which it will be united by the lateral lips.

vestibular lip of limb of spiral lamina   LABIUM LIMBI VESTIBULARE LAMINAE SPIRALIS.

lip-   LIPO-.

lipa-   LIPO-.

lipacidemia   The presence of fatty acid in blood.

lipaciduria [LIP- + ACIDURIA]   Urinary excretion of fatty acids, which is increased in ketoacidosis. A rarely used term.

lipaemia   A British spelling for LIPEMIA.

liparia [Gk *lipar(os)* fatty + -IA]   A condition of excess fat; obesity. A rarely used term.

liparocele   A hernia containing adipose tissue, such as an omental hernia.

liparodyspnea   Difficulty in breathing secondary to obesity.

liparomphalus [Gk *lipar(os)* oily, fat + *omphalos* the navel]   A lipoma of the umbilicus.

liparotrichia [Gk *liparo(s)* oily, greasy + TRICH- + -IA]   Seborrhoea of the scalp. An obsolete term.

liparous   Fat; obese.

lipase   Any enzyme that catalyzes the hydrolysis of a fat.

pancreatic lipase   The lipolytic digestive enzyme secreted by the exocrine pancreas. It is a triacylglycerol lipase (EC 3.1.1.3). Also called *pancreatolipase.*

lipasuria   Urinary excretion of lipase. Increased lipasuria reflects pancreatic disease, although it also may be present in diffuse renal diseases. It is not a practical diagnostic test.

lipectomy [LIP- + -ECTOMY]   The excision of a mass of subcutaneous adipose tissue. It is usually from the abdominal wall but it may be taken from any part of the body. Also called *adipectomy.*

suction lipectomy   A lipectomy performed by means of a vacuum device, usually utilized in the region of the hips and thighs. The device is applied through a metal cannula which is inserted into the subcutaneous tissue through a small incision.

submental lipectomy   A cosmetic operation for the removal of excessive fat beneath the chin.

lipedema   Chronic swelling caused by evenly distributed subcutaneous fat deposits and fluid. An imprecise and obsolete term.

lipemia [LIP- + -EMIA]   **1** An imprecise term for HYPERLIPIDEMIA.   **2** Greater than normal turbidity of plasma due to the presence of lipids.

alimentary lipemia   Transient lipemia developing after consumption of lipid-rich food. It is due largely to increase in the number of chylomicrons. Also called *postprandial lipemia.*

diabetic lipemia   Raised plasma values of triglycerides in uncontrolled diabetes mellitus. Many physiologic events combine to raise triglycerides, largely insulin lack, low levels of lipoprotein lipase, and low plasma postheparin lipolytic activity. Insulin repletion reverses these processes.

postprandial lipemia ALIMENTARY LIPEMIA.

lipemia retinalis A creamy or milky appearance of the retinal blood vessels due to marked hyperlipemia of any cause.

lipemic 1 Having increased concentration of lipids in serum or plasma. 2 Having a cloudy or milky appearance: used of a plasma or serum specimen.

lipfanogen Any substance which, when taken up by cells, results in formation of globules of fat in the cytoplasm of the cell.

lipid [LIP- + -ID^2] Any natural compound soluble in apolar but not in polar solvents. Lipids usually contain residues of fatty acids, one-chain alcohols, steroids, or sphingoids. Lipids therefore include fats and phospholipids. Also called *lipoid* (outmoded).

Gaucher lipid CEREBROSIDE.

Niemann-Pick lipid SPHINGOMYELIN.

skin surface lipid The lipid found on the skin surface. In the human this is composed mainly of sebum from the sebaceous glands, with a small contribution from the keratinizing epidermis and traces derived from exogenous sources, such as soaps and cosmetics.

lipid A The endotoxic component of lipopolysaccharide, consisting of a β-1,6-D-glucosamine disaccharide with all of its OH groups substituted (with two phosphates, a ketodeoxyoctonate trisaccharide link to the O antigen, and three fatty acids) and its NH$_2$ groups substituted with hydroxymyristic acid.

lipidemia [French *lipide* (from Gk *lipos* fat + French *-ide* -ID^1) fatty, fat + -EMIA] An imprecise term for HYPERLIPIDEMIA.

lipidolysis LIPOLYSIS.

lipidosis [LIPID + -OSIS] Any disorder of lipid metabolism in which abnormal amounts of lipid are stored within cells of the reticuloendothelial system. Also called *lipoid thesaurismosis, lipid storage disease.*

Bielschowsky type cerebral lipidosis BIELSCHOWSKY-DOL-LINGER SYNDROME.

cerebral lipidosis Any of a group of genetically determined disorders in which abnormal amounts of lipid are stored within brain neurons. Also called *familial cerebral lipidosis.*

familial cerebral lipidosis CEREBRAL LIPIDOSIS.

ganglioside lipidosis GANGLIOSIDOSIS.

glycolipid lipidosis An outmoded term for ANGIOKERA-TOMA CORPORIS DIFFUSUM.

hereditary dystopic lipidosis An outmoded term for AN-GIOKERATOMA CORPORIS DIFFUSUM.

neurovisceral lipidosis GM$_1$ GANGLIOSIDOSIS.

sphingomyelin lipidosis NIEMANN-PICK DISEASE.

sulfatide lipidosis METACHROMATIC LEUKODYSTROPHY.

lipiduria The presence of fat in the urine, as neutral fat bodies floating in the urine, oval fat bodies which appear yellow or black under reduced light and which may be single or aggregated, casts with inclusion fat or fatty cells, renal tubular epithelial cells containing neutral fat which stain red with Sudan III or oil red, or degenerating fatty vacuoles. It is characteristic of but not specific for the nephrotic syndrome. Also called *lipoiduria, lipuria, adiposuria* (obsolete).

Lipiodol An iodinated oil for use as a radiopaque contrast agent. A propietary name.

lipo- [Gk *lipos* animal grease, fat, lard, tallow, vegetable grease, oil] A combining form meaning fat or lipid. Also *lip-, lipa-.*

lipoadenoma [LIPO- + ADENOMA] A rare tumor, typically of the parathyroid, composed of an intimate admixture of glandular and fatty tissue. Also called *adenolipoma.*

lipoamide [LIPO- + AMIDE] The amide of lipoic acid, which is the cyclic disulfide formed by oxidation of 6,8-dimercaptooc-

tanoic acid. Since lipoic acid occurs in enzymes in amide combination with the side chain of a lysine residue, enzymes that catalyze conversions of the lipoyl group often act also on free lipoamide.

lipoamide reductase DIHYDROLIPOAMIDE DEHYDROGEN-ASE.

lipoarthritis Arthritis associated with any one of several types of lipid storage disorders or hyperlipidemia.

lipoatrophy 1 Atrophy of adipose tissue, as at subcutaneous sites of insulin injection. 2 LIPODYSTROPHY.

circumscribed lipoatrophy Focal areas of atrophy of subcutaneous adipose tissue, such as caused by repeated insulin injections.

lipoblast A cell, originating in connective tissue, which becomes a fat cell. The cell usually has a polyhedral shape and contains numerous small lipid droplets.

lipoblastoma [LIPO- + BLASTOMA] A localized lesion or form of lipoblastomatosis.

lipoblastomatosis [LIPO- + BLASTOMATOSIS] A benign lobulated tumor of fetal fat cells seen primarily in infants. It may be localized or diffuse.

lipocaic A hypothetical pancreatic hormone believed to influence fat metabolism. The controversial hypothesis derives from one of a number of possible interpretations of the evidence that depancreatized dogs given adequate doses of insulin develop fatty livers and this condition is relieved by the dogs' eating raw pancreas.

lipocardiac [LIPO- + CARDIAC] Pertaining to a fatty heart.

lipocatabolic Relating to the metabolic breakdown of fat.

lipocele [LIPO- + -CELE^1] A hernia containing fatty tissue. Also called *adipocele.*

lipochondrodystrophy An outmoded and inaccurate term for MUCOPOLYSACCHARIDOSIS IH.

lipochondroma [LIPO- + CHONDROMA] A chondroma with fat tissue.

lipochromemia A greater than normal concentration of carotenoid pigments in blood, as in hypercarotenemia.

lipoclasis LIPOLYSIS.

lipoclastic LIPOLYTIC.

lipocorticotrophic LIPOCORTICOTROPIC.

lipocorticotropic Describing a presumed hormonal activity of the adenohypophysis, believed to operate through the agency of the adrenal cortex to produce accumulation of fat in adipose tissue. Also *lipocorticotrophic.*

lipocrit [LIPO- + Gk *krit(os)* (verbal of *krinein* to separate) separated, to be separated] A device for determining the proportion of lipid in a fluid.

lipocyte [LIPO- + -CYTE] FAT CELL.

lipodermatosclerosis A brawny, pigmented fibrosis of the skin and subcutaneous tissues of the lower leg that results from chronic venous stasis. Also called *liposclerosis.*

lipodystrophia [LIPO- + DYSTROPHIA] LIPODYSTROPHY.

lipodystrophia intestinalis WHIPPLE'S DISEASE.

lipodystrophia progressiva PROGRESSIVE LIPODYSTROPHY.

lipodystrophy [LIPO- + DYSTROPHY] A condition characterized by abnormal fat metabolism. Also called *lipodystrophia.*

acquired generalized lipodystrophy A form of lipodystrophy that often develops after another illness or pregnancy. Characterized by loss of body fat (unlike the congenital form the face may be spared), accelerated linear growth, liver enlargement, nephrotic syndrome, hyperglycemia with insulin resistance, hypertriglyceridemia, and increased metabolic activity with normal thyroid function. Also called *Lawrence syndrome.*

acquired partial lipodystrophy PROGRESSIVE LIPODYSTROPHY.

lipodystrophy of Berardinelli SEIP SYNDROME.

cephalothoracic lipodystrophy Lipodystrophy involving the head and thorax.

congenital lipodystrophy SEIP SYNDROME.

congenital total lipodystrophy SEIP SYNDROME.

familial generalized lipodystrophy SEIP SYNDROME.

familial lipodystrophy of limbs and trunk A rare familial lipodystrophy of the limbs and lower trunk, sparing the face, neck, and upper trunk, inherited as a dominant trait. The condition chiefly affects women, with onset at puberty. Also called *reverse partial lipodystrophy, Köbberling-Dunnigan syndrome.*

generalized lipodystrophy SEIP SYNDROME.

inferior lipodystrophy Lipodystrophy involving the lower limbs.

insulin lipodystrophy Atrophy of subcutaneous fat at sites of insulin injection. Also called *insulin-induced lipodystrophy.*

insulin-induced lipodystrophy INSULIN LIPODYSTROPHY.

intestinal lipodystrophy WHIPPLE'S DISEASE.

progressive lipodystrophy The commonest form of lipodystrophy, usually characterized by a progressive symmetric loss of fat from the face and upper body and abnormal deposition of fat about the buttocks and thighs. Females are more often affected than males. Insulin resistance and endogenous hyperlipemia are generally present. Also called *lipodystrophia progressiva, acquired partial lipodystrophy, Barraquer-Simons syndrome.*

reverse partial lipodystrophy FAMILIAL LIPODYSTROPHY OF LIMBS AND TRUNK.

total lipodystrophy and acromegaloid gigantism SEIP SYNDROME.

trochanteric lipodystrophy RIDING BREECHES DEFORMITY.

lipoedema A chronic swelling of the legs that is associated with abundant subcutaneous fat.

lipoferous [LIPO- + -FEROUS] **1** Containing fat. **2** Capable of combining with fat for transport purposes.

lipofibroma [LIPO- + FIBROMA] FIBROLIPOMA.

lipofibromyxoma [LIPO- + FIBROMYXOMA] A lipoma with fibrous and myxomatous components.

lipofibrosarcoma [LIPO- + FIBROSARCOMA] A liposarcoma with a prominent fibrous component.

lipofuscin A brown pigment partially soluble in a fat, occurring in granules in cells, such as nerve or muscle cells, as a result of the fusion of a lysosome with an endocytic vesicle, the undigested material remaining being primarily lipofuscin. An estimate of the age of an animal can often be made based on the number of lipofuscin granules. Also called *age pigment.*

lipogenesis [LIPO- + GENESIS] The production of fat by the body. Also called *adipogenesis.*

lipogenetic LIPOGENIC.

lipogenic Of or relating to the production of fat. Also *adipogenic, adipogenous, lipogenous, lipoplastic, lipogenetic.*

lipogenous LIPOGENIC.

lipogranuloma A granulomatous inflammation of the subcutaneous fat. Also called *oleoma.*

lipogranulomatosis A rare metabolic disorder in which ceramides and gangliosides accumulate, as a result of ceramidase deficiency, within neurons and glial cells of the central nervous system, resulting in mental and motor retardation and a fatal outcome usually by the age of two years. Subcutaneous nodules and skin lesions are also seen. Also called *Farber's disease, disseminated lipogranulomatosis.*

disseminated lipogranulomatosis LIPOGRANULOMATOSIS.

lipohemangioma [LIPO- + HEMANGIOMA] A benign tumor of adipose and vascular elements.

lipohemarthrosis A joint abnormality characterized by synovial fluid containing both fat droplets and blood, as occurs in a bone fracture involving the joint.

lipohemia An imprecise term for HYPERLIPIDEMIA.

lipohistiodieresis [LIPO- + HISTIO- + DIERESIS] The loss of stored body fat.

lipohyalin Lipoid material sometimes found in hyalinized beta cells of the pancreatic islets of Langerhans in diabetes mellitus.

lipoic acid The acid formed by oxidation of the thiol groups of 6,8-dimercaptoocatanoic acid to a disulfide, so that a five-membered ring is formed. It is a component of the 2-oxo acid dehydrogenase complexes, and becomes reductively acylated in the course of the reaction in which, for example, pyruvate or 2-oxoglutarate is converted into acetyl-CoA or succinyl-CoA, respectively, with elimination of carbon dioxide, consumption of coenzyme A, and reduction of NAD. Lipoic acid occurs in amide linkage with lysine residues of one of the enzymes of the complex. Also called *thioctic acid.*

lipoid [LIP- + -OID] **1** Of or like fat. **2** An outmoded term for LIPID.

Forssman's lipoid FORSSMAN ANTIGEN.

lipoidemia An imprecise term for HYPERLIPIDEMIA.

lipoidosis [LIPOID + -OSIS] Any disturbance of fat metabolism. See also LIPIDOSIS.

arterial lipoidosis ATHEROSCLEROSIS.

lipoidosis corneae Fatty deposits within the cornea.

lipoidosis cutis et mucosae An outmoded term for LIPOID PROTEINOSIS.

kerasin lipoidosis An obsolete term for GAUCHER'S DISEASE.

renal lipoidosis A rarely used term for FATTY KIDNEY.

lipoidproteinosis LIPOID PROTEINOSIS.

lipoidsiderosis The deposit of iron pigments in adipose tissue. An obsolete term.

lipoiduria LIPIDURIA.

lipolipoidosis An obsolete term for FATTY INFILTRATION.

Lipo-Lutin A proprietary name for progesterone.

lipolysis [LIPO- + LYSIS] The hydrolysis of fat into free fatty acids and glycerol, often with release of free fatty acids into the plasma. Also called *adipolysis, steatolysis, lipidolysis, lipoclasis.*

lipolytic Of or relating to the breakdown of fat. Also called *adipolytic, lipoclastic, steatolytic.*

lipoma [LIP- + -OMA] A benign growth of mature adipose tissue cells showing no evidence of cellular atypia. It may occur at a variety of sites, such as skin and intestines. Also called *pimeloma, adipose tumor, fatty tumor, adipoma* (obsolete).

lipoma annulare colli Collarlike lipomatosis of the neck.

lipoma arborescens A lipomatous transformation of the synovium, producing a villous form.

calcified lipoma A lipoma containing deposits of calcium, usually the result of fat necrosis.

lipoma capsulare **1** A tumorlike accumulation of fat adjacent to the female breast. **2** A tumorlike accumulation of fat in the capsule of a joint.

lipoma cavernosum A lipoma containing large, blood-filled channels.

lipoma of corpus callosum A rare tumor of the corpus callosum which gives rise to a typical radiologic appearance because of calcification within the tumor.

diffuse lipoma An unencapsulated lipoma.

diffuse symmetrical lipomas of the neck A condition characterized by diffuse and symmetrical, benign adipose tumors in the neck and occasionally on the trunk. It occurs mostly in adult males and usually does not affect the general health. Also called *Madelung's disease.*

lipoma diffusum renis Replacement of atrophic or destroyed renal parenchyma by fatty tissue.

lipoma dolorosa A lipoma which is painful.

fetal fat cell lipoma HIBERNOMA.

lipoma fetalocellulare HIBERNOMA.

lipoma fibrosum FIBROLIPOMA.

infiltrating lipoma INTRAMUSCULAR LIPOMA.

intramuscular lipoma A benign proliferation of mature adipose tissue infiltrating striated muscle. Also called *infiltrating lipoma*.

lumbosacral lipoma A lipoma in the lumbosacral region, usually overlying a spina bifida.

lipoma myxomatodes MYXOLIPOMA.

nevoid lipoma ANGIOLIPOMA.

lipoma ossificans A lipoma with bone formation. Also called *lipoma petrificum ossificans*.

lipoma petrificans A lipoma with calcification.

lipoma petrificum ossificans LIPOMA OSSIFICANS.

renal lipoma A benign adipose tissue tumor of the renal cortex.

lipoma sarcomatodes LIPOSARCOMA.

lipoma of the spermatic cord A benign growth of adipose tissue of the spermatic cord which may show considerable swelling in the inguinal region and extend down to the scrotum, resembling an inguinal hernia.

spinal lipoma An intradural lipoma within the spinal cord, usually seen in association with spinal dysraphism and spina bifida.

telangiectatic lipoma ANGIOLIPOMA.

lipoma telangiectodes ANGIOLIPOMA.

lipomatoid [*lipomat(a)*, pl. of LIPOMA, + -OID] Resembling a lipoma.

lipomatosis [*lipomat(a)*, pl. of LIPOMA + -OSIS] **1** The presence of multiple or diffuse lipomas. **2** Replacement of atrophic or destroyed parenchyma of an organ, as the kidney, by adipose tissue. Also called *liposis*.

lipomatosis atrophicans Lipomatosis associated with atrophy of other structures or emaciation.

diffuse lipomatosis A diffuse, infiltrating proliferation of mature adipose tissue showing no evidence of cellular atypia. Large examples of this lesion may involve sizable portions of an extremity or the trunk. It chiefly affects children and is exceedingly rare during adult life.

lipomatosis dolorosa The presence of multiple painful lipomas. The pain often appears in one lipoma after another. Also called *lipomatosis neurotica*.

embryonal lipomatosis LIPOSARCOMA.

lipomatosis gigantea The presence of multiple, very large lipomas.

medullary lipomatosis Proliferation of renal hilar fat, a benign condition discovered incidentally on autopsy. Also called *lipomatosis renis*.

multiple symmetrical lipomatosis The presence of multiple, symmetrically distributed lipomas.

lipomatosis neurotica LIPOMATOSIS DOLOROSA.

nodular circumscribed lipomatosis The presence of multiple lipomas which are nodular and well delineated or encapsulated.

lipomatosis renis A rarely used term for MEDULLARY LIPOMATOSIS.

symmetrical lipomatosis See under MULTIPLE SYMMETRICAL LIPOMATOSIS.

visceral lipomatosis The replacement of atrophic or destroyed parenchyma of an organ, as the kidney, by fatty tissue.

lipomatous Pertaining to a lipoma. Also *steatomatous*.

lipomelanotic Characterized by melanin and intracellular lipid.

lipomeningocele [LIPO- + MENINGOCELE] A lipoma within the cauda equina. It is often associated with spina bifida.

lipomeria [Gk *leip(ein)* to leave, lack + *o* + *mer(o)*-¹ + IA] A congenital absence of one or more limbs. • A preferable term is *amelia*, modified by a specific designation of the missing limb(s).

lipometabolic Having to do with the metabolism of fat.

lipometabolism [LIPO- + METABOLISM] The metabolism of fat.

lipomicron CHYLOMICRON.

lipomphalus A fat hernia of the umbilicus.

lipomucopolysaccharidosis MUCOLIPIDOSIS.

lipomyohemangioma [LIPO- + MYO- + HEMANGIOMA] ANGIOMYOLIPOMA.

lipomyoma MYOLIPOMA.

lipomyosarcoma [LIPO- + MYO- + SARCOMA] A sarcoma with fat and muscle components.

lipomyxoma MYXOLIPOMA.

lipomyxosarcoma [LIPO- + MYXO- + SARCOMA] MYXOID LIPOSARCOMA.

Liponyssoides A genus of bloodsucking mites, ectoparasites of mammals. The mouse mite, *L. sanguineus*, transmits *Rickettsia akari* accidentally to humans, causing rickettsialpox. Also called *Allodermanyssus*.

Liponyssus [LIPO- + New L -*nyssus*, suffix formed from Gk *nyssein* or *nyttein* to prick, spur, pierce] ORNITHONYSSUS.

lipopectic Having to do with lipopexia. Also *lipopexic*.

lipopenia [LIPO- + -PENIA] A deficiency of fat occurring in the body.

lipopenic Having to do with lipopenia.

lipopexia The deposition of fat in the tissues.

lipopexic LIPOPECTIC.

lipophage A cell which takes in fat from its environment.

lipophagia LIPOPHAGY.

lipophagic Pertaining to or evidencing lipophagy.

lipophagy [LIPO- + -*phag(ia)* + -Y] The dissolution of adipose tissue and engulfment of the lipid by phagocytic cells. Also called *lipophagia*.

lipophanerosis FATTY DEGENERATION.

lipophilia An attraction for fat.

lipophilic Fat-soluble: used especially to describe the affinity of certain dyes for lipid substances.

lipophore [LIPO- + -PHORE] A pigmented cell whose color is caused by lipochrome pigment.

lipophrenia [Gk *leip(ein)* to leave, lack + *o* + -PHRENIA] Loss of mental capacity as a result of organic brain disorder, as in senile dementia. An outmoded term.

lipoplastic LIPOGENIC.

lipopolysaccharide Any substance of whose molecule part is a polysaccharide and part a lipid. Such substances are found as components of bacterial cell walls. They are frequently antigenic.

lipoprotein [LIPO- + PROTEIN] Any complex or compound of lipids with proteins. The lipoproteins of blood plasma are generally classified on the basis of density (lipid content) as very low density, low density, and high density lipoproteins, and are important in lipid transport. Other lipoproteins are important components of membranes.

high-density lipoprotein Any plasma lipoprotein of density in the range 1.06 1– 1.21 g/ml. Such lipoproteins contain about 50% protein, 25% phospholipid, 20% cholesterol, and 5% fat. They are longer lived than lipoproteins of lower density, with half-lives of some days. They originate in both liver and intestine. High concentrations have inverse correlation with cardiovascular disease, and this may be related to their function of cholesterol transport.

low-density lipoprotein   A lipoprotein containing relatively large amounts of cholesterol, average quantities of protein and phospholipid, and little triglyceride. Abbreviation: LDL

plasma lipoprotein   Any of the various complexes of lipid and protein which occur in blood plasma.

very-low-density lipoprotein   Any lipoprotein of the blood plasma of density below 1.006 g/ml. The lipid is about 55% fat, 25% cholesterol and its esters, and 20% phospholipid. Such lipoproteins are formed in both liver and intestinal mucosa, and are responsible for the transport of fat from these tissues. This fat can be converted, for utilization, into fatty acids by lipoprotein lipase.

lipoprotein-X   An abnormal plasma low-density lipoprotein that occurs in obstructive jaundice of any cause.

lipoprotein lipase   The enzyme (EC 3.1.1.34) that catalyzes the hydrolysis of fat to fatty acid and glycerol. It owes its ability to hydrolyze lipoprotein, e.g. very-low-density lipoprotein of the blood, rather than fat in other environments, to its activation by one of the apoproteins of blood lipoprotein. It is bound by glycosaminoglycan to capillary walls, and its action enables cells to obtain fatty acid from blood lipoproteins. Also called *clearing factor*.

lipoproteinosis   LIPOID PROTEINOSIS.

liposarcoma [LIPO- + SARCOMA]   A malignant tumor of adipose tissue. Atypical lipoblasts in varying stages of differentiation are characteristic. It may occur in a variety of sites but especially in soft tissue and retroperitoneum. Its behavior appears to vary with its degree of differentiation. It can be subtyped according to whether the predominant cell pattern is well-differentiated, myxoid (embryonal), round cell, pleomorphic (poorly differentiated), or mixed. Also called *lipoma sarcomatodes, embryonal lipomatosis, adipose sarcoma, lipomatous sarcoma, sarcoma lipomatodes*.

embryonal liposarcoma   MYXOID LIPOSARCOMA.

myxoid liposarcoma   A liposarcoma containing a predominant myxomatous component. Also called *embryonal liposarcoma, lipomyxosarcoma, myxoliposarcoma, myxolipofibrosarcoma*.

liposclerosis   LIPODERMATOSCLEROSIS.

lipose   Any lipase present in blood plasma. Also called *liposin*.

liposin   LIPOSE.

liposis   LIPOMATOSIS.

general liposis   Diffuse fatty infiltration of cells.

liposome   A small vesicular structure which forms spontaneously when phospholipids are placed in water. The phospholipids form bimolecular layers, with the hydrophobic portion of the molecules facing toward the middle of the layer and the hydrophilic portions of the molecules facing outward. The bilipid layers form multiple-layered spheres, the phospholipid bilayers being separated by an aqueous phase.

lipotamponade   Insertion of fatty tissue into the extrapleural space to collapse the lung; a treatment formerly used for pulmonary tuberculosis.

lipoteichoic acid   The type of teichoic acid found in bacterial membranes, as opposed to bacterial walls. It contains a lipid as a terminal part of the molecule. Also called *membrane teichoic acid*.

lipotrophic [LIPO- + -TROPHIC]   Stimulating the formation of fat.

lipotrophy [LIPO- + *troph-* + -Y]   An increase in fat content.

lipotropin   Any hormone that causes release of fatty acid from the fat of adipose tissue. Several pituitary hormones have this effect. Also called *lipotropic hormone, adipokinetic hormone* (older term).

β-lipotropin   A single-chain polypeptide hormone containing 91 amino acids, isolated from the anterior pituitary of several species, including man. It has weak lipolytic, melanophorotropic, and adrenocorticotropic properties, but its principal significance is its function as a prohormone for the endorphins, enkephalins, and melanocyte stimulating hormone.

γ-lipotropin   A single-chain polypeptide hormone containing 58 amino acids, isolated from the anterior pituitary of several species, including sheep and cattle. It has weak lipolytic properties. The physiologic role of the hormone is not yet known.

lipotuberculin   A tuberculin preparation containing in emulsion or solution the fatty component of the tubercle bacillus, *Mycobacterium tuberculosis*.

lipovaccine [LIPO- + VACCINE]   A vaccine prepared by suspending the microorganisms in vegetable oil. Absorption of antigenic material is thereby delayed.

lipovitellin   A lipoprotein of egg yolk.

lipoxenous   Relating to or characterized by lipoxeny.

lipoxeny [Gk *lip(ein)*, 2nd aorist inf. of *leipein* to desert in danger, forsake + *xen(os)* a host, guest + -Y]   The process or phenomenon of desertion of the host by a parasite upon completion of the parasite's development.

lipoxidase   An outmoded term for LIPOXYGENASE.

lipoxygenase   The enzyme (EC 1.13.11.12) that catalyzes the oxidation of linoleate, and of similar substances that contain the grouping $-CH=CH-CH_2-CH=CH-$, with uptake of molecular oxygen, to give the grouping $-CH(-O-OH)-CH=CH-CH=CH-$. Also called *lipoxidase* (outmoded).

lipoxysm [LIP- + OXY-[2] + -(i)sm]   A condition resulting from the ingestion of excessive amounts of fatty acids, such as oleic acid.

lippa [fem. sing. or neut. pl. of L *lippus* having inflamed or watery eyes]   BLEPHARITIS.

Lippes [Jacob *Lippes*, U.S. obstetrician, born 1924]   See under LOOP.

lipping   **1** A bony spur in the juxta-articular area secondary to degenerative arthritis.   **2** A seldom used term for CODMAN'S TRIANGLE.

lippitude [L *lippitud(o)* inflammation in the eyes]   BLEPHARITIS.

lip-print   An impression of the pattern of the ridges, cracks, and wrinkles of the lip surfaces, made by applying ink or other staining material to the lips which are then blotted on a white card or paper. As a method of identification, it has limited application since the lip surfaces change with age and season.

Lipschütz [Benjamin *Lipschütz*, Austrian dermatologist, 1878–1931]   **1** Lipschütz ulcer. See under DISEASE.   **2** Lipschütz bodies. See under BODY.

lipsis animi   SYNCOPE.

lipsotrichia [Gk *leips(is)* a leaving, omitting, want + *o* + TRICH- + -IA]   A loss of hair. An obsolete term. Also called *leipotrichia*, (obsolete), *trichomadesis* (seldom used).

lipuria   LIPIDURIA.

liq.   *liquor* (L, liquid).

liq dr   Symbol for the unit, liquid dram.

liq oz   Symbol for the unit, liquid ounce.

liq pt   Symbol for the unit, liquid pint.

liq qt   Symbol for the unit, liquid quart.

Liquaemin   64 sodium heparin.

Liquamar   A proprietary name for phenprocoumon.

liquefacient   1 Causing liquefaction.   **2** A substance that can bring about liquefaction.

liquefaction [Late L *liquefactio* (from L *liquefactus*, past part. of *liquefacere* to make fluid, from *liquere* to be fluid + *facere* to make) a making fluid]   The process of becoming or making liquid, often due to hydrolysis of structural macromolecules.

liquid [L *liquidus* (from *liquere* to be liquid, to be clear, akin to *lacus* a lake, *lacrima* a tear; Gk *lakkos* a hollow, pit, cistern, pond) liquid, fluid, clear, pure]   **1** Flowing or capable of flowing.   **2** A liquid substance consisting of molecules that lack the tendency to separate indefinitely; a substance that is neither a solid nor a gas.

Altmann's liquid   ALTMANN'S FLUID.

blistering liquid   LIQUOR EPISPASTICUS.

Cotunnius liquid   An obsolete term for PERILYMPHA.

Declat's liquid   A solution of carbolate of ammonia formerly used externally and internally in cases of cholera.

Flemming's liquid   FLEMMING'S FIXING FLUID.

Heidenhain's liquid   SUSA FIXATIVE.

Marchi's liquid   A solution of osmium tetroxide and potassium chlorate in acetic formaldehyde that is used in Marchi's method.

Pasteur's liquid   PASTEUR'S FLUID.

Scarpa's liquid   An outmoded term for ENDOLYMPHA.

Thoma's liquid   THOMA'S FLUID.

liquiform   Having the properties of a liquid.

liquogel   A gel whose liquified sol phase is of low viscosity.

liquor [L (from *liquere* to be liquid, to be clear, akin to *lacus* a lake, *lacrima* a tear; Gk *lakkos* a hollow, pit, cistern, pond), liquidity, fluidity, a liquid, fluid, liquor]   **1** A liquid or fluid.   **2** In anatomy, a fluid secretion that is produced by certain tissues, such as the antrum of an ovarian follicle and the choroid plexus of the brain. It is usually nutritive.   **3** In pharmacy, an aqueous solution of any nonvolatile substance, or an aqueous solution of a gas.

liquor amaranthi   AMARANTH SOLUTION.

liquor ammoniae dilutus   DILUTED AMMONIA SOLUTION.

liquor ammoniae fortis   STRONG AMMONIA SOLUTION.

liquor ammonii anisatus   An alcoholic solution containing ammonia and anise oil.

liquor amnii   AMNIOTIC FLUID.

liquor calcii hydroxidi   LIME WATER.

liquor calcis   LIME WATER.

liquor carbonis detergens   A liquid preparation containing coal tar in a soap solution.

liquor cerebrospinalis   [NA] A clear, colorless fluid that circulates within the four ventricles of the brain and the subarachnoid spaces surrounding the brain and spinal cord. An ultrafiltrate of the blood secreted by the choroid plexus in the lateral third and fourth ventricles, it is largely resorbed into the venous system via the arachnoid villi. Also called *cerebrospinal fluid, neurolymph* (seldom used).

liquor chloridorum trium isotonicus   RINGER SOLUTION.

liquor chorii   Fluid present in the early embryo within the confines of the chorion but outside the developing embryo and amniotic cavity.

liquor corneae   Fluid within the corneal lamellae.

liquor cotunnii   An obsolete term for PERILYMPHA.

liquor entericus   INTESTINAL JUICE.

liquor epispasticus   A solution containing cantharidin in a mixture of acetone, castor oil, and colophony. Also called *blistering liquid.*

liquor folliculi   FOLLICULAR FLUID.

liquor formaldehydi   FORMALDEHYDE SOLUTION.

liquor gastricus   GASTRIC JUICE.

liquor hepatis   A solution prepared from fresh liver.

liquor hydrogenii peroxidi   HYDROGEN PEROXIDE SOLUTION.

liquor iodi fortis   STRONG IODINE SOLUTION.

Morgagni's liquor   Fluid within a hypermature cataract.

mother liquor   The liquid that remains after a substance has crystallized from it.

liquor pancreaticus   PANCREATIC JUICE.

liquor pericardii   PERICARDIAL FLUID.

liquor pituitarii posterii   POSTERIOR PITUITARY INJECTION.

liquor plumbi subacetatis dilutus   DILUTED LEAD SUBACETATE SOLUTION.

liquor plumbi subacetatis fortis   Strong lead acetate solution.

liquor potassii hydroxidi   A solution of potassium hydroxide.

liquor prostaticus   SUCCUS PROSTATICUS.

liquor puris   The fluid, cell-free component of pus. An obsolete term.

liquor sanguinis   PLASMA.

liquor of Scarpa   ENDOLYMPHA.

liquor scarpae   An obsolete term for ENDOLYMPHA.

liquor seminis   The fluid component of semen.

liquor sodii chloridi isotonicus   A 0.9% solution of sodium chloride, which is isotonic with blood.

liquores   Plural of LIQUOR.

liquorice   GLYCYRRHIZA.

liquorrhea [*liquo(r)* + -RRHEA]   The excessive discharge of an otherwise normal secretion, for example, nasal mucus. A seldom used term.

Lisfranc [Jacques *Lisfranc*, French surgeon, 1790–1847]   **1** Lisfranc's joints. See under ARTICULATIONES TARSOMETATARSALES.   **2** See under DISLOCATION, LIGAMENT, FRACTURE.   **3** Lisfranc's operation. See under AMPUTATION.   **4** Lisfranc's tubercle, tuberculum scalenis lisfranci. See under TUBERCULUM MUSCULI SCALENI ANTERIORIS.

lisp [Middle English *lysp(en)*, *wlisp(en)* to lisp, from Old English *-wlispian*, from *wlisp*, *wlips* a lisping]   **1** Defective production of the sibilant sounds of speech such as *s* and *z*, which tend to be replaced by *th* sounds, with a tendency for the tongue tip to protrude past the upper central teeth.   **2** To speak with a lisp.

Lissauer [Heinrich *Lissauer*, German neurologist, 1861–1891]   **1** Lissauer's paralysis. See under LISSAUER TYPE OF GENERAL PARESIS(at *paresis*).   **2** Column of Lissauer, Lissauer's marginal zone, column of Spitzka-Lissauer. See under TRACTUS DORSOLATERALIS.

Lissencephala [Gk *liss(os)* smooth + New L *encephala*, pl. of *encephalon*, irreg. from Gk *enkephalos* the brain]   A group of placental mammals characterized by a cerebral cortex having few, if any, convolutions. Adjective: lissencephalic.

lissencephalia [Gk *liss(os)* smooth + ENCEPHAL- + -IA]   AGYRIA.

lissencephalic [Gk *liss(os)* smooth + ENCEPHAL- + -IC]   AGYRIC.

lissencephaly [Gk *liss(os)* smooth + ENCEPHAL- + -Y]   AGYRIA.

Lisser [Hans *Lisser*, U.S. physician, born 1888]   Escamilla-Lisser syndrome. See under SYNDROME.

lissive [Gk *liss(os)* smooth + -IVE]   Having the property of relieving muscle spasm.

list   A lateral deviation of the trunk.

listening / dichotic listening   An experimental procedure in which different stimuli or different messages are simultaneously presented to two ears as a means of examining selective attention.

Lister [Joseph *Lister*, English surgeon, 1827–1912]   **1** See under DRESSING.   **2** Lister's method. See under LISTERISM.   **3** Lister's tubercle. See under TUBERCULUM DORSALE RADII.

listerellosis LISTERIOSIS.

Listeria monocytogenes A small, Gram-positive, motile, aerobic to microaerophilic, asporogenous rod, tending to grow in chains, palisades, or filaments and easily mistaken for a diphtheroid. Several O and H antigenic types are recognized. It is a parasite in many vertebrates and invertebrates and is also found in soil and in rotting vegetation. In humans it most often causes a purulent meningitis (especially in debilitated patients), or intrauterine or perinatal infection.

listeriosis [*Listeri(a)* + -OSIS] Infection by *Listeria moncytogenes* in various animal species and birds. It is most common in adult ruminants and is characterized by encephalitis of the brainstem. Walking in circles is a frequent sign. Abortion and neonatal disease also occur but as a distinct and separate manifestation. In poultry and other animals, such as the dog, cat, pig, and rabbit, septicemia with focal liver necrosis is usual. The organism is transmissible to man by contact with infected tissues or fluids. Also called *listerellosis, circling disease.*

listerism [after Baron Joseph *Lister*, English surgeon, 1827–1912 + -ISM] The practice and procedures of aseptic and antiseptic surgery, developed originally by Joseph Lister. Also called *Lister's method.*

Listing [Johann Benedikt *Listing*, German physicist, 1808–1882] See under LAW, PLANE, EYE.

Liston [Robert *Liston*, English surgeon, 1794–1847] **1** See under OPERATION, KNIFE. **2** Liston scissors. See under SHEARS.

liter [French *litre* (from *litron* former measure of capacity containing a sixteenth of a bushel, irreg. from Med L and Gk *litra* a pound of twelve ounces) a liter, liter measure] A unit of volume or capacity equal to 10^3 cubic centimeters or 10^{-3} cubic meter: used in conjunction with SI units. A liter is equivalent to 1.0567 liquid quarts or 33.814 (US) fluid ounces. Also *litre.* Symbol: l, L ● In Great Britain and in international usage, the spelling *litre* is preferred, but in the United States *liter* is the usual spelling. The symbol l is preferred over L except in those instances where it might be confused with the numeral 1.
    liter per centimeter of water A unit of compliance and dynamic compliance equal to $1.019\ 72 \times 10^{-3}$ meter cubed per pascal: used especially in connection with respiratory ducts. Symbol: l/cmH₂O

liter-atmosphere A unit of energy equal to a volume of one cubic decimeter times a pressure of one standard atmosphere; 101.325 joules. Symbol: l·atm

lith- LITHO-.

-lith [Gk *lithos* stone] A combining form meaning (1) stone; (2) calculus.

lithaemia A British spelling for LITHEMIA.

lithagogectasia LITHECTASY.

lithagogue Any remedy that enhances the removal of concretions or calculi.

lithangiuria [LITH- + ANGI- + -URIA] The presence of calculi in the urinary tract.

lithecbole [LITH- + Gk *ekbolē* a throwing out, thrusting out, discharging] Passage of a calculus. A rarely used term.

lithectasy [LITH- + *ectas(ia)* + -Y] A surgical procedure in which a renal stone is extracted with a specially designed instrument through a surgically dilated urethra. Also called *lithagogectasia.*

lithectomy A seldom used term for LITHOTOMY.

lithemia [LITH- + -EMIA] HYPERURICEMIA.

lithemic Relating to, resulting from, or characterized by hyperuricemia.

lithiasis [LITH- + -IASIS] The development of calculi, usually in the gallbladder and kidneys. Formation of such calculi usually results from increased concentration in the bile or urine of substances contained within the stone, as well as favorable local physicochemical conditions. Also called *calculosis.* Adjective: lithiasic.
    appendicular lithiasis The formation of calcareous fecal concretions within the lumen of the vermiform appendix. A rarely used term.
    biliary lithiasis Gallstone formation in the gallbladder or biliary drainage system.
    lithiasis conjunctivae Calcifications of the conjunctival crypts.
    intestinal lithiasis The presence of calculi or concretions in the intestinal tract.
    pancreatic lithiasis The presence of concretions in the pancreas.
    renal lithiasis NEPHROLITHIASIS.

lithic Pertaining to calculi.

lithicosis PNEUMOCONIOSIS.

lithium Element number 3, having atomic weight 6.941. It is the lightest of all metals, with specific gravity 0.534. The first member of the alkali series, it is never found free in nature. There are numerous industrial applications and some pharmaceutical uses for the element. It does not appear to be essential to any organism. Symbol: Li

lithium antimoniothiomalate ANTHIOLIMINE.

lithium caffeine sulfonate A medication formerly used for the treatment of gout and rheumatism and as a diuretic. It has been replaced by more effective analgesics which do not contain the potentially toxic lithium ions.

lithium carbonate Li_2CO_3. A white, granular powder used as a source of lithium ions in the treatment of mania and the prophylaxis of manic depression and depression. Lithium ions compete with sodium ions, but the mechanism of its beneficial effects in depression is not known.

lithium salicylate A salt of salicylic acid with properties like those of sodium salicylate. It has been used in rheumatism and gout, but the preparation is not an optimal form of salicylate treatment because of the potential toxicologic effects of the lithium ion.

litho- [Gk *lithos* stone] A combining form meaning (1) stone; (2) calculus. Also *lith-.*

Lithobius A common genus of centipedes. They are characterized by 15 pairs of legs.

lithocenosis LITHOLAPAXY.

lithocholic acid 3α-Hydroxy-5β-cholanic acid. It is found in small amounts in mammalian bile, conjugated with glycine and taurine.

lithoclast LITHOTRITE.

lithoclasty LITHOLAPAXY.

lithoclysmia [LITHO- + Gk *klysm(os)* a washing out, esp. by a clyster + -IA] The instillation into the urinary bladder of single or multiple liquid agents to effect dissolution of stones. Also called *lithodialysis.*

lithoconion LITHOTRITE.

lithocystotomy A surgical procedure in which solitary or multiple stones are removed from the bladder through an incision and under direct vision.

lithodialysis LITHOCLYSMIA.

lithodialytic **1** Acting to dissolve or break up stones. **2** A liquid agent designed to be instilled into a body cavity, usually the urinary bladder, for the purpose of dissolving stones.

lithogenesis The formation of a calculus.

lithogenous [LITHO- + -GENOUS] Causing or capable of causing calculus formation.

lithoid Like a stone.

lithokelyphopedion A lithopedion with calcified membranes surrounding it.

lithokelyphos [LITHO- + Gk *kelyphos* a husk, shell] A retained fetus about which the fetal membranes have calcified.

lithokonion LITHOTRITE.

litholabe [LITHO- + Gk *labē* a grip, handle] A surgical instrument designed to hold a bladder calculus in order to aid in its removal or fragmentation.

litholapaxy [LITHO- + Gk *lapax(is)* (from *lapassein* to empty, evacuate) an emptying, evacuation + -Y] A surgical procedure consisting of crushing a stone or stones within the urinary system and immediately irrigating to remove the fragments. Also called *lithoclasty, lithotripsy, lithotrity, Civiale's operation, lithocenosis.*
Bigelow's litholapaxy A litholapaxy using a Bigelow lithotrite. Also called *Bigelow's operation.*

lithology [LITHO- + -LOGY] The science of the formation, effects, and treatment of calculi.

litholysis [LITHO- + LYSIS] Fragmentation or dissolution of stones in the urinary bladder.

litholyte An instrument designed to administer stone-dissolving agents directly inside the bladder.

litholytic Stone-dissolving; tending to dissolve calculi, especially in the bladder.

lithomyl LITHOTRITE.

lithonephria [LITHO- + NEPHR- + -IA] Any renal disease due to or related to calculi.

lithonephrotomy NEPHROLITHOTOMY.

lithontriptic LITHOTRIPTIC.

lithopaedion A British spelling for LITHOPEDION.

lithopedion [LITHO- + Gk *paidion* a young child, dim. of *pais* a child] A retained fetus, whether extrauterine or intrauterine, which has undergone calcification. Also called *calcified fetus, mummified fetus, stone child, osteopedion, lithopedium.*

lithopedium LITHOPEDION.

lithophagous [LITHO- + -PHAGOUS] **1** Eating gravel or pebbles, as certain birds. **2** Burrowing in rock, as some mollusks and echinoderms.

lithophone [LITHO- + Gk *phōnē* sound, voice] A device for detecting calculi by reflection of emitted sound, forerunner of current ultrasonic diagnostic devices.

lithoscope [LITHO- + -SCOPE] An instrument used for visual examination of calculi in the urinary bladder.

lithosis PNEUMOCONIOSIS.

lithosphere [LITHO- + SPHERE] The solid portion of the surface of earth. Also called *petrosphere.*

lithotome [LITHO- + -TOME] A knife specifically designed to perform lithotomies.

lithotomist A surgeon or other physician who removes stones, particularly from the bladder.

lithotomy [LITHO- + -TOMY] An incision into a duct or organ for the purpose of removing stones. Also called *lithectomy* (seldom used).
bilateral lithotomy A lithotomy in which a long, transverse perineal incision is made for the purpose of removing stones.
high lithotomy SUPRAPUBIC LITHOTOMY.
lateral lithotomy A lithotomy to remove urinary bladder stones employing an incision in the perineum immediately lateral to the raphe perinei. Also called *sectio lateralis.*
marian lithotomy MEDIAN LITHOTOMY.
median lithotomy A surgical incision into the raphe perinei for the purpose of removing bladder stones. Also called *marian lithotomy, prerectal lithotomy, Allarton's operation, sectio mediana.*

mediolateral lithotomy Any combination of incisions on or immediately lateral to the raphe perinei for the purpose of stone removal.
perineal lithotomy Any surgical incision into the perineum for the purpose of stone removal. Also called *celsian operation.*
prerectal lithotomy MEDIAN LITHOTOMY.
rectal lithotomy A surgical incision made within a dilated rectum for the purpose of retrieving bladder stones. Also called *rectovesical lithotomy.*
rectovesical lithotomy RECTAL LITHOTOMY.
suprapubic lithotomy The removal of a bladder calculus by an incision above the pubis.
vaginal lithotomy A surgical incision made through the vagina into the bladder for the purpose of stone removal. Also called *vesicovaginal lithotomy.*
vesicovaginal lithotomy VAGINAL LITHOTOMY.

lithotony [LITHO- + *ton(o)*- + -Y] A surgical procedure in which a bladder fistula is created for the purpose of urinary stone removal.

lithotresis [LITHO- + Gk *trēsis* a perforation] A surgical procedure in which holes are drilled into a calculus to facilitate its removal.
ultrasonic lithotresis A procedure in which ultrasonic waves are used to facilitate the removal of urinary stones.

lithotripsy [LITHO- + -TRIPSY] LITHOLAPAXY.
electrohydraulic lithotripsy The breaking up of kidney stones by using an electric discharge directly to the stone.
extracorporeal shock-wave lithotripsy Lithotripsy utilizing shock waves in a water-filled tub to pulverize kidney stones in a patient partially submerged in the tub. Surgery is avoided if the fragments pass spontaneously. The device utilizing this technique is usually called an extracorporeal shock-wave lithotriptor.

lithotriptic **1** Of or relating to lithotripsy. Also *lithontriptic.* **2** A device utilizing shock waves to break up kidney stones without surgical intervention.

lithotriptor LITHOTRITE.
extracorporeal shock-wave lithotriptor See under EXTRACORPOREAL SHOCK-WAVE LITHOTRIPSY.

lithotriptoscope A surgical instrument which is used to pulverize a bladder calculus under direct vision. Also called *cystoscopic lithotrite.*

lithotriptoscopy A surgical procedure in which bladder stones are crushed and flushed out under direct vision.

lithotrite [LITHO- + L *tritus*, past part. of *terere* to rub, wear away; Gk *teirein* to rub, rub away, wear away and *tribein* to rub, grind down] A surgical instrument designed to crush or to fragment stones and thereby facilitate spontaneous or operative removal. Also called *lithoclast, lithokonion, lithoconion, lithomyl, lithotriptor, brise-pierre* (obsolete).
Bigelow's lithotrite A surgical instrument designed to crush urinary bladder stones.
cystoscopic lithotrite LITHOTRIPTOSCOPE.
electrohydraulic lithotrite A flexible electrode placed next to a urinary calculus to fracture it into smaller pieces by applying a high-voltage spark.

lithotrity [LITHO- + L *trit(us)*, past part. of *terere* to rub + -Y] LITHOLAPAXY.

lithotroph [LITHO- + Gk *troph(ē)* nourishment] Any organism able to utilize inorganic compounds, such as hydrogen sulfide or Fe^{2+}, as an energy source. Adjective: lithotrophic.

lithous [LITH- + -OUS] Pertaining to or having the properties of a calculus.

lithoxiduria The occurrence of oxalate stones in the urine.

lithuresis [LITH- + URESIS] **1** Excess urinary excretion of uric acid. **2** The passage, usually painless, of tiny calculi (gravel) during urination.

lithureteria [LITH- + URETERIA] Calculi formation in the ureter.

litmus [Old Norse *litmose* (from *litr* color + *mosi* moss) a lichen used in dyeing] A natural pigment, obtained from lichens whose major principle is azolitmin. It is used primarily in paper strips as a pH indicator, being red at an acid pH below 4.5 and blue at an alkaline pH above 8.3. Also called *turnsol, lacmus.*

litrameter [Gk *litra* a pound of twelve ounces + -METER] An instrument for determining the specific gravity of liquids.

litre LITER.

Litten [Moritz *Litten*, German physician, 1845–1907] Litten's diaphragm phenomenon, Litten sign. See under DIAPHRAGM PHENOMENON.

litter [Middle English *litere*, from Old French *litiere* litter, from Med L *literia*, also *lectaria* litter, from L *lectus* bed] **1** A stretcher, cot, or bed adapted for transporting a sick or injured person. **2** The group of offspring that a multiparous mammal bears at one time. **3** The layer of decaying leaves and other organic debris that forms on the floor of a forest.

Little [Sir Ernest Gordon Graham *Little*, English physician, 1867–1950] Piccardi-Lassueur-Graham Little syndrome. See under LASSUEUR-LITTLE SYNDROME.

Little [James Lawrence *Little*, U.S. physician, 1836–1885] Little's area. See under KIESSELBACH'S AREA.

Little [William John *Little*, English surgeon, 1810–1894] **1** See under DISEASE. **2** Little's paralysis. See under ACUTE ANTERIOR POLIOMYELITIS.

Littoridina A genus of hydrobiid snails closely related to the genus *Amnicola.*

Littorina A genus of littoral water snails in the periwinkle family of prosobranch gastropods, the Littorinidae. They are heavy-shelled, imperforate, strongly conical snails with a pointed spire and horny operculum. Many are intermediate hosts of trematode parasites of shorebirds and other aquatic birds. Common species include *L. planaxis* of the western United States, *L. irrorata,* in brackish marshes of the eastern United States, *L. pintado* in Hawaii, *L. saxatalis* in eastern United States, and *L. littorea,* commonest Atlantic coast and northern European species.

Littorina planaxis The flat periwinkle, or eroded periwinkle, found on the west coast of the United States. It is the intermediate host of the bird schistome fluke, *Austrobilharzia variglandis,* an agent of cercarial dermatitis in humans.

Littorina saxatilis A species of snail that occurs along the Atlantic shore of the United States. It is an intermediate host of the New England gull echinostome *Himasthla littorinae.*

Littre [Alexis *Littre*, French anatomist, 1658–1726] **1** See under OPERATION, SPACE. **2** Littre's crypts, Littre's glands. See under GLANDULAE PREPUTIALES. **3** Littre's crypts, glandulae urethrales littrei, Littre's glands. See under GLANDULAE URETHRALES URETHRAE MASCULINAE. **4** Glandular foramina of Littre. See under FORAMEN.

littritis [after Alexis *Littre*, French anatomist and physician, 1658–1726 + -ITIS] Inflammation of Littre's glands, manifesting itself as an abscess which can open under the skin or in the urethra and result, in men, in a fistula of the urethra.

Litzmann [Karl Konrad Theodor *Litzmann*, German gynecologist, 1815–1890] Litzmann's obliquity. See under POSTERIOR ASYNCLITISM.

live [short for *alive*] **1** ALIVE. **2** Reverberant, as a room which has an unusually small amount of sound absorption.

live-born An infant that is born alive, in contradistinction to one that is stillborn.

livedo [L (from *livere* to be blue or bluish), lividness] A discoloration or erythema of the skin that follows the reticulate pattern of the cutaneous vascular network. Also called *suggillation* (obsolete).

livedo annularis LIVEDO RETICULARIS.

livedo calorica Livedo reticularis due to heat.

livedo frigore Livedo reticularis aggravated by cold.

inflammatory livedo A mottling of the skin of inflammatory origin.

livedo racemosa LIVEDO RETICULARIS.

livedo reticularis A mottled bluish or livid discoloration of the skin in a network pattern, an accentuation of the normal vascular pattern of the skin, with dilatation of the capillaries and small venules. It is a benign condition that may be due to either arterial and arteriolar constriction of diverse causation, aggravated by cold, or to external heat which selectively damages the dark part of the network with its more precarious blood supply. Also called *livedo annularis, livedo racemosa, asphyxia reticularis.*

livedo telangiectatica Livedo reticularis in which the small vessel dilatation is gross enough to cause visible telangiectases.

livedoid [*lived(o)* + -OID] **1** Resembling livedo. **2** Of or relating to livedo.

liver [Old English *lifer*] A large gland located in the upper right quadrant of the abdomen immediately beneath the diaphragm; hepar. As an exocrine gland it secretes bile. Its other major functions are the synthesis of plasma proteins, heparin, fibrinogen, and prothrombin; the destruction of red cells; detoxification; the metabolism of proteins, carbohydrates, and fats; and the storage of glycogen and other important substances. For a further discussion of the anatomy of the liver, see *hepar.*

albuminoid liver AMYLOID LIVER.

amyloid liver A liver infiltrated with amyloid. The liver becomes enlarged and appears pale gray and waxy. Microscopically, the deposits appear as an amorphous, eosinophilic substance deposited primarily in the space of Disse, between the hepatocytes and the sinusoidal endothelial cells. The continued accumulation of amyloid results in progressive atrophy of liver cells. Also called *albuminoid liver, lardaceous liver, sago liver, waxy liver.*

beavertail liver A liver with a large flat left lobe.

biliary cirrhotic liver A cirrhotic liver resulting from disease of the biliary tract. It is characteristically deeply bile-stained and nodular, and it may be caused by obstruction due to cancer or stone or by autoimmune damage to the small intrahepatic bile ducts, as in primary biliary cirrhosis.

brimstone liver The enlarged, bright yellow liver often seen in an individual with congenital syphilis or fulminant hepatitis.

bronze liver A liver that is bronze colored due to deposits of malarial pigment, mainly within Kupfer cells.

cirrhotic liver A liver affected by cirrhosis, a characteristic nodular transformation and scarring of the hepatic parenchyma. Externally, the normally smooth capsule shows multiple nodular protuberances which gives it the so-called hobnail appearance. Cirrhotic nodules range from 2 to 10 mm in diameter. Although not infrequently cirrhotic livers are of cryptogenic origin, alcoholism and viral hepatitis are common etiologies. Also called *hobnail liver, gin-drinkers' liver.*

desiccated liver Dried powder prepared from whole mammalian livers. It is a good source of riboflavin, nicotinic acid, choline, vitamin B_{12}, and iron, hence it is used as a nutritional supplement and is sometimes given in the treatment of macrocytic anemia.

fatty liver A liver with increased amounts of neutral fat in the cytoplasms of hepatocytes. This change results in a yellow, soft, and greasy liver. Microscopically, cytoplasmic fat vacuoles distend the hepatocyes. Although this condition may be caused by several systemic disorders such as diabetes mellitus, the most common cause is alcoholism. Also called *hepar adiposum*.

fatty liver of Brahmin children   An Indian term for KWASHI-ORKOR.

foamy liver   A putrefying liver commonly found in decomposing bodies and filled with variously sized gaseous cysts imparting a foamy or bubbly appearance to the capsular and cut surfaces. The cysts are formed by the putrefactive action of anaerobic bacilli, particularly *Clostridia* species.

frosted liver   A liver with hyaline thickening of its capsule, resulting in a white appearance that resembles cake icing. This is a non-specific and functionally unimportant change that is probably due to the organization of proteinaceous peritoneal exudates on the liver capsule. Also called *Curschmann's disease* (obsolete), *sugar-icing liver, sugar-frosting liver, icing liver, perihepatitis chronica hyperplastica*.

gin-drinkers' liver   CIRRHOTIC LIVER.

hobnail liver   CIRRHOTIC LIVER.

icing liver   FROSTED LIVER.

iron liver   A liver loaded with hemosiderin deposits. It is grossly chocolate brown and microscopically the pigment is found within hepatocytes, Kupfer cells, bile duct epithelium, and scar tissue. It may be caused by any disorder that results in excess iron in the body, such as hemolytic disorders, multiple transfusions, and hemochromatosis.

lardaceous liver   AMYLOID LIVER.

nutmeg liver   A liver affected by chronic vascular congestion that produces a characteristic alternating pattern of dark red centrilobular areas and paler peripheral lobular regions. This color pattern is reminiscent of the spice nutmeg. The condition is caused most often by right-sided heart failure. Also called *stasis liver*.

pigmented liver   A liver containing deposits of pigment, such as hemosiderin or malarial pigment.

polycystic liver   A liver affected with multiple congenital cysts, most often subcapsular in location. These cysts do not impair hepatic function. The condition is probably the result of defective formation of bile ducts, and may be associated with polycystic kidneys of the adult type.

sago liver   AMYLOID LIVER.

stasis liver   NUTMEG LIVER.

sugar-frosting liver   FROSTED LIVER.

sugar-icing liver   FROSTED LIVER.

syphilitic liver   The characteristic, contracted, nodular liver seen in chronic syphilitic hepatitis.

typhoid liver   A form of hepatitis that is seen in typhoid fever and characterized by intralobular collections of mononuclear cells.

waxy liver   AMYLOID LIVER.

liverwort [LIVER + *wort*, Old English *wyrt* plant, herb, root]   Any member of the class Hepaticae. They are generally less conspicuous than mosses, which comprise the class Musci, and which form the other member of the division Bryophyta.

American liverwort   *Hepatica nobilis*, an herb once held to be beneficial in treating ailments of the liver, a belief based on the doctrine of signatures. Also called *liver leaf*.

livid [L *livid(us)* leaden in color, bluish, black and blue]   Bluish black or deep purplish red, as a bruise; black-and-blue.

lividity [LIVID + -ITY]   **1** A black and blue discoloration of the skin, such as that caused by a contusion.   **2** A leaden or ashen hue, as occurring in cyanosis. Also called *livor*.

cadaveric lividity   LIVOR MORTIS.

postmortem lividity   LIVOR MORTIS.

Livierato [Panagino *Livierato*, Italian physician, 1860–1936]   See under SIGN.

livor [L, a bluish color, lividness, a blue or livid spot]   **1** LIVIDITY.   **2** LIVOR MORTIS.

livor mortis   The reddish blue to purple postmortem discoloration of the dependent, noncompressed skin surfaces, caused by the gravitational accumulation of reduced hemoglobin containing erythrocytes in subcutaneous capillaries. It begins forming immediately after death and is usually perceptible within two hours following the cessation of circulation. It is fully established after four hours but is absent in those areas where pressure, exerted by body weight on the supporting surface, compresses the capillary bed. Within 8 to 12 hours livor mortis becomes fixed, i.e., no blanching occurs when the skin surface is pressed. The fixation is caused by capillary obstruction, due to postmortem blood clotting, and by capillary constriction due to congealed adipose tissue. Therefore, finding fixed nondependent livor mortis may indicate that a body was moved following death. Also called *postmortem lividity, cadaveric lividity, livor*.

lixiviation [Late L *lixivi(um)* (from neut. sing. of L *lixivius* made into lye, from *lix* lye) a solution made by leaching + -ATION]   LEACHING.

lizard [Middle English *lesard*, from Old French *lesard* lizard, from L *lacerta*, also *lacertus* lizard, newt]   Any of the reptiles of the suborder Sauria.

LLL   left lower lobe (of lung).

Lloyd [Putnam C. *Lloyd*, U.S. physician, flourished early 20th century]   Lloyd syndrome. See under MULTIPLE ENDOCRINE NEOPLASIA.

Lloyd Morgan [Conway *Lloyd Morgan*, English zoologist and psychologist, 1852–1936]   See under CANON.

LLQ   left lower quadrant (of abdomen).

LM   **1** linguomesial.   **2** light minimum.

lm   Symbol for the unit, lumen.

LMA   left mentoanterior position (of a fetus). See under MENTUM ANTERIOR POSITION.

LMF   lymphocyte mitogenic factor.

lm/ft²   Symbol for the unit, lumen per square foot.

lm·ft⁻²   Symbol for the unit, lumen per square foot.

lm·h   Symbol for the unit, lumen-hour.

lm/m²   Symbol for the unit, lumen per square meter.

lm·m⁻²   Symbol for the unit, lumen per square meter.

LMP   left mentoposterior position (of a fetus). See under MENTUM POSTERIOR POSITION.

lm·s   Symbol for the unit, lumen-second.

LMT   left mentotransverse position (of a fetus). See under MENTUM TRANSVERSE POSITION.

lm/W   Symbol for the unit, lumen per watt.

lm·W⁻¹   Symbol for the unit, lumen per watt.

ln   natural logarithm.

LNPF   lymph node permeability factor.

LOA   left occipitoanterior position (of a fetus). See under OCCIPUT ANTERIOR POSITION.

Loa   A genus of filarial nematodes (family Onchocercidae) transmitted by blood-sucking flies. The adult nematodes wander in the subdermal spaces and the microfilariae are found in the bloodstream.

Loa loa   A filarial worm, the African eye worm, found in western equatorial Africa, and the etiologic agent of loiasis. Males average 25–35 mm long, females 50–60 mm. The sheathed microfilariae, which have nuclei that extend to the tip of the tail, can be found in peripheral blood primarily during the day, unlike *Wuchereria bancrofti*. Humans are the only known definitive hosts, with tabanid flies (genus *Chrysops*) serving as vectors. Infective larvae require from three years to mature following transmission, and the adults may live as long as 17 years in the subcutaneous connective tissues. Moving freely, they can sometimes be observed wriggling across the eye under the conjuctiva, hence the name eye worm. They are also responsible for Calabar swellings. Also called *Filaria diurna, Filaria extraocularis, Filaria lentis, Filaria loa, Filaria oculihumani.*

load [Old English *lād*] **1** The deviation from normal body content, as of salt, heat, or water. **2** The mechanical force, energy, or power a subject must expend during a stress test. **3** The impedance seen by the output of an electronic generator such as a pacemaker or defibrillator. **4** To enter data into the memory of a computer.

filtered load The amount of a substance that appears in the glomerular urinary space via filtration across the glomerular capillary wall per unit time. The load is calculated by multiplying the glomerular filtration rate by the concentration of the substance in glomerular filtrate.

genetic load **1** The reduction in health, longevity, or fitness of an individual or a population because of deleterious genes. Also called *mutational load.* **2** A formal genetic concept, developed by H.J. Muller in 1950. It specifies for any locus the proportion by which the genetic fitness of the individual or population is reduced because of deleterious alleles, when compared to the optimal genotype.

mutational load GENETIC LOAD.

occlusal load The total force on the teeth during mastication.

loader A computer program for loading other programs.

loading **1** The administration of a substance either in a quantity sufficient to saturate binding sites in the body or as a prelude to maintaining a constant plasma concentration. It facilitates measurement of the rate of metabolism or excretion of the substance. **2** An amount added to an insurance premium calculation to account for administrative costs.

loaiasis LOIASIS.

lobar Relating to or involving a lobe.

lobate Provided with or arranged in lobes. Also *lobose, lobous.*

lobation **1** The formation of lobes. **2** A lobe or lobate structure.

fetal lobation FETAL LOBULATION.

persistent lobation FETAL LOBULATION.

lobe [New L *lobus.* See LOBUS.] **1** A rounded projection or subdivision of an organ or structure demarcated by fissures, sulci, constrictions, or connective tissue septa; lobus. **2** A cusp on the crown of a tooth. An outmoded usage.

ansiform lobe That portion of the cerebellar hemisphere lying between the posterior superior fissure anteriorly and the gracile lobule posteriorly. The horizontal fissure divides it into the superior and inferior semilunar lobules (crus I and crus II, respectively).

anterior lobe of hypophysis ADENOHYPOPHYSIS.

anterior lobe of pituitary gland ADENOHYPOPHYSIS.

appendicular lobe A tongue-shaped downward extension of the right lobe of the liver. Also called *linguiform lobe, Riedel's lobe, lobus appendicularis, lobus linguiformis.*

azygos lobe A small accessory lobe at the apex of the right lung, marked off by a groove made by the azygos vein.

caudate lobe of cerebrum An obsolete term for INSULA.

caudate lobe of liver LOBUS CAUDATUS HEPATIS.

lobes of cerebrum LOBI CEREBRI.

cuneate lobe CUNEUS.

cuneiform lobe LOBULUS CUNEIFORMIS.

developmental lobe A protuberance on the crown of a developing tooth which is an independent center of initiation of enamel and dentin.

digastric lobe LOBULUS BIVENTER.

falciform lobe An outmoded term for LIMBIC LOBE.

flocculonodular lobe The smallest and phylogenetically old-

est division of the cerebellum, made up of a midline nodulus and two stalklike flocculi located on the posterior and ventral surface of the remainder of the cerebellum, from which it is almost entirely separated by the posterolateral fissure. It is functionally related to the vestibular nerve and nuclei. Also called *archicerebellum, flocculonodular complex.*

frontal lobe LOBUS FRONTALIS.

grand lobe limbique of Broca LIMBIC LOBE.

hepatic lobes LOBI HEPATIS.

Home's lobe SUBTRIGONAL GLAND.

inferior crescentic lobe of cerebellum An outmoded term for LOBULUS SEMILUNARIS INFERIOR.

inferior lobe of lung LOBUS INFERIOR PULMONIS.

inferior semilunar lobe LOBULUS SEMILUNARIS INFERIOR.

lateral lobes of prostate gland LOBUS PROSTATAE DEXTER ET SINISTER.

left lobe of liver LOBUS HEPATIS SINISTER.

limbic lobe The part of the brain situated on the medial surface of the hemisphere, surrounding the rostral brainstem and the interhemispheric commissures, and including the subcallosal, cingulate, and parahippocampal gyri, as well as the underlying hippocampal formation and dentate gyrus. It comprises the phylogenetically oldest portions of the cerebral cortex, and has maintained a remarkable constancy of gross and microscopic organization during the course of phylogeny. Also called *gyrus fornicatus, grand lobe limbique of Broca, circumvolutio cristata, gyrus limbicus, lobus falciformis* (outmoded), *falciform lobe* (outmoded). • The term *limbic lobe* was introduced in 1878 by the French neurologist, Paul Broca.

linguiform lobe APPENDICULAR LOBE.

lobes of liver LOBI HEPATIS.

lower lobe of lung LOBUS INFERIOR PULMONIS.

lobes of lung Major divisions of the lung, separated by fissures. The right lung has superior, middle, and inferior lobes, and the left lung has superior and inferior lobes.

lobes of mammary gland LOBI GLANDULAE MAMMARIAE.

median lobe of prostate LOBUS MEDIUS PROSTATAE.

middle lobe of cerebellum VERMIS CEREBELLI.

middle lobe of right lung LOBUS MEDIUS PULMONIS DEXTRI.

neural lobe LOBUS NERVOSUS NEUROHYPOPHYSEOS.

occipital lobe LOBUS OCCIPITALIS.

olfactory lobe LOBUS OLFACTORIUS.

optic lobes An obsolete term for CORPORA QUADRIGEMINA.

parietal lobe LOBUS PARIETALIS.

piriform lobe A portion of the anterior and ventromedial face of the temporal lobe composed of the terminal extensions of the lateral olfactory stria, the uncus, and the anterior part of the parahippocampal gyrus. It is demarcated laterally by the rhinal sulcus. Also *pyriform lobe.*

lobes of the placenta PLACENTAL COTYLEDON.

posterior lobe of hypophysis NEUROHYPOPHYSIS.

posterior lobe of pituitary gland NEUROHYPOPHYSIS.

prefrontal lobe The part of the frontal lobe of the cerebral hemispheres anterior to Brodmann's areas 6 and 8 (the motor and premotor zones), representing one of the latest phylogenetic developments of the brain. It is well developed only in primates, especially man.

lobes of prostate Lobus prostatae (dexter et sinister) and lobus medius prostatae.

pulmonary lobes See under LOBES OF LUNG.

pyramidal lobe of thyroid gland LOBUS PYRAMIDALIS GLANDULAE THYROIDEAE.

pyriform lobe PIRIFORM LOBE.

quadrangular lobe of cerebellum LOBULUS QUADRANGULARIS CEREBELLI.

quadrate lobe of cerebral hemisphere PRECUNEUS.

quadrate lobe of liver LOBUS QUADRATUS HEPATIS.

renal lobes LOBI RENALES.

Riedel's lobe APPENDICULAR LOBE.

right lobe of liver LOBUS HEPATIS DEXTER.

side lobe An undesired minor beam of sound traveling out in directions not included in the primary beam.

spigelian lobe LOBUS CAUDATUS HEPATIS.

superior crescentic lobe of cerebellum LOBULUS SEMILUNARIS SUPERIOR.

superior lobe of lung LOBUS SUPERIOR PULMONIS.

superior semilunar lobe LOBULUS SEMILUNARIS SUPERIOR.

supplemental lobe A protuberance on the crown which is not a typical morphologic feature of that tooth.

temporal lobe LOBUS TEMPORALIS.

lobes of thymus LOBUS THYMI DEXTER ET SINISTER.

lobes of thyroid gland LOBI GLANDULAE THYROIDEAE DEXTER ET SINISTER.

upper lobe of lung LOBUS SUPERIOR PULMONIS.

vermiform lobe VERMIS CEREBELLI.

lobectomy [Gk *lobos* the lobe of the ear, of the liver + -ECTOMY] The excision of a lobe, as of the brain, lung, or thyroid.

lobelia [after Matthias de *Lobel* or *L'Obel*, Flemish botanist, 1538–1616 + -IA] The dried leaves and flowering tops of *Lobelia inflata*, which contain the pyridine alkaloid lobeline. Lobelia has been used as an expectorant to treat asthma and bronchitis. Also called *asthma weed, Indian tobacco.*

lobeline $C_{22}H_{27}NO_2$. The major pyridine alkaloid obtained from the seeds and leaves of *Lobelia inflata*, lobelia. It resembles nicotine in action and stimulates respiration.

lobelism [*lobel(ine)* + -ISM] Poisoning from overdosage of lobeline, the chief alkaloid extracted from *Lobelia inflata*, Indian tobacco. Symptoms are increased respiration and blood pressure, and muscular fasciculations mimicking the nicotinic effects of acetylcholine.

lobi Plural of LOBUS.

lobite Designating or limited to a single lobe.

lobitis [*lob(e)* + -ITIS] Inflammation of a lobe of the lung.

Lobo [Jorge *Lobo*, Brazilian physician, flourished early 20th century] Lobo's disease. See under LOBOMYCOSIS.

Loboa loboi A species of yeastlike fungus which causes lobomycosis.

lobocyte POLYMORPHONUCLEAR LEUKOCYTE.

lobodontia [Spanish *lob(o)* wolf + -ODONTIA] A rare condition with multiple anomalies of the teeth including multituber-cular molar crowns, pointed buccal cusps on bicuspids, accentuation of cingula of incisors, and large diastemata in the canine region, resulting in a dentition resembling that of a carnivore.

lobomycosis [after Jorge *Lobo*, Brazilian physician, flourished 1931 + MYCOSIS] A localized, chronic, subepidermal fungal disease caused by *Loboa loboi*. It consists of keloidal, verrucoid, or nodular lesions. Also called *keloidal blastomycosis* (imprecise), *keloidal disease* (imprecise), *Lobo's disease, cheloidiform blastomycosis* (obsolete).

lobopod LOBOPODIUM.

lobopodia Plural of LOBOPODIUM.

lobopodium [Gk *lobo(s)* lobe + PODIUM] (*plural* lobopodia) A thick, lobed, pseudopodium of amebas containing ectoplasm and endoplasm, or only endoplasm. See also AXOPODIUM, FILOPODIUM, RHIZOPODIUM.

lobose LOBATE.

lobotomy [Gk *lobo(s)* the lobe of the ear, of the liver + -TOMY] The incision of a lobe, as of the brain or of a lung.

frontal lobotomy Lobotomy of the frontal lobe of the cerebrum in psychosurgery to sever the white connecting fibers. Also called *prefrontal lobotomy, leukotomy (chiefly British).*

prefrontal lobotomy FRONTAL LOBOTOMY.

transorbital lobotomy Division of the white fibers of the cerebrum by an instrument introduced through the orbit. Also called *transorbital leukotomy (used especially in the U.K.).*

lobous LOBATE.

Lobry de Bruyn [Cornelius Adriaan *Lobry de Bruyn*, Dutch chemist, 1857–1904] Lobry de Bruyn-van Ekenstein transformation. See under TRANSFORMATION.

Lobstein [Johann Georg C. F. M. *Lobstein*, German pathologist, 1777–1835] **1** Splanchnic ganglion of Lobstein, Lobstein's ganglion. See under GANGLION SPLANCHNICUM. **2** Lobstein's disease. See under SYNDROME.

lobular Pertaining to or resembling a lobule; composed of lobules.

lobulated Composed of or characterized by lobules.

lobulation The process of forming lobules or the state of being lobulated.

fetal lobulation A superficial lobular appearance on the surface of kidneys in postnatal life due to persistent shallow linear indentations characteristic of fetal kidneys. The lobulation may persist into adulthood. On roentgenograms the cortical indentations are seen to correspond to the regions of the renal columns. The lobulations are usually smooth and regular but at times may be confused with renal masses. Also called *persistent lobulation, fetal lobation, persistent lobation.*

glomerular lobulation LOBULAR GLOMERULONEPHRITIS.

persistent lobulation FETAL LOBULATION.

portal lobulation A pattern of regeneration seen in the liver following hepatic vein obstruction, characterized by periportal regenerative nodules.

lobule [LOBE + -ULE] LOBULUS.

ansiform lobule That portion of the lateral lobe (hemisphere) of the cerebellum between the posterior superior fissure and the gracile lobule.

anterior lunate lobule LOBULUS SEMILUNARIS SUPERIOR.

anterior quadrangular lobule PARS ANTERIOR LOBULI QUADRANGULARIS.

lobule of auricle LOBULUS AURICULAE.

biventral lobule LOBULUS BIVENTER.

caudal semilunar lobule LOBULUS SEMILUNARIS INFERIOR.

central lobule of cerebellum LOBULUS CENTRALIS CEREBELLI.

cerebellar lobule A subdivision of a cerebellar lobus, examples of which include the lobulus simplex, the paramedian lobule, and the superior and inferior semilunar lobules.

cortical lobules LOBULI CORTICALES RENIS.

cortical lobules of kidney LOBULI CORTICALES RENIS.

cranial semilunar lobule LOBULUS SEMILUNARIS SUPERIOR.

crescentic lobules of cerebellum Lobulus semilunaris inferior and lobulus semilunaris superior.

digastric lobule LOBULUS BIVENTER.

ear lobule LOBULUS AURICULAE.

lobules of epididymis LOBULI EPIDIDYMIDIS.

floccular lobule A small structure on the inferior ventral aspect of the cerebellum just above the roof of the fourth ventricle. With the adjacent nodulus, it comprises the flocculonodular complex or archicerebellum.

fusiform lobule GYRUS FUSIFORMIS.

glandular lobule A unit of glandular tissue that is supplied by a single duct and demarcated from adjacent glandular tissue by a connective tissue layer.

glomerular lobule One of several similar lobules of the renal glomerulus, formed by a peripheral capillary loop and its attached endothelial, epithelial, and mesangial structures. Normally, glomerular lobules are barely apparent, but in glomerular diseases a distinct lobular pattern often develops.

gracile lobule That portion of the cerebellar hemisphere situated anterior to the biventral lobule and posterior to the inferior semilunar lobule.

hepatic lobules   LOBULI HEPATIS.

inferior parietal lobule   LOBULUS PARIETALIS INFERIOR.

inferior semilunar lobule   LOBULUS SEMILUNARIS INFERIOR.

lobules of lung   1 LOBULI PULMONUM.   2 SEGMENTA BRONCHOPULMONALIA.

lobules of mammary gland   LOBULI GLANDULAE MAMMARIAE.

olfactory lobule   LOBUS OLFACTORIUS.

paracentral lobule   LOBULUS PARACENTRALIS.

paramedian lobule   A small gyrus on the medial surface of the cerebral hemisphere bounded by the sulcus cinguli below and by the superomedial border of the hemisphere above. The upper end of the central sulcus may penetrate it.

portal lobule of liver   A unit of liver tissue centering on one portal canal. In this concept, interlobular vessels are intra-acinar and several veins are at the periphery of the unit. Compare LOBULI HEPATIS.

posterior lunate lobule   LOBULUS SEMILUNARIS INFERIOR.

posterior quadrangular lobule   LOBULUS SIMPLEX.

primary lobule of lung   LOBULUS PULMONIS PRIMARIUS.

pulmonary lobules   1 LOBULI PULMONUM.   2 SEGMENTA BRONCHOPULMONALIA.

quadrangular lobule of cerebellum   LOBULUS QUADRANGULARIS CEREBELLI.

quadrate lobule   PRECUNEUS.

renal lobule   Any of several medullary rays of collecting ducts of the kidney, surrounded by the nephrons which drain into these ducts. Interlobular arteries demarcate the individual lobules.

secondary lobule of lung   LOBULUS PULMONIS SECUNDARIUS.

spermatic lobules   LOBULI TESTIS.

superior parietal lobule   LOBULUS PARIETALIS SUPERIOR.

superior semilunar lobule   LOBULUS SEMILUNARIS SUPERIOR.

lobules of testis   LOBULI TESTIS.

lobules of thymus   LOBULI THYMI.

lobules of thyroid gland   LOBULI GLANDULAE THYROIDEAE.

lobulette   1 A tiny lobule.   2 Any of the primary subdivisions of a lobule.

lobuli   Plural of LOBULUS.

lobulization [*lobul(e)* + -IZE + -ATION]   The process by which homogeneous tissue is changed into a lobulated state.

lobulose   Organized into, or having, lobules. Also *lobulous*.

lobulous   LOBULOSE.

lobulus [New L (from French or English *lobule*), a little lobe] (*plural* lobuli) A small lobe, or one of the parts into which a lobe is subdivided. Also called *lobule*.

lobulus auriculae [NA]   The soft, lowest part of the auricle of the ear, situated below the antitragus, devoid of cartilage and consisting of fatty and fibrous tissue; earlobe. Also called *lobule of auricle, ear lobule.*

lobulus biventer [NA]   A lobule on the posterior and inferior surface of the cerebellum, situated between the tonsilla of the cerebellum and the gracile lobule. Also called *digastric lobule, biventral lobule, digastric lobe.*

lobulus centralis cerebelli   An anterior portion of the vermis situated between the culmen and lingula and overlapping the anterior medullary velum. Also called *central lobule of cerebellum.*

lobulus clivi   DECLIVE.

lobuli corticales renis [NA]   Imperfectly separated portions of the renal cortex, each of which extends from the base of a renal pyramid to the fibrous capsule and comprises a pars radiata

and a pars convoluta. Interlobular blood vessels may partially demarcate the units. Also called *cortical lobules of kidney, cortical lobules, cortical arches of the kidney, cortical arches.*

lobulus culminis   CULMEN.

lobulus cuneiformis   The medial aspect of the occipital lobe bounded rostrally by the parieto-occipital sulcus, and inferiorly by the calcarine sulcus. Also called *cuneiform lobe.*

lobuli epididymidis [NA]   The conical masses forming the head of the epididymis and composed of dilated and highly convoluted efferent ductules of the testis. Also called *lobules of epididymis, coni epididymidis, vascular cones, coni vasculosi* (outmoded), *Haller's cones.*

lobulus folii   That portion of the vermis cerebelli lying in front of the lobus clivi and behind the fissura prima.

lobuli glandulae mammariae [NA]   The small glandular units forming the lobes of the mammary gland and consisting of clusters of saccular or tubulosaccular alveoli connected by areolar tissue and blood vessels. Each unit is drained by a duct which joins with adjacent ducts to form larger ducts which eventually terminate as the lactiferous duct draining each lobe of the gland. Also called *lobules of mammary gland, lobuli mammae* (outmoded).

lobuli glandulae thyroideae [NA]   Irregular subdivisions of each lobe of the thyroid gland formed by inward extensions of the investing connective tissue and composed of spherical follicles of varying size and number surrounded by very vascular connective tissue. Also called *lobules of thyroid gland.*

lobuli hepatis [NA]   Microscopic functional units of the liver tissue which comprise a central vein from which rows or plates of liver cells with intervening sinusoids radiate to the periphery of the units where the portal canals are situated. Also called *hepatic lobules.* Compare PORTAL LOBULE OF LIVER.

lobuli mammae   An outmoded term for LOBULI GLANDULAE MAMMARIAE.

lobulus paracentralis [NA]   A group of gyri on the superior part of the medial surface of the cerebral hemisphere, more or less continuous with the precentral and postcentral gyri of the frontal and parietal lobes, and bounded inferiorly by the cingulate sulcus. It surrounds the medial termination of the central sulcus of Rolando, and is composed of both sensory and motor cortex representing the lower leg and foot. Also called *paracentral lobule.*

lobulus parietalis inferior [NA]   That portion of the parietal lobe on the lateral surface of the cerebral hemisphere lying below the intraparietal sulcus, above the posterior ramus of the lateral cerebral fissure, and behind the postcentral sulcus. It includes the supramarginal and angular gyri, and in the dominant hemisphere is concerned with speech mechanisms. It overlaps but is not entirely congruent with the sensory speech area (Wernicke's center). Also called *inferior parietal lobule.*

lobulus parietalis superior [NA]   That portion of the parietal lobe on the lateral surface of the cerebral hemisphere situated between the postcentral sulcus anteriorly and the parieto-occipital fissure posteriorly, and above the intraparietal sulcus. It includes a group of association areas for somesthesia. Also called *superior parietal lobule.*

lobulus pulmonis primarius [NA]   A microscopic subdivision of the lung consisting of a respiratory bronchiole together with its associated alveolar ducts, alveolar sacs and alveoli. Also called *primary lobule of lung.*

lobulus pulmonis secundarius [NA]   A microscopic subdivision of the lung consisting of about fifty primary lobules and delineated by fibrous interlobular septa. Also called *secondary lobule of lung.*

lobuli pulmonum   1 Either primary or secondary lobules of the lung. An outmoded term. Also called *lobules of lung, pulmonary lobules.* See also LOBULUS PULMONIS PRIMARIUS, LOB-

ULUS PULMONIS SECUNDARIUS. **2** SEGMENTA BRONCHOPUL-
MONALIA.

lobulus quadrangularis cerebelli   The quadrangular lobule
of the cerebellum: those portions of the cerebellar hemisphere
that appear as lateral continuations of the culmen and declive
and lie on both sides of the primary fissure. Also called *quadrangular lobule of cerebellum, quadrangular lobe of cerebellum.*

lobulus semilunaris inferior   [NA] That portion of the cerebellar hemisphere appearing as the lateral continuation of the
tuber vermis. Also called *crus II, inferior crescentic lobe of
cerebellum, area lunata* (obsolete), *inferior semilunar lobule,
inferior semilunar lobe, caudal semilunar lobule, posterior lunate
lobule.*

lobulus semilunaris superior   [NA] That portion of the cerebellar hemisphere appearing as a lateral continuation of the
folium vermis. Also called *crus I, superior crescentic lobe of
cerebellum, superior semilunar lobule, anterior lunate lobule,
cranial semilunar lobule, superior semilunar lobe.*

lobulus simplex   [NA] That portion of the cerebellar hemisphere continuous with the declive of the vermis. Also called
*posterior quadrangular lobule, pars posterior lobuli quadrangu-
laris.*

lobuli testis   [NA] The cone-shaped subdivisions or units of
the glandular structure of the testis, numbering more than two
hundred and each containing up to four convoluted seminiferous
tubules supported by loose connective tissue with scattered
groups of interstitial cells. The units are incompletely separated
from each other by the septula testis, their apices converging on
the mediastinum testis while their bases are on the surface of
the testis. Also called *lobules of testis, spermatic lobules.*

lobuli thymi   [NA] The smaller subdivisions of the lobes of
the thymus gland, separated by trabeculae of connective tissue.
Also called *lobules of thymus.*

lobus [New L (from Gk *lobos* the lobe of the ear, of the liver), a
lobe] (*plural* lobi) Any rounded projection or subdivision of
an organ or structure demarcated by fissures, sulci, constrictions,
or connective tissue septa; a lobe.

lobus anterior hypophyseos   ADENOHYPOPHYSIS.

lobus appendicularis   APPENDICULAR LOBE.

lobus caudatus hepatis   [NA] A small elongated lobe situated
on the posterior part of the diaphragmatic surface and the
visceral surface of the liver between the fissure for the ligamentum venosum on the left and the groove for the inferior vena
cava on the right. It is bounded anteroinferiorly by the porta
hepatis just posterior to which the caudate process connects it
to the right lobe. Also called *caudate lobe of liver, lobus caudatus
spigeli* (outmoded), *spigelian lobe, lobus spigelii* (outmoded).

lobus caudatus spigeli   An outmoded term for LOBUS CAU-
DATUS HEPATIS.

lobus centralis   That portion of the anterior cerebellar vermis
between the lingula and culmen.

lobi cerebri   [NA] The major subdivisions of the cerebral pallium, defined by fissures, sulci, or arbitrary boundaries, and
named for the bones of the skull which overlie them. They
include frontal, parietal, occipital, and temporal lobes. Some
include the limbic lobe, an arc of pallium on the medial surface
of the hemisphere surrounding the corpus callosum, and continuations of the upper brainstem to the cerebrum. Also called
lobes of cerebrum.

lobus clivi   The posterior crescent-shaped lobes of the cerebellum. An outmoded term.

lobus falciformis   An outmoded term for LIMBIC LOBE.

lobus frontalis   [NA] The anterior portion of the cerebral
hemisphere, extending from the anterior pole to the sulcus centralis. Also called *frontal lobe.*

lobi glandulae mammariae   [NA] The fifteen to twenty major
subdivisions or lobes of the glandular substance of the breast.
They are distributed in a radial fashion around the nipple as the
central point. Each constitutes a separate modified sweat gland
of the apocrine type consisting of lobules and each is drained
by a lactiferous duct opening on the surface of the nipple. The
lobes are surrounded and held together by connective tissue,
fibrous strands of which attach them to the skin and to the
underlying pectoral fascia. Also called *lobes of mammary gland,
lobi mammae* (outmoded).

lobi glandulae thyroideae dexter et sinister   The right and
left cone-shaped lateral lobes of the thyroid gland, which are
connected across the midline by the narrow isthmus, surrounded
by the pretracheal fascia. They are in contact medially with the
thyroid cartilage, cricothyroid muscle, cricoid cartilage, and the
upper four or five tracheal cartilages, while laterally they are in
contact with the carotid sheath on each side. Also called *lobes
of thyroid gland.*

lobus glandularis of hypophysis   ADENOHYPOPHYSIS.

lobi hepatis   [NA] The morphological divisions of the liver
which, according to surface markings, are named lobus hepatis
dexter and lobus hepatis sinister, of which the former has two
further subdivisions, lobus caudatus and lobus quadratus. Their
internal structure is divided into segments according to the
distribution of the hepatic ducts, portal vein, and hepatic arteries. Also called *lobes of liver, hepatic lobes.*

lobus hepatis dexter   [NA] Morphologically, the right five-
sixths of the liver, separated from the left lobe anteriorly and
superiorly by the line of attachment of the falciform ligament,
and on the posterior and visceral surfaces by the fissure for
ligamentum venosum and the fissure for ligamentum teres. On
the visceral surface and the posterior part of the diaphragmatic
surface it has two subdivisions, the caudate and quadrate lobes.
Its substance is divided into anterior and posterior segments.
Also called *right lobe of liver.*

lobus hepatis sinister   [NA] Morphologically, the left one
sixth of the liver separated from the right lobe anteriorly and
superiorly by the line of attachment of the falciform ligament
and on the posterior and visceral surfaces by the fissure for
ligamentum venosum and the fissure for ligamentum teres. It is
thin and flattened superoinferiorly. Its substance is divided into
medial and lateral segments. Also called *left lobe of liver.*

lobus inferior pulmonis   [NA] The large lobe of the lung
situated below and behind the oblique fissure which separates it
from the superior lobe in the left lung and from the superior
and middle lobes in the right lung. In both lungs it comprises
five bronchopulmonary segments (VI through X). Its inferior
surface forms the base of the lung. Also called *inferior lobe of
lung, lower lobe of lung.*

lobus linguiformis   APPENDICULAR LOBE.

lobi mammae   An outmoded term for LOBI GLANDULAE
MAMMARIAE.

lobus medius prostatae   [NA] The slightly elevated portion
of the prostate, between the ejaculatory ducts and the urethra,
which forms the superior part of the posterior surface of the
prostate. Its size varies considerably and it usually only becomes
obvious when enlarged. Also called *median lobe of prostate,
Morgagni's caruncle, morgagnian caruncle.*

lobus medius pulmonis dextri   [NA] The small, wedge-
shaped lobe of the right lung which is separated from the superior lobe by the horizontal fissure and from the inferior lobe
by the oblique fissure. It varies in size and comprises the lateral
(IV) and medial (V) bronchopulmonary segments. Also called
middle lobe of right lung.

lobus nervosus neurohypophyseos   [NA] The body of the
neurohypophysis, the site of storage and release of oxytocin and
vasopressin. Along with the infundibulum (hypophysial stalk),

it constitutes the neurohypophysis. Also called *neural lobe, pars nervosa hypophyseos.*

lobus occipitalis [NA] The posterior portion of the cerebral hemisphere, extending from the posterior pole to an imaginary line connecting the parieto-occipital fissure superiorly and medially with the preoccipital notch inferiorly. Also called *occipital lobe.*

lobus olfactorius Those structures on the inferior surface of the frontal lobe of the cerebral hemisphere directly concerned with olfaction. It comprises the olfactory bulb, tract, trigone, and striae, and is maximally developed in macrosmatic animals. Also called *olfactory lobule, olfactory lobe.*

lobus parietalis [NA] The upper and central portion of the cerebral hemisphere, primarily on the lateral surface. It is separated anteriorly from the frontal lobe by the central sulcus, and inferiorly from the temporal lobe by the lateral sulcus, though there is some confluence at the posterior end of both lobes. It appears continuous behind with the occipital lobe on the lateral surface, but is separated from it on the medial surface by the parieto-occipital sulcus. For topographical purposes, division is made between the parietal and occipital lobes on the lateral surface by means of an imaginary line connecting the parieto-occipital sulcus (just visible at the vertex) with the preoccipital notch on the inferior surface. Also called *parietal lobe.*

lobus posterior hypophyseos NEUROHYPOPHYSIS.

lobus prostatae dexter et sinister The lateral portions, right and left, of the prostate below the transverse groove on the posterior surface, which is formed by the two ejaculatory ducts penetrating the gland and from which a median vertical furrow extends downward to demarcate the two lateral portions. They occupy the main mass of the gland, and are continuous behind the urethra and are connected in front of it by the isthmus. Also called *lateral lobes of prostate gland.*

lobus pyramidalis glandulae thyroideae [NA] A conical third lobe, present in about forty percent of thyroid glands, extending upwards from either the isthmus or the left lobe, and occasionally becoming continuous with a fibrous or fibromuscular band that attaches to the hyoid bone. It represents the distal remnant of the thyroglossal duct. Also called *pyramidal lobe of thyroid gland, pyramid of thyroid* (outmoded), *Lalouette's pyramid* (outmoded).

lobus quadratus hepatis [NA] A quadrilateral-shaped lobe on the visceral surface of the liver, structurally a part of the right lobe and bounded on the left by the fissure for ligamentum teres, on the right by the fossa of the gallbladder, anteriorly by the inferior margin of the liver, and posteriorly by the porta hepatis. Also called *quadrate lobe of liver.*

lobi renales [NA] The functional units of the kidney, each being a segment that drains through a renal papilla and containing several lobules. Up to six pyramids may be connected to a single papilla. In the normal human adult these units are not demarcated and the renal surface is smooth, but in fetuses and infants the surface is irregular and lobated. Also called *renal lobes.*

lobus spigelii An outmoded term for LOBUS CAUDATUS HEPATIS.

lobus superior pulmonis [NA] The large lobe of the lung situated above and in front of the oblique fissure in the left lung and the oblique and horizontal fissures in the right lung. Its upper limit forms the apex of the lung. In the right lung it contains bronchopulmonary segments I–III while in the left it includes I through V. Also called *superior lobe of lung, upper lobe of lung.*

lobus temporalis [NA] The ventral and lateral portion of the cerebral hemisphere. It lies below the lateral cerebral fissure lateral to the collateral fissure and merges with the occipital lobe posteriorly. Also called *temporal lobe.*

lobus thymi dexter et sinister The right and left lobes of the thymus. Also called *lobes of thymus.*

local Confined to a particular site or region of the body; limited in distribution or effect.

locality A specific area, usually geographically defined, such as that served by a health care facility.

type locality A geographic location from which the type specimen of a taxonomic group was first collected.

localization 1 The determination of the position of an object. 2 The determination of the confines of a phenomenon. 3 The process of confining to a limited area of extent.

auditory localization The determination by an organism of the position or direction of a sound source.

cerebral localization The concept that different regions of the cerebral cortex are specialized to express specific functional attributes.

germinal localization FATE MAP.

pneumotaxic localization Localization of cerebral structures as revealed by ventriculography. Modern noninvasive methods of visualization such as nuclear magnetic resonance radiography have replaced the method.

selective localization The specific accumulation of a radionuclide in an organ or tissue.

spatial localization 1 The directional and distance orientation of objects. 2 The ability to recognize the positioning of a stimulus on the body surface.

localized Confined to a particular region, as an infection.

localizer 1 COLLIMATOR. 2 An instrument used to identify the presence and position of a metallic foreign body in the eye.

locant [*loc(ation)* + -ANT] A number or letter added to a chemical name to show where substitution has been performed. Thus the numeral 6 in "glucose 6-phosphate", shows which hydroxyl group of glucose is phosphorylated.

locator Something used to mark the position or placement of a device or to detect the location of an object.

abutment locator A baseplate perforated so as to mark the positions of the abutments of a proposed implant.

Berman-Moorhead locator A type of electroacoustic locator for detecting metallic foreign objects embedded in body tissues.

electroacoustic locator A device that makes an audible signal when it comes in contact or approaches a metallic foreign object, used as a means of locating such objects embedded in body tissue.

loc. dol. *loco dolenti* (L, to the painful spot).

lochia [neut. pl. of Gk *lochios* (from *lochos* the act of lying in wait, an ambush, a lying-in, childbirth) pertaining to childbirth; as substantive *ta lochia* the discharge after childbirth] The uterine discharge that issues from the vagina postpartum. Adjective: lochial.

lochia alba A uterine discharge of a light color, usually the last of several uterine discharges after delivery. Lochia alba consists primarily of leukocytes. Also called *lochia purulenta.*

lochia cruenta LOCHIA RUBRA.

lochia purulenta LOCHIA ALBA.

lochia rubra A bright red uterine discharge that appears immediately after delivery. It consists primarily of blood. Also called *lochia cruenta.*

lochia sanguinolenta A thick, blood-tinged uterine discharge that usually appears several days after delivery.

lochia serosa A clear, serous uterine discharge that usually appears approximately five days after delivery.

lochial Pertaining to or characteristic of the lochia.

lochiocolpos [*lochi(a)* + *o* + Gk *kolpos* bosom, uterus, fold] Vaginal distension due to retained lochia.

lochiocyte A decidual cell contained in the lochia.

lochiometra [*lochi(a)* + *o* + Gk *mētra* the uterus]   Uterine distension due to retained lochia.

lochiometritis [Gk *lochio(s)* pertaining to childbirth + METRI-TIS]   PUERPERAL ENDOMETRITIS.

lochioperitonitis [*lochi(a)* + *o* + PERITONITIS]   Postpartum endometritis with associated peritonitis. Also called *lochoperitonitis.*

lochiopyra [*lochi(a)* + *o* + Gk *pyra*, pl. of *pyr* fire, fever heat]   A fever occurring in the early postpartum period. An older term.

lochiorrhagia [*lochi(a)* + *o* + -RRHAGIA]   LOCHIORRHEA.

lochiorrhea [*lochi(a)* + *o* + -RRHEA]   A profuse flow of the lochia. Also called *lochiorrhagia.*

lochioschesis [*lochi(a)* + *o* + Gk *schesis* a holding, retaining]   LOCHIOSTASIS.

lochiostasis [*lochi(a)* + *o* + -STASIS]   Retention of the lochia postpartum. Also called *lochioschesis.*

lochometritis [Gk *locho(s)* a lying in, childbirth + METRITIS]   PUERPERAL ENDOMETRITIS.

lochoperitonitis [Gk *locho(s)* a lying in, childbirth + PERITO-NITIS]   LOCHIOPERITONITIS.

loci   Plural of LOCUS.

lociation [*loc(al)* + *i* + -ATION]   A local variation in species composition within an association distinguished by the relative abundance of a dominant species.

lock / friction lock   A lower extremity prosthetic knee mechanism that dampens the swing phase of gait and provides increased stability when the prosthesis is extended during the stance phase.

   orthodontic lock   A spring device which enables an orthodontic arch wire to be removed from the anchor band and be replaced at will.

   transfer lock   In a controlled environment, opening in a laminar air flow tent that permits passage of materials to the patient.

Locke [Frank Spiller *Locke*, English physiologist, 1871–1949]   **1** Citrated Locke solution. See under SOLUTION. **2** Locke-Ringer solution. See under SOLUTION.

locking / head locking   INTERLOCKING.

lockjaw   **1** Trismus, especially as a manifestation of tetanus. A popular usage. **2** A popular term for TETANUS.

Lockwood [Charles Barrett *Lockwood*, English surgeon, 1858–1914]   **1** See under SIGN. **2** Lockwood's ligament, Lockwood suspensory ligament. See under SUSPENSORY LIGAMENT OF EYEBALL.

locoed   Poisoned by ingestion of the locoweed. A popular usage.

locoism [Spanish *loco* crazy + -ISM]   LOCOWEED POISONING.

locomotion [L *loc(us)* place + *o* + MOTION]   Movement from place to place effected or controlled by means of some mechanism within the moving object.

   brachial locomotion   BRACHIATION.

   fictive locomotion   Essentially normal locomotor activity produced through electric or pharmacologic stimulation of a central nervous structure.

locomotive   Relating to movement from one place to another. Also *locomotory.*

locomotor   Relating to locomotion or to the locomotive apparatus of the body.

locomotorial   Describing or pertaining to the locomotor system.

locomotory   LOCOMOTIVE.

Locorten   A proprietary name for flumethasone pivalate.

locular   Pertaining to a loculus or loculi.

loculate   Possessing or divided into a number of loculi.

loculation   The process of forming loculi or the state of having loculi.

locule [L *locul(us)* (dim. of *locus* a place, room) a small place, cavity]   **1** A cavity within a sporangium.   **2** A cavity of an ovary containing ovules.

loculi   Plural of LOCULUS.

Loculoascomycetidae [L *locul(us)* a small space, a cavity + *o* + *asc(us)* + *o* + *mycet(e)* + -IDAE]   An ascostromatic subclass of fungi, of which several members are economically important plant pathogens.

loculus (*plural* loculi)   A small chamber or cavity.

locum tenens [L *locum*, accus. of *locus* a place + *tenens*, pres. part. of *tenere* to hold. *Locum tenens* is the source of *lieutenant.*]   One filling in for or taking the place of another for a defined period of time, on a temporary basis, such as a physician covering or filling in for another physician.

locus [L, a place, position]   **1** A particular site or position, as of an anatomic part.   **2** In genetics, the position in the linkage map or in the chromosome of a gene, of a cluster of genes, or of a regulatory region that does not yield a product but that influences nearby genes.   **3** An imprecise term for GENE.

   locus ceruleus   [NA]   A deeply pigmented group of neurons in the superior angle of the floor of the fourth ventricle. The 3000–4000 cells in the paired nuclear complex generate a widespread axonal system that constitutes the major norepinephrine pathway of the central nervous system. Also called *locus cinereus, locus ferrugineus, nucleus pigmentosus pontis, substantia ferruginea.*

   locus cinereus   LOCUS CERULEUS.

   complex locus   A locus on a chromosome having more than one site at which recombination can occur.

   locus ferrugineus   LOCUS CERULEUS.

   H-2 locus   One of the principal components, along with the Ir gene, of the major histocompatibility complex in the mouse. It is comparable to the HLA loci in humans.

   histocompatibility locus   One of the genes located within the major histocompatibility complex that specifies transplantation antigens or immune response functions.

   locus minoris resistentiae   The site of least resistance; the region of the body in each individual that is most susceptible to disease.

   locus niger   SUBSTANTIA NIGRA.

   operator locus   A regulator locus that governs the transcription of adjacent structural genes through interaction with specific regulatory proteins. In bacterial genetics, the operator is proximal to the structural genes of the operon and is the binding site of a repressor protein molecule. Also called *operator.*

   locus perforatus anticus   SUBSTANTIA PERFORATA ANTERIOR.

   locus perforatus posticus   SUBSTANTIA PERFORATA POSTERIOR.

   PTC locus   A human gene which, by an unknown mechanism, determines whether the substance phenylthiocarbamide can be tasted or not. Also called *taster gene.*

   locus ruber   NUCLEUS RUBER.

   sex factor affinity locus   In bacterial conjugation, a surface locus on recipient cells to which the F pilus attaches. Also called *SFA locus.*

   SFA locus   SEX FACTOR AFFINITY LOCUS.

lodicules [L *lodicul(a)* a coverlet, dim. of *lodex*, gen. *lodicis*, a cover + English *-es*]   Small scales near the base of the stamens in most grass flowers. They swell with water and distend to separate the glumes, modified leaves or bracts between the groups of small flowers known as spikelets.

Loeb [Leo *Loeb*, U.S. pathologist, 1869–1959]   **1** See under

DECIDUOMA. **2** Loeb's decidual reaction. See under REAC-TION.

Loeffler [Friedrich August Johannes *Loeffler*, German bacteriologist, 1852–1915] **1** Loeffler medium. See under LOEFFLER'S BLOOD CULTURE MEDIUM (at CULTURE MEDIUM). **2** See under METHYLENE BLUE.

loeffleria [after Friedrich August Johannes *Loeffler*, German bacteriologist, 1852–1915 + -IA] A condition in which *Corynebacterium diphtheriae* are present but the characteristic symptoms of diphtheria are not. Also *löffleria*.

loemaemia A British spelling for LEMEMIA.

loemic A British spelling for LEMIC.

loempe BERIBERI.

Loenen [Johannes Jacobus Guilielmus van *Loenen*, Dutch physician, flourished 19th century] Loenen sign. See under HEGAR SIGN.

Loeschia A former genus of amebas that included the present genus *Entamoeba*.

Loevit [Moritz *Loevit*, Austrian pathologist, 1851–1918] Loevit cell. See under ERYTHROBLAST.

Loewenstein [Ludwig W. *Loewenstein*, German-born dermatologist, active in the United States, flourished 20th century] Tumor of Buschke-Loewenstein. See under TUMOR.

Loewi [Otto *Loewi*, German-born U.S. pharmacologist, 1873–1961] Loewi symptom, Loewi's test. See under REACTION.

Löffler [Friedrich August Johannes *Löffler*, German bacteriologist, 1852–1915] **1** Klebs-Löffler bacillus. See under *CORYNEBACTERIUM DIPHTHERIAE*. **2** See under SERUM.

Löffler [Wilhelm *Löffler*, Swiss physician, born 1887] **1** Löffler's parietal fibroplastic endocarditis, Löffler's disease. See under LÖFFLER'S ENDOCARDITIS. **2** Löffler's eosinophilia, Löffler's pneumonia, Löffler's disease. See under LÖFFLER SYNDROME.

löffleria LOEFFLERIA.

log logarithm; common logarithm.

log- LOGO-.

logadectomy [Gk *logad(es)* the whites of the eyes + -ECTOMY] Excision of a part of the conjunctiva.

logades [K *logades* the whites of the eyes] The white surfaces of the eye.

logaditis [Gk *logad(es)* the whites of the eyes + -ITIS] SCLERITIS.

logadoblennorrhoea [Gk *logad(es)* the whites of the eyes + o + BLENNO- + -RRHOEA] A conjunctivitis producing a serous or mucoid discharge.

logagnosia [LOG- + Gk *agnosia* ignorance, a not knowing] Inability to recognize spoken or written words. An obsolete term. Also called *alogognosia, asemognosia*.

logagraphia [LOG- + AGRAPHIA] Agraphia with particular inability to express meaning by the written word. Adjective: logographic.

logamnesia [LOG- + AMNESIA] Word deafness or word blindness.

Logan [William H. G. *Logan*, U.S. plastic surgeon, flourished 20th century] See under BOW.

logaphasia [LOG- + APHASIA] BROCA'S APHASIA.

logarithm [LOG- + Gk *arithmos* number, a number] The power to which a fixed number, called the base, must be raised to produce a given number. Thus, the logarithm of 10 000 to base 10 is 4, since 10^4 equals 10 000. Abbreviation: log

briggsian logarithm COMMON LOGARITHM.

common logarithm A logarithm with base 10. Also called *briggsian logarithm*. Abbreviation: log

naperian logarithm NATURAL LOGARITHM.

natural logarithm A logarithm with base *e*. Also called *naperian logarithm*. Abbreviation: ln

logasthenia An outmoded term for WERNICKE'S APHASIA.

Log Etronics A process for reproducing x-ray or photographic images with the use of electronic methods to change contrast or density or both. Also called *logetronography*.

logetronography LOG ETRONICS.

-logia -LOGY.

logic [Gk *logikē*, fem. of *logikos* (from *logos* word, reason + -*ikos* -IC) pertaining to speech or reason] **1** A discipline embodying sets of rules for determining the validity of an argument or a chain of reasoning without regard to empirical content. Formal (or symbolic) logic deals, in part, with certain relationships between statements. For example, if *A* and *B* are statements, the statement *A and B* is true if and only if both *A* and *B* are true, while the statement *A or B* is true if either *A* or *B* is true. Some of the principles of formal logic are incorporated in the design of computer logic circuits. **2** In a logic circuit, the physical realization of a particular type of logic or a particular principle of formal logic, as in *binary logic*, or *AND-gate logic*.

hard-wired logic A group of electronic logic circuits whose function is determined by the wiring that interconnects the circuits. In contrast the function of logic circuits in a microcomputer is determined by the program.

-logist [Gk *log(os)* word, speech, reason, + -IST] A combining form designating one who specializes in a science or study or adheres to a particular doctrine.

logit **1** In statistics, the natural logarithm of the odds corresponding to the probability *P* of a specified outcome given the existence of a stated attribute, for example, of a coronary attack given a diastolic blood pressure of 95 mmHg. Logit *P* = $\log_{\hat{e}}\left(\dfrac{P}{1-P}\right)$. The logarithm of the odds ratio is conveniently expressed as the difference of two logits. **2** In bioassay, a transformation based on a logistic model of the dose-response relationship such that the logit of the response is linearly dependent on the dose.

logo- [Gk *logos* word, speech, reason] A combining form meaning word or speech. Also *log-*.

logoclonia [LOGO- + Gk *klon(os)* confusion, tumult + -IA] Rhythmic and meaningless repetition of a word or of the last few syllables of a word, as seen particularly in presenile or senile dementia and in general paresis. Also called *logoklony*.

logoklony LOGOCLONIA.

logokophosis [LOGO- + Gk *kōphōsis* dumbness, deafness, dullness] An outmoded term for WERNICKE'S APHASIA.

logomania [LOGO- + -MANIA] Excessive, rapid speech, as in mania. Also called *lalorrhea, logorrhea, tachylogia, verbomania, tachyphemia, tachyphrasia, tachyphasia*.

logoneurosis Any kind of neurotically based speech disorder, especially stuttering. An older term.

logopaedics A British spelling for LOGOPEDICS.

logopathy [LOGO- + -PATHY] Any disorder of speech caused by disease of the central nervous system.

logopedia LOGOPEDICS.

logopedics [LOGO- + English *(ortho)pedics*, from ORTHO- + Gk *pais*, gen. *paidos*, a child] The study and treatment of speech disorders. Also called *logopedia*.

logophasia [LOGO- + *(a)phasia*] The dysarthria which occurs in some patients with motor or expressive aphasia, resulting in inability to pronounce words. An obsolete term.

logorrhea [LOGO- + -RRHEA] LOGOMANIA.

jargonaphasic logorrhea JARGON APHASIA.

logospasm [LOGO- + SPASM] Spasmodic and repeated utterance of certain words or syllables, noted in rare instances in epilepsy. An obsolete term. Also called *epileptic palilalia*.

logotherapy EXISTENTIAL PSYCHOTHERAPY.

-logy [Gk *logos* word, speech, reason] A combining form designating a (specified) science, study, doctrine, or treatise. Also *-logia*.

Löhlein [Max Hermann Friedrich *Löhlein*, German physician, 1877–1921] Baehr-Löhlein lesion. See under LÖHLEIN-BAEHR LESION.

Lohmann [Karl *Lohmann*, German biochemist, born 1898] **1** See under REACTION. **2** Lohmann's enzyme. See under CREATINE KINASE.

loiasis [*Lo(a)* + -IASIS] Filariasis caused by *Loa loa*, a nematode parasite widely distributed in western and central Africa. Calabar swellings are a classic manifestation caused by local inflammatory response to migration of adult worms in subcutaneous tissues. Adult worms occasionally migrate across the eye surface, hence the name eye worm. Microfilariae are found in the peripheral blood. Treatment is with diethylcarbamazine. Also called *loaiasis*.

loin LUMBUS.

loliism [*Loli(um temulentum)* + -ISM] Poisoning by seeds of *Lolium temulentum*, darnel ryegrass, which may contaminate grain made into flour and used for bread. Symptoms are tremors, blurred vision, vomiting and prostration. Also called *lolism*.

lolism LOLIISM.

Lombard [Etienne *Lombard*, French physician, 1869–1920] See under TEST.

lomosome A vesicular membranous structure lying between the fungal cell wall and the plasma membrane.

Lomotil A combination of diphenoxylate hydrochloride and atropine, used for the treatment of diarrhea. A proprietary name.

Londe [P. F. L. *Londe*, French neurologist, 1864–1944] **1** Fazio-Londe atrophy. See under ATROPHY. **2** Fazio-Londe syndrome, Fazio-Londe disease. See under INFANTILE PROGRESSIVE BULBAR PALSY.

longevity Length of life.

  ecological longevity The longevity of a population cohort under natural conditions.

longilineal Of tall and slender bodily form; dolichomorphic.

longimanous Having long and slender hands.

longipedate Having long and slender feet.

longiradiate Possessing long radiations, used especially of certain neuroglial cells. An obsolete term.

longitudinal Lying or directed lengthwise; parallel to the long axis of the body or of one of its organs or parts; longitudinalis.

longitypical DOLICHOMORPHIC.

longsightedness HYPEROPIA.

loop [Middle English *loupe*] **1** ANSA. **2** The characteristic shape of the arched dermal ridges in dermatoglyphics. **3** A curvature, varying from a gentle arch to an acute bend, in an anatomical structure.

  archoplasmic loop An inflammatory pseudomembrane. An obsolete term.

  Axenfeld's nerve loop An intrascleral nerve commonly associated with a small cuff of uveal pigment, usually occurring several millimeters above the upper limbus in heavily pigmented persons. Its clinical significance is that it may be mistaken for an imbedded foreign body.

  bulboventricular loop BULBOVENTRICULAR FOLD.

  capillary loops The capillaries in the dermal papillae.

  closed loop In an automatic control system, a signal path which includes a feedback path, which compares the controlled value with the desired value, and a forward path, which reduces any difference between the controlled value and the desired value. Also called *feedback mechanism, regulatory feedback loop*.

  epididymodeferential loop The flexure formed by the tail of the epididymis continuing as the ductus deferens behind the inferior pole of the testis. An outmoded term.

  gamma loop The reflex arc involving the gamma efferent fibers arising in the anterior horns and the sensory afferent fibers arising in the muscle spindles. It is involved in the control of muscle tone.

  loop of Henle A U-shaped portion of the nephron, the descending limb of which extends from the straight portion of the proximal convoluted tubule in the cortex to the medulla where it makes a U-turn into the ascending limb which extends towards the glomerulus to form the distal convoluted tubule. The lower parts of the limbs and the U-turn are often attenuated to form the thin segment, and are known as the tubulus attenuatus. The limbs run radially and are parallel in the medullary rays. There are numerous variations including loops of juxtaglomerular nephrons being long and thin and extending to the apex of the renal papilla, while loops of subcapsular nephrons are short, with the U-turn formed by a thick descending limb and extending only to the outer part of the medulla. Also called *nephronic loop, Henle's ansa, ansa nephroni, Henle's canal, canaliculus laqueiformis* (outmoded).

  loop of hypoglossal nerve ANSA CERVICALIS.

  Hyrtl's loop An occasional communication between the right and left hypoglossal nerves in the geniohyoid or genioglossus muscle. Also called *Hyrtl's anastomosis*.

  intestinal loop One of several U-shaped flexures formed by the jejunum and ileum, the convex surface of which is free while the concave surface is attached to the mesentery through which the gut receives its vessels and nerves. The free surfaces of the flexures are in contact with each other or with the anterior abdominal wall.

  lenticular loop ANSA LENTICULARIS.

  Lippes loop An S-shaped intrauterine contraceptive device.

  Meyer's loop The portion of the geniculocalcarine radiation that runs anterolaterally before looping around the inferior horn of the lateral ventricle and turning posteriorly. Due to its relatively wide-sweeping trajectory through the temporal lobe, it is a sensitive indicator of temporal lobe pathology, particularly for space-occupying lesions.

  nephronic loop LOOP OF HENLE.

  P loop The loop formed by atrial activity in the vectorcardiogram.

  loop of the pectoral nerves A common anastomotic loop between the medial pectoral and lateral pectoral nerves in front of the axillary artery and usually just below the origin of the thoracoacromial artery.

  peduncular loop ANSA PEDUNCULARIS.

  platinum loop A ring of platinum wire, mounted in a heat-resistant handle, that is used to transfer microbiologic material. Because it is highly resistant to solution and withstands very high temperatures, platinum can undergo repeated exposure to harsh sterilizing conditions.

  primitive intestinal loop The simple intestinal tube of a four-week human embryo. It lies in the median plane, loops ventrally from the stomach to the cloaca, and is continuous at midpoint with the stalk of the yolk sac. The segment above the midpoint is the cranial limb of the intestinal loop, that below is the caudal limb.

  QRS loop The loop formed by ventricular depolarization in the vectorcardiogram.

  loop of recurrent laryngeal nerve The anteroposterior loop formed by the recurrent laryngeal nerve after arising from the vagus nerve. The one on the right hooks around the front, lower, and posterior surfaces of the first part of the right subclavian artery, while that on the left hooks below the arch of the aorta and behind the attachment of the ligamentum arteriosum and then up the left side of the trachea. Developmentally the nerve turns under the sixth pair of aortic arches, the distal part of which on the left side forms the ligamentum arteriosum while on the right side this part and the fifth arch disappear so that the nerve ascends to the fourth arch, the right subclavian artery.

regulatory feedback loop   CLOSED LOOP.

Roux en Y loop   The structure that results from a surgical procedure in which a nonfunctioning loop of jejunum is anastomosed to the remaining proximal small bowel about 40 cm downstream. The procedure is undertaken to drain the pancreatic and/or biliary secretions following procedures.

Silastic loops   Silicon rubber fashioned into loops that, when passed once or twice around a vessel, can be used to occlude blood flow during surgery.

loops of spinal nerves   ANSAE NERVORUM SPINALIUM.

loop of Stoerck   Part of the primitive uriniferous tubule of the embryo which becomes the definitive loop of Henle and also a portion of the proximal convoluted tubule. Also called *Stoerck's loop*.

Stoerck's loop   LOOP OF STOERCK.

subclavian loop   ANSA SUBCLAVIA.

vector loop   The loop inscribed on a vectorcardiogram by cardiac electrical activity.

ventricular loop   A U-shaped loop resulting from the early bending on itself of the embryonic cardiac tube. The ventricle develops at the bottom of the loop.

loop of Vieussens   ANSA SUBCLAVIA.

loopful   The amount of fluid held by a platinum loop during the transfer of materials for microbiologic examination. It is used for estimating the concentration of organisms.

loosening   A disturbance of mental associations that renders thinking vague, diffuse, imprecise, and unfocused.

Looser   [Emil *Looser*, Swiss physician, 1877–1936]   **1** Looser's transformation zones. See under ZONE.   **2** Looser-Milkman syndrome. See under MILKMAN SYNDROME.

LOP   left occipitoposterior position (of a fetus). See under OCCIPUT POSTERIOR POSITION.

Lopez   [Jeanne A. *Lopez*, U.S. biochemist, flourished 20th century]   Lowry-Lopez-Bessey method. See under METHOD.

lophodont   [Gk *loph(os)* a ridge of ground + -ODONT]   Denoting a dentition in which the molar cusps fuse to form ridges, characteristic of horses and other grazing animals.

lophophorine $C_{13}H_{17}NO_3$. An extremely toxic alkaloid found in the cactus *Lophophora williamsii*. It has strychninelike effects if ingested.

lophotrichous   In bacteria, possessing multiple flagella at one pole only. Compare PERITRICHOUS.

Lorain   [Paul Joseph *Lorain*, French physician, 1827–1875]   **1** See under DISEASE.   **2** Lévi-Lorain infantilism, Lorain's infantilism, Lorain-Lévi syndrome, Lévi-Lorain type, Lorain type. See under HYPOPHYSIAL DWARFISM.   **3** Lévi-Lorain dwarf, Lorain-Lévi dwarf. See under HYPOPHYSIAL DWARF.

Lorand   [Lazlo *Lorand*, Hungarian-born U.S. physiologist, born 1923]   Laki-Lorand factor. See under FACTOR XIII.

lorazepam $C_{15}H_{10}Cl_2N_2O_2$. 7-Chloro-5-(2-chloro-phenyl)-1,3-dihydro-3-hydroxy-2*H*-1,4-benzodiazopin-2-one. A benzodiazepine drug with actions and uses like those of diazepam.

lorbamate $C_{12}H_{22}N_2O_4$. 2-(Hydroxymethyl)-2-methyl-pentyl cyclopropanecarbamate ester. It has been used as a muscle-relaxant drug.

lorchel   [German, lorel (a fungus)]   BEEFSTEAK FUNGUS.

lordoscoliosis   Increased lordosis in association with the lateral deviation of a scoliosis in the lumbar vertebrae.

lordosis   [Gk *lordōsis* (from *lordoun* to bend the body forward and inward + -*ōsis* -OSIS) a bending forward and inward]   **1** The anatomical anterior concavity of the cervical and lumbar vertebrae.   **2** An abnormally increased anatomical anterior concavity of the cervical and lumbar vertebrae. Also called *dorsal lordosis, cervical lordosis, hollow-back, backward curvature, saddle back, sway back.*

cervical lordosis   LORDOSIS.

compenstory lordosis   An increased anterior concave curvature of the lumbar spine taken up to balance the rest of the proximal spine or a pelvic obliquity deformity.

dorsal lordosis   LORDOSIS.

lordotic   **1** Of or relating to lordosis.   **2** Exhibiting lordosis.

lore   [L *lor(um)* a leather thong, string, or strap]   The space between the eye and the base of the bill of a bird or between the eye and the nasal area of fishes and reptiles.

Lorenz   [Adolf *Lorenz*, Austrian orthopedic surgeon, 1854–1946]   **1** Hoffa-Lorenz operation. See under LORENZ OPERATION.   **2** See under METHOD, SIGN, OSTEOTOMY.

Lorenzini   [Stefano *Lorenzini*, Italian physician, flourished 17th century]   Lorenzini ampullae. See under AMPULLA.

Loreta   [Pietro *Loreta*, Italian surgeon, 1831–1889]   See under OPERATION.

Lorfan   A proprietary name for levallorphan tartrate.

Lorrain Smith   See under SMITH.

loss / **anaphase lag loss**   SOMATIC NONDISJUNCTION.

autoimmune sensorineural hearing loss   Bilateral sensorineural hearing loss due to inflammatory changes produced by the deposition in the ear of autoimmune antigen-antibody complexes. It is usually confined to the inner ear and is progressive over weeks or months. Vestibular responses are diminished or lost and facial paralysis may occur. Consistent improvement has been reported with dexamethasone and cyclophosphamide therapy. Also called *immune complex associated deafness*.

birth loss   REPRODUCTIVE WASTAGE.

coincidence loss   Undercounting in a radiation detector due to the occurrence of ionizing events at a rate faster than the resolution time of the counting system.

conductive hearing loss   Hearing loss arising from causes in the external meatus or in the middle-ear cleft and its contained structures. Also called *conductive hearing impairment, transmission deafness*.

congenital hearing loss   Hearing loss present from birth or occurring in the perinatal period. It may arise from genetic or intrauterine causes.

dissociated sensory loss   Sensory impairment with one form of sensation, such as touch, pain or temperature, or position and joint sense, being affected more severely than the other forms. Also called *dissociation of sensation* (seldom used).

evaporative water loss   Water that is lost through the skin when the vapor pressure of the skin exceeds that of the ambient air. Such loss is about 500 ml per day in normal adults, and may be ten times greater in patients with severe burns.

hearing loss   **1** An increased auditory threshold above normal resulting in a diminished sense or acuity of hearing. The pure tone audiogram may show a raised threshold for one or two frequencies, or there may be a greatly increased threshold across the whole range of hearing. Also called *hearing impairment, amblyacusis, amblykusis, surdity*.   **2** DEAFNESS.

monaural hearing loss   UNILATERAL HEARING LOSS.

noise-induced hearing loss   Hearing loss resulting from exposure to high ambient noise levels. Also called *noise-induced deafness, acoustic-trauma deafness*.

nonorganic hearing loss   Hearing loss for which there is no structural or neurologic basis. It usually arises out of an acute or repeatedly stressful situation in which hearing plays an important role. It is to be distinguished from the assumed deafness of malingering. Also called *hysterical deafness*.

ototoxic drug-induced hearing loss   OTOTOXIC HEARING LOSS.

ototoxic hearing loss   Hearing loss arising from exposure to therapeutic agents which cause damage to the organ of Corti or related structures. Such agents include certain alkaloids and diuretics and the aminoglycoside antibiotics. Also called *ototoxic drug-induced hearing loss, ototoxic deafness, toxic deafness* (older term).

persistent hearing loss   Any form of hearing loss which does not improve spontaneously or as a result of treatment.

profound hearing loss   Hearing loss to such a degree that there may be no sensation of hearing for even the loudest environmental sounds. The pure tone audiogram is usually considered as showing a profound loss when the threshold is 90 dB HL or worse.

saddle sensory loss   Loss or impairment of sensation in the perineum and medial aspect of the buttocks, resulting usually from a low cauda equina lesion. The area affected is the part of the body which would come into contact with a saddle.

sensorineural hearing loss   Hearing loss arising out of pathologic changes affecting the biochemistry, electric potential, vascular supply and end organ structures within the cochlea, or its neural connections with the brainstem and the cochlear nuclei. Also called *sensorineural deafness, neural deafness, perceptive deafness* (outmoded), *acoustic paralysis*.

sudden hearing loss   Abrupt loss or deterioration of hearing. The loss usually arises unexpectedly in an ear which may have shown normal hearing, or may occur in an ear in which there was some degree of loss already present. Also called *apoplectiform deafness*.

unilateral hearing loss   Hearing loss affecting one ear while the hearing in the other ear remains normal. The hearing of the affected ear is often profoundly impaired. Also called *monaural hearing loss*.

water loss   Loss of water from the body in urine and stools, by insensible losses from the skin and expired air, and by sweating.

Lossen [Herman Friedrich *Lossen*, German surgeon, 1842–1909] See under RULE.

LOT   left occipitotransverse position (of a fetus). See under OCCIPUT TRANSVERSE POSITION.

lot.   *lotio* (L, lotion).

lota   PINTA.

lota tokelau   TINEA IMBRICATA.

Lotheissen [Georg *Lotheissen*, German surgeon, 1868–1941] See under OPERATION.

lotio [L (from *lotus*, a past part. of *lavare* to wash, bathe), a washing, lotion]   LOTION.

lotio acidi sulphurosi   A lotion containing sulfurous acid, tannic acid, and glycerin.

lotio acidi tannici   A lotion containing tannic acid and mercuric chloride, used in the past to treat burns.

lotio adstringens   A lotion containing sulfuric acid, alcohol, and turpentine.

lotio alba   WHITE LOTION.

lotio calaminae oleosa   OILY LOTION OF CALAMINE.

lotio calcii hydroxidi oleosa   An emulsion of linseed oil and lime water, used in the past to treat burns. Also called *carron oil*.

lotio cupri et zinci sulphati   A lotion containing copper sulfate and zinc sulfate.

lotio evaporans   EVAPORATING LOTION.

lotio phenolis   A lotion containing phenol and amaranth in water.

lotio plumbi et glycerini   A freshly prepared lotion containing lead subacetate and glycerin.

lotio potassae sulphuratae cum zinco   WHITE LOTION.

lotio sulphurata   A freshly prepared lotion containing potassium sulfate, acetone, glycerin, and lavender oil in water.

lotio sulphuris composita   A lotion composed of sulfur, alcohol, glycerin, tincture of quillaia, and a solution of calcium hydroxide.

lotio zinci sulphatis   LOTION OF ZINC SULFATE.

lotion [L *lotio*. See LOTIO.]   A liquid preparation for external application containing suspended or emulsified medicinal ingredients. Also called *lotio*.

benzyl benzoate lotion   A lotion containing a dilute aqueous solution of benzoyl benzoate.

calamine lotion   A lotion containing calamine, zinc oxide, glycerin, bentonite, and calcium hydroxide.

evaporating lotion   A lotion containing alcohol, ammonium chloride, and water. Also called *lotio evaporans*.

Goulard's lotion   A lotion containing a dilute solution of lead subacetate. Also called *lotion of lead*.

lotion of lead   GOULARD'S LOTION.

oily lotion of calamine   A lotion consisting of an oily emulsion of calamine, oleic acid, wool fat, arachis oil, and a solution of calcium hydroxide. Also called *lotio calaminae oleosa*.

phenolated calamine lotion   A modified preparation of calamine lotion containing 1% phenol.

white lotion   A lotion containing potassium sulfate and zinc sulfate in water. Also called *lotio alba, lotio potassae sulphuratae cum zinco*.

lotion of zinc sulfate   A lotion containing zinc sulfate and amaranth in water. Also called *lotio zinci sulphatis*.

Lotusate   A proprietary name for talbutal.

louchettes [French, formerly glasses worn to correct strabismus]   A monocular occlusion device for suppression amblyopia.

loudness   **1** The intensity of a sound or noise. It may be expressed in phons.   **2** The attribute of sound which enables the hearer to classify it by intensity of effect, one of the fundamental psychological qualities of auditory sensation. It has a nonlinear relation to the physical intensity of a sound, the relation being partly dependent on frequency.

Louis [Pierre-Charles-Alexandre *Louis*, French physician, 1787–1872]   **1** See under LAW.   **2** Angle of Louis. See under ANGULUS STERNI.

Louis-Bar [Denise *Louis-Bar*, European physician, flourished mid-20th century]   Louis-Bar disease, Louis-Bar syndrome. See under ATAXIA-TELANGIECTASIA.

loupe [French, a lens of biconvex glass for magnifying]   A small magnifying lens.

binocular telescopic loupe   A magnifying device for use with both eyes.

louping-ill [Middle English *loup(en)* to leap + -ING + English *ill*, a term for veterinary disease]   OVINE ENCEPHALOMYELITIS.

louse [Old English *lūs*]   (*plural* lice) A small, dorsoventrally flattened insect that is ectoparasitic on mammals or birds, belonging to the order Anoplura (sucking lice) or Mallophaga (biting or chewing lice).

biting louse   A member of the insect order Mallophaga. Also called *chewing louse*.

body louse   A louse of the subspecies *Pediculus humanus humanus*. Also called *clothes louse*.

chewing louse   BITING LOUSE.

clothes louse   BODY LOUSE.

crab louse   PUBIC LOUSE.

head louse A louse of the subspecies *Pediculus humanus capitis.*

pubic louse A louse of the species *Pthirus pubis.* Also called *crab louse*, *crab* (popular), *morpion* (popular French).

sucking louse A member of the insect order Anoplura.

lousicide [*lous(e)* + *i* + -CIDE] PEDICULICIDE.

lousiness PEDICULOSIS.

lousy [*lous(e)* + -Y] Infested with lice.

love / Dorian love An obsolete term for MALE HOMOSEXUALITY.

mother love Affection, possessiveness, devotion, and protectiveness which a mother has toward the child she has borne.

smother love Overprotectiveness, overpossessiveness, and total control that is exhibited under the guise of love and concern but which deprives the object of any possibility of achieving independence. Also called *maternal overprotection.*

transference love In psychiatry, feelings of love for and overestimation of the analyst, positive transference, based upon the subject's infantile or childhood relationship with parents or parental figures.

Lovelace [William Randolph *Lovelace* II, U.S. surgeon, 1907–1965] See under BLB MASK.

Loven [Otto Christian *Loven*, Swedish physician, 1835–1904] See under REFLEX.

Lovibond [Joseph Williams *Lovibond*, English physicist, 1833–1918] See under UNIT.

Løvset [Jorgen *Løvset*, Norwegian obstetrician, flourished 20th century] Løvset's method. See under MANEUVER.

Low [George C. *Low*, English physician, 1872–1952] Castellani-Low symptom. See under SYMPTOM.

low-cervical Denoting animal preparations in which a cervical transection of the neuraxis is made at the C₆ level or lower (i.e., with retention of diaphragmatic breathing). Attention is usually centered on nervous functions below the transection.

Lowe [Charles Upton *Lowe*, U.S. pediatrician, born 1921] **1** Lowe oculocerebrorenal syndrome. See under LOWE SYNDROME. **2** Lowe-Terrey-MacLachlan syndrome, Lowe's disease. See under OCULOCEREBRORENAL SYNDROME.

Löwe [Karl F. *Löwe*, German optician, 1874–1955] See under RING.

Löwenberg [Benjamin Benno *Löwenberg*, German-born French laryngologist, 1836–1905] **1** See under FORCEPS. **2** Löwenberg's canal, scala of Löwenberg. See under DUCTUS COCHLEARIS.

Löwenstein [Ernst *Löwenstein*, Austrian-born U.S. pathologist, 1878–1950] Löwenstein-Jensen agar, Löwenstein-Jensen medium. See under AGAR.

Löwenthal [Wilhelm *Lowenthal*, German physician, 1850–1894] Löwenthal's tract. See under TRACTUS TECTOSPINALIS.

Lower [Richard *Lower*, English physiologist, 1631–1691] **1** Lower's rings. See under ANNULI FIBROSI CORDIS. **2** See under SAC. **3** Fasciculus of Lower, Lower's tubercle, tuberculum lowerii, tuberculum intervenosum lowerii. See under TUBERCULUM INTERVENOSUM.

Lown [Bernard *Lown*, U.S. cardiologist, born 1921] Lown-Ganong-Levine syndrome. See under SHORT PR SYNDROME.

Lowry [Oliver Howe *Lowry*, U.S. pharmacologist and biochemist, born 1910] Lowry-Lopez-Bessey method. See under METHOD.

Lowsley [Oswald Swinney *Lowsley*, U.S. urologist, 1884–1955] See under OPERATION.

low-spin Denoting the state of a transition metal in which the electrons have as few unpaired spins as possible. They therefore leave some orbitals empty, and this is energetically favored if those orbitals are raised in energy by interaction with electrons of ligands. The iron of oxyhemoglobin is in the low-spin state, because the oxygen ligand raises the energy of one of its orbitals. The change in spin state on oxygenation allows the iron atom to fit more closely into the plane of the porphyrin, and this movement triggers the change of conformation that facilitates binding of oxygen molecules to the other heme groups of the molecule.

loxapine $C_{18}H_{18}ClN_3O.$ 2-Chloro-11-(4-methylpiperazinyl)dibenz[*b,f*][1,4]oxazepine. A tricyclic antipsychotic drug, also used for its tranquilizing properties.

loxapine succinate $C_{18}H_{18}ClN_3O\cdot C_4H_6O_4.$ A dibenzoxazepine drug with antipsychotic actions like the phenothiazines. It is used as a minor tranquilizer.

loxarthron [Gk *lox(os)* oblique, crosswise + *arthron* a joint, esp. the socket] A developmental deformity of a joint without dislocation of the bones involved, such as talipes and arthrogryposis. A seldom used term. Also called *loxarthrosis.*

loxarthrosis LOXARTHRON.

loxarthrus An individual afflicted with loxarthron.

loxia TORTICOLLIS.

loxocyesis [Gk *loxo(s)* slanting, crosswise + *kyēsis* pregnancy] Oblique displacement of the pregnant uterus.

loxophthalmus [Gk *lox(os)* slanting, crosswise + *ophthalmos* the eye] MANIFEST DEVIATION.

Loxosceles [Gk *loxo(s)* slanting, crosswise, oblique + *skelos* the leg] A genus of spiders in the family Loxoscelidae (or in some classifications, Scytodidae); the brown or fiddleback spiders. They are characterized by having six eyes (instead of the usual eight), tawny color, and a flattened, heavily sclerotized carapace, on which some species have a pattern suggestive of a violin. Certain species of the western hemisphere are often found in human dwellings and have a bite that can be seriously poisonous. See also LOXOSCELISM.

Loxosceles laeta The Chilean brown spider, which has a cytotoxic venom, medically important as a cause of loxoscelism in South America. The venom causes localized cellulitis and necrosis, hemorrhage, and a strong leukocytic and eosinophilic response. Some consider this severe clinical reaction to indicate an autopharmacologic response as well. About 5 percent of reported cases have resulted in death.

Loxosceles reclusa A species found principally in the south central United States; the brown recluse or violin spider. Its bite commonly results in local cutaneous necrosis and sometimes persistent ulceration. A number of deaths following systemic complications have been reported.

loxoscelism [*Loxoscel(es)* + -ISM] Poisoning from the bite of a spider of the genus *Loxosceles*, such as the South American *L. laeta* or the North American *L. reclusa*, the brown recluse. The hemolytic and necrotizing venom produces a long-lasting ulcerative lesion that often leaves a disfiguring scar at the site of the bite. Fever, muscle weakness, nausea, and vomiting are commonly observed.

viscerocutaneous loxoscelism Loxoscelism that progresses to serious systemic manifestations such as hemolytic anemia, thrombocytopenia, and sometimes death.

Loxosomatidae [Gk *loxo(s)* slanting, crosswise + *sōmat(a)*, pl. of *sōma* body + -IDAE] A family of sessile pseudocoelomates in the phylum Entoprocta. Members are solitary and attached to a substratum with a stalk. The pseudocoel of the calyx and stalk are continuous, and buds arise from the sides of the calyx.

Loxotrema ovatum METAGONIMUS YOKOGAWAI.

lozenge [Middle English *losenge*, from Middle French *losange* a diamond-shaped heraldic figure, prob. from Old French *lauze* a flat stone] A tablet containing a medication in a flavored and sweetened base. It is designed for local treatment of the mouth and throat by the steady release of the medicine while the mass slowly dissolves in the mouth. Also called *troche, trochiscus, morsulus, rotula.*

LP **1** lumbar puncture. **2** light perception.

LPF lymphocytosis-promoting factor.

LPH lipotropic hormone.

LPS lipopolysaccharide.

Lr **1** Symbol for the element, lawrencium. **2** Immunological symbol for limit of reachon. **3** Symbol for the Limes reacting dose of diphtheria toxin.

LRF luteinizing hormone releasing factor (gonadotropin releasing hormone).

LSA left sacroanterior position (of a fetus). See under SACRUM ANTERIOR POSITION.

LSD lysergic acid diethylamide.

LSH lutein-stimulating hormone.

LSP left sacroposterior position (of a fetus). See under SACRUM POSTERIOR POSITION.

LST left sacrotransverse position (of a fetus). See under SACRUM TRANSVERSE POSITION.

LT **1** labile toxin. **2** lymphotoxin.

LTH luteotropic hormone.

Lu Symbol for the element, lutetium.

lubb An onomatopoeic term used to represent the first heart sound on auscultation.

lubb-dupp The onomatopoeic syllables allegedly made during the first and second heart sounds on auscultation.

lubricant An agent used to reduce friction between two surfaces in contact.

Lubs [Herbert Augustus *Lubs*, Jr., U.S. physician, born 1929] See under SYNDROME.

Luc [Henri *Luc*, French laryngologist, 1855–1925] **1** See under FORCEPS. **2** Ogston-Luc operation. See under OPERATION. **3** Luc's operation. See under CALDWELL-LUC OPERATION.

Lucae [Johann Constantin August *Lucae*, German otologist, 1835–1911] Lucae's pressor. See under PROBE.

lucanthone hydrochloride $C_{20}H_{25}ClN_2OS$. 1-(2-Diethylaminoethylamino)-4-methylthiaxanthone hydrochloride. An antischistosomal drug used in the treatment of both urinary tract and intestinal schistosomiasis.

Lucas [Richard Clement *Lucas*, English anatomist and surgeon, 1846–1915] **1** Groove of Lucas. See under STRIA SPINOSA. **2** See under SIGN.

Lucatello [Luigi *Lucatello*, Italian physician, 1863–1926] See under SIGN.

lucent [L *lucens*, gen. *lucentis*, pres. part. of *lucere* to shine, light] **1** RADIOLUCENT. **2** TRANSLUCENT.

Lucherini [Tommaso *Lucherini*, Italian physician, born 1891] Lucherini-Giacobini syndrome. See under SYNDROME.

Luciani [Luigi *Luciani*, Italian physiologist, 1840–1919] See under TRIAD.

lucid **1** Easily understood; clear. **2** Able to think clearly.

luciferase An enzyme which catalyzes, in the presence of adenosine triphosphate, the transfer of an electron from luciferin to oxygen, with the emission of light. The reaction is the basis of the bioluminescence which occurs in fireflies, glowworms, certain bacteria, and some fungi.

luciferin Any of several substances involved in the emission of light by a living organism. Luciferins are chemically diverse, according to the organism. They are oxidized enzymatically (with luciferase) by molecular oxygen to form a product in an elec-

tronically excited state. This product can lose its excitation with emission of light.

Lucilia [New L, possibly from L *lux*, gen. *lucis*, light + *l* + -IA] A genus of blowflies (Calliphoridae) known popularly as greenbottle flies.

Lucilia caesar An Old World species of blowfly which normally breeds in decaying meat or carrion. The larvae were formerly used in treatment of septic wounds. Larvae sometimes cause traumatic and cutaneous myiasis in humans, while the adult, like *Musca domestica* and other filth flies, has been implicated as a carrier of the cholera vibrio. Accidental intestinal myiasis has also been reported.

Lucilia cuprina PHAENICIA CUPRINA.

Lucilia illustris A blowfly that normally deposits its eggs in the carcasses of animals. Occasionally they are found in sheep wool and may be responsible for traumatic or cutaneous myiasis. It is widely distributed in North America as an open woodland and meadow fly. The maggots may carry *Clostridium botulinum*, and chickens that eat them contract a fatal botulism manifested as limberneck.

Lucilia regina PHORMIA REGINA.

Lucilia sericata PHAENICIA SERICATA.

Lucio [R. *Lucio*, Mexican physician, 1819–1866] **1** See under PHENOMENON. **2** Diffuse Leprosy of Lucio and Latapí. See under LUCIO LEPROSY.

Lucké [Balduin *Lucké*, German-born U.S. pathologist, 1889–1954] See under VIRUS.

Lücke [George Albert *Lücke*, German surgeon, 1829–1894] See under TEST.

lückenschädel [German *Lücken* gaps, breaches + *Schädel* skull] CRANIOFENESTRIA.

Luckett [William Henry *Luckett*, U.S. surgeon, born 1872] See under OPERATION.

lucotherapy PHOTOTHERAPY.

Luder [Joseph *Luder*, English pediatrician, flourished 20th century] Luder-Sheldon syndrome. See under SYNDROME.

Ludloff [Karl *Ludloff*, German orthopedic surgeon, 1864–1945] See under SIGN, OPERATION.

Ludwig [Carl Friedrich Wilhelm *Ludwig*, German anatomist and physiologist, 1816–1895] **1** See under GANGLION. **2** Ludwig's theory of urine formation. See under THEORY. **3** Isaacs-Ludwig arteriole. See under ARTERIOLE. **4** Ludwig's labyrinths. See under LABYRINTH. **5** Ludwig's nerve, depressor nerve of Ludwig. See under AORTIC NERVE.

Ludwig [Daniel *Ludwig*, German anatomist, 1625–1680] Angle of Ludwig. See under ANGULUS STERNI.

Ludwig [Wilhelm Friedrich von *Ludwig*, German surgeon, 1790–1865] **1** Angina ludovici, angina Ludwigii. See under ANGINA. **2** Aryvocalis muscle of Ludwig, Ludwig's muscle. See under ARYVOCALIS.

lues [L (akin to *luere* to wash, purge, free, atone for and to Gk *lyein* to loose, set free, dissolve, hence *lysis* a loosing; also to *louein* to wash, esp. the body, bathe), a plague, pestilence, term of reproach to criminals, melted snow, a foul person, later syphilis] SYPHILIS. Adjective: luetic.

lues hepatis Syphilis of the liver.

lues nervosa NEUROSYPHILIS.

lues tarda LATE SYPHILIS.

lues venerea SYPHILIS.

luetic [L *lu(es)* plague, contagious disease + -*etica* English -*etic*] SYPHILITIC.

luetin An extract of *Treponema pallidum* formerly used as a skin test for syphilis.

luette UVULA.

Lieutaud's luette UVULA VESICAE.

Luft [Rolf *Luft*, Swedish endocrinologist, born 1914] **1** Luft syndrome. See under HYPERMETABOLIC MYOPATHY. **2** See under DISEASE.

lug [Middle English (Scottish) *lugge*, prob. from Middle English *luggen* to lug, of Scandinavian origin.] A projection from a dental casting.

occlusal lug OCCLUSAL REST.

retention lug A lug fixed to a tooth in order to provide an undercut for the retention of an appliance.

upright lug MINOR CONNECTOR.

vertical lug MINOR CONNECTOR.

luic [L *lu(es)* plague, contagious disease + -IC] SYPHILITIC.

LUL left upper lobe (of lung).

luliberin GONADOTROPIN RELEASING HORMONE.

lumbago [L, from *lumbus* loin] Pain in the lumbar, or loin, region. Also called *lumbar rheumatism, lumbodynia*.

ischemic lumbago Pain in the lumbar region as a consequence of arterial insufficiency.

lumbar Pertaining to the loin, or lumbus.

lumbarization [LUMBAR + -*iz(e)* + -ATION] A condition in which the last thoracic vertebra or the first vertebral segment of the sacrum displays anatomic characteristics similar to or identical with those of lumbar vertebrae. The change is particularly striking with the first sacral segment, which may exhibit a degree of independent movement.

lumbo- [L *lumbus* the loins] A combining form meaning the loins, lumbar.

lumboabdominal Pertaining to the lumbar region and the abdomen.

lumbocolostomy [LUMBO- + COLOSTOMY] A surgical procedure creating an opening for drainage of the fecal colonic contents through a fistula to the skin. It is performed through a flank incision.

lumbocolotomy A surgical incision into the large intestine using a flank approach.

lumbocostal Pertaining to the lumbar region, particularly the vertebrae, and the ribs. Also *costolumbar*.

lumbocrural **1** Pertaining to the lumbar and the crural regions. **2** LUMBOINGUINAL.

lumbodorsal Pertaining to the lumbar and the dorsal regions; dorsolumbar.

lumbodynia LUMBAGO.

lumboiliac **1** Pertaining to the lumbar and iliac regions. **2** LUMBOINGUINAL.

lumboinguinal Pertaining to the lumbar and inguinal regions. Also *lumboiliac, lumbocrural*.

lumboischial Pertaining to the lumbar vertebrae and the ischium.

lumbo-ovarian Pertaining to the lumbar region and the ovary.

lumbosacral Pertaining to the lumbar vertebrae and the sarum. Also *sacrolumbar*.

lumbovertebral Pertaining to the lumbar region and the vertebrae.

lumbrical **1** Any one of the musculi lumbricales. **2** Vermiform; earthwormlike; lumbricoid.

lumbrici Plural of LUMBRICUS.

lumbricide An obsolete term for ASCARICIDE.

lumbricoid [L *lumbric(us)* earthworm + -OID] Earthworm- or ascaridlike in appearance or form.

lumbricosis [L *lumbric(us)* earthworm, intestinal worm + -OSIS] An obsolete term for ASCARIASIS.

lumbricus A worm of the genus *Ascaris*.

lumbus [L, loin] The lower part of the back, between the lowest rib and the iliac crest on either side of the vertebral column. Also called *loin*.

lumen [L (akin to Gk *lampros* bright, clear and to Gaelic *laom* flame; also to L *lucere* to shine, from *lux* light), light, lamp, window, esp. a round one, pupil of the eye, any round opening] (*plural* lumina, lumens) **1** The cavity within a tubular structure, either natural or artificial. **2** The SI derived unit of luminous flux; the luminous flux emitted within the solid angle of one steradian by a point source having a uniform intensity of one candela. Also called *candela steradian*. Symbol: lm

lumen per square foot A unit of illuminance equal to 10.7639 lumens per square meter; 10.7639 lux. Also called *foot-candle* (obsolete). Symbol: lm/ft², lm.ft^{-2}

lumen per square meter **1** The SI derived unit of illuminance, more commonly referred to by the special name lux. **2** The SI derived unit of luminous exitance. Also called *luminous emittance* (outmoded). Symbol: lm/m², lm·m^{-2}

lumen per watt The SI derived unit of luminous efficacy and spectral luminous efficacy. Symbol: lm/W, lm·W^{-1}

residual lumen The remnants of Rathke's pouch, located between the pars intermedia and the pars distalis of the pituitary gland.

lumen-hour A unit of quantity of light equal to 3.6×10^3 lumen second. Symbol: lm·h

lumen-second The SI derived unit of quantity of light; the time integral of luminous flux. Symbol: lm·s

lumichrome 6,7-Dimethylalloxazine. It is formed from riboflavin in a photochemical reaction in which ribitol is split off.

lumiflavin A substance formed from riboflavin by a photochemical reaction, particularly in alkaline solution. It contains a methyl group in place of the ribitol residue originally present.

lumina Plural of LUMEN.

Luminal A proprietary name for phenobarbital.

luminescence [L *lumen*, gen. *luminis*, light, daylight + -ESCENCE] The emission of infrared, visible, or ultraviolet light by matter from any cause other than incandescence. It is subdivided according to the nature of the stimulus: photoluminescence, from light; radioluminescence, from ionizing radiation (x rays, gamma rays, electrons, or ions); electroluminescence, from electric fields or plasmas; chemiluminescence, from chemical reactions; bioluminescence, from biologic processes; and thermoluminescence, from thermal activation of a latent stimulus from another origin.

luminiferous [L *lumen*, gen. *luminis*, light + -FEROUS] Capable of transmitting light.

luminoscope An instrument which scans the surface of coalgasification workers suspected of contamination with toxic polycyclic aromatic hydrocarbons. Ultraviolet light at 365 nanometers is transmitted by fiberoptics and resultant fluorescent light is detected by a photomultiplier tube.

lumirhodopsin An intermediate photopigment in the degradation of rhodopsin.

lumisomes [*lumi(nescent)* + -*some*, combining form from Gk *sōma* body + *s*] Membrane-enclosed cytoplasmic vesicles, 0.1–0.2 µm in diameter, within which the bioluminescent reactions of certain cells occur.

lumisterol The sterol produced by the action of light on ergosterol. It differs from ergosterol by inversion of the configuration of the methyl group at C-10. Further illumination leads to breakage of ring B between C-9 and C-10, with the formation of ergocalciferol, a form of vitamin D.

lump Any localized swelling, mass, tumor, or protuberant part.

surfers' lumps Nodules, usually found on the shin, that are induced by surfboard injuries.

lumpectomy [English *lump* + -ECTOMY] A localized, surgical excision of a breast mass, usually cancer, and the surrounding tissue; a tylectomy used especially in the treatment of breast cancer.

Lumsden [Thomas William *Lumsden*, English physician, 1874–1953] Lumsden center. See under PNEUMOTAXIC CENTER.

lunacy [*luna(tic)* + -CY] An obsolete term for INSANITY.

lunar [L *lunar(is)* (from *lun(a)* the moon + *-aris* -AR) lunar] **1** Of or relating to the moon. **2** Crescent in shape.

lunare An outmoded term for OS LUNATUM.

lunate 1 Crescent-shaped or moon-shaped; semilunar. **2** OS LUNATUM.

lunatic [Middle English *lunatik*, from Late L *lunatic(us)* moonstruck, from L *luna* the moon] A person afflicted with insanity. An obsolete term.

lunatism [L *luna* the moon + *t* + -ISM] An obsolete term for SOMNAMBULISM.

lunatomalacia KIENBÖCK'S DISEASE.

Lund [Frederick Bates *Lund*, U.S. surgeon, born 1865] See under OPERATION.

lunella [L, dim. of *luna* moon] An outmoded term for HYPOPYON.

lung [Old English *lungen*] One of a pair of highly elastic cone-shaped organs of respiration occupying the thoracic cavity, where each is surrounded by a pleural sac and separated from the other by the heart and other contents of the mediastinum; pulmo.

arc-welders' lung A benign condition which occurs in arc welders who inhale iron oxide particles. X rays of the lungs reveal reticulation and nodulation. The condition causes no symptoms and no abnormal physical signs. A similar condition can occur among welders using the oxyacetylene torch. Also called *welders' lung, arc-welders' disease.*

artificial lung A tank ventilator, respirator, or other apparatus that provides respiration in the absense of normal lung action.

bird-breeders' lung BIRD-BREEDERS' DISEASE.

bird-fanciers' lung BIRD-BREEDERS' DISEASE.

black lung COAL WORKERS' PNEUMOCONIOSIS.

budgerigar-fanciers' lung BIRD-BREEDERS' DISEASE.

cardiac lung Chronic congestion of the lung resulting from left ventricular heart failure.

carnified lung Solid, airless, fibrotic lung tissue which resembles flesh in appearance.

coal miners' lung COAL WORKERS' PNEUMOCONIOSIS.

colliers' lung COAL WORKERS' PNEUMOCONIOSIS.

drowned lung A lung which is diffusely filled with exudate and contains no air. An obsolete term.

eosinophilic lung TROPICAL PULMONARY EOSINOPHILIA.

farmers' lung A common form of extrinsic allergic alveolitis, occurring among farmers from the inhalation of moldy hay. In its acute stage it is characterized by general malaise, slight fever, and dyspnea. Repeated exposure causes pulmonary fibrosis with emphysema. Also called *harvesters' lung, threshers' lung.*

fibroid lung A lung affected with chronic interstitial pneumonia and fibrosis. An obsolete term.

fluid lung WET LUNG.

harvesters' lung FARMERS' LUNG.

honeycomb lung A roentgenographic appearance of the lung, consisting of multiple small areas of radiolucency with intervening borders of soft-tissue density, seen in interstitial pulmonary disease with fibrosis.

hydrostatic lung The edematous lung seen in illnesses such as hypostatic pneumonia.

hyperlucent lung A lung which casts abnormally few shadows on chest radiograph, usually due to emphysema, overinfla-

tion, or reduction of blood flow.

iron lung A popular term for TANK VENTILATOR.

masons' lung STONEMASONS' DISEASE.

mushroom workers' lung MUSHROOM WORKERS' DISEASE.

pigeon-breeder's lung BIRD-BREEDERS' DISEASE.

pigeon-fanciers' lung BIRD-BREEDERS' DISEASE.

postperfusion lung A condition of atelectasis, pulmonary arterial venous shunting, and consolidation of the lung that is seen following cardiopulmonary bypass. Also called *pump lung.*

pump lung POSTPERFUSION LUNG.

quiet lung Collapse of a lung to facilitate chest surgery.

shock lung ADULT RESPIRATORY DISTRESS SYNDROME.

threshers' lung FARMERS' LUNG.

traumatic wet lung ADULT RESPIRATORY DISTRESS SYNDROME.

trench lung Hysterical dyspnea occurring in the trenches in the First World War.

uremic lung A complication of both acute and chronic renal failure characterized by dyspnea, orthopnea, and a perihilar vascular congestion and pulmonary edema yielding a "butterfly" pattern on roentgenograms. The etiology is controversial. Some believe it is due to uremic toxins, but most authorities believe it is due to circulatory overload. Also called *uremic pneumonitis* (imprecise).

vanishing lung Any condition in which the lung appears radiographically to become smaller or less opaque.

Vietnam lung ADULT RESPIRATORY DISTRESS SYNDROME.

welders' lung ARC-WELDERS' LUNG.

wet lung An edematous lung; pulmonary edema. Also called *fluid lung.*

white lung PNEUMONIA ALBA.

lungfish A fish of the order Dipnoi, having a swim bladder that functions as a lung.

lungmotor An obsolete apparatus for forcing gases into the lungs.

lungworm [English *lung* + *worm*] A parasitic nematode found in the lungs and airways of animals. Most are in the family Metastrongylidae, with genera such as *Metastrongylus, Neometastrongylus, Aelurostrongylus,* and *Crenosoma,* the family Dictyocaulidae which includes the genus *Dictyocaulus,* and the family Protostrongylidae, including such genera as *Protostrongylus, Pneumostrongylus,* and *Muellerius.*

red lungworm A lungworm of the species *Protostrongylus rufescens.*

lunula [L (from *luna* moon + -ULA -ULE) a little moon, half-moon-shaped ornament worn by women] (*plural* lunulae) **1** A small or narrow crescent-shaped or moon-shaped marking or structure; half-moon; demilune. Also called *lunule.* **2** [NA] An opaque white semilunar area at the proximal end of the body and the root of the nail where the papillae are less vascular. It is partially covered by the eponychium. Also called *lunula unguis, lunule of nail, selene unguium.*

lunulae of aortic valves LUNULAE VALVULARUM SEMILUNARIUM AORTAE.

lunulae of pulmonary trunk valves LUNULAE VALVULARUM SEMILUNARIUM TRUNCI PULMONALIS.

lunula of scapula An outmoded term for INCISURA SCAPULAE.

lunulae of semilunar valves of aorta LUNULAE VALVULARUM SEMILUNARIUM AORTAE.

lunulae of semilunar valves of pulmonary trunk LUNULAE VALVULARUM SEMILUNARIUM TRUNCI PULMONALIS.

lunula unguis LUNULA.

lunulae valvularum aortae An outmoded term for LUNULAE VALVULARUM SEMILUNARIUM AORTAE.

lunulae valvularum semilunarium aortae [NA] Crescentic

areas of thinning of the free edges of the three semilunar cusps, or valvules, of the aortic valve, one thin area being on each side of the thick nodule in the center of the margin of each cusp. Also called *lunulae of aortic valves, lunulae of semilunar valves of aorta, lunulae valvularum aortae* (outmoded).

lunulae valvularum semilunarium arteriae pulmonalis An outmoded term for LUNULAE VALVULARUM SEMILUNARIUM TRUNCI PULMONALIS.

lunulae valvularum semilunarium trunci pulmonalis [NA] Crescentic areas of thinning of the free edges of the three semilunar cusps, or valvules, of the pulmonary valve, one thin area being on each side of the thick nodule in the center of the margin of each cusp. Also called *lunulae of pulmonary trunk valves, lunulae of semilunar valves of pulmonary trunk, lunulae valvularum semilunarium arteriae pulmonalis* (outmoded).

lunulae Plural of LUNULA.

lunule LUNULA.

lunule of nail LUNULA.

lupia [L *lup(us)* a wolf, voracious fish, pike + -IA] A localized eyelid mass. An obsolete term.

lupiform LUPOID.

lupinine $C_{10}H_{19}NO$. Octahydroquinolizine-1-methanol, a solid alkaloid obtained from *Lupinus luteus* and other species.

lupoid Resembling lupus vulgaris. Also *lupiform*.

lupoma [L *lup(us)* a wolf + -OMA] A small granulomatous nodule characteristic of lupus vulgaris.

lupous Pertaining to lupus.

lupulin A yellowish brown powder made from the hairs, or glandular trichomes, separated from the catkin of the hop, *Humulus lupulus*. The powder contains an oil composed of the terpene humulene, esters of valeric acid and other acids, the bitter principle humulol, resins, and waxes. It is used as a tonic and mild hypnotic. Also called *humulin*.

lupus [L (akin to Gk *lykos* a wolf, in pl. spikes on a horse's bit), a wolf, voracious fish, hook or drag, bit with points like a wolf's teeth; later a corrosive ulcer, with *vulgaris* common, usual, a skin tuberculosis] **1** A popular term for LUPUS VULGARIS. **2** A popular term for LUPUS ERYTHEMATOSUS. • The term is used in combination with the designation of a specific disease and of itself has no specific meaning.

lupus atrophicus A circumscribed atrophy in a cutaneous lesion of lupus erythematosus.

bat's-wing lupus BUTTERFLY LUPUS.

butterfly lupus Lupus erythematosus that appears in a butterfly-shaped patch on the nose and cheeks. Also called *bat's-wing lupus, lupus sebaceus*.

chronic lupus erythematosus Lupus erythematosus that is of long duration and usually confined to the skin.

lupus crustosus Crusted lupus vulgaris.

discoid lupus erythematosus A form of lupus erythematosus in which only the skin is involved, with a characteristic rash but with no visceral involvement. It presents as plaques of erythema and telangiectasis with follicular plugging.

lupus discretus Disseminated lupus vulgaris with scattered small lesions.

disseminated lupus erythematosus SYSTEMIC LUPUS ERYTHEMATOSUS.

disseminated follicular lupus ACNE AGMINATA.

drug-induced lupus erythematosus An illness similar to spontaneous systemic lupus erythematosus, but occurring after exposure to any one of several drugs, such as procaine amide, which are capable of inducing this illness. The symptoms remit upon withdrawal of the offending drug.

lupus elephantiacus Lupus vulgaris associated with lymphedema.

lupus elevatus Lupus vulgaris marked by raised lesions.

lupus endemicus CUTANEOUS LEISHMANIASIS.

lupus erythematosus An inflammatory disorder in which immunological reactions give rise to widespread abnormalities of blood vessels and of connective tissue. Also called *lupus seborrhagicus* (obsolete), *Cazenave's disease* (obsolete), *lupus* (popular).

lupus erythematosus discoides A chronic form of lupus erythematosus, with plaques of persistent erythema and prominent plugged follicles. Also called *seborrhea congestiva* (obsolete).

lupus erythematosus hypertrophicus Chronic lupus erythematosus in which dense scarring and deep involvement of the dermis is evident.

lupus erythematosus hypertrophicus et profundus LUPUS ERYTHEMATOSUS PROFUNDUS.

lupus erythematosus migrans Lupus erythematosus marked by transitory lesions.

lupus erythematosus nodularis An unusual lupus erythematosus characterized by nodular lesions.

lupus erythematosus profundus An uncommon lupus erythematosus in which warty thickened plaques extend deep into the dermis and subcutis. Also called *lupus erythematosus hypertrophicus et profundus*.

lupus erythematosus tumidus Lupus erythematosus marked by raised, indurated lesions.

lupus erythematosus unguium mutilans The destruction of the nail in lupus erythematosus, caused by cyanosis of the nail area. Adherent scales and debris of the nail plate remain. A rarely used term.

lupus exfoliativus Lupus vulgaris in which scaling occurs during the healing process.

lupus exulcerans Lupus vulgaris characterized by ulcerations.

lupus fibrosus LUPUS SCLEROSUS.

lupus gangrenosus Lupus vulgaris characterized by severe ulceration.

Hilliard's lupus Tuberculous lupus vulgaris that affects the hands and arms.

hydralazine lupus A disorder resembling systemic lupus erythematosus provoked in a proportion of subjects by the prolonged administration of the drug hydralazine and dissappearing with its discontinuance. Hydralazine lupus, however, usually does not include nephritis or antidouble-stranded DNA antibodies. Also called *hydralazine lupus syndrome*.

lupus hypertrophicus Lupus vulgaris characterized by abundant scar formation.

keloidal lupus Lupus vulgaris with keloidal scars.

laryngeal lupus Lupus vulgaris spreading from the nose by way of the pharynx to reach the supraglottic larynx. This is a rare site, the epiglottis being more commonly involved.

lupus lymphaticus An obsolete term for LYMPHANGIOMA CIRCUMSCRIPTUM.

lupus maculosus The flat, macular lesions of incipient lupus vulgaris. Also called *lupus planus*.

lupus miliaris disseminatus faciei ACNE AGMINATA.

lupus mutilans Mutilating lupus vulgaris.

lupus nodosus The nodules characteristic of lupus vulgaris.

lupus oedematosus Edematous lesions often characteristic of lupus vulgaris.

lupus papillomatosus An obsolete term for WARTY LUPUS.

lupus pernio A form of sarcoidosis in which soft, bluish red plaques appear on the nose, cheeks, ears, fingers, and hands.

lupus phagedaenicus Destructive lupus vulgaris.

photosensitive lupus erythematosus Lupus erythematosus exacerbated by exposure to sunlight.

lupus planus LUPUS MACULOSUS.

postexanthematic lupus A disseminated form of lupus vulgaris occurring after acute specific fevers in children.

lupus profundus Deep-seated cutaneous lesions of lupus erythematosus.

lupus psoriasiformis Lupus vulgaris resembling psoriasis in appearance. Also called *lupus psoriasis*.

lupus psoriasis LUPUS PSORIASIFORMIS.

lupus rodens A destructive form of lupus vulgaris. Also called *lupus vorax*.

lupus rupioides Ulcerated lupus vulgaris marked by elevated crusting.

lupus sclerosus Thickened scars complicating lupus vulgaris. Also called *lupus fibrosus, lupus vulgaris fibromatosus*.

lupus sebaceus BUTTERFLY LUPUS.

lupus seborrhagicus An obsolete term for LUPUS ERYTHEMATOSUS.

lupus serpiginosus A spreading form of tuberculous lupus.

systemic lupus erythematosus A multisystem disease of unknown etiology characterized by vasculitis, serositis, synovitis, and involvement of the kidneys, skin, and nervous system. Women are affected much more frequently than men. There are a wide variety of autoantibodies in the serum of affected subjects, particularly to nonorgan-specific intracellular components. Antinuclear antibodies to double-stranded DNA and to native DNA nucleohistone are diagnostic. Immune complexes of autoantibodies and autoantigens play an important role in the pathogenesis of the disease. Certain species other than man, including dogs and several strains of inbred mice, are also susceptible to the disease. Also called *disseminated lupus erythematosus*. Abbreviation: SLE

telangiectatic lupus Lupus erythematosus marked by superficial lesions containing small dilated blood vessels. Also called *telangiectatic lupus erythematosus*.

telangiectatic lupus erythematosus TELANGIECTATIC LUPUS.

lupus tumidus Lupus vulgaris manifested as a soft, raised nodule.

lupus verrucosus WARTY LUPUS.

lupus vorax LUPUS RODENS.

lupus vulgaris A progressive chronic form of cutaneous tuberculosis that occurs as a postprimary infection in a subject with a moderate or high degree of immunity. Also called *lupus* (popular), *tuberculosis luposa, morbus vulpis, tuberculosis cutis luposa*.

lupus vulgaris erythematodes Superficial erythematous lesions seen in lupus vulgaris that resemble lupus erythematosus. Also called *lupus vulgaris erythematoides, LeLoir's disease*.

lupus vulgaris erythematoides LUPUS VULGARIS ERYTHEMATODES.

lupus vulgaris fibromatosus LUPUS SCLEROSUS.

warty lupus Lupus vulgaris characterized by wartlike eruptions. Also called *lupus verrucosus, lupus papillomatosus* (obsolete).

lupuscarcinoma A carcinoma arising from the lesions of lupus vulgaris.

LUQ left upper quadrant (of abdomen).

lura The constricted termination of the pituitary stalk or infundibulum. An outmoded term.

Luschka [Hubert von *Luschka*, German anatomist, 1820–1875] **1** Foramen of Luschka. See under APERTURA LATERALIS VENTRICULI QUARTI. **2** Luschka's fibers. See under FIBER. **3** Luschka's body, Luschka's gland, Luschka's ganglion. See under GLOMUS COCCYGEUM. **4** Luschka's ducts. See under LUSCHKA'S CRYPTS. **5** Luschka sinus. See under SINUS PETROSQUAMOSUS. **6** Luschka's tubercle. See under CARINA URETHRALIS VAGINAE. **7** Glandular foveae of Luschka. See under FOVEOLAE GRANULARES. **8** Luschka's bursa. See under BURSA PHARYNGEALIS. **9** Luschka subpharyngeal cartilage. See under CARTILAGE. **10** Luschka's crypts. See under ROKITANSKY-ASCHOFF SINUSES OF THE GALLBLADDER. **11** Internal coat of pharynx of Luschka. See under TELA SUBMUCOSA PHARYNGIS. **12** Joints of Luschka. See under JOINT. **13** Cricotracheal ligament of Luschka. See under LIGAMENT. **14** Luschka's fossa. See under RECESSUS ILEOCECALIS SUPERIOR. **15** Luschka's tonsil. See under TONSILLA PHARYNGEALIS. **16** Nerve of Luschka. See under RAMUS MENINGEUS NERVORUM SPINALIUM. **17** Nerve of Luschka. See under NERVUS ETHMOIDALIS POSTERIOR. **18** Laryngeal cartilage of Luschka, Luschka's cartilage, cartilago sesamoidea laryngis (Luschka). See under CARTILAGO SESAMOIDEA. **19** Liagments of Luschka. See under LIGAMENTA STERNOPERICARDIACA. **20** Luschka's muscles. See under MUSCULUS RECTOUTERINUS.

Lust [Franz Alexander *Lust*, German pediatrician, born 1880] Lust's phenomenon, Lust's reflex. See under SIGN.

lust Powerful craving or passion, often with the connotation of prurient or lascivious sexual desire.

Lustig [Alessandro *Lustig*, Italian pathologist and bacteriologist, 1857–1937] Lustig-Galeotti vaccine. See under VACCINE.

luteal [*lute(o)-* + *-AL*] Pertaining to, arising from, having the characteristics of, or involving the corpus luteum. Also *luteinic*.

luteectomy [*(corpus) lute(um)* + *-ECTOMY*] The surgical removal of the corpus luteum.

luteinic LUTEAL.

luteinization The transformation of granulosa cells into lutein cells in the formation of the corpus luteum of the ovary. Other cells may undergo luteinization, including theca cells, and coelomic and cervical cells.

luteinize To subject to the process of or undergo luteinization.

Lutembacher [René *Lutembacher*, French cardiologist, 1884–1916] Lutembacher's complex, Lutembacher's disease. See under SYNDROME.

luteo- [L *luteus* (from *lutum* yellow dye) golden yellow, saffron yellow, or orange yellow; *luteum* a yellow body] A combining form meaning yellow, yellowish.

luteogenic [LUTEO- + -GENIC] Inducing the growth, development, or hormonal secretion of the corpus luteum; luteinizing.

luteohormone [LUTEO- + HORMONE] An older term for PROGESTERONE.

luteoid **1** Like or acting like progesterone. **2** A luteoid substance.

luteolin A flavone pigment found in the mignonette (*Reseda luteola*) and foxglove, and used as a dye.

luteolysin A hypothetical hormonelike agent from the uterine endometrium that is believed to cause the dissolution of the corpus luteum.

luteolysis Destruction or natural involution of the corpus luteum.

luteoma [*lute(o)-* + *-OMA*] **1** A growth of hyperplastic nodules made up of lutein cells of the ovary, sometimes found in the third trimester of pregnancy, occurring most commonly in black women, and in some cases having the property of secreting androgenic hormones. They are not true tumors and they regress after parturition. Also called *luteoma of pregnancy*. **2** LIPOID CELL TUMOR OF OVARY.

luteoma of pregnancy LUTEOMA.

luteotrophic LUTEOTROPIC.

luteotrophin PROLACTIN.

luteotropic [LUTEO- + -TROPIC[2]] Promoting or stimulating the development, maturation, or hormonal secretion of the corpus luteum. Also *luteotrophic*.

luteotropin PROLACTIN.

lutetium Element number 71, having atomic weight 174.967. It is a silvery white metal of the lanthanide series. There are two natural isotopes, the stable lutetium 175 (97.4% natural abundance) and radioactive lutetium 176 (2.6%), having a half-life of 3×10^{10} years. Many synthetic unstable isotopes have been identified. Symbol: Lu

lutidine Any of the isomeric dimethylpyridines in which both methyl groups are on carbon atoms of the pyridine ring. 2,6-Lutidine is used as a basic solvent in organic synthesis when a base of low nucleophilic reactivity is required. The methyl groups flanking the nitrogen atom lower its reactivity by steric hindrance.

Lutocylol A proprietary name for ethisterone.

Lutrexin A proprietary name for lututrin.

Lutromone A proprietary name for progesterone.

lututrin A water soluble, relaxinlike factor from the corpus luteum of sow ovaries. It has been used as a uterine relaxant.

Lutz [Adolfo *Lutz*, Brazilian bacteriologist, 1855–1940] **1** Lutz-Jeanselme nodules. See under NODULE. **2** Lutz-Splendore-Almeida disease. See under SOUTH AMERICAN BLASTOMYCOSIS.

Lutz [Wilhelm *Lutz*, Swiss dermatologist, 1888–1958] Lewandowsky-Lutz disease. See under EPIDERMODYSPLASIA VERRUCIFORMIS.

Lutzomyia [origin unknown] A New World genus of sandflies, family Psychodidae, subfamily Phlebotominae, that includes a number of vectors of American cutaneous and visceral leishmaniasis (*Leishmania mexicana* and *L. brasiliensis* complexes and *L chagasi*). Sandflies of this genus play a role in New World leishmaniasis comparable to that of *Phlebotomus* species in the Old World disease.

Lutzomyia flaviscutellata The vector of *Leishmania mexicana amazonensis*, agent of a mild, nonulcerating form of cutaneous leishmaniasis in the Amazon basin and the state of Mato Grosso in Brazil. In this same area and in Venezuela, this sandfly has also been implicated as the probable vector of *L. pifanoi*, agent of diffuse cutaneous leishmaniasis. In Trinidad it has been implicated in the transmission of a subspecies of *L. mexicana*, causing a local form of cutaneous leishmaniasis. Also called *Phlebotomus flaviscutellatus*.

Lutzomyia intermedia A vector of *Leishmania braziliensis braziliensis*, agent of mucocutaneous leishmaniasis in the rainforests of Brazil, Peru, Ecuador, Bolivia, Venezuela, Paraguay, and Colombia. The role of this sandfly has been demonstrated by inoculating hamsters. Also called *Phlebotomus intermedius*.

Lutzomyia longipalpis The principal sandfly vector of *Leishmania chagasi* (or *L. donovani chagasi*), agent of kala-azar in northern Argentina, Paraguay, Bolivia, Brazil, Venezuela, Colombia, Guatemala, El Salvador, and Mexico.

Lutzomyia olmeca A sandfly vector of *Leishmania mexicana mexicana*, agent of chiclero ulcer, a form of cutaneous leishmaniasis found among woodcutters of the Yucatan and Guatemala. A different subspecies (*L. olmeca bicolor*) has been implicated as the probable intermediate host of *Leishmania mexicana aristedesi*, agent of Herrer's cutaneous leishmaniasis, occurring in Panama.

Lutzomyia peruensis The probable sandfly vector of *Leishmania peruviana*, agent of uta, a mild form of cutaneous leishmaniasis found in the mountains of Peru, along the arid western open slopes of the Andes.

Lutzomyia pessoai A vector of *Leishmania braziliensis braziliensis*, agent of Brazilian mucocutaneous leishmaniasis or espundia in the rainforests of central and northern South America. Also called *Phlebotomus pessoai*.

Lutzomyia verrucarum A species in Peru that transmits *Bartonella bacilliformis*, causal agent of Carrion's disease or bartonellosis in the Andes. Also called *Phlebotomus verrucarum*.

lux [L, the light, daylight] (*plural* lux) A special name for the SI derived unit of illuminance, an illuminance of one lumen per square meter. Symbol: lx

luxatio [L (from *luxatus*, past part. of *luxare* to dislocate, disjoint), a dislocating] DISLOCATION.

luxatio coxae congenita CONGENITAL DISLOCATION OF THE HIP.

luxatio erecta DISLOCATIO ERECTA.

luxatio perinealis A perineal dislocation of the femoral head.

luxation [L *luxatio*. See LUXATIO.] DISLOCATION.

luxation of the globe Displacement of the eye from its normal position within the orbit.

Malgaigne's luxation The dislocation of the radial head out of the annular ligament.

luxon [L *lux* light, brilliance + *-on* as in *photon*] TROLAND.

luxuriant Rich and abundant in growth.

luxus [L, luxury, voluptuousness, splendor] An excess.

Luys [Georges *Luys*, French urologist, 1870–1953] Luys segregator, Luys separator. See under SEGREGATOR.

Luys [Jules Bernard *Luys*, French physician, 1828–1895] **1** Syndrome of the corpus Luysii, body of Luys syndrome. See under HEMIBALLISMUS. **2** Nucleus of Luys, body of Luys. See under NUCLEUS SUBTHALAMICUS. **3** Centrum medianum of Luys. See under NUCLEUS MEDIALIS CENTRALIS THALAMI.

LVH left ventricular hypertrophy.

Lw Former symbol for the element, lawrencium.

lx Symbol for the unit, lux.

Ly See under LY ANTIGENS.

lyapolate sodium A synthetic heparinlike anticoagulant that has had limited use in ointments for the resolution of hematomas. Also called *ethenesulfonic acid homopolymer sodium salt, sodium polyethylene sulfonate*.

lyase Any enzyme that catalyzes the elimination of one molecule from another with formation of a double bond. Examples include isocitrate lyase, which catalyzes elimination of succinate from isocitrate and leaves glyoxylate, and fumarate hydratase, which catalyzes elimination of water from malate to leave fumarate.

Lyb See under LY ANTIGENS.

lycanthropy [Gk *lyk(os)* a wolf + *anthrop(o)-* + *-y*] The delusion that one can change himself or others into a wolf or some other animal. Also called *lycomania* (obsolete).

Lycine A proprietary name for betaine.

lycomania An obsolete term for LYCANTHROPY.

lycopene $C_{40}H_{56}$. A hydrocarbon found in tomatoes and responsible for their red color. The molecule consists of eight isoprene units, each a chain of 32 carbon atoms, with methyl groups at positions 2, 6, 10, 14, 19, 23, 27, and 31, with isolated double bonds at C-2 and C-30, and a system of conjugated double bonds from C-6 to C-27. It is the parent of the carotenes, which are formed from it by cyclization of one or both ends of the molecule.

lycopenemia An abnormally high level of lycopenes in the blood plasma or serum, resulting in yellowish discoloration of the skin resembling carotenemia. It is due to high dietary intake of tomatoes or tomato juice

Lycoperdales [Gk *lyko(s)* wolf + *perd(esthai)* to break wind + L *-ales*, pl. of *-alis* -AL] An order of fungi which includes puffballs and earthstars.

Lycoperdon A genus of fungi, the puffballs, characterized by two outer layers that encompass the inner, spore-bearing gleba.

lycoperdonosis A respiratory disease resulting from inhalation of the spores of puffballs (*Lycoperdon* sp.).

lycopersicin TOMATINE.

lycopodium The spores of various species of *Lycopodium*. They are used in the preparation of dusting powders and are valued for their absorbency. Their powdery texture has been employed in the preparation of pills and suppositories, where they serve as lubricants. Also called *vegetable sulfur*.

lycorexia BULIMIA.

lycorine $C_{16}H_{17}NO_4$. An alkaloid found in the bulb of *Narcissus* and *Lycorus* species. Also called *narcissine*.

Lycosa A genus of large wolf spiders (family Lycosidae).

Lycosa tarentula The European tarantula, whose bite was thought to induce tarantism, against which the hysterical frenzied dance, the tarantella, was employed in seventeenth-century southern Italy to ward off the imagined effects of the tarantula bite. It is now considered more or less harmless.

lydimycin $C_{10}H_{14}N_2O_3S$. An antibiotic from *Streptomyces lydicus* with antifungal activity.

Lyell [Alan *Lyell*, English dermatologist, flourished 20th century] Lyell's disease. See under TOXIC EPIDERMAL NECROLYSIS.

lygophilia [Gk *lyg(ē)* darkness + *o* + -PHILIA] Craving for or a need to be in dark or gloomy surroundings.

Lygranum Antigens derived from *Chlamydia trachomatis* grown on chick embryos and used in the complement-fixation test and the Frei test for lymphogranuloma venereum. A proprietary name.

lying / pathologic lying Lying usually with the intent to defraud or deceive others but sometimes as a way of denying to oneself one's true value, worth, achievements, or status. It is often an aspect of the antisocial personality. Also called *mendacity, mythomania, pseudologia fantastica, pseudoreminiscence*.

lying-in The period or state following childbirth; the postpartum period or state.

Lymnaea [irreg. from Gk *limnaios* (from *limnē* a large body of standing water, lake, esp. a marshy lake, a basin or reservoir for water) marshy, stagnant] A widespread genus of freshwater pulmonate snails, species of which are intermediate hosts for various trematodes, such as *Fasciola gigantica* (*L. natalensis, L. acuminata, L. auricularia* and others*)*, *Fasciola hepatica* (*L. rubiginosa, L. cubensis, L. swinhoei, L. philippinensis*, and others*)*, various mammal schistosomes, such as *Schistosoma nasale* and *S. incognitum* (*L. luteola*), *Schistosomatium douthitti* (*L. stagnalis*), *Orientobilharzia turkestanicum* (*L. tenera*), bird schistosomes such as *Trichobilharzia ocellata* (*L. stagnalis*), *T. yokogawai* (*L. swinhoe*). In addition, *L. rubiginosa* in southeastern Asia serves as the first intermediate host for species of *Trichobilharzia* and *Orientobilharzia,* and also as first and second intermediate host for various echinostome trematodes.

Lymnaeidae [*Lymnae(a)* + -IDAE] A large family of freshwater snails of the subclass Pulmonata. The principal genus is *Lymnaea*. Some groups such as *Pseudosuccinea, Bulimnea, Acella, Fossaria,* and *Stagnicola* are classified as separate genera by some malacologists and as subgenera of *Lymnaea* by others.

lymph [L *lymph(a)* (akin to *limus* soft mud, slime, moist earth, to Gk *lyma* dirt removed by washing, dirty water, from *louein* to wash the body, bathe, and to L *nympha* a bride, nymph, water and Gk *nympha*, also *nymphē* a bride, chrysalis) water, esp. clear water from springs, a nymph] A collection of tissue fluids which passes through the lymphatic vessels into the venous system. It is usually pale yellow and contains lymphocytes. When rich in fat it looks opalescent, and may be rose colored if red blood corpuscles are present. Also called *lympha*.

aplastic lymph Lymph with less fibrinogen and more lymphocytes than normal. Also called *corpuscular lymph*.

corpuscular lymph APLASTIC LYMPH.

euplastic lymph Lymph which tends to coagulate or has already coagulated. Also called *fibrinous lymph*.

fibrinous lymph EUPLASTIC LYMPH.

inflammatory lymph Lymph produced in response to inflammation or infection.

intercellular lymph INTERSTITIAL FLUID.

intravascular lymph Fluid within the lymphatic vessels.

Koch's lymph OLD TUBERCULIN.

plastic lymph BRAWNY EDEMA.

tissue lymph An outmoded term for INTERSTITIAL FLUID.

vaccine lymph Lymph containing vaccinia virus taken from vaccinial vesicles of a calf and used to immunize against smallpox.

lymph- LYMPHO-.

lympha LYMPH.

lymphaden NODUS LYMPHATICUS.

lymphadenectasia LYMPHADENECTASIS.

lymphadenectasis A combination of hyperplasia and increased lymph volume. An imprecise, obsolete term. Also called *lymphadenectasia*.

lymphadenectomy The surgical removal of one or more lymph nodes.

lymphadenhypertrophy Hypertrophy and hyperplasia of lymph nodes. An obsolete term.

lymphadenia Generalized lymph node hyperplasia. An obsolete term.

lymphadenism Any condition, or set of signs and symptoms, associated with lymph node hyperplasia. An obsolete term.

lymphadenitis [LYMPH- + ADENITIS] Inflammation of lymph nodes. Also called *adenolymphitis, lymphnoditis* (obsolete).

acute mesenteric lymphadenitis Inflammation of the lymph nodes of the mesentery of the large intestine or the vermiform appendix that may clinically resemble acute appendicitis.

acute suppurative lymphadenitis Acute inflammation of lymph nodes, accompanied by pus formation and usually due to bacterial infections. Occasionally the overlying skin may become involved, resulting in draining sinuses.

lymphadenitis calculosa Inflammation of lymph nodes associated with dystrophic calcification. An obsolete term.

caseous lymphadenitis 1 Caseating granulomatous inflammation of lymph nodes, usually due to tuberculosis. 2 PSEUDOTUBERCULOSIS.

dermatopathic lymphadenitis A reactive benign inflammation of the lymph nodes secondary to cutaneous disease.

mesenteric lymphadenitis MESENTERIC ADENITIS.

nonbacterial regional lymphadenitis CAT-SCRATCH DISEASE.

paracaseous lymphadenitis PARATUBERCULOUS LYMPHADENITIS.

paratuberculous lymphadenitis Nonspecific, reactive hyperplasia and chronic inflammation of lymph nodes associated with documented tuberculosis at other body sites, though tubercule bacilli are not demonstrable within the affected nodes. A seldom used term. Also called *paracaseous lymphadenitis*.

regional lymphadenitis 1 The inflammation of lymph nodes draining a nearby site of infection. 2 An imprecise and outmoded term for CAT-SCRATCH DISEASE.

satellite lymphadenitis Inguinal adenitis that accompanies a primary syphilitic chancre of the genitalia.

tuberculoid lymphadenitis An inflammation of the lymph nodes which resembles that occurring in tuberculosis but which results from other diseases such as sarcoidosis, leprosy, syphilis, or regional enteritis.

tuberculous lymphadenitis Tuberculosis of the lymph nodes, occurring either as a result of lymphatic spread from a primary focus of infection or as an aspect of the disseminated disease. Cervical and mediastinal nodes are the·most commonly affected. See also SCROFULA.

venereal suppurative benign lymphadenitis　An inflammation accompanied by a discharge of pus from the inguinal lymph glands that is caused by venereal disease, most often chancroid or lymphogranuloma venereum.

lymphadenocele　A cyst of a lymph node.

lymphadenocyst　A degenerating lymph node caused by obstruction or occlusion of the afferent lymphatic.

lymphadenography　LYMPHANGIOGRAPHY.

lymphadenoid　Resembling lymph node or lymphatic tissue.

lymphadenoma [LYMPH- + ADENOMA]　LYMPHOMA. Adjective: lymphadenomatous.

malignant lymphadenoma　LYMPHOMA.

multiple lymphadenoma　**1** LYMPHOMA.　**2** HODGKIN'S DISEASE.

lymphadenomatosis　LYMPHOMA.

lymphadenomatous　Pertaining to lymphadenoma.

lymphadenopathy [LYMPH- + ADENOPATHY]　Enlargement of lymph nodes due to uncertain or nonspecific causes. Also called *adenopathy, lymphadenosis.*

dermatopathic lymphadenopathy　A reactive benign enlargement of the local draining lymph nodes that is secondary to a cutaneous disease. Also called *dermopathic lymphadenopathy.*

dermopathic lymphadenopathy　DERMATOPATHIC LYMPHADENOPATHY.

giant follicular lymphadenopathy　NODULAR LYMPHOSARCOMA.

lipoplastic lymphadenopathy　Enlargement of lymph nodes due to an increase in adipose tissue, mainly in the hilum. A seldom used term.

lymphadenosis [LYMPH- + ADENOSIS]　LYMPHADENOPATHY.

acute lymphadenosis　Any acute generalized enlargement of lymph nodes; especially, infectious mononucleosis. An obsolete term.

acute epidemic lymphadenosis　INFECTIOUS MONONUCLEOSIS.

aleukemic lymphadenosis　Diffuse generalized hyperplasia of the lymphoid organs without accompanying leukemia. A seldom used term.

benign lymphadenosis　BENIGN LYMPHOCYTOMA CUTIS.

lymphadenosis benigna cutis　BENIGN LYMPHOCYTOMA CUTIS.

benign cutaneous lymphadenosis　BENIGN LYMPHOCYTOMA CUTIS.

chronic lymphadenosis　**1** Chronic hyperplasia of a lymph node. **2** Primary neoplasia of a lymph node.

leukemic lymphadenosis　**1** Infiltration of lymph nodes by leukemic cells. A rarely used term. **2** A rarely used term for CHRONIC LYMPHOCYTIC LEUKEMIA.

malignant lymphadenosis　LYMPHOMA.

lymphadenotomy [LYMPH- + ADENO- + -TOMY]　A surgical incision into one or more lymph nodes.

lymphadenovarix　Enlargement and varicose deformity of a lymph node resulting from lymphangiectasis. Also called *adenovarix.*

lymphagogue [LYMPH + -AGOGUE]　A stimulant of lymph formation.

lymphangeitis　LYMPHANGITIS.

lymphangial　Pertaining to a lymph vessel.

lymphangiectasia　LYMPHANGIECTASIS.

intestinal lymphangiectasia　Dilatation of the intestinal lymphatics with subsequent protein-losing enteropathy, steatorrhea and diarrhea. It may be congenital, due to hypoplasia of the thoracic duct, or acquired, due to inflammation or neoplasm of the lymphatics. Small bowel biopsy is characteristic, with dilated lacteals in intestinal villi.

lymphangiectasis [LYMPH- + ANGIECTASIS]　Dilatation of lymphatic vessels. Also called *lymphangiectasia, telangiectasis lymphatica* (obsolete), *lymphectasia* (seldom used). Adjective: lymphangiectatic.

cystic lymphangiectasis　CYSTIC LYMPHANGIOMA.

pericaliceal lymphangiectasis　Dilated lymph channels along the principal renal lymph ducts resulting in single or multiple cysts around the calices.

pulmonary lymphangiectasis　A congenital condition of the lung in which there are multiple small cystic dilatations in the lymphatic network, associated with neonatal respiratory distress and death.

lymphangiectasis of the scrotum　Idiopathic dilatation of the scrotal lymphatics probably due to a congenital or postinflammatory defect in the lymphatic system of the scrotum.

lymphangiectodes [*lymphangiect(asis)* + Gk -*ōdēs*, combining form denoting resembling]　LYMPHANGIOMA CIRCUMSCRIPTUM.

lymphangiectomy [LYMPH- + ANGIECTOMY]　The surgical removal of one or more lymphatic vessels.

lymphangiitis　LYMPHANGITIS.

lymphangioadenography　LYMPHANGIOGRAPHY.

lymphangioendothelioblastoma　LYMPHANGIOENDOTHELIOMA.

lymphangioendothelioma [LYMPH- + ANGIOENDOTHELIOMA]　A tumor of the lymphatic endothelium. These cells may form layers within the vascular channels. The tumor is considered malignant (lymphangiosarcoma) when cellular atypia is present. Also called *lymphangioendothelioblastoma, lymphendothelioma.*

malignant lymphangioendothelioma　LYMPHANGIOSARCOMA.

lymphangiofibroma [LYMPH- + ANGIOFIBROMA]　A lymphangioma containing a prominent component of fibrous tissue. A seldom used term.

lymphangiogram [LYMPH- + ANGIOGRAM]　A roentgenogram obtained during lymphangiography. Also called *lymphogram, lymphadenogram.*

lymphangiography [LYMPH- + ANGIOGRAPHY]　Radiographic study of the lymphatic channels and lymph nodes after their opacification by the injection of an oily radiopaque material into one or more small lymph channels in the foot, or, less commonly, in the hand. Also called *lymphography, lymphadenography, lymphangioadenography, hydrangiography* (rarely used).

indirect radionuclide lymphangiography　**1** Registration of emitted radioactivity from a radionuclide colloid preparation in lymph nodes. A radioactive colloid is injected, for example into the dorsum of the foot, and taken up into the lymphatic system. **2** Visualization of abnormal lymph nodes after the intravenous injection of a suitable radiotracer, such as gallium citrate.

pedal lymphangiography　Lymphangiography of the lower extremity, pelvis, and lower abdomen after injection of the contrast medium into a lymphatic vessel at the dorsum of the foot. It is usually done bilaterally.

lymphangioitis　An obsolete term for LYMPHANGITIS.

lymphangioleiomyomatosis　A proliferation of lymphatic vessels and smooth muscle. It typically affects the lungs and lymph nodes. It is a lesion of women of the reproductive age. Large cysts and a honeycomb appearance of the lung can occur, which leads to respiratory insufficiency.

lymphangiology　The study of the lymphatic vessels. Also

called *hydrangiology, lymphology.*

lymphangioma [LYMPH- + ANGIOMA]   A benign growth composed exclusively of lymph vessels of various size lined by a single layer of endothelial cells. The lesion is often congenital. Lymphangiomas can be subtyped as capillary, cavernous, or cystic. The cavernous and cystic forms (hygroma) are most frequent in the cervical, mediastinal, and retroperitoneal regions of infants and children. Capillary lymphangiomas are exceedingly rare and are difficult to distinguish from capillary hemangiomas. Also called *angiolymphoma, angioma lymphaticum, lymphangioma tuberosum multiplex* (seldom used).   ● *Angioma* is often used synonymously, but that term can also apply to a hemangioma.

lymphangioma capsulare varicosum   LYMPHANGIOMA CIRCUMSCRIPTUM.

lymphangioma cavernosum   CAVERNOUS LYMPHANGIOMA.

cavernous lymphangioma   A lymphangioma with large, dilated, thin-walled channels. Also called *lymphangioma cavernosum, cavernoma lymphaticum.*

lymphangioma circumscriptum   A circumscribed developmental defect of cutaneous and subcutaneous lymphatics presenting clinically as a yellowish cluster of thick-walled vesicles. Also called *lymphangiectodes, lymphangioma capulare varicosum, lymphangioma xanthelasoideum, lupus lymphaticus* (obsolete).

congenital lymphangioma   Any lymphangioma conspicuous at birth.

cystic lymphangioma   A lymphangioma characterized by large, lymph-filled cysts. It is seen most commonly in the regions of the neck and groin in children. Also called *lymphangioma cysticum, cystic lymphangiectasis.*

lymphangioma cysticum   CYSTIC LYMPHANGIOMA.

fissural lymphangioma   A lymphangioma at the site of a fetal skin fissure.

lymphangioma tuberosum multiplex   A seldom used term for LYMPHANGIOMA.

lymphangioma xanthelasmoideum   LYMPHANGIOMA CIRCUMSCRIPTUM.

lymphangiomatous   Pertaining to lymphangioma.

lymphangiomyoma [LYMPH- + ANGIO- + MYOMA]   A growth composed of bundles of smooth muscle tissue about cavernous or slitlike, endothelium-lined lymph spaces. Aggregates of lymphocytes may be found in association with the smooth muscle tissue. The tumor has been observed only in the mediastinum and retroperitoneum in close association with the thoracic duct and its tributaries. Chylothorax and pulmonary complications are common.

lymphangion   VAS LYMPHATICUM.

lymphangiophlebitis   Inflammation of both lymph vessels and blood vessels.

lymphangioplasty   The surgical replacement or repair of damaged or destroyed lymphatic vessels. Also called *lymphoplasty.*

Handley's lymphangioplasty   A surgical treatment for elephantiasis in which cotton wicks are inserted into the tissues to allow for external lymphatic drainage.

lymphangiosarcoma [LYMPH- + ANGIOSARCOMA]   A malignant tumor of lymphatic tissue, mainly associated with chronic lymph stasis, usually secondary to radical mastectomy. Also called *malignant lymphangioendothelioma, lymphangioendothelial sarcoma, lymphatic sarcoma.*

lymphangiotomy [LYMPH- + ANGIOTOMY]   A surgical incision into one or more lymphatic ducts.

lymphangitis [LYMPH- + ANGITIS]   Inflammation of lymphatic vessels, usually as a result of extension of an adjacent bacterial infection into or through their wall. Also called *lymphatitis* (obsolete), *angioleucitis, angioleukitis, angiolymphitis,*

lymphangeitis, lymphangiitis, lymphangioitis (obsolete), *lymphitis* (obsolete).

lymphangitis carcinomatosa   **1** The growth of carcinoma in lymphatics.   **2** The obstruction of lymphatics by carcinoma.

carcinomatous lymphangitis   The filling of lymphatic channels by metastatic cancer cells, particularly those of the lungs where the distended tumor-filled lymphatics are visible to the naked eye as whitish streaks or cords extending from the pleura to the hilum.

gummatous lymphangitis   An inflammation of lymphatic vessels that are associated with a gumma.

nonvenereal sclerosing lymphangitis   Inflammation and sclerosis of the lymphatics arising from or around the coronal sulcus of the penis.

lymphatic   **1** Relating to lymph.   **2** A lymph vessel; vas lymphaticum.

afferent lymphatic   A vessel carrying lymph to a lymph node.

efferent lymphatic   A vessel conducting lymph away from a lymph node.

gluteal lymphatics   Lymphatic vessels draining the gluteal region, the superficial group draining to the superficial inguinal lymph nodes while the deep vessels drain along the gluteal arteries and veins to the pelvic nodes along the internal iliac artery and vein.

ischial lymphatics   Deep lymph vessels of the ischial region following the course of corresponding arteries and veins.

obturator lymphatics   Deep lymphatic vessels along the obturator vessels which drain to the external and internal iliac lymph nodes either directly or through the obturator lymph nodes.

lymphaticosplenic   Pertaining to lymph nodes and the spleen.

lymphaticostomy [L *lymphatic(us)* watery, dropsical + *o* + -STOMY]   The surgical creation of an opening that establishes drainage from a large lymphatic duct, such as the thoracic duct.

lymphatism   STATUS LYMPHATICUS.

lymphatitis   An obsolete term for LYMPHANGITIS.

lymphatogenous   Originating from lymph.

lymphatology   The study of the lymphatic system.

lymphatolysin   A lysin that is effective on lymphatic cells and tissue.

lymphatolysis   Destruction of lymphatic vessels or lymphoid tissues. A seldom used term.

lymphatolytic   Capable of destroying lymphoid tissue or lymphatic vessels, as a serum.

lymphatome   LYMPHOTOME.

lymphectasia   A seldom used term for LYMPHANGIECTASIS.

lymphedema [LYMPH- + EDEMA]   The accumulation of interstitial fluid as a result of obstruction of lymphatic vessels, disorders of lymph nodes, or surgical removal of lymph nodes for cancer. Also called *lymphatic edema.*

congenital lymphedema   HEREDITARY LYMPHEDEMA TYPE I.

early-onset lymphedema   HEREDITARY LYMPHEDEMA TYPE I.

filarial lymphedema   Chronic edema and associated lymphangitis caused by the blockage by filariae of major lymphatics, such as those of the scrotum or lower extremities. Eventually fibrosis develops, leading to elephantiasis. *Wuchereria bancrofti* and *Brugia malayi* are the species usually responsible for these deformities.

hereditary lymphedema   Either hereditary lymphedema type I or type II. Also called *heredotrophedema.*

hereditary lymphedema, early-onset type   HEREDITARY LYMPHEDEMA TYPE I.

hereditary lymphedema type I   Congenital edema, predominantly affecting the legs, that is inherited as an autosomal dominant trait. It may be associated with intestinal protein loss and pleural effusion. Also called *Milroy's disease, Nonne-Milroy disease, hereditary lymphedema, early-onset type, trophedema, congenital trophedema, hereditary trophedema, trophoedema, congenital lymphedema, Nonne-Milroy-Meige syndrome, Milroy's edema, Nonne-Milroy lymphedema, early-onset lymphedema, congenital elephantiasis.*

hereditary lymphedema type II An autosomal dominant, variable, slowly progressive form of lymphedema with onset around puberty. Also called *Meige lymphedema, late-onset lymphedema, Meige's disease, trophoedema of Meige.*

late-onset lymphedema HEREDITARY LYMPHEDEMA TYPE II.

Meige lymphedema HEREDITARY LYMPHEDEMA TYPE II.

Nonne-Milroy lymphedema HEREDITARY LYMPHEDEMA TYPE I.

lymphedema praecox Lymphedema occurring in girls approaching puberty, and characterized by puffiness and swelling of the lower extremities.

secondary lymphedema Lymphedema due to radiotherapy, surgery, or other cause obstructing lymphatic drainage from a part.

lymphemia A rarely used term for CHRONIC LYMPHOCYTIC LEUKEMIA.

lymphendothelioma [LYMPH- + ENDOTHELIOMA] LYMPHANGIOENDOTHELIOMA.

lymphepithelioma LYMPHOEPITHELIOMA.

lymphitis An obsolete term for LYMPHANGITIS.

lymphization LYMPHOPOIESIS.

lymph node

lymph node NODUS LYMPHATICUS.

anterior bronchopulmonary lymph nodes Bronchopulmonary lymph nodes anterior to the structures in the root of the lung. An outmoded term.

anterior cecal lymph nodes NODI LYMPHATICI PRECECALES.

anterior cervical lymph nodes NODI LYMPHATICI CERVICALES ANTERIORES.

anterior jugular lymph nodes NODI LYMPHATICI JUGULARES ANTERIORES.

anterior mediastinal lymph nodes NODI LYMPHATICI MEDIASTINALES ANTERIORES.

anterior tibial lymph node NODUS TIBIALIS ANTERIOR.

anterior vesical lymph nodes Nodes of the nodi lymphatici vesicales laterales which are situated on the middle and inferior parts of the anterior wall of the urinary bladder.

apical lymph nodes NODI LYMPHATICI APICALES.

lymph node of arch of azygos vein NODUS ARCUS VENAE AZYGOS.

axillary lymph nodes NODI LYMPHATICI AXILLARES.

biliary lymph nodes Lymph nodes situated along the extrahepatic biliary ducts, including nodi lymphatici hepatici, nodus cysticus, and nodus foraminalis.

brachial lymph nodes NODI LYMPHATICI BRACHIALES.

bronchopulmonary lymph nodes NODI LYMPHATICI BRONCHOPULMONALES.

buccal lymph nodes See under NODI LYMPHATICI FACIALES.

buccal group of facial lymph nodes NODUS BUCCINATORIUS.

cecoappendicular lymph nodes The nodi lymphatici prece-

cales, nodi lymphatici retrocecales, and nodi lymphatici appendiculares considered together.

celiac lymph nodes NODI LYMPHATICI COELIACI.

central lymph nodes NODI LYMPHATICI CENTRALES.

circumflex iliac lymph nodes An inconstant group of one to four lymph nodes situated along the deep circumflex iliac artery. It is an outlying member of the external iliac group of lymph nodes.

common iliac lymph nodes NODI LYMPHATICI ILIACI COMMUNES.

cubital lymph nodes NODI LYMPHATICI CUBITALES.

lymph nodes of cubital fossa NODI LYMPHATICI CUBITALES.

deep cervical lymph nodes NODI LYMPHATICI CERVICALES PROFUNDI.

deep inguinal lymph nodes NODI LYMPHATICI INGUINALES PROFUNDI.

deep occipital lymph nodes A few nodi lymphatici occipitales which are situated along the occipital artery between the insertions of the splenius capitis and obliquus capitis superior muscles. An outmoded term.

deep parotid lymph nodes NODI LYMPHATICI PAROTIDEI PROFUNDI.

deep posterior lymph nodes of shoulder A group of three or four lymph nodes situated in the lateral part of the supraspinous fossa deep to the supraspinatus muscle and along the suprascapular artery and vein.

lymph nodes of deltopectoral groove Small lymph nodes along the course of the cephalic vein between the deltoid and pectoralis major muscles which drain into the infraclavicular nodes or the apical nodes.

diaphragmatic lymph nodes An outmoded term for NODI LYMPHATICI PHRENICI SUPERIORES.

epitrochlear lymph nodes NODI LYMPHATICI CUBITALES.

external iliac lymph nodes NODI LYMPHATICI ILIACI EXTERNI.

facial lymph nodes NODI LYMPHATICI FACIALES.

femoral lymph nodes Inconstant lymph nodes along the course of the femoral vein in the lower and middle parts of the thigh which receive the efferents of the popliteal nodes and send their lymph to the deep inguinal nodes.

lymph nodes of gastroduodenal artery NODI LYMPHATICI PYLORICI.

gastroepiploic lymph nodes The nodi lymphatici gastroomentales dextri and nodi lymphatici gastro-omentales sinistri.

lymph nodes of gastropancreatic fold An outmoded term for NODI LYMPHATICI SPLENICI.

hemal lymph node A lymph node in which blood flows through the sinusoidal system. Such structures have been identified in a number of experimental animals, particularly in the retroperitoneal position.

hepatic lymph nodes NODI LYMPHATICI HEPATICI.

lymph nodes of hepatic artery Four to eight nodi lymphatici hepatici situated along the ascending and horizontal segments of the course of the hepatic artery. An outmoded term.

ileoappendicular lymph nodes The lower nodes of the nodi lymphatici ileocolici which drain the lymph of the terminal ileum and the appendix. They are situated in the neighborhood of the base of the appendix. An outmoded term.

ileocecal lymph nodes The nodes of the nodi lymphatici ileocolici which are situated in the ileocecal angle. An outmoded term.

ileocolic lymph nodes NODI LYMPHATICI ILEOCOLICI.

iliac lymph nodes NODI LYMPHATICI ILIACI.

inferior auricular parotid lymph nodes NODI LYMPHATICI INFRA-AURICULARES.

inferior diaphragmatic lymph nodes NODI LYMPHATICI PHRENICI INFERIORES.

inferior epigastric lymph nodes   NODI LYMPHATICI EPIGAS-
TRICI INFERIORES.

inferior gastric lymph nodes   NODI LYMPHATICI GASTRO-
OMENTALES DEXTRI.

inferior mesenteric lymph nodes   NODI LYMPHATICI ME-
SENTERICI INFERIORES.

inferior tracheobronchial lymph nodes   NODI LYMPHATICI
TRACHEOBRONCHIALES INFERIORES.

infraclavicular lymph nodes 1 NODI LYMPHATICI API-
CALES.   2 One or two lymph nodes along the cephalic vein in
the infraclavicular fossa at the upper end of the deltopectoral
groove. Their efferents pierce the clavipectoral fascia to end in
the apical group of axillary nodes.

infrahyoid lymph nodes   A group of lymph nodes situated
on the front of the thyrohyoid membrane and deep to the investing layer of the deep cervical fascia. They receive afferents
from the anterior cervical nodes and their efferents end in the
deep lateral cervical nodes. Also called *thyrohyoid lymph nodes*
(outmoded).

infraorbital group of facial lymph nodes   A rarely occurring
group represented by one small lymph node situated along the
facial vein either just below the medial angle of the orbit or in
the canine fossa. An outmoded term.

inguinal lymph nodes   Nodi lymphatici inguinales superficiales and nodi lymphatici inguinales profundi.

intercostal lymph nodes   NODI LYMPHATICI INTERCOS-
TALES.

internal iliac lymph nodes   NODI LYMPHATICI ILIACI IN-
TERNI.

internal jugular lymph nodes   The nodi lymphatici jugulares
laterales and nodi lymphatici jugulares anteriores.

internal mammary lymph nodes   An outmoded term for
NODI LYMPHATICI PARASTERNALES.

internal thoracic lymph nodes   NODI LYMPHATICI PARA-
STERNALES.

intracapsular submandibular lymph nodes   Inconstant
nodes of the nodi lymphatici submandibulares embedded in the
submandibular gland and spread along its excretory duct. An
outmoded term.

jugulodigastric lymph node   NODUS JUGULODIGASTRICUS.

jugulo-omohyoid lymph node   NODUS JUGULO-OMOHYOI-
DEUS.

lateral aortic lymph nodes   NODI LYMPHATICI AORTICI LAT-
ERALES.

lateral axillary lymph nodes   NODI LYMPHATICI LATERA-
LES.

lateral cervical lymph nodes   NODI LYMPHATICI CERVI-
CALES LATERALES.

lateral jugular lymph nodes   NODI LYMPHATICI JUGULARES
LATERALES.

lateral lingual lymph nodes   Inconstant lymph nodes along
the lymphatic vessels accompanying the lingual artery and vein
on the external surface of the genioglossus and hyoglossus muscles. They receive afferents from the margins of the tongue.
Some of these nodes overlap with the nodi lymphatici submandibulares.

lateral retropharyngeal lymph nodes   The lateral group of
nodi lymphatici retropharyngeales, which is situated between
the fascia covering the posterolateral surface of the pharynx and
the prevertebral fascia and in front of the lateral mass of the
atlas along the outer margin of the longus capitis muscle on
each side.

lateral tracheal group of deep anterior cervical lymph nodes
NODI LYMPHATICI PARATRACHEALES.

lateral vesical lymph nodes   NODI LYMPHATICI VESICALES
LATERALES.

left anterior mediastinal lymph nodes   Nodes of the nodi

lymphatici mediastinales anteriores which extend from the nodus ligamenti arteriosi to the anterolateral surface of the left
common carotid artery and lie between the left phrenic nerve
and the arch of the aorta. They may be in contact with the
thymus.

left colic lymph nodes   NODI LYMPHATICI COLICI SINISTRI.

left gastric lymph nodes   NODI LYMPHATICI GASTRICI SIN-
ISTRI.

left gastroepiploic lymph nodes   NODI LYMPHATICI GAS-
TRO-OMENTALES SINISTRI.

left lateral tracheal lymph nodes   Four or five of the nodi
lymphatici paratracheales on the left side of the thoracic part
of the trachea. An outmoded term.

lymph nodes of lesser curvature   NODI LYMPHATICI GAS-
TRICI SINISTRI.

lingual lymph nodes   Small inconstant lymph nodes which lie
along the lymph vessels draining the tongue on the external
surfaces of the hyoglossus and genioglossus muscles and between
the latter muscles.

lumbar lymph nodes   NODI LYMPHATICI LUMBALES.

mandibular lymph nodes   See under NODI LYMPHATICI FA-
CIALES.

mastoid lymph nodes   NODI LYMPHATICI MASTOIDEI.

medial group of common iliac lymph nodes   Two to six of
the nodi lymphatici iliaci which are situated below the bifurcation of the aorta in front of the fifth lumbar vertebra or the
sacral promontory.

median retropharyngeal lymph nodes   Nodi lymphatici retropharyngeales situated in or near the midline of the back of
the posterior wall of the pharynx.

mesenteric lymph nodes   NODI LYMPHATICI MESENTERICI.

middle colic lymph nodes   NODI LYMPHATICI COLICI MEDII.

middle group of external iliac lymph nodes   An inconstant
group of two or three nodes of the nodi lymphatici iliaci externi
which are situated medial to the external iliac artery on the
anteromedial surface of the vein.

middle group of submental lymph nodes   Two to four nodes
of the nodi lymphatici submentales which are situated on the
inferior surface of the mylohyoid muscle and the two anterior
bellies of the digastric muscle equidistant from the mandible
and the hyoid bone. An outmoded term.

obturator lymph nodes   NODI LYMPHATICI OBTURATORII.

occipital lymph nodes   NODI LYMPHATICI OCCIPITALES.

pancreaticolienal lymph nodes   Nodi lymphatici splenici and
nodi lymphatici pancreatici considered together.

pancreaticosplenic lymph nodes   NODI LYMPHATICI PAN-
CREATICOLIENALES.

paracolic lymph nodes   NODI LYMPHATICI PARACOLICI.

parasternal lymph nodes   NODI LYMPHATICI PARASTER-
NALES.

paratracheal lymph nodes   NODI LYMPHATICI PARATRA-
CHEALES.

parotid lymph nodes   Nodi lymphatici parotidei superficiales
and nodi lymphatici parotidei profundi.

pectoral lymph nodes   NODI LYMPHATICI PECTORALES.

peritracheal lymph nodes   NODI LYMPHATICI PARATRA-
CHEALES.

popliteal lymph nodes   NODI LYMPHATICI POPLITEALES.

posterior auricular lymph nodes   NODI LYMPHATICI MAS-
TOIDEI.

posterior bronchopulmonary lymph nodes   The bronchopulmonary lymph nodes that are posterior to the bronchi in the
root of the lung. An outmoded term.

posterior cecal lymph nodes   NODI LYMPHATICI RETROCE-
CALES.

posterior group of submental lymph nodes   An inconstant group of nodi lymphatici submentales which is situated on the hyoid bone.

posterior intercostal lymph nodes   NODI LYMPHATICI INTERCOSTALES.

posterior mediastinal lymph nodes   NODI LYMPHATICI MEDIASTINALES POSTERIORES.

posterior tibial lymph nodes   Inconstant lymph nodes situated along the lymphatic vessels accompanying the posterior tibial vessels, mainly in the middle of the leg.

preaortic lymph nodes   NODI LYMPHATICI PREAORTICI.

preauricular lymph nodes   NODI LYMPHATICI PREAURICULARES.

precaval lymph nodes   NODI LYMPHATICI PRECAVALES.

pre-esophageal lymph nodes   Nodes of the nodi lymphatici juxta-esophageales pulmonales which are situated in front of the esophagus and on the diaphragm. An outmoded term.

prelaryngeal lymph nodes   NODI LYMPHATICI PRELARYNGEALES.

prepericardiac lymph nodes   NODI LYMPHATICI PREPERICARDIALES.

prethyroid group of deep anterior cervical lymph nodes   One or more nodes of the nodi lymphatici pretracheales which are situated in front of the isthmus of the thyroid gland. An outmoded term.

pretracheal lymph nodes   1 NODI LYMPHATICI PRETRACHEALES. 2 An outmoded term for NODI LYMPHATICI TRACHEOBRONCHIALES SUPERIORES.

pulmonary lymph nodes   NODI LYMPHATICI PULMONALES.

pulmonary lymph nodes proper   Lymph nodes situated along the ramifications of the intrapulmonary vessels and bronchi. They drain the lung substance and become continuous with the bronchopulmonary group in the hilum. An outmoded term.   •   The English nomenclature no longer distinguishes the more distal nodes ("proper") from those nearer the hilum within the lung substance.

pyloric lymph nodes   NODI LYMPHATICI PYLORICI.

renal group of lateral aortic lymph nodes   Lymph nodes which drain the deep capsular and parenchymatous lymphatics of the left kidney and are situated on and around the left renal vein. However, renal lymphatics may also drain to other nodes of the lumbar chain. An outmoded term.

retroaortic lymph nodes   NODI LYMPHATICI POSTAORTICI.

retroauricular lymph nodes   NODI LYMPHATICI MASTOIDEI.

retrocaval lymph nodes   NODI LYMPHATICI POSTCAVALES.

retropharyngeal lymph nodes   NODI LYMPHATICI RETROPHARYNGEALES.

retroxiphoid lymph nodes   A few inconstant nodes of the nodi lymphatici prepericardiales which are situated on the diaphragm behind the xiphoid process.

right anterior mediastinal lymph nodes   The nodes of the nodi lymphatici mediastinales anteriores which are situated anterior to the superior vena cava and the right brachiocephalic vein. An outmoded term.

right colic lymph nodes   NODI LYMPHATICI COLICI DEXTRI.

right gastric lymph nodes   NODI LYMPHATICI GASTRICI DEXTRI.

right gastroepiploic lymph nodes   NODI LYMPHATICI GASTRO-OMENTALES DEXTRI.

right lateral tracheal lymph nodes   Some nodes of the nodi lymphatici paratracheales which are situated on the right side, the lowest being continuous with the superior tracheobronchial nodes. An outmoded term.

sacral lymph nodes   NODI LYMPHATICI SACRALES.

lymph node of small saphenous vein   An inconstant node of the nodi lymphatici popliteales superficiales which is situated lateral to the small saphenous vein after it pierces the deep fascia of the popliteal fossa and medial to the common peroneal nerve.

sternal lymph nodes   NODI LYMPHATICI PARASTERNALES.

subaponeurotic occipital lymph nodes   A group of nodi lymphatici occipitales which is situated near the superior nuchal line on the splenius capitis muscle and deep to the investing layer of deep cervical fascia. An outmoded term.

subaponeurotic preauricular parotid lymph nodes   An outmoded term for NODI LYMPHATICI PREAURICULARES.

subduodenopyloric lymph nodes   An outmoded term for NODI LYMPHATICI PYLORICI.

submandibular lymph nodes   NODI LYMPHATICI SUBMANDIBULARES.

submental lymph nodes   NODI LYMPHATICI SUBMENTALES.

subscapular lymph nodes   NODI LYMPHATICI SUBSCAPULARES.

superficial cervical lymph nodes   NODI LYMPHATICI CERVICALES SUPERFICIALES.

superficial and deep parotid lymph nodes   The nodi lymphatici parotidei profunda and nodi lymphatici parotidei superficiales.

superficial inguinal lymph nodes   NODI LYMPHATICI INGUINALES SUPERFICIALES.

superficial occipital lymph nodes   A few of the nodi lymphatici occipitales which are situated on the epicranial aponeurosis over the superior nuchal line and related to the occipital artery and the greater occipital nerve. An outmoded term.

superficial parotid lymph nodes   NODI LYMPHATICI PAROTIDEI SUPERFICIALES.

superficial posterior axillary lymph node   A subcutaneous lymph node situated near the inferior angle of the scapula. An outmoded term.

superficial posterior scapular lymph nodes   Inconstant small subcutaneous lymph nodes which are situated on the back of the scapular region along afferent lymphatics of the subscapular nodes in the axilla.

superficial subaponeurotic parotid lymph nodes   An outmoded term for NODI LYMPHATICI PAROTIDEI SUPERFICIALES.

superficial supra-aponeurotic parotid lymph nodes   An outmoded term for NODI LYMPHATICI PAROTIDEI SUPERFICIALES.

superior bronchopulmonary lymph nodes   Bronchopulmonary lymph nodes which are situated above the root of the lung, those on the right being lateral to the superior branch of the right pulmonary artery while those on the left lie behind the superior branch of the left pulmonary artery. An outmoded term.

superior gastric lymph nodes   NODI LYMPHATICI GASTRICI SINISTRI.

superior group of pectoral lymph nodes   Pectoral lymph nodes situated in front of the lateral thoracic artery in the second and third intercostal spaces and on the third rib. An outmoded term.

superior mesenteric lymph nodes   NODI LYMPHATICI MESENTERICI SUPERIORES.

superior tracheobronchial lymph nodes   NODI LYMPHATICI TRACHEOBRONCHIALES SUPERIORES.

supraclavicular lymph nodes   NODI LYMPHATICI SUPRACLAVICULARES.

supratrochlear lymph nodes   NODI LYMPHATICI CUBITALES.

thyrohyoid lymph nodes   An outmoded term for INFRAHYOID LYMPH NODES.

thyroid lymph nodes   NODI LYMPHATICI THYROIDEI.

tracheal lymph nodes   NODI LYMPHATICI PARATRACHEALES.

tracheobronchial lymph nodes   NODI LYMPHATICI TRACHEOBRONCHIALES.

lymph node of Troisier   SENTINEL NODE.

uterovaginal lymph node   A lymph node situated at the junction of the uterus and vagina on each side. An outmoded term.

visceral lymph nodes of abdomen NODI VISCERALES AB-DOMINIS.

---

lymphnoditis An obsolete term for LYMPHADENITIS.

lympho- [L *lympha* (related to Gk *lyein* to loosen, dissolve, wash) water, clear spring water] A combining form denoting lymph or lymphatic tissue. Also *lymph-*.

lymphoblast An immature cell of the lymphocytic series that is 15–20 microns in diameter, with a nucleus that has a diffuse chromatin pattern and usually one or two nucleoli, and with rather scanty cytoplasm devoid of granules. The lymphoblast was formerly conceived as the precursor cell of the mature lymphocyte, but now is considered to be a lymphocyte that has been transformed from a resting state to a proliferating state by antigenic stimulation. Lymphoblasts occur in the blood in large numbers in acute lymphocytic leukemia. Also called *lympho-cytoblast, lymphogone.*

lymphoblasthemia LYMPHOBLASTOSIS.

lymphoblastic Of or relating to lymphoblasts.

lymphoblastoma [LYMPHO- + BLASTOMA] A lymphoblastic lymphoma. See under LYMPHOCYTIC LYMPHOMA.

giant follicular lymphoblastoma NODULAR LYMPHOSAR-COMA.

lymphoblastomatous Pertaining to lymphoblastoma.

lymphoblastomid [*lymphoblastom(a)* + -ID²] A cutaneous lesion of a lymphoma.

lymphoblastosis The presence of lymphoblasts in blood, as in acute lymphocytic leukemia. Also called *lymphoblasthemia.*

acute benign lymphoblastosis INFECTIOUS MONONUCLEO-SIS.

lymphocele [LYMPHO- + -CELE²] Any cystic structure that contains lymph. Also called *lymphocyst.*

lymphochloroma [LYMPHO- + CHLOROMA] A chloroma whose cells are thought to be of the lymphoid series.

lymphocinesia LYMPHOKINESIS.

lymphocyst [LYMPHO- + CYST] LYMPHOCELE.

lymphocystosis The development of multiple cystic lymphan-giomas.

lymphocyte [LYMPHO- + -CYTE] A leukocyte of blood, bone marrow, and lymphatic tissue that characteristically has a round nucleus with well-condensed chromatin, no identifiable nucleolus, and usually agranular cytoplasm that stains pale blue with Romanowsky dyes. A narrow lighter halo, or perinuclear clear zone, may surround the nucleus, and a few azurophilic granules may be seen in the cytoplasm. Lymphocytes play a major role in both cellular and humoral immunity, and thus several different functional and morphologic types must be recognized, i.e. the small, large, B-, and T-lymphocytes, with further morphologic distinctions being made among the B-lymphocytes. These distinctions are important in the classification of lymphocytic malignancies. Also called *lymphoid leukocyte, lymphoid corpuscle, lymphoid cell, lymph cell.*

atypical lymphocyte A large lymphocyte which by Romanowsky stain has abundant basophilic cytoplasm that often exhibits distinct paler cytoplasmic zones and an oval nucleus resembling that of a monocyte. Atypical lymphocytes, when numerous in blood, are characteristic of infectious mononucleosis, cytomegalovirus infection, viral hepatitis, and other viral infections. Also called *Downey cell, variant lymphocyte, virocyte.*

B lymphocyte One of the two major classes of lymphocytes having important immune regulatory functions. In birds, B lymphocytes pass through the bursa of Fabricius during their development. In mammals, the fetal liver is believed to be the equivalent of the bursa of Fabricius. B lymphocytes carry certain characteristic surface markers such as membrane-bound immunoglobulin. They recognize antigen independent of MHC molecules. When stimulated by antigens, they enlarge, develop very basophilic cytoplasm (from increase in RNA), and transform into plasma cells that secrete antibody. Also called *B cell, thymus-independent lymphocyte.* Compare T LYMPHOCYTE.

educated T lymphocyte A thymus-derived lymphocyte that has been exposed to antigen on an antigen-presenting cell and thus may be used in experiments of T lymphocyte-B lymphocyte cooperation to cause splenocytes from irradiated animals to respond to the antigen.

helper T lymphocyte HELPER CELL.

killer lymphocyte NATURAL KILLER CELL.

large lymphocyte A common lymphocyte in normal blood and lymph nodes. It is approximately 15 microns in diameter, having more cytoplasm than small lymphocytes. The nucleus occupies approximately one third of the cell volume.

NUL lymphocyte A lymphocyte which possesses neither T nor B cell markers on its surface. Also called *null cell.*

primed lymphocyte A lymphocyte which has been exposed to antigen and has thereby become more immunologically responsive. Upon further antigen exposure, it is capable of dividing rapidly, synthesizing antibody, or taking part in a cell-mediated immune reaction.

Rieder's lymphocyte A cell that has deep indentation, pseudolobulation, and cloverleaf formation of the nucleus, which is otherwise round or oval. This term has been applied to both the lymphocytes of chronic lymphocytic leukemia, and the myeloblasts of acute granulocytic leukemia. An imprecise and rarely used term.

small lymphocyte The predominant lymphocyte in normal blood and lymph nodes. It is approximately 10 microns in diameter, with a nucleus that is more than half the cell volume.

suppressor T lymphocyte SUPPRESSOR CELL.

T lymphocyte One of the two major classes of lymphocyte having important immune regulatory and effector functions. T lymphocytes must pass through the thymus during their development. T lymphocytes carry certain characteristic surface markers such as thy 1 and T3 antigens. They recognize antigen only in the context of MHC molecules, and they are responsible for the phenomena of cell-mediated immunity. Also called *T cell, thymus-dependent lymphocyte, thymus-dependent cell, thymus-derived cell.* Compare B LYMPHOCYTE.

thymus-dependent lymphocyte T LYMPHOCYTE.

thymus-independent lymphocyte B LYMPHOCYTE.

variant lymphocyte ATYPICAL LYMPHOCYTE.

lymphocythemia LYMPHOCYTOSIS.

lymphocytic Of or relating to lymphocytes.

lymphocytoblast LYMPHOBLAST.

lymphocytoid Resembling a lymphocyte.

lymphocytoma [LYMPHO- + CYTOMA] An obsolete term for LYMPHOCYTIC LYMPHOMA.

benign cutaneous lymphocytoma BENIGN LYMPHOCYTOMA CUTIS.

benign lymphocytoma cutis A nonmalignant aggregate of lymphoid cells in the dermis. On occastion it is found in follicular form. Also called *sarcoid of Spiegler-Fendt, benign cutaneous lymphadenosis, Bäfverstedt syndrome, benign cutaneous lumphocytoma, benign lymphocytic reticulosis, benign lymphadenosis, lymphadenosis benigna cutis.*

lymphocytopenia A fewer than normal number of lymphocytes in blood. Also called *lymphopenia, sublymphemia, lymphocytic leukopenia, hypolymphemia.*

lymphocytopoiesis LYMPHOPOIESIS.

lymphocytopoietic Characteristic of lymphocyte production.

lymphocytorrhexis   The disruption of lymphocytes.

lymphocytosis [LYMPHO- + CYTOSIS]   A greater than normal number of lymphocytes in blood. Also called *lymphocythemia*.

acute infectious lymphocytosis   An acute, benign, infectious disease of obscure, but presumably viral, etiology affecting children. Symptoms are mild, with fever, headache, and upper respiratory symptoms seen in most cases and abdominal pain and central nervous system involvement reported in some cases. Multiple cases occur in families and in institutional populations. The significant feature is a leukocytosis of one to two months duration in which small, mature lymphocytes account for 60–90 percent of the differential count. The heterophile antibody test is negative in all cases, and the illness is not associated with a rise in Epstein-Barr virus antibody.

relative lymphocytosis   An increase in the proportion of lymphocytes in the blood compared with other leukocytes, often the result of a decrease in the number of neutrophils.

lymphocytotic   Characterized by or pertaining to lymphocytosis.

lymphocytotoxin   A complement-fixing antilymphocyte antibody.

Lymphocytozoon   A postulated genus of intracellular parasites.

Lymphocytozoon cobayae   A postulated species of intracellular parasites seen in macrophages or large leukocytes of guinea pigs. See also KURLOFF BODIES.

lymphodermia [LYMPHO- + -DERMIA]   An abnormality in the lymphatic vessels in the skin. An obsolete term.

lymphodermia perniciosa   An obsolete term for LEUKEMIA CUTIS.

lymphoduct   VAS LYMPHATICUM.

lymphoedema   A British spelling for LYMPHEDEMA.

lymphoepithelioma   A carcinoma of the nasopharynx or oropharynx infiltrated by large numbers of lymphoid cells. The lymphoid cells are not neoplastic. Also called *lymphoepithelial carcinoma, lymphepithelioma*.

lymphogenesis   LYMPHOPOIESIS.

lymphogenous   1 LYMPHOPOIETIC. 2 Originating in the lymphatic system.

lymphoglandula   An outmoded term for NODUS LYMPHATICUS.

lymphogone   LYMPHOBLAST.

lymphogram [LYMPHO- + -GRAM]   LYMPHANGIOGRAM.

lymphogranuloma [LYMPHO- + GRANULOMA]   Any of several conditions characterized by lymphadenopathy and multiple granulomas in lymph nodes, such as sarcoidosis, lymphogranuloma venereum, and Hodgkin's disease.

lymphogranuloma benignum   An outmoded term for SARCOIDOSIS.

lymphogranuloma inguinale   LYMPHOGRANULOMA VENEREUM.

lymphogranuloma malignum   HODGKIN'S DISEASE.

lymphogranuloma venereum   A disease caused by microorganisms of the *Chlamydia trachomatis* group, transmitted by sexual contact, and characterized by transient genital ulcerations, systemic symptoms, and subsequent inguinal lymphadenopathy (bubo). Late complications include urethral and rectal strictures, genital lymphedema, and rectovaginal fistulas. Also called *adenitis tropicalis* (obsolete), *climatic bubo, strumous bubo, tropical bubo, Durand-Nicolas-Favre disease, Frei's disease, Nicolas-Favre disease, lymphogranuloma inguinale, lymphogranulomatosis inguinalis, lymphopathia venereum, poradenitis nostras, subacute inguinal poradenitis, poradenitis venerea, poradenolymphitis, fifth venereal disease* (outmoded), *sixth venereal*

disease (obsolete), *maladie de Nicolas et Favre, groin ulcer, Favre-Durand-Nicolas disease*.

lymphogranulomatosis [LYMPHO- + GRANULOMATOSIS]   A term used in Europe, but rarely in the U.S., for HODGKIN'S DISEASE. • Although this term might logically be used to embrace other conditions of lymphogranuloma, such as sarcoidosis, it is not, in practice, used that way.

benign lymphogranulomatosis   An outmoded term for SARCOIDOSIS.

lymphogranulomatosis cutis   Hodgkin's disease affecting the skin.

lymphogranulomatosis inguinalis   LYMPHOGRANULOMA VENEREUM.

lymphogranulomatosis maligna   HODGKIN'S DISEASE.

malignant lymphogranulomatosis   HODGKIN'S DISEASE.

lymphography   LYMPHANGIOGRAPHY.

lymphohistiocytic   Involving both lymphocytes and histiocytes.

lymphohistioplasmacytic   Involving lymphocytes, histiocytes, and plasma cells.

lymphoid   Pertaining to or resembling lymph or lymphatic tissue. Also *adenoid*.

lymphoidocyte   HEMOCYTOBLAST.

lymphokentric   Stimulating the production of lymphocytes.

lymphokine   Any of several soluble mediators produced by lymphocytes, usually in response to reaction with lectins or specific antigens, and which participate in inflammatory reactions or in the growth and differentiation of other lymphocytes.

lymphokinesis   1 The movement of lymph in the body. 2 The movement of endolymph within the membraneous labyrinth of the ear. A rarely used term. For defs. 1 and 2 also *lymphocinesia*.

lymphology   LYMPHANGIOLOGY.

lymphoma [LYMPH- + -OMA]   Any of various malignant neoplasms primarily affecting lymph nodes, including the lymphocytic lymphomas, histiocytic lymphoma, and Hodgkin's disease. All but the last are known as non-Hodgkin's lymphomas. Also called *malignant lymphoma, hematosarcoma* (rarely used), *lymphadenomatosis, malignant lymphadenoma, lymphadenoma, malignant lymphadenosis, lymphomatosis*. • Lymphomas have been variously classified over the years. For descriptions of the major classifications see under CLASSIFICATION.

African lymphoma   BURKITT'S LYMPHOMA.

B cell lymphoma   A lymphoma of B lymphocytes.

benign lymphoma of the rectum   BENIGN LYMPHOID POLYP.

Burkitt's lymphoma   A malignant lymphoma involving extranodal sites such as the jaws, orbit, abdominal viscera, and ovaries. The tumor contains large lymphoid cells with considerable cytoplasmic basophilia and lipid-containing vacuoles. Macrophages with pale cytoplasm are interspersed among the tumor cells to give a "starry sky" effect. It is the most common childhood tumor in parts of tropical Africa, usually affecting children between five and nine years of age. It also occurs in other tropical and, to a lesser extent, temperate countries, most commonly where mean monthly temperature is over 15.5°C and relative humidity is high. It is possibly caused by the Epstein-Barr virus, but is also associated with stable falciparum malaria. Also called *Burkitt's tumor, African lymphoma*.

centroblastic lymphoma   FOLLICULAR CENTER CELL LYMPHOMA.

centrocytic lymphoma   FOLLICULAR CENTER CELL LYMPHOMA.

convoluted cell lymphoma   A lymphoma with cells having pronounced nuclear convolutions.

cutaneous T cell lymphoma   SÉZARY SYNDROME.

diffuse lymphoma A lymphoma in which the histologic pattern is one of diffuse rather than of nodular growth.

fascicular lymphoma A lymphoma whose cells are arranged in rows separated by fine stromal fibers.

follicular lymphoma NODULAR LYMPHOMA.

follicular center cell lymphoma A lymphoma with cells derived from the follicular centers of lymphoid tissue. Also called *centroblastic lymphoma, centrocytic lymphoma, germinoblastic lymphoma.*

germinoblastic lymphoma FOLLICULAR CENTER CELL LYMPHOMA.

giant follicular lymphoma NODULAR LYMPHOSARCOMA.

granulomatous lymphoma HODGKIN'S DISEASE.

histiocytic lymphoma A form of malignant lymphoma that appears to be composed of histiocytes. Most of these cases are actually poorly differentiated lymphocytic lymphomas. Also called *histiocytic sarcoma, reticulum cell sarcoma, reticulosarcoma* (obsolete), *clasmocytoma* (obsolete).

immunoblastic lymphoma A diffuse lymphoma composed of large cells with basophilic cytoplasm and a single prominent nucleolus.

intestinal lymphoma A form of lymphoma arising in the small intestines and usually associated with alpha heavy-chain disease.

Lennert's lymphoma LYMPHOEPITHELIOID CELL LYMPHOMA.

lymphoblastic lymphoma See under LYMPHOCYTIC LYMPHOMA.

lymphocytic lymphoma A malignant lymphoma composed of lymphocytes. The pattern may be either nodular or diffuse, and the cells may be either well-differentiated small lymphocytes or poorly differentiated lymphocytes that are larger and have less-condensed nuclear chromatin and nucleoli. Poorly differentiated lymphocytic lymphoma has also been called lymphoblastic lymphoma in earlier classifications. Also called *lymphosarcoma* (obsolete), *lymphocytoma* (obsolete).

lymphocytic lymphoma of intermediate differentiation PROLYMPHOCYTIC LYMPHOMA.

lymphoepithelioid cell lymphoma A rare form of lymphoma characterized by replacement of lymph nodes by lymphocytes and aggregates of epithelioid cells. The condition as originally described was thought to be a form of Hodgkin's disease, but it is now thought to be a separate entity. It has poor prognosis, with median survival of one year. Also called *Lennert's lymphoma.*

lymphoplasmacytic lymphoma A rarely used term for WALDENSTRÖM'S MACROGLOBULINEMIA.

malignant lymphoma LYMPHOMA.

nodular lymphoma A lymphoma composed of cells arranged in groups somewhat like lymphoid follicles. Also called *Brill-Symmers disease, Symmers disease, giant follicular lymphadenopathy, giant follicular lymphoma, nodular malignant lymphoma, follicular lymphoma, giant follicular lymphoblastoma.*

nodular malignant lymphoma NODULAR LYMPHOSARCOMA.

non-Hodgkin's lymphoma Any malignant lymphoma other than Hodgkin's disease.

poorly differentiated lymphocytic lymphoma A lymphoma composed of immature lymphocytes. Also called *poorly differentiated lymphosarcoma.*

prolymphocytic lymphoma A malignant lymphoma composed of lymphocytes that are slightly larger and that have less condensed nuclear chromatin than the cells of well-differentiated lymphocytic lymphoma. Also called *lymphocytic lymphoma of intermediate differentiation.*

sclerosing lymphoma A lymphoma with a prominent stromal component.

signet-ring cell lymphoma A rare form of malignant lymphoma consisting of cells with a large cytoplasmic vacuole of immunoglobulin which displaces the nucleus to the periphery. It thus simulates signet-ring cell carcinoma and may be positive with the periodic acid-Schiff reaction. It gives negative results for mucin content with stains such as Alcian blue and mucicarmine.

stem cell lymphoma A lymphoma composed of large blastlike cells. Also called *undifferentiated malignant lymphoma.*

T cell lymphoma A lymphoma of T lymphocytes.

undifferentiated malignant lymphoma STEM CELL LYMPHOMA.

lymphomatoid [*lymphomat(a)*, pl of LYMPHOMA + -OID] Resembling lymphoma.

lymphomatosis [*lymphomat(a)*, pl. of LYMPHOMA + -OSIS] LYMPHOMA.

avian lymphomatosis AVIAN LEUKOSIS.

lymphomatosis of fowl AVIAN LEUKOSIS.

lymphomatosis granulomatosa HODGKIN'S DISEASE.

neural lymphomatosis An outmoded term for MAREK'S DISEASE.

ocular lymphomatosis An outmoded term for MAREK'S DISEASE.

osteopetrotic lymphomatosis A neoplastic disease of poultry characterized by thickening of bones, particularly the long bones of the legs. It belongs to the leukosis-sarcoma group of the avian leukosis complex. Also called *thick leg disease, osteopetrosis gallinarum, avian Paget's disease (outmoded and inaccurate).*

visceral lymphomatosis An outmoded term for LYMPHOID LEUKOSIS.

lymphomatous Pertaining to lymphoma.

lymphomonocyte A leukocyte that allegedly has features both of lymphocytic and of monocytic character. An archaic and rarely used term.

lymphomyeloma [LYMPHO- + MYELOMA] Lymphosarcoma in the marrow.

lymphonodi Plural of LYMPHONODUS.

lymphonodus [LYMPHO- + NODUS] (*plural* lymphonodi) NODUS LYMPHATICUS.

lymphonodi anorectales An outmoded term for NODI LYMPHATICI PARARECTALES.

lymphonodi retropharyngei An outmoded term for NODI LYMPHATICI RETROPHARYNGEALES.

lymphonodi submentales An outmoded term for NODI LYMPHATICI SUBMENTALES.

lymphopathia LYMPHOPATHY.

lymphopathia venereum LYMPHOGRANULOMA VENEREUM.

lymphopathy Any disorder of the lymphatic system. A seldom used term. Also called *lymphopathia.*

ataxic lymphopathy Swelling of the lymph nodes which may occur during a pain crisis of locomotor ataxia.

lymphopenia LYMPHOCYTOPENIA.

lymphoplasty LYMPHANGIOPLASTY.

lymphopoiesis The production of lymphocytes. Also called *lymphocytopoiesis, lymphogenesis, lymphization.*

lymphopoietic Characterized by lymphopoiesis. Also *lymphogenous.*

lymphopoietin A soluble factor required for the maturation of lymphocytes. Recent advances in the study of the growth and differentiation factors needed by lymphocytes make it clear that there are a substantial number of lymphopoietic molecules.

lymphoproliferative Pertaining to the proliferation of lymphoid cells.

lymphoreticular Of or relating to the lymphoid tissues and organs and their associated reticuloendothelial framework.

lymphoreticulosis Any proliferation of the constituent cells of lymphoid tissues.

benign lymphoreticulosis CAT-SCRATCH DISEASE.

lymphorrhage The escape of lymph from a ruptured lymphatic vessel.

lymphorrhagia [LYMPHO- + -RRHAGIA] LYMPHORRHEA.

lymphorrhea [LYMPHO- + -RRHEA] The flow of lymph from a disrupted lymphatic channel. Also called *lymphorrhagia*.

lymphorrhoid [LYMPHO- + -rrh(ea) + -OID] A local dilatation of perianal lymphatics, occurring in lymphogranuloma venereum. It is similar in appearance to a hemorrhoid.

lymphosarcoleukemia LYMPHOSARCOMA CELL LEUKEMIA.

lymphosarcoma [LYMPHO- + SARCOMA] An obsolete term for LYMPHOCYTIC LYMPHOMA.

cutaneous lymphosarcoma An aggregate of malignant lymphoid cells in the skin.

Murphy-Sturm lymphosarcoma A chemically induced, transplantable lymphocytic lymphoma of rats. Lymphoid leukemia also occurs.

pleomorphic lymphosarcoma An outmoded term for HODGKIN'S DISEASE.

poorly differentiated lymphosarcoma POORLY DIFFERENTIATED LYMPHOCYTIC LYMPHOMA.

lymphosarcomatosis [*lymphosarcomat(a)*, pl. of LYMPHOSARCOMA + -OSIS] A widely disseminated lymphosarcoma. An obsolete term.

lymphosarcomatous Related to or describing lymphosarcoma.

lymphoscrotum [LYMPHO- + SCROTUM] ELEPHANTIASIS SCROTI.

lymphosis An incorrect term for CHRONIC LYMPHOCYTIC LEUKEMIA.

lymphostasis The absence of flow within lymphatic vessels.

lymphotaxis [LYMPHO- + Gk *taxis* an arranging, ordering] The induction of lymphocyte movement.

lymphotome [LYMPHO- + -TOME] A surgical instrument designed to facilitate the excision of lymphoid tissue. Also called *lymphatome*.

lymphotoxemia Disease due to excessive amount of lymphatic tissue. An obsolete concept.

lymphotoxic Pertaining to any substance that is toxic to lymphoid tissue.

lymphotoxin 1 A substance which is toxic or destructive to lymphocytes. 2 A toxin produced by T lymphocytes during an immune response which causes membrane damage and death of certain target cells.

lymphotrophic 1 Relating to lymphotrophy. 2 Attracted to the lymphatic system. • Although widely used, in this sense it is linguistically incorrect.

lymphotrophy The carrying of nutrients by the lymphatic system to tissues which have a defective blood supply.

lymphous Pertaining to or containing lymph.

lymphuria [LYMPH + -URIA] CHYLURIA.

filarial lymphuria The presence of lymph in the urine due to lymphatic obstruction around a kidney, ureter, or bladder in some cases of filariasis. If chyle is present the urine appears milky. *Wuchereria bancrofti* and *Brugia malayi* are usually responsible.

lymph-vascular Pertaining to or having lymphatic vessels.

Lynchia maura *PSEUDOLYNCHIA CANARIENSIS.*

Lynen [Feodor *Lynen*, German biochemist, born 1911] See under CYCLE.

lynestrenol $C_{20}H_{28}O$. 19-Nor-pregn-4-en-20-yn-17α-ol. A semisynthetic progestin or progestogen.

Lynoral A proprietary name for ethynyl estradiol.

lyo- [Gk *lyein* to loosen, dissolve, wash] A combining form meaning dispersed, dissolved, loosened.

Lyon [Bethuel Boyd Vincent *Lyon*, U.S. physician, 1880–1953] Meltzer-Lyon test. See under TEST.

Lyon [Mary Frances *Lyon*, English geneticist, born 1925] Lyon-Russell hypothesis, Lyon hypothesis. See under LYON PHENOMENON.

lyonization LYON PHENOMENON.

lyophilic [LYO- + -PHILIC] Dispersing or dissolving easily because of having an affinity for the solvent: said of colloidal particles or macromolecules.

lyophilization [LYO- + -PHIL + -iz(e) + -ATION] The process of drying a sample by submitting it to a vacuum while frozen, so that ice sublimes out of it. Also called *freeze-drying*. • The term is somewhat misleading, as the process does not render materials lyophilic, but merely keeps them lyophilic to the extent that it avoids denaturing proteins.

lyophobic [LYO- + PHOBIC] Difficult to disperse because of having little affinity for the solvent: said of a colloidal material.

lyotropic Concerning the relative ability of ions to influence the medium in which they are dissolved. Hence ions high in a lyotropic series have great effect on solvent properties, particularly for colloidal substances, e.g. they are especially effective in salting out proteins.

Lyperosia irritans *HAEMATOBIA IRRITANS.*

Lyponyssus *ORNITHONYSSUS.*

lypressin Vasopressin with lysine in place of arginine at position 8, found in the supraopticoneurohypophysial unit of members of the pig family. The hippopotamus and domestic pig have lysine vasopressin only; the wart hog and peccary have both lysine and arginine vasopressin. The peptide is arranged into a five-member S-S bonded ring with a three-member side chain in which lysine occupies the position next to the terminal glycinamide. It is an antidiuretic and a vasopressor hormone, and is used as a nasal spray in the treatment of diabetes insipidus of central origin. Also called *vasopressin 8-lysine, lysine vasopressin.*

lyra [L (Gk *lyra*), a lyre, lute, harp] An anatomic structure suggestive of the shape of a lyre or lute. Also called *lyre.*

lyra davidis An obsolete term for COMMISSURA FORNICIS.

lyra uteri An outmoded term for PLICAE PALMATAE.

lyra uterina An outmoded term for PLICAE PALMATAE.

lyre LYRA.

lyre of David An obsolete term for COMMISSURA FORNICIS.

Lys Symbol for lysine.

lys- LYSO-.

lysate The product of lysis.

lyse [Back formation from LYSIS] To subject to lysis; to break up or rupture (a cell membrane).

lysemia Intravascular hemolysis with hemoglobinemia. A rarely used term.

lysenkoism A doctrine of genetics that embraced inheritance of acquired characteristics and denied the central role of genes and chromosomes. It was promulgated by T.D. Lysenko (1898–1976) and was the official position of the U.S.S.R. in the mid-twentieth century, but it wrought disastrous consquences on agronomy and the biological sciences in that country.

lysergic acid One of the ergot alkaloids, a component of the ergotamine molecule. Its molecule contains four rings, two of them containing nitrogen, and it is derived biosynthetically from tryptophan and dimethylallyl pyrophosphate.

lysergic acid diethylamide A hallucinogenic indole amine that is highly subject to abuse. Unlike the ergot alkaloids, this compound directly affects the central nervous system with effects resembling those of mescaline. It can induce temporary manifestations of schizophrenia, and it is suspected of causing chromosomal damage. Abbreviation: LSD, LSD-25

Lysholm [Erik Lorenz Rudolf *Lysholm*, Swedish radiologist, 1891–1947] See under PROJECTION.

lysidin 2-Methyl-2-imidazole. It was formerly used in the treatment of diseases characterized by high uric acid concentrations in the tissues because of its solvent effect on uric acid.

lysidin bitartrate A soluble white powder form of lysidin with considerably less solvent power for uric acid than lysidin itself. It has been used in the treatment of rheumatism.

lysin [LYS- + -IN] Any substance capable of causing lysis, especially a complement-fixing antibody: often used in combination to indicate the type of cell to which the action of the lysin is specifically directed, as hemolysin or bacteriolysin.

hot-cold lysin Any of those lysins that are activated only following incubation at 37°C followed by refrigeration, as β-hemolysin.

immune lysin An antibody detected by giving rise to complement-mediated cell lysis. An outmoded term.

lysine $NH_2—[CH_2]_4—CH(NH_2)COOH$. One of the twenty amino acids that are incorporated into proteins. It is important in human nutrition because it is essential. Diets may be deficient in it because, in general, plant proteins contain less lysine than do animal proteins. Lysine residues in proteins are usually on the outside of the molecules, providing positive charges, and lysine residues in enzymes sometimes form imines with carbonyl substrates or cofactors.

lysine vasopressin LYPRESSIN.

lysinosis An obsolete term for BYSSINOSIS.

lysis [Gk *lysis* (from *lyein* to loosen, dissolve, slacken, set free, weaken) a loosing, setting free, esp. of a prisoner; release, ransoming] **1** Any form of dissolution, particularly the breaking of membrane-bound structures such as cells. **2** A gradual reduction in strength of the symptoms of a disease, leading to its eventual disappearance. Compare CRISIS. Adjective: lytic.

bone lysis OSTEOLYSIS.

cell lysis Rupture of the cell membrane.

confluent lysis The total lysis of bacteria that are infected with a virulent bacteriophage, when growing as a lawn on an agar plate. This phenomenon is used in the preparation of transducing phage.

immune lysis The destruction of cells by immunologic mechanisms. These include lysis of antibody-sensitized cells by complement or killer cells and lysis of specific target cells by cytotoxic T lymphocytes.

osmotic lysis Rupture of the plasma membrane of a cell following immersion in a hypotonic solution.

lyso- [Gk *lysis* (from *lyein* to loosen, dissolve, wash) dissolution, loosing, decomposition] A combining form meaning lysis or dissolution. When applied to lipids, it signifies that one of the two acyl groups has been removed from the glycerol part of the molecule. Also *lys-*.

lysochrome A lipid-soluble pigment that is suitable for staining fats.

lysocythin A cytolytic substance formed by the reaction of body tissues to an animal venom.

lysogenic [LYSO- + -GENIC] Denoting a strain of bacterium that perpetuates a bacteriophage in the prophage state. The

lysogenic condition usually renders the bacteria immune to further infection by particles of the bacteriophage they carry, but not to particles of different phages.

lysogenization The process whereby a bacterium is rendered lysogenic by bacteriophage infection.

lysogeny [LYSO- + -GEN + -Y] A process whereby viral nucleic acid that has entered a cell does not initiate the synthesis of more viral material but becomes attached to specific sites in the chromosome, and is then both reproduced together with the chromosome and transmitted to daughter cells at each cell division: used particularly of viruses that infect bacteria (bacteriophages) and which, when in lysogeny, are described as being in the prophage state.

lysokinase TISSUE PLASMINOGEN ACTIVATOR.

lysolecithin LYSOPHOSPHATIDYLCHOLINE.

lysophosphatidylcholine A lipid in which phosphoric acid forms an ester link between a monoacylglycerol and choline. Also called *lysolecithin*.

lysophospholipase An enzyme that catalyzes hydrolysis of a lysophosphatidylcholine. Also called *lecithinase* (obsolete).

lysosomal Pertaining to or derived from a lysosome.

lysosome [LYSO- + Gk *sōma* the body] A membrane-limited cytoplasmic organelle containing hydrolytic enzymes which have a pH optimum in the acid range. Also called *cytolysome*.

primary lysosome A newly formed lysosome as it separates from the Golgi membranes.

secondary lysosome A cytoplasmic sac formed by the fusion of a primary lysosome and a phagosome containing material to be digested. Also called *digestive vacuole*.

lysostaphin An enzyme produced by *Staphylococcus staphylolyticus* that has antibacterial activity. The enzyme has specific action against staphylococci.

lysotype A type within a bacterial species as determined by its pattern of sensitivity to a set of test phages.

lysozyme The tear enzyme capable of killing some varieties of bacteria. Also called *muramidase* (obsolete).

lysozymuria Excretion of lysozyme in the urine. Greater than normal lysozymuria is characteristic of myeloproliferative disorders, especially chronic granulocytic leukemia and myelomonocytic leukemia.

lyssa [Gk *lyssa* rage, frenzy] An obsolete term for RABIES.

Lyssavirus A genus of the Rhabdoviridae family that includes rabies virus.

lyssic RABIC.

lyssoid [*lyss(a)* + -OID] RABIFORM.

lyssophobia [Gk *lyss(a)* a raving, frenzy + *o* + -PHOBIA] Pathologic fear of becoming insane or having a nervous breakdown.

Lyster [William John L. *Lyster*, U.S. surgeon, 1869–1947] See under BAG.

lysyl oxidase PROTEIN-LYSINE 6-OXIDASE.

Lyt See under LY ANTIGENS.

lytic Related to or capable of producing lysis.

Lytta A genus of blister beetles.

Lytta vesicatoria CANTHARIS VESICATORIA.

lyxose $CHO—[CHOH]_3—CH_2OH$. An aldopentose sugar having the opposite configuration to ribose at both C-2 and C-3. It is uncommon in living organisms.

M

M **1** A symbol widely used in chemistry to denote concentration in moles per liter. **2** Symbol for methionine. **3** Symbol for mega-: used with SI units.

M. **1** *mille* (L, thousand). **2** *misce* (L, mix). **3** *mistura* (L, mixture). **4** myopia. **5** mucoid (colony).

m **1** Symbol for milli-: used with SI units. **2** Symbol for the unit, meter.

m^{-1} Symbol for the unit, reciprocal meter.

m² Symbol for the unit, square meter.

m³ Symbol for the unit, cubic meter.

M Symbol for the quantities (1) bending moment, expressed in newton-meters; (2) molar mass, expressed in kilograms per mole; (3) moment of force, expressed in newton-meters; (4) mutual inductance, expressed in henrys; (5) radiant exitance, expressed in watts per square meter; (6) magnetization, expressed in amperes per meter; (7) luminous exitance, expressed in lumens per square meter.

M$_r$ Symbol for the quantity, relative molecular mass of a substance.

m Symbol for the quantities (1) mass, expressed in kilograms; (2) electron rest mass, expressed in kilograms or atomic mass units; (3) electromagnetic moment, expressed in ampere meters squared.

m- meta-.

m$_a$ Symbol for the quantity mass of an atom, or nuclidic mass, expressed in unified atomic mass units.

μ **1** Symbol for micro-: used with SI units. **2** Symbol for the unit, micrometer. An incorrect symbol. **3** Symbol for magnetic permeability.

μ Symbol for the quantities (1) coefficient of friction; (2) linear attenuation coefficient, expressed in reciprocal meters; (3) permeability, expressed in henrys per meter; (4) mobility, expressed in square meters per volt-second.

μ$_B$ Symbol for the quantity, Bohr magneton, expressed in ampere square meters.

μ$_N$ Symbol for the quantity, nuclear magneton, expressed in ampere square meters.

MA **1** Symbol for the unit, megaampere. **2** mental age. **3** meter angle.

Ma Mach number.

mA Symbol for the unit, milliampere.

mÅ Symbol for the unit, milliångström.

ma **1** Symbol for the obsolete combining form, myria-. **2** Symbol for milliampere. An incorrect symbol.

μA Symbol for the unit, microampere.

mabata A tick of the species *Ornithodoros moubata*.

MAC **1** maximum allowable concentration. **2** minimum alveolar concentration.

mac. *macerare* (L, macerate).

Macaca [New L, fem. of Portuguese *macaco* a monkey] A genus of the primate family Cercopithecidae; the macaques. They are characterized by stout bodies, powerful limbs, and a somewhat elongate snout. There are about 12 species distributed from Gibraltar to southeastern Asia. Several species of macaques are important subjects in medical and space research.

Macaca mulatta The rhesus monkey. It is widely used in medical and biological research.

macaque [French. See MACACA.] Any monkey of the genus *Macaca*.

crab-eating macaque CYNOMOLGUS.

Japanese macaque A primate of the species *Macaca fuscata*. This species breeds well in captivity and is used in some biomedical research.

MacCallum [William George *MacCallum*, Canadian pathologist active in the United States, 1874–1944] See under PATCH.

MacConkey [Alfred Theodore *MacConkey*, English bacteriologist, 1861–1931] See under AGAR.

Macdonald [George *Macdonald*, English malariologist, born 1903] See under INDEX.

Macdowel [Benjamin George *Macdowel*, Irish anatomist and surgeon, 1820–1885] Macdowel's frenum. See under FRENULUM.

Mace [contraction of *m(ethylchloroform chloro)ace(tophenone)*] C$_8$H$_7$ClO. A form of tear gas. It causes coughing, lacrimation, and vomiting, thus incapacitating its target.etary name. Also called *Chemical Mace*.

Chemical Mace MACE.

Mace [contraction of *m(ethylchloroform chloro)ace(tophenone)*] C$_8$H$_7$ClO. A form of tear gas. It causes coughing, lacrimation, and vomiting, thus incapacitating its target. A proprietary name. Also called *Chemical Mace*.

macerate [L *maceratus*, past part. of *macerare* to soften by steeping] To soften and disintegrate a mass of tissue, as by soaking in a fluid medium that contains acids or enzymes.

maceration [L *maceratio*, from *maceratus*. See MACERATE.] **1** In histology, the softening and disintegration of a mass of tissue by soaking in acids or enzymes. **2** The autolysis of fetal tissues, which develops when death occurs *in utero* and the fetus is retained.

macerative Of or related to maceration.

Macewen [Sir William *Macewen*, Scottish surgeon, 1848–1924] **1** See under SIGN. **2** Tibial spine of Macewen. See under SPINE. **3** Macewen's osteotomy. See under OPERATION. **4** Macewen's triangle. See under SUPRAMEATAL TRIANGLE.

Mach [Ernst *Mach*, Austrian physicist, 1838–1916] See under APPARATUS.

Mach [René Sigmund *Mach*, Swiss internist, born 1904] See under SYNDROME.

Mache [Heinrich *Mache*, Austrian physicist, 1876–1954] See under UNIT.

machine [L *machina* (from Gk *mēchanē* an instrument for lifting weights, engine of war, contrivance, means, from *mēchos* a means, expedient) a frame, stage, scaffold, engine of war, machine] A device for the production, conversion, or transmission of mechanical, electrical, or chemical energy or material.

anesthesia machine An apparatus used to supply anesthetic gases and vapors plus oxygen. It is capable of quantifying the volumes delivered, as well as delivering mixtures to a patient's breathing circuit for the inducement of general anesthesia. Also called *gas machine.*

casting machine A machine used in dentistry for forcing molten metal into a mold, usually by centrifugal force.

Clayton's machine An appliance that produces sulfur dioxide for fumigation, used chiefly on ships.

gas machine ANESTHESIA MACHINE.

heart-lung machine A combination of pump and oxygenator to effect extracorporeal circulation and oxygenation of blood during open-heart surgery.

Holtz machine An early form of high-voltage electrostatic generator.

panoramic rotating machine A type of x-ray equipment for dental pantomography, producing images of all the teeth and surrounding structures on one film. Its principle is the use of a reciprocating motion of the x-ray tube and a curved extraoral film.

static machine ELECTROSTATIC GENERATOR.

teaching machine A device for programed learning. Learners work at their own pace to master, in small steps, material presented to them automatically. The correctness of responses made to questions asked about the material presented determines the rate of progress in learning.

Van de Graaff machine VAN DE GRAAFF GENERATOR.

Wimshurst machine An early form of electrostatic generator.

macho A form of cutaneous leishmaniasis. An obsolete term.

Machover [Karen Alper *Machover*, U.S. psychologist, born 1902] Machover test. See under DRAW-A-PERSON TEST.

macies [L, leanness] WASTING.

Macintosh [Charles *Macintosh*, Scottish chemist, 1766–1843] See under SHEET.

MacKay [Ralph Stuart *MacKay*, U.S. biophysicist, born 1924] MacKay-Marg electronic tonometer. See under TONOMETER.

Mackenrodt [Alwin Karl *Mackenrodt*, German gynecologist, 1859–1925] **1** See under OPERATION. **2** Mackenrodt's ligament, transverse cervical ligament of Mackenrodt. See under LATERAL CERVICAL LIGAMENT.

Mackenzie [Sir James *Mackenzie*, Scottish physician, 1853–1925] **1** Mackenzie's disease. See under X DISEASE. **2** See under POLYGRAPH.

Mackenzie [Sir Stephen *Mackenzie*, English physician, 1844–1909] **1** Jackson-Mackenzie syndrome, Mackenzie syndrome. See under JACKSON'S PARALYSIS. **2** See under AMPUTATION.

MacLachlan [Elsie A. *MacLachlan*, U.S. medical researcher, flourished mid-20th century] Lowe-Terrey-MacLachlan syndrome. See under OCULOCEREBRORENAL SYNDROME.

MacLean [Charles *MacLean*, English physician, 1788–1824] MacLean-Maxwell syndrome. See under MACLEAN-MAXWELL DISEASE.

MacLeod [Roderick *MacLeod*, Scottish physician, 1795–1852] MacLeod's capsular rheumatism. See under RHEUMATOID ARTHRITIS.

Macleod [William Mathieson *Macleod*, English pneumologist, 1911–1977] Swyer-James-Macleod syndrome. See under SYNDROME.

macleyine PROTOPINE.

MacNeal [Ward J. *MacNeal*, U.S. bacteriologist, 1881–1946] MacNeal's tetrachrome stain. See under STAIN.

macr- MACRO-.

Macracanthorhynchus A genus of giant, thorny-headed, intestinal worms of the phylum Acanthocephala, order Archiacanthocephala.

Macracanthorhynchus hirudinaceus A common species of extremely large worms found in the small intestine of the pig and, rarely, in humans. The female is 25–60 cm long and the male, 5–10 cm. It is pink, pseudosegmented (transversely wrinkled), with a long, tapering, flattened body and a knoblike proboscis armed with five or six rows of thorns. The spiny proboscis induces development of nodules at the point of attachment. Soil-dwelling grubs of May beetles (*Cotinus*) and June beetles (*Phyllophaga*) serve as intermediate hosts, infecting pigs that root in the soil. Also called *Echinorhynchus gigas, Echinorhynchus hominis, Gigantorhynchus hirudinaceus.*

macracusia HYPERACUSIS.

macrencephalia MACROENCEPHALY.

macrencephalon MACROENCEPHALON.

macrencephaly MACROENCEPHALY.

macro- [Gk *makros* long, large] A combining form meaning (1) large or long; (2) abnormally or excessively large. Also *macr-, makro-.*

macroaggregate Any aggregate that is larger than normal.

macroaleuriospore [MACRO- + Gk *aleur(on)* wheaten flour + *io* + SPORE] An outmoded term for MACROCONIDIUM.

macroamylasemia [MACRO- + *amylas(e)* + -EMIA] The elevation of measured serum amylase due to the presence of macroamylase, a complex of amylase and globulin with a high molecular weight that does not pass through the glomerular filter. It may occur as a nonspecific laboratory abnormality in subjects with alcoholism, malabsorption, or other disorders of the digestive tract.

Macrobdella A genus of large leeches in the family Gnathobdellidae.

Macrobdella decora The American leech, a species found in the United States and Canada and formerly used for drawing blood in place of the European medicinal leech, *Hirudo medicinalis.*

macrobiota [MACRO- + BIOTA] The total visible flora and fauna of a biotic community.

macrobiote [MACRO- + Gk *biotē*, also *biotos* life, means of life] A long-lived organism, with special reference to prolonged survival in a dormant, resistant state, such as clostridial spores, eggs of *Ascaris*, or the survival qualities of certain ticks.

macrobiotic Of or relating to the macrobiota.

macroblast [MACRO- + -BLAST] Any unusually large normoblast. A rarely used term.

macroblast of Naegeli PRONORMOBLAST.

macroblepharia [MACRO- + BLEPHAR- + -IA] The condition of having abnormally large eyelids.

macrobrachia [MACRO- + *brach(ium)* + -IA] Excessive length or size in one or both arms.

macrocardia [MACRO- + -CARDIA] **1** Abnormal largeness of the heart in an infant or child with congenital cardiac disease. The increased size is usually the result of attempted functional compensation for circulatory inefficiency secondary to developmental defects. Also called *megalocardia.* **2** CARDIOMEGALY.

macrocardius [MACRO- + *cardi(a)* + New L -*us*, masc. noun suffix] An individual possessing an enlarged heart.

macrocephalia MACROCEPHALY.

macrocephalic MACROCEPHALOUS.

macrocephalous Exhibiting macrocephaly. Also *megacephalous, macrocephalic, megacephalic, megalocephalic.*

macrocephalus [MACRO- + -CEPHALUS] A fetus or postnatal individual with macrocephaly. Also called *megacephalus*.

macrocephaly [MACRO- + CEPHAL- + -Y] A disproportionate largeness of the head, either a general enlargement of the entire head or an increase in particular dimensions or parts. Also called *megacephaly, macrocephalia, megacephalia, megalocephaly, megalocephalia, megacephalum*.

macrocheilia [MACRO- + CHEIL- + -IA] An abnormal largeness of a lip, usually owing to a cavernous lymphangioma. Also called *macrolabia*. Also *macrochilia*.

macrocheiria [MACRO- + CHEIR- + -IA] CHEIROMEGALY.

macrochilia MACROCHEILIA.

macrochiria [MACRO- + CHIR- + -IA] CHEIROMEGALY.

macrochylomicron [MACRO- + CHYLOMICRON] A chylomicron of unusually large size.

macrochylomicronemia The presence of unusually large chylomicrons in blood.

macroclimate The climate experienced over a large geographical area, as a region, country, continent, or the entire earth.

macroclitoris [MACRO- + CLITORIS] Pathologic hypertrophy of the clitoris occurring in any virilizing disorder. Also called *clitorimegaly, megaloclitoris*.

macrocnemia [MACRO- + Gk *knēm(ē)* the leg + -IA] An abnormal largeness of one or both shins.

macroconidium [MACRO- + CONIDIUM] (*plural* macroconidia) A large fungal conidium, or asexually formed single-cell spore distinguished by its size from a microconidium produced by the same fungal organism. Also called *macrospore, macroaleuriospore* (outmoded), *megalospore, megaspore, fuseau*.

macrocornea [MACRO- + CORNEA] A pathologically large cornea.

macrocosm [French *macrocosme* (from Med L *macrocosmus* universe, from Gk *makro(s)* long, large + *kosm(os)* order, world, universe) the universe] A large natural environmental unit with open boundaries. Compare MICROCOSM.

macrocrania [MACRO- + *cran(i)-* + -IA] Disproportionate enlargement of the cranium compared to the face. It is seen in hydrocephalus. Compare MACROPROSOPIA.

macrocryoglobulinemia CRYOGLOBULINEMIA.

macrocyst [MACRO- + CYST] A large cyst. An outmoded term.

Macrocystis A genus of kelp (large, brown, marine algae) that belong to the order Laminariales of the Phaeophycophyta. The thalli of kelp species have been used as a source of a heparinlike substance.

macrocytase A cytase or complement which destroys tissue cells or blood cells and which is formed in large mononuclear leukocytes. An obsolete term.

macrocyte A large erythrocyte, usually more than nine micrometers in diameter or 100 femtoliters in volume, observed in the peripheral blood following recent hemorrhage, in hemolytic disorders, or as a result of deficiency of vitamin B_{12} or folic acid. Also called *macroerythrocyte, megalocyte*.

macrocythemia MACROCYTOSIS.

macrocytosis A greater than normal mean corpuscular volume of erythrocytes in blood, generally greater than 100 femtoliters. It is observed whenever there is accelerated formation of erythrocytes, as in hemolytic disorders or following hemorrhage. It is also characteristic of vitamin B_{12} or folate deficiency. Also called *macrocythemia, megalocythemia, megalocytosis*.

macrodactylia MACRODACTYLY.

macrodactylism MACRODACTYLY.

macrodactyly [MACRO- + DACTYL- + -Y] The abnormal largeness of one or more digits. Also called *macrodactylism,*

macrodactylia, giant finger, digital gigantism, megadactyly, megadactylia, megadactylism, megalodactylia, megalodactylism, megalodactyly, dactomegaly.

Macrodasyoidea [MACRO- + Gk *dasy(s)* shaggy + New L *-oidea*, from L *-oïdes* -OID + *-ea*, neut. pl. of *-eus* -EOUS] An order of small, wormlike marine invertebrates in the class Gastrotricha, found in mud or sand at the intertidal zone. They are hermaphroditic, have pharyngeal pores, and are usually furnished with anterior, lateral, and posterior adhesive tubules.

macrodont [MACR- + -ODONT] **1** Having abnormally large teeth. Also *megadontic, macrodontic*. **2** An abnormally large tooth, often bilateral. Its occurrence often follows familial or hereditary tendencies. Also called *megadont, megalodont*.

macrodontia [MACR- + -ODONTIA] Abnormal largeness of one or more teeth. Also called *macrodontism, megadontia, megalodontia, megadontism*.

macrodontic MACRODONT.

macrodontism MACRODONTIA.

macrodystrophia [MACRO- + DYSTROPHIA] The disproportionate overgrowth of any part.

macrodystrophia lipomatosa progressiva An overgrowth of adipose tissue in a part or a region resulting in partial or localized gigantism of the affected part.

macroencephalon [MACRO- + ENCEPHALON] An abnormally large brain. Also called *macrencephalon, megaloencephalon, megalencephalon*.

macroencephaly [MACRO- + ENCEPHAL- + -Y] The condition of having an excessively large brain. Also called *macrencephaly, megaloencephaly, megalencephaly, encephalauxe, macrencephalia*.

macroerythroblast MACRONORMOBLAST.

macroerythrocyte MACROCYTE.

macroesthesia [MACRO- + -ESTHESIA] A defect of tactile perception, in which objects felt or handled appear to be larger than they are. Also called *macrostereognosis, macrostereognosia*.

macroevolution [MACRO- + EVOLUTION] Evolution which gives rise to new species or other categories of organisms.

macrofauna Terrestrial animals in the size category of large insects, earthworms, and small centipedes.

macrofollicular Pertaining to large follicles.

macrogamete The larger, or egglike, gamete produced in anisogamy. It fuses with the microgamete, leading to zygote formation. Also called *megagamete*.

macrogametocyte The mother cell that produces macrogametes in anisogametic reproduction. Also called *macrogamont*.

macrogamont MACROGAMETOCYTE.

macrogenesis [MACRO- + GENESIS] The excessive growth of a part.

macrogenesy [MACRO- + *genes(is)* + -Y] A seldom used term for GIGANTISM.

macrogenitosomia [MACRO- + GENITO- + Gk *sōm(a)* the body + -IA] Excessive and untimely somatic and genital growth and development.

macrogenitosomia praecox A pathologic increase in growth and development of the body and genitals, occurring in early childhood, caused by untimely secretion of the sex steroids by the gonads or adrenal cortex.   • The term is sometimes incorrectly used to denote specifically the premature somatic and genital development associated with certain tumors of the pineal body, such as those associated with the Pellizzi syndrome.

macrogenitosomia praecox suprarenalis Premature somatic and genital growth and development, often occurring from infancy, in congenital adrenocortical hyperplasia with virilism in males and females.

macrogingiva [MACRO- + GINGIVA] GINGIVAL HYPERPLASIA.

macroglia [MACRO- + GLIA] The large neuroglial cells derived from neurectoderm, including astrocytes and oligodendrocytes. • The term is sometimes incorrectly used exclusively for astrocytes.

macroglial Of or pertaining to macroglia.

macroglobulin [MACRO- + GLOBULIN] Any globulin in serum of molecular mass above about 400 kDa. One of the most important is the versatile proteinase inhibitor called α_2-macroglobulin.

γ macroglobulin An obsolete term for IMMUNOGLOBULIN M.

macroglobulinemia [MACRO- + GLOBULINEMIA] A greater than normal concentration in plasma of macroglobulin.

primary macroglobulinemia WALDENSTRÖM'S MACROGLOBULINEMIA.

Waldenström's macroglobulinemia A lymphocytic lymphoma characterized by proliferation of lymphocytes, plasma cells, and cells that resemble both lymphocytes and plasma cells ("plasmacytoid lymphocytes") in association with high serum concentration of a monoclonal macroglobulin, or IgM. Also called *primary macroglobulinemia, lymphoplasmacytic lymphoma.*

macroglossia [MACRO- + GLOSS- + -IA] Diffuse enlargement of the tongue. It may be due, for example, to congenital muscular hypertrophy or lymphangioma, and occurs in certain endocrinopathies. Also called *megaloglossia.*

macrognathia [MACRO- + GNATH- + -IA] An abnormally large jaw. Either the upper or lower jaw may be or may become abnormally large in a variety of conditions ranging from acromegaly to mandibular prognathism. Also called *megagnathia.* Adjective: macrognathic.

macrogol A spectrum of polyethylene glycols, including both liquid and solid forms. The types are designated by numbers relating to the solidity of the substance; the higher the number, the harder the preparation. They are used as ointment bases and have many industrial uses.

macrogol 400 Polyethylene glycol with an average molecular weight of 380 to 420. It is a clear, hygroscopic, viscous liquid, used as a constituent of ointments and to stabilize emulsions.

macrogol 4000 Polyethylene glycol with an average molecular weight between 3100 and 3700. It is a solid, creamy-white, waxlike flaky material or a white powder. It is practically insoluble in water and not absorbed at all from the intestinal tract, but it is used as a vehicle of drugs to give a sustained release and slow absorption.

macrogyria [MACRO- + *gyr(us)* + -IA] Enlargement of the cerebral gyri.

macroinstruction A computer programing language instruction that produces a series of machine instructions.

macrolabia [MACRO- + L *labia* lip] MACROCHEILIA.

macrolecithal [MACRO- + LECITH- + -AL] MEGALECITHAL.

macrolide A natural lactone, whose ring is large, usually of about 14–20 atoms. Several antibiotics, including erythromycin, are macrolides. These inhibit protein biosynthesis.

macrolymphocyte A large lymphocyte.

macromania [MACRO- + MANIA] MACROMANIACAL DELIRIUM.

macromastia [MACRO- + MAST- + -IA] Excessive size of the breasts, usually not due to hormonal cause. Also called *megalomastia, macromazia* (rarely used).

macromazia A rarely used term for MACROMASTIA.

macromelia [MACRO- + MEL-¹ + -IA] An excessive size of one or more limbs. Also called *megalomelia, megamelia.*

macromelus An individual affected by macromelia.

macromere [MACRO- + -MERE] A large blastomere, as opposed to a micromere. In the eggs of batrachians, the macromeres situated at the inferior pole are well supplied with yolk and will supply especially the entoblastic elements. In mammals, provided that cleavage results in differences between the blastomeres, there exists at a certain time four micromeres and four macromeres. These last, after they have multiplied, become indistinct and form the inner cell mass.

macromerozoite A large merozoite. Also called *megamerozoite.*

macromethod Any analytical technique that uses standard quantities of reagents and of the specimen to be tested.

macromolecular Concerned with or possessing large molecules: in biology used especially of protein or nucleic acid.

macromolecule [MACRO- + MOLECULE] A very large molecule, such as a protein, nucleic acid, or polysaccharide molecule.

informational macromolecule A macromolecule which stores information for cellular structure and function, as the molecule of deoxyribonucleic acid or ribonucleic acid.

macromonocyte A monocyte which is larger than normal.

macromutation A major change in the genetic material which would give rise to a new species in a single generation.

macromyeloblast An unusually large myeloblast. A rarely used term.

macronodular Characterized by the presence of large nodules, as in macronodular cirrhosis.

macronormoblast A large normoblast. Also called *macroerythroblast, macronormochromoblast.*

macronormochromoblast MACRONORMOBLAST.

macronucleus [MACRO- + NUCLEUS] The larger of the two nuclei in ciliated protozoans, the smaller being the micronucleus. Macronuclei divide amitotically during fission and disappear during conjugation. They govern the metabolic functions of the vegetative cell. Also called *meganucleus, nutrition nucleus, somatic nucleus, trophic nucleus, vegetative nucleus.*

macronutrients [MACRO- + *nutrients,* pl. of NUTRIENT] **1** The fat, protein, and carbohydrate contents of the diet. **2** All nutrients required by the body in more than trace amounts, including the above plus the major minerals (calcium, magnesium, sodium, and potassium).

macronychia [*macr-* + ONYCH- + -IA] A condition marked by excessive size or thickness of fingernails or toenails. Also called *megalonychosis, megalonychia, macronychosis.*

macronychosis MACRONYCHIA.

macroparasite [MACRO- + PARASITE] A parasite visible to the naked eye, such as a tick or an intestinal worm.

macropathology The pathologic description and study of gross anatomic changes in disease. A seldom used term.

macropenis An excessive size or length of the penis. Also called *macrophallus, megalopenis, megalophallus.*

macrophage [MACRO- + Gk *phagein* to eat] A cell found in many tissues in the body which is derived from the blood monocyte and which has an important role in host defense mechanisms. It phagocytizes and kills many bacteria and is the site of infection for a number of intracellular parasites. Also called *macrophagocyte, clasmatocyte* (older term), *endothelial leukocyte, rhagiocrine cell.*

alveolar macrophage A phagocytic cell found in the alveoli of the lungs. It serves to eliminate foreign particles brought into the lungs in inspired air. Also called *alveolar phagocyte, dust cell.*

fixed macrophage A mononuclear phagocytic cell that is resident in one of several possible tissues of the body and does not migrate to various sites in response to stimuli. Also called *resting wandering cell.*

free macrophage   A mononuclear phagocytic cell, primarily found in the vascular system, which moves to various parts of the body, often in response to a chemotactic stimulus.

inflammatory macrophage   A mononuclear phagocytic cell found as one of the cellular components of inflammatory response, often as a result of bacterial invasion of the tissues.

tingible-body macrophage   A macrophage that has engulfed residual nuclear material from multiplying follicular center cells. The presence of tingible-body macrophages indicates follicular reactivity and distinguishes reactive follicles from the rounded cell masses of nodular lymphoma.

macrophagocyte   MACROPHAGE.

macrophagocytosis   The ingestion of foreign bodies by macrophages of the reticuloendothelial system.

macrophallus   MACROPENIS.

macrophthalmia [MACR- + OPHTHALMIA]   An excessive size of the eyeball. Also called *megalophthalmia, megalophthalmus, megalophthalmos, megophthalmos, ophthalmacrosis.*

macrophthalmous   Exhibiting macrophthalmia.

macropia   MACROPSIA.

macroplasia [MACRO- + -PLASIA]   Excessive growth of a tissue or organ. Also called *macroplastia.*

macroplastia   MACROPLASIA.

macropodal [MACRO- + -POD + -AL]   Having a large foot, stalk, or stem.

macropodia [MACRO- + -POD + -IA]   Abnormal largeness of the feet. Also called *megalopodia, pes gigas.*

macropolycyte   An abnormally large, hypersegmented polymorphonuclear leukocyte characteristic of pernicious anemia.

macropromyelocyte   An abnormally large promyelocyte, sometimes seen in pernicious anemia.

macroprosopia [MACRO- + PROSOP- + -IA]   A disproportionate largeness of the face, usually relative to the cranium. Also called *megaprosopia.* Compare MACROCRANIA.

macroprosopus   An individual having macroprosopia.

macropsia [MACR- + -OPSIA]   A visual fault which causes objects to appear magnified in size. Also called *macropia, megalopia, megalopsia.*

macropterous [MACRO- + PTER- + -OUS]   **1** Having large or long fins or wings.   **2** Having fully formed wings: said especially of insects. Compare BRACHYPTEROUS.

macrorhinia [MACRO- + RHIN- + -IA]   An abnormally large nose, whether of developmental or pathologic origin. A seldom used term. Also *macrorrhinia.*

macrorrhinia   MACRORHINIA.

macroscelia [MACRO- + Gk *skel(os)* the leg + -IA]   An abnormal girth or length of the legs.

macroscopic   Of ore relating to structures that are of sufficient size so as to be visible for study without the use of a microscope.

macroscopy [MACRO- + -SCOPY]   The study of structures by direct vision.

macrosis [MACR- + -OSIS]   An increase in size.

macrosmatic [MACR- + *osm(o)-* + -atic, English suffix]   Having an acute sense of smell.

macrosomatia [MACRO- + SOMAT- + -IA]   GIGANTISM.

macrosomia [MACRO- + Gk *sōm(a)* body + -IA]   GIGANTISM.

macrospore [MACRO- + SPORE]   MACROCONIDIUM.

macrostereognosia [MACRO- + STEREOGNOSIA]   MACROESTHESIA.

macrostereognosis [MACRO- + STEREO- + Gk *gnōsis* knowledge]   MACROESTHESIA.

macrostomia [MACRO- + STOM- + -IA]   A rare congenital defect resulting in abnormal elongation of the mouth. The defect may be unilateral or bilateral, partial or complete. In complete cases, the oral fissure extends as far as the ear. See also GENAL CLEFT.

macrostomic [MACRO- + Gk *stom(a)* mouth + -IC]   Having a very large mouth.

macrostructural   Pertaining to gross structure, as opposed to microscopic structure.

macrotia [MACR- + OT- + -IA]   Abnormally large external ears occurring as a rare congenital malformation.

macrotome [MACRO- + -TOME]   A slicing device for cutting large tissue sections for gross anatomic study.

macrotooth [MACRO- + TOOTH]   An abnormally large tooth.

macula [L (akin to *macere* to be lean, thin), a spot, stain, blemish] (*plural* maculae)   A small spot perceptibly different from the surrounding tissue.

acoustic maculae   MACULAE ACUSTICAE.

maculae acusticae   The macula sacculi and macula utriculi considered together. An outmoded term. Also called *maculae of membranous labyrinth, acoustic maculae.*

macula acustica sacculi   MACULA SACCULI.

macula acustica utriculi   MACULA UTRICULI.

macula adherens   DESMOSOME.

maculae albidae   An obsolete term for MILK SPOTS.

maculae atrophicae   MACULAR ATROPHY.

maculae caeruleae   Blue-gray macules sometimes seen on the abdominal wall and the thighs in pthiriasis pubis. Also called *taches bleuâtres, blue spot.*

cerebral macula   MENINGITIC STREAK.

macula communis   The epithelial ridge on the medial wall of the otocyst from which the maculae of the saccule and utricle and the ampullary cristae differentiate in the seventh week of embryonic life. An outmoded term.

macula corneae   A circular white scar of the cornea.

maculae cribrosae [NA]   Macula cribrosa inferior, macula cribrosa media, and macula cribrosa superior. Also called *cribriform spots.*

macula cribrosa inferior [NA]   The perforated area on the medial wall of the vestibule through which the branches of the vestibular division of the eighth cranial nerve pass to the posterior semicircular canal. Also called *inferior macula cribosa.*

macula cribrosa media [NA]   The perforated area on the wall of the vestibule through which branches of the vestibular division of the eighth cranial nerve pass to the sacculus. Also called *middle macula cribrosa.*

macula cribrosa superior [NA]   The perforated area on the wall of the vestibule through which branches of the vestibular division of the eighth cranial nerve pass to the utricle and to the anterior and lateral semicircular canals. Also called *superior macula cribrosa.*

macula densa   A short section of the distal tubule of the kidney in which the nuclei are larger and more closely packed than normal. It forms part of the juxtaglomerular apparatus.

false macula   The nonfoveal portion of the retina that has a straight-ahead directional value during binocular vision by a strabismic patient with abnormal retinal correspondence.

macula flava laryngis   A yellowish, occasionally cartilaginous, nodule at the anterior end of each vocal ligament in the larynx. An outmoded term.

macula flava retinae   An outmoded term for MACULA RETINAE.

macula folliculi   The point on the surface of an ovary at which a mature follicle ruptures and an ovum is extruded.

macula germinativa   EMBRYONIC DISK.

macula gonorrhoeica   A gonococcal inflammation of the orifice of a Bartholin gland duct. An obsolete term. Also called *Saenger's macula.*

inferior macula cribrosa   MACULA CRIBROSA INFERIOR.

maculae lacteae   A rarely used term for MILK SPOTS.

macula lutea   MACULA RETINAE.

macula lutea retinae   MACULA RETINAE.

maculae of membranous labyrinth   MACULAE ACUSTICAE.

middle macula cribrosa   MACULA CRIBROSA MEDIA.

mongolian macula   MONGOLIAN SPOT.

macula neglecta   A region of the embryonic saccule which has only a temporary existence.

macula occludens   See under TIGHT JUNCTION.

Reichert's macula cribrosa   An outmoded term for RECESSUS COCHLEARIS VESTIBULI.

macula retinae   [NA] An oval area, with the long axis placed horizontally, near the center of the posterior part of the retina. It is below and lateral to the optic disk and is characterized by a yellow pigment in the inner layers. In its center is the fovea centralis, an area modified for acute vision. Also called *macula lutea retinae, macula flava retinae* (outmoded), *macula lutea, yellow spot, limbus luteus retinae* (outmoded), *macular area, punctum luteum* (outmoded), *Bozzi's foramen* (outmoded), *neuroepithelium macularum, neuroepithelium of maculae, Soemmering spot.*

macula sacculi   [NA] An oval-shaped thickening of the epithelium of the anterior wall of the saccule which receives the saccular fibers of the vestibulocochlear nerve. Its plane is at right angles to that of the macula utriculi. The elongated columnar epithelium contains supporting cells and hair cells which project into the membrana statoconiorum and are concerned with equilibratory vestibular reflexes and possibly the reception of certain auditory stimuli. Also called *saccular spot, macula acustica sacculi.*

Saenger's macula   MACULA GONORRHOEICA.

macula solaris   FRECKLE.

superior macula cribrosa   MACULA CRIBROSA SUPERIOR.

macula utriculi   [NA] A thickening of the epithelium of the lateral part of the floor and adjoining lateral wall of the portion of the utricle that occupies the elliptical recess of the vestibule. It receives the utricular fibers of the vestibulocochlear nerve. Its plane is at right angles to that of the macula sacculi. The elongated columnar epithelium contains supporting cells and hair cells which project into the membrana statoconiorum and are concerned with equilibratory vestibular reflexes. Also called *macula acustica utriculi.*

maculae   Plural of MACULA.

macular   [*macul(a)* + -AR]   **1** Of, characterized by, or consisting of a macule or macules. Also called *maculate* (seldom used). **2** Relating to or denoting the macula retinae.

maculate   A seldom used term for MACULAR.

maculation   The process of macule formation. A rarely used term.

pernicious maculation   The development of purpura in cases of malaria.

macule   A small circumscribed area of discolored skin that is neither depressed nor elevated.

maculocerebral   Pertaining to disease affecting the central portion of the retina and the brain. Also *cerebromacular.*

maculoerythematous   Characterized by macules and erythema.

maculopapular   Marked by macules and papules.

maculopapule   A mark on the skin that combines the features of a macule and a papule.

maculopathy   [*macul(a lutea)* + *o* + -PATHY]   Any disorder of the macula lutea of the ocular fundus.

maculovesicular   Combining the features of a macule and a vesicle.

mad   [Middle English *medd, madd,* from Old English *gemæd,* past part. of *gemædan* to make mad]   An imprecise term for INSANE.

madarosis   [Gk *madaro(s)* bald + -SIS]   Loss of the eyelashes or eyebrows.

Maddox   [Ernest Edmund *Maddox,* English ophthalmologist, 1860–1933]   **1** See under PRISM.   **2** Maddox rods. See under ROD.

madefaction   [Late L *madefactio* a wetting, from L *madefactus,* past part. of *madefacere* (from *madere* to be or become wet + *facere* to make) to wet or moisten]   A process designed to make a subject or object wet or moist.

Madelung   [Otto Wilhelm *Madelung,* German surgeon, 1846–1926]   **1** Madelung syndrome. See under DEFORMITY.   **2** Madelung's disease. See under DIFFUSE SYMMETRICAL LIPOMAS OF THE NECK.   **3** Marfan-Madelung syndrome. See under MARFAN SYNDROME.

madidans   [Late L, pres. part. of *madidare* to moisten]   Moist, oozing: said of eczema. An obsolete term.

madisterion   MADISTERIUM.

madisterium   [New L, from Gk *madistērion* tweezers for pulling out hairs]   An instrument used for plucking hairs. An obsolete term. Also called *madisterion.*

Madlener   [Max *Madlener,* German gynecologist, 1868–1951]   See under OPERATION.

madness   [MAD + -NESS]   An imprecise term for INSANITY.

myxedema madness   Psychosis due to hypothyroidism, usually responsive to appropriate hormone replacement therapy. Also called *myxedematous madness, myxdematous dementia.*

myxedematous madness   MYXEDEMA MADNESS.

paralytic madness   An obsolete term for GENERAL PARESIS.

Madribon   A proprietary name for sulfadimethoxine.

Madurella   A genus of fungi implicated in maduromycosis.

Madurella mycetomi   One of several species of fungi known to cause mycetoma (maduromycosis). Also called *Oospora tozeuri* (obsolete), *Glenospora khartoumensis* (obsolete).

maduromycetoma   [after *Madur(a),* more recently *Madurai,* a city in southern India + *o* + MYCETOMA]   MYCETOMA.

maduromycosis   [after *Madur(a),* more recently *Madurai,* a city in southern India + *o* + MYCOSIS]   MYCETOMA.

maedi   [Icelandic, dispnea]   OVINE CHRONIC PROGRESSIVE PNEUMONIA.

MAF   macrophage activating factor.

mafenide $C_7H_{10}N_2O_2S$. An antibacterial sulfonamide used in the topical treatment of superficial infections, burns, and wounds.

Maffucci   [Angelo *Maffucci,* Italian physician, 1847–1903]   See under SYNDROME.

mag.   *magnus* (L, large).

magaldrate $Al_2H_{14}Mg_4O_{14}·2H_2O$. Aluminum magnesium hydroxide. A compound mixture of aluminum hydroxide and magnesium hydroxide. It is used as an oral antacid medication.

magdala red   A synthetic basic dye derived from naphthylamine.   • Magdala red has been incorrectly and confusingly used in the literature as a synonym for phloxine, an unrelated dye with different staining properties.

mageiric   [Gk *mageirik(ē)* cookery]   Related to the preparation of food.

magenblase   [German *Magen* the stomach + *Blase* bubble]   The stomach bubble, seen on erect roentgenogram of the abdomen as a radiolucency in the proximal stomach above the density of fluid in the stomach.

Magendie [François *Magendie*, French physiologist, 1783–1855] **1** Magendie symptom, Magendie-Hertwig sign, Magendie sign, Hertwig-Magendie sign, Hertwig-Magendie syndrome, Hertwig-Magendie phenomenon. See under SKEW DEVIATION. **2** Magendie's law. See under BELL-MAGENDIE LAW. **3** Magendie space. See under CAVUM SUBARACHNOIDEALE. **4** Foramen of Magendie. See under APERTURA MEDIANA VENTRICULI QUARTI.

magenstrasse CANALIS GASTRICUS.

magenta [after *Magenta*, a town in northern Italy discovered in a battle in 1859, from its fuchsia-red color suggesting the blood spilled in the fighting] BASIC FUCHSIN.

magenta II Triaminoditolylphenylmethane chloride, a consituent of basic fuchsin.

magersucht [German *mager* lean + *Sucht* a sickness] **1** The condition of being abnormally underweight. **2** Pathologic desire to be thin or underweight as in anorexia nervosa.

maggot [Middle English *maddock, magotte, mathek* grub, worm, maggot, akin to or from Old English *matha* maggot, worm, from the Scandinavian] The larva of a fly (order Diptera), a wormlike feeding stage. Blowfly maggots, for example, develop in carrion, flesh fly maggots, in necrotic or normal tissues of living hosts, and filth fly maggots live on excrement and decaying organic matter.

cheese maggot CHEESE SKIPPER.

Congo floor maggot A larva of the African fly *Auchmeromyia luteola*.

rat-tail maggot The larva of a fly of the genus *Eristalis* or the genus *Helophilus*, so called because of their long filiform, flexible and extendable respiratory process. These maggots may cause accidental nasal and intestinal myiasis in domestic animals and humans. Their presence in feces may also suggest intestinal parasitism, but the feces may also have been contaminated after passage. Also called *rat-tailed larva*.

sheep maggot WOOL MAGGOT.

surgical maggot The larva of a myiasis fly used in World War I to remove putrifying or necrotic tissue from battle wounds. The use of such maggots was discontinued after it was discovered that some normal flesh was also attacked.

wool maggot The larva of any of various species of blowflies causing myiasis through deposition of eggs (often called a strike) or of larvae on sheep. Death often results from destruction of flesh. Great losses occur in Australia from *Phaenicia cuprina*, which is also a source of damage, along with *Chrysomyia*, in South Africa. In New Zealand *Calliphora stygia* in the spring and *Phaenicia sericata* in the fall are causes of strike. The latter is also destructive in Europe. In the United States, maggots of *Phormia regina* and *Sarcophaga bullata* parasitize sheep and goats in southwestern states. Also called *fleece worm, sheep maggot*.

magistery **1** An unusual remedy or prescription. **2** A chemical precipitate. An outmoded usage.

magistral Prepared under the guidelines of a physician's prescription: used of medicines. Compare OFFICINAL.

Magitot [Emile *Magitot*, French oral surgeon, 1833–1897] Magitot's disease. See under CHRONIC PERIODONTITIS.

magma [L (from Gk *magma*, from *magm-*, perf. inf. root of *massein* to touch, handle, knead), a thin or soft mass or paste] **1** Finely divided material suspended in a small quantity of water. **2** A pastelike preparation of any organic substance.

magma reticulare MAGMA RETICULARIS.

magma reticularis The primary mesenchyme present in the cavity of the blastocyst of certain primates, including man, filling the space between the trophoblast externally, the amnion and the primary yolk sac. It forms a loose reticulum of cells, the origin and fate of which has been much discussed. Later, small cavities appear in it to form the extraembryonic coelom. Also called *magma reticulare*.

Magnacort A proprietary name for hydrocortamate.

Magnamycin A proprietary name for carbomycin.

Magnan [Valentin J. J. *Magnan*, French psychiatrist, 1835–1916] **1** Magnan's trombone movement. See under TROMBONE TONGUE. **2** Magnan sign, Magnan symptom. See under FORMICATION.

magnesemia HYPERMAGNESEMIA.

magnesia MgO. The oxide of magnesium. It is a solid of low solubility in water, but it neutralizes acids to give soluble magnesium salts.

citrate of magnesia MAGNESIUM CITRATE.

cream of magnesia An aqueous suspension of hydrated magnesium oxide containing the equivalent of 7.45–8.35% weight for weight of magnesium hydroxide. It is used as an antacid in small doses and as a laxative in high doses. Also called *magnesium hydroxide mixture*.

heavy magnesia MgO. A fine, white powder of magnesium oxide that is practically insoluble in water. It is used in powders and tablets as an antacid and mild laxative.

magnesia magma MILK OF MAGNESIA.

milk of magnesia A suspension of 7–8.5% weight for weight of magnesium hydroxide. It may also contain 0.1% citric acid and up to 0.05% of one or more essential oils as flavoring agents. Also called *magnesia magma*.

magnesite Naturally occurring magnesium carbonate, used like plaster of Paris or gypsum for bandages.

magnesium Element number 12, having atomic weight 24.312. There are three stable natural isotopes. Five radioactive isotopes have been identified, the longest lived being magnesium 28 with a half-life of 21 hours. Magnesium is the eighth most abundant element in the lithosphere. It is a silvery white metal, never found in the free state. The valence is 3. The magnesium ion is one of the principal cations governing the electrochemical properties of living systems. Magnesium is a constituent of the chlorophyll molecule, and it is required for the activity of many enzymes. Symbol: Mg

magnesium carbonate $Mg(OH)_2 \cdot 3MgCO_3 \cdot XH_2O$ ($X = 3$ or 4). A white, almost tasteless powder used as an antacid and laxative, often with other ingredients.

magnesium chloride $MgCl_2 \cdot 6H_2O$. Colorless flakes or a crystalline salt. It is used to replace electrolytes lost in peritoneal dialysis and blood dialysis.

magnesium citrate $C_{12}H_{10}Mg_3O_{14}$. A white, odorless, crystalline powder, used in solution as a mild cathartic. Also called *citrate of magnesia*.

effervescent magnesium citrate A powder containing a mixture of magnesium carbonate, citric acid, sodium bicarbonate, and sugar. It is used as a laxative.

magnesium hydroxide $Mg(OH)_2$. A white, amorphous, odorless, and tasteless powder almost insoluble in water. It is used as an antacid in the treatment of peptic ulcers, and it has mild laxative properties. It is used in tablets alone or in combination with other antacids, or as an aqueous suspension.

magnesium peroxide MgO_2. A white, tasteless powder, practically insoluble in water. It gradually decomposes, releasing oxygen. It is utilized medically as an antacid and anti-infective agent.

magnesium phosphate TRIBASIC MAGNESIUM PHOSPHATE.

tribasic magnesium phosphate $Mg_3(PO_4)_2 \cdot 5H_2O$. A white, odorless, tasteless powder, practically insoluble in water. It is an antacid and mild laxative, much like magnesium trisilicate, which has largely replaced it. Also called *magnesium phosphate, trimagnesium phosphate*.

magnesium stearate Magnesium compounded with stearic acid and palmitic acid in various proportions. It is insoluble in water and employed as a tablet lubricant in pharmaceutical preparations and dusting powders.

magnesium sulfate $MgSO_4 \cdot 7H_2O$. The heptahydrate, colorless crystals have been employed as an anticonvulsant agent, but its main medical uses are as a cathartic and as a local anti-inflammatory treatment. Also called *Epsom salts*.

effervescent magnesium sulfate A powder mixture of magnesium sulfate, sodium bicarbonate, tartaric acid, and citric acid, used as a laxative.

exsiccated magnesium sulfate Hydrated magnesium sulfate that has been dried at 100°C to reduce the weight by 25%. It is used as a paste for boils.

magnesium trisilicate A combination in various proportions of magnesium oxide, silicon dioxide, and water. It is used as a pharmaceutical aid and as an antacid.

magnet [Gk *(lithos) Magnētis* (fem. of *Magnētēs* a dweller in *Magnēsia* in Thessaly) a stone of Magnesia, lodestone] A body that attracts iron and certain other materials as a result of particular behavior of its atomic electrons.

giant magnet A large and powerful magnet used to extract iron and steel foreign bodies from within the eye.

Grüning's magnet A composite magnet made of a number of permanent magnets aligned in a bundle, used for the removal of intraocular foreign bodies.

Haab's magnet A giant magnet used for the removal of intraocular foreign bodies.

Hirschberg's magnet A powerful electromagnet used for the removal of intraocular foreign bodies.

lid magnets Tiny magnets implanted into the upper and lower eyelids, which serve to close the eyes when the levator palpebrae muscles relax. This is done to supplant the functionless orbicularis oculi muscles in facial nerve paralysis.

permanent magnet A body that possesses magnetism without need for an external influence to maintain this property.

temporary magnet A body that temporarily possesses the property of attracting iron by induction from a permanent magnet or from the effect of an electric current.

magnetic Of or related to magnets or magnetism.

magnetism [MAGNET + -ISM] **1** Magnetic force; the force exerted by a magnetic field. **2** The property of producing a magnetic field.

magnetization **1** The intensity of magnetism in a magnet. **2** The process of inducing magnetism.

magnetocardiogram A graphic record produced by a magnetocardiograph.

magnetocardiograph An instrument for recording the magnetic field of the heart, produced by the same ionic currents that generate the electrocardiogram.

magnetocardiography The process of recording using a magnetocardiograph.

magnetoelectricity Electricity produced by moving a conductor through a magnetic field.

magnetoencephalograph An instrument for recording the magnetic field of the brain, produced by the same ionic currents that generate the electroencephalogram.

magnetograph A recording magnetometer.

magnetoinduction MAGNETIC INDUCTION.

magnetometer An instrument for measuring the intensity and/or direction of a magnetic field or of a component of a magnetic field in one direction.

magneton [*magnet* + *-on*, suffix denoting a quantum unit, as in *photon*] A unit of magnetic moment used in atomic physics.

Bohr magneton A magneton referring to the electron, equal to $eh/2m_e$ where e is the elementary charge of an electron, h is the Planck constant/2π and m_e is the rest mass of an electron; equal to $(9.2732 \pm 0.0006) \times 10^{-24}$ ampere square meter. Also called *electron magneton*. Symbol: μ_B

electron magneton BOHR MAGNETON.

nuclear magneton A magneton referring to the proton, equal to $eh/2m_p$ where e is the elementary charge of a proton, h is the Planck constant/2π and m_p the rest mass of a proton; equal to $(5.0505 \pm 0.0004) \times 10^{-27}$ ampere squre meter. Symbol: μ_N

magnetostriction The contraction of a ferromagnetic rod when placed in a longitudinal magnetic field, a phenomenon utilized in loudspeakers.

magnetotherapy The use of magnets or magnetism for therapeutic purposes, as formerly practiced. See also ELECTROMAGNETIC FIELD THERAPY.

magnetron A vacuum tube in which electrons accelerating in a radial electric field are controlled by an axial magnetic field to produce power at microwave frequencies.

magnetropism The responsiveness of an organism to the direction of a magnetic field, as evidenced by movement or growth.

magnicellular Composed of large cells. Also *magnocellular*.

magnification Apparent increase of the image size of an object examined with a light or electron microscope.

biologic magnification BIOACCUMULATION.

magnify To increase the apparent image size of.

magnocellular MAGNICELLULAR.

Magnus [Rudolf *Magnus*, German physiologist, 1873–1927] Magnus and de Kleijn neck reflex. See under REFLEX.

Magovern [George Jerome *Magovern*, U.S. surgeon, born 1923] Magovern-Cromie prosthesis. See under PROSTHESIS.

Mahaim [I. *Mahaim*, French physician, flourished 20th century] Mahaim fibers. See under FIBER.

mahamari A form of plague which affects persons living in the southern Himalaya Mountains. A local name.

Mahler [Richter A. *Mahler*, German obstetrician, flourished 19th century] See under SIGN.

maidenhead An obsolete term for HYMEN.

Maier [Rudolf Robert *Maier*, German physician, 1824–1888] **1** Kussmaul-Maier disease. See under POLYARTERITIS NODOSA. **2** See under SINUS.

maieusiomania [Gk *maieusi(s)* delivery of a woman in childbirth + *o* + -MANIA] An obsolete term for POSTPARTUM PSYCHOSIS.

maieutics An older term for OBSTETRICS.

Maillard [Louis Camille *Maillard*, French biochemist, 1878–1936] See under COEFFICIENT.

maim [Middle English *maymen*, from Old French *mahaigner* to disable] To seriously wound, injure, disfigure, dismember, or disable.

main [French, the hand] [French, hand] Hand.

main d'accoucheur ACCOUCHEUR'S HAND.

main de singe MONKEY'S HAND.

main de squelette CORPSE HAND.

main des tranchées TRENCH HAND.

main en crochet A flexed position of the ring finger and little finger.

main en griffe CLAW HAND.

main en lorgnette OPERA-GLASS HAND.

main en pince **1** LOBSTER CLAW HAND. **2** CLEFT HAND.

main fourchée **1** LOBSTER CLAW HAND. **2** CLEFT HAND.

main succulente SUCCULENT HAND.

maintainer / orthodontic space maintainer A space maintainer designed to retain the space for an erupting tooth.

removable space maintainer A space maintainer which is

removed by the wearer for cleaning.

space maintainer   SPACE RETAINER.

maintenance   **1** The act or process of maintaining.   **2** Designed to maintain stable function or condition, as distinguished from remedial or prophylactic effect, as in *a maintenance dose of methadone, a maintenance ration to a laboratory animal.*

space maintenance   The provision of an appliance in orthodontics or pedodontics, where a tooth is missing or unerupted, to prevent the movement of adjacent teeth into the space.

maise   MAIZE.

maisin   [Spanish *maíz* Indian corn + -IN]   A protein found in the seeds of *Zea mays* (maize).

Maisonneuve   [Jules German François *Maisonneuve*, French surgeon, 1809–1897]   See under URETHROTOMY, URETHROTOME, SIGN, AMPUTATION.

maisonneuve   [after Jules Germain François *Maisonneuve*, French surgeon, 1809–1897]   MAISONNEUVE'S URETHROTOME.

Maissiat   [Jacques Henri *Maissiat*, French anatomist, 1805–1878]   Iliotibial ligament of Maissiat, ligament of Maissiat, Maissiat's band, Maissiat's tract. See under TRACTUS ILIOTIBIALIS.

maize   [Spanish *maíz*, from Taino (West Indies) *makiz* Indian corn]   A cereal grass of the species *Zea mays.* The preparations of this cereal used in human diets include corn on the cob, whole maize grain, whole maize meal, decorticated maize meal, degerminated maize meal, hominy and cerealine. The nutrient value of maize is similar to that of other cereals, except that yellow maize contains considerable amounts of β-carotene, and its protein, zein, lacks both lysine and tryptophan. The nicotinic acid present in maize is in an unavailable bound form. Hence, maize eating is associated with pellagra. Maize's composition is 9.5% protein, 4.3% fat, 2–3 mg iron, 2 mg nicotinic acid, and 100–800 μg Vitamin A per 100 g. *Zea mays* var. *indurata* (flint corn) and *Zea mays* var. *indentata* (dent corn) are the highest yielding varieties. Maize, or corn, oil, which is refined from the embryo of *Zea mays*, is used as a solvent for injections and in the preparation of food. Also called *corn, Indian corn.* Also *maise.* Adjective: zeistic.

Majocchi   [Domenico *Majocchi*, Italian dermatologist, 1849–1929]   **1** Granuloma of Majocchi, trichophytic granuloma of Majocchi. See under GRANULOMA.   **2** Majocchi's disease, Majocchi's purpura. See under PURPURA ANNULARIS TELANGIECTODES.

majoon   A confection prepared from the flowering tops of *Cannabis sativa.*

majority   The age at which a person becomes legally entitled to the full civil rights of an adult. The age varies by jurisdiction. In the United States, the age of 21 is most commonly used.   ● In Canada and India, the age of majority is 21. In Japan, it is 20 (although the term *majority* is not used), and there is a national day to celebrate it, January 15. The age of majority is 18 in the United Kingdom, South Africa, Australia, and New Zealand.

Makai   [Endre *Makai*, Hungarian surgeon, flourished 20th century]   Rothmann-Makai syndrome. See under SYNDROME.

make   The closing of a switch, relay, or other contact to complete an electric circuit and establish current flow.

Makeham   [William Matthew *Makeham*, English statistician, died 1892]   See under HYPOTHESIS.

makeshift   Denoting a shunt constructed from a large variceal collateral vessel to a systemic vein when a standard shunt cannot be employed. It is used in operations for portal hypertension.

Makkas   [M. *Makkas*, German surgeon, flourished 20th century]   See under OPERATION.

Maklakoff   [Aleksey *Maklakoff*, Russian ophthalmologist, 1837–1895]   See under TONOMETER.

makro-   MACRO-.

mal   [French (from L *malum* an evil, harm), an evil, pain, ache, illness]   **1** Disease; illness.   **2** Pain.

mal comitial   MAJOR EPILEPSY.

mal de caderas   A disease of horses due to *Trypanosoma equinum.* Common in some South American countries, it is manifested by remittent fever, emaciation, and weakness, especially of the hind quarters. The disease is usually fatal in horses, but cattle, sheep, and goats can be mildly affected. The capybara serves as a reservoir of infection.

mal de Cayenne   FILARIAL ELEPHANTIASIS.

mal de los pintos   A treponemal disease that produces dry, scaly, itchy skin lesions, usually on exposed parts of the body. Caused by *Treponema carateum* and usually transmitted by direct contact, it may be infectious for many years. Primary, secondary, and tertiary forms are recognized. The disease is endemic in Mexico, Cuba, and the upper Amazon basin. Treatment with penicillin and other antibiotics is effective.

mal del pinto   PINTA.

mal de Meleda   MELEDA DISEASE.

mal de mer   A French term for SEASICKNESS.

mal de rastrojos   ARGENTINIAN HEMORRHAGIC FEVER.   ● The Spanish word *rastrojos* refers to stubble in the grain fields, which may be contaminated with the virus from rodent urine and from which farm workers often contract the disease at harvest time.

grand mal   MAJOR EPILEPSY.   ● This term was once used to identify any convulsive epileptic attack with major manifestations, as opposed to petit mal.

haut mal   MAJOR EPILEPSY.

mal morado   ONCHOCERCIASIS.

mal perforant   PERFORATING ULCER OF THE FOOT.

petit mal   See under PETIT MAL.

mal rouge   A condition brought about by the ingestion of any substance which blocks the enzyme system responsible for conversion of ethanol to carbon dioxide and water, thus allowing the accumulation of acetaldehyde. Symptoms are nausea, vomiting, headache, flushing, palpitation, and marked fall in blood pressure.

mal-   [Old French *mal* (from L *malus* bad) bad; Old French *mal* (from L *male* badly, ill, from *malus* bad) badly]   A combining form meaning (1) bad, badly; (2) abnormally, defectively.

mala   [L, cheekbone, jawbone, cheek, jaw]   **1** BUCCA.   **2** OS ZYGOMATICUM.

malabsorption   [MAL- + ABSORPTION]   Impaired or incomplete absorption of nutrients by the intestine.

congenital malabsorption of cobalamin   IMERSLUND SYNDROME.

lactose malabsorption   A reduced capacity to absorb lactose arising as a result of lactase deficiency. This is the most frequently reported isolated enzyme deficiency in both children and adults, but is more common in adults. It is believed to be an inherited enzyme deficiency, but it can also be acquired secondary to diseases that result in mucosal damage. It does not seem to be induced in man through abstinence from milk. Estimates of lactase deficiency in North America range from 16–55% with the higher level found in blacks. In children under 11 years, 10% of Caucasians suffer and 35% of blacks. The frequency in children gradually increases with age due to a gradual decline in lactase activity. The majority of adults in the world have lower lactase activity than do children. Unhydrolyzed lactose is not absorbed, and remains in the gut lumen where it exerts a hyperosmolar effect. Large volumes of water are pulled into the gut lumen causing abdominal distension and discomfort. The flora of the lower bowel and colon metabolize the lactose to produce lactic, butyric, and other acids, causing cramps and diarrhea. A flat glucose curve is obtained in lactose intolerance when a 100 g load of lactose is ingested. However, the same patient when given equimolar amounts of glucose or galactose will show a rise of 20 mg of glucose per 100 ml of serum. Treatment involves the exclusion of lactose from the diet.

postgastrectomy malabsorption   Malabsorption secondary to partial gastrectomy.

Malacarne [Michele Vincenzo Giacinto *Malacarne*, Italian surgeon and anatomist, 1744–1816]   **1** See under PYRAMID.   **2** Malacarne's antrum, Malacarne space. See under SUBSTANTIA PERFORATA POSTERIOR.

malacia [Gk *malakia* a softness]   The pathologic softening of any tissue. Often used in combination to designate specific conditions, such as osteomalacia. Also called *malacosis*.

malacia cordis   Morbid softening of the heart.

metaplastic malacia   OSTEITIS FIBROSA CYSTICA.

myeloplastic malacia   OSTEOGENESIS IMPERFECTA.

malacia traumatica   TRAUMATIC SYRINGOMYELIA.

malacic   Characterized by softening.

malaco- [Gk *malakos* soft, gentle]   A combining form meaning soft, softness.

malacology [French *malacologie* (from Gk *malako(s)* soft + French *-logie* -LOGY) the study of mollusks]   The study of mollusks.

malacoma [*malac(o)-* + -OMA]   An abnormally soft spot or part. An obsolete term.

malacopathia [MALACO- + -PATHIA]   An obsolete term for EPIDERMOLYSIS BULLOSA.

malacoplakia   MALAKOPLAKIA.

malacosarcosis   The pathological softening of muscular tissue. An obsolete term.

malacosis   MALACIA.

malacosomous [MALACO- + Gk *sōm(a)* body + -OUS]   Characterized by a soft body.

malacosteon   OSTEOMALACIA.

Malacostraca   The largest class of the phylum Crustacea, containing about 19 100 species. Members occur in marine, freshwater and terrestrial habitats, and individual size ranges from a few millimeters to over three meters. Most members have an exoskeleton, fused head and thorax, and stalked compound eyes. The thorax usually consists of eight segments each bearing a pair of appendages. The anterior three pairs of appendages are modified for food gathering and the posterior five pairs of appendages are mainly used for locomotion. The abdomen generally consists of six segments, each with a pair of appendages modified for swimming, reproduction, or respiration. Adjective: malacostracan.

malacotic [MALACO- + *t* + -IC]   Softer than normal: said of teeth.

malacotomy [MALACO- + -TOMY]   A surgical incision into soft tissue, such as the anterior abdominal wall.

malactic   EMOLLIENT.

maladie [French, a disease, illness]   [French, illness, disease]   Disease.

maladie bleue   CYANOTIC HEART DISEASE.

maladie bronzée   ADDISON'S DISEASE.

maladie de Capdepont   DENTINOGENESIS IMPERFECTA.

maladie de Nicolas et Favre   LYMPHOGRANULOMA VENEREUM.

maladie de plongeurs   Inflammation and ulceration of the skin and subcutaneous tissues caused by stings of sea anemones. This condition is found among sea divers in the Mediterranean.

maladie de Roger   ROGER'S DISEASE.

maladie des jambes   A disease found in rice growers in Louisiana. It is very similar to beriberi and in severe cases progresses to peripheral polyneuritis with ankle drop, muscular atrophy, and difficulty in walking.

maladie des tics   GILLES DE LA TOURETTE SYNDROME.

maladie du sommeil   **1** GAMBIAN TRYPANOSOMIASIS.   **2** RHODESIAN TRYPANOSOMIASIS.

maladjustment [MAL + ADJUSTMENT]   An inability to cope adequately with the frustrations or stresses of living; a failure to adapt.

social maladjustment   Lack of or impaired ability to satisfy cultural and environmental demands, leading to an unsatisfactory relationship with other people or society as a whole.

malady [French *maladie* (from *malade*, earlier *malabde*, sick + *-ie* -Y; compare Old Provençal *malaptes*, *malaudes* sick; from L *male habitus* in bad condition, sick, from *male* badly + *habitus*, past part. of *habere* to have) sickness]   A disease; illness.

malagma [Gk *malagma*, a plaster, emollient, poultice]   An emollient or medicated poultice.

malaise [French (from *mal* bad, from L *malus* bad + French *aise* comfort, from L *adjacens*, pres. part. of *adjacere* to lie near), feeling of faintness or discomfort]   A feeling of untoward weakness, lethargy, or discomfort, as of impending illness.

malakoplakia   A form of chronic inflammation principally involving the urinary bladder and characterized by soft, pale or yellow plaques on its mucosa. The plaques are composed of macrophages and lymphocytes and an occasional multinucleated giant cell. Mineralized, laminated concretions (Michaelis Gutmann bodies) and altered bacteria may be present within the macrophages. A localized defect in macrophage function or an abnormal response to coliform bacteria is believed to be the cause. Also *malacoplakia*.

malalignment   **1** The healing of a fractured jaw with the parts incorrectly aligned.   **2** The state of having a tooth or teeth not in the normal position in the dental arch.

malar [L *mala* cheek]   **1** Pertaining to the cheek.   **2** Of or relating to the zygomatic bone.

malaria [Italian *mala*, fem. of *malo* (from L *malus* bad) bad + Italian *aria* air]   A febrile disease caused by infection with haemosporidian protozoa of the genus *Plasmodium* transmitted by the bites of infected female mosquitoes of the genus *Anopheles*. The four species in human malaria are *P. falciparum* (malignant tertian, subtertian), *P. vivax* (tertian), *P. ovale* (tertian), and *P. malariae* (quartan). The disease accounts for very great morbidity and mortality in tropical countries, especially in third-world populations. Children are particularly vulnerable. The parasite is inoculated into the human host as a sporozoite and undergoes an asymptomatic exoerythrocytic developmental cycle in the liver before large numbers of merozoites invade red blood cells, establishing the erythrocytic cycle which produces the characteristic symptoms of disease, including chills followed by rapid onset of high fever and sweating at regular intervals, varying with the species of parasite. Hemolytic anemia, jaundice, and splenomegaly may result. Severe cases of *P. falciparum* infection may be complicated by renal failure and cerebral involvement. Gametocytes produced during the erythrocytic cycle are ingested by mosquitoes with the blood meal, initiating the sexual developmental cycle. The sporozoites ultimately produced by nuclear division in the oocyst accumulate in the salivary glands of the mosquito, and are ready to infect a new host when the mosquito feeds, usually within 8–21 days. Diagnosis is made by demonstration of malaria parasites in blood films. Serodiagnosis is also of value. Although chloroquine has been the drug of choice in prophylaxis and treatment, malaria parasites in some regions have become resistant to this drug and others, and therapy of the disease has become complex. Also called *fever and ague* (obsolete), *Cameroon fever, Corsican fever, marsh fever, malarial fever, paludal fever, helodes, paludism.*

acute malaria   Malaria characterized by intermittent, remittent, or irregular but frequent paroxysms of chills, fever, and sweating, caused by the synchronous release of merozoites from red blood cells. The frequency of acute symptoms varies with the species of parasite. *Plasmodium falciparum* is responsible for the most severe disease, which if accompanied by renal and cerebral complications often leads to death. The acute disease is especially serious in children and during pregnancy. Rapid diagnosis and urgent treatment are vital if mortality is to be avoided. Compare CHRONIC MALARIA.

algid malaria   *Plasmodium falciparum* malaria with shock, cold skin, prostration, and visceral involvement, especially of the vessels of the gastrointestinal tract. Also called *cold malaria.*

autochthonous malaria   Endemic malaria acquired from sporozoites transmitted by local mosquitoes. Imported malarial organisms, passed to endemic mosquitoes in a new region, become a cause of autochthonous malaria when the parasites are transmitted within the newly invaded population.

avian malaria   Infection of wild and domestic birds with species of *Plasmodium,* which parasitizes red cells and is transmitted principally by culicine mosquitoes. Heavy infections are characterized by anemia.

benign subtertian malaria   A form of vivax malaria in which the 48-hour pattern of chills, fever, and sweats is irregular or modified.

benign tertian malaria   VIVAX MALARIA.

bilious remittent malaria   A form of intermittent falciparum malaria marked by occasional bilious attacks.

bovine malaria   BOVINE BABESIOSIS.

bromeliad malaria   Malaria transmitted by *Anopheles* mosquitoes that breed in bromeliad plants in South America and the West Indies.

cerebral malaria   A serious complication of *Plasmodium falciparum* infection, usually occurring in nonimmune subjects, frequently children. It is characterized by headache, irritability, hyperpyrexia, convulsions, and coma. Electroencephalographic abnormalities are also present. There is gross congestion with stasis in cerebral blood vessels as well as numerous petechial hemorrhages and intravascular coagulation. Although there is often a heavy parasitemia in the peripheral blood, that is not always the case. Even with adequate treatment, the condition carries a significant death rate. Also called *plasmodial meningitis.*

chronic malaria   Prolonged human infection with malaria parasites, *Plasmodium vivax, P. ovale,* and especially *P. malariae.* Serum globulin and IgG component are usually raised and malaria serology is usually positive. Chronic anemia and splenomegaly are usual, and there may be severe constitutional abnormalities. Chronic renal involvement (nephrotic syndrome) has been associated especially with *P. malariae* infections. An immune-complex basis seems likely, and treatment is unsatisfactory. Massive splenomegaly occasionally results from an aberrant immune mechanism, especially in tropical Africa and Papua New Guinea (tropical splenomegaly syndrome). Serum IgM concentration is high and hepatic sinusoidal lymphocytosis common. There is some evidence that chronic malaria increases the potential of the Epstein-Barr virus to cause Burkitt's lymphoma and to produce high HB$_s$Ag carrier rates. Also called *impaludism, malarial cachexia, limnemia* (rarely used). Compare ACUTE MALARIA.

cold malaria   ALGID MALARIA.

malaria comatosa   Falciparum malaria accompanied by coma. It is usually a manifestation of the dangerous cerebral form of falciparum malaria.

double tertian malaria   QUOTIDIAN MALARIA.

dysenteric malaria   Falciparum malaria marked by bloody diarrhea.

estivoautumnal malaria   Falciparum malaria with a summer-autumn onset, linked to the behavior of the *Anopheles* vectors. It was formerly endemic in parts of the United States. Also called *estivoautumnal fever.*

falciparum malaria   A form of malaria caused by *Plasmodium falciparum,* often characterized by paroxysms of fever occurring at 48-hour intervals and in severe cases sometimes by acute cerebral or renal manifestations attributable to the large number of red blood cells involved and by the tendency of infected cells to clump together or to adhere to the endothelial lining of blood vessels, resulting in blocked capillaries. The incubation period is 10–14 days but may be longer. Pyrexia of 40°C or more, hepatospenomegaly, tachycardia, hypotension, pallor, and sometimes hemolytic jaundice occur, especially in those with a high parasitemia. If untreated, mortality rates are high. Special clinical forms are called cerebral, algid, gastric, hemorrhagic, dysenteric, and comatose malaria, blackwater fever, and other descriptive terms. Also called *malignant tertian malaria, falciparum fever, malignant tertian ague, malignant tertian fever, malignant fever, subtertian malaria, jungle fever (East Indies).*

gastric malaria   Falciparum malaria marked by continual vomiting.

hemolytic malaria   BLACKWATER FEVER.

imported malaria   Malaria acquired outside and brought into a specified malaria-free area, such as the United States.

induced malaria   MALARIOTHERAPY.

intermittent malaria   Malaria in which there is a complete absence of fever and other symptoms in intervals between paroxysms, usually seen in the tertian (vivax) or quartan (malariae) types. Also called *intermittent malarial fever.*

introduced malaria   Malarial disease transmitted by mosquitoes from an imported case in an area ordinarily free of malaria.

latent malaria   Malarial infection in which there is a balance between the parasite and the body's defense mechanisms, so that no symptoms of the disease are produced.

malariae malaria   A form of malaria in which febrile paroxysms recur every 72 hours, caused by the release of merozoites of the parasite *Plasmodium malariae.* Also called *quartan malaria, quartan fever, quartan ague.*

malignant tertian malaria   FALCIPARUM MALARIA.

nonan malaria   A form of malaria in which febrile paroxysms occur every ninth day.

ovale malaria   A usually mild form of malaria caused by *Plasmodium ovale* which causes a benign tertian type of disease. Infection in conjunction with *P. falciparum* is not uncommon. Most cases occur in tropical Africa. latent periods of up to four years after infection have been documented. Relapses tend to occur after intervals of about three months. Treatment is with chloroquine and primaquine. Also called *ovale tertian malaria, tertian malaria.*

ovale tertian malaria   OVALE MALARIA.

pernicious malaria   Falciparum malaria characterized by severe symptoms accompanied by cerebral, hemorrhagic, or gastroenteric complications.

quartan malaria   MALARIAE MALARIA.

quintan malaria   A form of malaria in which febrile paroxysms recur every fifth day. Also called *quintan ague.*

quotidian malaria   A form of malaria characterized by daily febrile paroxysms. It is commonly due to simultaneous infection with two distinct groups of *Plasmodium vivax* parasites, but possibly with two species (e.g., *P. falciparum* and *P. vivax*), or with two forms of *P. falciparum.* Also called *quotidian ague, double tertian malaria.*

recrudescent malaria   A form of malarial resurgence, usually in disease caused by *Plasmodium malariae*, in which a latent or repressed erythrocytic infection begins to multiply rapidly and induces a clinical infection. This form of quartan malarial resurgence can continue for a long period, 30 years or more. In contrast, the shorter-lived relapsing malaria from *P. vivax* or *P. ovale* originates in the liver and rarely occurs more than five years after the initial mosquito-borne infection.

relapsing malaria Malaria characterized by the resurgence of clinical symptoms from a latent or delayed hepatic infection at an interval following the primary attack, usually within five years. The causative agent is usually *Plasmodium vivax* or *P. ovale.*

remittent malaria Malaria, usually of the falciparum type, in which the elevated body temperature falls somewhat but does not drop to normal in the interval between febrile attacks.

simian malaria An infection of red cells of monkeys with species of *Plasmodium,* transmitted principally by mosquitoes of the genus *Anopheles,* as in human malaria. Common in southeastern Asia and Africa, some of the parasitic species appear to be very similar to corresponding human forms and may be derived from them. The main signs of the disease are fever and anemia.

subtertian malaria FALCIPARUM MALARIA.

tertian malaria 1 VIVAX MALARIA. 2 OVALE MALARIA.

therapeutic malaria MALARIOTHERAPY.

vivax malaria A form of malaria in which paroxysms recur every 48 hours due to the release of merozoites from red blood cells infected by the parasite *Plasmodium vivax.* It is the most common and widespread form of human malaria, although it has been largely eradicated from temperate zone areas. It does not occur in most of tropical west Africa, being replaced there by ovale malaria. Also called *benign tertian malaria, tertian malaria, tertian ague, tertian fever, vivax fever.*

malariacidal MALARICIDAL.

malarial Of or pertaining to malaria.

malaricidal [*malari(a)* + *-cid(e)* + -AL] Destructive to malarial parasites. Also *malariacidal.*

malariology [*malari(a)* + *o* + -LOGY] The systematic study of malaria.

malariometry [*malari(a)* + *o* + -METRY] The use of quantitative methods in the epidemiological study or control of malaria.

malariotherapy Malaria produced through human agency, usually by inoculation with infective material, formerly a treatment for neurosyphilis and certain other conditions. Also called *therapeutic malaria, induced malaria, impf-malaria (German), malarial therapy, malarization therapy.*

malarious Affected by or marked by the presence of malaria.

malarticulation Impaired speech articulation.

Malassez [Louis Charles *Malassez,* French physiologist, 1842–1909] 1 Debris of Malassez. See under RESTS OF MALASSEZ. 2 Rests of Malassez. See under REST. 3 See under DISEASE, STAIN.

Malassezia [after Louis Charles *Malassez,* French physiologist, 1842–1910 + -IA] A form-genus of lipophilic yeasts of the normal skin flora. Also called *Pityrosporum.*

Malassezia furfur The form-species of fungus that causes pityriasis versicolor. Also called *Malassezia tropica, Malassezia macfadyeni.*

Malassezia macfadyeni MALASSEZIA FURFUR.

Malassezia ovale A form-species that is characteristically thick-walled and ovoid in form and that buds from a broad base. In man it is found especially on the scalp, face, and upper trunk. It may be identical to *M. furfur.*

Malassezia tropica MALASSEZIA FURFUR.

malassimilation [MAL- + ASSIMILATION] The defective incorporation of materials into the body tissues.

malate dehydrogenase Any of several enzymes that catalyze the dehydrogenation of malate with the concomitant reduction of NAD^+ or $NADP^+$. The most important (EC 1.1.1.37) is one that forms oxaloacetate in a step that is part of the citric acid cycle. Some enzymes of the group, designated "oxaloacetate decarboxylating," form pyruvate and carbon dioxide in place of oxaloacetate.

malate dehydrogenase (oxaloacetate decarboxylating) An enzyme that catalyzes the reaction of malate and $NADP^+$ to yield pyruvate, carbon dioxide, NADPH, and H^+. It is important in the supply of NADPH for fat synthesis, as well as in the cycle that allows acetyl groups to be exported from mitochondria as citrate for this purpose. Also called *malic enzyme.*

malate synthase An enzyme (EC 4.1.3.2) that catalyzes the formation of malate and coenzyme A from acetyl-CoA and glyoxylate. This is one of the enzymes of the glyoxylate cycle, not possessed by animals, whereby plants and microorganisms can convert fatty acids into carbohydrate.

malathion $C_{10}H_{19}O_6PS_2$. An organophosphate compound used to control a wide variety of insects, including aphids, spider mites, scale insects, houseflies, and mosquitoes, by inhibiting cholinesterase, thus interfering with nerve conduction.

malaxate To compound into a single mass; to mix up a medicinal preparation, as in the production of pharmaceuticals.

malaxation [Gk *malax(is)* a softening + -ATION] The act of working a mixture into a single mass; the process of mixing.

maldevelopment [MAL- + DEVELOPMENT] TERATISM.

maldigestion The impaired digestion of nutrients in the gastrointestinal tract.

male [L *masculus* (dim. of *mas* the male of humans, animals, and plants) male, masculine] 1 Of or belonging to the sex that in animals produces spermatozoa and begets young. 2 An individual of the male sex, as a man. 3 Producing pollen: used of a plant organ. 4 Designating a plant containing pollen-producing organs and no fruit-producing organs.

genetic male 1 A human possessing a normal male karyotype, 46,XY. 2 In any species, an individual possessing the karyotype that is usually present in the male.

Malécot [Achille-Etienne *Malécot,* French surgeon, 1852–1894] See under CATHETER.

maleic acid The *cis* form of the acid HOOC—CH=CH—COOH. Unlike the *trans* form, fumaric acid, it is not found in living matter. It readily forms an anhydride on heating.

maleic hydrazide 1,2-dihydro-3,6-pyridazine dione. Maleic acid hydrazide. A compound resulting from the reaction of maleic anhydride with hydrazine hydrate in alcohol. The compound is believed to selectively damage mitochondria in the cell. It also inhibits plant growth.

malemission [MAL- + EMISSION] Failure to ejaculate semen during sexual intercourse.

maleruption [MAL- + ERUPTION] The eruption of a tooth into a position of malalignment.

malethamer A polymer of maleic anhydride and ethylene, crosslinked with one or two percent vinyl crotonate. It is an antiperistalic agent.

maleylacetoacetate isomerase The enzyme (EC 5.2.1.2) that catalyzes the interconversion of the *cis* and *trans* isomers of HOOC—CH=CH—CO—CH$_2$—CO—CH$_2$—COOH, a reaction in the pathway of breakdown of phenylalanine and tyrosine in mammals and other organisms.

maleylpyruvate isomerase The enzyme (EC 5.2.1.4) that catalyzes *cis-trans* isomerization of the double bond in its substrate, which is an intermediate in the bacterial catabolism of *m*-cresol and gentisic acid. It acts by the transient addition of its thiol group to the double bonds.

malformation [MAL- + FORMATION] **1** Any product of abnormal development, particularly a structural defect. Also called *cacomorphosis.* **2** TERATISM. **3** MALFORMATION SEQUENCE.

Arnold-Chiari malformation ARNOLD-CHIARI DEFORMITY.

arteriovenous malformation A congenital failure of development of capillaries, resulting in a localized congeries of arteries and veins, the latter containing arterial blood. Also called *vascular malformation.*

congenital malformation CONGENITAL DEFECT.

Ebstein's malformation EBSTEIN'S ANOMALY.

Ebstein-like malformation of the mitral valve A lesion of the morphologically mitral valve in which the annular attachment of the mural (posterior) leaflet is displaced into the left ventricular cavity.

embryologic malformation A failure of proper or normal formation of any part of the body due to its defective development during the embryonic period. Also called *dysembryoplasia* (rarely used).

Klippel-Feil malformation The dominant feature of the Klippel-Feil syndrome in which malformation of the cervical spine results in a short, webbed neck.

major malformation A life-threatening malformation or one likely to cause significant impairment of health, longevity, or functional capacity. Malformations causing clinical disease or significant cosmetic problems are usually included. An imprecise usage.

minor malformation **1** A malformation not likely to cause clinical disease or significant cosmetic problem. An imprecise usage. **2** Any developmental variation (such as extra lobations on visceral organs, rudimentary accessory ribs, etc.) or developmental retardation (such as delayed ossification of certain bones). An incorrect usage.

Mondini malformation An abnormality of the cochlea present in a small proportion of congenitally deaf children. Only the first one and a half turns of the cochlea are normal, the remainder showing severe hypoplasia.

Taussig-Bing malformation A congenital malformation characterized by the aorta arising from the morphologically right ventricle and the pulmonary trunk overriding an anterior interventricular communication. The ventriculoarterial connection is usually double-outlet right ventricle but may be discordant (complete transposition). Also called *Taussig-Bing disease, Taussig-Bing syndrome.*

vascular malformation ARTERIOVENOUS MALFORMATION.

malfunction [MAL- + FUNCTION] A disordered or impaired function.

eustachian tube malfunction Failure of the eustachian tube to maintain normal middle-ear ventilation. This tends to produce middle-ear effusion and atelectasis.

Malgaigne [Joseph François *Malgaigne,* French surgeon, 1806–1865] **1** Malgaigne's fossa, Malgaigne's triangle. See under TRIGONUM CAROTICUM. **2** Malgaigne's hooks. See under HOOK. **3** See under HERNIA, APPARATUS, AMPUTATION, LUXATION.

Malherbe [Albert *Malherbe,* French surgeon, 1845–1915] Malherbe's epithelioma, Malherbe's tumor. See under PILOMATRIXOMA.

malic acid HOOC—CH₂—CHOH—COOH. The *S*-isomer of this compound, known as L-malic acid, is an intermediate in the citric acid cycle, being formed by hydration of fumarate, and being converted into oxaloacetate by malate dehydrogenase. It also has other metabolic roles, especially in plants.

malice [French (from L *malitia* bad quality, malice, from *malus* bad), propensity for doing ill] A harmful or evil intent.

malice aforethought A willful, predetermined, often malicious, intent to commit an unlawful act prior to its commission. There can be no legal justification or excuse for the act.

express malice The deliberate intent to commit an unlawful act, which can be demonstrated to have existed prior to the performance of the act, such as a verbal threat to take another's life, which is heard by others and later carried out by the individual who made the threat.

implied malice Circumstantially demonstrated or inferred proof that a deliberate intent to commit an unlawful act existed in an individual's mind before his performance of the act.

malignancy The state of being malignant.

malignant [Late L *malignans,* gen. *malignantis,* pres. part. of *malignare* (from L *malignus* wicked, malicious) to act wickedly or with malice] Tending to destroy, harm, or kill, particularly the last, as *malignant tumor, malignant hypertension.* Also *theriodic, cacoethic.*

malignogram [L *malign(us)* (from *malus* bad) bad, malicious, noxious + *o* + -GRAM] The quantitative evaluation of factors characterizing cancer cases.

mali-mali [Indonesian] A form of jumping chorea endemic in the Philippines. This condition, like latah and other similar disorders described in many parts of the world under different names, such as "the jumping Frenchmen of Maine," is now thought to be identical with Gilles de la Tourette syndrome.

malinger [French *malingre* (from *mal* badly + Old French *haingre, heingre* thin, prob. of Germanic origin) puny, stunted] To feign illness, or to exaggerate or prolong it.

malingering [*malinger,* from French *malingre* (from *mal* bad + Old French *haingre, heingre* thin, haggard) sickly + -ING] Simulation of illness or injury with conscious intent to deceive. Also called *pathomimesis, pathomimia, pathomimicry.*

Mall [Franklin P. *Mall,* U.S. anatomist, 1862–1917] **1** Mall's ridge. See under PULMONARY RIDGE. **2** See under FORMULA. **3** Periportal space of Mall. See under SPACE.

malleal Pertaining to the malleus. Also *mallear.*

mallear MALLEAL.

malleation [Med L *malleatio* (from *malleatus,* past part. of *malleare* to hammer, from L *malleus* a mallet, hammer) a hammering] Repetitive ticlike movements of the clenched hands beating against the thighs like a hammer.

malleiform Hammer-shaped.

mallein A skin test substance, analogous to tuberculin, prepared from *Pseudomonas mallei,* and used as a skin test in the diagnosis of glanders in horses.

malleoidosis MELIOIDOSIS.

malleoincudal Of the malleus and incus. Also *incudomalleal.*

malleolar Of or relating to a malleolus.

malleoli Plural of MALLEOLUS.

malleolus [L (dim. of *malleus* a hammer, mallet), a little hammer, fire dart] A rounded bony projection, as on either side of the ankle joint.

external malleolus An outmoded term for MALLEOLUS LATERALIS.

malleolus externus An outmoded term for MALLEOLUS LATERALIS.

malleolus fibulae An outmoded term for MALLEOLUS LATERALIS.

fibular malleolus An outmoded term for MALLEOLUS LATERALIS.

inner malleolus An outmoded term for MALLEOLUS MEDIALIS.

internal malleolus   An outmoded term for MALLEOLUS MEDIALIS.

malleolus internus   An outmoded term for MALLEOLUS MEDIALIS.

lateral malleolus   MALLEOLUS LATERALIS.

lateral malleolus of fibula   MALLEOLUS LATERALIS.

malleolus lateralis   [NA] The triangular, projecting lower end of the fibula. It presents four surfaces, the lateral being subcutaneous and the medial having an articular facet for the talus in the ankle joint. Its apex reaches a lower level than that of the medial malleolus. Also called *external malleolus* (outmoded), *malleolus externus* (outmoded), *malleolus fibulae* (outmoded), *fibular malleolus* (outmoded), *malleolus lateralis fibulae, outer malleolus* (outmoded), *lateral malleolus, lateral malleolus of fibula, extramalleolus* (outmoded).

malleolus lateralis fibulae   MALLEOLUS LATERALIS.

medial malleolus   MALLEOLUS MEDIALIS.

malleolus medialis   [NA] The short, expanded medial part of the lower end of the tibia that projects medially and downwards. Its lateral surface articulates with the medial aspect of the talus in the ankle joint, the medial surface is subcutaneous, while the posterior surface is grooved by the tendon of the tibialis posterior muscle. Also called *inner malleolus* (outmoded), *internal malleolus* (outmoded), *malleolus internus* (outmoded), *medial malleolus, malleolus medialis tibiae, medial malleolus of tibia, malleolus tibiae* (outmoded), *tibial malleolus* (outmoded).

malleolus medialis tibiae   MALLEOLUS MEDIALIS.

medial malleolus of tibia   MALLEOLUS MEDIALIS.

outer malleolus   An outmoded term for MALLEOLUS LATERALIS.

radial malleolus   An outmoded term for PROCESSUS STYLOIDEUS RADII.

malleolus radialis   An outmoded term for PROCESSUS STYLOIDEUS RADII.

malleolus tibiae   An outmoded term for MALLEOLUS MEDIALIS.

tibial malleolus   An outmoded term for MALLEOLUS MEDIALIS.

ulnar malleolus   An outmoded term for PROCESSUS STYLOIDEUS ULNAE.

malleolus ulnaris   An outmoded term for PROCESSUS STYLOIDEUS ULNAE.

Malleomyces   [L *malleus* glanders + Gk *mykēs* a mushroom, fungus]   PSEUDOMONAS.

Malleomyces whitmori   *PSEUDOMONAS PSEUDOMALLEI.*

malleotomy   Incision into the malleus. It may be performed to remove the malleus head as in modified radical mastoidectomy. Also called *sphyrotomy.* (seldom used).

mallet / automatic mallet   AUTOMATIC CONDENSER.

malleus   [L, a hammer, mallet]   (*plural* mallei) [NA] The largest of the auditory ossicles in the tympanic cavity resembling a club and consisting of a head, or caput; neck, or collum; handle, or manubrium; and two processes, anterior and lateral. It is attached to the tympanic membrane, and its head articulates posteriorly with the incus. Also called *hammer, plectrum* (outmoded).

mallochorion   [Gk *mallo(s)* a lock of wool or hair + *chorion* skin, leather]   The chorion in its early stage when it is covered with tufts of villi.

Mallophaga   [Gk *mallo(s)* a lock of hair or wool + New L *-phaga*, combining form denoting an eater]   An insect order of some 3000 species of biting or chewing lice, most of which are ectoparasites of birds and some, of mammals. Species that infest domestic mammals include *Bovicola, Felicola, Heterodoxus,* and *Trichodectes.* Bird lice that are pests of chickens include the shaft louse *Menopon gallinae,* the chicken body louse *Menacan-*

thus stramineus, the fluff louse *Goniocotes gallinae,* the brown chicken louse *Goniodes dissimilis,* the wing louse *Lipeurus caponis,* and the chicken head louse *Cuclotogaster heterographus.*

Mallory   [Frank Burr *Mallory*, U.S. pathologist, 1862–1941]   **1** Mallory's acid fuchsin. See under MALLORY'S TRIPLE STAIN. **2** Mallory's phosphotungstic acid hematoxylin stain. See under STAIN. **3** Mallory's bodies. See under BODY. **4** Councilman and Mallory blood serum. See under SERUM. **5** See under LEUKEMIA.

Mallory   [George Kenneth *Mallory*, U.S. pathologist, born 1900]   Mallory-Weiss syndrome. See under SYNDROME.

mallow   [Old English *mealwe*, from L *malva* the mallow; Gk *malachē* (from *malakos* soft, gentle, mild) the mallow]   The leaves of *Malva sylvestris* and *M. rotundifolia.* It is used to make cough syrups. Also called *high mallow.*

high mallow   MALLOW.

malnutrition   [MAL- + NUTRITION]   Any disorder resulting from a deficiency or an excess of one or more essential nutrients. This may arise as a result of an unbalanced diet or an inability to absorb or metabolize any nutrient. Also called *hypothrepsia, cacotrophy, kakotrophy.*

malignant malnutrition   KWASHIORKOR.

protein malnutrition   KWASHIORKOR.

protein-calorie malnutrition   Malnutrition resulting from an inadequate intake of sources of energy and/or protein which usually occurs in children under five years who are consuming a diet insufficient in these substances. People of any age may suffer from this disorder but in adults it is less common and the clinical symptoms less severe, because after growth ceases, the protein and energy needs are diminished. The spectrum of clinical manifestations range from marasmus, due to a chronic restriction of all nutrients, to kwashiorkor, due to a deficiency of protein without an accompanying inadequate intake of energy sources. Between these two extremes are a host of forms in which the clinical features are due to a combination of protein and energy deficiencies as well as deficiencies of vitamins and minerals and related infections. Also called *nutritional marasmus.*

malocclusion   [MAL- + OCCLUSION]   Any deviation from normal occlusion. Also called *patho-occlusion, odontoparallaxis.*

deflective malocclusion   A malocclusion caused by deflective occlusal contact or contacts.

malomaxillary   Of the malar bone and maxilla.

malonal   BARBITAL.

malonate   Any salt of malonic acid, a dicarboxylic acid that participates in many steps in intermediary metabolism.

malonic acid $HOOC—CH_2—COOH$. Propanedioic acid. It competitively inhibits the oxidation of succinate to fumarate by succinate dehydrogenase.

malonyl   The univalent 2-carboxyacetyl group, $HOOC—CH_2—CO—$. ● In strict chemical nomenclature this is the bivalent acyl group formed from malonic acid, namely $—CO—CH_2—CO—$.

malonyl-ACP   The thiol ester of malonic acid with acyl carrier protein, an intermediate in the biosynthesis of fatty acids in bacteria.

malonyl-coenzyme A   The thiol ester of malonic acid with coenzyme A, it is formed from acetyl-CoA by carboxylation in a reaction catalyzed by a biotinyl enzyme that hydrolyzes ATP and uses carbon dioxide. This is a step in the biosynthesis of fatty acids. The malonyl group is transferred onto the synthetic enzyme before condensation with another thiol ester group and release of carbon dioxide in the chain-lengthening step.

malonylurea   BARBITURIC ACID. ● This name is sometimes used because it is urea acylated on its nitrogen atoms with the two carboxyl groups of malonic acid.

maloplasty MELOPLASTY.

malouetine $C_{27}H_{52}N_2$. A teratogenic, steroidal alkaloid found in *Malouetia bequaertiana*.

Malpighi [Marcello *Malpighi*, Italian anatomist and physiologist, 1628–1694] **1** Malpighian tubes. See under MALPIGHIAN TUBULES. **2** Pyramid of Malpighi. See under RENAL PYRAMID. **3** Canal of Malpighi-Gartner. See under LONGITUDINAL DUCT OF EPOOPHORON. **4** Malpighi's vesicles. See under ALVEOLI PULMONIS. **5** Stratum germinativum epidermidis malpighii, stratum malpighii. See under GERMINATIVE LAYER OF EPIDERMIS.

malposed Abnormally placed, as teeth.

malposition [MAL- + POSITION] An abnormal position, as of teeth.

malpractice [MAL- + PRACTICE] Misconduct on the part of a professional practitioner while rendering a professional service, which results in injury or loss to the recipient of the service. See also NEGLIGENCE.

medical malpractice Negligent conduct on the part of a medical practitioner or health facility resulting in injury, loss, or damage to a patient. All of the following elements must be established to prove medical malpractice: a voluntary professional relationship must exist between the two parties, thereby obligating the physician or other provider of care to a duty of care to the patient; the provider of care must breach that duty of care by virtue of negligence; and the negligent act must be the proximate cause of the injury or loss sustained by the patient. In addition, the injury of loss must be compensable in monetary terms.

malpresentation [MAL- + PRESENTATION] An abnormal lie of the fetus during or preceding labor. • The term *malpresentation* is commonly used of all presentations other than the vertex presentation.

malrotation [MAL- + ROTATION] A developmental failure of rotation in the normal direction or to the normal degree. Such failure is seen mostly in the digestive tract, but sometimes in other structures that undergo a degree of rotation during embryogenesis, such as the heart, kidneys, and limbs.

maltase Any enzyme that hydrolyzes maltose to glucose. Such enzymes are usually called α-glucosidases, because they release glucose from the nonreducing ends of α1,4-linked oligosaccharides of glucose as well as from maltose itself.

Malthus [Thomas Robert *Malthus*, English economist and demographer, 1766–1834] Malthusian theory. See under MALTHUSIANISM.

malthusian [after Thomas Robert *Malthus*, English economist, 1766–1834] Malthusian law. See under LAW.

malthusianism [after Thomas Robert *Malthus*, English economist and demographer, 1766–1834 + -ian, adjectival suffix denoting characteristic of + -ISM] **1** Originally a social doctrine based on the theory that population increases by geometric progression while food production increases arithmetically, and leading to the conclusion that the number of births must be restricted by sexual continence or other means. Contrary to a widely held view, the theory is not based on any scientific analysis, but flows from *a priori* speculations. Also called *malthusian theory*. **2** NEOMALTHUSIANISM.

maltodextrin Any oligosaccharide of glucose residues, linked as in maltose, i.e. by α1-4 links.

maltose The disaccharide of glucose containing an α1-4 linkage. It is a hydrolysis product of starch and glycogen.

maltosuria [*maltos(e)* + -URIA] The appearance of maltose in the urine.

maltotriose The trisaccharide of glucose in which each of the

two links is like that of maltose, i.e. α1-4.

malum [L, an evil, harm, disease] A disease.

malum articulorum senilis OSTEOARTHRITIS.

malum coxae Arthritis of the hip, usually osteoarthritis.

malum coxae senilis Osteoarthritis of the hip. Also called *morbus coxarius* (obsolete).

malum perforans pedis PERFORATING ULCER OF THE FOOT.

malum senile OSTEOARTHRITIS.

malum venereum An outmoded term for SYPHILIS.

malum vertebrale suboccipitale Tuberculosis of the first and second cervical vertebrae.

malunion Union of a fracture in an abnormal position.

malvaria [L *malva* mallow + *r* + -IA] The presumed disorder of subjects whose urine showed a mauve factor when analyzed chromatographically.

mam Symbol for the obsolete unit, myriameter.

M + Am The combination of myopia and myopic astigmatism.

mamanpian [French *maman* mother + French *pian* yaw, from the Tupi and Guarani] MOTHER YAW.

mamba [Zulu *imamba* mamba] Any venomous snake of the genus *Dendroaspis* of the Elapidae family.

mamelon [French (dim. of *mamelle* woman's breast, from L *mamilla* the breast, from *mamma* the breast, a teat), nipple, any round protuberance] A small tubercle on the incisal edge of an unworn incisor tooth.

mamelonated An outmoded term for MAMILLATED.

mamelonation An outmoded term for MAMILLATION.

mamilla [L (dim. of *mamma* breast), breast, teat, nipple] (*plural* mamillae) **1** PAPILLA MAMMARIA. **2** Any nipplelike structure. Also *mammilla*.

mamillae Plural of MAMILLA.

mamillaria MILIARIA PROFUNDA.

mamillary Pertaining to or resembling a nipple. Also *mammillary*.

mamillated Covered with nipplelike protuberances. Also *mammillated, mamelonated* (outmoded), *mammillate*.

mamillation **1** A mamilliform protuberance. **2** The state of possessing nipples. For defs. 1 and 2 also *mamelonation* (outmoded), *mammillation*.

mamilliform Nipple-shaped. Also *mammilliform, mamilloid*.

mamilliplasty [L *mamill(a)*, dim. of *mamma* a woman's breast + *i* + -PLASTY] THELEPLASTY.

mamillitis [L *mamill(a)*, dim. of *mamma* a woman's breast + -ITIS] Inflammation of the nipple or teat. Also called *mammillitis, thelitis*.

bovine ulcerative mamillitis An ulcerative disease of cattle affecting the skin of the mammary gland, especially the teats. It is caused by a herpesvirus (Allerton virus). See also PSEUDOLUMPY SKIN DISEASE.

mamilloid MAMILLIFORM.

mamilloinfundibular Denoting connections between the mamillary body and the infundibular portion of the pituitary stalk.

mamillopeduncular Denoting the peduncles entering and exiting the mamillary bodies of the hypothalamus. These include the mamillary peduncle bringing afferent fibers from the reticular formation, and the mamillothalamic tract carrying efferents to the anterior mamillary nuclear complex.

mamillotegmental Denoting the mamillotegmental bundle. Also *mammillotegmental*.

mamillothalamic Denoting the tractus mamillothalamicus. Also *mammillothalamic*.

mamma [L, the breast, a female breast, teat, mother; Gk *mamma* or *mammē* a mother, a child's call to its mother; later a grandmother] (*plural* mammae) [NA] One of a pair of rounded subcutaneous protuberances on each side of the front of the chest. They are functional and developed in the female and rudimentary in the male, extending from the second to the sixth ribs vertically and from the side of the sternum to the midaxillary line horizontally. Protruding from approximately the center is the nipple, on which open 15–20 lactiferous ducts from the mammary gland proper; surrounding the nipple is the areola. The glandular portion comprises lobes, made up of lobules and acini, between and around which are connective tissue, blood vessels, lymphatics, nerves, and fat, which gives the organ its rounded contour. In the female it undergoes considerable development after puberty and during pregnancy, secreting milk during lactation after parturition. It alters in shape and size with aging. Also called *breast.*

mammae aberrantes   SUPERNUMERARY MAMMAE.

mammae accessoriae   SUPERNUMERARY MAMMAE.

accessory mammae   SUPERNUMERARY MAMMAE.

mamma areolata   An unusual degree of protuberance of the areola of the breast.

mamma erratica   Supernumerary mammae present at locations other than those corresponding to the embryonic milk line.

mamma masculina [NA] A mamma in a male, usually rudimentary throughout life and comprising only ducts that are usually solid, with some connective tissue and fat. The areola is developed but the papilla is small. In the adult male, it rarely develops beyond the female prepubertal stage. Also called *mamma virilis, male breast.*

supernumerary mammae   Mammary glands at sites other than the usual location of the breasts. They are most often along the embryonic milk lines extending from the axillae to the groin. Also called *mammae accessoriae, accessory mammae, mammae aberrantes, accessory mammary glands.*

mamma virilis   MAMMA MASCULINA.

mammae   Plural of MAMMA.

mammal [Late L *mammal(is)* (from L *mamm(a)* a woman's breast + *-alis* -AL) pertaining to the breasts]   Any member of the vertebrate class Mammalia.

mammalgia [*mamm(o)-* + -ALGIA]   MASTODYNIA.

Mammalia [New L (from Late L *mammal(is)* pertaining to the breasts, from L *mamma* breast, teat, + L *-ia* -IA)]   The class of homeothermic vertebrates characterized by hair and by milk-secreting mammary glands that nourish the young. The diaphragm is muscular, the heart four-chambered. The ramus of the mandible is composed of a single bone, the dentary, and the jaw articulates directly with the squamosal bone. There are three ear ossicles. Except for the egg-laying monotremes, all mammals are viviparous.

mammalogy [*mamma(l)* + -LOGY]   The study of mammals.

mammaplasty [MAMMA + -PLASTY]   MAMMOPLASTY.

mammary   Pertaining to the mamma or mammary gland.

mammectomy [*mamm(o)-* + -ECTOMY]   MASTECTOMY.

mammiferous   Bearing mammary glands.

mammiform   Shaped like a mamma. Also *mammose.*

mammilingus [*mamm(o)-* + *i* + L *-lingus*, combining form denoting licking, from *lingere* to lick]   Sucking on the breast, especially as an adult sexual activity of pathologic significance in the subject.

mammilla   **1** MAMILLA.   **2** PAPILLA MAMMARIA.

mammillary   MAMILLARY.

mammillate   MAMILLATED.

mammillated   MAMILLATED.

mammillation   MAMILLATION.

mammilliform   MAMILLIFORM.

mammilliplasty [See MAMILLIPLASTY.]   THELEPLASTY.

mammillitis   MAMILLITIS.

mammillotegmental   MAMILLOTEGMENTAL.

mammillothalamic   MAMILLOTHALAMIC.

mammiplasia   MAMMOPLASIA.

mammitis   MASTITIS.

mammo- [L *mamma* (from Gk *mammē* mother's breast) mother's breast]   A combining form denoting the breasts.

mammogen [MAMMO- + -GEN]   Any agent promoting or stimulating development of the breast.

mammogenesis   The hormonal and other processes that foster the growth and development of the breast and prepare it for lactation.

mammogram [MAMMO- + -GRAM]   A roentgenogram obtained during mammography. Also called *mastogram* (rarely used).

mammography [MAMMO- + -GRAPHY]   Radiographic examination of the breast. Also called *mastography* (rarely used).

mammoplasia [MAMMO- + -PLASIA]   The growth and development of the breast. Also called *mastoplasia, mammiplasia, mazoplasia.*

adolescent mammoplasia   The growth and development of the breast during puberty, especially the moderate development that often occurs transiently in the adolescent male.

mammoplasty [MAMMO- + -PLASTY]   Any plastic operation on the breast. Also called *mammaplasty, mastoplasty.*

augmentation mammoplasty   A mammoplasty performed to increase breast size, generally using alloplastic materials.

dermal pedicle mammoplasty   A mammoplasty in which the blood supply to the nipple is preserved through a pedicle of skin from which the epidermis has been removed, thus permitting burial of the pedicle beneath the skin.

reduction mammoplasty   A mammoplasty performed to reduce breast size, yet preserve a natural contour and a normal relationship of the nipple to the breast.

mammose   **1** Having full or large breasts.   **2** MAMMIFORM.

mammotomy [MAMMO- + -TOMY]   Incision into the breast.

mammotroph   MAMMOTROPIC CELL.

mammotropic [MAMMO- + -TROPIC¹]   **1** Stimulating the mammary gland.   **2** Pertaining to the development, milk production, and milk secretion of the mammary gland.

mammotropin [MAMMO- + *trop-* prefix denoting a turning, from Gk *tropos* a turn, from *trephein* to turn + -IN]   PROLACTIN.

mampirra   A tropical bloodsucking ceratopogonid gnat that causes considerable skin irritation and itching. Also called *merutu.*

man [Old English]   **1** A male adult human being.   **2** Humanity or mankind including especially the species *Homo sapiens* but extended also to include other species of the genus *Homo* known from the fossil record.   • Some human fossils, Peking man, for example, were originally assigned to other genera of the family Hominidae but have mostly been reclassified as species of *Homo.* Hominids currently classified in other genera are usually not called "man" or "human."

Cro-Magnon man   An upper Pleistocene, European "race" of man typified by a group of skeletons found at Cro-Magnon in France by L. Lartet in 1868. The cranium is sometimes described as dolichopentagonal: large, long, and five-sided as seen from above. The postcranial skeleton is that of modern humans in all respects and indicates tall, slender, and muscular people.

Folsom man   A partial skeleton recovered from Holocene deposits at a point on the Cimarron River, 8 miles east of Folsom, New Mexico in 1935. Initially regarded as a new species of man in the New World, it is now widely regarded as falling within the range of *Homo sapiens* and probably represents early American Indians.

Heidelberg man A human fossil represented by a mandible recovered in 1908 from a sand pit near the village of Mauer near Heidelberg, West Germany. The deposits contain a fauna that suggest the climate was warm-temperate, perhaps during the first European interglacial period. Initially attributed to a separate human species, *Homo heidelbergensis*, it is now more commonly regarded as a European pre-Neandertal form.

Java man Any of a group of fossil human remains recovered in Java since 1891 from various sites all of which are probably less than 1 000 000 but more than 500 000 years old. Initially assigned to a new genus and species of "ape-man," *Pithecanthropus erectus*, the Java fossils are now widely regarded as belonging to an archaic species of man known as *Homo erectus*.

Neandertal man See under *HOMO NEANDERTHALENSIS*.

Ngandong man A human population represented by a group of skulls and leg bones recovered from Pleistocene deposits in Java at Ngandong in the valley of the Solo river. Initially regarded as a new species of man, *Homo soloensis*, it was later regarded as being more properly attributed to *Homo sapiens*, and yet again, most recently, as a late example of *Homo erectus*.

Peking man An extinct human population represented by a group of fossil remains recovered from Choukoutien (Zhoukoudian), near Peking, China, since 1927. The fossils consist of skulls, jaws, teeth, and a few postcranial bones. Initially regarded as a new genus and species, *Sinanthropus pekinensis*, it was later recognized as belonging to *Homo erectus*.

reference man A hypothetical man whose anatomy, physiology, biochemistry, clinical chemistry, and hematologic values are within normal limits, and with whom all other men may be compared. Also called *standard man*.

Rhodesian man An extinct human population represented by a group of fossil remains recovered from Broken Hill, Zambia (formerly Northern Rhodesia), comprising a skull and postcranial remains from several individuals. The remains are dated as more than 100 000 years old. Initially assigned to a separate species, *Homo rhodesiensis*, they were later classified as belonging to an archaic subspecies of modern man, *Homo sapiens rhodesiensis*.

spinal man A patient with complete transection of the spinal cord at any level.

standard man REFERENCE MAN.

man. *manipulus* (L, a handful).

manaca The dried root of *Brunfelsia hopeana*. It has been used to treat syphilis. Also called *vegetable mercury*.

management / case management The handling of a case of disease, injury, or other medical abnormality, with the end of achieving through care and/or treatment a result that is satisfactory under the circumstances. Also called *patient management*.

patient management CASE MANAGEMENT.

risk management A course of action that may be taken to control, reduce, or eliminate a risk; in health care institutions, efforts specifically directed to prevent or control possible liability such as from medical malpractice or personal injury.

manager / unit manager The administrator of a patient care unit in a health care facility such as a hospital.

mandama The equivalent in the East Indies of PHRYNODERMA.

Mandelamine A proprietary name for methenamine mandelate.

mandelic acid Ph—CHOH—COOH. 2-Hydroxy-2-phenylacetic acid. Both enantiomers are found in nature. It occurs, often combined, in plants.

mandible [L *mandibula*. See MANDIBULA.] **1** The bone of the

lower jaw of mammals; mandibula. **2** A member of the anterior pair of mouthparts in some invertebrates.

Mauer mandible A hominid mandible found in 1907 in a sandpit at the village of Mauer, near Heidelberg, West Germany. The mandible is of possibly middle Pleistocene age and is associated with an extinct fauna. It is large and robust with a parabolic dental arcade and no chin. It may belong to a European example of *Homo erectus* or to a pre-Neanderthal variety of *H. sapiens*.

Piltdown mandible A mandible discovered at Piltdown in Sussex, England. First thought to be hominid, it was named *Eoanthropus dawsoni*. It was later proved to be part of an elaborate hoax, the jaw being actually that of a modern orangutan. It had been artificially aged.

mandibula [Late L (from L *mandere* to chew, akin to *mala* the cheekbone, jaw and to Gk *masasthai*, first aorist inf. of root *maō* strive for, to touch), the lower jaw] [NA] The large, arched, movable bone of the lower part of the face, consisting of a curved horizontal body on each side, fused in the midline at the symphysis menti. It is continuous posteriorly with a vertical ramus, the upper border of which ends posteriorly in a condyle that articulates with the temporal bone at the temporomandibular joint. The upper, or alveolar, border of the body supports the lower teeth. Its functions include protection of the tongue, and involvement in mastication and speech. Also called *mandible*, *lower jaw*, *inferior jaw*, *jaw bone*, *submaxilla* (outmoded), *inferior maxilla* (outmoded), *lower jaw bone*, *inferior maxillary bone* (outmoded).

mandibulae Plural of MANDIBULA.

mandibular Pertaining to the mandible.

mandibulectomy The excision of the lower jaw.

mandibulofacial Pertaining to the mandible and the facial bones.

mandibuloglossus An occasional muscle bundle that extends from the posterior border of the mandible, above the angle, to the side of the tongue.

mandibulomarginalis One of the accessory slips of the platysma muscle, extending forward from the mastoid process over the angle of the mandible to the main body of the muscle.

mandibulopharyngeal Of or relating to the mandible and the pharynx: used especially of the anatomic area between them.

mandioca [Spanish and Portuguese (from the Tupi), manioc, cassava, tapioca] CASSAVA.

mandrake [Middle English; Old English *mandragora* (from L and Gk *mandragoras* mandrake) the mandrake] A plant of the species *Posophyllum peltatum*, the roots of which are used to make podophyllum resin. Also called *May apple*, *mayapple*, *Indian apple*.

mandrel [prob. alteration of French *mandrin* mandrel, of obscure origin, possibly from Gk *mandra* the setting for a seal, a bezel. The German is *Mandrel*.] A rotating shaft used in a dental handpiece to hold abrasive instruments by means of a screw, chuck, or pin. Also *mandril*.

disk mandrel A mandrel used for abrasive disks in operative dentistry.

Morgan's mandrel A disk mandrel with a split head, grooved to hold a disk with a square central hole.

mandril MANDREL.

mandrin [prob. French. See MANDREL.] A stylet used to help introduce soft catheters.

manducate [L *manducat(us)*, past part. of *manducare* to chew + *e*] To chew or masticate. An obsolete term.

maneuver [French *manoeuvre* (from L *manus* hand and *operari* to work, from *opus*, gen. *operis*, a work) a maneuver] A manual procedure, especially a skillful one.

Adson maneuver   See under ADSON'S TEST.

Allen maneuver   A maneuver to confirm the presence of the scalenus anterior syndrome by testing for the obliteration of the radial pulse when compressing the subclavicular artery against the scalenus muscle as the head is rotated to the opposite shoulder and the arm is extended and externally rotated.

Bracht maneuver   A procedure used in assisting a breech delivery. The fetus is allowed to be delivered to the umbilicus. Then, while the fetal arms are held against the sides, the fetal body is elevated anteriorly toward the symphysis pubis. The maneuver usually results in delivery of the vertex.

Brandt-Andrews maneuver   A procedure used in assisting delivery of the placenta. While exerting traction on the umbilical cord with one hand, the other is placed on the abdomen to displace the uterus upwards. Also called *Brandt-Andrews method.*

Buzzard's maneuver   A method of facilitating elicitation of the knee jerk, in which the patient points his toe to the ground or to a fixed point. A seldom used term. Also called *Buzzard's reflex.*

Chassard-Lapiné maneuver   A special roentgenographic projection in which the patient sits at the edge of the table, bending far forward with the head near the knees, and the x-ray beam is directed from above, centered to the pelvis, penetrating the spine. This projection is used to demonstrate the pelvic inlet and also during barium enema examination to display the loops of the sigmoid with diminished overlapping.

Credé's maneuver   **1** Placenta expulsion by manual pressure on the uterus by the abdominal wall. **2** The instillation of a solution of 0.1 percent silver nitrate in the eyes of newborns. **3** Urine expulsion by pressure on the bladder through the abdominal wall. For defs. 1, 2, and 3 also called *Credé's method.*

DeLee's maneuver   A procedure used in obstetrics of converting a face presentation to a brow presentation.

Engel-Lysholm maneuver   A radiographic technique used to demonstrate the retrogastric region with regard to size or mass impressions. A translateral horizontal beam film of the abdomen is taken with the patient prone, after gaseous distention of the stomach, such as by effervescent powders. A posteroanterior vertical beam projection is also obtained.

Fowler maneuver   A test for contracted intrinsic musculature with ulnar deviation at the metacarpophalangeal joint. The test is performed by flexing the wrists. In normal subjects the fingers can be extended. In intrinsic muscle contraction the fingers remain in flexion at the proximal interphalangeal joint.

Halstead maneuver   A maneuver to confirm the presence of the scalenus anterior syndrome by the obliteration of the radial pulse when the head is rotated contralaterally and and examiner applies downward pressure on the extended limb of the involved side.

Hampton maneuver   A radiographic technique during gastrointestinal series, designed to demonstrate the duodenal cap with a combination of barium coating and air distention, as in an air-contrast examination. The supine patient is placed in the left posterior oblique position. This maneuver is helpful for the roentgenographic demonstration of a posterior-wall ulcer.

Heimlich maneuver   A procedure designed to clear the airway of a bolus, especially food, in an emergency by exerting a sudden, intense pressure inward on the abdomen immediately below the diaphragm, thus forcing the victim to expel air from the lungs. If the victim is standing, the rescuer places his or her arms around the victim, placing a fist just below the sternum, and, with the other open hand around the fist, thrusts the fist inward and upward. This forces an explosive release of air which, it is hoped, will dislodge the blockage. Variations of the maneuver can accommodate victims who are sitting or supine.

Hippocratic maneuver   A maneuver used to restore to proper position a dislocated shoulder. The operator's foot is placed in the patient's axilla and the patient's arm is pulled downward.

Hodge maneuver   A means of assisting vaginal delivery of a fetus. The obstetrician aids flexion of the fetal head by exerting pressure on the fetal brow with each uterine contraction.

Hoguet's maneuver   A surgical procedure in which the sac of an inguinal hernia is passed beneath the deep epigastric vessels to facilitate its removal.

Jendrassik's maneuver   A procedure for facilitation or reinforcement of the patellar reflex: the patient is asked to pull on his hands which are clasped together in claw fashion, while the patellar tendon is percussed. Also called *reinforcement of tendon reflexes.*

key-in-lock maneuver   A method of rotating the fetal head using obstetric forceps. After an initial arc of rotation, the forceps are reapplied in order to complete the rotation. Most frequently, this method is utilized to convert a fetal head from a transverse or posterior position to an anterior position.

Kocher's maneuver   A method of reducing a dislocated shoulder by internally rotating and adducting the flexed involved limb across the trunk.

Kristeller's maneuver   An obstetric procedure in which pressure is maintained on the uterine fundus in an effort to express the infant. The procedure is not always successful and carries a risk of uterine rupture.

Lasègue's maneuver   NERI SIGN.

Leadbetter maneuver   A method of reducing a fractured femoral neck by applying a vertical force on the flexed femur and then extending it into abduction.

Leopold's maneuvers   A series of four steps in palpating the abdomen of a pregnant woman in order to ascertain the position and presentation of the fetus.

Levret maneuver   A type of internal fetal version utilizing rotation in an effort to disimpact a fetus from the pelvic brim.

Løvset's maneuver   A method of extracting the arms in a breech delivery by rotating the trunk of the fetus after it has delivered to the level of the umbilicus. Also called *Løvset's method.*

Marie and Foix maneuver   A maneuver in which firm pressure behind the ascending ramus of the mandible produces facial contraction. This contraction is absent in peripheral facial paralysis. A seldom used term.

Mauriceau maneuver   A method of delivering the head in a breech delivery.

Mauriceau-Smellie-Veit maneuver   A modified Mariceau maneuver utilized to deliver the head in a breech delivery.

McDonald maneuver   A method of estimating the duration of a pregnancy by measuring the distance from the symphysis pubis to the top of the gravid uterus with a tape measure.

McMurray's circumduction maneuver   A test for a tear in a knee meniscus in which the acutely flexed knee is extended and a varus or valgus strain is applied. The examiner will feel a click or catch, and the subject will experience pain, if a tear is present.

modified Ritgen maneuver   A procedure to assist delivery of the head in a vertex presentation by producing extension through pressure on the brow, maxilla, and chin in succession, using the tips of the fingers placed on the perineum just behind the anus.

Müller's maneuver   MÜLLER'S EXPERIMENT.

Müller-Hillis maneuver   A means of assessing the size of the fetal head in relation to the maternal pelvis in order to determine whether or not there is cephalopelvic disproportion.

Munro Kerr maneuver   A means of assessing the size of the fetal head in relation to the maternal pelvis in order to determine whether or not there is cephalopelvic disproportion.

oath-taking maneuver   OATH-TAKING SIGN.

Pajot maneuver   The application of traction with both hands to facilitate vaginal delivery of a fetus with forceps. Also called *Saxtorph's maneuver.*

Phalen's maneuver   A method of bringing out or accentuating the symptoms of a carpal tunnel syndrome by forced flexion of the affected wrist for 30–60 seconds or by applying a sphygmomanometer cuff to the arm at above arterial pressure for one minute.

Pinard maneuver   A procedure to identify and deliver a foot during a breech delivery.

Prague maneuver   A procedure used in a breech delivery in which a finger is hooked over the shoulder of the fetus to exert traction and allow engagement of the head, facilitating subsequent delivery.

Proust-Lichtheim maneuver   A way to demonstrate that an aphasic patient knows and recognizes a word he is unable to say, by having him gesture or tap out with a finger the number of letters or syllables the word contains.

Ritgen maneuver   A means of facilitating delivery of the fetal head in a vertex presentation. Originally described in 1855, the initial method has been replaced by the modified Ritgen maneuver. Also called *Ritgen's method.*

Saxtorph's maneuver   PAJOT MANEUVER.

Scanzoni maneuver   A method of midforceps rotation of the fetal head from a posterior to an anterior position.

Schatz maneuver   A method of converting a face presentation to a brow presentation in order to facilitate vaginal delivery.

Sellick's maneuver   The application of pressure on the cricoid cartilage to occlude the esophagus posteriorly, thereby preventing regurgitation and aspiration of gastric contents. It is used for a patient with a full stomach during rapid induction of anesthesia and tracheal intubation.

Thorn maneuver   A method of converting a face presentation to a vertex presentation in order to facilitate vaginal delivery.

Toynbee's maneuver   The production of alterations in intratympanic pressure by swallowing with the mouth closed and the nose pinched. These alterations are assessed by listening to the sounds produced using an auscultation tube.

Valsalva maneuver   **1** The forcible inflation of the middle ear by a strong expiratory effort made with the mouth closed and the nostrils pinched. It is frequently adopted by patients to gain relief from the discomfort in the ears and impaired hearing caused by negative pressure consequent on obstruction of the eustachian tubes. It is used by otologists as a test of tubal patency. Also called *Valsalva's procedure, Valsalva's experiment, auto inflation.* **2** A forceable exhalation against a closed glottis. The increased pressure which develops within the thorax causes a change in venous return and in heart rate. Compare MÜLLER'S EXPERIMENT.

Van Hoorn maneuver   A modification of the Prague maneuver in which transabdominal pressure is appled to the fetal brow with one hand in order to facilitate engagement of the fetal head.

Westphal maneuver   The use of movements of the head and/or the eyes by dyslexic patients to trace out the outline of letters or symbols which they cannot read at a glance.

Wigand's maneuver   An external transabdominal palpatory maneuver to convert a transverse lie of a fetus to a vertex presentation. Also called *Wigand-Martin maneuver.*

Wigand-Martin maneuver   WIGAND'S MANEUVER.

manganese   Element number 25, having atomic weight 54.9380. It is a hard, brittle metal resembling iron. Its compounds are widely distributed in the lithosphere and the ocean floor in spots is strewn with nodules containing about 24% manganese. A single stable isotope, manganese 55, occurs in nature. Nine radioactive isotopes and an isomer have been described. Manganese is a reactive element, with valences 1, 2, 3, 4, 6, and 7. Biologically, small amounts are essential constituents of several enzymes. Large amounts are toxic. Symbol: Mn

manganese 52   A radioisotope of manganese emitting a positron, a characteristic chromium x ray of 5.4 keV, and a gamma ray. It has been used for irradiation of lymph nodes. Physical half-life is 5.7 days. Symbol: ^{52}Mn

manganese 54   A radioisotope of manganese, emitting by electron capture a gamma photon at 835 keV and a characteristic chromium x ray of 5.4 keV. It has been used for local irradiation of lymph nodes. It has a half-life of 291 days. Symbol: ^{54}Mn

manganese glycerophosphate $C_3H_7MnO_6P$. A white or pink powder, utilized formerly as a nerve tonic and hematinic.

manganese hypophosphite $Mn(H_2PO_2)_2 \cdot H_2O$. It was formerly used as a hematinic but is now used as a nutritional supplement or source of manganese.

manganese peptonate   A solution of iron peptonate and manganese chloride. It has been used as a source of iron in the treatment of microcytic anemia. The manganese is presumed to increase the efficiency of iron absorption.

manganese saccharate   A preparation of manganese that has been used to increase the efficiency of iron absorption in the treatment of microcytic anemia.

manganic   Of manganese in its tervalent state.

manganic acid H_2MnO_4. An acid that does not exist in the free state. Its salts are manganates.

manganism   [*mangan(ese)* + -ISM]   MANGANESE POISONING.

manganous   Of manganese in its bivalent state.

mange   [Middle English *manjewe*; Old French *mangeue* an appetite, itching, eating, from *mangier* (from L *manducare* to chew, from *mandere* to chew) to eat]   A contagious skin disease of domestic animals, caused by infestation with any of several species of mange mites of such genera as *Chorioptes, Demodex, Notoedres, Psoroptes,* and *Sarcoptes,* causing chorioptic, demodectic, notoedric, psoroptic, or sarcoptic mange. The mites burrow into the skin causing multiple vesicular and papular lesions and intense itching. The agents are called scab mites. Also called *gafeira (Portuguese).*

chorioptic mange   Mange caused by *Chorioptes bovis.* It especially affects the legs of cattle, sheep, goats, horses, and rabbits. In rams, the scrotal skin is often affected. Also called *chorioptic acariasis, chorioptic sarcoptidosis, chorioptosis.*

demodectic mange   See under DEMODECTIC ACARIASIS.

follicular mange   See under DEMODECTIC ACARIASIS.

foot mange   Mange caused by *Chorioptes bovis* infestation between the claws of sheep. Also called *foot scab.*

notoedric mange   Mange caused by *Notoedres cati,* and occurring especially in cats, dogs, rabbits, and certain rodents, but apparently not humans.

otodectic mange   Mange of the skin of the external ear canal, caused by *Otodectes cynotis.* It occurs mainly in dogs, cats, foxes, rabbits, and ferrets. The mites may swarm in the external ear, causing severe itching, tenderness, twisting of the neck, and paroxysms.

psoroptic mange   Mange caused by scab mites such as *Psoroptes ovis* of sheep, cattle, and horses. It affects any part of the body, including the external ear canal. It damages sheep wool, causing it to become rough, ragged, and matted. Also called *psoroptic acariasis, psorootosis, psoroptic scab, psoroptic sarcoptidosis, psoroptic itch.*

red mange   Mange in dogs, caused by the follicular mite of dogs, *Demodex canis,* often associated with bacterial infection, such as *Staphylococcus pyogenes albus,* the probable cause of hair loss; canine demodectic mange.

sarcoptic mange   Mange caused by *Sarcoptes scabiei* or other scabies mites or itch mites. Host-adapted variants are found on man (scabies), dogs, horses, pigs, and other mammalian hosts. Also called *sarcoptic acariasis.*

mangosteen   The pericarp of *Garcinia mangostana*, which has astringent properties.

mangrove [Portuguese *mangue* (from Spanish *mangle* the mangrove tree, from the Taino) mangrove, marshy ground by the sea + English *grove*]   A woody plant that stabilizes marine coastal shorelines in tropical and semitropical areas. The black mangrove *(Avicennia nitida)* is a shrub. The red mangrove *(Rhizophora mangle)* is the dominant, indigenous species in mangrove swamps from Florida to South America and along the African Atlantic shore. These plants have viviparous fruit.

mania [Gk *mania.* See -MANIA.]   **1** A syndrome consisting of elated although unstable mood, hyperactivity, and mental overactivity expressed in garrulousness. As part of manic-depressive psychosis or bipolar disorder, mania is sometimes classified on the basis of intensity as hypomania, acute mania, or delirious mania. Also called *psycheclampsia* (obsolete), *psychlampsia* (obsolete).   **2** Any type of mental disorder, especially if symptoms have an impulsive, compulsive, or repetitive quality.

acute mania   The second most severe form of manic-depressive psychosis.

akinetic mania   A manic syndrome in which relative immobility replaces hyperactivity.

alcoholic mania   PATHOLOGIC INTOXICATION.

mania à poter   PATHOLOGIC INTOXICATION.

mania à potu   PATHOLOGIC INTOXICATION.

Bell's mania   DELIRIOUS MANIA.

brooding mania   OBSESSIVE RUMINATION.

chronic mania   Mania which, unlike other forms, has episodes that persist, sometimes for years. In degree, it is similar to acute mania.

collecting mania   COLLECTING COMPULSION.

dancing mania   CHOREOMANIA.

delirious mania   The most severe form of mania, seen in manic-depressive psychosis, with such intense psychomotor excitement that physical collapse and death may ensue. Partial or complete disorientation is usually a prominent feature. Also called *Bell's mania, collapse delirium, delirium grave, hypermania, Bell's delirium.*

depressive mania   A state of mania seen in manic-depressive psychosis in which some symptoms of depression intrude into the manic state.

doubting mania   FOLIE DU DOUTE.

epileptic mania   **1** A state of mania occurring during or after an attack of epilepsy. Seldom used in this sense.   **2** An epileptic attack which may, in rare cases, occur in the phase of postmanic exhaustion in a patient with acute mania.

monopolar mania   UNIPOLAR MANIA.

periodical mania   Mania which occurs in an episodic fashion. Also called *recurrent mania.*

puerperal mania   Postpartum psychosis that takes a manic form.

questioning mania   FOLIE DU POURQUOI.

Ray's mania   A seldom used term for MORAL INSANITY.

reactive mania   An episode of mania that appears to be precipitated by an external event, typically a loss, failure, business reversal, etc. Also called *reactive excitation.*

reasoning mania   A state characterized by hyperactivity, euphoria, and impulsivity, with maintenance of intellectual function but a disregard for accepted social standards. An imprecise and outmoded term.

recurrent mania   PERIODICAL MANIA.

religious mania   **1** Excessive religiosity.   **2** An acute state of excitement accompanied by hallucinations or delusions with a religious content.

rhyming mania   Mania in which there is a tendency to use clang associations, puns, rhymes, and other types of sound associations rather than considering the meaning of the words spoken.

stuporous mania   UNPRODUCTIVE MANIA.

transitory mania   Mania with incoherence and varying degrees of disturbances of consciousness that remits spontaneously within hours or a few days. A seldom used term.

unipolar mania   A rare form of major affective disorder in which the episodes are only of the manic type, with no history of depressive episodes. Also called *monopolar mania.* Compare UNIPOLAR DEPRESSION.

unproductive mania   A manic episode in which the patient becomes mute. Also called *stuporous mania, manic stupor, stupemania.*

-mania [Gk *mania* (from *mainesthai* to rage in war, rave with anger, be mad with wine) madness, frenzy, rage, enthusiasm]   A combining form meaning a morbid preference or irresistible impulse for behaving (in a specified way), a morbid fondness for or attachment to (something specified).

maniac [Med L *maniac(us)* (from Late Gk *maniakos*, from Gk *mani(a)* mania + *-akos* -AC) maniac]   A person with mania or any kind of mental illness. An imprecise usage.

maniacal   Characterized by mania.

maniaphobia   Pathologic fear of becoming insane.

manic   Of, characterized by, or suffering from mania.

manic-depressive   See under MANIC-DEPRESSIVE PSYCHOSIS.

manie de perfection [French *manie* (from Gk *mania* madness, enthusiasm) mania + French *de* of + *perfection* perfection]   SCRUPULOSITY.

manie de rumination [French *manie* (from Gk *mania* madness, enthusiasm) mania + French *de* of + *rumination* rumination. See RUMINATION.]   OBSESSIVE RUMINATION.

manifestation [Late L *manifestatio* (from *manifestatus*, past part. of *manifestare* to make evident, make clear, from L *manus* the hand + *-festus* as in *infestus* hostile, aggressive) a making clear, revealing]   Something manifested, especially an observable sign or symptom of disease.

behavioral manifestation   The expression of an illness through abnormal behavior.

ictal epileptic manifestations   Electroencephalographic or clinical manifestations indicative of an epileptic attack. Also called *critical epileptic phenomena.*

interictal epileptic manifestations   Electroencephalographic or clinical manifestations occurring in epileptic patients between clinically overt attacks. Also called *intercritical epileptic phenomena, interictal epileptic phenomena.*

neurotic manifestation   Any symptom of psychogenic origin.

postictal epileptic manifestations   Electroencephalographic or clinical manifestations which may occur in epileptic patients immediately after an attack. Electroencephalographically, they usually comprise focal or diffuse slow waves. Clinical features include coma, confusion, and automatism. Also called *postcritical epileptic phenomena.*

preictal epileptic manifestations   Electroencephalographic or clinical manifestations which occur in epileptic patients and may presage an impending attack. These symptoms can often be carefully differentiated from those which herald the onset of the attack (the aura). Electroencephalographically, there are usually more and more frequent generalized or focal subclinical epileptic discharges. Clinically, the precritical epileptic symptoms are generally vague and ill-defined and are sometimes called prodromal epileptic symptoms. Also called *precritical epileptic phenomena.*

psychophysiologic manifestation   The expression of a psychologic conflict through the altered functioning of one or more organ systems of the body, characteristic of psychosomatic disorders.

psychotic manifestation   The expression of a severe mental disorder; any of the symptoms of psychosis.

manifold   A series of interconnected units engineered to deliver or receive, in a series, gases or liquids, as in oxygen delivery systems or sampling of blood.

manihot [French (from the Tupi), cassava]   CASSAVA.

manikin [Dutch *manneken* a little man, dim. of *man* man]   An anatomical model of the human body, usually with movable and detachable parts. It is made of plastic, plaster of Paris, ceramic, or other materials, and used for various teaching purposes.

manioc [French (from the Tupi, akin to MANDIOCA), cassava]   CASSAVA.

maniphalanx   A phalanx of any finger. Compare PEDIPHALANX.

maniple   MANIPULUS.

manipulation [French (from *manipul(e)* an apothecary's handful, from L *manipul(us)* handful + *-ation* -ATION) a performing of manual operations in chemistry or pharmaceutics]   **1** Any manual operation.   **2** The application of a passive change in position by a skillful hand maneuver.

conjoined manipulation   An obstetric maneuver performed with both hands.

manipulative   Directive, controlling, or exploitative of others as a way to gain one's own ends.

manipulus [L, a handful]   A handful. Also called *maniple*.

Mann [Frank Charles *Mann*, U.S. surgeon and physiologist, 1887–1962]   **1** Mann-Williamson ulcer. See under MANN-WILLIAMSON OPERATION.   **2** Mann-Bollman fistula. See under FISTULA.

Mann [Gustav *Mann*, German physiologist active in England and the United States, born 1864]   Mann stain. See under METHOD.

Mann [Henry Berthold *Mann*, Austrian-born U.S. mathematician, born 1905]   Mann-Whitney U test. See under TEST.

Mann [John Dixon *Mann*, English physician, 1840–1912]   Dixon Mann sign. See under MANN SIGN.

Mann [Ludwig *Mann*, Polish neurologist, 1866–1936]   Wernicke-Mann hemiplegia. See under HEMIPLEGIA.

manna   The dried saccharine juice exuded from the stems of the flowering ash tree. It contains mannitol, mucilage, and sugar, and has been used as a laxative.

mannan   A polysaccharide composed of mannose residues. Such polysaccharides occur in plant cell walls.

manner of death   In forensic pathology, one of the means by which death occurs. There are four etiologic categories of manner of death relating to the circumstances and events surrounding death. The four categories are natural, suicide, homicide, and accident. In instances where accurate, unequivocal determination of manner of death cannot be made, a fifth category, undetermined, is used.

mannitol $CH_2OH-[CHOH]_4-CH_2OH$. The alcohol formed by chemical reduction of mannose. It may also be formed by enzymatic reduction of fructose, or, together with sorbitol, by chemical reduction of fructose.

mannitol hexanitrate $C_6H_8N_6O_{18}$. It is a vasodilator, prepared by the nitration of mannitol. It is slower in its actions than nitroglycerin.

Mannkopf [Emil Wilhelm *Mannkopf*, German physician, 1836–1918]   See under SIGN.

mannose   One of the aldohexose sugars, the 2-epimer of glucose. Its residues occur widely in glycolipids and glycoproteins.

mannosidase   An enzyme that catalyzes the hydrolysis of the glycoside mannoside to form an alcohol and D-mannoside. There are two forms, α- and β-mannosidase, which are responsible for degrading α-D mannoside and β-D mannoside.

mannoside   A glycoside of mannose.

mannosidosis   A rare disease characterized by the accumulation of mannoside in the tissues caused by the absence of D-mannosidase.

mannosidostreptomycin   A naturally occurring derivative of streptomycin in which the latter is combined in glycosidal linkage to a *D*-mannose molecule.

man-of-war / Portuguese man-of-war   A colonial marine jellyfish of the genus *Physalia*, class Scyphozoa, phylum Cnidaria. Its nematocysts contain a neurotoxic poison used to capture its prey, and are capable of causing a painful sting or paralysis upon contact.

manometer [Gk *manos* thin, scanty + -METER]   An instrument for measuring pressures of liquids and gases. Also called *pressometer*.

airway pressure manometer   An apparatus for measuring the pressure of gas in the airways.

aneroid manometer   A manometer comprising a pointer attached to a diaphragm which forms the end of an evacuated box. Changes of pressure may be recorded directly by movement of the pointer.

flame manometer   An apparatus which uses a flame to measure variations of gas pressure.

Koenig's manometer   An instrument for detecting pressure variations associated with sound waves of different frequency.

spring manometer   A manometer comprising a coiled tube into which gas or liquid is introduced, the extent of uncoiling of the tube indicating the pressure of the contents.

manometric   Relating to measurements obtained with a manometer.

manometry [Gk *mano(s)* thin, scanty + -METRY]   The measurement of pressure of fluids and gases.

Cartesian diver manometry   A gasometric technique for measuring the metabolic activity of small quantities of respiring tissue.

manoptoscope [L *man(us)* hand + OPTO- + -SCOPE]   A device in the shape of a hollow cone with an opening at its apex, used for determining ocular dominance by sighting with both eyes toward the apex.

man. pr.   *mane primo* (L, early in the morning).

manslaughter   The unlawful killing of one human being by another under circumstances devoid of premeditation, deliberation, and express or implied malice.

involuntary manslaughter   **1** The unintentional killing of another by an individual committing an unlawful but not felonious act or an unlawful act not usually associated with potentially lethal injury, such as striking and killing a pedestrian while operating a vehicle in excess of the speed limit.   **2** The unintentional killing of another by an individual committing a lawful act in which the requisite skills or necessary precautions associated with the act have not been employed, such as the intraoperative or postoperative death of a patient undergoing surgery performed by an intoxicated surgeon or one under the influence of drugs, if no extenuating circumstances existed.

voluntary manslaughter   The unpremeditated killing of one individual by another in a sudden heat of passion, as when a quarrel between two individuals leads to a fight resulting in one person's death. A lack of previous intent to kill must be proven.

Manson [Sir Patrick *Manson*, British physician and parasitologist 1844–1922]   **1** See under HEMOPTYSIS, TAPEWORM, WORM.   **2** Manson's disease, Manson schistosomiasis. See under SCHISTOSOMIASIS MANSONI. **3** Pyosis of Manson. See under PEMPHIGUS CONTAGIOSUS.

Mansonella A genus of filarial parasites of primates, characterized by unsheathed microfilariae, a narrow, poorly formed esophagus (as contrasted with the well-developed muscular and glandular esophagus of *Dipetalonema*), and four terminal lobes in the female (contrasted with two in *Dipetalonema*). The human parasites *Mansonella perstans* and *M. streptocerca* have been transferred to this genus from *Dipetalonema* and from the synonymized genus *Tetrapetalonema*.

Mansonella ozzardi A filarial nematode occurring in the visceral fat and mesentery of humans and found in Panama, Colombia, Argentina, Guyana, Surinam, and Yucatan. The microfilariae are unsheathed, and nuclei are absent in the tail. Humans are the only known definitive host, punkies or midges (*Culicoides* spp.) serving as intermediate hosts. The parasite is not known to cause any serious disease. Also called *Filaria demarquayi, Filaria juncea, Filaria ozzardi.*

Mansonella perstans A species found in humans and other primates in Africa and Central and South America, transmitted by biting midges of the genus *Culicoides* and chiefly of the species *C. austeni.* Generally considered nonpathogenic, the adult worms live in pleural and peritoneal cavities, the pericardium, or on mesenteries and retroperitoneal tissues. Also called *Dipetalonema perstans, Acanthocheilonema perstans.*

Mansonella streptocerca A filarial nematode found in the corium of the skin of humans in west Africa; the cause of streptocerciasis. Nonhuman primates probably serve as reservoir hosts. The microfilariae are sometimes confused with those of *Onchocerca volvulus*, which are also found in the skin. The vector of *M. streptocerca* is the biting midge, *Culicoides grahami.* Also called *Dipetalonema streptocerca, Acanthocheilonema streptocerca, Filaria streptocerca, Agamofilaria streptocerca.*

mansonelliasis [*Mansonell(a)* + -IASIS] A usually asymptomatic infection with the filarial worm *Mansonella ozzardi*, infecting human mesenteries and visceral fat in the American tropics.

Mansonia A genus of mosquitoes whose larvae obtain air from the roots or stems of aquatic plants. They are important as vectors of *Brugia malayi,* and also transmit viral equine encephalomyelitis in the Orient. Also called *Taeniorhynchus.*

Mansonia annulifera An important vector of *Brugia malayi* in India.

Mansonioides A subgenus of *Mansonia.*

mantissa [L (prob. from the Etruscan), a trifling addition] The fractional part of a logarithm. For example, the logarithm (to base 10) of 234 is 2.3692159, and 0.3692159 is the mantissa.

mantle [L *mantel(um)*, also *mantellum* a cloak, mantle, cover] **1** A covering or surrounding layer. **2** A popular term for CORTEX CEREBRI.

blue mantles of Manasse Basophilic bone deposited in the perivascular spaces produced by the resorption of enchondral bone in otosclerosis. It is one of the principal histologic features of the disease.

brain mantle CORTEX CEREBRI.

chordomesodermal mantle The continuous epithelial sheet of notochordal and mesodermal material which forms on the dorsal side of the amphibian embryo during gastrulation.

myoepicardial mantle The mesodermal wall of the embryonic pericardial cavity. It later surrounds the heart tube and gives rise to the myocardium and epicardium of the heart. Also called *epimyocardium.*

Mantoux [Charles *Mantoux*, French physician, 1887–1947] **1** See under CONVERSION. **2** Mantoux reaction. See under TEST.

manual [L *manual(is)* (from *manu(s)* hand + *-alis* -AL) pertaining to the hand] Of or done by the hands.

manubria Plural of MANUBRIUM.

manubrial **1** Pertaining to the manubrium sterni. **2** Shaped like the manubrium sterni.

manubriate Possessing a handle-shaped process.

manubriosternal Pertaining to the manubrium and the corpus of the sternum.

manubrium [New L (from L MANUS + L *hibrium* a holding, hold, from *habere* to have), a handle, haft] (*plural* manubria) **1** A structure or part resembling a handle or hilt. **2** MANUBRIUM STERNI.

manubrium mallei [NA] The large, elongated process that extends downward, posteriorly, and medially below the neck of the malleus and is attached to the inner surface of the tympanic membrane by its lateral margin. The tensor tympani muscle is inserted into its upper end. Also called *manubrium of malleus, handle of malleus.*

manubrium of malleus MANUBRIUM MALLEI.

manubrium sterni [NA] A flattened, irregularly shaped bone that is broader superiorly than inferiorly where it joins the body of the sternum and the second costal cartilages at the sternal angle. Superolaterally it articulates with the clavicles and the first costal cartilages. The notched and thick superior border forms the lower limit of the neck in the midline, and its anterior surface is subcutaneous. Also called *manubrium of sternum, presternum* (outmoded), *manubrium.*

manubrium of sternum MANUBRIUM STERNI.

manuduction [L *manu*, ablative of *manus* hand + *ductio* a conveying, pulling, or drawing] Any surgical or obstetrical procedure in which the unaided hands are used.

manudynamometer An instrument which measures the force exerted by a manual dental instrument.

manus [L (akin to Gk *mare* the hand), the hand] [NA] The extremity of the upper limb distal to the forearm; hand. It comprises a bony skeleton of eight carpal bones forming the wrist; five metacarpal bones forming the palm and the dorsum; and three phalanges for each finger except the thumb, which only has two; as well as a series of intrinsic and extrinsic muscles. It is a prehensile organ capable of grasping, precise and/or coarse manipulation by the fingers, and a variety of movements. ● In naming the different deformities of the hand, reference is given to the deviation from the general plane of the forearm.

manus cava Excessive concavity of the palm of the hand.

manus curta TALIPOMANUS.

manus extensa A club hand with deviation or fixation in the direction of extension, particularly at the wrist. Also called *manus superextensa.*

manus flexa A club hand with deviation or fixation in the direction of flexion.

manus plana The appearance of the hand when all the intrinsic muscles and those forearm muscles which move the fingers are paralyzed and atrophic. Also called *flat hand.*

manus superextensa MANUS EXTENSA.

manus valga A club hand with deviation toward the ulna and adduction at the wrist.

manus vara A club hand with deviation toward the radius and adduction at the wrist.

manyplies A seldom used term for OMASUM.

Manz [Wilhelm *Manz*, German ophthalmologist, 1833–1911] Manz glands. See under GLAND.

Manzullo [Alfredo *Manzullo*, Argentinian immunologist, born 1909] Manzullo's test. See under TELLURITE TEST.

MAO monoamine oxidase.

MAOI monoamine oxidase inhibitor.

map [Med L *mappa* (from L *mappa* a napkin, akin to Hebrew *mĕnaphā* a fan) a map] **1** A graphic representation on a flat surface of the relative positions of particular units or parts; chart for locating position in a configuration or in three-dimensional space. **2** A linkage map. See under CHROMOSOME MAP, LINKAGE MAP.

chromosome map The linear arrangement of genes along the chromosomes of an organism. It is usually presented graphically, with the location of each gene determined by one or more of a variety of mapping techniques. Also called *cytogenetic map, genetic map*.

cognitive map A hypothesized representation in the mind of the environment, which serves as an organizing schema for establishing relationships between the events that occur in a learning situation. Once a mental picture of this kind is complete, responses quite different from those made during the original learning can be initiated in order to attain the goal.

complementation map The determination of the arrangement of genes on chromosomes using complementation.

cytogenetic map CHROMOSOME MAP.

fate map A plan which shows areas of prospective fate in normal embryonic development, principally applied to regional localization at the blastula or early gastrula stage. Also called *germinal localization*.

genetic map **1** LINKAGE MAP. **2** CHROMOSOME MAP.

heat map THERMOGRAM.

linkage map The linear arrangement of genetic loci as determined by linkage analysis. Loci within linkage groups are ordered by a variety of family, biochemical, and cytogenetic techniques and, similarly, are ordered into syntenic groups that correspond to individual chromosomes. The linkage map is most often represented graphically as the linear array of loci along each chromosome, and genes close together will combine less frequently than those further apart. Also called *genetic map*.

Mapharsen A proprietary name for oxophenarsine hydrochloride.

mapping / cytologic mapping The process by which identifiable chromosome changes, such as deletions and inversions, are used to order genes on the chromosome map. The technique is used to particular advantage in organisms with polytene chromosomes.

deletion mapping The process by which spontaneous or induced deletions of portions of a chromosome are used in cytologic, linkage, or biochemical analysis to order genes in the chromosome map. Also called *deletion method*.

fine structure genetic mapping The process of determining the order of nucleotide sequences around individual genes, especially those of functional significance such as introns, exons, promoters, and enhancers. It may be achieved by a variety of methods including restriction enzyme analysis, deletion mapping, and direct nucleotide sequencing.

genetic mapping The process by which a chromosome map is constructed. It involves a variety of techniques, such as cytologic, deletion, complementation, and linkage mapping; *in situ* hybridization; pedigree analysis; recombinant DNA studies; and somatic cell genetics.

maprotiline $C_{20}H_{23}N$. *N*-Methyl-9,10-ethananthracene-9-(10*H*)-propylamine. It is used clinically as an antidepressant agent.

Maraglas An epoxy resin that is used as an embedding medium in electron microscopy. A proprietary name.

Maragliano [Edoardo *Maragliano*, Italian physician, 1849–1940] See under BODY, TUBERCULIN.

Marañón [Gregorio *Marañón*, Spanish endocrinologist, 1887–1960] **1** Marañón sign. See under REACTION. **2** See under SYNDROME.

maranta [after Bartolomeo *Maranta*, Italian physician and botanist, died 1571] ARROWROOT.

marantic MARASMIC.

marasmatic MARASMIC.

marasmic Of or relating to marasmus. Also *marantic, marasmatic*.

marasmoid Resembling marasmus.

marasmus [Late L (from Gk *marasmos*, a dying away, withering, from *marainein* to quench, extinguish, die away, burn low), a dying out. Galen and Aristotle used Gk *maransis*, which later became *marasmos*.] Starvation occurring in children. It occurs most frequently in infants under one year of age and is more often found in urban populations. In this environment, there may be a rapid succession of pregnancies and early and abrupt weaning followed by dirty and inadequate bottle feeding consisting of very small amounts of dilute milk serving as a low source of energy and protein. The unsterile foods cause repeated infections, especially of the gastrointestinal tract, which the mother treats by long periods of fasting. The clinical symptoms are growth retardation (weight more so than height), abnormal behavior (irritability), dehydration, diarrhea, extreme hunger or anorexia, weak musculature, dry and atrophic skin and mucous membranes, absence of subcutaneous fat, and presence of vitamin deficiencies. If a child is exposed to marasmus for only a short period, complete recovery is possible. If the disease is severe and of long duration, the prognosis is often poor and the child may become mentally retarded and growth retarded. Also called *athrepsia, marcor, infantile atrophy, Parrot's atrophy of the newborn, pedatrophia*.

enzootic marasmus Anemia and wasting, which develop in cattle and sheep raised on pastures deficient in cobalt. An outmoded term.

nutritional marasmus PROTEIN-CALORIE MALNUTRITION.

marbleization The state of being veined as a marble stone. Also called *marmorization, marmoration*.

Marburg [Otto *Marburg*, German neurologist, born 1878] See under TRIAD.

marc The residue remaining after extraction of the juice or oil from a vegetable source.

march [French *marcher* to march] The progressive spread of abnormal electrical discharge to contiguous areas of the motor cortex in patients with focal motor epilepsy.

jacksonian march The spread of focal convulsive phenomena, whether motor or sensory, from one part of the body to another, in the order in which these areas are represented in those parts of the cerebral motor and/or sensory cortex contiguous with the area in which the discharge originates. Also called *jacksonism* (seldom used), *protospasm* (outmoded).

Marchand [Felix Jacob Marchand, German pathologist, 1846–1928] **1** Marchand's organ. See under MARCHAND'S ADRENAL. **2** See under CELL.

Marchant [Gerard T. Joseph *Marchant*, French surgeon, 1850–1903] Marchant's detachable zone. See under ZONE.

marche à petits pas A slow, shuffling gait with very short steps, as seen in parkinsonism. Also called *Petren gait*.

Marchesani [Oswald *Marchesani*, German ophthalmologist, 1900–1952] Marchesani syndrome. See under WEILL-MARCHESANI SYNDROME.

Marchetti [Andrew A. *Marchetti*, U.S. obstetrician and gynecologist, 1901–1970] Marshall-Marchetti operation. See under OPERATION.

Marchi [Vittorio *Marchi*, Italian physiologist, 1851–1908] **1** Marchi's tract. See under TRACTUS TECTOSPINALIS. **2** See under LIQUID, REACTION, METHOD. **3** Marchi's globule. See under BALL.

Marchiafava [Ettore *Marchiafava*, Italian pathologist, 1847–1935] **1** Marchiafava's disease, Marchiafava Bignami disease.

See under MARCHIAFAVA-BIGNAMI SYNDROME. **2** Marchiafava-Micheli disease, Marchiafava-Micheli syndrome. See under PAROXYSMAL NOCTURNAL HEMOGLOBINURIA.

marcid [L *marcid(us)* withered, languid, feeble] Wasted; emaciated.

marcor MARASMUS.

Marcus Gunn [Robert *Marcus Gunn*, English ophthalmologist, 1850–1909] **1** Marcus Gunn phenomenon, Gunn's phenomenon, Gunn syndrome. See under MARCUS GUNN SYNDROME. **2** Marcus Gunn inverse syndrome, inverse Marcus Gunn phenomenon, inverted Marcus Gunn phenomenon. See under MARIN AMAT SYNDROME. **3** Gunn's pupillary phenomenon, Gunn's pupillary sign, Marcus Gunn pupillary sign. See under MARCUS GUNN PUPILLARY PHENOMENON. **4** Gunn's crossing sign. See under GUNN SIGN. **5** Gunn's dots. See under DOT.

mare [Old English *mere*, fem. of *mearh* horse, akin to Irish *marc* horse and Icelandic *merr* mare] A female horse or other equine animal.

Marek [Josef *Marek*, Hungarian veterinarian and pathologist, 1867–1952] See under DISEASE.

mareo de la cordillera MOUNTAIN SICKNESS.

Marey [Etienne Jules *Marey*, French physiologist, 1830–1904] See under LAW, REFLEX, TAMBOUR.

Marfan [Antonin Bernard Jean *Marfan*, French pediatrician, 1858–1942] **1** Marfan's epigastric puncture. See under EPIGASTRIC PUNCTURE. **2** See under SIGN, METHOD. **3** Marfan-Madelung syndrome. See under MARFAN SYNDROME.

marfanoid [*Marfan (syndrome)* + *-OID*] Having some or all of the physical characteristics of the Marfan syndrome.

Marg [Elwin *Marg*, U.S. scientist, born 1918] MacKay-Marg electronic tonometer. See under TONOMETER.

margaric acid CH_3—$[CH_2]_{15}$—COOH. Heptadecanoic acid. Like other fatty acids with an odd number of carbon atoms, it is rare in natural sources.

margarid Resembling a pearl in color or shape.

margaritoma A seldom used term for CHOLESTEATOMA.

Margaropus [New L (from Gk *margaros* a pearl oyster, from *margaron*, also *margaritēs* a pearl + New L *-pus* relating to a foot, from Gk *pous* a foot)] A genus of inornate ticks (family Ixodidae) characterized by enlarged back legs and a prolonged median plate. The genus is thought to represent relict boophilids. A species probably normally infesting zebras and giraffes in Africa, *M. winthemi*, is now found also on domestic horses in winter and sometimes on cattle and sheep as well in South America and southern Africa.

Margaropus annulatus BOOPHILUS ANNULATUS.

margin

margin [L *margo*, gen. *marginis*, a brink, brim, edge, border, margin] The edge or border of a structure or organ.

alveolar margin of mandible ARCUS ALVEOLARIS MANDIBULAE.

alveolar margin of maxilla ARCUS ALVEOLARIS MAXILLAE.

anterior margin of fibula MARGO ANTERIOR FIBULAE.

anterior margin of lung MARGO ANTERIOR PULMONIS.

anterior margin of pancreas MARGO ANTERIOR PANCREATIS.

anterior margin of parietal bone MARGO FRONTALIS OSSIS PARIETALIS.

anterior margin of scapula An outmoded term for MARGO LATERALIS SCAPULAE.

anterior margin of spleen MARGO SUPERIOR SPLENIS.

anterior margin of testis MARGO ANTERIOR TESTIS.

anterior margin of tibia MARGO ANTERIOR TIBIAE.

anterior margin of ulna MARGO ANTERIOR ULNAE.

axillary margin of scapula MARGO LATERALIS SCAPULAE.

cartilaginous margin of acetabulum An outmoded term for LABRUM ACETABULARE.

cavity margin The edge surrounding a prepared dental cavity.

cervical margin The part of a cavity margin adjacent to the gingiva.

ciliary margin of iris MARGO CILIARIS IRIDIS.

convex margin of testis An outmoded term for MARGO ANTERIOR TESTIS.

coronal margin of frontal bone An outmoded term for MARGO PARIETALIS OSSIS FRONTALIS.

coronal margin of parietal bone An outmoded term for MARGO FRONTALIS OSSIS PARIETALIS.

crenate margin of spleen MARGO SUPERIOR SPLENIS.

cristate margin of spleen MARGO SUPERIOR SPLENIS.

dentate margin PECTINATE LINE.

dorsal margin of radius MARGO POSTERIOR RADII.

dorsal margin of ulna MARGO POSTERIOR ULNAE.

external margin of scapula MARGO LATERALIS SCAPULAE.

external margin of testis An outmoded term for MARGO ANTERIOR TESTIS.

falciform margin of fascia lata An outmoded term for MARGO FALCIFORMIS HIATUS SAPHENUS.

falciform margin of saphenus hiatus MARGO FALCIFORMIS HIATUS SAPHENUS.

falciform margin of white line of pelvic fascia An outmoded term for ARCUS TENDINEUS FASCIAE PELVIS.

fibular margin of foot An outmoded term for MARGO LATERALIS PEDIS.

free margin of eyelid The anterior margin of each eyelid where the anterior and posterior surfaces meet. Each margin bears eyelashes and has a rounded anterior edge and a sharp posterior edge. Also called *margo palpebrae* (outmoded).

free gingival margin GINGIVAL MARGIN.

free gum margin GINGIVAL MARGIN.

free margin of nail MARGO LIBER UNGUIS.

free margin of ovary MARGO LIBER OVARII.

frontal margin of greater wing of sphenoid bone MARGO FRONTALIS ALAE MAJORIS.

frontal margin of parietal bone MARGO FRONTALIS OSSIS PARIETALIS.

gingival margin The edge of the gingiva which is not directly attached to tooth or bone. Also called *free gingival margin, gum margin, free gum margin*.

gum margin GINGIVAL MARGIN.

hidden margin of nail MARGO OCCULTUS UNGUIS.

margin incisalis INCISAL EDGE.

inferior margin of liver MARGO INFERIOR HEPATIS.

inferior margin of lung MARGO INFERIOR PULMONIS.

inferior margin of suprarenal gland FACIES RENALIS GLANDULAE SUPRARENALIS.

infraorbital margin Either margo infraorbitalis orbitae or margo infraorbitalis maxillae.

infraorbital margin of maxilla MARGO INFRAORBITALIS MAXILLAE.

infraorbital margin of orbit MARGO INFRAORBITALIS ORBITAE.

internal margin of testis An outmoded term for MARGO POSTERIOR TESTIS.

interosseous margin of fibula MARGO INTEROSSEUS FIBULAE.

interosseous margin of tibia MARGO INTEROSSEUS TIBIAE.
interosseous margin of ulna MARGO INTEROSSEUS ULNAE.
lacrimal margin of maxilla MARGO LACRIMALIS MAXILLAE.
lambdoid margin of occipital bone MARGO LAMBDOIDEUS SQUAMAE OCCIPITALIS.
lambdoid margin of parietal bone An outmoded term for MARGO OCCIPITALIS OSSIS PARIETALIS.
lateral margin of foot MARGO LATERALIS PEDIS.
lateral margin of humerus MARGO LATERALIS HUMERI.
lateral margin of kidney MARGO LATERALIS RENIS.
lateral margin of nail MARGO LATERALIS UNGUIS.
lateral margin of scapula MARGO LATERALIS SCAPULAE.
lateral margin of tongue MARGO LINGUAE.
lateral margin of uterus MARGO UTERI DEXTER ET SINISTER.
left margin of heart An outmoded term for FACIES PULMONALIS CORDIS.
malar margin An outmoded term for MARGO ZYGOMATICUS ALAE MAJORIS.
mamillary margin An outmoded term for MARGO MASTOIDEUS SQUAMAE OCCIPITALIS.
mastoid margin **1** MARGO MASTOIDEUS SQUAMAE OCCIPITALIS. **2** ANGULUS MASTOIDEUS OSSIS PARIETALIS.
mastoid margin of occipital bone MARGO MASTOIDEUS SQUAMAE OCCIPITALIS.
mastoid margin of parietal bone ANGULUS MASTOIDEUS OSSIS PARIETALIS.
medial margin of foot MARGO MEDIALIS PEDIS.
medial margin of forearm MARGO MEDIALIS ANTEBRACHII.
medial margin of humerus MARGO MEDIALIS HUMERI.
medial margin of kidney MARGO MEDIALIS RENIS.
medial margin of suprarenal gland MARGO MEDIALIS GLANDULAE SUPRARENALIS.
medial margin of tibia MARGO MEDIALIS TIBIAE.
mesovarial margin of ovary MARGO MESOVARICUS OVARII.
mesovarian margin of ovary MARGO MESOVARICUS OVARII.
nasal margin of frontal bone MARGO NASALIS OSSIS FRONTALIS.
obtuse margin of spleen MARGO INFERIOR SPLENIS.
occipital margin of parietal bone MARGO OCCIPITALIS OSSIS PARIETALIS.
occipital margin of temporal bone MARGO OCCIPITALIS OSSIS TEMPORALIS.
orbital margin MARGO ORBITALIS.
parietal margin of frontal bone MARGO PARIETALIS OSSIS FRONTALIS.
parietal margin of great wing of sphenoid bone MARGO PARIETALIS ALAE MAJORIS.
parietal margin of occipital bone MARGO LAMBDOIDEUS SQUAMAE OCCIPITALIS.
parietal margin of parietal bone MARGO SAGITTALIS OSSIS PARIETALIS.
parietal margin of temporal bone MARGO PARIETALIS OSSIS TEMPORALIS.
parietofrontal margin of great wing of sphenoid bone MARGO FRONTALIS ALAE MAJORIS.
posterior margin of fibula MARGO POSTERIOR FIBULAE.
posterior margin of testis MARGO POSTERIOR TESTIS.
posterior margin of ulna MARGO POSTERIOR ULNAE.
pupillary margin of iris MARGO PUPILLARIS IRIDIS.
radial margins of fingers FACIES LATERALES DIGITORUM MANUS.
radial margin of forearm MARGO LATERALIS ANTEBRACHII.
red margin VERMILION BORDER.
margin of safety A measure of drug safety based upon the dose required to produce an effective, therapeutic response in most people, versus the dose required to produce toxic effects in a few individuals. The LD_1/ED_{99}, rather than the LD_{50}/ED_{50} is preferred for this purpose. The margin of safety is similar to, but not the same as, the therapeutic index. See also EFFECTIVE DOSE, LETHAL DOSE.
sagittal margin of parietal bone MARGO SAGITTALIS OSSIS PARIETALIS.
sphenoidal margin of parietal bone ANGULUS SPHENOIDALIS OSSIS PARIETALIS.
sphenoidal margin of temporal bone MARGO SPHENOIDALIS OSSIS TEMPORALIS.
sphenotemporal margin of parietal bone MARGO SQUAMOSUS OSSIS PARIETALIS.
squamous margin of greater wing of sphenoid bone MARGO SQUAMOSUS ALAE MAJORIS.
squamous margin of parietal bone MARGO SQUAMOSUS OSSIS PARIETALIS.
straight margin of testis An outmoded term for MARGO POSTERIOR TESTIS.
superior margin of pancreas MARGO SUPERIOR PANCREATIS.
superior margin of parietal bone MARGO SAGITTALIS OSSIS PARIETALIS.
superior margin of scapula MARGO SUPERIOR SCAPULAE.
superior margin of spleen MARGO SUPERIOR SPLENIS.
superior margin of suprarenal gland MARGO SUPERIOR GLANDULAE SUPRARENALIS.
supraorbital margin of frontal bone MARGO SUPRAORBITALIS OSSIS FRONTALIS.
supraorbital margin of orbit MARGO SUPRAORBITALIS ORBITAE.
temporal margin of parietal bone MARGO SQUAMOSUS OSSIS PARIETALIS.
tibial margin of foot MARGO MEDIALIS PEDIS.
margin of tongue MARGO LINGUAE.
ulnar margins of fingers FACIES MEDIALES DIGITORUM MANUS.
ulnar margin of forearm MARGO MEDIALIS ANTEBRACHII.
vertebral margin of scapula MARGO MEDIALIS SCAPULAE.
volar margin of radius An outmoded term for MARGO ANTERIOR RADII.
volar margin of ulna An outmoded term for MARGO ANTERIOR ULNAE.
zygomatic margin of greater wing of sphenoid bone MARGO ZYGOMATICUS ALAE MAJORIS.

---

marginal Of or relating to a margin.
margination [L *marginatus*, past part. of *marginare* to make a margin or border to something] The collection of leukocytes on blood vessel walls early in the injury response.
margines Plural of MARGO.
marginoplasty [MARGIN + *o* + -PLASTY] Any plastic operation on an anatomic border or margin.

margo

---

margo [L, a brink, brim, edge, border, margin] (*plural* margines) The edge or border of an organ or a structure; margin.
margo alveolaris **1** An outmoded term for ARCUS ALVEOLARIS MANDIBULAE. **2** An outmoded term for ARCUS ALVEOLARIS MAXILLAE.
margo anterior fibulae [NA] The anterior border of the fibula

extending from the head down to a point proximal to the lateral malleolus where it divides into two, surrounding a triangular subcutaneous area. The anterior intermuscular septum of the leg is attached to it. Also called *anterior margin of fibula, crista anterior fibulae, anterior crest of fibula, oblique line of fibula* (outmoded).

margo anterior hepatis   MARGO INFERIOR HEPATIS.

margo anterior lienis   An outmoded term for MARGO SUPERIOR SPLENIS.

margo anterior pancreatis   [NA] The border of the pancreas that separates the anterior from the inferior surface and over which the transverse mesocolon separates onto the two surfaces. Also called *anterior margin of pancreas, anterior border of pancreas.*

margo anterior pulmonis   [NA] The thin anterior border of the lung that overlaps the pericardium and separates the costal and mediastinal surfaces. On the right side it is vertical while on the left the curved cardiac notch indents it laterally between the levels of the fourth and sixth costal cartilages. Also called *anterior margin of lung.*

margo anterior radii   [NA] A ridge of bone that extends inferolaterally from the radial tuberosity to the lateral margin of the anterior surface, along which it runs to the anterior margin of the styloid process, separating the anterior from the lateral surfaces. The proximal third, often called the anterior oblique line, gives origin to the radial head of the flexor digitorum superficialis muscle. Also called *anterior border of radius, margo volaris radii* (outmoded), *volar margin of radius* (outmoded).

margo anterior splenis   MARGO SUPERIOR SPLENIS.

margo anterior testis   [NA] The convex anterior border, between the medial and lateral surfaces, of the testis. It is invested by the visceral layer of the tunica vaginalis and free of attachments. Also called *anterior margin of testis, convex margin of testis* (outmoded), *external margin of testis* (outmoded).

margo anterior tibiae   [NA] The subcutaneous sinuous crest extending from the lateral edge of the tuberosity of the tibia to the anterior border of the medial malleolus; shin. It provides attachment for the deep fascia of the leg. Also called *anterior margin of tibia, anterior border of tibia, crista anterior tibiae, tibial crest, anterior crest of tibia.*

margo anterior ulnae   [NA] The rounded anterior border of the ulna extending downward and posteriorly from the medial side of the ulnar tuberosity to the base of the styloid process. It provides origin for the flexor digitorum profundus and pronator quadratus muscles. Also called *anterior margin of ulna; margo volaris ulnae* (outmoded), *volar margin of ulna* (outmoded).

margo axillaris scapulae   An outmoded term for MARGO LATERALIS SCAPULAE.

margo ciliaris iridis   [NA] The peripheral border of the iris, where it becomes continuous with the ciliary body and also connected to the cornea by the pectinate ligament. Also called *ciliary margin of iris, peripheral border of iris, base of iris, iridociliary junction.*

margo dexter cordis   [NA] The rounded, vertical right surface of the heart formed by the right atrium and extending from the termination of the superior vena cava to the point of entry of the inferior vena cava into the right atrium. Also called *right border of heart.*

margo dorsalis radii   An outmoded term for MARGO POSTERIOR RADII.

margo dorsalis ulnae   An outmoded term for MARGO POSTERIOR ULNAE.

margo falciformis fasciae latae   An outmoded term for MARGO FALCIFORMIS HIATUS SAPHENUS.

margo falciformis hiatus saphenus   [NA] The sharp, arched, well-defined lateral margin of the saphenous opening in the fascia lata of the upper thigh. It is continuous superiorly with the superior cornua and inferiorly with the inferior cornua, and it lies anterior to the femoral vessels. The cribriform fascia is attached to it. Also called *falciform margin of saphenus hiatus, margo falciformis fasciae latae* (outmoded), *falciform margin of fascia lata* (outmoded), *Hey's ligament, Burns ligament, falciform incisure of fascia lata, falciform fold of fascia lata.*

margo fibularis pedis   MARGO LATERALIS PEDIS.

margo frontalis alae magnae   An outmoded term for MARGO FRONTALIS ALAE MAJORIS.

margo frontalis alae majoris   [NA] A triangular sutural edge formed by the superior margins of the cerebral, orbital and temporal surfaces of the greater wing of the sphenoid bone and articulating with the orbital plate of the frontal bone. Also called *frontal margin of greater wing of sphenoid bone, margo frontalis alae magnae* (outmoded), *parietofrontal margin of great wing of sphenoid bone.*

margo frontalis ossis parietalis   [NA] The markedly serrated and beveled anterior border of the parietal bone articulating with the frontal bone and forming one half of the coronal suture on each side. Also called *frontal margin of parietal bone, anterior margin of parietal bone, coronal margin of parietal bone* (outmoded).

margo inferior cerebri   [NA] The inferior lateral margin of the cerebral hemisphere. Also called *margo inferolateralis cerebri.*

margo inferior hepatis   [NA] The sharp border of the liver that separates the diaphragmatic surface and visceral surface anteriorly. It is notched by the ligamentum teres just to the right of the median plane and by the fossa of the gallbladder to the right of that. Also called *inferior border of liver, inferior margin of liver, margo anterior hepatis, anterior border of liver.*

margo inferior lienis   MARGO INFERIOR SPLENIS.

margo inferior pancreatis   [NA] The inferior border of the pancreas which separates the inferior from the posterior surface. At its right end the superior mesenteric vessels pass between it and the uncinate process of the pancreas. Also called *inferior border of pancreas, margo posterior pancreatis* (outmoded).

margo inferior pulmonis   [NA] The lower border of the lung, which is thin and sharp between the costal and the diaphragmatic surfaces and rounded between the mediastinal and the diaphragmatic surfaces. Also called *inferior margin of lung.*

margo inferior splenis   [NA] The straight and rounded margin of the spleen which separates the renal impression of the visceral surface from the diaphragmatic surface. Normally it lies at the level of the lower margin of the left eleventh rib. Also called *inferior border of spleen, margo inferior lienis, margo posterior lienis* (outmoded), *obtuse margin of spleen.*

margo inferolateralis cerebri   MARGO INFERIOR CEREBRI.

margo inferomedialis cerebri   MARGO MEDIALIS CEREBRI.

margo infraglenoidalis tibiae   The ill-defined rim at the proximal end of the tibia just below the articular surfaces of the condyles. An outmoded term.

margo infraorbitalis maxillae   [NA] The rounded anterior margin of the orbital surface of the maxilla, forming a portion of the circumference of the orbit at its junction with the anterior surface of the body of the maxilla and being continuous medially with the lacrimal crest on the frontal process. Also called *infraorbital margin of maxilla.*

margo infraorbitalis orbitae   [NA] The sharp lower margin of the circumference of the orbital opening. It is formed medially by the infraorbital margin of maxilla meeting the orbital margin of the zygomatic bone laterally. Also called *infraorbital margin of orbit.*

margo interosseus fibulae   [NA] A sharp ridge medial to the anterior margin of the fibula for the attachment of the interosseous membrane. It extends from the anterior aspect of the head of the fibula to a point proximal to the articular surface of the malleolus, where it splits around a rough triangular area to which the interosseous ligament is attached. Also called *interosseous margin of fibula, interosseous border of fibula, interosseous crest of fibula, interosseous ridge of fibula, crista interossea fibulae, medial border of fibula* (outmoded).

margo interosseus radii [NA] The conspicuous ridge on the medial side of the radius, between the anterior and the posterior surfaces. It commences proximally at the posterior part of the radial tuberosity, where it is rounded, and terminates distally by dividing and becoming continuous with the anterior and posterior borders of the ulnar notch. The interosseous membrane is attached to its lower three fourths while the oblique cord attaches proximally. Also called *interosseous border of radius, interosseous ridge of radius, interosseous crest of radius, crista interossea radii, radial crest.*

margo interosseus tibiae [NA] A prominent longitudinal ridge on the lateral side of the tibia extending from the front of the fibular articular surface proximally to the fibular notch, above which it divides around a rough triangular area for the interosseous ligament. Attached to it is the interosseous membrane, except proximally where the anterior tibial vessels pass between the tibia and the fibula. Also called *interosseous margin of tibia, interosseous border of tibia, interosseous crest of tibia, interosseous ridge of tibia, crista interossea tibiae, angulus lateralis tibiae, lateral angle of border of tibia, external angle of border of tibia.*

margo interosseus ulnae [NA] The prominent, sharp, middle two fourths of the lateral margin of the ulna. It is continuous proximally with two or more distinct lines, one of which passes anterior to the radial notch and another passes posterior as the supinator crest. The interosseous margin separates the anterior and posterior surfaces of the ulna and provides attachment for the interosseous membrane. Also called *interosseous border of ulna, interosseous margin of ulna, crista interossea ulnae, interosseous ridge of ulna, crista ulnae, ulnar crest, interosseous crest of ulna.*

margo lacrimalis maxillae [NA] The posterior border of the upper end of the frontal process of the maxilla that articulates with the lacrimal bone. Also called *lacrimal border of maxilla, lacrimal margin of maxilla, inferior maxillary incisure* (outmoded).

margo lambdoideus squamae occipitalis [NA] The serrated superolateral border on either side of the squamous part of the occipital bone, extending from the superior to the lateral angle and articulating with the occipital border of the parietal bone to form one half of the lambdoid suture. Also called *lambdoid margin of occipital bone, lambdoid border of occipital bone, parietal margin of occipital bone.*

margines laterales digitorum pedis An outmoded term for FACIES LATERALES DIGITORUM PEDIS.

margo lateralis antebrachii [NA] The outer, or radial, border of the forearm. Also called *radial margin of forearm, margo radialis antebrachii, margo radialis antibrachii* (outmoded), *radial antebrachial region* (outmoded), *regio antibrachii radialis* (outmoded).

margo lateralis humeri [NA] The outer border of the humerus, extending from the posteroinferior part of the greater tubercle to the lateral epicondyle. It is prominent only in its distal third where it provides attachment for the lateral intermuscular septum, anterior to which the brachioradialis and the extensor carpi radialis longus muscles are attached. Posteriorly is the attachment of the medial head of triceps. The middle third is interrupted by the wide, shallow sulcus for the radial nerve. Also called *lateral margin of humerus, lateral border of humerus, margo radialis humeri* (outmoded), *lateral angle of humerus.*

margo lateralis linguae MARGO LINGUAE.

margo lateralis pedis [NA] The outer, or fibular, border of the foot, extending from the heel to the fifth toe. Also called *fibular margin of foot* (outmoded), *lateral margin of foot, margo pedis lateralis* (outmoded), *margo fibularis pedis.*

margo lateralis renis [NA] The narrow convex outer border of the kidney separating the anterior or visceral surface from the posterior or parietal surface. Also called *lateral margin of kidney.*

margo lateralis scapulae [NA] The thick outer border of the scapula, extending from the lower margin of the glenoid cavity to the inferior angle. The upper two thirds is grooved anteriorly along its length for part of the origin of the subscapularis muscle. The long head of the triceps muscle arises from a tubercle at its upper extremity. Also called *margo axillaris scapulae* (outmoded), *lateral border of scapula, anterior margin of scapula* (outmoded), *axillary margin of scapula, external margin of scapula, lateral margin of scapula, pila scapulae* (outmoded), *pillar of scapula* (outmoded).

margo lateralis unguis [NA] The edge on either side of a nail, extending from the proximal edge to the free border and partially covered by the nail wall. Also called *lateral margin of nail.*

margo lateralis uteri An outmoded term for MARGO UTERI DEXTER ET SINISTER.

margo liber ovarii [NA] The rounded, free border of the ovary directed into the rectouterine pouch of peritoneum and towards the ureter. It is on the side opposite the mesovarian border. Also called *free margin of ovary.*

margo liber unguis [NA] The distal free border of a nail that overlaps the tip of a digit. Also called *free margin of nail.*

margo linguae [NA] The free lateral border on each side of the tongue that separates the dorsum from the inferior surface and meets the opposite border at the apex. It is in contact with the gums and the teeth. Also called *margin of tongue, lateral margin of tongue, margo lateralis linguae.*

margo mastoideus squamae occipitalis [NA] The margin of the squamous part of the occipital bone. It extends from the lateral angle to the jugular process and articulates with the occipital margin of the petrous part of the temporal bone to form the occipitomastoid suture. Also called *mastoid margin of occipital bone, mastoid margin, mamillary margin* (outmoded).

margines mediales digitorum pedis An outmoded term for FACIES MEDIALES DIGITORUM PEDIS.

margo medialis antebrachii [NA] The inner, or ulnar, border of the forearm. Also called *medial margin of forearm, ulnar margin of forearm, medial border of forearm, margo ulnaris antibrachii* (outmoded), *margo ulnaris antebrachii, ulnar antebrachial region* (outmoded), *regio antibrachii ulnaris* (outmoded).

margo medialis cerebri [NA] The medial and inferior margin of the cerebral hemisphere. Also called *margo inferomedialis cerebri.*

margo medialis glandulae suprarenalis [NA] The paravertebral border of the suprarenal gland. That of the left gland is convex and related to the left celiac ganglion and the left inferior phrenic and the left gastric arteries, while that of the right gland is thin, paralleling the posterolateral border of the adjacent inferior vena cava, and related to the right celiac ganglion and right inferior phrenic artery. Also called *medial margin of suprarenal gland.*

margo medialis humeri [NA] The inner border of the humerus. It commences at the lesser tubercle, continuing as the medial lip of the intertubercular sulcus for the attachment of the teres major muscle, and extends to the medial epicondyle. In its lower half it has a sharp edge for attachment of the medial intermuscular septum, anterior to which is the origin of the brachialis muscle and posteriorly is the medial head of the triceps muscle attachment. Also called *medial margin of hu-*

merus, medial border of humerus, margo ulnaris humeri, medial angle of humerus, inner angle of humerus.

margo medialis pedis [NA] The inner, or tibial, border of the foot, extending from the heel to the great toe. Also called *medial margin of foot, medial border of foot, margo tibialis pedis, tibial margin of foot, margo pedis medialis* (outmoded).

margo medialis renis [NA] The medial border of each kidney. It is concave in the center and convex over each pole above and below. The concavity is fissured by the hilum which contains the renal pelvis, vessels, and nerves. It separates the anterior from the posterior surface of the kidney medially. Also called *medial margin of kidney.*

margo medialis scapulae [NA] The medial, and longest, border of the scapula, extending from the superior to the inferior angle. It is divided into three unequal portions by the triangular medial end of the spine of the scapula where the rhomboideus minor muscle is attached. Above it the levator scapulae muscle is attached, while below it the rhomboideus major muscle is attached. Also called *margo vertebralis scapulae* (outmoded), *vertebral margin of scapula.*

margo medialis tibiae [NA] The inner border of the tibia. It is rounded proximally and distally but sharp in the middle, extending from the posterior part of the medial condyle to the posterior margin of the medial malleolus. The soleus muscle is attached to its middle third. Also called *medial margin of tibia, medial border of tibia, angulus medialis tibiae, medial angle of tibia, internal angle of tibia.*

margo mesovaricus ovarii [NA] The straight border of the ovary which is attached to the back of the broad ligament of the uterus by the mesovarium and is directed towards the obliterated umbilical artery. It is on the side opposite to the free margin of the ovary and contains the hilum of the ovary. Also called *mesovarian margin of ovary, mesovarial margin of ovary.*

margo nasalis [NA] The curved margin of the frontal bone that articulates with the nasal bones at the frontonasal suture. Also called *margo nasi* (outmoded).

margo nasalis ossis frontalis [NA] The curved inferior edge of the nasal part of the frontal bone, on either side of the nasal spine, that articulates with the nasal bones and the frontal process of the maxilla. Also called *nasal margin of frontal bone, nasal incisure of frontal bone.*

margo nasi An outmoded term for MARGO NASALIS.

margo occipitalis ossis parietalis [NA] The serrated posterior border of the parietal bone. It extends from the occipital angle to the mastoid angle and articulates with the parietal margin of the occipital bone to form one half of the lambdoid suture. Also called *occipital margin of parietal bone, lambdoid margin of parietal bone* (outmoded).

margo occipitalis ossis temporalis [NA] A portion of the inferior margin of the posterior surface of the petrous part of the temporal bone that articulates with the occipital squama along the occipitomastoid suture. Also called *occipital margin of temporal bone.*

margo occultus unguis [NA] The irregular, thin proximal edge of a nail that is completely covered by the nail wall. Also called *hidden margin of nail.*

margo orbitalis The quadrangular base, or anterior boundary, of the orbital cavity. It comprises four margins, namely, margo supraorbitalis, margo infraorbitalis, margo lateralis, and margo medialis. Also called *orbital margin.*

margo palpebrae An outmoded term for FREE MARGIN OF EYELID.

margo parietalis alae majoris [NA] The superior extremity of the greater wing of the sphenoid bone that articulates with the sphenoidal angle of the parietal bone. Also called *angulus parietalis ossis sphenoidalis, parietal margin of great wing of sphenoid bone, parietal angle of sphenoid bone.*

margo parietalis ossis frontalis [NA] The thick, serrated posterior border of the frontal bone, semicircular in shape and beveled on its inner aspect. It articulates with the parietal bone to form the coronal suture and with the greater wing of the sphenoid bone inferiorly on each side. Also called *parietal margin of frontal bone, coronal margin of frontal bone* (outmoded).

margo parietalis ossis temporalis [NA] The arched superior border of the squamous part of the temporal bone, beveled internally and overlapping the inferior border of the parietal bone to form the squamosal suture. Also called *margo parietalis squamae temporalis* (outmoded), *parietal margin of temporal bone.*

margo parietalis squamae temporalis An outmoded term for MARGO PARIETALIS OSSIS TEMPORALIS.

margo pedis lateralis An outmoded term for MARGO LATERALIS PEDIS.

margo pedis medialis An outmoded term for MARGO MEDIALIS PEDIS.

margo posterior fibulae [NA] A ridge, ill-defined proximally, that extends from the back of the head of the fibula to the medial margin of the peroneal groove on the distal extremity. It provides attachment for the posterior intermuscular septum. Also called *posterior margin of fibula, crista lateralis fibulae, posterior border of fibula, lateral crest of fibula.*

margo posterior lienis An outmoded term for MARGO INFERIOR SPLENIS.

margo posterior pancreatis An outmoded term for MARGO INFERIOR PANCREATIS.

margo posterior partis petrosae ossis temporalis The border or margin on the petrous portion of the temporal bone that separates the inferior from the posterior surfaces. It is intermediate in length between the superior border and anterior angle. Its medial half helps to form the sulcus for the anterior petrosal sinus behind which and laterally is the jugular fossa that helps to form the jugular foramen. Also called *angulus superior pyramidis ossis temporalis, angulus posterior pyramidis ossis temporalis, posterior border of petrous portion of temporal bone, posterior angle of petrous portion of temporal bone.*

margo posterior radii [NA] A ridge on the posterior aspect of the radius that is clearly marked in its middle third only where it separates the posterior from the lateral surface, extending from the posteroinferior part of the radial tuberosity to the region of the dorsal tubercle on the posterior aspect of the distal end of the radius. Also called *posterior border of radius, margo dorsalis radii* (outmoded), *dorsal margin of radius.*

margo posterior testis [NA] The flattened posterior border of the testis, separating the medial and lateral surfaces and attached to the epididymis and spermatic cord laterally. In its upper two thirds is the mediastinum testis for the blood vessels and lymphatics of the testis. Also called *posterior margin of testis, internal margin of testis* (outmoded), *straight margin of testis* (outmoded), *dorsum of testis.*

margo posterior ulnae [NA] A thick, rounded crest that extends in a sinuous course from the apex of the posterior aspect of the subcutaneous olecranon to the styloid process and separates the posterior from the medial surface of the ulna. It is subcutaneous and provides attachment for the flexor carpi ulnaris, extensor carpi ulnaris, and flexor digitorum profundus muscles. Also called *posterior margin of ulna, dorsal margin of ulna, margo dorsalis ulnae* (outmoded).

margo pupillaris iridis [NA] The inner margin of the iris which surrounds the circular aperture of the pupil. It rests upon the front surface of the lens, which elevates it slightly, and it is edged by a finely notched, dark seam. Also called *pupillary margin of iris.*

margines radiales digitorum manus An outmoded term for FACIES LATERALES DIGITORUM MANUS.

margo radialis antebrachii MARGO LATERALIS ANTEBRACHII.

margo radialis antibrachii An outmoded term for MARGO LATERALIS ANTEBRACHII.

margo radialis humeri An outmoded term for MARGO LATERALIS HUMERI.

margo sagittalis ossis parietalis [NA] The markedly serrated, thick medial edge of the parietal bone that articulates with the corresponding border of the opposite bone to form the sagittal suture. Also called *sagittal margin of parietal bone, superior margin of parietal bone, parietal margin of parietal bone.*

margo sphenoidalis ossis temporalis [NA] The anterior, serrated border of the squamous part of the temporal bone that articulates with the posterior margin of the greater wing of the sphenoid bone. Also called *margo sphenoidalis squamae temporalis* (outmoded), *sphenoidal margin of temporal bone.*

margo sphenoidalis squamae temporalis An outmoded term for MARGO SPHENOIDALIS OSSIS TEMPORALIS.

margo squamosus alae magnae An outmoded term for MARGO SQUAMOSUS ALAE MAJORIS.

margo squamosus alae majoris [NA] The border of the greater wing of the sphenoid bone that extends forwards from the sphenoidal spine and is serrated and thinned to articulate with the squamous part of the temporal bone. Also called *squamous margin of greater wing of sphenoid bone, margo squamosus alae magnae.* (outmoded).

margo squamosus ossis parietalis [NA] The lateral or inferior edge of the parietal bone that is divided into three portions: a thin, short anterior portion that is overlapped by the parietal margin of the greater wing of the sphenoid bone; an arched, beveled middle portion overlapped by the squamous part of the temporal bone; and a short, thick and serrated posterior part that articulates with the mastoid portion of the temporal bone. Also called *squamous margin of parietal bone, sphenotemporal margin of parietal bone, temporal margin of parietal bone.*

margo superior cerebri [NA] The superior and medial margin of the cerebral hemisphere. Also called *margo superomedialis cerebri.*

margo superior glandulae suprarenalis [NA] The curved superolateral border of the suprarenal gland which joins the upper extremities of the medial border and the renal surface and separates the anterior from the posterior surface. On the right suprarenal gland it is related to the right lobe of the liver and on the left to the diaphragm. Also called *superior margin of suprarenal gland, superior border of suprarenal gland.*

margo superior lienis MARGO SUPERIOR SPLENIS.

margo superior pancreatis [NA] The upper border of the pancreas which separates the anterior from the posterior surface. It is thin near the tail and flattened towards the right side. The splenic artery runs along it to the left and at its right extremity is the omental tuberosity. Also called *superior border of pancreas, superior margin of pancreas.*

margo superior partis petrosae ossis temporalis [NA] The border or margin that separates the anterior and posterior surfaces of the petrous portion of the temporal bone, of which it is the longest border. It has a groove for the superior petrosal sinus to which the dura mater of the tentorium cerebelli is attached. Also called *superior border of petrous portion of temporal bone, superior angle of petrous portion of temporal bone.*

margo superior scapulae [NA] The short, thin, upper border of the scapula extending from the coracoid process to the superior angle. Laterally it has the scapular notch, bridged over by the superior transverse scapular ligament, to the edges of which the inferior belly of the omohyoid muscle is attached. Also called *superior margin of scapula, superior border of scapula.*

margo superior splenis [NA] The rounded, upper border of the spleen which separates the diaphragmatic surface from the gastric impression of the visceral surface. Near the lateral extremity it may have a few notches, representing the persistence of lobulations characteristic of the spleen in early fetal life. Also called *superior margin of spleen, margo superior lienis, margo anterior splenis, superior border of spleen, margo anterior lienis* (outmoded), *anterior margin of spleen, crenate margin of spleen, cristate margin of spleen.*

margo superomedialis cerebri MARGO SUPERIOR CEREBRI.

margo supraorbitalis Either margo supraorbitalis orbitae or margo supraorbitalis ossis frontalis.

margo supraorbitalis orbitae [NA] The sharp, arched upper margin of the circumference of the orbital opening formed by the supraorbital margin of the frontal bone and extending from its nasal margin to the zygomatic process. Also called *supraorbital margin of orbit.*

margo supraorbitalis ossis frontalis [NA] The curved anterior edge of the frontal bone at the junction of its external and orbital surfaces, articulating medially at its nasal margin with the frontal process of the maxilla and laterally at its zygomatic process with the zygomatic bone. It is interrupted by the supraorbital notch. Also called *supraorbital margin of frontal bone, geisoma, geison, orbital crest, supraorbital arch of frontal bone, orbital arch of frontal bone.*

margo tibialis pedis MARGO MEDIALIS PEDIS.

margines ulnares digitorum manus An outmoded term for FACIES MEDIALES DIGITORUM MANUS.

margo ulnaris antebrachii MARGO MEDIALIS ANTEBRACHII.

margo ulnaris antibrachii An outmoded term for MARGO MEDIALIS ANTEBRACHII.

margo ulnaris humeri MARGO MEDIALIS HUMERI.

margo uteri dexter et sinister [NA] The convex junction between the anterior and posterior surfaces on each side of the body of the uterus. It extends as far as the lateral angles where the uterine tubes enter the uterine wall, below which the broad ligament is attached as well as the round ligament of the uterus and the ligament of the ovary between its folds on each side. Also called *lateral margin of uterus, margo lateralis uteri* (outmoded).

margo vertebralis scapulae An outmoded term for MARGO MEDIALIS SCAPULAE.

margo volaris radii An outmoded term for MARGO ANTERIOR RADII.

margo volaris ulnae An outmoded term for MARGO ANTERIOR ULNAE.

margo zygomaticus alae magnae An outmoded term for MARGO ZYGOMATICUS ALAE MAJORIS.

margo zygomaticus alae majoris [NA] The anterior border of the greater wing of the sphenoid bone. It separates its orbital and temporal surfaces and articulates inferiorly with the free edge of the orbital surface of the zygomatic bone, and often with the maxilla. Also called *zygomatic margin of greater wing of sphenoid bone, margo zygomaticus alae magnae* (outmoded), *malar margin* (outmoded), *zygomatic crest of great wing of sphenoid bone, malar crest of great wing of sphenoid bone, jugular crest of great wing of sphenoid bone* (outmoded).

---

mariculture [L *mare*, gen. *maris*, the sea + CULTURE] The cultivation of oysters or fish for human food in a marine habitat.

Marie [Pierre *Marie*, French physician, 1853–1940] **1** Marie sign, Brissaud-Marie syndrome. See under BRISSAUD-MARIE SIGN. **2** Bamberger-Marie disease, Marie-Bamberger disease, Marie-Bamberger syndrome, Marie's disease. See under HYPERTROPHIC PULMONARY OSTEOARTHROPATHY. **3** Marie-Strümpell arthritis, Marie-Strümpell spondylitis, Marie-Strümpell disease, Strümpell-Marie disease, Marie's disease. See under ANKYLOSING SPONDYLITIS. **4** Marie-Strümpell disease, Strümpell-Marie disease. See under ACUTE INFANTILE HEMIPLEGIA. **5** Quadrilateral space of Marie. See under SPACE. **6** See under MYOPATHY, HYPERTROPHY. **7** Pierre Marie cerebellar heredoataxia, Nonne-Marie syndrome, Marie sclerosis, Marie's disease. See under MARIE'S HEREDITARY CEREBELLAR ATAXIA. **8** Marie-Strümpell encephalitis. See under ENCEPHALITIS. **9** Marie-Foix sign. See under SIGN. **10** Marie and Foix maneuver. See under MANEUVER. **11** Marie-Tooth disease, Charcot-Marie atrophy, Charcot-Marie-Tooth atrophy, Charcot-Marie-Tooth-Hoffmann syndrome. See under CHARCOT-MARIE-TOOTH DISEASE. **12** Marie-Sainton disease. See under CLEIDOCRANIAL DYSPLASIA. **13** Marie's disease, Marie syndrome. See under ACROMEGALY.

marihuana [Mexican Spanish *marihuana*, also *mariguana*] The dried leaves, stems, and flowers of *Cannabis sativa*. It is smoked or used in foods. It produces distorted perception and sometimes hallucinogenic effects. Also called *ganja, guaza, subjee, churganja*. Also *marijuana*.

marijuana MARIHUANA.

Marin Amat [Manuel *Marin Amat*, Spanish ophthalmologist, born 1879] Marin Amat phenomenon. See under SYNDROME.

marine [L *marin(us)* (from *mar(e)* the sea + *-inus* -INE) pertaining to the sea] Pertaining to the ocean or sea.

Marinesco [Georges *Marinesco*, Rumanian pathologist, 1863–1938] **1** Marinesco's hand. See under SUCCULENT HAND. **2** Marinesco-Garland syndrome, Marinesco-Sjögren-Garland syndrome. See under MARINESCO-SJÖGREN SYNDROME. **3** See under SIGN.

marinobufagin A toxin produced by the skin glands of *Bufo marinus*, a marine toad, which secretes an extremely toxic venom. Its action is similar to that of the cardiac glycosides.

marinotherapy [*marin(e)* + *o* + THERAPY] A form of climatotherapy involving exposure to seaside environments. In Europe, various seaside resorts are reputed to have differing therapeutic value depending on the prevailing local climatic conditions. A North Sea environment, for example, is recommended for invigoration and the Mediterranean, for sedation.

Marion [Georges *Marion*, French urologist, 1869–1932] See under DISEASE.

Mariotte [Edmé *Mariotte*, French physicist, 1620–1684] **1** See under EXPERIMENT. **2** Mariotte spot. See under BLIND SPOT. **3** Mariotte's law. See under BOYLE'S LAW.

mariposia [L *mare*, gen. *maris*, the sea + Gk *pos(is)* a drink, drinking + -IA] THALASSOPOSIA.

marital Pertaining to marriage.

maritonucleus [L *marit(us)* married, tied together + *o* + NUCLEUS] In the zygote, the nucleus of the ovum after the spermatozoon has entered the ovum to provide the male pronucleus.

Marjolin [Jean Nicolas *Marjolin*, French physician, 1780–1850] Marjolin's ulcer. See under BURN SCAR CARCINOMA.

mark [Old English *mearc*; akin to L *margo* margin] **1** A sign or spot on a surface, as a circumscribed area of skin visibly different from the surrounding skin. **2** To signify one's attachment to (territory), as by the deposit of an odorous substance: said of animals.

beauty mark A melanocytic pigmented nevus commonly found in the skin overlying the maxilla.

birth mark See under BIRTHMARK.

current mark A cutaneous lesion produced by the passage of electrical current through the skin, a sign that may be useful in forensic pathology. However, current marks may or may not cause death and cannot be uniformly distinguished from similar appearing lesions produced by other causes. Not all contacts

with electrical current produce current marks. They do not appear in circumstances in which the current contacts a large surface area of the body, lasts only a few seconds, and is of low amperage.

hesitation marks See under HESITATION WOUNDS.

lightning mark An erythematous line, usually 2–8 cm wide, and extending continuously or discontinuously in a craniocaudal direction on the skin surface of a person struck by lightning. It is essentially identical to a first degree thermal burn except for the pattern which is fernlike and arborescent. It may not be visible until several hours after the lightning strikes.

longing mark NEVUS.

mulberry mark A dark-colored variety of strawberry nevus. Also called *nevus morus*.

pock mark See under POCKMARK.

Pohl's mark A constricted zone in the hair shaft coinciding in time of formation with an episode of acute illness, acute and severe hypoprotinemia, or the administration of cytotoxic drugs. Also called *Pohl-Pinkus mark*.

Pohl-Pinkus mark POHL'S MARK.

port-wine mark PORT-WINE STAIN.

quillon mark An abrasion adjacent to a stab wound which is produced by the impact of the quillon or guard separating the blade from the handle of the knife.

raspberry mark STRAWBERRY NEVUS.

strawberry mark STRAWBERRY NEVUS.

suture marks Small scars across the line of a surgical or traumatic scar, caused by stitches which are too tight or left in too long.

Unna's mark A port-wine stain on the nape of the neck. Also called *nevus flammeus nuchae, nape nevus*.

washerman's mark DHOBIE MARK DERMATITIS.

marker [MARK + -ER] **1** Something used to mark. **2** ANTIGENIC DETERMINANT.

Amsler's marker A device formerly used to locate retinal tears upon the scleral surface with respect to their geometric position, as determined by a perimeter.

Crane-Kaplan pocket marker A modified form of dental tweezer for marking the depth of a pocket on the oral surface of the gingiva prior to gingivectomy.

genetic marker Any distinct phenotype, determined by a single gene or mutant allele, that can be used in experimental genetics for such purposes as estimating the linkage distance between two loci in recombination analysis.

time marker On a graphic recorder, an instrument that marks the time at regular intervals such as every second.

marking / directive markings Markings on a predator that serve to confuse the prey as to the location of the predator's mouth.

Fontana's markings Fine, superficial, transverse indentations seen on branching peripheral nerves.

Marlow [Frank William *Marlow*, U.S. ophthalmologist, 1858–1942] See under TEST.

marmorated [L *marmorat(us)*, past part. of *marmorare* to decorate with marble, + English *-ed*] Characterized by a variegated patterning of the skin that suggests the appearance of marble.

marmoration MARBLEIZATION.

marmoreal [L *marmore(us)* (from *marmor* marble + *-eus* English *-eous*) made of or pertaining to marble + -AL] Resembling marble: said of a bone in cases of osteopetrosis.

marmorization MARBLEIZATION.

Marmosa monodelphus domestica A gray, short-tailed opossum of Brazil, used in biological research especially for the study of early embryonic development. Adults become sexually mature in 4–5 months and have a gestation period of about 2 weeks.

Maroteaux [Pierre *Maroteaux*, French physician, born 1926] **1** Maroteaux-Lamy disease. See under DISEASE. **2** Maroteaux-Lamy syndrome. See under MUCOPOLYSACCHARIDOSIS VI.

Marplan A proprietary name for isocarboxazid.

marriage / companionate marriage A form of marriage where the prime objective is companionship between two persons of opposite sex rather than procreation or sexual gratification.

Marriott [Williams McKim *Marriott*, U.S. physician, 1885–1936] Levy, Rowntree, and Marriott method. See under METHOD.

marrow MEDULLA.

bone marrow The soft mesenchymal tissue occupying the cavities within bone, consisting of a reticular meshwork filled with fat, blood cells, and their precursors; medulla ossium. Also called *medulla of bone, medullary substance of bone, myeloid tissue.*

depressed marrow Bone marrow with abnormally decreased production of blood cells.

fat marrow YELLOW BONE MARROW.

gelatinous marrow Marrow that has lost its normal cellular elements and fat. It resembles gelatin in gross appearance, due to a relative increase in glycosaminoglycan-rich ground substance.

hemopoietic marrow RED BONE MARROW.

primary marrow RED BONE MARROW.

red marrow RED BONE MARROW.

red bone marrow Bone marrow that produces formed blood elements. Also called *red marrow, red medullary substance of bones, primary marrow, hemopoietic marrow, medulla ossium rubra.*

spinal marrow MEDULLA SPINALIS.

yellow marrow YELLOW BONE MARROW.

yellow bone marrow Adipose tissue in which the connective tissue supports predominantly fat cells and only a few primitive blood cells. It is found mostly in long bones. Also called *yellow marrow, fat marrow, medulla ossium flava, yellow medullary substance of bones.*

marrowbrain An obsolete term for MYELENCEPHALON.

marrubiin $C_{21}H_{28}O_4$. The bitter element found in horehound, *Marrubium vulgare.* It has been utilized as an expectorant and stomach tonic in the past, but is not used now.

Marsh [Sir Henry *Marsh*, Irish physician, 1790–1860] Marsh disease. See under GRAVES DISEASE.

Marshall [Don *Marshall*, U.S. ophthalmologist, born 1905] See under SYNDROME.

Marshall [John *Marshall*, English anatomist, 1818–1891] **1** Marshall's fold. See under PLICA VENAE CAVAE SINISTRAE. **2** Accompanying artery of vein of Marshall. See under ARTERY. **3** Vein of Marshall, Marshall's oblique vein. See under VENA OBLIQUA ATRII SINISTRI.

Marshall [Victor F. *Marshall*, U.S. urologist, born 1913] Marshall-Marchetti operation. See under OPERATION.

Marshallagia marshalli A stomach worm of the family Trichostrongylidae found in the abomasum of sheep, goats, camels, and several kinds of wild ruminant.

Marshall Hall [*Marshall Hall*, English physiologist, 1790–1857] Marshall Hall's facies. See under FACIES.

marshmallow ALTHEA.

marsupia Plural of MARSUPIUM.

marsupial [L *marsupi(um)* a purse or bag for carrying money + -AL] Any member of the order Marsupialia.

Marsupialia [MARSUPIAL + -IA] A diverse order of pouched mammals, the marsupials. Members of the order are characterized by a skull with a small cranial cavity and a large facial area, marsupial bones on the pelvic girdle, a marsupium containing mammary glands on the abdomen of females, and viviparous reproduction with only brief uterine development. Marsupials occur in Australia and adjacent islands, and in North and South America.

marsupialization [L *marsupi(um)* a purse or bag for carrying money + -AL + -*iz(e)* + -ATION] A method of treating a dental or other large cyst when complete removal of the cyst lining is not possible. A wide opening is made and it is maintained by the use of an obturator which is gradually reduced in depth as the cyst cavity becomes shallower. Also called *Partsch's operation.*

marsupium [L (from Gk *marsipion, marsypion* a small bag or pouch, dim. of *marsipos, marsypos* a bag or pouch), a purse, pouch] (*plural* marsupia) **1** The abdominal pouch of a female marsupial. It contains the teats and is the site of extensive postgestation development of the young. **2** SCROTUM.

marsupia patellaris An outmoded term for PLICAE ALARES.

Martin [August E. *Martin*, German gynecologist, 1847–1933] See under PELVIMETER.

Martin [Henry Austin *Martin*, U.S. surgeon, 1824–1884] See under OPERATION, DISEASE.

Martinotti [Giovanni *Martinotti*, Italian physician, 1857–1928] See under CELL, NEURON.

Martius [Karl Alexander *Martius*, German chemist, 1838–1920] See under YELLOW.

Martorell [Fernando *Martorell*, Spanish physician, born 1906] Martorell syndrome. See under TAKAYASU'S ARTERITIS.

masc. mass concentration (obsolete).

maschaladenitis Inflammation of the axillary lymph nodes. An obsolete term.

maschale FOSSA AXILLARIS.

maschalephidrosis [Gk *maschal(ē)* the armpit + *ephidrōsis* a perspiring, perspiration] Hyperhidrosis of the axillary region.

maschaloncus [Gk *maschal(ē)* the armpit + -ONCUS] A tumor in the axillary area. An obsolete term.

masculine [L *masculinus* (from *masculus* male, masculine, from *mas* the male of humans, animals, and plants) masculine, manly, male] Of or relating to the male sex; having the qualities characteristic of men.

masculinism An older term for VIRILISM.

masculinity The state of being masculine; possession of the normal characteristics of men. Also called *virilism.*

masculinization [*masculiniz(e)* + -ATION] **1** VIRILIZATION. **2** Normal development of secondary sex characters in the male.

masculinize [L *masculin(us)* pertaining to the male + -IZE] **1** To induce the development in the male of male secondary sex characters. **2** VIRILIZE.

masculinizing **1** Inducing male qualities, especially male secondary sex characters. **2** VIRILIZING.

masculinoma [L *masculin(us)* male, masculine + -OMA] A tumor, usually ovarian, causing masculinization. A seldom used term.

masculinovoblastoma [L *masculin(us)* male, masculine + -OVO + BLASTOMA] An ovarian tumor causing masculinization.

masculonucleus [L *mascul(inus)* male, masculine + *o* + NUCLEUS] MALE PRONUCLEUS.

maser [*m(icrowave) a(mplification by) s(timulated) e(mission of) r(adiation)*] A device that generates or amplifies microwave radiation and that produces an intense, nearly nondivergent, beam.

masfr.   mass fraction (obsolete).

mask [French *masque* (from Italian *máschera* a mask, cover, from Med L *masca* a witch) a false face with cartoon painting] **1** A gauze covering for the nose and mouth to preserve antiseptic conditions or to prevent the spread of infection. **2** A patient's facial expression or characteristic facial appearance as affected by disease, such as Parkinson's facies. **3** A metal frame covered with gauze placed over the face of a patient for the administration of inhalation anesthesia. **4** To cover metal parts of (a denture) with an opaque material.

BLB mask   An oxygen mask used at high altitudes, having a combined inspiratory and expiratory valve in a rebreathing bag. • The mask is named after its designers, Boothby, Lovelace, and Bulbulian.

Curschmann's mask   A mask formerly used to inhale turpentine vapors. An obsolete term.

death mask   A reproduction of the face of a corpse, by the postmortem application of plaster of Paris to form a cast of the face. Secondary castings in bronze or other metals may be made from the plaster cast.

ecchymotic mask   Cyanosis of the head and neck resulting from traumatic asphyxia.

full-face mask   A device fitting tightly over the nose and mouth and used for general inhalation anesthesia or respiratory assistance.

gravidic mask   MELASMA.

Hutchinson's mask   TABETIC MASK.

Kuhn's mask   A mask used formerly in the treatment of pulmonary tuberculosis to obstruct exhalation through the nose and mouth, supposedly thus causing a therapeutic hyperemia of the lung tissues.

leutic mask   A masklike pigmentation and depigmentation of the upper face that is associated with the late stages of syphilis.

meter mask   A mask which is attached to a meter to measure volume of gases.

nonrebreathing mask   A tight-fitting mask placed over the nose and mouth in order to permit the inhalation of fresh gas during general anesthesia or respiratory assistance, while allowing for the elimination of expired gas without rebreathing.

Parkinson's mask   The expressionless face that is characteristic of parkinsonism.

partial rebreathing mask   An oxygen mask which permits some of the exhaled air to be rebreathed.

mask of pregnancy   MELASMA.

surgical mask   An appliance, made of cloth or paper, that covers the nose and mouth of the members of an operating team during surgical procedures.

tabetic mask   A sense of tightness of the skin of the face experienced by some patients with tabes dorsalis. Also called *Hutchinson's mask.*

tracheostomy mask   A mask placed over a tracheostomy for delivery of oxygen or humidity.

tropical mask   Chloasma intensified by tropical sunshine.

uterine mask   MELASMA.

Venturi mask   A mask that delivers a constant concentration of oxygen, using the Venturi principle of entrainment of air to dilute the flow of pure oxygen.

masked   Disguised or hidden by unrelated symptoms or organisms, as when a reducing diet conceals signs of a wasting disease.

masker / tinnitus masker   A device, resembling an ear-level hearing aid, for use in the treatment of tinnitus. An extraneous noise is produced by the instrument and adjusted with the aim of masking the subjective noise experienced by the patient.

masking   **1** The process by which one perceptible event or ac-

tivity is rendered imperceptible by another. In audiology it refers to the process by which a sound of a particular frequency is rendered inaudible by a louder sound the frequency spectrum of which includes the frequency of the occluded or masked sound. It is of special importance in determining the auditory threshold of a deafened ear in the presence of normal hearing in the other ear: the normal ear must be exposed to an appropriate level of masking noise of the appropriate frequency spectrum in order to avoid a spurious result. That is, the level of hearing in the deafened ear might be assessed as better than it should be, owing to the test sound's being picked up by the better hearing ear. **2** A phenomenon demonstrated during the analysis of EEG frequencies showing that in a particular tracing there are two different basic rhythms, although only one is apparent visually in the recording. This rhythm has masked the other one. **3** The covering of metal parts of a denture with opaque material.

central masking   The masking effect on heard sounds that is induced by the central, neural interaction between the two ears.

Maslow [Abraham Harold *Maslow*, U.S. psychologist, 1908–1970] **1** Maslow's motivational hierarchy. See under HIERARCHY. **2** Maslow's theory of human motivation. See under THEORY.

masochism [after Leopold von Sacher-*Masoch*, 1835–1895, Austrian novelist, who introduced masochism into his stories, + -ISM] **1** A paraphilia in which the individual has a preference for or need to be humiliated, beaten, or otherwise subjected to suffering in order to achieve sexual arousal. Also called *algophilia* (obsolete), *algophily* (obsolete), *passive algolagnia.* **2** A general pattern of self-destructive behavior that invites abuse, exploitation, or mistreatment by others.

moral masochism   A need for punishment stemming from infantile conflicts. It may be expressed as extreme passivity, total subjection to others' demands, or provocation of others to retaliate by injuring or destroying the subject. Also called *fate neurosis, neurosis of destiny.*

masochist   A person having an inclination toward masochism.

Mason [James Tate *Mason*, U.S. surgeon, 1882–1936]   See under INCISION.

mas. pil.   *massa pilularum* (L, pill mass).

mass [L *massa*. See MASSA.]   **1** The quantitative measure of inertia, that is, of resistance to acceleration. **2** A collection of tissue; body; massa.

achromatic mass   A nonstaining mass of protoplasm which surrounds the chromosomes during mitosis and meiosis.

appendiceal mass   A right lower quadrant abdominal mass associated with acute appendicitis, often with appendiceal rupture and abscess formation. Also called *appendix mass.*

appendix mass   APPENDICEAL MASS.

apperceptive mass   The body of knowledge or schema already existing within the mind that is instrumental in determining the way in which the properties of a new object will be perceived and understood. A rarely used term.

atomic mass   The mass of a neutral atom of a given species, categorized as physical or chemical. Also called *atomic weight (imprecise but customary).* Symbol: m, m_a • The International Organization for Standardization (ISO) recommends that the term *atomic mass* be applied only to the value in SI units, i.e., kilograms. A separate term, *relative atomic mass*, is to be used for the dimensionless number obtained by dividing the mass of an atom in atomic mass units. This distinction, however, is rarely observed.

atrioventricular cushion mass   SEPTUM INTERMEDIUM.

blue mass   MERCURY MASS.

body cell mass   The weight of all body cells that take part in body functions.

cell mass 1 The active metabolizing tissue in the body. In an active lean healthy individual, it represents approximately 55% of the total body weight. In an obese person, the figure is much less. It may be calculated by multiplying cell water by 100/70. Since 70% of the whole cell mass is water, cell water is calculated by subtracting extracellular water from total body water. Cell mass may also be measured from an assessment of total potassium 40 in the body using a whole-body counter. 2 INNER CELL MASS.

chemical atomic mass The average atomic mass of the naturally occurring isotopes of an atom, weighted according to their relative abundances.

critical mass The minimum mass of fissionable material capable of maintaining a chain reaction.

electronic mass The mass of an electron, 9.1×10^{-28} gram.

embryonic mass INNER CELL MASS.

epithelial mass The primitive cells of the indifferent gonad.

injection mass A solution that is injected into vascular or other spaces of a tissue or organ to form a permanent cast of that structure. The surrounding tissue is subsequently either dissolved or rendered transparent.

inner cell mass The initial small group of cells which segregates within the enveloping trophoblast at one pole of the hollow mammalian blastocyst and which is destined to develop into the embryo. Also called *embryonic mass, cell mass.*

intermediate mass ADHESIO INTERTHALAMICA.

intermediate cell mass A mass of mesoderm in early embryos situated between the medially placed paraxial mesoderm and the lateral plate mesoderm. In human embryos it becomes fused from the eighth somite caudally into an unsegmented column, termed the nephrogenic cord. The nephrotomes develop in the metameric segments of the cord to give rise to three embryonic kidney systems: pronephros, mesonephros, and metanephros.

isotopic mass PHYSICAL ATOMIC MASS.

lateral mass of atlas MASSA LATERALIS ATLANTIS.

lateral mass of ethmoid bone LABYRINTHUS ETHMOIDALIS.

lateral mass of occipital bone PARS LATERALIS OSSIS OCCIPITALIS.

lateral mass of sacrum PARS LATERALIS OSSIS SACRI.

lateral mass of vertebra An outmoded term for PEDICLE OF VERTEBRAL ARCH.

lean body mass The weight of the fat-free component of the body.

mercury mass A mixture of mercury oleate, mercury, honey, glycerin, and other ingredients formerly used for the treatment of pediculosis pubis. Also called *blue mass, massa hydrargyri.*

molecular mass The mass of a molecule of given chemical species, equal to the sum of the masses of the atoms of which the molecule is composed. The numerical value of the molecular mass in atomic mass units (or daltons) is equal to the relative molecular mass.

muscle mass The total amount of muscle found in the body of a human or other animal. Urinary excretion of creatinine is often used as an estimate of muscle mass in the presence of normal renal function. However, this is subject to a twofold error as muscle creatine concentrations vary from 0.3%–0.5%.

physical atomic mass Atomic mass of a single isotope. Its value in atomic mass units is very nearly equal to the mass number of the isotope. Also called *isotopic mass, isotopic weight (rare and imprecise).*

pill mass PILULAR MASS.

pilular mass A soft, solid drug of a consistency suitable for being made into pills. Also called *pill mass.*

premuscle mass The mesodermal precursor of developing muscle.

Priestley's mass A green or brown stain on anterior teeth, caused by chromogenic bacteria. An outmoded term.

relative atomic mass The mass of a nuclide in atomic mass units, where the atomic mass unit is defined as 1/12 the mass of the nuclide carbon 12.

relative molecular mass The quantity characteristic of a substance obtained by dividing the mass of its molecule by the atomic mass unit or dalton. It is therefore a dimensionless number, equal to the numerical part of the molar mass of the substance in g/mol and to that of the molecular mass in daltons. Symbol: M_r. • *Molecular weight* is the common usage, although *relative molecular mass* is more accurate.

relativistic mass The increased mass of a body due to its velocity. Change in mass is negligible until the velocity approaches that of light.

sarcoplasmic masses Masses of undifferentiated sarcoplasm not containing myofibrils as seen in transverse sections of skeletal muscle in the periphery of some muscle fibers, especially in patients with dystrophia myotonica.

Schultze's granular mass Agglutinated fragments of damaged blood platelets seen on stained smears which exhibit a granular appearance.

Stent's mass STENT DRESSING.

tigroid masses NISSL SUBSTANCE.

total red cell mass The total volume of erythrocytes in the blood.

ventrolateral mass A ventrolateral, hypaxial, division of the myotome which gives rise to the ventral and lateral trunk muscles, supplied by the anterior primary rami of the spinal nerves. Also called *hypomere.*

massa [L from Gk *maza* barley bread, barley cake, from *massein* to knead), a lump, mass] [NA] A cohesion of tissue.

massa hydrargyri MERCURY MASS.

massa innominata PARADIDYMIS.

massa intermedia ADHESIO INTERTHALAMICA.

massa lateralis atlantis One of two bulky portions of the atlas, each with superior and inferior articular facets. They are connected to each other by the anterior and the posterior arches. On the medial aspect of each is a small tubercle for the transverse ligament and on the lateral aspect is the transverse process. Also called *lateral mass of atlas.*

massa lateralis ossis ethmoidalis An outmoded term for LABYRINTHUS ETHMOIDALIS.

massa lateralis ossis sacri An outmoded term for PARS LATERALIS OSSIS SACRI.

massa lateralis vertebrae An outmoded term for PEDICLE OF VERTEBRAL ARCH.

massa mollis An obsolete term for ADHESIO INTERTHALAMICA.

massae Plural of MASSA.

massage [French (from *masser* to press and knead the body with the hand, from Arabic *mass* pressure on the body muscles; Gk *massein* to knead and *maza* barley bread, barley cake), a massaging] Therapeutic stimulation of soft tissue by manual or mechanical means.

cardiac massage Rhythmic manual compression of the heart either through a thoracotomy (open cardiac massage) or by pressure applied to the sternum (closed cardiac massage), used as a means of resuscitation when the heart has stopped beating or is beating very feebly. Also called *cardiac compression, heart massage.*

carotid sinus massage Massage of the carotid sinus by firm stroking in the region of the sinus, a technique used to cause reflex slowing of the heart, particularly for the identification or correction of supraventricular tachycardias.

electrovibratory massage Superficial stimulation of the skin and underlying muscles by use of an electrical device that produces mechanical vibration.

gingival massage   Rubbing of the gingiva as a form of treatment. Removal of dental plaque is probably the only beneficial effect.

heart massage   CARDIAC MASSAGE.

nerve-point massage   Deep friction massage localized to points of tenderness as described by Alfons Cornelius in Berlin in 1909. It might be considered a precursor of modern trigger point massage.

spray massage   Spray application of a vapo-coolant such as ethyl chloride for the relief of muscle spasm and myofascial pain.

trigger point massage   Focal massage directed to the "breaking up" of trigger points, that is, local diminution of pain probably related to vasodilation. See also NERVE-POINT MASSAGE.

vapor massage   An obsolete treatment of pulmonary tuberculosis by administration of a nebulized vapor by positive pressure.

vibratory massage   Massage carried out with the aid of a vibrating device.

massc.   mass concentration.

Masselon   [Julien *Masselon*, French ophthalmologist, 1844–1917]   Masselon spectacles. See under SPECTACLES.

masseter   [irreg. from Gk *masētēr* (from *masasthai* to chew) a chewer, muscle of the lower jaw used in chewing]   MUSCULUS MASSETER.

masseteric   Of or relating to the masseter muscle.

masseur   [French, from *mass(er)* (from Arabic *mass(a)* to paipate, stroke + French *-er*, inf. termination) to massage + *-eur* -ER]   A person trained in, or who practices, the art and techniques of massage.   • In current usage *masseur* may refer either to a man or a woman, and usually designates a lay practitioner or one whose profession is limited to massage.

masseuse   [French, fem. of MASSEUR]   A female masseur.

massfr.   mass fraction.

Masson   [Claude Laurent Pierre *Masson*, French-born Canadian pathologist, 1880–1959]   **1** Masson stain, Masson's trichrome method. See under MASSON'S TRICHROME STAIN.   **2** See under BODY.

mast-   MASTO-.

mastadenitis   [MAST- + ADENITIS]   MASTITIS.

mastadenoma   [MAST- + ADENOMA]   A tumor of the breast. An outmoded term.

mastadenovirus   [MAST- + ADENOVIRUS]   A member of the genus *Mastadenovirus* in the family Adenoviridae, which includes all adenovirus species isolated from mammalian hosts. Most viruses of the genus, except some bovine strains, share a common antigen absent in the aviadenoviruses. Over 50 serotypes have been described. The virions are naked, ether-resistant, icosahedral particles, 70–80 nm in diameter. They contain a linear, double-stranded DNA genome with a mass of 20–25 million daltons.

mastalgia   [MAST- + -ALGIA]   MASTODYNIA.

mastatrophia   [MAST- + ATROPHIA]   MASTATROPHY.

mastatrophy   [MAST- + ATROPHY]   Atrophy or shrinkage of the breast. Also called *mastatrophia*.

mastauxe   [MAST- + Gk *auxē* growth, increase]   Enlargement of the breast.

mastecchymosis   [MAST- + ECCHYMOSIS]   Subcutaneous hemorrhage in the breast, which creates a blue or purple patch.

mastectomy   [MAST- + -ECTOMY]   Removal of the breast. Also called *mammectomy*.

  Halsted radical mastectomy   RADICAL MASTECTOMY.

  radical mastectomy   A mastectomy involving the pectoral

muscles, axillary lymph nodes, and associated skin and subcutaneous tissue, in breast cancer. Also called *Halsted radical mastectomy, Meyer's operation, Halsted's operation.*

  simple mastectomy   Removal of the breast only. Compare RADICAL MASTECTOMY.

  subcutaneous mastectomy   A mastectomy wherein the areola and sufficient skin are preserved in preparation for reconstruction of the breast by means of a mammary implant. It is used for mastodynia and for the prophylaxis of breast cancer, but not in the treatment of breast cancer.

Master   [Arthur Matthew *Master*, U.S. cardiologist, 1895–1973]   See under TEST.

Masterone   A proprietary name for dromostanolone propionate.

masthelcosis   [MAST- + HELCOSIS]   Ulceration of the breast.

mastic   A resinous exudate from *Pistacia lentiscus*, composed primarily of mastichic acid and masticin. It has been used as a carminative, as an ingredient in temporary dental fillings and cavity varnishes, and in commercial varnishes and perfumes. Also called *mastiche*.

masticate   [Late L *masticat(us)*, past part. of *masticare* (from Gk *mastichan* to gnash the teeth, from *mastax* the jaws, a mouthful) to chew]   To chew (food) in preparation for swallowing.

mastication   [Late L *masticatio*, from *masticatus*, past part. of *masticare* to chew. See MASTICATE.]   The act or process of chewing food.

masticatory   [Late L *masticat(us)*, past part. of *masticare* (from Gk *mastichan* to gnash the teeth) to chew + -ORY]   **1** Of or used for chewing.   **2** A preparation designed to be chewed.

mastiche   MASTIC.

Mastigophora   A subphylum of protozoa characterized by having one or more flagella, particularly in the trophozoite stage of development. Most species are free-living but many are found as parasites of invertebrates and vertebrates, including humans. The taxon includes the classes Phytomastigophorea and Zoomastigophorea. Also called *Flagellata* (former name), *Euflagellata* (former name).

mastigophoran   **1** Pertaining or belonging to the subphylum Mastigophora.   **2** A member of the subphylum Mastigophora; a mastigote or flagellate.

mastigophorous   Pertaining to or characteristic of the subphylum Mastigophora.

mastigote   [irreg. from Gk *mastix*, gen. *mastigos*, a whip, scourge]   A member of the subphylum Mastigophora; a flagellate.

mastitis   [MAST- + -ITIS]   Inflammation of the mammary gland or breast. Also called *mastadenitis, mammitis, St. Agatha's disease* (obsolete).

  acute mastitis   Inflammation or infection of the breast with rapid onset.

  bovine mastitis   Inflammation of the mammary gland of cattle, caused by various infectious agents, mainly bacterial but also mycoplasmal and viral. The inflammation varies from the acute and suppurative to the nonsuppurative, from the gangrenous to the chronic and indurative. The condition is a cause of serious economic losses in the dairy industry worldwide.

  chronic cystic mastitis   CYSTIC MASTOPATHY.

  gargantuan mastitis   Chronic inflammation and excessive enlargement of the breast.

  glandular mastitis   Inflammatory disease of the breast that involves the lactiferous tubules. Also called *parenchymatous mastitis*.

  interstitial mastitis   An inflammatory disease of the breast in which bacteria gain access to the connective tissue through a crack or deep fissure. Also called *phlegmonous mastitis*.

lactation mastitis   Inflammation of the breast occurring during lactation.

mastitis neonatorum   **1** An infection of the breast tissue in neonates.   **2** The enlargement and secretory activity of the breasts (witch's milk) which is common in infants of both sexes in the first days of life.

parenchymatous mastitis   GLANDULAR MASTITIS.

periductal mastitis   Inflammation of tissues about the ducts of the breast.

phlegmonous mastitis   INTERSTITIAL MASTITIS.

plasma cell mastitis   Mastitis in which inspissation and stasis are present, making this a chemical rather than a bacterial inflammation. Those affected are usually multiparas.

puerperal mastitis   Postpartum inflammation of the breast.

retromammary mastitis   SUBMAMMARY ABSCESS.

stagnation mastitis   Inflammation or local engorgement in a galactocele in a lactating woman.

submammary mastitis   SUBMAMMARY ABSCESS.

suppurative mastitis   Inflammation of the breast due to infection by pyogenic bacteria.

masto-   [Gk *mastos* (from earlier *mazos* a woman's breast) a woman's breast]   A combining form denoting (1) the breast or mammary glands; (2) the mastoid process. Also *mast-*.

mastocarcinoma   [MASTO- + CARCINOMA]   A carcinoma of the breast. An outmoded term.

mastoccipital   MASTO-OCCIPITAL.

mastochondroma   [MASTO- + CHONDROMA]   A chondroma of the breast. An outmoded term. Also called *mastochondrosis*.

mastochondrosis   [MASTO- + CHONDROSIS]   **1** MASTOCHONDROMA.   **2** Deposits of cartilage in the breast.

mastocyte   MAST CELL.

mastocytogenesis   The development and maturation of mast cells.

mastocytoma   A tumor of mast cells.

solitary mastocytoma   An isolated cutaneous tumor that consists of an aggregate of mast cells.

mastocytosis   [MASTO- + CYTOSIS]   **1** Infiltration of tissues by mast cells.   **2** An increased number of mast cells in bone marrow. For defs. 1 and 2 also called *mast cell disease*. See also URTICARIA PIGMENTOSA.

cutaneous mastocytosis   A localized increase in the number of mast cells in the dermis.

diffuse cutaneous mastocytosis   A benign but widespread increase in the number of mast cells in the dermis. Thickening and pigmentation of the overlying epidermis is common.

malignant mastocytosis   MAST CELL LEUKEMIA.

systemic mastocytosis   A widespread form of mast cell proliferation with involvement of skin (urticaria pigmentosa), liver, lymph nodes, intestinal tract, bone, and bone marrow.

mastodynia   [MAST- + -ODYNIA]   Pain in the breast. Also called *mammalgia, mastalgia, mazodynia*.

mastogram   [MASTO- + -GRAM]   A rarely used term for MAMMOGRAM.

mastography   [MASTO- + -GRAPHY]   A rarely used term for MAMMOGRAPHY.

mastoid   [MAST- + -OID]   **1** Resembling a nipple or breast in shape.   **2** PROCESSUS MASTOIDEUS OSSIS TEMPORALIS.   **3** Of or relating to the mastoid process, the mastoid antrum, or the mastoid cells. Also *mastoidal*.

acellular mastoid   SCLEROTIC MASTOID.

diploic mastoid   The mastoid process of the temporal bone in the early stage of development, when it is occupied by bone marrow, that is, before pneumatization has occurred. In some individuals this diploic pattern persists into adult life.

ivory mastoid   SCLEROTIC MASTOID.

pneumatic mastoid   PNEUMATIZED MASTOID.

pneumatized mastoid   The mastoid process of the temporal bone in its normal cellular state, that is, honeycombed with air cells of variable size. Also called *pneumatic mastoid*.

sclerotic mastoid   The mastoid process of the temporal bone when neither air cells nor marrow spaces are found and the process throughout is of the consistency of ivory. Also called *acellular mastoid, ivory mastoid*.

mastoidal   MASTOID.

mastoidale   In craniometry, the lowest point of the mastoid process.

mastoidalgia   [MASTOID + -ALGIA]   Pain in the region of the mastoid process. Pain, when it occurs in cases of mastoid disease, will as a rule be experienced as earache (otalgia). A seldom used term.

mastoidea   An outmoded term for PROCESSUS MASTOIDEUS OSSIS TEMPORALIS.

mastoidectomy   [MASTOID + -ECTOMY]   Any operation requiring removal of part of the mastoid process of the temporal bone, with the object of eradicating disease and/or gaining access to deeper parts, especially the middle-ear spaces. Also called *mastoid operation*.

Bondy mastoidectomy   MODIFIED RADICAL MASTOIDECTOMY.

combined approach mastoidectomy   Radical or modified radical mastoidectomy in which access is gained to the sites of disease by both the transmastoid and transmeatal routes, leaving intact the posterosuperior bony canal wall so as to facilitate subsequent tympanoplasty.

conservative mastoidectomy   SIMPLE MASTOIDECTOMY.   • The operation is conservative in the sense that it avoids interference with the sound-conduction apparatus of the middle ear, thus conserving the potential for normal hearing.

cortical mastoidectomy   SIMPLE MASTOIDECTOMY.   • The operation was designed to provide access to the diseased air cells by removal of a portion of the cortical bone of the mastoid process.

modified mastoidectomy   An imprecise term for MODIFIED RADICAL MASTOIDECTOMY.

modified radical mastoidectomy   An operation undertaken as an alternative to radical mastoidectomy, when it is judged that certain middle-ear structures may be safely and advantageously conserved, for example the pars tensa of the tympanic membrane and the attached malleus handle. Also called *modified mastoidectomy* (imprecise), *Bondy mastoidectomy, Bondy operation*.

radical mastoidectomy   The excision of all diseased tissues in the tympanic portion (tympanectomy) as well as the mastoid portion of the middle-ear cleft. Access to the tympanum is gained by removing a large part of the bone of the posterior meatal and outer attic walls and preserved by creating suitable flaps of the posterior meatal skin. The usual indication is cholesteatoma. Currently, intact canal wall techniques are often preferred. Also called *mastoidotympanectomy*.

Schwartze mastoidectomy   SIMPLE MASTOIDECTOMY.

simple mastoidectomy   The classical operation for the relief of acute mastoiditis, intended to achieve exenteration of all infected mastoid air cells, to exclude spread of disease to important adjacent structures, such as the meninges, and to restore normal hearing. Also called *Schwartze mastoidectomy, Schwartze's operation, cortical mastoidectomy, conservative mastoidectomy*.

mastoideocentesis   MASTOIDOTOMY.

mastoideum   An outmoded term for PROCESSUS MASTOIDEUS OSSIS TEMPORALIS.

mastoiditis   [MASTOID + -ITIS]   Inflammation of the mastoid process of the temporal bone involving at first the mucoendosteum of the air cells but in more severe cases resulting in osteitis and sometimes a subperiosteal abscess behind or beneath the ear. It occurs as a complication of acute suppurative otitis media. Also called *otitis mastoidea* (obsolete).

Bezold's mastoiditis Mastoiditis leading to destruction of the mastoid tip on its medial aspect, and abscess formation (Bezold's abscess) deep to the upper fibers of the sternomastoid muscle.

coalescent mastoiditis Mastoiditis in a cellular mastoid process where destruction of the cell walls results in more or less extensive cavitation.

mastoiditis externa Mastoiditis presenting externally, as when there is a subperiosteal abscess. An obsolete term.

mastoiditis interna Mastoiditis which does not spread beyond the mastoid process. An obsolete term. Also called *endomastoiditis*.

masked mastoiditis Mastoiditis in the absence of overt physical signs such as swelling and tenderness over the mastoid process. It is a potentially dangerous condition, usually occurring as a consequence of inadequate antibiotic treatment. Also called *silent mastoiditis*.

sclerosing mastoiditis Recurrent low-grade mastoiditis which, occurring at an early age, was once considered to result in a sclerotic mastoid. This was probably an erroneous interpretation, the likely cause of sclerosis being malfunction of the eustachian tube. An ambiguous usage.

silent mastoiditis MASKED MASTOIDITIS.

tuberculous mastoiditis A rare manifestation of tuberculous otitis media, with its highest incidence in childhood. It is usually diagnosed only after laboratory reports on granulation tissue are obtained at mastoidectomy.

zygomatic mastoiditis Acute mastoiditis spreading forward into zygomatic air cells and presenting as a swelling in front of the ear over the zygomatic process of the temporal bone.

mastoidotomy [MASTOID + *o* + -TOMY] Surgical incision of the mastoid process for the purpose of exploration or other procedures. A seldom used term. Also called *mastoideocentesis*.

mastoidotympanectomy RADICAL MASTOIDECTOMY.

mastology [MASTO- + -LOGY] The scientific study of the breast.

mastomenia [MASTO- + Gk *mēn* month + -IA] Vicarious menstruation from the breast.

Mastomys natalensis A species of rat which is widely distributed in Africa. In west Africa it is a host of Lassa virus. Bluetongue virus has also been isolated from it.

mastoncus [MAST- + -ONCUS] A tumor the breast. An outmoded term.

masto-occipital Of or relating to the mastoid process of the temporal bone and the occipital bone. Also *mastoccipital*.

mastoparietal PARIETOMASTOID.

mastopathia [MASTO- + -PATHIA] MASTOPATHY.

mastopathia cystica CYSTIC MASTOPATHY.

mastopathy [MASTO- + -PATHY] Any disease of the mammary glands. Also called *mastopathia*.

cystic mastopathy A breast condition in which cysts are formed and the breast has an indurated consistency primarily in the upper quadrants. Also called *shotty breast, cystic breast, adenocystic disease, Bloodgood's disease, cystic disease of breast, fibrocystic disease of breast, Schimmelbusch disease, mammary dysplasia, cystic hyperplasia of the breasts, chronic cystic mastitis, mastopathia cystica, mastosis*.

mastopexy [MASTO- + -PEXY] A plastic operation on the breast to eliminate ptosis and restore a youthful contour. This usually requires relocation of the nipple. Also called *mazopexy*.

Mastophora A genus of spider in the family Araneidae (Ar-

giopidae). Also called *Glyptocranium*.

Mastophora gasteracanthoides The cat-headed spider of Argentina, Chile, and Peru, whose bite causes necrotic sores among vineyard workers.

mastoplasia MAMMOPLASIA.

mastoplastia [MASTO- + -*plast(y)* + -IA] Hyperplasia and hypertrophy of the breast.

mastoplasty [MASTO- + -PLASTY] MAMMOPLASTY.

mastoptosis [MASTO- + PTOSIS] Dropping of the breasts.

mastorrhagia [MASTO- + -RRHAGIA] Hemorrhage from a breast.

mastoscirrhus [MASTO- + SCIRRHUS] Hardening of the breast, usually as the effect of a carcinoma.

mastosis [MASTO- + -SIS] CYSTIC MASTOPATHY.

mastospargosis [MASTO- + Gk *sparg(an)* to swell + -OSIS] Enlargement of the breast during lactation secondary to excessive secretion of milk.

mastosquamous Of or relating to the mastoid and squamous parts of the temporal bone.

mastostomy [MASTO- + -STOMY] Incision of the breast for drainage of blood or pus. Also called *mastotomy*.

mastosyrinx [MASTO- + Gk *syrinx* a pipe, windpipe, fistula, nostrils, trachea] A fistula of the breast.

mastotic Pertaining to mastosis (cystic mastopathy).

mastotomy [MASTO- + -TOMY] MASTOSTOMY.

mastous [MAST- + -OUS] Having unusually large breasts.

masturbation [L *masturbatus*, past part. of *masturbari* (prob. from *ma(nus)* hand + *stuprare* to defile, deflower) to masturbate] Self-manipulation of the genitals to achieve sexual gratification. In the adolescent and adult, masturbation is usually accompanied by frankly sexual fantasies. Also called *ipsation* (seldom used).

Masugi [Matazo *Masugi*, Japanese pathologist, flourished 20th century] See under NEPHRITIS.

masurium [New L (after *Masuria*, a region in northern Poland + suffix -*ium*), former name of chemical element 43] An outmoded term for TECHNETIUM.

mat / gingival mat The densely fibrous connective tissue which attaches the gingiva to the tooth and to the crest of the alveolar bone. An outmoded term.

Matas [Rudolph *Matas*, U.S. surgeon, 1860–1957] See under TEST, TREATMENT, BAND, OPERATION.

matching **1** Comparison, selection, or adjustment for compatibility or similarity. **2** A reduction in the effects of an impedance difference at a boundary by inserting a material of intermediate impedance value.

impedance matching Assistance to the passage of sound waves across an interface between media of different acoustic impedance such as is provided by the transformer mechanism of the middle ear to the passage of sound waves from air to the inner ear fluids.

suprathreshold matching In psychophysical testing, the selection of similar stimuli, both of which are of an intensity above that at which the stimulus can first be perceived.

Mátéfy [Ladislaus *Mátéfy*, Hungarian physician, born 1889] Mátéfy's reaction. See under TEST.

materia [L (from *mater* mother; Gk *mētēr* mother), matter, stuff, wood, timber, source; also MATERIES] Matter; substance.

materia alba A soft whitish deposit on the teeth consisting of food debris, desquamated cells, and unorganized microorganisms. It is easily washed away with a water spray. This deposit has been confused with dental plaque. Also called *rhyparia* (outmoded).

materia dentica The medicinal substances used in dentistry.

materia medica   The medical science that deals with the origin and preparation of drugs, their administration, and mode of action; pharmacology.

material [MATERIA + L *-alis* -AL]   The substance of which something is made or composed.

air-equivalent material   In radiology, any material having the same effective atomic number as air in respect to the absorption of x rays.

base material   Substance used for the base of an artificial denture, such as acrylic resin, or chrome-cobalt alloy.

cross-reacting material   A mutated form of an enzyme or other biologically active molecule that has lost biological activity but can be detected and quantitated by antibody to the native molecule. Such products have been very important in relating biological function to protein structure. Abbreviation: CRM

disclosing material   A silicone paste or a wax applied to the fitting surface of a denture to identify areas of pressure.

fissionable material   Material containing, as a major component, one or more elements whose nuclei are capable of dividing into two very roughly equal fragments, or of being stimulated to do so by bombardment with suitable subatomic projectiles (usually neutrons). The process entails conversion of some mass into a relatively huge amount of energy. The most important of the fissionable nuclides are uranium 235 and plutonium 239.

genetic material   **1** An imprecise term for GENE.   **2** DEOXYRIBONUCLEIC ACID.

impression material   One of the many substances used for taking impressions, such as plaster of Paris, alginate, hydrocolloid, compound, or elastomeric.

membranoid material   ARGYROPHILIC DEPOSIT.

plastic filling material   Any material used for filling a prepared dental cavity. It is inserted into the cavity in a plastic state and subsequently hardens.

target material   That material which is the object of bombardment by high energy subatomic particles for the purpose of producing nuclear reactions within the material.

tissue equivalent material   A material whose properties are similar in some manner, as in radiation absorption, to average human tissue.

trace material   An element which exists in extremely minute amounts in tissues or other materials.

materialization   PAIR PRODUCTION.

materies [see MATERIA.]   Substance.

materies morbi   The cause of a disease and the cause of the pathological changes it produces. An obsolete term.

maternal [Med L *maternal(is)* (from L *matern(us)* pertaining to a mother + *-alis* -AL) maternal]   **1** Of or pertaining to a mother; motherly.   **2** Derived or received from a mother.

maternity [Med L *maternitas* (from L *maternus* maternal, motherly, from *mater* mother; Gk *mētēr* mother; + L *-itas* -ITY) maternity, motherhood]   **1** The condition of being a mother; motherhood.   **2** An obstetric hospital.

flat maternity   Characterizing health insurance which provides a single reimbursement fee or benefit for all maternity-related services.

swap maternity   Characterizing health insurance which provides maternity benefits to new enrollees but terminates coverage on pregnancies in progress for enrollees whose coverage has ended.

switch maternity   Characterizing health insurance which provides maternity benefits only to employees who have husbands covered under their plan as a dependent.

maternohemotherapy [*matern(al)* + *o* + HEMO- + THERAPY]   The injection of infants with blood from their mothers, with the intention of transferring immunity to such diseases as tetanus, measles, or poliomyelitis.

Mathews [Joseph McDowell *Mathews*, U.S. physician, born 1847]   See under SPECULUM.

Mathieu [Albert *Mathieu*, French physician, 1855–1917]   Lancereaux-Mathieu disease, Mathieu's disease. See under ICTERIC LEPTOSPIROSIS.

matico   The leaves of *Piper angustifolium*, which have properties of an aromatic and stimulant. The leaves have been used as a hemostatic.

mating   **1** The union of a pair of individuals for the purpose of sexual reproduction. Mating usually involves individuals of different sex, but it may involve pairs of hermaphroditic forms.   **2** In bacteriology, the process in which a plasmid transfers part of the bacterial chromosome from donor to recipient cell; bacterial conjugation.

assortative mating   NONRANDOM MATING.

assorted mating   NONRANDOM MATING.

assortive mating   NONRANDOM MATING.

backcross mating   BACKCROSS.

disassortative mating   Nonrandom mating based on individual differences.

dissortative mating   Nonrandom mating based on the phenotypic differences in individuals.

half-sib mating   In experimental genetics, the mating of a male and female who have one common parent.

interrupted mating   A microbiologic technique used to demonstrate the order of entry of genes from an Hfr cell in bacterial conjugation, and also to map distances between genes directly, in units of time. Mating may be interrupted by using a blender or a vortex mixer, or by repeated passage through the narrow orifice of a pipette.

nonrandom mating   A mating situation in which the pairing combinations between individuals in a population are directed or controlled in some manner. Also called *assortative mating, assorted mating, assortive mating, assortment.*

random mating   A mating situation with no element of selectivity, a condition that occurs when mates are chosen at random, the probability of mating is the same for all members, all couples are equally fecund, and all offspring are equally viable. For statistical purposes these conditions may be accepted as being fulfilled in large human populations but not for small or isolated groups. Also called *panmixia, panmixis.*

matlazahuatl [Aztec (Mexican Indian)]   A Mexican term for EPIDEMIC LOUSE-BORNE TYPHUS.

matrass [French *matras* (from Middle French *matras* an arrow, from Gaulish *mataris* a javelin) a vase with long neck, used in chemistry]   A long-necked glass container that holds dry materials for heating.

matrical   Of or relating to a matrix. Also *matricial.*

matricaria   The flowering heads of *Matricaria chamomilla*, which contain an essential oil composed of ozulene and sesquiterpenes, and a bitter principle. The heads were previously used against worm infections, and their oil has been used for flavoring cigarette tobacco. Also called *chamomilla.*

matrices   Plural of MATRIX.

matricial   MATRICAL.

matricide [L *mater* (gen. *matris*) mother + -CIDE]   The act of killing one's mother.

matriclinous   MATROCLINOUS.

matrilineal   In cytoplasmic inheritance, the transmission of traits only through females.

matrix [L (from *mater* mother, in archaic L the uterus; Gk *mētēr* mother, in archaic Gk the uterus), a mold, bed, enclosing mass in which a thing is formed, female animal kept for breeding] (*plural* matrices) **1** The intercellular substance in a tissue. **2** A mold, for a dental restoration, in the form of a thin steel or plastic strip surrounding a tooth. **3** In dentistry, the female component of a precision attachment. Compare PATRIX. Adjective: matrical, matricial.

amalgam matrix A steel matrix used when inserting amalgam into a prepared dental cavity.

bone matrix The ground substance of bony tissue, which is composed of protein and mucopolysaccharide. As the bony tissue matures the content of collagen fibers and bone salt increases.

cartilaginous matrix A basic, homogeneous basophil substance of embryonic skeletal tissue in the center of which articular cartilage develops.

cytoplasmic matrix The fluid portion of the cytoplasm interspersed between the organelles, filaments, and tubules.

direct platinum matrix A platinum matrix which is made on a crown preparation in the mouth rather than on a die.

fluid matrix Any of the fluids that bathe tissue, including blood plasma and lymph.

hair matrix The germinative layer of the epithelium of the hair follicles. Also called *hair germ.*

interterritorial matrix The general cartilage matrix except for the more basophilic areas around groups of cartilage cells.

mesangial matrix A mesh in the space between the renal glomerular capillary loops, formed from material similar to that of the capillary basement membrane. Mesangial cells are scattered in the matrix, which is made up of a homogeneous substance probably composed of mucopolysaccharides and glycoproteins. The matrix also contains filaments related to collagen. The mesangial cells are phagocytic, while the matrix is permeable to substances of large molecular size or to aggregates which may become localized in the matrix as deposits.

mitochondrial matrix The contents of the inner compartment of the mitochondrion. The cristae of the inner membrane partially divide the matrix into compartments. The composition of the matrix is maintained by selective pumps in the inner membrane. Soluble enzymes of the citric acid cycle are contained within the matrix.

nail matrix MATRIX UNGUIS.

nuclear matrix The translucent material between the various chromatin granules and filaments within the nucleus.

plastic matrix A matrix made of transparent, flexible plastic material. It is used when inserting a silicate cement or composite filling material.

platinum matrix A base of platinum foil, usually made on a die, used in the firing of a porcelain complete veneer crown. It is removed from the finished crown by solution in strong acid.

sarcoplasmic matrix The fluid portion of the cytoplasm of a muscle cell, containing the soluble enzymes.

T-band matrix A steel mold for fillings in the form of an elongated T. The short arms are folded to make a slot into which the long arm is inserted so that no matrix holder is required.

territorial matrix The basophilic cartilage matrix around a group of cartilage cells.

matrix unguis [NA] The modified corium and the germinative zone upon which the body and root of the nail rest. It has longitudinal vascular ridges homologous to dermal papillae. Also called *nail matrix, nail bed, lactulum unguis, keratogenous membrane* (outmoded), *onychostroma.*

matroclinous Of, pertaining to, or designating an offspring influenced by matrocliny or exhibiting inheritance as in matrocliny. Also *matriclinous.*

matrocliny Any mode of inheritance in which the offspring predictably resemble the female parent more than the male parent, as in hologynic inheritance. Compare PATROCLINY.

matron [L *matron(a)* (from *mater,* gen. *matris,* a mother) a wife, matron] The chief nursing officer in a small hospital with total responsibility for nursing services and supervisory responsibility for services other than medical services which directly affect patient care, such as catering and domestic services.

Matson [Donald Darrow *Matson,* U.S. neurosurgeon, 1913–1969] See under OPERATION.

matter [Old French *matere* or *matiere* (from L *materia* matter, stuff, wood, timber, source, from *mater* mother) substance] **1** Material substance. **2** Pus.

gelatinous matter SUBSTANTIA GELATINOSA. See under SUBSTANTIA GELATINOSA MEDULLAE SPINALIS ROLANDI.

gray matter SUBSTANTIA GRISEA.

gray matter of spinal cord SUBSTANTIA GRISEA MEDULLAE SPINALIS.

medullary white matter SUBSTANTIA ALBA.

organic matter **1** In ecology, the hydrocarbons which are formed and transformed in the food chain. **2** Material that is derived from plants and animals and is in the process of decomposition.

white matter SUBSTANTIA ALBA.

Mattioli-Foggia [Cesare *Mattioli-Foggia,* Italian pathologist, flourished mid-20th century] Mattioli-Foggia and Raso syndrome. See under FIBROLIPOCALCAREOUS MYOPATHY.

mattress / alternating pressure mattress RIPPLE MATTRESS.

divided mattress A mattress that is split, generally in the perineal area, so that excrement can be collected and removed.

ripple mattress A mattress consisting of transverse, inflatable tubes which are usually 5–12 cm in diameter. Alternate tubes are linked in series to a pump working on a fixed cycle so that each alternate tube is inflating while the tube next to it is deflating. Thus the area of compression between skin and mattress changes on a regular cycle, helping to prevent the formation of decubitus ulcers or bed sores. Also called *alternating pressure mattress.*

water mattress See under WATER BED.

maturant **1** An agent that promotes maturation. **2** An agent that brings about a maturation, or ripening, of a boil or an ovarian follicle.

maturate To suppurate or to come close to the point of spontaneous drainage of pus.

maturation [L *maturatio* (from *maturatus,* past part. of *maturare* to ripen, hasten, mature, from *maturus* ripe, mature, akin to *madidus* wet, steeped, tender, sufficiently cooked, to *mitis* tender, mellow, ripe, and to Gk *madan* to be moist, melt away) a hastening, ripening] **1** The division of gonadal cells to produce an ovum or sperm cells, which have half the chromosome number characteristic of the somatic cells of the species. **2** The process of reaching full development or maturity. See also MATURATION-DEVELOPMENT.

biologic maturation The structural and functional development of a biologic system, as the central nervous system, the sensory organs, the musculoskeletal system, and the reproductive organs.

maturation of the fetus The morphologic and physiologic development of the fetus up to the time of birth. A fetus is called "mature" when all such processes have reached certain stages in their completion compatible with the independent existence of the neonate, and "immature" when they have not. Immaturity of the neonate should be related to its age, but certain adverse conditions may also affect development.

maturation-development The process by which children, concomitant with the biologic maturation of the body, pass by stages, at predictable times, from the condition of newborn helplessness to independence, with socialization and the power of abstract reasoning. The infant moves in one year from primitive type of motor response when newly born to the complex pattern required for upright posture, and then to highly complex skills in the next three years, acquiring at the same time fluent use of language, control of bowel and bladder, control of aggression, use of memory, and ability to solve problems. Developmental attainment can be assessed at any age by tests and reference to norms. Brain-damaged children mature at a much slower rate and cease developing earlier than normal children. Also called *postnatal development.*

mature   **1** Fully developed, as an ovum following meiosis; ripe. **2** To reach full development; ripen.   **3** Having reached puberty.

maturity [L *matur(itas)*, from *matur(us)* ripe, mature + *-itas* -ITY. See MATURATION.] **1** Puberty.   **2** The state of completed growth.   **3** The gestational age or stage of development of a fetus or newborn infant.

matut.   *matutinus* (L, in the morning).

Mauchart [Burkhard David *Mauchart*, German anatomist, 1696–1751] Mauchart's ligaments. See under LIGAMENTA ALARIA.

Maunoir [Jean Pierre *Maunoir*, Swiss surgeon, 1768–1861] Maunoir's hydrocele. See under BRANCHIAL CYST.

Maurer [Georg *Maurer*, German physician active in Sumatra] Maurer's clefts, Maurer spots, Maurer stippling. See under MAURER'S DOTS.

Mauriac [Leonard Pierre *Mauriac*, French physician, born 1882] See under SYNDROME.

Mauriceau [François *Mauriceau*, French obstetrician, 1637–1709] **1** See under MANEUVER, LANCE.   **2** Mauriceau-Smellie-Veit maneuver. See under MANEUVER.

Mauthner [Ludwig *Mauthner*, Austrian ophthalmologist, 1840–1894] **1** See under CELL, FIBER, TEST.   **2** Mauthner's membrane, Mauthner sheath. See under AXOLEMMA.

MAVIS   mobile artery and vein imaging system.

max   maximum.

Maxcy [Kenneth Fuller *Maxcy*, U.S. bacteriologist, 1889–1966] Maxcy's disease. See under FLEA-BORNE TYPHUS.

maxicell   A cell in which the chromosomal genes have been inactivated by irradiation and the products of plasmids can then be selectively formed.

maxilla [L (dim. of *mala* the cheekbone, jawbone), the jawbone, jaw (upper and lower)]   (*plural* maxillae) [NA] One of a pair of facial bones that is irregular in shape, supports the upper teeth, and takes part in the formation of the orbit, nasal cavity and hard palate, as well as the infratemporal and pterygopalatine fossae. The central body contains a sinus. Superiorly, the frontal and zygomatic processes project; inferiorly are the palatine and alveolar processes. Also called *myle* (outmoded), *upper jaw, upper jaw bone, superior maxillary bone, maxillary bone, supermaxilla* (outmoded), *supramaxilla* (outmoded).

first maxillae   The most anterior pair of head appendages of annelids, arthropods, and related phyla, part of the oral complex used for food grasping and feeding. In crustaceans, they occur usually as the third pair of appendages, in millipedes as the fourth pair.

inferior maxilla   An outmoded term for MANDIBULA.

maxillae   Plural of MAXILLA.

maxillary   Pertaining to the maxilla.

maxillectomy [*maxill(a)* + -ECTOMY]   The surgical removal of the maxilla or part of it.

maxillitis   An inflammation of the maxilla.

maxillodental   Pertaining to the maxilla and the upper teeth.

maxillofacial [*maxill(a)* + *o* + FACIAL]   Relating to both the face and the jaws, but more particularly to the face and upper jaw.

maxillofrontale [L *maxill(a)* (dim. of *mala* cheekbone, jawbone) jawbone, jaw + *o* + New L *frontale*, neut. sing. of *frontalis* frontal]   A craniometric point situated at the sutural junction of the maxilla and the frontal and lacrimal bones.

maxillojugal   Pertaining to the maxilla and the cheek, or zygomatic bone.

maxillolabial   Of or relating to the maxilla and the lip.

maxillolacrimal   Pertaining to the maxilla and the lacrimal bone.

maxillomandibular   Pertaining to the maxilla and the mandible.

maxillopalatine   Of or relating to the maxilla and the palatine bone.

maxillopharyngeal   PHARYNGOMAXILLARY.

maxillotomy [*maxill(a)* + *o* + -TOMY]   MAXILLARY OSTEOTOMY.

maxima   Plural of MAXIMUM.

maximal   Being or related to a maximum; greatest or most. Also *maximum.*

Maximow [Alexander Alexandrovich *Maximow*, Russian-born histologist active in Germany and the United States, 1874–1928] **1** See under FIXATIVE.   **2** Maximow's method. See under HEMATOXYLIN-EOSIN-AZURE II STAIN.

maximum [L (neut. of *maximus* the greatest, most; superl. of *magnus* great), the largest amount]   (*plural* maximums, maxima) **1** The greatest or greatest possible degree or quantity. Abbreviation: max   **2** MAXIMAL.

excretory tubular transport maximum   The greatest quantity of a substance that can be excreted in unit time by the renal tubular excretory mass.

glucose transport maximum   The greatest quantity of glucose that can be transported across a biological membrane in unit time.

reabsorptive tubular transport maximum   The greatest quantity of a substance that can be reabsorbed in unit time by the total of the renal tubules.

transport maximum   The maximum rate at which the renal tubules can secrete or reabsorb a substance. Symbol: Tm

tubular maximum   The greatest rate at which the renal tubules can excrete or reabsorb substances.

tubular reabsorption maximum   The maximum rate in milligrams per minute at which a substance filtered by the glomerulus can be actively reabsorbed by the renal tubules. For example, as the plasma glucose level increases so does the filtered glucose load, and the rate of tubular glucose reabsorption is exceeded. The reabsorption maximum is calculated by the difference between glucose filtered per minute and the amount excreted in the bladder urine per minute. The reabsorption maximum for glucose reflects the proximal convoluted tubular mass. Inorganic sulfate, inorganic phosphate, and some amino acids also have reabsorption maxima.

Maxipen   A proprietary name for phenethicillin potassium.

Maxitate   A proprietary name for mannitol hexanitrate.

Maxwell [Alice Freeland *Maxwell*, U.S. obstetrician and gynecologist, 1890–1961] Goldberg-Maxwell syndrome. See under TESTICULAR FEMINIZATION.

Maxwell [James Laidlow *Maxwell*, English physician active in Formosa, 1836–1921] MacLean-Maxwell syndrome. See under MACLEAN-MAXWELL DISEASE.

Maxwell [Patrick William *Maxwell*, Irish ophthalmologist, 1856–1917] See under RING, SPOT.

maxwell [after James Clerk *Maxwell*, Scottish physicist, 1831–1879]   A CGS electromagnetic unit of magnetic flux, equal to

10^{-8} weber. An obsolete unit. Symbol: Mx

May [Richard *May*, German physician, 1863–1936] **1** May-Hegglin anomaly. See under ANOMALY. **2** May-Grünwald stain. See under STAIN.

mayapple   MANDRAKE.

Maydl [Karel *Maydl*, Czech surgeon, 1853–1903]   See under OPERATION.

Mayer [Carl *Mayer*, Austrian neurologist, 1862–1932]   Mayer's reflex. See under FINGER-THUMB REFLEX.

Mayer [Karl Wilhelm *Mayer*, German gynecologist, 1795–1868] See under PESSARY.

Mayer [Paul *Mayer*, German chemist, 1848–1923]   **1** Mayer solution. See under MAYER'S HEMALUM.   **2** See under MUCI-HEMATEIN.   **3** Mayer mucicarmine stain. See under STAIN.   **4** Mayer's mucicarmine. See under MUCICARMINE.

mayer [after Julius Robert von *Mayer*, German physicist, 1814–1878]   A unit of specific heat capacity equal to one joule per gram-degree or 10^3 joules per kilogram kelvin. An obsolete unit. Symbol: mayer

mayfly [*May* + *fly*]   An insect of the order Ephemeroptera. These abundant insects breed in fresh water and represent significant elements of the food of birds, bats, trout, and other insectivorous animals. See also EPHEMERIDAE.

mayhem [Middle English *maym, mayme, maheym*, from Middle French *mahaing, main, mahaim* a disabling, maiming]   **1** The violent act or acts committed by one person against another resulting in actual or functional loss of any organ, limb, or member, such that the loss rendered the injured person less able to fight. An outmoded legal usage, but of historic importance. **2** An act resulting in disfigurement of survivors of violence or postmortem mutilation of nonsurvivors.

mayidism [irreg. from Spanish *maíz* maize + ISM]   An obsolete term for PELLAGRA.

Mayo [Charles Horace *Mayo*, U.S. physician, 1865–1939] Mayo's treatment. See under METHOD.

Mayo [William James *Mayo*, U.S. surgeon, 1861–1939]   **1** Quénu-Mayo operation. See under OPERATION.   **2** Mayo's operation. See under OPERATION.   **3** Mayo's vein. See under VENA PREPYLORICA.

Mayor [Mathias Louis *Mayor*, Swiss surgeon, 1775–1847]   See under SCARF.

Mayo-Robson [Sir Arthur William *Mayo-Robson*, English surgeon, 1853–1933]   Mayo-Robson position. See under ROBSON'S POSITION.

Mayou [Marmaduke Stephen *Mayou*, English ophthalmologist, 1876–1934]   Batten-Mayou disease. See under BATTEN DISEASE.

maypop   PASSION FLOWER.

maza [New L, placenta, from Gk *maza* (from *massein* to knead) barley bread, barley cake]   PLACENTA. Adjective: mazic.

maze [Middle English *maze, mase*]   A labyrinth for observing learning in human or animal subjects. It consists of a series of pathways between a starting point and a goal, usually with only one path leading from the start to the finish, all alternate branches being blind alleys. Learning is measured by the time needed to reach the goal, or by the number of errors made, or by some combination of those two over a series of trials until performance becomes error-free.

radiation maze   An arrangement of protective walls and corridors leading to a room containing a radiation source.

T maze   A device for observing learning in animal or human subjects consisting of a starting point and a pathway from it in the shape of the letter T. A turn in the correct direction leads to the goal and a reward, while choosing the other arm is an error leading only into a blind alley. Multiple T mazes combine

a series of such units, each in the shape of a T.

mazindol $C_{16}H_{13}ClN_2O$. 5-(4-Chlorophenyl)-2,5-dihydro-3*H*-imidazo[2,1-*a*]isoindol-5-ol. A compound that stimulates the central nervous system and has properties similar to those of amphetamine. It is used as an anorexic drug in the treatment of obesity.

mazo- [Gk *mazos* a woman's breast]   A combining form denoting the breast.

mazodynia [*maz(o)-* + *-ODYNIA*]   MASTODYNIA.

mazopexy   MASTOPEXY.

mazoplasia   MAMMOPLASIA.

Mazzini [Louis Y. *Mazzini*, U.S. serologist, born 1894]   See under TEST.

Mazzoni [Vittorio *Mazzoni*, Italian physiologist, 1880–1940]   **1** Golgi-Mazzoni corpuscles. See under GOLGI-MAZZONI ENDINGS.   **2** See under CORPUSCLE.

M.B.   *Medicinae Baccalaureus* (L, Bachelor of Medicine).

mb   Symbol for the unit, millibar, used especially in meteorology.

m.b.   *misce bene* (L, mix well).

μb   Symbol for the unit, microbar. An incorrect symbol.

mbar   Symbol for the unit, millibar.

μbar   Symbol for the unit, microbar.

MBC   maximum breathing capacity.

MBD   minimal brain dysfunction.

MBP   mean blood pressure.

MBq   Symbol for the unit, megabecquerel.

MC   **1** Symbol for the unit, metric carat. A British usage.   **2** Symbol for the unit, megacoulomb.

mC   Symbol for the unit, millicoulomb.

μC   Symbol for the unit, microcoulomb.

μc.   Symbol for the unit, microcurie. An outmoded symbol.

McAlpine [Douglas *McAlpine*, English neurologist, born 1890]   Lhermitte-McAlpine syndrome. See under SYNDROME.

McArdle [Brian *McArdle*, English neurologist, flourished 20th century]   McArdle's disease, McArdle's syndrome. See under GLYCOGEN STORAGE DISEASE.

McArthur [Louis Linn *McArthur*, U.S. surgeon, 1858–1934]   See under INCISION.

McBurney [Charles *McBurney*, U.S. surgeon, 1845–1913]   See under OPERATION, SIGN, INCISION, POINT.

McCarthy [Daniel J. *McCarthy*, U.S. neurologist, 1874–1958]   **1** McCarthy's reflex. See under SUPRAORBITAL REFLEX.   **2** See under SIGN.

McCarthy [Joseph Francis *McCarthy*, U.S. urologist, 1874–1965]   **1** McCarthy's panendoscope. See under PANENDOSCOPE.   **2** McCarthy's electrotome. See under MCCARTHY'S RESECTOSCOPE.

McClintock [Alfred Henry *McClintock*, Irish physician, 1822–1881]   See under SIGN.

McCollum [Estel Bertrum *McCollum*, U.S. physician, born 1903]   See under TUBE.

McCune [Donovan James *McCune*, U.S. pediatrician, born 1902]   McCune-Albright syndrome, Albright-McCune-Sternberg syndrome. See under ALBRIGHT'S DISEASE.

McDonald [Ellice *McDonald*, U.S. gynecologist, 1876–1955]   See under MANEUVER, RULE.

MCF   macrophage chemotactic factor.

McGill [A. F. *McGill*, English surgeon, 1846–1890]   McGill's operation. See under SUPRAPUBIC TRANSVESICAL PROSTATECTOMY.

McGoon [Dwight Charles *McGoon*, U.S. heart surgeon, born 1925]   See under TECHNIQUE.

MCH   mean corpuscular hemoglobin.

mc-h   Symbol for the unit, millicurie-hour. An outmoded symbol.

mc.h.   Symbol for the unit, millicurie-hour. An outmoded symbol.

MCHC   mean corpuscular hemoglobin concentration.

MCHg   mean corpuscular hemoglobin.

mc-hr   Symbol for the unit, millicurie-hour. An outmoded and incorrect symbol.

MCi   Symbol for the unit, megacurie.

mCi   Symbol for the unit, millicurie.

mCiδ   Symbol for the unit, millicurie destroyed.

μCi   Symbol for the unit, microcurie.

mCi·h   Symbol for the unit, millicurie-hour.

μCi·h   Symbol for the unit, microcurie-hour.

McKee [George Kenneth *McKee*, British orthopedic surgeon, born 1930] See under LINE.

McKesson [Elmer Isaac *McKesson*, U.S. anesthetist, 1881–1935] See under APPARATUS.

McKinnon [Neil E. *McKinnon*, Canadian physician, born 1894] See under TEST.

MCL   midclavicular line.

McLean [Franklin Chambers *McLean*, U.S. physician, born 1888] McLean and Van Slyke method. See under METHOD.

McLean [John Milton *McLean*, U.S. ophthalmologist, born 1909] See under TONOMETER.

McLean [Malcolm *McLean*, U.S. obstetrician, 1848–1924] Tucker-McLean forceps. See under FORCEPS.

McMurray [Thomas Porter *McMurray*, English orthopedic surgeon, 1887–1949] **1** McMurray's circumduction maneuver. See under MANEUVER. **2** McMurray's test. See under SIGN.

McNeal [Ward J. *McNeal*, U.S. bacteriologist, 1881–1946] **1** Novy, McNeal and Nicolle medium. See under MEDIUM. **2** Novy and MacNeal blood agar. See under AGAR.

McNemar [Quinn *McNemar*, U.S. psychologist and statistician, born 1900] See under TEST.

mcoul   Symbol for the unit, millicoulomb. An incorrect symbol.

McPhail [Murchie Kilburn *McPhail*, Canadian physiologist, born 1907] See under TEST.

McPheeters [Herman Oscar *McPheeters*, U.S. surgeon, born 1891] See under TREATMENT.

Mc.p.s.   Symbol for the unit, megacycle per second. An incorrect symbol.

MCR   metabolic clearance rate.

Mc/s   Symbol for the unit, megacycle per second.

MCT   mean circulation time.

MCV   mean corpuscular volume.

McVay [Chester Bidwell *McVay*, U.S. surgeon, born 1911] See under OPERATION.

M.D.   *Medicinae Doctor* (L, Doctor of Medicine).

Md   Symbol for the element, mendelevium.

MDA   **1** mentum dexter anterior (a fetal position). **2** methylenedioxyamphetamine.

MDR   minimum daily requirement.

Mdyn   Symbol for the unit, megadyne.

Me   methyl.

MEA   multiple endocrine adenomatosis (multiple endocrine neoplasia).

meal [Old English *mæl* mealtime] A given quantity of foods taken at set times during the day.

    barium meal An emulsion or suspension of barium sulfate taken orally by a patient undergoing roentgenography of the upper gastrointestinal tract.

    bismuth meal An outmoded opaque meal, containing a bismuth salt.

    Boyden test meal A motor meal for testing the evacuation time of the gallbladder: it contains three or four egg yolks combined with milk and seasoning.

    butter meal A highly nutritious food containing butter, milk, flour, and sugar.

    Ewald's test meal A meal for testing gastric function: it consists of two rolls or slices of dry bread and 270 to 360 ml of water.

    Knoepfelmacher's butter meal A food consisting of butter, flour, milk, and sugar and which is given to children.

    liver meal A preparation consisting of dessicated beef liver, malted milk, and powdered cinnamon.

    motor meal A test meal administered to determine the progress of substances through some part of the digestive tract. It usually contains radiopaque material for roentgenographic observation.

    opaque meal A light solid or liquid meal containing a radiopaque contrast medium, usually barium sulfate, for roentgenographic examination of the stomach and intestinal tract.

    Schmidt's meal A meal consisting primarily of raw chopped meat, formerly used as a test of digestive function of the stomach based upon the fact that when gastric secretion is greatly diminished, connective tissue masses appear in the stool after eating raw chopped meats.

    test meal A meal containing specified amounts of specified substances which is used in the diagnostic evaluation of the stomach or small intestine, either radiographically or by later analysis of the gastric or intestinal contents obtained by peroral intubation and aspiration.

meals-on-wheels A program to provide meals to individuals in their homes who are unable to cook for themselves and might otherwise require institutional care. A term used chiefly in the U.S., Canada, the United Kingdom, Australia, and New Zealand.

mean An average of a set of values. • Without qualification, the term always refers to the arithmetic mean.

    arithmetic mean The ratio of the sum of the terms in a statistical series to their number. Also called *average*.

    geometric mean A value indicating the central tendency of a statistical series of *n* terms, equal to the positive *n*th root of their product. The geometric mean cannot be calculated if the series contains a negative or a zero term. The geometric mean is less than the arithmetic mean.

    harmonic mean For a given set of values, the reciprocal of the mean of the reciprocals of the individual values. Thus, the harmonic mean of the set 10, 20, 50 is

$$\cfrac{1}{\dfrac{1}{3} + \left(\dfrac{1}{10} + \dfrac{1}{20} + \dfrac{1}{50}\right)} = 17.65 \ .$$

    weighted mean WEIGHTED ARITHMETIC MEAN.

    weighted arithmetic mean The ratio of the sum of the products of each term in a statistical series and an appropriate factor, or weight, to the sum of the weights. The use of weights in calculating the mean takes into account the relative importance of each term. Also called *weighted mean*.

Means [James H. *Means*, U.S. physician, 1885–1967] **1** See under SIGN. **2** Lerman-Means scratch. See under SCRATCH.

means / best practicable means A requirement, according to applicable legislation of the United Kingdom and some other countries, that industrial establishments use the most effective method available to reduce the discharge of pollutants, subject to economic and technical feasibility.

measle [See MEASLES.]   CYSTICERCUS.

measles [Middle English *meseles*, pl. of *mesel* measles; Dutch *maselen*, dim. of *masa* a spot]   **1** A highly contagious viral disease caused by a paramyxovirus (measle virus) and occurring chiefly in young children. An incubation period of 10–14 days precedes the prodrome in which fever, coryza, cough, conjunctivitis, and malaise occur. Koplik spots, blue-gray spots with a red areola, appear on the buccal membranes at the end of the prodrome and are virtually pathognomonic of measles. An erythematous, maculopapular rash spreading downward from the head and face to the trunk and limbs then erupts and lasts about five days. Complications include pneumonia, otitis media, and subacute sclerosing panencephalitis. The disease is especially severe in tropical regions of west Africa and Central and South America, and malnourished children living in these areas may be most seriously affected. Recovery from measles confers immunity. A live measles vaccine is available. Also called *rubeola, morbilli*.   **2** Infection of cattle or swine by encysted larval tapeworms, producing measly meat.

bastard measles   RUBELLA.

black measles   HEMORRHAGIC MEASLES.

confluent measles   Measles in which the lesions of the rash merge.

French measles   RUBELLA.

German measles   RUBELLA.

hemorrhagic measles   A severe form of measles in which the rash is extremely dark and petechial due to hemorrhages into the skin. Also called *black measles*.

three-day measles   RUBELLA.

measly [*measl(e)* + -Y]   Infected with cysticerci, the larval stage of the cestode *Taenia*, as in *measly pork* (infected with *T. solium* larvae) and *measly beef* (with *T. saginata*).

measurand   A physical quantity, property, or condition that is to be measured.

measure [L *mensura* (from *mensus*, past part. of *metiri* to measure, akin to Gk *metron* a measure, rule) a measuring, amount]   **1** To ascertain the magnitude of (a physical quantity) by comparison to some accepted standard or by calculation.   **2** A specified or standard magnitude of a physical quantity.   **3** A graduated instrument used to measure an object or substance.

input measure   A measure of the quality of health services based on the number, type, and quality of resources used in the production of the services.

outcome measure   A measure of the quality of health care in which the standard of judgment is the attainment of specified results from the care, such as changes in health status, recovery from illness, or change in ability to function.

output measures   Qualitative or quantitative indicators of the results of producing health care services, often in relation to the resources used in providing care.

photometric measure   Any measure of the energy of light that is expressed in terms of its relative effect on the visual receptors, rather than in purely physical units, or by the magnitude of the sensation evoked.

process measure   An indicator of the quality of health care which measures or documents the activities of health care providers and programs in managing patient care.

structural measure   An indicator of the quality of health care which measures or documents the organization, administrative arrangements and relationships, and physical setup for providing health care services.

measurement   **1** The act or process of measuring.   **2** A result of measuring, as a dimension of something measured.

azimuth measurement   The ability of a subject to identify the angular location of a suprathreshold sound stimulus at points around the circumference of a horizontal circle centered on the head. Also called *localization audiometry* (incorrect).

end-point measurement   The quantitation of a substance performed by measuring the change in a variable after the completion of the chemical reaction. Compare KINETIC MEASUREMENT.

kinetic measurement   The quantitation of a substance, usually an enzyme, performed by monitoring the changes in absorbance over time, either continuously or at frequent intervals. Compare END-POINT MEASUREMENT.

mental measurement   The measurement of mental phenomena, or the externally observable behavior representing such events, by an application either of mental tests or of psychophysical methods. It is used most often to describe individual differences, with responses of different subjects assigned a position on a common quantitative scale.

real-time measurement   **1** A measurement made at the actual time that a physical process takes place. This is required in a control system so that no delay occurs in supplying corrective action.   **2** A measurement made at normal system operating speed or frequency as distinguished from slowed down operation.

skinfold measurements   Determinations of the thickness of a fold of skin using calipers. The skin is pinched into a fold with the sides parallel and calipers exerting a pressure of ten grams per square millimeter are applied. Measurements at four specified sites are used to assess body fat content: the triceps, at a point midway between the tip of the acromion and the olecranon; subscapular, immediately beneath the inferior angle of the scapular; the biceps, at the midpoint of the muscle with the arm hanging vertically; and, suprailiac, over the iliac crest in the midaxillary line. Standard tables are available relating skinfold thickness to body fat as a percentage of body weight according to age and sex. Measurements at a single site provide less accurate assessment of body fat.

meatal   Of or relating to a meatus.

meatitis   Inflammation of the tissues of a meatus.

ulcerative meatitis   A common affection of the urinary meatus caused by various microorganisms, resulting in reddening of the meatus with vesiculation.

meato- [L *meatus* a going, passage, passing]   A combining form denoting meatus.

meatome   MEATOTOME.

meatometer [MEATO- + -METER]   An apparatus devised to measure a meatus, especially the urinary meatus.

meatoplasty [MEATO- + -PLASTY]   Reconstructive surgery of the meatus, usually the external auditory meatus. The procedure requires the use of flaps of meatal skin.

Körner's meatoplasty   A modification of Stacke's meatoplasty in which a rectangular flap composed of meatal and conchal skin, hinged proximally, is turned in to line the outer aspect of the mastoid cavity and enlarge the entrance to the meatus.

Panse's meatoplasty   A modification of Stacke's meatoplasty in which the skin of the posterior meatal wall is fashioned into two flaps, one hinged superiorly and the other inferiorly.

Siebenmann's meatoplasty   A modification of Stacke's meatoplasty in which three flaps are raised by incising the posterior meatal wall in the form of a Y, the diverging limbs extending into the concha.

Stacke's meatoplasty   A type of meatoplasty used as the final stage of the radical mastoidectomy operation. A large rectangular flap of meatal skin, hinged inferiorly, is turned back to line the floor of the mastoid cavity.

meatorrhaphy [MEATO- + -RRHAPHY] The suturing of the urethral membrane to the glans penis following surgery to enlarge the urinary meatus.

meatoscope [MEATO- + -SCOPE] An instrument used to inspect the urinary meatus.

meatoscopy [MEATO- + -SCOPY] Meatus examination with a meatoscope.

ureteral meatoscopy Examination of the ureteral orifice with a cystoscope.

meatotome [MEATO- + -TOME] A surgical instrument used to incise and enlarge the urinary meatus. Also called *meatome*.

meatotomy [MEATO- + -TOMY] An incision of a meatus, as the urinary meatus, to increase its diameter. Also called *porotomy*.

meatus [L (from *meatus*, past part. of *meare* to go, pass), a going, motion, path, way] An opening to a canal or passage in the body.

acoustic meatus 1 MEATUS ACUSTICUS EXTERNUS. **2** MEATUS ACUSTICUS INTERNUS.

meatus acusticus externus [NA] The S-shaped canal of the external ear leading from the concha of the auricle to the tympanic membrane. It comprises an outer cartilaginous portion and an inner bony portion, and it has constrictions about midway and near the membrane. It is lined by skin which continues on to the tympanic membrane. Also called *external acoustic meatus, external auditory meatus, meatus auditorius externus* (outmoded), *auricular canal, acoustic meatus, external auditory foramen, acoustic duct, external auditory canal, external acoustic canal, auricular tube* (outmoded).

meatus acusticus externus cartilagineus [NA] The outer one third of the external acoustic meatus, composed of fibrocartilage and shaped like a trough, the deficient posterosuperior part being filled by collagen and the anterior part having two or more fissures. Laterally it is continuous with the auricular cartilage and medially it is attached to the bony part by fibrous tissue. The lining skin contains fine hairs and sebaceous and ceruminous glands. Also called *cartilaginous external acoustic meatus, meatus auditorius externus cartilagineus* (outmoded), *cartilaginous external auditory meatus*.

meatus acusticus externus osseus The medial two thirds of the external acoustic meatus, located in the temporal bone and connecting the cartilaginous portion, to which it is attached by fibrous tissue, to the tympanic cavity. At its narrow, oblique, medial end is the incomplete tympanic sulcus to which the circumference of the tympanic membrane is attached. The adherent lining skin is devoid of hair and glands. Also called *bony external acoustic meatus, meatus auditorius externus osseus* (outmoded), *bony external auditory meatus*.

meatus acusticus internus [NA] A short canal above the anterior part of the jugular foramen in the petrous part of the temporal bone transmitting the facial, intermediate and vestibulocochlear nerves and the labyrinthine vessels, and extending from the internal acoustic opening near the apex of the posterior surface of the bone to the fundus, where a plate of bone pierced by foramina separates the meatus from the internal ear. Also called *internal acoustic meatus, meatus auditorius internus, internal auditory meatus, acoustic meatus, internal auditory canal, internal acoustic canal.*

meatus acusticus internus osseus The canal leading from the opening, or porus, on the posterior surface of the petrous part of the temporal bone near its apex. Through it passes the facial, intermediate, and vestibulocochlear nerves and the labyrinthine vessels. It ends at the fundus, where it is separated by the cribriform plate from the vestibule of the internal ear. Also called *bony internal acoustic meatus, meatus auditorius internus osseus* (outmoded), *bony internal auditory meatus*.

meatus auditorius externus An outmoded term for MEATUS ACUSTICUS EXTERNUS.

meatus auditorius externus cartilagineus An outmoded term for MEATUS ACUSTICUS EXTERNUS CARTILAGINEUS.

meatus auditorius externus osseus An outmoded term for MEATUS ACUSTICUS EXTERNUS OSSEUS.

meatus auditorius internus MEATUS ACUSTICUS INTERNUS.

meatus auditorius internus osseus An outmoded term for MEATUS ACUSTICUS INTERNUS OSSEUS.

bony common nasal meatus MEATUS NASI COMMUNIS OSSEUS.

bony external acoustic meatus MEATUS ACUSTICUS EXTERNUS OSSEUS.

bony external auditory meatus MEATUS ACUSTICUS EXTERNUS OSSEUS.

bony inferior nasal meatus MEATUS NASI INFERIOR OSSEUS.

bony internal acoustic meatus MEATUS ACUSTICUS INTERNUS OSSEUS.

bony internal auditory meatus MEATUS ACUSTICUS INTERNUS OSSEUS.

bony middle nasal meatus MEATUS NASI MEDIUS OSSEUS.

bony nasopharyngeal meatus MEATUS NASOPHARYNGEUS OSSEUS.

bony superior nasal meatus MEATUS NASI SUPERIOR OSSEUS.

cartilaginous external acoustic meatus MEATUS ACUSTICUS EXTERNUS CARTILAGINEUS.

cartilaginous external auditory meatus MEATUS ACUSTICUS EXTERNUS CARTILAGINEUS.

common meatus of nose MEATUS NASI COMMUNIS.

meatus conchae ethmoturbinalis minoris An outmoded term for MEATUS NASI SUPERIOR.

meatus conchae maxilloturbinalis An outmoded term for MEATUS NASI INFERIOR.

meatus conchae turbinalis majoris An outmoded term for MEATUS NASI INFERIOR.

external acoustic meatus MEATUS ACUSTICUS EXTERNUS.

external auditory meatus MEATUS ACUSTICUS EXTERNUS.

fish-mouth meatus An inflamed and inverted urinary meatus evident in gonorrhea.

inferior nasal meatus MEATUS NASI INFERIOR.

internal acoustic meatus MEATUS ACUSTICUS INTERNUS.

internal auditory meatus MEATUS ACUSTICUS INTERNUS.

middle nasal meatus MEATUS NASI MEDIUS.

meatus nasi communis The space between the nasal conchae and the nasal septum into which the nasal meatuses open. An outmoded term. Also called *common meatus of nose.*

meatus nasi communis osseus The space between the bony nasal septum medially and the superior and medial nasal conchae of the ethmoid bone and the inferior nasal concha laterally into which the bony nasal meatuses open. An outmoded term. Also called *bony common nasal meatus.*

meatus nasi inferior [NA] The space between the arched inferior nasal concha superiorly and the floor of the nose inferiorly. The nasolacrimal duct opens into the anterior portion of its lateral wall. Also called *inferior nasal meatus, meatus conchae maxilloturbinalis* (outmoded), *meatus conchae turbinalis majoris* (outmoded).

meatus nasi inferior osseus The space between the bony inferior nasal concha and the floor of the nose, formed by the palatine process of the maxilla and the horizontal plate of the palatine bone. In the anterior part of its lateral wall is the inferior opening of the nasolacrimal canal. Also called *bony inferior nasal meatus.*

meatus nasi medius [NA] The passage under cover of the middle nasal concha, deeper anteriorly than posteriorly and continuous anteriorly with the atrium. On its lateral wall is the rounded bulla ethmoidalis, anterior and inferior to which is the curved hiatus semilunaris and the openings of the anterior and middle ethmoidal sinuses. Into the anterior end, or infundibulum, the frontonasal duct opens while near the roof is the opening of the maxillary sinus. Also called *middle nasal meatus.*

meatus nasi medius osseus   The bony passage between the middle and inferior nasal conchae which contains a curved groove (the hiatus semilunaris) bounded by the bulla ethmoidalis above, the uncinate process of the ethmoid bone below, and continuous anteriorly with the ethmoidal infundibulum. The anterior and middle ethmoidal sinuses, the inferior opening of the frontal sinus, and the maxillary sinus open into the passage. Also called *osseous middle meatus of nose, bony middle nasal meatus.*

meatus nasi superior   [NA] A short, narrow passage located partly under the superior nasal concha and extending above the middle nasal concha for about half its length. The posterior ethmoidal sinuses open into the anterior end, usually by way of a single aperture. Also called *superior nasal meatus, meatus conchae ethmoturbinalis minoris* (outmoded), *ethmoid fissure* (outmoded).

meatus nasi superior osseus   The short, narrow passage between the bony superior and middle nasal conchae into which open the posterior cells of the ethmoidal sinus, usually by a single opening. Also called *bony superior nasal meatus, osseous superior meatus of nose.*

nasopharyngeal meatus   MEATUS NASOPHARYNGEUS.

meatus nasopharyngeus   [NA] The posterior part of the nasal cavity, extending from the posterior ends of the middle and inferior nasal conchae to the choanae and situated between the adjacent lateral and medial walls of the nasal fossa. Also called *nasopharyngeal meatus, posterula* (outmoded).

meatus nasopharyngeus osseus   The posterior part of the nasal cavity behind the bony middle and inferior conchae. Posterior to the middle concha in the lateral wall is the sphenopalatine foramen, which links the nasal cavity with the pterygopalatine fossa. Also called *bony nasopharyngeal meatus.*

meatus of nose   The passages in the lateral wall of the nose, such as meatus nasi superior, meatus nasi medius, and meatus nasi inferior.

osseous middle meatus of nose   MEATUS NASI MEDIUS OSSEUS.

osseous superior meatus of nose   MEATUS NASI SUPERIOR OSSEUS.

posterior meatus of urethra   The beginning of the spongy urethra in the bulbus penis after its narrowing as the membranous urethra. An outmoded term.

superior nasal meatus   MEATUS NASI SUPERIOR.

meatus of urethra   OSTIUM URETHRAE EXTERNUM.

meatus urinarius   An outmoded term for OSTIUM URETHRAE EXTERNUM.

urinary meatus   An outmoded term for OSTIUM URETHRAE EXTERNUM.

Mebaral   A proprietary name for mephobarbital.

mebendazole $C_{16}H_{13}N_3O_3$.   5-Benzoyl-2-benzimidazolecarbamic acid methyl ester. An agent given by oral administration as an anthelmintic in the treatment of trichuriasis, enterobiasis, hookworm, and ascariasis.

mebeverine   hydrochloride $C_{25}H_{35}NO_5 \cdot HCl$.   4-[Ethyl(*p*-methoxy-α-methylphenethyl)amino]butyl veratrate hydrochloride. A smooth muscle relaxant agent used to treat disorders affecting the gastrointestinal tract.

mebutamate $C_{10}H_{20}N_2O_4$.   2-Methyl-2-(1-methylpropyl)-1,3-propanediol dicarbamate. A drug used to treat hypertension, often in combination with diuretics or other hypotensive agents. It is given orally.

mecamine   Mecamylamine. See under MECAMYLAMINE HYDROCHLORIDE.

mecamylamine   hydrochloride $C_{11}H_{22}ClN$.   *N*,2,3,3-Tetramethylbicyclo[2.2.1]-heptan-2-amine hydrochloride. A ganglionic blocking agent which has been used orally for the treatment of severe hypertension.

mechanical   **1** Done by machine.   **2** Being or relating to a machine or machinery.

mechanicoreceptor   MECHANORECEPTOR.

mechanicotherapeutics   MECHANOTHERAPY.

mechanicotherapy   MECHANOTHERAPY.

mechanics   [MECHANO- + -ICS]   The branch of physics concerned with the interaction of force and matter.

animal mechanics   BIOMECHANICS.

body mechanics   Kinesiologic principles of body movement and posture.

developmental mechanics   The mechanisms of development as revealed principally by the techniques of experimental embryology.

mechanics of labor   MECHANISM OF LABOR.

quantum mechanics   The mechanics of subatomic particles as formulated in quantum theory.

mechanism   **1** A contrivance or machinelike device.   **2** A process or technique by which some result is achieved.

catch mechanism   A muscle contraction in which the shortened state continues for a protracted time after the initial excitatory process with little expenditure of additional energy. It is seen in muscles of some invertebrates.

compulsory-order mechanism   ORDERED MECHANISM.

coping mechanism   Any of the conscious or unconscious ways that a person uses to adjust to environmental demands.

countercurrent multiplier mechanism   The mechanism by which the loop of Henle contributes to the production of a concentrated urine. Small osmolar concentration differences established between the fluid contents of the two limbs at each level of the loop are enhanced by the flow of fluid in opposite directions in the descending and ascending limbs. The gradient of increasing osmolarity in the renal medulla between the corticomedullary junction and the tips of the renal papillae is established by the active pumping of sodium chloride out of the ascending limb of the loop of Henle which is believed to be water impermeable.

defence mechanism   A British spelling for DEFENSE MECHANISM.

defense mechanism   Any of the mechanisms developed by the ego to control impulses that if left unchecked would cause conflict between the ego and id. Various defenses have been described, including repression, displacement, identification, dissociation, introjection, isolation, postponement of affect, projection, reaction formation, regression, undoing, and sublimation.

diluting mechanism   The mechanism in the nephron by which urine is diluted. As glomerular filtrate passes down the nephron, two thirds is reabsorbed isotonically in the proximal tubule. More water is reabsorbed and solute is added as the remainder of the glomerular filtrate passes down the descending limb of the loop of Henle, resulting in hypertonic urine fluid. The remainder of the nephron represents the diluting area and is almost impermeable to water during conditions of dilute urine formation when active and passive reabsorption of solutes in this area, therefore, leads to the formation of dilute urine. Normally in humans, up to one sixth of the glomerular filtrate theoretically could be excreted as free water after a large water load. However, excretion of free water is limited by solutes which require water for their excretion and by the minimal urinary osmolarity.

Douglas mechanism   The spontaneous movement of a fetus from a transverse lie to a vertex presentation.

Duncan mechanism   Delivery of the placenta with the maternal surface appearing first at the vaginal introitus.

escape mechanism   The ego's method of dealing with unbearable suffering by fleeing from its source through the development of a psychosis or neurosis.

feedback mechanism   CLOSED LOOP.

Frank-Starling mechanism   The alteration of the energy of cardiac muscle contraction that accompanies changes in the fiber length at the start of contraction. See also STARLING'S LAW.

hysterical defense mechanisms   **1** The symptoms of hysteria.   **2** The main defense mechanisms that produce the symptoms of hysteria, such as repression, conversion, and dissociation.

immunological mechanisms of tissue damage   A system for classifying immunological reactions that can produce damage to host tissues, in which the initiating immunological event provides the basis of the classification. It was devised by R. R. A. Coombs and P. G. H. Gell. Four types of reactions are distinguished. Type 1 reactions (anaphylactic reactions, immediate hypersensitivity) are initiated by antigens reacting with cell-bound antibody, usually IgE. Release of mediators, mainly from basophils and mast cells, provide the pathogenic mechanism. Type 2 reactions (cytotoxic reactions) are initiated by antibody reacting with cell-bound antigen. Type 3 reactions are initiated by antigen-antibody complexes formed either at the site of tissue damage (Arthus reactions) or localizing from the circulation (soluble immune complex reactions). Type 4 reactions (delayed hypersensitivity) are initiated by antigen-reactive T cells reacting with specific antigen. These four types of reactions are also referred to as Type 1–4 hypersensitivity reactions.

investing mechanism   An arrangement of tissues, including the periodontium and gingiva, which retain and support a tooth in the jaw.

ion-exchange mechanism   **1** A mechanism affecting passive or active transport of ions across a biologic membrane in such a way that the movements of ions in opposite directions are related quantitatively.   **2** The replacement of ions in solution by ions of similar charge present in materials such as synthetic resins with which the solution is brought into contact. This technique has been used in water softening and in the removal of unwanted ions from the body.

isolating mechanism   A natural means whereby a species population is divided into distinct subunits that allow population differences to evolve.

mechanism of labor   The succession of factors and forces which lead to delivery of the products of conception during labor. Also called *mechanics of labor.*

middle-ear transformer mechanism   The mechanism provided by the tympanic membrane acting together with the ossicular chain which, by reason of the ossicular lever ratio along with the middle-ear areal ratio, greatly increases the force of the sound arriving at the oval window compared with the force incident on the tympanic membrane.

mote-beam mechanism   A mechanism by which an individual becomes oblivious to the presence of an undesirable trait in himself but is acutely aware of its existence in others.

oculogyric mechanism   Those structures contributing to movement of the eye about the anteroposterior axis, including the extrinsic muscles of the eyeball, their innervating nerves, and the nuclei of origin in the brainstem.

ordered mechanism   A mechanism of enzyme-catalyzed reactions in which the substrates only bind to the enzyme in a certain order, i.e. the second substrate cannot bind until the first has done so. Also called *compulsory-order mechanism.*

ping-pong mechanism   The mechanism of an enzymic reaction in which an enzyme E first reacts with one substrate A to form a modified enzyme E' and a product P, this process being followed by a subsequent reaction of E' with the second substrate B to form the second product Q and to re-form the original enzyme E. It is distinguished from mechanisms with ternary complexes, in which the two reactants A and B bind simultaneously to the enzyme.

pressoreceptive mechanism   A mechanism sensitive to blood pressure changes, such as a carotid sinus receptor.

reentrant mechanism   A fundamental mechanism of arrhythmogenesis in which cardiac tissue is reexcited by the same impulse for one or more cycles. The prerequisites for this arrhythmia mechanism are: an area, anatomic or functional, of unidirectional conduction; a pathway, anatomic or functional, with a conduction time long enough to permit reexcitation; and an initiating impulse. See also REENTRY.

scapegoat mechanism   **1** A method of rationalizing for one's failures by blaming them on another.   **2** A mechanism by which all the emotions that a family cannot accept as originating from themselves are attributed to one member of the family, typically the one identified as sick or disturbed.

Schultze mechanism   Delivery of the placenta with the smooth fetal surface appearing first at the vaginal opening.

somatic mechanism   The structures and tissues that form the framework or walls of the body, excluding the viscera, and that are considered to be a functional entity.

splanchnic mechanism   The internal organs of the body considered as a functional entity.

suspensory mechanism   An arrangement of collagen fibers in the periodontal membrane which appears to suspend a tooth in its socket.

mechano- [Gk *mēchanē* instrument, machine]   A combining form meaning machine, mechanical.

mechanocardiography   The recording of the pulsatile waveforms that result from cardiac contraction such as the apexcardiogram and carotid pulse waveforms.

mechanogymnastics   Gymnastic exercises done with mechanical devices such as Zander apparatus.

mechanoreceptor   Any of a variety of tactile end organs responsive to low-amplitude cutaneous displacement. Also called *tactile receptor, touch receptor, contact receptor, contact ceptor, mechanicoreceptor.*

mechanotherapy   The use of mechanical devices to aid in the performance of exercises for therapeutic purposes. Also called *mechanicotherapy, mechanicotherapeutics.*

mechanothermy [MECHANO- + THERM- + -Y]   Local or general increase in body heat as a result of exercise or massage.

Mecholyl   A proprietary name for methacholine chloride.

mecism [Gk *mēk(os)* length, height + -ISM]   The abnormal length of a part of the body or of the body as a whole.

Mecistocirrus digitatus   A nematode found chiefly in Asia that is parasitic in the abomasum of a wide variety of ruminants. It can cause severe anemia. Cases of human infection have also been reported. The genus *Mecistocirrus* is monotypic and is the only genus in the subfamily Mecistocirrhinae of the family Trichostrongylidae. Also called *Nematodirus gibsoni, Nematodirus fordi.*

Meckel [Johann Friedrich *Meckel,* the elder, German anatomist, 1724–1774]   **1** Meckel's ganglion. See under GANGLION PTERYGOPALATINUM.   **2** Lesser ganglion of Meckel. See under GANGLION SUBMANDIBULARE.   **3** Meckel's cavity, cavum mecklii, Meckel's cave, Meckel's space. See under CAVUM TRIGEMINALE.   **4** Meckel's ligament. See under BAND.

Meckel [Johann Friedrich *Meckel,* the younger, German anatomist and surgeon, 1781–1833]   **1** Meckel's rod. See under MECKEL'S CARTILAGE.   **2** See under DIVERTICULUM, PLANE.   **3** Meckel-Gruber syndrome. See under MECKEL SYNDROME.

meckelectomy [after Johann Friedrich *Meckel*, the elder, German anatomist, 1724–1774 + -ECTOMY] Excision of Meckel's ganglion.

meclizine dihydrochloride $C_{25}H_{29}Cl_3N_2$. 1-(*p*-Chloro-α-phenylbenzyl)-4-(*m*-methylbenzyl)piperazine dihydrochloride. It is an antihistaminic agent used in the management of nausea and vomiting caused by motion sickness. It may also be effective in the treatment of vertigo caused by diseases affecting the vestibular apparatus. It is given orally.

meclocycline $C_{22}H_{21}ClN_2O_8$. 7-Chloro-6-methylene-5-hydroxy-tetracycline. A topically applied antibiotic closely related to chlortetracycline. It is used as a dermatologic anti-infective agent.

mecloqualone $C_{15}H_{11}ClN_2O$. 3-(2-Chlorophenyl)-2-methyl-4(3*H*)-quinazolinone. A compound with hypnotic and sedative properties.

mecocephalic DOLICHOCEPHALIC.

mecometer [Gk *mēko(s)* height, length + -METER] A form of caliper designed to measure newborn infants.

meconalgia [Gk *mēkōn* the poppy + -ALGIA] Spontaneous neuralgic pain occurring after the withdrawal of opiate remedies to which the individual has become addicted.

meconeuropathia [Gk *mēkō(n)* the poppy + NEURO- + -PATHIA] Any of the nervous symptoms which develop in opium addicts. An outmoded term.

meconic acid A plant acid whose molecules possess a 6-membered ring which contains an oxygen atom, two double bonds, and a carbonyl group, and which also possess a hydroxyl group and two carboxyl groups. Alkaloids are often found as their salts with meconic acid.

meconin The lactone of 2,3-dimethoxy-6-hydroxymethylbenzoic acid. It is found in combination as part of several opium alkaloids.

meconism Opium addiction or opium poisoning.

meconium [L, from Gk *mēkōnion* juice of the poppy, opium, discharge from the bowels of newborn children] The black or greenish black, odorless, sticky, semisolid material that fills the lower bowel of the newborn infant. Meconium stools are replaced by feces within the first two or three days of life.

mecystasis A state in which muscle shows unchanged characteristics of tension contraction and relaxation despite an increase in initial length.

MED 1 minimal effective dose. 2 minimal erythema dose.

medallion [French *médaillon* (from Italian *medaglione* a medallion, augmentative of *medaglia* a medal, coin, from Late L *medialis* middle, from L *medi(us)* middle + -*alis* -AL) a medallion, locket] The circumscribed red scaly patch that is the characteristic lesion of pityriasis rosea.

medazepam hydrochloride $C_{16}H_{15}ClN_2\cdot HCl$. 7-Chloro-2,3-dihydro-1-methyl-5-phenyl-1*H*-1,4-benzodiazepine monohydrochloride. It is used as a weak tranquilizer and antianxiety medication.

Medex [shortened form of French *médecin extension* physician extension] A physician assistant training program used in the United States, originally developed to adapt former military corpsmen for civilian duty but more recently expanded to train other individuals for medical care duties under the supervision of a physician.

medi- MEDIO-.

media Plural of MEDIUM.

mediad Toward a median line or plane.

medial 1 Of, at, or toward the middle. 2 Relatively near the midline or median plane of the body, as compared with other structures or parts situated farther to the right or left. Compare LATERAL. 3 Relating to a tunica media or any middle layer.

medialecithal [L *media*, fem. of *medius* middle, middling + LECITH- + -AL] Having a moderate quantity of yolk: said of an ovum. Also *mesolecithal*.

medialis [NA] Medial.

median 1 The term in an ordered statistical series such that the number of observations which are less than it is the same as the number that exceed it. 2 Lying in the middle or in the vertical plane at the midline dividing a structure bilaterally.

mediaometer [L *media*, pl. of *medium* the middle + *o* + -METER] A device for measuring the dioptric power of the eye.

mediastina Plural of MEDIASTINUM.

mediastinal Pertaining to the mediastinum.

mediastinitis [*mediastin(um)* + -ITIS] Inflammation of the mediastinum.

fibrous mediastinitis MEDIASTINAL FIBROSIS.

indurative mediastinitis MEDIASTINAL FIBROSIS.

mediastinogram [*mediastin(um)* + *o* + -GRAM] A radiograph of the mediastinum after introduction of an opaque medium or gas.

mediastinography [*mediastin(um)* + *o* + -GRAPHY] Roentgenography of the mediastinal structures.

gas mediastinography Radiographic study of the mediastinum after injection of a gas, such as nitrous oxide, into the mediastinum via a needle introduced behind the sternum or behind the trachea. Also called *pneumomediastinography*.

opaque mediastinography Radiographic study of the mediastinum after injection of an opaque medium into the mediastinum.

mediastinopericarditis Inflammation of the pericardium and adjacent mediastinal tissues that usually results in the formation of fibrous adhesions between the parietal pericardium and surrounding structures.

mediastinoscope [*mediastin(um)* + *o* + -SCOPE] An endoscope used to visualize structures in the superior mediastinum. It is usually inserted through a small suprasternal cervical incision.

mediastinoscopy The examination of structures of the superior mediastinum by the use of a mediastinoscope.

mediastinotomy [*mediastin(um)* + *o* + -TOMY] Surgical incision of the mediastinum.

mediastinum [New L (from neut. of *mediastinus* medial; as substantive, a drudge, kitchen slave, from *medius* middle + *stare* to stand)] (*plural* mediastina) 1 A median septum or partition between two parts of a cavity or an organ. 2 [NA] The interval between the right and left pleural sacs, extending from the thoracic inlet above to the diaphragm below, and from the sternum in front to the thoracic vertebrae behind. It contains the heart, pericardium, great vessels, and all other thoracic viscera lying between the pleural sacs. It is divided into superior, anterior, middle, and posterior mediastina. Also called *septum mediastinale, interpulmonary septum, mediastinal septum, interpleural space, mediastinal space*.

anterior mediastinum MEDIASTINUM ANTERIUS.

mediastinum anterius [NA] A shallow space between the pericardium and the body of the sternum above the level of the fourth costal cartilages. It is narrow because of the close approximation near the midline of the left and the right mediastinal pleurae, and contains loose connective tissue, the lower part of the thymus gland, the sternopericardial ligaments, lymph nodes and vessels, and a few mediastinal branches of the internal thoracic vessels. Also called *anterior mediastinum, cavum mediastinale anterius, anterior mediastinal cavity*.

mediastinum cerebelli FALX CEREBELLI.

mediastinum cerebri A seldom used term for FALX CEREBRI.

mediastinum medium [NA] The large central portion of the lower part of the mediastinal space occupied by the pericardium, heart, ascending aorta, the pulmonary trunk dividing into left and right pulmonary arteries, the bifurcation of the trachea and the bronchi, the arch of the azygos vein, the lower part of the superior vena cava, the left and right pulmonary veins, the phrenic nerves and accompanying vessels, tracheobronchial lymph nodes, and the deep part of the cardiac plexus. Also called *middle mediastinum*.

middle mediastinum MEDIASTINUM MEDIUM.

posterior mediastinum MEDIASTINUM POSTERIUS.

mediastinum posterius [NA] The mediastinal space bounded by the lower eight thoracic vertebrae posteriorly; the mediastinal pleura on each side; and the pericardium, bifurcation of trachea, pulmonary vessels, and the upper surface of the diaphragm anteriorly. It is continuous superiorly with the posterior part of the superior mediastinum, and it contains the esophagus, descending thoracic aorta, azygos and hemiazygos veins, thoracic duct, vagus and splanchnic nerves, and lymph nodes. Also called *posterior mediastinum, cavum mediastinale posterius, posterior mediastinal cavity, postmediastinum*.

superior mediastinum MEDIASTINUM SUPERIUS.

mediastinum superius [NA] The mediastinal space bounded posteriorly by the upper four thoracic vertebrae and longus colli muscles, anteriorly by the manubrium sterni and sternohyoid and sternothyroid muscles, laterally by the mediastinal pleurae, superiorly by the thoracic inlet, and inferiorly by the plane between the sternal angle and the lower border of the body of the fourth thoracic vertebra, below which its posterior part is continuous with the posterior mediastinum. It contains connective tissue; part of the thymus gland; the arch of the aorta and its branches; the brachiocephalic veins; the upper part of the superior vena cava; lymph nodes; and the vagus, cardiac, phrenic and left recurrent laryngeal nerves. Also called *superior mediastinum*.

mediastinum testis [NA] The incomplete vertical septum formed by the projection of the tunica albuginea into the testis through its posterior border along its upper two thirds. Through it pass the blood vessels and lymphatics of the testis. It also contains the rete testis. Also called *septum of testis, body of Highmore, corpus highmori, corpus highmorianum*.

mediate [L *mediat(us)*, past part. of *mediare* to be in the middle, from *medi(us)* middle] **1** Acting or occurring indirectly through an agent. **2** To be such an agent for effecting (a result). **3** Intermediate; intervening.

mediation The act or result of mediating.

chemical mediation The linking of related functions by a chemical intermediary, especially used of the transmission of nerve impulses between presynaptic and postsynaptic elements.

mediator Something that mediates; an agent that effects a result.

chemical mediator An intermediary agent which is chemical in nature.

Medibank Formerly, the Australian national program of health insurance. In 1984 it was replaced by Medicare.

medicable Capable of being treated medically and with the expectation of effective cure.

Medicaid [*medic(al)* + *-aid*] A federally aided, state-operated and administered program in the United States which provides medical care benefits for certain low-income, medically indigent individuals through a governmental insurance type of entitlement program.

medical Of or relating to medicine or to the practice of medicine.

major medical Insurance designed to offset high medical expenses resulting from catastrophic or prolonged illness or injury.

Medical Assistance Program The health care program in the United States authorized by title XIX of the Social Security Act, known generally as Medicaid, for aiding the poor in obtaining health care.

medicament [French *médicament* (from L *medicament(um)* medicine, remedy, from *medica(ri)* to heal, cure + *-mentum* -MENT) substance used for curing illness] A medicinal agent or any substance used as a therapeutic material. Adjective: medicamentous.

medicamentosus MEDICAMENTOUS.

medicamentous Referring to a medication, or related to the use of a therapeutic agent. Also *medicamentosus*.

Medicare [*medi(cal)* + *care*] A nationwide, federally funded and administered insurance program in the United States for individuals aged 65 and over and certain others, which provides funding for a number of specified health care services, but is not all-inclusive. • A similar national program of health insurance of the same name exists in Australia.

medicaster [Italian *medicastro* (from *medic(o)* physician + *-astro* English *-aster*, suffix denoting inferiority) a quack] QUACK.

medicate **1** To impregnate or permeate with a medicinal substance. **2** To treat by administering a drug.

medicated Treated or impregnated with a medicinal substance.

medication [L *medicatio* (from *medicatus*, past part. of *medicari* to heal, cure; Gk *medein*, archaic verb to rule) a healing] **1** A medicinal substance; a medicine. **2** Treatment by the administration of medicines. **3** Impregnation or permeation with a medicinal substance.

arrhenic medication A treatment employing arsenic to cure disease.

conservative medication Medication intended to preserve or to restore to full strength or capacity.

hypodermatic medication Treatment with a medicinal substance that is introduced beneath the skin, as by injection.

intracanal medication The use of drugs in the root canals of teeth as part of endodontic treatment.

ionic medication IONTOPHORESIS.

preanesthetic medication Medication administered prior to local or general anesthesia, as sedatives or tranquilizers for anxiety, analgesics (such as opioids), and vagolytic agents (such as atropine and scopolamine) to block vagal-induced, excessive airway secretion or bradycardia. Also called *preanesthesia, premedication*.

sublingual medication Treatment with a medicinal substance that is placed under the tongue.

medicator An instrument for applying a medicine locally, especially within a body cavity.

medicephalic Of or relating to the median cephalic vein. An outmoded term.

medicerebellar Denoting to the central portion of the cerebellum. A seldom used term.

medicerebral Denoting to the central portion of the cerebrum.

medicinal **1** Having healing properties. **2** Of or relating to medicine.

medicine [L *medicina* (fem., as substantive, of *medicinus*, pertaining to the art of healing, from *medicus* wholesome, healing, medicinal, from *mederi* or *medicari* to heal, cure; Gk archaic verb *medein* to rule) the art of healing] **1** The art and science dealing with the maintenance and restoration of health, including the prevention and treatment of disease. **2** The branch of medicine that employs nonsurgical methods of treatment. **3** Any substance used to treat disease or alleviate pain.

adolescent medicine The branch of medicine dealing with the care and treatment of individuals from the onset of puberty to about age 19. Also called *ephebiatrics, hebiatrics*.

aerospace medicine SPACE MEDICINE.

aviation medicine A specialized branch of medicine dealing with the physiologic, pathologic, and psychologic conditions which occur in professional fliers and people transported by air. It includes the selection, maintenance, and treatment of aircraft personnel, advising on the design of aircraft and related equipment, and dealing with the transport of the sick and wounded. Also called *aeromedicine*.

Ayurvedic medicine Traditional Indian medicine, based upon Hindu scriptures and the use of plants and drugs indigenous to India. Also called *Ayurvedism*.

behavioral medicine The application of the principles of learning and learning theory to treat those disorders, caused at least in part by psychologic factors, as if they were behaviors. Specific techniques are applied to reverse the expressions of maladaptive functioning, whether purely psychologic, as in a phobia, or partly physiologic, as in faulty patterns of learned autonomic nervous system response leading to cardiovascular disease.

clinical medicine Medical practice or instruction involving and based on direct observation of patients as opposed to theoretical study, laboratory investigation, or classroom teaching.

community medicine The practice of medicine or the study of health care services focusing on community needs and care rather than on the individual. Examples include public health services and preventive medicine.

defensive medicine Aspects of medical practice in which fear or concern over the threat of professional liability, including possible malpractice suits, affects how the provider practices.

diagnostic nuclear medicine The *in vivo* study of distribution of radioactive materials, which are preferably gamma-emitting.

domestic medicine The treatment of illness or injury in the home, without the advice or assistance of a physician.

dosimetric medicine The administration of drugs or medicines by an exact and standardized system of dosages.

emergency medicine A branch of medicine that specializes in providing immediate diagnosis and treatment of those who are acutely and often suddenly ill or severely injured, such that any considerable delay would likely result in deterioration or death.

environmental medicine 1 The study of the environmental aspects related to the etiology and prevention of disease as well as specific environmental aspects of the promotion of good health. 2 An imprecise term for ENVIRONMENTAL HYGIENE.

experimental medicine Medical research based on experimentation with animals, especially for the study of disease processes and therapies.

family medicine A popular term for FAMILY PRACTICE.

fetal-maternal medicine A subspecialty of obstetrics and gynecology dealing with the care of the pregnant mother and her fetus with particular emphasis on managing high-risk situations.

folk medicine The treatment of illness or injury based on tradition, especially an oral tradition passed from one generation to the next, rather than on scientific practice. It often utilizes indigenous flora as remedies.

forensic medicine The application of theoretical and practical medical knowledge and skill to the solution of problems encountered in the administration of justice. Also called *legal medicine, medical jurisprudence, juridical medicine* (outmoded). • The term was first used in Scotland and England.

genitourinary medicine A British term for VENEREOLOGY.

geographical medicine A branch of medicine concerned with geographical differences in the clinical manifestations and pathology of diseases, their incidence, and their economic impact.

geriatric medicine A medical specialty concerned with the diagnosis, prevention, and treatment of physical and mental disorders and diseases of the elderly. Also called *geriatrics* (popular), *gerontotherapy* (seldom used), *presbyatrics*.

group medicine Medicine practiced by a group of associates. See also GROUP PRACTICE.

holistic medicine An approach to health care based on the theory that health is the result of harmony between body, mind, and spirit and that stress of any kind, including physical, psychological, and social pressure, is inimical to health. Also called *whole person medicine*.

humanistic medicine Medicine practiced with a concern for the value and worth of mankind, and with regard for the physical and mental well-being of the entire patient, rather than with a purely clinical perspective.

hyperbaric medicine Medical treatment under conditions exceeding normal atmospheric pressure. 〈"Hyperbaric medicine's origin as a therapy for divers with decompression sickness still hasn't been left behind, though. The field's professional association is named the Undersea Medical Society." —*Medical World News*, 28 Feb. 1983, 29.〉

industrial medicine An outmoded term for OCCUPATIONAL MEDICINE.

integrated medicine The practice of medicine characterized by close cooperation of the physician and paramedical colleagues, such as social workers and therapists. A term seldom used in the U.S.

internal medicine The branch of medicine which deals with the diagnosis and nonsurgical treatment of diseases and disorders affecting internal parts or systems of the body. • The English term was apparently borrowed from the German, *Innere Medizin*, which became common in Germany in the early 1880s. (William B. Bean, *New England Journal of Medicine*, 21 Jan. 1982, 182–183). *Internal medicine* is used in the U.S., Canada, India, New Zealand, the United Kingdom (where *general medicine* is preferred), and Japan, where *Innere Medizin* is also used. The corresponding term in South Africa is simply *medicine*; *internal medicine* is not used.

juridical medicine An outmoded term for FORENSIC MEDICINE.

legal medicine FORENSIC MEDICINE.

manipulative medicine Medical practice based on manipulative therapy; chiropractic.

mental medicine PSYCHIATRY.

neonatal medicine NEONATOLOGY.

nuclear medicine The branch of medicine dealing with the diagnostic, therapeutic (exclusive of sealed radiation sources), and investigative use of radionuclides. Also called *nuclear radiology*.

occupational medicine A branch of medicine dealing with prevention of disease and injury among people at work. It has two main functions: to ensure the suitability of an individual for particular kinds of work in order to protect the health and safety of that individual, fellow workers, and, where appropriate, the public; and to identify and control health and safety hazards in the workplace. Also called *industrial medicine* (outmoded).

oral medicine The study and treatment of diseases of the soft tissues of the mouth.

osteopathic medicine OSTEOPATHY.

patent medicine A medicine protected by a trademark, often with the composition not completely made known.

perinatal medicine A specialized branch of medicine dealing with the management of mother and fetus during pregnancy and of the infant immediately after delivery. In contrast to general obstetrics, special emphasis is placed on managing high-risk pregnancies.

physical medicine A field of medical practice that utilizes physical modalities such as light, heat, sound, electricity, mechanical devices, and exercise for therapeutic purposes. Developed during the late nineteenth century, it originally also included radium and x-ray modalities. Physical medicine in more recent times has evolved into the specialty known as physical medicine and rehabilitation, or physiatrics. • See note at PHYSICAL MEDICINE AND REHABILITATION, under MEDICINE.

physical medicine and rehabilitation The branch of medicine concerned with the use of physical agents and modalities including electricity, light, heat, sound, mechanical devices, and physical activity in the diagnosis, treatment, and prevention of disease. In the last several decades this medical specialty has been increasingly focused on the diagnosis, treatment, and prevention of physical disabilities, including pain. Also called *physiatrics (used chiefly in the U.S. and Canada), physiatry (used chiefly in the U.S. and Canada).* • Originally and still known in many countries as *physical medicine,* the specialty was broadened in the United States in 1949 to include *rehabilitation* as part of its formal name. *Physical medicine* is the term by which this specialty is known in the United Kingdom, South Africa, India, New Zealand, and Australia, although in Australia *rehabilitation medicine* appears to be gaining ground. In Japan, *rehabilitation* is preferred. *Physiatrics* and *physiatry* are widely used only in the United States and Canada.

preclinical medicine 1 Medical science and practice that deals with the prevention or treatment of illness prior to the point at which clinical measures become necessary or advisable. 2 The part of the medical curriculum that precedes, and prepares the student for, clinical instruction and training, and which typically includes the study of biology, anatomy, physiology, pharmacology, and related sciences.

preventive medicine The branch of medicine concerned with the prevention of disease, injury, and disability, and with the promotion of safety and of practices aimed at lessening the probability of disease, with regard to individuals and whole populations, as distinguished from remedial or curative measures.

proprietary medicine A drug or medicine the manufacture or composition of which is controlled by an owner through patent rights or copyrights previously obtained.

psychological medicine PSYCHIATRY.

psychosomatic medicine The branch of medicine devoted to psychosomatic disorders. Also called *psychopneumatology* (obsolete).

rehabilitation medicine The branch of medicine specializing in the treatment of the disabled to restore normal function. When applied to the restoration of physical function, it is generally identified with the specialty known as physical medicine and rehabilitation. • See note at PHYSICAL MEDICINE AND REHABILITATION, under MEDICINE.

social medicine The study and use of ways and means whereby disease is prevented, new cases discovered, the public educated in health matters, and the provision of health care facilitated.

socialized medicine 1 STATE MEDICINE. 2 Any medical care system which is administered or controlled predominantly by government or other public agencies and in which private practice is limited in scope or significance.

space medicine A special branch of aviation medicine which deals with the stresses imposed on man by projection through and beyond the earth's atmosphere, flight in interplanetary space, and return to earth. Such stresses include the agravic state, exposure to radiation, and isolation. Also called *aerospace medicine.*

sports medicine A subspecialty of clinical practice concerned with the injuries and disorders resulting from athletics and other sporting activities.

state medicine A medical care system in which the organization and provision of care is under the direct control of gov-

ernment and in which the providers are employed directly or through contractual arrangements by the government. Also called *socialized medicine.*

tropical medicine The medical specialty concerned with those diseases and disorders that are contracted chiefly in a hot or warm climate, or which exhibit unique characteristics in tropical countries. See also TROPICAL DISEASE. • In common medical use, *tropical medicine* refers not only to diseases associated with hot climates but also to diseases common in tropical countries because of poor socioeconomic conditions prevalent there.

veterinary medicine The branch of medicine that deals with the diagnosis and treatment of disease in all animals other than man. Also called *theriatrics* (obsolete).

whole person medicine HOLISTIC MEDICINE.

medicinerea The gray matter constituting the putamen and claustrum of the forebrain. An outmoded term.

medico- [L *medicus* physician, surgeon] A combining form meaning medical.

medicobiologic Medical and biologic.

medicochirurgic Relating to the practice of medicine and surgery.

medicodental Relating to both the practice of medicine and the practice of dentistry.

medicolegal [MEDICO- + LEGAL] Pertaining to forensic medicine or to that which involves both medicine and law.

medicomechanical Involving both medicinal and mechanical therapeutic modalities.

medicopsychology [MEDICO- + PSYCHOLOGY] PSYCHIATRY.

medicosocial [MEDICO- + SOCIAL] Pertaining to or involving both medical and social factors. Also called *sociomedical.*

medicostatistical [MEDICO- + STATISTICAL] Pertaining to the statistical aspects of medicine.

medifrontal MIDFRONTAL.

Medin [Oskar *Medin,* Swedish physician, 1847–1927] Medin's disease, Heine-Medin disease. See under ACUTE ANTERIOR POLIOMYELITIS.

medio- [L *medius* middle] A combining form meaning middle. Also *medi-.*

mediocarpal MIDCARPAL.

medioccipital MIDOCCIPITAL.

mediodorsal Pertaining to the median plane and the dorsum.

mediofrontal MIDFRONTAL.

mediolateral Pertaining to the median plane and one side.

medionecrosis Necrosis of the tunica media of an artery, usually the aorta.

medionecrosis of the aorta CYSTIC MEDIAL NECROSIS.

mediopalatine Pertaining to the middle of the palate.

mediopeduncle A seldom used term for PEDUNCULUS CEREBELLARIS MEDIUS.

medioplantar Pertaining to the middle of the sole of the foot.

mediopontine Denoting the central portion of the pons.

mediosuperior Both above and toward the middle.

mediosylvian Denoting that portion of the lateral cerebral fissure of Sylvius which is closer to midline.

mediotarsal MIDTARSAL.

mediotemporal Denoting the central portion of the temporal lobe of the cerebrum.

mediotrusion [MEDIO- + *(trans)trusion*] Inward transtrusion.

mediotype MESOMORPH.

mediscalenus An outmoded term for MUSCULUS SCALENUS MEDIUS.

medisect [MEDI- + *sect(ion)*] A surgical procedure in which tissues are dissected free and divided medially.

meditation / transcendental meditation A variant of yoga practice, in which a relaxed meditative state is induced by the constant repetition of a mantra, a special phrase or sound selected for that individual.

medium [L (substantive from *medium*, neut. of *medius* middle, midmost, akin to Gk *mesos* middle), the middle] **1** A material in which a substance, an impulse, or information is transported. **2** A material in which interactions take place. **3** CULTURE MEDIUM. See also AGAR, BROTH, CULTURE, CULTURE MEDIUM.

Apathy's medium An aqueous medium for mounting slide preparations directly from water. It is used when dehydration with alcohol and xylene would be detrimental.

Bavister's medium A simple culture medium in which hamster and human eggs may be fertilized *in vitro* in the laboratory. The medium, a modification of the Tyrode solution, contains bovine serum albumin. Also called *Tyrode-B.*

brain-heart infusion medium 1 A liquid culture medium containing peptone and infusion solids of calf brain and beef heart. It is used in cultivating many microorganisms, especially fastidious bacteria. **2** BRAIN-HEART INFUSION AGAR.

Bruns glucose medium A mixture of glycerine, glucose, and camphor in an aqueous solution that was once used for clearing biological specimens. It has been superceded by methyl salicylate.

Cary-Blair transport medium A medium used for the collection and transport of clinical specimens intended for microbiologic examination.

clearing medium A medium used to make histologic specimens transparent or translucent.

complete medium Any medium for the *in vitro* culture of cells, tissues, or organisms that contains, in addition to basic nutrients, supplemental nutrients to support growth of fastidious or mutant cells or organisms.

contrast medium In radiology, a substance of different radiopacity from that of the organ or tissues being studied, to allow roentgenographic demonstration of the contours of a lumen or structure. When the substance is more radiopaque than the tissues, it is called a positive contrast medium, for example, a substance containing barium or iodine. When the substance is less radiopaque than the tissues, it is called a negative contrast medium, for example, air. Also called *radiopaque medium.*

culture medium See under CULTURE MEDIUM.

deoxycholate-citrate medium DEOXYCHOLATE-CITRATE AGAR.

dioptric media REFRACTING MEDIA.

Dubos medium A culture medium containing oleic acid and albumin for growing the tubercle bacillus.

Farrant's medium An aqueous medium that contains gum arabic and is used for mounting slide preparations directly from water.

ionizing medium A material capable of being ionized by collision with charged particles, such as the gas in a Geiger-Müller counter that is ionized when a particle or ray passes through the counter.

Littman ox-gall medium A medium used to isolate fungi from a mixed culture. The selectively active ingredients are crystal violet, streptomycin, and bile salts.

Loeffler medium LOEFFLER'S BLOOD CULTURE MEDIUM.

Löwenstein-Jensen medium LÖWENSTEIN-JENSEN AGAR.

marking medium A material used for marking occlusal contacts or pressure points on the fitting surface of a denture.

minimal medium Any medium for the *in vitro* culture of cells, tissues, or organisms that contains only those nutrients needed for growth of wild types or otherwise normal cells or organisms, the only carbon and nitrogen sources being salts and pure and defined chemicals.

motility test medium A nutrient medium prepared with a low concentration of agar so that the consistency is less solid than usual and allows motile organisms to establish growth in parts of the medium away from the line of inoculation. It is used in differentiating species of bacteria. Also called *semisolid culture medium.*

mounting medium Any substance used to mount objects on slides for microscopic study, usually a resin, glycerol, or polymer. Also called *mountant.*

NNN medium NOVY, MCNEAL AND NICOLLE MEDIUM.

Novy, McNeal and Nicolle medium A saline rabbit's blood medium suitable for the culturing of *Leishmania donovani*. Also called *NNN medium, N.N.N. culture medium.*

radiopaque medium CONTRAST MEDIUM.

refracting media The portions of the eye able to change the vergence of light. Also called *dioptric media.*

separating medium In dentistry, a material such as oil, petroleum jelly, soft soap, or alginate solution, used to prevent the adhesion of one surface to another, as of freshly mixed plaster of Paris to the surface of a set mix.

Stuart transport medium A non-nutritive medium of soft consistency containing thioglycollate, glycerophosphate, and cysteine, used to transport specimens and prevent the death of fastidious organisms before the specimen is planted on appropriate culture media. See also STUART BROTH.

support medium An inert material in which or on which a reaction takes place.

Thayer-Martin medium THAYER-MARTIN AGAR.

transparent media of the eye The cornea, lens, aqueous humor, and vitreous body.

MEDLARS [Acronym formed from *Med(ical) L(iterature) A(nalysis and) R(etrieval) S(ystem)*] A computerized system providing on-line search and retrieval services to the extensive medical bibliography of the U.S. National Library of Medicine by means of various databases, including MEDLINE, the database devoted to worldwide coverage of recent biomedical literature.

MEDLINE [Acronym formed from *MED(LARS) (on-)line*] See under MEDLARS.

Medomin A proprietary name for heptabarbital.

medorrhea [Gk *mēd(ea)* the genitals + *o* + -RRHEA] Discharge from the urethra.

medphalan D-3-[*p*[Bis(2-chloroethyl)amino]-phenyl]-alanine. A mustard-type antineoplastic drug.

Medrol A proprietary name for methylprednisolone.

medroxyprogesterone acetate $C_{24}H_{34}O_4$. 17α-Hydroxy- 6α-methylpregn-4-ene-3,20-dione 17-acetate, a progestin widely used as a contraceptive and to treat precocious puberty in the female, functional uterine bleeding, dysmenorrhea, endometriosis, and threatened abortion, and to suppress postpartum lactation.

medulla [L (from *medius* middle), the inmost part, marrow of bones, pith of plants, heart] (*plural* medullae) **1** [NA] The innermost or middle part of an organ or structure. Also called *marrow, medullary substance.* **2** MEDULLA OBLONGATA.

adrenal medulla MEDULLA GLANDULAE SUPRARENALIS.

medulla of bone BONE MARROW.

medulla glandulae suprarenalis The internal reddish or reddish brown layer of the suprarenal, or adrenal, gland that is composed of groups of nerve cells and a network of cords and groups of chromaffin cells with large anastomosing venous sinusoids between them. Also called *adrenal medulla, medulla of suprarenal gland, suprarenal medulla, substantia medullaris glandulae suprarenalis.*

medulla of hair shaft The central core of the hair shaft, present in all but the finest hairs. Also called *hair pulp.*

medulla of kidney MEDULLA RENALIS.

medulla of lymph node MEDULLA NODI LYMPHATICI.

medulla nodi lymphatici The darker central portion of a lymph node that extends to the surface at the hilum where it is continuous with the efferent lymph vessels. It has a trabecular meshwork containing a well defined fibrocellular reticulum and cords of cells, such as lymphocytes, and lymph sinuses around the cords. Also called *medulla of lymph node, substantia medullaris lymphoglandulae.*

medulla oblongata [NA] The caudal portion of the brainstem that extends between the pons and the most rostral part of the cervical spinal cord. It lies anterior to the cerebellum, and its upper posterior part forms the floor of the lower half of the fourth ventricle. The medulla oblongata contains large cellular groups of neurons that form the central nuclei of the glossopharyngeal, vagus, accessory, and hypoglossal nerves, and it is importantly related to the reflex functions of the pharynx, larynx, and tongue and in the regulation of life-sustaining respiratory and cardiovascular reflexes as well as consciousness. Through the medulla oblongata course the long ascending afferent tracts to the cerebellum and thalamus and the descending pathways from higher brain centers that control motor activity. Also called *spinal bulb, medulla, oblongata* (seldom used).

medulla ossium [NA] The soft tissue found in the cavities of bones; bone marrow. It differs in composition in different bones and at different ages, and usually as two types, red marrow and yellow marrow. The basic meshwork of connective tissue contains blood vessels and cells, such as fat cells and various blood cells. See also CAVITAS MEDULLARIS OSSIUM.

medulla ossium flava YELLOW BONE MARROW.

medulla ossium rubra RED BONE MARROW.

medulla ovarii [NA] The central, vascular portion of the ovary which consists of loose connective tissue with elastin fibers, smooth muscle fibers, and a mass of contorted blood vessels. It is surrounded by the thick cortex except at the hilum where strands of smooth muscle fibers extend into it from the mesovarium. Also called *zona vasculosa, zona vasculosa of Waldeyer, medulla of ovary.*

medulla of ovary MEDULLA OVARII.

medulla renalis [NA] The inner part of the kidney, comprising a number of striated pyramidal masses (the renal pyramids), the bases of which face outward abutting on the cortex while their apices are directed to the renal sinus, where they appear as the renal papillae projecting into the minor calices. Each pyramid is composed of renal tubules. Also called *medulla of kidney, substantia medullaris renis* (outmoded), *medullary zone, medullary substance of kidney.*

spinal medulla MEDULLA SPINALIS.

medulla spinalis [NA] The elongated cylindrical part of the central nervous system, located in the vertebral canal and covered by three membranes. It extends from the upper border of the atlas, where it is continuous with the medulla oblongata, to the first or second lumbar vertebra (in the adult human), where it forms the tapered conus medullaris from which the filum terminale extends downward. The vertebral level of the conus medullaris varies with species and developmental age. Also called *spinal cord, spinal medulla, spinal marrow, chorda spinalis* (obsolete), *funis argenteus* (obsolete), *myelon* (obsolete).

suprarenal medulla MEDULLA GLANDULAE SUPRARENALIS.

medulla of suprarenal gland MEDULLA GLANDULAE SUPRARENALIS.

medullae Plural of MEDULLA.

medullar MEDULLARY.

medullary **1** Pertaining to a medulla. **2** Resembling marrow. For defs. 1 and 2 also *medullar.*

medullated **1** Having a lipoprotein (myelin) sheath; myeli-

nated: said of a nerve fiber. **2** Having a medulla.

medullation [*medull(a)* + -ATION] The formation of a medulla or marrow, especially the formation of the myelin (medullary) sheath around a nerve fiber.

medullectomy [*medull(a)* + -ECTOMY] A surgical procedure in which the medulla, or most central portion of a body part, is removed.

medulliadrenal MEDULLOADRENAL.

medullispinal Pertaining to the spinal cord.

medullitis [*medull(a)* + -ITIS] **1** MYELITIS. **2** Inflammation of the medulla oblongata. **3** OSTEOMYELITIS.

medullization The process of widening of the haversian canals until they become marrow spaces in chronic osteomyelitis. A rarely used term.

medulloadrenal Pertaining to the medulla of the adrenal gland. Also *medulliadrenal.*

medulloarthritis [*medull(a)* + *o* + *arthritis*] An inflammation of the marrow space juxtaposed to a joint. This concept does not have medical validity as a separate diagnosis.

medulloblast A cell derived from a germinal cell of the inner ependymal layer, rounded, poor in cytoplasm and without processes, found in the middle (mantle) layer of the embryonic neural tube. According to some embryologists, it will be bipotent and able to differentiate into either a glioblast or a neuroblast. Others maintain this bipotentiality does not exist except for medulloblasts of the cerebellum. Elsewhere, the medulloblasts will already correspond to two cell types, apolar neuroblasts and apolar glioblasts.

medulloblastoma [*medull(a)* + *o* + BLASTOMA] A malignant brain tumor composed of small, poorly differentiated cells which tend to form pseudorosettes. The main site of growth is the midline of the cerebellum and in the roof of the fourth ventricle. Children are affected mostly. Also called *glioblastoma isomorphe, glioma sarcomatoides* (obsolete).

desmoplastic medulloblastoma A variant form of medulloblastoma, with similar tumor cells but with an abundant network of reticulin fibers in a fibrous stroma. It affects older patients, and is often lateral on the cerebellar surface. Also called *circumscribed cerebellar arachnoidal sarcoma.*

medulloepithelioma [*medull(a)* + *o* + *epitheli(o)* + -OMA] **1** A tumor of the eye, primarily of children, characterized by the formation of multilayered sheets of undifferentiated cells resembling the primitive medullary epithelium of the optic vesicle. Benign and malignant forms occur. The latter resemble retinoblastoma. Medulloepitheliomas are mainly found at the ciliary body and rarely in the retina. Also called *dictyoma, diktyoma.* **2** A very rare malignant tumor of the central nervous system composed of undifferentiated columnar cells forming tubular or papillary patterns resembling primitive neural epithelium. Also called *embryonal medulloepithelioma, neurocytoma.*

embryonal medulloepithelioma MEDULLOEPITHELIOMA.

medulloid Any adrenergic agent having an effect mimicking that of the hormones of the adrenal medulla.

medullosis An obsolete term for LEUKEMIA.

medullosuprarenoma [*medull(a)* + *o* + SUPRA- + REN + -OMA] **1** PHEOCHROMOCYTOMA. **2** An adrenal medullary tumor.

medullotherapy A prophylactic treatment for rabies introduced by Pasteur, utilizing emulsions of fixed virus from the spinal medulla of rabbits.

medusa [after *Medusa* (from Gk *Medousa*) a Gorgon in Gk mythology slain by Perseus] A free-swimming jellyfish, a stage in the life of organisms in the classes Hydrozoa and Scyphozoa of the phylum Cnidaria. Many have nematocysts which upon contact release a fine thread with a toxin or a sticky material. The scyphozoan jellyfish *Rhizostoma cuvieri* bears tentacles which release a toxic substance that, upon contact with a swimmer, can cause congestion of the splanchnic vessels.

medusocongestin A toxic agent obtained from the tentacles of the jellyfish *Rhizostoma cuvieri* and causing intense congestion of the splanchnic vessels. It is thought to be identical to congestin.

Meeh [K. *Meeh*, German physiologist, flourished late 19th century] See under FORMULA.

Mees [R. A. *Mees*, Dutch scientist, flourished 20th century] Bands of Mees, Mees stripes. See under MEES LINES.

mefenamic acid $C_{15}H_{15}NO_2$. 2-[2,3-Dimethylphenyl)amino]benzoic acid. An agent with analgesic, anti-inflammatory, and antipyretic properties. It is administered orally to relieve mild pain.

mefexamide $C_{15}H_{24}N_2O_3$. *N*-[2-(Diethylamino)ethyl]-2-(4-methoxyphenoxy)-acetamide. A stimulant having specific actions on the central nervous system. It has been used to treat fatigue and depression.

mefruside $C_{13}H_{19}ClN_2O_5S_2$. 4-Chloro-*N*'-methyl-*N*'-(tetrahydro-2-methyl-furfuryl)-*m*-benzenedisulfonamide. A substance with uses similar to those of chlorothiazide.

MEG magnetoencephalograph.

mega- [Gk *megas* great, large] A combining form denoting 10^6, one million: used with SI units. Symbol: M

mega-ampere [MEGA- + AMPERE] A unit of electric current equal to 10^6 amperes. Also called *megampere*. Symbol: MA

megabecquerel [MEGA- + BECQUEREL] A unit of activity of a radionuclide equal to 10^6 becquerel. Symbol: MBq

megabladder MEGALOCYSTIS.

megacalix [MEGA- + L *calix* cup, chalice] An abnormally large calix either congenital or secondary to obstruction.

megacardia CARDIOMEGALY.

megacaryoblast MEGAKARYOBLAST.

megacaryocyte MEGAKARYOCYTE.

megacecum A greatly enlarged or distended cecum.

megacephalia [MEGA- + CEPHAL- + -IA] MACROCEPHALY.

megacephalic MACROCEPHALOUS.

megacephalous [MEGA- + CEPHAL- + -OUS] MACROCEPHALOUS.

megacephalum MACROCEPHALY.

megacephalus [MEGA- + -CEPHALUS] MACROCEPHALUS.

megacephaly [MEGA- + CEPHAL- + -Y] MACROCEPHALY.

megacholedochus A greatly enlarged or distended common bile duct.

megacin A bacteriocin of *Bacillus megaterium*.

megacolon [MEGA- + -COLON] Enlargement of the colon, either segmental or total, marked by clinical manifestations of constipation or obstipation. Also called *giant colon* (seldom used).

  acquired megacolon Enlargement of the colon either secondary to an associated disease or of psychogenic origin. There is neither aganglionosis nor any other congenital motor abnormality.

  acute megacolon TOXIC MEGACOLON.

  aganglionic megacolon The absence of ganglion cells in the myenteric plexus. It results in dilatation of the affected bowel segment, which is most often the distal colon and rectum. It is the major feature of congenital megacolon, and it is also found in the Down syndrome, Waardenburg syndrome, familial piebaldness, and Chagas disease.

  congenital megacolon An autosomal recessive condition characterized by a marked dilatation of the colon proximal to

a "narrowed" segment in which intramural ganglion cells are absent (aganglionosis) in the submucosal (Meissner's) and myenteric (Auerbach's) plexuses. This aganglionic intestine does not enter into normal propulsion of colonic contents, and the dilatation of the normally innervated areas is secondary to the distal obstruction. The condition is more common in males, and it is usually a multifactorial trait. Also called *Hirschsprung's disease, Ruysch disease, congenital aganglionic megacolon*.

  congenital aganglionic megacolon CONGENITAL MEGACOLON.

  idiopathic constitutional megacolon Megacolon of unknown etiology thought to be related to chronic laxative abuse.

  secondary megacolon Megacolon due to an identifiable underlying condition, most often ulcerative colitis.

  toxic megacolon Gross distention of the colon not due to mechanical obstruction and associated with systemic signs of illness such as fever, tachycardia, or hypotension. Usually associated with severe ulcerative colitis, it has been seen with granulomatous colitis, infectious colitis, colitis related to antibiotics, and even to lymphoma of the colon. It is thought to be due at least in part to impairment of muscular or neuromuscular function in the colon wall, leading to progressive dilatation. Also called *acute megacolon*.

megacoulomb [MEGA- + COULOMB] A unit of quantity of electricity, electric charge, or electric flux equal to 10^6 coulombs. Symbol: MC

megacurie [MEGA- + CURIE] A unit of activity of a radionuclide or of a radioactive source equal to 10^6 curies; 3.7×10^{16} becquerels exactly. Symbol: MCi

megacycle A popular but incorrect term for MEGACYCLE PER SECOND.

  megacycle per second A unit of frequency equal to 10^6 cycles per second; 10^6 hertz or one megahertz. Also called *megacycle (popular but incorrect)*. Symbol: Mc/s ● The term *megahertz* is now commonly employed.

megacystis MEGALOCYSTIS.

megadactyl MEGALODACTYLOUS.

megadactylia MACRODACTYLY.

megadactylism MACRODACTYLY.

megadactyly MACRODACTYLY.

megadolichocolon A distended and elongated colon.

megadont MACRODONT.

megadontia [MEGA- + -(o)dontia] MACRODONTIA.

megadontic MACRODONT.

megadontism [MEGA- + -(o)dont + -ISM] MACRODONTIA.

megaduodenum A distended duodenum.

megadyne [MEGA- + DYNE] A unit of force equal to 10^6 dynes; 10 newtons. Symbol: Mdyn

megaelectronvolt [MEGA- + ELECTRONVOLT] A unit of energy equal to 10^6 electronvolts; $1.602\ 19 \times 10^{-13}$ joule; 160.219 petajoules. Symbol: MeV

megaesophagus Enlarged esophagus as commonly found in achalasia. Also called *megaloesophagus*.

megafarad [MEGA- + FARAD] A unit of electrical capacitance equal to 10^6 farads. Symbol: MF

megafauna Terrestrial animals such as large snails, small mammals, reptiles, and amphibians that are slightly larger than the macrofauna.

megagamete MACROGAMETE.

megagnathia MACROGNATHIA.

megahertz A unit of frequency equal to 10^6 hertz. Symbol: MHz

megajoule [MEGA- + JOULE] A unit of energy, work, or quantity of heat equal to 10^6 joules. Symbol: MJ

megakaryoblast A large bone-marrow cell with an unsegmented nucleus and abundant, usually granular, cytoplasm. It is the precursor of the megakaryocyte. Also *megacaryoblast.*

megakaryocyte A very large bone-marrow cell, usually with multiple nuclear lobes and copious granular cytoplasm, which releases membrane-enclosed fragments of its cytoplasm as platelets. Also called *megalokaryocyte, megalocaryocyte.* Also *megacaryocyte.*

basophilic megakaryocyte PROMEGAKARYOCYTE.

lymphoid megakaryocyte PROMEGAKARYOCYTE.

stage II megakaryocyte PROMEGAKARYOCYTE.

megakaryocytopenia An abnormal decrease in the number of megakaryocytes in the bone marrow.

megakaryocytosis 1 An increase in the number of megakaryocytes in the bone marrow. 2 The occurrence of megakaryocytes in the peripheral blood.

megakaryophthisis Reduced platelet production due to a decreased number of megakaryocytes in the bone marrow.

megalakria A seldom used term for ACROMEGALY.

megalecithal [MEGA- + LECITH- + -AL] Full of yolk: said of an ovum. Also *macrolecithal, polylecithal.*

megalencephalon MACROENCEPHALON.

megalencephaly MACROENCEPHALY.

megalerythema ERYTHEMA INFECTIOSUM.

megalgia A severe pain of sudden onset: usually applied to muscular rheumatism.

megalo- [Gk *megas* (feminine *megalē*) large, big] A combining form meaning of abnormally large size.

megaloblast Any of a series of abnormally large, nucleated erythrocyte precursors seen in the bone marrow in pernicious anemia or other disorders of vitamin B_{12} or folic acid metabolism.

megaloblast of Sabin PRONORMOBLAST.

megaloblastic Exhibiting the morphologic features of megaloblasts: said of erythrocyte precursors. Compare NORMOBLASTIC.

megaloblastoid Having some features resembling megaloblastic maturation of the erythrocytic series. An erythrocyte precursor is said to be megaloblastoid when nuclear chromatin condensation is in clumps, as it is normally, but parachromatin is prominent: i.e., open, transparent, unstained clefts are prominent in the nucleus and the contours of the nucleus are irregular.

megaloblastosis The presence of megaloblasts in the bone marrow.

megalocardia CARDIOMEGALY.

megalocaryocyte MEGAKARYOCYTE.

megalocephalia [MEGALO- + CEPHAL- + -IA] MACROCEPHALY.

megalocephalic [MEGALO- + CEPHALIC] MACROCEPHALOUS.

megalocephaly [MEGALO- + CEPHAL- + -Y] MACROCEPHALY.

megalocheiria CHEIROMEGALY.

megaloclitoris [MEGALO- + CLITORIS] MACROCLITORIS.

megalocornea [MEGALO- + CORNEA] A sex-linked recessive condition in which the corneal diameter is enlarged, without increased intraocular pressure. Also called *keratoglobus, cornea globata, cornea globosa.*

megalocystis An abnormally enlarged or distended bladder. Also called *megacystis, megabladder.*

megalocyte MACROCYTE.

megalocythemia MACROCYTOSIS.

megalocytosis MACROCYTOSIS.

megalodactylia MACRODACTYLY.

megalodactylism MACRODACTYLY.

megalodactylous Exhibiting macrodactyly. Also *megadactyl.*

megalodactyly MACRODACTYLY.

megalodont MACRODONT.

megalodontia [*megal(o)-* + -ODONTIA] MACRODONTIA.

megaloencephalic Exhibiting macroencephaly.

megaloencephalon MACROENCEPHALON.

megaloencephaly MACROENCEPHALY.

megaloenteron Abnormal largeness of the intestinal tract or segment thereof; enteromegaly.

megaloesophagus MEGAESOPHAGUS.

megalogastria [MEGALO- + GASTR- + -IA] Abnormal enlargement or distention of the stomach.

megaloglossia MACROGLOSSIA.

megalohepatia HEPATOMEGALY.

megalokaryoblastoma An obsolete term for HODGKIN'S DISEASE.

megalokaryocyte MEGAKARYOCYTE.

megalomania [MEGALO- + -MANIA] A delusion of grandeur characterized by belief in one's unsurpassed power, greatness, or eminence, as in some field of endeavor.

megalomastia [MEGALO- + MAST- + -IA] MACROMASTIA.

megalomelia [MEGALO- + MEL-[1] + -IA] MACROMELIA.

megalonychia MACRONYCHIA.

megalonychosis MACRONYCHIA.

megalopenis MACROPENIS.

megalophallus MACROPENIS.

megalophthalmia MACROPHTHALMIA.

megalophthalmos MACROPHTHALMIA.

megalophthalmus MACROPHTHALMIA.

megalopia MACROPSIA.

megaloplastocyte GIANT PLATELET.

megalopodia [MEGALO- + -POD + -IA] MACROPODIA.

megalopsia MACROPSIA.

Megalopyge A genus of flannel moths (family Megalopygidae).

Megalopyge opercularis A species of flannel moth whose larvae have hairs that carry an urticating toxic substance and can pierce the skin, causing caterpillar dermatitis.

megalosplanchnic Having abnormal largeness of some or all viscera, particularly of major cavity organs.

megalosplenia SPLENOMEGALY.

megalospore [MEGALO- + SPORE] MACROCONIDIUM.

Megalosporon An obsolete term for *TRICHOPHYTON.*

megalosyndactylia MEGALOSYNDACTYLY.

megalosyndactyly [MEGALO- + SYNDACTYLY] A condition characterized by the abnormally large size and fusion of two or more digits. Also called *megalosyndactylia.*

megaloureter In an infant, an abnormally large size of a ureter occurring in the absence of evident obstruction or infection. It is presumed to be of developmental origin. Also called *megaureter.*

megalourethra [MEGALO- + URETHRA] In an infant, an abnormally large urethra occurring in the absence of obstruction or infection. It is presumed to be of developmental origin.

-megaly [Gk *megaleios* (from *megas,* feminine *megalē,* large, big) magnificent] A combining form meaning of abnormally large size.

megamelia [MEGA- + MEL-[1] + -IA] MACROMELIA.

megamerozoite MACROMEROZOITE.

megampere MEGA-AMPERE.

meganewton [MEGA- + NEWTON] A unit of force equal to 10^6 newtons. Symbol: MN

Meganthropus palaeojavanicus A taxonomic designation that has been applied to some fossil hominids of Java represented by mandibular fragments. They are now commonly classified as early *Homo erectus*.

meganucleus [MEGA- + NUCLEUS] MACRONUCLEUS.

megaohm MEGOHM.

megapascal [MEGA- + PASCAL] A unit of pressure or stress equal to 10^6 pascals. Symbol: MPa

megaprosopia [MEGA- + PROSOP- + -IA] MACROPROSOPIA.

megaprosopous [MEGA- + PROSOP- + -OUS] Exhibiting macroprosopia.

megarectum Marked distension of the rectum.

Megarhininae TOXORHYNCHITINAE.

Megarhinus TOXORHYNCHITES.

megaroentgen [MEGA- + ROENTGEN] A unit of ionization exposure equal to 10^6 roentgen; 2.58×10^2 coulomb per kilogram. Symbol: MR

Megaselia A genus of flies some species of which have produced myiasis in humans from larvae in wounds. *M. scalaris (Apiochaeta ferruginea)* has also been reported as a cause of human intestinal myiasis.

megaseme [MEGA- + Gk *sēm(a)* a sign, mark] Having an orbital index of more than 89.

megasigmoid Marked distension and elongation of the sigmoid colon.

megasoma GIGANTISM.

megasome [MEGA- + Gk *sōm(a)* body] An individual with gigantism. Also called *giant*.

megasomia [MEGA- + Gk *sōm(a)* body + -IA] GIGANTISM.

megaspore [MEGA- + SPORE] MACROCONIDIUM.

megasthenic [MEGA- + STHEN- + -IC] Enormously strong.

megatherm [MEGA- + Gk *therm(ē)* heat] An organism that is dependent upon high temperatures for its normal development.

megatonne [MEGA- + TONNE] A unit of mass or weight equal to 10^6 tonnes, or 10^9 kilograms: used especially to describe the equivalent explosive power of nuclear weapons in terms of tonnes of TNT. Symbol: Mt

megaunit [MEGA- + UNIT] A quantity equal to 10^6 units. Symbol: MU

megaureter MEGALOURETER.

megavolt [MEGA- + VOLT] A unit of electrical potential, potential difference, or electromotive force equal to 10^6 volts. Symbol: MV

megavoltage Voltage of more than a million volts. Megavoltage radiation may refer to x rays or gamma rays having photon energies greater than a million electron volts.

megavolt-ampere A unit of electrical power equal to 10^6 volt-amperes. Symbol: MV·A

megawatt [MEGA- + WATT] A unit of power equal to 10^6 watts. Symbol: MW

megestrol acetate $C_{25}H_{32}O_4$. 17-(Acetyloxy)-6-methyl-16-methylene-pregna-4,6-diene-3,20-dione. A synthetic progentin used as an antineoplastic agent in the palliative management of metastatic endometrial carcinoma. It is given orally.

Megimide A proprietary name for bemegride.

Méglin [Jean Antoine *Méglin*, French physician, 1756–1824] See under POINT.

meglumine diatrizoate A methylglucamine salt of diatrizoic acid, used as a water-soluble positive contrast medium for intravascular administration, as in angiography and urography.

meglumine iodipamide 3,3-Adipoly-bis(3-amino-2,4,6-triiodobenzoic acid), the methylglucamine salt of iodipamic acid, used as a contrast medium for intravenous cholangiography. Also called *methylglucamine iodipamide*.

meglumine iothalamate A methylglucamine salt of iodothalamic acid, used as a radiopaque medium administered intravascularly, as in angiography and urography.

megohm A unit of electric resistance equal to 10^6 ohms. Also called *megaohm*. Symbol: MΩ

megophthalmos MACROPHTHALMIA.

megrim [Middle English *migrene, migrein*, from Middle French *migraine*. See MIGRAINE.] MIGRAINE.

Mehlis [Karl Friedrich Eduard *Mehlis*, German physician, 1796–1832] Mehlis glands. See under GLAND.

mehlnährschaden [German *Mehl* meal, flour + *nähr(en)* to feed, nourish + *Schaden* damage, injury] A disorder similar to kwashiorkor that arises in children as a result of protein malnutrition. It is characterized by growth failure, despite a normal fat skinfold thickness, muscle wasting, edema, and psychomotor disturbances.

Meibom [Heinrich *Meibom*, German anatomist, 1638–1700] **1** Meibomian glands. See under GLANDULAE TARSALES. **2** Meibomian stye. See under STYE.

meibomianitis Inflammation of the tarsal glands (Meibomian glands). Also called *meibomitis*.

meibomitis MEIBOMIANITIS.

Meige [Henry *Meige*, French physician, 1866–1940] **1** Meige's disease, trophoedema of Meige. See under LYMPHEDEMA. **2** Nonne-Milroy-Meige syndrome. See under HEREDITARY LYMPHEDEMA TYPE I.

Meigs [Arthur Vincent *Meigs*, U.S. physiologist, 1850–1912] **1** See under TEST. **2** Meigs capillaries. See under CAPILLARY.

Meigs [Joe Vincent *Meigs*, U.S. gynecologist, 1892–1963] See under SYNDROME.

meio- MIO-.

meiogenic [MEIO- + -GENIC] Promoting or causing meiosis.

meiosis [Gk *meiōsis* (from *meioun* to lessen) a lessening, diminution] The process of genetic recombination and division of diploid germ cells to produce haploid gametes occurring in gonadal tissue. The functional steps are DNA replication; pairing of homologous chromosomes; crossing-over (recombination); meiotic division I, in which each diploid daughter cell receives one duplicated homologue (two sister chromatids); and meiotic division II, in which each haploid gamete receives one sister chromatid of each chromosome of the set. Adjective: meiotic.

meiospore A spore formed as a result of meiosis.

meiosporangium [MEIO- + SPORANGIUM] (*plural* meiosporangia) An oval, thick-walled, sculptured, resistant, generally overwintering, fungal sporangium which produces diploid zoospores.

meiotic Pertaining to or resulting from meiosis.

Meirowsky [Emil *Meirowsky*, U.S. dermatologist, 1876–1960] See under PHENOMENON.

Meissner [Georg *Meissner*, German histologist, 1829–1905] **1** See under GANGLION. **2** Meissner's plexus. See under PLEXUS SUBMUCOSUS. **3** Meissner's corpuscles. See under CORPUSCULA TACTUS.

mel [Gk *mel(i)* honey] Honey, especially the refined, clarified honey used in pharmaceutical preparations.

mel-¹ [Gk *melos* limb] A combining form meaning limb. Also called *melo-¹*.

mel-² MELO-².

mel-³ MELI-.

melagra [MEL-¹ + -AGRA] Muscle pain occurring in the extremities. An obsolete term.

melalgia [MEL-¹ + -ALGIA] Pain in the extremities.

melamine A heterocyclic compound, derived from cyanuric acid, whose molecules consist of six-membered rings, each comprising three —N=C(—NH$_2$)— groups.

melamine formaldehyde A plastic made from melamine and formaldehyde, in which melamine units are joined by methylene bridges between their amino groups.

melan- MELANO-.

melancholia [Late L (from MELAN- + Gk *cholē* gall, bile + -IA), melancholy] **1** DEPRESSION. **2** ENDOGENOUS DEPRESSION. **3** A condition characterized by severe depression as manifested by loss of pleasure in all activities, early morning awakening, marked agitation or retardation, severe anorexia with weight loss, intensification of symptoms in the morning, and excessive or inappropriate guilt feelings. Also called *athymia* (obsolete), *cafard, monomoria, tristimania.*

acute melancholia The second most severe form of depression in manic-depressive psychosis.

affective melancholia A depressive form of manic-depressive psychosis. An older term.

melancholia agitata INVOLUTIONAL MELANCHOLIA.

agitated melancholia INVOLUTIONAL MELANCHOLIA.

melancholia attonita Depression marked by immobility, as in depressive stupor or catatonic withdrawal.

climacteric melancholia INVOLUTIONAL MELANCHOLIA.

melancholia hypochondriaca Depression accompanied by somatic delusions of a hypochondriacal nature.

involutional melancholia A major depression occurring for the first time in the involutional period, between 40 and 55 years in females and 50 to 65 years in males. Its characteristic triad of symptoms are delusions of guilt or poverty, obsession with death, and delusional fixation on gastrointestinal functioning all within a setting of agitation and depression. In some, paranoid delusions of persecution also occur. Also called *climacteric psychosis, agitated depression, involutional depression, climacteric insanity* (obsolete), *involutional psychosis, climacteric melancholia, affective paraphrenia* (obsolete), *degenerative insanity* (obsolete), *agitated melancholia, melancholia agitata, involutional psychotic reaction, involutional paraphrenia.*

paranoid melancholia Depression with paranoid delusions, usually a form of involutional melancholia.

paretic melancholia Depression accompanying parenchymatous syphilis of the central nervous system.

melancholia religiosa Depression with delusions of having committed an unpardonable sin.

melancholia simplex The least severe form of depression in manic-depressive psychosis.

stuporous melancholia DEPRESSIVE STUPOR.

melanedema [MELAN- + EDEMA] COAL WORKERS' PNEUMOCONIOSIS.

melanemesis An obsolete term for COFFEE-GROUND VOMIT.

melanemia The presence of melanin in blood.

melanephidrosis The production of black-brown sweat.

Melania [MELAN- + -IA] A genus of snails in the family Thiaridae that serve as hosts for several genera of parasitic trematodes.

melanic [MELAN- + -IC] Black in color.

melanicterus WINCKEL'S DISEASE.

melanidrosis [MELAN- + *(h)idrosis*] Black sweat. It is usually apocrine in origin.

melaniferous Containing melanin.

melanin [MELAN- + -IN] The natural pigment of hair and skin, also found in other parts of the body. It is formed by the oxidation of tyrosine via dopa and dopaquinone to a complex polymeric material.

melanism [MELAN- + -ISM] Excessive melanin pigmentation.

metallic melanism ARGYRIA.

melanistic Affected by melanism.

melano- [Gk *melas* (genitive *melanos*) black, dark] A combining form meaning black, dark. Also *melan-*.

melanoacanthoma A seborrheic keratosis in which a high melanin content is present within melanocytes.

melanoameloblastoma [MELANO- + AMELOBLASTOMA] MELANOTIC NEUROECTODERMAL TUMOR.

melanoblast A derivative of the neural crest which differentiates in an embryo into a melanocyte.

amelanotic melanoblast A precursor of the melanocyte that does not contain demonstrable melanin.

melanoblastoma [MELANO- + BLASTOMA] MALIGNANT MELANOMA.

melanoblastosis [MELANO- + BLAST- + -OSIS] MELANOTIC NEUROECTODERMAL TUMOR.

melanocancroid A pigmented epithelial ulcer. An imprecise and obsolete term.

melanocarcinoma [MELANO- + CARCINOMA] MALIGNANT MELANOMA.

melanochroic Pertaining to Caucasians having dark hair and a pale complexion.

melanocomous Having black hair. An obsolete term.

melanocyte A cell bearing or capable of forming melanin. Also called *pigment cell of skin, Merkel-Ranvier cell.*

melanocytoma [MELANO- + CYT- + -OMA] A benign pigment deposit upon the optic disk, occurring especially in black persons.

compound melanocytoma A benign tumor that arises from epidermal melanocytes and is characterized both by junctional activity and nevus cells in the dermis.

dermal melanocytoma A cutaneous lesion arising from a proliferation of dermal melanocytes.

melanocytosis A condition characterized by the presence of excessive numbers of melanocytes.

melanoderm [MELANO- + -DERM] A dark-skinned individual.

melanoderma [MELANO- + DERMA] An excess of melanin pigmentation in the skin.

melanoderma cachecticorum CHLOASMA OF CACHEXIA.

parasitic melanoderma VAGRANTS' DISEASE.

racial melanoderma Dark pigmentation resulting from genetic factors associated with race.

senile melanoderma Hyperpigmentation of the skin that appears with advancing age.

melanodermatitis [MELANO- + DERMATITIS] Dermatitis associated with melanosis.

melanodermatitis toxica lichenoides The melanosis, atrophy, telangiectasia, and lichenoid papules that result from exposure to a combination of coal-tar products and sunlight.

melanodermic Affected by or pertaining to melanoderma.

melanodes MELANOID.

melanoepithelioma [MELANO- + EPITHELIOMA] **1** A carcinoma containing melanin. **2** An obsolete term for MALIGNANT MELANOMA.

melanogen A colorless intermediate in the metabolic pathway of tyrosine to melanin that may be nonenzymatically converted to melanin under certain circumstances.

melanogenemia [MELANO- + -GEN + -EMIA] The presence of melanin precursors, such as 3,4-dihydroxyphenylalanine, or related substances, in the blood. This phenomenon may occur in persons with disseminated malignant melanoma.

melanogenesis [*melan(in)* + *o* + GENESIS] The process of melanin formation. Adjective: melanogenic.

melanoglossia [MELANO- + GLOSS- + -IA] BLACKTONGUE.

melanoid 1 Dark in color. **2** A pigment resembling melanin. Also called *melanodes*.

Melanoides THIARA.

melanokinesis Melanin turnover.

Melanolestes A genus of reduviid bugs. Their bite may cause a severe skin reaction.

Melanolestes picipes A species of kissing bug, the black corsair, common in parts of the United States. Its bite is said to have an effect like that of a wasp's sting.

melanoleukoderma Patchy and irregular increased and decreased melanosis. It is usually postinflammatory. Also called *leukomelanoderma*.

melanoleukoderma colli VENEREAL COLLAR.

melanoma [MELAN- + -OMA] Any benign or malignant melanocytic tumor.

acral lentiginous melanoma A malignant melanoma occurring on the palms, soles, or nailbeds and characterized by a lentiginous growth of atypical melanocytes in the epidermis, elongated rete ridges, and acanthosis.

amelanotic melanoma A melanoma without pigment. • This term is usually applied to a malignant melanoma and not to a nonpigmented nevus.

benign melanoma NEVUS.

benign juvenile melanoma EPITHELIAL AND/OR SPINDLE CELL NEVUS.

Cloudman melanoma S91 A spontaneous, transplantable, malignant melanoma of mice.

melanoma de novo A malignant melanoma arising from an area where no previous nevus or lesion has been.

Harding-Passey melanoma A spontaneous, transplantable, malignant melanoma of mice.

juvenile melanoma EPITHELIOID AND/OR SPINDLE CELL NEVUS.

malignant melanoma A highly malignant tumor of melanocytic cells. The tumor most often occurs in the skin. It may arise de novo, from a pre-existing nevus or from a precancerous melanosis (Hutchinson's melanotic freckle). It appears to be more frequent in light-skinned people than in the heavily pigmented races. It is rare in children. The eye is the second most frequent site. Here melanoma typically arises from uveal structures. As in skin, darkly pigmented peoples are not commonly affected. Among other sites for primary malignant melanoma are the oral mucosa, nose, vagina, lung, and meninges. All are rare and highly malignant. Metastases are typically widespread, at unusual sites, for example, the heart and small bowel, and may appear after long quiescent periods. Also called *melanomalignancy, melanoblastoma, anthracina* (obsolete), *cancer anthracinus* (obsolete), *melanocarcinoma, black cancer* (obsolete), *melanotic cancer, chromoma* (obsolete), *melanosarcoma* (obsolete), *melanotic carcinoma, carcinoma melanodes, melanoepithelioma* (obsolete), *carcinoma nigrum, chromatophoroma* (obsolete), *nevocarcinoma, nevomelanoma, melanotic sarcoma*. • Melanoma is often used without modification as a synonym of malignant melanoma. However this may be ambiguous, as some call a nevus a benign melanoma.

spindle cell melanoma A malignant melanoma with fusiform tumor cells: used more for ocular than dermal melanomas. Spindle cell melanomas of the eye are often less aggressive than epithelioid cell melanomas.

subungual melanoma A malignant melanoma arising under a fingernail.

melanoma suprarenale ADDISON'S DISEASE.

melanomalignancy [MELANO- + MALIGNANCY] MALIGNANT MELANOMA.

melanomatosis [*melanomat(a)*, pl. of MELANOMA + -OSIS] Widespread malignant melanomas.

melanomatous [*melanomat(a)*, pl. of MELANOMA + -OUS] Pertaining to melanoma.

melanonychia [MELAN- + ONYCH- + -IA] Black or brown discoloration of the nails. It may appear as diffuse, longitudinal, or transverse streaking.

melanopathy [MELANO- + -PATHY] Any disorder of melanin pigmentation.

melanophage A cell which contains melanin pigment due to phagocytosis but which is unable to synthesize melanin.

melanophore A pigment cell containing melanin. Melanophores contribute to rapid color changes in some organisms due to the movement of melanosomes within the melanophores.

melanophorin A chemical which can cause the dispersion of the pigment in a melanophore.

melanoplakia The presence of pigmented patches on the oral or genital mucous membrane.

melanoptysis The expectoration of black-tinged sputum containing carbon pigment due to the repeated inhalation of great amounts of coal dust, as in coal mining.

melanorrhagia [MELANO- + -RRHAGIA] The passage of melenic and bloody stool.

melanosarcoma [MELANO- + SARCOMA] An obsolete term for MALIGNANT MELANOMA.

melanosarcomatosis [MELANO- + *sarcomat(a)*, pl. of SARCOMA + -OSIS] Multiple or disseminated malignant melanomas. An obsolete term.

melanoscirrhus [MELANO- + SCIRRHUS] A firm malignant melanoma. An outmoded term.

melanosis [MELAN- + -OSIS] The abnormal black-brown pigmentation of tissues due to the deposition of melanin or melaninlike substances. Adjective: melanotic.

melanosis coli The presence of a brown to black mucosal discoloration in the colon or a segment thereof that has no clinical significance and is due to the accumulation of macrophages within the lamina propria containing a melanin-like pigment. The pigment is histochemically similar to melanin and lipofuscin. Also called *melanosis of the colon*.

melanosis of the colon MELANOSIS COLI.

melanosis of the eyelids PERIOCULAR HYPERPIGMENTATION.

oculocutaneous melanosis OTA'S NEVUS.

melanosis of Ordoñez A generalized, reversible hypermelanosis that occurs among malnourished subjects who live at high elevations.

precancerous melanosis of Dubreuilh HUTCHINSON'S MELANOTIC FRECKLE.

Riehl's melanosis Melanosis that affects primarily the forehead and temples and is possibly caused by external contact with photodynamic agents.

melanosis sclerae Congenital pigmented flecks in the sclera.

tar melanosis Melanosis due to contact with tar.

toxic melanosis of Hoffmann and Habermann Melanosis associated with follicular hyperkeratosis of the hands and forearms. It is caused by contact with tar and mineral oil.

melanosity [New L *melanos(is)* abnormal deposit of dark pigments in tissues, from Gk *melan*, neut. of *melas* dark, black + New L *-os(is)* -OSIS + -ITY] A darkness of the skin.

melanosome [MELANO- + Gk *sōm(a)* body] A discrete melanin-containing organelle, usually located near a Golgi body. The melanosome appears uniformly electron-dense and without demonstrable tyrosinase activity. Also called *melanin granule*.

compound melanosome   The precursor of the mature melanin granule. It has a spiral or laminar structure contained within an oval vesicle.

melanotic   Affected with melanosis.

melanotrichia [MELANO- + TRICH- + -IA]   A darkness of the hair.

melanotrichia linguae   BLACK HAIRY TONGUE.

melanotropic [MELANO- + -TROPIC¹]   Possessing an attraction to melanin.

melanotropin   The pituitary hormone that stimulates melanin-granule dispersion in amphibian and fish melanocytes, as well as melanin synthesis in mammalian melanocytes. Two forms exist, α-melanotropin, an *N*-acylated tridecapeptide amide, and β-melanotropin, a peptide of 18 residues. Both are formed by proteolysis of larger molecules. The sequence of α-melanotropin is included within the corticotropin molecule, and β-melanotropin has several residues in common with it.

melanous [MELAN- + -OUS]   Of or relating to a dark skin.

melanthin   A toxic glycoside found in the seeds of *Nigella sativa*.

melanuresis   MELANURIA.

melanuria [MELAN- + -URIA]   The excretion of melanin in the urine as seen in patients with widely metastatic malignant melanoma. Melanin is excreted as a colorless precursor that becomes dark when the urine stands at room temperature for several hours. Also called *melanuresis*. Adjective: melanuric.

melanuric   Characterized by or pertaining to melanuria.

melarsoprol $C_{12}H_{15}AsN_6OS_2$. A narrow-spectrum antiprotozoal drug containing trivalent arsenic (melarsen oxide) and dimercaprol. It is used for treating advanced African trypanosomiasis with central nervous system involvement. Also called *Mel B*.

melasma [Gk *melasma* (from *melas* black) a black spot]   Hypermelanosis affecting the cheeks, forehead, and chin. Also called *chloasma, melasma gravidarum, gravidic mask, mask of pregnancy, uterine mask*.

melasma addisonii   An older term for ADDISON'S DISEASE.

melasma gravidarum   MELASMA.

melasma suprarenale   An older term for ADDISON'S DISEASE.

melasma universale   A generalized darkened pigmentation.

melatonin   *N*-Acetyl-5-methoxytryptamine. A natural substance formed by methylation and acetylation of serotonin. It is nearly uniquely synthesized in and secreted by the pineal gland, and in amphibia it has an action opposite to that of melanocyte stimulating hormone. It stimulates the aggregation of melanosomes in melanophores, thus lightening the skin. Postulated to be the pineal hormone, its physiologic role in man is unknown. Also called *melanocyte inhibiting factor*.

melatrophy   Atrophy of the extremities. A seldom used term.

Mel B   MELARSOPROL.

melena [Gk *melaina*, fem. of *melas* black]   The passage of dark or blackish, tarry stools stained with altered blood. Compare HEMATOCHEZIA.

melena neonatorum   Melenic stool in the newborn.

melena spuria   Melena produced from blood resulting from bleeding other than in the gastrointestinal tract, such as deglutition from a nose bleed, or produced by ingestion of other substances that can cause black stools, such as bismuth.

melena vera   True melena; dark stool due to the presence of blood derived from bleeding into the intestinal tract.

melenemesis [Gk *melain(a)*, fem. of *melas* black + *emesis* a vomiting]   COFFEE-GROUND VOMIT.

Meleney [Frank Lamont *Meleney*, U.S. surgeon, 1889–1963]   **1** Meleney synergistic gangrene. See under PROGRESSIVE POSTOPERATIVE GANGRENE.   **2** See under ULCER.

melenic   Relating to or characterized by melena. Also *melenotic*.

melenotic   MELENIC.

melezitose   A trisaccharide found in gymnosperm trees, such as larch and fir, and consisting of sucrose glucosylated on C-3 of its fructose residue. It cannot be digested by bees, and often crystallizes from their honey.

meli- [Gk *meli* (genitive *melitos*) honey]   A combining form meaning honey, sweet. Also *mel-³*.

melibiose   The disaccharide consisting of galactose bearing an α-glucosyl group on O-6. It occurs naturally as a digestion product of raffinose.

melicera [Gk *melikēra* (from *meli* honey + *kēros* wax) a virulent eruption on the head]   A cyst containing viscous, sticky, semi-solid material.

melilotic acid   3-(2-Hydroxyphenyl)propionic acid. An acid found in plants, often glycosylated.

melilotoxin   DICUMAROL.

melioidosis [Gk *mēli(s)* a distemper of asses + -OID + -OSIS]   An infectious disease primarily of rodents that occurs occasionally in farm and pet animals and man. It resembles equine glanders and is caused by *Pseudomonas pseudomallei*. The portal of entry is probably via open skin lesions and by inhalation. The severity of illness ranges from inapparent infection to overwhelming septicemia. The disease has a protean clinical spectrum, including acute or chronic localized suppurative infection, acute pneumonitis with abscess formation, and septicemia. Hepatic and splenic abscesses may also be present. It occurs most commonly in India, Malaysia, Burma, Thailand, and Indonesia. Isolation of the organism from urine, blood, or skin pustules is the best method of diagnosis in the acute disease. In the chronic form, serologic tests are of value. *P. pseudomallei* is usually sensitive to chloramphenicol, tetracycline, sulfadiazine, and novobiocin. Also called *pseudoglanders, malleoidosis, Whitmore's fever, Stanton's disease*.

melissic   Derived from honey or beeswax.

melissic acid CH_3—$[CH_2]_{28}$—COOH. A long-chain fatty acid, found in beeswax.

melissotherapy   APIOTHERAPY.

melitensis [after *Melit(a)*, ancient L name of Malta + L -*ensis* English -*ese*]   MALTA FEVER.

melitin   A preparation of soluble antigen of *Brucella melitensis*, used in the diagnosis of undulant fever. When injected intradermally in the arm a skin reaction may develop, indicating that a *Brucella* infection has occurred previously.

melitis [MEL-² + -ITIS]   Inflammation of the cheek.

melitococcosis [L *Melit(a)* Malta + *o* + L *cocc(us)* the scarlet berry, kermes berry + -OSIS]   BRUCELLOSIS.

melitoptyalon   Sugar, especially glucose, in the saliva.

melituria [Gk *meli* (gen. *melitos*) honey + -URIA]   The presence of sugar in the urine. Also *mellituria*. Adjective: melituric.

melituria inosita   INOSITURIA.

melituric   Pertaining to or having melituria.

Melkersson [Ernst Gustaf *Melkersson*, Swedish physician, 1898–1932]   Melkersson syndrome. See under MELKERSSON-ROSENTHAL SYNDROME.

Mellaril   A proprietary name for thioridazine hydrochloride.

mellitic acid   Benzenehexacarboxylic acid. It occurs as an aluminum salt in coal.

mellitum [L, substantive from *mellitum*, neut. sing. of *mellitus* pertaining to honey]   Any sweet pharmaceutical preparation containing honey.

mellituria   MELITURIA.

Melnick [John Charles *Melnick*, U.S. roentgenologist, born

1928] Melnick-Needles syndrome. See under SYNDROME.

melo-¹ MEL-¹.

melo-² [Gk *mēlon* apple, fruit of a tree, cheek] A combining form meaning cheek. Also *mel-²*.

melocervicoplasty [MELO- + CERVICO- + -PLASTY] FACE-LIFT.

melodidymia [MELO- + -*didym(us)* + -IA] The existence of an extra limb. An imprecise and obsolete term.

melodidymus [MELO- + -DIDYMUS] An individual with an extra limb. An imprecise and obsolete term.

melomania [Gk *melo(s)* a song + -MANIA] Psychosis in which the main manifestation is incessant singing. An obsolete term.

melomelia [MELO-¹ + MEL-¹ + -IA] A condition of unequal conjoined twins in which both normal limbs and rudimentary accessory limbs are present.

melomelus Unequal conjoined twins with melomelia.

melon 1 A large, berrylike fruit with a firm covering. 2 A plant of the species *Cucumis melo* or *Citrullus lanatus.* The fruit of the plant is borne on a vine.

meloncus [MEL-² + -ONCUS] A tumor of the cheek. An outmoded term.

melonoplasty MELOPLASTY.

Melophagus A genus of wingless parasitic louse flies of the dipteran family Hippoboscidae. *M. ovinus,* the ked, or so-called sheep tick, is a bloodsucking ectoparasite of sheep and goats widely distributed in the cool temperate parts of the world.

meloplastic Pertaining to meloplasty.

meloplasty [MELO- + -PLASTY] Any plastic operation on the cheeks. Also called *melonoplasty, maloplasty.*

melorheostosis [Gk *melo(s)* limb + *rhe(o)-* + -OST- + -OSIS] A rare abnormality of long bone growth in which the cortex becomes thickened and irregular to resemble the appearance of a candle with melted wax that has flowed down the sides. Also called *Leri's disease, candle wax disease, rheostosis, flowing hyperostosis, osteopathia hyperostotica congenita.*

melosalgia [Gk *melos* limb + -ALGIA] Pain in the lower extremities.

meloschisis [MELO- + -SCHISIS] A congenital facial cleft in which a groove or fissure crosses the cheek. It may run obliquely upward toward the lower eyelid (oblique facial cleft) or it may cross the face transversely from the corner of the mouth (genal cleft).

melotia [MEL-² + OT- + -IA] The congenital displacement of the external ears, as in low-set ears.

melotrophosis [Gk *melo(s)* a limb + TROPH- + -OSIS] Any trophic disorder of the extremities, especially of the hand. A rarely used term.

traumatic melotrophosis Any of a variety of trophic disorders involving the hand, once thought to be of sympathetic origin, and attributed to the aftereffects of a cut on a finger. No such identifiable disease or syndrome exists. An obsolete term.

Melotte [George W. *Melotte,* U.S. dentist, 1835–1915] See under METAL.

melotus [MEL-² + OT- + New L *-us,* masc. noun suffix] An individual with displaced, usually low-set, external ears.

melphalan $C_{13}H_{18}Cl_2N_2O_2$. 4-[Bis(2-chloroethyl)amino]-L-phenylalanine. A phenylalanine analogue of the nitrogen mustards, used as an antineoplastic agent. It is given orally.

melting 1 The transition of solid to liquid, in which ions or molecules leave ordered positions and acquire random motions. 2 Any of several processes in which molecules or parts of molecules acquire greater random movement, such as the tumbling motion of lipid hydrocarbon chains within a biologic membrane and the disruption of base stacking in nucleic acid on heating.

Meltzer [Samuel James *Meltzer,* U.S. physiologist, 1851–1920] 1 See under REACTION. 2 Meltzer's anesthesia. See under METHOD. 3 Meltzer's law. See under LAW OF CONTRARY INNERVATION. 4 Meltzer-Lyon test. See under TEST.

member A constituent or part of a body; a limb or appendage; membrum.

inferior member MEMBRUM INFERIUS.

virile member PENIS.

memberment The way in which parts of the body are arranged.

membra Plural of MEMBRUM.

membrana

membrana [L (from *membrum* a member, limb, part; akin to *fibra* fiber, filament of a plant, *fimbria* a thread, and *barba* a beard), a thin skin, web of fibers, membrane, film] (*plural* membranae) [NA] A thin layer of tissue that covers a surface of a part, cavity, or organ; that connects two structures; or that divides a space or an organ. Also called *membrane.*

membrana abdominis An outmoded term for PERITONEUM.

membrana adamantina NASMYTH'S MEMBRANE.

membrana adventitia 1 An outmoded term for TUNICA ADVENTITIA. 2 An outmoded term for DECIDUA CAPSULARIS.

membrana agnina AMNION.

membrana atlanto-occipitalis anterior [NA] A sheet of dense fibers extending from the anterior surface and upper margin of the anterior arch of the atlas to the anterior margin of the foramen magnum and the inferior aspect of the basilar part of the occipital bone. The thicker central fibers, attached to the anterior tubercle, are continuous inferiorly with the anterior longitudinal ligament. Also called *anterior atlanto-occipital membrane, anterior atlanto-occipital ligament, atlanto-occipital obturator ligament* (outmoded), *anterior obturator membrane of atlas* (outmoded), *deep atlanto-occipital ligament, obturator ligament of atlas* (outmoded).

membrana atlanto-occipitalis posterior [NA] A broad, flaccid sheet extending from the posterior surface and upper margin of the posterior arch of the atlas to the posterior margin of the foramen magnum between the two condyles. It corresponds to the position of the ligamenta flava and is adherent to the dura mater anteriorly. It forms part of the floor of the suboccipital triangle and is pierced by the vertebral artery and the posterior ramus of the first cervical nerve. Also called *posterior atlanto-occipital membrane, posterior obturator membrane of atlas* (outmoded), *posterior atlanto-occipital ligament.*

membrana basalis ductus semicircularis [NA] The homogeneous basement membrane contained in the internal lining of the simple epithelium of the internal ear's semicircular duct. Also called *basal membrane of semicircular duct.*

membrana basalis glomeruli corpusculi renalis GLOMERULAR BASEMENT MEMBRANE.

membrana basilaris ductus cochlearis An outmoded term for LAMINA BASILARIS DUCTUS COCHLEARIS.

membranae caducae An outmoded term for MEMBRANAE DECIDUAE.

membrana capsularis 1 An outmoded term for CAPSULA ARTICULARIS. 2 The posterior part of the capsula lentis. An outmoded term.

membrana capsulopupillaris The segment of the embryonic membrana pupillaris that extends sideways between the pupil and the anterior surface of the lens.

membrana carnosa An outmoded term for TUNICA DARTOS.

membrana choriocapillaris LAMINA CHOROIDOCAPILLARIS.

membrana cordis PERICARDIUM.

membrana cricovocalis CONUS ELASTICUS LARYNGIS.

membranae deciduae [NA] The layers of the altered endometrium, or decidua, of the uterus that become continuous with the placenta and are shed after parturition. Also called *deciduous membranes, membranae caducae* (outmoded), *decidual membranes, anhistous membranes.*

membrana eboris The layer of odontoblasts at the periphery of the pulp of a tooth. An outmoded term.

membrana elastica externa EXTERNAL ELASTIC LAMINA.

membrana elastica interna INTERNAL ELASTIC LAMINA.

membrana elastica laryngis An outmoded term for MEMBRANA FIBROELASTICA LARYNGIS.

membrana fenestrata elastica A membrane characterized by a large number of irregular round and oval openings, such as in the elastic membranes of the tunica intima and tunica media of certain arteries. Also called *fenestrated membrane.*

membrana fibroelastica laryngis [NA] A layer of fibrous and elastic tissue beneath the mucous membrane of the larynx that is interrupted on each side by the gap between the vocal and the vestibular ligaments. Thus it consists of an upper part, the quadrangular membrane, and a lower part, the conus elasticus. A middle portion lies opposite the ventricle of the larynx. Also called *membrana elastica laryngis* (outmoded), *fibroelastic membrane of larynx.*

membrana fibrosa capsulae articularis [NA] The outer layer of the articular capsule of a synovial joint. It is composed of white fibrous tissue and some elastic fibers, varying in thickness and often strengthened either by fiber bundles forming ligaments or by incorporation of tendons of muscles. It attaches to bone by blending with the periosteum. Also called *fibrous membrane of articular capsule, stratum fibrosum capsulae articularis* (outmoded), *fibrous articular capsule, fibrous membrane, fibrous layer of articular capsule.*

membrana flaccida PARS FLACCIDA MEMBRANAE TYMPANI.

membrana fusca LAMINA FUSCA SCLERAE.

membrana germinativa BLASTODERM.

membrana gliae superficialis The fine, closely adherent outer membrane of the brain and spinal cord made up of the pia arachnoid and adherent neuroglial end feet. Also called *pialglial membrane.*

membrana granulosa STRATUM GRANULOSUM FOLLICULI OVARICI SECUNDARII.

membrana hyaloidea An outmoded term for MEMBRANA VITREA.

membrana hyothyreoidea An outmoded term for MEMBRANA THYROHYOIDEA.

membrana intercostalis externa [NA] An aponeurotic layer that replaces the anterior portion of an external intercostal muscle between the costal cartilages as far as the sternum. It is usually absent in the tenth and eleventh spaces and occasionally in the first. Also called *external intercostal membrane, ligamenta intercostalia externa* (outmoded), *external intercostal aponeurosis* (outmoded), *external intercostal ligament, proper ligament of costal cartilage* (outmoded), *anterior intercostal membrane, interchondral ligament* (outmoded).

membrana intercostalis interna [NA] An aponeurotic layer that replaces the posterior portion of an internal intercostal muscle. It extends backward from the posterior costal angle, where it is continuous anteriorly with the fascia between the external and internal intercostal muscles and posteriorly with the superior costotransverse ligaments and the subcostal muscle. Also called *internal intercostal membrane, ligamenta intercostalia interna* (outmoded), *internal intercostal ligament, internal intercostal aponeurosis* (obsolete), *internal interchondral aponeurosis* (obsolete).

membrana interossea antebrachii [NA] A thin fibrous sheet, the fibers of which run obliquely downward and medially from the interosseous border of the radius to that of the ulna. It holds the two bones together and increases the surface area for the attachment of the deep muscles of the forearm. Also called *interosseous membrane of forearm, membrana interossea antibrachii* (outmoded), *radioulnar interosseous membrane* (outmoded), *radioulnar interosseous ligament* (outmoded).

membrana interossea antibrachii An outmoded term for MEMBRANA INTEROSSEA ANTEBRACHII.

membrana interossea cruris [NA] A thin aponeurotic layer, the fibers of which run obliquely connecting the interosseous borders of the tibia and fibula. It separates the deep muscles on the front and on the back of the leg and serves as an attachment for some muscles. The anterior tibial artery pierces it proximally while the perforating branch of the peroneal artery pierces it distally. It is continuous inferiorly with the interosseous ligament of the tibiofibular syndesmosis. Also called *interosseous membrane of leg, crural interosseous membrane, interosseous ligament of leg* (outmoded), *ligamentum tibiofibulare medium* (outmoded).

membrana limitans Either stratum limitans externum or stratum limitans internum of the retina.

membrana mucosa nasi An outmoded term for TUNICA MUCOSA NASI.

membrana mucosa vesicae felleae An outmoded term for TUNICA MUCOSA VESICAE BILIARIS.

membrana nictitans 1 PLICA SEMILUNARIS CONJUNCTIVAE. 2 NICTITATING MEMBRANE.

membrana obturatoria [NA] A fibrous sheet attached to the pelvic aspect of the bony margin of the obturator foramen, closing it except superiorly where the membrane is deficient, forming the lower boundary of the obturator canal. The obturator externus and internus muscles arise partly from its external and pelvic surfaces, respectively. Also called *obturator membrane, membrana obturatrix* (outmoded), *obturator ligament of pelvis* (outmoded).

membrana obturatoria stapedis An outmoded term for MEMBRANA STAPEDIS.

membrana obturatrix An outmoded term for MEMBRANA OBTURATORIA.

membrana orbitalis musculosa An outmoded term for MUSCULUS ORBITALIS.

membrana oronasalis BUCCONASAL MEMBRANE.

membrana perinei [NA] A strong, somewhat triangular fibrous sheet that spans the pubic arch between the ischiopubic rami. The posteriorly directed base is attached centrally to the perineal body, while it is attached superiorly to the endopelvic fascia and inferiorly to the membranous layer of the superficial fascia of the perineum behind the superficial transverse perineal muscle. The anteriorly directed apex is flattened and thickened to form the transverse perineal ligament. It is pierced by the urethra and nerves and vessels to the external genitalia in both sexes and by the ducts of the bulbourethral glands in the male and the vagina in the female. Inferiorly it is related to the superficial perineal pouch and the external genitalia in both sexes and to the bulb of the penis in the male, while superior to it is the deep perineal region containing the sphincter urethrae muscle and the prostate gland in the male and musculus transversus perinei profundus in both sexes. Also called *perineal aponeurosis, superficial layer of triangular ligament, perineal ligament of Carcassonne, fascia diaphragmatis urogenitalis inferior, deep perineal fascia* (outmoded), *deep fascia of perineum* (outmoded), *lateral prostatic aponeurosis* (outmoded), *ischioprostatic aponeurosis* (outmoded), *ischioprostatic fascia, Carcassonne's ligament, superficial layer of urogenital diaphragm, perineal membrane, inferior layer of urogenital diaphragm, ligamentum triangulare* (outmoded), *triangular ligament of Colles.*

membrana pituitosa An outmoded term for TUNICA MUCOSA NASI.

membrana preformata MEMBRANA PREFORMATIVA.

membrana preformativa An apparent thickening of the basement membrane between the inner enamel epithelium and the dental papilla which precedes the initial formation of dentin. Also called *membrana preformata, dentinoenamel membrane.*

membrana propria An outmoded term for LAMINA PROPRIA MUCOSAE.

membrana propria ductus semicircularis [NA] The layer of fibrous tissue, which contains blood vessels and pigment cells, that forms the outer of the three layers of the membranous semicircular ducts of the internal ear. It lines the endosteum of the bony labyrinth and may be adherent to it. Also called *proper membrane of semicircular duct.*

membrana pupillaris PUPILLARY MEMBRANE.

membrana quadrangularis [NA] The upper portion of the fibroelastic membrane of the larynx, extending between the side of the epiglottic cartilage anteriorly and the arytenoid cartilage posteriorly. Its upper edge is within the aryepiglottic fold, which it supports, and anteroinferiorly it is attached in the angle of the thyroid cartilage, the inferior free margin forming the vestibular ligament within the vestibular fold. Also called *quadrangular membrane.*

membrana reticularis ductus cochlearis [NA] A netlike lamina in which the apertures contain the free ends of the rows of outer hair cells of the spiral organ of Corti. These hair cells are lateral to the outer rods. Also called *reticular membrane, membrana reticulata* (outmoded), *Kölliker's membrane, reticular lamina, reticular membrane of organ of Corti, reticulated membrane.*

membrana reticulata An outmoded term for MEMBRANA RETICULARIS DUCTUS COCHLEARIS.

membrana ruyschiana An outmoded term for LAMINA CHOROIDOCAPILLARIS.

membrana sacciformis RECESSUS SACCIFORMIS ARTICULATIONIS RADIOULNARIS DISTALIS.

membrana serosa 1 TUNICA SEROSA. 2 CHORION.

membrana serotina An outmoded term for DECIDUA BASALIS.

membrana spiralis ductus cochlearis PARIES TYMPANICUS DUCTUS COCHLEARIS.

membrana stapedis [NA] A thin mucosal lamina filling the space between the two crura and the base of the stapes. Also called *stapedial membrane, membrana obturatoria stapedis* (outmoded).

membrana statoconiorum MEMBRANA STATOCONIORUM MACULARUM.

membrana statoconiorum macularum [NA] A flattened gelatinous layer between and upon the projecting sensory hairs of the maculae of the utricle and the saccule. It contains, superficially, numerous minute granules of calcite and protein, called otoconia, otoliths, or statoconia. The gelatinous material is secreted by the supporting cells. Also called *statoconic membrane of maculae, otolithic membrane, membrana statocornium.*

membrana sterni [NA] A dense fibrous layer investing the sternum. It is formed by interweaving of the periosteum with fibers of the radiate sternocostal ligaments and, anteriorly, tendinous fibers of the pectoralis major muscle. Also called *sternal membrane.*

membrana succingens An outmoded term for PLEURA.

membrana suprapleuralis [NA] A domelike expansion of endothoracic fascia that is attached anteriorly to the inner border of the first rib and posteriorly to the transverse process of the seventh cervical vertebra. It strengthens the cervical pleura over the apex of the lung. On its superior surface are strengthening muscle fibers from the scalene muscles. Also called *suprapleural membrane, Sibson's fascia, Sibson's aponeurosis, scalene fascia, vertebropleural ligament* (outmoded).

membrana synovialis capsulae articularis The inner layer of the articular capsule of synovial joints, consisting of loose connective tissue, elastic fibers, and a varying amount of fat. It is coextensive with the outer fibrous layer and usually attached to bone at or near the peripheral border of the articular cartilage. Occasionally it forms folds or pouches or is continuous with the lining of bursae. It produces synovial fluid, and its inner smooth surface faces the joint cavity. Also called *synovial membrane of articular capsule, stratum synoviale capsulae articularis* (outmoded), *synovial layer of articular capsule, synovial capsule, synovium* (outmoded), *synovial membrane.*

membrana tectoria [NA] The cranial prolongation of the anterior layer of the posterior longitudinal ligament inside the vertebral canal, extending from the posterior surfaces of the bodies of the third and second cervical vertebrae to the inner aspect of the basilar part of the occipital bone where it blends with dura mater. Also called *tectorial membrane, long occipitoaxial ligament, posterior occipitoaxial ligament, apparatus ligamentosus colli, apparatus ligamentosus colli weitbrechti, ligamentous membrane* (outmoded), *long occipitoaxial membrane, cervicobasilar ligament* (outmoded), *occipitoaxial ligament, anterior cervical ligament* (outmoded).

membrana tectoria ductus cochlearis [NA] A flexible gelatinous membrane that is attached to the limbus laminae spiralis osseae and that covers the sensory receptive mechanism of the spiral organ of Corti, including the inner and outer hair cells and rods. Also called *tectorial membrane of cochlear duct, Corti's membrane.*

membrana tensa PARS TENSA MEMBRANAE TYMPANI.

membrana thyrohyoidea [NA] A broad fibroelastic sheet that extends from the upper margin of the thyroid cartilage and the front of the superior cornua to the upper margin of the posterior surface of the body and greater cornua of the hyoid bone, being separated from the hyoid body by a bursa. Also called *thyrohyoid membrane, membrana hyothyreoidea* (outmoded), *hyothyroid membrane, obturator membrane of larynx* (outmoded).

membrana tympani [NA] The thin, ellipsoid, semitransparent membranous partition between the external acoustic meatus and the tympanic cavity. The thick border of the larger inferior portion, the pars tensa, is attached by a fibrocartilaginous ring to the tympanic sulcus of the temporal bone, while the triangular anterosuperior portion, the pars flaccida, is attached directly to the bone at the tympanic notch. It is obliquely set and comprises three layers: an outer stratum corneum, an intermediate fibrous layer having outer radiate fibers and inner circular fibers, and an inner stratum mucosum. The manubrium of malleus is attached to its inner surface. Also called *tympanic membrane, eardrum, drum membrane, drumhead, myrinx, myringa, drum head, drum, tegmentum auris* (outmoded).

membrana tympani secundaria [NA] The fibrous mucosa-covered sheet that closes the fenestra cochleae. It is situated posteroinferior to the promontory on the medial wall of the tympanic cavity. Also called *secondary tympanic membrane, Scarpa's membrane.*

membrana versicolor of Fielding An obsolete term for TAPETUM.

membrana vestibularis PARIES VESTIBULARIS DUCTUS COCHLEARIS.

membrana vestibularis reissneri An outmoded term for PARIES VESTIBULARIS DUCTUS COCHLEARIS.

membrana vibrans An outmoded term for PARS TENSA MEMBRANAE TYMPANI.

membrana vitellina VITELLINE MEMBRANE.

membrana vitrea   [NA] The condensation of the gel and fibrillar framework at the periphery of the vitreous body of the eyeball. It is attached to the ciliary epithelium and processes and to the margin of the optic disk. Also called *vitreous membrane, membrana hyaloidea* (outmoded), *hyaloid membrane, hydatoid* (outmoded), *tunica hyaloidea* (outmoded).

membranaceous   MEMBRANOUS.

membranae   Plural of MEMBRANA.

membranal   Pertaining to or having the characteristics of the cell membrane.

membranate   Having the properties of a membrane.

membrane

membrane [L *membrana.* See MEMBRANA.]   MEMBRANA.

abdominal membrane   An outmoded term for PERITONEUM.

accidental membrane   An obsolete term for PSEUDOMEMBRANE.

adamantine membrane   NASMYTH'S MEMBRANE.

adventitious membrane   A congenitally aberrant membrane, usually obstructing an orifice or a lumen.

adventitious hyaloid membrane   A new-formed tissue layer upon the surface of the vitreous humor.

allantoid membrane   ALLANTOIS.

alveolocapillary membrane   The composite structure of an alveolar lining cell, basement membrane, and pulmonary capillary wall through which respiratory exchange takes place.

alveolodental membrane   PERIODONTIUM.

anal membrane   In the embryo, the posterior part of the cloacal membrane after the transverse division of the latter into two portions by the urorectal (cloacal) septum at about the seventh week. The membrane breaks down during the ninth week and the anal canal comes to open into the amniotic cavity.

anhistous membranes   MEMBRANAE DECIDUAE.

animal membrane   A dialysis or diffusion membrane of animal origin.

anterior atlanto-occipital membrane   MEMBRANA ATLANTO-OCCIPITALIS ANTERIOR.

anterior intercostal membrane   MEMBRANA INTERCOSTALIS EXTERNA.

anterior obturator membrane of atlas   An outmoded term for MEMBRANA ATLANTO-OCCIPITALIS ANTERIOR.

aponeurotic membrane   APONEUROSIS.

arachnoid membrane   ARACHNOIDEA.

Ascherson's membrane   A casein film assumed to surround the fat droplets in milk, preventing their coalescence.

asphyxial membrane   The membrane covering the terminal segments of the respiratory tree in respiratory distress syndrome of newborn. Also called *pulmonary hyaline membrane.*

Baer's membrane   A surgical dressing composed of a treated pig's bladder. It is most often applied over freshly cut bone surfaces.

basal membrane   BASEMENT MEMBRANE.

basal membrane of semicircular duct   MEMBRANA BASALIS DUCTUS SEMICIRCULARIS.

basement membrane   A condensation of glycoprotein and tropocollagen that is formed by and closely applied to the surfaces of Schwann cells, muscle cells, endothelial cells, and all epithelial cells. In the latter case, the basement membrane is most apparent at the interface with the underlying connective tissue. Also

called *basement tissue, basement layer, basement lamina, basilemma, basal membrane.*

basilar membrane   LAMINA BASILARIS DUCTUS COCHLEARIS.

basilar membrane of cochlear duct   LAMINA BASILARIS DUCTUS COCHLEARIS.

Bichat's membrane   HENLE'S FENESTRATED MEMBRANE.

birth membranes   The amnion and the placenta. A seldom used term.

black lipid membrane   An artificial bimolecular lipid membrane made between two liquid compartments for the study of membrane phenomena, e.g. the effects of ionophores on electrical conductance. It is called black because it is too thin to show interference effects with light in the visible wavelength range.

Bogros serous membrane   A serous membrane that lines the space of Tenon and separates it from the posterior pole of the eyeball.

Bowman's membrane   LAMINA LIMITANS ANTERIOR CORNEAE.

brood membrane   The germinal layer of the hydatid cyst of *Echinococcus granulosus.*

Bruch's membrane   COMPLEXUS BASALIS CHOROIDEAE.

Brunn's membrane   The epithelium of the nasal olfactory region.

bucconasal membrane   In the embryo, the membrane which separates the olfactory pit from the primitive buccal cavity towards the sixth week of development. It then breaks down to mark the position of the primitive posterior naris. Also called *bucconasal septum, membrana oronasalis, oronasal membrane.*

buccopharyngeal membrane   A transitory membrane in the embryo formed where the anterior part of the primitive intestine makes contact with the outer wall of the body. Composed of ectoderm, it separates the external depression of the stomodeum from the future pharynx. It breaks down in man in the middle of the fourth week to establish communication between these cavities. No trace of the membrane is found in the adult. Also called *oral membrane, pharyngeal membrane, stomatodeal plate, oral plate.*

capsular membrane   CAPSULA ARTICULARIS.

capsulopupillary membrane   PUPILLARY MEMBRANE.

cell membrane   PLASMA MEMBRANE.

chorioallantoic membrane   CHORIOALLANTOIS.

chromatic membrane   A layer of chromatin located on the interior surface of the nuclear membrane.

cloacal membrane   A transitory membrane in the embryo where the posterior part of the primitive intestine makes contact with the caudal region of the body. Endoderm of the intestine becomes opposed to ectoderm with no intervening mesoderm. The membrane breaks down to form the urogenital and anal orifices. Also called *cloacal plate.*

complex membrane   COMPOUND MEMBRANE.

compound membrane   A membrane that is formed from two or more differing tissue layers. Also called *complex membrane.*

Corti's membrane   MEMBRANA TECTORIA DUCTUS COCHLEARIS.

costocoracoid membrane   FASCIA CLAVIPECTORALIS.

coxofemoral synovial membrane   An outmoded term for HIP JOINT SYNOVIAL MEMBRANE.

cribriform membrane   FASCIA CRIBROSA.

cricothyroid membrane   CONUS ELASTICUS LARYNGIS.

cricotracheal membrane   LIGAMENTUM CRICOTRACHEALE.

cricovocal membrane   CONUS ELASTICUS LARYNGIS.

croupous membrane   The false membrane occurring in diphtheria. An outmoded term.

crural interosseous membrane   MEMBRANA INTEROSSEA CRURIS.

Cuprophan membrane   A cellulose membrane widely used in hemodialysis. It is highly permeable to substances with molecular weights of 100–200, much less permeable in the range of 1000–2000, and almost impermeable to substances with molecular weight greater than 5000. A proprietary name.

cyclitic membrane An inflammatory layer of tissue across the pupil.

cytoplasmic membrane PLASMA MEMBRANE.

Debove's membrane The basement membrane of the tracheal, bronchial, and intestinal epithelia. Also called *subepithelial endothelium*.

decidual membranes MEMBRANAE DECIDUAE.

deciduous membranes MEMBRANAE DECIDUAE.

Demours membrane LAMINA LIMITANS POSTERIOR CORNEAE.

dendritic membrane The portion of the plasma membrane of the nerve cell that covers the dendritic processes. It is usually the site of the highest concentrations of synaptic terminals. Some types of neuronal dendritic membrane are characterized by protruding structures or spines that serve as specialized postsynaptic receptive sites.

dentinoenamel membrane MEMBRANA PREFORMATIVA.

Descemet's membrane LAMINA LIMITANS POSTERIOR CORNEAE.

dialysis membrane A semipermeable membrane which separates the blood compartment from the dialysate compartment of the hemodialyzer. The membrane usually is made of cellulose but a large variety of other substances with differing permeability to substances of varying molecular weights has been used. In general, a membrane is most permeable to substances of small molecular weight, such as water, electrolytes, urea, and creatinine, and decreasingly permeable to substances of greater molecular weight, becoming impermeable, or almost so, to large molecules such as protein molecules and the formed elements of blood. Diffusion of substances across the semipermeable membrane according to the concentration gradient between blood and dialysate is the fundamental principle underlying hemodialysis.

differentially permeable membrane A membrane which allows some substances to pass, and prevents the passage of other substances, such as the plasma membrane.

diphtheritic membrane The characteristic pseudomembrane of diphtheria that covers the mucous membranes of the nasopharynx, oropharynx, and laryngopharynx.

drum membrane MEMBRANA TYMPANI.

Duddell's membrane LAMINA LIMITANS POSTERIOR CORNEAE.

egg membranes Coverings, varying in structure and number and additional to the vitelline membrane, that can be demonstrated in all eggs. Primary membranes are created by the ovum, secondary ones by the cells of the corona radiata, and tertiary ones are added on the outside of the ovum from secretions of the uterine tube or the uterus. The zona pellucida is an example of a mammalian egg membrane, probably of the secondary type, and an avian eggshell is a tertiary membrane. Also called *egg envelopes*.

elastic membrane ELASTIC LAMELLA.

enamel membrane NASMYTH'S MEMBRANE.

endoneural membrane NEURILEMMA.

excitable membrane A cell membrane which can generate action potentials and transmit them along its surface. Membranes on nerve and muscle cells are excitable.

exocoelomic membrane A thin layer of cells, possibly delaminated from the inner surface of the cytotrophoblast, that lies between the cytotrophoblast and the primary yolk sac in early human embryos. Other sites of origin, such as extraembryonic mesoderm and disk endoderm, have been suggested for various primate species. The layer soon disappears as the yolk sac develops. Also called *Heuser's membrane*.

external elastic membrane EXTERNAL ELASTIC LAMINA.

external intercostal membrane MEMBRANA INTERCOSTALIS EXTERNA.

external limiting membrane An ill-defined layer formed by the outermost terminations of the glial cells in the retina between the rod and cone processes and their cell bodies. Also called *stratum limitans externum*.

extraembryonic membrane Any of the membranous structures surrounding or pertaining to an embryo which protect it, provide it with oxygen and nutritive substances, and remove waste, and some of which may produce hormones. They are the chorion, amnion, yolk sac, and allantois. At a later stage in development, they are called fetal membranes.

false membrane PSEUDOMEMBRANE.

fenestrated membrane MEMBRANA FENESTRATA ELASTICA.

fertilization membrane A modification which takes place in the properties of the vitelline membrane of the recently fertilized egg in some species of animals. This change tends to inhibit additional sperm penetration, and is therefore involved in the block to polyspermy. It is brought about following the release of the contents of the cortical granules into the perivitelline space.

fetal membrane Any of the extraembryonic structures that provide protection, nutrition, respiration, excretion, or hormonal secretion to aid or affect the fetus. They include the chorion, amnion, yolk sac, allantois, and all parts of the functional placenta.

fibroelastic membrane of larynx MEMBRANA FIBROELASTICA LARYNGIS.

fibrous membrane MEMBRANA FIBROSA CAPSULAE ARTICULARIS.

fibrous membrane of articular capsule MEMBRANA FIBROSA CAPSULAE ARTICULARIS.

Fielding's membrane An obsolete term for TAPETUM.

flaccid membrane of Shrapnell PARS FLACCIDA MEMBRANAE TYMPANI.

filtration slit membrane of glomerulus A fine membranous layer between the glomerular basement membrane and the slit pores of the epithelial cell foot processes. This membrane is covered by material continuous with the surface of the foot processes, a material which has the staining characteristics of polysaccharides and which represents glycoproteins. Also called *filtration slit diaphragm of glomerulus*.

germinal membrane BLASTODERM.

glassy membrane ZONA PELLUCIDA.

glial cell membrane The surface or cytoplasmic membrane of a macroglial cell.

glomerular basement membrane The thick basal membrane that separates the podocytes of the visceral wall of the renal glomerulus from the endothelium of the glomerular capillaries. It is involved with selective filtration between these structures. Also called *membrana basalis glomeruli corpusculi renalis, lamina densa* (outmoded), *glomerular capillary basement membrane, dense layer*.

glomerular capillary basement membrane GLOMERULAR BASEMENT MEMBRANE.

gradocol membranes Thin films of collodion that are made with pore sizes of controlled diameter, usually 3–10 μ. They are used in ultrafiltration to determine the size of particulate elements, especially viruses.

Haller's membrane LAMINA VASCULOSA CHOROIDEAE.

Hannover's intermediate membrane NASMYTH'S MEMBRANE.

Held's limiting membrane BLOOD-BRAIN BARRIER.

Henle's membrane COMPLEXUS BASALIS CHOROIDEAE.

Henle's elastic membrane EXTERNAL ELASTIC LAMINA.

Henle's fenestrated membrane The thick membrana elastica interna beneath the endothelium. It is characterized by a number of irregular, rounded openings and is found in the wall of large arteries. Also called *Bichat's membrane*.

Heuser's membrane   EXOCOELOMIC MEMBRANE.

hip joint synovial membrane   An extensive synovial membrane that lines the neck of the femur within the fibrous capsule of the hip joint and is attached to both surfaces of the labrum acetabulare and lines the ligament of the head of the femur and a pad of fat within the acetabular fossa. Also called *coxofemoral synovial membrane* (outmoded).

homogeneous membrane   A thin layer or deposits of fibrinoid found in the boundary zone between fetal and maternal tissues from early in human pregnancy. It is also found on the surface of the syncytiotrophoblast of the chorionic villi.

Hovius membrane   COMPLEXUS BASALIS CHOROIDEAE.

Huxley's membrane   HUXLEY'S LAYER.

hyaline membrane   Any membrane with a relatively clear, untextured appearance, particularly the membrane lining the pulmonary alveoli implicated in the respiratory distress syndrome of newborn.

hyaloid membrane   MEMBRANA VITREA.

hymenal membrane   HYMEN.

hyoepiglottic membrane   LIGAMENTUM HYOEPIGLOTTICUM.

hyoglossal membrane   A strong fibrous sheet that extends from the body of the hyoid bone to the undersurface of the root of the tongue. It receives some fibers of the genioglossus muscle anteriorly.

hyothyroid membrane   MEMBRANA THYROHYOIDEA.

inner nuclear membrane   The inner layer of a double-walled sac that encloses the nucleus of a cell.

internal elastic membrane   INTERNAL ELASTIC LAMINA.

internal intercostal membrane   MEMBRANA INTERCOSTALIS INTERNA.

internal limiting membrane   The innermost layer of the retina that separates the nerve fiber layer from the vitreous body. It is formed by the innermost terminations of the retinal glial cells. Also called *stratum limitans internum*.

interosseous membrane of forearm   MEMBRANA INTEROSSEA ANTEBRACHII.

interosseous membrane of leg   MEMBRANA INTEROSSEA CRURIS.

interspinal membranes   An outmoded term for LIGAMENTA INTERSPINALIA.

intersutural membrane   SUTURAL LIGAMENT.

intrachoroidal membrane   A layer of ependyma just below the embryonic choroidal fissure.

ion-selective membrane   A cell membrane that impedes the transmission of certain ions and facilitates the passage of others.

Jackson's membrane   A seldom used term for PERICOLIC MEMBRANE.

Jacob's membrane   STRATUM NEUROEPITHELIALE RETINAE.

keratogenous membrane   An outmoded term for MATRIX UNGUIS.

Kölliker's membrane   MEMBRANA RETICULARIS DUCTUS COCHLEARIS.

Krause membrane   An obsolete term for Z BAND.

ligamentous membrane   An outmoded term for MEMBRANA TECTORIA.

limiting membrane   A membrane that forms the boundary, or limit, of a tissue or structure.

long occipitoaxial membrane   MEMBRANA TECTORIA.

Mauthner's membrane   AXOLEMMA.

meconic membrane   A desquamated epithelial film covered with mucus and stained with bile. It is formed in the fetal intestine and voided shortly after birth.

medullary membrane   ENDOSTEUM.

mucocutaneous membrane   A compound membrane with a

modified cutaneous layer on one side and a mucous membrane on the other.

mucous membrane   TUNICA MUCOSA.

mucous membrane of colon   TUNICA MUCOSA COLI.

mucous membrane of esophagus   TUNICA MUCOSA ESOPHAGI.

mucous membrane of gallbladder   TUNICA MUCOSA VESICAE BILIARIS.

mucous membrane of mouth   TUNICA MUCOSA ORIS.

mucous membrane of pharynx   TUNICA MUCOSA PHARYNGIS.

mucous membrane of rectum   TUNICA MUCOSA RECTI.

mucous membrane of small intestine   TUNICA MUCOSA INTESTINI TENUIS.

mucous membrane of stomach   TUNICA MUCOSA GASTRICA.

mucous membrane of tongue   TUNICA MUCOSA LINGUAE.

mucous membrane of ureter   TUNICA MUCOSA URETERIS.

mucous membrane of urinary bladder   TUNICA MUCOSA VESICAE URINARIAE.

Nasmyth's membrane   An integument consisting of the primary enamel cuticle and the reduced enamel epithelium which covers the completed enamel of an unerupted tooth. Also called *enamel cuticle, enamel membrane, Hannover's intermediate membrane, adamantine membrane, membrana adamantina*.

nictitating membrane   A transparent inner eyelid that can be drawn over the cornea to moisten and protect it. It is generally present in birds and reptiles and in grazing mammals. It is vestigial in humans. Also called *palpebra tertius, membrana nictitans*.

membrane of Nitabuch   A fibrinoid layer which, from the third or fourth month of gestation, separates the decidual from the trophoblastic elements within the basal plate of the placenta. The layer is thought by some to originate from degenerating cytotrophoblast. It tends to thicken as pregnancy advances and, near term, the trophoblast cells only make contact with it as discontinuous islands. This fibrinoid material is actually present elsewhere in the placenta. It unites the anchoring villi to the basal plate, and is encountered in many places in the intervillous spaces (fibrinoid substance of Rohr) or forms islands on the chorionic plate (fibrinoid substance of Langhans). Also called *striae of Nitabuch, layer of Nitabuch, zone of Nitabuch*.

nuclear membrane   1 The inner membrane of the nuclear envelope.   2 An older term for NUCLEAR ENVELOPE.

oblique membrane of forearm   CHORDA OBLIQUA.

obturator membrane   MEMBRANA OBTURATORIA.

obturator membrane of larynx   An outmoded term for MEMBRANA THYROHYOIDEA.

olfactory membrane   TUNICA MUCOSA OLFACTORIA.

olfactory mucous membrane   TUNICA MUCOSA OLFACTORIA.

oral membrane   BUCCOPHARYNGEAL MEMBRANE.

oronasal membrane   BUCCONASAL MEMBRANE.

otolithic membrane   MEMBRANA STATOCONIORUM MACULARUM.

outer membrane   A membrane outside the peptidoglycan layer in Gram-negative bacteria, and connected to the inner membrane at intervals by localized junctions through gaps in the peptidoglycan. The inner leaflet contains phospholipids and the lipid termini of lipoproteins. In the outer leaflet the lipid A portion of lipopolysaccharide may be the only lipid. The number of different proteins is much smaller than in the inner membrane; the matrix protein provides a molecular sieve whose pores exclude molecules larger than 800–900 daltons. Abbreviation: OM

outer nuclear membrane   The outer layer of a double-walled sac that encloses the nucleus of a cell. It is this outer layer that is contiguous with the rough-surfaced endoplasmic reticulum of the cell cytoplasm.

ovular membrane VITELLINE MEMBRANE.

palatine membrane PALATINE MUCOSA.

pericolic membrane An occasional delicate, fibrous layer of additional vascularized peritoneum or membrane that extends inferomedially from the lateral abdominal wall to the anterior surface of the ascending colon and cecum. It is usually associated with a congenitally mobile ascending colon. By kinking the intestine, it may produce obstruction. Also called *pericolonic membrane, Jackson's membrane* (seldom used), *Jackson's veil.*

pericolonic membrane PERICOLIC MEMBRANE.

peridental membrane PERIODONTIUM.

perineal membrane MEMBRANA PERINEI.

periodontal membrane PERIODONTIUM.

periorbital membrane PERIORBITA.

pharyngeal membrane BUCCOPHARYNGEAL MEMBRANE.

pharyngobasilar membrane FASCIA PHARYNGOBASILARIS.

pia-arachnoid membrane Collectively, the pia mater and the arachnoidea.

pial-glial membrane MEMBRANA GLIAE SUPERFICIALIS.

pituitary membrane of nose An outmoded term for TUNICA MUCOSA NASI.

placental membrane The anatomic barrier in the placenta which lies between the fetal and maternal bloodstreams. It varies in thickness and in the number of layers of which it is composed, depending on the order, or even the species, involved. Terms such as epitheliochorial, endotheliochorial, and hemochorial indicate the layers present respectively in ungulates, Carnivora, and man.

plasma membrane The three-layered membrane surrounding the cytoplasm. It is composed of a phospholipid layer coated with proteins on the outer and inner surfaces, the outer surface also having associated glycoproteins which form the glycocalyx. Also called *cytoplasmic membrane, cell membrane, plasmalemma, cytomembrane, cytolemma, ectosarc.*

platelet demarcation membrane The membrane that outlines a newly-formed platelet as it buds from a megakaryocyte.

pleuropericardial membrane A membrane on each side of the embryo which helps to separate the pericardial and pleural cavities. Within its substance are the common cardinal vein and the phrenic nerve. Also called *pericardiopleural septum.*

pleuroperitoneal membrane PLEUROPERITONEAL FOLD.

polyacrylonitrile membrane A membrane used for hemodialysis and hemofiltration, characterized by high permeability to molecules of medium to large molecular weight.

posterior atlanto-occipital membrane MEMBRANA ATLANTO-OCCIPITALIS POSTERIOR.

posterior obturator membrane of atlas An outmoded term for MEMBRANA ATLANTO-OCCIPITALIS POSTERIOR.

postsynaptic membrane That portion of the plasma membrane of a neuron in closest apposition to an impinging afferent presynaptic terminal, from which it is separated only by a synaptic cleft. It represents the target structure upon which neurotransmitter molecules (in a chemogenic synapse) or current fluxes (in an electrogenic synapse) are directed.

presynaptic membrane The portion of the plasma membrane of a neuron in closest apposition to its target element, from which it is separated only by a synaptic cleft. In chemogenic synapses its highly complex molecular substructure allows for the selective release of neurotransmitter molecules, usually by discharge of synaptic vesicles, and the subsequent uptake of inactivated neurotransmitter fragments following termination of the synaptic process.

proligerous membrane CUMULUS OOPHORUS.

proper mucous membrane The innermost layer of the gut wall. It is composed of epithelium, the lamina propria, and the muscularis mucosae. Also called *tunica propria mucosa.*

proper membrane of semicircular duct MEMBRANA PRO-PRIA DUCTUS SEMICIRCULARIS.

prophylactic membrane PYOPHYLACTIC MEMBRANE.

pseudoserous membrane A membrane that is macroscopically similar to a serous membrane but that microscopically lacks the flattened layer of epithelial cells.

pulmonary hyaline membrane ASPHYXIAL MEMBRANE.

pupillary membrane The delicate, vascular mesodermal membrane, part of the embryonic lens capsule, on the anterior surface of the lens epithelium which closes the pupil until about the sixth month of human development. If the capsule is not completely resorbed it can persist to give rise to congenital atresia of the pupil. Also called *capsulopupillary membrane, membrane pupillaris, Wachendorf's membrane.*

purple membrane The membrane of halophilic bacteria containing rhodopsin and capable of pumping hydrogen ions in response to illumination.

purpurogenous membrane The epithelium of the retinal pigment.

pyogenic membrane PYOPHYLACTIC MEMBRANE.

pyophylactic membrane The inner lining of an organizing abscess, characterized by granulation tissue, fibrin, and intact polymorphonuclear leukocytes. An obsolete term. Also called *prophylactic membrane, pyogenic membrane.*

quadrangular membrane MEMBRANA QUADRANGULARIS.

radioulnar interosseous membrane An outmoded term for MEMBRANA INTEROSSEA ANTEBRACHII.

Ranvier's membrane A hyaline membrane at the dermoepidermal junction.

Reichert's membrane LAMINA LIMITANS ANTERIOR CORNEAE.

Reissner's membrane PARIES VESTIBULARIS DUCTUS COCHLEARIS.

respiratory membrane The alveolar membrane through which gas exchange in the lung takes place.

reticular membrane MEMBRANA RETICULARIS DUCTUS COCHLEARIS.

reticular membrane of organ of Corti MEMBRANA RETICULARIS DUCTUS COCHLEARIS.

reticulated membrane MEMBRANA RETICULARIS DUCTUS COCHLEARIS.

Rivinus membrane PARS FLACCIDA MEMBRANAE TYMPANI.

ruffle membrane A thin cytoplasmic fold that extends out from a macrophage and is capable of engulfing large particulate matter.

Ruysch membrane LAMINA CHOROIDOCAPILLARIS.

ruyschian membrane LAMINA CHOROIDOCAPILLARIS.

Scarpa's membrane MEMBRANA TYMPANI SECUNDARIA.

schneiderian membrane TUNICA MUCOSA NASI.

Schwann's membrane NEURILEMMA.

secondary membrane Residual opacity following extracapsular cataract extraction.

secondary tympanic membrane MEMBRANA TYMPANI SECUNDARIA.

semipermeable membrane A membrane that allows the free passage of water or other solvent but restricts the movement of certain solutes or colloidally dispersed material.

serous membrane TUNICA SEROSA.

serous membrane of epididymis TUNICA VAGINALIS TESTIS.

shell membrane A two layered, parchmentlike envelope made of protein fibers that fits snugly about the contents of a bird's egg. The inner, or egg membrane (membrana putaminis), surrounds the albumen of the egg. It is firmly cemented to the inside of the outer membrane except at the blunt end of the egg where the air cell usually lies. The outer, or "true" shell membrane (membrana testae) is so closely adherent to the inner surface of the eggshell that it cannot be separated without tearing it. The double-layered membrane is thin but tough, pinkish white due to porphyrin pigmentation, pliable when wet but brittle when dry. It is porous and allows passage of gases and liquids by diffusion and osmosis. Each of the membranes can be further subdivided into more or less distinct but thin layers with a network arrangement of interwoven fibers.

Shrapnell's membrane   PARS FLACCIDA MEMBRANAE TYM-PANI.

membrane of Slavianski   ZONA PELLUCIDA.

spiral membrane of cochlear duct   PARIES TYMPANICUS DUCTUS COCHLEARIS.

stapedial membrane   MEMBRANA STAPEDIS.

membrane of stapes   PLICA STAPEDIS.

statoconic membrane of maculae   MEMBRANA STATOCONI-ORUM MACULARUM.

sternal membrane   MEMBRANA STERNI.

striated membrane   ZONA PELLUCIDA.

subepithelial membrane   A basement membrane on the deep surface of an epithelium.

subimplant membrane   The layer of fibrous tissue which forms between the framework of a subperiosteal implant and the bone.

submucous membrane   TELA SUBMUCOSA.

submucous membrane of stomach   TELA SUBMUCOSA GAS-TRICA.

subzonal membrane   The outermost layer of the amnion.

suprapleural membrane   MEMBRANA SUPRAPLEURALIS.

sutural membrane   SUTURAL LIGAMENT.

synaptic membrane   The portion of plasma membrane separating one neuron from another at a point of synapse. Also called *synaptolemma*.

synovial membrane   MEMBRANA SYNOVIALIS CAPSULAE AR-TICULARIS.

synovial membrane of articular capsule   MEMBRANA SYN-OVIALIS CAPSULAE ARTICULARIS.

synovial membrane of round ligament   The synovial membrane of the hip joint that usually ensheathes the ligament of the head of the femur.

tarsal membrane   SEPTUM ORBITALE.

tectorial membrane   MEMBRANA TECTORIA.

tectorial membrane of cochlear duct   MEMBRANA TECTO-RIA DUCTUS COCHLEARIS.

tendinous membrane   An outmoded term for APONEUROSIS.

Tenon's membrane   VAGINA BULBI.

thyrohyoid membrane   MEMBRANA THYROHYOIDEA.

tibiotarsal synovial membrane   The synovial membrane lining the capsule of the talocrural joint that ascends for a short distance between the distal ends of the tibia and fibula. An outmoded term.

Toldt's membrane   The anterior layer of the fascia of the kidney.

tympanic membrane   MEMBRANA TYMPANI.

undulating membrane   **1** A membrane that runs, finlike, along the body of certain flagellate parasites such as trypanosomes and trichomonads. The margin of the membrane is formed by the flagellum, which in some cases extends free beyond the membrane. A rippling movement is characteristic of the undulating membrane and serves to propel the organism. **2** An organelle found in the oral groove of some ciliates (protozoan phylum Ciliophora), formed by the fusion of one or more longitudinal rows of cilia. For defs. 1 and 2 also called *undulatory membrane*. See also MEMBRANELLE.

undulatory membrane   UNDULATING MEMBRANE.

unit membrane   A model of membrane structure in which a phospholipid layer is coated on its outer and inner surfaces by proteins in the extended β-configuration. This membrane shows a trilaminar (dark-light-dark) pattern of electron density.

urogenital membrane   The anterior part of the cloacal membrane in the embryo, formed by the transverse division of the membrane into two parts by the downgrowth of the cloacal (urorectal) septum at about the seventh week in man. It closes off the end of the urogenital sinus and is prolonged forwards in forming a temporary cover (until the ninth week) for the urogenital groove on the inferior aspect of the genital tubercle, later to form the penis in the male.

urorectal membrane   CLOACAL SEPTUM.

uteroepichorial membrane   DECIDUA PARIETALIS.

vaginal synovial membrane   VAGINA SYNOVIALIS TENDINIS.

vascular membrane of viscera   An outmoded term for TELA SUBMUCOSA.

vernix membrane   The pulmonary membrane of respiratory distress syndrome of newborn. An obsolete term. • The term is so named because it was originally thought to be the result of fetal inhalation of the vernix caseosa, which accumulates on the surface of the fetus during the latter part of pregnancy.

vestibular membrane of cochlear duct   PARIES VESTIBU-LARIS DUCTUS COCHLEARIS.

virginal membrane   An outmoded term for HYMEN.

vitelline membrane   The cell membrane of an ovum, produced by the cytoplasm of the ovum. Also called *membrana vitellina, ovular membrane, yolk membrane*.

vitreous membrane   **1** LAMINA LIMITANS POSTERIOR COR-NEAE. **2** MEMBRANA VITREA. **3** COMPLEXUS BASALIS CHO-ROIDEAE.

Volkmann's membrane   A thin membrane containing numerous caseating granulomas that lines the interior of a tuberculous cavity. A seldom used term.

Wachendorf's membrane   PUPILLARY MEMBRANE.

yolk membrane   VITELLINE MEMBRANE.

Zinn's membrane   The anterior layer of the iris, comprising a layer of flattened endothelial cells.

---

membranectomy [*membran(e)* + -ECTOMY]   The surgical removal of part or all of a membrane.

membranelle [from New L *membranella*, dim. of MEMBRANA]   A minute membrane in certain ciliate protozoa formed by the fusion of two or more transverse rows of cilia. It is often a part of the cytostome complex.

membraniform   Having the appearance of a membrane.

membranocartilaginous   Of or relating to both membranous and cartilaginous tissue.

membranocranium [*membran(e)* + *o* + RANIUM]   The primitive precursor of the skull in the embryo. It is made of membranous material and precedes the bony and other elements which eventually form the fetal skull proper.

membranoid   Like a membrane, as in appearance or quality.

membranous   Being or having the properties of a membrane. Also *membranaceous*.

membroid   A capsule of membranous composition which is resistant to the actions of gastric secretions but dissolves in the lumen of the small intestine. It is a type of enteric coating for drugs to be delivered to the intestinal portion of the gastrointestinal tract.

membrum [L (akin to *fibra* fiber, filament of a plant, *fimbria* a thread, and *barba* a beard), a member, limb, part]   (*plural* membra) A limb or appendage.

membrum inferius   The lower limb of the human body, including the hip, thigh, leg and foot. Also called *inferior limb, lower extremity, inferior extremity, extremitas inferior, inferior member, pelvic limb, lower limb*.

membrum muliebre   An outmoded term for CLITORIS.

membrum superius   [NA] The upper limb of the human body, including the shoulder, arm, forearm, wrist and hand. Also called *superior limb, extremitas superior* (outmoded), *superior extremity, upper extremity, thoracic limb, upper limb.*

membrum virile   An outmoded term for PENIS.

memory [Middle French *memorie* (from L *memori(a)* memory, from *memor* mindful, from *meminisse* to remember) memory] **1** The persistence of the effects of experience on the behavior of living organisms. Memory includes several stages; learning, retaining, recognizing, and recalling.   **2** The recall of one's past or of a particular object or event.   **3** Equipment or media in which information for a computer can be stored and retrieved. **4** That portion of a computer in which instructions and data are stored.   **5** A tendency to retain effects as a result of past treatment, as a permanent deformation in a plastic after a load is removed.

affect memory   The emotion that accompanies recall of a significant experience.

biologic memory   Inherited engram, such as an instinct or the collective unconscious of jungian psychology.

coast memory   TROPICAL AMNESIA.

external memory   A data storage medium that is external to a computer's internal memory, such as a floppy disk, magnetic tape, or punch tape.

iconic memory   The hypothesized first stage of visual memory formation, in which a faint copy of a visual input persists very briefly in the sensory register, allowing a longer interval for the extraction of information.

immediate memory   SHORT-TERM MEMORY.

immunologic memory   The capacity of the immune system to mount an increased and more sustained response to a subsequent exposure to a particular antigen than was mounted to the initial exposure. Immunologic memory is produced by the expansion of clones of antigen-reactive lymphocytes as a result of the first contact with antigen. These cells (memory cells) can then be stimulated to proliferate and differentiate when antigen is encountered again.

kinesthetic memory   Memory for movements rather than events.

long-term memory   The hypothesized substage of the memory process in which information is stored in a relatively permanent way, possibly for the lifetime of the organism, and which can be retrieved for use as required.

physiologic memory   Learning displayed by physiologic processes that are not under conscious control, such as conditioning of an autonomic nervous system reaction. A seldom used term.

primary memory   A process likened to memory hypothesized to occur even among the lowest animate organisms to account for the fact that their behavior is modified by experience. A seldom used term.

racial memory   The postulation that there is an inherited or biologic memory of phylogenetic origin, such as the collective unconscious of jungian psychology.

random access memory   A computer memory, usually using a semiconductor, that permits immediate access for writing data into any storage location or reading data from any storage location. Also called *read/write memory.* Abbreviation: RAM

read-only memory   A computer memory, usually using a semiconductor, that contains unalterable programs or data. Like a dictionary, data are easily accessed, cannot be changed, and are not lost when the power turns off. Abbreviation: ROM

read/write memory   RANDOM ACCESS MEMORY.

recent memory   In clinical usage, the ability to recall events that have occurred within the past hours, days, or weeks.

remote memory   In clinical usage, the ability to recall events that occurred several years, or many years, ago. Also called *palinmnesis.*

retrograde memory   The memory for events prior to a trauma

or other incident that has affected one's memory.

rote memory   The memorizing or learning of a body of material without regard to understanding its meaning but only with the intent to reproduce it later in the exact form in which it has been memorized.

screen memory   The memory of a real event that covers or blurs the memory of an allied event.

short-term memory   A hypothesized substage of the memory process assumed to be of short duration, and in any event not exceeding 25 minutes, and to possess a distinctly limited capacity, possibly of five to nine items. Although material is thought to be held only very briefly in the short-term memory stage, this may suffice to allow processing of the information into the long-term memory store for later use. Also called *immediate memory.*

subconscious memory   Mental impressions of an event that are not ordinarily or readily recalled but are retained and can be reproduced under certain conditions.

virtual memory   A computer technique that permits the programmer to treat external memory, such as a floppy disk, as an extension of random access memory, thus giving the virtual appearance of a larger random access memory.

MEN   multiple endocrine neoplasia

menacme [Gk *mēn* month + *akmē* a point, the highest point, bloom]   **1** The height of menstrual activity.   **2** The years between menarche and menopause.

menadiol   2-Methylnaphthalene-1,2-diol. The reduced form of menadione.

menadiol sodium diphosphate   2-Methyl-1,4-naphthalenediol bis(dihydrogen phosphate) tetra-sodium salt hexahydrate. A synthetic derivative of menadione (vitamin K_3) that is biologically transformed into an active metabolite with vitamin K activity. It is used for the same indications as menadione and is given orally, intravenously, or subcutaneously.

menadione   2-Methyl-1,4-naphthoquinone. It is the parent substance of the various forms of vitamin K, which differ in the nature of the substituent at C-3. 3-Substituted menadiones are collectively called menaquinones, and the substituent is a chain of isoprene units. Also called *vitamin K_3.*

menadione sodium bisulfite   The water-soluble, sodium bisulfite form of menadione, used as a source of vitamin K in the treatment of hemorrhagic conditions associated with hypoprothrombinemic states. It has the same actions and uses as menadione.

menalgia [*men(o)-* + -ALGIA]   DYSMENORRHEA.

menaquinone   Any of several 3-substituted manadiones, which vary in the length of the polyisoprenoid substituent. All have vitamin K activity. Also called *vitamin K_2, farnoquinone* (obsolete).

menarche [Gk *mēn* month + *archē* a beginning, origin]   The appearance of the first menstrual period. Also called *menophania.* Adjective: menarchal, menarcheal, menarchial.

delayed menarche   PRIMARY AMENORRHEA.

mendacity [Late L *mendacitas* (from L *mendax*, stem *mendac-*, deceitful, lying + *-itas* -ITY) mendacity]   PATHOLOGICAL LYING.

Mendel [Felix *Mendel*, German physician, 1862–1912]   Mendel's test. See under MANTOUX TEST.

Mendel [Johann Gregor *Mendel*, Austrian botanist, 1822–1884] **1** Mendelian inheritance. See under INHERITANCE.   **2** Mendelian law. See under MENDEL'S LAWS.   **3** Mendelian disorder. See under DISORDER.   **4** Mendelism. See under MENDELIAN THEORY.   **5** Mendelian rate. See under MENDELIAN RATIO.

Mendel [Kurt *Mendel*, German neurologist, 1874–1946]   **1** Mendel-Bekhterev sign. See under SIGN.   **2** Bekhterev-Mendel reflex, Mendel's reflex, Mendel's dorsal reflex of foot. See under

MENDEL-BEKHTEREV REFLEX.

mendelevium A synthetic element of the actinide series, having atomic number 101. Mendelevium 256 was discovered in 1952, produced by bombarding einsteinium with alpha particles. Its half-life is approximately 1.25 hours. Four isotopes are recognized. The longest lived, mendelevium 258, has a half-life of 2 months. Symbol: Md

mendelian Associated with the work of or developed by Gregor Mendel, as *mendelian theory.*

mendelism MENDELIAN THEORY.

mendelizing Displaying an inheritance that is in accordance with mendelian theory.

Mendelsohn [Martin *Mendelsohn,* German physician, 1860–1930] See under TEST.

Mendelson [Curtis Lester *Mendelson,* U.S. obstetrician and gynecologist, born 1913] See under SYNDROME.

Ménétrier [Pierre *Ménétrier,* French physician, 1859–1935] See under DISEASE.

Menformon A proprietary name for estrone.

Menge [Karl *Menge,* German gynecologist, 1864–1945] See under PESSARY.

mengovirus MENGO VIRUS.

menhidrosis [Gk *mēn* month + HIDROSIS] A form of vicarious menstruation characterized by monthly extrusion of sweat, sometimes bloody, at the expected time of menses. Also called *menidrosis.*

menidrosis MENHIDROSIS.

Menière [Prosper *Menière,* French physician, 1799–1862] Menière syndrome. See under DISEASE.

mening- MENINGO-.

meningeal Describing, pertaining to, or affecting the meninges.

meningematoma A hematoma involving the dura mater. Also called *meninghematoma.*

meningeocortical MENINGOCORTICAL.

meningeoma MENINGIOMA.

meningeorrhaphy [Gk *mēnenge(s),* pl. of *mēninx* membrane + *o* + -RRHAPHY] Suture of the dura mater.

meninges [See MENINX.] (*singular* meninx) [NA] The three membranes that envelop the brain and spinal cord, comprising a dense, fibrous outer cover (dura mater), a thin inner layer adhering closely to the underlying neural tissue (pia mater), and a trabeculated middle layer (the arachnoidea). The last two are usually grouped together as the leptomeninges.

meninghematoma MENINGEMATOMA.

meningi- MENINGO-.

meningina An obsolete term for LEPTOMENINGES.

meninginitis [*meningin(a)* (term coined by François Chaussier, French physician, 1746–1828, for the pia-arachnoid; irreg. from Gk *mēninx,* gen. *mēningos,* membrane) + -ITIS] LEPTOMENINGITIS.

meningioma [MENINGI- + -OMA] A tumor of the cellular elements of the meninges. It is most often attached to the dura, especially where arachnoid villi are numerous. It is typically benign, but may compress the brain, erode and extend into bone and, on rare occasions, become malignant through transformation into a sarcoma. A number of morphologic subtypes are recognized, but their behavior does not seem to differ greatly from one another. Also called *exothelioma* (obsolete), *meningoma, mesothelioma of meninges.* Also *meningeoma.*

anaplastic meningioma A recognizable meningioma with anaplastic features. This differs from a meningeal sarcoma, which does not contain features of a meningioma. Also called *meningoblastoma.*

angioblastic meningioma HEMANGIOBLASTIC MENINGIOMA.

angiomatous meningioma A meningioma with many large and small vascular channels predominating.

arachnotheliomatous meningioma MENINGOTHELIOMATOUS MENINGIOMA.

clinoidal meningioma A meningioma localized near the median part of the sphenoidal ridge and therefore producing ocular symptoms, olfactory hallucinations, and personality changes.

endotheliomatous meningioma MENINGOTHELIOMATOUS MENINGIOMA.

fibroblastic meningioma FIBROUS MENINGIOMA.

fibrous meningioma A meningioma in which fibroblastlike cells predominate. Collagen and reticulin are abundant. Also called *meningeal fibroblastoma, fibroblastic meningioma, meningofibroblastoma.*

hemangioblastic meningioma A meningioma which closely resembles a capillary hemangioblastoma of the cerebellum. Also called *angioblastic meningioma, dural endothelioma.*

hemangiopericytic meningioma A meningioma with the histologic appearance of a hemangiopericytoma.

meningothelial meningioma MENINGOTHELIOMATOUS MENINGIOMA.

meningotheliomatous meningioma A meningioma composed of cells with poorly defined cell membranes, which result in a syncytial appearance. Also called *arachnotheliomatous meningioma, endotheliomatous meningioma, meningothelial meningioma, syncytial meningioma, meningothelioma.*

mixed meningioma TRANSITIONAL MENINGIOMA.

myxomatous meningioma A meningioma with a myxomatous appearance histologically.

meningioma of olfactory groove A meningioma developing in the olfactory groove in relation to the undersurface of one frontal lobe, usually giving rise to unilateral anosmia and other variable neurologic symptoms and signs.

parasagittal meningioma A meningioma arising in the parasagittal region between the two cerebral hemispheres and often becoming evident first with spastic weakness of both legs and feet.

psammomatous meningioma A meningioma, usually spinal, in which psammoma bodies are a predominant feature.

meningioma of the sphenoid sinus A meningioma located at the base of the skull, that has invaded the sphenoid bone and encroached upon the sphenoid sinus. The characteristic lesion is a bony boss within the sinus where new bone formation marks the site of the intracranial tumor.

suprasellar meningioma A meningioma in the suprasellar region.

syncytial meningioma MENINGOTHELIOMATOUS MENINGIOMA.

transitional meningioma A meningioma composed of a mixture of syncytial and fibroblastic elements. Also called *mixed meningioma.*

meningiomatosis [*meningiomat(a),* pl. of MENINGIOMA, + -OSIS] The presence of multiple meningiomas.

meningion An obsolete term for ARACHNOIDEA.

meningism [*mening(itis)* + -ISM] A group of symptoms and signs suggesting meningitis which may occur in the absence of any identifiable pathologic lesion of the meninges. The major manifestations are headache and neck stiffness. The syndrome usually occurs in children suffering from febrile infections such as pneumonia, tonsillitis, and systemic viral infections. Also called *pseudomeningitis Dupré syndrome* (obsolete), *meningismus, Dupré's disease.*

meningismus MENINGISM.

meningitic [*meningit(is)* + -IC] Describing or pertaining to meningitis.

meningitides Plural of MENINGITIS.

meningitiform [*meningiti(s)* + -FORM] Resembling meningitis or its effects.

meningitis

meningitis [MENING- + -ITIS] (*plural* meningitides) Any inflammation of the meninges. Meningitis has been termed cerebral, spinal, or cerebrospinal, according to whether the inflammation affects principally the meninges over the brain alone, those investing the spinal cord alone, or the whole cerebrospinal complex. This distinction has little validity in clinical practice, since there is usually though not invariably some spread of inflammation from one compartment to the other. Two principal forms can be distinguished on pathologic grounds, pachymeningitis, which involves the dura mater, and leptomeningitis, which affects the arachnoid and the pia mater. The latter is much commoner, and by common usage meningitis is usually taken to mean leptomeningitis. The major manifestations include headache, vomiting, fever, and neck stiffness. The condition can result from many kinds of microorganism, including bacteria, fungi, spirochetes, viruses, and parasites. It can also be aseptic, due to irritation of the meninges by chemical or physical agents, or to tumor metastasizing in the meninges. Adjective: meningitic.

abacterial meningitis Meningitis due to an organism or agent other than a bacterium.

acute aseptic meningitis Acute meningitis, usually with a lymphocytic pleocytosis and usually viral in origin.

acute benign lymphocytic meningitis LYMPHOCYTIC CHORIOMENINGITIS.

acute purulent meningitis ACUTE SEPTIC MENINGITIS.

acute pyogenic meningitis Acute meningitis resulting from infection with any pus-forming organism.

acute septic meningitis Any form of bacterial meningitis resulting in pus formation in the subarachnoid space, whether due to a primary meningitic illness, as in most cases of meningococcal or pneumococcal meningitis, or due to spread of infection from the brain, in cerebral abscess, from the ears or paranasal sinuses, or from some other more distant infective focus, as from the lungs in bronchiectasis. Also called *acute purulent meningitis.*

African meningitis Meningitis occurring in African trypanosomiasis. An ambiguous and seldom used term.

amebic meningitis Meningitis due to infection with an ameba.

aseptic meningitis Inflammation of the meninges resulting from aseptic processes, and resulting from a variety of infectious, toxic, chemical, or physical agents, including, for example, that secondary inflammatory process which may result from bleeding or from the injection or release of air, drugs, or other foreign substances into the subarachnoid space. No bacterial organisms can be identified in or isolated from the cerebrospinal fluid, but studies often reveal viral etiology. Also called *sterile meningitis.*
• *Aseptic meningitis* is sometimes used to refer to meningitides of viral origin, but *viral meningitis* is preferred in this sense.

Bacteroides meningitis Meningitis due to anaerobic fusiform bacilli of the genus *Bacteroides.*

basal meningitis Meningitis largely restricted to the meninges over the base of the brain. This may occur in subacute, chronic, or inadequately treated bacterial meningitis, or in granuloma-

tous processes such as tuberculosis or sarcoidosis. Also called *basilar meningitis, meningitis of the base.*

meningitis of the base BASAL MENINGITIS.

basilar meningitis BASAL MENINGITIS.

benign lymphocytic meningitis See under LYMPHOCYTIC MENINGITIS.

benign recurrent endothelioleukocytic meningitis A form of acute meningitis of undetermined etiology characterized by an abrupt onset, a marked pleocytosis in the cerebrospinal fluid with initially a high proportion of endothelial cells in the fluid, rapid spontaneous remission, and frequent relapses. A virus has been isolated in one case. Also called *Mollaret's meningitis.*

brucellar meningitis Meningitis which may arise as a complication of brucellosis. It is seen either as a typical meningeal syndrome or else as a simple pleocytosis in the cerebrospinal fluid. Many and various neurologic syndromes have been attributed to infection with *Brucella* species.

meningitis carcinomatosa Widespread or diffuse metastatic carcinoma in the meninges.

cerebral meningitis Inflammation of the meninges overlying the brain.

cerebrospinal meningitis An infectious and at times epidemic disease caused by a variety of microorganisms, but usually meningococci, transmitted by direct human contact, often with asymptomatic carriers who harbor the organisms in the nasopharynx. The onset is typically abrupt, with fever, headache, and vomiting, followed almost immediately by neck stiffness, and leading to drowsiness, delirium, and ultimately coma if untreated. The Kernig and Brudzinski signs are positive in about 50% of cases. In acute cases, especially in childhood, there may be a purpuric rash on the skin, and in some cases there is an associated septicemia. The pressure of the cerebrospinal fluid is raised, and it is purulent at this time, containing many abnormal polymorphonuclear leukocytes and bacteria, which are often surprisingly scanty. The protein level is raised and the glucose content reduced or absent. With appropriate antibiotics the prognosis is usually good in adults and older children, but the condition can still be more serious in young children. Also called *epidemic meningitis, meningococcal meningitis, meningococcic meningitis, petechial fever, tetanoid fever, spotted sickness, cerebrospinal fever, stiffneck fever.*

chemical meningitis Aseptic meningitis due to irritation of the meninges resulting from the presence of any foreign chemical substance in the subarachnoid space.

chronic posterior basic meningitis A form of indolent meningitis largely confined to the basal meninges. The usual cause is inadequate resolution or treatment of pyogenic meningitis due to the meningococcus or pneumococcus. Since the introduction of antibiotics this condition has become very rare. Also called *posterior meningitis, posterior basic meningitis.*

meningitis circumscriptaspinalis Localized spinal meningitis due to any cause.

cryptococcal meningitis A form of meningitis, sometimes occurring acutely but much more often in a subacute or chronic form, due to *Cryptococcus neoformans.* It may occur spontaneously but often develops in cachectic patients, especially those with reticulosis or carcinomatosis. The causal fungus usually can be grown from the cerebrospinal fluid on Sabouraud's medium. Once almost universally fatal, the condition can now be effectively treated in many cases with amphotericin B and 5-fluorocytosine. Also called *torula meningitis, torular meningitis.*

curable serous meningitis LYMPHOCYTIC CHORIOMENINGITIS.

eosinophilic meningitis A disorder of the human central nervous system due either to parasitic infection or, rarely, to malignancy and characterized by headache, nuchal rigidity, vomiting or decreased sensorium, a predominance of eosinophils in the cerebrospinal fluid, and, possibly, low-grade fever and cranial nerve defects. It is most often a benign, self-limited illness resulting from infection with the rat lungworm, *Angiostrongylus cantonensis*, although other parasitic infections, including paragonimiasis, schistosomiasis, and gnathostomiasis, can give rise to a very similar clinical picture. The illness is seen almost exclusively in the Far East and Pacific islands, where the parasites may be ingested accidentally by persons eating contaminated raw vegetables, snails, or shellfish. While human angiostrongyliasis is usually a subclinical illness, in some cases the larvae migrate to the central nervous system where they provoke eosinophilic meningitis. Rarely, eosinophilic meningitis develops in persons with malignancies, especially Hodgkin's disease and lymphomas. In these instances, the illness, if untreated, is associated with high mortality. Also called *eosinophilic meningoencephalitis*.

epidemic meningitis   CEREBROSPINAL MENINGITIS.

epidemic serous meningitis   LYMPHOCYTIC CHORIOMENINGITIS.

external meningitis   PACHYMENINGITIS.

fulminating adrenal meningitis   Meningococcal septicemia accompanied by adrenocortical failure and hypotension (Waterhouse-Friderichsen syndrome). Extensive purpura and gangrene of the extremities may follow and, if untreated, death is usual.

gonococcal meningitis   A rare form of purulent meningitis complicating gonococcal septicemia, occasionally confused with meningococcal meningitis after examination of the cerebrospinal fluid because of the resemblance between meningococci and gonococci on Gram stain. The course is less acute than that of meningococcal meningitis, and there is a marked tendency towards loculation of the infection in the meninges.

granulomatous meningitis   Any form of meningitis producing granulomatous changes in the subarachnoid space. The commonest causes include tuberculosis, syphilis, and sarcoidosis.

gummatous meningitis   Meningitis occurring in the tertiary stage of syphilis, marked pathologically by gummata scattered either in the pia mater or alternatively in the dura mater. These are particularly abundant over the base of the skull. Clinically the condition produces either signs of increased intracranial pressure or a picture of subacute meningitis. Also called *sclerogummatous meningitis* (obsolete).

hemophilus meningitis   Meningitis caused by *Haemophilus influenzae*, occurring most often in infants and children. Also called *Pfeiffer's bacillary meningitis* (outmoded).

herpetic meningitis   Meningitis caused by the infection with any of the human herpes virus, such as herpes simplex virus or herpes zoster virus, complicating the skin rash or preceding it by a few hours or days. It produces a meningeal syndrome, with clear cerebrospinal fluid containing abundant lymphocytes and an increased protein content. The meningeal signs usually disappear within a few days, and recovery is generally complete. An imprecise usage.

influenzal meningitis   Meningitis due to *Hemophilus influenzae*.

internal meningitis   Meningitis involving the internal aspect of the dura mater.

leptospiral meningitis   Meningitis due to *Leptospira* species.

localized tuberculous meningitis   A form or stage of tuberculous meningitis in which the inflammation is or becomes localized to some part of the subarachnoid space such as the basal meninges, the fourth ventricle and basal cisterns, or the spinal canal.

lymphocytic meningitis   Any form of meningitis in which the cerebrospinal fluid shows lymphocytic pleocytosis. • The term *benign lymphocytic meningitis* is often used to identify a group of self-limiting viral meningitides which usually recover spontaneously.

malarial meningitis   The presence of meningeal symptoms in cerebral malaria, usually due to *Plasmodium falciparum* infestation. • This seldom-used term is a misnomer. The cerebrospinal fluid is sometimes under increased pressure and contains a moderate increase in lymphocytes and sometimes protein. Although the meninges may be grossly congested, the major pathology involves the brain. Capillaries are congested and blocked by parasitized erythrocytes, and petechial hemorrhages are present. In a minority of cases of cerebral malaria, cerebral edema is present.

meningococcal meningitis   CEREBROSPINAL MENINGITIS.

meningococcic meningitis   CEREBROSPINAL MENINGITIS.

metastatic meningitis   Meningitis caused by the spread of a pathogen from a site of infection outside the nervous system via the blood or lymphatic system.

Mollaret's meningitis   BENIGN RECURRENT ENDOTHELIOLEUKOCYTIC MENINGITIS.

mumps meningitis   Meningitis complicating mumps, resulting from the invasion of the subarachnoid space by the virus, and sometimes preceding involvement of the parotid glands, or even being the sole manifestation of the infection. The onset is typically abrupt, but the course of the condition is usually short, the meningeal signs disappearing towards the end of the first week. In some cases the meningeal symptoms are associated with manifestations of encephalitis. The cerebrospinal fluid is often under increased pressure. It shows a lymphocytic pleocytosis and contains a modest increase in protein content, and the mumps virus can usually be isolated.

mycotic meningitis   Meningitis complicating any mycotic infection, such as cryptococcosis, aspergillosis, and others, and the bacterial infection, actinomycosis.

meningitis necrotoxica reactiva   Meningitis associated with multiple areas of focal cerebral cortical softening. An imprecise and outmoded term.

neonatal meningitis   Meningitis in the newborn infant. The infecting agent is commonly Gram-negative bacteria such as *Escherichia coli*. The illness is frequently fatal, especially if infection develops within the first three days of life.

occlusive meningitis   Meningitis leading to communicating hydrocephalus.

meningitis ossificans   Ossification or calcification in the meninges in chronic meningitis. Also called *ossifying meningitis* (seldom used).

ossifying meningitis   A seldom used term for MENINGITIS OSSIFICANS.

otitic meningitis   OTOGENIC MENINGITIS.

otogenic meningitis   Any type of meningitis complicating acute or chronic otitis media. Also called *otitic meningitis*.

Pfeiffer's bacillary meningitis   An outmoded term for HEMOPHILUS MENINGITIS.

plague meningitis   Meningitis caused by *Yersinia pestis*.

plasmodial meningitis   CEREBRAL MALARIA.

pneumococcal meningitis   A severe purulent form of meningitis, occurring at any age but commoner in young children. It sometimes complicates infection in some other part of the body, such as sinusitis, otitis, pneumonia, empyema, endocarditis, or peritonitis, but more often develops in the absence of any evident focus elsewhere of pneumococcal infection. Modern chemotherapy and antibiotic treatment have improved the prognosis, but unless treatment is started early prognosis is still poor.

posterior meningitis   CHRONIC POSTERIOR BASIC MENINGITIS.

posterior basic meningitis   CHRONIC POSTERIOR BASIC MENINGITIS.

post-traumatic meningitis   Meningitis following head injury due usually to skull fracture involving the middle ear or paranasal sinuses thus allowing organisms to enter the cranial cavity.

purulent meningitis　Meningitis caused by pyogenic bacteria, such as meningococci, pneumococci, staphylococci, streptococci, *Haemophilus influenzae*, or coliforms, and characterized by large numbers of polymorphonuclear leukocytes in the cerebrospinal fluid. Also called *pyogenic meningitis, suppurative meningitis.*

purulent otogenic meningitis　Acute septic meningitis complicating otitis media and caused by a variety of organisms, particularly pneumococci, streptococci, *Bacillus proteus*, or anaerobic bacteria.

pyogenic meningitis　PURULENT MENINGITIS.

Quincke's meningitis　Acute noninfective or aseptic meningitis. An imprecise and obsolete term.

rheumatic meningitis　Meningitis complicating any rheumatic illness, such as systemic lupus erythematosus, the Behçet syndrome, and, rarely, rheumatoid arthritis.

sarcoid meningitis　Granulomatous meningitis due to sarcoidosis.

saturnine meningitis　The meningeal reaction which may occur as a manifestation of lead encephalopathy. An obsolete term.

sclerogummatous meningitis　An obsolete term for GUMMATOUS MENINGITIS.

septicemic meningitis　An acute inflammation of the meninges following an episode of septicemia.

meningitis serosa　SEROUS MENINGITIS.

meningitis serosa circumscripta　Localized arachnoiditis. Also called *serous circumscribed meningitis.*

meningitis serosa circumscripta cystica　Localized arachnoiditis with arachnoidal cyst formation.

serous meningitis　Any of various forms of meningitis, such as arachnoiditis of undetermined cause and the syndromes of otitic hydrocephalus and benign intracranial hypertension. An imprecise and obsolete term. Also called *meningitis serosa.*

serous circumscribed meningitis　MENINGITIS SEROSA CIRCUMSCRIPTA.

serum meningitis　A meningeal reaction occurring as one manifestation of serum sickness, usually developing about seven or eight days after the injection of foreign serum. • The term is a misnomer, as the cerebrospinal fluid is usually normal, or else it shows a minimal pleocytosis with a modest increase in protein content. The clinical manifestations are those of an encephalopathy and not of a true meningitis.

spinal meningitis　Inflammation of the spinal meninges. This may occur as a result of loculation of an inflammatory process in the spinal canal in any form of meningitis, but rare forms of staphylococcal and tuberculous meningitis largely restricted to the spinal meninges have been described. Also called *spinitis* (obsolete).

staphylococcal meningitis　A severe type of purulent meningitis which can arise as a complication of staphylococcal septicemia, or by infection of the meninges, either as a result of a compound skull fracture or through spread of infection from a staphylococcal cranial or spinal osteomyelitis. A rare variety of primary spinal staphylococcal meningitis has been described.

sterile meningitis　ASEPTIC MENINGITIS.

streptococcal meningitis　A severe type of purulent meningitis, usually resulting from the introduction of streptococci into the subarachnoid space either as a consequence of trauma, of otitis media or sinusitis, or through metastatic spread from a distant septic focus in septicemia or acute endocarditis.

suppurative meningitis　PURULENT MENINGITIS.

meningitis sympathica　A non-specific, aseptic, reactive inflammation of the meninges caused by the presence of an adjacent, specific inflammatory focus. A rarely used term.

syphilitic meningitis　Meningitis occurring as a manifestation of either secondary syphilis, in which case it is an acute, self-limiting lymphocytic type, or in meningovascular syphilis, in which case the meningitis is usually subacute and granulomatous in type.

torula meningitis　CRYPTOCOCCAL MENINGITIS.

torular meningitis　CRYPTOCOCCAL MENINGITIS.

toxic meningitis　A meningeal reaction occurring in various forms of metabolic and toxic encephalopathy. An imprecise and seldom used term.

traumatic meningitis　A meningeal reaction complicating physical injury to the head or spine. An imprecise and seldom used term.

trypanosomal meningitis　Meningitis complicating African trypanosomiasis. An acute meningitis may occur in the course of the disease, with lymphocytosis and a moderately raised albumen level in the cerebrospinal fluid. In advanced disease, high IgM concentrations are present in cerebrospinal fluid. Lymphocytes, mononuclear cells, eosinophils, morula cells, and trypanosomes may also be present. In the later states, meningoencephalomyelitis may occur.

tubercular meningitis　TUBERCULOUS MENINGITIS.

tuberculous meningitis　Meningitis due to the tubercle bacillus. This usually complicates primary or miliary tuberculosis but can develop in patients with tuberculosis at any stage and is generally due to the rupture of a cortical tuberculoma into the subarachnoid space. The onset may be acute but more often the illness runs a subacute or chronic course, and a few days or weeks of general malaise, mild fever, and headache may presage the development of more typical symptoms of meningitis. This form of meningitis is often complicated by variable manifestations of encephalomyelopathy, by cranial nerve palsies, by neurologic signs resulting from cerebral ischemia due to endarteritis of basal vessels, and by communicating hydrocephalus or by other manifestations resulting from the formation of adhesions in the subarachnoid space with consequent loculation of the inflammatory process. A chronic spinal form has been described, often giving rise to paraparesis. The cerebrospinal fluid is under increased pressure and is often clear or only faintly turbid, but a fine fibrin web often forms after the specimen has been allowed to stand overnight. The fluid invariably contains an increase in cells (polymorphonuclear in the early stages, lymphocytes and other mononuclears later), the cell count usually varying from 50–1000 white cells per cubic millimeter. Its protein content is raised and its sugar content moderately reduced. Tubercle bacilli may be isolated by culture or, rarely, identified in the cerebrospinal fluid by microscopy. Also called *tubercular meningitis, cerebral tuberculosis.*

tuberculous exudative meningitis　Tuberculous meningitis with chronic exudative granulomatous change in the basal subarachnoid space, often with local caseation. An obsolete term.

tuberculous follicular meningitis　A form or stage of tuberculous meningitis in which small follicular tubercles may be found scattered throughout the leptomeninges. An obsolete term.

typhoid meningitis　**1** A clinical meningeal syndrome sometimes seen in typhoid fever as a manifestation of an aseptic meningeal reaction or a secondary infection.　**2** An unusual form of meningitis due to invasion of the subarachnoid space by *Salmonella typhi*. In most cases this complication develops towards the end of the course of typhoid fever.

verminal meningitis　Acute meningitis complicating an intestinal parasitic infestation, usually with ascariasis, less frequently taeniasis (cysticercosis), and characterized by a slight increase in the cerebrospinal fluid pressure, with a rise in protein and mild lymphocytosis, and by meningeal symptoms and signs of moderate intensity. A seldom used term.

vertical meningitis　Meningitis in which the inflammatory exudate is most striking over the superior aspect of the cerebral hemispheres. This is seen particularly in pneumococcal meningitis. An older term.

viral meningitis Meningitis caused by a virus infection and characterized by fever, headache, stiffness of the neck, nausea, malaise, and the presence of lymphocytes in the cerebrospinal fluid. Viruses that commonly produce this disorder include enteroviruses, mumps virus, lymphocytic choriomeningitis virus, and herpes simplex virus type 2. See also LYMPHOCYTIC MENINGITIS.

Wallgren's aseptic meningitis LYMPHOCYTIC CHORIOMENINGITIS.

yeast meningitis Meningitis due to yeasts such as *Cryptococcus* or *Blastomyces.*

---

meningitophobia 1 Pathologic fear of contracting meningitis. 2 A state marked by meningitislike conversion symptoms.

meningium An obsolete term for ARACHNOIDEA.

meningo- [Gk *mēninx* (gen. *mēningos*) membrane] A combining form denoting the meninges. Also *mening-, meningi-.*

meningoarteritis [MENINGO- + ARTERITIS] Meningitis associated with or causing inflammation of the arteries in the subarachnoid space.

meningoblast [MENINGO- + -BLAST] A primitive or precursor cell that contributes toward the formation of the meninges.

meningoblastoma [MENINGO- + BLASTOMA] ANAPLASTIC MENINGIOMA.

meningocele [MENINGO- + -CELE¹] The protrusion of the dura mater and the arachnoid meningeal layers surrounding the brain or the spinal cord through a developmental defect in the osseoligamentous coverings of these organs. It is usually manifested as a fluid-filled sac covered by modified skin on the midline of the cranium or back. Rarely, an acquired meningocele can follow trauma or surgery.

cerebral meningocele A meningocele involving cranial meninges and appearing on the surface of the head or, rarely, in the orbital, nasal, or nasopharyngeal cavities.

spurious meningocele TRAUMATIC MENINGOCELE.

traumatic meningocele The protrusion of a fluid-filled sac through an acquired defect in the cranial cavity or spinal canal as a result of trauma. Also called *Billroth's disease.*

meningocephalitis MENINGOENCEPHALITIS.

meningocerebral Of or pertaining to the meninges and cerebral cortex.

meningocerebritis MENINGOENCEPHALITIS.

meningococcemia [*meningococc(us)* + -EMIA] The presence of meningococci in the bloodstream. It is often associated with a diffuse petechial rash and, at times, disseminated intravascular coagulation, shock, and death.

acute fulminating meningococcemia Severe meningococcal sepsis with or without meningitis and often associated with purpura, disseminated intravascular coagulation, bilateral adrenal hemorrhages, collapse, and death. See also WATERHOUSE-FRIDERICHSEN SYNDROME.

chronic meningococcemia A syndrome of persistent or recurrent meningococcal bacteremia and low-grade fever which may be associated with rash and arthritis.

meningococci Plural of MENINGOCOCCUS.

meningococcin A skin-test antigen prepared from *Neisseria meningitidis* that was once used in intradermal testing for the meningococcal carrier state.

meningococcosis [*meningococc(us)* + -OSIS] Any meningococcal infection or disease.

meningococcus [MENINGO- + L *coccus* the kermes berry, scarlet berry] (*plural* meningococci) A microorganism of the species *Neisseria meningitidis.*

meningocortical Of or pertaining to the meninges and the cerebral cortex. Also called *meningeocortical.*

meningoencephalitis [MENINGO- + ENCEPHALITIS] Inflammation of the brain and meninges. Also called *cerebromeningitis, encephalomeningitis, meningocephalitis, meningocerebritis, periencephalitis, periencephalomeningitis, cephalomeningitis* (seldom used). Adjective: meningoencephalitic.

biundulant meningoencephalitis The central European subtype of tick-borne encephalitis. See under TICK-BORNE ENCEPHALITIS.

chronic meningoencephalitis 1 Any meningoencephalitis running a chronic course. 2 GENERAL PARESIS.

demyelinating meningoencephalitis PERIVENOUS MENINGOENCEPHALITIS.

eosinophilic meningoencephalitis EOSINOPHILIC MENINGITIS.

mumps meningoencephalitis Meningoencephalitis due to mumps virus.

perivenous meningoencephalitis Meningoencephalitis in which the areas of inflammatory cell infiltration and demyelination are largely perivenous in distribution. Many forms of postinfective meningoencephalitis can be so described but this is a pathologic description and not a diagnosis. Also called *demyelinating meningoencephalitis.*

primary amebic meningoencephalitis Meningoencephalitis caused by free-living soil or freshwater pathogenic strains of *Naegleria* or *Acanthamoeba* species. Infection usually is via the cribriform plate, death occurring in three to five days following onset.

syphilitic meningoencephalitis 1 Acute or subacute meningoencephalitis in meningovascular syphilis. 2 GENERAL PARESIS.

taiga tick meningoencephalitis RUSSIAN SPRING-SUMMER ENCEPHALITIS.

trypanosomal meningoencephalitis A subacute or chronic meningoencephalitis involving the base of the brain predominantly, caused by the highly pathogenic flagellate protozoa *Trypanosoma gambiense* or *T. rhodesiense.* The complications occur in weeks to a few months with *T. rhodesiense* and in months or years with *T. gambiense.* Onset is insidious in most cases. The condition leads to progressive mental deterioration and classic sleeping sickness. See also TRYPANOSOMIASIS.

Tüga's meningoencephalitis A rickettsial disease of the Far East, transmitted by the tick *Haemaphysalis cincinna,* and giving rise to meningoencephalitic symptoms and benign recurrent fever.

meningoencephalocele ENCEPHALOCELE.

meningoencephalomyelitis [MENINGO- + ENCEPHALOMYELITIS] Inflammation of the meninges and of the brain and spinal cord.

meningoencephalomyelopathy [MENINGO- + ENCEPHALO- + MYELOPATHY] Any disease involving the brain, meninges, and spinal cord.

meningoencephalomyeloradiculoneuritis [MENINGO- + ENCEPHALO- + MYELO- + RADICULONEURITIS] Inflammation of the brain, meninges, spinal cord, nerve roots, and peripheral nerves.

meningoencephalopathy [MENINGO- + ENCEPHALOPATHY] Any of a large group of diffuse disorders of function of the brain and meninges not due to inflammation. • The term is somewhat imprecise and is used infrequently, but many varieties of toxic and metabolic encephalopathy have been described.

meningoependymitis Any disorder causing inflammation of the meninges and ependyma.

meningofibroblastoma [MENINGO- + FIBROBLASTOMA] FI-BROUS MENINGIOMA.

meningoma [MENING- + -OMA] MENINGIOMA.

meningomalacia Softening of a membrane, particularly the meninges, as a result of necrosis. A seldom used term.

meningomyelitis [MENINGO- + MYELITIS] Inflammation of the spinal cord and of its covering membranes, usually of the arachnoid and pia mater, less frequently of the dura mater. Also called *myelomeningitis* (seldom used).
   blastomycotic meningomyelitis Meningomyelitis due to one of the several known systemic, human, pathogenic, blastomycotic fungi, *Paracoccidioides brasiliensis, Histoplasma capsulatum, H. capsulatum* var. *duboisii, Coccidioides immitis,* and *Blastomyces dermatitidis.*
   sporotrichotic meningomyelitis Meningomyelitis due to *Sporothrix schenkii.*
   torular meningomyelitis Meningomyelitis due to *Cryptococcus neoformans.* • *Torular* refers to the genus *Torula,* an earlier name for *Cryptococcus.*

meningomyelocele A protrusion of the spinal cord and associated meninges through a developmental defect in the spinal canal, resulting in exposure at the surface along the midline of the back. Also called *myelomeningocele.* • This is a nonspecific term that is often used regardless of the presence or absence of a cystlike lesion or of demonstrated cord tissue in the herniated parts.

meningomyeloencephalitis [MENINGO- + MYELO- + EN-CEPHALITIS] Inflammation of the meninges, spinal cord, and brain.

meningomyeloradiculitis [MENINGO- + MYELO- + RADI-CULITIS] Inflammation of the meninges, of the spinal cord, and of the spinal nerve roots. Also called *meningoradiculomyelitis.*

meningo-osteophlebitis Periostitis that is associated with inflammation of the venous sinuses of a bone.

meningopathy [MENINGO- + -PATHY] Any disease or disorder affecting the meninges.

meningorachidian [MENINGO- + RACHIDIAN] Of or pertaining to the meninges and spinal cord.

meningoradicular [MENINGO- + RADICULAR] Of or pertaining to the meninges and the roots of the spinal and cranial nerves.

meningoradiculitis [MENINGO- + RADICULITIS] Inflammation of the spinal meninges and of the spinal nerve roots.

meningoradiculomyelitis MENINGOMYELORADICULITIS.
   progressive meningoradiculomyelitis **1** A rare and late spinal complication of cerebrospinal meningitis, resulting in progressive paraparesis. **2** Any of several distinct varieties of progressive myelitis, such as subacute necrotic myelitis.

meningorecurrence A temporary exacerbation of syphilitic meningitis induced by treatment. It is one form of the Jarisch-Herxheimer reaction.

meningorrhagia [MENINGO- + -RRHAGIA] Extravasation of blood within the cerebral or spinal meninges. Also called *meningorrhea.*

meningorrhea MENINGORRHAGIA.

meningosis A union of bones by the formation of membranous attachments, as seen in the neonatal skull. A rarely used term.

meningothelioma [MENING- + THEL- + *i* + -OMA] MEN-INGOTHELIOMATOUS MENINGIOMA.

meningothelium [MENINGO- + *(epi)thelium*] Epithelial-like cells of the arachnoidea that line the inner aspect of the dura mater.

meningotropism [MENINGO- + TROPISM] An affinity for the meninges.

meningovascular [MENING- + VASCULAR] Of or pertaining to the meninges and blood vessels.

meninguria [MENING- + -URIA] The excretion of shreds of membrane in the urine.

meninx [Gk *mēninx* membrane] **1** A membrane. **2** Singular of MENINGES.
   meninx fibrosa An obsolete term for DURA MATER.
   meninx primitiva ECTOMENINX.
   meninx serosa An obsolete term for ARACHNOIDEA.
   meninx tenuis An obsolete term for LEPTOMENINGES.
   meninx vasculosa An obsolete term for PIA MATER.

meniscal Pertaining to a meniscus.

meniscectomy [*menisc(us)* + -ECTOMY] The surgical excision of a semilunar cartilage of the knee.
   arthroscopic meniscectomy The removal of all or part of a damaged semilunar cartilage of the knee through an arthroscope.

menischesis MENOSCHESIS.

menisci Plural of MENISCUS.

meniscitis Inflammation of a meniscus.

meniscocyte SICKLE CELL.

meniscocytosis SICKLE CELL ANEMIA.

meniscopathy [*menisc(us)* + *o* + -PATHY] Any abnormality of a meniscus.

meniscopexy The surgical repositioning of a displaced meniscus.

meniscotomy An incision of semilunar cartilage in the knee.

meniscus [Late L (from Gk *mēniskos* a crescent, from *mēnē* a crescent, the moon, from *mēn* a month), a crescent or crescent-shaped body] (*plural* menisci) A crescent-shaped structure. • The term is often used alone to refer to one of the semilunar fibrocartilaginous disks in the knee joint.
   meniscus of acromioclavicular joint An outmoded term for DISCUS ARTICULARIS ARTICULATIONIS ACROMIOCLAVICU-LARIS.
   articular meniscus MENISCUS ARTICULARIS.
   meniscus articularis [NA] A crescentic wedge of fibrocartilage or dense fibrous tissue found in certain synovial joints, such as the knee. Its broad convex base is usually attached to the articular capsule, while the two sides are in contact with apposing articular surfaces of the bones, deepening a flat or shallow articular surface and usually adding to the stability of the joint. Also called *articular meniscus, articular crescent, joint meniscus, intra-articular disk.*
   converging meniscus A concavoconvex lens, oriented with the convex side away from the eye. Also called *positive meniscus.*
   discoid meniscus A congenital abnormality in which the semilunar cartilage of the knee is rounded in shape.
   discoid lateral meniscus A congenital abnormality of a disk-shaped lateral meniscus. It is seen more frequently than a similar abnormality in the medial compartment of the knee joint.
   diverging meniscus A convexoconcave lens, oriented with the concave side away from the eye. Also called *negative meniscus.*
   meniscus of inferior radioulnar joint An outmoded term for DISCUS ARTICULARIS ARTICULATIONIS RADIOULNARIS DIS-TALIS.
   joint meniscus MENISCUS ARTICULARIS.
   Kuhnt's meniscus The neuroglial layer on the anterior surface of the optic disk.
   lateral meniscus MENISCUS LATERALIS ARTICULATIONIS GE-NUS.
   meniscus lateralis articulationis genus A near-complete ring of fibrocartilage situated on the circumferential part of the

superior articular surface of the tibia. Its anterior end is attached anterior to the lateral intercondylar tubercle of the tibia behind the anterior cruciate ligament, and its posterior end is attached behind the tubercle where it blends with the posterior cruciate ligament behind it. It is less firmly attached to the articular capsule than the medial meniscus. The popliteus tendon lies between it and the fibular collateral ligament. The transverse ligament is attached to its anterior portion. Also called *lateral meniscus of knee joint, external semilunar fibrocartilage, external semilunar cartilage of knee joint, lateral meniscus.*

lateral meniscus of knee joint   MENISCUS LATERALIS ARTICULATIONIS GENUS.

medial meniscus   MENISCUS MEDIALIS ARTICULATIONIS GENUS.

meniscus medialis articulationis genus   [NA] An oval crescent of fibrocartilage situated on the circumferential part of the superior articular surface of the tibia. Its broad anterior end is attached to the anterior intercondylar area of the tibia in front of the anterior cruciate ligament and continuous with the transverse ligament, while its posterior end is attached to the posterior intercondylar area between the posterior end of lateral meniscus and posterior cruciate ligament. Its outer margin is adherent to the fibrous articular capsule and the tibial collateral ligament. Also called *medial meniscus of knee joint, internal semilunar fibrocartilage, internal semilunar cartilage of knee joint, medial meniscus.*

medial meniscus of knee joint   MENISCUS MEDIALIS ARTICULATIONIS GENUS.

negative meniscus   DIVERGING MENISCUS.

periscopic meniscus   A curved lens without dioptric strength.

positive meniscus   CONVERGING MENISCUS.

slipped meniscus   A torn medial meniscus of the knee joint.

meniscus of sternoclavicular joint   An outmoded term for DISCUS ARTICULARIS ARTICULATIONIS STERNOCLAVICULARIS.

tactile meniscus   MENISCUS TACTUS.

meniscus tactus   Any of the concave neurofibrillar disks forming the terminal expansions of nerve fiber in the deeper portions of the germinative layers of the skin. Each disk is closely applied to a modified epithelial cell and acts as a touch receptor. Also called *Merkel cell, Merkel's disk, tactile disk, tactile meniscus.*

meniscus of temporomandibular joint   DISCUS ARTICULARIS ARTICULATIONIS TEMPOROMANDIBULARIS.

meniscus of temporomaxillary joint   An outmoded term for DISCUS ARTICULARIS ARTICULATIONIS TEMPOROMANDIBULARIS.

Menkes [John H *Menkes*, Austrian-born U.S. pediatric neurologist, born 1928]   Menkes disease. See under SYNDROME.

Mennell [James Beaver *Mennell*, English physician, born 1880] Mennell's test. See under SIGN.

meno- [Gk *mēn* (genitive *mēnos*) month]   A combining form denoting the menses.

menoctone   2-(8-Cyclohexyloctyl)-3-hydroxy-1,4-naphthoquinone. A compound with antimalarial properties.

menolipsis [MENO- + Gk *leipsis* a ceasing, failing]   **1** A seldom used term for AMENORRHEA.   **2** A temporary cessation of menstruation.

menometrorrhagia [MENO- + METRO- + -RRHAGIA]   Abnormal uterine bleeding characterized both by occurrence between menstrual periods and increased flow during menstrual periods. Also called *metromenorrhagia.*

menopause [French *ménopause* (from MENO- + Gk *pausis* a cessation, from *pauein* to cease, bring to an end) the menopause] The immediate postreproductive phase of a woman's life, when menstrual function ceases due to failure to form ovarian follicles and ova. It is usually of several years' duration, with onset usually between age 45–50, and is accompanied by a variety of physiologic alterations. Irregularity of the menses usually occurs at the onset of menopause, leading to cessation. Symptoms include sudden sensations of heat and flushing (known popularly as hot flashes) of the face and torso, and vaginal dryness. Osteoporosis is a common postmenopausal symptom. Also called *menostasis, menostasia.* Adjective: menopausal.

artifical menopause   Menopause caused by hypophysectomy, ovariectomy, radiation, or chemotherapy.

male menopause   CLIMACTERIC.

menopause praecox   PREMATURE MENOPAUSE.

premature menopause   Premature failure of cyclic ovarian function. In the United States and other countries, ovarian failure before the age of 38 is considered premature menopause. When not due to systemic illness, severe malnutrition, or discernible endocrine cause, as a destructive pituitary tumor, the etiology is unknown. Also called *menopause praecox, climacterium praecox.*

menophania [MENO- + Gk *phan(ō)*, fut. of *phainein* to appear + -IA]   MENARCHE.

menoplania [MENO- + Gk *plan(ē)* a wandering, error + -IA] VICARIOUS MENSTRUATION.

Menopon [possibly from Gk *menein* to abide, linger + *ponos* pain, toil]   An economically important genus of poultry lice of the order Mallophaga.

Menopon gallinae   The shaft louse, an important mallophagan parasite of the feather shafts of chickens, and of ducks, turkeys, and guinea fowl, especially when they are housed with chickens. Horses living near infected chickens occasionally harbor the lice.

menorrhagia [MENO- + -RRHAGIA]   Excessive or prolonged menstruation. Also called *cyclic hemorrhage.*

functional menorrhagia   Menorrhagia not due to detectable organic cause, but the result of disordered ovarian function involving the normal cyclic secretion of estrogen and progesterone. Also called *primary menorrhagia.*

primary menorrhagia   FUNCTIONAL MENORRHAGIA.

menorrhalgia [MENO- + -*rrh(ea)* + -ALGIA]   DYSMENORRHEA.

menorrhea [MENO- + -RRHEA]   Normal menstruation. Adjective: menorrheal.

menoschesis [MENO- + Gk *schesis* a holding, retention] Suppression of menstruation. Also *menischesis.*

menosepsis   Septicemia resulting from endometritis caused by retention of menstrual discharge.

menostasia   MENOPAUSE.

menostasis   MENOPAUSE.

menostaxis [MENO- + Gk *staxis* a dripping]   AMENORRHEA.

menotropins   The purified and standardized extract human postmenopausal urine, which contains almost exclusively follicle stimulating hormone with only a trace of luteinizing hormone. It is used with human chorionic gonadotropin to induce fertility in anovulatory women.

menouria [MENO- + -URIA]   The discharge of menses into the urinary bladder secondary to a pre-existing vesicouterine fistula.

menoxenia [MENO- + Gk *xen(os)* a stranger + -IA]   Any abnormality of menstruation. A seldom used term.

menses [L, pl. of *mensis* month]   MENSTRUATION.

mens rea [L *mens* the mind, intention + *rea*, fem. of *reus* answerable for, guilty]   CRIMINAL INTENT.

menstrual   Of, relating to, or characteristic of menstruation; pertaining to the menses. Also *menstruous.*

menstruant [Late L *menstruans*, gen. *menstruatis*, pres. part of *menstruari* (from L *menstruus* monthly) to menstruate]   **1** Menstruating or capable of menstruating.   **2** A woman capable of menstruating.

menstruate [Late L *menstruatus*, past part. of *menstruari* (from L *menstruus* monthly) to menstruate]   To have menstruation.

menstruation [Late L *menstruatus*, past part. of *menstruari* to menstruate, from L *menstrua* (pl. of *menstruum* rations for a month, from *menstruum*, neut. of *menstruus* monthly, from *mensis* a month, akin to Gk *mēn* a month) menses]   The physiologic cyclic shedding of the uterine endometrium at a mean interval of 28 days, unless pregnancy intervenes, and characterized by vaginal bleeding of three to seven days' duration in the mature human female and in other higher primates. The hormonal basis is cyclic hypothalamic-adenohypophysial secretion of gonadotropic hormones, including a sharp midcycle surge of luteinizing hormone releasing hormone and of luteinizing hormone, resulting normally in ovulation. These hormonal rhythms are reflected in cyclic variations of ovarian secretion of estrogen and progesterone with consequent formation of first proliferative, then secretory endometrium. Also called *menses, menstrual period, monthly period, terms, emmenia, catamenia, metremia, regel (German), metrorrhea* (obsolete), *monthly sickness* (popular).

anovular menstruation   ANOVULATORY MENSTRUATION.

anovulatory menstruation   Periodic uterine bleeding occurring in the absence of ovulation. Also called *anovular menstruation, nonovulational menstruation, anovulatory cycle.*

delayed menstruation   The absence of menstruation at the time it is expected to appear.

infrequent menstruation   OLIGOMENORRHEA.

nonovulational menstruation   ANOVULATORY MENSTRUATION.

regurgitant menstruation   RETROGRADE MENSTRUATION.

retained menstruation   HEMATOCOLPOS.

retrograde menstruation   A flow of menstrual blood through the fallopian tubes. Also called *regurgitant menstruation.*

scanty menstruation   Menses of a smaller than usual amount or lasting less than two days.

supplementary menstruation   Menstruation accompanied by vicarious menstruation from certain areas such as the urinary tract or the umbilicus. It is usually associated with endometriosis.

vicarious menstruation   Bleeding from any surface other than the endometrium occurring periodically at the time when normal menstruation takes place. It is usually caused by endometriosis. Also called *menoplania.*

menstruous   MENSTRUAL.

menstruum [Med. L (from neut. sing. of L *menstruus* monthly, menstruous), menses]   **1** The menstrual blood. **2** The liquid vehicle used to extract the active ingredients from a crude source of a drug and prepare an official tincture of the drug.

Pitkin menstruum   A mixture of gelatin, dextrose, glacial acetic acid, and water, that has been used as a medium for certain drugs, such as heparin, to delay diffusion of the drug and prolong the drug action.

mensual   Monthly.

mensuration [Late L *mensuratio* (from *mensuratus*, past part. of *mensurare* to measure, from L *mensus*, past part. of *metiri* to measure) a measuring]   The act or process of measuring.

-ment [French (from L *-mentum,* noun suffix), suffix forming nouns from verbs signifying action, concrete result, state, or condition]   A noun suffix denoting action, state, or result.

mentagrophyton   Any fungus of the species *Trichophyton mentagrophytes.*. An obsolete term.

mental¹ [Late L *mental(is)* (from L *mens,* gen. *mentis,* the mind + *-alis* -AL) pertaining to the mind]   Pertaining to mind or to the activities or processes of the mind.

mental² [L *ment(um)* chin, beard + -AL]   Of or pertaining to the chin; genial.

mentality [MENTAL + -ITY]   The powers or capacity of mind characteristic of an individual. A rarely used term.

Menten [Maud Lenore *Menten,* U.S. physician, 1879–1960]   **1** Michaelis-Menten equation. See under EQUATION. **2** Michaelis-Menten kinetics. See under MICHAELIS KINETICS.

menthene carbonate $(C_{10}H_{18})CO_3$. A white compound similar to menthol in its medicinal uses.

menthol   2-Isopropyl-5-methylcyclohexanol, with the isopropyl group *trans* and the methyl group *cis* to the hydroxyl group. It is a terpene alcohol, found in *Mentha piperita* and other mint species and also produced synthetically. It is used as a nasal decongestant, antiseptic, anesthetic, counterirritant, and topical antipruritic. Also called *peppermint camphor.*

menthyl anthranilate $C_8H_9NO_2$. 2-Aminobenzoic acid methyl ester. A natural constituent of neroli, bergamot, jasmine, and some other essential oils. It is also prepared synthetically as artificial neroli oil. It is used in ointments and perfumes.

menti- [L *mens,* gen. *mentis,* the mind]   A combining form meaning the mind.

menticide [L *mens,* gen. *mentis,* the mind + -CIDE]   BRAINWASHING.

mento- [New L, from L *mentum* the chin]   A combining form denoting the chin.

mentoanterior [MENTO- + ANTERIOR]   In a face presentation, having the fetal chin pointing anteriorly in relation to the maternal pelvis.

mentobregmatic   Pertaining to the chin and the bregma.

mentolabial   Of or relating to the chin and the lip.

menton [French (from L *mentum* chin), chin]   A cephalometric point situated at the lowest point of the chin in the midline.

mentoparietal   Of or relating to the chin and the parietal bone.

mentoplasty [MENTO- + -PLASTY]   Any plastic operation performed on the chin.

mentoposterior [MENTO- + POSTERIOR]   In a face presentation, having the fetal chin pointing posteriorly in relation to the maternal pelvis.

mentotransverse [MENTO- + TRANSVERSE]   In a face presentation, having the fetal chin pointing laterally in relation to the maternal pelvis.

mentula   An outmoded term for PENIS.

mentulagra [L *mentul(a)* the penis + -AGRA]   PRIAPISM.

mentulate [L *mentul(a)* the penis + -ATE]   Having a large penis.

mentum [L, the chin]   The anterior prominence of the mandible that is produced by the mental protuberance; chin. The fleshy muscles and connective tissues covering it are separated from the lower lip by a groove.

Meonine   A proprietary name for methionine.

mepacrine hydrochloride   QUINACRINE HYDROCHLORIDE.

meparfynol $C_6H_{10}O$. A colorless or pale yellow liquid with an unpleasant burning taste. It is used as a short-acting hypnotic.

mepazine $C_{19}H_{22}N_2S$.   10-[(-methyl-3-piperidinyl)methyl]-10*H* phenothiazine. A tranquilizer employed as a sedative in the treatment of a variety of anxiety states. It is also used as a preoperative or postoperative sedative. It is administered orally or intramuscularly. Also called *pecazine.*

mepenzolate bromide $C_{21}H_{26}BrNO_3$. 3-[(Hydroxydiphenylacetyl)oxy]-1,1-dimethyl-piperidinium bromide. An anticholinergic agent used in the treatment of disorders where hypermotility of the colon is of concern. It is given orally.

meperidine hydrochloride $C_{15}H_{21}NO_2 \cdot HCl$. Ethyl-1-methyl-4-phenylpiperidine-4-carboxylate hydrochloride. A synthetic white, odorless powder, soluble in water and alcohol. It is a narcotic analgesic with spasmolytic properties. Its continued use may lead to addiction. It is usually given orally or intramuscularly. Also called *pethidine hydrochloride, isonipecaine.*

mephenamine ORPHENADRINE.

mephenesin $C_{10}H_{14}O_3$. 3-(2-Methylphenoxy)-1,2-propanediol. It is a white, crystalline powder employed as a skeletal muscle relaxant agent. It is given orally. Also called *stilalgin, cresoxypropanediol, cresoxydiol.*

mephenoxalone $C_{11}H_{13}NO_4$. 5-[(*o*-Methoxyphenoxy)methyl]-2-oxazolidinone. It possesses mild tranquilizing properties, and is used as a skeletal muscle relaxant.

mephentermine sulfate $(C_{11}H_{17}N)2 \cdot H_2SO_4$. $N\alpha,\alpha$-Trimethylbenzeneethanamine. A white, crystalline powder with adrenergic properties. It is used for its vasopressor effects in the treatment of certain hypotensive states. It can be given orally, intramuscularly, or intravenously, and may be applied topically to the nasal mucosa as a decongestant drug.

mephenytoin $C_{12}H_{14}N_2O_2$. 5-Ethyl-3-methyl-5-phenyl-2,4-imidazolidinedione. It is used as an anticonvulsant drug in the control of focal, jacksonian, grand mal, and psychmotor seizures that are not responsive to other drugs. It is given orally.

mephitic Pertaining to or characteristic of a foul or noxious odor. A rarely used term.

mephitis [L (earlier *mefitis*, from the Oscan), a noxious, pestilential exhalation from the earth] Exhalation of a foul smelling odor. A rarely used term.

mephobarbital $C_{13}H_{14}N_2O_3$. 5-Ethyl-1-methyl-5-phenyl-2,4,6(1*H*,3*H*,5*H*)-pyrimidinetrione. A barbiturate with prolonged actions, used as a sedative in the treatment of anxiety. It is also employed as an anticonvulsant in the treatment of grand mal and petit mal epilepsy. It is given orally. Also called *phemitone.*

Mephyton A proprietary name for vitamin K_1.

mepivacaine $C_{15}H_{22}N_2O$. *N*-(2,6-Dimethylphenyl)-1-methyl-2-piperidine-carboxamide. A white, crystalline powder which is administered as the hydrochloride salt. It is an analogue of lidocaine, used to produce local anesthesia by infiltration injection, peripheral nerve block, and epidural block.

Meprane A proprietary name for promethestrol.

meprednisone $C_{22}H_{28}O_5$. 17-α, 21-Dihydroxy-16β-methylpregna-1,4-diene-3,11,20-trione. A synthetic glucocorticoid which occurs as a white powder. It is used in the treatment of inflammatory, rheumatic, and allergic conditions, and is also used to treat corticosteroid-responsive diseases, such as certain connective tissue disorders and some neoplastic diseases. It is given orally.

meprobamate $C_9H_{18}N_2O_4$. 2-Methyl-2-propyl-1,3-propanediol dicarbamate. A white powder with activity as a tranquilizer and muscle relaxant, and with anticonvulsant properties. It is used orally as a sedative and antianxiety medication, and to promote sleep in tense patients. It is used intramuscularly as an adjunct treatment for tetanus.

meprylcaine hydrochloride $C_{14}H_{21}NO_2 \cdot HCl$. 2-Methyl-2-(propylamino)-1-propanol benzoate (ester) hydrochloride. A white, crystalline powder, used as a local anesthetic for infiltration and nerve block anesthesia.

mepyramine maleate PYRILAMINE MALEATE.

mepyrapone METYRAPONE.

mEq Symbol for the quantity, milliequivalent.

mequidox $C_{10}H_{10}N_2O_3$. 3-Methyl-2-quinoxalinemethanol 1,4-dioxide. It is employed as an antibacterial agent.

meractinomycin ACTINOMYCIN D.

meralein sodium $C_{19}H_9HgI_2NaO_7S$. 2,7-Diiodo-4-hydroxy-mercuriresorcinsulfonphthalein monosodium salt. A water-soluble, topically applied, anti-infective agent.

meralgia [*mer(o)-*[2] + -ALGIA] A pain in the thigh.

meralgia paresthetica A benign but troublesome syndrome resulting from compression of the lateral cutaneous nerve of the thigh as it passes beneath or through the fibers of the inguinal ligament just medial to the anterior superior iliac spine. It may develop spontaneously, often in obese subjects, but sometimes first appears in pregnancy. Pain and paresthesiae are felt, particularly on standing for long periods, on the outer aspect of the thigh, and blunting of cutaneous sensation is usually noted in this area. Also called *neuralgia of the cutaneous nerve of the thigh, Bernhardt's disease, Roth-Bernhardt syndrome, Bernhardt-Roth disease, Bernhardt's paresthesiae, Rot's disease, Roth's disease, Rot-Bernhardt disease, Bernhardt-Rot syndrome, Rot syndrome, Roth syndrome, Rot-Bernhardt syndrome, Roth-Bernhardt disease, Bernhardt syndrome.*

meralluride $C_{16}H_{22}HgN_6O_7$. *N*-[[2-Methoxy-3-[(1,2,3,6-tetrahydro-1,3-dimethyl-2,6-dioxopurin-7-yl)mercuri]propyl]carbamoyl]succinamic acid. A diuretic agent used in the treatment of edema secondary to congestive heart failure, nephrosis, and ascites of liver disease. It is given intramuscularly or subcutaneously.

meralopia MEROPIA.

meramaurosis Incomplete amaurosis.

Meratran A proprietary name for pipradrol.

merbromin $C_{20}H_8Br_2HgNa_2O_6$. 2'7'-Dibromo-3',6'-dihydroxy-3-oxospiro[isobenzofuran-1(3*H*),9'[9*H*]xanthene]-4'-yl) hydroxomercury disodium salt. It is used clinically as a topical antibacterial drug.

mercaptalbumin The form of serum albumin that has one thiol group per molecule, in distinction from the form in which this group exists as the mixed disulfide with a thiol of low molecular mass. A seldom used term.

mercaptan An obsolete term for THIOL.

mercaptide An obsolete term for THIOLATE.

mercapto- [Med L *mer(curium)*, accus. of *mercurius* mercury, after *Mercurius* Roman messenger of the gods + L *capt(ans)*, pres. part. of *captare* to seize + *o*] A combining form denoting substitution of a hydrogen atom by a thiol group. See also SULFHYDRYL.

mercaptoethanol $HS-CH_2-CH_2OH$. One of the most commonly used reagents containing a thiol group, often added to cell extracts to prevent or reverse the formation of $-S-S-$ bonds from thiol groups by materials in these extracts. It is of particular utility because the hydroxyl group lowers its volatility and gives it considerable solubility in water.

mercaptoethylamine C_2H_7NS. A compound prepared from ethanolamine and carbon disulfide via 2-mercaptothiazoline. It has been used in treating radiation sickness and chronic leukemia. It is a component of the coenzyme A molecule. Also called *cysteamine.*

2-mercaptoimidazole An antithyroid agent of the thiouricil family. It is considered to be about five times more potent than methylthiouricil.

mercaptomerin sodium $C_{16}H_{25}HgNNa_2O_6S$. *N*-[3-(Carboxymethylthiomercuri)-2-methoxypropyl]-α-camphoramate. A mercurial diuretic drug that is given subcutaneously or intramuscularly.

mercaptopurine 6-Purinethiol. A hypoxanthine and adenine analogue that serves as a purine antagonist. It is utilized primarily as an antineoplastic agent since it is a potent inhibitor of DNA synthesis.

mercapturic acid An *S*-aryl-*N*-acetylcysteine. It is found in the urine after ingestion of aromatic halogen compounds.

Mercier [Louis Auguste *Mercier*, French urologist, 1811–1882] **1** Mercier's operation. See under PROSTATECTOMY. **2** See under CATHETER, VALVE. **3** Mercier's barrier, Mercier's bar. See under PLICA INTERURETERICA. **4** Mercier's barrier. See under MEDIAN BAR.

Mercuhydrin   A proprietary name for meralluride.

mercupurin   An outmoded term for MERCUROPHYLLINE.

mercuramide   MERSALYL SODIUM.

mercurial   **1** Of, relating to, or resembling mercury. **2** Denoting a preparation of mercury or one containing mercury, as in *mercurial diuretic.*

mercurialentis   [English *mercuria(l)* + L *lens*, gen. *lentis*, a lentil] A bilateral and symmetric, light gray or brownish discoloration of the anterior capsule of the crystalline lens due to the deposition of mercury. It is a sign of chronic exposure to low levels of inorganic mercury or its compounds.

mercurialism   MERCURY POISONING.

***p*-mercuribenzoate**   The substance formed from the anion of benzoic acid by substitution of the *p*-hydrogen by Hg^+-. The mercury atom normally bears an anionic ligand such as Cl^- or OH^-, but this is exchangeable, and easily replaced by a thiolate. This gives mercuribenzoate a high affinity for thiols, and its use in titrating thiol groups and as an inhibitor of enzymes depends on this property.

mercuric   [*mercur(y)* + -IC] Concerning mercury in its Hg(II) form. Mercuric salts are toxic because of their high affinity for the thiol groups of proteins.

mercuric chloride $HgCl_2$. A water-soluble salt of mercury. It is highly toxic owing to the Hg^{2+} ions it contains. It is used as a secondary fixative where preservation of proteins is particularly important. Also called *corrosive sublimate.* (obsolete), *hydrargyri perchloridum.*

mercuric cyanide $Hg(CN)_2$. A poisonous mercuric salt formerly used as an antiseptic and for the treatment of syphilis.

mercuric imidosuccinate   MERCURIC SUCCINIMIDE.

mercuric oxycyanide $3Hg(CN)_2 \cdot HgO$. A white, crystalline powder, formerly used in solution as an antiseptic for some types of conjunctivitis. Also called *hydrargyi oxycyanidum.*

mercuric salicylate $(OH \cdot C_6H_4 \cdot CO_2)_2Hg$. A white, insoluble powder formerly used in the treatment of syphilis. Also called *hydrargyri salicylas.*

mercuric succinimide $C_8H_8HgN_2O_4$. A white powder, soluble in water. It was formerly used in the treatment of syphilis. Also called *mercuric imidosuccinate.*

mercuric sulfate $HgSO_4$. The sulfate of bivalent mercury. It is a very dense white powder. It is anhydrous, darkens in light, is slightly soluble in water, and is toxic. It is the starting material for making mercuric chloride and basic mercuric sulfate and is used as a catalyst in organic synthesis.

mercuric sulfide HgS. A bright red powder that has been used in an ointment base as a treatment for chronic skin diseases. Also called *cinnabar.*

Mercurio   [Geronimo Scipione *Mercurio*, Italian obstetrician, flourished late 16th century] See under POSITION.

Mercurochrome   A proprietary name for merbromin.

mercurophylline   An organic mercurial diuretic agent in combination with theophylline in approximately equimolecular amounts. It is given by intramuscular or intravenous injection. Also called *mercupurin* (outmoded).

mercurous   Concerning the ion Hg^+-Hg^+. Its chloride, calomel, has very low solubility in water.

mercurous chloride   CALOMEL.

mercurous sulfate Hg_2SO_4. Sulfate of univalent mercury. It is a crystalline yellowish white powder becoming grey on exposure to light. It is slightly soluble in water and soluble in dilute nitric acid. It is used in the manufacture of electric batteries.

mercury   [after *Mercurius* (Mercury) son of Jupiter and Maia, and messenger of the gods; his name was given to the planet and later to the metal, possibly because his swiftness was deemed characteristic of mercury (quicksilver)] A metallic element of atomic number 80, atomic weight 200.59, specific gravity 13.5, and boiling point $-38.842°C$. It is the only common metal that is liquid (and volatile) at ordinary temperatures. It does not occur in the free state but is readily freed from its principal ore, cinnabar, by heat. Natural mercury consists of seven stable isotopes. Numerous radioactive isotopes have been identified, all of them relatively short lived. Valences are 1 and 2. In an electric discharge, mercury combines with the so-called inert gases argon, krypton, neon, and xenon. Though relatively rare in the lithosphere, mercury is universally familiar through its use in thermometers, barometers, and the like. It is indispensable in many industrial and research operations. It is commonly used in dental amalgams and has several other medical applications. But its vapor and some of its compounds are virulent poisons. The vapor is readily absorbed through mucous membrane or unbroken skin. Methyl mercury is a dangerous environmental pollutant. It is elaborated by anaerobic bacteria in many rivers and streams where mercury-containing waste has been discharged, and thence it can enter the food chain via fishes, insects, and birds. Also called *quicksilver, hydrargyrum.* Symbol: Hg See also MERCURY POISONING.

ammoniated mercury $HgNH_2Cl$. A substance occurring as a white, amorphous powder or as small, white granules. It is applied topically in an ointment base as an anti-infective medication. Also called *hydrargyrum ammoniatum.*

mercury with chalk   A powder produced by mixing mercury with chalk to obtain a uniform gray color, with no metallic globules of mercury visible under a magnifying glass. It has been used as a laxative, but its use in children may cause acrodynia. Also called *gray powder.*

vegetable mercury   MANACA.

mercury oleate   A composition of yellow mercuric oxide and oleic acid. It has been used topically for some chronic skin diseases. Also called *hydrargyrum oleatum.*

Mercuzanthin   A preparation of mercurophylline. A proprietary name.

-mere   [Gk *meros* a part] A combining form meaning a part.

Merendino   [Alvin Aurelius *Merendino*, U.S. surgeon, born 1914] See under TECHNIQUE.

merergasia   [*mer(o)-*[1] + Gk *ergasia* work, occupation] Any disorder which results in a partial inability to work or function, as may occur in the neuroses. Also called *kakergasia.* Adjective: merergastic.

merethoxylline   Dehydro-2-[*n*-(3″-hydroxymercuri-2″-methoxyethoxy)propylcarbamoyl]phenoxyacetic acid.

merethoxylline procaine   A combination of merethoxylline, theophylline, and procaine. It is used in the treatment of edema secondary to congestive heart failure and the nephrotic syndrome. It is given intramuscularly or subcutaneously.

meridian   [L *meridianus.* See MERIDIANUS.] MERIDIANUS.

meridian of cornea   A line perpendicular to the optic axis at the corneal plane.

meridians of eyeball   MERIDIANI BULBI OCULI.

horizontal meridian   An imaginary line that passes through the point of visual fixation and is oriented horizontally in the frontal plane.

interpalpebral meridian   An imaginary line oriented parallel to the opening between upper and lower eyelids.

vertical meridian   A line that passes through the point of visual fixation and is oriented vertically in the frontal plane.

meridiani Plural of MERIDIANUS.

meridianus [L (from *meri-*, alteration of *medi-* mid-, from *medius* middle + *dies* day + *-anus* adjectival suffix), of or at midday] [NA] An imaginary line on the surface of a spherical body passing along the plane of its axis. Also called *meridian*.

meridiani bulbi oculi Circumferential lines joining the poles of the eyeball. Also called *meridians of eyeball*.

meridional Pertaining to a meridian.

merisis HYPERPLASIA.

merism [*mer(o)-*[1] + -ISM] The occurrence of regular, equal segmentation. Compare AMERISM.

merisoprol Hg 197 CHLORMERODRIN 197.

merispore A secondary spore resulting from the segmentation of a compound or septate spore.

meristem [Gk *merist(os)* (from *merizein* to divide into parts, from *meris* a part) divided + *-ēm(a)* noun suffix] Undifferentiated plant tissue from which new cells proliferate. Adjective: meristematic.

  apical meristem The growing region of a vascular plant stem or root tip, which is composed of meristematic tissue.

  ground meristem The large, thin-walled cells that form the greatest part of the meristematic tissue in the shoot tip.

  lateral meristems The vascular and cork cambium meristematic tissue in a vascular plant which produces the secondary tissues: secondary phloem, secondary xylem, and periderm.

méristème d'attente [French *méristème* MERISTEM + *d(e)* of + *attente* (from L *attentus*, past part. of *attendere* to give attention to) a wait] A quiescent region or a waiting meristem of certain plant shoots that is believed to give rise to most of the floral reproductive structures.

meristic [Gk *meristik(os)* (from *meris* a part + *t* + *-ikos* -IC) suitable for dividing] Indicating symmetry or serial division in the arrangement of parts.

meristoma [*merist(em)* + -OMA] An abnormal growth or tumor occurring in the meristem of a plant.

Merkel [Friedrich S. *Merkel* German anatomist and physiologist, 1845–1919] **1** Merkel's disk, Merkel cell. See under MENISCUS TACTUS. **2** Grandry-Merkel corpuscles, Merkel's corpuscles. See under GRANDRY'S CORPUSCLES. **3** Merkel cell carcinoma. See under CARCINOMA. **4** Merkel's corpuscles. See under CORPUSCLE. **5** Merkel-Ranvier cell. See under MELANOCYTE.

Merkel [Karl Ludwig *Merkel*, German anatomist and laryngologist, 1812–1876] **1** Merkel's filtrum, Merkel's fossa. See under FILTRUM VENTRICULI. **2** Merkel's muscle. See under MUSCULUS CERATOCRICOIDEUS.

Mermis [Gk *mermis* a cord, rope] A common genus of nematodes of the family Mermithidae, superfamily Mermithoidea, a group of unusual nematodes in which only the larvae are parasitic (in insects) and the adults are nonfeeding and free-living, sometimes reaching a considerable length (up to 50 cm).

mermithid [Gk *mermis*, gen. *mermithos*, a cord, rope + -ID[1]] **1** Relating or belonging to the family Mermithidae. **2** A member of the family Mermithidae.

Mermithidae [Gk *mermis*, gen. *mermithos*, a cord, rope + -IDAE] A family of nematodes in the superfamily Mermithoidea, characterized by adults that are free-living and generally nonfeeding, and larvae that are parasitic in the hemocoel of various insects, especially orthopterans such as crickets and grasshoppers. Larvae have occassionally been found in the human digestive tract as a result of ingesting contaminated water and possibly food.

mero-[1] [Gk *meros* part] A combining form meaning part, partial.

mero-[2] [Gk *mēros* upper part of the thigh, the ham] A com-

bining form denoting the thigh.

meroacrania The developmental absence of a part of the cranium. Also called *merocrania*.

meroanencephalia MEROANENCEPHALY.

meroanencephaly [MERO-[1] + ANENCEPHALY] Anencephaly in which less than the usual erosion of cerebral tissue has occurred during intrauterine life and identifiable parts of the cerebrum such as peduncles and thalamus may remain. Also called *meroanencephalia*.

meroblastic [MERO-[1] + BLAST- + -IC] See under MEROBLASTIC CLEAVAGE.

merocele [MERO-[2] + -CELE[2]] FEMORAL HERNIA.

merocoxalgia Any painful condition of the hip and thigh.

merocrania MEROACRANIA.

merocrine [MERO-[1] + Gk *krin(ein)* to separate, put apart] Denoting or characterized by secretion that involves the discharge of the secretory product from an intact cell. Compare HOLOCRINE.

merocyte [MERO-[1] + -CYTE] An incompletely isolated cell found in the vicinity of the yolk of a fertilized ovum during segmentation. Its nucleus is generally derived from accessory spermatozoa. Ova with abundant yolk often manifest this phenomenon (physiologic polyspermy).

merodiastolic Pertaining to a part of diastole.

meroencephaly [MERO-[1] + ENCEPHAL- + -Y] The developmental absence of a part of the brain, such as the cerebellum or the corpus callosum.

meroergasia NEUROSIS.

merogastrula [MERO-[1] + GASTRULA] A gastrula that develops from a meroblastic ovum.

merogenesis [MERO-[1] + GENESIS] CLEAVAGE.

merogenetic Relating to or characterized by merogenesis or cleavage. Also *merogenic*.

merogenic MEROGENETIC.

merogonic Resulting from or pertaining to merogony.

merogony [MERO-[1] + -GONY] **1** The development of only a portion of an egg. If the egg contains only the male pronucleus, the development is termed andromerogony, and if only the female pronucleus, gynomerogony. **2** SCHIZOGONY.

  diploid merogony Development of a portion of an egg containing the combined products of the male and female pronuclei.

merology [MERO-[1] + -OLOGY] The study of the rudimentary tissues.

meromelia [MERO-[1] + MEL-[1] + -IA] The developmental absence of a part of one or more limbs. Also called *limb reduction defect*. See also HEMIMELIA, PEROMELIA, MICROMELIA, ECTRODACTYLY, AMELIA.

meromicrosomia [MERO-[1] + MICRO- + *som(ato)-* + -IA] The developmental smallness of a part of the body. ● The term is used in reference to a part not readily described by the prefix *micro*, as with specific organs or regions.

meromorphosis [MERO-[1] + MORPH- + -OSIS] The partial regeneration of a lost part.

meromyarial Designating a type of nematode musculature in which there are only a few platymyarial muscle bands in each quadrant below the cuticle and hypodermis and between the dorsal or ventral and a lateral chord. It is characteristic of smaller nematodes such as *Enterobius*. Compare POLYMYARIAL.

meromyosin [MERO-[1] + MYOSIN] One of two proteins, heavy meromyosin and light meromyosin, formed by enzymatic digestion of myosin. The region of myosin susceptible to the proteolysis lies near the "head" of the molecule, i.e. the region that protrudes from the fibril and interacts with actin. Heavy meromyosin molecules contain these heads and have the ability to interact with actin and to hydrolyze ATP. Light meromyosin molecules interact with each other to form fibrils. The separation of these substances and the characterization of their properties led to increased understanding of the mechanism of muscular contraction.

meront [*mer(o)*[1] + Gk *ont(os)*, gen. of *ōn*, pres. part. of *eimi* to be] A schizont that produces merozoites.

meroparesthesia [MERO-[2] + PARESTHESIA] Paresthesia involving the thighs and legs.

meropelagic [MERO-[1] + PELAGIC] Pertaining to the pelagic larval stages of certain benthic marine organisms that are only temporary members of the plankton community.

meropia [MERO-[1] + -OPIA] Loss of sight in one or more meridians of the visual field.

meroplankton [MERO-[1] + PLANKTON] Organisms in marine coastal areas that spend only part of their life cycle as plankton, being at other times benthic dwellers.

merorachischisis [MERO-[1] + RACHISCHISIS] Rachischisis limited to a short segment of the spinal cord. Also called *mesorachischisis, mesorrhachischisis, mesorrhaschisis, rachischisis partialis*. Also *merorrhachischisis*.

merorrhachischisis MERORACHISCHISIS.

meros [Gk *mēros* upper part of the thigh, the ham] **1** The femur. **2** The thigh.

merosmia [*mer(o)-*[1] + *osm(o)-*[2] + -IA] A disturbance of olfaction in which the patient claims to be able to smell some odors but not others.

merosome [MERO-[1] + Gk *sōm(a)* body] SOMITE.

merostotic Relating to the femur.

merotomy [MERO-[1] + -TOMY] Dissection into parts, particularly the dissection of a cell, in order to study the capacity for growth and development of the separate parts.

merozoite [MERO-[1] + *zo(o)*- + -ITE] A motile form of a sporozoan that results from the asexual division of the schizont during schizogony. In the life cycle of the malarial plasmodium in man, the merozoite is released into the blood from the exoerythrocytic stage in the liver or from the erythrocytic stages in infected red cells, from which it invades new erythrocytes. Also called *endoxocyte* (obsolete), *enhemospore* (obsolete), *enhematospore* (obsolete), *schizozoite, zoite*.

merozygote A bacterium that is diploid for a portion of its genome through transduction, F-duction, or some other process that introduces exogenous DNA. Processes that introduce a DNA fragment rather than a replicon (conjugation, transformation) yield a transient merozygote.

merphalan A racemic mixture of melphalan and medphalan. It is used as an antineoplastic drug.

Merphenyl A proprietary name for basic phenylmercuric nitrate.

Merritt [Katharine Krom *Merritt*, U.S. pediatrician, born 1886] Kasabach-Merritt syndrome. See under SYNDROME.

mersalyl acid A mixture of *o*-carboxymethylsalicyl-(3-hydroxymercuric-2-methoxypropyl)-amide and its anhydride. It is used for the same indications as mersalyl sodium.

mersalyl sodium $C_{13}H_{16}HgNNaO_6$. [3-[[2-Carboxymethoxy)-benzoyl]amino]-2-methoxy-propyl]hydroxymercury monosodium salt. A diuretic used in combination with theophylline in the treatment of edema secondary to such conditions as cardiorenal disease, nephrosis, and hepatic cirrhosis. It is given intramuscularly or intravenously. Also called *mercuramide*.

mersalyl sodium and theophylline Mersalyl sodium mixed with theophylline for administration together to lessen the degree of decomposition of the former.

Merthiolate A proprietary name for thimerosal.

Merulius An obsolete term for SERPULA.

merutu MAMPIRRA.

Merzbacher [Ludwig *Merzbacher*, German neurologist active in Argentina, born 1875] Merzbacher-Pelizaeus disease, Pelizaeus-Merzbacher sclerosis, Pelizaeus-Merzbacher type diffuse sclerosis. See under PELIZAEUS-MERZBACHER DISEASE.

mes- MESO-.

mesaconic acid HOOC—CH=C(CH₃)—COOH. One of the acids that is formed by fungi, or, by the action of heat and then alkali, from citric acid. It is the *trans* isomer of the formula shown, the *cis* isomer being citraconic acid.

mesad MESIAD.

mesal MESIAL.

mesangial Pertaining to the mesangium.

mesangiolysis Degeneration of mesangial cells and matrix secondary to radiation and some snake toxins.

mesangium The framework of the glomerulus, which arises from the vascular pole and extends into the intercapillary spaces, forming lobule centers. The mesangium contains matrix and mesangial cells in communication with the capillary lumen. The mesangial cells are phagocytic, while large molecules and aggregates may accumulate in the matrix. Adjective: mesangial.

Mesantoin A preparation of mephenytoin. A proprietary name.

mesaortitis MESOAORTITIS.

mesaraic An outmoded term for MESENTERIC.

mesarteritis Inflammation localized to the media, or muscular layer, of an artery.

    Mönckeberg's mesarteritis MÖNCKEBERG SCLEROSIS.

mesaticephalic MESOCEPHALIC.

mesatikerkic [Gk *mesat(os)* midmost + *i* + *kerk(is)* radius of the forearm + -IC] Having a radiohumeral index in the range 75–80.

mesatipellic MESATIPELVIC.

mesatipelvic [Gk *mesat(os)* midmost + *i* + PELVIC] Having a transverse pelvic diameter equal to that of the true conjugate diameter. Also *mesatipellic*.

mesaxon The contact interface between pairs of parallel membranes formed by the concentric growth of the Schwann cell enfolding an axon.

    internal mesaxon The innermost portion of the mesaxon which is adjacent to the axon itself. Also called *inaxon*.

mescal **1** PEYOTE. **2** A liquor distilled from the fermented sap of *Agave* species.

mescaline 3,4,5-Trimethoxyphenethylamine. It is a hallucinogenic alkaloid found in the peyote cactus (mescal button).

mesectoblast [MES- + ECTOBLAST] ECTOMESOBLAST.

mesectoderm [MES- + ECTODERM] The part of the middle layer of the embryo arising from the ectoderm through the intermediary of the neural plate, or more specifically, directly from the neural crest. It is sometimes contrasted with mesentoderm and with mesentoblast, but it is more properly distinguished from true mesoderm. Also called *mesohypoblast*.

mesembrine $C_{17}H_{23}NO_3$. A tropane-like alkaloid presumed to be the hallucinogenic compound of *Mesembryanthemum expansum* of the plant family Aizoaceae.

mesencephal MESENCEPHALON.

mesencephalic Pertaining to the mesencephalon.

mesencephalitis [MES- + ENCEPHALITIS] Encephalitis affecting the midbrain especially severely.

mesencephalohypophysial Pertaining to the mesencephalon and the hypophysis cerebri, or pituitary gland.

mesencephalon [MES- + New L *encephalon* the brain, irreg.

from Gk *enkephalos* the brain] **1** That portion of the brainstem that lies between the pons and the diencephalon in the fully developed brain. **2** The middle of the three expansions which develop in the early embryo at the front of the primitive neural tube. These expansions are called the primitive brain vesicles. It gives rise to the colliculi, the tegmentum, and the crura cerebri. Also called *midbrain vesicle*. For defs. 1 and 2 also called *midbrain, mesocephalon, mesencephale.*

mesencephalotomy [*mesencephalo(n)* + -TOMY]   An incision into the mesencephalon, such as division of pain tracts for the relief of intractable pain.

mesenchyma   MESENCHYME.

mesenchyme [MES- + Gk *enchyma* infusion, juice, from EN- + Gk *chymos* juice, from *cheein* to pour, spill]   Primitive embryonic connective or packing tissue originating from mesoderm and developing into the supporting tissues. It consists of widely separated stellate cells surrounded by ground substance and some reticular fibers. Also called *mesenchyma, embryonal connective tissue, mesenchymal tissue, desmohemoblast.* Adjective: mesenchymal, mesenchymatous.

interzonal mesenchyme   A plate of homogenous mesenchymatous tissue which separates the centers of chondrification at the joints formed from the fifth week of human embryonic development. In the synovial joints, this zone includes three regions: two chondrogenic layers, each in continuity with the perichondrium of the future skeletal elements, and an intermediate avascular layer continuous at the periphery with the synovial mesenchyme. It is within this intermediate layer that a cleft will appear to become the future joint cavity.

primary mesenchyme   Mesenchyme appearing at an early stage between the trophoblast on one side, and the amnion and the yolk sac on the other, while the embryo is still two-layered. Its origin is still not certain.

secondary mesenchyme   Intraembryonic mesenchyme essentially derived from dissociation of the mesoblast.

mesenchymoma [MESENCHYME + -OMA]   A rare, benign or malignant tumor consisting of two or more clearly identifiable mesenchymal elements in addition to fibrous tissue. The mixed mesodermal tumors of the genitourinary tract are not included in this group.

benign mesenchymoma   A mesenchymoma whose component tissues are mature and without evidence of aggressive growth.

malignant mesenchymoma   A mesenchymoma one or more of whose component tissues shows malignant characteristics. This may appear as a fibrosarcoma, liposarcoma, leiomyosarcoma, osteosarcoma, etc. Also called *mixed cell sarcoma, polymorphous sarcoma.*

mesenterectomy [*mesenter(y)* + -ECTOMY]   The surgical removal of part or all of a mesenteric attachment.

mesenteric   Pertaining to mesentery. Also *mesaraic* (outmoded).

mesentericomesocolic   Relating to the mesentery and mesocolon.

mesenteriolum [dim. of MESENTERIUM. See MESENTERIUM.]   A mesentery of small size.

mesenteriolum appendicis vermiformis   An outmoded term for MESOAPPENDIX.

mesenteriolum processus vermiformis   An outmoded term for MESOAPPENDIX.

mesenteriopexy   A surgical procedure in which a torn or ptotic redundant mesentery is resuspended and repaired. Also called *mesopexy.*

mesenteriorrhaphy   A surgical procedure in which sutures are used to repair or resuspend a damaged or redundant mesentery.

Also called *mesorrhaphy, mesentorrhaphy.*

mesenteriplication   A surgical procedure in which a redundant mesentery is shortened by folding it upon itself and then suturing the folds into place.

mesenteritis   Mesenteric inflammation. Adjective: mesenteritic.

retractile mesenteritis   A chronic inflammation of the mesentery resulting in progressive fibrosis and nodular thickening with retraction and distortion of the intestinal loops. A condition of uncertain etiology, it is believed to be similar to and related to retroperitoneal fibrosis.

mesenterium [New L (from Gk *mesenterion* or *mesenteron* mesentery, from MES- + Gk *enteron* a piece of gut, pl. *entera* the intestines), mesentery]   **1** A fold of peritoneum that encloses an abdominal viscus while anchoring it to the abdominal wall, and that carries between its two layers blood vessels, lymphatics, and nerves to and from the viscus.   **2** [NA] The extensive peritoneal fold attaching the jejunum and ileum to the posterior abdominal wall and extending obliquely from the duodenojejunal junction to the ileocecal junction. For defs. 1 and 2 also called *mesentery, mesostenium* (outmoded).

mesenterium commune   COMMON DORSAL MESENTERY.

mesenterium dorsale commune   COMMON DORSAL MESENTERY.

mesenteron [MES- + Gk *enteron* a piece of gut]   MIDGUT.

mesentery [New L *mesenterium.* See MESENTERIUM.]   MESENTERIUM.

mesentery of ascending part of colon   MESOCOLON ASCENDENS.

caval mesentery   A fold of dorsal body wall tissue, just to the right of the main dorsal mesentery, bridging the cephalic pole of the right mesonephros and the liver. Vessels in this fold differentiate to form the infrahepatic segment of the interior vena cava. Also called *caval fold.*

common mesentery   COMMON DORSAL MESENTERY.

common dorsal mesentery   A double-layered partition of visceral splanchnic mesoderm which divides the embryonic coelom into halves, suspends the primitive digestive tube from the posterior body wall, and carries the blood supply to the tube. The covering coelomic epithelium is continuous with the parietal splanchnic mesoderm, and together they will form the future peritoneum, its folds, ligaments, and mesenteries. Initially, there is also a ventral mesentery related to the gastroduodenal portion of the tube from which the lesser omentum is derived. The common dorsal mesentery, at first called the primitive mesentery, applies to all of the embryonic dorsal mesentery. It stretches the entire length of the primitive digestive tube and takes part in the complex development of the latter. Also called *common mesentery, dorsal mesentery, mesenterium commune, mesenterium dorsale commune, lamina mesenterii propria* (outmoded), *proper lamina of mesentery* (outmoded). See also PERSISTENT COMMON MESENTERY.

mesentery of descending part of colon   MESOCOLON DESCENDENS.

dorsal mesentery   COMMON DORSAL MESENTERY.

persistent common mesentery   A condition in which the embryonic dorsal mesentery or parts thereof retain the primitive attachments between the mid-dorsal body wall and the gastrointestinal tract. During normal embryogenesis the dorsal mesentery is either lost by fusion with the body wall or by repositioning, as the various segments of the gastrointestinal tract undergo rotation while the midgut is withdrawn from the umbilical stalk. In malrotation or incomplete rotation of the tract the mesentery retains some of its embryonic relationships.

primitive mesentery   Double-layered embryonic membrane formed by the union of the two opposing splanchnopleuric layers when the abdominal wall closes off and the peritoneal cavity develops. It has dorsal and ventral parts in relation to the gut which it encloses. The dorsal part of the primitive mesentery will become the common dorsal mesentery.

mesentery of rectum   MESORECTUM.

mesentery of sigmoid colon   MESOCOLON SIGMOIDEUM.

mesentery of transverse part of colon   MESOCOLON TRANS-VERSUM.

ventral mesentery   A fold of peritoneum which extends from the ventral wall of the foregut toward the diaphragm and anterior abdominal wall as far down as the umbilicus. It is probably derived from the septum transversum and it contributes to the definitive lesser omentum and the falciform ligament.

mesentery of vermiform appendix   MESOAPPENDIX.

mesentoderm [MES- + ENTODERM]   True mesoderm as opposed to mesectoderm. An imprecise usage.

mesentorrhaphy   MESENTERIORRHAPHY.

mesepithelium   MESOTHELIUM.

mesh   One of the spaces in a screen or sieve, or the intersecting wires which form such spaces.

suspending mesh   In dentistry, a retaining mesh attached to the intraosseous magnet of a magnetic implant.

tanner mesh   A skin graft that has been expanded by mesh grafting with the Tanner Vanderput Dermatome.

meshwork   NETWORK.

trabecular meshwork   RETICULUM TRABECULARE SCLERAE.

mesiad   Directed or proceeding toward the median sagittal plane of the body or, specifically, following the dental arch toward the center line. Also *mesad*.

mesial [MESI(O)- + -AL]   Nearer or nearest the midline in the dental arch: used especially of the surface of a tooth. Also *mesal*. Compare DISTAL.

mesic [MES- + -IC]   Characterized by or pertaining to temperate environmental conditions, especially those including moderate moisture.

mesio- [Gk *mesos* (adjective) middle, in the middle, between] A combining form meaning mesial.

mesioclusion [MESIO- + *oc(c)lusion*]   MANDIBULAR PROGNATHISM.

mesiodens [MESIO- + L *dens* tooth]   A centrally placed upper supernumerary tooth.

mesiodentes   Plural of MESIODENS.

mesiodistal [MESIO- + DISTAL]   Relating to the line joining the midpoints of the mesial and distal surfaces of a tooth.

mesiogression [MESIO- + L *gress(us)* (past part. of *gradi* to step) a step + *-io* -ION]   The condition of having the teeth forward of the normal position in the arch.

mesion   MEDIAN PLANE.

mesio-occlusal [MESIO- + OCCLUSAL]   Relating to both the mesial and occlusal surfaces of a tooth: said of cavities and restorations involving these surfaces. Abbreviation: MO

mesio-occlusion   MANDIBULAR PROGNATHISM.

mesio-occlusodistal [MESIO- + OCCLUSODISTAL]   Relating to all the mesial, occlusal, and distal surfaces of a tooth: said of cavities and restorations involving these surfaces. Abbreviation: MOD

mesioplacement [MESIO- + *placement*]   MESIOVERSION.

mesioversion [MESIO- + VERSION]   **1** A position of a tooth nearer the median line than normal. **2** A more than normally anterior position of a jaw. Also called *mesial displacement, mesioplacement*.

mesiris   STROMA IRIDIS.

mesitylene   1,3,5-Trimethylbenzene. It can be formed by the condensation of acetone.

mesitylenic acid   3,5-Dimethylbenzoic acid. It can be prepared by the oxidation of mesitylene.

mesityl oxide $(CH_3)_2C{=}CH{-}CO{-}CH_3$. A condensation product of acetone.

mesmerism [after Franz Friedrich Anton *Mesmer*, Austrian physician, 1734–1815 + -ISM]   HYPNOTISM.

meso- [Gk *mesos* (adjective) middle, in the middle, between]   **1** A prefix meaning intermediate or connective, or denoting a means of attachment to a designated organ. Also *mes-*. **2** In stereochemistry, a prefix denoting an isomer of dissymmetric compounds that possesses dissymmetric carbon atoms but is not itself dissymmetric because of internal compensation. **3** In chemistry, a prefix denoting substitution of a bridging atom.

mesoaortitis   Inflammation localized to the middle, or muscular, layer of the aorta. Also called *mesaortitis*.

mesoaortitis syphilitica   Inflammation of the media of the ascending aorta due to syphilitic infection. It is a chronic process characterized by loss of elastic fibers and their replacement by fibrous scars that cause the aorta to dilate and even rupture.

mesoappendicitis   Inflammation of the mesoappendix.

mesoappendix   [NA]   A triangular fold of peritoneum around the vermiform appendix, one side being attached for varying distances along the appendix and the other side attaching the latter to the posterior surface of the mesentery of the ileum. The artery to the appendix runs along the free margin of the fold. Also called *mesentery of vermiform appendix, mesenteriolum processus vermiformis* (outmoded), *mesenteriolum appendicis vermiformis* (outmoded).

mesoarial   Pertaining to the mesovarium. An outmoded term.

mesoarium   An outmoded term for MESOVARIUM.

mesobiota [MESO- + BIOTA]   Small soil organisms, including such animals as mites, nematodes, and springtails, present in a biotic community that typically does not include plant species.

mesoblast [MESO- + -BLAST]   MESODERM.

mesoblastema [MESO- + BLASTEMA]   All the cells comprised in the mesoderm. Adjective: Mesoblastemic.

mesobranchial [MESO- + BRANCHIAL]   Pertaining to the medial aspect of the branchial arches.

mesocardia [MESO- + -CARDIA]   Displacement of the heart so that the apex is in the midline.

mesocardiac   Pertaining to or characterized by mesocardia.

mesocardium [New L, from MESO- + Gk *kardia* the heart]   A double-layered dorsal or posterior serous membrane which suspends the embryonic heart tube from the dorsal wall of the pericardial cavity. It fenestrates very soon, leaving a gap (the transverse pericardial sinus). There is also a ventral or anterior mesocardium but it disappears immediately after its appearance. Also called *dorsal mesocardium*.

arterial mesocardium   The tube of visceral pericardium reflected along the pulmonary trunk and the ascending aorta. An outmoded term.

dorsal mesocardium   MESOCARDIUM.

lateral mesocardium   PULMONARY RIDGE.

venous mesocardium   The serous pericardium reflected over the roots of the pulmonary veins and of the venae cavae. An outmoded term.

mesocarpal   MIDCARPAL.

mesocecal   Relating to the mesocecum.

mesocecum   The mesentery of the cecum, which is seldom present.

mesocephalic   Having head proportions intermediate between dolichocephalic and brachycephalic, with a cephalic index between 76 and 80.9. Also *mesaticephalic, mesocranic, normocephalic*.

mesocephalon MESENCEPHALON.

mesocephaly [MESO- + CEPHAL- + -Y] Intermediate length-breadth proportions of the head, with a cephalic index between 76 and 80.9.

Mesocestoides A large genus of cyclophyllidean tapeworms (family Mesocestoididae) characterized by a ventrally located genital aperture. The adults are found in the intestines of carnivores, including cats, dogs, and raccoons, and in meat-eating birds and humans. Larvae, known as tetrathyridia, occur in the peritoneum or coelom of snakes, mice, dogs, cats, and other vertebrates. A first intermediate host, not yet identified, is probably required for infection of the vertebrate intermediate host. See also TETRATHYRIDIUM.

Mesocestoides variabilis A North American species found in dogs, cats, and wild carnivores. The adult worm inhabits the small intestine and is up to 150 cm long. It was once reported in a child.

Mesocestoididae [MESO- + L *cest(us)* a girdle, strap + -OID + -IDAE] A family of tapeworms (order Cyclophyllidea, subclass Cestoda) found in carnivorous birds and mammals.

mesochondrium The cartilaginous tissue matrix, which is composed of mucopolysaccharides such as chondroitin sulfate. Depending on the type of cartilage, various fibers may be laid down within the matrix.

mesochord MESOCORD.

mesochoroidea An outmoded term for LAMINA CHOROIDO-CAPILLARIS.

mesocoelia An obsolete term for AQUEDUCTUS CEREBRI.

mesocolic Of or relating to the mesocolon.

mesocolon [MESO- + COLON] [NA] The peritoneal fold attaching the various parts of the colon to the posterior abdominal wall. Only the transverse colon and the sigmoid colon usually have actual mesenteries connecting them to the abdominal wall.

mesocolon ascendens [NA] The short peritoneal fold that, in about one in four adults, surrounds the ascending colon and attaches it to the posterior abdominal wall. Usually the ascending colon is covered by peritoneum only anteriorly and on the sides. Also called *mesentery of ascending part of colon, ascending mesocolon, right mesocolon* (outmoded).

ascending mesocolon MESOCOLON ASCENDENS.

mesocolon descendens The short peritoneal fold that, in approximately one in three adults, surrounds the descending colon and attaches it to the posterior abdominal wall. Usually the descending colon is covered by peritoneum only anteriorly and on the sides. Also called *mesentery of descending part of colon, descending mesocolon, left mesocolon* (outmoded).

descending mesocolon MESOCOLON DESCENDENS.

iliac mesocolon An outmoded term for MESOCOLON SIGMOIDEUM.

left mesocolon An outmoded term for MESOCOLON DESCENDENS.

pelvic mesocolon MESOCOLON SIGMOIDEUM.

right mesocolon An outmoded term for MESOCOLON ASCENDENS.

sigmoid mesocolon MESOCOLON SIGMOIDEUM.

mesocolon sigmoideum [NA] A peritoneal fold securing the sigmoid colon to the pelvic wall in the shape of an inverted V. The apex is near the bifurcation of the left common iliac vessels, the left limb passes medial to the left psoas major muscle, and the right limb descends to the left of the midline to end at the middle of the third sacral vertebra. Also called *pelvic mesocolon, iliac mesocolon* (outmoded), *mesentery of sigmoid colon, mesosigmoid* (outmoded), *sigmoid mesocolon.*

transverse mesocolon MESOCOLON TRANSVERSUM.

mesocolon transversum [NA] A broad peritoneal fold that connects the transverse colon to the structures on the posterior abdominal wall, especially the head of pancreas and the anterior border of the body of the pancreas. Within the two layers are the middle colic artery and vein, nerves, and lymphatics. The upper layer is adherent to the greater omentum, while the lower passes down over the pancreas to the front of the third and fourth parts of the duodenum. Also called *transverse mesocolon, mesentery of transverse part of colon.*

mesocolopexy A surgical procedure in which the mesocolon is fixed or resuspended to prevent ptosis or torsion of the transverse colon.

mesocoloplication A surgical procedure in which the mesocolon is folded back on itself and then sutured into place in order to control the mobility of the transverse colon.

mesocord [MESO- + CORD] An umbilical cord, a segment of which is bound to the placenta by an accessory fold. Also *mesochord.*

mesocornea An outmoded term for SUBSTANTIA PROPRIA CORNEAE.

mesocortex [MESO- + CORTEX] **1** The cerebral cortex of the cingulate and retrospenial gyri that does not pass through a six-layered developmental stage, but approximates the appearance of isocortex in the adult. **2** GYRUS CINGULI.

mesocranic MESOCEPHALIC.

mesocranium VERTEX.

Mesocricetus [MESO- + New L *cricetus* (of Slavic origin) hamster] A monotypic genus of the rodent family Cricetidae; the golden hamsters. They are found in the wild in southeastern Europe and southwestern Asia. Golden hamsters have become widely domesticated as house pets and used frequently for laboratory research. It appears that all domesticated strains can be traced to a single female and 12 young which were imported into Israel from Syria in 1930.

mesocuneiform OS CUNEIFORME INTERMEDIUM.

mesocyst A rare peritoneal fold that suspends the gallbladder from its fossa on the liver. Usually only its posteroinferior surface and sides are covered by peritoneum.

mesocytoma [MESO- + CYTOMA] A tumor of connective tissue. An outmoded term.

mesoderm [MESO- + -DERM] One of the three primary germ layers, formed between the ectoderm (outermost layer) and endoderm (innermost layer) of the embryo. From this layer are derived the majority of the skeletal system, the circulatory system, the musculature, the excretory system and most of the reproductive system of vertebrates. Also called *mesoblast.*

axial mesoderm PARAXIAL MESODERM.

enterocoelic mesoderm Embryonic mesoderm formed as an outpouching of the archenteron. The mesoderm subsequently obliterates the blastocoel and lines a new cavity, the coelom. It occurs in Chaetognatha, Brachiopoda, Echinodermata, Hemichordata, and Chordata.

extraembryonic mesoderm The mesoderm that develops outside the embryo and separates the primary yolk sac from the trophoblast. In human embryos, it appears to be derived from trophoblast. It increases in amount and forms the loose magma reticulare. Also called *primary mesoderm.*

gastral mesoderm In comparative embryology, true mesoderm, the part of the middle germ layer differentiating at the end of gastrulation or a homologous process. In lower vertebrates it is invaginated during gastrulation and subsequently constricted from the roof of the archenteron or yolk sac.

head mesoderm Mesoderm situated cranially to the somites.

intermediate mesoderm A continuous longitudinal tract of mesoderm in the embryo, lying between the paraxial and the lateral plate mesoderm from which the nephrogenic cord will develop. Also called *intermediate cell mass, mesomere.*

intraembryonic mesoderm Mesoderm formed within the boundaries of the early embryo almost entirely from the primitive streak.

lateral mesoderm LATERAL PLATE MESODERM.

lateral plate mesoderm That part of the intraembryonic, or secondary, mesoderm which develops lateral to the paraxial mesoderm of the embryo. It is continuous with the extraembryonic, or primary, mesoderm beyond the margins of the embryonic disk. Also called *lateral mesoderm*.

paraxial mesoderm The part of the mesoblast forming a thickened mass of tissue at the level of the head region of the embryo in the immediate neighborhood of and at each side of the neural groove. Also called *axial mesoderm*.

peristomal mesoderm Mesoderm that develops from the ventral aspect of the blastoporal lips.

primary mesoderm EXTRAEMBRYONIC MESODERM.

prochordal mesoderm The part of the mesoderm derived from division of the cells of the prochordal plate. It plays an inductive role in causing formation of various structures anteriorly in the head and gives rise, probably conjointly with ectomesenchyme, to several facial skeletal elements.

prospective head mesoderm PRECHORDAL PLATE.

prostomial mesoderm Mesoderm that arises in lower vertebrates by continued proliferation from the lateral lips of the blastopore.

schizocoelic mesoderm Embryonic mesoderm formed as solid masses of cells budding from a posterior body region. Body cavities then form by a cleavage within the masses of mesoderm. It occurs in mollusks and annelid worms.

secondary mesoderm Mesoderm formed from the primitive streak of the embryonic disk which spreads laterally and forward between the ectoderm and underlying endoderm. Secondary mesoderm for the head region is contributed from the prochordal plate and, at least in lower vertebrates, from the cranial end of the neural crest. This type of mesoderm gives rise to connective and supporting tissue, muscle, blood, and lymphatic tissues, part of the urogenital system, and the mesothelium lining the serous cavities.

somatic mesoderm The outer layer formed as a result of the splitting of the lateral plate mesoderm when the intraembryonic coelom is formed. Together with the overlying ectoderm, it becomes the somatopleure.

splanchnic mesoderm The inner layer formed as a result of the splitting of the lateral plate mesoderm when the intraembryonic coelom appears. Together with the underlying endoderm, it becomes the splanchnopleure. Also called *visceral plate*.

mesodiastole [MESO- + DIASTOLE] A period in the middle of diastole.

mesodiastolic In the middle of cardiac diastole; pertaining to mesodiastole.

mesodont [MES- + -ODONT] Having medium-sized teeth.

mesodontia [MES- + -ODONTIA] The condition of having medium-sized teeth.

mesodontic Having medium-sized teeth, with a dental index between 42 and 44.

mesoduodenal Relating to the mesoduodenum.

mesoduodenitis Inflammation of the mesentery of the duodenum.

mesoduodenum [MESO- + DUODENUM] A part of the primitive midline dorsal mesentery in relation to the embryonic duodenum. After the rotation of the gut and the development of the pancreas between the two layers of the mesoduodenum, the latter becomes adherent on its posterior surface to the primitive posterior parietal peritoneum. Later, both layers are absorbed, and so the duodenum becomes retroperitoneal. The suspensory muscle (of Treitz) and its fascia develop in this region, and

extend from the right crus of the diaphragm retroperitoneally to the terminal part of the duodenum.

mesoepididymis An occasional fold of tunica vaginalis that connects the testis to the epididymis.

mesoesophagus [MESO- + ESOPHAGUS] That part of the primitive dorsal mesentery attached to the esophagus. It persists in the adult only at the lower end near its junction with the stomach below the diaphragm.

mesofauna The organism size category between microfauna and macrofauna that includes such ground-dwelling animals as mites, some insects and their larvae, and springtails.

mesogaster [MESO- + -GASTER] MESOGASTRIUM.

mesogastric Relating to the mesogastrium.

mesogastrium [MESO- + -GASTER + -ium, New L noun suffix] That part of the primitive dorsal mesentery which is related to the developing stomach in an embryo and which becomes the greater omentum. Also called *mesogaster*.

dorsal mesogastrium The part of the primitive, midline dorsal mesentery which connects the embryonic stomach to the posterior abdominal wall. It is concerned with development of a large sacculation, the omental bursa, or lesser sac of peritoneum, and finally forms the greater omentum. The body of the pancreas and the spleen develop in its thickened portions.

ventral mesogastrium The primitive midline mesentery which in the embryo connects the stomach and the superior part of the loop of the duodenum to the anterior abdominal wall as far as the umbilicus. The liver develops between the two layers of this mesentery and the ligamentum teres. The falciform ligament and the lesser omentum of the adult are derived from it.

mesoglea [MESO- + Gk *gloia* glue] The layer of cells between the epidermis and the gastrodermis of cnidarians.

mesoglia [MESO- + *(neuro)glia*] Nonastrocytic neuroglia, i.e., oligodendroglia and microglia. A seldom used term.

mesoglioma [MESO- + GLIOMA] An outmoded term for OLIGODENDROGLIOMA.

mesogluteal Of or relating to the gluteus medius muscle.

mesogluteus An outmoded term for MUSCULUS GLUTEUS MEDIUS.

mesognathic Having an average jaws-to-head relationship or a gnathic index of between 98 and 103. Also *mesognathous*.

mesognathion The lateral segment of the os incisivum, or premaxilla, bearing the lateral incisor. It is located lateral to the medial segment, or endognathion, and considered to derive from a separate center of ossification.

mesognathous MESOGNATHIC.

Mesogonimus A former genus that included a polyphyletic group of trematodes now transferred to the genera *Heterophyes* and *Paragonimus*.

Mesogonimus heterophyes *HETEROPHYES HETEROPHYES*.

mesohyloma [MESO- + HYLOMA] A tumor of mesoderm. An outmoded term.

mesohypoblast [MESO- + HYPO- + -BLAST] MESECTODERM.

mesoileum That portion of the mesentery that attaches the ileum to the posterior abdominal wall.

mesojejunum That portion of the mesentery attaching the jejunum to the posterior abdominal wall.

mesokurtic [MESO- + Gk *kyrt(os)* curved, convex + -IC] Of or relating to a normal distribution of data.

mesolecithal [MESO- + LECITH- + -AL] MEDIALECITHAL.

mesolepidoma [MESO- + LEPIDOMA] **1** A tumor of mesoderm. **2** A tumor of mesothelium. An outmoded term.

mesolobus An outmoded term for CORPUS CALLOSUM.

mesolymphocyte A lymphocyte of intermediate size, in contrast to a small lymphocyte and a large lymphocyte. A seldom used term.

mesomelia **1** The relative shortening of the middle segment of the limbs. **2** MESOMELIC DWARFISM.

mesomelic Pertaining to the midportion of the upper or lower limb.

mesomere [MESO- + -MERE] **1** A blastomere of a size intermediate between a macromere and a micromere. **2** INTERMEDIATE MESODERM. **3** SOMITE.

mesomeric Pertaining to or exhibiting mesomerism.

mesomerism [MESO- + -mer(e) + -ISM] An obsolete term for RESONANCE.

mesometritis [mesometr(ium) + -ITIS] Inflammation of the mesometrium.

mesometrium **1** [NA] The portion of the broad ligament below the mesovarium. **2** An outmoded term for TUNICA MUSCULARIS UTERI.

mesomorph [MESO- + -MORPH] An individual with the characteristics of mesomorphy. Also called *mediotype, midrange somatotype* (seldom used).

mesomorphic Characterized by mesomorphy.

mesomorphy [MESOMORPH + -Y] A type of human body conformation with characteristics between those of the ectomorph and the endomorph. In contrast to these the physique is usually muscular and well proportioned. Compare ENDOMORPHY, ECTOMORPHY.

mesomula An early embryonic stage when there is only ectoderm and endoderm with a mass of mesoderm in between.

meson [MES- + -on, suffix denoting an elementary particle] Any of several kinds of short-lived elementary particles belonging to the class that takes part in the strong nuclear interaction, and having intrinsic angular momentum (spin) equal to the integral multiple of Planck's constant divided by 2π. They may be positively or negatively charged or neutral. Their masses range from about 275 times the mass of the electron to as much as about 10 times the mass of the proton. Also called *mesotron, barytron* (outmoded).

mesonasal Located in or pertaining to the middle of the nose.

mesonephroi Plural of MESONEPHROS.

mesonephroid Resembling the mesonephros.

mesonephroma [MESO- + NEPHR- + -OMA] WOLFFIAN DUCT CARCINOMA.

  benign mesonephroma WOLFFIAN ADENOMA.

mesonephron [MESO- + NEPHRON] A unit of the mesonephros. Also called *deutonephron* (obsolete).

mesonephros [MESO- + Gk *nephros* a kidney] The part of renal tissue situated between the pronephros anteriorly and the metanephros posteriorly. It appears just after the first month of embryonic development. It consists of a series of nephrotomes communicating through nephric tubules with the wolffian duct. In mammals the mesonephros is functional for part of the fetal period but eventually it involutes, leaving some vestigial remnants. In the male these remnants include the efferent ductules of the testis while in the female they form tubules of the epoophoron. Also called *wolffian body, corpus Wolffi, Oken's body, corpus of Oken, middle kidney.*

  caudal mesonephros The caudal part of the mesonephros, which forms the tubules of the paroophoron.

  cranial mesonephros A part of the mesonephros anterior of the gonad. It atrophies as development advances.

  genital mesonephros That part of the mesonephros which gives rise to the ductuli efferentes and is opposite to the gonad.

mesopallium An obsolete term for PALEOPALLIUM.

mesopause [MESO- + PAUSE] The discontinuity in the earth's

upper atmosphere separating the mesosphere from the thermosphere.

mesopelagic Pertaining to the layer of ocean waters between the epipelagic and the bathypelagic, usually with reference to marine organisms that live in darkness at moderate ocean depths.

mesopexy MESENTERIOPEXY.

mesopharynx An outmoded term for PARS ORALIS PHARYNGIS.

mesophile [MESO- + -PHILE] An organism adapted to an intermediate temperature range. Compare THERMOPHILE, PSYCHROPHILE. Adjective: mesophilic.

mesophlebitis An inflammation localized to the media of a vein.

mesophryon **1** GLABELLA. **2** The midpoint of the glabella.

mesophyll [MESO- + Gk *phyll(on)* a leaf] The photosynthetic tissue, made up of parenchyma cells, located between the epidermal layers of a leaf.

mesophyte [MESO- + Gk *phyton* a plant, tree] A plant that grows in areas of moderate moisture. Adjective: mesophytic.

mesopia [MES- + -OPIA] Ability to see in the twilight range, between photopic and scotopic vision. Adjective: mesopic.

mesopic Pertaining to mesopia.

Mesopin A proprietary name for homatropine methylbromide.

mesopneumon The visceral pleura that covers the root of the lung proximally, anteriorly, and posteriorly where it becomes continuous with the mediastinal pleura. Also called *mesopneumonium.*

mesopneumonium MESOPNEUMON.

mesoporphyrin The porphyrin whose ring substituents are: methyl, ethyl, methyl, ethyl, methyl, 2-carboxyethyl, 2-carboxyethyl, methyl. It differs from the protoporphyrin that is found in hemoglobin by hydrogenation of the two vinyl groups to form ethyl groups.

mesoprosopic Having a face of medium width, the facial index being about 90.

mesopterygium [MESO- + *pteryg(o)-* + L *-ium*, neut. noun suffix] The middle of three cartilaginous rods which attaches to the paired fins of cartilaginous fishes, between the propterygium and the metapterygium.

mesopterygoid **1** Pertaining to a process of the pterygoid bone of the bird. **2** The mesopterygoid bone. **3** The space between the pterygoid bones of mammals.

mesopulmonon [MESO- + PULMON- + -on, arbitrary suffix] The root of the mesentery for each developing lung, derived from the dorsal thoracic mesentery or mediastinum, The tissue is drawn outwards as the lung grows and forms the visceral pleura.

mesorachischisis MERORACHISCHISIS.

mesorchium [MES- + *orch(i)-* + L *-ium*, neut. noun suffix] A thick fold of peritoneum which in the male embryo connects the developing testis to the mesonephric fold. It contains the testicular vessels and nerves and some undifferentiated mesenchyme. Also called *mesotestis.*

mesorectum The peritoneum that almost surrounds the upper portion of the rectum. The middle portion of the rectum has peritoneum on the front and sides, and the lower portion in front only. Also called *mesentery of rectum.* ● The term is a misnomer in that the rectum has no mesentery.

mesoretina The middle layer of the retina. An outmoded term.

mesoridazine $C_{21}H_{26}N_2OS_2$. 10-[2-(1-Methyl-2-piperidinyl)ethyl]-2-(methylsulfinyl)-10*H*-phenothiazine. A metabolite of thioridazine that has activity as an antipsychotic agent.

mesoropter [MES- + Gk *(h)or(os)* a measure, boundary + *op-*

tēr(ios) pertaining to sight] The normal, centrally aligned position of the eye. Also called *muscular mesoropter.*

muscular mesoropter   MESOROPTER.

mesorrhachischisis   MERORACHISCHISIS.

mesorrhaphy   MESENTERIORRHAPHY.

mesorrhaschisis   MERORACHISCHISIS.

mesorrhine [MESO- + Gk *rhis,* gen. *rhinos,* the nose] Having a nasal index between 48 and 53.

mesosalpinx   [NA] The portion of the broad ligament of the uterus that lies above the mesovarium and the ligament of the ovary, and extends to the free border. The uterine tube is located in it.

mesoscapula   An outmoded term for SPINA SCAPULAE.

mesoseme [MESO- + Gk *sēm(a)* a sign, mark] Having an orbital index in the range between 83 and 89.

mesosigmoid   An outmoded term for MESOCOLON SIGMOIDEUM.

mesosigmoiditis   Inflammation of the sigmoid mesocolon.

mesosigmoidopexy   A surgical procedure in which the mesocolon of the sigmoid colon is suspended from the abdominal wall in order to prevent sigmoid volvulus or rectal prolapse.

mesoskelic [MESO- + Gk *skel(os)* the leg + -IC] Having legs of medium length.

mesosoma   MESOSOMIA.

mesosomatous   Being of medium height.

mesosome [MESO- + Gk *sōm(a)* body] A convoluted membranous body formed by involution of the bacterial plasma membrane. It functions in cellular respiration and septum formation.

mesosomia [MESO- + Gk *sōm(a)* body + -IA] Medium stature. Also called *mesosoma.*

mesosphere [MESO- + SPHERE] The stratum of the earth's upper air that extends beyond the stratosphere to an altitude of about 85 km above the earth's surface. In this stratum, the temperature decreases as altitude increases.

mesostaphyline [MESO- + STAPHYL- + -INE] Having a palatal index in the middle range, between 84 and 84.9.

mesostenium   An outmoded term for MESENTERIUM.

mesosternal   Pertaining to the mesosternum.

mesosternale [MESO- + New L *stern(um)* (from Gk *sternon* the chest) breastbone + L -*ale,* neut. sing. of -*alis* -AL] An anthropometric point situated on the anterior surface of the chest in the midline at the level of the fourth sternochondral junction.

mesosternum   An outmoded term for CORPUS STERNI.

mesosthenic [MESO- + STHEN- + -IC] Moderately strong.

mesostomia [MESO- + STOM- + -IA] The condition of having an oral fissure of medium size.

mesostroma   Fine, fibrillar, reticular tissue in the embryo of a type resembling that from which the vitreous of the eye develops.

mesosyphilis   SECONDARY SYPHILIS.

mesosystolic   In the middle of cardiac systole; pertaining to the middle period of systole.

mesotarsal   MIDTARSAL.

mesotendineum   A threadlike band of vascular connective tissue covered by synovial membrane that extends between a tendon within its synovial sheath and an osseous groove or adjacent connective tissue structure. It is located at the point of invagination of a tendon into its sheath and is essentially the junction of the visceral and parietal layers. It is homologous to a mesentery and conveys blood vessels and nerve fibers, and it may be quite extensive. Specialized cordlike forms are called vincula tendinum. Also called *mesotendon, mesotenon.*

mesotendon   MESOTENDINEUM.

mesotenon   MESOTENDINEUM.

mesotestis [MESO- + TESTIS]   MESORCHIUM.

mesothelioma [MESO- + THELIOMA]   A benign or malignant tumor arising from the mesothelial lining of one of the coelomic cavities, usually the pleura or perineum, and consisting of epitheloid and spindle cell elements. It is usually subtyped by predominance as epithelioid, fibrous (spindle cell), or biphasic. Benign mesotheliomas are usually localized. Malignant mesotheliomas grow in a diffuse manner. Epithelioid tumors show tubular and/or papillary growth patterns. The fibrous type may resemble a fibroma or fibrosarcoma. Mesotheliomas associated with exposure to asbestos fibers are invariably malignant. Also called *celioma, celiothelioma, celothelioma.*

mesothelioma of meninges   MENINGIOMA.

pleural mesothelioma   A mesothelioma arising from the pleura. Localized forms are usually benign. Diffuse growth indicates malignancy but widespread metastases are not common. The tumor may encase the lung. Malignant mesotheliomas of the pleura are associated with exposure to asbestos.

mesothelium   1 Epithelial cells of mesodermal origin which come to line the serous cavities such as the peritoneal, pleural, and pericardial cavities, and are also found as the secretory epithelium in the kidney and the mesothelium of the anterior chamber of the eye. Also called *celothel, coelothel, celothelium, coelothelium, coelarium, mesepithelium.*   2 An incorrect term for MESENCHYMAL EPITHELIUM. See also COELOMIC EPITHELIUM. Adjective: mesothelial.

mesothenar   An outmoded term for MUSCULUS ADDUCTOR POLLICIS.

mesotherm [MESO- + Gk *thermē* heat]   An organism that requires moderate temperatures for its development.

mesothorium 1   RADIUM 228. Symbol: MsTh1

mesothorium 2   ACTINIUM 228. Symbol: MsTh2

mesotocin   A posterior pituitary hormone found in birds, reptiles, amphibia and lung fishes. It differs from mammalian oxytocin by possessing an isoleucine residue in place of leucine at position 8.

mesotron   MESON.

mesotropic   Located toward the median plane of a cavity, as the abdomen.

mesoturbinal   CONCHA NASALIS MEDIA.

mesoturbinate   CONCHA NASALIS MEDIA.

mesotympanum   SYMPLECTIC BONE.

mesouranic   MESURANIC.

mesovarium   [NA] A short, thick, peritoneal fold that attaches the straight mesovarian border of the ovary to the posterior layer of the broad ligament just below its superior border. Between its two layers blood vessels and nerves pass to the hilum of the ovary. Also called *mesoarium* (outmoded).

mesoxalic acid   HOOC—CO—COOH. An unstable acid, easily decarboxylated to yield carbon dioxide and glyoxylic acid. Its ureide is alloxan, a pyrimidine derivative.

mesoxalyl urea   ALLOXAN.

Mesozoa [MESO- + Gk *zōa,* pl. of *zōon* a living being, animal]   A small group of multicellular endoparasites of extremely simple organization whose phyletic origins are little understood. The few species known are divided into two orders, Dicyemida, parasitic in the kidneys of cephalopods, with an incompletely known life cycle, and Orthonectida, with species parasitic in tissue spaces of a variety of invertebrates (turbellarians, nemerteans, annelids, brittle stars, gastropods, bivalves), and a known life cycle, involving a free-living sexual and parasitic asexual stage.

messenger   1 Designating the RNA that carries the information encoded in a DNA sequence to the site of protein biosynthesis, where it specifies the order of amino-acid residues. **2** The mediator of an effect, e.g. a hormone secreted in one part of an organism and having an effect on distant cells, sometimes operating via a second messenger.

second messenger   A substance produced when a hormone acts on a cell and mediating the response of the cell to that hormone. The hormone itself is regarded as the first messenger. An example is cAMP produced in response to epinephrine.

Mestinon   A proprietary name for pyridostigmine bromide.

mestranol   3-Methoxy-19-nor-17α-pregna-1,3,5(10)-triene-20-yne-17α-ol. An estradiol derivative used as an estrogenic component in some progestin-estrogenic oral contraceptives.

mesuranic [MES- + *uran(o)*- + -IC]   Having a maxilloalveolar index of between 110 and 114.9. Also *mesouranic*.

mesurpine hydrochloride $C_{19}H_{26}N_2O_5S \cdot HCl$. 2″-Hydroxy-5′-[1-hydroxy-2-[*p*-methoxyphenethyl)amino]propyl]-methanesulfonanilide monohydrochloride. A compound used as a vasodilator and as a smooth muscle relaxant agent.

mesyl   The methylsulfonyl group $CH_3—SO_2—$.

mesylate   The ion $CH_3—SO_3{}^-$ or the group $CH_3—SO_3—$. The group is often used in organic synthesis as the means by which oxygen in a molecule can be replaced. Thus a hydroxyl group may be converted into $CH_3—SO_2—O—$, and this is easily displaced as the mesylate ion by nucleophiles, in one instance leaving carbon over 10 000 times faster than does chloride.

Met   Symbol for methionine.

met-   META-.

meta- [Gk *meta* (*meth-* as prefix before Gk aspirated vowel) after, among, between, with, by means of, during, back again, over]   **1** A prefix meaning changed in form or position, transformed.   **2** A prefix meaning after, behind, following.   **3** A prefix meaning with, next to.   **4** A prefix meaning above, beyond, transcending. For defs. 1–4 also *met-*, *meth-*.   **5** A prefix indicating the position of a substituent in benzene as being on C-3 when the numbering is defined in relation to a reference substituent on C-1. Symbol: *m-*

metabasidium [META- + BASIDIUM]   The portion of the fungal basidium in which meiosis occurs.

metabasis   An alteration in the natural course of any disease process. An obsolete term.

metabiosis   A relationship between two organisms characterized by the dependence of the welfare of one upon the presence and preceding activities of the other.

metabisulfite   The ion $S_2O_5{}^{2-}$, which reacts with water to form two bisulfite ions, $HSO_3{}^-$.

metabolic   Of or related to metabolism.

metabolimeter [*metaboli(sm)* + -METER]   An instrument for measuring basal metabolism.

metabolimetry [*metaboli(sm)* + -METRY]   The measurement of basal metabolism.

metabolism [Gk *metabolē* (from META- + Gk *bolē* a throw, from *ballein* to throw) a change + -ISM]   The totality of the chemical processes occurring in a living organism, especially those associated with the exchange of matter and energy between a cell and its environment.

acid-base metabolism   The processes influencing the hydrogen ion concentration in the body.

aerobic metabolism   Metabolic activity that is dependent upon the presence of gaseous oxygen. Also called *respiratory metabolism*.

ammonotelic metabolism   Those chemical changes taking place within the body that produce ammonia.

anaerobic metabolism   Metabolism occurring in the absence of molecular oxygen.

basal metabolism   The state of minimal metabolic activity associated with the maintenance of body function at its normal temperature in the postabsorptive state at mental and physical rest.

carbohydrate metabolism   The chemical reactions associated with the production and utilization of carbohydrates in the body.

electrolyte metabolism   The processes influencing the concentrations of electrolytes in the body.

endergonic metabolism   Metabolic activity associated with a positive standard free-energy change.

endogenous metabolism   **1** The chemical changes associated with the nitrogenous components of the body tissues.   **2** The chemical changes associated with the turnover of body tissues as distinct from the turnover of ingested food materials.

energy metabolism   Metabolic activity associated with energy production or utilization.

excess metabolism of exercise   The increase in metabolic activity during exercise and recovery over that during sleep.

exergonic metabolism   Metabolic activity associated with a negative standard free-energy charge.

exogenous metabolism   The chemical changes associated with ingested food materials not incorporated as constituents of body tissues.

fat metabolism   The chemical changes associated with the production and utilization of fats in the body.

intermediary metabolism   The chemical changes associated with the synthesis of cellular components from food materials and their degradation.

protein metabolism   The chemical changes associated with the production and utilization of proteins in the body.

respiratory metabolism   AEROBIC METABOLISM.

metabolite   A substance taking part in or produced by metabolic activity.

essential metabolite   An indispensable component of a metabolic process.

secondary metabolite   Any of the compounds produced by many microorganisms under conditions (idiophase) in which foodstuffs are no longer converted into the primary metabolites of growth but are converted into other products, which vary widely in different organisms. The antibiotics are a subclass.

metabolizable   Capable of being metabolized.

metabolize [Gk *metabol(ē)* a change, changing + -IZE]   To subject to metabolic change.

metabutethamine hydrochloride $C_{13}H_{21}ClN_2O_2 \cdot HCl$. 2-[(2-Methylpropyl)amino]ethanol 3-aminobenzoate(ester)monohydrochloride. It is used in dentistry as a local anesthetic, producing infiltration and nerve block anesthesia.

metacarpal   **1** Pertaining to the metacarpus.   **2** Any one of ossa metacarpalia I-V.

metacarpale ulnare   The most lateral point of the hand, over the head of the fifth metacarpal bone. It is used in somatometry for measuring hand breadth.

metacarpectomy [*metacarp(al)* + -ECTOMY]   The surgical removal of a part or all of one or more metacarpal bones.

metacarpophalangeal   Of or relating to the metacarpus and the phalanges.

metacarpus [NA]   A series of five cylindrical bones articulating with the carpus proximally and with the proximal phalanges distally. See also OSSA METACARPALIA I-V.

metacentric   In cytogenetics, having the centromere near the middle of a chromosome, resulting in nearly equal lengths of the arms. In humans, this is characteristic of chromosomes of groups A and F.

metacercaria [META- + CERCARIA]   (*plural* metacercariae)

The encysted stage of a digenetic trematode, which occurs in the tissues or on the surface of its intermediate host, such as a snail, aquatic arthropod, amphibian, or fish, or on vegetation. This stage is the usual infective or transfer stage to the definitive host.

metacercariae Plural of METACERCARIA.

metachromasia [New L, from Gk *meta-* with + *chrōma* color + *s* + *-ia* -IA] A phenomenon in which a histologic stain reacts with certain tissue elements, such as sulfated polysaccharides and sialic acid mucins, to give a different color from that of surrounding structures. The color change is normally toward the shorter wavelength of the visual spectrum and is thought to be due to polymerization of dye molecules. Also called *metachromia, metachromatism.*

metachromatic Possessing metachromasia. Also *metachromic.*

metachromatin Basophilic nuclear chromatin.

metachromatism METACHROMASIA.

metachromatophil METACHROMOPHIL.

metachromia METACHROMASIA.

metachromic METACHROMATIC.

metachromophil A cell that contains substances exhibiting metachromasia. Also called *metachromophile, metachromatophil.*

metachromophile METACHROMOPHIL.

metacinesis METAKINESIS.

metacism [irreg. from Gk *mytakism(os)* (from *my* the letter *m*, the sound of murmuring with closed lips) the making of *m* sounds, murmuring] A disorder of speech in which the letter *m* or its sound is used incorrectly or to excess in speaking or writing.

metacoele [META- + -COELE] The cavity of the metencephalon in the embryo, which eventually contributes to the fourth ventricle.

metacoeloma [META- + Gk *koilōma* a hollow] That portion of the coelom in an embryo which forms the pleuroperitoneal canal.

metacone [META- + CONE] The distobuccal cusp of the trigonid; the outer posterior of the mammalian upper molar tooth.

metaconid [*metacon(e)* + -ID¹] The distolingual cusp of the trigonid; the inner anterior cusp of the mammalian lower molar tooth.

metaconule [META- + CONULE] A small cusp situated between the metacone and the protocone on the upper molar teeth of early and primitive mammals.

metacortandracin PREDNISONE.

metacortandralone PREDNISOLONE.

metacryptomerozoite METACRYPTOZOITE.

metacryptozoite [META- + CRYPTO- + *zo(o)-* + -ITE] A merozoite of the second generation of the exoerythrocytic cycle in the development of malarial parasites in the liver. Also called *metacryptomerozoite.*

metacyesis [META- + Gk *kyēsis* pregnancy] An older term for ECTOPIC PREGNANCY.

metaduodenum [META- + DUODENUM] That part of the embryonic duodenum which is derived from the midgut. It is the distal part beyond the entry of the papilla.

metadysentery An outmoded term for BACILLARY DYSENTERY.

metaerythrocytic EXOERYTHROCYTIC.

metafemale Any genetic female possessing one or more extra female sex-determining chromosomes in addition to the normal diploid set of autosomes. The most common example of a human metafemale is the triple-X syndrome associated with a 47,XXX karyotype. Also called *superfemale* (outmoded).

metagaster [META- + -GASTER] The intestinal canal of the embryo when the canal's outline is finally determined.

metagastrula [META- + GASTRULA] A gastrula resulting from a cleavage process other than that giving rise to the usual form.

metagenesis [META- + GENESIS] ALTERNATION OF GENERATIONS.

metageria [META- + *ger(o)-* + -IA] A genetically determined syndrome characterized by the almost total absence of subcutaneous fat, a thin face with a prominent beaked nose, and atrophy, telangiectasia, and mottled pigmentation of the skin of the limbs and upper trunk.

metaglobulin A derived protein resulting from the partial degradation of albumin, usually due to action of an acid or an alkali (acid or alkali albuminate).

metagnathous [META- + GNATH- + -OUS] **1** Having the mandible tips crossed, as in the crossbills, whose bills are adapted for extraction of pine nuts. **2** Having larvae with biting mouth parts and adults with sucking mouth parts, as in certain insects.

metagonimiasis Infection with trematodes of the genus *Metagonimus.*

Metagonimus [New L (from META- + Gk *gonimos* fruitful, productive, from *gonos* that which is begotten, a child, race, birth, descent)] A genus of heterophyid trematodes that encyst on fish, infecting fish-eating animals, including humans.

Metagonimus ovatus METAGONIMUS YOKOGAWAI.

Metagonimus yokogawai An intestinal heterophyid fluke found in the Far East, the Balkans, and the Near East. It occurs in the small intestine, the smallest trematode infecting man (1 to 2.5 mm in length), transmitted by snails of the genus *Semisulcospira* to various fish, and subsequently to fish-eating mammals and birds, as well as to humans eating raw or undercooked fresh or brackish-water fish. Also called *Loxotrema ovatum, Metagonimus ovatus.*

metagranulocyte METAMYELOCYTE.

metagrippal Occurring consequent upon influenza (grippe).

metaherpes [META- + HERPES] METAHERPETIC KERATITIS.

metainfective [META- + INFECTIVE] Occurring as a sequel to infection or during the convalescent stage of an infectious disease: said especially of a fever.

metakentrin An older term for LUTEINIZING HORMONE.

metakinesis The separation during mitosis of the two chromatids of a chromosome and their movement toward the opposite spindle poles. Also *metacinesis.*

metal [L *metallum* a metal, gold, silver, iron, a mine, quarry, from Gk *metallon* a mine, quarry] Any of several chemical elements that share, more or less, a group of characteristic properties: they are good conductors of electricity or heat, are malleable, often have a shiny appearance, are generally basic, form oxides, and liberate cations.

Babbitt's metal An alloy composed of tin, copper, and antimony, used in dental technology.

cliche metal A low-fusing alloy of tin, lead, antimony, and bismuth, used in dentistry.

heavy metal A metal which is at least five times denser than water. Some heavy metals, such as mercury, copper, lead, and cadmium, are toxic, but the degree of toxicity varies. The toxicity of their cations is often due to their tight binding to essential proteins of the body.

Melotte's metal An alloy composed of bismuth, lead, and tin, used in dental technology. Also called *Newton's alloy.*

noble metal A metal difficult to oxidize to its salts, and easily produced from them. Examples are gold, silver, and platinum.

metallaxis [Gk *metallaxis* a change, exchange] Transformation of the structure of an organ or tissue caused by a pathologic process. An obsolete term.

metallesthesia The recognition of metals through the sense of touch.

metalloenzyme Any enzyme which has metal atoms as its prosthetic group, such as the cytochromes (Fe^{2+} or Fe^{3+}), cytochrome oxidase (Cu^{2+} or Cu^+), or alcohol dehydrogenase (Zn^{2+}).

metalloflavodehydrogenase Any of a class of dehydrogenase enzymes which are active only if a flavin nucleotide, as a coenzyme, and metal ions, as iron or copper, are available.

metalloflavoprotein An enzyme which functions as a dehydrogenase by the reduction of the prosthetic group. The enzyme is composed of a metal, a flavin, and a protein.

metallophil A cell or tissue which stains with metallic salts, such as silver salts, generally the reticular cells.

metallophilia The binding of certain metal ions by various cells and tissues.

metallophilic Having an affinity for metallic stains: said of cells or tissues.

metalloprotein A protein with a metal ion bound to it. Normally this ion is a bi- or tervalent ion that is chelated by the protein and hence fairly firmly bound. Many enzymes are metalloproteins.

metalloscopy Observation of the effects of application of metals to the skin.

metallothionein A cadmium-binding protein originally isolated from equine kidney. Its major distinctive features are the absence of aromatic amino acids, high cysteine content, and a high affinity for certain metals, especially cadmium, zinc, mercury, silver, and tin. It is found in many tissues of both man and animals, having been isolated from kidney, spleen, liver, intestine, heart, brain, lung, and skin.

metaluetic METASYPHILITIC.

metamale In *Drosophila*, a fly with one X chromosome and 3 sets of autosomes.

metamere [META- + -MERE] Any one of a series of similarly constructed segments forming the body of an animal. Metameres are seen best in segmented forms such as the annelid earthworm, but they are a feature of all vertebrate embryos. In most terrestrial vertebrates and in man metameric segmentation is obscured. Also called *body segment*. See also SOMITE.

metameric 1 Pertaining to metamerism. 2 Arising from a metamere.

metamerism [META- + *mer(o)*¹- + -ISM] The repetition of similar parts or segments in the body of an animal. Also called *metameric segmentation*.

  complete metamerism Full segmentation or strobilization, as in tapeworms, arthropods, and other metameric animals.

  cutaneous metamerism An area of the skin surface corresponding to a primitive spinal segment or neurotome.

  incomplete metamerism Partial segmentation, as in acanthocephalans or larval cestodes which show external segments that do not correspond to internal body divisions.

Metamine A proprietary name for trolnitrate phosphate.

metamorphic Of or relating to metamorphosis.

metamorphopsia [META- + MORPH- + -OPSIA] Distortion of the visual image, which may be due to physical displacement of the macular portion of the retina, usually by small amounts of subretinal fluid, or which may result from central lesions such as parietal lobe disorders or from intoxication with drugs such as mescaline or lysergic acid. Also called *anorthopia, visus defiguratus*.

metamorphopsia varians A continual changing of the size and shape of the visual image.

metamorphosis [Gk *metamorphōsis* (from *metamorphoun* to transform, from META- + Gk *morphē* form, shape + *-ōsis* -OSIS) a transformation] The transformation of shape or structure: used especially in relation to the forms an organism passes through during its various stages of development from egg to adult, as illustrated, for example, by the life cycle of the holometabolous orders of insects. Adjective: metamorphic.

  fatty metamorphosis FATTY CHANGE.

  regressive metamorphosis RETROGRADE METAMORPHOSIS.

  retrograde metamorphosis 1 A degenerative change in which cells or tissues seem to revert to an earlier or less differentiated type. 2 Metamorphosis of insects or other life forms which reverses the normal course of development; retromorphosis. For defs 1 and 2 also called *retrogressive metamorphosis, regressive metamorphosis*.

  retrogressive metamorphosis RETROGRADE METAMORPHOSIS.

  structural metamorphosis A transformation in the structure of a cell or organism.

  tissue metamorphosis Any change in the structure or habits of a tissue.

metamorphotic Relating to, or characterized by, metamorphosis.

Metamucil A proprietary name for psyllium hydrophilic mucilloid.

metamyelocyte An intermediate form in neutrophil maturation, between myelocyte and band neutrophil, that has an indented or "kidney-bean" nucleus with condensed chromatin, no identifiable nucleoli, and neutrophilic cytoplasmic granules. Also called *metagranulocyte, rhabdocyte* (rarely used), *juvenile cell*.

metamyxovirus Any of a subgroup of viruses of the Paramyxoviridae family that includes respiratory syncytial virus and pneumonia virus of mice.

Metandren A proprietary name for methyltestosterone.

metanephridium [META- + NEPHRIDIUM] A type of nephridium with the nephridial tubule having a ciliated, funnel-like internal opening (nephrostome) in the coelom and an external opening (nephridiopore) on the surface of the body. It acts as an excretory and osmoregulatory structure in certain phyla, such as Annelida and Mollusca.

metanephrogenic Having to do with the formation of the metanephros.

metanephroi Plural of METANEPHROS.

metanephron [META- + NEPHRON] A unit of the metanephros.

metanephros [META- + Gk *nephros* a kidney] The tubular system in the embryo, caudal to the mesonephros and developing after it, which gives rise to the definitive kidney of reptiles, birds, and mammals. The metanephros is formed from two parts: from mesenchymatous tissue corresponding to fused nephrotomes of the sacral region, and from an outgrowth of the mesonephric duct called the ureteric bud or diverticulum. Also called *definitive kidney, hind-kidney*.

metaniline yellow METANIL YELLOW.

metanil yellow An acid dye that is used as a pH indicator, changing from red at a pH of 1.2 to yellow at pH 2.3. Also called *metaniline yellow, tropaeolin G*.

metanucleus [META- + NUCLEUS] The nucleus of an ovum while it is undergoing maturation.

metaphase The stage of mitosis or meiosis during which the chromosomes are aligned on the equatorial plate.

Metaphen A proprietary name for nitromersol.

metaphosphate   Any of several phosphate species, notionally formed from orthophosphate by loss of water. The highly reactive ion PO_3^{2-}, transferred from ATP when it phosphorylates compounds, is monomeric metaphosphate. Trimetaphosphate refers to the cyclic triphosphate ion, $P_3O_9^{3-}$.

metaphosphoric acid $(HPO_3)_n$. A transparent, deliquescent solid that is soluble in water or alcohol. It is used as a phosphorylating agent or dehydrating agent and in precipitation tests for urinary protein. It is also used in the manufacture of dental cements. Also called *glacial phosphoric acid.*

metaphrenia [META- + -PHRENIA]   A condition marked by self-aggrandizement and withdrawal of interest from the social group and onto oneself.

metaphrenon   The dorsum, especially the region associated with the kidneys. An outmoded term.

metaphyseal   Pertaining to the metaphysis. Also *metaphysial.*

metaphyses   Plural of METAPHYSIS.

metaphysial   METAPHYSEAL.

metaphysis (*plural* metaphyses) [NA] The actively growing zone at each end of the diaphysis adjacent to the epiphysial cartilage in a growing long bone. In the adult, with the cessation of growth, the bony metaphysis is indistinguishably fused to the epiphysis and diaphysis.

metaphysitis [*metaphys(is)* + -ITIS]   Inflammation, usually with infection, of a metaphysis of a long bone.

metaplasia [META- + -PLASIA]   The abnormal transformation from one differentiated, adult tissue form to another type of adult tissue within a given organ. It is an acquired condition, usually representing an adaptative response of tissues to many forms of injury.

agnogenic myeloid metaplasia   Extramedullary hematopoiesis, especially of the spleen, associated with myelofibrosis. It presents insidiously or in the context of one of the myeloproliferative syndromes. The spleen is markedly enlarged and may weigh several pounds. The extramedullary hematopoiesis affects primarily the red pulp with erythroid, myeloid, and megakaryocytic precursors being represented. The liver and, rarely, the lymph nodes also show metaplasia. Also called *myeloid metaplasia, primary myeloid metaplasia, nonleukemic myelosis, chronic nonleukemic myelosis.*

apocrine metaplasia   A metaplasia of the epithelium of the breast to apocrine sweat gland epithelium, commonly seen in fibrocystic disease.

autoparenchymatous metaplasia   Metaplasia involving the parenchymal cells of an organ. An obsolete term.

intestinal metaplasia   The transformation of gastric mucosa into a glandular epithelium reminiscent of that of the small intestines. It contains goblet and Paneth cells, and is typically seen in chronic atrophic gastritis.

myeloid metaplasia   AGNOGENIC MYELOID METAPLASIA.

primary myeloid metaplasia   AGNOGENIC MYELOID METAPLASIA.

pseudopyloric metaplasia   A histologic variant of atrophic gastritis characterized by replacement of acid and pepsinogen-secreting glands by simple glands of the pyloric type. It does not carry an increased incidence of malignant change.

metaplasia of pulp   A change in the dental pulp to nonspecialized connective tissue incapable of producing dentin.

squamous metaplasia   The transformation of an epithelium, usually mucosal or glandular, to a stratified squamous epithelium. It is a common adaptation to injury such as occurs to the ciliated, columnar, respiratory epithelium under the prolonged effect of cigarette smoking. Also called *keratoid degeneration* (obsolete).

metaplasis [Gk *metaplasis* transformation]   The state of completed growth or development.

metaplasm [META- + -PLASM]   The nonliving inclusions within the protoplasm, as vacuoles or yolk. Also called *metaplastic substance, metaplasma.*

metaplasma   METAPLASM.

metaplastic   Characterized by metaplasia.

metaplexus   The choroid plexus of the fourth ventricle of the medulla oblongata. An obsolete term. Also called *metatela.*

metapneumonic   Subsequent to, or secondary to, pneumonia or pneumococcal infection.

metapodialia   The bones of either the metacarpus, the metatarsus, or both collectively. Also called *metapodials.*   • The term is usually used in comparative anatomy and paleontology.

metapodials   METAPODIALIA.

metapodium [META- + PODIUM]   (*plural* metapodia) **1** The bones of the foot located between the tarsus and the digits.   **2** The posterior part of the foot of a mollusk. Adjective: metapodial.

metapophysis   PROCESSUS MAMMILLARIS VERTEBRARUM LUMBALIUM.

metapore   An obsolete term for APERTURA MEDIANA VENTRICULI QUARTI.

metaprotein [META- + PROTEIN]   A protein obtained when an acid or a base acts upon a natural protein. Metaproteins are generally soluble in weak acids or bases but insoluble at a neutral pH.

metaproterenol sulfate $C_{22}H_{36}N_2O_{10}S$. A potent β-adrenergic stimulant with a rapid onset of action and a longer duration than isoproterenol. It is used as a bronchodilator in the treatment of bronchial asthma, bronchitis, and emphysema.

metapsyche   METENCEPHALON.

metapsychology   A philosophical and speculative analysis of the relationship between mind and body.

metapterygium [META- + *pteryg(o)-* + L *-ium*, neut. noun suffix]   The posterior cartilaginous rods supporting the base of the pectoral and pelvic girdles in recent elasmobranchs.

metapyretic   POSTFEBRILE.

metapyrone   METYRAPONE.

metaraminol $C_9H_{13}NO_2$. *m*-Hydroxyphenylpropanolamine. A compound with vasopressor activity that is given parenterally to elevate the blood pressure, usually in the form of the bitartrate salt.

metaraminol bitartrate $C_{13}H_{19}NO_8$. The bitartrate salt of metaraminol, freely soluble in water. It is a potent sympathomimetic amine that increases the systolic and diastolic pressures. It is used to prevent or treat acute hypotension due to spinal anesthesia, surgical complications, and hemorrhage or brain damage.

metarchon [*met(a)-* + Gk *archōn* (from *archōn*, pres. part. of *archein* to rule) a ruler]   A biologic control agent, such as a confusing pheromone or sex attractant, by which the feeding or reproductive behavior of insect pests may be altered and their population reduced.

metarhodopsin   An intermediate formed in the retina of the eye as the unstable lumirhodopsin degrades. Metarhodopsin is also unstable and degrades to scotopsin and *trans*-retinene.

metarteriole   That part of the terminal arteriole that is surrounded by an additional layer of smooth muscle cells and acts as the final control of blood flow into the capillary bed. Also called *central channel* (outmoded), *arteriola precapillaris, junctional capillary, arterial capillary, precapillary, arteriolar capillary, precapillary arteriole.*

metarubricyte   ORTHOCHROMATIC NORMOBLAST.

metasomatome [META- + SOMATOME]   The constriction between two somites in an embryo.

metastable   Denoting a substance that has a negligible rate of breakdown to a specified product, but for which the Gibbs energy change for such breakdown is negative. It is therefore unstable from a thermodynamic viewpoint, but stable kinetically, since there is no facile pathway for the breakdown.

metastasectomy [*metastas(is)* + -ECTOMY]   The resection of a metastatic lesion, such as a metastasized malignant tumor.

metastases   Plural of METASTASIS.

metastasis [Gk *metastasis* (from *methistanai* to place in another way, change, remove, from META- + Gk *histanai* to place, set) a removal from one place to another, change]   (*plural* metastases)   **1** The transfer of a disease from one body site to another: said especially of cancers and infectious diseases.   **2** A secondary growth of a malignant tumor at a site separate from the primary from which it was derived. It is usually the result of blood-borne or lymphatic spread, although it may occur through the cerebrospinal fluid circulation or along other channels. The metastasis usually shows histologic features similar to that of the primary growth. Also called *metastatic cancer, metastatic neoplasm, metastatic tumor.*   **3** The process of developing metastases.

metastasis ad nervos   A reflexly induced disorder of nervous function. A seldom used term.

calcareous metastasis   METASTATIC CALCIFICATION.

cannonball metastasis   Metastatic cancer in the lung producing a round radiographic image similar in appearance to a cannonball. Also called *cotton-ball metastasis.*

cerebral metastasis   Metastatic spread of disease to the cerebrum.

contact metastasis   Metastasis from one surface to another following contact.

cotton-ball metastasis   CANNONBALL METASTASIS.

crossed metastasis   Metastasis following transfer of the agent or cells from the venous to the arterial circulation, bypassing the pulmonary vasculature.

direct metastasis   Metastasis in the same direction as the flow of blood or lymph.

extradural metastasis   A metastasis in the cranial cavity or spinal canal lying between the dura mater and the overlying bone.

implantation metastasis   A form of metastasis in which the tumor cells are brought to the site by fluid, usually along a serosal surface.

osteoblastic metastasis   An osseous metastasis in which an increase in bone formation is associated with the tumor cells. It is most typical of carcinoma of the prostate. Also called *osteoplastic metastasis.*

osteolytic metastasis   An osseous metastasis which produces destruction of the invaded bone.

osteoplastic metastasis   OSTEOBLASTIC METASTASIS.

paradoxical metastasis   Metastasis in a direction other than that of the expected flow of blood or lymph. It may be due to reflux from obstruction of lymphatics, lymph nodes, or blood vessels. Also called *retrograde metastasis.*

pulsating metastasis   A highly vascularized metastasis which pulsates.

retrograde metastasis   PARADOXICAL METASTASIS.

transplantation metastasis   Metastasis from one organ to another.

metastasize [*metastas(is)* + -IZE]   To spread lesions by metastasis.

metastatic   Pertaining to metastasis.

metasternum   An outmoded term for PROCESSUS XIPHOIDEUS.

metastrongyle   **1** Belonging to or characteristic of the family Metastrongylidae.   **2** A nematode worm of the family Metastrongylidae.

Metastrongylidae [META- + STRONGYL- + -IDAE]   A family of bursate nematodes in the superfamily Metastrongyloidea, order Strongylida, which includes the genera *Metastrongylus* in various mammals and *Neometastrongylus* in ungulates. Other genera, such as *Protostrongylus, Dictyocaulus, Muellerius, Filaroides,* and *Angiostrongylus* were formerly in this family, but have been given separate family status in the families Protostrongylidae, Dictyocaulidae, and Angiostrongylidae, although some workers consider them to belong to subfamilies (Dictyocaulinae, Metastrongylinae, Filaroidinae, Vogeloidinae, Skrjabingylinae, and Protostrongylinae) of a larger grouping within the family Metastrongylidae.

Metastrongylus [New L, from META- + Gk *strongylos* round]   A genus of lungworms in the family Metastrongylidae, infecting pigs. Four species are known, *M. apri, M. salmi, M. pudendotectus,* and *M. madagascariensis.*

Metastrongylus apri   A common lungworm found in the trachea, bronchi, and bronchioles of wild and domestic pigs, causing bronchitis, pneumonia, unthriftiness, and retarded growth. It is suspected of transmitting hog cholera and swine influenza. Other, less common hosts include oxen, sheep, goats, dogs, and man. The life cycle is indirect, the eggs being taken up by various earthworms which serve as intermediate hosts.

Metastrongylus elongatus   *METASTRONGYLUS SALMI.*

Metastrongylus pudendotectus   A common lungworm of domestic and wild pigs, smaller than *M. apri,* and important in the transmission of swine influenza and hog cholera.

Metastrongylus salmi   A species found in the trachea and small airways of wild and domestic pigs in Europe. The larvae develop to the infectious third stage in earthworms. Also called *Metastrongylus elongatus, Strongylus longevaginatus, Strongylus paradoxus.*

metastructure   The structural organization of the protoplasm which is not resolved by the microscope; structure at the molecular level.

metasynapsis   The abnormal end-to-end joining of homologous chromosomes during meiosis. Also called *metasyndesis.*

metasyncrisis [META- + SYN- + Gk *krisis* a separating, putting apart]   The discharge of waste material.

metasyndesis   METASYNAPSIS.

metasyphilis   The manifestations associated with syphilis.

metasyphilitic   Pertaining to manifestations associated with syphilis. Also *metaluetic.*

metatarsal   **1** Pertaining to the metatarsus.   **2** Any one of the five bones of the metatarsus.

metatarsalgia   Pain in the metatarsal region. It usually arises beneath the metatarsal heads in the transverse plantar arch.

metatarsectomy   The surgical removal of one or more metatarsal bones.

metatarsomegaly   Enlargement of one or more metatarsal bones.

metatarsometatarsal   Pertaining to the relationships of the metatarsal bones to each other.

metatarsophalangeal   Pertaining to the metatarsal bones and the phalanges of the foot.

metatarsus [META- + Gk *tarsos* flat of the foot, the foot]   [NA]   A series of five cylindrical bones in the distal part of the foot articulating with the tarsus proximally and with the phalanges distally. They lie almost parallel to each other and are numbered from the medial side. Each bone is a miniature long bone with a base, shaft, and head.

metatarsus adductocavus   Talipes varus associated with talipes cavus; talipes with abnormal adduction at the ankle and excessive curvature of the arch.

metatarsus adductovarus   Talipes varus in which the distal foot is rotated in extreme adduction.

metatarsus adductus   A fixed deformity in which the distal foot is bent on the longitudinal axis of the foot as a whole so that the digits to a degree turn inward toward the midsagittal plane of the body.

metatarsus atavicus   An abnormal degree of shortness of the first metatarsal bone.

metatarsus latus   BROAD FOOT.

metatarsus primus varus   An abnormal angulation of the first metatarsal bone toward the sagittal plane of the body. Hallux valgus and bunion formation inevitably result from the malformation.

metatarsus varus   A fixed deformity in which the distal part of the foot is rotated on the longitudinal axis of the foot so that the plantar surfaces of the ball and toes tend to face the sagittal plane of the body.

metatela   METAPLEXUS.

metathalamus [META- + THALAMUS]   That portion of the thalamus composed of the medial and lateral geniculate bodies.

metathesis   **1** The deliberate moving of a pathologic process to a site where it will be less troublesome.   **2** DOUBLE DECOMPOSITION.

metathrombin   A thrombin-antithrombin complex that is formed during clotting and is inactive.

metatroph   HETEROTROPH.

metatrophic   HETEROTROPHIC.

metatypic   METATYPICAL.

metatypical   Characterized by tissue that is typical of its site with respect to its component elements, but atypical in the way those elements are arranged: used in reference to tumors. Also *metatypic.*

metaxalone $C_{12}H_{15}NO_3$. 5-[(3,5-Dimethylphenoxy)methyl]-2-oxazolidinone. It is used therapeutically as a skeletal muscle relaxant in the treatment of severe musculoskeletal conditions. It is given orally.

metaxeny   HETERECISM.

metaxylem [META- + XYLEM]   The last xylem to form from the initial plant body.

Metazoa [META- + Gk *zōa*, pl. of *zōon*, a living being, animal] A subkingdom of the kingdom Animalia comprising all multicellular organisms having specialized cells arranged in tissues and, in the higher forms, into organ systems. The Metazoa include all phyla except those in the subkingdom Protozoa.

metazoan (*plural* metazoa, metazoans)   **1** Any member of the Metazoa; any multicellular animal.   **2** Of or pertaining to members of the Metazoa.

metazonal   Located after or distal to a sclerozone.

metazoonosis [META- + ZOONOSIS]   A type of zoonosis requiring both an invertebrate and a vertebrate host stage in the life cycle of the causative organism, as, for example, human helminth infections that involve a snail intermediate host or an insect vector.

Metchnikoff [Elie *Metchnikoff*, Russian-born bacteriologist and zoologist active in France, 1845–1916]   See under THEORY.

metecious   HETERECIOUS.

metempiric [MET- + Gk *empeirik(os)* experienced]   Proceeding from one's interpretations of or deductions from experience rather than from experience itself.

metencephal   An obsolete term for METENCEPHALON.

metencephalic   Of or pertaining to the metencephalon.

metencephalon [*met(a)*- + ENCEPHALON]   The more rostral of the two parts that develop from the rhombencephalon in the embryo. It develops into the cerebellum and pons. The caudal part (myelencephalon) forms the medulla oblongata. Also called *afterbrain, metapsyche, metencephal* (obsolete).

metencephalospinal   Of or pertaining to the metencephalon (cerebellum and pons) and the spinal cord. A seldom used term.

meteorism   TYMPANITES.

meteoropathology   The study of ill effects on the body caused by climatic conditions.

meteoropathy   Any morbid condition, disease, or ill health caused by climatic conditions.

meteororesistant   Unaffected by or relatively insensitive to climatic conditions.

meteorosensitive   **1** Exhibiting a sensitivity to climatic conditions.   **2** Affected by climatic conditions.

meteorotropic   **1** Affected by meteorologic conditions or events: said especially of certain diseases.   **2** Pertaining to meteorotropism.

meteorotropism   The innate or involuntary tendency of an organism to be influenced by meteorologic factors.

metepa   The triamide of phosphoric acid in which the amine component is 2-methylaziridine, so that the compound contains three 3-membered ethyleneimine rings. It is used as a sterilant for water and for flameproofing fabrics.

metepencephalon   An obsolete term for MYELENCEPHALON.

meter [French *mètre* (from Gk *metron* a measure, rule, standard) unit of length equaling one ten-millionth of a quarter of a terrestrial meridian]   The SI base unit of length, approximately equal to 39.37 inches, 3.28 feet, or 1.09 yards. The meter is equal to the distance traveled by electromagnetic radiation through a vacuum in 1/299 792 458 second, a measure based on the speed of light. Between 1960 and 1983, the meter was defined as being equal to 1 650 763.73 wavelengths in vacuum of the radiation corresponding to the transition between the levels $2p_{10}$ and $5d_5$ of the krypton-86 atom. Symbol: m • In Great Britain and in international usage, the spelling *metre* is preferred, but in the United States *meter* is the usual spelling.

acuity meter   ACOUMETER.

candle meter   METER CANDLE.

constancy meter   An instrument that monitors a controllable quantity to keep it at a desired value.

counting-rate meter   A device that indicates the average rate of arrival of random pulses put out by a radiation detector. The usual readout is by milliammeter, whose reading may be unsteady if the pulse rate is low.

cubic meter   The SI derived unit of volume equal to the volume of a cube having sides of length one meter; 1.308 cubic yards. Symbol: m^3

cubic meter per second   The SI derived unit of volume rate of flow equal to one cubic meter flowing in one second. Also called *cumec* (popular). Symbol: m^3/s, $m^3 \cdot s^{-1}$

Cutie Pie survey meter   A battery-operated ionization chamber suitable for surveying radiation hazard.

D O meter   An apparatus for determining the amount of dissolved oxygen taken up by an effluent.

dosage meter   DOSIMETER.

dose-rate meter   In radiology, an instrument which displays the radiation dose rate.

electronic pH meter   A device that determines the pH of a solution by measuring the voltage differences generated at the surface of a pH-responsive electrode.

exposure meter   A photoelectric cell calibrated so as to convey the camera settings appropriate for the intensity of the light reflected from an object to be photographed.

flicker meter   FLICKER PHOTOMETER.

Geiger-Müller survey meter   A portable instrument used for the detection of radiation, commonly used for radiation protection. The instrument is based on the Geiger-Müller counter principle.

hot-wire meter An instrument that measures current by passing it through a fine wire. The wire heats and changes length, moving a pointer.

integrating dose meter Any dose meter that displays the total dose received rather than the dose rate.

light meter An instrument, often small and portable, that measures the intensity of illumination.

peak flow meter A device for measuring peak expiratory flow.

meter per second The SI derived unit of speed and velocity. Symbol: m/s, $m{\cdot}s^{-1}$.

meter per second per second METER PER SECOND SQUARED.

meter per second squared The SI derived unit of acceleration. Also called *meter per second per second*. Symbol: m/s^2, $m{\cdot}s^{-2}$.

potential acuity meter An optical system for measuring the acuity of a cataract patient. It focuses the standard visual-acuity letter chart down to a diameter of 150 nm and beams it through a clear window in the cataract to the retina.

meter to the power minus one RECIPROCAL METER.

rate meter Any instrument designed to show or measure the speed of some function or phenomenon, as a radiation detector which continually shows radiation intensity.

reciprocal meter The SI derived unit of wave number, absorption coefficient, attenuation coefficient, and linear ionization of a particle. Also called *meter to the power minus one*. Symbol: m^{-1}.

smoke meter An instrument designed for measuring the amount of smoke in stack or exhaust gases.

sound level meter An acoustic instrument which measures the very small oscillations of atmospheric air pressure induced by sound producing activity. The result is displayed in dB SPL. See also A-WEIGHTED SOUND LEVEL, WEIGHTING NETWORK.

square meter The SI derived unit of area equal to the area of a square having sides one meter in length; 10.764 square feet or 1.196 square yards. Symbol: m^2

survey meter A portable device used for the detection and measurement of radiation.

ventilation meter An apparatus for measuring the volume of air breathed in unit time.

zero-crossing meter A component of Doppler devices that produces an analog waveform by converting into voltage the number of flow directional changes within an artery.

-meter [Gk *metron* measure, rule, standard] A combining form meaning (1) measure, measurement; (2) instrument for measuring. Also *-metre (British spelling)*.

metergasis [MET- + *ergasis*, irreg. from Gk *ergasia* (from *ergaseiein* to be about to do) work, business] An alteration in function.

metestrum METESTRUS.

metestrus The period intermediate between estrus and diestrus in the estrous cycle. Also called *metestrum*.

metformin $C_4H_{11}N_5$. 1,1-Dimethylbiguanide. It is a structural analogue of phenformin and is also an oral hypoglycemic agent that has been used in the treatment of diabetes.

meth- META-.

methacetin ACETANISIDINE.

methacholine The β-methyl derivative of acetylcholine, usually administered in the form of its chlorine or bromide salt. It is much more stable than acetylcholine and has only muscarinic actions. It has some clinical use in the treatment of paroxysmal tachycarditis. Also called *methylacetylcholine, acetyl-β-methylcholine*.

methacholine bromide $C_8H_{18}BrNO_2$. A white, crystalline powder with the same pharmacological properties as methacholine chloride. It is very hygroscopic.

methacholine chloride $C_8H_{18}ClNO_2$. A colorless, crystalline powder that has been used as a cholinergic drug, particularly for its muscarinic properties on the cardiovascular system. Also called *acetyl-β-methylcholine chloride*.

methacrylate METHYL METHACRYLATE.

methacrylic acid $CH_2{=}C(CH_3){-}COOH$. 2-Methylacrylic acid. It is used as a substrate for polymerization in the manufacture of plastics.

methacycline $C_{22}H_{22}N_2O_8$. 6-Methyleneoxytetracycline. A semisynthetic antibiotic of the tetracycline family of drugs. It is effective against a wide spectrum of bacterial species. It is given orally as the hydrochloride.

methadone $C_{21}H_{27}NO$. 6-Dimethylamino 4,4-diphenyl-3-heptanone. A synthetic narcotic analgesic with morphinelike effects. It is used in opiate withdrawal and as maintenance treatment of heroin addicts, and is a drug of abuse. It is usually given as the hydrochloride.

methadyl acetate ACETYLMETHADOL.

methaemalbumin A British spelling for METHEMALBUMIN.

methaemoglobin A British spelling for METHEMOGLOBIN.

methallenestril $C_{18}H_{22}O_3$. β-Ethyl-6-methoxy-χ,χ-dimethyl-2-naphthalenepropionic acid. A synthetic, nonsteroidal estrogenic agent used orally for its estrogenic activity.

methallibure $C_7H_{14}N_4S_2$. 1-Methyl-6-(1-methylallyl)-2,5-dithiobiurea. This compound has the ability to activate the anterior pituitary gland and stimulate the production of hormones in swine.

methalthiazide 3-[(Allylthio)-methyl]-6-chloro-3,4-dihydro-2-methyl-2H-1,2,4-benzothiadiazine-7-sulfonamide-1,1-dioxide. A diuretic agent which has been used to treat essential hypertension.

methamphetamine $C_{10}H_{15}N$. (S)-N,α-Dimethylbenzeneethanamine. A sympathomimetic amine that is a structural analogue of amphetamine. It is used as a general central nervous system stimulant.

methamphetamine hydrochloride $C_{10}H_{16}ClN$. The hydrochloride salt of methamphetamine, having the same actions and uses as the parent compound.

methandriol $C_{20}H_{32}O_2$. 17α-Methyl-5-androstene-3β,17β-diol. A steroid with anabolic activity. It is used therapeutically for this purpose. Also called *5,6-dehydroandrosterone*.

methandrostenolone Δ'-17α-Methyltestosterone. A steroid with strong anabolic and androgenic properties.

methane CH_4. The simplest hydrocarbon, it is a constituent of natural gas. It is sometimes known as marsh gas, because it is formed by anaerobic microorganisms that live in marshes.

Methanobacteriaceae A family of strictly anaerobic autotrophic bacteria that use hydrogen to reduce carbon dioxide to methane and water, thereby obtaining energy for carbon dioxide fixation. They are widely distributed in nature, including the vertebrate gut. The unusual composition of their macromolecules has led to their designation as Archaebacteria.

methanogen Any of a group of strictly anaerobic bacteria that derive energy from the reaction $CO_2 + 4H_2 \rightarrow CH_4 + 2H_2O$. See also METHANOBACTERIACEAE.

methanol $CH_3{-}OH$. A colorless, inflammable liquid, miscible with water, ethanol, ether, and gasoline. Its freezing point is $-97.8°C$, and the boiling point is $64.65°C$. Once prepared by distillation of wood, it is now obtained synthetically. It is toxic, and can quite often cause damage to the eyes if drunk. It is a general solvent. Also called *methyl alcohol, wood alcohol, carbinol* (obsolete).

methanolysis The decomposition of a compound with methanol, with scission of a bond in the molecule so that the parts of methanol are added to either side of the bond broken.

methantheline bromide $C_{21}H_{26}BrNO_3$. β-Diethylamino-ethyl-9-xanthenecarboxylate bromide. An anticholinergic agent used to supress gastric motility and secretions.

methapyrilene $C_{14}H_{19}N_3S$. N,N-Dimethyl-N'-2-pyridinyl-N'-(2-thienylmethyl)-1,2-ethanediamine, an antihistaminic agent of relatively short duration and moderate potency. It has some sedative activity. It is given orally, and it is also available as the fumarate and hydrochloride salts.

methapyrilene fumarate $(C_{14}H_{19}N_3S)_2\cdot3C_4H_4O_4$. The fumarate salt of methapyrilene, having the same properties and uses as the parent drug. It is given orally.

methapyrilene hydrochloride $C_{14}H_{20}ClN_3S$. N,N-Dimethyl-N'-2-pyridinyl-N'-(2-thienylmethyl)-1,2-ethanediamine hydrochloride. An effective antihistaminic agent, used therapeutically for that purpose. It is given orally or parenterally.

methaqualone $C_{16}H_{14}N_2O$. 2-Methyl-3-(2-methylphenyl)-4(3H)-quinazolinone. An agent used therapeutically as a sedative and a hypnotic. Chronic use has been reported to lead to psychological and physical dependence.

metharbital $C_9H_{14}N_2O_3$. 5,5-Diethyl-1-methyl-2,4,6(1H,3H,5H)pyridinetrione. A barbiturate employed as an anticonvulsant drug in the treatment of various forms of seizures, as of grand mal, petit mal, or myoclonic seizure. It is given orally.

methazolamide $C_5H_8N_4O_3S_2$. N-[5-(Aminosulfonyl)-3-methyl-1,3,4-thiadiazol-2(3H)-ylidene]-acetamide. A white, crystalline powder used as a carbonic anhydrase inhibitor to reduce intraocular pressure for the treatment of glaucoma. It is given orally.

MetHb methemoglobin.

methdilazine $C_{18}H_{20}N_2S$. 10-[(1-Methyl-3-pyrrolidinyl)methyl]-phenothiazine, an antihistaminic agent used to treat pruritus of allergic or nonallergic origin. It is given orally as tablets or a syrup. It is also available as the hydrochloride salt.

Methedrine A proprietary name for methamphetamine hydrochloride.

methelepsia METHILEPSIA.

methemalbumin A complex of plasma albumin with heme, in the Fe(III) state, released from hemoglobin. It occurs in small amounts in plasma when there is intravascular hemolysis.

metheme Heme that has its iron in the Fe(III) state.

methemoglobin A derivative of hemoglobin in which the iron component has been oxidized from the Fe(II) to the Fe(III) state. Methemoglobin imparts a brownish color to blood and is unable to transport oxygen. Also called *oxidized hemoglobin, ferrihemoglobin.*

methemoglobinemia [*met(a)-* + HEMOGLOBINEMIA] The presence of methemoglobin in blood in greater than normal concentration, i.e. greater than 1% of the total hemoglobin pigments. Methemoglobinemia is a cause of cyanosis.

congenital methemoglobinemia HEREDITARY METHEMOGLOBINEMIA.

enterogenous methemoglobinemia Methemoglobinemia that results from intestinal absorption of nitrite following reduction of ingested nitrate to nitrite by bacteria of the intestinal tract. Nitrite rapidly oxidizes hemoglobin to methemoglobin.

hereditary methemoglobinemia A rare type of methemoglobinemia that is life-long in duration and of genetic transmission. The principal manifestation is cyanosis, which may be very slight or quite marked. Most often, hereditary methemoglobinemia is an autosomal recessive disorder due to deficiency of erythrocyte

methemoglobin reductase. Autosomal dominant hereditary methemoglobinemia may be due to inheritance of one of several very rare hemoglobinopathies, such as Hb M-Saskatoon, Hb M-Boston, Hb M-Iwate, among others. Also called *congenital methemoglobinemia, primary methemoglobinemia.*

primary methemoglobinemia HEREDITARY METHEMOGLOBINEMIA.

secondary methemoglobinemia Methemoglobinemia that is induced rather than due to an intrinsic abnormality of the erythrocyte or of hemoglobin.

toxic methemoglobinemia Methemoglobinemia that results from exposure of hemoglobin to drugs or their metabolites or to nitrites. The drugs most commonly responsible are phenacetin, sulfones (especially dapsone), and chemically related substances such as acetanilid and phenazopyridine.

methemoglobinemic Having methemoglobinemia.

methemoglobin reductase An erythrocyte enzyme that converts methemoglobin to hemoglobin while oxidizing NADPH. Also called *NADPH diaphorase.*

methemoglobinuria HEMOGLOBINURIA. • Hemoglobin in the urine is usually methemoglobin. The distinction is not made in practice, so the term is redundant.

methenamine $C_6H_{12}N_4$. Hexamethylenetetramine. A colorless or white crystalline solid that is soluble in water and alcohol and very slightly soluble in ether. Its molecules contain four nitrogen atoms arranged in a tetrahedron and bridged by methylene groups. It is a mild disinfectant, probably because of its slow hydrolysis to formaldehyde, and it was formerly used in treating bacterial infections of the urinary tract. Also called *hexamine, acetoform, hexamethylenaminesalicylsulfonic acid.*

methenamine hippurate $C_6H_{12}N_4,C_9H_9NO_3$. Hexamethylenetetramine hippurate. A white crystalline powder, soluble in water and alcohol. It has the same antimicrobial action as methenamine, though hippuric acid, a bacteriostatic agent, may contribute to the effect. It is used to treat urinary tract infections. Also called *hexamine hippurate.*

methenamine mandelate $C_6H_{12}N_4,C_8H_8O_3$. Hexamethylenetetramine mandelate. A white crystalline solid, very soluble in water and alcohol. It is used to treat urinary tract infections. The salt has the same antimicrobial spectrum of activity as methenamine, plus the bacteriostatic contribution of mandelic acid. Also called *hexamine mandelate.*

Methergine A proprietary name for methylergonovine maleate.

methestrol PROMETHESTROL.

methetoin $C_{12}H_{14}N_2O_2$. 5-Ethyl-1-methyl-5-phenyl-2,4-imidazoleidinedione. An analogue of phenytoin used as an anticonvulsant agent in the treatment of various forms of epileptic seizures. It is given orally.

methexenyl HEXOBARBITAL.

methicillin sodium $C_{17}H_{19}N_2NaO_6S$. 6-(2,6-Dimethoxybenzamido)-3,3-dimethyl-7-oxo-4-thia-1-azabicyclo[3.2.0]heptane-2-carboxylic acid sodium salt. A semisynthetic antibiotic derived from penicillin. It is used in the treatment of infections due to organisms resistant to penicillin G, due to penicillinase production. It is given intramuscularly or intravenously. Also called *dimethoxyphenyl penicillin sodium, sodium methicillin.*

methilepsia [Gk *meth(ē)* strong drink, drunkenness + *i* or *methy* wine + -LEPSIA] A morbid craving for alcohol. An older term. Also called *methomania.* Also *methelepsia, methylepsia.*

methimazole $C_4H_6N_2S$. 1-Methyl-2-mercaptoimidazole, a potent and widely used antithyroid agent, used in the treatment of hyperthyroidism (Graves disease). It acts by interfering with the incorporation of iodine into an organic form, thus inhibiting the biosynthesis of the thyroid hormones.

methine The group ═CH—.

methiodal sodium CH_2INaO_3S. Iodomethanesulfonic acid sodium salt. An iodine-containing compound used as a contrast medium to visualize the urinary-tract structures by intravenous urography and retrograde pyelography.

methionine $CH_3—S—CH_2—CH_2—CH(NH_3^+)—COO^-$. One of the twenty amino acids that can be incorporated into proteins. It is essential in mammalian diet. It is converted by methionine adenosyltransferase into the sulfonium salt *S*-adenosylmethionine, which is the main biologic donor of methyl groups. Symbol: Met, M

active methionine An outmoded term for *S*-ADENOSYL-METHIONINE.

methionine adenosyltransferase The enzyme (EC 2.5.1.6) that converts methionine into *S*-adenosylmethionine using ATP, and forming also orthophosphate and pyrophosphate (diphosphate). This reaction activates methionine for methyl donation.

methionine sulfoximine The compound formed by changing the group —S— in methionine into —S(O)(NH)—.It is formed from methionine residues in flour when this is treated with nitrogen trichloride, as was once done to bleach it. The compound is highly toxic.

methisazone 2-(1,2-Dihydro-1-methyl-2-oxo-3*H*-indol-3-ylidene)hydrazinecarbothioamide. A synthetic antiviral agent of little clinical use. It has been reported to confer short-term protection against smallpox, but is ineffective once the disease has developed. Also called *thiosemicarbazone*.

Methium A proprietary name for hexamethonium chloride.

methixene hydrochloride $C_{20}H_{23}N_5HCl \cdot H_2O$. 1-Methyl-3-(9*H*-thioxanthen-9-yl-methyl)piperidine hydrochloride. An anticholinergic agent utilized therapeutically in the treatment of gastrointestinal hypermotility and spasm. It is given orally.

methocarbamol $C_{11}H_{15}NO_5$. 3-(*o*-Methoxyphenoxy)-1,2-propanediol-1-carbamate. A muscle relaxant agent administered orally, intramuscularly, or intravenously.

method

method [META- + Gk *hodos* way, path, road] A way or manner of performing an action or of accomplishing a result. For terms not found under *method*, see also under *procedure, technique, stain,* and *test.*

Abbott's method A technique for the correction of scoliosis in which the patient is placed on a special frame and a plaster body jacket is applied while the patient is undergoing traction.

A.B.C. method An obsolete method of treating sewage, using alum, blood, clay, charcoal, or other substances to precipitate the sludge and deodorize the effluent. Also called *A.B.C. process.*

Abell-Kendall method An analytical technique for quantifying total serum cholesterol. The cholesterol and cholesteryl esters are first extracted from the serum and hydrolyzed, thus avoiding interferences from protein and nonspecific chromogens. Acetic anhydride and sulfuric acid are then combined with the serum to obtain the final color reaction.

absorption method The use of adsorption onto a solid medium to separate materials from a mixed solution or suspension. Either the antigen or antibody can be removed by attachment to the solid phase, using adsorbing material which can be either an intrinsic part of the solid phase surface or can be artifically bound to a surface.

acid hematin method A procedure for estimation of the hemoglobin concentration of blood, based on the formation of hematin from hemoglobin upon mixing a small quantity of blood with a 0.1 mol/l HCl solution. The intensity of the brown color of the solution so formed is compared with precalibrated tinted glass standards. This method is now rarely used. Also called *Sahli's method.*

Adams method A method in which the fat content of milk is measured by extracting, drying, and weighing the fat from a fixed volume of milk that has been dried on filter paper.

Addis method An obsolete method of evaluating renal disease by quantifying the cells, formed elements, and protein present in a 12-hour urine specimen.

Adelmann's method Flexion of an extremity by force as a first aid measure to control hemorrhage. An obsolete term.

agar diffusion method A method of estimating drug sensitivity or concentration by determining the diameter of the area of growth inhibition around a deposit of the drug on a heavily seeded plate. The method is also used for bioassay of a nutrient required by an auxotrophic test organism. Also called *auxanographic method.*

Ahlfeld's method Disinfection of the hands with hot water followed by a rinse with alcohol, an old-fashioned method.

alkaline hematin method Measurement of hemoglobin concentration after treating blood with a sodium hydroxide solution of 0.1 mol/l. This method is now obsolete.

alternate case method A method of testing the value of a form of therapy by applying it to other patients having the disease or injury under investigation.

alternate paired-case method A method of evaluating the efficacy of a drug or procedure. Patients are paired according to the extent of the disease present and other characteristics. A different drug is used on each member of the pairs.

Altmann's method A histologic staining technique that uses acid fuchsin and picric acid to demonstrate mitochondria.

Altmann-Gersh method A method of freeze-drying tissue in a vacuum for histologic examination.

aniline-fuchsin-methyl green method A staining method for mitochondria utilizing acid fuchsin dissolved in aniline water, followed by a methyl green counterstain.

arch bar method Intermaxillary reduction and splinting of a fracture by rubber bands attached to labial arch wires which are themselves attached to the teeth.

Aronson's method A method of producing gaseous formaldehyde by heating trioxymethylene.

Ashby method A technique for measuring the survival of transfused red cells without using radionuclide labeling. Compatible cells that possess a surface antigen absent from the host's cells are injected into the host. An agglutinating antibody specific for that surface antigen is then added. The proportion of transfused cells present in an aliquot of blood is determined by counting cell agglutinates. Also called *differential agglutination method.*

auxanographic method AGAR DIFFUSION METHOD.

Baer's method A technique once performed to prevent the formation of intra-articular adhesions in a joint in which oil was injected into the joint.

Bangerter's method PLEOPTICS.

Baréty's method A technique of lower limb traction that is used in the treatment of hip disorders.

Barraquer's method Cataract extraction performed with a suction cup.

Bass method A vibratory toothbrushing technique in which an attempt is made to clean the gingival sulcus. The bristles of a soft brush are directed at 45° into the gingival sulcus, and the brush head vibrated with a very small circular movement.

bathophenanthroline method An analytical technique for

measuring iron in serum. Ferric iron is dissociated from serum proteins, reduced to the ferrous state, and reacted with the disodium salt of bathophenanthroline (4,7-diphenyl-1,10-phenanthroline) sulfonate to yield a red-colored complex which can be measured spectrophotometrically.

Beck's method 1 A surgical treatment of tuberculosis of bone that involves scraping all infected material from the cavity and then packing the cavity with Beck's paste. 2 BECK'S GASTROSTOMY.

Bell method A vertical toothbrushing technique in which the bristles of a soft multituft brush are swept from the teeth to gums. Also called *physiologic method.*

Benedict's method A method for detecting glucose and other reducing substances in urine, based on the reduction of copper (II) ions to the copper (I) state.

Benedict and Newton method Preparation of a protein-free filtrate following precipitation of blood proteins by use of a tungstomolybdic acid reagent.

Berger's method The repair of a transverse fracture of the patella with bridging sutures.

Bethe's method A fixation method that employs ammonium molybdate and osmium tetroxide and is used prior to staining peripheral nerve endings with methylene blue.

Bethea's method A method of detecting reduced movement of one side of the thorax by palpation of movement of the ribs.

Bielschowsky's method BIELSCHOWSKY STAIN.

bipolar method A method of recording the electrical activity of the brain underlying two electrodes which are connected to a single channel of the electroencephalograph. There is usually one electrode which is common to two successive channels, three electrodes in series being connected, in pairs, to each of the two channels.

Bivine's method Treatment of the convulsions of strychnine poisoning by administering chloral hydrate.

Blanchard's method BLANCHARD'S TREATMENT.

Bliss method The transformation into probits of the relative frequency of responses obtained in a bioassay. Also called *Bliss transformation.*

Bloch's method for dopa oxidase A histochemical method used to demonstrate dopa oxidase activity in cells, usually undertaken to identify melanoblasts. A dark brown pigment localizes the sites where dopa oxidase acts upon the substrate L-dopa.

Bodian method A method of staining nerve cells and fibers with silver in paraffin sections.

Born method of wax plate reconstruction The construction of a series of wax plates of equal thickness cut out according to the scaled enlargements of serial sections of the part or structure being reconstructed. The plates are placed on top of each other to produce a three-dimensional model of the part or structure.

Brandt-Andrews method BRANDT-ANDREWS MANEUVER.

breath alcohol method A method for measuring the alcohol concentration in expired alveolar air, as of a motor vehicle operator suspected of being impaired by the influence of alcohol. Various tests are used, but all are based on an equation derived from Henry's law: the weight of alcohol in 2100 mls of expired alveolar air equals the weight of alcohol in one ml of blood.

brine flotation method A method to concentrate parasitic ova from feces. Ova rise to the top and solid fecal material sinks to the bottom in a solution with a relative density of 1.16 to 1.18. The method is seldom used today.

bromcresol green method A dye-binding method for quantification of serum albumin. A bromcresol green solution buffered to pH 4.2 is mixed with the serum sample, and the absorbance change is read at 628 nm. The method may conveniently be automated and is not subject to bilirubin or salicylate inter-

ference. It may, however, give erroneously high readings at very low albumin concentrations.

Brunninghausen's method An obsolete means of inducing labor by manual dilatation of the uterine cervix.

Butler and Tuthill method WEINBACH'S METHOD.

C method A chromosome banding technique which stains the centric regions and other constitutive heterochromatic regions of the chromosome. Also called *centric heterochromatin method.*

Cajal method A histologic technique for demonstrating the presence of astrocytes in nervous tissue that uses gold chloride impregnation.

Cajal's double method ACHUCÁRRO STAIN.

caliper method A method for estimating body fat content by using calipers to measure the skin fold thickness at selected points on the body surface.

Calkins method Following delivery of the infant, delay in delivering the placenta until the uterus assumes a globular shape, indicating placental separation.

Callahan's method CHLOROPERCHA METHOD.

Carrel's method Anastomosis of two blood vessels end to end with no compromise of the lumen. An obsolete term.

cartesian diver method A method of measuring pressure fluctuations at the surface of a liquid by monitoring the vertical position of a gas-filled chamber floating in the liquid.

Castañeda's method A procedure for visualizing rickettsiae and viral inclusion bodies in smears. A thin smear is made in a phosphate buffer, then is stained with methylene blue solution and counterstained with safranine solution. Rickettsiae and inclusion bodies stain pale blue while tissue cells stain red.

Castel method 1 A histochemical method to demonstrate arsenic in tissue, which is fixed in formalin containing 2.5% cupric acetate. Arsenic, if present, produces bright green cupric acetoarsenite. 2 A histochemical method to demonstrate the presence of bismuth in frozen sections of formalin-fixed tissue. A positive reaction is the formation of red quinine iodobismuthate.

cathartic method CATHARSIS.

Cathelin's method SPINAL ANESTHESIA.

centric heterochromatin method C METHOD.

Chandler's method Fibrinogen determination by nitrogen assay of clot precipitated from plasma by calcium chloride.

Chaput's method A surgical procedure for treatment of osteomyelitis consisting of scraping all necrotic tissue from the cavity and then packing with a free graft of fat.

Charter's method A vibratory toothbrushing technique in which the bristles of a hard two-rowed brush are applied at 45° to the long axes of the teeth directed toward the biting surfaces. The head of the brush is rotated in small circles with the bristles forced between the teeth and exerts a massaging action on the gingiva.

Chervin's method CHERVIN'S TREATMENT.

Chèvremont-Combaire method A histochemical method used to estimate riboflavin, involving the reduction of riboflavin to leucoriboflavin and reoxidation to rhodoflavin.

chloropercha method A method of filling a root canal with gutta percha cones partially dissolved in chloroform. Also called *Callahan's method, Johnston's method.*

Choman's method for nickel A histochemical method to demonstrate nickel in frozen tissue sections. A positive reaction is indicated by the formation of red needle-shaped crystals when nickel-containing tissue is stained with dimethylglyoxime after exposure to ammonia fumes.

Ciaccio's method A histologic staining technique for demonstrating the presence of neutral fat by using an acid dichromate fixative followed by an oil-soluble stain such as Sudan III. Also called *Ciaccio stain.*

Clark-Collip method A classic reference method, now seldom used, for measuring serum calcium. Calcium is precipitated as calcium oxalate, which is converted to oxalic acid by solution in sulfuric acid. The oxalic acid is measured by titration against potassium permanganate.

Clausen's method A colorimetric method to measure lactate in body fluids. Currently available enzymatic techniques have rendered this procedure obsolete.

closed-plaster method The immobilization of a wound, fracture, or infected part by means of a circumferential plaster cast.

confrontation method Visual field measurement with handheld test objects and no background perimeter or campimeter.

Conway method 1 A diffusion technique for the measurement of volatile materials or substances that can be converted quantitatively to volatile analytes. The material to be volatized is placed in the outer ring of a sealed chamber; a central chamber contains material that will both trap and quantify or titrate the diffused analyte. The technique was used originally for determination of ammonia and urea nitrogen, and it is still employed for analysis of volatile toxic substances. **2** An obsolete method for measuring chloride.

Coons fluorescent antibody method The use of fluoresence labeling to identify the location of antibody on a slide. An antibody conjugated to a fluorochrome can be used in direct immunofluorescent techniques, in which a labeled antibody reacts with its specific antigen, or in indirect immunofluorescent techniques, in which a fluorochrome-labeled antiglobulin serum attaches to and allows visualization of an unlabeled antibody that has reacted with an antigen in cells or tissues.

Copenhagen method A technique of artificial respiration developed in the Danish army. With the patient in prone position, inspiration is produced by extension of the arms and expiration by pressure on the scapulae. Also called *Holger Nielsen method.*

copper sulfate method Determination of the specific gravity of blood or plasma by observing the rise, fall, or motionless suspension of drops of blood or other assay fluid in a series of copper sulfate solutions having specific gravity increments of 0.004.

Corning's method SPINAL ANESTHESIA.

coupling method A technique used in transmitting ultrasound from the transducer surface into the body without significant loss of ultrasonic energy. Typically a gel fills the space between the transducer and the skin to exclude the film of air that would cause large reflections.

Coutard's method A method of roentgentherapy consisting of the administration of small doses of irradiation at intervals over a prolonged time.

Cox modification of Golgi's corrosive sublimate method A modern variant of Golgi's method for staining nervous tissue that uses mercuric chloride.

Cox yolk-sac method Cultivation of *Rickettsia prowazeki* in the yolk sac of eggs with subsequent formalin treatment for production of a vaccine against typhus. Newer live vaccines are more effective.

Crane method The use of a skin flap to transfer tissue to a distant recipient site, after which the flap is returned to its original location.

Credé's method CREDÉ'S MANEUVER.

Credé method of expressing placenta Application to the uterus of pressure down into the pelvis while massaging the uterine fundus.

Cronin method A method often used to lengthen the nasal columella, especially the short columella associated with bilateral cleft lip.

cross-sectional method A method of research in psychology which focuses on a given process, such as intelligence or psychomotor coordination. This may be measured in two or more groups of subjects at different stages of development, but at a given time. Contrasts between the groups can then be made and some inferences attempted about the form and development that particular process would have taken if the same individuals could have been followed at intervals over a lifetime. Also called *cross-sectional study.*

Cuignet's method The measurement of refractive error by retinoscopy.

cyanmethemoglobin method Determination of hemoglobin concentration of blood by conversion of all forms of hemoglobin (except sulfhemoglobin) to cyanmethemoglobin and measuring absorbence at 540 nm relative to known standards.

Dakin-Carrel method CARREL'S TREATMENT.

Dare's method Determination of hemoglobin concentration by visual comparison with a color standard. This method is now obsolete but was once widely used.

Davenport's alcoholic silver nitrate method A silver impregnation technique for the differential staining of nerve cells and nerve fibers. Also called *Davenport stain.*

Defer's method Evacuation and cauterization of a hydrocele sac with silver nitrate.

definitive method An analytic method whose precision, specificity, and freedom from systematic error have been studied and expressed in an uncertainty statement, which shows the method to be optimally compatible with the goals of the analysis. The midpoint of the overall bounds of error can be taken as the true value.

deletion method DELETION MAPPING.

Delore's method The performance of manual osteoclasis in order to correct genu valgum. It was originally used primarily to correct the deformity in cases of rickets.

Demme's method Iodine injection for hydrocele.

Diamond's method The application of Ehrlich's test for urobilinogen to serial dilutions of urine. Also called *Wallace-Diamond method.*

Dick's method DICK TEST.

Dickinson method A technique to control postpartum hemorrhage. The uterus is lifted superiorly out of the pelvis and compressed against the vertebral column.

Dieffenbach's method DIEFFENBACH'S OPERATION.

differential agglutination method ASHBY METHOD.

diffraction method The determination of average erythrocyte diameter by measuring the diffraction of light through a blood smear.

direct method The use of a direct ophthalmoscope.

direct aeration method The determination of blood urea by urease conversion to ammonium carbonate, acid aeration of ammonia, treatment with Nessler's reagent, and colorimetric comparison.

direct centrifugal flotation method A method of concentrating nonoperculated helminth eggs and protozoan cysts by suspending filtered fecal matter in a saturated saline solution, which is then centrifuged. The supernatant is picked up with a bacterial loop or by touching it with a coverslip. This suspension is then examined microscopically for parasites. Also called *Lane method.*

disk sensitivity method The antimicrobial susceptibility test performed with drug-impregnated disks placed on an agar culture medium.

Domagk's method A technique for demonstrating the presence of phagocytic cells of the reticuloendothelial system in which a bacterial culture is injected intravenously into a rat, which is then killed. The tissues are subsequently stained with Gram stain and borax carmine.

Douglas method The spontaneous conversion of a fetal transverse lie to a breech presentation through intrauterine rotation.

Drinker's method A technique of artificial respiration in which a second person assists in inspiration by raising the patient's arms.

Dubois method DUBOIS TREATMENT.

Dubois-Brachet method A histochemical reaction used to show the localization of ribonucleic acid. It is based upon the disappearance of the basophilic staining properties following digestion with ribonuclease.

Duke's method DUKE BLEEDING TIME TEST.

Duplay's method DUPLAY'S OPERATION.

Eicken's method A method for examining the larynx and hypopharynx using a special esophageal speculum.

Erlangen method A method of radiation therapy consisting of the delivery of a large dose of irradiation through multiple portals at one treatment session.

Esbach's method A method for semiquantitative measurement of protein in the urine. It involves precipitation with picric acid, followed by measuring the volume of the precipitate. Although rarely used now, for many years this was one of the useful methods for estimating the degree of proteinuria.

excess lime method LIME TREATMENT.

method of extinct generations A method of estimating annual mortality rates at very advanced ages for the purpose of constructing life tables.

Fahraeus method A method for determination of the erythrocyte sedimentation rate.

falling-drop method A means of determining specific gravity by adding drops of a liquid to cylinders containing solutions of known specific gravity. By observing the specific gravity of the solutions in which the drop falls, remains stationary, or rises, one can infer the specific gravity of the test material, precision being dependent upon the gradations of known specific gravities used. This method is most often used as a rapid means of ascertaining acceptable hemoglobin levels in the blood of prospective blood donors.

Faust's method A centrifugal concentration method for detecting helminth eggs or larvae or protozoan cysts, in which zinc sulfate solution (relative density 1.18) is the suspending medium.

Fell-O'Dwyer method A technique of artificial respiration, introduced in the late nineteenth century, utilizing a bellows to force air into an intubated patient.

Feulgen method A histologic technique used to demonstrate the presence of DNA. Mild acid hydrolysis releases aldehyde groups which can then be demonstrated using the periodic acid-Schiff stain. The appearance of a purple color indicates a positive reaction, or the presence of DNA. Also called *Feulgen procedure, Feulgen's test.*

Fick's method A technique for measuring cardiac output using the Fick principle.

Fishberg's method FISHBERG CONCENTRATION TEST.

Fiske and Subbarow method **1** Determination of acid-soluble phosphorus by heating with nitric and sulfuric acids to denature organic matter, precipitating phosphorus as magnesium ammonium phosphate, reducing precipitate with *p*-aminonaphthylsulfonic acid, and colorimetric comparison with known phosphate standards. **2** Determination of inorganic phosphate by precipitating as ammonium phosphomolybdate, followed by reduction and colorimetric assay as above.

Fitz Gerald method ZONE THERAPY.

flash method A process used for pasteurizing milk in which the temperature of the milk is raised to 74°C for a few seconds and then quickly cooled. In the normal pasteurization procedure a temperature of 60°C is used. However, in the flash method, the length of time of heating is much reduced below the 30 seconds normally used. This leads to less development of a "cooked" flavor.

flotation method Any of a number of methods for separating

helminth ova and protozoan cysts from other components of feces, based on using a solution of a density (specific gravity usually 1.180) intermediate between that of parasitic ova and cysts, which float, and the remainder of the stool that is heavier and is deposited as sediment following centrifugation or direct flotation.

fogging method Refraction of hyperopia by use of excessive plus lens strength.

Folin and Svedberg method The determination of blood urea by urease conversion to ammonium carbonate, addition of Nessler's reagent, distillation of ammonia, and colorimetric measurement.

Folin and Wright's method A modification of Kjeldahl's test for nitrogen in the urine.

Fones method A toothbrushing technique with the teeth in occlusion and the head of the brush describing large circles over the teeth and gums. With the teeth apart smaller circles are used for lingual surfaces and an anteroposterior scrub for the occlusal aspects. Also called *Fones technique.*

Forsgren method A histochemical technique to demonstrate the presence of bile acids in tissue sections. The tissue is treated with barium chloride, acid fuchsin, phosphomolybdic acid, and aniline blue-orange G. If the tissue assumes a reddish blue color, the reaction is positive. The procedure is now seldom used in the United States.

Freiburg method A seldom-used approach to analgesia and anesthesia during labor and delivery in which a variety of drugs are used to produce amnesia. An obsolete term.

Fridericia's method A method of measuring the concentration of carbon dioxide in a gas, such as expired air, by measuring the decrease in volume after absorption in a solution of potassium hydroxide.

Friedemann and Graeser method The determination of lactic acid by glucose removal and conversion of lactic acid to acetaldehyde, which is combined with sodium bisulfite and measured by iodimetry. Also called *Graeser's method.*

Fülleborn's method A flotation method for detecting parasite eggs in feces that involves grinding 1 gm of stool, mixing it with 20 ml of a saturated solution of salt and, after an hour, placing a coverglass on the surface of the mixture, transferring the adherent liquid and parasitic material directly to a slide for microscopic examination. Also called *Hung's method, Wilson's method.*

G method GIEMSA METHOD.

Gerota's method A technique of injecting lymphatics for anatomical purposes with prussian blue dissolved in chloroform, ether, or alcohol.

Giemsa method A method of chromosome banding in which chromosomes are treated with trypsin, which denatures chromosomal protein, and are then stained with Giemsa stain. The chromosomes take the stain in a pattern of dark and light bands (G bands). Also called *G method.*

Gilmer method Intermaxillary wiring of teeth in occlusion. A wire is twisted around the neck of each tooth, and then with another similar wire on the opposing tooth.

Girard's method GIRARD'S TREATMENT.

glucose oxidase method A highly specific analytical method for the detection of glucose in which the enzyme glucose oxidase acts on glucose to yield gluconic acid and hydrogen peroxide. The attendant oxygen consumption may be measured directly, or a second peroxidase step may be added to yield a colored end product.

Golgi's method A histologic technique for differentiating nervous tissue that uses potassium dichromate followed by silver nitrate impregnation. It is used to demonstrate a selection of neurons and neuroglial cells.

Gomori's method **1** A histologic silver impregnation technique for reticulin fibers. **2** An aldehyde fuchsin method for distinguishing elastic fibers. **3** Any of several histochemical techniques for identifying acid and alkaline phosphatase. For defs. 1, 2, and 3 also called *Gomori stain.*

Gordon and Sweet method A histologic silver impregnation technique for the demonstration of reticulin fibers.

Graeser's method Friedemann and Graeser method.

Graff method Indophenol test.

Gram's method Gram stain.

Greenberg's method The determination of serum proteins by separation with sodium sulfate, treatment with a phenol reagent, and colorimetric comparison.

Greenwald and Lewman method Determination of titratable alkali of blood by precipitating protein with excess picric acid, determining free and total picric acid in filtrate, and attributing the difference to binding by titratable alkali.

Greenwood-Yule method A statistical technique to test whether the occurrence of a disease or abnormality is dependent on birth order. The procedure is not subject to bias due to associations between risk and sibship size and is therefore less subject to disturbance from factors influencing the latter. It has the disadvantage that sibships must be complete before the analysis can be undertaken.

Grossich's method The use of tincture of iodine as a topical antiseptic agent preparatory to a surgical procedure.

Gruber's method A technique used for inflation of the middle ear. It is a modification of politzerization where, instead of swallowing as the bag is compressed, the patient says "hik" or "huk."

Habel's method A test for potency of rabies vaccines made from inactivated rabies virus, in which lethality of a standard virus preparation is compared in vaccinated and nonvaccinated mice.

Haden-Hausser method The determination of hemoglobin concentration of blood by dilution in a white-cell pipette, conversion to acid hematin, and colorimetric comparison by microscopic examination via a specially designed dilution chamber. Also called *Hausser method.*

Hagedorn and Jensen method Determination of blood sugar by precipitating protein with zinc hydroxide, heating filtrate with potassium ferricyanide, and determining ferricyanide reduction by addition of iodide followed by sodium thiosulfate titration of the free iodine produced.

Hamilton's method A technique to control postpartum hemorrhage. One hand maintains pressure on the uterine fundus while the other hand is placed as a fist in the vagina.

Hammerschlag's method Determination of the specific gravity of blood by observing the rise, fall, or motionless suspension of a sample in mixtures of benzene and chloroform of known proportions and therefore of calculable specific gravity.

Handley's method Handley's lymphangioplasty.

Harris method A method of staining tissue to demonstrate the presence of Negri bodies.

Hart's method An old method of measuring casein in milk by precipatation and titration.

Hartel's method A technique of injecting the gasserian ganglion which involves approaching the foramen ovale from inside the mouth.

Hausser method Haden-Hausser method.

Hellige method An obsolete method for determination of hemoglobin concentration by conversion to acid hematin and visual comparison with color standards.

hematoxylin-safranin method A double stain that uses the metachromatic property of safranin to demonstrate the presence of mucin and cartilage.

Heublein method A method of whole-body irradiation using low doses for many hours each day for several days.

hexokinase method An analytical method for detecting the presence of glucose in which the enzyme hexokinase acts on glucose and ATP to yield glucose 6-phosphate and ADP. A second enzyme, glucose-6-phosphate dehydrogenase, converts the glucose 6-phosphate and NADP to 6-phosphogluconate and NADPH, which can be measured spectrophotometrically.

Hilton's method The division of sensory nerves supplying the region of an ulcer.

hip lift-prone pressure method An artificial respiration technique in which expiration is assisted by lifting of the hips.

hip roll-prone pressure method An artificial respiration technique in which expiration is assisted by rolling of the hips to one side or the other.

Hirschberg's method Estimation of ocular deviation by observing the corneal light reflex.

Hirschfeld's method A vibratory toothbrushing technique with the bristles approximately at right angles to the teeth. For the inner aspects of the dental arches, the brush is held as nearly vertical as possible.

holding method A method involving the heating of milk to 65°C and maintaining it at that temperature for 35–45 minutes, as a means of pasteurization.

Holger Nielsen method Copenhagen method.

horizontal scrub method A toothbrushing technique in which the teeth and gums are brushed with short horizontal strokes.

Hortega method A histologic technique that uses silver carbonate impregnation of nervous tissue to demonstrate the presence of glial cells.

Hotchkiss method Schiff's test.

Howard's method An artificial respiration technique in which the patient is prone with the head lower than the abdomen and the hands under the head. Respiration is effected by pressure applied to both sides of the thoracic cage.

Howell's method Determination of clotting time of blood by measuring the time required for 5 ml of whole blood to clot in a 21 mm test tube that is being tilted every two minutes.

Howe silver precipitation method A method of precipitating silver within the hard tissues of a tooth by applying silver nitrate solution followed by reduction with eugenol or formalin.

Hung's method Fülleborn's method.

Hunt's method A bioassay using mice that was developed to measure the activity of thyroid preparations, based upon the reduction in toxicity of a test dose of acetonitrile after a 10-day administration of the test material (thyroid preparation).

impedance method The use of electrical impedance measurements for localizing brain structures.

India ink method A method for visualizing spirochetes and yeasts or other fungi. A smear is made using a loopful of the material to be examined with a loopful of India ink. The organisms appear white against a black background. Also called *India ink stain, negative stain.*

indirect method A method of making a gold inlay or other gold casting by first taking an impression of the prepared tooth and making a die from it. A wax pattern is built up on the die, and after removal from the die it is invested, heated and cast in gold. It is returned to the die for finishing and polishing and is then ready to be cemented to the prepared tooth.

indophenol method A quantitative method used in the calculation of the vitamin C content of plant and animal tissues. Vitamin C, in acid solution, is used to reduce a standard indophenol solution to a colorless compound.

introspective method A technique of psychological experimentation making use of systematic self-observation. The subject gives a verbal report on all conscious experience or feelings that may be related to a stimulus situation, usually without any attempt at discovering meaning or interpretation but only to provide an objective report on the contents, elements, or processes of consciousness.

Italian method ITALIAN RHINOPLASTY.

Ivy's method IVY BLEEDING TIME TEST.

Japanese method A technique to improve adherence of tissue sections to glass slides by using Mayer's albumin.

Johnson's modification method A modification of Callahan's method of root canal treatment. The main canal is filled with solid gutta percha.

Johnston's method CHLOROPERCHA METHOD.

Kaiserling's method A TECHNIQUE FOR PRESERVING THE NATURAL COLORS OF MUSEUM SPECIMENS. See under KAISERLING'S FLUID.

Karr's method Determination of urea in blood by enzymatic conversion to ammonium carbonate, treatment with Nessler's reagent, and colorimetric comparison with known standards similarly prepared.

Keating-Hart method Fulguration of a surface cancer.

Kenny's method A poliomyelitis rehabilitation technique extensively used in the early twentieth century. Hot wet packs and passive range-of-motion exercises and muscle reeducation are utilized in the acute stage of the disease.

Kety-Schmidt method A method of measuring cerebral blood flow using inhalation of nitrous oxide.

Kittrich method A straining method for detecting epidermal cells of fetal origin in amniotic fluid discharged per vaginam. They stain red after application of dilute Nile blue sulfate.

Kjeldahl's method KJELDAHL'S TEST.

Klapp's method KLAPP'S CREEPING TREATMENT.

Klüver-Barrera method A histologic technique that uses Luxol fast blue to stain myelin a blue-green color.

Korotkoff's method The determination of blood pressure using auscultation. See also KOROTKOFF SOUNDS.

Krause's method FULL-THICKNESS GRAFT.

Kristeller's method An old-fashioned maneuver to assist expulsion of the fetus. Manual pressure is applied to the uterine fundus when the fetal head is on the perineum. Also called *Kristeller technique*.

Laborde's method Treatment of asphyxiation by rhythmical traction of the tongue to stimulate spontaneous respiration.

Lamaze method A technique utilized by women in labor in which concentration is shifted from the discomfort of uterine contractions to relaxing maneuvers in order to reduce or eliminate the need for analgesia. In addition, the method requires antenatal practice of exercises and provides detailed information about labor and delivery so that couples are fully prepared for childbirth.

Lane method DIRECT CENTRIFUGAL FLOTATION METHOD.

Langendorff's method LANGENDORFF PREPARATION.

lateral condensation method A method of filling a root canal with a number of gutta percha cones one after the other, space being made for each addition by spreading the others apart with a special instrument called a root canal spreader. Also called *multiple cone method*.

lead dioxide method LEAD DIOXIDE CANDLE.

lead peroxide method LEAD DIOXIDE CANDLE.

Leake and Guy method The enumeration of platelets using light microscopy and a counting chamber of known volume after careful dilution in an aqueous solution of formalin, sodium oxalate and crystal violet. Although the test is seldom used now, it is historically important.

method of least squares A statistical procedure involving the substitution of some function of the variable from each observed value such that the sum of the squares of the differences between the pairs of observed and calculated values is a minimum. The technique is used for calculating a line of best fit in linear regression.

Leboyer method A method of conducting labor and delivery in which the newborn is handled as gently as possible by avoiding obstetric forceps, not using bright lights, and by placing the infant in a warm bath immediately after delivery.

Letonoff and Reinhold method A colorimetric method for determination of inorganic sulfate in serum after deproteinization, precipitation and redissolution.

Levaditi's method A histologic staining method for detecting spirochetes in which a block of tissue is impregnated with silver nitrate and sectioned after reducing the silver with pyrogallol.

Levy, Rowntree, and Marriott method Determination of the hydrogen ion concentration of blood by dialysis against physiologic saline, addition of phenolsulfonphthalein to the dialysate, and colorimetric comparison with known standards.

Lewisohn's method A technique of treating blood with sodium citrate, thereby making indirect transfusion possible.

light-field method A method for counting dust particles on a slide by using a light microscope.

lime method A technique to generate gaseous formaldehyde by adding 10% sulfuric acid and 40% formaldehyde to calcium oxide.

Lindemann's method An obsolete but historical technique of direct blood transfusion utilizing a system of cannula and syringe connecting the venous circulations of the donor and recipient.

Ling's method SWEDISH GYMNASTICS.

linguistic-kinesic method The study of language and movement disturbances as one expression of behavior or mental disorder.

Linser's method The injection of mercuric chloride into varicose veins to obliterate the varices. An obsolete term.

Lister's method LISTERISM.

longitudinal method A method of research in psychology which studies the same individual, or group of individuals, over a considerable period of time, making periodic measurements of a given process at critical stages of developmental change or over the entire life span. Also called *longitudinal study*.

Looney and Dyer method for potassium in blood A colorimetric method for determination of serum potassium after deproteinization, precipitation as a metallic nitrite complex, and redissolution.

Lorenz method A manipulation technique for the reduction of a congenitally dislocated hip.

Lorthiore's method The repair of an inguinal hernia by dissecting the sac to free it and then removing it without incising the inguinal canal directly.

Lowry-Lopez-Bessey method A spectrophotometric method to measure ascorbic acid in plasma in which ascorbic acid is oxidized, combined with 2,4-dinitrophenylhydrazine, and added to sulfuric acid to yield a red compound.

Løvset's method LØVSET'S MANEUVER.

MacLachlan method MACLACHLAN'S PROCESS.

macro-Kjeldahl method KJELDAHL'S TEST.

Majorström method The use of a vacuum extractor, a suction device applied to the fetal head, to effect vaginal delivery of an infant.

Malloy-Evelyn method A diazo reaction used to measure bilirubin. Conjugated bilirubin reacts directly with diazotized sulfanilic acid, forming purple azobilirubin. The addition of methanol to the specimen allows unconjugated bilirubin to react.

Manchester method A method of repairing a bilateral congenital cleft lip.

Mann's method A histologic staining technique that uses a mixture of methyl blue and eosin to distinguish nerve cells, Negri bodies, and amebas. Also called *Mann stain*.

Mantel-Haenszel method A method of statistical analysis of data from case-control studies to estimate the odds ratio and its standard error both when matched pairs are compared and when there is more than one matched control per case. ⟨Mantel, M. and Haenszel, W. *Journal of the National Cancer Institute* 22:719, 1959⟩

Marchi's method   A histologic technique that uses osmium tetroxide and potassium chlorate to differentiate normal from degenerating myelin.

Marfan's method   The technique of aspirating a pericardial effusion by epigastric puncture.

marking-recapture method   A method for the determination of the size of an animal population by marking a number of members of the population and releasing the marked individuals, then sampling a number of marked and unmarked individuals from the population. The number of marked individuals (percent recaptured) and the ratio of marked to unmarked individuals in the sample are used to estimate the number of animals in the population.

Masson's trichrome method   MASSON'S TRICHROME STAIN.

Maximow's method   HEMATOXYLIN-EOSIN-AZURE II STAIN.

Mayo's method   An obsolete method for treating trigeminal neuralgia in which the nerve is resected and then a silver screw is inserted in the foramen ovale. Also called *Mayo's treatment.*

McLean and Van Slyke method   An obsolete method for measuring chlorides in plasma.

Meltzer's method   The continuous tracheal insufflation of air or oxygen containing anesthetic vapor, a technique formerly used in thoracic surgery. Also called *Meltzer's anesthesia.*

metatrophic method   The alteration or modification of a patient's nutrition to increase the effectiveness of a drug being given at the same time.

Meulengracht's method   Estimation of the bilirubin concentration of serum by serially diluting the specimen until it matches a yellow standard. An obsolete procedure.

micro-Astrup method   A technique to determine partial pressure of carbon dioxide (PCO_2) in the blood by extrapolation from pH measurements. The measured pH of the specimen is plotted on a line constructed from the pH values determined on reference specimens of known PCO_2.

micro-Kjeldahl method   A modification of Kjeldahl's test that is designed to measure quantities of protein nitrogen in the range of a few milligrams.

Millard method   A method of repairing a bilateral congenital cleft lip. Also called *Millard operation.*

Minkowski's method   A technique of kidney palpation following gas dilatation of the colon. Also called *Naunyn-Minkowski method.*

monopolar method   An electroencephalographic method in which the activity of the brain occurring beneath a single electrode is recorded. As current can only flow between two electrodes, there must always be a second register or indifferent electrode, and the channel to which each electrode pair is connected records the electrical activity passing between the active and the register electrodes. As it is virtually impossible to find a point on the skull where a register electrode can be placed without recording underlying cerebral activity, this method is now little used.

Monte Carlo method   The analysis of system behavior done by randomly changing system parameters, observing system output, and then simulating the system on a computer.

Morestin's method   MORESTIN'S OPERATION.

Morison's method   Wound treatment by débridement and application of a thin layer of B.I.P. paste. This method is useful in preserving viability of exposed tendons in a wound not suitable for closure.

multiple cone method   LATERAL CONDENSATION METHOD.

Murphy method   **1** An obsolete method of vascular suture in which the vessel ends are invaginated over a small metal tube. **2** MURPHY DRIP.

Myers method   Estimation of the urea concentration of blood by conversion of urea to ammonium carbonate through the action of uricase. Ammonium is converted to ammonia, which is collected and measured by reaction with Nessler's reagent.

Naunyn-Minkowski method   MINKOWSKI'S METHOD.

Nègre and Bretey method   BCG vaccination by means of cutaneous scarifications, the number and dimension of which vary with the age of the subject.

nigrosin method   The use of the dye nigrosin as a negative stain to delineate microorganisms in a smear of unstained material, especially spirochetes or diphtheria bacilli. Organisms appear clear against a black background.

Nikiforoff's method   Fixation of blood films by immersion in pure ethanol or pure ether or in a 1:1 mixture of ethanol and ether.

Nimeh's method   A radiological technique of evaluating liver and spleen size by appropriate flat plates of the abdomen with or without carbon dioxide gas insufflation of the retroperitoneal space.

Nissl's method   A histologic technique that demonstrates the presence of aggregated RNA or Nissl granules in the cytoplasm of neurons.

no-touch method   **1** A technique used in cancer surgery for excision of a tumor whereby the blood and lymph supply is divided before the tumor itself is touched. This method is said to decrease the likelihood of disseminating tumor cells. **2** In a surgical procedure or in the treatment of wounds, a method of cleaning and dressing without the introduction of the sterile gloved hand or fingers into the wound or incision, all manipulation being performed by the use of sterile instruments.

Nové-Josserand method of reconstruction of urethra   In the treatment of hypospadias, the use of a tubed split-thickness skin graft to provide additional length to the urethra. The graft is secured from within by a rubber catheter and from without by a metal cannula.

nutritional table method   The calculation of food intake using food composition tables.

Ogino-Knaus method   A modification of the rhythm birth control method.

Ombrédanne method   A method of correcting hypospadias by reconstructing the urethra with a long rectangular turnover flap based at the receded urethral meatus. The resultant skin defect on the ventral shaft of the penis is then covered with another turnover flap fashioned from the prepuce. This second turnover flap must have a small slit incised in its center to accommodate the glans.

one-stage method   ONE-STAGE PROTHROMBIN TIME TEST.

optical density method   A method for measuring the concentration of a substance, or the density of a cell population in a fluid by directing a light of specific wavelength through the fluid and measuring the amount of light absorbed by the solution or suspension.

Orr method   ORR TREATMENT.

Orsi-Grocco method   A method of palpatory percussion of the heart.

Oudin's method   OUDIN TECHNIQUE.

ovulation method   A method of contraception in which intercourse is avoided during the fertile midmenstrual cycle time period, which is identified by monitoring changes in the cervical or vaginal mucus.

Pachon's method   An oscillometric method for assessing the patency of arteries. An obsolete term.

Pajot's method   An old-fashioned maneuver in which the head of a dead fetus is decapitated in order to facilitate vaginal delivery.

panoptic method   G BANDING.

Paracelsian method The treatment of diseases only by chemicals.

parallax method A radiologic method of localization, as of a radiopaque foreign structure within the body, by measuring the shift in position of the structure caused by a predetermined shift in the position of the x-ray tube.

part method A method of memorizing a large amount of material by first reducing it to small sections, each to be mastered in turn and then combined into the whole.

Pavlov's method The technique for studying conditioned reflex activity by measuring gastric or salivary secretion in awake dogs.

Payr's method An archaic method of vascular anastomosis that uses absorbable magnesium cylinders.

Perdrau's method A silver impregnation technique for the demonstration of reticulin fibers in tissue.

Pfiffner and Myers method Measurement of quanidine in blood by its reaction with ferricyanide and nitroprusside.

physiologic method BELL METHOD.

Pickrell's method PICKRELL SPRAY.

Pickworth method A stain for hemoglobin, using benzidine and nitroprussic acid. A rarely used term.

picture completion method A method of evaluating mental capacity in which the subject is asked to identify a missing part of a simple line drawing.

point source method A method of radiation therapy to the wall of the urinary bladder, consisting of a point source of radiation at the center of a Foley catheter bag, which is then distended with a solution, such as water, saline, or contrast medium.

Power and Wilder method An obsolete method for measuring urine glucose that uses alkaline ferricyanide.

Price-Jones method Determination of the distribution of erythrocyte diameters in a blood specimen.

probit method A statistical method of displaying the distribution of responses in biological assays that is based upon normal equivalent deviation units. The resulting plot of cumulative probability units versus the logarithm of the dose can be used to calculate the ED_{50} value and the dispersion of the population about the mean.

Prochownick's method A method of resuscitating a newborn by chest compression while the infant's head is in a hyperextended position.

projective method A psychological assessment technique utilizing unstructured tests that give minimal clues as to the appropriate responses and thus elicit interpretations based on the subject's needs, impulses, defenses, and drives. The Rorschach inkblot test and the ambiguous pictures of the thematic apperception test are examples of the use of the projective method.

Pryce slide-culture method A microculture technique to demonstrate *Mycobacterium tuberculosis*. The material is placed on a slide, dried, treated with acid, then washed and incubated with hemolyzed blood for seven days. It is then examined directly for the presence of acid-fast bacilli.

psychometric method The application of standardized tests for measuring one or more aspects of the mental ability of an individual, such as intelligence, aptitudes, interests, or personality characteristics.

psychophysical method Any of several standard procedures devised for investigating the relation between systematic variations in physical energies and the experience reported, or behavior evoked, in an experimental subject.

pulse reflection method PULSE ECHO TECHNIQUE.

Purmann's method A method of obliterating an aneurysmal sac.

Q method QUINACRINE FLUORESCENT METHOD.

quinacrine fluorescent method A chromosome banding technique in which chromosomes are treated with quinacrine mustard compounds which produce fluorescent bands, or Q bands, across the chromosomes. Also called *Q method*.

R method REVERSE GIEMSA METHOD.

radioactive balloon method A method of radiation therapy applied to the wall of the urinary bladder, consisting of the intravesical placement of a Foley catheter, the bag of which is then filled with a radioactive solution or suspension.

recall method A method employed in the quantitative study of memory: the number of items learned, to an agreed-upon criterion of mastery, that can be successfully reproduced following an elapsed interval of time provides a measure of the degree of retention.

recognition method A method employed in the quantitative study of memory: the subject is required to select those items to which he has been previously exposed in the experiment from among several other items to which he has not been exposed.

Reed-Merrell method A shortcut method for constructing abridged life tables, that is, life tables with entries only at five-year or ten-year intervals, using a set of standard conversion tables to derive mortalities from the death rates over the five-year or ten-year age ranges.

Reed and Muench method A method for determining the median lethal dose by interpolation.

reference method An analytic technique that is used as a standard against which other measurement procedures are compared or that is used to define reference materials that can be used to standardize other procedures. It is highly accurate but usually is too tedious or demanding for routine analysis.

Regaud method A radiotherapy technique for cancer of the cervix, using intracavitary irradiation by probe and irradiation of the parametria by colpostat.

Rehfuss method REHFUSS TEST.

Reichert's method The crystallization of oxyhemoglobin in ammonium oxalate.

retrofilling method A method of filling the apical part of a root canal or its equivalent after apicoectomy from the apical end, usually with dental amalgam.

Reverdin's method REVERDIN GRAFT.

reverse Giemsa method A chromosome banding technique in which the chromosomes are pretreated with heat followed by Giemsa staining. The resulting dark and light bands (R bands) are the reverse of the G and Q bands. Also called *R method*.

rhythm method A means of contraception by avoiding sexual intercourse just prior to and after ovulation in the middle of the menstrual cycle. Also called *rhythm contraception, periodic abstinence*.

Ricord's method An obsolete technique of circumcision.

Ritchie's formol-ether method A method for detecting parasitic cysts and ova in fecal material. The specimen is fixed in formol-saline solution and extracted with ether. The washed residue is then examined microscopically.

Ritgen's method RITGEN MANEUVER.

roll method A toothbrushing technique in which the bristles are placed on the gums and swept toward the biting surfaces of the teeth by rotation of the toothbrush.

Roughton-Scholander method SYRINGE-CAPILLARY METHOD.

Sahli's method ACID HEMATIN METHOD.

savings method A method used for the quantitative study of memory. A body of material is first learned, then an interval is allowed to elapse that is sufficient to assure partial or complete forgetting, followed by an opportunity to relearn the same material. The difference between the time, or the number of trials, needed to achieve the same degree of mastery provides an index of the amount of the original material that has been retained. Also called *relearning*.

Sayre's method SAYRE'S OPERATION.

Schales and Schales method An obsolete method for measurement of serum chloride concentration, based on titration of the serum specimen with a solution of mercuric nitrate of known concentration. Diphenylcarbazone, used as an indicator, turns purple when there is excess mercuric ion, unbound by chloride.

method of Schmidt and Thannhauser A method for the determination of RNA and DNA in a sample. The nucleic acids are precipitated with trichloroacetic acid and washed to remove all phosphorus compounds of low molecular size. The residue is warmed with alkali, which hydrolyzes RNA but not DNA, thanks to attack by the 2'-oxygen (when it is deprotonated) on the phosphorus atom. Subsequent acidification with trichloroacetic acid precipitates DNA but leaves the phosphorus originally present in RNA in solution, so that phosphorus analysis of the precipitate and of the supernatant gives the amounts of DNA and RNA originally present.

Schoenheimer and Sperry method A procedure for measurement of serum cholesterol in which cholesterol is first extracted from serum with a mixture of acetone and ethanol, and then the cholesterol is precipitated from solution by digitonin. The cholesterol purified in this manner is then treated with a mixture of concentrated sulfuric acid and acetic anhydride, with which it undergoes the Liebermann-Burchard reaction, resulting in a blue-green color, the intensity of which is proportional to the cholesterol concentration. The method has been largely supplanted by the Abell-Kendall method, which is also based on the Liebermann-Burchard reaction.

Schroeder's method An old-fashioned method of resuscitating a newborn in which the thorax is compressed by bending the infant's body over its abdomen from the supine position.

Schultz method A histochemical technique that uses iron alum and acetic sulfuric acid to identify cholesterol and cholesterol esters.

Schweninger's method The treatment of obesity by the reduction of fluid intake.

sectional method SEGMENTATION METHOD.

sedimentation method Any separation technique based on differential density of substances relative to the solution in which they are suspended.

segmentation method A method of filling a root canal with gutta percha cones in stages, with a short segment starting at the apex. Also called *sectional method.*

self-report method Any attempt to have individuals describe their own behaviors, traits, interests, or personality characteristics, usually by marking on a questionnaire each of the preselected alternatives that best describe them.

Shaffer's method A modification of Jaffe's test for creatinine, that is used for analysis of very dilute solutions.

Shock and Hastings method A procedure for measurement of plasma pH and plasma carbon dioxide content, the latter by use of a manometer.

Shohl and Pedley method A quantitative technique for measuring urinary calcium. Calcium is precipitated as calcium oxalate and treated with sulfuric acid to produce oxalic acid. The product is then titrated with potassium permanganate.

Sicka method An obsolete procedure for measurement of the hemoglobin concentration of blood, in which oxyhemoglobin is reduced to deoxyhemoglobin and the resulting lavender color is compared with a calibrated tinted glass standard.

silver cone method A method of filling a root canal with a single silver cone.

Sippy method See under SIPPY DIET.

Skoog's method A method of repairing a bilateral congenital cleft lip. Also called *Skoog's operation.*

Sluder's method **1** Treatment of sphenopalatine neuralgia by injecting the ganglion, via the sphenopalatine foramen, with local anesthetic. **2** A method of guillotine enucleation of the tonsils used in the early part of the 20th century. An obsolete term.

Smellie's method A technique of delivering the aftercoming head in a breech presentation by resting the baby's trunk on the obstetrician's forearm.

Somogyi method **1** A copper reduction method for demonstrating the presence of glucose and other reducing sugars in body fluids. **2** A saccharogenic method for measuring serum amylase. A copper reduction test is applied to the reducing substances released from starch by action of the amylase.

Souligoux-Morestin method ETHER LAVAGE.

Spina's method A method of repairing a congenital bilateral cleft lip.

split cast method SPLIT CAST MOUNTING.

Staffieri's method An operation to create a phonatory neoglottis to enable the patient to speak after total laryngectomy. A low tracheostome is established and the larynx is removed so as to conserve several tracheal rings above this level. A fistulous opening into the hypopharynx is created just above the laryngeal stump and the hypopharyngeal musculature surrounding the fistula is sutured to the top of the trachea so that the fistula becomes the neoglottis.

Stammer's method Measurement of blood glucose concentration by boiling and filtering blood, and determining the length of time required for the filtrate to decolorize methylene blue when mixed together and boiled. This method is now obsolete.

St. Clair's method A system for classifying neutrophils according to the number of lobes of the nucleus. See also ARNETH CLASSIFICATION, COOKE'S CRITERION.

Steinach's method STEINACH'S OPERATION.

Stillman's method A vibratory toothbrushing technique with the bristles at a 45° angle to the long axis of the teeth, directed toward the apices. A modified version of the method adds a vertical sweep toward the biting surfaces at the end of each vibratory phase.

Stoll's method A method for quantifying helminth ova in feces, calculated by counting the eggs in a known volume of feces diluted and suspended in 0.1 normal solution of sodium hydroxide and then multiplying to determine the number present per gram of feces. A correction factor is used to relate fecal consistency to weight.

Stout's method A method of reducing and fixing fractures of the jaws by means of steel wire loops made by passing one continuous length of wire in and out of the interdental spaces. Also called *Stout wiring.*

Stratmann method A method of measuring atmospheric sulfur dioxide based on the absorption of the gas by silica gel.

method of successive approximations SHAPING.

suction method A gynecologic procedure in which the uterine contents are removed by aspiration through a cannula, using a device to produce negative pressure. Most commonly the procedure is used to carry out abortion during the first one-third of pregnancy.

suspension method A method of radiation therapy to the wall of the urinary bladder, consisting of the instillation of a radioactive solution or suspension into the vesical lumen, usually via a urethral catheter.

symptothermal method A method of contraception in which intercourse is avoided during the fertile midmenstrual cycle time period, which is identified by monitoring changes in the cervical or vaginal mucus and symptoms suggesting ovulation, including a plot of basal body temperatures.

syringe-capillary method A micromethod for measurement of the volume of gases in blood, in which a graduated capillary tube serves as the manometer. Also called *Roughton-Scholander method.*

Terry's method A method for rapid diagnosis in which the freehand sectioning of tissue with a sharp razor is followed by staining with polychrome methylene blue. Also called *Terry stain*.

Thane's method The locating of the upper end of the central sulcus of the brain by finding the midpoint of a line that is drawn between the glabella and the inion.

Theden's method The treatment of aneurysm in a limb by compression of the entire limb with a roller bandage.

thick-film method An examination of several drops of hemolyzed blood (fixed in methyl alcohol and stained in Giemsa's or other Romanowski-type blood stains) for the gross detection of intraerythrocytic parasites, as the malarial parasites. Species diagnosis is based on a subsequent study of a standard thin blood smear, which can conveniently be placed on the same slide.

thin-film method The preparation of a film of blood on a glass microscope slide, so that a single layer of cells may be observed microscopically.

transparent-chamber method A method for studying cells or tissues in a living organism, usually an animal, by means of a clear plastic chamber implanted in a suitable area, such as a rabbit's ear.

Tuffier's method SPINAL ANESTHESIA.

turbidity method The demonstration of the presence of protein in a body fluid by precipitating the fluid with sulfosalicylic acid or other additives.

Tuthill's method WEINBACH'S METHOD.

urease method Any of several methods for measuring urea that is based on the quantity of ammonia produced following hydrolysis of urea by urease.

van Gehuchten's method A rapid fixation technique that uses van Gehuchten's fixative.

Van Slyke and Cullen method **1** A seldom-used gasometric method for quantifying the amount of carbon dioxide in blood. **2** A urease method for measuring urea in which the ammonia is titrated into a standard acid.

Van Slyke and Meyer method An obsolete procedure in which the nitrogen content of blood amino acid is measured by first precipitating proteins with alcohol, then liberating nitrogen with nitrous acid, and measuring the volume of gas released.

Van Slyke and Neill method The measurement of the volume of oxygen or other gases in blood or other fluids by use of a manometer.

Wade's method A method of detecting *Mycobacterium leprae*. A small sample of tissue pulp and lymph from a leprosy lesion are obtained by pinching a fold of skin, inserting a scalpel, and rotating the blade to scrape the sides of the incision. The sample is stained with carbolfuchsin and examined for the presence of *M. leprae*.

Wade-Fite method A staining method to demonstrate acid-fast bacilli in paraffin tissue sections which are dewaxed in rectified turpentine and heavy paraffin oil, stained with carbolfuchsin, decolorized in sulfuric acid, and stained with picric acid and acid fuchsin. Acid-fast organisms appear dark blue to blue-black.

Wade-Fite-Faraco method A staining method to demonstrate acid-fast bacilli in paraffin tissue sections after the sections are dewaxed with a mixture of paraffin oil and rectified turpentine or paraffin oil and aviation gasoline. They are then stained with carbolfuchsin, decolorized with hydrochloride and ethanol, and counterstained with methylene blue. The acid-fast organisms appear red against a light blue background.

Walgren's method Intradermal vaccination with bacille Calmette-Guérin.

Walker's method A method for estimating the ferric iron content of food. The food to be analyzed is completely burned and the ash cooled and dissolved in dilute nitric acid. The resulting solution is filtered and the filtrate oxidized with hydrogen peroxide. Potassium thiocyanate is added and the blood-red color produced is compared with a standard solution of iron that has been similarly treated. In the case of ferrous iron no pronounced color is produced by this reaction.

Walker-Reisinger method A microcolorimetric method for reducing substances in blood or urine, based on the ability of glucose and other reducing sugars to convert dinitrosalicylic acid to a colored compound.

Wallace-Diamond method DIAMOND'S METHOD.

Wardill four-flap method A method of closing a cleft palate using four mucoperiosteal flaps.

Wardill two-flap method A method of closing clefts of the palate utilizing two mucoperiosteal flaps. This procedure is used if the defect involves less than half of the hard palate.

Watson's method An old-fashioned approach to induction of labor whereby castor oil, quinine, and Pituitrin were administered successively to the pregnant woman.

Weed-McKibben method Treatment of increased intracranial pressure by the parenteral injection or oral ingestion of hypertonic solutions such as sucrose or magnesium sulfate.

Weigert-Pal method A modification of Weigert's myelin sheath stain that is particularly useful for demonstrating large areas of demyelination within the nervous system. An oxalic acid-potassium sulfite mixture is used for differentiation. Also called *Weigert-Pal technique*.

Weil-Hallé method Subcutaneous vaccination with bacille Calmette-Guérin in which half of the 0.05 mg dose is injected into the loose skin under each armpit. The vaccination usually gives rise to a cutaneous reaction within one to two months.

Weinbach's method An obsolete method for measurement of serum sodium concentration by deproteinization, followed by precipitation as sodium uranyl zinc acetate, in turn followed by titration with a sodium hydroxide solution of known concentration. Also called *Tuthill's method, Butler and Tuthill method*.

Welcker's method A measurement of purines, in which phosphates are first removed with magnesium oxides, then the purine bases are precipitated with ammonium hydroxide and silver nitrate, and then the nitrogen content of the precipitate is determined by the Kjeldahl method.

Welker and Marsh method A method utilizing aluminum hydroxide to clarify milk.

Westergren method A procedure for measurement of erythrocyte sedimentation rate that employs a column 20 cm long, with 2 mm internal diameter, graduated in millimeters. Anticoagulated blood is introduced into this "Westergren tube," which is then supported in a vertical position, and at one hour, the number of millimeters between the upper level of plasma and the upper level of erythrocytes is recorded. The normal erythrocyte sedimentation rate for men is 0–15 mm/hr, for women 0–20 mm/hr.

West-Gaeke method A method of measuring atmospheric sulfur dioxide by the reaction between the gas and a solution of dipotassium tetrachloromercurate (1-).

Whipple's method The administration of liver as treatment for pernicious anemia, an obsolete form of treatment.

Whitehorn's method An obsolete method of measuring blood chloride concentration, based on its reaction with silver ion.

Wiechowski and Handovsky method A method for isolating and quantifying allantoin in urine. Urine, cleared of chlorides, ammonia and basic compounds, is treated with mercuric and sodium acetate to precipitate the allantoin, which is then measured by gravimetric, titrimetric, or Kjeldahl techniques.

Wilson's method **1** A technique used in experimental teratology to diagnose soft tissue and other internal malformations in fetal and newborn laboratory animals. A fixed specimen is cut transversely into 1 mm sections with a razor blade and examined with a dissecting microscope. **2** FÜLLEBORN'S METHOD.

Wintrobe method   The determination of hematocrit, using a glass tube, called a Wintrobe tube, with 2.5 × 115 nm bore. The tube is calibrated from 0 to 100 nm.

Wintrobe and Landsberg method   The determination of erythrocyte sedimentation rate by measurement of sedimentation at one hour and correction for hematocrit value by a standard table.

Wright's method   A seldom-used method of treating wounds, consisting of débridement followed by washing with hypertonic saline and then with isotonic saline.

Wynn method   A method of repairing a cleft lip by lengthening the prolabium on the side of the cleft by means of a superiorly based triangular transposition flap taken from a segment of the lateral part of the lip.

---

methodology   The methods used in a particular field.

methohexital   A methyl-substituted barbiturate used for intravenous induction of general anesthesia characterized by rapid onset and recovery.

methohexital sodium $C_{14}H_{17}N_2NaO_3$. 5-Allyl-1-methyl-5-(1-methyl-2-pentynyl)barbituric acid sodium salt. A very short-acting barbiturate used intravenously to produce anesthesia of short duration or for induction of general anesthesia. It is used like sodium thiopental.

methomania   [Gk *meth(ē)* strong drink, drunkenness + *o* + -MANIA]   METHILEPSIA.

methopromazine   METHOXYPROMAZINE.

methotrexate $C_{20}H_{22}N_8O_5$. 4-Amino-10-methylfolic acid. A very potent folic acid antagonist which has been used as a cytotoxic drug in the treatment of neoplastic diseases and as an immunosuppressant agent. Also called *amethopterin*.

methotrimeprazine   10-(3-Dimethylamino-2-methyl-propyl) 2-methoxyphenothiazine. A phenothiazine with potent analgesic properties. It is used as an analgesic for severe pain, for obstetric analgesic effects without respiratory depression, and as a preanesthetic medication.

methoxamine hydrochloride $C_{11}H_{17}NO_3 \cdot HCl$. α-(1-Aminoethyl)-2,5-dimethoxybenzoyl alcohol hydrochloride. A white crystalline compound, used as an adrenergic vasopressor in hypotensive states and to end attacks of paroxysmal atrial tachycardia.

methoxsalen $C_{12}H_8O_4$. 9-Methoxy-7H-furo[3,2-g][1]benzopyran-7-one. A psoralen compound occurring in the plant, *Amni majus*. This agent may be used in association with ultraviolet light exposure to enhance repigmentation after idiopathic vitiligo. It is also used to precipitate a phototoxic response in treatment of psoriasis. It has the capacity to accelerate suntan and functions as a sun screen. It is used both topically and orally. Also called *xanthotoxin, 8-methoxypsoralen*.

methoxy-   A combining form indicating the presence of a methoxyl radical (CH_3—O—) in a molecule.

methoxy acetanilide   ACETANISIDINE.

methoxychlor $Cl_3CCH(C_6H_4OCH_3)_2$. 2,2-bis(p-Methoxyphenyl)-1,1,1-trichloroethane. An insecticide that is used to control mosquito larvae and flies.

methoxyflurane   A volatile, nonflammable fluoride and other halogen-substituted ether used as a general anesthetic. It has been virtually abandoned because of nephrotoxicity.

methoxyindoles   Indoles containing a methoxy group of the class of melatonin, the secretory product of the pineal, having in experimental animals actions on sodium balance, light-dark

adaptation, dermal melanin pigmentation and possibly upon gonadotropin release by the adenohypophysis. Their physiologic role and their importance in man are not known.

methoxyl   The univalent group CH_3—O—.

methoxyphenamine $C_{11}H_{17}NO \cdot HCl$. 2-Methoxy-N,α-dimethylbenzeneethanamine hydrochloride. An adrenergic agent with actions pharmacologically as a bronchodilator. It is used chiefly in the treatment of bronchial asthma and given orally.

methoxypromazine $C_{18}H_{22}N_2OS$. 2-Methoxy-N,N-dimethyl-10H-phenothiazine-10-propanamine. A phenothiazine with actions typical of that class of compounds. It is usually used clinically as the maleate salt as a tranquilizer. Also called *methopromazine*.

8-methoxypsoralen   METHOXSALEN.

methscopolamine bromide $C_{18}H_{24}BrNO_4$. 6β-7β-Epoxy-3α-hydroxy-8-methyl-1αH,5αH-tropanium tropate (ester). A quaternary derivative of scopolamine with anticholinergic actions like scopolamine but absorbed less rapidly and having less effect on the central nervous system. It is used for gastrointestinal spasm and as a preoperative medication. Also called *hyoscine methobromide, epoxymethamine bromide*.

methsuximide $C_{12}H_{13}NO_2$. 1,3-Dimethyl-3-phenyl-2,5-pyrrolidinedione. An anticonvulsant agent employed therapeutically in the treatment of psychomotor and petit mal epilepsy. It is given orally.

methyclothiazide $C_9H_{11}Cl_2N_3O_4S_2$. 6-Chloro-3-(chloromethyl)-3,4-dihydro-2-methyl-2H-1,2,4-benzothiadiazine-7-sulfonamide 1,1-dioxide. A thiazide antihypertensive, diuretic agent. It is employed in the treatment of edema secondary to congestive heart failure, chronic renal disease, pregnancy, premenstrual syndrome, cirrhosis, and obesity and in steroid therapy. It is given orally for edema and hypertension.

methyl   The univalent group CH_3-.

   angular methyl   A methyl group attached to the atom that forms the junction between two rings in a molecule. There are two such groups in cholesterol.

methyl-   [English *methyl*, back formation from French *methyl(ène)* methylene, from Gk *meth(y)* wine + *(h)yl(ē)* wood, matter + *-ēnē*, fem. patronymic suffix]   A combining form denoting the presence of the methyl (—CH_3) group in a chemical compound.

methylacetylcholine   METHACHOLINE.

methylal $CH_2(OCH_3)_2$. Dimethoxymethane. A colorless liquid used as an anesthetic and hypnotic drug. It is also used as a reagent in some organic syntheses and as an ingredient in perfumes.

methyl alcohol   METHANOL.

methylamine CH_3—NH_2. The simplest primary amine, it is a gas but readily dissolves to give an alkaline solution (pK = 10.6). Together with glyoxylate it can be formed biologically from sarcosine by an oxidation catalyzed by glycine oxidase. Its characteristic smell is readily detected in water in which fish has been stored.

methyl amyl ketone $C_7H_{14}O$. A volatile substance contained in oil of cloves.

methylaspartate ammonia-lyase   An enzyme (EC 4.3.1.2) which catalyzes the removal of ammonia from 3-methylaspartate with the formation of a double bond. The reaction is a step in the fermentation of glutamate by some bacteria.

methylated   Containing the methyl group or having it attached.

methylation   The reaction of introducing a methyl group into a substance, either in replacement of a hydrogen atom or with gain of a positive charge. Hydroxyl groups of sugars are methylated, often with methyl sulfate, in determining which are free and which masked by ring formation or intersugar bonds. In living beings methylation is usually by transmethylation from the $CH_3—S^+R_1R_2$ group of S-adenosylmethionine. Methylation determines the susceptibility of certain nucleotide sequences to restriction by site-specific nucleases and influences or even controls gene activity.

biologic methylation　The addition of a methyl group to a substance as a result of biologic action. This reaction is of particular importance in facilitating the incorporation of mercury in aquatic food chains and subsequently in the human diet.

methylatropine hydrobromide　$C_{18}H_{25}O_3NHBr$. An anticholinergic agent with actions similar to those of atropine. It is employed as a mydriatic drug as well as in the treatment of pyloric stenosis in infants. Also called *atropine methylbromide*.

methylatropine nitrate　ATROPINE METHYL NITRATE.

methylbenzenethonium chloride　$C_{28}H_{44}ClNO_2$. Benzyldimethyl-[2-[2-(p-1,1,3,3-tetramethylbutylcresoxy)-ethoxy]ethyl] ammonium chloride. It is used as a topical anti-infective medication to decrease bacterial proliferation in preparations to treat diaper rash and ammonia dermatitis.

methyl bromide　CH_3Br. A highly toxic, colorless gas, usually odorless, with a sweetish, chloroformlike odor. Its principal uses are as an insect fumigant in mills, ships, and freight cars, and as a soil fumigant. It is also used in fire extinguishers, but because of its toxicity, this use is being discouraged in smaller devices. It is dangerous because symptoms of illness from exposure are delayed. After inhalation convulsions may occur without warning or may be preceded by giddiness, numbness of limbs, weakness, drowsiness, and headache. Patients who survive the convulsions may suffer permanent brain damage. Also called *bromomethane*.

3-methylbutyl　The chemical group $(CH_3)_2CH—[CH_2]_2—$. Also called *isoamyl* (outmoded).

(24S)-methylcalciol　VITAMIN D_4.

methylcatechol　GUAIACOL.

methylcellulose　A methyl ether of cellulose prepared from wood pulp or cotton. It is a white, odorless, tasteless granular material which forms a colorless liquid after being dissolved in water or other solvents. It is used as a bulk laxative and as a colloidal constituent in emulsions and as a suspending agent.

methyl chloride　CHLOROMETHANE.

methyl chloroform　A chemical solvent, extensively used in industry, that has been found in the stratosphere, where it may damage the ozone layer and possibly cause harmful effects on the earth's climate.

methyl chloroformate　$CH_3—O—CO—Cl$. A reagent used for substituting amines and alcohols with the methoxycarbonyl group. It can be regarded as the half acid chloride and half methyl ester of carbonic acid.

methylcholanthrene　One of the carcinogenic polycyclic hydrocarbons found in coal tar.

methyl cyanide　ACETONITRILE.

methyl cyanoacetate　$N≡C—CH_2—CO—O—CH_3$. A colorless liquid, soluble in water and organic solvents, having a freezing point of $-22.5°C$ and a boiling point of $203°C$. It is an important reagent in organic synthesis, because its methylene group is slightly acidic, and it is used in making dyes and medicaments.

methyldopa　$C_{10}H_{13}NO_4$. 3-Hydroxy-α-methyl-L-tyrosine. An antihypertensive agent used to treat essential hypertension. It acts centrally via α-methylnorepinephrine on α-adrenergic receptors to inhibit sympathetic activity. The drug is given orally.

methylene　The bivalent radical of formula $—CH_2—$.

methylene azure　A trimethylated thiazin dye used in the Giemsa stain. Also called *azure I*.

methylene blue　A blue dyestuff, once widely used in biochem-

ical investigations of dehydrogenases, which is easily reduced to a colorless compound. It is a thiazine. Its reduced form is related to bis(p-dimethylaminophenyl)amine by fusion of the two benzene rings through a sulfur atom at the position *ortho* to the bridging nitrogen and *meta* to the dimethylamino groups. On oxidation, one ring becomes quinonoid.

Loeffler's methylene blue　A stain used to detect polymetaphosphate granules, particularly in corynebacteria.

polychrome methylene blue　A mixture of methylene blue, methylene green, methylene azure, and methylene violet.

Unna's alkaline methylene blue　A stain for plasma cells that employs methylene blue in a strongly basic solution.

methylene chloride　METHYLENE DICHLORIDE.

methylenecitrylsalicylic acid　$C_3H_2O_3$ $(CH_2COOC_6H_4CO-OH)_2$. A white powder with antirheumatic and antiseptic properties. Also called *anhydromethylenecitric acid*.

methylene dichloride　Dichloromethane, a substance frequently used as a solvent in chemical synthesis and as a refrigerant. Also called *methylene chloride*.

methylene green　A synthetic metachromatic dye that can be used to distinguish mast cell granules.

methylene iodide　An alcohol-soluble yellow liquid with a relative density of 3.33. It is insoluble in water and used in separation procedures and density determinations. Also called *diiodomethane*.

methylenetetrahydrofolate dehydrogenase　One of two enzymes that catalyze the dehydrogenation of 5,10-methylenetetrahydrofolate, a complex of formaldehyde with tetrahydrofolate, to form 5,10-methenyltetrahydrofolate. One of them (EC 1.5.1.5) uses $NADP^+$ as the hydrogen acceptor, and the other (EC 1.5.1.15) uses NAD^+.

methylene violet　$(CH_3)_2NC_6H_3(SN)CH_3O$. A violet dye that is used as a component of stains for biologic tissue.

methylenophil　**1** Capable of being stained by methylene blue. Also *methyleneophilous*. **2** Any cell or tissue constituent stained by methylene blue.

methylenophilous　METHYLENOPHIL.

methylepsia [See METHILEPSIA.]　**1** METHILEPSIA. **2** Hypersexuality due to alcoholic intoxication. An imprecise and old-fashioned usage.

methylergonovine maleate　$C_{24}H_{29}N_3O_6$. N-[α-(Hydroxymethyl)propyl]-D-lysergamide maleate. It is an oxytocic agent used to induce uterine contractions to shorten the third stage of labor. It is also used after delivery to combat postpartum atony and hemorrhage from the uterus. The drug can be given orally, intramuscularly, or intravenously.

methyl eugenol　$C_3H_5·C_6H_3(OCH_3)_2$. A volatile oil found in oil of bay.

methylglucamine　1-Deoxy-1-(methylamino)-D-glucitol.　A compound used in the synthesis of certain pharmaceuticals. It is prepared from methylamine and D-glucose.

methylglucamine iodipamide　MEGLUMINE IODIPAMIDE.

methylglyoxal　$CH_3—CO—CHO$. A reactive compound, once thought to be a major intermediate, produced by some aerobic bacteria from dihydroxyacetone phosphate with elimination of inorganic orthophosphate. It is also an intermediate in one pathway of threonine catabolism.

methyl green　A cytochemical dye used to detect undenatured DNA.

methylguanosine　A type of nucleoside found in tRNA, consisting of guanosine methylated on N-1 or on N-7.

methylhexaneamine　$C_7H_{17}N$. 1,3-Dimethylamylamine. It is an adrenergic agent used primarily in inhalers to relieve congestion of the nasal airways.

methylide A compound resulting from combination of an element with the methyl group.

methylidyne The tervalent group CH.

methylinosine A nucleoside sometimes present in a tRNA molecule. It is a rare base.

methyl iodide CH_3I. Iodomethane. A liquid of boiling point 43 °C. It is a methylating agent widely used in organic synthesis, and it is highly toxic. Symptoms of exposure include nausea, vomiting, slurred speech, visual disturbances, drowsiness, and coma. It is also likely to be carcinogenic because of its ability to methylate nucleic acid.

ϵ-N-methyllysine Lysine methylated on its side-chain nitrogen. This amino acid occurs in many proteins, such as myosin, and is produced by methylation of lysine residues already incorporated into the protein. It is subject to further methylation, which may give di- and trimethyllysines. The same compounds can also be produced by treating proteins with formaldehyde and a reducing agent such as borohydride. Since the residues remain positively charged, the modification does not usually alter protein conformation, but it prevents the lysine from entering some chemical reactions.

methylmalonicaciduria An abnormal elevation of methylmalonic acid in the blood. It may be caused by inborn errors in the metabolism of methylmalonic acid which have varying clinical presentations and therapeutic responses to vitamin B_{12}. Enzyme defects that produce the condition include methylmalonyl-CoA racemase, methylmalonyl-CoA mutase, and several enzymes involved in B_{12} metabolism. The condition also occurs in the dietary B_{12} deficiency caused by the reduced activity of methylmalonyl-CoA mutase.

methylmalonyl-CoA carboxyltransferase The enzyme (EC 2.1.3.1) that catalyzes the reaction of propionyl-CoA with oxaloacetate to form (S)-methylmalonyl-CoA and pyruvate. This is a step in the pathway of utilization of fatty acids that contain an odd number of carbon atoms. Also called *transcarboxylase*.

methylmalonyl-CoA epimerase The enzyme (EC 5.1.99.1) that interconverts (R)-methylmalonyl-CoA, which is interconvertible with succinyl-CoA, and (S)-methylmalonyl-CoA, which is interconvertible with propionyl-CoA. It thus catalyzes a step in the pathway by which propionic acid, and hence all fatty acids containing an odd number of carbon atoms, may be used. Also called *methylmalonyl-CoA racemase* (outmoded).

methylmalonyl-CoA mutase The enzyme (EC 5.4.99.2) that isomerizes (R)-methylmalonyl-CoA to form succinyl-CoA. This exchange of hydrogen and carboxyl groups requires a cobamide coenzyme, and probably the reversible breaking of a carbon-cobalt bond. It is the one well-characterized reaction in mammals that involves coenzyme B_{12}, and it is part of the pathway by which propionyl-CoA can be metabolized.

methylmalonyl-CoA racemase An outmoded term for METHYLMALONYL-COA EPIMERASE. • This name is incorrect because the reaction does not interconvert enantiomers, since it changes the chirality of the methylmalonyl group, but not that of coenzyme A.

methylmalonyl-coenzyme A The substance formed from propionyl-CoA by the enzyme methylmalonyl-CoA carboxyltransferase, which forms the S-isomer. This is then epimerized to the R-isomer before isomerization to give succinyl-CoA. These reactions place it on the pathway of utilization of fatty acids with an odd number of carbon atoms.

methyl mercury An alkyl mercury compound formed by aquatic anaerobes in the presence of metallic mercury. Used as a fungicide, it has seen limited production and use in the United States because of its adverse effects on the central nervous system.

methyl methacrylate $CH_2:C(CH_3)COOCH_3$. An acrylic resin derived from methyl acrylic acid. It occurs as a monomer, which is a liquid, and a polymer, which is a solid. The two forms are mixed to make a plastic substance which sets into a rigid material by virtue of the polymerization of the monomer. It is used to make denture bases, artificial teeth, crowns, and restorations. Also called *methacrylate*.

methyl orange A weakly acidic aminobenzene dye that is widely used as a pH indicator, turning from red to yellow at pH 3.0 to 4.4. Also called *helianthin, tropaeolin D, orange III*.

methylpentose Any of the 6-deoxyhexoses, such as rhamnose or fucose.

methylphenidate hydrochloride $C_{14}H_{19}NO_2 \cdot HCl$. Methyl-α-phenyl-2-piperidineacetate hydrochloride salt. It is used in the treatment of hyperkinetic children because of its actions as a mild central nervous system psycomotor stimulant. It is given orally.

methylprednisolone $C_{20}H_{30}O_5$. 11β,17α,21-Trihydroxy-6α-methyl-1,4-pregnadiene-3,20-dione.It is a methylated analogue of prednisolone, maintaining the same actions and uses as the parent compound. It is given orally.

methylpurine Any methylated purine, especially one formed from adenine and guanine by methylation in tRNA.

methyl red A dye used as an indicator. It is red in acid and yellow in alkali, with a pK of 5.0.

methyl salicylate $C_8H_8O_3$. 2-Hydroxybenzoic acid methylester. An ester naturally present in leaves of *Gaultheria procumbens* and in *Betula lenta*. It is a colorless, oily liquid with a strong, pleasant odor. It is used in perfumes and as a flavoring for candies, and it is applied in preparations externally as a counterirritant. Also called *wintergreen oil, sweet birch oil, teaberry oil*.

methyltestosterone $C_{25}H_{38}O_2$. 17α-Methyl-4-androstene-17(β)-ol-one. An androgenic steroidal agent generally used as a replacement therapy for androgen-deficiency disease states. It is given orally.

N^5-methyltetrahydrofolic acid An intermediate in the conversion of formaldehyde and its donors into methyl groups. It is formed under the action of 5,10-methylenetetrahydrofolate reductase, and it transfers its methyl group e.g. to homocysteine under the action of the cobamide-containing enzyme tetrahydropteroylglutamate methyltransferase to form methionine, and, in some anaerobic bacteria, to a C_1-unit to form acetate.

methylthio- [METHYL- + THIO-] A combining form denoting the group CH_3—S—, which may substitute for either hydrogen or hydroxyl in the compound whose name follows, since the term *thio* can mean either the bivalent group —S—, or substitution of sulfur for oxygen.

methyltransferase Any of many enzymes, classified as EC 2.1.1, that transfer methyl groups. Most of them use S-adenosylmethionine as donor. Also called *transmethylase*.

5-methyluracil THYMINE.

methyl violet A synthetic metachromatic basic dye composed of crystal violet and two other pararosanilins with lesser degrees of methylation and correspondingly redder shades of violet. Methyl violet is used as a stain for amyloid. Also called *Paris violet*.

methysergide $C_{21}H_{27}N_3O_2$. 1-Methyl-d-lysergic acid butanolamide. It is a serotonin receptor antagonist used therapeutically as a vasoconstrictor in the treatment of severe vascular headaches, such as migraine. It is given orally.

methysergide maleate $C_{21}H_{27}N_3O_2 \cdot C_4H_4O_4$. N-[1-(Hydroxymethyl)propyl]-4-methyl-(+)-lysergamide hydrogen maleate.

A serotonin antagonist that, like the parent drug, is used to prevent severe migraine headaches. It is given orally.

Meticortelone   A proprietary name for prednisolone.

Meticorten   A proprietary name for prednisone.

MetMb   metmyoglobin.

metmyoglobin   Myoglobin oxidized to the iron(III) state.

metocurine iodide $C_{39}H_{46}I_2N_2O_6$. d-Tubocurarine iodine dimethyl ether. A derivative of tubocurarine that is more potent and longer acting than tubocurarine. Also called *dimethyltubocurarine iodide*.

metoecious   HETERECIOUS.

metoestrum   A British spelling for METESTRUM.

metoestrus   A British spelling for METESTRUS.

metonymy   [Gk *metōnymia* (from *meta* over + *onym(a)* name + -*ia* -IA) change of name]   A disorder in which the patient uses an approximate but related term in place of the specific or idiomatic term, a form of loosening.

metopagus   [New L (from Gk *metō(pon)* the forehead, from *meta* between + *ōps* the eye, + *pagos* a thing fixed)]   Equal conjoined twins with union at the forehead. Also called *metopopagus*.

metopantritis   [Gk *metōp(on)* (from *met(a)* between and *ōps*, gen. *ōpos*, eye) + *antr(on)* cave + -ITIS]   An obsolete term for FRONTAL SINUSITIS.

metopantron   An outmoded term for SINUS FRONTALIS.

metopantrum   SINUS FRONTALIS.

metopic   Pertaining to the forehead.

metopion   The craniometric point at which a line joining the frontal eminences intersects the median sagittal plane.

metopism   The persistence in the adult of the frontal, or metopic, suture.

metopodynia   [Gk *metōp(on)* (from *met(a)*- between + *ōps* the eye) the space between the eyes, forehead + -ODYNIA]   Headache in the frontal region. An obsolete term.

metopon   [Gk *metōpon* (from *met(a)*- between + *ōps*, gen. *ōpos*, the eye) the space between the eyes, forehead]   The anterior part of the frontal lobe of the cerebral hemisphere. An obsolete term.

metopopagus   METOPAGUS.

metopoplasty   [Gk *metōpo(n)* the forehead + -PLASTY]   Any plastic operation on the forehead.

Metorchis conjunctus   A species of opisthorchid fish-borne flukes parasitic in the gallbladder of dogs, foxes, cats, mink, and raccoons over a wide area of eastern Canada. They are also found occasionally in humans.

metoxenous   HETERECIOUS.

metoxeny   HETERECISM.

metr-   METRO-.

metra   [Gk *mētra* uterus]   An outmoded term for UTERUS.

metra-   METRO-.

metralgia   [METR- + -ALGIA]   UTERALGIA.

metranastrophe   [METR- + Gk *anastrophē* a turning about]   INVERSION OF UTERUS.

metraterm   [METRA- + TERM]   The terminal portion of the uterus of a trematode, which is equipped with special muscular walls that serve to eject ova.

metratomy   [METRA- + -TOMY]   HYSTEROTOMY.

metratonia   [METRA- + ATONIA]   Atony of the uterus.

metratresia   [METR- + ATRESIA]   Metratrophia.

metratrophia   [METR- + ATROPHIA]   Uterine atrophy. Also called *metratresia*.

Metrazol   A proprietary name for pentylenetetrazol.

metre   A British spelling for METER.

-metre   A British spelling for -METER.

metrectasia   [METR- + ECTASIA]   Dilatation of a nonpregnant uterus.

metrectomy   [METR- + -ECTOMY]   HYSTERECTOMY.

metrectopia   [METR- + ECTOPIA]   Any type of uterine displacement. An older term.

metremia   [METR- + -EMIA]   MENSTRUATION.

metreurynter   [METR- + Gk *eurynein* to widen]   A soft bag that is inserted into the cervix and inflated in order to dilate the cervical canal. Also called *colpeurynter, hysteurynter*.

metreurysis   [METR- + EURY- + -SIS]   Dilatation of the cervical canal by means of an inflatable bag which is inserted through the cervical os.

metria   [METR- + -IA]   An inflammatory or infectious condition occurring during the postpartum period. An older term.

metric   Of or relating to a decimal system of measures, especially to the metric system.

metrifonate $C_4H_8Cl_3O_4P$. A schistosomicidal drug that is particularly effective against the bladder blood fluke, *Schistosoma haematobium*.

metriocephalic   Having a moderately vaulted skull, the altitudinal index being between 72 and 77.

metritic   Pertaining to or characteristic of metritis.

metritis   [METR- + -ITIS]   An inflammation of the uterus.

  metritis dissecans   An obsolete term for DISSECTING METRITIS.

  dissecting metritis   An acute inflammatory process of the uterus that extends along interstitial planes in the myometrium. Also called *metritis dissecans* (obsolete).

  puerperal metritis   Any postpartum infection of the uterus.

metrizamide   A nonionic radiographic contrast agent found to be significantly less toxic than standard contrast media.

metrizoate sodium   The sodium salt of metrizoic acid. It is used as a contrast medium for diagnostic purposes such as coronary arteriography.

metrizoic acid $C_{12}H_{11}I_3N_2O_4$.   3-(Acetylamino)-5-(acetylmethylamino)-2,4,6-triiodobenzoic acid, a compound used as a contrast medium in diagnostic procedures. It is most often used in its sodium or *N*-methylglucamine salt form.

metro-   [Gk *mētra* uterus]   A combining form denoting the uterus. Also *metr-, metra-*.

metrocarcinoma   [METRO- + CARCINOMA]   Carcinoma of the uterus. An outmoded term.

metrocele   [METRO- + -CELE¹]   HYSTEROCELE.

metrocolpocele   [METRO- + COLPO- + -CELE¹]   A hernia containing the uterus and the vagina.

metrocystosis   [METRO- + CYSTOSIS]   Cystic changes in the uterus. It is not specific for endometrium or myometrium, hence could be secondary to cystic hyperplasia or adenomyosis.

metrodynamometer   [METRO- + DYNAMOMETER]   An old-fashioned instrument designed to measure the strength of uterine contractions.

metrodynia   [METR- + -ODYNIA]   UTERALGIA.

metrodystocia   [METRO- + DYSTOCIA]   Dystocia secondary to inadequate or inefficient uterine contractions.

metroendometritis   ENDOMYOMETRITIS.

metrofibroma   [METRO- + FIBROMA]   Fibroma of the uterus. An outmoded term.

metrogenous   Arising from the uterus.

metrography   [METRO- + -GRAPHY]   An obsolete term for HYSTEROGRAPHY.

metroleukorrhea   [METRO- + LEUKORRHEA]   A white discharge from the uterus.

metrology [METRO- + -LOGY] The science or study of units of measurement.

metroloxia [METRO- + Gk *lox(os)* slanting, crosswise, oblique + -IA] Oblique displacement of the uterus.

metrolymphangitis [METRO- + LYMPHANGITIS] Inflammation of the uterine lymphatic vessels.

metromalacia Necrosis and softening of the uterus, especially the myometrium.

metromenorrhagia [METRO- + MENORRHAGIA] MENOMETRORRHAGIA.

metronania [METRO- + *nan(o)*- + -IA] Unusually small size of the uterus.

metroncus [METR- + -ONCUS] A tumor of the uterus. An outmoded term.

metronidazole $C_6H_9N_3O_3$. 1-(β-Hydroxyethyl)-2-methyl-5-nitroimidazole. It has trichomonacidal and amebicidal activity against *Trichomonas vaginalis* and *Endomoeba histolytica*. It is used to treat acute intestinal amebiasis and amebic liver abscess. It is also used to treat trichomoniasis in males and females. It is given orally and it is well absorbed. The drug has been reported to be carcinogenic in rodents, and it should be reserved for those special conditions in which it is particularly effective.

metronoscope [Gk *metron* a measure + *o* + -SCOPE] A reading device that exposes text at a controlled rate.

metroparalysis [METRO- + PARALYSIS] Paralysis or cessation of uterine contractions.

metropathia METROPATHY.

    metropathia hemorrhagica A condition of the uterus characterized by hemorrhage, usually accompanied by hypertrophy of the uterine mucous membranes and ovarian cystic disease.

metropathy [METRO- + -PATHY] Any disease of the uterus. Also called *metropathia, hysteropathy*. Adjective: metropathic.

    syncytiotrophoblastic metropathy Trophoblastic neoplasm of the uterus.

metroperitoneal Of or relating to the uterus and the peritoneum.

metroperitonitis Inflammation of the myometrium and surrounding peritoneum.

metropexy [METRO- + -PEXY] HYSTEROPEXY.

metrophlebitis Inflammation of the veins of the uterus.

metrophyma [METRO- + Gk *phyma* a thing that grows upon the body, tumor] A tumor of the uterus.

Metropine A proprietary name for atropine methyl nitrate.

metroplasty [METRO- + -PLASTY] UTEROPLASTY.

metropolis [Gk *mētropolis* (from *mētēr* mother + *polis* city, state) the mother state, home] The home area of an organism.

metroptosis [METRO- + PTOSIS] PROLAPSE OF UTERUS.

metrorrhagia [METRO- + -RRHAGIA] Uterine bleeding occurring at times other than the expected menses. Also called *endometrorrhagia*.

    metrorrhagia myopathica Postpartum hemorrhage secondary to uterine musculature atony. An older term.

metrorrhea [METRO- + -RRHEA] An obsolete term for MENSTRUATION.

metrorrhexis [METRO- + -RRHEXIS] Rupture of the uterus. Also called *hysterorrhexis*.

metrosalpingitis [METRO- + SALPINGITIS] Inflammation of the uterus and one or both of the fallopian tubes.

metrosalpingography [METRO- + SALPINGO- + -GRAPHY] A rarely used term for HYSTEROSALPINGOGRAPHY.

metrosalpinx TUBA UTERINA.

metroscirrhus [METRO- + Gk *skiros* or *skirrhos* gypsum, stucco, tumor] A scirrhous carcinoma of the uterus. An outmoded term.

metroscope [METRO- + -SCOPE] HYSTEROSCOPE.

metrostasis The isometric state.

metrostaxis [METRO- + Gk *staxis* a dripping] A small but persistent hemorrhage from the uterus.

metrostenosis Stenosis of the uterine cavity, as may occur in synechiae of the uterus.

metrotomy [METRO- + -TOMY] HYSTEROTOMY.

metrotoxin [METRO- + TOXIN] A postulated substance originating in the pregnant uterus, believed to inhibit ovarian function. An obsolete term.

metrotubography [METRO- + TUBO- + -GRAPHY] A rarely used term for HYSTEROSALPINGOGRAPHY.

-metry [Gk *metrein* to measure] A combining form meaning the act or process of measuring.

m. et sig. *misce et signa* (L, mix and write a label).

Metubine A proprietary name for metocurine iodide.

Metubine Iodide A proprietary name for dimethyltubocurarine iodide.

Metycaine A proprietary name for piperocaine.

metyrapone $C_{14}H_{14}N_2O$. 2-Methyl-1,2-di-3-pyridyl-1-propanone. It is used as a diagnostic aid in the detection of abnormalities in pituitary function. It reduces the levels of cortisol by inhibition of adrenal 11-β-hydroxylase. In normal individuals this is followed by an increase in ACTH release from the pituitary, followed by an increase in the release of 17-hydroxycorticoids. Also called *metapyrone, mepyrapone*.

Meulengracht [Einar *Meulengracht*, Danish internist, born 1887] See under METHOD.

Meunier [Leon *Meunier*, French physician, born 1856] See under SIGN.

MeV Symbol for the unit, megaelectronvolt.

mevaldic acid $H—CO—CH_2—C(OH)(CH_3)—CH_2—COOH$. The aldehyde formed by the dehydrogenation of the hydroxymethyl group of mevalonic acid. An enzyme has been found that catalyzes this dehydrogenation.

mevalonate kinase The enzyme (EC 2.7.1.36) that catalyzes the phosphorylation of the 5-hydroxyl group of mevalonic acid, with ATP acting as the phosphate donor. This is the first step in the biosynthetic pathway from mevalonic acid to steroids and terpenes.

mevalonic acid (3R)-3,5-Dihydroxy-3-methylvaleric acid. It is produced by reduction of 3-hydroxy-3-methylglutaryl-CoA in the pathway of biosynthesis of sterols and isoprenoids in plants and animals.

Meyenburg [Hans von *Meyenburg*, Swiss pathologist, born 1877] 1 Meyenburg's disease, Meyenburg-Altherr-Uehlinger syndrome. See under RELAPSING POLYCHONDRITIS. 2 Meyenburg's complexes. See under COMPLEX.

Meyer [Adolf *Meyer*, Swiss-born U.S. psychiatrist and neurologist, 1866–1950] 1 See under LOOP. 2 Meyer system, Meyer's theory. See under PSYCHOBIOLOGY.

Meyer [Georg Hermann von *Meyer*, German anatomist, 1815–1892] 1 See under ORGAN, LINE. 2 Meyer sinus. See under SINUS MEYERI.

Meyer [Hans Horst *Meyer*, German pharmacologist, 1853–1939] Meyer-Overton theory. See under LIPOID THEORY OF NARCOSIS.

Meyer [Hans Wilhelm *Meyer*, Danish otologist, 1824–1885] Meyer's disease. See under ADENOIDISM.

Meyer [Victor *Meyer*, German chemist, 1848–1897] See under LAW.

Meyer [Willy *Meyer*, U.S. surgeon, 1859–1932] Meyer's operation. See under RADICAL MASTECTOMY.

Meyer-Betz [Friedrich *Meyer-Betz*, German physician, flourished early 20th century] Meyer-Betz disease. See under FAMILIAL MYOGLOBINURIA.

Meyerhof [Otto Fritz *Meyerhof*, German biochemist, 1884–1951] Embden-Meyerhof cycle. See under EMBDEN-MEYERHOF PATHWAY.

Meyer-Schwickerath [Gerhard *Meyer-Schwickerath*, German ophthalmologist, born 1920] Meyer-Schwickerath and Weyer syndrome. See under OCULODENTODIGITAL DYSPLASIA.

Meynert [Theodor Hermann *Meynert*, German-born physician active in Austria, 1833–1892] **1** Meynert's bundle, Meynert's fasciculus, Meynert's tract, fibers of Meynert. See under FASCICULUS RETROFLEXUS. **2** Meynert's commissure. See under VENTRAL SUPRAOPTIC COMMISSURE. **3** Meynert's cells. See under CELL. **4** See under NUCLEUS. **5** Meynert's layer. See under INTERNAL PYRAMID LAYER.

Meynet [Paul C. H. *Meynet*, French physician, 1831–1892] Meynet's nodes. See under NODE.

mezereon MEZEREUM.

mezereum The dried bark of shrubs in the genus *Daphne*, family Thymelaeaceae. It has vesicatory and purgative properties. Also called *mezereon, spurge flax, olive spurge.*

MF **1** microscopic factor. **2** mitotic figure. **3** multiplying factor. **4** mycosis fungoides.

mF Symbol for the unit, millifarad.

μF Symbol for the unit, microfarad.

MFD minimal fatal dose.

m. ft. *mistura fiat* (L, let a mixture be made).

Mg Symbol for the element, magnesium.

mg Symbol for the unit, milligram.

mg% Symbol for the concentration of a solution expressed in milligrams per 100 milliliters.

mγ Symbol for the obsolete unit, milligamma.

μg Symbol for the unit, microgram.

μγ Symbol for the obsolete unit, microgamma.

mg/dl Symbol for the unit, milligram per deciliter.

mg·dl⁻¹ Symbol for the unit, milligram per deciliter.

mg·h Symbol for the obsolete unit, milligram-hour.

mg/l Symbol for the unit, milligram per liter.

mg·l⁻¹ Symbol for the unit, milligram per liter.

μg/l Symbol for the unit, microgram per liter.

μg·l⁻¹ Symbol for the unit, microgram per liter.

mgm Symbol for the unit, milligram. An incorrect symbol.

mgr Symbol for the unit, milligram. An incorrect symbol.

MGS metric gravitational system.

MGUS monoclonal gammopathy of undetermined significance.

mGy Symbol for the unit, milligray.

μGy Symbol for the unit, microgray.

mH Symbol for the unit, millihenry.

μH Symbol for the unit, microhenry.

MHC major histocompatibility complex.

mHg Symbol for the unit, millimeter of mercury (conventional millimeter of mercury).

μHg Symbol for the unit, micron of mercury.

mho A unit of electric conductance, the reciprocal of the ohm, now replaced by the siemens. An obsolete term.

MHz Symbol for the unit, megahertz.

mi Symbol for the unit, mile.

miasmology [Gk *miasm(a)* defilement, pollution + *o* + -LOGY] The study of unwholesome or noxious atmospheres, effluvia, or emanations. An obsolete term.

Mibelli [Vittorio *Mibelli*, Italian dermatologist, 1860–1910] **1**

See under POROKERATOSIS. **2** Angiokeratomas of Mibelli. See under ANGIOKERATOMA.

mic A unit of inductance, equal to one microhenry. A popular usage.

mica [L, a crumb, morsel (sense later altered by influence of *micare* to glitter)] A mineral occurring in fine transparent sheets, easily cleavable and flexible, composed of a mixture of silicates of aluminum, iron, and alkali metals. It is found in many crystalline rocks. It is used as an insulator because of its high resistance to heat, and in the manufacture of various optical components and instruments.

mication [L *micatus*, past part. of *micare* to move quickly, flicker, glance] A rapid motion, such as blinking.

micatosis [MICA + *t* + -OSIS] Pneumoconiosis due to inhalation of particles of mica.

mice Plural of MOUSE.

micelle [French (from L *mica* crumb, morsel, particle), a particle formed from an aggregate of similar molecules] **1** A submicroscopic unit of protoplasm. **2** A molecular aggregate as that of a colloid, often formed by the action of detergents on a hydrocarbon in water. It usually has a hydrocarbon interior and a surface of charged groups.

Michaelis [Gustav Adolph *Michaelis*, German obstetrician, 1798–1848] See under RHOMBOID.

Michaelis [Leonor *Michaelis*, German-born U.S. chemist, 1875–1949] **1** See under CONSTANT, STAIN. **2** Michaelis equation. See under MICHAELIS-MENTEN EQUATION. **3** Michaelis-Menton kinetics. See under MICHAELIS KINETICS. **4** Michaelis-Gutmann bodies. See under BODY.

Michel [Gaston *Michel*, French surgeon, 1875–1937] Michel's clip. See under SKIN CLIP.

Michel [J. von *Michel*, German ophthalmologist, 1943–1911] Michel's flecks. See under FLECK.

Micheli [Ferdinando *Micheli*, Italian physician, 1872–1937] **1** Marchiafava-Micheli disease, Marchiafava-Micheli syndrome. See under PAROXYSMAL NOCTURNAL HEMOGLOBINURIA. **2** Microelliptopoikilocytic anemia of Rietti, Greppi, and Micheli. See under ANEMIA.

miconazole $C_{18}H_{14}Cl_4N_2O \cdot HNO_3$. 1-[2,4-Dichloro-β-[(2,4-dichlorobenzyl)oxy]phenethyl]imidazole mononitrate. An antifungal agent.

micr- MICRO-.

micra Plural of MICRON.

micracoustic **1** Relating to faint sounds. **2** Amplifying faint sounds to make them audible. Also *microcoustic.*

micranatomy HISTOLOGY.

micrangiopathy MICROANGIOPATHY.

micrangium [MICR- + *ang(i)-* + L *-ium*, neut. sing. noun termination] A group of small blood vessels, such as capillaries and arterioles.

micrencephalia MICRENCEPHALY.

micrencephalon [MICR- + Gk *encephalos* brain] **1** An obsolete term for CEREBELLUM. **2** An abnormally small brain. Also called *microencephalon.*

micrencephalous Possessing an abnormally small brain.

micrencephaly [MICR- + ENCEPHAL- + -Y] An abnormal smallness of the brain. Also called *microencephaly, micrencephalia.*

micro- [Gk *mikros* small, little] A combining form meaning (1) very small, minute; (2) abnormally small; (3) acting to enlarge an image; (4) depending on or relating to microscopy, microscopic; (5) 10^{-6}, one millionth: used with SI units. Also *micr-, mikro-.* Symbol: μ

microabscess [MICRO- + ABSCESS] A small abscess, usually a millimeter or less in diameter and often multiple, seen in multiple organs during septicemia.

Munro's microabscesses   One of the characteristic lesions of psoriasis, consisting of focal accumulations of polymorphonuclear leukocytes in the upper layer of the epidermis. Also called *Munro's abscesses.*

Pautrier's microabscesses   Focal collections of atypical T lymphocytes in the epidermis of patients with mycosis fungoides. Also called *Pautrier's abscesses.*

microadenoma [MICRO- + ADENOMA]   A small, nonmalignant, glandular tumor, such as those associated with Cushing's disease.

microadenopathy   A disorder of small lymphatics.

microaerophil   An anaerobe that can tolerate or requires a low oxygen tension. Adjective: microaerophilic.

microaerosol   A suspension in the air of minute particles, the maximum diameter of which is variously taken as 1 to 10 μ.

microaerotonometer   An instrument for determining the amount of gases dissolved in the blood.

microalbuminuria   Excretion in the urine of less than 100 μg per minute of albumin but more than 15 μg per minute. A sensitive radioimmunoassay technique is necessary to measure albumin in this range. Microalbuminuria is an early sign of diabetic glomerulopathy.

microaleuriospore [MICRO- + Gk *aleur(on)* flour + *io* + -SPORE]   An outmoded term for MICROCONIDIUM.

microammeter   An instrument calibrated to measure the magnitude of electric current in microamperes.

microampere [MICRO- + AMPERE]   A unit of electric current equal to 10^{-6} ampere. Symbol: μA

microanalysis   Analysis using small amounts of material, particularly by modern methods that are much more sensitive than the classical methods of chemical analysis that involved weighing precipitated material.

microanatomist   HISTOLOGIST.

microanatomy   HISTOLOGY.

microaneurysm   An aneurysmal dilitation affecting small arteries, arterioles, or capillaries. Capillary microaneurysms in the retina are a feature of diabetes mellitus. Microaneurysms also occur in other disorders, including thrombotic thrombocytopenic purpura.

diabetic microaneurysm   Multiple, small (10–200 μ in diameter) aneurysms arising from retinal capillaries, a sign that is virtually diagnostic of diabetes mellitus and, together with the associated exudates and hemorrhage, constitute the characteristic feature of diabetic retinopathy.

microangiography [MICRO- + ANGIOGRAPHY]   Magnification roentgenography of small blood vessels which have been opacified by the injection of a contrast medium.

microangiopathic   Pertaining to or characterized by microangiopathy.

microangiopathy [MICRO- + ANGIOPATHY]   A disease process affecting small blood vessels. Also called *micrangiopathy.*

diabetic microangiopathy   Thickening of the basement membrane in capillaries at many sites in diabetes mellitus, as in the retina and kidney. It is a major cause of severe pathologic complications contributing to disability. The pathogenesis is poorly understood, but appears to be related to poor control of hyperglycemia.

diabetic renal microangiopathy   Disease of the small blood vessels of the kidney, including the afferent and efferent arterioles, in long-standing diabetes mellitus, characterized by thickening of the basement membrane and, often, associated microaneurysms. It is associated with the Kimmelstiel-Wilson syndrome.

dietetic microangiopathy   A disease of small blood vessels in pigs, particularly affecting the vessels of the heart. It is probably caused by a deficiency of selenium and vitamin E. Also called *mulberry heart disease.* (outmoded).

thrombotic microangiopathy   Microangiopathy associated with or due to clots in arterioles and capillaries.

microangioscopy   CAPILLARIOSCOPY.

microaudiphone   An instrument that amplifies faint sounds to make them audible.

microbalance   An analytical balance used for weighing in increments as small as 1 μg.

microbar [MICRO- + BAR]   A unit of pressure equal to 10^{-6} bar; 0.1 pascal. Symbol: μbar

microbe [MICRO- + -*be*, combining form from Gk *bi(os)* life]   MICROORGANISM.

microbemia   SEPTICEMIA.

microbial   Pertaining to or caused by a microbe or microbes. Also *microbic.*

microbic   MICROBIAL.

microbicidal   Lethal to microbes.

microbicide [*microb(e)* + *i* + -CIDE]   An agent that kills microbes.

microbid   A widespread eruption in a sensitized subject that is attributed to the dissemination of bacterial allergens from a focus of infection.

microbiemia   SEPTICEMIA.

microbioassay   A nonquantitative analytical technique for demonstrating the presence of biologically active materials, based on the effect exerted on the growth of cultured microorganisms.

microbiologist   A specialist in the study of microbiology.

microbiology [MICRO- + BIOLOGY]   The branch of science concerned with microorganisms. It can be divided variously into branches, either by content (bacteriology, virology, mycology, protozoology, phycology) or by area of application (medical, soil, etc.). Adjective: microbiologic.

microbion   An obsolete term for MICROORGANISM.

microbiota   Minute organisms, such as bacteria, fungi, algae, and protozoa, that comprise the microflora and microfauna of a biotic community.

microbiotic   **1** Having to do with microscopic organisms. **2** Relating to the microbiota.

microbism   The state of being infected with microbes.

latent microbism   The asymptomatic presence of certain pathogenic microorganisms in the body; a carrier state.

microblast   A small nucleated erythroid precursor, often having a diameter less than that of mature erythrocytes.

microblepharia   MICROBLEPHARY.

microblepharism   MICROBLEPHARY.

microblepharon   An abnormally small eyelid.

microblephary [MICRO- + BLEPHAR- + -Y]   An abnormal smallness of the eyelids, often associated with smallness of the palpebral fissure. Also called *microblepharia, microblepharism.*

microbody [MICRO- + BODY]   A membrane-bound cytoplasmic particle, approximately 0.5–1.0 μm in diameter, containing enzymes. See also PEROXISOME, GLYOXISOME.

microbrachia [MICRO- + L *brachia* arms]   Abnormal smallness of one or both arms.

microbrachius [New L (from MICRO- + Gk *brachiōn* arm)]   An embryo, fetus, or postnatal individual with abnormally small or foreshortened arms.

microbrenner [MICRO- + German *Brenner* burner]   An electric cautery with a needlelike point.

microburet   A buret for measuring or delivering small aliquots of fluids or gases in increments ranging from 0.001 to 0.02 ml.

microcalculus [MICRO- + CALCULUS]   A very small calculus formed in the lumen of a renal tubule and which may serve as a focus for calcification of the tubule. Also called *microlith*.

microcalorie   An outmoded term for 15°C CALORIE.

microcalorimetry   The measurement of heat absorption or production in minute systems.

microcapsule   A layer too thin to be visualized but providing a bacterium with the surface antigen characteristic of a capsule.

microcardia [MICRO- + -CARDIA]   An abnormal small size of the heart.

microcardius [New L (from MICRO- + Gk *kardia* heart)]   An individual possessing an abnormally small heart.

microcarriers   Miniature beads that multiply the surface area and hence the yield for anchorage-dependent cells during cell culture.

microcaulia [MICRO- + Gk *kaul(os)* stem, stalk, penis + -IA]   An abnormal smallness of the penis.

microcavitation   The formation of very small abscess cavities.

microcentrum [MICRO- + CENTRUM]   CENTROSOME.

microcephalia   MICROCEPHALY.

microcephalic   MICROCEPHALOUS.

microcephalism   MICROCEPHALY.

microcephalous   Exhibiting microcephaly. Also *leptocephalous, leptocephalic, microcephalic*.

microcephalus   A fetus or postnatal individual with microcephaly. Also called *leptocephalus*.

microcephaly [MICRO- + Gk *kephalē* the head + -Y]   Abnormal smallness of the brain case specifically, or of the head as a whole. Also called *microcephalia, microcephalism, microcrania, leptocephaly*.

   encephaloclastic microcephaly   Microcephaly associated with congenital growth deficiencies in localized parts of the brain.

   schizencephalic microcephaly   Microcephaly associated with specific developmental defects of the brain, particularly those of an aplastic nature.

microcercous [MICRO- + Gk *kerk(os)* tail + -OUS]   Having a very short tail.

microcheilia [MICRO- + CHEIL- + -IA]   The abnormal smallness of one or both lips. Also *microchilia*.

microcheilus   A fetus or postnatal individual with microcheilia.

microcheiria [MICRO- + CHEIR- + -IA]   An abnormal smallness of one or both hands. Also *microchiria*.

microcheirus   A fetus or postnatal individual with microcheiria.

microchemistry   The branch of chemical practice dealing with small quantities of substance, about 20mg–10 mg. It includes two types of operation: the preparation of traces of substances by special apparatus such as micromanipulators, and the measurement of small quantities of substance (microanalysis). Adjective: microchemical.

microchilia   MICROCHEILIA.

microchiria   MICROCHEILIA.

microcinematography   The use of motion pictures of microscopic specimens, revealing movement and growth. Time-lapse microcinematography can greatly compress the time scale.

microcirculation [MICRO- + CIRCULATION]   The circulation in the small vessels (arterioles, capillaries, and venules).

microclimate [MICRO- + CLIMATE]   The climate of a small portion of the environment as that adjacent to a surface or in a small area such as that in a room or plant community.

Micrococcaceae [MICRO- + L *cocc(us)* the scarlet berry, kermes berry + -ACEAE]   A family of Gram-positive spherical bacteria that characteristically divide in more than one plane to yield irregular clusters. The family includes the aerobic micrococci found in the environment and the facultative staphylococci found on animals. However, the two are biologically distant, the G + C content being 65–70% and 30–35%, respectively.

micrococci   Plural of MICROCOCCUS.

micrococcin   A naturally occurring antibiotic obtained from a particular strain of *Micrococcus*. It has antitubercular activity.

Micrococcus [New L, from MICRO- + L *coccum* or *coccus* (from Gk *kokkos* a kernel, berry, esp. the kermes berry) the kermes berry, scarlet berry, scarlet dye, a scarlet coat]   A genus of the family Micrococcaceae that is found in the environment. They resemble staphylococci morphologically but differ in other fundamental respects.

micrococcus (*plural* micrococci)   Any organism of the genus *Micrococcus*.

microcolon   An abnormally small colon.

microcolony   A colony so small as to require magnification for ready observation.

microcomedo [MICRO- + COMEDO]   An early stage in the formation of a comedo in which the hair follicle becomes dilated by impacted keratin.

microcomputer   A computer that has the central processing unit, timing, control, and memory on one or a few integrated-circuit chips.

microconidia   Plural of MICROCONIDIUM.

microconidium [MICRO- + CONIDIUM]   (*plural* microconidia)   A consistently small fungal conidium, asexually formed, that often serves as a spermatium. It is distinguished by its size from a macroconidium produced by the same fungal organism. Also called *microspore, microaleuriospore* (outmoded).

microcoria [MICRO- + *cor(e)-* + -IA]   An abnormal smallness of the pupil, particularly as seen in congenital constriction of the pupil.

microcornea [MICRO- + CORNEA]   An abnormally small cornea, associated with relatively normal size of the rest of the eye.

microcosm [French *microcosme* (from Gk *mikro(s)* little + *kosm(os)* order, world, universe) a little world, microcosm]   A local ecosystem with discrete boundaries that is often viewed as a miniature world or balanced biologic system for experimental purposes or for use as a model of the functioning of larger and more complex environmental units. Compare MACROCOSM.

microcoulomb [MICRO- + COULOMB]   A unit of quantity of electricity, electric charge, or electric flux, equal to 10^{-6} coulomb. Symbol: μC

microcoustic   MICRACOUSTIC.

microcrania   MICROCEPHALY.

microcrystalline   Describing the state of matter in which the material is in small, randomly orientated crystals. It therefore appears amorphous, and a single crystal cannot be isolated for study.

microcurie   A unit of activity of a radionuclide or of a radioactive source equal to 10^{-6} curie; 3.7×10^4 becquerels exactly. Symbol: μCi

microcurie-hour   A unit of total number of nuclear transformations or transitions, equal to 10^{-6} curie-hour; 1.332×10^8 transformations. Symbol: μCi·h

microcyst   A very small cyst.

microcystometer [MICRO- + CYSTO- + -METER]   A small device to measure pressure in the urinary bladder.

microcyte   An erythrocyte of less than normal volume. Also called *microerythrocyte*.

microcythemia   MICROCYTOSIS.

microcytosis   A predominance of microcytes in the blood. Also called *microcythemia*.

microdactylia   MICRODACTYLY.

microdactylous   Characterized by microdactyly.

microdactyly [MICRO- + DACTYL- + -Y]   An abnormal smallness of one or more fingers or toes. Also called *microdactylia*.

microdentism   MICRODONTIA.

microdissection   The dissection of tissue using a dissecting microscope for visualization and very fine instruments for manipulation. Also called *microvivisection*.

microdont [MICR- + -ODONT]   Having abnormally small teeth. Also *microdontic*.

microdontia [MICR- + -ODONTIA]   The condition of having abnormally small teeth. Also called *microdentism, microdontism*.

microdontic   MICRODONT.

microdontism   MICRODONTIA.

microdrepanocytic   Pertaining to hemoglobin S-β-thalassemia.

microdrepanocytosis   HEMOGLOBIN S-β-THALASSEMIA. Adjective: microdrepanocytic.

microecology   That aspect of parasite ecology that deals with the mutual effects of the host-parasite relationship.

microecosystem   A small ecosystem, either naturally occurring or contrived by man for experimental purposes.

microelectrode   In electroencephalography, an electrode with a very small tip diameter (less than 100 μm) which is placed in direct contact with the surface of the brain, or which is inserted into the brain substance in an attempt to record the activity of a single neuron.

microelectrophoresis   An analytic technique in which the direction and velocity of electrophoretic migration of charged particles is observed and measured microscopically.

microelectrophoretic   Pertaining to or derived from microelectrophoresis.

microembolus (*plural* microemboli) An embolus which occludes a small vessel.

microencephalon   MICRENCEPHALON.

microencephaly   MICRENCEPHALY.

microenvironment [MICRO- + ENVIRONMENT]   The area immediately surrounding an individual, such as a patient's bed, bedside locker, and chair in a hospital.

microerythrocyte   MICROCYTE.

microesthesia [MICRO- + ESTHESIA]   A defect of sensation in which the patient underestimates the weight and volume of an object held in the hand.

microevolution   Organismal evolution that is concerned with speciation.

microfarad [MICRO- + FARAD]   A unit of electric capacitance equal to 10^{-6} farad. Symbol: μF

microfauna   Microscopic animals or protozoa.

microfibril   FIBRIL.

microfibroadenoma [MICRO- + FIBROADENOMA]   A minute fibroadenoma visible only with a microscope.

microfilament   A cytoplasmic filament 4–6 nm in diameter, composed of the protein actin and often associated with cellular movement. Microfilaments are present in most eukaryotic cells.

microfilaremia [*microfilar(iae)* + -EMIA]   The presence of microfilariae in the peripheral blood.

microfilaria [MICRO- + FILARIA]   (*plural* microfilariae) A prelarval parasite of the superfamily Filarioidea, family Onchocercidae, found extracellularly in the blood or tissue fluids of the

human host and in the tissues of the vector.   • The term has sometimes been used as a pseudo-genus name, but it has no taxonomic significance, and when combined with species epithets as in the subentries below, it is better not capitalized or italicized.

microfilaria bancrofti   The sheathed, blood-inhabiting microfilaria of *Wuchereria bancrofti*, found only at night in the peripheral blood of the nocturnally periodic strains.

microfilaria diurna   An obsolete term for MICROFILARIA LOA.

microfilaria loa   The sheathed microfilaria of *Loa loa*, found diurnally in the peripheral blood of its human or other primate host. Also called *microfilaria diurna* (obsolete).

microfilaria malaya   The sheathed microfilaria of *Brugia malayi* found in peripheral blood, appearing at night in the nocturnally periodic strains.

sheathed microfilaria   A microfilaria encased in a stretched vitelline membrane that extends beyond either end of the organism. Species that have sheathed microfilariae found in human blood include *Wuchereria bancrofti, Brugia malayi,* and *Loa loa*.

microfilaria streptocerca   The skin-inhabiting, unsheathed microfilaria of *Mansonella streptocerca*.

microfilaria volvulus   The unsheathed microfilaria of *Onchocerca volvulus*, found in dermal tissue fluids.

microfilariasis   The presence of microfilariae in the blood or tissue fluids of the host.

microfilm   **1** A photographic film bearing greatly reduced images of printed records.   **2** To record on microfilm.

microflora   The bacteria and fungi that inhabit an area.

microfollicular   Composed of very small follicles.

microfracture   HAIRLINE FRACTURE.

microfungus [MICRO- + FUNGUS]   A small fungus, usually best observed using a microscope. The majority of fungi other than some Ascomycetes and Basidiomycetes fall into this category.

microgamete   The smaller, or spermlike, motile gamete produced in anisogamy. It fuses with the macrogamete, leading to zygote formation.

microgametocyte   The mother cell that produces microgametes in anisogametic reproduction. Also called *microgamont*.

microgamma [MICRO- + GAMMA]   A unit of mass or weight equal to 10^{-12} gram or one picogram. An obsolete unit. Symbol: $\mu\gamma$

microgamont   MICROGAMETOCYTE.

microgamy [MICRO- + GAM- + -Y]   ISOGAMY.

microgasometer / Natelson microgasometer   An instrument for manometric measurement of gases in quantities of fluid as small as 0.03 ml, using the measurement of gas partial pressures in a closed system before and after the absorption of carbon dioxide.

microgastria [MICRO- + GASTR- + -IA]   An abnormal smallness of the stomach.

microgastric [MICRO- + GASTRIC]   Having a small abdomen: said of animals, particularly insects.

microgenesis   HYPOPLASIA.

microgenia [MICRO- + Gk *gen(eion)* the chin + -IA]   An abnormal smallness of the chin.

microgenitalism [MICRO- + GENITAL + -ISM]   **1** The occurrence of abnormally small genitalia in relation to the overall developmental stage.   **2** The presence of infantile genitalia in an adolescent or adult individual.

microglia [MICRO- + GLIA]   Small cells of nonectodermal origin that form the third of the three major families of neuroglia in the central nervous system. Microglia are believed to be of mesodermal origin and may have several sources, such as circulating monocytes and perivascular pericytes. Following infection or damage to brain tissue, they become actively phagocytic (gitter cells), rounded with phagocytized material, and are usually carried away and destroyed. Also called *microglial cells, perivascular glial cells, Hortega cells.*

microgliacyte   MICROGLIOCYTE.

microglial   Of or pertaining to microglia.

microgliocyte [MICRO- + GLIOCYTE]   A microglial cell. See under MICROGLIA. Also *microgliacyte.*

microglioma [MICRO- + GLIOMA]   A primary lymphoma of the central nervous system.

microgliomatosis cerebri   A diffuse neoplastic process originating in the microglial cells and spreading widely through the brain. Also called *cerebral reticulum cell sarcoma.*

microgliosis [*microgli(a)* + -OSIS]   An excess or proliferation of microglia.

microglobulin [MICRO- + GLOBULIN]   Any serum or urinary globulin of molecular mass below about 40 kDa, including especially Bence-Jones proteins.

β-microglobulin   A polypeptide of 11 600 daltons that forms the light chain of class 1 major histocompatibility antigens and can therefore be detected on all cells bearing these antigens. Free β2-microglobulin is found in the blood and in particular the urine of patients with certain diseases, such as Wilson's disease, cadmium poisoning, and renal tubular acidosis.

microglossia [MICRO- + GLOSS- + -IA]   An abnormally small tongue. It is often seen in hypomicrognathus and agnathia.

microglossic   1 Of or characterized by microglossia.   2 Having a short tongue: said particularly of certain insects.

micrognathia [MICRO- + GNATH- + -IA]   Abnormal smallness of either the upper or lower jaw, particularly the lower. Congenital or acquired varieties occur. The condition may be apparent only, due to the abnormal position of the jaws.

microgonioscope   A device to observe the anterior chamber angle under magnification.

microgram [MICRO- + GRAM]   A unit of mass or weight equal to 10^{-6} gram, or 10^{-9} kilogram. Also called *gamma (obsolete and informal)*. Symbol: μg

microgram per liter   A unit of mass concentration equal to 10^{-6} gram per liter. Symbol: μg/l, μg·l⁻¹

micrograph [MICRO- + -GRAPH]   1 PHOTOMICROGRAPH.   2 An instrument that converts pressure fluctuations, such as those from the arterial pulse, to minute deviations of a diaphragm. The deviations are magnified by a reflected light beam and recorded on moving film.

acoustic micrograph   The image produced by an acoustic microscope.

electron micrograph   The photographic image that is produced by an electron microscope. Also called *electronograph.*

micrographia [MICRO- + GRAPH- + -IA]   Writing in very small letters, often decreasing progressively in size, as often seen in patients with Parkinson's disease.

micrography   1 MICROSCOPY.   2 A description of materials observed by microscopic examination.

microgray [MICRO- + GRAY]   A unit of absorbed dose in the field of ionizing radiation equal to 10^{-6} gray. Symbol: μGy

microgyri   Plural of MICROGYRUS.

microgyria [MICRO- + GYR- + -IA]   The abnormal smallness or narrowness of cerebral convolutions, usually associated with polygyria.

microgyrus   A fetus or postnatal individual with microgyria.

microhabitat   The local or immediate part of the environment of an organism. It is the smallest unit of the biosphere.

microhaematocrit   A British spelling for MICROHEMATOCRIT.

microhemagglutination   The agglutination of small quantities of red blood cells in multiple-well plates. It is used as the end point in many immunologic procedures performed in these microtiter plates.

microhematocrit   Use of a capillary tube to determine by centrifugation the packed cell volume of a small sample of blood.

microhenry [MICRO- + HENRY]   A unit of inductance equal to 10^{-6} henry. Symbol: μH

microhepatia [MICRO- + HEPAT- + -IA]   An abnormal smallness of the liver. It can result from developmental or pathologic causes.

microheterogeneity   The occurrence of molecules that are not identical, but whose differences are very limited. A glycoprotein, for example, might have molecules all of which possessed the same polypeptide chain, glycosylated on the same amino-acid residues, but by oligosaccharides that differed slightly in numbers of monosaccharide residues.

microhistology   HISTOLOGY.

microhm [MICR- + OHM]   A unit of electrical resistance equal to 10^{-6} ohm. Also called *microohm*. Symbol: μΩ

micro-inch [MICRO- + INCH]   A unit of length equal to 10^{-6} inch; 0.0254 micrometer or 25.4 nanometers. Symbol: μin

microincineration   The reduction to ashes of very small pieces of tissue or other material prior to the identification of their constituent elements.

microincision [MICRO- + INCISION]   A small opening into a cell, usually made to remove or destroy a cellular organelle. Microincisions can be made with a laser beam.

microinfarct   An infarct resulting from occlusion of a small vessel.

microinjection [MICRO- + INJECTION]   The injection of small quantities of material into a cell, usually using a micromanipulator and a microneedle.

microinjector   A device permitting the delivery, by infusion, of a very small quantity of drug or other medicinal agent.

microinvasion [MICRO- + INVASION]   Invasion by a cancer too short a distance to be detected without a microscope. The term usually applies to squamous cell carcinoma of the cervix invading the underlying stroma.

microkatal [MICRO- + KATAL]   A unit of catalytic activity equal to 10^{-6} katal; 10^{-6} mole per second. Symbol: μkat

microkeratome [MICRO- + KERATOME]   A surgical instrument for precise cutting of the cornea.

microkymatotherapy   MICROWAVE THERAPY.

microlaryngoscopy   Suspension laryngoscopy using a specially designed laryngoscope through which the surgeon may inspect a magnified image of the interior of the larynx with the operating microscope and carry out any necessary surgery with correspondingly greater precision.

microlecithal [MICRO- + LECITH- + -AL]   MIOLECITHAL.

microlens [MICRO- + LENS]   A very small, thin, contact lens.

microlentia   SPHEROPHAKIA.

microlesion [MICRO- + LESION]   A lesion of minute size.

microleukoblast   MYELOBLAST.

microliter [MICRO- + LITER]   A unit of volume or capacity equal to 10^{-6} liter, 10^{-9} cubic meter, or 10^{-3} cubic centimeter. Symbol: μl

microlith [MICRO- + Gk *lith(os)* a stone]   MICROCALCULUS.

microlithiasis [MICRO- + LITHIASIS]   Small mineral concretions present within an organ, such as those seen in pulmonary alveoli and prostatic glands.

microlithiasis alveolaris pulmonum   PULMONARY ALVEOLAR MICROLITHIASIS.

pulmonary alveolar microlithiasis   A condition of unknown cause in which innumerable small hard calcium-containing nodules are present in the alveoli of both lungs. Also called *microlithiasis alveolaris pulmonum*.

micromandible   An abnormal shortness of the mandible. Also called *brachygnathia*.

micromania   MICROMANIACAL DELIRIUM.

micromanipulation   The handling or management of extremely small pieces of tissue or cells or parts of cells, as in removing a defective gene from a cell and replacing it with a normal gene. Also called *micrurgy*.

micromanipulator   Any device used to hold and control the instruments used in microdissection.

micromanometer   A device for measuring pressure of minute amounts of gas or vapor. It is used especially in measuring gas generated by metabolic activity of small tissue specimens.

micromanometric   Pertaining to or derived from use of a micromanometer.

micromastia [MICRO- + MAST- + -IA]   Abnormally small breasts. Also called *micromazia*.

micromaxilla [MICRO- + MAXILLA]   An extremely small maxilla.

micromazia [MICRO- + *maz(o)*- + -IA]   MICROMASTIA.

micromegalopsia [MICRO- + *megal(o)*- + -OPSIA]   The abnormal perception of objects as changing in size, becoming alternately larger and smaller than in normal perception.

micromegaly [MICRO- + -MEGALY]   PROGERIA.

micromelia [MICRO- + MEL-[1] + -IA]   A disproportionate shortness or smallness of one or more limbs.

   rhizomelic micromelia   A developmental deformity of a limb in which the limb is shortened because of the absence or deficient development of the proximal segments.

micromelic   Displaying micromelia.

micromelus   A fetus or postnatal individual with micromelia.

micromere [MICRO- + -MERE]   A small blastomere resulting from unequal cleavage of a developing zygote.

micromerozoite [MICRO- + MEROZOITE]   An extremely small type of merozoite.

micrometastasis [MICRO- + METASTASIS]   (*plural* micrometastases) A metastatic deposit of cancer of microscopic size.

micrometeorology   The study of meteorology in a restricted zone, usually within a shallow layer of atmosphere close to the earth.

micrometer[1] [MICRO- + -METER]   A unit of length equal to 10^{-6} meter. Also called *micron* (obsolete). Symbol: μm

   conventional micrometer of mercury   A unit or pressure equal to 10^{-3} conventional millimeter of mercury; 0.133 322 pascal. Also called *micron of mercury* (popular). Symbol: μmHg

   micrometer of mercury   See under CONVENTIONAL MICROMETER OF MERCURY.

micrometer[2] [French *micromètre*, from *micro*- MICRO- + -*mètre* -METER]   1 An instrument containing a microscope for accurate linear measurement of very small units of length.   2 A caliper having a spindle moved by a screw for measuring minute distances.

   caliper micrometer   A caliper that is driven by a finely threaded screw (micrometer screw) and used to measure extremely thin objects.

   eyepiece micrometer   A calibrated scale for linear measurement that is inserted into the eyepiece of a compound microscope and used for direct determination of the size of objects viewed. Also called *ocular micrometer*.

   filar micrometer   An eyepiece micrometer consisting of two parallel wires and a graduated distance scale. Measurement is made by moving one of the two wires across the graduated scale away from the fixed wire.

   ocular micrometer   EYEPIECE MICROMETER.

   screw micrometer   A device for measuring circumferential distance and the angle subtended.

   slide micrometer   A measuring scale marked on a glass slide and intended for use in a microscope field of view.

   stage micrometer   A micrometer ruled on a microscope stage, which is usually movable. It is often in the form of a vernier to allow accurate measurement of very small movements of the viewing field.

   vernier-scale micrometer   A slide micrometer or stage micrometer that uses a vernier for measuring increments of distance.

micromethod   Any laboratory procedure that uses much smaller quantities of test materials and reagents than a standard method.

micrometre   A British spelling for MICROMETER.

micrometry   The use of a micrometer and microscope to measure minute objects.

micromicro- [MICRO- + MICRO-]   A combining form denoting 10^{-12}: formerly used with SI units, now replaced by *pico*-. Symbol: $\mu\mu$

micromicrocurie [MICROMICRO- + CURIE]   An outmoded term for PICOCURIE. Symbol: $\mu\mu$Ci

micromicrofarad [MICROMICRO- + FARAD]   An outmoded term for PICOFARAD. Symbol: $\mu\mu$F

micromicrogram [MICROMICRO- + GRAM]   An outmoded term for PICOGRAM. Symbol: $\mu\mu$g

micromicron [MICRO- + Gk *mikron*, neut. of *mikros* small, little]   An obsolete term for PICOMETER. Symbol: $\mu\mu$

micromil [contraction of MICROMIL(LIMETER)]   An obsolete term for NANOMETER.

micromilli- [MICRO- + MILLI-]   A combining form denoting 10^{-9}: formerly used with SI units, now replaced by *nano*-. Symbol: μm

micromilligram [MICROMILLI- + GRAM]   An outmoded term for NANOGRAM. Symbol: μmg

micromillimeter [MICROMILLI- + METER]   An obsolete term for NANOMETER. Symbol: μmm

micromolar   A unit of concentration equal to 10^{-6} molecular weight in grams (10^{-6} mole) dissolved in one liter of solution. An obsolete unit. Symbol: μM

micromole [MICRO- + MOLE[3]]   A unit of amount of substance equal to 10^{-6} mole. Symbol: μmol

Micromonospora   A genus of actinomycete that has yielded a few antibiotics, designated by the suffix -*micin*.

micromonosporin   A naturally occurring antibiotic produced by cultures of *Micromonospora*. It is active against a wide variety of Gram-positive bacterial species.

micromotor [MICRO- + MOTOR]   A miniaturized high-speed electric motor attached directly to the handpiece of a dental drill.

micromotoscope [MICRO- + *moto*-, combining form denoting motion, from *mo(tion)* + *(mo)to(r)* + -SCOPE]   A device to observe, measure, or record the movement of objects viewed with a microscope.

micromyelia [MICRO- + MYEL- + -IA]   A disproportionate smallness or shortness of the spinal cord.

micromyeloblast   A small myeloblast sometimes seen in acute myelogenous leukemia. Because of its small size, the micromyeloblast may be mistaken for a lymphocyte or lymphoblast.

micromyelolymphocyte   An obsolete term for MYELOBLAST.

micron [neut. of Gk *mikros* small]   1 An obsolete term for

MICROMETER. **2** A unit of time equal to the period of vibration of an ether wave which has a wavelength of one micrometer. An obsolete unit. Symbol: μ

micron of mercury A popular term for CONVENTIONAL MICROMETER OF MERCURY. Symbol: μHg

microneedle A thin glass needle used in microdissection or microsurgery.

microneme [MICRO- + -neme, combining form from Gk *nēma* thread, yarn, tissue] A small, rod-shaped organelle in the anterior portion of certain stages of sporozoa of the phylum Apicomplexa. It is a characteristic structure of merozoites and sporozoites and helps to define the phylum Apicomplexa. Also called *sarconeme, toxoneme*.

micronemous Having a fine, threadlike structure.

micronephridium [MICRO- + NEPHRIDIUM] (*plural* micronephridia) An excretory system in which the nephridia are very small, often lacking a nephrostome, as in certain oligochaetes.

micronewton [MICRO- + NEWTON] A unit of force equal to 10^{-6} newton. Symbol: μN

micronic Having the size of one micron (10^{-6} meter).

micronize [MICRON + -IZE] To pulverize or reduce material to particles of very small size, often to size that will pass through mesh of 400 to 1000 gauge.

micronodular Composed of small nodules.

micronodulation The state of being formed of many small nodules.

micronormoblast An erythrocyte precursor that is smaller than normal. The nucleus is pyknotic, and the cytoplasm contains some hemoglobin and forms a small rim around the nucleus. Micronormoblasts are present in the bone marrow in iron deficiency anemia.

micronucleus **1** The smaller of the two types of nuclei found in ciliate protozoa, the one involved in sexual or genetic exchange rather than in the vegetative functions of the macronucleus. Also called *reproductive nucleus, karyogonad, gonad nucleus, gametic nucleus*. **2** A small nucleus. **3** NUCLEOLUS.

micronutrient [MICRO- + NUTRIENT] Any essential dietary constituent, such as the vitamins and trace minerals, required by the body in small quantities.

micronychia [MICR- + ONYCH- + -IA] An abnormal smallness of one or more nails. Also called *micronychosis*.

micronychosis MICRONYCHIA.

micronystagmus Very small spontaneous movements of the eye, occurring normally in all persons.

microohm MICROHM.

micro-orchidia MICRORCHIDIA.

micro-orchism MICRORCHIDIA.

microorganism [MICRO- + ORGANISM] Any single-celled organism, formally assigned to the kingdom Protista. Also called *microbe, microbion* (obsolete).

    pyogenic microorganism A pus-producing microorganism, such as *Staphylococcus aureus* and *Streptococcus pyogenes*.

micropapular Consisting of small papules.

microparasite [MICRO- + PARASITE] A parasitic microorganism.

micropathological Pertaining to lesions or tissue changes visible with the light microscope. A rarely used term.

micropathology A rarely used term for HISTOPATHOLOGY.

micropenis [MICRO- + PENIS] A disproportionate smallness or shortness of the penis. Also called *microphallus*.

microperfusion The perfusion of small quantities of material.

microphage A small phagocyte, specifically a polymorphonuclear leukocyte. Microphages engulf and digest bacteria, whereas macrophages, such as monocytes, engulf and digest dead or senescent cells and cellular debris. Also called *microphagocyte, microphagus*.

microphagocyte MICROPHAGE.

microphagus MICROPHAGE.

microphakia SPHEROPHAKIA.

microphallus [MICRO- + L *phallus* (from Gk *phallos* penis) penis] MICROPENIS.

microphobia Pathologic fear of small objects or animals.

microphone A transducer that causes sound waves to generate or modulate an electric current, usually for recording or transmitting speech or music.

microphonia LEPTOPHONIA.

microphonics / cochlear microphonics Electrical potentials generated in the cochlea by the passage of sound waves across the middle ear. Also called *electrophonic effect* (seldom used), *Wever-Bray phenomenon*.

microphonograph A device to amplify and simultaneously to record, used in speech therapy for the hearing-impaired.

microphonoscope A stethoscope equipped with a membrane for amplification of the sound.

microphotograph PHOTOMICROGRAPH.

microphthalmia [MICR- + OPHTHALMIA] Abnormal smallness of one or both eyeballs. This is a recessive trait in humans. Also called *nanophthalmia, microphthalmos, nanophthalmos, microphthalmus, nanophthalmus*.

microphthalmic [MICR- + OPHTHALMIC] Having abnormally small eyes.

microphthalmos MICROPHTHALMIA.

microphthalmoscope A device for examination of the ocular fundus at high magnification.

microphthalmus MICROPHTHALMIA.

micropia MICROPSIA.

micropipet **1** A pipet calibrated for accurate delivery of very small quantities, usually less than 0.5 ml. **2** A pipet with a fine tip used in microinjection.

microplankton Plankton between 60 and 500 μm in size.

microplasia [MICRO- + -PLASIA] Abnormally limited growth, as in dwarfism.

microplastocyte A very small platelet. An obsolete term.

microplethysmography A sensitive technique for measuring very small changes in volume of an organ or part.

microplicae (*singular* microplica) Ridgelike folds on the surface of a cell. They are especially evident on epithelial cells from the inner cheek.

micropodia [MICRO- + POD- + -IA] An abnormal smallness of one or both feet.

micropolariscope A polariscope that is used in conjunction with a microscope for the polariscopic examination of microscopic materials.

micropollutant [MICRO- + POLLUTANT] A pollutant present in very small quantities.

micropolygyria POLYGYRIA.

micropore [MICRO- + PORE] A submicroscopic break in the membrane of a protozoan cell or microbe through which exchange of material, pinocytosis or other minute forms of flow may occur. It is seen in electron micrographs of *Eimeria* and *Plasmodium*. Also called *micropyle* (outmoded), *cytostome* (imprecise), *ultracytostome* (rarely used).

micropredation The act of feeding by an organism on some of the fluids or tissues of a larger organism without destroying the organism.

micropredator An organism that engages in micropredation.

microprobe An ultrafine probe used for exploration and fixation of tissues in microsurgical procedures.

laser microprobe   A diagnostic device consisting of a very fine laser beam that vaporizes a small region of tissue. The vapor is then analyzed by emission spectroscopy. Also called *laser microscope.*

microprogram   **1** A sequence of computer machine cycles necessary to execute a single program instruction. **2** A special-purpose program stored in read-only memory that is initiated by a single program instruction.

microprojection   A projection upon a screen of the visual field of a microscope.

microprojector   A device used for microprojection.

microprosopus [MICRO- + New L *prosopus* face, irreg. from Gk *prosōpon* face]   A fetus or postnatal individual with small or underdeveloped facial region.

micropsia [MICR- + -OPSIA]   Perception of objects as being much smaller than they would normally appear. It may result from stretching of the retina, as in retinal detachment, or occur as a visual hallucination in temporal lobe epilepsy, in intoxication from drugs, in febrile deliriums, and in other systemic or central nervous system disorders. Also called *visual diminutus, micropia, lilliputian hallucination, microptic hallucination.* Adjective: microptic.

micropterous   BRACHYPTEROUS.

microptic   Pertaining to micropsia.

micropuncture [MICRO- + PUNCTURE]   An experimental technique involving the insertion of a micropipet into the lumen of a renal tubule to collect tubular fluid in order to analyze functions of specific portions of the tubule.

micropus [New L (from MICRO- + New L *-pus*, combining form denoting foot, from Gk *pous* foot)]   A fetus or postnatal individual with abnormally small feet.

micropyknometer   A device used to measure the relative density of very small quantities of liquid.

micropyle [MICRO- + Gk *pylē* gate, entrance]   **1** A minute opening in the outer covering of teleost eggs, allowing the entry of the spermatozoa.   **2** An outmoded term for MICROPORE.

microquantity   A very small quantity, expressed in microgram units.

microradiogram   MICRORADIOGRAPH.

microradiograph   A recorded image obtained by microradiography, used for high-resolution imaging of thin objects such as tissue sections. Also called *microradiogram.*

microradiography   A technique by which a radiograph of a thin object, as a tissue section, is produced on fine-grained film and can be examined microscopically or enlarged with a resolution approaching the resolution of the photographic emulsion.

microrchidia [MICR- + *orchid(o)*- + -IA]   An abnormal smallness of one or both testicles. Also called *micro-orchism, microorchidia.*

microrefractometer   An instrument for studying the fine structure of cells as indicated by variations in optical properties of cell components.

microrespirometer   An apparatus for measuring the respiratory activity of minute amounts of tissue.

microrhinia [MICRO- + RHIN- + -IA]   The disproportionate smallness of the nose.

microroentgen [MICRO- + ROENTGEN]   A unit of ionization exposure equal to 10^{-6} roentgen; 2.58×10^{-10} coulomb per kilogram. Symbol: μR, μr

microrupture   A microscopic rupture.

microscelous   Having abnormally short legs.

microscope [MICRO- + -SCOPE]   An optical instrument having one or more lenses, used to view magnified images of small objects.

acoustic microscope   A device in which ultrasound distorts a reflective surface, which is then optically scanned to produce an image. Also called *ultrasonic microscope.*

binocular microscope   A microscope with two eyepieces, intended for binocular viewing.

capillary microscope   A microscope used for examining the capillaries, particularly those of the nail bed.

centrifuge microscope   An optical device located within a centrifuge that permits observation of material undergoing high-speed centrifugation. The objective rotates and projects the image onto a stationary ocular located at the axis.

color-contrast microscope   A dark-field microscope in which the condenser stop is colored instead of opaque. With the annulus a complementary color, the object appears in the color of the annulus against a complementary field. Also called *Rheinberg microscope.*

comparator microscope   COMPARISON MICROSCOPE.

comparison microscope   An optical device that allows the simultaneous viewing, through a single set of eyepieces, of images transmitted by two different objectives. Also called *comparator microscope.*

compound microscope   A microscope with more than one lens system. The magnified image transmitted by the system nearest the object is further magnified by passage through lenses near the eye of the viewer.

corneal microscope   SLIT LAMP.

dark-field microscope   A microscope that employs dark-field illumination. Unstained objects appear bright against a dark background.

dissecting microscope   A compound microscpe with two sets of eyepieces and objectives, constructed to present a nonreversed, stereoscopic image of three-dimensional objects. The distance between the objective lenses and the object stage is great enough to allow manipulation of the object examined.

electron microscope   A microscope that uses a beam of electrons to visualize particles too small to be resolved by a light microscope. Also called *ultramicroscope, supermicroscope.*

fluorescence microscope   A compound microscope in which ultraviolet or violet-blue visible light is used to produce a fluorescence of the examined object, which may have natural fluorescence or may have been treated with a fluorochrome.

flying spot microscope   A microscope in which the object is subjected to light from an optical scanning device.

hypodermic microscope   A system for examining the microscopic detail of tissues that uses a fiberoptic probe which can be passed through a hollow needle.

infrared microscope   A microscope used for examining opaque, particulate objects in which the image is obtained by observing or measuring the absorption of infrared light waves.

interference microscope   A microscope used to examine unstained, transparent, or reflecting specimens. Incident and diffracted waves from a single light source are recombined at the plane of image, where their interference effects cause the differences in refraction and light transmission to become visible.

ion microscope   A device that is used to etch surfaces, using a beam of atoms passing through a vacuum. The final preparation is then examined in an electron microscope.

laser microscope   LASER MICROPROBE.

light microscope   A device used to obtain a magnified image of very small objects, viewed with light in the visible range. Also called *optical microscope.*

ocular microscope   A microscope with a single lens system.

opaque microscope   A microscope used to examine opaque objects. The object is illuminated by light incident from a condenser that surrounds the object.

operating microscope   A microscope specially designed to be used by surgeons when operating on very small structures. It helps to improve visibility and precision. Its essential features are an adequate working distance between objective lens and operative field, brilliant illumination and ease of adjustment. Also called *surgical microscope*.

optical microscope   LIGHT MICROSCOPE.

phase microscope   A microscope in which light is transmitted at slightly different phases, so that differences in refraction within the object examined become visible as contrasting areas of different intensity. It is used especially to examine living cells or unstained material. Also called *phase-contrast microscope*.

phase-contrast microscope   PHASE MICROSCOPE.

polarizing microscope   A microscope in which the specimen is illuminated by polarized light. It is used to examine birefringent specimens, which cause the refractive index to vary with the direction of light transmission.

projection microscope   A microscope in which the image is projected upon a screen, rather than being viewed directly through the eyepieces.

projection x-ray microscope   A high resolution microscope using low-energy x rays, with the resultant images being observed on a fluorescent screen or recorded on film.

reflecting microscope   A compound microscope in which the objective lens system is replaced by a concave and a convex mirror, creating an image system free of chromatic aberration at any wavelength of visible light.

Rheinberg microscope   COLOR-CONTRAST MICROSCOPE.

scanning electron microscope   A microscope that produces a detailed surface view of an object by scanning a narrow electron beam over its surface. The secondary electrons given off from the surface are then used to build up a composite picture in an image analyzer.

schlieren microscope   A microscope that uses schlieren optics so that differences in the density of the examined object become visible as differences in the refraction of transmitted light.

simple microscope   A magnifying device consisting of a single lens.

slit lamp microscope   SLIT LAMP.

stereoscopic microscope   A microscope with dual eyepieces and objectives, arranged so that the separate images combine to give a stereoscopic or three-dimensional image.

stroboscopic microscope   A microscope that is used to examine and analyze moving objects of microscopic size by subjecting the object to illumination flashing at a constant rate.

surgical microscope   OPERATING MICROSCOPE.

television microscope   A projecting microscope that uses a television camera to display the magnified image.

trinocular microscope   A microscope fitted with a third ocular system. It is used for photography or other optical manipulation.

ultrapaque microscope   A microscope that is designed to examine the surface structure of opaque organs by using an incident light source instead of a transmitted light source.

ultrasonic microscope   ACOUSTIC MICROSCOPE.

ultraviolet microscope   A microscope whose energy source is electromagnetic radiation with a wavelength of 180–400 nm. The image is visualized by reflecting optics, fluorescence optics, or crystal objectives that transmit ultraviolet wavelengths.

x-ray microscope   A microscope which uses a beam of x rays instead of light, with the image usually being recorded on photographic film.

microscopic   **1** Extremely small; specifically, of a size that can be seen only with the aid of a microscope.   **2** Of or relating to microscopes or their use.

microscopist   An individual with special skills in microscopy.

microscopy [MICRO- + -SCOPY]   The study of both animate and inanimate objects using the magnifying power of a microscope. Also called *micrography, microtechnic*.

bright-field microscopy   Microscopy in which there is direct, vertical illumination.

clinical microscopy   **1** The use of microscopic examinations for clinical diagnosis.   **2** Clinical laboratory tests not readily classified in other disciplines, such as an analysis of gastric acidity, examination of feces, and amniotic fluid analysis.

corneal microscopy   Observation of the cornea with a slit lamp.

dark-field microscopy   Microscopy that uses a condenser, resulting in a dark background and illumination from the side so that microorganisms appear light in a dark field.

electron microscopy   The preparation of material and the subsequent examination in an electron microscope. Also called *ultramicroscopy*.

fundus microscopy   Observation of the ocular fundus with a slit lamp.

immersion microscopy   A microscopic examination in which the objective lens and the cover glass are both immersed in a liquid with the same refractive index as glass.

immune electron microscopy   The use of an electron microscope to study a specimen that has been stained with a labeled specific antibody capable of identifying a particular protein. Abbreviation: IEM

immunofluorescent microscopy   Fluorescence microscopy in which antigens are identified by use of antibodies to which are attached fluorescent dyes.

phase-contrast microscopy   The use of a microscope which changes the phase relationships of light passing through and around an object so that staining and other special preparations are not necessary for visualization of the object.

scanning transmission electron microscopy   The process of examining a specimen by both transmission and scanning electron microscopy within the same instrument.

television microscopy   The use of a television camera to project an image obtained by a flying spot microscope or standard compound microscope.

transmission electron microscopy   The use of a microscope in which an electron beam is passed through an ultrathin section of tissue to provide a detailed image of cell and tissue components according to their capacity to permit or obstruct the flow of electrons.

microsecond [MICRO- + SECOND]   A unit of time equal to 10^{-6} second. Symbol: μs

microsection   A thin slice of tissue that is prepared for examination with a microscope.

microsere [MICRO- + SERE]   A sere that occurs on a microhabitat such as a decaying log or a boulder.

microshock   A mild immunologic reaction that occurs following the injection of a small amount of a substance given to avoid the possibility of a severe reaction when a larger therapeutic dose is given.

Microsiphonales [MICRO- + Gk *siphōn* reed, tube, siphon + L *-ales*, pl. of *-alis* -AL]   TRICHOMYCETES.

microsomal   Of or relating to microsomes.

microsomatia   MICROSOMIA.

microsome [MICRO- + Gk *sōm(a)* body]   A fragment of endoplasmic reticulum with associated ribosomes. Such fragments are usually obtained by homogenizing cells and centrifuging them at high speed. Also called *cytomicrosome*.

microsomia [MICRO- + Gk *sōma* body + -IA]   A general smallness of the body, as seen in dwarfism. Also called *microsomatia*.

microsomia fetalis An abnormally small-sized fetus in relation to fetal age.

microspectrography The study of the composition of an object, especially of cellular constituents, using a spectroscope that makes a photographic record of the spectrum.

microspectrophotometer An instrument used to measure the absorption, reflection, or emission of light by objects under a microscope. It is used especially for spectral analysis of constituents of individual cells.

microspectrophotometry The analysis of the absorption spectrum of a single cell's constituents, a process used especially for characterizing nucleoproteins.

microspectroscope A spectroscope designed for use in the eyepiece of a compound microscope. It is used especially to analyze the spectrum of living cells.

microspherocyte SPHEROCYTE.

microspherocytosis SPHEROCYTOSIS.

microspherulation ERYTHROCYTORRHEXIS.

microspherule A spherule of natural or synthetic origin, having a diameter of a few microns.

microsphygmia [MICRO- + SPHYGM- + -IA] A weak or small pulse; weakness or smallness of the pulse. Also called *microsphygmy*.

microsphygmy MICROSPHYGMIA.

microsplanchnia Abnormal smallness of a viscus or viscera, particularly abdominal viscera.

microsplanchnic **1** Possessing small abdominal viscera. **2** Of or relating to a body constitution in which the horizontal diameters are less developed than the vertical ones and in which the abdominal portion is relatively smaller than the thoracic. For defs. 1 and 2 also *microsplanchnous*.

microsplanchnous MICROSPLANCHNIC.

microsplenia [MICRO- + SPLEN- + -IA] The abnormal smallness of the spleen, as is often seen in the presence of accessory splenic tissue.

microsplenic Characterized by microsplenia.

Microspora [MICRO- + Gk *spora* a sowing, seed] A phylum of protozoa characterized by unicellular spores containing a long tubular polar filament and polar cap as an extrusion apparatus, which lack mitochondria, and are found as obligatory intracellular parasites of most major animal groups. These protozoa were formerly placed in an order Microsporidia, or Microsporida.

microspore [MICRO- + SPORE] MICROCONIDIUM.

microsporid Dermatophytid that is provoked by a *Microsporum* species. Also called *microsporide*.

Microsporida See under MICROSPORA.

microsporide MICROSPORID.

Microsporidia See under MICROSPORA.

microsporidian **1** Pertaining to the former order Microsporidia. **2** A member of the former order Microsporidia, now reclassified as the phylum Microspora.

microsporosis Ringworm, especially ringworm of the scalp, that is caused by a *Microsporum* species.

Microsporum [New L (from MICRO- + New L -*sporum*, combining form denoting spore, from Gk *spora* a sowing, seed)] A genus of fungi that causes various dermatophytoses, including tinea corpus and tinea capitis.

Microsporum audouini A form-species of fungus identified as one of the etiologic agents of tinea capitis. Also called *Cercosphaera addisoni, Trichophyton microsporon* (obsolete).

Microsporum canis The form-species of fungus which causes animal ringworm, a condition occasionally transmitted to humans.

Microsporum cookei A form-species of keratinophilic soil

fungus. It is not a human pathogen.

Microsporum distortum A form-species of fungus which causes tinea capitis, especially of children.

Microsporum ferrugineum A form-species of fungus which is an agent of tinea capitis in eastern Europe and Asia. It appears to be clinically identical with *Microsporum audouini* in the West. Both cause epidemics of ringworm in children.

Microsporum fulvum A form-species of fungus which is one of the etiologic agents of ringworm of the scalp and skin.

Microsporum gypseum A species of fungus causing inflammatory tinea capitis or tinea corporis.

microstereognosia [MICRO- + STEREO- + Gk -*gnōsia*, combining form from *gnōs(is)* knowledge + -*ia* -IA] An abnormality of tactile sensation in which objects seem abnormally small when touched or felt.

microstethophone [MICRO- + STETHO- + Gk *phōnē* sound, voice] A stethoscope utilizing an amplifying device which may be electronic.

microsthenic Referring to a person with generally reduced muscle strength; feeble.

microstomia [MICRO- + STOM- + -IA] A disproportionate smallness of the oral orifice.

microstrabismus [MICRO- + STRABISMUS] A very small angle of manifest ocular deviation.

microsurgery [MICRO- + SURGERY] Surgery performed with the aid of an enlarging lens or dissecting microscope.

microsuture A very fine monofilament used in microsurgery. The diameter of the suture is usually 40 μ or less.

microsyringe A syringe whose piston is controlled by a micrometer screw. It is finely graduated for accurate delivery of very small quantities of liquid. Also called *micrometer syringe*.

microtechnic MICROSCOPY.

microthelia [MICRO- + THEL- + -IA] An abnormal smallness of one or both nipples.

microthrombosis Thrombosis in many small vessels.

microthrombus (*plural* microthrombi) A thrombus of very small size.

microtia [MICR- + OT- + -IA] The abnormal smallness of the pinna or auricle of the ear. The external auditory meatus may be reduced in bore, end blindly, or be absent.

microtitrimetry Analysis, by titration procedures, of small-volume specimens.

microtome [MICRO- + -TOME] A mechanical device used for preparing histologic sections for microscopic examination. Also called *histotome, section cutter.*

freezing microtome A mechanical device for cutting frozen sections of tissue without a temperature control cabinet. It usually includes a device for quick freezing of unfixed or unprocessed tissue. Also called *cryotome.*

rocking microtome A microtome in which the block of tissue to be sectioned is rocked up and down against a horizontal knife blade.

rotary microtome A microtome in which the block of tissue to be sectioned is moved up and down against a horizontal knife blade, using a rotary hand action.

sliding microtome A microtome in which the block of tissue to be sectioned is pushed along a track toward the microtome knife.

microtomization The use of a microtome to obtain a section for examination.

microtomography A technique for rotating a small sample in an electron microscope through 90 degrees, processing the data by computer, and displaying three-dimensional images, as of the changes within living cells.

microtomy [MICRO- + -TOMY] The cutting of tissue sections so as to make them suitable for examination with a microscope.

microtonometer An instrument for measuring the partial pressure of gases in minute quantities of material.

microtoposcopy A three-dimensional technique of displaying the electroencephalographic waveform derived from different parts of the brain.

microtrauma [MICRO- + TRAUMA] A tiny or microscopically visualized injury.

microtrichia [MICRO- + TRICH- + -IA] An unusual fineness of the hair, with a reduced mean diameter of the individual hairs.

Microtrombidium akamushi See under *LEPTOTROMBIDIUM.*

Microtrombidium wichmanni A mite found in New Guinea that is an ectoparasite of human skin, causing severe itching.

microtubule [MICRO- + TUBULE] A small, hollow, cylindrical structure found in the cytoplasm of nearly all eukaryotic cells. It has an outside diameter of 250 Å, with a wall thickness of 50 Å, and hence an inside diameter of 150 Å. The wall is a polymer composed of equal numbers of units of α-tubulin and β-tubulin. Microtubles function as a cellular skeleton and are also involved in the phenomena of cell movement.

chromosomal microtubule CHROMOSOMAL SPINDLE FIBER.
kinetochore microtubule CHROMOSOMAL SPINDLE FIBER.
spindle microtubule Any of the microtubules which form the mitotic spindle. The spindle fibers are composed of bundles of microtubules.

subpellicular microtubule A microtubule found in certain sporozoa in various stages of their development. In coccidian sporozoites and merozoites such microtubules originate at the polar ring and extend to the nucleus in a regular subpellicular pattern from anterior to posterior regions.

microtus A fetus or postnatal individual displaying microtia.

microunit [MICRO- + UNIT] A quantity equal to 10^{-6} unit. Symbol: μu.

microvasculature The total of all arterioles, capillaries, and venules in the body.

microvilli Plural of MICROVILLUS.

microvillosity The state of having numerous microvilli.

microvillus [MICRO- + L *villus* a long hair, shaggy hair] A minute fingerlike process from a cell surface that is visible under an electron microscope. Microvilli are often arranged together in a closely packed form to provide a brush border.

placental microvillus A minute extension from a trophoblastic cell of the placenta.

microviscosimeter A viscosimeter which can be used to measure viscosity in small quantities of blood or plasma.

microvivisection MICRODISSECTION.

microvolt [MICRO- + VOLT] A unit of electrical potential, potential difference, or electromotive force equal to 10^{-6} volt. Symbol: μV.

microvoltometer A device for measuring the very small changes in electric potential that occur in cellular physiology and pathology.

microwatt [MICRO- + WATT] A unit of power equal to 10^{-6} watt. Symbol: μW.

microwave An electromagnetic wave of short wavelength, especially between 100 and 1 cm. Sources of emission include radar, cathode-ray tubes, induction furnaces, and electrotherapy devices. There is evidence that microwave exposure can cause cataract and thermal damage to the eye. Also called *microelectric wave.*

microwelding A procedure whereby two or more minute objects are brought together and fused by heat.

microxycyte MICROXYPHIL.

microxyphil [MICR- + OXY-² + -PHIL] A cell that contains small acidophilic granules. Also called *microxycyte.*

microzoa Plural of MICROZOON.

microzoon [MICRO- + Gk *zoön* living being, animal] (*plural* microzoa) Any microscopic multicellular animal.

micrurgy MICROMANIPULATION.

Micruroides A genus of venomous snakes of the Elapidae family; coral snakes.

Micruroides euryoxanthus A species of coral snake of the southwestern United States. It is a burrower and feeds on lizards, other snakes, and insects. It has prominent rings of black, yellow, and red around the body. The venom is neurotoxic.

Micrurus A genus of venomous snakes of the Elapidae family; coral snakes. Also called *Elaps.*

Micrurus fulvius A species of coral snake of the family Elapidae, found in the southern United States and Central America, having a pattern of prominent red, black, and yellow rings around the body. It is nocturnal, and it feeds on lizards and other snakes. The venom is highly neurotoxic.

miction [Late L *mictio,* from L *mictus,* past part. of *meiere,* later *mingere* to urinate] URINATION.

micturate [L *mictur(ire)* to urinate + -ATE] URINATE.

micturition [L *micturitus,* past part. of *micturire,* desiderative verb from *mictus,* past part. of *meiere,* later *mingere* to urinate] URINATION.

MID 1 minimal infective dose. 2 minimal inhibiting dose.

midbody An accumulation of electron-dense material at the peripheral spindle fibers associated with the process of furrowing during cytokinesis. As constriction proceeds to pinch the cell in two, the midbody becomes smaller, usually disappearing before cleavage is complete.

midbrain MESENCEPHALON.

midcarpal 1 Pertaining to the center of the carpus. 2 Between the proximal and distal rows of the carpal bones. For defs. 1 and 2 also *mediocarpal, mesocarpal.*

midclavicular Pertaining to the central point or portion of the clavicle.

Middeldorpf [Albrecht Theodor von *Middeldorpf,* German surgeon, 1824–1868] See under TRIANGLE.

middlepiece MIDDLE PIECE. See under PIECE.

midepigastric Pertaining to the middle of the epigastrium in the transverse plane.

midfoot The central portion of the foot in the region of the cuboid, navicular, and cuneiform bones.

midfrontal 1 Of or relating to the middle of the frontal bone, or forehead. 2 Both median and frontal. For defs. 1 and 2 also *mediofrontal, medifrontal.*

midge [Middle English *migge,* from Old English *mycg,* akin to Gk *myia* a fly and L *musca* a fly] Any of the small flies of the families Chironomidae, Ceratopogonidae, and others. They often appear in great numbers and the Ceratopogonidae give painful bites. Some species are vectors of the filarial worms *Mansonella ozzardi, Dipetalonema perstans, D. streptocerca,* and other parasites.

midget [dim. of *midge,* from Middle English *migge,* from Old English *mycg*] An abnormally small but normally proportioned individual. A popular usage.

midgut 1 The middle segment of the embryonic intestine, precursor of the stomach, of the small intestine, and of the colon with the exception of the sigmoid colon and the rectum. It connects with the yolk sac through the vitellointestinal duct at the level of the umbilical ring. 2 The region of the arthropod gut derived from endoderm, between the ectodermal, chitin-lined foregut and hindgut. Also called *mesenteron.*

midhead CENTRICIPUT.

Midicel A proprietary name for sulfamethoxypyridazine.

midline 1 MEDIAN PLANE. 2 The central axis of a part or organ. 3 Any line that bisects a structure along its axis.

midmenstrual [English *mid* + L *menstrual(is)* (from *menstru(a)* menses + *-alis* -AL) menstrual] In the middle of the menstrual cycle around the time of ovulation.

midoccipital Pertaining to the central portion or point of the occiput. Also *medioccipital*.

midpain [*mid* + *pain*] MITTELSCHMERZ.

midperiphery The equatorial portion of the ocular fundus.

midphalangeal 1 Of or relating to the middle phalanx. 2 Of or relating to the middle of a phalanx.

mid-piece 1 A globulin fraction of complement which precipitates when electrolytes are removed from serum. It unites with sensitized erythrocytes but produces hemolysis only if another complement fraction, the end-piece, is also present. 2 The region of a sperm cell between the head and the tail region; middle piece.

midplane PELVIC PLANE OF LEAST DIMENSIONS.

midriff DIAPHRAGMA.

midsection A slice or cut through the middle of an organ or a structure.

mid-stance The interval in the stance phase of the gait cycle between heel strike and push-off.

midsternum CORPUS STERNI.

midtarsal 1 Pertaining to the center of the tarsus. 2 Between the calcaneus and talus proximally and the cuboid and navicular bone distally. For defs. 1 and 2 also *mediotarsal, mesotarsal*.

midtegmentum The middle or central portion of the tegmentum, particularly that of the pons and mesencephalon.

midventral Pertaining to the middle part of a ventral surface.

midvesical Of or relating to the middle of a bladder.

midwife [Middle English *midwif, midwyf*, from Middle and Old English *mid* with + Middle English *wif* a woman, from Old English *wif, wīf* a woman] A health care worker, who may or may not be formally trained and is not a physician, that delivers babies and provides associated maternal care. Also called *accoucheuse, sage femme*.

midwifery The practice of obstetrics by a midwife.

Mierzejewski [Johann Lucian *Mierzejewski*, Russian neurologist and psychiatrist, 1839–1908] See under EFFECT.

Miescher [Guido *Miescher*, Swiss dermatologist, 1877–1961] 1 Miescher's granuloma. See under CHRONIC PROGRESSIVE DISCIFORM GRANULOMATOSIS. 2 Miescher's disease. See under SYNDROME. 3 Miescher syndrome. See under GRANULOMATOMA CHEILITIS.

Miescher [Johann Friedrich *Miescher*, Swiss pathologist, 1811–1887] Miescher's tube, Miescher's tubule. See under SARCOCYST.

Miescheria *SARCOCYSTIS.*

MIF 1 migration inhibition factor (of macrophages). 2 melanocyte stimulating hormone inhibiting factor.

migraine [French (from Late L *hemicrania* pain in one side of the head, from Gk *hēmi-* half + *kranion* the upper part of the head, the skull), pain in one side of the head] A common syndrome characterized by recurrent paroxysmal attacks of headache, often throbbing in character and sometimes, but not invariably, unilateral in distribution. The attacks, which often last for hours, less commonly for several days, are often preceded by visual phenomena, such as hemianopia, scotoma, teichopsia, or fortification spectra, or by sensory phenomena such as paresthesiae, and are usually accompanied by nausea or vomiting,

and photophobia. The aura or warning is due to arterial constriction, the headache to extracranial and intracranial dilatation. Often the headache occurs without an aura, less commonly the aura is not followed by headache. Also called *hemicrania, megrim*.

abdominal migraine Episodic abdominal symptoms such as pain and nausea or vomiting occurring in migraine sufferers. They are believed to represent migrainous equivalents.

cervical migraine 1 An attack of migraine in which the headache, whether unilateral or bilateral, is predominantly occipital or nuchal in distribution. Seldom used in this sense. 2 An episode of posterior cervical and occipital pain, accompanied by variable neurologic manifestations and attributed to cervical spondylosis. A misleading and obsolete usage. Also called *Bärtschi-Rochaix syndrome, cervicocephalic syndrome*.

classic migraine Migraine in which all of the typical or classic features occur, including a visual or sensory aura, unilateral headache, and nausea or vomiting.

common migraine Paroxysmal attacks of headache typical of migraine occurring without other specific distinguishing features such as the typical aura.

complicated migraine An attack of migraine in which the manifestations of the aura, such as hemianopia, hemiplegia, aphasia, etc., are unusually severe or long-lasting or in which the attack is accompanied by exceptional manifestations such as syncope or epilepsy.

epileptic migraine 1 The concurrence of epilepsy and migraine in the same individual. 2 Headache resembling that of migraine preceding or following an attack of epilepsy. 3 Any of various visual or sensory hallucinatory phenomena resembling those of an aura of migraine but occurring as a manifestation of focal or partial epilepsy. An obsolete and imprecise term.

facioplegic migraine Unilateral and transient facial palsy occurring in an attack of migraine.

fulgurating migraine Migraine in which the attacks of headache are exceptionally violent and of explosive onset.

hemiplegic migraine Migraine in which recurrent episodes of hemiplegia occur during the attacks. This disorder is often familial and probably of dominant inheritance.

menstrual migraine Migraine in which the attacks occur at or about the time of the menstrual periods.

ophthalmic migraine Any of several visual symptoms, such as transient amblyopia, hemianopia, photophobia, scintillating scotomata, and teichopsia, occurring as manifestations of the aura of migraine. In rare cases visual field defects may remain permanent, due to occlusion of retinal arteries or of one posterior cerebral artery.

ophthalmoplegic migraine Paresis or paralysis of one of the cranial nerves which innervate the external ocular muscles (usually the oculomotor, less often the abducens or trochlear) occurring during an attack of migraine. Some afflicted patients are found to have an intracranial aneurysm of the internal carotid artery, but in the majority, who suffer recurrent attacks, no such physical cause is demonstrated. Also called *Charcot's disease, Möbius disease, Möbius syndrome, relapsing periodic oculomotor paralysis, relapsing ophthalmoplegia*.

migrainoid [French *migraine* (from Gk *hēmi-* half + *kranion* the upper part of the skull, head) an ache affecting only one side of the head + -OID] Resembling migraine.

migrainous Relating to migraine.

migrate [L *migrat(us)*, past part. of *migrare* to quit a place, move to a place] To move from place to place, as cells, parasitic organisms, large populations of animals, or individually perceived sensations.

migration [L *migratio* (from *migratus*, past part. of *migrare* to leave a place), a removal, changing of habitation] Movement from one place to another.

anodic migration A movement of negatively charged particles in an electrical field toward the positive electrode.

cathodic migration The movement of positively charged particles in an electrical field toward the negative electrode.

epithelial migration **1** The gradual spread of epithelial cells from the junctional epithelium over the surface of a tooth root in periodontitis, as the normal structure of the periodontal ligament breaks down. **2** A similar spread from the oral epithelium over the surface of the buried framework of an implant, which eventually becomes entirely covered.

external migration of ovum TRANSPERITONEAL MIGRATION.

internal migration of ovum The passage of an ovum to the contralateral fallopian tube following ovulation. The ovum passes through the oviduct on the same side as ovulation and into the uterus, followed by entry into the other tube.

migration of ovum The passage of the ovum through the fallopian tube following ovulation.

retrograde migration Movement of foreign bodies from the urethra into the upper urinary tract.

return migration A migration pattern in which an animal travels great distances from its point of origin or hatching to mature, or in response to seasonal climatic conditions, returning to its specific place of origin to lay eggs or rear its young.

tooth migration DRIFTING.

transperitoneal migration The passage of an ovum to the contralateral fallopian tube following ovulation without passing through the uterus. Also called *external migration of ovum*.

Mikedimide A proprietary name for bemegride.

Mikity [Victor G. *Mikity*, U.S. radiologist, born 1919] Wilson-Mikity syndrome. See under SYNDROME.

mikro- MICRO-.

Mikulicz [Johannes von *Mikulicz*-Radecki, Polish surgeon active in Germany, 1850–1905] **1** See under CLAMP, PROCEDURE, RESECTION, CELL, OPERATION. **2** Heineke-Mikulicz operation. See under HEINEKE-MIKULICZ PYLOROPLASTY. **3** Mikulicz aphthae. See under PERIADENITIS MUCOSA NECROTICA RECURRENS. **4** Mikulicz angle. See under ANGLE OF FEMORAL TORSION. **5** Mikulicz-Sjögren syndrome, Mikulicz-Radecki syndrome, Mikulicz syndrome. See under VON MIKULICZ SYNDROME.

mil [L *mil(le)* a thousand] **1** A unit of length equal to 10^{-3} inch, or 25.4 micrometers. A popular unit. **2** A unit of volume, used epecially in pharmaceutical work, equal to one milliliter. An obsolete, popular unit. **3** A unit of circular measure equal to 10^{-3} radian.

circular mil A unit of area, especially of cross-sectional area of wire, equal to the area of a circle having a diameter of 10^{-3} inch; $7.853\ 98 \times 10^{-7}$ square inch; 506.707 square micrometers. The unit is used especially to measure electric conductors.

milammeter MILLIAMMETER.

mildew [Old English *meledēaw, mildēaw*] Any of various ascomycetous fungi, several of which are very important economically as plant pathogens. They are initially observed on the plant leaf surface, and they penetrate into the leaf interior.

downy mildew A disease of plants caused by fungi of the class Oomycetes.

powdery mildew **1** A disease condition of plants brought about by the growth of fungi of the family Erysiphaceae. **2** The fungus causing this condition.

mile [L *mil(ia passuum)* (pl. of *mille passus* a thousand paces) thousands of paces] A unit of length equal to 1760 yards or 5280 feet; 1.6093 kilometers or 1609.344 meters. Symbol: mile

n mile Symbol for the unit, nautical mile.

nautical mile A unit of length for measuring distances at sea, in international usage, equal to 1852 meters or approximately 6076 feet. In Great Britain, a nautical mile equals 6080 feet or approximately 1853 meters. An obsolete unit. Symbol: n mile

square mile A unit of area equal to a square of one mile per side; 640 acres; $2.589\ 99 \times 10^6$ square meters; 2.589 99 square kilometers. Symbol: mile²

Miles [William Ernest *Miles*, English surgeon, 1869–1947] See under OPERATION.

milfoil *Achillea millefolium*, an herb used in folk medicine. Its volatile oil, achillein, acts as a diaphoretic, astringent, tonic, stimulant, and mild aromatic. Also called *yarrow*.

milia Plural of MILIUM.

Milian [Gaston *Milian*, French dermatologist, 1871–1945] **1** Milian's erythema. See under ERYTHEMA OF THE NINTH DAY. **2** See under SIGN.

miliaria [L, fem. of *miliarius* (from *milium* millet; Gk *melinē* millet) pertaining to millet] An eruption of minute vesicles, papules, or nodules, each of which is related to a sweat duct. It results from the obstruction of the duct at various levels and is associated with prolonged sweating. Also called *sweat fever, summer eruption, miliaria tropicalis*.

miliaria alba MILIARIA CRYSTALLINA.

miliaria crystallina An eruption of minute, very superficial vesicles, each related to a sweat pore. It is caused by the obstruction of the sweat duct within the stratum corneum and is associated with profuse sweating. Also called *sudamina, miliaria alba, crystal rash*.

miliaria papulosa Miliaria characterized mainly by papules. Also called *miliary papulosis*.

miliaria profunda Miliaria marked by an eruption of skin-colored dermal papules or nodules due to the obstruction of the sweat duct within the dermis. It is often not itchy but may lead to anhidrosis and anhidrotic heat exhaustion. Also called *mamillaria*.

miliaria propria MILIARIA RUBRA.

pustular miliaria Miliaria rubra or miliaria profunda in which the vesicles are purulent and are the result of bacterial infection. Also called *miliary impetigo*.

miliaria rubra Miliaria caused by the obliteration of the sweat duct within the epidermis. It manifests itself as minute erythematous papules or vesicles. Also called *prickly heat, wildfire rash,* (popular), *summer rash, miliaria propria, bedouin itch, lichen strophulosus* (obsolete), *lichen infantum* (obsolete), *lichen tropicus*.

miliaria tropicalis MILIARIA.

miliaria vesiculosa Miliaria rubra or miliaria crystallina that is clinically evidenced by vesicle formation.

miliary [*miliar(ia)* + -Y] **1** Characterized by the presence of numerous, small lesions resembling millet seeds as in pulmonary tuberculosis. **2** Resembling a millet seed.

Milibis A proprietary name for glycobiarsol.

milieu [French (from *mi* middle, from L *medius* middle + French *lieu* place, from L *locus* place), center, middle, environment] **1** Surroundings; environment. **2** In psychiatry, an integrated and stable socioenvironmental context, such as a hospital, designed for the patient because it provides a setting in which the treatment can be best provided to meet the patient's particular needs.

milieu extérieur EXTERNAL ENVIRONMENT.

milieu intérieur INTERNAL ENVIRONMENT.

milium [L (Gk *melinē* millet), millet] (*plural* milia) A white nodule in the skin, composed of densely packed keratin which forms a globular lesion. Also called *acne albida* (obsolete), *acne* *punctata albida* (obsolete), *whitehead, closed comedo, sebaceous tubercle, strophulus albidus, grutum* (obsolete).

colloid milium A degenerative disorder of the dermal connective tissue, characterized clinically by the development of yellowish translucent plaques or papules on skin exposed to light. Also called *colloid acne, colloid atrophy of the skin, Wagner's disease, colloid pseudomilium, pseudomilium.*

milium congenitale Small, white, horny, follicular papules that are present at birth and are usually found on the central area of the face.

milium of the eyelids A mass of firmly packed lamellated keratin presenting as a pearly white globular lesion on the eyelid.

milia neonatorum Minute yellowish dots visible on a newborn infant's face, marking the orifices of sebaceous glands. Also called *milium of the newborn.*

milium of the newborn MILIA NEONATORUM.

milk [Old English *milc, meolc, meoluc*] **1** The secretion of the mammary glands used for feeding infants. Milk from different animals varies in composition. All types contain water, protein (caseinogen, lactoalbumin, and lactoglobulin), carbohydrate (lactose and small quantities of other sugars), and fats (glycerides of palmitic, myristic, and oleic acids as well as smaller quantities of stearic acid and C_4–C_{24} fatty acids). Sterols and phosphatides in the form of lecithin and cephalin are also present. Mineral salts present include calcium, potassium, and sodium as cations and phosphate and chloride as anions. Small quantities of iron, magnesium, citrate, and lactate are also present. Vitamins A, B_1 and B_2, niacin, and pantothenic acid are also present in significant amounts. Milk is low in vitamins C and D. Cow, buffalo, goat, ass, mare, and ewe milks are often used as food, but bovine milk is most frequently used. **2** An aqueous suspension resembling milk in appearance, as *milk of magnesia.*

acidophilus milk A milk soured by *Lactobacillus acidophilus.* It contains 0.1–2.0% fat with increased quantities of the other milk constituents. It is similar to soured buttermilk with a slightly acid flavor. It is used therapeutically in patients with gastrointestinal disorders as a means of changing the composition of the bacterial flora existing in the gastrointestinal tract. Also called *lactic acid milk.*

adapted milk Cows' milk which has been adapted to make it more similar to human milk. This usually involves reducing the proportion of protein, particularly casein, and increasing the ration of unsaturated to saturated fatty acid in the fat.

after-milk The milk taken from the breast at the end of a feed. It has been suggested that the fat content of breast milk increases during a feed. Thus the after-milk should contain more fat than the milk removed from the breast at the beginning of a feed. Also called *hind milk.*

albumin milk PROTEIN MILK.

bitter milk **1** A bitter-tasting milk obtained from cows that have eaten bitter herbs. **2** Milk that has become bitter as a result of bacterial action.

breast milk Milk produced by the mammary gland, especially that from a mother used to nourish an infant. Between 600–800 ml of milk can be produced by a woman daily for a period after she has given birth. The composition and daily output are little influenced by maternal diet except in starvation situations. However, the type of fat present in the milk and its quantitative content of water-soluble vitamins are affected by maternal food intake. Approximately 900 kcal are needed to produce each liter. One third comes from maternal energy stores laid down in pregnancy, and the rest comes from daily food intake. In comparison to cow's milk, breast milk contains less protein, minerals, and vitamins except C, D, and nicotinic acid, and the

form of vitamin D present in breast milk is more easily absorbed. Breast milk has a higher percentage of lactoalbumin and lactose. The initial milk produced (colostrum) is rich in certain antibodies such as IgA.

Budd milk BUDDEIZED MILK.

buddeized milk Milk that has been sterilized using hydrogen peroxide followed by heating to break down the peroxide and liberate the oxygen. Also called *Budd milk.*

Bulgarian milk BULGARICUS MILK.

bulgaricus milk Milk treated with *Lactobacillus bulgaricus.* Also called *Bulgarian milk.*

cancer milk A milky substance on the surface of a cancer.

casein milk PROTEIN MILK.

certified milk Milk that has been designated as being pure by a board of physicians or a medical milk commission.

certified pasteurized milk Milk that is certified as having no more than 10 000 bacteria per ml before pasteurization and not more than 500 bacteria per ml after pasteurization. After processing it must be cooled to 7°C or below and maintained at that temperature until sold.

citric acid milk Milk treated with 4 g dehydrated citric acid per quart or liter.

condensed milk Milk that has been evaporated to one third of its original volume and sweetened with sugar. The sugar acts as a preservative. Condensed milk is available as full cream or skimmed milk. Also called *lactein, lactolin.*

diabetic milk Milk that has had most of its lactose removed.

dialyzed milk Milk that has been dialyzed through a parchment membrane to remove the sugar.

dried milk Milk in a state of dryness resulting from evaporation of its water content using either spray-drying or roller-drying.

evaporated milk Milk that has been reduced to approximately 45% of its original volume through evaporation of its water content. It contains not less than 7–8% fat and 25.5% total solids.

fat milk Any type of milk modified to contain at least as much fat as human milk.

fore-milk **1** The first milk produced by the mammary gland at any one milking. It usually has a lower fat content than the after-milk. **2** COLOSTRUM.

fortified milk Milk which has been supplemented with some nutrient such as vitamin D, cream, or egg-white and so has a higher nutrient content than in the natural state.

fortified vitamin D milk Milk that contains 400 IU per quart or liter. It is obtained by adding vitamin D directly to the milk.

grade A milk Milk which contains no more than 30 000 bacteria per milliliter.

grade B milk Milk which contains no more than 100 000 bacteria per milliliter.

hind milk AFTER-MILK.

homogenized milk Milk treated mechanically after pasteurization to break down the fat globules into very small droplets of approximately equal size, which are evenly distributed throughout the milk. These globules absorb much of the milk protein, which stabilizes the emulsion and prevents the cream from rising to the top.

humanized milk Cow's milk that has been modified to resemble human milk. The main changes are a reduction in the protein content from 3–4% to 0.9–1.0% and an increase in the lactose content from 5% to 7%. Also called *modified milk.*

hydrochloric acid milk A preparation made by adding 5 ml of one-tenth normal hydrochloric acid to 100 ml of milk.

irradiated vitamin D milk Cow's milk that has been exposed to ultraviolet light in order to increase its vitamin D content. The milk is irradiated in a thin film and standardized such that its vitamin D content is raised to 400 IU per quart or liter.

kefir milk   See under KEFIR FUNGUS.

laboratory milk   Milk prepared to meet given specifications.

lactic acid milk   ACIDOPHILUS MILK.

lactobacillary milk   Milk injected with lactic-acid-producing organisms such as *Bacillus acidophilus* and *B. bulgaricus*.

lemon-juice milk   A soured milk produced by adding 3/4 ounce (2.2 g) of lemon juice to approximately 1 quart or liter of cow's milk.

milk of magnesia   See under MAGNESIA.

metabolized vitamin D milk   Milk produced by cows fed irradiated yeast. This product is standardized to contain at least 400 IU per quart or liter.

metallized milk   Milk that has been supplemented with copper, iron, and magnesium so as to provide an ideal food for one suffering from a deficiency of hemoglobin.

modified milk   HUMANIZED MILK.

pasteurized milk   Milk that has been heated at low temperatures in order to destroy all its inherent pathogens. However, it still contains benign bacteria, such as the lactic acid bacteria and so sours within a few days. To be considered pasteurized, milk must be maintained at 63–66°C for 30 minutes and then immediately cooled, or heated for 15 seconds at 72°C, or flash pasteurized at 74°C for a few seconds. Since flash pasteurization involves heating the milk for such a short interval, little flavor loss occurs with this method.

peptonized milk   Milk that has been treated with an acid or an enzyme in order to cause partial hydrolysis of the casein and so facilitate digestion of the milk. The peptonized milk comes in a light brown powder that is soluble in water and is used as a nutrient for patients who are convalescing.

perhydrase milk   Milk that has been treated with hydrogen dioxide for sterilization purposes.

protein milk   A milk having a lower fat and carbohydrate content but a higher protein content than ordinary milk. It is produced by partially skimming sour milk and supplementing it with milk curd. It is believed to be more easily digested by those with disorders of the digestive tract. Also called *albumin milk, casein milk*.

roller-dried milk   Milk that has been dried by pouring it over the surface of internally heated rollers. The milk is spread over the rollers in a very thin layer and dries in a few seconds. It is then scraped off by rotating the rollers against a blade. The milk is subject to minimal damage but greater losses of vitamins B and C result than in the spray-drying procedure.

Schloss milk   Milk that has been modified so as to contain exactly the same ratio of salts and fat as human milk.

skimmed milk   Milk that has had the cream removed. In all other respects it is the same as whole milk.

soft curd milk   Milk having a soft and homogeneous curd produced by boiling or by the addition of cream or sodium citrate.

sour milk   Milk that contains lactic acid which gives it a characteristic sour flavor. On standing, lactic acid is produced by fermentation of lactobacilli which are indigenous to milk.

spray-dried milk   Dried milk resulting from evaporation of its water content using a spray dryer. The milk is sprayed in a fine jet into a chamber containing hot air. As it enters, it dries and falls to the bottom as a dry powder. The milk is heated for a short period of time and so damage is limited.

sterilized milk   Milk that has been homogenized and maintained at a temperature of 104–116°C for 20–40 minutes to precipitate all the albumin contained in it. The albumin is filtered off and the milk is tested for turbidity before it is certified as sterilized. Ammonium sulfate is added to the milk and if any albumin is present it will be precipitated and the milk will become cloudy. If it has been properly sterilized no albumin

remains and the milk will stay clear.

tuberculin-tested milk   Milk from cows that have been examined by a veterinary inspector and have been found free from tuberculin.

uterine milk   A whitish liquid, resembling milk, containing nutritious substances (proteins, fats, and carbohydrates have been identified) derived from secretion of uterine glands and by transudation through the uterine wall. It is present in the uterine cavity before implantation and is a source of nutrition for the blastocyst. It is also found between the chorion and the uterine epithelium in pigs and ruminants exhibiting epitheliochorial placentas. See also EMBRYOTROPHE.

uviol milk   Milk that has been sterilized by the use of ultraviolet light.

vegetable milk   Artificial milk made out of vegetables such as soya. It is sometimes used to feed infants who are allergic to milk or suffer from lactose intolerance.

vinegar milk   Sour milk prepared by adding vinegar to milk.

vitamin D milk   Cow's milk that has been supplemented with vitamin D through irradiation by ultraviolet light, direct addition of the vitamin, or feeding of the cows with irradiated yeast.

witch's milk   A few drops of milk that may be expressed from a newborn infant's nipples during the first few days of life. Also called *hexenmilch*.

yeast milk   Milk rich in vitamin D produced by cows fed irradiated yeast.

milking   A manual or mechanical technique for removing fluid from a body part. It can be used for reduction of local edema, or to obtain specimens of secretions such as might accumulate in the urethra.

Milkman   1 Louis Arthur *Milkman*, U.S. physician, 1895–1951. 2 Looser-Milkman syndrome. See under MILKMAN SYNDROME.

milkpox   ALASTRIM.

Millar   [John *Millar*, Scottish physician, 1733–1805]   Millar's asthma. See under LARYNGISMUS STRIDULUS.

Millard   [Auguste *Millard*, French internist, 1830–1915]   Millard-Gubler paralysis, Gubler-Millard paralysis. See under MILLARD-GUBLER SYNDROME.

Miller   [Thomas Grier *Miller*, U.S. physician, born 1886]   Abbott-Miller tube. See under MILLER-ABBOTT TUBE.

Miller Fisher   See under FISHER.

Milles   [George *Milles*, U.S. pathologist, born 1902]   See under SYNDROME.

milli-   [L *mille* a thousand]   A combining form denoting 10^{-3}, one thousandth: used with SI units. Symbol: m

milliammeter   An instrument calibrated to measure the magnitude of electric current in milliamperes. Also called *milammeter, milliamperemeter*.

milliampere   [MILLI- + AMPERE]   A unit of electric current equal to 10^{-3} ampere. Symbol: mA

milliampere-hour   In radiotherapy, the product of tube current in milliamperes and the exposure time in hours.

milliamperemeter   MILLIAMMETER.

milliångström   [MILLI- + ÅNGSTRÖM]   A unit of length equal to 10^{-13} meter; 0.1 picometer; 100 femtometers. Symbol: mÅ

millibar   [MILLI- + BAR]   A unit of pressure equal to 10^{-3} bar; 100 pascals. A popular unit. Symbol: mbar, mb • The symbol *mb* is used especially in meteorology.

millicoulomb   [MILLI- + COULOMB]   A unit of quantity of electricity, electric charge, or electric flux, equal to 10^{-3} coulomb. Symbol: mC

millicurie   [MILLI- + CURIE]   A unit of activity of a radionuclide or of a radioactive source equal to 10^{-3} curie; 3.7×10^6 becquerels exactly. Symbol: mCi, mc. (outmoded)

millicurie destroyed   A unit of x-ray dosage; a dose equivalent to a drop of one millicurie in the radioactivity of a brachytherapy source. An obsolete unit. Symbol: mCiδ

intensity millicurie   The intensity of gamma radiation existing one centimeter from a one milligram point source of radium filtered by 0.5 millimeter of platinum, equal to 8.4 roentgens per hour; 3.612×10^{-5} coulomb per kilogram second. An obsolete unit.

millicurie-hour   A unit of total number of nuclear transformations or transitions equal to 10^{-3} curie hour; 1.332×10^{11} transformations. Symbol: mCi·h, mc.h. (outmoded), *mc-h* (outmoded)

milliequivalent   **1** A quantity equal to 10^{-3} of the equivalent weight of an element or compound. **2** The amount of substance in one milliliter of normal solution. Symbol: mEq

millifarad [MILLI- + FARAD]   A unit of electric capacitance equal to 10^{-3} farad. Symbol: mF

milligamma [MILLI- + GAMMA]   A unit of mass or weight equal to 10^{-9} gram; 1 nanogram. An obsolete unit. Symbol: mγ

milligram [MILLI- + GRAM]   A unit of mass or weight equal to 10^{-3} gram or 10^{-6} kilogram; 0.0154 grain. Symbol: mg

milligrams percent   The concentration of a solution expressed in milligrams per 100 milliliters. Also called *milligram-percent.* Symbol: mg%

milligram per deciliter   A unit of mass concentration equal to 0.01 gram per liter. Symbol: mg/dl, mg·dl^{-1}

milligram per liter   A unit of mass concentration equal to 10^{-3} gram per liter. Symbol: mg/l, mg·l^{-1}

milligramage   MILLIGRAM-HOUR.

milligram-hour   A unit of radiation dose equal to the radiation emission in one hour from a source having an equivalent radium content of one milligram. An obsolete unit. Also called *milligramage.* Symbol: mg·h

milligram-percent   MILLIGRAMS PERCENT. See under MILLIGRAM.

milligray [MILLI- + GRAY]   A unit of absorbed dose in the field of ionizing radiation equal to 10^{-3} gray. Symbol: mGy

millihenry [MILLI- + HENRY]   A unit of inductance equal to 10^{-3} henry. Symbol: mH

Millikan [Clark Harold *Millikan*, U.S. neurologist, born 1915] Millikan-Siekert syndrome. See under SYNDROME.

Millikan [Robert Andrews *Millikan*, U.S. physicist, 1868–1954] Millikan rays. See under COSMIC RAYS.

millikatal [MILLI- + KATAL]   A unit of catalytic activity equal to 10^{-3} katal; 10^{-3} mole per second. Symbol: mkat

millikatal per liter   A unit of catalytic concentration or concentration of enzymic activity equal to 10^{-3} katal per liter; one mole per meter cubed second. Symbol: mkat/l, mkat·l^{-1}

millilambert [MILLI- + LAMBERT]   A unit of illuminance equal to 10^{-3} lambert; 10 lux. Symbol: mLa

milliliter [MILLI- + LITER]   A unit of volume or capacity equal to 10^{-3} liter, 10^{-6} cubic meter, or one cubic centimeter; 0.034 fluid ounce. Symbol: ml

millilitre   A British spelling for MILLILITER.

millilux [MILLI- + LUX]   A unit of illuminance equal to 10^{-3} lux. Symbol: mlx

millimeter [MILLI- + METER]   A unit of length equal to 10^{-3} meter; 0.039 37 inch. Symbol: mm

conventional millimeter of mercury   A unit of pressure equal to 13.5951 conventional millimeters of water; 133.322 pascals. Symbol: mmHg

conventional millimeter of mercury minute per liter   A unit of vascular resistance to flow; 79.9934×10^6 pascals second per meter cubed; 79.9934 kilopascals second per liter. Symbol: mmHg·min/l, mmHg·min·l^{-1}

conventional millimeter of water   A unit of pressure, the pressure due to an ideal column of water of height one millimeter, of uniform density one gram per cubic centimeter, and under the action of the standard acceleration of 9.806 65 meters per second squared; 9.806 65 pascals. Symbol: mmH$_2$O

cubic millimeter   A unit of volume equal to 10^{-9} cubic meter, or one microliter. Symbol: mm^3

millimeter of mercury   See under CONVENTIONAL MILLIMETER OF MERCURY.

millimeter of mercury minute per liter   See under CONVENTIONAL MILLIMETER OF MERCURY MINUTE PER LITER.

square millimeter   A unit of area equal to 10^{-6} square meter; 10^{-2} square centimeter. Symbol: mm^2

millimeter of water   See under CONVENTIONAL MILLIMETER OF WATER.

millimetre   A British spelling for MILLIMETER.

millimicro- [MILLI- + MICRO-]   A combining form denoting 10^{-9}: formerly used with SI units, now replaced by *nano-.* Symbol: mμ

millimicrocurie [MILLIMICRO- + CURIE]   An outmoded term for NANOCURIE. Symbol: mμCi

millimicrogram [MILLIMICRO- + GRAM]   An outmoded term for NANOGRAM. Symbol: mμg

millimicrometer [MILLIMICRO- + METER]   An obsolete term for NANOMETER.

millimicron [MILLI- + Gk *mikron*, neut. of *mikros* little, small] An obsolete term for NANOMETER.

millimicrosecond [MILLIMICRO- + SECOND]   An outmoded term for NANOSECOND.

millimole [MILLI- + MOLE³]   A unit of amount of substance equal to 10^{-3} mole. Symbol: mmol

millimole per liter   A unit of substance concentration equal to 10^{-3} mole per liter; one mole per cubic meter. Symbol: mmol/l, mmol·l^{-1}

millimu [MILLI- + μ symbol for micron]   An obsolete term for NANOMETER.

millinewton [MILLI- + NEWTON]   A unit of force equal to 10^{-3} newton. Symbol: mN

milling-in   GRINDING-IN.

millinormal 10^{-3} normal: said of a solution.

milliohm [MILLI- + OHM]   A unit of electric resistance equal to 10^{-3} ohm. Symbol: mΩ

million / standard million   In demography, a group of one million representing proportionately the age and sex distribution of the total population being analyzed. It is used for standardization, as of mortality rates.

milliosmole [MILLI- + OSMOLE]   A unit of osmolality equal to 10^{-3} osmole. Symbol: mosm

millipede [MILLI- + L *pes* (gen. *pedis*) foot]   Any member of the arthropod class Diplopoda. The body is cylindrical and segmented, each segment having two pairs of short legs, of which there may be several hundred altogether in some species. Millipedes are vegetarian and, in contrast with centipedes, lack poison glands, although most kinds produce irritating fluids that repel predation by birds.

milliphot [MILLI- + PHOT]   A unit of illuminance equal to 10^{-3} phot; 10 lux. Symbol: mphot

millipièze [MILLI- + PIÈZE]   A unit of pressure or stress equal to 10^{-3} pièze; one pascal. An obsolete unit. Symbol: mpz

millipond [MILLI- + POND]   A unit of force equal to 10^{-3} pond; $9.806\ 65 \times 10^{-6}$ newton; 9.806 65 micronewtons. Symbol: mp

millirad   A unit of absorbed dose of ionizing radiation equal to 10^{-3} rad; 10^{-5} gray. Symbol: mrad

millirem   A unit of radiation dose equal to 10^{-3} rem; 10^{-5}

joule per kilogram; 10^{-5} sievert or 10 microsievert. Symbol: mrem

milliroentgen   A unit of ionization exposure equal to 10^{-3} roentgen; 2.58×10^{-7} coulomb per kilogram. Symbol: mR

millisecond [MILLI- + SECOND]   A unit of time equal to 10^{-3} second. Symbol: ms

milliunit [MILLI- + UNIT]   A quantity equal to 10^{-3} unit. Symbol: mU

millival [MILLI- + *(equi)val(ent)*]   milliequivalent. Symbol: mval

millivolt [MILLI- + VOLT]   A unit of electrical potential difference, or electromotive force, equal to 10^{-3} volt. Symbol: mV

millivolt-ampere   A unit of electrical power equal to 10^{-3} volt-ampere. Symbol: mV·A

millivolt-second   A unit of magnetic flux equal to 10^{-3} volt second, 10^{-3} weber; one milliweber. Symbol: mV·s

milliwatt [MILLI- + WATT]   A unit of power equal to 10^{-3} watt. Symbol: mW

milliweber [MILLI- + WEBER]   A unit of magnetic flux equal to 10^{-3} weber. Symbol: mWb

Mills [Charles Karsner *Mills*, U.S. neurologist, 1845–1931]   See under DISEASE, TEST.

Mills [Hiram Francis *Mills*, U.S. engineer, 1836–1921]   Mills-Reincke phenomenon. See under PHENOMENON.

Milontin   A proprietary name for phensuximide.

Milpath   A combination of meprobamate and tridihexethyl chloride, a medication for antispasmodic treatment of gastrointestinal disorders responding to anticholinergic treatment. A proprietary name.

Milroy [William Forsyth *Milroy*, U.S. physician, 1855–1942]   Milroy's edema, Milroy's disease, Nonne-Milroy disease, Nonne-Milroy lymphedema, Nonne-Milroy-Meige syndrome. See under HEREDITARY LYMPHEDEMA TYPE I.

Milton [John Laws *Milton*, English dermatologist, 1820–1898]   Milton's edema, Milton-Quincke edema. See under HEREDITARY ANGIOEDEMA.

Miltown   A proprietary name for meprobamate.

milzbrand [German, anthrax, from *Milz* spleen + *Brand* a burning, fire, gangrene, necrosis]   ANTHRAX.

Mima   A former genus of aerobic Gram-negative diplococci, now included in *Acinetobacter*.

mimesis [Gk *mimēsis* imitation]   **1** The resemblance of one disease or condition to another.   **2** The simulation of an organic disorder by nonorganic symptoms, as in conversion hysteria or factitious disorders. For defs. 1 and 2 also called *mimosis*.

mimetic   **1** Of or relating to mimesis.   **2** An agent that affects mimesis. Also called *mimic*.

mimic [Gk *mimos* an imitator, mime + -IKOS *-ic*]   **1** To initiate.   **2** MIMETIC.
    genetic mimic   **1** A species that exhibits, through evolution of a genetically determined phenotype, a resemblance to selectively advantageous characteristics of another species.   **2** GENOCOPY.

mimicry [MIMIC + -RY]   The imitation of one species by another in an adaptation tending to improve its survival chances.
    antigenic mimicry   The antigenic similarity seen between unrelated macromolecules, especially with respect to the antigenic cross-reaction between components of group A streptococci and tissue-specific mammalian antigens. Such antigenic mimicry is believed to play a part in the pathogenesis of diseases such as rheumatic fever. Also called *molecular mimicry*.
    batesian mimicry   The imitation of an unpalatable species by a palatable one, especially when the latter is the more abundant.
    molecular mimicry   ANTIGENIC MIMICRY.

    müllerian mimicry   A mimicry, seen especially in insects, in which both model and mimic are unpalatable to potential predators and together gain survival advantage against predation.

mimosis   MIMESIS.

min   **1** Symbol for the unit, minute (of time).   **2** In Great Britain, symbol for the obsolete unit, minim.   **3** minimum.

μin   Symbol for the unit, microinch.

Mincard   A proprietary name for aminometradine.

mind [Middle English *minde, mynde*, from Old English *(ge)mynd* memory, akin to L *mens* mind and Gk *menos* spirit, temper]   The organized total of psychological processes and contents that allow the individual to respond to external and internal stimuli in an integrated and dynamic way, relating response of the present to both the past and the future of the individual. The processes of perceiving, learning, thinking, remembering, feeling, and behaving with intelligence are its principal processes. The contents of the mind vary with experience. Adjective: mental.

Minderer [Raymond *Minderer* (Mindererus), German physician, 1570–1621]   Spirit of Mindererus. See under AMMONIUM ACETATE SOLUTION.

mineral [Med L *mineralis* (from *miner(a)* ore, a mine, from Old French *miniere* pertaining to mines, from *mine* a mine, + *-alis* -AL) pertaining to mines]   Any substance of nonbiologic origin, including inorganic constituents of living matter. The meaning is extended to include petroleum, as its biologic origin is only remote.
    trace minerals   Minerals needed by the body in very small amounts. These include iodine, copper, manganese, magnesium, iron, cobalt, zinc, and chromium. Iodine is usually the only one lacking in the diet, although zinc deficiency is sometimes encountered in the United States, especially in children.

mineralization   The conversion of organic material into inorganic material. Examples include the deposition of salts in living organisms, e.g. calcium phosphate in bone formation, and the complete oxidation of organic compounds, so that their carbon and hydrogen are oxidized to carbon dioxide and water, and other elements present to inorganic oxidation products, whose amounts may be measured comparatively easily.

mineralocorticoid   Any of the class of corticosteroids that act principally on the renal retention of sodium and the excretion of potassium, such as aldosterone.

minicell [*mini(ature)* + CELL]   A small cell, produced frequently by some mutants by an abnormal cell division, that lacks a chromosome but contains all the constituents of the cytoplasm. The inclusion of plasmids makes these cells useful for obtaining the products of their transcription and translation.

minicomputer [*mini-*, combining form from *mini(ature)* + *computer*]   A medium sized computer larger than a microcomputer and smaller than a mainframe computer, suitable for a laboratory or business.

minifilm   A small-sized radiographic film, usually of the chest, used for economy in large surveys.

minify   To make smaller.

minim [L *minim(us)* least, smallest]   **1** In the United States, a unit of capacity for liquid measure only, equal to 1/480 (US) fluid ounce or 0.061 611 5 milliliter. Symbol: minim   **2** In Great Britain, a unit of capacity equal to 1/480 (UK) fluid ounce or 0.059 193 9 milliliter. An obsolete unit. Symbol: min

minima   Plural of MINIMUM.

minimal   Being or relating to a minimum; least or slightest.

minimum [L (neut. sing. of *minimus*, least, smallest, superl. of *parvus* little, small), the smallest amount or size; as adv., very little]   (*plural* minimums, minima)   **1** The least or least possible degree or quantity. Abbreviation: min Adjective: minimal.

2 Least in quantity, range, or extent.

minimum audibile AUDITORY THRESHOLD.

minimum discernible 1 In psychophysics, denoting the smallest discriminable stimulus increment. **2** Denoting the minimum energy required for stimulus detection.

light minimum The least amount of light visible under the given conditions. Also called *minimum visibile*.

minimum separabile The smallest angular distance visible between two objects.

minimum visibile LIGHT MINIMUM.

Minin [A. V. *Minin*, Russian surgeon, flourished early 20th century] See under LIGHT.

minipill An oral contraceptive consisting of progestin only or progestin and very low doses of estrogen.

minipolymyoclonus [L *mini(mus)* least, smallest + POLY- + MYO- + CLONUS] A type of action tremor of the limbs described in some patients with spinal muscular atrophy.

Minkowski [Oskar *Minkowski*, Russian pathologist active in Germany, 1858–1931] **1** Naunyn-Minkowski method. See under MINKOWSKI'S METHOD. **2** Minkowski-Chauffard syndrome. See under HEREDITARY SPHEROCYTOSIS.

minocycline $C_{23}H_{27}N_3O_7$. 4,7-Bis(dimethylamino)-1,4α, 4$a\alpha$, 5α, 5$a\alpha$, 6, 11, 12$a\alpha$-octahydro-3, 10, 12, 12a-tetrahydroxy-1,11-dioxo-2-naphthacenecarboxamide. A semisynthetic antibiotic belonging to the tetracycline group of agents. It has a wide range of actions and uses. The hydrochloride salt may be given orally or by intravenous infusion for infections, chiefly staphylococcal, that are responsive to tetracyclines as well as others that do not respond to them.

minometer [*min(ute)*, from L *minut(us)*, past part. of *minuere* to make less or smaller + *o* + -METER] A device capable of detecting small amounts of radiation, such as that received by persons working with x rays or radioactive substances.

Minor [Lazar Salomovich *Minor*, Russian pathologist, 1855–1942] **1** Minor-Oppenheim syndrome. See under MINOR'S DISEASE. **2** See under SIGN.

minor 1 Lesser or smaller: usually denoting the lesser of two similar structures. **2** One who has not yet reached the legal age (the age of majority) for being accorded the full civil rights of an adult. The age varies by jurisdiction. • See note at MAJORITY.

Minot [George Richards *Minot*, U.S. physician, 1885–1950] Minot-Murphy treatment. See under TREATMENT.

Mintezol A proprietary name for thiabendazole.

minute [L *minut(us)* (past part. of *minuere* to lessen) small, minute] **1** A unit of time equal to 60 seconds. Symbol: min **2** A unit of plane angle equal to 1/60 degree; π/10 800 radian. Symbol: ′

new minute A unit of plane angle equal to 0.01 grade; 10^{-4} right angle. Symbol: ^{c}

minuthesis [irreg. from Gk *minythēsis* decrease] The fatigue of a sensory organ brought about by persistent stimulation.

MIO minimal identifiable odor.

mio- [Gk *meiōn* (comparative of *mikros* small, little and of *oligos* few, little) smaller, less, fewer] A combining form meaning less, fewer. Also *meio-*.

miocardia SYSTOLE.

miodidymus [New L (from Gk *meiō(n)* smaller, less + *didymos* a twin)] CRANIOPAGUS PARASITICUS.

miodymus [New L (from Gk *meiō(n)* smaller, less + *(di)dymos* a twin)] CRANIOPAGUS PARASITICUS.

miolecithal [MIO- + LECITH- + -AL] Having little or no yolk, as the ova of placental mammals. Also *alecithal, isolecithal, oligolecithal, microlecithal*.

mioplasmia Reduction in the plasma volume of circulating blood. A seldom used term.

miopragia [MIO- + *prag*, a root of Gk *prassein* to achieve, manage + -IA] Reduced functional activity.

miopus [New L (from Gk *mei(ōn)* smaller, less + *ōps*, gen. *ōps*, eye)] Unequal conjoined twins united at the head in such fashion that the face of one member is rudimentary.

miosis [Gk *meiōsis* (from *meiōn*, comparative of *mikros* small and *oligos* small) a lessening, diminishing] Marked constriction of the pupil. Also *myosis*. Adjective: miotic.

irritative miosis Smallness of the pupil due to inflammation or excessive stimulation of its parasympathetic innervation.

paralytic miosis Smallness of the pupil due to paralysis of the dilator muscle of the iris.

senile miosis Smallness of the pupil occurring normally with age.

spastic miosis Smallness of the pupil due to excessive contraction of the iris sphincter.

spinal miosis Smallness of the pupil due to cervical sympathetic damage.

miotic 1 Pertaining to or causing miosis. **2** A medication, such as a parasympathomimetic drug or morphine, that causes constriction of the pupil. Also *myotic*.

miracidia Plural of MIRACIDIUM.

miracidium [New L (from Gk *meirax* boy, girl + New L -*idium*, diminishing suffix)] (*plural* miracidia) The first-stage ciliated larva that emerges from the egg of a trematode. After hatching it moves rapidly in search of a specific snail intermediate host, which it must penetrate to continue its life cycle. In some groups (families Opisthorchiidae, Heterophyidae) the minute eggs are eaten by the snail. When they hatch, the larvae penetrate the snail's tissues from within to initiate the sporocyst-rediacercaria series of ontogenetic and multiplicative stages.

Miracil D A proprietary name for lucanthone hydrochloride.

miraculin A glycoprotein found in the fruit of *Synsepalum dulcificum*, miracle berry. When the pulp of the fruit is placed on the tongue, sour materials taste sweet. It is used as a sweetening substance.

Mirault [Germanicus *Mirault*, French surgeon, 1796–1879] See under OPERATION.

mire [French (from L *mirari* to look at), line of sight. French *se mirer* means to look at oneself in a reflecting surface.] A luminous pattern used to measure curvature by reflection.

mirestrol A natural estrogenic substance extracted from the tuberous roots of the Asiatic vine, *Pueraria mirifica*. Given parenterally, it equals estradiol in potency, and it is more potent than diethylstilbestrol when administered by mouth.

mirror [Middle English *mirour* (from Old French *mireour* mirror, from *mirer* to gaze at one's reflection in, from L *mirari* to wonder at, admire) mirror] A polished surface, as of glass, capable of reflecting images under illumination.

concave mirror A mirror having a concave reflecting surface.

convex mirror A mirror having a convex reflecting surface.

dental mirror MOUTH MIRROR.

frontal mirror HEAD MIRROR.

Glatzel mirror A polished surface, such as that provided by a metal spatula, used to study the volume and other characteristics of air expired through the nose by approximating the cold surface to the nares and observing the patches of condensed moisture. Certain inferences about the nasal airway may thus be reached. Also called *nasographic mirror*.

head mirror A concave mirror, worn on a headband or spectacle frame, used for focusing a beam of light from an outside source onto a small area to be examined. The observer looks through a hole in the center of the mirror into a well-illuminated, shadow-free field. Also called *frontal mirror.*

laryngeal mirror A circular plane mirror used to examine the interior of the larynx and hypopharynx. It is around 2.5 cm in diameter, mounted at an angle of about 120 degrees on a slender shank and handle, and altogether some 22 cm in length.

mouth mirror A small mirror, attached to a handle, used in the examination of teeth and the mouth. It may be made of glass and sterilizable, or of plastic and disposable. Also called *dental mirror, odontoscope, dental reflector* (obsolete).

nasographic mirror GLATZEL MIRROR.

nasopharyngeal mirror A small laryngeal mirror, around 1 cm in diameter, used to examine the nasopharynx. Also called *postnasal mirror.*

plane mirror A mirror having a flat reflecting surface.

postnasal mirror NASOPHARYNGEAL MIRROR.

van Helmont's mirror An outmoded term for CENTRUM TENDINEUM.

miryachit MYRIACHIT.

mis- MISO-.

misanthropia MISANTHROPY.

misanthropy [MIS- + *anthrop(o)*- + -Y] Hatred or profound distrust of people in general. Also called *misanthropia.*

miscarriage [English *mis*-, prefix denoting badly + *carriage* (from Middle English *cariage* carriage, from Old North French *carier* to transport)] A popular term for SPONTANEOUS ABORTION.

miscarry [MIS- + *carry*] To abort the products of conception spontaneously. A popular usage.

misce [L, 2nd person sing. imperative of *miscere* to mix] Mix: a direction used in pharmacy.

miscegenation [L *misce(re)* to mix, intermingle + *gen(us)* race, stock, nation + -ATION] Interbreeding, marriage, or cohabitation of persons of different races.

miscible [Med L *miscibilis* (from L *misc(ere)* to mix + -*ibilis* English -*ible*) capable of being mixed] Capable of being mixed, without forming separate phases, as ethanol and water.

miscoding MISTRANSLATION.

misdiagnose To diagnose wrongly.

misdiagnosis An incorrect diagnosis.

mismatch / acoustic mismatch A significant difference in acoustic impedance between two materials at the interface between them, which increases reflections and decreases transmission.

miso- [Gk *misos* hatred] A combining form meaning hatred. Also *mis-.*

misocainia [MISO- + *cain(o)*- + -IA] Pathologic fear of anything new or different. Also called *misoneism.*

misogamy [MISO- + GAM- + -Y] Hatred or abhorrence of marriage.

misogyny [MISO- + GYN- + -Y] Hatred or abhorrence of women.

misoneism MISOCAINIA.

misreading MISTRANSLATION.

mist [Middle English, from Old English] Condensed water vapor present in the lower layers of the atmosphere in quantities sufficient to reduce visibility.

mist. *mistura* (L, a mixture).

mister In the United Kingdom, a title of address prefixed to the name of a surgeon. Abbreviation: Mr. • Usage in Australia accords with that of Britain. In South Africa the usage is obsolescent, with *doctor* replacing it. *Mister* is still used of surgeons in New Zealand but is regarded by some as pretentious and is not used in universities. The title is never used in the United States, Canada, or Japan.

mistranslation The incorporation into a protein of an amino acid other than the one specified by the codon. In bacteria and their extracts, such misreading of genetic information is stimulated by aminoglycoside antibiotics and by ram (ribosomal ambiguity) mutations. Also called *misreading, miscoding.*

mistura [L (from *mistus*, also *mixtus*, past part. of *miscere* to mix; Gk *mixai*, first aorist inf. of *mignynai* to mix, mingle), a mixture] Mixture: used in pharmacy.

mistura cretae CHALK MIXTURE.

mistura glycyrrhizae composita BROWN MIXTURE.

mistura oleobalsamica OLEOBALSAMIC MIXTURE.

mistura pectoralis EXPECTORANT MIXTURE.

mit. *mitte* (L, send).

mitapsis [*mit(o)*- + Gk *(h)apsis*, Ionic Gk *apsis* a joining] The fusion of chromatin granules occurring in the final stage of cell conjugation.

Mitchell See under WEIR MITCHELL.

mite [Old English *mite* a small insect] A very small arachnid of the subclass Acari. The mites are an extremely large and varied group and occupy many different habitats. Most are under 1 mm long and many are microscopic. Most kinds of mite are free-living, predatory soil dwellers, feeding on various invertebrates, soil microbes, insect eggs, and other organisms. Many are parasitic for at least part of their life cycles, feeding on skin and blood of vertebrates. Others are permanent obligate parasites living within the skin. The abdomen and the cephalothorax are broadly joined, and segmentation is often difficult to discern. Four pairs of legs are present in nymphs and adults, but are reduced in follicular and scabies mites. Larvae have three pairs of legs. The ticklike mesostigmatic mites possess a hypostome while the others do not. Some 200 families are recognized. The current classification places the mesostigmatic mites and ticks in the order Parasitiformes, and the other mites in the order Acariformes and Opilioacariformes. Also called *acarus.*

auricular mite A mite of the species *Otodectes cynotis.*

burrowing mite A mite that forms burrows in the skin, as the female of the human scabies mite.

cheese mite A mite of the species *Tyrophagus longior.*

chigger mite A trombiculid mite; a chigger.

clover mite A small mite of the genus *Bryobia.* It infests clover plants.

copra mite A meal or grain mite causing copra itch, usually *Tyrophagus putrescentiae.*

face mite A mite of the species *Demodex folliculorum.*

flour mite A grain mite of the genus *Tyrophagus,* especially *T. farinae.*

follicle mite A mite of the genus *Demodex.*

food mite A mite of the genus *Glycyphagus.*

grain mite Any of various mites that are pests on grain crops. Many of them can cause dermatitis among workers handling these crops or their products. Also called *meal mite.* See also *TYROPHAGUS.*

grain itch mite A mite of the genus *Pyemotes.*

hair follicle mite A mite of the genus *Demodex.*

harvest mite A mite of the species *Trombicula autumnalis.* Also called *harvest bug, aoûtat* (French).

itch mite Any of various skin-infesting mites that cause an itching dermatitis, such as those of the genera *Notoedres, Sarcoptes, Pyemotes, Cheyletiella,* and *Psorergates.*

kedani mite A trombiculid mite, especially one of the species *Leptotrombidium* (or *Trombicula*) *akamushi.*

louse mite A mite of the genus *Pyemotes.*

mange mite Any mite that causes mange, such as those of the genera *Chorioptes, Knemidokoptes, Psoroptes,* and *Sarcoptes.*

meal mite GRAIN MITE.

onion mite A mite of the species *Acarus rhyzoglypticus hyacinthi*.

red mite An adult mite of the family Trombiculidae, the chigger mites. The mature mites, oval or figure eight in shape, are usually covered with a dense coat of bright red, velvety hairlike setae. Also called *red bug*.

spider mite A web-spinning mite of the family Tetranychidae that is a pest on various crops. A temporary itching dermatitis may develop in hop-pickers and other harvesters who become sensitized to the mites. Also called *spinning mite*.

spinning mite SPIDER MITE.

straw mite A mite belonging to any of several genera of the family Pyemotidae, which is commonly found as a predator of insects, and which may produce skin lesions in humans associated with straw, hay, grains, or grasses.

mitella [L (dim. of *mitra* an Oriental headdress), a female headdress, a sling] An arm sling.

mithramycin $C_{52}H_{72}O_{24}$. An antibiotic used chiefly as an antineoplastic agent. It is produced by *Streptomyces argillaceus, S. tanashienis*, and *S. plicatus*, and is a yellow, crystalline powder. It is used therapeutically in the treatment of various testicular carcinomas which cannot be removed surgically. The agent is also used in the treatment of various forms of hypercalcemia secondary to carcinomas. It is given intravenously.

mithridatism [after *Mithridates*, King of Pontus (died 63 B.C.), who is said to have practiced this method] Development of tolerance for a poison by ingestion of small but gradually increasing doses of it.

miticidal [*mit(e)* + *i* + *-cid(e)* + *-AL*] Destructive to mites.

miticide Any chemical that is used to control mite populations.

mitigate To make or become milder; moderate.

mitis Mild: used in prescription writing to denote the weaker of two available preparations.

mito- [Gk *mitos* thread, web of the loom] A combining form meaning (1) thread, threadlike; (2) mitosis.

mitocarcin An antibiotic used chiefly as an antineoplastic agent. It is derived from various species of *Streptomyces*.

mitochondria Plural of MITOCHONDRION.

mitochondrion [MITO- + Gk *chondrion* (dim. of *chondron*, also *chondros* a grain) a small grain, granule] (*plural* mitochondria) A cytoplasmic organelle of eukaryotic cells, enclosed by a double membrane. The inner membrane infolds to form cristae which partially divide the inner compartment. Mitochondria may be rod-shaped, branched, spherical, or donut-shaped. The mitochondria represent the site of aerobic respiration in the cell. Mitochondria contain ribosomes and possess extranuclear genes. Division is by binary fission. Also called *Altmann's granule, electrosome, plastiosome* (outmoded), *bioblast (early name), chondriome* (older term), *chondriosome* (older term).

giant mitochondrion An unusually large mitochondrion, which is produced as a consequence of nutritional deficiencies, toxic influences, or the effects of electromagnetic fields.

mitochondrion of hemoflagellates The single, extremely large mitochondrion characteristic of hemoflagellates, extending through much of the length of the body. Its structure varies with the biochemical activity at different developmental stages of the flagellate, being most elaborate in the midgut stage of the insect vector, and relatively simple, with few short and tubular cristae, in the blood-inhabiting, elongate stages in which the energy sources of the vertebrate host are utilized and the biochemical independence of the parasite is minimal.

mitocromin An antibiotic employed chiefly as an antineoplastic agent. It is produced by the species *Streptomyces viridochromogenes*.

mitogen [MITO- + -GEN] An agent which promotes mitosis.

pokeweed mitogen A mitogen acting mainly on B cells derived from the plant *Phytolacca americana*.

mitogenesia MITOGENESIS.

mitogenesis [MITO- + GENESIS] 1 The initiation of mitosis. 2 Formation as a result of division by mitosis. For defs. 1 and 2 also called *mitogenesia*.

mitogenetic MITOGENIC.

mitogenic Stimulating or promoting mitosis. Also *mitogenetic*.

mitogillin An antibiotic with antineoplastic activity. It is generated by the species *Aspergillus restrictus*.

mitomalcin An antibiotic agent used chiefly for its antineoplastic activity. It is a product of the species *Streptomyces malayensis*.

mitome A thread contained in the protoplasm of a cell, either a cytomitome or a karyomitome.

mitomycin A group of antibiotic substances produced by species of *Streptomyces* and differentiated as mitomycin A, B, and C. Mitomycin C inhibits cell division by blocking the crosslinking of DNA strands, thus preventing DNA synthesis. It is used as an antineoplastic agent.

mitoplasm [MITO- + -PLASM] The threadlike chromatin in the nucleus of the cell.

mitoschisis [MITO- + Gk *schisis* a cleaving, division] KARYOKINESIS.

mitoses Plural of MITOSIS.

mitosis [MITO- + -OSIS] (*plural* mitoses) The division of the nucleus of a cell to produce two daughter nuclei, each having a genome identical with that of the parent nucleus. Mitosis is a genetically controlled process and is usually followed by cytokinesis. Mitosis is divided into four phases beginning with prophase during which the reduplicated chromosomes appear in species-specific number. At the beginning of prophase the chromosomes appear as long threads consisting of two chromatids each. During prophase the chromosomes become progressively shorter and more compact. Prophase ends with the disruption of the nuclear envelope, the formation of the spindle, and the movement of chromosomes toward the metaphase plate. During metaphase, the second phase of mitosis, the chromosomes reach the metaphase plate with all centromers aligned at the spindle equator. Anaphase follows metaphase with the separation of the sister chromatids and their movement toward the opposite poles of the spindle. During telophase, which commences as the chromatids arrive at the poles, the nuclear envelope is reformed, and the chromatin is uncoiled. Also called *karyomitosis, mitotic cycle, indirect nuclear division* (older term).

abortive mitosis PATHOLOGIC MITOSIS.

anastral mitosis Mitosis in which asters are not present.

astral mitosis Mitosis characterized by the presence of centrioles, asters, and a spindle, as generally observed in animal cells.

asymmetrical mitosis A mitotic division in which the two daughter cells have unequal chromosome numbers, a result of an irregular chromosome distribution or a reduction in chromosome number in one nucleus.

heterotypic mitosis Mitosis in which the sister chromatids are united at their ends, forming ring structures.

homeotypic mitosis Mitosis in which two asters are present, daughter chromosomes separate, and one daughter chromosome of each type moves to each aster. This is the typical mitotic sequence.

multicentric mitosis MULTIPOLAR MITOSIS.

multipolar mitosis Mitosis in which three or more asters are present at the poles of the spindle resulting in the formation of a nucleus at each aster. The result is an aberrant chromosome distribution. It is a mechanism by which polyploid cells reduce ploidy. Also called *multicentric mitosis.*

pathologic mitosis   Mitosis in which the chromosome numbers of the daughter cells are not equal. Also called *abortive mitosis.*

pluripolar mitosis   Mitotic division in which there are more than two centrioles. Such division results in more than two daughter cells.

mitosome [MITO- + -*some*, combining form denoting body, from Gk *sōma* body]   A cytoplasmic body which originates from the spindle of a previous mitosis. Also called *spindle remnant.*

mitosper   An antineoplastic agent derived from the mold *Aspergillus glaucus.*

mitospore   A diploid spore, as in fungi of the class Chytridiomycetes, which serves to repeat the diploid generation by producing more sporothalli.

mitotic   Of or pertaining to mitosis. Also *karyomitotic.*

mitragynine $C_{23}H_{30}N_2O_4$. A white amorphous powder. It is the major alkaloid of *Mitragyna speciosa.*

mitral   **1** Denoting a structure in the shape of a turban or of a bishop's miter. **2** Pertaining to the mitral valve of the heart.

mitralism [*mitral (valve)* + -ISM]   A disorder affecting the mitral valve apparatus.

mitralization   A configuration of the heart shadow, consisting of straightening of the left cardiac border, often resulting from stenosis of the mitral valve with enlargement of the left atrial appendage and the pulmonary artery.

mitroid   Having the shape of a miter.

Mitsuda [Kensuke *Mitsuda*, Japanese physician, born 1876]   **1** Mitsuda reaction, Mitsuda test. See under LEPROMIN TEST. **2** Mitsuda lepromin. See under LEPROMINUM INTEGRALE (MITSUDA TYPE). **3** Mitsuda antigen. See under LEPROMIN.

mittelschmerz [German *mittel* middle + *Schmerz* pain]   Pain in the lower abdomen at the time of ovulation. Also called *midpain, dysmenorrhea intermenstrualis, intermenstrual pain.*

Mittendorf [William F. *Mittendorf*, U.S. physician, flourished late 19th century]   See under DOT.

mittor [L *mitt(ere)* to make go, send + -OR]   An obsolete term for NEUROMITTOR.

mix / case mix   The composition of the practice of a health care provider, program, or organization according to types of case, as specified by diagnoses. Also *case-mix.*

patient mix   The composition of the practice of a health care provider, program, or organization according to the number and types of patients served.

mixer / amalgam mixer   A machine for mixing dental alloy and mercury. They are placed in a capsule with a steel ball and vigorously vibrated.

mixing / vacuum mixing   The mixing of plaster of Paris and water in a state of partial vacuum in order to reduce the size of air bubbles in the final mixture.

mixoploid   POIKILOPLOID.

mixoploidy   POIKILOPLOIDY.

mixoscopia [Gk *mix(is)* intercourse + *o* + *skop(ein)* to look at, contemplate + -IA]   A paraphilia in which sexual gratification depends upon watching the loved one have sexual intercourse with another person. Also called *mixoscopy.*

mixoscopy   MIXOSCOPIA.

mixotrophic   Able to oxidize inorganic substrates, and therefore lithotrophic, but also able to use organic substrates and often showing enhanced growth with them.

Mixter [Samuel Jason *Mixter*, U.S. surgeon, 1855–1926]   See under DILATOR.

mixture [L *mistura.* See MISTURA.]   A combining or blending of two or more substances without chemical reaction, so that the properties of the components are retained. Pharmaceutical mixtures usually contain a solid component dispersed as a suspension in a liquid containing gum acacia, sugar, or some other viscid substance. Also called *admixture.*

ACE mixture   A mixture of alcohol, chloroform, and ether, formerly used as an inhalation anesthetic.

Agazotti's mixture   A mixture of oxygen and carbon dioxide formerly used for relief of air sickness.

Aldrich mixture   A solution of one percent gentian violet formerly used in treating burns.

Arkövy's mixture   A mixture of phenol (2 g), camphor (1 g) and eucalyptus oil (1 ml), used in the treatment of septic root canals.

Biedert's cream mixture   An infant food preparation consisting of cream, water, and lactose.

Bordeaux mixture   A plant fungicide that is composed of 5 parts copper sulfate and 400 parts water, to which 5 parts calcium oxide is added.

brown mixture   A mixture composed of liquid extract of licorice, antimony potassium tartrate, camphorated tincture of opium, spirit of nitrous ether, glycerin, and water. It is used in the treatment of fevers, coughs, and colds. Also called *mistura glycyrrhizae composita, compound opium and glycyrrhiza mixture.*

carminative mixture   Any mixture that relieves epigastric distress and gas. Many of these mixtures contain opiates.

Castellani's mixture   A mixture of tartar emetic, sodium salicylate, potassium iodide, sodium bicarbonate, and water. It was formerly used to treat yaws, but is now obsolete.

C-E mixture   E-C MIXTURE.

chalk mixture   A mixture containing aromatic chalk powder, chalk, tragacanth, and cinnamon water. It is used as an antacid and in the treatment of diarrhea. Also called *mistura cretae.*

compound opium and glycyrrhiza mixture   BROWN MIXTURE.

compound mixture of senna   A liquid extract of senna, magnesium sulfate, extract of licorice, tincture of cardamom, and aromatic spirit of ammonia. It has been used as a laxative. Also called *black draft, haustus niger.*

E-C mixture   The combination of diethyl ether and chloroform, yielding the more favorable effects of both general anesthetics. Also called *C-E mixture.*

Elzholz mixture   A solution of eosin in glycerol and water, used in an obsolete procedure for the quantitative estimation of leukocytes in a blood sample.

expectorant mixture   A mixture of ammonium carbonate, fluid extract of senega and squill, camphorated tincture of opium, syrup of tolu, and water. It is used to loosen and increase bronchial secretions. Also called *pectoral mixture, mistura pectoralis.*

extemporaneous mixture   A mixture prepared at the time ordered from a prescription, rather than from a stock supply.

Gregory's mixture   COMPOUND POWDER OF RHUBARB.

Gunning's mixture   A mixture of sulfuric acid, copper sulfate, and potassium sulfate used in the measurement of nitrogen in urine. An obsolete term.

kaolin mixture with pectin   A mixture containing kaolin, pectin, tragacanth, benzoic acid, saccharin, glycerin, and peppermint oil in purified water. It is used as an adsorbant medication and as a lenitive agent.

magnesium hydroxide mixture   CREAM OF MAGNESIA.

oleobalsamic mixture   An alcoholic solution of balsam of Peru and aromatic oils. It is used as a skin stimulant. Also called *mistura oleobalsamica.*

pectoral mixture   EXPECTORANT MIXTURE.

Ringer's mixture   RINGER SOLUTION.

toxin-antitoxin mixture   See under TOXIN-ANTITOXIN.

Vincent's mixture **1** A combination of one part stearin and two parts each of paraffin and petrolatum. It is used to line tubes and vessels that transport blood in transfusions. **2** A combination of sodium hypochlorite and boric acid that has been used to cover surgical or traumatic wounds.

Miyagawa [Yoneji *Miyagawa*, Japanese bacteriologist, 1885–1959] Miyagawa bodies. See under BODY.

Miyagawanella An obsolete term for *CHLAMYDIA*.

Mizuo [Gentaro *Mizuo*, Japanese ophthalmologist, 1876–1913] See under PHENOMENON.

MJ Symbol for the unit, megajoule.

MK monkey lung cells (as used in tissue culture).

mkat Symbol for the unit, millikatal.

μkat Symbol for the unit, microkatal.

mkat/l Symbol for the unit, millikatal per liter.

mkat·l⁻¹ Symbol for the unit, millikatal per liter.

MKS meter-kilogram-second (system).

ML midline.

ml Symbol for the unit, milliliter.

μl Symbol for the unit, microliter.

MLA mentoclaeva anterior (a fetal position).

mLa Symbol for the unit, millilambert.

MLC mixed lymphocyte culture.

MLD **1** median lethal dose. **2** minimal lethal dose.

MLP mentolaeva posterior (a fetal position).

MLT mentolaeva transversa (a fetal position).

mlx Symbol for the unit, millilux.

MM **1** mucous membrane. **2** myeloid metaplasia (agnogenic myeloid metaplasia).

mm **1** Symbol for the unit, millimeter. **2** muscle.

mm² Symbol for the unit, square millimeter.

mm³ Symbol for the unit, cubic millimeter.

mμ **1** Symbol for millimicro-. **2** Symbol for the obsolete unit, millimicron.

μM Symbol for the obsolete unit, micromolar.

μm **1** Symbol for the unit, micrometer. **2** Symbol for micromilli-.

μμ Symbol for micromicro-.

mμc. Symbol for the unit, millimicrocurie.

μμF Symbol for the unit, micromicrofarad.

mμg Symbol for the unit, millimicrogram (nanogram).

μmg Symbol for the unit, micromilligram (nanogram).

μμg Symbol for the unit, micromicrogram (picogram).

mmHg Symbol for the unit, conventional millimeter of mercury.

μmHg Symbol for the unit, conventional micrometer of mercury.

mmHg·min/l Symbol for the unit, conventional millimeter of mercury minute per liter.

mmHg·min·l⁻¹ Symbol for the unit, conventional millimeter of mercury minute per liter.

mmH₂O Symbol for the unit, conventional millimeter of water.

MMI **1** macrophage migration inhibition. **2** methylmercaptoimidazole.

μmm Symbol for the unit, micromillimeter (nanometer).

mmol Symbol for the unit, millimole.

μmol Symbol for the unit, micromole.

mmol/l Symbol for the unit, millimole per liter.

mmol·l⁻¹ Symbol for the unit, millimole per liter.

MMPI Minnesota multiphasic personality inventory.

mmpp millimeters partial pressure (partial pressure as expressed in conventional millimeters of mercury).

mμs Symbol for the unit, millimicrosecond.

MMTV mouse mammary tumor virus.

MN Symbol for the unit, meganewton.

Mn Symbol for the element, manganese.

mN Symbol for the unit, millinewton.

μN Symbol for the unit, micronewton.

M'Naghten [Daniel *M'Naghten*, British criminal, died 1865] M'Naghten test. See under M'NAGHTEN RULE.

mnemoderma [Gk *mnēm(ē)* a remembering, record + *o* + -DERMA] The tendency for certain skin eruptions to recur at the same site. An obsolete term.

mnemonic [Gk *mnēmonik(os)* (from *mnēmōn* remembering, from *mnasthai* to remember, + -*ikos* -IC) pertaining to memory] Aiding the recall of verbal or numerical materials from memory.

mnemonics [Gk *mnēmon(ika)*, neut. pl. of *mnēmon(ikos)* (from *mnēmōn* mindful + -*ikos* -IC) pertaining to memory + -ICS] The use, or devising, of techniques to facilitate memory and rote learning. Also called *mnemotechnics*.

mnemotechnics MNEMONICS.

MO mesio-occlusal.

Mo Symbol for the element, molybdenum.

MΩ Symbol for the unit, megohm.

mΩ Symbol for the unit, milliohm.

μΩ Symbol for the unit, microhm.

mobbing A group reaction to a predator by a number of small birds, a defensive counteraggression in which a predator is harassed. Many species of birds are known to engage in the practice.

mobility [L *mobilitas* (from *mobilis* movable, from *movere* to move + -*itas* -ITY) mobility] The capacity for movement.
  electrophoretic mobility The velocity at which ions of a substance migrate in an electric field. It has the dimensions of velocity divided by potential gradient. Relative values are often stated rather than absolute ones.
  tooth mobility The loosening of a tooth. It may occur in periodontal disease, increased occlusal stress, and acute inflammatory conditions of the periodontium.

mobilization A process or an operation whereby an object or a substance is freed or made mobile, as, for example, a physical therapy technique to restore the normal range of motion to a joint or body part whose movement has become restricted.
  chromosome mobilization The conjugative transfer of part or all of a bacterial chromosome, resulting from integration of a plasmid that codes for transfer of itself.
  stapes mobilization The transmeatal operative mobilization of the stapes ankylosed by otosclerosis. It is intended to restore the impaired hearing. It has been almost entirely superseded by stapedectomy. Also called *stapediolysis, stapes mobilization operation*.

mobilize To make movable a part or parts that had been fixed and immovable.

mobilizer / patient mobilizer An electric device for transferring an immobile patient from a bed to a gurney. A thin sheet of rollers moves under the patient and, in conveyer belt fashion, retracts back to the gurney, bringing the patient along with it.

Mobitz [Woldemar *Mobitz*, German cardiologist, born 1889] Mobitz-type atrioventricular dissociation. See under BLOCK.

Möbius [Paul Julius *Möbius*, German neurologist, 1853–1907] **1** See under SIGN, SYNDROME. **2** Möbius disease, Möbius syndrome. See under OPHTHALMOPLEGIC MIGRAINE. **3** Leyden-Möbius muscular dystrophy. See under LEYDEN-MÖBIUS MYOPATHY. **4** Leyden-Möbius syndrome. See under SYNDROME. **5** Ledyen-Möbius dystrophy. See under LIMB-GIRDLE MUSCULAR DYSTROPHY.

moccasin [from the Algonquian]   Any venomous snake of the crotaline genus *Agkistrodon.*

water moccasin   A semiaquatic venomous snake of the species *Agkistrodon piscivorous.* Also called *cottonmouth.*

mock-up   A full-sized structural model of an apparatus, used for study, testing, or improvement of design.

MOD   mesio-occlusodistal.

modality [French *modalité* (from Med L *modal(is)* modal + French *-ité* -ITY, from L *mod(us)* measure + *-alis* AL) form, mode]   **1** A specific type of sensation.   **2** A therapeutic method, especially one employed in physical therapy.

mode [L *modus* a measure, standard, manner, mode]   **1** The most frequent value of the variable in a frequency distribution.   **2** A specific manner of operation or presentation. Adjective: modal.

A mode   A mode of ultrasonic imaging in which the horizontal axis in the display represents depth and the vertical axis represents echo amplitude.

B mode   A mode of ultrasonic imaging in which the display presents a two-dimensional image of a slice through the body with brightness contours determined by echo amplitude.

isocontour mode   In radiation therapy, a display mode in which contours are plotted, each representing the locus in space of a preselected level of radiation intensity, often defined by count rate.

list mode   A data collection technique in nuclear medicine in which the position information of each detected radioactive event is recorded, together with its time of collection relative to other pulses collected during the study. It is a particularly helpful method of collecting dynamic data since images and activity curves in time mode can be constructed.

M mode   A mode of ultrasonic imaging in which the display records a spot brightening for each echo received, producing a one-dimensional display of reflector position and motion versus time. Also called *TM mode.*

radial mode   Oscillation of an ultrasound transducer in the radial direction.

TM mode   M MODE.

model [French *modèle* (from Italian *modello* a model, pattern, from L *modus* a measure, standard + *-ulus* -ULE) an object that is reproduced by imitation]   **1** A means by which something else can be visualized or represented, as an object fashioned on the same or a smaller scale after something else (as of anatomic parts) or a representation in a different form, as in mathematical symbols or computer codes, to provide a basis for analysis or experimentation.   **2** CAST.

animal model   A pathologic condition or physiologic event occurring in an animal species but analogous to or illuminative of an event occurring in humans.

articulating model   A cast in a dental articulator.

casting model   A cast made of a refractory material and used as part of the mold for making a cast-metal denture base.

copy-choice model   A model, now abandoned, used to explain genetic recombination, in which it was proposed that DNA synthesis moved back and forth between two chromosomes.

Danielli-Davson model   A representation of the molecular arrangement of the components of the cellular membranes in which a lipid layer separates two protein layers. The lipids are phospholipids and are arranged in two monomolecular layers with their hydrophobic tails toward the inside of the membrane and their hyrophilic phosphates toward the surface protein.

deterministic model   A model of a system which contains no random elements, so that the future course of the system is determined by its state at a given point in time. Early attempts to develop a mathematical theory of epidemics relied on deterministic models.

fluid mosaic model   A theoretical model of cell membrane structure. It implies a degree of dynamic change, with molecules being exchanged continuously while providing a stable envelope to maintain a constant internal environment.

Hassell-Varley model   A mathematical model found useful in describing certain host-parasite and predator-prey population interactions.

implant model   A cast of the bony surface on which a subperiosteal implant will rest.

linear model   A statistical model of the relationship between two or more variables in which one is treated as a linear function of the other or others.

mathematical model   A simplified representation of a problem, process, system, or situation in the form of a set of equations or a computer program. Such a model might, for example, simulate the operation of the pressure-flow relationships in the cardiovascular system.

metabolic model   An analysis and reconstruction of the way in which a specific substance is dealt with in the body. It includes data on the proportion of the intake which is absorbed, the proportion stored in the body, and the tissues in which it is stored; the mechanism of its subsequent release or relocation; the proportion which is broken down in the body; and the subsequent dispersal of the products, the proportion of the substance excreted, and the rate of excretion by the various organs concerned.

rolling circle model   A form of DNA replication, observed in some circular virus genomes, in which the replication does not terminate after completing the circle but continues in additional rounds, producing a long continuous chain that is then cleaved to appropriate lengths.

stochastic model   A model of a system incorporating one or more random variables, so that the future state of the system can be predicted only in terms of probabilities. Stochastic models have been developed for population growth, the theory of epidemics, etc.

study model   STUDY CAST.

Watson-Crick model   A molecular model which represents the structure of deoxyribonucleic acid as a double helix with a right-handed coiling. The two strands of the helix are composed of antiparallel strands of polynucleotides. See also DEOXYRIBONUCLEIC ACID.

modeling   The normal process by which a child comes to acquire appropriate social and cognitive behaviors by observing and imitating the behavior observed by significant others, such as parents or older sibs. This copying is in its turn rewarded and positively reinforced by members of the social group. Modeling thus serves as an important mechanism for the socialization of new members.

modelling   A British spelling for MODELING.

modem [*mo(dulator-)dem(odulator)*]   An electronic device that transmits computer data over telephone lines. It converts the voltage levels that represent binary 0 and 1 to different frequency tones and vice versa.

Moderil   A proprietary name for rescinnamine.

modification [L *modificatio* (from *modus* a measure, standard + *-ficatio* -FICATION) the measuring of a thing]   A change in an organism that is acquired or learned and does not involve heredity.

behavior modification   The use of conditioning or other learning techniques to alter human behavior in desired ways. See also BEHAVIOR THERAPY.

weather modification   An alteration of the climate that is caused by human activity such as the polluting of the air or attempting to seed clouds to produce rainfall.

modifier   MODIFYING GENE.

modiolus [L (dim. of *modius* a measuring vessel), a drinking vessel, hub of a wheel, instrument for cutting out bone] **1** [NA] The conical central bony axis of the cochlea which is tunneled by longitudinal canals and a spiral canal for the conduction of nerves and vessels, while projecting outward throughout its length is the osseous spiral lamina. Its broad base is at the lateral end of the internal acoustic meatus. Also called *columella cochleae* (outmoded). **2** MODIOLUS LABII.

modiolus labii A nodular mass just lateral to the angle of the mouth where muscle fibers of the upper and lower lips decussate with each other and with those of several other facial muscles, such as the zygomaticus major and minor, levator anguli oris, depressor anguli oris, and buccinator muscles. Also called *modiolus*.

mod. praesc. *modo praescripto* (L, in the manner prescribed).

modulation [L *modulatio* (from *modulatus*, past part. of *modulari* to measure, modulate) a rhythmical measure] **1** The functional and morphologic adaptation of cells to changes in environment. **2** The change in amplitude or pitch of the voice. **3** Variation of the amplitude, frequency, or phase of a single-frequency wave (carrier wave) in order to transmit a message such as in radio.

amplitude modulation Modulation of the amplitude, usually of a carrier radio wave by an audio signal wave. Abbreviation: AM

frequency modulation Modulation of the frequency, usually of a radio carrier wave by an audio signal wave. Abbreviation: FM

intensity modulation Variation of the electron beam current in a cathode ray tube to achieve variation in brightness of the image, as for example in a television or ultrasonic monitor.

modulator In embryology, an inductor that specifically produces features related to definite regions during development.

module [L *modul(us)*, dim. of *modus* a measure, quantity, size] An assembly of interconnected components contained in one package which can be tested as a unit or removed and replaced with a spare.

modulus [L (dim. of *modus* a measure), a small measure] **1** A numerical constant or coefficient expressing the degree to which a substance possesses a given property. **2** The absolute value of a complex number. **3** The ratio between the logarithm of a number to one base (especially the Naperian logarithm) and the logarithm of that number to another base.

bulk modulus A coefficient of elasticity of a substance, pertaining to the change in volume under hydrostatic pressure, measured in pascals. It is defined as the ratio of the applied pressure to the resulting fractional change in volume. It is the reciprocal of the compressibility. Symbol: K

modulus of elasticity The factor of proportionality in the mathematical equation expressing the experimental law that when a body is subjected to a mechanical stress, the resulting fractional deformation (called strain) is up to a point, proportional to the applied stress.

Young's modulus A coefficient of elasticity of a substance, as a bone, pertaining to the change in dimension under unidirectional tension or compression, expressed in pascals. It is defined as the ratio of the tensile or compressional stress (force per unit cross-sectional area) to the fractional change in dimension parallel to the stress. Symbol: E

Modumate A proprietary name for arginine glutamate.

Moe [John H. *Moe*, U.S. surgeon, born 1905] See under PLATE.

Moeller [Alfred *Moeller*, German bacteriologist, born 1868] Moeller's operation. See under RHINOREACTION.

Moeller [Julius Otto Ludwig *Moeller*, German physician, 1819–1887] **1** Moeller's glossitis. See under CHRONIC SUPERFICIAL GLOSSITIS. **2** Moeller-Barlow disease. See under INFANTILE SCURVY.

Moentjang tina In Indonesia, intoxication by the use in food preparation of an oil from a tropical tree. It is intended to be used only in lamps.

Moersch [Frederick Paul *Moersch*, U.S. neurologist, born 1889] Moersch-Woltman syndrome. See under STIFF-MAN SYNDROME.

mogi- [Gk *mogis* with difficulty] A combining form meaning with difficulty.

mogiarthria [MOGI- + ARTHR- + -IA] A form of dysarthria in which spasm, similar to that of writer's cramp in the hand, involves the muscles of articulation.

mogigraphia [MOGI- + -GRAPH + -IA] A seldom used term for WRITERS' CRAMP.

mogilalia Any of various disorders of articulation, including stuttering or stammering. An imprecise and outmoded term. Also called *molilalia*.

mogiphonia [MOGI- + PHON- + -IA] Difficulty in production of voiced laryngeal sounds while talking.

mogitocia [MOGI- + *toc(o)*- + -IA] An older term for DYSTOCIA.

Mohrenheim [Baron Joseph Jakob Freiherr von *Mohrenheim*, Austrian surgeon, 1759–1799] Mohrenheim's fossa. See under FOSSA INFRACLAVICULARIS.

Mohs [Frederic Edward *Mohs*, U.S. surgeon, born 1910] See under CHEMOSURGERY.

moiety [Middle English *moite* (from Middle French *moité*, also *moitié* a half, from L *medietas* the middle, mean, from *medius* middle) half] **1** A half. **2** A portion or part.

mol Symbol for the unit, mole.

molal molality.

molality The amount of substance of a solute divided by the mass of the solvent, expressed in moles per kilogram. Abbreviation: molal

molar[1] **1** Divided by amount of substance: divided by mole. **2** Having a concentration of one mole per liter. See also MOLE[3].

molar[2] [L *molar(is)* (from *mola* a mill, millstone) pertaining to a mill, millstone; as substantive, a millstone, huge stone, grinding tooth, molar] Any of the most posterior teeth in each jaw, two per quadrant in the human deciduous dentition and three per quadrant in the human permanent dentition. Also called *molar tooth, multicuspid tooth, multicuspidate*.

bicuspidized molar A molar which has been divided buccolingually so as to obtain access to the furcation area for home-care cleaning in periodontal treatment.

dome-shaped molar See under SYPHILITIC TOOTH.

first molar The most anterior tooth of the molar series.

Moon's molar See under SYPHILITIC TOOTH.

mulberry molar See under SYPHILITIC TOOTH.

second molar The second tooth from the front in the molar series.

sixth-year molar The human first permanent molar which erupts at about six years of age.

third molar The third tooth from the front of the molar series; the most posterior tooth of the human permanent dentition. Also called *wisdom tooth, dens sapientiae, dens serotinus*.

twelfth-year molar The human second permanent molar which erupts at about 12 years of age.

molariform [MOLAR + *i* + -FORM] Shaped like a molar.

molarity The concentration of a substance expressed in moles per liter.

molasses The syrupy residue produced by washing raw sugar. This solution is boiled and the sugar that becomes crystallized is removed. The remaining solution is rich in nonsugars and minerals, especially iron.

mold **1** Any fungus having a cottony appearance, abundant in damp, dark locations, that is highly destructive to stored materials though an essential element of recycling of organic material and soil formation. **2** A hollow form in which a plastic material is shaped or cast. **3** To shape or cast in a mold. **4** That which is cast in a mold. **5** The shape of a molded object, such as an artificial tooth. For defs. 1–5 also *mould (British spelling).*

bread mold A fungus of the species *Rhizopus nigricans.*

ear mold A plastic fitting molded to the contours of the entrance to the external auditory meatus, forming part of an electrical hearing aid.

refractory mold A mold for dental casting that can withstand high temperature.

slime mold Any of a heterogeneous group of eukaryotic organisms, with both ameboid and moldlike phases in their life cycles. They include the acellular slime molds (myxomycetes) and the cellular slime molds (acrasiae).

snow mold A fungus, *Calonectria graminicola,* which, under certain environmental conditions, kills grass in parks, lawns, and golf courses.

sooty mold Fungi of the subclass Loculoascomycetidae which grow on the "honeydew" or excreta of a variety of plant-feeding insects. The fungal growth, although epiphytic, becomes so dense and dark that photosynthetic activity is greatly reduced. It is found on leaves and needles, stems, twigs, and fruit.

water mold Any fungus of the class Oomycetes.

white mold Any fungus having a white, cottony appearance in the vegetatively growing portion, the mycelium.

molding **1** A process whereby an object or a mass is caused by surrounding objects or pressures to assume a certain shape. **2** The shaping of the fetal head during labor and delivery that facilitates passage through the birth canal.

border molding The shaping of the borders of a dental impression by the action of the adjacent soft tissues in function or by manipulation. Also called *tissue molding, muscle-trimming.*

compression molding Forming a cast by using a mold of which the two parts are first separated and a mass of plastic material, such as acrylic resin in the "dough" stage of setting, is placed between them. They are then forced together and the material sets, usually with the application of heat, to the shape of the mold. This is the method used most frequently in the making of dentures.

injection molding Forming a cast by injecting a fluid material into a mold through tunnels. The material then sets, usually by the cooling of previously heated thermoplastic material, to the shape of the mold.

tissue molding BORDER MOLDING.

mole¹ [Old Englih *māl, māēl,* possibly from L *macula* a spot, stain, possibly akin to Gk *miainein* to stain, defile] A circumscribed, pigmented lesion of the skin, often slightly elevated; nevus pigmentosus. Also called *soft nevus, nevocytic nevus, nevus-cell nevus.*

cellular mole A cutaneous mole composed of nevus cells, some of which contain melanin.

hairy mole NEVUS PILOSUS.

pigmented mole A benign cutaneous nevus derived from the melanocyte system.

warty mole A raised cutaneous lesion that is usually derived from the melanocyte system and that bears a superficial resemblance to a viral wart.

white mole A mole or nevus that is devoid of melanin. It may resemble neural tissue or a neurofibroma.

mole² [L *mola* (from Gk *mylē* a mill) salt cake, a mill, millstone,

mooncalf, mole, false conception] An amorphous mass or tumor that forms in the uterus after degeneration of the conceptus. It usually consists of blood clots and remnants of the placenta and fetal membranes, but it may be calcified or develop cysts, as a hydatidiform mole.

blood mole CARNEOUS MOLE.

Breus mole A hematoma, or cluster of hematomas, of the decidua that protrude through the chorionic plate, resulting in fetal death due to compression of the intervillous circulation. This occurs in cases of missed abortion resulting in the formation of an organized, fleshy mass. A rarely used term.

carneous mole A spontaneous abortion in which the ovum is surrounded by a capsule of clotted blood. Also called *blood mole, hemorrhagic mole.*

cystic mole HYDATIDIFORM MOLE.

false mole A uterine tumor resembling a hydatidiform mole.

fleshy mole A degenerated retained placenta having a fleshy appearance. Also called *maternal mole.*

grape mole HYDATIDIFORM MOLE.

hemorrhagic mole CARNEOUS MOLE.

hydatid mole HYDATIDIFORM MOLE.

hydatidiform mole A trophoblastic lesion characterized by large grapelike, edematous, avascular chorionic villi. Trophoblastic cells may show signs of proliferation, but the lesion is benign. Also called *grape mole, cystic mole, hydatid mole, vesicular mole.*

invasive mole CHORIOADENOMA DESTRUENS.

invasive hydatidiform mole CHORIOADENOMA DESTRUENS.

malignant mole CHORIOADENOMA DESTRUENS.

malignant hydatidiform mole CHORIOADENOMA DESTRUENS.

maternal mole FLESHY MOLE.

metastasizing mole CHORIOADENOMA DESTRUENS.

placental mole Degeneration of the placenta to form a variety of intrauterine mole.

stone mole A hydatidiform mole which has become calcified.

true mole A mole derived from a degenerating ovum.

tubal mole The residue of a conceptus, comprising clotted blood and degenerating chorionic villi, in a tubal pregnancy.

tuberous mole A type of missed abortion in which only chorionic vesicles surrounded by blood clot, placenta, and decidua are expelled. Also called *tuberous subchorial hematoma, subchorial tuberous hematoma of the placenta, hematomole.*

vesicular mole HYDATIDIFORM MOLE.

mole³ [*(gram) mole(cule)* or German *Mole(kulargewicht)* molecular weight] The SI base unit of amount of substance, equal to that amount of substance of a system which contains as many elementary entities as there are atoms in 0.012 kilogram of carbon 12. When the mole is used, the elementary entities must be specified and may be atoms, molecules, ions, electrons, other particles, or specified groups of such particles. Also called *gram molecular weight* (obsolete). Symbol: mol

mole per cubic meter The SI derived unit of substance concentration. Symbol: mol/m^3, $mol·m^{-3}$

mole per kilogram The SI derived unit of molality, or of substance content. Symbol: mol/kg, $mol·kg^{-1}$

mole per liter A unit of substance concentration equal to 10^3 mole per cubic meter. Symbol: mol/l, $mol·l^{-1}$

mole per second The SI derived unit of catalytic (or enzymatic) activity. Symbol: mol/s, $mol·s^{-1}$

molecular **1** Concerned with molecules, as with the mass or structure of a single molecule. **2** Relating to the study of structures and processes occurring at the molecular level, especially of the macromolecules that are components of living matter, as in *molecular biology.*

molecule [Late L *molecula,* dim. of L *moles* a mass, shapeless mass, trouble, burden] The smallest entity of a substance. It is composed of atoms.

effector molecule **1** A cell or organ that responds to a stimulus, such as a nervous impulse, by an active process, such as secretion or contraction. **2** In the operon model of genetic regulation, a molecule that interacts with and either enhances or inhibits the action of the repressor. **3** A metabolite of a biochemical pathway that interacts with and modifies the activity of an enzyme catalyzing a reaction in the pathway.

molfr. mole fraction.

molilalia MOGILALIA.

molimen [L (from *moliri* to struggle, labor), a great exertion] The effort exerted in the performance of a bodily function: sometimes applied to the discomfort associated with menstruation.

molimen climactereium virile A reduction in sexual desire or responsivity in the involutional male, generally occurring from 50 to 65 years of age. An older term.

menstrual molimen Perimenstrual symptoms, such as swelling and cramps.

molimina Plural of MOLIMEN.

Molisch [Hans *Molisch*, Austrian botanist and chemist, 1836–1937] See under REACTION, TEST.

mol/kg Symbol for the unit, mole per kilogram.

mol·kg⁻¹ Symbol for the unit, mole per kilogram.

Moll [Jakob Anthoni *Moll*, Dutch anatomist and ophthalmologist, 1832–1914] Moll's glands, glandulae ciliares molli. See under GLANDULAE CILIARES PALPEBRARUM.

mol/l Symbol for the unit, mole per liter.

mol·l⁻¹ Symbol for the unit, mole per liter.

Mollaret [Pierre *Mollaret*, French neurologist, born 1898] Mollaret's meningitis. See under BENIGN RECURRENT ENDOTHELIOLEUKOCYTIC MENINGITIS.

Mollicutes [L *mollis* soft + *cutis* skin] The class of bacteria commonly referred to as mycoplasmas. It has two families, Mycoplasmataceae, which require sterols for growth, and Acholeplasmataceae, which do not. Genera include *Mycoplasma, Acholeplasma, Ureaplasma, Spiroplasma, Thermoplasma,* and *Anaeroplasma.*

mollin A form of soft soap containing glycerin and fats, used for the topical delivery of drugs or medicinal preparations externally.

mollities [L (from *mollis* soft, tender, pliant, mild), softness, pliancy, flexibility, weakness, effeminacy. Also *mollitia.*] Abnormal softening, denoting a portion of an organ or part of the body softened by necrosis. An obsolete term.

mollities ossium OSTEOMALACIA.

mollities unguium A softness of the nail. A rarely used term.

mollusc MOLLUSK.

Mollusca [New L, from neut. pl. of L *molluscus* rather soft. See MOLLUSCUM.] A major phylum of invertebrate animals constituting some 45 000 extant species in seven classes, and including a variety of marine, freshwater and terrestrial types, ranging from microscopic specimens to those quite large in size. Examples include snails, slugs, clams, whelks, limpets, octopuses, and squids.

molluscicidal [L *mollusc(a),* neut. pl. of *molluscus* soft + *i* + *-cid(e)* + -AL] Toxic to mollusks.

molluscicide Any agent that is toxic to mollusks.

molluscoid Resembling a mollusk.

molluscous Of or relating to molluscum.

molluscum [L (neut. of *molluscus* rather soft, from *mollis* soft, tender, pliant, mild), a fungus growing on a maple tree] **1** An

eruption of soft cutaneous nodules. **2** MOLLUSCUM CONTAGIOSUM.

molluscum contagiosum A benign infectious disease of the skin caused by a poxvirus and characterized by small, rounded, pearly white, umbilicated papules which yield basophilic, Feulgen-positive, intracytoplasmic inclusion bodies. The lesions appear most often on the trunk and anogenital area. Infection is transmitted by direct contact and by fomites. Venereal spread has been suggested. Also called *molluscum sessile, molluscum epitheliale, molluscum verrucosum, molluscum varioliformis, condyloma subcutaneum, Paterson's nodules* (seldom used), *molluscum, Bateman's disease.*

molluscum epitheliale MOLLUSCUM CONTAGIOSUM.

molluscum fibrosum NEUROFIBROMATOSIS.

molluscum giganteum Molluscum contagiosum with large lesions.

molluscum pendulum A polypoid soft tumor of the skin.

molluscum sessile MOLLUSCUM CONTAGIOSUM.

molluscum varioliformis MOLLUSCUM CONTAGIOSUM.

molluscum verrucosum MOLLUSCUM CONTAGIOSUM.

mollusk A member of the phylum Mollusca. Also *mollusc.* Adjective: molluscan.

mol/m³ Symbol for the unit, mole per cubic meter.

mol·m⁻³ Symbol for the unit, mole per cubic meter.

Moloney [Paul Joseph *Moloney*, Canadian physician, 1870–1939] Moloney reaction. See under TEST.

Moloy [Howard Carman *Moloy*, U.S. obstetrician and gynecologist, 1903–1953] Caldwell-Moloy classification. See under CLASSIFICATION.

mol/s Symbol for the unit, mole per second.

mol·s⁻¹ Symbol for the unit, mole per second.

molt [Middle English *mouten*, from Old English *mutian* to change, from L *mutare* to change] **1** To shed the exoskeleton, allowing an increase in size. Molting occurs periodically in many invertebrates, such as arthropods and nematodes. **2** In birds, to lose and replace feathers. **3** The process of molting.

molugram An obsolete term for GRAM-MOLECULE.

mol wt molecular weight.

molybdate Any anion with a central molybdenum atom, especially MoO_4^{2-}, or a salt containing such an anion. Molybdate is used in biochemistry to test for phosphate and to test for reducing agents, especially tyrosine residues in proteins, in the Folin test. Phosphate and molybdate can react to form the ion $PMo_{12}O_{40}^{3-}$, and its partial reduction to a mixture of Mo(V) and Mo(VI) gives an intensely blue complex.

molybdenosis MOLYBDENUM POISONING.

molybdenum Element number 42, having atomic weight 95.94. A silvery white, very hard metal, which is never found native but is widely distributed in various ores of other metals. It is an important alloying element in steel and has other technologic applications. Biologically, it is an essential trace element in plant nutrition and is required for activity of several animal enzymes. Symbol: Mo

molybdenum 99 One of the ten radioactive isotopes of molybdenum with a half-life of 66.7 hours, used in generators for the production of technetium 99m by decay. Symbol: ⁹⁹Mo

moment [L *moment(um)* (for *movimentum*, from *mov(ere)* to move + *i* + *-mentum* -MENT) that which moves the balance, a minute thing, motion, moment, change] In statistics, a cumulative function of the deviations of a set of observations from the mean of the series. The first moment, being the algebraic sum of the deviations, is by definition zero. The second moment, the sum of the squares of the deviations, is related to the standard deviation. The third moment, the sum of the cubes of the deviations, is related to skewness; while the sum of the fourth power of the deviations is related to kurtosis.

moment of death   That point in time when an individual is declared dead. This determination is based upon criteria which are defined by law and which differ according to the situation. For autopsy or burial purposes, criteria include the clinical judgment that respiration and circulation have ceased as well as the appearance of a secondary indication of death, such as livor or algor mortis. If tissues are to be obtained for organ transplantation, a criterion such as brain death is employed even though functional circulatory and respiratory activities may persist.

dipole moment   A system comprising two point charges, one positive and one negative, separated by a distance *l*. The electric dipole moment is the product *ql*, where *q* is the positive charge in electrostatic units of charge and *l* is the distance in centimeters between the two charges. Dipole moments are expressed in debye units (D), one unit beingequal to 10^{-18} electrostatic units of charge $\times$ centimeters.

magnetic moment   A measure of the torque exerted on a magnetic system when placed in a magnetic field, expressed as a vector quantity.

momentum   [L, that which moves the balance, weight, movement, motion]   The product of the mass and velocity of a body, an index of the "quantity of motion." In a collision, total momentum is conserved.

angular momentum   A vector quantity expressing the quantity of angular motion, depending on the rotational speed and the distribution of mass relative to the axis of rotation.

angular momentum of particle   The moment of momentum of the particle relative to a specified origin; the product of its (linear) momentum by the perpendicular distance of its line of motion from the origin.

mon-   MONO-.

monad   **1** A solitary unicellular organism, especially a free-swimming flagellate such as one of the genus *Monas*. **2** A single chromatid or member of a tetrad in meiosis.

springing monad   A flagellate protozoan of the species *Bodo saltans*.

Monakow   [Constantin von *Monakow*, Russian-born Swiss neurologist, 1853–1930]   **1** Monakow's theory. See under DIASCHISIS. **2** Striae of Monakow, striae of von Monakow. See under STRIAE MEDULLARES VENTRICULI QUARTI. **3** See under SYNDROME. **4** Monakow's bundle, fasciculus aberrans of Monakow, Monakow's fasciculus, Monakow's fibers, Monakow's tract, von Monakow's fibers. See under TRACTUS RUBROSPINALIS. **5** Clarke-Monakow nucleus, Monakow's nucleus. See under NUCLEUS CUNEATUS ACCESSORIUS.

Monaldi   [Vincenzo *Monaldi*, Italian physician, born 1899]   See under DRAINAGE.

monaminuria   MONOAMINURIA.

monangle   [MON- + ANGLE]   Having only one angle in the shaft: said of dental instruments.

monarthric   MONOARTICULAR.

monarthritis   [MON- + ARTHRITIS]   Arthritis of a single joint. Compare DIGARTHRITIS, POLYARTHRITIS.

monarthritis deformans   Severe, deforming arthritis, usually osteoarthritis, of a single joint. An obsolete term.

traumatic deforming monarthritis   Degenerative osteoarthrosis affecting a joint that was previously damaged by injury.

monarticular   MONOARTICULAR.

monaster   An aberrant spindle apparatus which may arise by the suppression of centriole division. When a monaster forms, the chromosomes fail to separate.

monathetosis   [MON- + ATHETOSIS]   Athetosis confined to a single limb.

monatomic   Composed of a single atom: used especially of the molecules of a noble gas. Such molecules do not have rotations available to them, and this gives characteristic values to the specific heats of gases composed of them. They also have characteristic absence of vibrations.

monauchenos   [MON- + Gk *auchēn*, gen. *auchenos*, the neck]   **1** Equal conjoined twins with complete union in all parts except the head, resulting in a single trunk with two heads on a single neck. Also called *dicephalus monauchenos*. **2** Single-necked.

monaural   Using only one ear or, in sound amplification, only one channel of transmission.

monavitaminosis   [MON- + Gk *a-* priv. + VITAMIN + -OSIS]   A nutrient deficiency disease caused by a diet lacking in one specific vitamin.

monaxial   **1** Of or denoting a neuron possessing only one axon. **2** Denoting a structure organized around a single axis, as a monaxial filament.

monaxon   A neuron possessing only one axon. A seldom used term.

monaxonic   Having a single axon.

Mönckeberg   [Johann Georg *Mönckeberg*, German pathologist, 1877–1925]   Mönckeberg's arteriosclerosis, Mönckeberg's degeneration, Mönckeberg's mesarteritis, Mönckeberg's medial sclerosis. See under MÖNCKEBERG'S SCLEROSIS.

Mondor   [Henri Jean Justin *Mondor*, French surgeon, 1885–1962]   See under DISEASE.

monellin   A two-chain, 94-residue protein found in the fruit of an African shrub, *Dioscoreophyllum cumminsii*, and exhibiting a sweetness 10^5 times greater than that of sucrose on a molar basis. It is temperature-sensitive and easily spoiled.

moner   A non-nucleated protoplasmic mass.

monerula   [New L, from *monēr(ēs)* single + -ULA, L fem. dim. suffix]   A fertilized ovum in the state before clevage has begun.

monesthetic   [MON- + ESTHETIC]   Describing, relating to, or affecting a single sense or variety of sensation.

monestrous   Characterized by the occurrence of estrus once each year; having one mating period a year.

Monge   [Carlos *Monge*, Peruvian physician, 1884–1970]   Monge's disease. See under MOUNTAIN SICKNESS.

mongol   A person with the Down syndrome. An imprecise and outmoded term.

Mongolian   **1** Belonging to the Mongoloid race. An outmoded usage. **2** Characterized by mongolism or the Down syndrome. An obsolete and incorrect usage.

mongolism   An outmoded term for DOWN SYNDROME.

translocation mongolism   An outmoded term for TRANSLOCATION DOWN SYNDROME.

Mongoloid   **1** Characterized by or similar to the physical features of the peoples of eastern Asia. **2** An individual having such physical features.   • The term *mongoloid* (not capitalized in this sense) was formerly much used in reference to the Down syndrome. This usage is not recommended.

Moniezia   A genus of tapeworms (family Anoplocephalidae) that are parasitic in cattle, sheep, goats, and other ruminants. As with other members of this cestode family, soil-dwelling oribatid mites serve as the sole intermediate host.

Moniezia expansa   The broad tapeworm of sheep. The most common sheep tapeworm, it is found in the small intestine and attains a length of about 3.5 to 4.5 meters (12 to 15 feet). Larval forms (cysticercoids) develop in various oribatid mites which are ingested with grass. Infections are usually nonpathogenic in normal hosts but heavy infestations in lambs may predispose them to enterotoxemia.

monilated   MONILIFORM.

monilethrix [L *monile* a necklace, collar + Gk *thrix* hair] A developmental defect of the hair shaft in which it becomes beaded and brittle. Elliptical nodes, 0.7–1 mm apart, are separated by internodes at which the medulla is lacking.

Monilia [L, pl. of *monile* a collar, necklace] An obsolete term for CANDIDA.

Moniliaceae [*monili(a)* + -ACEAE] A form-family of fungi which includes many saprobes, but in addition has included numerous plant and animal parasites, including human pathogens. Also called *Perisporiaceae* (obsolete).

monilial 1 Pertaining to the form-family Moniliaceae. 2 An incorrect term for CANDIDAL.

Moniliales [*Monili(a)* + L -*ales*, pl. of -*alis* -AL] A form-order of imperfect fungi which is subdivided into the form-families Moniliaceae, Dematiaceae, Tuberculariaceae, and Stilbellaceae. It includes a number of dermatophytes. Also called *Conidiosporales* (obsolete), *Thallosporales* (obsolete).

moniliasis [MONILIA + -SIS] An older term for CANDIDIASIS.

cutaneous moniliasis An incorrect term for CUTANEOUS CANDIDIASIS.

oral moniliasis THRUSH.

monilide An outmoded term for CANDIDIDE.

moniliform [L *monili(a)*, pl. of *monile* collar, necklace + -FORM] Having a structure suggestive of a string of beads. Also *monilated*.

Moniliformis [L *monile* a necklace, collar + -*formis*, suffix denoting a form, from *forma* form] A genus of acanthocephalan worms infecting mammals, chiefly rodents. Two common species are *M. dubius,* infecting rats and *M. moniliformis,* infecting squirrels and other rodents. Single reports of human infection have come from Italy, Sudan, Java, Israel, and the United States. Adult worms inhabit the small intestine, where they have little effect unless the infection is heavy.

moniliid An outmoded term for CANDIDIDE.

moniliosis [*monili(a)* + -OSIS] An older term for CANDIDIASIS.

monism [MON- + -ISM] The philosophic theory that there is but one kind of ultimate reality, since the universe consists of but a simple ultimate substance, and that mind and matter are, therefore, modes or aspects of the same substance.

monitor [L (from *monitus,* past part. of *monere* to remind, warn, foretell, chastise, akin to *monstrare* to show, demonstrate and to *meminisse* to remember; + -*or* OR), an adviser, admonisher] 1 To keep close watch over; check carefully and continually. 2 An apparatus used to record or display data, as of physiologic signs of a patient under continuous surveillance. See also under MONITORING.

apnea monitor An alarm system for alerting attendants to the occurrence of apnea, usually in a premature infant. Two types are in common use. One consists of an air mattress in which the breathing or any other slight movement causes a flow of air across a thermistor, producing resistance changes which can operate an electrical alarm if they cease. The other type is an impedance pneumograph which detects changes in electrical impedance through the chest during breathing.

monitoring [MONITOR + -ING] 1 The maintenance of close and sometimes continuous supervision, especially over patients considered at risk, often utilizing electronic equipment to monitor vital functions. 2 Periodic or continuous surveillance of a radioactive source or area, including the people in it, to provide early warning of adverse changes. The instruments used are designed to detect low-level ionizing radiation of various kinds, especially neutrons and gamma rays.

biological monitoring BIOASSAY.

cardiac monitoring The continuing observation of the func-

tions of the heart, notably the electrocardiogram and vascular pressures.

electronic fetal monitoring A method whereby patterns of fetal heart rate and uterine contractions are recorded utilizing an electronic instrument. Prolonged depression of heart rate following a contraction is predictive of an increased likelihood of fetal death.

wound monitoring A periodic surveillance of a burn or other open wound using bacterial cultures. Increasing colony counts predict impending infection. High colony counts (generally considered greater than 100 000 organisms per gram of tissue) make successful wound closure less likely. See also QUANTITATIVE CULTURE.

monkey [prob. of Germanic origin, akin to Old Spanish *mona* monkey] Any member of the families Cebidae and Cercopithecidae.

rhesus monkey A large macaque, *Macaca mulatta*, distributed over a large area including northern India, southern China, and all of southeast Asia. Because it is plentiful and easily raised in captivity, it is widely used in medical and biological research.

monkey-paw MONKEY'S HAND.

monkeypox A disease of Old and New World monkeys and anthropoid apes, caused by a poxvirus and characterized by cutaneous and mucosal lesions that progress from macules to pustules that form dry scabs in the healing stages.

Monks [George Howard *Monks*, U.S. surgeon, 1853–1933] Monks-Esser island flap. See under FLAP.

Monneret [Jules Auguste Edward *Monneret*, French physician, 1810–1868] See under PULSE.

mono- [Gk *monos* single, only, standing alone] 1 A combining form meaning one, single. 2 A combining form denoting the presence of a single atom of a specified element in a molecule or a single grouping within a molecule. Also *mon-*.

monoamine Any amine containing only one amino group.

monoamine oxidase The flavin-containing amine oxidase (EC 1.4.3.4). It oxidizes primary amines with dioxygen, and forms an aldehyde, hydrogen peroxide and ammonia. It also acts on secondary and tertiary amines with small substituents. It is important in the catabolism of epinephrine and tyramine. The traditional name. Also called *tyraminase* (obsolete), *tyramine oxidase*.

monoamino acid An amino acid with only one amino group, usually an amino acid without a basic group in its side chain.

monoaminodicarboxylic acid Any amino acid that has one amino group and two carboxyl groups. Of the amino acids that can be incorporated into proteins, aspartic and glutamic acids are such, and hence have overall acidity, or negative charge at neutral pH.

monoaminomonocarboxylic acid Any amino acid that has one amino group and one carboxyl group. Most of the commoner amino acids are of this type, but not the basic and the acidic amino acids.

monoaminuria [MONO- + AMINURIA] Urinary excretion of monoamino acids. Also called *monaminuria*.

monoamniotic [MONO- + AMNIOTIC] Possessing a single amnion, as in a certain type of twinning. See also MONOZYGOTIC TWINS.

monoarticular [MONO- + ARTICULAR] Pertaining to a single joint. Also *monarthric, monarticular, uniarticular, uniarticulate*.

monoauricular Of or relating to only one auricle.

monobacillary Pertaining to or caused by a single species of bacillus: said especially of an infection.

monobacterial Pertaining to or caused by a single species of bacteria: said especially of an infection.

monoballism [MONO- + Gk *ballism(os)* (from *ballizein* to dance, jump about) a dancing, jumping about] Hemiballismus confined to either the upper or the lower limb.

monobasic   Having only one acidic group in its molecule: said of an acid.

monobenzone $C_{13}H_{12}O_2$. 4-(Phenylmethoxy)phenol, the monobenzyl ether of hydroquinone. It has been used in ointment form to produce irreversible depigmentation of skin areas.

monoblast   The precursor of mature monocytes. It is not normally present in blood or bone marrow.

monoblastoma   MONOCYTIC LEUKEMIA.

monoblepsia [MONO- + Gk *bleps(is)* sight + -IA]   The ability to see better with one eye than with both together.

monobrachia [mono- + *brach(i)-* + -IA]   A condition marked by having one arm or forelimb. Also called *unilateral brachial agenesis, unilateral brachial amelia.*

monobrachius   A fetus or postnatal individual with monobrachia.

monocarboxylic   Having only one carboxyl group in its molecule: used of a compound.

monocardian [MONO- + *cardi(a)* + -*an* adjectival suffix]   Having a heart with one atrium and one ventricle, as in hemicardia.

monocellular   UNICELLULAR.

monocentric   **1** Having one center. **2** Of or relating to a chromosome that has one centromere.

monocephalus   CEPHALOPAGUS.

Monocercomonas   A genus of parasitic flagellates characterized by a piriform body that is rounded anteriorly, presence of a pelta and a parabasal body, with an anterior nucleus and cytostome. There are four flagella, usually three anterior and one trailing. Species have been described from mammals, birds, reptiles, amphibians, fish, and insects and other arthropods.

Monocercomonas cuniculi   A flagellate commonly found in the cecum of rabbits. Also called *Trichomastix cuniculi.*

monochord   An instrument with a single string stretched over a sounding board, used at one time for the study of musical intervals but subsequently adapted for testing hearing.

Schultze monochord   A monochord designed for testing high tone hearing, particularly the upper limit thereof. It has been rendered obsolete by electrical audiometers.

monochorea [MONO- + CHOREA]   Choreic movements restricted to a single limb.

monochorial   MONOCHORIONIC.

monochorionic [MONO- + CHORIONIC]   Possessing a single chorion, as in a certain type of twinning. Also *monochorial.*

monochroic   MONOCHROMATIC.

monochromasy [MONO- + Gk *chrōma* color + *s* + -Y]   COMPLETE COLOR BLINDNESS.

monochromat [MONO- + Gk *chrōma* (gen. *chrōmatos*) color]   A subject affected with total color blindness.

monochromatic   **1** Having or producing a single color. **2** Pertaining to total color blindness. For defs. 1 and 2 also *monochroic, monochromic.*

monochromatism [MONO- + CHROMAT- + -ISM]   COMPLETE COLOR BLINDNESS.

monochromatophil   **1** A cell or a tissue element that readily combines with a single stain. **2** The property of combining with only one stain.

monochromatophilic   Capable of combining with or being stained by only a single dye: said of cells present in tissue sections. Also *monochromophilic.*

monochromator   A spectograph that is adapted to allow isolation of a specific band of wavelengths for analysis or manipulation.

monochromic   MONOCHROMATIC.

monochromophilic   MONOCHROMATOPHILIC.

monoclinic   Describing crystals having all three axes of the unit cell of unequal length, and in which two of them are not at right angles, although the third is at right angles to the plane containing these two.

monoclonal   Pertaining to or originating in a single clone of cells. All of the cells in such a clone would have identical products, such as specific antibodies or proteins. Compare POLYCLONAL.

monocont [MONO- + L *cont(us)* a pole, shaft]   A seldom used term for UNIFLAGELLATE.

monocontaminated   Infected by or contaminated with a single species of organism: said of an animal that is otherwise germfree. Also *monoxenic.*

monocontamination   The introduction of a single infecting species into a previously germ-free animal.

monocontous [MONOCONT + -OUS]   A seldom used term for UNIFLAGELLATE.

monocorditis   Laryngitis confined to one vocal cord only. A rarely used term.

monocotyledon   A member of the class Monocotyledoneae, whose embryos have one cotyledon.

monocranius   CEPHALOPAGUS.

monocrotaline $C_{16}H_{23}NO_6$. A pyrrolizidine alkaloid found in *Crotalaria* species. Ingestion by fowl, cattle, horses, and swine has resulted in poisoning and death.

monocrotic   Characterized by a single wave uninterrupted by notches: said of a pulse. Compare DICROTIC, TRICROTIC.

monocrotism [MONO- + Gk *krot(os)* the sound of striking, a beat + -ISM]   The characteristic of a pulse in which there is a single wave uninterrupted by notches.

monocular [MON- + OCULAR]   Pertaining to one eye only.

monoculture   The repeated culture or production of only one or, at best, a very few domesticated species of organisms, especially plants.

monoculus [MON- + L *oculus* the eye]   **1** CYCLOPS. **2** A bandage over one eye.

monocyclic [MONO- + CYCLIC]   Containing one ring of atoms in its molecule: used of a substance.

monocyesis [MONO- + Gk *kyēsis* pregnancy]   Pregnancy with a single fetus. An older term.

monocystic   Characterized by or containing a single cyst or solitary cysts.

Monocystis [MONO- + CYSTIS]   A genus of sporozoan protozoa in the subclass Gregarinia, order Eugregarinida, species of which are found in the seminal vesicles of the earthworm.

monocytangina   INFECTIOUS MONONUCLEOSIS.

monocyte [MONO- + -CYTE]   A leukocyte which differs from the granular leukocytes by its larger size (12–20μm in diameter), and by a round or indented (kidney-shaped) nucleus. Its cytoplasm has no granules and on staining has a basophil blue-gray frosted glass appearance. It is related to the tissue macrophages. Monocytes make up 3–6% of the circulating leukocyte population and are also found in marrow, lymphatic tissues, lung, and liver. Also called *hyaline leukocyte* (obsolete), *endothelial phagocyte, transitional leukocyte* (obsolete).

monocytic   Relating to monocytes.

monocytoid   Resembling a monocyte.

monocytoma   Monocytic leukemia.

monocytopenia   A less than normal number of monocytes in the circulating blood. Also called *monopenia, monocytic leukopenia.*

monocytopoiesis   The formation of monocytes in the bone marrow.

monocytosis [MONO- + CYTOSIS] A greater than normal number of monocytes in blood.

avian monocytosis A transient disease of chickens, most severe in pullets, with high morbidity and low mortality. Sudden onset of inappetence, depression, and diarrhea is characteristic. Monocytosis is common. Other signs include lowered egg production and cyanosis of comb and wattles. The cause is unknown. Also called *bluecomb disease of chickens, pullet disease*.

monodactylia MONODACTYLY.

monodactylism MONODACTYLY.

monodactyly [MONO- + DACTYL- + -Y] The occurrence of a single digit on a hand or a foot. Also called *monodactylism, monodactylia*.

monodal Connected to one terminal of a coil of wire so that high-frequency resonating current passes through the capacitance formed by the patient and ground.

monodermoma [MONO- + DERM- + -OMA] A tumor arising from one germinal layer.

monodidymus [MONO- + Gk *didymos* double; as substantive, a twin brother] An individual that is one of twins.

monodiplopia [MONO- + DIPLOPIA] Double vision with only one eye.

monodisperse Occurring as suspended particles of uniform size.

Monodon A monotypic genus of the cetacean family Monodontidae; the narwhals. They have only two teeth, both in the upper jaw, and one of them develops in the male into a long, spiraling tusk. Members of the genus occur around the pack ice in the Arctic realm.

monodont [MON- + -ODONT] Having a single tooth, as the narwhal.

Monodral bromide A proprietary name for penthienate bromide.

monodromic UNIDIRECTIONAL.

monoesterase Any enzyme that catalyzes the hydrolysis of a monoester of an acid, usually phosphoric acid, that can form diesters.

monoestrous A British spelling for MONESTRUS.

monofactorial Relating to a single factor.

monofilament A single filament, as of a synthetic material, used as a suture.

monofilm MONOLAYER.

monogamous [MONO- + GAM- + -OUS] Having one spouse only, or, in the case of animals, one mate.

monogamy [MONO- + GAM- + -Y] The state of having one spouse only, or, in the case of animals, one mate.

monoganglial Describing, pertaining to, or affecting a single ganglion.

monogenesis 1 The production of offspring that are all of one type, or all of one sex, in each generation. 2 The production of uniparental progeny, as in nonsexual generation or in parthenogenesis. 3 MONOXENY.

monogenetic Pertaining to or characterized by monogenesis. Also *monogenous*.

monogenic Pertaining to a phenotype or biologic process that is determined primarily by a single gene.

monogenism [MONO- + Gk *gen(os)* race, descendant + -ISM] An anthropological theory which holds that all the major races of modern man were derived from a single primitive stock. Compare POLYGENISM.

monogenous [MONO- + -GENOUS] 1 Derived from a single source. 2 MONOGENETIC.

monogerminal [MONO- + GERMINAL] MONOZYGOTIC.

monoglyceride A glycerol molecule acylated on one of its

hydroxyl groups; a monoacylglycerol. An outmoded term.

monogonia Plural of MONOGONIUM.

monogonium [New L (from MONO- + -GON² + -*ium*, noun suffix)] (*plural* monogonia) Any of the asexual forms of malarial parasites in the blood. An obsolete term.

monograph [MONO- + -GRAPH] A book, paper, or treatise devoted to a single subject.

monogyny [MONO- + GYN- + -Y] The practice of a male having only one female mate.

monohybrid An offspring of two parents differing only in that each is homozygous for a different allele at a specific locus. The offspring is thus heterozygous at that locus.

monohydrate A substance with one molecule of water added per molecule of substance. This water may be bound, or may have crystallized together with the substance.

monohydrated Having one molecule of water associated per molecule of substance.

monohydric Containing one hydroxyl group in its molecule: said of an alcohol.

monoideism [MONO- + *ide(a)* + -ISM] 1 The focusing of one's attention on a single idea or sensory stimulus, as a way to increase suggestibility in hypnotic induction. 2 A condition marked by harping on one idea or senseless repetition of the same train of thought. For defs. 1 and 2 also called *monomania (An imprecise and outmoded term)*.

monoinfection [MONO- + INFECTION] An infection caused by a single kind of organism.

monoiodomethanesulfonic acid CH_2ISO_3H. An acid which, in the form of its sodium salt, was formerly used as a contrast medium for intravenous urography.

monoiodotyrosine Tyrosine that is iodinated, usually on C-3, in distinction from tyrosine doubly iodinated, on C-3 and C-5, which is also a precursor in the biosynthesis of thyroxin.

monolayer 1 A layer of molecules a single molecule thick. Such layers may form through the attraction of nonpolar parts of the molecules for each other, and the attraction of a polar end of each for the solvent. They are commonly encountered in studies of phospholipids. Also called *monofilm, monomolecular layer*. 2 A cell culture preparation in which a single layer of uniformly contiguous cells completely covers the surface.

monolepsis The appearance in offspring of the characteristics of one, but not the other, parent. A seldom used term.

monolobular Pertaining to or possessing one lobule.

monolocular Composed of a single cavity.

monomania [MONO- + -MANIA] 1 Partial insanity in which only one area of functioning is disrupted or a single concept is abnormal. Also called *monopsychosis* (obsolete), *oligomania* (obsolete). 2 An impulsive act without clear or comprehensible motive. 3 An imprecise and outmoded term for MONOIDEISM.

intellectual monomania An obsolete term for PARANOIA.

monomanie incendiaire [French *monomanie* (from *mono-* MONO- + Gk *mania* madness, enthusiasm) monomania + French *incendiaire* incendiary] PYROMANIA.

monomastigote [MONO- + MASTIGOTE] A mastigote with a single flagellum.

monomaxillary Involving one jaw. An outmoded term.

monomelic Pertaining to, affecting, or possessing one limb.

monomer [MONO- + Gk *mer(os)* part] A single unit or molecule which can polymerize with similar units to form a chain or polymer.

fibrin monomer The monomer that results at the instant that fibrinogen loses its fibrinopeptides A and B. Such monomers promptly polymerize.

monomeric Containing a single unit in its molecule, in contrast with substances in which two or more such units are joined.

monomethylmorphine   CODEINE.

monomicrobic   Pertaining to or characterized by the presence of a single species of a microorganism.

monomoria [MONO- + Gk *mōr(os)* dull, sluggish, slow + -IA] MELANCHOLIA.

monomorphic [MONO- + MORPH- + -IC] Having one form only; unchangable in form throughout development.

monomorphism [MONO- + MORPH- + -ISM] Possession of a single body form throughout the life cycle.

monomorphous   Composed of cells or lesions of the same type.

monomphalus [New L (from MON- + Gk *omphalos* navel)] OMPHALOPAGUS.

monomyoplegia [MONO- + MYO- + -PLEGIA] Paralysis of a single muscle.

Mononchus [New L (from MON- + New L *-onchus*, combining form denoting a barb or hook, irreg. from Gk *onkos* the barb of an arrow, a hook)] A genus of free-living nematodes found in moist soil and fresh water. A reported occurrence in human urine was probably an example of spurious parasitism.

mononephrous [MONO- + NEPHR- + -OUS] Related to or affecting only one kidney.

mononeural   **1** Pertaining to or receiving connections from a single neuron or nerve.   **2** Possessing a single neuron. For defs. 1 and 2 also *mononeuric*.

mononeuralgia [MONO- + NEURALGIA] Neuralgia in the region supplied by a single nerve.

mononeuric   MONONEURAL.

mononeuritis [MONO- + NEURITIS] Neuritis affecting a single peripheral nerve.

  mononeuritis multiplex   A syndrome of concurrent lesions of several individual peripheral nerves, as distinct from the syndrome of polyneuritis or polyneuropathy in which various components of the peripheral nervous system are diffusely involved in a disease process. Multiple involvement of peripheral nerves is usually of vascular origin, as in polyarteritis nodosa or the other collagen or connective tissue disorders, or due to inflammatory processes such as leprosy. • *Multiple neuritis* can also be used, but is better avoided as it has been used by some authors as a synonym of polyneuropathy.

mononeuropathy [MONO- + NEUROPATHY] Disease or dysfunction of a single nerve, as in the neuropathy of diabetes mellitus or carcinoma.

  cranial mononeuropathy   Disease or dysfunction of a single cranial nerve.

monont [MON- + Gk *-ont*, combining form from *ōn*, gen. *ontos*, pres. part. of *einai* to be] An obsolete term for SCHIZONT.

mononuclear [MONO- + NUCLEAR] Having a single nucleus: used especially of a cell. Also called *mononucleate, uninuclear, uninucleate*.

mononucleate   MONONUCLEAR.

mononucleosis [MONO- + NUCLEOSIS] A greater than normal number of mononuclear leukocytes in the blood. Lymphocytes, monocytes, metamyelocytes, and more immature cells of the granulocytic, lymphocytic, and monocytic series are all mononuclear cells.

  infectious mononucleosis   An acute infectious disease caused by the Epstein-Barr virus and most often affecting adolescents and young adults. It is usually characterized by fever, sore throat, malaise, fatigue, weakness, lymphadenopathy, hepatosplenomegaly, a mononuclear leukocytosis, atypical lymphocytes, and high titers of sheep erythrocyte agglutinins. The acute and convalescent phases of the disease may persist for months, and, rarely, the disease follows a chronic, relapsing course. An illness resembling infectious mononucleosis may be caused by other microbial agents, including *Toxoplasma gondii* and cytomegalovirus. Also called *glandular fever, acute benign lymphoblastosis, acute epidemic lymphadenosis, acute infectious adenitis, kissing disease* (popular), *monocytic angina (ambiguous and seldom used), monocytangina, kagami fever, Tokushima fever, Pfeiffer's disease, Pfeiffer's glandular fever, influenza lymphatica, Filatov's disease.*

  post-transfusion mononucleosis   An acute febrile illness that may follow transfusion, accompanied by lymphadenopathy, often by splenomegaly, and by the presence of numerous atypical lymphocytes in the blood. The condition is due to transmission of a virus, such as Epstein-Barr virus or cytomegalovirus. Also called *postperfusion syndrome, post-transfusion syndrome.*

mononucleotide   A nucleotide composed of a phosphorylated nucleoside, in distinction from one in which two or more such units are combined, as in nucleic acids.

mono-osteitic   Denoting inflammation localized to a single bone.

monoparesis [MONO- + PARESIS] Paresis of a single limb or part of a limb.

monoparesthesia [MONO- + PARESTHESIA] Paresthesia involving a single limb.

monopathophobia   Pathologic fear of contracting some specific disease. An obsolete term.

monopathy   A pathologic process localized to a single organ or part of the body. An obsolete term.

monopenia   MONOCYTOPENIA.

monophagia [MONO- + -PHAGIA] Pathologic desire for only one kind of food. An outmoded term. Also called *monophagism*.

monophagism   MONOPHAGIA.

monophagous [MONO- + -PHAGOUS] Consuming but one food species: used especially of herbivores. Monophagous insects respond to specific chemical stimuli in the selection of food. Also *monotrophic*.

monophasia [MONO- + *(a)phasia*] A manifestation of motor or expressive aphasia in which the patient is able to pronounce only one word or phrase, which he repeats constantly. A seldom used term.

monophasic   **1** Presenting only one phase or variation.   **2** In electroencephalography, denoting a deflection of the trace to one side of the baseline only.   **3** Exhibiting or characterized by monophasia.

monophenol monooxygenase   A group of copper-containing enzymes (EC 1.14.18.1) that oxidize phenols such as tyrosine using dioxygen as oxidant, forming an *o*-quinone. They can use benzene-1,2-diols as substrates. Also called *tyrosinase, monophenol oxidase* (outmoded).

monophenol oxidase   An outmoded term for MONOPHENOL MONOOXYGENASE.

monophobia [MONO- + -PHOBIA] Pathologic fear of being alone.

monophosphate   A compound bearing one phosphate group, in distinction from a diphosphate, which bears one residue of diphosphoric acid, or from a bisphosphate, which bears two separate phosphate groups.

monophthalmia [MON- + OPHTHALMIA] CYCLOPIA.

monophthalmus [New L (from MON- + Gk *ophthalmos* the eye)] CYCLOPS.

monophyletic   Originating from a single ancestral type.

monophyletism [MONO- + Gk *phylet(ēs)* one of the same tribe + -ISM]   **1** The hypothesis that all blood cells originate from a common ancestral cell type.   **2** The hypothesis that all living organisms are descended from a common ancestor.

monophyletist An individual who holds to the theory of the monophyletic origin of living organisms or of cells, such as blood cells.

monophyodont [Gk *monophy(ēs)* (from *monos* only, sole + *phyē* one's natural powers or parts) of simple nature, of one piece + -ODONT] Having a single set of teeth of which none are replaced.

monopia [MON- + -OPIA CYCLOPIA.

Monoplacophora [New L (from MONO- + Gk *plax*, gen. *plakos*, anything flat and broad + New L -*phora*, combining form denoting carrying, from Gk *pherein* to carry)] A primitive class of the invertebrate phylum Mollusca, comprising the single extant genus *Neopilina*. Members are characterized by a single symmetrical shell that bears three to eight muscle scars on its underside. They are believed to be ancestral to gastropods, bivalves, and cephalopods.

monoplasmatic Formed of a single substance.

monoplast [MONO- + -PLAST] A single cell unit. Also called *monoplastid*.

monoplastic UNICELLULAR.

monoplastid MONOPLAST.

monoplegia [MONO- + -PLEGIA] Paralysis restricted to a single limb or part of a limb. Adjective: monoplegic.

   monoplegia facialis Unilateral facial palsy.

   monoplegia masticatoria Paralysis of the mucles of mastication on one side only.

monoploid HAPLOID.

monopodal Having one pseudopodium, as in certain ameba.

monopodia **1** The presence of a single foot, as in those forms of sirenomelus in which a symmetrical footlike structure is present at the distal end of the fused lower extremity. Also called *sirenoid monopodia*. **2** A limb reduction deformity in which one foot is present and one missing, as in unilateral transverse hemimelia or unilateral apodia.

   sirenoid monopodia MONOPODIA.

monopodial Characterized by monopodia.

monopolar Relating to the use of a single electrical pole, positive or negative.

monops [MON- + Gk *ōps* eye] CYCLOPS.

monopsychosis An obsolete term for MONOMANIA.

Monopsyllus A genus of fleas common on rodents.

   Monopsyllus anisus A species of rat flea in Japan and northern China.

monoptychial Formed from a single layer of epithelium that is attached to its basement membrane.

monopus [New L (from MONO- + New L -*pus*, combining form denoting foot, from Gk *pous* foot)] SYMPUS MONOPUS.

monopyramidal Having a single pyramid and papilla: said of kidneys found in a few species of mammals.

monoradicular [MONO- + RADICULAR] Possessing one root.

monorchia MONORCHIDISM.

monorchid MONORCHIS.

monorchidic **1** MONORCHIS. **2** Exhibiting monorchidism.

monorchidism [MON- + *orchid(o)*- + -ISM] The condition of having one testis or the appearance of one testis when the other is undescended, as in cryptorchidism. Also called *monorchia*, *monorchism*.

monorchis [MON- + Gk *orchis* testicle] A fetus or postnatal individual having or appearing to have only one testis. Also called *monorchid, monorchidic*.

monorchism MONORCHIDISM.

Monorchotrema [New L (from MONO- + *orch(i)*- + *o* + Gk *trēma* a hole, aperture)] *HAPLORCHIS*.

monorecidive CHANCRE REDUX.

monorhinal MONORHINE.

monorhine [MONO- + Gk *rhis* (gen. *rhinos*) nose] Having a single nasal cavity only, as in lampreys. Also *monorhinal, monorhinic*.

monorhinic MONORHINE.

monosaccharide A simple sugar, in contrast with carbohydrates formed by glycosylation of one sugar by another.

monoscelous Possessing only one leg.

monosexual [MONO- + SEXUAL] Displaying the characteristics of a single sex.

monosodium glutamate The sodium salt of glutamic acid, with only one sodium ion per molecule of glutamic acid. Its solutions are neutral. It is used for enhancing the flavor of food, and in large doses it may cause discomfort to some people (Chinese restaurant syndrome).

monosomatous DICEPHALOUS.

monosome [MONO- + Gk *sōma* body] **1** In a normally diploid cell or organism, any chromosome of the usual set lacking a homologue. This routinely occurs in the sex chromosomes of the heterogametic sex. For example, in the human male, the X and the Y chromosomes are monosomes. It also occurs whenever an aberrant meiosis or mitosis results in loss of an autosome. **2** A single ribosome bound to mRNA. Compare POLYSOME.

monosomia [MONO- + Gk *sōm(a)* body + -IA] DICEPHALY.

monosomian DICEPHALOUS.

monosomic Pertaining to or characterized by monosomy.

monosomous DICEPHALOUS.

monosomy **1** Aneuploidy in which a normally diploid cell or organism lacks one chromosome of a homologous pair. **2** The chromosome complement of the heterogametic sex in which neither sex chromosome has a complete homologue. Each sex chromosome can be considered a monosome. A seldom used term.

monospasm [MONO- + SPASM] Muscular spasm limited to a single muscle, muscle group, or limb.

monospermy [MONO- + SPERM + -Y] Fertilization effected by a single spermatozoon.

Monosporium A genus of ascomycetous fungi that causes mycetoma. Its perfect (sexual) stage is *Allescheria*.

   Monosporium apiospermum An obsolete term for *ACEDOSPORIUM APIOSPERMUM*.

Monostoma [MONO- + Gk *stoma* mouth] A former genus of trematodes having a single sucker. The species formerly included are of polyphyletic origin and are now placed in several families.

   Monostoma lentis A monostome fluke of uncertain identification reported to have been taken from the crystalline lens of the eye of a man.

monostome [MONO- + -*stome*, combining form denoting mouth, from Gk *stoma* mouth] **1** Having a single sucker: said of certain digenetic trematodes. **2** A digenetic trematode with a single sucker.

Monostomum *PARAMPHISTOMUM*.

monostotic Pertaining to or involving a single bone. Compare POLYOSTOTIC.

monostratal MONOSTRATIFIED.

monostratified Arranged in a single layer or sheet. Also *monostratal*.

monosymptom A symptom occurring in isolation.

monosymptomatic [MONO- + SYMPTOMATIC] Characterized by a single symptom.

monosynaptic Denoting or pertaining to a neuronal pathway, such as a reflex arc, containing only a single synapse.

monosyphilid Syphilis that is manifested by a solitary skin lesion. Also called *monosyphilide*.

monosyphilide   MONOSYPHILID.

monoterpene   A substance whose molecules are composed of two isoprene residues, and have the general formula $C_{10}H_{16}$. It is found in plant oils.

Monotheamin   A proprietary name for theophylline ethanolamine.

monothermia   A state of constant body temperature throughout the day.

monotic   Pertaining to one ear only. Also *uniaural*.

monotocia   [Gk *monotokia* (from *mono(s)* without others + *tok(os)* a bringing forth + *-ia* -IA) a bringing forth only one at a time]   The state or characteristic of being monotocous. A seldom used term.

monotocous   Producing only singleton offspring.

Monotremata   [MONO- + Gk *trēma*, pl. *trēmata*, a hole, aperture]   An order of the class Mammalia that includes the platypus and the echidna. The female lays eggs that incubate and hatch outside the body of the mother. Their body temperature is low and sometimes fluctuating, and they possess a cloaca. These features are unique among mammals. The monotremes have more features in common with reptiles than with other mammals. They occur in Australia, Tasmania, and New Guinea.

monotreme   [MONO- + Gk *trēm(a)* a hole, aperture]   Any member of the mammalian order Monotremata.

monotrichate   MONOTRICHOUS.

monotrichous   [MONO- + TRICH- + -OUS]   Possessing a single flagellum. Also *monotrichate*.

monotrophic   MONOPHAGOUS.

monotropic   [MONO- + -TROPIC[1]]   **1** Having only one directional tendency or attraction.   **2** Affecting only one kind of tissue or microorganism. An obsolete term.

monotypic   Represented by only one example, as a genus containing a single species.

monovalent   UNIVALENT.

monovular   [MON- + OVULAR]   Developed from a single ovum, as monozygotic twins.

monovulatory   [MON- + OVULATORY]   Liberating a single ovum at each ovulation in the reproductive cycle. This is usually characteristic of the human female.

monoxenic   MONOCONTAMINATED.

monoxenous   [MONO- + *xen(o)*- + -OUS]   Requiring only one host to complete the life cycle; autecious.

monoxeny   [MONO- + *xen(o)*- + -Y]   A life cycle pattern, characteristic of many parasites, in which only one host is required for the organism to complete the cycle. Also called *monogenesis*.

monoxide   Signifying the addition of one atom of oxygen per atom, or specified number of atoms, of another element, as in *carbon monoxide*, CO.

monozygosity   [MONO- + ZYGO- + *s* + -ITY]   Development from a single fertilized ovum, as in certain twins.

monozygotic   [MONO- + ZYGOTIC]   Developed from a single fertilized ovum, as in *monozygotic twins*. Also *monogerminal, enzygotic*.

Monro   [Alexander Secundus *Monro*, Scottish anatomist, 1733–1817]   **1** Foramen of Monro. See under FORAMEN INTERVENTRICULARE.   **2** Monro-Kellie doctrine. See under DOCTRINE.   **3** Fissure of Monro, sulcus of Monro. See under SULCUS HYPOTHALAMICUS.   **4** Monro's bursa. See under BURSA INTRATENDINEA OLECRANI.   **5** Monro's line. See under MONRO-RICHTER LINE.

mons   [L, gen. *montis*, mountain]   In anatomy, a prominence or an elevation.

mons pubis   [NA]   The rounded prominence in front of the symphysis pubis formed by a varying mass of subcutaneous fatty tissue and covered by coarse hair at puberty. It is continuous inferiorly with the commissura labiorum anterior. Also called *mons veneris*.

mons ureteris   A slight mucosal elevation around the ostium ureteris in the urinary bladder. An outmoded term.

mons veneris   MONS PUBIS.

Monson   [George S. *Monson*, U.S. dentist, 1869–1933]   **1** See under CURVE.   **2** Anti-Monson curve. See under REVERSE CURVE.

monster   [L *monstrum* (from *monere* to warn, foretell) a thing shown, omen, monster]   A congenitally deformed individual, particularly one whose malformations are severe.   • This is a popular but archaic term that has much of the connotation of "sideshow freak."

endocymic monster   ENDOCYMA.

Gila monster   The venomous lizard *Heloderma suspectum*, found mainly in the arid regions of Arizona and New Mexico.

monstriparity   [*monstr(um)* + *i* + English *parity*]   The condition of having given birth to a fetal monster.   • A nonspecific, rarely used term that is best avoided.

montage   [French (from *mont(er)* to mount, from L *mons*, gen. *montis*, a mountain, + French *-age* -AGE), a combining of various pictures, an assembling, mounting]   In electroencephalography, an arrangement of electrodes applied to the scalp in such a way that the electrical activity of the entire brain or of a particular area of the brain can be recorded simultaneously. When using the bipolar technique, there is usually one electrode common to two successive leads, the three electrodes being in series, that is, connected in pairs to two amplifying channels, the common electrode being linked in opposite polarity to the two channels.

montanylic alcohol CH_3—$[CH_2]_{27}$—CH_2OH. Nonacosan-1-ol. A fatty alcohol present as esters in waxes.

Monteggia   [Giovanni Battista *Monteggia*, Italian surgeon, 1762–1815]   Monteggia's fracture, Monteggia's dislocation. See under FRACTURE-DISLOCATION.

Montgomery   [William Fetherston *Montgomery*, Irish gynecologist, 1797–1859]   **1** Montgomery's tubercles. See under TUBERCLE.   **2** Montgomery's follicles. See under FOLLICLE.   **3** Montgomery's cups. See under CUP.   **4** Montgomery's cups. See under NABOTHIAN CYSTS.

monticulus   A small eminence or elevation.

monticulus cerebelli   The eminence formed by the central portion of the cerebellar vermis.

mood   [Middle English *mod, mood*, from Old English *mōd* spirit, akin to L *mos*, gen. *moris*, manner, custom, whence English *morae*]   An enduring but not permanent emotional predisposition to react in a certain way, as with sadness or anger.

mood-congruent   In harmony with the prevailing affect, as are delusions or hallucinations whose content is consistent with the manic's ideas of inflated worth, or with the depressive subject's feelings of worthlessness, guilt, and need for retribution.

Moon   [Henry *Moon*, English dental surgeon, 1845–1892]   Moon's tooth. See under SYPHILITIC TOOTH.

Moon   [Robert Charles *Moon*, U.S. ophthalmologist, 1844–1914]   Laurence-Moon syndrome. See under SYNDROME.

Moore   [Edward Mott *Moore*, U.S. surgeon, 1814–1902]   See under FRACTURE.

Moore   [Matthew Thibaud *Moore*, U.S. neuropsychiatrist, born 1901]   Moore syndrome. See under ABDOMINAL EPILEPSY.

Moore   [Robert Foster *Moore*, English ophthalmologist, 1878–1963]   Moore's lightning streaks. See under STREAK.

Moorehead   [Frederick Brown *Moorehead*, U.S. oral surgeon, born 1875]   See under RETRACTOR.

Mooren [Albert *Mooren*, German oculist, 1828–1899] See under ULCER.

Mooser [Hermann *Mooser*, Swiss pathologist active in Mexico, born 1891] **1** Neill-Mooser reaction. See under SCROTAL REACTION. **2** Neill-Mooser bodies. See under MOOSER BODIES. **3** See under CELL.

MOPP The anticancer chemotherapeutic combination of nitrogen mustard (mechlorethamine), vincristine (Oncovin), procarbazine, and prednisone. It is especially effective in Hodgkin's disease.

Morand [Sauveur François *Morand*, French surgeon, 1697–1773] **1** See under FOOT. **2** Morand's spur. See under CALCAR AVIS. **3** Morand's foramen. See under FORAMEN CAECUM LINGUAE. **4** Vein of calcar avis of Morand. See under VEIN.

Morat [Jean-Pierre *Morat*, French physiologist, 1846–1920] Dastre-Morat law. See under LAW.

Morawitz [Paul Oskar *Morawitz*, German physiologist, 1879–1936] See under THEORY.

Morax [Victor *Morax*, French ophthalmologist, 1866–1935] **1** Morax-Axenfeld bacillus. See under BACILLUS. **2** Morax-Axenfeld conjunctivitis. See under ANGULAR CONJUNCTIVITIS.

Moraxella lacunata A Gram-negative coccobacillus (family Neisseriaceae) that is parasitic on mucous membranes and occasionally causes conjunctivitis.

morbi [L, gen. of *morbus* disease] Of a disease; of the disease.

morbid [L *morbid(us)* (from *morbus* disease, sickness, akin to *mors* death) diseased, causing disease] **1** Affected by disease; in a diseased state; pathologic. **2** Causing or capable of causing disease; pathogenic.

morbidity [L *morbid(us)* a disease, malady, akin to *mors* death, + -ITY] **1** A diseased state or character; ill health. **2** The result of exposing a person or group of persons to the causes of disease. **3** Within a given population, the number of sick persons or cases of disease recorded as of a stated point in time or over a stated period. Thus, morbidity may be expressed as the number of new cases arising (incidence) or the number of cases existing whether old or newly arisen (prevalence).

puerperal morbidity A temperature of 100.4°F (38°C) occurring on any two of the first 10 postpartum days with the exception of the first 24 hours. The temperature must be taken by a standard oral technique at least four times a day.

morbidostatic Capable of halting the progress of disease.

morbific PATHOGENIC.

morbigenous An obsolete term for PATHOGENIC.

morbilli [Med L, pl. of *morbillus* pustule, dim. of L *morbus* disease] MEASLES.

morbilliform [Med L *morbilli*, pl. of *morbillus* (dim. of l *morbus* disease, malady) spot on the skin + -FORM] Resembling the eruption characteristic of measles.

Morbillivirus A genus of the Paramyxoviridae family that includes measles virus.

morbillous [Med L *morbill(i)* spots on the skin + -OUS] Pertaining to measles.

morbus [L, a disease, sickness, grief] A disease.

morbus addisonii ADDISON'S DISEASE.

morbus apoplectiformis An obsolete term for MENIÈRE'S DISEASE.

morbus basedowii GRAVES DISEASE.

morbus caducus An obsolete term for EPILEPSY.

morbus cardiacus HEART DISEASE.

morbus celsi An obsolete term for EPILEPSY.

morbus comitialis An obsolete term for EPILEPSY.

morbus cordis HEART DISEASE.

morbus coxae senilis Degenerative arthritis of the hip joint, especially of the aged.

morbus coxarius An obsolete term for MALUM COXAE SENILIS.

morbus cucullaris PERTUSSIS.

morbus divinus An obsolete term for EPILEPSY.

morbus dormitivus **1** GAMBIAN TRYPANOSOMIASIS. **2** RHODESIAN TRYPANOSOMIASIS.

morbus elephas FILARIAL ELEPHANTIASIS.

morbus errorum VAGRANTS' DISEASE.

morbus gallicus SYPHILIS.

morbus herculeus **1** FILARIAL ELEPHANTIASIS. **2** DUCHENNE TYPE MUSCULAR DYSTROPHY.

morbus maculosus neonatorum HEMORRHAGIC DISEASE OF THE NEWBORN.

morbus maculosus werlhofii IDIOPATHIC THROMBOCYTOPENIC PURPURA.

morbus magnus An obsolete term for MAJOR EPILEPSY.

morbus major An obsolete term for MAJOR EPILEPSY.

morbus miseriae Any disease associated with deprivation and neglect.

morbus moniliformis lichenoides LICHEN RUBER MONILIFORMIS.

morbus morsus muris RAT-BITE FEVER.

morbus nauticus An obsolete term for SEASICKNESS.

morbus navalis An obsolete term for SEASICKNESS.

morbus naviticus An obsolete term for SEASICKNESS.

morbus pediculosus PEDICULOSIS.

morbus sacer An obsolete term for EPILEPSY.

morbus saltatorius CHOREA.

morbus senilis An obsolete term for OSTEOARTHRITIS.

morbus Skerljevo SCHERLIEVO.

morbus strangulatorius DIPHTHERIA.

morbus tuberculosis pedis Mycetoma of the foot; Madura foot. An imprecise and rarely used term.

morbus vagabondus VAGRANTS' DISEASE.

morbus vesicularis An obsolete term for PEMPHIGUS VULGARIS.

morbus virgineus Pallor in adolescent girls or young women, most likely due to iron deficiency anemia. An archaic term, of historical interest only.

morbus vulpis LUPUS VULGARIS.

morbus werlhofii IDIOPATHIC THROMBOCYTOPENIC PURPURA.

morcel [French *morcel(er)* (from L *morsus* a bite, biting) to divide into pieces or parts] To remove in section rather than en bloc, as a tissue mass.

morcellation [French *morcel(er)* (from *morceau* a piece, from L *morsus* a bite) to divide into parts + *l* + English -ATION] The division of a mass into many small sections in order to facilitate its surgical removal. Also called *morcellement*.

morcellement MORCELLATION.

mordacious [L *mordax*, gen. *mordacis* (from *mordere* to bite, sting) biting, stinging + English -ious] Caustic; biting.

mordant [French, pres. part. of *mordre* & (from L *mordere* to bite) to bite] **1** An agent that combines with dye to form an insoluble compound. It is used to fix and intensify stains in tissue or cell preparations, or dyestuffs in textiles. Alum, anilines, and phenol are the most common histologic mordants. **2** To subject to the action of a mordant.

mor. dict. *more dicto* (L, in the manner directed).

Morel [Augustin Benoit *Morel*, French psychiatrist, 1809–1873] **1** See under EAR. **2** Morel-Kraepelin disease. See under SCHIZOPHRENIA.

Morel [Ferdinand *Morel*, Swiss psychiatrist and neurologist, 1888–1957] **1** Morel-Wildi syndrome. See under SYNDROME.

2 Stewart-Morel syndrome, Morgagni-Stewart-Morel syndrome, Morel syndrome. See under HYPEROSTOSIS FRONTALIS INTERNA.

morel [French *morille* (from the Germanic) a woodland mushroom] Any of several edible ascomycetous fungi of the genus *Morchella.*

    false morel A fungal fruiting body of the genus *Gyromitra,* which, when consumed, may cause gastrointestinal upset due to monomethylhydrazine poisoning.

Morelli [F. *Morelli,* Italian physician, died 1918] See under TEST.

Morerastongylus A genus of metastrongyle nematodes that are principally parasitic in rodents in tropical America.

    Morerastrongylus costaricensis A species of nematode worm that ordinarily infects the mesenteric arteries of wild rodents such as the cotton rat *Sigmodon hispidus* of tropical America. Human infection, reported usually in children in Mexico, Costa Rica, and Brazil, probably results from accidental ingestion of infected snails or slugs. Thickening of the intestinal wall of the cecum and appendix, with necrosis and heavy eosinophilic infiltration, is caused by blockage of intestinal arterioles by juvenile worms and eggs. Symptoms include intestinal pain and high fever. Also called *Angiostrongylus costaricensis.*

mores [L, pl. of *mos,* gen. *moris,* manner, custom] **1** A behavior norm of persons belonging to a given culture. **2** The accepted customs of a social group which are regarded as essential for group survival.

Moreschi [Carlo *Moreschi,* Italian pathologist, 1876–1921] Moreschi phenomenon. See under COMPLEMENT FIXATION.

Morestin [Hippolyte *Morestin,* French surgeon, 1869–1919] **1** Souligoux-Morestin method. See under ETHER LAVAGE. **2** Morestin's method. See under OPERATION.

Morgagni [Giovanni Battista *Morgagni,* Italian physician, 1682–1771] **1** See under LIQUOR, CATARACT, PROLAPSE, CRYPT, FORAMEN, SINUS. **2** Morgagni-Adams-Stokes syndrome. See under ADAMS-STOKES SYNDROME. **3** Morgagni's globules. See under GLOBULE. **4** Morgagni spheres. See under SPHERE. **5** Morgagni's glands. See under GLANDULAE URETHRALES URETHRAE MASCULINAE. **6** Fossa navicularis urethrae morgagnii, fovea of Morgagni, crypt of Morgagni, fossa of Morgagni. See under FOSSA NAVICULARIS URETHRAE. **7** Glandular foramen of Morgagni. See under FORAMEN CAECUM LINGUAE. **8** Appendix of laryngeal ventricle of Morgagni. See under SACCULUS LARYNGIS. **9** Morgagni's tubercle. See under MONTGOMERY'S TUBERCLE. **10** Morgagni's tubercle. See under BULBUS OLFACTORIUS. **11** Vesicular appendages of epoöphoron of Morgagni, morgagnian cysts. See under APPENDICES VESICULOSAE EPOÖPHORI. **12** Morgagni's concha. See under CONCHA NASALIS SUPERIOR. **13** Columns of Morgagni, columnae rectales morgagnii. See under COLUMNAE ANALES. **14** Pedunculated hydatid of Morgagni. See under HYDATID. **15** Pedunculated hydatid of Morgagni. See under APPENDIX OF THE EPIDIDYMIS. **16** Morgagni's disease, Morgagni's hyperostosis, Morgagni-Stewart-Morel syndrome, Morgagni syndrome. See under HYPEROSTOSIS FRONTALIS INTERNA. **17** Cartilage of Morgagni. See under CARTILAGO CUNEIFORMIS. **18** Morgagni's caruncle. See under LOBUS MEDIUS PROSTATAE. **19** Urethral lacunae of Morgagni. See under LACUNAE OF MORGAGNI. **20** Lacunae morgagnii urethrae muliebris. See under LACUNA. **21** Hydatid of Morgagni. See under APPENDIX MORGAGNII. **22** Hydatid of Morgagni. See under APPENDIX TESTIS. **23** Frenulum of Morgagni, frenum of Morgagni. See under FRENULUM VALVAE ILEALIS. **24** Morgagni's foramen. See under FORAMEN SINGULARE. **25** Morgagni's foramen. See under FORAMEN CAECUM LINGUAE. **26** Morgagni's nodules. See under NODULI VALVULARUM SEMILUNARIUM VALVAE AORTAE. **27** Semilunar valves of Morgagni. See under SINUS ANALES. **28** Morgagni's ventricle, sinus of Morgagni. See under VENTRICULUS LARYNGIS. **29** Morgagni's valves. See under VALVULAE ANALES. **30** Sinus of Morgagni. See under SINUS AORTAE. **31** Sinus of Morgagni. See under PROSTATIC UTRICLE. **32** Papilla of Morgagni. See under ANAL PAPILLA.

Morgan [Thomas Hunt *Morgan, U.S. geneticist, 1866–1945*] Morgan unit. See under MORGAN.

morgan [after Thomas Hunt *Morgan,* U.S. geneticist, 1866–1945] The standard unit of genetic map length, equal to the map distance between two loci that experience, on average, one cross-over during each meiosis. Distances between loci are usually expressed in centimorgans and are determined by the recombination fraction. Also called *morgan unit.* Abbreviation: M

morgue [French] **1** A building or a room designated for the purpose of retaining unidentified or unclaimed bodies pending identification and disposition of the remains. **2** A building or room where dead bodies are retained for the purpose of autopsy and subsequent burial or cremation. For defs. 1 and 2 also called *mortuary.*

moria [Gk *mōria* (from *mōr(os)* silly + *-ia* -IA) silliness, folly] WITZELSUCHT.

moribund [L *moribund(us)* (from *mori,* also *moriri* to die) dying, ready to die] In the process of dying; close to death.

Morison [James Rutherford *Morison,* English surgeon, 1853–1939] **1** See under METHOD. **2** Morison-Talma operation. See under MORISON-TALMA OPERATION. **3** Morison's paste. See under BISMUTH IODOFORM PASTE. **4** Morison's pouch. See under RECESSUS HEPATORENALIS.

Mörner [Karl Axel Hampus *Mörner,* Swedish chemist, 1854–1917] Mörner's body. See under NUCLEOALBUMIN.

Mornidine A proprietary name for pipamazine.

Moro [Ernst *Moro,* German pediatrician, 1874–1951] **1** Moro's reagent, Moro's test. See under REACTION. **2** Moro's reagent. See under TUBERCULIN. **3** See under TEST. **4** Moro's embrace reflex. See under MORO'S REFLEX.

moron [neut. sing. of Gk *mōros* dull, stupid] A mildly mentally retarded individual, defined by an IQ in the range of 50–70, or by a mental age of approximately 7–12. Most are educable and do not require institutionalization but need some supervision in working at some simple job by which they can become self-sustaining members of society. An obsolete term.

morph- MORPHO-.

-morph [Gk *morphē* form, appearance] A combining form meaning an organism or part characterized by a specified form.

morphea [Med L] A circumscribed form of scleroderma, presenting as a central atrophic lesion with a pigmented border. It does not progress to systemic scleroderma. Also called *localized scleroderma, kelis* (obsolete), *Addison's keloid.*

    acroteric morphea SCLERODACTYLY.

    morphea acroterica An obsolete term for SCLERODACTYLY.

    morphea atrophica The atrophic skin of a morphea lesion.

    morphea guttata GUTTATE MORPHEA.

    guttate morphea Morphea with small discrete lesions. This condition may be confused with lichen sclerosus. Also called *morphea guttata, white spot disease.*

    herpetiform morphea MORPHEA HERPETIFORMIS.

    morphea herpetiformis Morphea in a distribution similar to that of the rash of herpes zoster. Also called *herpetiform morphea.*

    linear morphea LINEAR SCLERODERMA.

    morphea linearis LINEAR SCLERODERMA.

morphea pigmentosa The pigmented component of a morphea lesion.

morphea tuberosa Morphea characterized by thickened nodular lesions.

morphia MORPHINE.

morphina MORPHINE.

morphine $C_{17}H_{19}NO_3 \cdot H_2O$. The white, crystalline, principle alkaloid of opium. Morphine is almost insoluble in water, alcohol, or ether, and it is levorotatory. It is a potent narcotic analgesic. It also causes drowsiness, respiratory depression, decreased gastrointestinal motility, nausea, vomiting, and changes in mood, including euphoria. Repeated use leads to tolerance, physical dependence, and addiction. Also called *morphinium, morphina, morphia, morphium*.

morphine sulfate $(C_{17}H_{19}NO_3)_2 \cdot H_2SO_4 \cdot H_2O$. A white, crystalline salt of morphine soluble in water. This form of morphine is commonly used for various parenteral preparations.

morphine tartrate $(C_{17}H_{19}NO_3)_2 \cdot C_4H_6O_6 \cdot 3H_2O$. A white, crystalline powder form of morphine, much more soluble in water than morphine base and used for various parenteral preparations.

morphinia MORPHINISM.

morphinic Relating to morphine.

morphinism [*morphin(e)* + -ISM] 1 A diseased state brought on by the prolonged use of morphine. Also called *morphinia.* 2 Addiction to morphine.

morphinist One who is addicted to morphine.

morphinistic Pertaining to morphinism.

morphinium MORPHINE.

morphinization Subjection to the effects of morphine.

morphiometry The determination of the proportion or the amount of morphine in a narcotic preparation.

morphium MORPHINE.

morpho- [Gk *morphē* form, appearance] A combining form meaning form, structure. Also *morph-*.

morphobiometry MORPHOMETRICS.

morphocytology The science dealing with the morphology of the cell.

morphodifferentiation [MORPHO- + DIFFERENTIATION] The emergence of shape and form in a developing embryo, or in any of its parts or organs.

morphoea A British spelling for MORPHEA.

morphogenesia MORPHOGENESIS.

morphogenesis [MORPHO- + GENESIS] The development or evolutionary appearance of structural form or shape in an organism. It can be considered from both phylogenetic and ontogenetic viewpoints. It involves differentiation of cells and tissues coordinated spatially and at specific times in a definite order, and results in all parts and organs reaching specific relationships with one another and attaining the right cellular constitution and cell number and thus overall size. Also called *morphogenesia, morphogeny, morphosis, topogenesis*. Adjective: morphogenetic.

morphogenetic Relating to or effecting morphogenesis, as *morphogenetic hormone*. Also *morphotic*.

morphogeny MORPHOGENESIS.

morpholine The base whose molecule consists of a six-membered ring, composed of two —CH_2—CH_2— groups, joined at one end through an oxygen atom, and at the other through an —NH— group.

morphologic Pertaining to morphology.

morphology [MORPHO- + -LOGY] The study of the form, shape, and structure of animals and plants. Also called *tectology.*

colonial morphology The form of a bacterial colony, including such important features as size, shape, color, surface texture, opacity, and friability. These features are of considerable diagnostic significance. Observation requires well-isolated colonies in order to avoid changes due to inadequate nutrition or to interaction with products of neighboring colonies.

tooth morphology The study of tooth shape.

morpholysis Destruction of the normal architecture of an organ or tissue. An obsolete term.

morphometrics The use of comparative measurements of form in the classification or analysis of relationships among organisms. Also called *morphometry, morphobiometry, anatometry* (outmoded).

morphometry MORPHOMETRICS.

morphoplasm The protoplasm which makes up the cellular reticulum.

morphosis MORPHOGENESIS.

morphosynthesis The activity performed in the cerebral cortex of the parietal lobes in integrating concepts of shapes, sizes, and interrelationships of parts of the body so as to produce a body image.

morphotic MORPHOGENETIC.

morphotype [MORPHO- + TYPE] The type specimen for one form of a polymorphic species.

-morphous [Gk *morphē* form, appearance + English suffix -*ous*] A combining form meaning characterized by a specified form.

morpion [French *mor(ds)*, imperative of *mordre* to bite + *pion* infantryman] A popular French term for PUBIC LOUSE.

Morquio [Louis *Morquio*, Uruguayan physician, 1867–1935] 1 See under SIGN. 2 Morquio's disease, Morquio's dystrophy, Morquio-Ullrich disease, Morquio syndrome, Morquio-Ullrich syndrome. See under MUCOPOLYSACCHARIDOSIS IV.

morrhuate sodium The sodium salt of morrhuic acid, the oily yellow liquid that represents the fatty acids of codliver oil. The salt is used as a sclerosing material and is injected into varicose veins.

Morris [John McLean *Morris*, U.S. surgeon, born 1914] Morris syndrome. See under TESTICULAR FEMINIZATION.

Morrison [Ashton B. *Morrison*, U.S. pathologist, born 1922] Verner-Morrison syndrome. See under SYNDROME.

mors [L, death] Death.

mors putativa APPARENT DEATH.

mors subita SUDDEN DEATH.

mors thymica Sudden and unexpected death of an infant or child thought to be in some way connected with enlargement of the thymus gland (status lymphaticus). An obsolete term.

morsal [L *mors(us)* a bite, biting + -AL] OCCLUSAL.

morselize [*morsel* + -IZE] To divide into small bits or pieces, such as is done with larger fragments of bone or cartilage used to reshape an area of the skeleton. It is also used in treating premature closure of skull sutures.

mor. sol. *more solito* (L, in the usual way).

morsulus LOZENGE.

morsus [L, a bite, biting] A bite or sting. A seldom used term.

morsus diaboli An outmoded term for FIMBRIAE TUBAE UTERINAE.

morsus humanus A bite by a human. A seldom used term.

mortal [L *mortal(is)* (from *mors*, gen. *mortis*, death + -*alis* -AL) subject to death, causing death] 1 Subject to death. 2 Resulting in or causing death.

mortality [L, *mortalitas* (from *mortalis* subject to death, mortal, from *mors* death; + -*itas* -ITY) mortality, mankind] 1 The fact of being subject to death. 2 DEATH RATE.

actual mortality The number of deaths occurring among 1000 insured persons over a specified period of time.

annual actual mortality The number of deaths that occurred during a stated year per 1000 insured persons.

mortality associated with maternity Mortality of a woman not directly attributed to pregnancy or childbearing but certified as being associated therewith, as the death from chronic rheumatic heart disease of a woman far advanced in pregnancy.

ecological mortality The death of individuals occurring as a natural phenomenon. Also called *realized mortality*.

fetal mortality STILLBIRTH RATE.

infant mortality Mortality under the age of one year.

maternal mortality Mortality of women attributable to complications of pregnancy, confinement, or the puerperium.

neonatal mortality Mortality during the first month or four weeks of life.

perinatal mortality The combined mortality from stillbirths and deaths in the first week of life.

postnatal mortality An incorrect term for POSTNEONATAL MORTALITY.

postneonatal mortality Mortality occurring between the end of the first month (neonatal period) and the age of one year. Also called *postnatal mortality* (incorrect).

proportionate mortality PROPORTIONATE MORTALITY RATIO.

realized mortality ECOLOGICAL MORTALITY.

reproductive mortality The total mortality related to the reproductive function, including, in addition to deaths directly attributable to the complications of pregnancy, confinement, and the puerperium, associated deaths of pregnant or parturient women from other diseases such as diabetes and chest disease as well as deaths connected with the use of any form of contraception, temporary or permanent.

specific mortality A death rate specific for age, sex, ethnic group, cause of death, or other defined characteristic or combination of characteristics, such as the death rate from tuberculosis of males aged 25–29 years.

tabular mortality The death rates set out in a table of mortalities such as a life table.

mortalogram A graph of human mortality for a specific cause, showing time period and median age at death. A seldom used term.

mortar A vessel with a rounded interior that is used for the crushing of drugs and other substances with a pestle.

mortician One who arranges and manages funerals; an undertaker.

Mortierella A genus of fungi of the class Zygomycetes. *Mortierella wolfii* has been found to cause abortion and fatal pneumonia of cattle.

Mortierellaceae [Possibly from French *mortier* a bowl for pounding substances, also mortar of sand and cement + *-ella*, L fem. diminishing suffix + -ACEAE] A family of fungi belonging to the order Mucorales, class Zygomycetes, which are occasional etiologic agents of mucormycosis.

mortification [Late L *mortificatio* (from *mortificatus*, past part. of *mortificare* to kill, mortify, from L *mors*, gen. *mortis*, death + *-ficare* -FY) a killing, mortification] Gangrene or necrosis; death of a part.

Mortimer [Mrs. *Mortimer*, English patient of Sir Jonathan Hutchinson, flourished 19th century] Mortimer's disease. See under SARCOIDOSIS.

mortinatality [L *mors*, gen. *mortis* death + NATALITY] STILLBIRTH RATE.

mortise / ankle mortise The space occupied by the talus in the talocrural joint.

mortisemblant Seemingly dead.

Morton [Dudley J. *Morton*, U.S. orthopedic surgeon, 1884–1960] See under SYNDROME.

Morton [Richard *Morton*, English physician, 1637–1698] See under COUGH.

Morton [Samuel George *Morton*, U.S. physician and anthropologist, 1799–1851] See under PLANE.

Morton [Thomas George *Morton*, U.S. surgeon, 1835–1903] **1** Morton's foot, Morton's disease, Thomas Morton's disease, Morton's neuralgia, Morton's toe. See under NEUROMA. **2** See under TEST.

Morton [William Thomas Green *Morton*, U.S. physician, 1819–1868] See under INHALER.

mortuary [L *mortuar(ius)* (from *mortu(us)*, past part. of *mori*, also *moriri* to die, + *-arius* -ARY) pertaining to burial] **1** Pertaining to death. **2** MORGUE.

morula [L *morum* mulberry, so-called because of its resemblance to a mulberry] A solid mass of cells formed by the cleavage of the fertilized egg. The arrangement of the blastomeres in the morula varies in different groups, the arrangement being orderly in some groups, such as batrachians, but more complex in others, such as mammals. Also called *embryotic sphere, yolk sphere, vitelline sphere, segmentation sphere.*

morulation [MORULA + *-(a)tion*] The formation of a morula.

moruloid [*morul(a)* + -OID] Having the shape of a mulberry.

morulus [L (dim. of *morum* a blackberry), blackberry-colored, blackish] The lesion characteristic of yaws, resembling a mulberry or raspberry.

Morvan [Augustin Marie *Morvan*, French physician, 1819–1897] **1** Morvan's fibrillar chorea, Morvan's chorea. See under FIBRILLARY CHOREA. **2** Morvan's disease. See under SYNDROME.

mosaic [Late Middle English *musyche*, from French *mosaïque* mosaic work, from Late L *musaicus* (adj.) mosaic, from L *musæum* (opus) mosaic (work), from Gk *mouseion* (neut. sing. of *mouseios* pertaining to the muses, from Gk *mousa* a muse) mosaic work] **1** In genetics, an individual whose cells consist of at least two genotypically distinct populations that arose after fertilization through somatic mutation or somatic nondisjunction. **2** Of or pertaining to such an individual. **3** A protein that contains multiple domains, some of which are shared with other proteins. It arises through gene duplication, exon shuffling, or other mechanisms that are obscure.

chromosomal mosaic The state of being mosaic for a morphologic variation in karyotype. A common example in humans is an individual with one chromosomally normal cell line and another lacking (or having an additional) sex chromosome, such as 46,XY/45,X.

mosaicism The state or situation of being mosaic.

erythrocyte mosaicism The presence of two distinct populations of erythrocytes in the blood of one individual, when not the result of blood transfusion or chimerism. Mosaicism usually occurs in erythrocytes (and all other cells) of women who are heterozygous for an X-chromosome-linked genetic trait such as glucose-6-phosphate dehydrogenase deficiency. Males, who have but one X-chromosome, do not exhibit mosaicism.

gonadal mosaicism In genetics, the presence in a gonad of a germ-cell line that is genotypically distinct from that comprising the rest of the individual. One potential result is the appearance in multiple offspring of a dominant phenotype not present in the parent.

haploid-diploid mosaicism A situation in which some of the component cells of an originally haploid individual have diploidized while others have remained haploid, so that both haploid and diploid cells of a genetically identical pedigree are present within the same individual. Compare HAPLODIPLOIDY.

Moschcowitz [Alexis Victor *Moschcowitz*, U.S. surgeon, 1865–1933] See under OPERATION.

Moschcowitz [Eli *Moschcowitz*, U.S. physician, 1879–1964] **1** Moschcowitz sign. See under TEST. **2** Moschcowitz disease, Moschcowitz syndrome. See under THROMBOTIC THROMBO-CYTOPENIC PURPURA.

Mosenthal [Herman Otto *Mosenthal*, U.S. physician, 1878–1954] See under TEST.

Mosetig-Moorhof [Albert von *Mosetig-Moorhof*, Austrian surgeon, 1838–1907] Mosetig-Moorhof bone wax. See under WAX.

Mosher [Harris Payton *Mosher*, U.S. surgeon and laryngologist, 1867–1954] Air cells of Mosher. See under CELL.

Mosler [Karl Friedrich *Mosler*, German physician, 1831–1911] **1** Mosler's diabetes. See under INOSITURIA. **2** See under SIGN.

mosm Symbol for the unit, milliosmole.

mosquiticidal Lethal or destructive to mosquitoes. Also *mosquitocidal*.

mosquiticide [*mosquit(o)* + *i* + -CIDE] An agent that is toxic or destructive to mosquitoes. Also *mosquitocide*.

mosquito [Spanish (dim. of *mosca* a fly, from L *musca* a fly; Gk *myia* a fly), a gnat, mosquito] Any insect of the dipteran family Culicidae. The eggs are generally laid on water, and larvae and pupae are aquatic. Most larvae feed on organic debris but some are predators. In the adult, females are bloodsuckers and are vectors of some important viral, protozoan, and filarial pathogens. Most species of medical importance belong to the genera *Aedes*, *Anopheles*, *Culex*, and *Stegomyia*.

anautogenous mosquito A mosquito unable to produce viable eggs without taking a blood meal.

autogenous mosquito A mosquito that is able to produce viable eggs without having had a blood meal.

eurygamous mosquito A mosquito that requires extensive outdoor space for breeding.

house mosquito Any of the abundant and widespread mosquitoes, such as *Culex pipiens*, that are commonly found living and feeding in human dwellings.

stenogamous mosquito A mosquito able to breed in captivity or in limited space.

tiger mosquito A mosquito of the species *Aedes aegypti*.

mosquitocidal MOSQUITICIDAL.

mosquitocide MOSQUITICIDE.

Moss [Melvin Lionel *Moss*, U.S. anatomist, born 1923] Gorlin-Chaudhry-Moss syndrome. See under SYNDROME.

Moss [William Lorenzo *Moss*, U.S. physician, 1876–1957] See under CLASSIFICATION.

moss [Middle English *mos, moss* a swamp, akin to Old English *meoss* moss and L *muscus* moss] Any low, green bryophytic plant of the class Musci. True mosses consist of three subclasses: Bryideae, Sphagnideae, and Andreaeideae. The class is distinguished by the presence of leafy gametophytes, sporophytes with complex forms of dehiscence, and multicellular rhizoids.

Iceland moss *Cetraria islandica*, a lichen of the Parmeliaceae family. It has demulcent, nutritive, and tonic properties.

Irish moss CARRAGEEN.

muskeag moss SPHAGNUM MOSS.

peat moss SPHAGNUM MOSS.

sphagnum moss A moss of the genus *Sphagnum* which was once used as an absorbent dressing. Also called *peat moss, muskeag moss*.

Mosse [Max *Mosse*, German physician, born 1873] See under SYNDROME.

Mosso [Angelo *Mosso*, Italian, physiologist, 1846–1910] See under ERGOGRAPH, PLETHYSMOGRAPH.

Motais [Ernst *Motais*, French ophthalmologist, 1845–1913] See under OPERATION.

moth [Old English *moththe*] Any of numerous lepidopteran insects characterized by filamentous, often plumate antennae and usually nocturnal habits, in contrast with butterflies, which have smooth, knobbed antennae and are usually diurnal.

brown-tail moth A moth of the species *Euproctis chrysorrhoea*.

flannel moth A moth of the family Megalopygidae, especially one of the genus *Megalopyge*. The stout, hairy caterpillars have stinging hairs that can cause a painful urticaria.

Io moth A moth of the species *Automeris io*.

meal moth A moth of the species *Asopia farinalis*. See also MEAL WORM.

tussock moth A moth of the genus *Hemerocampa*.

mother [Old English *mōdor*, akin to L *mater* a mother and Gk *mētēr* a mother] **1** A woman who has borne a child; a female parent. **2** A pregnant woman, considered as distinct from her developing fetus. • This sense is commonly used in obstetrics, where a distinction between the fetus and the woman carrying it is often important. In such contexts, *mother* is equivalent to *expectant mother*. **3** The original model or central source from which similar units are derived. **4** A cell which divides to give rise to two daughter cells. Adjective: maternal.

Colles mother A clinically asymptomatic mother of a child with congenital syphilis.

elderly mother ELDERLY PRIMIGRAVIDA.

expectant mother A pregnant woman.

phallic mother The male child's belief that his mother possesses a penis.

schizophrenogenic mother A mother whose own psychopathology and handling of her child is a basic determinant in the subsequent development of schizophrenia in that child.

surrogate mother **1** A woman who bears the offspring of another, typically infertile woman, whose partner's sperm is utilized, usually by artificial insemination, to achieve conception. *In vitro* development of the conceptus followed by early implantation in the uterus of the surrogate mother has also been successfully employed. **2** MOTHER SURROGATE. See under MOTHER SURROGATE.

mothering / surrogate mothering The medicolegal practice by which a surrogate mother bears offspring for another woman and her male partner, by whose sperm she is impregnated, usually by artificial insemination, and relinquishes the offspring to the father and his partner following parturition. See also SURROGATE MOTHER.

mother surrogate An object or animal that performs or is perceived as performing one or more of the functions normally executed by the natural mother of a young animal, as a person acting as a substitute or deputy mother for an infant or child, or an animal of one species acting as a substitute for the offspring of an animal of a different species. Objects identified with warmth have also been used in experimental studies as mothers surrogate. Also called *surrogate mother*. See also SURROGATE MOTHER.

motile [L *mot(us)* (past part. of *movere* to move, stir, put in motion) + *-ilis*, -ILE[1]] Capable of self-generated movement, an important diagnostic criterion in bacteria.

motilin A gastrointestinal polypeptide of 22 amino acids and molecular weight 2700, located in the enterochromaffin cells, chiefly of the duodenum and upper jejunum, having the effects of increasing gastric and colonic motility. It is released by changes in the pH of small intestinal contents.

motility [MOTILE + -ITY] The capacity for spontaneous movement.

automatic motility SPONTANEOUS MOVEMENT.

segmental motility Regularly spaced ring-like contractions of the small intestine that, as they disappear, are replaced by similar contractions in the segments of the intestine between those previously contracted. Also called *segmentation movement, pendular movement.*

voluntary motility VOLUNTARY MOVEMENT.

motion [L *motio* (from L *motus*, past part. of *movere* to move, stir, put in motion, akin to *pavere* to tremble, be afraid, *vivere* to live, and Gk *ameusasthai* to surpass) movement, motion] **1** A change of place or position; movement in space. **2** The process of defecation. **3** Matter defecated.

active motion ACTIVE MOVEMENT.

passive motion PASSIVE MOVEMENT.

wave motion The mechanism by which a periodic disturbance or vibration passes through a medium or empty space.

motivation [MOTIVE + -ATION] The hypothesized inner state of a person or animal that serves to arouse, maintain, and guide behavior toward a goal.

extrinsic motivation Motivation evidently based not on satisfaction inherent in the activity itself but on the possibility of receiving a reward.

intrinsic motivation Motivation based on satisfaction found in behaviors or activities, such as exploration or game playing, in and of themselves rather than in achieving any external goal.

motive [Med L *motiv(us)* (from *motus*, past part. of *movere* to move, stir, put in motion + -*ivus* -IVE) anything that moves] **1** An energizing condition arising within an organism that serves to initiate, maintain, or direct a sequence of behavior toward a goal. **2** The reason assigned by a person to account for some aspect of his or her behavior. A less technical usage.

achievement motive The tendency to invest oneself in task performance and to increase self-esteem by improvement in performance. An individual with a strong achievement motive will strive to do difficult tasks quickly and well for their own sake, and not necessarily for fame or with a concern for getting ahead.

motoceptor [*moto(r)* + *(re)ceptor*] A muscle sense receptor, such as a muscle spindle or Golgi tendon organ, located in muscle. A seldom used term.

motofacient Causing movement.

motoneuron [*moto-* (from English *motor*) prefix denoting the imparting of motion + NEURON] A central neuron whose target organ is an effector structure such as a muscle or gland; an efferent neuron conveying motor impulses. Also called *motor neuron, motor cell, exciter neuron, peripheral motor neuron.*

α-motoneurons Neurons of the anterior horn of the spinal cord which give rise to α-efferents innervating skeletal muscles. Neuron soma sizes vary from about 20–100 μm, the larger ones innervating large pale muscle fibers, and the smaller supplying red muscle fibers.

β-motoneurons Neurons which give rise to β-efferents innervating both extrafusal and intrafusal fibers of muscle spindles. The axons are of the size of smaller α-motoneuron axons and contribute to the α-wave of an evoked neurogram recorded from the ventral root.

γ-motoneurons Small neurons of the anterior horn of the spinal cord that give rise to γ-efferents (fusimotor fibers) innervating the intrafusal fibers of a muscle spindle.

heteronymous motoneurons Motor cells supplying muscles which do not directly supply them with afferent impulses.

homonymous motoneurons Motor cells supplying the muscle that is the source of the afferent impulses.

lower motoneurons Motor cell bodies in the anterior horn of the spinal cord or in the cranial nuclei whose axons terminate in skeletal muscles.

peripheral motoneurons Neurons participating in peripheral reflex arcs that receive impulses from interneurons and transmit them to voluntary muscles. Such cells are found in the anterior horn of the spinal cord and in the motor components of cranial nerve nuclei.

upper motoneurons Cerebral cortical nerve cells whose axons project upon motor nuclei of cranial nerves or the anterior horn of the spinal cord. Most of these cells are found in the posterior portion of the frontal lobe along the anterior wall of the central sulcus.

motoneuronitis [L *mot(us)* a moving, motion + *o* + NEURONITIS] Polyneuritis predominantly involving motor nerves.

motor [L (from *motus*, past part. of *movere* to move, stir, put in motion + -*or* -OR), a person or thing that imparts motion] **1** Carrying or transmitting an impulse to a peripheral effector organ of the nervous system, either to elicit a response or to inhibit it. **2** A mechanism that imparts motion.

air motor An air-driven, medium-speed motor attached directly to the handpiece of a dental drill.

club motor A plastic motor in which the attachment is by means of a knob or club of tissue.

loop motor A plastic motor in which the attachment is by means of a loop of tissue.

plastic motor An arrangement of muscles and tendons used in kineplasty whereby muscle tissue of the stump is used to provide power to the prosthetic limb.

motorgraphic KINETOGRAPHIC.

motorial Describing or pertaining to a movement or to a motor pathway in the nervous system.

motoricity The ability to initiate or to perform movement. Also called *motricity.*

motorium [Late L, neut. of *motorius* in motion, from L *mot(us)*, past part. of *movere* to move, + -*orium* -ORY] The central neural centers and pathways which control movement. An obsolete term.

motorius an obsolescent and rarely used term for MOTOR NERVE.

motormeter Any of various devices capable of measuring the strength, speed, and intensity of movement of a muscle or limb.

motorogerminative [*motor* + *o* + *germinative*] Giving rise to muscle, as does the myotome of an embryo.

motricity MOTORICITY.

mottling Patchy and irregular spots of color.

mouches volantes MUSCAE VOLITANTES.

Mouchet [Albert *Mouchet*, French surgeon, born 1869] See under DISEASE.

moulage [French (from *moule* a cast, mold, from L *modulus*, dim. of *modus* a measure + French -*age* -AGE), the making of a cast or mold] **1** A molded impression made by applying a wax or other plastic material directly to a lesion or body part. **2** The making of a mold or model, as in dentistry.

mould A British spelling for MOLD.

moulding A British spelling for MOLDING.

moult A British spelling for MOLT.

mounce [*m(etric)* + OUNCE] A unit of mass or weight equal to 25 grams. An obsolete unit. Also called *metric ounce.*

mound / anal mound A small, midline swelling in front of the anal opening of an embryo. It is formed by the union of the anal tubercles.

mounding MYOEDEMA.

Mount [Lester Adran *Mount*, U.S. neurosurgeon, born 1910]

Mount-Reback syndrome. See under MOUNT SYNDROME.

mount **1** To prepare for microscopic or gross examination. **2** A material prepared for microscopic or gross examination.

mountant MOUNTING MEDIUM.

mounting **1** The preparation of slides or specimens for examination. **2** The attachment to an an articulator of casts of the jaws.

split cast mounting A method of mounting in dentistry which permits accurate remounting of the cast on the same articulator. Grooves are cut in the base of the cast before mounting, or special metal plates may be used. Also called *split cast method.*

mourning Grief as a normal reaction to the death or loss of a loved one.

mouse [Old English *mūs,* akin to L *mus* a mouse, rat and to Gk *mys* a mouse, muscle] A small rodent, *Mus musculus,* which weighs about 30 g and has a sleek body, smooth hair coat, long hairless tail, and erect rounded ears. Vast numbers are used throughout the world in laboratory research for which numerous defined strains have been developed.

B mouse A mouse subjected to an experimental procedure that destroys both T and B lymphocytes, followed by a second procedure replacing the B lymphocytes. Also called *deprived mouse.*

BALB/c mouse An inbred strain of white mice commonly used in experimental immunology. It has a low incidence of mammary tumors and leukemia and is extremely sensitive to radiation. Arteriosclerosis is common in both males and females and amyloidosis of the spleen is usual in males by 20 months.

CBA mouse An inbred strain of white mice of which one substrain carries an easily recognizable chromosomal marker.

deprived mouse B MOUSE.

joint mouse A free cartilaginous fragment within the joint space.

multimammate mouse A member of a form of the genus *Rattus* having eight to twelve pairs of mammae, formerly classified in the separate genus *Mastomys.*

New Zealand black mouse An inbred strain of mouse characterized by autoimmune hemolytic anemia, extramedullary hematopoiesis, and lupuslike nephritis with glomerular and tubular damage. Also called *NZB mouse.*

nude mouse A hairless mouse with a mutant gene on chromosome 11 characterized by congenital absence of the thymus, reduction in number of T cells, inability to reject allogeneic or xenogeneic skin grafts, a deficient supply of immunoglobulins, antinuclear autoantibody, and glomerulonephritis. Such mice have proved a valuable tool for investigating the role of the thymus in the development of immune responses. Also called *nu nu mouse.*

nu nu mouse NUDE MOUSE.

NZB mouse NEW ZEALAND BLACK MOUSE.

peritoneal mouse A discrete, small, calcific density seen on an abdominal roentgenogram, representing an appendix epiploica or small piece of omentum which has twisted, become necrotic, and, lying free in the peritoneal cavity, has been encrusted with calcium.

pleural mouse A soft-tissue density, usually round, seen on a chest roentgenogram, representing a fibrin body in the pleural space. Such a fibrin body may be secondary to pneumothorax, pleural fluid, or other pleural disease.

Snell-Bagg mouse An inbred strain of mice, some of which have abnormalities of the pituitary and thymus with resultant lack of thymic tissue and depressed cell-mediated immunity. A recessive gene causes a deficiency of pituitary hormones and thus the appearance of dwarf mice in Snell-Bagg litters. Such mice have a life-span of about five months, one quarter that of normal littermates.

mousepox INFECTIOUS ECTROMELIA.

mouth [Old English *mūth,* akin to L *mandere* to chew, eat and to Gk *masasthai* to touch, chew] **1** OS[1]. **2** OSTIUM.

Ceylon sore mouth An outmoded term for TROPICAL STOMATITIS.

denture sore mouth DENTURE STOMATITIS.

dry mouth XEROSTOMIA.

tapir mouth The characteristic pouting appearance of the lips seen in facioscapulohumeral muscular dystrophy. Also called *tapir lips, bouche de tapir.*

trench mouth NECROTIZING ULCERATIVE GINGIVITIS.

white mouth An older term for THRUSH.

mouth-to-mouth See under MOUTH-TO-MOUTH RESUSCITATION.

mouthwash A solution for rinsing the mouth, having antibacterial, palliative, astringent, or deodorant properties.

alkaline mouthwash of phenol A solution containing phenol, potassium hydroxide, and amaranth. It is used as a medicinal gargle. Also called *collutorium phenolis alkalinum.*

compound mouthwash of sodium chloride A mouthwash or gargling solution containing sodium chloride, sodium carbonate, and peppermint water. Also called *collutorium sodii chloridi compositum.*

mouthwash of zinc sulfate and zinc chloride A mouthwash composed of a solution of zinc sulfate and zinc chloride in dilute hydrochloric acid with tartrazine and chloroform water.

movement

movement The act or process of moving; activity causing a change in position.

active movement A movement produced by a subject's own action; a voluntary action. Also called *active motion.*

adversive movement A turning or beginning or progression to the side on which a sensory or electrical stimulus to a central nervous structure has been applied or which a lesion has been made.

ameboid movement Locomotion of cells such as leukocytes or amebas resulting from protoplasmic streaming into pseudopodia. The relative degree of protoplasmic rigidity determines the rate and direction of flow, and the presence of microtubules is required for the movement to take place. Also called *streaming movement.*

angular movement A movement associated with a change in angle, as that of a joint.

apparent movement The subjective impression that physically stationary stimuli, when exposed in quick succession, are actually moving, as, for example, in cinematic motion pictures. The illusion is most often perceived in response to visual stimuli, but it can occur in other sensory modes as well. Also called *delta movement, phi phenomenon.*

assistive movement A physical therapy technique in which the therapist assists the patient in carrying out the movement of a paralyzed limb through a greater range of motion than would be possible unaided. It may be active, with the patient's own muscle power being brought into play as far as possible, or passive, with the therapist supplying all the power for range-of-motion exercise in a totally paralyzed limb.

associated movement The involuntary movement of one part of the body that accompanies movement of another part of the body.

associated contralateral movement In a hemiplegic patient, an involuntary movement occurring on the affected side that is induced by a corresponding voluntary movement on the normal side.

athetoid movements Movements resembling those seen in athetosis.

automatic movements Movements occurring in a state of automatism.

autonomic movement Any movement associated with stimulation by the autonomic division of the nervous system.

Bennett movement A lateral shift of the head of the condyle of the mandible towards the working side as the mandible is lowered and swung outwards in preparation for chewing on that side.

bodily movement The lateral movement of a tooth without tipping. Also called *translatory movement*.

border movement Extreme movement of the muscles of mastication, muscles of facial expression, and of the tongue.

border tissue movements Movements of the soft tissues in border molding.

bowel movement 1 An act of defecation. 2 The feces produced by an act of defecation; stool.

brownian movement The rapid random motion of small particles suspended in a liquid that is caused by the unequal impact of the molecules of the liquid on the particles. Also called *molecular movement, brunonian movement, Brownian-Zsigmondy movement.*

brownian-Zsigmondy movement BROWNIAN MOVEMENT.

brunonian movement BROWNIAN MOVEMENT.

cardinal movements The six cardinal positions of the eye: up lateral, straight lateral, and down lateral, to each side.

choreic movements The disorganized involuntary movements of chorea.

choreiform movements Movements occurring in or resembling those of chorea. They are involuntary, abrupt, rapid, arrhythmic, and variable in location, often involving the whole body but sometimes predominating on one side. They are more marked in the face and arms. They are increased by fatigue, emotion, and effort, and cease when the patient is asleep. They take the form of aimless, wild gestures. In the arms they comprise flexion, extension, and abduction movements, adduction of the hands and fingers, flinging out the arms, and shrugging of the shoulders. The facial movements cause the patient to grimace and he may protrude his tongue intermittently. The movements may be transient or persistent.

ciliary movement Action of cilia on a nonattached single-celled or acellular organism, providing its motility; ciliary actions of attached cells that function as a ciliated surface, providing a means of transporting food, waste, or other materials along that surface.

circus movement 1 A gait involving circumduction of both legs, as in bilateral hemiparesis. 2 Electrical activation of part of the heart occurring over a circular pathway, thought to be responsible for atrial flutter.

communicated movement Movement produced by the application of an external force.

corrective fusion movements Vergence alignments for the purpose of binocular synthesis of the visual images.

curtain movement The sideways movement of the posterior pharyngeal wall seen in cases of unilateral paralysis of the superior constrictor muscle of the pharynx when the patient gags, says "Ah," etc. The movement, like the pulling aside of a curtain, is in a direction away from the paralyzed side. Also called *Vernet's rideau phenomenon* (obsolete).

cytoplasmic movement PROTOPLASMIC MOVEMENT.

delta movement APPARENT MOVEMENT.

disjugate movement of the eyes A turning of the two eyes in opposite directions. Also called *disjunctive movement.*

disjunctive movement DISJUGATE MOVEMENT OF THE EYES.

diurnal movement The daily movement of a plant or plant part in response to the position of the sun.

dystonic movement A slow and often bizarre involuntary movement, resembling in some respects those of athetosis but generally associated with a fixed alteration in posture of the affected part of the body.

eccentric movement Movement of the mandible to an eccentric position.

excursive movement Any mandibular movement during mastication.

fetal movement Intrauterine changes in fetal position or limb activity that are perceptible to the mother.

forced movement 1 INVOLUNTARY MOVEMENT. 2 PASSIVE MOVEMENT.

free mandibular movement A movement of the mandible not affected by occlusion or by food.

Frenkel's movements A system of exercises used in the treatment of parkinsonism and ataxia to increase precision and spontaneity of movement by cortical reinforcement. Footprints are painted or pasted on the floor at appropriate intervals and the patient is encouraged to walk on them.

functional mandibular movement Any physiologic movement of the mandible.

gliding movement of the mandible MANDIBULAR GLIDE.

hinge movement Movement of the mandible around the hinge axis.

index movement Cephalic movement about the fixed caudal part of a body.

intermediary movement INTERMEDIATE MOVEMENT.

intermediate movement An excursive movement not reaching its limit. Also called *intermediary movement.*

involuntary movement Involuntary contraction of one or more muscle groups or rarely of a single muscle, producing movement of a limb or of some other part of the body. This may be due to a variety of neurologic disorders, including principally focal motor seizures, clonus and myoclonus, tremor, chorea, athetosis, dystonia, hemiballismus, and facial dyskinesia. Involuntary contraction of bundles of muscle fibers not producing movement at a joint (fasciculation) is not usually so classified, nor are tics (habit spasm), as the latter are initially under voluntary control. Also called *forced movement*. Compare VOLUNTARY MOVEMENT.

jaw movement Any movement of the mandible.

labial movement Movement of a tooth toward the lip.

lingual movement Movement of a tooth toward the tongue.

Magnan's trombone movement TROMBONE TONGUE.

masticatory movement Any one of the movements of the mandible during the masticatory cycle.

mirror movement ALLOKINESIS.

molecular movement BROWNIAN MOVEMENT.

morphogenetic movement The changes in position and displacements of cells and groups of cells, the folding and rearrangement of layers of cells, and any alteration in position of structures or organs during the development of the embryo. Gastrulation eventually establishes the three germ layers, ectoderm, endoderm and mesoderm which move into the positions where they will subsequently develop into particular parts and features of the embryo.

nucleopetal movement 1 Movement of entities in the cytoplasm toward the nucleus of the cell. 2 Movement of male pronucleus towards female pronucleus after fertilization.

opening movement Any mandibular movement increasing the distance between the upper and lower anterior teeth.

passive movement Movement imposed by external force rather than by muscular contraction, as on a paralyzed limb or a nonresponsive patient for purposes of exercise and maintenance of joint mobility. Also called *forced movement, passive motion.*

pedal movement   A type of repetitive movement of the feet, which make pedaling or paddling movements. In rare cases, this is seen in Parkinson's disease, but it may be a result of treatment with levodopa.

pendular movement   SEGMENTAL MOTILITY.

percussion movements   Rapid, short blows used in massage. Various methods involve the fingertips or the side of the hand in different positions. Also called *tapotement.*

perverted mandibular movement   A habitual, nonfunctional movement, as in bruxism.

posterior opening movement   An opening movement about the hinge axis.

protoplasmic movement   Movement of a mass of protoplasm, usually effected by the action of microtubules or microfilaments. Also called *cytoplasmic movement.*

rapid eye movement   **1** The jerky ocular movements observed in deep sleep. Abbreviation: REM.   **2** SACCADE.

reflex movement   Any involuntary movement evoked by stimulation of sensory receptors or an afferent pathway.

resistive movement   Movement in which a muscle or limb is obliged to work against external weight or resistance, as used, for example, in progressive resistive exercises.

rotatory movement   Torsion of the eyes upon an anteroposterior axis.

running movements   STEPPING.

saccadic eye movement   SACCADE.

scissors movement   Opposing directional change of the retinoscopic reflex, indicating irregular astigmatism.

segmentation movement   SEGMENTAL MOTILITY.

spontaneous movement   Movement occurring without voluntary or apparent external stimulation. Also called *automatic motility.*

stepping movements   STEPPING.

streaming movement   AMEBOID MOVEMENT.

Swedish movement   SWEDISH GYMNASTICS.

synkinetic movement   An involuntary movement that accompanies more gross voluntary activity, such as the grimace associated with physical exertion.

tipping movement   The lateral movement which occurs when a force is applied to one point of a crown. The tooth rotates in the vertical plane about an imaginary fulcrum near the apex, which moves in the opposite direction to the crown.

translatory movement   BODILY MOVEMENT.

vermicular movements   PERISTALSIS.

voluntary movement   Activity that occurs as a consequence of a conscious decision. Also called *voluntary motility.* Compare INVOLUNTARY MOVEMENT.

---

mover / prime mover   A muscle that constantly initiates and maintains a particular movement of a part, such as the brachialis muscle in flexion of the elbow joint; an agonist.

moxa [New L (from Japanese *mogusa* a soft mass of wormwood leaves burned and used as a cautery)]   A cone or cylinder of cotton, wool, or other combustible material, ignited and placed on the skin, formerly used especially in Japanese folk medicine to produce a counterirritation or cautery.

moxalactam $C_{20}H_{20}N_6O_9S$.   7-[[Carboxy(4-hydroxyphenyl)acetyl]amino]-7-methoxy-3-[[(1-methyl-1H-tetrazol-5-yl)thio]-methyl]-8-oxo-5-oxal-azabicyclo[4.2.0]oct-2-ene-2-carboxylic acid. An anti-infective agent like the cephalosporins, with a broad antibiotic spectrum much like that of cefotaxime. It is given parenterally, usually as the sodium salt (latamoxef sodium).

moxibustion [*mox(a)* + *i* + *(com)bustion*]   The former practice especially in Japanese folk medicine of producing cautery or counterirritation by igniting a cone or cylinder (moxa) of cotton, wool, or other combustible material and placing it on the skin. Also called *byssocausis* (obsolete).

moyamoya [Japanese, misty, foggy, hazy, gloomy, from duplicated *moya* a mist, fog, haze]   See under MOYAMOYA DISEASE.

Mozart [Wolfgang Amadeus *Mozart*, Austrian composer, 1756–1791]   See under EAR.

mp   **1** Symbol for the unit, millipond.   **2** melting point.

MPa   Symbol for the unit, megapascal.

MPD   maximum permissible dose.

mphot   Symbol for the unit, milliphot.

MPO   minimum perceptible odor.

MPS   **1** mucopolysaccharidosis.   **2** multiphasic screening.

MPV   mean platelet volume.

mpz   Symbol for the obsolete unit, millipièze.

MR   Symbol for the unit, megaroentgen.

Mr.   mister (used as a title of address prefixed to a name).   ● See note at MISTER.

mR   Symbol for the unit, milliroentgen.

μR   Symbol for the unit, microroentgen.

μr   Alternative symbol for the unit, microroentgen.

μ/ρ   Symbol for the quantity, mass attenuation coefficient, expressed in square meters per kilogram.

mrad   Symbol for the unit, millirad.

MRD   minimal reacting dose.

mrem   Symbol for the unit, millirem.

MRI   magnetic resonance imaging (nuclear magnetic resonance).

mRNA   messenger ribonucleic acid.

MRO   minimum recognizable odor (minimal identifiable odor).

MS   **1** multiple sclerosis.   **2** mitral stenosis.

ms   Symbol for the unit, millisecond.

m/s   Symbol for the unit, meter per second.

m/s²   Symbol for the unit, meter per second squared.

m·s⁻²   Symbol for the unit, meter per second squared.

m³/s   Symbol for the unit, cubic meter per second.

m·s⁻¹   Symbol for the unit, meter per second.

m³·s⁻¹   Symbol for the unit, cubic meter per second.

μs   Symbol for the unit, microsecond.

MSB   most significant bit.

msec   Symbol for the unit, millisecond. An incorrect symbol.

μsec   Symbol for the unit, microsecond. An incorrect symbol.

MSH   melanocyte stimulating hormone.

MSH/ACTH   **4–10**   Met-Glu-His-Phe-Arg-Trp-Gly. An amino acid common to the adrenocorticotropic hormone (ACTH) and β-melanocyte stimulating hormone (MSH) molecules, which functions as an endogenous psychoactive drug in having anti-anxiety effects in normal subjects and in improving visual memory in senile patients.

MSH-IF   melanocyte stimulating hormone inhibiting factor.

MSHRF   melanocyte stimulating hormone releasing factor (melanocyte stimulating hormone releasing hormone).

MSHRH   melanocyte stimulating hormone releasing hormone.

MSL   midsternal line.

MT   **1** empty.   **2** medical technologist.   **3** membrana tympani.   **4** metatarsal.

Mt   Symbol for the unit, megatonne.

MTBF   mean time between (or before) failures.

MTF   modulation transfer function.

MTU   methylthiouracil.

MTX   methotrexate.

MU   **1** Symbol for the quantity, megaunit.   **2** In medicine, mouse unit.

M.u.   Mache unit.

mU   Symbol for milliunit.

mu   The name of the twelfth letter of the Greek alphabet. Symbol: μ

μU   Symbol for microunit.

mucanain   A proteolytic enzyme found in the seed pod spines of *Mucuna pruriens*. In contact with the skin this enzyme is extremely irritating.

Much [Hans Christian R. *Much*, German physician, 1880–1932] **1** Much reaction. See under MUCH-HOLZMANN REACTION.   **2** Schrön-Much granules. See under MUCH'S GRANULES.

Mucha [Viktor *Mucha*, Austrian dermatologist, 1877–1919] Mucha's disease, Mucha-Habermann disease, Mucha-Habermann syndrome. See under PITYRIASIS LICHENOIDES.

mucic acid   HOOC—[CHOH]$_4$—COOH. Galactaric acid. The dicarboxylic acid that can be formed by oxidation of galactose at C-1 and C-6.

mucicarmine   A staining solution containing carmine and aluminum chloride or aluminum hydroxide in water or alcohol. It is used in tissue sections to demonstrate mucin and as a stain for fungi. Also called *Mayer's mucicarmine*.

Mayer's mucicarmine   MUCICARMINE.

mucid   A rarely used term for MUCILAGINOUS.

muciferous   Secreting mucus.

mucification [*muc(o)*- + *i* + -FICATION] A progesterone-induced change in the superficial cells of the vaginal epithelium. Instead of being squamous, the cells become filled with mucus. This leads to the production of copious amounts of mucus in the vagina during the progestational stage of the estrous cycle.

muciform   Like mucus in appearance and consistency.

mucigenous   Mucus-producing. Also *muciparous, blennogenic, blennogenous*.

mucigogue [*muc(us)* + *i* + -*(a)gogue*] **1** An agent that stimulates the secretion of mucus.   **2** Provoking the secretion of mucus.

mucihematein / Mayer's mucihematein   A staining solution that is based on hematein, the oxidized form of hematoxylin, and is used to demonstrate the presence of the connective tissue mucin.

mucilage [Late L *mucilago*. See MUCILAGO.] **1** A gumlike plant cell product composed of sulfate esters of complex polysaccharides.   **2** An aqueous solution of a gum utilized for suspending rather insoluble substances in mixtures. Another use is to increase the viscosity of oil-in-water emulsions, such as those used for dermatologic preparations and lubricating medications. For defs. 1 and 2 also called *mucilago*.

mucilaginous   Having a viscous, mucoid, or slimy consistency. Also *mucid* (rarely used).

mucilago [Late L (from L *mucus* mucus) a musty fluid, gelatinous substance] MUCILAGE.

mucilago tragacanthae   GUM TRAGACANTH.

mucilloid   A thick, sticky, gluelike preparation resembling mucilage.

mucin   Any mucoprotein secreted by cells which raises the viscosity of the medium around them.

mucinase   Any of several enzymes that break down glycosaminoglycans. They break glycoside bonds either by hydrolysis or by elimination reactions.

mucinemia   The presence of mucin in blood, a condition that may occur in metastatic malignancies of the gastrointestinal tract or the ovaries. Also called *myxemia*.

mucinoblast   A precursor of a mucin-secreting cell.

mucinolytic   Capable of breaking down mucoproteins or glycosaminoglycans.

mucinosis [MUCIN + -OSIS] An abnormal accumulation of mucopolysaccharides in the skin.

follicular mucinosis   An inflammatory disorder characterized clinically by infiltrated cutaneous plaques, with scaling and loss of hair. Histologically it is manifested by the accumulation of acid mucopolysaccharides in the sebaceous glands and the outer root sheath of the hair follicle.

papular mucinosis   LICHEN MYXEDEMATOSUS.

mucinous   Characterized by or containing mucin.

mucinuria [MUCIN + -URIA] The presence of mucin in the urine, a condition which may reflect contamination from the vagina.

muciparous   MUCIGENOUS.

mucitis   MUCOSITIS.

mucivorous [*muc(o)*- + *i* + L *vor(are)* to devour, swallow + -OUS] Subsisting on mucus, as microbes.

Muckle [Thomas James *Muckle*, Canadian pediatrician, flourished 20th century] Muckle-Well syndrome. See under SYNDROME.

muco- [L *mucus*] A combining form meaning mucus, mucous.

mucoalbuminous   Having both a watery and mucoid consistency.

mucoantibody   Antibody present on a mucous surface, as of the bronchial tree or in the intestinal lumen. These antibodies are predominantly secretory IgA and are found mixed with the mucous secretion of the membrane concerned. They form the immunologic component of the mucosal barrier protecting the mucosal surfaces from infectious agents. A seldom used term.

mucobuccal   Pertaining to the mucous membrane lining the cheek.

mucocartilage   Cartilaginous tissue with a soft mucoid matrix, as is found in the central nucleus pulposus of the intervertebral disk.

mucocele [MUCO- + -CELE[1]] **1** A retention cyst of a mucous gland.   **2** Distension with mucus of a mucous membrane-lined organ or compartment of the body (for example, the gallbladder, appendix, frontal sinus) as the result of acquired atresia of its duct or lumen.

ethmoid sinus mucocele   A mucocele seeming to have its origin in the ethmoid air cells. It is among the more common paranasal sinus mucoceles.

frontal sinus mucocele   A mucocele of the frontal sinus. It is the most common of the paranasal sinus mucoceles and, in neglected cases, liable to reach such a size as to displace an eye or even destroy the function of that eye.

frontoethmoid mucocele   A large mucocele occupying both the frontal sinus and the anterior part of the ethmoid labyrinth. It probably arises in the frontal sinus and expands into the adjacent ethmoid cells by destroying the intervening bony walls. The majority of large mucoceles in the frontal region, particularly those which displace the orbital contents, fall into this category.

lacrimal mucocele   A mucocele of the lacrimal sac, presenting as a swelling at the inner canthus of the eye under the medial palpebral ligament. It must be distinguished from a mucocele of the anterior ethmoidal cells which presents above the medial palpebral ligament.

maxillary sinus mucocele   Mucocele of the maxillary sinus, a rare variety of paranasal sinus mucocele. Also called *antracele, antrocele*.

nasolacrimal duct mucocele   A mucocele expanding the nasolacrimal duct but not involving the lacrimal sac. It is an exceedingly rare occurrence.

paranasal sinus mucocele　A mucocele arising in any one of the paranasal sinuses. It is a rare occurrence of uncertain cause, and includes the frontal sinus and frontoethmoidal mucoceles as the more common varieties, in which acquired atresia of the frontonasal duct is a constant finding. Also called *serous sinusitis* (incorrect).

sphenoid sinus mucocele　Mucocele of the sphenoid sinus. It is an exceptionally rare paranasal sinus mucocele.

suppurating mucocele　A mucocele containing pus.

mucoclasis [MUCO- + -CLASIS]　The surgical removal or destruction of the inner lining of any hollow organ.

mucocolpos [MUCO- + Gk *kolpos* bosom, uterus, fold]　The accumulation of mucus in the vagina.

mucocutaneous [MUCO- + CUTANEOUS]　Pertaining to the skin and mucous membranes. Also *cutaneomucosal*.

mucocyst [MUCO- + CYST]　A saclike extension below the pellicle of certain ciliates with a mucoid content that is expelled upon stimulation to form a protective covering. The mucocyst originates in the endoplasm.

mucocyte [MUCO- + -CYTE]　An amorphous extracellular basophilic, metachromatic mass averaging 100 μ in diameter found in the white matter of normal and abnormal brains. It is believed to be artefactual and derived from precipitation of a component of myelin in the process of tissue fixation.

mucoderm [MUCO- + -DERM]　LAMINA PROPRIA MUCOSAE.

mucodermal　Of or relating to the lamina propria mucosae.

mucoepidermoid　Showing characteristics of both a mucussecreting and an epidermal cell type of epithelial structure: used especially in describing tumor differentiation.

mucofibrous　MYXOID.

mucoflocculent　Of or relating to a colloidal suspension in which mucus constitutes the semisolid phase.

mucogingival [MUCO- + GINGIVAL]　Pertaining to the junction between the gingival mucosa and the alveolar mucosa.

mucohemorrhagic　MUCOSANGUINEOUS.

mucoid　**1** Resembling or having the characteristics of mucus. **2** Describing the glistening appearance of a bacterial colony, often associated with excessive uptake of water by the polysaccharides in the cell envelope. **3** An acid-soluble glycoprotein. An obsolete term.

mucolemma [MUCO- + Gk *lemma* husk, skin, scale]　A layer of mucin 65–130 micrometers thick, that covers the fertilized ovum of the rabbit during its passage along the fallopian tube.

mucolipidosis [MUCO- + LIPIDOSIS]　Any inborn error of metabolism that has clinical and cytologic characteristics of both the mucopolysaccharidoses and the sphingolipidoses. Four distinct conditions, designated mucolipidoses I through IV, have been labeled on the basis of a classification first proposed by Spranger and Wiedemann in 1970. The distinctions have limited utility, however, because of extensive biochemical and pathogenic diversity. Also called *lipomucopolysaccharidosis*. Abbreviation: ML

mucolipidosis I　A now largely abandoned entity based on disorders of glycoprotein metabolism that were seen in patients who had clinical features of both mucopolysaccharide and glycolipid storage disease.

mucolipidosis II　An inborn error of post-translational modification of lysosomal enzymes. The autosomal recessive phenotype is obvious in infancy and is characterized by coarse facies, severe growth and mental retardation, dysostosis multiplex, and death by age 5 years. The basic defect involves UDP-*N*-acetylglucosamine:lysosomal enzyme *N*-acetylglucosaminylphosphotransferase, an enzyme that attaches sugar groups to enzymes

stored in lysosomes. Also called *I-cell disease*.

mucolipidosis III　An inborn error in the post-translational modification of multiple lysosomal enzymes. The phenotype is similar to but milder than those of mucopolysaccharidosis IH and mucolipidosis II (ML II). Patients have an intracellular deficit and an increased serum level of most lysosomal hydrolases. The basic defect in some patients is the same as in ML II, suggesting that the defects are allelic. Genetic heterogeneity has been found *in vitro* among patients with this condition. Also called *pseudo-Hurler polydystrophy, pseudo-Hurler's disease*.

mucolipidosis IV　A diverse group of conditions that share features of mucopolysaccharide and glycolipid storage diseases, often accompanied by an autosomal recessive defect in a ganglioside-specific, nonlysosomal neuraminidase. An imprecise usage.

mucolytic　Having the property of liquifying or breaking down mucus.

mucomembranous　Of or relating to a mucous membrane.

muconic acid　HOOC—CH=CH—CH=CH—COOH.　A compound found in the urine of animals, such as rabbits and dogs, after experimental ingestion of benzene.

mucopeptide　Any glycosylated peptide derived from a mucoprotein. Its carbohydrate component normally has alternate residues of aminosugars and uronic acids.

mucoperiosteum　A mucous membrane that is applied directly to a layer of periosteum, as is seen in the petrous temporal bone, nasal cavities, and air sinuses. Adjective: mucoperiosteal.

mucopoiesis [MUCO- + -POIESIS]　The formation of mucus. Also called *myxopoiesis*.

mucopolysaccharide　GLYCOSAMINOGLYCAN.

mucopolysaccharidoses　Plural of MUCOPOLYSACCHARIDOSIS.

mucopolysaccharidosis [MUCO- + POLYSACCHARIDE + -OSIS]　Any of the inborn errors of mucopolysaccharide metabolism, each of which is due to deficiency of a specific degradative, lysosomal enzyme and characterized by mucopolysacchariduria, short stature, and dysostosis multiplex. Also called *polydystrophic dwarfism*.

mucopolysaccharidosis I　An autosomal recessive inborn error of mucopolysaccharide metabolism due to a deficiency of α-iduronidase. Depending on the severity of the symptoms, the syndrome is designated mucopolysaccharidosis IH, mucopolysaccharidosis IH/S, or mucopolysaccharidosis IS.

mucopolysaccharidosis IH　An autosomal recessive inborn error of mucopolysaccharide metabolism due to a deficiency of α-iduronidase and characterized by progressive mental retardation and physical deterioration, short stature, coarse facies, corneal clouding, dysostosis multiplex, restricted joint mobility, and death by the mid-second decade as a result of pulmonary or cardiac complications. Also called *Hurler syndrome, gargoylism* (outmoded), *lipochondrodystrophy (outmoded and inaccurate), Hurler-Pfaundler syndrome* (outmoded). Abbreviation: MPS IH

mucopolysaccharidosis IH/S　An autosomal recessive inborn error of mucopolysaccharide metabolism caused by a deficiency of α-iduronidase and characterized by a phenotype intermediate to those of MPS IH and MPS IS. Intelligence is usually subnormal and death due to pulmonary complications occurs in the third or fourth decade. Some cases may represent genetic compounds between MPS IH and MPS IS alleles while others are homozygotes for other alleles at the α-iduronidase locus on chromosome 22. Also called *Hurler-Scheie syndrome, Hurler-Scheie compound*. Abbreviation: MPS IH/S

mucopolysaccharidosis IS　An autosomal recessive inborn error of mucopolysaccharide metabolism due to deficiency of α-iduronidase and characterized by corneal clouding, progressive arthropathy that particularly affects the hip, mild dysostosis multiplex, and aortic valvular disease. Although biochemically indistinguishable from MPS IH, its features are much milder and intelligence is often normal. Also called *Scheie syndrome.* Abbreviation: MPS IS

mucopolysaccharidosis II An X-linked recessive inborn error of mucopolysaccharide metabolism caused by a deficiency of iduronate-sulfate sulfatase, with a phenotype distinguishable from MPS IH only by the absence of affected females and the absence of corneal clouding. There is a mild form, with normal intelligence, which is presumably due to an allelic mutation. Also called *Hunter syndrome, X-linked recessive gargoylism* (outmoded).

mucopolysaccharidosis III A group of autosomal recessive inborn errors of mucopolysaccharide metabolism that are all characterized by coarse facies, hirsutism, mild dysostosis multiplex, and profound mental retardation. The four types, which can be distinguished only by enzyme assay, are: IIIA, a deficiency of heparan sulfate sulfatase; IIIB, a deficiency of *N*-acetyl-α-D-glucosaminidase; IIIC, a deficiency of acetyl-CoA:α-glucosaminidase *N*-acetyltransferase; and IIID, a deficiency of *N*-acetyl-glucosamine-6-sulfate sulfatase. Also called *Sanfilippo syndrome.*

mucopolysaccharidosis IV An autosomal recessive inborn error of mucopolysaccharide metabolism characterized by corneal clouding, short stature particularly involving the vertebral column, keratosulfaturia, odontoid hypoplasia, and aortic valvular disease. At least two distinct enzyme deficiencies produce this phenotype: galactosamine-6-sulfatase deficiency results in enamel hypoplasia, and β-galactosidase deficiency results in a milder phenotype with normal enamel. Also called *Morquio syndrome, Morquio-Suarez syndrome, Morquio-Ullrich syndrome, familial osteochondrodystrophy, eccentrochondro-osteodystrophy, osteochondrodystrophia, osteochondrodystrophia deformans, eccentro-osteochondrodysplasia, Morquio's disease, Morquio-Ullrich disease, Morquio's dystrophy.*

mucopolysaccharidosis V A mucopolysaccharidosis that is no longer considered to be a distinct entity. See under MUCOPOLYSACCHARIDOSIS IS.

mucopolysaccharidosis VI An autosomal recessive inborn error of mucopolysaccharide metabolism due to deficiency of arylsulfatase B, characterized by severe dysostosis multiplex, corneal clouding, aortic valvular disease, and urinary excretion of chondroitin sulfate. Severe, mild, and intermediate forms occur, presumably due to allelic variation at the arylsulfatase locus on chromosome 5. Also called *Maroteaux-Lamy syndrome.*

mucopolysaccharidosis VII An autosomal recessive inborn error of mucopolysaccharide metabolism due to deficiency of β-glucuronidase. The phenotype is variable, but dysostosis multiplex, hepatosplenomegaly, mental retardation, and granular inclusions in polymorphonuclear leukocytes have been consistent features. Also called *Sly syndrome.*

mucopolysacchariduria [*mucopolysaccharid(e)* + -URIA] The excretion of mucopolysaccharides in the urine, a feature of mucopolysaccharidosis.

mucoprotein One of several substances whose solutions are highly viscous and which often have lubricant function. They are glycoproteins, more specifically proteoglycans, i.e. ones whose carbohydrate parts are polysaccharides, usually composed of alternate resides of hexosamine and of uronic acid, and often esterified with sulfate.

Tamm-Horsfall mucoprotein A large glycoprotein produced by the renal epithelial cells lining Henle's loop, the distal convoluted tubule, and the collecting ducts. A normal constituent of urine, it precipitates in conditions of retarded flow, high urine

concentration, and abnormal concentrations of albumin, and it constitutes the matrix of most urinary casts.

mucopurulent Denoting an exudate composed of pus and mucus. Also *puromucous* (obsolete).

mucopus An exudate composed of pus and mucus. Also called *mycopus* (obsolete).

Mucor [L (from *mucere* to be moldy), mold] A genus of zygomycetous fungi which grow saprophytically on a variety of substrates, including foodstuffs and soil, and some of which are human pathogens that cause mucormycosis.

Mucor corymbifer An obsolete term for *ABSIDIA CORYMBIFERA.*

Mucor mucedo A species best known for causing food deterioration.

Mucor pusillus A species known to cause mucormycosis.

Mucor racemosus A species isolated from mucormycosis lesions but not considered the primary etiologic agent.

Mucor ramosus A species reported from human infections but rarely seen.

Mucor rhizopodiformis A species of fungus known to cause mucormycosis when experimentally introduced in animals and also known as a natural cause of bovine abortion. Natural infection is either by ingestion or inhalation of spores from moldy feed. Many animal species, including birds, are susceptible.

Mucoraceae [MUCOR + -ACEAE] A family of fungi, some of which are causal agents of mucormycosis and otomycosis. Important genera include *Mucor, Chlamydomucor, Actinomucor, Absidia, Zygorhynchus, Rhizopus, Circinella,* and *Phycomyces.*

mucoraceous Related to or encompassed by the fungal family, Mucoraceae.

Mucorales [MUCOR + L *-ales,* pl. of *-alis* -AL] An order of mainly saprophytic fungi, a few of which are known for synthesizing commercially usable products such as acids. A few genera are known to cause mucormycosis of humans and domestic animals.

mucormycosis [L *mucor* moldiness, mustiness + MYCOSIS] An infection by one of several genera of fungi, notably *Rhizopus, Mucor,* and *Absidia.* The disease is most often manifested in the head including the nose and sinuses, and in the facial and cranial areas. Also called *zygomycosis, phycomycosis, phycomycetosis, phycomycotic infection.*

mucosa [L (fem. of *mucosus* mucous, from *mucus* mucus), alone or with *membrana* membrane: mucous membrane] TUNICA MUCOSA.

alveolar mucosa The nonkeratinized mucosa which covers the alveolar process of the mandible or maxilla apical to the attached gingiva.

buccal mucosa The stratified squamous epithelium and underlying connective tissue layer that lines the inner aspect of the cheek.

endocervical mucosa The mucus-secreting columnar epithelium and underlying connective tissue layer that lines the cervical canal of the uterus.

gingival mucosa The mucosa of the gingiva.

labial mucosa The stratified squamous epithelium and underlying connective tissue layer that covers the inner surface of both lips and extends as far forward as the vermilion border.

laryngeal mucosa A respiratory epithelium and underlying connective tissue layer that lines the larynx.

masticatory mucosa Mucous membrane involved in masticatory activity, comprising the hard palate, gingivae, edentulous ridges, and the dorsum of the tongue.

muscular mucosa A thin layer of smooth muscle that marks the deep margin of the mucosa in the stomach, small intestine, and large intestine.

olfactory mucosa The mucous membrane that lines the roof of the nasal cavity and contains the olfactory cells and their supporting cells.

oral mucosa   The moist integument lining of the oral cavity.

palatine mucosa   The mucosa which covers the roof of the mouth. Also called *palatine membrane*.

pharyngeal mucosa   A nonkeratinizing stratified squamous epithelium and underlying connective tissue layer that lines the pharynx.

respiratory mucosa   A ciliated columnar cell epithelium, which contains goblet cells, and an underlying connective tissue layer that line the respiratory tract.

tracheal mucosa   A respiratory epithelium and its underlying connective tissue layer that line the trachea.

mucosa of the vagina   The stratified squamous mucosal lining of the vagina.

mucosal   Pertaining to the tunica mucosa.

mucosalpinx [MUCO- + Gk *salpinx* tube]   A dilated, closed fallopian tube containing mucus.

mucosanguineous   Containing both mucus and blood. Also *mucohemorrhagic*.

mucosedative   A drug or therapeutic agent that produces a soothing effect on mucus-bearing surfaces.

mucoserous   Of or relating to the production of both mucin and proteinaceous secretions.

mucosin   Mucus of a particularly sticky or tenacious variety that is found especially in the upper respiratory tract and uterine cervix.

mucositis [*mucos(a)* + -ITIS]   An inflammation localized to a mucous membrane. An obsolete term. Also called *mucitis*.

mucositis necroticans agranulocytica   Inflammation of a mucous membrane accompanied by marked necrosis and associated with agranulocytosis. An obsolete term.

radiation mucositis   Mucous membrane inflammation following exposure to ionizing radiation. For example, inflammation of the rectal mucosa may follow pelvic irradiation.

mucosocutaneous   Of or related to the transition from a mucous membrane to the skin.

mucostatic   Having the effect of reducing or arresting the secretion of mucus.

mucotome [MUCO- + -TOME]   An instrument similar to a dermatome, used to harvest mucous membrane for transplantation.

Castroviejo mucotome   A small, electrically powered dermatome used to harvest mucosal grafts from the inner surface of the lips or cheeks. It has shims which are used to adjust the thickness of the graft. Also called *Castroviejo dermatome*.

mucous   Of or relating to mucus or to the production of mucin. Also *muculent*.

mucoviscidosis   CYSTIC FIBROSIS.

mucro [L (gen. *mucronis*, akin to *pugio* a dagger and to Gk *amyssein* to tear, wound), a sharp point, point or edge of a sword, sword]   In anatomy, the pointed end, or tip, of a structure or an organ.

mucro baseos cartilaginis arytaenoideae   An outmoded term for PROCESSUS VOCALIS.

mucro cordis   An outmoded term for APEX CORDIS.

mucro sterni   An outmoded term for PROCESSUS XIPHOIDEUS.

mucronate   Possessing or pertaining to a sharp pointed tip or end.

mucroniform [L *mucro*, gen. *mucronis*, a sharp point, sword + -FORM]   Pointed or spinelike.

muculent   MUCOUS.

mucus [L (akin to *emunctus*, past part of *emungere* to blow the nose, and to Gk *myxa* mucus, phlegm), mucus]   A viscid secretion of mucous membranes. Also called *blenna*.

cervical mucus   The secretion from the columnar epithelium

lining the upper portion of the uterine cervical canal.

nasal mucus   The secretions of the glands and goblet cells of the mucous membrane lining the nose and paranasal sinuses.

Muellerius [after Fritz *Mueller*, German zoologist, 1882–1897]   A genus of hair lung-worms (phylum Nematoda) in the family Protostrongylidae. *M. capillaris* is an important species frequently found in sheep, goats, and deer. It is found in the smaller bronchi and lung parenchyma, and is relatively nonpathogenic to its host. Also *Müllerius*.

Muench [Hugo *Muench*, U.S. physician and statistician, 1894–1972]   Reed and Muench method. See under METHOD.

muffle   A chamber used in a furnace or other heating apparatus to protect material from direct contact with the flame or other heat source.

muguet   A French term for THRUSH.

muhinyo   A local name used in Uganda for BRUCELLOSIS.

mulaire [L *mul(us)* mule + French *-aire* -AR]   A skin lesion, seen in cases of verruga peruana, that begins subcutaneously and leads to the breakdown of the overlying tissue, forming an ulcer.

Mulder [Johannes *Mulder*, Dutch anatomist, 1769–1810]   See under ANGLE.

mule [L *mul(us)* mule]   **1** The sterile hybrid offspring that results from crossing a male ass and a female horse.   **2** Any sterile hybrid.

Mules [Philip Henry *Mules*, English ophthalmologist, 1843–1905]   **1** See under OPERATION.   **2** Mules scoop. See under EVISCERATION SCOOP.

muliebria [L (substantive from *muliebria*, neut. pl. of *muliebris* female, pertaining to women), female genitalia]   The female genitalia. An outmoded term.

muliebris   Pertaining to a female; feminine.

muliebrity [Late L *muliebr(itas)* (from *muliebr(is)* pertaining to womanhood + *-itas* -ITY) the state of being a woman]   **1** The sum of the attributes peculiar to the female sex; femininity.   **2** The taking on of female characteristics by the male; effemination.

mull [Short for *mulmul*, an Indian term for muslin, from Hindi *malmal* muslin, probably from Persian]   A thin cloth made of cotton or similar material and impregnated with ointment or other medication for dressings.

plaster mull   A sheet of muslin coated with gutta-percha. It is used as a dressing in the treatment of skin conditions.

salve mull   Soft cotton or muslin cloth impregnated with an ointment.

Müller [Friedrich von *Müller*, German physician, 1858–1941]   See under SIGN.

Müller [Fritz *Müller*, German naturalist, 1821–1897]   Müller-Haeckel law. See under RECAPITULATION THEORY.

Müller [Heinrich *Müller*, German anatomist, 1820–1864]   **1** See under MUSCLE.   **2** Müller's fibers. See under FIBER.   **3** Müller cells. See under SUSTENTACULAR CELLS.

Müller [Hermann F. *Müller*, German histologist, 1866–1898]   **1** See under FLUID.   **2** Formol-Müller fluid. See under ORTH SOLUTION.

Müller [Johann Friedrich Theodor *Müller*, German zoologist, 1821–1897]   Müllerian mimicry. See under MIMICRY.

Müller [Johannes Peter *Müller*, German anatomist, physiologist, and pathologist, 1801–1858]   **1** Müller's tubercle. See under MÜLLERIAN TUBERCLE.   **2** Ganglion of Müller. See under GANGLION SUPERIUS NERVI GLOSSOPHARYNGEI.   **3** Müllerian duct, ductus Mülleri, Müller's canal. See under PARAMESONEPHRIC DUCT.   **4** See under TUMOR.   **5** Müller's law. See under LAW OF SPECIFIC IRRITABILITY.   **6** Vieth-Müller horopter. See under HOROPTER.   **7** Müller capsule, müllerian capsule. See under CAPSULA GLOMERULI.   **8** Müller's maneuver. See under EXPERIMENT.

Müller [Peter *Müller*, German obstetrician, 1836–1922] Müller-Hillis maneuver. See under MANEUVER.

Müller [Walther *Müller*, German physicist, flourished 20th century]   **1** Geiger-Müller counter. See under GEIGER COUNTER. **2** Geiger-Müller survey meter. See under METER.   **3** Side-window Geiger-Müller tube. See under TUBE.   **4** Halogen-quenched Geiger-Müller tube. See under TUBE.   **5** Geiger-Müller tube. See under TUBE.

muller   A type of pestle with a flattened bottom that is used to crush drugs on a flat surface or slab of the same type of material as the pestle.

müllerianoma [*müllerian (duct)* + -OMA]   A tumor arising from the müllerian duct.

Müllerius   MUELLERIUS.

mulling [MULL¹ + -ING]   The kneading of a dental amalgam to complete the mixing process after the dental alloy and mercury have been ground in a mortar. It is not necessary if an amalgam mixer is used.

multangular   Having many angles.

multangulum [neut. of L *multangulus* (from *multus* much, in pl. many + *angulus* a corner, angle) many-cornered, many-angled]   A bone possessing numerous angles.
 multangulum majus   An outmoded term for OS TRAPEZIUM.
 multangulum minus   An outmoded term for OS TRAPEZOIDEUM.

multi- [L *multus* many, much]   A combining form meaning many, more than one, much.

multiallelic   Characterized by multiple allelic variants, as a genetic locus.

multiarticular   Of or pertaining to many joints. Also *polyarticular*.

multicapsular   Encased by many layers of outer coat.

multicell   A tissue or organism which is composed of many cells.

multicellular   Composed of many cells. Also *polycellular*.

Multiceps [MULTI- + L *-ceps*, combining form of *caput* the head]   A genus of tapeworms of the family Taeniidae. The larval forms (coenuri) are found in herbivores, and those of some species occasionally infect humans. The mature worms generally inhabit the intestines of carnivores.
 Multiceps multiceps   A species of tapeworm which in the adult form is found in the intestines of dogs, foxes, and jackals. The cyst (sometimes called *Coenurus cerebralis*) occurs in the brains of sheep, cattle, horses, and other herbivorous animals, where it causes motor defects, or staggers. There have been reports of human infection in subcutaneous tissues and muscles and of space-occupying lesions in the brain and spinal cord. It is likely that some of these infections may involve *M. serialis* or other *Multiceps* species.
 Multiceps serialis   A species which in the mature form is found in the intestines of dogs. The coenurus larvae occur in the tissues of rabbits, and occasional reports of tissue infection of humans are recorded.

multicipital   Possessing many heads, as of origins of a muscle.

multiclonal   POLYCLONAL.

multicontaminated   Contaminated by more than one kind of contaminant or infective agent.

multicore / multicores in muscle   A variant of central core disease of muscle in which many skeletal muscle fibers contain several cores. See also CENTRAL CORE DISEASE OF MUSCLE.

multicostate   Possessing many ribs.

multicuspidate   **1** Possessing more than two cusps.   **2** MOLAR².

multidentate   Possessing many teeth or toothlike processes.

multidetermination   OVERDETERMINATION.

multidigitate   Possessing many digits or digitate processes.

multifactorial   Relating to many factors and their interactions.

multifetation [MULTI- + FETATION]   The development of more than one fetus within the uterus.

multifid   Divided into many parts or segments.

multiflagellate   Having more than two flagella.

multifocal   Pertaining to or arising from many foci. Also *plurifocal*.

multiform   Having many shapes.

multiganglionate   Having many ganglia.

multiganglionic   Relating to, characterized by, or affecting many ganglia.

multigesta [MULTI- + L *gesta*, fem. of *gestus*, past part. of *gerere* to produce, bear]   MULTIGRAVIDA.

multiglandular   PLURIGLANDULAR.

multigravida [MULTI- + L *gravida* (fem. of *gravidus* laden, full) pregnant; as substantive, a woman with child]   A woman who has been pregnant more than once. Also called *multigesta, plurigravida*.
 grand multigravida   A woman who has been pregnant six or more times.

multihallucalism   MULTIHALLUCISM.

multihallucism   A form of polydactyly characterized by the presence of more than one great toe on one or both feet. Also called *multihallucalism*.

multihematinic   A medication promoting formation of red blood cells and containing several components effective for this purpose, such as various iron salts, certain vitamins, and trace metals that facilitate iron absorption.

multi-infarct   A number of areas of cell death resulting directly from impairment of blood supply, usually due to vascular disease.

multi-infection [MULTI- + INFECTION]   An infection caused by more than one kind of organism; mixed infection.

multilobar   Possessing many lobes.

multilobular   Possessing many lobules. Also *polylobular*.

multilocular   Possessing many compartments or cells. Also *plurilocular, multiloculate*.

multiloculate   MULTILOCULAR.

multimammae   POLYMASTIA.

multimer [MULTI- + Gk *mer(os)* part]   A substance whose molecule consists of many identical units.

multinodal   Possessing many nodes.

multinodular   Possessing many nodules.

multinuclear [MULTI- + NUCLEAR]   Having two or more nuclei in a common protoplasmic mass. Also *multinucleated, plurinuclear, polynuclear, polynucleated*.

multinucleated   MULTINUCLEAR.

multipara [MULTI- + L *par(ere)* to bear or bring forth young + *a*]   A woman who has carried more than one pregnancy to a stage of viability, regardless of whether all gestations resulted in a live-born infant. Also called *pluripara*.
 grand multipara   A woman who has carried at least six pregnancies to a viable stage.

multiparity [MULTIPAR(A) + -ITY]   The condition of being multiparous. Also called *pluriparity*.

multiparous [*multipar(a)* + -OUS]   **1** Having carried more than one pregnancy to a viable stage.   **2** Producing more than one offspring during the same gestation.

multipartite Composed of or having many parts or lobes; multilobar. Also *pluripartite*.

multipenniform MULTIPENNATE MUSCLE.

multiphasic Composed of or performed in several separate phases.

multiple 1 Involving more than one, as *multiple birth*. 2 Existing concurrently in several or numerous parts of the body.

multiplexer A device which permits transmission of two or more signals over one line. A time-division multiplexer uses a multiposition electronic switch for time-sharing by alternating the signals. A frequency-division multiplexer transmits signals simultaneously in different frequency bands.

multiplicitas [Late L (from L *multiplex*, gen. *multiplicis*, manifold + *-itas* -ITY), multiplicity] A developmental defect characterized by supernumerary organs or parts.

multiplicitas cordis The presence of one or more accessory or supernumerary hearts.

multiplier 1 An instrument that performs arithmetic multiplication by digital or analog means. 2 An instrument that increases mechanical force or electrical current or voltage.

photoelectric multiplier PHOTOMULTIPLIER TUBE.

multipolar 1 Denoting a cell having a mitotic spindle with more than two poles. This may result from polyspermy and usually results in aberrant chromosome distribution. 2 Denoting a cell having a number of cytoplasmic processes, as a neuron with an axon and numerous dendrites. For defs. 1 and 2 also *pluripolar*.

multipollicalism MULTIPOLLICISM.

multipollicism [MULTI- + L *pollex*, gen. *pollicis*, the thumb, great toe + -ISM] A form of polydactyly characterized by the presence of more than one thumb on one or both hands. Also called *multipollicalism*.

multipolypoid Pertaining to or characterized by multiple polyps.

multiprocessor A computer network of two or more processors capable of simultaneous execution of two or more programs as in a time-sharing operation.

multirooted Denoting teeth with two or more roots.

multisensitivity A state of sensitivity to more than one allergen.

multiseptate Having several septa or crosswalls: used especially of complex fungal conidia.

multisynaptic Denoting a physiological event or neuroanatomical pathway involving more than two neurons.

multisystem Involving more than one bodily system, as a disease.

multiterminal Having several terminals for accommodating several electrodes.

multituberculate Possessing many tubercles.

multivalent 1 Possessing a valence of a fairly high value, at least two. 2 Denoting the repression of the biosynthesis of a protein by several substances, all of which are needed for maximal repression. For defs. 1 and 2 also *polyvalent*.

mumbling In neurology, any of various movements of the lips, tongue, and jaws, such as chewing, often producing indefinable sounds. It is seen in orofacial dyskinesia or in the attacks of temporal lobe epilepsy.

mu-meson A subatomic particle having a mass equal to 207 times the mass of the electron, and a charge of either plus or minus one. Also called *muon*.

mummification [*mummy* (from French *momie* preserved corpse, from Arabic *moumia, mūmiyah* mummy, bitumen) + L *-ficatio* -FICATION] Dessication of the whole or a part such that it resembles a mummy, as in dry gangrene.

fetal mummification The process of absorption of fluid from a dead fetus and its conversion to a dried state suggesting mummification. Also called *mummification of the fetus*.

mummification of the fetus FETAL MUMMIFICATION.

mummification of pulp 1 Dry gangrene of the pulp of a tooth. 2 A method of endodontic treatment in teeth of which the radicular pulp cannot be completely removed because of extreme curvature or other obstruction. The parts of the pulp which cannot be removed are treated with paraformaldehyde or other mummifying agents.

mummying An outmoded technique of physical restraint in which the entire body is enveloped by a sheet.

mumps [pl. of English dialect *mump* a grimace] An acute generalized infection with a paramyxovirus, which occurs most frequently in school-age children and is characterized by fever, malaise, and parotitis. Complications include aseptic meningitis, encephalitis, pancreatitis, and in postpubertal patients, epididymoorchitis or oophoritis. The disease is endemic world-wide and often occurs epidemically, especially in closed communities. A live attenuated mumps vaccine is available. Also called *epidemic parotitis, angina parotidea* (obsolete).

iodine mumps A toxic hypersensitivity or idiosyncratic reaction to iodine therapy resulting in enlargement of salivary and lacrimal glands.

metastatic mumps A complication of mumps in which the virus infects various glands and organs of the body, particularly the meninges, testes, ovaries, pancreas, or mammary glands.

mumu [Samoan, red] Acute recurrent episodes of inflammation of the tissues of the spermatic cord, sometimes with swelling of the scrotum, epididymis, and testicle, probably occurring as an allergic manifestation of microfilarial infection.

Münchhausen [Baron Karl Friedrich Hieronymus Freiherr von *Münchhausen*, German hunter and soldier, 1720–1797] See under MUNCHAUSEN SYNDROME.

Münchmeyer [Ernst *Münchmeyer*, German physician, 1846–1880] Münchmeyer's disease, Münchmeyer syndrome. See under MYOSITIS OSSIFICANS PROGRESSIVA.

Munch-Peterson [Carl J. *Munch-Peterson*, Danish neurologist, born 1896] Munch-Peterson encephalomyelitis. See under REDLICH'S ENCEPHALOMYELITIS.

mundificant Having the ability to cleanse or heal.

munity [Middle English *munitie*, shortened from *immunitie*, from L *immunitas* exemption from a public duty, immunity] A condition of particular susceptibility to infection.

Munro [John Cummings *Munro*, U.S. surgeon, 1858–1910] See under POINT.

Munro [William John *Munro*, Australian dermatologist, flourished late 19th century] Munro's abscesses. See under MUNRO'S MICROABSCESSES.

Munro Kerr [John Martin *Munro Kerr*, U.S. gynecologist and obstetrician, born 1868] See under MANEUVER.

Munsell [Albert Henry *Munsell*, U.S. painter, 1858–1918] Munsell's colors. See under COLOR.

muon [contraction of *mu-(mes)on*] MU-MESON.

mural [L *mural(is)* (from *mur(us)* wall + *-alis* -AL) pertaining to a wall] In anatomy, of or relating to the wall of a cavity.

muramic acid 2-Amino-3-]($1R$)-1-carboxyethyl]-2-deoxyglucose. An ether formed between lactic acid and glucosamine. It occurs in bacterial cell walls, usually *N*-acetylated, in a β1-4-linked structure alternating with residues of *N*-acetylglucosamine, and cross-linked through peptides attached to the carboxyl group of the lactic acid residue.

muramidase An obsolete term for LYSOZYME.

Murat [Louis *Murat*, French physician, born 1874] See under SIGN.

Murchison [Charles *Murchison*, English physician, 1830–1879]
Murchison-Pel-Ebstein fever. See under PEL-EBSTEIN FEVER.

murein The rigid layer of the bacterial cell wall, consisting of a single sacculus in which the peptidoglycan chains are covalently cross-linked both within a layer and between layers. In some Gram-negative organisms a lipoprotein of the outer membrane is also covalently linked to peptidoglycan. Also called *basal wall* (outmoded).

murein hydrolase An enzyme that hydrolyzes the bond between the lactyl carboxyl of muramic acid and the N terminus of the tetrapeptide in murein. The enzyme has been useful in analyzing peptidoglycan structure, and it plays a role in shaping the cell.

Murel A proprietary name for valethamate bromide.

Muret [Paul-Louis *Muret*, French physician, born 1878] Quénu-Muret sign. See under SIGN.

Murex [L, a sharp-pointed shellfish from which Tyrian dye was obtained] A genus of mollusks that produces an acetylcholine-related neurotoxin.

Murex purpurea A mollusk, the source of a neurotoxic substance, tyrian purple, once used as a remedy for uterine diseases.

murexide The purple-red ammonium salt of purpuric acid, a pyrimidine dimer formed by the action of nitric acid on purines, especially uric acid. A seldom used term. See also MUREXIDE TEST.

murexine β-(4-Imidazolyl)acrylcholine. A potent nicotinic and curariform compound present in the hypobranchial body of the marine gastropod *Murex trunculus* and related species.

muriate An ionic chloride. An obsolete term.

muriatic acid HYDROCHLORIC ACID.

Muridae [L *mus*, gen. *muris*, mouse + -IDAE] The large and diverse family of rodents that includes Old World rats and mice. Characteristic features are a long, scaly tail and absence of premolars. They are generally nocturnal. They are widely distributed in the tropical and temperate Old World.

murine [L *mus*, gen. *muris*, mouse + -INE] Of or pertaining to the rodent family Muridae, comprising rats and mice, as in *murine pneumonia*.

Murless [Brian Charles *Murless*, South African obstetrician, flourished 20th century] See under EXTRACTOR.

murmur

murmur [L, a murmur] A prolonged or continuous auscultatory sound, particularly one deriving from the heart or cardiovascular system. Also called *susurrus, susurration*.

accidental murmur A transient murmur of no pathological significance. Also called *incidental murmur*.

amphoric murmur A sound as of air blowing over the neck of a jar heard during auscultation over a lung cavity.

anemic murmur Cardiac murmur heard in anemia, usually a pulmonary midsystolic murmur. Also called *blood murmur, hemic murmur*.

aneurysmal murmur A murmur heard over an aneurysm.

aortic murmur A murmur arising from a disorder of the aortic valve or aorta.

apical murmur A murmur heard in the apical region of the heart.

apical diastolic murmur A diastolic murmur in the apical region of the heart.

arterial murmur A murmur or bruit heard over an artery, often associated with stenosis or aneurysm.

atriosystolic murmur A murmur caused by atrial systole, usually presystolic in timing.

attrition murmur PERICARDIAL RUB.

Austin Flint murmur An apical mid-diastolic or presystolic murmur in aortic regurgitation. Austin Flint originally described the murmur as presystolic and "blubbering." Also called *Flint's murmur*.

basal diastolic murmurs Murmurs heard at the base of the heart due to aortic or pulmonary regurgitation.

bellows murmur A systolic-diastolic murmur suggestive of the sound of a bellows. Also called *to-and-fro murmur*.

blood murmur ANEMIC MURMUR.

brain murmur Murmur heard over the skull in cases of cerebrovascular abnormalities.

bronchial murmur See under BRONCHIAL BREATHING.

Cabot-Locke murmur An early diastolic murmur heard at the left lower sternal edge in anemia.

cardiac murmur A murmur arising from the heart.

cardiopulmonary murmur A sound heard during auscultation of the chest which is related to breathing but is modified by the beating of the heart. Also called *cardiorespiratory murmur*.

cardiorespiratory murmur CARDIOPULMONARY MURMUR.

Carey Coombs murmur An apical mid-diastolic murmur occurring in the acute phase of rheumatic fever but disappearing thereafter and not due to mitral stenosis.

Cole-Cecil murmur The diastolic murmur of aortic regurgitation when heard, particularly or predominantly, in the left axilla.

continuous murmur A murmur which continues from a systole into diastole. Most characteristic of persistent ductus arteriosus, it occurs in other disorders in which there is an arteriovenous shunt, such as arteriovenous fistulae and aortopulmonary septal defect, and also when there is prolonged flow through a stenosis as in some cases of coarctation of the aorta and pulmonary arterial stenosis.

cooing murmur A murmur resembling the cooing of a dove.

crescendo murmur A murmur which increases in loudness and is then abruptly terminated, such as the presystolic murmur of mitral stenosis which terminates with the onset of the first heart sound.

Cruveilhier-Baumgarten murmur A venous murmur heard over the veins in the abdominal wall when there are anastomoses between the veins of the portal and caval systems.

diamond-shaped murmur A murmur of the ejection type which increases and decreases in such a way as to produce a diamond-shaped appearance on the phonocardiogram.

diastolic murmur A murmur occurring at some time in the interval between the second heart sound and the first heart sound.

double murmur of Duroziez DUROZIEZ MURMUR.

Duroziez murmur A to-and-fro murmur heard over a major peripheral artery, particularly the femoral, in cases of aortic regurgitation. Also called *double murmur of Duroziez*.

dynamic murmur A murmur of functional type, such as that encountered in anemia or other high-flow states, as opposed to organic murmurs such as those caused by valvular abnormalities.

ejection murmur A murmur caused by the ejection of blood from one or the other ventricle into the related great artery.

exocardial murmur EXTRACARDIAC MURMUR.

expiratory murmur A sound heard during exhalation in auscultation of the lungs.

extracardiac murmur A murmur arising outside the heart, as in a pericardial murmur or cardiorespiratory murmur. Also called *exocardial murmur*.

Flint's murmur   AUSTIN FLINT MURMUR.

Fraentzel murmur   The mid-diastolic and presystolic murmur of mitral stenosis, in which the middle portion is softer than the beginning and end.

friction murmur   PERICARDIAL RUB.

functional murmur   A murmur occurring in a structurally normal heart, either in the absence of any abnormality or as a result of such conditions as anemia, thyrotoxicosis, or pregnancy. Also called *physiologic murmur.*

Gibson's murmur   The continuous murmur of a persistent ductus arteriosus.

Graham Steell's murmur   The murmur of pulmonary regurgitation, usually associated with pulmonary hypertension, particularly as a consequence of mitral stenosis. Also called *Steell's murmur.*

Hamman's murmur   A rough crunching sound heard with the heartbeat over the precordium in the presence of mediastinal emphysema or pneumopericardium during auscultation of the chest. Also called *Hamman sign.*

hemic murmur   ANEMIC MURMUR.

Hodgkin-Key murmur   The early diastolic murmur heard in prolapse of an aortic cusp.

holodiastolic murmur   A murmur occupying the whole of diastole.

holosystolic murmur   A murmur lasting the whole of systole, that is, from the first heart sound to the second heart sound. Also called *pansystolic murmur.*

hourglass murmur   A murmur which on a phonocardiographic record has an hourglass appearance, being loud at onset and at termination but softer in between.

humming-top murmur   VENOUS HUM.

incidental murmur   ACCIDENTAL MURMUR.

innocent murmur   Murmur occurring in the absence of organic heart disease. Also called *inorganic murmur.*

inorganic murmur   INNOCENT MURMUR.

inspiratory murmur   A sound heard during inspiration on auscultation of the lungs.

late systolic murmur   A murmur occurring in the latter part of systole, often associated with a click and due to mitral valve prolapse.

machinery murmur   A continuous, machinelike, rumbling murmur such as is encountered in persistent ductus arteriosus.

mid-diastolic murmur   A murmur occurring in the mid-portion of diastole, characteristically appearing in mitral stenois immediately after the opening snap. It may also occur in atrial myxoma and in conditions in which there is a high flow through the mitral valve shortly after its opening, as in some cases of mitral regurgitation and ventricular septal defect.

mill wheel murmur   A splashing auscultatory sound heard in the chest, suggestive of that made by a mill wheel. It may be of cardiac, pericardial, or pleural origin. Also called *waterwheel murmur, waterwheel sound, bruit de moulin.*

mitral murmur   A murmur heard in the mitral area.

muscle murmur   The sound produced by a contracting muscle.

musical murmur   A cardiac murmur having a musical quality.

nun's murmur   VENOUS HUM.

obstructive murmur   A murmur heard in the presence of valvular stenosis.

organic murmur   A murmur resulting from organic disease of the heart or a blood vessel.

pansystolic murmur   HOLOSYSTOLIC MURMUR.

pericardial murmur   PERICARDIAL RUB.

physiologic murmur   FUNCTIONAL MURMUR.

presystolic murmur   A murmur occurring immediately before the first heart sound, that is, during atrial systole but immediately prior to ventricular systole. It is particularly associated with mitral stenosis and tricuspid stenosis.

pulmonary murmur   PULMONIC MURMUR.

pulmonic murmur   A murmur occurring as a consequence of a disorder of the pulmonary valve or pulmonary artery. Also called *pulmonary murmur.*

regurgitant murmur   A murmur occurring in association with regurgitation through a valvular orifice.

Roger's murmur   A murmur occurring in the maladie de Roger; a holosystolic murmur at the left sternal edge due to a small ventricular septal defect.

sea gull murmur   A murmur suggesting the raucous call of a gull, occurring in some cases of aortic regurgitation associated with prolapse or rupture of an aortic cusp.

seesaw murmur   A to-and-fro murmur, likened to the sound of a seesaw.

short systolic murmur   A murmur occurring in only a small part of systole.

Steell's murmur   GRAHAM STEELL'S MURMUR.

stenosal murmur   A murmur resulting from stenosis of an artery or cardiac valve.

Still's murmur   An innocent murmur of twanging quality, heard to the left of the sternum in children.

systolic murmur   A murmur occurring during a part or the whole of systole. Also called *systolic bruit.*

to-and-fro murmur   BELLOWS MURMUR.

transmitted murmur   A sound conducted to a location remote from the site of production.

Traube's murmur   GALLOP RHYTHM.

tricuspid murmur   A murmur deriving from disease at the tricuspid valve.

vascular murmur   A murmur heard over a blood vessel.

venous murmur   A murmur heard over a vein.

vesicular murmur   The normal sound of breathing heard during auscultation of the chest.

waterwheel murmur   MILL WHEEL MURMUR.

Murphy [James Bumgardner *Murphy*, U.S. pathologist, 1884–1950] Murphy-Sturm lymphosarcoma. See under LYMPHOSARCOMA.

Murphy [John Benjamin *Murphy*, U.S. surgeon, 1857–1916] See under DRIP, PUNCH, SIGN, METHOD, BUTTON, TEST, TREATMENT.

Murphy [William Parry *Murphy*, U.S. physician, born 1892] Minot-Murphy treatment. See under TREATMENT.

Murri [Augusto *Murri*, Italian physician, 1841–1932] See under DISEASE.

murrina [Spanish *morriña* murrain] A South American form of animal trypanosomiasis corresponding to what is more generally known as surra. It is caused by *Trypanosoma evansi* and is transmitted by vampire bats as well as by the tabanid vectors that are usual elsewhere. Also called *derrengadera.*

Mus [L, a mouse, rat; akin to Gk *mys* a mouse, muscle] A cosmopolitan genus of rodents of the Muridae family; the house mice. Characteristic features are a flat skull, sparse hair on the tail, fur that is soft to rough and light brown to dark gray, and 10 or 12 mammae. It is a common experimental animal.

Musca [L, a fly; akin to Gk *myia* a fly] A genus of flies of the family Muscidae in which the mouth parts are adapted for sponging and lapping. They are generally dull in color and of small to medium size. They are synanthropic in habits and noxious as filth feeders and as mechanical spreaders of bacterial and other infectious agents of human and animal disease. They include the houseflies.

Musca autumnalis The face fly, a common housefly pest in Europe, parts of Asia, Africa, and North America. In North

America it causes irritation and reduces feeding in domestic animals by its habit of hovering about the face.

Musca domestica The common housefly, which is predominantly gray, has four dark stripes on the dorsal thorax and is 6 to 9 mm long. It occurs wherever humans congregate and human waste and debris are found. Breeding in organic waste and filth, it is a mechanical vector of many pathogens.

Musca domestica nebulo An Indian subspecies of the housefly.

Musca domestica vicina A subspecies that is found in Egypt, the Middle East, and India, and is a notorious pest frequently seen on the faces of children. Also called *Musca vicina*.

Musca luteola *AUCHMEROMYIA LUTEOLA*.

Musca sorbens A species common in Africa, southern Asia, Indonesia, and many Pacific islands. It is thought to transmit conjunctivitis, trachoma, and other fly-borne infections.

Musca vicina *MUSCA DOMESTICA VICINA*.

Musca vomitoria *CALLIPHORA VOMITORIA*.

musca (*plural* muscae) A fly; a housefly. A Latin term.

muscae hispanicae CANTHARIDES.

muscae volitantes Entoptic floating spots perceived visually due to opacities, suspended within the vitreous humor, which cast shadows on the retina. Also called *mouches volantes, opplotentes*.

muscacide MUSCICIDE.

muscae Plural of MUSCA.

muscarine [L *muscarius* relating to flies, from *musca* a fly + -*in*, -INE] A toxic alkaloid derived from *Amanita muscaria* and other fungi. Its molecules consist of a tetrahydrofuran ring carrying methyl, hydroxyl, and trimethylammoniomethyl substituents. It binds to some of the receptors for acetylcholine in the nervous system (muscarinic receptors), mainly in the autonomic nervous system.

muscarinic Denoting the biologic actions of acetylcholine that mimic those of muscarine.

muscarinism [*muscarin(e)* + -ISM] Poisoning from ingestion of muscarine, a poisonous alkaloid present in *Amanita muscaria* in minute amounts, and in *Inocybe* and *Clitocybe* in larger amounts. It causes nausea, vomiting, lacrimation, bradycardia, circulatory collapse, coma, and occasionally death.

muscegenetic [L *musc(a)e*, pl. of *musca* a fly + GENETIC] Producing muscae volitantes.

muscicide [*Musci(dae)* + -CIDE] An agent destructive to flies. Also called *muscacide*.

Muscidae [*Musc(a)* + -IDAE] A family of flies (order Diptera) that includes the genera *Musca* (houseflies), *Stomoxys* (stable flies), *Fannia* (lesser house flies, latrine flies), *Muscina* (false stable flies), *Hydrotaea, Atherigona, Ophyra, Morella* (sweat flies), and others.

Muscina A genus of dung-breeding, nonbiting stable flies in the family Muscidae, related to the houseflies *(Musca)* and having similar habits.

Muscina stabulans A species of fly that is a generalized feeder, utilizing decomposing organic matter and dead and living insects; the false stable fly. It is a facultative parasite implicated in traumatic myiases, including sheep strike.

muscle

muscle [French, from L *musculus* muscle. See MUSCULUS.] A basic tissue of the body, the cells of which are characteristically contractile, enabling movement to take place; musculus. Three types are usually described: striated muscle, cardiac muscle, and nonstriated muscle. See also MUSCULUS SKELETI, CARDIAC MUSCLE, SMOOTH MUSCLE.

abductor muscle of great toe MUSCULUS ABDUCTOR HALLUCIS.

abductor muscle of little finger MUSCULUS ABDUCTOR DIGITI MINIMI MANUS.

abductor muscle of little toe MUSCULUS ABDUCTOR DIGITI MINIMI PEDIS.

accessory muscle An additional muscle slip not usually present, often being a variant of the usual attachments of a muscle. Occasionally it represents a muscle better developed in animals other than humans.

accessory flexor muscle MUSCULUS QUADRATUS PLANTAE.

accessory zygomaticus minor muscle An occasional muscle fasciculus of the musculus orbicularis oculi that joins the musculus zygomaticus minor.

adductor muscle of great toe MUSCULUS ADDUCTOR HALLUCIS.

adductor muscle of thumb MUSCULUS ADDUCTOR POLLICIS.

Aeby's muscle 1 A muscle located in the lips of the mouth and composed of fibers passing obliquely between the skin and the mucous membrane of the inner margin and somewhat at right angles to the fibers of musculus orbicularis oris. It is better developed in infants than in adults. Also called *musculus cutaneomucosus, compressor muscle of lip, Bovero's muscle, Klein's muscle, cutaneomucous muscle*. 2 MUSCULUS DEPRESSOR LABII INFERIORIS.

agonistic muscle AGONIST.

Albinus muscle 1 MUSCULUS RISORIUS. 2 MUSCULUS SCALENUS MINIMUS. 3 A triangular muscle band extending between the side of the nose and the nasolabial furrow.

anconeus muscle MUSCULUS ANCONEUS.

antagonistic muscle A muscle that either opposes the action of a prime mover or initiates and maintains an opposite movement, thereby either controlling the action of the prime mover, neutralizing its contraction, or stabilizing or fixating a joint so that other prime movers may act on it. Also called *antagonist*.

anterior auricular muscle MUSCULUS AURICULARIS ANTERIOR.

anterior intertransverse muscles An outmoded term for MUSCULI INTERTRANSVERSARII THORACIS.

anterior intertransverse muscles of neck MUSCULI INTERTRANSVERSARII ANTERIORES CERVICIS.

anterior papillary muscle of left ventricle MUSCULUS PAPILLARIS ANTERIOR VENTRICULI SINISTRI.

anterior papillary muscle of right ventricle MUSCULUS PAPILLARIS ANTERIOR VENTRICULI DEXTRI.

anterior sacrococcygeal muscle MUSCULUS SACROCOCCYGEUS VENTRALIS.

anterior scalene muscle MUSCULUS SCALENUS ANTERIOR.

anterior serratus muscle MUSCULUS SERRATUS ANTERIOR.

anterior tibial muscle MUSCULUS TIBIALIS ANTERIOR.

antigravity muscles Muscles whose tonic state opposes the force of gravity and maintains the posture of an animal. Also called *postural muscles*.

muscle of antitragus MUSCULUS ANTITRAGICUS.

appendicular muscle Any one of the skeletal muscles of a limb.

arrector muscles of hair MUSCULI ARRECTORES PILORUM.

articular muscle MUSCULUS ARTICULARIS.

articular muscle of elbow MUSCULUS ARTICULARIS CUBITI.

articular muscle of knee MUSCULUS ARTICULARIS GENUS.

aryepiglottic muscle MUSCULUS ARYEPIGLOTTICUS.

aryvocalis muscle of Ludwig ARYVOCALIS.

muscles of auditory ossicles MUSCULI OSSICULORUM AUDITUS.

axial muscle Any one of the skeletal muscles of the trunk or head.

Bell's muscle A band of oblique muscle fibers arising behind each ostium ureteris in the base of the bladder, descending along each side of the trigone towards the dorsum of the prostate, and inserting into the median lobe of the prostate by a fibrous band.

biceps muscle of arm MUSCULUS BICEPS BRACHII.

biceps muscle of thigh MUSCULUS BICEPS FEMORIS.

bicipital muscle A muscle with two heads of origin, such as the biceps brachii.

bipennate muscle MUSCULUS BIPENNATUS.

bipenniform muscle MUSCULUS BIPENNATUS.

Bochdalek's muscle MUSCULUS TRITICEOGLOSSUS.

Bovero's muscle AEBY'S MUSCLE.

Bowman's muscle MUSCULUS CILIARIS.

brachial muscle MUSCULUS BRACHIALIS.

brachioradial muscle MUSCULUS BRACHIORADIALIS.

Braune's muscle MUSCULUS PUBORECTALIS.

bronchoesophageal muscle MUSCULUS BRONCHOESOPHAGEUS.

Brücke's muscle The external part of the ciliary muscle, composed of meridional, or longitudinal, fibers. Also called *Crampton's muscle.*

buccinator muscle MUSCULUS BUCCINATOR.

buccopharyngeal muscle PARS BUCCOPHARYNGEA MUSCULI CONSTRICTORIS PHARYNGIS SUPERIORIS.

bulbar muscles MUSCULI BULBI.

bulbocavernous muscle MUSCULUS BULBOSPONGIOSUS.

canine muscle MUSCULUS LEVATOR ANGULI ORIS.

cardiac muscle The involuntary but striated muscle constituting the myocardium of the heart and situated in all its walls and in those of the pulmonary veins and superior vena cava. The muscle fibers are composed of several individual cells joined end to end by cell junctions, or intercalated disks, and usually containing a single nucleus. In addition, they consist of myofibrils, sarcoplasm, and sarcolemma. Between the fibers is the endomysium, containing small blood vessels and lymphatics. The fibers contract rhythmically and automatically. Also called *textus muscularis striatus cardiacus.*

Casser's muscle LIGAMENTUM MALLEI ANTERIUS.

casserian muscle LIGAMENTUM MALLEI ANTERIUS.

Casser's perforated muscle MUSCULUS CORACOBRACHIALIS.

ceratocricoid muscle MUSCULUS CERATOCRICOIDEUS.

ceratopharyngeal muscle PARS CERATOPHARYNGEA MUSCULI CONSTRICTORIS PHARYNGIS MEDII.

cervicopubic muscle Smooth muscle fibers in the pelvic fascia connecting the cervix of the uterus to the pubis, and probably to part of musculus pubovaginalis. An outmoded term.

cervicorectal muscle An outmoded term for MUSCULUS RECTOUTERINUS.

Chassaignac's axillary muscle A variation of the pectorodorsalis muscle in which a muscle slip extends from the lower border of the latissimus dorsi muscle across the axilla and over the coracobrachialis muscle to either the brachial fascia or the lower border of the pectoralis minor muscle.

cheek muscle MUSCULUS BUCCINATOR.

chondroglossus muscle MUSCULUS CHONDROGLOSSUS.

chondrohumeralis muscle An accessory muscular slip occasionally found arising either from one or two rib cartilages, from the thoracic fascia deep to the pectoralis major muscle, or from its lower margin, and extending down the inner side of the arm to either the brachial fascia, the intertubercular groove, or the medial epicondyle. It is commonly found in many lower mammals.

chondropharyngeal muscle PARS CHONDROPHARYNGEA MUSCULI CONSTRICTORIS PHARYNGIS MEDII.

ciliary muscle 1 MUSCULUS CILIARIS. 2 RIOLAN'S MUSCLE.

circular Santorini's muscles The innermost circular fibers of the sphincter urethrae muscle. An outmoded term.

circumpennate muscle A muscle in which the fasciculi arise from surrounding bones and fasciae and converge obliquely towards a centrally situated tendon in a fanlike fashion. Also called *circumpennate.*

coccygeal muscle MUSCULUS COCCYGEUS.

coccygeal muscles MUSCULI COCCYGEI.

coccygeofemoralis muscle An uncommon variant of the gluteus maximus muscle in which some fasciculi may extend from the coccyx to the linea aspera, or from the sacrotuberous ligament to the fascia lata.

Coiter's muscle MUSCULUS CORRUGATOR SUPERCILII.

common extensor muscle of digits An outmoded term for MUSCULUS EXTENSOR DIGITORUM.

common extensor muscle of thumb and index finger An inconstant muscle that results from a doubling of the extensor indicis muscle, one tendon inserting on the dorsum of the index finger and the other on the dorsum of the thumb.

compressor bulbi proprius muscle The middle fibers of the bulbospongiosus muscle that encircle the bulb and adjacent posterior part of the corpus spongiosum penis. An outmoded term.

compressor muscle of lip AEBY'S MUSCLE.

compressor muscle of naris PARS TRANSVERSA MUSCULI NASALIS.

congenerous muscles Muscles that perform the same function.

coracobrachial muscle MUSCULUS CORACOBRACHIALIS.

costocervicalis muscle MUSCULUS ILIOCOSTALIS CERVICIS.

cowl muscle MUSCULUS TRAPEZIUS.

Crampton's muscle BRÜCKE'S MUSCLE.

cremaster muscle MUSCULUS CREMASTER.

cricoarytenoid muscle Either musculus cricoarytenoideus lateralis or musculus cricoarytenoideus posterior.

cricopharyngeal muscle PARS CRICOPHARYNGEA MUSCULI CONSTRICTORIS PHARYNGIS INFERIORIS.

cricothyroid muscle MUSCULUS CRICOTHYROIDEUS.

cutaneomucous muscle An outmoded term for AEBY'S MUSCLE.

cutaneous muscle MUSCULUS CUTANEUS.

dartos muscle of scrotum MUSCULUS DARTOS.

deep flexor muscle of fingers MUSCULUS FLEXOR DIGITORUM PROFUNDUS.

deep stylohyoid muscle of Sappey An occasional fasciculus of the stylohyoid muscle that extends from the lateral side of the styloid process near its tip to the lesser cornu of the hyoid bone. It has the same action and nerve supply as the stylohyoid muscle.

deep transverse muscle of perineum MUSCULUS TRANSVERSUS PERINEI PROFUNDUS.

deltoid muscle MUSCULUS DELTOIDEUS.

depressor muscle of angle of mouth MUSCULUS DEPRESSOR ANGULI ORIS.

depressor muscle of lower lip MUSCULUS DEPRESSOR LABII INFERIORIS.

depressor muscle of nasal septum MUSCULUS DEPRESSOR SEPTI NASI.

dermal muscle MUSCULUS CUTANEUS.

detrusor urinae muscle MUSCULUS DETRUSOR VESICAE.

detrusor muscle of urinary bladder MUSCULUS DETRUSOR VESICAE.

diaphragmatic muscle DIAPHRAGMA.

digastric muscle MUSCULUS DIGASTRICUS.

dilator muscle of nose PARS ALARIS MUSCULI NASALIS.

dilator muscle of pupil MUSCULUS DILATOR PUPILLAE.

dorsal muscles MUSCULI DORSI.

dorsal interosseous muscles of foot MUSCULI INTEROSSEI DORSALES PEDIS.

dorsal interosseous muscles of hand MUSCULI INTEROSSEI DORSALES MANUS.

dorsal sacrococcygeal muscle MUSCULUS SACROCOCCYGEUS DORSALIS.

Dupré's muscle MUSCULUS ARTICULARIS GENUS.

Duverney's muscle PARS LACRIMALIS MUSCULI ORBICULARIS OCULI.

emergency muscles Muscles that contract to assist prime movers when considerable force is needed.

epicranial muscle MUSCULUS EPICRANIUS.

epimeric muscle A muscle derived from the dorsal part of a myotome, or epimere, and innervated by the dorsal ramus of a spinal nerve.

epitrochleoanconeus muscle An occasional fasciculus, found in about 25% of humans, extending from the back of the medial epicondyle of the humerus to the olecranon process of the ulna by arching over the ulnar nerve, which innervates it by a small branch. It represents an adductor of the olecranon of lower mammals. Also called *musculus epitrochleoanconaeus* (outmoded), *epitrochleo-olecranonis muscle.*

epitrochleo-olecranonis muscle EPITROCHLEOANCONEUS MUSCLE.

erector muscle of penis An outmoded term for MUSCULUS ISCHIOCAVERNOSUS.

erector muscle of spine MUSCULUS ERECTOR SPINAE.

eustachian muscle An outmoded term for MUSCULUS TENSOR TYMPANI.

extensor muscle of fingers MUSCULUS EXTENSOR DIGITORUM.

extensor muscle of index finger MUSCULUS EXTENSOR INDICIS.

extensor muscle of little finger MUSCULUS EXTENSOR DIGITI MINIMI.

external intercostal muscles MUSCULI INTERCOSTALES EXTERNI.

external oblique muscle of abdomen MUSCULUS OBLIQUUS EXTERNUS ABDOMINIS.

external obturator muscle MUSCULUS OBTURATORIUS EXTERNUS.

external pterygoid muscle An outmoded term for MUSCULUS PTERYGOIDEUS LATERALIS.

external sphincter muscle of anus MUSCULUS SPHINCTER ANI EXTERNUS.

extraocular muscles MUSCULI BULBI.

extrinsic muscle A muscle inserted into a structure, part, or organ from without.

muscles of eye MUSCULI BULBI.

facial muscle Any one of the several muscles of the face and scalp that affect the movements of the eyelids, nose, lips, ears, and scalp and are able to produce the various expressions of the face.

muscles of fauces MUSCULI PALATI ET FAUCIUM.

femoral muscle An outmoded term for MUSCULUS VASTUS INTERMEDIUS.

fibulotibialis muscle An accessory variant of the popliteus muscle that occasionally (less than 10%) arises from the medial side of the head of the fibula and is inserted into the posterior surface of the tibia deep to popliteus. Also called *peroneotibialis.*

fixation muscles FIXATOR MUSCLES.

fixator muscles Prime movers and antagonistic muscles acting together either to stabilize the position of a joint or part or to permit other prime movers to act on the joint or part. Also called *fixation muscles.*

fixator muscle of base of stapes MUSCULUS FIXATOR BASEOS STAPEDIS.

Folius muscle An outmoded term for LIGAMENTUM MALLEI LATERALE.

frontal muscle VENTER FRONTALIS MUSCULI OCCIPITOFRONTALIS.

frontalis muscle VENTER FRONTALIS MUSCULI OCCIPITOFRONTALIS.

fusiform muscle MUSCULUS FUSIFORMIS.

gastrocnemius muscle MUSCULUS GASTROCNEMIUS.

Gavard's muscle FIBRAE OBLIQUAE GASTRICAE.

Gegenbaur's muscle AURICULOFRONTALIS.

genioglossus muscle MUSCULUS GENIOGLOSSUS.

geniohyoid muscle MUSCULUS GENIOHYOIDEUS.

glossopalatine muscle MUSCULUS PALATOGLOSSUS.

glossopharyngeal muscle PARS GLOSSOPHARYNGEA MUSCULI CONSTRICTORIS PHARYNGIS SUPERIORIS.

gracilis muscle MUSCULUS GRACILIS.

great adductor muscle MUSCULUS ADDUCTOR MAGNUS.

greater pectoral muscle MUSCULUS PECTORALIS MAJOR.

greater psoas muscle MUSCULUS PSOAS MAJOR.

greater rhomboid muscle MUSCULUS RHOMBOIDEUS MAJOR.

greater zygomatic muscle MUSCULUS ZYGOMATICUS MAJOR.

greatest gluteal muscle MUSCULUS GLUTEUS MAXIMUS.

Gruber's muscle A peroneus accessorius that extends from the peroneus brevis muscle to an insertion on the calcaneus. Also called *peroneocalcaneus externus.*

Guthrie's muscle MUSCULUS SPHINCTER URETHRAE.

Hall's muscle A band of muscle fibers occasionally arising from the ischial tuberosities in common with musculus transversus perinei superficialis and passing forwards and medially to join the bulbospongiosus muscle.

hamstring muscle One of the muscles at the back of the thigh: the semimembranosus, semitendinosus, or biceps femoris.

muscle of Henle MUSCULUS AURICULARIS ANTERIOR.

Hilton's muscle MUSCULUS ARYEPIGLOTTICUS.

Horner's muscle PARS LACRIMALIS MUSCULI ORBICULARIS OCULI.

Houston's muscle **1** Compressor venae dorsalis of the penis. **2** A fasciculus of the ischiocavernosus muscle that occasionally is inserted into the fascia on the dorsum of the penis.

hyoglossal muscle MUSCULUS HYOGLOSSUS.

hyoglossus muscle MUSCULUS HYOGLOSSUS.

muscles of hyoid bone Musculi infrahyoidei and musculi suprahyoidei.

hypaxial muscles The muscles ventral to the vertebral column, such as longus capitis, longus colli, the vertebral portion of the diaphragm, and sacrococcygeus anterior. Also called *subvertebral muscles.*

hypomeric muscle A muscle derived from the ventral, or hypaxial, region of a myotome that migrates anteriorly in the body wall, or somatopleure, and is innervated by a ventral ramus of a spinal nerve.

iliac muscle MUSCULUS ILIACUS.

iliococcygeal muscle MUSCULUS ILIOCOCCYGEUS.

iliocostal muscle MUSCULUS ILIOCOSTALIS.

iliocostal muscle of loins MUSCULUS ILIOCOSTALIS LUMBORUM.

iliocostal muscle of neck MUSCULUS ILIOCOSTALIS CERVICIS.

iliocostal muscle of thorax MUSCULUS ILIOCOSTALIS THORACIS.

iliopsoas muscle MUSCULUS ILIOPSOAS.

incisive muscles of inferior lip MUSCULI INCISIVI LABII IN-
FERIORIS.
incisive muscles of lower lip MUSCULI INCISIVI LABII IN-
FERIORIS.
incisive muscles of superior lip MUSCULI INCISIVI LABII
SUPERIORIS.
incisive muscles of upper lip MUSCULI INCISIVI LABII SU-
PERIORIS.
muscle of incisure of helix MUSCULUS INCISURAE HELICIS.
inferior constrictor muscle of pharynx MUSCULUS CON-
STRICTOR PHARYNGIS INFERIOR.
inferior gemellus muscle MUSCULUS GEMELLUS INFERIOR.
inferior longitudinal muscle of tongue MUSCULUS LONGI-
TUDINALIS INFERIOR LINGUAE.
inferior oblique muscle of eyeball MUSCULUS OBLIQUUS
INFERIOR BULBI.
inferior oblique muscle of head MUSCULUS OBLIQUUS CAP-
ITIS INFERIOR.
inferior pharyngeal constrictor muscle MUSCULUS CON-
STRICTOR PHARYNGIS INFERIOR.
inferior posterior serratus muscle MUSCULUS SERRATUS
POSTERIOR INFERIOR.
inferior rectus muscle of bulb MUSCULUS RECTUS INFERIOR
BULBI.
inferior straight muscle MUSCULUS RECTUS INFERIOR
BULBI.
inferior tarsal muscle MUSCULUS TARSALIS INFERIOR.
inferior thyroarytenoid muscle An outmoded term for MUS-
CULUS VOCALIS.
infrahyoid muscles MUSCULI INFRAHYOIDEI.
infraspinous muscle MUSCULUS INFRASPINATUS.
innermost intercostal muscles MUSCULI INTERCOSTALES
INTIMI.
inspiratory muscles The muscles taking part in quiet, deep
and forced inspiration, including the diaphragm, intercostal,
scalene, pectoral, and erector spinae muscles.
interarytenoid muscles The musculus arytenoideus obliquus
and the musculus arytenoideus transversus.
interbranchial muscle A broad flat deep muscle which is
attached to the outer surface of the elements of the gill bars in
sharks.
intercostal muscle Any of the short voluntary muscles between adjacent ribs.
interfoveolar muscle LIGAMENTUM INTERFOVEOLARE.
internal intercostal muscles MUSCULI INTERCOSTALES IN-
TERNI.
internal oblique muscle of abdomen MUSCULUS OBLIQUUS
INTERNUS ABDOMINIS.
internal obturator muscle MUSCULUS OBTURATORIUS IN-
TERNUS.
internal pterygoid muscle An outmoded term for MUSCULUS
PTERYGOIDEUS MEDIALIS.
internal sphincter muscle of anus MUSCULUS SPHINCTER
ANI INTERNUS.
interspinal muscles MUSCULI INTERSPINALES.
interspinal muscles of loins MUSCULI INTERSPINALES LUM-
BORUM.
interspinal muscles of neck MUSCULI INTERSPINALES CER-
VICIS.
interspinal muscles of thorax MUSCULI INTERSPINALES
THORACIS.
intertransverse muscles MUSCULI INTERTRANSVERSARII.
intertransverse muscles of thorax MUSCULI INTERTRANS-
VERSARII THORACIS.
intra-auricular muscles Musculus stapedius and musculus
tensor tympani.
intraocular muscles The intrinsic muscles of the eyeball, such

as the musculus ciliaris, musculus dilator pupillae, and musculus
sphincter pupillae.
intratympanic muscle Either musculus tensor tympani or
musculus stapedius.
intrinsic muscle A muscle in which both origin and insertion
are contained within the same part or organ.
involuntary muscle Collectively, muscles that are not usually
under the direct control of the will, such as those in the walls
of the alimentary and urogenital tracts and blood vessels. Although cardiac muscle is involuntary it is different in structure
from both skeletal and nonstriated muscle. Also called *nonstriated muscle, smooth muscle, plain muscle, organic muscle*
(outmoded), *visceral muscle, textus muscularis nonstriatus, unstriated muscle.*
iridic muscles The muscles that regulate the iris, namely the
musculus dilator pupillae and the musculus sphincter pupillae.
ischiocavernous muscle MUSCULUS ISCHIOCAVERNOSUS.
Jarjavay's muscle An anomalous muscle derived from the
bulbospongiosus muscle that fuses with the sphincter of the
vagina and may depress the urethra.
Jung's muscle MUSCULUS PYRAMIDALIS AURICULAE.
Klein's muscle AEBY'S MUSCLE.
Landström's muscle Minute peribulbar smooth muscle bundles around the anterior aspect of the eyeball that are attached
to the orbital septum and the palpebral muscles.
Langer's muscle A variation of the pectorodorsalis muscle,
or axillary arch, in which a slip from the tendon of the pectoralis
major muscle extends across the axilla to the insertion of the
latissimus dorsi muscle.
muscles of larynx MUSCULI LARYNGIS.
lateral anconeus muscle An outmoded term for CAPUT LAT-
ERALE MUSCULI TRICIPITIS BRACHII.
lateral cricoarytenoid muscle MUSCULUS CRICOARYTENOI-
DEUS LATERALIS.
lateral gastrocnemius muscle An outmoded term for CAPUT
LATERALE MUSCULI GASTROCNEMII.
lateral intertransverse muscles of loins MUSCULI INTER-
TRANSVERSARII LATERALES LUMBORUM.
lateral pterygoid muscle MUSCULUS PTERYGOIDEUS LATE-
RALIS.
lateral rectus muscle of bulb MUSCULUS RECTUS LATERALIS
BULBI.
lateral straight muscle MUSCULUS RECTUS LATERALIS
BULBI.
latissimus muscle of back MUSCULUS LATISSIMUS DORSI.
latissimus dorsi muscle MUSCULUS LATISSIMUS DORSI.
least gluteal muscle MUSCULUS GLUTEUS MINIMUS.
left pleuroesophageus muscle of Hyrtl A bundle of smooth
muscle that connects the esophagus with the left mediastinal
pleura behind the aorta at the level of the crossing of the esophagus by the left principal bronchus.
lesser rhomboid muscle MUSCULUS RHOMBOIDEUS MINOR.
lesser zygomatic muscle MUSCULUS ZYGOMATICUS MINOR.
levator muscle of angle of mouth MUSCULUS LEVATOR AN-
GULI ORIS.
levator ani muscle MUSCULUS LEVATOR ANI.
levator muscle of prostate MUSCULUS LEVATOR PROSTA-
TAE.
levator muscles of ribs MUSCULI LEVATORES COSTARUM.
levator muscle of scapula MUSCULUS LEVATOR SCAPULAE.
levator muscle of thyroid gland MUSCULUS LEVATOR GLAN-
DULAE THYROIDEAE.
levator muscle of upper eyelid MUSCULUS LEVATOR PAL-
PEBRAE SUPERIORIS.
levator muscle of upper lip MUSCULUS LEVATOR LABII SU-
PERIORIS.
levator muscle of upper lip and ala of nose MUSCULUS

LEVATOR LABII SUPERIORIS ALAEQUE NASI.

levator muscle of velum palatinum MUSCULUS LEVATOR VELI PALATINI.

long abductor muscle of thumb MUSCULUS ABDUCTOR POLLICIS LONGUS.

long adductor muscle MUSCULUS ADDUCTOR LONGUS.

long extensor muscle of great toe MUSCULUS EXTENSOR HALLUCIS LONGUS.

long extensor muscle of thumb MUSCULUS EXTENSOR POLLICIS LONGUS.

long extensor muscle of toes MUSCULUS EXTENSOR DIGITORUM LONGUS.

long fibular muscle MUSCULUS PERONEUS LONGUS.

long flexor muscle of great toe MUSCULUS FLEXOR HALLUCIS LONGUS.

long flexor muscle of little toe The fasciculus of the flexor digitorum longus muscle destined for the little toe that is occasionally separated from the rest of the origin of the muscle on the posterior surface of the tibia and gives the appearance of a separate muscle.

long flexor muscle of thumb MUSCULUS FLEXOR POLLICIS LONGUS.

long flexor muscle of toes MUSCULUS FLEXOR DIGITORUM LONGUS.

long muscle of head MUSCULUS LONGUS CAPITIS.

longissimus muscle MUSCULUS LONGISSIMUS.

longissimus muscle of back An outmoded term for MUSCULUS LONGISSIMUS THORACIS.

longissimus muscle of head MUSCULUS LONGISSIMUS CAPITIS.

longissimus muscle of neck MUSCULUS LONGISSIMUS CERVICIS.

longissimus muscle of thorax MUSCULUS LONGISSIMUS THORACIS.

longitudinal muscle A muscle or muscle mass in which the fibers extend in a lengthwise direction.

long levator muscles of ribs MUSCULI LEVATORES COSTARUM LONGI.

long muscle of neck MUSCULUS LONGUS COLLI.

long palmar muscle MUSCULUS PALMARIS LONGUS.

long peroneal muscle MUSCULUS PERONEUS LONGUS.

long rotator muscles MUSCULI ROTATORES LONGI.

Ludwig's muscle ARYVOCALIS.

lumbrical muscles of foot MUSCULI LUMBRICALES PEDIS.

lumbrical muscles of hand MUSCULI LUMBRICALES MANUS.

Luschka's muscles MUSCULUS RECTOUTERINUS.

muscle of Macallister A medial variant of fibulocalcaneus.

masseter muscle MUSCULUS MASSETER.

masticatory muscle A muscle which is attached to the mandible and moves it during mastication.

medial anconeus muscle An outmoded term for CAPUT MEDIALE MUSCULI TRICIPITIS BRACHII.

medial gastrocnemius muscle An outmoded term for CAPUT MEDIALE MUSCULI GASTROCNEMII.

medial intertransverse muscles of loins MUSCULI INTERTRANSVERSARII MEDIALES LUMBORUM.

medial pterygoid muscle MUSCULUS PTERYGOIDEUS MEDIALIS.

medial rectus muscle of bulb MUSCULUS RECTUS MEDIALIS BULBI.

medial straight muscle MUSCULUS RECTUS MEDIALIS BULBI.

Merkel's muscle MUSCULUS CERATOCRICOIDEUS.

mesothenar muscle An outmoded term for MUSCULUS ADDUCTOR POLLICIS.

middle constrictor muscle of pharynx MUSCULUS CONSTRICTOR PHARYNGIS MEDIUS.

middle gluteal muscle MUSCULUS GLUTEUS MEDIUS.

middle pharyngeal constrictor muscle MUSCULUS CONSTRICTOR PHARYNGIS MEDIUS.

middle scalene muscle MUSCULUS SCALENUS MEDIUS.

Müller's muscle 1 FIBRAE CIRCULARES MUSCULI CILIARIS. 2 MUSCULUS TARSALIS SUPERIOR. 3 MUSCULUS ORBITALIS.

multicipital muscle A muscle with several heads of origin.

multifidus muscles MUSCULI MULTIFIDI.

multipennate muscle A muscle with several tendons between which the fasciculi run obliquely in featherlike fashion, as in the deltoid muscle. Also called *multipenniform, multipenniform muscle.*

multipenniform muscle MULTIPENNATE MUSCLE.

multi-unit muscle A type of smooth muscle in which many cells receive motor terminals from nerve plexuses that initiate contraction, such as in the muscle of the iris and the walls of larger arteries. Compare UNITARY MUSCLE.

mylohyoid muscle MUSCULUS MYLOHYOIDEUS.

mylopharyngeal muscle PARS MYLOPHARYNGEA MUSCULI CONSTRICTORIS PHARYNGIS SUPERIORIS.

nasal muscle MUSCULUS NASALIS.

muscles of neck MUSCULI COLLI.

nonstriated muscle INVOLUNTARY MUSCLE.

oblique arytenoid muscle MUSCULUS ARYTENOIDEUS OBLIQUUS.

oblique muscle of auricle MUSCULUS OBLIQUUS AURICULAE.

obturator externus muscle MUSCULUS OBTURATORIUS EXTERNUS.

obturator internus muscle MUSCULUS OBTURATORIUS INTERNUS.

occipital muscle VENTER OCCIPITALIS MUSCULI OCCIPITOFRONTALIS.

occipitofrontal muscle MUSCULUS OCCIPITOFRONTALIS.

Ochsner's muscle An inconstant circular thickening of the muscular coat of the duodenum just below the opening of the common bile duct into the lumen. It is doubtful if it is a normal structure.

ocular muscles MUSCULI BULBI.

Oddi's muscle MUSCULUS SPHINCTER AMPULLAE HEPATOPANCREATICAE.

Oehl's muscles Muscle fibers occasionally located in the chordae tendineae of the mitral valve.

omohyoid muscle MUSCULUS OMOHYOIDEUS.

opposing muscle of little finger MUSCULUS OPPONENS DIGITI MINIMI.

opposing muscle of thumb MUSCULUS OPPONENS POLLICIS.

orbicular muscle MUSCULUS ORBICULARIS.

orbicular muscle of eye MUSCULUS ORBICULARIS OCULI.

orbicular muscle of mouth MUSCULUS ORBICULARIS ORIS.

orbital muscle MUSCULUS ORBITALIS.

organic muscle An outmoded term for INVOLUNTARY MUSCLE.

muscles of ossicles MUSCULI OSSICULORUM AUDITUS.

muscles of palate and fauces MUSCULI PALATI ET FAUCIUM.

palatoglossus muscle MUSCULUS PALATOGLOSSUS.

palatopharyngeal muscle MUSCULUS PALATOPHARYNGEUS.

palatouvularis muscle An outmoded term for MUSCULUS UVULAE.

palmar interosseous muscles MUSCULI INTEROSSEI PALMARES.

papillary muscles MUSCULI PAPILLARES.

pectinate muscles MUSCULI PECTINATI.

pectineal muscle MUSCULUS PECTINEUS.

pectorodorsalis muscle One of the accessory muscles of the pectoral region of which there are several variants, the more common being Langer's muscle and Chassaignac's axillary muscle. It consists of a slip from the pectoralis major muscle that may either fuse with either the latissimus dorsi or teres major muscle, or extend from latissimus dorsi either to the long tendon of the biceps brachii muscle, to the axillary fascia, or to the coracoid process. It is innervated by one of a number of nerves. Also called *axillary arch, Langer's axillary arch.*

pennate muscle A muscle in which the fasciculi are oblique to the line of pull of the tendon in featherlike patterns that are categorized as unipennate, bipennate, circumpennate, or multipennate. Also called *penniform muscle.*

penniform muscle PENNATE MUSCLE.

perineal muscles MUSCULI PERINEI.

muscles of perineum MUSCULI PERINEI.

peroneus digiti quinti muscle MUSCULUS PERONEUS DIGITI QUINTI.

pharyngopalatine muscle An outmoded term for MUSCULUS PALATOPHARYNGEUS.

Phillips muscle A very inconstant slip of muscle extending from the radial collateral ligament of the wrist and the styloid process of the radius to the phalanges of the thumb.

piriform muscle MUSCULUS PIRIFORMIS.

plain muscle INVOLUNTARY MUSCLE.

plantar muscle MUSCULUS PLANTARIS.

plantar interosseous muscles MUSCULI INTEROSSEI PLANTARES.

platysma muscle PLATYSMA.

pleuroesophageal muscle MUSCULUS PLEUROESOPHAGEUS.

popliteal muscle MUSCULUS POPLITEUS.

postaxial muscle A muscle located caudal to the axial line of an extremity.

posterior auricular muscle MUSCULUS AURICULARIS POSTERIOR.

posterior cricoarytenoid muscle MUSCULUS CRICOARYTENOIDEUS POSTERIOR.

posterior intertransverse muscles of neck MUSCULI INTERTRANSVERSARII POSTERIORES CERVICIS.

posterior papillary muscle of left ventricle MUSCULUS PAPILLARIS POSTERIOR VENTRICULI SINISTRI.

posterior papillary muscle of right ventricle MUSCULUS PAPILLARIS POSTERIOR VENTRICULI DEXTRI.

posterior sacrococcygeal muscle MUSCULUS SACROCOCCYGEUS DORSALIS.

posterior scalene muscle MUSCULUS SCALENUS POSTERIOR.

posterior tibial muscle MUSCULUS TIBIALIS POSTERIOR.

postural muscles ANTIGRAVITY MUSCLES.

Pozzi's muscle MUSCULUS EXTENSOR DIGITORUM BREVIS MANUS.

preaxial muscle A muscle located cranial to the axial line of an extremity.

prevertebral muscles A deep group of muscles situated on the anterior surface of the cervical and first three thoracic vertebrae. They are symmetrically placed on each side of the median plane and comprise the musculus longus capitis, musculus longus colli, musculus rectus capitis anterior, and musculus rectus capitis lateralis. Together they flex the head and the neck. They are innervated by the ventral rami of the cervical nerves. Some authorities also include the scalene muscles in this group.

principal thyroarytenoid muscle An outmoded term for MUSCULUS THYROARYTENOIDEUS.

procerus muscle MUSCULUS PROCERUS.

proper extensor muscle of fifth digit An outmoded term for MUSCULUS EXTENSOR DIGITI MINIMI.

pterygopharyngeal muscle PARS PTERYGOPHARYNGEA MUSCULI CONSTRICTORIS PHARYNGIS SUPERIORIS.

pubicoperitoneal muscle An outmoded term for LIGAMENTUM INTERFOVEOLARE.

pubococcygeal muscle MUSCULUS PUBOCOCCYGEUS.

puboprostatic muscle MUSCULUS PUBOPROSTATICUS.

puborectal muscle MUSCULUS PUBORECTALIS.

puborectalis muscle MUSCULUS PUBORECTALIS.

pubovaginal muscle MUSCULUS PUBOVAGINALIS.

pubovesical muscle MUSCULUS PUBOVESICALIS.

pyramidal muscle MUSCULUS PYRAMIDALIS.

pyramidal muscle of auricle MUSCULUS PYRAMIDALIS AURICULAE.

quadrate muscle of lower lip An outmoded term for MUSCULUS DEPRESSOR LABII INFERIORIS.

quadrate pronator muscle MUSCULUS PRONATOR QUADRATUS.

quadrate muscle of sole MUSCULUS QUADRATUS PLANTAE.

quadrate muscle of thigh MUSCULUS QUADRATUS FEMORIS.

quadrate muscle of upper lip An outmoded term for MUSCULUS LEVATOR LABII SUPERIORIS.

quadriceps femoris muscle MUSCULUS QUADRICEPS FEMORIS.

quadriceps muscle of thigh MUSCULUS QUADRICEPS FEMORIS.

radial flexor muscle of wrist MUSCULUS FLEXOR CARPI RADIALIS.

rectococcygeus muscle MUSCULUS RECTOCOCCYGEUS.

rectourethral muscle MUSCULUS RECTOURETHRALIS.

rectouterine muscle MUSCULUS RECTOUTERINUS.

rectovesical muscle MUSCULUS RECTOVESICALIS.

red muscle Skeletal muscle of dark color, rich in myoglobin and containing numerous mitochondria, characterized by slow contractability. Compare WHITE MUSCLE.

Reisseisen's muscles The smooth muscle fibers of the smallest bronchi and the bronchioles.

retractor muscle Any muscle that draws a limb or body part in toward the body.

ribbon muscles MUSCULI INFRAHYOIDEI.

riders' muscles The adductor muscles of the thigh, used to grip the saddle during horseback riding.

right pleuroesophageus muscle of Treitz A bundle of smooth muscle that connects the lower third of the esophagus with the right mediastinal pleura.

Riolan's muscle **1** The portion of the orbicularis oculi nearest to the eyelid margin. Also called *ciliary muscle.* **2** MUSCULUS CREMASTER.

risorius muscle MUSCULUS RISORIUS.

rotator muscles MUSCULI ROTATORES.

rotator muscles of neck MUSCULI ROTATORES CERVICIS.

rotator muscles of thorax MUSCULI ROTATORES THORACIS.

Rouget's muscle FIBRAE CIRCULARES MUSCULI CILIARIS.

round pronator muscle MUSCULUS PRONATOR TERES.

Ruysch's muscle The musculature of the uterus.

sacrospinal muscle An outmoded term for MUSCULUS ERECTOR SPINAE.

salpingopharyngeal muscle MUSCULUS SALPINGOPHARYNGEUS.

Santorini's muscle **1** MUSCULUS RISORIUS. **2** MUSCULUS INCISURAE HELICIS. **3** A partial band of smooth muscle fibers under the sphincter urethrae.

muscle of Sappey MUSCULUS TEMPOROPARIETALIS.

sartorius muscle MUSCULUS SARTORIUS.

scalene muscles Those muscles that pass from cervical vertebral transverse processes to the first rib. They have been implicated in the development of thoracic outlet syndrome.

Sebileau's muscle The deeper fibers of the tunica dartos that bend inward at the raphe of the scrotum to help form the septum of the scrotum.

semimembranous muscle MUSCULUS SEMIMEMBRANOSUS.

semispinal muscle MUSCULUS SEMISPINALIS.

semispinal muscle of head MUSCULUS SEMISPINALIS CAPITIS.

semispinal muscle of neck   MUSCULUS SEMISPINALIS CERVICIS.

semispinal muscle of thorax   MUSCULUS SEMISPINALIS THORACIS.

semitendinous muscle   MUSCULUS SEMITENDINOSUS.

septal papillary muscles of right ventricle   MUSCULI PAPILLARES SEPTALES VENTRICULI DEXTRI.

shawl muscle   An outmoded term for MUSCULUS TRAPEZIUS.

short abductor muscle of thumb   MUSCULUS ABDUCTOR POLLICIS BREVIS.

short adductor muscle   MUSCULUS ADDUCTOR BREVIS.

short anconeus muscle   An outmoded term for CAPUT LATERALE MUSCULI TRICIPITIS BRACHII.

short extensor muscle of great toe   MUSCULUS EXTENSOR HALLUCIS BREVIS.

short extensor muscle of thumb   MUSCULUS EXTENSOR POLLICIS BREVIS.

short extensor muscle of toes   MUSCULUS EXTENSOR DIGITORUM BREVIS.

short fibular muscle   An outmoded term for MUSCULUS PERONEUS BREVIS.

short flexor muscle of great toe   MUSCULUS FLEXOR HALLUCIS BREVIS.

short flexor muscle of little finger   MUSCULUS FLEXOR DIGITI MINIMI BREVIS MANUS.

short flexor muscle of little toe   MUSCULUS FLEXOR DIGITI MINIMI BREVIS PEDIS.

short flexor muscle of thumb   MUSCULUS FLEXOR POLLICIS BREVIS.

short flexor muscle of toes   MUSCULUS FLEXOR DIGITORUM BREVIS.

short levator muscles of ribs   MUSCULI LEVATORES COSTARUM BREVES.

short palmar muscle   MUSCULUS PALMARIS BREVIS.

short peroneal muscle   MUSCULUS PERONEUS BREVIS.

short radial extensor muscle of wrist   MUSCULUS EXTENSOR CARPI RADIALIS BREVIS.

short rotator muscles   MUSCULI ROTATORES BREVES.

shunt muscles   See under SHUNT MUSCLE THEORY.

Sibson's muscle   MUSCULUS SCALENUS MINIMUS.

skeletal muscle   MUSCULUS SKELETI.

smaller pectoral muscle   MUSCULUS PECTORALIS MINOR.

smaller psoas muscle   MUSCULUS PSOAS MINOR.

smallest adductor muscle   MUSCULUS ADDUCTOR MINIMUS.

smallest scalene muscle   MUSCULUS SCALENUS MINIMUS.

smooth muscle   INVOLUNTARY MUSCLE.

Soemmering's muscle   MUSCULUS LEVATOR GLANDULAE THYROIDEAE.

soleus muscle   MUSCULUS SOLEUS.

somatic muscle   An outmoded term for MUSCULUS SKELETI.

sphincter muscle   MUSCULUS SPHINCTER.

sphincter muscle of bile duct   MUSCULUS SPHINCTER DUCTUS CHOLEDOCHI.

sphincter muscle of hepatopancreatic ampulla   MUSCULUS SPHINCTER AMPULLAE HEPATOPANCREATICAE.

sphincter muscle of membranous urethra   MUSCULUS SPHINCTER URETHRAE.

sphincter muscle of pancreatic duct   MUSCULUS SPHINCTER DUCTUS PANCREATICI.

sphincter muscle of pupil   MUSCULUS SPHINCTER PUPILLAE.

sphincter muscle of pylorus   MUSCULUS SPHINCTER PYLORICUS.

sphincter muscle of urethra   MUSCULUS SPHINCTER URETHRAE.

sphincter muscle of urinary bladder   MUSCULUS SPHINCTER VESICAE URINARIAE.

spinal muscle   MUSCULUS SPINALIS.

splenius muscle of head   MUSCULUS SPLENIUS CAPITIS.

splenius muscle of neck   MUSCULUS SPLENIUS CERVICIS.

spurt muscles   See under SHUNT MUSCLE THEORY.

stapedius muscle   MUSCULUS STAPEDIUS.

sternal muscle   MUSCULUS STERNALIS.

sternocleidomastoid muscle   MUSCULUS STERNOCLEIDOMASTOIDEUS.

sternohyoid muscle   MUSCULUS STERNOHYOIDEUS.

sternomastoid muscle   MUSCULUS STERNOCLEIDOMASTOIDEUS.

sternothyroid muscle   MUSCULUS STERNOTHYROIDEUS.

strap muscles   MUSCULI INFRAHYOIDEI.

striated muscle   MUSCULUS SKELETI. ● Cardiac muscle, though involuntary, is also striated.

striped muscle   MUSCULUS SKELETI.

styloglossus muscle   MUSCULUS STYLOGLOSSUS.

stylohyoid muscle   MUSCULUS STYLOHYOIDEUS.

stylopharyngeus muscle   MUSCULUS STYLOPHARYNGEUS.

subanconeus muscle   MUSCULUS ARTICULARIS CUBITI.

subarcual muscle   A ventral muscle of the gill arch in teleost fishes.

subclavius muscle   MUSCULUS SUBCLAVIUS.

subcostal muscles   MUSCULI SUBCOSTALES.

subcrural muscle   An outmoded term for MUSCULUS ARTICULARIS GENUS.

subquadricipital muscle   An outmoded term for MUSCULUS ARTICULARIS GENUS.

subscapular muscle   MUSCULUS SUBSCAPULARIS.

subvertebral muscles   HYPAXIAL MUSCLES.

superciliary corrugator muscle   MUSCULUS CORRUGATOR SUPERCILII.

superciliary depressor muscle   MUSCULUS DEPRESSOR SUPERCILII.

superficial flexor muscle of fingers   MUSCULUS FLEXOR DIGITORUM SUPERFICIALIS.

superficial transverse muscle of perineum   MUSCULUS TRANSVERSUS PERINEI SUPERFICIALIS.

superior auricular muscle   MUSCULUS AURICULARIS SUPERIOR.

superior constrictor muscle of pharynx   MUSCULUS CONSTRICTOR PHARYNGIS SUPERIOR.

superior gemellus muscle   MUSCULUS GEMELLUS SUPERIOR.

superior longitudinal muscle of tongue   MUSCULUS LONGITUDINALIS SUPERIOR LINGUAE.

superior oblique muscle of eyeball   MUSCULUS OBLIQUUS SUPERIOR BULBI.

superior oblique muscle of head   MUSCULUS OBLIQUUS CAPITIS SUPERIOR.

superior pharyngeal constrictor muscle   MUSCULUS CONSTRICTOR PHARYNGIS SUPERIOR.

superior posterior serratus muscle   MUSCULUS SERRATUS POSTERIOR SUPERIOR.

superior rectus muscle of bulb   MUSCULUS RECTUS SUPERIOR BULBI.

superior tarsal muscle   MUSCULUS TARSALIS SUPERIOR.

superior thyroarytenoid muscle   An occasional narrow muscle that is situated on the lateral surface of the main mass of the thyroarytenoid muscle and extends obliquely from the angle of the thyroid cartilage to the muscular process of the arytenoid cartilage. It helps to regulate the tension of the vocal ligaments and to adduct the vocal cords.

supinator muscle   MUSCULUS SUPINATOR.

supraclavicular muscle   MUSCULUS STERNOCLAVICULARIS.

suprahyoid muscles   MUSCULI SUPRAHYOIDEI.

supraspinous muscle   MUSCULUS SUPRASPINATUS.

suspensory muscle of duodenum   MUSCULUS SUSPENSORIUS DUODENI.

synergic muscle SYNERGISTIC MUSCLE.

synergistic muscle A muscle that complements a prime mover acting across a multiaxial joint or a number of joints by serving as a partial antagonist and permitting the prime mover to maximize its action. For example, in flexion of the fingers, the prime movers act maximally when the carpal extensors contract simultaneously, serving as synergists. Also called *synergic muscle*.

temporal muscle MUSCULUS TEMPORALIS.

temporoparietal muscle MUSCULUS TEMPOROPARIETALIS.

tensor muscle of the choroid FIBRAE MERIDIONALES MUSCULI CILIARIS.

tensor muscle of fascia lata MUSCULUS TENSOR FASCIAE LATAE.

tensor tympani muscle MUSCULUS TENSOR TYMPANI.

tensor muscle of tympanic membrane MUSCULUS TENSOR TYMPANI.

tensor muscle of tympanum MUSCULUS TENSOR TYMPANI.

tensor muscle of velum palatini MUSCULUS TENSOR VELI PALATINI.

teres major muscle MUSCULUS TERES MAJOR.

teres minor muscle MUSCULUS TERES MINOR.

thenar muscles The muscles forming the thenar eminence, namely, abductor pollicis brevis, flexor pollicis brevis, and opponens pollicis.

third fibular muscle An outmoded term for MUSCULUS PERONEUS TERTIUS.

third peroneal muscle MUSCULUS PERONEUS TERTIUS.

thyroarytenoid muscle MUSCULUS THYROARYTENOIDEUS.

thyroepiglottic muscle MUSCULUS THYROEPIGLOTTICUS.

thyrohyoid muscle MUSCULUS THYROHYOIDEUS.

thyropharyngeal muscle PARS THYROPHARYNGEA MUSCULI CONSTRICTORIS PHARYNGIS INFERIORIS.

Tod's muscle MUSCULUS OBLIQUUS AURICULAE.

muscles of the tongue MUSCULI LINGUAE.

tracheal muscle MUSCULUS TRACHEALIS.

trachelomastoid muscle An outmoded term for MUSCULUS LONGISSIMUS CAPITIS.

muscle of tragus MUSCULUS TRAGICUS.

transverse muscle of abdomen MUSCULUS TRANSVERSUS ABDOMINIS.

transverse arytenoid muscle MUSCULUS ARYTENOIDEUS TRANSVERSUS.

transverse muscle of auricle MUSCULUS TRANSVERSUS AURICULAE.

transverse muscle of chin MUSCULUS TRANSVERSUS MENTI.

transverse muscle of nape MUSCULUS TRANSVERSUS NUCHAE.

transverse muscle of thorax MUSCULUS TRANSVERSUS THORACIS.

transverse muscle of tongue MUSCULUS TRANSVERSUS LINGUAE.

transversospinal muscles MUSCULI TRANSVERSOSPINALES.

transversus abdominis muscle MUSCULUS TRANSVERSUS ABDOMINIS.

trapezius muscle MUSCULUS TRAPEZIUS.

muscle of Treitz MUSCULUS SUSPENSORIUS DUODENI.

triangular muscle MUSCULUS DEPRESSOR ANGULI ORIS.

triceps muscle of arm MUSCULUS TRICEPS BRACHII.

triceps muscle of calf MUSCULUS TRICEPS SURAE.

tricipital muscle A muscle with three heads of origin, as the triceps brachii.

ulnar flexor muscle of wrist MUSCULUS FLEXOR CARPI ULNARIS.

unipennate muscle MUSCULUS UNIPENNATUS.

unitary muscle A type of smooth muscle with relatively scanty motor innervation, so that its rhythmic contraction is myogenic in origin, such as in the walls of the uterus, intestines, stomach, and ureter. Compare MULTI-UNIT MUSCLE.

unstriated muscle INVOLUNTARY MUSCLE.

muscle of uvula MUSCULUS UVULAE.

Valsalva's muscle MUSCULUS TRAGICUS.

ventral sacrococcygeal muscle MUSCULUS SACROCOCCYGEUS VENTRALIS.

vertical muscle of tongue MUSCULUS VERTICALIS LINGUAE.

vestigial muscle A muscle that is rudimentary or incompletely developed in humans but fully developed and functional in some lower mammals.

visceral muscle INVOLUNTARY MUSCLE.

vocal muscle MUSCULUS VOCALIS.

volar interosseous muscles An outmoded term for MUSCULI INTEROSSEI PALMARES.

voluntary muscle A muscle that is usually under the direct control of the will. This type of muscle is usually skeletal, and its myofibrils are striated, except for cardiac muscle which, though striated, is involuntary.

white muscle Skeletal muscle of pale color, having little myoglobin and few mitochondria, characterized by fast contractability. Compare RED MUSCLE.

Wilson's muscle Longitudinal bundles of the musculus sphincter urethrae that are not generally accepted to be present.

zygomatic muscle MUSCULUS ZYGOMATICUS MAJOR.

---

muscle-bound Possessing an excessive physical musculature that is functionally suboptimal.

muscle-trimming BORDER MOLDING.

muscoid Of or belonging to the dipteran superfamily Muscoidea, suborder Cyclorrhapha, which includes the many disease-bearing and pestiferous flies of the family Muscidae.

muscular [*muscul(us)* + -AR] Of or relating to structures that have a highly developed contractile function.

muscularis Pertaining to a muscle or muscles, particularly the muscular coat of a tubular structure or hollow organ.

muscularity The state of being muscular or of possessing strong muscles.

muscularize To form into muscle.

musculation The contraction of a muscle.

musculature [French (from L *musculus* a little mouse, a muscle, dim. of *mus* a mouse, rat + L *-atus*, adjectival suffix after verbs ending in *-are* + French *-ure* -URE), the muscular system] **1** The muscle system as a whole or of a part. **2** The arrangement of muscles in a part or an organ.

epaxial musculature The dorsal trunk muscles of a vertebrate.

hypaxial musculature The ventrolateral musculature of the trunk, including the subvertebral flank and ventral abdominal muscles, of most vertebrates.

musculi Plural of MUSCULUS.

musculoaponeurotic Pertaining to a structure that is composed of both muscle and an aponeurosis.

musculocutaneous Pertaining to muscles and skin, especially in reference to certain nerves supplying both muscle and skin. Also *musculodermic* (outmoded), *myocutaneous*.

musculodermic An outmoded term for MUSCULOCUTANEOUS.

musculoelastic Pertaining to or possessing both muscle and elastic tissues.

musculofascial Composed of both muscular and fascial tissues.

musculofibrous Pertaining to tissue that is both muscular and fibrous.

musculointestinal   Pertaining to the muscles and the intestines.

musculomembranous   Pertaining to or possessing both muscle fibers and membrane.

musculophrenic   Pertaining to or supplying muscles and the diaphragm.

musculoplasty [L *muscul(us)* a little mouse, a muscle + *o* + -PLASTY] **1** MASTOID MYOPLASTY. **2** Any operation in which muscle flaps are used for reconstruction.

musculorachidian   Pertaining to the spinal muscles.

musculoskeletal   Pertaining to muscles and the skeleton, as *musculoskeletal system*.

musculospiral   Pertaining to muscles and a spiral direction, especially with reference to nervus radialis.

musculospiralis   A seldom used term for NERVUS RADIALIS.

musculotegumentary   Pertaining to muscle and the integument.

musculotendinous   Pertaining to or comprising both muscle and tendinous fibers.

musculotonic   Denoting the sustained contraction and active tension of a muscle.

musculotropic   Directed to or attracted by muscle tissue.

musculus

musculus [L (dim. of *mus* a mouse, rat; Gk *mys* a mouse, muscle), a little mouse, a muscle] (*plural* musculi) An organ of the body composed of tissue the contraction of which produces motion; muscle. See also MUSCULUS SKELETI, CARDIAC MUSCLE, SMOOTH MUSCLE.

musculi abdominis [NA] The muscles forming the walls, roof, and floor of the abdominal cavity.

musculus abductor digiti minimi Either the musculus abductor digiti minimi manus or the musculus abductor digiti minimi pedis.

musculus abductor digiti minimi manus [NA] A muscle originating from the pisiform bone, pisohamate ligament and the tendon of the flexor carpi ulnaris muscle. It is inserted onto the medial side of proximal phalanx of little finger and the medial border of dorsal expansion of extensor digiti minimi. It is supplied by the ulnar nerve, and abducts the extended little finger. Also called *abductor muscle of little finger, musculus abductor digiti quinti manus* (outmoded).

musculus abductor digiti minimi pedis [NA] A muscle originating from the medial and lateral processes of the calcanean tuberosity and the bone between them, the central portion of plantar aponeurosis, and the lateral intermuscular septum. It is inserted onto the lateral surface of the proximal phalanx of fifth toe. It is supplied by the lateral plantar nerve and abducts and flexes the proximal phalanx of little toe. Also called *abductor muscle of little toe, musculus abductor digiti quinti pedis* (outmoded).

musculus abductor digiti quinti manus An outmoded term for MUSCULUS ABDUCTOR DIGITI MINIMI MANUS.

musculus abductor digiti quinti pedis An outmoded term for MUSCULUS ABDUCTOR DIGITI MINIMI PEDIS.

musculus abductor hallucis [NA] A muscle originating from flexor retinaculum, medial process of calcaneal tuberosity, plantar aponeurosis, and medial intermuscular septum. It is inserted with tendon of flexor hallucis brevis into the base of the proximal phalanx of the great toe. It is supplied by the medial plantar nerve, abducts and flexes the proximal phalanx of hallux, and helps to maintain the medial longitudinal arch. Also called *abductor muscle of great toe.*

musculus abductor pollicis brevis [NA] A muscle originating from flexor retinaculum, and from the tubercles of the trapezium and scaphoid bones. Its medial fibers are inserted into the lateral side of the base of the proximal phalanx of thumb, and its lateral fibers into the dorsal expansion of the extensor pollicis longus muscle. Supplied by the median nerve, it abducts the thumb, rotating it medially; flexes the proximal phalanx; and extends the terminal phalanx. Also called *short abductor muscle of thumb.*

musculus abductor pollicis longus [NA] A muscle originating from the upper middle portion of the lateral part of the posterior surface of the ulna, the adjacent interosseous membrane, and the middle third of the posterior surface of the radius. It is inserted into the lateral side of the base of the first metacarpal bone and the trapezium, and supplied by the posterior interosseous nerve. It abducts the thumb; helps to extend the thumb; and helps to abduct the hand. Also called *long abductor muscle of thumb.*

musculus accelerator urinae An outmoded term for MUSCULUS BULBOSPONGIOSUS.

musculus accessorius gluteus minimus MUSCULUS SCANSORIUS.

musculus adductor brevis [NA] A muscle originating from the medial part of the outer aspect of the body and inferior ramus of pubis. It is inserted by aponeurotic bands into the lower part of the pectineal line and upper third of the linea aspera of femur, behind the insertion of the pectineus and adductor longus muscles. It is supplied by the obturator nerve, and adducts and helps to flex and laterally rotate the thigh. Also called *short adductor muscle, short head of triceps femoris muscle* (outmoded), *breviductor* (obsolete).

musculus adductor hallucis [NA] A muscle of which the caput obliquum originates from the bases of the second, third, and fourth metatarsals, and from the sheath of the tendon of the peroneus longus muscle; and caput transversum from the plantar metatarsophalangeal ligaments of the lateral three toes and deep transverse metatarsal ligaments between them. It is inserted into the lateral part of base of proximal phalanx of hallux and onto the lateral sesamoid bone. It is supplied by the lateral plantar nerve, and adducts and flexes the proximal phalanx of the great toe. Also called *adductor muscle of great toe.*

musculus adductor longus [NA] A muscle originating at the front of the pubis in the angle between the crest and the symphysis pubis. It is inserted into the middle third of linea aspera of femur, fused with the medial intermuscular septum. It is supplied by the anterior division of the obturator nerve, and adducts, flexes, and medially rotates the thigh. Also called *long adductor muscle, long head of triceps femoris muscle* (outmoded), *long head of adductor triceps muscle* (outmoded).

musculus adductor magnus [NA] A muscle originating from the inferior pubic ramus, the ramus of the ischium, and the inferolateral portion of the ischial tuberosity. It is inserted into the medial margin of the gluteal ridge, the distal three-fourths of the linea aspera, the proximal portion of the medial supracondylar line, and the adductor tubercle. It is supplied by the posterior division of the obturator nerve and the tibial division of the sciatic nerve. It adducts, extends, and medially rotates the thigh; and acts synergistically with the other adductors in locomotion and in controlling erect posture. Also called *great adductor muscle, great head of triceps femoris muscle* (outmoded).

musculus adductor minimus The superior portion of the adductor magnus muscle that arises from the inferior pubic ramus and inserts into the medial margin of the gluteal ridge and the upper part of linea aspera. It is supplied by the nerve to quadratus femoris or the obturator nerve. Also called *smallest adductor muscle, third part of quadriceps femoris muscle* (outmoded).

musculus adductor pollicis [NA] A muscle of which the caput obliquum originates from the bases of the second and third metacarpal bones, the capitate, and the palmar ligaments of the carpus; and caput transversum from the distal two-thirds of the palmar ridge of the third metacarpal bone. It is inserted onto the ulnar side of the palmar surface of the base of the proximal phalanx of thumb. It is supplied by the deep branch of the ulnar nerve, adducts and flexes the first metacarpal bone, and flexes the proximal phalanx of the thumb, especially in gripping movements. Also called *adductor muscle of thumb, mesothenar muscle, mesothenar* (outmoded).

musculus anconeus [NA] A muscle originating from the posterior surface of the lateral epicondyle of humerus and the adjacent capsule of the elbow joint. It is inserted into the lateral side of the olecranon and the adjacent posterior surface of the shaft of the ulna. It is supplied by the radial nerve, helps the triceps brachii muscle to extend the elbow joint, and may abduct the ulna in pronation. In many nonhuman primates it is a part of the triceps muscle. Also called *anconeus muscle.*

musculus antitragicus A muscle originating from the outer part of the antitragus and inserted into the cauda helicis and antihelix. It is supplied by the temporal and posterior auricular branches of the facial nerve, and produces very slight, if any, modification of the shape and position of the ear in humans. Also called *muscle of antitragus, antitragicus.*

musculi arrectores pilorum [NA] The muscles that cause the erection of the hairs. Also called *arrector muscles of hair, arrectores pilorum.*

musculus articularis [NA] A muscle that inserts, either partly or completely, into the capsule of a joint, usually in order to lift the capsule in certain movements. Also called *articular muscle.*

musculus articularis cubiti [NA] A muscle that originates by a slip of muscle from the deep surface of the lower part of the triceps brachii muscle. It is inserted into the back of the fibrous capsule of the elbow joint. It is supplied by the radial nerve, and lifts up the back of the capsule of the elbow joint during extension of the forearm. Also called *articular muscle of elbow, subanconeus muscle.*

musculus articularis genu An outmoded term for MUSCULUS ARTICULARIS GENUS.

musculus articularis genus [NA] A muscle originating from the anterior surface of the lower part of the shaft of the femur, and inserted into the upper portion of the synovial membrane of the knee joint. It is supplied by the femoral nerve, and draws up the synovial membrane during extension of the knee joint. Also called *articular muscle of knee, Dupré's muscle, subcrural muscle* (outmoded), *subquadricipital muscle* (outmoded), *musculus articularis genu* (outmoded).

musculus aryepiglotticus [NA] Some fibers of musculus arytenoideus obliquus that extend beyond the lateral side of the apex of the arytenoid cartilage and insert into the aryepiglottic fold. It assists the oblique arytenoid muscle as a sphincter of the inlet of the larynx. It is innervated by the recurrent laryngeal nerve. Also called *aryepiglottic muscle, aryepiglotticus, Hilton's muscle.*

musculus arytenoideus obliquus [NA] Two bands of muscle fibers that cross each other in the form of an X superficial to the transverse arytenoid muscle, each arising from the posterior aspect of the muscular process of an arytenoid cartilage and inserting into the apex of the adjacent arytenoid cartilage. It is supplied by the recurrent laryngeal nerve, and serves as a sphincter of the inlet of the larynx with the help of the aryepiglottic

muscles. Also called *oblique arytenoid muscle.*

musculus arytenoideus transversus [NA] A single muscle arising from the posterior aspect of the muscular process and lateral margin of one arytenoid cartilage and inserting into corresponding parts of the other arytenoid cartilage. It is supplied by the recurrent laryngeal nerve, and by bringing the two arytenoid cartilages together it helps to close the rima glottidis. Also called *transverse arytenoid muscle.*

musculus aryvocalis Some of the deeper fibers of the vocalis muscle that are attached to the vocal ligament, especially posteriorly. An outmoded term.

musculus attollens aurem An outmoded term for MUSCULUS AURICULARIS SUPERIOR.

musculus attollens auriculam An outmoded term for MUSCULUS AURICULARIS SUPERIOR.

musculus attrahens aurem An outmoded term for MUSCULUS AURICULARIS ANTERIOR.

musculus attrahens auriculam An outmoded term for MUSCULUS AURICULARIS ANTERIOR.

musculus auricularis anterior [NA] A muscle originating from the lateral margin of the epicranial aponeurosis, and inserted into the spine of the helix of external ear. It is supplied by the temporal branch of the facial nerve, and pulls the auricle forwards and upwards. Also called *anterior auricular muscle, musculus attrahens aurem* (outmoded), *musculus attrahens auriculam* (outmoded), *attrahens aurem* (outmoded), *muscle of Henle.*

musculus auricularis posterior [NA] A muscle originating from the mastoid process of the temporal bone and inserted into the ponticulus of eminentia conchae. It is supplied by the posterior auricular branch of the facial nerve, and pulls back the auricle. Also called *posterior auricular muscle, musculus retrahens aurem, musculus retrahens auriculam, retrahens aurem* (outmoded).

musculus auricularis superior [NA] A muscle originating from the epicranial aponeurosis and inserted into the upper part of the cartilage of the auricle. It is supplied by the temporal branch of the facial nerve, and pulls the auricle upward. Also called *superior auricular muscle, musculus attollens aurem* (outmoded), *musculus attollens auriculam* (outmoded), *attollens aurem* (outmoded).

musculus biceps brachii [NA] A muscle of which the caput breve originates from the tip of the coracoid process of scapula, and caput longum from the supraglenoid tubercle and the glenoid labrum within the fibrous capsule. It is inserted into the posterior half of the tuberosity of the radius and, by the bicipital aponeurosis, into the deep fascia on the upper medial side of the forearm. It is supplied by the musculocutaneous nerve, supinates and flexes the forearm, and slightly flexes the shoulder joint. Also called *biceps muscle of arm, biceps brachii.*

musculus biceps femoris [NA] A muscle of which the caput longum originates from the superomedial aspect of the ischial tuberosity and the sacrotuberous ligament, and caput breve from the lower half of the lateral lip of linea aspera, the upper two-thirds of the lateral supracondylar line of the femur, and the lateral intermuscular septum. It is inserted into the head of the fibula, the lateral condyle of the tibia, and the fibular collateral ligament. Its caput longum is supplied by the tibial part of the sciatic nerve, and caput breve by the common peroneal. It laterally rotates the leg when the knee is partly flexed, laterally rotates the thigh when the hip is extended, and together with the semitendinosus and semimembranosus it flexes the leg and extends the hip joint. Also called *biceps muscle of thigh, biceps femoris.*

musculus bipennatus [NA] A muscle in which the fasciculi converge obliquely on a central tendon from two sides in a featherlike pattern, as in the rectus femoris and the dorsal interossei. Also called *bipennate muscle, bipenniform muscle.*

musculus brachialis [NA] A muscle originating from the lower half of the front of the humerus, and from the intermuscular septa. It is inserted onto the tuberosity of the ulna and the front of the coronoid process of the ulna. It is supplied by the musculocutaneous and radial nerves, and flexes the forearm. Also called *brachial muscle.*

musculus brachioradialis [NA] A muscle originating from the upper two-thirds of the lateral supracondylar ridge of the humerus and the front of the lateral intermuscular septum. It is inserted into the lateral aspect of the base of the styloid process of the radius and supplied by a branch of the radial nerve containing fibers of the fifth and sixth cervical nerves. It flexes the forearm, especially in the semiprone position, is active in rapid extension of the forearm, and helps in pronation when the forearm is supine and flexed. Also called *brachioradial muscle.*

musculus bronchoesophageus [NA] Inconstant muscle fasciculi extending from the back of the left bronchus to the esophagus. Also called *bronchoesophageal muscle.*

musculus buccinator [NA] A muscle originating from the outer surface of the molar area of the alveolar process of the maxilla and of the mandible, and from the anterior aspect of the pterygomandibular raphe. It is inserted into the orbicularis oris muscle at the angle of the mouth. It is supplied by buccal branches of the facial nerve, flattens the cheeks, and pulls the angle of the mouth laterally. Also called *buccinator muscle, cheek muscle, alveolabialis* (outmoded), *buccinator.*

musculus buccopharyngeus PARS BUCCOPHARYNGEA MUSCULI CONSTRICTORIS PHARYNGIS SUPERIORIS.

musculi bulbi [NA] The muscles inside the orbit that move the eyeball. They include the superior rectus, inferior rectus, lateral rectus, medial rectus, orbital, superior oblique, inferior oblique, and levator palpebrae superioris muscles. Also called *extraocular muscles, muscles of eye, ocular muscles, bulbar muscles, musculi oculi* (outmoded).

musculus bulbocavernosus MUSCULUS BULBOSPONGIOSUS.

musculus bulbospongiosus [NA] A muscle that is located anterior to the anus and composed of symmetrical right and left halves, the attachments of which differ in the two sexes. In the male, it originates from a median raphe that joins the two halves and the central tendon of the perineum, and is inserted into the perineal membrane, an aponeurosis on the superior surfaces of the bulbus penis and corpus spongiosum penis; and the sides of corpus spongiosum penis anterior to the ischiocavernosus muscle and an expansion superficial to the dorsal vessels of the penis. It is supplied by the perineal branch of the pudendal nerve. It compresses the urethra, expelling urine at the end of micturition, and assists in erection of the penis and in ejaculation. In the female, it originates from the central tendon of perineum, blending with the external anal sphincter. It is inserted into the perineal membrane on each side of the vagina lateral to the vestibular bulbs and the sides of corpora cavernosa clitoridis and an expansion dorsal to them and superficial to the deep dorsal vein of clitoris. It is supplied by the perineal branch of the pudendal nerve, compresses the orifice of the vagina, and helps in erection of the clitoris. Some authorities reverse the above origins and insertions. Also called *bulbospongiosus, bulbocavernosus, accelerator urinae* (outmoded), *musculus ejaculator seminis* (outmoded), *bulbocavernous muscle, musculus bulbocavernosus, musculus accelerator urinae, urinaccelerator* (outmoded), *musculus compressor urethrae* (outmoded).

musculus caninus An outmoded term for MUSCULUS LEVATOR ANGULI ORIS.

musculi capitis [NA] The muscles of the head, including the muscles of mastication, muscles of expression, and the suboccipital muscles.

musculus ceratocricoideus [NA] An occasional band of the lower margin of the posterior cricoarytenoid muscle that attaches to the inferior horn of the thyroid cartilage and the adjacent cricoid lamina. Also called *ceratocricoid muscle, Merkel's muscle, ceratocricoideus.*

musculus ceratopharyngeus PARS CERATOPHARYNGEA MUSCULI CONSTRICTORIS PHARYNGIS MEDII.

musculus cervicalis ascendens An outmoded term for MUSCULUS ILIOCOSTALIS CERVICIS.

musculus chondroglossus [NA] A muscle originating from the medial side and base of the lesser horn and the adjacent part of the body of the hyoid bone, and inserted into the intrinsic muscles of the tongue between the genioglossus and hyoglossus muscles. It is supplied by the hypoglossal nerve, and assists in depressing the tongue. Also called *chondroglossus muscle, chondroglossus.*

musculus chondropharyngeus PARS CHONDROPHARYNGEA MUSCULI CONSTRICTORIS PHARYNGIS MEDII.

musculus ciliaris [NA] The nonstriated muscle mass that forms the bulk of the ciliary body of the eye and comprises three portions which are mostly attached to the scleral spur from which they run in various directions. They are the outermost fibrae meridionales extending into the stroma of the choroid and ciliary processes (also called meridional or longitudinal fibers, Brücke's muscle, or tensor muscle of choroid); the innermost fibrae circulares extending in a circumferential fashion near the periphery of the lens (also called circular fibers, Rouget's muscle, or Müller's muscle); and the intermediate fibrae radiales (also called radiating fibers) which run obliquely forming an interlacing network. It is innervated by the short ciliary nerves and its action produces changes in the shape of the lens in the process of accommodation. Also called *ciliary muscle, Bowman's muscle, ciliary ligament* (outmoded), *ciliaris.*

musculus cleidomastoideus The lateral, or clavicular, portion of the sternocleidomastoid muscle. It is occasionally distinct from the sternomastoid part in humans, but usually separated from it in many lower mammals.

musculi coccygei [NA] The muscles attached to the coccyx, including the coccygeus and the dorsal and ventral sacrococcygeal muscles. Also called *coccygeal muscles.*

musculus coccygeus [NA] A muscle originating from the pelvic aspect of the ischial spine and from the sacrospinous ligament, and inserted onto the lateral margin of the coccyx and of the fourth and fifth sacral vertebrae. It is supplied by the third and fourth or fourth and fifth sacral nerves, flexes the coccyx, and supports it, especially after defecation and parturition. Also called *coccygeal muscle, ischiococcygeus, coccygeus.*

musculi colli [NA] The anterolateral muscles of the neck, including the sternocleidomastoid, suprahyoid, infrahyoid, scalene, longus colli, and platysma muscles. Also called *muscles of neck.*

musculus compressor naris PARS TRANSVERSA MUSCULI NASALIS.

musculus compressor urethrae **1** An outmoded term for MUSCULUS SPHINCTER URETHRAE. **2** Musculus sphincter urethrae and musculus transversus perinei profundus considered together. An outmoded term. Also called *musculus constrictor urethrae, transversourethralis.* **3** [NA] Some deep fibers of musculus sphincter urethrae arising from the ramus of the ischium. **4** An outmoded term for MUSCULUS BULBOSPONGIOSUS.

musculus constrictor pharyngis inferior [NA] The lowest of the three constrictor muscles of the pharynx that consists of two parts, pars cricopharyngea and pars thyropharyngea, arising from the cricoid and thyroid cartilages. Their fibers run posteriorly and medially to be inserted with the fibers from the opposite side into a fibrous raphe in the midline posteriorly. The lowest muscle fibers are continuous with the circular muscle of the esophagus, while the upper fibers overlap the middle constrictor of the pharynx. It is supplied by the pharyngeal plexus and branches of the external and recurrent laryngeal nerves, and takes part in constriction of the pharynx and propulsion of its contents during swallowing. Also called *inferior constrictor muscle of pharynx, musculus laryngopharyngeus, inferior pharyngeal constrictor muscle, infraconstrictor* (outmoded), *laryngopharyngeus.*

musculus constrictor pharyngis medius [NA] The middle of the three constrictor muscles of the pharynx that consists of two parts, pars chondropharyngea and pars ceratopharyngea, arising from the lesser and greater horns of the hyoid bone and the stylohyoid ligament. Their fibers run posteriorly and medially and are inserted with the fibers of the opposite side in a fibrous raphe in the midline posteriorly. The lowest fibers are overlapped by the inferior constrictor and the upper fibers overlap the superior constrictor muscle of the pharynx. It is supplied by the pharyngeal plexus, and constricts the pharynx during swallowing. Also called *middle constrictor muscle of pharynx, middle pharyngeal constrictor muscle, musculus hyopharyngeus* (outmoded).

musculus constrictor pharyngis superior [NA] The highest of the three constrictor muscles of the pharynx that consists of four parts, namely, pars pterygopharyngea from the medial pterygoid plate, pars buccopharyngea from the pterygomandibular raphe, pars mylopharyngea from the back of the mylohyoid line of the mandible, and pars glossopharyngea from the side of the tongue. Their fibers run posteriorly and medially to be inserted with the fibers from the opposite side into the fibrous raphe in the midline posteriorly as well as in the pharyngeal tubercle on the basilar part of the occipital bone. Its lowest fibers are overlapped by the middle constrictor muscle, while the upper fibers are separated from the base of the skull by a space through which pass the auditory tube and the levator veli palatini muscle. It is supplied by the pharyngeal plexus, and constricts the pharynx during swallowing. Also called *superior constrictor muscle of pharynx, superior pharyngeal constrictor muscle, cephalopharyngeus* (outmoded).

musculus constrictor urethrae **1** An outmoded term for MUSCULUS SPHINCTER URETHRAE. **2** MUSCULUS COMPRESSOR URETHRAE.

musculus coracobrachialis [NA] A muscle originating from the tip of the coracoid process of the scapula with the tendon of the short head of biceps brachii muscle, and inserted onto the middle of the medial surface of the humerus. It is supplied by the musculocutaneous nerve, and flexes and adducts the arm. Also called *coracobrachial muscle, coracobrachialis, Casser's perforated muscle.*

musculus corrugator supercilii [NA] A muscle originating from the medial end of the superciliary arch of the frontal bone, and inserted into the skin above the medial part of the supraorbital margin. It is supplied by temporal branches of the facial nerve, and pulls the eyebrow downward and medially producing the vertical furrows above the nasal bridge, as in frowning. Also called *superciliary corrugator muscle, Coiter's muscle.*

musculus cremaster [NA] A muscle well developed in the male, arising from the inguinal ligament and the lower part of the internal oblique and transversus abdominis muscles. It forms loosely arranged loops around the spermatic cord as far as the tunica vaginalis, helps to form the cremasteric fascia, and is inserted into the pubic tubercle. It is supplied by the genital branch of the genitofemoral nerve, and lifts the testis towards the superficial inguinal ring. Also called *cremaster muscle, Riolan's muscle, cremaster, suspensorium testis.*

musculus cricoarytenoideus lateralis [NA] A muscle originating from the superior margin of the arch of the cricoid cartilage and the adjacent conus elasticus, and inserted into the

anterior surface of the muscular process of the arytenoid cartilage. It is supplied by the recurrent laryngeal nerve, and approximates the vocal processes and closes the rima glottidis. Also called *lateral cricoarytenoid muscle.*

musculus cricoarytenoideus posterior [NA] A muscle originating from the posterior surface of the cricoid lamina on each side of the median crest, and inserted into the posterior surface and tip of the muscular process of the arytenoid cartilage. It is supplied by the recurrent laryngeal nerve, widens the rima glottidis, and tenses the vocal ligaments. Also called *posterior cricoarytenoid muscle.*

musculus cricopharyngeus PARS CRICOPHARYNGEA MUSCULI CONSTRICTORIS PHARYNGIS INFERIORIS.

musculus cricothyreoideus An outmoded term for MUSCULUS CRICOTHYROIDEUS.

musculus cricothyroideus [NA] A muscle originating from the anterior and lateral surfaces of the cricoid cartilage. Its pars obliqua is inserted into the anterior margin of the inferior horn of the thyroid cartilage, and pars recta into the posterior part of the lower margin of the lamina of the thyroid cartilage. It is supplied by the external laryngeal branch of the superior laryngeal nerve, and tenses and elongates the vocal ligaments. Also called *cricothyroid muscle, musculus cricothyreoideus* (outmoded).

musculus cutaneomucosus An outmoded term for AEBY'S MUSCLE.

musculus cutaneus [NA] A striated muscle inserted into the skin. Also called *dermal muscle, cutaneous muscle.*

musculus dartos [NA] A thin layer of smooth muscle fibers in the superficial fascia of the scrotum, the more superficial fibers being attached to the skin, while the deeper fibers in the sagittal plane take part in the formation of a septum that divides the scrotum into two cavities by attaching to the inferior surface of the radix of the penis. The fibers produce the transverse ridges on the surface of the scrotum. It is innervated by the genitofemoral nerve. When it contracts, it wrinkles and tightens the scrotum. Also called *dartos muscle of scrotum, dartos, suspensory apparatus of scrotum* (outmoded), *tunica carnea* (outmoded).

musculus deltoides clavicularis The clavicular portion of the deltoid muscle when it is separated from the rest of the muscle. In reptiles, it is the equivalent of the pars clavicularis musculi deltoidei of some mammals. An outmoded term.

musculus deltoideus [NA] A muscle originating from the anterior margin and superior surface of the lateral third of the clavicle, the lateral margin and superior surface of the acromion, and the inferior border of the crest of the spine of the scapula. It is inserted onto the deltoid tuberosity on the lateral side of the shaft of the humerus. It is supplied by the axillary nerve and abducts the arm 90°. The anterior fibers can flex and medially rotate the arm, while the posterior fibers can extend and laterally rotate it. Also called *deltoid muscle, deltoid.*

musculus depressor anguli oris [NA] A muscle originating from the oblique line of the mandible, and inserted into the skin of the angle of the mouth, and into the orbicularis oris muscle and other muscles at the angle of mouth. It is supplied by the buccal branch or mandibular branch of the facial nerve, and pulls the angle of the mouth downwards and laterally. Also called *depressor muscle of angle of mouth, triangular muscle, musculus triangularis, depressor anguli oris, triangularis.*

musculus depressor labii inferioris [NA] A muscle originating from the oblique line of the mandible between the mental protuberance and the mental foramen, and inserted into the orbicularis oris muscle, the depressor muscle from the opposite side, and the skin and mucosa of the lower lip. It is supplied by the mandibular branch of the facial nerve, and pulls down and everts the lower lip. Also called *depressor muscle of lower lip, Aeby's muscle, quadrate muscle of lower lip, musculus quadratus* *labii inferioris, depressor labii inferioris.*

musculus depressor septi nasi [NA] A muscle originating from the incisive fossa of the maxilla, and inserted into the cartilaginous part of the nasal septum and the ala of the nose. It is supplied by the buccal branch of the facial nerve, pulls the ala of nose downward, and helps the nasalis in widening the nostrils in deep inspiration. Some consider the muscle to be a portion of the alar part of the nasalis muscle. Also called *depressor muscle of nasal septum, depressor alae nasi* (outmoded).

musculus depressor supercilii [NA] The upper fasciculi of the orbital part of the orbicularis oculi muscle that insert into the skin and subcutaneous tissue of the eyebrow. Also called *superciliary depressor muscle.*

musculus detrusor urinae MUSCULUS DETRUSOR VESICAE.

musculus detrusor vesicae [NA] The three layers of the tunica muscularis vesicae urinariae considered as a single functional unit. The term has been applied, incorrectly, to either the external longitudinal layer alone or the musculus pubovesicalis. Also called *detrusor muscle of urinary bladder, detrusor urinae, musculus detrusor urinae, detrusor urinae muscle, detrusor vesicae.*

musculus digastricus [NA] A muscle of which the venter anterior originates from the digastric fossa on each side of the midline on the base of the mandible; and venter posterior from the mastoid notch of the temporal bone. Its intermediate tendon is attached by a fibrous loop to the body and greater cornu of the hyoid bone. Its venter anterior is supplied by the mylohyoid branch of the inferior alveolar nerve, and venter posterior by the facial nerve. It depresses the mandible and elevates the hyoid bone. Also called *digastric muscle, biventer mandibulae.*

musculus dilatator An outmoded term for MUSCULUS DILATOR.

musculus dilator A muscle that expands or opens the orifice or lumen of an organ, tube, or space. Also called *musculus dilatator.*

musculus dilator iridis MUSCULUS DILATOR PUPILLAE.

musculus dilator naris PARS ALARIS MUSCULI NASALIS.

musculus dilator pupillae [NA] A thin layer of radially arranged nonstriated muscle fibers with myoepithelial cells that extends from the sphincter pupillae almost to the base of the iris. Superficial and posterior to this layer are the pigmented cells of the posterior epithelium. It is innervated by the short and long ciliary nerves and its function is to dilate the pupil. Also called *dilator muscle of pupil, musculus dilator iridis, iridodilator.*

musculus dilator pylori gastroduodenalis Some of the superficial fibers of the longitudinal fibers of the stomach's tunica muscularis that either extend into the duodenum or end in the pyloric sphincter. An outmoded term.

musculus dilator pylori ilealis The longitudinal muscle fibers of the tunica muscularis of the terminal ileum that extend into the ileocecal valve. An outmoded term.

musculi dorsi [NA] The muscles of the back, including the trapezius, latissimus dorsi, rhomboid, serratus posterior, levator scapulae, erector spinae, transversospinalis, interspinal, and intertransverse muscles. Also called *dorsal muscles.*

musculus ejaculator seminis An outmoded term for MUSCULUS BULBOSPONGIOSUS.

musculus epicranius [NA] The muscular layer of the scalp, comprising musculus occipitofrontalis, musculus temporoparietalis, and the galea aponeurotica. Also called *epicranial muscle.*

musculus epitrochleoanconaeus An outmoded term for EPITROCHLEOANCONEUS MUSCLE.

musculus erector clitoridis An outmoded term for MUSCULUS ISCHIOCAVERNOSUS.

musculus erector penis An outmoded term for MUSCULUS ISCHIOCAVERNOSUS.

musculus erector spinae [NA] The superficial longitudinal muscle mass on either side of the spines of the vertebral column that splits in the upper lumbar region into three columns, namely, a medial, or spinalis, group; an intermediate, or longissimus, group; and a lateral, iliocostalis or iliocostocervicalis group. Its tendinous origin attaches to the median sacral crest, the spines and supraspinous ligaments of all the lumbar and the twelfth and eleventh thoracic vertebrae, the medial surface of the posterior part of the iliac crest, and the adjacent sacrotuberous and dorsal sacroiliac ligaments. It is supplied by the dorsal rami of the lumbar, thoracic, and cervical spinal nerves, and is a powerful extensor as well as a lateral flexor of the vertebral column. Also called *sacrospinal muscle, musculus sacrospinalis* (outmoded), *erector muscle of spine.*

musculus extensor carpi radialis brevis [NA] A muscle originating from the lateral epicondyle of the humerus, the radial collateral ligament of the elbow joint, and the intermuscular septa; and inserted onto the posterior surface of the base of the third metacarpal bone and the adjacent part of the second metacarpal bone. It is supplied by the posterior interosseous nerve, extends the wrist, abducts the hand and, acting synergistically with the finger flexors, steadies the wrist when they act. Also called *short radial extensor muscle of wrist.*

musculus extensor carpi radialis longus [NA] A muscle originating from the lower third of the lateral supracondylar ridge of the humerus and the lateral intermuscular septum, and inserted into the lateral aspect of the posterior surface of the base of the second metacarpal bone. It is supplied by the radial nerve; extends the wrist, abducts the hand and, acting synergistically with the finger flexors, steadies the wrist when they act. Also called *long radial extensor of wrist.*

musculus extensor carpi ulnaris [NA] A muscle of which the caput humerale originates from the lateral epicondyle of the humerus and the antebrachial fascia, and caput ulnare from the proximal three fourths of the posterior margin of the ulna. It is inserted into the medial side of the base of the fifth metacarpal bone, supplied by the posterior interosseous nerve, and adducts the hand medially and extends it. Also called *ulnar extensor of wrist.*

musculus extensor coccygis An outmoded term for MUSCULUS SACROCOCCYGEUS DORSALIS.

musculus extensor digiti minimi [NA] A muscle originating from the lateral epicondyle of the humerus with the common extensor tendon and the intermuscular septa, and inserted into the dorsal digital expansion of the fifth digit. It is supplied by the posterior interosseous nerve, extends the little finger and, with musculus extensor digitorum, extends the wrist. Also called *extensor muscle of little finger, proper extensor muscle of fifth digit, musculus extensor digiti quinti proprius* (outmoded).

musculus extensor digiti quinti proprius An outmoded term for MUSCULUS EXTENSOR DIGITI MINIMI.

musculus extensor digitorum [NA] A muscle originating from the lateral epicondyle of the humerus by the common extensor tendon, the intermuscular septa, and the antebrachial fascia. It is inserted by four tendons into the dorsal digital expansion of each of the medial four fingers, the intermediate slip of which attaches to the base of the middle phalanx while the two collateral slips reunite to attach to the back of the base of the distal phalanx. It is supplied by the posterior interosseous nerve, extends the fingers at the metacarpophalangeal and interphalangeal joints, and then extends the wrist. Also called *extensor muscle of fingers, common extensor muscle of digits* (outmoded), *musculus extensor digitorum communis* (outmoded).

musculus extensor digitorum brevis [NA] A muscle originating from the anterior part of the superolateral surface of the calcaneus and the stem of the inferior extensor retinaculum. It is inserted by four tendons, the most medial being the extensor hallucis brevis, while the lateral three are attached to the lateral margins of the tendons of the extensor digitorum longus with slips to the bases of the proximal phalanges. It is supplied by the deep peroneal nerve, and extends the phalanges of the middle three toes. Also called *short extensor muscle of toes.*

musculus extensor digitorum brevis manus   A rarely occurring short extensor muscle of the fingers similar to the short extensor muscle of the toes. It arises either from the dorsum of the carpus or from the lower end of the radius and ulna, and divides distally into a varying number of tendons inserting into tendons of musculus extensor digitorum. Also called *Pozzi's muscle.*

musculus extensor digitorum communis   An outmoded term for MUSCULUS EXTENSOR DIGITORUM.

musculus extensor digitorum longus   [NA] A muscle originating from the lateral condyle of the tibia, the upper three fourths of the medial surface of the fibula, the upper anterior surface of the interosseous membrane, the anterior crural intermuscular septum, and the fascia cruris. It is inserted by four tendons into the dorsal digital expansion of each of the lateral four toes, the intermediate slip of which attaches to the base of the middle phalanx, while the two collateral slips reunite and attach to the dorsum of the base of the distal phalanx. It is supplied by the deep peroneal nerve, extends the toes, and dorsiflexes the foot. Also called *long extensor muscle of toes.*

musculus extensor hallucis brevis   [NA] The large, medial belly of musculus extensor digitorum brevis that is inserted into the dorsum of the base of the proximal phalanx of the great toe. It is supplied by the deep peroneal nerve, and extends the proximal phalanx of the great toe. Also called *short extensor muscle of great toe.*

musculus extensor hallucis longus   [NA] A muscle originating from the middle two fourths of the medial surface of the fibula and the front of the interosseous membrane. It is inserted onto the dorsum of the base of the distal phalanx of the great toe. It is supplied by the deep peroneal nerve, dorsiflexes the foot, and extends the phalanges of the great toe. Also called *long extensor muscle of great toe.*

musculus extensor indicis   [NA] A muscle originating from the proximal part of the distal third of the posterior surface of the ulna and from the interosseous membrane. It is inserted into the medial side of the tendon of the extensor digitorum muscle to the index finger. It is supplied by the posterior interosseous nerve, and helps to extend the index finger and the wrist. Also called *extensor muscle of index finger, musculus extensor indicis proprius* (outmoded), *indicator.*

musculus extensor indicis proprius   An outmoded term for MUSCULUS EXTENSOR INDICIS.

musculus extensor pollicis brevis   [NA] A muscle originating from the distal part of the middle third of the posterior surface of the radius, and from the interosseous membrane; and inserted into the dorsal surface of the base of the proximal phalanx of the thumb. It is supplied by the posterior interosseous nerve, and extends the thumb. Also called *short extensor muscle of thumb.*

musculus extensor pollicis longus   [NA] A muscle originating from the middle third of the lateral part of the posterior surface of the ulna and from the interosseous membrane, and inserted into the dorsum of the base of the distal phalanx of the thumb. It is supplied by the posterior interosseous nerve; extends the thumb; adducts the extended thumb, rotating it laterally; and helps to adduct the hand. Also called *long extensor muscle of thumb.*

musculi extremitatis inferioris   An outmoded term for MUSCULI MEMBRI INFERIORIS.

musculi extremitatis superioris   An outmoded term for MUSCULI MEMBRI SUPERIORIS.

musculus fibularis brevis   MUSCULUS PERONEUS BREVIS.

musculus fibularis longus   MUSCULUS PERONEUS LONGUS.

musculus fibularis tertius   MUSCULUS PERONEUS TERTIUS.

musculus fixator baseos stapedis   The muscle fibers of the stapedius that oppose the action of the tensor tympani muscle and prevent the base of the stapes from being pushed too tightly into the fenestra vestibuli. An outmoded term. Also called *fixator muscle of base of stapes.*

musculus flexor accessorius   MUSCULUS QUADRATUS PLANTAE.

musculus flexor carpi radialis   [NA] A muscle originating from the medial epicondyle of humerus by the common flexor tendon, the antebrachial fascia, and the intermuscular septa; and inserted onto the base of the second metacarpal and usually by a slip to the third metacarpal. It is supplied by the median nerve, and helps to flex and abduct the hand. Also called *radial flexor muscle of wrist, radiocarpus* (outmoded).

musculus flexor carpi ulnaris   [NA] A muscle of which the caput humerale originates from the medial epicondyle of humerus by the common flexor tendon; and caput ulnare from the medial side of the olecranon and the upper two thirds of the posterior margin of the ulna. It is inserted onto the pisiform bone and by the pisohamate and pisometacarpal ligaments to the hamate bone and the base of fifth metacarpal bone respectively. It is supplied by the ulnar nerve, and helps to flex and adduct the hand. Also called *ulnar flexor muscle of wrist.*

musculus flexor digiti minimi brevis manus   [NA] A muscle originating from the hook of the hamate bone and the flexor retinaculum, and inserted onto the medial side of the base of the proximal phalanx of the little finger. It is supplied by the deep branch of the ulnar nerve, and flexes the proximal phalanx of the little finger. Also called *short flexor muscle of little finger, musculus flexor digiti quinti brevis manus* (outmoded).

musculus flexor digiti minimi brevis pedis   [NA] A muscle originating from the sheath of the peroneus longus muscle and from the plantar aspect of the base of the fifth metatarsal bone, and inserted onto the lateral side of the base of the proximal phalanx of the little toe. It is supplied by the superficial branch of the lateral plantar nerve, and flexes the proximal phalanx of the little toe. Also called *short flexor muscle of little toe, musculus flexor digiti quinti brevis pedis* (outmoded).

musculus flexor digiti quinti brevis manus   An outmoded term for MUSCULUS FLEXOR DIGITI MINIMI BREVIS MANUS.

musculus flexor digiti quinti brevis pedis   An outmoded term for MUSCULUS FLEXOR DIGITI MINIMI BREVIS PEDIS.

musculus flexor digitorum   A muscle which flexes the digits on either the front or hind foot of certain tetrapods.

musculus flexor digitorum brevis   [NA] A muscle originating from the medial process of the calcaneal tuberosity, the central part of the plantar aponeurosis, and the medial and lateral intermuscular septa. It is inserted by four tendons into the sides of the middle phalanges of the lateral four toes after splitting to allow the corresponding long flexor tendons through, then rejoining, decussating, and dividing again. It is supplied by the medial plantar nerve, and flexes the middle and proximal phalanges of the lateral four toes. Also called *short flexor muscle of toes.*

musculus flexor digitorum longus   [NA] A muscle originating from the medial part of the posterior surface of the tibia below the soleal line. It is inserted by four tendons into the base of the terminal phalanx of the lateral four toes after passing through a gap in the corresponding tendon of flexor digitorum brevis. It is supplied by the tibial nerve, flexes the toes and foot when the foot is off the ground, and acts synergistically with other plantar muscles to stabilize the foot when it is on the ground. Also called *long flexor muscle of toes.*

musculus flexor digitorum profundus [NA] A muscle originating from the upper three fourths of the posterior margin and of the medial and anterior surfaces of the ulna, and from the anterior surface of the adjacent interosseous membrane. It is inserted by four tendons into the base of the distal phalanx of the medial four fingers after passing through an opening in the corresponding tendon of flexor digitorum superficialis. It is supplied by the ulnar nerve and the anterior interosseous branch of the median nerve, flexes the distal phalanges, and helps to flex the wrist. Also called *deep flexor muscle of fingers, perforans manus* (outmoded).

musculus flexor digitorum sublimis An outmoded term for MUSCULUS FLEXOR DIGITORUM SUPERFICIALIS.

musculus flexor digitorum superficialis [NA] A muscle of which the caput humeroulnare originates from the medial epicondyle of humerus by the common flexor tendon, and from the ulnar collateral ligament of the elbow joint, the medial margin of the coronoid process of ulna, and the intermuscular septum between it and overlying muscles; and caput radiale from the oblique line of radius and the anterior margin below it. It is inserted by four tendons that divide over the proximal phalanges of the medial four fingers to allow passage of the corresponding tendons of flexor digitorum profundus, and then reunite, decussate and divide again to attach to the sides of the middle phalanges. It is supplied by the median nerve, flexes the middle and proximal phalanges, and helps to flex the wrist. Also called *superficial flexor muscle of fingers, musculus flexor digitorum sublimis* (outmoded).

musculus flexor hallucis brevis [NA] A muscle originating from the medial side of the plantar surface of the cuboid bone and the lateral cuneiform bone, and inserted by medial and lateral parts into corresponding sides of the base of the proximal phalanx of the great toe, each containing a sesamoid bone and each blending with adjacent muscles. It is supplied by the medial plantar nerve, and flexes the proximal phalanx of the great toe. Also called *short flexor muscle of great toe.*

musculus flexor hallucis longus [NA] A muscle originating from the distal two thirds of the posterior surface of the fibula, the adjacent interosseous membrane, and posterior crural intermuscular septum; and inserted into the base of the terminal phalanx of great toe. It is supplied by the tibial nerve, flexes the great toe, and helps to invert the foot and to plantiflex the ankle joint. Also called *long flexor muscle of great toe.*

musculus flexor palmaris profundus In amphibians, a muscle that flexes the palm and is the homologue of the musculus flexor digitorum profundus and musculus flexor pollicis longus, considered together, in humans.

musculus flexor pollicis brevis [NA] A muscle of which the caput superficiale originates from the tubercle of trapezium and the adjacent part of flexor retinaculum; and caput profundum from the trapezoid and capitate bones and palmar ligaments. It is inserted onto the lateral side of the base of proximal phalanx of thumb. It is supplied by the recurrent branch of the median nerve and the deep branch of the ulnar nerve, flexes the proximal phalanx of thumb, and flexes and medially rotates the first metacarpal bone. Also called *short flexor muscle of thumb.*

musculus flexor pollicis longus [NA] A muscle originating from the anterior surface of the radius from the radial tuberosity to the upper margin of attachment of the pronator quadratus muscle; and from the adjacent interosseous membrane; and inserted onto the anterior aspect of the base of the distal phalanx of thumb. It is supplied by the anterior interosseous branch of the median nerve, flexes the thumb, and helps to flex the wrist. Also called *long flexor muscle of thumb.*

musculus flexor tarsi In certain tetrapods, a muscle on the upper surface of the hindfoot which flexes the foot.

musculus flexor tibialis In reptiles, a pair of ventral hind leg muscles. The externus is homologous with the musculus biceps femoris in humans and the internus with musculus semimembranosus and musculus semitendinosus together.

musculus frontalis An outmoded term for VENTER FRONTALIS MUSCULI OCCIPITOFRONTALIS.

musculus fusiformis [NA] A spindle-shaped muscle in which the longitudinal fasciculi of its fleshy belly are parallel and taper to a tendon at one or both ends. Also called *fusiform muscle.*

musculus gastrocnemius [NA] A muscle of which the caput laterale originates from the posterolateral surface of the lateral condyle of femur, the lower part of the lateral supracondylar line, and the capsule of the knee joint; and caput mediale from the posterosuperior part of the medial condyle of femur behind the adductor tubercle, the popliteal surface superolateral to this, and the capsule of the knee joint. It is inserted with the soleus muscle by tendo calcaneus into the middle of the posterior surface of the calcaneus. It is supplied by the tibial nerve; plantiflexes the foot, raising the heel off the ground; and flexes the knee. Also called *gastrocnemius muscle, gastrocnemius.*

musculus gemellus inferior [NA] A muscle originating from the upper part of the inner surface of the ischial tuberosity and sacrotuberous ligament, and inserted into the tendon of the obturator internus muscle and the medial aspect of the greater trochanter of femur. It is supplied by the nerve to quadratus femoris and, with the obturator internus and superior gemellus muscles, laterally rotates the extended thigh and abducts the flexed thigh. Also called *inferior gemellus muscle.*

musculus gemellus superior [NA] A muscle originating from the posterior surface of the ischial spine and the adjacent part of the lesser sciatic notch and inserted into the tendon of the obturator internus muscle and the medial surface of the greater trochanter of femur. It is supplied by the nerve to obturator internus and, with the obturator internus and inferior gemellus muscles, it laterally rotates the extended thigh and abducts the flexed thigh. Also called *superior gemellus muscle.*

musculus genioglossus [NA] A muscle originating from the upper genial tubercle of the mental spine on the lingual surface of the symphysis menti, and inserted onto the anterior surface of the body of the hyoid bone and the inferior surface of the tongue. It is supplied by the hypoglossal nerve, pulls forward the tongue and protrudes the apex, and depresses the tongue. Also called *genioglossus muscle, genioglossus, geniohyoglossus.*

musculus geniohyoideus [NA] A muscle originating from the lower genial tubercle of the mental spine behind the symphysis menti, and inserted onto the anterior surface of the body of the hyoid bone. It is supplied by the first cervical spinal nerve via the hypoglossal nerve, elevates and draws forward the hyoid bone, and depresses the mandible when the hyoid is fixed. Also called *geniohyoid muscle, geniohyoideus.*

musculus glossopalatinus An outmoded term for MUSCULUS PALATOGLOSSUS.

musculus glossopharyngeus PARS GLOSSOPHARYNGEA MUSCULI CONSTRICTORIS PHARYNGIS SUPERIORIS.

musculus gluteus maximus [NA] A muscle originating from the outer surface of the ilium posterior to the posterior gluteal line and the adjacent iliac crest, the aponeurosis of the erector spinae muscle, the posterior surface of the fourth and fifth sacral vertebrae, the coccyx and the sacrotuberous ligament, and the gluteal fascia, and inserted into the gluteal tuberosity of femur and the iliotibial tract. It is supplied by the inferior gluteal nerve, extends and laterally rotates the thigh, tenses the fascia lata and steadies the knee joint, abducts the thigh, steadies the trunk during locomotion, and rotates the pelvis backwards on the femur. Also called *greatest gluteal muscle.*

musculus gluteus medius [NA] A muscle originating from the outer surface of the ilium between the anterior and posterior gluteal lines and the iliac crest above this area, and from the gluteal fascia; and inserted into the posterosuperior angle and oblique ridge on the outer surface of the greater trochanter of femur. It is supplied by the superior gluteal nerve. It abducts the thigh, anterior fibers medially rotate and flex the thigh, posterior fibers laterally rotate and extend the thigh, and it tends to pull down and stabilize the pelvis when the opposite leg is off the ground, thereby maintaining the trunk upright. Also called *middle gluteal muscle, mesogluteus* (outmoded).

musculus gluteus minimus [NA] A muscle originating from the outer surface of the ilium between the anterior and inferior gluteal lines, and from the margin of the greater sciatic notch; and inserted onto the anterolateral surface of the greater trochanter of femur. It is supplied by the superior gluteal nerve, and agrees with the gluteus medius in all of its actions. Also called *least gluteal muscle.*

musculus gluteus quartus MUSCULUS SCANSORIUS.

musculus gracilis [NA] A muscle originating from the medial margin of the inferior pubic ramus and the adjoining ischial ramus and inserted onto the upper part of the medial surface of the tibia, below the condyle and behind the insertion of the sartorius muscle. It is supplied by the obturator nerve, flexes and medially rotates the leg, and adducts the thigh. Also called *gracilis muscle.*

musculus helicis major [NA] A muscle originating from the spine of the helix of the pinna and inserted into the anterosuperior margin of the helix, where it turns posteriorly. It is supplied by the temporal branch of the facial nerve.

musculus helicis minor [NA] A slender muscle fasciculus extending from the anterior margin of the helix to the concha of the pinna and covering the crus helicis.

musculus hyoglossus A muscle originating from the greater horn and lateral part of the body of the hyoid bone, and inserted into the side of the tongue between the inferior longitudinal and styloglossus muscles. It is supplied by the hypoglossal nerve. It depresses the tongue. Also called *hyoglossal muscle, hyoglossus muscle.*

musculus hyopharyngeus An outmoded term for MUSCULUS CONSTRICTOR PHARYNGIS MEDIUS.

musculus iliacus [NA] A muscle originating from the upper two thirds of the iliac fossa, the adjacent inner lip of the iliac crest, the iliolumbar ligament, the ventral sacroiliac ligaments, and the ala of sacrum; and inserted into the tendon of the psoas major muscle and the femur below the lesser trochanter. It is supplied by the femoral nerve and, with the psoas major muscle, it flexes the thigh and also flexes the pelvis on the thigh. Also called *iliac muscle.* See also MUSCULUS PSOAS MAJOR, MUSCULUS ILIOPSOAS.

musculus iliacus minor One of the variations of the musculus iliacus, either a separate lamina attached to the iliac fascia, or a separate small slip from the anterior inferior iliac spine to either the intertrochanteric line or the iliofemoral ligament. Also called *musculus iliocapsularis, iliocapsularis.*

musculus iliocapsularis MUSCULUS ILIACUS MINOR.

musculus iliococcygeus [NA] A morphological subdivision of the levator ani muscle that arises from the ischial spine and the posterior part of the tendinous arch of the obturator fascia and inserts into the coccyx and the median raphe behind the anus. For nerve supply and action, see musculus levator ani. Also called *iliococcygeal muscle, iliococcygeus.*

musculus iliocostalis [NA] The lateral column of the erector spinae muscle that separates in the upper lumbar region into iliocostalis lumborum, iliocostalis thoracis, and iliocostalis cervicis. It is supplied by dorsal rami of lower cervical, thoracic, and upper lumbar spinal nerves; and extends and laterally flexes the vertebral column. Also called *iliocostal muscle, musculus iliocostocervicalis.*

musculus iliocostalis cervicis [NA] A muscle originating from the angles of the third to sixth ribs, and inserted onto posterior tubercles of the transverse processes of the fourth, fifth, and sixth cervical vertebrae. It is supplied by dorsal rami of the lower cervical spinal nerves. Also called *iliocostal muscle of neck, musculus cervicalis ascendens* (outmoded), *costocervicalis muscle, costocervicalis.*

musculus iliocostalis dorsi An outmoded term for MUSCULUS ILIOCOSTALIS THORACIS.

musculus iliocostalis lumborum [NA] A muscle originating from the erector spinae muscle in the upper lumbar region and inserted onto the inferior margins of the angles of the lower six or seven ribs. It is supplied by dorsal rami of the upper lumbar spinal nerves. Also called *iliocostal muscle of loins.*

musculus iliocostalis thoracis [NA] A muscle originating from the superior margins of the angles of the lower six or seven ribs, and inserted onto the superior margins of the angles of the upper six ribs and the transverse process of the seventh cervical vertebra. It is supplied by dorsal rami of the thoracic spinal nerves. Also called *iliocostal muscle of thorax, musculus iliocostalis dorsi* (outmoded).

musculus iliocostocervicalis MUSCULUS ILIOCOSTALIS.

musculus iliofemoralis externus In birds, a large dorsal muscle on the outer side of the leg. It may be homologous with the musculus gluteus medius and musculus gluteus minimus, in part, in mammals.

musculus iliofemoralis internus In birds, a large dorsal muscle on the inner side of the leg. It is possibly a homologue of the musculus iliopsoas in some mammals.

musculus iliopsoas [NA] A compound muscle comprising musculus iliacus and musculus psoas major. It is a powerful flexor of the thigh. When the muscles on both sides act together from below, they pull the trunk and pelvis forward against resistance, as on rising from the supine position to a sitting position. Also called *iliopsoas muscle, iliopsoas.*

musculus iliotibialis In amphibians and reptiles, a slender dorsal muscle of the hind leg which is the homologue of the musculus rectus femoris in mammals. It extends from the ilium to the tibia and is the most anterior of the superficial muscles.

musculus iliotrochantericus In birds, a dorsal muscle that is part of the deep gluteal sheet of muscles.

musculi incisivi labii inferioris Fibers of the orbicularis oris muscle that arise on either side of the midline from the mandible, lateral to the mentalis muscle, and then curve to the angle of the mouth where it intermingles with other muscle fibers. Also called *incisive muscles of inferior lip, incisive muscles of lower lip.*

musculi incisivi labii superioris Fibers of the orbicularis oris muscle that arise from the alveolar border of the maxilla above the lateral incisor tooth on either side and curve to the lateral angle of the mouth, where they intermingle with other muscle fibers. Also called *incisive muscles of superior lip, incisive muscles of upper lip.*

musculus incisurae helicis [NA] A small muscle occasionally present in the auricle extending anteriorly from the musculus tragicus across the incisure of the cartilaginous meatus. It is supplied by the temporal branch of the facial nerve. Also called *muscle of incisure of helix, musculus incisurae helicis santorini* (outmoded), *Santorini's muscle.*

musculus incisurae helicis santorini An outmoded term for MUSCULUS INCISURAE HELICIS.

musculi infracostales An outmoded term for MUSCULI SUBCOSTALES.

musculi infrahyoidei [NA] The group of muscles attached to the hyoid bone from below and serving as antagonists to the suprahyoid muscles in depressing the hyoid bone. They include the sternohyoid, omohyoid, sternothyroid, and thyrohyoid muscles. Also called *infrahyoid muscles, strap muscles, ribbon muscles.*

musculus infraspinatus [NA] A muscle originating from the medial three fourths of the infraspinous fossa of the scapula, the inferior surface of the spine of scapula, and the infraspinous fascia, and inserted onto the middle facet on the greater tubercle of humerus. It is supplied by the suprascapular nerve, laterally rotates the arm, and helps adjacent muscles to steady the head of the humerus, especially in abduction. Also called *infraspinous muscle.*

musculi intercostales externi [NA] Muscles, eleven on each side, originating from the inferior border of the rib between the tubercle posteriorly and the costal cartilage anteriorly, and inserted onto the superior border of the rib below between the tubercle and the costal cartilage. They are supplied by the intercostal nerves, elevate the ribs during inspiration, and may act with internal intercostals during forced respiration. Also called *external intercostal muscles.*

musculi intercostales interni [NA] Muscles, eleven on each side, originating from the floor of the costal groove and the corresponding costal cartilage, and inserted onto the superior border of the rib below. They are supplied by the intercostal nerves, draw adjacent ribs together, may depress the ribs during expiration, and act with external intercostals during forced inspiration. Also called *internal intercostal muscles.*

musculi intercostales intimi [NA] The deepest layer of the internal intercostal muscles, separated from the latter by the intercostal vessels and nerves. They are usually not clearly developed in the upper intercostal spaces, but in the lower spaces they extend over the middle two fourths of the space, being continuous posteriorly with the corresponding subcostal muscle. Their innervation and action are identical to those of the internal intercostal muscles. Also called *innermost intercostal muscles.*

musculi interossei dorsales manus [NA] Four bipennate muscles in each hand, originating from the adjacent sides of two metacarpal bones and inserted onto the bases of proximal phalanges and dorsal digital expansions, the first on the radial side of the index finger, the second and third on radial and ulnar sides, respectively, of the middle finger, and the fourth on the ulnar side of the ring finger. They are supplied by the ulnar nerve; abduct the second, third and fourth fingers from the midline axis of the middle finger; flex the proximal phalanges; and extend the middle and distal phalanges. Also called *dorsal interosseous muscles of hand.*

musculi interossei dorsales pedis [NA] Four bipennate muscles, originating from the adjacent sides of two metacarpal bones and inserted onto the bases of the proximal phalanges and dorsal digital expansions, the first on the medial side of the second toe, and the second, third, and fourth on the lateral sides of the second, third, and fourth toes. They are supplied by the deep branch of the lateral plantar nerve; abduct the second, third, and fourth toes from the midline axis of the second toe; flex the proximal phalanges; and extend the middle and distal phalanges. Also called *dorsal interosseous muscles of foot.*

musculi interossei palmares [NA] Four muscles, though often only three are recognized, the first being considered a part of either flexor pollicis brevis or adductor pollicis. The first originates from the medial side of the palmar surface of the first metacarpal bone near the base, the second from the medial side of the second metacarpal, the third from the lateral side of the fourth metacarpal, and the fourth from the lateral side of the fifth metacarpal. The first is inserted onto the medial side of the base of the proximal phalanx and the dorsal digital expansion of thumb, the second into the medial side of the digital expansion of the index finger, the third into the lateral side of the digital expansion of the ring finger, and the fourth into the lateral side of the digital expansion and base of the proximal phalanx of the

little finger. They are supplied by the deep branch of the ulnar nerve; adduct the fingers toward the axial midline of the middle finger; and flex the proximal phalanges and extend the middle and distal phalanges of the medial four fingers, while the first flexes and adducts the proximal phalanx of thumb. Also called *musculi interossei volares* (outmoded), *volar interosseous muscles* (outmoded), *palmar interosseous muscles.*

musculi interossei plantares [NA] Three muscles originating from the bases and medial surfaces of the third, fourth, and fifth metatarsal bones, inserted onto the medial sides of the bases of the proximal phalanges of the third, fourth, and fifth toes and their dorsal digital expansions. They are supplied by the deep branch of lateral plantar nerve, adduct the lateral three toes towards the axial midline of the second toe, flex proximal phalanges, and extend the middle and distal phalanges. Also called *plantar interosseous muscles.*

musculi interossei volares An outmoded term for MUSCULI INTEROSSEI PALMARES.

musculi interspinales [NA] Short muscle bundles between the spines of adjacent vertebrae, one on each side of the interspinous ligaments, divided into three groups for the cervical, thoracic, and lumbar regions. They are innervated by dorsal rami of spinal nerves, and extend the vertebral column. Also called *interspinal muscles.*

musculi interspinales cervicis [NA] Six pairs of distinct muscle bundles extending between the adjacent bifid spines of the seven cervical and first thoracic vertebrae. They are supplied by dorsal rami of the cervical spinal nerves. Also called *interspinal muscles of neck.*

musculi interspinales lumborum [NA] Four pairs of short muscle bundles extending between the spines of adjacent lumbar vertebrae on either side of the interspinous ligaments. They are supplied by dorsal rami of the lumbar spinal nerves. Also called *interspinal muscles of loins.*

musculi interspinales thoracis [NA] Short muscle bundles extending between the spines of adjacent thoracic vertebrae, usually poorly developed except between the first two, the second and third, and the last two thoracic vertebrae. They are supplied by dorsal rami of the thoracic spinal nerves. Also called *interspinal muscles of thorax.*

musculi intertransversarii [NA] A deep group of small muscle bundles extending between the transverse processes of the vertebrae in the lumbar, thoracic, and cervical regions, and subdivided into anterior and posterior groups in the neck, and lateral and medial groups in the lumbar region. They act with other muscles to produce lateral flexion of the vertebral column and serve as postural muscles. Also called *intertransverse muscles.*

musculi intertransversarii anteriores An outmoded term for MUSCULI INTERTRANSVERSARII THORACIS.

musculi intertransversarii anteriores cervicis [NA] Seven pairs of small muscle bundles extending between the anterior tubercles of contiguous cervical vertebrae, and separated from the posterior intertransverse muscles by the ventral rami of the spinal nerves, which innervate the former. Also called *anterior intertransverse muscles of neck.*

musculi intertransversarii laterales An outmoded term for MUSCULI INTERTRANSVERSARII LATERALES LUMBORUM.

musculi intertransversarii laterales lumborum [NA] The lateral set of intertransverse muscles of the lumbar region that are subdivided into anterior and posterior parts, the anterior bundles extending between the transverse processes of adjacent lumbar vertebrae, while each posterior bundle extends between the accessory process of one vertebra and the transverse process of the next. They are homologous with the intercostal muscles, and supplied by anterior primary rami of lumbar spinal nerves. Also called *lateral intertransverse muscles of loins, musculi in-*

tertransversarii laterales (outmoded).

musculi intertransversarii mediales An outmoded term for MUSCULI INTERTRANSVERSARII MEDIALES LUMBORUM.

musculi intertransversarii mediales lumborum [NA] The medial set of intertransverse muscles of the lumbar region, each extending between the accessory process of one lumbar vertebra and the mamillary process of the next on each side. They are homologous with the levatores costarum, and represent the true intrinsic musculature of the back. They are supplied by medial divisions of posterior primary rami of lumbar spinal nerves. Also called *medial intertransverse muscles of loins, musculi intertransversarii mediales* (outmoded).

musculi intertransversarii posteriores An outmoded term for MUSCULI INTERTRANSVERSARII POSTERIORES CERVICIS.

musculi intertransversarii posteriores cervicis [NA] Seven pairs of small muscle bundles extending between the posterior tubercles of contiguous cervical vertebrae and separated from the anterior intertransverse muscles by the ventral rami of the spinal nerves. They are subdivided into medial and lateral parts, supplied by the dorsal and ventral rami of the cervical spinal nerves respectively. Also called *posterior intertransverse muscles of neck, musculi intertransversarii posteriores* (outmoded).

musculi intertransversarii thoracis [NA] Single muscle bundles extending between the adjacent transverse processes of the lowest three thoracic and first lumbar vertebrae. In the remaining thoracic region they are poorly developed or represented by ligamentous bands. They are supplied by dorsal rami of thoracic spinal nerves. Also called *intertransverse muscles of thorax, anterior intertransverse muscles* (outmoded), *musculi intertransversarii anteriores* (outmoded).

musculus ischiocavernosus [NA] A muscle originating from the medial surface of the ischial tuberosity behind the crus penis or crus clitoridis and the ramus of the ischium, and inserted into the sides and inferior surface of crus penis or crus clitoridis. It is supplied by the perineal branch of the pudendal nerve, and compresses the crus penis or crus clitoridis. Also called *ischiocavernous muscle, musculus erector penis* (outmoded), *musculus erector clitoridis* (outmoded), *erector muscle of penis* (outmoded), *erector clitoridis.*

musculi laryngis [NA] The intrinsic muscles of the larynx that act on the vocal cords, including the cricothyroid, posterior and lateral cricoarytenoid, transverse and oblique arytenoid, aryepiglottic, thyroarytenoid, vocalis, and thyroepiglottic muscles. All except the transverse arytenoid muscle are paired, and all except the cricothyroid muscle are innervated by the recurrent laryngeal nerve. Also called *muscles of larynx.*

musculus laryngopharyngeus MUSCULUS CONSTRICTOR PHARYNGIS INFERIOR.

musculus latissimus dorsi [NA] A muscle originating from the spines and interspinous ligaments of the lower six thoracic and upper lumbar vertebrae, the thoracolumbar fascia, the posterior third of the outer lip of iliac crest, and the outer surface of the lower three or four ribs; and inserted onto the floor of the intertubercular sulcus of humerus. It is supplied by the thoracodorsal nerve; adducts, extends, and medially rotates the arm; and pulls the trunk up and forwards when the arms are fixed, as in climbing. Also called *latissimus muscle of back, latissimus dorsi muscle.*

musculus levator alae nasi The alar insertion of musculus levator labii superioris alaeque nasi. An outmoded term.

musculus levator anguli oris [NA] A muscle originating from the canine fossa of maxilla, inferior to the infraorbital foramen; and inserted into the skin and muscles of the angle of the mouth. It is supplied by the zygomatic branch of the facial nerve, and raises the angle of the mouth, pulling it medially and accentuating the nasolabial furrow. Also called *levator muscle*

of angle of mouth, canine muscle, musculus caninus (outmoded), *caninus.*

musculus levator ani [NA] A broad muscle sheet attached to the inner aspect of the wall of the true pelvis and meeting the opposite muscle centrally to form most of the pelvic diaphragm, or floor, of the pelvis. Morphologically it is divisible into musculus pubococcygeus, musculus levator prostatae, musculus puborectalis, and musculus iliococcygeus. It originates from the inner surface of the body of the pubis lateral to the symphysis, and from the arcus tendineus of the obturator fascia and the inner aspect of the ischial spine. It inserts onto the lateral margin of the lower two coccygeal segments, the anococcygeal raphe, sphincter ani externus, and the perineal body; and is supplied by the fourth sacral nerve and the inferior rectal, or perineal, branch of the pudendal nerve. It supports and raises the pelvic floor, resisting increased intra-abdominal pressure, and constricts the anorectal junction and vagina. Also called *levator ani muscle.*

musculi levatores costarum [NA] Twelve small muscle bundles on each side of the thorax. They originate from the tip and lower margin of a transverse process of the seventh cervical and upper eleven thoracic vertebrae, and are inserted onto the upper margin and posterior surface of the rib below the vertebra from which it takes origin, from the tubercle to the angle. The lower four muscles have two fasciculi of insertion, the one attaching as above and the other missing the rib below and attaching to the second rib below the vertebra of origin. They are supplied by the intercostal nerves, and elevate the ribs. Also called *levator muscles of ribs.*

musculi levatores costarum breves [NA] The levatores costarum muscles, each of which inserts on the upper margin and external surface of the rib, between the tubercle and the angle, below the vertebra from which it takes origin. Also called *short levator muscles of ribs.*

musculi levatores costarum longi [NA] One of the two fasciculi of insertion of the lower four levatores costarum muscles that misses the rib below and attaches to the second rib below the vertebra from which it takes origin. Also called *long levator muscles of ribs.*

musculus levator glandulae thyreoideae An outmoded term for MUSCULUS LEVATOR GLANDULAE THYROIDEAE.

musculus levator glandulae thyroideae [NA] A muscular or fibromuscular band that occasionally extends from the body of the hyoid bone to either the isthmus of the thyroid gland or its pyramidal lobe, when present. It is located more often on the left side of the midline. Also called *levator muscle of thyroid gland, Soemmering's muscle, musculus levator glandulae thyreoideae* (outmoded).

musculus levator labii superioris [NA] A muscle originating from the infraorbital margin of the maxilla and from the zygomatic bone just above the infraorbital foramen. It is inserted into the skin and muscles of the upper lip medial to the angle of the mouth. It is supplied by the facial nerve, and raises and everts the upper lip. Also called *levator muscle of upper lip, caput infraorbitale musculi quadrati labii superioris, infraorbital head of quadratus labii superioris muscle* (outmoded), *quadrate muscle of upper lip* (outmoded).

musculus levator labii superioris alaeque nasi [NA] A muscle originating from the middle of the frontal process of the maxilla. Its medial fasciculus is inserted into the skin and alar cartilage of the nose, and its lateral fasciculus into the skin and muscles of the lateral part of the upper lip. It is supplied by the facial nerve. Its medial fasciculus dilates the nostril, and its lateral fasciculus raises and everts the upper lip, elevating the nasolabial furrow. Also called *levator muscle of upper lip and ala of nose, caput angulare musculi quadrati labii superioris, nasal head of levator labii superioris alaeque nasi muscle, angular* *head of quadratus labii superioris muscle* (outmoded).

musculus levator palpebrae superioris [NA] A muscle originating from the inferior surface of the lesser wing of the sphenoid bone, above and in front of the optic canal. Its lamina superficialis is inserted into the anterior surface of the superior tarsus and the skin of the upper eyelid, and lamina profunda (superior tarsal muscle) onto the upper margin of the superior tarsus, and by fascia to the superior conjunctival fornix. It is supplied by the oculomotor and cervical sympathetic nerves, and raises the upper eyelid. Also called *levator muscle of upper eyelid.*

musculus levator prostatae [NA] The most anterior fibers of the levator ani muscle that pass backwards, downwards, and medially across the side of the prostate to insert into the central tendon of the perineum in the male. Also called *levator muscle of prostate, elevator of prostate.*

musculus levator scapulae [NA] A muscle that originates from the posterior tubercles of transverse processes of the first four cervical vertebrae and is inserted onto the medial margin of scapula between the superior angle and the medial end of the spine. It is supplied by the third and fourth cervical and the dorsal scapular nerves, helps to elevate and retract the scapula, and helps to rotate and depress the scapula. Also called *levator muscle of scapula.*

musculus levator veli palatini [NA] A muscle originating from the inferior surface of the petrous part of the temporal bone and the inferior surface of the cartilaginous part of the auditory tube, and inserted onto the upper surface of the palatine aponeurosis. It is supplied by the pharyngeal plexus, and elevates the soft palate. Also called *levator muscle of velum palatinum, staphylinus internus* (outmoded), *petrostaphylinus* (outmoded), *petrosalpingostaphylinus* (outmoded).

musculi linguae [NA] The extrinsic and intrinsic muscles that form and move the tongue and change its shape, the former including the genioglossus, hyoglossus, chondroglossus, and styloglossus muscles, and the latter including the superior and the inferior longitudinal, the transverse, and the vertical muscles. Also called *muscles of tongue.*

musculus longissimus [NA] The intermediate, and largest, column of the musculus erector spinae, extending from the sacral region to the mastoid process of the temporal bone and divided into musculus longissimus capitis, musculus longissimus cervicis, and musculus longissimus thoracis. Also called *longissimus muscle.*

musculus longissimus capitis [NA] A muscle originating from the transverse processes of the upper three or four thoracic vertebrae and from the articular processes of the lower three or four cervical vertebrae, and inserted ontothe posterior margin of the mastoid process. It is supplied by the dorsal rami of the lower cervical spinal nerves, extends the head, and rotates the head to the same side. Also called *longissimus muscle of head, trachelomastoid muscle* (outmoded), *trachelomastoid* (outmoded).

musculus longissimus cervicis [NA] A muscle originating from the transverse processes of the upper four or five thoracic vertebrae, and inserted onto the posterior tubercles of the transverse processes of the middle cervical vertebrae. It is supplied by the dorsal rami of the lower cervical and upper thoracic spinal nerves, and helps to extend and laterally flex the vertebral column. Also called *longissimus muscle of neck.*

musculus longissimus dorsi An outmoded term for MUSCULUS LONGISSIMUS THORACIS.

musculus longissimus thoracis [NA] A muscle that, blended with the iliocostalis lumborum, originates from the posterior surfaces of the transverse processes and accessory processes of the lumbar vertebrae, and from the thoracolumbar fascia; and

is inserted onto the tips of the transverse processes of all the thoracic vertebrae, and onto the lower eight or nine ribs lateral to the tubercles. It is supplied by the dorsal rami of the lumbar and thoracic spinal nerves, and helps to extend the vertebral column and to bend and rotate the trunk to one side. Also called *longissimus muscle of thorax, longissimus muscle of back* (outmoded), *musculus longissimus dorsi* (outmoded).

musculus longitudinalis inferior linguae [NA] A narrow intrinsic muscle of the tongue extending on each side along the inferior surface from the base to the apex. Some posterior fibers may be attached to the body of the hyoid bone. It is supplied by the hypoglossal nerve, helps to shorten the tongue, and pulls the apex downward. Also called *inferior longitudinal muscle of tongue.*

musculus longitudinalis superior linguae [NA] A thin, superficial intrinsic muscle of the tongue extending along the dorsum from the base to the apex just deep to the lingual aponeurosis, to which some fibers are attached. It is supplied by the hypoglossal nerve, helps to shorten the tongue, and turns the margins and apex upwards, making the dorsum concave. Also called *superior longitudinal muscle of tongue.*

musculus longus capitis [NA] A muscle originating from the anterior tubercles of the transverse processes of the third to sixth cervical vertebrae and inserted onto the inferior surface of the basilar portion of the occipital bone, anterolateral to the pharyngeal tubercle. It is supplied by the ventral rami of the first to fourth cervical nerves, flexes the head, and rotates the head to the same side. Also called *long muscle of head.*

musculus longus colli [NA] A triangular muscle comprising three parts: the superior oblique, or superolateral, part, originating from the anterior tubercles of the transverse processes of the third to sixth cervical vertebrae, and inserted onto the anterior tubercle of atlas; the inferior oblique, or inferolateral, part, originating from the anterolateral parts of the bodies of the first three thoracic vertebrae, and inserted onto the anterior tubercles of the transverse processes of the fifth and sixth cervical vertebrae; and the vertical, or medial, part, originating from the anterolateral parts of the bodies of the first three thoracic and last three cervical vertebrae, and inserted onto the anterolateral surfaces of the bodies of the second to fourth cervical vertebrae. It is supplied by the ventral rami of the second to sixth cervical nerves. It flexes the neck; the superior oblique part flexes the neck laterally and rotates it to the same side; and the inferior oblique part rotates the neck to the opposite side. Also called *long muscle of neck.*

musculi lumbricales manus [NA] Four small muscles in each hand, of which the first and second originate from the lateral sides and palmar surfaces of the flexor digitorum profundus tendons to the index and middle fingers, and the medial two originate from adjacent sides of the deep flexor tendons to the middle and ring fingers and ring and little fingers respectively. They are inserted onto the lateral margin of the dorsal digital expansions of the extensor digitorum tendons to the medial four fingers. The lateral two are supplied by the median nerve, and the medial two by the deep branch of the ulnar nerve. They help to flex the proximal phalanges and extend the middle and distal phalanges of the medial four fingers. Also called *lumbrical muscles of hand, fidicinales* (outmoded).

musculi lumbricales pedis [NA] Four small muscles in each foot, of which the first originates from the medial margin of the flexor digitorum longus tendon to the second toe, and the lateral three from adjacent sides of the long flexor tendons to the third, fourth, and fifth toes. They are inserted into the medial sides of the dorsal digital expansions of the lateral four toes. The first is supplied by the medial plantar nerve, and the lateral three by the deep branch of the lateral plantar nerve. They flex the proximal phalanges of the lateral four toes, and slightly extend the other phalanges of those toes. Also called *lumbrical muscles of foot.*

musculus masseter   [NA] A muscle of which pars superficialis originates from the anterior two thirds of the inferior margin of zygomatic arch and from the zygomatic process of maxilla, and pars profunda from the inferior margin and deep surface of the zygomatic arch. Pars superficialis is inserted onto the lower half of the lateral surface of the ramus, and onto the angle and the adjacent part of the body of mandible; and pars profunda onto the upper half of the lateral surface of the ramus and the coronoid process of the mandible. It is supplied by the mandibular nerve, elevates the mandible, and participates in protraction and retraction and side-to-side movements of the mandible. Also called *masseter muscle, masseter.*

musculi membri inferioris   [NA] The muscles of the various segments of the lower limb, namely, thigh, leg, and foot. Also called *musculi extremitatis inferioris* (outmoded).

musculi membri superioris   [NA] The muscles of the various segments of the upper limb, namely, shoulder, arm, forearm, and hand. Also called *musculi extremitatis superioris.*

musculus mentalis   [NA] A muscle originating from the incisive fossa of mandible; inserted into the skin of the chin, fusing with the muscle of the opposite side; and supplied by the mandibular branch of the facial nerve. It draws up and wrinkles the skin of the chin, protruding the lower lip.

musculi multifidi   [NA] The second layer of the transversospinalis group of muscles of the back. They originate from the back of the sacrum, the aponeurosis of erector spinae muscle, the posterior superior iliac spine, dorsal sacroiliac ligaments, mamillary processes of lumbar vertebrae, transverse processes of thoracic vertebrae, and articular processes of the lower four cervical vertebrae. They are inserted onto the spines of vertebrae from fifth lumbar to axis, either onto the contiguous one above or spanning two to four vertebrae. They are supplied by the dorsal rami of the spinal nerves. They extend, laterally flex, and rotate the vertebral column; and participate in general control of posture. Also called *multifidus muscles.*

musculus mylohyoideus   [NA] A muscle originating from the mylohyoid line on the inner surface of the body of the mandible. It is inserted onto the front of the body of the hyoid bone and into a median fibrous raphe between it and its opposite fellow. It is supplied by the mylohyoid branch of the inferior alveolar nerve, elevates the floor of the mouth at the beginning of the act of swallowing, elevates the hyoid bone, and depresses the mandible. Also called *mylohyoid muscle, diaphragm of mouth, oral diaphragm, diaphragma oris.*

musculus mylopharyngeus   PARS MYLOPHARYNGEA MUSCULI CONSTRICTORIS PHARYNGIS SUPERIORIS.

musculus nasalis   A muscle of which pars transversa originates from the maxilla lateral to the lower part of the nasal notch, and pars alaris from the maxilla, medial to pars transversa. Pars transversa is inserted into an aponeurosis across the bridge of the nose in common with the part of the opposite side; and pars alaris is inserted into the cartilage of the ala nasi. It is supplied by the buccal branch of the facial nerve. Pars transversa compresses the nasal aperture, and pars alaris pulls the ala downwards and laterally, dilating the anterior nasal opening. Also called *nasal muscle.*

musculus obliquus auriculae   [NA] A muscle originating from the posterosuperior aspect of eminentia conchae of the auricle of the external ear, inserted onto the eminentia triangularis, and supplied by the posterior auricular branch of the facial nerve. It helps to modify the shape and position of the ear. Also called *Tod's muscle, oblique muscle of auricle.*

musculus obliquus capitis inferior   [NA] A muscle originating from the spine and adjacent lamina of the axis, inserted onto the back of the tip of transverse process of atlas, and supplied by the dorsal ramus of the first cervical nerve. It pulls the head to the same side. Also called *inferior oblique muscle of head.*

musculus obliquus capitis superior   [NA] A muscle originating from the upper surface of the transverse process of atlas, inserted onto the lateral part of the area between the superior and inferior nuchal lines of the occipital bone, and supplied by the dorsal ramus of the first cervical nerve. It extends the head and rotates it to the same side. Also called *superior oblique muscle of head.*

musculus obliquus externus abdominis   [NA] A muscle originating on the outer surfaces of the lower eight ribs lateral to the costal cartilages. It inserts onto the anterior two thirds of the outer lip of the iliac crest; by an aponeurosis into linea alba, upper border of pubic symphysis, and pubic crest; by the inguinal ligament to pubic tubercle and anterior superior iliac spine; and by the lacunar ligament to the pecten pubis. It is supplied by the ventral rami of the lower six thoracic spinal nerves. It supports and compresses abdominal viscera, depresses and compresses the lower part of the thorax during expiration, flexes the trunk when the pelvis is fixed, rotates the trunk to the opposite side, and flexes and rotates the pelvis when the thorax is fixed. Also called *external oblique muscle of abdomen.*

musculus obliquus inferior bulbi   [NA] A muscle that originates on the orbital surface of the maxilla lateral to the nasolacrimal groove. It is inserted onto the outer surface of the sclera behind the equator of the eyeball, between the insertions of the superior rectus and lateral rectus muscles. It is supplied by the oculomotor nerve, and serves to rotate the eyeball so as to turn the cornea upward and outward. When the cornea is deviated medially, it elevates the cornea. Also called *inferior oblique muscle of eyeball, musculus obliquus inferior oculi* (outmoded).

musculus obliquus inferior oculi   An outmoded term for MUSCULUS OBLIQUUS INFERIOR BULBI.

musculus obliquus internus abdominis   A muscle that originates in the lateral two thirds of the inguinal ligament, the anterior two thirds of the intermediate line of the iliac crest, and the thoracolumbar fascia. It inserts onto the lower three or four ribs, the conjoint tendon, and the linea alba and seventh, eighth, and ninth costal cartilages through the rectus sheath. It is supplied by the ventral rami of the lower six thoracic and first lumbar spinal nerves. It supports and compresses the abdominal viscera, depresses the lower thorax during expiration, flexes the trunk forwards and laterally, rotates the trunk to the same side, and flexes and rotates the pelvis when the thorax is fixed. Also called *internal oblique muscle of the abdomen.*

musculus obliquus superior bulbi   [NA] A muscle of the eyeball that originates on the body of the sphenoid bone above and medial to the optic canal within the orbit. It is inserted onto the outer surface of the sclera behind the equator of the eyeball and between the insertions of the superior rectus and lateral rectus muscles. It is supplied by the trochlear nerve, and it rotates the eyeball so as to turn the cornea downward and outward. When the cornea is deviated medially, it turns the cornea downward. Also called *superior oblique muscle of eyeball, musculus obliquus superior oculi* (outmoded).

musculus obliquus superior oculi   An outmoded term for MUSCULUS OBLIQUUS SUPERIOR BULBI.

musculus obturator externus   An outmoded term for MUSCULUS OBTURATORIUS EXTERNUS.

musculus obturator internus   An outmoded term for MUSCULUS OBTURATORIUS INTERNUS.

musculus obturatorius externus   [NA] A muscle that arises from the lateral surface of the pubic and ischial rami adjacent to the obturator foramen and of the obturator membrane. It is inserted onto the trochanteris fossa of the femur. Supplied by the posterior branch of the obturator nerve, it rotates the thigh laterally and serves as a postural muscle in steadying the hip joint. Also called *external obturator muscle, musculus obturator externus* (outmoded), *obturator externus muscle.*

musculus obturatorius internus [NA] A leg muscle that arises from the medial part of the pelvic surface of the obturator membrane, and the pubic rami and ischial ramus adjacent to the obturator foramen. It is inserted onto the anterior part of the medial surface of the greater trochanter of the femur. Supplied by the nerve to the obturator internus, it laterally rotates the extended thigh and abducts the flexed thigh. Also called *internal obturator muscle, obturator internus muscle, musculus obturator internus* (outmoded).

musculus occipitalis VENTER OCCIPITALIS MUSCULI OCCIP-ITOFRONTALIS.

musculus occipitofrontalis [NA] A muscle of the scalp with two venters, or bellies. Its venter occipitalis originates from the lateral two thirds of the supreme nuchal line and mastoid process on each side. Its venter frontalis originates from the galea aponeurotica. The venter occipitalis inserts onto the galea aponeurotica, whereas the venter frontalis inserts onto the skin and muscles of the eyebrows and the root of the nose. The venter occipitalis is supplied by the posterior auricular branch of the facial nerve; and the venter frontalis, the temporal branches of the facial nerve. The venter frontalis raises the eyebrows and skin above the nose and wrinkles the forehead, and the venter occipitalis pulls the scalp back and tenses the galea aponeurotica. Also called *occipitofrontal muscle, occipitofrontalis.*

musculi oculi An outmoded term for MUSCULI BULBI.

musculus omohyoideus [NA] A muscle that consists of an inferior and a superior belly, united at an angle by an intermediate tendon that is encircled by deep cervical fascia that attaches it to the clavicle and first rib. Its origin, by the inferior belly, is at the superior margin of the scapula adjacent to the scapular notch. It inserts, by the superior belly, onto the inferior margin of the body of the hyoid bone. The inferior belly is innervated by the ansa cervicalis, and the superior belly is innervated by the superior ramus of the ansa cervicalis. The muscle helps to pull down and steady the hyoid bone, as during swallowing and phonation. Also called *omohyoid muscle, coracohyoid, omohyoid.*

musculus opponens digiti minimi [NA] A muscle of the little finger that originates at the distal margin of the hook of the hamate bone and its adjacent flexor retinaculum. It is inserted onto the medial margin of the fifth metacarpal bone. It is supplied by the deep branch of the ulnar nerve and serves to pull the fifth metacarpal anteriorly and rotate it laterally, helping to cup the hand. Also called *opposing muscle of little finger, musculus opponens digiti quinti manus* (outmoded).

musculus opponens digiti quinti manus An outmoded term for MUSCULUS OPPONENS DIGITI MINIMI.

musculus opponens pollicis [NA] A muscle of the thumb that originates at the flexor retinaculum and tubercle of the trapezium and inserts onto the whole lateral half of the anterior surface of the first metacarpal bone. It is supplied by the median nerve and serves to flex, abduct, and medially rotate the first metacarpal in opposition. Also called *opposing muscle of thumb.*

musculus orbicularis [NA] A muscle in which the fibers are arranged in a circular fashion around an opening, such as the mouth or orbit. Also called *orbicular muscle, orbicularis.*

musculus orbicularis oculi [NA] A muscle of which the pars orbitalis originates from the frontal process of maxilla, the nasal portion of the frontal bone, and the medial palpebral ligament; pars palpebralis from the medial palpebral ligament and adjacent bone; and pars lacrimalis from the posterior lacrimal crest and lacrimal fascia. Of pars orbitalis, many fibers are inserted into

the skin of the eyebrows and others blend with the venter frontalis musculi occipitofrontalis; pars palpebralis is inserted into the lateral palpebral raphe; and pars lacrimalis into the tarsi of eyelids and lateral palpebral raphe. It is supplied by the temporal and zygomatic branches of the facial nerve and closes the eyelids tightly when all parts act together, as well as pulling the skin of the forehead and the skin lateral to the eye towards the inner canthus of eye. The pars palpebralis alone can close the eyelids, while the pars lacrimalis pulls the eyelids and lacrimal papillae medially. Also called *orbicular muscle of eye, sphincter oculi* (outmoded), *sphincter of eye.*

musculus orbicularis oris [NA] A composite, sphincterlike muscle surrounding the oral orifice and comprising two superficial layers, pars marginalis and pars labialis, and a deep layer composed of some fibers of musculus buccinator, musculus incisivus labii superioris, and musculus incisivus labii inferioris. The fibers of pars marginalis blend with eight or nine surrounding muscles that converge and interlace in the modiolus at each angle of the mouth. The fibers of pars labialis are those confined to the lips, and include oblique fibers of the compressor muscle of lip extending between the skin and the mucous membrane. It is supplied by the buccal, and mandibular branches of the facial nerve. It closes the mouth, compresses the lips against the teeth, and protrudes the lips. Also called *orbicular muscle of mouth, sphincter oris* (outmoded), *orbicularis oris.*

musculus orbitalis [NA] A thin layer of nonstriated muscle that bridges the inferior orbital fissure and the infraorbital groove posteriorly. It is innervated by sympathetic nerves. The actions are obscure. Also called *orbital muscle, Müller's muscle, membrana orbitalis musculosa* (outmoded).

musculi ossiculorum auditus [NA] The muscles attached to and acting on the ossicles in the middle ear, namely, musculus tensor tympani and musculus stapedius. Also called *muscles of auditory ossicles, muscles of ossicles.*

musculi ossis hyoidei Musculi infrahyoidei and musculi suprahyoidei considered together. An outmoded term.

musculi palati et faucium [NA] The muscles of the soft palate and the palatoglossal and palatopharyngeal arches, namely, musculus levator veli palatini, musculus tensor veli palatini, musculus uvulae, musculus palatoglossus, and musculus palatopharyngeus. Also called *muscles of palate and fauces, muscles of fauces.*

musculus palatoglossus [NA] A muscle that originates on the inferior surface of the palatine aponeurosis of the soft palate and inserts onto the side of the tongue. It is innervated by the pharyngeal plexus, and it serves to elevate the root of the tongue and pull the palatoglossal arch medially, closing off the oral cavity from the oropharynx. Also called *palatoglossus muscle, glossopalatine muscle, musculus glossopalatinus* (outmoded), *constrictor isthmi faucium* (outmoded), *glossopalatinus.*

musculus palatopharyngeus [NA] A muscle that originates on the superior surface of the palatine aponeurosis of the soft palate and the posterior margin of the osseous palate. It inserts onto the posterior margin of the thyroid cartilage and the pharyngobasilar fascia of the pharyngeal wall. Supplied by the pharyngeal plexus, it elevates the pharynx during swallowing. Acting with the opposite side it brings together the arches narrowing the pharyngeal isthmus. It also depresses the soft palate. Also called *palatopharyngeal muscle, musculus pharyngopalatinus* (outmoded), *pharyngopalatine muscle* (outmoded).

musculus palmaris brevis [NA] A muscle that originates on the medial edge of the palmar aponeurosis and flexor retinaculum. It inserts onto the skin on the medial margin of the hand. Supplied by the superficial branch of the ulnar nerve, it pulls the skin on the medial side of the hand toward the hollow of the palm, deepening the palm. Also called *short palmar muscle, caro quadrata manus* (outmoded).

musculus palmaris longus A muscle that originates on the common flexor tendon on the medial epicondyle of the humerus, and on the antebrachial fascia. It is inserted onto the distal part of the flexor retinaculum and the palmar aponeurosis, and it is supplied by the medial nerve. It flexes the hand and tenses the palmar aponeurosis. Also called *long palmar muscle*.

musculi papillares [NA] Conical portions of the trabeculae carneae that are attached by their bases to the ventricular walls while their apices project inward and are continuous with the chordae tendineae, which are attached to the triangular cusps of the atrioventricular valves. In each ventricle there are two papillary muscles, anterior and posterior, while in the right ventricle there are also some small septal papillary muscles. Each papillary muscle is usually attached by chordae tendineae to more than one cusp. Also called *papillary muscles*.

musculi papillares septales ventriculi dextri Some small papillary muscles arising from the interventricular septum in the right ventricle of the heart and attached by chordae tendineae to the septal and anterior cusps of the tricuspid valve. An outmoded term. Also called *septal papillary muscles of right ventricle*.

musculus papillaris anterior ventriculi dextri [NA] The anterior and larger of the two papillary muscles in the right ventricle, the chordae tendineae of which connect it to the anterior and posterior cusps of the tricuspid valve. It is attached to the sternocostal wall of the ventricle. Also called *anterior papillary muscle of right ventricle*.

musculus papillaris anterior ventriculi sinistri [NA] The large anterior papillary muscle attached to the sternocostal wall of the left ventricle and connected by chordae tendineae to both cusps of the mitral valve. Also called *anterior papillary muscle of left ventricle*.

musculus papillaris posterior ventriculi dextri [NA] The posterior and smaller of the two papillary muscles in the right ventricle which is attached to the diaphragmatic wall. Occasionally it consists of several parts and its chordae tendineae connect it to the posterior and septal cusps of the tricuspid valve. Also called *posterior papillary muscle of right ventricle*.

musculus papillaris posterior ventriculi sinistri [NA] One of the two papillary muscles of the left ventricle of the heart which arises from the diaphragmatic wall of the ventricle. Its rounded free extremity gives attachment to chordae tendineae which extend to both cusps of the mitral valve. Also called *posterior papillary muscle of left ventricle*.

musculi pectinati [NA] Prominent ridges of myocardium forming a network on the internal walls of the auricles of the heart. In the right auricle they extend into a portion of the right atrium as parallel ridges on the lateral side of the crista terminalis. Also called *pectinate muscles*.

musculus pectineus A muscle that originates from the pecten of the pubis and the bone in front of it, and from the pectineal fascia. It is inserted onto the upper part of the pectineal line behind and below the lesser trochanter of the femur. The femoral or, occasionally, the obturator nerve supplies the muscle, which adducts and flexes the thigh. Also called *pectineal muscle*.

musculus pectoralis major [NA] A muscle of which pars clavicularis originates from the medial half of anterior surface of the clavicle; pars sternocostalis from the anterior surface of sternum down to sixth costal cartilage and the anterior surface of second to sixth costal cartilages; and pars abdominalis from the aponeurosis of obliquus externus abdominis. It is inserted onto the lateral lip of intertubercular sulcus of humerus, and is supplied by the medial and lateral pectoral nerves. It flexes, adducts, and medially rotates the arm when the thorax is fixed; and pulls the chest upwards when arms are fixed, as in climbing or in forced inspiration. Also called *greater pectoral muscle, ectopectoralis* (outmoded).

musculus pectoralis minimus An occasional accessory pectoral muscle that extends from the first costal cartilage and adjacent sternum to the coracoid process of the scapula.

musculus pectoralis minor [NA] A muscle originating from the second to fifth ribs near the costal cartilages. It is inserted onto the medial margin and upper surface of the coracoid process of scapula, and supplied by the medial and lateral pectoral nerves. It helps serratus anterior to pull the scapula forwards, and depresses and rotates the scapula. Also called *smaller pectoral muscle*.

musculi perinei [NA] The muscles occupying the inferior pelvic aperture, including those of the pelvic diaphragm, urogenital diaphragm, and external genitals. Also called *muscles of perineum, perineal muscles*. • Common usage limits the muscles of the perineum mainly to those of the latter two, which are divided into anal and urogenital groups.

musculus peroneocalcaneus A rare variant of musculus flexor hallucis longus in which a slip arises from the back of the fibula, passes under the sustentaculum tali, and inserts into the calcaneus. Also called *peroneocalcaneus internus*.

musculus peroneus brevis [NA] A muscle that originates from the distal two thirds of the lateral surface of the fibula, and the anterior and posterior crural intermuscular septa. It inserts onto the lateral aspect of the base of the fifth metatarsal bone. Supplied by the superficial peroneal nerve, it everts and plantar flexes the foot. Also called *short peroneal muscle, musculus fibularis brevis, short fibular muscle* (outmoded).

musculus peroneus digiti quinti An occasional accessory peroneal muscle that arises from the distal fourth of the fibula, either separate from or fused with the peroneus brevis muscle, and is inserted by a tendon into the fifth toe. It is normally present in monkeys. In humans, it is extremely variable when it occurs, especially with respect to its insertion. Also called *musculus peroneus of fifth toe* (outmoded), *peroneus digiti quinti muscle*.

musculus peroneus of fifth toe An outmoded term for MUSCULUS PERONEUS DIGITI QUINTI.

musculus peroneus longus [NA] A leg muscle that originates at the head and proximal two thirds of the lateral surface of the fibula, the anterior and posterior crural intermuscular septa, and lateral condyle of the tibia. It is inserted on the inferior surface of the medial cuneiform bone and lateral side of the base of the first metatarsal bone. Supplied by the superficial peroneal nerve, it everts and plantarflexes the foot as well as supports the transverse arch of the foot. Also called *long peroneal muscle, musculus fibularis longus, long fibular muscle*.

musculus peroneus tertius [NA] A muscle of the leg that originates at the distal third of the medial surface of the fibula and adjacent interosseous membrane. It is inserted onto the dorsal surface of the base and part of the medial margin of the shaft of the fifth metatarsal bone. Supplied by the deep peroneal nerve, it dorsiflexes and everts the foot. Also called *third peroneal muscle, musculus fibularis tertius, third fibular muscle* (outmoded).

musculus pharyngopalatinus An outmoded term for MUSCULUS PALATOPHARYNGEUS.

musculus piriformis [NA] A muscle that originates from the lateral part of the anterior surface of the second, third, and fourth sacral vertebrae, the areas between the pelvic sacral foramina, and the posterior margin of the greater sciatic notch. It is inserted onto the anteromedial part of the upper margin of the greater trochanter of the femur. It is innervated by the fifth lumbar and first and second sacral nerves. It serves to laterally rotate the extended thigh and abduct the flexed thigh. Also called *piriform muscle*. Also *musculus pyriformis*.

musculus plantaris [NA] A muscle that originates from the distal part of the lateral supracondylar line and oblique popliteal ligament. It is inserted onto the middle of the posterior surface of the calcaneus with the tendo calcaneus. Supplied by the tibial nerve, it plantarflexes the foot. Also called *plantar muscle, plantaris*.

musculus pleuroesophageus [NA] An accessory slip of smooth muscle fibers that occasionally connects the left mediastinal pleura to the esophagus, helping to fix it. Also called *pleuroesophageal muscle*.

musculus popliteus [NA] A muscle that originates from a facet at the anterior end of the groove on the lateral aspect of the lateral condyle of the femur and arcuate popliteal ligament. It is inserted onto the posterior surface of the shaft of the tibia above the soleal line, and it is supplied by the tibial nerve. It rotates the tibia medially and flexes it, and laterally rotates the femur when the tibia is fixed. Also called *popliteal muscle, popliteus*.

musculus procerus [NA] A muscle of the face that originates from the upper part of the lateral nasal cartilage and the fascia over the nasal bone. It is inserted into the skin just above the root of the nose and the frontal part of the occipitofrontalis muscle. It is supplied by the buccal branches of the facial nerve. It pulls down the medial end of the eyebrows and skin of the forehead, producing transverse wrinkles above the root of the nose. Also called *procerus muscle, procerus*.

musculus procoracohumeralis A muscle of the pectoral girdle in urodeles that originates laterally on the procoracoid cartilage, inserts on the lateral surface of the humerus, and moves the humerus anteriorly.

musculus pronator profundus In comparative anatomy, the homologue of the musculus pronator quadratus in the pectoral limb and, in reptiles, of the musculus tibialis posterior in the hind or pelvic limb.

musculus pronator quadratus [NA] A muscle of the forearm that originates from the medial side of the anterior surface of the distal fourth of the ulna. It is inserted onto the lower fourth of the anterior surface and anterior margin of the radius and into a small area above the ulnar notch of radius. It is innervated by the anterior interosseous branch of the median nerve, and it serves to pronate the forearm and hand. Also called *quadrate pronator muscle, quadratipronator* (outmoded).

musculus pronator teres [NA] A muscle of the forearm that has two heads. The caput humerale originates from the upper part of the anterior surface of the medial epicondyle and the common flexor tendon, whereas the caput ulnare originates from the medial margin of the coronoid process of the ulna. The muscle is inserted onto the middle third of the lateral surface of the radius. It is supplied by the median nerve, and it serves to pronate the forearm and hand as well as to help flex the forearm. Also called *round pronator muscle*.

musculus prostaticus An outmoded term for SUBSTANTIA MUSCULARIS PROSTATAE.

musculus psoas major [NA] A muscle of the back that originates from the intervertebral disks between the twelfth thoracic and fifth lumbar vertebrae and adjacent margins of the bodies of these vertebrae, the anterior surfaces and lower borders of the transverse processes of the lumbar vertebrae, and the fibrous arches over the lateral aspects of the bodies of the lumbar vertebrae. It inserts onto the lesser trochanter of the femur, and it is supplied by the ventral rami of the first, second, and third lumbar nerves. It acts with the iliacus muscle to flex the thigh upon the pelvis, to flex the pelvis and trunk on the thigh, to laterally flex the vertebral column, and medially rotate the free lower limb. Also called *greater psoas muscle*.

musculus psoas minor [NA] A muscle that originates from the sides of the bodies of the twelfth thoracic and first lumbar vertebrae and the disk between them. It is inserted onto the iliopectineal eminence and pecten pubis. It is supplied by the

first lumbar nerve, and it weakly flexes the trunk. Also called *smaller psoas muscle*.

musculus pterygoideus externus An outmoded term for MUSCULUS PTERYGOIDEUS LATERALIS.

musculus pterygoideus internus An outmoded term for MUSCULUS PTERYGOIDEUS MEDIALIS.

musculus pterygoideus lateralis [NA] A muscle whose upper head originates from the infratemporal crest and infratemporal surface of the greater wing of the sphenoid bone and whose lower head originates from the lateral surface of the lateral pterygoid plate. It is inserted onto the front of the neck of the mandibular condyle and the articular disk and capsule of the temperomandibular joint. It is innervated by the mandibular nerve, and it serves to open the mouth and protrude the mandible when both sides act with the medial pterygoids. It can also rotate the jaw to the opposite side. Also called *lateral pterygoid muscle, musculus pterygoideus externus* (outmoded), *external pterygoid muscle* (outmoded), *ectopterygoid* (outmoded).

musculus pterygoideus medialis [NA] A muscle of the jaw that originates from the medial surface of the lateral pterygoid plate, the pyramidal process of the palatine bone, and the tuberosity of the maxilla. It is inserted onto the lower half of the medial surface of the ramus and the angle of the mandible. Supplied by the mandibular nerve, it elevates the mandible, protrudes the mandible when acting with both lateral pterygoids, and produces side-to-side movements of the mandible when the two sides act alternately. Also called *medial pterygoid muscle, musculus pterygoideus internus* (outmoded), *internal pterygoid muscle* (outmoded).

musculus pterygopharyngeus PARS PTERYGOPHARYNGEA MUSCULI CONSTRICTORIS PHARYNGIS SUPERIORIS.

musculus pterygospinosus An accessory muscle slip that occasionally extends between the spine of the sphenoid bone and the posterior margin of the lateral pterygoid plate.

musculus pubococcygeus [NA] A morphologic subdivision of the levator ani muscle that originates from the pelvic surface of the pubis and anterior part of the arcus tendineus. It is inserted onto the anterior sacrococcygeal ligament, the anococcygeal ligament, and the rectum. Also called *pubococcygeal muscle, pubococcygeus*.

musculus puboischiofemoralis externus A ventral muscle on the hind leg of reptiles which pulls the femur downward. Its origin is on the outer surface of the pubis and ischium, and its insertion is on the side of and near the head of the femur.

musculus puboischiotibialis A hind-limb muscle of reptiles and urodeles that originates ventrally on the ischium, inserts on the proximal end of the tibia, and acts to draw the hind limb toward the body and flex the leg.

musculus puboprostaticus [NA] Smooth muscle fibers of the external longitudinal layer of the urinary bladder that are located in the medial puboprostatic ligament. Also called *puboprostatic muscle*.

musculus puborectalis [NA] A thick portion of musculus levator ani that arises from the back of the pubis below the origin of pubococcygeus, the obturator fascia, and the pelvic surface of the urogenital diaphragm. It then extends on each side of the rectum, where some fibers blend with its longitudinal layer of muscle and descend to the anal canal between the internal and external sphincters of the anus, even extending to the skin. Other fibers loop behind the anorectal junction to end in the anococcygeal ligament. Also called *puborectal muscle, Braune's muscle, puborectalis muscle*.

musculus pubovaginalis [NA] The most anterior fibers of the levator ani muscle in the female that pass backwards and medially across the sides of the vagina to end in the central tendon of the perineum, serving as a sphincter of the vagina. It is homologous to the levator prostatae in the male. Also called *pubovaginal muscle*.

musculus pubovesicalis [NA] Some smooth muscle fibers of the external longitudinal layer of the urinary bladder that extend into the pubovesical ligaments in the female. It is homologous to musculus puboprostaticus in the male. Also called *pubovesical muscle*.

musculus pyramidalis [NA] A muscle that originates from the front of the body of the pubis and pubic symphysis. It is inserted onto the linea alba about midway between the pubis and the umbilicus. Supplied by the subcostal nerve, it tenses the linea alba. Also called *triangular fascia of Macalister* (outmoded), *pyramidal muscle, pyramidalis*.

musculus pyramidalis auriculae [NA] A small muscle of the external ear that is occasionally present as an upward extension of some fibers of musculus tragicus to the spine of the helix. Also called *pyramidal muscle of auricle, Jung's muscle*.

musculus pyriformis MUSCULUS PIRIFORMIS.

musculus quadratus femoris [NA] A muscle that originates from the upper part of the lateral margin and adjacent surface of the ischial tuberosity. It is inserted onto a tubercle about midway along the intertrochanteric crest of the femur and a short distance below. It is supplied by a branch from the fifth lumbar and first sacral nerves, and serves to rotate the thigh laterally. Also called *quadrate muscle of thigh*.

musculus quadratus labii inferioris An outmoded term for MUSCULUS DEPRESSOR LABII INFERIORIS.

musculus quadratus labii superioris A muscle with three heads now designated as three separate muscles, namely, musculus levator labii superioris, musculus levator labii superioris alaeque nasi, and musculus zygomaticus minor. An outmoded term.

musculus quadratus lumborum [NA] A muscle that originates from the iliolumbar ligament and adjacent inner lip of the iliac crest and the transverse processes of the lower three or four lumbar vertebrae. It is inserted onto the medial part of the lower margin of the twelfth rib and the transverse processes of the upper three or four lumbar vertebrae. It is innervated by the ventral rami of the twelfth thoracic and upper three or four lumbar nerves. It acts to depress and fix the twelfth rib, especially in inspiration; flex the trunk laterally; and, when both sides act together, to assist in the extension of the vertebral column.

musculus quadratus plantae [NA] A muscle of the foot that originates by lateral and medial heads from the inferior surface of the calcaneus anterior to the lateral and medial processes, respectively. It is inserted onto the tendon or tendons of the musculus flexor digitorum longus, and it is supplied by the lateral plantar nerve. It exerts traction on the tendon of the flexor digitorum longus so as to flex the toes along their axes and helps to maintain the longitudinal arches of the foot. Also called *plantar head of flexor digitorum pedis longus muscle* (outmoded), *quadrate head of flexor digitorum pedis longus muscle* (outmoded), *caro quadrata sylvii* (outmoded), *musculus flexor accessorius, quadrate muscle of sole, accessory flexor muscle*.

musculus quadriceps femoris [NA] A muscle that originates by four heads: musculus rectus femoris, musculus vastus medialis, musculus vastus intermedius, and musculus vastus lateralis. It is inserted onto the base of the patella by a common tendon, the tuberosity of the tibia by the ligamentum patellae, and the medial and lateral patellar retinacula. Supplied by the femoral nerve, it extends the leg. Also called *quadriceps muscle of thigh, quadriceps femoris muscle, quadriceps femoris*.

musculus rectococcygeus [NA] Two nonstriated muscle bundles that arise from the front of the second and third coccygeal vertebrae where they blend with fibers of the levator ani muscle and extend anteriorly to join the longitudinal muscle fibers on the posterior wall of the anal canal and the perirectal fascia. It helps to elevate and retract the lower part of the rectum and the anal canal. Also called *rectococcygeal muscle*.

musculus rectourethralis [NA] Some fasciculi of the anterior longitudinal muscle of the rectal ampulla that extend anteriorly to the central tendon of the perineum and the membranous urethra in the male. Also called *rectourethral muscle*.

musculus rectouterinus [NA] A band of longitudinal muscle fibers of the uterus that passes backwards from the cervix in the rectouterine fold, helping to form the uterosacral ligament, to blend with longitudinal muscle fibers of the rectum. Also called *rectouterine muscle, Luschka's muscles, cervicorectal muscle* (outmoded).

musculus rectovesicalis Some muscle fibers of the external longitudinal layer of the urinary bladder that extend from the base to the front of the rectum. Also called *rectovesical muscle, rectovesicalis*.

musculus rectus abdominis [NA] A muscle that originates from the crest of the pubis, the front of the pubic symphysis, and the lower part of the linea alba. It is inserted onto the fifth, sixth, and seventh costal cartilages and the xiphoid process. It is supplied by the ventral rami of the lower six or seven thoracic spinal nerves. The muscle serves to flex the trunk forward when the pelvis is fixed, helps to compress the abdominal viscera, and acts to flex the pelvis when the thorax is fixed.

musculus rectus anticus femoris An outmoded term for MUSCULUS RECTUS FEMORIS.

musculus rectus capitis anterior [NA] A muscle that originates from the anterior surface of the lateral mass and part of the transverse process of the atlas. It is inserted onto the inferior surface of the basilar part of the occipital bone in front of the condyle. Supplied by the first and second cervical nerve, it serves to flex the head forward and rotate the head toward the same side.

musculus rectus capitis lateralis [NA] A muscle that originates from the upper surface of the transverse part of the atlas and is inserted onto the inferior surface of the jugular process of the occipital bone. Supplied by the first and second cervical nerves, it serves to bend the head to the same side.

musculus rectus capitis posterior major [NA] A muscle whose origin is on the spine of the axis and whose insertion is located on the lateral half of the inferior nuchal line of the occipital bone. It is supplied by the dorsal ramus of the first cervical nerve, and it serves to extend the head and rotate the head to the same side.

musculus rectus capitis posterior minor [NA] A muscle that originates from the tubercle on the posterior arch of the atlas. It is inserted onto and below the medial third of the inferior nuchal line of the occipital bone. Supplied by the dorsal ramus of the first cervical nerve, it serves to extend the head.

musculus rectus externus MUSCULUS RECTUS LATERALIS BULBI.

musculus rectus femoris [NA] A muscle of which the straight head originates from the anterior inferior iliac spine and the reflected head from the groove above the acetabulum. It is inserted onto the upper margin of the patella, the tendon of the quadriceps femoris muscle, and onto the tuberosity of tibia by the ligamentum patellae. It is supplied by the femoral nerve, extends the leg, and flexes the thigh. Also called *musculus rectus anticus femoris* (outmoded).

musculus rectus inferior bulbi [NA] A muscle that originates from the lower part of the annulus tendineus communis and is inserted onto the lower aspect of the outer surface of the sclera behind the corneal margin. Supplied by the oculomotor nerve, it rotates the visual axis, downward about the transverse axis and medially about the vertical axis. It also extorts the eye. Also called *inferior straight muscle, inferior rectus muscle of* *bulb, musculus rectus inferior oculi* (outmoded), *deprimens oculi* (outmoded).

musculus rectus inferior oculi   An outmoded term for MUS-CULUS RECTUS INFERIOR BULBI.

musculus rectus internus   MUSCULUS RECTUS MEDIALIS BULBI.

musculus rectus lateralis bulbi   [NA] A muscle that originates from the lateral side of the annulus tendineus communis and the orbital surface of the greater wing of the sphenoid bone, just lateral to the tendon. It is inserted onto the lateral aspect of the sclera behind the corneal margin. Supplied by the abducent nerve, the muscle rotates the eyeball laterally. Also called *lateral straight muscle, musculus rectus externus, lateral rectus muscle of bulb, abducens oculi, musculus rectus lateralis oculi* (outmoded), *extrarectus* (outmoded).

musculus rectus lateralis oculi   An outmoded term for MUS-CULUS RECTUS LATERALIS BULBI.

musculus rectus medialis bulbi   [NA] A muscle that originates from the medial aspect of the annulus tendineus communis and is inserted onto the medial aspect of the scleral surface behind the corneal margin. Supplied by the oculomotor nerve, it rotates the eyeball medially. With the lateral rectus, it can act on both eyes together to produce convergence or divergence. Also called *medial straight muscle, medial rectus muscle of bulb, musculus rectus internus, musculus rectus medialis oculi* (outmoded).

musculus rectus medialis oculi   An outmoded term for MUS-CULUS RECTUS MEDIALIS BULBI.

musculus rectus superior bulbi   [NA] A muscle of the eye that originates from the upper part of the annulus tendineus communis and is inserted onto the upper part of the sclera behind the corneal margin. Supplied by the oculomotor nerve, it acts in the elevation, medial rotation, and intorsion of the eyeball. Also called *superior rectus muscle of bulb, musculus rectus superior oculi* (outmoded).

musculus rectus superior oculi   An outmoded term for MUS-CULUS RECTUS SUPERIOR BULBI.

musculus retrahens aurem   MUSCULUS AURICULARIS POSTERIOR.

musculus retrahens auriculam   MUSCULUS AURICULARIS POSTERIOR.

musculus rhomboatloideus   A rare variant of the rhomboid muscles that extends from the cervical and thoracic vertebrae to the atlas.

musculus rhomboideus   Either the musculus rhomboideus major or the musculus rhomboideus minor.

musculus rhomboideus major   [NA] A muscle that originates from the spines of the second to fifth thoracic vertebrae and their supraspinous ligaments. It is inserted onto the medial margin of the scapula from the root of the spine to the inferior angle. Supplied by the dorsal scapular nerve, it elevates and retracts the scapula and helps to rotate the scapula and depress the point of the scapula. Also called *greater rhomboid muscle.*

musculus rhomboideus minor   [NA] A muscle originating from the lower part of the ligamentum nuchae and the spines of the seventh cervical and first thoracic vertebrae. It is inserted onto the medial margin of the scapula opposite the root of the spine. Supplied by the dorsal scapular nerve, it elevates and retracts the scapula and helps to rotate and depress the point of the scapula. Also called *lesser rhomboid muscle.*

musculus risorius   [NA] A muscle of the face that originates from the parotid fascia and is inserted into the skin and mucosa at the angle of the mouth. Supplied by the buccal branches of the facial nerve, it pulls the angle of the mouth laterally. Also called *risorius muscle, Santorini's muscle, Albinus muscle.*

musculi rotatores   [NA] The deepest layer of transversospinal muscles comprising small muscles between the transverse and spinous processes of the vertebrae and extending from the sacrum to the spinous process of the axis. They are divided into three morphologic units: the musculi rotatores cervicis, musculi rotatores thoracis, and musculi rotatores lumborum. They are supplied by the dorsal rami of the spinal nerves in their respective regions. They rotate the vertebral column, help to laterally flex and extend the vertebral column, and help to control posture, especially in steadying the vertebral column during body movements. Also called *rotator muscles.*

musculi rotatores breves   Those rotator muscles arising from transverse processes and inserting on the laminae of the next vertebra above. Also called *short rotator muscles.*

musculi rotatores cervicis   [NA] Variable muscle bundles that connect the transverse process of a cervical vertebra to the lamina of the vertebra next above, extending as far as the root of its spine. Also called *rotator muscles of neck.*

musculi rotatores longi   Those rotator muscles that arise from transverse processes and insert on the laminae of the second vertebra above. Also called *long rotator muscles.*

musculi rotatores lumborum   [NA] Variable and irregular muscle bundles that each connect the transverse process of a lumbar vertebra to the lamina of the vertebra next above, extending as far as the root of its spine.

musculi rotatores thoracis   [NA] A series of eleven muscles on each side that each connects the upper part of a transverse process of a thoracic vertebra to the outer surface of the lamina of the vertebra next above, extending as far as the root of its spine. Also called *rotator muscles of thorax.*

musculus sacrococcygeus anterior   MUSCULUS SACROCOC-CYGEUS VENTRALIS.

musculus sacrococcygeus dorsalis   [NA] An inconstant accessory muscle composed of a few fasciculi extending behind the sacrococcygeal joint, from the posterior surface of lower sacral vertebrae or from the posterior inferior iliac spine to the posterior aspect of the coccyx. It is a vestigial representation of an elevator muscle of tailed mammals. Also called *dorsal sacrococcygeal muscle, musculus sacrococcygeus posterior, musculus extensor coccygis* (outmoded), *posterior sacrococcygeal muscle.*

musculus sacrococcygeus posterior   MUSCULUS SACROCOC-CYGEUS DORSALIS.

musculus sacrococcygeus ventralis   [NA] An inconstant muscle that arises from the sides of the fourth and fifth sacral vertebrae, the front of the first coccygeal vertebra, and the sacrospinous ligament, and that is inserted into the second to fourth coccygeal vertebrae and anterior sacrococcygeal ligament. It is a vestigial representation of a depressor muscle of tailed mammals. Also called *coccygerector* (outmoded), *musculus sacrococcygeus anterior, ventral sacrococcygeal muscle, anterior sacrococcygeal muscle.*

musculus sacrospinalis   An outmoded term for MUSCULUS ERECTOR SPINAE.

musculus salpingopharyngeus   [NA] A muscle that originates from the inferior surface of the cartilage of the auditory tube near its opening in the pharynx and fuses with the palatopharyngeus muscle in the wall of the pharynx. Supplied by the pharyngeal plexus, it elevates the upper part of the pharynx and aids in opening the auditory tube during swallowing. Also called *salpingopharyngeal muscle.*

musculus sartorius   [NA] A muscle that originates from the anterior superior iliac spine and the surface just below it. It is inserted onto the upper end of the medial surface of the tibia and into the fascia cruris. It is supplied by the femoral nerve, and it flexes, abducts, and laterally rotates the thigh as well as flexes and medially rotates the leg. Also called *sartorius muscle.*

musculus scalenus anterior   [NA] A muscle that originates from the anterior tubercles of the transverse process of the third to sixth cervical vertebrae and is inserted onto the scalene tubercle and the upper surface of the first rib. It is supplied by the ventral rami of the third to sixth cervical nerves. Acting from above, it elevates the first rib; acting from below, it flexes the cervical vertebrae forward and sideways and rotates them to the opposite side. Also called *anterior scalene muscle, musculus scalenus anticus* (outmoded), *scalenus anticus* (outmoded).

musculus scalenus anticus An outmoded term for MUSCULUS SCALENUS ANTERIOR.

musculus scalenus medius [NA] A muscle that originates from the transverse processes of the axis, and often of the atlas, and the posterior tubercles of the transverse processes of the lower five cervical vertebrae. It is inserted onto the upper surface of the first rib behind the subclavian groove. It is supplied by the ventral rami of the third to eighth cervical nerves. Acting from above, it raises the first rib. Acting from below it flexes the cervical vertebrae to the same side. Also called *middle scalene muscle, mediscalenus.*

musculus scalenus minimus [NA] A separate muscle band occasionally present between the scalenus anterior and medius muscles. It arises from the anterior tubercles of the transverse processes of the sixth and seventh cervical vertebrae and is inserted on the inner border of first rib and to the dome of the pleura, which it tenses on contraction. Some authorities consider the suprapleural membrane to be the flattened tendon of this muscle. Also called *smallest scalene muscle, Sibson's muscle, Albinus muscle.*

musculus scalenus posterior [NA] A muscle that arises from the posterior tubercles of the transverse processes of the fourth, fifth, and sixth cervical vertebrae. It is inserted onto the lateral surface of the second rib, and it is supplied by the ventral rami of the sixth, seventh, and eighth cervical spinal nerves. Acting from above, it elevates the second rib; acting from below, it flexes the lower cervical vertebrae to the same side. Also called *posterior scalene muscle.*

musculus scansorius An inconstant muscle slip deep to the gluteus minimus muscle that is derived either from the latter or the piriformis muscle and is inserted into the capsule of the hip joint. Also called *musculus accessorius gluteus minimus, musculus gluteus quartus.*

musculus semimembranosus [NA] A muscle that arises from the superolateral impression on the upper part of the ischial tuberosity. It is inserted onto the back of the medial condyle of the tibia, the lateral femoral condyle by the oblique popliteal ligament, and the capsule of the knee joint. Supplied by the tibial nerve, it flexes the leg and medially rotates the flexed leg as well as extends the thigh and medially rotates the extended thigh. Also called *semimembranous muscle.*

musculus semispinalis [NA] The superficial mass of the transversospinal group of muscles, extending from the thorax to the occipital bone and divided into three morphological units: the musculus semispinalis capitis, musculus semispinalis cervicis, and musculus semispinalis thoracis. It is supplied by the dorsal rami of the cervical and thoracic spinal nerves. Also called *semispinal muscle, semispinalis.*

musculus semispinalis capitis [NA] A muscle that arises from the transverse processes of the upper six or seven thoracic and seventh cervical vertebrae and the articular processes of the lower four cervical vertebrae. It is inserted onto the medial part of the area between the superior and inferior nuchal lines of the occipital bone. Supplied by the dorsal rami of the cervical spinal nerves, it extends the head and rotates it to the opposite side. Also called *semispinal muscle of the head, complexus.*

musculus semispinalis cervicis [NA] A muscle that arises from the transverse processes of the upper five or six thoracic vertebrae. It is inserted onto the spines of the second to sixth cervical vertebrae, and it is supplied by the dorsal rami of the cervical and thoracic spinal nerves. It extends the cervical and

thoracic vertebrae and rotates the vertebral column to the opposite side. Also called *semispinal muscle of neck.*

musculus semispinalis dorsi An outmoded term for MUSCULUS SEMISPINALIS THORACIS.

musculus semispinalis thoracis [NA] A muscle of the back that arises from the transverse processes of the sixth to tenth thoracic vertebrae and is inserted onto the spines of the upper four thoracic and lower two cervical vertebrae. It is supplied by the dorsal rami of the cervical and thoracic spinal nerves. It extends the cervical and thoracic vertebrae and rotates them to the opposite side. Also called *semispinal muscle of thorax, musculus semispinalis dorsi* (outmoded).

musculus semitendinosus [NA] A muscle that arises from the inferomedial impression on the upper part of the ischial tuberosity. It is inserted onto the upper part of the medial surface of the tibia behind and below the insertion of the gracilis muscle. Supplied by the tibial nerve, it flexes the leg and medially rotates the flexed leg. It also extends the thigh and medially rotates the extended thigh. Also called *semitendinous muscle.*

musculus serratus anterior [NA] A muscle that arises by digitations from the outer surfaces of the anterior angles of the upper eight or nine ribs. It is inserted onto the costal surface of the superior and inferior angles and intervening medial margin of the scapula. Supplied by the long thoracic nerve, it draws the shoulder girdle forward and laterally and helps to rotate the scapula, especially in lifting the arm above shoulder level. The upper part helps to pull the scapula downward and forward. Also called *anterior serratus muscle, costoscapularis* (outmoded), *serratus magnus* (outmoded).

musculus serratus posterior inferior [NA] A muscle that arises from the spines of the lower two thoracic and first two lumbar vertebrae and the supraspinous ligament. It is inserted onto the lower margins of the last four ribs lateral to their angles. Supplied by the ventral rami of the ninth to twelfth thoracic spinal nerves, it depresses the ribs. Also called *inferior posterior serratus muscle.*

musculus serratus posterior superior [NA] A muscle that arises from the lower part of the ligamentum nuchae, the spines of the lower two cervical and upper two thoracic vertebrae, and the supraspinous ligament. It is inserted onto the outer surfaces of the second to fifth ribs lateral to their angles. Supplied by the second to fifth intercostal nerves, it elevates the ribs. Also called *superior posterior serratus muscle.*

musculus skeleti A muscle attached to the axial and appendicular skeleton and crossing at least one joint on which it acts. It consists of long, thin multinucleated fibers containing myofibrils with regularly spaced alternate dark and light striations, lying in semifluid sarcoplasm and enclosed in a sheath, the sarcolemma. The fibers are organized in bundles, or fasciculi. Also called *skeletal muscle, striated muscle, striped muscle, somatic muscle* (outmoded), *textus muscularis striatus.*

musculus soleus [NA] A muscle that arises from the upper fourth of the posterior surface of the shaft and back of the head of the fibula, the soleal line and middle third of the medial margin of the tibia, and the fibrous arch between the tibia and fibula. It is inserted onto the middle of the posterior surface of the calcaneus by the tendo calcaneus. Supplied by the tibial nerve, it plantarflexes and inverts the foot and raises the heel off the ground. Also called *soleus muscle.*

musculus sphincter [NA] A ring of muscle fibers that surround a tube, duct, or orifice which is diminished or closed by their contraction. Also called *sphincter, sphincter muscle.*

musculus sphincter ampullae hepatopancreaticae [NA] The thickened circular muscle of the wall of the descending part of the duodenum that forms a compound sphincter comprising the circular muscle around the terminal part of the common bile duct (the musculus sphincter ductus choledochus), of the pancreatic duct (the musculus sphincter ductus pancreatici), and around the ampulla hepatopancreatica. They are continuous with one another but one or both of the latter two may be absent or weakly formed. Also called *Oddi sphincter, Oddi's muscle, Glisson sphincter, sphincter muscle of hepatopancreatic ampulla, sphincter of hepatopancreatic ampulla, duodenal sphincter.*

musculus sphincter ani externus [NA] A voluntary muscle which surrounds the anal canal and extends from the central tendon of the perineum and the skin to the coccyx. It is divided into three parts that are imperfectly separated, namely, pars profunda, pars subcutanea, and pars superficialis. It is innervated by the inferior rectal branch of the pudendal nerve and the perineal branch of the fourth sacral nerve. Also called *external sphincter muscle of the anus, external sphincter of anus.*

musculus sphincter ani internus [NA] The annular thickening of the circular fibers of the tunica muscularis recti. It extends from the anorectal junction to the intersphincteric groove just above the anal orifice. It is separated from the deep part of the external sphincter by the longitudinal muscle of the rectum and anal canal and from the subcutaneous part by the anal intermuscular septum derived from the longitudinal muscle. Also called *internal sphincter muscle of the anus, internal sphincter of anus.*

musculus sphincter colli A thin, flat superficial muscle circling the neck ventrally and laterally in tetrapods.

musculus sphincter ductus choledochi [NA] A thickening of the circular muscle fibers of the wall of the descending part of the duodenum around the lower part of the common bile duct just before it joins the pancreatic duct. Also called *choledochal sphincter, sphincter muscle of bile duct, sphincter of common bile duct, sphincter of Boyden, Giordano sphincter, sphincter of bile duct, sphincter choledochus* (outmoded).

musculus sphincter ductus pancreatici [NA] An inconstant thickening of the circular muscle fibers of the wall of the descending part of the duodenum around the terminal part of the pancreatic duct just before it joins the common bile duct in the ampulla. Also called *sphincter muscle of pancreatic duct, sphincter of duct of Wirsung.*

musculus sphincter pupillae [NA] A circular flattened band of nonstriated muscle fibers in the stroma iridis, near the periphery of the pupil to which they run parallel. Posteriorly it is attached by collagen fibers to the dilator pupillae. It is innervated by the short ciliary nerves. Also called *sphincter muscle of pupil, sphincter pupillae, sphincter iridis* (outmoded).

musculus sphincter pylori MUSCULUS SPHINCTER PYLORICUS.

musculus sphincter pyloricus [NA] A ring of thickened circular muscle fibers of the tunica muscularis around the pyloric canal of the stomach. Also called *sphincter muscle of pylorus, pyloric sphincter, musculus sphincter pylori.*

musculus sphincter urethrae [NA] A group of striated muscle fibers that surrounds the membranous urethra and rises on the prostate almost to the base of the bladder. It arises from the transverse perineal ligament and the fascial sheath of the pudendal vessels and is inserted onto the central tendon of the perineum and around the membranous urethra. It is supplied by the perineal branch of the pudendal nerve. In the male it compresses the membranous urethra and takes part in ejaculation. In the female it encircles the lower end of the urethra, and some fibers end in the vaginal wall. Also called *constrictor urethrae* (outmoded), *musculus sphincter urethrae membranaceae* (outmoded), *musculus constrictor urethrae* (outmoded), *sphincter muscle of membranous urethra, sphincter muscle of urethra, Guthrie's muscle, sphincter urethrae, musculus compressor urethrae* (outmoded).

musculus sphincter urethrae membranaceae An outmoded term for MUSCULUS SPHINCTER URETHRAE.

musculus sphincter vesicae urinariae A group of smooth muscle fibers of the circular layer of the urinary bladder that encircle the internal urethral orifice and are continuous with the levator prostatae muscle surrounding the proximal part of the urethra. It is innervated by the vesical plexus and it helps in controlling micturition. Also called *sphincter muscle of urinary bladder, annulus urethralis* (outmoded), *urethral ring.*

musculus spinalis [NA] The medial column of the musculus erector spinae, comprising the musculus spinalis capitis, musculus spinalis cervicis, and musculus spinalis thoracis. It is supplied by the dorsal rami of the lower cervical and thoracic spinal nerves, and it extends the vertebral column. Also called *spinal muscle.*

musculus spinalis capitis [NA] An inconstant prolongation of musculus spinalis cervicis to the medial part of the area between the superior and inferior nuchal lines of the occipital bone, and usually blended with the musculus semispinalis capitis. Also called *biventer cervicis.*

musculus spinalis cervicis [NA] An inconstant muscle, often absent, that arises from the spines of the lower two cervical and upper two thoracic vertebrae. It is inserted onto the spines of the second and third cervical vertebrae.

musculus spinalis dorsi An outmoded term for MUSCULUS SPINALIS THORACIS.

musculus spinalis thoracis [NA] A muscle that arises from the tips of the spines of the two upper lumbar and lower two thoracic vertebrae and is inserted onto the spines of the upper thoracic vertebrae. It is usually fused to the musculus semispinalis thoracis. Also called *musculus spinalis dorsi* (outmoded).

musculus splenius capitis [NA] A muscle that arises from the lower part of the ligamentum nuchae and the spines of the seventh cervical and upper three or four thoracic vertebrae. It is inserted onto the mastoid process and the lateral part of the superior nuchal line of the occipital bone. It is supplied by the dorsal rami of the middle cervical spinal nerves, and it helps to extend the head, pull it to one side, and rotate it to the same side. Also called *splenius muscle of head.*

musculus splenius cervicis [NA] A muscle that arises from the spines of the lower cervical and upper thoracic vertebrae. It is inserted onto the posterior tubercles of the transverse processes of the upper two or three cervical vertebrae. Supplied by the dorsal rami of the lower cervical spinal nerves, it helps to extend the head and neck as well as rotate the head to the same side. Also called *splenius muscle of neck.*

musculus stapedius [NA] A muscle that arises from within the pyramidal eminence on the posterior wall of the middle ear. It is inserted onto the posterior surface of the neck of the stapes and is supplied by the facial nerve. It reflexly aids the tensor tympani muscle in dampening the intensity of sounds reaching the internal ear. Also called *stapedius muscle.*

musculus sternalis [NA] An inconstant muscle slip on the surface of the musculus pectoralis major, running parallel to the sternum and extending from the rectus sheath and lower costal cartilages to either the sternal origin of the musculus sternocleidomastoideus or the pectoral fascia. It is innervated by nerves to the sternocleidomastoid or pectoral muscles. Also called *sternal muscle, sternalis.*

musculus sternochondroscapularis An inconstant accessory muscle slip that extends from the first costal cartilage and adjacent sternum to the coracoid process of the scapula.

musculus sternoclavicularis An occasional accessory muscle slip that extends from the upper margin of the manubrium sterni to the upper surface of the clavicle near its midpoint. Also called *musculus supraclavicularis, supraclavicular muscle.*

musculus sternocleidomastoideus [NA] A muscle of the neck that has a sternal or medial head arising from the upper anterior surface of the manubrium sterni below the clavicular notch and a clavicular or lateral head arising from the medial third of the upper surface of the clavicle. It is inserted onto the anterior margin and lateral surface of the mastoid process and the lateral part of the superior nuchal line of the occipital bone. It is supplied by the accessory nerve and the ventral rami of the second and third cervical nerves. It flexes the head laterally and rotates it to the opposite side, flexes the head forward when both sides act together, and, when both sides act together from above, helps to elevate the thorax in forced inspiration. Also called *sternomastoid muscle, sternocleidomastoid muscle.*

musculus sternofascialis An occasional muscle slip extending from the upper anterior surface of the manubrium sterni to the fascia of the omohyoid muscle. It is posterior to the sternocleidomastoid muscle.

musculus sternohyoideus [NA] A muscle that arises from the posterosuperior aspect of the manubrium sterni and the posterior surface of the medial end of the clavicle. It is inserted onto the inferior margin of the body of the hyoid bone. Supplied by the ansa cervicalis, it depresses the hyoid bone. Also called *sternohyoid muscle.*

musculus sternothyreoideus An outmoded term for MUSCULUS STERNOTHYROIDEUS.

musculus sternothyroideus [NA] A muscle that arises from the posterior surface of the manubrium sterni and the first costal cartilage. It is inserted onto the oblique line on the lamina of the thyroid cartilage. Supplied by the ansa cervicalis, it pulls the thyroid cartilage downward after it has been elevated. Also called *sternothyroid muscle, musculus sternothyreoideus* (outmoded), *sternothyreoideus.*

musculus styloglossus [NA] A muscle originating from the anterolateral surface of the styloid process of the temporal bone near its apex and from the contiguous part of the stylomandibular ligament. It is inserted into the side of the tongue, is supplied by the hypoglossal nerve, and pulls the tongue backwards and upwards. Also called *styloglossus muscle, styloglossus.*

musculus stylohyoideus [NA] A muscle that arises from the posterior surface of the styloid process of the temporal bone near its base and is inserted onto the body of the hyoid bone at the junction with the greater cornu. Supplied by the facial nerve, it elevates and pulls back the hyoid bone. Also called *stylohyoid muscle, stylohyoid.*

musculus stylolaryngeus The fibers of the stylopharyngeus muscle that are inserted on the posterior margin of the thyroid cartilage. An outmoded term.

musculus stylopharyngeus [NA] A muscle that originates from the medial side of the base of the styloid process of the temporal bone. It is inserted onto the posterior margin of the thyroid cartilage with the palatopharyngeus muscle, the lateral glossoepiglottic fold, and the pharyngeal constrictor muscles. Supplied by the glossopharyngeal nerve, it elevates the pharynx. Also called *stylopharyngeus muscle.*

musculus subclavius [NA] A muscle that arises from the upper surface of the junction of the first rib and its cartilage. It is inserted onto the inferior surface of the middle third of the clavicle and is supplied by the fifth and sixth cervical nerve. It acts to depress the clavicle and point of the shoulder when the first rib is fixed. It also helps in forced inspiration when the clavicle is fixed and steadies the clavicle against the sternum in movements of the shoulder. Also called *subclavius muscle.*

musculus subcoracoscapularis A deep muscle associated with the insertion of the latissimus in the pectoral girdle of reptiles.

musculi subcostales [NA] A series of muscle fibers on the internal aspect of the thoracic wall that are closely associated with the lower internal intercostal muscles, each one extending from the inner surface of a rib near its angle to the inner surface of the second or third rib below. The lateral margin of each is continuous with the posterior margin of adjacent intercostales intimi. They depress the ribs. Also called *subcostal muscles, musculi infracostales.*

musculus subcutaneus colli An outmoded term for PLATYSMA.

musculus subscapularis [NA] A muscle that arises from the medial two thirds of the subscapular fossa of the scapula and the intermuscular septa. It is inserted onto the capsule of the shoulder joint and lesser tubercle of the humerus. Supplied by the upper and lower subscapular nerves, it medially rotates the arm and helps to steady the head of the humerus in the glenoid cavity during movements of the shoulder joint. Also called *subscapular muscle.*

musculus supinator [NA] A muscle that arises from the lower part of the posterior surface of the lateral epicondyle of the humerus, the radial collateral ligament of the elbow joint, the area below the radial notch and supinator crest of the ulna. It is inserted onto the proximal third of the lateral surface of the radius. Supplied by the posterior interosseous nerve, it laterally rotates the forearm to turn the palm of the hand to face forward. Also called *supinator muscle, supinator.*

musculus supraclavicularis MUSCULUS STERNOCLAVICULARIS.

musculus supracoracoideus A large muscle which arises from the coracoid plate and runs to the underside of the humerus in reptiles. There is no homologue in the mammal.

musculi suprahyoidei [NA] The muscles that connect the upper margin of the hyoid bone to the base of the skull and the mandible, namely, the stylohyoid, digastric, mylohyoid, and geniohyoid muscles. They elevate the hyoid bone and the larynx, and the latter three also depress the mandible. Also called *suprahyoid muscles.*

musculus supraspinalis One of several muscle bundles between the tips of the spines of adjacent cervical vertebrae.

musculus supraspinatus [NA] A muscle of the scapula that arises from the medial two thirds of the supraspinous fossa of the scapula and the supraspinous fascia. It is inserted onto the highest of three facets on the greater tubercle of the humerus. Supplied by the suprascapular nerve, it helps to initiate abduction of the arm and helps to steady the head of the humerus and to prevent downward sliding in the glenoid cavity. Also called *supraspinous muscle.*

musculus suspensorius duodeni [NA] A fibromuscular band that extends from the right crus of the diaphragm near the esophageal hiatus to the back of the upper part of the duodenojejunal flexure as well as to the horizontal and ascending portions of the duodenum. Its contraction maintains and increases the angle of the flexure, tending to prevent obstruction. Also called *suspensory muscle of duodenum, muscle of Treitz, ligament of Treitz, retention band, suspensory ligament of duodenum.*

musculus tarsalis inferior [NA] A layer of smooth muscle extending between the fascial sheath of the inferior rectus muscle and the inferior tarsus, and serving to depress the lower eyelid. It is innervated by sympathetic fibers. Also called *inferior tarsal muscle.*

musculus tarsalis superior [NA] A layer of smooth muscle in the inferior lamella of the musculus levator palpebrae superioris that is attached to the upper anterior margin of the superior tarsus and serves to elevate the upper eyelid. It is innervated by sympathetic fibers. Also called *superior tarsal muscle, Müller's muscle, lamina profunda musculi levatoris palpebrae superioris.*

musculus temporalis [NA] A muscle that originates from the temporal fossa and fascia. It is inserted onto the apex, margins, and medial surface of the coronoid process of the mandible and the anterior margin of the ramus of the mandible, and supplied by deep temporal branches of the mandibular nerve. It elevates the mandible and closes the mouth, its posterior fibers retract the mandible, and it helps in side-to-side movements of the mandible. Also called *temporal muscle, temporalis.*

musculus temporoparietalis [NA] A variable sheet of muscle extending between the frontal part of the musculus occipitofrontalis and the anterior and superior auricular muscles. It is supplied by the temporal branches of the facial nerve. Also called *temporoparietal muscle, muscle of Sappey.*

musculus tensor fasciae latae [NA] A muscle that arises from the anterior part of the outer lip of the iliac crest, on the outer surface of the anterior superior iliac spine and the area below it. It is inserted into the upper anterior part of the iliotibial tract and supplied by the superior gluteal nerve. It extends and laterally rotates the leg, medially rotates the thigh when the foot is off the ground, and helps to steady and flex the pelvis when the foot is on the ground and the leg is fixed. Also called *tensor muscle of fascia lata.*

musculus tensor tarsi PARS LACRIMALIS MUSCULI ORBICULARIS OCULI.

musculus tensor tympani [NA] A muscle that arises from the cartilaginous part of the auditory tube, the adjacent part of the greater wing of the sphenoid bone, and the bony semicanal in which it lies. It is inserted onto the manubrium of the malleus, and it is supplied by the nerve to the medial pterygoid. The muscle tenses the tympanic membrane and helps to dampen sound vibrations. Also called *tensor ligament* (outmoded), *tensor tympani muscle, tensor muscle of tympanic membrane, tensor muscle of tympanum, eustachian muscle* (outmoded).

musculus tensor veli palatini [NA] A muscle that arises from the scaphoid fossa of the pterygoid process, the spine of the sphenoid bone, and the lateral lamina of the cartilage of the auditory tube. It is inserted into the palatine aponeurosis of the soft palate and the transverse ridge on the inferior surface of the horizontal plate of the palatine bone. Supplied by the mandibular nerve, it tightens the soft palate and opens the auditory tube. Also called *tensor muscle of velum palatini, palatosalpingeus* (outmoded), *staphylinus externus* (outmoded).

musculus teres major [NA] A muscle that originates from the posterior surface of the inferior angle of the scapula and from the intermuscular septa, is inserted into the medial lip of the intertubercular groove of the humerus and supplied by the lower subscapular nerve. It adducts, medially rotates, and extends the arm. Also called *teres major muscle.*

musculus teres minor [NA] A muscle that arises from the upper two thirds of the posterior surface of the lateral margin of the scapula. It is inserted onto the lowest of the three facets on the greater tubercle of the humerus and about one inch below it. Supplied by the axillary nerve, it helps to rotate the arm laterally, adducts the arm, and helps to steady the head of the humerus in the glenoid cavity during movements of the shoulder joint. Also called *teres minor muscle.*

musculus tetragonus PLATYSMA.

musculi thoracis [NA] The muscles of the walls of the thorax, including the pectoral, subclavius, serratus anterior, levatores costarum, intercostal, subcostal, and transversus thoracis muscles.

musculus thyreoarytaenoideus externus An outmoded term for MUSCULUS THYROARYTENOIDEUS.

musculus thyreopharyngeus PARS THYROPHARYNGEA MUSCULI CONSTRICTORIS PHARYNGIS INFERIORIS.

musculus thyroarytenoideus [NA] A muscle that arises from the lower part of the inner surface of the angle of the thyroid cartilage and is inserted onto the lateral margin of the arytenoid cartilage. Supplied by the recurrent laryngeal nerve, it pulls forward and rotates the arytenoid cartilage to relax the vocal ligament. Also called *thyroarytenoid muscle, principal thy-*

roarytenoid muscle (outmoded), *musculus thyreoarytaenoideus externus* (outmoded).

musculus thyroepiglotticus [NA] A muscle that arises from the inner surface of the angle of the thyroid cartilage at the upper margin of the thyroarytenoid muscle. It is inserted onto the lateral margin of the epiglottis. Supplied by the recurrent laryngeal nerve, it widens the inlet of the larynx. Also called *thyroepiglottic muscle.*

musculus thyrohyoideus [NA] A muscle that arises from the oblique line on the lamina of the thyroid cartilage. It is inserted onto the inferior margin of the lateral third of the body and the lateral surface of the greater cornu of the hyoid bone. It is supplied by the first cervical spinal nerve via the hypoglossal nerve, and it serves to depress the hyoid bone and elevate the larynx. Also called *thyrohyoid muscle.*

musculus tibialis anterior [NA] A muscle that arises from the lower part of the lateral condyle and the upper two thirds of the lateral surface of the tibia, the interosseous membrane, and the fascia cruris. It is inserted onto the medial surface of the medial cuneiform bone and the base of the first metatarsal bone. Supplied by the deep peroneal nerve, it dorsiflexes and inverts the foot, increases the medial longitudinal arch, and pulls the leg forward when acting from below. Also called *anterior tibial muscle.*

musculus tibialis posterior [NA] A muscle that arises from the lateral part of the middle third of the posterior surface of the tibia below the soleal line, from the interosseous membrane, and from the medial part of the upper two thirds of the posterior surface of the fibula. Its superficial or medial division is inserted onto the tuberosity of the navicular bone and the inferior surface of the medial cuneiform bone, and its deep or lateral division is inserted onto the intermediate and lateral cuneiform and cuboid bones and the plantar surface of the bases of the second, third, and fourth metatarsal bones. Supplied by the tibial nerve, it inverts and plantarflexes the foot. Also called *posterior tibial muscle.*

musculus tibialis secundus An occasional accessory muscle that arises from the back of the tibia deep to the flexor digitorum longus and inserts into the capsule of the ankle joint, serving as a tensor of the capsule.

musculus tibiofascialis anterior An occasional tendinous slip of the musculus tibialis anterior that inserts in the dorsal fascia of the foot. Also called *musculus tibiofascialis anticus.*

musculus tibiofascialis anticus MUSCULUS TIBIOFASCIALIS ANTERIOR.

musculus trachealis [NA] The tunica muscularis of the trachea, extending transversely between the free ends of the tracheal cartilages in the posterior wall of the trachea. It pulls together the ends and diminishes the lumen of the trachea. Also called *tracheal muscle.*

musculus tracheloclavicularis A rare muscle that extends from the cervical vertebrae to the lateral end of the clavicle.

musculus tragicus [NA] A short, flattened band of muscle fibers running vertically on the outer surface of the tragus of the external ear. It is innervated by temporal branches of the facial nerve. Also called *muscle of tragus, Valsalva's muscle.*

musculi transversospinales [NA] A system of deep muscles of the back whose fibers run obliquely upward and medially from the transverse process of a vertebra to the spine or lamina of a vertebra at a higher level, spanning up to six vertebrae. The system is subdivided according to the number of vertebrae crossed, the semispinalis group spanning more than four vertebrae, the multifidus group spanning two to four vertebrae. The short and long rotators, the deepest group, attach to the next vertebra or the one above that. Also called *transversospinal muscles.*

musculus transversus abdominis [NA] A muscle that arises from the inner surfaces of the lower six costal cartilages, the thoracolumbar fascia, the inner lip of the anterior two thirds of the iliac crest, and the lateral third of the inguinal ligament. It is inserted into the upper two thirds of the linea alba through the posterior lamella of the rectus sheath, the lower third of the linea alba through the anterior lamella of the rectus sheath, the crest and pecten of the pubis by the conjoint tendon, and the superior pubic ramus by the interfoveolar ligament. Supplied by the ventral rami of the lower six thoracic and first lumbar spinal nerves, it supports and compresses the abdominal viscera and helps to compress the thorax during expiration. Also called *transverse muscle of abdomen, transversus abdominis muscle.*

musculus transversus auriculae [NA] A small group of muscle and tendinous fibers on the cranial aspect of the auricle connecting the eminentia conchae to the eminentia scaphae. It is supplied by the posterior auricular branch of the facial nerve. Also called *transverse muscle of auricle.*

musculus transversus linguae [NA] An intrinsic muscle of the tongue that is positioned transversely between the superior and the inferior longitudinal muscles, arising from the septum linguae and being inserted into the lingual aponeurosis at the lateral margins of the tongue. Supplied by the hypoglossal nerve, it narrows and elongates the tongue. Also called *transverse muscle of tongue.*

musculus transversus menti [NA] An occasional fibromuscular band of the musculus depressor anguli oris that crosses the midline to interdigitate with the muscle of the other side below the chin. Also called *transverse muscle of chin.*

musculus transversus nuchae [NA] An occasional muscular slip arising from either the external occipital protuberance or the superior nuchal line and inserting either with the posterior auricular muscle or into the posterior margin of the sternocleidomastoid muscle. It is located either superficial or deep to the trapezius muscle. Also called *transverse muscle of nape.*

musculus transversus perinei profundus [NA] A muscle that arises from the inner aspect of the ramus of the ischium and is inserted into the medial raphe and perineal body. Supplied by the perineal branch of the pudendal nerve, it pulls back and stabilizes the perineal body. Also called *deep transverse muscle of perineum.*

musculus transversus perinei superficialis [NA] A poorly developed and occasionally absent thin muscular slip that arises from the anteromedial part of the ischial tuberosity and is inserted into the perineal body. Supplied by the perineal branch of the pudendal nerve, it pulls back and stabilizes the perineal body. Also called *superficial transverse muscle of perineum.*

musculus transversus thoracis [NA] A muscle that arises from the lower part of the posterior surface of the body of the sternum and the posterior surface of the xiphoid process. It is inserted onto the posterior surface of the cartilages of the second to sixth ribs. Supplied by the second to sixth intercostal nerves, it pulls down the costal cartilages, especially in expiration. Also called *transverse muscle of thorax, musculus triangularis sterni* (outmoded), *sternocostalis.*

musculus trapezius [NA] A muscle that arises from the medial part of the superior nuchal line of the occipital bone, the external occipital protuberance, the ligamentum nuchae, and the spines of the seventh cervical and all thoracic vertebrae and their supraspinous ligaments. It is inserted onto the posterosuperior aspect of the lateral third of the clavicle, the medial margin of the acromion, the upper margin of the spine of the scapula, and the tubercle at the medial end of the spine of the scapula. It is supplied by the accessory nerve and the ventral rami of the third and fourth cervical nerves. It elevates the scapula and point of the shoulder, helps to rotate the scapula forward and the glenoid cavity upward, retracts the scapula, extends the head and bends it to the same side when the shoulder

is fixed, and helps to control the scapula in movements of the upper limb. Also called *cucullaris* (outmoded), *trapezius muscle, shawl muscle* (outmoded), *cowl muscle.*

musculus triangularis An outmoded term for MUSCULUS DEPRESSOR ANGULI ORIS.

musculus triangularis sterni An outmoded term for MUSCULUS TRANSVERSUS THORACIS.

musculus triceps brachii [NA] A muscle of the arm. Its caput longum arises from the infraglenoid tubercle of the scapula; its caput laterale arises from the upper lateral part of the posterior surface of the humerus, the lateral margin of the humerus, and the lateral intermuscular septum; and its caput mediale arises from the posterior surface of the humerus below the radial groove and the medial and lateral intermuscular septa. It is inserted onto the upper surface of the olecranon, and the antebrachial fascia posterolaterally. Supplied by the radial nerve, it extends the forearm. Its caput longum helps to extend and adduct the arm. Also called *triceps muscle of arm.*

musculus triceps femoris In certain tetrapods, a muscle on the anterior surface of the thigh that is inserted on the front of the tibia just below its head but that arises from the pelvic girdle as three separate muscles, the rectus femoris, vastus lateralis or gluteus maximus, and the vastus medialis or crureus. It serves to straighten the leg.

musculus triceps surae [NA] The gastrocnemius and soleus muscles considered as one muscle mass, inserting by the tendo calcaneus into the middle of the posterior surface of the calcaneus. Also called *triceps muscle of calf, triceps surae.*

musculus triticeoglossus An occasional muscle fasciculus connecting the root of the tongue with the cartilago triticea. An outmoded term. Also called *Bochdalek's muscle.*

musculus unipennatus [NA] A muscle in which the fibers attach obliquely to the long axis of the muscle along one side of the tendon, as in the flexor pollicis longus. Also called *unipennate muscle.*

musculus uvulae [NA] A muscle that arises from the posterior nasal spine of the palatine bone and the palatine aponeurosis of the soft palate. It is inserted into the mucous membrane of the uvula and is supplied by the pharyngeal plexus. It raises and contracts the uvula. Also called *muscle of uvula, staphylinus medius* (outmoded), *palatouvularis* (outmoded), *palatouvularis muscle* (outmoded).

musculus vastus externus An outmoded term for MUSCULUS VASTUS LATERALIS.

musculus vastus intermedius [NA] A muscle that arises from the upper two thirds of the anterior and lateral surfaces of the shaft of the femur and the lateral intermuscular septum. It is inserted onto the tendon of the quadriceps femoris muscle, the upper and lateral margins of the patella, and the tuberosity of the tibia by the ligamentum patellae. Supplied by the femoral nerve, it extends the leg. Also called *crureus, femoral muscle* (outmoded).

musculus vastus internus An outmoded term for MUSCULUS VASTUS MEDIALIS.

musculus vastus lateralis [NA] A muscle that arises from the upper part of the intertrochanteric line of the femur, the anteroinferior margin of the greater trochanter, the gluteal tuberosity, the upper part of the lateral lip of the linea aspera, and the lateral intermuscular septum. It is inserted onto the tendon of the quadriceps femoris muscle, the upper and lateral margins of the patella, the tibial tuberosity by the ligamentum patellae, and the lateral condyle of the tibia by an expansion. Supplied by the femoral nerve, it extends the leg and helps to stabilize the knee joint. Also called *musculus vastus externus* (outmoded).

musculus vastus medialis [NA] A muscle that arises from the lower part of the intertrochanteric line, the spiral line, the medial lip of the linea aspera, the upper part of the medial supracondylar line, and the medial intermuscular septum. It is inserted onto the tendon of the quadriceps femoris muscle, the upper and medial margins of the patella, the tibial tuberosity by the ligamentum patellae, and the medial condyle of the tibia by an expansion. Supplied by the femoral nerve, it extends the leg and stabilizes the patella on the patellar surface of the femur during extension of the knee joint. Also called *musculus vastus internus* (outmoded).

musculus ventricularis A few fibers of the thyroarytenoid muscle that pass around the laryngeal saccule to enter the vestibular fold. An outmoded term.

musculus verticalis linguae [NA] A group of muscle fibers that extends vertically from the aponeurosis of the dorsum to the inferior surface of the front part of the tongue and decussates with the transverse muscle fibers. Supplied by the hypoglossal nerve, it flattens and widens the tongue. Also called *vertical muscle of tongue.*

musculus viscerum The nonstriated muscle of an internal organ. An outmoded term.

musculus vocalis [NA] The upper and deeper fibers of the thyroarytenoid muscle that lie parallel and lateral to the vocal ligament and extend from the angle of the thyroid cartilage to the vocal process and oblong fovea of the arytenoid cartilage. Many fibers are attached to the vocal ligament. Supplied by the recurrent laryngeal nerve, it draws forward the arytenoid cartilage and relaxes the ligament, as well as helping to control the tension of the vocal ligament. Also called *vocal muscle, inferior thyroarytenoid muscle* (outmoded).

musculus zygomaticus An outmoded term for MUSCULUS ZYGOMATICUS MAJOR.

musculus zygomaticus major [NA] A muscle that arises from the lateral surface of the zygomatic bone behind the inferolateral margin of the orbit. It is inserted into the muscles, skin, and mucosa at the angle of the mouth. Supplied by the buccal branches of the facial nerves, it pulls the angle of the mouth upward and laterally. Also called *greater zygomatic muscle, zygomatic muscle, musculus zygomaticus* (outmoded).

musculus zygomaticus minor A muscle that arises from the lateral surface of the zygomatic bone just behind the zygomaticomaxillary suture. It is inserted into the skin and muscle of the upper lip medial to the angle of the mouth. Supplied by the buccal branches of the facial nerve, it raises the outer part of the upper lip and accentuates the nasolabial furrow. Also called *lesser zygomatic muscle, distortor oris* (outmoded), *zygomatic head of quadratus labii superioris muscle* (outmoded), *caput zygomaticum musculi quadrati labii superioris.*

---

musenna [Amharic, a language of Ethiopia] The bark of the tree *Albizia anthelmintica,* a decoction from which is used as an anthelmintic and purgative in Africa. Overdoses have resulted in death.

mushbite [*mush* + *bite*] An obsolete and inaccurate method of obtaining a maxillomandibular record using a single mass of soft wax.

mushroom [Middle English *muscheron,* from French *mousseron* a small edible mushroom, from Late L *mussirio* an edible fungus] A fleshy, sometimes tough, umbrellalike basidiocarp of certain Basidiomycetes.

fly mushroom FLY AGARIC.

musicogenic Caused or triggered by music, as *musicogenic epilepsy.*

musicolepsy [L *music(us)* (from Gk *mousikos* devoted to the Muses; as substantive, a musician; from *Mousa* a Muse) musical, pertaining to music + *o* + -LEPSY] MUSICOGENIC EPILEPSY.

musicomania Obsessive preoccupation with music to the ex-

tent that the subject can think of nothing else. An obsolete term.

musicotherapy The use of music as a therapeutic adjunct.

musk [Middle English *muske* (from Old French *musc* musk, from Late L *muscus* musk, from Persian mushk)] An odorous material obtained from the musk glands of animals such as the male musk deer. It is sometimes used as a perfume base.

musophobia [L *mus* a mouse + *o* + -PHOBIA] Pathologic fear of mice.

Musset [Alfred de *Musset,* French poet, 1810–1857] Musset sign. See under DE MUSSET SIGN.

mussitation [L *mussitatus,* past part. of *mussitare* to mutter, murmur, be silent, say in a low tone] Movement of the lips as in speaking, but without the production of sounds, as seen in some patients with various types of severe brain disease.

must [L *must(um)* (from *mustum,* neut. sing. of *mustus* wet, juicy) new wine] The mechanically expressed, settled, unfermented juice of grapes and other fruits.

mustard [Old French *moutarde* (from *moust* must, from L *mustum* new wine, from L *mustum,* neut. sing of *mustus* juicy, wet, new) mustard] A plant of the genus *Brassica,* which includes asparagus, broccoli, Brussels sprouts, cabbage, cauliflower, kale, kohlrabi, and mustard. The crushed seeds of many species are used as a pungent condiment, rubefacient, and counterirritant. Volatile mustard oil, from the dried ripe seeds of *B. nigra,* black mustard, is a strong irritant that can blister the skin. Expressed mustard oil is obtained by pressure from the seeds of *B. nigra* as a byproduct in the manufacture of volatile mustard oil.

nitrogen mustard Any bis(2-chloroalkyl)amine. Such compounds react intramolecularly to form derivatives of ethyleneimine, whose molecules contain a three-membered ring containing nitrogen. These are powerful alkylating agents, and their ability to alkylate nucleic acids probably explains their carcinogenic and mutagenic properties as well as their use in treating cancers.

Mustargen hydrochloride A proprietary name for mechlorethamine hydrochloride.

mutafacient An outmoded term for MUTAGENIC.

mutagen [*muta(tion)* + -GEN] Any physical or chemical agent that acts on chromosomes to alter their genetic information.

mutagenesis The process by which a change in genetic information either occurs in nature or is induced experimentally.

directed mutagenesis In experimental genetics, the creation of genetic change at a specific nucleotide sequence by means of recombinant DNA techniques.

insertional mutagenesis The creation of genetic change and, as a result, altered expression of a host cell's genome, by insertion of a foreign segment of DNA.

mutagenic Of or relating to a mutagen. Also *mutafacient* (outmoded).

mutagenicity The effectiveness of an agent in inducing mutation, usually relative to other agents.

mutagenize To experimentally treat an organism or colony with a mutagen.

mutant [L *mutans,* gen. *mutantis,* pres. part. of *mutare* to move, shift, change] **1** In classical genetics, an organism that carries an alteration in its genotype capable of exerting a detectable effect on its phenotype. **2** In molecular genetics, an organism or cell with an alteration in its genotype that is detectable by analysis of protein or nucleic acid sequence, but that may not grossly alter the phenotype. **3** Designating an organism or the part of the genome (chromosome, locus, gene) so altered.

amber mutant See under AMBER CODON.

auxotrophic mutant A mutant with an additional growth requirement, resulting from loss of a biosynthetic enzyme. Such mutants are conveniently selected by exposure of growing bacteria, in minimal medium, to an agent (e.g., penicillin) that kills only growing cells. They have been useful in analyzing biosynthetic pathways and as markers in genetic studies.

cryptic mutant An organism or cell line that contains a nucleotide alteration from the wild type in one or more of its chromosomes not expressed in the phenotype.

leaky mutant An incompletely blocked auxotrophic mutation, whose growth is stimulated by but does not require a particular nutrient.

polarity mutant POLAR MUTATION.

R mutant ROUGH MUTANT.

R$_e$ mutants Extreme rough mutants. Among rough mutants of salmonella, blocked at various stages in lipopolysaccharide synthesis, R$_e$ mutants retain the least amount of core polysaccharide (ending with ketodeoxyoctonate) compatible with viability.

rough mutant A mutant that forms a rough colony, because it no longer makes a surface constituent, such as lipopolysaccharide side chains in Gram-negative bacteria or certain lipids in mycobacteria, required for forming a smooth colony. Also called *R mutant.*

temperature-sensitive mutant A mutant strain of bacteria or viruses unable to grow at certain temperatures that permit growth of the parent. The term is usually applied to strains that can grow at 34°C or less but not at 37°C, those exhibiting the reverse effect being designated "cold-sensitive." Also called *ts* mutant.

ts **mutant** TEMPERATURE-SENSITIVE MUTANT.

mutarotation [L *muta(re)* to change + English *rotation*] The phenomenon of a change in the optical rotation of a sugar after it has been dissolved. This is due to equilibration between its α and β hemiacetal forms, via opening of the ring to give the chain form with a free carbonyl group. Some equilibration between pyranose and furanose forms may also be involved.

mutase Any enzyme that catalyzes an isomerization involving the transfer of a group from one part of a molecule to another.

mutation [L *mutatio* (from *mutatus*, past part. of *mutare* to move, shift, change) a change, changing, alteration] **1** In classical genetics, any change within a genotype that can be detected by its effect on the phenotype. **2** Any change in the nucleotide sequence of the DNA in a chromosome, which may or may not affect the phenotype. **3** A change in chromosomes that is recognized as morphologically abnormal. For defs. 1, 2, and 3 also called *genomic mutation, transgenation.*

amber mutation A nonsense mutation which results in production of an amber codon (UAG) in the reading frame of messenger RNA, causing premature termination of transcription. In prokaryotes this process is suppressible by amber suppressors.

back mutation Any change in nucleotide sequence of the DNA of a chromosome that results in re-establishing a function of a phenotype that had been lost through a forward mutation. A true back mutation exactly reverses the original mutation. Compare FORWARD MUTATION. See also REVERSION.

cold sensitive mutation A genetic mutation that expresses a wild-type phenotype on the culture or growth of the cells or organism at a permissive temperature and a mutant phenotype at a lower, restrictive, temperature.

conditional lethal mutation Any mutation which is lethal under only certain environmental or genetic conditions.

constitutive mutation Any change in the genome resulting in the loss of metabolic regulation of a gene product, such as a mutation that results in the synthesis of constant amounts of an enzyme which is, in the wild type, inducible.

forward mutation Any mutation that is subsequently completely or partially corrected at the level of the phenotype by another mutation. Compare BACK MUTATION.

frame-shift mutation An insertion or deletion of nucleotides that results in an alteration in the sequence in which nucleotides are grouped, or read, as codons (the reading frame). The sequence distal to the mutation contains missense, nonsense, and sense codons. The resulting polypeptide chain will therefore have an altered amino acid sequence and be either too short or too long.

genomic mutation MUTATION.

heat sensitive mutation Any change in the genome that causes no change in wild-type phenotype at one range of temperatures, known as the permissive temperatures, but results in an altered phenotype at a higher temperature, the restrictive temperature.

homoeotic mutation A genetic change recognized by the appearance of homoeosis. Identification of the mutation suggests that the nucleotide sequence involved is part of a gene that participates in development.

induced mutation A mutation caused by an external mutagen. It often occurs by design in experimental genetics. Compare NATURAL MUTATION.

lethal mutation Any alteration in the genotype, such as a point mutation or a chromosome aberration, that prevents reproduction of the affected organism. For example, the organism may die before reproducing, never become sexually mature, or be infertile.

missense mutation A change in DNA nucleotide sequence that alters one or more codons such that different amino acids are inserted in a polypeptide.

natural mutation A change in DNA nucleotide sequence that occurs spontaneously (as through a mistake by a polymerase, or because of ultraviolet light). Also called *spontaneous mutation.* Compare INDUCED MUTATION.

neutral mutation A mutation that has no effect on the adaptability of the organism and does not alter selection.

nonsense mutation A mutation that alters the sequence of a codon such that no amino acid is encoded; the polypeptide chain therefore prematurely terminates. The three nonsense codons in mRNA are UAG (amber codon), UAA (ochre codon), and UGA (umber codon).

ochre mutation A nonsense mutation which results in production of an ochre codon (UAA) in the reading frame of messenger RNA, causing premature termination of transcription.

opal mutation UMBER MUTATION.

point mutation **1** A change in a single nucleotide in the DNA of the genome. **2** In classical genetics, a small alteration in the genome, recognized phenotypically but not cytogenetically, which is capable of recombining with many other small mutations in the same region of the genome.

polar mutation Any mutation that affects the expression of genes distal to the altered nucleotide sequence. Also called *polarity mutant.*

reverse mutation A mutation that reverses the effect of another mutation. A true reversion would restore the original DNA sequence, but more often phenotypic reversion is achieved by genetic changes that suppress the first mutation.

silent mutation **1** A mutation that has no effect on phenotype. **2** A mutation that has no effect on the amino acid sequence of the gene product because of redundancy of the genetic code.

somatic mutation Any change in the genome of a nongerm line cell. If the mutation is perpetuated in a clone of cells, the organism becomes a mosaic with respect to the altered locus, loci, or chromosome. Somatic mutations can be transmitted to progeny if the change occurs early enough in embryogenesis and occurs in a cell destined to be a progenitor of the gonads, in which case germinal mosaicism occurs.

spontaneous mutation NATURAL MUTATION.

suppressor mutation A change in the genome that reverses or mitigates the phenotype produced by a mutation at another gene (intergenic suppressor mutation) or within the same gene (intragenic or intracistronic suppressor mutation). The suppressor mutation thus serves phenotypically as a back mutation. Examples are a frameshift mutation that re-establishes the correct reading frame distal to a primary frameshift mutation, and a mutation that generates a suppressor tRNA that misreads the primary mutation.

temperature sensitive mutation Any change in the genome that is expressed as an altered phenotype only at certain temperatures. Also called *TS mutation.*

TS mutation TEMPERATURE SENSITIVE MUTATION.

umber mutation A nonsense mutation which results in production of an umber codon (UGA) in the reading frame of messenger RNA, causing premature termination of transcription. Also called *opal mutation.*

mutational Pertaining to or characterized by a mutation.

mute [L *mutus* (akin to *mu* the sound of grumbling and to Gk *my* the sound of muttering or murmuring with closed lips) dumb, mute, inarticulate, silent] **1** Unable to speak. Also *dumb.* **2** One who cannot talk. The cause may be deafness or severe, primary expressive disorder or it may be a deliberate cessation as the result of psychogenic disorder.

deaf mute One who has such a severe degree of hearing impairment that he is unable to hear the sounds of speech and therefore cannot learn to talk normally, without special help. The deafness is usually congenital or arises in early childhood before the full development of speech and language has taken place. Also called *partimute, surdimute.* Also *deaf-mute.*

mutilate [L *mutilat(us)*, past part. of *mutilare* to crop or cut off, maim] **1** In criminal law, to subject to any injury that totally destroys or removes an organ, limb, or other essential body part, thus rendering less capable of fighting. **2** To subject to such extreme injury as to render grotesque or, in death, often unidentifiable.

mutilation [Late L *mutilatio* (from L *mutilatus*, past part. of *mutilare* to cut or lop off, maim) a cutting off, maiming, mutilating] The infliction of an injury upon a person which totally destroys or removes, or permanently and severely damages, an organ, limb, or other essential body part. In forensic medicine, mutilation is most often inflicted upon the face and fingers of murder victims in order to render the body unidentifiable. Mutilation also applies to injuries sustained by survivors of criminal violence.

mutisia Any plant belonging to the genus *Mutisia. M. viciae-folia,* vetchleaf mutisia, has been used as a sedative and as a medicine to treat diseases of the heart and of the respiratory and nervous systems.

mutism [*mut(e)* + -ISM] The state of being mute. Also called *St. Zachary's disease, mutitas.*

akinetic mutism A state of severely disordered consciousness, usually due to a midbrain lesion, in which the subject is mute and immobile although the eyes are open and may move randomly. Also called *Cairns stupor.*

deaf mutism The condition of being a deaf mute. Also called *partimutism, surdimutism, surdimutitas* (obsolete), *mutitas surdorum* (obsolete). Also *deaf-mutism.*

elective mutism Self-imposed silence by a child in all his interpersonal contacts except for a few close friends and family members. At times it may constitute a symptom of a school phobia and be related to actual or threatened separation from the family.

hysterical mutism Mutism as a conversion symptom. Also called *Kussmaul's aphasia, hysterical pseudoaphasia.*

mutitas MUTISM.

mutitas atonica Dumbness due to paralysis of the tongue. An outmoded term.

mutitas organica Mutism resulting from an organic disorder which may be auditory, neurologic, or laryngeal in nature.

mutitas surdorum An obsolete term for DEAF MUTISM.

muton The smallest unit of deoxyribonucleic acid which is capable of undergoing a mutation.

mutualism A form of symbiosis in which the association between two or more species populations is beneficial to the well-being of all.

mutualist One of two individuals of different species in an interaction that is beneficial to both species.

muzzle [Middle English *mosel,* from Old French *musel, muzel,* dim. of *mus, muse* snout, muzzle, from Med. L *musus, musum* snout, muzzle] The projecting jaws and nose of an animal; snout.

MV Symbol for the unit, megavolt.

Mv Symbol for the element, mendelevium.

mV Symbol for the unit, millivolt.

μV Symbol for the unit, microvolt.

MV·A Symbol for the unit, megavolt-ampere.

mV·A Symbol for the unit, millivolt-ampere.

mval Symbol for millival.

mV·s Symbol for the unit, millivolt-second.

MVV maximum voluntary ventilation.

MW Symbol for the unit, megawatt.

mW Symbol for the unit, milliwatt.

μW Symbol for the unit, microwatt.

mWb Symbol for the unit, milliweber.

Mx Symbol for the unit, maxwell.

My. myopia.

my- MYO-.

Mya A genus of commercially important clams including the soft-shell clam, *M. arenaria.*

myalgia [MY- + -ALGIA] Pain in the muscles. Also called *myosalgia.*

myalgia abdominis Pain in the muscles of the abdominal wall.

myalgia capitis Pain in the muscles attached to the scalp.

myalgia cervicalis Pain in the muscles of the back of the neck.

epidemic myalgia EPIDEMIC PLEURODYNIA.

lumbar myalgia Pain in the muscles of the lumbar region.

spastic myalgia Pain in muscles affected by spasticity.

myalgia thermica HEAT CRAMP.

myalgic Pertaining to myalgia.

Myambutol A proprietary name for ethambutol dihydrochloride.

Myanesin A proprietary name for mephenesin.

myasis MYIASIS.

myasthenia [MY- + ASTHENIA] Abnormal muscle fatigue; reduction of muscle power. Also called *amyosthenia, muscle asthenia, myoasthenia.* Adjective: myasthenic.

angiosclerotic myasthenia An outmoded term for INTERMITTENT CLAUDICATION.

angiosclerotic paroxysmal myasthenia INTERMITTENT CLAUDICATION.

carcinomatous myasthenia LAMBERT-EATON SYNDROME.

myasthenia cordis Weakness of the heart. An obsolete term.

myasthenia gastrica Weakness and loss of tone in the muscular coats of the stomach; gastric atony.

myasthenia gravis A neuromuscular disorder of autoimmune origin in which weakness occurs in certain muscle groups or, less often, throughout the skeletal musculature and is greatly increased by exertion or repeated contraction of the affected muscles. In some cases the disease is limited to the external ocular muscles, resulting in ptosis, diplopia, and variable strabismus, but more often the weakness is evident in the muscles of swallowing and chewing and to a variable extent in those of the limbs and trunk. In some patients there is thymic enlargement or even a thymoma, and there is an association with hyperthyroidism and to a lesser extent with other autoimmune disorders. Myasthenic crises may occur and may be fatal if untreated, due to respiratory paralysis. There is evidence of a defect of neuromuscular transmission due to the formation of autoantibodies against the acetylcholine receptors on the surface of the muscle fibers. Diagnosis is made by noting the improvement in muscle power produced by intravenous edrophonium. Spontaneous remissions may occur. Treatment with pyridostigmine, with thymectomy, or with steroids is effective, depending upon the circumstances of the individual case. Also called *Erb-Goldflam syndrome, bulbospinal paralysis, myasthenia gravis pseudoparalytica, Hoppe-Goldflam syndrome, Erb syndrome, Erb-Oppenheim-Goldflam syndrome, Erb-Goldflam disease, Wilks symptom complex, Wilks syndrome, Goldflam's disease, Goldflam-Erb disease, asthenobulbospinal paralysis* (incorrect), *asthenic bulbar paralysis* (incorrect), *bulbospinal asthenia* (incorrect).

myasthenia gravis pseudoparalytica MYASTHENIA GRAVIS.

myasthenia laryngis Weakness of the muscles of phonation, particularly the thyroarytenoid and interarytenoid muscles. It occurs chiefly as the result of excessive use of the voice as is seen in professional singers, actors, etc. The condition often occurs as a complication in other laryngeal disorders. It manifests itself in weak and unreliable vocalization. Also called *phonasthenia*.

neonatal myasthenia Myasthenia gravis in the newborn infant of a myasthenic mother.

myasthenic Pertaining to or suffering from myasthenia.

myatonia [MY- + ATONIA] Reduction in or absence of muscle tone. Also called *muscle atony, amyotonia, myatony*. Adjective: *myatonic*.

myatonia congenita A syndrome of severe congenital hypotonia of the skeletal musculature. Also called *Oppenheim's disease, amyotonia congenita, Oppenheim's amyotonia, congenital atonic pseudoparalysis, Oppenheim syndrome*. • The condition was once thought to represent a disorder in which the infantile hypotonia was benign and was generally followed by improvement or even recovery, but subsequently it became apparent that most such patients were suffering from acute infantile spinal muscular atrophy (Werdnig-Hoffmann disease). Hence the term is now obsolete in this sense, though there are many other disease processes which cause infantile hypotonia, some of which are benign, and these may still sometimes be described as *myatonia congenita* or *myatonia congenita syndrome*.

periodic myatonia An outmoded term for PERIODIC PARALYSIS.

myatony MYATONIA.

myatrophy AMYOTROPHY.

myautonomy [MY- + AUTONOMY] A state of a muscle characterized by abnormally protracted delay in contraction following excitation.

myc- MYCO-.

mycelial Of or pertaining to a mycelium. Also *mycelian*.

mycelian MYCELIAL.

myceliate Covered by a mycelium.

mycelioid Appearing mycelial and radiating outward from a central point, as with certain fungal colonies.

mycelium [MYC- + Gk *hēlos* nail, wart, callus, corn + New L

noun suffix *-ium*] (*plural* mycelia) The mass of hyphae that constitutes the body of a fungus.

aerial mycelium The mass of hyphae extending above the surface of the solid or liquid substrate.

coenocytic mycelium A mycelium in which the hyphae are uninterrupted by crosswalls and the nuclei are embedded in the common cytoplasm. Also called *nonseptate mycelium*.

nonseptate mycelium COENOCYTIC MYCELIUM.

primary mycelium A monoploid mycelium produced from germinating spores and unable to form sexually induced spores.

reproductive mycelium That portion of the mycelium having undergone sexual reproduction and eventually giving rise to sexually produced spores. In a strict sense, all mycelium is reproductive, at least vegetatively.

secondary mycelium Mycelium which has sexually fused and is binucleate in every cell.

septate mycelium A mycelium having hyphae with regular crosswalls which separate the cellular contents from cell to cell.

substrate mycelium VEGETATIVE MYCELIUM.

tertiary mycelium The organized, specialized tissues composing sporophores of the complex fungi. Tertiary mycelium usually has diploid nuclei.

vegetative mycelium A mycelium located in the solid or liquid substrate and which grows vegetatively. It supplies nutrients to all parts of the fungus plant. Also called *substrate mycelium*.

-myces [Gk *mykēs* a mushroom, fungus] A combining form meaning fungus or funguslike.

mycet- MYCO-.

mycete [Gk *mykēs*, gen. *mykētos*, mushroom, fungus] Any fungus.

-mycetes [Gk *mykētes*, pl. of *mykēs* mushroom, fungus] A combining form designating fungal classes.

mycethemia The presence of fungi in blood. Also called *mycohemia, fungemia*.

mycetism [MYCET- + -ISM] An older term for MUSHROOM POISONING.

mycetismus [New L (MYCET- + New L *-ismus* -ISM)] An older term for MUSHROOM POISONING.

mycetismus cerebris Mushroom intoxication characterized by hallucinations. Mushrooms in the genera *Psilocybe, Paneolus*, and *Conocybe* are known to be hallucinogenic.

mycetismus choleriformis A form of mushroom poisoning following the ingestion of *Amanita phalloides, A. verna, A. virosa*, or *A. bisporagera*, or several species of *Galerina*. The chief toxicologic effect is severe gastroenteritis, as evidenced by bloody diarrhea and persistent vomiting which may be so severe as to result in shock, coma, and death. The onset of symptoms is usually delayed for several hours.

mycetismus gastrointestinalis A mild form of poisoning marked by nausea, vomiting, and diarrhea, due to the ingestion of certain species of mushroom such as *Clitocybe illudens*.

mycetismus nervosus Poisoning caused by the ingestion of any of several species of *Amanita*, especially *A. muscaria*, a mushroom containing muscarine. The signs are characteristic of stimulation of the parasympathetic nervous system and include salivation, lacrimation, miosis, nausea, vomiting, defecation, and bradycardia, terminating in convulsions. The effects can be completely reversed by atropine.

mycetismus sanguinarius Poisoning resulting from the ingestion of mushrooms of the *Gyromitra* species, especially *Gyromitra esculenta*. The toxin, gyromitrin (monomethyl hydrazine), may cause symptoms of nausea, vomiting, diarrhea, cramps, weakness, headaches, and develop to convulsions, coma, and even death.

myceto- MYCO-.

mycetogenic [MYCETO- + -GENIC] Produced or brought about by a fungus or fungi, as a disease. Also *mycetogenous*.

mycetogenous MYCETOGENIC.

mycetoid [MYCET- + -OID] FUNGOID.

mycetoma [*mycet(o)*-- + -OMA] **1** A chronic infection of the subcutaneous and deeper tissues caused by any of various fungi (*Eumycetes*) such as *Madurella* or by actinomycetes such as *Nocardia* and *Streptomyces*. It is characterized by local swelling, necrosis, sinus formation, and suppuration. Infection is usually by puncture of the skin by infected thorns. Mycetoma occurs worldwide but is seen most often in tropical and subtropical areas of northwest and central Africa, Asia, and Central and South America. Mycetoma of the foot (the most common site) is called Madura foot or foot fungus. Historically, some types of mycetoma were named according to the color of the granules in the pus. Staining affinities are of value in differentiation. Also called *maduromycetoma, maduromycosis, Madura boil, Ballingall's disease.* **2** A nodule or non-neoplastic tumor made up largely of mycelial elements, such as an aspergilloma.

Bouffard's black mycetoma A mycetoma containing black granules, caused by *Madurella mycetomatis* and *M. grisea*, occurring in tropical Africa, North and South America, and southest Asia.

Bouffard's white mycetoma A mycetoma containing white granules, caused by *Streptomyces somaliensis*, occurring in north and west Africa and South America. Also called *Brumpt's white mycetoma.*

Brumpt's white mycetoma BOUFFARD'S WHITE MYCETOMA.

Carter's black mycetoma A mycetoma containing black granules, caused by *Madurella mycetomatis,* and found in tropical Africa, India, southeast Asia, and parts of North and South America.

Nicolle's white mycetoma An exceptionally rare eumycotic mycetoma caused by *Aspergillus nidulans* and characterized by white grain or granule color.

Raynier's white mycetoma A fairly common actinomycotic mycetoma thought to be caused by *Streptomyces somaliensis* and characterized by yellow to brown grain or granule color.

Vincent's white mycetoma A mycetoma containing white granules.

white mycetoma A mycetoma occurring in many tropical countries in which the granules in the suppurative material are white, caused by *Petriellidium boydii, Acremonium falciforme, Nocardia brasiliensis, Steptomyces somaliensis*, and other organisms.

mycetophagous [MYCETO- + -PHAGOUS] Feeding on fungi.

Mycetozoa [MYCETO- + Gk *zōa*, pl. of *zōon* a living being, animal] EUMYCETOZOEA.

Mycetozoida [*Mycetozo(a)* + New L -*ida*, combining form, neut. in form, from L -*ides*, patronymic suffix] EUMYCETOZOEA.

mycetozoon [*myceto*- + Gk *zōon* a living being, animal] (*plural* mycetozoa) A motile cell of a slime mold. An obsolete term.

mycid [MYC- + -ID²] An obsolete term for DERMATOPHYTID.

-mycin [Gk *myk(ēs)* fungus, mushroom + -*in*, from French -*ine*, from L -*ina*, fem. of -*inus*, suffix denoting of or belonging to] A combining form meaning something derived from a fungus.

myco- [Gk *mykēs* (genitive *mykētos*) fungus, mushroom] A combining form denoting fungus. Also *myc-, mycet-, myceto-, myko-*.

mycoagglutinin An agglutinin capable of agglutinating fungi.

mycobacidin ACTITHIAZIC ACID.

mycobacteria Plural of MYCOBACTERIUM.

mycobacteriosis Any infection caused by mycobacteria.

Mycobacterium [MYCO- + BACTERIUM] A genus of bacteria of the family Mycobacteriaceae, order Actinomycetales. The cardinal characteristic is acid-fast staining, due to the large amount of lipid in the outer layer of the wall. Corynebacteria and nocardiae share some of the same special lipids, such as mycolic acids. Growth is slow. They are obligate aerobes, and are straight or curved, slender rods, occasionally mycelial.

Mycobacterium avium A bacillus that produces tuberculosis in birds and pigs and occasionally in humans. It forms smooth colonies and has a higher temperature optimum (41°C) than *M. tuberculosis*. It closely resembles *M. intracellulare* immunologically. Also called *Mycobacterium tuberculosis avium.*

Mycobacterium bovis A species that is the cause of bovine tuberculosis and of milk-borne tuberculosis in humans. More microaerophilic than *M. tuberculosis*, it differs slightly immunologically, and is more pathogenic in rabbits. Also called *Mycobacterium tuberculosis bovis.*

Mycobacterium chelonei A species of fast-growing mycobacteria very similar to *M. fortuitum*, originally isolated from turtles.

Mycobacterium fortuitum A relatively fast-growing mycobacterium that is abundant in soil and occasionally causes abscesses in humans. It includes the former species *M. ranae*. No pigment has been found in this species.

Mycobacterium intracellulare A species closely related immunologically to *Mycobacterium avium* but less pathogenic for birds and having a lower temperature optimum. It is considered by some to be an intermediate form of *M. avium*. It has been isolated from human lesions, but is also found in the soil. Also called *Battey bacillus.*

Mycobacterium johnei MYCOBACTERIUM PARATUBERCULOSIS.

Mycobacterium kansasii A photochromogen that is a common cause of human mycobacterial disease other than that due to *M. tuberculosis*.

Mycobacterium leprae The species that causes human leprosy. Though found in great numbers in lesions and morphologically almost indistinguishable from *M. tuberculosis*, it has not been cultivated and experimental transmission to man has been unsuccessful. It can be propagated in the foot pads of mice and in the nine-banded armadillo. Generation time is 12 to 13 days.

Mycobacterium lepraemurium A species that causes rat leprosy. Like the human leprosy bacillus, it cannot be cultivated.

Mycobacterium marinum A photochromogen that causes disease in fish and chronic human skin lesions which are acquired through abrasions in a marine environment. The optimum growth temperature is 33°C.

Mycobacterium microti A mycobacterium that causes natural tuberculosis in voles. It is similar immunologically to *M. tuberculosis* and *M. bovis*.

Mycobacterium paratuberculosis An obligate parasite that causes a chronic enteritis (paratuberculosis) in cattle and sheep. The tuberculin, johnin, cross-reacts with that of *M. tuberculosis*. It requires mycobactin for growth in artificial culture. Also called *Johne's bacillus, Mycobacterium johnei.*

Mycobacterium phlei A saprobic mycobacterium found on timothy hay.

Mycobacterium scrofulaceum A scotochromogenic species that is a common cause of lymphadenitis in children. It has some antigens in common with *M. avium* and *M. intracellulare*.

Mycobacterium smegmatis A saprobic mycobacterium found in smegma and in butter.

Mycobacterium thamnopheos A species isolated from snakes that resembles a nocardia more than a mycobacterium.

Mycobacterium tuberculosis A very slow-growing mycobacterium species (generation time at least 12 hours) that causes granulomatous lesions in man; the tubercle bacillus. There is no reservoir in nature. Cells are hydrophobic and disperse poorly in liquid media. They form rough colonies, virulent strains aggregating more than avirulent strains and growing as serpentine cords. Growth requirements are simple. A heat-stable protein (tuberculin) from culture filtrates is used in a delayed reaction skin test. Also called *Mycobacterium tuberculosis hominis*.

Mycobacterium tuberculosis avium M*YCOBACTERIUM AVIUM*.

Mycobacterium tuberculosis bovis M*YCOBACTERIUM BOVIS*.

Mycobacterium tuberculosis hominis M*YCOBACTERIUM TUBERCULOSIS*.

Mycobacterium ulcerans A mycobacterium that causes cutaneous ulcers in humans. It grows only below 33°C.

Mycobacterium xenopi A thermophilic scotochromogen, first isolated from a toad and then also from water storage tanks and from chronic human pulmonary lesions.

mycobacterium [MYCO- + BACTERIUM] (*plural* mycobacteria) Any of a group of bacteria characterized by a hydrophobic waxy coat that results in acid-fast staining.

  anonymous mycobacteria An outmoded term for ATYPICAL MYCOBACTERIA.

  atypical mycobacteria A wide variety of mycobacteria, with reservoirs in soil and water or in lower animals, that may cause disease in humans, usually less severe than classical tuberculosis. The importance of these agents has been recognized increasingly as infection with *Mycobacterium tuberculosis* and *M. bovis* has waned. Also called *anonymous mycobacteria* (outmoded).

mycobactin A siderophore containing hydroxamic acid, formed by most mycobacteria and required for growth by *Mycobacterium paratuberculosis*.

Mycocandida [MYCO- + L *candida*, fem. sing. of *candidus* glowing, shining white] An older term for *CANDIDA*.

mycocide A seldom used term for FUNGICIDE.

Mycoderma [MYCO- + Gk *derma* skin] An obsolete genus of pathogenic fungi now classified in the genera *Candida* and *Paracoccidioides*.

  Mycoderma aceti A grouping of yeasts and bacteria which, in combination, ferment a substrate to acetic acid. An obsolete and incorrect term.

  Mycoderma dermatitidis An obsolete term for *BLASTOMYCES DERMATITIDIS*.

mycoderma TUNICA MUCOSA.

mycodermatitis [MYCO- + DERMATITIS] An outmoded term for TINEA.

mycodermomycosis An obsolete term for TINEA.

mycodermosis An obsolete term for TINEA.

mycogonose [*mycogon(e)* + New L -*os(is)*, suffix denoting a disease caused by a fungus] A diseased condition of commercial mushrooms, caused by growth of the white mold, *Mycogone*, upon their sporophores. The invaded mushroom is often misshapen or reduced in size, making it less desirable commercially. Also called *mycogonosis*.

mycogonosis MYCOGONOSE.

mycohemia MYCETHEMIA.

mycoid [MYC- + -OID] FUNGOID.

mycologist [MYC- + -OLOGIST] An individual who studies or is knowledgeable about fungi.

mycology [MYCO- + -LOGY] The science or study of fungi. Adjective: mycologic.

mycomyringitis MYRINGOMYCOSIS.

mycopathogen [MYCO- + PATHOGEN] Any fungus that causes disease.

mycopathology The study of fungal diseases.

mycophage [MYCO- + *phage* (from Gk *phagein* to eat)] Any phage which causes lysis of fungi.

mycophagy [MYCO- + -PHAGY] The act or practice of eating mushrooms.

mycophenolic acid $C_{17}H_{20}O_6$. A bacteriostatic and fungostatic antibiotic derived from cultures of *Penicillium brevi-compactum* and related species.

mycophthalmia [MYC- + OPHTHALMIA] A fungus infection of the eye.

Mycoplasma [MYCO- + PLASMA] A major genus in the group of mycoplasma. Unlike *Acholeplasma*, it requires a sterol for growth.

  Mycoplasma hominis A commensal species of mycoplasma found occasionally in the mouth and frequently in the genital tract. It may be responsible for some cases of salpingitis.

  Mycoplasma hyorhinis A species of mycoplasma that often contaminates tissue cultures. It may grow on artificial media and is usually identified by immunofluorescence.

  Mycoplasma mycoides The organism that causes contagious bovine pleuropneumonia. This was the first of the mycoplasmas to be recognized.

  Mycoplasma orale An anaerobic mycoplasma widely present as a commensal in the human mouth.

  Mycoplasma pneumoniae The agent of mycoplasmal pneumonia (primary atypical pneumonia), long thought to be a virus because it is filterable.

mycoplasma Any of the bacteria of the class Mollicutes, which lack a rigid cell wall. This feature and their small size permit them to pass through 450 nm filters. They slowly form very small colonies, which tend to burrow into the agar. They are found widely in nature and also cause human mycoplasmal pneumonia and a wide variety of serious diseases in animals. Some mycoplasmas have a specialized terminal structure that plays a role in attachment and in gliding motility. Also called *pleuropneumonialike organism* (outmoded).

  T mycoplasma A group of mycoplasmas that cause nonspecific urethritis.

mycoprecipitin An antibody which is detected by precipitation of antigens present in extracts prepared from fungi.

mycopus An obsolete term for MUCOPUS.

mycorrhiza [MYCO- + Gk *rhiza* a root] (*plural* mycorrhizae) A symbiotic association between the hyphae of certain fungi and the absorptive organs, typically the roots, of plants. Also called *root-fungi association, fungus root* (older term).

mycoses Plural of MYCOSIS.

mycosis [MYC- + New L -*osis*, suffix denoting a disease caused by a fungus] (*plural* mycoses) Any disease brought on by a fungus. Adjective: mycotic.

  cutaneous mycosis TINEA.

  mycosis cutis chronica Any chronic fungal disease of the skin. An obsolete term.

  mycosis framboesioides YAWS.

  mycosis fungoides A malignant neoplasm of lymphoid cells that arises in the upper dermis. The cells spread to the epidermis as aggregates. Lymph nodes and viscera may subsequently be involved. Also called *fibroma fungoides, granuloma sarcomatodes, inflammatory fungoid neoplasm, granuloma fungoides, granulosarcoid* (obsolete), *granulosarcoma* (obsolete).

  mycosis fungoides en plaques A skin condition that is characterized by the appearance of erythematous pruritic plaques on the skin. Histologically, a lymphoid infiltrate in the epidermis develops into small dermal papillae. It may present with large fungating tumors, but it is more often preceded, sometimes by several years, by plaques of erythema and fine scaling which later show poikilodermatous atrophy. This precedes the onset of mycosis fungoides. Despite its name, the condition is not fungal.

Gilchrist's mycosis BLASTOMYCOSIS.

mycosis interdigitalis A fungal infection of the webs between the toes or, occasionally, between the fingers.

mycosis pemphigoides A yeast infection of the skin that bears a superficial resemblance to pemphigus vulgaris.

Posada mycosis COCCIDIOIDOMYCOSIS.

mycostasis The prevention of fungal growth and reproduction.

mycostat FUNGISTAT.

mycostatic FUNGISTATIC.

Mycostatin A proprietary name for nystatin.

mycosubtilin A naturally occurring antibiotic obtained from one strain of *Bacillus subtilis*. It has both antifungal and anti-yeast activity *in vitro*.

mycotic Pertaining to mycosis.

-mycotina [MYCO- + *t* + -INA] A combining form designating fungal subdivisions.

mycotization Introduction, growth, and development of a fungus infection on a preexisting lesion.

mycotonic acid A poisonous narcotic substance derived from tropical American shrubs of the genus *Palicourea* belonging to the family Rubiaceae.

Mycotoruloides [MYCO- + *torul(a)* + L -*oïdes* -OID] An obsolete term for *CANDIDA*.

mycotoxicology [MYCO- + TOXICOLOGY] The study of the actions, detection, and treatment of fungal poisons.

mycotoxicosis [MYCO- + TOXICOSIS] Poisoning caused by the ingestion of any fungal toxin such as, for example, aflatoxin.

mycotoxin A toxin produced by a fungus under special conditions of moisture and temperature.

mycotoxinization Introduction of a fungal toxin into an organism or environment.

mycteroxerosis [Gk *myktēr*, gen. *myktēros*, the nose, nostrils + XERO- + -SIS] Dryness of the nose or nares. A rarely used term. Also called *xeromycteria*.

mydaleine A poisonous ptomaine formed in putrified viscera.

mydatoxine A ptomaine from decaying flesh.

mydesis An obsolete term for PUTREFACTION.

Mydriacyl A proprietary name for tropicamide.

mydriasis [Gk *mydriasis* undue enlargement of the pupil of the eye] Enlargement of pupil size. Adjective: mydriatic.

alternating mydriasis Dilatation of first one pupil, then the other. Also called *springing mydriasis, bounding mydriasis*.

bounding mydriasis ALTERNATING MYDRIASIS.

paralytic mydriasis Dilatation of the pupil because of paralysis of the iris sphincter muscle.

spasmodic mydriasis SPASTIC MYDRIASIS.

spastic mydriasis Dilatation of the pupil due to excessive activity of the iris dilator muscle. Also called *spasmodic mydriasis*.

spinal mydriasis Dilatation of the pupil because of increased activity in the cervical sympathetic outflow.

springing mydriasis ALTERNATING MYDRIASIS.

mydriatic 1 Pertaining to or causing mydriasis. 2 A sympathomimetic drug capable of dilating the pupil, but without cycloplegic effect.

myectomy [MY- + -ECTOMY] The surgical removal of part or all of a muscle or a group of muscles.

myectopia MYECTOPY.

myectopy Displacement of a muscle from its usual position. Also called *myectopia*.

myel- MYELO-.

myelalgia [MYEL- + -ALGIA] Pain due to disease of the spinal cord.

myelanalosis 1 An outmoded term for MYELATROPHY. 2 An outmoded term for TABES DORSALIS.

myelapoplexy Spontaneous hemorrhage occurring within the substance of the spinal cord. A seldom used term.

myelasthenia [MYEL- + ASTHENIA] Muscular weakness resulting from spinal cord disease. An imprecise and obsolete term.

myelatelia [MYEL- + Gk *ateleia* incompleteness] MYELODYSPLASIA.

myelatrophy Atrophy of the spinal cord, usually resulting from trauma. A rarely used term. Also called *myelanalosis*.

myelauxe [MYEL- + Gk *auxē* growth, increase] An abnormal increase in size of the spinal cord.

myelemia A rarely used term for CHRONIC GRANULOCYTIC LEUKEMIA.

myelencephalitis [MYEL- + ENCEPHALITIS] ENCEPHALOMYELITIS.

myelencephalon 1 The posterior of the two brain vesicles formed in the developing embryo by the maturative division of the primitive hindbrain, or rhombencephalon. 2 [NA] The most posterior portion of the brainstem, including the medulla oblongata and the caudal half of the fourth vesicle. Also called *metepencephalon* (obsolete), *marrowbrain* (obsolete).

myelencephalospinal Of or pertaining to the myelencephalon and spinal cord.

myelic [MYEL- + -IC] Pertaining to or affecting the spinal cord.

myelin [MYEL- + -IN] An insulating, multilaminar sheath around axons formed from the cell membranes of either an oligodendroglial or Schwann cell.

myelinated Having a myelin sheath: said of a nerve fiber.

myelination [MYELIN + -ATION] The process by which the nerve fibers acquire myelin sheaths, which enhance the conduction of nerve impulses. For peripheral axons, myelinization is brought about by neurilemmal, or Schwann, cells and for central nervous system axons by oligodendrocytes. It commences during fetal life and in humans continues through the first two or three years after birth. Also called *myelinization, myelogenesis, myelinogenesis*.

myelinic Of or relating to myelin.

myelinization MYELINATION.

myelinoclasis [MYELIN + Gk *klasis* a breaking, from *klan* to break, break in pieces] An obsolete term for DEMYELINATION.

acute perivascular myelinoclasis ACUTE DISSEMINATED ENCEPHALOMYELITIS.

central pontine myelinoclasis CENTRAL PONTINE MYELINOLYSIS.

postinfection perivenous myelinoclasis POSTINFECTIOUS ENCEPHALOMYELITIS.

myelinogenesis MYELINATION.

dystopic cortical myelinogenesis The appearance of the cerebral cortex in the Alpers syndrome. Also called *driftwood cortex*.

myelinogenetic Forming myelin by the process of myelinization.

myelinogeny MYELOGENY.

myelinolysin A hypothetical substance allegedly present in the serum of patients with multiple sclerosis and capable of destroying myelin. An obsolete term.

myelinolysis DEMYELINATION.

central pontine myelinolysis Massive demyelination of the central part of the pons, giving rise to progressive dysarthria and spastic quadriplegia. This disorder may complicate alcoholism, liver disease, or uremia. Also called *pontine myelinosis, central pontine myelinoclasis.*

myelinoma [MYELIN + -OMA] A tumor of myelin-forming cells.

myelinopathy [MYELIN + *o* + -PATHY] Any disease or dysfunction of myelin.

myelinosis Fat necrosis with formation of myelin.

  pontine myelinosis CENTRAL PONTINE MYELINOLYSIS.

myelitic Relating to myelitis.

myelitis [MYEL- + -ITIS] **1** Inflammation of the spinal cord. • The term is also used in certain contexts to denote chronic and noninflammatory changes in the spinal cord. Also called *medullitis, notomyelitis* (obsolete). **2** An inflammatory condition of the bone marrow. Rarely used in this sense. Adjective: myelitic.

  acute syphilitic myelitis Transverse myelitis occurring in meningovascular syphilis, partly as a result of inflammation but more often due to endarteritis and vascular occlusion, and giving rise to flaccid paraplegia, often of abrupt onset, and associated with a well-defined upper level of sensory loss on the trunk and with sphincter paralysis.

  acute transverse myelitis Acute inflammation of the spinal cord usually due to a postinfective demyelinating process and giving rise either to a clinical picture suggesting a transverse cord lesion or to acute ascending paralysis.

  amyotrophic syphilitic myelitis Syphilitic meningomyelitis giving rise to a clinical picture resembling that of amyotrophic lateral sclerosis.

  anemic myelitis An incorrect term for SUBACUTE COMBINED DEGENERATION OF THE SPINAL CORD.

  angiohypertrophic spinal myelitis SUBACUTE NECROTIC MYELITIS.

  apoplectiform myelitis HAYEM'S DISEASE.

  ascending myelitis Myelitis which extends progressively upwards from the lower part of the spinal cord. There are many different causes of such a process, including multiple sclerosis, syphilis, and subacute necrotic myelitis.

  bulbar myelitis Myelitis ascending to involve the brainstem.

  cavitary myelitis SYRINGOMYELIA.

  cavitating myelitis An obsolete term for SYRINGOMYELIA.

  central myelitis Inflammation of the spinal cord restricted chiefly to the gray matter. A seldom used term.

  cervical myelitis Myelitis restricted to the cervical region of the spinal cord.

  chronic myelitis A slowly progressive or smoldering form of myelitis.

  compression myelitis An outmoded term for COMPRESSION MYELOPATHY.

  cornual myelitis Myelitis principally involving the horns of gray matter.

  descending myelitis Myelitis which extends progressively downwards from the upper part of the spinal cord to the conus. A seldom used term.

  diffuse myelitis DISSEMINATED MYELITIS.

  disseminated myelitis Myelitis in which many discrete affected areas are found in different parts of the spinal cord. Multiple sclerosis is the commonest cause. Also called *diffuse myelitis.*

  focal myelitis Myelitis localized to one part of the spinal cord.

  foudroyant myelitis Acute myelitis.

  funicular myelitis **1** Myelitis predominantly involving the white matter of one or more spinal tracts. Seldom used in this sense. **2** An obsolete term for FUNICULAR MYELOSIS.

  hemorrhagic myelitis HEMATOMYELITIS.

  interstitial myelitis Myelitis in which supposedly the supporting structures and glia rather than the nerve cells and myelin

of the spinal cord are predominantly involved. There is no evidence that this occurs. An obsolete term.

  metastatic myelitis Myelitis caused by microorganisms derived from a distant site of infection. Also called *intramedullary spinal abscess.*

  neuro-optic myelitis NEUROMYELITIS OPTICA.

  parenchymatous myelitis PARENCHYMATOUS MYELOPATHY.

  periependymal myelitis Myelitis affecting principally that part of the spinal cord around the ependymal canal. A seldom used term.

  peripheral myelitis A type of myelitis affecting principally the white matter of the spinal cord, as seen particularly in the postinfectious demyelinating variety, known as acute disseminated encephalomyelitis. A seldom used term.

  postvaccinal myelitis Myelitis of the postinfectious demyelinating type following smallpox vaccination.

  pressure myelitis COMPRESSION MYELOPATHY.

  pseudotumoral myelitis A type of myelitis in which there is severe edema of the inflamed segments of the spinal cord giving a myelographic appearance which simulates that of intramedullary tumor.

  radiation myelitis RADIATION MYELOPATHY.

  sclerosing myelitis Myelitis in which there is marked proliferation of neuroglial elements and of connective tissue in the spinal cord. • This is an imprecise and outmoded term, as this type of pathologic change can occur in any form of subacute myelitis, irrespective of etiology.

  subacute necrotic myelitis A type of myelitis progressing gradually over the course of about two years, and resulting in paraplegia, sensory loss, and sphincter disturbance of increasing severity. Generally, there is a marked increase in the protein content of the cerebrospinal fluid. The condition may be associated with cor pulmonale or other chronic respiratory disease. In most cases occluded and distended veins are found over and within the cord at autopsy, and many authorities believe that the primary cause is a venous angioma. A different form of subacute necrotizing myelitis has been described as a remote manifestation of malignant disease. Also called *Foix-Alajouanine disease, Foix-Alajouanine syndrome, angiodysgenetic myelomalacia, angiohypertrophic spinal myelitis, Spiller syndrome.*

  systemic myelitis SYSTEMIC MYELOPATHY.

  transverse myelitis Myelitis in which the inflammatory process principally involves one or more restricted spinal cord segments, showing the manifestations of a transverse cord lesion which usually develops acutely. Initially there is a flaccid paraplegia with sphincter paralysis and total loss of sensation below the level of the lesion, but as the acute spinal shock passes off the paraplegia later becomes spastic. Acute multiple sclerosis and postinfective myelitis are among the commonest causes of this syndrome, which must be distinguished from spinal cord infarction due to anterior spinal artery occlusion. In the latter, posterior column sensibility is usually comparatively spared.

  traumatic myelitis Myelitis following injury to the spinal cord, usually following fracture dislocation of the spine. Direct physical injury to the cord does not produce a myelitis.

  tuberculous myelitis Myelitis due to tuberculosis, usually developing as a complication of spinal tuberculous meningitis. Also called *caseous osteitis.*

  myelitis vaccinia Postvaccinal myelitis, occurring as one manifestation of postvaccinal encephalomyelitis.

myelo- [Gk *myelos* marrow, core, the brain] A combining form meaning (1) bone marrow; (2) the spinal cord. Also *myel-.*

myeloarchitecture The organization of nerve fibers and fiber tracts in the cerebral hemispheres, brainstem, cerebellum, and spinal cord, as revealed by staining techniques selective for myelin sheaths.

myeloblast [MYELO- + -BLAST]   The earliest precursor of granulocytes. The cell is usually 15–20 μm diameter, with a nucleus that has fine, nonaggregated chromatin and 2–5 pale nucleoli, and with absence of granules in the cytoplasm. Myeloblasts normally comprise 1–3% of bone marrow cells. When present in blood they usually signify acute myelogenous leukemia. Also called *microleukoblast, micromyelolymphocyte* (obsolete), *type I myeloblast, premyeloblast.*

type I myeloblast   MYELOBLAST.

type II myeloblast   A cell that is intermediate in maturation between a typical myeloblast (type I myeloblast) without cytoplasmic granules and a typical progranulocyte with numerous prominent primary granules. The type II myeloblast has a small number of primary granules. Also called *early progranulocyte.*

myeloblastemia   The presence of myeloblasts in blood, as in acute myelogenous leukemia. Also called *myeloblastosis.*

myeloblastic   Having to do with, or characterized by an excessive number of myeloblasts.

myeloblastoma   GRANULOCYTIC SARCOMA.

myeloblastosis   MYELOBLASTEMIA.

myelocele [MYELO- + -CELE¹]   A neural tube defect in which the embryonic neural plate fails to close in some part of the spinal cord, with the result that the persisting neural plate is not subsequently covered by cutaneous and mesodermal structures. The unclosed neural tissue and the laterally continuous epidermis enclose a sac of cerebrospinal fluid that protrudes on the back as fluid pressure rises.

myelocerebellar   Denoting the spinal cord and cerebellum. A seldom used term.

myeloclast [MYELO- + -CLAST]   A cell which lyses or degrades the coverings of medullated nerve fibers.

myelocoele [MYELO- + -COELE]   The central canal of the spinal cord, especially in the embryo.

myelocyst   A malformation of the spinal cord characterized by dilatation of the central canal which is lined by ependymal cells. It is caused by defective lamination of the posterior vertebral arches. Adjective: myelocystic.

myelocystocele [MYELO- + CYSTO- + -CELE¹]   A myelocele which becomes a prominent cystlike protrusion on the back.

myelocystography [MYELO- + CYSTO- + -GRAPHY]   The examination to demonstrate an intramedullary spinal cord cyst, either by roentgenography after percutaneous injection of air or contrast material into the cyst, or by scanning after injection of a radionuclide into the cyst.

myelocystomeningocele [MYELO- + CYSTO- + MENINGO-CELE]   A myelocystocele in which meninges are thought to be or are demonstrated to be present in association with the protruding neural plate. If the sac of neural tissue and modified skin remain intact, meninges only line the underlying fluid-filled cyst.

myelocyte [MYELO- + -CYTE]   A polymorphonuclear leukocyte at the earliest recognizable stage of differentiation, with a nucleus that exhibits chromatin condensation, that contains no recognizable nucleoli, and is round, oval or slightly indented, and a ctyoplasm that contains secondary (specific) granules which permit the myelocyte to be identified as belonging to the neutrophilic, eosinophilic, or basophilic series.

myelocythemia   MYELOCYTOSIS.

myelocytic   Pertaining to or characterized by myelocytes.

myelocytosis   The presence in blood of a much greater than normal number of myelocytes. Also called *myelocythemia.*

myelodiastasis [MYELO- + DIASTASIS]   Necrosis of the spinal cord. Also called *myelodiastema.*

myelodiastema   MYELODIASTASIS.

myelodysplasia [MYELO- + DYSPLASIA]   **1** Any developmental defect of the spinal cord. Also called *myelatelia.* **2** Abnormal formation of blood cell precursors in bone marrow. Adjective: myelodysplastic.

myeloencephalic   Denoting the spinal cord and brain.

myeloencephalitis   ENCEPHALOMYELITIS.

epidemic myeloencephalitis   ACUTE ANTERIOR POLIOMYELITIS.

myelofibrosis   The presence of fibrous tissue in bone marrow, as may occur following radiotherapy to adjacent structures, in some cases of Hodgkin's disease, as a late stage of polycythemia vera, or in the absence of any known cause. Also called *myelosclerosis* (ambiguous), *osteomyelofibrotic syndrome, osteomyelosclerosis.* See also AGNOGENIC MYELOID METAPLASIA.

acute myelofibrosis   A malignant disorder characterized by rapidly progressing pancytopenia and fibrosis of the bone marrow. The disorder appears to be the result of a malignant transformation of megakaryocytes analogous to an acute leukemia.

osteosclerosis myelofibrosis   An obliteration of the bone marrow by new bone formation, seen in some advanced myeloproliferative syndromes. Also called *centro-osteosclerosis, centrosclerosis.*

myelofugal   Denoting an efferent pathway from the spinal cord. A seldom used term.

myelogenesis   MYELINATION.

myelogenic   MYELOGENOUS.

myelogenous [MYELO- + -GENOUS]   Originating in bone marrow. Also *myelogenic.*

myelogeny [MYELO- + -GEN + -Y]   The development of myelin sheaths throughout the central nervous system to their final state. Also called *myelinogeny.*

myelogone   HEMATOGONE.

myelogram [MYELO- + -GRAM]   A roentgenogram obtained during myelography.

myelography [MYELO- + -GRAPHY]   Roentgenography of the spinal canal after injection of a contrast medium into the subarachnoid space, usually of the lumbar spine. Also called *perimyelography.*

air myelography   Myelography with the use of air as the contrast medium.

oxygen myelography   Myelography with oxygen as the contrast medium.

myeloid [MYEL- + -OID]   **1** Resembling or pertaining to the spinal cord. **2** Resembling or pertaining to the bone marrow. **3** Pertaining to granulocytes.

myeloidosis   A condition of growth and hyperplasia of tissue of the spinal cord. An ambiguous usage.

myelokentric   Stimulatory to the formation of leukocytes of the granulocytic series.

myeloleukemia   GRANULOCYTIC LEUKEMIA.

myelolipoma [MYELO- + LIPOMA]   A benign tumor composed of hematopoietic and adipose tissues. It occurs in the adrenal gland and, less frequently, in the retroperitoneum and pelvis. It is not associated with hematopoietic abnormalities.

myelolymphangioma   FILARIAL ELEPHANTIASIS.

myelolymphocyte   An abnormal lymphocyte of marrow origin. An imprecise and seldom used term.

myelolysis   The degradation and dissolution of myelin.

myelolytic   Causing or referring to myelolysis.

myeloma [MYEL- + -OMA]   A neoplastic proliferation of plasma cells, characterized by bone tumors and often complicated by pathologic fractures. Diffuse infiltration as well as tumors may also occur in the bone marrow and viscera. Uncommonly, solitary myeloma tumors of bone may show very slow progression and only become generalized after several years. The generalized disease is usually associated with IgA, or light-chain (Bence-Jones) monoclonal immunoglobulin production, and a monoclonal protein is detectable in the serum and/or urine by immunochemical techniques. Occasionally the anomalous immunoglobulin is IgD or very rarely IgE. Such protein abnormalities are not a feature of solitary myelomas. Also called *Kahler's disease* (obsolete), *lymphomyeloma, multiple myeloma, plasma cell tumor, sarcomatous osteitis* (obsolete), *myelomatosis, multiple myelomatosis, myelomatosis multiplex, plasma cell myeloma, malignant osteomyelitis, plasmacytic myeloma, plasmacytoma, extramedullary plasmacytoma, multiple plasmacytoma of bone, disseminated myelomatosis, peripheral plasmacytoma, solitary plasmocytoma, plasmoma.*

endothelial myeloma EWING SARCOMA.

extramedullary myeloma An extraskeletal plasmacytoma.

giant-cell myeloma GIANT CELL TUMOR OF BONE.

mouse myeloma A disease occurring in mice and characterized by neoplastic proliferation of plasma cells in the bone marrow. It may occur spontaneously or following injection of nonspecific adjuvants or various antigens. Myeloma proteins isolated from these mice may exhibit all five immunoglobulin types.

multiple myeloma MYELOMA.

osteogenetic myeloma GIANT CELL TUMOR OF BONE.

peripheral plasma cell myeloma An extraskeletal plasmacytoma.

plasma cell myeloma MYELOMA.

plasmacytic myeloma MYELOMA.

myelomalacia Pathologic softening of the spinal cord, usually resulting from recent infarction.

angiodysgenetic myelomalacia SUBACUTE NECROTIC MYELITIS.

myelomatoid [*myelomat(a)*, pl. of MYELOMA + -OID] Resembling myeloma.

myelomatosis [*myelomat(a)*, pl. of MYELOMA + -OSIS] MYELOMA.

disseminated myelomatosis MYELOMA.

multiple myelomatosis MYELOMA.

myelomatosis multiplex MYELOMA.

myelomenia [MYELO- + *men(o)-* + -IA] Endometriosis involving the spinal cord.

myelomeningitis A seldom used term for MENINGOMYELITIS.

myelomeningocele MENINGOMYELOCELE.

myelomeninx The membranes surrounding the spinal cord.

myelomere [MYELO- + -MERE] A segmental portion of the developing central nervous system.

myelomonocyte A leukocyte that appears to resemble both myelocytes and monocytes, in that nuclear chromatin is less condensed than in the myelocyte, and the cytoplasm has few neutrophilic granules. Enzyme cytochemistry may also identify the cell as being of either monocytic or neutrophilic lineage. Such cells represent aberrant maturation, as occurs in myelomonocytic leukemia.

myelomyces [MYELO- + Gk *mykēs* fungus, mushroom] A soft cancer. An obsolete term.

myelon An obsolete term for MEDULLA SPINALIS.

myeloneuritis [MYELO- + NEURITIS] Inflammation of the spinal cord and peripheral nerves.

myelonic [MYELO- + *n* + -IC] Pertaining to or affecting the spinal cord. An obsolete term.

myelo-opticoneuropathy [MYELO- + OPTICO- + NEUROPATHY] Any disease or dysfunction of the spinal cord and the optic and peripheral nerves. Also called *myelopticoneuropathy.*

subacute myelo-opticoneuropathy A syndrome characterized by a sensorimotor polyneuropathy involving the arms and legs and sometimes the oculomotor nerves, combined often with signs of optic atrophy and of corticospinal tract dysfunction, indicative of spinal cord involvement. It is the result of excessive and long-continued self-medication with clioquinol and its derivatives, taken for prophylaxis or treatment of intestinal affections, especially chronic diarrhea. Withdrawal of the causative drug is generally followed by recovery in one to two years, but occasional fatal cases have been described, and some patients have shown evidence of permanent neurologic sequelae. Abbreviation: SMON

myeloparalysis Paralysis due to disease of the spinal cord.

myelopathy [MYELO- + -PATHY] Any disease or dysfunction of the spinal cord. Adjective: myelopathic.

apoplectiform myelopathy Any myelopathy of very sudden onset.

arteriosclerotic myelopathy Ischemic myelopathy resulting from arteriosclerosis.

ascending myelopathy Any myelopathy in which symptoms and signs begin in the lower limbs and later spread upwards.

cervical myelopathy Compression myelopathy in the cervical region due to spondylosis or other causes.

compression myelopathy Any myelopathy resulting from compression of the spinal cord. Also called *compression myelitis* (outmoded), *pressure myelitis.*

descending myelopathy Any myelopathy in which symptoms and signs begin in the upper limbs and later spread to the lower limbs.

diabetic myelopathy Damage to the spinal cord in diabetes mellitus, consisting of segmentally localized degeneration in the posterior columns and localized necrosis and degenerative changes in the lateral columns. This is a rare complication, possibly due to diabetic angiopathy of arterioles in the affected areas.

focal myelopathy The clinical syndrome produced by any focal lesion of the spinal cord.

funicular myelopathy A myelopathy confined to one or more specific spinal tracts.

hemorrhagic myelopathy Any myelopathy associated with hemorrhage into the spinal cord.

interstitial myelopathy SCLEROSING MYELOPATHY.

ischemic myelopathy NEUMAYER'S AMYOTROPHIC LATERAL PSEUDOSCLEROSIS.

necrotic myelopathy SUBACUTE NECROTIC MYELOPATHY.

parenchymatous myelopathy Any myelopathy predominantly involving the neurons of the spinal cord. An outmoded term. Also called *parenchymatous myelitis.*

radiation myelopathy A progressive myelopathy which usually begins from six months to two years after inadvertent exposure to excessive doses of ionizing radiation incidental to radiotherapy for neoplastic lesions in the neck, thorax, or abdomen. Also called *radiation myelitis.*

sclerosing myelopathy Any myelopathy in which there is a marked proliferation of glial cells and fibers. An outmoded term. Also called *interstitial myelopathy.*

subacute necrotic myelopathy A progressive ascending myelopathy in which there is necrosis of the lower spinal cord segments with slow upward extension. It may occur in subjects with malignant disease outside the nervous system or in those with cor pulmonale in whom there is venous infarction of the spinal cord. Also called *necrotic myelopathy.*

systemic myelopathy Any myelopathy affecting predominantly one or more specific tracts and pathways. Also called *systemic myelitis.*

toxic myelopathy   Myelopathy due to exogenous or endogenous toxins.

transverse myelopathy   Any myelopathy producing a transverse lesion of the spinal cord. Transverse myelitis is one example.

myeloperoxidase   A peroxidase obtained from human leukocytes. Also called *verdoperoxidase.*

myelopetal   Traveling towards the spinal cord, as a nerve impulse.

myelophage [MYELO- + *phage* (from Gk *phagein* to eat)]   A macrophage which phagocytoses myelin. Adjective: myelophagous.

myelophthisis [MYELO- + PHTHISIS]   Any myelopathy involving cavitation of the spinal cord.

myeloplaque   MYELOPLAX.

myeloplasm [MYELO- + PLASM]   Material of which the wall of the primitive neural tube in the embryo is composed. It is derived from neurectoderm and is similar to a primitive syncytium either lacking, or with very thin, plasma membranes.

myeloplax   A giant multinucleated cell found in bone marrow. An obsolete term. Also called *myeloplaque.*

myeloplegia [MYELO- + -PLEGIA]   SPINAL PARALYSIS.

myelopoiesis [MYELO- + -POIESIS]   The formation, growth, and maturation of blood cells in the bone marrow. Adjective: myelopoietic.

    ectopic myelopoiesis   Formation of granulocytes in a location other than bone marrow. Also called *extramedullary myelopoiesis.*

    extramedullary myelopoiesis   ECTOPIC MYELOPOIESIS.

myelopore [MYELO- + PORE]   Any opening into the spinal cord.

myeloproliferative   Characterized by an increased rate of formation of leukocytes of the granulocytic series. Any of several neoplastic conditions affecting principally granulocytes, megakaryocytes, and erythroblasts are myeloproliferative disorders, including chronic granulocytic leukemia, polycythemia vera, myelofibrosis, erythroleukemia, and essential thrombocythemia.

myelopticoneuropathy   MYELO-OPTICONEUROPATHY.

myeloradiculitis   Inflammation of the spinal cord and the spinal nerve roots.

myeloradiculodysplasia [MYELO- + RADICULO- + DYSPLASIA]   Any developmental defect of the spinal cord and spinal nerve roots.

myeloradiculopathy   Any disease affecting the spinal cord and spinal nerve roots.

myeloradiculopolyneuronitis [MYELO- + RADICULO- + POLYNEURONITIS]   Inflammation of the spinal cord, spinal roots, and peripheral nerves.

myelorrhagia [MYELO- + -RRHAGIA]   Hemorrhage into the spinal cord.

myelosarcoma   A seldom used term for GRANULOCYTIC SARCOMA.

    erythroblastic myelosarcoma   A rare form of myeloid sarcoma containing a preponderant number of cells of the erythroid series. Also called *erythrosarcoma.*

myelosarcomatosis   An obsolete term for GRANULOCYTIC SARCOMA.

myeloschisis [MYELO- + Gk *schisis* a cleaving, division]   Any developmental defect of the spinal cord in which the embryonic neural tube fails to close, in part or in toto, or in which the neural tube reopens after having closed, if indeed such ever occurs.

myeloscintogram   The image obtained by myeloscintography.

myeloscintography   External imaging of the spinal cord and

canal and of the kinetics of the spinal fluid, following the intrathecal administration of a radiolabeled substance.

myelosclerosis   **1** Sclerosis of the spinal cord.   **2** Multiple sclerosis restricted to the spinal cord.   **3** An ambiguous term for MYELOFIBROSIS.

myelosclerotic   Denoting or pertaining to myelosclerosis.

myelosis [MYEL- + -OSIS]   **1** Any kind of abnormal proliferation of cells in the bone marrow, including various leukemias, myelofibrosis, and myeloma.   **2** Abnormal proliferation of medullary cells in the spinal cord.

    aplastic myelosis   APLASTIC ANEMIA.

    chronic myelosis   CHRONIC GRANULOCYTIC LEUKEMIA.

    chronic nonleukemic myelosis   AGNOGENIC MYELOID METAPLASIA.

    erythremic myelosis   A neoplastic disorder of erythropoiesis, characterized by megaloblastoid and dyserythropoietic erythroid hyperplasia, varying myeloid dysplasia, anemia with immature erythrocytes in the circulating blood, and hepatosplenomegaly. The acute form is erythroleukemia, and there is also a chronic form.

    funicular myelosis   Degeneration of the spinal cord white matter. An imprecise and outmoded term.

    leukopenic myelosis   SUBLEUKEMIC LEUKEMIA.

    nonleukemic myelosis   AGNOGENIC MYELOID METAPLASIA.

myelospasm [MYELO- + SPASM]   Muscular spasm resulting from spinal cord disease. An obsolete term.

myelospongium [MYELO- + SPONGIUM]   A network made by the interconnections of spongioblasts in the neural tube of the embryo.

myelosyphilis [MYELO- + SYPHILIS]   Any disorder of the spinal cord due to syphilis. Also called *myelosyphilosis.*

myelosyphilosis   MYELOSYPHILIS.

myelosyringocele   SYRINGOMYELIA.

myelosyringosis   SYRINGOMYELIA.

myelotome   A knife for making incisions in the spinal cord.

myelotomy [MYELO- + -TOMY]   **1** Incision into the spinal cord or into the medulla oblongata.   **2** Division of a tract as the spinothalamic tract for relief of pain.

    Bischof's myelotomy   COMMISSURAL MYELOTOMY.

    commissural myelotomy   A longitudinal incision through the midline of the spinal cord in order to divide pain fibers. Also called *midline myelotomy, Bischof's myelotomy, commissurotomy.*

    midline myelotomy   COMMISSURAL MYELOTOMY.

myelotoxicity   The capability to destroy bone marrow.

myelotoxin   Any substance that causes the death of bone marrow cells. Adjective: myelotoxic.

myelotropic   Showing a selective affinity for the spinal cord.

myentasis   MYOTASIS.

myenteric [MY + ENTERIC]   Relating to the muscular coat of the intestine.

myenteron   TUNICA MUSCULARIS INTESTINI TENUIS.

Myers [Victor Caryl *Myers*, U.S. biochemist, born 1883]   **1** See under METHOD.   **2** Pfiffner and Myers method. See under METHOD.

myesthesia [MY- + ESTHESIA]   Sensations, exclusive of pain, that arise in a muscle, particularly during contraction. Also called *mesoblastic sensibility.* Also *myoesthesia.*

Myhrman [Gustaf Christofer *Myhrman*, Swedish physician, born 1903]   Myhrman-Zetterholm disease. See under EPIDEMIC NEPHROPATHY.

myiasis [Gk *myia* a fly + -IASIS]   Infection, usually of the skin and subcutis, by fly larvae. Also called *myiosis, myasis.*

    aural myiasis   Infestation of the external ear by the larvae of various species of fly, a disease becoming increasingly rare.

creeping myiasis   CUTANEOUS LARVA MIGRANS.

creeping cutaneous myiasis   CUTANEOUS LARVA MIGRANS.

cutaneous myiasis   Infestation of the skin by the larvae of dipterous flies. Also called *dermal myiasis, myiasis dermatosa.*

dermal myiasis   CUTANEOUS MYIASIS.

myiasis dermatosa   CUTANEOUS MYIASIS.

furuncular myiasis   Cutaneous myiasis that is marked by single or grouped vesicles in which larvae are contained.

genitourinary myiasis   A rare form of primary myiasis due to maggots of the genera *Fannia* or *Calliphora,* believed to occur when eggs are laid in the vicinity of the urethra.

intestinal myiasis   Infestation of the intestine by fly maggots. Also called *enteromyiasis.*

myiasis linearis   CUTANEOUS LARVA MIGRANS.

nasal myiasis   Infestation of one or both nasal cavities with larvae of flies of the species *Musca domestica* and the genera *Calliphora, Lucilia* and others. Also called *peenash (Indian).*

ocular myiasis   Invasion of the conjunctival sac or eyeball by larvae of any of various species of flies, such as warble flies (*Hypoderma bovis, H. lineata*), blow flies (*Sarcophaga* species), and bot flies (*Gasterophilus intestinalis* and others). Also called *ophthalmomyiasis.*

myiasis oestrosa   Myiasis caused by botflies or gadflies (family Oestridae).

subcutaneous myiasis   CUTANEOUS LARVA MIGRANS.

subcutaneous myiasis with migrating nodules   Creeping myiasis that is manifested by migratory nodules, one or more of which ultimately ulcerates.

traumatic myiasis   An infection of a necrotic lesion by fly larvae that normally breed in carrion or rotting meat. Blowflies of various species (family Calliphoridae) are usually involved, including *Calliphora vicina, Phaenicia sericata, P. cuprina, Lucilia illustris, L. caesar, Phormia regina, Cochliomyia macellaria,* and *Chrysomyia* species. Flies of other families also may be involved, such as *Sarcophaga haemorrhoidalis,* the phorid *Megaselia scalaris,* or even the housefly, *Musca domestica.* Also called *wound myiasis.*

wound myiasis   TRAUMATIC MYIASIS.

myiocephalon   An outmoded term for IRIDOCELE.

myiocephalum   An outmoded term for IRIDOCELE.

myiodesopsia [Gk *myiōdēs* like a fly + -OPSIA]   The condition of seeing muscae volitantes before the eyes. Also called *myodesopsia, myopsis.*

myiosis   MYIASIS.

myitis   MYOSITIS.

myko-   MYCO-.

mylacris   An outmoded term for PATELLA.

myle [Gk *mylē* a mill, nether millstone]   **1** An outmoded term for PATELLA.   **2** An outmoded term for MAXILLA.

Myleran   A proprietary name for busulfan.

mylohyoid   Pertaining to the molar teeth, or the bony region related to them, and the hyoid bone.

myo- [Gk *mys* mouse, muscle]   A combining form denoting muscle. Also *my-.*

myoalbumin   An albumin component of muscle.

myoarchitectonic   Of or relating to the structure of muscle.

myoasthenia   MYASTHENIA.

myoatrophy   AMYOTROPHY.

myoblast [MYO- + -BLAST]   Each of the primitive cells forming the mass of a muscle (myotome) during development. The myoblasts multiply by mitosis and then elongate to become multinucleated myocytes. Myofibrils develop as rows of granules which fuse and eventually exhibit cross-striation. Also called *myogenic cell, sarcoblast, sarcogenic cell.*

myoblastoma [MYO- + BLASTOMA]   GRANULAR CELL TUMOR.

granular cell myoblastoma   GRANULAR CELL TUMOR.

myoblastomyoma [MYO- + BLASTO- + MYOMA]   GRANULAR CELL TUMOR.

myobradia   In certain generalized metabolic disease, the slowed muscle contraction that follows electric stimulation.

myocardiac   MYOCARDIAL.

myocardial   Pertaining to the myocardium. Also *myocardiac.*

myocardiogram   A record obtained by a myocardiograph.

myocardiograph   An instrument for recording the movements of the heart muscle.

myocardiolysis [MYO- + CARDIO- + LYSIS]   Necrosis of myocardial fibers with replacement by scar tissue.

myocardiopathy [MYO- + CARDIOPATHY]   CARDIOMYOPATHY.

alcoholic myocardiopathy   ALCOHOLIC CARDIOMYOPATHY.

chagasic myocardiopathy   A myocardiopathy induced by Chagas disease, characterized in its severe form by saccular apical ventricular aneurysm.

myocardiorrhaphy   Suture of the myocardium.

myocardiosis   CARDIOMYOPATHY.

myocarditic   Pertaining to or characterized by myocarditis.

myocarditis [MYO- + CARDITIS]   Inflammation of the muscle of the heart.

acute bacterial myocarditis   Myocarditis due to infection by bacteria, usually pyogenic.

acute isolated myocarditis   Interstitial myocarditis, without associated endo- or pericarditis. It is an acute illness of unknown cause, sometimes fatal. Also called *Fiedler's myocarditis, idiopathic myocarditis.*

acute rheumatic myocarditis   Myocarditis occurring as a complication of rheumatic fever, characterized by foci of inflammation (Aschoff's bodies) with accumulation of multinucleate giant cells and mononuclear leucocytes and swelling of collagen fibrils.

Chagas myocarditis   Subacute or chronic interstitial myocarditis occurring in Chagas disease.

chronic myocarditis   **1** Chronic inflammation of the myocardium, often following acute myocarditis, and characterized by much fibrosis as well as inflammatory cell infiltration. **2** Chronic myocardial damage or destruction from any cause with replacement by collagen.

chronic interstitial myocarditis   Chronic inflammation of heart muscle with collections of leucocytes and some collagen between the often damaged muscle fibers, as may occur following acute rheumatic fever or in Chagas disease. Also called *fibrous myocarditis.*

Coxsackie myocarditis   Acute or chronic myocarditis due to infection with coxsackievirus, especially group B.

degenerative myocarditis   **1** Degeneration of heart muscle due to toxins, as for example diphtheria toxin. **2** Ischemic damage to the myocardium. An imprecise usage.

diphtherial myocarditis   DIPHTHERITIC MYOCARDITIS.

diphtheritic myocarditis   An acute cardiomyopathy, often leading to necrosis, with reactive inflammation, due to toxin absorbed from a diphtheria infection elsewhere. It is often fatal, but recovery is usually complete in survivors. Also called *diphtherial myocarditis.*

fibrous myocarditis   CHRONIC INTERSTITIAL MYOCARDITIS.

Fiedler's myocarditis   ACUTE ISOLATED MYOCARDITIS.

giant cell myocarditis   Myocarditis with multinucleated giant cells as well as leukocytes, as in rheumatic fever, granulomatous diseases, and immunoreactive diseases.

idiopathic myocarditis   ACUTE ISOLATED MYOCARDITIS.

interstitial myocarditis Myocarditis with exudate, diffuse or focal, between the muscle fibers, which are damaged secondarily. There are many causes, including rheumatic fever.

local myocarditis Myocarditis confined to one or to relatively few areas, usually due to bacterial infection, adjacent or blood-borne.

nutritional myocarditis A cardiomyopathy due to under-nutrition, including protein deficiency as in kwashiorkor, or thiamin deficiency as in beriberi.

parenchymatous myocarditis A cardiomyopathy with inflammatory changes secondary to heart muscle fiber damage, especially by bacterial toxins as in diphtheria, typhoid fever, or pneumonia.

rheumatic myocarditis Interstitial myocarditis due to rheumatic fever. It may be acute, subacute, or chronic.

suppurative myocarditis A focal form of myocarditis with abscesses, usually due to infection by pyogenic bacteria.

syphilitic myocarditis Myocarditis due to syphilis giving rise usually to one or more gummas, or more rarely, to diffuse inflammation.

toxic myocarditis Myocarditis caused by toxicity from exogenous sources such as drugs, or from bacterial toxins such as that of diphtheria.

tuberculous myocarditis Myocarditis associated with foci of tuberculous infection of the myocardium.

typhic myocarditis 1 Myocarditis which sometimes occurs in typhus. 2 Myocarditis which sometimes occurs in typhoid fever.

virus myocarditis Myocarditis due to infection by a virus, such as type B coxsackievirus.

myocardium [NA] The intermediate, contractile muscular layer of the heart wall, constituting cardiac muscle, and comprising atrial and ventricular fibers separated by fibrous rings.

myocardosis CARDIOMYOPATHY.

myocele [MYO- + -CELE¹] A muscle hernia whereby the fleshy belly protrudes through a gap in its fascial covering.

myocelialgia A painful muscle hernia.

myocelitis The inflammation of a herniated muscle.

myocellulitis Cellulitis that involves muscle.

myoceptor MOTOR ENDPLATE.

myocerosis A waxy degeneration of muscle. Also called *myokerosis.*

Myochrysine A proprietary name for sodium aurothiomalate.

myocinesimeter MYOKINESIMETER.

myoclonia [MYO- + Gk *klonos* a violent motion, tumult, throng + -IA] MYOCLONUS.

myoclonia epileptica EPILEPTIC MYOCLONUS.

myoclonia fibrillaris multiplex PARAMYOCLONUS MULTIPLEX.

fibrillary myoclonia PARAMYOCLONUS MULTIPLEX.

infantile myoclonia An incorrect term for INFANTILE MASSIVE SPASM.

infectious myoclonia SYDENHAM'S CHOREA.

massive flexion myoclonia An incorrect term for INFANTILE MASSIVE SPASM.

massive infantile myoclonia An incorrect term for INFANTILE MASSIVE SPASM.

pseudoglottic myoclonia Hiccuping; singultation.

Unverricht's myoclonia PROGRESSIVE MYOCLONIC EPILEPSY.

myoclonic Characterized by myoclonus.

myoclonus [MYO- + -CLONUS] A brief, shocklike contraction of a single muscle or of one or more muscle groups, rarely of part of a muscle. The phenomenon may be physiologic, as in nocturnal myoclonus, or pathologic, as a manifestation of many brain diseases, in which it can occur sporadically but repetitively. Myoclonus may also occur repetitively in many widespread muscle groups throughout the body in response to startle, in hereditary essential myoclonus (paramyoclonus multiplex). Also called *myoclonic attack, myoclonic contraction, myoclonia, tic nondouloureux* (outmoded), *myoclonic jerk.* Adjective: myoclonic.

action myoclonus Myoclonus of one part of the body, particularly of one limb, which does not occur when the patient is completely relaxed, but which appears when he undertakes muscular activity, such as maintaining a position or attitude (postural or attitudinal myoclonus), the automatic execution of a movement, or, in particular, purposive voluntary movement (intention myoclonus). This is an important sequel of diffuse cerebral anoxia. Also called *intention myoclonus, postural myoclonus.*

diaphragmatic myoclonus EPIDEMIC HICCUP.

encephalitic myoclonus Myoclonic jerking in encephalitis lethargica.

epileptic myoclonus Myoclonus occurring in association with generalized epilepsy, with progressive myoclonic epilepsy, and with a variety of inflammatory or degenerative brain diseases. Also called *myoclonia epileptica.*

facial myoclonus FACIAL HEMISPASM.

focal myoclonus Myoclonus involving one limb, part of a limb, or some other restricted part of the body, as the lips, eyeball, palate, or tongue. Usually such myoclonus is an epileptic phenomenon (focal epileptic myoclonus) but in rare cases it is physiologic, occurring in patients who demonstrate no other manifestations of epilepsy, or else it results from a focal cerebral or spinal lesion, in which event its epileptic character is uncertain.

focal epileptic myoclonus Localized myoclonus involving one limb or a restricted part of the body, usually associated with focal spike or other epileptic discharges seen in the EEG, and arising in the appropriate part of the opposite cerebral hemisphere. Also called *localized epileptic myoclonus.*

hereditary essential myoclonus An uncommon and benign disorder of dominant inheritance in which there are frequent myoclonic jerks of the extremities, often elicited by a sudden noise or other sensory stimulus, but there is no association with epilepsy or other neurologic manifestation. See also PARAMYOCLONUS MULTIPLEX.

intention myoclonus ACTION MYOCLONUS.

localized epileptic myoclonus FOCAL EPILEPTIC MYOCLONUS.

massive epileptic myoclonus Epileptic myoclonus involving virtually the entire body and resulting from a hypersynchronous neuronal discharge arising in the brainstem. In the EEG there is usually simultaneous discharge of multispikes, or of multi-spike-waves, less frequently of spike-wave or spike-slow wave complexes.

myoclonus multiplex PARAMYOCLONUS MULTIPLEX.

nocturnal myoclonus Transient myoclonic jerks of the limbs and trunk which commonly occur in normal people during the early or slow wave stage of sleep, less often at other times in sleep.

palatal myoclonus Myoclonus of the soft palate, either unilateral or bilateral, a variety of palatopharyngeal myoclonus where only the palatal muscles are seen to be involved; often responsible for a clicking tinnitus, audible in some cases to others close to the patient. Also called *velopalatine myoclonus, palatal nystagmus.*

palatopharyngolaryngeal myoclonus Myoclonus of the soft palate, pharynx, and larynx, which may also involve the tongue, facial muscles, and diaphragm. The myoclonus is rhythmic (100 to 200 per minute) and does not stop when the patient is asleep.

It is usually associated with a lesion of unknown etiology in the olivary bodies, the dentate nucleus, and sometimes in the central tegmental tract of the midbrain. Also called *velopalatine myoclonic syndrome, myoclonic skull syndrome* (obsolete).

petit mal myoclonus   Transient generalized myoclonus occurring during attacks of petit mal or in patients who also suffer from petit mal.

postural myoclonus   ACTION MYOCLONUS.

segmental myoclonus   Myoclonic jerks, either isolated or repetitive, involving the muscles of one or more adjacent metameric bodily segments (that part innervated by one or more contiguous anterior roots). This is, in rare cases, an epileptic phenomenon, but more often it is a manifestation of spinal myoclonus.

spinal myoclonus   Myoclonic jerking limited to the muscles of the abdominal wall and trunk or less often of the legs and resulting from spinal cord disease.

sporadic myoclonus   Myoclonus in which the jerking movements of the musculature involve the various parts of the body in an episodic, irregular, and asynchronous manner, and in which any multispike or spike-wave discharges which may be seen in the EEG do not necessarily occur in time with the jerks. Such a pattern of myclonus may occur in hereditary essential myoclonus, which is probably not an epileptic condition in the usual sense of the term, but is also seen in progressive myoclonic epilepsy and various other degenerative brain diseases.

startle myoclonus   Myoclonic jerks elicited by startle.

velopalatine myoclonus   PALATAL MYOCLONUS.

myocoele [MYO- + -COELE]   The cavity inside a myotome. Also called *somite cavity.*

myocolpitis   Inflammation of the uterus and vagina.

myocrismus   The sound heard over a contracting muscle.

myoctonine $C_{72}H_{84}N_4O_{20}$. A poisonous alkaloid from wolfsbane, *Aconitum lycoctonum.*

myoculator [MY- + L *oculat(us)* (from *ocul(us)* eye + *-atus* -ATE) having eyes, seeing]   An orthoptic device that presents a target that moves laterally, vertically, and in rotation and also permits fusion.

myocutaneous   MUSCULOCUTANEOUS.

myocyst   A cystic tumor in muscle tissue.

myocyte [MYO- + -CYTE]   MUSCLE CELL.

Anichkov's myocyte   CARDIAC HISTIOCYTE.

myocytolysis   The absence of myofibrils and concomitant vacuolar change of the cytoplasm of cardiac muscle cells. It commonly occurs in the subendocardial region of the myocardium and at the periphery of old scars. Although a nonspecific change, it is believed by some to result from and be indicative of chronic ischemia.

focal myocytolysis of heart   A form of chronic, principally ischemic damage to the myocardial cells characterized by almost complete disappearance of sarcomeres with preservation of sarcolemmal membranes and nuclei. Because this change is typically found next to old infarcts and subendocardially, it is thought to represent a state of adaptation of myocardial cells to chronic ischemia, and the cells so affected to be viable though not capable of contraction.

myocytoma   A rare benign tumor consisting of bundles of myocytes.

myodegeneration   A deteriorating of muscle, either due to prior muscle disease or secondary to interruption of the nerve supply to the muscles.

myodemia   Fatty change of muscle. An obsolete term.

myodesopsia   MYIODESOPSIA.

myodiastasis   The separation of a muscle from its bony origin.

myodiopter   The force of ciliary muscle contraction required

to produce one diopter of accommodation.

myodynamic   Pertaining to force production in a muscle.

myodynamics   The subject concerned with the production and translation of force within a muscle.

myodynamometer   Any of a variety of instruments adapted for measuring the strength of particular muscles or muscle groups.

myodynia [MY- + -ODYNIA]   Pain originating in a muscle.

hysterical myodynia   Muscular tenderness, often over the ovarian region, as a conversion symptom.

myodysplasia [MYO- + DYSPLASIA]   Impaired development of skeletal muscle.

myodysplasia fibrosa multiplex   PROGRESSIVE MYOSCLEROSIS.

myodystonia   Any disorder that gives rise to abnormal muscle tone. Also called *myodystony.*

myodystony   MYODYSTONIA.

myodystrophia   MUSCULAR DYSTROPHY.

myodystrophia fetalis   CONGENITAL MULTIPLE ARTHROGRYPOSIS.

myodystrophy   MUSCULAR DYSTROPHY.

myoedema   Edema of a muscle. Also called *mounding, myoidem.*

myoelastic   Pertaining to a combination of smooth muscle fibers with elastic fibers, as is seen in the walls of blood vessels.

myoelectric   Denoting the potentials exhibited by a muscle during contraction, or its other electrical characteristics. A seldom used term.

myoendocarditis   Inflammation of the myocardium and the endocardium, especially that over the valves.

myoepithelial   Of or relating to myoepithelium.

myoepithelioma [MYO- + EPITHELIOMA]   A tumor of myoepithelial cells.

myoepithelium   Epithelial tissue possessing contractile properties. Also called *muscle epithelium.*

myoesthesia   MYESTHESIA.

myofascial   Of or relating to the connective tissue that is associated with muscle.

myofascitis   The inflammation of a muscle and its fascia. It often leads to interstitial fibrosis and induration of the muscle.

myofiber   A seldom used term for MUSCLE FIBER.

myofibril   One of the parallel bundles of myofilaments running longitudinally in a muscle fiber. The myofibrils are one to two micrometers in diameter. Also called *myofibrilla, muscle rod, muscle fibril, muscular fibril.*

myofibrilla   MYOFIBRIL.

myofibrillae   Plural of MYOFIBRILLA.

myofibroblast   A fibroblast which, when viewed in electron microscopy, has certain features characteristic of a smooth muscle cell. Believed to be caused by myofibroblasts, wound contraction can be inhibited experimentally by the administration of smooth muscle antagonists. Also called *contractile fibroblast.*

myofibroma [MYO- + FIBROMA]   LEIOMYOMA.

myofibrosarcoma [MYO- + FIBROSARCOMA]   A sarcoma containing muscular and fibrous components.

myofibrosis   Fibrous replacement, focal or interstitial, of muscle.

myofibrosis cordis   Interstitial fibrosis of the myocardium. A seldom used term.

myofibrositis   Interstitial inflammation and fibrosis of skeletal muscle.

myofilament   Any of the individual thick or thin filaments of the myofibril. The thick filaments are composed of the protein myosin, the thin filaments of actin associated with tropomyosin and troponin.

myofunctional   Relating to normal muscular function: said of forces applied to the teeth by the physiologic action of the orofacial muscles.

myogaster   VENTER MUSCULI.

myogelosis   A localized hardening in a muscle, most commonly seen in the gluteus maximus.

myogen [MYO- + -GEN]   A particular fraction of muscle extract, consisting largely of glycolytic enzymes. An obsolete term.

myogenesis [MYO- + GENESIS]   Formation of muscular tissue in the embryo.

myogenic [MYO- + -GENIC]   Developing into muscle.

myogenous   Arising from muscle tissue.

myoglia   Fine connective tissue fibrils attached to the external aspects of a muscle cell.

myoglobin [MYO- + L *glob(us)* ball, sphere, globe + -IN]   A respiratory pigment which is seen in muscle cells. It binds reversibly with molecular oxygen, thus functioning in oxygen storage. Myoglobin contains a globular protein of molecular weight 16 900, containing 153 amino-acid residues and a prosthetic (heme) group. Also called *myohemoglobin, muscle hemoglobin.*

myoglobinemia   The presence of myoglobin in the blood plasma or serum.

myoglobinuria [MYOGLOBIN + -URIA]   Excretion of myoglobin in the urine. It may follow muscle trauma or severe muscular exercise, extreme hyperthermia, extensive infarction when the main artery of a limb is occluded, or it may be associated with polymyositis, Haff disease, alcoholic polymyopathy, or McArdle disease. Some cases are familial, usually of unknown pathogenesis. Large amounts of myoglobin impart a burgundy red color to the urine, but since myoglobin is cleared rapidly by the kidneys, the serum usually is normal, in contrast to the early phases of hemoglobinuria where the serum is pink. Severe myoglobinuria may result in acute renal failure. Myoglobin and hemoglobin in urine are distinguished by differential absorption. Ammonium sulfate precipitates out hemoglobin and does not affect myoglobin.

familial myoglobinuria   Any heritable condition that results in abnormal skeletal muscle lysis and myoglobinuria. It is a feature of acute recurrent rhabdomyolysis, carnitine palmityltransferase deficiency, and muscle phosphorylase deficiency.

idiopathic myoglobinuria   Myoglobinuria of unknown cause, as in familial myoglobinuria (Meyer-Betz disease). Also called *spontaneous myoglobinuria.*

paralytic myoglobinuria   An exertional or nutritional myopathy of working horses or horses in training, characterized by myoglobinuria. It is usually of rapid onset during or soon after work or exercise. Severely affected horses go down and are unable to rise because of the extent of muscle damage. The condition is not truly paralytic, since the nervous system is unaffected. Also called *Monday morning sickness, azoturia, azoturia of horses, Monday morning disease of horses, hemoglobinemia paralytica* (incorrect).

paroxysmal myoglobinuria   IDIOPATHIC RHABDOMYOLYSIS.

paroxysmal idiopathic myoglobinuria   IDIOPATHIC RHABDOMYOLYSIS.

spontaneous myoglobinuria   IDIOPATHIC MYOGLOBINURIA.

traumatic myoglobinuria   The presence of myoglobin in the urine resulting from disruption of muscle cells following a crush injury, overly strenuous exercise, or deep thermal burn. Acute renal failure is a common consequence.

myoglobulin   A globulin component of muscle.

myognathus [New L (from MYO- + Gk *gnathos* jaw, esp. the lower jaw)]   Unequal conjoined twins in which the parasitic member is attached to the lower jaw of the host. Also called *gnathopagus parasiticus, hypognathus* (incorrect).

myogram [MYO- + -GRAM]   A record of muscular contraction.

myograph [MYO- + -GRAPH]   An apparatus for recording muscular contraction.

palate myograph   PALATOMYOGRAPH.

torsion-wire myograph   An instrument for recording muscle tension, consisting of a stiff wire, fixed at one or both ends, that is rotated slightly by force applied to a lever arm fixed vertical to the wire and to the line of applied force. The rotation may be amplified and visualized through reflection of a light beam by a mirror fixed to the wire.

myographic   Pertaining to the recording of muscular contraction.

myography   **1** The recording of the activity of a muscle during rest or contraction by means of a special apparatus. **2** The detailed description of muscles.

myohemoglobin   MYOGLOBIN.

myohypertrophia   Hypertrophy of muscle.

myohypertrophia kymoparalytica   A paralyzing muscular dystrophy.

myohysterectomy [MYO- + HYSTERECTOMY]   HYSTERECTOMY.

myoid [MY- + -OID]   **1** Resembling muscle; musclelike. **2** A substance resembling muscle. **3** A filamentous protoplasmic thread seen in epithelial cells of some invertebrates.

cone myoid   The contractile inner cone segment in the retina of birds and fishes.

rod myoid   The contractile inner rod segment in the retina of birds and fishes.

myoidem   MYOEDEMA.

myoidema [MY- + Gk *oidēma* a swelling]   A phenomenon in which a sharp tap upon the belly of a voluntary muscle, especially deltoid, biceps brachii, or gastrocnemius, produces a localized linear ridge which is electrically silent on electromyography and which gradually disappears within a few seconds. The cause of the phenomenon is unknown. It usually occurs in malnourished or cachectic patients, occasionally in hypothyroidism.

myoideum   MUSCULAR TISSUE.

myoidism [MY- + -OID + -ISM]   A state of unusual responsiveness of muscles to mechanical stimulation.

myoischemia   A localized loss of the blood supply to muscle tissue.

myokerosis   MYOCEROSIS.

myokinase   An older term for ADENYLATE KINASE.

myokinesimeter   A device for measuring, and usually recording, the time course and amplitude of a muscle's contraction. A seldom used term. Also called *myocinesimeter.*

myokinesiogram   A record of muscle contraction, expressed either as change in tension or angular excursion of a joint, as recorded by a myokinesimeter.

myokinesiography   The use and interpretation of records taken with a myokinesimeter.

myokinesis   The subject concerned with movements of whole muscles, their constituent heads and motor units and, by extension, the body parts acted upon.

myokinetic   Pertaining to the movements of a muscle or the subject of myokinesis.

myokymia [MYO- + Gk *kym(a)* anything swollen, a wave + -IA]   **1** Any of several syndromes characterized by involuntary contraction of skeletal muscle, as benign myokymia of the lower eyelid or facial myokymia. An ambiguous usage. **2** A syndrome of widespread, benign, coarse fasciculation of the voluntary muscles, often associated with hyperhidrosis and anxiety symptoms. **3** A rare syndrome of widespread muscular fasciculation with manifestations of myotonia, spasm of muscles, and contractures in the extremities. Also called *neuromyotonia, live flesh, Isaacs syndrome, kymatism.*

benign myokymia of the lower eyelid An irregular, repetitive, twitching movement of the lower eyelid, commonly experienced by normal individuals, especially when fatigued.

facial myokymia A continuous or intermittent, wavelike or rippling movement of the facial muscles, usually unilateral and often of unknown cause though it may occur in multiple sclerosis.

hereditary myokymia A rare inherited disorder in which myokymia, hypoglycemia, and hypothyroidism occur.

myoleiotic Of or relating to smooth muscle.

myolemma SARCOLEMMA.

myolipoma [MYO- + LIPOMA] A benign tumor composed of muscle and fatty tissue. Also called *lipomyoma.*

myologia [MYO- + -LOGIA] **1** [NA] The nomenclature dealing with muscles, bursae, and synovial sheaths. **2** MYOLOGY.

myologic Pertaining to myology.

myology [MYO- + -LOGY] The study of muscles and associated structures. Also called *myologia.*

myolysis [MYO- + LYSIS] The disintegration and liquifaction of muscle tissue. It may follow atrophy or fatty degeneration.

myolysis cardiotoxica Destruction of heart muscle fibers by blood-borne toxins such as diphtheria toxin.

myoma [MY- + -OMA] A benign tumor of muscle tissue. Also called *muscular tumor.*

ball myoma A round myoma.

myoma levicellulare LEIOMYOMA.

mydartoic myoma A neoplasm arising from subcutaneous muscle tissue.

myoblastic myoma GRANULAR CELL TUMOR.

myoma previum A myoma which obstructs the uterine canal in pregnancy.

myoma sarcomatodes MYOSARCOMA.

myoma striocellulare RHABDOMYOMA.

myoma telangiectodes A highly vascular myoma.

myomagenesis [MYOMA + GENESIS] The formation or causation of myomas.

myomalacia An abnormal softening of muscle tissue.

myomalacia cordis Necrosis and softening of heart muscle, most often due to coronary artery occlusion, sometimes to severe poisoning.

myomata Plural of MYOMA.

myomatectomy MYOMECTOMY.

myomatosis [MYOMA, pl. *myomata* + -OSIS] Numerous myomas.

myomatous Pertaining to myomas.

myomectomy [*myom(a)* + -ECTOMY] The surgical excision of a uterine fibromyoma or leiomyoma. Also called *myomatectomy.*

abdominal myomectomy The surgical removal of one or more tumors of muscular tissue from within or about the abdominal cavity. Also called *celiomyomectomy, laparomyomectomy.*

vaginal myomectomy The surgical removal of a leiomyoma of the cervix or uterus via the vagina. Also called *colpomyomotomy, colpomyomectomy.*

myomelanosis An abnormal black pigmentation of muscle.

myomere [MYO- + -MERE] **1** The part of a somite which forms the elements of the musculature after other elements have differentiated to form the sclerotome. Together they demon-

strate metameric segmentation (metamerism) in that the two elements establish the somites. **2** One of the series of muscle segments on the body wall of fishes and lancelets.

myometer [MYO- + -METER] An instrument that measures changes in length of muscle.

myometritis [MYO- + METRITIS] Inflammation of the myometrium usually secondary to endometritis. Also called *idiometritis.*

acute myometritis Abrupt onset of or the first episode of an inflammatory condition of the myometrium.

myometrium TUNICA MUSCULARIS UTERI.

myomitochondrion (*plural* myomitochondria) SARCOSOME.

myomohysterectomy [New L *myomo-*, combining form from *my-* MY- + *-oma* -OMA + HYSTERECTOMY] The surgical removal of a uterus with one or more leiomyomas attached.

Myomorpha [New L (from Gk *mys*, gen. *myos*, a mouse, muscle + *-morpha*, fem. sing. or neut. pl. of New L *-morphus* combining form denoting shape, form)] The most flourishing of the three suborders of the order Rodentia; the ratlike rodents. Species possess a complex of masseter muscles distinctly divided into three parts and elongated due to a combination of movement of origin of the complex anteriorly and movement of the muscles through a broadened infraorbital canal.

myomotomy [*myom(a)* + *o* + -TOMY] An incision into one or more muscular tumors. A seldom used term.

myon [MY- + *-on*, suffix denoting a unit] A group of muscle cells that together form a single, functional, contractile unit.

myonecrosis [MYO- + NECROSIS] Necrosis of muscular tissue.

myoneme A contractile fibril found in certain protozoa.

myonephropexy [MYO- + NEPHRO- + -PEXY] Surgical fixation of a movable kidney to muscle tissue to prevent its movement.

myoneural [MYO- + NEURAL] **1** Of or denoting both muscle and nerve. **2** Denoting the highly specialized junction between motor nerve terminals and muscle fibers.

myoneuralgia Neuralgic pain in the muscles. An imprecise and obsolete term.

postural myoneuralgia A pain in a muscle caused by the fatigue produced when maintaining a fixed position.

myoneurasthenia Muscle weakness occurring in conjunction with neurasthenia.

myoneure [MYO- + *neur(on)*] A nerve cell that communicates with a muscle cell.

myoneuroma A tumor that consists of proliferating Schwann cells together with myocytes.

myoneurosis [MYO- + -NEUROSIS] Complaints centered on the muscles as the major manifestation of neurotic conflict. An outmoded term.

myonicity A rarely used term for MYOTILITY.

myonitis MYOSITIS.

myonosus MYOPATHY.

myonymy The nomenclature of muscles.

myopachynsis Muscle hypertrophy.

myopalmus Muscle twitching.

myoparalysis Paralysis of one or more skeletal muscles.

myoparesis [MYO- + PARESIS] Weakness of one or more skeletal muscles.

myopathia [MYO- + -PATHIA] MYOPATHY.

Biemond's myopathia distalis juvenilis hereditaria A disease with clinical manifestations similar to those of Welander's myopathia distalis tarda hereditaria, but with an earlier onset. This condition is not a myopathy but a neuropathy, almost certainly one form of peroneal muscular atrophy.

myopathia cordis CARDIOMYOPATHY.

myopathia infraspinata The development of sudden pain about the shoulder, accompanied by tenderness of the infraspinatus muscle.

Welander's myopathia distalis tarda hereditaria LATE DISTAL HEREDITARY MYOPATHY.

myopathic Pertaining to or characteristic of myopathy.

myopathy [MYO- + -PATHY] Any disease of skeletal or voluntary muscle. Also called *myopathia, myonosus*. Adjective: myopathic. • In clinical parlance, this term has often been used in the past as a synonym of muscular dystrophy, but this incorrect usage is becoming less frequent.

acromegalic myopathy A presumably specific weakness and wasting of skeletal muscles occurring late in the course of acromegaly, due to some deleterious effect of growth hormone on muscle.

ACTH myopathy A myopathy associated with increased levels of circulating ACTH following bilateral adrenalectomy for Cushing's disease.

acute necrotizing myopathy Any acute myopathy in which there are areas of necrosis of skeletal muscle fibers.

acute thyrotoxic myopathy Myopathy occurring acutely during the course of Graves disease.

alcoholic myopathy Myopathy due to the toxic effects of alcohol occurring in alcoholic subjects. Both acute and subacute forms occur. Also called *alcoholic paralysis.*

arachnodactyly nemaline myopathy Nemaline myopathy occurring in subjects showing some features of arachnodactyly.

Barnes myopathy An uncommon, dominantly inherited variant of distal myopathy of late onset or muscular dystrophy in which the disease was once said to progress through hypertrophic and atrophic phases. The question as to whether this is a specific disease entity is still unresolved. Also called *Barnes muscular dystrophy.*

benign congenital myopathy Any of a group of myopathies which are present from birth and run a benign course.

carcinomatous myopathy A myopathy associated with a carcinoma. It is a paraneoplastic phenomenon.

centronuclear myopathy A benign congenital myopathy in which many muscle fibers show central nuclei and resemble fetal myotubes. Also called *myotubular myopathy.*

corticosteroid-induced myopathy Myopathy due to prolonged treatment with corticosteroid drugs, involving first the limb girdle muscles and later the distal musculature. It also occurs in spontaneously occurring Cushing syndrome. It is characterized histochemically by type II fiber atrophy. Removal of the excessive corticosteroid restores muscular structure and function to normal. Also called *steroid myopathy.*

Cushing's disease myopathy Myopathy complicating Cushing's disease. See also STEROID MYOPATHY.

diabetic myopathy Proximal muscular weakness in association with diabetes mellitus. The nature of the relation between diabetes and the myopathy is not clear.

distal myopathy Myopathy beginning in the distal muscles of the upper and lower limbs, especially in the small muscles of the hands.

distal myopathy of late onset LATE DISTAL HEREDITARY MYOPATHY.

Duchenne's myopathy DUCHENNE TYPE MUSCULAR DYSTROPHY.

Erb's juvenile myopathy SCAPULOHUMERAL MUSCULAR DYSTROPHY.

Erb's primary progressive myopathy SCAPULOHUMERAL MUSCULAR DYSTROPHY.

fibrolipocalcareous myopathy A rare type of myopathy characterized by progressive muscular atrophy in limb muscles, with the formation of indurated painless nodules as a result of lipofibrous degeneration followed by calcification. Also called *Mattioli-Foggia and Raso syndrome.*

fingerprint body myopathy A benign congenital myopathy in which electron microscopy of sections of skeletal muscle reveals structures resembling fingerprints.

granulomatous myopathy A subacute inflammatory myopathy in which there are large collections of inflammatory cells, often with giant cells resembling multiple granulomas, in sections of affected skeletal muscle.

hypermetabolic myopathy A rare form of mitochondrial myopathy in which there is a greatly increased basal metabolic rate but without hyperthyroidism. Also called *Luft syndrome.*

hyperparathyroid myopathy A mild disorder of proximal limb muscles in primary and secondary hyperparathyroidism, characterized by muscular weakness and fatigue, atrophy of muscles, and pressure tenderness of bones. The exact relation of muscle involvement to hypercalcemia is not clear.

hypothyroid myopathy MYXEDEMATOUS MYOPATHY.

Landouzy-Dejerine myopathy FACIOSCAPULOHUMERAL MUSCULAR DYSTROPHY.

late distal hereditary myopathy A dominantly inherited form of muscular dystrophy beginning in middle or late life and involving first the muscles of the hands and of the forearms and later the distal muscles of the legs. Many cases have been described in Sweden, few in other countries. The course of the disease is indolent. Also called *distal myopathy of late onset, slow hereditary distal myopathy, Welander's myopathy, Welander's myopathia distalis tarda hereditaria.*

Leyden-Möbius myopathy A form of primary progressive myopathy, sometimes beginning in infancy, sometimes in later life, which starts in the pelvifemoral muscles and subsequently involves the trunk and eventually the upper limbs. It now seems likely that patients once so diagnosed were suffering from either limb-girdle muscular dystrophy or from Kugelberg-Welander disease. Also called *Leyden-Möbius muscular dystrophy.*

Marie's myopathy A rare type of muscular dystrophy involving the levators of the upper lids and the muscles of mastication. It now seems that this syndrome would be embraced by the modern concept of ocular or oculopharyngeal muscular dystrophy, though similar features can be seen in dystrophia myotonica. An obsolete term.

megaconial myopathy A form of mitochondrial myopathy in which the mitochondria in skeletal muscle are greatly enlarged and many contain paracrystalline inclusions.

metabolic myopathy Any myopathy resulting from a metabolic disorder.

mitochondrial myopathy Any of a group of metabolic myopathies in which the mitochondria are structurally and biochemically abnormal. The attendant biochemical abnormalities include in different cases impaired oxidative phosphorylation, hypermetabolism, metabolic acidosis, and disorders of the electron transport chain.

myogranular myopathy An obsolete term for NEMALINE MYOPATHY.

myotonic myopathy DYSTROPHIA MYOTONICA.

myotubular myopathy CENTRONUCLEAR MYOPATHY.

myxedematous myopathy Weakness, myxedema, and slowed speed of contractility and relaxation of proximal limb muscles in hypothyroidism with myxedema. Serum values of creatine phosphokinase are greatly elevated, but muscle biopsies are often normal with the occasional presence of a mucoid substance within muscle fibers; the clinical picture is reversed with thyroid hormone. Also called *hypothyroid myopathy.*

nemaline myopathy A rare benign congenital myopathy in which the clinical features sometimes suggest arachnodactyly and in which muscle fibers often show collections of structures like rods or threads lying beneath the sarcolemma. Also called *rod myopathy.*

Nevin's late-onset progressive myopathy LATE-ONSET PSEUDOMYOPATHIC POLYMYOSITIS.

nutritional myopathy A noninflammatory degeneration of skeletal and cardiac muscle, associated with a deficiency of selenium and vitamin E. It occurs in lambs, calves, foals, pigs, and many other animal species. Also called *white muscle disease* (imprecise).

ocular myopathy Progressive muscular dystrophy of the external ocular muscles. Also called *Kiloh-Nevin syndrome.*

pleoconial myopathy A mitochondrial myopathy in which an abnormally large number of mitochondria are seen in sections of skeletal muscle.

primary progressive myopathy MUSCULAR DYSTROPHY.

progressive atrophic myopathy MUSCULAR DYSTROPHY.

Raymond and Guillain myopathy RAYMOND AND GUILLAIN LUMBOPELVIFEMORAL MYOPATHY.

Raymond and Guillain lumbopelvifemoral myopathy A syndrome once considered a form of muscular dystrophy of pelvifemoral distribution of late onset. However, the cases described probably included limb-girdle muscular dystrophy, spinal muscular atrophy, and other disease entities. An obsolete term. Also called *Raymond and Guillain myopathy.*

rod myopathy NEMALINE MYOPATHY.

sarcoid myopathy Granulomatous myopathy due to sarcoidosis.

scapuloperoneal myopathy Progressive muscular dystrophy beginning in the peroneal and anterior tibial muscles of the lower limbs and in serratus and other muscles around the scapulae in the upper limbs.

senile myopathy A progressive weakness of the legs occurring in the elderly, which is due to many causes but rarely, if ever, to myopathy. An imprecise and outmoded term.

slow hereditary distal myopathy LATE DISTAL HEREDITARY MYOPATHY.

steroid myopathy Corticosteroid-induced myopathy.

thyrotoxic myopathy A disorder of skeletal muscle in hyperthyroidism or Graves disease, affecting more than half of patients. The shoulder and pelvic girdle are commonly weak and atrophied, and, less often, the extraocular muscles and the bulbar musculature are afflicted. The disorder is reversible when a euthyroid state is restored.

uremic myopathy Myopathy of the proximal limb muscles resulting from chronic uremia, usually in cases of renal failure.

Welander's myopathy LATE DISTAL HEREDITARY MYOPATHY.

myope A nearsighted individual.

myopericarditis [MYO- + PERICARDITIS] Inflammation of both myocardium and pericardium. Also called *cardiopericarditis.*

myophage A phagocyte which destroys muscle tissue.

myophagia MUSCULAR ATROPHY.

myophagism MUSCULAR ATROPHY.

myophone [MYO- + Gk *phōnē* sound, voice] A microphone used to pick up sounds produced during the contraction of a muscle for amplification and projection over a speaker and recording.

myopia [MY- + -OPIA] The refractive error requiring correction with a concave lens in order to see clearly in the distance. Also called *nearsightedness, shortsightedness, brachymetropia, near sight, short sight, hypometropia* (seldom used), *plesiopia, visus brevior.* Adjective: myopic.

chromic myopia Inability to recognize colors at a distant location.

curvature myopia Myopia due to a steeper than normal contour of the cornea or lens.

high myopia A large amount of nearsightedness; severe myopia.

index myopia Myopia due to denser optical media. Also called *indicial myopia.*

indicial myopia INDEX MYOPIA.

low myopia A small amount of nearsightedness; moderate myopia.

malignant myopia Degenerative myopia, causing pathologic structural changes. Also called *pernicious myopia.*

pernicious myopia MALIGNANT MYOPIA.

prodromal myopia The development of myopia as an early stage of nuclear cataract.

progressive myopia Myopia that increases in severity with aging.

progressive myopia of children Myopia beginning in early life and increasing in severity as the individual ages.

myopic Pertaining to or affected by myopia. Also *nearsighted, brachymetropic, shortsighted.*

myoplasm SARCOPLASM.

myoplastic Pertaining to myoplasty.

myoplasty [MYO- + -PLASTY] Any plastic operation on muscle.

mastoid myoplasty A variety of the mastoid obliteration operation in which a pedicled flap of temporalis muscle is turned down to occupy the mastoid excavation. Also called *musculoplasty.*

myoplegia [MYO- + -PLEGIA] Muscular paralysis. An obsolete term.

familial myoplegia PERIODIC PARALYSIS.

myoporthosis [*myop(ia)* + ORTHO- + -SIS] The correction of myopia.

myoprotein Any protein found within muscle cells.

myopsis [Gk *my(ia)* a fly + -OPIS] MYIODESOPSIA.

myopsychopathy Neuromuscular disease associated with mental dysfunction. Also called *myopsychosis.*

myopsychosis MYOPSYCHOPATHY.

myoreceptor An obsolete term for MUSCLE RECEPTOR.

myorrhaphy [MYO- + -RRHAPHY] The rejoining of transected muscle, usually with suture material. Also called *myosuture.*

myorrhexis [MYO- + -RRHEXIS] The rupture of a muscle.

myorrhythmia Slow, regular, involuntary contraction of the limb muscles, giving rise to rhythmic movements as one sees particularly in patients with postencephalitic parkinsonism.

myosalgia MYALGIA.

myosalpingitis [MYO- + SALPINGITIS] Inflammation of muscle of the salpinx. It is associated with endosalpingitis.

myosalpinx TUNICA MUSCULARIS TUBAE UTERINAE.

myosarcoma A malignant tumor of muscle tissue. Also called *myoma sarcomatodes.*

myoschwannoma [MYO- + SCHWANNOMA] GRANULAR CELL TUMOR.

myosclerosis An abnormal hardening of muscle tissue.

familial myosclerosis A rare familial disorder, probably of autosomal recessive inheritance, in which progressive muscular weakness and contractures involving many limb muscles result from widespread proliferation of fibrous tissue within the muscles.

progressive myosclerosis A neuromuscular disorder which is sometimes sporadic, sometimes familial, in which progressive muscular weakness and wasting is accompanied by marked intramuscular proliferation of connective tissue leading to increasingly severe contractures. This is probably a syndrome of multiple etiology. In many reported cases the individuals have been found to be suffering from spinal muscular atrophy. Also called *myodysplasia fibrosa multiplex.*

myoscope [MYO- + -SCOPE] An orthoptic instrument that produces a moving fixation target.

myoseism The irregular spasmodic contraction of muscle.

myoseptum [MYO- + SEPTUM] (*plural* myosepta) A thin mesenchymatous septum which in the embryo separates the muscular masses derived from myotomes. Myosepta are also common in fishes.

myoserum SARCOPLASM.

myosin [MYO- + *s* + -IN] The component of muscle that forms the thicker fibrils. Myosin molecules have two components: heads, which stick out from the fibril, have ATPase activity, and are responsible for interaction with the actin fibrils; and tails, which associate together and are responsible for fibril formation.

myosinuria [MYOSIN + -URIA] Excretion of myosin in the urine. Also called *myosuria.*

myosis **1** MIOSIS. **2** A condition affecting muscular tissue.
endolymphatic stromal myosis A uterine tumor resembling endometrial stroma which permeates the myometrium, usually by way of vascular spaces. It is typically of low-grade malignancy. Also called *interstitial endometriosis.*

myositic Of or relating to myositis.

myositis [MYO- + *s* + -ITIS] The inflammation of a muscle. Also called *myonitis, myitis, sarcitis* (obsolete).
acute disseminated myositis PRIMARY MULTIPLE MYOSITIS.
acute progressive myositis A rare inflammatory disease of the muscle in which all muscle groups become involved and result ultimately in death from respiratory failure.
cervical myositis Acute stiff neck. An outmoded and inaccurate term.
Coxsackie myositis Myositis resulting from infection with one of the Coxsackie group of viruses. Epidemic pleurodynia is one example.
epidemic myositis EPIDEMIC PLEURODYNIA.
myositis fibrosa A syndrome of widespread muscular contractures with proliferation of connective tissue in the affected muscles, developing usually in childhood in a subject with polymyositis. Also called *Froriep's induration* (seldom used).
myositis a frigore Muscular pain after exposure to cold. An outmoded term.
generalized myositis ossificans A rare progressive disorder, often familial, in which there is progressive calcification and sometimes ossification within certain skeletal muscles, often beginning in those around the scapula and in the back and cervical region.
infectious myositis An inflammation of skeletal muscle that is characterized by pain and swelling. It is most commonly seen in the upper limbs and shoulders.
interstitial myositis An inflammatory and sometimes proliferative process involving the interstitial connective tissue of a muscle with relative sparing of the myofibers. A seldom used term.
ischemic myositis Infarction of muscle occurring as a result of vasculitis, or in polyarteritis nodosa. • The term is a misnomer as the myositis is not due to ischemia.
localized myositis ossificans Localized areas of calcification followed by ossification in muscles subjected to trauma, such as the thigh adductors in horseback riders or after surgery. A similar syndrome can develop in lower limb muscles as a complication of spastic paraparesis.
multiple myositis POLYMYOSITIS.
ocular myositis ORBITAL MYOSITIS.
orbital myositis Myositis limited to the external ocular mus-

cles, usually resulting in pain, proptosis, and ophthalmoplegia. The process is generally autoimmune and steroid-responsive. Also called *ocular myositis.*
myositis ossificans Bone formation in muscle, whether localized or generalized.
myositis ossificans circumscripta Localized dystrophic calcification and ossification occurring within a muscle, most often associated with persistent trauma.
myositis ossificans progressiva A rare, familial disease of unknown etiology in which the skeletal tissue of muscles, tendons, fasciae, and ligaments becomes edematous and progressively calcified and ossified. Onset is usually in childhood, and the condition is commoner in males. Congenital skeletal abnormalities such as malformed fingers and toes are often associated features. Eventually, large sheets of bone splint the trunk and lead to death from respiratory complications. Also called *fibrositis ossificans progressiva, Münchmeyer's disease, Münchmeyer syndrome, fibrodysplasia, progressive ossifying myositis* (rarely used).
myositis ossificans traumatica The presence of bonelike calcium deposits within muscle following injury, as in the triceps tendon at the elbow following a severe burn. The metabolic cause is unknown, and it can occur in muscles remote from the injury.
parenchymatous myositis An inflammatory process predominantly affecting the myofibers. An obsolete term.
postparaplegic myositis ossificans PARAPLEGIC PARAOSTEOARTHROPATHY.
primary multiple myositis An inflammatory disease of acute onset that is characterized by foci of inflammation of muscles and overlying skin. The condition appears identical to dermatomyositis. Also called *acute disseminated myositis.*
progressive ossifying myositis A rarely used term for MYOSITIS OSSIFICANS PROGRESSIVA.
myositis purulenta SUPPURATIVE MYOSITIS.
myositis purulenta tropica TROPICAL PYOMYOSITIS.
rheumatoid myositis FIBROSITIS.
myositis serosa Muscle edema in polymyositis. An outmoded term.
suppurative myositis Inflammation and suppuration in muscles resulting from infection with pyogenic microorganisms such as streptococci and staphylococci. The inflammation may be diffuse, spreading, localized, or abscess-forming, and general symptoms of septic infection may be apparent. Also called *myositis purulenta.* See also TROPICAL PYOMYOSITIS.
trichinous myositis The changes occurring in skeletal muscle following hematogenous dissemination of *Trichinella spirallis.* Initially there are acute inflammatory changes with eosinophilic infiltrates followed by encapsulation and formation of cysts containing the microorganisms.
tropical myositis TROPICAL PYOMYOSITIS.

myospasia PARAMYOCLONUS MULTIPLEX.

myospasm A condition that gives rise to spasmodic contraction, which may be prolonged, in the voluntary muscles.
facial myospasm FACIAL HEMISPASM.

myospasmia Any disease or disorder giving rise to myospasm.

myostasis A fixed muscle length, as occurs after prolonged splintage.

myostatic **1** Related to the resting tension of a muscle. **2** Generated by the stretching of a muscle at rest as in myostatic reflex. For defs. 1 and 2 also *myotatic.*

myosteoma A benign tumor of muscle containing bony elements.

myosthenic Of or relating to the strength of a muscle.

myosthenometer [MYO- + STHENO- + -METER] An apparatus for measuring muscle strength.

myostroma   The connective tissue framework of muscular tissue.

myosuria   MYOSINURIA.

myosuture   MYORRHAPHY.

myosynizesis   Muscle adhesions.

myosynovitis [MYO- + SYNOVITIS]   Inflammation of muscle and joint synovia.

myotactic   Denoting any reflex or phenomenon evoked by tapping the belly or tendon of a skeletal muscle; related to proprioceptive function.

myotamponade   An obsolete method of pulmonary collapse in treatment of tuberculosis in which the extrapleural space is packed with muscle.

myotasis [MYO- + Gk *tasis* a stretching]   The stretching of muscle. Also called *myentasis*.

myotatic [MYO- + Gk *tatik(os)* (from *teinein* to stretch) exerting tension]   MYOSTATIC.

myotendinitis [MYO- + TENDINITIS]   Inflammation of a muscle and its attached tendon. Also called *myotenositis*.

myotendinous   Of or relating to a muscle and tendon unit.

myotenontoplasty   TENOMYOPLASTY.

myotenositis   MYOTENDINITIS.

myotenotomy   The surgical excision of part of a muscle and its tendon. Also called *tenomyotomy, tenontomyotomy*.

myothermic   Relating to the alteration in the temperature of muscles as a result of contraction.

myotic   MIOTIC.

myotility   The contractile property of muscle. A rarely used term. Also called *myonicity* (rarely used).

myotome [MYO- + -TOME]   **1** That part of a somite in an embryo that is formed from paraxial mesoderm and gives rise to skeletal muscle. It appears to be derived from the edges of the dermatome and is at first made up of closely packed, flattened cells. Also called *muscle segment*.   **2** All of the voluntary or striated muscles that are supplied by neurons within a single segment of the spinal cord.   **3** A surgical instrument for performing myotomy; a knife.

myotomy [MYO- + -TOMY]   An incision into muscle tissue.

cricopharyngeal myotomy   The surgical division of the fibers of the cricopharyngeal muscle, indicated in three unrelated conditions: (1) for the symptomatic relief of dysphagia in certain pharyngeal palsies, (2) as a step towards preventing recurrence after the excision of hypopharyngeal diverticula, and (3) to assist voice production in certain cases after laryngectomy.

myotone   Muscular tone; tonus.

myotonia [MYO- + Gk *ton(os)* tension, stretching, tightening + -IA]   A phenomenon characterized by an apparent delay in relaxation after a muscular contraction, accompanied by an electrical afterdischarge in the electromyogram after voluntary innervation ceases. The condition is due to an abnormality of the muscular fiber membrane, and the diagnosis can be confirmed by the occurrence of typical spontaneous discharges in the electromyogram. When an affected patient grasps an object there is difficulty in letting go, and the fingers uncurl slowly. A brisk tap upon a muscle belly evokes either a contraction of the whole muscle, if small, followed by slow relaxation, or else formation of a dimple, which slowly disappears (mechanical myotonia). This phenomenon is seen in three dominantly inherited disorders, myotonia congenita, paramyotonia congenita, and dystrophia myotonica. Also called *myotony*. Adjective: myotonic.

myotonia acquisita   Acquired, as distinct from congenital, myotonia. Most patients formerly so described were probably suffering from dystrophia myotonica, some possibly from pseu-

domyotonia due to hypothyroidism. An obsolete term. Also called *Talma's disease*.

myotonia atrophica   DYSTROPHIA MYOTONICA.

chondrodystrophic myotonia   A rare disorder of infancy characterized by generalized myotonia, dwarfism, a typical appearance of the face with puckered lips and narrow palpebral fissures, as well as widespread skeletal abnormalities. Also called *Schwartz-Jampel syndrome*.

myotonia congenita   A dominantly inherited myotonia that is generalized throughout the skeletal muscles from birth, often causing difficulty in feeding and a "strangled" cry. The myotonia is temporarily relieved by exercise and worsened by cold. A gradual improvement takes place as the subject ages, widespread muscular hypertrophy is common, and dystrophic features do not develop. Also called *Thomsen's disease, congenital myotonia, myotonia hereditaria*.

myotonia congenita intermittens   PARAMYOTONIA CONGENITA.

congenital myotonia   MYOTONIA CONGENITA.

myotonia dystrophica   DYSTROPHIA MYOTONICA.

myotonia hereditaria   MYOTONIA CONGENITA.

mechanical myotonia   A myotonic aftercontraction or myotonic activity in the electromyogram evoked by tapping a muscle.

myotonia neonatorum   TETANISM.

myotonia paradoxa   Myotonia which appears to be worsened rather than relieved by repeated contraction of the affected muscle.

myotonic   **1** Characterized by or pertaining to myotonia.   **2** Pertaining to muscle tone. Seldom used in this sense.

myotonoid   Resembling myotonia.

myotonometer   Any apparatus capable of gauging the degree of muscle tone. A seldom used term.

myotonus   MUSCLE SPASM.

myotony   MYOTONIA.

myotrophic   **1** Concerning the stimulation of muscle growth.   **2** Of or relating to myotrophy.

myotrophy [MYO- + TROPH- + -Y]   The nutrition of muscle.

myotropic   Directed toward or acting upon a muscle.

myotube   A developing skeletal muscle cell in which the centrally positioned nuclei cause the sarcoplasm to assume a tubular appearance. Also called *myotubule*.

myotubule   MYOTUBE.

myovascular   **1** Of or relating to the heart and its blood vessels.   **2** Pertaining to the anatomical unit that consists of a muscle and its blood supply.

myria- [Gk *myrios* countless, huge in size, endless in time; pl. *myrioi* as substantive, ten thousand]   A combining form denoting 10^4, 10 000. An obsolete form. Symbol: ma

myriachit [Russian, from Gk *myrios* countless]   A form of bizarre repetitive and widespread habit spasm affecting many members of a community, often in an imitative way. It has been described in Java, Borneo, and in parts of Russia. Also *miryachit*.

myriameter [MYRIA- + METER]   A unit of length equal to 10^4 meter. An obsolete unit. Symbol: mam

Myriangiales [*myri(a)* + ANGI- + L *-ales*, pl. of *-alis* -AL]   An order of ascomycetous fungi which are mainly plant parasites but also include some that utilize insects and human hair, in the latter case resulting in piedra.

myriapod [MYRIA- + -POD]   Any of a large assortment of terrestrial mandibulate arthropods having a body consisting of a head and an elongate trunk with many leg-bearing segments, and including millipedes, (Diplopoda), centipedes (Chilopoda), pauropods (Pauropoda), and symphylans (Symphyla). These classes were formerly grouped into a superclass Myriapoda, but the alliance of these groups is now considered an artificial one.

myrica The dried root bark of *Myrica cerifera*, bayberry or wax myrtle. It was once used as an emetic, an astringent, and a tonic. Also called *wax myrtle bark*.

myricin 1 $C_{30}H_{61} \cdot C_{16}H_{31}O_2$. Myricyl palmitate. A substance extracted from beeswax by crystallization. 2 A medicinal agent prepared by concentration of the principle of the dried bark of the root *Myrica cerifera*. It was formerly used as an emetic and astringent and in the treatment of indolent ulcers.

myricyl The group $C_{31}H_{63}$, systematically hentricontyl. Myricyl alcohol occurs as its esters in plant waxes.

myring- MYRINGO-.

myringa [New L (alteration of Med. L *miringa* membrane, alteration of Late L *mininga*, also *meninga* membrane, from Gk *mēninx*, gen. *mēningos*, membrane] MEMBRANA TYMPANI.

myringectomy [MYRING- + -ECTOMY] Excision of the tympanic membrane, unlikely to be performed except as a step in radical mastoidectomy. A seldom used term. Also called *myringodectomy*.

myringitis [MYRING- + -ITIS] Inflammation of the tympanic membrane. • The tympanic membrane, serving as the wall separating the external ear from the middle ear, will usually share in inflammatory processes affecting either compartment. However, it is unusual to describe the inflamed membrane typical, for example, of acute suppurative otitis media as an example of myringitis.

myringitis bullosa BULLOUS MYRINGITIS HEMORRHAGICA.
myringitis bullosa hemorrhagica Otitis externa hemorrhagica in which the bullae are confined to the surface of the tympanic membrane. Also called *bullous myringitis, myringitis bullosa*.
bullous myringitis MYRINGITIS BULLOSA HEMORRHAGICA.

myringo- [New L *myringa* tympanic membrane, from late L *meninga* membrane, from Gk *mēninx* (genitive *mēningos*) membrane] A combining form denoting the membrana tympani. Also *myring-*.

myringodectomy MYRINGECTOMY.

myringodermatitis Otitis externa when confined chiefly to the deep meatus and the tympanic membrane. A rarely used term.

myringomycosis A variety of otomycosis in which the fungus, often a saprophyte, is confined to the tympanic membrane. Also called *mycomyringitis*.
myringomycosis aspergillina Myringomycosis caused by one of a number of fungi of the genus *Aspergillus*, especially *A. niger*.

myringoplasty [MYRINGO- + -PLASTY] The surgical repair of a perforated tympanic membrane. It may be performed as part of a tympanoplasty. Adjective: myringoplastic.
inlay myringoplasty A variation of underlay myringoplasty.
onlay myringoplasty A technique of myringoplasty in which a fascial graft is applied to the outer surface of the tympanic membrane after the surface epithelium has been removed.
underlay myringoplasty A method of performing myringoplasty in which a fascial graft is applied to the inner aspect of the perforated tympanic membrane.

myringorupture A rarely used term for RUPTURE OF THE TYMPANIC MEMBRANE.

myringostapediopexy A variety of tympanoplasty in which the tympanic membrane, or the graft needed to repair it, is applied directly to the stapes, because the incus has been destroyed or so damaged by disease that its removal is unavoidable.

myringotome [MYRINGO- + -TOME] The fine lancet used for myringotomy.

myringotomy [MYRINGO- + -TOMY] Incision of the tympanic

membrane. Before the advent of chemotherapy and antibiotics, it was the obligatory treatment for acute suppurative otitis media with a bulging drumhead. At present, it is frequently employed to treat cases, usually in children, of secretory otitis media. In most instances it is performed in order to insert ventilation tubes. Also called *paracentesis tympani, auripuncture* (obsolete), *tympanotomy*.

myrinx [See MYRINGA.] MEMBRANA TYMPANI.

myristica The dried, ripe seed of *Myristica fragrans* that has been deprived of its seed coat and aril, with or without a coating of lime. It is used in pharmaceutical preparations and as a condiment and carminative. Myristica oil (nutmeg oil) is obtained by distilling the seed, and it is used as a flavoring and carminative. Also called *nutmeg, nux moschata*.

myristic acid $CH_3-[CH_2]_{12}-COOH$. Tetradecanoic acid, a natural fatty acid.

myristicene $C_{10}H_{14}$. A fragrant principle obtained from nutmeg oil.

myristicin A toxic, crystalline, safrole derivative present in star anise, parsley seed oil, and nutmeg oil. When ingested in large quantities, it can cause convulsions, hallucinations, tachycardia, and possibly death.

myristoleic acid *cis*-Tetradec-9-enoic acid. The homologue of oleic acid, four carbon atoms shorter, and with the double bond at the same distance from the carboxyl group.

myristyl alcohol $CH_3-[CH_2]_{12}-CH_2OH$. Tetradecan-1-ol. A fatty alcohol present as esters in waxes.

myrmalgia [Gk *myrm(ēx)* the ant + -ALGIA] Painful pins and needles. A seldom used term.

myrmecology [Gk *myrmēx*, gen. *myrmēkos*, an ant + *o* + -LOGY] The study of ants.

myronic acid A thioglucoside, present, as its salt, in black mustard seeds and having the structure GLc—S—C(—O—SO₃H)=N—CH₂—CH=CH₂. It is hydrolyzed under the action of thioglucosidase to form glucose, sulfate, and allyl isothiocyanate, $CH_2=CH-CH_2-N=C=S$.

myrosin An outmoded term for THIOGLUCOSIDASE.

myrosinase An outmoded term for THIOGLUCOSIDASE.

myrrh [Middle English *mirre*, from Old English *myrre*, from L *myrrha*, also *murrha*, from Gk *myrrha* the balsamic juice of the Arabian myrtle, from Arabic *murr* myrrh, bitter] A gum resin obtained from cuts made in the bark of trees of the genus *Commiphora*, especially *C. myrrha*, the common myrrh tree. It is widely used in incense, perfume, salves, medicines, disinfectants, and embalming mixtures and has carminative, tonic, and astringent properties. It has been compounded in mouthwashes and also used as a local stimulant to the mucous membranes.

myrrholin A mixture of myrrh and fat, combined in equal parts. It is employed as a vehicle for administering creosote.

myrtenol $C_{10}H_{16}O$. A terpene alcohol found in plant oils. It is related to α-pinene by replacement of CH_3 by CH_2OH.

Myrtus A genus of tropical and subtropical shrubs or rarely trees in the Myrtaceae family. The leaves of *M. communis*, common myrtle, have antiseptic and astringent properties.

Mysoline A proprietary name for primidone.

mysophilia [Gk *myso(s)* filth, defilement + -PHILIA] A paraphilia in which dirt or filth is essential for sexual arousal. It is often associated with coprophilia and urophilia.

mysophobia [Gk *myso(s)* filth, defilement + -PHOBIA] Pathologic fear of dirt, uncleanliness, or contamination, often manifested as compulsive handwashing.

Mytelase A proprietary name for ambenonium chloride.

mythomania PATHOLOGIC LYING.

mythophobia Pathologic fear of stories or myths, sometimes expressed as an inability to believe anything one is told.

mytilocongestin A toxin from mussels of the species *Mytilus edulis*, which causes congestion and hemorrhage when injected into the viscera of laboratory animals.

mytilotoxin SAXITOXIN.

mytilotoxism [Gk *mytilo(s)* + TOX- + -ISM] Poisoning from ingestion of mussels contaminated with mytilotoxin.

myx- MYXO-.

myxadenitis Inflammation of mucous glands.

myxadenitis labialis CHEILITIS GLANDULARIS.

myxadenoma [MYX- + ADENOMA] A tumor of mucous gland cells. An obsolete term. Also called *myxoadenoma*.

myxameba An ameboid cell of a slime mold.

myxasthenia [MYX- + ASTHENIA] Diminished secretion of mucus with consequent drying of the affected mucosa.

myxedema [MYX- + EDEMA] The condition that accompanies severe hypothyroidism characterized by yellowish pallor and nonpitting edema, especially obvious in the face, with scanty hair in the eyebrows, periorbital puffiness, and thick lips. The tongue is large, movements are sluggish, and the voice is hoarse. Anemia is usually present, and the heart may be seriously affected. The mucoid deposits that constitute the edema and the clinical syndrome are both corrected by thyroid hormone. Also called *mucous edema* (outmoded), *solid edema* (rarely used). Adjective: myxedematous.

circumscribed myxedema Myxedema associated with the thyrotoxicosis of Graves disease and almost invariably accompanied by exophthalmos. The edematous lesions are localized, typically in the pretibial region, less often on the face or the dorsa of the feet or hands. The lesions appear as subcutaneous swellings, the overlying skin being shiny, violaceous, and resembling orange peel in texture.

circumscribed plane myxedema A rarely used term for PRETIBIAL MYXEDEMA.

congenital myxedema CRETINISM.

hypothalamic myxedema HYPOTHALAMIC HYPOTHYROIDISM.

infantile myxedema Myxedema resulting from hypothyroidism in an infant. A seldom used term. Also called *Brissaud's infantilism* (outmoded), *Brissaud's dwarfism* (outmoded).

internal myxedema ESCAMILLA-LISSER SYNDROME.

juvenile myxedema Hypothyroidism in a child or adolescent. The thyroid deficiency is usually of mild degree. The effects develop insidiously and are characterized by marked stunting of growth, a sallow complexion, supraclavicular pads of fat, potbelly, placidity, and often little or no impairment of intelligence. The condition is rare in countries with adequate diagnostic services.

nodular myxedema TUBEROUS MYXEDEMA.

operative myxedema POSTOPERATIVE MYXEDEMA.

papular myxedema LICHEN MYXEDEMATOSUS.

pituitary myxedema Myxedema associated with thyroprivic hypothyroidism.

postoperative myxedema Myxedema resulting from removal of all or part of the thyroid gland and the consequent loss of thyroid function. Also called *surgical myxedema, operative myxedema*.

pretibial myxedema Circumscribed myxedema occurring in the pretibial region. Also called *circumscribed plane myxedema* (rarely used). See under CIRCUMSCRIBED MYXEDEMA.

surgical myxedema POSTOPERATIVE MYXEDEMA.

tertiary myxedema HYPOTHALAMIC HYPOTHYROIDISM.

tuberous myxedema A nodular form of circumscribed myxedema. The mucin-containing nodules are about the size of a bean or a pea. They may be isolated or in bunches and occur in reddish or waxy plaques, especially on hairy skin, in the pre-

patellar region, the forearm, or in the intergluteal crease. Also called *nodular myxedema*.

myxedematoid Resembling or simulating myxedema.

myxedematous Of, relating to, or characterized by myxedema.

myxemia MUCINEMIA.

myxidiocy [*myx(edema)* + IDIOCY] Myxedema associated with defective mental development, as in cretinism. A seldom used term. Also called *myxidiotie* (seldom used).

myxidiotie A seldom used term for MYXIDIOCY.

myxiosis [MYX- + *i* + -OSIS] Mucus discharge. A rarely used term.

myxo- [Gk *myxa* discharge from the nose, mucus, phlegm] A combining form meaning mucus or slime. Also *myx-*.

myxoadenoma MYXADENOMA.

myxobacteria (*singular* myxobacterium) Rod-shaped bacteria found in soil and decomposing vegetation, embedded in a slime layer and capable of a gliding movement. They can aggregate to form a large fruiting body, in which the cells become resting myxospores.

myxoblastoma 1 MYXOMA. 2 MYXOSARCOMA.

Myxobolus [MYXO- + Gk *bōlos* a clod, lump, mass] A genus of myxozoan protozoa (class Myxosporea) that are parasites of fish. *M. cyprini* is the cause of carp pox. *M. pfeifferi* causes boil disease in barbels.

myxochondrofibrosarcoma [MYXO- + CHONDRO- + FIBROSARCOMA] A sarcoma with myxoid, chondroid, and fibrous components.

myxochondroma [MYXO- + CHONDROMA] A benign tumor with myxoid and chondroid components.

myxochondrosarcoma [MXYO- + CHONDRO- + SARCOMA] A sarcoma with myxoid and chondroid components.

myxocylindroma CYLINDROMA.

myxocystitis [MYXO- + CYSTITIS] Inflammation of the mucous membrane of the urinary bladder.

myxocystoma MUCINOUS CYSTADENOMA.

myxocyte [MYXO- + -CYTE] An angulated or stellate connective tissue cell that is responsible for the production of myxoid connective tissue.

myxoenchondroma [MYXO- + ENCHONDROMA] A chondroma with myxoid areas.

myxoendothelioma [MYX- + ENDOTHELIOMA] An endothelioma containing myxomatous tissue.

myxofibrochondrosarcoma [MYXO- + FIBRO- + CHONDROSARCOMA] A variety of chondrosarcoma containing myxoid, fibrous, and cartilaginous components. A rarely used term.

myxofibroma FIBROMYXOMA.

myxofibrosarcoma [MYXO- + FIBROSARCOMA] A fibrosarcoma containing myxomatous areas.

myxoglioma [MYXO- + GLIOMA] A glioma with myxoid areas.

myxoid [MYX- + -OID] Having the consistency and appearance of mucus: used especially of a connective tissue with a high content of mucoproteins and mucopolysaccharides. Also *mucofibrous*.

myxoinoma [MYXO- + Gk *is*, gen. *inos*, a sinew, nerve, fiber, muscle + -OMA] FIBROMYXOMA.

myxolipofibrosarcoma [MYXO- + LIPO- + FIBROSARCOMA] MYXOID LIPOSARCOMA.

myxolipoma A lipoma with myxoid components. This must be distinguished from a well-differentiated myxoid liposarcoma. Also called *fibromyxolipoma, lipomyxoma, lipoma myxomatodes, lipomatous myxoma*.

myxoliposarcoma [MYXO- + LIPOSARCOMA] MYXOID LI-POSARCOMA.

myxoma [MYX- + -OMA] A benign but often infiltrating growth of unknown histogenesis, characterized by rather small, inconspicuous, round, spindle, or stellate cells within a matrix containing abundant mucoid material, chiefly hyaluronic acid, a loose meshwork of reticulin and collagen fibrils, and scant vascularity. The large muscles of the shoulder and thigh are the most common sites. Except in the jaws true myxomas of bone rarely occur. Also called *myxoblastoma, myxoma gelatinosum, gelatinous tumor.*

atrial myxoma A soft gelatinous mobile tumor, more often found in the left then the right atrium of the heart, usually tethered by a narrow stalk to the interatrial septum. The symptoms and signs often mimic those of mitral stenosis, but vary more from time to time.

myxoma cavernosum CYSTIC MYXOMA.

cystic myxoma A myxoma containing cysts. Also called *myxoma cavernosum.*

enchondromatous myxoma A myxoma containing cartilage.

erectile myxoma TELANGIECTATIC MYXOMA.

myxoma fibrosum FIBROMYXOMA.

myxoma gelatinosum MYXOMA.

giant mammary myxoma CYSTOSARCOMA PHYLLODES.

myxoma of the heart A benign gelatinous tumor of the heart occurring especially in the cavity of the left atrium, and derived from primitive mucoid connective tissue (mesenchyme) with scanty polyhedral cells. See also ATRIAL MYXOMA.

intracanalicular myxoma INTRACANALICULAR FIBROADENOMA.

lipomatous myxoma MYXOLIPOMA.

odontogenic myxoma A myxoma of odontogenic type.

myxoma sarcomatosum MYXOSARCOMA.

telangiectatic myxoma A myxoma containing numerous blood vessels. Also called *erectile myxoma, vascular myxoma.*

vascular myxoma TELANGIECTATIC MYXOMA.

myxomatosis [*myxomat(a)*, pl. of MYXOMA + -OSIS] **1** The presence of multiple myxomas. **2** A disease in domestic rabbits caused by a poxvirus transmitted by certain mosquitoes and biting flies and by direct contact. It can result in high mortality. The virus has been used to control wild rabbits in Australia. Conjunctivitis, fever, swelling of the head and subcutaneous nodules (myxomas) are common signs of the infection. See also MYXOMA VIRUS.

myxomatous Pertaining to myxoma.

Myxomycetes [MYXO- + -MYCETES] A class of fungi forming one group of slime molds.

myxomyoma [MYXO- + MYOMA] A leiomyoma with myxomatous areas.

myxoneuroma [MYXO- + NEUROMA] A neuroma with a myxomatous component.

myxoneurosis [MYXO- + NEUROSIS] Conversion hysteria marked by mucous discharge from the respiratory or intestinal mucosas. An older term.

myxopapilloma [MYXO- + PAPILLOMA] **1** A papilloma with myxomatous stroma. **2** A papilloma with mucinous epithelium.

myxopoiesis MUCOPOIESIS.

myxorrhea [MYXO- + -RRHEA] Mucinous discharge. A seldom used term.

gastric myxorrhea Excessive production of mucus by the stomach; gastromyxorrhea.

intestinal myxorrhea The increased secretion of mucus by the intestine. Also called *myxorrhea intestinalis.*

myxorrhea intestinalis INTESTINAL MYXORRHEA.

myxosarcoma [MYXO- + SARCOMA] The malignant counterpart of a myxoma. Most so-called myxosarcomas are probably myxoid liposarcomas. Also called *myxoblastoma, myxoma sarcomatosum, sarcoma myxomatodes.* Adjective: myxosarcomatous.

Myxospora [MYXO- + Gk *spora* a sowing, seed] A subphylum of protozoa characterized by myxospores. Because of the multicellular origin of the myxospores, many protozoologists do not consider these organisms to be true protozoans, but place them in a distinct phylum, Myxozoa, and class, Myxosporea. The spore membrane of the myxospore has from two to six valves, the number of valves serving to distinguish the orders Bivalvulida and Multivalvulida. Common genera include *Leptotheca, Ceratomyxa, Myxidium, Hanneguya, Myxobolus,* and *Myxosoma. Myxosoma squamalis* is a parasite of trout and salmon, and *M. cerebralis,* which causes the whirling disease of salmonids, is a particularly destructive parasite of young brook and rainbow trout in hatcheries.

myxosporangium [MYXO- + SPORANGIUM] The sporangium of myxomycetes.

myxospore A resting cell of a myxobacterium.

Myxosporidia [MYXO- + New L *sporidium* a small spore] An order of protozoan, spore-bearing parasites that infect lower vertebrates such as fish, reptiles, and amphibians. More recent classifications place this group in the order Bivalvulida, class Myxosporea, plylum Myxozoa.

myxovirus [MYXO- + VIRUS] **1** ORTHOMYXOVIRUS. **2** Any virus of the Orthomyxoviridae or Paramyxoviridae families.

Myxozoa [MYXO- + Gk *zōa,* pl. of *zōon* a living being, animal] See under MYXOSPORA.

Myzomyia A subgenus of *Anopheles* including species that transmit malaria.

Myzorhynchus A subgenus of *Anopheles* including species that transmit malaria.

Myzostoma [New L (from Gk *myz(ein)* to suck in + *o* + Gk *stoma* mouth)] A genus of polychaete worms in the family Myzostomidae; myzostomes. These worms are closely associated with echinoderms, either commensally or as a parasite.

N

N **1** Symbol for the unit, newton. **2** Symbol for the element, nitrogen. **3** Symbol for the unit, neper. **4** Symbol for normal. **5** Symbol for asparagine. **6** Symbol for radiance.

n **1** Symbol for nano-: used with SI units. **2** Symbol for normal. **3** refractive index.

n_D refractive index.

N Symbol for the quantities (1) Avogadro's constant or number; (2) loudness; (3) neutron number; (4) number of molecules or particles.

N_A Symbol for Avogadro's constant.

n Symbol for the quantities (1) amount of substance, expressed in moles; (2) neutron number density, expressed in reciprocal cubic meters; (3) refractive index; (4) rotational frequency, expressed in reciprocal seconds or revolutions per minute.

n- normal; used in organic chemistry.

ν **1** Symbol for the quantity, frequency, expressed in hertz. **2** Symbol for the quantity, kinematic velocity, expressed in meters squared per second.

NA **1** Nomina Anatomica. **2** numerical aperture.

Na Symbol for sodium.

nA Symbol for the unit, nanoampere.

Naboth [Martin *Naboth*, German anatomist and physician, 1675–1721] Naboth's ovules, Naboth's vesicles, nabothian glands, ovula nabothi, nabothian follicles, vesiculae nabothi. See under NABOTHIAN CYSTS.

Nacton A proprietary name for poldine methylsulfate.

NAD **1** Symbol for nicotinamide adenine dinucleotide. **2** no appreciable disease, nothing abnormal detected.

NADH Symbol for the reduced form of nicotinamide adenine dinucleotide.

nadide NICOTINAMIDE ADENINE DINUCLEOTIDE.

NAD kinase An enzyme (EC 2.7.1.23) which catalyzes the transfer of a phosphate in the following reaction: $ATP + NAD^+ \rightleftharpoons ADP + NADP^+$.

NADP Symbol for nicotinamide adenine dinucleotide phosphate. It usually represents both oxidized and reduced forms of the compound, which are distinguished by the symbols $NADP^+$ and NADPH, respectively. Occasionally, however, it is used for the oxidized form, with the reduced form being represented as $NADPH_2$.

NADPH Symbol for the reduced form of NADP.

NADPH diaphorase METHEMOGLOBIN REDUCTASE.

Naegeli [Karl *Naegeli*, Swiss organic chemist, 1895–1942] Naegeli test. See under SCRATCH-PATCH TEST.

Naegeli [Oskar *Naegeli*, Swiss dermatologist, 1885–1959] See under SYNDROME.

Naegeli [Otto *Naegeli*, Swiss hematologist, 1871–1938] **1** See under LAW. **2** Naegeli leukemia. See under NAEGELI TYPE ACUTE MYELOMONOCYTIC LEUKEMIA. **3** Macroblast of Naegeli. See under PRONORMOBLAST.

Naegleria A genus of free-living amebas having both an ameboid and a flagellate stage. They are found primarily in stagnant waters, and as coprozoites in feces. Also called *Dimastigamoeba*.

Naegleria fowleri A species of ameba that has been isolated and cultured from cerebrospinal fluid and brain tissue suspensions of patients who died of an acute meningoencephalitis. Infection has been associated with swimming in stagnant, warm freshwater lakes or ponds, with entry of amebas via the olfactory mucosa and cribriform plate. It now appears that exposure is frequent but penetration leading to the disease is extremely rare.

naevus A British spelling for NEVUS.

nafcillin sodium $C_{21}H_{21}N_2NaO_5S\cdot H_2O$. Sodium 6-(2-ethoxy-1-naphthamido)penicillanate monohydrate. A penicillin with antimicrobial activity like that of cloxacillin. It is used intramuscularly to treat severe infections by organisms resistant to benzylpenicillin, or orally for less serious infections.

Naffziger [Howard Christian *Naffziger*, U.S. surgeon, 1884–1961] **1** See under DECOMPRESSION, OPERATION, TEST. **2** Naffziger syndrome. See under SCALENUS ANTERIOR SYNDROME.

nagana [Zulu (a Bantu language) *u-nakane*] Trypanosomiasis affecting animals, usually domestic mammals, and transmitted by tsetse flies (*Glossina* spp.). It commonly takes a rapidly fatal course and effectively eliminates the raising of cattle and certain other animals in the tsetse belt of Africa. The main pathogens are *Typanosoma brucei*, *T. congolense*, *T. vivax*, *T. uniforme*, *T. simiae*, and *T. suis*. Also called *n'gana*.

nagarse [Originally a trade name] SUBTILISIN.

Nagel [Willibald *Nagel*, German physiologist, 1870–1911] See under TEST.

Nägele [Franz Karl *Nägele*, German obstetrician, 1777–1851] **1** Nägele's obliquity. See under ANTERIOR ASYNCLITISM. **2** See under RULE, PELVIS.

Nageotte [Jean *Nageotte*, French histologist, 1866–1948] Babinski-Nageotte syndrome. See under SYNDROME.

Nagler [F. P. O. *Nagler*, Australian bacteriologist, flourished 20th century] See under REACTION.

naiad [Gk *naïas*, gen. *naïados* (from *nan* to flow) a river nymph, water nymph] The nymphal stage of development of certain aquatic insects such as dragonflies, stoneflies, and mayflies. Also called *nyad*.

nail [Old English *nægl*, *nægel*] **1** A rigid, wirelike piece of metal or other substance often with a pointed end that can be driven into bone fragments to fix them in place. **2** A horny keratin structure that covers the dorsal aspect of the terminal phalanx of each digit; unguis.

cloverleaf nail An orthopedic device, shaped like a cloverleaf when viewed in cross-section, that is used for internal fixation of fractures.

eggshell nail A thin nail that assumes a semitransparent, bluish white hue resembling the color of an egg. It is sometimes seen in vitamin A deficiencies.

nail en raquette A congenital abnormality of the thumb, inherited as an autosomal dominant trait, that is characterized by one or both distal phalanges and their nails being shorter and wider than normal. The lateral curvature of the nail is lost, so that the nail resembles a tennis racket. It is more common among women.

fracture nail A rod of metal or other rigid material that is used to provide internal fixation to one or more fracture fragments.

hippocratic nail A loss of the normal angle between the nail and the posterior nail fold that is characteristic of hippocratic fingers.

ingrowing nail A painful inflammation of the perionychial area that is caused by the overlapping of the nail by adjacent tissues, producing granulation and ulceration. It usually affects the great toe. Also called *incarnatio, incarnatio unguis, ingrown nail, acronyx, unguis incarnatus, unguis aduncus, onyxis.*

ingrown nail INGROWING NAIL.

Jewett nail A rod of metal and attached plate that are used to provide internal fixation for an intratrochanteric femoral fracture.

Küntscher nail A long, metal, hollow nail, trefoil-shaped in cross section, that is passed down the medullary cavity of a large long bone such as a femur.

Neufeld nail A rod of metal with plate attached at an angle of 130°. It provides internal fixation of an intratrochanteric femoral fracture.

parrot-beak nail The symmetrical overcurvature of the free margin of the fingernails, simulating the beak of a parrot.

pitted nails Nails marked by small depressions in the surface of the nail plate. The condition is seen in psoriasis and alopecia areata. Occasionally, pits are seen in normal nails.

racket nail A congenitally broad, short thumbnail.

ram's-horn nail A nail that displays the thickening and curvature of onychogryposis.

reedy nail A nail that is marked by longitudinal ridges.

Smith-Petersen nail A rigid rod with a large flange that is used to provide internal fixation in fractures of the neck of the femur.

spoon nail KOILONYCHIA.

Thornton nail A metallic orthopedic nail used to provide internal fixation of intertrochanteric femoral fractures.

turtle-back nail A nail marked by a curvature in all directions to produce a humplike appearance. A rarely used term.

nailing The internal fixation of fractured bone by insertion of a rigid rodlike device to stabilize the fragments.

intramedullary nailing A surgical procedure in which a rigid nail or rod is placed in the marrow cavity of a fractured bone in order to provide internal fixation following an open reduction. Also called *marrow nailing, medullary nailing.*

marrow nailing INTRAMEDULLARY NAILING.

medullary nailing INTRAMEDULLARY NAILING.

Naja A genus of venomous snakes of the Elapidae family; the cobras. The venom is neurotoxic and the teeth are proteroglyphic. Six species are distributed in Africa and Asia.

Najjar [Victor Assad *Najjar*, Lebanese-born U.S. pediatrician, born 1914] Crigler-Najjar disease. See under SYNDROME.

naked [Old English *nacod*, akin to Old High German *nackot*, L *nudus*, Gk *gymnos*, all meaning naked, unclad] Without a lipid envelope: said of certain viruses.

nalidixic acid $C_{12}H_{12}N_2O_3$. 1-Ethyl-1,4-dihydro-7-methyl-4-oxo-1,8-naphthyridine-3-carboxylic acid. An antibiotic with antibacterial activity against Gram-negative bacteria. It is used orally against urinary-tract infections caused by susceptible microorganisms such as *Proteus* strains, *Klebsiella, Enterobacter,* and *Escherichia coli.*

Nalline A proprietary name for nalorphine.

nalorphine hydrochloride $C_{19}H_{21}NO_3 \cdot HCl$. *N*-Allylnormorphine hydrochloride. A narcotic antagonist given intravenously to reverse the respiratory depression produced by narcotics, such as morphine, methadone, and meperidine. Also called *allorphine hydrochloride.*

naloxone hydrochloride $C_{19}H_{21}NO_4 \cdot HCl$. 17-Allyl-4,5-epoxy-3,14-dihydroxymorphinan-6-one hydrochloride. The prototype narcotic antagonist. It is structurally related to morphine, and is used parenterally as an antidote to narcotic overdosage, or for an overdose of pentazocine.

name / brand name A recognized, sometimes trademarked, name for a product such as a drug.

nonproprietary name A shortened, commonly used name of a chemical or drug, which is not protected by trademark rights. It is not identical to the generic name of a drug.

official name A name for a product or item that is authorized or approved by a governmental or other recognized authority.

scientific name The name of an organism which includes the generic name and the specific epithet. The first letter of the generic name is capitalized; the species name is in lower-case letters. Both names are italicized. A subspecies name may also be included. See also BINOMIAL NOMENCLATURE.

semisystematic name The name of a chemical which is partly a systematic designation and partly a trivial name. For example, *benzoylcholine* includes the systematic *benzoyl* for C_6H_5CO, and the trivial *choline* for (2-hydroxyethyl)trimethylammonium. Many generic and nonproprietary drug names are semisystematic but are said to be trivial names even if not entirely so. Also called *semitrivial name.*

semitrivial name SEMISYSTEMATIC NAME.

special name A name for an SI derived unit, usually eponymous, such as *newton,* that can be used to form other derived units. See under SI DERIVED UNIT.

systematic name The name for a chemical based upon the structure and substituents present so that the chemical structure can be deduced from the name using specific, conventional rules.

trivial name A chemical name that gives no systematic indication of the structural components present in the molecule. Examples are *aspirin, insulin*, and *quinine*. Many chemical names are said to be trivial that are in fact partly trivial, or semitrivial, because a portion of the name does indicate something of its chemical structure, e.g., methylglycine. Frequently, a portion of the name indicates some important systemic feature of the chemical structure of the compound. The assignment of trivial names is often arbitrary, and usually rather short, for convenience.

vernacular name Any name, other than the official taxonomic designation, that is used to identify an organism.

naming An association disorder seen in schizophrenia in which the subject's only response and contact with the outside world consists of naming and touching objects, or stating the action he is performing, such as saying "now he is standing up.".

nandrolone decanoate $C_{28}H_{44}O_3$. 17β-[(1-Oxodecyl)oxy]-estr-4-en-3-one, an ester with anabolic properties that is administered by intramuscular injection.

nanism [*nan(o)-* + *-ism*] DWARFISM.

Paltauf's nanism Small stature accompanying status lymphaticus, the supposed pathologic entity in which excessive growth of lymphatic tissue is associated with slow and defective somatic development.

renal nanism RENAL DWARFISM.

senile nanism PROGERIA.

symptomatic nanism Dwarfism associated with poor teeth and bone formation along with sexual underdevelopment.

Nannizzia The genus of the perfect (sexual) state of fungi of the genus *Microsporum,* a fungus previously known only in the imperfect state.

nano- [Gk *nanos* dwarf] **1** A combining form meaning dwarf, dwarfish. **2** A combining form denoting 10^{-9}, one billionth: used with SI units. Symbol: n

nanoampere [NANO- + AMPERE] A unit of electric current equal to 10^{-9} ampere. Symbol: nA

nanocephalia NANOCEPHALY.

nanocephalic Displaying nanocephaly. Also *nanocephalous.*

nanocephalous NANOCEPHALIC.

nanocephalus [NANO- + -CEPHALUS] An embryo, fetus, or postnatal individual with nanocephaly.

nanocephaly [NANO- + CEPHAL- + -Y] **1** Extreme smallness of the head, often accompanied by specific malformations of the face or cranium. Also called *nanocephalia.* **2** An inexact and outmoded term for SECKEL SYNDROME.

nanocormia [NANO- + Gk *korm(os)* trunk of a tree, log + -IA] An abnormal smallness of the trunk as compared with the head and limbs.

nanocormus [NANO- + Gk *kormos* the trunk of a tree with branches lopped off, a log] An individual exhibiting nanocormia.

nanocoulomb [NANO- + COULOMB] A unit of quantity of electricity, electric charge or electric flux equal to 10^{-9} coulomb. Symbol: nC

nanocurie [NANO- + CURIE] A unit of activity of a radionuclide or of a radioactive source equal to 10^{-9} curie; 37 becquerels exactly. Also called *millimicrocurie* (outmoded). Symbol: nCi

nanofarad [NANO- + FARAD] A unit of electric capacitance equal to 10^{-9} farad. Symbol: nF

nanogram [NANO- + GRAM] A unit of mass or weight equal to 10^{-9} gram. Also called *micromilligram* (outmoded), *millimicrogram* (outmoded). Symbol: ng

nanoid [*nan(o)-* + -OID] Possessing the characteristics of a dwarf.

nanokatal [NANO- + KATAL] A unit of catalytic activity equal to 10^{-9} katal; 10^{-9} mole per second. Symbol: nkat

nanoliter [NANO- + LITER] A unit of volume or capacity equal to 10^{-9} liter; 10^{-12} cubic meter; 10^{-6} cubic centimeter. Symbol: nl

nanomelia [NANO- + MEL-[1] + -IA] A disproportionate smallness of the limbs compared with the head and trunk.

nanomelous Displaying nanomelia.

nanomelus A fetus or postnatal individual with nanomelia.

nanometer [NANO- + METER] A unit of length equal to 10^{-9} meter. Also called *micromil* (obsolete), *micromillimeter* (obsolete), *millimicrometer* (obsolete), *millimicron* (obsolete), *millimu* (obsolete). Symbol: nm

　reciprocal nanometer A unit of wave number equal to $1/10^{-9}$ meter.

nanometre A British spelling for NANOMETER.

nanomole [NANO- + MOLE[3]] A unit of amount of substance equal to 10^{-9} mole. Symbol: nmol

nanophthalmia MICROPHTHALMIA.

nanophthalmos MICROPHTHALMIA.

nanophthalmus MICROPHTHALMIA.

Nanophyetus A genus of digenetic flukes of the family Nanophyetidae (formerly placed in the family Troglotrematidae) that parasitize fish-eating mammals, including man. It was formerly included in the genus *Troglotrema.*

Nanophyetus salmincola A species found along the northwestern coast of North America in dogs and other fish-eating mammals. It is important in the transmission of *Neorickettsia*

helminthoeca, the rickettsial agent of salmon poisoning, via infected metacercariae encysted in salmonid intermediate hosts. Also called *Troglotrema salmincola.*

nanoplankton Aquatic organisms, such as protozoa, bacteria, and fungi, that are less than 0.06 mm in size.

nanosecond [NANO- + SECOND] A unit of time equal to 10^{-9} second. Also called *millimicrosecond* (outmoded). Symbol: ns

nanosoma [NANO- + Gk *sōma* body] DWARFISM.

nanosome [NANO- + Gk *sōm(a)* body] DWARF.

nanosomia [NANO- + Gk *sōm(a)* body + -IA] DWARFISM.

nanosomus [NANO- + Gk *sōm(a)* body + New L -us, masc. sing. suffix] DWARF.

nanounit [NANO- + UNIT] A quantity equal to 10^{-9} unit. Symbol: nU

nanous [Gk *nan(os)* dwarf + -OUS] Dwarfish; undersized.

Nanta [A. *Nanta,* French physician, flourished early 20th century] Gandy-Nanta disease. See under SIDEROTIC SPLENOMEGALY.

nanukayami [Japanese *nanu-,* combining form denoting seven + *-ka,* combining form denoting day + *-yami,* combining form denoting illness] A form of leptospirosis of man caused by *Leptospira hebdomadis* and transmitted by the field vole. First reported in Japan, the disease is characterized by fever and jaundice. Also called *akiyami, autumn fever, gikiyami, seven-day fever, nanukayami fever, leptospirosis hebdomadis.*

nanus [Gk *nanos* dwarf] DWARF.

NAP nasion, point A, pogonion. (The three points forming the angle of convexity, used as a measure of prognathism).

nape [Middle English *knappe* a knob, akin to Old English *cnæp* top of a hill] NUCHA.

napelline $C_{22}H_{33}NO_3$. A racemic mixture of alkaloids derived from aconite and possessing analgesic properties.

napex [Prob. formed from nape, which originally may have referred to the external occipital protuberance] That part of the scalp just below the external occipital protuberance.

naphazoline hydrochloride $C_{14}H_{14}N_2HCl$. 4,5-Dihydro-2-(1-naphthalenyl methyl)-1*H*-imidazole monohydrochloride. A white, crystalline powder utilized as an adrenergic agent to produce vasoconstriction. It may be applied topically to the nasal or ocular surfaces.

naphtha [Gk *naphtha* (akin to Arabic *naft* naphtha and to Persian *neft* naphtha) naphtha] Any of the hydrocarbon fractions, usually derived from petroleum or coal tar, that boil between 70°C and 140°C.

naphthalene $C_{10}H_8$. The compound whose molecule consists of two benzene rings fused together. It is a white solid obtained from coal tar, and is used for chemical syntheses and, domestically, as moth balls.

　chlorinated naphthalene Any of the compounds of naphthalene in which the hydrogenations in the naphthalene are replaced by chlorine. Some of these compounds are waxes which have special insulating and water-resistant properties. Occupational exposure causes a severe form of pruritic acne, which itches, and toxic jaundice. Chlorinated naphthalenes are also used in combination with chlorinated diphenyls, which have similar toxic effects. Also called *perna, perchloronaphthalene.*

naphthaleneacetic acid $C_{12}H_{10}O_2$. A synthetic auxin used to induce the formation of adventitious roots in plant cuttings and to reduce fruit drop in commercial crops. Also called *naphthylacetic acid.*

naphthalic acid Naphthalene-1,8-dicarboxylic acid. This compound is somewhat similar in its properties to phthalic acid, because of the closeness of its two carboxyl groups.

naphthionic acid $NH_2C_{10}H_6SO_3H$. A compound obtained from the sulfonation of α-naphthylamine. It is used in the treatment of urinary infections and as a constituent of dyestuffs. Also called *naphthylaminosulfonic acid.*

naphthoic acid   Either of the two isomeric naphthalenecarboxylic acids.

naphthol   Either of the two isomeric phenols derived from naphthalene by substitution of a hydroxyl group for a hydrogen atom.

naphtholism [*naphthol* + -ISM]   Poisoning from acute or chronic exposure to excessive amounts of naphthol. Ingestion of large amounts may cause abdominal pain, vomiting, diarrhea, circulatory failure, convulsions, and death. External application may cause nephritis, hematuria, hemolytic anemia, jaundice, convulsions, and death.

α-naphthol phthalein   A dyestuff used as a pH indicator, changing from pinkish yellow at a pH of 7.3 to greenish blue at a pH of 8.7.

naphthol yellow   An acid synthetic dye that is used for specific staining of basic proteins.

naphthol yellow S   The sodium or potassium salt of flavianic acid, used in microspectrophotometry to localize basic proteins.

naphthoquinone   One of the two substances related to naphthalene by replacement of two of the CH groups in one of its rings by CO groups. These groups may be in the 1 and 2 or in the 1 and 4 positions. Substances with vitamin K activity are substituted naphtho-1,4-quinones, bearing a methyl group on C-2 and a polyisoprene side chain on C-3.

naphthyl   The group formed from naphthalene by removal of one hydrogen atom. It may be α or β, according to whether H-1 or H-2 is removed.

naphthylacetic acid   NAPHTHALENEACETIC ACID.

naphthylamine   One of two amines formed by replacing H-1 or H-2 of naphthalene with an amino group. When H-2 is so replaced, the compound, which may be designated β-naphthylamine, is carcinogenic.

naphthylaminosulfonic acid   NAPHTHIONIC ACID.

α-naphthylthiourea   A common rodenticide. It is poisonous for many other animals, particularly dogs. Abbreviation: ANTU

Napier [Lionel Everard *Napier*, English physician active in India, born 1888]   Napier serum test. See under FORMOL-GEL TEST.

naprapath   A practitioner of naprapathy.

naprapathy   A Bohemian folk medicine regimen using manipulation, diet, and massage.

naproxen $C_{14}H_{14}O_3$.   (+)-6-Methoxy-α-methyl-2-naphthaleneacetic acid. A white, crystalline powder employed as an anti-inflammatory, antipyretic agent, and as an analgesic. It can be given orally for the treatment of rheumatoid arthritis.

Naqua   A proprietary name for trichlormethiazide.

naranol hydrochloride $C_{18}H_{21}NO_2 \cdot HCl$.   8,9,10,11,11*a*,12-hexahydro-8,10-dimethyl-7*aH*-naphtho[1,2:5,6]pyrano-[3,2*c*]pyridin-7*a*-ol. It has been used clinically as a tranquilizer.

Narcan   A proprietary name for naloxone hydrochloride.

narceine $C_{23}H_{27}NO_8$. An isoquinoline alkaloid related to nicotine and isolated from *Papaver somniferum*, opium poppy, in extremely small amounts. Its properties are similar to those of papaverine.

narcism   NARCISSISM.

narcissine   LYCORINE.

narcissism [*narciss(us)* + -ISM. See NARCISSUS.]   **1** The stage in development of object relationships that follows the autoerotic or somatogenic stage. The child does not differentiate between self and nonself and believes he is omnipotent.   **2** As applied to the adult, hypercathexis of the self or self-love. Also called *autophilia, amor sui* (obsolete).   **3** Genital love of the self,

sometimes expressed as a need to watch oneself masturbating in front of a mirror. For defs. 1, 2, and 3 also called *narcism.*

disease narcissism   Hypercathexis of one or more parts of the self that are not affected by but do coexist with a disease or injury. A seldom used term.

primary narcissism   The most primitive type of object relationship, where all available libido is stored in the ego and has not yet been directed onto representations of objects external to oneself. An imprecise usage.

secondary narcissism   Narcissism in which the psychic force involved is directed toward the ego after having been attached to objects. Somatic overconcern that develops in association with diminution in object relationships is an example.

narcissistic   Relating to or manifesting narcissism. Also *egotropic.*

narco- [Gk *narkē* numbness, stupor]   A combining form meaning stupor, numbness, narcosis.

narcoanalysis   See under NARCOTHERAPY.

narcocatharsis   See under NARCOTHERAPY.

narcodiagnosis   See under NARCOTHERAPY.

narcohypnia [MARCO- + HYPN- + -IA]   SLEEP PARALYSIS.

narcohypnosis   See under NARCOTHERAPY.

narcolepsy   A disorder characterized by an irresistible tendency to fall asleep in circumstances which would be normally conducive to relaxation, as during a lecture or during the performance of a semiautomatic, monotonous task, such as driving a car. The sufferer can be aroused as from physiologic sleep, and the attacks may last for minutes or for hours. The etiology is unknown. The pattern of sleep in narcoleptic subjects is immediately of the paradoxical (REM) type. Most narcoleptic subjects also suffer from cataplexy, and some also experience sleep paralysis and hypnagogic hallucinations. Also called *Gélineau syndrome, sleeping disease, hypnolepsy, pyknolepsy, paroxysmal sleep, Friedmann's disease, sleep epilepsy* (incorrect), *narcoleptic epilepsy* (inaccurate and obsolete). Adjective: narcoleptic.

narcoleptic   Relating to narcolepsy.

narcoma [*narc(o)-* + -OMA]   Coma or stupor induced by hypnotic drugs.

narcomatous   Denoting, pertaining to, inducing, or affected by narcoma.

narcose [NARC(O)- + -*ose*, suffix denoting full of]   In a state of stupor. Also *narcous.*

narcosine   NOSCAPINE.

narcosis [Gk *narcōsis* (from *narkoun* to make numb or *narkan* to grow stiff or numb, from *narkē* stiffness, numbness + -*ōsis* -OSIS) an act of benumbing]   An alteration in consciousness, ranging from mere sleep to deep, unresponsive coma. It can be produced by sedatives, narcotics, anesthetics, or physical means.

basal narcosis   BASAL ANESTHESIA.

basis narcosis   BASAL ANESTHESIA.

carbon dioxide narcosis   Coma or stupor due to abnormally high levels of carbon dioxide in arterial blood.

insufflation narcosis   INSUFFLATION ANESTHESIA.

intravenous narcosis   INTRAVENOUS ANESTHESIA.

medullary narcosis   SPINAL ANESTHESIA.

nitrogen narcosis   Confusion, stupefaction, or unconsciousness resulting from breathing the nitrogen of atmospheric air at increased barometric pressures, as during depth diving.

prolonged narcosis   CONTINUOUS SLEEP TREATMENT.

narcospasm [NARCO- + SPASM]   Any spasmodic or recurrent disorder inducing stupor. An outmoded term.

narcostimulant   An agent with both narcotic and stimulant properties.

narcosynthesis   See under NARCOTHERAPY.

narcotherapy [NARCO- + THERAPY]   In psychotherapy, the

use of intravenous barbiturates to enhance relaxation, to facilitate communication, and to render the subject more responsive to the suggestions of the therapist. In any particular narcotherapeutic session, the focus may be on reassurance (narcohypnosis), on uncovering repressed material (narcoanalysis), on encouraging expression of repressed affects (narcocatharsis), on eliciting data for later assimilation (narcosynthesis), or on obtaining data to provide more adequate evaluation (narcodiagnosis). Also called *narcosis therapy.*

narcotic 1 Relating to or producing narcosis. 2 A sleep-producing or pain-relieving agent, commonly an opioid. Also called *drug.* • Because almost all known agents capable of relieving severe pain also tend to induce sleep, they are often called narcotics even when their primary purpose is relief from pain. Such drugs are usually addictive. See also the note at HYPNOTIC.

narcoticoirritant 1 Having both narcotic and irritant properties. 2 A narcoticoirritant drug or agent.

narcotine NOSCAPINE.

narcotize [*narcot(ic)* + -IZE] To subject to the effect of a narcotic agent to diminish consciousness, as in the administration of general anesthesia or sedation.

narcous NARCOSE.

nard The aromatic root of *Nardostachys jatamansi*. Its volatile oil, known as spikenard, is used as a deodorant, carminative, and stimulant for the skin. Also called *nardus root.*

Nardil A proprietary name for phenelzine dihydrogen sulfate.

nares [L, the nostrils] (*singular* naris) [NA] The rounded external openings of the nasus externus, on either side of the septal cartilage and bounded laterally by the alae. Also called *nostrils, prenares.*

naringin $C_{27}H_{32}O_{14}$. A bitter flavonoid present in grapefruit.

naris [L (usu. in pl. *nares*, gen. *narium*, nostrils), a nostril] Singular of NARES.

　anterior naris Either of the two external openings of the nasal cavity. Also called *external naris.*

　external naris ANTERIOR NARIS.

　internal naris An outmoded term for CHOANA.

　posterior naris CHOANA.

naristillae [L *nari(s)* a nostril + *stillae*, pl. of *stilla* a drop] An outmoded term for NOSE DROPS.

Narone A proprietary name for dipyrone.

narrowing / **aortic narrowing of esophagus** A normal constriction of the esophagus produced by the right side of the arch of the aorta at the level of the fourth thoracic vertebra. Also called *aortic indentation of esophagus.*

　bronchial narrowing of esophagus A normal constriction of the esophagus that is produced by the left principal bronchus crossing in front of it at the level of the fifth thoracic vertebra.

　cardiac narrowing of esophagus A ventral concavity of the esophagus due to its passage behind the left atrium of the heart.

　cricoid narrowing of esophagus A normal constriction of the commencement of the esophagus at the distal border of the cricoid cartilage opposite the sixth cervical vertebra.

　diaphragmatic narrowing of esophagus A normal constriction of the esophagus at the site of its passage through the diaphragm into the abdominal cavity and at the level of the tenth thoracic vertebra.

　iliac narrowing of ureter A normal narrowing of the lumen of the ureter at the level where it crosses the brim of the pelvis anterior to either the common or the external iliac vessels.

　sternal narrowing of esophagus An occasional impression on the esophagus stated to be produced by the incisura jugularis in obese subjects.

nasal [Late L *nasal(is)* (from L *nas(us)* nose + -alis -AL) per-

taining to the nose] Of or relating to the nose. Also *rhinal, nasalis.*

nasalis [Late L (from L *nas(us)* nose + -alis -AL), pertaining to the nose] NASAL.

nasality [NASAL + -ITY] The quality of speech associated with nasal emission.

nascent [L *nascens*, gen. *nascentis*, pres. part. of *nasci* to be born] 1 Being in the process of formation. 2 Having just been born.

nasiform Resembling a nose in appearance.

nasion [L *nas(us)* the nose + Gk -*ion*, dim. suffix] A craniometric point situated at the midpoint of the nasofrontal suture. Also called *nasal point.*

Nasmyth [Alexander *Nasmyth*, Scottish dentist and anatomist, died 1847] See under MEMBRANE.

naso- [L *nasus* nose, sense of smell] A combining form meaning nose, nasal.

nasoalveolar Pertaining to or joining nasion and prosthion.

nasoantral Pertaining to the nose and the maxillary sinus. Also *nasomaxillary.*

nasoantritis [NASO- + *antr(o)*- + -ITIS] Rhinitis complicated by maxillary sinusitis.

nasobronchial Pertaining to the nasal cavity and the bronchi.

nasobuccal Pertaining to the nose and the cheek.

nasobuccopharyngeal Pertaining to the nose, cheek, and pharynx.

nasociliary Pertaining to the nose and the eyelids, as the nasociliary nerve.

nasocular Pertaining to the nose and the eye.

nasoendoscope An instrument inserted through one of the nostrils to examine the nasal cavity.

nasoendoscopy Examination of the interior of the nose, nasopharynx, or larynx using an endoscope passed through one of the anterior nares.

nasofacial Pertaining to the nose and the face.

nasofrontal FRONTONASAL.

nasogastric [NASO- + GASTRIC] Relating to the nose and the stomach: applied principally to stomach tubes inserted via the nose and esophagus.

nasograph [NASO- + -GRAPH] An anthropometric instrument used for measuring nose shape.

nasolabial Of or relating to the nose and the upper lip.

nasolacrimal 1 Pertaining to the nasal cavity and the lacrimal apparatus. 2 Of or relating to the nasal and lacrimal bones.

nasomalar Having to do with both the external nose and the malar bone or the malar region of the face.

nasomanometer RHINOMANOMETER.

nasomaxillary 1 Of or relating to the nasal and maxillary bones. 2 NASOANTRAL.

nasomental Pertaining to the nose and the chin.

naso-occipital Pertaining to the nose and the occiput: said especially of craniometric dimensions.

naso-oral Pertaining to the nose and the mouth.

naso-orbital ORBITONASAL.

nasopalatine Pertaining to the nose and the palate.

nasopalpebral Pertaining to the nose and the eyelids.

nasopharyngeal Pertaining to the nasopharynx. Also *epipharyngeal, pharyngonasal.*

nasopharyngitis Postnasal pharyngitis, a common accompaniment of many upper respiratory infections including the common cold. Also called *epipharyngitis, rhinopharyngitis.*

nasopharyngoscope Any optical instrument used for nasopharyngoscopy, rhinoscopy, or laryngoscopy. For these purposes, flexible fiberscopes with controllable tips have replaced rigid electrical endoscopes that used distal illumination.

nasopharyngoscopy Examination of the nasopharynx either indirectly through the mouth using a nasopharyngeal mirror or directly through the nose using a nasopharyngoscope. Also called *posterior rhinoscopy.*

nasopharynx PARS NASALIS PHARYNGIS.

nasorostral Of or relating to the nasal cavity and the rostrum of the sphenoid bone.

nasoscope [NASO- + -SCOPE] RHINOSCOPE.

nasoscopy [NASO- + -SCOPY] A rarely used term for RHINOS-COPY.

nasoseptal Pertaining to the septum of the nose.

nasosinusitis Inflammation of the nasal lining which has spread to involve one or more of the paranasal sinuses.

nasospinale [NASO- + Late L *spinale,* neut. sing. of *spinalis* (from L *spin(a)* spine + -*alis* -AL) spinal] A craniometric point situated at the intersection of a horizontal line tangential to the lower margins of the piriform aperture and the median plane.

nasostenosis NASAL STENOSIS.

nasoturbinal Pertaining to the nasal cavity and a nasal concha.

Nassarius [New L (from L *nass(a)* fish trap + -*arius,* noun suffix)] A genus of small, carnivorous, brackish-water and marine snails of the subclass Prosobranchiata, order Neogastropoda, family Nassariidae, that serve as the initial hosts of a number of digenetic trematodes that infect birds and mammals.

Nassarius obsoletus A widespread North American mudflat species that serves as host of a number of trematodes, including the avian schistosome *Austrobilharzia variglandis,* which causes dermatitis in humans, the lepocreadiid fish parasite *Lepocreadium setiferoides,* the acanthocolpid fish parasite *Stephanostomum tenuis,* and the echinostome *Himasthla quissetensis,* a parasite of birds.

nasus [L, the nose] The centrally located facial structure that serves as the peripheral organ of smell and a part of the respiratory system; nose. It is located above the roof of the mouth and comprises the external nose and the nasal cavity.

nasus cartilagineus An outmoded term for CARTILAGINES NASI.

nasus duplex A rarely used term for CLEFT NOSE.

nasus externus [NA] The external, projecting portion of the nose. It is formed above by bones attached to the forehead between the eyes and below by hyaline cartilages on each side which are covered by muscles and skin. Internally it is lined by periosteum and perichondrium covered by mucous membrane. It is divided into two compartments by a median cartilaginous septum that is attached posteriorly to the bony septum of the nasal cavity. It extends from the root, where the bones form the bridge, to the apex or tip. The intervening portion constitutes the dorsum and is continuous on either side with the alae, the distal openings of which being the nostrils. Also called *external nose, nose, promontorium faciei* (outmoded).

nasus incurvus An obsolete term for SADDLE NOSE.

nasus osseus The bony framework of the nose.

natal[1] [L *natalis* (from *natus,* past part. of *nasci,* for *gnasci,* to be born; Gk *gignesthai* to be, be born + -*alis* -AL) natal, native] Relating to birth.

natal[2] Pertaining to the nates, or buttocks.

natality [NATAL[1] + -ITY] **1** In demography, the role of births in population change. **2** In ecology, birth as a phenomenon of recruitment in a population.

absolute natality MAXIMUM NATALITY.

ecological natality A natality increment to a population under natural environmental conditions. Also called *realized natality.*

maximum natality The greatest production of new individuals possible under ideal environmental conditions. It is regarded as a constant for a given population. Also called *absolute natality, physiologic natality.*

physiologic natality MAXIMUM NATALITY.

realized natality ECOLOGICAL NATALITY.

nates [L, the buttocks] The two rounded prominences that are formed by the gluteal muscles, fat, and other tissues behind the hips and are separated from each other by a cleft; the buttocks. Also called *clunes, natiform protuberance.*

natimortality [L *nat(us),* past part. of *nasci* to be born + *i* + English *mortality*] STILLBIRTH RATE.

National Ambient Air Quality Standards A series of air quality standards issued by the Environmental Protection Agency following passage of the 1970 Clean Air Act Amendments to the 1963 Clean Air Act. They established goals for the control of air quality in the United States.

National Formulary An official compendium of standards for particular pharmaceuticals and preparations that are not listed in the United States Pharmacopeia. It is revised every five years. Abbreviation: NF

National Health Service The publicly operated health care system in the United Kingdom. The National Health Service Act was enacted by Parliament in 1946 and has been modified by subsequent legislation.

natis [L (usu. in pl. *nates,* gen. *natium,* the buttocks) a buttock] Singular of NATES.

native [L *nativus* (from *natus,* past part. of *nasci* to be born) native, natural, inborn] **1** Naturally originating in an area, as populations of flora and fauna. **2** Unaltered from the natural state. **3** Not combined with other substances: used of a chemical element.

nativism [L *nativ(us)* (from *natus* born) native, inbred + -ISM] **1** The philosophic doctrine that certain, and perhaps all, of the important physical and mental functions of the human organism, particularly the perception of space and time, are inborn and thus not dependent on external stimulation or experience for their expression. **2** Any tendency to attach greater importance to the influence of heredity as opposed to environment on the expression of abilities, such as intelligence.

Natolone A proprietary name for pregnenolone.

natriuresis [New L *natri(um)* (from French *natron* carbonate of sodium, from Arabic *natrūn* carbonate of soda, from Gk *nitron* soda, carbonate of soda) sodium + -URESIS] Increased excretion of sodium in the urine. It occurs in tubulointerstitial disease and cystic renal disease, the Bartter syndrome, the diuretic recovery phase of acute renal failure, and during spontaneous or diuretic-induced reduction of edema. Also called *natruresis.* Adjective: natriuretic.

natriuretic **1** Pertaining to or causing increased urinary excretion of sodium. **2** A drug that promotes urinary excretion of sodium. Also *natruretic.*

natruresis NATRIURESIS.

natruretic NATRIURETIC.

natural Not dependent on prior experience, as in *natural immunity.*

nature-nurture The controversial problem of determing the relative contribution made by hereditary factors (nature), as opposed to that made by environmental factors (nurture), to the development and expression of adult characteristics or abilities, as in an attempt to account for individual differences in intelligence or personality.

Naturetin A proprietary name for bendroflumethiazide.

naturopath A practitioner of naturopathy.

naturopathic Pertaining to naturopathy.

naturopathy [*natur(e)* + *o* + -PATHY] A system of folk medicine utilizing the forces of nature such as air, light, water, heat, cold, physical activity, and massage, and eschewing all drugs.

Naunyn [Bernard *Naunyn*, German physician, 1839–1925] Naunyn-Minkowski method. See under MINKOWSKI'S METHOD.

naupathia [Gk *nau(s)* a ship + -PATHIA] An obsolete term for SEASICKNESS.

nausea [L (from Gk *nausia* seasickness, retching, from *naus* a ship + -IA), seasickness] An unpleasant sensation of needing to vomit. Also called *sicchasia* (rarely used).

    nausea epidemica ACUTE EPIDEMIC NONBACTERIAL GASTROENTERITIS.

    nausea gravidarum MORNING SICKNESS.

    nausea marina SEASICKNESS.

    nausea navalis A seldom used term for SEASICKNESS.

nauseant An agent that induces or precipitates nausea.

nauseate To cause to feel nausea.

nauseous 1 Causing an urge to vomit. 2 Feeling an urge to vomit; nauseated.

nautilus [L (from Gk *nautilos* a seaman; the nautilus, a shellfish having a membrane for sail, from *naus* ship), the nautilus] A mollusk of the class Cephalopoda having gas-filled chambers which give it buoyancy. It is used in neurobiological research.

navel [Old English *nafela*] UMBILICUS.

    blue navel CULLEN SIGN.

    enamel navel An indentation in the external enamel epithelium of the junction of a tooth germ and the dental lamina.

navicular SCAPHOID.

naviculocuboid CUBOIDEONAVICULAR.

naviculocuneiform CUNEONAVICULAR.

naviculoid SCAPHOID.

Nb Symbol for the element, niobium.

NBS National Bureau of Standards.

nC Symbol for the unit, nanocoulomb.

nc Symbol for the unit, nanocurie. An outmoded symbol.

NCA 1 neurocirculatory asthenia. 2 nonspecific cross-reacting antigen.

NCF neutrophil chemotactic factor.

NCI National Cancer Institute.

nCi Symbol for the unit, nanocurie.

NCV 1 noncholera vibrios. 2 nerve conduction velocity.

Nd Symbol for the element, neodymium.

Ne Symbol for the element, neon.

nealogy [Gk *nea(lēs)* (from *neos* young, new) fresh with youth + -LOGY] The study of the young of animals after birth and during early immaturity; in man, the study of infants.

Neanderthal See under *HOMO NEANDERTHALENSIS.*

neanderthaloid Exhibiting characteristics of Neandertal man. See also *HOMO NEANDERTHALENIS.*

nearsighted MYOPIC.

nearsightedness MYOPIA.

nearthrosis NEOARTHROSIS.

nebenkern [German *neben* near + *Kern* kernel, grain] 1 A mitochondrial mass formed by the coalescence of numerous smaller mitochondria, located near the nucleus in the spermatid and around the axial filament of the flagellum in the spermatozoon. 2 A basophilic granular mass located in the cytoplasm near the nucleus, usually composed of ribonucleic acid; a paranucleus.

nebenkörper [German *naben* near, accessory + *Körper* body] (*plural* nebenkörper) An extranuclear "accessory body" in the cytoplasm of the marine ameba *Paramoeba* which elongates and divides when the nucleus divides. It is now recognized as a protistan hyperparasite. See also *PARAMOEBA.*

nebramycin A mixture of semisynthetic aminoglycoside antibiotics closely related to kanamycin B.

nebula [L, mist, fog, vapor, cloud] 1 A minimal corneal opacity. 2 A liquid preparation for use in atomizer sprays.

    nebula epinephrinae hydrochloridi A preparation of epinephrine hydrochloride in an aqueous or alcoholic solution containing sodium metabisulfite in an atomizer, suitable for spraying the throat or intranasally.

nebulization [*nebul(a)* + -*iz(e)* + -ATION] The conversion of a liquid into a mist or cloud.

nebulize [L *nebul(a)* (Gk *nephelē* a cloud, cloud mass) mist, fog, vapor + -IZE] To convert (a liquid) into a mist or cloud.

nebulizer [NEBULIZE + -ER] A device for converting liquid into a mist or cloud, used primarily for permeating the atmosphere of an enclosed space or for direct inhalation.

    jet nebulizer A nebulizer that operates by utilizing a stream of air to break up fluid into particles.

    spinning disk nebulizer A nebulizer that disperses a liquid into small particles centrifugally by means of a spinning disk.

    ultrasonic nebulizer A nebulizer in which a high-frequency oscillator drives a piezoelectric transducer. The high-frequency vibrations at the air-water surface break the water into droplets 0.5 to 3 micrometers in diameter for inhalation therapy.

Necator [L (from *necatus*, past part. of *necare* to kill + -*or* -OR; Gk *nekros* a dead body), a murderer] A genus of hookworms of the family Ancylostomatidae, subfamily Necatorinae, characterized by cutting plates rather than teeth in the buccal cavity and by fused copulatory spicules in the male.

    Necator americanus The New World or tropical hookworm, a species common in humans in tropical areas of Central and South America, central and southern Africa, southern Asia, and Polynesia. Adult worms live in the small intestine, causing disease through their blood-sucking activities. In heavy, long-term infections, severe weight loss and hypochromic microcytic anemia may result. Infection occurs through penetration of the skin by third-stage filariform larvae, that migrate via blood vessels into the alveoli, where they molt and move, a week later, into the bronchioles, up the ciliated air passages to the trachea, and downward to the jejunum where they mature. Also called *Ancylostoma americanum, Uncinaria americana.*

    Necator suillus A species found in the intestine of pigs in Central America and Trinidad.

necatoriasis [*Necator* genus of hookworms + -IASIS] Infection by hookworms of the genus *Necator,* especially *N. americanus.* The symptoms are similar to those of ancylostomiasis.

necessity [L *necessitas* (from *necesse* necessary, indispensable + -*itas* -ITY) necessity]

    pharmaceutic necessity A substance having little or no therapeutic value, but used in the preparation of various drugs or medicinals. Examples are preservatives, solvents, ointments, flavorings, colorings, emulsifying agents, and suspending agents. Also called *pharmaceutic aid.*

neck [Old English *hnecca*] 1 A narrowing or constriction. 2 COLLUM. 3 CERVIX.

    anatomical neck of humerus COLLUM ANATOMICUM HUMERI.

    neck of ankle bone COLLUM TALI.

    big neck A popular term for GOITER.

    bison neck BUFFALO HUMP.

    buffalo neck BUFFALO HUMP.

    bull neck Massive swelling of the upper cervical lymph nodes, particularly as seen in cases of pharyngeal diphtheria.

    neck of condyle NECK OF CONDYLAR PROCESS OF MANDIBLE.

neck of condylar process of mandible A slender region of bone which unites the condylar head to the rest of the condylar process of the mandible. Also called *neck of condyle*.

dental neck NECK OF TOOTH.

Derbyshire neck A popular term for GOITER.

false neck of humerus An outmoded term for COLLUM CHIRURGICUM HUMERI.

neck of femur COLLUM OSSIS FEMORIS.

fibrous neck of bulb A transverse fibrous loop that elevates the inferior wall of the membranous urethra at its entry into the bulb of the penis, producing a narrowing of the lumen. An outmoded term.

neck of gallbladder COLLUM VESICAE BILIARIS.

neck of glans penis COLLUM GLANDIS PENIS.

neck of hair follicle The part of the hair follicle between the hair bulb and the follicular orifice. Also called *collum folliculi pili*.

neck of humerus COLLUM ANATOMICUM HUMERI.

neck of implant substructure The vertical projection, from the framework, which carries the abutment and is surrounded by oral mucosa. Also called *implant post, post of implant substructure*.

lateral neck of vertebra An outmoded term for PEDICLE OF VERTEBRAL ARCH.

Madelung's neck Multiple symmetrical lipomatosis affecting the neck.

neck of malleus COLLUM MALLEI.

neck of mandible COLLUM MANDIBULAE.

Nithsdale neck A popular term for GOITER.

neck of pancreas An ill-defined constricted area between the head and the body of the pancreas. It corresponds to a groove on its posterior surface that is formed by the termination of the superior mesenteric vein and the portal vein.

neck of penis COLLUM GLANDIS PENIS.

neck of radius COLLUM RADII.

neck of rib COLLUM COSTAE.

neck of scapula COLLUM SCAPULAE.

neck of seminal vesicle The constriction at the lower, anteromedial end of the seminal vesicle. It becomes a duct that joins with the ductus deferens to form the ejaculatory duct. An outmoded term.

stiff neck A popular term for MYOGENIC TORTICOLLIS.

surgical neck of femur A narrow segment of the femur, difficult to define, that is situated just below the lesser trochanter and that separates the upper extremity of the femur from its shaft. An outmoded term.

surgical neck of humerus COLLUM CHIRURGICUM HUMERI.

neck of talus COLLUM TALI.

neck of tooth A region of a tooth, often slightly constricted, where the crown and the root unite. Also called *collum dentis, cervix dentis, dental neck*.

true neck of humerus COLLUM ANATOMICUM HUMERI.

tubular neck A short segment of the nephron connecting the tubular pole of the glomerulus to the proximal convoluted tubule, characterized by low epithelial cells. In humans, the lumen of the tubular neck is slightly constricted over a very short segment.

turkey gobbler neck Vertical skin folds on the front of the neck.

neck of urinary bladder CERVIX VESICAE.

uterine neck CERVIX UTERI.

neck of uterus CERVIX UTERI.

neck of vertebra An outmoded term for PEDICLE OF VERTEBRAL ARCH.

neck of vertebral arch An outmoded term for PEDICLE OF VERTEBRAL ARCH.

webbed neck A neck that appears to be unusually broad because of bilateral folds of skin extending from the regions of the clavicles to the lower lateral parts of the head.

wry neck TORTICOLLIS.

necklace A band, usually rashlike in character, that surrounds the neck.

Casal's necklace The erythema and pigmentation that characteristically encircles the neck in pellagra. Also called *Casal's collar*.

necr- NECRO-.

necrectomy NECRONECTOMY.

necrencephalus [NECR- + Gk *enkephalos* the brain] Necrosis or softening of the brain.

necro- [Gk *nekros* (adjective) dead, (noun) dead body] A combining form meaning (1) dead body, corpse; (2) death; (3) dead, necrotic. Also *necr-, nekro-*.

necrobacillosis [NECRO- + *bacill(us)* + -OSIS] Infection with *Fusobacterium necrophorum*, an anaerobic microorganism which occurs in the normal flora of man and animals and is implicated in a variety of infections in them. It is always associated with necrosis of the affected tissue by virtue of its necrotizing endotoxin. Also called *bacillary necrosis*.

necrobiosis [NECRO- + BIOSIS] **1** Physiologic, or normal, cell death in the midst of living tissue. Also called *bionecrosis*. **2** A pathologic process of incomplete or circumscribed tissue necrosis, especially of the dermis.

necrobiosis lipoidica An inflammatory disorder characterized by necrobiosis and chronic inflammation. It usually appears on the lower legs and arises as a rounded, firm, dull red papule which may slowly spread to form large areas with an atrophic, waxy yellow center. It is classically but uncommonly associated with diabetes mellitus, and atypical forms do occur. Also called *Urbach-Oppenheim disease, necrobiosis lipoidica diabeticorum, granulomatosis disciformis chronica et progressiva*.

necrobiosis lipoidica diabeticorum NECROBIOSIS LIPOIDICA.

necrobiotic Of or relating to necrobiosis.

necrocytosis A seldom used term for NECROSIS.

necrocytotoxin A toxin that causes cellular necrosis.

necrodermatitis An inflammation of the skin that accompanies necrosis.

necrogenic Capable of causing cell or tissue death. Also *necrogenous*.

necrogenous NECROGENIC.

necrologic Of or relating to necrology.

necrologist A specialist in necrology.

necrology [NECRO- + -LOGY] A list of dead persons, especially the recent dead; an obituary.

necrolysis [NECRO- + LYSIS] Dissolution, separation, or exfoliation of dead tissue. A seldom used term.

epidermal necrolysis Necrosis accompanied by the disappearance of keratinocytes.

toxic epidermal necrolysis A syndrome in which most of the body surface becomes erythematous and the inflamed and necrotic epidermic strips off. The appearance resembles scalding. In infancy and childhood staphylococci, phage type 71 (Group 2), are often the causative organisms. In adults most cases are due to drug reactions, although staphylococci are occasionally incriminated and in some the etiology is unknown. Also called *scalded skin syndrome, Lyell's disease, toxic bullous epidermolysis* (obsolete), *epidemic exfoliative dermatitis, dermatitis exfoliativa neonatorum, exfoliative dermatitis of the newborn, keratolysis neonatorum, Ritter's disease*.

necromania [NECRO- + -MANIA] An obsolete term for NECROPHILIA.

necromimesis   The delusion that one is dead.

necronectomy [NECRO- + *n* + -ECTOMY]   A surgical procedure in which necrotic tissue is removed or débrided. Also called *necrectomy.*

necroparasite   SAPROTROPH.

necropathy   A condition or disease process principally characterized by tissue death or gangrene. An obsolete term.

necrophilia [NECRO- + -PHILIA]   A paraphilia in which sexual arousal is possible only if the sexual object, whether of the same or opposite sex, is dead. Also called *necromania* (obsolete).

necrophilous [NECRO- + -PHIL + -OUS]   **1** Tending towards or exhibiting necrophilia. **2** Growing on dead tissue.

necrophobia [NECRO- + -PHOBIA]   Pathologic fear of dead bodies or of death.

necropneumonia   Gangrene in the lung.

necropsy   AUTOPSY.

necrosadism   A paraphilia in which sexual excitement depends upon beating or defiling a corpse.

necroscopy   A seldom used term for AUTOPSY.

necrose   To undergo or to cause necrosis.

necroses   Plural of NECROSIS.

necrosin   A mediator of inflammation released from dead tissue. An obsolete term.

necrosis [NECR- + -OSIS]   The morphologic changes that follow cell death, characterized most frequently by nuclear changes. These include pyknosis, karyolysis, and karyorrhexis. Cytoplasmic changes that may be seen include increased eosinophilia, vacuolated cytoplasm, and increased cytoplasmic homogeneity. The changes seen are variable and depend on the tissues involved, the causative factors, and the magnitude of the accompanying inflammatory response. Also called *necrocytosis* (seldom used).

acute tubular necrosis   Severe damage to the epithelial cells of renal tubules, especially those of the proximal convoluted tubules, characterized by loss of microvilli, endoplasmic reticulum, and often by disruption of the tubular basement membrane. Clinically the condition is characterized by acute renal failure and may follow severe trauma or major surgery, hemorrhagic shock, or toxic drugs or chemicals. In ischemic tubular necrosis, tubular damage may be represented by scattered foci of tubular necrosis. Also called *tubular necrosis, necrotizing nephrosis, Bywaters syndrome, lower nephron necrosis* (outmoded and imprecise).

arteriolar necrosis   Necrosis of arterioles as seen in malignant hypertension. The lesion is accompanied by fibrinoid necrosis and characteristically affects the afferent glomerular arterioles.

aseptic necrosis   Tissue death that is secondary to any pathologic process other than infection. It is most commonly due to ischemia. Also called *spontaneous necrosis, quiet necrosis, bland necrosis.*

aseptic necrosis of bone   The destruction of bone tissue that is usually secondary to interruption of its blood supply, with resulting ischemia.

avascular necrosis   Necrosis due to inadequate blood supply, frequently used in the context of infarction of the head of the femur.

bacillary necrosis   NECROBACILLOSIS.

Balser's fatty necrosis   Fat necrosis due to acute pancreatitis. An obsolete term.

bilateral renal cortical necrosis   Diffuse ischemic necrosis of both renal cortices due to disseminated intravascular coagulation. Microscopically, fibrin thrombi occlude glomerular capillaries and afferent arterioles, resulting in confluent microinfarcts. Also called *cortical necrosis.*

bland necrosis   ASEPTIC NECROSIS.

caseous necrosis   The characteristic lesion of tuberculosis, it appears grossly as friable, gray-white areas that resemble cheese. Microscopically, the necrotic cells are not totally liquefied, resulting in eosinophilic, amorphous, granular debris seen within confluent granulomas. Also called *cheesy degeneration, caseous degeneration* (seldom used), *cheesy necrosis, caseation.*

central necrosis   Coagulation necrosis of the central part of an organ or tissue. This term is almost exclusively used to describe necrosis of the liver cells adjacent to the central vein of a lobule, most often due to ischemia resulting from cardiac failure or shock.

cerebrocortical necrosis   A British and European term for POLIOENCEPHALOMALACIA.

cheesy necrosis   CASEOUS NECROSIS.

chemical necrosis   Tissue destruction caused by a chemical substance.

colliquative necrosis   LIQUEFACTION NECROSIS.

cortical necrosis   BILATERAL RENAL CORTICAL NECROSIS.

coumarin necrosis   A rare and often lethal form of disseminated intravascular coagulation that occurs following ingestion of a coumarin anticoagulant drug such as warfarin. Gangrene of extremities, breasts, genitalia, or large areas of skin is characteristic.

cystic medial necrosis   A degenerative condition of the media of the aorta of unknown cause. It tends to give rise to dissecting aneurysm. Also called *mucoid medial degeneration, medionecrosis of the aorta, Erdheim's cystic medial necrosis, Erdheim syndrome.*

dental necrosis   An obsolete term for DENTAL CARIES.

diphtheritic necrosis   Local epithelial necrosis caused by infection with *Corynebacterium diphtheriae* and resulting from the inhibition of the normal inflammatory response by the exotoxin produced by the organism. The necrotic tissue, along with an exudate rich in fibrin and a great many bacteria, forms the characteristic pseudomembrane.

dry necrosis   A rarely used term for DRY GANGRENE.

embolic necrosis   Ischemic necrosis due to embolic occlusion of an artery.

epiphysial aseptic necrosis   EPIPHYSIAL ISCHEMIC NECROSIS.

epiphysial ischemic necrosis   Necrosis due to inadequate blood supply of the articular end of a long bone, such as the femoral head. Also called *epiphysial aseptic necrosis.*

Erdheim's cystic medial necrosis   CYSTIC MEDIAL NECROSIS.

fat necrosis   Abnormal destruction of fat cells due to extracellular lipases as in acute pancreatitis. The enzymes convert the adipose cells' triglycerides into free fatty acids which then complex with calcium to form calcium soaps. Thus, foci of fat necrosis appear chalky white grossly. Also called *adiponecrosis.*

fibrinoid necrosis   Necrosis in which the affected tissue stains deeply eosinophilic, homogeneous, and refractile, resembling fibrin. Most often used in referring to necrosis of blood vessel walls, as in immune complex vasculitis. Here the fibrinoid material represents fibrinogen and other plasma proteins that accumulate due to increased permeability of the damaged vessel wall. Also called *fibrinous degeneration, fibrinoid change.*

focal necrosis   Necrosis of a circumscribed area of an organ or tissue.

gangrenous necrosis   A clinical term for the combination of coagulation and liquefaction necrosis, most often seen in a lower limb that has become ischemic and secondarily infected. Either coagulation necrosis (dry gangrene) or liquefaction necrosis (wet gangrene) may predominate.

glomerular necrosis   Necrosis of all or part of a glomerulus, characterized by karyorrhexis and the presence of debris. Total necrosis of a glomerulus follows occlusion of the afferent arteriole, and is characterized by glomerular hemorrhage.

gummatous necrosis Coagulative necrosis within the granulomatous inflammatory lesions of tertiary syphilis (gummas). Also called *syphilitic necrosis.*

hyaline necrosis Segmental necrosis of muscle cells characterized by the eosinophilic, glassy, homogeneous appearance of the affected fibers. It may be seen in prolonged infections such as typhoid fever and hepatitis. This change can be artificially induced by mechanical injury such as that caused by handling of live muscle with dissecting tools. Also called *Zenker's necrosis, Zenker's degeneration.*

ischemic necrosis Coagulative necrosis due to interruption of blood flow.

laminar cortical necrosis Necrosis localized to one or more specific layers of the cerebral cortex, as seen in anoxia.

liquefaction necrosis Necrosis characterized by softening and liquefaction of the affected tissue as the result of the action of hydrolytic enzymes released by polymorphonuclear leukocytes in the course of pyogenic bacterial infections. It is also the characteristic type of necrosis seen in brain infarcts. Also called *colliquation* (seldom used), *colliquefaction* (seldom used), *colliquative necrosis.*

mandibular necrosis PHOSSY JAW.

massive hepatic necrosis Necrosis of confluent areas of hepatocytes involving entire lobules, usually due to fulminant acute viral hepatitis, hepatotoxins, or drug hypersensitivity. It is accompanied by acute hepatic failure and is almost always fatal.

mechanical necrosis Tissue destruction by the forceful disruption of cells or of the blood supply to the tissue. Also called *physical necrosis.*

medial necrosis Necrosis of the media of an artery. It may lead to rupture.

mummification necrosis DRY GANGRENE.

nephrotoxic tubule necrosis Acute tubular necrosis due to a toxic agent.

Paget's quiet necrosis A small area of necrosis in the articular surface of a bone that becomes separated from the adjacent healthy bone as a sequestrum. This is usually seen in the lower end of the femur. A rarely used term.

papillary necrosis RENAL PAPILLARY NECROSIS.

peripheral necrosis Necrosis of the outer aspect of an organ or structure. • May be used to describe necrosis of the periportal areas of the liver lobule as it occurs in eclampsia and phosphorus poisoning.

phosphorus necrosis PHOSSY JAW.

physical necrosis MECHANICAL NECROSIS.

postpartum pituitary necrosis The adenohypophysial lesion causing the Sheehan syndrome.

pressure necrosis Necrosis of a tissue due to interference with its blood supply by external pressure. It is seen especially in decubitus ulcers.

progressive emphysematous necrosis GAS GANGRENE.

quiet necrosis ASEPTIC NECROSIS.

radiation necrosis Tissue death following exposure to injurious doses of ionizing radiation.

radium necrosis Necrosis of bones, as of fingers and jaws, from radium. In the past, the manufacture and use of radium compounds for luminous dials on watches, clocks, and meters was a serious hazard. The jaw was at risk because workers would use their lips to make their brushes pointed before painting the dials.

renal coagulation necrosis Coalescing areas of opacification and condensation of cytoplasm with nuclear pyknosis, karyolysis, or karyorrhexis. The cells may desquamate resulting in denuded basement membrane, which is often thickened and sometimes fragmented. Coagulation necrosis may follow renal ischemia or severe trauma.

renal medullary necrosis RENAL PAPILLARY NECROSIS.

renal papillary necrosis Necrosis of one or more pyramids, characterized clinically by renal colic, pyuria, and acute or chronic renal failure. Roentgenography may show a characteristic appearance. Papillary necrosis may result from pyelonephritis, diabetes mellitus, excessive analgesic drug intake, obstructive uropathy, sickle cell disease, or cyclophosphamide toxicity. Renal papillae may be passed in the urine. Also called *papillary necrosis, renal medullary necrosis, necrotizing renal papillitis, papillary erosion, necrotizing papillitis.*

septic necrosis Necrosis occurring as a result of infection, usually bacterial.

simple necrosis Coagulative necrosis in an aseptic area of the body.

spontaneous necrosis ASEPTIC NECROSIS.

subcutaneous fat necrosis Ischemic damage to the subcutaneous fat cells in the newborn by trauma, such as pressure of a forceps blade on the cheek or pressure on other parts, resulting in cell necrosis with release of the fat, at first in a solid state. Indurated plaques can be felt in the skin. Later the fat may liquefy or calcify. It is finally dispersed and absorbed. Also called *subcutaneous adiponecrosis in infants, pseudosclerema* (obsolete), *cytosteatonecrosis.*

subendocardial necrosis Diffuse, laminar necrosis of the myocardium subjacent to the endocardial lining. It occurs primarily in the left ventricle, and is due to either hypoperfusion, as in shock, or partial stenosis of a coronary artery.

superficial necrosis Death of the outermost layers of an organ or tissue.

syphilitic necrosis GUMMATOUS NECROSIS.

total necrosis Necrosis of an entire organ or part.

transmural necrosis Necrosis through the entire wall of a hollow viscus, a blood vessel, or the heart, as the necrosis following a transmural myocardial infarct.

tubular necrosis ACUTE TUBULAR NECROSIS.

necrosis ustilaginea Gangrene caused by ergot poisoning. A rarely used term.

x-ray necrosis The death of tissue caused by the administration of x rays.

Zenker's necrosis HYALINE NECROSIS.

necrospermia [NECRO- + SPERM + -IA] A condition in which the sperm in the seminal fluid are nonliving. Also called *necrozoospermia.*

necrospermic Pertaining to or exhibiting necrospermia.

necrosteon Necrosis of bone.

necrosteosis The pathological processes involved in bone necrosis.

necrotaxis [NECRO- + Gk *taxis* an ordering, arranging] The attraction of neutrophil polymorphs and macrophages by the autolysis of necrotic cells.

necrotic Characterized by or pertaining to necrosis. Also *necrobiotic* (obsolete).

necrotize To cause necrosis.

necrotomy [NECRO- + -TOMY] **1** A seldom used term for AUTOPSY. **2** An operative procedure in which a bone sequestrum is removed.

osteoplastic necrotomy The removal of a sequestrum of dead bone followed by replacement of the overlying living bone.

necrotoxin The alpha toxin of *Staphylococcus aureus.* An obsolete term.

necrozoospermia [NECRO- + ZOOSPERMIA] NECROSPERMIA.

nectar [L, from Gk *nektar* the drink of the gods] A sugary fluid secreted by the nectaries of angiosperm flowers. It attracts insects that pollinate the flowers.

nectareous Like nectar; pleasant to the taste.

nectary [New L *nectar(ium)* (from L *nectar* nectar + L *-ium*, neut. sing. noun suffix) nectary + -Y] A gland in flowering plants that secretes a sugary fluid, nectar, which pollinators use for food.

Necturus [Gk *nēkt(os)*, verbal of *nēchein* to swim + New L *-urus* suffix denoting tail, from Gk *oura* tail] A genus of neotenic aquatic salamanders of the Proteidae family. Members of the genus have large external gills. They are commonly used as laboratory specimens.

need A lack or want of some substance or condition which, if present, would help to preserve the well-being, health, or life of the individual. The deficiency, whether arising from internal processes or as the result of the action of external forces, impels seeking behavior by the organism to relieve the tension and restore equilibrium by satisfying the particular lack.

dependency needs Those supports required for adequate development and adaptation, including mothering, love, affection, shelter, protection, security, food and warmth.

needle [Old English *nædl*, from a prehistoric Germanic noun akin to L *nere* to spin and to Gk *nēn* or *nein* to spin] **1** Any of various long, thin, surgical instruments, hollow or solid, used for aspiration, injection, or suturing. **2** To pierce with a needle, as for the diagnostic or therapeutic aspiration.

Abrams needle A long, thin, hollow structure designed to obtain material for biopsy without introducing air.

aneurysm needle A large tapered needle that once was used to oversew aneurysms on large blood vessels.

aspirating needle A long, thin, hollow instrument designed to permit safe removal of fluid or gas from a body cavity.

atraumatic needle A surgical needle that permits suturing with minimal damage to the tissues being sutured. Its diameter in cross section is smaller than that of the suture material, thus minimizing tissue damage.

biopsy needle A long, thin, hollow instrument with a sharp point designed to obtain small cores of tissue for diagnostic purposes.

butterfly needle A small-gauge, thin-walled metal needle with flanges, used for introduction into small veins such as a scalp vein in an infant.

cataract needle KNIFE NEEDLE.

Cope's needle A long, thin, hooked instrument designed to obtain biopsy samples of membranes such as the peritoneum, pericardium, and pleura.

cutting needle A long, thin, sharp instrument with triangular or honed edges to permit easy penetration of firm structures.

discission needle KNIFE NEEDLE.

electrosurgical needle A needle equipped with a handle and attached to an electric cautery for incising, destroying, or coagulating tissue by means of an electric current.

exploring needle A surgical needle, sometimes calibrated, with an opening near the tip. It is introduced into a tissue mass or body cavity to determine the presence of abnormal resistance or to aspirate fluid if it is encountered.

fascia needle A large suturing needle with a large eye which can accommodate strips of fascia for use as suture material.

Fischer's needle A needle used to induce therapeutic artificial pneumothorax in the treatment of tuberculosis.

Francke's needle A small, thin, sharp, lancet-shaped needle formerly used to drain small quantities of subcutaneous fluid. An obsolete term.

Hagedorn's needle A curved surgical needle with two cutting edges and a sharp point that was formerly used for suturing.

harelip needle A needle at one time employed in an operation formerly used for the correction of congenital cleft lip. Several needles were used to skewer the defect of the lip and they were held in place with suture material wound in a figure-of-eight

fashion around the two ends of each needle.

hypodermic needle A needle suitable for an injection under the skin.

knife needle A thin and small surgical knife for incision of the lens capsule. Also called *cataract needle, discission needle.*

lumbar puncture needle A hollow needle used principally for introduction into the spinal subarachnoid space for the purpose of measuring pressure, withdrawing fluid, or injecting a liquid. Also called *spinal needle.*

malleable spinal needle A needle made of a material, such as platinum, that can be bent without danger of breaking.

Menghini needle A long, thin, hollow surgical instrument that is designed to take core samples for biopsy, specifically of the liver, without the need of rotating the device.

radium needle A needle-pointed tube, 12 mm in diameter and 15 cm in length, in which is sealed a few milligrams of radium. It is used for interstitial radiation treatments.

Reverdin's needle A surgical needle with an eye at the end that may be opened or closed by means of a movable slide. It was formerly used for placing sutures.

round needle A surgical needle which is perfectly round in cross section.

Silverman needle A long, thin, hollow surgical instrument with two moving parts. It is used to take core samples of tissue for biopsy without the need to rotate the device.

spinal needle LUMBAR PUNCTURE NEEDLE.

stop needle A long, thin, sharp surgical instrument with a flange that prevents insertion beyond the flange.

surgical needle A long, thin, sharp, rodlike instrument that is used during surgical procedures, especially for suturing.

swaged needle A sharp, thin, rodlike surgical device to which suture material is permanently attached for use during an operative procedure.

University of Illinois needle A needle used for bone marrow aspiration. It is characterized by a locking stylet and an adjustable guard that protects against excessively deep penetration.

ventriculopuncture needle A semisharp, calibrated needle designed for introduction into the cerebral ventricle.

vicat needle A device used to determine the time required for plaster or other materials to set.

Vim-Silverman needle A split hollow needle used to obtain a core of tissue from the liver for histologic study.

Needles [Carl F. *Needles*, U.S. pediatrician, born 1935] Melnick-Needles syndrome. See under SYNDROME.

needling Incision of the lens capsule with a knife needle.

needy / categorically needy Characterizing the population group that meets officially established criteria for receipt of services under governmental health care programs for the medically and sometimes economically indigent.

medically needy Lacking adequate resources to provide for one's health care needs, the criteria for which may be officially defined by governmental authorities.

Neef [Christopher Ernst *Neef*, German physician, 1782–1849] Neef's hammer. See under WAGNER'S HAMMER.

Neel [Axel Valdemar *Neel*, Danish physician, 1878–1952] Bing-Neel syndrome. See under SYNDROME.

Neelsen [Friedrich Carl Adolf *Neelsen*, German pathologist, 1854–1894] **1** Ziehl-Neelsen technique. See under TECHNIQUE. **2** Ziehl-Neelsen carbolfuschin. See under ZIEHL-NEELSEN STAIN.

neem *Melia azadirachta*, a tree of the Meliaceae family. The oil, neem oil or margosa oil, that is extracted from the seeds has both inflammatory and healing properties and has been used in the treatment of skin diseases.

neencephalon [*ne(o)-* + ENCEPHALON] The phylogenetically newer parts of the brain, especially the cerebral cortices. A seldom used term. Also called *neoencephalon* (seldom used).

NEEP   negative end-expiratory pressure.

NEFA   nonesterified fatty acids.

nefrens [L *ne* not + *frendere* to gnash the teeth]   Edentate, or without erupted teeth.

Neftel [William Basil *Neftel*, U.S. neurologist, 1830–1906]   See under DISEASE.

Negatan   A proprietary name for negatol.

negation   The act of denying; denial.

negative [L *negativ(us)* (from *negat(us)*), past part. of *negare* to deny + *-ivus* -IVE) expressing a negation, inhibiting]   **1** Lacking positive or affirmative character.   **2** Characterized by or signifying the absence of a condition, especially one being tested, or the failure of a particular response to occur.   **3** A negative finding or result.

false negative   A test result that is negative when the correct result would be positive.

negative G   The pull of gravity toward the head when one is in an upside-down position.

negativism   In psychiatry, behavior that is characterized as being resistant or in opposition to what is expected.

active negativism   Negativism in which the subject does the opposite of what is asked or demanded.

passive negativism   Negativism in which the subject, without any prompting, fails to do what is expected.

negatol   A colloidal product obtained from the reaction of metacresolsulfonic acid with formaldehyde. It is applied topically to the cervix as a germicidal antiparasital, or bacteriostatic agent.

negatoscope [*negat(ive)* + *o* + -SCOPE]   An apparatus, now obsolete, to display roentgenograms.

negatron [contraction of *neg(ative) (elec)tron*, as distinguished from positive electron (positron)]   ELECTRON.

neglect / senile neglect   DIOGENES SYNDROME.

negligence [L *negligentia* (from *negligens*, gen. *negligentis*, pres. part. of *negligere* to neglect + *-ia* -IA) negligence, neglect]   **1** An unintentional failure to perform a legally recognized duty, causing foreseeable injury or loss to another.   **2** In medical practice, the failure of a physician to exercise the degree of skill, prudence, and care that would usually and customarily be exercised by other reputable physicians treating the patient in question or a similar patient. Negligence is the basis for most claims of medical malpractice. It includes both acts of commission and omission.

comparative negligence   In negligence law, the practice of comparing proven contributory negligence with proven professional negligence to assess degrees of responsibility and determine the proportion of damages. In medical malpractice cases involving proven negligence by both physician and patient, percentages are used to express the relative degree of each party's responsibility. If contributory negligence is responsible for 60% of the injury or loss, then the physician would be responsible for paying 40% of the total assessed damages.

contributory negligence   In negligence law as it pertains to medical malpractice, the negligent conduct on the part of the patient concurrent with that of the physician's negligence and constituting a part of the proximate cause of the injury or loss for which damages are being sought.

Negri [Adelchi *Negri*, Italian pathologist, 1876–1912]   Negri bodies. See under BODY.

Negri [Silvio *Negri*, Italian physician, flourished 20th century]   Jacod-Negri syndrome. See under PETROSPHENOID SYNDROME.

Negro [Camillo *Negro*, Italian neurologist, 1861–1927]   **1** Negro's phenomenon. See under COGWHEEL SIGN.   **2** See under SIGN.

Negroid   Characterized by or similar to the physical features of the "black" races of man.   • The term is usually applied to the major race of Africa but on occasion has been applied to both Africans and to the spiral-haired peoples of southern Asia and Oceania.

Negus [Victor Ewings *Negus*, English otorhinolaryngologist, born 1887]   **1** See under TUBE, ESOPHAGOSCOPE.   **2** Negus hydrostatic dilator. See under DILATOR.

negrophobia [Spanish and Portuguese negro (from L *niger*, gen. *nigri*, black, dusky, dark) black, dark; as substantive, Negro, black color + -PHOBIA]   **1** Pathologic fear of darkness or blackness.   **2** Fear of people with dark or black skin.

neighborwise   In embryology, in a manner similar to that prevailing locally: said of the development of transplanted cells when they adopt the behavior prevalent in their new surroundings.

Neill [James Maffett *Neill*, U.S. bacteriologist, born 1894]   Van Slyke and Neill method. See under METHOD.

Neill [Mather Humphrey *Neill*, U.S. physician, 1882–1930]   Neill-Mooser reaction. See under SCROTAL REACTION.

Neisser [Max *Neisser*, German bacteriologist, 1869–1938]   Neisser-Wechsberg phenomenon. See under COMPLEMENT DEVIATION.

Neisseria [after Albert Ludwig Siegmund *Neisser*, German bacteriologist and physician, 1855–1916 + -IA]   A genus of aerobic, fastidious, small, Gram-negative diplococci whose cultivation requires elevated concentrations of carbon dioxide and protection (by serum, starch, or charcoal) against inhibitory traces of detergents and ions of heavy metals. The major pathogens are *N. gonorrhoeae* and *N. meningitidis*. Related nonpathogens or rare pathogens, also in the family Neisseriaceae, include species of *Acinetobacter*, *Moraxella*, and *Veillonella*.

Neisseria catarrhalis   A frequent and nonpathogenic inhabitant of the nasopharynx, easily mistaken for the meningococcus. Also called *Branhamella catarrhalis* (obsolete).

Neisseria gonorrhoeae   The species that causes gonorrhea; the gonococcus. There are many types based on heterogeneity in the outer membrane proteins, pili, and lipopolysaccharide. Piliated strains enter and multiply in cells of the epithelial mucosae. In purulent discharges the organisms are directly recognized as Gram-negative intracellular diplococci, in leukocytes.

Neisseria lactamica   A nonpathogenic species often found in the nasopharynx of children. It closely resembles *N. meningitidis* except that it ferments lactose.

Neisseria meningitidis   A species of a Gram-negative diplococci frequently present in the normal nasopharynx; the meningococci. There are several groups based on a polysaccharide capsule, and several types based on a surface protein. Group A is the main cause of epidemics of meningitis. Groups B and C cause endemic cases.

neisseria (*plural* neisseriae) Any organism of the genus *Neisseria*.

neisseriology [*Neisseri(a)* + *o* + -LOGY]   The scientific study of gonorrhea.

neisserosis   Infection with *Neisseria*, especially *N. gonorrhoeae*. An older term.

nekro-   NECRO-.

nekton [Gk *nēkton*, neut. of *nēktos*, verbal of *nēchein* to swim]   Free-swimming marine animals, such as fish, dolphins, and whales, that move largely independent of currents and waves.

Nélaton [Auguste *Nélaton*, French surgeon, 1807–1873]   **1** Nélaton's catheter. See under FLEXIBLE CATHETER.   **2** See under TUMOR, DISLOCATION, LINE, OPERATION.   **3** Nélaton's sphincter. See under FOLD.   **4** Nélaton's fibers. See under FIBER.

nelavane **1** GAMBIAN TRYPANOSOMIASIS. **2** RHODESIAN TRYPANOSOMIASIS.

Nelson [Don H. *Nelson*, U.S. internist, born 1925] See under SYNDROME.

Nelson [Warren Otto *Nelson*, U.S. endocrinologist, 1906–1964] Heller-Nelson syndrome. See under SYNDROME.

nem [German *Nahrungs Einheit Milch* nutritional unit milk] A unit of nutrition; the amount of an infant food equivalent in nutritional value to 1 gram of breast milk.

Nema A proprietary name for tetrachloroethylene.

nema [Gk *nēma*, gen. *nēmatos*, thread, yarn, tissue] A nematode, especially one of the free-living forms. • The term is commonly used in agricultural nematology.

nemaline [Gk *nēma* thread, yarn + *l* + -INE] Threadlike: used especially of the subsarcolemmal rodlike structures seen with the electron microscope in nemaline myopathy.

nemat- NEMATO-.

nemathelminth [NEMAT- + HELMINTH] NEMATODE.

Nemathelminthes [NEMAT- + Gk *helminthes*, pl. of *helmins* worm] NEMATODA.

nemathelminthiasis [NEMATHELMINTH + -IASIS] NEMATODIASIS.

nematicide NEMATOCIDE.

nematization Infection by nematodes: used chiefly in reference to plant infection.

nemato- [Gk *nēma* (genitive *nematos*) thread, yarn, tissue] A combining form meaning (1) thread, threadlike; (2) nematode. Also *nemat-*.

nematoblast [NEMATO- + -BLAST] SPERMATID.

Nematocera [NEMATO- + Gk *kera(s)* horn] A suborder of the order Diptera comprising the most primitive flies, characterized by antennae with numerous segments. It includes gnats, mosquitoes, midges, blackflies, crane flies, and gallflies.

nematocide [NEMATO- + -CIDE] An agent that kills nematodes. Also called *nematicide*.

nematocyst [NEMATO- + CYST] The stinging barb of a jellyfish or other coelenterate. Exposure to multiple such barbs can inflict painful lesions and occasionally cause death to an unwary swimmer. Also called *cnida*.

Nematoda [NEMAT- + New L *-oda*, irreg. from *-oidea*, neut. pl. suffix, from L *-oid(es)* -OID + *-ea*, neut. pl. of *-eus* English *-eous*] A phylum of helminths characterized by an extremely protective cuticular wall, a tapered cylindrical shape, muscles oriented longitudinally, and a triradiate esophagus. It includes both parasitic and nonparasitic species, the latter being the more common and including both soil and aquatic forms. The two major taxonomic groups are based on the presence or absence of olfactory caudal organs called phasmids. Roundworms such as *Ancylostoma, Ascaris, Enterobius,* and the blood and tissue filarial roundworms are placed in the phasmidial class Secernentea (formerly called Phasmidia) while the nonphasmidial nematodes, which include *Trichinella, Trichuris, Capillaria,* and *Dioctophyma,* are in the class Adenophorea (formerly called Aphasmidia). Also called *Nemathelminthes*.

nematode [Gk *nēma*, gen. *nēmatos*, thread, yarn, tissue + English *-ode*, suffix denoting resemblance] **1** Of or belonging to the phylum Nematoda. **2** A member of the phylum Nematoda; a roundworm. Also called *nemathelminth*.

nematodiasis [*nematod(e)* + -IASIS] Infection by a nematode. Also called *nemathelminthiasis, nematodosis, nematosis*.

nonpatent nematodiasis VISCERAL LARVA MIGRANS.

Nematodirella longispiculata A thread-necked trichostrongyle nematode in the subfamily Nematodirinae, family Trichostrongylidae, found in the small intestine of goats, sheep, musk

ox, moose, pronghorn, and reindeer in circumpolar north latitudes. Little disease is noted, except in heavily infected young animals.

Nematodirus [NEMATO- + -*dirus*, prob. from Gk *deirē* the neck] A genus of thread-necked nematodes of the family Trichostrongylidae found in many herbivorous animals. Normally they occur in the small intestine where they are relatively nonpathogenic, though in heavy infections or in malnourished or immunosuppressed animals the infection can be overwhelming.

Nematodirus abnormalis A species common in the United States, found in goats, sheep, pronghorn, mule deer, and camels.

Nematodirus filicollis A cosmopolitan species found in goats, sheep, oxen, and many wild ruminants.

Nematodirus fordi *MECISTOCIRRUS DIGITATUS.*

Nematodirus gibsoni *MECISTOCIRRUS DIGITATUS.*

Nematodirus helvetianus A species found in the small intestine of sheep, goats, cattle, and camels in Asia, the Americas, and Europe.

Nematodirus lanceolatus A species found in the small intestine of domestic and bighorn sheep and pronghorn in the Americas.

Nematodirus leporis A species found in the duodenum of rabbits in North America.

Nematodirus spathiger The most common *Nematodirus* species, found in sheep, goats, camels, alpacas, llamas, and many other domestic and wild ruminants throughout the world. Most infections are light and insignificant but heavy infections may cause profuse diarrhea and death, especially of lambs, within a few days of onset of signs.

nematodosis NEMATODIASIS.

nematoid [*nemat(ode)* + -OID] **1** Resembling a nematode. **2** A nematoid; a member of the Nematoidea (Nematoda).

nematologist A specialist in nematology.

nematology [NEMATO- + -LOGY] The scientific study of nematode worms, including subspecialties related to agriculture, medicine, genetics, and biological control.

Nematomorpha [NEMATO- + New L *-morpha*, neut. pl. of *-morphus*, suffix denoting form, from Gk *morphē* form, appearance] A phylum of long, slender, blunt-ended cylindrical worms known as hairworms or horsehair worms, parasitic as juveniles in insects and free-living in fresh water as adults. Adults, which are commonly from one-half to one meter long, lack a functional gut, lateral cords, and an excretory system. Feeding and respiration are by diffusion across the body wall. Worms of this phylum were formerly regarded as constituting a class of the phylum Aschelminthes. Also called *Gordiacea*.

nematosis NEMATODIASIS.

nematospermia [NEMATO- + SPERM- + -IA] A trait, possessed by man, of producing spermatozoa with long, slender tails.

Nembutal A proprietary name for pentobarbital sodium.

Nemertea RHYNCHOCOELA.

nemertean NEMERTINE.

Nemertina [New L (from Gk *Nēmert(ēs)* Nemertes, a Nereid, and *nēmertēs* unerring + L *-ina*, fem. of *-inus*, suffix denoting belonging to)] RHYNCHOCOELA.

nemertine [Gk *Nēmert(ēs)* a Nereid + -INE] **1** Any member of the phylum Nemertina. Also called *proboscis worm, ribbon worm, rhynchocoelan, nemertean*. **2** Pertaining to any member of the phylum Nemertinea (or Rhynchocoela).

Nemertinea [See NEMERTINA.] RHYNCHOCOELA.

Nemertini [See NEMERTINA.] RHYNCHOCOELA.

nemic [*nem(atode)* + -IC] Relating to nematodes.

neo- [Gk *neos* new, youthful] A combining form meaning new.

Neo-Antergan A proprietary name for pyrilamine maleate.

neoantigen Antigenic determinants that are produced when a protein (or other antigenic substance) is chemically attached to another protein (or to a cell) but that are not found in either of the two components of the reaction when not chemically combined.

neoantimosan STIBOPHEN.

neoarsphenamine $C_{13}H_{13}As_2N_2NaO_4S$. [5-[(3-Amino-4 hydroxy-phenol)arseno]-2-hydroxyanilino]methonol sulfoxylate sodium. A soluble compound containing arsphenamine, formerly used as a major antisyphilitic medication. Also called *novarsenobenzene, novarsenobenzol.*

neoarthrosis A new joint, as a pseudarthrosis or a surgically placed artificial joint. Also called *nearthrosis.*

Neoascaris A genus of ascaridoid nematodes (family Toxocaridae) parasitic in the intestines of mammals and possessing an esophagus with a posterior ventriculus.

Neoascaris vitulorum The large roundworm of cattle that is parasitic in the small intestine. Although uncommon in the United States, it is an important cattle parasite in many other countries. Young animals may be severely affected if infestation is heavy. Also called *Ascaris vitulorum.*

neoblastic Of or relating to the development of new tissue.

neocerebellum The largest and phylogenetically newest part of the cerebellum, including all of the cerebellum between the primary fissure anteriorly and the posterolateral fissure posteriorly. • Although the midline vermis is included, the term is used most often in reference to the cerebellar hemispheres, which are especially related to the coordination of skilled movements initiated at cortical levels.

neochymotrypsinogen Chymotrypsinogen from which the peptide Thr-Asn in positions 1478 has been removed by the action of chymotrypsin. Splitting of the bond between Arg-15 and Ile-16 by trypsin is required to convert a chymotrypsinogen into a chymotrypsin.

neocinetic NEOKINETIC.

Neo-Cobefrin A proprietary name for levonordefrin.

neocortex ISOCORTEX.

neocystostomy [NEO- + CYSTOSTOMY] The creation of a new opening in the urinary bladder to permit drainage.

ureteral neocystostomy The creation of a new connection between a ureter and the urinary bladder.

ureteroileal neocystostomy A surgically created opening between the urinary bladder and one or both ureters, utilizing a segment of defunctionalized ileum for drainage from the bladder.

neocyte An immature erythrocyte, especially a reticulocyte.

neocytosis The presence of immature erythrocytes, especially reticulocytes, in the circulating blood.

neodarwinism A blending of the darwinian concept of the survival of the fittest and mendelian laws of heredity. This is a modern view of natural selection and survival of the fittest.

neodentatum That portion of the dentate nucleus of the cerebellum which exclusively receives fibers from the cerebellar hemisphere.

neodymium An element of the lanthanide series, having atomic number 60 and atomic weight 144.24. It has limited use, chiefly in manufacturing colored glass. Its compounds are moderately toxic. Symbol: Nd

neoencephalon A seldom used term for NEENCEPHALON.

neofetus [NEO- + FETUS] The fetus when it has just been formed at the end of the embryonic period at about the eighth week of human intrauterine development. Adjective: neofetal.

neoformation [NEO- + FORMATION] NEOPLASM.

neoformative Pertaining to a newly formed structure or to a neoplasm.

Neofrakt A system of pouring polyurethane foam into a cotton stocking to produce casts, splints, braces, and temporary artificial limbs. A proprietary name.

neogala [NEO- + Gk *gala* milk] COLOSTRUM.

neogenesis New formation or growth; regeneration. Adjective: neogenetic.

neoglottis PHONATORY NEOGLOTTIS.

phonatory neoglottis A hypopharyngeal fistula constructed at the upper end of the trachea after total laryngectomy and serving as a new glottis. Also called *neoglottis.*

Neognathae [NEO- + New L -*gnathae*, fem. pl. of -*gnathus*, combining form denoting the jaw] A superorder of the vertebrate class Aves. It includes almost all modern birds, except the ratites. Most species are capable of flight and all possess a sternum with a prominent keel, wings, and a pygostyle. Their distribution is world-wide, except for the Antarctic region.

Neohetramine A proprietary name for thonzylamine hydrochloride.

Neo-Hombreol A proprietary name for testosterone propionate.

Neohydrin A proprietary name for chlormerodrin.

neohymen An obsolete term for PSEUDOMEMBRANE.

Neo-Iopax A proprietary name for sodium iodomethamate.

neokinetic Describing or pertaining to the pyramidal (corticospinal) motor system which controls voluntary movement. Also *neocinetic.*

neolalia [NEO- + -LALIA] The use of neologisms in speech, especially as seen in some psychiatric disorders. Also called *neolalism, allegorization.*

neolalism NEOLALIA.

neologism 1 A newly coined word or phrase. 2 In psychiatry, the practice of using neologisms that are typically obscure or incomprehensible to others, thus constituting an impediment to communication.

neomalthusianism [NEO- + *Malthusianism*, theory that population increases faster than food supplies and is checked only by famine, disease, and war, after Thomas Robert *Malthus*, English political economist, 1766–1834] A doctrine which advocates birth control, abortion, and sterilization, together or separately, in order to curb population growth. Also called *malthusianism.*

neomembrane PSEUDOMEMBRANE.

neomimia [Gk *neo(s)* new, strange + *mim(os)* an imitator, copyist + -IA] The stereotypical repetition of a gesture or movement that is senseless to the observer and meaningful only to the subject.

neomin NEOMYCIN.

neomorph [NEO- + -MORPH] An entirely new feature or characteristic that has recently appeared in the course of evolutionary development.

neomorphism [NEO- + -MORPH + -ISM] The appearance of an entirely new feature in the course of recent evolutionary development.

neomycin An antibacterial substance obtained from the metabolic products of *Streptomyces fradiae* and active against a variety of Gram-negative and Gram-positive microorganisms. The sulfate salt is administered orally and applied topically. The drug may produce ototoxicity and nephrotoxicity. Also called *nyacyne, neomin.*

neomycin palmitate The palmitate salt of neomycin. It is applied topically as an antibacterial agent in the treatment of skin infections, burns, wounds, and ulcers.

neomycin sulfate The sulfate salt of neomycin. It is a white or slightly yellow powder, used as an anti-infective agent for the treatment of urinary tract, skin, eye, ear, and enteric infections. It is also used for preoperative disinfection. It may be administered orally, topically, or intramuscularly.

neomycin undecenoate The undecenoic acid derivative of neomycin. It has the same properties and uses as the sulfate, and it is used primarily in ear drops for the treatment of otitis externa. Also called *neomycin undecylenate*.

neomycin undecylenate NEOMYCIN UNDECENOATE.

neon Element number 10, having atomic weight 20.179. Neon is a colorless, odorless gas, occurring uncombined in the atmosphere in a ratio of about 15 parts per million. Three stable isotopes occur, and five radioactive isotopes have been described. The valence is 0. Symbol: Ne

neonatal [NEO- + NATAL] Of or relating to a newborn infant from birth to the 28th day, or to this period of life.

neonate [New L *neonatus.* See *neonatus.*] An infant during the first four weeks of life. Also called *newborn, newborn infant, newborn child, neonatus.* ● Although the first 28 days of life comprise the usual period designating a *neonate* or *newborn,* for statistical purposes some have reckoned the period as the first 7 days. The term *early neonate* has been used to describe the first week of life.

neonaticide [*neonat(e)* + *i* + -CIDE] The killing of a neonate.

neonatologist [NEO- + L *nat(us)* born + -OLOGIST] A physician specializing in neonatology.

neonatology [NEO- + L *nat(us)* born + *o* + -LOGY] The branch of medicine dealing with the newborn infant and its diseases, as well as its physical and psychological care, assessment, and development. Also called *neonatal medicine.*

neonatorum [L, genitive pl. of *neonatus* newborn infant] Of the neonate.

neonatus [New L (from Gk *neo(s)* new + L *natus,* past part. of *nasci* to be born) a newborn child] NEONATE.

neo-olive The largest and phylogenetically newest portion of the inferior olivary nucleus of the medulla oblongata, comprising the lateral two thirds of the principal olivary nucleus.

neopallium ISOCORTEX.

Neoparamonostomum parvum PARAMONOSTOMUM PARVUM.

neopathy [NEO- + -PATHY] 1 A new or newly discovered disease. 2 A disease or complication of disease newly present in a patient.

neopentane The hydrocarbon 2,2-dimethylpropane.

neopentyl The group $(CH_3)C—CH_2—$. 2,2-Dimethylpropyl. Its compounds are inert to nucleophilic substitutions, because they are sterically hindered and because the group cannot form a stable carbocation.

neophasia The invention of one or more new languages by a subject who alone knows the grammar, syntax, or vocabulary of the invented tongue. It is a rare phenomenon that has been reported in expansive paranoia and mania.

neophobia [NEO- + -PHOBIA] Pathologic fear of anything new or of any alteration in the status quo. Also called *misocainia, misoneism.*

Neopilina A surviving genus of the most primitive class of mollusks, the Monoplacophora. They are bilaterally symmetrical, with a saucer-shaped shell and five pairs of gills around the foot. The surviving species of the class is *N. galathea,* specimens of which have been taken at 3600 meters off the west coast of Mexico. Paired structures and other segmental features show either an evolutionary venture into linear replication of parts and pseudosegmentation or the primitive nature of this genus and its role as a link in the relationship between mollusks and annelids.

neoplasia [NEO- + -PLASIA] The process of tumor formation.

multiple endocrine neoplasia Any of a group of uncommon syndromes characterized by benign or malignant tumors of more than one endocrine gland. Type I (MEN I, sometimes called Lloyd syndrome) includes lesions of the parathyroids, the adenohypophysis (hypopituitarism or acromegaly), the pancreas (β cells and non-β cells, hypoglycemia, hypergastrinemia) and, less commonly, the adrenal cortex and thyroid. Zollinger-Ellison syndrome is often associated. The familial form of MEN I is known as the Wermer syndrome. Type II (MEN II) comprises tumors of the thyroid (medullary carcinoma) and the adrenal medulla (pheochromocytoma) and chief cell hyperplasia of the parathyroids. The familial form of MEN II is known as the Sipple syndrome. Type III, sometimes considered part of Type II, includes thyroid carcinoma (medullary), pheochromocytoma, and associated neurologic abnormalities, mucosal neuromas, and hyperplastic corneal nerves. Also called *multiple endocrine adenomatosis, polyendocrine adenomatosis, pluriglandular adenomatosis, pluriglandular syndrome, endocrine adenomatosis, familial polyendocrine adenomatosis, multiple endocrine adenomas, polyendocrinoma, endocrine polyglandular syndrome, polyglandular syndrome.* Abbreviation: MEN

neoplasm [NEO- + -PLASM] A benign or malignant expanding lesion composed of proliferating cells; a tumor. Also called *neoformation, new growth, histioma* (obsolete), *histoma* (obsolete), *true tumor, oncoma.*

benign neoplasm A neoplasm that cannot metastasize. It typically grows in an expansile manner, displacing or compressing surrounding tissues rather than invading them.

histoid neoplasm A neoplasm which resembles the tissue in which it arises. An outmoded term.

inflammatory fungoid neoplasm MYCOSIS FUNGOIDES.

malignant neoplasm CANCER.

metastatic neoplasm 1 A primary neoplasm which has metastasized. 2 METASTASIS.

organoid neoplasm A neoplasm which resembles an organ.

trophoblastic neoplasm Any of a group of biologically and morphologically interrelated tumors of trophoblastic tissue that arise either from pregnancy (gestational) or from ovary, testes, or extragonadal tissues (nongestational).

neoplasmatic Having the properties of a neoplasm.

neoplastic [NEO- + -PLAST + -IC] Pertaining to a tumor or tumor formation.

neoplastigenic [NEO- + -PLAST + *i* + -GENIC] ONCOGENIC.

neoprene A synthetic rubber formed by polymerization of 2-chlorobutadiene (CH_2=CCl—CH=CH_2). It is more resistant to oil than is natural rubber.

Neopsylla A genus of fleas parasitizing rodents.

Neorickettsia helminthoeca The species responsible for poisoning dogs and other mammals that eat raw salmon infected with the metacercariae of a nanophyetid fluke (*Nanophyetes salmincola*) that harbors the rickettsial organisms. About 90 percent of infected dogs die, but those that recover usually have a life-long immunity.

Neornithes [Gk *ne(os)* new, recent + *ornis,* pl. *ornithes,* bird] One of the two avian subclasses; true birds. It includes all modern birds and fossil birds, but excludes the ancestral bird Archaeopteryx. Distribution is worldwide, except for the Antarctic region.

Neoschoengastia A genus of chigger mites (family Trombiculidae) that affects birds.

Neoschoengastia americana The turkey chigger mite, a species infesting turkey poults and quail and probably other birds in the southeastern United States.

neosensibility Sensory information perceived in phylogenetically newer parts of the cerebral cortex. A seldom used term.

neostigmine bromide   The bromide salt of neostigmine. It is a white, crystalline powder, used as a cholinergic drug in the symptomatic treatment of myasthenia gravis. It is also used as a miotic, and may be given orally or applied topically to the conjunctiva.

neostigmine methylsulfate   The methylsulfate salt of neostigmine. It is a white, crystalline powder, used as a reversible cholinesterase inhibitor in the symptomatic treatment of myasthenia gravis. It is also used for urinary retention and as an antidote for excessive treatment with curare. It is given either intravenously or subcutaneously.

neostomy [NEO- + -STOMY]   The creation of an artificial opening into any organ or body cavity.

neostriatum   The phylogenetically newest parts of the corpus striatum that share a common origin, including the caudate nucleus and the putamen. Also called *striatum*.

neostrophingic [NEO- + Gk *stroph(ē)* a turning + English *(h)ing(e)* + -IC]   Of or relating to the surgical relief of mitral stenosis by rehinging the septal leaflet. The procedure is performed by extending the arcuate line of valve closure.

Neo-Synephrine   A proprietary name for phenylephrine hydrochloride.

neotenin   JUVENILE HORMONE.

neoteny [NEO- + New L *-ten(ia)*, combining form from Gk *teinein* to extend + -Y]   The extension of the larval state, such as occurs in certain termite castes which hold larvae as future replacements of the queen. This condition can be induced under laboratory conditions by injection of the juvenile hormone neotenin into developing insects, which inhibits the maturation process stimulated by the opposing growth and differentiation hormone, ecdysone. Compare PEDOGENESIS.

neothalamus   The phylogenetically newest part of the thalamus, especially the ventrolateral and dorsolateral nuclei. • These were formerly contrasted with the so-called paleothalamus, or medial and midline nuclei, which were not believed to project to the neocortex. Reciprocal connections between these medial thalamic structures and the neocortex are now known to exist, so that the term has essentially lost its significance.

Neothylline   A proprietary name for dyphylline.

Neotoma lepida   The desert wood rat, found in the western parts of North America, from which *Brucella neotomae* has been isolated.

neovascular   Pertaining to or characterized by newly formed vessels.

neovascularization   The formation of new blood vessels in abnormal locations, as in diabetic retinopathy, or in abnormal tissues, as in tumors.

nepenthic   **1** Producing peace, tranquillity, or forgetfulness. **2** A nepenthic drug or agent.

neper [after John *Napier,* Scottish mathematician, 1550–1617]   A unit, used especially in telecommunications, expressing the ratio between powers P_1 and P_2 equal to $\log_e P_1/P_2$. Symbol: Np, N

nephablepsia [Gk *neph(os)* a cloud + *ablepsia* blindness]   Reduced vision due to reduced transparency of the cornea. Also called *nephelopia*.

nephalism [Gk *nēphal(ios)* drinking no wine + -ISM]   Abstinence from alcoholic beverages.

nephela [Gk *nephelē* cloud, cloud mass]   **1** A cloudy appearance of urine.   **2** A white scar of the cornea.

nephelometer [Gk *nephel(ē)* a cloud + *o* + -METER]   A photometer designed to estimate the amount of particulate matter

in a turbid medium, measuring light-scattering properties to make comparisons with a series of standard suspensions. Also called *suspensiometer.*

photoelectric nephelometer   A nephelometer in which the scattered light falls upon and is measured by a photoelectric cell.

nephelometry [Gk *nephel(ē)* a cloud + *o* + -METRY]   The estimation of the concentration of particles in a suspension by means of a nephelometer. Also called *nephalometric analysis.*

nephelopia [Gk *nephel(ē)* a cloud + -OPIA]   NEPHABLEPSIA.

nephr-   NEPHRO-.

nephradenoma [NEPHR- + ADENOMA]   An adenoma of the kidney.

nephralgia [NEPHR- + -ALGIA]   Pain in the renal area. Adjective: nephralgic.

nephranuria [NEPHR- + ANURIA]   Scanty or absent excretion of urine.

nephrasthenia [NEPHR- + ASTHENIA]   Mild renal disease. An obsolete term.

nephrauxe [NEPHR- + Gk *auxē* an increase]   NEPHROMEGALY.

nephrectasia [NEPHR- + ECTASIA]   Distension of the renal pelvis, usually secondary to obstruction. Also called *nephrectasis, sacciform kidney.*

nephrectasis   NEPHRECTASIA.

nephrectomize   To perform a nephrectomy on.

nephrectomy [NEPHR- + -ECTOMY]   The resection of one or both kidneys.

abdominal nephrectomy   A nephrectomy using an anterior, transperitoneal approach. Also called *anterior nephrectomy.*

anterior nephrectomy   ABDOMINAL NEPHRECTOMY.

lumbar nephrectomy   A nephrectomy using a posterior, retroperitoneal approach through a flank incision. Also called *paraperitoneal nephrectomy, posterior nephrectomy.*

paraperitoneal nephrectomy   LUMBAR NEPHRECTOMY.

partial nephrectomy   Surgical removal of a portion of the kidney.

posterior nephrectomy   LUMBAR NEPHRECTOMY.

radical nephrectomy   Total removal of the kidney and surrounding tissues, usually as a surgical treatment of cancer of the kidney.

simple nephrectomy   Surgical removal of the kidney without the removal of surrounding tissues characteristic of radical nephrectomy.

transthoracic nephrectomy   The resection of one or both kidneys by making an incision in the chest and exposing the kidneys through the diaphragm.

nephredema [NEPHR- + EDEMA]   Edema or congestion of the kidney. Also called *nephremia.*

nephrelcosis   Ulceration of the mucous membrane of the kidney pelvis or calices of the kidney.

nephremia [NEPHR- + -EMIA]   NEPHREDEMA.

nephresia   Any pathological disorder of a kidney. An obsolete term.

nephric [NEPHR- + -IC]   Pertaining to or related to the kidney.

nephridium [NEPHR- + -IDIUM]   A segmental excretory tubule present in some invertebrates. It extends from an opening in the coelom to one on the exterior of the animal.

nephritic   Of, relating to, or affected by nephritis.

nephritides   Plural of NEPHRITIS.

nephritis

nephritis [NEPHR- + -ITIS] Inflammation of the kidney, involving the parenchyma, interstitium, or vascular system of the organ.

acute nephritis ACUTE DIFFUSE GLOMERULONEPHRITIS.

acute focal nephritis An acute process involving the glomeruli or the renal interstitium in a focal distribution.

acute serum sickness nephritis Acute nephritis occurring in the course of serum sickness. It is characterized clinically by the acute nephritic syndrome with oliguria and hematuria; and pathologically by acute diffuse proliferative glomerulonephritis, with immunofluorescent and electromicroscopic evidence of immune complex pathogenesis. Serum complement is reduced. This form of nephritis can be readily produced in experimental animals by two appropriately spaced injections of a foreign protein. Immune complex reaction to penicillin may be a close approximation of serum sickness nephritis.

acute suppurative nephritis RENAL ABSCESS.

allergic nephritis 1 Acute renal parenchymal, interstitial, or vascular hypersensitivity reaction to a drug or food. 2 An inflammatory reaction produced in the kidney by an immunologic mechanism.

anaphylactoid purpura nephritis SCHÖNLEIN-HENOCH PURPURA NEPHRITIS.

antiglomerular basement membrane antibody nephritis GOODPASTURE SYNDROME.

antitubular basement membrane tubulointerstitial nephritis Tubulointerstitial nephritis due to antibodies directed against tubular basement membrane material. Such antibodies and disease may be produced in experimental animals. Antitubular basement membrane antibodies have been demonstrated in association with antiglomerular basement membrane antibodies in the Goodpasture syndrome, methicillin poisoning, and renal transplant rejection, or alone in some instances of tubulointerstitial nephritis.

arteriosclerotic nephritis ARTERIONEPHROSCLEROSIS.

ascending nephritis Acute or chronic infection of renal parenchyma secondary to urinary tract infection.

azotemic nephritis Any nephritis associated with nitrogen retention due to inadequate glomerular filtration.

bacterial nephritis PYELONEPHRITIS.

Balkan nephritis A chronic progressive interstitial nephritis characterized by focal tubular atrophy, and interstitial edema and infiltration leading to interstitial fibrosis and contracted kidneys. The disease occurs only in the area where Yugoslavia, Rumania, and Bulgaria meet. The geographical distribution suggests some toxin but the etiology remains unknown. Clinically, the disease is characterized by impaired concentrating ability, mild proteinuria, tubular acidosis, and progressive renal failure, along with high incidence of papillary transition cell carcinoma in the renal pelvis and upper ureter. Also called *Balkan nephropathy.*

capsular nephritis A rarely used term for EXTRACAPILLARY GLOMERULONEPHRITIS.

caseous nephritis Renal abscesses with caseous deposits. Also called *cheesy nephritis.*

catarrhal nephritis Desquamation of renal tubule epithelial cells. A seldom used term.

cheesy nephritis CASEOUS NEPHRITIS.

chronic nephritis Slowly progressive nephritis with persistent proteinuria and often microscopic hematuria and cylinduria.

Progressive renal insufficiency eventually is complicated by uremia, hypertension, edema, and visual disturbances. Renal functions are decreased. Anatomically, the kidneys usually are small with a granular surface. Microscopically, hyalinized glomeruli are associated with vascular sclerosis, interstitial fibrosis, and tubule degeneration. Chronic nephritis may follow acute nephritis or a number of other renal diseases, or may be idiopathic. Most instances of chronic nephritis are glomerular or vascular in origin.

chronic interstitial nephritis Renal insterstitial cellular infiltration, fibrosis, and tubular damage. Glomerular involvement occurs only in the late stages. Clinical manifestations include little or no proteinuria, minimal pyuria, impaired concentrating ability, and slowly progressive renal failure with acidosis and inability to conserve sodium. The condition may occur in infections, ischemia, analgesic abuse, sickle cell anemia, urinary tract obstruction, and Balkan nephritis.

chronic parenchymatous nephritis Any chronic involvement of the renal parenchyma.

chronic suppurative nephritis Chronic abscesses in one or both kidneys.

congenital nephritis Nephritis present at birth. It is often a result of congenital syphilis.

degenerative nephritis An obsolete term for LIPOID NEPHROSIS.

diffuse nephritis Nephritis characterized by lesions involving all nephrons.

diffuse suppurative nephritis Multiple abscesses in one or both kidneys.

nephritis dolorosa Painful thickening of the renal capsule due to inflammation of unknown etiology.

dropsical nephritis Nephritis associated with the nephrotic syndrome.

embolic nephritis FOCAL EMBOLIC GLOMERULONEPHRITIS.

embolic nonsuppurative focal nephritis The original term for FOCAL EMBOLIC GLOMERULONEPHRITIS.

epidemic nephritis Acute nephritis which occurs in epidemics. Former epidemics were of unknown etiology, but in recent years epidemics of poststreptococcal acute glomerulonephritis have been associated with nephritogenic group A hemolytic streptococcal infections of the skin or pharynx.

epimembranous nephritis MEMBRANOUS NEPHRITIS.

exudative nephritis Any renal lesion with leukocytic infiltration.

familial nephritis HEREDITARY NEPHRITIS.

familial hemorrhagic nephritis HEREDITARY NEPHRITIS.

fibrolipomatous nephritis Perinephritis in which the perirenal fat is fibrosed and scarred.

fibrotic nephritis NEPHROSCLEROSIS.

fibrous nephritis NEPHROSCLEROSIS.

focal embolic nephritis FOCAL EMBOLIC GLOMERULONEPHRITIS.

glomerular nephritis GLOMERULONEPHRITIS.

glomerulocapsular nephritis A rarely used term for EXTRACAPILLARY GLOMERULONEPHRITIS.

nephritis gravidarum NEPHRITIS OF PREGNANCY.

hemorrhagic nephritis Nephritis in which the predominant symptom is hematuria.

hemotogenous nephritis Acute, rapidly progressive, or chronic nephritis in which an infectious or toxic agent is the cause of the nephritis or in which the agent reaches the kidney via the bloodstream.

hereditary nephritis A genetically heterogenous group of disorders characterized by familial nephropathy of various types, with or without other organ involvement. It includes the Alport syndrome and familial nephropathy with and without gout. Also called *familial nephritis, familial hemorrhagic nephritis, familial nephropathy, hereditary hematuria.*

hereditary nephritis and nerve deafness A genetically heterogenous group of disorders characterized by progressive nephritis, variable sensorineural deafness, and variable ocular abnormalities. X-linked and, perhaps, autosomal recessive forms occur, as well as an autosomal dominant form known as the Alport syndrome.

Heymann's nephritis HEYMANN'S NEPHROSIS.

hydremic nephritis An outmoded term for NEPHROTIC SYNDROME.

hydropigenous nephritis An outmoded term for NEPHROTIC SYNDROME.

indurative nephritis A scarred and contracted condition of a kidney. A rarely used term.

interstitial nephritis 1 Acute or chronic nephritis characterized by primary or secondary inflammation of the renal interstitium. The acute form presents as the nephrotic syndrome and is due to an adverse reaction to a drug, acute deposition of uric acid, a remote reaction to an infection, or to direct pyogenic suppuration. The chronic form involves variable degrees of interstitial cellular infiltration and fibrosis with early damage to the lower tubules and late glomerular damage. Proteinuria is usually minimal. Hypertension is a late development. The chronic form is common in many conditions including analgesic abuse, drug hypersensitivities, infections, ischemia, sickle-cell anemia, hypokalemia, hyperkalemia, and urinary-tract obstruction. Also called *tubulointerstitial nephritis.* 2 NEPHROSCLEROSIS.

interstitial granulomatous nephritis Nephritis characterized by focal distribution of granulomas in the renal interstitium. It may be caused by a variety of chronic infections such as tuberculosis, syphilis, brucellosis, or mycoses, by accumulations of urate crystals, or by surrounding casts in distal tubules in multiple myeloma. Granulomas are characterized by giant cells, mononuclear cells, and increased fibrous tissue.

interstitial nonsuppurative nephritis Nephritis characterized by infiltration of the renal interstitium by inflammatory cells and edema fluid in the acute stage. Later, interstitial fibrosis may develop. The disease may develop acutely in the course of an infection or as a reaction to a drug. The chronic form may follow as the acute phase subsides or may develop insidiously. Differentiation from chronic pyelonephritis is difficult if not impossible.

interstitial scarlatinal nephritis An acute, nonsuppurative, interstitial nephritis, once a common complication of scarlet fever. It has almost disappeared since the advent of antibiotic therapy.

interstitial suppurative nephritis Infection of the renal parenchyma, either of hematogenous origin or secondary to ascending extension of a urinary tract infection.

interstitial syphilitic nephritis 1 Nephritis of congenital syphilis characterized by periglomerular and periarterial fibrosis. 2 Nephritis of syphilis in infants, characterized by gummas in the renal interstitium.

Lancereaux's nephritis Interstitial nephritis formerly attributed to rheumatic fever. An outmoded term.

latent nephritis The asymptomatic phase of chronic glomerulonephritis.

leptospiral nephritis Leptospirosis involving the kidney with distal convoluted tubule dilatation, necrosis, and basement membrane rupture in the early stages, and later with interstitial edema and infiltration with lymphocytes, neutrophils, plasma cells and histiocytes. Glomerular lesions occur late and are nonspecific. Hemorrhages into the renal parenchyma characterize the later phases of severe cases, and acute tubular necrosis is a serious complication. Clinically, renal involvement is man-

ifested by proteinuria, hematuria, pyuria, and rapidly progressive renal failure. Recovery of renal function in survivors is the rule, although some permanent impairment of concentrating ability is common. Leptospira may be recovered from the blood and urine in the acute phase.

lipomatous nephritis A rarely used term for LIPOID NEPHROSIS.

Löhlein's nephritis FOCAL EMBOLIC GLOMERULONEPHRITIS.

lupus nephritis Any of the several forms of glomerulonephritis that may occur during the course of systemic lupus erythematosus. Focal glomerulonephritis is associated with little proteinuria, microscopic hematuria, and little impairment of renal function. The prognosis usually is good, but the condition may become more diffuse and lead to renal failure. Diffuse proliferative glomerulonephritis is more serious and is characterized by more proteinuria, hematuria, cylinduria, and renal functional impairment. A third variety of lupus nephritis is diffuse membranous glomerulopathy and a fourth is membranoproliferative glomerulonephritis. Both have an intermediate prognosis. These forms are mesangial IgA/IgG glomerulonephritis and arteritis. The pathogenesis of all forms of lupus nephritis is assumed to be related to circulating immune complexes. IgG, other immunoglobulins, and complement components are easily demonstrable in glomeruli by immunofluorescent techniques. Serum complement fractions are reduced in active forms of proliferative lupus nephritis. Treatment with steroid hormones and immunosuppressive agents appears to be effective. Recently, plasmapheresis plus immunosuppression have appeared promising.

Masugi nephritis An experimental glomerulonephritis produced in rats by injections of heterologous antibodies against glomerular basement membrane material. The lesion is characterized by continuous accumulation of immunoglobulins and complement components along the glomerular capillary basement membranes. This was the original model for immunologically produced glomerulonephritis. Also called *nephrotoxic nephritis.*

membranous nephritis A renal lesion in which immune deposits are seen on the subepithelial side of the glomerular basement membrane. Also called *epimembranous nephritis.*

nephrotoxic nephritis MASUGI NEPHRITIS.

parenchymatous nephritis Any acute or chronic disease involving the renal parenchyma.

pneumococcal nephritis Acute nephritis following a pneumococcal infection. It has been described clinically in a few cases but only rarely has concomitant group A hemolytic streptococcal infection been ruled out.

poststreptococcal nephritis POSTSTREPTOCOCCAL ACUTE GLOMERULONEPHRITIS.

potassium-losing nephritis Any chronic nephritis in which deficient tubular reabsorption of potassium leads to a negative potassium balance. Only moderate impairment of renal function may be present, proteinuria usually is minimal, and muscle weakness and characteristic electrocardiographic changes reflect potassium deficiency.

nephritis of pregnancy Any nephritic condition occuring during pregnancy, excluding toxemia of pregnancy. Also called *nephritis gravidarum.*

radiation nephritis Interstitial nephritis and arteriolar lesions with chronic progressive renal failure and often hypertension resulting from irradiation of a kidney exceeding 2300 rads.

salt-losing nephritis A syndrome in patients with chronic nephritis who lose excess amounts of sodium chloride in the urine, characterized by polyuria, hyponatremia, dehydration, asthenia, muscle cramps, nausea, and vomiting. Diagnostic criteria include appearance of symptoms of dehydration on normal salt intake, and control of symptoms by saline administration. Also called *salt-wasting nephritis.*

salt-wasting nephritis   SALT-LOSING NEPHRITIS.

saturnine nephritis   Nephritis due to chronic lead poisoning.

scarlatinal nephritis   Acute glomerulonephritis secondary to scarlet fever.

Schönlein-Henoch purpura nephritis   Glomerulonephritis in the form of glomerular lesions associated with Schönlein-Henoch purpura. The disease is commoner and usually less severe in young persons than in adults. By immunofluorescent techniques IgA and C3, and sometimes IgG, can be demonstrated in a granular pattern in the mesangium. The lesions are similar to those of IgA nephropathy. Also called *anaphylactoid purpura nephritis.*

shunt nephritis   A glomerulonephritis probably of immune complex pathogenesis secondary to infection of a ventriculoatrial, ventriculojugular, or ventriculoperitoneal shunt established in a child or, sometimes, an adult to correct internal hydrocephalus, and consisting of membranous or mesangiocapillary lesions. The clinical findings include proteinuria, microhematuria, and renal function impairment. Serum C3 levels usually are low and rheumatoid factor and cryoglobulins often are present. The infecting organism most frequently is a coagulase-negative staphylococcus, but numerous other organisms have been implicated. Early recognition and appropriate antibiotic therapy are important and may lead to healing of the glomerular lesions.

Steblay nephritis   AUTOIMMUNE GLOMERULONEPHRITIS.

subacute nephritis   RAPIDLY PROGRESSIVE GLOMERULONEPHRITIS.

suppurative nephritis   Abscesses in one or both kidneys.

suppurative cortical nephritis   Multiple abscesses in the renal cortex, usually due to staphylococci.

syphilitic nephritis   Glomerular lesions which may develop with or without the nephrotic syndrome in both congenital and secondary syphilis. The lesions usually are membranous, often with some degree of proliferation. Granular deposits of IgG and complement suggest an immune-complex pathogenesis. Elution of antitreponemal antibody from the glomeruli of a man with acquired syphilis supports this hypothesis. The lesions in this patient and in several others have been reported to resolve after penicillin therapy. However, spontaneous resolution also has been reported. Gummas of the kidney may develop in tertiary syphilis.

transfusion nephritis   Acute tubular necrosis and renal failure secondary to intravascular hemolysis in a mismatched blood transfusion.

trench nephritis   WAR NEPHRITIS.

tubal nephritis   TUBULAR NEPHRITIS.

tuberculous nephritis   RENAL TUBERCULOSIS.

tubular nephritis   Renal disease affecting the renal tubules. It occurs in renal tubular acidosis, the Fanconi syndrome, acute renal failure, and tubulointerstitial nephritis. Also called *tubal nephritis.*

tubulointerstitial nephritis   INTERSTITIAL NEPHRITIS.

vascular nephritis   NEPHROSCLEROSIS.

war nephritis   Acute epidemic nephritis occurring under war conditions as in the American Civil War and in World War I, presumably due to group A hemolytic streptococci. Also called *trench nephritis.*

water-losing nephritis   NEPHROGENIC DIABETES INSIPIDUS.

---

nephritogenic [*nephrit(is)* + *o* + -GENIC]   Causing nephritis: said of conditions, or of agents such as strains of group A hemolytic streptococci that cause acute glomerulonephritis.

nephro- [Gk *nephros* kidney]   A combining form denoting the kidney. Also *nephr.*

nephroangiosclerosis   NEPHROSCLEROSIS.

nephroblastoma [NEPHRO- + BLASTOMA]   A malignant renal tumor of nephroblastic tissue forming structures which resemble embryonic kidney. It is typically a tumor of childhood. Also called *Wilms tumor, adenosarcoma, embryonal adenosarcoma* (outmoded), *embryonal nephroma, malignant nephroma, hamartoblastoma of the kidney* (outmoded), *embryonal sarcoma, embryonal mixed tumor of the kidney, embryoma of kidney, blastomal tumor, embryonal carcinosarcoma.*

nephrocalcinosis   The presence of calcium deposits in the renal interstitium, tubule cells and lumen, and occasionally the glomeruli, but most commonly in the medulla. Calcium deposition in the proximal tubule cells is due to renal tubular acidosis, or to calcium mobilization and hypercalcemia of any origin, including hyperparathyroidism, excessive vitamin D intake, the milk-alkali syndrome, and sarcoidosis. Nephrocalcinosis also may be drug-induced. Nephrocalcinosis may cause renal calculi, renal tubule dysfunction, or chronic renal failure. Local calcification may occur in renal tuberculosis, infarction, and malignant tumor. Also called *renal calcification.*

drug-induced nephrocalcinosis   Nephrocalcinosis secondary to administration of such drugs as calciferol, the milk-alkali syndrome encountered in the long-term intake of excessive amounts of milk, oxalate deposition following methoxyflurane anesthesia, or crystal formation in the kidneys due to sulfonamide therapy. Phosphate loading may also cause nephrocalcinosis, especially in the presence of hypercalcemia, resulting in renal failure.

nephrocapsectomy   NEPHROCAPSULECTOMY.

nephrocapsulectomy   The removal of the renal capsule from one or both kidneys; decapsulation of the kidney. Also called *nephrocapsectomy.*

nephrocapsulotomy   An incision into the renal capsule of one or both kidneys for the purpose of exploration or decompression.

nephrocarcinoma [NEPHRO- + CARCINOMA]   A carcinoma of the kidney.

nephrocele [NEPHRO- + -CELE[1]]   A hernia containing a kidney.

nephrochalazosis   The small and granular kidney seen in chronic nephritis and arteriosclerosis. An obsolete term.

nephrocirrhosis   CIRRHOSIS OF THE KIDNEY.

nephrocoele [NEPHRO- + -COELE]   The cavity of the nephrotome in an embryo.

nephrocolic   **1** RENAL COLIC. **2** Pertaining to both colon and kidney.

nephrocolopexy   A surgical procedure in which the kidney and colon are sutured to the nephrocolic ligament for the purpose of suspension or prevention of ptosis.

nephrocoloptosis   Displacement of the kidneys and colon toward the pelvic area.

nephrocystanastomosis [NEPHRO- + CYST- + ANASTOMOSIS]   A surgical connection between the kidney and the bladder.

nephrocystitis [NEPHRO- + CYSTITIS]   Inflammation of the kidneys and bladder.

nephrocystosis   The presence of renal cysts.

nephroerysipelas   Erysipelas complicated by nephritis.

nephrogastric [NEPHRO- + GASTRIC]   Pertaining to the kidneys and stomach.

nephrogenesis [NEPHRO- + GENESIS]   The formation of a kidney or of renal tissue.

nephrogenic [NEPHRO- + -GENIC]   Developing kidney tissue. Also *renogenic, nephropoietic.*

nephrogenous [NEPHRO- + -GENOUS] Pertaining to or originating in the kidneys.

nephrogram [NEPHRO- + -GRAM] The appearance of renal parenchymal opacification during intravenous urography or renal angiography.

nephrography [NEPHRO- + -GRAPHY] Radiography of the kidney whose parenchyma has been opacified by appropriate iodinated contrast medium intravascularly administered.
isotope nephrography An inaccurate term for RADIORENOGRAPHY.

nephrohemorrhagia [NEPHRO- + HEMO- + -RRHAGIA] Bleeding from the kidneys.

nephrohypertrophy [NEPHRO- + HYPERTROPHY] RENAL HYPERTROPHY.

nephroid Resembling the shape or nature of a kidney. Also *reniform*.

nephrolith RENAL CALCULUS.

nephrolithiasis The presence of renal calculi. Calcareous stones account for approximately 90 percent of cases, and usually are secondary to hypercalciuria due to excess resorption of bone, increased intestinal absorption of calcium, or impaired renal tubule reabsorption of calcium. Hyperuricemia hyperoxaluria also may lead formation of calcareous stones. Noncalcareous stones may be formed by uric acid, cystine, or xanthine. Also called *renal lithiasis*.
uric acid nephrolithiasis Nephrolithiasis caused by uric acid stones, usually a consequence of hyperuricemia.

nephrolithotomy An incision into the renal parenchyma for the purpose of removing one of more renal calculi. Also called *lithonephrotomy*.

nephrologic 1 Pertaining to the kidneys. 2 Related to nephrology.

nephrologist [NEPHR- + -OLOGIST] A specialist in nephrology.

nephrology [NEPHRO- + -LOGY] A subspecialty of internal medicine comprising the study of the kidney, its structure, function, and diseases, and of hypertensive and fluid electrolyte disorders.

nephrolysin NEPHROTOXIN.

nephrolysis [NEPHRO- + LYSIS] Surgical separation of a kidney from perinephric adhesions. Adjective: nephrolytic.

nephrolytic Pertaining to or causing nephrolysis.

nephroma [NEPHR- + -OMA] A tumor of the kidney. Also called *nephroncus*.
congenital mesoblastic nephroma MESOBLASTIC NEPHROMA.
embryonal nephroma NEPHROBLASTOMA.
malignant nephroma 1 NEPHROBLASTOMA. 2 Carcinoma of the kidney.
mesoblastic nephroma A tumor of the kidney composed of tissue resembling smooth muscle. Cartilage and cysts may be present. It is typically present in infants and is considered benign. Also called *leiomyomatous hamartoma, fetal hamartoma, congenital mesoblastic nephroma, infantile mesenchymal hamartoma*.
multilocular cystic nephroma A rare congenital and benign unilateral multilocular lesion which contains dysontogenetic mesenchymatous tissues including cartilage and smooth and striated muscle. It is enclosed in a capsule.

nephromalacia A softening or dystrophy of the kidney. A rarely used term.

nephromegaly [NEPHRO- + -MEGALY] Enlargement of a kidney, usually as a result of compensatory hypertrophy after surgical removal or disease of the other kidney. Also called *nephrauxe, renomegaly*.

nephromere [NEPHRO- + -MERE] NEPHROTOME.

nephron [German, from Gk *nephros* kidney] The functional unit of the kidney, consisting of a glomerulus and attached tubule. A human kidney has approximately one million nephrons.
lower nephron The distal convoluted tubule and collecting ducts of the nephron.

nephroncus [NEPHR- + ONCUS] NEPHROMA.

nephronophthisis MEDULLARY CYSTIC DISEASE.
familial juvenile nephronophthisis Medullary cystic disease inherited as an autosomal recessive. It is usually fatal during childhood.

nephro-omentopexy An antiquated surgical procedure in which the greater omentum is used to cover a decapsulated ischemic kidney or kidneys. It was originally proposed as a means of establishing a new blood supply and thus treat hypertension.

nephropathia NEPHROPATHY.
nephropathia epidemica EPIDEMIC NEPHROPATHY.
nephropathia scandinavica EPIDEMIC NEPHROPATHY.

nephropathic [NEPHRO- + -PATH + -IC] Causing organic renal disease or impairment of renal function.

nephropathy [NEPHRO- + -PATHY] Any organic disease of the kidneys. Also called *nephropathica, renopathy, nephropathia*.
acute hypokalemic nephropathy Reversible histologic changes in the kidney, including vacuolization of proximal convoluted tubule cells and expansion of the subbasilar extracellular compartments, due to short-term potassium deficiency.
acute urate nephropathy Rapid deposition of urates in the interstitium and collecting tubules of the kidneys characterized clinically by acute renal failure. It usually follows effective chemotherapy of certain malignant disease such as leukemias and lymphomas when large amounts of nucleoprotein are released and converted to uric acid.
amphotericin B nephropathy The primary reaction to the toxicity of amphotericin B, with cylindruria as the first sign, soon followed by proteinuria, microhematuria, renal tubular acidosis with increasing urine pH, and then decrease of glomerular filtration rate to less than half of the pretreatment level. Focal necrosis of both proximal and distal tubules is interspersed with regenerative foci of epithelial cells. Calcification of tubule casts and the interstitium is a common feature. Diuresis and alkali administration should be maintained during amphotericin B therapy. If azotemia develops amphotericin B should be reduced or discontinued, and mannitol may be helpful. Usually renal function will return to normal.
analgesic nephropathy Kidney damage resulting from long-term analgesic ingestion, especially of phenacetin, although salicylates and other analgesics also have been implicated. The nephropathy is characterized by papillary necrosis and secondary obstructive changes in the cortex. Papillary necrosis may have a characteristic roentgenologic appearance, and sloughed necrotic papillae may cause renal colic. Impairment of concentrating ability is an early clinical feature, and hematuria and pyuria are common. Slowly progressive renal failure is usual.
bacitracin nephropathy Acute tubular necrosis and acute renal failure produced by systemic administration of bacitracin. This antibiotic is therefore limited to topical use.
Balkan nephropathy BALKAN NEPHRITIS.
bismuth nephropathy Renal tubule damage, caused by soluble bismuth salts and characterized by proteinuria, glycosuria, cylindruria, desquamation of tubule epithelial cells, and hyposthenuria. Anuria or the nephrotic syndrome may develop. This condition has become uncommon since the abandonment of bismuth therapy for syphilis. Also called *bismuth toxicity, bismuth nephrotoxicity*.

cadmium nephropathy   Proteinuria with little or no histologic changes following ingestion of or exposure to cadmium. It may also be accompanied by glycosuria, hypercalciuria, aminoaciduria, and increased uric acid excretion with hypouricemia. Characteristic of cadmium toxicity in humans and animals is excretion of a protein of low molecular weight (20 000–30 000) which differs electrophoretically from protein excreted in other metal intoxications.

carbon tetrachloride nephropathy   Acute tubular necrosis and acute renal failure due to ingestion, inhalation, or dermal absorption of carbon tetrachloride.

chronic hypokalemic nephropathy   Progressive chronic interstitial nephritis characterized by hyposthenuria and nocturia and renal failure, which are reversible in the early stages, due to prolonged potassium deficiency.

chronic urate nephropathy   Very slowly progressive renal failure associated with chronic hyperuricemia. Even after focal changes in the medulla and interstitium develop, renal function may remain normal. Proteinuria and impaired concentrating ability are the first signs of chronic urate nephropathy, followed by decreasing glomerular filtration rate. The passage of urate stones or gravel may occur, but is not necessary to make the diagnosis.

copper nephropathy   Intravascular hemolysis and acute tubular necrosis, especially of the ascending limb of the loop of Henle and the distal convoluted tubules, due to acute copper poisoning, usually from ingestion of copper sulfate.

diabetic nephropathy   Any renal disease related to diabetes mellitus, including diabetic glomerulosclerosis, arterionephrosclerosis, arteriolonephrosclerosis, and papillary necrosis and pyelonephritis.

dropsical nephropathy   Any nephropathy associated with the nephrotic syndrome.

epidemic nephropathy   A febrile illness, found in northern Scandinavia and Finland, which is followed by heavy proteinuria, oliguria, and moderate renal failure. Recovery is prompt and complete. It has been established that this disease is caused by a virus either identical to or closely related to that responsible for epidemic hemorrhagic fever (Hantaan virus). Clinically, however, it is considerably milder and carries a lower mortality. Also called *Myhrman-Zetterholm disease, nephropathia epidemica, nephropathia scandinavica.* See also EPIDEMIC HEMORRHAGIC FEVER.

ethylene glycol nephropathy   The precipitation of calcium oxalate crystals in the renal tubules, with necrosis of the epithelial cells and acute renal failure, following the ingestion of ethylene glycol. The effects of this common automobile antifreeze on the central nervous system resemble those of ethanol. Metabolism of ethylene glycol produces oxalic acid. Metabolic acidosis may be severe due to the combination of oxalic acid and renal failure. A dose of 100 milliliters of ethylene glycol is fatal, and for lesser doses the fatality rate is high. Also called *ethylene glycol nephrotoxicity, glycol nephrotoxicity.*

familial nephropathy   HEREDITARY NEPHRITIS.

gold nephropathy   Proteinuria followed by the nephrotic syndrome developing in a small percentage of cases of rheumatoid arthritis treated with organic gold salts. Immune deposits or gold deposits or both may appear in the lysosomes of the proximal tubules, and immune subendothelial deposits may occur in the glomeruli. The lesions and clinical manifestations usually disappear when gold therapy is discontinued.

gouty nephropathy   Urate nephropathy or nephrosclerosis developing during the course of gout. Also called *gouty kidney.*

hypazoturic nephropathy   Nephropathy with nitrogen retention. An outmoded term.

hypercalcemic nephropathy   Functional and histologic abnormalities of the kidneys due to hypercalcemia from any cause, the severity being related to the duration of the hypercalcemia. Impairment of renal concentrating ability is an early sign which may be followed rapidly by decreased glomerular filtration rate and renal failure.

hyperuricemic nephropathy   URATE NEPHROPATHY.

hypokalemic nephropathy   Renal functional impairment and renal lesions due to potassium deficiency. Also called *kaliopenic nephropathy, nephropathy of potassium depletion, hypokalemic nephrosis.*

iodide nephropathy   Nephropathy related to the iodide in contrast media used in radiography of vasculature and of urinary or biliary tracts. Nephrotoxicity may result in direct cellular toxicity, decreased renal blood flow, obstructive uric acid crystalluria, or an idiosyncratic reaction. Dose-related decrease in renal function or acute tubular, medullary, or cortical necrosis may develop. Dehydration prior to radiography and excessive contrast dosage should be avoided.

iron nephropathy   Acute tubular necrosis and acute renal failure in children as a result of large doses of ferrous sulfate. Hemochromatosis and severe hemosiderosis may result in iron pigment deposition, interstitial fibrosis, and chronic renal failure.

kaliopenic nephropathy   HYPOKALEMIC NEPHROPATHY.

kanamycin nephropathy   Proteinuria, microscopic hematuria, and cylindruria resulting from kanamycin therapy. At a dosage of 25–50 mg/kg/day it develops in 10–20 percent of patients. Two to three weeks on this dose causes significant decrease in glomerular filtration rate and concentrating ability in half the patients. The incidence of kanamycin nephropathy is greater in cases of pre-existing renal disease and of concomitant streptomycin or viomicin therapy.

lead nephropathy   An interstitial nephritis resulting from chronic ingestion of lead. Two types of renal effects have been observed in man: damage to the proximal tubules with a decrease in the tubular reabsorption of glucose, amino acids, and phosphate; and interstitial fibrosis, sclerosis of blood vessels, and glomerular atrophy.

malarial nephropathy   Clinical or histopathologic renal disorders associated with *Plasmodium malariae* malarial infections, sometimes leading to the nephrotic syndrome and progressive renal failure. Glomerular lesions may be proliferative, membranous, or mesangiocapillary. Most commonly found in Africa, especially among adolescents. In all varieties, response to steroid and other therapies has been poor or absent. Falciparum malaria is a rare cause of proliferative glomerulonephritis, in addition to being associated with blackwater fever and acute renal failure.

membranous nephropathy   MEMBRANOUS GLOMERULONEPHRITIS.

mercury nephropathy   Acute tubular necrosis and acute renal failure following ingestion or inhalation of organic or inorganic mercury compounds. In chronic mercury nephropathy, proteinuria may result in the nephrotic syndrome.

mesangial nephropathy   MESANGIAL IGA/IGG GLOMERULONEPHRITIS.

mesangial IgA/IgG nephropathy   MESANGIAL IGA/IGG GLOMERULONEPHRITIS.

neomycin nephropathy   Acute tubular necrosis and acute renal failure resulting from parenteral administration or following large oral doses of neomycin, especially in the presence of pre-existing renal or gastrointestinal disease. For this reason, neomycin is usually restricted to topical applications.

obstructive nephropathy   Nephropathy due to obstruction of the urinary tract.

oxalate nephropathy   Any of variety of renal diseases possibly related to excess oxalate production or gastrointestinal absorption, which may result in oxalate deposition, calcium oxalate calculi, or nephrocalcinosis. Causes of oxalate nephropathy include excess intake of foods high in oxalic acid, such as rhubarb and beets, ethylene and other glycol exposure, and primary or acquired increases of oxalate excretion, as in primary or secondary hyperoxaluria.

phenacetin nephropathy See under ANALGESIC NEPHROPATHY.

polymyxin nephropathy Renal tubular necrosis, with proteinuria and decreased concentrating ability, related to dosage in polymixin therapy.

nephropathy of potassium depletion HYPOKALEMIC NEPHROPATHY.

quartan malarial nephropathy Nephrotic syndrome of immune-complex type, associated with *Plasmodium malariae* infection in children in west and east Africa. It has been reported to have a characteristic glomerular lesion consisting of thickening of the capillary wall with a focal or diffuse double contour appearance with subendothelial deposits and lacunae in the basement membrane on electron microscopy. By immunofluorescent study IgG, IgM, and often C3 granular deposits are distributed along the glomerular basement membrane. Most studies have been made in Nigeria and Uganda. Malarial nephropathy caused by *P. malariae* responds poorly or not at all to steroid therapy, and the prognosis is poor.

salt-losing nephropathy Any renal disease that results in excess salt excretion in the urine, usually related to tubulointerstitial disease or advanced renal failure. Salt-losing nephropathy is characterized by polyuria, hypovolemia and often hyponatremia. Dehydration and postural hypotension are common clinical features. The condition responds to salt and water replacement.

sickle cell nephropathy Chronic renal disease occurring in a person with sickle cell anemia and due to repeated infarctions of kidney tissue by intravascular sickling of erythrocytes. Such chronic renal disease is nearly universal in patients with homozygous sickle cell disease after several years of life, and may lead to severe azotemia and death.

silver nephropathy Acute renal failure due to silver salts. The condition has been reported in photo developers. In rabbits intraperitoneal silver salts cause tubular degeneration and silver deposits and edema in the renal interstitium.

streptomycin nephropathy Proteinuria and cylindruria consequent to streptomycin therapy. The condition occurs in up to 20 percent of patients on streptomycin. Only a few have decreased glomerular filtration rate and acute tubular necrosis is rare.

sulfonamide nephropathy Renal complications following sulfonamide therapy, usually caused by precipitation of insoluble crystals of such compounds as sulfapyridine, sulfadiazine, and sulfathiazole in the renal tubules and urinary tract. Symptoms are flank pain, hematuria, cylindruria, crystalluria, and renal failure. Although such side effects were common and serious in the first decade of sulfonamide therapy, they have been greatly reduced by the use of sulfonamide mixtures and more soluble congeners, and more effective antibiotics. The few instances of sulfonamide crystallization at present are due to overdosage. Hypersensitivity reaction to a sulfonamide may cause an acute interstitial nephritis and renal failure. Steroid therapy may be effective, and complete recovery is possible.

tetracycline nephropathy A toxic nephropathy due to degradation products of outdated tetracycline which appears after three or four days of administration as a reversible Fanconi syndrome or as Bence Jones proteinuria, transient hyperglycemia, and a maculopapular skin rash. Histopathologically, there may be tubular necrosis, desquamated epithelial cells and regenerative foci. Both new and outdated tetracyclines block protein synthesis and thus cause increased azotemia in persons whose renal function is already impaired.

toxic nephropathy Any disease of the kidney resulting from a toxic agent or from an adverse reaction to a drug. The primary damage usually is to the tubules. In severe instances either acute or chronic renal failure may develop.

tubular nephropathy Any disease of the renal tubules.

uranium nephropathy Necrosis of the proximal convoluted tubules and acute renal failure following administration of uranium to experimental animals. Proteinuria and cylindruria have been demonstrated in human volunteers with terminal cancer who received uranyl nitrate intravenously.

urate nephropathy Renal impairment consequent to the progressive decrease in glomerular filtration rate and tubule function which occurs in hyperuricemia as urate is deposited in the distal convoluted and collecting tubules where concentration and acidification are greatest. Resultant obstruction, dilatation, and subsequent atrophy of renal tubules proximal to the obstruction lead to necrosis and fibrosis. Urate deposits also occur in the interstitium, where they initiate an inflammatory reaction with lymphocytic infiltration and fibrosis. Large interstitial crystalline deposits distinguish urate from other forms of interstitial nephritis. Hyalinization and thickening of the intima and media of the renal arterioles and small arteries contribute to the renal ischemia of urate nephropathy. Also called *uric acid nephropathy, hyperuricemic nephropathy.*

uric acid nephropathy URATE NEPHROPATHY.

vascular nephropathy Any nephropathy associated with vasculitis, such as arteriolonephrosclerosis or arterionephrosclerosis.

nephropexy [NEPHRO- + -PEXY] A surgical procedure in which one or both floating kidneys are sutured to the abdominal wall for the purposes of suspension and prevention of ptosis.

nephrophagiasis [NEPHRO- + *phag(o)-* + -IASIS] The destruction of the kidney by parasitic infection.

nephropoietic [NEPHRO- + Gk *poiētik(os)* capable of making] NEPHROGENIC.

nephroptosis [NEPHRO- + PTOSIS] Abnormal mobility of a kidney, usually asymptomatic but occasionally responsible for renal colic. The kidneys are displaced toward the pelvis. Also called *movable kidney, floating kidney* (popular), *wandering kidney* (popular).

nephropyelitis [NEPHRO- + PYELITIS] Inflammation of the kidney and renal pelvis.

nephropyelography [NEPHRO- + PYELOGRAPHY] Radiography of the kidney after its pelvis and parenchyma have been opacified by the intravascular administration of an appropriate contrast medium. A seldom used term.

nephropyelolithotomy A surgical incision into the renal parenchyma for the purpose of removing one or more stones from the renal pelvis.

nephropyeloplasty [NEPHRO- + PYELO- + -PLASTY] The surgical reconstruction of a deformed or injured renal pelvis.

nephropyosis [NEPHRO- + PYO- + -SIS] Renal abscess.

nephrorrhagia [NEPHRO- + -RRHAGIA] Bleeding from a kidney.

nephrorrhaphy [NEPHRO- + -RRHAPHY] The insertion of single or multiple sutures in the kidney for the purpose of reconstruction after surgical intervention or trauma.

nephrosclerosis [NEPHRO- + SCLEROSIS] Interstitial fibrosis of the renal cortex and glomerulosclerosis due to renal arterial or arteriolar disease. Also called *nephroangiosclerosis, vascular nephritis, fibrotic nephritis, fibrous nephritis, interstitial nephritis, sclerotic kidney.* Adjective: nephrosclerotic.

arterial nephrosclerosis ARTERIONEPHROSCLEROSIS.

arteriolar nephrosclerosis ARTERIOLONEPHROSCLEROSIS.

benign nephrosclerosis ARTERIONEPHROSCLEROSIS.

congenital nephrosclerosis FOCAL GLOMERULOSCLEROSIS.

hyaline arteriolar nephrosclerosis Nephrosclerosis associated with hyaline thickening of the walls of the afferent arterioles in hypertension or diabetes.

hyperplastic arteriolar nephrosclerosis A marked thickening of the intima of interlobular and arcuate renal arteries in malignant hypertension, often associated with fibrinoid necrosis and an "onion skin" appearance of the arterioles and rapidly progressive renal failure.

intercapillary nephrosclerosis DIABETIC GLOMERULOSCLEROSIS.

malignant nephrosclerosis Nephrosclerosis associated with malignant hypertension and rapidly progressive renal failure.

senile nephrosclerosis Arterionephrosclerosis associated with aging and with slowly progressive renal failure.

nephrosclerotic [NEPHRO- + SCLEROTIC] Related to or pertaining to nephrosclerosis.

nephroses Plural of NEPHROSIS.

nephrosiderosis Iron deposition in the kidneys in hemosiderosis, or associated with frequent blood transfusions.

nephrosis [NEPHRO- + -SIS] NEPHROTIC SYNDROME. Adjective: nephrotic.

acute nephrosis Nephrotic syndrome of sudden onset. In severe cases it may cause hypovolemia, hypotension, and decreased glomerular filtration rate.

amyloid nephrosis Renal amyloidosis associated with the nephrotic syndrome.

cholemic nephrosis Nephropathy associated with obstructive jaundice or other hepatic or biliary dysfunction. An outmoded term.

chronic nephrosis Persistent or recurrent nephrotic syndrome.

congenital nephrosis Nephrotic syndrome developing in infancy in association with hematuria, cylinduria, hypertension, and progressive renal failure. Immunoglobulins and complement components may be demonstrated along the glomerular capillary basement membranes. Therapy is almost always ineffective, with death before age two.

glycogen nephrosis The presence of glycogen inclusions (Armanni-Ebstein lesions) in the pars recta of the proximal convoluted tubules in poorly controlled diabetes.

hemoglobinuric nephrosis Acute tubular necrosis and acute renal failure associated with acute intravascular hemolysis and hemoglobinuria. An outmoded term.

Heymann's nephrosis An experimental disease in rats produced by injection of homologous kidney extract and Freund's adjuvant. The disease is due to deposition of circulating complexes of autoantibodies and autologous antigens from renal tubular epithelial cells. Also called *Heymann's nephritis*.

hydropic nephrosis The presence of vacuoles in epithelial cells of the convoluted tubules. These may be related to physiologic processes or to disease, as in glycogen nephrosis.

hypokalemic nephrosis HYPOKALEMIC NEPHROPATHY.

hypoxic nephrosis Acute renal failure due to ischemic tubular necrosis.

larval nephrosis LIPOID NEPHROSIS.

lipemic nephrosis A rarely used term for LIPOID NEPHROSIS.

lipid nephrosis LIPOID NEPHROSIS.

lipoid nephrosis A primary glomerular disease characterized by heavy proteinuria and the nephrotic syndrome. The disease is most common in children but may occur at any age. The glomeruli appear normal by light and immunofluorescent microscopy but on electron microscopy the foot processes of the epithelial cells appear smudged. The proteinuria usually is highly selective and renal function remains normal. Remissions occur spontaneously or may be induced by steroid hormones or immunosuppressive agents. However, relapses are common. Also called *glomerular epithelial cell disease, larval nephrosis,*

lipid nephrosis, foot process disease, minimal lesion glomerulonephritis, minimal change disease, minimum change glomerulopathy, minimal change glomerular disease, pure nephrosis, lipomatous nephritis (rarely used), *nil disease, minimal lesion disease, lipemic nephrosis, degenerative nephritis.*

lower nephron nephrosis An outmoded and imprecise term for ACUTE TUBULAR NECROSIS. ● This term was introduced during World War II to describe the renal lesions noted in soldiers suffering from acute renal failure due to crush and other severe trauma.

mercurial nephrosis Membranous nephropathy and the nephrotic syndrome due to prolonged exposure to mercurial diuretics or to ingestion or absorption through the skin of small amounts of mercury.

necrotizing nephrosis A rarely used term for ACUTE TUBULAR NECROSIS.

nephritic nephrosis The nephrotic syndrome associated with any form of glomerulonephritis.

osmotic nephrosis Marked dilatation of renal tubules with vacuolization of the pars recta of the proximal tubule. The condition may develop in severe glycosuria due to diabetes mellitus. Similar lesions may develop in patients given intravenous hypertonic sucrose to treat cerebral edema or mannitol to induce diuresis. The renal cortex is congested after administration of mannitol and the diameter of the tubule lumen is decreased. The lesions are reversible within 96 hours. No functional disorders accompany the histologic lesions. However, the infusion of dextrons of low molecular weight to treat peripheral vascular disorders has been followed by florid osmotic nephrosis, and oliguria secondary either to toxic effects on tubule cell function or to narrowing of the tubule lumens by swollen cells.

pure nephrosis LIPOID NEPHROSIS.

toxic nephrosis Acute tubular necrosis following ingestion, inhalation, or skin absorption of toxic agents, such as bichloride of mercury.

vacuolar nephrosis The nephrotic syndrome associated with vacuolization of the renal tubule epithelial cells. A rarely used term.

nephrosonephritis [NEPHROS(IS) + *o* + NEPHRITIS] **1** The renal syndrome characteristic of epidemic hemorrhagic fever. A rarely used term. **2** A rarely used term for EPIDEMIC HEMORRHAGIC FEVER.

hemorrhagic nephrosonephritis EPIDEMIC HEMORRHAGIC FEVER.

nephrospasis [NEPHRO- + Gk *span* to draw, draw out; in passive, to be dislocated] A highly moveable kidney that hangs by its pedicle.

nephrosplenopexy The suspension of the left kidney and the spleen from the abdominal wall in order to prevent ptosis of a floating kidney or spleen.

nephrostogram [*nephrosto(my)* + -GRAM] A roentgenogram of the kidney after its pelvis has been opacified by instillation of contrast medium via a nephrostomy tube.

nephrostoma [NEPHRO- + Gk *stoma* mouth] A primitive arrangement, exhibited by some lower vertebrates, whereby a nephric tubule opens into the coelomic cavity. Such an opening may be seen in relation to pronephric tubules and early mesonephric tubules, but few mesonephric and no metanephric tubules possess a nephrostoma. Also called *nephrostome*.

nephrostome NEPHROSTOMA.

nephrostomy [NEPHRO- + -STOMY] A form of urinary diversion involving placement of a tube within the kidney pelvis or calyces in order to provide urinary drainage directly to an external urinary collection appliance. The nephrostomy tube may be temporary or permanent, and is used to provide urinary drainage in a kidney which has become obstructed. A nephrostomy tube may be established by open surgical exposure of the kidney, or by use of a technique wherein the tube is passed directly through the skin in to the kidney (percutaneous nephrostomy).

nephrotic [NEPHR- + -OTIC[1]]   Related to or associated with the nephrotic syndrome (nephrosis).

nephrotome [NEPHRO- + -TOME]   One of a series of segmental units in the intermediate mesoderm from which the nephric tubules differentiate. They comprise the three successive renal organs during development: pronephros, mesonephros, and metanephros. Also called *nephromere.*

nephrotomogram [NEPHRO- + -tom(e) + o + -GRAM]   A roentgenogram obtained during nephrotomography.

nephrotomography [NEPHRO- + -tom(e) + o + -GRAPHY]   Body section roentgenography of the kidney whose parenchyma has been opacified by intravascularly administered appropriate iodinated contrast medium.

nephrotomy [NEPHRO- + -TOMY]   A surgical incision into one or both kidneys.

abdominal nephrotomy   An incision into the kidney, utilizing a transperitoneal or anterior approach.

lumbar nephrotomy   An incision into one or both kidneys utilizing a retroperitoneal flank approach.

nephrotoxic [NEPHRO- + TOXIC]   Causing renal lesions or impairing renal function.

nephrotoxicity [NEPHRO- + TOXICITY]   The ability of an agent or drug to produce renal lesions or functional impairment.

antibiotic nephrotoxicity   The ability of an antibiotic to produce renal lesions, usually tubulointerstitial, or renal functional impairment.

bismuth nephrotoxicity   BISMUTH NEPHROPATHY.

ethylene glycol nephrotoxicity   ETHYLENE GLYCOL NEPHROPATHY.

glycol nephrotoxicity   ETHYLENE GLYCOL NEPHROPATHY.

salicylate nephrotoxicity   See under ANALGESIC NEPHROPATHY.

nephrotoxin [NEPHRO- + TOXIN]   Any agent or substance that causes renal lesions or impairment of renal function. Also called *nephrolysin.*

nephrotresis [NEPHRO- + Gk *trēsis* a boring, piercing, hole]   The surgical creation of a fistula by suturing the edges of a nephrostomy to the muscles of the abdominal wall.

nephrotrophic   Having an effect on the kidneys: said of a substance. Also *nephrotropic, renotrophic, renotropic.*

nephrotrophin   Any substance that has an effect on the kidneys. Also called *renotrophin.*

nephrotropic   NEPHROTROPHIC.

nephroureteral   Referring to the kidney and ureter.

nephroureterectomy   The resection of one or both kidneys and ureters.

nephroureterocystectomy   Surgical extirpation of the kidney, the ureter, and all or part of the bladder wall.

nephrydrosis   HYDRONEPHROSIS.

neptunium   Element number 93, having atomic weight 237.0482. First discovered as a synthetic product of neutron bombardment of uranium 238, traces also exist in uranium ores. Thirteen isotopes are known, of which the most stable is neptunium 237, an energetic emitter of alpha radiation with a half-life of 2.4×10^6 years. This isotope is produced in gram quantities in nuclear reactors as a by-product of plutonium production. Symbol: Np

Neri [Vincenzo *Neri*, Italian neurologist, born 1882]   See under SIGN.

neritic [Gk *Nērei(s)*, also *Nērēi(s)* a Nereid or Nymph of the sea + *t* + -IC]   Pertaining to the waters of the continental shelf.

Nernst [Walther Hermann *Nernst*, German chemist, 1864–1941]   See under POTENTIAL, LAW, EQUATION.

nerol $(CH_3)_2C=CH-[CH_2]_2-C(CH_3)=CH-CH_2OH$.   A terpene alcohol formed from two isoprene units. It is the *cis*-isomer of geraniol. Its diphosphate is formed from geranyl diphosphate as an intermediate in the biosynthesis of several terpenes.

nerval   NEURAL.

nerve

nerve [L *nervus.* See NERVUS.]   A cordlike structure, visible to the naked eye, made up of nerve fibers conveying impulses between a part of the central nervous system and some other region of the body. A nerve is made up of individual nerve fibers with their sheaths and supporting cells, small blood vessels, and a surrounding connective tissue sheath. Each nerve fiber (axon) is surrounded by a cellular sheath (neurilemma) from which it may or may not be separated by a laminated lipo-protein layer (myelin sheath) derived from the neurilemma (Schwann) cells. A number of such nerve fibers, making up a fasciculus, are surrounded by a sheet of connective tissue (perineurium), leaflets of which also surround each individual nerve fiber (endoneurium). All of the fasciculi and the nourishing blood vessels are bound together by a thicker investment of connective tissue (epineurium). Also called *nervus.*

abdominal splanchnic nerves   The nervus splanchnicus major, nervus splanchnicus minor, and nervus splanchnicus imus considered together. An outmoded term.

abducent nerve   NERVUS ABDUCENS.

accelerator nerves   The cardiac sympathetic nerves, whose stimulation increases the rate of cardiac contraction. Also called *Gaskell's nerves* (seldom used).

accessory nerve   NERVUS ACCESSORIUS.

accessory deep peroneal nerve   NERVUS PERONEUS PROFUNDUS ACCESSORIUS.

accessory obturator nerve   NERVUS OBTURATORIUS ACCESSORIUS.

accessory phrenic nerves   NERVI PHRENICI ACCESSORII.

acoustic nerve   NERVUS VESTIBULOCOCHLEARIS.

nerve to adductor brevis muscle   A branch of the anterior ramus of the obturator nerve. When this branch is absent, the muscle receives a branch from the posterior ramus.

nerve to adductor longus muscle   A branch of the anterior ramus of the obturator nerve. Occasionally the muscle may receive a branch from the accessory obturator nerve when present.

nerve to adductor magnus muscle   1 A branch of the posterior ramus of the obturator nerve.   2 Any of the branches (L_{2-4}) of the tibial division of the sciatic nerve.

adrenergic nerve   The sympathetic postganglionic axons that liberate epinephrine or norepinephrine at their terminals.

afferent nerve   A nerve fiber or bundle that conducts towards the central nervous system or to a given neuron. Also called *centripetal nerve, esodic nerve* (outmoded).   ● See note at AFFERENT.

ampullary nerves   The branches of the vestibular nerve that convey afferent impulses from the ampullae of the semicircular ducts of the internal ear to the brain, namely, the nervus ampullaris anterior, nervus ampullaris lateralis, and nervus ampullaris posterior.

anabolic nerve An autonomic nerve that conserves or supports synthetic metabolic processes, such as the vagus nerve.

Andersch nerve NERVUS TYMPANICUS.

anococcygeal nerves NERVI ANOCOCCYGEI.

anterior ampullary nerve NERVUS AMPULLARIS ANTERIOR.

anterior auricular nerves NERVI AURICULARES ANTERIORES.

anterior crural nerve NERVUS FEMORALIS.

anterior cutaneous nerve of abdomen RAMUS CUTANEUS ANTERIOR PECTORALIS ET ABDOMINALIS NERVORUM INTERCOSTALIUM.

anterior cutaneous nerve of neck NERVUS TRANSVERSUS COLLI.

anterior ethmoidal nerve NERVUS ETHMOIDALIS ANTERIOR.

anterior gastric nerve TRUNCUS VAGALIS ANTERIOR.

anterior interosseous nerve of forearm NERVUS INTEROSSEUS ANTEBRACHII ANTERIOR.

anterior labial nerves NERVI LABIALES ANTERIORES.

anterior palatine nerve NERVUS PALATINUS MAJOR.

anterior scrotal nerves NERVI SCROTALES ANTERIORES.

anterior superior alveolar nerves RAMI ALVEOLARES SUPERIORES ANTERIORES NERVI INFRAORBITALIS.

anterior supraclavicular nerves NERVI SUPRACLAVICULARES MEDIALES.

anterior thoracic nerve The medial and lateral pectoral nerves. An obsolete term.

anterior vagal nerve TRUNCUS VAGALIS ANTERIOR.

aortic nerve A branch of the vagus nerve which supplies afferent fibers to the aortic arch and base of the heart. Its stimulation results in cardiac slowing, peripheral vascular dilatation, and a fall in blood pressure. Also called *Ludwig's nerve, depressor nerve of Ludwig, Cyon's nerve.*

Arnold's nerve RAMUS AURICULARIS NERVI VAGI.

articular nerve NERVUS ARTICULARIS.

nerve to articularis genus muscle A filament of one of the muscular branches of the femoral nerve to the vastus intermedius muscle that pierces the latter to reach the articularis genus muscle.

association nerve A communication between the abducens nerve and the nerve of the pterygoid canal.

auditory nerve NERVUS VESTIBULOCOCHLEARIS.

augmentor nerves Nerve fibers of sympathetic origin which increase the rate and force of contraction of the heart.

auricular nerve of vagus RAMUS AURICULARIS NERVI VAGI.

auriculotemporal nerve NERVUS AURICULOTEMPORALIS.

autonomic nerves Any of the peripheral nerves of the sympathetic and parasympathetic nervous systems.

axillary nerve NERVUS AXILLARIS.

Bell's nerve NERVUS THORACICUS LONGUS.

Bock's nerve RAMUS PHARYNGEUS GANGLII PTERYGOPALATINI.

brachial plexus nerve A component of the brachial plexus.

nerve to brachioradialis muscle A branch of the radial nerve given off in front of the lateral intermuscular septum of the arm.

buccal nerve NERVUS BUCCALIS.

buccinator nerve NERVUS BUCCALIS. • The term is misleading, since the nervus buccalis has no direct connection with the buccinator muscle.

caroticotympanic nerves NERVI CAROTICOTYMPANICI.

cavernous nerves of clitoris NERVI CAVERNOSI CLITORIDIS.

cavernous nerves of penis NERVI CAVERNOSI PENIS.

celiac nerves RAMI CELIACI NERVI VAGI.

centrifugal nerve EFFERENT NERVE.

centripetal nerve AFFERENT NERVE.

cerebral nerves An outmoded term for NERVI CRANIALES.

cervical nerves NERVI CERVICALES.

cholinergic nerves Nerves that release the neurotransmitter acetylcholine at their terminations, including all autonomic preganglionic nerves, parasympathetic postganglionic nerves, and somatic motor nerves.

chorda tympani nerve CHORDA TYMPANI.

circumflex humeral nerve NERVUS AXILLARIS.

coccygeal nerve NERVUS COCCYGEUS.

cochlear nerve **1** PARS COCHLEARIS NERVI OCTAVI. **2** RADIX INFERIOR NERVI VESTIBULOCOCHLEARIS.

common digital nerve NERVUS DIGITALIS COMMUNIS.

common fibular nerve NERVUS PERONEUS COMMUNIS.

common peroneal nerve NERVUS PERONEUS COMMUNIS.

common plantar digital nerves NERVI DIGITALES PLANTARES COMMUNES.

conarial nerves Two nerves constituting the primary neural supply to the pineal body in the rat. They pass to the dorsal aspect of the organ from the tentorium cerebelli. Most or all the fibers are sympathetic with the cell bodies in the superior cervical ganglia. Also called *nervi conarii.*

nerve of Cotunnius NERVUS NASOPALATINUS.

cranial nerves NERVI CRANIALES.

crotaphitic nerve An outmoded term for NERVUS MAXILLARIS.

cubital nerve NERVUS ULNARIS.

cutaneous nerve NERVUS CUTANEUS.

Cyon's nerve AORTIC NERVE.

deep fibular nerve NERVUS PERONEUS PROFUNDUS.

deep peroneal nerve NERVUS PERONEUS PROFUNDUS.

deep petrosal nerve NERVUS PETROSUS PROFUNDUS.

deep radial nerve NERVUS INTEROSSEUS ANTEBRACHII POSTERIOR.

deep temporal nerves NERVI TEMPORALES PROFUNDI.

deep vidian nerve NERVUS PETROSUS PROFUNDUS.

dental nerve Either nervus alveolaris inferior or one of the nervi alveolares superiores.

depressor nerve A nerve which upon stimulation lowers the blood pressure, especially the carotid sinus nerve.

depressor nerve of Ludwig AORTIC NERVE.

descending cervical nerve RADIX INFERIOR ANSAE CERVICALIS.

diaphragmatic nerve NERVUS PHRENICUS.

digastric nerve RAMUS DIGASTRICUS NERVI FACIALIS.

digital nerves NERVI DIGITALES.

dorsal nerve of clitoris NERVUS DORSALIS CLITORIDIS.

dorsal cutaneous nerve of forearm NERVUS CUTANEUS ANTEBRACHII POSTERIOR.

dorsal digital nerves NERVI DIGITALES DORSALES.

dorsal digital nerves of foot NERVI DIGITALES DORSALIS PEDIS.

dorsal nerve of penis NERVUS DORSALIS PENIS.

dorsal nerve of scapula NERVUS DORSALIS SCAPULAE.

dorsal scapular nerve NERVUS DORSALIS SCAPULAE.

effector nerve A peripheral efferent nerve to muscles or glands.

efferent nerve A nerve conducting away from a central neuronal aggregate, mainly to muscles and glands. Also called *centrifugal nerve, exodic nerve.*

eighth cranial nerve NERVUS VESTIBULOCOCHLEARIS.

nerve of Eisler The greater coccygeal perforating nerve arising from the fourth and fifth sacral nerves. The nerve is inconstant.

eleventh cranial nerve NERVUS ACCESSORIUS.

esodic nerve An outmoded term for AFFERENT NERVE.

ethmoidal nerve Either nervus ethmoidalis anterior or nervus ethmoidalis posterior.

exciter nerve A nerve that upon stimulation increases the impulse discharge for functional activity of postsynaptic cells.

excitoreflex nerve   A nerve which upon stimulation elicits an autonomic reflex action.

exodic nerve   An outmoded term for EFFERENT NERVE.

nerve to extensor carpi radialis brevis muscle   A branch of the deep terminal branch of the radial nerve that occasionally arises from the beginning of the superficial branch of the radial nerve.

nerve to extensor carpi radialis longus muscle   A branch of the radial nerve that arises in front of the lateral intermuscular septum of the arm.

nerve of external acoustic meatus   NERVUS MEATUS ACUSTICI EXTERNI.

external carotid nerves   NERVI CAROTICI EXTERNI.

external laryngeal nerve   RAMUS EXTERNUS NERVI LARYNGEI SUPERIORIS.

external palatine nerve   NERVUS PALATINUS MEDIUS.

external pterygoid nerve   NERVUS PTERYGOIDEUS LATERALIS.

external respiratory nerve of Bell   An imprecise term for NERVUS THORACICUS LONGUS.

external saphenous nerve   NERVUS SURALIS.

external spermatic nerve   RAMUS GENITALIS NERVI GENITOFEMORALIS.

external superficial petrosal nerve   A twig leaving the sympathetic plexus on the middle meningeal artery to pass along the auriculotemporal nerve and up the facial canal as far as the geniculate ganglion.

extrinsic nerve   A peripheral nerve that connects any structure to the central nervous system.

facial nerve   NERVUS FACIALIS.

femoral nerve   NERVUS FEMORALIS.

fifth cranial nerve   NERVUS TRIGEMINUS.

first cranial nerve   NERVI OLFACTORII.

nerve to flexor digitorum longus muscle   A muscular branch of the tibial nerve that arises deep to the soleus muscle in the leg and supplies the flexor digitorus longus muscle.

nerve to flexor hallucis longus muscle   A muscular branch of the tibial nerve that arises deep to the soleus muscle and accompanies the peroneal vessels to supply the flexor hallucis longus muscle.

fourth cranial nerve   NERVUS TROCHLEARIS.

frontal nerve   NERVUS FRONTALIS.

furcal nerve   NERVUS FURCALIS.

Galen's nerve   RAMUS COMMUNICANS NERVI LARYNGEI SUPERIORIS CUM NERVO LARYNGEO INFERIORE.

gangliated nerve   Any nerve of the sympathetic division of the autonomic nervous system.

ganglioglomerular nerves   Nerve filaments that pass from the superior cervical sympathetic ganglion to the carotid sinus.

Gaskell's nerves   A seldom used term for ACCELERATOR NERVES.

gastric nerves   Truncus vagalis anterior and truncus vagalis posterior.

nerve to gemellus inferior and quadratus femoris muscles   NERVUS MUSCULI QUADRATI FEMORIS.

nerve to gemellus superior muscle   A branch of the nerve to the obturator internus muscle that is given off below the piriformis muscle in the gluteal region and enters the posterior surface of the gemellus superior muscle.

nerve to geniohyoid muscle   A branch of the hypoglossal nerve that consists of fibers of the first cervical spinal nerve destined for the geniohyoid muscle.

genitofemoral nerve   NERVUS GENITOFEMORALIS.

glossopalatine nerve   That portion of the seventh cranial (facial) nerve made up of the nervus intermedius and including the geniculate ganglion, chorda tympani and greater superficial petrosal nerve, in addition to the parasympathetic part including the submaxillary and sphenopalatine ganglia and their branches.

glossopharyngeal nerve   NERVUS GLOSSOPHARYNGEUS.

nerve to gracilis muscle   A branch of the anterior branch of the obturator nerve that is given off behind the pectineus muscle and in front of the adductor longus muscle. It proceeds medially to innervate the gracilis muscle.

great auricular nerve   NERVUS AURICULARIS MAGNUS.

greater cavernous nerve   NERVUS CAVERNOSUS PENIS MAJOR.

greater occipital nerve   NERVUS OCCIPITALIS MAJOR.

greater palatine nerve   NERVUS PALATINUS MAJOR.

greater petrosal nerve   NERVUS PETROSUS MAJOR.

greater splanchnic nerve   NERVUS SPLANCHNICUS MAJOR.

greater superficial petrosal nerve   NERVUS PETROSUS MAJOR.

great sciatic nerve   NERVUS ISCHIADICUS.

Hering's nerve   RAMUS SINUS CAROTICI NERVI GLOSSOPHARYNGEI.

Hirschfeld's nerve   An inconstant lingual branch derived from the nervus facialis.

nerves to hyoglossus and styloglossus muscles   Lingual branches of the hypoglossal nerve which arise on the lateral surface of the hyoglossus muscle and supply the hyoglossus and styloglossus muscles.

hypogastric nerve   NERVUS HYPOGASTRICUS DEXTER ET SINISTER.

hypogastric nerve of Latarjet   NERVUS HYPOGASTRICUS DEXTER ET SINISTER.

hypoglossal nerve   NERVUS HYPOGLOSSUS.

iliohypogastric nerve   NERVUS ILIOHYPOGASTRICUS.

ilioinguinal nerve   NERVUS ILIOINGUINALIS.

nerves to iliopsoas muscle   Branches to the iliacus muscle and the psoas major muscle that arise from the second and third, and occasionally the fourth, lumbar nerves of the lumbar plexus.

inferior alveolar nerve   NERVUS ALVEOLARIS INFERIOR.

inferior ampullar nerve   NERVUS AMPULLARIS POSTERIOR.

inferior cardiac nerve   NERVUS CARDIACUS CERVICALIS INFERIOR.

inferior cervical cardiac nerve   NERVUS CARDIACUS CERVICALIS INFERIOR.

inferior clunial nerves   NERVI CLUNIUM INFERIORES.

inferior dental nerve   NERVUS ALVEOLARIS INFERIOR.

inferior gluteal nerve   NERVUS GLUTEUS INFERIOR.

inferior hemorrhoidal nerves   NERVI RECTALES INFERIORES.

inferior laryngeal nerve   NERVUS LARYNGEUS INFERIOR.

inferior lateral brachial cutaneous nerve   NERVUS CUTANEUS BRACHII LATERALIS INFERIOR.

inferior lateral cutaneous nerve of arm   NERVUS CUTANEUS BRACHII LATERALIS INFERIOR.

inferior rectal nerves   NERVI RECTALES INFERIORES.

inferior splanchnic nerve   NERVUS SPLANCHNICUS MINOR.

inferior vesical nerves of pudendal plexus   NERVI VESICALES INFERIORES PLEXUS PUDENDI.

inferior vesical nerves of vesical plexus   NERVI VESICALES INFERIORES PLEXUS VESICALIS.

infraoccipital nerve   NERVUS SUBOCCIPITALIS.

infraorbital nerve   NERVUS INFRAORBITALIS.

infratrochlear nerve   NERVUS INFRATROCHLEARIS.

inhibitory nerve   A nerve that upon stimulation decreases the discharge or functional activity of postsynaptic cells.

intercostal nerves   See under RAMI VENTRALES NERVORUM THORACICORUM.

intercostobrachial nerves   NERVI INTERCOSTOBRACHIALES.

intermediary nerve   NERVUS INTERMEDIUS.

intermediate dorsal cutaneous nerve   NERVUS CUTANEUS DORSALIS INTERMEDIUS.

intermediate supraclavicular nerves NERVI SUPRACLAVICULARES INTERMEDII.

intermediate nerve of Wrisberg NERVUS INTERMEDIUS.

internal auricular nerve RAMUS POSTERIOR NERVI AURICULARIS MAGNI.

internal carotid nerve NERVUS CAROTICUS INTERNUS.

internal cutaneous nerve NERVUS CUTANEUS BRACHII MEDIALIS.

internal laryngeal nerve RAMUS INTERNUS NERVI LARYNGEI SUPERIORIS.

internal occipital nerve NERVUS OCCIPITALIS MAJOR.

internal popliteal nerve NERVUS TIBIALIS.

internal pterygoid nerve NERVUS PTERYGOIDEUS MEDIALIS.

internal superior laryngeal nerve RAMUS INTERNUS NERVI LARYNGEI SUPERIORIS.

interosseous nerve of leg NERVUS INTEROSSEUS CRURIS.

intrinsic nerve The ultimate ramifications of an autonomic nerve in the organ it supplies. A seldom used term.

ischiadic nerve NERVUS ISCHIADICUS.

Jacobson's nerve NERVUS TYMPANICUS.

joint nerve NERVUS ARTICULARIS.

jugular nerve NERVUS JUGULARIS.

jugular nerve of Arnold NERVUS JUGULARIS.

kinesodic nerve MOTOR NERVE.

lacrimal nerve NERVUS LACRIMALIS.

nerves of Lancisi Stria longitudinalis lateralis corporis callosi and stria longitudinalis medialis corporis callosi. Also called *longitudinal nerves of Lancisi.*

Langley's nerve PILOMOTOR NERVES.

laryngeal nerve Any one of several nerves that supply portions of the intrinsic musculature and/or lining of the larynx. They include external, internal, inferior, and superior components.

lateral ampullary nerve NERVUS AMPULLARIS LATERALIS.

lateral antebrachial cutaneous nerve NERVUS CUTANEUS ANTEBRACHII LATERALIS.

lateral cutaneous nerve of calf NERVUS CUTANEUS SURAE LATERALIS.

lateral cutaneous nerve of forearm NERVUS CUTANEUS ANTEBRACHII LATERALIS.

lateral cutaneous nerve of thigh NERVUS CUTANEUS FEMORIS LATERALIS.

lateral dorsal cutaneous nerve of foot NERVUS CUTANEUS DORSALIS LATERALIS.

lateral femoral cutaneous nerve NERVUS CUTANEUS FEMORIS LATERALIS.

lateral pectoral nerve NERVUS PECTORALIS LATERALIS.

lateral plantar nerve NERVUS PLANTARIS LATERALIS.

lateral popliteal nerve NERVUS PERONEUS COMMUNIS.

lateral pterygoid nerve NERVUS PTERYGOIDEUS LATERALIS.

lateral superior cutaneous nerve of arm NERVUS CUTANEUS BRACHII LATERALIS SUPERIOR.

lateral supraclavicular nerves NERVI SUPRACLAVICULARES LATERALES.

lateral sural nerve A general sensory nerve formed by union of the medial sural cutaneous branch of the tibial nerve and the peroneal communicating branch of the common peroneal nerve. Distribution includes skin on back of leg and side of foot.

lateral nerves of uterus Branches of the uterovaginal plexus that enter the base of the broad ligament of the uterus and accompany the uterine arteries on either side of the uterus, supplying branches to the body of the uterus and the uterine tubes and communicating with tubal nerves of the inferior hypogastric plexus and branches of the ovarian plexus. The branches to the body of the uterus end in the myometrium and endometrium.

least occipital nerve NERVUS OCCIPITALIS TERTIUS.

least splanchnic nerve NERVUS SPLANCHNICUS IMUS.

lesser occipital nerve NERVUS OCCIPITALIS MINOR.

lesser palatine nerves NERVI PALATINI MINORES.

lesser petrosal nerve NERVUS PETROSUS MINOR.

lesser splanchnic nerve NERVUS SPLANCHNICUS MINOR.

lesser superficial nerve NERVUS PETROSUS MINOR.

lesser superficial petrosal nerve NERVUS PETROSUS MINOR.

nerves to levator ani muscle A branch from the fourth sacral spinal nerve and a branch from the perineal division of the pudendal nerve that supply the levator ani muscle on each side. It may also receive a branch from the inferior rectal nerve.

lingual nerve NERVUS LINGUALIS.

long buccal nerve NERVUS BUCCALIS.

long ciliary nerves NERVI CILIARES LONGI.

nerve to long head of biceps brachii muscle A branch of the musculocutaneous nerve that arises after the nerve has pierced the coracobrachialis muscle. It supplies the long head of the biceps brachii muscle.

nerve to long head of triceps muscle One of the medial muscular branches of the radial nerve that innervates the long head of the triceps muscle before the nerve enters the radial sulcus behind the humerus.

longitudinal nerves of Lancisi NERVES OF LANCISI.

long thoracic nerve NERVUS THORACICUS LONGUS.

lowest splanchnic nerve NERVUS SPLANCHNICUS IMUS.

Ludwig's nerve AORTIC NERVE.

lumbar nerves NERVI LUMBALES.

lumbar splanchnic nerves NERVI SPLANCHNICI LUMBALES.

lumboinguinal nerve RAMUS FEMORALIS NERVI GENITOFEMORALIS.

nerve of Luschka 1 RAMUS MENINGEUS NERVORUM SPINALIUM. 2 NERVUS ETHMOIDALIS POSTERIOR.

major splanchnic nerve NERVUS SPLANCHNICUS MAJOR.

mandibular nerve NERVUS MANDIBULARIS.

masseteric nerve NERVUS MASSETERICUS.

maxillary nerve NERVUS MAXILLARIS.

medial antebrachial cutaneous nerve NERVUS CUTANEUS ANTEBRACHII MEDIALIS.

medial cutaneous nerve of arm NERVUS CUTANEUS BRACHII MEDIALIS.

medial cutaneous nerve of calf NERVUS CUTANEUS SURAE MEDIALIS.

medial cutaneous nerve of forearm NERVUS CUTANEUS ANTEBRACHII MEDIALIS.

medial dorsal cutaneous nerve of foot NERVUS CUTANEUS DORSALIS MEDIALIS.

nerve to medial head of triceps and anconeus A long branch of the radial nerve that is given off in the radial sulcus behind the humerus and descends through the medial head of the triceps muscle, supplying it, and ending in the anconeus muscle after crossing behind the elbow joint. It is accompanied by the middle collateral branch of the profunda brachii artery.

medial pectoral nerve NERVUS PECTORALIS MEDIALIS.

medial plantar nerve NERVUS PLANTARIS MEDIALIS.

medial popliteal nerve NERVUS TIBIALIS.

nerve to medial pterygoid muscle NERVUS PTERYGOIDEUS MEDIALIS.

medial supraclavicular nerves NERVI SUPRACLAVICULARES MEDIALES.

medial sural cutaneous nerve NERVUS CUTANEUS SURAE MEDIALIS.

median nerve NERVUS MEDIANUS.

meningeal nerve RAMUS MENINGEUS NERVI VAGI.

mental nerve NERVUS MENTALIS.

middle alveolar nerve RAMUS ALVEOLARIS SUPERIOR MEDIUS NERVI INFRAORBITALIS.

middle cardiac nerve NERVUS CARDIACUS CERVICALIS MEDIUS.

middle cervical cardiac nerve NERVUS CARDIACUS CERVICALIS MEDIUS.

middle clunial nerves NERVI CLUNIUM MEDII.

middle deep temporal nerve The middle branch of the nervi temporales profundi of the mandibular nerve which traverses the porus crotaphitico-buccinatorius behind the nerve to the masseter muscle and passes between the lateral pterygoid muscle and the greater wing of the sphenoid bone to end in the middle part of the temporalis muscle. It is occasionally absent.

middle gluteal nerves NERVI CLUNIUM MEDII.

middle palatine nerve NERVUS PALATINUS MEDIUS.

middle subscapular nerve NERVUS THORACODORSALIS.

middle superficial petrosal nerve NERVUS PETROSUS MINOR.

middle supraclavicular nerves NERVI SUPRACLAVICULARES INTERMEDII.

minor splanchnic nerve NERVUS SPLANCHNICUS MINOR.

mixed nerve A peripheral nerve containing both afferent and efferent axons. Also called *sensorimotor nerve.*

motor nerve An efferent nerve to skeletal muscle. Also called *motorius (obsolescent and rarely used), neuromotor nerve, kinesodic nerve.*

motor nerve of tongue NERVUS HYPOGLOSSUS.

nerve to muscle of malleus NERVUS MUSCULI TENSORIS TYMPANI.

musculocutaneous nerve NERVUS MUSCULOCUTANEUS.

musculocutaneous nerve of arm NERVUS MUSCULOCUTANEUS.

musculocutaneous nerve of foot NERVUS PERONEUS SUPERFICIALIS.

musculocutaneous nerve of leg NERVUS PERONEUS PROFUNDUS.

musculospiral nerve NERVUS RADIALIS.

mylohyoid nerve NERVUS MYLOHYOIDEUS.

nasociliary nerve NERVUS NASOCILIARIS.

nasopalatine nerve NERVUS NASOPALATINUS.

neuromotor nerve MOTOR NERVE.

ninth cranial nerve NERVUS GLOSSOPHARYNGEUS.

obturator nerve NERVUS OBTURATORIUS.

nerve to obturator externus A branch of the posterior branch of the obturator nerve. The posterior branch pierces and supplies the obturator externus muscle at the upper part of the obturator foramen before it continues between the adductor brevis and adductor magnus muscles. An outmoded term.

oculomotor nerve NERVUS OCULOMOTORIUS.

olfactory nerves NERVI OLFACTORII.

ophthalmic nerve NERVUS OPHTHALMICUS.

ophthalmic recurrent nerve RAMUS TENTORII NERVI OPHTHALMICI.

ophthalmic nerve of Willis NERVUS OPHTHALMICUS.

optic nerve NERVUS OPTICUS.

orbital nerves RAMI ORBITALES GANGLII PTERYGOPALATINI.

pain nerve A peripheral axon activated by a nociceptor and whose activation results in a sensory report of pain. Also called *nociceptive afferent.*

palatine nerves NERVI PALATINI.

palmar digital nerves NERVI DIGITALES PALMARES.

paracervical nerve The cervical portion of the sympathetic trunk. An obsolete term.

parasympathetic nerve Any of the nerves of the parasympathetic division of the autonomic nervous system.

parotid nerves RAMI PAROTIDEI NERVI AURICULOTEMPORALIS.

pathetic nerve NERVUS TROCHLEARIS.

nerve to pectineus muscle The nerve supplying the pectineus muscle that arises from the femoral nerve above the inguinal ligament and passes behind the femoral sheath to enter the muscle. It may also be innervated by a branch from either the obturator or the accessory obturator nerve.

nerves to pectoralis major muscle The nervus pectoralis lateralis and nervus pectoralis medialis.

pelvic splanchnic nerves NERVI SPLANCHNICI PELVICI.

perineal nerves NERVI PERINEALES.

peripheral nerves **1** All nerves whose distribution is to the skin or peripheral parts of the body. **2** Any nerves that enter or leave the central nervous system.

peroneal communicating nerve RAMUS COMMUNICANS PERONEUS NERVI PERONEI COMMUNIS.

peroneal cutaneous nerve An outmoded term for NERVUS CUTANEUS SURAE LATERALIS.

nerves to peroneus longus muscle Muscular branches of the superficial peroneal nerve that supply the peroneus longus muscle as the nerve descends deep to the muscle in the lateral compartment of the leg.

nerve to peroneus tertius A branch of the deep peroneal nerve that is given off in the lower part of the leg.

petrosal nerve The nervus petrosus major, nervus petrosus minor, nervus petrosus profundus, or nervus petrosus superficialis.

phrenic nerve NERVUS PHRENICUS.

phrenicoabdominal nerves RAMI PHRENICOABDOMINALES NERVI PHRENICI.

pilomotor nerves Peripheral axons innervating the arrectores pilorum muscles of cutaneous hairs. Also called *Langley's nerve.*

nerve to piriformis muscle NERVUS PIRIFORMIS.

plantar digital nerves NERVI DIGITALES PLANTARES.

nerve to plantaris muscle A branch to the plantaris muscle that is given off by the tibial nerve as it passes between the two heads of the gastrocnemius muscle.

pneumogastric nerve NERVUS VAGUS.

nerve to popliteus muscle A branch of the tibial nerve that is given off between the two heads of the gastrocnemius muscle and then descends laterally and obliquely across the popliteal vessels to the lower margin of the popliteus muscle. Around the popliteus muscle it bends to enter the anterior surface of the muscle.

posterior ampullary nerve NERVUS AMPULLARIS POSTERIOR.

posterior antebrachial cutaneous nerve NERVUS CUTANEUS ANTEBRACHII POSTERIOR.

posterior auricular nerve NERVUS AURICULARIS POSTERIOR.

posterior brachial cutaneous nerve NERVUS CUTANEUS BRACHII POSTERIOR.

posterior cutaneous nerve of arm NERVUS CUTANEUS BRACHII POSTERIOR.

posterior cutaneous nerve of forearm NERVUS CUTANEUS ANTEBRACHII POSTERIOR.

posterior cutaneous nerve of thigh NERVUS CUTANEUS FEMORIS POSTERIOR.

posterior deep temporal nerve NERVUS TEMPORALIS PROFUNDUS POSTERIOR.

posterior ethmoidal nerve NERVUS ETHMOIDALIS POSTERIOR.

posterior femoral cutaneous nerve NERVUS CUTANEUS FEMORIS POSTERIOR.

posterior gastric nerve TRUNCUS VAGALIS POSTERIOR.

posterior interosseous nerve of forearm NERVUS INTEROSSEUS ANTEBRACHII POSTERIOR.

posterior labial nerves NERVI LABIALES POSTERIORES.

posterior palatine nerve NERVUS PALATINUS POSTERIOR.

posterior scrotal nerves NERVI SCROTALES POSTERIORES.

posterior supraclavicular nerves NERVI SUPRACLAVICU-LARES LATERALES.

posterior thoracic nerve NERVUS THORACICUS LONGUS.

posterior vagal nerve TRUNCUS VAGALIS POSTERIOR.

post-trematic nerve The main nerve of a branchial (pharyngeal) arch. It lies just behind the preceding pharyngeal pouch and in some instances gives off a pretrematic branch which contributes to the innervation of the preceding arch. The post-trematic nerves are: the mandibular division of the trigeminal for the first arch, the facial nerve for the second, the glossopharyngeal for the third, the superior laryngeal branch of the vagus for the fourth, and inferior laryngeal branch of the vagus for the sixth. The post-trematic nerve for the fifth arch is not known, but it could be the pharyngeal branch of the vagus.

presacral nerve PLEXUS HYPOGASTRICUS SUPERIOR.

pressor nerve An afferent nerve which upon stimulation elevates blood pressure.

pretrematic nerve The branch of the main post-trematic nerve in each pharyngeal arch which loops over the adjacent pouch to supply part of the preceding arch. For example, the chorda tympani which supplies structures in the first arch is a pretrematic branch of the facial nerve, the nerve of the second arch.

profundus nerve The first of the three trunks of the trigeminal nerve. It innervates the snout region of most vertebrates. In lower vertebrates it is independent, with some indication of once having been a branchial nerve associated with a gill slit now lost in extant vertebrates. Also called *nervus ophthalmicus profundus*.

proper digital nerve NERVUS DIGITALIS PROPRIUS.

proper palmar digital nerves NERVI DIGITALES PALMARES PROPRII.

nerve of pterygoid canal NERVUS CANALIS PTERYGOIDEI.

pterygopalatine nerves NERVI PTERYGOPALATINI.

pudendal nerve NERVUS PUDENDUS.

pudic nerve NERVUS PUDENDUS.

nerve to quadratus femoris muscle NERVUS MUSCULI QUADRATI FEMORIS.

nerves to quadratus lumborum The ventral rami of the twelfth thoracic and the upper third and fourth lumbar spinal nerves.

radial nerve NERVUS RADIALIS.

nerves to rectus capitis anterior muscle Branches from the loop between the ventral rami of the first and second cervical spinal nerves.

recurrent nerve NERVUS LARYNGEUS RECURRENS.

recurrent laryngeal nerve NERVUS LARYNGEUS RECURRENS.

renal nerve NERVUS SPLANCHNICUS IMUS.

respiratory nerve Either of two nerves supplying important muscles of respiration; the internal one is the nervus phrenicus, and the external is the nervus thoracicus longus.

nerve to rhomboids NERVUS DORSALIS SCAPULAE.

saccular nerve NERVUS SACCULARIS.

sacral nerves NERVI SACRALES.

sacral splanchnic nerves NERVI SPLANCHNICI SACRALES.

saphenous nerve NERVUS SAPHENUS.

Scarpa's nerve NERVUS NASOPALATINUS.

sciatic nerve NERVUS ISCHIADICUS.

second cranial nerve NERVUS OPTICUS.

secretomotor nerves SECRETOMOTORIC FIBERS.

secretory nerves SECRETOMOTORIC FIBERS.

segmental nerve Any nerve supplying structures from one of the original body somites, as an intercostal nerve.

nerve to semimembranosus A branch of the tibial portion of the sciatic nerve that arises in common with the branch to the ischial head of the adductor magnus muscle in the upper portion of the back of the thigh and supplies the semimembranosus muscle.

sensorimotor nerve MIXED NERVE.

sensory nerve A peripheral axon or bundle of axons conveying activity from sense organs to the central nervous system.
● See note at AFFERENT.

nerve to serratus anterior NERVUS THORACICUS LONGUS.

seventh cranial nerve NERVUS FACIALIS.

short ciliary nerves NERVI CILIARES BREVES.

short saphenous nerve NERVUS SURALIS.

sinus nerve RAMUS SINUS CAROTICI NERVI GLOSSOPHARYNGEI.

sinuvertebral nerve RAMUS MENINGEUS NERVORUM SPINALIUM.

sixth cranial nerve NERVUS ABDUCENS.

skin nerve NERVUS CUTANEUS.

small deep petrosal nerves NERVI CAROTICOTYMPANICI.

small sciatic nerve NERVUS CUTANEUS FEMORIS POSTERIOR.

Soemmering's nerve NERVUS PUDENDUS.

nerve to soleus muscle A branch that arises from the tibial nerve as it passes between the two heads of the gastrocnemius muscle. It enters the posterior surface of the soleus muscle.

somatic nerves Nerves that supply muscle and somatic tissue with motor and sensory fibers.

somatic efferent nerve **1** Each of the nerves which in the embryo corresponds with a somite. They are the evidence of the original metamerism and conserve their primitive theoretical disposition in the region of the spinal cord, where the nerve roots have a typical segmental arrangement. The intercostal nerves in the thoracic region are the most characteristic. In the regions of the cervical, brachial, lumbar, and sacral plexuses the intermingling of the various somites and their nerves makes their segmental arrangement less schematic. **2** Any of certain cranial nerves developing in the somitic territories of the head (muscles of the eye and the tongue), as opposed to the brachial nerves corresponding to each of the brachial arches which take part in the construction of the head and the neck. The somitic cranial nerves are: the oculomotor (third cranial nerve), the trochlear (fourth cranial nerve), the abducent (sixth cranial nerve) and the hypoglossal (twelfth cranial nerve). Also called *somitic nerve.*

somitic nerve SOMATIC EFFERENT NERVE.

space nerve A branch of the auditory nerve which innervates the semicircular canals.

sphenoid-palatine nerve An outmoded term for NERVUS NASOPALATINUS.

spinal nerves NERVI SPINALES.

spinal accessory nerve NERVUS ACCESSORIUS.

splanchnic nerves The nerves supplying viscera and blood vessels, especially the visceral branches of the thoracic, lumbar, and pelvic portions of the sympathetic trunks. They represent axons of preganglionic neurons that pass through the paravertebral ganglion and the sympathetic trunk en route to the celiac and mesenteric ganglia.

stapedial nerve NERVUS STAPEDIUS.

stapedius nerve NERVUS STAPEDIUS.

stylohyoid nerve RAMUS STYLOHYOIDEUS NERVI FACIALIS.

stylopharyngeal nerve RAMUS MUSCULI STYLOPHARYNGEI NERVI GLOSSOPHARYNGEI.

subclavian nerve NERVUS SUBCLAVIUS.

nerve to subclavius muscle NERVUS SUBCLAVIUS.

subcostal nerve NERVUS SUBCOSTALIS.

subcutaneous temporal nerves RAMI TEMPORALES SUPERFICIALES NERVI AURICULOTEMPORALIS.

sublingual nerve NERVUS SUBLINGUALIS.

submaxillary nerves RAMI GLANDULARES GANGLII SUBMANDIBULARIS.

suboccipital nerve NERVUS SUBOCCIPITALIS.

subscapular nerves NERVUS SUBSCAPULARIS.

sudomotor nerves Autonomic nerves controlling the activity of sweat glands.

superficial cervical nerve NERVUS TRANSVERSUS COLLI.

superficial ciliary nerves Sensory fibers of the ophthalmic and long ciliary nerves that participate in the annular plexus at the periphery of the cornea from which filaments enter the substantia propria and radiate towards the center. An outmoded term.

superficial fibular nerve NERVUS PERONEUS SUPERFICIALIS.

superficial peroneal nerve NERVUS PERONEUS SUPERFICIALIS.

superficial radial nerve RAMUS SUPERFICIALIS NERVI RADIALIS.

superior alveolar nerves NERVI ALVEOLARES SUPERIORES.

superior ampullary nerve NERVUS AMPULLARIS ANTERIOR.

superior cardiac nerve NERVUS CARDIACUS CERVICALIS SUPERIOR.

superior cervical cardiac nerve NERVUS CARDIACUS CERVICALIS SUPERIOR.

superior clunial nerves NERVI CLUNIUM SUPERIORES.

superior dental nerves NERVI ALVEOLARES SUPERIORES.

superior gluteal nerve NERVUS GLUTEUS SUPERIOR.

superior laryngeal nerve NERVUS LARYNGEUS SUPERIOR.

superior lateral cutaneous nerve of arm NERVUS CUTANEUS BRACHII LATERALIS SUPERIOR.

superior vesical nerves of vesical plexus NERVI VESICALES SUPERIORES PLEXUS VESICALIS.

supraclavicular nerves NERVI SUPRACLAVICULARES.

supraorbital nerve NERVUS SUPRAORBITALIS.

suprascapular nerve NERVUS SUPRASCAPULARIS.

supratrochlear nerve NERVUS SUPRATROCHLEARIS.

supreme cardiac nerves RAMI CARDIACI CERVICALES SUPERIORES NERVI VAGI.

sural nerve NERVUS SURALIS.

sympathetic nerve 1 One of the nerves of the sympathetic division of the autonomic nervous system. 2 TRUNCUS SYMPATHICUS. See also SYSTEMA NERVOSUM AUTONOMICUM.

temporal facial nerve RAMI TEMPORALES NERVI FACIALIS.

nerve of tensor tympani muscle NERVUS MUSCULI TENSORIS TYMPANI.

nerve of tensor veli palatini NERVUS TENSORIS VELI PALATINI.

tenth cranial nerve NERVUS VAGUS.

tentorial nerve RAMUS TENTORII NERVI OPHTHALMICI.

nerve to teres minor muscle A branch of the posterior branch of the axillary nerve that arises as the nerve passes through the quadrangular space where it enters the teres minor muscle. It often possesses a pseudoganglion.

terminal nerve NERVUS TERMINALIS.

third cranial nerve NERVUS OCULOMOTORIUS.

third occipital nerve NERVUS OCCIPITALIS TERTIUS.

thoracic nerves NERVI THORACICI.

thoracic cardiac nerves NERVI CARDIACI THORACICI.

thoracodorsal nerve NERVUS THORACODORSALIS.

nerve to thyrohyoid muscle RAMUS THYROHYOIDEUS ANSAE CERVICALIS.

tibial nerve NERVUS TIBIALIS.

nerves to tibialis anterior muscle Branches of the deep peroneal nerve that enter the tibialis anterior muscle near the middle of the leg. Occasionally a branch from the common peroneal nerve enters the proximal portion of the muscle.

nerves to tibialis posterior muscle Small branches of the tibial nerve that supply the tibialis posterior muscle near the middle of the leg.

Tiedemann's nerve The plexus of sympathetic nerve fibrils surrounding the central artery of the retina. A seldom used term.

tonsillar nerves RAMI TONSILLARES NERVI GLOSSOPHARYNGEI.

transverse cervical nerve NERVUS TRANSVERSUS COLLI.

transverse cutaneous nerve of neck NERVUS TRANSVERSUS COLLI.

transverse nerve of neck NERVUS TRANSVERSUS COLLI.

nerves to trapezius Branches from a plexus formed by the termination of the accessory nerve and the ventral rami of the third and fourth cervical spinal nerves that is situated deep to the trapezius muscle.

trifacial nerve NERVUS TRIGEMINUS. • The nerve is so called because of its three major branches.

trigeminal nerve NERVUS TRIGEMINUS.

trochlear nerve NERVUS TROCHLEARIS.

trophic nerve 1 Any nerve that sustains the function of a given structure. 2 Any nerve concerned with the control of nutrition, digestion, and growth.

twelfth cranial nerve NERVUS HYPOGLOSSUS.

twelfth thoracic nerve NERVUS SUBCOSTALIS.

tympanic nerve NERVUS TYMPANICUS.

tympanic nerve of Jacobson NERVUS TYMPANICUS.

ulnar nerve NERVUS ULNARIS.

ulnar collateral nerve of Krause The muscular branch of the radial nerve to the medial head of the triceps that arises on the medial side of the arm at the base of the axilla. It is accompanied by the ulnar nerve and superior ulnar collateral artery as far as the distal third of the arm.

upper lateral cutaneous nerve of arm NERVUS CUTANEUS BRACHII LATERALIS SUPERIOR.

uterine nerves PLEXUS UTERINUS.

utricular nerve NERVUS UTRICULARIS.

utriculoampullar nerve NERVUS UTRICULOAMPULLARIS.

vagal accessory nerve RADICES CRANIALES NERVI ACCESSORII.

vaginal nerves NERVI VAGINALES.

vagus nerve NERVUS VAGUS.

Valentin's nerve The nerve that connects the pterygopalatine ganglion with the abducent nerve.

vascular nerve NERVUS VASCULARIS.

vasoconstrictor nerve Any autonomic nerve which upon stimulation causes constriction of blood vessel walls.

vasodilator nerve Any autonomic nerve which upon stimulation causes increased lumen size and flow in blood vessels.

vasomotor nerves The autonomic nerves that control the smooth muscle walls of blood vessels. Also called *nervi vasorum.*

vasosensory nerve Any nerve containing afferent axons arising from blood vessel walls.

nerve to vastus lateralis muscle A large branch of the posterior division of the femoral nerve that runs laterally and downwards with the descending branch of the lateral circumflex femoral artery deep to the rectus femoris muscle. It ends in the lower part of the vastus lateralis muscle. It sends a branch to the knee joint.

nerve to vastus medialis muscle A large branch of the posterior division of the femoral nerve that descends along the surface of the vastus medialis muscle in the upper part of the adductor canal to end in the middle of the muscle. It sends a branch to the knee joint.

vertebral nerve NERVUS VERTEBRALIS.

vestibular nerve PARS VESTIBULARIS NERVI OCTAVI.

vestibulocochlear nerve NERVUS VESTIBULOCOCHLEARIS.

visceral nerve Any peripheral sensory or motor nerve supplying a visceral structure.

volar interosseous nerve NERVUS INTEROSSEUS ANTEBRACHII ANTERIOR.

vomeronasal nerve Nerve fibers originating in a diverticulum on the nasal septum called the vomeronasal organ (of Jacobson) and ending in an accessory olfactory bulb, located dorsomedial to the main bulb, found in non-primate mammals, submammals, and in a small proportion of human embryos, in which the nerve is present but degenerates with maturity.

nerve of Willis NERVUS ACCESSORIUS.

nerve of Wrisberg 1 NERVUS INTERMEDIUS. **2** NERVUS CUTANEUS BRACHII MEDIALIS.

zygomatic nerve NERVUS ZYGOMATICUS.

zygomaticofacial nerve RAMUS ZYGOMATICOFACIALIS NERVI ZYGOMATICI.

zygomaticotemporal nerve RAMUS ZYGOMATICOTEMPORALIS NERVI ZYGOMATICI.

---

nerve-plate / terminal nerve-plate of Rouget An obsolete term for MOTOR ENDPLATE.

nervi Plural of NERVUS.

nervimotility NEURIMOTILITY.

nervimotor NEURIMOTOR.

nervimuscular Pertaining to the axonal supply of muscle. Also *nervomuscular*.

nervomuscular NERVIMUSCULAR.

nervone The cerebroside formed from sphingosine by acylation of its amino group with nervonic acid and glycosylation of its hydroxyl group with galactose.

nervonic acid The C_{24} unsaturated acid of structure CH_3—$[CH_2]_7$—CH=CH—$[CH_2]_{13}$—$COOH$. It is found in the cerebroside nervone, in which it acylates the amino group of the sphingosine part of the molecule.

nervosism NEURASTHENIA.

nervous 1 Of or relating to a nerve or nerves, as *nervous tissue, central nervous system*. **2** Marked by a feeling of acute and agitated sensitivity. A popular usage.

nervus

nervus [L (akin to Gk *neuron* a sinew, tendon, nerve, string; pl. *neura* the tendons of the feet), a sinew, tendon, nerve, ligament, string] (*plural* nervi) [NA] NERVE.

nervus abducens [NA] The sixth cranial nerve, originating in the caudal pons beneath the floor of the fourth ventricle, emerging anteriorly at the junction of the medulla and pons, and supplying the lateral rectus muscle of the eye. Also called *abducent nerve, sixth cranial nerve, abducens*.

nervus accessorius [NA] The eleventh cranial nerve which arises from cranial roots emerging from the ventrolateral surface of the medulla and from spinal roots emerging from the upper 3–5 cervical segments. The roots unite, forming a nerve which divides into a cranial or internal branch and a spinal or external branch. The cranial portion runs with the vagus nerve and innervates the palate, pharynx, larynx, and thoracic viscera. The spinal branch supplies the sternocleidomastoid and trapezius muscles. The nerves include general somatic efferent and general visceral efferent (parasympathetic) components. Also called *accessory nerve, eleventh cranial nerve, spinal accessory nerve, nerve of Willis*.

nervus acusticus NERVUS VESTIBULOCOCHLEARIS.

nervi alveolares superiores [NA] Branches arising from the maxillary nerve in the pterygopalatine fossa or infraorbital canal that supply innervation to the teeth and gingiva of the upper jaw. Posterior, middle and anterior nerves are recognized. Also called *superior alveolar nerves, superior dental nerves*.

nervus alveolaris inferior [NA] The direct continuation of the posterior division of the mandibular nerve that descends deep to the lateral pterygoid muscle to pass between the sphenomandibular ligament and ramus of the mandible, where, after giving off the mylohyoid nerve, it enters the mandibular foramen. Within the mandibular canal, branches supply motor and premolar teeth and the adjacent gum, and at the mental foramen gives rise to the mental nerve to the cutaneous and mucosal surfaces of the lower lip. The nerve continues in the canal as the incisive branch. Also called *inferior alveolar nerve, inferior dental nerve*.

nervus ampullaris anterior [NA] Fibers of the vestibular nerve that supply the crista ampullaris of the anterior semicircular canal. They travel in the utriculoampullary division of the nerve. Also called *anterior ampullary nerve, superior ampullary nerve, nervus ampullaris superior*.

nervus ampullaris inferior NERVUS AMPULLARIS POSTERIOR.

nervus ampullaris lateralis [NA] Component of the utriculoampullary nerve leading from the ampulla of the lateral semicircular canal. Also called *lateral ampullary nerve*.

nervus ampullaris posterior [NA] A branch of the vestibular nerve that runs through the foramen singulare at the bottom of the internal auditory meatus and divides into filaments supplying the posterior semicircular canal. Also called *posterior ampullary nerve, nervus ampullaris inferior, inferior ampullary nerve*.

nervus ampullaris superior NERVUS AMPULLARIS ANTERIOR.

nervi anococcygei [NA] An offshoot of the coccygeal plexus ($S_{4,5}Co$) which, after piercing the sacrotuberous ligament, supplies the coccyx and overlying skin. Also called *anococcygeal nerve*.

nervus articularis [NA] A nerve to an articulation. It may arise from the nerve to a muscle acting on the joint or from a cutaneous nerve. Also called *articular nerve, joint nerve*.

nervi auriculares anteriores [NA] Two small branches of the auriculotemporal nerve which supply the skin over the tragus of the ear. Also called *anterior auricular nerves*.

nervus auricularis magnus [NA] A sensory branch of the cervical plexus that passes around the posterior margin of the sternocleidomastoid muscle and ascends beneath the platysma to the level of the parotid gland, where it divides into an anterior branch distributed to skin over the gland and a posterior branch to skin over the mastoid process, back of the auricle, and ear lobe. A filament pierces the cartilage of the auricle to innervate the concha. It carries fibers from C_2 and $_3$ segmental levels. Also called *great auricular nerve*.

nervus auricularis posterior [NA] A branch of the facial nerve that ascends between the external acoustic meatus and mastoid process to supply the auricularis posterior and intrinsic auricular muscles via an auricular branch, and the occipitalis muscle through its occipital branch. Also called *posterior auricular nerve*.

nervus auriculotemporalis [NA] A sensory branch from the posterior trunk of the mandibular nerve. It arises from two roots that embrace the middle meningeal artery, and then runs backward deep to the lateral pterygoid and between the sphenomandibular ligament and the neck of the mandible. Emerging from behind the temporomandibular joint, it crosses the root of the zygoma and divides into superficial temporal branches. It supplies anterior auricular branches to the tragus, external meatus, and tympanic membrane; temporal branches to the temple and scalp; twigs to the temporomandibular joint; and relays otic ganglion and sympathetic fibers to the parotid gland. Also called *auriculotemporal nerve.*

nervus axillaris [NA] One of the five major terminal branches of the brachial plexus. Composed of C_5 and $_6$ axons from the posterior cord, it winds around the humerus by passing backward through the quadrangular space. Its branches supply the deltoid and teres minor muscles, and form the upper lateral cutaneous nerve of the arm. Also called *axillary nerve, circumflex humeral nerve.*

nervus buccalis [NA] A branch of the anterior trunk of the mandibular nerve. After passing forward between the two heads of the lateral pterygoid, it courses downward to cross the pterygomandibular raphe and join with branches of the facial nerve that ramify on the buccinator muscle. It supplies the skin and mucosa of the cheek near the mouth and the buccal surface of the gums, and sends a motor branch to the lateral pterygoid. Also called *buccal nerve, long buccal nerve, buccinator nerve, nervus buccinatorius.*

nervus buccinatorius NERVUS BUCCALIS.

nervus canalis pterygoidei [NA] A nerve formed in the foramen lacerum by the joining of parasympathetic and sensory fibers of the greater petrosal nerve (from the facial nerve) with sympathetic fibers of the deep petrosal nerve. It passes through the pterygoid canal, at the rostral end of which it enters the pterygopalatine fossa. The parasympathetic fibers synapse in the pterygopalatine ganglion, while sympathetic and sensory axons simply pass through for distribution over the ganglion's branches. Also called *nerve of pterygoid canal.*

nervi cardiaci cervicale Nerves that arise at three levels along the cervical sympathetic trunk and descend through the thoracic inlet to end in the cardiac plexuses. Their sympathetic fibers ultimately reach the lungs and other thoracic viscera, as well as the heart. Afferent fibers mediating pain travel in the middle and inferior cervical cardiac nerves, but not in the superior one.

nervi cardiaci thoracici [NA] Filaments that arise from the second to fourth thoracic sympathetic ganglia and end in the deep cardiac plexus. They have an acceleratory influence on the heart equal to that of the cervical cardiac nerves, and carry visceral afferent fibers. Also called *thoracic cardiac nerves.*

nervus cardiacus cervicalis inferior [NA] A nerve that arises from the cervicothoracic ganglion of the sympathetic trunk to descend behind the subclavian artery and join the deep cardiac plexus. Also called *nervus cardiacus inferior, inferior cardiac nerve, inferior cervical cardiac nerve.*

nervus cardiacus cervicalis medius [NA] The largest of the sympathetic nerves to the heart. It arises from the middle cervical sympathetic ganglion or nearby trunk, and ends in the deep cardiac plexus. Also called *middle cervical cardiac nerve, middle cardiac nerve, nervus cardiacus medius.*

nervus cardiacus cervicalis superior [NA] A cardiac nerve arising from the lower pole of the superior cervical sympathetic ganglion. On the right side it enters the deep cardiac plexus and, on the left, the superficial part of the plexus. Also called *nervus cardiacus superior, superior cardiac nerve, superior cervical cardiac nerve.*

nervus cardiacus inferior NERVUS CARDIACUS CERVICALIS INFERIOR.

nervus cardiacus medius NERVUS CARDIACUS CERVICALIS MEDIUS.

nervus cardiacus superior NERVUS CARDIACUS CERVICALIS SUPERIOR.

nervi carotici externi [NA] Twigs bridging over to the superior cervical sympathetic ganglion from the external carotid plexus. Their axons are distributed via branches of the artery. Also called *external carotid nerves.*

nervi caroticotympanici [NA] Two tiny filaments that leave the internal carotid sympathetic plexus to pass through openings in the posterior wall of the carotid canal and enter the middle ear, where they join the tympanic plexus. Inferior and superior nerves are distinguished. Also called *caroticotympanic nerves, small deep petrosal nerves.*

nervus caroticus internus [NA] A fine nerve passing upward from the superior cervical sympathetic ganglion to join the internal carotid plexus. Also called *internal carotid nerve.*

nervi cavernosi clitoridis [NA] Bundles, composed of sympathetic, parasympathetic, and sensory fibers, that supply the erectile tissue of the clitoris. They are forward continuations of the uterovaginal plexus. Also called *cavernous nerves of clitoris.*

nervi cavernosi penis [NA] Nerves that supply the erectile tissue of the corpora cavernosa and corpus spongiosum. They arise as offshoots from the front of the prostatic plexus, are joined by branches of the pudendal nerve, and carry postganglionic sympathetic, parasympathetic, and sensory fibers. Also called *cavernous nerves of penis.*

nervi cavernosi penis minores Cavernous nerves that pierce the tunic of the corpus spongiosum near the root of the penis.

nervus cavernosus penis major A cavernous nerve that derives from the plexus prostaticus and runs forward on the dorsum of the penis for distribution to the corpora cavernosum penis and corpus spongiosum. Also called *plexus cavernosus penis, cavernous plexus of penis, greater cavernous nerve.*

nervi celiaci RAMI CELIACI NERVI VAGI.

nervi cerebrales An outmoded term for NERVI CRANIALES.

nervi cervicales [NA] Spinal nerves arising from cervical segments of the spinal cord. There are eight, including the suboccipital nerve (C_1) and the nerve (C_8) passing through the foramen between the last cervical and first thoracic vertebrae. Each divides into a dorsal and ventral primary ramus. The ventral primary rami at levels C_1–C_4 form the cervical plexus, and at levels C_5–C_8 contribute to the brachial plexus. Also called *cervical nerves.*

nervus cervicalis superficialis NERVUS TRANSVERSUS COLLI.

nervi ciliares breves [NA] Filaments that leave the ciliary ganglion carrying postganglionic parasympathetic fibers as well as transient sympathetic and general sensory axons to the eyeball. Ten to twelve nerves leave the ganglion, and subdivide into 15-20 strands that pierce the sclera around the optic nerve and travel forward in impressions on the sclera to supply the sphincter pupillae and ciliaris muscles and blood vessels and sensory endings of the choroid and iris. Also called *short ciliary nerves.*

nervi ciliares longi [NA] Two or three slender branches of the nasociliary nerve that penetrate the sclera near the optic nerve and run forwards between the sclera and choroid to terminals in the ciliary body, iris, and cornea. They carry superior cervical sympathetic post-ganglionic fibers to the dilator pupillae and the sensory innervation of the cornea. Also called *long ciliary nerves.*

nervi clunium inferiores [NA] Several branches of the posterior femoral cutaneous nerve that round the inferior border of the gluteus maximus to supply the skin over the lower part of that muscle. Also called *inferior clunial nerves.*

nervi clunium medii [NA] Two or three branches of the lateral divisions of the dorsal primary rami that pierce the gluteus maximus to innervate the skin over the adjacent gluteal and sacral area. A gap separates the segmental representation, S_{1-3}, of these nerves from that of the superior gluteal nerves, L_{1-3}. Also called *middle clunial nerves, middle gluteal nerves.*

nervi clunium superiores [NA] Lateral branches of the L_{1-3} dorsal primary rami that appear at the outer border of the erector spinae and cross the iliac crest to supply the skin over the upper and lateral gluteal region. Also called *superior clunial nerves.*

nervus coccygeus   One of the pair of nerves that emerge from the coccygeal segment of the spinal cord to supply the region of the coccyx. Also called *coccygeal nerve.*

nervus cochleae   PARS COCHLEARIS NERVI OCTAVI.

nervi conarii   CONARIAL NERVES.

nervi craniales   The twelve pairs of nerves which are connected with the intracranial portion of the central nervous system, consisting of the nervi olfactorii (I), opticus (II), oculomotorius (III), trochlearis (IV), trigeminus (V), abducens (VI), facialis (VII), vestibulocochlearis (VIII), glossopharyngeus (IX), vagus (X), accessorius (XI), and hypoglossus (XII). Nervus accessorius is also derived in part from the upper portion (C_1–C_4) of the spinal cord. Also called *cranial nerves, nervi cerebrales* (outmoded), *cerebral nerves* (outmoded).

nervus cutaneus   [NA] A nerve supplying an area of skin and its underlying fascia. It carries sympathetic fibers to the glands, blood vessels, and arrectores pili and other smooth muscle, as well as sensory axons. Also called *cutaneous nerve, skin nerve.*

nervus cutaneus antebrachii dorsalis   NERVUS CUTANEUS ANTEBRACHII POSTERIOR.

nervus cutaneus antebrachii lateralis   [NA] The cutaneous component ($C_{5,6}$) of the musculocutaneous nerve. It sends an anterior branch along the volar aspect of the forearm and a posterior branch down the dorsal surface, both reaching as far as the thenar eminence. Also called *lateral antebrachial cutaneous nerve, lateral cutaneous nerve of forearm.*

nervus cutaneus antebrachii medialis   [NA] A nerve (C_8, T_1) arising from the medial cord of the brachial plexus. It supplies the skin over the anteromedial aspect of the elbow and forearm to the wrist, and an adjoining strip on the dorsal aspect of the forearm. Also called *medial antebrachial cutaneous nerve, medial cutaneous nerve of forearm.*

nervus cutaneus antebrachii posterior   [NA] A branch ($C_{5,6,7,8}$) of the radial nerve that pierces the lateral head of the triceps to supply an extensive area of skin along the dorsolateral side of the arm, elbow, and forearm down to the wrist. Also called *posterior antebrachial cutaneous nerve, posterior cutaneous nerve of forearm, nervus cutaneus antebrachii dorsalis, dorsal cutaneous nerve of forearm.*

nervus cutaneus brachii lateralis inferior   [NA] A branch ($C_{5,6}$) of the radial nerve that pierces the lateral head of the triceps to supply the skin over the lateral part of the lower half of the arm. Anteriorly the distribution adjoins that of the medial brachial cutaneous nerve. Also called *inferior lateral brachial cutaneous nerve, inferior lateral cutaneous nerve of arm.*

nervus cutaneus brachii lateralis superior   [NA] A branch of the axillary nerve that passes around the posterior margin of the deltoid muscle to supply the skin over the insertion of that muscle and the adjacent triceps. Also called *upper lateral cutaneous nerve of arm, superior lateral cutaneous nerve of arm, lateral superior cutaneous nerve of arm.*

nervus cutaneus brachii medialis   [NA] A small offshoot (C_8, T_1) of the medial cord of the brachial plexus that supplies the skin over the medial side of the lower third of the arm. It is usually joined by the intercostobrachial nerve (T_2), or may be replaced by that nerve. Also called *medial cutaneous nerve of arm, internal cutaneous nerve, nerve of Wrisberg.*

nervus cutaneus brachii posterior   [NA] A nerve ($C_{5,6,7,8}$) that, in the axilla, leaves the radial nerve to supply a small area of skin over the dorsum of the middle third of the arm. Also called *posterior brachial cutaneous nerve, posterior cutaneous nerve of arm.*

nervus cutaneus colli   NERVUS TRANSVERSUS COLLI.

nervus cutaneus dorsalis intermedius   [NA] The smaller of two terminal branches of the superficial peroneal nerve. It sup-

plies the skin on the lateral aspect of the ankle and on contiguous sides of the lateral three toes, as well as nearby joints. Also called *intermediate dorsal cutaneous nerve.*

nervus cutaneus dorsalis lateralis   [NA] The continuation of the sural nerve along the lateral border of the foot (L_5, $S_{1,2}$). Also called *lateral dorsal cutaneous nerve of foot.*

nervus cutaneus dorsalis medialis   [NA] The branch of the superficial peroneal nerve supplying the skin and joints along the medial side of the great toe and the cleft between the second and third toes. Also called *medial dorsal cutaneous nerve of foot.*

nervus cutaneus femoris lateralis   [NA] A nerve supplying the skin over the lateral and anterior aspects of the thigh from the inguinal ligament to the knee. It arises from posterior divisions of the L_2 and L_3 anterior primary rami, and leaves the pelvis by passing beneath the inguinal ligament near the anterior superior iliac spine. Also called *lateral femoral cutaneous nerve, lateral cutaneous nerve of thigh.*

nervus cutaneus femoris posterior   [NA] A large contribution of the sacral plexus to cutaneous innervation of the thigh. Arising from S_{1-3} levels, it lies dorsomedial to the sciatic nerve as the latter passes out the infrapiriform aperture of the sciatic foramen. Below the gluteus maximus it becomes cutaneous and runs down the middle of the thigh and onto the calf. It supplies the skin along this zone, and sends inferior cluneal branches over the lower portion of the gluteus maximus and a long perineal branch to the lateral extent of the perineum. The medial and lateral branches of the trunk derive respectively from anterior and posterior divisions of the sacral plexus; i.e., the nerve marks the postaxial border of the limb. Also called *posterior femoral cutaneous nerve, small sciatic nerve, posterior cutaneous nerve of thigh.*

nervus cutaneus surae lateralis   [NA] A branch ($L_{4,5}$ S_1) of the common peroneal nerve that supplies the skin over the anterior, posterior, and lateral surfaces of the proximal leg. It gives rise to the sural communicating branch. Also called *lateral cutaneous nerve of calf, peroneal cutaneous nerve* (outmoded).

nervus cutaneus surae medialis   [NA] The tibial nerve component of the sural nerve. It descends between the heads of the gastrocnemius and is then joined by the communicating branch of the lateral sural to form the sural nerve. Also called *medial sural cutaneous nerve, medial cutaneous nerve of calf.*

nervus descendens cervicalis   RADIX INFERIOR ANSAE CERVICALIS.

nervi digitales   One of the four nerves that course along the dorsolateral and ventrolateral aspects of a digit to supply its joints, skin, and nailbed. It may arise directly from a major parent nerve, e.g., ulnar, or through bifurcation of a common digital nerve. Also called *digital nerves.*

nervi digitales dorsales   [NA] Small nerves that extend varying distances along the dorsolateral surfaces of a digit to give cutaneous and articular innervation. In the human hand those to the radial $2^1/_2$ fingers arise from common or proper digital branches of the superficial radial nerve (nervi digitales dorsales nervi radiales) while nerves to the remaining fingers arise from comparable branches of the dorsal carpal branch of the ulnar nerve (nervi digitales dorsales nervi ulnaris). Also called *dorsal digital nerves.*

nervi digitales dorsales pedis   [NA] Branches of the deep and superficial peroneal nerves that supply a single side of toe, i.e., proper digital nerves, or split to supply adjacent sides of two toes, i.e., common digital nerves. Also called *dorsal digital nerves of foot.*

nervi digitales palmares   Digital nerves that course along the ventral aspect of a finger. They arise from the ulnar and median nerves. Also called *palmar digital nerves.*

nervi digitales palmares communes   [NA] Sensory nerves of the palmar surface of the hand which, as they approach the cleft between two fingers, divide into proper digital nerves supplying adjacent surfaces of the digits. Two arise from the median nerve and one from the ulnar nerve.

nervi digitales palmares proprii [NA] Small nerves coursing along the two sides of a digit on its volar aspect. In the human hand six usually arise through bifurcation of common digital nerves, while single branches arising directly from the ulnar and median nerve trunks travel along the ulnar side of the little finger, radial side of the index finger, and both sides of the thumb. They innervate the joints, the skin over the volar surfaces, the nail bed, and generally, via dorsal branches, the skin over the middle and distal phalanges. Also called *proper palmar digital nerves, nervi digitales volares proprii.*

nervi digitales plantares Digital nerves that course along the ventral aspect of a toe. They arise from the medial and later plantar nerves. Also called *plantar digital nerves.*

nervi digitales plantares communes [NA] The nervi digitales plantares communes nervi plantaris lateralis and the nervi digitales plantares communes nervi plantaris medialis. Also called *common plantar digital nerves.*

nervi digitales plantares communes nervi plantaris lateralis The two digital nerves into which the superficial branch of the lateral plantar nerve divides. The lateral of these supplies the flexor digiti minimi brevis muscle and two interosseous muscles in the fourth intermetatarsal space, and then continues along the lateral aspect of the little toe as the sensory nerve to that region. The more medial nerve divides into two proper branches that serve as the sensory nerves, each supplying one of the adjacent surfaces of the fourth and fifth toes. Also called *common plantar digital nerves of lateral plantar nerve.*

nervi digitales plantares communes nervi plantaris medialis The three digital nerves into which the medial plantar nerve divides. Each splits into two proper digital nerves that supply cutaneous innervation to the four medial toes. The most medial of these supplies proper plantar digital nerves to the adjacent sides of the great toe and the second toe; the intermediate nerve supplies the adjacent sides of the second and third toes; and the most lateral supplies the adjacent sides of the third and fourth toes. Also called *common plantar digital nerves of medial plantar nerve.*

nervi digitales plantares proprii nervi plantaris lateralis [NA] Proper digital branches of the lateral plantar nerve. They are distributed to adjacent sides of the digits IV and V, and to the lateral side of the fifth digit.

nervi digitales plantares proprii nervi plantaris medialis [NA] Proper digital branches of the medial plantar nerve. They are distributed to the medial three toes and one side of the fourth toe, each branch supplying one side of a toe. Several arise through bifurcation of common digital nerves destined for adjacent sides of two toes.

nervi digitales volares proprii NERVI DIGITALES PALMARES PROPRII.

nervus digitalis communis A digital nerve which as it approaches the cleft between two fingers divides into two proper digital nerves supplying the adjacent surfaces of the digits. Also called *common digital nerve.*

nervus digitalis proprius A digital nerve which arises directly from a major nerve without being associated with nerves to other digits. Also called *proper digital nerve.*

nervus dorsalis clitoridis [NA] The main continuation of the pudendal nerve. It passes forward along the pubic ramus, enters the urogenital diaphragm, and courses along the dorsum of the clitoris to end in the glans. It supplies the deep transverse perineal muscle, sphincter urethra, corpus cavernosum, and glans with motor and general sensory innervation. Also called *dorsal nerve of clitoris.*

nervus dorsalis penis [NA] The continuation of the internal pudendal nerve, which runs on the deep surface of the inferior layer of the urogenital diaphragm and then on the dorsum of the penis to supply the corpus cavernosum and glans. Also called *dorsal nerve of penis.*

nervus dorsalis scapulae [NA] A branch of the fifth cervical nerve that, after piercing the scalenus medius to reach the deep surfaces of the rhomboid muscles, supplies these muscles and sometimes the levator scapulae. Also called *dorsal scapular nerve, nerve to rhomboids, dorsal nerve of scapula.*

nervi erigentes NERVI SPLANCHNICI PELVICI. • The term is not preferred, since these nerves not only innervate the erectile tissue of the genitalia, but other pelvic organs as well.

nervus ethmoidalis anterior [NA] The continuation of the nasociliary nerve beyond its entry in the anterior ethmoid foramen and canal. Within the cranial cavity but deep to the dura mater the nerve runs forward on the cribiform plate to an aperture at the side of the crista galli, through which it descends into the nasal cavity. Lying on the inner surface of the nasal bone, it supplies internal nasal branches to the septum and lateral wall of the nasal cavity, and then emerges at the distal border of the nasal bone as the external nasal branch supplying the skin over the bridge, apex, ala, and vestibule of the nose. Also called *anterior ethmoidal nerve.*

nervus ethmoidalis posterior [NA] A twig of the nasociliary nerve that exits the orbit through the posterior ethmoid foramen to supply posterior ethmoidal air cells and the sphenoid sinus. Also called *posterior ethmoidal nerve, nerve of Luschka.*

nervus facialis [NA] The seventh cranial nerve and a derivative of the second branchial arch. Arising anteriorly to the inferior cerebellar peduncle at the caudal border of the pons as a motor root and a distinct nervus intermedius bearing sensory and parasympathetic preganglionic fibers, it traverses the internal acoustic meatus and enters the facial canal, where the geniculate ganglion of its sensory fibers is located. The main nerve leaves the canal at the stylomastoid foramen and in the parotid gland separates into branches distributed to muscles of the scalp, auricle and face, the platysma, stylohyoid muscles and posterior belly of the digastric. Other branches given off in the facial canal are the greater superficial petrosal nerve, chorda tympani and nerve to the stapedius. Through these branches taste receptors of the soft palate and presulcal surface of the tongue are supplied, and motor fibers reach glands of the nasal and palative mucosae, and the submandibular, sublingual and labial glands. Also called *seventh cranial nerve, facial nerve, portio dura paris septimi* (outmoded).

nervus femoralis [NA] The sensorimotor nerve to an extensive anteromedial region of the lower leg. Contributions from L_{2-4} spinal nerves join within the belly of the psoas muscle to form the nerve trunk which, still resting on the muscle surface, leaves the abdomen by passing beneath the inguinal ligament. Within the femoral trigone it splits into several muscular and cutaneous branches, of which the saphenous nerve is the direct continuation. The nerve supplies the sartorius, quadriceps femoris, and pectineus muscles, the skin over the anterior and medial surfaces of the limb from the inguinal ligament to the big toe, and nearby sectors of joints. Derived from posterior divisions of the lumbar plexus, it supplies, in the embryo, the dorsal, extensor aspect of the limb. Also called *femoral nerve, anterior crural nerve.*

nervus fibularis communis NERVUS PERONEUS COMMUNIS.

nervus fibularis profundus NERVUS PERONEUS PROFUNDUS.

nervus fibularis superficialis NERVUS PERONEUS SUPERFICIALIS.

nervus frontalis [NA] The largest branch of the ophthalmic nerve. It enters the orbit through the superior orbital fissure, and coursing between the levator palpebrae and periorbita separates into a supraorbital nerve and a smaller, more medially located supratrochlear nerve. Also called *frontal nerve*.

nervus furcalis The lumbar spinal nerve whose anterior primary ramus bifurcates to contribute to both the lumbar and sacral plexuses. Generally it is the L_4 nerve, but it may be L_3 or L_5. Also called *furcal nerve*.

nervus genitocruralis NERVUS GENITOFEMORALIS.

nervus genitofemoralis [NA] A mixed nerve arising from L_1 and $_2$ levels of the lumbar plexus. It passes obliquely downwards through and on the psoas major muscle to divide above the inguinal ligament into an external spermatic nerve that enters the deep inguinal ring and a femoral branch that descends beneath the inguinal ligament to the femoral trigone. Also called *genitofemoral nerve, nervus genitocruralis.*

nervus glossopharyngeus [NA] The ninth cranial nerve, innervating structures derived from the third branchial arch, including the mucosa of the oropharynx, tonsil, and the postsulcal part of the tongue, as well as one muscle, the stylopharyngeus. All the general and the special sensory fibers have their cell bodies in the inferior and superior ganglia located in the jugular foramen. Centrally the fibers of general sensibility synapse in the nucleus of the spinal tract of the trigeminal nerve, while the taste fibers end in the nucleus of the tractus solitarius. The motor fibers arise in the nucleus ambiguus. The nerve's parasympathetic fibers come from the inferior salivatory nucleus, and pass through the lesser petrosal branch to the otic ganglion, which gives off postsynaptic fibers to the parotid gland. Also called *glossopharyngeal nerve, glossopharyngeus, ninth cranial nerve.*

nervus gluteus inferior [NA] A nerve arising from ventral rami of the L_5, $S_{1,2}$ nerves that leaves the pelvis below the piriformis muscle to supply the gluteus maximus. Also called *inferior gluteal nerve.*

nervus gluteus superior [NA] The superior ($L_{4,5}$ S_1) of two nerves supplying the main gluteal muscles. It leaves the pelvis through the suprapiriform portion of the greater sciatic foramen to enter the gluteal region. A superior branch ends in the gluteus medius, and an inferior branch supplies this muscle, the gluteus minimus, and farther anteriorly the tensor fasciae latae. The latter branch also supplies the hip joint. Also called *superior gluteal nerve.*

nervi haemorrhoidales inferiores NERVI RECTALES INFERIORES.

nervi haemorrhoidales medii An obsolete term for PLEXUS RECTALES MEDII.

nervus hypogastricus dexter et sinister [NA] The bundle of nerve filaments between the point of bifurcation of the superior hypogastric plexus and the more expanded inferior hypogastric plexus of one side. Also called *hypogastric nerve, hypogastric nerve of Latarjet.*

nervus hypoglossus [NA] The twelfth cranial nerve, providing innervation to all the muscles of the tongue except the palatoglossus. The fibers arise in cell columns of the medulla homologous in position with the anterior column in the cord at lower levels, an indication of their origin from four occipitocervical somites. Rootlets surface in the centerolateral sulcus between the pyramid and olive and, after gathering into one or more bundles, pass forward through the hypoglossal canal. A recurrent branch passes to meninges of the posterior fossa. Fibers from the first cervical nerve join the true hypoglossal fibers, to pass on to the geniohyoid and thyrohyoid muscles and, via the descendens hypoglossi branch, to strap muscles of the neck. A sensory ganglion (Froriep's) found on the nerve in the embryo, is generally absent in adult man. Also called *hypoglossal nerve, hypoglossus, motor nerve of tongue, twelfth cranial nerve.*

nervus iliohypogastricus [NA] The main trunk of the first lumbar nerve. In its course between the transversalis abdominis and internal oblique muscles above the iliac crest, it divides into a lateral cutaneous branch that supplies the skin over the pos-

terolateral gluteal region, and an anterior trunk that sends branches to the two muscles and then perforates the external oblique aponeurosis to supply the skin above the pubis. The lateral cutaneous branch is homologous with the iliac branch of the twelfth cranial nerve, and consequently has a more caudal (posterior) distribution over the gluteal region. Also called *iliohypogastric nerve.*

nervus ilioinguinalis [NA] The major continuation of the first lumbar spinal nerve which, in an oblique course across the abdomen, supplies the abdominal muscles, the skin and peritoneum over the pubis symphysis, and the anterior scrotum or labia. It is homologous with the collateral branch of an intercostal nerve. The nerve emerges from behind the psoas major muscle, and crosses the posterior abdominal wall to pass through the deep inguinal ring and inguinal canal. A lateral branch supplies the skin over a superomedial area of the thigh. Also called *ilioinguinal nerve.*

nervus infraorbitalis The continuation of the maxillary nerve beyond its entry into the infraorbital groove and canal. After exiting from the infraorbital foramen, it divides into branches spreading to the alae of the nose, the lower eyelid, and the skin and mucous membrane of the cheek and upper lip. Also called *infraorbital nerve.*

nervus infratrochlearis [NA] A branch of the nasociliary nerve. It runs forward along the upper border of the medial rectus muscle, and just below the trochlea pierces the orbital septum to supply the skin of the eyelids, conjunctiva, lacrymal sac, duct and caruncle, and an adjacent portion of the nose. Also called *infratrochlear nerve.*

nervi intercostobrachiales [NA] The particularly large lateral cutaneous branch of the second intercostal nerve. It crosses the axilla to supply the skin over medial and posterior aspects of the upper arm. The homologous third intercostal branch supplying the axilla and medial aspect of the arm is sometimes distinguished as a second intercostobrachial nerve. Also called *intercostobrachial nerves.*

nervus intermedius The smaller root of the seventh cranial (facial) nerve which contains special sensory fibers for taste to the anterior two thirds of the tongue and parasympathetic fibers supplying secretomotor impulses to the submaxillary, sublingual, lacrimal, nasal, and palatine glands. Also called *intermediate nerve of Wrisberg, nerve of Wrisberg, nervus intermedius of Wrisberg, intermediary nerve, portio intermedia nervi acustici* (outmoded).

nervus intermedius of Wrisberg NERVUS INTERMEDIUS.

nervus interosseus antebrachii anterior [NA] A major branch of the median nerve that courses along the interosseous membrane deep to the flexor pollicis longus, flexor digitorum profundus, and pronator quadratus muscles, supplying these muscles, sensory receptors on the interosseous membrane, and distally the radioulnar, radiocarpal, and carpal joints. Also called *anterior interosseous nerve of forearm, volar interosseous nerve, nervus interosseus antebrachii volaris.*

nervus interosseus antebrachii posterior [NA] A motor branch of the radial nerve that innervates the majority of muscles on the dorsal aspect of the forearm. It separates from the superficial radial nerve in the lateral part of the popliteal fossa, sends branches to the extensor carpi radialis brevis and supinator, and then winds laterally around the radius between layers of the latter muscle. In its further deep course down the extensor compartment it gives short branches to the extensores digitorum, digiti minimi and carpi ulnaris; a lateral branch to the abductor pollicis longus and extensor pollicis brevis; and a medial branch ot the extensores pollicis longus and indicis. The remaining nerve then runs down the interosseous membrane and dorsum of the carpus, supplying nearby joints as far as the carpometacarpal level. Also called *posterior interosseous nerve of forearm, ramus* *profundus nervi radialis, deep radial nerve, deep branch of radial nerve.*

nervus interosseus antebrachii volaris NERVUS INTEROSSEUS ANTEBRACHII ANTERIOR.

nervus interosseus cruris [NA] A branch of the popliteus muscle nerve (from the tibial nerve) that descends alongside the fibula as far as the inferior tibiofibular joint. It supplies this joint and sensory receptors on the interosseous membrane. Also called *interosseous nerve of leg.*

nervus ischiadicus [NA] The major contribution of the sacral plexus (L_4-S_3) to innervation of the lower extremity. The largest nerve in the body, it typically enters the gluteal region through the infrapiriform aperture of the greater sciatic foramen, though its peroneal (dorsal) division often pierces the piriformis, or may be separated by the entire muscle from the tibial (ventral) division. The latter gives rise to branches to the hamstring muscles, including the ischial head of the adductor magnus, while the peroneal division supplies the short head of the biceps femoris. A sprig is sent to the hip joint. The nerve divides at the upper limit of the popliteal fossa into the tibial and common peroneal nerves. Also called *sciatic nerve, great sciatic nerve, ischiadic nerve.*

nervus jugularis [NA] A nerve that leaves the superior cervical sympathetic ganglion to ascend toward the base of the skull, where it sends branches to the inferior ganglion of the glossopharyngeal nerve and the superior ganglion of the vagus, as well as filaments to the jugular bulb and meninges. Also called *jugular nerve, jugular nerve of Arnold.*

nervi labiales anteriores [NA] Sensory branches of the ilioinguinal nerve supplying the anterior extent of the labium major. Its segmental supply, $L_{1,2}$, contrasts sharply with that of the adjoining posterior labial branches of the pudendal nerve, $S_{3,4}$. Also called *anterior labial nerves.*

nervi labiales posteriores [NA] Medial and lateral branches of the perineal nerve that, after piercing the inferior fascia of the urogenital diaphragm, innervate a major portion of the labia majora. Also called *posterior labial nerves.*

nervus lacrimalis [NA] The smallest branch of the ophthalmic nerve. It enters the orbit through the superior orbital fissure, runs along the upper border of the rectus lateralis, and after piercing the orbital septum supplies the skin of the upper eyelid. It is joined by secretomotor fibers from the zygomaticotemporal nerve, which are given off to the lacrimal gland and nearby conjunctiva. Also called *lacrimal nerve.*

nervus laryngeus inferior [NA] The continuation of the recurrent laryngeal nerve beyond its point of entrance into the larynx deep to the inferior constrictor muscle and posterior to the cricothyroid articulation. It is distributed to the mucosa and glands of the larynx below the vocal cord, and the laryngeal musculature except for the cricothyroid. Also called *inferior laryngeal nerve.*

nervus laryngeus recurrens [NA] A branch of the vagus nerve distributed to those structures derived from the sixth branchial arch, namely portions of the larynx, trachea, and esophagus. It supplies sensory and autonomic innervation to the cervical esophagus, the trachea, and the larynx up as far as the vocal cords, as well as motor fibers to all the skeletal muscles of the larynx except the cricothyroid. At its origin from the vagus, it sends branches to the deep cardiac plexus that are distributed to thoracic viscera. After leaving the main vagus trunk on the right side it winds around the subclavian artery, and on the left side winds around the arch of the aorta just distal to the ligamentum arteriosum. Thereafter it travels up the groove between esophagus and trachea to enter the larynx posterior to the inferior horn of the thyroid cartilage. Also called *recurrent laryngeal nerve, recurrent nerve, ramus laryngeus recurrens nervi vagi, nervus recurrens, ramus laryngei inferior nervi vagi.*

nervus laryngeus superior [NA] A branch of the vagus nerve that, after arising from the inferior vagal ganglion, splits into the internal and external laryngeal nerves, which give sensory and autonomic innervation to the hypopharynx and the larynx above the vocal cord, as well as motor fibers to the inferior constrictor and cricothyroid muscles. Also called *superior laryngeal nerve.*

nervus lingualis [NA] The sensory nerve to the mucous membrane of the floor of the mouth, the lingual aspect of the mandibular gums, and the two-thirds of the tongue anterior to the terminal sulcus, exclusive of the taste receptors. It arises from the posterior division of the mandibular nerve, and is joined by the chorda tympani, whose parasympathetic outflow leaves the lingual nerve by a short root to synapse in the submandibular ganglion, and then rejoins the nerve for distribution to sublingual and lingual salivary glands. Also called *lingual nerve.*

nervi lumbales [NA] The five anterior primary rami of spinal nerves that appear through intervertebral foraminae below respective lumbar vertebrae. The four more cranial rami join the lumbar plexus and two join the sacral plexus, the fourth nerve (the furcal nerve) generally contributing to both plexuses. They also connect with the sympathetic trunk by gray and, at the upper first or second levels, white rami. Also called *lumbar nerves.*

nervus lumboinguinalis RAMUS FEMORALIS NERVI GENITOFEMORALIS.

nervus mandibularis [NA] The largest division of the trigeminal nerve. It is formed from a sensory root from the lateral third of the semilunar ganglion and a motor root, which join after passing through the foramen ovale. The nerve divides into anterior and posterior trunks whose branches supply the skin of the temporal region, the auricle, the lower lip and face, the mucosa of the pre-sulcal part of the tongue and floor of the mouth, and the teeth and gums of the mandible. The motor component supplies all the muscles of mastication. Sprigs from the main trunk reach the internal pterygoid nerve and the meninges. Also called *mandibular nerve.*

nervus massetericus [NA] The nerve supply of the masseter muscle. It arises from the anterior trunk of the mandibular nerve and passes through the mandibular notch, giving a twig en route to the temporomandibular joint. Also called *masseteric nerve.*

nervus masticatorius An obsolete term for RADIX MOTORIA NERVI TRIGEMINI.

nervus maxillaris [NA] The intermediate division of the trigeminal nerve, supplying derivatives of the embryonic maxillary and frontonasal processes. Arising in the semilunar ganglion, it passes through the cavernous sinus, exits the foramen rotundum, crosses the pterygopalatine fossa, and continues as the infraorbital nerve after entering the inferior orbital fissure. Branches go to the meninges of the middle fossa, the teeth, skin and mucosal linings of the upper jaw, and the palate, lip, cheek, lower lid, and nasal and sinus cavities. Also called *maxillary nerve, crotaphitic nerve* (outmoded).

nervus meatus acustici externi [NA] The sensory branch of the auriculotemporal nerve supplying the tympanic membrane and the skin lining the external auditory meatus. Also called *nerve of external acoustic meatus, nervus meatus auditorii externi.*

nervus meatus auditorii externi NERVUS MEATUS ACUSTICI EXTERNI.

nervus medianus [NA] The major nerve (C_5-T_1) to flexor aspects of the forearm and hand. It arises as two roots springing from lateral and medial cords of the brachial plexus, and courses deep within the medial bicipital furrow to the cubital fossa, where it passes between two heads of the pronator teres. It then descends deep to the flexor digitorum superficialis and flexor retinaculum, finally dividing into palmar digital nerves to the radial $3^1/_2$ digits and a stout muscular branch. The latter is of major functional importance, since it innervates the flexor pollicis brevis, abductor pollicis brevis, and opponens pollicis. In the forearm the median nerve gives rise to the nervus interosseous antebrachii, which supplies most flexor muscles in the forearm. Also called *median nerve.*

nervus meningeus medius RAMUS MENINGEUS MEDIUS NERVI MAXILLARIS.

nervus mentalis [NA] The continuation of the inferior alveolar nerve after it emerges from the mental foramen. It sends separate branches to the skin over the chin, the skin of the lip, and the mucosa. Also called *mental nerve.*

nervus musculi quadrati femoris [NA] A nerve arising from the ventral branches of the ventral rami of the fourth and fifth lumbar and first sacral nerves and passing through the greater sciatic foramen below the piriform muscle to run deep to the sciatic nerve, obturator internus, and gemelli muscles. It supplies branches to the anterior surface of the gemellus inferior muscle and the hip joint, and it ends in the quadratus femoris muscle. Also called *nerve to gemellus inferior and quadratus femoris muscles, nerve to quadratus femoris muscle.*

nervus musculi tensoris tympani [NA] Fibers of the nerve to medial pterygoid muscle which pass through the otic ganglion without synapsing with its cells and run posteriorly to provide motor and proprioceptive innervation to the tensor tympani muscle. Also called *nervus tensoris tympani* (outmoded), *nerve of tensor tympani muscle, nerve to muscle of malleus.*

nervus musculocutaneus [NA] A major terminal branch (C_{5-7}) of the lateral cord of the brachial plexus, innervating flexor aspects of the upper limb. It perforates and supplies the coracobrachialis, sends branches to the brachialis and biceps as it courses distalward between these muscles, and emerges as the lateral cutaneous nerve supplying the skin along the radial forearm as far as the thenar eminence. Branches are sent into the elbow joint and nutrient foramen of the humerus. Also called *musculocutaneous nerve, musculocutaneous nerve of arm.*

nervus mylohyoideus [NA] A branch of the inferior alveolar nerve that descends along the medial aspect of the mandible to reach the inferior surface of the mylohyoid muscle. It innervates this muscle and the anterior belly of the digastric. Also called *mylohyoid nerve.*

nervus nasociliaris A branch of the ophthalmic division of the fifth cranial (trigeminal) nerve. It supplies sensory innervation to the mucous membrane of the nasal cavity and sinuses and to the skin of the ala and apex of the nose. Also called *nasociliary nerve.*

nervus nasopalatinus A branch of the maxillary division of the fifth cranial (trigeminal) nerve, supplying sensory innervation to the roof of the nasal cavity and septum. Also called *nasopalatine nerve, nerve of Cotunnius, Scarpa's nerve, sphenoid-palatine nerve* (outmoded).

nervi nervorum Filaments supplying sensory and sympathetic innervation to the sheath and endoneurium of a peripheral nerve.

nervus obturatorius [NA] The major nerve to the adductor group of leg muscles. It arises from anterior divisions of the L_{2-4} anterior primary rami, assembles in the belly of the psoas major muscle, and passes along the lateral pelvic wall to the entrance of the obturator canal. Within the canal it splits into an anterior branch that sends branches to the gracilis, adductores longus and brevis, and often the pectineus; and a posterior branch deep to the brevis that supplies this muscle and more anterior portions of the adductor magnus. Filaments are sent to the hip and knee joints. Also called *obturator nerve.*

nervus obturatorius accessorius [NA] A fairly constant nerve that arises from the ventral branches of the ventral rami of the third and fourth lumbar nerves and accompanies the obturator nerve along the medial border of the psoas major muscle into the pelvis. There it crosses the superior pubic ramus behind the pectineus muscle and divides into branches. One supplies the pectineus, a second reaches the hip joint, and a third joins the anterior branch of the obturator nerve to supply the adductor longus muscle. Also called *accessory obturator nerve.*

nervus obturatorius internus [NA] A nerve that is formed by the ventral branches of the ventral rami of the fifth lumbar and first and second sacral nerves. It leaves the pelvis through the greater sciatic foramen below the piriformis muscle, and, after crossing the ischial spine, it re-enters the pelvis through the lesser sciatic foramen and ends in the pelvic surface of the obturator internus muscle. Above the ischial spine it also gives a branch to the gemellus superior muscle.

nervus occipitalis major [NA] A nerve which, passing upward around the inferior oblique muscle (i.e., outside the occipital triangle) and semispinalis capitis, pierces the latter and fibers of the trapezius to ramify in the scalp as far forward as the vertex. A motor branch is given to the semispinalis. It represents the medial branch of the dorsal primary ramus of the C_2 spinal nerve. Also called *greater occipital nerve, internal occipital nerve.*

nervus occipitalis minor [NA] A branch arising from the anterior primary ramus of the second cervical nerve and sometimes the third, that supplies the scalp between the territories of the greater occipital and great auricular nerves, and through an auricular branch the skin over the cranial surface of the upper third of the pinna. Also called *lesser occipital nerve, mastoid branch of cervical plexus* (outmoded).

nervus occipitalis tertius [NA] A nerve that pierces the trapezeus to supply the skin of the suboccipital and low occipital areas medial to the zone supplied by the greater occipital nerve. It represents the medial branch of the posterior primary ramus at C_3. Also called *third occipital nerve, least occipital nerve.*

nervus octavus NERVUS VESTIBULOCOCHLEARIS.

nervus oculomotorius [NA] The third cranial nerve, originating in the cell groups of the oculomotor nucleus in the rostral two thirds of the midbrain, containing somatic efferent fibers for the ocular muscles and parasympathetic fibers for the ciliary ganglion, and innervating the medial, inferior, and superior rectus muscles, the levator palpebrae superioris, and the sphincter muscles of the pupil and the muscles of accommodation in the iris. Also called *oculomotor nerve, third cranial nerve.*

nervi olfactorii [NA] The first cranial nerve, consisting of approximately ten million very fine, slowly conducting fibers which are the central processes of the olfactory receptors. They run from the upper part of the nasal cavity through the cribriform plate of the ethmoid bone, enter the ventral surface of the olfactory bulb, and terminate in axodendritic tufts (glomeruli). Also called *olfactory nerve, first cranial nerve, olfactory fibers, fila olfactoria.*

nervus ophthalmicus [NA] The superior division of the trigeminal nerve, providing sensory supply to the forehead, the eyes and orbit, the nasal cavity, and the skin over the nose. Commencing in the anteromedial part of the trigeminal ganglion, the nerve passes through the cavernous sinus, enters the orbit through the superior orbital fissure, and divides into three branches, the lacrimal, frontal, and nasociliary. Also called *ophthalmic nerve, ophthalmic nerve of Willis.*

nervus ophthalmicus profundus PROFUNDUS NERVE.

nervus opticus [NA] The cranial nerve mediating vision. Forming through concentration at the optic disc of axons from retinal ganglion cells, it takes a sinuous course through the orbit to the optic foramen. At the intracranial end of the optic canal it separates at the optic chiasma into bundles of fibers that cross to the opposite optic tract and those that remain ipsilateral. The extent of crossing differs among species; in man the division is approximately equal. Embryonically the nerve is a protrusion of the brain rather than a proper nerve. Also called *optic nerve, second cranial nerve, opticus.*

nervi palatini Two, or sometimes three, maxillary nerve branches that supply the palate and posterior portions of the nasal cavity. They arise from the pterygopalatine ganglion and descend in the greater and lesser palatine canals to exit through foramina on the inferior surface of the bony palate. Included are general sensory fibers from the maxillary nerve, postganglionic parasympathetic fibers from the pterygopalatine ganglion, and postganglionic sympathetic and facial nerve taste fibers. Also called *palatine nerves.*

nervi palatini minores [NA] Palatine nerves that, after leaving the lesser palatine canal and foramen, supply the soft palate, uvula, and tonsil. They carry some taste fibers. Also called *lesser palatine nerves.*

nervus palatinus anterior NERVUS PALATINUS MAJOR.

nervus palatinus major [NA] The larger of the palatine nerves. A branch of the maxillary nerve, it descends in the palatine canal and exits through the greater palatine foramen to appear on the inferior surface of the bony palate. It then runs forward, supplying in its course the gums, mucosa, and glands of the hard palate and a small zone of the soft palate. While in the palatine canal, posterior inferior and nasal branches are given off to the middle and inferior meatuses and the inferior concha. Also called *greater palatine nerve, anterior palatine nerve, nervus palatinus anterior.*

nervus palatinus medius A nerve containing fibers of the maxillary nerve and sphenopalatine ganglion that descends in the pterygopalatine canal and emerges from a lesser palatine foramen to supply the tonsil and soft palate. Also called *middle palatine nerve, external palatine nerve.*

nervus palatinus posterior The more posterior and larger of the nervi palatini minores. Also called *posterior palatine nerve.*

nervus patheticus NERVUS TROCHLEARIS.

nervus pectoralis lateralis [NA] A branch (C_{5-7}) arising from the lateral cord or upper and medial trunks of the brachial plexus that innervates clavicular and upper sternal sections of the pectoralis major. Some of its fibers reach the pectoralis minor through a communication with the nervus pectoralis medialis. Also called *lateral pectoral nerve.*

nervus pectoralis medialis [NA] A branch (C_8, T_1) of the medial cord of the brachial plexus that, after entering and supplying the pectoralis minor, continues on to innervate costal and lower sternal portions of the pectoralis major. Also called *medial pectoral nerve.*

nervi perineales [NA] Branches of the perineal nerve that supply muscles in the superficial perineal pouch, portions of the external anal sphincter and levator ani, the bulb and bulbar urethra of the penis and, through posterior scrotal and labial nerves, posterior portions of the scrotum and labia major. Also called *perineal nerves, nervi perinei.*

nervi perinei NERVI PERINEALES.

nervus peroneus communis [NA] The terminal component of the sciatic nerve arising from the posterior divisions of the lumbosacral plexus (L_4–S_2) and destined to supply extensor aspects of the embryonic limb bud. Separating from the tibial division of the sciatic nerve high in the popliteal fossa, it descends obliquely to the head of the fibula, where it divides into the superficial and deep peroneal nerves. In the fossa it gives rise to the lateral cutaneous nerve of the calf and a communicating branch to the sural nerve, as well as branches to the knee and tibiofibular joints. The nerve to the short head of the biceps

arises from the peroneal division of the sciatic before it separates from the tibial division. Also called *common peroneal nerve, nervus fibularis communis, common fibular nerve, lateral popliteal nerve.*

nervus peroneus profundus [NA] A nerve supplying the muscles of the peroneal compartment, deep structures on the dorsum of the ankle, and a small area of skin on the toes. Arising from the common peroneal nerve lateral to the fibula, it sends branches to the peroneus longus, extensor digitorum longus, extensor hallucis longus, and peroneus tertius, and then continues down the interosseous membrane and across the tarsus before bifurcating. The lateral branch supplies the extensor digitorum brevis, tarsal and metatarsal joints of digits II and III. The medial branch supplies the metatarsophalangeal joint of the hallux, and the skin on adjacent sides of the great and second toes. Also called *deep peroneal nerve, nervus fibularis profundus, deep fibular nerve, musculocutaneous nerve of leg.*

nervus peroneus profundus accessorius An anomalous nerve to the extensor digitorum brevis and adjacent talar region arising from the peroneus branch of the superficial peroneal nerve. Also called *accessory deep peroneal nerve.*

nervus peroneus superficialis [NA] A branch of the common peroneal nerve that, as it descends in the lateral compartment of the leg, supplies the peroneus longus and brevis muscles, then sends medial and lateral branches to the skin and joints of the dorsal surfaces of the ankle, tarsus, and most toes. It does not supply the cleft between the great and second toes or the lateral surface of the little toe. The medial branch (L_{4-5}) communicates with the saphenous nerve, and the lateral (L_5 S_1) with the sural nerve. Also called *nervus fibularis superficialis, superficial fibular nerve, superficial peroneal nerve, musculocutaneous nerve of foot.*

nervus petrosus major [NA] An intracranial derivative of the nervus intermedius portion of the cranial nerve carrying sensory and parasympathetic innervation destined for orbital, nasal, nasopharyngeal, and palatine areas. It arises from the genicular ganglion, appears along a groove on the anterior side of the petrous pyramid, and crosses the foramen lacerum beneath the trigeminal ganglion. There it is joined by the deep petrosal nerve to form the nerve of the pterygoid canal for eventual distribution by branches of the pterygopalatine ganglion to the lacrimal gland, nasal and palatine glands, and taste receptors on the soft palate. Phylogenetically the nerve represents the pretrematic branch of the nerve to the second branchial arch. Also called *greater petrosal nerve, greater superficial petrosal nerve, nervus petrosus superficialis major.*

nervus petrosus minor [NA] A branch of the ninth cranial nerve bringing preganglionic parasympathetic fibers to the otic ganglion. Arising in the tympanic plexus, it travels along a canal inferior to the tensor tympani to enter the middle cranial fossa, and then passes out of the cranium via the foramen ovale or innominatus to reach the ganglion. Also called *lesser petrosal nerve, lesser superficial petrosal nerve, nervus petrosus superficialis minor, middle superficial petrosal nerve, lesser superficial nerve.*

nervus petrosus profundus [NA] A bundle of nerve fibers that leave the internal carotid artery plexus in the vicinity of the foramen lacerum to join the greater petrosal nerve and form the nerve of the pterygoid canal. It carries postganglionic fibers from the superior cervical sympathetic ganglion destined for lacrimal, nasal, and palatine glands and vessels. Also called *deep petrosal nerve, deep vidian nerve.*

nervus petrosus superficialis major NERVUS PETROSUS MAJOR.

nervus petrosus superficialis minor NERVUS PETROSUS MINOR.

nervi phrenici accessorii [NA] The contribution made by

the C_5 spinal nerve to the phrenic nerve when at cervical levels it courses at a distance from the main nerve. It is usually associated with the subclavian nerve. Also called *accessory phrenic nerves.*

nervus phrenicus [NA] The motor nerve to the diaphragm. It arises from branches of the C_3, C_4 and C_5 levels of the cervical plexus which joining in front of the anterior scalene muscle, enter the thoracic inlet, pass anterior to the root of the lung, and pierce the diaphragm to innervate it on its inferior surface. Sprigs are sent to the pericardium (ramus pericardiacus) and celiac plexus (ramus phrenicoabdominalis). Also called *phrenic nerve, diaphragmatic nerve.*

nervus piriformis [NA] A nerve that is formed by the dorsal branches of the ventral rami of the first and second sacral nerves. It ends in the anterior surface of the piriformis muscle. Also called *nerve to piriformis muscle.*

nervus plantaris lateralis [NA] The smaller of two terminal branches of the tibial nerve. It innervates the quadratus plantae, abductor and flexor digitorum minimi, adductor hallucis, all the interossei and the lateral three lumbrical muscles. Branches also go to the joints and skin of the lateral sole, little toe, and adjacent surface of the fourth toe. Also called *lateral plantar nerve.*

nervus plantaris medialis [NA] The more medial of the two branches into which the posterior tibial nerve splits deep to the flexor retinaculum. It supplies the abductor pollicis muscle, the flexores hallucis and digitorum brevis, the first lumbrical muscle, and the joints and skin of the instep and medial $3^1/_2$ toes. Also called *medial plantar nerve.*

nervus presacralis PLEXUS HYPOGASTRICUS SUPERIOR.

nervus pterygoideus externus NERVUS PTERYGOIDEUS LATERALIS.

nervus pterygoideus internus NERVUS PTERYGOIDEUS MEDIALIS.

nervus pterygoideus lateralis [NA] A branch to the lateral pterygoid muscle arising from the anterior division of the mandibular nerve. Also called *lateral pterygoid nerve, nervus pterygoideus externus, external pterygoid nerve.*

nervus pterygoideus medialis [NA] A slender branch that separates from the mandibular nerve just below the foramen ovale to innervate the medial pterygoid muscle. Other sprigs, after passing through the otic ganglion, supply the tensor tympani and tensor veli palatini. Also called *nerve to medial pterygoid muscle, nervus pterygoideus internus, internal pterygoid nerve.*

nervi pterygopalatini [NA] Two short nerves passing between the maxillary nerve and the pterygopalatine ganglion lying beneath it. They carry sensory axons passing through the ganglion and postganglionic axons traveling to destinations of the maxillary nerve. Also called *pterygopalatine nerves, nervi sphenopalatini.*

nervus pudendus [NA] The principal nerve to the skin and muscles of the anal and perineal regions. Derived from S_{2-4} levels, it leaves the pelvis through the infrapiriform aperture to enter the gluteal region, and immediately passes through the lesser sciatic foramen to enter the pudendal canal on the wall of the ischiorectal fossa. After giving off inferior rectal nerves, it ends at the posterior margin of the urogenital diaphragm by dividing into a perineal nerve and a dorsal nerve of the penis or clitoris. Also called *pudendal nerve, pudic nerve, Soemmering's nerve, pudendal plexus.*

nervus radialis [NA] The major nerve (C_{5-8}) supplying extensor aspects of the upper limb. The largest terminal branch of the brachial plexus, it arises from the posterior cord and winds posteriorly around the humerus in the radial groove to appear along the lateral side of the cubital fossa, where it separates into the deep and superficial radial nerves. In the arm, it supplies the heads of the triceps, anconeus, brachioradialis, and

extensor digitorum longus, and sends sprigs to the brachialis and the elbow joint. Arising above the level of the elbow are also the posterior and lower lateral cutaneous nerves of the arm and the posterior cutaneous nerve to the forearm. Together these branches provide sensibility over the dorsal surface from the level of the deltoid insertion to the dorsum of the wrist. Also called *radial nerve, musculospiral nerve, musculospiralis* (seldom used).

nervi rectales inferiores [NA] Several branches of the pudendal nerve that pierce the wall of the pudendal canal and cross the ischiorectal fossa to innervate the external anal sphincter, ectodermal mucosa of the anal canal, and perianal skin. The latter area ($S_{3,4}$) dorsally adjoins that of the anococcygeal nerve (S_5C_1). Also called *inferior rectal nerves, nervi haemorrhoidales inferiores, inferior hemorrhoidal nerves.*

nervus recurrens NERVUS LARYNGEUS RECURRENS.

nervus saccularis [NA] The inferior branch of the vestibular nerve which as filaments traverses foramina in the inferior vestibular area of the internal acustic meatus to end on receptors of the macula in the saccule. Also called *saccular nerve.*

nervi sacrales 1 [NA] The five anterior primary rami that pass through anterior sacral foramina and between the sacrum and coccyx to join the sacral and coccygeal plexuses. **2** The nerve of this sacral series, usually the fourth nerve, that splits to contribute to both plexuses. Also called *sacral nerves.*

nervus saphenus [NA] The largest cutaneous branch ($L_{3,4}$) of the femoral nerve. It descends in the adductor canal, emerging at the lower end to take a subcutaneous course on the medial aspect of the knee and leg, where it splits into two branches. One of these ends at the ankle, while the other passes in front of the ankle to reach the base of the big toe. An infrapatellar branch runs in front of the patella, where it joins in the patellar plexus. Also called *saphenous nerve.*

nervi scrotales anteriores [NA] Branches of the ilioinguinal nerve that supply the skin over the root of the penis and anterosuperior portions of the scrotum. The segmental levels represented ($L_{1,2}$) contrast sharply with those of the adjacent territory of the posterior scrotal nerve (S_{2-4}). Also called *anterior scrotal nerves.*

nervi scrotales posteriores [NA] Two branches of the perineal nerve, medial and lateral, that pierce the inferior fascia of the urogenital diaphragm and pass forward to innervate posterior aspects of the scrotum. Also called *posterior scrotal nerves.*

nervus spermaticus externus RAMUS GENITALIS NERVI GENITOFEMORALIS.

nervi sphenopalatini NERVI PTERYGOPALATINI.

nervi spinales [NA] The nerves on each side of the spinal column formed by the union of dorsal (posterior) and ventral (anterior) spinal roots. Shortly after emerging from an intervertebral foramen, each nerve splits into dorsal and ventral primary rami that bring sensory and motor innervation to the trunk, limbs, and viscera. Also called *spinal nerves.*

nervus spinosus An obsolete term for RAMUS MENINGEUS NERVI MANDIBULARIS.

nervi splanchnici lumbales [NA] Four branches leaving the sympathetic chain to join respectively the celiac, renal, and intermesenteric plexuses; the lower part of the intermesenteric plexus; the superior mesenteric plexus via a route anterior to the common iliac vessels; and the superior mesenteric plexus via a route deep to these vessels. Also called *lumbar splanchnic nerves.*

nervi splanchnici pelvici [NA] Branches of the anterior primary rami of sacral nerves 2, 3 and 4 that, joining the inferior hypogastric plexus, bring preganglionic sympathetic innervation to pelvic viscera and, via the superior hypogastric plexus, to the rectum and descending colon. The ganglia are located both in the plexuses and in walls of the viscera. The nerves also carry sensory fibers from the viscera. Also called *pelvic splanchnic nerves, nervi erigentes.*

nervi splanchnici sacrales   [NA] Branches passing between the sacral sympathetic trunk and the superior and inferior hypogastric plexuses. They contain pre– and postganglionic sympathetic fibers and sensory axons from pelvic viscera. Also called *sacral splanchnic nerves.*

nervus splanchnicus imus   [NA] The lowermost of visceral branches given off by the thoracic sympathetic trunk. Recognizable in 50% of bodies, it enters the abdomen alongside the sympathetic trunk and ends in the renal plexus. Also called *lowest splanchnic nerve, renal nerve, least splanchnic nerve, minor splanchnic nerve, nervus splanchnicus minimus* (outmoded).

nervus splanchnicus major   [NA] The largest of the nerves to abdominal viscera formed by the joining of offshoots from the thoracic sympathetic trunk. It arises from the fifth to ninth or tenth thoracic ganglia, perforates the crus of the diaphragm, and ends in the celiac and aorticorenal ganglia and in the medulla of the suprarenal gland. A splanchnic ganglion of variable size is present on the nerve above the diaphragm, and at this level a few filaments pass to the aorta. The nerve carries preganglionic myelinated sympathetic axons from roots T1 to 8, especially T4, and afferent fibers from the viscera. Also called *greater splanchnic nerve, major splanchnic nerve.*

nervus splanchnicus minimus   An outmoded term for NERVUS SPLANCHNICUS IMUS.

nervus splanchnicus minor   [NA] A nerve formed by filaments leading off from the 9th and 10th, or 10th and 11th ganglia of the thoracic sympathetic trunk. It perforates the crus of the diaphragm to join the aorticorenal ganglion. Also called *lesser splanchnic nerve, inferior splanchnic nerve.*

nervus stapedius   [NA] The motor nerve to the stapedius muscle. It arises from the facial nerve in the facial canal to pass forward and sharply upward in a minute canal leading to the pyramidal eminence and muscle. Also called *stapedius nerve, stapedial nerve.*

nervus statoacusticus   NERVUS VESTIBULOCOCHLEARIS.

nervus subclavius   [NA] A branch ($C_{5,6}$) from the superior trunk of the brachial plexus that supplies the subclavius muscle. It is often accompanied by the C_5 contribution to the phrenic nerve. Also called *subclavian nerve, nerve to subclavius muscle.*

nervus subcostalis   [NA] The anterior primary ramus of the spinal nerve that passes between the last thoracic and first lumbar vertebrae. In man, it ravels below the 12th rib and beyond to supply lower portions of the abdominal musculature, including the pyramidalis muscle, and a strip of skin and mucosa culminating above the pubis. A gluteal branch homologous to a lateral cutaneous branch of an intercostal nerve supplies the skin over the anterolateral aspect of the thigh. Also called *subcostal nerve, twelfth thoracic nerve.*

nervus sublingualis   [NA] A branch of the lingual nerve supplying parasympathetic fibers to the sublingual glands and sensory fibers to adjacent mucosa in the floor of the mouth. Also called *sublingual nerve.*

nervus suboccipitalis   [NA] A nerve representing the posterior primary ramus of the first spinal nerve. Leaving the spinal canal between the skull and the neural arch of the atlas vertebra, it enters the suboccipital triangle where branches pass to the rectus capitis major and minor muscles, the obliquus superior and inferior, and a sector of the semispinalis capitis. It has no cutaneous, nor generally even any proprioceptive component. Also called *suboccipital nerve, infraoccipital nerve.*

nervus subscapularis   [NA] The nervous contributions of the posterior cord to innervation of the subscapularis and teres major muscles. The NA recognizes only a single nerve, but a superior subscapular nerve to the cranial portion of the subscapular muscle, and an inferior subscapular nerve supplying the

caudal portion and teres major are always distinguishable. They are separated by the thoracodorsal nerve, which sometimes is called the middle subscapular nerve because of its location rather than its innervation. Also called *subscapular nerves.*

nervi supraclaviculares   [NA] Three nerves or nerve bundles that arise by a common trunk from C_3 and C_4 cervical nerves to supply the skin over the lower neck, uppermost thorax, and shoulder. Also called *supraclavicular nerves.*

nervi supraclaviculares anteriores   NERVI SUPRACLAVICULARES MEDIALES.

nervi supraclaviculares intermedii   [NA] The middle of the three supraclavicular nerve bundles. It supplies the skin over the clavicle, pectoralis major, and deltoid to the level of the second rib. Also called *intermediate supraclavicular nerves, middle supraclavicular nerves.*

nervi supraclaviculares laterales   [NA] A nerve bundle supplying the skin over the lateral and posterior aspects of the shoulder and upper arm. Also called *lateral supraclavicular nerves, nervi supraclaviculares posteriores, posterior supraclavicular nerves.*

nervi supraclaviculares mediales   [NA] A nerve bundle supplying the skin over the insertion of the sternocleidomastoid muscle, the first intercostal space, and the manubrium. A twig goes to the sternoclavicular joint. Also called *nervi supraclaviculares anteriores, anterior supraclavicular nerves, medial supraclavicular nerves.*

nervi supraclaviculares posteriores   NERVI SUPRACLAVICULARES LATERALES.

nervus supraorbitalis   [NA] The major continuation of the frontal nerve. Separating from the supratrochlear nerve between the levator palpebrae and the roof of the orbit, it passes through the supraorbital notch and, via medial and lateral branches, extends backwards nearly to the lambdoid suture. Branches are given to the frontal sinus, conjunctiva and eyelid, pericranium, and scalp. Also called *supraorbital nerve.*

nervus suprascapularis   [NA] A branch ($C_{5,6}$) of the superior trunk of the brachial plexus that innervates the supraspinatus and infraspinatus muscles, and gives twigs to the shoulder and acromiclavicular joints. It passes beneath the ligament that bridges the suprascapular notch. Also called *suprascapular nerve.*

nervus supratrochlearis   [NA] A branch of the frontal nerve that passes forward above the trochlea of the superior oblique and then curves around the orbital margin to continue upward deep to the corrugator and frontalis muscles. Branches are given off to the conjunctiva and skin of the upper eyelid, the root of the nose, and the skin over the forehead near the midline. Also called *supratrochlear nerve.*

nervus suralis   [NA] A nerve formed midway down the calf by the union of the medial sural cutaneous nerve and the communicating branch of the common peroneal nerve. Accompanying the small saphenous vein, it descends along the tendo calcaneus to round the lateral malleolus and continue along the side of the foot and little toe. The nerve marks the watershed between anterior and posterior divisions of the L_5, $S_{1,2}$ spinal nerves. Named branches are the rami calcanei laterales to the heel and sole, and the nervus cutaneus dorsalis, the latter being the continuation along the lateral aspect of the foot. The term is sometimes used for the branch arising from the tibial nerve, relegating the peroneal contribution to a mere communication. Also called *sural nerve, short saphenous nerve, external saphenous nerve.*

nervi temporales profundi   [NA] Branches of the anterior trunk of the mandibular nerve that supply the temporalis muscle. Two, often three, branchesround the infratemporal crest of the skull, above the lateral pterygoid, to enter the deep surface of the muscle. Also called *deep temporal nerves.*

nervus temporalis profundus anterior The more anterior and larger of the deep temporal nerves.

nervus temporalis profundus posterior The deep temporal nerve located toward the posterior limit of the temporal fossa. Also called *posterior deep temporal nerve.*

nervus tensoris tympani An outmoded term for NERVUS MUSCULI TENSORIS TYMPANI.

nervus tensoris veli palatini [NA] A branch of the mandibular nerve that supplies the tensor of the palate. Below the foramen ovale, it is included in the nerve to the medial pterygoid, but shortly separates, passing through the otic ganglion en route to the muscle. Also called *nerve of tensor veli palatini.*

nervus tentorii RAMUS TENTORII NERVI OPHTHALMICI.

nervus terminalis [NA] A small nerve lying between the olfactory bulb and crista galli that receives unmyelinated filaments from the nasal mucous membrane, and caudally enters the anterior perforated substance where its fibers pass into the lamina terminalis and anterior hypothalamus. A ganglion terminal is located along the nerve. It has been suggested that it mediates special osmoreception or supplies blood vessels and glands of the nasal mucosa. In the latter role, the nerve and ganglion have been likened to a cranial extension of the sympathetic trunk. In man, the nerve is poorly developed and it has not been recognized as one of the enumerated cranial nerves. Also called *terminal nerve.*

nervi thoracales NERVI THORACICI.

nervi thoracales anteriores The medial and lateral pectoral nerves. An obsolete and seldom used term.

nervi thoracales posteriores The dorsal scapular nerve, together with the long thoracic nerves. An obsolete term.

nervus thoracalis longus NERVUS THORACICUS LONGUS.

nervi thoracici [NA] The thoracic spinal nerves, including eleven pairs of intercostal nerves and one pair of subcostal nerves. Each is designated by the number of the vertebra beneath which it appears. Also called *thoracic nerves, nervi thoracales.*

nervus thoracicus longus [NA] The nerve supplying the serratus anterior. It originates from branches of the C_5 and C_6 nerves that pierce the scalenus medius and pass behind the axillary artery and brachial plexus to descend near the midaxillary line. Twigs are given off to each digitation of the serratus. In 40 percent of bodies it receives a C_7 contribution. Also called *long thoracic nerve, posterior thoracic nerve, nerve to serratus anterior, external respiratory nerve of Bell* (imprecise), *nervus thoracalis longus, Bell's nerve.*

nervus thoracodorsalis [NA] The nerve to the latissimus dorsi. Carrying $C_{6,7,8}$ fibers, it arises from the posterior cord between the upper and lower subscapular nerves. Also called *the thoracodorsal nerve, middle subscapular nerve.*

nervus tibialis [NA] The larger terminal branch of the sciatic nerve. Representing dorsal divisions of L_4-S_3 components of the lumbosacral plexus, it supplies muscles of the dorsal aspect of the thigh (except the short head of the biceps femoris), the calf, and the plantar aspect of the foot, as well as the skin over the calf and sole of the foot and a number of joints. After giving rise to muscle, crural interosseous, medial sural cutaneous, and medial calcaneal branches, the tibial nerve terminates by bifurcating into the medial and lateral plantar nerves. Also called *tibial nerve, medial popliteal nerve, internal popliteal nerve.*

nervus transversus colli [NA] A cutaneous nerve that, arising from C_2 and C_3 cervical nerves, turns around the sternocleidomastoid to supply anterolateral regions of the neck extending from mandible to sternum. Also called *transverse cervical nerve, transverse cutaneous nerve of neck, anterior cutaneous nerve of neck, transverse nerve of neck, nervus cervicalis superficialis, superficial cervical nerve, nervus cutaneus colli.*

nervus trigeminus [NA] The largest of the cranial nerves, emerging from the lateral surface of the pons and containing both sensory and motor components, together with some intermediate fibers. Cell bodies of origin of the sensory root are located in the trigeminal ganglion of Gasser, from which the three divisions of the nerve (n. ophthalmicus, n. maxillaris, and n. mandibularis) arise. The sensory components supply the face, teeth, mouth, and nasal cavity, and the motor components supply the muscles of mastication. Also called *trigeminal nerve, fifth cranial nerve, trifacial nerve.* • The name derives from the nerve's three divisions, or roots.

nervus trochlearis [NA] The motor nerve to the superior oblique muscle of the eyeball, taking origin from a cell cluster in the ventral part of the central gray substance just lateral to the midline and dorsal to the medial longitudinal fasciculus. The fibers run dorsally and laterally, then cross the midline in the superior medullary velum to emerge from the dorsolateral aspect of the midbrain below the inferior colliculi. The nerve runs forward in the lateral wall of the cavernous sinus and traverses the superior orbital fissure, forming the longest intracranial trajectory of any cranial nerve. Also called *trochlear nerve, fourth cranial nerve, nervus patheticus, pathetic nerve.*

nervus tympanicus [NA] A nerve arising from the inferior, or petrosal, ganglion of the glossopharyngeal nerve and ascending via the inferior tympanic canaliculus to the tympanic cavity, where it divides into the tympanic plexus, which supplies branches to the mucous membrane of the tympanic cavity, the auditory tube, and the mastoid air cells; the lesser petrosal nerve; and the greater petrosal nerve. It is thought to be general sensory and parasympathetic in function. Also called *tympanic nerve, Jacobson's nerve, Andersch nerve, tympanic nerve of Jacobson.*

nervus ulnaris [NA] A mixed peripheral nerve that originates in the medial cord of the brachial plexus, (C_8 and T_1, though often receiving fibers from C_7). Descending through the axilla and along the medial side of the brachial artery, it then traverses a groove on the dorsum of the medial epicondyle and reaches the wrist along the medial surface of the forearm. Its branches are articular, muscular, palmer cutaneous, dorsal, superficial terminal, and deep terminal. Its distribution is largely to the skin on the front and back of the medial portion of the hand, some flexor muscles on the front of the forearm, and many short muscles of the hand, elbow joint, and joints of the hand. Also called *ulnar nerve, cubital nerve.*

nervus utricularis [NA] The branch of the vestibular portion of the eighth cranial nerve that innervates the macula of the utricle. Also called *utricular nerve.*

nervus utriculoampullaris [NA] A nerve that arises from the vestibular portion of the eighth cranial nerve and supplies the utricle and ampullae of the semicircular canals. Also called *utriculoampullar nerve.*

nervi vaginales [NA] Nerves arising from the lower parts of the inferior hypogastric and uterovaginal plexuses and following the vaginal arteries to be distributed to the vaginal walls, the clitoris, and the urethra. The nerves contain many parasympathetic fibers that facilitate the vasodilation of erectile tissue. Also called *vaginal nerves, plexus vaginalis.*

nervus vagus [NA] The tenth cranial nerve, a mixed nerve emerging from the lateral aspect of the medulla oblongata between the inferior olive and the inferior cerebellar peduncle. It exits the skull via the jugular foramen and continues through the neck and thorax into the abdomen. It supplies sensory fibers to the ear, tongue, pharynx, and larynx; motor fibers to the pharynx, larynx, and esophagus; and parasympathetic and visceral afferent fibers to thoracic and abdominal viscera as far as the splenic flexure of the colon. Its major branches include the superior and recurrent laryngeal nerves; the meningeal, auricular, pharyngeal, cardiac, bronchial, gastric, hepatic, celiac, and renal rami; and the pharyngeal, pulmonary, and esophageal plexuses. As the largest single contributor to the parasympathetic division of the autonomic nervous system, its range of functions can be thought of as largely anabolic, synthetic, and/or supportive of body activities. Also called *vagus nerve, tenth cranial nerve, pneumogastric nerve.*

nervus vascularis [NA] Any nerve branch supplying the adventitia of a blood vessel. Also called *vascular nerve.*

nervi vasorum VASOMOTOR NERVES.

nervus vertebralis [NA] A nerve originating from cervicothoracic and vertebral ganglia. Each component ascends along the vertebral artery, forming part of a sympathetic plexus that supplies the spinal meninges, cervical nerves, and the posterior cranial fossa. Also called *vertebral nerve.*

nervi vesicales inferiores plexus pudendi A small group of nerve fibers thought to arise from the pudendal plexus and innervating the bladder. An obsolete term. Also called *inferior vesical nerves of pudendal plexus.*

nervi vesicales inferiores plexus vesicalis The nerve fibers reaching the vesical plexus by way of the inferior vesical artery. An obsolete term. Also called *inferior vesical nerves of vesical plexus.*

nervi vesicales inferiores systematis sympathici The sympathetic nerve fiber components in the inferior vesical nerves, now included in the more general term plexus vesicales.

nervi vesicales superiores plexus vesicalis The nerve fibers reaching the vesical plexus via the superior vesical artery. An obsolete term. Also called *superior vesical nerves of vesical plexus.*

nervi vesicales superiores systematis sympathici The sympathetic nerve fiber components in the superior vesical nerves, now included in the more general term plexus vesicales.

nervus vestibularis PARS VESTIBULARIS NERVI OCTAVI.

nervus vestibuli The vestibular portion of the eighth cranial nerve.

nervus vestibulocochlearis [NA] The eighth cranial nerve, emerging in the groove between pons and medulla behind the facial nerve and in front of the inferior cerebellar peduncle. It consists of two components, both of which are concerned with transmission of afferent impulses from the inner ear. The vestibular root arises from cells of the vestibular ganglion and conveys information about position and movement in space from the semicircular canals, utricle, and saccule. The cochlear root originates from cells of the spinal ganglion and transmits auditory information from the cochlea. Also called *vestibulocochlear nerve, eighth cranial nerve, auditory nerve, acoustic nerve, nervus acusticus, nervus statoacusticus, auditorius, portio mollis paris septimi* (outmoded), *nervus octavus.*

nervus zygomaticus [NA] A nerve originating in the maxillary branch of the fifth cranial nerve in the pterygopalatine fossa, entering the orbit via the inferior orbital fissure, and dividing into the zygomaticotemporal and zygomaticofacial nerves. It supplies the skin on the temple and the prominence of the cheek. Also called *zygomatic nerve.*

Nesacaine A proprietary name for chloroprocaine hydrochloride.

nesidiectomy [Gk *nēsidi(on)* an islet, dim. of *nēsos* an islet + -ECTOMY] The excision of the pancreatic islands of Langerhans.

nesidioblast [Gk *nēsidio(n)*, dim. of *nēsos* an islet + -BLAST] One of the precursor cells that give rise to the cells of the pancreatic islets.

nesidioblastoma [Gk *nēsidio(n)* (dim. of *nēsos* an island) an islet + BLASTOMA] ISLET CELL TUMOR.

malignant nesidioblastoma ISLET CELL CARCINOMA.

nesidioblastosis [Gk *nēsidio(n)* (dim. of *nēsos* an island) an islet + BLAST + -OSIS] Hyperplasia of the pancreatic islet cells.

-ness [Old English suffix denoting condition, quality, or degree] A noun suffix denoting state or quality.

Nessler [Julius *Nessler*, German chemist, 1827–1905] Nessler solution. See under REAGENT.

nesslerization The use of Nessler's reagent in testing for the nitrogen content of proteins, urea, or ammonia.

nest [Old English, akin to L *nidus* a nest] A small group or collection, as of cells within a tissue.

Brunn's epithelial nests Cell clusters found in the normal ureter.

cell nest A collection of densely packed cells, usually epithelial, surrounded by connective tissue, such as those seen in carcinomas.

egg nest The envelope of epithelial granulosa cells and the enclosed oogonium or primary oocyte. See also PRIMORDIAL FOLLICLE.

epithelial nests Small aggregates of epithelial cells in an abnormal location.

Walthard's cell nests Nests of epithelial cells found in the subserosal region of the ovary or fallopian tubes. They are thought to originate from squamous metaplasia of mesothelial cells, and may be a factor in the development of Brenner's tumor of the ovary. Also called *Walthard's inclusions.*

nesteostomy [See NESTIOSTOMY.] JEJUNOSTOMY.

nestia [Gk *nēsteia* a fast] Abstaining from sustenance; fasting. Also called *nestis.*

nestiatria LIMOTHERAPY.

nestiostomy [Gk *nēsti(s)* not eating, fasting; as substantive, *intestinum jejunum*, from its always being found empty; + *o* + -STOMY] JEJUNOSTOMY.

nestis NESTIA.

nestitherapy LIMOTHERAPY.

nestotherapy LIMOTHERAPY.

net [Old English *net, nett*, akin to L *nodus* a knot] NETWORK.

achromatic net The part of a cell structure that does not take up histologic stains.

Chiari's net An embryonic vestige consisting of anastomosing strands of fibrous tissue in the right atrium that are a result of incomplete or less than the usual resorption of the embryonic septum spurium.

chromidial net A network of material within the cell cytoplasm that stains with basic dyes and corresponds to cytoplasmic RNA.

nerve net A loose, intersecting assemblage of fine nerves arranged for the most part in a plane. They may or may not be functionally interconnected by synaptic or electrically inductive contacts.

Trolard's net A seldom used term for PLEXUS VENOSUS CANALIS HYPOGLOSSI.

Netherton [Earl Weldon *Netherton*, U.S. dermatologist, born 1893] See under SYNDROME.

Netterhynchus armillatus *ARMILLIFER ARMILLATUS.*

nettle [Old English *netle, netel, netele*] A plant of the genus *Urtica.*

horse nettle SOLANUM.

stinging nettle *Urtica dioica*, a perennial of the Urticaceae family. It has stimulant, diuretic, and hemostatic properties, and it has been used in homeopathic medicine to treat skin disease. The plant's covering of stinging hairs, which contain histamine-like substances, can cause irritant dermatitis.

network An arrangement of interconnecting fibers or vessels that resembles a meshed fabric in a reticulum, rete, plexus, or anastomosis. Also called *net, meshwork.*

acquaintance network The direct personal contacts made by an individual in the course of employment, recreation, or social intercourse, which may be causally relevant to the individual's development and/or transmission of an infectious disease.

acromial network An arterial anastomosis on the superior surface of the acromion process of the scapula that is formed by the acromial branches of the thoracoacromial artery and the suprascapular artery and the posterior circumflex humeral artery. Also called *rete acromiale, acromial rete.*

arterial network RETE ARTERIOSUM.

calcanean network RETE CALCANEUM.

cell network CYTORETICULUM.

Chiari's network A specialized route for carrying impulses from the sinuatrial node to the atrioventricular node via the crista terminalis of the right ventricle. Also called *Chiari's reticulum, posterior internodal tract.*

chromatin network The threadlike network of chromatin observed in the nucleus of the cell. Also called *nucleoreticulum.*

community health network A community health system for delivering health care to defined population groups.

Gerlach's network The apparent but illusory interlacing of the dendritic processes of large neurons in the spinal cord, formerly regarded as evidence in support of the reticular concept of neural organization.

network of Gesvelst A reticulated appearance in the myelin sheath of an axon, occasionally seen but of unknown significance. An obsolete term.

lateral malleolar network RETE MALLEOLARE LATERALE.

medial malleolar network An arterial anastomosis on the medial malleolus of the tibia, formed by the anterior medial malleolar branch of the anterior tibial artery, the malleolar and calcaneal branches of the posterior tibial artery, the medial tarsal branches of the dorsalis pedis artery, and branches of the medial plantar artery. Also called *medial malleolar rete, rete malleolare mediale.*

neurofibrillar network A plexus of the fine, threadlike structures running throughout the cell body, axon, and dendrites of a neuron. They were originally discovered during examination of reduced silver sections with the light microscope, but they are studied to best advantage with the electron microscope, which shows that they are composed of much finer, tubelike structures, the neurotubules, microtubules, and microfilaments.

peritarsal network A deep plexus of lymphatic vessels in front of and behind the tarsal plates of the eyelids, most of which drain to the superficial and deep parotid lymph nodes. Those of the medial half of the lower eyelid and of the medial angle drain to the submandibular nodes.

periterminal network A network of delicate fibrils and end knobs seen with metallic staining of the motor endplate. The appearances are largely artifactual. An obsolete term.

Purkinje's network JUNCTIONAL TISSUE.

subpapillary network RETE ARTERIOSUM SUBPAPILLARE.

trabecular network RETICULUM TRABECULARE SCLERAE.

venous network RETE VENOSUM.

weighting network The electronic circuitry in a sound level meter which filters the acoustic input and shapes it so that usually the response is no longer linear but gives greater emphasis to the range of frequencies at which human hearing is most sensitive.

neu A seldom used term for NEURILEMMA.

Neubauer [Johann Ernst *Neubauer*, German anatomist, 1742–1777] Neubauer's artery. See under ARTERIA THYROIDEA IMA.

Neuber [Gustav Adolf *Neuber*, German surgeon, 1850–1932] See under OPERATION, TUBE, TREATMENT.

Neuberg [Carl *Neuberg*, German biochemist, 1877–1956] See under ESTER.

Neufeld [Alonzo John *Neufeld*, U.S. orthopedic surgeon, born 1906] See under NAIL.

Neufeld [Fred *Neufeld*, German bacteriologist, 1861–1945] **1** See under PHENOMENON. **2** Neufeld reaction. See under QUELLUNG REACTION.

Neuhauser [Edward B. *Neuhauser*, U.S. radiologist, born 1908] See under SIGN.

Neumann [Alfred *Neumann*, German physician, flourished 20th century] Charcot-Neumann crystals. See under CHARCOT-LEYDEN CRYSTALS.

Neumann [Ernst F. C. *Neumann*, German pathologist, 1834–1918] **1** Neumann syndrome. See under PEMPHIGUS VEGETANS. **2** See under SHEATH. **3** Neumann cell. See under NUCLEATED RED BLOOD CELL. **4** Rouget-Neumann sheath. See under SHEATH.

Neumann [Isidor Edler von Heilwart *Neumann*, U.S. dermatologist, 1832–1906] See under APHTHOSIS.

neur- NEURO-.

neurad [NEUR- + -AD] Moving toward or closer to a neural structure.

neuradynamia NEURASTHENIA.

neuragmia [NEUR- + Gk *agm(os)* breakage + -IA] The physical tearing or disruption of a nerve.

neural [NEUR- + -AL] **1** Denoting or pertaining to the structure or function of nerves and their connections. **2** Denoting or pertaining to the nervous system or any part of it. Also *nerval.*

neuralgia [NEUR- + -ALGIA] Pain occurring in the area served by a sensory nerve, either because of compression or disease of that nerve, or else occurring without any apparent organic cause. Neuralgia is often paroxysmal and, in some cases, attacks may be precipitated by various stimuli applied over the course of the nerve or in its area of cutaneous innervation. Also called *neurodynia.* Adjective: neuralgic.

abdominolumbar neuralgia Neuralgic pain caused by damage to the L_1 and L_2 spinal nerves or roots or to the genitoabdominal and genitofemoral nerves and involving the lumbar region, the lower abdominal wall, and the external genitalia. It may be due to root compression in disease of upper lumbar intervertebral disks, but can also be caused by pelvic disease (of the cecum or sigmoid colon), inguinal, femoral or obturator hernia, epididymitis, or varicocele. An imprecise and seldom used term.

Arnold's neuralgia An obsolete term for OCCIPITAL SYNDROME.

atypical facial neuralgia A type of chronic facial pain, occurring most often in young and middle-aged women. The pain is constant, dull, and aching in character and often affects predominantly the upper jaw region, though it may spread to other parts of the head and neck, and it may persist for months or years. While local physical disease, as of the teeth, sinuses, etc., must be excluded, in most cases the pain is a manifestation of chronic tension and anxiety and/or depression. Also called *atypical facial pain, facial sympathalgia.*

auriculotemporal neuralgia Neuralgic pain involving the region of the ear and temple, sometimes resulting from temporomandibular joint dysfunction.

brachial neuralgia Recurrent neuralgic pain in the arm. See also CERVICOBRACHIAL NEURALGIA.

brachial plexus neuralgia Recurrent neuralgic pain in the arm due to irritation or compression of the brachial plexus.

cardiac neuralgia An obsolete term for ANGINA PECTORIS.

cervical neuralgia Recurrent neuralgic pain in the neck, corresponding to the distribution of the sensory cervical neurons.

cervicobrachial neuralgia Recurrent pain in the arm. This symptom has many causes, cervical radiculopathy due to spondylosis being one of the commonest.

cervico-occipital neuralgia Neuralgic pain occurring in the posterior cervical and occipital regions, often with associated stiffness of the neck and muscular tenderness, and usually but not invariably resulting from cervical spondylosis.

ciliary neuralgia Periodic migrainous neuralgia in which the pain is located behind the eye.

cranial neuralgia Any neuralgic syndrome involving the head and/or the face and the neck.

neuralgia of the cutaneous nerve of the thigh MERALGIA PARESTHETICA.

degenerative neuralgia Neuralgia resulting from degenerative changes in a cranial or peripheral nerve or at its origin. An imprecise and outmoded term.

facial neuralgia Any form of facial pain, including trigeminal neuralgia, tic douloureux, including supraorbital neuralgia, and sometimes pain of dental or other origin. An obsolete term. Also called *opalgia, opsialgia.*

neuralgia facialis vera TRIGEMINAL NEURALGIA.

femoral neuralgia Neuralgic pain over the anteromedial aspect of the thigh and knee, usually caused by irritation of the femoral nerve from various causes, such as compression by hernia or tumor, injury to the pelvis, or uterine disease, but also occurring commonly in diabetes mellitus, along with atrophy of the quadriceps (diabetic amyotrophy).

Fothergill's neuralgia An obsolete term for TRIGEMINAL NEURALGIA.

geniculate neuralgia GENICULATE GANGLION NEURALGIA.

geniculate ganglion neuralgia Facial pain involving the retro-orbital, retromaxillary, and palatine regions, once believed to be identifiable as a separate variety and resulting, it was thought, from dysfunction of the geniculate ganglion. This concept is no longer tenable. Most patients formerly so diagnosed were probably suffering from periodic migrainous neuralgia (cluster headache). An obsolete term. Also called *Ramsay Hunt neuralgia* (obsolete), *geniculate neuralgia, otic neuralgia, tympanic neuralgia, Hunt's neuralgia.*

glossopharyngeal neuralgia A paroxysmal episode of neuralgic pain, similar to that of trigeminal neuralgia, but involving the back of the throat on one side and sometimes the ear and precipitated by swallowing. Surgical division of the glossopharyngeal nerve may be required to afford relief in the more severe cases. Also called *Sicard-Robineau syndrome* (rarely used), *pharyngotympanic cephalalgia, Legal's disease.*

Harris migrainous neuralgia MIGRAINOUS NEURALGIA.

herpetic neuralgia POSTHERPETIC NEURALGIA.

Hunt's neuralgia GENICULATE GANGLION NEURALGIA.

idiopathic neuralgia Any neuralgia occurring without recognizable pathologic change in the affected nerve or nerves.

intercostal neuralgia Recurrent neuralgic pain, often in girdle distribution, following the course of an intercostal nerve. Also called *intercostal neuropathy.*

mammary neuralgia Neuralgic pain in one or both breasts.

mandibular joint neuralgia Neuralgic pain in or around the temporomandibular joint or considered to arise from a disorder of this joint, as in temporomandibular joint syndrome.

migrainous neuralgia An attack of severe burning pain occurring in or around one eye, and lasting from half an hour up to two hours, usually recurring once or twice in each twenty-four hour period, often at the same time of the day or night. Often there is ipsilateral lacrimation and blockage of the nose. The attacks usually occur in bouts lasting for a few weeks or months, separated by intervals of freedom. Also called *cluster headache, vasculosympathetic facial pain, histamine headache, Horton's vascular headache, Horton's disease, Bing-Horton syndrome* (obsolete), *Harris migrainous neuralgia, histamine cephalalgia, periodic migrainous neuralgia.*

Morton's neuralgia MORTON'S NEUROMA.

nasociliary neuralgia Migrainous neuralgia in which the pain is located in the nose and behind the eye.

obturator neuralgia Neuralgic pain radiating down the upper and medial aspect of the thigh and resulting from compression or irritation of the obturator nerve due to lesions in the pelvis or in the region of the obturator foramen, where an obturator hernia may be the cause.

occipital neuralgia OCCIPITAL SYNDROME.

otic neuralgia GENICULATE GANGLION NEURALGIA.

Parsonage and Turner amyotrophic neuralgia SHOULDER GIRDLE SYNDROME.

periodic migrainous neuralgia MIGRAINOUS NEURALGIA.

peripheral neuralgia Neuralgic pain along the course of a sensory peripheral nerve.

phrenic neuralgia A rare type of neuralgia described as radiating along the course of the phrenic nerve from the diaphragm to the cervical region and exacerbated by diaphragmatic movement, as coughing or breathing, and by swallowing hot or cold liquids. It is unlikely that the so-called idiopathic type exists, even though pain resembling that described may occur in patients with pericarditis, pleurisy, and aortitis, but more especially in cases of hiatus hernia. An obsolete term.

posterior auricular neuralgia Neuralgic pain behind the ear, following the distribution of the posterior auricular nerve.

postherpetic neuralgia Continuous neuralgic pain in the distributions of the affected sensory roots (dermatomes) following an attack of herpes zoster. Also called *herpetic neuralgia.*

pudendal plexus neuralgia Neuralgic pain in the perineum, scrotum, penis, and/or testes.

Ramsay Hunt neuralgia An obsolete term for GENICULATE GANGLION NEURALGIA.

red neuralgia ERYTHROMELALGIA.

retrobulbar neuralgia Any neuralgic pain occurring behind the eye. An imprecise and outmoded term.

sciatic neuralgia SCIATICA.

Seeligmüller's neuralgia Bilateral auriculotemporal neuralgia formerly seen in some patients with syphilis. An obsolete term.

segmental neuralgia Neuralgic pain involving a precisely defined segmental area, for example the region innervated by an intercostal nerve.

Sluder's neuralgia SPHENOPALATINE NEURALGIA.

sphenopalatine neuralgia Periodic migrainous neuralgia in which pain occurs in the nose and pharynx, and sometimes also in the tongue, side of the neck, and upper jaw. The cause is unknown and the connection with the sphenopalatine ganglion debatable. Also called *Sluder's neuralgia, vidian neuralgia, Sluder syndrome, sphenopalatine ganglion neurosis.*

stump neuralgia Recurrent neuralgic pain in an amputation stump.

supraorbital neuralgia Neuralgia in the distribution of the supraorbital nerve. Also called *brow ague* (obsolete), *brow pang.*

symptomatic neuralgia Any neuralgic pain resulting from, or associated with a disease not primarily involving the nervous system.

symptomatic trigeminal neuralgia Trigeminal neuralgia occurring as a symptom of a structural lesion such as posterior fossa tumor or multiple sclerosis. The possibility that the syndrome may be symptomatic may be suspected if there is sensory loss in the distribution of the affected trigeminal nerve or diminution of the appropriate corneal reflex.

trifacial neuralgia TRIGEMINAL NEURALGIA.

trigeminal neuralgia A common form of paroxysmal facial neuralgia, usually occurring in late middle life or old age, but occasionally seen in young people, when it may be associated with multiple sclerosis. The pain is confined to the skin areas supplied by the trigeminal nerve and never crosses the midline. It is momentary, sharp, and lancinating, but a faint, dull ache may be present between paroxysms and it is often provoked by more than one trigger, such as touching or washing the face, especially in a "trigger" zone, or speaking, laughing, or chewing. The pain is so severe that it often appears to elicit an involuntary contraction of facial muscles on the affected side (which is why the condition is also called tic douloureux). Physical signs are generally absent. The cause is uncertain but is believed to be due to pressure on the nerve root by an adjacent artery or by an organic lesion such as a posterior fossa tumor or multiple sclerosis. Spontaneous remissions lasting weeks or months sometimes occur. Also called *tic douloureux, tortua facies, Fothergill's disease* (obsolete), *Fothergill's neuralgia* (obsolete), *trismus dolorificus, Trousseau's disease* (obsolete), *face ague* (obsolete), *neuralgia facialis vera, trifacial neuralgia, prosopalgia, prosoponeuralgia.*

trigeminal sympathetic neuralgia   Trigeminal neuralgia accompanied by ipsilateral Horner syndrome. An obsolete term.

tympanic neuralgia   GENICULATE GANGLION NEURALGIA.

vidian neuralgia   SPHENOPALATINE NEURALGIA.

visceral neuralgia   Pain stemming from an internal organ, as the liver, stomach, uterus, etc. A seldom used term.

Wartenberg's paresthetic neuralgia   CHEIRALGIA PARESTHETICA.

neuralgic   Denoting, pertaining to, or affected by neuralgia.

neuralgiform [*neuralgi(a)* + -FORM]   Resembling neuralgia.

neuraminic acid   5-Amino-4,6,8,9-pentahydroxy-2-oxononanoic acid. Its *N*-acetyl derivative is formed by reaction of *N*-acetylmannosamine, i.e. 2-acetamido-2-deoxymannose, which provides C-4 to C-9 of the product, with phosphoenolpyruvate, which provides C-1 to C-3, with splitting off of orthophosphate. It normally occurs in the pyranose form, with C-2 linked to O-6. Its acylated derivatives are known as sialic acids, and they occur in both glycoproteins (including those of the cell surface) and glycolipids.

neuraminidase   SIALIDASE.

neuranagenesis [NEUR- + ANA- + GENESIS]   Regeneration in the nervous system.

neurangiosis [NEUR- + ANGIO- + -SIS]   Blood vessel proliferation in the nervous system.

neurapophysis [NEUR- + APOPHYSIS]   Each of the portions of the posterior (neural) arch of an embryonic vertebra.

neurapraxia [NEUR- + APRAXIA]   A peripheral nerve lesion in which there is temporary failure of conduction in the affected nerve fibers, often resulting from compression, but without actual division of axons. Also called *axonapraxis.*

neurarchy [NEUR- + Gk *arch(ē)* sovereignty, dominion + -Y]   The dominant, controlling influence of the nervous system over other bodily systems.

neurarthropathy [NEUR- + ARTHROPATHY]   NEUROGENIC ARTHROPATHY.

neurasthenia [NEUR- + ASTHENIA]   A condition characterized by fatigability, weakness, multiple aches and pains, and insomnia, often with symptoms focused on a particular organ or body system. Because the accompanying affect is typically one of disaffection or unhappiness, current classifications group such syndromes among the affective disorders as a form of neurotic depressive disorder. Also called *aneuria* (obsolete), *neurotic asthenia, neuropathic diathesis* (obsolete), *Beard's disease, nervosism, neuradynamia, fatigue neurosis* (obsolete), *neurasthenic neurosis, neurosthenia, nervous prostration (imprecise and old-fashioned), somasthenia* (seldom used), *somatasthenia* (seldom used).

acoustic neurasthenia   Neurasthenia with prominent symptoms involving the hearing.

angioparalytic neurasthenia   Obsessively intrusive awareness of one's pulse beat. An outmoded term.

aviators' neurasthenia   AEROASTHENIA.

cardiac neurasthenia   Neurasthenia with prominent symptoms involving heart function. Also called *cardiac neurosis, disordered action of the heart.*

cardiovascular neurasthenia   Neurasthenia with prominent symptoms involving the heart, blood pressure, or other vascular function.

gastric neurasthenia   Neurasthenia with prominent symptoms involving stomach function.

sexual neurasthenia   Neurasthenia with complaints of sexual debility as a predominant feature.

traumatic neurasthenia   Anxiety or emotional distress following an emotional crisis or an injury. An outmoded term.

neurasthenic   Pertaining to or characterized by neurasthenia.

neuratrophia   NEURATROPHY.

neuratrophy [NEUR- + ATROPHY]   Atrophy of muscle or other tissue due to disease or dysfunction of a nerve. Also called *neuratrophia.* Adjective: neuratrophic.

neuraxial   Denoting or pertaining to the neuraxis.

neuraxis [NEUR- + AXIS]   **1** SYSTEMA NERVOSUM CENTRALE. **2** A seldom used term for AXON. Adjective: neuraxial.

neuraxitis [*neurax(is)* + -ITIS]   Inflammation of the neuraxis. Adjective: neuraxitic.

epidemic neuraxitis   ENCEPHALITIS LETHARGICA.

multilocular neuraxitis   MULTIPLE SCLEROSIS.

neuraxon   AXON.

neure   NEURON.

neurectasia [NEUR- + ECTASIA]   A surgical procedure employed for lengthening the proximal portion of a divided nerve to facilitate closure of a gap when performing neuroanastomosis. Also called *neurectasis, neurectasy, neurodiastasis, neurotension, neurotony.*

neurectasis   NEURECTASIA.

neurectasy   NEURECTASIA.

neurectoderm   NEUROBLAST.

neurectomy [NEUR- + -ECTOMY]   Excision of a nerve.

gastric neurectomy   Resection of the vagus nerve. Also called *vagectomy, vagotomy.*

opticociliary neurectomy   A surgical severing of the ciliary nerves behind the eye, as to relieve discomfort caused by a blind, painful eye.

presacral neurectomy   Excision of the unpaired hypogastric sympathetic nerve plexus lying retroperitoneally at the promontory of the sacrum.

retrogasserian neurectomy   Excision of the root of the trigeminal nerve, usually by avulsion.

tympanic neurectomy   Surgical excision of part of the tympanic nerve, where it passes across the promontory as a component of the plexus tympanicus, with the object of interrupting the secretomotor nerve supply of the parotid gland. Tympanic neurectomy is used as a means of diminishing parotid secretion when ligating the parotid duct for chronic or recurrent parotid sialadenitis and for the relief of the crocodile tear syndrome.

neurectopia   NEURECTOPY.

neurectopy [NEUR- + ECTOPY]   The occurrence of neural tissue which is displaced from its normal position, is found in an abnormal anatomical situation, or is abnormally distributed as a nerve or nerve trunk. Also called *neurectopia.*

neurenteric [NEUR- + ENTERIC]   Pertaining to the neural tube and the archenteron, or primitive gut. Also called *neuroenteric.*

neurepithelial   NEUROEPITHELIAL.

neurepithelium   NERVE EPITHELIUM.

neurergic   Dependent upon nervous action or innervation.

neurexeresis [NEUR- + EXERESIS]   NERVE AVULSION.

neuriatry [NEUR- + -IATRY]   The treatment of diseases of the nervous system.

neuricity   Nervous energy; the excitable property found in all neural tissue.

neurilemma [NEUR- + *i* + Gk *lemma* (from *lepein* to strip off, peel) a peel, husk, skin, scale]   A sheath of flattened cells whose plasma membranes and accompanying basement membrane invest the myelin of larger peripheral nerve fibers. It also provides a thin layer surrounding the axoplasm of unmyelinated nerves. Also called *Schwann's membrane, sheath of Schwann, endoneural membrane, neurilemmal sheath, nucleated sheath, primitive sheath* (seldom used), *neurolemma* (older term), *inner endoneurium* (obsolete), *neu* (seldom used).

neurilemmitis [*neurilemm(a)* + -ITIS]   Inflammation of a neurilemma. Also called *neurolemmitis.*

neurilemmoma [*neurilemm(a)* + -OMA]   A benign and usually well-demarcated or encapsulated tumor, arising from the Schwann cells of the neurolemma. Hemorrhage, thrombosis, hemosiderin, and perivascular hyalinization are common within the tumor. There are two typical growth patterns: Antoni type A with organized cell arrangements, and Antoni type B with loosely structured tissue. Also called *schwannoma, neurinoma, schwannoglioma, perineural glioma* (outmoded), *peripheral glioma* (outmoded), *lemmocytoma, neurolemmoma, Schwann cell tumor.* Also *neurilemoma.*

acoustic neurilemmoma   A neurilemmoma of the acoustic nerve. Also called *acoustic neurofibroma, acoustic neuroma.*

malignant neurilemmoma   MALIGNANT SCHWANNOMA.

neurilemmosarcoma [*neurilemm(a)* + *o* + SARCOMA]   MALIGNANT SCHWANNOMA.

neurilemoma   NEURILEMMOMA.

neurility [NEUR- + ILE-¹ + -ITY]   The inherent electrical conductive property of nervous tissue.

neurimotility   Neuromuscular activity. Also called *nervimotility.*

neurimotor   Pertaining to motor nerves. Also *nervimotor.*

neurinoma [NEUR- + INO- + -OMA]   NEURILEMMOMA.

malignant neurinoma   MALIGNANT SCHWANNOMA.

neurite   A long process of a neuron.   • The term usually denotes the process of an axon, but is occasionally used collectively to include dendritic processes.

neuritic   **1** Relating to nerves, or acting upon the nervous system, as *neuritic poison.* **2** Relating to neuritis.

neuritis [NEUR- + -ITIS]   Inflammation of a nerve. Adjective: neuritic.

adult nonfamilial progressive hypertrophic neuritis   A disease marked by progressive thickening of peripheral nerve trunks, initially giving rise to intermittent autonomic and sensory defects in the hands and feet, and subsequently to distal muscular weakness and atrophy. Hypertrophy of peripheral nerves may occur in many different forms of familial and acquired demyelinating peripheral neuropathy. An imprecise and outmoded term. Also called *Roussy-Cornil syndrome.*

adventitial neuritis   Neuritis once thought to be due to inflammation of the interstitial tissue of one or more peripheral nerves. Most cases so designated were later proved to be due to irritation or compression of the nerve. An obsolete term.

alcoholic neuritis   Neuritis, or more correctly neuropathy or polyneuropathy, complicating chronic alcoholism.

amyloid neuritis   AMYLOID NEUROPATHY.

arsenical neuritis   Peripheral neuritis following acute or chronic exposure to arsenic.

ascending neuritis   Neuritis in which the inflammatory process ascends the affected nerve or nerves. An obsolete term.

brachial neuritis   SHOULDER GIRDLE SYNDROME.

central neuritis   **1** PARENCHYMATOUS NEURITIS. **2** Neuritis attributed to degeneration of the corresponding central spinal neuron. An obsolete and inaccurate concept.

compression neuritis   Neuropathy or neuritis caused by pressure on a nerve from circumferential swelling, swelling of a compartment, or wrapping applied too tightly. Also called *pressure neuritis.*

degenerative neuritis   Degeneration and progressive fragmentation of the axon and myelin sheath of a peripheral nerve.

descending neuritis   A form of neuritis in which the neuritic process was once thought to progress towards the periphery of the nerve. An obsolete and inaccurate term.

dietetic neuritis   BERIBERI.

diphtheritic neuritis   Neuritis caused by the effects of the toxins produced by *Corynebacterium diphtheriae* and affecting the cranial nerves or any of the peripheral nerves. Neuritis may occur during the course of diphtheria or it may appear two to six weeks or more after the onset of diphtheria, and usually first or exclusively affects muscles supplied by nerves adjacent to the site of infection. In some cases the neuritis is localized from the outset, while in other cases it begins as a generalized polyneuritis.

disseminated neuritis   An obsolete term for SEGMENTAL NEURITIS.

Eichhorst's neuritis   An obsolete term for INTERSTITIAL NEURITIS.

endemic neuritis   Polyneuropathy due to vitamin B_1 deficiency (beriberi). An obsolete term.

experimental allergic neuritis   An autoimmune disease produced in various animal species following injection of preparations of peripheral nerve incorporated in complete Freund's adjuvant. The disease is characterized by focal perivascular accumulation of mononuclear cells and by demyelination of peripheral nerves and resembles the human Guillain-Barré syndrome.

exudative neuritis   The combined pathologic changes of edema of the myelin sheaths with leukocytic infiltration of peripheral nerves, as sometimes seen in the Guillain-Barré syndrome. An obsolete term.

facial neuritis   An outmoded term for BELL'S PALSY.

fallopian neuritis   Facial nerve neuritis due to inflammation in the fallopian canal.

familial hypertrophic neuritis   HEREDITARY HYPERTROPHIC INTERSTITIAL NEUROPATHY.

femoral neuritis   An isolated neuropathy of the femoral nerve.

Gombault's neuritis   HEREDITARY HYPERTROPHIC INTERSTITIAL NEUROPATHY.

influenzal neuritis   A peripheral neuritis attributed to influenza virus infection.

interstitial neuritis   Neuritis or neuropathy thought to be due to inflammation in and around the peripheral nerves, giving rise to degeneration of the myelin sheath. Many cases of compression neuropathy and of inflammatory and demyelinating neuropathy were probably included under this title in the past. An obsolete term. Also called *Einchorst's neuritis* (obsolete).

interstitial hypertrophic neuritis   HEREDITARY HYPERTROPHIC INTERSTITIAL NEUROPATHY.

intraocular neuritis   Optic neuritis visible ophthalmoscopically.

ischemic neuritis   Nerve damage causing pain, numbness, or paralysis due to impairment of a nerve's blood supply.

jake neuritis   JAMAICA JAKE PARALYSIS.

latent neuritis   Inflammation of one or more peripheral nerves without producing overt clinical manifestations.

lead neuritis   NEURITIS SATURNINA.

lepromatous neuritis   Neuritis occurring in the lepromatous form of leprosy. Also called *tuberculoid neuritis*.

leprous neuritis   Any one of the forms of neuritis due to leprosy.

Leyden's neuritis   Fatty infiltration of a peripheral nerve. An obsolete term.

malarial neuritis   Mononeuropathy or polyneuropathy occurring as a complication of malaria.

malarial multiple neuritis   Polyneuropathy occurring as a complication of malaria.

neuritis migrans   MIGRATING NEURITIS.

migrating neuritis   Mononeuritis multiplex spreading from one nerve to another. Also called *neuritis migrans*.

multiple neuritis   **1** POLYNEUROPATHY.   **2** See under MONONEURITIS MULTIPLEX.

neuritis multiplex endemica   BERIBERI.

neuritis nodosa   Neuritis in which hypertrophic nodules are formed along the nerve trunks, presumably indicating hypertrophic neuropathy with focal areas of thickening. An obsolete term.

optic neuritis   Inflammation of the second cranial nerve. Also called *postocular neuritis, retrobulbar neuritis, fasciculitis optica* (outmoded), *ophthalmoneuritis*.

orbital optic neuritis   Inflammation of the second cranial nerve external to the eye.

paralytic brachial neuritis   SHOULDER GIRDLE SYNDROME.

parenchymatous neuritis   Any neuropathy in which degeneration of the axons and/or myelin sheaths occurs. An obsolete term. Also called *central neuritis* (obsolete).

periaxial neuritis   Any form of neuropathy in which there are segmental lesions of the myelin sheaths and Schwann cells while the axons are spared. An obsolete term. Also called *demyelinating neuropathy, periaxial neuropathy, segmental neuropathy*.

peripheral neuritis   Polyneuritis or polyneuropathy.

porphyric neuritis   Polyneuropathy in acute porphyria.

postfebrile neuritis   Polyneuropathy following any acute febrile disorder.

postocular neuritis   OPTIC NEURITIS.

pressure neuritis   COMPRESSION NEURITIS.

progressive hypertrophic interstitial neuritis   HEREDITARY HYPERTROPHIC INTERSTITIAL NEUROPATHY.

neuritis puerperalis traumatica   Obstetric pressure palsy of the lumbosacral plexus.

radiation neuritis   Neuropathy due to ionizing radiation.

radicular neuritis   RADICULITIS.

retrobulbar neuritis   OPTIC NEURITIS.

rheumatic neuritis   Neuritis associated with musculoskeletal complaints. This term has no precise diagnostic implications.

neuritis saturnina   Neuropathy or neuritis due to chronic exposure to lead. Also called *lead neuritis*.

sciatic neuritis   SCIATICA.

segmental neuritis   A form of neuropathy in which there are focal areas of demyelination or axonal degeneration in peripheral nerves separated by relatively unaffected areas. This may be seen in compression neuropathies but otherwise the term has little pathologic validity. Also called *disseminated neuritis* (obsolete).

senile neuritis   Polyneuropathy occurring in the aged. An imprecise and outmoded term.

serum neuritis   SERUM NEUROPATHY.

shoulder girdle neuritis   SHOULDER GIRDLE SYNDROME.

spinal neuritis   Neuritis or neuropathy involving the spinal nerves.

syphilitic neuritis   Any form of neuropathy due to syphilis. Also called *tabetic neuritis* (obsolete).

tabetic neuritis   An obsolete term for SYPHILITIC NEURITIS.

terminal neuritis   An outmoded term for ERYTHROMELALGIA.

toxic neuritis   Neuritis or neuropathy due to endogenous or exogenous toxic agents, including bacterial and chemical toxins.

traumatic neuritis   Neuropathy due to physical injury or compression of a nerve trunk. An obsolete term.

tuberculoid neuritis   LEPROMATOUS NEURITIS.

neuro-   [Gk *neuron* nerve, sinew, tendon]   A combining form meaning (1) nerve, neural; (2) relating to the nervous system. Also *neur-*.

neuroabiotrophy   Loss of vitality and function of neurological cells that is not due to known disease and may be caused by aging. An obsolete term.

neuroallergy   Allergy manifested in nervous tissue.

neuroamebiasis   [NEURO- + AMEBIASIS]   Infection of the nervous system by amebas.

neuroanastomosis   [NEURO- + ANASTOMOSIS]   A surgical joining of the cut ends of two nerves.

neuroanatomy   [NEURO- + ANATOMY]   The branch of neurology concerned with the anatomy of the nervous system. With the development of new research techniques, the field now includes gross descriptive anatomy; the study of tracts and pathways, i.e., tractology or hodology; the microscopic and ultramicroscopic study of neural tissue, i.e., histology; the study and identification of cell fiber systems on the basis of contained transmitter substances, i.e., histofluorescence; and the examination of living neural tissue *in vivo* or *in vitro*, i.e., tissue culture, among others.

neuroanemia   An obsolete term for PERNICIOUS ANEMIA.

neuroarthropathy   NEUROGENIC ARTHROPATHY.

neuroasthenia   [NEURO- + ASTHENIA]   Neurasthenia with neurologic complaints, as in sciatica, as the most prominent.

neuroastrocytoma   [NEURO- + ASTROCYTOMA]   GANGLIOGLIOMA.

neuroataralgesia   NEUROLEPTANALGESIA.

neuroavitaminosis   [NEURO- + AVITAMINOSIS]   Any neurologic disorder resulting from vitamin deficiency.

neurobiology   [NEURO- + BIOLOGY]   The study of the biology of the nervous system; cellular neuroscience.

neurobiotaxis   The migration of a nerve cell in the direction from which it habitually receives stimuli. A nerve cell tends to remain close to its source of stimulation but development of neighboring structures may prevent the maintenance of such proximity and migration follows. Examples of such shifting in position of groups of nerve cells in the embryo are furnished by the lateral migration of the visceral motor nuclei of the cranial nerves, and in particular by the curious course of the fibers arising from the facial nucleus.

neuroblast   [NEURO- + -BLAST]   **1** That part of the ectoderm which invaginates and then differentiates into the neural tube and neural crest with their derivatives.   **2** An embryonic nerve cell which will give rise to a neuron. Also called *neurectoderm*.

sympathetic neuroblast   SYMPATHOBLAST.

neuroblastoma   [NEURO- + BLASTOMA]   A highly malignant tumor of undifferentiated neuroblasts. The cells are small with dark-staining nuclei and indistinct cytoplasm. Arrangement of the cells in spheroid groups about a central tangle of fibrillary material (Homer-Wright rosettes) is a characteristic feature. The tumor occurs predominantly in children under the age of four years, usually in close association with the adrenal medulla or the sympathetic chain. Also called *sympathoblastoma, sympathicoblastoma, neurocytoma, sympathogonioma, sympathicogonioma, sympathicocytoma, sympathotropic cell tumor*.

neuroblastoma of the brain   A rare cerebral tumor which resembles the neuroblastoma of the adrenal and sympathetic nervous system.

Hutchison type neuroblastoma　A neuroblastoma whose metastases are mainly in the brain.

olfactory neuroblastoma　A malignant nasal tumor of olfactory neural tissue with cells showing pleomorphism and only scant amounts of neurofibrillar matrix. Also called *esthesioneuroblastoma* (rarely used).

Pepper type neuroblastoma　Neuroblastoma of the right adrenal gland with metastases mostly confined to the liver.

neuroblastomatosis [NEURO- + *blastomat(a)*, pl. of *blastoma* + -OSIS]　**1** Widespread neuroblastomas.　**2** An obsolete term for NEUROFIBROMATOSIS.

neurocanal　An obsolete term for CANALIS VERTEBRALIS.

neurocardiac　Denoting, pertaining to, or affecting the nervous system and the heart.

neurocentrum [NEURO- + CENTRUM]　A relatively dense part of the vertebral primordium in an embryo. It gives rise to the centrum of a vertebra and the neural arch. Adjective: neurocentral.

neuroceptor　**1** A terminal element of a neuron that is specialized to receive stimuli. Peripherally, neuroceptors act as transducers, converting physical or chemical stimuli of many types into discrete electrical signals (action potentials) which then enter the central nervous system.　**2** A dendrite within the central nervous system serving as a receptive structure that is postsynaptic to impinging presynaptic axons from other neurons.

neuroceratin　NEUROKERATIN.

neurochemistry　The chemistry of the nervous system, including that of the passage of the nervous system and its transmission across synapses.

neurochitin　A fibrous substance thought to form the supportive framework for nerve fibers. An obsolete term.

neurochondrite [NEURO- + CHONDR- + -ITE]　A cartilaginous element in the embryo which becomes the neural arch of a vertebra.

neurochorioretinitis [NEURO- + CHORIO- + RETINITIS]　Inflammation of the optic disk and the fundus.

neurochoroiditis [NEURO- + CHOROIDITIS]　Inflammation of the optic disk and the choroid.

neurocirculatory　Denoting, pertaining to, or affecting the nervous and circulatory systems.

neurocladism [NEURO- + Gk *klad(os)* a young branch, slip, or shoot + -ISM]　Regeneration of axons in peripheral nerves following division, and the process by which these regenerating axons eventually become connected to the peripheral end organ. Also called *odogenesis*.

neuroclonic [NEURO- + CLONIC]　Denoting or pertaining to clonic spasms of neural origin.

neurocoele [NEURO- + -COELE]　NEURAL CANAL.

neurocranial　Pertaining to the neurocranium.

neurocranium　The part of the embryonic skull that surrounds the brain; braincase. Constituted initially of a dense mesenchyme, it includes the base of the skull (chondrocranium), which undergoes endochondral ossification, and the cranial vault of flat bones, which undergoes intramembranous ossification. Compare SPLANCHNOCRANIUM.

neurocrine　NEUROENDOCRINE.

neurocutaneous　**1** Of or relating to nerves and the skin.　**2** Pertaining to nerves of the skin.

neurocyte [NEURO- + -CYTE]　NEURON.

neurocytology　The study of the cellular components of the nervous system.

neurocytolysin　A toxin that destroys nerve cell membranes, occurring especially in snake venoms, usually in low concentrations. Higher concentrations are found in venoms of North American coral snakes and in the water moccasin (cottonmouth) of the eastern United States.

neurocytolysis [NEURO- + CYTOLYSIS]　Destruction, or lysis, of the cells of the nervous system.

neurocytoma [NEURO- + CYTOMA]　**1** NEUROEPITHELIOMA.　**2** MEDULLOEPITHELIOMA.　**3** NEUROBLASTOMA.

olfactory neurocytoma　A rare nasal tumor, corresponding clinically to the olfactory neuroblastoma but displaying histologic differences, the cells appearing uniform with prominent neurofibrillar matrix. Pseudorosettes are frequent. Also called *esthesioneurocytoma* (rarely used).

neurodealgia [Gk *neurōdē(s)* the retina + -ALGIA]　Pain in the retina.

neurodeatrophia [Gk *neurōdē(s)* the retina + ATROPHIA]　Degeneration of the retina.

neurodegenerative　Characterized by or relating to degeneration of the nervous tissue.

neurodendrite　DENDRITE.

neurodendron　DENDRITE.

neuroderm　NEURAL TUBE.

neurodermatitis [NEURO- + DERMATITIS]　A skin disorder of psychosomatic genesis or in which psychological factors play an important part, as when rubbing and scratching induce circumscribed patches of thickened skin. Also called *cutaneous neurosis*.　● In some countries the term is applied more generally to atopic dermatitis. This use is imprecise, since it falsely implies that nervous factors are always present.

circumscribed neurodermatitis　LICHEN SIMPLEX.

generalized neurodermatitis　A form of extensive constitutional eczema which is exacerbated by psychological stress.

neurodermatomyositis　Neuromyositis with skin involvement.

neurodermatrophia　Atrophy of skin due to denervation or any other disorder of its nerve supply.

neurodes　RETINA.

neurodiagnosis [NEURO- + DIAGNOSIS]　Diagnosis of disorders of the nervous system.

neurodiastasis [NEURO- + DIASTASIS]　NEURECTASIA.

neurodynamia　Nervous power or force. An outmoded term. Adjective: neurodynamic.

neurodynia　NEURALGIA.

neurodystonia　A disorder of function attributable to disturbance of autonomic visceral regulation. An imprecise and seldom used term.

neuroectoderm [NEURO- + ECTODERM]　Ectodermal cells which become neuroepithelial cells. Adjective: neuroectodermal.

neuroelectricity　The electrical activity generated in nervous system tissues.

neuroelectrotherapeutics　The use of electricity in treatment of diseases of the nervous system. An obsolete term.

neuroencephalomyelopathy [NEURO- + ENCEPHALO- + MYELO- + -PATHY]　ENCEPHALOMYELOPATHY.

optic neuroencephalomyelopathy　NEUROMYELITIS OPTICA.

neuroendocrine　Of or relating to neuroendocrinology; relating to the interactions between the nervous and endocrine systems. Also *neurocrine*.

neuroendocrinology [NEURO- + ENDOCRINOLOGY]　The study of the interactions between the nervous and endocrine systems.

neuroenteric　NEURENTERIC.

neuroepidermal Giving rise to or pertaining to neural and epidermal cells.

neuroepithelial Of or relating to the neuroepithelium. Also *neurepithelial.*

neuroepithelioma [NEURO- + EPITHELIOMA] **1** A tumor of primitive neural tissue arising in the central nervous system. **2** A form of olfactory neurogenic tumor; olfactory neuroepithelioma. Also called *esthesioneuroepithelioma, neurocytoma, neuroepithelial tumor.*

neuroepithelium [NEURO- + EPITHELIUM] NERVE EPITHELIUM.

neuroepithelium of ampullary crest The sensory epithelium that covers the ampullary crests of the semicircular canals in the membranous labyrinth of the inner ear. Also called *neuroepithelium cristae ampullaris.*

neuroepithelium cristae ampullaris NEUROEPITHELIUM OF AMPULLARY CREST.

neuroepithelium of maculae MACULA RETINAE.

neuroepithelium macularum MACULA RETINAE.

neurofibril A fine, threadlike structure visible within the cytoplasm of a neuron with light microscopy. Electron microscopy reveals that it corresponds to a bundle of neurofilaments. Also called *nerve fibril, neurofibrilla.*

neurofibrilla NEUROFIBRIL.

neurofibrillae Plural of NEUROFIBRILLA.

neurofibrillar Of or relating to a neurofibril.

neurofibroma [NEURO- + FIBROMA] A benign localized or diffuse tumor, consisting of a mixture of Schwann cells and fibroblasts accompanied by loosely arranged collagen fibers and mucinous material. Plexiform neurofibromas are the result of growth within and about a preformed nerve, giving the nerve trunk a tortuous, thickened, and plexiform appearance. Neurites can be frequently demonstrated within these tumors. Malignant transformation of neurofibromas may occur. Also called *endoneural fibroma, neurofibromyxoma.*

acoustic neurofibroma ACOUSTIC NEURILEMMOMA.

dumbbell neurofibroma HOURGLASS TUMOR.

neurofibroma gangliocellulare GANGLIONEUROMA.

neurofibroma ganglionare GANGLIONEUROMA.

granular cell neurofibroma GRANULAR CELL TUMOR.

malignant neurofibroma MALIGNANT SCHWANNOMA.

symmetrical bundle neurofibromas HEREDITARY HYPERTROPHIC INTERSTITIAL NEUROPATHY.

neurofibromatosis [NEURO- + FIBROMATOSIS] Any of various clinically and genetically heterogeneous disorders associated with multiple neurofibromata. The vast majority of cases are von Recklinghausen's disease, and are characterized by café-au-lait skin macules, axillary freckling, fibromatous tumors, Lisch nodules of the iris, scoliosis, and autosomal dominant inheritance. The severity of the condition is extremely variable, and a predisposition of malignancy exists. Other neurofibromatosis syndromes involve acoustic neuromas with rare or nonexistent cutaneous signs, or multiple intestinal neurofibromata. Also called *neuroblastomatosis* (obsolete), *neurofibrophacomatosis, sarcoma molluscum, multiple fibroma, molluscum fibrosum.*

abortive neurofibromatosis INCOMPLETE NEUROFIBROMATOSIS.

incomplete neurofibromatosis Neurofibromatosis with few clinical manifestations. Also called *abortive neurofibromatosis.*

neurofibromyxoma [NEURO- + FIBRO- + MYXOMA] NEUROFIBROMA.

neurofibrophacomatosis NEUROFIBROMATOSIS.

neurofibrosarcoma [NEURO- + FIBROSARCOMA] MALIGNANT SCHWANNOMA.

neurofibrositis [NEURO- + FIBROSITIS] Inflammation of nerves and fibrous tissue. An obsolete term.

neurofilament An elongate, tubular protein chain of indefinite length and approximately 100 å in diameter observed in the soma, dendrites, and axons of neurons with the electron microscope. Bundles of neurofilaments can be impregnated with metallic salts to form the neurofibrils of light microscopy.

neurofixation [NEURO- + FIXATION] The development of neurosyphilis following treatment of early symphilitic infection with arsenical preparations. The condition is no longer seen.

neuroganglioma GANGLIONEUROMA.

neuroganglioma myelinicum verum GANGLIONEUROMA.

neuroganglion GANGLION.

neuroganglionitis [NEURO- + GANGLIONITIS] Inflammation of nerves and ganglia. Also called *neuroganglitis.*

neuroganglitis NEUROGANGLIONITIS.

neurogastric Of or involving the nervous system and the stomach; relating to the innervation of the stomach.

neurogen [NEURO- + -GEN] **1** A chemical substance essential to neural plate formation. **2** An obsolete term for NEUROTRANSMITTER.

neurogenesis [NEURO- + GENESIS] The development of a nervous system.

neurogenetics The field of knowledge concerned with genetic mechanisms underlying early embryonic development, as well as cell differentiation, patterns of neural organization, and genetic disorders of the nervous system.

neurogenic [NEURO- + -GENIC] **1** Originating in the nervous system. Also *neurogenous.* **2** In embryology, having the property of forming neural tissue: said of undifferentiated cells.

neurogenous NEUROGENIC.

neuroglia [NEURO- + GLIA] Collectively, the non-neuronal cellular components of the central nervous system that, together with the fine tissue web they generate, make up the structural and functional support system of the brain and spinal cord. Neuroglial cells are usually divided into two major categories, macroglia and microglia. The macroglia consists of astrocytes and oligodendrocytes (oligodendroglia), which are of ectodermal origin. Astrocytes may be of protoplasmic or fibrillary type, the latter developing particularly in later life or in response to neural tissue injury. Oligodendrocytes frequently surround neurons closely as satellite cells or lie among myelinated axon bundles as interfascicular oligodendroglia. All of these types may be involved in the control of the ionic and molecular medium and in the synthesis of important neurally active materials. Interfascicular oligoglia are also concerned with the formation and maintenance of myelin. The microglia, of mesodermal origin, are believed to be derived from blood vessels, and they form wandering phagocytes. Also called *glia, nerve cement* (obsolete), *Kölliker's reticulum.*

interfascicular neuroglia Collectively, oligodendrocytes of white matter found along the myelin sheaths and concerned with the formation and maintenance of myelin. See also OLIGODENDROGLIA.

protoplasmic neuroglia PROTOPLASMIC ASTROCYTE.

neuroglial Pertaining to neuroglia. Also *neurogliar.*

neurogliar NEUROGLIAL.

neurogliocyte A neuroglial cell.

neurogliocytoma [NEURO- + GLIO- + CYTOMA] GLIOMA.

neuroglioma [NEURO- + GLIOMA] GLIOMA.

neuroglioma ganglionare GANGLIOGLIOMA.

neurogliomatosis [*neurogliomat(a),* pl. of NEUROGLIOMA + -OSIS] Diffuse involvement of brain tissue by glioma.

central neurogliomatosis A condition in which neurilemmomas of nerve roots are associated with gliomas of the central nervous system.

neurogliosis [*neurogli(al)* + -OSIS] Diffuse hyperplasia of neuroglial tissue.

neurogliosis gangliocellularis diffusa Tuberous sclerosis.

neurogram [NEURO- + -GRAM] **1** A recording of the action potential of nerves. **2** Persistent effects of past events that participate in personality formation. An outmoded usage.

neurohemal Denoting or relating to systems of axon terminals of neurons in contact with small blood vessels which characteristically synthesize, store, and release their secretions (neurohormones) into the circulation.

neurohistochemistry The microscopic study of neural tissue using chemical markers, generally enzymes and antibodies to specific antigens.

neurohistology The study of the microscopic structure of the nervous system. Also called *histoneurology* (obsolete).

neurohormonal Designating or pertaining to hormones originating in the nervous system.

neurohormone [NEURO- + HORMONE] A secretory product of a neuron which enters the bloodstream and acts as a hormone, such as vasopressin or thyrotropin-releasing hormone. Also called *neurohumor* (older term).

neurohumor An older term for NEUROHORMONE.

neurohumoral An older term for NEUROHORMONAL.

neurohumoralism The theory that autonomic nervous system effects are mediated by the release of specific neurotransmitters.

neurohypnologist A student of neurohypnology.

neurohypnology [NEURO- + HYPNO- + -LOGY] The study of hypnotism. Also called *neurypnology*.

neurohypophyseal NEUROHYPOPHYSIAL.

neurohypophysectomy [NEURO- + *hypophys(is)* + -ECTOMY] The surgical removal of the posterior lobe of the hypophysis.

neurohypophysial Describing or pertaining to the neurohypophysis. Also called *neurohypophyseal*.

neurohypophysis [NEURO- + HYPOPHYSIS] [NA] The posterior lobe of the pituitary gland (hypophysis), which develops in the embryo as an evagination from the floor of the diencephalon. Its major afferent nerve supply is the supraoptico-hypophysial tract. Also called *lobus posterior hypophyseos, posterior lobe of hypophysis, posterior lobe of pituitary gland, pituitarium posterius, hypophysis sicca* (outmoded), *infundibular body, neural lobe* (obsolete), *posthypophysis* (rarely used). See also PITUITARY GLAND.

neuroid Resembling neural tissue.

neuroinidia Impaired nutrition of neurons.

neurokeratin The artifactitious network of pseudokeratin seen in histologic sections of nerve in which myelin is inadequately preserved. Also called *neuroceratin*.

neurokinet [NEURO- + Gk *kinētēs* a mover] An outmoded apparatus for mechanical tap excitation of nerve.

neurokyme [NEURO- + Gk *kym(a)* a seething, wave, surge] Nervous action or activity. An outmoded term.

neurolabyrinthitis Inflammation of the vestibular sense organs and the vestibular nerve. It has been postulated as the cause in certain cases of epidemic vertigo when a viral agent is suspected.

neurolathyrism [NEURO- + LATHYRISM] LATHYRISM.

neurolemma An older term for NEURILEMMA.

neurolemmitis NEURILEMMITIS.

neurolemmoma NEURILEMMOMA.

neuroleptanalgesia [NEURO- + LEPT- + ANALGESIA] The effects achieved by the combined administration of a neuroleptic and of an analgesic drug. Also called *ataralgesia*.

neuroleptanalgesic **1** Denoting, pertaining to, or producing neuroleptanalgesia. **2** A neuroleptanalgesic agent.

neuroleptanesthesia [NEURO- + LEPT- + ANESTHESIA] A technique in which the pain relief of neuroleptanalgesia is combined with general anesthesia induced by nitrous oxide and oxygen. It is stress-free, causes relative hypotension, and requires neuromuscular blockers for relaxation of muscles during surgery. Also called *neuroleptoanesthesia, neuroataralgesia*.

neuroleptanesthetic **1** Relating to neuroleptanesthesia. **2** Any substance resulting in the state characterizing neuroleptanesthesia.

neuroleptic **1** Acting to prevent or alleviate mental disorders, as a drug. **2** A neuroleptic chemical or drug. For defs. 1 and 2 also *antipsychotic*.

neuroleptoanesthesia NEUROLEPTANESTHESIA.

neurolipomatosis [NEURO- + *lipomat(a)*, pl. of *lipoma* + -OSIS] NEUROLIPOMATOSIS DOLOROSA.

neurolipomatosis dolorosa A disorder largely restricted to females which produces localized painful accumulations of subcutaneous fat. Also called *Dercum's disease, neurolipomatosis, adiposis dolorosa*.

neurologia NEUROLOGY.

neurologic Pertaining to neurology.

neurologist [NEURO- + -LOGIST] A physician who specializes in neurology. Also called *neuropathist* (obsolete).

neurology [NEURO- + -LOGY] That branch of medicine dealing with diseases of the nervous system. Also called *neurologia*.

clinical neurology The study of the clinical manifestations of neurologic disorders.

neurolues NEUROSYPHILIS.

neurolymph [NEURO- + LYMPH] A seldom used term for LIQUOR CEREBROSPINALIS.

neurolymphomatosis [NEURO- + LYMPHOMATOSIS] Invasion of nerves by malignant lymphoma.

neurolymphomatosis gallinarum An outmoded term for MAREK'S DISEASE.

peripheral neurolymphomatosis Involvement of peripheral nerves by deposits of lymphoma or other reticuloses or by leukemic infiltrations.

neurolysis [NEURO- + LYSIS] **1** Destruction or dissolution of nervous tissue. **2** A surgical procedure in which a nerve is freed from compression by scar tissue or other compressive agents. **3** Destruction of a nerve by injecting alcohol or phenol into it.

neurolytic Causing lysis of neural structures.

neuroma [NEUR- + -OMA] A benign tumor or tumorlike lesion composed of a mass of nerve fibers. It may be congenital or arise after trauma. The nerve fibers may be myelinated or unmyelinated, and cyst formation may occur.

acoustic neuroma ACOUSTIC NEURILEMMOMA.

amputation neuroma TRAUMATIC NEUROMA.

amyelinic neuroma A neuroma of unmyelinated nerves.

appendical neuroma APPENDICEAL NEUROMA.

appendiceal neuroma A tumorlike lesion composed of proliferated nerve fibers in a chronically inflamed vermiform appendix. Also called *appendical neuroma*.

neuroma cutis A neuroma in the skin. Also called *dermal neuroma*.

cystic neuroma A neuroma with cysts.

dermal neuroma NEUROMA CUTIS.

false neuroma **1** A neuroma which does not contain nerve fibers, and is made up wholly of proliferating Schwann cells and fibrous tissue. **2** TRAUMATIC NEUROMA.

fascicular neuroma MYELINIC NEUROMA.

ganglionated neuroma GANGLIONIC NEUROMA.

ganglion-celled neuroma　GANGLIONIC NEUROMA.

ganglionic neuroma　**1** A neuroma containing nerve cells. Also called *ganglionated neuroma, ganglion-celled neuroma.* **2** GANGLIONEUROMA. **3** GANGLIONEUROFIBROMA.

malignant neuroma　**1** A malignant tumor of nerves. **2** MALIGNANT SCHWANNOMA. Also called *neurosarcoma.*

medullated neuroma　MYELINIC NEUROMA.

Morton's neuroma　A painful tumorlike lesion of an interdigital plantar nerve, usually between the second and third toes, that is characterized by the proliferation of perineural tissues with the degeneration of axons and myelin. It is caused by pressure on the nerve at the metatarsophalangeal joint. Also called *Morton's neuralgia, Thomas Morton's disease, Morton's foot, Morton's toe, Morton's disease.*

multiple neuroma　NEUROMATOSIS.

myelinic neuroma　A neuroma arising from myelinated nerves and containing myelin. Also called *fascicular neuroma, medullated neuroma.*

nevoid neuroma　TELANGIECTATIC NEUROMA.

plexiform neuroma　A neuroma in which there are interlacing neural elements resembling a plexus. Also called *Verneuil's neuroma.*

post-traumatic neuroma　TRAUMATIC NEUROMA.

telangiectatic neuroma　A neuroma with numersous blood vessels. Also called *neuroma telangiectodes, nevoid neuroma.*

neuroma telangiectodes　TELANGIECTATIC NEUROMA.

traumatic neuroma　A benign, nonneoplastic overgrowth of nerve fibers, Schwann cells, and scar tissue occurring at the proximal end of a severed nerve trunk. Also called *amputation neuroma, post-traumatic neuroma, false neuroma.*

true neuroma　A neoplastic growth of nerve fibers.

Verneuil's neuroma　PLEXIFORM NEUROMA.

neuroma verum　GANGLIONEUROMA.

neuromalacia　Softening and cavitation in the nervous system. Also called *neuromalakia.*

neuromalakia　NEUROMALACIA.

neuromatoid [NEUROMA + *t* + -OID]　Resembling a neuroma.

neuromatosis [*neuromat(a)*, pl. of NEUROMA + -OSIS]　The presence of multiple neuromas. Also called *multiple neuroma.*

neuromatous　Pertaining to a neuroma.

neuromechanism　A functional property dependent upon the nervous system.

neuromelanin　Pigment granules within the cytoplasm of neurons in the substantia nigra.

neuromeningeal　Denoting, pertaining to, or affecting the central nervous system and meninges.

neuromere [NEURO- + -MERE]　Each of the segments of the neural tube. Also called *neural segment, neurotome.*

neuromery [NEURO- + *mer(o)*-¹ + -Y]　Segmentation of the embryonic neural tube exhibited by localized enlargments (neuromeres) separated from one another by constrictions. It is especially obvious in fish embryos and at the level of the rhombencephalon, but it is only temporary, leaves no trace, and is not correlated with metameric segmentation.

neuromimesis　The simulation of some disorder of the nervous system performed either consciously and willfully or unconsciously.

neuromittor　A terminal structure at the peripheral end of a neuronal process that transfers a stimulus to the receptor terminal of the adjoining neuron. A seldom used term. Also called *mittor* (obsolete).

neuromodulator　One of the numerous substances contained in neurons that do not serve as neurotransmitters at synapses but modulate neuronal membrane events, including hormones, nucleotides, and a variety of peptides.

neuromotor [NEURO- + MOTOR]　NEUROMUSCULAR.

neuromuscular [NEURO- + MUSCULAR]　Denoting, pertaining to, or affecting the lower motor neurons and muscles. Also *neuromyal, neuromyic, neuromotor.*

neuromyal　NEUROMUSCULAR.

neuromyasthenia　Neurasthenia in which emotional lability and muscular weakness are the predominant symptoms. An older term.

epidemic neuromyasthenia　BENIGN MYALGIC ENCEPHALOMYELITIS.

neuromyelitis [NEURO- + MYELITIS]　Myelitis associated with neuritis, especially that form of demyelinating myelitis occurring in neuromyelitis optica (Devic's disease).

neuromyelitis hyperalbuminotica　GUILLAIN-BARRÉ SYNDROME.

neuromyelitis optica　Demyelination involving one or both optic nerves and the spinal cord. Some such cases ultimately prove to be suffering from multiple sclerosis. Also called *Devic's disease, neuro-optic myelitis, opthalmoneuromyelitis, optic neuroencephalomyelopathy.*

neuromyic　NEUROMUSCULAR.

neuromyoarterial　Of, pertaining to, or affecting the neuromuscular and arterial systems.

neuromyocardium　The myocardial tissues that constitute the conduction system of the heart.

neuromyology　The classification of muscles according to their innervation.

neuromyon [NEURO- + MYON]　The intramuscular motor and sensory nerves. An obsolete term.

neuromyopathic　Relating to a disorder which affects both the voluntary muscles and the central or peripheral nervous system.

neuromyopathy　Any disease process which involves both the peripheral or central nervous system and the voluntary muscles. Adjective: neuromyopathic.

carcinomatous neuromyopathy　Any paraneoplastic syndrome giving rise to disease of the central nervous system but more often of the peripheral nerves in association with a myopathy. Often the causative neoplasm is an oat cell bronchial carcinoma.

neuromyositis [NEURO- + MYOSITIS]　**1** Polymyositis and polyneuritis occurring together in the same patient. An imprecise usage. **2** POLYNEUROMYOSITIS.

neuromyotonia　MYOKYMIA.

neuron [Gk *neuron* a sinew, tendon, nerve, string]　**1** The basic cellular conducting element of the central and peripheral nervous systems. A typical neuron consists of a cell body, or perikaryon, containing a nucleus and cytoplasm, and several radiating processes of varying shape and length. The axon, usually a long, thin cytoplasmic structure, conducts impulses away from the cell body. Dendrites, ordinarily consisting of multiple branching protoplasmic extensions that greatly extend the surface area of the receptive membrane of the cell body, generally serve as the receptive pole of the neuron. The cell body cytoplasm in most cases contains a dense, multilaminate, membranous system, the endoplasmic reticulum, which is concerned with protein synthesis and helps to maintain the extended structure of the cell. The neuron also contains an extensive endocellular skeleton of microtubules and microfilaments, the neurofibrillar network, which may be involved in structural support and transport roles throughout the nerve cell. Also called *nerve cell, neure, neurocyte, nerve unit.* **2** An obsolete term for AXON.

afferent neuron　A neuron whose axon conducts impulses towards another neuron or a central neuronal aggregate.

alpha motor neuron　A central neuron whose peripheral axon innervates skeletal muscle fibers and conducts at the highest velocities.

autonomic neuron Any preganglionic or postganglionic neuron controlling smooth or cardiac muscle or glands.

bipolar neuron A neuron with two major neurofibril-containing processes. During maturation, one process usually becomes the axon, or central process, and the other becomes the dendrite, or peripheral process. Bipolar neurons are usually sensory in function and subserve impulses generated by olfactory, visual, auditory, and vestibular receptor endings.

central neuron A neuron whose cell body lies within the central nervous system.

central sensory neuron Any neuron of the central nervous system synaptically activated by peripheral sense organs. Also called *secondary sensory neuron*.

connector neuron INTERNEURON.

correlation neuron A neuron that receives input and integrates activity from diverse sources.

effector neuron A neuron that carries impulses toward an effector.

efferent neuron A neuron in a pathway leading from the central nervous system to a peripheral effector organ.

exciter neuron MOTONEURON.

first-order neuron PRIMARY NEURON.

fusimotor neuron GAMMA MOTOR NEURON.

gamma neuron GAMMA MOTOR NEURON.

gamma motor neuron A central neuron whose peripheral axon innervates the intrafusal muscle fibers of muscle spindles and conducts impulses at velocities in the range of gamma efferent nerve fibers. Also called *gamma neuron, fusimotor neuron*.

Golgi type I neurons Nerve cells having long axons that leave the local neuropil area of the parent cell body, enter the white matter, and project to other parts of the nervous system. Compare GOLGI TYPE II NEURONS. ● The two major neuronal types were originally distinguished by Camillo Golgi on the basis of axonal length.

Golgi type II neurons Nerve cells having axons with short trajectories, typified by the stellate cells of the cerebral and cerebellar cortex. Axonal length and trajectory may vary. In some cases, the axon system is contained entirely within the confines of the dendrite system of the parent cell. In others, such as the cerebellar granules cell, the axon may run for 1–3 mm. Many authorities include all neurons whose axons do not enter the white matter, thereby remaining within the local neuropil. Also called *cells of van Gehuchten*. Compare GOLGI TYPE I NEURONS.

horizontal neurons HORIZONTAL CELLS.

intercalary neuron INTERNEURON.

intercalated neuron INTERNEURON.

internuncial neuron INTERNEURON.

long neuron A neuron possessing a long axonal process.

Martinotti neuron Small local circuit neurons of the cerebral cortex whose axons characteristically ascend toward the cortical surface.

motor neuron MOTONEURON.

multiform neuron POLYMORPHIC NEURON.

multipolar neuron A neuron with many processes issuing from the cell body. Most of the nerve cells in the central nervous system are of this type.

peripheral motor neuron MOTONEURON.

peripheral sensory neuron PRIMARY SENSORY NEURON.

phasic motor neuron An alpha motor neuron whose peripheral axon controls skeletal muscles initiating rapid movements.

polymorphic neuron A nerve call of irregular shape usually characterized by multipolar configuration with dendrites emerg-

ing at many points along the cell body. Also called *muliform neuron*.

postganglionic neuron A neuron in a peripheral autonomic ganglion whose axon controls smooth or cardiac muscle or glands.

preganglionic neuron Any neuron of the spinal cord or brainstem whose peripheral axon terminates on autonomic ganglia.

premotor neuron UPPER MOTOR NEURON.

primary neuron In a neural pathway, a neuron, as a sensory receptor, whose axon forms a synapse with another neuron (second-order neuron) for the transmission of an impulse. Also called *first-order neuron*.

primary sensory neuron A dorsal root ganglion cell possessing one neurite extending to a peripheral sense organ and a neurite entering the central nervous system. Also called *sensory neuron, peripheral sensory neuron*.

projection neuron **1** A neuron that transmits activity from the cerebral cortex to motor neurons. **2** A neuron that transmits activity from sense organs to the cerebral cortex.

pyramidal neuron PYRAMIDAL CELL.

secondary sensory neuron CENTRAL SENSORY NEURON.

second-order neuron In a neural pathway, the neuron on which the axon of a primary (first-order) neuron synapses, as for example the spinothalamic neurons serving to relay impulses from axons of sensory receptors, or in sympathetic ganglia, the postganglionic neuron contacted by the sympathetic motoneuron whose cell body is the spinal cord.

sensory neuron **1** Any neuron of the central nervous system synaptically activated by peripheral sense organs. **2** PRIMARY SENSORY NEURON.

short neuron A neuron whose axon breaks up into terminal branches in the local grey matter without entering the white matter. See also GOLGI TYPE II NEURONS.

superior motor neuron UPPER MOTOR NEURON.

sympathetic neuron An autonomic ganglion cell of the thoracolumbar prevertebral or paravertebral ganglia of the sympathetic system.

tonic motor neuron An alpha motor neuron whose peripheral axon controls postural muscle tone.

unipolar neuron A neuron with only one process, usually the axon. Such cells are unusual in the central nervous system, where the best-known examples, the cells of the dorsal root spinal ganglia and of the mesencephalic root of the fifth nerve, are actually of bipolar derivation, having become unipolar through subsequent fusion of the two processes. Such neurons are also called T-shaped unipolar cells. Also called *unipolar cell*.

upper motor neuron A neuron that controls activity in motor neurons. Also called *superior motor neuron, premotor neuron*.

neuronagenesis [NEURON + Gk *a-* priv. + GENESIS] A failure of neuron development.

neuronal Of, pertaining to, or affecting a neuron. Also *neuronic* (seldom used).

neurone A British spelling for NEURON.

neuronephric [NEURO- + NEPHRIC] Of, pertaining to, or affecting the nervous and renal systems.

neuronevus A nevus composed of cells that exhibit neural characteristics.

neuronic A seldom used term for NEURONAL.

neuronitis [NEURON + -ITIS] CELLULONEURITIS.

infective neuronitis An outmoded term for GUILLAIN-BARRÉ SYNDROME.

myoclonic spinal neuronitis A rare and poorly understood syndrome in which spinal myoclonus occurs and inclusion bodies may be found in the anterior horn cells of the spinal cord.

vestibular neuronitis A form of vertigo of acute onset, causing prostration, nausea, and vomiting, and lasting often for several days during which any movement of the head induces severe vertigo. Recovery is eventually complete. The condition may occur in epidemics and is believed to be due to a viral infection involving the vestibular nuclei of the brainstem. Also called *Gerlier's disease, Gerlier syndrome, paralytic vertigo, paralyzing vertigo, kubisagari (Japanese)*.

neuronography [NEURON + *o* + -GRAPHY] 1 The study of connections among neurons, originally used with reference to microanatomic techniques that allowed for visual tracing of connections. 2 A physiologic method of mapping connections within the cerebral cortex by recording electrical discharges elicited in various cortical zones following the local application of strychnine. Also called *physiologic neuronography*.

physiologic neuronography NEURONOGRAPHY.

strychnine neuronography An electrophysiological technique for tracing connections in the central nervous system based on the capability of strychnine to synchronize neuronal firing patterns.

neuronopathy A rarely used term for NEUROPATHY.

neuronophage Any phagocytic, usually microglial, cell which has ingested dead neurons or neuronal debris. Also called *neurophage* (rarely used).

neuronophagia The ingestion of dead neurons or neuronal debris by phagocytes. Also called *neuronophagy* (rarely used).

neuronophagy A rarely used term for NEURONOPHAGIA.

neuronosis A seldom used term for NEUROPATHY.

neuronotropic Possessing a selective affinity for neurons.

neuronymy [NEUR- + Aeolian Gk *onym(a)* for Gk *onoma* a name + -Y] The systematic naming of the parts of the nervous system. A seldom used term.

neuronyxis [NEURO- + Gk *myxis* a puncturing, pricking] Puncture of a nerve. A seldom used term.

neuro-ophthalmology [NEURO- + OPHTHALMOLOGY] The science or study of relationships between the central nervous system and the eyes, including the nervous control of vision and ocular movement. Also called *neurophthalmology*.

neuro-optic [NEURO- + OPTIC] Pertaining to the brain and eye.

neuro-otology The study of phenomena, particularly diseases, of concern both to neurologists and otologists; the mutual management of patients with such diseases. Also called *neurotology, otoneurology*.

neuropacemaker [NEURO- + PACEMAKER] An implanted electrical nerve stimulator that helps to relieve intractable pain.

neuropapillitis [NEURO- + PAPILLITIS] PAPILLEDEMA.

neuroparalysis [NEURO- + PARALYSIS] Paralysis attributable to peripheral nerve damage. A seldom used term.

neuroparalytic 1 Relating to neuroparalysis. 2 Designating any of a wide variety of neurological disorders giving rise to paralysis. Seldom used in this sense.

neuroparasite [NEURO- + PARASITE] 1 A parasite whose development takes place exclusively in the nervous system of the host. 2 A parasite of the nervous system. Adjective: neuroparasitic.

neuropath [NEURO- + -PATH] One who suffers from any nervous or mental disorder. An imprecise and outmoded term.

neuropathic [NEURO- + -PATH + -IC] Pertaining to, inducing, or caused by neuropathy.

neuropathist [NEURO- + -PATH + -IST] An obsolete term for NEUROLOGIST.

neuropathogenesis [NEURO- + PATHOGENESIS] Pathogenesis of nervous system disease. A seldom used term.

neuropathogenicity The production of pathologic changes in the nervous system or the ability to induce them.

neuropathology The study of pathologic changes in the nervous system.

neuropathy [NEURO- + -PATHY] 1 Any disease of the central or peripheral nervous system. 2 A disorder of the peripheral nerves, as distinct from myelopathy or encephalopathy in which the central nervous system is involved. Also called *neuronosis* (seldom used), *neuronopathy* (rarely used).

a-alphalipoproteinemic neuropathy ANALPHALIPOPROTEINEMIA.

abetalipoproteinemic neuropathy ABETALIPOPROTEINEMIA.

acrodystrophic neuropathy Any peripheral neuropathy producing severe trophic changes, including sometimes painless ulceration or destruction of tissue in the extremities.

acute autonomic neuropathy A rare syndrome of sudden onset in children and adults, characterized by postural hypotension, paralysis of accommodation, anhidrosis, loss of lacrimation, and urinary and fecal retention. Spontaneous recovery is usual in a few weeks or months. Also called *pandysautonomia*.

alcoholic neuropathy Polyneuropathy complicating alcoholism and resulting as a rule from associated thiamine deficiency. Also called *alcoholic paralysis, alcoholic polyneuritis, alcoholic polyneuropathy, polyneuritis potatorum* (obsolete), *alcoholic pseudotabes* (obsolete).

amyloid neuropathy Polyneuropathy due to deposition of amyloid (amyloidosis) in peripheral nerves. Portuguese, Iowa, and Indiana types have been described. See under AMYLOIDOSIS. Also called *amyloid neuritis, amyloid polyneuropathy*.

Andrade type amyloid neuropathy PORTUGUESE TYPE AMYLOIDOSIS.

ascending neuropathy Polyneuropathy first affecting the feet and legs and only later the trunk and upper limbs.

asymmetric motor neuropathy Any motor neuropathy in which the clinical manifestations are asymmetric, involving the two sides of the body unequally.

autonomic neuropathy Polyneuropathy principally or wholly involving autonomic nerves. Also called *vasoneuropathy*.

axonal neuropathy Any neuropathy in which the primary pathologic change is one involving axons rather than their myelin sheaths.

carcinomatous neuropathy Polyneuropathy developing as a complication of carcinoma without direct invasion of peripheral nerves by malignant cells.

congenital peripheral neuropathy Polyneuropathy present at birth. It has been postulated as one cause of arthrogryposis multiplex congenita.

demyelinating neuropathy PERIAXIAL NEURITIS.

Denny-Brown sensory neuropathy A paraneoplastic disorder, usually associated with oat cell carcinoma of the bronchus, giving rise to paresthesiae and sensory loss in the distal parts of the limbs and progressive sensory ataxia, resulting from progressive degeneration of posterior root ganglia, sensory fibers in peripheral nerves and secondary degeneration in ascending sensory tracts in the spinal cord. Motor function is unaffected. Also called *Denny-Brown syndrome*.

descending neuropathy Polyneuropathy first affecting the upper limbs and later spreading to the trunk, legs, and feet.

diabetic neuropathy The distal, bilateral, usually symmetrical, and predominantly sensory polyneuropathy associated with diabetes mellitus. The chief symptoms are hyperesthesia of hands and feet with signs of trophic changes in the extremities, such as coldness, loss of hair, thinness of skin, and disorders of sweating.

dying-back neuropathy Polyneuropathy, such as that due to triorthocresylphosphate, in which the degeneration of axons begins at the periphery and spreads centripetally.

entrapment neuropathy   Neuropathy, usually limited to a single peripheral nerve, in which the nerve is entrapped or compressed within a bony or fibrous canal. Also called *pressure neuropathy.*

giant axonal neuropathy   Neuropathy in which the principal pathologic finding is a massive swelling or enlargement of affected axons.

glue-sniffers' neuropathy   Polyneuropathy due to the accidental or more often deliberate sniffing of the vapor given off by certain glues used, for example, in plastic modeling kits. The toxic agent appears to be *n*-hexane.

hereditary hypertrophic interstitial neuropathy   A disease, often familial, with onset in infancy, marked by symmetrical muscular atrophy of the extremities, with severe sensory disorders and ataxia, arising from ascending neuritis with an associated spinal cord lesion. This form of familial hypertrophic neuropathy, sometimes dominantly inherited, sometimes due to an autosomal recessive trait, is characterized clinically by distal muscular weakness and sensory loss in the limbs and pathologically by demyelination of peripheral nerves with Schwann cell proliferation giving rise to concentric "onion bulb" formation. Spinal cord compression may result from massive hypertrophy of motor and sensory roots within the spinal canal. Pupillary abnormalities, resembling the Argyll Robertson pupil, and/or optic atrophy have been described in some affected individuals and families. It is closely related to peroneal muscular atrophy (Charcot-Marie-Tooth disease) and must be distinguished from the nonfamilial forms of hypertrophic neuropathy, some of which are due to autoimmunity and may be steroid-responsive. Also called *Gombault-Mallet hereditary muscular atrophy, neuritic amyotrophy, Gombault's neuritis, interstitial hypertrophic neuritis, hypertrophic interstitial radiculoneuropathy, progressive hypertrophic interstitial polyneuropathy, symmetrical bundle neurofibromas, Gombault-Mallet disease, Schwann hyperplasia, familial hypertrophic neuritis, Dejerine-Sottas syndrome, Dejerine-Sottas disease, Dejerine disease, Dejerine-Sottas atrophy, Gombault's degeneration, Dejerine-Ceillier syndrome, progressive hypertrophic interstitial neuritis, progressive hypertrophic interstitial neuropathy, progressive hypertrophic polyneuritis.*

hereditary sensorimotor neuropathy types I-III   CHARCOT-MARIE-TOOTH DISEASE.

hereditary sensory neuropathy   A form of genetically determined neuropathy of autosomal recessive inheritance characterized histologically by degeneration of posterior root ganglia and clinically by severe sensory impairment, usually with painless ulceration, in the extremities. Also called *hereditary sensory radicular neuropathy.*

hereditary sensory radicular neuropathy   HEREDITARY SENSORY NEUROPATHY.

hypertrophic neuropathy   Any neuropathy associated with hypertrophy of peripheral nerves. Some forms are inherited, others inflammatory, with repeated cycles of demyelination and remyelination giving the so-called onion-bulb hypertrophy of the affected nerves. Also called *hypertrophic interstitial neuropathy.*

hypertrophic interstitial neuropathy   HYPERTROPHIC NEUROPATHY.

Indiana type amyloid neuropathy   INDIANA TYPE AMYLOIDOSIS.

intercostal neuropathy   INTERCOSTAL NEURALGIA.

intestinal neuropathy   ENTERONEUROPATHY.

Iowa type amyloid neuropathy   IOWA TYPE OF AMYLOIDOSIS.

ischemic neuropathy   Local or diffuse lesions of peripheral nerves resulting either from restriction of blood supply to a single peripheral nerve, often due to compression or from diffuse arterial disease.

isoniazid neuropathy   ISONIAZID POLYNEUROPATHY.

Jamaican neuropathy   JAMAICA JAKE PARALYSIS.

lead neuropathy   Mononeuropathy or polyneuropathy due to exposure to lead. Principal symptoms are wristdrop and weakness of the extensor muscles. Hyperesthesia and analgesia may also occur. Also called *lead paralysis, lead palsy.*

myxedematous neuropathy   Polyneuropathy developing in patients with hypothyroidism.

obscure nutritional neuropathy   Polyneuropathy due to a nutritional deficiency or to a toxic substance in food which cannot be precisely defined.

periaxial neuropathy   PERIAXIAL NEURITIS.

peripheral neuropathy   POLYNEUROPATHY.

plexus neuropathy   Neuropathy of nerves which form part of either the brachial or sacral plexus.

Portuguese type amyloid neuropathy   PORTUGUESE TYPE AMYLOIDOSIS.

postirradiation neuropathy   Localized neuropathy occurring as a late sequel of therapeutic ionizing radiation.

pressure neuropathy   ENTRAPMENT NEUROPATHY.

progressive hypertrophic interstitial neuropathy   HEREDITARY HYPERTROPHIC INTERSTITIAL NEUROPATHY.

radiation neuropathy   Damage to nerves, especially peripheral nerves, caused by radiation.

retrobulbar neuropathy   Inflammation or demyelination of the optic nerve behind the eye, causing no visible ophthalmoscopic changes.

segmental neuropathy   PERIAXIAL NEURITIS.

sensorimotor neuropathy   Any neuropathy or polyneuropathy involving motor and sensory nerves or fibers.

sensory neuropathy   Any neuropathy or polyneuropathy involving only sensory nerves or fibers.

serum neuropathy   Mononeuropathy or polyneuropathy following the injection of foreign serum. Also called *serum neuritis, serum paralysis.*

symmetric distal neuropathy   Any polyneuropathy involving distal muscles equally on the two sides of the body.

tomaculous neuropathy   A pathologic change observed in which affected peripheral nerves show sausage-shaped swellings. An imprecise usage.

trigeminal neuropathy   A neuropathy restricted to one or both trigeminal nerves.

triorthocresyl phosphate neuropathy   The severe and irreversible sensorimotor axonal neuropathy which may result from intoxication with triorthocresyl phosphate. An outbreak of Jamaica jake paralysis in 1930 was caused by contamination of ginger extract with cresyl phosphates. Other incidents have occurred since then due to unintentional contamination of food by triorthocresyl phosphate or contaminated fuel oil improperly sold for cooking purposes. Also called *triorthocresyl phosphate polyneuritis.*

tropical ataxic neuropathy   Neuropathy due to cyanide intoxication and giving rise to optic atrophy, ataxia, and polyneuropathy in varying combinations. It is endemic in Nigeria and in other parts of Africa, where it results from the dietary ingestion of cassava root. Also called *nutritional spinal ataxia.*

uremic neuropathy   UREMIC POLYNEUROPATHY.

neurophage   A rarely used term for NEURONOPHAGE.

neuropharmacology   The branch of pharmacology dealing with the action of drugs on the nervous system and its functions.

neurophil   NEUROSPONGIUM.

neurophilic   NEUROTROPIC.

neurophonia   Attacks in which the subject produces abrupt harsh or high-pitched cries as the result of intermittent spasm of the laryngeal and respiratory musculature. A seldom used term.

neurophrenia [NEURO- + -PHRENIA] A seldom used term for MINIMAL BRAIN DYSFUNCTION.

neurophthalmology NEURO-OPHTHALMOLOGY.

neurophthisis Atrophy of neural tissue. An obsolete term.

neurophysin One of two proteins of low molecular mass (10 kDa) of the neurohypophysis. It is capable of binding oxytocin or vasopressin. It is believed to be a carrier protein for the hormones and may play a role in their storage in the posterior pituitary.

neurophysiology [NEURO- + PHYSIOLOGY] The study of the relation of structure and function in the nervous system.

neurophysis spinalis caudalis UROHYPOPHYSIS.

neuropil [NEURO- + Gk *pil(os)* wool or hair wrought into felt] The dense feltwork of cytoplasmic processes of nerve cells and neuroglia that constitutes the basic stroma of the central nervous system. It generally corresponds to the gray matter, and includes virtually all zones where synaptic interactions may occur, in contradistinction to the long tracts, or white matter (substantia alba). Also called *neuropilem* (obsolete), *neuropile (a chiefly British spelling)*.

neuropile A chiefly British spelling of NEUROPIL.

neuropilem An obsolete term for NEUROPIL.

neuroplasm The unstructured cytoplasm of a nerve cell of neuron. Adjective: neuroplasmic.

neuroplasty [NEURO- + -PLASTY] Surgical repair of a damaged nerve.

neuroplegia [NEURO- + -PLEGIA] **1** Paralysis of any function of the nervous system. **2** A depressive action exerted by various drugs upon the functions of the peripheral and central nervous system.

neuroplexus A plexus or network of nerve cells or fibers.

neuropodia Plural of NEUROPODIUM.

neuropodion END FOOT.

neuropodium END FOOT.

neuropore [NEURO- + Gk *poros* a passage, way through, pore] An opening which temporarily allows communication between the canal within the neural tube of an embryo of protochordates and vertebrates with the outside. An anterior neuropore is always present, but the existence of the posterior neuropore in every form is debatable.

anterior neuropore An opening at the cranial end of the embryonic neural tube leading into the amniotic cavity. Its closure occurs at the 20-somite stage, about the 26th day of intrauterine life in man.

posterior neuropore An opening at the caudal end of the embryonic neural tube communicating with the amniotic cavity. Its closure occurs at about the 25-somite stage, around the 28th day of intrauterine life in man.

neuroprobasia [NEURO- + Gk *probas(is)* (from *probainein* to step forward) a stepping forward + -IA] Progression along nerves, a characteristic of certain viral disease processes.

neuroprosthesis Any prosthetic device applied to a peripheral nerve or implanted in a central nervous structure for purposes of chronic stimulation.

neuropsychiatrist [NEURO- + PSYCHIATRIST] A specialist in neuropsychiatry.

neuropsychiatry [NEURO- + PSYCHIATRY] That branch of medicine which embraces both neurology and psychiatry.

neuropsychic [NEURO- + PSYCHIC] Relating to the functions of the nervous system and of the mind. A seldom used term.

neuropsychology [NEURO- + PSYCHOLOGY] The study of the relationship between the central nervous system and behavior, centering on the integrative functioning of the brain as principal mediator of all mental processes and behavioral reactions.

neuropsychopathic [NEURO- + PSYCHOPATHIC] Relating to disorders of both nervous and mental function.

neuropsychopathy [NEURO- + PSYCHOPATHY] Any disorder which affects the nervous system and the mind.

neuropsychopharmacology The branch of pharmacology dealing with the effects of drugs on psychiatric illnesses and the mechanism of action of these agents.

neuropsychosis [NEURO- + PSYCHOSIS] An obsolete term for PSYCHOSIS.

neuroradiology [NEURO- + RADIOLOGY] A subspecialty of radiology dealing with the diagnosis of diseases of the nervous system. Also called *neuroroentgenography* (seldom used).

neurorecidive [NEURO- + L *recidiv(us)* recurring] NEURO-RECURRENCE.

neurorecurrence [NEURO- + *recurrence*] A recurrence or relapse of nervous illness. Also called *neurorecidive*.

neuroregulation The control of physiological processes by the nervous system.

neuroretinitis [NEURO- + RETINITIS] Inflammation of optic disk and retina.

neuroretinopathy [NEURO- + RETINOPATHY] A disorder of the optic disk and retina.

hypertensive neuroretinopathy Hypertensive damage of optic disk and retina.

neuroroentgenography [NEURO- + ROENTGENOGRAPHY] A seldom used term for NEURORADIOLOGY.

neurorrhaphy [NEURO- + -RRHAPHY] Approximation by suture of a divided nerve. Also called *neurosuture, nerve suture*.

neurorrhexis [NEURO- + -RRHEXIS] Rupture of a nerve.

Neurorrhyctes hydrophobiae An obsolete term for NEGRI BODIES.

neurosal Pertaining to neurosis. An outmoded term.

neurosarcokleisis [NEURO- + SARCO- + -KLEISIS] The release of a confined or compressed nerve by opening its canal or by altering its position.

neurosarcoma [NEURO- + SARCOMA] **1** MALIGNANT NEUROMA. **2** MALIGNANT SCHWANNOMA.

neurosclerosis Hardening, or gliosis, of neural tissue. An obsolete term.

neurosecretion **1** The sum of the processes by which neurons elaborate substances that are released or secreted into the bloodstream and act as hormones. **2** A substance so produced and having an effect or influence on other cells.

neurosecretory Of or relating to neurosecretion.

neurosegmental Denoting a spinal division or segment served by a dorsal and ventral root pair.

neurosensory Describing, pertaining to, or affecting sensory components of the nervous system.

neuroses Plural of NEUROSIS.

neurosis [NEUR- + -OSIS] Any of various functional disorders of behavior characterized by excessive anxiety or by behavior distorted by an exaggerated use of avoidance behaviors or by other recognized mechanisms for defending against anxiety. In psychoanalytic usage, neurosis is the symptomatic expression of conflict between the id's sexual and aggressive impulses and the ego's need to cope with and adapt to reality. One or more distressing and ego-dystonic symptoms develop as a result of the ego's attempt to defend itself against the id. Also called *psychoneurosis, neurotic disorder, defense neurosis, meroergasia, defense psychoneurosis*. • Although DSM-III has discarded *neurosis* in favor of *neurotic disorder*, the former term is still widely used.

accident neurosis COMPENSATION NEUROSIS.

actual neurosis According to Freud, those symptoms arising from present-day disturbances of sexuality in contrast to neuroses which arise from infantile conflicts. Neurasthenia, hypochondriasis, and anxiety neurosis were considered actual neuroses. Also called *true neurosis, physioneurosis.*

air neurosis   AEROASTHENIA.

anankastic neurosis   OBSESSIVE-COMPULSIVE NEUROSIS.

anxiety neurosis   According to Freud, an actual neurosis manifested in general irritability, anxious expectation and excessive free-floating anxiety, pangs of conscience, and exaggerated fear of common dangers such as snakes, mice, or vermin. Also called *anxiety syndrome.*

artificial neurosis   EXPERIMENTAL NEUROSIS.

association neurosis   SHARED DELUSION.

cardiac neurosis   CARDIAC NEURASTHENIA.

character neurosis   CHARACTER DISORDER.

combat neurosis   A post-traumatic stress disorder occurring as a reaction to active warfare. Also called *combat fatigue, military neurosis, war neurosis, battle fatigue, operational fatigue, combat exhaustion, traumatic war neurosis.*

compensation neurosis   A neurosis that develops or persists in a person who has suffered injury from an accident while a tort claim is pending. It tends to prolong the illness (a manifestation of epinosic gain) and delay recovery. Also called *pension neurosis, accident neurosis.*

compulsion neurosis   OBSESSIVE-COMPULSIVE NEUROSIS.

conversion neurosis   CONVERSION HYSTERIA.

craft neurosis   Occupational cramp.

cutaneous neurosis   NEURODERMATITIS.

defense neurosis   NEUROSIS.

depressive neurosis   NEUROTIC DEPRESSIVE DISORDER.

neurosis of destiny   MORAL MASOCHISM.

expectation neurosis   A neurosis characterized by the fear that one will be inadequate in performing the anticipated task. It is often a symptom of agoraphobia.

experimental neurosis   A neurosis created in animals by altering the experimental conditions to which they have adapted. They can no longer discriminate between the different stimuli presented and therefore cannot supply what has been learned as the correct response to a specific stimulus. Also called *artificial neurosis.*

fate neurosis   MORAL MASOCHISM.

fatigue neurosis   An obsolete term for NEURASTHENIA.

fixation neurosis   Any neurosis that develops on the basis of the subject's failure to transfer energy from primitive levels to higher levels during the course of development. An imprecise and old-fashioned term.

fright neurosis   An older term for TRAUMATIC NEUROSIS.

housewife's neurosis   **1** An obsessive-compulsive neurosis characterized by preoccupation with cleanliness and orderliness of the household. Also called *housewife's psychosis.* **2** A syndrome of homemakers characterized by chronic dissatisfaction and feelings of stagnation and emptiness because marriage and parenthood have eliminated the stimulation of employment and freedom of movement among active and accomplishing adults. Also called *tired housewife syndrome.*

hypochondriacal neurosis   HYPOCHONDRIASIS.

hysterical neurosis   HYSTERIA.

military neurosis   COMBAT NEUROSIS.

neurasthenic neurosis   NEURASTHENIA.

obsessional neurosis   OBSESSIVE-COMPULSIVE NEUROSIS.

obsessive-compulsive neurosis   A neurosis characterized by intruding, ego-dystonic, anxiety-provoking thoughts and repetitive impulses to perform actions that are often distasteful or unwanted but are the only way to achieve a temporary surcease of the anxiety. Also called *obsessional neurosis, compulsion neurosis, anankastic neurosis, substitution neurosis, ruminative tension state, obsessive-ruminative state, compulsive-obsessive psy-*

choneurosis, obsessive-compulsive reaction, compulsive state, compulsive insanity.*

occupational neurosis   OCCUPATIONAL CRAMP.

organ neurosis   PSYCHOSOMATIC DISORDER.

pension neurosis   COMPENSATION NEUROSIS.

phobic neurosis   ANXIETY HYSTERIA.

phobic anxiety-depersonalization neurosis   A state in which the individual feels symptoms of both anxiety and depersonalization. It is characterized by giddiness, mood changes, and other symptoms of depersonalization as well as fear of collapse or loss of control in public. Also called *pseudoschizophrenic neurosis.*

postconcussion neurosis   A traumatic neurosis following head injury.

professional neurosis   OCCUPATIONAL CRAMP.

promotion neurosis   A neurosis characterized by an inability to function when given added responsibility or authority.

pseudo-schizophrenic neurosis   Phobic anxiety-depersonalization neurosis.

regression neurosis   A neurosis involving the exhibition of childish attitudes which betoken a desire to return to a lower and easier level of functioning rather than attempting to meet current demands for responsible coping. Symptoms include distressing visceral tensions and wish-fulfilling fancies and postures. An older term.

sphenopalatine ganglion neurosis   SPHENOPALATINE NEURALGIA.

substitution neurosis   OBSESSIVE-COMPULSIVE NEUROSIS.

neurosis tarda   Neurotic symptoms arising as a consequence of organic brain disease in the elderly.

traumatic neurosis   A neurosis brought on by physical injury and triggered by the threat of subsequent harm or actual physical injury. This leads to intrusive recollections of the stressful event, recurrent frightening dreams about it, contraction of the general level of functioning, general irritability, and proclivity to explosive aggressive reactions. Also called *fright neurosis* (older term).

traumatic war neurosis   COMBAT NEUROSIS.

true neurosis   ACTUAL NEUROSIS.

vagabond neurosis   WANDERLUST.

vasomotor neurosis   Neurasthenia with prominent vegetative, autonomic, and vasomotor complaints.

vegetative neurosis   PINK DISEASE.

war neurosis   COMBAT NEUROSIS.

neuroskeletal   **1** Pertaining to the neuroskeleton. **2** Pertaining to nervous and skeletal muscle tissues.

neuroskeleton   **1** The bony parts surrounding the brain, or neurocranium, and spinal cord, or vertebral column. **2** ENDOSKELETON.

neurosome   [NEURO- + Gk *sōm(a)* body]   The main cytoplasmic mass of a neuron, which contains the cell nucleus.

neurosonology   ECHOENCEPHALOGRAPHY.

neurospasm   [NEURO- + SPASM]   Any muscular spasm caused by dysfunction of a motor nerve.

neurosplanchnic   Of, pertaining to, or affecting the autonomic nerves innervating the viscera. Also *neurovisceral.*

neurospongioma   [NEURO- + SPONGI- + -OMA]   GLIOMA.

neurospongium   [NEURO- + New L *-spongium*, combining form from L *spongia* sponge]   An intricate meshwork of axons, dendrites, and neuroglial processes within the central nervous system. Also called *neurophil.*

Neurospora   [NEURO- + Gk *spora* seed]   A genus of ascomycetous, mainly saprobic fungi which have been reported to cause mycotic keratitis.

Neurospora crassa   A species of ascomycetous fungus used extensively in the development of biochemical genetics.

neurostatus   [NEURO- + STATUS]   The relative importance in a case history of symptoms relating to the nervous system.

neurostearic Of, pertaining to, or affecting nervous and fatty tissues.

neurosthenia NEURASTHENIA.

neurostimulator An implantable electric stimulator similar to a pacemaker with output electrodes that encircle a nerve to effect muscle contraction or block pain.

neurosurgeon [NEURO- + SURGEON] One who performs surgery on the nervous system.

neurosurgery [NEURO- + SURGERY] Surgery of the nervous system and its supporting structures, as the vascular supply to the brain and spine.

neurosuture NEURORRHAPHY.

neurosyphilid CIRCINATE SYPHILITIC ERYTHEMA.

neurosyphilis Any of the forms of syphilis of the central nervous system, including secondary syphilis, late syphilis, and tabes dorsalis. Also called *lues nervosa, neurolues, vérole nerveuse.*

juvenile neurosyphilis Neurosyphilis occurring in early adolescence with symptoms similar to general paresis in adults except that delusions are more puerile, the dementia is more complete, and the course is more prolonged. It is a subtype occurring in not more than one percent of congenital syphilitics.

latent neurosyphilis Asymptomatic neurosyphilis that is revealed only by examination of the cerebrospinal fluid. Also called *preparetic neurosyphilis.*

meningeal neurosyphilis Syphilis of the coverings of the brain and spinal cord.

meningovascular neurosyphilis Syphilitic involvement of the meninges and cerebral blood vessels, frequently with involvement of cranial nerves. Also called *mesodermogenic neurosyphilis* (obsolete).

mesodermogenic neurosyphilis MENINGOVASCULAR NEUROSYPHILIS.

paretic neurosyphilis GENERAL PARESIS.

preparetic neurosyphilis LATENT NEUROSYPHILIS.

tabetic neurosyphilis TABES DORSALIS.

neurosystemitis epidemica ENCEPHALITIS LETHARGICA.

neurotabes TABES DORSALIS.

neurotendinal NEUROTENDINOUS.

neurotendinous [NEURO- + TENDINOUS] Of, pertaining to, or affecting nerves and tendons. Also *neurotendinal.*

neurotension [NEURO- + TENSION] NEURECTASIA.

neuroterminal END ORGAN.

neurothecitis [NEURO- + *thec(a)* + -ITIS] Inflammation of a nerve sheath. An outmoded term.

neurothele [NEURO- + Gk *thēlē* a nipple] NERVE PAPILLA.

neurothelion [NEURO- + New L *thelion* (from Gk *thēl(ē)* nipple + -ion, New L dim. suffix) a small nipple, center of a nipple] A small neural papilla.

neurotherapeutics [NEURO- + THERAPEUTICS] NEUROTHERAPY.

neurotherapy [NEURO- + THERAPY] Treatment of disorders of the nervous system. A seldom used term. Also called *neurotherapeutics.*

neurotic [NEUR- + -otic, suffix forming adjectives from -osis nouns] 1 Relating to or characterized by neurosis. 2 A patient suffering from neurosis. • In popular usage, the term in this sense is often used perjoratively to indicate that the subject does not act consistently in the way others expect or want, or that the subject's complaints are imaginary and without foundation.

neurotica [New L (from Gk *neur(on)* nerve + -*otica*, neut. pl. noun suffix formed from nouns ending in -*osis*, as NEUROSIS)]

Functional nervous disorders of emotional as distinct from physical origin. A seldom used term.

neuroticism [*neur(osis)* + -*otic* as in *narcotic* + -ISM] The state of suffering from neurosis.

neurotigenic NEUROTOGENIC.

neurotization [NEURO- + *t* + -*iz(e)* + -ATION] 1 Implantation of nerve into muscle. 2 Regeneration of a nerve.

neurotmesis [NEURO- + Gk *tmēsis* (from *temnein* to cut) a cutting, division] A lesion of a peripheral nerve in which there is actual division of axons, so that regeneration will be needed for recovery to take place.

neurotogenic Productive of neurosis. Also *neurotigenic.*

neurotology NEURO-OTOLOGY.

neurotome [NEURO- + -TOME] 1 A narrow-bladed knife for cutting nerves. 2 NEUROMERE.

neurotomy [NEURO- + -TOMY] 1 The dissection of nerves. 2 Division of a nerve.

retrogasserian neurotomy TRIGEMINAL RHIZOTOMY.

neurotonia [NEURO- + *ton(o)-* + -IA] Instability of autonomic tone. An imprecise and obsolete term.

neurotonic Possessing a stimulating or tonic effect upon nerves. An obsolete term.

neurotonogenic Producing increased nervous tone. An obsolete term.

neurotony [NEURO- + *ton(o)-* + -Y] NEURECTASIA.

neurotoxia [NEURO- + TOX- + -IA] A state induced in the nervous system by exposure to a toxin.

neurotoxic [NEURO- + TOXIC] Having a toxic effect on the nervous system.

neurotoxicity [NEURO- + TOXICITY] The quality of having a toxic effect upon the nervous system.

neurotoxin [NEURO- + TOXIN] Any toxin which acts directly upon neurons, sometimes affecting the cell body but more often acting at synapses, whether excitatory or inhibitory, and thus giving rise to disordered neuronal function. For example, some neurotoxins act at the neuromuscular junction, causing paralysis, while others, such as tetanus toxin, act upon interneuronal connections in the spinal cord causing hyperexcitability of neurons.

neurotransmitter Any chemical substance released at a nerve terminal as a result of the nerve impulse and capable of transmitting that impulse across a synapse by binding to receptors in another cell, thereby exciting it. Also called *transmitter substance, neurogen* (obsolete).

neurotrauma [NEURO- + TRAUMA] Any injury to a nerve. Also called *neurotrosis.*

neurotrophasthenia Inadequate nutrition of neuronal tissue. An obsolete term.

neurotrophic [NEURO- + -TROPHIC] 1 Relating to neurotrophy. 2 Describing trophic disorders of nervous origin.

neurotrophy The maintenance of the nutrition and of the structural and functional integrity of nervous tissue.

neurotropic Having an affinity or attraction for nervous tissue. Also *neurophilic.*

neurotropism The possession of neurotropic qualities. Also called *neurotropy, neutropism.*

neurotropy NEUROTROPISM.

neurotrosis [NEURO- + Gk *trōsis* (from *titrōskein* to wound) a wound] NEUROTRAUMA.

neurotubule Long microtubules of fixed ≈20–30 nm diameter seen in the axons of neurons with the electron microscope. The long axes of the microtubules are parallel to the long axis of the axon. The neurotubules are involved in growth and axonal transport of intracellular materials.

neurovaccine   A vaccine prepared by utilizing the brain of a rabbit for the growth of the virus.

neurovascular   Of, pertaining to, or affecting the nervous and vascular systems.

neurovegetative   Pertaining to or affecting the autonomic nervous system.

neurovirulence [NEURO- + VIRULENCE]   Pathogenicity of an infective agent for tissue of the central nervous system.

neurovirulent   Pathogenic for nerve tissue of the central nervous system: said of infective agents.

neurovirus   NEUROTROPIC VIRUS.

neurovisceral   NEUROSPLANCHNIC.

neurovoltometer   A device for measuring nerve potentials. An obsolete term.

neurula [NEUR- + L -*ula* -ULE]   The embryonic stage following that of the gastrula during which a portion of the ectoderm forms the neural plate, from which the neural tube, the precursor of the central nervous system, will be fashioned.

neurulation [*neurul(a)* + -ATION]   The development of the embryonic neural plate, the neural folds, and then the neural tube from which the central nervous system arises.

neururgic [NEUR- + New L -*urg(ia)*, combining form from Gk *ergon* work, + -IC]   Denoting, pertaining to, or stimulating activity in nerves.

neurypnology   NEUROHYPNOLOGY.

neuston [Gk *neuston*, neut. of *neustos* swimming, verbal of *nein* to swim]   The community of aquatic organisms, such as water striders and mosquito larvae, that are associated with the surface film of water.

neutral [L *neutralis* (from *neuter*, gen. *neutri*, neither of two, from *ne-* negative + *uter* whether) neutral, neuter]   **1** Being neither acidic nor basic, but having a pH near 7: used of a solution.   **2** Having neither acidic nor basic properties: used of a substance.

neutralism   A relationship between two or more species' populations that is devoid of interaction.

neutrality   The state of being neutral, especially the acidity of water when the concentrations of H$^+$ and OH$^-$ ions are equal, i.e. pH 7.

neutralization   **1** The addition of an acid to a base in solution, or vice-versa, so as to obtain a neutral solution.   **2** The addition to water of chemical substances in order to adjust the pH to 7.   **3** Removal of energy from the aggressive or sexual impulse with which it was originally associated to a make it available as instinct-free energy for use by the ego. Neutralization includes desexualization and deaggressivation.

neutralized   **1** Describing an acid which has been converted into a salt by adding a base, or a base converted into a salt by adding an acid.   **2** Rendered ineffective by combination with a reagent: said of a property of a group or molecule.   **3** In crystallography and geology, describing mineral acids, rich in silica, that have been more or less completely converted into their salts.

Neutrapen   A proprietary name for penicillinase.

neutrino   A subatomic particle postulated to account for energy discrepancies in beta decay. It has no charge and, at most, one percent of the mass of an electron. It takes part in only the weak nuclear interaction (and possibly gravitation), and so has enormous penetrating power.

neutroclusion [L *neuter*, gen. *neutri*, neutral, neuter + *o* + *(oc)clusion*]   Normal anatomic relation between the dental arches.

neutrocyte   NEUTROPHIL.

neutrocytopenia   NEUTROPENIA.

neutrocytophilia   NEUTROPHILIA.

neutrocytosis   NEUTROPHILIA.

neutron [*neutr(al)* + -*on*, suffix denoting an elementary particle]   A nuclear particle with no electric charge, with a mass about 1.0014 times that of a proton and with $1/2$ unit of spin. Apart from the lighter elements, neutrons contribute roughly 40% to a typical nuclear mass. A free neutron decays (with a half-life of 15 minutes) into a proton, an electron, and an antineutrino.

delayed neutron   A neutron emitted by radioactive fission products over a time span of seconds or minutes after fission has occurred. Delayed neutrons account for less than 1% of all neutrons produced by fission, but they must be taken into account in the design and control of reactors.

epithermal neutron   A neutron with an energy between a few hundredths of an electron volt and about 100 electron volts, directly above the range of thermal neutrons.

fast neutron   Any neutron having a high kinetic energy, of the order of 1 MeV or more.   ● Some authorities call any neutron "fast" if its energy is greater than 100 KeV.

fission neutron   Any neutron emitted during nuclear fission in a nuclear reactor.

high-energy neutron   A neutron that has an energy exceeding 10^5 eV.

instant neutron   PROMPT NEUTRON.

intermediate neutron   A neutron with an energy between that of a slow neutron and a fast neutron, or between about 1 and 100 000 electron volts.

primary neutron   A neutron projected at a fissionable target or other susceptible target, as distinguished from neutrons that the fission process or other nuclear reaction would project from the target.

prompt neutron   A neutron emitted no more than a few milliseconds after the fission event that produced it. More than 99% of fission neutrons are prompt. Also called *instant neutron.*

slow neutron   A neutron having kinetic energy of 1eV or less.

thermal neutron   Any neutron in thermal equilibrium with the environment, thus having low kinetic energy, about 0.025 eV.

neutrontherapy [NEUTRON + THERAPY]   Radiotherapy using either fast or slow neutrons.

neutropenia [*neutro(phil)* + -PENIA]   A decreased number of neutrophils in the circulating blood. Also called *neutrocytopenia, neutrophilopenia, neutrophilic leukopenia.*

chronic benign neutropenia   An uncommon condition of unknown cause in which neutrophils are much lower than normal in the blood and all other blood elements are normal. The bone marrow is usually normal. Mouth ulcers or respiratory infections may occur when the number of neutrophils is very low.

chronic hypoplastic neutropenia   A rare syndrome of granulocytic hypoplasia in the marrow, chronic neutropenia in the circulating blood, mild to moderate splenomegaly, and recurrent infections especially involving the skin and oral cavity.

congenital neutropenia   A rare and usually lethal disorder that is probably of autosomal recessive genetic transmission, characterized by onset in infancy of recurrent cutaneous infections, aphthous ulcers, severe neutropenia of blood, hyperplasia of early granulocyte precursors in bone marrow, and paucity of later stages of granulocyte maturation. Also called *infantile genetic agranulocytosis, infantile lethal agranulocytosis, Kostmann's disease, congenital aleukia, congenital leukopenia.*

cyclic neutropenia   A syndrome of neutropenia regularly recurring at intervals of 12–35 days and lasting 4–10 days, accompanied by fever, malaise, infections, and arthralgias. Also called *periodic neutropenia.*

familial benign chronic neutropenia   A rare syndrome of autosomal-dominant inheritance, characterized by mild neutropenia and impaired granulocytic maturation beyond the myelocyte, but with few infections or symptoms.

hypersplenic neutropenia A condition marked by neutropenia, myeloid hyperplasia of the marrow, splenomegaly, and frequent bacterial infections, and which responds to splenectomy. Also called *primary splenic neutropenia*.

idiopathic neutropenia Neutropenia of obscure cause.

malignant neutropenia AGRANULOCYTOSIS.

periodic neutropenia CYCLIC NEUTROPENIA.

primary splenic neutropenia HYPERSPLENIC NEUTROPENIA.

toxic neutropenia Neutropenia resulting from exposure to drugs, chemicals or physical agents which decrease neutrophil production by the bone marrow.

transitory neonatal neutropenia Severe neutropenia in infants born of mothers with neutropenia of autoimmune origin, attributed to the passage of maternal antibody against neutrophils across the placenta. Neutropenia abates as antibody titre declines after delivery, and it seldom lasts over 21 days.

neutrophil [*neutro*-, combining form (from L *neuter* neither, neuter) denoting neither, neuter + -PHIL] **1** A polymorphonuclear leukocyte that has numerous minute cytoplasmic granules that are "neutral" in their tinctorial properties, i.e. that stain a pale pink or rose color with Romanowsky dyes. An increase in the number of neutrophils in blood is commonly observed in systemic bacterial infections or inflammatory disorders. Also called *neutrophil leukocyte, heterophil leukocyte, heterophil granulocyte, neutrophil granulocyte, neutrophilic cell, neutrocyte, orthoneutrophil.* **2** Any cell or histologic structure that is stainable by neutral dyes or by both acid and basic dyes. **3** Readily stainable by both acid and basic dyes; neutrophilic.

band neutrophil A neutrophil in which the nucleus is elongated but not segmented into distinct lobes. Band neutrophils are intermediate in maturation between metamyelocytes and mature neutrophils. Also called *juvenile neutrophil, stab neutrophil, stab, stab cell, staff cell, band cell, rod neutrophil, nonfilamented neutrophil.*

filamented neutrophil SEGMENTED NEUTROPHIL.

giant neutrophil An abnormally large, hypersegmented neutrophil; a macropolycyte. It is seen in deficiency of vitamin B_{12} or folic acid.

hypersegmented neutrophil Any neutrophil having six or more nuclear lobes, seen in deficiencies of vitamin B_{12} or folic acid, in some chronic myeloproliferative disorders, and, rarely, through inheritance.

immature neutrophil A neutrophilic granulocyte which has not matured sufficiently to have a segmented nucleus.

juvenile neutrophil BAND NEUTROPHIL.

mature neutrophil SEGMENTED NEUTROPHIL.

nonfilamented neutrophil BAND NEUTROPHIL.

rod neutrophil BAND NEUTROPHIL.

segmented neutrophil A mature granular neutrophil displaying a nucleus of two to five lobes joined by fine chromatin threads and a cytoplasm containing fine granules and displaying chemotaxis, phagocytosis, and immune complex binding. Also called *mature neutrophil, filamented neutrophil, polymorphonuclear granulocyte, polymorph, poly, segmented cell.*

stab neutrophil BAND NEUTROPHIL.

neutrophilia An increased number of neutrophils in the peripheral blood. Also called *neutrocytophilia, neutrocytosis.*

neutrophilic **1** Having the property of staining equally with acid and basic stains, or of staining with neutral dyes. **2** Characterized by the presence of neutrophilic granulocytes.

neutrophilopenia NEUTROPENIA.

neutropism NEUROTROPISM.

neutrotaxis The phenomenon of neutrophil movement toward (positive neutrotaxis) or away from (negative neutrotaxis) various substances.

nevi Plural of NEVUS.

Nevin [Samuel *Nevin*, English neurologist, born 1905] **1** See under SYNDROME. **2** Kiloh-Nevin syndrome. See under SYNDROME.

nevocarcinoma [L *naev(us)* a mole or other natural mark on the body + *o* + CARCINOMA] MALIGNANT MELANOMA.

nevocytic **1** Of or relating to a nevus cell. **2** Pertaining to clusters of melanocytes.

nevoid [*nev(us)* + -OID] Of or relating to a nevus.

nevolipoma [*nev(us)* + *o* + LIPOMA] A deposit of fatty tissue in the dermis with characteristics of a nevus. Also called *nevus molluscum, nevus mollusciformis.*

nevomelanoma [L *naev(us)* a birthmark, mole + *o* + MELANOMA] MALIGNANT MELANOMA.

nevose [*nev(us)* + -OSE¹] Spotted or macular; having nevi.

nevous Of or relating to a nevus or its structures.

nevoxanthoendothelioma [L *naev(us)* a mole on the body + *o* + XANTHO- + ENDOTHELIOMA] JUVENILE XANTHOMA.

nevus

nevus [L *naevus* a mole or mark on the body] **1** A localized cutaneous malformation of the skin or mucous membranes, congenital in origin, and involving either an excess or relative deficiency of any one of the normal cutaneous structures. Also called *mother spot, longing mark, spilus.* **2** A benign proliferation of melanocytic cells. Also called *benign melanoma.*

achromic nevus A pale nevus characterized by the relative absence or poor functional capacity of cutaneous capillaries.

nevus acneiformis An epidermal nevus characterized by the presence of dilated pilar sebaceous follicles and comedones, or blackheads.

nevus acneiformis unilateris A linear epidermal nevus distinguished by the presence of comedones. Also called *nevus unilateralis comedonicus.*

alopecic nevus A nevus seen on the scalp and characterized by an absence of normal hair follicles in the area.

amelanic nevus AMELANOTIC NEVUS.

amelanotic nevus A nevus characterized by the presence of melanocytic nevus cells that do not produce normal quantities of melanin pigment. Also called *nonpigmented nevus, amelanic nevus.*

nevus anemicus A nevus characterized by the presence of pale macules on the skin surface. It is caused by a relative absence of local capillary vessels or by the inability of the vessels to dilate.

nevus angiectodes VASCULAR NEVUS.

nevus angiomatodes VASCULAR NEVUS.

angiomatous nevus VASCULAR NEVUS.

nevus à pernione ANGIOKERATOMA.

nevus aplasticus A nevus comprising a depressed, smooth cutaneous surface and a relative absence of adnexal skin structures.

nevus arachnoideus SPIDER TELANGIECTASIS.

nevus araneosus SPIDER TELANGIECTASIS.

nevus araneus SPIDER TELANGIECTASIS.

atrophic nevus A connective tissue nevus characterized by an absence of normal collagen tissue.

balloon cell nevus A nevus many of whose cells have abundant amounts of clear cytoplasm.

basal-cell nevus   BASAL CELL NEVUS SYNDROME.

bathing trunk nevus   A large congenital melanocytic nevus that frequently contains terminal hairs and is characterized by a tendency to malignant change. It is usually located on skin of the pelvic and thigh regions, areas formerly covered by bathing trunks.

Becker's nevus   A nevus that comprises a large number of tan macules. It is frequently seen on the shoulder area or the hips and forms after prolonged sun exposure. Onset commonly occurs during childhood or adolescence as one or more brown patches. As they enlarge, new patches develop beyond the spreading edge, to which they eventually become attached. At puberty, hypertrichosis develops in the same region as the pigmentation but is not coextensive with it. The increase in pigment is caused by an increase in melanocyte activity without an increase in the number of melanocytes. Also called *nevus spilus tardus.*

blue nevus   A circumscribed intradermal nevus of blue-black color composed of dermal melanocytes that are bipolar dendritic cells and that usually contain large quantities of melanin pigment. The nevi develop as discrete nodular growths 2–15 mm in diameter on the face, forearms, and hands during childhood. Also called *Jadassohn-Tièche nevus.*

blue rubber bleb nevus   The presence of multiple bluish cutaneous hemangiomas resembling nevi on the skin surface. It is usually inherited by the autosomal dominant transmission pattern.

capillary nevus   CAPILLARY HEMANGIOMA.

nevus cavernosus   CAVERNOUS HEMANGIOMA.

cellular nevus   A nevus characterized by the presence of melanocytic nevus cells.

cellular blue nevus   A rare blue nevus that is most often found on the wrists or buttocks and is characterized by interlacing foils of bipolar dendritic cells.

cerebriform nevus   A melanocytic nevus that has a surface topography resembling cerebral tissue. It occurs in the scalp.

cobblestone nevus   A nevus characterized by a hyperkeratotic papular surface that resembles paving stones or cobblestones. Also called *paving-stone nevus.*

comedo nevus   An epidermal nevus characterized by the presence of comedones or blackheads. Also called *nevus comedonicus.*

nevus comedonicus   COMEDO NEVUS.

compound nevus   A melanocytic nevus characterized by the presence of both junctional activity and melanocytic nevus cells within the dermis.

connective tissue nevus   A nevus comprising only dermal elements and characterized by changes in the normal elastic tissue, collagen, or other structures within the dermis.

dermoepidermal nevus   A nevus in which the abnormalities are present both in the epidermis and dermis of the skin site. Also called *epidermic-dermic nevus.*

nevus elasticus   A connective tissue nevus characterized by excessive amounts of elastic tissue.

nevus elasticus of Lewandowsky   A dermal nevus composed of connective tissue elements and characterized by smooth white papules. It is usually seen on the trunk.

nevus elasticus regionis mammariae   A connective tissue nevus that appears as a yellow raised plaque on the chest and contains excessive elastic tissue. Also called *nevus sclerodermicus thoracis* (outmoded).

epidermal nevus   A nevus comprising only abnormalities of epidermal tissue.

epidermic-dermic nevus   DERMOEPIDERMAL NEVUS.

epithelial and/or spindle cell nevus   A compound nevus with abundant elongated and/or epithelioid cells. Melanin is usually minimal or absent. It is benign and commonly occurs on the face, mostly in children. Also called *benign juvenile melanoma, Spitz nevus, spindle cell and/or epithelioid nevus, juvenile melanoma.*

epithelioid cell nevus   A nevus with large epithelial-like cells. Giant cells may be present.

nevus epitheliomatocylindromatosus   ECCRINE DERMAL CYLINDROMA.

nevus epitheliomatosis multiplex   BASAL CELL NEVUS SYNDROME.

erectile nevus   STRAWBERRY NEVUS.

fatty nevus   NEVUS LIPOMATOSUS.

nevus fibrosus   A soft nevus composed of fibrous tissues.

nevus flammeus   PORT-WINE STAIN.

nevus flammeus nuchae   UNNA'S MARK.

nevus foliaceus   A port-wine stain with sharply demarcated edges.

nevus follicularis   HAIR FOLLICLE NEVUS.

nevus follicularis keratosus   A hyperkeratotic nevus that contains large numbers of hair follicles in the dermis and epidermis.

nevus fragarius   STRAWBERRY NEVUS.

nevus fuscoceruleus acromiodeltoideus   NEVUS OF ITO.

nevus fuscoceruleus ophthalmomaxillaris   OTA'S NEVUS.

giant pigmented nevus   A large, congenital skin lesion, usually darkly pigmented, which contains both superficial and deep components. The deep part extends into the subcutaneous tissue. The meninges may also be affected by melanocytic lesions in affected patients. Malignant melanoma develops in a significant number of affected patients.

hair follicle nevus   A nevus characterized by the presence of excessive numbers of hair follicles. Also called *nevus follicularis.*

hairy nevus   A nevus marked by excessive growth of body hair. It is usually associated with excessive pigmentation and the presence of melanocytic nevus cells in the dermis and epidermis. Most hairy nevi are congenital in origin.

halo nevus   A nevus characterized by the presence of melanocytic cells in the center and surrounded by a depigmented white halo. Also called *Sutton's nevus.*

hard nevus   An epidermal nevus that appears as an overgrowth. It may form in infancy.

honeycomb nevus   ULERYTHEMA OPHRYOGENES.

hypertrophic nevus   A nevus characterized by an excessive, hyperkeratotic, warty surface. It is usually confined to the epidermis.

nevus ichthyosiformis systematisatus   NEVUS UNIUS LATERIS.

intradermal nevus   A nevus characterized by the presence of melanocytic nevus cells in the dermis.

nevus of Ito   A dermal nevus composed of excessive numbers of bipolar dendritic pigment-containing nevus cells. Such nevi are found in those areas innervated by the posterior supraclavicular and lateral cutaneous brachial nerves. Also called *nevus fuscoceruleus acromiodeltoideus.*

Jadassohn-Tièche nevus   BLUE NEVUS.

junction nevus   JUNCTIONAL NEVUS.

junctional nevus   A melanocytic nevus characterized by the presence of large numbers of melanocytes at the dermoepidermal junction. Also called *marginal nevus, junction nevus.*

keratoid nevus   An epidermal nevus with conspicuous thickening of the horny layer.

keratotic nevus   An epidermal nevus marked by hyperkeratosis and surface irregularities.

nevus keratoticus papillomatosus   ICHTHYOSIS HYSTRIX.

nevus lichenodes   A nevus that bears a superficial resemblance to lichen planus.

linear nevus   A nevus that arises in the epidermis and consists of linear hyperkeratotic streaks.

nevus lipomatodes superficialis A cutaneous nevus that arises from a proliferation of fat cells. Clinically it is seen most often on the buttocks and appears as a large yellowish plaque. Also called *nevus lipomatosus cutaneus superficialis.*

nevus lipomatosus A nevus characterized by excessive amounts of fatty tissue and fat cells in the dermis. Also called *fatty nevus.*

nevus lipomatosus cutaneus superficialis NEVUS LIPOMATODES SUPERFICIALIS.

nevus lymphangiectodes LYMPHATIC NEVUS.

lymphatic nevus A nevus characterizd by an excessive number of lymphatic vessels in the dermis. Also called *nevus lymphangiectodes, nevus lymphaticus.*

nevus lymphaticus LYMPHATIC NEVUS.

nevus maculosus A flat, macular, melanocytic nevus.

malignant blue nevus A malignant melanoma arising in a blue nevus. These appear to be less aggressive than the usual malignant melanomas despite the fact that they lie deeply in the skin.

marginal nevus JUNCTIONAL NEVUS.

melanocytic nevus A nevus characterized by an excessive number of melanocytes in the dermis or epidermis.

mixed nevus A nevus formed by more than one type of cell, such as an epidermal nevus derived in part from apocrine sweat glands and in part from sebaceous glands.

nevus mollusciformis NEVOLIPOMA.

nevus molluscum NEVOLIPOMA.

nevus morus MULBERRY MARK.

multiplex nevus SEBACEOUS NEVUS.

nape nevus UNNA'S MARK.

nevus nervosus NEVUS UNIUS LATERIS.

nevocytic nevus 1 MOLE[1]. 2 A melanocytic nevus composed of melanocytic nevus cells that are found at the dermoepidermal junction and in the dermis. Also called *nevus-cell nevus.*

nevus-cell nevus 1 MOLE[1]. 2 NEVOCYTIC NEVUS.

nodular connective tissue nevus A nevus, commonly seen in children, that is clinically composed of raised yellow nodules on the trunk and histologically evidenced by a thickening of collagen fibers and abnormalities in the quantity of elastic tissue.

nonpigmented nevus AMELANOTIC NEVUS.

oral epithelial nevus WHITE SPONGE NEVUS.

Ota's nevus A dermal nevus comprising dermal melanocytes that involve the ocular tissues and the facial skin in a unilateral pattern. Also called *nevus fuscoceruleus ophthalmomaxillaris, oculocutaneous melanosis.*

pachydermic nevus An epidermal nevus characterized by gross hyperkeratinization.

nevus papillaris PAPILLOMATOUS NEVUS.

papillomatous nevus A nevus having a raised hyperkeratotic papillary surface. Also called *nevus papillaris.*

paving-stone nevus COBBLESTONE NEVUS.

pigmented nevus NEVUS PIGMENTOSUS.

pigmented hairy epidermal nevus An epidermal nevus marked by an increase in melanin pigmentation and some terminal hair growth.

nevus pigmentosus A nevus containing excessive melanin that arises as a result of proliferation of melanocytes or nevus cells; in common usage, a mole. Also called *pigmented nevus.*

pilose nevus NEVUS PILOSUS.

nevus pilosus A nevus characterized by the outgrowth of terminal hair from the lesion. Also called *pilose nevus, hairy mole.*

plane nevus A nevus that does not protrude above the level of the surrounding tissue. Also called *nevus planus.*

nevus planus PLANE NEVUS.

nevus porokeratodes A nevus unius lateris with excessive hyperkeratosis and prominent pilosebaceous follicles.

port-wine nevus PORT-WINE STAIN.

nevus profundus A vascular nevus that extends deeply into the underlying dermis.

raspberry nevus STRAWBERRY NEVUS.

nevus sanguineus VASCULAR NEVUS.

nevus sclerodermicus thoracis An outmoded term for NEVUS ELASTICUS REGIONIS MAMMARIAE.

sebaceous nevus An epidermal nevus characterized by an excessive number of sebaceous glands. These lesions are most commonly seen on the scalp. Throughout childhood they appear as slightly raised yellow areas with hypotrichosis. At puberty the sebaceous component enlarges in response to the circulating androgen. Transformation to basal cell carcinoma may occur in adult life. Also called *congenital sebaceous gland hyperplasia, nevus sebaceus, multiplex nevus, sebaceous nevus of Jadassohn.*

sebaceous nevus of Jadassohn SEBACEOUS NEVUS.

nevus sebaceus SEBACEOUS NEVUS.

seborrheic nevus SEBORRHEIC KERATOSIS.

segmental nevus A cutaneous nevus following the distribution of one or more dermotomes. Also called *zoniform nevus.*

soft nevus MOLE[1].

spider nevus SPIDER TELANGIECTASIS.

nevus spilus A flat, congenital melanocytic nevus that is spotted with areas of darker pigmentation.

nevus spilus tardus BECKER'S NEVUS.

spindle cell nevus A nevus with elongated cells.

spindle cell and/or epithelioid nevus EPITHELIAL AND/OR SPINDLE CELL NEVUS.

Spitz nevus EPITHELIOID AND/OR SPINDLE CELL NEVUS.

nevus spongiosus albus mucosae WHITE SPONGE NEVUS.

stellar nevus SPIDER TELANGIECTASIS.

straight-hair nevus A circumscribed area of the scalp in which straight hair replaces the type of hair normal for that site.

strawberry nevus A superficial type of cavernous hemangioma consisting of a red, raised lesion appearing in the newborn period, and often growing rapidly at first before starting to regress. Spontaneous and complete healing occurs in five years or less. Also called *strawberry angioma, strawberry mark, strawberry birthmark, nevus fragarius, raspberry nevus, raspberry mark, erectile nevus.*

subcutaneous nevus A vascular nevus, most often a cavernous angioma, comprising abnormalities of the deeper capillary plexus. The overlying epidermis is relatively normal.

Sutton's nevus HALO NEVUS.

nevus syringocystadenosus papilliferus A nevus arising from the apocrine sweat gland apparatus.

systematized nevus A nevus comprising multifocal deposits throughout several parts of the body.

nevus tardus A nevus that is not present at birth. It may develop after prolonged exposure to the sun, as a Becker's nevus.

nevus unilateralis comedonicus NEVUS ACNEIFORMIS UNILATERIS.

nevus unius lateris An epidermal nevus having a linear distribution and commonly involving a limb. Also called *nevus ichthyosiformis systematisatus, nevus nervosus.*

Unna's nevus An obsolete term for PORT-WINE STAIN.

vascular nevus A nevus that aries as a result of an excess of dermal capillaries. Also called *nevus sanguineus, nevus angiomatodes, angiomatous nevus, nevus angiectodes, nevus vascularis.*

nevus vascularis VASCULAR NEVUS.

nevus vascularis fungosus A pedunculated cavernous angioma, which is usually red or purple in color.

nevus vasculosus Any cutaneous nevus characterized by the presence of excessive capillaries in the skin and subcutis.

nevus venosus A nevus comprising a circumscribed area of excessive cutaneous venules.

venous nevus A superficial venous hemangioma.

verrucoid nevus VERRUCOUS NEVUS.

nevus verrucosus VERRUCOUS NEVUS.

verrucous nevus A nevus with an irregular, superficial brown warty appearance. Also called *verrucoid nevus, nevus verrucosus*.

nevus vinosus PORT-WINE STAIN.

white sponge nevus A nevus arising on the oral mucous membrane. It is frequently a familial condition that is believed to be inherited by autosomal dominant transmission. Also called *white folded gingivostomatitis, nevus spongiosus albus mucosae, white folded gingivostomatosis, oral epithelial nevus*.

zoniform nevus SEGMENTAL NEVUS.

zosteriform nevus A pigmented nevus that arises as a result of an excessive number of melanocytes or nevus cells, has a cutaneous dermal distribution, and resembles herpes zoster in appearance.

---

newborn 1 NEONATE. **2** NEONATAL.

Newton [Isaac *Newton*, English mathematician and astronomer, 1642–1727] **1** See under DISK. **2** Newton's rings. See under RING. **3** Newton's alloy. See under MELOTTE'S METAL. **4** Newtonian aberration. See under CHROMATIC ABERRATION. **5** Newtonian constant. See under GRAVITATIONAL CONSTANT. **6** Non-newtonian fluid. See under FLUID. **7** Newton's law of gravitation. See under LAW.

newton [after Sir Isaac *Newton,* English mathematician and physicist, 1642–1727] Special name for the SI derived unit of force, equal to the force which, applied to a mass of one kilogram, gives to it an acceleration of one meter per second squared; one newton equals one kilogram times one meter per second squared. Symbol: N

newton per square meter The SI derived unit of pressure or stress, equal to the pressure or stress produced by a force of one newton applied uniformly distributed over an area of one square meter, more commonly referred to by the special name pascal. Symbol: N/m^2, $N \cdot m^{-2}$

newton-meter 1 The SI derived unit of work generally known by the special name joule. Symbol: $N \cdot m$ **2** The SI derived unit of moment of a force or torque. Symbol: $N \cdot m$

newton-meter per second The SI derived unit of power, generally known by the special name watt. Symbol: $N \cdot m/s$, $N \cdot m \cdot s^{-1}$

newton-second per square meter The SI derived unit of dynamic viscosity, more commonly referred to as the pascal-second. Symbol: $N \cdot s/m^2$, $N \cdot s \cdot m^{-2}$

nexus [L (from *nexus*, past part. of *nectere* to tie, bind, fasten), a binding, tying together] **1** GAP JUNCTION. **2** A bond or an interlacing.

nexus stamineus oculi An obsolete term for CORPUS CILIARE.

Neyman [Jerzy *Neyman*, Rumanian-born U.S. statistician, born 1894] See under BIAS.

Nezelof [C. *Nezelof*, French pathologist, born 1922] See under SYNDROME.

NF *National Formulary.*

nF Symbol for the unit, nanofarad.

ng Symbol for the unit, nanogram.

n'gana NAGANA.

NGF nerve growth factors.

NHC 1 National Health Council. **2** neonatal hypocalcemia.

NHL non-Hodgkin's lymphoma.

NHS 1 National Health Service (United Kingdom). **2** normal human serum.

Ni Symbol for the element, nickel.

niacin Nicotinic acid: used especially in nutritional contexts. Niacin is a member of the B complex vitamins and is needed for the synthesis of the coenzyme nicotinamide adenine dinucleotide, which is the hydrogen acceptor for many dehydrogenases. It can be made in the body from tryptophan, 60 mg of tryptophan being equivalent to 1 mg of niacin. A deficiency of niacin gives rise to pellagra. The dietary requirement is 6.6 mg per 1000 dietary kcals. Also called *antipellagra vitamin, pellagramin, anti-black-tongue factor, antipellagra factor, pellagra-preventive factor*.

niacinamide NICOTINAMIDE.

niacinamidosis PELLAGRA.

nialamide $C_{16}H_{18}N_4O_2$. 4-Pyridinecarboxylic acid 2-[3-oxo-3-[(phenylmethyl)amino]propyl]hydrazine. An antidepressant drug that acts as an inhibitor of monoamine oxidase. It is given orally.

Niamid A proprietary name for nialamide.

nib [Old English *neb, nebb* beak] The tip of a dental condenser. The face of the tip which compresses the amalgam or foil is flat and may be smooth or serrated. Also called *condenser point*.

niche [French (from Italian *nicchia* niche, from L *nidificare* or *nidulari* to nest, from *nidus* a nest), recess in a wall for a statue] **1** In radiology, a depression in the wall of a hollow organ, best demonstrated as a localized projection when the lumen of the organ is filled with contrast medium, as *the niche of a peptic ulcer*. **2** The functional role of an organism or species in a community. Also called *ecological niche*.

Barclay's niche A small ulcer projection of the duodenal cap as seen on gastrointestinal series.

ecological niche NICHE.

enamel niche A funnel-shaped depression between the lingual and buccal parts of the dental lamina.

fundamental niche The maximum niche that a given species is capable of occupying when not restrained by competition.

Haudek's niche A crater of a penetrating gastric ulcer which, on the erect projection during gastrointestinal series, has triple layering consisting of barium at the bottom, gastric fluid above it, and air at the top. Also called *Haudek sign, niche sign*.

realized niche The niche that an organism is able to occupy in the face of the constraints of interaction with other species populations.

temporal niche A separation in time of potentially competing species.

Nichols [Ernest Fox *Nichols*, U.S. physicist, 1869–1924] See under RADIOMETER.

nick 1 A break in a protein chain that permits subsequent separation of the resulting polypeptides (e.g., polypeptides A and B of diphtheria toxin, whose separation is important for its action). Also called *single chain break, single strand break*. **2** To cause such a break.

nickel Element number 28, having atomic weight 58.71. It is a hard, malleable metal used chiefly as a constituent of stainless steel and other alloys. Symbol: Ni

nickel carbonyl C_4NiO_4. A colorless, volatile liquid with high vapor pressure at room temperature, used to refine impure nickel powder. It is highly poisonous, causing acute symptoms of headache, giddiness, shortness of breath, and vomiting. The highly insoluble vapor penetrates to the alveoli, causing pulmonary edema.

nicking AV NICKING.

AV nicking Apparent indentation of a retinal vein by the overlying arteriole, due to opacity of the arteriolar wall. Also called *nicking*.

Nickkrampf [German *Nick* a nod + *Krampf* a cramp, spasm] INFANTILE MASSIVE SPASM.

niclosamide $C_{13}H_8Cl_2N_2O_4$. 2′,5-Dichloro-4′-nitrosalicylanilide, an antiparasitic agent effective against tapeworm infections. It is incapable of destroying tapeworm ova, however, and cysticercosis may follow inadequate treatment to remove the tapeworm segments.

Nicol [William *Nicol*, Scottish physicist and geologist, 1768–1851] See under PRISM.

Nicolas [Joseph *Nicolas*, French physician, born 1868] Durand-Nicolas-Favre disease, maladie de Nicolas et Favre, Nicolas-Favre disease, Favre-Durand-Nicolas disease. See under LYMPHOGRANULOMA VENEREUM.

Nicolle [Charles Jules Henri *Nicolle*, French bacteriologist, 1866–1936] **1** See under MYCETOMA. **2** Novy, McNeal and Nicolle medium. See under MEDIUM. **3** Nicolle stain for capsules. See under STAIN.

Niconyl A proprietary name for isoniazid.

nicotinamide A biologically active amide of nicotinic acid that forms needlelike, white, bitter crystals, soluble in water and alcohol. It is a member of the vitamin B complex, differing from niacin in that it lacks vasodilator action. It occurs naturally in the body and is interconvertible with niacin. It is used in the treatment of pellagra. Also called *nicotinic acid amide, niacinamide.*

nicotinamide adenine dinucleotide A hydrogen acceptor for many dehydrogenases. Its molecule consists of *N*-(5-phosphoribosyl)nicotinamide joined by a pyrophosphate bond to the phosphate group of adenosine 5′-phosphate. In the course of its reduction, a hydride ion is accepted by the pyridine ring of the nicotinamide, on C-4, to give a dihydropyridine derivative. The respiratory chain of mitochondria, aerobic microorganisms, etc. can reoxidize the reduced form at the expense of molecular oxygen. Also called *factor V (the letter V), coenzyme I* (obsolete), *cozymase* (obsolete), *diphosphopyridine nucleotide* (obsolete), *nadide.* Symbol: NAD

nicotinamide adenine dinucleotide phosphate Nicotinamide adenine dinucleotide phosphorylated on O-2′ of the adenosine group. It is hydrogen acceptor for some dehydrogenases. Its reduced form is the hydrogen donor for many biosyntheses, including fat synthesis. Also called *coenzyme II* (obsolete), *phosphocozymase* (obsolete), *triphosphopyridine nucleotide* (outmoded). Symbol: NADP

nicotinamidemia The presence of nicotinamide in the blood.

nicotinamide mononucleotide Nicotinamide bearing a 5-phosphoribosyl group on its ring nitrogen atom; an intermediate in NAD formation.

nicotine $C_{10}H_{14}N_2$. 1-Methyl-2-(3-pyridyl)pyrrolidine, a colorless, toxic liquid obtained from leaves of the tobacco plant. It is responsible for many of the effects derived from the smoking or chewing of tobacco and is also used as a botanical insecticide.

nicotinehydroxamic acid methiodide An agent with the capacity to reactivate cholinesterase inhibited by organophosphates. Its actions are like those of pralidoxime.

nicotinic Of or relating to nicotine or to effects resembling those produced by nicotine.

nicotinic acid Pyridine-3-carboxylic acid. It is a vitamin, being needed for the formation of NAD and NADP. It can be made by oxidizing 3-methylpyridine, which is a constituent of coal tar.

nicotinic acid amide NICOTINAMIDE.

nicotinism [*nicotin(e)* + -ISM] Poisoning due to chronic exposure to excessive amounts of nicotine through inhalation or ingestion. The smoking or chewing of tobacco causes stimulation, followed by depression, of the central and autonomic nervous systems, vasoconstriction in the hands and feet, and a slight rise in blood pressure and heart rate. In middle age, chronic smokers often develop slowly progressive fogginess of vision and inability to do fine work.

nicotinolytic Blocking the action of nicotine.

nicotinomimetic Mimicking the action of nicotine; nicotinic.

nicotinuric acid The amide formed by acylation of glycine with nicotinic acid. It is a minor metabolite of nicotinic acid and is found in urine.

nicotyrine $C_{10}H_{10}N_2$. 3-(1-Methyl-2-pyryl) pyridine, an oily, odoriferous alkaloid produced by the catalytic dehydrogenation of nicotine. It has insecticidal properties.

Nicozide A proprietary name for isoniazid.

nictation NICTITATION.

nictatio spastica SPASMUS NUTANS.

nictitate [Med L *nictitat(us)*, past part. of *nictitare*, alteration of L *nictare* to wink, blink] To blink.

nictitation [from Med L *nictitatus*, past part. of *nictitare*, frequentative of L *nictare* to wink, blink] **1** The act of blinking or winking. Also called *nictation.* **2** The contracture of the nictitating membrane in reptiles, birds, and certain mammals (including the carnivores) that possess such a membrane over the medial aspect of the cornea.

nidal Pertaining to a nidus.

nidation [L *nid(us)* nest + English -ATION] IMPLANTATION.

NIDDM non-insulin-dependent diabetes mellitus.

nidi Plural of NIDUS.

nidicolous [L *nid(us)* nest + *i* + L *col(ere)* to inhabit + -OUS] Designating birds that are hatched naked, blind, and too weak to stand or feed themselves, thus remaining confined to the nest during maturation.

nidifugous [L *nid(us)* nest + *i* + *fug(ere)* to flee + OUS] Designating birds that are hatched with down, well-developed legs, open eyes, the capacity to feed themselves, and the ability to leave the nest shortly after hatching.

nidulariaceous Having a resemblance to a bird's-nest fungus.

nidulate [L *nidul(us)* a little nest + -ATE] Having the appearance of a nest or a nestlike fungus.

nidulus [L, a little nest, dim. of *nidus* a nest] A nucleus of neurons.

nidus [L, nest] **1** A focus of origin, such as a collection of bacteria in infections or the point of precipitation in calculus formation. **2** The nucleus of a nerve in the central nervous system.

nidus avis A depression in the surface of the cerebellum between the posterior velum and the uvula. An obsolete term. Also called *nidus hirundinis.*

nidus hirundinis NIDUS AVIS.

Niemann [Albert *Niemann*, German surgeon, 1880–1921] **1** Niemann-Pick lipid. See under SPHINGOMYELIN. **2** Niemann's disease, Niemann splenomegaly. See under NIEMANN-PICK DISEASE. **3** Niemann-Pick cell. See under CELL.

Nigella A genus of annual herbs indigenous to western Asia and the Mediterranean area belonging to the family Ranunculaceae. The seeds of *N. sativa*, fennel flower or love-in-a-mist, are noted for their carminative, diuretic, antispasmodic, emmenagogue, and antihelminthic properties.

nigerine $C_{12}H_{16}N_2$. *N,N*-dimethyltryptamine, an alkaloid found in the leaves of plants that have hallucinogenic properties, especially *Mimosa hostilis* and *Prestonia amazonica*. It is believed to be the active ingredient that brings about the psychologic effect.

nightmare [*night*, from Middle English and Old English *niht* + English *mare*, from Middle English and Old English, akin to

Old Norse *mar* incubus] A reaction of fright or a terrifying dream occurring during **REM** sleep, usually within an hour or two after falling asleep. It is much more frequent in children than adults. Also called *ephialtes* (older term).

epileptic nightmare A group of symptoms resembling a nightmare (or night terrors in childhood), including fear and frightening visual hallucinations, which may, in rare cases, occur in nocturnal attacks of temporal lobe epilepsy, and which may cause the patient to be wakened from sleep. Some authorities have suggested, on the other hand, that a genuine nightmare may on occasion precipitate an epileptic attack, but this is uncertain. An imprecise and seldom used term. Also called *epileptic incubus* (obsolete).

nightshade / deadly nightshade BELLADONNA.

nigra [L, fem. of *niger* black] SUBSTANTIA NIGRA.

nigral [L *nigr(a)*, fem. sing. of *niger* black, dusky, dark + -AL] Pertaining to the substantia nigra.

nigredo NIGRISMUS.

nigricans [L, pres. part. of *migricare* (from *niger* black) to be blackish, shade into black] Blackish in color.

nigrismus [L *nigr-*, stem of *niger* black + *-ismus* -ISM] The pigmentation of the skin by melanin. Also called *nigredo*.

nigrismus linguae A seldom used term for BLACK HAIRY TONGUE.

nigrities [L (from *niger* black), blackness] Blackness of pigmentation.

nigrities linguae A rarely used term for BLACK HAIRY TONGUE.

nigroreticular Denoting connections between the substantia nigra and the reticular formation.

nigrorubral Denoting connections between the substantia nigra and the nucleus ruber.

nigrosin NIGROSINE.

nigrosine Any of a group of dyes made by heating aromatic amines and nitro compounds with iron filings. It is used as a background stain or counterstain. Also *nigrosin*, *benzalin*.

nigrostriatal Denoting the substantia nigra and corpus striatum, especially the fine-fibered but functionally significant dopaminergic tract between them (strionigral tract), now known to be causally involved in Parkinson's disease.

NIH National Institutes of Health.

nihilism [L *nihil* nothing + -ISM] In psychiatry, the delusion of nonexistence of the self or the world, in whole or in part.

therapeutic nihilism Disbelief in or extreme skepticism about the curative powers of drugs or other therapies.

nikethamide $C_{10}H_{14}N_2O$. *N,N*-Diethyl-3-pyridinecarboxamide, a centrally acting stimulant of the respiratory and cardiovascular centers. The margin between the dose required to obtain stimulation of these centers and the dose producing convulsions is narrow. Other, safer stimulants have supplanted such older stimulants.

Nikiforoff [Mikhail Nikiforovich *Nikiforoff*, Russian dermatologist, 1858–1915] See under METHOD.

Nikolsky [Pyotr Vasilyevich *Nikolsky*, Russian dermatologist, 1858–1940] See under SIGN.

Nilevar A proprietary name for norethandrolone.

nimazone $C_{11}H_9ClN_4O$. 3-(4-Chlorophenyl)-4-imino-2-oxo-1-imidazolideneacetonitrile. A compound with anti-inflammatory activity.

Nimeh [William *Nimeh*, Lebanese gastroenterologist, born 1891] See under METHOD.

NIMH National Institute of Mental Health.

nimiety [L *nimietas* (from *nimie-*, combining form from *nimius* above measure, too much, + *-tas* English *-ty*) superfluity] The

point at which an excessive consumption of water results in an aversion to fluid intake. An obsolete term.

ninhydrin The substance whose molecule consists of the group —CO—C(OH)$_2$—CO— substituted for hydrogen on adjacent atoms of a benzene ring. It is essentially a triketone, but the central carbonyl group is rendered so reactive by the electron attraction of the others that it normally exists in the hydrated state. Ninhydrin is used to detect and determine amino acids and peptides. When it is heated with an amino acid R—CH(NH$_2$)COOH in an appropriate medium, imine formation leads to decarboxylation of the amino acid, and release of the aldehyde R—CHO leaves the triketone group of the ninhydrin in the form —C(—O$^-$)=C(NH$_2$)—CO—. The compound so produced forms an imine with a second molecule of ninhydrin, whose delocalized charges give it a deep purple color, absorbing maximally at 570 nm. When the reaction is applied to peptides, it is largely the N-terminus that reacts, and the color is roughly proportional to the total peptide concentration, irrespective of the lengths of the peptides present. Also called *triketohydrindene hydrate* (obsolete).

niobium Element number 41, having atomic weight 92.9064. It is a soft, lustrous white metal with numerous technologic applications, most notably as an alloying element. Also called *columbium (a term used mostly in commerce and technology)*. Symbol: Nb

Nionate A proprietary name for ferrous gluconate.

niphablepsia [Gk *niph(a)* snow + *ablepsia* blindness] SNOW BLINDNESS.

niphotyphlosis [Gk *niph(a)* snow + *o* + TYPHLO- + -SIS] SNOW BLINDNESS.

nippers [Middle English *nipp(en)* to nip + -ER + *s*] A surgical instrument in the form of pliers with cutting beaks used for cutting small amounts of either soft tissue or bone.

bone nippers A surgical instrument designed to cut away small amounts of cartilage or bone.

nipple [prob. dim. of Middle English *neb* beak, nose] The pigmented, blunted, conical projection at the apex of the breast. The lactiferous ducts open into it; papilla mammaria. Also called *papillula*.

cracked nipple The superficial fissuring of the skin of the nipple, a problem sometimes noted in breast-feeding mothers.

crater nipple A nipple that has remained in the fetal state. Its lactiferous ducts open normally on its surface, which is, however, invaginated below the level of the areola.

herniated nipple A deformity of the breast wherein the nipple and areola bulge out from the surface of the breast.

inverted nipple A nipple that has retracted behind the areola, leaving a pucker where the nipple usually presents. It is usually a benign condition, but if it occurs in a previously normal nipple it may be a sign of underlying breast cancer.

retracted nipple A nipple whose contour is deformed due to scarring or to an underlying carcinoma.

Nippostrongylus [New L (from *Nippo(n)* + Gk *strongylos* round)] A monotypic genus of hookworms (subfamily Viannaiinae, family Trichostrongylidae). Its single species, the rat hookworm, *N. brasiliensis,* occurs in the anterior portion of the small intestine of domiciliated rats and the house mouse throughout the world. It is far commoner in rats than in mice, in which the more common hookworm is *Nematospiroides dubius). N. brasiliensis* is widely used as a model for parasite immunologic research.

Nisentil A proprietary name for alphaprodine hydrochloride.

nisin A 34-residue peptide antibiotic produced by *Streptococcus lactis*. It contains residues of lanthionine and 3-methyllanthionine, which provide thioether cross-linking between different parts of the chain. They are derived by reaction of cysteine residues with residues of 2-aminoacrylic acid (derived by dehydration of serine) and 2-aminocrotonic acid (derived by dehydration of threonine), respectively. The peptide also contains unreacted residues of 2-aminoacrylic and 2-aminocrotonic acids.

Nissl [Franz *Nissl*, German neurologist, 1860–1919] **1** Primary reaction of Nissl. See under AXON REACTION. **2** Nissl's degeneration. See under AXONAL DEGENERATION. **3** Primary degeneration of Nissl. See under DEGENERATION. **4** See under METHOD. **5** Nissl bodies, Nissl granules. See under SUBSTANCE.

Nisulfazole A proprietary name for para-nitrosulfathiazole.

nisus [L, also *nixus* (from *nixus*, past part. of *niti* to strive, labor), effort, endeavor] **1** The display of power in performance; an effort or exertion; an endeavor, molimen. **2** The seasonal sexual urge manifested by certain species.

nit^1 [Middle English *nite, nitte*, from Old English *hnitu*] The egg of a louse, especially of the human louse (*Pediculus humanus*) or the pubic louse (*Pthirus pubis*). The lice secrete a gluelike chitinous substance which they use to attach the nits to the base of hairs or to clothing.

nit^2 A unit of luminance equal to 1 candela per square meter. An obsolete term.

Nitabuch [Raissa *Nitabuch*, German physician, flourished 19th century] Zone of Nitabuch, striae of Nitabuch, layer of Nitabuch. See under MEMBRANE.

nitr- NITRO-.

Nitranitol A proprietary name for mannitol hexanitrate.

nitratase An obsolete term for NITRATE REDUCTASE.

nitrate **1** The anion NO_3^- derived from nitric acid, or a salt containing it, or an ester of nitric acid. Nitrate is one of the main sources of nitrogen available to plants. Plants and many microorganisms can reduce it to ammonia, which they can incorporate into amino acids for protein biosynthesis. **2** To substitute with a nitro group.

nitrate reductase Any of several enzymes that catalyze the reduction of nitrate to nitrite. They use various reductants and they vary in chemical nature, some containing molybdenum. The reaction allows some bacteria to use nitrate as a terminal electron acceptor, and it allows plants to use nitrate as a source of nitrogen for protein synthesis, since the nitrite formed can be further reduced. Also called *nitratase* (obsolete).

nitrazepam $C_{15}H_{11}N_3O_3$. 1,3-Dihydro-7-nitro-5-phenyl-2*H*-1,4-benzodiazepin-2-one, an antianxiety drug used to produce hypnosis and sedation. It is also used as an anticonvulsant drug. It is given orally.

nitremia AZOTEMIA.

Nitretamin A proprietary name for trolnitrate phosphate.

nitric acid HNO_3. An acid obtained industrially by catalytic oxidation of ammonia. It is a colorless liquid which fumes in air. The anhydrous acid boils at 83°C, with decomposition, particularly if illuminated. With water it gives a negative azeotrope, 68% acid, boiling at 120.5°C. It is a strong acid and a strong oxidizing agent, and its salts (nitrates) are almost all soluble in water. It is used for preparing nitrated derivatives which contain the NO_2 group. It is dangerous to breathe and colors the skin yellow (xanthoproteic reaction) by nitrating tyrosine residues. *o*-Nitrophenols are appreciably dissociated at neutral pH and their anions are yellow. Also called *spirit of nitre, aqua fortis*.

nitride Any binary compound of nitrogen with another element.

nitrification The oxidation of ammonia to nitrite and nitrate. This reaction is an essential part of the nitrogen cycle, preserving fixed nitrogen in the soil in a nonvolatile form. The main nitri-

fying organisms are *Nitrosomonas*, which oxidizes only to nitrite, and *Nitrobacter*.

nitrifier Any organism, as a soil bacterium of the family Nitrobacteraceae, that oxidizes ammonium salts to nitrites and nitrates.

nitrilase The enzyme (EC 3.5.5.1) that catalyzes the hydrolysis of a nitrile R—CH to form R—COOH and ammonia. It is found in plants and acts on a number of aromatic nitriles.

nitrile Any compound of general formula R—C≡N. It can be considered as derived from the ammonium salts of carboxylic acids by loss of two molecules of water.

nitrilo- [from *nitrile* from Gk *nitron* soda, carbonate of soda + *-ile* English suffix used in making certain names, especially diketones] A combining form signifying the tervalent nitrogen atom, as in nitrilotriacetic acid, $N(—CH_2—COOH)_3$.

nitrite The ion NO_2^- derived from nitrous acid, or a salt containing it, or an ester of nitrous acid. Nitrites are added as preservatives to foods, such as cooked meats. Since, however, they react slowly with secondary amines to form nitrosamines, some of which are carcinogenic, this practice may not be without danger.

nitrite reductase One of several enzymes that reduce nitrite, using various reductants, to nitric oxide or hydroxylamine. The reaction is on the pathway of reduction of nitrate to ammonia in plants and microorganisms.

nitrituria The excretion of nitrites in the urine, usually an index of bacterial proliferation. A rarely used term.

nitro- [L *nitrum* from Gk *nitron*] A combining form denoting the presence of the nitro group, —NO_2, in a molecule. It is a strongly electron-withdrawing group. Also *nitr-*.

nitroaniline $C_6H_6N_2O_2$. One of the several aromatic nitro compounds used in the chemical industry. Exposure can cause anemia and cyanosis. This gives rise to the characteristic anoxia symptoms of headache, fatigue, nausea, vertigo, chest pain, air hunger, and irrational behavior.

Nitrobacter The major genus of chemolithotrophic bacteria that oxidize nitrite to nitrate.

nitrobenzene C_6H_5—NO_2. A substance produced by nitration of benzene. It is a raw material for the production of aniline dyes and explosives. It is toxic, with poisoning occurring most often through skin absorption. Symptoms of acute poisoning include fatigue, headache, vomiting, and vertigo, which may be followed by unconsciousness. Cyanosis and pronounced anemia may follow with jaundice due to excessive destruction of blood cells. In chronic poisoning anemia and hemolytic jaundice are the leading features. Also called *oil of mirbane*.

***m*-nitrobenzoic acid** NO_2—C_6H_4—COOH. An acid of pK 3.5, forming monoclinic plates, having a bitter taste, and slightly soluble in water. It is used in syntheses and as a gravimetric reagent for thorium and for alkaloids.

***p*-nitrobenzoic acid** NO_2—C_6H_4—COOH. An acid of pK 3.4, forming monoclinic platelets. It is slightly soluble in water and more soluble in acetone and methanol. It is the starting point for the synthesis of procaine and of esters of *p*-hydroxybenzoic acid.

nitrocellulose Cellulose whose hydroxyl groups have been partially esterified with nitric acid. It was once used as the basis of transparent plastics, but it is highly inflammable and its use has diminished for that reason.

nitrochloroform CHLOROPICRIN.

nitrofuran Any of a group of antibacterial agents such as furazolidone, nitrofurazone, and nitrofurantoin, each having actions on a wide variety of bacteria.

nitrofurantoin $C_8H_6N_4O_5$. 1-[[(5-Nitro-2-furanyl)methylene]amino]-2,4-imidazolidinedione, a synthetic antibacterial agent. It is effective against some Gram-negative and Gram-positive organisms, including *Escherichia coli, Staphylococcus pyogenes, S. aureus*, and some strains of *Proteus* and *Pseudomonas*. It is given orally to treat urinary tract infections.

nitrofurazone 5-Nitro-2-furaldehyde semicarbazone. An antibacterial agent used in the treatment of burns and infections of the skin, otitis, and ophthalmic conditions. It is also used in the treatment of trypanosomiasis.

nitrogen [French *nitrogène* (from L *nitrum* natron, natural soda, niter, saltpeter + French *-gène*, noun suffix from Gk *-gen*, noun suffix from *gennan* to beget, produce, bring forth) nitrogen, azote] Element number 7, having atomic weight 14.0067. It is a colorless, odorless gas forming 78% of the volume of the atmosphere. It is obtained from liquid air by fractional distillation. There are two natural isotopes, having mass numbers 14 and 15, the former comprising over 99.6% of the total. Five radioactive isotopes are known. Valences are 3 and 5. Elemental nitrogen is fairly inert but its compounds are very reactive and are a constituent of food, fertilizers, and many explosives and poisons. It is a key element in the substance of all living organisms. See also NITROGEN CYCLE. Symbol: N

amide nitrogen The fraction of nitrogen in a material that is in the form of amide groups. Usually unsubstituted amides are meant, and hence this nitrogen is released as ammonia on hydrolysis. Its determination can indicate the content of asparagine and glutamine in a protein.

amino nitrogen The amount of nitrogen in a sample that is in unsubstituted amino groups. This was once commonly determined, e.g. to find the degree to which protein hydrolysis had proceeded, by measuring the volume of dinitrogen released under the action of nitrous acid.

blood urea nitrogen The amount of nitrogen in plasma or serum deriving from the urea molecule, expressed in mg/dl or mmol/l. The two atoms of nitrogen per molecule of urea constitute 46.64% of urea mass. Normal levels depend somewhat upon the analytical method used, but approximate 7–18 mg/dl or 5–13 mmol/l. Abbreviation: BUN

Kjeldahl nitrogen See under KJELDAHL'S TEST.

nitrogen fixation See under FIXATION.

nonprotein nitrogen The amount of nitrogen in a sample that does not belong to protein. It was once commonly determined by nitrogen analysis after protein precipitation, often as a check on the individual components of blood, such as urea, creatinine, amino acids, and ammonia. Also called *rest nitrogen* (seldom used).

rest nitrogen A seldom used term for NONPROTEIN NITROGEN.

urea nitrogen The portion of urea composed of nitrogen, representing approximately half the urea molecule. In the United States blood or serum levels are reported in terms of urea nitrogen, but in the United Kingdom urea levels are reported. In the past, urea nitrogen was usually measured in whole blood, but with currently available automatic analyzers urea nitrogen is measured in serum. Since urea is distributed throughout body water, the results in blood and serum are very close.

nitrogen 13 A cyclotron-produced radioisotope of nitrogen, decaying by positron emission. It can be used for study of the metabolism of many nitrogen-containing compounds. Physical half-life is 10 minutes. Symbol: ^{13}N

nitrogen 15 A stable isotope of nitrogen comprising 0.37 percent of natural nitrogen. It may be separated by mass spectrography and used as a metabolic tracer. Symbol: ^{15}N

nitrogenase One of two enzymes responsible for bacterial nitrogen fixation. Both catalyze the reduction of dinitrogen, N_2, to ammonia. Nitrogenase (EC 1.18.2.1) uses reduced ferredoxin as the hydrogen donor, whereas nitrogenase (flavodoxin) (EC

1.16.2.1) uses reduced flavodoxin.

nitrogenous Containing nitrogen, usually in combined form.

nitrogen trichloride NCL_3. An explosive liquid, decomposed by water to form ammonia and hypochlorous acid. It was once used to decolorize flour, and this treatment converted the methionine residues of proteins into the sulfoximine, containing the —S(O)(NH)— group, which is toxic.

nitroglycerin Any ester of glycerol with nitric acid, particularly glycerol trinitrate, which is used as an explosive. Nitroglycerin is also used medicinally as a vasodilator for treating angina pectoris. Exposed workers in factories manufacturing explosives may suffer headaches, nausea, vomiting, and lowered pulse pressures. They usually develop a tolerance, which may be lost during weekends. Such workers may have a higher than expected sudden death rate from coronary heart disease. Nitroglycerin is also a skin irritant. Also called *trinitrin, trinitroglycerol, trinitroglycerin*. See also DYNAMITE HEADACHE.

Nitroglyn A proprietary name for nitroglycerin.

Nitrol A proprietary name for nitroglycerin.

nitromersol $C_7H_5HgNO_3$. 5-Methyl-2-nitro-7-oxa-8-mercurabicyclo[4.2.0]octa-1,3,5-triene, a synthetic organic mercurial compound used as an antiseptic for the skin and mucous membranes.

nitrometer [*nitro(gen)* + -METER] An apparatus for collecting and quantifying nitrogen evolved in chemical reactions.

nitromethane CH_3—NO_2. A liquid of boiling point 101°C, used as an aprotic polar solvent. Strong bases remove a proton from it to form a carbanion, which is used in organic syntheses.

nitron The molecular weight of emanation from radium. An obsolete term.

nitrophenol Any of the disubstituted benzene compounds in which a nitro group and a hydroxyl group may be in the ortho-, para-, or meta- configuration. They are used as pH indicators and as intermediates in organic synthesis.

p-nitrophenyl phosphate An ester of *p*-nitrophenol with phosphoric acid, or any of its salts. It is used as a substrate for phosphatases, because the release of *p*-nitrophenol is easily followed due to the bright yellow color of its quinonoid anion.

nitroprusside The ion $[Fe(CN)_5NO]^{2-}$ or a salt that contains it. It is systematically named pentacyanonitrosylferrate(2-). It is reddish brown, and gives a purple color with sulfide or with thiol groups, and also with acetone and acetoacetate.

nitrosamine Any nitrosylated secondary amine, of general formula RR′N—NO. Many are carcinogenic and mutagenic, especially if R or R′ is acyl, because they can decompose to form alkylating agents.

nitroso- [L *nitrosus* (from Gk *nitron* soda, carbonate of soda) nitrous] A combining form denoting the presence of the univalent radical —N=O in a molecule. Also *nitros-*.

Nitrosomonas The major genus of chemolithotrophic bacteria that oxidize ammonia to nitrite.

nitrosugar Any of a group of nitrite-containing substances used in the treatment of angina pectoris.

p-nitrosulfathiazole $C_9H_7N_3O_4S_2$. *p*-Nitro-*N*-2-thiazolylbenzenesulfonamide. A very insoluble sulfonamide antibacterial agent used in the treatment of ulcerative colitis.

nitrosyl Any of the chemical species NO: used to designate it as a ligand for metal atoms and to name simple compounds, as *nitrosyl chloride*, NOCl.

nitrous acid The unstable acid HNO_2, produced by acidifying a nitrite. It is used as a reagent to convert primary amines into diazonium compounds, which easily liberate nitrogen and allow the original amino group to be replaced by other substituents. It is also used to convert secondary amines into nitrosamines.

nitrous oxide N_2O. A fairly inert gas, used as an anesthetic. Also called *dinitrogen monoxide, laughing gas.*

nitryl The cation NO_2^+, a species active as a nitrating agent in solutions of nitric acid. Its concentration is increased by the addition of sulfuric acid.

Nivemycin A proprietary name for neomycin.

njovera A Zimbabwean term for BEJEL.

NK Nomenklatur Kommission. (A Committee of the Anatomical Society in Germany appointed to revise and supplement the Basle Nomina Anatomica.).

nkat Symbol for the unit, nanokatal.

nl Symbol for the unit, nanoliter.

NM 1 nuclear medicine. 2 neuromuscular.

N/m² Symbol for the unit, newton per square meter.

N·m Symbol for the unit, newton-meter.

N·m⁻² Symbol for the unit, newton per square meter.

nm Symbol for the unit, nanometer.

n_c/m_s Symbol for the quantity, substance content, expressed in moles per kilogram.

NMN nicotinamide mononucleotide.

nmol Symbol for the unit, nanomole.

NMR nuclear magnetic resonance.

N·m/s Symbol for the unit, newton-meter per second.

N·m·s⁻¹ Symbol for the unit, newton-meter per second.

nn. *nervi* (L, nerves).

NND neonatal death.

No Symbol for the element, nobelium.

no number.

nobelium A synthetic element of the actinide series, having atomic number 102. Seven isotopes are recognized, the longest lived having atomic mass 255. Half-lives range from 2.3 seconds to 3 minutes. Symbol: No

Noble [Charles Percy *Noble*, U.S. gynecologist, 1863–1935] See under POSITION.

nocardamin $C_{27}H_{48}N_6O_9$. An antibiotic substance produced by a strain of *Nocardia*. It is bacteriostatic against mycobacteria, and bacteriocidal only at very high concentrations.

Nocardia [after Edmond Isidore Étienne *Nocard*, French veterinarian and biologist, 1850–1903 + -IA] A genus of Gram-positive, weakly acid-fast, aerobic actinomycetes of the family Nocardiaceae. These organisms are found in the soil. Two species, *N. asteroides* and *N. brasiliensis*, may cause severe pulmonary lesions (pulmonary nocardiosis), or spreading subcutaneous abscesses (mycetomas), much like those caused by *Actinomyces* species. The presence of mycolic acids in the cell wall relates the organisms to mycobacteria.

Nocardia asteroides An aerobic actinomycete, found in soil, and intermediate in staining between Gram-positive and acid-fast bacilli. It forms granulating and suppurative pulmonary lesions, and chronic subcutaneous abscesses (mycetomas).

Nocardia brasiliensis An actinomycete closely resembling *N. asteroides*, found mostly in Mexico.

nocardial Of or pertaining to organisms of the genus *Nocardia* or closely related genera.

nocardiasis NOCARDIOSIS.

nocardin An antibiotic substance derived from *Nocardia coeliaca*. It has activity against tubercle bacilli.

nocardiosis [*Nocardi(a)* + -OSIS] Infection with microorganisms of the genus *Nocardia*. Also called *nocardiasis.*

granulomatous nocardiosis An atypical inflammatory response to Nocardia, characterized by ill-defined granulomas instead of the usual abscesses.

Nochtia A monotypic genus of small nematodes (family Trichostrongylidae, subfamily Nochtiinae) parasitic in primates. The single species is *N. nochti*, found in the stomach of the rhesus monkey, *Macaca mulatta*. Gastric tumors have been produced in experimental infections of the Javanese macaque, *M. fascicularis mordax.*

noci- [L *nocere* to injure] A combining form meaning pain or injury.

nociassociation [NOCI- + *association*] Uncoordinated nervous discharge either following injury or while in shock.

nociception [NOCI- + *(per)ception*] PAIN SENSE.

nociceptive [NOCI- + *(per)ceptive*] Denoting responsiveness or sensitivity to noxious stimuli capable of eliciting pain.

nociceptor [NOCI- + *(re)ceptor*] A class of sense organs uniquely excited by noxious stimuli that threaten or produce frank tissue damage. Also called *pain ending, pain receptor, algoceptor, nocifensor.*

nocifensor NOCICEPTOR. • The term is used from the point of view of its role in protecting tissue from injury.

noci-influence Anything having a damaging effect, or the effect itself.

nociperception [NOCI- + PERCEPTION] The recognition by the nervous system or organism of a traumatic or hurtful stimulus.

noct. *nocte* (L, at night).

noctalbuminuria A pathologic increase of albumin in urine excreted during the evening, a very rarely observed event.

noctambulation SOMNAMBULISM.

noctambulic [French *noctambule* (from L *nox*, gen. *noctis*, night + *ambulare* to walk) one who goes about at night + -IC] Pertaining to somnambulism.

Noctec A proprietary name for chloral hydrate.

noctiphobia NYCTOPHOBIA.

noct. maneq. *nocte maneque* (L, at night and in the morning).

nocturia [L *nox* (gen. *noctis*) night + -URIA] Urination during normal sleeping hours. The interruption of sleep to urinate may reflect a large fluid intake before retiring, decreased concentrating ability, or bladder overflow in obstructive disease such as prostatic hypertrophy. Also called *nycturia.*

nocturnal Pertaining to night, especially to a night-time period of animal activity. Also *nycterine.* Compare DIURNAL.

nocuity [L *nocu(us)* hurtful + -ITY] Harmfulness; noxiousness. An obsolete term.

nocuous [L *nocu(us)* hurtful + -OUS] Injurious; poisonous; harmful.

nodal Like, consisting of, or having a node.

node [L *nodus*. See NODUS.] NODUS.

anterior auricular nodes NODI LYMPHATICI PAROTIDEI SUPERFICIALES.

node of anterior border of epiploic foramen NODUS FORAMINALIS.

Aschoff's node NODUS ATRIOVENTRICULARIS.

node of Aschoff and Tawara NODUS ATRIOVENTRICULARIS.

atrioventricular node NODUS ATRIOVENTRICULARIS.

Auerbach's node AUERBACH'S GANGLION.

A-V node NODUS ATRIOVENTRICULARIS.

Babès nodes BABÈS TUBERCLES.

Bouchard's nodes Osteophytic swellings around the proximal interphalangeal joints of the fingers in osteoarthrosis. Also called *Bouchard's nodules.*

Cloquet's node The highest of the deep inguinal lymph nodes, situated either in the femoral canal or the femoral ring. Also called *Cloquet's gland, Rosenmüller's gland, Rosenmüller's node.*

coronary node The highest part or extension of the atrioventricular node, closest to the orifice of the coronary sinus in the right atrium of the heart.

cystic node   NODUS CYSTICUS.

Delphian node   A lymph node situated in the pretracheal fascia in the midline in front of either the isthmus or the pyramidal lobe of the thyroid gland.

Dürck's nodes   Nodes occurring in human trypanosomiasis, caused by an infiltration of perivascular lymphatic tissue of the brain, spinal cord, and meninges.

enamel node   ENAMEL KNOT.

epitrochlear nodes   NODI LYMPHATICI CUBITALES.

Ewald's node   SENTINEL NODE.

external nodes of internal jugular chain   An outmoded term for NODI LYMPHATICI JUGULARES LATERALES.

Féréol's nodes   RHEUMATIC NODULES.

Flack's node   NODUS SINUATRIALIS.

gouty node   Palpable swelling due to tophus.

Haygarth's nodes   Joint swellings seen in rheumatoid arthritis.

Heberden's nodes   Bony swellings of the distal interphalangeal joints of the hands, characteristic of osteoarthritis. Also called *Heberden sign, Heberden's arthropathy.*

hemal node   A lymphoid structure, organized like a spleen, that has lymphatic tissue with erythrocytes occurring normally in the lymphatic sinuses. It is commonly found in many mammals, especially ruminants, but its presence in humans is debatable. Also called *hemal gland, hemal lymph gland, vascular gland.*

hemolymph node   A lymph node that contains erythrocytes in its sinuses due to hemorrhage in its tributary field. Also called *hemolymph gland.*

Hensen's node   A specialized area at the cephalic extremity of the primitive streak present in embryos of higher vertebrates. An invagination or pit (blastopore) forms in the region of the node and the invaginating cord of cells migrates forwards to give origin to the notochordal or head process. This is essentially the precursor of the notochord which is itself the primary organizer and precursor of the axial skeleton. The node of Hensen can bear an orifice as in certain birds, which can, as in man, continue as a true canal (notochordal canal) opening into the endoderm. Also called *primitive node, primitive knot, node of Hensen.*

node of Hensen   HENSEN'S NODE.

His-Tawara node   NODUS ATRIOVENTRICULARIS.

juxta-articular node   A lymph node near a joint, usually an abnormally enlarged node, as the epitrochlear node. Also called *juxta-articular nodule.*

Keith's node   NODUS SINUATRIALIS.

Keith-Flack node   NODUS SINUATRIALIS.

Koch's node   NODUS ATRIOVENTRICULARIS.

lymph node   NODUS LYMPHATICUS.

lymphatic node   NODUS LYMPHATICUS.

Meynet's nodes   Tendon nodules seen in juvenile arthritis and rheumatic fever.

node of neck of gallbladder   NODUS CYSTICUS.

Osler nodes   Tender, swollen, erythematous areas that are 2–15 mm in size. They may be seen on the pads of the fingers or toes, the palms of the hands, or the soles of the feet and are associated with infective endocarditis.

Parrot's node   PARROT SIGN.

pectoral axillary nodes   NODI LYMPHATICI PECTORALES.

preachers' nodes   VOCAL NODULES.

preauricular nodes   NODI LYMPHATICI PAROTIDEI SUPERFICIALES.

primitive node   HENSEN'S NODE.

nodes of Ranvier   The periodic constrictions of the myelin sheath surrounding large axons. They demarcate the junctions

between adjacent Schwann cells, and are the sites for impulse generation. Also called *constrictions of Ranvier* (obsolete).

Rosenmüller's node   **1** PARS PALPEBRALIS GLANDULAE LACRIMALIS.   **2** CLOQUET'S NODE.

Rotter's nodes   Lymph nodes between the pectoralis major and pectoralis minor muscles which may contain metastatic cancer from a primary carcinoma of the breast.

node of Rouviere   The lateral retropharyngeal node of the retropharyngeal group, which drains the auditory tube.

S-A node   NODUS SINUATRIALIS.

Schmidt's node   The myelinated interannular segment of a nerve fiber.

Schmorl's node   A radiographic circumscribed lucency in a vertebral body that is adjacent to an intervertebral disk. It is caused by the intrusion of disk material into the vertebral body, as can occur in cases of increased bone fragility. Also called *Schmorl's disease.*

sentinel node   A palpable, usually left, supraclavicular lymph node containing metastatic cancer from a frequently undisclosed deep-seated primary site. Also called *signal node, Troisier's node, Virchow's node, Virchow's gland, Ewald's node, Troisier sign, lymph node of Troisier.*

signal node   SENTINEL NODE.

singers' nodes   VOCAL NODULES.

sinoatrial node   NODUS SINUATRIALIS.

sinuatrial node   NODUS SINUATRIALIS.

sinuatrial node of Keith and Flack   NODUS SINUATRIALIS.

syphilitic node   A subcutaneous, hard, fibrous swelling occurring around the joints or on tendon sheaths, especially on the fingers, during late syphilis. The condition is only rarely seen.

node of Tawara   NODUS ATRIOVENTRICULARIS.

teachers' nodes   VOCAL NODULES.

triticeous node   CARTILAGO TRITICEA.

Troisier's node   SENTINEL NODE.

Virchow's node   SENTINEL NODE.

vital node   NOEUD VITAL.

vocal nodes   VOCAL NODULES.

nodi   Plural of NODUS.

nodose   Characterized by nodes or localized swellings. Also *nodulated, nodulous.*

nodositas   A rarely used term for NODOSITY.

nodosity   A knoblike swelling or node. Also called *nodositas* (rarely used).

nodular   **1** Pertaining to or resembling a node or a nodule.   **2** Characterized by nodules. For defs. 1 and 2 also *toruloid.*

nodulated   NODOSE.

nodulation   The formation of nodules.

nodule   [L *nodulus.* See NODULUS.]   **1** A small node.   • This term is commonly used in referring to circumscribed, solid, elevated skin lesions greater than 5 mm in diameter, as compared to papules, which are less than 5 mm in diameter.   **2** NODULUS.

accessory thymic nodules   Minute aggregations of thymic tissue left behind during the migration of the thymus from the primitive pharyngeal region to its adult position within the upper thoracic region. Also called *noduli thymici accessorii.*

aggregate nodule   FOLLICULI LYMPHATICI AGGREGATI.

aggregated lymphatic nodules of appendix   AGGREGATED LYMPHOID FOLLICLES OF VERMIFORM APPENDIX.

Albini's nodules   Small gray nodules occasionally seen on the free margins of atrioventricular valvular cusps. Also called *Cruveilhier's nodule.*

nodules of aortic valve   NODULI VALVULARUM SEMILUNARIUM VALVAE AORTAE.

apple jelly nodules   The epithelioid tubercles characteristic of lupus vulgaris. They are best displayed by diascopic examination.

nodules of Arantius   NODULI VALVULARUM SEMILUNARIUM VALVAE AORTAE.

Aschoff's nodules   ASCHOFF BODIES.

Babès nodules   BABÈS TUBERCLES.

benign vocal nodules   VOCAL NODULES.

Bianchi's nodules   NODULI VALVULARUM SEMILUNARIUM VALVAE AORTAE.

Bohn's nodules   BOHN'S EPITHELIAL PEARLS.

Bouchard's nodules   BOUCHARD'S NODES.

Busacca nodules   Lymphoid deposits in an inflamed iris.

Caplan's nodules   See under CAPLAN SYNDROME.

cold nodule   Any space-occupying lesion in the substance of the thyroid gland that fails to take up administered radiotracer, usually iodine or technetium. It is generally held to be compatible with but not diagnostic of a malignant neoplasm.

cortical nodule   NODULUS LYMPHATICUS.

Cruveilhier's nodule   ALBINI'S NODULES.

Dalen-Fuchs nodules   The aggregation of epithelioid cells in the choroid, characteristic of sympathetic ophthalmia.

enamel nodule   ENAMEL PEARL.

Fraenkel's nodules   Nodules forming on the cutaneous blood vessels as a result of vascular endothelial proliferation. They are characteristic lesions of typhus.

Gamna nodules   GAMNA-GANDY BODIES.

Gandy-Gamna nodules   GAMNA-GANDY BODIES.

Guatamahri's nodules   Nodules found on the face and scalp in human onchocerciasis. An obsolete term.

hot nodule   Any space-occupying lesion in the substance of the thyroid gland that takes up administered radiotracer, usually iodine or technetium. It is generally held to indicate the presence of a benign thyroidal lesion rather than a malignant neoplasm. Also called *warm nodule.*

Jeanselme's nodules   LUTZ-JEANSELME NODULES.

juxta-articular nodule   JUXTA-ARTICULAR NODE.

nodules of Kerckring   NODULI VALVULARUM SEMILUNARIUM VALVAE AORTAE.

Koeppe nodules   Lymphoid nodules of the iris in iritis.

Koester's nodule   A granuloma consisting of a double layer of cells enclosing a single giant cell, as seen in granulomatous inflammation.

Leishman's nodules   Pinkish nodules seen in cutaneous leishmaniasis.

lentiform nodule   An outmoded term for PROCESSUS LENTICULARIS INCUDIS.

lumbar-sacral nodules   Nodules composed of subcutaneous adipose tissue herniated through the fascia of the lumbar-sacral region. They are believed by some to explain the pain associated with non-articular rheumatism in this part of the body.

Lutz-Jeanselme nodules   Syphilitic gummata on joint capsules or tendons. Also called *Jeanselme's nodules.*

lymphatic nodule   NODULUS LYMPHATICUS.

lymphatic nodule of stomach   LYMPHOID FOLLICLE OF STOMACH.

malpighian nodules   FOLLICULI LYMPHATICI SPLENICI.

Morgagni's nodules   NODULI VALVULARUM SEMILUNARIUM VALVAE AORTAE.

Paterson's nodules   A seldom used term for MOLLUSCUM CONTAGIOSUM.

periosteal nodules   Palpable swellings along a bony prominence, occurring between periosteum in bone.

preachers' nodules   VOCAL NODULES.

prehyoid nodule   A nodule with a cartilaginous consistency in the most posterior part of the lingual septum, slightly in front of the hyoid bone in the fetus before term. It is no longer present in the neonate. It is a temporary organ only of vestigial interest.

primary nodule   NODULUS PRIMARIUS.

pulmonary nodules   Small solid lumps within the lung substance, or small opacities seen on the chest radiograph.

nodules of pulmonary trunk valves   NODULI VALVULARUM SEMILUNARIUM VALVAE TRUNCI PULMONALIS.

pulp nodule   DENTICLE.

rabic nodules   BABÈS TUBERCLES.

rheumatic nodules   Cutaneous nodules present in the skin in rheumatic disease that consist of noncaseating, pallisading granulomata. Also called *rheumatoid nodules, Féréol's nodes.*

rheumatoid nodules   RHEUMATIC NODULES.

root nodules   Tumorlike growths occurring chiefly on the roots of legumes and caused by nitrogen fixing bacteria of the genus *Rhizobium.*

Schmorl's nodule   A localized depression of a vertebral plate due to herniation of the nucleus pulposus into the bone. The appearance is most easily seen on a lateral roentgenogram of the spine. Also called *Schmorl body.*

secondary nodule   GERMINAL CENTER.

siderotic nodules   GAMNA-GANDY BODIES.

singers' nodules   VOCAL NODULES.

solitary lymphatic nodules of large intestine   SOLITARY LYMPHOID FOLLICLES OF LARGE INTESTINE.

solitary lymphatic nodule of small intestine   An isolated collection of normal and reactive lymphoid cells in the lamina propria of the small intestine. Also called *folliculus lymphaticus solitarius intestinus tenuis, solitary gland of small intestine, nodulus lymphatici solitarii intestini tenuis.*

splenic lymph nodules   FOLLICULI LYMPHATICI SPLENICI.

subcutaneous nodule   Any of several different types of swellings that occur beneath skin and are not attached to underlying bone. Subcutaneous nodules are commonly found in rheumatic diseases, such as rheumatoid arthritis, rheumatic fever, and gout.

surfers' nodules   SURFERS' KNOTS.

teachers' nodules   VOCAL NODULES.

triticeous nodule   CARTILAGO TRITICEA.

tubal lymphatic nodules   TONSILLA TUBARIA.

typhoid nodule   An aggregation of hypertrophied reticuloendothelial cells in the spleen resulting from typhoid fever.

typhus nodule   A focal collection of mononuclear cells surrounding the small vessel lesions of ricksettsial diseases, especially typhus fever. Although they may occur in any tissue, they are most commonly seen in skin and brain.

nodule of vermis   NODULUS VERMIS.

vestigial nodule   TUBERCULUM AURICULAE.

vocal nodules   Small, white, symmetrically placed nodules, somewhat pyramidal in shape, occurring at the junction of the anterior with the middle one-third of the vocal cords. They occur as the result of misuse or overuse of the voice, particularly in susceptible individuals such as singers, preachers, and teachers. The early complaint is slight huskiness and, in soprano singers, difficulty in singing high notes softly. Surgical treatment should be the last resort. Also called *vocal nodes, benign vocal nodules, singers' nodules, singers' nodes, preachers' nodules, preachers' nodes, teachers' nodules, teachers' nodes, nodules of the vocal cords, chorditis nodosa.*

nodules of the vocal cords   VOCAL NODULES.

warm nodule   HOT NODULE.

noduli   Plural of NODULUS.

nodulous   NODOSE.

nodulus   [dim. of NODUS. See NODUS.]   (*plural* noduli) A small nodus; a very small knotlike mass of tissue or cells. Also called *nodule.*

noduli aggregati processus vermiformis   An outmoded term for AGGREGATED LYMPHOID FOLLICLES OF VERMIFORM APPENDIX.

nodulus cerebelli   NODULUS VERMIS.

nodulus intercaroticus   An outmoded term for GLOMUS CA-ROTICUM.

noduli lymphatici aggregati appendicis vermiformis   AG-GREGATED LYMPHOID FOLLICLES OF VERMIFORM APPENDIX.

noduli lymphatici aggregati cavitatis laryngis   Accumulations of lymphocytes scattered in the lamina propria of the larynx. Also called *noduli lymphatici laryngei* (outmoded), *laryngeal lymphatic follicles, folliculi lymphatici laryngei*.

noduli lymphatici aggregati peyeri   An outmoded term for FOLLICULI LYMPHATICI AGGREGATI.

noduli lymphatici aggregati tubae auditivae   TONSILLA TUBARIA.

noduli lymphatici bronchiales   Small accumulations of lymphocytes in the lamina propria of the extrapulmonary bronchi.

noduli lymphatici conjunctivales   Aggregations of lymphocytes in the lamina propria of the conjunctiva at the edge of the cornea. An outmoded term.

noduli lymphatici laryngei   An outmoded term for NODULI LYMPHATICI AGGREGATI CAVITATIS LARYNGIS.

noduli lymphatici lienales malpighii   An outmoded term for FOLLICULI LYMPHATICI SPLENICI.

noduli lymphatici solitarii intestini crassi   SOLITARY LYMPHOID FOLLICLES OF LARGE INTESTINE.

noduli lymphatici solitarii recti   FOLLICULI LYMPHATICI RECTI.

noduli lymphatici tubarii tubae auditivae   An outmoded term for TONSILLA TUBARIA.

noduli lymphatici vesicales   Lymphocytes that are found rarely in the wall of the urinary bladder.

nodulus lymphaticus   [NA] One of the densely packed spherical masses of lymphocytes embedded in a relatively scanty reticular meshwork of any lymphatic tissue. It varies in appearance according to the stage of lymphocytopoietic activity. When responding to an antigen its germinal center or secondary nodule actively produces new lymphocytes and is surrounded by a densely packed peripheral zone or corona. In the cortex of lymph nodes the trabeculae tend to separate these masses from each other. They are also located in the tonsils and spleen. Solitary masses are found in the walls of the alimentary canal, although in the intestine they may aggregate into loosely organized structures or Peyer's patches. Also called *lymphatic nodule, folliculus lymphaticus, cortical nodule, lymphatic follicle*.

nodulus lymphaticus gastricus   LYMPHOID FOLLICLE OF STOMACH.

nodulus lymphaticus solitarius intestini tenuis   SOLITARY LYMPHOID NODULE OF SMALL INTESTINE.

nodulus primarius   A lymphatic nodule, such as in the cortex of a lymph node, in which the secondary nodule or germinal center either has not yet appeared, as in the first few months after birth, or has become mitotically inactive. Also called *primary nodule*.

nodulus secundarius   GERMINAL CENTER.

noduli thymici accessorii   ACCESSORY THYMIC NODULES.

noduli valvularum aortae   An outmoded term for NODULI VALVULARUM SEMILUNARIUM VALVAE AORTAE.

noduli valvularum semilunarium   An outmoded term for NO-DULI VALVULARUM SEMILUNARIUM VALVAE TRUNCI PULMONALIS.

noduli valvularum semilunarium arantii   An outmoded term for NODULI VALVULARUM SEMILUNARIUM VALVAE AORTAE.

noduli valvularum semilunarium valvae aortae   The small, dense fibrous tubercle at the center of the free margins of the three semilunar valvules or cusps of the aortic valve from which tendinous fibers radiate to the attached margins. Also called *noduli valvularum aortae* (outmoded), *noduli valvularium semi-*

lunarium arantii (outmoded), *Morgagni's nodules, nodules of Kerckring, Bianchi's nodules, nodules of Arantius, nodules of aortic valve, bodies of Arantius, corpora arantii*.

noduli valvularum semilunarium valvae trunci pulmonalis   The small, dense fibrous tubercle at the center of the free margins of the three semilunar valvules or cusps of the valve of the pulmonary trunk from which tendinous fibers radiate to the attached margins. Also called *noduli valvularum semilunarium* (outmoded), *noduli valvularum semilunarium ventriculi dextri* (outmoded), *nodules of pulmonary trunk valves*.

noduli valvularum semilunarium ventriculi dextri   An outmoded term for NODULI VALVULARUM SEMILUNARIUM VALVAE TRUNCI PULMONALIS.

nodulus vermis   **1** That portion of the cerebellar vermis on the ventral surface, to which the inferior medullary velum is attached.   **2** The midline portion of the archicerebellum whose afferent and efferent connections are primarily with the vestibular nuclei. Also called *nodule of vermis, nodulus cerebelli*.

nodus

nodus   [L (akin to *nectere* to tie, bind, fasten), a knot, knob on the joint of an animal, knot in the wood of plants, tie, bond] (*plural* nodi)   **1** A knotlike mass of tissue or cells.   **2** A small knoblike protuberance or organ.   **3** A swelling. For defs. 1, 2, and 3 also called *node*.

nodus arcus venae azygos   [NA] A large lymph node that belongs either to the superior tracheobronchial or to the paratracheal nodes of the right side. It is related to the arch of the azygos vein anterior to the origin of the right principal bronchus. Also called *lymph node of arch of azygos vein*.

nodus atrioventricularis   [NA] A collection of specialized cardiac muscle fibers located in the atrial septum just above the coronary sinus of the right atrium. It is composed of a dense network of Purkinje fibers enmeshed with connective tissue. The fibers are continuous with the surrounding atrial muscle fibers and the atrioventricular bundle. It is supplied by the right coronary artery. Also called *atrioventricular node, Aschoff's node, node of Aschoff and Tawara, node of Tawara, A-V node, His-Tawara node, Koch's node, cardiomotor center* (outmoded).

nodus buccinatorius   [NA] Any of the one or more lymph nodes that are part of the nodi lymphatici faciales and are situated along the facial vein overlying the buccinator muscle. Also called *buccal group of facial lymph nodes*.

nodus cordis   Either trigonum fibrosum dextrum or trigonum fibrosum sinistrum. An outmoded term.

nodus cysticus   [NA] A constant constituent of the nodi lymphatici hepatici that is situated at the junction of the cystic and common hepatic ducts. Also called *cystic node, node of neck of gallbladder*.

nodus foraminalis   [NA] A constant constituent of the nodi lymphatici hepatici which is situated along the upper part of the common bile duct in the lesser omentum. Also called *node of anterior border of epiploic foramen*.

nodus jugulodigastricus   [NA] A large node in a group of superior deep cervical lymph nodes that is situated between the internal jugular vein, the facial vein, and the posterior belly of the digastric muscle, just below the angle of the mandible and at the level of the greater cornu of the hyoid bone. It receives lymph from the posterior third of the tongue and the palatine tonsil. Also called *jugulodigastric lymph node*.

nodus jugulo-omohyoideus   [NA] One of the inferior deep cervical lymph nodes that is situated on or above the intermediate tendon of the omohyoid muscle where it crosses the internal jugular vein. It receives lymph from the tongue both directly and indirectly. Also called *jugulo-omohyoid lymph node.*

nodus ligamentis arteriosi [NA] The most inferior node of the left group of anterior mediastinal lymph nodes which is situated in front of the ligamentum arteriosum and below the left pulmonary artery. Also called *ganglion of duct of Botallo.*

nodi lymphatici anorectales NODI LYMPHATICI PARARECTALES.

nodi lymphatici aortici laterales [NA] The group of nodi lymphatici lumbales sinistri that are situated along the left side of the abdominal aorta. They drain the viscera and other structures, mainly on the left side, that are supplied by the lateral and posterior branches of the aorta, such as the left suprarenal gland, kidney, ureter, testis, ovary, and some pelvic viscera. They also receive efferents from outlying groups related to the left common iliac arteries and their branches. Also called *lateral aortic lymph nodes.*

nodi lymphatici apicales The apical group of six to twelve axillary lymph nodes situated in the apex of the axilla medial to the axillary vein and behind the clavipectoral fascia. They drain all the lymph nodes in the axilla, the infraclavicular nodes along the cephalic vein, and lymphatics directly from the upper outer quadrant of the breast. Most of the efferents drain into the subclavian lymph trunk but some end in the lower inferior deep cervical lymph nodes. Also called *apical lymph nodes, infraclavicular lymph nodes.*

nodi lymphatici axillares A large group of 20 to 30 lymph nodes situated in and along the walls of the axilla, draining the whole upper limb, most of the breast, and part of the side and back of the trunk. It is subdivided into five groups: a lateral group (nodi lymphatici laterales), an anterior or pectoral group (nodi lymphatici pectorales), a posterior or subscapular group (nodi lymphatici subscapulares), a central group (nodi lymphatici centrales), and an apical group (nodi lymphatici apicales). Also called *axillary lymph nodes, pectoral glands, axillary glands.*

nodi lymphatici brachiales [NA] A few lymph nodes situated along the brachial vessels in the arm. They receive lymph from the deep nodes in the forearm as well as from the supratrochlear lymph nodes that are situated superficial to the deep fascia above the medial epicondyle of the humerus. They drain into the axillary lymph nodes, specifically the lateral group. Also called *brachial glands, brachial lymph nodes.*

nodi lymphatici bronchopulmonales One of the five main groups of tracheobronchial lymph nodes situated in the hilum of each lung. It drains and is continuous with the pulmonary nodes on the one side and continuous with the superior and inferior tracheobronchial nodes on the other. Also called *bronchopulmonary lymph nodes.*

nodi lymphatici buccales See under NODI LYMPHATICI FACIALES.

nodi lymphatici centrales The central group of four or five axillary lymph nodes through which the intercostobrachial nerve passes. Its afferents come mainly from the pectoral, lateral, and subscapular groups of nodes as well as the cubital nodes, while the efferents end in the apical group of axillary nodes. Also called *central lymph nodes.*

nodi lymphatici cervicales anteriores [NA] An inconstant group of lymph nodes situated in the midline of the neck anteriorly and divided into a superficial and a deep series. The superficial nodes lie along the anterior jugular veins, their efferents ending in deep cervical nodes on both sides. The deep group comprises prelaryngeal nodes on the conus elasticus and cricovocal membrane, pretracheal nodes, thyroid nodes, and paratracheal nodes. They drain the lower part of the larynx,

thyroid gland and the upper part of the trachea and their efferents end in adjacent superior deep cervical nodes. Also called *anterior cervical lymph nodes.*

nodi lymphatici cervicales laterales [NA] The vertical chains of lymph nodes that are situated on the lateral side of the neck and that can be divided into superficial, deep, and retropharyngeal groups. The superficial group includes the submandibular nodes and a few nodes along the external jugular vein. Their lymph drains into the upper nodes of the deep group. The deep group comprises many large nodes lying along and around the carotid sheath and includes the nodi lymphatici jugulares laterales, nodi lymphatici jugulares anteriores, nodi lymphatici supraclaviculares, nodus jugulodigastricus, and nodus jugulo-omohyoideus. They are also arbitrarily divided into superior and inferior groups, above and below the omohyoid muscle, respectively, and they drain all the deep and superficial tissues of the neck, either directly or indirectly through superficial and outlying nodes. The retropharyngeal group comprises the nodi lymphatici retropharyngeales and drains the nasal cavity, paranasal sinuses, soft and hard palate, nasopharynx, oropharynx, and middle ear. Also called *lateral cervical lymph nodes.*

nodi lymphatici cervicales profundi [NA] A large chain of lymph nodes situated along the internal jugular vein and the subclavian vein, draining all the lymphatics of the head and neck either directly or through intermediate groups of nodes. They are arbitrarily divided into superior deep cervical nodes, which lie above the point of crossing of the omohyoid muscle over the internal jugular vein, and inferior deep cervical nodes below that point. Their efferents form the jugular trunk. Also called *deep cervical lymph nodes.*

nodi lymphatici cervicales superficiales [NA] A few lymph nodes along the external jugular vein superficial to the sternocleidomastoid muscle. They drain part of the external ear, the lower parotid area, and the skin over the angle of the mandible. The efferents end either in the superior or the inferior deep cervical nodes. Also called *superficial cervical lymph nodes.*

nodi lymphatici coeliaci [NA] A group of lymph nodes adjacent to the celiac trunk in front of the abdominal aorta. They drain the liver, gallbladder, stomach, duodenum, pancreas, and spleen via the gastric, hepatic, pancreatic, and splenic lymph nodes. Also called *celiac lymph nodes, celiac glands.*

nodi lymphatici colici dextri [NA] Lymph nodes situated along the right colic artery and its branches. They drain the ascending colon and part of the cecum, and send efferents to the superior mesenteric lymph nodes in front of the aorta. Also called *right colic lymph nodes.*

nodi lymphatici colici medii [NA] Lymph nodes along the middle colic artery and its branches that drain the right colic flexure and the proximal two thirds of the transverse colon and send efferents to the superior mesenteric nodes in front of the aorta. Also called *middle colic lymph nodes.*

nodi lymphatici colici sinistri [NA] Lymph nodes that are situated along the left colic artery and its branches. They receive lymphatics from the distal third of the transverse colon and from the descending and sigmoid parts of the colon, and they send efferents to the inferior mesenteric nodes in front of the aorta. Also called *left colic lymph nodes.*

nodi lymphatici cubitales [NA] A group of one or two lymph nodes situated above the medial epicondyle of the humerus in the superficial fascia along the basilic vein just before it pierces the deep fascia. Its afferents drain the medial side of the forearm and hand while its efferents end in the lateral and central groups of axillary lymph nodes. In addition, a few lymph nodes are situated deep in the cubital fossa at the confluence of the radial and ulnar veins. These nodes are included, by some authorities, under this term. Some of their efferents may end in the above nodes, while most extend along the brachial veins to the axillary nodes. Also called *cubital lymph nodes, supratrochlear lymph nodes, epitrochlear lymph nodes, epitrochlear nodes, lymph nodes of cutibal fossa, Sigmund's glands.*

nodi lymphatici epigastrici inferiores [NA] A few small lymph nodes, situated along the inferior epigastric vessels, that receive afferents from the lower anterior abdominal wall and send efferents to the external iliac lymph nodes. Also called *inferior epigastric lymph nodes.*

nodi lymphatici faciales [NA] The nodi lymphatici buccales (buccal lymph nodes) and the nodi lymphatici mandibulares (mandibular lymph nodes) considered together. These nodes are situated along the facial vein and comprise the nodus buccinatorius, nodus nasolabialis, nodus malaris, and nodus mandibularis, and are located on the buccinator muscle, in the nasolabial furrow, in the infraorbital area, and on the lower margin of the mandible, respectively. They receive afferents from some of the skin and mucous membrane of the nose, cheek, and lips; from the medial part of the eyelids and conjunctiva, and also from some parotid nodes. The efferents drain to the submandibular nodes. Also called *facial lymph nodes.*

nodi lymphatici gastrici dextri [NA] Two or three lymph nodes along the right gastric artery that drain the pyloric portion adjacent to the lesser curvature of the stomach and send efferents to the hepatic nodes around the common hepatic artery. Also called *right gastric lymph nodes.*

nodi lymphatici gastrici sinistri [NA] A chain of lymph nodes situated along the left gastric artery and divided into three groups: an upper, on the stem of the artery; a lower, in the lesser omentum along the cardiac half of the lesser curvature; and a paracardial group around the esophagogastric junction. They drain the cardia, the lesser curvature and adjacent half of the stomach, and the abdominal part of the esophagus, while their efferents follow the course of the artery to end in the celiac lymph nodes. Also called *left gastric lymph nodes, superior gastric lymph nodes, lymph nodes of lesser curvature.*

nodi lymphatici gastroepiploici dextri NODI LYMPHATICI GASTRO-OMENTALES DEXTRI.

nodi lymphatici gastroepiploici sinistri NODI LYMPHATICI GASTRO-OMENTALES SINISTRI.

nodi lymphatici gastro-omentales dextri [NA] A short chain of about six lymph nodes that are situated along the right gastro-omental artery in the greater omentum along the pyloric part of the greater curvature of the stomach. They receive afferents from the lower part of the left half of the stomach and send efferents to the pyloric nodes. Also called *right gastroepiploic lymph nodes, inferior gastric lymph nodes, nodi lymphatici gastroepiploici dextri.*

nodi lymphatici gastro-omentales sinistri [NA] A few lymph nodes that are situated along the greater curvature of the stomach in the greater omentum along the left gastro-omental artery. They drain the adjacent surfaces of the stomach and greater omentum. They are usually associated with and included among the nodi lymphatici pancreatici. Also called *nodi lymphatici gastroepiploici sinistri, left gastroepiploic lymph nodes.*

nodi lymphatici hepatici [NA] A small chain of lymph nodes extending along the hepatic artery between the layers of the lesser omentum to the porta hepatis. It includes nodus cysticus inthe curve of the neck of the gallbladder and nodus epiploicus along the upper part of the common bile duct. Afferents are received from some deep lymphatics of the liver, parts of the visceral surface and lower anterior part of the diaphragmatic surface of the liver, the gallbladder, the right gastroepiploic lymph nodes, and part of the pyloric portion of the stomach. Efferents proceed to the celiac lymph nodes. Also called *hepatic lymph nodes.*

nodi lymphatici ileocolici [NA] Clumps of lymph nodes situated along the ileocolic artery and its branches. They receive lymph from the cecal nodes along the anterior and posterior cecal arteries and the appendicular nodes along the appendicular artery, as well as afferents from the terminal ileum via the ileal node and from the commencement of the ascending colon. Efferents end in the superior mesenteric lymph nodes. Also called *ileocolic lymph nodes.*

nodi lymphatici iliaci The groups of lymph nodes associated with the iliac arteries, namely, the common, external, and internal iliac arteries and their branches. They receive lymphatics from the pelvis, most of the pelvic viscera, the anterior and lateral parts of the abdominal wall, and the lower limbs, and their efferents end in the lumbar lymph nodes. An outmoded term. Also called *iliac lymph nodes.*

nodi lymphatici iliaci communes [NA] A group of lymph nodes situated around the common iliac vessels and below the bifurcation of the aorta, the afferents being lymphatics from the external and internal iliac lymph nodes while the efferents proceed to the lumbar lymph nodes. Also called *common iliac lymph nodes.*

nodi lymphatici iliaci externi [NA] Several lymph nodes, located lateral, medial, and anterior to the external iliac vessels, that receive lymphatics from the inguinal nodes; the deep layers of the anterior abdominal wall below the umbilicus, including efferents from the inferior epigastric and circumflex iliac nodes; as well as lymphatics from the prostate gland, fundus of the bladder, the membranous urethra, the cervix, and part of the uterus and vagina. Efferents run to the common iliac nodes but lymphatics also connect with the internal iliac nodes. Also called *external iliac lymph nodes.*

nodi lymphatici iliaci interni [NA] Lymph nodes located around the internal iliac vessels and the junctions of their branches, receiving afferents either directly or via intermediate nodes, from all the pelvic viscera, the deeper aspects of the perineum, the gluteal region, and back of the thigh. The efferents proceed to the common iliac lymph nodes and connect with the external iliac nodes. Also called *internal iliac lymph nodes.*

nodi lymphatici infra-auriculares [NA] One or two nodes of the nodi lymphatici parotidei superficiales that are situated below the ear and outside the parotid gland but deep to its fascia in the region of the commencement of the external jugular vein. Also called *inferior auricular parotid lymph nodes.*

nodi lymphatici inguinales profundi [NA] One to three lymph nodes medial to the femoral vein at the base of the femoral triangle. When three are present, the lowest is at the junction of the great saphenous vein with the femoral vein, the middle one is in the femoral canal, and the highest is in the femoral ring. They receive deep lymphatics of the lower limb that accompany the femoral vein, some lymphatics from the superficial inguinal nodes, and those from the glans penis or clitoridis. Their efferents pass through the femoral canal to end in the external iliac lymph nodes. Also called *deep inguinal lymph nodes.*

nodi lymphatici inguinales superficiales [NA] A large number of lymph nodes, arranged in a T shape, superficial to the deep fascia below the inguinal ligament and divided into upper and lower groups. The upper group is parallel to the inguinal ligament and receives lymphatics from the anterior abdominal wall below the umbilicus, the gluteal region, the external genitalia, the perianal area, and lower part of anal canal. The lower group lies vertically along the terminal part of the great saphenous vein and receives superficial lymphatics from the whole limb except the back and lateral side of the leg. Most of the efferents pass through the femoral sheath directly to the external iliac lymph nodes, but a few end in the deep inguinal nodes.

Also called *superficial inguinal lymph nodes.*

nodi lymphatici intercostales   [NA] One or two lymph nodes at the back of each intercostal space near the heads of the ribs that drain the posterolateral parts of the thoracic wall and parietal pleura. The efferents of the nodes in the upper spaces end in the thoracic duct on the left and the right lymphatic duct on the right, whereas those of the lower spaces unite to form a trunk that ends either in the cisterna chyli or into the commencement of the thoracic duct. Also called *intercostal lymph nodes, posterior intercostal lymph nodes.*

nodi lymphatici jugulares anteriores   [NA] Lymph nodes of the deep group of nodi lymphatici cervicales laterales that are situated anterior to the internal jugular vein, especially above the level where it is crossed by the omohyoid muscle. The jugulodigastric node may be included in this group. Also called *anterior jugular lymph nodes.*

nodi lymphatici jugulares laterales   [NA] Lymph nodes of the deep group of nodi lymphatici cervicales laterales that lie lateral to the internal jugular vein. Their drainage pattern cannot be separated from that of the deep group as a whole. Also called *lateral jugular lymph nodes, external nodes of internal jugular chain* (outmoded).

nodi lymphatici laterales   Three to six lymph nodes around the axillary vein, the afferents of which drain most of the upper limb and the efferents end in the central and apical groups of axillary lymph nodes. Also called *lateral axillary lymph nodes.*

nodi lymphatici linguales   Small and inconstant lymph nodes situated between the genioglossus muscles and on the lateral surface of the hyoglossus muscle, draining to the superior deep cervical nodes.

nodi lymphatici lumbales   [NA] A large number of prominent lymph nodes situated around the whole length of the abdominal aorta and part of the inferior vena cava. They are divided into right, left, and intermediate groups. The left group includes the lateral aortic, pre-aortic, and postaortic nodes lying lateral, anterior, and posterior to the aorta respectively. The right group includes the left caval, precaval, and postcaval nodes in relation to the inferior vena cava. Afferents are received from the common iliac nodes, the organs and tissues supplied by the paired branches of the aorta, and by the inferior mesenteric artery. The efferents of the uppermost nodes form a lumbar trunk on each side that terminates in the cisterna chyli. Also called *lumbar lymph nodes.*

nodi lymphatici mandibulares   See under NODI LYMPHATICI FACIALES.

nodi lymphatici mastoidei   [NA] A few lymph nodes behind the auricle on the mastoid insertion of the sternocleidomastoid muscle and deep to the posterior auricular muscle. They receive afferents from the scalp above the ear, the cranial surface of the upper part of the auricle, and the posterior wall of the external acoustic meatus, and they send efferents to the superior deep cervical nodes. Also called *nodi lymphatici retroauriculares* (outmoded), *retroauricular lymph nodes, posterior auricular lymph nodes, subauricular glands, mastoid lymph nodes.*

nodi lymphatici mediastinales anteriores   [NA] A number of small lymph nodes located in the superior mediastinum in front of the brachiocephalic veins and the arch of the aorta. They receive lymphatics from the thymus and thyroid glands, the upper part of the pericardium and pleura, superior lobe of left lung, and the right side of the heart. The efferents unite with those of the tracheobronchial and parasternal lymph nodes to form the bronchomediastinal lymph trunks. Also called *anterior mediastinal lymph nodes.*

nodi lymphatici mediastinales posteriores   [NA] A number of lymph nodes located behind the pericardium and adjacent to the esophagus and thoracic aorta. They receive afferents from the esophagus, the back of the pericardium and diaphragm, and some intercostal spaces. Most of the efferents end in the thoracic duct, whereas a few end in the tracheobronchial lymph nodes. Also called *posterior mediastinal lymph nodes.*

nodi lymphatici mesenterici   **1** [NA] A large number of small lymph nodes situated between the two layers of the mesentery in three groups: a peripheral group along the vasa recta close to the wall of the intestine; an intermediate group among the primary arcades and intestinal arteries; and a third group along the upper part of the stem of the superior mesenteric artery. Also called *mesenteric lymph nodes, mesocolic glands.* **2** An outmoded term for NODI LYMPHATICI MESENTERICI SUPERIORES.

nodi lymphatici mesenterici inferiores   [NA] Lymph nodes situated in front of the abdominal aorta around the main trunk of the inferior mesenteric artery, draining the distal third of the transverse colon, the descending colon, the sigmoid colon, and upper part of the rectum via the left colic, sigmoid, and superior rectal nodes, respectively. The efferents end in the superior mesenteric and left lateral aortic groups of lymph nodes. Also called *inferior mesenteric lymph nodes.*

nodi lymphatici mesenterici superiores   [NA] Lymph nodes situated in front of the duodenum and head of pancreas around the main trunk of the superior mesenteric artery and its origin from the aorta. They receive afferents from the mesenteric, ileocolic, right colic, and middle colic nodes that drain the jejunum, ileum, cecum, appendix, ascending colon, and proximal two thirds of the transverse colon, as well as afferents from some of the pyloric nodes and part of the duodenum and the head of the pancreas. Efferents pass to the celiac lymph nodes and intestinal lymph trunks. Also called *superior mesenteric lymph nodes, nodi lymphatici mesenterici* (outmoded).

nodi lymphatici mesocolici   [NA] Lymph nodes that drain the ascending, transverse, and descending colon. They are divided into paracolic nodes, which lie along the mesenteric border of the colon, and colic nodes, which lie along the right, middle, and left colic arteries. Their efferents drain into nodes lying around the trunks of the superior and inferior mesenteric arteries that are continuous with the corresponding preaortic lymph nodes. Also called *mesocolic glands.*

nodi lymphatici obturatorii   [NA] Lymph nodes along the obturator vessels that drain the lymphatics of the adductor region of the thigh. A constant node is present on the obturator nerve in the sulcus of the obturator foramen. Their efferents end in the external iliac nodes, while the node on the obturator nerve may occasionally drain into the internal iliac nodes. Also called *obturator lymph nodes.*

nodi lymphatici occipitales   [NA] A small group of lymph nodes located along the occipital artery at the apex of the posterior triangle of the neck, between the proximal attachments of the trapezius and sternocleidomastoid muscles. They drain the occipital region of the scalp and the superficial tissues of the upper part of the neck. Some efferents drain to the superior deep cervical nodes while most end in nodes along the accessory nerve in the posterior triangle of the neck. Also called *occipital lymph nodes.*

nodi lymphatici pancreatici   [NA] Lymph nodes, including the nodi lymphatici gastro-omentales, that are situated along the splenic artery on the posterosuperior surface of the pancreas. They receive afferents from the fundus and upper part of the body of the stomach and the pancreas. The efferents end in the celiac group of nodes.

nodi lymphatici pancreaticolienales   The nodi lymphatici pancreatici and nodi lymphatici splenici. Also called *pancreaticosplenic lymph nodes.*

nodi lymphatici paracolici   [NA] Lymph nodes situated

along the medial borders of the ascending and descending colon and the mesenteric borders of the transverse and sigmoid colon. They drain the epicolic nodes in the wall of the gut and their efferents pass to the intermediate colic nodes. Also called *paracolic lymph nodes.*

nodi lymphatici pararectales [NA] Numerous lymph nodes that lie in the wall of the rectum next to the muscular coat. Most drain to the superior rectal nodes and then to the preaortic nodes at the origin of the inferior mesenteric artery. Others drain to the internal iliac and common iliac lymph nodes. Also called *nodi lymphatici anorectales, lymphonodi anorectales* (outmoded).

nodi lymphatici parasternales [NA] Lymph nodes situated along the internal thoracic artery at the anterior ends of the upper three or four intercostal spaces. They receive lymphatics from the medial part of the mammary gland, the deeper part of the anterior thoracic wall and the anterior abdominal wall above the umbilicus, and the upper surface of the liver. The efferents may join those of the tracheobronchial and brachiocephalic nodes to form the bronchomediastinal lymph trunk. Also called *parasternal lymph nodes, sternal lymph nodes, internal thoracic lymph nodes, internal mammary lymph nodes* (outmoded).

nodi lymphatici paratracheales **1** [NA] One of the five groups of tracheobronchial lymph nodes that is located on each side of the thoracic part of the trachea and receives afferents from the superior tracheobronchial nodes. Its efferents terminate in the bronchomediastinal lymph trunks. Also called *peritracheal lymph nodes, tracheal lymph nodes.* **2** [NA] A group of deep anterior cervical lymph nodes that is situated along the recurrent laryngeal nerve on each side between the trachea and the esophagus. Their efferents end either in the lowest deep cervical nodes, in the jugular trunk, or in the thoracic duct. They may become enlarged in the presence of metastatic thyroid cancer. Also called *lateral tracheal group of deep anterior cervical lymph nodes, paratracheal lymph nodes. For defs. 1 and 2 also called nodi lymphatici tracheales.*

nodi lymphatici parotidei profundi [NA] Intraglandular lymph nodes embedded in the substance of the parotid gland and deep to the gland on the lateral wall of the pharynx. Some of the lymph from the external acoustic meatus and eyelids draining to the superficial parotid nodes also reaches the deep nodes, as well as lymph from the gland, the middle ear, auditory tube, soft palate, and the posterior part of the floor of the nasal cavity. Their efferents join the adjacent upper deep cervical nodes. Also called *deep parotid lymph nodes.*

nodi lymphatici parotidei superficiales [NA] Lymph nodes superficial or deep to the parotid fascia that include the preauricular group in front of the tragus of the ear, draining the temporal and frontal regions of the scalp, the lateral surface of the auricle, the external wall of the external acoustic meatus and the lateral parts of the eyelids and conjunctiva. Their efferents end in the upper deep cervical nodes. A few infra-auricular glands are situated on the external jugular vein just below the parotid gland. Also called *superficial parotid lymph nodes, preauricular nodes, anterior auricular nodes, superficial subaponeurotic parotid lymphnodes* (outmoded), *superficial supraaponeurotic parotid lymph nodes* (outmoded).

nodi lymphatici pectorales Three to five lymph nodes lying along the lateral thoracic artery at the junction of the anterior and medial walls of the axilla. The efferents join the central and apical groups of axillary nodes. Also called *pectoral lymph nodes, pectoral axillary nodes.*

nodi lymphatici phrenici inferiores [NA] A series of lymph nodes located on the abdominal surface of the diaphragm along the right inferior phrenic artery. They receive lymphatics from the posterior surface of the right lobe of the liver and adjacent diaphragm, and their efferents end in the right lateral caval

nodes. Also called *inferior diaphragmatic lymph nodes.*

nodi lymphatici phrenici superiores [NA] A series of lymph nodes located on the thoracic surface of the diaphragm and comprising three sets. The anterior nodes are situated behind the xiphisternal joint and seventh costal cartilages, receiving afferents from the diaphragmatic surface of the liver, the adjacent diaphragm, and anterior abdominal wall. They send efferents to the parasternal nodes. The middle nodes are adjacent to the phrenic nerves, receiving lymphatics from the middle part of the diaphragm and part of the liver surface and sending efferents to the anterior phrenic nodes. The posterior nodes lie behind the crura of the diaphragm, draining that area and connecting with the lumbar and posterior mediastinal nodes. Also called *diaphragmatic lymph nodes* (outmoded).

nodi lymphatici popliteales [NA] A number of lymph nodes located in the fat of the popliteal fossa and divided into superficial and deep groups. A superficial node is situated at the termination of the small saphenous vein, receiving lymphatics from the superficial region at the back and lateral side of the leg. A deep group is related to the popliteal vessels, receiving lymphatics from the knee joint as well as deep lymphatics accompanying the anterior tibial, posterior tibial, and peroneal vessels. Their efferents end in the deep inguinal nodes. Also called *popliteal lymph nodes.*

nodi lymphatici postaortici [NA] Lumbar lymph nodes that are situated behind the abdominal aorta and are essentially members of both the right and the left lumbar groups of nodes, as they have no defined area of drainage. Also called *retroaortic lymph nodes.*

nodi lymphatici postcavales [NA] Lumbar lymph nodes that are situated behind the inferior vena cava along the medial border of the psoas major muscle and on the right crus of the diaphragm. Also called *retrocaval lymph nodes.*

nodi lymphatici preaortici [NA] Lymph nodes that are situated immediately in front of the abdominal aorta and drain outlying intermediate nodes of the gastrointestinal tract, liver, spleen, and pancreas. Their efferents end in the intestinal trunks that help to form the cisterna chyli. They are divided into three groups surrounding the origins of corresponding arteries, namely, celiac, superior mesenteric, and inferior mesenteric. Also called *preaortic lymph nodes.*

nodi lymphatici preauriculares [NA] Some nodes of the nodi lymphatici parotidei profundi that are located deep to the fascia of the parotid gland in front of the tragus of the auricle. Some authorities include them in the nodi lymphatici parotidei superficiales. They receive efferents from the latter nodes or directly from the external acoustic meatus, the lateral portions of the eyelids, the auricle, and skin of the temporal and frontal regions. Also called *preauricular lymph nodes, subaponeurotic preauricular parotid lymph nodes* (outmoded).

nodi lymphatici precavales [NA] Those right lateral aortic lymph nodes that are situated in front of the inferior vena cava from its origin as far as the renal veins. One constant node is situated at the level of the bifurcation of the aorta. They receive afferents from structures supplied by lateral and posterior branches of the aorta and from outlying nodes of the iliac arteries. Also called *precaval lymph nodes.*

nodi lymphatici prececales [NA] Several lymph nodes that lie along the anterior cecal arteries and drain lymphatics on the front of the cecum and root of the vermiform appendix. Their efferents pass to the ileocolic nodes. Also called *anterior cecal lymph nodes.*

nodi lymphatici prelaryngeales [NA] A group of deep cervical lymph nodes lying on the conus elasticus and the median cricothyroid ligament and deep to the investing layer of deep fascia. They receive afferents from the walls of the larynx and from the thyroid gland. Their efferents pass to lower deep cervical nodes. Also called *prelaryngeal lymph nodes.*

nodi lymphatici prepericardiales [NA] Lymph nodes situated behind the xiphoid process and the sixth and seventh costal cartilages on each side. They constitute the anterior group of the superior phrenic nodes and receive afferents from the liver and the front of the diaphragm. The efferents end in the parasternal nodes. Also called *prepericardiac lymph nodes.*

nodi lymphatici pretracheales [NA] One of the deep groups of the anterior cervical lymph nodes lying anterior to the trachea and along the inferior thyroid vessels. They receive afferents from the upper, cervical part of the trachea and the thyroid gland, and send efferents to the inferior deep cervical nodes. Also called *pretracheal lymph nodes.*

nodi lymphatici pulmonales One of the five groups of tracheobronchial lymph nodes that is situated along the larger branches of the principal bronchi in the lung substance. It receives the lymphatics draining the deep plexus in the bronchial submucosa and the peribronchial connective tissue, and its efferents pass to the contiguous bronchopulmonary nodes. Also called *pulmonary lymph nodes.* • Some authorities combine this group with the bronchopulmonary nodes under the single latter term.

nodi lymphatici pylorici [NA] Some lymph nodes around the termination of the gastroduodenal artery in front and behind the groove between the junction of the first and second parts of the duodenum and the head of pancreas. They receive lymphatics from the right gastroepiploic nodes, the duodenum, and the pyloric part of the stomach, and they send efferents up to the hepatic nodes and down to the superior mesenteric nodes of the preaortic group. Also called *pyloric lymph nodes, subduodenopyloric lymph nodes* (outmoded), *lymph nodes of gastroduodenal artery.*

nodi lymphatici retroauriculares An outmoded term for NODI LYMPHATICI MASTOIDEI.

nodi lymphatici retrocecales [NA] Several lymph nodes that lie along the posterior cecal arteries and drain lymphatics on the back of the cecum and root of the vermiform appendix. Their efferents pass to the ileocolic nodes. Also called *posterior cecal lymph nodes.*

nodi lymphatici retropharyngeales [NA] A few lymph nodes of each deep cervical lymph chain situated between the fascia of the pharynx and the prevertebral fascia along the lateral margin of the longus capitis muscle. They receive afferents from the nasal fossae, paranasal sinuses, nasopharynx, auditory tube, oropharynx, and adjacent vertebral joints. The efferents end in the superior deep cervical nodes. Also called *retropharyngeal lymph nodes, lymphonodi retropharyngei* (outmoded).

nodi lymphatici sacrales [NA] Two or three peripheral nodes of the internal iliac lymph nodes located along the median and lateral sacral vessels in front of the second and third sacral foramina. They receive afferents from the rectum, uterus, vagina, prostate gland, and posterior pelvic wall. Also called *sacral lymph nodes.*

nodi lymphatici splenici [NA] Lymph nodes situated along the terminal part of the splenic artery and in the gastrosplenic ligament. Afferents derive from the spleen and efferents pass to the celiac lymph nodes. Also called *lymph nodes of gastropancreatic fold* (outmoded).

nodi lymphatici submandibulares [NA] Three or more lymph nodes deep to the deep cervical fascia in or around the submandibular salivary gland and related to the facial artery below the inferior margin of the mandible. They receive afferents from the facial and submental lymph nodes, thereby receiving much of the lymph from the central portion of the face, as well as lymphatics from the submandibular and sublingual salivary glands. The efferents pass to both the superior and the inferior deep cervical nodes. Also called *submandibular lymph nodes.*

nodi lymphatici submentales [NA] Two to four lymph nodes situated on the external surface of the mylohyoid muscle, between the anterior bellies of the right and left digastric muscles. They receive afferents from the middle portion of the lower lip and gums, floor of the mouth, and tip of the tongue. The efferents end in both the submandibular and jugulo-omohyoid lymph nodes. Also called *submental lymph nodes, lymphonodi submentales* (outmoded).

nodi lymphatici subscapulares The posterior group of axillary lymph nodes located along the subscapular vessels and their branches. Their efferents drain to the central and apical groups of axillary nodes. Also called *subscapular lymph nodes.*

nodi lymphatici supraclaviculares [NA] A group of inferior deep cervical lymph nodes situated above the clavicle just behind the clavicular attachment of the sternocleidomastoid muscle and in close relation to the junction of the internal jugular and subclavian veins. They receive lymph from the superior deep cervical nodes as well as from nodes and lymphatics along the subclavian vessels. Their efferents enter the jugular trunk. Also called *jugular glands, supraclavicular lymph nodes.*

nodi lymphatici thyroidei [NA] Small lymph nodes on the course of the lymphatics draining the thyroid gland, which tend to follow the blood vessels of the gland, as well as a large node occasionally located in front of the middle of the thyroid cartilage. Also called *thyroid lymph nodes.*

nodi lymphatici tracheales NODI LYMPHATICI PARATRACHEALES.

nodi lymphatici tracheobronchiales [NA] A large number of lymph nodes forming a continuous chain along the bronchi, both inside and ouside the lungs, and the trachea, and divided into five groups; paratracheal, superior tracheobronchial, inferior tracheobronchial, bronchopulmonary, and pulmonary. The afferents drain the lungs, visceral pleura, bronchi, the thoracic part of trachea, the heart, and the posterior mediastinal lymph nodes. The efferents unite with those of the parasternal and anterior mediastinal nodes to form the left and right bronchomediastinal trunks. Also called *tracheobronchial lymph nodes.*

nodi lymphatici tracheobronchiales inferiores [NA] One of the five groups of tracheobronchial lymph nodes that is situated in the angle between the two bronchi just below the bifurcation of the trachea. They receive afferents from the bronchopulmonary nodes and send efferents to the superior tracheobronchial nodes. Also called *inferior tracheobronchial lymph nodes.*

nodi lymphatici tracheobronchiales superiores [NA] One of the five groups of tracheobronchial lymph nodes, situated in the angle between the trachea and the brochus on each side just above the bifurcation of the trachea. They receive afferents from the inferior tracheobronchial nodes and send efferents to the paratracheal lymph nodes. Also called *superior tracheobronchial lymph nodes, pretracheal lymph nodes* (outmoded).

nodi lymphatici vesicales laterales [NA] Small lymph nodes that are located along the lymph vessels running upward on each lateral aspect of the urinary bladder. They drain the region of the trigone and base as well as the sides of the bladder. Most of their efferents end in the external iliac nodes, but a few may pass directly to the internal or common iliac nodes. Also called *lateral vesical lymph nodes.*

nodus lymphaticus [NA] Any of the small rounded or oval masses of lymphoid tissue that are irregularly placed along the course of lymphatic vessels and through which the lymph of those vessels passes. They vary in size and shape and have a hilum on one side where blood vessels enter and leave and efferent lymphatic vessels leave. Each is an organ surrounded by a fibrous capsule from which collagenous trabeculae extend inward. It consists of a cortex through which afferent lymphatic vessels enter and a medulla arranged in cords that extend to the surface at the hilum. A fibrocellular reticular meshwork occupies the spaces between the trabeculae and contains lymphocytes, macrophages, and lymph sinuses. The cortex contains lymphatic nodules. Also called *lymph node, lymphatic node, lymphonodus, lymphoglandula* (outmoded), *lymphatic gland, absorbent gland* (outmoded), *globate gland* (outmoded), *conglobate gland, lymph gland, lymphaden, ganglion lymphaticum.*

nodus malaris [NA] One of the nodi lymphatici faciales that is situated along the facial vein anterior to the zygomatic bone near the nasal bridge.

nodus mandibularis [NA] One of the nodi lymphatici faciales that is situated along the facial vein at the inferior margin of the body of the mandible just anterior to its angle. There are usually more than one node.

nodus nasolabialis [NA] One of the nodi lymphatici faciales that is situated along the facial vein in the nasolabial furrow.

nodus sinuatrialis [NA] A narrow, U-shaped collection of specialized cardiac muscle situated at the upper end of the sulcus terminalis of the right atrium near the junction of the entrance of the superior vena cava and the right auricle. It comprises slender fusiform fibers that contract more rapidly than the surrounding cardiac muscle and it is considered to initiate the cardiac cycle of contraction. Hence it is called the pacemaker of the heart. Also called *S-A node, sinoatrial node, sinuatrial node, Keith's node, sinuatrial node of Keith and Flack, Keith-Flack node, Flack's node, Keith's bundle, atrionector, sinoatrial bundle* (outmoded).

nodus tibialis anterior [NA] An inconstant lymph node that drains some of the deep lymphatics accompanying the anterior tibial vessels and is located along their upper third. Its efferents end in the deep group of popliteal nodes. Also called *anterior tibial lymph node.*

nodi viscerales abdominis Lymph nodes situated along the efferent lymphatics of the abdominal viscera. They lie along the celiac artery and its branches, the superior mesenteric artery, the inferior mesenteric artery, and the biliary tract. Also called *visceral lymph nodes of abdomen.*

---

noeud vital The respiratory centers of the brain. An obsolete term. Also called *vital node.*

no-fault Referring to insurance compensation to the insured for specified damages regardless of who caused the loss.

nogalamycin An anticancer antibiotic, the product of *Streptomyces nogalater.*

noise [Middle English, from L *nausea* seasickness] **1** Sound usually of a random nature the spectrum of which does not exhibit any clearly defined frequency components. **2** An unpleasant or undesired sound. **3** Electric oscillations of an undesired or random nature such as the 60-cycle frequency wave in an electrocardiogram.

pink noise White noise which has been shaped so that the energy is not distributed evenly but is inversely proportional to frequency.

steady-state noise Noise in which the acoustic characteristics show little or no variation over a specified time.

thermal noise The small fluctuations of voltage across a resistor due to the random motion of thermally agitated electrons.

transient noise Sounds of extremely short duration such as clicks and impulse noise and certain speech sounds.

white noise Nonperiodic sound in which there is an equal distribution of acoustic energy throughout the audible range of frequencies and beyond. It is used in otology for masking one ear while the other is being tested. Also called *white sound.*

Noludar A proprietary name for methyprylon.

noma [Gk *nomē* (from *nemein* to devour, pasture, feed on; of ulcers, to spread) a pasture, feeding on, spreading, spreading ulcer] Spreading gangrene, usually of the facial tissues in and around the mouth (cancrum oris) but sometimes of the female external genitalia, (noma vulvae) occurring in the severely malnourished, chiefly children, and as a complication of the exanthemata.

noma pudendi A gangrenous condition of the vulva, affecting young girls. An obsolete term. Also called *noma vulvae, phlegmonous vulvitis.*

noma vulvae NOMA PUDENDI.

nomadic Not fixed or stabilized; moving or apt to move freely.

nomen [L] (*plural* nomina) A name.

nomen conservandum A scientific name which does not follow the rules of nomenclature, but which has been accepted for continued use.

nomen dubium A proposed taxonomic name which is invalid because it is not accompanied by a definition or description of the taxon to which it applies.

nomen nudum A proposed taxonomic name which is invalid either because the name was previously used for another species, or because the accompanying description cannot be interpreted satisfactorily.

nomen rejectum A proposed taxonomic name which is rejected, and should not be used for the organism in question.

nomenclature [L *nomenclatura* (from *nomenclator* a slave who tells his master the names of persons he has met, from *nomen* a name + *calare* to call, call out, summon, from Gk *kalein* to call, call by name) a naming, listing of names, terminology] A system for naming or the names assigned to particular types that can be usefully distinguished from others in a science or other discipline, as of animals or plants or their structures.

binomial nomenclature The system developed by Linnaeus for naming flora and fauna. A species is designated by a unique combination of two names, a generic name and a specific epithet.

Nomina Anatomica The standard anatomical terminology, which was adopted by the German Anatomical Society at Basle (later *Basel*, abbreviated *BNA*), Switzerland, in 1895. It was revised in 1933 (Birmingham Revision) and in 1936 (Jena Nomina Anatomica). In 1955 a completely revised Nomina Anatomica, First Edition (abbreviated *NA*), was published, and since then several revisions have been issued. The fourth edition, published in 1977, also included a Nomina Histologica and a Nomina Embryologica, as have subsequent editions. Abbreviation: NA

nomo- [Gk *nomos* law, usage, custom] A combining form meaning law, custom, usage.

nomogenesis [NOMO- + GENESIS] The theory that the course of evolution is entirely fixed and determined by natural law, without random variation.

nomogram [NOMO- + -GRAM] A diagram representing the relationships between variables in a given system. For example, if the system consists of three variables, the value taken by one of them is represented in the nomogram for each pair of values taken by the other two, in a graphical manner.

blood volume nomogram A nomogram that indicates the normal blood volume for a person's height and weight.

Friedenwald's nomogram A table correlating readings on the Schiøtz tonometer with the intraocular pressure.

Radford nomogram A graphic presentation of the tidal volume required during artificial ventilation of the lungs computed according to the characteristics and condition of the patient.

nomograph [NOMO- + -GRAPH] NOMOGRAM.

nomography [NOMO- + -GRAPHY] The construction of nomograms.

nomothetic   Relating to general or universal laws based on the observation of many cases.

nomotopic   Occurring in the normal place. Also *normotopic* (obsolete).

non- [L *non* (from early *noenum, noenu* none, no one, from *ne* not + *unum* one) not]   A prefix meaning not.

nona [prob. a corruption of Italian *coma* (from Gk *kōma* deep sleep) lethargy]   A condition resembling encephalitis lethargica which appeared in Italy during an influenza epidemic in 1889–90. An obsolete term.

nona- [L *nonus* (feminine *nona*) ninth]   A combining form meaning nine.

nonaccess   The lack of an opportunity to engage in sexual intercourse or the absence of sexual intercourse. In cases of disputed paternity, nonaccess is a common defense used by a putative father.

nonacosane $C_{29}H_{60}$. The hydrocarbon whose molecule is a chain of 29 carbon atoms saturated with hydrogen.

nonactin   An antibiotic ionophore containing a tetralactone ring of 32 atoms.

nonadherent   Not attached to or connected with contiguous structures.

nonan [L *nonan(a)* (from *nona*, fem. of *nonus* for *novenus* ninth, from *novem* nine) pertaining to the Roman Ninth Legion]   Recurring or characterized by attacks every ninth day, as *nonan malaria*.

nonane C_9H_{20}. The hydrocarbon whose molecule is a chain of nine carbon atoms saturated with hydrogen.

nonarticular   Not occurring in a joint: used especially with reference to periarticular complaints.

nonbursate   Lacking a copulatory bursa: applied primarily to nonstrongyloid nematodes. An outmoded term.

noncariogenic [NON- + CARIOGENIC]   Not causing dental decay.

nonchromaffin   Not staining with chromium salts: said especially of cells of the adrenal medulla, carotid body, or paraganglia that do not secrete epinephrine.

noncomitance [NON- + COMITANCE]   A misalignment of the eyes in which the angle of the deviation changes with different directions of gaze. Adjective: noncomitant.

non compos mentis [L *non* not + *compos* master of + *mentis*, gen. of *mens* reason]   Not of sound mind; in legal usage, not competent to manage one's affairs or to execute specified actions or judgments independently. Compare COMPOS MENTIS.

nonconductor   A material that transmits heat, electricity, or sound poorly.

nondepolarizer   A muscle relaxant agent that causes striatal muscular paralysis by competitively blocking neurotransmission at the myoneural junction. An example is *d*-tubocurarine.

nondisjunction   The failure of normal segregation of chromosomes to daughter cells during cell division.

primary nondisjunction   Nondisjunction that occurs during the first meiotic division in which both chromosomes of a homologous pair segregate to a secondary gametocyte.

secondary nondisjunction   Nondisjunction occurring during the second stage of meiosis, in which both chromatids of a chromosome segregate to a gamete during anaphase.

somatic nondisjunction   Nondisjunction occurring during mitosis in which one daughter cell receives both, and the other cell receives neither, chromosome of an homologous pair. Also called *anaphase lag loss*.

nonencapsulated   Not surrounded by a containing capsule: used of a swelling, such as a tumor or abscess.

nongranular   AGRANULAR.

nongranulocyte   A blood leukocyte that does not contain granules in its cytoplasm. Lymphocytes and monocytes are nongranulocytes.

nonhomogeneity   A lack of uniformity in a structure or population.

nonhomologues   NONHOMOLOGOUS CHROMOSOMES.

nonigravida [L *non-* ninth + *i* + GRAVIDA]   A woman who has been pregnant nine times.

noninfectious   Incapable of spreading or causing disease.

noninvasive   Not involving the penetration of a body cavity or the skin: used especially of a therapeutic or diagnostic procedure.

noninvolution [NON- + INVOLUTION]   Failure of the uterus to return to its normal shape and size following a pregnancy.

nonionic   Not containing charges in its molecule, as in detergents whose hydrophilic groups are not ionized.

nonipara [L *non-* ninth + *i* + PARA]   A woman who has produced viable fetuses in nine pregnancies.

nonlamellar   Not arranged in layers: said of immature bony tissue in which the collagen bundles are not arranged in regular layers and consequently do not give a lamellar pattern with polarized light microscopy.

nonmedullated   UNMYELINATED.

nonmetal   **1** Not possessing the properties of a metal.   **2** An electronegative element.

nonmyelinated   UNMYELINATED.

Nonne [Max *Nonne*, German neurologist, 1861–1939]   **1** Nonne-Froin syndrome. See under FROIN SYNDROME.   **2** Nonne-Marie syndrome. See under MARIE'S HEREDITARY CEREBELLAR ATAXIA.   **3** Nonne-Milroy disease, Nonne-Milroy lymphedema, Nonne-Milroy-Meige syndrome. See under HEREDITARY LYMPHEDEMA TYPE I.   **4** Nonne syndrome. See under SCALENUS ANTERIOR SYNDROME.

non-nucleated   ANUCLEAR.

nonnutritive   **1** Not assimilable as food.   **2** Not of nutritive value.

nonocclusion [NON- + OCCLUSION]   The failure of a tooth or teeth to contact antagonists.

nonoliguric [NON- + OLIGURIC]   Producing urine in normal volume: usually said of acute renal failure that is without the usual oliguria.

nononcogenic [NON- + ONCOGENIC]   Not capable of causing tumors.

nonopaque [NON- + OPAQUE]   In radiology, easily pervious to x ray and thus on a roentgenogram not distinguishable as a discrete shadow.

nonose [*non(a)-* + *-OSE*^{2}]   Any aldose sugar of nine carbon atoms.

nonosteogenic [NON- + OSTEOGENIC]   Failing or unable to give rise to bone.

nonovulatory [NON- + OVULATORY]   Characterized by the absence of ovulation, usually associated with absence of menstruation.

nonoxynol-9   Nonylphenoxypolyethoxyethanol, with 9 oxyethylene groups in the polyoxyethylene, $(OCH_2CH_2)n$, chain. It is used as a spermicidal component in some contraceptive materials, including aerosol foams.

nonparous [NON- + PAROUS]   NULLIPAROUS.

nonpathogen   A microorganism that does not normally cause disease.

nonpenetrant   In genetics, pertaining to a trait which is not apparent or evident on assay despite the presence of a particular genotype capable of determining the trait. It usually refers to monogenic traits, such as a heterozygote for a completely recessive trait.

nonpermissive Allowing a conditionally lethal mutation to block formation of a required gene product: said of environmental conditions, such as temperature.

nonpolar Having molecules that possess no charges or dipole moments: used of substances such as paraffins. When applied to solvents it suggests that they will not dissolve polar compounds and will not favor chemical reactions whose mechanism involves charge separation. The term is also applied to an environment without charges or dipoles.

nonradiable [NON- + RADIABLE] Not allowing passage of rays, such as x rays.

nonrandom [NON- + RANDOM] Having a statistical pattern, such as uniformity or coherence, as opposed to being without a discernable pattern.

non rep. *non repetatur* (L, do not repeat; no refill).

nonrespondent [NON- + RESPONDENT] One who does not respond to an inquiry, such as an interview or questionnaire. Nonresponse may be due to an individual's refusal to give information or to failure on the part of the inquirer to contact the person. Without adequate collateral evidence as to the relevant characteristics of nonrespondents it cannot be assumed that their response pattern would have been the same as that of respondents.

nonrotation Failure of a structure during embryonic life to rotate to its normal position.

nonrotation of the intestine Lack of rotation of the embryonic intestine when normally it should rotate from a sagittally aligned loop to take up its adult relationships in the abdominal cavity.

nonsecretor An individual who lacks the inherited ability to secrete substances A, B, H in his body fluids while being able to express these substances on his tissue cells.

nonsegmented Lacking body segments; nonmetameric: often used to describe exceptions to a generally segmented group of organisms, such as the Cestodaria, the nonsegmented cestodes.

nonself [NON- + SELF] Those antigens that are not a normal constituent of the body of a given individual and to which antibodies can be formed. Being foreign to the self, such antigens are recognized by the immune system. Also called *not-self*. Compare SELF.

nonspecific 1 Not caused by one particular microorganism: said of an infection or disease. 2 Denoting a general effect of a drug, in contrast to its effect from specific interaction at a designated site of action or receptor.

nonstriated UNSTRIATED.

nonsuppurative Not accompanied by pus formation.

nonsurgical Not requiring operative intervention: used especially of a therapeutic or diagnostic procedure.

nontaster 1 In a linkage between loci, an individual incapable of tasting a specific substance when the ability to taste is a mendelian trait. 2 An individual incapable of tasting phenylthiocarbamide (PTC), due to homozygosity of an allele at the PTC locus. Such an inability is an autosomal recessive trait.

nonunion The failure of a fractured bone to heal with new bone formation. Also called *faulty union*.

established nonunion Stabilization of the healing process of a fracture without evidence that eventual union will take place.

nonus [L, ninth] The hypoglossal (twelfth) cranial nerve, once thought erroneously to be the ninth. An obsolete term.

nonvenereal [NON- + VENEREAL] Not caused or spread by sexual contact.

nonviability [NON- + VIABILITY] The state or quality of being nonviable.

nonviable [NON- + VIABLE] Describing a fetus that has not yet reached that stage of intrauterine development at which it could survive birth. A fetus of less than five months' gestation is generally regarded as being nonviable.

nonvisualization [NON- + VISUALIZATION] In radiology, the failure to demonstrate in an organ an administered radiopaque contrast medium normally excreted by that organ, as during intravenous urography.

Noon [Leonard *Noon*, English physician, 1878–1913] Noon pollen unit. See under UNIT.

Noonan [Jacqueline Anne *Noonan*, U.S. cardiologist, born 1921] See under SYNDROME.

Noorden [Carl Harko von *Noorden*, German physician, 1858–1944] Noorden treatment. See under OATMEAL TREATMENT.

noosphere [Gk *noo(s)* mind + SPHERE] ANTHROPOSPHERE.

nootropic Activating or stimulating to mental activity; causing cerebral or intellectual activity.

nopalin G An eosin dye which has a bluish color.

nor- [shortened from *normal*. See NORMA.] 1 A prefix signifying the removal of a methylene group, —CH$_2$—, from a named compound. Thus for example, norepinephrine contains —NH— where epinephrine contains —N(—CH$_3$)—. 2 A prefix denoting the isomer of the amino acid that has an unbranched chain: used in this sense only in the names *norvaline* and *norleucine*.

noradrenalin NOREPINEPHRINE.

noradrenaline The British term for NOREPINEPHRINE.

noradrenalin N-methyltransferase The enzyme (EC 2.1.1.28) responsible for the conversion of norepinephrine into epinephrine. The donor of the methyl group is *S*-adenosylmethionine.

norbiotin A compound homologous to biotin but with one fewer CH$_2$ grouping in its side chain. In some bacteria, it acts antagonistically to biotin. In other organisms, it can carry out some of the functions of biotin.

norbornane The hydrocarbon formed by bridging C-1 and C-4 of cyclohexane with a methylene group. It differs from the terpene bornane by lacking two methyl groups on the bridging atom, and one on a bridgehead atom. The peculiar chemistry of displacement of groups from substituted norbornane is explained by postulating a novel "nonclassical" structure for the norbornyl carbocation. Also called *norcamphane* (obsolete).

norcamphane An obsolete term for NORBORNANE.

Nordau [Max Simon *Nordau*, German physician and author, 1849–1923] See under DISEASE.

norepinephrine A catecholamine, *l*-β-[3,4-dihydroxyphenyl]-α-aminoethanol, a major adrenergic neurotransmitter liberated by postganglionic adrenergic nerve endings, and secreted also by the chromaffin granules of the adrenal medulla in response to splanchnic stimulation. Acting chiefly upon the α adrenergic receptors of effector organs, its chief property is to induce arteriolar constriction with raised systolic and diastolic arterial blood pressure, venoconstriction, and increased peripheral resistance. Also called *arterenol, levarterenol, arterenol, noradrenalin, noradrenaline (British usage), sympathin E* (outmoded).

norethandrolone C$_{20}$H$_{30}$O$_2$. 17-Hydroxy-19-norpregn-4-en-3-one. A synthetic androgenic steroid similar in structure to testosterone. It has similar pharmacologic effects and is used primarily as an anabolic steroid.

norethindrone C$_{20}$H$_{26}$O$_2$. 17-Hydroxy-19-nor-17α-pregn-4-en-20-yn-3-one. A progestational steroid with some estrogenic and androgenic activity. It is used as a substitute for progesterone and it is combined with an estrogenic agent as an oral contraceptive medication.

norethindrone acetate C$_{22}$H$_{28}$O$_3$. The acetate salt of norethindrone. It has the same actions and uses as the parent compound.

norethynodrel $C_{20}H_{26}O_2$. 17-Hydroxy-19-nor-17α-pregn-5(10)-en-20-yn-3-one. A progestational steroid used in combination with ethynylestradiol 3-methyl ether as an oral contraceptive agent.

Norflex A proprietary name for orphenadrine citrate.

norleucine CH_3—$[CH_2]_3$—$CH(NH_3{}^+)$—COO^-. 2-Aminohexanoic acid, the isomer of leucine with an unbranched carbon chain. It is somewhat misleading as a name, because the prefix *nor-* does not have its usual meaning of removal of a methylene group. It is used as a standard in amino-acid analysis, as it does not normally occur in biologic material. Symbol: Nle

Norlutate A proprietary name for norethindrone acetate.

Norlutin A proprietary name for norethindrone.

norm [L *norm(a)*. See NORMA.] A statistical measure of usual observed performance.

developmental norm The level of behavioral functioning established as usual, typical, or characteristic of children at any specified chronological age. This is often described in tabular or graphic form.

norma [L (akin to *gnoscere* or *noscere* to know, examine; also akin to *gnarus* knowing, expert and to Gk *gnōrimos* well-known), a carpenter's square, rule of any kind, standard] In anatomy, an aspect of the cranium or skull from a particular viewpoint, often as seen in outline.

norma anterior NORMA FACIALIS.

norma basalis NORMA BASILARIS.

norma basilaris 1 The outline of the inferior surface of the base of the skull. It extends from the front of the dental arch to the superior nuchal lines of the occipital bone. Also called *norma inferior* (outmoded), *norma ventralis* (outmoded), *norma basalis, basis cranii externa* (imprecise). 2 An imprecise term for BASIS CRANII EXTERNA.

norma facialis [NA] The outline of the skull as viewed from the front. Also called *norma frontalis, norma anterior.*

norma frontalis NORMA FACIALIS.

norma inferior An outmoded term for NORMA BASILARIS.

norma lateralis [NA] The outline of the skull as viewed from either side. Also called *norma temporalis* (outmoded).

norma occipitalis [NA] The outline of the skull as viewed from behind. It resembles a broad arch with a flat base. Its features include the external occipital protuberance, the nuchal lines, and the lambdoid suture. Also called *norma posterior* (outmoded).

norma posterior An outmoded term for NORMA OCCIPITALIS.

norma sagittalis The outline of a sagittal section through the skull. An outmoded term.

norma superior An outmoded term for NORMA VERTICALIS.

norma temporalis An outmoded term for NORMA LATERALIS.

norma ventralis An outmoded term for NORMA BASILARIS.

norma verticalis [NA] The outline of the skull as viewed from above. Anteriorly it is continuous with the norma facialis. It varies considerably, and the coronal, sagittal, and lambdoid sutures are exposed. Also called *norma superior* (outmoded).

normal [L *normal(is)* (from *norm(a)* a carpenter's square, rule of any kind, standard + *-alis* -AL) according to rule] 1 Conforming to a standard or norm; specifically, considered to be substantially free from defect, such that no intervention or correction is warranted, as *normal pulse, normal hearing.* 2 Being of satisfactory or average health. 3 Not exposed to an infective agent, as an experimental animal; not immunized. 4 Having a linear carbon chain: used of an alcohol or alkyl radical. 5 Describing the concentration of a solution one liter of which

yields or reacts with one mole of the unitary entities involved in a specified reaction, usually a titration, such as protons in acidimetry, or electrons in oxidation-reduction reactions. 6 Referring to standard conditions of temperature, 0°C (273.15K exactly), or of pressure, one atmosphere (101.325 kPa exactly).

normalize To adjust the values in a determination to an arbitrary standard, usually by multiplying them all by the same factor so that their total comes to a value known by an independent determination.

Norman [Ronald Melville *Norman*, English physician, flourished mid-20th century] Norman-Wood syndrome. See under SYNDROME.

normergic Concerning normal responsiveness to stimulation.

normetanephrine An intermediate in the catabolism of norepinephrine, from which it is produced by methylation of the phenolic hydroxyl *meta* to the carbon side chain.

normo- [L *norma* rule, law, standard] A combining form meaning normal.

normobaric [NORMO- + *bar(o)*- + -IC] Pertaining to a barometric pressure equivalent to sea-level pressure.

normoblast [NORMO- + -BLAST] Any erythrocyte precursor that exhibits normal characteristics of nuclear chromatin and cytoplasm, in contradistinction to the megaloblast. Several stages of maturation of the normoblast are recognized: pronormoblast, basophilic normoblast, polychromatophilic normoblast, and the penultimate stage, orthochromatic normoblast. Also called *hemonormoblast.*

acidophilic normoblast ORTHOCHROMATIC NORMOBLAST.

basophilic normoblast A stage of maturation of erythrocyte precursors in which the nucleus exhibits slight chromatin condensation, no nucleolus is identifiable, the nucleus occupies about half the volume of the cell, and the cytoplasm is free of granules and is a deep blue color when stained by Romanowsky dyes. Also called *basophilic erythroblast, early erythroblast, early normoblast, prorubricyte.*

early normoblast BASOPHILIC NORMOBLAST.

eosinophilic normoblast ORTHOCHROMATIC NORMOBLAST.

intermediate normoblast POLYCHROMATOPHILIC NORMOBLAST.

late normoblast ORTHOCHROMATIC NORMOBLAST.

orthochromatic normoblast The final stage in maturation of erythrocyte precursors before extrusion of the nucleus and release of the cell from bone marrow to blood. The cell is slightly larger than an erythrocyte, and the nucleus is small, about one fourth of the cell volume or less, with dense chromatin. The cytoplasm is red-orange, tinctorially identical with a mature erythrocyte, when stained with Romanowsky dyes. Also called *acidophilic erythroblast, eosinophilic erythroblast, late erythroblast, orthochromatic erythroblast, oxyphilic erythroblast, metarubricyte, acidophilic normoblast, eosinophilic normoblast, late normoblast, oxyphilic normoblast.*

oxyphilic normoblast ORTHOCHROMATIC NORMOBLAST.

polychromatophilic normoblast A stage of maturation of erythrocyte precursors, following the basophilic stage and preceding the orthochromatic stage, in which the nucleus exhibits prominent chromatin condensation and parachromatin, often resembling a checkerboard, and no nucleoli are identifiable. The nucleus occupies approximately one-third of the cell volume, and the cytoplasm is slate gray to lavender when stained by Romanowsky dyes. The color of the cytoplasm reflects the presence of both hemoglobin and abundant RNA in the cytoplasm. This is the last maturation stage at which cell division still occurs. Also called *intermediate erythroblast, polychromatophilic erythroblast, intermediate normoblast, rubricyte.*

normoblastic Having the morphologic characteristics of the normal maturation of erythrocyte precursors. Also *erythroblastic.* Compare MEGALOBLASTIC.

normoblastosis　The presence of nucleated erythrocyte precursors (normoblasts) in blood.

normocalcemia　A normal concentration of calcium in blood or serum.

normocalcemic　Exhibiting normocalcemia.

normocapnia　A normal concentration of carbon dioxide (and carbonic acid) in blood. Also called *eucapnia.*

normocapnic　Exhibiting normocapnia.

normocephalic　MESOCEPHALIC.

normocholesterolemia　A normal concentration of cholesterol in blood plasma or serum.

normocholesterolemic　Exhibiting normocholesterolemia.

normochromasia　NORMOCHROMIA.

normochromatic　Having normal color in stained blood films: used of erythrocytes or erythrocyte precursors. In Wright-stained blood films the cytoplasm exhibits no bluish tinge.

normochromia　A normal concentration of hemoglobin in erythrocytes. Also called *normochromasia.*

normochromic　Having normal concentration of hemoglobin in erythrocytes. Also *orthochromatic.*

normocrinic　Pertaining to normal hormonal secretion or to normal hormonal action.

normocyte　An erythrocyte of normal volume, usually 82–99 fl. Also called *normoerythrocyte.*

normocytic　Having erythrocytes of normal volume.

Normocytin　A proprietary name for vitamin B_{12}.

normocytosis　The state of having erythrocytes of normal volume. Also *normo-orthocytosis.*

normoerythrocyte　NORMOCYTE.

normoglycemia [NORMO- + GLYC- + -EMIA]　The presence of glucose in normal concentration in the blood.

normoglycemic　Characterized by or having blood glucose concentration within the accepted normal range.

normokalemia　A normal concentration of plasma or serum potassium. • As used, this term is not meant to apply to whole blood. Red cell K^+ concentration is much higher than that of serum.

normokalemic　Having normal plasma or serum potassium concentration.

normo-orthocytosis　NORMOCYTOSIS.

normoproteinemia　A normal concentration of proteins in serum.

normoreflexia [NORMO- + REFLEX + -IA]　Reflexes within the range of normal variation.

normosexual　Having all of the characteristics typical for a given genetic sex.

normosthenuria　The state of normal urine production.

normotension [NORMO- + TENSION]　Normal arterial blood pressure.

normotensive [NORMO- + *tens(ion)* + -IVE]　Characterized by normal arterial blood pressure.

normothermia [NORMO- + THERM- + -IA]　A state of normal body temperature.

normothermic　Of or relating to normothermia.

normothymotic　Mood-normalizing: used of drugs that restore abnormal moods to normal but do not affect a preexisting normal mood.

normotonia [NORMO- + *ton(o)-* + -IA]　**1** Normal muscle tone. **2** Normal blood pressure; normotension.

normotonic　**1** Characterized by normal muscle tone. **2** Characterized by normal blood pressure; normotensive.

normotopia　A state in which structures are normally positioned. An obsolete term.

normotopic　An obsolete term for NOMOTOPIC.

normotrophic [NORMO- + -TROPHIC]　Concerning normal growth and development.

normouricemia　A normal concentration of uric acid in serum or plasma.

normouricemic　Characterized by normouricemia.

normovolemia　Normal blood volume.

normovolemic　Having a normal blood volume.

nornicotine　$C_9H_{12}N_2$. A toxic pyridine alkaloid present in plant species of the genera *Duboisia, Nicotiana, Salpiglossis* and *Zinnia.* It is used in agriculture as an insecticide.

Norodin　A proprietary name for methamphetamine.

norophthalmic acid　The tripeptide γ-glutamylalanylglycine, found in the lens of the eye. It differs from ophthalmic acid, which occurs with it, in having —CH_3 rather than —CH_2—CH_3 as the side chain of its central residue, where glutathione has —CH_2SH.

norpseudoephedrine　$C_9H_{13}NO$. A central nervous system stimulant present in the dried leaves of *Catha edulis.* It has had limited use as an anorectic agent. Also called *cathine.*

Norrie [Gordon *Norrie*, Danish ophthalmologist, 1855–1941]　Norrie syndrome. See under DISEASE.

nortriptyline　$C_{19}H_{21}N$. 3-(10,11-Dihidro-5*H*-dibenzo[*a,d*]cyclohepten-5-ylidene)-*N*-methyl-1-propanamine. A tricyclic antidepressant drug. The mechanism by which these agents exert their mood elevation effect is not known. It is generally given orally as the hydrochloride salt.

nosazontology　NOSETIOLOGY.

noscapine　$C_{22}H_{22}NO_7$. An isoquinoline alkaloid which has cough-suppressing properties and aids respiration. It occurs in the capsules of *Papaver somniferum* and hence in opium. It is used in treating whooping cough and bronchitis. Also called *narcotine, narcosine, opian, opianine.*

nose [Old English *nosu,* from L *nasus,* also *nasum* the nose]　**1** NASUS EXTERNUS.　**2** The nasus externus and cavitas nasi considered together; nasus.

brandy nose　RHINOPHYMA.

cleft nose　The appearance as of duplicated nose due to persistence of the embryonic frontonasal groove or improper union of the medial nasal processes. Various degrees of this congenital deformity are seen. Rarely it is associated with other anomalies such as optic hypertelorism or hypotelorism, cleft lip and cleft palate. Also called *double nose* (rarely used), *nasus duplex* (rarely used).

collie nose　ECZEMA NASI OF DOGS.

copper nose　RHINOPHYMA.

dog nose　GOUNDOU.

double nose　A rarely used term for CLEFT NOSE.

external nose　NASUS EXTERNUS.

familial hump nose　A condition of the nose where there is a conspicuous hump in the bridge line, usually a familial trait. Also called *rhinokyphosis.*

Funke's nose　In the myogram of a muscle exhibiting fatigue after repeated contraction, a rounding of the transition from the plateau of tension during tetanus to the abrupt fall after the stimulus terminates. In a fresh muscle the transition takes the form of a sharp angle.

hammer nose　RHINOPHYMA.

potato nose　RHINOPHYMA.

rum nose　RHINOPHYMA.

saddle nose　A nose deformed by the collapse of the support of the dorsum between the tip and the nasal bones normally provided by the cartilage of the nasal septum. The resultant deformity is characterized by a saddle-shaped depression of the nasal dorsum. The causes are many and include trauma (accidental or surgical), septal infection (abscess, syphilis, etc.), and congenital deformity. Also called *nasus incurvus* (obsolete).

strawberry nose   RHINOPHYMA.

Swedish nose   A device for helping to maintain the humidity of the lower airways in cases of tracheostomy. It consists of wire mesh disks in a plastic container fitted to the tracheostomy tube. During expiration water vapor condenses on the wire mesh, which acts as a humidifier when the patient breathes in.

telescope nose   Atrophy of the septum and vomer causing a depression below the root of the nose. This condition is seen in leprosy.

toper's nose   RHINOPHYMA.

whisky nose   RHINOPHYMA.

nosebleed   EPISTAXIS.

nosebrain [NOSE + BRAIN]   An obsolete term for RHINENCEPHALON.

nosegay   In anatomy, a structure or structures resembling a small bunch of flowers. A rarely used term.

Riolan's nosegay   The group of muscles and ligaments attached to the styloid process of the temporal bone. Also called *bouquet of Riolan*.

Nosema   A genus of sporozoan parasites of many invertebrate and some vertebrate hosts, belonging to the family Nosematidae in the phylum Microspora. Schizogony in host cells produces spores, which consist of an external wall, sporoplasm, and a coiled polar filament within a polar capsule. A closely related and possibly synonymous genus is *Encephalitozoon*.

Nosema cuniculi   ENCEPHALITOZOON CUNICULI.

nosema [Gk *nosēma* sickness, disease, plague]   A disease or illness. An obsolete term.

Nosematidae [Gk *nosēmat(a)*, pl. of *nosēma*, sickness, disease + -IDAE]   A family of parasites in the protozoan phylum Microspora, characterized by oval spores that multiply intracellularly by schizogony with eventual production of infective spores. The spore has a characteristic wall enveloping a sporoplasm and a coiled filament within a polar capsule.

nosencephalus [*nos(o)-* + Gk *enkephalos* the brain]   An older term for ANENCEPHALUS.

nosencephaly [*nos(o)-* + ENCEPHAL- + -Y]   An outmoded term for ANENCEPHALY.

nosepiece   In a compound microscope, the mounting to which the objective lens is attached. It is often in the form of a pivoting plate on which are mounted several interchangeable objectives.

nosetiology   The study of the causes of disease. A seldom used term. Also called *nosazontology*.

noso- [Gk *nosos* sickness, disease]   A combining form meaning disease.

nosochthonography [NOSO- + Gk *chthōn* the earth + *o* + -GRAPHY]   A seldom used term for GEOMEDICINE.

nosocomial [New L *nosocomialis* (from Gk *nosokomei(on)* a hospital, from *nosokomos* a sick-nurse, from *noso(s)* sickness + *-komos*, combining form from *kamnein* to be sick; + *-alis* -AL)]   Pertaining to or acquired in a hospital or other health facility: used especially in reference to hospital-acquired infections and diseases.

nosogenesis   A seldom used term for PATHOGENESIS.

nosogenic   An obsolete term for PATHOGENIC.

nosogeny   A seldom used term for PATHOGENESIS.

nosogeography [NOSO- + GEOGRAPHY]   A seldom used term for GEOMEDICINE.

nosographer   One who practices nosography.

nosographic   Relating to nosography.

nosography [NOSO- + -GRAPH + -Y]   A classification or description of diseases.

nosointoxication [NOSO- + INTOXICATION]   A toxic condition produced by the products or processes of a disease.

nosologic   Pertaining to nosology.

nosologist [NOSO- + -LOGIST]   One specializing in nosology.

nosology [NOSO- + -LOGY]   **1** The science of the systematic classification of diseases.   **2** A systematic classification or list of diseases.

psychiatric nosology   The study of mental disorders from the point of view of their classification, grouping, ordering, and relationship to one another.

nosomania [NOSO- + -MANIA]   An obsolete term for HYPOCHONDRIASIS.

nosometry [NOSO- + -METRY]   The quantification of the amount of disease in a population. A seldom used term.

nosomycosis [NOSO- + MYCOSIS]   Any fungal disease or infection.

nosonomy [*nos(o)-* + Gk *onom(a)* a name + -Y]   The naming of diseases. A seldom used term.

nosoparasite [NOSO- + PARASITE]   **1** An organism associated with a particular disease and able to modify its course, but not serving as the actual causal agent.   **2** A pathogenic parasite that attacks only already diseased tissues.

nosophilia [NOSO- + -PHILIA]   An obsolete term for HYPOCHONDRIASIS.

nosophobia [NOSO- + -PHOBIA]   Pathologic fear of disease, maintained despite lack of credible evidence. Also called *pathophobia*.

nosophyte [NOSO- + Gk *phyt(on)* a plant, tree]   A plant microorganism that can give rise to pathologic conditions in humans or other hosts.

nosopoietic   An obsolete term for PATHOGENIC.

Nosopsyllus   A genus of fleas, normally ectoparasites of rodents.

Nosopsyllus fasciatus   The northern or European rat flea, a species that transmits the plague bacillus between rats and rarely to man. It is also a suspected vector of murine typhus. Also called *Ceratophyllus fasciatus*, *Pulex fasciatus*.

nosotaxy [NOSO- + -TAXY]   The ordering of diseases into a classification. A seldom used term.

nosotherapy [NOSO- + THERAPY]   The use of one disease to treat another, such as malaria-induced fever for the treatment of central nervous system syphilis.

nosotoxic   Of or pertaining to a nosotoxin.

nosotoxicity   The property of being nosotoxic.

nosotoxicosis   TOXICOSIS.

nosotoxin   Any toxin causing or associated with a disease.

nosotrophy [Gk *nosotrophi(a)* (from *noso(s)* sickness, disease + *treph(ein)* to nourish + *-ia* -Y) care of the sick]   The care of the sick.

nosotropic [NOSO- + -TROPIC[1]]   Directed against the manifestations or symptoms of a disease: said of a treatment or medication. Compare ETIOTROPIC.

nostology [Gk *nosto(s)* a return home + -LOGY]   An obsolete term for GERONTOLOGY.

nostrate [L *nostras*, gen. *nostratis* (from *noster* ours) pertaining to our own country or nation; in pl. *nostrates*, as substantive, our countrymen]   An older term for ENDEMIC.

nostrils   NARES.

nostrum [L, neut. sing. of *noster* our, ours]   A quack medication, usually a preparation made with a private, secret formula and promoted with exaggerated claims about its healing powers for a variety of diseases.

Nostyn A proprietary name for ectylurea.

notal Pertaining to the back; dorsal.

notalgia DORSALGIA.

  notalgia paresthetica Pain and paresthesiae in the back following the distribution of the posterior primary rami of the lumbar nerves. It is thought to be due to entrapment of one or more of these nerves.

notalysin An antibacterial substance obtained from the fungus *Penicillium notatum*.

notancephalia [*not(o)-* + Gk *an-* priv. + *kephal(ē)* the head + -IA] A congenital deficiency in the posterior part of the skull.

notanencephalia [*not(o)-* + Gk *an-* priv. + ENCEPHAL- + -IA] A congenital absence or deficiency of the cerebellum. A seldom used term.

notatin An obsolete term for GLUCOSE OXIDASE.

notch

notch INCISURA.

  acetabular notch INCISURA ACETABULI.

  anacrotic notch A notch on the upstroke of an arterial pulse tracing. Also called *anacrotic incisura*.

  angular notch INCISURA ANGULARIS GASTRICA.

  antegonial notch A shallow depression in the lower border of the mandible at the anterior edge of the insertion of the masseter muscle. Also called *pregonium*.

  anterior cerebellar notch INCISURA CEREBELLI ANTERIOR.

  anterior notch of ear INCISURA ANTERIOR AURIS.

  aortic notch DICROTIC NOTCH.

  notch of apex of heart INCISURA APICIS CORDIS.

  auricular notch Either incisura anterior auris or incisura terminalis auris.

  buccal notch A notch in the flange of a denture where it crosses the buccal frenum.

  cardiac notch of left lung INCISURA CARDIACA PULMONIS SINISTRI.

  cardiac notch of stomach INCISURA CARDIACA GASTRICA.

  catacrotic notch A notch, or one of the notches, additional to the dicrotic notch on the downstroke of an arterial pulse tracing.

  clavicular notch of sternum INCISURA CLAVICULARIS STERNI.

  coracoid notch INCISURA SCAPULAE.

  costal notches of sternum INCISURAE COSTALES STERNI.

  cotyloid notch INCISURA ACETABULI.

  craniofacial notch An occasional defect in the bony partition separating the orbital and nasal cavities.

  dicrotic notch The notch preceding the dicrotic wave in the downstroke of an arterial pulse tracing, marking the closure of the semilunar valve. Also called *aortic notch.*

  digastric notch INCISURA MASTOIDEA OSSIS TEMPORALIS.

  duodenal notch of pancreas A slight groove between the cranial border of the head of the pancreas and the superior border of its body where the gastroduodenal artery and the superior portion of the duodenum overlap it. It is situated at the superior border of the neck of the pancreas.

  notch of ethmoid INCISURA ETHMOIDALIS OSSIS FRONTALIS.

  ethmoidal notch INCISURA ETHMOIDALIS OSSIS FRONTALIS.

  ethmoidal notch of frontal bone INCISURA ETHMOIDALIS OSSIS FRONTALIS..

  fibular notch INCISURA FIBULARIS TIBIAE.

  fibular notch of tibia INCISURA FIBULARIS TIBIAE.

  frontal notch INCISURA FRONTALIS.

  notch of frontal bone INCISURA FRONTALIS.

  notch of gallbladder FOSSA VESICAE BILIARIS.

  gastric notch INCISURA ANGULARIS GASTRICA.

  notch of glenoid cavity INCISURA GLENOIDALIS.

  greater ischiatic notch INCISURA ISCHIADICA MAJOR.

  greater sacrosciatic notch An outmoded term for INCISURA ISCHIADICA MAJOR.

  greater sciatic notch INCISURA ISCHIADICA MAJOR.

  hamular notch SULCUS HAMULI PTERYGOIDEI.

  Hutchinson's crescentic notch A notch in the incisal edge of a permanent incisor tooth, caused by congenital syphilis.

  iliosciatic notch An outmoded term for INCISURA ISCHIADICA MAJOR.

  inferior notch of neck of pancreas INCISURA PANCREATIS.

  inferior thyroid notch INCISURA THYROIDEA INFERIOR.

  inferior vertebral notch INCISURA VERTEBRALIS INFERIOR.

  infrasternal notch A surface depression at the lower end of the body of the sternum between the sternal attachments of the seventh costal cartilages and just above the fossa epigastrica.

  interarytenoid notch INCISURA INTERARYTENOIDEA LARYNGIS.

  interclavicular notch INCISURA JUGULARIS STERNI.

  intercondylar notch FOSSA INTERCONDYLARIS FEMORIS.

  intercondylar notch of femur FOSSA INTERCONDYLARIS FEMORIS.

  interlobar notch INCISURA LIGAMENTI TERETIS.

  intertragic notch INCISURA INTERTRAGICA.

  intervertebral notch Either the incisura vertebralis superior or incisura vertebralis inferior.

  jugular notch Any of three notches: (1) incisura jugularis ossis occipitalis; (2) incisura jugularis ossis temporalis; (3) incisura jugularis sterni.

  jugular notch of occipital bone INCISURA JUGULARIS OSSIS OCCIPITALIS.

  jugular notch of sternum INCISURA JUGULARIS STERNI.

  jugular notch of temporal bone INCISURA JUGULARIS OSSIS TEMPORALIS.

  labial notch A notch in the flange of a denture where it crosses the labial frenum.

  lacrimal notch INCISURA LACRIMALIS MAXILLAE.

  lacrimal notch of maxilla INCISURA LACRIMALIS MAXILLAE.

  lesser ischiatic notch INCISURA ISCHIADICA MINOR.

  lesser sacrosciatic notch An outmoded term for INCISURA ISCHIADICA MINOR.

  lesser sciatic notch INCISURA ISCHIADICA MINOR.

  notch of ligamentum teres INCISURA LIGAMENTI TERETIS.

  mandibular notch INCISURA MANDIBULAE.

  marsupial notch An obsolete term for INCISURA CEREBELLI POSTERIOR.

  mastoid notch INCISURA MASTOIDEA OSSIS TEMPORALIS.

  median prostatic notch A well marked notch at the terminal end of the vertical median sulcus. It is located on the posterior border of the base of the prostate, just anterior to which is a deep depression for the entrance of the ejaculatory ducts.

  nasal notch INCISURA NASALIS MAXILLAE.

  nasal notch of maxilla INCISURA NASALIS MAXILLAE.

  palatine notch INCISURA PTERYGOIDEA.

  palatine notch of palatine bone INCISURA SPHENOPALATINA OSSIS PALATINI.

  pancreatic notch INCISURA PANCREATIS.

  parietal notch INCISURA PARIETALIS OSSIS TEMPORALIS.

  parietal notch of temporal bone INCISURA PARIETALIS OSSIS TEMPORALIS.

parotid notch The space occupied by the parotid gland, between the ramus of the mandible and the mastoid process of the temporal bone.

popliteal notch A groove in the extreme posterior part of the area intercondylaris posterior on the tibia where the posterior cruciate ligament is attached.

postcondylar notch An outmoded term for FOSSA CONDYLARIS.

posterior cerebellar notch INCISURA CEREBELLI POSTERIOR.

preoccipital notch INCISURA PREOCCIPITALIS.

presternal notch INCISURA JUGULARIS STERNI.

pterygoid notch INCISURA PTERYGOIDEA.

radial notch of ulna INCISURA RADIALIS ULNAE.

rivinian notch INCISURA TYMPANICA.

notch of Rivinus INCISURA TYMPANICA.

sacrococcygeal notch A space that is lateral to the sacrococcygeal joint and medial to the inferior lateral angle of the sacrum.

scapular notch INCISURA SCAPULAE.

semilunar notch of mandible An outmoded term for INCISURA MANDIBULAE.

semilunar notch of scapula An outmoded term for INCISURA SCAPULAE.

Sibson's notch An upward and medial extension of the area of cardiac dullness to percussion: a clinical sign of pericardial effusion.

sigmoid notch An outmoded term for INCISURA MANDIBULAE.

sphenopalatine notch INCISURA SPHENOPALATINA OSSIS PALATINI.

sphenopalatine notch of palatine bone INCISURA SPHENOPALATINA OSSIS PALATINI.

spinoglenoid notch The arched gap between the concave lateral margin of the spine of the scapula and the dorsal surface of the neck of the scapula.

sternal notch INCISURA JUGULARIS STERNI.

superior thyroid notch INCISURA THYROIDEA SUPERIOR.

superior vertebral notch INCISURA VERTEBRALIS SUPERIOR.

supraorbital notch **1** INCISURA SUPRAORBITALIS. **2** INCISURA FRONTALIS.

suprascapular notch INCISURA SCAPULAE.

suprasternal notch INCISURA JUGULARIS STERNI.

tentorial notch INCISURA TENTORII.

terminal notch of auricle INCISURA TERMINALIS AURIS.

trigeminal notch A depression in the superior margin of the petrous part of the temporal bone that is produced by the impressio trigeminalis.

trochlear notch of ulna INCISURA TROCHLEARIS ULNAE.

tympanic notch INCISURA TYMPANICA.

ulnar notch of radius INCISURA ULNARIS RADII.

umbilical notch INCISURA LIGAMENTI TERETIS.

---

notched Having one or more notches; emarginate.

notching / rib notching Localized erosions of the undersurfaces of ribs by enlarged and tortuous intercostal arteries, most commonly demonstrated radiologically and typically seen in patients with coarctation of the aorta.

note A sound, as one heard on auscultation.

bell note COIN SOUND.

cracked-pot note See under CRACKED-POT SOUND.

percussion note A sound produced by percussion, as of the chest.

Notechis A genus of active, aggressive, and fast-moving venomous snakes of the Elapidae family, occurring in Australia.

They are considered extremely dangerous.

notencephalocele [*not(o)*- + ENCEPHALOCELE] A protrusion of the brain through a developmental defect in the posterior part of the skull.

notencephalus [*not(o)*- + Gk *enkephalos* the brain] A fetus or postnatal individual with notencephalocele.

Nothnagel [Carl Wilhelm Hermann *Nothnagel*, Austrian physician, 1841–1905] **1** See under SIGN, SYNDROME, ACROPARESTHESIA. **2** Nothnagel's bodies. See under BODY.

nothrous [Gk *nōthr(os)* + -OUS] **1** Languid. **2** Stupid. An outmoded term.

notifiable Requiring notification by statute or regulation to a competent authority, as a government health department or local health officer, of a newly diagnosed case of a specified disease, an industrial injury, or other specified event.

notification The act of making an official record of an event.

notification of birth The legal requirement to inform a competent authority, usually a local health officer, of the occurrence of a birth. In some countries, notification of birth is required by law in addition to a legal obligation to register the birth with a registration officer.

notification of disease The legal requirement that the appropriate authority be informed of each patient newly diagnosed as suffering from one of a list of specified diseases.

not-me Denoting an experience that is foreign, unreal, and uncanny.

noto- [Gk *nōton* the back] A combining form denoting the back.

notochord [NOTO- + CHORD] A rod-shaped body composed of cells derived from the mesoblast, below the primitive groove of the embryo, found in all species of the phylum Chordata. It extends from the tail region cranially to the caudal edge of the thickened prochordal plate. The constituent cells become vacuolated and turgid. It is, to a variable extent in different vertebrates, incorporated within the vertebral column. In adult mammals it probably only persists as the nucleus pulposus, within the intervertebral disk. The notochord probably acts as the inductor for the axial nervous system. The vertebral bodies develop around the notochordal tissue. A bony arch then extends around the spinal cord to close off the vertebral canal. Also called *chorda dorsalis, notochordal rod*.

notochordoma [NOTO- + CHORDOMA] CHORDOMA.

Notoedres A genus of mites of the family Sarcoptidae. *N. cati* is the cause of notoedric mange of cats and rabbits.

notogenesis [NOTO- + GENESIS] The formation of the notochord in the early embryo.

notomelus [NOTO- + Gk *melos* a limb] Unequal conjoined twins in which the parasitic member is principally represented by one or more accessory lower limbs attached to the back of the host.

notomyelitis [NOTO- + MYELITIS] An obsolete term for MYELITIS.

not-self NONSELF.

nourishment [Middle English *norysshement*, from Old French *norissement* (from *norrir* to nourish, from L *nutrire* to suckle, feed, + *-ment* -MENT) nourishment] Food and the process of taking in food.

Novaldin A proprietary name for dipyrone.

novarsenobenzene NEOARSPHENAMINE.

novarsenobenzol NEOARSPHENAMINE.

novaurantia ORANGE G.

Nové-Josserand [Gabriel *Nové-Josserand*, French surgeon, flourished 20th century] See under METHOD.

novobiocin A toxic antibiotic with a narrow spectrum of activity. It is no longer used, but it is of value in research because it inhibits DNA gyrase. Also called *cardelmycin.*

Novocain A proprietary name for procaine hydrochloride.

novoscope [L *nov(us)* new + *o* + -SCOPE] An instrument formerly used for auscultatory percussion.

Novrad A proprietary name for levopropoxyphene napsylate.

Novy [Frederick George *Novy,* U.S. bacteriologist, 1864–1957] **1** Novy, McNeal and Nicolle medium. See under MEDIUM. **2** Novy and MacNeal blood agar. See under AGAR.

noxa [L, an injury, harm] (*plural* noxae) An injurious influence. A seldom used term.

noxious [L *noxius* (from *noxa* harm, injury, akin to *nocere* to injure) hurtful, injurious] Harmful or injurious to health.

noxious thing In forensic medicine, a substance unlawfully administered to another or taken by oneself with a deliberate intent to cause ill effects or death. It may be a poison or any substance capable of producing injury. The amount administered, the form of administration, and an individual's response must be considered before a substance can be designated a noxious thing.

noy A unit of perceived noisiness equal to the perceived noisiness of random noise in the frequency band 910–1090 Hz at a sound pressure level of 40 dB above 0.0002 microbar.

Np **1** Symbol for the element, neptunium. **2** Symbol for the unit, neper.

NPH neutral protamine Hagedorn (insulin). See under ISOPHANE INSULIN SUSPENSION.

NPH Iletin A proprietary name for isophane insulin suspension.

NPN nonprotein nitrogen.

NRC normal retinal correspondence.

ns Symbol for the unit, nanosecond.

n.s. not significant (i.e., statistically, or, in common usage, having a P value greater than 0.05).

nsec Symbol for the unit, nanosecond. An incorrect symbol.

NSHD nodular sclerosing Hodgkin's disease.

NSILA nonsuppressible insulinlike activity.

N·s/m² Symbol for the unit, newton-second per square meter.

N·s·m⁻² Symbol for the unit, newton-second per square meter.

NSR normal sinus rhythm.

nt Symbol for the obsolete unit, nit.

N-terminal Denoting the end of a polypeptide chain in which the amino acid has a free NH_2 group. Also *amino-terminal.*

NTP Symbol for normal temperature and pressure (usually 0°C and 1 standard atmosphere).

nU Symbol for nanounit.

nubecula [L (dim. of *nubes* a cloud), a little cloud, a dark spot] Cloudiness, as of the cornea or the urine. An obsolete term.

nubility [L *nubil(is)* (from *nubere* to marry, from Gk *nympheuein* to marry) ripe for marriage + -ITY] The condition of female sexual maturity; fitness of the female to marry.

nucha [Med. L, nape of the neck, from Arabic *nukhā'* spinal marrow] The back of the neck. It extends vertically between a horizontal line through the external occipital protuberance and one through the spine of the seventh cervical vertebra, and is bounded laterally approximately by the lateral margin of trapezius muscle on each side. Also called *nape.*

nuchal Pertaining to the nucha.

nucin An acid from the bark of the butternut, *Juglans cinerea.* It is one of the constituents of juglone, and is a cathartic,

hepatic stimulant, and antispasmodic. Also called *juglandic acid.*

Nuck [Anton *Nuck,* Dutch anatomist, 1650–1692] **1** Nuck's hydrocele. See under HYDROCELE FEMINAE. **2** Canal of Nuck. See under PERITONEOVAGINAL CANAL. **3** See under DIVERTICULUM.

nuclear [*nucle(us)* + -AR] **1** Pertaining to a nucleus. **2** Pertaining to the specialty of nuclear medicine.

nuclease Any enzyme that catalyzes the hydrolysis of nucleic acid.

micrococcal nuclease An enzyme (EC 3.1.31.1) from *Micrococcus* which hydrolyzes a polynucleotide, by endonucleolytic cleavage, to 3′-phosphomono- and oligonucleotide products.

nucleated Having a nucleus, as a eukaryotic cell.

nucleation [*nucle(us)* + -ATION] The process of formation of nuclei; specifically, the formation of small crystals in a saturated solution, a process necessary before crystal growth can occur.

nuclei Plural of NUCLEUS.

nucleic acid A nucleotide polymer composed of subunits which are either deoxyribonucleotides or ribonucleotides, joined to each other by phosphodiester bridges between (usually) the 5′-hydroxyl group of one nucleotide and the 3′-hydroxyl group of another. It is one of a group of long linear molecules found in chromosomes, mitochondria, ribosomes, bacteria, and viruses. The molecule may be DNA or various types of RNA. Upon hydrolysis it yields purine and pyrimidine bases, phosphoric acid, and a pentose sugar. Also called *nucleinic acid.*

infectious nucleic acid A nucleic acid which by itself is capable of initiating a viral replication cycle in a cell.

yeast nucleic acid RIBONUCLEIC ACID.

nucleiform Having the general form of a cell nucleus.

nuclein An aggregate of protein and nucleic acid. An obsolete term.

nucleinic acid NUCLEIC ACID.

nucleo- [L *nucleus* (for *nuculeus;* from *nux,* gen. *nucis,* nut) kernel of a nut, stone of a fruit] A combining form meaning nucleus, nuclear.

nucleoalbumin A complex of a nucleic acid with albumin. Also called *Mörner's body.*

nucleocapsid A unit of viral structure which consists of a nucleic acid encapsulated in a protein coat. A simple virus may be a single nucleocapsid, or nucleocapsids may be only part of the structure of a more complex virus.

nucleochylema [NUCLEO- + Gk *chylos* juice, chyle] KARYOLYMPH.

nucleocytoplasmic Pertaining to both the nucleus and the cytoplasm of a cell.

nucleofugal Moving away from the nucleus.

nucleography DISKOGRAPHY.

nucleohistone [NUCLEO- + HIST- + Gk *-ōnē,* fem. patronymic suffix] A complex of histone proteins and deoxyribonucleic acid found in the cell nucleus.

nucleoid [*nucle(us)* + -OID] **1** Having the appearance of a nucleus; resembling a nucleus. **2** A structure of variable shape in prokaryotes, containing the genetic material of the cell. Unlike the eukaryotic nucleus, the prokaryotic nucleoid does not have a membrane.

nucleolar Pertaining to the nucleolus.

nucleoli Plural of NUCLEOLUS.

nucleoliform Having the appearance and shape of a nucleolus. Also *nucleoloid.*

nucleolin The constituents of the nucleolus, primarily deoxyribonucleic acid, ribonucleic acid, and proteins.

nucleoloid NUCLEOLIFORM.

nucleololus NUCLEOLAR ORGANIZER.

nucleolonema A threadlike network composed of granules arranged in irregular rows in the nucleolus of the cell. The network is composed of nucleolar genes involved in the transcription of ribosomal RNA.

    reticular nucleolonema A pattern of nucleolar structure in which the pars granulosa forms an open framework.

nucleolonucleus NUCLEOLUS.

nucleolus [dim. of NUCLEUS. See NUCLEUS.] (*plural* nucleoli) A dense spherical accumulation of fibers and granules found in the nucleus of most eukaryotic cells. It is the site of transcription of ribosomal ribonucleic acid and of the production of ribosomes. The size of the nucleolus and the number of nucleoli varies with the requirement of a given cell for ribosomes and protein synthesis. Also called *nucleolonucleus, micronucleus, plasmosome* (obsolete). Adjective: nucleolar.

    chromatin nucleolus KARYOSOME.

    false nucleolus KARYOSOME.

    secondary nucleolus A small granular mass located near and resembling the nucleolus.

nucleolymph [NUCLEO- + LYMPH] KARYOLYMPH.

nucleomicrosome NUCLEOSOME.

nucleon [*nucle(us)* + *(prot)on*] One of the building blocks of an atomic nucleus, especially a proton or a neutron.

nucleonic Referring to the atomic nucleus or its constituent nucleons.

nucleonics [*nucle(us)* + *-on*, noun suffix denoting an elementary particle + -ICS] The branch of physics concerned with the phenomena of the atomic nucleus.

nucleopetal Tending to move toward the nucleus of a cell.

Nucleophaga A genus of chytrid fungus parasites of many protozoans that destroys the nucleus of the host.

nucleophile [NUCLEO- + -PHILE] A chemical species that is reactive owing to the availability of its electrons. It contributes both the electrons of the new bond formed between it and another species on reaction. It is so named because it has affinity for the positively charged nucleus of an atom.

nucleophilic Having an affinity for the nucleus of a cell, as a stain.

nucleoplasm The protoplasm of the cell nucleus. Also called *karyoplasm.*

nucleoprotein A complex of protein and nucleic acid, such as chromatin.

nucleoreticulum CHROMATIN NETWORK.

nucleorrhexis [NUCLEO- + -RRHEXIS] Degradation of a cell nucleus in which the nuclear material forms irregular cytoplasmic granules which are excreted from the cell. Also called *karyorrhexis, karyoclasis.*

nucleosidase **1** The enzyme (EC 3.2.2.1) that hydrolyzes an *N*-ribosylpurine to ribose and a purine. **2** Any enzyme that catalyzes the hydrolysis of a nucleoside.

nucleoside A molecule formed by bonding a purine or pyrimidine base with a pentose sugar, with an *N*-glycoside bond.

nucleoside deaminase An enzyme which catalyzes the deamination of the purine of a nucleoside, adenosine forming inosine, and guanosine forming xanthosine.

nucleosidediphosphatase The enzyme (EC 3.6.1.6) that catalyzes the hydrolysis of a nucleoside 5'-diphosphate to orthophosphate and a nucleoside 5'-phosphate. It is found preferentially at the forming face of the Golgi body in the cell cytoplasm

and serves as an indicator of the inner face. Also called *thiamin pyrophosphatase.*

nucleoside diphosphate A nucleoside esterified on one of its hydroxyl groups, nearly always on O-5', with diphosphoric acid. Such compounds are formed by transfer of phosphate groups from nucleoside triphosphates, which are common biologic phosphate donors.

nucleoside diphosphate kinase Any of a class of enzymes (EC 2.7.4.6) which catalyze the conversion of adenosine triphosphate and a nucleoside diphosphate to adenosine diphosphate and a nucleotide triphosphate. Also called *nucleoside diphosphokinase.*

nucleoside diphosphate sugars Any of the compounds consisting of nucleoside diphosphate with a simple, or complex, sugar bonded to the 5'-diphosphate group. Examples are uridine diphosphoglucose, and guanosine diphosphomannose.

nucleoside diphosphokinase NUCLEOSIDE DIPHOSPHATE KINASE.

nucleoside monophosphate Any nucleoside esterified with phosphoric acid on one of its hydroxyl groups. Unless otherwise indicated, the position of substitution is usually O-5'.

nucleosidemonophosphate kinase The enzyme (EC 2.7.4.4) that catalyzes the transfer of a group from ATP to a nucleoside 5'-phosphate to form ADP and a nucleoside 5'-diphosphate. This is usually a prelude to the building of a nucleoside 5'-triphosphate.

nucleoside phosphate PENTOSE NUCLEOTIDE.

nucleoside triphosphate A nucleoside esterified, usually on O-5', with triphosphoric acid. Nucleoside triphosphates are the precursors of nucleic acids, and they also act as phosphate donors and as the precursors of cyclic nucleotides.

nucleosin THYMOPOIETIN.

nucleosis The proliferation of nuclei within a single cell, such as that occurring in subsarcolemmal nuclei during regeneration of injured skeletal muscle cells. A seldom used term.

nucleosome The fundamental packing unit of chromatin. It is composed of a core particle and a unit of linker DNA for a total of about 200 base pairs of DNA. Also called *nucleomicrosome, nu body.*

nucleospindle The achromatic mitotic spindle formed during division of a cell nucleus.

nucleotidase **1** Any enzyme that catalyzes the hydrolysis of a nucleotide. **2** The enzyme (EC 3.1.3.31) that catalyzes the hydrolysis of many nucleoside 2'-, 3'- and 5'-phosphates to the nucleoside and orthophosphate. Also called *phosphonuclease.*

nucleotide A molecule formed from the combination of one nitrogenous base (purine or pyrimidine), a sugar (ribose or deoxyribose), and a phosphate group. It is a hydrolysis product of a nucleic acid.

nucleotide pyrophosphatase The enzyme (EC 3.6.1.9) that catalyzes the hydrolysis of a dinucleotide in which there is a residue of diphosphate (pyrophosphate) with breakage of the anhydride bond in this group, so that two molecules of mononucleotide are formed.

nucleotidyl The group formed by removing hydroxyl from the phosphorus atom of a nucleotide.

nucleotidyltransferase Any enzyme transferring a nucleotidyl group, usually using a nucleoside 5'-triphosphate as the donor. Such enzymes include DNA and RNA polymerases.

nucleotoxin [NUCLEO- + TOXIN] **1** Any substance which is toxic to the cell nucleus. **2** A toxic material which is produced by the cell nucleus.

nucleotropic Denoting antimicrobial or antiviral agents that alter nucleic acids.

nucleus

nucleus [L (for *nuculeus*; from *nux*, gen. *nucis*, nut, akin to Old English *hnutu* nut), kernel of a nut, stone of a fruit] (*plural* nuclei) **1** A membrane-bounded compartment in a eukaryotic cell which contains the genetic material and the nucleoli. The nucleus represents the control center of the cell. The nucleus divides by mitosis or meiosis. **2** The inner or central part of any structure; core. **3** In neuroanatomy, an aggregate of neurons. **4** The positively charged central core of the atom, consisting of protons and neutrons, except in the ordinary hydrogen atom, where there is a proton only. Over 99.9% of an atom's mass is in the nucleus.

abducens nucleus NUCLEUS NERVI ABDUCENTIS.

nucleus of abducens nerve NUCLEUS NERVI ABDUCENTIS.

nucleus abducentis NUCLEUS NERVI ABDUCENTIS.

nucleus accessorius NUCLEUS OCULOMOTORIUS ACCESSORIUS.

accessory nucleus NUCLEUS OCULOMOTORIUS ACCESSORIUS.

accessory nucleus of auditory nerve NUCLEI COCHLEARES VENTRALIS ET DORSALIS.

accessory cuneate nucleus NUCLEUS CUNEATUS ACCESSORIUS.

accessory medial nucleus A cell mass located at the border of the central grey matter in the rostral midbrain, dorsal and medial to the nucleus ruber. A seldom used term.

nucleus of accessory nerve NUCLEUS NERVI ACCESSORII.

accessory oculomotor nucleus NUCLEUS OCULOMOTORIUS ACCESSORIUS.

accessory olivary nucleus Nucleus olivaris accessorius medialis or nucleus olivaris accessorius lateralis.

acetabular nucleus OS ACETABULI.

nuclei of acoustic nerve NUCLEI NERVI VESTIBULOCOCHLEARIS.

nucleus acusticus Any of the nuclei comprising the nuclei nervi vestibulocochlearis.

nucleus acusticus inferior et lateralis NUCLEI COCHLEARES VENTRALIS ET DORSALIS.

nucleus acusticus superior NUCLEUS VESTIBULARIS SUPERIOR.

Aitken nuclei AITKEN PARTICLES.

nucleus alae cinereae NUCLEUS DORSALIS NERVI VAGI.

ambiguous nucleus NUCLEUS AMBIGUUS.

ambiguous nucleus of Quain An obsolete term for NUCLEUS NERVI HYPOGLOSSI.

nucleus ambiguus [NA] A column of cells in the lower half of the medulla oblongata, approximately halfway between the spinal nucleus of the trigeminal nerve and the inferior olivary complex. The nucleus receives afferents from the corticobulbar system and from the pharyngeal and laryngeal muscles and mucosa via the vagal, glossopharyngeal, and trigeminal nerves. Efferent fibers join the vagal, glossopharyngeal, and cranial part of the spinal accessory nerves. Also called *ambiguous nucleus, laryngeal nucleus, vagoglossopharyngeal nucleus* (seldom used).

nucleus amygdalae CORPUS AMYGDALOIDEUM.

nucleus amygdaliformis of J. Stilling NUCLEUS SUBTHALAMICUS.

amygdaloid nucleus CORPUS AMYGDALOIDEUM.

nucleus angularis NUCLEUS VESTIBULARIS SUPERIOR.

nucleus of the ansa lenticularis Small groups of neurons scattered along the course of the ansa lenticularis in the subthalamus.

anterior cochlear nucleus See under NUCLEI COCHLEARES VENTRALIS ET DORSALIS.

nuclei anteriores thalami [NA] Three groups of neurons lying beneath the dorsal surface of the rostral pole of the thalamus, where they form a distinct swelling, the tuberculum anterius thalami. The cell complex comprises a large principle nucleus, the anteroventral, and two accessory cell groups, the anterodorsal and anteromedial. The major afferent fiber source is the mamillary body, and all of the nuclei appear to project to the cingulate gyrus, Brodmann's areas 23, 24 and 32. These cell groups and their input and output connections form the thalamic portion of the Papez circuit. Also called *anterior nuclei of thalamus.*

anterior median nucleus The most rostral cell contingent of the paired visceral nuclei collectively referred to as the Edinger-Westphal nucleus. This portion of the oculomotor nerve nucleus lies on each side of the raphe and gives rise to uncrossed preganglionic parasympathetic fibers that emerge with the somatic root fibers.

anterior olfactory nucleus NUCLEUS NERVI OLFACTORII.

anterior nuclei of thalamus NUCLEI ANTERIORES THALAMI.

anterior ventral nucleus of thalamus NUCLEI ANTEROVENTRALIS.

nucleus anterodorsalis [NA] One of three components of the nuclei anteriores thalami. It contains small round cell bodies that receive afferents from the lateral mamillary nucleus and send efferents to the cingulate gyrus via the anterior limb of the internal capsule. See also NUCLEI ANTERIORES THALAMI.

anterolateral ventral nucleus NUCLEUS VENTRALIS ANTEROLATERALIS.

nucleus anteromedialis [NA] One of the three components of the nuclei anteriores thalami. It contains small round cells that receive afferents from the medial mamillary nucleus and send efferents to the cingulate gyrus. See also NUCLEI ANTERIORES THALAMI.

nucleus anteroventralis [NA] One of the three components of the nuclei anteriores thalami. It contains small round cells that receive afferents from the medial mamillary nucleus and fornix and send efferents to the cingulate gyrus. See also NUCLEI ANTERIORES THALAMI. Also called *anterior ventral nucleus of thalamus.*

nuclei arciformes NUCLEI ARCUATI.

arcuate nucleus NUCLEUS VENTRALIS POSTEROMEDIALIS.

arcuate nuclei of medulla oblongata NUCLEI ARCUATI.

nuclei arcuati [NA] Small irregular masses of grey matter found along the ventromedial aspect of the pyramid of the medulla oblongata. Afferent fibers are derived from the cerebral cortex, while efferent fibers project to the cerebellum as the crossed external arcuate fibers. Also called *arcuate nuclei of medulla oblongata, nuclei arciformes.*

auditory nuclei NUCLEI NERVI VESTIBULOCOCHLEARIS.

nuclei of auditory nerve NUCLEI NERVI VESTIBULOCOCHLEARIS.

autonomic nucleus of oculomotor nerve NUCLEUS OCULOMOTORIUS ACCESSORIUS.

Balbiani's nucleus BALBIANI'S BODY.

basal nucleus **1** A seldom used term for NUCLEUS OLIVARIS. **2** Basal ganglia: used in the plural.

nucleus basalis A seldom used term for NUCLEUS OLIVARIS.

basal olfactory nuclei Cell masses on the ventral and medial aspects of the cerebral hemisphere related to olfactory function. They include the nucleus of the olfactory tract, olfactory trigone, olfactory area, gyrus paraterminalis, and parolfactory area.

Béclard's nucleus BÉCLARD'S OSSIFICATION CENTER.

Bekhterev's nucleus NUCLEUS VESTIBULARIS SUPERIOR.

Blumenau's nucleus The lateral portion of the cuneate nucleus. A seldom used term.

nucleus of Burdach's column NUCLEUS CUNEATUS.

nucleus caudalis centralis [NA] A midline group of cells in the caudal third of the oculomotor nucleus. It gives rise to fibers, both crossed and uncrossed, that innervate the levator palpebrae muscle. Also called *central caudal nucleus.*

caudal vestibular nucleus NUCLEUS VESTIBULARIS INFERIOR.

caudate nucleus NUCLEUS CAUDATUS.

nucleus caudatus [NA] An elongated, arched mass of gray matter that forms one of the basal ganglia located deep to the cerebral cortex and bordering the lateral ventricle. It consists of a pear-shaped head lying rostral and lateral to the thalamus, a more slender body extending along the dorsolateral border of the thalamus, and a long curved tail that tapers around the roof of the ventricular temporal horn as far as the central nucleus of the amygdaloid body. The caudate nucleus, together with the putamen, from which it is separated by the internal capsule, form a functional unit known as the neostriatum of the basal ganglia. Major sources of afferent fibers are the cerebral cortex, medial thalamic nuclei, and substantia nigra. Most of its efferent fibers project to the putamen and globus pallidus. The caudate and lentiform nuclei are usually grouped together as the corpus striatum, and they help form the extrapyramidal system that influences the motor functions of the cerebral cortex, brainstem, and spinal cord. Also called *caudate nucleus, caudate, caudatum* (seldom used), *intraventricular nucleus of corpus striatum* (outmoded).

central caudal nucleus NUCLEUS CAUDALIS CENTRALIS.

nucleus centralis thalami A group of small and medium-sized neurons lying close to the wall of the third ventricle between the medial and posterior ventral complex of nuclei. They occupy the medial half of the intralaminar nuclei and are considered part of the intralaminar or nonspecific nuclei of the thalamus. Their connections are not completely understood, but they are believed to receive afferents from various cortical areas, the basal ganglia, more laterally-lying thalamic nuclei, and the brainstem. Efferent fibers probably project back upon most of these sites. Also called *central nucleus of thalamus.*

central nucleus of thalamus NUCLEUS CENTRALIS THALAMI.

centrodorsal nucleus NUCLEUS PROPRIUS OF POSTERIOR HORN.

nucleus centromedianus thalami NUCLEUS MEDIALIS CENTRALIS THALAMI.

nucleus cerebelli NUCLEUS DENTATUS CEREBELLI.

nucleus cerebelloacusticus A group of nerve cells in the lateral wall of the fourth ventricle. The relationship of these neurons to cell organization in the dorsomedial portion of the medulla oblongata is uncertain. An outmoded term.

cervical nucleus NUCLEUS LATERALIS CERVICALIS.

nucleus cinereum The central gray substance of the spinal cord. An obsolete term.

nucleus of circumolivary bundle of the pyramid See under CIRCUMOLIVARY BUNDLE OF THE PYRAMID.

Clarke's nucleus NUCLEUS THORACICUS.

nucleus of Clarke's column NUCLEUS THORACICUS.

clavate nucleus NUCLEUS GRACILIS.

Clarke-Monakow nucleus NUCLEUS CUNEATUS ACCESSORIUS.

cleavage nucleus A nucleus formed in the fertilized ovum after the union of the male and female pronuclei. It takes part in the first stage of cleavage. Also called *segmentation nucleus.*

cochlear nuclei NUCLEI COCHLEARES VENTRALIS ET DORSALIS.

nuclei cochleares ventralis et dorsalis [NA] The ventral, or anterior, and dorsal, or posterior, nuclei of the cochlear division of the eighth cranial nerve. These structures form a more or less continuous cell mass lateral and dorsolateral to the inferior cerebellar peduncle near the pontomedullary junction, but each contains distinctive cell types and cytoarchitectural organization. The dorsal cochlear nucleus forms an eminence (the acoustic tubercle) on the most lateral portion of the ventricular floor. Both nuclei receive axons that are the central processes of cells in the spiral ganglion. Efferent fibers from both nuclei are grouped into three acoustic striae, which are distributed bilaterally to several auditory processing centers in the brainstem, including the superior olive, the internal and external preolivary nuclei, the nucleus of the trapezoid body, and the nucleus of the lateral lemniscus. Also called *accessory nucleus of auditory nerve, nucleus acusticus inferior et lateralis, nuclei nervi cochlearis, nuclei of cochlear nerve, cochlear nuclei.*

nuclei of cochlear nerve NUCLEI COCHLEARES VENTRALIS ET DORSALIS.

nucleus colliculi inferioris [NA] A mass of nerve cell bodies comprising most of the substance of the inferior colliculus. They are divided into three groups: an ovoid cell mass, the central nucleus; a thin dorsal layer of cells, or cortex; and a pericollicular tegmentum surrounding the central nucleus on its ventral, lateral, and medial aspects and containing most of the myelinated fibers entering and leaving the colliculus. Afferent fibers come from the lateral lemniscus, the opposite inferior colliculus, the reticular formation, the ipsilateral medial geniculate body, and the auditory cortex. Efferent fibers project to the medial geniculate body, the contralateral inferior colliculus, the superior colliculus, and to more caudal relay nuclei in the auditory system. Also called *nucleus of inferior colliculus.*

commissural nucleus The right and left dorsal motor nuclei, when they merge at the midline to form a single cell cluster.

compact nucleus A cell nucleus in which the granular chromatin is packed in a smaller than normal volume. The condition occurs in a typical sperm nucleus.

conjugation nucleus ZYGOTE NUCLEUS.

nucleus conterminalis RETROPYRAMIDAL NUCLEUS.

nucleus corporis geniculati lateralis The nucleus of the lateral geniculate body, composed of a large, horseshoe-shaped, laminated mass of cells dorsally and a less defined ventral component. The dorsal complex consists of six concentric cell layers separated by intervening fiber bands. Crossed fibers from the optic tract terminate in laminae 1, 4, and 6, and uncrossed fibers end in laminae 2, 3, and 5. Corticogeniculate afferents arise from visual area 18. Efferent fibers project mainly to the primary visual cortex (area 17). The ventral nucleus is believed to represent a subthalamic structure related to the zona incerta. Also called *nucleus of lateral geniculate body.*

nucleus corporis geniculati medialis [NA] A neuron complex composed of small cells dorsally and large cells ventrally. Afferent fibers originate in a number of secondary auditory nuclei and the inferior colliculus, entering via the brachium of the inferior colliculus. Efferent fibers project to the superior temporal convolution via the auditory (geniculotemporal) radiation. Also called *nucleus of medial geniculate body, medial geniculate nucleus, nucleus of internal geniculate body.*

nuclei corporis mamillaris [NA] The nuclei of the mamillary body, which is located on the ventral surface of the posterior hypothalamus. There are three major cell groups: medial, intermediate, and lateral, of which the medial group is largest in man. The nuclei receive fibers from basal olfactory areas, septum, and fornix, and project to the anterior thalamus and mesencephalic tegmentum via mamillothalamic and mamillotegmental fasciculi. Also called *nuclei of mamillary body.*

nuclei corporis trapezoidei [NA] Several groups of nerve cells scattered among the fibers of the trapezoid body, medial to the superior olive in the tegmentum of the lower pons. These large, globular neurons receive thick axons from the contralateral cochlear nuclei that terminate on the trapezoidal cell bodies by means of large calixes in a one-to-one relationship. The cells project to the lateral superior olive on the same side.

cortical nucleus of amygdala PERIAMYGDALOID CORTEX.

nuclei of cranial nerves NUCLEI NERVORUM CRANIALIUM.

cuneate nucleus NUCLEUS CUNEATUS.

nucleus cuneatus [NA] A wedge-shaped mass of neurons on the dorsolateral aspect of the posterior medulla oblongata just above the spinobulbar junction. It is one of two major nuclei of the posterior funiculi and receives the ascending, heavily myelinated axonal branches of dorsal root ganglia, which transmit sensory impulses from the upper six thoracic and all cervical dermatomes. These fibers ascend in the fasciculus cuneatus and end in oblique serial laminae on the cells of the nucleus cuneatus. Efferent axons project ventromedially as internal arcuate fibers, cross the midline, and continue rostrally toward the thalamus as the medial lemnisci. Also called *cuneate nucleus, nucleus of Burdach's column, nucleus funiculi cuneati.*

nucleus cuneatus accessorius A group of nerve cells lying lateral to the nucleus cuneatus on the dorsolateral aspect of the caudal medulla oblongata. It receives heavily myelinated axons from dorsal root ganglia transmitting impulses from the first cervical through first thoracic dermatomes. It relays information from muscle spindles, group II fibers, and cutaneous afferents, and gives rise to cuneocerebellar fibers which enter the cerebellum via the inferior cerebellar peduncle. This nucleus is the medullary equivalent of the dorsal nucleus of Clarke. Also called *lateral cuneate nucleus, accessory cuneate nucleus, external cuneate nucleus, Monakow's nucleus, Clarke-Monakow nucleus.*

nucleus of Darkschewitsch One of three accessory oculomotor nuclei lying inside the ventrolateral border of the periaqueductal gray matter and lateral to the somatic cell columns of the oculomotor (III) complex. It is believed to receive fibers from the medial longitudinal fasciculus and superior colliculus. Its efferent fibers enter the posterior commissure, but do not reach the oculomotor complex or lower brain stem. Also called *Darkschewitsch's ganglion.*

daughter nucleus Either of the two nuclei resulting from mitosis. Each daughter nucleus has the same genetic information as the mother nucleus.

nucleus of Deiters NUCLEUS VESTIBULARIS LATERALIS.

dental nucleus DENTAL PULP.

dentate nucleus NUCLEUS DENTATUS CEREBELLI.

dentate nucleus of cerebellum NUCLEUS DENTATUS CEREBELLI.

nucleus dentatus cerebelli [NA] The largest of the deep, or roof, nuclei of the cerebellum, situated in the cerebellar white matter just lateral to the nucleus emboliformis. It receives axons from the Purkinje cells of the neocerebellum and collaterals from cerebellopetal mossy fibers. Its efferent fibers form most of the superior cerebellar peduncle and project mainly to the contralateral red nucleus and the ventrolateral nucleus of the thalamus. Also called *dentate nucleus, dentate nucleus of cerebellum, nucleus cerebelli, dentatum, nucleus oliva cerebellaris, corpus dentatum cerebelli* (obsolete), *dentate body of cerebellum* (obsolete), *corpus rhomboidale* (obsolete).

nucleus of descending fifth nerve NUCLEUS TRACTUS SPINALIS NERVI TRIGEMINI.

descending vestibular nucleus NUCLEUS VESTIBULARIS INFERIOR.

diploid nucleus A nucleus which contains two haploid sets of chromosomes, typical of the somatic cells of most animals.

disseminate nucleus An obsolete term for NUCLEUS PROPRIUS OF ANTERIOR HORN.

dorsal accessory olivary nucleus NUCLEUS OLIVARIS ACCESSORIUS DORSALIS.

dorsal nucleus of Clarke NUCLEUS DORSALIS CLARKII.

dorsal cochlear nucleus See under NUCLEI COCHLEARES VENTRALIS ET DORSALIS.

dorsal nucleus of glossopharyngeal nerve NUCLEUS DORSALIS NERVI GLOSSOPHARYNGEI.

nucleus dorsalis clarkii A column of neurons located in the medial part of spinal cord lamina VII at the base of the dorsal horn, and extending from C_8 through L_2 or L_3. Afferent fibers convey impulses from stretch, touch, and pressure receptors located in the lower extremities, abdomen, and trunk. Efferent fibers constitute the posterior spinocerebellar tract and project rostrally to the cerebellum. Also called *dorsal nucleus of Clarke, Clarke's column of spinal cord, nucleus dorsalis stillingi.*

nucleus dorsalis corporis trapezoidei A seldom used term for NUCLEUS OLIVARIS SUPERIOR.

nucleus dorsalis nervi glossopharyngei [NA] The rostral portion of the cell column forming the dorsal nucleus of the vagus (X) nerve. It is believed to contribute some fibers to the glossopharyngeal nerve. Also called *dorsal nucleus of glossopharyngeal nerve.*

nucleus dorsalis nervi vagi [NA] The dorsal motor nucleus of the vagus nerve, situated dorsal or dorsolateral to the nucleus intercalatus. It receives afferents from sensory nuclei of the glossopharyngeal and vagus nerves and gives origin to parasympathetic fibers, many of which are secretomotor in function. Also called *nucleus alae cinereae, dorsal nucleus of vagus nerve.*

nucleus dorsalis stillingi NUCLEUS DORSALIS CLARKII.

dorsal lateral nucleus NUCLEUS DORSOLATERALIS.

dorsal tegmental nuclei NUCLEI TEGMENTI MESENCEPHALICI.

dorsal nucleus of trapezoid body NUCLEUS OLIVARIS SUPERIOR.

dorsal nucleus of vagus nerve NUCLEUS DORSALIS NERVI VAGI.

dorsolateral nucleus NUCLEUS DORSOLATERALIS.

nucleus dorsolateralis [NA] A dorsally situated cell group in the lateral part of the oculomotor nuclear complex that innervates the inferior rectus muscle. Also called *dorsolateral nucleus, dorsal lateral nucleus.*

dorsomedial nucleus of hypothalamus NUCLEUS DORSOMEDIALIS HYPOTHALAMI.

nucleus dorsomedialis hypothalami The more dorsal of two cell groups in the medial part of the tuberal region of the hypothalamus. Also called *nucleus hypothalamicus dorsomedialis, dorsomedial nucleus of hypothalamus.*

dorsomedial nucleus of thalamus A prominent nuclear mass lying between the periventricular gray matter and the internal medullary lamina. It is composed of a magnocellular zone lying medially and a larger, more lateral, parvicellular zone. Extensive two-way connections exist with the cortex, basal forebrain, and amygdala, hypothalamus, and other areas of the thalamus. Connections between the parvicellular area and the prefrontal cortex are especially prominent in man. Also called *medial nucleus of thalamus, nucleus medialis thalami* (seldom used).

droplet nucleus The dried or partially dried residue, 0.1–3 μm in diameter, of an air-borne droplet that results from coughing, sneezing, or spraying.

Duval's nucleus A group of multipolar neurons in the medulla oblongata ventrolateral to the hypoglossal nucleus.

Edinger's nucleus NUCLEUS OCULOMOTORIUS ACCESSORIUS.

Edinger-Westphal nucleus NUCLEUS OCULOMOTORIUS ACCESSORIUS.

nucleus of the eleventh cranial nerve NUCLEUS NERVI ACCESSORII.

emboliform nucleus of cerebellum NUCLEUS EMBOLIFORMIS CEREBELLI.

nucleus emboliformis cerebelli [NA] A deep cerebellar (roof) nucleus found in great apes and man, lying between the nucleus globosus medially and the nucleus dentatus laterally. It receives fibers from Purkinje cells in the cerebellar hemispheres, and collaterals from cerebellopetal afferents. Its efferents project to the mesencephalon and thalamus via the superior cerebellar peduncle. Also called *embolus, emboliform nucleus of cerebellum.*

end nuclei   A seldom used term for NUCLEI TERMINATIONIS NERVORUM CRANIALIUM.

entopeduncular nucleus   NUCLEUS INTERPEDUNCULARIS.

even-even nucleus   A nucleus having an even number of protons and an even number of neutrons.

even-odd nucleus   A nucleus having an even number of protons and an odd number of neutrons.

external cuneate nucleus   NUCLEUS CUNEATUS ACCESSORIUS.

nucleus facialis   NUCLEUS NERVI FACIALIS.

nucleus of facial nerve   NUCLEUS NERVI FACIALIS.

family nucleus   NUCLEAR FAMILY.

fastigial nucleus of cerebellum   NUCLEUS FASTIGII CEREBELLI.

nucleus fastigii cerebelli   [NA] The most medial and phylogenetically oldest of the deep cerebellar nuclei, near the midline in the roof of the fourth ventricle. It receives fibers from Purkinje cells in the cerebellar vermis, and collaterals from olivocerebellar afferents. Efferent fibers reach the brainstem via the uncinate bundle (of Russell) and the juxtarestiform body. Also called *fastigial nucleus of cerebellum, nucleus tecti, nucleus of roof of cerebellum.*

fertilization nucleus   ZYGOTE NUCLEUS.

nucleus fibrosus linguae   An outmoded term for SEPTUM LINGUAE.

fibrous nucleus of tongue   An outmoded term for SEPTUM LINGUAE.

free nucleus   A nucleus isolated from a living cell.

nucleus funiculi cuneati   NUCLEUS CUNEATUS.

nucleus funiculi gracilis   NUCLEUS GRACILIS.

gametic nucleus   MICRONUCLEUS.

nucleus gelatinosus   NUCLEUS PULPOSUS DISCI INTERVERTEBRALIS.

germ nucleus   PRONUCLEUS.

germinal nucleus   PRONUCLEUS.

gingival nucleus   A cerebellar nucleus appearing during the fourth month of fetal life.

globose nucleus   NUCLEUS GLOBOSUS CEREBELLI.

nucleus globosus cerebelli   [NA] A deep cerebellar nucleus peculiar to the great apes and man, located between the emboliform nucleus laterally and the fastigial nucleus medially. It receives afferents from Purkinje cells of the paravermal cerebellar cortex, and collaterals from many cerebellar afferent fiber systems. Its axons leave the cerebellum primarily via the superior cerebellar peduncle, and project to various brainstem and thalamic nuclei. Also called *globose nucleus, spherical nucleus* (seldom used).

nucleus of Goll's column   NUCLEUS GRACILIS.

gonad nucleus   MICRONUCLEUS.

gracile nucleus   NUCLEUS GRACILIS.

nucleus gracilis   [NA] A column of neurons in the caudal portion of the medulla oblongata at the rostral end of the fasciculus gracilis of the spinal cord. This nucleus, which serves as the site of the initial synapse for the long ascending branches of cells in the dorsal root ganglia, also receives collaterals from the brainstem reticular formation and the pyramidal tract. Its efferent fibers exit the nucleus ventromedially, decussate, and turn rostrally to form the medial lemniscus, which projects to the nucleus ventrobasolateralis of the thalamus. Also called *gracile nucleus, clavate nucleus, nucleus funiculi gracilis, nucleus of Goll's column.*

gray nucleus   SUBSTANTIA GRISEA MEDULLAE SPINALIS.

gustatory nucleus   The enlarged rostral portion of the nucleus tractus solitarii in the medulla oblongata, which receives special visceral afferent (taste) fibers from the facial and glossopharyngeal nerves.

nucleus of habenula   NUCLEI HABENULAE.

nuclei habenulae   [NA] Two cell groups within the habenular trigone of the epithalamus that receive terminals from the stria medullaris thalami and give rise to the habenulointerpeduncular tract (fasciculus retroflexus). Also called *nuclei of habenula, habenular nuclei.*

habenular nuclei   NUCLEI HABENULAE.

haploid nucleus   A nucleus containing only a single set of chromosomes, as the nucleus of a gamete.

hypoglossal nucleus   NUCLEUS NERVI HYPOGLOSSI.

nucleus hypoglossalis   NUCLEUS NERVI HYPOGLOSSI.

nucleus of hypoglossal nerve   NUCLEUS NERVI HYPOGLOSSI.

hypothalamic nucleus   NUCLEUS SUBTHALAMICUS.

nucleus hypothalamicus dorsomedialis   NUCLEUS DORSOMEDIALIS HYPOTHALAMI.

India ink nucleus   The presence of hyperchromatic spots resembling droplets of India ink in nuclei in cytological specimens.

nucleus of inferior colliculus   NUCLEUS COLLICULI INFERIORIS.

inferior olivary nucleus   NUCLEUS OLIVARIS.

inferior salivatory nucleus   NUCLEUS SALIVATORIUS INFERIOR.

inferior vestibular nucleus   NUCLEUS VESTIBULARIS INFERIOR.

infundibular nucleus   Infundibulum hypothalami.

nucleus intercalatus   [NA] A group of neurons lying between the hypoglossal nucleus and the dorsal nucleus of the vagus nerve and forming part of the perihypoglossal nuclear complex. The cerebellum constitutes a primary source of afferent fibers, and efferents have been traced to several portions of cerebellum including the flocculus, nodulus, vermis, and anterior lobe. Also called *nucleus of Staderini.*

intermediate ventral nucleus of thalamus   NUCLEUS VENTRALIS INTERMEDIUS.

nucleus intermediolateralis   COLUMNA INTERMEDIOLATERALIS.

nucleus intermediomedialis   A column of small and medium-sized neurons lying in the most medial portion of lamina VII of the spinal cord, lateral to the central canal. The nucleus, which extends throughout almost the entire length of the spinal cord, receives small numbers of dorsal root fibers at all levels and may serve as a relay in the transmission of impulses to visceral motor neurons.

nucleus of internal geniculate body   NUCLEUS CORPORIS GENICULATI MEDIALIS.

nucleus interpeduncularis   [NA] An unpaired nuclear mass in the raphe of the ventral mesencephalic tegmentum, dorsal to the interpeduncular fossa and between the cerebral peduncles. It receives afferents from the stria medullaris thalami and habenular nuclei via the fasciculus retroflexus. Efferents project into the adjacent dorsal tegmental nucleus. Also called *entopeduncular nucleus, interpeduncular ganglion, intercrural ganglion, Ganser's ganglion* (obsolete), *corpus interpedunculare* (obsolete), *ganglion isthmi* (obsolete).

interstitial nucleus of Cajal   NUCLEUS INTERSTITIALIS.

nucleus interstitialis   [NA] A small collection of multipolar neurons near the rostral end of the medial longitudinal fasciculus in the mesencephalon. Afferent fibers come from various sources, largely via the medial longitudinal fasciculus. Efferent fibers are distributed to several nuclei of the oculomotor complex, the trochlear nuclei, the ipsilateral medial vestibular nucleus, and the spinal cord. Also called *interstitial nucleus of Cajal.*

nuclei intralaminares [NA] The nuclei within the internal medullary lamina of the thalamus. The include the centromedian and parafascicular nuclei and a group of smaller, more rostrally situated cell groups, such as the paracentral, central lateral, and central median nuclei. The connections of this system are not fully understood. Afferent fibers come from the spinal cord, brainstem, basal ganglia, and cortex, and efferents may be equally broadly distributed. Also called *intralaminar nuclei of thalamus.*

intralaminar nuclei of thalamus NUCLEI INTRALAMINARES.

intraventricular nucleus of corpus striatum An outmoded term for NUCLEUS CAUDATUS.

Kaiser's nuclei Spinal motor cells in the cervical and lumbar enlargements, arranged longitudinally between the nucleus intermediolateralis and the median column. An outmoded term.

Kölliker's nucleus SUBSTANTIA INTERMEDIA CENTRALIS MEDULLAE SPINALIS.

nucleus lacrimalis A poorly delineated group of neurons near the superior salivatory nucleus thought to project through the facial nerve to the pterygopalatine ganglion, where they synapse with neurons that then supply the lacrimal gland. Also called *lacrimatory nucleus.*

lacrimatory nucleus NUCLEUS LACRIMALIS.

large cell auditory nucleus NUCLEUS VESTIBULARIS LATERALIS.

laryngeal nucleus NUCLEUS AMBIGUUS.

lateral cervical nucleus NUCLEUS LATERALIS CERVICALIS.

lateral cuneate nucleus NUCLEUS CUNEATUS ACCESSORIUS.

nuclei laterales thalami [NA] A complex nuclear mass occupying the lateral half of the thalamus between the internal medullary lamina and the internal capsule, dorsal to the ventral nuclear group. Constituent cell masses include, from anterior to posterior, the lateral dorsal, lateral posterior, and pulvinar nuclei. Afferent connections are poorly understood, and efferent fibers project mainly to parieto-occipital neocortex.

nucleus of lateral geniculate body NUCLEUS CORPORIS GENICULATI LATERALIS.

nucleus lateralis NUCLEUS LATERALIS THALAMI.

nucleus lateralis cervicalis The lateral cervical nucleus of the spinal cord. A small longitudinal column of neurons in the lateral funiculus of the first and second cervical segments, serving as a relay center in the spinocervicothalamic pathway. Uncrossed afferent fibers come from cells in the posterior horn, reach the nucleus via the spinocervical tract, and transmit low-threshold cutaneous stimuli. Efferent fibers cross to the opposite side of the spinal cord, ascend in association with the contralateral medial lemniscus and terminate in the ventral posterolateral nucleus of the thalamus. Also called *lateral cervical nucleus, cervical nucleus.*

nucleus lateralis dorsalis [NA] A group of neurons located in the dorsolateral aspect of the thalamus that forms one of the nuclei in the lateral thalamic nuclear complex. In addition to having connections with other thalamic nuclei, this nuclear group appears to project to the cingulate gyrus as well as to the supralimbic cortex of the parietal lobe above that gyrus.

nucleus lateralis medullae oblongatae [NA] A small group of neurons in the ventrolateral portion of the medulla oblongata, dorsal to the inferior olive. It receives afferents from cerebral cortex, red nucleus, and spinal cord. Efferent fibers project almost exclusively to the anterior lobe and vermis of the cerebellum. Also called *lateral reticular nucleus.*

nucleus lateralis thalami The cell masses occupying the lateral half of the thalamus. Also called *nucleus lateralis, lateral nucleus of thalamus.* See also NUCLEI LATERALES THALAMI. • Because of the complexity of the area, the term is seldom used in its singular form.

nucleus of lateral lemniscus NUCLEUS LEMNISCI LATERALIS.

lateral posterior nucleus A large, thalamic association nucleus in the dorsolateral portion of the posterior thalamus.

lateral reticular nucleus NUCLEUS LATERALIS MEDULLAE OBLONGATAE.

lateral sympathetic nucleus COLUMNA INTERMEDIOLATERALIS.

lateral nucleus of thalamus NUCLEUS LATERALIS THALAMI.

lateral tuberal nuclei NUCLEI TUBERALES.

lateral vestibular nucleus NUCLEUS VESTIBULARIS LATERALIS.

nucleus lemnisci lateralis [NA] Diffuse groups of cells situated along the medial face of the lateral lemniscus during its course through the pons and caudal mesencephalon. Also called *nucleus of lateral lemniscus.*

nucleus of lens NUCLEUS LENTIS.

nucleus lenticularis NUCLEUS LENTIFORMIS.

lentiform nucleus NUCLEUS LENTIFORMIS.

nucleus lentiformis [NA] That portion of the corpus striatum consisting of the globus pallidus and putamen. In frontal sections it appears wedge-shaped, and is located adjacent to the inferolateral border of the internal capsule, which separates it from the caudate nucleus rostrally and the thalamus caudally. Also called *nucleus lenticularis, lenticular body* (obsolete), *lenticula, lentiform nucleus, lentiform.* • Though considered an anatomical entity because of its roughly lens-shaped configuration, the embryological derivation and connections of its two component nuclei differ.

nucleus lentis [NA] The hard central core of the substance of the lens of the eye. Also called *nucleus of lens, central cartilage* (outmoded).

lower sensory nucleus of trigeminal nerve An obsolete term for NUCLEUS TRACTUS SPINALIS NERVI TRIGEMINI.

nucleus of Luys NUCLEUS SUBTHALAMICUS.

nucleus magnocellularis An obsolete term for NUCLEUS VESTIBULARIS LATERALIS.

magnocellular vestibular nucleus NUCLEUS VESTIBULARIS LATERALIS.

nuclei of mamillary body NUCLEI CORPORIS MAMILLARIS.

medial accessory olivary nucleus NUCLEUS OLIVARIS ACCESSORIUS MEDIALIS.

medial geniculate nucleus NUCLEUS CORPORIS GENICULATI MEDIALIS.

nucleus of medial geniculate body NUCLEUS CORPORIS GENICULATI MEDIALIS.

nucleus medialis centralis thalami [NA] The largest, most caudal, and most easily defined of the thalamic intralaminar nuclei, lying between the dorsomedial nucleus above and the ventral posteromedial nucleus below, and composed of several cell types, both large and small. Its medial border interfaces with the parafascicular nucleus, and its edges are swept by fibers of the internal medullary lamina. Its connections are not fully understood, but it is known to receive afferent fibers from a number of sites, including Brodmann's area 4 of the cerebral cortex, the basal ganglia, thalamus, brainstem reticular formation, spinothalamic tract, globus pallidus, and spinal cord. Efferent fibers project to more lateral thalamic nuclei, the caudate nucleus, putamen, and cerebral cortex. Also called *nucleus centromedianus thalami, centrum medianum of Luys.*

nucleus medialis dorsalis A thalamic nucleus consisting of a rostral magnocellular and a caudal parvocellular part. It has interconnecting fibers with many other thalamic nuclei and receives input from the amygdaloid nuclei and the piriform cortex; this nucleus sends fibers to the corpus striatum, the hypothalamus, and the frontal cortex. Also called *nucleus mediodorsalis.*

nucleus medialis thalami [NA] A seldom used term for DOR-

SOMEDIAL NUCLEUS OF THALAMUS.

nucleus medialis ventralis Part of the thalamic midline nuclei, or central commissural system. Also called *nucleus reuniens.*

medial mamillary nucleus The largest component of the nuclei corporis mamillaris containing the neurons contributing axons principally to the mamillothalamic and mamillotegmental tracts.

medial thalamic nuclei An ambiguous term for the nuclei of the medial, but not midline, thalamus, the largest component of which in man is the huge nucleus medialis dorsalis, the neurons of which project to frontal lobe association cortex.

medial nucleus of thalamus NUCLEUS MEDIALIS THALAMI.

medial vestibular nucleus NUCLEUS VESTIBULARIS MEDIALIS.

nucleus mediodorsalis NUCLEUS MEDIALIS DORSALIS.

nucleus medullaris cerebelli An obsolete term for CORPUS MEDULLARE CEREBELLI.

medullary nucleus of cerebellum An obsolete term for CORPUS MEDULLARE CEREBELLI.

merocyte nucleus An additional nucleus inside a fertilized ovum, resulting from either polyspermia or deliberate experimental introduction.

nucleus of mesencephalic tract of trigeminal nerve NUCLEUS TRACTUS MESENCEPHALICI NERVI TRIGEMINI.

nucleus mesencephalicus nervi trigemini NUCLEUS TRACTUS MESENCEPHALICI NERVI TRIGEMINI.

mesoblastic nucleus The nucleus of a mesoblastic, or mesodermal, cell.

metastable nucleus An atomic nucleus between the stable and unstable state, in a state of excitation but unable to release energy and return to the normal state until it is involved in another collision or other influence.

nucleus of Meynert Groups of neurons located in the basal forebrain surrounding the diagonal band, anterior commissure, and the ventral border of the anterior half of the globus pallidus. These cells, which are rich in acetylcholine and choline acetyltransferase, project widely upon cerebral neocortex and undergo extensive degenerative changes in Alzheimer's disease.

Monakow's nucleus NUCLEUS CUNEATUS ACCESSORIUS.

mother nucleus The cell nucleus prior to mitosis, which generally divides to produce two daughter nuclei.

motion nucleus KINETOPLAST.

motor nucleus Any collection of nerve cells of the central nervous system giving rise to the motor fibers of a nerve.

nucleus motorius nervi trigemini [NA] The nucleus of origin of the motor fibers of the fifth cranial nerve, located in the dorsolateral portion of the pons just medial to the entering sensory root and the main sensory nucleus. Efferent fibers innervate the muscles of mastication, the tensor tympani, and the tensor veli palatini. Also called *motor nucleus of trigeminal nerve.*

motor nucleus of spinal cord A group of somatic motor cells located in the anterior horn whose axons project to striated voluntary muscles. It includes large alpha motor neurons (40–100 mm) and small gamma motor neurons (10–25 mm).

motor nucleus of trigeminal nerve NUCLEUS MOTORIUS NERVI TRIGEMINI.

nucleus nervi abducentis [NA] The nucleus of the abducens of the sixth cranial nerve, lying in the caudal part of the pontine tegmentum, forming the lateral portion of the facial colliculus in the floor of the fourth ventricle. Efferent fibers innervate the lateral rectus muscle of the eye. Discrete unilateral lesions there characteristally produce conjugate weakness or paralysis of lateral gaze toward the side of the lesion. Also called *nucleus abducentis, abducens nucleus, nucleus of abducens nerve, nucleus of the sixth cranial nerve.*

nucleus nervi accessorii [NA] The nucleus of the eleventh cranial nerve, the most caudal of all the cranial nerves. It is divided into cranial and spinal portions, which form, respectively, the internal and external branches of the nerve. The cranial root arises from neurons in the caudal portion of the nucleus ambiguus. The spinal portion arises from a cell column in the anterior horn extending from the fifth cervical segment to the level of the pyramidal decussation. The cranial root joins the vagus nerve and, as motor fibers of the inferior (recurrent) laryngeal nerve, supplies the intrinsic muscles of the larynx. The spinal root supplies the sternocleidomastoid and upper parts of the trapezius muscles. Also called *nucleus of accessory nerve, nucleus of the eleventh cranial nerve.*

nuclei nervi acustici NUCLEI NERVI VESTIBULOCOCHLEARIS.

nuclei nervi cochlearis NUCLEI COCHLEARES VENTRALIS ET DORSALIS.

nucleus nervi facialis **1** [NA] A collection of multipolar neurons in the ventrolateral tegmentum of the caudal pons dorsal to the superior olivary nucleus. Its efferent fibers innervate the muscles of facial expression, the platysma, the buccinator, and the posterior belly of the digastric and stapedius muscles. The emergent fibers first ascend into the dorsomedial portion of the tegmentum, where they turn sharply from medial to lateral around the rostral pole of the abducens nucleus, forming the internal genu of the facial nerve. They then descend to emerge from the ventrolateral aspect of the pons. Also called *nucleus of facial nerve, nucleus facialis.* **2** Collectively, the superior salivatory nucleus and the nucleus of the tractus solitarius, in conjunction with the motor nucleus.

nucleus nervi facialis of Arnold COLLICULUS FACIALIS.

nucleus nervi glossopharyngei [NA] The nuclear complex serving as origin and termination of the glossopharyngeal or ninth cranial nerve. Located in the medulla oblongata, it consists of sensory and motor, somatic and visceral elements served by the inferior salivatory nucleus, the rostral part of the nucleus ambiguus, and the rostrolateral, or gustatory, portion of the nucleus of the tractus solitarius.

nucleus nervi hypoglossi [NA] The nucleus of origin of the hypoglossal or twelfth cranial nerve, consisting of a column of large somatic motor cells in the dorsomedial portion of the caudal half of the medulla oblongata. The fibers supply the extrinsic muscles of the tongue. Also called *ambiguous nucleus of Quain* (obsolete), *nucleus hypoglossalis, nucleus of hypoglossal nerve, hypoglossal nucleus.*

nucleus nervi oculomotorii [NA] Several cell masses located in the dorsal part of the mesencephalic tegmentum immediately ventral to the central gray matter and lying between the medial longitudinal fasciculi. The nuclear complex is made up of lateral paired somatic cell groups, a median, unpaired somatic nucleus found only in the caudal third of the complex, and paired visceral cell masses (nucleus oculomotorius accessorius, also known as the Edinger-Westphal nucleus), which is parasympathetic in function. The somatic groups innervate the levator palpebrae superioris and all of the extraocular muscles except the lateral rectus and superior oblique. The visceral nuclei supply the sphincter pupillae and ciliary muscle via the ciliary ganglion and the short ciliary nerves. Also called *nucleus of oculomotor nerve.*

nucleus nervi olfactorii The neuronal region at the caudal end of the olfactory bulb, embedded in the olfactory tract to which it contributes axons. Also called *anterior olfactory nucleus, nucleus of olfactory tract.*

nucleus nervi pneumogastrici An obsolete term for FLOCCULUS.

nuclei nervi trigemini [NA] The complex of nuclei serving as origin and termination of the trigeminal nerve. The component nuclei extend from high cervical spinal cord levels to the mesencephalon, and include the spinal (descending) tract of the trigeminal nerve, the motor nucleus, the main sensory nucleus, and the mesencephalic root. Also called *nuclei of trigeminal nerve.*

nucleus nervi trochlearis [NA] A small compact group of cells constituting the nucleus of origin of the fourth cranial nerve. It lies close to the midline in the ventral part of the central grey matter of the caudal mesencephalon, indenting the dorsal surface of the medial longitudinal fasciculus. The emergent fibers have a long intracranial course, decussating dorsally in the superior medullary vellum, and innervate the superior oblique muscle of the eye. Also called *nucleus of trochlear nerve.*

nucleus nervi vagi [NA] The nuclear complex constituting the origin and termination of the vagus nerve. Situated in the floor of the fourth ventricle and in the dorsal third of the medulla oblongata, it includes the nucleus dorsalis, the nucleus ambiguus and the nucleus of the tractus solitarius. Also called *nuclei of vagus nerve, vagal nuclei.*

nuclei nervi vestibularis VESTIBULAR NUCLEI.

nuclei nervi vestibulocochlearis [NA] The nuclei of termination of the sensory fibers of the vestibular and cochlear divisions of the eighth cranial nerve, located in the dorsolateral portion of the medulla oblongata, and comprising the ventral and dorsal cochlear nuclei and the four vestibular nuclei, medial, lateral, inferior, and superior. Also called *vestibulocochlear nuclei* (seldom used), *nuclei of acoustic nerve, nuclei nervi acustici, nuclei of auditory nerve, auditory nuclei.*

nuclei nervorum cerebralium NUCLEI NERVORUM CRANIALIUM.

nuclei nervorum cranialium [NA] Those nerve cell groups whose axons form the twelve pairs of cranial nerves. With the exception of the spinal portion of the nucleus accessorius (XI), all are located within the cranial cavity. They include the nucleus nervi olfactorii (I), optici (II), oculomotorii (III), trochlearis (IV), trigemini (V), abducentis (VI), facialis (VII), vestibulocochlearis (VIII), glossopharyngei (IX), vagi (X), accessorii (XI), and hypoglossi (XII). Also called *nuclei of cranial nerves, nuclei nervorum cerebralium.*

nutrition nucleus MACRONUCLEUS.

nucleus oculomotorius accessorius [NA] A cluster of neurons located dorsal to the rostral part of the main oculomotor nucleus in the midbrain. It contains the preganglionic neuron cell bodies of the parasympathetic visceromotor nerve fibers that course in the oculomotor nerve and synapse in the ciliary ganglion. Also called *accessory oculomotor nucleus, nucleus accessorius, autonomic nucleus of oculomotor nerve, accessory nucleus, Edinger-Westphal nucleus, Westphal's nucleus, Edinger's nucleus.*

nucleus of oculomotor nerve NUCLEUS NERVI OCULOMOTORII.

odd-even nucleus A nucleus having an odd number of protons and an even number of neutrons.

odd-odd nucleus A nucleus having an odd number of protons and an odd number of neutrons.

nucleus of olfactory tract NUCLEUS NERVI OLFACTORII.

nucleus oliva cerebellaris NUCLEUS DENTATUS CEREBELLI.

nucleus olivaris [NA] A folded and convoluted band of gray matter enclosing a white core (the hilum nuclei olivaris), located in the ventral portion of the medulla oblongata just lateral and dorsal to the pyramidal tract. The largest nuclear mass of the medulla, it receives afferents from the spinal cord, mesencephalon, subthalamus, and cerebral cortex, and sends all of its efferents to the contralateral cerebellum, both vermis and hemisphere, via the inferior cerebellar peduncle. Also called *olivary nucleus, inferior olivary nucleus, nucleus olivaris inferior, nucleus basalis* (seldom used), *basal nucleus* (seldom used), *dentate body of medulla oblongata* (obsolete), *corpus dentatum olivae* (obso-

lete), *inferior olive, dentoliva* (obsolete).

nucleus olivaris accessorius dorsalis [NA] The band of cells lying dorsal to the primary nucleus of the inferior olive. It receives afferents mainly from the spinal cord, and sends efferents to the contralateral cerebellum, particularly the vermis. Also called *dorsal accessory olivary nucleus.*

nucleus olivaris accessorius medialis [NA] The band of gray matter lying between the olivary nucleus and the midline that projects fibers to the contralateral portion of the cerebellum, mainly the vermis. Also called *medial accessory olivary nucleus, pyramidal nucleus.*

nucleus olivaris inferior NUCLEUS OLIVARIS.

nucleus olivaris superior A column of nerve cells in the caudal portion of the ventrolateral pontile tegmentum, just dorsal to the trapezoid body. It receives afferents from the cochlear nuclei and sends efferents to the trapezoid body and lateral lemniscus. Also called *superior olivary nucleus, nucleus dorsalis corporis trapezoidei* (seldom used), *dorsal nucleus of trapezoid body* (seldom used), *superior olive.*

olivary nucleus NUCLEUS OLIVARIS.

ootid nucleus Any one of the four haploid nuclei that are produced by oocyte maturation through meiosis. In humans, three of the nuclei are polar bodies which degenerate.

nucleus of origin Any group of nerve cells giving origin to some or all of the fibers of a nerve tract or peripheral nerve.

nuclei of origin of cranial nerves NUCLEI ORIGINIS NERVORUM CRANIALIUM.

nuclei originis nervorum cerebralium NUCLEI ORIGINIS NERVORUM CRANIALIUM.

nuclei originis nervorum cranialium [NA] Groups of nerve cells in the central nervous system that give rise to axons exiting as the efferent fibers of the various cranial nerves. Also called *nuclei originis nervorum cerebralium, nuclei of origin of cranial nerves.*

Pander's nucleus An outmoded term for NUCLEUS SUBTHALAMICUS.

parabducent nucleus A group of neurons believed to lie in the reticular formation adjacent to or within the abducens nucleus that may give rise to efferents directed to the oculomotor nucleus for controlling horizontal eye movements. Also called *pontine center for lateral gaze.*

parabigeminal nucleus A group of cells lying between the lateral lemniscus and the periphery in the caudal half of the mesencephalon. Its connections are still obscure but it is believed to send efferents to the lateral nuclei of the pons.

paracentral nucleus of the thalamus A small cell group associated with the internal medullary lamina and constituting one of the intralaminar nuclei. It lies along the lateral border of the dorsomedial nucleus, fusing with the lateral central nucleus dorsolaterally and the medial central nucleus ventromedially. Its connections are uncertain, but it probably receives afferents from the brainstem reticular formation and frontal cortex, and sends efferents to the caudate nucleus.

parafascicular nucleus of the thalamus A group of cells in the caudal third of the thalamus lying medial to the centromedian nucleus and ventral to the dorsomedial nucleus. The fasciculus retroflexus of Meynert almost bisects it from dorsal to ventral. Its connections are not yet clear, but it appears to receive afferents from the spinothalamic tract, the brainstem reticular formation, and Brodmann's area 6 of cerebral cortex, and send efferents to the striatum, cerebral cortex, and possibly the mesencephalic tegmentum.

paramedian reticular nuclei Cell clusters located in the medullary reticular formation, dorsal to the inferior olive. Their major axonal projection is to the cerebellum.

nuclei paraventriculares anteriores et posteriores Rather distinct clusters of neurons located in the dorsomedial ventricular wall of the thalamus that are classified as belonging to the median or midline group of thalamic nuclei.

paraventricular nucleus of hypothalamus NUCLEUS PARAVENTRICULARIS HYPOTHALAMI.

nucleus paraventricularis hypothalami [NA] A well-defined cell group in the wall of the third ventricle in the supraoptic portion of the hypothalamus. Many of the cells are neurosecretory in function and send efferent fibers to the posterior lobe of the hypophysis. Also called *paraventricular nucleus of hypothalamus.*

perifornical nucleus Scattered cell groups found along the course of the fornix. A seldom used term.

perihypoglossal nuclei The nuclei adjacent to the hypoglossal nucleus, including the nucleus intercalatus, nucleus prepositus, and nucleus of Roller.

nucleus of Perlia A group of cells in the midline of the oculomotor nuclear complex. It is believed to be associated with ocular convergence. Also called *Spitzka's nucleus* (seldom used). See also CONVERGENCE CENTER.

nucleus pigmentosus pontis LOCUS CERULEUS.

polymorphic nucleus A nucleus with an irregular shape and having a number of lobes connected by strands of nucleoplasm.

pontine nuclei NUCLEI PONTIS.

nuclei pontis [NA] Groups of nerve cells among the fiber bundles of the pyramidal tract in the ventral portion of the pons upon which the fibers of the corticopontine system synapse. Efferent axons project largely, though not completely, upon the contralateral brachium pontis and thence to the cerebellum. Also called *pontine nuclei.*

pontobulbar nucleus A cell column located along the lateral and ventral aspects of the inferior cerebellar peduncle. It is believed to be a caudal continuation of the ventral pontine nuclei.

posterior cochlear nucleus See under NUCLEI COCHLEARES VENTRALIS ET DORSALIS.

nucleus posterior hypothalami [NA] A group of nerve cells in the posterior portion of the hypothalamus dorsal to the mamillary bodies. The nucleus has a number of afferent and efferent connections with the brainstem via the periventricular fibers and the dorsal longitudinal bundle. The area is sensitive to conditions of decreasing body temperature, and controls mechanisms for conservation and increased production of heat. Also called *posterior nucleus of hypothalamus.*

posterior nucleus of hypothalamus NUCLEUS POSTERIOR HYPOTHALAMI.

nucleus posterior thalami [NA] The large, caudal, pillowlike expansion constituting the posterior pole of the thalamus, generally divided, in man, into three main nuclei. Although its connections are not fully understood, it is known to receive afferents from the upper brainstem, thalamus, and cortex and to send efferents to occipital, parietal, and temporal parts of the cerebral cortex. Parts of this nucleus receiving tectothalamic projections may transmit visual information to the extrastriate visual cortex. Also called *pulvinar, pulvinar thalami, gibber inferior thalami, posterior nucleus of thalamus, posterior tubercle of thalamus, tuberculum posterius thalami.*

posterior nucleus of thalamus NUCLEUS POSTERIOR THALAMI.

posterior ventral nucleus of thalamus NUCLEUS VENTRALIS THALAMI POSTERIOR.

posterolateral ventral nucleus of thalamus NUCLEUS VENTRALIS POSTEROLATERALIS.

posteromarginal nucleus A thin layer of large nerve cells covering the tip of the dorsal horn and constituting lamina 1 of the spinal gray matter. Afferent fibers probably include many pain-transmitting axons from the lateral division of the dorsal root. Efferents enter the lateral white funiculus as ascending and descending fibers of the propriospinal system. They are known

to be activated by stimuli causing tissue injury, and to be inhibited by descending serotonergic fibers from the raphe nuclei of the brainstem.

premamillary nucleus A small group of hypothalamic cells lying near the anterosuperior surface of the medial mamillary nucleus.

preolivary nuclei Small groups of nerve cells lying ventromedial and ventrolateral to the superior olive. They probably serve as intercalated nuclei in the secondary auditory pathways.

nuclei preoptici medialis et lateralis Groups of small and medium-sized neurons located in the preoptic region of the basal forebrain, rostral to the anterior hypothalamic nuclei and dorsal to the supraoptic and suprachiasmatic nuclei. The medial preoptic nucleus lies immediately lateral to the preoptic periventricular nucleus, and the lateral preoptic nucleus is located adjacent but lateral to the medial preoptic nucleus.

nucleus prepositus An elongated group of nerve cells in the medulla oblongata extending from the oral pole of the hypoglossal nucleus almost to the abducens nucleus, and constituting one of the perihypoglossal nuclei. Afferent fibers come principally from the cerebellum, with smaller numbers from the midbrain and the face region of the sensorimotor cortex. Efferent fibers project to the cerebellum and to the ocular motor nuclei.

nucleus pretectalis [NA] A group of cells with indistinct boundaries lying rostral to the superior colliculi at the level of the posterior commissure. It receives afferents from the optic tract, the lateral geniculate body, several cortical areas, and the posterior thalamic nuclei, and sends efferents to the visceral nuclei of the oculomotor complex. It is thought to function as the principal midbrain center involved in the pupillary light reflex.

principal sensory nucleus of trigeminal nerve NUCLEUS SENSORIUS SUPERIOR NERVI TRIGEMINI.

nucleus proprius of anterior horn Small cells scattered among the large alpha motor neurons of the ventral horn of the spinal cord. They probably represent a mixture of gamma motoneurons and spinal interneurons such as Renshaw cells. A seldom used term. Also called *disseminate nucleus* (obsolete).

nucleus proprius of posterior horn A rather poorly defined column of cells of diverse morphology located in laminae III, IV, and V of the dorsal horn of the spinal cord. It is found at all levels of the cord, but the cells are most numerous in the lumbosacral area. Also called *centrodorsal nucleus, sensibilus proprius nucleus* (obsolete).

nucleus pulposus disci intervertebralis [NA] The inner, semifluid core of the intervertebral disks, composed at birth of soft, gelatinous mucoid material that is gradually replaced by fibrocartilage as it loses its elasticity and water-binding property with age, so that it merges with the surrounding annulus fibrosus. It is better developed in the cervical and lumbar regions than in the thoracic, and it is situated nearer the posterior than the anterior part of the disk. It is derived from the embryonic notochord, but all the notochordal cells disappear by the end of the second decade of life. Also called *pulpy nucleus, nucleus gelatinosus.*

pulpy nucleus NUCLEUS PULPOSUS DISCI INTERVERTEBRALIS.

pulvinar nucleus The thalamic nucleus that forms a caudal bulge (or "pillow") adjacent to the lateral geniculate nucleus. In the human brain it is a nuclear complex with its several nuclei comprising the largest thalamic region dominating the posterolateral thalamus.

pyknotic nucleus The shrunken, deeply basophilic appearance of the nucleus following cell death, due to clumping of the chromatin.

pyramidal nucleus NUCLEUS OLIVARIS ACCESSORIUS MEDIALIS.

nucleus radicis descendentis nervi trigemini NUCLEUS TRACTUS MESENCEPHALICI NERVI TRIGEMINI.

red nucleus NUCLEUS RUBER.

reproductive nucleus MICRONUCLEUS.

nucleus reticularis tegmenti A medial tegmental extension of pontine nuclear cells receiving afferents from the frontal and parietal cortex and from the cerebellum via the brachium conjunctivum, and sending efferents to the cerebellum via the middle cerebellar peduncle. Also called *reticulotegmental nucleus*.

nucleus reticularis thalami [NA] A thin sheet of multipolar nerve cells on the lateral surface of the thalamus within the external medullary lamina. Afferents are received from almost all of the thalamic specific nuclei, mesencephalic reticular cells, and the cerebral cortex. Virtually all of the efferents project back upon the thalamus, thereby providing powerful inhibitory modulation of thalamocortical activity. Also called *reticular nucleus of thalamus*.

reticular nucleus of subthalamus Groups of neurons scattered along the thalamic and lenticular fasciculi and the tegmental field of Forel and probably functioning as bed nuclei for these largely thalamopetal tracts. A seldom used term. Also called *nucleus of tegmental field*.

reticular nucleus of thalamus NUCLEUS RETICULARIS THALAMI.

reticulotegmental nucleus NUCLEUS RETICULARIS TEGMENTI.

retropyramidal nucleus Highly variable masses of nerve cells located between the dorsal surface of the pyramid and the inferior olive. Also called *nucleus conterminalis*.

nucleus reuniens NUCLEUS MEDIALIS VENTRALIS.

Roller's nucleus A group of large nerve cells in the medulla oblongata lying ventral to the rostral pole of the hypoglossal nucleus and adjacent to its root fibers. Like the other perihypoglossal nuclei of which it is considered part, its principal connections are with the cerebellum. Also called *sublingual nucleus*.

nucleus of roof of cerebellum NUCLEUS FASTIGII CEREBELLI.

roof nuclei of cerebellum The deep nuclei of the cerebellum, lying in the roof of the fourth ventricle and comprising the dentate, emboliform, globose, and fastigial nuclei.

nucleus rotundus A cellular mass of large multipolar neurons found in the diencephalon of reptiles and birds that may be homologous with some portion of the mammalian nucleus ventralis medialis in the thalamus.

nucleus ruber [NA] A paired, red ovoid mass in the anterior part of the midbrain, forming a part of the extrapyramidal system. Also called *red nucleus, tectorial nucleus, locus ruber, nucleus of Sappey* (seldom used).

sacral nucleus The extension into the lumbosacral spinal cord of the nucleus thoracicus. Also called *Stilling's sacral nucleus, Stilling's nucleus*.

nucleus salivatorius caudalis NUCLEUS SALIVATORIUS INFERIOR.

nucleus salivatorius cranialis NUCLEUS SALIVATORIUS SUPERIOR.

nucleus salivatorius inferior [NA] The caudal portion of the column of scattered cells in the dorsolateral part of the reticular formation in the upper pons and lower medulla oblongata whose axons constitute the general visceral efferent (parasympathetic) outflow of the glossopharyngeal nerve which, via the otic ganglion, supplies the parotid gland. Also called *inferior salivatory nucleus, nucleus salivatorius caudalis*.

nucleus salivatorius superior [NA] A group of scattered visceral neurons in the dorsolateral reticular formation of the upper medulla oblongata and the lower pons that constitutes the general visceral efferent (parasympathetic) outflow of the facial nerve (via the nervus intermedius), supplying the lacrimal, nasal, palatine, submandibular, and sublingual glands. The more caudal elements of this cell group constitute the nucleus salivatorius interior. Also called *superior salivatory nucleus, nucleus salivatorius cranialis*.

nucleus of Sappey A seldom used term for NUCLEUS RUBER.

Schwalbe's nucleus NUCLEUS VESTIBULARIS MEDIALIS.

Schwann's nucleus The nucleus of a Schwann cell.

secondary nucleus SUBNUCLEUS.

segmentation nucleus CLEAVAGE NUCLEUS.

semilunar nucleus NUCLEUS VENTRALIS POSTEROMEDIALIS.

sensibilus proprius nucleus NUCLEUS PROPRIUS OF POSTERIOR HORN.

nucleus sensorius inferior nervi trigemini NUCLEUS TRACTUS SPINALIS NERVI TRIGEMINI.

nucleus sensorius principalis nervi trigemini NUCLEUS SENSORIUS SUPERIOR NERVI TRIGEMINI.

nucleus sensorius superior nervi trigemini [NA] The primary receptive nucleus for afferent fibers carrying impulses for sensations of touch and pressure from all three divisions of the trigeminal nerve, located in the dorsolateral part of the medial pons. The neurons are characterized by large receptive fields, show high levels of spontaneous activity, and respond to a wide range of pressure stimuli with little adaptation. Also called *principal sensory nucleus of trigeminal nerve, superior sensory nucleus of trigeminal nerve, nucleus sensorius principalis nervi trigemini*.

sensory nucleus Any aggregate of neurons which receives the terminals of afferent (sensory) fibers entering the nervous system via a peripheral (spinal or cranial) nerve.

septal nuclei The paired medial and lateral nuclei continuous with septum pellucidum, near the base of the pillars of the fornix and overlying the nucleus of the diagonal band. Its connections are diverse but principally with the hippocampal formation via the fornix.

Setchenow's nuclei SETCHENOW CENTER.

shadow nucleus A cell nucleus in a stage of dissolution where it has lost its chromatin and does not stain with a nuclear stain.

Siemerling's nucleus One of the components of the oculomotor nuclear complex. A seldom used term.

nucleus of the sixth cranial nerve NUCLEUS NERVI ABDUCENTIS.

sole nuclei A collection of nuclei within a skeletal muscle cell at the myoneural junction.

nucleus solitarius NUCLEUS TRACTUS SOLITARII.

nucleus of solitary tract NUCLEUS TRACTUS SOLITARII.

somatic nucleus MACRONUCLEUS.

sperm nucleus MALE PRONUCLEUS.

spherical nucleus A seldom used term for NUCLEUS GLOBOSUS CEREBELLI.

spinal nucleus of accessory nerve NUCLEUS SPINALIS NERVI ACCESSORII.

nucleus spinalis nervi accessorii [NA] The groups of nerve cells in the anterior horn of the spinal cord at levels C_1 through C_5 or C_6 that contribute to the formation of the spinal roots of the accessory nerve. Also called *spinal nucleus of accessory nerve*.

nucleus of spinal tract of trigeminal nerve NUCLEUS TRACTUS SPINALIS NERVI TRIGEMINI.

spinal nucleus of trigeminal nerve NUCLEUS TRACTUS SPINALIS NERVI TRIGEMINI.

spinal vestibular nucleus NUCLEUS VESTIBULARIS INFERIOR.

spinocerebellar nucleus NUCLEUS THORACICUS.

Spitzka's nucleus A seldom used term for NUCLEUS OF PERLIA.

nucleus of Staderini NUCLEUS INTERCALATUS.

Stilling's nucleus 1 NUCLEUS THORACICUS. 2 SACRAL NUCLEUS.

Stilling's sacral nucleus SACRAL NUCLEUS.

striate nucleus Any of the components of the corpus striatum. An imprecise usage.

subependymal nucleus The dorsal cochlear nucleus. A seldom used term. See under NUCLEI COCHLEARES VENTRALIS ET DORSALIS.

sublingual nucleus ROLLER'S NUCLEUS.

submedial nucleus of thalamus Nucleus submedius: a small cell group lying along the internal medullary lamina in the anterior portion of the thalamus, ventral to the paracentral nucleus and dorsal to the nucleus medialis ventralis. It is considered part of the nonspecific or diffusely projecting nuclei of the medial thalamus.

nucleus subthalamicus [NA] A lens-shaped mass of gray matter on the inner surface of the peduncular portion of the internal capsule. Afferent fibers come primarily from the lateral segment of the globus pallidus via the subthalamic fasciculus, and efferents traverse the internal capsule and project primarily to the caudal portions of the medial segment of the globus pallidus. In man, discrete lesions of the nucleus result in forceful chorealike movements (hemiballismus). Also called *hypothalamic nucleus, corpus subthalamicum, nucleus of Luys, corpus luysii, nucleus amygdaliformis of J. Stilling, corpus hypothalamicum* (obsolete), *discus lentiformis* (obsolete), *Pander's nucleus* (outmoded), *body of Luys* (outmoded).

superior nucleus NUCLEUS VESTIBULARIS SUPERIOR.

superior olivary nucleus NUCLEUS OLIVARIS SUPERIOR.

superior salivatory nucleus NUCLEUS SALIVATORIUS SUPERIOR.

superior sensory nucleus of trigeminal nerve NUCLEUS SENSORIUS SUPERIOR NERVI TRIGEMINI.

superior vestibular nucleus NUCLEUS VESTIBULARIS SUPERIOR.

suprachiasmatic nucleus The small hypothalamic nucleus lying on the optic chiasm. It receives optic nerve fibers and it has been implicated in the control of circadian rhythms.

suprageniculate nucleus A triangular-shaped group of neurons extending dorsomedially from the medial geniculate nucleus between the pretectal area and the pulvinar. A seldom used term.

supramamillary nucleus A group of cells lying dorsal to the mamillary nucleus and thought to be a rostral extension of the tegmental gray matter.

supraoptic nucleus of hypothalamus NUCLEUS SUPRAOPTICUS HYPOTHALAMI.

nucleus supraopticus NUCLEUS SUPRAOPTICUS HYPOTHALAMI.

nucleus supraopticus hypothalami [NA] A sharply defined group of hypothalamic cells lying just above the optic chiasm that send their axons to the posterior lobe of the hypothalamus in the supraopticohypophysial tract. The cells are clearly neurosecretory in function and probably produce both vasopressin and oxytocin. Also called *nucleus supraopticus, supraoptic nucleus of hypothalamus.*

supraspinal nucleus Small clusters of somatic motor neurons in the ventral horn of the first cervical segment of spinal cord that extend a short distance into the lower medulla. Also called *nucleus supraspinalis of Jacobsohn.*

nucleus supraspinalis of Jacobsohn SUPRASPINAL NUCLEUS.

supratrigeminal nucleus A group of neurons near the motor nucleus of the trigeminal nerve. A seldom used term.

nucleus sympathicus lateralis COLUMNA INTERMEDIOLATERALIS.

nucleus taeniaeformis An obsolete term for CORPUS AMYGDALOIDEUM.

nucleus tecti NUCLEUS FASTIGII CEREBELLI.

tectorial nucleus NUCLEUS RUBER.

tegmental nuclei NUCLEI TEGMENTI MESENCEPHALICI.

nucleus of tegmental field RETICULAR NUCLEUS OF SUBTHALAMUS.

tegmental nuclei of Gudden NUCLEI TEGMENTI MESENCEPHALICI.

nuclei tegmenti mesencephalici [NA] Several cell groups in the rostral pons and caudal mesencephalon that lie close to the course of the superior cerebellar peduncle. Afferent fibers probably come from the precentral gyrus and the globus pallidus, while efferent projections are still uncertain. Also called *tegmental nuclei, dorsal tegmental nuclei, tegmental nuclei of Gudden.*

terminal nuclei NUCLEI TERMINATIONIS NERVORUM CRANIALIUM.

nuclei terminales NUCLEI TERMINATIONIS NERVORUM CRANIALIUM.

nuclei of termination of cranial nerves NUCLEI TERMINATIONIS NERVORUM CRANIALIUM.

nuclei terminationis nervorum cranialium [NA] Groups of cells within the central nervous system upon which the centripetal axons of the various cranial nerves synapse. Also called *nuclei of termination of cranial nerves, nuclei terminales, terminal nuclei, end nuclei* (seldom used).

nucleus thoracicus [NA] A column of large nerve cells found in the medial part of the base of the dorsal horn of the spinal cord just lateral to the central canal, extending from the seventh or eighth cervical to the second or third lumbar segment. The cells receive large-caliber primary afferent fibers primarily from muscle spindles, and efferents give rise to the ipsilateral dorsal spinocerebellar tract, which terminates ipsilaterally in the cerebellar vermal cortex as mossy fibers. Also called *nucleus of Clarke's column, Clarke's nucleus, Stilling's nucleus, spinocerebellar nucleus, posterovesicular column of Clarke.*

nucleus tractus mesencephalici nervi trigemini [NA] A slender cell column in the dorsolateral portion of the rostral pons and caudal mesencephalon. The cell bodies are unique in being monopolar primary sensory neurons, and resemble dorsal root ganglion cells. The peripheral processes of the cells form the mesencephalic tract, and carry proprioceptive impulses from the muscles of mastication. The central processes have widespread connections with brainstem and cerebellum, including the motor nucleus of the trigeminal nerve. Also called *nucleus of mesencephalic tract of trigeminal nerve, nucleus radicis descendentis nervi trigemini, nucleus mesencephalicus nervi trigemini.*

nucleus tractus solitarii [NA] A column of nerve cells lying in the dorsolateral aspect of the medulla oblongata to which course primary visceral afferent fibers from the facial, glossopharyngeal, and vagus nerves. These fibers include special sensory afferents conveying taste impulses from the tongue and palate, as well as general visceral afferents from the pharynx, esophagus, and gastrointestinal organs. Prior to entering the nucleus, the primary afferent fibers course longitudinally in the adjacent tractus solitarius. Neurons in the nucleus of the tractus solitarius project rostrally to the pons and to diencephalic levels. Also called *nucleus of solitary tract, nucleus solitarius.*

nucleus tractus spinalis nervi trigemini [NA] A column of nerve cells that extends from the site of entry of the trigeminal nerve in the pons caudally through the medulla oblongata to about the second cervical level of the spinal cord. It lies along the medial border of the descending or spinal tract of the trigeminal nerve, and primary afferent nerve fibers from this tract terminate within the nucleus throughout its extent. It is usually divided into an oral part, an interpolar part, and a caudal part and pain impulses and thermal and tactile sensations from most of the head and face are relayed from this nucleus to the reticular formation and the thalamus by way of secondary trigeminal tracts. Also called *spinal nucleus of trigeminal nerve, nucleus of descending fifth nerve, nucleus of spinal tract of trigeminal nerve, nucleus sensorius inferior nervi trigemini, lower sensory nucleus of trigeminal nerve.*

nucleus of trapezoid body NUCLEUS VENTRALIS CORPORIS TRAPEZOIDEI.

nucleus triangularis NUCLEUS VESTIBULARIS MEDIALIS.

nuclei of trigeminal nerve NUCLEI NERVI TRIGEMINI.

nucleus of trochlear nerve NUCLEUS NERVI TROCHLEARIS.

trophic nucleus Macronucleus.

tuberal nuclei NUCLEI TUBERALES.

nuclei tuberales [NA] Two or three well-delimited cell groups in the middle part of the lateral hypothalamus near the tuber cinereum. They contain small multipolar neurons arranged in round or oval clusters surrounded by a delicate fiber capsule. They often produce small elevations on the basal surface of the hypothalamus. Their functions and connections are unknown. Also called *nuclei tuberis, lateral tuberal nuclei, tuberal nuclei.*

nuclei tuberis NUCLEI TUBERALES.

vagal nuclei NUCLEUS NERVI VAGI.

vagoglossopharyngeal nucleus A seldom used term for NUCLEUS AMBIGUUS.

nuclei of vagus nerve NUCLEUS NERVI VAGI.

vegetative nucleus MACRONUCLEUS.

ventral cochlear nucleus See under NUCLEI COCHLEARES VENTRALIS ET DORSALIS.

nucleus ventralis anterolateralis [NA] The rostral subdivision of the ventral nucleus of the thalamus. It contains clusters of multipolar neurons arranged in distinct magnocellular and parvocellular portions. It receives input from the substantia nigra and globus pallidus, and projects to the cerebral cortex. Also called *nucleus ventralis thalami anterior, anterolateral ventral nucleus.*

nucleus ventralis corporis trapezoidei [NA] A group of nerve cells situated among the transverse auditory fibers crossing the pontine tegmentum as the trapezoid body. It acts as a relay for some fibers from the opposite cochlear nuclei, and contributes fibers to the lateral lemniscus. Also called *ventral nucleus of trapezoid body, nucleus of trapezoid body.*

nucleus ventralis intermedius [NA] The median subdivision of the ventral nucleus of the thalamus. It is subdivided into pars oralis, medialis, and caudalis, and receives projections from the contralateral half of the cerebellum and from the ipsilateral substantia nigra and globus pallidus. It projects to Brodmann's areas 4 and 6 of the precentral cortex. Also called *nucleus ventralis lateralis, nucleus ventralis thalami intermedius, intermediate ventral nucleus of thalamus.*

nucleus ventralis lateralis NUCLEUS VENTRALIS INTERMEDIUS.

nucleus ventralis posterolateralis [NA] The lateral portion of the nucleus ventralis thalami posterior, subdivided into pars oralis and caudalis. It receives sensory fibers of the spinothalamic tract and medial lemniscus, and projects to the postcentral cortex. Also called *posterolateral ventral nucleus of thalamus.*

nucleus ventralis posteromedialis [NA] The medial portion of the nucleus ventralis thalami posterior, receiving sensory data from the head via secondary trigeminal fibers and projecting to the postcentral cortex. Also called *arcuate nucleus, semilunar nucleus, posterior ventral nucleus of thalamus.*

nucleus ventralis thalami The ventral portion of the lateral nuclear mass of the thalamus, containing specific relay nuclei that project to motor and sensory areas of cerebral cortex. It is subdivided into a rostral nucleus ventralis anterolateralis, an intermediate nucleus ventralis intermedius, and a caudal nucleus ventralis thalami posterior. Also called *ventral nucleus of thalamus.*

nucleus ventralis thalami anterior NUCLEUS VENTRALIS ANTEROLATERALIS.

nucleus ventralis thalami intermedius NUCLEUS VENTRALIS INTERMEDIUS.

nucleus ventralis thalami posterior The largest and most caudal part of the nucleus ventralis thalami. It is subdivided into nucleus ventralis posterolateralis and nucleus ventralis posteromedialis, which relay sensory data to the postcentral gyrus.

ventral nucleus of thalamus NUCLEUS VENTRALIS THALAMI.

ventral nucleus of trapezoid body NUCLEUS VENTRALIS CORPORIS TRAPEZOIDEI.

nucleus ventrobasolateralis The lateral segment of the thalamic ventrobasal nuclear complex, receiving its principal lemniscal input from the nucleus gracilis; nucleus ventrobasalis, pars externa; and nucleus ventralis posterolateralis.

ventromedial nucleus of hypothalamus NUCLEUS VENTROMEDIALIS HYPOTHALAMI.

nucleus ventromedialis [NA] Neurons in the ventral part of the oculomotor (III) nucleus. A seldom used term.

nucleus ventromedialis hypothalami A cluster of small neurons situated ventrally in the tuberal region of the medial hypothalamus. It functions in the regulation of food and water intake. Also called *ventromedial nucleus of hypothalamus.*

vesicular nucleus A cell nucleus in which there are large unstained areas between the stained chromatin threads and granules.

vestibular nuclei A group of four relay nuclei found in the floor of the fourth ventricle. They receive primary vestibular fibers from the cristae of the semicircular canals and maculae of the saccule and utricle. They give rise to secondary vestibular projections to cerebellum, spinal cord, and motor nuclei of cranial nerves III, IV, and VI. The nuclei comprise the nucleus vestibularis inferior, lateralis, medialis, and superior. Also called *nuclei nervi vestibularis.*

nucleus vestibularis caudalis NUCLEUS VESTIBULARIS INFERIOR.

nucleus vestibularis cranialis NUCLEUS VESTIBULARIS SUPERIOR.

nucleus vestibularis inferior [NA] A group of neurons located in the dorsolateral aspect of the medulla oblongata that extends from the rostral limit of the nucleus gracilis to the pontomedullary junction adjacent to the point of entrance of the vestibular nerve. It receives fibers from the descending root of the vestibular nerve and gives rise to vestibulocerebellar fibers that project to the cerebellum, and descending fibers that join the medial longitudinal fasciculus. Also called *spinal vestibular nucleus, descending vestibular nucleus, caudal vestibular nucleus, nucleus vestibularis caudalis, inferior vestibular nucleus.*

nucleus vestibularis lateralis [NA] A group of nerve cells located laterally in the floor of the fourth ventricle at the caudal border of the pons, immediately rostral to the nucleus vestibularis inferior. It receives incoming primary afferent nerve fibers from the vestibular division of the vestibulocochlear nerve and axons from the cerebellar cortex and the fastigial nucleus of the cerebellum, and it gives rise to fibers that form the vestibulospinal tract, which exerts important facilitating influences on extensor muscle tone and spinal reflex activity. Also called *nucleus of Deiters, magnocellular vestibular nucleus, lateral vestibular nucleus, large cell auditory nucleus, nucleus magnocellularis* (obsolete).

nucleus vestibularis medialis [NA] A group of nerve cells located in the floor of the fourth ventricle medial to the lateral and inferior vestibular nuclei. The rostral part of the nucleus receives ascending branches of the bifurcated primary vestibular afferent fibers, while the more caudal part receives primary vestibular fibers by way of the descending root of the vestibular nerve. Also called *Schwalbe's nucleus, nucleus triangularis, medial vestibular nucleus.*

nucleus vestibularis superior [NA] A small aggregate of nerve cell bodies, the most rostrally located of the vestibular nuclei, lying in the pons at the angle formed by the floor and lateral wall of the fourth ventricle, cranial to the medial and lateral vestibular nuclei. Primary vestibular afferent fibers terminate in its central region. Also called *nucleus vestibularis cranialis, superior vestibular nucleus, nucleus angularis, Bekhterev's nucleus, nucleus acusticus superior, superior nucleus.*

vestibulocochlear nuclei A seldom used term for NUCLEI NERVI VESTIBULOCOCHLEARIS.

Voit's nucleus A cluster of small neurons that is accessory to the dentate nucleus of the cerebellum. A rarely used term.

Westphal's nucleus NUCLEUS OCULOMOTORIUS ACCESSORIUS.

yolk nucleus BALBIANI'S BODY.

zygote nucleus The nucleus of the fertilized ovum when the male and female pronuclei first unite. Also called *conjugation nucleus, fertilization nucleus, zygotic nucleus, synkaryon.*

zygotic nucleus ZYGOTE NUCLEUS.

---

nuclide [*nucl(eo)-* + *-ide,* irreg. from Gk *eid(os)* form, shape, species] A nuclear species as characterized by its atomic number (number of protons) and either its mass number or (less commonly) the number of neutrons.

radioactive nuclide RADIONUCLIDE.

stable nuclide Any nuclide which is not radioactive.

unstable nuclide RADIONUCLIDE.

Nuel [Jean-Pierre *Nuel,* Belgian physician, 1847–1920] See under SPACE.

NUG necrotizing ulcerative gingivitis.

Nuhn [Anton *Nuhn,* German anatomist, 1814–1899] Nuhn's gland, Blandin and Nuhn gland, anterior lingual gland of Blandin and Nuhn. See under GLANDULA LINGUALIS ANTERIOR.

nuisance In forensic medicine, any activity or condition caused by one or more individuals, that potentially or in fact offends public or private sensibilities, violates precepts of common decency, or endangers life and health. The resulting discomfort, annoyance, or inconvenience must be of sufficient magnitude that the law will presume resulting damage.

nulligravid [*null(us)* no one, none, no + *i* + *gravid(a)* pregnant] Having never been pregnant.

nulligravida [L *null(us)* no one, none, no + *i* + GRAVIDA] A woman who has never been pregnant.

nullipara [L *null(us)* no one, none, no + *i* + PARA] A woman who has never given birth to a viable infant.

nulliparity [L *null(us)* not any + *i* + *par(a)* + -ITY] The condition of being nulliparous.

nulliparous Having never given birth to a viable infant. Also *nonparous.*

nullisomic Lacking both members of a particular pair of homologous chromosomes.

numb [Middle English *nomen,* past part. of *nimen* to seize, take] Being without sensation.

number [French *nombre* (from L *numerus* a number, measure, akin to *nomen* a name and to Gk *nemein* to deal out, distribute) a number] **1** The sum total of a collection of units. **2** Relative place in a sequence of units determined by assigning a unique designation to each unit according to a system of count-

ing. **3** A symbol or word used to designate number.

atomic number The number of protons in an atomic nucleus. This number determines the normal number of orbiting electrons, and therefore the chemical properties of the atom and its position in the periodic table. Symbol: Z

Avogadro's number The number of specified particles in one mole of substance. It is about 6.023×10^{23}.

basic number HAPLOID NUMBER.

Brinell hardness number A rating that denotes the hardness of a substance. It is measured by the spherical surface area of indentation produced when a steel ball 1 cm in diameter is applied with a standard force, and it is expressed in kg/mm^2.

chromosome number The number of chromosomes normally present in the somatic cell of an organism. This number is the diploid or $2n$ chromosome number. One set of chromosomes (n) is contributed by each gamete in the formation of a zygote ($2n$). The chromosome number in human somatic cells is 46.

copy number The characteristic average number of copies of each bacterial plasmid per cell genome, determined by the genes that regulate replication. Small plasmids often have a much larger number than large plasmids.

dibucaine number A figure indicating the extent to which the enzyme pseudocholinesterase can be inhibited by dibucaine. Normal forms of the enzyme are inhibited to 75% or above. The variant form of the enzyme, associated with clinical conditions of excessive susceptibility to the effects of succinyl choline, is resistant to dibucaine. Homozygotes for the atypical enzyme have inhibition levels below 25%, and heterozygotes for the gene determining atypical enzyme activity usually have 40 to 60% inhibition.

expected number The number predicted according to a statistical hypothesis or mathematical model.

gametic number HAPLOID NUMBER.

haploid number The number of chromosomes that comprise a set. Also called *basic number, monoploid number, gametic number.*

iodine number An expression of the degree of unsaturation of fatty acids in a fat. It is derived from the quantity of iodine, in grams, that combine with 100 grams of the fat. Also called *iodine value.*

isotopic number The number obtained by subtracting the atomic number from the number of neutrons, giving the number of excess neutrons. The isotopic number is usually an important indication of the radioactivity of the nucleus.

Knoop hardness number A rating expressing hardness of a substance as determined by the indentation produced by a diamond indenter with a rhombic base and apical angles of 130° and 172°30′. It is used especially on very hard substances.

linkage number LINKING NUMBER.

linking number The number of superhelical turns present in a topographically constrained piece or region of DNA; designated α. The relaxed linking number ($α_0$) is the number of turns present in a topographically defined, but unconstrained, piece or region of DNA. A "+" sign indicates right-hand winding. Also called *linkage number, winding number.*

Mach number The ratio of the speed of a moving object to the speed of sound in the surrounding medium.

mass number The sum of the number of protons and the number of neutrons in the nucleus of a nuclide. It is the integer closest to the physical atomic mass of the nuclide. Symbol: A

monoploid number HAPLOID NUMBER.

neutron number The number of neutrons in a nucleus, obtained by subtracting the number of protons from the mass number. Symbol: N

quantum number An integer or half-integer used to designate one of the values of a dynamical variable which according to quantum theory can take on only discrete values, such as the energy of an atomic electron.

random number In statistics, a number expressed by a sequence of randomly chosen digits, from 0 to 9, each digit being such that any other might have been chosen with equal probability. Such numbers may be generated either by resort to irrational mathematical functions or to a mechanism that operates in an essentially random fashion. Tables of random numbers are available, and by their use an unbiased selection of a sample is assured, resulting in a random sample.

saponification number The number of milligrams of potassium hydroxide required to neutralize the fatty acids, free or combined, in one gram of fat. This number used to be determined by titrating the excess of potassium hydroxide, after the fat had been hydrolyzed with this reagent, as a method of determining the mean molecular mass of the fatty acids present.

transport number The fraction of the current carried by a specified ion when electric current passes through a solution.

turnover number A measure of enzyme activity equal to the number of molecules of substrate modified by one molecule of enzyme per unit time, usually when the enzyme is saturated with substrate. It is therefore equal to the rate constant for breakdown to products of the enzyme-substrate complex.

viable number The number of bacteria in a preparation that are capable of forming colonies when placed on an adequate culture medium. With bacteria that do not separate regularly on cell division, such as streptococci, the usual procedure measures the number of clumps and not of cells.

wave number The number of electromagnetic waves in unit length, measured as a reciprocal of length.

winding number LINKING NUMBER.

numbering The assignment of numbers, as to atoms in a molecule, for identifying position, sequence, or quantity.

series numbering In anatomy, the sequential numbering of parts, from proximal or cephalic to distal or caudal, such as of metameric segments, spinal nerves, etc.

numbness The condition of being numb.

waking numbness Transient numbness of the extremities on awakening.

numc. number concentration.

nummiform [L *numm(us)*, *numus* a coin + *i* + -FORM] Shaped like a coin; disk-shaped.

nummular [French *nummulaire* (from L *nummul(us)*, dim. of *nummus* a coin, from Gk *nomimos* legal, + French *-aire* -AR) a plant with coin-shaped leaves] **1** Having or tending to assume the shape of a coin; discoid. See also NUMMULAR SPUTUM. **2** Having or tending to assume the shape of a rouleau or stack of coins, as erythrocytes in small blood vessels.

nummulation The formation of a nummular arrangement, especially by erythrocytes. See also ROULEAU.

Numorphan A proprietary name for oxymorphone hydrochloride.

Nunn [Thomas William *Nunn*, English surgeon, born 1825] Nunn's gorged corpuscles. See under CORPUSCLE.

nunnation [New L *nunnatio* (from Arabic *nūn*, the letter *n* + L *-atio* -ATION) the adding of a final *n* in the declining of Arabic nouns] **1** Undue use of the sound of the letter "n" during speech. **2** The faulty production of the sound of the letter "n" which leads to the substitution of another sound such as that of the letter "d." An imprecise usage.

Nupercaine A proprietary name for dibucaine hydrochloride.

nuptiality [L *nuptial(is)* (from *nupti(ae)* nuptials, from *nuptus*, past part. of *nubere* to be wedded; + *-alis* -AL) pertaining to marriage + English -ITY] The frequency of marriages in a given population. The nuptiality rate is usually expressed as the number of marriages per 1000 population. Also called *marriage rate*.

nurse [French *nourrice* (from L *nutricia*, fem. of *nutricius* nourishing, akin to *nutrix*, gen. *nutricis*, a nurse, foster mother and to *nutrire* or *nutriri* to suckle, nourish, bring up) a wet nurse] **1** A health care professional trained to perform the duties and to assume the responsibilities of assisting the sick or disabled and of maintaining health; a practitioner of nursing. See also NURSING CARE. **2** A person charged with the duties of taking care of an infant or small child; a nursemaid.

attending nurse The nurse who is responsible for the care of a specified patient in a health care institution, especially in hospitals.

baccalaureate nurse A nurse who is a graduate of a baccalaureate nursing program.

chairside nurse A British term for DENTAL NURSE.

charge nurse The nurse in charge of patient care for an individual or an organizational unit.

community nurse A British term for PUBLIC HEALTH NURSE.

community health nurse A nurse who is responsible for providing or organizing care for a community or region, often involving public health services. A term used only in the U.S.

dental nurse A person who assists a dentist by passing instruments and materials to the dentist. A term used in Britain and New Zealand. Also called *chairside nurse (British usage)*.

district nurse **1** A nurse who is responsible for providing or organizing care for a health district. **2** In the United Kingdom, a registered nurse employed by a health authority to nurse patients in their own homes.

domiciliary nurse A British term for VISITING NURSE.

dry nurse A woman engaged to care for another's infant but does not breast-feed it. Compare WET NURSE.

factory nurse A nurse who, unlike a fully trained occupational health nurse, undertakes limited duties comprising provision of first-aid treatment at the workplace of acute illness and injuries and continued treatment of persons who stay at work. A term not used in the U.S.

general duty nurse A nurse whose duties are not specialized.

graduate nurse A nurse who has completed a nursing degree program.

head nurse The nurse who is in charge of an administrative unit.

hospital nurse A nurse who is employed by a hospital.

licensed practical nurse A nurse who is licensed by the government as a practical nurse.

licensed vocational nurse A nurse who is licensed by the government as a vocational nurse.

monthly nurse A nurse who attends women who have recently given birth. An older term.

occupational health nurse A nurse who has been trained in occupational health to promote and maintain health, to prevent disease and injury, and to provide treatment for injury and disease where necessary, for industrial workers.

office nurse A nurse who works in the office of a physician or other health care practitioner.

operating room nurse OR NURSE.

OR nurse A member of the operating room nursing staff specially trained to provide assistance to the operating team of surgeons. Also called *operating room nurse, theater nurse (used in India)*.

practical nurse A nurse who performs certain nursing functions but is not a graduate of a degree program in nursing and who may or may not be licensed.

preclinical student nurse A student nurse who has not yet entered the clinical component of training.

private nurse PRIVATE DUTY NURSE.

private duty nurse A nurse who is employed by or for a private patient. Also called *private nurse.*

psychiatric nurse A nurse with specialized postgraduate training in psychiatric theory and the management of patients with different types of psychiatric disorders.

public health nurse **1** A nurse who is employed by a public health agency or is involved in the provision of public health services. Also called *community nurse (British).* **2** In the United Kingdom, an unofficial term for HEALTH VISITOR.

registered nurse A nurse who has graduated from a formal training program and has been licensed by the appropriate governmental authority to practice nursing. Abbreviation: RN

registered general nurse In the United Kingdom and South Africa, a nurse with at least three years of training and who has passed the appropriate examination. Also called *state registered nurse* (outmoded). Abbreviation: RGN

scrub nurse A member of the operating room nursing staff who is in attendance at the operating table, having completed a surgical scrub and donned gown and gloves.

state registered nurse An outmoded term for REGISTERED GENERAL NURSE. Abbreviation: SRN

student nurse A nurse who is in training and has not been awarded a degree or certificate.

theater nurse **1** In Britain, the first assistant to the operating theater sister. **2** A term used in India for OR NURSE. • The sense of def. 1 is also found in South Africa and New Zealand.

trained nurse A nurse who has received formal training.

visiting nurse A nurse who visits and cares for patients in their homes or in other residential facilities. Also called *domiciliary nurse (British).*

wet nurse A woman engaged to breast-feed the infant of another. Also called *nutrix.* Compare DRY NURSE.

nurse aide NURSE'S AIDE. See under AIDE.

nurse-anesthetist A trained nurse who administers anesthetic agents to patients.

nurse-midwife A nurse who provides care to pregnant women including performing deliveries and associated services.

nurse-practitioner A nurse who usually has additional specialty training and who provides primary care or specialized services, usually under the supervision of a physician.

nursery [Middle English *norserie,* from *norse* (from Old French *norice* a nurse, from Late L *nutricia* a nurse, from L *nutrix,* gen. *nutricis,* a wet nurse, from *nutrire* to nourish) a nurse + *-rie* -RY] An area in a hospital where newborn infants are cared for.

day nursery A place where preschool children may be left under supervision during the day.

premature nursery A hospital nursery that provides specialized care to premature infants.

nurse specialist A nurse who usually has additional training beyond the nursing degree and who provides specialized services, often under the supervision of and in assistance to a physician.

nursing The health care profession devoted to the provision of nursing care and the training of nurses. Most training takes the form of a four-year degree program or a three-year diploma program. Nurses with additional training beyond the minimum requirements may assume a greater independent clinical role in providing health care. See also NURSING CARE.

foster nursing The nursing of a young animal by one other than the natural mother.

Nussbaum [Moritz *Nussbaum,* German histologist, 1850–1915] See under EXPERIMENT.

nut [Old English *hnutu,* akin to L *nux,* gen. *nucis,* a nut] A dry, indehiscent, hard, one-seeded fruit. It is generally produced by fusion of more than one carpel. Also called *nux.*

betel nut ARECA.

bissy nuts COLA.

kola nuts COLA.

poison nut NUX VOMICA.

nutation [L *nutatio* (from *nutatus,* past part. of *nutare* to nod, wag the head) a nodding] Involuntary or repetitive nodding of the head. Adjective: nutatory.

nutatory [L *nutat(us),* past part. of *nutare* to nod, wag the head + English *-ory,* a characterizing suffix] Denoting or pertaining to nutation.

nutgall OAK GALL.

nutmeg MYRISTICA.

nutrient [L *nutriens,* gen. *nutrientis,* pres. part. of *nutrire* or *nutriri* to suckle, nourish, bring up] Any substance in the diet which furnishes nourishment to the body.

available soil nutrient The nutrient that is available to a plant in a given growing season for growth, as contrasted to the total fertility or nutrient content of a soil.

essential nutrients Essential dietary substances that cannot be made in the body, such as vitamins, minerals, carbohydrate, some amino acids, and some fatty acids.

secondary nutrient A substance that stimulates the gut flora to produce other nutrients.

trace nutrient Any nutrient that is required by the body in quantities of a few milligrams or less.

nutrilite A specific growth factor required by a bacterium.

nutriment [L *nutriment(um)* food, nutriment] That which gives nourishment; food.

nutriology [*nutri(tion)* + *o* + -LOGY] NUTRITION.

nutrition [Late L *nutritio* (from L *nutritus,* past part. of *nutrire* or *nutriri* to suckle, nourish, bring up) nourishment, the act of nourishing or being nourished] **1** The process by which animals and plants assimilate and utilize exogenous substances for synthesis of new tissue and production of energy. Also called *threpsis.* **2** The study of the dietary requirements of human beings and other animals in a variety of normal and pathologic states. Also called *nutriology, threpsology, trophology.*

adequate nutrition Nutrition which supplies the body with all the essential nutrients in adequate amounts to maintain functioning.

hemotrophic nutrition The supply of nutritive substances through the placenta to the embryo by means of the circulation of the maternal bloodstream.

parasitic nutrition Nutrition obtained by an organism that lives in or on another organism and obtains its food from the substance or energy of this host organism.

parenteral nutrition The provision of nutritional requirements by a parenteral route. It is usually done intravenously, by means of a peripheral vein cannula or a central vein catheter.

rectal nutrition Administration of nutritive substances by way of the rectum.

saprophytic nutrition The absorption through the cell membrane of essential nutrients liberated from nonliving organic matter by extracellular digestion. This form of nutrition is characteristic of protozoa, yeast, molds, and some bacteria. Also called *saprophytism.*

total parenteral nutrition The provision of all nutritional requirements by a parenteral route, usually by infusion of a solution containing all the essential nutrients by way of a central or peripheral venous catheter. This method is used when oral or tube feeding is inadequate to prevent starvation or for hyperalimentation of a malnourished patient.

nutritional Pertaining or contributing to nutrition. Also *nutritive, nutritory.*

nutritiongram [NUTRITION + -GRAM] Five tests sometimes used to assess nutritional status. Total lymphocyte count, serum albumin analysis, and delayed hypersensitivity skin tests are used to measure visceral proteins and immune response. Triceps skinfold and midarm circumference measurements are used to assess body fat and muscle mass respectively.

nutritionist   One who has specialized knowledge in the professional study of the effects of food on the body in health and disease.

nutritious   Having nutritional value.

nutritive   NUTRITIONAL.

nutritory   NUTRITIONAL.

nutriture [*nutrit(ion)* + -URE]   The nutritional status of the body with regard to all nutrients or just one, such as a specific vitamin.

nutrix [L, wet nurse, nurse]   WET NURSE.

nutrose   A dried nutrient preparation made from milk and consisting mainly of sodium caseinate.

Nuttall [John Michael *Nuttall*, English physicist, died 1958] Geiger-Nuttall law. See under LAW.

Nuttallia [Babesia (Nuttallia); after George Henry Falkiner *Nuttall*, American-born English biologist, 1862–1937 + -IA]   BABESIA.

nux [L, a nut]   NUT.

nux moschata   MYRISTICA.

nux vomica   The poisonous dried ripe fruit of *Strychnos nux-vomica*. The cell wall and cell contents contain alkaloids, including strychnine and brucine. It is used as a bitter tonic and a central nervous system stimulant. Also called *quaker button, dog button, poison nut.*

nyacyne   NEOMYCIN.

nyad   NAIAD.

nychthemeral [Gk *nyx*, gen. *nyktos*, night + *hēmer(a)* day + -AL]   Of or relating to the alternation of day and night, particularly a single night followed by day. Also *nycterohemeral, nyctohemeral.*

nyct-   NYCTO-.

nyctalgia [NYCT- + -ALGIA]   Any recurrent nocturnal pain. An outmoded term.

nyctalope [Gk *nyktalōp(s)* (from *nyx*, gen. *nyktos*, night + *al(aos)* blind + *ōps* eye) one afflicted with night blindness]   An individual who is unable to see under scotopic (dark) conditions; one affected by nyctalopia.

nyctalopia [Gk *nyktalōp(s)* (see NYCTALOPE) + -*ia* -Y]   The inability to see well under scotopic (dark) conditions, due to faulty rod function. Also called *night blindness, nyctotyphlosis.*

nyctaphonia [NYCT- + APHONIA]   Nocturnal loss of voice or difficulty in speaking. Also called *nyctophonia.*

nycterine   NOCTURNAL.

nycterohemeral   NYCHTHEMERAL.

nycto- [Gk *nyx* (genitive *nyktos*) night, darkness]   A combining form meaning night, nocturnal. Also *nyct-.*

nyctohemeral   NYCHTHEMERAL.

nyctophilia [NYCTO- + -PHILIA]   Abnormal preference for darkness or night. Also called *scotophilia.*

nyctophobia [NYCTO- + -PHOBIA]   Pathologic fear of night or darkness. Also called *noctiphobia, scotophobia.*

nyctophonia   NYCTAPHONIA.

Nyctotherus   A genus of spirotrich ciliates in the family Plagiotomidae, order Heterotrichida, parasitic in the intestine of amphibians, fish, and invertebrates. As a sporozoic ciliate, it occasionally is found in human feces. *N. cordiformis* occurs in frogs and tadpoles, and *N. ovalis* in cockroaches and millipedes. *Nyctotherus*-like ciliates have been found in feces of elk and sheep in Wyoming after storage at 4°C for about 30 days.

nyctotyphlosis [NYCTO- + TYPHLO-² + -SIS]   NYCTALOPIA.

nycturia [NYCT- + -URIA]   NOCTURIA.

NYD   not yet diagnosed.

Nydrazid   A proprietary name for isoniazid.

Nyhan [William Leo *Nyhan*, U.S. physician, born 1926]   Lesch-Nyhan disease. See under LESCH-NYHAN SYNDROME.

nylon   A lightweight plastic polymer, frequently used for non-absorbable sutures.

nymph [Gk *nymph(ē)* a bride, wife, marriageable young woman]   A developmental stage in certain acarines and hemimetabolous insects, in which the developing juvenile resembles the adult, lacking mature genitalia and (in insects) fully developed wings, and in which growth occurs without any intermediate stages into the adult form.

nymph-   NYMPHO-.

nympha [Gk *nymphē* bride, chrysalis; in pl. *nymphai* part of the female genitalia.]   (*plural* nymphae) LABIUM MINUS PUDENDI.

nymphae   Plural of NYMPHA.

nymphal   **1** Relating to a nymph.   **2** Relating to the nymphae or labia minora.

nymphectomy [NYMPH- + -ECTOMY]   The excision of one or both labia minora.

nymphitis [NYMPH- + -ITIS]   An inflammation of the labia minora. An obsolete term.

nympho- [Gk *nymphē* bride, married woman]   A combining form denoting the nymphae (labia minora). Also *nymph-.*

nymphocaruncular   Of or relating to the labia minora and the carunculae hymenales.

nymphohymeneal   Pertaining to the labia minora and the hymen.

nymphoid [NYMPH + -OID]   Resembling a nymph; nymphlike.

nympholabial   Pertaining to the labia minora and the labia majora, especially to the furrow between them on each side.

nymphomania [NYMPHO- + -MANIA]   Hypersexuality in a woman. Also called *hysteromania, andromania* (obsolete), *clitoromania* (obsolete), *cytheromania* (obsolete), *estromania* (obsolete), *furor femininus, furor uterinus, lascivia* (obsolete).

nymphomaniac   A woman with nymphomania.

nymphoncus [NYMPH- + -ONCUS]   A swelling or hypertrophy of the labia minora. An obsolete term.

nymphotomy [NYMPHO- + -TOMY]   An incision into one or both of the labia minora.

Nyssen [René *Nyssen*, Belgian neurologist, flourished 20th century]   Van Bogaert-Nyssen-Peiffer disease. See under METACHROMATIC LEUKODYSTROPHY.

Nyssorhynchus   A subgenus of *Anopheles* mosquitoes, many species of which are medically important as malaria vectors in tropical America.

nystagmic   Pertaining to or having the characteristics of nystagmus.

nystagmiform   NYSTAGMOID.

nystagmogram   A recording of the eye movements in nystagmus.

nystagmograph   A device to record eye movements in nystagmus.

photoelectric nystagmography   The recording of nystagmic movements electronically.

nystagmoid   Resembling nystagmus; characteristic of or similar to nystagmus. Also *nystagmiform.*

nystagmus [Gk *nystagmos* (akin to *nystazein* to nod, esp. in sleep, to slumber, sleep, to be sleepy) a nodding, esp. in sleep, drowsiness]   Spontaneous, rapid, rhythmic movement of the eyes, occurring either on fixation or on ocular movement, and often due to faulty supranuclear or internuclear innervation. It may, however, be oscillatory or pendular due to poor fixation resulting from impaired visual acuity and is sometimes congenital. Also called *nystaxis, talantropia, ocular ataxia.* Adjective: nystagmic.

nystagmus against the rule A manifestation of miners' nystagmus, in which the characteristic eye movements occur when the eyes are looking down. When miners' nystagmus is not constantly present these movements can usually be elicited by looking upwards.

ataxic nystagmus Internuclear ophthalmoplegia due to a lesion of the medial longitudinal fasciculus, giving rise to nystagmus in the abducting eye appearing on lateral movement of the eyes, associated with impairment of medial movement of the adducting eye. Also called *anterior internuclear ophthalmoplegia, Harris sign, medial longitudinal fasciculus syndrome.*

aural nystagmus VESTIBULAR NYSTAGMUS.

Barany's nystagmus The vestibular nystagmus resulting from rotation of the body in the planes of the semicircular canals.

benign positional nystagmus The nystagmus accompanying paroxysms of benign positional vertigo.

caloric nystagmus Nystagmus occurring as the result of chilling or warming the inner ear by way of the external auditory meatus as in the caloric test.

cervical torsion nystagmus A form of vestibular nystagmus induced by asymmetric impairment of arterial blood flow to the inner ears by rotation of the head and neck causing distortion of a vestibular artery.

Cheyne's nystagmus CHEYNE-STOKES NYSTAGMUS.

Cheyne-Stokes nystagmus Nystagmus in which the timing of the ocular movements resembles that of Cheyne-Stokes respiration. Also called *Cheyne's nystagmus.*

congenital nystagmus Nystagmus that is present at or soon after birth. It may be the result of a birth injury or of a sex-linked inheritance without associated neurologic lesions.

deviational nystagmus NYSTAGMOID JERKS.

disjunctive nystagmus Repetitive ocular movements consisting of recurring convergence and divergence of the eyes.

dissociated nystagmus Any nystagmus in which the range of movement is different in the two eyes. Also called *incongruent nystagmus.*

down-beat nystagmus Vertical nystagmus occurring on downward gaze.

nystagmus of eccentric fixation Nystagmus in which the abnormal eye movement lessens or ceases at some position of the eyes, usually when directed to one side.

end-point nystagmus NYSTAGMOID JERKS.

end-position nystagmus NYSTAGMOID JERKS.

fixation nystagmus Nystagmus occurring when attention is directed towards an object.

incongruent nystagmus DISSOCIATED NYSTAGMUS.

jerking nystagmus PHASIC NYSTAGMUS.

labyrinthine nystagmus VESTIBULAR NYSTAGMUS.

latent nystagmus Nystagmus that occurs only when one eye is covered or receives reduced illumination.

lateral nystagmus Nystagmus in which the rhythmic movements are in a side to side direction.

miners' nystagmus Nystagmus caused by inefficient lighting which prevents stimulation of the macula sufficient to support reflex macular fixation. Movements of the eyeball are undulatory or rotary. This condition used to occur among coal miners, but with improved lighting in coal mines it is now rarely found. The condition is presently associated with psychoneurotic symptoms.

monocular nystagmus Nystagmus occurring in only one eye.

myopathic nystagmus Nystagmus caused by weakness of a muscle or by a defect of its innervation.

occupational nystagmus A condition resulting from prolonged deficient illumination and retinal fatigue. It used to be common among coal miners, but it has also been described among sewermen, ceiling plasterers, train dispatchers, and telegraphers. See also MINERS' NYSTAGMUS.

ocular nystagmus Nystagmus occurring only under conditions of difficulty or handicap in seeing.

opticokinetic nystagmus OPTOKINETIC NYSTAGMUS.

optokinetic nystagmus Nystagmus induced by looking at a moving pattern, such as houses observed from the window of a train or vertical stripes on a rotating drum. This can be induced on examination to test the integrity of ocular and vestibular mechanisms. Also called *opticokinetic nystagmus, railroad nystagmus, train-dispatchers' nystagmus, optomotor nystagmus.*

optomotor nystagmus OPTOKINETIC NYSTAGMUS.

oscillating nystagmus Any nystagmus in which the movements of the eyes in each direction are similar in speed and amplitude. Also called *undulatory nystagmus, vibratory nystagmus.*

palatal nystagmus PALATAL MYOCLONUS.

paretic nystagmus Nystagmus occurring in the field of action of a weakened extraocular muscle.

pendular nystagmus Oscillating nystagmus with slow, smooth, to-and-fro movements of the eyes like the swing of a long pendulum.

phasic nystagmus Nystagmus evoked by ocular movement in which there is a rapid repetitive movement of the eyes towards the direction of gaze followed each time by a slow recoil. Also called *jerking nystagmus, resilient nystagmus, rhythmic nystagmus.*

positional nystagmus Nystagmus induced by movement of the head in a particular direction or by any change in position of the head. It is often associated with positional vertigo. Also called *postural nystagmus.*

postrotational nystagmus The nystagmus observed in a subject immediately following rotation, as for example, after pirouetting or, in test conditions, rotating in the Bárány chair. It is due to the inertia of the endolymph in the semicircular canals resulting in a continuing flow relative to the now static fixed labyrinthine structure. Also called *secondary nystagmus.*

postural nystagmus POSITIONAL NYSTAGMUS.

provocation nystagmus Nystagmus provoked either by rapid side-to-side movements of the head or by the variety of cervical posture tests. The condition is best observed if the subject wears Frenzel glasses.

railroad nystagmus OPTOKINETIC NYSTAGMUS.

rebound nystagmus An uncommon variety of nystagmus seen in some patients with cerebellar degeneration in whom phasic nystagmus occurs on lateral gaze but fatigues in about 20 seconds. When the eyes return to the midline, phasic nystagmus to the opposite side develops but also fatigues rapidly.

resilient nystagmus PHASIC NYSTAGMUS.

retraction nystagmus Retraction of the globe of the eyes toward the orbit with each voluntary or spontaneous movement of the eyes. It is a sign of disease in the midbrain. Also called *nystagmus retractorius.*

nystagmus retractorius RETRACTION NYSTAGMUS.

rhythmic nystagmus PHASIC NYSTAGMUS.

rotatory nystagmus Nystagmus in which the rhythmic ocular movements show a rotatory component rather than to-and-fro movement in a horizontal or vertical plane.

secondary nystagmus POSTROTATIONAL NYSTAGMUS.

seesaw nystagmus A rare form of nystagmus in which one eye moves upward while the other moves downward repetitively. It usually results from lesions in the third ventricle or the pons.

train-dispatchers' nystagmus OPTOKINETIC NYSTAGMUS.

undulatory nystagmus OSCILLATING NYSTAGMUS.

unilateral nystagmus Nystagmus evoked by movement of the eyes to one side only and not to the other.

up-beat nystagmus   Nystagmus in which the rhythmic movements are in an up and down direction.

vertical nystagmus   Nystagmus occurring only in a vertical as distinct from a horizontal direction.

vestibular nystagmus   Nystagmus arising from disturbance of function of the vestibular end organs subserving the various balance mechanisms located within the bony labyrinth. Also called *aural nystagmus, labyrinthine nystagmus.*

vibratory nystagmus   OSCILLATING NYSTAGMUS.

visual nystagmus   Pendular nystagmus due to poor vision and impaired ocular fixation, as in albinism.

voluntary nystagmus   Nystagmus that can be initiated by the individual at will.

nystagmus-myoclonus   A rare form of congenital nystagmus that is associated with abnormal involuntary movements of the limbs and trunk.

nystatin $C_{46}H_{77}NO_{19}$. An antibiotic produced by *Streptomyces nowsei*. Specific actions on *Candida albicans* account for its use in the treatment of vaginal, intestinal, oral, and dermatologic infections by the latter. It is given orally or by topical application. Also called *fungicidin.*

nystaxis   NYSTAGMUS.

Nysten [Pierre Humbert *Nysten*, Belgian physician active in France, 1771–1818]   See under LAW.

nyxis [Gk *nyxis* a puncture, piercing]   PARACENTESIS.

O

O Symbol for the element, oxygen.

O. **1** Symbol for the nonmotile strain of an organism. **2** oculus. **3** occiput.

O₂ oxygen (diatomic form).

O₃ ozone.

o- ortho-.

Ω Symbol for the unit, ohm.

Ω⁻¹ Symbol for the unit, reciprocal ohm.

ω Symbol for the quantities (1) angular velocity, expressed in radians per second; (2) circular frequency, angular frequency, or pulsatance, expressed in reciprocal seconds; (3) solid angle, expressed in steradians.

OAF osteoclast activating factor.

oak [Old English *āc*] Any deciduous, semi-evergreen or evergreen tree or shrub of the genus *Quercus*.

poison oak **1** Either of two species of *Toxicodendron* shrub or vine. *T. diversilobum*, western poison oak, and *T. quercifolium*, eastern poison oak, can cause contact dermatitis as well as severe reactions in the oral cavity and gastrointestinal tract if ingested. An extract of the plant is used as an inhibitor of allergic reactions. **2** Dermatitis resulting from contact or exposure to the toxin of the poison oak plant.

oario- OOPHORO-.

oasis [Gk *oasis*, a word for the fertile islets in the Libyan desert, probably from Egyptian; Coptic *wahe*] A focus of normal tissue within a diseased area.

oath [Old English *āth*] A solemn assertion, declaration, or affirmation.

hippocratic oath See under HIPPOCRATES.

OB obstetrics.

ob- [L *ob* (assimilated before *c*, *f*, *g*, and *p* as *oc-*, *of-*, *og-*, and *op-*) against, in front of, before, on account of] A prefix meaning (1) towards, facing; (2) against, opposed to; (3) inverse, opposite. Also *oc-*, *of-*, *og-*, *op-*.

obcecation [OB- + L *caec(us)* blind + -ATION] Partial blindness.

obclavate [OB- + English *clavate*, from L *clavatus* club-shaped, from *clav(a)* a club + -*atus* -ATE] Having the shape of a bowling pin: used especially of fungal cells.

obdormition [Late L *obdormitio* (from L *obdormitus*, past part. of *obdormire* to sleep, sleep soundly) a sleeping soundly] Numbness and paresthesiae in any extremity or part of the body due to pressure upon a peripheral nerve.

obduction [L *obductio* (from *obductus*, past part. of *obducere* to cover, draw over) a veiling, covering over] A seldom used term for MEDICOLEGAL AUTOPSY.

obedience / automatic obedience The execution of another person's order blindly without regard for possible harmful consequences to oneself. It is particularly likely to occur in catatonic states and in mental retardation.

deferred obedience The execution of a prohibition or command the subject believes to have been issued in childhood many years earlier, occurring as part of an adult neurosis.

O'Beirne [James *O'Beirne*, Irish surgeon, 1786–1862] **1** See under EXPERIMENT. **2** O'Beirne's valve. See under SPHINCTER.

obeliac Of or relating to the obelion.

obeliad Toward the obelion.

obelion [Gk *obel(os)* a spit, obelisk + -*ion*, diminishing suffix] A craniometric point situated on the sagittal suture on a line joining the two parietal foramina.

Ober [Frank Roberts *Ober*, U.S. surgeon, 1881–1960] **1** Ober's test. See under SIGN. **2** See under OPERATION.

Obermayer [Friedrich *Obermayer*, Austrian physician, 1861–1925] See under TEST.

Obersteiner [Heinrich *Obersteiner*, Austrian neurologist, 1847–1922] **1** Obersteiner-Redlich area. See under OBERSTEINER-REDLICH ZONE. **2** Obersteiner-Redlich Line. See under OBERSTEINER-REDLICH SPACE.

obese [L *obesus* (from OB- + L *esus*, past part. of *edere* to eat, swallow, eat up, waste; Gk *edein* to eat, akin to German *essen* to eat) eaten away, meager, lean; fat, gross] Characterized by an excess accumulation of body fat; marked by or relating to obesity. Also *polysarcous*.

obesitas OBESITY.

obesity [OBESE + -ITY] A state of excess accumulation of body fat. Obesity is often defined specifically as an increase in body weight of more than 20% above the standard weight for a person's height, adjusted for age, sex, and race, although some authorities recommend that an excess of 10% is cause for treatment. Obesity has been associated etiologically with genetic, hypothalamic, and endocrine factors, and physical and psychologic trauma. Obese individuals have increased morbidity and mortality from respiratory diseases, hypertension, and endocrine and metabolic disorders. The usual treatments consists of diet therapy and behavior modification. Also called *obesitas, ventrosity, polysarcia, polypionia, hyperadiposis, hyperadiposity, adiposis*.

adrenocortical obesity The obesity characteristic of Cushing syndrome. There is a typical distribution of fat deposits in the cheeks, the nape of the neck, the supraclavicular fossae, and the trunk, the extremities being spared. Also called *centripetal obesity, hyperinterrenal obesity*.

alimentary obesity EXOGENOUS OBESITY.

buffalo obesity BUFFALO HUMP.

centripetal obesity ADRENOCORTICAL OBESITY.

endocrine obesity Obesity associated with any of several endocrine diseases, such as Cushing syndrome with hypercortisolism, eunuchoidism, and hyperinsulinism.

endogenous obesity Adiposity due to a metabolic or hormonal cause.

exogenous obesity Obesity resulting from overindulgence in food. Also called *alimentary obesity, simple obesity*.

hyperinsulinar obesity OBESITY OF HYPERINSULINISM.

obesity of hyperinsulinism Obesity due to excessive secretion of insulin, with hypoglycemia and gross increase of appetite. It is frequently observed in cases of islet cell adenoma of the pancreas. Also called *hyperinsulinar obesity*.

hyperinterrenal obesity An older term for ADRENOCORTI-CAL OBESITY.

hypogonad obesity HYPOGONADAL OBESITY.

hypogonadal obesity Obesity associated with deficient secretion of sex hormones. It is especially notable in cases of male hypogonadism. Also called *hypogonad obesity*.

hypothalamic obesity Adiposity due to any lesion affecting those centers of the hypothalamus that are involved in the control of appetite. Also called *pituitary obesity* (incorrect).

hypothyroid obesity A condition associated with myxedema, in which the accumulation of mucoid material and water subcutaneously and elsewhere gives a misleading appearance of obesity, whereas fat synthesis is actually diminished. Also called *myxedematous obesity*.

myxedematous obesity HYPOTHYROID OBESITY.

pituitary obesity An incorrect term for HYPOTHALAMIC OBESITY.

plethoric obesity Adrenocortical obesity with associated florid facies resulting from thin facial skin and polycythemia.

simple obesity EXOGENOUS OBESITY.

obesogenous Conducive to obesity.

obex [L (for *objex* a barrier, from *objectus*, past part. of *objicere* to put before), what is put before, hindrance, barrier] [NA] The midline apex of the V-shaped inferior boundaries of the fourth ventricle.

obfuscation [Late L *obfuscatio* (from OB- + L *fuscatus*, past part. of *fuscare* to darken, blacken, make swarthy or tawny) a making obscure] A process that involves darkening and thus making obscure.

object / anxiety object The object or situation that is feared and avoided in anxiety hysteria or phobic disorder.

bad object Any of the objects cathected with aggressive energy which are subsequently internalized and either become part of the critical, punishing superego or if too terrifying are split off and relegated to deeper layers of the unconscious.

good object Any of the objects cathected with libidinal energy which are subsequently internalized to support the ego's binding of the death instinct with libido.

libidinal object LOVE OBJECT.

love object 1 The external object whose representation is cathected with libido. Also called *libidinal object*. 2 The person to whom one is sexually attracted or whom one loves. Also called *sex object*.

partial object 1 A love object with whom the subject's relationship is based on immature or pregenital impulses. 2 A portion of the love object that is able to satisfy the subject's desire for the object, such as a fetish.

object of regard The point at which the eye looks; fixation point.

sex object LOVE OBJECT.

transitional object Any material thing such as a sheet or security blanket that soothes and reduces anxiety in the infant under stress, and particularly when going to sleep. Attachment to the object is made directly by the infant rather than by passive acceptance of a pacifier thrust upon him.

objectivation In psychiatry, the projection of one's unacceptable mechanisms followed by a readiness to recognize and overemphasize their significance in others.

objective [L *objectus* (from *objectus*, past part. of *objicere* to throw or put before, proffer, offer) a placing before, an object + *-ivus* -IVE] 1 Verifiably perceptible to the senses. 2 In psychology, existing outside the observer's body and thus measurable by physical instruments. 3 In a compound microscope, the lens system nearest the object to be viewed, functioning to focus the rays coming from or through the viewed object. Also called *object glass*.

achromatic objective An objective lens system that is corrected for axial (chromatic) aberration for two colors.

apochromatic objective A combination of fluorite lenses that allows correction for chromatic aberration in three wavelengths and for spherical aberration in two wavelengths. Also called *apochromat*.

binocular objectives A pair of objectives used to provide a stereoscopic image in dissecting microscopes.

dry objective Any microscope objective intended for use with air alone between the lens and the object examined.

fluorite objective Any objective system that employs fluorite lenses instead of glass.

immersion objective Any microscope objective intended for use with a liquid that bathes both the lens and the object examined.

oil-immersion objective An objective lens intended for use with immersion oil in contact with the lens and the cover glass over the object examined.

quartz objective A system of quartz lenses that permits the use in microscopy of ultraviolet light waves.

semiapochromatic objective A system of fluorite and optical glass lenses in which chromatic aberration is corrected for three wavelengths, but correction of spherical aberration is less than that possible with apochromatic objectives. Also called *semiapochromat*.

obligate [L *obligat(us)*, past part. of *obligare* (from *ob* against + *ligare* to bind) to tie to, bind] Having no alternative way of living, as, for example, an obligate parasite, an organism that can live only as a parasite. Compare FACULTATIVE.

oblique [French (from L *obliquus* slanting, sideways, from OB- + L *-liquus*, suffix akin to *liquis* oblique), on the bias, inclined from the perpendicular] Slanting rather than horizontal or perpendicular.

obliquity [OBLIQUE + -ITY] Oblique character or condition; inclination from the vertical or horizontal.

biparietal obliquity ASYNCLITISM.

Litzmann's obliquity POSTERIOR ASYNCLITISM.

Nägele's obliquity ANTERIOR ASYNCLITISM.

obliquity of pelvis An abnormal tilt of the pelvis in relation to the vertebral column, as seen in structural scoliosis of the lumbar spine.

Roederer's obliquity A fetal position in normal labor such that the occiput presents and flexion of the head will be likely.

obliquus Oblique.

obliteration The complete loss of a space or solid part of the body, by disease, irradiation, or surgery.

percutaneous transhepatic obliteration of varices An embolization of the coronary vein to halt bleeding from gastroesophageal varices. A catheter is inserted percutaneously into a portal vein radicle within the liver, then into the main portal vein, and finally into the coronary vein.

oblongata [New L, fem. of *oblongatus*, past part. of *oblongare* (from L *oblongus* oblong, rather long) to lengthen] A seldom used term for MEDULLA OBLONGATA.

oblongatal Denoting the medulla oblongata.

obmutescence The condition of being mute.

obnubilation [Late L *obnubilatio* (from L *obnubilatus*, past part. of *obnubilare* to make cloudy or obscure) a making clouded, darkened, obscure] STUPOR.

observerscope An endoscope with two eyepieces so that two persons can observe the image at the same time.

obsession [L *obsessio* (from *obsessus*, past part. of *obsidere* to beset, sit down near, blockade, from OB- + L *sedere* to sit, stay fixed) a blockade, a besetting] An idea or sensory image, usually experienced as senseless or repugnant, that repetitively and insistently forces itself into consciousness even though the subject tries his best to ignore or suppress it. Obsessions are a prominent feature of obsessive-compulsive neurosis. Also called *imperative idea, ruminative idea.*

brooding obsession An obsession with the metaphysical questions about the purpose of life, the goal of existence, etc. Also called *intellectual obsession.*

hallucinatory obsession An obsession that appears as an auditory or visual hallucination.

inhibiting obsession An obsession centering around doubts or scruples about one's actions, sometimes so intense as to restrict any and every activity.

intellectual obsession BROODING OBSESSION.

somatic obsession Preoccupation with one's body or one of its organs or parts.

obsessive **1** Manifesting an obsession. **2** Exhibiting a tendency to become preoccupied with details.

obsessive-compulsive Having the characteristics seen in obsessive-compulsive neurosis or obsessive-compulsive personality.

obsolescence [English *obsolesc(ent)*, from L *obsolescens*, gen. *obsolescentis*, pres. part. of *obsolescere* to become antiquated + -ENCE] A process of becoming or the state of being useless, as a physiologic function; otioseness.

glomerular obsolescence Loss of glomerular function due to sclerosis, hyalinization, or fibrosis.

obsolete No longer used, as a procedure or a word.

obstetric [L *obstetr(ix)* (from *obstare* to stand against) a midwife + -IC] Relating to the care of women during pregnancy, labor, delivery, and postpartum. Also *obstetrical.*

obstetrical OBSTETRIC.

obstetrician [OBSTETRIC + L *-ianus* -IAN] A physician who specializes in obstetrics. Also called *accoucheur, obstetrist.*

obstetrics [L *obstetr(ix)* a midwife + -ICS] The field of medicine dealing with the care of women during pregnancy, labor and delivery, and the postpartum period. Also called *maieutics* (older term), *tictology* (older term), *tocology* (older term). Adjective: obstetric, obstetrical.

obstetrist OBSTETRICIAN.

obstipation [Late L *obstipatio* (from L *obstipatus*, past part. of *obstipare* to press against) close pressure] An extreme degree of constipation.

obstruction [L *obstructio* (from *obstructus*, past part. of *obstruere* to build against, block, stop, from OB- + *struere* to put together, build, devise, akin to Gk *storennynai* to spread, make level) a hindrance, a closing up by building] Blockage to the normal flow of a hollow viscus, a duct, or a blood vessel.

false colonic obstruction OGILVIE SYNDROME.

female prostatic obstruction Obstruction of the bladder neck due to inflammation and/or hypertrophy of the proximal urethral glands which surround the posterior neck of the female urethra.

idiopathic ureteropelvic junction obstruction Obstruction of the renal pelvis outlet by extrinsic fibrous bands, intrinsic stenosis, or high insertion of the ureter in the renal pelvis. The conditions usually are congenital, and may or may not cause hydronephrosis.

intestinal obstruction Partial or complete blockage of the passage of contents through the intestine. See also ILEUS.

pyloric obstruction Blockage of the stomach at the junction of stomach and duodenum.

renal pelvic obstruction Obstruction of the renal pelvis by calculi, tumor, or idiopathic ureteropelvic junction obstruction. Hydronephritis and secondary infections with loss of renal function are common.

ureteral obstruction Obstruction of the ureter by a calculus, tumor, extrinsic fibrous bands, localized intrinsic stenosis, or retroperitoneal fibrosis. One or both ureters may be involved. Calculi may be associated with renal colic, and hydronephrosis and secondary infections are common.

ureteropelvic obstruction Obstruction of the renal pelvic outlet by a calculus, tumor, or idiopathic ureteropelvic junction obstruction. Hydronephrosis and secondary infections are common.

ureterovesical obstruction Obstruction of the ureter at the uretervesicular junction due to calculus or tumor. Hydronephrosis and secondary infection are common.

urinary obstruction A blockage of the urinary tract.

urinary tract obstruction Obstruction due to calculi, tumor, or other abnormalities anywhere in the urinary tract, including the renal pelvis, ureter, bladder, and urethra.

uteropelvic obstruction A stenosis or a blockage at the renal pelvis and ureteral junction.

obstructive Tending or acting to obstruct; causing or apt to cause obstruction.

obstruent [L *obstruens*, gen. *obstruentis*, pres. part. of *obstruere* to build against, block or wall up, hinder. The past part. is *obstructus.*] **1** Causing obstruction. **2** An agent causing obstruction.

obstupefacient [L *obstupefaciens*, pres. part. of *obstupefacere* (from *ob-* against, in front of + *stupefacere* to stupefy, astonish) to stupefy, astonish] Possessing the ability to stupefy; narcotic or soporific.

obtainer / space obtainer A device used to enlarge the space between two teeth.

obtund [L *obtund(ere)* to beat, blunt, dull. Past part. is *obtusus*, whence obtuse.] To cause to be semiconscious; to cause to have dulled or blunted senses.

obtundation [L *obtund(ere)* (from *ob* against + *tundere* to beat or strike repeatedly, stun) to beat, belabor, blunt, dull + -ATION] Any general depression of cerebral function ranging from sedation to coma; a clouding of consciousness.

obtundent [L *obtundens*, gen. *obtundentis*, pres. part. of *obtundere* to blunt, make dull] **1** Acting to dull sensation or consciousness, as a drug. **2** An obtundent drug or agent.

obtundity [L *obtund(ere)* to beat, blunt, dull + -ITY] A state of dulled or blunted consciousness.

obturation [from L *obturatus*, past part. of *obturare* to stop or close up] **1** Closure or occlusion of an opening or cleft. **2** Intestinal obstruction by a foreign body or by impaction. A seldom used term.

obturator [New L (from L *obturat(us)*, past part. of *obturare* to stop or close up + *-or* -OR)] **1** A device for closing or occluding an opening or cavity. **2** A prosthetic appliance closing a congenital or acquired opening in the palate. **3** In radiotherapy, a device that blocks a part of an area being irradiated without interrupting the emission of the rays.

buccofacial obturator A mechanical device for closing a pathological opening of the cheek to facilitate speech and feeding.

obtusion [L *obtusus* (past part. of *obtundere* to beat, blunt) blunt, dull, weakened] A state of diminished sensibility or consciousness.

Obwegeser [Hugo *Obwegeser*, Swedish oral surgeon, flourished 20th century] See under OPERATION.

oc- OB-.

Occam [William of *Occam*, English philosopher, c. 1285–c. 1349] See under RAZOR.

occasion of service A single occasion in which a health care service is rendered.

occipital Of or relating to the occiput.

occipitalis VENTER OCCIPITALIS MUSCULI OCCIPITOFRONTALIS.

occipitalization The fusion of the atlas with the occiput by synostosis.

occipito- [L *occiput* (genitive *occipitis*) back of the head] A combining form meaning occiput, occipital.

occipitoanterior [OCCIPITO- + ANTERIOR] Having the occiput directed towards the mother's symphysis pubis: said of a fetal position.

occipitoatloid Pertaining to the occipital bone and the atlas.

occipitoaxoid Pertaining to the occipital bone and the axis.

occipitobasilar Pertaining to the occiput and the base of the skull.

occipitobregmatic Pertaining to the occiput and the bregma.

occipitocalcarine Denoting axons of the occipital cerebral cortex traced to the calcarine sulcus.

occipitocervical Pertaining to the occiput and the neck.

occipitofacial Pertaining to the occiput and the face.

occipitofrontal Pertaining to the occiput and the forehead or frontal bone.

occipitofrontalis MUSCULUS OCCIPITOFRONTALIS.

occipitomastoid Pertaining to the occipital bone and the mastoid process.

occipitomental Pertaining to the occiput and the chin.

occipitoparietal PARIETO-OCCIPITAL.

occipitopontine Denoting the occipital cortex and pons, or connections between them.

occipitoposterior [OCCIPITO- + POSTERIOR] Having the occiput directed towards the mother's sacrum: said of a fetal position.

occipitoscapularis An occasional accessory slip of the rhomboid muscles that passes between the trapezius and spenius capitis muscles to the occipital bone. It corresponds to the rhomboideus capitis muscle commonly found in some mammals. Also called *rhomboideus occipitalis*.

occipitotemporal Pertaining to the occipital and the temporal bones or lobes of the cerebrum. Also *temporo-occipital*.

occipitothalamic Denoting the nerve fibers between the caudal thalamus (lateral geniculate body) and occipital lobe cerebral cortex.

occiput [L, from *oc-* OC- + *caput* head] The back part of the skull or head. Compare SINCIPUT.

occlude 1 To close off or stop up; obstruct. 2 To bring or come into a state of occlusion, as upper and lower teeth.

occluder ARTICULATOR.

occlusal [L *occlus(us)* (past part. of *occludere* to shut) closed, shut + -AL] Describing the surface of a tooth which faces or contacts a tooth in the opposite jaw. Also *morsal*.

occlusion [L *occlusus* (past part. of *occludere* to shut, close, from *oc-* + *claudere* to shut; Gk *kleiein* to shut) closed, shut + -*io* -ION] 1 The act of occluding or the condition of being occluded. 2 The relation between upper and lower antagonistic teeth in contact with each other. Also called *syncleisis*. 3 The spacial overlap of central neural excitation in a reflex event where the sum of two or more inputs together is less than the sum of their effects individually.

acentric occlusion ECCENTRIC OCCLUSION.

acquired eccentric occlusion Eccentric occlusion with maximum contact of teeth. It is caused by a deflecting premature contact. Also called *convenience occlusion, convenience bite, convenience relation of teeth, habitual occlusion*.

afunctional occlusion A malocclusion which prevents mastication.

anatomic occlusion An occlusion with the teeth arranged in their correct positions in the arches and occluding correctly in centric occlusion.

anterior occlusion MANDIBULAR PROGNATHISM.

balanced occlusion An occlusion that provides even contact throughout the dental arch in centric and eccentric positions. Also called *balanced articulation, balanced bite*.

bilateral balanced occlusion An occlusion that is balanced during lateral movements of the mandible.

buccal occlusion An occlusion in which the position of posterior tooth is buccal to the line of the dental arch.

capsular occlusion The surgical closure of the perinephric capsule. This procedure has been proposed as a treatment for a floating or ptotic kidney.

central occlusion CENTRIC OCCLUSION.

centric occlusion Occlusion with maximal tooth contacts and the mandible in centric position. Also called *normal occlusion, centric relation occlusion, central occlusion, centric contact*.

centrically balanced occlusion An occlusion which is balanced only in centric position.

centric relation occlusion CENTRIC OCCLUSION.

convenience occlusion ACQUIRED ECCENTRIC OCCLUSION.

coronary occlusion Occlusion of a coronary artery or its branches, most often due to thrombosis, less often to spasm or embolism, and often causing myocardial infarction.

distal occlusion DISTOCLUSION.

dynamic occlusion DENTAL ARTICULATION.

eccentric occlusion The occlusion when the mandible is in any eccentric position. Also called *acentric occlusion*. Also *excentric occlusion*.

edge-to-edge occlusion An occlusion in which the tips of the upper and lower anterior teeth meet instead of overlapping. Also called *end-to-end occlusion, edge-to-edge bite, end-to-end bite*.

end-to-end occlusion EDGE-TO-EDGE OCCLUSION.

enteromesenteric occlusion Occlusion of the superior mesenteric artery.

equilibrated occlusion An occlusion which has been brought into balance.

excentric occlusion ECCENTRIC OCCLUSION.

faulty centric occlusion Centric occlusion which does not correspond with a centric jaw relationship.

functional occlusion An incompletely balanced occlusion which functions satisfactorily without causing abnormal stress.

gliding occlusion DENTAL ARTICULATION.

habitual occlusion ACQUIRED ECCENTRIC OCCLUSION.

handheld centric occlusion The occlusion of casts obtained by locating the posterior cusps in their anatomic relationship.

hepatic vein occlusion Occlusion of one or both hepatic veins, most often due to thrombosis and giving rise to the Budd-Chiari syndrome.

hyperfunctional occlusion TRAUMATIC OCCLUSION.

ideal occlusion An anatomic occlusion which is also balanced.

labial occlusion An occlusion in which the position of an anterior tooth is labial to the line of the dental arch.

lateral occlusion Occlusion of the teeth with the lower jaw on the right or left of centric position.

lingual occlusion An occlusion in which a tooth is lingual to the line of the dental arch.

locked occlusion An occlusion with very limited eccentric movements, as a deep overbite or scissors crossbite. Also called *locked bite*.

malfunctional occlusion An occlusion which reduces masticatory efficiency.

mechanically balanced occlusion An occlusion which has been balanced on an articulator rather than physiologically.

mesenteric artery occlusion Cessation of flow in the mesenteric artery, especially of the superior mesenteric artery, due to embolism or thrombosis.

mesial occlusion An occlusion in which a lower tooth is positioned mesial to its equivalent in the upper jaw. Also called *prenormal occlusion.*

neutral occlusion NORMAL OCCLUSION.

normal occlusion 1 CENTRIC OCCLUSION. 2 Normal anatomic relation of dental arches and of teeth within each arch. Also called *normal bite, neutral occlusion.*

pathogenic occlusion A malocclusion which is likely to cause disorders of the masticatory system.

physiologic occlusion An occlusion in harmony with the condyle paths and the neuromuscular system.

physiologic normal occlusion An occlusion which is in harmony in centric relation.

posterior occlusion MANDIBULAR RETRUSION.

postnormal occlusion DISTOCLUSION.

prenormal occlusion MESIAL OCCLUSION.

protrusive occlusion MANDIBULAR PROGNATHISM.

puerperal tubal occlusion Physiologic closure of the uterine tubes which sometimes occurs during the six-week period after delivery of a child.

occlusion of the renal artery Complete obliteration of the lumen of the renal artery or one of its branches due to embolism or thrombosis. It may cause hypertension, and if bilateral, may produce renal failure.

retrusive occlusion MANDIBULAR RETRUSION.

spherical form of occlusion A pattern of occlusion corresponding to the surface of a sphere.

static occlusion Occlusion with teeth interdigitated.

terminal occlusion Occlusion when the teeth are in maximum contact.

torsive occlusion TORSIOCCLUSION.

traumatic occlusion An occlusion causing injury to the periodontium, to an edentulous ridge, or to the teeth. Also called *hyperfunctional occlusion.*

traumatogenic occlusion An occlusion considered to be capable of causing injury to the periodontium, the teeth, the temporomandibular joints, or the residual ridge.

working occlusion Occlusion on the working side. Also called *working bite.*

occlusive 1 Pertaining to dental occlusion. 2 Sealing against exposure to air, as a dressing.

occlusometer [*occlus(ion)* + *o* + *-METER*] GNATHODYNAMOMETER.

occlusorehabilitation OCCLUSAL REHABILITATION.

occult [L *occult(us)*, past part. of *occulare* to cover, hide] Not readily apparent or detectable; hidden or disguised, as an infection, the presence of blood, or a tumor, as, for example, a cancer whose primary site is hidden but whose metastases are evident.

occupancy The period during which a unit quantity of a substance, administered in a particular fashion, is present in a specific part of the body or at certain sites, before it is excreted or metabolized.

bed occupancy The ratio, relating to a specified period and usually expressed as a percentage, of the average number of beds occupied daily in a hospital or other institution to the average number of beds available daily for use in that hospital or institution. Both averages are usually derived from a daily census of the hospital, the sums over the period of the number of beds occupied and the number available each day being divided by the number of days in the period.

occupation / prescribed occupation An activity prescribed for specific therapeutic purposes, such as weaving with a loom to exercise the elbow and upper extremity.

oceanic Pertaining to that portion of the open ocean beyond the continental shelf waters.

ocellus [L, a little eye, an eye] (*plural* ocelli) 1 EYESPOT. 2 The simple eye found in some insects and other arthropods. 3 One of the units of a compound eye of an insect. 4 An eyelike color patch.

Ochlerotatus A subgenus of *Aedes* mosquitoes.

ochlesis [Gk *ochlēsis* a disturbance, annoyance] Any diseased or unhealthful state due to or exacerbated by overcrowding.

ochletic Pertaining to ochlesis.

ochratoxicosis The disease state caused by the toxic metabolites of the fungus *Aspergillus ochraceus.* The principal toxin is ochratoxin A, which is also produced by *Penicillium viridicatum.* Various animal species, including poultry, may be affected if fed cereal grains or prepared food contaminated with these mycotoxins.

Ochrogaster contraria A species of caterpillar whose hairs cause an allergic reaction characterized by urticaria and a papular pruritic eruption in susceptible individuals.

ochrometer [Gk *ōchro(s)* paleness, wanness + *-METER*] An instrument for determining capillary blood pressure by measuring the pressure necessary to cause blanching of the skin.

Ochromonadidae [Gk *ōchro(s)* yellow, pale + *monas*, gen. *monados*, single + IDAE] A family of chlorophyll-bearing flagellate protozoa (class Phytomastigophorea, order Chrysomonadina) with one long and one short flagellum. They are free-swimming and form colonies. The family includes the genera *Uroglena* and *Uroglenopsis.* Some lack chlorophyll or chromatophores, such as the colorless members of the genus *Monas.*

Ochromyia CORDYLOBIA.

ochronosis [Gk *ōchros* pale, sallow, yellow + *-nosis* irreg. (influenced by new L *-osis*) from Gk *nosos* sickness, disease] Chronic joint disease associated with the deposition of pigment within articular cartilage and found in patients with alkaptonuria. Also *ochronosus.* Adjective: ochronotic.

exogenous ochronosis A discoloration of the skin and other tissues, as that allegedly caused by exposure to phenol or phenolic compounds.

ocular ochronosis Scleral pigmentation associated with alkaptonuria.

ochronosus OCHRONOSIS.

ochronotic Pertaining to ochronosis.

Ochsner [Albert John *Ochsner*, U.S. surgeon, 1858–1925] See under SPHINCTER, RING, MUSCLE.

oct- OCTA-.

octa- [Gk *octō* eight] A combining form meaning eight. Also *oct-, octi-, octo-.*

octacosanol $C_{28}H_{58}O$. A solid alcohol that is found in wheat germ oil and vegetable waxes.

octacosyl alcohol CH_3—$[CH_2]_{26}$—CH_2OH. Octacosan-1-ol. A fatty alcohol present as esters in waxes.

octahedral 1 Having the symmetry of an octahedron. 2 Denoting a molecular configuration in which six ligands are regularly arranged around a center.

octahedron [Gk *oktaedron* (from neut. of *oktaedros* eight-sided, from *oct(ō)* eight + *a* + *(h)edra* a seat, base) an octahedron] The regular polyhedron with eight faces, which are equilateral triangles, and six vertices.

octan [L *oct(o)* eight + English *-an*, as in *quartan*] Recurring every eighth day, as certain febrile paroxysms.

octane 1 CH_3—$[CH_2]_6$—CH_3. The hydrocarbon whose molecules are saturated chains of eight carbon atoms. 2 Any of the isomers of this hydrocarbon.

octanoic acid CH_3—$[CH_2]_6$—COOH. One of the fatty acids, occurring in butter as its esters. Also called *caprylic acid* (outmoded).

octanol CH_3—$[CH_2]_6$—CH_2OH. Octan-1-ol. A fatty alcohol present as esters in some natural oils, and used in the perfume industry. Both it and octan-2-ol, CH_3—$[CH_2]_5$—CHOH—CH_3, prevent foaming of protein solutions. Also called *capryl alcohol*.

octaploidy [OCT- + *(h)aploidy*] The state of having eight times the haploid number of chromosomes.

octarius [L *octo* eight] A measure of volume equal to a pint, or one-eighth of a gallon.

octave [Middle English, from L *octava*, fem. of *octavus* eighth from *octo* eight] The interval between two frequencies or sounds having a frequency ratio of 2:1.

octi- OCTA-.

octigravida [OCTI- + GRAVIDA] A woman experiencing her eighth pregnancy.

Octin A proprietary name for isometheptene.

octipara [OCTI- + PARA] A woman who has produced viable fetuses in eight pregnancies.

octo- OCTA-.

Octomitus *HEXAMITA.*

Octomitus hominis *PENTATRICHOMONAS HOMINIS.*

Octomyces [Gk *oktō* eight + *mykēs*, fungus, mushroom] An obsolete term for *SACCHAROMYCES*.

octopine N^2-(1-Carboxyethyl)arginine. A substance related to both arginine and alanine. It is found in the muscles of many marine invertebrates, such as the octopus.

octopod [OCTO- + -POD] Any individual of the order Octopoda.

Octopoda [New L (from Gk *oktō* eight + New L *-poda*, neut. pl. of *-pod*, suffix denoting foot)] A marine order in the molluscan class Cephalopoda. The finless body has eight arms and sessile suckers.

Octopus [New L (from Gk *oktōpous* octopod, from *oktō* eight + *pous*, gen. *podos*, foot)] The type genus of the order Octopoda. Members are adapted for bottom dwelling in the intertidal or rocky littoral zone of the marine habitat, usually occupying a den or hiding place except for brief feeding forays.

Octopus vulgaris A common Mediterranean species of octopus. It is the host of the first virus or viruslike particle reported from a mollusk. The virus causes edematous nodular tumors on the tentacles and self-mutilation, with a fatal outcome. It is also the host of a parasitic copepod, *Octopicola superbus*. In addition, nearly all individuals have dicyemid mesozoan parasites in their renal organ.

octose [OCT- + -OSE^2] Any aldose sugar with eight carbon atoms.

Octoson An automatic ultrasound imaging system employing a series of eight transducers mounted in a water bath in such a way that the image lies in the focal zone of each transducer. The transducers are moved mechanically in an arc, each producing a scan which is integrated into a single picture.

octyl gallate Octyl 3,4,5-trihydroxybenzoate. It has been employed as an antioxidizing agent in pharmaceutic preparations, particularly fat-soluble compounds.

ocular [L *ocul(us)* (akin to Gk *osse* the two eyes and to Arabic *uc* the eye) the eye + *-aris* -AR] 1 Pertaining to the eye. 2 EYEPIECE.

Huygen's ocular HUYGENIAN EYEPIECE.

Ramsden's ocular An eyepiece with two planoconvex lenses

of approximately equal focal length placed with convex surfaces facing each other. The separation between the lenses is approximately two thirds the focal length of the lenses. Also called *Ramsden's eyepiece.*

telaugic oculars An optical device with an exit pupil positioned a considerable distance from the viewing lenses of the instrument.

wide-field ocular WIDEFIELD EYEPIECE.

oculentum [L *ocul(us)* eye + *-entum* English *-ent*] An ointment for use in or around the eye.

oculi Plural of OCULUS.

oculist [*ocul(o)-* + -IST] OPHTHALMOLOGIST.

oculistics [*ocul(o)-* + -IST + -ICS] The science of treatment of ocular disease.

oculo- [L *oculus* the eye] A combining form denoting the eye.

oculocephalic [OCULO- + CEPHALIC] Pertaining to or affecting the eyes and brain.

oculocephalogyric [OCULO- + CEPHALO- + GYR- + -IC] Pertaining to abnormal movements of both head and eyes, as in the oculogyric crises of Parkinson's disease.

oculocompressor An instrument once used to study physiologic variations in the oculocardiac reflex. It comprised two metallic cups padded with rubber, with a calibrated spring by means of which variable pressure could be exerted. The instrument was placed on the eyeballs and fastened by a headband.

oculocutaneous [OCULO- + CUTANEOUS] Pertaining to conditions affecting both skin and eyes.

oculofacial Pertaining to the eyes and the face.

oculofrontal Of or relating to the eyes and the forehead.

oculography [OCULO- + -GRAPHY] The recording of extraocular muscle movements of the position of the eye.

photosensor oculography The recording of movements of the eye as measured by an infrared sensor that detects movements of the limbus.

oculogyria [OCULO- + GYR- + -IA] Movement of the eyes.

oculogyric [OCULO- + GYR- + -IC] Describing, pertaining to, or producing spontaneous and sustained ocular movements, usually in an upward direction as in parkinsonism. Also *ophthalmogyric.*

oculomandibulodyscephaly with hypotrichosis HALLERMANN-STREIFF SYNDROME.

oculometroscope [OCULO- + *-metr(y)* + *o* + -SCOPE] A retinoscope in which the trial lenses are rotated automatically by the instrument.

oculomotor [OCULO- + MOTOR] Pertaining to or affecting ocular movement.

oculomycosis [OCULO- + MYCOSIS] Any fungous disease of the eye.

oculonasal Pertaining to the eyes and the nose.

oculopalpebral Pertaining to the eye and the eyelid.

oculopathy [OCULO- + -PATHY] Any disorder of the eye.

oculopharyngeal Pertaining to the eye and the pharynx.

oculoplethysmography A diagnostic technique whereby the presence of critical internal carotid artery stenosis or occlusion is indirectly inferred by demonstrating an ipsilateral delay in the arrival of ocular pressures transmitted from branches of the ophthalmic artery, when compared with arrival of the ipsilateral external carotid artery pulse as manifested by an ear lobe photocell.

oculopneumoplethysmography An indirect test for demonstrating the presence of a critical carotid artery stenosis or occlusion by measuring the negative pressure, when applied to the eye, that is required to obliterate pulsations due to the pulse pressure in branches of the ophthalmic artery. Also called *pneumoplethysmography*.

oculopupillary Pertaining to the pupil of the eye.

oculoreaction OPHTHALMIC REACTION.

oculosensory [OCULO- + SENSORY] Pertaining to or affected by stimuli to the eye.

oculospinal Pertaining to the eye and the spinal cord.

oculozygomatic Pertaining to the eye and the zygomatic bone or process.

oculus [L (akin to Gk *ōps*), the eye] (*plural* oculi) [NA] The organ of vision comprising bulbus oculi and nervus opticus; eye.

  oculus caesius GLAUCOMA.

  oculus dexter The right eye. Abbreviation: OD

  oculus laevus The left eye. Abbreviation: OL

  oculus leporinus LAGOPHTHALMOS.

  oculus purulentus Purulent discharge in the anterior chamber of the eye.

  oculus sinister The left eye. Abbreviation: OS

ocyodinic OXYTOCIC.

OD **1** oculus dexter. **2** optical density (absorbance). **3** (drug) overdose. A popular usage. **4** outside diameter.

odaxesmus [Gk *odaxēsmos* (from *odaxein* to bite, sting) a sharp biting] Biting of the tongue, lip, or cheek in a major epileptic attack.

odaxetic [Gk *odax(ein)* to bite, sting + *-etik(os)* adjectival suffix] Producing a sense of itching or of being bitten.

Oddi [Ruggero *Oddi*, Italian physician, 1864–1913] Oddi's muscle. See under MUSCULUS SPHINCTER AMPULLAE HEPATOPANCREATICAE.

odditis [*(sphincter of) Odd(i)* + -ITIS] Inflammation of the sphincter of Oddi, which lies at the junction of the common bile duct and the duodenum. A rarely used term.

odds / relative odds ODDS RATIO.

odiferous ODORIFEROUS.

odogenesis [Gk *(h)odo(s)* a way, path + GENESIS] NEUROCLADISM.

odont- ODONTO-.

-odont [Gk *odous* or Ionic variant *odōn* (gen. of both, *odontos*) tooth] A combining form meaning having teeth (of a specified kind). Also *-dont*.

odontalgia [ODONT- + -ALGIA] TOOTHACHE.

  phantom odontalgia A toothache felt in an edentulous part of the mouth.

odontatrophy [ODONT- + ATROPHY] Hypoplasia of the teeth.

odontectomy [ODONT- + -ECTOMY] Removal of a tooth or roots requiring an incision in the oral mucosa.

odonterism [ODONT- + Gk *erism(a)* a quarreling] Chattering of the teeth. A seldom used term.

odontexesis [ODONT- + *e* + Gk *xesis* a polishing by scraping or planing] Scaling and polishing of the teeth.

-odontia [Gk *odous* or Ionic variant *odōn* (gen. of both, *odontos*) tooth + *-ia* L and Gk feminine-noun termination denoting state or condition] A combining form meaning state or condition of the teeth.

odontiatria [ODONT- + Gk *iatreia* a treatment, healing] DENTISTRY.

odontic [ODONT- + -IC] Relating to the teeth.

odontinoid ODONTOID.

odonto- [Gk *odous* (genitive *odontos*) tooth] A combining form denoting tooth or teeth. Also *odont-*.

odontoameloblastoma [ODONTO- + AMELOBLASTOMA] A very rare neoplasm characterized by the presence of enamel, dentine, and an odontogenic epithelium resembling that of an ameloblastoma both in structure and behavior.

odontoameloblastosarcoma AMELOBLASTIC ODONTOSARCOMA.

odontoamelosarcoma [ODONTO- + AMELO- + SARCOMA] AMELOBLASTIC ODONTOSARCOMA.

odontoatlantal ATLANTOAXIAL.

odontoblast [ODONTO- + -BLAST] One of the specialized connective tissue cells which take part in the formation of the dentin of a tooth. They form a layer of columnar cells on the outer part of the dental pulp and each cell leaves a dentinal fiber within a dentinal tubule as the dentin is deposited on the outer aspect of the odontoblast layer. Odontoblasts persist throughout the life of a tooth. Also called *dentinoblast, odontoplast, dentin cell, fibrilloblast* (outmoded).

odontoblastoma [ODONTO- + BLASTOMA] A tumor of odontoblasts.

odontobothrion [ODONTO- + Gk *bothrion*, dim. of *bothros* a pit, trench] A bony trough for accommodating the teeth within the alveolar process of the jaw.

odontobothritis [ODONTO- + Gk *bothr(ion)* a small pit or trench + -ITIS] An inflammation in the alveolar bone. A seldom used term.

odontocele [ODONTO- + -CELE²] An outmoded term for APICAL PERIODONTAL CYST.

odontoceramic [ODONTO- + CERAMIC] Relating to porcelain crowns or artificial teeth.

odontochirurgic ODONTOCHIRURGICAL.

odontochirurgical [ODONTO- + L *chirurgic(us)* (from *chirurgia* surgery, from Gk *cheirourgia* a working by hand, from *cheir* the hand + *-ourg(os)* suffix denoting working + *-ia* -IA) surgical + *-alis* -AL] Relating to dental surgery. Also *odontochirurgic*.

odontoclamis [ODONTO- + Gk *chlamys* a horseman's short cloak or mantle] DENTAL OPERCULUM.

odontoclast [ODONTO- + -CLAST] A cell, indistinguishable from an osteoclast, which is involved in the resorption of the roots of deciduous teeth.

odontodynia [ODONT- + -ODYNIA] TOOTHACHE.

odontodysplasia [ODONTO- + DYSPLASIA] A developmental anomaly affecting both dentin and enamel production. Also called *ghost teeth*.

odontogenesis [ODONTO- + GENESIS] The initiation and development of teeth. Also called *odontogeny*. Adjective: odontogenetic.

  odontogenesis imperfecta DENTINOGENESIS IMPERFECTA.

odontogenic [ODONTO- + -GENIC] **1** Capable of giving rise to teeth. **2** Denoting the zone of predentin.

odontogenous [ODONTO- + -GENOUS] Originating within or around the teeth.

odontogeny ODONTOGENESIS.

odontogram [ODONTO- + -GRAM] The linear record produced by an odontograph.

odontograph [ODONTO- + -GRAPH] A device for magnifying the profile of a tooth surface.

odontoiatry [ODONTO- + -IATRY] DENTAL THERAPEUTICS.

odontoid [ODONT- + -OID] Toothlike in structure or function. Also *odontinoid*.

odontolith [ODONTO- + Gk *lithos* a stone] DENTAL CALCULUS.

odontolithiasis [ODONTO- + LITHIASIS] The condition of having calculus on the teeth.

odontologist [ODONT- + -OLOGIST] DENTIST.

odontology [ODONTO- + -LOGY] DENTISTRY.

  forensic odontology FORENSIC DENTISTRY.

odontoloxia [ODONTO- + Gk *lox(os)* slanting, crosswise + -IA] Slanting or irregular teeth.

odontolysis [ODONTO- + LYSIS] Resorption of dental hard tissue.

odontoma [ODONT- + -OMA] **1** A malformative odontogenic tumorlike lesion in which a mixture of dental tissues, particularly enamel and dentine, is present. Also called *odontome.* **2** An exostosis on a tooth. An outmoded usage. **3** Any odontogenic tumor. An outmoded usage.

odontoma adamantinum An odontoma composed mainly of enamel. Also called *osteo-odontoma.*

ameloblastic odontoma An odontoma with ameloblastic epithelium.

calcified odontoma A calcified tumor arising from odontogenic cells, such as cementoma, complex odontoma, compound odontoma, dentinoma, and enameloma.

complex odontoma A tumorlike malformative lesion of the jaw in which all dental tissues are present. The components are well formed, but arranged in a disorderly manner. Also called *composite odontoma.*

composite odontoma **1** COMPLEX ODONTOMA. **2** COMPOUND ODONTOMA.

compound odontoma A tumorlike malformative lesion of the jaw in which all dental tissues are present and in a more orderly manner than in a complex odontoma, so that the relations between the components resemble that seen in the normal tooth. Also called *composite odontoma.*

coronal odontoma **1** An odontoma affecting the crown of a tooth. **2** An odontoma occurring when the crown is developing. Also called *coronary odontoma.*

coronary odontoma CORONAL ODONTOMA.

cystic odontoma An odontoma with an associated follicular cyst.

dilated odontoma DENS INVAGINATUS.

dilated composite odontoma DENS INVAGINATUS.

epithelial odontoma An odontoma of ectodermal origin, such as ameloblastoma, adenoameloblastoma, calcifying epithelial odontogenic tumor, and calcifying epithelial odontogenic cyst.

fibrous odontoma ODONTOGENIC FIBROMA.

geminated composite odontoma A tumorlike lesion composed of two fused dental germ units. Also called *connate tooth, fused teeth, geminate tooth, geminated tooth.*

gestant odontoma DENS INVAGINATUS.

mixed odontoma An odontoma composed of more than one of the tooth structures.

radicular odontoma **1** An odontoma affecting the root of a tooth. **2** An odontoma occurring when the root is developing.

simple odontoma An odontogenic tumor composed of only one element of dental germ tissue.

odontome ODONTOMA.

odontoneuralgia [ODONTO- + NEURALGIA] Facial neuralgia caused by dental decay.

odontonomy [ODONT- + Gk *onom(a)* a name + -Y] The terminology relating to the teeth.

odontonosology [ODONTO- + NOSOLOGY] The study of dental diseases.

odontoparallaxis [ODONTO- + PARALLAXIS] MALOCCLUSION.

odontopathy [ODONTO- + -PATHY] Any disease or disorder of the teeth.

odontoperiosteum PERIODONTIUM.

odontophobia [ODONTO- + -PHOBIA] Pathologic fear of teeth.

odontoplast ODONTOBLAST.

odontoplasty [ODONTO- + -PLASTY] Reshaping the crown and/or root surface of teeth, mainly to improve accessibility for oral hygiene.

odontoprisis [ODONTO- + Gk *prisis* (from *priein* to saw, gnash or grind the teeth) a sawing] BRUXISM.

odontoptosis [ODONTO- + PTOSIS] Overeruption of an upper tooth.

odontoradiograph [ODONTO- + RADIOGRAPH] A roentgenogram of teeth.

odontorrhagia [ODONTO- + -RRHAGIA] Hemorrhage following tooth extraction. An outmoded term.

odontorthosis [ODONT- + ORTHOSIS] ORTHODONTICS.

odontosarcoma [ODONTO- + SARCOMA] AMELOBLASTIC ODONTOSARCOMA.

ameloblastic odontosarcoma A very rare malignant tumor similar to the ameloblastic fibrosarcoma but containing dysplastic dentine and enamel. Also called *odontoameloblastosarcoma, odontoamelosarcoma.*

odontoschism [ODONTO- + Gk *schisma* a thing cloven or parted, a cleft] A partial or complete fission of a tooth.

odontoscope [ODONTO- + -SCOPE] MOUTH MIRROR.

odontoscopy [ODONTO- + -SCOPY] The making of casts of the teeth for personal identification.

odontoseisis [ODONTO- + Gk *seisis* a shaking, moving to and fro] Looseness of teeth. A seldom used term.

odontosis [ODONTO- + -SIS] The formation or the eruption of teeth. An outmoded term.

odontotechny [ODONTO- + Gk *technē* an art, skill] DENTISTRY.

odontotheca DENTAL FOLLICLE.

odontotomy [ODONTO- + -TOMY] The procedure of cutting into a tooth, especially into fissures.

prophylactic odontotomy The cutting out and filling of the pits and fissures of the teeth as a preventive measure against caries.

odontotripsis [ODONTO- + TRIPSIS] Loss of tooth substance from wear. A seldom used term.

odor [L (akin to *olere* to emit an odor, and to Gk *ozein* to have a smell and *odmē* a smell, scent, sweet or bad odor), an odor] The property of something that excites the sense of smell.

butcher shop odor A smell like that of a butcher shop, said to be characteristic of patients with yellow fever. An obsolete term.

minimal identifiable odor MINIMUM RECOGNIZABLE ODOR.

minimum recognizable odor The lowest concentration of a substance in the atmosphere which enables it to be identified by the sense of smell. Tests are usually conducted on a group of people and any obviously extreme value due to personal idiosyncrasy is excluded before determining a mean value. Also called *minimal identifiable odor.*

odorant **1** Producing an odor; odoriferous. **2** Any substance producing an odor.

odoriferous Characterized by or disseminating an odor, particularly an agreeable odor. Also *odorous, odiferous* (seldom used).

odorimeter A means of attempting to assess the strength and other characteristics of odorants.

odorimetry The performance of tests using an odorimeter.

odorivection [L *odor* scent, smell + *i* + *vectio* a carrying, riding] The transmission of an odor.

odorivector [L *odor* + *i* + *vector* a bearer, carrier] A substance which emits or conveys an odor.

odorogram OLFACTORY SPECTROGRAM.

odorography [ODOR + *o* + -GRAPHY] Literature pertaining to odors or odorants.

odorous ODORIFEROUS.

O'Dwyer [Joseph P. *O'Dwyer*, U.S. physician, 1841–1898] **1** Fell-O'Dwyer method. See under METHOD. **2** See under TUBE.

odynacousis ODYNACUSIS.

odynacusis [*odyn(o)*- + ACU-² + -SIS] Pain in the ear induced by sound. Also *odynacousis*.

-odynia [Gk *odynē* pain, distress] A combining form meaning pain.

odyno- [Gk *odynē* pain, distress] A combining form meaning pain.

odynometer [ODYNO- + -METER] An instrument designed to measure pain.

odynophagia [ODYNO- + -PHAGIA] Pain on swallowing.

odynopoeia [ODYNO- + Gk *poiein* to make, produce] The induction or strengthening of uterine contractions in labor.

odynuria [ODYN- + -URIA] Pain while urinating.

Oe Symbol for the obsolete unit, oersted.

oe- For words beginning *oe*-, see also under E-.

Oeciacus A genus of bugs of the family Cimicidae, distinguished from bedbugs by their hairiness. Normally ectoparasites of birds, both the Old World swallow bug *O. hirundinis* and its New World counterpart *O. vicarius* occasionally infest humans.

oeco- ECO-.

oecosite ECOSITE.

oedema A British spelling for EDEMA.

oedematous A British spelling for EDEMATOUS.

oedipal Relating to the Oedipus complex or the age period during which the complex reaches its heights.

oedipism [after *Oedip(us)*, legendary king of Thebes, who mistakenly killed his father, married his mother, and tore out his own eyes in anguish + -ISM] The act of inflicting injury upon one's own eyes. An older term. Also *edipism*.

Oehl [Eusebio *Oehl*, Italian anatomist, 1827–1903] **1** Oehl's layer. See under STRATUM LUCIDUM EPIDERMIDIS. **2** Oehl's muscles. See under MUSCLE.

Oehler [Johannes *Oehler*, German physician, born 1879] See under SYMPTOM.

oersted [after Hans Christian *Oersted*, Danish physicist, 1777–1851] A CGS electromagnetic unit of magnetic field strength, equivalent to $10^3/4\pi$ amperes per meter, 79.5775 amperes per meter. An obsolete unit. Symbol: Oe

oesophagitis A British spelling for ESOPHAGITIS.

oesophago- A British spelling for ESOPHAGO-.

oesophagocele A British spelling for ESOPHAGOCELE.

oesophagoscope A British spelling for ESOPHAGOSCOPE.

oesophagoscopy A British spelling for ESOPHAGOSCOPY.

oesophagostomiasis [*Oesophagostom(um)* + -IASIS] A disease caused by infection with *Oesophagostomum* nematodes in sheep, cattle, goats, swine, and subhuman primates. In heavy infections young animals may have diarrhea and become unthrifty. After repeated infections the larvae which inhabit the intestinal mucosa incite a granulomatous reaction and the formation of nodules which calcify. Also called *nodule disease, nodular disease*. Also *esophagostomiasis*.

Oesophagostomum [ESOPHAGO- + New L -*stomum*, combining form from Gk *stoma* the mouth] A genus of nematodes (family Strongylidae), the nodular worms, in which adults are parasitic in the lumen of the large intestine of primates and herbivores. The larvae encyst in the intestinal wall of the host, stimulating a reaction that results in the formation of nodules, in which the larvae develop. Related genera in the subfamily Oesophagostominae include *Chabertia* and *Ternidens*, the bowel worms.

Oesophagostomum apiostomum A species commonly parasitic in monkeys and apes in central Africa, India, the Philippines, China, and Brazil. The larvae can encyst in the human intestine, sometimes causing a form of dysentery. Tumorlike lesions of the ileocecal region with eosinophilic infiltration have been reported in Uganda. The worms leave the nodules to become adults in the lumen of the large intestine. Treatment is with intestinal anthelmintics. Also called *Oesophagostomum brumpti*.

Oesophagostomum bifurcum A species found in monkeys and sometimes in humans in the Philippines and Africa. It is considered by some to be identical with *O. apiostomum*.

Oesophagostomum brevicaudum A species found in the colon and cecum of pigs in North America and India. Also called *Oesophagostomum suis*.

Oesophagostomum brumpti OESOPHAGOSTOMUM APIOSTOMUM.

Oesophagostomum columbianum A species of nodular worm that infects goats, sheep, cattle, deer, and African antelopes. It appears to be relatively nonpathogenic except in heavy infections. Also called *Oesophagostomum venulosum*.

Oesophagostomum dentatum The type species of the genus, cosmopolitan in distribution, found in the colon of swine. It causes nodular lesions similar to those found in sheep infected with *O. columbianum*.

Oesophagostomum georgianum A species found in the cecum and colon of pigs in the United States.

Oesophagostomum inflatum OESOPHAGOSTOMUM RADIATUM.

Oesophagostomum quadrispinulatum A species found in the cecum and colon of pigs in North America, South America, southeastern Asia, and Europe. It is sometimes considered to be a subspecies of *O. dentatum*.

Oesophagostomum radiatum A cosmopolitan species found in cattle and in the water buffalo. It causes a nodular disease similar to that caused by *O. venulosum (O. columbianum)* in sheep. Also called *Oesophagostomum inflatum*.

Oesophagostomum stephanostomum A species found in Africa, parasitic in monkeys, chimpanzees, and gorillas. One human case has been reported from Brazil.

Oesophagostomum suis OESOPHAGOSTOMUM BREVICAUDUM.

Oesophagostomum venulosum OESOPHAGOSTOMUM COLUMBIANUM.

oesophagostomy A British spelling for ESOPHAGOSTOMY.

oesophagotomy A British spelling for ESOPHAGOTOMY.

oesophagus A British spelling for ESOPHAGUS.

oestradiol A British spelling for ESTRADIOL.

oestriasis [*Oestr(us)* + -IASIS] Infestation of sheep by maggots of the genus *Oestrus*. Also *estriasis*.

oestrid [*oestr(us)* + -ID¹] **1** Of or belonging to the family Oestridae. **2** A member of the family Oestridae.

Oestridae [*oestr(us)* + -IDAE] A family of true flies (order Diptera) containing some economically important myiasis flies, the head maggots. Members have hairy bodies and rudimentary mouth parts. Genera include *Oestrus*, the sheep botfly; *Rhinocephalus*, the head maggots of horses; *Gedoelstia*, the nasal bot of antelopes; and *Cephenomyia*, the head maggots of deer. Also *Estridae*.

oestriol A British spelling for ESTRIOL.

oestrogen A British spelling for ESTROGEN.

oestrone A British spelling for ESTRONE.

oestrous A British spelling for ESTROUS.

oestrum A British spelling for ESTRUM.

Oestrus [L (Gk *oistros* the gadfly, a sting, agony, tormentor, vehement passion, frenzy), the gadfly, horsefly, inspiration, frenzy] A genus of head maggots or botflies (family Oestridae) that cause tissue-invading myiasis in mammals. Also called *Cephalomyia*.

Oestrus hominis OESTRUS OVIS.

Oestrus ovis The sheep botfly or head maggot, a now cosmopolitan species of botfly that was originally imported into North America from Europe. The adult deposits larvae in the sheep's nostrils. The larvae develop in the nasal cavities and sinuses, disrupting feeding and causing irritation and a mucous discharge. They can cause serious problems, if present in large numbers, particularly in weak, old, or very young animals. Occasionally they cause myiasis in humans, especially ocular myiasis. Also called *Oestrus hominis*.

oestrus A British spelling for ESTRUS.

of- OB-.

OFD I OROFACIODIGITAL SYNDROME I.

OFD II OROFACIODIGITAL SYNDROME II.

office A room or suite of rooms in which a medical or other health professional regularly receives patients and treats them insofar as more extensive facilities are not required. • This usage of *office* is established in the United States and to some extent in Canada and New Zealand. In the United Kingdom and elsewhere, *surgery* is preferred, though it is somewhat more specific and is distinguished, for example, from *consulting room*.

officer / district nursing officer In the United Kingdom, a nurse responsible for nursing services in a district of the National Health Service. Compare DISTRICT NURSE.

divisional nursing officer In the United Kingdom, a nurse responsible for a certain type of nursing within a district of the National Health Service.

house officer A health care professional, usually a physician, who is in training in a hospital; a member of the house staff.

official Recognized by, and meeting the requirements of, an authoritative body such as the National Formulary, the U.S. Pharmacopeia, or the British Pharmaceutical Codex.

officinal Denoting a chemical or drug kept regularly in stock in a pharmacy, as opposed to those preparations compounded as requested, as specified by a prescription. Compare MAGISTRAL.

off-line **1** Not under the direct control of a central computer processing unit: used of equipment such as a printer. **2** Designating the operative of input/output devices not under direct control of a system. **3** Designating a system in which an aliquot is withdrawn from the stream and conveyed to the detector.

og- OB-.

Ogilvie [Sir William Heneage *Ogilvie*, English physician, flourished 20th century] See under SYNDROME.

Ogino [Kyusaka *Ogino*, Japanese physician, born 1881] Ogino-Knaus method. See under METHOD.

ogive [Middle French] The curve of an unimodal frequency distribution with variate values on the abscissa and cumulative frequency on the ordinate. The curve has the shape of a drawn-out letter S.

ogo GANGOSA.

Ogston [Sir Alexander *Ogston*, Scottish surgeon, 1844–1929] **1** Ogston-Luc operation. See under OPERATION. **2** See under OPERATION, LINE.

Oguchi [Chuta *Oguchi*, Japanese ophthalmologist, 1875–1945] See under DISEASE.

O'Hara [Michael *O'Hara*, Jr., U.S. surgeon, 1869–1926] See under FORCEPS.

Ohara [Hachiro *Ohara*, Japanese physician, born 1882] Ohara's disease. See under TULAREMIA.

Ohlmacher [Albert Philip *Ohlmacher*, U.S. physician, 1865–1916] See under SOLUTION.

Ohm [Georg Simon *Ohm*, German physicist, 1787–1854] See under LAW.

ohm [after Georg Simon *Ohm*, German physicist, 1787–1854] The special name for the SI derived unit of electric resistance; the electric resistance between two points of a conductor when a constant potential difference of one volt, applied at those points, produces in the conductor a current of one ampere, the conductor not being the seat of any electromotive force; 1 ohm = 1 volt/1 ampere. Symbol: Ω

reciprocal ohm A unit of electrical conductance, now generally referred to by the special name siemens. Symbol: Ω^{-1}

ohmammeter A combined ohmmeter and ammeter.

ohmmeter An instrument for directly indicating electrical resistance in ohms.

-oic [o + -IC] A suffix replacing the final -e of the suffix -*ane* of a hydrocarbon to convert its name into that of a carboxylic acid.

-oid [Gk *eidos* form, shape] A suffix meaning having the form of, like, resembling.

Oidiomycetes [New L (from *oidi(um)* a genus of fungi, from Gk *ō(on)* egg + New L -*idi(um)*, diminishing suffix + *o* + -*mycetes*, suffix denoting fungi, from Gk *mykētes*, pl. of *mykēs* fungus, mushroom)] An obsolete genus of powdery mildews which have been reclassified in the genus *Erysiphe* and related genera of the order Erysiphales.

oidiomycosis [*Oidium*, an earlier genus name + MYCOSIS.] A disease caused by fungi of the form-genus *Acrosporium*. Adjective: oidiomycotic.

Oidium [New L (from Gk *ō(on)* egg + New L -*idium*, diminishing suffix)] An obsolete form-genus of fungi which have been implicated in dermatomycosis, candidosis, and blastomycosis, and which have been reclassified under various form-genera.

oidium [$o(o)$- + -IDIUM] (*plural* oidia) A thin-walled, free, hyphal cell derived from the fragmentation of somatic hypha into its component cells or from an oidiophore. This cell serves as a spore or a spermatium.

oiko- ECO-.

oikology [OIKO- + -LOGY] ECOLOGY.

oikosite [OIKO- + Gk *sit(os)* food] ECOSITE.

oil [Old French *oile* (from L *oleum* olive oil, oil, from Gk *elaion* olive oil, oil) oil] Any viscous, combustible liquid, often a petroleum fraction, insoluble in water and soluble in ether. Also called *oleum*.

ajowan oil An essential oil extracted from the dried, ripe fruits of *Trachyspermum ammi*. It is used as a carminative and antispasmodic agent.

allspice oil See under PIMENTA.

oil of amber A pale yellow or brownish yellow oil with a penetrating odor and a sharp, burning taste, obtained by the destructive distillation of certain resins. It was formerly obtained from amber. It has properties like those of turpentine oil and is used in liniments. Also called *oleum succini*.

aromatic castor oil A mixture of castor oil with cinnamon oil, clove oil, saccharin, vanilla, and alcohol. It is used as a laxative. Also called *oleum ricini aromaticum*.

artificial essential oil of almond BENZALDEHYDE.

benne oil SESAME OIL.

oil bergamot An expressed oil from the inedible fresh fruit of *Citrus aurantium*. It is used in perfume, in hair tonics, and in other external preparations.

birch tar oil A pyroligneous oil obtained by the dry distillation of bark and wood of *Betula alba* and related *Betula* species, and rectified by steam distillation (rectified birch tar oil). It is used in lotions as a counterirritant and as an antiseptic for some skin diseases.

bitter almond oil   A volatile oil obtained from the ripe kernels of bitter almond, peach, apricot, and other kernels that contain amygdalin. It is composed primarily of benzaldehyde, and it can be extremely poisonous if any trace of its hydrogen cyanide component remains after processing.

burbot liver oil   Oil extracted from the liver of the burbot, *Lota maculosa*, which is a freshwater fish related to the cod. The oil is rich in vitamin D.

cade oil   JUNIPER TAR.

camphorated oil   CAMPHOR LINIMENT.

caraway oil   A volatile oil distilled from the seed of *Carum carvi*, caraway. Its main constituent is carvone, and it is used as a flavoring agent and a carminative.

carbolic oil   PHENOLATED OIL.

carron oil   LOTIO CALCII HYDROXIDI OLEOSA.

cassia oil   CINNAMON OIL.

castor oil   A fixed oil cold-pressed from the kernel of the seeds of *Ricinus communis*. Its principal constituent is triricinolein. It also contains isoricinolein, palmitin, and dihydroxystearin. The mild purgative property of ricinoleic acid and its isomer is produced in the duodenum by hydrolysis. It has been used in the treatment of hemorrhoids, during pregnancy, as an ointment for irritated skin, a solvent for alkaloids in treating the conjunctiva, and as an ingredient of soaps. The seeds also contain a highly toxic substance. Also called *oleum ricini, ricinus oil, oil of Palma Christi, tangantangan oil*.

cedar oil   A volatile oil obtained from the distillation of the wood of various species of cedar, principally *Juniperus virginiana*. The oil consists almost entirely of cedrene, a liquid sesquiterpene, and cedral. It is used in microscopy as a clearing agent and immersion medium with oil-immersion objectives, and also in perfumery.

chaulmoogra oil   A fatty oil expressed from the fresh ripe seeds of *Hydnocarpus wightiana, H. anthelmintica*, and *Taraktogenos kurzii*. It contains glycerides of chaulmoogric and hydnocarpic acids. It is a powerful rubefacient and has been used in treating leprosy. Also called *hydnocarpus oil*.

oil of cherry laurel   An extremely poisonous volatile oil obtained from the leaves of *Prunus laurocerasus* which contains hydrogen cyanide. It is similar in odor and taste to bitter almond oil.

chloriodized oil   A vegetable oil containing iodine and chlorine, formerly used as an opaque medium in bronchography and hysterosalpingography.

cinnamon oil   A volatile oil obtained from the distillation of leaves and twigs of *Cinnamomum cassia*, with subsequent rectification. Its chief ingredient is cinnamaldehyde, with an admixture of terpenes and other compounds. It is used as a flavoring agent, a carminative, and a pungent aromatic. Also called *cassia oil*.

clove oil   An oil obtained by the distillation of the dried, highly aromatic, unopened flower buds and twig tips of the clove tree, *Eugenia caryophyllata*. Its chief constituent is eugenol. Taken internally, it is used as an antispasmodic and a carminative. It is used externally as a rubefacient, counterirritant, and a mild analgesic, and it is used in histology as a clearing agent.

distilled oil   VOLATILE OIL.

essential oil   VOLATILE OIL.

ethereal oil   VOLATILE OIL.

ethiodized oil   A poppyseed oil containing organically combined iodine, used as a contrast medium for bronchography and laryngography.

eucalyptus oil   A volatile oil from the oil distilled from the fresh leaves of various *Eucalyptus* species. It is used as an antiseptic, deodorant, diaphoretic, expectorant, and in the synthesis of menthol.

fusel oil   Any of the liquid products of alcoholic fermentation other than ethanol and glycerol. It is a source of higher alcohols.

geranium oil   A volatile oil distilled from the leaves of *Pelargonium capitatum, P. odoratissimum*, and *P. radula*, having a roselike scent. It has been used in the production of dentifrices and ointments. Also called *oil of pelargonium, oil of rose geranium*.

gingilli oil   SESAME OIL.

Haarlem oil   JUNIPER TAR.

halibut liver oil   Oil obtained from the liver of the halibut, *Hippoglossus hippoglossus*. The oil is used as a convenient way of administering vitamins A and D, as it contains 100 times as much vitamin A as cod liver oil and 250 times as much vitamin D. It has only a slight fishy odor and taste. Also called *oleum hippoglossi*.

hydrocarpus oil   CHAULMOOGRA OIL.

immersion oil   In immersion microscopy, the oil that is interposed between the objective lens and the cover slip over the object being examined. Cedarwood or cedar oil, from *Juniperus virginiana*, is often used.

Indian melissa oil   LEMON GRASS OIL.

Indian oil of verbena   LEMON GRASS OIL.

iodized oil   A vegetable oil containing organically combined iodine and used as a contrast medium in radiologic examinations, such as bronchography, hysterosalpingography and laryngography.

jojoba oil   A liquid derived from the crushed seeds of *Simmindsia chinensis* and *S. californica*, shrubs indigenous to the Southwestern U.S. and Northern Mexico. It is used mainly as a lubricant.

juniper tar oil   JUNIPER TAR.

kernel oils   Oils extracted or expressed from the seeds of plants.

lemon grass oil   An oil obtained by distillation from the grasses *Cymbopogon flexuosus* and *C. citratus* from India. It was formerly used as a flavoring agent and carminative, but is now primarily used as a source of citral, which is important in vitamin A synthesis, and in perfumery. It also contains traces of geraniol, citronellal, and dipentene. Also called *Indian oil of verbena, Indian melissa oil*.

mineral oil   **1** A petroleum fraction of fairly high boiling point, usually purified to the standards necessary for medicinal use. It is not absorbed from the gut and is therefore sometimes used as a laxative. Also called *liquid paraffin*. **2** PETROLEUM.

oil of mirbane   NITROBENZENE.

neroli oil   ORANGE FLOWER OIL.

nondestearinated cod liver oil   The fixed oil separated from the fresh livers of *Gadus morrhua* and other species of *Gadus*. It is a pale yellow oil with a pronounced fishy odor and taste. It is used as a source of vitamins A and D. The oil consists of the glycerides of the fatty acids palmitoleic, oleic, linoleic, gadoleic, and clupadonicand so is a rich source of unsaturated fatty acids. It also contains lesser quantities of the saturated fatty acids myristic, palmitic, and stearic.

olive oil   A fixed oil expressed from the ripe fruit of *Olea europaea*, olive. It is used in foods, as a demulcent, and as a laxative.

orange oil   A volatile oil expressed from the peel of the fruit of *Citrus aurantium*, orange. Bitter orange oil, obtained from the dried rind of an unripe fruit, is used in flavoring pharmaceuticals.

orange flower oil   A yellow oil with a characteristic, sweet aromatic odor and taste, obtained by distilling flowers of the bitter orange tree, *citrus aurantium*. The methyl ester of anthranilic acid is believed to be the main aromatic component.

It is used as a flavoring agent and in perfumes. Also called *neroli oil.*

palm oil   A red oil produced from the nuts of *Elaeis guineensis.* The oil is extracted from the mesocarp or pericarp which is the fibrous pulp found just under the surface of the nut's skin. The color is due to its high content of β-carotene and other carotenoids. It is used for margarine and cooking fats, especially in Africa.

oil of Palma Christi   CASTOR OIL.

oil of pelargonium   GERANIUM OIL.

percomorph oil   An oil rich in vitamins A and D, obtained from the livers of percomorph fishes. Also called *oleum percomorphum.*

phenolated oil   A 5% weight per volume solution of phenol in arachis oil. It was formerly used as local anesthetic on the skin, but dizziness and fever sometimes followed its use. Dilution of phenolic solutions with water are caustic, and glycerine should be used instead. Also called *carbolic oil.*

pimenta oil   See under PIMENTA.

ricinus oil   CASTOR OIL.

rose oil   ATTAR OF ROSES.

oil of rose geranium   GERANIUM OIL.

safflower oil   A fixed, unsaturated oil that is extracted from the seeds of *Carthamus tinctorius.* The oil is rich in linoleic compounds which are not conducive to serum cholesterol buildup. It is used principally in the production of margarine, salad oils, and mayonnaise.

sassafras oil   A volatile oil obtained by the distillation of the root of *Sassafras albidum* and other species of *Sassafras.* It has carminative properties, and is used in flavoring medicaments.

sesame oil   A fixed oil obtained by expression from the seeds of one or more varieties of *Sesamum indicum.* It has nutritive, laxative, and emollient properties. The oil is used as a solvent for injections and in the preparation of ointments. Also called *benne oil, gingilli oil, teel oil.*

sweet birch oil   METHYL SALICYLATE.

tangantangan oil   CASTOR OIL.

tansy oil   An oil obtained from the leaves and flowering tops of the herb *Tanacetum vulgare,* tansy. It consists of thujone, borneol, camphor, and resins, and it has been used as an anthelmintic.

teaberry oil   METHYL SALICYLATE.

teel oil   SESAME OIL.

theobroma oil   A yellowish white edible fat expressed from the crushed and roasted seeds of *Theobroma cacao,* containing glycerides of stearic, palmitic, arachic, and oleic acids. It is used in the production of chocolate, and in suppositories, pessaries, bougies, ointments, and lubricants. Also called *cocoa butter, cacao butter.*

tuna-liver oil   An oil rich in vitamin D_3 obtained from the fresh liver of the tuna fish.

turpentine oil   The volatile oil obtained by the distillation of the oleoresin from *Pinus palustris* and other species of *Pinus.* It consists almost entirely of pinene. Rectified turpentine oil has been used as a local irritant and externally as a mild antiseptic. Also called *spirit of turpentine, terebenthene.*

volatile oil   An odorous principle found in different parts of plants which evaporates when exposed to air at ordinary temperatures. Volatile oils represent the essences or active principle in plants. Although differing greatly in their chemical composition, they have several physical properties in common. They have characteristic odors due to the presence of oxygenated derivatives of terpenes and sesquiterpenes. They have high refractive indices. Most are optically active. Generally, they are not miscible with water but are soluble in alcohol, ether, and most organic solvents. The oils are obtained by steam distillation, enzymatic hydrolysis, expression, enfleurage, and destruc-

tive distillation. Also called *distilled oil, essential oil, ethereal oil.*

wintergreen oil   METHYL SALICYLATE.

wood oil   GURJUN BALSAM.

oiling   The spraying of gasoline or heavier oils on the surface of bodies of water in areas infested with mosquitoes in order to kill the larvae.

oinomania   An obsolete term for DIPSOMANIA.

ointment

ointment [Old French *oignement* (irreg. from L *unguentum* an ointment, perfume, akin to *unctus,* past part. of *ungere* to wet, anoint, smear; Gk *hygros* wet, soft) an ointment]   A semisolid preparation of one or more medicinal substances in a suitable base. There are hydrocarbon bases for emollient effects, water-in-oil emulsion bases for good absorption, creams that can be washed off for cosmetic reasons, and greaseless ointment bases. Also called *salve, unction, unguent, unguentum, uncture, aliptic.*

ammoniated mercury ointment   An ointment containing ammoniated mercury, usually at about a 5% concentration, in a suitable oily base. It has been used in the past for external application for some skin conditions but has been generally replaced with other medications. The danger of mercury poisoning is too serious, to use such mercurial agents. Also called *white precipitate ointment, unguentum hydrargyri ammoniati.*

ointment of ammonium ichtholsulfonate   ICHTHAMMOL OINTMENT.

anthralin ointment   An ointment containing anthralin in a soft paraffin or other suitable base, used for the treatment of psoriasis and a number of other chronic dermatoses. Also called *dithranol ointment (British usage).*

bacitracin ointment   A preparation of bacitracin in an ointment base containing 500 units of bacitracin per gram. It is used topically and in the eye.

benzocaine ointment   A preparation of benzocaine used as a topical anesthetic. Also called *ethylaminobenzoate ointment.*

benzoic and salicylic acid ointment   An ointment containing 6% benzoic acid and 3% salicylic acid. Also called *Whitfield's ointment, unguentum acidi benzoici compositum.*

boric acid ointment   An ointment containing 1% boric acid in white petrolatum. Also called *unguentum acidi borici.*

calamine ointment   An ointment containing 15% calamine in white petrolatum. Also called *Turner cerate, unguentum calaminae.*

calomel ointment   MILD MERCUROUS CHLORIDE OINTMENT.

candicidin ointment   An ointment containing about 0.6 mg/g of candicin, an antifungal antibiotic obtained from *Streptomyces grisens.*

ointment of capsicum   An ointment containing capsicum oleoresin. Also called *unguentum capsici.*

carbolic acid ointment   PHENOL OINTMENT.

chloramphenicol ophthalmic ointment   A sterile eye ointment containing 1% chloramphenicol.

chrysarobin ointment   An ointment containing 4% chrysarobin. Also called *unguentum chrysarobini.*

coal tar ointment   An ointment containing coal tar, polysorbate 80, and zinc paste. It is used in the treatment of eczema. Also called *unguentum picis carbonis.*

ointment of colophony   An ointment containing pine resin, formerly used as a protective dressing for blisters and wounds. Also called *unguentum colophonii, unguentum resinae.*

compound ointment of calamine   An ointment containing calamine and zinc oxide in white petrolatum combined in solution with coal tar in hydrous wool fat. Also called *unguentum calaminae compositum, unguentum sedativum.*

compound ointment of capsicum   An ointment containing capsicum oleoresin, menthol, chloral hydrate, camphor, and petrolatum. Also called *chillie paste, unguentum capsici compositum, unguentum oleoresinae capsici compositum.*

compound menthol ointment   An ointment containing menthol, methyl salicylate, white wax, and lanolin. It is used as a local irritant. Also called *unguentum mentholis compositum, inunctum mentholis compositum.*

compound ointment of methyl salicylate   An ointment containing methyl salicylate, menthol, eucalyptol, cajuput oil in beeswax, and lanolin. Also called *unguentum betulae compositum, unguentum methylis salicylatis compositum.*

compound resorcinol ointment   An ointment containing resorcinol, bismuth subnitrate and zinc oxide. It is used to treat certain skin diseases. Also called *unguentum resorcini compositum, unguentum resorcinolis compositum.*

compound undecylenic acid ointment   An ointment containing 20% zinc undecylenate and 5% undecylenic acid. It is used topically as an antifungal agent in the treatment or prevention of dermatophytoses. Also called *unguentum acidi undecylenici compositum.*

Danish ointment   POTASSIUM POLYSULFIDE OINTMENT.

dexamethasone sodium phosphate ophthalmic ointment   A sterile ointment containing 0.05% of dexamethasone phosphate. It is applied to the conjunctiva as an anti-inflammatory medication.

dimethisoquin hydrochloride ointment   An ointment containing 0.5% dimethisoquin hydrochloride. It is used as a surface anesthetic agent.

dithranol ointment   A British term for ANTHRALIN OINTMENT.

emulsifying ointment   An ointment composed of emulsifying wax, white petrolatum, and mineral oil. Also called *unguentum emulsificans.*

epinephrine bitartrate ophthalmic ointment   An eye ointment containing approximately 1% epinephrine bitartrate in a hydrophilic petrolatum base. Also called *unguentum epinephrinae bitartratis ophthalmicum.*

eserine ointment   PHYSOSTIGMINE OINTMENT.

ethylaminobenzoate ointment   BENZOCAINE OINTMENT.

flurandrenolide ointment   An ointment containing 0.025 or 0.05% flurandrenolide. It is used as a topical preparation to provide glucocorticoid therapy in certain dermatoses as an anti-inflammatory agent.

ointment of gall   An ointment containing powdered gall and lard. It contains tannic acid, and has been used to treat hemorrhoids. Also called *unguentum gallae.*

ointment of gall and opium   An ointment of gall with powdered opium as the additional ingredient. Also called *unguentum gallae et opio.*

gentamicin sulfate ointment   A preparation containing 0.1% gentamicin in a suitable ointment base. It is applied topically to the conjunctiva as an antibacterial medication.

ointment of glycerin of lead subacetate   An ointment containing lead subacetate glycerin in white petrolatum. Also called *unguentum glycerini plumbi subacetatis.*

golden ointment   YELLOW MERCURIC OXIDE OPHTHALMIC OINTMENT.

hamamelis ointment   An ointment containing witch hazel extract in anhydrous lanolin and petrolatum base. Also called *unguentum hamamelidis.*

hydrocortisone ointment   A preparation of hydrocortisone in an ointment base, containing 90–110% of the labeled 0.5, 1.0,

or 2.5% hydrocortisone. These products are employed as anti-inflammatory corticosteroid medications. Also called *unguentum hydrocortisoni.*

hydrocortisone acetate ointment   A 1.0–1.25% preparation of hydrocortisone acetate in a suitable ointment base. It is used topically as an adrenocortical steroid. Also called *unguentum hydrocortisoni acetatis.*

hydrocortisone acetate ophthalmic ointment   An ointment base containing 90–110% of the labeled 0.5% hydrocortisone acetate. It is utilized as an anti-inflammatory remedy and is applied topically to the conjunctiva.

hydrophilic ointment   An emulsion of water in oil containing methylparaben, propylparaben, sodium lauryl sulfate, propylene glycol, stearyl alcohol, white petrolatum, and purified water. It is used as a base for ointments. Also called *unguentum hydrophilicum.*

hydroquinone ointment   A preparation of 2% or 4% hydroquinone in a suitable ointment base. It is used as a depigmenting agent on the skin to inhibit the formation of melanin.

ointment of hydrous wool fat   An ointment composed of equal parts of lanolin and petrolatum. Also called *unguentum adipis lanae hydrosi.*

ichthammol ointment   An ointment containing 10% ammonium ichthosulfonate, wool fat, and yellow soft paraffin. It is used to treat chronic skin diseases. Also called *ointment of ammonium ichthosulfonate, unguentum ichthammollis.*

idoxuridine ophthalmic ointment   A preparation containing 0.45–.55% idoxuridine in a suitable petrolatum base. It is applied topically to the conjunctivae as an antiviral agent, and is used in the treatment of herpes simplex keratitis.

iodine ointment   Iodine in arachis oil and yellow soft paraffin in ointment form. It is used externally for its potent microbicidal actions. Also called *unguentum iodi.*

iodochlorhydroxyquin ointment   Iodochlorhydroxyquin in a suitable ointment base, containing 90–110% of the labeled 3% iodochlorhydroxyquin. It is used in the treatment of some dermatoses, such as eczema, as an anti-infective medication.

iodochlorhydroxyquin and hydrocortisone ointment   An ointment preparation containing 90–110% of the labeled 3 and 5% or 3 and 1% of iodochlorhydroxyquin and hydrocortisone. It is used as a local anti-infective agent and a glucocorticoid medication.

isoflurophate ophthalmic ointment   A 0.0225–0.0275% preparation of isoflurophate in a suitable anhydrous base. It is used in the treatment of glaucoma, and is applied to the conjunctiva as a cholinergic agent that acts by inhibition of acetylcholinesterase.

ointment of kaolin   An ointment containing kaolin in a hard paraffin base. It has been used to protect abraded skin. Also called *unguentum kaolini.*

lanolin ointment   An ointment containing a mixture of lanolin and soft paraffin. It is used as a skin emollient and as a general ointment base. Also called *unguentum lanolini.*

ointment of lead subacetate   An ointment containing 12.5% lead subacetate in a base of lanolin and petrolatum. Also called *unguentum plumbi subacetis.*

lidocaine ointment   A preparation of lidocaine in a hydrophilic base containing 95–105% of the labeled 5% lidocaine hydrochloride. It is applied topically as a local anesthetic.

Löwenstein's ointment   An ointment prepared from a culture of diphtheria bacteria containing the killed organisms and toxin. It was used in the past to attempt to induce immunization against diphtheria.

ointment of menthol and camphor   An ointment composed of menthol and camphor in soft paraffin. It is used on the chest to relieve symptoms of bronchitis and other respiratory conditions.

mercury bichloride ointment An ointment containing mercuric chloride. It is of limited application because of the potential hazard of systemic toxicity from absorption of mercury. Also called *unguentum hydrargyri bichloridi.*

methyl salicylate ointment An ointment containing 50 g methyl salicylate, 25 g white beeswax, and 25 g of lanolin. It has been used as a skin dressing to relieve pain of rheumatic and deep muscle origin. Also called *wintergreen ointment.*

mild mercurous chloride ointment An ointment containing mercurous chloride, hydrous wool fat, and petrolatum. It was formerly used to treat skin diseases and infections. Also called *calomel ointment, unguentum hydrargyri subchloridi.*

monobenzone ointment An ointment preparation containing 94–106% of the labeled 20% monobenzone in a water-soluble base. It has been used as a depigmenting agent on the skin.

neomycin sulfate ointment A suitable ointment base containing 3.5 mg of neomycin per gram. It is applied topically as an antibacterial medication.

nitrofurazone ointment An ointment containing 0.2% nitrofurazone in a suitable water-miscible base. It is used as an antibacterial treatment in the care of burns, but is not applied for more than a few days, as sensitization and allergic reactions are then likely to be encountered. Also called *unguentum nitrofurazoni.*

nystatin ointment A suitable ointment base containing in each gram 90–130% of the labeled 100 000 units of nystatin activity. It is applied topically as an antifungal medication.

ointment of oil of cade An ointment composed of 25 gms of cade oil, 12.5 gms of yellow beeswax, and 62.5 gms of yellow soft paraffin. It is used in the treatment of eczema and psoriasis.

oily cream hydrous ointment An ointment consisting of 50 g of wool alcohol ointment, 1 g of phenoxyethanol, 500 mg of dried magnesium phosphate, and 48.5 g of water. It is used as a base for water-and-oil emulsions.

Pagenstecher's ointment YELLOW MERCURIC OXIDE OPHTHALMIC OINTMENT.

paraffin ointment An ointment composed of beeswax, paraffin wax, and white and yellow soft paraffin. It is used mainly as a stable base for emulsions and creams. Also called *unguentum paraffini.*

penicillin ointment An ointment base containing calcium penicillin, crystalline penicillin, or procaine penicillin. Also called *unguentum penicillini.*

petrolatum rose water ointment An ointment containing spermaceti, white wax, mineral oil, sodium borate, rose water, and rose oil, an emollient and ointment base. Also called *unguentum aquae rosae petrolatum.*

phenol ointment An ointment of phenol in lard and paraffin. It is used topically for its antipruritic action. Also called *carbolic acid ointment, unguentum acidi carbolici, unguentum phenolis.*

physostigmine ointment A preparation containing physostigmine salicylate and chloroform in a yellow soft paraffin base. It is used in the eye as a miotic medication. Also called *eserine ointment, unguentum physostigminae.*

pine tar ointment An ointment containing pine tar, yellow wax, and yellow ointment. Also called *unguentum picis pini.*

polyethylene glycol ointment A water-soluble ointment base containing a mixture of polyethylene glycol 4000 and polyethylene glycol 400. Also called *unguentum glycolis polyethyleni.*

polymyxin B sulfate ointment A topical antibacterial medication composed of polymyxin B sulfate in an anhydrous petrolatum base. It contains 90–120% of the labeled 20 000 polymyxin B sulfate units per gram.

potassium polysulfide ointment An ointment containing polysulfides of potassium, zinc hydroxide, and benzaldehyde in a wool fat and paraffin base. It was used to treat scabies. Also called *Danish ointment, unguentum potassi polysulphidi.*

ointment of resorcinol $C_6H_6O_2$. Benzene-1,3-diol. 2–5% resorcinol in a suitable ointment base, utilized as a keratolytic agent in the treatment of acne and seborrheic dermatitis. It is also applied to the skin for its antipruretic and exfoliative properties. Also called *unguentum resorcini, unguentum resorcinolis.*

rose water ointment An ointment containing rose water, beeswax, borax, almond oil, and rose oil. Also called *unguentum aquae rosae.*

ointment of salicylic acid and sulfur An ointment containing 2–3% salicylic acid and 2–3% sulfur. Also called *unguentum acidi salicyli et sylphuris.*

scarlet red ointment An ointment containing scarlet red, olive oil, anhydrous lanolin, and petrolatum. It is used topically as a protective medication. Also called *unguentum rubri scarlatini, unguentum rubrum.*

simple ointment An ointment composed primarily of white petrolatum with various amounts of lanolin and white beeswax. Also called *unguentum simplex.*

sodium perborate ointment An ointment containing sodium perborate in a paraffin base. It is used as an antiseptic to quicken healing. Also called *unguentum sodii perboratis.*

sodium sulfacetamide ophthalmic ointment A sterile ointment of sodium sulfacetamide in a suitable base, which can be applied topically to the conjunctiva as an antibacterial medication for sulfonamide-responsive eye infections. Also called *unguentum sulfacetamidi sodici.*

ointment of spermaceti An ointment containing spermaceti, white beeswax, and mineral oil. Also called *unguentum cetacei.*

sulfur ointment Precipitated sulfur mixed with mineral oil and white ointment. It is used as a scabicide. Also called *unguentum sulfuris.*

ointment of tannic acid An ointment containing tannic acid and glycerin, formerly used for the treatment of burns. Also called *unguentum acidi tannici.*

ointment of tar An ointment consisting of tar, lard, and yellow beeswax. It has been used on the skin for antipruritic effects in treating chronic skin diseases. Also called *unguentum picis liquidae.*

tetracaine ophthalmic ointment A white petrolatum ointment base containing 0.45–0.55% added tetracaine. It is used as a local anesthetic agent.

thymol ointment An ointment containing thymol dissolved in soft paraffin. It is used in the treatment of eczema and other skin diseases. Also called *unguentum thymolis.*

triamcinolone acetonide ointment $C_{24}H_{31}FO_6$. A suitable ointment base containing triamcinolone acetonide. It is a corticosteroid preparation that is applied topically in the treatment of diseases of the skin.

triclobisonium chloride ointment A suitable ointment base containing triclobisonium chloride that is applied topically as an anti-infective agent, mainly in combating gynecologic infections.

Wertheim's ointment An ointment compounded of ammoniated mercury and bismuth in glycerin. It was formerly used to treat chloasma.

white ointment An ointment containing 5% white beeswax and 95% white petrolatum. Also called *unguentum album.*

white precipitate ointment AMMONIATED MERCURY OINTMENT.

Whitfield's ointment BENZOIC AND SALICYLIC ACID OINTMENT.

wintergreen ointment METHYL SALICYLATE OINTMENT.

wool alcohols ointment An ointment containing wool alcohols, petrolatum, and other ingredients to obtain a suitable water-in-oil emulsion. Also called *unguentum alcoholium lanae.*

yellow ointment An ointment base containing yellow wax and petrolatum. Also called *unguentum flavum.*

yellow mercuric oxide ophthalmic ointment   An ointment containing finely powdered yellow mercuric oxide, liquid petrolatum, and white ointment, the concentration of mercuric oxide being 0.9–1.1%. It is used as a topical anti-infective agent in the eye. Also called *golden ointment, Pagenstecher's ointment, unguentum hydrargyri oxidi flavi.*

zinc ointment   ZINC OXIDE OINTMENT.

zinc and castor oil ointment   A preparation containing zinc oxide and castor oil in benzoinated lard. It is used as a protective medication for the skin. Also called *unguentum zinci et olei ricini.*

zinc oxide ointment   A medication containing zinc oxide and mineral oil in a white ointment base. It is used topically as an astringent and protective product. Also called *zinc ointment, unguentum zinci oxidi.*

ointment of zinc oxide with benzoin   An ointment containing tincture of benzoin in zinc oxide ointment. It is used to aid in the healing of minor injuries to the skin. Also called *unguentum zinci oxidi cum benzoino.*

zinc undecenoate ointment   A mixture of zinc undecenoate and undecenoic acid in an emulsifying ointment base. It is used primarily in the treatment of mycotic infections. Also called *unguentum undecylenati.*

Oken   [Lorenz *Oken*, German naturalist and philosopher, 1779–1851]   **1** Canal of Oken. See under MESONEPHRIC DUCT. **2** Corpus of Oken, Oken's body. See under MESONEPHROS.

OL   oculus laevus.

ol.   *oleum* (L, oil).

-ol [*(alcoh)ol.* See ALCOHOL.]   A suffix designating the presence of a hydroxyl group, —OH. It replaces the final -e in the name of an alkane, e.g., *ethane* yields *ethanol.*

-ole [L *-olus* suffix diminishing nouns]   A suffix meaning a small or little one.

oleaginous   Having the consistency of oil; oily.

oleandomycin $C_{35}H_{61}NO_{12}$. A macrolide antibiotic produced by *Streptomyces antibioticus* no. ATCC 11891. Its structure is like that of erythromycin, and it is given parenterally for the treatment of staphylococci and some other Gram-positive bacteria. It is usually administered as its phosphate, or triacetyl derivative, troleandomycin.

oleandrin $C_{32}H_{48}O_9$. A cardiac glycoside obtained from *Nerium oleander*, oleander. In therapeutic amounts it is used to treat cardiac insufficiency, but in cases of excess ingestion, it may be fatal.

oleandrism [*oleand(e)r* + -ISM]   Poisoning from ingestion of a cardiac glycoside contained in the roots, flowers, seeds, or bark of oleander, *Nerium oleander*. It may result in nausea, vomiting, bradycardia, heart block, cardiac arrhythmia, and cardiac arrest.

olecranal   Of or relating to the olecranon.

olecranarthritis [*olecran(on)* + ARTHRITIS]   Inflammation of the olecranon bursa and elbow joint.

olecranarthrocace [*olecran(on)* + ARTHRO- + Gk *kakē* badness]   An inflammation, often tuberculous in nature, of the elbow joint. An older term.

olecranarthropathy [*olecran(on)* + ARTHROPATHY]   Abnormality of the olecranon bursa, olecranon, and elbow joint.

olecranoid   Resembling or shaped like the olecranon.

olecranon   [NA]   The proximal part of the upper end of the ulna, bent forward at its highest point so that its concave anterior surface forms the upper part of the trochlear notch. The quadrangular-shaped superior surface has a rough posterior part for the insertion of the tendon of the triceps muscle and a smooth anterior part related to the subtendinous bursa. The junction of the superior and posterior surfaces forms the angular tip of the elbow. The latter surface is triangular and subcutaneous, its apex being continuous distally with the posterior margin of the shaft of the ulna. The anterior margins provide attachment for the capsule of the elbow joint. Also called *olecranon process of ulna, gibber ulnae* (outmoded), *anconeal process of ulna* (outmoded).

olefin   A hydrocarbon containing a double bond.

oleic acid CH_3—$[CH_2]_7$—CH=CH—$[CH_2]_7$—$COOH$. The *cis* form of octadec-9-enoic acid. It occurs in fats and phospholipids. Its compounds in membranes increase their fluidity in comparison with saturated fatty acids. Unlike some other unsaturated fatty acids, it can be made in the mammalian body.

olein $(C_{17}H_{33}COO)_3C_3H_5$. Glyceryl trioleate, an unsaturated, liquid fat occurring in many natural fats and oils. Also called *triolein.*

olenitis [Gk *ōlen(ē)* elbow + -ITIS]   Arthritis of the elbow joint. An obsolete term.

oleo- [L *oleum* olive oil, oil]   A combining form denoting oil.

oleoarthrosis   Injection of oil into a joint cavity.

oleochrysotherapy   Treatment with gold salts in a fat or oily base.

oleoetherization   Etherization involving the use of oil as a conduit for the ether.

rectal oleoetherization   GWATHMEY'S OIL-ETHER ANESTHESIA.

oleogranuloma [OLEO- + GRANULOMA]   PARAFFINOMA.

oleoinfusion   A medicinal preparation obtained by extraction of the active components of a crude drug into an oil.

oleoma   LIPOGRANULOMA.

oleometer   A device that measures the purity of an oil by determining its relative density. Also called *eleometer.*

oleoperitoneography [OLEO- + PERITONEOGRAPHY]   Roentgenographic study of the peritoneal cavity after its being injected percutaneously with iodized oil.

oleoresin [L *oleoresina.* See OLEORESINA.]   **1** A combination of a resin and a volatile oil present in some plants. **2** A semisolid pharmaceutical product obtained by removing the volatile oils and resins from a plant or plant part with a solvent and then evaporating the solvent.

aspidium oleoresin   An extract made from aspidium. It has been used in the treatment of tapeworm infection. Also called *aspidum oleoresin.*

capsicum oleoresin   A thick, dark, reddish brown liquid containing not less than 8% capsicin, obtained by extraction of capsicum with hot acetone or alcohol, evaporating the solvent, and extracting the residue with cold 90% alcohol, followed by evaporation of the alcohol. It is used as a carminative agent in very dilute solutions and externally as an irritant.

oleotherapy   Medicinal use of oil, as in oleoarthrosis.

oleothorax   The injection of oil into the thoracic cavity to effect partial or complete collapse of the lung. This procedure, now obsolete, was originally proposed to treat tuberculosis. Also called *eleothorax.*

oleovitamin [OLEO- + VITAMIN]   A dietary supplement consisting of one or more of the fat-soluble vitamins or their derivatives in solution in fish-liver oil or vegetable oil.

oleovitamin A   A preparation of fish-liver oil or vegetable oil containing natural or synthetic vitamin A.

oleovitamin A and D   A preparation containing natural or synthetic vitamins A and D in fish-liver oil or vegetable oil.

oleovitamin D_2   A preparation of fish-liver oil or vegetable oil containing natural vitamin D_2 (calciferol). It is often used as a dietary supplement.

oleovitamin D_3   A preparation containing 7-dehydrocholesterol in fish-liver oil or vegetable oil.

oleum **1** OIL. **2** Fuming sulfuric acid.

oleum camphorae essentiale RECTIFIED CAMPHOR OIL.

oleum camphorae rectificatum RECTIFIED CAMPHOR OIL.

oleum hippoglossi HALIBUT LIVER OIL.

oleum iodisatum IODIZED OIL.

oleum percomorphum PERCOMORPH OIL.

oleum ricini CASTOR OIL.

oleum ricini aromaticum AROMATIC CASTOR OIL.

oleum succini OIL OF AMBER.

olfact [L *olfact(us)*, past part. of *olfacere* (from *ol(ere)* to emit an odor + *facere* to make) to smell] The mean minimal perceptible odor as measured by the Proetz olfactometer. See also PROETZ OLFACTOMETER.

olfactie The unit of olfactory acuity measured by the olfactometer of Zwaardemaker, expressed as the distance on the centimeter scale at which the subject just perceives the test odor.

olfaction [OLFACT + -ION] **1** The process of smelling. Also called *osmesis* (seldom used). **2** The sense of smell. Also called *osphresis* (seldom used).

olfactism [L *olfact(us)*, past part. of *olfacere* (from *ol(ere)* to smell, scent + *facere* to make) to smell, scent + -ISM] A sensation of smell produced by a sensory stimulus which is not normally olfactory.

olfactology [OLFACT + *o* + -LOGY] The science concerned with the study of the sense of smell. Also called *osmics* (rarely used).

olfactometer [OLFACT + *o* + -METER] An instrument or arrangement, as of various odorants, for assessing the acuity of the sense of smell or for measuring the olfactory threshold for a selected range of odors. Also called *ophresiometer* (rarely used).

blast olfactometer An olfactometer for injecting into the nose a measured volume of air containing a constant concentration of the odorant under test.

Proetz olfactometer An olfactometer consisting of a rack of one-hundred small bottles arranged in ten rows. Each row across is concerned with one particular odorant, the concentration of which increases from left to right. The results are recorded in units called "olfacts," corresponding to the concentration in grams of the odorant per liter of the diluent.

olfactometer of Zwaardemaker An olfactometer consisting of two tubes, one sliding within the other, the outer one being impregnated with one of a variety of odorants. The inner tube of glass, calibrated in centimeters, was designed to enable the subject to breathe through it, using one side of the nose or the other. According to the length of outer tube exposed, by sliding out the inner tube, the intensity of the odor in the inspired air could be varied and represented as so many centimeters. It is no longer used.

olfactory [L *olfactori(us)*, from *olfact(us)*, past part. of *olfacere* (from *ol(ere)* to emit a smell + *facere* to make, do) to smell (a thing); + -*orius* -ORY] **1** Of or relating to the sense of smell. **2** Possessing a sense of smell. For defs. 1 and 2 also *osmatic, osphretic.*

olig- OLIGO-.

oligaemia A British spelling for OLIGEMIA.

oligemia An obsolete term for ANEMIA.

oligergasia An outmoded term for MENTAL RETARDATION.

olighidria HYPOHIDROSIS.

olighydria HYPOHIDROSIS.

oligidria HYPOHIDROSIS.

oligo- [Gk *oligos* few, little] A combining form meaning (1) small, few; (2) abnormally small or few. Also *olig-*.

oligoamnios The presence of a less than normal amount of amniotic fluid.

oligoarthritis [OLIGO- + ARTHRITIS] Arthritis of a few joints. Compare MONARTHRITIS, POLYARTHRITIS.

oligoastrocytoma [OLIGO- + ASTROCYTOMA] A glioma with a conspicuous mixture of oligodendroglial and astrocytic components.

oligoblast [OLIGO- + -BLAST] A primitive macroglial cell that differentiates into an oligodendrocyte. Also called *oligodendroblast.*

oligoblennia [OLIGO- + BLENN- + -IA] A state of abnormally reduced mucus secretion.

oligocardia [OLIGO- + -CARDIA] BRADYCARDIA.

Oligochaeta [OLIGO- + Gk *chaitē* long flowing hair] An order of worms in the phylum Annelida that includes the common earthworm, *Lumbricus*, and related forms, as well as many freshwater annelids.

oligocholia [OLIGO- + CHOL- + -IA] A state of insufficient bile secretion. An outmoded term.

oligochromasia Hypochromia.

oligochylia [OLIGO- + CHYL- + -IA] A state of insufficient gastric secretion. An outmoded term.

oligochymia [OLIGO- + *chym(e)* + -IA] A state of insufficient chyme. An outmoded term.

oligocystic Containing but a few cysts.

oligocythemia An obsolete term for ANEMIA.

oligocytosis An obsolete term for ANEMIA.

oligodacrya [OLIGO- + Gk *dakrya*, pl. of *dakryon* a tear] A deficiency in tearing of the eyes.

oligodactylia ECTRODACTYLY.

oligodactyly ECTRODACTYLY.

oligodendria A seldom used term for OLIGODENDROGLIA.

oligodendroblast OLIGOBLAST.

oligodendroblastoma [OLIGO- + Gk *dendro(n)* a tree (usu. a fruit tree) + BLASTOMA] **1** OLIGODENDROGLIOMA. **2** A tumor of immature oligodendrocytes.

oligodendrocyte Any cell of the oligodendroglia.

oligodendroglia A group of macroglial cells that is subdivided into perineuronal, interfascicular, and juxtavascular types. Most cells are characterized by thin, flat processes that envelop axons to form segments of their myelin sheaths. Also called *oligodendria* (seldom used), *oligoglia* (seldom used), *interfascicular oligoglia.*

oligodendroglioma [*oligodendrogli(al)* + -OMA] A tumor composed predominantly of oligodendroglial cells. The cells are usually uniform, with round nuclei, clear cytoplasm and well-defined cell membranes giving a halo appearance. Calcification is often present. This is typically a slow-growing tumor but an anaplastic form is recognized. Also called *mesoglioma, oligodendroma, oligodendroblastoma.*

oligodendrogliomatosis [OLIGO- + Gk *dendro(n)* a tree + GLIOMATOSIS] Diffuse neoplastic growth of oligodendroglia.

oligodendrogliomatosis cerebri GLIOMATOSIS CEREBRI.

oligodendroma [OLIGO- + Gk *dendr(on)* a tree + -OMA] OLIGODENDROGLIOMA.

oligodipsia [OLIGO- + DIPSIA] HYPODIPSIA.

oligodontia [*olig(o)*- + -ODONTIA] HYPODONTIA.

oligoencephalon MICRENCEPHALON.

oligogalactia [OLIGO- + GALACT- + -IA] Abnormally low secretion of breast milk.

oligogenesis [OLIGO- + GENESIS] The condition of having borne few children.

oligogenic   Controlled by more than one, but relatively few, genetic loci.

oligogenics [OLIGO- + -GEN + -ICS]   Birth control by means of contraceptives. An obsolete term.

oligoglia   A seldom used term for OLIOGODENDROGLIA.

    interfascicular oligoglia   OLIGODENDROGLIA.

oligohemia   An obsolete term for ANEMIA.

oligohidrosis   HYPOHIDROSIS.

oligohydramnios [OLIGO- + HYDR- + *amnio(n)* + s]   A deficiency in the amount of amniotic fluid.

oligohydruria [OLIGO- + HYDR- + -URIA]   Abnormally high specific gravity of the urine. It may result from heavy glycosuria or intravenous administration of mannitol or radiographic contrast agents.

oligohypermenorrhea [OLIGO- + HYPER- + MENORRHEA]   Infrequent episodes of menstrual bleeding characterized by a heavy flow.

oligohypomenorrhea [OLIGO- + HYPO- + MENORRHEA]   Infrequent episodes of menstrual bleeding associated with scant flow.

oligolecithal [OLIGO- + LECITHAL]   MIOLECITHAL.

oligoleukocythemia   LEUKOPENIA.

oligoleukocytosis   LEUKOPENIA.

oligomania [OLIGO- + -MANIA]   An obsolete term for MONOMANIA.

oligomenorrhea [OLIGO- + MENORRHEA]   A reduction in the frequency of menstruation, with cycle lengths usually exceeding 40 days. Also called *relative amenorrhea, infrequent menstruation.*

oligomer [*oligo-* + *-mer(e)*]   A substance whose molecules are formed by combination of a few simpler molecules, usually identical.

oligomeric   Containing two or more polypeptides, which may be the same or different: used of a protein.

oligomycin   Any of several macrolide antibiotics produced by an actinomycete similar to *Streptomyces* and having specific actions against fungi. Oligomycin A shows activity against fungi such as *Blastomyces dermatitides*, and Oligomycin B is a potent inhibitor of mitochondrial oxidative phosphorylation.

oligonatality [OLIGO- + NATALITY]   A relative scarcity of births. A seldom used term.

oligonucleotide   A compound whose molecules consist of a few nucleoside-phosphate residues joined together. Such compounds are obtained on partial hydrolysis of nucleic acids.

oligo-ovulation [OLIGO- + OVULATION]   A reduction in the number of oocytes maturing or in the frequency of ovulation.

oligopepsia [OLIGO- + Gk *peps(is)* digestion + -IA]   A state of insufficient digestion. An outmoded term.

oligopeptide   A peptide whose molecule contains a few amino-acid residues, up to about 20.

oligophagous [OLIGO- + -PHAGOUS]   Having a limited choice or preference of foods, as a parasite with few acceptable hosts.

oligophagy [OLIGO- + -PHAGY]   The condition of having a very limited range of preferred foods.

oligophrenia [OLIGO- + -PHRENIA]   An older term for MENTAL RETARDATION.

    phenylpyruvic oligophrenia   PHENYLKETONURIA.

    oligophrenia phenylpyruvica   PHENYLKETONURIA.

    polydystrophic oligophrenia   An outmoded term for PHENYLKETONURIA.

    uric acid disorder oligophrenia   LESCH-NYHAN SYNDROME.

oligophrenic   Pertaining to mental retardation.

oligoplasmia   An abnormal reduction in the amount of plasma in the blood. See also HEMOCONCENTRATION.

oligoplastic   Possessing an abnormally reduced capacity for repair.

oligopnea   HYPOPNEA.

oligoposia [OLIGO- + Gk *pos(is)* a drinking, drink + -IA]   An abnormal self-imposed reduction in fluid intake. An outmoded term. Also called *oligoposy.*

oligoposy   OLIGOPOSIA.

oligopyrene   Having a reduced chromosome complement, especially in a sperm. Also *oligopyrous.*

oligopyrous   OLIGOPYRENE.

oligosaccharide   A compound whose molecule consists of a few sugar residues joined by glycoside links.

oligosialia [OLIGO- + SIAL- + -IA]   HYPOSALIVATION.

oligosideremia   HYPOFERREMIA.

oligospermatic [OLIGO- + SPERMATIC]   Characterized by an abnormally low number of sperm in semen.

oligospermatism   OLIGOSPERMIA.

    oligospermia   An abnormally low number of sperm in semen. Also called *oligozoospermia, oligozoospermatism, oligospermatism.*

oligosteatosis   Dryness of the skin caused by insufficient sebum excretion. Also called *asteatosis, asteatosis cutis, asteatodes, hyposteatosis.*

oligosymptomatic   Having or producing few symptoms.

oligosynaptic   Denoting a neural pathway that includes only one or two interneurons, i.e., a di- or trisynaptic connection.

oligothymia [OLIGO- + THYM-² + -IA]   A condition marked by a poverty of affectivity.

oligotrichy   HYPOTRICHOSIS.

oligotrophia   OLIGOTROPHY.

oligotrophic   Providing very little nutrition.

oligotrophy [OLIGO- + TROPH- + -Y]   A state of nutrient scarcity or insufficiency. Also called *oligotrophia.*

oligozoospermatism   OLIGOSPERMIA.

oligozoospermia   OLIGOSPERMIA.

oliguresis   OLIGURIA.

oliguria [OLIG- + -URIA]   Scanty urine excretion. It may occur in acute renal failure, dehydration, shock, congestive heart failure, and urinary tract obstruction in the urethra, in bilateral ureteral obstruction, or in unilateral renal obstruction if only one kidney is functional. Also called *oliguresis.* Adjective: oliguric.

olisthe   OLISTHY.

olistherochromatin   The components of the constricted region of a chromosome.

olisthy [Gk *olisthan(ein)* to slip, slide + -Y]   A slipping of the bones of a joint so that they remain in an abnormal relationship to each other. Also *olisthe.*

oliva [L, olive, olive tree]   [NA] A prominent oval elevation, located on the ventrolateral aspect of the medulla oblongata and produced by the underlying inferior olivary nucleus. Also called *olivary body, olivary eminence, olive, medullary olive.*

olivae   Plural of OLIVA.

olivary   Denoting the olivary nuclei.

olive [L *oliv(a)* (from Gk *elaia* the olive tree, olive) the olive tree, olive]   **1** OLIVA. **2** The smooth, rounded, elliptical tip on the end of an internal vein stripper, so placed to avoid piercing the vein wall while the stripper is passed through the vein.

    inferior olive   NUCLEUS OLIVARIS.

    medullary olive   OLIVA.

    superior olive   NUCLEUS OLIVARIS SUPERIOR.

Oliver [William Silver *Oliver*, English physician, 1836–1908]   See under SIGN.

olive spurge MEZEREUM.

olivifugal Originating in and projecting from the inferior olive.

olivipetal Converging upon the inferior olive.

olivocerebellar Denoting the inferior olive and cerebellum, as the olivocerebellar fibers connecting them, which form the largest component of the restiform body projecting to the cerebellar cortex.

olivocortical Pertaining to nerve fibers that arise in the inferior olive and terminate in the cerebellar cortex.

olivonuclear Pertaining to nerve fibers passing from the inferior olive to the deep cerebellar nuclei.

olivopontocerebellar Denoting the inferior olivary nucleus, ventral pons, and the cerebellar cortex, and especially denoting the course of fibers entering the middle cerebellar peduncle, as well as olivopontocerebellar atrophy, ataxia, or degeneration, which is a heredodegenerative disease involving the middle cerebellar peduncles and pontine, arcuate, and olivary nuclei.

olivospinal Denoting the inferior olivary nucleus and the spinal cord, and especially denoting fibers that originate in the olivary nucleus and descend in a tract located near the anterolateral surface of the spinal cord.

Ollendorff [Helene *Ollendorff*, German dermatologist, flourished early 20th century] Buschke-Ollendorff syndrome. See under DISSEMINATED LENTICULAR DERMATOFIBROSIS.

Ollier [Léopold *Ollier*, French surgeon, 1830–1900] **1** Ollier's layer. See under STRATUM OSTEOGENETICUM. **2** See under LAW. **3** Ollier's osteochondromatosis. See under UNILATERAL CHONDRODYSPLASIA.

Ollier [Louis Xavier Edouard *Ollier*, French surgeon, 1830–1900] **1** See under OPERATION. **2** Ollier's disease. See under UNILATERAL CHONDRODYSPLASIA.

ololiuqui IPOMOEA.

olophonia [Gk *olo(os)* destroyed, undone + PHON- + -IA] An impediment of speech due to maldevelopment of any of the organs of speech. A rarely used term.

Olsen [Olaf *Olsen*, Swedish ophthalmologist, flourished 20th century] Alström-Olsen syndrome. See under ALSTRÖM SYNDROME.

Olshausen [Robert von *Olshausen*, German obstetrician, 1835–1915] See under OPERATION.

Olshevsky [Dimitry Eugene *Olshevsky*, U.S. physicist, born 1900] See under TUBE.

Olszewski [Jerzy *Olszewski*, Polish-born Canadian neurologist, 1913–1966] Steele-Richardson-Olszewski syndrome. See under PROGRESSIVE SUPRANUCLEAR PALSY.

oltipraz A 1,2-dithiole synthetic antischistosomal compound effective against *Schistosoma mansona* and *S. haematobium*.

OM **1** outer membrane. **2** otitis media.

o.m. *omni mane* (L, every morning).

-oma [Gk suffix *-ōma* denoting morbid condition, usually swelling or tumor] A suffix meaning tumor or neoplasm.

omacephalus [*om(o)-* + Gk *a-* priv. + *kephalē* head] ABRACHIOCEPHALUS.

omagra [*om(o)-* + -AGRA] Gout in the shoulder. An obsolete term.

omalgia [*om(o)-* + -ALGIA] OMODYNIA.

omarthralgia [*om(o)-* + ARTHR- + -ALGIA] OMODYNIA.

omarthritis [*om(o)-* + ARTHRITIS] Arthritis in the shoulder joint. An obsolete term.

omasitis Inflammation of the omasum.

omasum [L, bullock's tripe, ox's thick, fat gut] The third of the stomach chambers in a ruminant animal, situated between the reticulum and the most posterior chamber, the abomasum. Also called *manyplies* (seldom used), *psalterium*.

Ombrédanne [Louis *Ombrédanne*, French physician, 1871–1956] See under OPERATION, METHOD.

ombrophore [Gk *ombro(s)* rain, water + -PHORE] A device for administering a douche of carbonated water.

omega The name of the 24th and last letter of the Greek alphabet. Symbol: ω

omega melancholicum A wrinkling of the skin above the nose and between the eyebrows that takes the shape of the Greek letter omega (ω). It occurs as frowning, and as a persisting facial expression in depression. Also called *Schüle sign*.

omenta Plural of OMENTUM.

omental Of or relating to the omentum.

omentectomy The partial or complete removal of the greater omentum and sometimes the lesser omentum, either partially or completely, as well. Also called *epiploectomy, omentumectomy.*

omentitis [*oment(um)* + -ITIS] Inflammation of the omentum. Also called *epiploitis.*

omentofixation OMENTOPEXY.

omentopexy [*oment(um)* + *o* + -PEXY] **1** A surgical procedure in which the greater omentum is used as a graft to serve either as a mechanical patch or as a vascular supply to damaged tissues. **2** The surgical fixation of the omentum. Also called *epiplopexy, omentofixation, epiplopexia.*

omentoplasty [*oment(um)* + *o* + -PLASTY] Any plastic operation on omentum. Also called *epiploplasty.*

omentoportography [*oment(um)* + *o* + *port(al)* + *o* + -GRAPHY] Roentgenography of the portal veins in the liver after the injection of a radiopaque, water-soluble contrast medium into an omental vein.

omentorrhaphy [*oment(um)* + *o* + -RRHAPHY] The rejoining, by suture, of lacerated or transected omentum. Also called *epiplorrhaphy.*

omentosplenopexy A surgical procedure in which the omentum and the spleen are suspended from the abdominal wall to prevent ptosis or torsion.

omentotomy [*oment(um)* + *o* + -TOMY] A surgical incision into the omentum.

omentovolvulus A volvulus involving torsion of the omentum.

omentum [L, fat skin, fat, the caul of the entrails, the bowels] A double layer of peritoneum that connects the stomach to another abdominal organ. Also called *epiploon.*

colic omentum An outmoded term for OMENTUM MAJUS.

gastric omentum OMENTUM MAJUS.

gastrocolic omentum OMENTUM MAJUS.

gastrohepatic omentum An outmoded term for OMENTUM MINUS.

gastrosplenic omentum An outmoded term for LIGAMENTUM GASTROSPLENICUM.

greater omentum OMENTUM MAJUS.

lesser omentum OMENTUM MINUS.

omentum majus [NA] A double layer of peritoneum that is folded on itself in front of the small intestine to form four layers. Two layers are attached to the greater curvature of the stomach and the beginning of the duodenum, which, after descending and forming a fold, ascend to the anterosuperior margin of the transverse colon to fuse with the anterior layer of the transverse mesocolon. Along the greater curvature it contains the right and left gastroepiploic vessels and lymph nodes, while elsewhere it contains fat and macrophages. Also called *greater omentum, colic omentum* (outmoded), *gastrocolic omentum, gastric omentum, colic part of omentum, great epiploon* (outmoded).

omentum minus [NA] The double layer of peritoneum that extends, on the one side, from the abdominal portion of the esophagus, the lesser curvature of the stomach, and the commencement of the duodenum to the porta hepatis and the bottom of the fissure for the ligamentum venosum on the other side. Along its right free margin it encloses the hepatic artery, portal vein, and bile duct as well as lymph nodes and vessels and the hepatic plexus of nerves. Along the lesser curvature of the stomach it encloses the right and left gastric vessels, lymph nodes, and nerves. Also called *lesser omentum, gastrohepatic omentum* (outmoded), *hepatogastroduodenal ligament, lesser epiploon* (outmoded), *Willis pouch* (outmoded).

pancreaticosplenic omentum A portion of the ligamentum splenorenale that occasionally unites the tail of the pancreas with the lower part of the visceral surface of the spleen. An outmoded term.

splenogastric omentum An outmoded term for LIGAMENTUM GASTROSPLENICUM.

omentumectomy OMENTECTOMY.

omitis [om(o)- + -ITIS] Inflammation of the shoulder. An obsolete term.

ommatidium [Gk *omma,* gen. *ommatos,* the eye + -IDIUM] (*plural* ommatidia) The functional unit of the compound eye of an arthropod.

ommochrome [Gk *omm(a)* the eye + *o* + *chrōm(a)* color] Any of a group of pigments occurring in insects' eyes. They are polycyclic compounds derived from 3-hydroxykynurenine, itself derived from tryptophan.

omn. bih. *omni bihora* (L, every two hours).

omn. hor. *omni hora* (L, every hour).

omnipotence 1 The state or condition of being all-powerful. 2 The condition of believing that one is all-powerful.

omnipotence of thought The conviction that one's thoughts control the outside world, that wishing does in fact make it so. It is normal in the infant, usually expressed only symbolically in the adult neurotic, but may appear as a delusion in the psychotic.

omnivore [L *omni(s)* all + *vor(are)* to eat, swallow] Any animal that feeds on both animals and plants.

omnivorous [L *omni(s)* all + *var(are)* to eat, swallow + -OUS] Characterized by a diet of both plants and animals.

omn. noct. *omni nocte* (L, every night).

omo- [Gk *ōmos* shoulder, shoulder with upper part of arm] A combining form denoting the shoulder.

omocephalus [OMO- + -CEPHALUS] An embryo, fetus, or newborn infant with severe malformation of the head associated with agenesis of the upper extremities.

omocervicalis LEVATOR CLAVICULAE.

omoclavicular Pertaining to the shoulder and the clavicle.

omodynia [om(o)- + -ODYNIA] Pain in the shoulder. An obsolete term. Also called *omalgia, omarthralgia.*

omohyoid 1 Pertaining to the shoulder and the hyoid bone. 2 MUSCULUS OMOHYOIDEUS.

omophagia [Gk *ōmo(s)* raw, undressed + -PHAGIA] The consumption of uncooked food.

omophagic [Gk *ōmophag(os)* (from *ōmo(s)* raw + *phagein* to eat) eating raw flesh + -IC] Eating raw food, or raw flesh.

omoplata An outmoded term for SCAPULA.

omosternal 1 Of or relating to the shoulder and the sternum. 2 Pertaining to the omosternum.

omosternum The articular disk of the sternoclavicular joint.

omothyroid An occasional muscle slip that extends between the omohyoid muscle and the superior horn of the thyroid cartilage.

omovertebral Of or relating to the scapula and the vertebrae.

omphal- OMPHALO-.

omphalectomy [OMPHAL- + -ECTOMY] A partial or total resection of the umbilicus.

omphalelcosis Ulceration of the umbilicus. An obsolete term.

omphalic UMBILICAL.

omphalitis [OMPHAL- + -ITIS] Inflammation of the umbilicus.

omphalo- [Gk *omphalos* navel] A combining form denoting the umbilicus. Also *omphal-.*

omphaloangiopagus [OMPHALO- + ANGIO- + -PAGUS] ALLANTOIDOANGIOPAGOUS TWINS.

omphalocele [OMPHALO- + -CELE[1]] Herniation of intra-abdominal viscera into the umbilical cord. The herniated viscera are contained in a thin translucent sac of peritoneum and amnion. The condition may present with membranes (peritoneum and amnion) ruptured. Also called *exomphalos, exumbilication, exomphalos hernia.* Compare UMBILICAL HERNIA.

omphalochorion [OMPHALO- + CHORION] CHORIOVITELLINE PLACENTA.

omphalodidymus [OMPHALO- + Gk *didymos* a twin] OMPHALOPAGUS.

omphaloenteric Relating to or involving the umbilicus and the intestine.

omphalogenesis [OMPHALO- + GENESIS] Development of the umbilicus in the embryo.

omphaloma [OMPHAL- + -OMA] A tumor of the umbilicus. Also called *omphaloncus.*

omphalomesaraic OMPHALOMESENTERIC.

omphalomesenteric Pertaining to the umbilicus and the mesentery. Also *omphalomesaraic.*

omphaloncus [OMPHAL- + ONCUS] OMPHALOMA.

omphalopagus [OMPHALO- + Gk *pagos* a thing fixed or hardened] Conjoined twins linked at the umbilicus. Also called *monomphalus, omphalodidymus.*

omphalophlebitis [OMPHALO- + PHLEBITIS] Inflammation or infection of the umbilical veins.

omphalorrhagia [OMPHALO- + -RRHAGIA] Hemorrhage from the umbilicus. An outmoded term.

omphalorrhea [OMPHALO- + -RRHEA] A fluid discharge from the umbilicus. An outmoded term.

omphalorrhexis [OMPHALO- + -RRHEXIS] Rupture of the umbilicus. An outmoded term.

omphalos UMBILICUS.

omphalosite [OMPHALO- + Gk *sit(os)* food] The parasitic member of unequal monochorial twins that derives its blood supply from the placental vessels of the autosite. The omphalosite is not capable of independent existence after birth. Also called *placental parasitic twin, chorioangiopagus parasiticus.*

omphalosoter [OMPHALO- + Gk *sōtēr* a savior, preserver] An obsolete obstetric instrument used to replace loops of umbilical cord that have prolapsed from the amniotic cavity.

omphalospinous Pertaining to the umbilicus and the anterior superior iliac spine, especially with reference to the line connecting these points on the right side as used to locate McBurney's point.

omphalotaxis [OMPHALO- + Gk *taxis* an arranging, ordering] Replacement of a prolapsed umbilical cord into the uterine cavity.

omphalotomy [OMPHALO- + -TOMY] Severance of the umbilical cord after childbirth.

Omphalotus olearius A species of luminescent mushroom; the jack-o-lantern. It produces a neurologic toxin and can result in death. See also FOXFIRE.

omphalus UMBILICUS.

om. quar. hor. *omni quadrante hora* (L, every quarter of an hour).

omunono YAWS.

onanism [after Judah's son *Onan,* who spilled his seed on the ground so as not to give it to his dead brother's wife (Genesis 38:9) + -ISM] COITUS INTERRUPTUS.

onc- [Gk *onkos* the barb of an arrow, a hook] A combining form meaning barb, hook, hooklike. Also *onch-, oncho-, onci-, onco-.*

onch- ONC-.

oncho-[1] ONCO-[1].

oncho-[2] ONC-.

Onchocerca [properly *Oncocerca.* See ONCOCERCA.] A genus of long, threadlike filarial nematodes of the family Onchocercidae. They are found in subcutaneous and connective tissue, or confined within tough, fibrous cysts. The most important species, *O. volvulus,* is the cause of human onchocerciasis. Other species cause cutaneous diseases among domestic and wild herbivores. Also *Oncocerca.*

Onchocerca caecutiens ONCHOCERCA VOLVULUS.

Onchocerca cervicalis A species found in the ligamentum nuchae of horses and other equids. These worms have been implicated as a predisposing cause of fistulous withers and poll evil but their effect, if any, is slight.

Onchocerca gibsoni A species found in cattle, sheep, and buffalo in India, southeast Asia, Egypt, and Australia. It forms hard nodules in the hides of cattle, thereby greatly reducing their commercial value.

Onchocerca lienalis A species found in cattle and buffalo in various sites in connective tissue, including the cervical or tibiofemoral ligament and the spleen capsule. It is distributed throughout most of the world but is not common in the United States.

Onchocerca volvulus A species of filarial worm that causes human onchocerciasis. It is widely distributed in western, central, and, less commonly, eastern Africa, and in Guatemala and the Yucatan peninsula. It is transmitted by the bite of blackflies of the genus *Simulium,* such as *S. damnosum* and *S. neavei* in Africa and *S. ochraceum, S. metallicum, S. callidum,* and *S. exiguum* in Central America. Also called *Onchocerca caecutiens, Filaria volvulus.*

onchocerciasis [*Onchocerc(a)* + -IASIS] A disease caused by infection with filarial worms of the genus *Onchocerca,* primarily *O. volvulus,* transmitted by the bite of female blackflies of the genus *Simulium.* The disease is characterized by nodular swellings formed by fibrous cysts containing the worms. Microfilariae are found both in the nodules and in intercellular lymph in the skin. Onchocerciasis often results in blindness after a long period, because lesions occur in all parts of the eye as a result of the presence of microfilariae. The passage of microfilariae through the dermal tissues causes breakdown of elastic fibers resulting in conditions known by such descriptive names as elephant skin and hanging groin. Other dermatologic manifestations are known as lizard skin and leopard skin. There may be an eosinophilia. Filarial serology is positive; histological examination of the skin samples (skin-snips) is diagnostic. Treatment is with diethylcarbamazine and suramin, both of which cause serious systemic and ocular side effects. Mebendazole is an alternative. The disease is common near fast-flowing rivers in western, central, and, less commonly, eastern Africa and in Guatemala and the Yucatan peninsula. Twenty to fifty million people are affected. In some areas 15 percent of the population is rendered blind by the parasite. Also called *onchocercosis, volvulosis, blinding disease, blinding filarial disease, Robles disease, mal morado.* Also *oncocerciasis.*

ocular onchocerciasis Ocular complication of chronic oncho-cerciasis, including iridocyclitis, retrobulbar neuritis, keratitis, choroiditis, glaucoma, and blindness (river blindness) due to prolonged presence of microfilariae of *Onchocerca volvulus.*

onchocercid 1 Of or belonging to the family Onchocercidae. 2 A member of the family Onchocercidae.

Onchocercidae [ONCHO-[1] + Gk *kerk(os)* tail + -IDAE] A family of filarial worms in the superfamily Onchocercoidea, suborder Filarina. It includes most of the important filarial parasites of humans and domestic animals, including such genera as *Wuchereria, Brugia, Loa, Onchocerca, Dipetalonema, Elaeophora,* and *Litomosoides.*

onchocercoma [*Onchocerc(a)* + -OMA] A subcutaneous nodule or lesion, usually situated near a bony prominence, that contains the adult worms in infections caused by *Onchocerca* species, especially *O. volvulus.* It is composed of a dense mass of connective tissue with cystic areas containing adult worms and microfilariae.

onchocercosis ONCHOCERCIASIS.

onchodermatitis [ONCHO-[2] + DERMATITIS] The skin lesions in onchocerciasis, caused by migratory movements of the *onchocerca* microfilariae. Also called *elephant skin (local African term), leopard skin (local African term).*

onci- ONC-.

Oncicola A genus of the phylum Acanthocephala, order Archiacanthocephala, parasitic in mammals. *O. canis* is a parasite of dogs in the southern United States, and larvae are found in armadillos and in the esophagus of turkeys, which are probably facultative transport hosts. As is the case with most acanthocephalans, the first intermediate host is undoubtedly an arthropod and probably an insect.

onco-[1] [Gk *onkos* mass, bulk] A combining form meaning tumor or mass. Also *oncho-.*

onco-[2] ONC-.

Oncocerca [Gk *onkos* a barb + *kerkos* the tail of an animal] ONCHOCERCA.

oncocerciasis ONCHOCERCIASIS.

oncocyte [ONCO-[1] + -CYTE] A large cell with abundant, granular, eosinophilic cytoplasm, found in a variety of glandular tissues, such as salivary glands, thyroid, and parathyroids. By electron microscopy the cells are shown to contain large numbers of mitochondria. The significance of the cell is unknown, and some consider it to be involuted. In the thyroid, oncocytes are known as Hürthle cells, and may be components of follicular adenomas or follicular carcinomas (Hürthle-cell carcinoma).

oncocytoma ONCOCYTIC ADENOMA.

salivary gland oncocytoma See under ONCOCYTIC ADENOMA.

oncocytosis [ONCO-[1] + CYT- + -OSIS] Extensive oncocytic metaplasia.

oncogene A viral gene that produces a substance capable of transforming a cell to the malignant state.

oncogenesis [ONCO-[1] + GENESIS] The formation of tumors.

oncogenetic [ONCO-[1] + GENETIC] Pertaining to the cause, origin, or formation of tumors.

oncogenic [ONCO-[1] + -GENIC] Pertaining to the causation of a tumor, as *oncogenic virus.* Also *neoplastigenic.* ● *Carcinogenic* and *cancerogenic* refer to malignant tumors, whereas *oncogenic* refers to both benign and malignant tumors.

oncogenicity The ability to cause the formation of tumors.

oncogenous [ONCO-[1] + -GENOUS] Having origin from a tumor.

oncography [ONCO-[1] + -GRAPHY] A record of the size of an organ that is obtained with an oncometer.

oncoides [*onc(o)-*[1] + L *-oïdes* -OID] Turgor, or intumescence. An obsolete term.

oncologic Related to oncology.

oncologist [ONCO-[1] + -LOGIST] A specialist in oncology. Also called *cancerologist*.

oncology [ONCO-[1] + -LOGY] The study of tumors.

clinical oncology The study of tumors in human patients, particularly in relation to therapy.

experimental oncology The study of tumors by laboratory experiments, particularly in laboratory animals.

oncolysis [ONCO-[1] + LYSIS] Destruction of tumors or tumor cells.

oncolytic [ONCO-[1] + LYTIC] Able to destroy tumors or tumor cells.

oncoma [ONCO-[1] + -OMA] NEOPLASM.

Oncomelania [possibly ONCO-[1] + MELAN- + -IA] A genus of prosobranch (operculated) snails, one species of which is important in the transmission of schistosomiasis japonica. The genus has been transferred from the family Hydrobiidae to the family Pomatiopsidae along with *Tricula* and other genera of importance as hosts of trematodes of medical interest. Snails of the genus are amphibious, small, dextrally coiled, with conical shells. They are found along moist weedy banks, often in large numbers, their small size and conical form rendering them inconspicuous. Control of these snails is made difficult by their amphibious habit, which allows them to escape molluscicides placed in the water. Also called *Katayama*.

Oncomelania hupensis The single species of the genus, includes as subspecies the formerly recognized species *O. hupensis, O. quadrasi, O. formosana, O. lindoensis,* and *O. nosophora,* each being a morphologically distinct regional host of *Schistosoma japonicum*. The five subspecies readily interbreed in the laboratory, an important factor in considering them to be a single species.

Oncomelania hupensis formosana A subspecies of *O. hupensis* which serves as intermediate host only for the zoophilic strain of *Schistosoma japonicum,* which infects animals and not humans.

Oncomelania hupensis hupensis A subspecies of *O. hupensis,* a rib-shelled variant that serves as the intermediate host for *Schistosoma japonicum* infecting humans and other mammals in China. Other forms from China described as separate species include *O. fausti* and *O. tangi,* which are probably identical with *O. hupensis hupensis.*

Oncomelania hupensis lindoensis A subspecies of *O. hupensis* from Sulawesi (Celebes), where it serves as the intermediate host of a localized form of *Schistosoma japonicum* in the Lake Lindu area.

Oncomelania hupensis nosophora A smooth-ribbed subspecies of *O. hupensis* found in Japan and some parts of southern China. It serves as the intermediate host of human and animal *Schistosoma japonicum* in these areas.

Oncomelania hupensis quadrasi A subspecies of *O. hupensis* in the Philippines where it is the intermediate host of *Schistosoma japonicum* infecting humans and animals. It is characterized by small size (height, 3–5 mm compared with 5–10 mm in other subspecies) and a smooth shell with five axial growth lines. Also called *Oncomelania hydrobiopsis.*

Oncomelania hydrobiopsis *ONCOMELANIA HUPENSIS QUADRASI.*

oncometer [ONCO-[1] + -METER] An apparatus used to encapsulate an organ for the purpose of determining changes in its size.

oncometric Of or relating to oncometry.

oncometry [ONCO-[1] + -METRY] The procedure of determining changes in the size of an organ by the use of an oncometer.

Oncornavirinae A subfamily of the Retroviridae family which includes the oncoviruses.

oncornavirus ONCOVIRUS.

oncosis [ONCO-[1] + -SIS] The development of tumors.

oncosphere [ONCO-[2] + SPHERE] The six-hooked embryo formed within the eggshell of cestodes of the subclass Eucestoda, which usually penetrates the gut wall of its host and forms the infective larval stage (procercoid, cysticercus, cysticercoid, strobilicercus, coenurus, or hydatid, depending on the kind of tapeworm). Also called *hexacanth.*

oncotherapy Treatment of tumors.

oncothlipsis [ONCO-[1] + Gk *thlipsis* a pressing, pressure] Pressure or compression caused by a tumor.

oncotic **1** Capable of causing volume changes across a membrane. **2** Pertaining to or caused by a neoplasm.

oncotomy [ONCO-[1] + -TOMY] A surgical incision into a tumor.

oncotropic Having an affinity for neoplastic cells.

Oncovin A proprietary name for vincristine.

oncovirus [ONCO-[1] + VIRUS] Any of various tumor-producing viruses of the Retroviridae family. They are grouped into three genera or types. Type B includes mouse mammary tumor viruses. Type C viruses produce leukemias and sarcomas in various birds, mammals, and reptiles. Type D viruses produce tumors in primates. Also called *oncornavirus.*

-oncus [New L (from Gk *onkos* mass, bulk)] A combining form meaning a tumor, mass.

ondometer [French *ondemètre* (from L *unda* a wave + French *mètre* meter) an apparatus for measuring electromagnetic wavelengths] An instrument for measuring the frequency of high-frequency oscillations in a circuit.

-one [Gk suffix *-ōnē* denoting female descendant; chemical suffix] A combining form indicating replacement of CH_2 by CO in a molecule so that the substance is a ketone. Thus propane, CH_3—CH_2—CH_3, gives propanone, CH_3—CO—CH_3, the systematic name for acetone.

oneiric [*oneir(o)* + -IC] Pertaining to or resembling a dream. Also *oniric.*

oneirism [*oneir(o)-* + -ISM] A dreamlike state occurring while one is awake.

oneiro- [Gk *oneiros* dream] A combining form meaning dream. Also *onir-, oniro-.*

oneiroanalysis [ONEIRO- + English *analysis*] The analysis of dreams as an important part of psychoanalytic treatment. Also called *oneiroscopy* (outmoded).

oneirodelirium [ONEIRO- + DELIRIUM] SOMNAMBULISM.

oneirogenic [ONEIRO- + -GENIC] Giving rise to a dreamlike state. Also *onirogenic.*

oneirogmus [Gk *oneirōgmos* (from *oneiros* a dream) nocturnal emission] An obsolete term for NOCTURNAL EMISSION.

oneirology [ONEIRO- + -LOGY] The study of dreams.

oneirophrenia [ONEIRO- + PHREN- + -IA] Schizophreniform psychosis with clouding of the sensorium.

oneiroscopy [ONEIRO- + -SCOPY] An outmoded term for ONEIROANALYSIS.

onir- ONEIRO-.

oniric ONEIRIC.

oniro- ONEIRO-.

onirogenic ONEIROGENIC.

-onium [*(amm)onium.* See AMMONIUM.] A suffix indicating that an atom has acquired a positive charge by addition of a hydrogen ion. It is frequently used for substituted derivatives, thus R_3S^+ is a sulfonium cation.

onkinocele A swelling of a tendon sheath.

onlay [*on* + *lay*] **1** ONLAY GRAFT. **2** A cast metal restoration covering the cusps of a tooth, but not the entire crown.

bone onlay ONLAY BONE GRAFT.

epithelial onlay Any epithelial graft that is applied as an onlay graft, usually without suture. Also called *epithelial outlay.*

onobaio [Cushitic] An arrow poison formerly used in parts of Somaliland. It has powerful cardiac depressant action.

onomatomania [Gk *onoma,* gen. *onomatos,* a word, name + -MANIA] A state in which obsessions are expressed through the use of certain words or phrases of a sentence that invade the subject's thinking.

onomatophobia [Gk *onoma,* gen. *onomatos,* a word, name + -PHOBIA] Pathologic fear of hearing a certain sound or a particular name.

onomatopoiesis The practice of forming words (as *swish* or *fizz*) whose meanings represent the sounds made in pronouncing the words. It is sometimes seen in schizophrenics.

onset of labor See under LABOR.

Onthophagus A genus of beetles of the family Scarabeidae (scarabs). Some species, such as *O. bifasciatus* and *O. unifasciatus,* are occasionally found in the rectum of children in India, Sri Lanka and South Africa, causing diarrhea and debilitation. *O. granulatus* perforates the stomach of horses and calves in Australia in cases of scarabiasis.

ontoanalysis [Gk *onto(s),* gen. sing. masc. or neut. of *ōn,* pres. part. of *einai* to be, exist + ANALYSIS] EXISTENTIAL ANALYSIS.

ontocline [*onto-,* combining form from Gk *ōn,* gen. *ontos,* pres. part. of *einai* to be + *klin(ein)* to make slope or slant] A gradient in developmental phenotypes, such as body form or pigmentation, that appears at varying times in the life cycle of individuals within a population.

ontogenesis ONTOGENY.

ontogeny The development of an individual member of a species. Also called *ontogenesis, henogenesis.* Compare PHYLOGENY.

ontomutation [Gk *ont(o),* masc. and neut. gen. of *ōn* being + English *mutation*] Sudden and profound transformation in the organization of the cytoplasm of the ovum.

onyalai A form of thrombocytopenic purpura encountered in East, Central, and South Africa, characterized by bloody vesicles affecting oral mucous membranes. Also called *chilopa, kafindo, akembe.*

onych- ONYCHO-.

onychalgia [ONYCH- + -ALGIA] Extremely sensitive nails. Also called *onychalgia nervosa, hyperesthesia unguium.*

onychalgia nervosa ONYCHALGIA.

onychatrophia A congenital or acquired reduction in the size and thickness of the nail plate, often accompanied by fragmentation and splitting. The nail may be replaced by scar tissue.

onychectomy [ONYCH- + -ECTOMY] The partial or complete removal of a nail and/or a nail bed.

onychexallaxis [ONYCH- + Gk *exallaxis* a changing] A degeneration of the nails. A rarely used term.

onychia [ONYCH- + -IA] An inflammation of the nail matrix, either following trauma or accompanying paronychia. Also called *onyxitis, onychitis.*

onychia craquelé A fragility and cracking of the nails. A rarely used term.

onychia lateralis PARONYCHIA.

onychia maligna A rare ulceration of the nail matrix that produces discoloration and shedding of the nail. The condition is seen in debilitated persons. A rarely used term.

monilial onychia An inflammation of the nail matrix that is caused by a *Monilia* or *Candida albicans* infection. It may be associated with paronychia.

onychia periungualis PARONYCHIA.

onychia punctata A pitting of the nail plate. A rarely used term.

onychia sicca A dry brittleness of the nails.

onychia simplex An inflammation of the nail matrix that is accompanied by the loss of the nail plate. A rarely used term.

onychia superficialis undulata A waving and rippling of the nail plate that is seen rarely in secondary syphilis.

syphilitic onychia A syphilitic inflammation of the nail matrix.

onychitis ONYCHIA.

onycho- [Gk *onyx* (genitive *onychos*) talon, claw, nail] A combining form denoting nail or claw. Also *onych-.*

onychoarthro-osteodysplasia / hereditary onychoarthroosteodysplasia NAIL-PATELLA SYNDROME.

onychoclasis [ONYCHO- + -CLASIS] A breaking of the nails. A rarely used term.

onychodystrophy Any disorder of the nails.

onychogenic **1** Producing nail substance. **2** Of or relating to nail production.

onychogram A recording made by an onychograph.

onychograph [ONYCHO- + -GRAPH] An instrument for recording the blood pressure in the capillaries beneath the nails.

onychography [ONYCHO- + -GRAPHY] The procedure of recording the blood pressure in the capillaries beneath the nails.

onychogryphosis ONYCHOGRYPOSIS.

onychogryposis [ONYCHO- + Late Gk *grypōsis* (from Gk *gryp(ousthai)* to become bent or hooked + -*ōsis* -OSIS) excessive curvature] A thickening and curvature of the nail which is associated with an increase in length such that the nail resembles a ram's horn. Also called *gryposis unguium, gryposis, gryphosis, onychogryphosis.*

onychohelcosis [ONYCHO- + HELCOSIS] An ulceration of the nail.

onychoid [ONYCH- + -OID] Resembling a nail of the finger or toe.

onychology [ONYCHO- + -LOGY] A study of the nails and their disorders.

onycholysis [ONYCHO- + LYSIS] A separation of the nail plate from the nail bed.

favic onycholysis Onycholysis that is caused by a favus infection.

onycholysis partialis A partial separation of the nail plate from the nail bed.

trichophytic onycholysis The separation of the nail plate from the nail bed as a result of an infection by a dermatophyte such as *Trichophyton rubrum.*

onychomadesis [ONYCHO- + Gk *madēsis* a becoming bald] A spontaneous shedding of the nail, starting at the base and extending forward. Also called *piptonychia, defluvium unguium.*

onychomalacia A softening of the nails.

onychomycosis [ONYCHO- + MYCOSIS] Any fungal infection of the nails. Usually, invasion of the nail plate rather than just the nail fold is implied, but the distinction between damage caused by the fungus, as in ringworm, and harmless colonization of an already damaged nail, as occurs with aspergilli, is often unclear.

onychonosus ONYCHOPATHY.

onycho-osteodysplasia NAIL-PATELLA SYNDROME.

onychopacity LEUKONYCHIA.

onychopathic Of or relating to a disease of the nails.

onychopathology   The study of diseases of the nails.

onychopathy [ONYCHO- + -PATHY]   Any disease of the nails. Also called *onychonosus.*

onychophagia [ONYCHO- + -PHAGIA]   Nail-biting. Also called *onychophagy.*

onychophagy   ONYCHOPHAGIA.

Onychophora [ONYCHO- + New L -*phora*, pl. of -*phorum*, suffix denoting a carrying, bearing]   A phylum of invertebrates having features of both annelid worms and arthropods.

onychophosis [ONYCHO- + PHOSIS]   A condition marked by a horny epithelial growth in the nailbed.

onychophyma [ONYCHO- + Gk *phyma* a growth, inflamed swelling]   A disease of the nails that is marked by hypertrophy.

onychoptosis   A downward displacement of the nails.

onychorrhexis [ONYCHO- + -RRHEXIS]   The presence of longitudinal striations in the nail plate.

onychorrhiza   RADIX UNGUIS.

onychoschizia [ONYCHO- + SCHIZ- + -IA]   The splitting of the nail plate into layers.

onychosis [ONYCHO- + -SIS]   Any disease or malformation of the nails.

onychostroma   MATRIX UNGUIS.

onychotomy [ONYCHO- + -TOMY]   Incision through a fingernail, usually for the release of pus or blood.

onyx [Gk *onyx* talon, claw, nail]   A fingernail or toenail.

onyxis [New L, irreg. from Gk *onyx* talon, claw, nail]   INGROWING NAIL.

onyxitis   ONYCHIA.

oo- [Gk *ōon* egg]   A combining denoting egg or ovum.

ooblast [OO- + -BLAST]   **1** OOGONIUM. **2** OOCYTE.

oocenter [OO- + CENTER]   The centrosome of a fertilized ovum. Also called *ovocenter.*

Oochoristica [OO- + Gk *chōristika* (from *chōris* separately, apart) separable]   A genus of cyclophyllidean tapeworms of the family Linstowiidae, similar to the Davaineidae but with unarmed scolices. They are parasites of insectivorous birds, mammals, and reptiles. The plerocercoids develop in beetles.

oocinesia   OOKINESIS.

oocinete   OOKINETE.

oocyesis [OO- + CYESIS]   An older term for OVARIAN PREGNANCY.

oocyst [OO- + CYST]   The encysted form of the zygote in the sporozoan life cycle, in which multiplication occurs by sporogony, resulting in the formation of sporozoites. In some forms, as among the coccidia, the oocyst contents first form sporocysts within which the sporozoites form. Examples are seen in *Eimeria, Isospora, Toxoplasma,* and *Sarcocystis.*

oocyte [OO- + -CYTE]   A female germ cell situated in the thickened ovarian cortex, resulting from the transformation of an oogonium at the end of the multiplicative phase of the primordial oogonia. This transformation consists of a relatively slow increase in cytoplasmic volume, the formation of a peripheral envelope of ovarian follicular cells to form a primordial follicle, and above all, within the oocyte's nucleus, a series of divisions (both meiotic or reduction, and maturation divisions) which result in the halving of the chromosome number. The oocyte thus passes through a veritable maturation process in both nucleus and cytoplasm, for a period that varies with the species and which in man can take up to four decades. Also called *ovocyte, ooblast, ovigerm.*

primary oocyte   A female germ cell resulting from the proliferation of the primordial ovogonia before the phases of growth and maturation in oogenesis. Its essential characteristic is the presence, centered in the nucleus, of changes related to the process of meiosis and thus a reduction by half in the number of chromosomes of each species. Proliferation before, at, and just after birth results in female neonates possessing a definitive stock of primary oocytes. In each human ovary this stock consists of 300 000–400 000 oocytes. The oocytes are protected by an envelope of follicular cells, but their development is retarded for many years at the last stage of prophase of the first meiotic division. The greater proportion of the primary oocytes will degenerate (atresia) without being utilized. Only 200–300 reach the final phase of maturation, which will come about, every 28–30 days, from puberty to the menopause, when each becomes a secondary oocyte capable of being fertilized after ovulation.

secondary oocyte   A female germ cell arising from a primary oocyte during the second phase of maturation in oogenesis, which starts at puberty. From then on, at an age that varies according to the species, some of the primary oocytes of the original neonatal stock will, one by one, following a rhythm also characteristic of the species, undergo a particularly complex maturation in the space of only a few days. In mammals, the envelope of cells surrounding and nourishing the oocyte enlarges into a graafian follicle. The oocyte included within this follicle undergoes a considerable enlargement in volume, from some 30 μm to 140 μm in diameter in less than 30 days. The nucleus of the oocyte passes through the final stages of the reduction division initiated since before birth. After extrusion of the first polar body, it has only half the original number of chromosomes. The final reduction division occurs only after ovulation, then only after fertilization, with the extrusion of the second polar body. The haploid chromosomal constitution of the secondary oocyte usually includes a single female x chromosome.

oogamous   Of or characterized by oogamy.

oogamy   Fertilization of a nonmotile oocyte by a motile gamete.

oogenesis [OO- + GENESIS]   The formation and development of the female germ cells. Oogenesis comprises three phases: a phase of proliferation, in which the oogonia in the ovarian cortex divide several times, usually during fetal life or just after birth to produce numerous primary oocytes; a phase of growth, in which the oocytes increase in size and accumulate yolk as a food reserve; and a phase of maturation, in which the primary oocyte undergoes a reduction division which results in two daughter cells, one very small (the first polar body), destined to degenerate, the other (the secondary oocyte) which may grow to a size larger than the parent cell but with a haploid chromosome number. The secondary oocyte divides into two unequal cells, the second polar body, which degenerates, and the ovum (ootid) ready for fertilization. However, in most mammals it is a secondary oocyte which is shed at ovulation, and the final maturation division occurs only after penetration of the secondary oocyte by a spermatozoon. The final maturation division results, therefore, in the extrusion of the second polocyte (polar body) and the formation of the female pronucleus within an ovum already containing a spermatozoon. Also called *ovogenesis, ovigenesis.*

oogenetic   Pertaining to oogenesis. Also *ovigenetic.*

oogenic [OO- + -GENIC]   Producing ova. Also *oogenous, ovigenic, ovigenous.*

oogenous   OOGENIC.

oogonium [OO- + New L *gonium* (from GON- suffix denoting seed + L -*ium*, neut. sing. noun suffix)]   (*plural* oogonia)   **1** The precursor in the ovary of an oocyte. It is derived from a primordial female germ cell, which in mammals probably arises from the primitive endoderm and in man has been identified in the endoderm of the yolk sac. The primordial cells migrate into the embryo and pass via the dorsal mesentery to reach the genital ridge from which the ovary will develop. They proliferate in the ovarian cortex by mitosis to form oogonia, and the full number for each individual is reached just before or shortly after parturition. Also called *ooblast, ovigerm, ovoblast, ovogonium.* **2** In fungi, a female gametangium containing one or more eggs. Also called *oosporangium.*

ookinesis [OO- + KINESIS] Divisions which occur in the maturation of an ovum. Also called *oocinesia.*

ookinete [OO- + Gk *kinēt(os)* moving] The motile, fertilized macrogamete, or zygote, of a malarial parasite. It moves to the outer lining of the gut wall of the vector mosquito and there forms the oocyst, in which masses of sporozoites are produced. Also called *oocinete, pseudovermicule, pseudovermiculus, traveling vermicule.*

oolemma [OO- + LEMMA] ZONA PELLUCIDA.

Oomycetes [OO- + New L *-mycetes,* suffix denoting fungi, from Gk *mykētes,* pl. of *mykēs* fungus, mushroom] A class of aquatic fungi; the water molds. These fungi are characterized by having two flagella. None are known human pathogens.

oomycetous Of or pertaining to the fungi of the class Oomycetes.

oomycosis [OO- + MYCOSIS] (*plural* oomycoses) Any infection or disease caused by a fungus of the class Oomycetes.

oophagia OOPHAGY.

oophagy [OO- + *-phag(ia)* + -Y] The eating of eggs, as by certain insects and mites that feed primarily upon the eggs of other arthropods. Also called *oophagia.*

oophor- OOPHORO-.

oophoralgia [OOPHOR- + -ALGIA] OVARIALGIA.

oophorectomize [*oophorectom(y)* + -IZE] To perform an oophorectomy upon.

oophorectomy [*oophor(o)-* + -ECTOMY] Removal of one or both ovaries. Also called *ovariectomy, ovariosteresis, oothecectomy, oothectomy.*

　bilateral partial oophorectomy Removal of tissue from each ovary.

oophoritis [OOPHOR- + -ITIS] Inflammation of an ovary, usually associated with salpingitis. Also called *ovaritis.*

　oophoritis parotidea Oophoritis resulting from infection with the mumps virus and occurring during, before, or as the only manifestation of mumps.

oophoro- [Gk *ōophoron* (from *ōon* egg + *-phoros* bearing) ovary] A combining form denoting the ovary. Also *oario-, oophor-.*

oophorocystectomy [OOPHORO- + CYST- + -ECTOMY] The surgical removal of one or more ovarian cysts.

oophorocystosis The formation of ovarian cysts. A seldom used term. Also called *oothecocystosis.*

oophorocystostomy [OOPHORO- + CYSTO- + -STOMY] A surgical excision into one or more ovarian cysts for purposes of drainage.

oophoroepilepsy [OOPHORO- + EPILEPSY] A reflex epilepsy once incorrectly thought to be induced by disordered ovarian function. An obsolete term. Also called *ovarian epilepsy.*

oophorogenous [OOPHORO- + -GENOUS] OVARIOGENIC.

oophorohysterectomy [OOPHORO- + HYSTER- + -ECTOMY] A surgical procedure in which one or both ovaries are removed along with the uterus. Also called *oothecohysterectomy, ovariohysterectomy.*

oophoroma [OOPHOR- + -OMA] A tumor of the ovary.

　oophoroma folliculare BRENNER TUMOR.

oophoromalacia Softening of the ovary. An obsolete term.

oophoron OVARIUM.

oophoropathy [OOPHORO- + -PATHY] Any disease of the ovary. Also called *ovariopathy, oothecopathy* (obsolete).

oophoropexy [OOPHORO- + -PEXY] The surgical attachment of the ovary to the lateral pelvic wall, sometimes carried out to

protect the ovary when pelvic radiation therapy is needed. Also called *ovariopexy, oothecopexy* (outmoded), *oothecorrhaphy* (outmoded).

oophoroplasty [OOPHORO- + -PLASTY] Any plastic operation on an ovary.

oophorosalpingectomy SALPINGO-OOPHORECTOMY.

oophorosalpingitis SALPINGO-OOPHORITIS.

oophorostomy [OOPHORO- + -STOMY] A surgical opening into an ovary or an ovarian cyst to permit drainage. Also called *oothecostomy, ovariostomy.*

oophorotomy [OOPHORO- + -TOMY] A surgical incision into one or both ovaries. Also called *ovariotomy.*

oophorrhagia [*oopho(r)-* + -RRHAGIA] Bleeding from an ovary.

oophyte [OO- + Gk *phyt(on)* a plant, a tree] GAMETOPHYTE.

ooplasm [OO- + -PLASM] **1** The cytoplasm of the egg. Also called *ovoplasm.* **2** In oomycetous fungi, the oosphere protoplasm, as differentiated from the periplasm.

oosome [OO- + *-some,* suffix denoting body, from Gk *sōma* body] GERM-CELL DETERMINANT.

oosperm [OO- + SPERM] ZYGOTE.

oosphere [OO- + SPHERE] A large, naked, nonmotile, female fungal gamete.

Oospora [OO- + New L *-spora,* pl. of *-sporum,* suffix denoting seed, from Gk *spora* seed] An obsolete term for *GEOTRICHUM.*

　Oospora tozeuri An obsolete term for *MADURELLA MYCETOMI.*

oosporangium An outmoded term for OOGONIUM.

oospore [OO- + SPORE] A thick-walled fungal spore that develops from an oosphere through either fertilization or parthenogenesis.

oothec- OOTHECO-.

ootheca [OO- + Gk *thēkē* case, box] (*plural* oothecae) An egg case produced by certain insects and crustaceans.

oothecectomy OOPHORECTOMY.

ootheco- [Modern L *ootheca* (from Gk *ōon* egg + *thēkē* case, box) egg case, ovary] A combining form denoting the ovary. Also *oothec-.*

oothecocyesis [OOTHECO- + CYESIS] Intraovarian pregnancy resulting from implantation of the blastocyst within ovarian tissue. See also ECTOPIC PREGNANCY.

oothecocystosis An obsolete term for OOPHOROCYSTOSIS.

oothecohysterectomy OOPHOROHYSTERECTOMY.

oothecoma [OOTHEC- + -OMA] **1** An ovarian tumor. **2** THECOMA.

oothecopathy [OOTHECO- + -PATHY] An obsolete term for OOPHOROPATHY.

oothecopexy [OOTHECO- + -PEXY] An outmoded term for OOPHOROPEXY.

oothecorrhaphy [OOTHECO- + -RRHAPHY] An outmoded term for OOPHOROPEXY.

oothecosalpingectomy SALPINGO-OOPHORECTOMY.

oothecostomy OOPHOROSTOMY.

oothectomy OOPHORECTOMY.

ootherapy [OO- + THERAPY] The use of ovarian extract in treatment. An older term. Also called *ovotherapy, ovariotherapy, ovarotherapy.*

ootid [OO- + *t* + -ID[1]] A mature ovum, a product of meiosis in the ovary. In most mammals fertilization occurs prior to the completion of meiosis, thus the ootid contains male and female pronuclei.

ootomy [OO- + -TOMY] Incision in a fertilized ovum, carried out for experimental reasons, particularly in order to study the development of its various parts.

ootype [OO- + TYPE]   An egg-processing structure in the center of the female reproductive system of cestodes and trematodes. It is the site of fertilization, after which yolk material is compressed around the ovum and shell material is laid down. Then the egg is passed into the uterus and the shell is tanned and hardened.

ooze   Soft mud on the bottom of the sea floor.

oozooid   Any individual developed from an ovum.

op-   OB-.

opacification [*opaci(fy)* + -FICATION]   A loss of transparency; the process of becoming opaque.

opacify [L *opac(us)* (akin to *umbra* shadow, shade) shaded, dark + *i* + *-fy*]   To lose transparency; be in the process of becoming opaque.

opacity [L *opacitas* shadiness]   The condition of being opaque, as that resulting from the loss of transparency.

Caspar's ring opacity   A circular corneal opacity due to injury.

opalescent   Pertaining to the scattering of light through translucent media. Also *opaline*.

opalgia [OP- + -ALGIA]   FACIAL NEURALGIA.

Opalina [L *opal(us)* opal + -INA]   A genus of multinucleated protozoa with organelles resembling cilia in oblique rows over the body surface. The cytostome is absent, reproduction is by interkinetal binary fission and after syngamy with anisogamous flagellated gametes. They are parasitic in the colon of frogs and toads. Formerly thought to be primitive ciliates, they are now considered to be in the Sarcomastigophora, but still distinct enough to be classified as a separate subphylum Opalinata.

opaline   OPALESCENT.

Opalski [Adam *Opalski*, Polish physician, 1897–1963]   See under CELL.

opaque [French, from L *opacus* shaded, dark]   Impervious to the transmission of light or other electromagnetic energy, such as x rays.

OPD   outpatient department.

-ope [Gk *ōps*, gen. *ōpos*, eye]   One having a (specified) visual defect.

opeidoscope [Gk *op(a)*, accus. of *ops* a voice + *eido(s)* image + -SCOPE]   An apparatus for studying voice vibrations in which a mirror, attached to a fine membrane, is used to reflect light onto a screen.

open   **1** Not covered with intact skin, as an injury to deeper tissues.   **2** In group psychotherapy, admitting new members after the group has been formed, in distinction to therapy in which no new members may be added.

opening   An orifice, aperture or entrance in or to a structure, organ, cavity, or tube.

anterior opening of aqueduct of Sylvius   The orifice of the aqueductus mesencephali in the posteroinferior wall of the third ventricle below the posterior commissure. Also called *opening of Vieussens, orifice of Vieussens.*

anterior opening of orbital cavity   ADITUS ORBITAE.

anterior opening of stomach   An outmoded term for OSTIUM PYLORICUM.

aortic opening   **1** OSTIUM AORTAE.   **2** HIATUS AORTICUS.

aortic opening in diaphragm   HIATUS AORTICUS.

bite opening   Increasing of the vertical relation when the teeth are in occlusion.

cardiac opening   OSTIUM CARDIACUM.

opening of coronary sinus   OSTIUM SINUS CORONARII.

cutaneous opening of male urethra   OSTIUM URETHRAE EXTERNUM MASCULINAE.

duodenal opening of stomach   An outmoded term for OSTIUM PYLORICUM.

esophageal opening in diaphragm   HIATUS ESOPHAGEUS.

opening of esophagus   HIATUS ESOPHAGEUS.

external opening of aqueduct of cochlea   APERTURA EXTERNA CANALICULI COCHLEAE.

femoral opening   HIATUS TENDINEUS.

ileocecal opening   OSTIUM ILEOCAECALE.

ileocolic opening   OSTIUM ILEOCAECALE.

opening in adductor magnus muscle   HIATUS TENDINEUS.

inferior openings of caroticotympanic canaliculi   The tiny openings in the carotid canal in the petrous part of the temporal bone through which filaments of the carotid sympathetic plexus and branches of the internal carotid artery enter the canaliculi caroticotympanici.

inferior opening of Hunter's canal   An outmoded term for HIATUS TENDINEUS.

inferior opening of pelvis   APERTURA PELVIS INFERIOR.

inferior opening of sacral canal   HIATUS SACRALIS.

inferior thoracic opening   APERTURA THORACIS INFERIOR.

opening of inferior vena cava   **1** OSTIUM VENAE CAVAE INFERIORIS.   **2** FORAMEN VENAE CAVAE.

interauricular opening   **1** An outmoded term for OSTIUM PRIMUM.   **2** An outmoded term for OSTIUM SECUNDUM.

internal urethral opening   OSTIUM URETHRAE INTERNUM.

interventricular opening   FORAMEN INTERVENTRICULARE.

opening to lesser sac of peritoneum   FORAMEN OMENTALE.

opening for lesser superficial petrosal nerve   HIATUS CANALIS NERVI PETROSI MINORIS.

lower thoracic opening   APERTURA THORACIS INFERIOR.

nasal opening of facial skeleton   APERTURA PIRIFORMIS.

opening of omental bursa   FORAMEN OMENTALE.

orbital opening   ADITUS ORBITAE.

ovarian opening of uterine tube   OSTIUM ABDOMINALE TUBAE UTERINAE.

opening of parotid duct   The opening in the tip of the papilla parotidea in the oral vestibule opposite the upper second molar tooth.

pharyngeal opening of auditory tube   OSTIUM PHARYNGEUM TUBAE AUDITIVAE.

pharyngeal opening of eustachian tube   OSTIUM PHARYNGEUM TUBAE AUDITIVAE.

piriform opening   APERTURA PIRIFORMIS.

opening of pulmonary trunk   OSTIUM TRUNCI PULMONALIS.

pyloric opening   OSTIUM PYLORICUM.

saphenous opening   HIATUS SAPHENUS.

semilunar opening of ethmoid bone   HIATUS SEMILUNARIS.

opening for smaller superficial petrosal nerve   HIATUS CANALIS NERVI PETROSI MINORIS.

opening of sphenoidal sinus   APERTURA SINUS SPHENOIDALIS.

superior opening of pelvis   APERTURA PELVIS SUPERIOR.

superior thoracic opening   APERTURA THORACIS SUPERIOR.

superior opening of tympanic canal   The upper opening of the tympanic canaliculus through which the tympanic branch of the glossopharyngeal nerve enters the tympanic cavity.

tendinous opening   HIATUS TENDINEUS.

tympanic opening of auditory tube   OSTIUM TYMPANICUM TUBAE AUDITIVAE.

opening for tympanic branch of glossopharyngeal nerve   The inferior opening of the tympanic canaliculus, located on the ridge between the jugular fossa and the opening of the carotid canal on the inferior surface of the petrous part of the temporal bone. It transmits the tympanic branch of the glossopharyngeal nerve.

upper thoracic opening   APERTURA THORACIS SUPERIOR.

uterine opening of uterine tube   OSTIUM UTERINUM TUBAE UTERINAE.

opening for vena cava   FORAMEN VENAE CAVAE.

opening of vermiform appendix   OSTIUM APPENDICIS VERMIFORMIS.

vertical opening   VERTICAL RELATION.

vesicourethral opening   OSTIUM URETHRAE INTERNUM.

opening of Vieussens   ANTERIOR OPENING OF AQUEDUCT OF SYLVIUS.

operability   The state of susceptibility to successful surgical treatment.

operable [L oper(ari) to work, take pains with + -abilis English -able]   Susceptible to treatment by surgical means with a significant degree of safety and success.

operant [L operans, gen. operantis, pres. part. of operari to work, take pains with]   1 Describing a response or pattern of responses defined by its effects on the environment, and by its effectiveness in achieving reward or reinforcement. An operant response is identified by its known consequences in a definable situation rather than in terms of the stimulus which may have given rise to that behavior.   2 An operant response considered as a unit of behavior.   3 Designating a method of conditioning based on the control of operant responses.

operate [L operat(us), past part. of operari to work, labor, operate. See OPERATION.]   1 To perform a surgical procedure.   2 A patient who has undergone surgery in an experimental situation, as distinguished from the control. Rarely used in this sense.

operation

operation [L operatio (from operatus, past part. of operari to work, labor, from opus, gen. operis, work, labor) a working, laboring, operation]   1 A surgical procedure.   2 The act of carrying out a task, especially in an orderly way according to established practice.

Abbe's operation   The repair of a lip defect making use of an Abbe flap.

Abbe-Estlander operation   An operation utilizing a cross-lip flap of either the Abbe or Estlander type.

Adams operation   1 A percutaneous intracapsular division of the femoral neck that was previously performed in cases of ankylosis.   2 The percutaneous division of the palmar fascia to relieve Dupuytren's contracture.   3 Excision of a wedge of tissue from the eyelid margin, used to treat ectropion.   4 An operation once performed for the correction of traumatic deformities of the nose and nasal septum by forcibly refracturing and repositioning the septum and, if necessary, the nasal bones, using a special forceps (Adams forceps). It was superseded by such procedures as submucous resection of the nasal septum and, more recently, septorhinoplasty.

Adelmann's operation   The disarticulation of a finger together with the metacarpal head.

Albee's operation   1 An operation to correct ankylosis of the hip in which the femoral head is divided and the cartilage of the acetabulum is removed.   2 A spinal fusion procedure that uses a tibial bone graft. The graft is keyed into the split spinous processes of the vertebrae.

Albert's operation   The excision of the knee to create an arthrodesis in cases of a flail knee joint.

Aldridge operation   The use of a fascial sling to elevate the posterior urethrovesical angle to correct urinary stress incontinence.

Allarton's operation   MEDIAN LITHOTOMY.

Allingham's operation   1 A surgical procedure in which the rectum is excised by a circumferential incision into the ischiorectal space that is extended back to the coccyx.   2 The creation of an inguinal colostomy through an incision parallel to the inquinal ligament.

Alouette's operation   ALOUETTE'S AMPUTATION.

Ammon's operation   DACRYOCYSTOTOMY.

Amussat's operation   A surgical procedure in which a long transverse incision is made for purposes of exploring the intraperitoneal colon.

Anagnostakis operation   A surgical procedure for the correction of an inturned eyelid or for posterior misdirection of the eyelashes.

anastomotic operation   A surgical procedure which consists, at least in part, of the creation of a connection between two vessels or organs.

Anderson's operation   1 The longitudinal splitting of a tendon, followed by a pulling along one of the cut edges in order to gain length.   2 A method of lengthening a limb, using an external fixation device along with the gradual distraction of a step osteotomy. For defs. 1 and 2 also called Anderson's amputation.

Anel's operation   Probing and irrigation of the nasolacrimal duct.

Annandale's operation   1 A method of suturing displaced menisci in the knee.   2 An obsolete procedure to correct a genu valgum deformity in which the femoral condyle is excised.

Arlt's operation   Surgical fracture of the tarsus for trachomatous entropion.

Arlt-Jaesche operation   A surgical displacement of the eyelashes forward for the correction of corneal irritation resulting from an anomalous double row of eyelashes.

Asch operation   An operation once used for correction of deviation of the nasal septum, but since superseded by the submucous resection operation. A cruciate mucosal incision was made, flaps raised, and the deflected cartilage or bone removed.

Babcock's operation   The stripping of varicose veins by the use of olive-tipped sounds that are passed through the veins via a small skin incision. Also called Jackson-Babcock operation.

Badal's operation   An obsolete procedure supposed to relieve ocular pain by severing the infratrochlear nerve.

Baldy's operation   An old-fashioned surgical procedure to fix the uterus from a retrodisplaced position in the pelvis to an anterior position. Also called Baldy-Webster operation, Webster's operation.

Baldy-Webster operation   BALDY'S OPERATION.

Bardeleben's operation   Subperiosteal resection of a portion of the vomer in the management of the protruding premaxilla in cases of bilateral cleft lip and palate.

Barkan's operation   GONIOTOMY.

Barker's operation   1 An excision of the hip joint using an anterior approach.   2 A talectomy in which the incision is made from the lateral malleolus to the dorsum of the foot.

Barraquer's operation   A technique of intracapsular cataract extraction utilizing a suction device to grasp the capsular surface.

Barsky's operation   A method of repairing a congenital cleft hand.

Barton's operation   A method of achieving an arthrodesis of a joint by removing V-shaped segments of bone and cartilage from either side of the joint, thus creating an interlocking continuity.

Barwell's operation   A method of correcting a genu valgum deformity in children by dividing the upper tibia below its proximal epiphysis and the lower tibia above its distal epiphysis.

Basset's operation   Inguinal lymph node dissection for cancer of the vulva.

Bassini's operation   A surgical repair of an inguinal hernia in which the entire length of the posterior wall of the inguinal canal is incised and reconstructed by suturing the medial structures—the transverse fascia and aponeurosis, the transverse abdominal muscle, and the internal oblique muscle—laterally to the reflected edge of the inguinal ligament. This procedure is often performed today without incising the posterior wall.

Bates operation   The cutting of a stricture of the urethra from within by a urethrotome.

Battle's operation   A surgical procedure in which normal ovaries are removed to treat certain hormone-dependent conditions, such as uterine fibroids.

Beck I operation   An obsolete operation to revascularize the ischemic heart in which the collateral blood supply is stimulated by pericardial poudrage, epicardial abrasion, and partial occlusion of the coronary sinus.

Beck II operation   An obsolete operation once used to revascularize the ischemic heart. It is performed to two stages, the first of which creates an anastomosis between the coronary sinus and the descending thoracic aorta. The second procedure forms a partial occlusion of the coronary sinus to direct aortic blood retrograde into the coronary veins.

Beer's operation   Cataract extraction performed with a relatively large cataract knife of steep triangular shape.

Belfield's operation   VASOTOMY.

Bent's operation   An excision of the arm at the shoulder using a flap from the deltoid region.

Bergenhem's operation   A surgical procedure in which the ureter is implanted in the rectum.

Berger's operation   An interscapulothoracic amputation of the upper limb. Also called *Berger's amputation.*

Bergmann's operation   Surgical incision of the tunica vaginalis testis for hydrocele.

Berke's operation   The correction of ptosis by levator resection approached via a skin incision.

Berke-Motais operation   The correction of ptosis by suspension of the eyelid upon the superior rectus muscle.

Bernard's operation   A method of reconstructing the lower lip utilizing sliding flaps taken from the cheeks.

Bevan's operation   A surgical procedure in which an undescended testicle is brought into the scrotum.

Bier's operation   BIER'S AMPUTATION.

Bigelow's operation   BIGELOW'S LITHOLAPAXY.

Billroth's operation   1 A surgical procedure in which a gastroenterostomy or gastroduodenostomy is performed following a distal gastric resection. Also called *Billroth anastomosis.* 2 Glossectomy by way of a curved submental incision.

Bissell's operation   An obsolete gynecolgic operation to treat uterine retroversion.

Blalock's operation   An operation to palliate diminished pulmonary artery blood flow secondary to valvular or infundibular pulmonary stenosis by anastomosing the subclavian or innominate artery to the ipsilateral pulmonary artery; a form of systemic-pulmonary artery shunt for palliation of diminished pulmonary artery blood flow. Also called *Blalock-Taussig operation.*

Blalock-Hanlon operation   An operation in which a portion of the atrial septum is excised to enable more adequate mixing of left and right atrial blood to palliate transposition of the great arteries. The operation is done employing vascular occlusion techniques rather than using cardiopulmonary bypass.

Blalock-Taussig operation   BLALOCK'S OPERATION.

Blaskovics operation   An outmoded method for the surgical correction of epicanthus.

bloodless operation   A surgical procedure in which little or no blood is lost.

Boari's operation   Implantation of the ureter into a tube of bladder tissue to obtain more length when the ureter is short.

Böhm's operation   Correction of strabismus by tenotomy.

Bondy operation   MODIFIED RADICAL MASTOIDECTOMY.

Bonzel's operation   A technique of iridodialysis utilizing a small hook.

Bose operation   A superior tracheotomy in which a cruciate skin incision is made at the level of the cricoid cartilage and the soft tissues are retracted downwards to expose the upper tracheal rings, which may then be incised safely.

Bottini's operation   Repair of an enlarged prostate through which a channel is made with galvanocautery.

Bozeman's operation   HYSTEROCYSTOCLEISIS.

Brailey's operation   An obsolete procedure supposed to relieve ocular pain by damaging the supratrochlear nerve.

Brenner's operation   A surgical procedure to treat inguinal hernias by suturing abdominal wall musculature to the cremaster muscle.

Bricker's operation   A surgical procedure in which an ileal conduit for urine is created as a substitute for the bladder.

Brock's operation   TRANSVENTRICULAR CLOSED VALVOTOMY.

Brophy's operation   An obsolete operation for cleft palate, involving wire compression sutures across the gap in the alveolus.

Brunschwig's operation   1 The surgical removal of the duodenum and a portion of the pancreas, with reconstitution of intestinal continuity.   2 TOTAL PELVIC EXENTERATION.

Bryant's operation   A lumbar colotomy performed through an incision between the eleventh rib and the iliac crest.

Buck's operation   1 A method of excising the patella and proximal ends of the tibia and fibula.   2 An operation for repairing the defect in spondylolysis in which a compression screw is passed across the defect in the pars interarticularis.

Buie's operation   A hemorrhoidectomy performed with the patient in a prone position on the operating table.

Burckhardt's operation   An operation to drain a chronic retropharyngeal abscess by way of a neck incision along the anterior border of the sternomastoid muscle.

buttonhole operation   A small surgical incision or counterincision usually made to provide drainage through a separate wound. Also called *boutonnière.*

Buzzi's operation   A needling technique for creating a pupillary opening.

Caldwell-Luc operation   An operation for the relief of chronic maxillary sinusitis. The maxillary sinus is opened by a sublabial incision, diseased sinus mucosa is removed, and a counter-opening is made from the interior of the sinus into the inferior meatus of the nose. Also called *radical maxillary antrostomy, Luc's operation.*

Calot's operation   The forcible manipulation and correction of tuberculous kyphosis followed by immobilization of the spine in a plaster cast.

Canfield's operation   A modification of an intranasal antrostomy in which, by removing the angle of bone between the inferior nasal meatus and the canine fossa, the antrostome is brought further forward than in an antrostomy. This provides easier postoperative access.

capital operation   Any surgical procedure of such magnitude that it may represent a significant threat to the patient's life.

Carnochan's operation   An operation on the gasserian ganglion and nerve through an opening in the maxillary antrum, for the relief of facial pain.

Carpue's operation   INDIAN RHINOPLASTY.

Carter's operation   A technique for optical iridotomy.

Cassells operation The permeatal removal of exostoses of the external auditory meatus.

Cecil's operation An operation for urethral stricture which is performed in three stages.

celsian operation PERINEAL LITHOTOMY.

Charles operation A surgical procedure for lymphedema in which lymphedematous skin and subcutaneous tissue are excised and the operative site is covered by skin grafts.

Cheever's operation An external operation for malignant disease of the tonsil, undertaken by way of a cervical skin incision.

Cheselden operation A technique of enlarging an abnormal ocular pupil by making a linear cut in the iris.

Chevalier Jackson's operation VENTRICULOCORDECTOMY.

Chiene's operation A wedge osteotomy to correct genu valgum.

Chopart's operation 1 CHOPART'S AMPUTATION. 2 MEDIOTARSAL AMPUTATION.

cinch operation A shortening of the extraocular muscles for strabismus correction by means of a form of tucking.

Civiale's operation LITHOLAPAXY.

Clark's operation A plastic procedure for repair of a urethral fistula.

Coakley's operation An operation once used for the relief of chronic maxillary sinusitis. Through a long sublabial incision, the anterolateral wall of the sinus was extensively removed and an attempt was made to remove every trace of the lining membrane. The cavity was packed with iodoform gauze for several days and repacked at intervals over a period of three to six months with the object being the eventual obliteration of the sinus. The operation has since been replaced by less radical procedures.

Cock's operation A form of perineal urethrotomy.

Codivilla's operation 1 A method of treating a pseudarthrosis by surrounding the region with slivers of osteoperiosteal bone taken from the anteromedial surface of the tibia. 2 The original surgical method of obtaining an increase in limb length by cutting the bone and applying traction.

Collis operation An operation for the repair of unilateral congenital cleft lip. It is rarely, if ever, used, but it was the first operation designed to correct the deformed alar base and nasal floor.

Colonna's operation 1 An arthroplasty of the hip joint used in neglected cases of congenital dysplasia or dislocation of the hip. 2 A now obsolete reconstruction operation for intracapsular fracture of the femoral neck.

commando operation An operation in which resection of a primary malignant tumor of the floor of the mouth, cheek, tongue, tonsillar area, pharynx, or larynx is combined with radical dissection of the lymph nodes in the neck. • It was named after the Allied commando raid on Dieppe, a famous combined operation undertaken in 1942.

compensating operation A strabismus procedure that weakens the direct antagonist of a paretic extraocular muscle.

cosmetic operation An operation designed to correct an undesirable bodily feature so that the feature will more closely match that which is generally considered normal. Also called *esthetic surgery, featural surgery.*

Cotte's operation The excision of presacral nerves.

Cotting's operation An operation for the removal of the nail fold and the side of the nail. It is performed to treat an ingrowing toenail.

crescent operation Surgical repair of a lacerated perineum, secondary to an obstetrical delivery.

Critchett's operation A form of evisceration.

Crosby-Cooney operation The drainage of ascites through a flanged glass tube inserted into the peritoneal cavity.

Cushing's operation SUBTEMPORAL DECOMPRESSION.

Dana's operation POSTERIOR RHIZOTOMY.

Dandy's operation Division at the pons of the sensory root of the trigeminal nerve for the relief of facial pain.

Daniel's operation Exploratory scalene lymphadenectomy when the nodes are not palpable.

Daviel's operation Cataract extraction performed by expression of the lens through a corneal incision.

Davies-Colley operation The removal of a laterally based wedge of bone from the tarsus for correction of talipes equinovarus.

decompression operation The surgical removal of structures confining an organ that is under pressure, as in subtemporal decompression of the brain or decompression laminectomy of the spinal cord.

Dees operation A pyelolithotomy performed by entrapping the stones and debris in an artificial coagulum and removing the solidified mass of coagulum and stones from the renal pelvis.

de Grandmont's operation A corrective procedure for eyelid ptosis.

Delorme's operation The lysis or excision of pericardial adhesions in constrictive or fibrosing pericarditis.

Del Toro's operation Thermal flattening of a keratoconus.

Denis Brown operation 1 A method of correction of hypospadias, in which a strip of skin is separated, extending from the urethral meatus to the end of the penis, the adjacent skin is closed, and then a catheter is placed between the skin strip and the closed skin. The skin strip then becomes a tube by epithelialization. 2 A variation of the Swenson anal pull-through procedure used for primary resection and anastomosis in the treatment of congenital megacolon. This procedure varies in that the rectosigmoid is completely mobilized and pulled through before the bowel is divided.

Denker's operation A modification of the Caldwell-Luc operation intended to afford easier postoperative access from the nose to the interior of the maxillary antrum by bringing the antrostome further forward.

Denonvilliers operation Partial, lateral rhinoplasty for the reconstruction of the ala nasi.

Dieffenbach's operation An amputation of a lower limb through the hip that uses a circular incision in which bleeding is controlled by an elastic tourniquet and ligature of the vessels. After hemostasis is achieved, a lateral incision is made from above the greater trochanter to the lateral margin of the initial circular incision. Also called *Dieffenbach's amputation, Dieffenbach's method.*

Dittel's operation A surgical procedure for enucleation of the lateral lobes of an enlarged prostate.

Dohlman's operation An endoscopic operation to relieve the symptoms of hypopharyngeal diverticulum. The wall separating the diverticulum from the esophagus is exposed with a special speculum and divided using diathermy.

Doléris operation A surgical operation to treat uterine retroversion by shortening the round ligaments by fixing them to the rectus sheath.

Doppler's operation The destruction of nerves supplying gonads, an obsolete procedure to increase hormonal production. Also called *sympathicodiaphtheresis.*

Dorrance operation PALATAL PUSHBACK OPERATION.

Doyen's operation Relief of hydrocele by eversion of the sac.

Dufourmentel-Mouly operation A surgical procedure in which a composite graft is taken from the lower lip and is transplanted to the upper lip.

Duhamel operation A surgical procedure designed to correct congenital megacolon in which a longitudinal anastomosis is created between the normal proximal colon and the aganglionic rectum.

Dührssen's operation A seldom-used obstetrical operation in which one or more radial incisions are made into the cervix to expedite delivery of the fetal head.

Duplay's operation A method of reconstructing the urethra in congenital hypospadias. Also called *Duplay's method.*

Dupuy-Dutemps operation Repair of an eyelid defect by transplantation of tissue from the opposing eyelid.

Dupuytren's operation DUPUYTREN'S AMPUTATION.

Eagleton's operation An operation designed to drain infected air cells in cases of petrositis. It utilizes an extrapetrosal approach to the apex of the petrous portion of the temporal bone, with the site of disease being reached by elevating the dura mater of the middle fossa.

Edebohls operation A rarely used surgical procedure undertaken to increase renal blood flow by decapsulating the kidney, thus permitting the development of collateral circulation.

Edmonds operation for correction of chordee A rarely used, two-stage method of correcting chordee, utilizing a bipedicle flap fashioned from the prepuce.

Elliot's operation Corneoscleral trephination for glaucoma.

Eloesser's operation A method of draining empyema by an open technique in which a flap of pleura is used to create an open communication with the skin.

Emmet's operation 1 TRACHELORRHAPHY. 2 A procedure for repair of a lacerated perineum. 3 Surgical formation of a vesicovaginal fistula for bladder drainage in cystitis.

equilibrating operation Correction of an ocular imbalance due to muscle paralysis by severing the opposite muscle tendon from the sclera.

Esser's operation An outmoded term for INLAY GRAFT.

Estes operation A procedure for infertility in which the ovary is placed into the interstitial portion of the uterine tube.

Estlander's operation An operation in which a cross-lip flap is transferred from the lateral portion of one lip to a defect in the ipsilateral side of the other lip. Its pedicle receives its blood supply from the coronary artery and vein at the new corner of the mouth. The pedicle need not be severed, and the mouth can be opened and closed immediately.

face-lift operation FACE-LIFT.

Fasanella-Servat operation An operation for correcting minor degrees of ptosis of the upper eyelid. The lid is everted and then up to three millimeters is excised of the tarsus, conjunctiva, Müller's muscle and levator muscle.

fenestration operation An operation for the relief of deafness due to ankylosis of the stapes, in which a fistula from the middle ear into the inner ear is made at the site of the lateral semicircular canal in order to provide alternative sound access. The procedure is now outmoded. Also called *fenestration.*

Fick operation SACCULOTOMY.

Filatov's operation An operation utilizing a tubed flap.

filtering operation A procedure for glaucoma that creates a passage permitting the aqueous humor to escape from the anterior chamber into the subconjunctival space.

Findlay's operation A surgical procedure designed to close a gastroenteric fistula.

Finney's operation FINNEY PYLOROPLASTY.

Finzi-Harmer operation An operation once regularly employed for carcinoma of the larynx, involving the use of a palisade of radium needles inserted into a window created by resection of part of the ala of the thyroid cartilage adjacent to the tumor. It is now largely superseded by teletherapy.

Flajani's operation A technique of iridodialysis utilizing a knife needle.

flap operation A periodontal surgical procedure in which mucoperiosteal flaps are reflected to allow better access for root planing and bone reshaping.

Fontan operation A surgical procedure designed to treat tricuspid valve atresia, in which right atrial blood is shunted

through a valved conduit to the pulmonary artery.

forceps operation Any manipulation with obstetric forceps to effect the delivery of an infant.

Förster's operation Posterior spinal rhizotomy for the treatment of spastic paralysis.

Förster-Penfield operation Excision of a cerebral cortical scar for the relief of convulsions.

Fothergill operation A surgical operation to correct uterine prolapse by amputation of the cervix followed by attachment of the cardinal ligaments to the anterior uterus.

Fothergill-Donald operation MANCHESTER OPERATION.

four-point operation A procedure for correction of a pupil block glaucoma by double transfixion (entry and exit) of both sides of the iris.

Franco's operation SUPRAPUBIC CYSTOTOMY.

Frank's operation The creation of a gastrostomy by utilizing a mushroom-shaped section of anterior gastric wall that is sutured to the abdominal wall. Also called *Ssabanejew-Frank operation.*

Franke's operation Excision of thoracic nerves, formerly performed for the relief of tabetic pain.

Frazier-Spiller operation Selective trigeminal rhizotomy for the relief of trigeminal neuralgia.

Freckner's operation An operation designed to drain infected air cells for relief of petrositis, utilizing an intrapetrosal surgical approach working inward under the arch of the superior semicircular canal.

Fredet-Ramstedt operation PYLOROMYOTOMY.

Freyer's operation Suprapubic enucleation of an enlarged prostate.

Frommel's operation An old-fashioned gynecologic operation in which the uterosacral ligaments are shortened to correct deviations of uterine position.

frontalis suspension operation A procedure that corrects ptosis by an attachment of the upper eyelid to the frontalis muscle.

Frost-Lang operation Reconstitution of the orbital volume with a gold ball after ocular enucleation.

Fukala's operation Removal of a clear lens for the correction of high myopia, an obsolete procedure.

Fuller's operation An incision of the seminal vesicles to effect drainage.

Gant's operation An osteotomy of the femoral shaft distal to the lesser trochanter to effect ankylosis of the hip joint.

Geraghty's operation A form of partial prostatectomy. It is a modification of Young's operation.

Gersuny's operation A rarely used method of urinary diversion in which the rectum is divided from the sigmoid, the proximal end of the rectum is closed, and the ureters are anastomosed to the rectum. The free end of the sigmoid is then brought to the skin anterior to the anus as a perineal colostomy.

Gifford's operation An attempt to prevent progression of a corneal ulcer by cutting the stroma at the border of the ulcer.

Gigli's operation A seldom-used obstetric operation to allow vaginal delivery in instances of cephalopelvic disproportion, whereby a ramus of the pubic bone is divided with a wire saw.

Gill operation 1 A procedure for a drop foot deformity in which a wedge of bone from the os calcis is inserted into the posterior part of the ankle joint. 2 An operative procedure to relieve the symptoms of spondylolisthesis in which the loose lamina and spinous processes are removed.

Gillespie's operation An excision of the wrist by way of a longitudinal dorsal incision.

Gilliam's operation A surgical operation used to suspend the uterus and correct retrodisplacement, whereby the round ligaments are shortened by suturing a loop of the ligament which has been brought through the anterior peritoneum to the rectus fascia.

Gillies operation The surgical reduction of a fractured zygoma, utilizing an incision in the temple.

Giraldes operation A long-outmoded method of repairing a unilateral congenital cleft lip. • This technique was once erroneously thought to be the forerunner of the Millard method.

Glenn's operation An anastomosis of the superior vena cava to the right pulmonary artery for palliation of cyanotic congenital cardiac defects such as tricuspid atresia, certain tetralogy of Fallot lesions, and pulmonary atresia.

Gonin's operation Surgical correction of retinal detachment.

Graber-Duvernay operation A surgical method of relieving arthritic symptoms by drilling small holes in the head of the femur to increase the blood supply.

Graefe's operation Peripheral iridectomy for angle-closure glaucoma.

Graham operation A surgical procedure in which a perforated duodenal ulcer is plicated with an overlying duodenal omental patch.

Grant's operation A method of excising a lip tumor by which triangular flaps are created for suturing by making oblique incisions from the angles of a square tumor bed.

Gritti's operation GRITTI'S AMPUTATION.

Grondahl-Finney operation Enlargement of the esophagogastric junction by esophagogastroplasty.

Grossmann's operation An obsolete technique for retinal detachment in which saline solution was injected intravitreally to restore the normal retinal position.

Gussenbauer's operation The cutting of an esophageal stricture exposed by a proximal esophagotomy.

Guyon's operation GUYON'S AMPUTATION.

Hacker's operation A surgical procedure for treatment of balanitic hypospadias.

Hagedorn's operation An early method of correcting unilateral congenital cleft lip with a rectangular flap.

Hagner's operation Incision of the epididymis for drainage of pus in gonorrheal epididymitis.

Hahn's operation The dilatation of a pyloric stricture in direct view through a gastrotomy.

Hajek's operation A radical osteoplastic operation for the relief of chronic frontal sinusitis. Through an L-shaped incision above the eye, a triangular osteoplastic flap is created from the front wall of the sinus and hinged above so as to provide good access to the interior of the sinus and the upper end of the frontonasal duct. It has been superseded by the modern osteoplastic frontal sinus operation.

Halpin's operation Removal of the lacrimal gland via an eyebrow incision.

Halsted's operation **1** RADICAL MASTECTOMY. **2** A type of inguinal hernioplasty.

Hancock's operation HANCOCK'S AMPUTATION.

Harrington's operation A surgical procedure in which the left phrenic nerve is temporarily rendered nonfunctional by crushing to facilitate repair of a large diaphragmatic hernia.

Hartley-Krause operation Excision of the gasserian ganglion, using an extradural temporal approach, for the relief of facial neuralgia. An outdated procedure.

Haultaim's operation A modification of the Küstner operation for chronic inversion of the uterus.

Haynes operation Surgical drainage of the cisterna magna, an obsolete treatment for meningitis.

Heath's operation Mastoidectomy in which drainage of the mastoid cavity was provided by the creation of a fistula between the cavity and the external auditory meatus adjacent to the tympanic annulus. This operation is no longer practiced.

Heaton's operation A surgical procedure used to treat inguinal hernias.

Heine's operation Attempted control of elevated intraocular pressure by cyclodialysis.

Heineke's operation A surgical type of pyloroplasty, similar to a Heineke-Mikulicz pyloroplasty.

Heineke-Mikulicz operation HEINEKE-MIKULICZ PYLOROPLASTY.

Heisrath's operation Removal of redundant or misaligned trachomatous tarsal tissue.

Heller's operation CARDIOMYOTOMY.

Herbert's operation A transscleral filtering operation for glaucoma.

Hey's operation HEY'S AMPUTATION.

Hibbs operation An obsolete procedure for Pott's disease of the spine in which the spinous processes of the vertebrae are fractured and pushed against the decorticated lamina below. The technique has been modified for use in spinal fusion operations to correct scoliosis.

high forceps operation The application of obstetric forceps before the fetal head is engaged. This procedure is condemned by modern obstetricians.

Hochenegg's operation A surgical treatment of carcinomas of the middle and distal rectum.

Hoffa's operation LORENZ OPERATION.

Hoffa-Lorenz operation LORENZ OPERATION.

Hofmeister operation A method of anastomosing the stomach to the jejunum. It involves the closure of a portion of the lesser curvature side of the divided stomach and the implantation of the greater curvature side of the divided stomach into the side of the jejunum.

Hoke's operation **1** Arthrodesis of the hindfoot that involves both the talocalcaneal and talonavicular junctures. **2** The surgical correction of talipes planus that involves lengthening of the tendo calcaneus and fusing the tarsal bones on the medial border of the foot.

Holmes operation A method of excising the os calcis via an incision on the upper outer border of the foot and another across the plantar surface of the heel.

Holth's operation Sclerocorneal excision for open-angle glaucoma.

Horgan's operation TRANSANTRAL ETHMOIDECTOMY.

Horsley's operation Excision of the motor cortex for the relief of adventitious movement in the upper limbs.

Horton-Devine operation A method of correcting hypospadias, utilizing a tube-shaped full-thickness skin graft taken from the prepuce to provide the additional length needed for the urethra.

Hotchkiss operation A method for removal of a carcinoma of the buccal surface with resections of portions of maxilla and mandible and plastic reconstruction from tongue and cervical tissues.

Huggins operation Resection of testes for carcinoma of the prostate.

Humphry's operation The surgical removal of a mandibular condyle.

Huntington's operation A gynecologic operation for chronic inversion of the uterus. From the abdominal approach, the operator successively grasps the walls of the inverted uterus with tenacula and exerts traction in an effort to reverse the uterus to its normal position.

Indian operation INDIAN RHINOPLASTY.

interposition operation WATKINS OPERATION.

interval operation A surgical procedure performed in the period between the cessation and expected recurrence of an acute attack, as in appendicitis.

iris inclusion operation A procedure for relief of glaucoma, consisting of incarceration of a piece of iris within a limbal incision, so as to maintain an open leak of aqueous humor to the subconjunctival space.

Irving sterilization operation A surgical sterilization procedure in which the medial cut end of the oviduct is buried in the myometrium posteriorly and the distal cut end is buried in the mesosalpinx.

Italian operation ITALIAN RHINOPLASTY.

Jaboulay's operation INTERPELVIABDOMINAL AMPUTATION.

Jackson-Babcock operation BABCOCK'S OPERATION.

Jacobaeus operation The division of pleural adhesions by cauterization using a thoracoscope.

Jansen's operation An external operation for the relief of frontal sinusitis.

Jarvis operation The removal of part of a nasal concha, usually of the middle or inferior concha, or of a hyperplastic portion of one of these. This operation was once commonly performed but has long since been superseded by other procedures.

Jelks operation A surgical procedure designed to treat anorectal strictures caused by perirectal fibrosis. The fibrotic material is divided by parallel anterior and posterior incisions.

Jewett operation A form of surgical anastomosis between the ureter and the sigmoid colon.

Jonnesco's operation Cervical sympathectomy for the relief of exophthalmos.

Joseph's operation A reduction rhinoplasty performed subcutaneously through intranasal incisions.

Kader's operation KADER-SENN OPERATION.

Kader-Senn operation A surgical procedure in which a gastrostomy is created by imbricating a section of the gastric cardia with a glass cone. Also called *Kader's operation.*

Kahn's operation Division of the dentate ligaments in decompressing the spinal cord.

Kanavel's operation The use of full-thickness skin grafts on the palm and/or fingers following palmar fasciectomy in the treatment of Dupuytren's contracture.

Kazanjian's operation A surgical procedure to extend the vestibular sulcus.

Keegan's operation A variety of Indian rhinoplasty, in which a new nose is built from a flap taken from either side of the forehead.

Kelly's operation 1 A surgical procedure to correct urinary incontinence in women. 2 A variety of arytenoidectomy for the relief of bilateral abductor paralysis of the larynx. A square window was excised in the posterior part of the thyroid ala, through which the arytenoid cartilage was removed. It was soon superseded by Woodman's operation. An outmoded term.

Key's operation A lateral lithotomy performed using a straight staff.

Killian's operation KILLIAN FRONTAL SINUS OPERATION.

Killian frontal sinus operation An operation for the relief of chronic frontal sinusitis requiring the removal of most of the front wall and floor of the sinus but the preservation of the upper orbital arch to avoid deformity. Also called *Killian's operation.*

King's operation An arytenoidopexy utilized to improve the airway in cases of bilateral abductor paralysis of the larynx. The object is to abduct one of the paralyzed cords by fixing the arytenoid with the vocal process rotated outward.

Knapp's operation Use of roller forceps to express trachomatous follicles.

Kocher's operation An excision of the ankle joint via an incision below the lateral malleolus and division of the perioneal tendons, with resuture of the tendons after joint débridement.

Kocks operation A gynecologic vaginal operation to treat uterine prolapse by shortening the cardinal ligaments.

Kolomnin's operation The electrocautery of the diseased tissues in hip-joint disease.

Kondoleon operation A procedure to relieve elephantiasis by removing strips of subcutaneous connective tissue.

König's operation An acetabuloplasty performed to correct congenital dislocation of the hip whereby an osteoperiosteal flap is created from the outer border of the ilium to deepen the floor of the acetabulum. Also called *shelf operation, shelving operation, shelf procedure.*

Körte-Ballance operation Anastomosis of the facial and spinal accessory nerves for the relief of facial paralysis.

Kortzeborn's operation A seldom used method for repositioning a thumb in an individual who suffers from intrinsic muscle paralysis as a result of motor palsy of the median nerve.

Kraske's operation A rectal resection following freeing of the coccyx and left sacral wing to provide posterior exposure.

Krimer's operation An operation once used for the repair of cleft palate. Mucoperiosteal flaps from either side were sutured together in the midline.

Kronlein operation Removal of the outer wall of the orbit to provide operative access to the orbital contents.

Kuhnt-Szymanowski operation A method of correcting ectropion of the lower eyelid wherein the lid is split along its free margin into a tarsoconjunctival layer and a skin-muscle layer. Sections of tissue that are offset one from the other are then removed from each layer and the layers are closed independently. Also called *Kuhnt-Szymanowski procedure.*

Küstner operation A gynecologic operation to correct chronic inversion of the uterus. The myometrium is incised posteriorly to expose the fundus and traction is then applied to restore the uterus to its normal position.

Lagrange's operation Sclerectomy for glaucoma.

Landolt's operation Reconstruction of the lower eyelid with a bridge flap of skin brought down from the upper lid.

Lange's operation An operation in which a gap in a tendon is bridged with alloplastic, nonabsorbable suture material. This procedure is no longer in practice.

Lanz operation An operative procedure for treating elephantiasis of the leg in which strips of the fascia lata femoris are inserted into an opening in the femur.

Larrey's operation LARREY'S AMPUTATION.

laryngeal drop operation LARYNGEAL RELEASE.

Latzko's operation A gynecologic operation to repair genital tract fistulas. A flap of vaginal mucosa is utilized to cover the fistula tract.

Laurens operation An operation for the repair of postauricular fistulas persisting after mastoidectomy. The cicatricial circumference of the fistula is excised, vertical extensions are incised upwards and downwards from the opening, and the skin widely elevated as anterior and posterior flaps are carefully sutured together.

Lawson's operation A submucous resection of the vocal cord performed by way of the laryngofissure approach. Through a mucosal incision along the cord, the arytenoid cartilage along with the thyroarytenoid and cricoarytenoid muscles are removed.

Le Fort's operation A gynecologic operation to treat uterine prolapse whereby the anterior and posterior walls of the vagina are sutured together, obliterating most of the vagina. Also called *Le Fort-Neugebauer operation.*

Le Fort-Neugebauer operation LE FORT'S OPERATION.

LeMesurier operation A method of correcting unilateral congenital cleft lip wherein the additional length needed for the medial lip segment is provided by interposing a rectangular flap from the lateral segment at the lower end of the repair.

lip adhesion operation The first of two operations to repair a congenital cleft lip and palate where the width of the cleft in the palate is great. A temporary incomplete closure of the lip is carried out with the object of providing continuous traction by the joined muscles of the lip on the components of the cleft palate in the hope of narrowing the cleft ahead of a later definitive operation.

Lisfranc's operation LISFRANC'S AMPUTATION.

Liston's operation Excision of the upper jaw, once used for the removal of certain kinds of tumors. By means of skin incisions alongside the nose, through the upper lip, and from the angle of the mouth to the temple, a large cheek flap was raised to expose the tumor and facilitate division of its bony attachments.

Littre's operation The creation of a colostomy in the left inguinal region.

Longuet's operation An operation for correction of testicular hydrocele, involving extraserous placement of a testicle. Also called *Longuet's incision.*

Lorenz operation An operation for congenital dislocation of the hip in which the head of the femur is fixed against the rudimentary acetabulum until a socket is formed. Also called *Hoffa-Lorenz operation, Hoffa's operation.*

Loreta's operation The dilatation of a pyloric stenosis by digital manipulation through a prepyloric gastrostomy.

Lotheissen's operation McVAY'S OPERATION.

low forceps operation The application of obstetric forceps when the head of the fetus is on the pelvic floor and the sagittal suture lies in the anteroposterior diameter of the pelvic outlet.

Lowsley's operation A surgical procedure for correction of epispadias.

Luc's operation CALDWELL-LUC OPERATION.

Luckett operation An operation for the correction of congenital lop ears in which excisions are made of a crescent-shaped portion of skin from the posteromedial aspect of the pinna and a smaller subjacent strip of cartilage, to restore the antihelical fold. It was the basis of subsequent procedures to correct this defect.

Ludloff's operation An oblique osteotomy of the first metatarsal bone for the correction of the metatarsus primus varus deformity of hallux valgus.

Lund's operation A talectomy performed to correct talipes.

Macewen's operation A supracondylar osteotomy of the femur for correction of a genu valgum deformity. Also called *Macewen's osteotomy.*

Mackenrodt's operation An old-fashioned gynecologic operation whereby the round ligaments are fixed to the vagina in an effort to correct a retroflexed uterus.

Madlener operation A surgical sterilization procedure in which a knuckle of the oviduct is crushed and then ligated without resection.

magnet operation Extraction of a magnetic intraocular foreign body with a magnet.

Makkas operation An operation for treatment of ectopia of the bladder.

Manchester operation A gynecologic operation to correct uterine prolapse whereby the cervix is amputated, the cardinal ligaments are attached anteriorly to the upper cervix, and an anterior colporraphy is performed. Also called *Fothergill-Donald operation, Manchester-Fothergill operation.*

Manchester-Fothergill operation MANCHESTER OPERATION.

Mann-Williamson operation An experimental surgical procedure that is used to study ulceration in the small intestine in dogs. The duodenum is separated from the stomach at the pylorus and the severed ends are closed. The ileum is then connected to the stomach by a side to side anastomosis. Ulcers develop in the ileal mucosa.

Marian's operation A surgical procedure to treat bladder stones in which a transperitoneal medial incision is used. Also called *Mariano's operation.*

Mariano's operation MARIAN'S OPERATION.

Marshall-Marchetti operation An operation for the correction of stress incontinence in which the urethra and bladder are attached to the pubic bone.

Martin's operation A procedure for radical cure of hydrocele.

mastoid operation MASTOIDECTOMY.

mastoid obliteration operation Any operation for obliterating the cavity remaining after mastoidectomy, especially after radical mastoidectomy and, before it became outmoded, the fenestration operation. A number of techniques have been employed using cancellous bone, bone paste, acrylic resin, fat and, particularly, pedicled fascia and muscle flaps. In general, such operations have fallen out of favor.

Matas operation Any of several types of endoaneurysmorrhaphy.

Matson's operation Anastomosis between the proximal end of a ureter and the spinal arachnoid. The operation is performed for relief of increased intracranial pressure such as in the communicating type of hydrocephalus. The subarachnoid ureterostomy requires the sacrifice of a kidney and mobilization of its ureter.

Maydl's operation A surgical procedure in which a colostomy is created and the wound is left open until adhesions form to fix the colon in place.

Mayo's operation **1** A surgical repair of an umbilical hernia, utilizing a two-layer, overlapping closure. **2** A surgical procedure in which the duodenum is excluded by pyloric excision and a posterior gastrojejunostomy performed. **3** Removal of varicose veins of the lower extremity, using an external stripper.

McBurney's operation A surgical procedure to treat inguinal hernias by excising the sac and securing the overlying imbricated skin to underlying musculature.

McGill's operation SUPRAPUBIC TRANSVESICAL PROSTATECTOMY.

McKissock's operation A reduction mammoplasty in which the blood supply to the nipple is preserved by means of a bipedicled vertical de-epithelized skin flap.

McVay's operation A groin hernioplasty in which the repair involves the pectineal ligament. Also called *Lotheissen's operation, Cooper's ligament hernioplasty.*

Meller's operation A technique of dacryocystectomy.

Mercier's operation PROSTATECTOMY.

Meyer's operation RADICAL MASTECTOMY.

midforceps operation The application of obstetric forceps after the fetal head has become engaged but is not on the pelvic floor and/or the sagittal suture is not in the anteroposterior diameter of the pelvic outlet.

mika operation Creation of a fistula in the male urethra in order to prevent reproduction.

Mikulicz operation **1** An excision of the sternocleidomastoid muscle for the correction of congenital torticollis. **2** An excision of the hindfoot in which the talus and the os calcis are excised together with the articular surfaces of the tibia, fibula, and the cuboid and navicular bones. The foot is then brought into alignment with the leg.

Miles operation Abdominoperineal resection of rectal carcinoma.

Millard operation **1** MILLARD METHOD. **2** MILLARD ROTATION-ADVANCEMENT OPERATION.

Millard rotation-advancement operation A popular method for the repair of unilateral congenital cleft lip wherein the cupid's bow on the medial side of the cleft is rotated into anatomic position by means of a curved convex incision along the medial border of the cleft, usually with the assistance of a back cut at the superior end. The lateral lip segment is then formed onto an advancement flap and joined to the repositioned medial segment. Many modifications and refinements have been described. Also called *Millard operation.*

Millin-Read operation An operation for the correction of urinary stress incontinence in which fascial strips from the anterior abdominal wall are used for a suprapubic sling which passes around the urethra.

Mingazzini-Förster operation Intentional surgical injury of the lens with the purpose of hastening liquefaction of the cortex, thereby facilitating a subsequent extracapsular extraction.

Mirault's operation A method for the repair of unilateral congenital cleft lip, wherein the necessary additional length on the medial side of the cleft is achieved by paring the medial edge to a sufficient distance, and applying to the raw surface a triangular-shaped full-thickness flap taken from the free border of the lateral side.

modified flap operation A flap operation that is extended horizontally to allow adequate access without the need for vertical incisions.

Morestin's operation A disarticulation at the knee with division of the femur through the condyles. Also called *Morestin's method.*

Morison-Talma operation A rarely performed surgical procedure in which peritoneal and visceral adhesions are induced in order to treat ascites stemming from portal hypertension by increasing portosystemic shunting. Also called *Talma's operation.*

Moschcowitz's operation A surgical procedure designed to treat femoral hernias using an inguinal approach.

Motais operation An obsolete technique of ptosis surgery utilizing the superior rectus tendon.

Mules operation Implantation of a sphere into the muscle cone after enucleation of the eye.

Müller's operation A method of completing vaginal hysterectomy by splitting the uterus in the midline into halves and then resecting each half separately.

Mustard's operation MUSTARD PROCEDURE.

Naffziger operation Intracranial decompression of the orbit for the relief of exophthalmos.

Nélaton's operation An excision of the shoulder joint via a transverse incision.

Neuber's operation An operation utilizing the central portion of a skin flap to fill a cavity in a bone.

Ober's operation The division of a joint capsule for the correction of contractures.

Obwegeser's operation A method of surgically splitting the rami of the mandible in a sagittal plane in order to reposition the body of the mandible with respect to the rami.

Ogston's operation A wedge osteotomy through the tarsus to correct a flat foot deformity.

Ogston-Luc operation An operation once used for the relief of frontal sinusitis. The sinus was approached by a midline incision above the root of the nose and the anterior wall was trephined. It has since been superseded by other procedures.

Ollier's operation 1 The transfer of a thin split-skin graft. 2 An operation for the repair of a defect in the lower lip with a flap obtained from the submental region. 3 Decortication of the nose in cases of rhinophyma.

Olshausen's operation An old-fashioned gynecologic operation whereby the uterus is suspended by suturing it to the anterior abdominal wall.

Ombrédanne's operation A surgical procedure for correction of hypospadias, wherein the preputial skin is opened upon itself, leaving a dorsal attachment. The flap thus created is then folded onto the ventral surface of the penis, and the glans penis passed

through a small incision in the center of the flap.

open operation A surgical procedure by which, as a result of the incision, internal organs and tissues become exposed to view.

open flap operation A flap operation with one or more vertical relieving incisions.

Ord's operation A method of breaking down recent joint adhesions.

osteoplastic frontal sinus operation An operation for the relief of chronic frontal sinusitis. The principal feature is the turning down, as an osteoplastic flap, of the anterior wall of the frontal sinuses, previously marked out using an x-ray template. With access to the interior of the sinuses so afforded, the lining mucosa is meticulously removed and drainage established into the nose by creating a passage through the ethmoidal air cells from above.

Owen cleft lip operation A method of repairing unilateral congenital cleft lip that has long been in disuse because it involved the considerable sacrifice of tissue and consequent distortion.

Paci's operation A modification of the Lorenz operation for congenital dislocation of the hip.

palatal pushback operation 1 An operation for the repair of cleft palate, now superseded by the Wardill V-Y pushback operation. Palatal pushback is a two-stage operation in which the palatal soft tissues are raised and the anterior palatine arteries ligated and, two or three weeks later, the delayed flap is moved backwards and the repair completed. Also called *Dorrance operation.* 2 An operation to correct velopharyngeal insufficiency by the posterior repositioning of the soft palate. For defs. 1 and 2 also called *pushback procedure.*

Panas operation A type of frontalis suspension operation for ptosis of the upper eyelid.

Partsch's operation MARSUPIALIZATION.

Péan's operation An obsolete method of performing a vaginal hysterectomy entirely by morcellation.

Peet's operation A supradiaphragmatic sympathectomy for vascular hypertension.

Petersen's operation A lithotomy in which a suprapubic approach is used.

Phelps operation A soft tissue release operation through the medial aspect of the foot to correct a talipes deformity.

Phemister operation The insertion of a cancellous bone graft for a delayed union or nonunion of a stable fracture.

Physick's operation A technique of optical iridectomy.

plastic operation An operation to improve form or function, primarily by molding, shifting, or adding tissues. Also called *plastic surgery.*

Politzer's operation 1 A former method of producing a perforation of the tympanic membrane in such a way as to delay healing. The opening was created by the brief application of electric cautery to the chosen site. The technique was used as a diagnostic procedure in cases of suspected chronic adhesive otitis media. 2 The division of the anterior ligament of the malleus in cases of severe retraction of the tympanic membrane due to chronic adhesive otitis media. Using a small curved knife, the anterior malleolar fold was divided, the knife advanced 2 mm and an upward incision made as far as the edge of the notch of Rivinus. This procedure is no longer utilized.

Pollock's operation An amputation of the lower limb through the knee joint using a long anterior flap and retaining the patella.

Polya's operation A surgical reconstruction following a distal gastrectomy in which a retrocolic gastrojejunostomy is not preceded by a Hofmeister operation.

Pomeroy's operation A simple method of achieving sterilization whereby a loop of fallopian tube is ligated with catgut suture without crushing it and the loop is then resected.

Poncet's operation   The surgical lengthening of the Achilles tendon in order to correct a talipes deformity.

Portmann interposition operation   A variety of stapedectomy in which the stapes superstructure is left intact and attached to the incus while only the foot-plate is removed. A vein graft is interposed between the stapedial crura and the patent oval window. No prosthesis is required. Also called *platinectomy*.

Potts operation   The creation of an anastomosis between the descending aorta and pulmonary artery in patients with severe pulmonary stenosis, as seen especially in the tetralogy of Fallot. Also called *Potts-Smith-Gibson operation*.

Potts-Smith-Gibson operation   POTTS OPERATION.

Power's operation   An early attempt at corneal transplantation, utilizing a heterograft obtained from a rabbit.

punch operation   Prostatectomy employing punches and a resectoscope.

Puussepp's operation   A posterior longitudinal incision in the spinal cord, for the treatment of syringomyelia.

Quaglino's operation   A technique of sclerotomy with a small knife.

Quénu-Mayo operation   A radical surgical treatment for rectal malignancies in which all of the rectum and the tissues bearing lymph nodes are removed.

Ramadier's operation   An operation for the relief of petrositis involving an intrapetrosal surgical approach to the apex of the petrous portion of the temporal bone. The procedure entails retraction of the carotid artery forward to gain access to the site of infection through the posterior wall of the bony carotid canal.

Ramstedt operation   PYLOROMYOTOMY.

Rastelli's operation   The correction of various forms of cyanotic congenital cardiac anomalies, such as truncus arteriosus, pulmonary artery atresia, and transposition of the great arteries with pulmonary stenosis by the use of a valved prosthetic or allograft conduit between the right ventricle and the pulmonary artery.

reconstructive operation   RECONSTRUCTIVE SURGERY.

Reverdin's operation   REVERDIN GRAFT.

Riedel's operation   A radical operation once used for the relief of frontal sinusitis. The entire floor and anterior wall of the sinus were removed, resulting in an unsightly deformity.

Ries-Clark operation   A type of radical hysterectomy for treatment of invasive carcinoma of the cervix.

Rigaud's operation   Plastic correction for a urethral fistula, utilizing a combination of turnover and advancement flaps.

Rose's operation   GASSERECTOMY.

Rosenthal's operation   The closure of a congenital cleft palate by utilizing the procedures of von Langenbeck's operation but using an inferiorly based pharyngeal flap in closure of the defect.

Rose-Thompson operation   A method of repairing minimal degrees of congenital cleft lip, wherein the additional length required on the medial side of the cleft is obtained by means of curved concave incisions on either side. When the curved edges are approximated as a straight line, the necessary extra length is automatically provided.

Roux en Y operation   A surgical procedure in which a defunctionalized limb of the small bowel is created by an end-to-end enteroenterostomy. The end of this loop may be used for a number of types of biliary, enteric, gastric, or pancreatic anastomoses.

Royle's operation   Lumbar sympathectomy, for improving the blood supply to the lower limb.

saccus operation   Any one of several operations intended to relieve the symptoms of Menière's disease by decompressing the saccus endolymphaticus. Over the years, this has included incision of the saccus, the use of an endolymphatic shunt, and the exposing of the saccus without opening it.

Saemisch's operation   A corneal section supposed to limit the spread of infection.

Sayoc's operation   A method of creating a supratarsal fold in the Oriental upper eyelid.

Sayre's operation   A nonsurgical treatment of spondylitis or Pott's disease by use of a plaster body cast. Also called *Sayre's method*.

Scanzoni's operation   An operation utilizing obstetrical forceps to rotate a fetal head from the posterior to the anterior position. After the fetus is rotated, the forceps are reapplied so that they are aligned with the pelvic axis.

Scarpa's operation   A surgical procedure in which the femoral artery is ligated within the trigonum femorale (Scarpa's triangle).

Schauta's operation   SCHAUTA-AMREICH VAGINAL OPERATION.

Schauta-Amreich vaginal operation   A method of treating carcinoma of the uterine cervix by performing a radical or extended vaginal hysterectomy whereby the uterus is removed close to its attachments to the pelvic wall. Also called *Schauta's operation*.

Schauta-Wertheim operation   WERTHEIM-SCHAUTA OPERATION.

Scheie's operation   A thermal shrinkage of the scleral edge of a limbal incision to permit aqueous drainage to the subconjunctival space as a treatment for glaucoma.

Schlatter's operation   A total gastrectomy performed with an esophagoenterostomy.

Schmalz operation   Use of a thread to maintain patency of an occluded nasolacrimal duct.

Schönbein's operation   PALATOPHARYNGOPLASTY.

Schwartze's operation   SIMPLE MASTOIDECTOMY.

Schwartze-Stacke operation   A modification of Stacke's operation, the principal feature of which is preservation of the outer attic wall so as to protect the malleus and incus and conserve hearing. Usually the limited approach was inadequate for the removal of all the existing disease and the operation has long been abandoned.

Sédillot's operation   A method for reconstruction of the upper lip utilizing full-thickness flaps from the cheeks.

Semb's operation   A surgical method of extrapleural collapse therapy of the apex of the lung in pulmonary tuberculosis.

Senn's operation   An intestinal anastomosis accomplished by lateral approximation between a pair of bone plates.

Serré's operation   A Z-plasty performed for correction of skin contractures occurring at the commissure of the lips of the mouth. Utilizing a Z-flap, the triangular flap containing the commissure is interposed with the triangular flap containing skin and subcutaneous tissue.

seton operation   A filtering operation for glaucoma, in which the drain site is kept open by the presence of some type of foreign substance.

Sewall operation   A surgical method of decompressing the optical orbit, in cases of severe exophthalmos, by removing the medial orbital wall through an incision beneath the eyebrow.

shelf operation   KÖNIG'S OPERATION.

shelving operation   KÖNIG'S OPERATION.

Siebold's operation   An old-fashioned technique of pubiotomy.

Sistrunk operation   A method for removal of thyroglossal cysts and sinuses. Because the thyroglossal tract is intimately related to the body of the hyoid bone and may be identified as far as the foramen cecum, it was advocated that the central portion of the hyoid bone together with a core of lingual muscle should be excised to ensure against recurrence.

Sjöquist's operation   Medullary section of the tract of the trigeminal nerve, for the relief of trigeminal neuralgia.

Skoog's operation 1 A technique of repairing unilateral congenital cleft lip wherein the additional length needed is obtained on the medial side of the cleft by the interposition of two small triangular flaps from the lateral side. 2 SKOOG'S METHOD.

Smith's operation Intracapsular delivery of a cataract by pressure applied to the inferior sclera.

Smith-Robinson operation A cervical spine fusion using an anterior approach that is effected by the removal of an intervertebral disk and the grafting of bone.

Smithwick's operation LUMBODORSAL SPLANCHNICECTOMY.

Socin's operation Enucleation of a thyroid tumor to preserve functioning thyroid tissue.

Spinelli's operation An operation to correct chronic uterine inversion in which the anterior myometrium is incised and traction is exerted on the exposed fundus in order to restore the uterus to its normal status.

Spivack's operation Cystostomy in which a tube is fashioned from a flap of subcutaneous tissue on the anterior abdominal wall.

Ssabanejew-Frank operation FRANK'S OPERATION.

Stacke's operation A variety of radical mastoidectomy advocated in cases where the mastoid is sclerotic and the mastoid antrum hard to find. A tympanectomy is performed first and then the antrum is opened working upwards and backwards from the meatus.

stapes mobilization operation STAPES MOBILIZATION.

State operation The surgical correction of congenital megacolon in which the normal colon is anastomosed to the aganglionic distal rectum in an end-to-end communication.

Stein operation A rarely used method of reconstructing a defect in the central portion of the lower lip, utilizing paired, laterally based flaps from the central portion of the upper lip.

Steinach's operation Ligation of the vas deferens to promote proliferation of the testicular interstitial tissue with a resultant increase in production of testicular hormones. Also called *Steinach's method.*

Steindler's operation 1 An arthrodesis of the elbow performed by using a cortical bone graft extending from the lower end of the humerus to the olecranon. 2 A method of correcting talipes cavus by stripping all muscle and fascia from the plantar surface of the heel.

Stoffel's operation Division of motor nerves for the relief of spasticity.

Stokes operation GRITTI-STOKES AMPUTATION.

Stone operation WREDEN OPERATION.

Stookey-Scarff operation The creation of an opening between the third ventricle and the pontine cistern for a cerebrospinal fluid shunt. This operation is used in the treatment of a ventricular obstruction at a point distal to the third ventricle.

string operation The dilatation of an esophageal stricture in which the patient swallows a string and esophageal dilatators are then passed, using the string as a guide.

Strombeck's operation A reduction mammoplasty wherein the blood supply to the nipple is preserved by means of a bipedicled horizontal de-epithelized skin flap.

Sturmdorf's operation Excision of the squamocolumnar junction of the uterine cervix by making a conical incision to excise the tissue and then suturing flaps of adjacent vaginal mucosa into the area of excision to control bleeding and encourage healing.

subcutaneous operation An operation performed through a small stab incision.

Swenson's operation A surgical treatment for congenital megacolon in which the normal colon is pulled through the aganglionic rectum and sutured into place.

Syme's operation 1 SYME AMPUTATION. 2 A method for performing external urethrotomy.

Szymanowski operation An operation for the repair of a defect of the upper lip by using a rotation flap from the cheek, which is brought as far as the midline.

Taarnhøj's operation Decompression of the ganglion and root of the trigeminal nerve, for the relief of trigeminal neuralgia.

tack operation An operation for the relief of the symptoms of Menière's disease by intermittent decompression of the saccule. It is a modification of sacculotomy. A stainless steel tack is inserted through the stapes foot-plate so as to puncture the saccule whenever it should become distended.

tagliacotian operation An outmoded term for ITALIAN RHINOPLASTY.

talc operation PERICARDIAL POUDRAGE.

Talma's operation MORISON-TALMA OPERATION.

Tanner's operation The surgical ligation of the portal azygos connections and the division and resuturing of the stomach immediately below the gastroesophageal junction to correct bleeding esophageal varices.

Tansini's operation 1 Mastectomy followed by use of a skin flap from the back to cover the defect. 2 A method of resecting a hepatic cyst.

Tanzer's operation A method of reconstructing a congenitally absent external ear, utilizing costal cartilage grafts for the framework and skin grafts and local skin flaps for the integument.

Teale's operation TEALE'S AMPUTATION.

Tennison-Randall operation A method for repairing congenital cleft lip deformities wherein a triangular flap from the lateral segment affords additional vertical height necessary for correction.

Tessier's operation The surgical repositioning of the frontal bone, the bony orbits, and sometimes the maxilla and zygomata, in the treatment of craniofacial anomalies.

Thiersch operation 1 A procedure in which a silver subcutaneous stitch inserted around the anus is used in the treatment of rectal prolapse. 2 A procedure used for the repair of epispadias. 3 OLLIER-THIERSCH GRAFT.

three-snip operation Incision of the lacrimal punctum and canaliculus for relief of obstruction of tear flow.

Torek operation An operation formerly used for correction of an undescended testicle, in which the testicle is temporarily attached to the inner thigh through an incision in the scrotum. An obsolete term.

Torkildsen's operation TORKILDSEN SHUNT.

Toti's operation A variety of external dacryocystorhinostomy, no longer used. After removing the inner wall of the lacrimal sac, bone was resected to expose the nasal lining adjacent to the front end of the middle concha. A portion of nasal mucosa was then removed to encourage fistula formation between the sac and the nasal cavity.

Trauner's operation A method of repairing congenital cleft lip by attaining the extra length necessary on the medial side of the cleft through the utilization of a long, narrow triangular flap in the upper part of the repair and a smaller, broader one in the lower part.

Trendelenburg's operation 1 Pulmonary embolectomy, especially without the use of cardiopulmonary bypass. 2 The surgical removal of a varicose vein. 3 The ligation of a saphenous vein. 4 SYNCHONDROSEOTOMY.

Treves operation An operation to evacuate the abscessed psoas muscle associated with spinal tuberculosis.

Tuttle operation A single-stage procedure utilized to treat carcinoma of the rectum.

uterine suspension operation Any operative procedure utilized to reposition the uterus from retroversion to anteversion.

vacuum extraction operation The use of a suction cup placed on the fetal head to facilitate vaginal delivery. The suction device takes the place of obstetric forceps and is used for the same indications.

van Hook's operation   URETEROURETEROSTOMY.

Verhoeff's operation   A technique for management of expulsive hemorrhage during cataract surgery, in which the blood is released via a posterior sclerotomy.

Vermale's operation   An amputation followed by the transfixion of two flaps from the sides of the limb.

Vidal's operation   A multiple, subcutaneous, venous ligation used to treat a varicocele.

Vineberg's operation   An operation to revascularize an ischemic heart by implanting a divided internal mammary artery into a myocardial tunnel.

Volkmann's operation   Incision of the tunica vaginalis testis for treatment of hydrocele.

von Langenbeck's operation   An operation for the closure of a cleft palate utilizing von Langenbeck's bipedicled mucoperiosteal flaps. Flaps are raised on each side of the cleft and then sutured together near the midline.

Voronoff's operation   Transplantation of anthropoid ape testes into a man.

Wagner's operation   A craniotomy in which a window of bone is resected from the skull and the bone section remains attached to muscle.

Walton's operation   **1** A surgical procedure used to treat a gastric ulcer of the lesser curvature which has resulted in an hourglass stomach.   **2** The reconstruction of the extrahepatic biliary tree.

Wardill's V-Y pushback operation   A pharyngoplasty for velopharyngeal incompetence, performed by gathering the fibers of the superior constrictor muscle and suturing them into a mound on the posterior wall of the pharynx. Two V-shaped flaps are raised and moved back toward the pharynx, the line of repair of the soft palate forming the stem of the letter Y.

Waters operation   A method of performing an extraperitoneal cesarean section.

Watkins operation   A vaginal operation used to treat uterine and vaginal prolapse. The uterine fundus is brought forward and is transposed to lie against the base of the bladder in order to prevent futher prolapse. Also called *interposition operation*.

Webster's operation   BALDY'S OPERATION.

Weir's operation   APPENDICOSTOMY.

Wertheim's operation   A hysterectomy consisting of excision at the origin of the uterine attachments and removal of the upper portion of the vagina. This operation is employed in treating carcinoma of the cervix and is often performed in conjunction with a pelvic lymphadenectomy.

Wertheim-Schauta operation   Radical hysterectomy carried out through a primary vaginal incision. Also called *Schauta-Wertheim operation*.

Wheelhouse's operation   A form of external urethrotomy.

Whipple's operation   PANCREATICODUODENECTOMY.

White's operation   Castration for prostatic hypertrophy.

Whitehead's operation   The treatment of severe rectal hemorrhoids by excising a ring of abnormal mucosa and closing the defect with normal rectal mucosa drawn down from above.

Whitman's operation   An obsolete arthroplasty of the hip that was performed following a fracture of the femoral neck in which avascular necrosis of the femoral head followed. The femoral head was removed and the greater trochanter and its attached muscles were advanced distally.

Winiwarter's operation   The surgical establishment of a communication between the gallbladder and the small intestine. It is usually performed to bypass the distal bile duct or periampullary neoplasms.

Witzel's operation   A surgical procedure in which a tube jejunostomy is created for enteric feeding by way of a jejunal tunnel.

Wladimiroff's operation   A tarsectomy similar to that of the Mikulicz operation.

Wolfe-Krause operation   FULL-THICKNESS GRAFT.

Wölfler's operation   The surgical creation of an anterior gastroenterostomy to reestablish intestinal continuity following a distal gastric resection.

Woodman's operation   A variety of arytenoidectomy and cordopexy used for the relief of bilateral abductor paralysis of the larynx. Through a skin incision along the anterior border of the sternomastoid muscle, the inferior constrictor muscle is separated from the thyroid cartilage, permitting elevation of the thyroid ala and exposure of the arytenoid cartilage where it articulates with the cricoid cartilage. The arytenoid cartilage is removed and the posterior end of the vocal cord stitched to the inferior horn of thyroid cartilage.

Wreden operation   The restoration of anal sphincter control by plastic surgery. Also called *Stone operation, Wreden-Stone operation*.

Wreden-Stone operation   WREDEN OPERATION.

Wützer's operation   A surgical procedure for inguinal hernia.

Wyeth's operation   A disarticulation of the lower limb through the hip joint in which bleeding is controlled by an elastic cord that is passed around large needles (Wyeth pins) to transfix the tissues on each side of the articulation.

Young's operation   A partial prostatectomy employing a punch.

Ziegler's operation   A cautery of the eyelid to correct malposition by shrinking the tissue.

Z-plastic relaxing operation   Z-PLASTY.

---

operative [Middle French *operatif* (from L *operat(us)*, past part. of *operari* to work, take pains with) pertaining to a work]   **1** Pertaining to surgical procedures.   **2** Active or effective; not passive or inert.

operator   **1** One who performs an operation.   **2** One who operates equipment.   **3** OPERATOR LOCUS.

gene operator   A segment of a chromosome which is located adjacent to a structural gene and which controls transcription of the structural gene.

operatory [Med L *operatori(um)* (from L *operat(us)*, past part. of *operari* to work, + *-orium* -ORY) a room for medical work]   The room in which a dentist carries out dental operations on patients. A British usage.

opercle   OPERCULUM.

opercula   Plural of OPERCULUM.

opercular   The posterior bone of the operculum of a fish, forming a gill cover and framing the cheek region posteriorly.

operculate   OPERCULATED.

operculated   Possessing an operculum, or lid. Also *operculate*.

operculectomy [*opercul(um)* + *-ECTOMY*]   The surgical removal of the operculum of the insula.

operculitis [*opercul(um)* + *-ITIS*]   PERICORONITIS.

operculum [L (from *opertus*, past part. of *operiri* to cover, from OP- + L *partus*, past part. of *parere* to bring forth, bear), a lid, cover]   (*plural* opercula)   **1** A covering membrane or lid, such as occurs in a wide variety of vertebrate and invertebrate animals. It varies in form from a membranous flap to a horny lid, and generally serves as a movable, protective covering that can seal off an internal organ or system. Also called *opercle*.   **2** The cortical lid or cover on the insula, formed by those portions of the frontal, parietal, and temporal lobes bordering the lateral (sylvian) fissure.   • The plural form *opercula insulae* is often used when referring to the folds comprising this cover.

cartilaginous operculum　An outmoded term for DISCUS ARTICULARIS ARTICULATIONIS TEMPOROMANDIBULARIS.

cortical operculum　**1** Generically, the "apron" of cortex hidden within a deep cerebral fissure.　**2** Specifically, the operculum of the lateral sulcus overlying the insula.

dental operculum　The flap of oral mucosa partially or completely covering an erupting or impacted tooth. Also called *tooth hood, odontoclamis, occlusal pad.*

frontal operculum　OPERCULUM FRONTALE.

operculum frontale　[NA] The part of the inferior frontal gyrus that forms the anterior part of the cortical covering of the insula. It borders the lateral sulcus, and is subdivided into orbital, triangular, and opercular portions. In the left (or dominant) hemisphere, the triangular and opercular portions constitute Broca's motor speech area. Also called *frontal operculum, operculum orbitale, pars frontalis operculi, pars triangularis.*

frontoparietal operculum　OPERCULUM FRONTOPARIETALE.

operculum frontoparietale　[NA] The part of the cortical covering of the insula lying along the superior border of the lateral sulcus between the ascending and posterior branches of that sulcus. It includes the opercular portion of the inferior frontal gyrus, the lower ends of the precentral and postcentral gyri, and the supramarginal gyrus of the inferior parietal lobule. Also called *frontoparietal operculum, pars parietalis operculi.*

opercula insulae　See under OPERCULUM.

occipital operculum　The portion of the occipital lobe forming the posterior wall of the simian fissure, or sulcus lunatus, when this fissure is present in the human brain.

operculum orbitale　OPERCULUM FRONTALE.

parietal operculum　The inferior portions of the precentral, postcentral, and supramarginal gyri bordering the lateral sulcus and overlying the insula. Stimulation of the parietal operculum produces gustatory sensations.

temporal operculum　OPERCULUM TEMPORALE.

operculum temporale　[NA] The part of the superior temporal gyrus forming the lower margin of the lateral sulcus and overlying the insula. The transverse gyri of Heschel lie on its superior surface, and the most anterior of these gyri is the auditory area. Also called *temporal operculum, pars temporalis operculi.*

trophoblastic operculum　The lid of trophoblast which closes over the point of implantation on the endometrial surface.

operon　A functional unit of DNA that includes one or more structural genes, an adjacent promoter that can initiate transcription, and an operator locus whose interaction with regulatory molecules modulates the activity of the promoter.

lac operon　A region of the chromosome of *Escherichia coli* consisting of three adjacent structural genes plus an operator and a promoter, the promoter being the site to which ribonucleic acid polymerase first binds. The structural genes of the lac operon code for the enzymes β-galactosidase, galactoside permease, and galactoside transacetylase, which allow utilization of the sugar lactose.

transfer operon　The operon in a conjugative plasmid that codes for the components of the F pilus.

ophi-　OPHIO-.

ophiasis　[Gk *ophiasis* a bald place on the head, winding in form] OPHIASIC ALOPECIA AREATA.

Ophidia　[OPHI- + *d* + -IA]　SERPENTES.

ophidiasis　OPHIDISM.

ophidic　[OPHI- + *d* + -IC]　Of or pertaining to snakes.

ophidiophobia　[Gk *ophidio(n)*, dim. of *ophis* a serpent, snake + -PHOBIA]　Pathologic fear of snakes.

ophidism　[OPHI- + *d* + -ISM]　Poisoning from snake venom. Also called *ophidiasis, ophitoxemia, ophiotoxemia.*

ophio-　[Gk *ophis* a serpent, snake]　A combining form meaning snake, snakelike. Also *ophi-.*

Ophiophagus hannah　A venomous snake of the Elapidae family; the king cobra.

ophiotoxemia　OPHIDISM.

ophiotoxin　[OPHIO- + TOXIN]　The poison found in snake venom.

ophitoxemia　OPHIDISM.

ophryitis　[Gk *ophry(s)* the eyebrow + -ITIS]　Dermatitis of the eyebrow region. Also called *ophrytis.*

ophryon　[Gk *ophry(s)* the brow, eyebrow + *(i)on*, diminishing suffix]　A craniometric point situated on the frontal bone at the midpoint of the minimum frontal diameter. Also called *supranasal point.*

Ophryoscolecidae　[Gk *ophry(s)* the brow, eyebrow + *o* + *skōlēx*, gen. *skōlēkos*, a worm + -IDAE]　A family of highly specialized parasitic ciliates found in the rumen of cattle and other ruminants. Some of the species (*Entodinium* and *Diplodinium*) can utilize bacteria as food. Some of the latter group possess cellulase and contain cellulytic bacteria, and can thereby aid their hosts in digesting cellulose. It is likely that many of these ciliates can properly be considered mutualists as well as commensal inhabitants of the host stomach, where they are often found in tremendous numbers and significant volume.

ophryosis　[Gk *ophry(s)* the eyebrow + -OSIS]　Spasm of the muscles of the face causing movement or displacement of the eyebrows.

ophryphtheiriasis　[Gk *ophry(s)* eyebrow + *phtheir* louse + -IASIS]　Infestation of the eyebrows and eyelashes by lice. See also *PTHIRUS PUBIS.*

ophrytic　Of or relating to the eyebrow; superciliary.

ophrytis　OPHRYITIS.

Ophthaine　A proprietary name for proparacaine hydrochloride.

ophthalm-　OPHTHALMO-.

ophthalmacrosis　MACROPHTHALMIA.

ophthalmagra　OPHTHALMALGIA.

ophthalmalgia　[OPHTHALM- + -ALGIA]　An acute pain in the eye. Also called *ophthalmagra.*

ophthalmatrophia　[OPHTHALM- + ATROPHIA]　PHTHISIS BULBI.

ophthalmecchymosis　[OPHTHALM- + ECCHYMOSIS]　Hemorrhage in the subconjunctival region.

ophthalmectomy　[OPHTHALM- + -ECTOMY]　The surgical enucleation of the eye.

ophthalmedema　[OPHTHALM- + EDEMA]　Swelling of the conjunctiva.

ophthalmencephalon　[OPHTHALM- + ENCEPHALON]　The visual pathway, including the retina, the optic nerve and tract, the lateral geniculate nucleus of the thalamus, and thalamocortical projections (optic radiations) to visual areas of the occipital lobe. A seldom used term.

ophthalmia　[OPHTHALM- + -IA]　Inflammation of the eye.

actinic ray ophthalmia　ACTINIC CONJUNCTIVITIS.

catarrhal ophthalmia　A viral form of conjunctivitis.

caterpillar ophthalmia　OPHTHALMIA NODOSA.

ophthalmia eczematosa　Keratoconjunctivitis associated with allergic skin disease.

Egyptian ophthalmia　TRACHOMA.

electric ophthalmia　ACTINIC CONJUNCTIVITIS.

flash ophthalmia　WELDERS' CONJUNCTIVITIS.

gonococcal ophthalmia of newborn　Purulent conjunctivitis due to *Neisseria gonorrhoeae.* The infection is derived from the mother's birth canal, and generally becomes evident about the third day of life. It may be unilateral or bilateral. Infant-to-infant infection may also occur in an infant nursery. Because the conjunctival infection can spread to other structures within the eye, the condition was at one time a major cause of blindness. Prophylactic treatment of the eyes at birth with drops (for example, one percent silver nitrate) has therefore often been routinely applied.

gonorrheal ophthalmia GONOCOCCAL CONJUNCTIVITIS.

granular ophthalmia Conjunctivitis causing surface follicles or papillae.

jequirity ophthalmia Severe inflammation of the eye and its deeper structures due to self-mutilation by placing the toxic seeds of jequirity, *Arbus precatorius,* in the conjunctival sac.

ophthalmia lenta BEHÇET SYNDROME.

metastatic ophthalmia Infection reaching the eye via the bloodstream.

migratory ophthalmia The supposed transmission of sympathetic ophthalmia via channels in the optic nerves, an erroneous concept.

mucous ophthalmia A conjunctivitis associated with a proteinaceous discharge.

ophthalmia neonatorum INFANTILE PURULENT CONJUNCTIVITIS.

neuroparalytic ophthalmia NEUROPARALYTIC KERATITIS.

ophthalmia nivialis SNOW BLINDNESS.

ophthalmia nodosa Toxic and mechanical irritation of the conjunctiva due to imbedded caterpillar hairs or vegetable fibers. Also called *caterpillar ophthalmia, caterpillar conjunctivitis, nodular conjunctivitis.*

phlyctenular ophthalmia Keratoconjunctivitis with focal elevated vascularized nodules. Also called *strumous ophthalmia.*

purulent ophthalmia Keratoconjunctivitis eliciting a leukocytic response.

scrofulous ophthalmia Keratoconjunctivitis occurring in conjunction with tuberculosis.

solar ophthalmia GLARE CONJUNCTIVITIS.

spring ophthalmia VERNAL KERATOCONJUNCTIVITIS.

strumous ophthalmia PHLYCTENULAR OPHTHALMIA.

sympathetic ophthalmia A severe post-traumatic uveitis due to autoimmunity to uveal pigment, affecting both eyes even if the original injury damaged only one eye. Also called *sympathetic uveitis.*

transferred ophthalmia Inflammation of the uninjured eye in sympathetic ophthalmia.

ultraviolet ray ophthalmia ACTINIC CONJUNCTIVITIS.

varicose ophthalmia Ophthalmia associated with a varicose condition of the conjunctival veins.

ophthalmiac [OPHTHALM- + *i* + -AC] A person suffering from ocular inflammation.

ophthalmiatric Pertaining to the medical treatment of ocular diseases.

ophthalmiatrics [OPHTHALM- + -IATRICS] The medical treatment of ocular diseases.

ophthalmic [OPHTHALM- + -IC] Pertaining to the eye.

ophthalmic acid A tripeptide first isolated from the eye. It is the analogue of glutathione in which the thiol group is replaced by a methyl group.

ophthalmitic Pertaining to inflammation of the eye.

ophthalmitis [OPHTHALM- + -ITIS] Inflammation of the eye. Adjective: ophthalmitic.

sympathetic ophthalmitis An inflammatory condition of the eye following a traumatic injury to the other eye. It is characterized by mononuclear cell infiltration and granuloma formation secondary to a postulated cell-mediated immunity to antigens normally sequestered in the eye which have been liberated after injury to the opposite eye.

ophthalmo- [Gk *ophthalmos* eye] A combining form denoting the eye. Also *ophthalm-.*

ophthalmoblennorrhea [OPHTHALMO- + BLENNORRHEA] A discharge from the eye.

ophthalmocarcinoma [OPHTHALMO- + CARCINOMA] Carcinoma of the eye.

ophthalmocele [OPHTHALMO- + -CELE¹] A rarely used term for EXOPHTHALMOS.

ophthalmocentesis [OPHTHALMO- + -CENTESIS] Surgical drainage of the eye.

ophthalmocopia [OPHTHALMO- + Gk *kop(os)* weariness + -IA] ASTHENOPIA.

ophthalmodiaphanoscope A device using transillumination to view the ocular fundus.

ophthalmodiastimeter A device to measure the separation of the visual axes at the distance eyeglasses are positioned.

ophthalmodonesis [OPHTHALMO- + Gk *donēsis* a trembling] Flickering or trembling of the eyes and eyelids.

ophthalmodynamometer A device that measures the intraocular blood pressure by measuring the external pressure required to stop the circulation of blood.

ophthalmodynamometry [OPHTHALMO- + Gk *dynam(is)* + *o* + -METRY] A technique of measuring the blood pressure in the ophthalmic artery by applying an ophthalmodynamometer to the globe of the eye.

ophthalmodynia [OPHALM- + -ODYNIA] Ocular pain.

ophthalmoeikonometer A device that measures the difference in size between the two ocular images.

ophthalmogram [OPHTHALMO- + -GRAM] A recording of eye movements during reading.

ophthalmograph [OPHTHALMO- + -GRAPH] A device to record eye movements during reading.

ophthalmography [OPHTHALMO- + -GRAPHY] The recording of eye movements during reading.

ophthalmogyric OCULOGYRIC.

ophthalmoiconometry [OPHTHALMO- + Gk *eikōn* figure, image + *o* + -METRY] Measurement of differences in image size perceived by the two eyes.

ophthalmoleukoscope A device for evaluating color vision by mixing spectral colors to produce white light.

ophthalmolith [OPHTHALMO- + Gk *lith(os)* a stone] A concretion in the lacrimal apparatus.

ophthalmologic Pertaining to ophthalmology.

ophthalmologist [OPHTHALMO- + -LOGIST] A physician specializing in the care and treatment of the eye; a specialist in ophthalmology. Also called *oculist.*

ophthalmology [OPHTHALMO- + -LOGY] The medical and surgical specialty of eye care, including treatment of diseases of the eye and the correction of refractive error. Adjective: ophthalmologic, ophthalmological.

ophthalmolyma [OPHTHALMO- + Gk *lymē* destruction] Total loss of an eye.

ophthalmomacrosis [OPHTHALMO- + MACRO- + -SIS] A pathologic increase in size of the eye.

ophthalmomalacia Infarction or necrosis of the eye. Also called *ophthalmophthisis.*

ophthalmometer KERATOMETER.

ophthalmometroscope An ophthalmoscope used to determine the refractive error of the eye.

ophthalmometry [OPHTHALMO- + -METRY] KERATOMETRY.

ophthalmomycosis [OPHTHALMO- + MYCOSIS] A fungal infection of the eye or adnexa.

ophthalmomyiasis [OPHTHALMO- + MYIASIS] OCULAR MYIASIS.

ophthalmomyitis OPHTHALMOMYOSITIS.

ophthalmomyositis [OPHTHALMO- + MYOSITIS] Inflammation of the extraocular muscles. Also called *ophthalmomyitis.*

ophthalmomyotomy [OPHTHALMO- + MYOTOMY] A surgical severing of an extraocular muscle.

ophthalmoneuritis [OPHTHALMO- + NEURITIS] OPTIC NEURITIS.

ophthalmoneuromyelitis NEUROMYELITIS OPTICA.

ophthalmoparalysis OPHTHALMOPLEGIA.

ophthalmopathy [OPHTHALMO- + -PATHY] Any disorder of the eye or its adnexa.

    endocrine ophthalmopathy EXOPHTHALMIC OPHTHALMOPLEGIA.

    external ophthalmopathy Any disorder of the surface of the eye or the eyelids.

    hyperthyroid ophthalmopathy EXOPTHALMIC OPHTHALMOPLEGIA.

    infiltrative ophthalmopathy EXOPHTHALMIC OPHTHALMOPLEGIA.

    internal ophthalmopathy Any disorder of the structures within the eye.

    thyrotoxic ophthalmopathy EXOPHTHALMIC OPHTHALMOPLEGIA.

ophthalmophacometer A device for measuring the curvatures of the lens and cornea and the distances separating these surfaces.

ophthalmophasmatoscopy A device for evaluating the spectral colors of the interior of the eye.

ophthalmophlebotomy [OPHTHALMO- + PHLEBOTOMY] Incision into the conjunctiva with the intent of relieving vascular stasis; drainage of venous blood from the eye. Also called *phlebophthalmotomy.*

ophthalmophthisis OPHTHALMOMALACIA.

ophthalmoplasty A plastic operation on the eye or its adnexa.

ophthalmoplegia [OPHTHALMO- + -PLEGIA] Paralysis of ocular muscles. Also called *ophthalmoparalysis.* Adjective: ophthalmoplegic.

    anterior internuclear ophthalmoplegia ATAXIC NYSTAGMUS.

    basal ophthalmoplegia Ophthalmoplegia due to any pathologic process, such as meningitis or arachnoiditis, involving the meninges at the base of the brain.

    congenital ophthalmoplegia The paralysis of one or more motor nerves of the eye from birth.

    diabetic ophthalmoplegia Ocular palsy associated with diabetes mellitus, particularly, involvement of the third cranial nerve by diabetic neuropathy with resulting paresis of extraocular muscle.

    exophthalmic ophthalmoplegia Swelling of the external ocular muscles and orbital contents in Graves disease, usually presenting with diplopia (often due initially to weakness of one superior rectus muscle) and with exophthalmos, either unilateral or bilateral. The latter may become very severe. Also called *ophthalmic Graves disease, infiltrative ophthalmopathy, thyrotoxic ophthalmopathy, thyrotoxic ophthalmoplegia, hyperthyroid ophthalmopathy, hyperthyroid ophthalmoplegia, endocrine ophthalmopathy.*

    ophthalmoplegia externa EXTERNAL OPHTHALMOPLEGIA.

    external ophthalmoplegia Paralysis of the extraocular muscles. Also called *ophthalmoplegia externa, Ballet's disease.*

    fascicular ophthalmoplegia Internuclear ophthalmoplegia due to a lesion of the medial longitudinal bundle.

    hyperthyroid ophthalmoplegia EXOPHTHALMIC OPHTHALMOPLEGIA.

    hysterical ophthalmoplegia Strabismus or diplopia or both, resembling oculomotor of abducens paralysis, and resulting from a psychologic cause.

    infectious ophthalmoplegia Ophthalmoplegia due to any infective process such as encephalitis.

    ophthalmoplegia interna INTERNAL OPHTHALMOPLEGIA.

    internal ophthalmoplegia Ophthalmoplegia of the iris or ciliary body. Also called *ophthalmoplegia interna.*

    internuclear ophthalmoplegia Ophthalmoplegia due to a lesion of any of the nerve fiber tracts, such as the medial longitudinal bundle, which connect the nuclei of the third, fourth, and sixth cranial nerves. Also called *internuclear paralysis.*

    nuclear ophthalmoplegia Ophthalmoplegia due to a lesion or lesions of one or more of the nuclei of the third, fourth, and sixth cranial nerves.

    orbital ophthalmoplegia Paralysis of the extraocular muscles caused by a condition within the orbit.

    painful ophthalmoplegia 1 SUPERIOR ORBITAL FISSURE SYNDROME. 2 TOLOSA-HUNT SYNDROME.

    Parinaud's ophthalmoplegia PARINAUD SYNDROME.

    ophthalmoplegia partialis An incomplete paralysis of function of the extraocular muscles.

    posterior internuclear ophthalmoplegia Paralysis of lateral movement of one eye with normal adduction of the other due to a lesion immediately rostral to the sixth nerve nucleus on the affected side.

    ophthalmoplegia progressiva Progressive paralysis of the ocular musculature.

    progressive ophthalmoplegia Progressive paralysis of the external ocular muscles causing bilateral ptosis and ultimately inability to move the eyes in any direction. Some cases may be due to nuclear degeneration, but most result from a progressive myopathy of the external ocular muscles.

    relapsing ophthalmoplegia OPHTHALMOPLEGIC MIGRAINE.

    Sauvineau's ophthalmoplegia Paralysis of the medial rectus of one eye and overaction of the lateral rectus of the other eye, as may occur when the paretic eye is used for fixation.

    sensorimotor ophthalmoplegia A seldom used term for ORBITAL APEX SYNDROME.

    thyrotoxic ophthalmoplegia EXOPHTHALMIC OPHTHALMOPLEGIA.

    ophthalmoplegia totalis A complete paralysis of all the ocular musculature, both internal and external.

ophthalmoplegic Pertaining to ophthalmoplegia.

ophthalmoptosis EXOPHTHALMOS.

ophthalmoreaction CALMETTE'S REACTION.

    Calmette's ophthalmoreaction CALMETTE'S REACTION.

ophthalmorrhagia [OPHTHALMO- + -RRHAGIA] Hemorrhage from the eye.

ophthalmorrhea [OPHTHALMO- + -RRHEA] An ocular discharge.

ophthalmorrhexis [OPHTHALMO- + -RRHEXIS] Rupture of the eyeball.

ophthalmoscope [OPHTHALMO- + -SCOPE] A device for viewing the fundus of the eye. Also called *funduscope* (imprecise).

    binocular ophthalmoscope A device that permits use of both eyes to examine the ocular fundus.

    direct ophthalmoscope An ophthalmoscope that causes the retinas of subject and observer to be directly conjugate with each other without an intervening real image.

    ghost ophthalmoscope A device for observing the fundus of the eye and simultaneously providing a view for another person by means of a partially transmitting mirror.

    indirect ophthalmoscope An ophthalmoscope that forms an inverted real image between the fundus and the observer.

    luminous ophthalmoscope A self-lighted ophthalmoscope.

reflecting ophthalmoscope An ophthalmoscope using the reflection of an external light as its source of illumination.

ophthalmoscopic Pertaining to ophthalmoscopy.

ophthalmoscopy [OPHTHALMO- + -SCOPY] The clinical examination of the interior of the eye by means of an ophthalmoscope. Also called *funduscopy* (imprecise), *fundoscopy* (imprecise). Adjective: opthalmoscopic.

direct ophthalmoscopy Observation of the retina with an ophthalmoscope that images the retina directly upon the observer's retina, without the interposition of an inverted aerial real image.

indirect ophthalmoscopy Observation of the retina with an ophthalmoscope that projects an inverted real image between the patient's retina and the observer.

medical ophthalmoscopy The performance of an ophthalmoscopic examination of the retina as part of a physician's examination for diagnostic purposes.

metric ophthalmoscopy Use of the direct ophthalmoscope to determine the approximate refractive error of the eye.

ophthalmospintherism [OPHTHALMO- + Gk *spinthēr* a spark + -ISM] The occurrence of unformed visual hallucinations like sparks or flashes of light. An outmoded term.

ophthalmostasis [OPHTHALMO- + -STASIS] The relative position of the eye in the orbit.

ophthalmostat EXOPHTHALMOMETER.

ophthalmostatometer EXOPHTHALMOMETER.

ophthalmosteresis [OPHTHALMO- + Gk *sterēsis* (from *ster(ein)* to deprive + *-ēsis* -ESIS) deprivation, loss] Absence or loss of one or both eyes.

ophthalmosynchysis [OPHTHALMO- + SYNCHYSIS] Liquefaction of the interior of the eye.

ophthalmothermometer [OPHTHALMO- + THERMOMETER] A device to determine the temperature of the eye or its parts.

ophthalmotomy [OPHTHALMO- + -TOMY] A surgical incision into the eye.

ophthalmotonometer A device to measure intraocular pressure.

ophthalmotonometry The measurement of intraocular pressure.

ophthalmotoxin [OPHTHALMO- + TOXIN] Any toxin exerting a deleterious effect upon the eye.

ophthalmotrope [OPHTHALMO- + -TROPE] A model of the eye and attached muscles for the demonstration of ocular movements resulting from contraction of the extraocular muscles.

ophthalmotropometer [OPHTHALMO- + *trop(e)-* + *o* + -METER] A device for measuring the amount of strabismus.

ophthalmovascular Concerning the blood vessels of the eye.

ophthalmoxerosis [OPHTHALMO- + XEROSIS] XEROPHTHALMIA.

ophthalmoxyster [OPHTHALMO- + XYSTER] A surgical instrument intended for obtaining conjunctival scrapings.

ophthalmula [OPHTHALM- + Gk *oulē* a scar] An ocular scar.

-opia [Gk *ōps*, gen. *ōpos*, eye + -IA] A combining form meaning having vision (of a specified kind). Also *-opsia*.

opian NOSCAPINE.

opianic acid 2,3-Dimethoxy-6-formylbenzoic acid. It is obtained by chemical degradation of alkaloids.

opianine NOSCAPINE.

opiate A medicinal agent containing opium or an alkaloid obtained from opium.

opilação [Portuguese, *oppilation*. See OPPILATION.] CHAGAS DISEASE.

opinion / second opinion A judgment independently arrived at by a practitioner not previously consulted on a case as to the correctness of a diagnosis or, especially, as to the advisability of a proposed medical or surgical treatment.

opiophagism OPIOPHAGY.

opiophagy [Gk *opio(n)* opium, dim. of *opos* juice from trees or plants, gum + -PHAGY] The oral ingestion of opiates. Also called *opiophagism*.

Opisocrostis A genus of rodent fleas, some of which transmit sylvatic plague.

opisth- OPISTHO-.

opisthe [Gk *opisthe* to the rear, backward] The posterior daughter of transverse division of certain protozoans, such as gregarines. Compare PROTER.

opisthenar The dorsum of the hand.

opisthencephalon A rarely used term for CEREBELLUM.

opisthiobasial Pertaining to the opisthion and the basion, especially the line or distance between them as used in craniometry.

opisthion [Gk *opisthion*, neut. sing. of *opisthios* (from *opisthe* (adverb) behind) pertaining to the back or hinder parts] A point on the posterior margin of the foramen magnum in the midline.

opisthionasial Pertaining to the opisthion and the nasion, especially the distance between them as measured in craniometry.

opistho- [Gk *opisthe* (*opisthen* before vowel) to the rear, backward] A combining form meaning backward, posterior, dorsal. Also *opisth-*.

opisthocheilia [OPISTHO- + CHEIL- + -IA] The condition of having lips which are thin, inverted, less prominent than normal, or in extreme cases, actually inverted.

opisthocoelous [OPISTHO- + COEL- + -OUS] Designating or characterized by a vertebral centrum in which the anterior face is convex and the posterior face is concave, as in some anurans.

opisthocranion [Late Gk *opisthokranion* (from Gk *opisth(e)* (adverb) behind + *o* + *kranion* the skull)] A craniometric point situated on the occipital bone at its most posterior point in the midline when the skull is orientated in the Frankfort horizontal plane. Also called *occipital point*.

opisthogenia [OPISTHO- + Gk *gen(ys)* the chin + -IA] Recession of the chin as may be seen when the lower jaw fails to develop normally.

opisthoglyphic [OPISTHO- + Gk *glyph(ein)* to carve + -IC] Having two to three pairs of grooved poison fangs at the rear of the upper jaw: used of snakes. The fangs are held in the wound after striking to permit the infusion of venom. Because this mechanism for delivering venom is relatively inefficient, opisthoglyphic snakes are generally less dangerous than other venomous snakes. Compare SOLENOGLYPHIC, PROTEROGLYPHIC.

opisthognathism [OPISTHO- + GNATH- + -ISM] The condition of having receding jaws.

opisthomastigote [OPISTHO- + MASTIGOTE] A stage of development of certain trypanosomatid flagellates characterized by the flagellum arising from the kinetoplast located behind the nucleus and emerging from the anterior end, with no undulating membrane. This stage is limited to members of the genus *Herpetomonas*.

opisthoporeia [OPISTHO- + Gk *poreia* a walking, going] RETROPULSION.

opisthorchiasis Infection with flukes of the genus *Opisthorchis*. *O. viverrini* is a normal parasite of dogs and cats, and *O. felineus* of dogs, cats, and pigs. Human infection is common in northern Thailand, eastern Europe, and the USSR. Eggs are passed in feces by the definitive host into water. Following development in intermediate snail hosts, metacercariae encyst in the flesh of fish which if eaten raw infects man. They are free in the small intestine and travel up the biliary system, where they become adult flukes. Biliary obstruction, abscess formation, and adenocarcinoma of the biliary system result. Treatment is with praziquantel. Also called *opisthorchosis*.

opisthorchid [OPISTH- + *orch(i)*- + -ID¹] **1** Of or belonging to the genus *Opisthorchis* or the family Opisthorchiidae. **2** A member of the genus *Opisthorchis* or the family Opisthorchiidae.

Opisthorchiidae [OPISTH- + ORCHI- + -IDAE] A family of digenetic trematodes in the superfamily Opisthorchioidea infecting the liver and bile ducts of fish-eating mammals, birds, and fish.

Opisthorchis [OPISTH- + Gk *orchis* a testicle] A genus of digenetic flukes of the family Opisthorchiidae, species of which are parasitic in the livers of fish-eating carnivores, including cats, dogs, foxes, pigs, and man. The eggs hatch in snails, the first intermediate hosts, and metacercariae encyst in the muscles and subcutaneous tissues of fresh-water fish, the second intermediate hosts. Carnivorous mammals, the definitive hosts, acquire infection when they ingest infected, uncooked fish. The young flukes excyst in the intestine and migrate to the liver, where they mature.

Opisthorchis felineus *OPISTHORCHIS TENUICOLLIS*.

Opisthorchis sinensis *CLONORCHIS SINENSIS*.

Opisthorchis tenuicollis A species of fluke that is parasitic in the gallbladder and bile ducts of cats, dogs, pigs, and humans in India, Japan, southeast Asia, Siberia, and Europe; the cat liver fluke. The eggs are ingested by snails of the genus *Bithynia*, which release cercariae that encyst in fish. Human infection is acquired by eating raw or undercooked fish. Infection without clinical disease is common, but biliary cirrhosis, chronic pancreatitis, and cholangitis have been reported. Also called *Opisthorchis felineus, Distoma felineum* (obsolete).

Opisthorchis viverrini A species common in humans in Thailand and closely related to *O. tenuicollis*. It infects various fish-eating animals as well as humans.

opisthorchosis OPISTHORCHIASIS.

opisthotic Located behind the ear.

opisthotonoid Resembling opisthotonos.

opisthotonos [OPISTHO- + Gk *tonos* tension, stretching, tightening] Spasmodic contraction of the muscles of the neck and back with arching of the body. When severe, the subject may rest only on his head and heels. This may occur in tetanus, in some brainstem lesions, or in far-advanced meningitis in infants and children. Also *opisthotonus*. Compare EMPROSTHOTONOS. Adjective: opisthotonic.

opisthotonos fetalis A hyperextended position of the fetus during labor in which the head is bent backward and the back is arched.

opisthotonus OPISTHOTONOS.

Opitz [John Marius *Opitz*, German-born U.S. pediatrician, born 1935] Smith-Lemli-Opitz syndrome. See under SYNDROME.

opium [L (from Gk *opion* poppy juice, opium, from *opos* juice, esp. of trees or plants; milky juice, resin, gum), the dried juice of the poppy] A gummy exudate of the poppy *Papaver album* or *P. somniferum*. It yields various alkaloids, of which morphine is the most important and abundant. Other significant alkaloids isolated are codeine, narcotine, thebaine, narceine, and papaverine. Opium is primarily a narcotic, but preparations have been used as aphrodisiacs, as diaphoretics, and as sedatives. Also called *gum opium*.

denarcotized opium Opium powder that has been extracted with pure petroleum benzene in order to remove certain constituents that cause nausea. Also called *opium deodoratum, deodorized opium*.

opium deodoratum DENARCOTIZED OPIUM.

deodorized opium DENARCOTIZED OPIUM.

granulated opium Opium pulverized to a coarse powder

form. Also called *opium granulatum*.

opium granulatum GRANULATED OPIUM.

lettuce opium LACTUCARIUM.

powdered opium Opium that has been dried and reduced to a fine powder at a temperature not in excess of 70°C. This product contains not less than 10% nor more that 10.5% anhydrous morphine, and may be used in the composition of products with any of the dilutants of powdered extracts, except for starch. Also called *opium pulveratum*.

opium pulveratum POWDERED OPIUM.

opobalsamum TOLU BALSAM.

opocephalus [Gk *ōps*, gen. *ōpos*, eye, face + -CEPHALUS] An embryo, fetus, or newborn infant with various serious malformations of the head including agenesis of mouth and nose, a rudimentary jaw, fused ears, and a single eye.

opodidymus [Gk *ōps*, gen. *ōpos*, eye, face + *didymos* double, a twin] Equal conjoined twins with a single body, a normal complement of limbs, and two heads united in the neck and occipital regions but more or less separate in the facial regions. Also called *opodymus*.

opodymus OPODIDYMUS.

opotherapy [Gk *opo(s)* vegetable juice, milky juice from a plant, sap + THERAPY] Treatment with juices, especially extracts of endocrine glands of animals.

Oppenheim [Hermann *Oppenheim*, German neurologist, 1858–1919] **1** See under GAIT. **2** Oppenheim's reflex. See under SIGN. **3** Erb-Oppenheim-Goldflam syndrome. See under MYASTHENIA GRAVIS. **4** Minor-Oppenheim syndrome. See under MINOR'S DISEASE. **5** Oppenheim syndrome, Oppenheim's amyotonia, Oppenheim's disease. See under MYOTONIA CONGENITA. **6** Ziehen-Oppenheim disease. See under DYSTONIA MUSCULORUM DEFORMANS.

Oppenheim [Maurice Oppenheim, U.S. dermatologist, 1876–1949] Urbach-Oppenheim disease. See under NECROBIOSIS LIPOIDICA.

oppilation [L *oppilatio* (from *oppilatus*, past part. of *oppilare* to stop up, from *op-* against + *pilare* to thrust down, from *pila* a mortar) an obstruction] Obstruction to secretion or to flow; especially, constipation. A rarely used term.

oppilative [L *oppilat(us)*, past part. of *oppilare* to stop up + -IVE. See OPPILATION.] Obstructive to secretion or flow; especially, constipating. A rarely used term.

opplotentes [Gk *ōps*, gen. *ōpos*, the eye + *plōtos* sailing, floating, swimming] MUSCAE VOLITANTES.

opponens [L, pres. part. of *opponere* to place against] Opposing or placing against: in anatomy, designating those muscles of the thumb and little finger that move these digits so as to touch each other or other digits.

opportunist A normally harmless organism that becomes pathogenic in a host with reduced resistance.

opportunistic [L *opportun(us)* (from *op-* against + *portus* a port, place of refuge) + -IST + -IC] **1** Denoting a microorganism which produces disease only in a host whose immunological status has been compromised by other infections, disease processes, or drugs. In a host with normal immune function, the organism may be present but does not cause disease. Thus *Pneumocystis carinii*, which causes pneumonitis almost exclusively in immunocompromised or debilitated persons, although antibody to the organism is present in up to two-thirds of the general population, is called opportunistic. **2** Denoting a disease or infection produced by an opportunistic pathogen. ⟨"such opportunistic infections as disseminated mycobacteria and herpes simplex, central-nervous-system toxoplasmosis, and cryptococcal meningitis." — *Medical World News*, 23 Nov. 1981, 57.⟩

oppositionism [*opposition* + -ISM] Involuntary contraction of the antagonists of those muscles participating in a passive movement, lasting for several moments before disappearing abruptly. This phenomenon may be seen in various extrapyramidal disorders including torsion dystonia but can also be an hysterical phenomenon. A seldom used term.

-opsia -OPIA.

opsialgia [Gk *ōps* the eye, face + *i* + -ALGIA] FACIAL NEURALGIA.

opsigenes [Gk *opsigonos* (from *opse* late + *genesthai* to be born) late-born] Late born: used especially of third molar teeth.

opsin The protein that combines with retinal to form a visual pigment.

opsinogen An antigenic substance which can induce the production of opsonin. Also called *opsonogen, opsogen*.

opsinogenous Capable of producing opsonin.

opsiometer OPTOMETER.

-opsis [Gk *opsis* sight, vision, appearance] A combining form denoting an organism or part likened to or resembling (something specified).

opsiuria [Aeolian Gk *opsi* (Hellenic Gk *opse*) late + -URIA] A condition characterized by the excretion of more urine in the fasting state than in the fed state.

opsoclonia OPSOCLONUS.

opsoclonus [Gk *ōps* the eye + *o* + CLONUS] A sudden, shocklike, clonic movement of the eyes. Such movements are sometimes irregularly repetitive. They may occur as a manifestation of myoclonic encephalopathy in childhood. Also called *opsoclonia*.

opsogen OPSINOGEN.

opsomania [Gk *opso(n)* rich or dainty food + -MANIA] A great desire for a specific food, especially sweets. A seldom used term.

opsone OPSONIN.

opsonic Relating to or having the action of an opsonin; inducing opsonization.

opsoniferous Containing opsonin.

opsonification OPSONIZATION.

opsonify OPSONIZE.

opsonin [Gk *opson* (akin to *epsein* to boil, seethe, and to *opsōnion* provisions and *opsōnein* to buy fish or victuals) boiled meat, flesh, meat, sauce, seasoning + -IN] Any of various substances capable of binding to the surfaces of bacteria or other cells to make them more susceptible to phagocytosis. Opsonins occur in blood plasma and may be antibodies, fragments of complement components, or enzymes such as lysozyme. Also called *opsone*.

immune opsonin OPSONIZING ANTIBODY.

normal opsonin The opsonin normally present in blood. It is more easily denatured by heat than is the specific opsonin that appears in response to bacterial infection. Also called *thermolabile opsonin*.

thermolabile opsonin NORMAL OPSONIN.

opsonization The modification of bacteria and other cells, most usually by coating them with antibody and/or complement, to make them more susceptible to phagocytosis. Also called *opsonification*.

opsonize [*opson(in)* + -IZE. See OPSONIN.] To modify (bacteria and other cells) to make them more susceptible to phagocytosis. Also *opsonify*.

opsonocytophagic Relating to phagocytosis of bacteria coated with opsonin.

opsonogen OPSINOGEN.

opsonometry 1 A measurement of opsonic activity. 2 The measurement of the level of opsonins that are present in a fluid.

opsonophilic Pertaining to or exhibiting opsonophilia.

opsonophoric Conveying opsonin. An outmoded term.

opsonotherapy Therapeutic treatment of infection by inducing an increase of opsonins in the blood, as by the use of a bacterial vaccine.

-opsy -OPIA.

opt- OPTO-.

optesthesia [OPT- + ESTHESIA] Visual sensibility. A seldom used term.

optic [Gk *optikos* pertaining to the eye or to vision] Of or relating to the eye.

optical [OPTIC + -AL] Of or relating to vision or to means of enhancing vision, especially lenses.

optician [French *opticien* (from *optique* relating to sight, from Gk *optika* optics + French *-ien* English *-ian*) a maker of and dealer in optical items. See OPTICS.] One who practices opticianry; one who fills ophthalmic prescriptions for spectacles and dispenses them. Also called *dispensing optician (British and South African usage)*. • See note at OPTOMETRIST.

dispensing optician The British and South African term for OPTICIAN. • See note at OPTOMETRIST.

ophthalmic optician In Great Britain, an optician who also tests vision and prescribes corrective lenses. • See note at OPTOMETRIST.

opticianry The science or practice of preparing ophthalmic prescriptions, such as spectacle lenses and contact lenses, and fitting them.

optico- OPTO-.

Wernicke subcortical opticoagnosia PURE WORD BLINDNESS.

opticochiasmatic Pertaining to the crossing of optic nerve fibers at the optic chiasm. Also called *opticochiasmic* (seldom used), *optochiasmic* (seldom used).

opticochiasmic A seldom used term for OPTICOCHIASMATIC.

opticociliary Pertaining to or affecting the optic and ciliary nerves.

opticocinerea [OPTICO- + L *cinerea*, fem. sing. of *cinereus* ashy] The gray matter in or in relation to the optic tract.

opticoele [OPT- + *i* + -COELE] The space within the optic vesicle.

opticofacial Relating to or affecting the optic and facial nerves.

opticokinetic [OPTICO- + KINETIC] Pertaining to eye movements mediated through the cerebral cortex as part of the following reflex.

opticonasion [OPTICO- + NASION] A cephalometric measure of the linear distance from the posterior margin of the optic canal to the nasion.

opticopupillary Relating to or affecting the optic nerve and the pupil.

optics [Gk *optika* (neut. pl. of *optikos* optical, from *optomai*, root of *oran* to see, look; akin to *ōps* the eye) optics] The science that deals with light, including its origin, propagation, and use.

electron optics The physical principles that influence the passage of an electron beam through an electron microscope and the formation of an image on a fluorescent screen or photographic plate.

physiological optics The science of visual perception.

schlieren optics An optical technique in which density gradients in a fluid flow are determined by the diffraction pattern cast in the optical system. Light passes, in sequence, through a slit, the first lens, the flow model, and the second lens, which focuses it on a knife edge from which the diffraction pattern passes to a screen or photographic film.

opticus [Gk *optikos* (from *opt(izesthai)*, also *opt(azesthai)* to be seen + *-ikos* -IC) pertaining to sight] NERVUS OPTICUS.

optimeter   OPTOMETER.

optimism   A cheerful habit of mind characterized by an inclination to believe that the uncertainties of the present will be resolved favorably.

oral optimism   A character trait associated with oral satisfaction in infancy and marked by self-assurance and a positive attitude toward taking and receiving.

therapeutic optimism   An inclination to believe that a particular method of treatment will be successful. Compare THERAPEUTIC PESSIMISM.

optimization   [L *optim(us)* (superl. of *bonus* good) best + *-iz(e)* + -ATION]   **1** The selection of principles or components during the design of a system to maximize or minimize some performance index.   **2** The adjustment of parameters during the operation of a system to obtain the best operating conditions.

optimum   The best set of conditions for a particular activity or function, as for obtaining the best or most reliable results.

optist   OPTOMETRIST.

opto-   [Gk *optos* seen or *optikos* (from *ōps*, genitive *ōpos*, eye) pertaining to the eye]   A combining form meaning sight, vision, optical. Also *opt-, optico-*.

optoacoustic   Perceived by or relating to both vision and hearing.

optoblast   A retinal ganglion cell, with a large cell body suggestive of a primitive or blast cell.

optochiasmic   A seldom used term for OPTICOCHIASMATIC.

Optochin   A proprietary name for ethyl hydrocuprein chloride.

optogram   [OPTO- + -GRAM]   The retinal image produced by a visual stimulus.

optokinetic   [OPTO- + KINETIC]   Pertaining to movement of the eye.

optomeninx   RETINA.

optometer   [OPTO- + -METER]   A device for measurement of the refractive error of the eye. Also called *opsiometer, optimeter*.

coincidence optometer   A device for measurement of refractive error by means of aligning an image projected upon the patient's retina.

hair optometer   A device to measure the near point of accommodation.

skiascope optometer   A device to measure refractive error by means of retinoscopy.

optometrist   [*optometr(y)* + -IST]   One who practices optometry; a practitioner skilled in the measurement of visual defect and in the prescription and fitting of corrective lenses. Also called *optist*.   ● The term is used in the U.S., Australia, New Zealand, and India. In the United Kingdom and South Africa, the equivalent term is *optician* (also sometimes used in New Zealand). In Britain, *optician* is often qualified by *ophthalmic* if used in the sense described above, and by *dispensing* if used in the sense of one who fills prescriptions for spectacles. In the U.S., such a person is simply called an optician.

optometry   [OPTO- + -METRY]   **1** The practice of nonmedical eye care, dealing primarily with the testing of vision for refractive error and with the prescription and fitting of corrective lenses.   **2** The measurement of refractive error by means of an optometer.   ● *Optometry* (def. 1) is used throughout the English-speaking world, in spite of the variety of terms applying to the sense of optometrist. See the note at OPTOMETRIST.

optomyometer   A device for measuring eye muscle balance and vergence.

optophone   [OPTO- + Gk *phōnē* sound, voice]   An assistive device for the blind which converts variations in light intensity to variations in sound.

optotype   [OPTO- + TYPE]   TEST TYPE.

OR   operating room.

-or   [L, a suffix denoting an agent, doer, performer]   A suffix denoting a person or thing performing an action.

ora¹   [L, edge, border]   Margin; edge.

ora serrata retinae   [NA]   The anterior crenated margin of the pars optica retinae that marks the junction between the posterior periphery of the ciliary body and the choroid and the site where the sensory part of the retina is abruptly reduced to two layers of epithelial cells. The cell layers continue anteriorly as the pars ciliaris retinae. The serrated appearance is produced by dentate processes extending from the retina along grooves in the orbiculus ciliaris.

ora²   Plural of OS¹.

Orabilex   A proprietary name for buniodyl.

Oracon   An oral contraceptive agent containing dimethisterone and ethinyl estradiol. A proprietary name.

orad   Toward the mouth.

orae   Plural of ORA¹.

oral   [L *os*, gen. *oris*, mouth + -AL]   **1** Of, for, or with the mouth. Also called *stomatic, stomal*.   **2** Pertaining to the developmental phase in infancy during which the locus of satisfaction of the subject's drives is the mouth.

orale   [L *os*, gen. *oris*, mouth + *-ale*, neut. sing. of *-alis* -AL]   In craniometry, the midpoint of a line drawn tangential to the posterior margins of the sockets of the upper central incisor teeth.

orality   The oral components of psychic development, including signs of their persistence into adult life. See also PSYCHOSEXUAL DEVELOPMENT.

oralogy   A rarely used term for STOMATOLOGY.

Oram   [Samuel *Oram*, English cardiologist, born 1913]   Holt-Oram syndrome. See under SYNDROME.

orange   [L *aurentium* orange tree; or from Middle French *orange, orenge* orange, from Old Provençale *(n)auranja* (with loss of *n* due to confusion with article *une*) orange, from Arabic *nāranj* orange, from Persian *nārang* orange, from Sanskrit *nāranga* orange tree, of Dravidian origin]   An evergreen tree of the genus *Citrus. C. aurantium*, the Seville or bitter orange, is a source of fruit, fruit juice, bitter orange peel, orange oil, orange flower oil, and orange flower water. *C. sinensis*, the sweet orange, is valued for its fruit and fruit juice.

orange II   An orange acid dye of the monoazo group that is sometimes used as a pH indicator, turning from yellow at a pH of 11.0 to red at 13.0. It is used occasionally to stain sections of plant or animal tissue. Also called *gold orange*.

orange III   METHYL ORANGE.

orange G   An acid azo dye often used as a cytoplasmic counterstain in histologic preparations, particularly in Mallory's triple stain. It is also used in the Papanicolaou stain for cytology preparations. Also called *wool orange, novaurantia*.

gold orange   ORANGE II.

wool orange   ORANGE G.

Oranixon   A proprietary name for mephenesin.

orb   [French *orbe* (from L *orb(is)* a ring, disk, circle, socket of the eye, the eye) orbit]   **1** A sphere.   **2** An outmoded term for BULBUS OCULI.

Orbeli   [Leon Abgarovich *Orbeli*, Russian physiologist, 1882–1958]   Orbeli phenomenon. See under EFFECT.

orbicular   Circular; spherical. Also *orbicularis*.

orbiculare   An outmoded term for PROCESSUS LENTICULARIS INCUDIS.

orbicularis   **1** ORBICULAR.   **2** MUSCULUS ORBICULARIS.

orbicularis oris   MUSCULUS ORBICULARIS ORIS.

orbiculi   Plural of ORBICULUS.

orbiculus [L (dim. of *orbis* a ring, disk, coil, wheel), a small disk] A small, disk-shaped structure.

orbiculus ciliaris [NA] The smooth, annular posterior two thirds of the internal aspect of the ciliary body. It is continuous anteriorly with the corona ciliaris and ends posteriorly at the ora serrata. The dentate processes of the ora serrata extend along it to meet the striae of the ciliary zonule, producing meridional grooves in it. Also called *ciliary disk, annulus ciliaris* (outmoded), *pars plana corporis ciliaris* (outmoded), *ciliary ring.*

orbit [L *orbit(a)*. See ORBITA.] ORBITA.

orbita [L (from *orbis* a ring, disk, coil, wheel), the track of a wheel, path, course] (*plural* orbitae) [NA] The pyramidal bony cavity in the skull that contains the eyeball and its accessory organs and comprises a roof, a floor, medial and lateral walls, and the orbital opening which forms the base anteriorly. The apex is directed posteromedially and leads into the middle cranial fossa. Also called *orbit, orbital cavity, eye socket, concha of eye* (outmoded), *arcula* (outmoded).

orbitae Plural of ORBITA.

orbital 1 Pertaining to the orbit or its contents. 2 Denoting an electron confined to its orbit in an atom, as distinguished from a free electron.

delocalized orbital An electronic orbital that is spread over several atoms and is formed by combination of several atomic orbitals.

orbitale [Med L *orbita* (from L *orbita* path of a wheel, path, from *orbis* a wheel, discus) orbit + *-ale*, neut. sing. of *-alis* -AL] A craniometric point situated at the lowest point on the orbital margin.

orbitalis Referring to one or both orbits.

orbitonasal Pertaining to the orbit and the nose. Also *naso-orbital.*

orbitonometer A device for measuring the ease of displacement of the eye into the orbital tissue, of value in the study of exophthalmos.

orbitonometry [ORBIT + *o* + -METRY] Measurement of the ease of displacement of the eye into the orbital tissue. This is of value in the study of exophthalmos.

orbitopagus [English orbit + *o* + Gk *pagos* anything fixed or hardened] Unequal conjoined twins in which the parasitic member, usually very poorly formed, is attached in the orbital region of the host. Also called *teratoma orbitae.*

orbitosphenoid Pertaining to the orbit and the sphenoid bone.

orbitostat [*orbit(al)* + *o* + -STAT] A craniometric instrument used for measuring the orbital axis.

orbitotemporal Of or relating to the orbit and the temporal bone region.

orbitotomy [ORBIT + *o* + -TOMY] Any operation creating an opening into the orbit. The approach may be either anterior or lateral.

orbivirus A member of the *Orbivirus* genus of the Reoviridae family. Viruses of this genus have two protein capsids and double-stranded RNA. They include bluetongue virus and Colorado tick fever virus.

orcein A brown stain that is used to demonstrate the presence of elastic fibers. Originally obtained from lichens, it is now prepared synthetically.

orchalgia ORCHIALGIA.

orchectomy ORCHIDECTOMY.

orchi- ORCHIO-.

orchialgia [ORCHI- + -ALGIA] Pain affecting the testis. Also called *didymalgia, didymodynia, orchalgia, orchidalgia, orchiodynia, orchioneuralgia, testalgia.*

orchiatrophy [ORCHI- + ATROPHY] TESTICULAR ATROPHY.

orchic ORCHIDIC.

orchichorea Repetitive elevation of the testicle because of clonic spasm of the cremaster muscle.

orchidalgia ORCHIALGIA.

orchidatrophia [*orchid(o)*- + ATROPHIA] TESTICULAR ATROPHY.

orchidatrophy [*orchid(o)*- + ATROPHY] TESTICULAR ATROPHY.

orchidectomy [*orchid(o)*- + -ECTOMY] Surgical excision of one testis. The operation may be performed through an incision in the scrotal wall (simple orchidectomy), or through an inguinal approach (inguinal orchidectomy). When the testis is found to have a tumor, both the testis and the spermatic cord are removed through an inguinal incision (radical orchidectomy). Also called *orchiectomy, orchectomy, testectomy.*

orchidic Referring to one or both testes. Also *orchic.*

orchidion [Gk *orchidion*, dim. of *orchis* a testicle] A testis that is smaller than normal.

orchiditis ORCHITIS.

orchido- [erroneous form for genitive Gk *orchis* testicle] ORCHIO-.

orchidoepididymectomy Surgical excision of a testis and the epididymis. Operative removal of the testis (orchidectomy), either simple or radical, implies simultaneous excision of the epididymis.

orchidoepididymitis ORCHIEPIDIDYMITIS.

orchidometer [ORCHIDO- + -METER] Any device for measuring the size of a testicle, especially the Prader orchidometer. **Prader orchidometer** Plastic beads, graded in size, which enable an examiner to gauge by comparison the size of a testicle.

orchidoncus [*orchid(o)*- + -ONCUS] A testicular tumor.

orchidopathy ORCHIOPATHY.

orchidopexy ORCHIOPEXY.

orchidoplasty [ORCHIDO- + -PLASTY] A plastic operation on the testicle. Also called *orchioplasty.*

orchidoptosis [ORCHIDO- + PTOSIS] Testicular prolapse due to either a lax scrotum or a varicocele.

orchidorrhaphy ORCHIOPEXY.

orchidoscheocele ORCHIOSCHEOCELE.

orchidospongioma [ORCHIDO- + SPONGI- + -OMA] A tumorlike testicular mass due to tuberculosis.

orchidotherapy Therapeutic administration of testicular extracts.

orchidotomy ORCHIOTOMY.

orchidotyloma [ORCHIDO- + Gk *tyl(os)* a knot, callus, lump, knob + -OMA] A hard testicular nodule.

orchiectomy ORCHIDECTOMY.

orchiencephaloma [ORCHI- + ENCEPHALOMA] A soft tumor of the testis. An obsolete term.

orchiepididymitis [ORCHI- + EPIDIDYMITIS] Inflammation of the testis and epididymis. Also called *orchidoepididymitis.*

orchil CUDBEAR.

orchilytic [ORCHI- + LYTIC] Destructive of the tissue of the testis. Also *orchitolytic.*

orchio- [Gk *orchis* (genitive *orchios*) testicle] A combining form denoting the testes. Also *orchi-, orchido-.*

orchiocatabasis The descent of the testes.

orchiocele [ORCHIO- + -CELE¹] 1 Herniation of a testis. 2 SCROTAL HERNIA.

orchiodynia [ORCHI- + -ODYNIA] ORCHIALGIA.

orchiomyeloma [ORCHIO- + MYELOMA] Plasmacytoma occurring in the testis.

orchioncus [ORCHI- + -ONCUS] A tumor of the testis.

orchioneuralgia [ORCHIO- + NEURALGIA] ORCHIALGIA.

orchiopathy [ORCHIO- + -PATHY] Disease of the testes. Also called *orchidopathy, testopathy.*

orchiopexy [ORCHIO- + -PEXY] The surgical repositioning of a testicle usually performed to place an undescended testicle within the scrotum. Also called *orchidopexy, orchiorrhaphy, orchidorrhaphy, cryptorchidopexy.*

orchioplasty ORCHIDOPLASTY.

orchiorrhaphy ORCHIOPEXY.

orchioscheocele [ORCHI- + OSCHEO- + CELE¹] A scrotal tumor associated with scrotal hernia. Also called *orchidoscheocele.*

orchioscirrhus Fibrosis of the testis. An obsolete term.

orchiotomy [ORCHIO- + -TOMY] Incision into a testis, as to allow drainage. Also called *orchotomy, orchidotomy.*

orchis [Gk *orchis* a testicle, the testicles] TESTIS.

orchitic Pertaining to or exhibiting orchitis.

orchitis [orch(i)- + -ITIS] Inflammation of the testis, manifested by swelling and tenderness and usually of infectious origin, as in tuberculosis, mumps, syphilis, or certain fungal diseases. Also called *testitis, didymitis, orchiditis.*

acute pyogenic orchitis Acute purulent inflammation of the testes.

acute syphilitic orchitis An acute, rare form of testicular infection usually occurring during the second stage of syphilis and clinically resembling acute pyogenic orchitis.

metastatic orchitis The spread of infection to the testis via the bloodstream, as may occur in mumps in postpubertal males.

mumps orchitis ORCHITIS PAROTIDEA.

orchitis parotidea Orchitis resulting from infection with the mumps virus and occurring before, during, or as the only manifestation of mumps. Also called *mumps orchitis.*

spermatogenic granulomatous orchitis Nontuberculous granulomatous inflammation of a testis, most often seen in middle-aged men after trauma to the testis. It is believed to be due to an autoimmune response to the extravasation of sperm.

traumatic orchitis Inflammation of a testicle following injury to the testicle or other part of the male genital system. It can follow surgical procedures as well as direct mechanical trauma.

orchitis variolosa Orchitis occurring as a complication of smallpox.

orchitolytic ORCHILYTIC.

orchotomy ORCHIOTOMY.

orcinol A phenol, 5-methylresorcinol, found combined in depsides. The name β-orcinol is applied to its derivative, 2,5-dimethylresorcinol.

ORD optical rotatory dispersion.

Ord [William Miller *Ord*, English surgeon, 1834–1902] See under OPERATION.

order 1 A hierarchical rank or category. 2 A taxonomic group ranking between class and family.

birth order 1 In demography, the number of children born alive to the mother, including the present child. 2 The serial ranking of the members of a sibship according to date of birth.

form-order See under FORM.

peck order A pervasive system of dominance and subordination within a group of similar individuals, often taking the form of a hierarchy. Also called *pecking order.*

pecking order PECK ORDER.

orderliness / organic orderliness A compulsively meticulous or stereotyped approach to the environment characteristic of some persons with organic brain disease, whose clothing must always be arranged in the same order, whose daily routine must

be rigidly maintained, and who allow no deviation from the status quo.

orderly An assistant or health worker who performs a wide range of services in a hospital, generally involving patient care or institutional operations, but not at the level of nursing care.

ordinate [New L *(linea) ordinate (applicata)* a line applied in an orderly manner. L *ordinate* is an adverb formed from *ordinatus,* past part. of *ordinare* to arrange, regulate] The value measured on the vertical axis (the y-axis) in a system of coordinates. Compare ABSCISSA.

Ordoñez [J. Hernando *Ordoñez,* Colombian physician, born 1910] See under MELANOSIS.

ordure [Middle English, excrement, from Old French *ord* filthy, from L *horrid(us)* horrid] Filth or excrement.

orectic [Gk *orektik(os)* (from *orekt(os)* stretched out, from *oregein* to reach or stretch out, desire, + -*ikos* -IC) having an appetite] 1 Having an appetite. 2 A substance that enhances the appetite.

Oreopithecus bambolii A species of fossil primate derived from the lower Pliocene or upper Miocene from lignite deposits in Tuscany, Italy. It bears some resemblances to small modern apes, having a short face and long arms that may indicate arboreal locomotor specialization.

Oretic A proprietary name for hydrochlorothiazide.

Oreton A proprietary name for testosterone propionate.

orexia Appetite.

orexigenic [Gk *orexi(s)* a yearning after, desire for + -GENIC] Serving to stimulate the appetite.

oreximania [Gk *orexi(s)* a yearning for a thing + -MANIA] The consumption of enormous quantities of food motivated by a fear of losing weight. An older term.

orexis Appetite.

orf [alteration of dialectal *hurf,* prob. from the Scandinavian] A highly contagious disease of sheep and goats due to the orf virus, a parapoxvirus, and causing watery, papillomatous lesions of the cornea, mucous membranes, and lips of young animals. Man can be infected by close or direct contact with an infected animal. In man, one or several lesions develops at the sites of inoculation as hypertrophic bullae. Also called *contagious ecthyma, contagious pustular dermatitis, ecthyma infectiosum, soremouth* (popular), *contagious pustular stomatitis* (popular), *ulcerative stomatitis of sheep* (rarely used).

organ [L *organum* (Gk *organon* an instrument, tool, engine, musical instrument, work) an implement, instrument, esp. a musical instrument] Any differentiated part or structure that is adapted for one or more special functions of an organism; organum.

absorbent organ The tissue, containing odontoclasts, which resorbs the root of a deciduous tooth as the successor erupts.

accessory organs of eye ORGANA OCULI ACCESSORIA.

acoustic organ ORGANUM SPIRALE.

adipose organ A localized collection of adipose tissue, such as the greater omentum.

Bidder's organ A rudimentary ovary that occurs in male toads. It develops into a functional ovary upon removal of the testis.

cell organ ORGANELLE.

cement organ A tissue composed of cementoblasts, which gives rise to the cement substance of a tooth.

organ of Chievitz An ectodermal outgrowth from embryonic cheek epithelium behind the site of origin of the parotid salivary gland. Present from the second to fourth month of fetal life in man, it may contribute to the parotid or represent a vestigial salivary gland. Although it can give rise to a tumor, it usually disappears completely.

organ of Corti   ORGANUM SPIRALE.

critical organ   The organ showing adverse effects at the lowest dose, with no reference to the severity of the effects. Other organs may be markedly affected but only at higher doses.

cutaneous sense organs   The variety of mechanical, thermal, and nociceptive afferent organs in the skin, most terminating in the dermal papillary layer and overlying basal epidermis.

digestive organs   APPARATUS DIGESTORIUS.

effector organ   EFFECTOR.

enamel organ   One of the series of knoblike thickenings which develop from the dental lamina and which produce the enamel of the teeth. The enamel organ forms an invaginated bell-shaped cap over the dental papilla. It has an inner enamel layer composed of ameloblasts, which produce enamel at the surfaces situated against the dental papilla. It also plays an important part in molding the final shape of a tooth.

end organ   The encapsulated ending of the peripheral part of a sensory nerve fiber. These comprise exteroceptors, enteroceptors, and proprioceptors. Also called *neuroterminal.*

essential organ of thalamus   The part of the thalamus that functions as an integrating center in lower animals lacking a cerebral cortex.

external genital organs   The labia majora, labia minora, and clitoris in the female, and the penis and scrotum in the male.

female genital organs   The organa genitalia feminina externa and organa genitalia feminina interna.

female reproductive organs   The various structures in the female related to reproduction, including the external genital organs, the vagina, the uterus, the fallopian tubes, and the ovaries. Also called *organa genitalia muliebria.*

organ of generation   Any anatomic structure that takes part in reproduction.

genital organs   ORGANA GENITALIA.

organ of Giraldès   PARAGENITAL DUCTS.

Golgi tendon organ   TENDON ORGAN. Abbreviation: GTO

gustatory organ   ORGANUM GUSTUS.

hydrostatic organ   An organ used for buoyancy, such as the swim bladder of the bony fishes.

internal reproductive organs   The vagina, uterus, fallopian tubes, and ovaries in the female, and the prostate, seminal vesicles, and testes in the male.

intromittent organ   A male organ which introduces sperm into the female reproductive tract.

organ of Jacobson   VOMERONASAL ORGAN.

lateral line organs   A sensory system for orienting and balancing fish. The sensory endings are located as a longitudinal line on each side of the body.

male genital organs   ORGANA GENITALIA MASCULINA.

male reproductive organs   The testes, epididymis, ductus deferens, seminal vesicles, ejaculatory duct, prostate, bulbourethral gland, and penis.

Marchand's organ   MARCHAND'S ADRENAL.

organs of mastication   MASTICATORY APPARATUS.

Meyer's organ   A cluster of vallate papillae on each side of the pharyngeal part of the tongue. An outmoded term.

motorial end organ   An obsolete term for MOTOR ENDPLATE.

neurotendinous organ   TENDON ORGAN.

olfactory organ   ORGANUM OLFACTUS.

parietal organ   A median eye occurring on the middorsal aspect of the head and brain in many fish, amphibians, and reptiles.

pineal organ   CORPUS PINEALE.

primitive fat organ   INTERSCAPULAR GLAND.

reproductive organs   GENITALIA.

respiratory organ   Any of various specialized organs, such as lungs or gills, in which occurs the exchange of oxygen and carbon dioxide between the organism and the environment.

Rosenmüller's organ   EPOÖPHORON.

rudimentary organ   An undeveloped or uncompleted organ.

organ of Ruffini   BRUSHES OF RUFFINI.

segmental organ   HOLONEPHROS.

sense organs   ORGANA SENSUUM.

sensory end organs   ORGANA SENSUUM.

sex organ   One of the reproductive organs.

organ of smell   ORGANUM OLFACTUS.

organs of special sense   ORGANA SENSUUM.

spiral organ   ORGANUM SPIRALE.

subcommissural organ   A group of specialized columnar ciliated ependymal cells that line the dorsal aspect of the cerebral aqueduct just caudal to the posterior commissure. The function of these cells is uncertain.

subfornical organ   A glomoid neurosecretory structure in the third ventricle, attached below the descending columns of the fornix, that has been described in various mammals. It is believed by some researchers to play a role in electrolyte balance.

target organ   An organ, as in a patient, toward which diagnostic, therapeutic, or experimental procedures are directed.

taste organ   ORGANUM GUSTUS.

tendon organ   An encapsulated receptor lying at the musculotendinous junction or within the tendon, hence in series with the muscle fibers and sensitive to tension developed either during contraction or passive stretch of the muscle. The discharge elicits the lengthening reaction. Also called *Golgi tendon organ, Golgi corpuscle, neurotendinous organ, tendon spindle, fusus neurotendineus, neurotendinous spindle.*

terminal organ   A sense organ or muscle; the organ at either end of a neural reflex arc.

touch organs   1 CORPUSCULA TACTUS. 2 PINKUS-IGGO RECEPTOR.

urinary organs   The differentiated parts of the urinary tract, including the kidneys, renal pelvis, ureter, bladder and urethra. A popular usage. Also called *uropoietic system, urinary system, organa urinaria, urinary apparatus.*

vestibular organ   LABYRINTHUS VESTIBULARIS.

vestibular end organ   An outmoded term for GANGLION VESTIBULARE.

vestibulocochlear organ   ORGANUM VESTIBULOCOCHLEARE.

vestigial organ   Any organ which today is seen only in undeveloped or rudimentary form but which in the evolutionary past was well developed and functional.

organ of vision   ORGANUM VISUS.

visual organ   ORGANUM VISUS.

vomeronasal organ   A rudimentary diverticulum on the median wall of each nasal fossa in higher vertebrates. At 8 mm stage in man it forms a groove, supported by special cartilages and supplying nerve fibers to join the olfactory nerve. It begins to regress after the sixth month of intrauterine life but may persist into adult life. In many tetrapods it functions as a supplementary olfactory organ. Also called *organ of Jacobson, organum vomeronasale.*

Weber's organ   PROSTATIC UTRICLE.

organs of Zuckerkandl   CORPORA PARA-AORTICA.

organa   Plural of ORGANUM.

organella (*plural* organellae) ORGANELLE.

organellae   Plural of ORGANELLA.

organelle [New L organell(a) (from L organ(um) organ + -ella, diminishing suffix] An intracellular structure having a specialized function, such as a mitochondrion, lysosome, or chloroplast. Also called *cell organ, organoid, organella.*

paired organelle   RHOPTRY.

organic   1 Relating to or of the nature of animals and plants. 2 Of or relating to an organ. 3 Structural in nature or origin, as *organic defect.* ⟨"His condition [paralysis] was not organic (*i.e.*, it must have been learned) because under pentothal narcosis he was able to move his arm in all directions with ease." — John Dollard and Neal E. Miller, *Personality and Psychotherapy*, 1950, p. 165.⟩ **4** Containing carbon other than that occurring in carbon dioxide or its salts or in carbon monoxide: used of a chemical compound. **5** Derived from or relating to the use of fertilizer of plant or animal origin rather than that of artificially produced substances.

organicism **1** The belief that each organ of the body has a unique constitution. **2** The theory that all symptoms are due to organic disease, whether physical or psychologic in nature.

organicist A proponent of organicism. Also called *somatist*.

organisin A hypothetical substance thought to be secreted by embryonic cells of an organizing center and responsible for the inductive action of the center.

organism [ORGAN + -ISM] Any living individual considered as a whole, whether plant or animal, viral or microbial.

pleuropneumonialike organism An outmoded term for MY-COPLASMA.

target organism The species that is the object of a pest-control program.

organization [Med L *organizatio* (from *organizatus*, past part. of *organizare* to organize, from L *organum* an implement, instrument; + *-io* -ION) an act of organizing] **1** A group of individuals functioning as a system in a collective enterprise or of things contributing to a result that depends on their participation. **2** The transformation of a pathological state into vascularized connective tissue by the ingrowth of fibroblasts and capillary buds. • This sense is most often applied to the resolution of a thrombus or of a fibrinous exudate.

health maintenance organization An organization that provides prepaid health care services to an enrolled clientele, using its own facilities or those contracted for in the community in which it operates. It generally offers comprehensive coverage including preventive care. There are usually few if any copayments on the part of the enrollee beyond a contribution to the premium that is required in some plans. Abbreviation: HMO • The term *health maintenance organization* was originally used in United States federal legislation passed in the early 1970s to promote prepaid forms of practice, and has been more extensively used in recent years. The term is also used in Australia.

preferred provider organization In the United States, a health-care insurer that offers benefits through an arrangement of contractual commitments by community-based providers who usually agree to a preferential negotiated rate of payment for specific services offered to individuals enrolled in the insurance. Abbreviation: PPO

pregenital organization Libidinal organization during the years preceding the genital instinctual level.

tonotopic organization The spatial arrangement of neurons within the nuclei of the auditory nervous system so as to correspond to specific tones, most clearly demonstrated in the cochlear nuclei.

organizer **1** A part or region of an embryo which is capable of evoking and controlling the morphologic differentiation of other groups of cells within the embryo. The groups of cells therefore act as an evocator which is capable of determining the fate of other cell groups with which it comes into contact. Also called *activating agent, inductor, organizer zone.* **2** See under PRIMARY ORGANIZER. **3** INDUCTOR.

mesodermic organizer The early notochord in its capacity to act as an inductor region which stimulates the differentiation of the adjacent mesoderm into somites.

nucleolar organizer A site on the chromosome containing multiple copies of ribosomal ribonucleic acid genes where the nucleolus originates. Also called *nucleololus*.

primary organizer The region of the dorsal lip of the blastopore in lower vertebrates and Hensen's node in higher vertebrates that differentiates without prior induction. This region acts as an inductor and is capable of evoking the formation of the medullary plate and adjacent ectoderm.

secondary organizer A part previously formed as a result of induction, that is in turn capable of providing a morphogenetic stimulus on an adjacent part or parts of the embryo. An example is the induction of the lens by the underlying optic vesicle. Also called *organizer of the second grade.*

tertiary organizer A part of the embryo that has developed as a result of induction by a secondary organizer, which is in turn capable of providing morphogenetic stimulus on an adjacent part or parts. An example is the tympanic ring which exerts influences on the tympanic membrane. Also called *organizer of the third grade.*

organo- [Gk *organon* organ] A combining form meaning organ.

organoaxial Pertaining to the long axis of an organ.

organofaction ORGANOGENESIS.

organogenesis [ORGANO- + GENESIS] Formation and development of the different organs of an animal or plant. Although the greater part occurs during the embryonic period, that of some organs, such as those of the special senses and the central nervous system, continue to be developed during the fetal period and in man even after birth. Also called *organofaction, morphologic synthesis, organogeny.* Adjective: organogenetic.

organogenic [ORGANO- + -GENIC] Having origin within an organ.

organogeny ORGANOGENESIS.

organography The visualization of organs using radiographic techniques.

organoid [ORGAN + -OID] **1** Resembling an organ in appearance. **2** An organlike substance or structure. **3** ORGANELLE.

organoleptic Capable of being perceived by one or more sense organs.

organoma [ORGAN + -OMA] A tumor containing elements arranged in an organlike manner, as in teratomas. An obsolete term.

organomegaly SPLANCHNOMEGALY.

organometallic **1** Denoting compounds that contain a bond between organic carbon and metal atoms, such as the carbon-cobalt bond in methylcobalamin. **2** Of or relating to the chemistry of such compounds.

organon [Gk (akin to *ergon* work), an instrument, tool, engine, musical instrument, work] An outmoded term for ORGANUM.

organon auditus An outmoded term for ORGANUM VESTIBULOCOCHLEARE.

organa genitalia muliebria FEMALE REPRODUCTIVE ORGANS.

organon gustus An outmoded term for ORGANUM GUSTUS.

organon olfactus An outmoded term for ORGANUM OLFACTUS.

organon spirale An outmoded term for ORGANUM SPIRALE.

organon visus An outmoded term for ORGANUM VISUS.

organopathy A disease which affects one organ system within the body. A rarely used term.

organopexia [ORGANO- + -pex(y) + -IA] A surgical procedure in which an organ is fixed or resuspended to increase its support. Also called *organopexy.*

organopexy ORGANOPEXIA.

organophilic [ORGAN + o + -PHILIC] ORGANOTROPIC.

organophilism ORGANOTROPISM.

organoscopy [ORGAN + *o* + -SCOPY]   Inspection of internal organs with an endoscope. A rarely used term.

organotaxis [ORGANO- + Gk *taxis* an arranging, order]   A migration towards or attraction to a particular organ.

organotherapy [ORGANO- + THERAPY]   The use of extracts of animal endocrine glands or other organs for therapeutic purposes. Also called *Brown-Séquard treatment, organ treatment, cellular therapeutics, organic therapy.*

   heterologous organotherapy   The use of organ extracts to treat diseases of a different or unrelated organ.

   homologous organotherapy   The use of animal organ extracts to treat human diseases of the same organ system.

organotrope [ORGANO- + -TROPE]   An agent or substance that has an affinity for a particular organ or organ system.

organotrophic   Pertaining to the nutrition of an organ or organs of the body.

organotropic [ORGAN + *o* + -TROPIC²]   Having an affinity for or an effect on particular organs or organ systems; characterized by organotropism. Also *organophilic.*

organotropism [ORGANO- + TROPISM]   An affinity for particular organs or organ systems, such as that exhibited by certain chemical agents, drugs, and pathogens. Also called *organotropy, organophilism.*

organotropy   ORGANOTROPISM.

organ-specific   Found in or having an action directed to a particular organ, as that of certain antigens or antibodies.

organule   An encapsulated ending of a sensory nerve receptor. An outmoded term.

organum [L (Gk *organon* an instrument, tool, engine, musical instrument, work), an implement, instrument, esp. a musical instrument]   (*plural* organa) Any differentiated part or structure that is adapted for one or more special functions of an organism; organ. Also called *organon* (outmoded).

   organum auditus   An outmoded term for ORGANUM VESTIBULOCOCHLEARE.

   organa genitalia   The reproductive organs of the urogenital apparatus, subdivided into organa genitalia masculina interna, organa genitalia masculina externa, organa genitalia feminina interna, and organa genitalia feminina externa. Also called *genital organs.*

   organa genitalia feminina externa   The external genital organs of the female, including the pudendum feminum, or vulva, the clitoris, and the urethra feminina. Also called *partes genitales femininae externae* (outmoded), *partes genitales externae muliebres* (outmoded).

   organa genitalia feminina interna   [NA] The internal genital or reproductive organs and ducts of the female, including ovarium, tuba uterina, uterus, and vagina.

   organa genitalia masculina   The organa genitalia masculina externa and organa genitalia masculina interna. Also called *male genital organs, organa genitalia* (outmoded), *virilia.*

   organa genitalia masculina externa   [NA] The external genital organs of the male, including penis, scrotum and urethra masculina. Also called *partes genitales masculinae externae* (outmoded), *partes genitales externae viriles* (outmoded).

   organa genitalia masculina interna   [NA] The internal genital or reproductive organs and ducts of the male, including the testis, epididymis, ductus deferens, vesicula seminalis, funiculus spermaticus, prostata, and glandula bulbourethralis.

   organa genitalia virilia   An outmoded term for ORGANA GENITALIA MASCULINA.

   organum gustus   [NA] A number of microscopic taste buds, or caliculi gustatorii, that comprise the organ of taste. They are located mostly in the tongue epithelium of the vallate papillae or fungiform papillae and in the surface between them, whereas

a few are found in the lingual surface of the soft palate and on the epiglottis. Also called *taste organ, gustatory organ, organon gustus* (outmoded).

   organa oculi accessoria   [NA] The structures associated with the eyeball in the orbit, namely, the bulbar muscles, orbital fasciae, eyebrows, eyelids, conjunctiva, and lacrimal apparatus. Also called *accessory organs of the eye, adnexa oculi* (outmoded), *appendages of the eye.*

   organum olfactus   [NA] The organ of smell which comprises the specialized epithelium on the superior nasal concha, the opposing part of the nasal septum, and the roof of the nasal cavity as well as its nervous connections. Also called *olfactory organ, organ of smell, organon olfactus* (outmoded).

   organa sensuum   [NA] End organs derived from neurectoderm that translate various forms of energy into neural activity leading to sensations. Also called *organs of special sense, sensory end organs, sense organs, sensory apparatus.*

   organum spirale   [NA] The specialized structures in the internal ear subserving the function of hearing and comprising a series of epithelial structures that rest upon the zona arcuata of the basilar membrane in the cochlear duct. In the center are the inner and outer rods of Corti, or pillar cells, separated from each other by the inner tunnel of Corti. On the medial side of the tunnel of Corti is a single row of inner hair cells. On the lateral side of the outer rods are four rows of outer hair cells and supporting cells, namely, the phalangeal cells of Deiters and the cells of Hensen and of Claudius. The free ends of the outer hair cells protrude through the netlike reticular membrane, and the whole complex is covered by the tectorial membrane. The basal ends of the hair cells are in synaptic contact with the fibers of the cochlear nerve. Also called *spiral organ, acoustic organ, organ of Corti, organon spirale* (outmoded), *papilla spiralis* (outmoded).

   organa urinaria   [NA] URINARY ORGANS.

   organum vestibulocochleare   [NA] The anatomical structures outside the central nervous system that serve the functions of hearing and balance and that comprise the external, middle, and internal ear. Also called *vestibulocochlear organ, organum auditus* (outmoded), *organon auditus* (outmoded).

   organum visus   [NA] The organ that controls vision and conducts visual stimuli to and from the central nervous system. It comprises the optic nerve; the bulbus oculi, including its fibrous, vascular, and internal coats; blood vessels, chambers, and the lens, as well as the organa oculi accessoria. Also called *organ of vision, organon visus* (outmoded), *visual organ.*

   organum vomeronasale   VOMERONASAL ORGAN.

orgasm [Gk *orgasm(os)* (from *organ* to swell, be lustful or passionate, akin to *orgē* a violent passion, anger) luxuriant fullness, appetite]   The peak of genital excitation; sexual climax.

   alimentary orgasm   The infant's feeling of bliss and the rapid reduction in tension that occurs at the height of breast feeding.

   inhibited male orgasm   EJACULATIO RETARDATA.

orgasmolepsy [ORGASM + *o* + -LEPSY]   **1** An attack of epilepsy occurring during orgasm. An obsolete usage. **2** An attack of epilepsy resulting from a discharge arising in the lobulus paracentralis or, more frequently, in the temporal lobe, producing erotic sensations simulating orgasm.

orientation [L *oriens* (gen. *orientis*, pres. part. of *oriri* to rise) rising + -ATION]   **1** The conscious mental ability to determine one's position in time and space. **2** In psychiatry, one's philosophy or point of view, as the body of theory to which one subscribes, as *psychoanalytic orientation, behavioristic orientation.*

   double orientation   The maintenance of two attitudes about the self that would logically appear to be mutually exclusive, such as the bus driver who has worked dutifully for many years even as he is convinced that he is a prime minister.

goal orientation　The tendency to direct both posture and action toward a particular goal. An animal in an experimental maze-learning situation moves in the general direction of the goal, not away from it, even though some blind alleys continue to be entered while searching for the correct path.

oral orientation　A view of the world from the perspective of orality, characteristic of the infant, whose mouth is his most differentiated organ and chief perceptive apparatus, and of the adult oral character.

personal orientation　An orientation toward an appreciation of one's self, of one's own personality, of one's psychic self, and of the identity of the people who are part of one's usual environment.

reality orientation　A form of therapy intended to promote awareness of time, space, person, and identity in persons who are confused or disoriented from any cause. It is most often used with severely regressed schizophrenics and patients with organic dementia.

social orientation　**1** The general direction of behavior of a group or of a member of a group.　**2** The attitude toward and degree of conformity with the customs and ethics of a group to which the subject belongs.

Orientobilharzia [L *oriens* (gen. *orientis*, pres. part. of *oriri* to rise) + *Bilharzia*, after Theodor *Bilharz*, German helminthologist and physician, 1825–1862 + -IA]　A genus of schistosomes parasitic in mammals.

Orientobilharzia dattae　The type species of this genus of schistosomes, found in the vascular system of water buffalos in India.

Orientobilharzia turkestanicum　A schistosome infecting mammals and of veterinary significance in cattle. It is sometimes responsible for spurious parasitism, leading to confusion and misdiagnosis, when the eggs from infected beef are passed in human feces.

orifice [L *orificium*. See ORIFICIUM.]　Any opening to or from an organ, cavity, tube, or structure, including any foramen, meatus, or ostium. Also called *orificium*.

abdominal orifice of uterine tube　OSTIUM ABDOMINALE TUBAE UTERINAE.

aortic orifice　**1** OSTIUM AORTAE.　**2** HIATUS AORTICUS.

atrioventricular orifice　Either the ostium atrioventriculare dextrum or ostium atrioventriculare sinistrum. Also called *auriculoventricular orifice* (outmoded).

auriculoventricular orifice　An outmoded term for ATRIO-VENTRICULAR ORIFICE.

buccal orifice　RIMA ORIS.

cardiac orifice　OSTIUM CARDIACUM.

duodenal orifice of stomach　OSTIUM PYLORICUM.

epiploic orifice　FORAMEN OMENTALE.

esophagogastric orifice　OSTIUM CARDIACUM.

orifice of external acoustic meatus　PORUS ACUSTICUS EXTERNUS.

external orifice of aqueduct of vestibule　APERTURA EXTERNA AQUEDUCTUS VESTIBULI.

external orifice of female urethra　OSTIUM URETHRAE EXTERNUM FEMININAE.

external orifice of male urethra　OSTIUM URETHRAE EXTERNUM MASCULINAE.

external orifice of uterus　OSTIUM UTERI.

gastroduodenal orifice　OSTIUM PYLORICUM.

golf-hole ureteral orifice　A ureteral orifice (the ostium ureteris) which has taken on a funnel shape, commonly associated with vesicoureteral reflux.

hymenal orifice　OSTIUM VAGINAE.

internal orifice of urethra　OSTIUM URETHRAE INTERNUM.

left atrioventricular orifice　OSTIUM ATRIOVENTRICULARE SINISTRUM.

orifice of maxillary sinus　HIATUS MAXILLARIS.

mitral orifice　OSTIUM ATRIOVENTRICULARE SINISTRUM.

pharyngeal orifice　OSTIUM PHARYNGEUM TUBAE AUDITIVAE.

pilosebaceous orifice　The opening at the skin surface of the pilosebaceous follicle.

pulmonary orifice　OSTIUM TRUNCI PULMONALIS.

pyloric orifice　OSTIUM PYLORICUM.

right atrioventricular orifice　OSTIUM ATRIOVENTRICULARE DEXTRUM.

tricuspid orifice　OSTIUM ATRIOVENTRICULARE DEXTRUM.

orifice of ureter　OSTIUM URETERIS.

uterine orifice of uterine tube　OSTIUM UTERINUM TUBAE UTERINAE.

vaginal orifice　OSTIUM VAGINAE.

vesicourethral orifice　OSTIUM URETHRAE INTERNUM.

orifice of Vieussens　**1** ANTERIOR OPENING OF AQUEDUCT OF SYLVIUS.　**2** One of the foramina venarum minimarum cordis.

orificia　Plural of ORIFICIUM.

orificial　Pertaining to an orifice.

orificialist　One who claims to treat disease by manipulating, dilating, or operating on external body orifices.

orificium [L (from *os*, gen. *oris*, mouth + -*ficium*, noun suffix from *facere* to make), orifice]　ORIFICE.

orificium externum isthmi　An outmoded term for OSTIUM UTERI.

orificium externum uteri　An outmoded term for OSTIUM UTERI.

orificium internum isthmi　OS UTERI INTERNUM.

orificium internum uteri　An outmoded term for OS UTERI INTERNUM.

orificium ureteris　An outmoded term for OSTIUM URETERIS.

orificium urethrae externum muliebris　An outmoded term for OSTIUM URETHRAE EXTERNUM FEMININAE.

orificium urethrae externum virilis　An outmoded term for OSTIUM URETHRAE EXTERNUM MASCULINAE.

orificium urethrae internum　OSTIUM URETHRAE INTERNUM.

orificium vaginae　OSTIUM VAGINAE.

oriform　Shaped like a mouth.

origin [L *origo* (gen. *originis*; from *oriri* to rise, akin to Gk *ornynai* to make to arise, rouse) origin]　**1** The more fixed attachment of a muscle from which it exerts its action on the more mobile part on which it is inserted. Under certain circumstances this direction of action may be reversed.　**2** The parent stem from which a nerve or vessel arises or branches off.　**3** The first site or manifestation in the embryo or fetus of a structure, tissue, or organ.

Orinase　A proprietary name for tolbutamide.

orinotherapy　Living at high altitudes as a form of therapy.

ormetoprim　$C_{14}H_{18}N_4O_2$.　2,4-diamino-5-(6-methylveratryl)pyrimidine, an antibacterial agent.

Ormond [John Kelso *Ormond*, U.S. urologist, born 1886]　Ormond's disease. See under IDIOPATHIC RETROPERITONEAL FIBROSIS.

Orn　Symbol for ornithine.

ornithine　NH_2—$[CH_2]_3$—$CH(NH_2)$—COOH. An amino acid not incorporated into proteins, it is an intermediate in the urea cycle. It is formed together with urea on hydrolysis of arginine by arginase, and it is converted into citrulline by the action of ornithine carbamoyltransferase. It is present in blood. Birds excrete aromatic (benzoic, nicotinic) acids as diacyl ornithines. Symbol: Orn

ornithine acetyltransferase An enzyme which catalyzes the transfer of an acetyl group from α-*N*-acetylornithine to glutamate.

ornithine carbamoyltransferase The enzyme (EC 2.1.3.3) that catalyzes the transfer of the carbamoyl group from carbamoyl phosphate to ornithine in the synthesis of citrulline. This is a step in urea synthesis in the liver.

ornithine decarboxylase An enzyme (EC 4.1.1.17) which catalyzes the decarboxylation of ornithine to form putrescine.

ornithinemia A rare inherited deficiency of ornithine aminotransferase resulting in greatly elevated blood ornithine levels. It is usually accompanied by gyrate atrophy of the choroid and retina. It is not associated with hyperammonemia or any other known disturbances.

Ornithodoros [Gk *ornis* (gen. *ornithos*) a bird + *doros* a leather bag] A genus of soft-bodies ticks of the family Argasidae. They are characterized by a subterminal capitulum hidden by the dorsum, a well-developed hypostome, and a patterned integument. About 90 species, placed in seven subgenera, are known, some of which infest mammals and some, birds. Many species are involved in transmission of pathogenic agents, the most important of which are spirochetes that cause relapsing fever.

Ornithodoros coriaceus A species found in the mountains and coastal areas of California and Mexico; the pajaroello or tlalaja tick. The adults are parasitic on cattle and deer and will also attack humans. Their bite is painful and irritating.

Ornithodoros hermsi A species found on rodents and an important vector of spirochetes such as *Borrelia hermsii*, a cause of relapsing fever. The geographic distribution includes the western United States and parts of Canada.

Ornithodoros lahorensis A species thought to transmit *Borrelia persica*, an agent of relapsing fever in Iran, *Rickettsia sibirica*, the agent of Siberian tick typhus, and an enzootic abortion agent of sheep. This tick is reported to have caused extensive losses of sheep in the southern Soviet Union.

Ornithodoros marocanas A species considered the probable vector of *Borrelia hispanica*, the agent of Spanish relapsing fever.

Ornithodoros moubata A group of African ticks originally considered a single species, now recognized as including four species and one subspecies, which transmit agents of relapsing fever. *O. moubata* proper, the tampan tick, is found on a variety of hosts domestic and wild, and is widely distributed in arid regions of Africa. *O. compactus* is a parasite of South African tortoises. *O. apertus,* a large and rare tick, is found in the burrows of porcupines. *O. porcinus,* an ectoparasite of warthogs, is widely distributed as several subspecies in burrows and lairs and in hollow baobab trees in east, central, and southern Africa and Madagascar. This species carries African swine fever virus. *O. Porcinus domesticus* is common in human dwellings in east Africa. Distinct races are described that feed on humans and fowls in different ecotypes.

Ornithodoros pappilipes A species that transmits *Borrelia persica*, an agent of relapsing fever in Iran. Known as the Persian bug, it is found in the Near East and the Soviet Union.

Ornithodoros parkeri A species found in the western United States that transmits *Borrelia parkeri*, an agent of relapsing fever.

Ornithodoros rudis A species important as a vector of *Borrelia venezuelensis*, an agent of relapsing fever in Central and South America. It is thought to form a species complex similar to that of *O. moubata* and to include the form known as *O. venezuelensis.*

Ornithodoros savigni A species that is a vector of *Borrelia kochii*, an agent of relapsing fever in eastern Africa, the south of Egypt, Ethiopia, and southwestern Asia. In addition, the bite

itself can be toxic. Bovines have been reported to die overnight from attacks of the tick, which has proteinlike toxins in the saliva.

Ornithodoros talaje A species found on wild rodents and domestic animals in Mexico, Central America, and South America. It also attacks humans, causing extreme pain and irritation by its bite, and transmitting *Borrelia mazzottii*, a spirochete that causes relapsing fever. Also called *Alectorobius talaje.*

Ornithodoros tholozani A species that transmits *Borrelia persica*, an agent of relapsing fever. Records kept for 16 to 30 years of tick-borne spirochetosis in uninhabited areas of Turkmenistan suggest long periods of transovarial transmission.

Ornithodoros turicata A species found in the western United States and Mexico that transmits *Borrelia turicatae,* an agent of relapsing fever.

Ornithodoros venezuelensis A species belonging to the *O. rudis* complex that transmits *Borrelia venezuelensis,* an agent of relapsing fever in Venezuela and Colombia as well as in other mountainous areas of Central and South America. It is chiefly a human parasite but will feed also on other animals.

Ornithodoros verrucosus A species that transmits *Borrelia caucasica* in the Caucasus.

ornithology [Gk *ornis*, gen. *ornithos*, bird + o + -LOGY] The branch of science concerning birds.

Ornithonyssus [New L (from Gk *ornis*, gen. *ornithos*, a bird + *nyssa* a starting post or turning post on a racetrack or *nyssein* to spur, pierce, prick)] A genus of mites in the family Macronyssidae (formerly listed in the family Dermanyssidae). They are morphologically homogeneous and chiefly tropical in distribution. Also called *Liponyssus, Lyponyssus.*

Ornithonyssus bacoti The tropical rat mite, a cosmopolitan species particularly closely associated with the roof rat, *Rattus rattus*. Its bite may cause a painful form of dermatitis known as rat-mite dermatitis. It is the intermediate host of the cotton rat filaria *Litomosoides carinii* in a host-vector-filaria system widely used for testing antifilarial drugs. There are no reports of natural transmission of human disease, though experimental transmission of various pathogens has taken place in the laboratory (murine typhus, plague, rickettsialpox). Also called *Leiognathus bacoti.*

Ornithonyssus bursa The tropical fowl mite, an ectoparasite of poultry and wild birds on all continents, chiefly in tropical and subtropical regions. Humans are only temporary hosts, as the mite can survive for only ten days away from an avian host.

Ornithonyssus sylviarum The northern fowl mite, found on many species of domestic and wild fowl. It causes itching and annoyance in humans, especially among poultry and egg handlers. It can survive away from an avian host for three to six weeks.

ornithophobia [Gk *ornis*, gen. *ornithos*, a bird + -PHOBIA] Pathologic fear of birds.

ornithosis PSITTACOSIS.

ornithuric acid N^2,N^5-Dibenzoylornithine, a compound found in bird urine.

oro-[1] [L *os* (genitive *oris*) mouth] A combining form meaning mouth, oral.

oro-[2] ORRHO-.

oroantral Situated between the inside of the mouth and the interior of the maxillary antrum: applied particularly to fistulas.

orofacial Pertaining to the mouth and the face.

orolingual Of or relating to the mouth and the tongue.

oromaxillary Pertaining to the mouth and the maxilla.

oromeningitis ORRHOMENINGITIS.

oronasal Relating to both the mouth and the nose.

oronosus MOUNTAIN SICKNESS.

oropharyngeal Pertaining to the oropharynx. Also *pharyngo-oral.*

oropharynx PARS ORALIS PHARYNGIS.

orophilic [Gk *oro(s)* a mountain + -PHILIC] Thriving in mountainous regions: said of an animal organism, especially an insect.

Oropsylla [Gk *oros* a mountain or L *os* (gen. *oris*) mouth + Gk *psylla* a flea] A genus of fleas that infest rodents.

Oropsylla idahoensis A species found on rodents in the western United States that is involved in the transmission of sylvatic plague.

Oropsylla montana See under *DIAMANUS.*

Oropsylla silantiewi A species found on *Marmota sibirica,* the Manchuria marmot, or tarabagan, that can transmit plague from animal to animal. Trappers of these valuable fur animals suffered from a plague outbreak in the Transbaikalian region of Siberia, initiating the last major pandemic of plague reported. The pathogens were spread from humans to commensal rat fleas along trade routes, causing the Hong Kong epidemic of 1894, and thence over much of the globe.

orosomucoid ACID GLYCOPROTEIN.

orotate The salt of orotic acid. It is the biological precursor of orotidylic acid.

orotate phosphoribosyltransferase An enzyme (EC 2.4.2.10) which catalyzes the conversion of orotidine-5'-phosphate and pyrophosphate to orotate and 5-phospho-α-D-ribose 1-diphosphate.

orotate reductase DIHYDROOROTATE DEHYDROGENASE.

orotherapy The medicinal use of whey, either by ingestion or bathing.

orotic acid 6-Carboxyuracil. A pyrimidine synthesized in the cell from carbamoyl phosphate and aspartic acid via condensation, dehydration, and oxidation. It reacts with 5-phosphoribosylpyrophosphate to form inorganic pyrophosphate and orotidine 5'-phosphate, whose decarboxylation leads to the pyrimidine nucleotides uridylic acid, UTP, and (after its amination) CTP.

oroticaciduria OROTIC ACIDURIA.

orotidine N^1-Ribosylorotic acid, the nucleoside of orotic acid. Its 5'-phosphate, is an intermediate in pyrimidine biosynthesis.

orotidylic acid Orotidine 5'-phosphate. Its decarboxylation to uridylic acid is the final step in pyrmidine biosynthesis. It is made biologically from orotate and 5-phosphoribose 1-diphosphate by transfer of the 5-phosphoribosyl group.

orphenadrine $C_{18}H_{23}NO.$ *N,N*-Dimethyl-2-(*o*-methyl-α-phenylbenzyl)oxy-ethylamine. An antispasmodic, antitremor agent that has antihistaminic properties. It is used in the treatment of painful musculoskeletal disorders. Also called *mephenamine.*

orphenadrine citrate $C_{18}H_{23}NO\cdot C_6H_8O_7.$ The citrate salt form of orphenadrine. It is used as a skeletal muscle relaxant in treating acute spasms of voluntary muscles, regardless of location. Post-traumatic and tension muscle spasms also respond to this drug. It can be given intramuscularly, intravenously, or orally.

orphenadrine hydrochloride $C_{18}H_{23}NO\cdot HCl.$ The hydrochloride salt form of orphenadrine. It serves as a muscle relaxant agent and antispasmodic drug in the treatment of parkinsonism and drug-induced extrapyramidal tract diseases.

Orr [Hiram Winnett *Orr,* U.S. orthopedic surgeon, 1877–1956] Orr method, Orr technique. See under TREATMENT.

orrho- [Gk *orrhos* whey, serum] A combining form meaning serum. Also *oro-².*

orrhology [ORRHO- + -LOGY] SEROLOGY.

orrhomeningitis Inflammation of a serous membrane such as the peritoneum. An obsolete term. Also *oromeningitis.*

orrhoreaction SEROREACTION.

orrhorrhea [ORRHO- + -RRHEA] A thin, watery, or serous discharge. An obsolete term. Also called *seriflux.*

orrhotherapy [ORRHO- + THERAPY] An obsolete term for SEROTHERAPY.

orris The rhizome of *Iris florentina.* It is ground into a powder and used in dentifrices, cosmetics, and perfumes. Also called *iridis rhizoma.*

orsellinic acid 2,4-Dihydroxy-6-methylbenzoic acid, a compound found combined in depsides. Its decarboxylation yields orcinol.

Orsi [Francesco *Orsi,* Italian physician, 1828–1900] Orsi-Grocco method. See under METHOD.

Orth [Johannes J. *Orth,* German pathologist, 1847–1923] Orth stain. See under SOLUTION.

orth- ORTHO-.

orthergasia EUERGASIA.

orthesis ORTHOSIS.

orthetic ORTHOTIC.

orthetics ORTHOTICS.

orthetist ORTHOTIST.

ortho- [GK *orthos* straight, upright] **1** A combining form meaning (1) straight, correct, or normal; (2) designed to correct, corrective. Also *orth-.* **2** A prefix signifying substitution on the atom of a benzene ring adjacent to the reference atom, which is usually one already substituted. This prefix is italicized and joined to what follows by a hyphen. Abbreviation: *o-* **3** A combining form signifying an ester of the structure R—C(—OR')₃, where R—CO—OR' would be the normal ester of the same acid R—COOH. **4** A combining form signifying a particular state of hydration of an inorganic oxoacid, e.g. H_3PO_4 rather than HPO_3.

orthoaminosalicylic acid $CH_3(NH_2)OHCOOH.$ An insoluble analogue of salicylic acid. It is used in the treatment of chronic rheumatism.

orthobiosis A healthy way of life.

orthocardiac Concerning the effects on the heart from assuming an upright posture.

orthocephalic Having a head with an altitudinal index between 70.1 and 75. Also *orthocephalous.*

orthocephalous ORTHOCEPHALIC.

orthocheilia [ORTHO- + CHEIL- + -IA] The state of having lips which are of average shape and prominence.

orthochorea [ORTHO- + CHOREA] Chorea in which the characteristic movements only appear or are greatly accentuated when the patient is standing up. A seldom used term.

orthochromatic NORMOCHROMIC.

orthochromatin A region of chromatin that contains stable structural genes. A seldom used term.

orthochromia The tinctorial characteristic of a mature erythrocyte, in staining red with Romanowsky dyes and exhibiting no degree of basophilia.

orthochromic Having the expected affinity for histochemical reagents.

orthochromophil A cell that possesses normal staining properties. Also called *isochromatophil.*

orthocrasia [ORTHO- + Gk *kras(is)* a mixing, compounding (of drugs), close union + -IA] A physiologic mechanism in the body which ensures that the administration of drugs or the ingestion of food substances will not alter the body's homeostasis.

orthocresol phthalein A phthalein derivative used as a pH indicator. A one-color indicator like phenolphthalein, it changes from colorless at an acid pH to red over the pH range of 8.2 to 9.8.

orthocytosis The absence of any nucleated erythrocyte precursors in human blood, i.e. the normal condition. A rarely used term.

orthodactylous Characterized by straight fingers or toes.

orthodentin Dentin containing tubules within which are extensions of the odontoblasts.

orthodiagram [ORTHO- + DIAGRAM] A drawing of the image obtained in orthodiascopy. Also called *orthoradiogram, orthoskiagram.*

orthodiagraph [ORTHO- + DIA- + -GRAPH] A radiographic device for recording the size and shape of internal organs without the distortion of ordinary roentgenography. Also called *orthoskiagraph, orthodiascope.*

orthodiagraphy [ORTHO- + DIA- + -GRAPHY] A method by which the exact outlines of an organ, especially the heart, can be measured by using a fluoroscopic image. Also called *orthoroentgenography.*

orthodiascope ORTHODIAGRAPH.

orthodiascopy A radiologic method of obtaining a nonmagnified image of the heart or other structures, by direct tracing of its silhouette as projected on a fluoroscopic screen. Also called *orthoradioscopy, orthoskiagraphy.*

orthodigita The correction of deformities of the fingers or toes.

orthodont [ORTHO- + -DONT] Possessing an ideal arrangement of teeth.

orthodontia [ORTH- + -ODONTIA] The study of irregularities in position of the teeth and of malocclusion, and their treatment.

orthodontics [ORTH- + -ODONT + -ICS] The putting into practice of orthodontia. Also called *odontorthosis, orthodontology, dental orthopedics, dentofacial orthopedics.*

interceptive orthodontics Early orthodontic treatment to the primary or mixed dentitions.

preventive orthodontics The prevention of tooth migration by space maintenance. Also called *prophylactic orthodontics.*

prophylactic orthodontics PREVENTIVE ORTHODONTICS.

surgical orthodontics Correction of malocclusion by the surgical repositioning of the jaw, or segments of the jaw.

orthodontist A dentist who specializes in orthodontics.

orthodontology ORTHODONTICS.

orthodromic Concerning movement of impulses in their normal direction.

orthoendocrine [ORTHO- + ENDOCRINE] Capable of secreting products which are normal for a given cell in its specific anatomic location: used especially of apudomas.

orthogenesis [ORTHO- + GENESIS] The evolution of organisms along unbranching phyletic lines. Also called *determinate evolution, bathmic evolution.*

orthogenics EUGENICS.

orthoglycemic Denoting the state of normal blood sugar concentration.

orthognathia [ORTHO- + GNATH- + -IA] A specialty dealing with the etiology and treatment of abnormal relationships between the bones of the jaws.

orthognathic Having a gnathic index of less than 98. Also *orthognathous.*

orthognathism The characteristic of having nonprojecting jaws, the gnathic index being below 98.

orthognathous ORTHOGNATHIC.

orthogonal Situated at right angles; intersecting in perpendicular planes.

orthograde Characterized by walking in a direction perpendicular to the long axis of the body; walking upright. Compare PRONOGRADE.

orthokeratosis [ORTHO- + KERATOSIS] Normal keratinization of tissue.

orthokinetics The dynamic use of an orthotic device to facilitate movement of one muscle while inhibiting its antagonist, as a treatment for spasticity.

orthomelic Relating to the correction of limb deformities.

orthometer [ORTHO- + -METER] EXOPHTHALMOMETER.

orthomolecular Concerning the maintenance of optimal quantities of bodily substances.

orthomorphia The correction of structural deformities.

Orthomyxoviridae [ORTHO- + MYXO- + *vir(us)* + -IDAE] A family of RNA-containing enveloped viruses which includes the influenza viruses.

orthomyxovirus Any virus of the Orthomyxoviridae family. Also called *myxovirus.*

orthoneuron In the organ of Corti, a nerve filament that, leaving its contact with a hair cell, passes straight across the basilar membrane to the spiral ganglion in the modiolus.

orthoneutrophil NEUTROPHIL.

Ortho-Novum An oral contraceptive tablet containing norethindrone and mestranol. A proprietary name.

orthopaedic A British spelling for ORTHOPEDIC.

orthopaedics A British spelling for ORTHOPEDICS.

Orthopantomograph [ORTHO- + PAN- + TOMO- + -GRAPH] A proprietary type of x-ray apparatus used in dental radiology to make orbiting panoramic radiographs.

orthopedic Of or relating to orthopedics.

orthopedics [ORTHO- + Gk *pais* (gen. *paidos*) a child + -ICS] A branch of surgery which deals with the preservation and restoration of function in the musculoskeletal system, particularly the joints and bones, including the alleviation of pain in these structures.

dental orthopedics ORTHODONTICS.

dentofacial orthopedics ORTHODONTICS.

orthopedist ORTHOPEDIC SURGEON.

orthopercussion A method of percussion in which the pleximeter (percussing) finger is held perpendicular to the chest wall.

orthophenanthrolene $C_{12}H_8N_2$. An indicator used in oxidation-reduction measurements.

orthophenolase An enzyme occurring in sweet potatoes and having the ability to oxidize catechol and orthocresol.

orthophony [ORTHO- + PHON- + -Y] The accurate and correct production of the various sound components during speech.

orthophoria [ORTHO- + -PHORIA] Spontaneous accurate alignment of the eyes for a given distance of fixation, without the aid of fusion stimuli.

asthenic orthophoria Precise spontaneous alignment of the eyes in the absence of good fusional convergence amplitude.

orthophoric Pertaining to spontaneous precise alignment of the eyes upon the object of fixation.

orthophosphate Any of the anions, or a salt containing one of them, of orthophosphoric acid, H_3PO_4, or of its esters: used to distinguish the phosphate from those derived from other phosphoric acids, e.g. from diphosphoric acid, $H_4P_2O_7$.

orthophosphoric acid PHOSPHORIC ACID. ● This term is used to distinguish H_3PO_4, the commonest form, from its condensed forms, such as diphosphoric acid, $H_4P_2O_7$, or from its dehydrated form, HPO_3, which is very unstable and exists only as a reaction intermediate.

orthopia [ORTH- + -OPIA] The condition of normal vision and alignment of the eyes.

orthoplast [ORTHO- + -PLAST] A plastic that becomes flexible when heated and rigid when cooled. It is used to make splints that conform to the affected part.

orthoplastocyte   A normal blood platelet.

orthoplessimeter   An instrument previously used in place of the pleximeter finger in orthopercussion.

orthopnea [ORTHO- + -PNEA]   Shortness of breath experienced when lying down. Compare PLATYPNEA.

   two-pillow orthopnea   Orthopnea of sufficient degree to require two pillows during sleep.

orthopneic   Affected by or relating to orthopnea.

orthopnoea   A British spelling for ORTHOPNEA.

orthopoxvirus   A virus of the *Orthopoxvirus* genus of the Poxviridae. Viruses of this genus infect mammals and most of them cause generalized infection with rash. Variola, vaccinia, cowpox, ectromelia, rabbitpox, and monkeypox viruses are included in the genus. The virions are large, enveloped, and brick-shaped. They contain double-stranded DNA and are 90 percent protein with at least 30 recognized polypeptides, including a numer of enzymes. Suspensions of virus agglutinate erythrocytes. The different viruses of the genus are serologically closely related but fine descrimination between species and strains can be made. Vaccinia virus is the type species.

orthopraxis   ORTHOPRAXY.

orthopraxy [ORTHO- + Gk *prax(is)* a doing, action + -Y]   Correction of body and limb deformities by mechanical means. Also called *orthopraxis.*

orthopsychiatry   The division of psychiatry concerned with mental hygiene, prevention of mental disorder, and early detection of developmental deviations.

Orthoptera [ORTHO- + Gk *ptera* (pl. of *pteron* feather) feathers, wings]   A major order of hemimetabolous insects that includes grasshoppers, locusts, katydids, crickets, mantises, and the like.

orthoptic   Designed to improve ocular motility and binocular function; pertaining to orthoptics.

orthoptics [ORTH- + OPTICS]   A method of therapy intended to train the eyes to achieve improved muscle balance and binocular vision.

orthoptist [ORTH- + OPT- + -IST]   A technician who measures ocular motility and binocular function and provides therapy to improve them.

orthoptoscope   A device for presenting various images to the two eyes at various angles.

orthoradiogram [ORTHO- + RADIOGRAM]   ORTHODIAGRAM.

orthoradioscopy   ORTHODIASCOPY.

orthoroentgenography   ORTHODIAGRAPHY.

orthorrhachic   Denoting a lumbar spine held straight by muscle spasm as opposed to exhibiting the normal lordotic curvature.

orthoscope [ORTHO- + -SCOPE]   A stereoscope used for evaluation of relative image size of the two eyes.

orthoscopic   Pertaining to a distortion-free optical system.

orthoscopy [ORTHO- + -SCOPY]   Examination of the eye for visual distortion.

orthoselection   A directional trend in natural selection or evolution.

orthosis [ORTHO- + -SIS]   (*plural* orthoses) A device or appliance worn on the body to correct or prevent joint deformity, provide support for ambulation, reduce pain, diminish weight-bearing force, or assist motion. Also called *orthesis, orthotic.* Adjective: orthotic.

   balanced forearm orthosis   An orthosis that facilitates motion of a weakened shoulder or elbow. It supports the forearm and is attached to a wheelchair through a swivel mechanism.

   double adjustable ankle orthosis   An ankle orthosis with adjustable dorsiflexion and plantar flexion.

   dynamic orthosis   An orthosis that includes movable components activated by the patient or by external power. Also called *lively orthosis.*

   flexible orthosis   An orthosis made of flexible material that provides some support and flexibility.

   functional orthosis   An orthosis constructed to enhance function.

   inductive orthosis   An orthosis used to correct postural problems by causing the patient to assume a better posture.

   lively orthosis   DYNAMIC ORTHOSIS.

   passive orthosis   STATIC ORTHOSIS.

   powered orthosis   Any type of orthosis that utilizes external power to activate movable components.

   spiral foot-ankle orthosis   A plastic spiral orthosis that winds around the leg, from just below the knee to the foot, ending as an arch support.

   standing orthosis   An orthosis that supports the entire lower limb and pelvis to allow standing.

   static orthosis   An orthosis with nonmovable components. Also called *passive orthosis.*

orthoskiagram [ORTHO- + SKIA- + -GRAM]   ORTHODIAGRAM.

orthoskiagraph   ORTHODIAGRAPH.

orthoskiagraphy   ORTHODIASCOPY.

orthostatic   Relating to the erect posture.

orthostatism   The erect position of the torso when standing.

orthostereoscope [ORTHO- + STEREOSCOPE]   An apparatus for viewing stereograms.

orthosympathetic   Pertaining to the sympathetic or thoracolumbar division of the autonomic nervous system as distinct from the parasympathetic or craniosacral division. An outmoded term.

orthotast   An apparatus used for straightening bent bones.

orthoterion   An obsolete instrument used for straightening deformed bones.

orthothanasia   PASSIVE EUTHANASIA.

orthotherapy   Treatment aimed at correcting postural abnormalities.

orthotic   **1** Relating to the use of orthoses or other devices for improving or restoring function in the musculoskeletal system. Also *orthetic.* **2** ORTHOSIS.

orthotics   The speciality relating to orthoses and their use. Also called *orthetics.*

orthotist   A practitioner of orthotics. Also called *orthetist.*

orthotonus   A spasmodic or tetanic contraction of axial muscles causing the body to be held rigid in a straight line.

orthotopia [ORTHO- + *top(o)-* + -IA]   The occurrence of body parts in their usual and normal positions.

orthotopic   **1** Occurring in the normal or usual place; not heterotopic or ectopic. **2** Describing a graft of tissue of a type normally found in the recipient site.

orthotropism   An upward or downward vertical growth response or tropism of organs to a given stimulus.

orthovoltage [ORTHO- + VOLTAGE]   High voltage, as used for x-ray production, in the range of 200 to 300 kilovolts.

Orthoxine   A proprietary name for methoxyphenamine.

orthropsia [Gk *orthr(os)* dawn, early morning + -OPSIA]   Keener vision during dawn or twilight than in bright sunlight, a characteristic of the human eye.

orthuria [ORTH- + -URIA]   Urination at normal, regular intervals.

Ortolani [Marius *Ortolani*, Italian orthopedic surgeon, flourished 20th century]   See under SIGN.

-ory [L -orium, neut. of -orius, suffix denoting a place for] A suffix meaning a place or instrument for (performing an action).

oryzenin A glutelin extracted from rice bran.

OS oculus sinister (left eye).

Os Symbol for the element, osmium.

os¹ [L (gen. oris), the mouth, an opening, the face, speech] (plural ora) **1** [NA] The proximal end of the digestive tract, comprising the oral cavity (cavitas oris), teeth, tongue and palate and communicating externally through the space or fissure between the lips and internally with the oropharynx through the isthmus of the fauces. **2** [NA] The lips and the space between them. For defs. 1 and 2 also called *mouth*. **3** [NA] OSTIUM.

external os of uterus OSTIUM UTERI.

incompetent cervical os An acquired or congenital weakness of the uterine cervix such that a pregnancy cannot be carried beyond the second trimester.

internal os of uterus OS UTERI INTERNUM.

Scanzoni second os PATHOLOGIC RETRACTION RING.

os uteri externum An outmoded term for OSTIUM UTERI.

os uteri internum The opening in the supravaginal part of the cervix uteri communicating with the cavity of the uterus. It corresponds to the surface constriction at the isthmus uteri. An outmoded term. Also called *orificium internum isthmi* (outmoded), *orificium internum uteri* (outmoded), *internal os of uterus*.

os²

os² [L (gen. ossis; akin to Gk osteona bone), a bone, heart, stone] (plural ossa) [NA] A specialized connective tissue in which lamellae of helically arranged collagen fibers are held together by a ground substance impregnated with inorganic salts, providing hardness and rigidity to the tissue, which yet remains plastic; bone. It forms the skeletal framework of the body, supporting and protecting vital organs, serving as a store for calcium, and providing attachment to muscles and ligaments involved in locomotion. The defined units, or bones, consist of an outer compact layer and an inner spongy layer containing marrow, and they are surrounded by a vascular layer, or periosteum. Bones are classified into long, short, flat, and irregular bones.

os acetabuli Either of two secondary centers of ossification appearing in the triradiate cartilage of the acetabulum of the hip bone at about the twelfth year. One may appear anteriorly between pubis and ilium, and another posteriorly between ilium and ischium, becoming fused with each other and with the rest of the ossifying triradiate cartilage. Also called *cotyloid bone, Krause's bone, acetabular nucleus, acetabular bone*.

os acromiale An acromion separated from the spine of the scapula due to failure of fusion, occurring in about five percent of individuals. Also called *acromiale os*.

os acromiale secundarium A rounded structure seen on x ray above the greater tubercle of the humerus. Also called *acromiale os secundarium*.

os basilare **1** The basisphenoid and basioccipital bones considered together. **2** PARS BASILARIS OSSIS OCCIPITALIS.

os basioticum An accessory ossicle resulting from the development of a separate center of ossification between the basioccipital and sphenoid bones. Also called *os prebasioccipitale*.

os breve [NA] A type of bone the three dimensions of which are approximately equal and that is characterized by compactness, many articular surfaces, and limited mobility, as those of the carpus and tarsus. Also called *short bone*.

os calcis CALCANEUS.

os capitatum [NA] The largest bone of the carpus, situated in the distal row between the trapezoid and hamate bones and presenting a rounded proximal and lateral portion, or head, for articulation with the lunate and scaphoid bones, and a distal cubical portion for the bases of the second, third, and fourth metacarpal bones. Also called *capitate, capitate bone, os magnum* (outmoded), *os carpale distale tertium* (outmoded), *capitatum, third carpal bone, great carpal bone* (outmoded), *capitate* (imprecise).

os carpale distale primum An outmoded term for OS TRAPEZIUM.

os carpale distale quartum An outmoded term for OS HAMATUM.

os carpale distale secundum An outmoded term for OS TRAPEZOIDEUM.

os carpale distale tertium An outmoded term for OS CAPITATUM.

ossa carpalia OSSA CARPI.

ossa carpi [NA] The eight bones of the carpus, or wrist, arranged in two rows and including os scaphoideum, os lunatum, os triquetrum, os pisiforme, os trapezium, os trapezoideum, os capitatum, and os hamatum. Also called *carpal bones, ossa carpalia*.

os centrale [NA] An additional cartilaginous nodule occasionally found in the wrist of a two month old fetus that usually fuses with the cartilaginous scaphoid but may remain separate as a bony nodule on the dorsum of the wrist between the trapezoid, capitate, and scaphoid bones. It occurs normally in many mammals. Also called *central bone, accessory multangular bone, central carpal bone, os centrale of wrist*.

os centrale tarsi An outmoded term for OS NAVICULARE.

os centrale of wrist OS CENTRALE.

os clitoridis A heterotopic bone in the clitoris of some mammals, analogous to the os penis in the male.

os coccygis [NA] A small triangular bone, the base of which articulates with the apex of the sacrum at the distal end of the vertebral column. It comprises four, and sometimes five, rudimentary vertebrae fused in the adult to form a curved bone, the apex of which is directed distally and anteriorly. It represents the skeleton of the tail in humans. Also called *coccyx, coccygeal bone, cuckoo bone, coccygeal column* (outmoded).

os cordis A three-pronged, heterotopic bone found in the heart of deer and bovids.

os coronae CORONARY BONE.

os coronale CORONARY BONE.

os costale [NA] One of the 24 curved, narrow bones that are arranged in 12 pairs on either side of the thoracic vertebrae; rib. Each comprises a head, neck, and body, the latter presenting a tubercle at its junction with the neck, an angle posteriorly, and a groove along its inferior margin internally. They extend anteriorly from the thoracic vertebrae to the sternum to form the skeletal thorax. Also called *costal bone, costa*.

os coxae [NA] A large irregularly-shaped bone articulating posteriorly with the sacrum and anteriorly with its opposite fellow to form the bony walls of the pelvis. It is composed of three bones, the pubis, ilium, and ischium that are fused in the adult at a central constriction, the acetabulum, which articulates with the head of the femur in the hip joint. Also called *hip bone, innominate bone* (outmoded), *os innominatum* (outmoded), *pelvic bone, coxa, innominatum*.

ossa cranii [NA] The eight bones of the cerebral cranium, comprising an occipital, two parietal, two temporal, a frontal, a sphenoid, and an ethmoid bone. Also called *cranial bones, bones of cranium, bones of cerebral cranium, bones of skull*.

os cuboideum [NA] An irregular cubical bone on the lateral side of the distal row of the tarsus, articulating with the calcaneus proximally, the fourth and fifth metatarsal bones distally, and the lateral cuneiform and navicular bones medially. Also called *cuboid bone, os tarsale distale quartum* (outmoded), *cuboides.*

os cuneiforme intermedium [NA] A wedge-shaped bone of the distal row of the tarsus, possessing a square dorsal surface and lying between the medial and the lateral cuneiform bones while it articulates proximally with the navicular bone and distally with the base of the second metatarsal bone. Also called *intermediate cuneiform bone, os cuneiforme secundum* (outmoded), *mesocuneiform bone, middle cuneiform bone, second cuneiform bone, second tarsal bone, os tarsale distale secundum* (outmoded), *mesocuneiform.*

os cuneiforme laterale [NA] A wedge-shaped bone in the distal row of the tarsus situated between the intermediate cuneiform and cuboid bones while it articulates proximally with the navicular bone and distally with the base of the third metatarsal bone. Its dorsal surface is rectangular, and the plantar surface forms a narrow edge. Also called *lateral cuneiform bone, os cuneiforme tertium* (outmoded), *third cuneiform bone, ectocuneiform bone, external cuneiform bone, third tarsal bone, os tarsale distale tertium* (outmoded), *ectocuneiform* (outmoded), *ectosphenoid* (outmoded).

os cuneiforme mediale [NA] The medial bone of the distal row of the tarsus, shaped like a large wedge with its base plantarward and its apex dorsal and situated between the navicular bone proximally and the base of the first metatarsal bone distally. Lateral to it is the intermediate cuneiform bone. Also called *medial cuneiform bone, os cuneiforme primum* (outmoded), *first cuneiform bone, entocuneiform bone* (outmoded), *internal cuneiform bone, first tarsal bone, os tarsale distale primum* (outmoded), *entocuneiform.*

os cuneiforme primum An outmoded term for OS CUNEIFORME MEDIALE.

os cuneiforme secundum An outmoded term for OS CUNEIFORME INTERMEDIUM.

os cuneiforme tertium An outmoded term for OS CUNEIFORME LATERALE.

ossa digitorum manus [NA] The fourteen bones, or phalanges, that constitute the skeleton of the digits of the hand. Each finger has a proximal, middle, and distal phalanx, except the thumb, which only has a proximal and a distal phalanx. Also called *phalanges of fingers, phalanges digitorum manus* (outmoded), *phalangeal bones of hand, bones of fingers.*

ossa digitorum pedis [NA] The fourteen bones, or phalanges, that constitute the skeleton of the digits of the foot. Each toe has a proximal, middle, and distal phalanx, except the great toe, which only has a proximal and a distal phalanx. Also called *phalanges of toes, phalanges digitorum pedis* (outmoded), *bones of toes, phalangeal bones of foot.*

os entomion A sutural bone occurring at the entomion.

os epitympanicum The occasional separate posterior portion of the ossification center of the squamous part of the temporal bone. It forms some mastoid air cells that may be separated by a plate of bone from the deeper cells in the petrous part. An outmoded term.

os ethmoidale [NA] A cube-shaped bone situated in the base of the skull anteriorly between the orbital parts of the frontal bone below the ethmoidal notch, which is occupied by the cribriform plate that roofs the ethmoid bone. It takes part in the formation of the medial walls of the orbits, as well as of the roof, lateral walls, and septum of the nasal cavity and the anterior cranial fossa. It comprises the cribriform plate, the perpendicular plate, and two lateral masses, or labyrinths, enclosing air cells. Also called *ethmoid bone, cribriform bone, ethmoid.*

ossa extremitatis inferioris An outmoded term for OSSA MEMBRI INFERIORIS.

ossa extremitatis superioris An outmoded term for OSSA MEMBRI SUPERIORIS.

ossa faciei The bones forming the skeleton of the facial part of the skull or visceral cranium and surrounding the orbits (in part), the nose, and the mouth. They include the paired maxilla, zygomatic, lacrimal, palatine, nasal, and inferior nasal concha and the unpaired mandible and vomer, as well as the hyoid bone and the malleus, incus, and stapes of the tympanic cavity. Also called *facial bones, bones of face.*

os falciforme A crescent-shaped heterotopic bone that supports the extra digit in the forelimb of moles.

ossa fonticulorum Sutural bones located at the sites of fetal fontanels or fonticuli.

os frontale [NA] The large, curved bone that has a vertical portion, or squama, forming the forehead above the skeleton of the face while its horizontal, or orbital, portion extends posteriorly from the inferior or supraorbital margin of the squama on each side to form most of the roof of each orbital cavity. The central part of the inferior margin is the nasal portion that articulates with the nasal bones and forms part of the roof of the nasal cavity. The posterior, or parietal, margin of the squama articulates with the parietal bones and the greater wings of the sphenoid bone, while the posterior margin of the orbital portion articulates with the lesser wings of the sphenoid bone. Between the orbital portions and behind the nasal portion is the ethmoidal notch. Also called *frontal bone.*

os hamatum [NA] A wedge-shaped carpal bone with a hook-like process, or hamulus, projecting from its palmar surface. It is located at the medial side of the distal row of carpal bones, its triangular proximal aspect lying between the triquetrum medially and the capitate laterally, while the apex articulates with the lunate. The broad distal surface articulates with the bases of the fourth and fifth metacarpal bones. The laterally directed concave surface of the hamulus bounds the carpal tunnel, while the deep branch of the ulnar nerve grooves its base distally. Also called *hamate bone, unciform bone, uncinate bone, os carpale distale quartum, fourth carpal bone, hamatum, hamate, uncinatum* (outmoded), *unciforme* (outmoded), *unciform.*

os hyoideum [NA] A U-shaped bone situated in the anterior part of the neck between the base of the tongue and the larynx and suspended from the styloid processes of the temporal bones by the stylohyoid ligaments. Below, it is connected to the thyroid cartilage by the thyrohyoid membrane. It is divided into a body and two pairs of processes, the greater and lesser cornua. Also called *hyoid bone, lingual bone, tongue bone, hyoid.*

os ilii [NA] The quadrangular upper blade of the hip bone that is divided into an upper curved and flattened wing, or ala, and a body, or corpus, inferiorly, forming the upper two-fifths of the acetabulum. The ala presents three surfaces, namely, gluteal, sacropelvic, and the iliac fossa. It is a separate bone at birth but later fuses with the pubis and the ischium. Also called *ilium, iliac bone, flank bone.*

os incae An outmoded term for OS INTERPARIETALE.

os incisivum [NA] A paired and separate bone anterior to the maxilla in most vertebrates, but in humans one secondary center of ossification appears above the incisor tooth germs and becomes overgrown by bone from the rest of the maxilla that fuses anteriorly with the alveolar process so that no separate bone is apparent after the third month of fetal life. In postnatal life, suturelike grooves may be apparent passing from the floor of the nasal cavity medially on each side of the incisive canal as well as from the incisive fossa to the alveolar bone between the lateral incisor and canine teeth, thus delimiting the area representing the separate bone. Also called *incisive bone, premaxilla, premaxillary bone, os intermaxillare* (outmoded), *intermaxillary* *bone, os premaxillare, Goethe's bone, intermaxilla.*

os innominatum An outmoded term for OS COXAE.

os in os The radiographic pattern, seen most often in osteopetrosis, formed by continuous lines of radiodensity within bone and resembling a miniature model of the bone concentric to the cortex. An outmoded term.

os intercuneiforme An additional bone occasionally situated between the medial and the intermediate cuneiform bones.

os interfrontale An occasional sutural bone located in the lower part of the metopic suture.

os intermaxillare An outmoded term for OS INCISIVUM.

os intermedium An outmoded term for OS LUNATUM.

os intermetatarseum An occasional additional bone occurring on the dorsum of the foot in the angle between the medial cuneiform and the first and second metatarsal bones.

os interparietale [NA] The interparietal portion of the occipital squama above the highest nuchal line when it remains separated from the rest of the occipital bone throughout life. Also called *interparietal bone, os incae* (outmoded), *incarial bone, proper epactal bone* (outmoded), *inca bone, superior occipital squama* (outmoded).

os ischii [NA] The posteroinferior portion of the hip bone, comprising a body, or corpus, and a ramus. It is a separate bone at birth but later fuses with the pubis and the ilium. Also called *ischium, ischial bone, chancebone.*

os japonicum A zygomatic bone that is divided into two or three parts, a condition stated to occur more commonly (about 7%) among Japanese than other populations.

os lacrimale [NA] One of two delicate bones, the smallest in the face, which is quadrilateral in shape and situated at the front end of the medial wall of each orbit. It has a lateral, or orbital, surface and a medial, or nasal, surface as well as four borders, namely, anterior, posterior, superior, and inferior. They articulate with the frontal process of the maxilla, the orbital plate of the ethmoid bone, the frontal bone, and the orbital surface of the maxilla, respectively. Also called *lacrimal bone, os unguis* (outmoded).

os longum [NA] Any of the elongated bones of the limbs in which the length exceeds the breadth, reflecting the degree of power and speed in movement. It consists of a tubular shaft, or diaphysis, containing a medullary cavity, and two expanded ends, or epiphyses, which develop from separate centers of ossification and are usually articular. Also called *long bone.*

os lunatum [NA] A crescent-shaped bone in the middle of the proximal row of the carpal bones lying between the scaphoid on the lateral side and the triquetral on its medial side. Its convex proximal surface articulates with the radius and the articular disk of the inferior radioulnar joint, while its concave distal surface articulates with the head of the capitate bone. Also called *lunate bone, intermediate bone* (outmoded), *intermediate carpal bone* (outmoded), *semilunar bone, os intermedium, semilunare* (outmoded), *lunare* (outmoded), *lunate.*

os magnum An outmoded term for OS CAPITATUM.

os mastoideum An outmoded term for PARS MASTOIDEA OSSIS TEMPORALIS.

ossa membri inferioris [NA] The skeleton of the lower limb including the pelvic girdle, composed of the hip bones, and the bones of the free inferior limb, namely, os femoris, patella, tibia, fibula, tarsals, metatarsals, and the phalanges of the digits. Also called *bones of lower limb, ossa extremitatis inferioris* (outmoded).

ossa membri superioris [NA] The skeleton of the upper limb, composed of the pectoral girdle, comprising the clavicle and the scapula, and the bones of the free superior limb, namely, humerus, radius, ulna, carpals, metacarpals, and phalanges of digits. Also called *bones of upper limb, ossa extremitatis superioris* (outmoded).

ossa metacarpi I-V [NA] The five cylindrical miniature long bones forming the skeleton of the palm of the hand, numbered from lateral to medial side, each having a rounded head or caput at the distal extremity, a shaft, or corpus, and an expanded base, or basis, at the proximal extremity. The bases articulate with the carpal bones, while each head articulates with the base of a proximal phalanx. The heads produce the prominent knuckles when the hand is clenched. Also called *metacarpal bones, basalia* (rarely used).

ossa metatarsi I-V [NA] The five cylindrical miniature long bones at the front end of the foot, numbered from medial to lateral side, each having a rounded head, or caput, at the distal extremity, a shaft, or corpus, and an expanded base at the proximal extremity. The heads articulate with the proximal phalanges of their respective digits, while the bases articulate with each other and with the distal row of tarsal bones. Also called *metatarsal bones, metacarpal bones.*

os multangulum majus An outmoded term for OS TRAPEZIUM.

os multangulum minus An outmoded term for OS TRAPEZOIDEUM.

os nasale [NA] One of two small oblong bones that lie parallel to each other contiguously between the frontal processes of the maxillae and below the nasal part of the frontal bone to form the bridge of the nose. Inferiorly each is attached to the lateral nasal cartilage. Also called *nasal bone.*

os naviculare [NA] A flattened, oval bone interposed on the medial side between the proximal and distal rows of tarsal bones, that is, between the head of talus proximally and the cuneiform bones distally. The dorsal surface is convex from side to side, while the plantar surface is concave and ends in the enlarged prolongation or tuberosity of the medial surface. Also called *navicular bone, os centrale tarsi* (outmoded), *os naviculare pedis* (outmoded), *navicular bone of foot, scaphoid bone of foot* (outmoded).

os naviculare manus An outmoded term for OS SCAPHOIDEUM.

os naviculare pedis An outmoded term for OS NAVICULARE.

os naviculare pedis retardatum KÖHLER'S DISEASE.

os novum New bone formed from implanted periosteum.

os occipitale [NA] A curved, trapezoidal bone forming a large part of the back and base of the cranium and comprising four parts, namely, the squamous part above and behind the foramen magnum, the basilar part in front of the foramen magnum, and a lateral part on each side of the foramen magnum. The external surface is convex and the internal surface is concave. It articulates with the two parietal and the two temporal bones on either side, with the sphenoid bone anteriorly, and by its condyles with the atlas inferiorly. Also called *occipital bone.*

os odontoideum The dens of the axis that does not fuse with and remains separated from the body of the axis.

os orbiculare 1 An outmoded term for PROCESSUS LENTICULARIS INCUDIS. 2 An outmoded term for OS PISIFORME.

os orbitale The upper portion of a bipartite zygomatic bone.

os palpebrae A heterotopic bone embedded in the eyelids of crocodilians.

os palatinum [NA] One of a pair of L-shaped bones that helps to form the back of the hard palate and floor of the nasal cavity with its horizontal plate, the lateral wall of the nasal cavity with its perpendicular plate that lies between the maxilla and the medial plate of pterygoid process, and the back of the floor of the orbit with its orbital process. At the junction of the horizontal and the perpendicular plates is the pyramidal process, while at the top of the perpendicular plate are the orbital and sphenoidal processes with the sphenopalatine notch between them. Also called *palatine bone, palate bone.*

os parietale [NA] One of two irregularly quadrangular bones forming a large part of the vault and sides of the cranium, each having a convex external surface and a concave internal surface. There are four margins, namely, sagittal, frontal, occipital, and squamosal; and four angles, namely, frontal, sphenoidal, occipital, and mastoid. Also called *parietal bone, bregmatic bone.*

os pedis PEDAL BONE.

os penis A heterotopic bone that supports the penis in many mammals. Also called *baculum.*

os peroneum A sesamoid bone occasionally found in the tendon of peroneus longus either behind the lateral malleolus or adjacent to the calcaneus or the cuboid bone.

os pisiforme [NA] A small pea-shaped bone with a flattened dorsal surface with which it articulates with the triquetral bone. Its rough palmar surface provides attachment for the flexor retinaculum and abductor digiti minimi muscles and the tendon of flexor carpi ulnaris and its extensions, the pisohamate and pisometacarpal ligaments of which give it the appearance of being a sesamoid bone. Also called *pisiform bone, lentiform bone* (outmoded), *lenticular bone of hand* (outmoded), *postulnar bone* (outmoded), *os orbiculare* (outmoded), *pisiform.*

os planum **1** [NA] A type of bone that is platelike, such as some of the bones of the cranium that comprise an inner and an outer compact layer, or table, between which is a layer of trabecular bone, the diploë. However, in the scapula, sternum, and ribs the two layers of compact bone enclose a thin marrow space. Also called *flat bone, tabular bone.* **2** An outmoded term for LAMINA ORBITALIS OSSIS ETHMOIDALIS.

os pneumaticum Any bone containing air-filled cavities or sinuses. Also called *pneumatic bone.*

os prebasioccipitale OS BASIOTICUM.

os premaxillare OS INCISIVUM.

os priapi OS PENIS.

os pubis [NA] The anteroinferior portion of the hip bone, comprising a body, or corpus, from which the superior ramus extends backward and upward and the inferior ramus extends backward and downward. The medial surface of the body meets that of the opposite side at the symphysis pubis. It is a separate bone at birth but later becomes fused with os ilium and os ischii. Also called *pubic bone, pubis.*

os purum Bone detached from surrounding connective tissue suitable for bone grafting.

os radiale An outmoded term for OS SCAPHOIDEUM.

os sacrum [NA] A large triangular bone formed by the fusion of the five sacral vertebrae at the base of the vertebral column and lying between the hip bones at the posterosuperior aspect of the pelvic cavity. Its broad base articulates superiorly with the fifth lumbar vertebra, while its apex articulates inferiorly with the coccyx. The auricular surface at the anterosuperior end of the lateral surface articulates with the ilium at the sacroiliac joint. In the erect posture it is directed posteroinferiorly and its convex posterior surface provides attachment for powerful muscles and ligaments, while its concave pelvic surface has four pairs of pelvic sacral foramina that communicate with the sacral canal. Also called *sacrum, sacral bone, resurrection bone, great terminal vertebra* (outmoded), *vertebra magnum* (outmoded), *sacral column* (outmoded).

os scaphoideum [NA] The largest bone in the proximal row of the carpal bones, situated on the lateral side with its convex proximal surface articulating with the radius and its convex distal surface articulating with the trapezium and trapezoid bones. The medial surface has a concave facet for the capitate bone as well as a crescentic facet for the lunate bone. The palmar surface has a tubercle for the attachment of the flexor retinaculum and abductor pollicis brevis muscle. The radial collateral ligament of the wrist is attached to its lateral surface. Also called *scaphoid bone, os naviculare manus* (outmoded), *navicular bone of hand, scaphoid bone of hand, radial carpal bone, os radiale*

(outmoded), *shuttle bone* (outmoded), *navicular bone* (outmoded), *scaphoid.*

os sedentarium An outmoded term for TUBER ISCHIADICUM.

ossa sesamoidea [NA] Ovoid nodules of varying sizes and shapes that are partly or completely ossified and found usually in tendons passing over either articular surfaces or sharply angulated bones. The surface of the nodule in relation to these surfaces is covered by articular cartilage, thereby modifying pressure, diminishing friction and possibly affecting the direction of action of the muscle. These nodules may also occur in the capsule of a joint or in a tendon unrelated to a joint or bony surface. They tend to ossify late, often only postpubertally. Also called *sesamoid bones.*

ossa sesamoidea manus [NA] Sesamoid bones in the hand that are usually limited to tendons passing over the palmar aspects of joints, as in the adductor pollicis and flexor pollicis brevis muscles over the head of the first metacarpal bone, where nodules are also present in the capsule. They may also be encountered in front of the metacarpophalangeal joints of the other fingers. Also called *sesamoid bones of hand.*

ossa sesamoidea pedis [NA] Sesamoid bones that are usually found, analogously to those in the hand, articulating with the plantar aspect of the head of a metatarsal or, less commonly, of a phalanx, such as the pair of nodules in the tendons of the flexor hallucis brevis muscle on the plantar aspect of the metatarsophalangeal joint of the great toe, as well as in the capsules over the other metatarsophalangeal joints and the interphalangeal joint of the great toe. Sesamoid bones may also occur in the tendons of peroneus longus adjacent to the calcaneus and the cuboid bones, of the tibialis anterior muscle over the medial cuneiform bone, and of tibialis posterior over the medial surface of the head of the talus. Also called *sesamoid bones of foot.*

os sphenoidale [NA] An irregular bone occupying a central position in the base of the skull in front of the temporal bones and the basilar part of the occipital bone and taking part in the formation of the floor of the anterior, middle, and posterior cranial fossae, as well as of the nasal cavity and orbit and of the infratemporal and temporal fossae. It consists of a central portion or body, two greater and two lesser wings, which extend outward from the sides of the body, and two pterygoid processes that hang down from the junctions of the body and the greater wings. Also called *sphenoid bone, alar bone, azyges, suprapharyngeal bone* (outmoded), *cavilla* (outmoded), *sphenoid.*

os styloideum The prominent styloid process of the third metacarpal bone when it occasionally develops a separate center of ossification and persists as a distinct ossicle not fusing with the base of the metacarpal bone.

os subtibiale An additional small bone, rarely found, in the region of the tip of the medial malleolus of the tibia.

os suffraginis The first or proximal phalanx, phalanx proximalis, of the horse. An outmoded term.

ossa suprasternalia [NA] Ossicles that occasionally develop in the ligaments of the sternoclavicular articulation along the upper margin of the manubrium sterni. Also called *suprasternal bones, Breschet's bones, episternal bones, episternal ossicles.*

ossa suturalia [NA] Irregular, isolated bones or ossicles situated in the course of the sutures of the skull, the lambdoid suture being the most commonly involved, and over the sites of fetal fontanels. They develop from extra centers of ossification, and are often symmetrical on the two sides. Also called *ossa suturarum, sutural bones, epactal bones, wormian bones, ossa wormi* (outmoded), *Andernach's ossicles* (outmoded), *epactal ossicles* (outmoded), *intercalcar ossicles* (outmoded), *wormian ossicles* (outmoded), *true wormian bones* (outmoded), *wormian bones of the sutures.*

ossa suturarum OSSA SUTURALIA.

os tarsale distale primum An outmoded term for OS CU-NEIFORME MEDIALE.

os tarsale distale quartum An outmoded term for OS CU-BOIDEUM.

os tarsale distale secundum An outmoded term for OS CU-NEIFORME INTERMEDIUM.

os tarsale distale tertium An outmoded term for OS CUNEI-FORME LATERALE.

ossa tarsalia An outmoded term for OSSA TARSI.

ossa tarsi [NA] The bones of the ankle, or tarsus, that are grouped in a proximal row consisting of talus and calcaneus, and a distal row consisting of the medial, intermediate, and lateral cuneiform bones and the cuboid bone, while interposed between the rows on the medial side is the navicular bone. Their shapes vary greatly, partly dependent on their functions in weight bearing and maintenance of the arches of the foot. Also called *tarsal bones, ossa tarsalia* (outmoded).

os tarsi fibulare An outmoded term for CALCANEUS.

os tarsi tibiale An outmoded term for TALUS.

os temporale [NA] One of a pair of bones located at the side and the base of the cranium and composed of three parts: the anterosuperior thin squamous part (pars squamosa) forming part of the lateral wall of the cranium; the dense pyramidal petrous part (pars petrosa) wedged between the sphenoid and occipital bones at the base of the skull; and the curved quadri-lateral platelike tympanic part (pars tympanica) situated below the squamous part and in front of the mastoid process and contributing to the wall of the tympanic cavity and the external acoustic meatus. In addition, the styloid process develops from the back of the hyoid bone in association with the petrous part and fuses with the floor of the tympanic cavity. The three parts are distinct at birth but fuse later to form one bone. Also called *temporal bone*.

os tibiale externum OS TIBIALE POSTERIUS.

os tibiale posterius A sesamoid bone that may occur in the tendon of the tibialis posterior muscle, where it plays over the medial side of the head of the talus. It usually occurs late in life and may fuse with the tuberosity of the navicular. Also called *os tibiale posticum, tibiale externum, tibiale posticum, os tibiale externum*.

os tibiale posticum OS TIBIALE POSTERIUS.

os trapezium [NA] An irregular oblong bone situated lat-erally in the distal row of the carpal bones and articulating proximally with the scaphoid and distally by a saddle-shaped facet with the base of the first metacarpal. Its medial surface articulates with the trapezoid bone. It is characterized by a tubercle for the attachment of muscles and the flexor retinacu-lum and by a groove for the flexor carpi radialis tendon on its palmar surface. Also called *trapezium bone, os multangulum majus* (outmoded), *greater multangular bone, trapezoid bone of Lyser, os carpale distale primum, first carpal bone, trapezium, multangulum majus* (outmoded).

os trapezoideum [NA] A small triangular bone in the distal row of the carpal bones wedged between the trapezium laterally, the capitate medially, the base of the second metacarpal distally and the scaphoid proximally. Also called *trapezoid bone, os multangulum minus* (outmoded), *lesser multangular bone* (out-moded), *trapezium bone of Lyser, lesser trapezium bone, os car-pale distale secundum, second carpal bone, trapezoid, multan-gulum minus* (outmoded).

os triangulare **1** OS TRIGONUM. **2** OS TRIQUETRUM.

os tribasilare A synostotic bone resulting from fusion of the occipital, temporal, and sphenoid bones at the base of the skull in infancy, which may eventuate in shortening of the base.

os trigonum [NA] A small accessory bone in the foot that occasionally develops when an additional primary center of ossification forms in the lateral tubercle of the posterior process

of the talus and remains separate from the rest of the talus or joined to it by cartilage. Also called *triangular bone of tarsus, os triangulare*.

os triquetrum [NA] A pyramidal bone on the medial side of the proximal row of the carpal bones, the base of which is directed proximally to articulate with the lunate, while the distal apex is rough for the attachment of the ulnar collateral ligament of the wrist joint. The medial surface moves against the articular disk in full adduction, and the lateral surface articulates with the hamate. On its palmar surface is the characteristic oval facet for articulation with the pisiform bone. Also called *triquetral bone, os triangulare, triangular bone, cubital bone, cuneiform bone of carpus, pyramidal bone, ulnar carpal bone, cubitale* (outmoded), *pyramidale* (outmoded), *triquetrum, ulnare* (out-moded).

os unguis An outmoded term for OS LACRIMALE.

os vesalianum An accessory bone sometimes located in the angle between the base of the fifth metacarpal and the hamate. Also called *vesalian bone*.

os vesalianum pedis An occasional additional ossicle in the foot produced by separation of the tuberosity of the base of a fifth metatarsal bone in which a separated center of ossification had developed. Also called *vesalian bone, vesalianum*.

ossa wormi An outmoded term for OSSA SUTURALIA.

os zygomaticum [NA] A roughly quadrilateral bone forming the prominence of the cheek and completing the zygomatic arch. Its frontal process articulates with the zygomatic process of the frontal bone, thereby completing part of the margin, floor, and wall of the orbit. Besides an orbital surface, it also presents a convex external, or lateral, and a temporal surface. Also called *zygomatic bone, yoke bone* (outmoded), *jugal bone, mala, malar bone, cheek bone, zygoma, orbital bone* (outmoded), *cheekbone*.

---

osazone A compound formed by reaction of a reducing sugar, aldose or ulose, with phenylhydrazine. In the reaction C-2 of the aldose and C-1 of the ulose are oxidized to give a second carbonyl group, and both carbonyl groups then form hydra-zones, so that the product contains the grouping —C(=N—NH—Ph)—CH=N—NH—Ph. Osazones have characteristic crystal forms and were previously much used in identifying particular sugars.

oscedo YAWN.

osch- OSCHEO-.

oschea SCROTUM.

oscheal Referring to the scrotum.

oscheitis [Gk *osche(o)*- + -ITIS] Inflammation of the scrotum. Also called *oschitis*.

oschelephantiasis [OSCH- + ELEPHANTIASIS] Elephantiasis affecting the scrotum.

oscheo- [Gk *oscheon* scrotum] A combining form denoting the scrotum. Also *osch-*.

oscheocele [OSCHEO- + -CELE¹] **1** A tumor affecting the scro-tum. **2** SCROTAL HERNIA. **3** OSCHEOMA.

oscheohydrocele SCROTAL HYDROCELE.

oscheolith [OSCHEO- + -LITH] A calculous mass in the seba-ceous glands of the scrotum.

oscheoma [*osche(o)*- + -OMA] A tumor of the scrotum. Also called *oscheocele, oscheoncus*.

oscheoncus OSCHEOMA.

oscheoplasty [OSCHEO- + -PLASTY] A reconstructive, repar-ative, or plastic operation of the scrotum.

oschitis OSCHEITIS.

oscillation [L *oscillatio* (from *oscillatus*, past part. of *oscillare* to swing) a swinging] **1** A regular back and forth movement, as of a pendulum, in a periodic sequence. Also called *vibration*. **2** A variation or perturbation, as a periodic change in population density. **3** A variance between extremes which might be periodic, as in an electric oscillator. See also CYCLE.

bradykinetic oscillation Choreiform movements occurring in encephalitis lethargica.

damped oscillation An oscillation whose amplitude decreases with time because of dissipation of energy in the system.

oscillator An electrical circuit for producing alternating current, especially at audio and radio frequencies.

oscillogram A record of the display from an oscillograph or oscilloscope.

oscillograph [L *oscill(are)* (from *oscillum* a swing) to swing + *o* + -GRAPH] A measuring instrument that permanently records voltage variations as a function of time. It usually contains a galvanometer, which deflects a light beam or a direct-writing pen, and moving paper, as in an electrocardiograph.

oscillometer [L *oscill(um)* a swing + *o* + -METER] An instrument for measuring oscillations, especially those recorded from blood-pressure fluctuations during sphygmomanometry.

oscillometric Relating to oscillometry or to the use of an oscillometer.

oscillometry [L *oscill(are)* to swing + *o* + -METRY] The measurement of oscillations.

oscillopsia A condition in which the visual image is seen to move rapidly from side to side or vertically.

oscilloscope [L *oscill(are)* (from *oscillum* a swing) to swing + *o* + -SCOPE] A measuring instrument that transiently displays voltage variations, usually as a function of time. The voltage deflects a cathode-ray beam, which causes illumination of the fluorescent screen.

Oscinidae CHLOROPIDAE.

Oscinis pallipes HIPPELATES PALLIPES.

oscitancy [L *oscitans*, pres. part. of *oscitare* (from *os* mouth + *citare* to impel) to yawn + -Y] YAWNING.

oscitant [L *oscitans*, gen. *oscitantis*, pres. part. of *oscitare* to yawn] Concerning yawning.

oscitate YAWN.

oscitation [L *oscitatio* (from *oscitatus*, past part. of *oscitare* to yawn) a yawning] YAWNING.

osculum [L, a little mouth, dim. of *os* mouth] A small aperture or pore.

-ose[1] [L *-osus*, a combining form meaning full of, possessing] A suffix meaning having, characterized by, or full of.

-ose[2] [French *(gluc)ose* (alteration of Gk *gleukos* sweet new wine, from *glykys* sweet) a glucide of sweet taste contained in certain fruits] A combining form designating a sugar. If applied directly to a numerical prefix, as in *octose*, it signifies the aldose sugar with the specified number of carbon atoms. The ending is modified to indicate various derivatives; for example, its replacement with *-itol* signifies the sugar alcohol obtained by reduction of the —CHO group in an aldose to —CH_2OH, or the —CO— group in a ketose to —CHOH—. Thus D-mannitol can be formed by the reduction of D-mannose or of D-fructose.

Oseretsky [N. I. *Oseretsky*, Russian psychologist, flourished 20th century] Lincoln-Oseretsky Motor Development Scale. See under SCALE.

Osgood [Robert Bayley *Osgood*, U.S. orthopedic surgeon, 1873–1956] Schlatter-Osgood disease. See under OSGOOD-SCHLATTER DISEASE.

Osiander [Johann Friedrich *Osiander*, German obstetrician, flourished early 19th century] See under SIGN.

-osis [Gk suffix *-sis* denoting state or condition] A suffix meaning (1) state, condition, or process; (2) diseased or abnormal

condition; (3) formation, production, or increase.

osladin A steroid saponin occurring in the rhizomes of *Polypodium vulgare* that is a sugar substitute.

Osler [Sir William *Osler*, Canadian-born physician active in the United States and England, 1849–1919] **1** Osler nodes, Osler sign. See under NODE. **2** Rendu-Osler-Weber syndrome, Rendu-Osler-Weber disease, Osler's disease, Osler-Weber-Rendu disease. See under HEREDITARY HEMORRHAGIC TELANGIECTASIA. **3** See under TRIAD. **4** Osler's disease, Osler-Vasquez disease. See under POLYCYTHEMIA VERA.

osm Symbol for the unit, osmole.

osmatic OLFACTORY.

osmesis A seldom used term for OLFACTION.

osmesthesia [*osm(o)-*[2] + -ESTHESIA] The sense of smell.

osmic acid OsO_4. Osmium tetroxide, which can form salts with alkali. It is used to oxidize alkenes to 1,2-diols in organic chemistry.

osmicate To treat with osmium tetroxide, as in preparation for electron microscopy.

osmication The process of treating with osmium tetroxide. Also called *osmification*.

osmics A rarely used term for OLFACTOLOGY.

osmidrosis BROMHIDROSIS.

osmification OSMICATION.

osmiophilic Having the property of reducing osmium tetroxide to its black, lower oxide.

osmiophobic Descriptive of a substance that does not reduce osmium tetroxide.

osmium Element number 76, having atomic weight 190.2. Found associated with platinum and other metals, osmium is one of the heaviest elements known (specific gravity, 22.61). The metal in solid form is not affected by air, but the powdered and sintered metal gives off exceedingly toxic fumes of osmium tetroxide. Symbol: Os.

osmium tetroxide An expensive, toxic chemical that is used for both its staining and fixative properties in electron microscopy. It is reduced to the black lower oxide by both protein and lipid substances. Also called *perosmic acid*.

osmo-[1] [Gk *ōsmos* (from *ōthein* push) impulsion] A combining form denoting osmosis.

osmo-[2] [Gk *osmē* odor, smell, scent] A combining form meaning smell, scent.

osmoceptor OSMORECEPTOR.

osmoconformer A cell having an internal osmotic pressure that varies with the osmotic pressure of its environment. Compare OSMOREGULATOR.

osmol Symbol for osmole.

osmolagnia [OSMO-[2] + Gk *lagneia* lust, desire] OSPHRESIOLAGNIA.

osmolal [*osmol(e)* + -AL] Having a concentration of one osmole per kilogram of solution.

osmolality [OSMOLAL + -ITY] The concentration of a solution in osmolal units.

calculated serum osmolality A figure for serum osmolality derived from the measured levels of solutes which determine osmolality, especially the electrolytes, glucose, urea, and the serum proteins. Different formulas can be used according to the degree of accuracy desired and the number of measurements available.

osmolar Having a concentration of one osmole per liter.

osmolarity The concentration of a solution in osmolar units.

osmole [*os(mo)-*[1] + MOLE[3]] **1** A mole of particles that exist as separate entitites in solution. Hence one osmole of sodium chloride is half a mole of NaCl, since 0.5 mol of Na^+ and 0.5

mol of Cl⁻ summate to 1 mol of total particles, which is what determines the osmotic pressure of the solution. **2** The amount of ideal solute that has the same effect on osmotic pressure as the actual amount of solute present. Symbol: osmol

osmology [OSMO-¹ + -LOGY] **1** The science of osmosis. Also called *osmosology*. **2** A rarely used term for OSPHRESIOLOGY.

osmometer [OSMO-¹ + -METER] **1** An instrument used to determine the osmolal concentration of a solution. **2** An instrument used to determine osmotic pressure.

freezing-point osmometer An instrument used to determine the osmolal concentration of a solution by measuring the depression of freezing point.

membrane osmometer An apparatus that uses a semipermeable membrane to determine osmotic pressure effects created by solutions.

osmometry [OSMO-¹ + -METRY] A process of measuring molecular weights based on the osmotic pressure derived when molecules diffuse through a semipermeable membrane.

osmonosology The study of disorders of olfaction. A rarely used term.

osmophilic Having an affinity for osmium, and thus having a black appearance under the light microscope, or being electron dense when examined electronmicroscopically. Osmium tetroxide is used both as a fixative and stain in the preparation of tissues for electron microscopy.

osmophobia [OSMO-² + -PHOBIA] OSPHRESIOPHOBIA.

osmophore [OSMO-² + -PHORE] The group of atoms in a compound whose arrangement is responsible for its characteristic odor.

osmoreceptor **1** A specialized peripheral sense organ or a neuron in the brain whose electrical activity is altered by local changes in fluid ionic concentration. Also called *osmoceptor*. **2** An outmoded term for OLFACTORY RECEPTOR.

osmoregulator A cell that can utilize energy to control the concentration of salts in the intracellular fluid and therefore maintain an osmotic pressure independent of the environment. Compare OSMOCONFORMER.

osmose [Gk *ōsmos* (from *ōthein* to thrust, push) an impulsion] To move in consequence of osmotic forces.

osmosis [OSMO-¹ + -SIS] The movement of solvent through a membrane from a lower solute concentration to a higher solute concentration. The membrane is impermeable or semipermeable to the solute but permeable to the solvent.

reverse osmosis The passage of solvent across a semipermeable membrane from an area of higher solute concentration to an area of lower solute concentration, the reverse of usual osmotic flow. The direction of flow is reversed by application of hydrostatic pressure to the compartment with higher solute concentration.

osmosology OSMOLOGY.

osmotaxis [OSMO-¹ + Gk *taxis* an arranging] Cell movement induced by the density of its fluid environment.

osmotherapy The use of hypertonic solutions by intravenous injection to reduce edema and dehydrate body tissues.

osmotic Of or relating to osmosis.

osmotroph SAPROTROPH.

osone The 1,2-dicarbonyl compound formed by oxidizing C-2 of an aldose or C-1 of a ulose. It is obtained by hydrolysis of an osazone.

osphradium [New L (from Middle Gk *osphrad(ion)* a nosegay, dim. of late Gk *osphra* a smell, equivalent to Gk *osmē* a smell, earlier *odmē* a smell, + *-ium*, L neut. sing. suffix)] A structure located at the base of the siphon in mollusks which is believed to be a chemosensitive forward-seeking exploratory organ, or perhaps it tests the quality of the water in the oral cavity. In

carnivorous mollusks, it serves to locate living and dead animal food. It is particularly well developed in whelks of the genus *Buccinum*, being pectinate and resembling a small gill.

osphresiolagnia [Gk *osphrēsi(s)* a smelling, sense of smell + *o* + *lagneia* lust] A paraphilia characterized by a dependency on specific odors for sexual arousal. Also called *osmolagnia*.

osphresiology [Gk *osphrēsi(s)* a smelling, smell + *o* + -LOGY] The study of the nature and associations of odorants and of the sense of smell. Also called *osmology* (rarely used).

osphresiometer A rarely used term for OLFACTOMETER.

osphresiophobia [Gk *osphrēsi(s)* a smelling, sense of smell + *o* + -PHOBIA] Pathologic fear of odors or of emitting a bad odor oneself. Also called *osmophobia*.

osphresis A seldom used term for OLFACTION.

osphretic OLFACTORY.

osphyarthrosis An inflammation of the hip joint. An obsolete term.

osphyitis An inflammation of the loin.

osphyomyelitis An inflammation of the lumbar region of the spinal cord.

osphyotomy [Gk *osphys*, gen. *osphyos*, hip, loin + -TOMY] A surgical incision into the loin.

ossa Plural of OS².

ossature [L *ossa*, pl. of *os* bone + *t* + -URE] The bony arrangement of the body or parts thereof.

ossein Bone collagen. Also called *ostein*.

osseo- [L *osseus* of bone, bony] A combining form meaning bone, osseous.

osseoaponeurotic Relating both to bone and to muscle fascial covering.

osseocartilaginous Relating to or consisting of bone and cartilage. Also *osteocartilaginous*.

osseofibrous Pertaining to or composed of bone and fibrous tissue.

osseoligamentous Relating to ligament and bone.

osseomucin The ground substance of bone that is present between the fibrous and cellular elements.

osseomucoid A mucin that is present within bone. Also called *osteomucoid*.

osseosonometer An instrument used to measure the conduction of sound through bone.

osseosonometry The measurement of sound waves conducted through bone.

osseous [L *osseus* (from *os*, gen. *ossis*, bone + *-eus* English *-eous*) bony] Consisting of or resembling bone; bony.

ossicle [L *ossiculum*. See OSSICULUM.] OSSICULUM.

Andernach's ossicles An outmoded term for OSSA SUTURALIA.

auditory ossicles OSSICULA AUDITUS.

Bertin's ossicles CONCHA SPHENOIDALIS.

dermal ossicle A bone embedded in the skin, as in certain reptiles.

epactal ossicles An outmoded term for OSSA SUTURALIA.

episternal ossicles OSSA SUPRASTERNALIA.

intercalcar ossicles An outmoded term for OSSA SUTURALIA.

Kerckring's ossicle An occasional center of ossification that appears in the posterior margin of the foramen magnum about the sixteenth week of embryonic life and usually unites with the adjacent squamous parts before birth.

pterion ossicle EPIPTERIC BONE.

Riolan's ossicles Small sutural bones occasionally located between the occipital bone and the petrous part of the temporal bone.

sclerotic ossicles SCLEROTIC BONES.

sphenoturbinal ossicles   CONCHA SPHENOIDALIS.

wormian ossicles   An outmoded term for OSSA SUTURALIA.

ossicula   Plural of OSSICULUM.

ossicular   Pertaining to an ossicle or ossicles.

ossiculectomy [L *ossicul(um)* an ossicle, dim. of *os*, gen. *ossis*, a bone + -ECTOMY]   The surgical removal of one or more of the auditory ossicles, usually in the course of mastoidectomy and because of damage by cholesteatoma. It is often followed by attempts at repair, employing one of the various tympanoplasty techniques.

ossiculoplasty [L *ossicul(um)* a little bone, dim. of *os* a bone + *o* + -PLASTY]   The surgical reconstruction of the ossicular chain when this is congenitally deficient or has been damaged or destroyed by injury or disease. The operation is usually undertaken in the course of tympanoplasty with the aim of improving the hearing. A number of techniques have been favored, including the use of autograft or allograft bone, cartilage or remodeled ossicle and, more recently, prostheses made from a range of alloplastic materials such as high density polyethylene sponge, aluminum or calcium phosphate, or special glass.

ossiculotomy [L *ossicul(um)* a small bone + *o* + -TOMY]   Cutting of one of the auditory ossicles, usually the malleus, to remove the diseased head in the course of modified radical mastoidectomy.

ossiculum [L (dim. of *os*, gen. *ossis*, a bone), a small bone]   [NA]   A small bone or bony nodule, especially one of the small bones in the tympanic cavity. Also called *ossicle*.

ossicula auditus   [NA]   The three small movable bones in the middle ear, namely, malleus, incus, and stapes, stretching chainlike from the tympanic membrane, to which the handle of the malleus is attached, to the fenestra vestibuli, to the circumference of which the base of the stapes is attached. Because of the synovial joints between the bones, they act collectively like a bent lever, converting the vibrations of the tympanic membrane into thrusts of the stapes against the perilymph, which in turn affects the secondary tympanic membrane occupying the fenestra cochleae. Also called *auditory ossicles, ear bones, ossicular chain* (outmoded), *phonophores* (outmoded).

ossidesmosis   OSTEODESMOSIS.

ossiferous   Possessing the ability to produce bone.

ossific   Pertaining to the formation of bone.

ossification [L *os* (gen. *ossis*) a bone + *-ficatio* -FICATION]   The process by which other tissues are converted to bone.

cartilaginous ossification   Ossification that takes place in a cartilage model.

endochondral ossification   Ossification that occurs at the metaphyseal side of the cartilaginous growth plate. Also called *endochondral bone formation.*

heterotopic ossification   The formation of bone in a site where bone does not normally occur.

intramembranous ossification   The development of bone from connective tissue, as distinct from a cartilage model. Such a process is seen in the skull.

membranous ossification   The formation of bony tissue directly within fibrocellular, vascular connective tissue without the development of a cartilage precursor.

metaplastic ossification   The formation of bone in pathological tissues such as those of heart valves, blood vessels, and old scars.

perichondral ossification   Bone that is formed on the surface of cartilage beneath the perichondrium.

ossifluence   The softening of bone.

ossiform   Resembling bone. Also *ossteoid.*

ossify   To convert to bony tissue.

ossiphone [*oss(eo)-* + *i* + Gk *phōnē* sound, voice]   The me-

chanical precursor of the bone conduction hearing aid.

ost-   OSTEO-.

ostalgia   OSTEALGIA.

ostalgitis   Bone pain due to an inflammatory process.

ostarthritis   OSTEOARTHRITIS.

oste-   OSTEO-.

osteal   Bony; osseous.

ostealgia [OSTE- + -ALGIA]   Pain arising from bone. Also called *ostalgia, osteodynia*. Adjective: ostealgic.

osteanabrosis   OSTEOPOROSIS.

osteanagenesis   OSTEOANAGENESIS.

osteanaphysis   OSTEOANAGENESIS.

ostearthritis   OSTEOARTHRITIS.

ostearthrotomy   The excision of an articular surface of bone. Also called *osteoarthrotomy.*

ostectomy [OST- + -ECTOMY]   Removal of bone around a tooth in the treatment of chronic periodontitis. Also called *osteectomy, osteoectomy.*

osteectomy   OSTECTOMY.

osteectopia   The state of having a bone in an abnormal position within the body. Also called *osteectopy, osteoectopia.*

osteectopy   OSTEECTOPIA.

Osteichthyes [OSTE- + Gk *ichthyes*, pl. of *ichthys* fish]   A class of fishes of the subphylum Vertebrata; the bony fishes, comprising the ray-finned and lobe-finned fishes. Their marine and freshwater habitats are worldwide.

ostein   OSSEIN.

osteite   An isolated center of ossification.

osteitic   **1** Relating to an osteite.   **2** Of or relating to osteitis.

osteitis [OSTE- + -ITIS]   An inflammation of bone that is characterized by bone enlargement, with local tenderness and continuous pain. Also called *ostitis.*

osteitis albuminosa   Osteomyelitis accompanied by the formation of albuminous fluid.

alveolar osteitis   Osteomyelitis of a tooth socket, which may occur after a tooth extraction.

apical osteitis   Osteitis adjacent to the apex of a tooth.

benign necrotizing osteitis of the external auditory meatus   An uncommon infection of the external auditory meatus characterized by the insidious occurrence of shallow ulceration of the deep meatal floor, where bone becomes exposed. A small sequestrum may separate before healing takes place. The pathogenesis is uncertain, but some cases follow exposure to irradiation.

carious osteitis   OSTEOMYELITIS.

osteitis carnosa   OSTEITIS FUNGOSA.

caseous osteitis   TUBERCULOUS MYELITIS.

central osteitis   Osteomyelitis affecting chiefly the medullary cavity.

chronic osteitis   Chronic inflammation of a bone, most commonly due to infection.

chronic nonsuppurative osteitis   SCLEROSING OSTEITIS.

osteitis condensans   CONDENSING OSTEITIS.

osteitis condensans generalisata   OSTEOPOIKILOSIS.

osteitis condensans ilii   Pain in the sacroiliac joint that is caused by a thickening of the iliac bone adjacent to the joint.

condensing osteitis   Chronic osteitis in the alveolar bone manifested by reduction of bone marrow space and increase in radiopacity. Also called *osteitis condensans, osteitis ossificans, productive osteitis, proliferative osteitis.*

cortical osteitis   PERIOSTITIS.

osteitis deformans   A bone disease of unknown etiology marked by episodes of bone resorption followed by repair, resulting in excessive bone turnover. The subsequent destruction of the normal bony architecture can cause weakness, which can lead to bowing of the long bones and pathologic fractures. Also called *Paget's disease, Paget's disease of bone, pagetoid osteitis*.

fibrocystic osteitis   OSTEITIS FIBROSA CYSTICA.

osteitis fibrosa circumscripta   Monostotic fibrous dysplasia. See under FIBROUS DYSPLASIA.

osteitis fibrosa cystica   A radiographically visible lesion of long bones, marked by large bone cysts filled with fibrous tissue. It is characteristic and virtually pathognomonic of the excessive secretion of parathyroid hormone in primary hyperparathyroidism. Also called *osteitis fibrosa osteoplastica, parathyroid osteitis, necrotic osteitis, osteodystrophia fibrosa, osteodystrophia cystica, metaplastic malacia, osteoplastica, fibrocystic osteitis, chronic hemorrhagic osteomyelitis, hemorrhagic osteomyelitis, Recklinghausen's disease of bone, fibrocystic disease of bone, Engel-Recklinghausen disease.*

osteitis fibrosa cystica generalisata   PARATHYROID OSTEODYSTROPHY.

osteitis fibrosa disseminata   MULTIFOCAL OSTEITIS FIBROSA.

osteitis fibrosa localisata   Monostotic fibrous dysplasia. See under FIBROUS DYSPLASIA.

osteitis fibrosa osteoplastica   OSTEITIS FIBROSA CYSTICA.

formative osteitis   An obsolete term for SCLEROSING OSTEITIS.

osteitis fragilitans   An obsolete term for OSTEOGENESIS IMPERFECTA.

osteitis fungosa   Chronic osteitis marked by bony cavities filled with granulation tissue. Also called *osteitis carnosa, osteitis granulosa*.

Garré's osteitis   NONSUPPURATIVE OSTEOMYELITIS.

osteitis granulosa   OSTEITIS FUNGOSA.

gummatous osteitis   A chronic form of osteitis that is seen in syphilitic infections.

hematogenous osteitis   Hematogenous osteitis that is seen as a complication of septicemia. It usually occurs in children and is typically located in the metaphyses of the long bones.

multifocal osteitis fibrosa   The polyostotic form of fibrous dysplasia. Also called *osteitis fibrosa disseminata*.

necrotic osteitis   OSTEITIS FIBROSA CYSTICA.

osteitis ossificans   CONDENSING OSTEITIS.

pagetoid osteitis   OSTEITIS DEFORMANS.

parathyroid osteitis   OSTEITIS FIBROSA CYSTICA.

polycystic osteitis   An inflammatory condition of bone that is characterized by the development of cystic cavities. It is symptomatic of sarcoidosis and hyperparathyroidism.

productive osteitis   CONDENSING OSTEITIS.

proliferative osteitis   CONDENSING OSTEITIS.

osteitis pubis   **1** A painful inflammatory condition of the pubic symphysis which may follow genitourinary surgery, urinary tract infection, rheumatoid arthritis, or pregnancy. It is characterized by lytic areas with surrounding bony sclerosis. **2** Sclerosis of bone adjacent in the pubic symphysis which may be seen as an incidental finding on radiographs.

sarcomatous osteitis   An obsolete term for MYELOMA.

sclerosing osteitis   **1** Any osteitis that causes a condensation of bony tissue as is seen in osteitis condensans ilii. Also called *chronic nonsuppurative osteitis, formative osteitis* (obsolete). **2** NONSUPPURATIVE OSTEOMYELITIS.

secondary hyperplastic osteitis   HYPERTROPHIC PULMONARY OSTEOARTHROPATHY.

typhoid osteitis   TYPHOID OSTEOMYELITIS.

osteitis tuberculosa cystica   SARCOIDOSIS.

osteitis tuberculosa multiplex cystoides   SARCOIDOSIS.

vascular osteitis   Bone inflammation characterized by osteoporosis and a proliferation of vascular channels in the bone.

ostemia   OSTEOPOROSIS.

ostempyesis   Suppurative osteomyelitis.

osteo-   [Gk *osteon* a bone]   A combining form denoting bone. Also *ost-, oste-*.

osteoacusis   [OSTEO- + ACU² + -SIS]   Hearing by bone conduction.

osteoanabrosis   OSTEOPOROSIS.

osteoanagenesis   The regeneration of bone. Also called *osteanagenesis, osteanaphysis*.

osteoanesthesia   The insensitivity to pain that is seen in bone.

osteoaneurysm   An aneurysm within a bone.

osteoarthrectomy   Excision of a joint including the adjacent bone.

osteoarthritis   [OSTEO- + ARTHRITIS]   A form of chronic arthritis characterized by cartilage degradation, mildly inflammatory or noninflammatory joint fluid, joint-space narrowing and bone sclerosis, and absence of abnormalities in blood tests of the sedimentation rate or in tests for rheumatoid factor. Osteoarthritis generally occurs in an older age group, or in those whose joints have been previously deformed for any reason. Also called *osteoarthrosis, atrophic arthritis, degenerative arthritis, senescent arthritis, arthrosis deformans, degenerative joint disease, malum articulorum senilis, malum senile, morbus senilis* (obsolete), *ostarthritis, ostearthritis, Heberden's rheumatism*.

osteoarthritis deformans   Osteoarthritis of a severe degree causing deformity, especially of the knees or back.

osteoarthritis deformans endemica   ENDEMIC OSTEOARTHRITIS.

endemic osteoarthritis   Osteoarthritis occurring at a high frequency in a given population. Also called *osteoarthritis deformans endemica*.

erosive osteoarthritis   A subset of osteoarthritis, in which the onset is often inflammatory, and x rays demonstrate erosive changes as well as the typical features of osteoarthritis.

hypertrophic osteoarthritis   Osteoarthritis marked by osteophyte formation.

interphalangeal osteoarthritis   Osteoarthritis occurring in the proximal or distal interphalangeal joints of the fingers.

ochronotic osteoarthritis   Secondary osteoarthritis due to and associated with ochronosis.

primary generalized hypertrophic osteoarthritis   A form of osteoarthritis in which the onset is primarily inflammatory and involves multiple joints within a short period of time. It usually occurs in middle-aged women with a positive family history.

osteoarthropathy   [OSTEO- + ARTHROPATHY]   Any abnormality involving both bones and joints.

familial osteoarthropathy of fingers   THIEMANN'S DISEASE.

hypertrophic pneumic osteoarthropathy   HYPERTROPHIC PULMONARY OSTEOARTHROPATHY.

hypertrophic pulmonary osteoarthropathy   A condition caused by chronic lung or heart disease that is marked by arthritis, subperiosteal new bone formation, an often malignant pulmonary lesion, and, occasionally, skin changes. Localized swellings of the terminal phalanges and the long bones of the forearm and leg result from symmetrical osteitis that appears secondarily. The condition may also be associated with nonpulmonary diseases. Also called *Marie's disease* (obsolete), *tuberculous polyarthritis, pulmonary osteoarthropathy, hypertrophic pneumic osteoarthropathy, pneumogenic osteoarthropathy, pulmonary hypertrophic osteoarthropathy, Marie-Bamberger syndrome, Marie-Bamberger disease, Bamberger-Marie disease, osteopulmonary arthropathy, secondary hyperplastic osteitis, secondary hypertrophic osteoarthropathy*.

idiopathic hypertrophic osteoarthropathy   A condition similar to hypertrophic pulmonary osteoarthropathy but occurring in the absence of a defined primary cause. It is often familial.

pneumogenic osteoarthropathy HYPERTROPHIC PULMONARY OSTEOARTHROPATHY.

pulmonary osteoarthropathy HYPERTROPHIC PULMONARY OSTEOARTHROPATHY.

pulmonary hypertrophic osteoarthropathy HYPERTROPHIC PULMONARY OSTEOARTHROPATHY.

secondary hypertrophic osteoarthropathy HYPERTROPHIC PULMONARY OSTEOARTHROPATHY.

tabetic osteoarthropathy TABETIC ARTHROPATHY.

osteoarthrosis OSTEOARTHRITIS.

osteoarthrotomy OSTEARTHROTOMY.

osteoarticular Pertaining to both bones and joints.

osteoblast [OSTEO- + -BLAST] A cell capable of forming bone and located on the surface of bony trabeculae and within lacunae. Also called *osteoplast, osteogenic cell, Gengenbaur cell, skeletogenous cell.*

osteoblastic [OSTEO- + -BLAST + -IC] Forming bone: used especially of radiographically visible bone sclerosis, as seen in certain types of tumors. Also *osteoplastic.*

osteoblastoma [OSTEO- + BLASTOMA] A benign lesion with a histologic structure similar to that of osteoid osteoma, but characterized by its large size, usually more than 1 cm, and by the usual absence of any surrounding zone of reactive bone formation. Osteoblastomas are less frequent than osteoid osteomas. They usually occur in the vertebrae, ilium, ribs, and the bones of the hand or foot. They do not, as a rule, seem to produce the intense pain commonly associated with osteoid osteoma. In some cases, the histologic distinction from osteosarcoma may be difficult. Osteoid osteoma and osteoblastoma are clearly related. There are differences in the size, site, radiologic appearance, and clinical presentation of the tumors, and differences in the surrounding bony reaction. It is possible that these differences are related to the respective sites of the two groups of lesion, cortical for osteoid osteoma and medullary for benign osteoblastoma. Also called *benign osteoblastoma, giant osteoid osteoma, osteogenic fibroma.*

benign osteoblastoma OSTEOBLASTOMA.

osteocachexia Cachexia secondary to chronic bone disease. Adjective: osteocachectic.

osteocamp A surgical instrument used for straightening a bent femur after an osteotomy.

osteocampsia The abnormal curvature of a bone. Also called *osteocampsis.*

osteocampsis OSTEOCAMPSIA.

osteocarcinoma [OSTEO- + CARCINOMA] **1** An osteoblastic metastatic carcinoma in bone. **2** A carcinoma with osseous metaplasia.

osteocartilaginous OSSEOCARTILAGINOUS.

osteocele [OSTEO- + -CELE¹] A bony nodule in a hernia sac.

osteocementum CELLULAR CEMENTUM.

osteocephaloma [OSTEO- + CEPHAL- + -OMA] A soft sarcoma of bone. An obsolete term. Also called *osteoencephaloma.*

osteochondral Of or relating to a bone and its articular cartilage or growth plate.

osteochondritis [OSTEO- + CHONDRITIS] An inflammatory process affecting bone and its cartilage simultaneously.

adolescent osteochondritis Osteochondritis dissecans of the medial femoral condyle occurring in adolescents. It is similar to the osteochondrosis of the proximal femoral epiphysis (Perthes disease) seen in children, and is of unknown etiology.

calcaneal osteochondritis 1 ACHILLES BURSITIS. **2** SEVER'S DISEASE.

osteochondritis deformans juvenilis PERTHES DISEASE.

osteochondritis deformans juvenilis dorsi SCHEUERMANN'S KYPHOSIS.

osteochondritis dissecans An osteochondritic process resulting in the separation of pieces of cartilage and the underlying bone into a joint cavity. It most often affects the convex surfaces of the knee, shoulder, or ankle joints. Also called *König's disease, osteochondrosis dissecans, osteochondrolysis.*

osteochondritis ischiopubica A radiographic feature sometimes seen in children, that appears to be fragmentation of the junction of the pubis and ischium.

osteochondritis necroticans The fragmentation of the sesamoid bone of the great toe.

syphilitic osteochondritis WEGNER'S DISEASE.

osteochondritis of the tarsal navicular KÖHLER'S DISEASE.

osteochondroarthropathy A joint disease brought on by the disease of its associated bone and cartilage.

osteochondrodysplasia A developmental disorder of cartilage and bone. More than 100 heritable disorders have been so labeled, and most are characterized by skeletal deformities and short stature. Also called *osteochondrodystrophy, skeletal dysplasia, hereditary bone dysplasia, chondro-osteodystrophy.*

osteochondrodystrophia MUCOPOLYSACCHARIDOSIS IV.

osteochondrodystrophia deformans MUCOPOLYSACCHARIDOSIS IV.

osteochondrodystrophy OSTEOCHONDRODYSPLASIA.

familial osteochondrodystrophy MUCOPOLYSACCHARIDOSIS IV.

osteochondrofibroma A benign tumor containing bone, cartilage, and fibrous elements. Also called *fibrosing osteochondroma, osteofibrochondroma.*

osteochondrolysis OSTEOCHONDRITIS DISSECANS.

osteochondroma [OSTEO- + CHONDROMA] A cartilage-capped, bony projection on the external surface of a bone. This is a frequent type of bone lesion. It may be solitary or part of the generalized condition, as in hereditary multiple exostoses. Osteochondromas are commonly located in the metaphyseal regions of long bones, particularly the lower femur, upper tibia, and upper humerus, but may also be found in other bones, such as the scapula or ilium. Solitary lesions may have either a broad or a narrow base, that is, they may be either sessile or pedunculated, while in the multiple lesions the whole metaphysis of a bone may be involved. They occur most frequently in children, and their growth usually ceases at the time of skeletal maturation. They are probably disorders of growth rather than true neoplasms. Malignant change is rare in solitary osteochondromas, but it occurs more frequently in cases of hereditary multiple exostoses. Also called *cartilaginous exostosis, chondro-osteoma, chondrosteoma, ecchondroma, enchondroma petrificum, ecchondrosis, osteocartilaginous exostosis, osteochondrophyte, osteoenchondroma.*

fibrosing osteochondroma OSTEOCHONDROFIBROMA.

osteochondromatosis The presence of multiple osteochondromas. Also called *Henderson-Jones disease.*

Ollier's osteochondromatosis UNILATERAL CHONDRODYSPLASIA.

synovial osteochondromatosis SYNOVIAL CHONDROMATOSIS.

osteochondromyxoma OSTEOMYXOCHONDROMA.

osteochondromyxosarcoma [OSTEO- + CHONDRO- + MYXO- + SARCOMA] An osteosarcoma with cartilaginous and myxoid elements.

osteochondropathia OSTEOCHONDROPATHY.

osteochondropathia cretinoidea LÄWEN-ROTH SYNDROME.

osteochondropathy Any disease or injury affecting both bone and articular or growth plate cartilage. Also called *osteochondropathia.*

familial endocrine osteochondropathy LUCHERINI-GIA-COBINI SYNDROME.

osteochondrophyte OSTEOCHONDROMA.

osteochondrosarcoma [OSTEO- + CHONDROSARCOMA] A malignant bone tumor showing both osteosarcomatous and chondrosarcomatous components. This is now believed to be basically an osteosarcoma with a cartilaginous component. The behavior is that of an osteosarcoma. An obsolete term.

osteochondrosis [OSTEO- + CHONDROSIS] A disease of growth cartilage in children involving secondary centers of ossification which become necrotic and fragmented.

osteochondrosis deformans tibiae An osteochondrotic process of the medial tibial condyle that leads to tibia vara deformity. Also called *Blount's disease, nonrachitic bowleg.*

osteochondrosis dissecans OSTEOCHONDRITIS DISSECANS.

osteochondrous Consisting of cartilage and bone.

osteoclasia The absorption of bone tissue by osteoclasts.

traumatic osteoclasia A type of cementoma in which the alveolar bone adjacent to a tooth apex is first replaced by fibrous tissue and then by cementum.

osteoclasis [OSTEO- + -CLASIS] The controlled surgical fracture of bone, a procedure used to correct bony deformity. Also called *diaclasis, osteoclasty.*

osteoclast [OSTEO- + Gk *klastos* broken in pieces, from *klan* to break, break in pieces] **1** A multinuclear giant cell responsible for bone absorption and destruction. Also called *osteophage.* **2** An instrument once used to perform osteoclasis.

Collin's osteoclast An instrument used for fracturing a long bone at a precise level.

Rizzoli's osteoclast An obsolete instrument that was used to fracture a bone at any desired point. It consists of a rod with two adjustable padded rings, between which is a firm pad. The pad can be screwed down upon the limb to create a fracture.

osteoclastic Capable of bone destruction as exhibited by an osteoclast.

osteoclastoma GIANT CELL TUMOR OF BONE.

osteoclastoma innocens A benign giant cell tumor of bone.

osteoclasty OSTEOCLASIS.

osteocomma A segment or member of a group of bony structures, such as a vertebra.

osteocope Severe bone pain. It often may be a symptom of syphilitic disease of bone. Also called *osteocopic pain.*

osteocopic Related to osteocope.

osteocranium [OSTEO- + CRANIUM] The fetal skull after its ossification has begun.

osteocystoma BONE CYST.

osteocyte [OSTEO- + -CYTE] An effete osteoblast that has become embedded in a bone lacuna. It forms a contact with other osteocytes via canaliculi that contain fine cytoplasmic processes. Also called *bone corpuscle, osseous cell, bone cell.*

osteodentin Dentin that resembles bone histologically. It is the normal dentin of some fish, but may occur pathologically in many species, including man. It may be the result of rapid secondary dentin formation with the inclusion of cells.

osteodentinoma [OSTEO- + DENTIN + -OMA] A tumor containing both bone and dentin. Also called *dentinosteoid.*

osteodermatoplastic Of or relating to the pathologic ossification of cutaneous structures.

osteodermatous Pertaining to the pathologic ossification of the skin.

osteodermia [OSTEO- + -DERMIA] OSTEOSIS CUTIS.

osteodesmosis The formation of bone within a tendon. Also called *ossidesmosis.*

osteodiastasis The separation of two bones that normally lie adjacent to each other.

osteodynia OSTEALGIA.

osteodysplasia Any disorder characterized by abnormal bone development.

osteodysplastic Pertaining to abnormal development of bone.

osteodysplasty MELNICK-NEEDLES SYNDROME.

osteodystrophia [OSTEO- + DYSTROPHIA] OSTEODYSTROPHY.

osteodystrophia cystica OSTEITIS FIBROSA CYSTICA.

osteodystrophia fibrosa OSTEITIS FIBROSA CYSTICA.

osteodystrophy [OSTEO- + DYSTROPHY] Abnormal bone formation. Also called *osteodystrophia.*

Albright's hereditary osteodystrophy An inherited disease in which patients evince, at about age 8, the clinical features of pseudohypoparathyroidsm with nonresponse to parathyroid hormone, or of pseudopseudohypoparathyroidism with the skeletal characteristics but not the biochemical abnormalities of pseudohypoparathyroidism. Manifestations are any combination of mental retardation, short stature, round face, ectopic bone formation, and short metacarpals. The basic abnormality may be a defective parathyroid hormone receptor-adenyl cyclase system in bone, kidney and elsewhere. Inheritance is thought to be sex-influenced autosomal dominance or genetic heterogeneity. Also called *Albright syndrome, Albright's dystrophy.*

azotemic osteodystrophy RENAL OSTEODYSTROPHY.

parathyroid osteodystrophy A condition consisting of bone demineralization, paracortical erosions, fractures, and, occasionally, brown tumors, which occurs in states of prolonged and severe parathyroid hormone excess. The most common cause is chronic renal failure. Also called *osteitis fibrosa cystica generalisata.*

renal osteodystrophy Skeletal pathology secondary to chronic renal failure, including osteomalacia, osteitis fibrosa, osteosclerosis, osteoporosis, or any combination of these. Associated calcification of soft tissue is common. Etiologies include secondary or tertiary hyperparathyroidism, acidosis, and defects in vitamin D metabolism. Renal osteodystrophy may exist for several years before becoming symptomatic. Also called *osteonephropathy* (rarely used), *azotemic osteodystrophy, pseudorickets, renal rickets, renal osteosis.*

osteoectomy OSTECTOMY.

osteoectopia OSTEECTOPIA.

osteoencephaloma OSTEOCEPHALOMA.

osteoenchondroma OSTEOCHONDROMA.

osteoepiphysis EPIPHYSIS.

osteofibrochondroma OSTEOCHONDROFIBROMA.

osteofibrochondrosarcoma [OSTEO- + FIBRO- + CHONDROSARCOMA] An osteosarcoma containing prominent fibrous and cartilagenous components. The distinction from osteosarcoma is not considered of pratical use. An obsolete term.

osteofibrolipoma [OSTEO- + FIBRO- + LIPOMA] A benign tumor containing bone, fibrous, and fatty tissue.

osteofibroma [OSTEO- + FIBROMA] OSSIFYING FIBROMA.

periapical osteofibroma CEMENTOMA.

osteofibromatosis The presence of multiple ossifying fibromas.

cystic osteofibromatosis Polyostotic fibrous dysplasia having a cystic appearance due to a thin cortical shell of bone and a cavity filled with fibrous tissue containing trabeculae of immature bone.

osteofibrosarcoma An osteosarcoma containing a prominent component of fibrous tissue. An obsolete term.

osteofibrosis Fibrosis of the bone, principally entailing the red bone marrow.

periapical osteofibrosis CEMENTOMA.

osteofluorosis A metabolic disorder of the bone, manifested as osteosclerosis and osteomalacia, that is caused by excess consumption of fluoride.

osteogen [OSTEO- + -GEN] A material or layer from which bone is formed.

osteogenesis [OSTEO- + GENESIS] The process by which bone tissue and the bones of the skeleton are formed, including all stages of bone formation, not just mineralization. Also called *osteogeny, ostosis.* Adjective: osteogenic, osteogenetic.

endochondral osteogenesis The process of forming bone from cartilage through osteoblastic activity. Also called *intracartilaginous bone formation.*

osteogenesis imperfecta Any of the several heritable disorders of connective tissue that are marked by bone fragility. Individual syndromes are distinguishable clinically by the presence or absence of blue sclerae, opalescent teeth, and hearing loss; by mode of inheritance; and by biochemical definition of defects in collagen. One classification scheme includes four major types (osteogenesis imperfecta types I, II, III, and IV), whereas older schemes include the designations *tarda* and *congenita.* Also called *osteitis fragilitans* (obsolete), *myeloplastic malacia, hereditary fragility of bone, fragilitas ossium, brittle bone, Durante's disease, brittle bone syndrome, osteopsathyrosis.*

osteogenesis imperfecta congenita The severest form of osteogenesis imperfecta in which intrauterine fractures of long bones are manifested at birth. Also called *Vrolik's disease.*

osteogenesis imperfecta cystica A condition characterized by growths of myxomatous fibroid tissue within the marrow spaces. On x rays the growths appear to be cysts.

periosteal osteogenesis The formation of new bony tissue on the surface of a bone by the deeper layer of periosteal tissue.

osteogeny OSTEOGENESIS.

osteogram A graphic representation of the spine that is used to record the presence and nature of bony lesions.

osteography A description of the bones.

osteohalisteresis OSTEOMALACIA.

osteohydatidosis A hydatid disease affecting bone.

osteohypertrophic Pertaining to any condition in which bony overgrowth is a feature.

osteoid [OSTE- + -OID] **1** The collagenous matrix of bone that precedes mineralization. **2** OSSIFORM.

osteolathyrism A disease characterized chiefly by abnormalities in connective tissue that has been induced in experimental animals fed a diet containing seeds of *Lathyrus odoratus,* the sweet pea, whose active principle is β-aminoproprionitrile. See also LATHYRISM.

osteolipochondroma A benign tumor containing bone, fat, and cartilaginous tissue.

osteolipoma A lipoma containing osseous elements. This may represent metaplastic bone.

osteolith [OSTEO- + -LITH] A stonelike osseous fragment found in an ectopic (nonbony) site.

osteologia [NA] The nomenclature dealing with bones.

osteologist A person professionally involved in the study of bone and bones.

osteology The study of bones including the morphological, physical, and chemical properties and functions of bone.

osteolysis [OSTEO- + LYSIS] The resorption of bone, especially its mineralized component. Also called *bone lysis.*

essential osteolysis The inevitable loss of bone associated with immobility and disuse.

osteolytic Of or relating to osteolysis.

osteoma [OSTE- + -OMA] A benign lesion consisting of well-differentiated mature bone tissue with a predominantly lamellar structure, and showing very slow growth. These lesions are regarded by some as hamartomas rather than true neoplasms. They are almost entirely restricted to the skull and the mandible and sometimes grow into paranasal sinuses as dense, ivorylike, bony masses. Also called *osteoncus.*

cavalrymen's osteoma An osteoma at the insertion of the adductor femoris longus.

compact osteoma An osteoma made of dense bone with little medullary space. Also called *osteoma eburneum, osteoma durum, ivory osteosis, ivorylike tumor.*

osteoma cutis An osteoma in the dermis.

dental osteoma Exostosis from a root of a tooth.

osteoma durum COMPACT OSTEOMA.

osteoma eburneum COMPACT OSTEOMA.

ethmoid sinus osteoma An osteoma arising from the ethmoid bone, usually from the ethmoidal labyrinth. It is the site of some 25% of osteomas involving the paranasal sinuses.

frontal sinus osteoma An osteoma within the frontal sinus. Approximately 70% of paranasal sinus osteomas occur in this location where they are usually discovered on routine radiology. They may reach a large size, making their removal difficult.

giant osteoid osteoma OSTEOBLASTOMA.

intranasal osteoma An osteoma, usually an ethmoid sinus osteoma, presenting in the nasal cavity. It is a rare condition.

ivory osteoma An osteoma with a dense structure simulating ivory. It is typically found in paranasal sinuses.

maxillary osteoma An osteoma arising from the maxilla, a rare site but significant since a proportion of these tumors are cancellous, in contrast with the commoner ivory osteomas of the frontal and ethmoidal bones.

osteoma medullare An osteoma with conspicuous medullary spaces.

osteoid osteoma A benign osteoblastic lesion characterized by its small size, usually less than 1 cm, its clearly demarcated outline, and the usual presence of a surrounding zone of reactive bone formation. Histologically, it consists of cellular, highly vascularized tissue made up of immature bone and osteoid tissue. Osteoid osteomas mostly occur in the shafts of long bones, particularly the tibia and femur. The patient is usually an adolescent or young adult, and males are more frequently affected than females. The lesions are generally painful. They do not appear to enlarge, as judged by clinical observation. See also OSTEOBLASTOMA.

osteoma sarcomatosum OSTEOSARCOMA.

sphenoidal sinus osteoma A variety of paranasal sinus osteoma occurring in the sphenoidal sinus. It is extremely rare but important as a sometimes unsuspected cause of headache and because orbital involvement may be an eventual consequence.

osteoma spongiosum An osteoma made of spongy bone.

osteomalacia [OSTEO- + MALACIA] An impairment of bone mineralization that is characterized by the excess deposition of osteoid tissue. It leads to a gradual softening and deformation of the bones, particularly those that are weight-bearing. Also symptomatic are muscle weakness and poor appetite. It is caused by a vitamin D and/or calcium deficiency or by renal tubular dysfunction. The condition is seen more often in females than in males. Also called *osteohalisteresis, tardy rickets, mollities ossium, avitaminosis D, late rickets, adult rickets, malacosteon, rachitis tarda, Miller's disease, halisteresis* (obsolete), *acute adolescent osteomalacia, halisteretic atrophy, halosteresis.*

acute adolescent osteomalacia OSTEOMALACIA.

anticonvulsant osteomalacia Osteomalacia developing in patients under treatment with anticonvulsant drugs.

bovine osteomalacia Osteomalacia due to dietary phosphorus deficiency. A rarely used term.

familial hypophosphatemic osteomalacia FAMILIAL HY-POPHOSPHATEMIC BONE DISEASE.

infantile osteomalacia RICKETS.

juvenile osteomalacia RICKETS.

puerperal osteomalacia Osteomalacia that follows repeated pregnancies and periods of lactation, with marked depletion of the calcium phosphate complexes of the skeleton.

renal tubular osteomalacia Osteomalacia that results from a deficiency in the production of ammonia by the renal tubules, with consequent acidosis and hypercalciuria.

senile osteomalacia Osteomalacia in the elderly. It may result from a dietary calcium deficiency or from kidney disease.

osteomalacic Relating to or characterized by osteomalacia.

osteomatoid Having the appearance of an osteoma.

osteomatosis HEREDITARY MULTIPLE EXOSTOSES.

osteomere One of a series of similarly formed segments of bone, as the vertebrae.

osteometric Relating to osteometry.

osteometry [OSTEO- + -METRY] The measurements of bones.

osteomiosis A breakdown of bone structure.

osteomucoid OSSEOMUCOID.

osteomyelitic Relating to or characteristic of osteomyelitis.

osteomyelitis [OSTEO- + MYELITIS] An inflammation of bone that is caused by a pathogenic organism, such as staphylococci, and that involves all elements of bone from the periosteum to the marrow. Also called *medullitis, bone abscess, ossifluent abscess* (seldom used), *carious osteitis.*

chronic hemorrhagic osteomyelitis OSTEITIS FIBROSA CYSTICA.

chronic sclerosing osteomyelitis CONDENSING OSTEITIS.

Garré's osteomyelitis NONSUPPURATIVE OSTEOMYELITIS.

hemorrhagic osteomyelitis OSTEITIS FIBROSA CYSTICA.

juvenile osteomyelitis Osteomyelitis occurring in a growing child.

malignant osteomyelitis MYELOMA.

nonsuppurative osteomyelitis Chronic osteomyelitis that is not accompanied by suppuration but is evidenced by a marked thickening of the cortices of the long bones. Also called *sclerosing nonsuppurative osteomyelitis, Garré's osteomyelitis, Garré's disease, sclerosing osteitis, Garré's osteitis.*

sclerosing nonsuppurative osteomyelitis NONSUPPURATIVE OSTEOMYELITIS.

subacute pyogenic osteomyelitis Subacute osteomyelitis caused by a pyogenic bacterium.

tuberculous spinal osteomyelitis TUBERCULOUS SPONDYLITIS.

typhoid osteomyelitis Osteomyelitis due to *Salmonella typhi* and occurring during the course of or consequent to typhoid fever. Also called *typhoid osteitis.*

osteomyelitis variolosa Osteomyelitis arising as a complication of a generalized smallpox infection.

osteomyelodysplasia An inflammatory disease marked by intermittent fever, leukopenia, vascular enlargement of the marrow spaces, and thinning of the overlying cortices.

osteomyelography Radiography of the bone marrow after the injection of contrast material into the marrow. This is a rarely used technique.

osteomyelosclerosis MYELOFIBROSIS.

osteomyxochondroma [OSTEO- + MYXO- + CHONDROMA] An osteochondroma with myxoid elements. Also called *osteochondromyxoma.*

osteon The basic unit of compact bone. It is composed of a central core (the haversian canal) containing blood vessels and nerve endings, surrounded by a variable number (approximately six) of concentric osseous lamellae, which are each 3–7 mm thick. The osteons are arranged longitudinally to follow the axis of the bone and communicate with one another. Also called *haversian system.* Also *osteone.*

osteoncus OSTEOMA.

osteone OSTEON.

osteonecrosis Death of the mass of bone.

osteonephropathy A rarely used term for RENAL OSTEODYSTROPHY.

osteoneuralgia Bone pain.

osteonosus OSTEOPATHY.

osteo-odontoma ODONTOMA ADAMANTINUM.

osteopath [OSTEO- + -PATH] A practitioner who specializes in osteopathy.

osteopathia [OSTEO- + -PATHIA] OSTEOPATHY.

osteopathia condensans OSTEOPOIKILOSIS.

osteopathia condensans disseminata OSTEOPOIKILOSIS.

osteopathia condensans generalisata OSTEOPOIKILOSIS.

osteopathia hemorrhagica infantum An obsolete term for INFANTILE SCURVY.

osteopathia hyperostotica congenita MELORHEOSTOSIS.

osteopathia hyperostotica multiplex infantilis PROGRESSIVE DIAPHYSEAL DYSPLASIA.

osteopathia striata A developmental, asymptomatic condition in which segmental lines of condensed bone form as a result of the failure of remodeling in the metaphyseal-diaphyseal cancellous areas. Also called *Vorrhoeve's disease.*

osteopathic Relating to osteopathy.

osteopathology Bone pathology.

osteopathy [OSTEO- + -PATHY] 1 Any disease or pathology of bone. Also called *osteonosus, osteopathia.* 2 A system or method of medical practice in which accepted diagnostic and therapeutic measures of treatment are used with emphasis placed on the importance of maintaining normal body mechanics and posture and the use of manipulative methods to detect and correct faulty physical structure. This system was postulated by A.T. Still (1828–1917), who stated that the body—when "in correct adjustment" with its own structural relationship, normal nutrition, and favorable environment—has the capacity to make its own remedies against disease and other toxic conditions. Also called *osteopathic medicine.*

alimentary osteopathy HUNGER OSTEOPATHY.

disseminated condensing osteopathy OSTEOPOIKILOSIS.

hunger osteopathy Any disease of the bones arising as a result of inadequate nutrition, and frequently found in populations subject to famine. It is characterized by impaired bone calcification usually resulting from inadequate intakes of vitamin D. Also called *alimentary osteopathy.* See also RICKETS, OSTEOMALACIA.

myelogenic osteopathy A disease in which an abnormality exists in the myelogenous content of the medullary cavity and the bone.

scorbutic osteopathy INFANTILE SCURVY.

starvation osteopathy Any disease of bones resulting from starvation. Such diseases include rickets and osteomalacia both of which result from vitamin D and/or calcium deprivation.

osteopecilia OSTEOPOIKILOSIS.

osteopedion [OSTEO- + Gk *paidion* a young child, dim. of *pais* a child] LITHOPEDION.

osteopenia [OSTEO- + -PENIA] 1 A reduction in bone mass that is caused by decreased osteoid formation in the presence of normal bone resorption. 2 Any decrease in bone density or mass below normal amounts.

disuse osteopenia A reduction in bone density caused by disuse.

hyperthyroid osteopenia Osteoporosis and high rate of bone turnover associated with thyrotoxicosis. Radiographic evidence of generalized bone demineralization is often best seen in the skull. Osteitis fibrosa and wide osteoid seams are frequently found histologically.

osteoperiosteal Of or relating to bone and periosteum.

osteoperiostitis [OSTEO- + PERIOSTITIS] An inflammation of bone and adjacent periosteum. Also called *periostosteitis*.

alveolodental osteoperiostitis PERIODONTITIS.

osteopetrosis A heterogeneous group of hereditary disorders that share generalized sclerosis and fragility of the skeleton and elevated serum acid phosphatase. In the autosomal dominant form, cranial nerve palsies and "bone-within-bone" radiologic appearance occur, and longevity is usually unimpaired. In one autosomal recessive form, macrocephaly, blindness, and severely impaired hematopoiesis occur in infancy and cause early death. Bone marrow transplantation to provide normal osteoclasts has been successful in treating the condition. A mild recessive form and one with renal tubular acidosis also occur. Also called *Albers-Schönberg disease, marble bone disease, ivory bones, chalky bones, marble bones, osteosclerosis fragilis generalisata, Albers-Schönberg marble bones, osteosclerosis fragilis.*

osteopetrosis gallinarum OSTEOPETROTIC LYMPHOMATOSIS.

osteophage OSTEOCLAST.

osteophagia 1 The osteoclastic erosion of bone. 2 The eating of bones by cattle with a calcium or phosphorus deficiency.

osteophlebitis An inflammation of osseous veins.

osteophone An instrument that measures the sound conducting capability of bone.

osteophore A bone-crushing forceps.

osteophyma OSTEOPHYTE.

osteophyte A bony outgrowth, seen most often in osteoarthrosis of a joint, that forms at a location adjacent to the eroded articular cartilage. It can arise either by endochondral or intramembranous ossification. Also called *osteophyma*.

osteophytosis [OSTEO- + PHYTOSIS] A condition characterized by the formation of osteophytes.

spinal osteophytosis The presence of osteophytes around the intervertebral joints, as is seen in degenerative spondylosis.

subperiosteal osteophytosis A bone outgrowth arising from intramembranous ossification.

osteoplaque Any layer of bone.

osteoplasia Bone formation that results from osteoblastic activity.

osteoplast OSTEOBLAST.

osteoplastic OSTEOBLASTIC.

osteoplastica OSTEITIS FIBROSA CYSTICA.

osteoplasty [OSTEO- + -PLASTY] The reshaping of marginal alveolar bone in periodontal surgery in order to improve the gingival contour, and not necessarily to eliminate pockets.

osteopoikilosis [OSTEO- + POIKILO- + -SIS] An autosomal dominant condition marked by mottled or spotted bones. It is seen most often in compact bones and the ends of the long bones as multiple sclerotic foci or stippled areas of dense bone. The condition is benign. Also called *osteopathia condensans disseminata, osteopathia condensans generalisata, osteopathia condensans, disseminated condensing osteopathy, osteitis condensans generalisata, osteopecilia.* Adjective: osteopoikilotic.

osteoporosis [OSTEO- + POROSIS] A reduction in the quantity and quality of bone by the loss of both bone mineral and protein content. It can be primary, as is seen in postmenopausal women or elderly men, or secondary, as a consequence of thyrotoxicosis, hypersteroidism, or prolonged immobilization. Also called *bone atrophy, osteoanabrosis, osteanabrosis, ostemia.* Adjective: osteoporotic.

adipose osteoporosis Osteoporosis in which the interstices are filled with fat.

osteoporosis circumscripta cranii Circumscribed lytic lesions of the skull that occur in osteitis deformans (Paget's disease of bone). Also called *Schüller's disease* (seldom used).

osteoporosis of disuse A demineralization of bone, usually of a limb, that follows prolonged immobilization of the part.

postmenopausal osteoporosis Primary osteoporosis that is seen in postmenopausal women. It most often involves the thoracolumbar spine and causes pain, the crushing of vertebral bodies, and pathologic fractures.

post-traumatic osteoporosis Demineralization of bone that is caused by disuse resulting from injury. The disease may result either from direct damage to the area or from disuse because of severe pain. Also called *traumatic osteoporosis, post-traumatic atrophy of bone, Sudeck's disease, Sudeck's atrophy, Leriche's disease, fracture disease, Sudeck-Leriche syndrome.*

osteoporosis with renal diabetes GLUCOPHOSPHATEMIC DIABETES.

traumatic osteoporosis POST-TRAUMATIC OSTEOPOROSIS.

osteopsathyrosis OSTEOGENESIS IMPERFECTA.

osteoradionecrosis The destruction of bone tissue following irradiation.

osteorrhaphy The suturing or wiring together of bone fragments. Also called *osteosuture.*

osteosarcoma [OSTEO- + SARCOMA] A highly malignant tumor characterized by the direct formation of bone or osteoid tissue by the tumor cells. Osteosarcoma is the most common of the primary malignant tumors of bone. Most of them occur in patients between the ages of 10 and 20 years, and males are more frequently affected than females. Many of the tumors developing after middle age are associated with Paget's disease. The metaphyses of the long bones, particularly the lower end of the femur, the upper end of the tibia, and the upper end of the humerus, are common sites. The usual osteosarcoma, in contrast to the juxtacortical variety, arises centrally and expands and invades the surrounding tissue as it grows. Osteosarcomas show a considerable variation in histologic pattern, differing greatly in the amount of tumor bone or osteoid present and in the pleomorphism of the tumor tissue. In addition to bone and osteoid, the tumor cells may produce cartilage, fibrous tissue, or myxoid tissue, and many areas of tumor tissue may have an undifferentiated spindle-celled structure without any specific type of intercellular material. Subdivision of the osteosarcoma group on the basis of a predominantly osteoblastic, chondroblastic, or fibroblastic structure does not seem to be useful as far as prognosis is concerned. Also called *osteogenic sarcoma, osteoma sarcomatosum, osteogenic osteosarcoma, malignant bone cyst, malignant hemorrhagic bone cyst, sarcoma of bone, osteoblastic sarcoma, osteoid sarcoma, osteolytic sarcoma.*

juxtacortical osteosarcoma A distinct type of osteosarcoma, characterized by an origin on the external surface of a bone and a high degree of structural differentiation. This tumor grows relatively slowly, and has a better prognosis than the ordinary type of osteosarcoma. It usually occurs in young adults, and involves the shafts of long bones, most commonly the lower part of the femur and the upper part of the humerus. It is a circumscribed and sometimes lobulated lesion, adherent to or surrounding the cortex of the bone. The central marrow cavity is involved only at a late stage. It is relatively infrequent compared with the usual type of osteosarcoma. Histologically, the tumor tissue is often mature, merging with the adjacent cortical bone. The cells of the tumor usually show little anaplasia or mitotic activity, except when there is invasion of adjacent tissues. The distinction from myositis ossificans may be difficult, especially when a juxtacortical osteosarcoma is at an early stage of development. Also called *parosteal osteosarcoma.*

osteoblastic osteosarcoma   An osteosarcoma forming large amounts of bone.

osteogenic osteosarcoma   OSTEOSARCOMA.

parosteal osteosarcoma   JUXTACORTICAL OSTEOSARCOMA.

telangiectatic osteosarcoma   A highly vascularized osteosarcoma. Also called *osteotelangiectasia* (outmoded).

osteosarcomatous   Pertaining to osteosarcoma.

osteoscirrhus [OSTEO- + Gk *skiros* or *skirrhos* gypsum, stucco, tumor]   A scirrhous cancer of bone. An outmoded term.

osteosclerosis [OSTEO- + SCLEROSIS]   Any abnormal thickening of bone that results in increased density on radiography. It may take the form of eburnation or condensing osteitis. Also called *centrosclerosis* (obsolete). Adjective: osteosclerotic.

osteosclerosis congenita   ACHONDROPLASIA.

osteosclerosis fragilis   OSTEOPETROSIS.

osteosclerosis fragilis generalisata   OSTEOPETROSIS.

myelofibrosis osteosclerosis   See under MYELOFIBROSIS.

osteoscope [OSTEO- + -SCOPE]   A device for evaluating the performance of radiologic equipment by making roentgenograms of a standard bone specimen.

osteoseptum   The bony part of the nasal septum, formed almost entirely by the vomer and the perpendicular plate of the ethmoid. A seldom used term.

osteosis [OSTE- + -OSIS]   The abnormal deposition of bone salt complexes in connective tissues. Also called *ostosis.*

osteosis cutis   The presence of bony deposits in the skin. Also called *osteodermia.*

ivory osteosis   COMPACT OSTEOMA.

parathyroid osteosis   Any of several bone abnormalities due to hyperfunction or hypofunction of the parathyroid gland.

renal osteosis   RENAL OSTEODYSTROPHY.

osteospongioma   A thinning of cortical bone tissue by an expanding neoplasm.

osteosuture   OSTEORRHAPHY.

osteosynthesis   A closing up and apposing of bony fragments by surgical, mechanical means. Also called *synthetism.*

osteotabes   The atrophy of the bone marrow cells. An obsolete term.

osteotelangiectasia   An outmoded term for TELANGIECTATIC OSTEOSARCOMA.

osteothrombophlebitis   A spreading thrombosis of small veins or venules in a bone that has become infected. It is frequently seen in the mastoid. Also called *osteothrombosis.*

osteothrombosis   OSTEOTHROMBOPHLEBITIS.

osteotome   A surgical instrument that is used to cut bone.

osteotomoclasia   OSTEOTOMOCLASIS.

osteotomoclasis   The partial division of a bony curvature, using an osteotome, followed by the manual fracturing of the bone to achieve the final correction. Also called *osteotomoclasia.*

osteotomy [OSTEO- + -TOMY]   The sectioning, cutting, or perforation of bone.

block osteotomy   An osteotomy performed to remove a segment of bone.

cuneiform osteotomy   An osteotomy in which a wedge of bone is removed.

cup-and-ball osteotomy   An osteotomy in which the end of one bone fragment is rounded and recessed and the end of the other bone fragment is curved to fit into the rounded, recessed end.

dome osteotomy   The surgical division of bone in which the distal fragment is pointed and the proximal fragment is recessed, thus permitting long bone realignment without a reduction in length.

hinge osteotomy   A curved osteotomy combined with bending of the bone.

innominate osteotomy   A division of the innominate bone joint, with its downward displacement. It is usually performed over a dysplastic or shallow hip joint.

intertrochanteric osteotomy   The division of the femur between the lesser and greater trochanter to allow reorientation of the hip joint. It is most commonly performed to relieve osteoarthrosis of the hip joint.

Le Fort I osteotomy   An operation in which the tooth-bearing portion of the maxilla is separated from its bony attachments by cutting transversely with saw or chisel in order to reposition the maxilla.

Le Fort II osteotomy   An operation in which the entire maxilla and the contiguous nasal bones are freed *en bloc* from their bony attachments in order to reposition them.

Le Fort III osteotomy   An operation in which the maxilla, the nasal bones, and both zygomata are freed *en bloc* from their bony attachments for the purpose of repositioning.

linear osteotomy   A straight cut through bone.

Lorenz osteotomy   A V-shaped osteotomy through the neck of the femur to provide weight bearing support around the hip joint.

Macewen's osteotomy   MACEWEN'S OPERATION.

maxillary osteotomy   An incision into the maxilla. Also called *maxillotomy.*

Mitchell's osteotomy   An osteotomy of the first metatarsal to correct metatarsus primus varus.

pelvic osteotomy   An osteotomy performed through the innominate or pubic bones.

perforation osteotomy   Perforation of alveolar bone over a root apex by driving a dental bur through the mucosa and then the bone in order to provide surgical drainage.

sagittal split osteotomy   An operation for repositioning the mandible by means of osteotomies, usually bilateral, in the sagittal plane of the mandibular rami.

segmental alveolar osteotomy   The separation of blocks of alveolar bone and teeth, as a preliminary to repositioning them.

step osteotomy   A surgical division of bone in which a lateral shift of the two fragments obliterates all cortical continuity.

subtrochanteric osteotomy   The correction of a deformity of the upper femur by dividing the femur below the level of the lesser trochanter.

transtrochanteric osteotomy   An osteotomy between the trochanters of the upper femur.

osteotribe   A grinding instrument used for the removal of abnormal bone. Also called *osteotrite.*

osteotrite   OSTEOTRIBE.

osteotrophy   The nutrition of bone tissue.

osteotylus   The expanded end of a healing bone resulting from callus formation.

Ostertagia [after Robert von *Ostertag*, German veterinarian and parasitologist, 1864–1940 + -IA]   A genus of nematodes of the family Trichostrongylidae, occurring in the abomasum, infrequently the small intestine, of cattle, goats, sheep, and other ruminants; the medium, or brown, stomach worms. The larvae penetrate the mucosa, causing nodules or cysts on the wall of the abomasum and hyperplasia of the surface mucous cells. There is concomitant diarrhea, hypoproteinema, and loss of weight.

Ostertagia bisonis   A North American species found in bison, deer, and cattle.

Ostertagia circumcincta   A cosmopolitan species nematode found in the abomasum and occasionally small intestine of sheep. It is an economically important parasite in all sheep-raising areas. Goats, vicuñas, camels, wild deer, and other ruminants are also infected. Heavy infestation causes hyperplasia of the abomasal mucosa and a protein-losing gastroenteropathy with resultant loss of weight. Also called *Strongylus vicarius, Strongylus cervicornis, Strongylus instabilis.*

Ostertagia lyrata   A species found in the abomasum of cattle and wild ruminants such as alpacas, bighorn sheep, and deer.

Ostertagia occidentalis   A species found in the abomasum and, rarely, the small intestine of sheep, goats, pronghorn, mule deer, and other ruminants in the western United States, northern Africa, the Soviet Union, India, and Australia.

Ostertagia orloffi   A species found in sheep, including Barbary sheep, and in cattle and deer in North America, Europe, and the Soviet Union. It has not been found in sheep in North America, however.

Ostertagia ostertagi   An important worldwide parasite of cattle, the principal host, and occasionally found in sheep and goats and in various wild ruminants, particularly deer. Sheep may be affected but they are generally resistant. Young cattle are most susceptible to infection. The typical lesion is hyperplasia of the abomasal mucosa with the formation of nodules or diffuse irregular thickening. Hypoproteinemia and persistent diarrhea are common in heavy infections. Also called *Strongylus convolutus, Strongylus cervicornis.*

Ostertagia trifurcata   A worldwide species found in sheep, goats, and wild ruminants. It was also found in the marmot *Marmota baibacina* in China in an area containing infected sheep.

osthexia   OSTHEXY.

osthexy   Any process of abnormal ossification. Also called *osthexia.*

ostia   Plural of OSTIUM.

ostial   Pertaining to an ostium or orifice. Also *ostiary* (obsolete).

ostiary   An obsolete term for OSTIAL.

ostiole   [New L *ostiol(um)*, dim. of L *ostium* door, entrance, mouth]   **1** A necklike structure in an ascocarp, lined with periphyses and terminating in a pore.   **2** The opening of a pycnidium.

ostitis   [OST- + -ITIS]   OSTEITIS.

ostium   [L (from *os* the mouth), a door, entrance]   (*plural ostia*) A small orifice or opening, especially into a cavity or a tubular organ or structure. Also called *os*[1], *mouth.* Adjective: ostial.

ostium abdominale tubae uterinae   [NA] The narrow lateral opening of the uterine tube situated at the bottom of the expanded infundibulum, the margins of which extend out to form the fingerlike branching fimbriae. The opening communicates with the pelvic peritoneal cavity adjacent to the ovary. Also called *abdominal orifice of uterine tube, ovarian opening of uterine tube.*

ostium aortae   [NA] The circular opening in the left ventricle that lies immediately in front and to the right of the left atrioventricular orifice, from which it is separated by the anterior cusp of the mitral valve. It is guarded by the aortic valve, which separates it from the ascending aorta. Also called *aortic orifice, aortic opening.*

ostium appendicis vermiformis   [NA] The orifice between the vermiform appendix and the cecum. It is situated below and behind the ileocecal opening, and may be partially covered by a semilunar valve formed by a fold of mucous membrane. Also called *opening of vermiform appendix.*

ostium arteriosum cordis   An outmoded term for OSTIUM ATRIOVENTRICULARE SINISTRUM.

ostium atrioventriculare dextrum   [NA] The large rounded orifice situated between the right atrium and the right ventricle of the heart. It is surrounded by a fibrous ring to which is attached the right atrioventricular, or tricuspid, valve which closes the orifice during systole. Also called *right atrioventricular*

orifice, tricuspid orifice, ostium venosum cordis (outmoded).

ostium atrioventriculare sinistrum   [NA] The oval orifice, smaller than the tricuspid orifice, situated between the left atrium and the left ventricle of the heart a little below and to the left of the aortic orifice. It is surrounded by a fibrous ring to which the left atrioventricular, or mitral, valve is attached. Also called *left atrioventricular orifice, mitral orifice, ostium arteriosum cordis* (outmoded).

ostium cardiacum   [NA] The opening leading from the esophagus into the cardiac part of the stomach, situated on the left of the median plane behind the seventh costal cartilage. Also called *cardiac opening, esophagogastric orifice, cardia ventriculi* (outmoded), *cardia, cardiac orifice.*

ostium commune   The single atrioventricular canal in the embryo. It may persist in certain cardiac abnormalities such as hemicardia.

ostium ileocaecale   [NA] The opening between the terminal part of the ileum and the large intestine at the junction of the cecum and the ascending colon. It is surrounded by the ileocecal papilla into which the fibers of the tunica muscularis of the ileum project to form a sphincterlike valve. Also called *ileocecal opening, ileocolic opening, ostium ileocaecocolicum* (outmoded).

ostium ileocaecocolicum   An outmoded term for OSTIUM ILEOCAECALE.

ostium internum uteri   An outmoded term for OSTIUM UTERINUM TUBAE UTERINAE.

ostium maxillare   HIATUS MAXILLARIS.

persistent ostium primum   A persistence of the embryonic interatrial foramen primum that results in an abnormal communication between the cardiac atria through the interatrial septum immediately above and posterior to the atrioventricular valves.

ostium pharyngeum tubae auditivae   [NA] The triangular opening of the pharyngeal end of the cartilaginous part of the auditory tube, located on the lateral wall of the nasopharynx behind and below the posterior end of the inferior nasal concha. Superiorly it is bounded by the prominent tubal elevation, from the lower part of which the salpingopharyngeal fold passes vertically downward behind the orifice. Also called *pharyngeal orifice, pharyngeal opening of auditory tube, pharyngeal opening of eustachian tube.*

ostium primum   An orifice which exits transitorily in the anteroinferior part of the septum primum of the embryonic heart and which allows communication between the two developing atria. It is obliterated early in development when the septum fuses with the atrioventricular cushions. Also called *foramen primum, primitive interatrial foramen, foramen subseptale, interatrial foramen primum, interauricular opening* (outmoded).

ostium pyloricum   [NA] The opening between the stomach and the duodenum which lies at the distal end of the pyloric canal and is surrounded by the pyloric sphincter. Its position is marked on the surface of the stomach by the pyloric constriction and the prepyloric vein. Also called *pyloric opening, pyloric orifice, gastroduodenal orifice, duodenal orifice of stomach, duodenal opening of stomach* (outmoded), *anterior opening of stomach* (outmoded).

ostium secundum   An orifice which appears in the cranial part of the septum primum of the embryonic heart just before the ostium primum is obliterated. It allows communication between the right and left atria even when overlapped on its right side by the septum secundum on formation of the foramen ovale. Also called *foramen secundum, interatrial foramen secundum, foramen ovale cordis, oval foramen of fetus.*

ostium sinus coronarii   [NA] The opening for the termination of the coronary sinus, which is located in the sinus venarum of the right atrium of the heart between the orifice of the inferior vena cava and the atrioventricular orifice. It is guarded by the valve of the coronary sinus which covers its lower part. Also called *opening of coronary sinus.*

sinusoidal ostium Any of the orifices of the anterior cardiac veins in the right atrium of the heart.

ostium trunci pulmonalis [NA] The circular opening between the right ventricle and the origin of the pulmonary trunk, located at the top of the infundibulum of the right ventricle of the heart near the ventricular septum and guarded by the pulmonary valve, which is closed during diastole. Also called *opening of pulmonary trunk, pulmonary orifice.*

ostium tubae In vertebrates, the opening of the oviduct into the coelomic cavity.

ostium tympanicum tubae auditivae The opening of the bony part of the auditory tube in the superior part of the anterior wall of the tympanic cavity just below the orifice of the canal for the tensor tympani muscle. Also called *tympanic opening of auditory tube.*

ostium ureteris [NA] The ureteral opening into the bladder, situated at each posterolateral angle of the trigone and connected to each other by the interureteric crest. Also called *orificium ureteris* (outmoded), *ureterostoma* (outmoded), *orifice of ureter.*

ostium urethrae externum Either the ostium urethrae externum femininae or the ostium urethrae externum masculinae. Also called *urinary meatus* (outmoded), *meatus urinarius* (outmoded), *meatus of urethra.*

ostium urethrae externum femininae [NA] The external orifice of the female urethra in the vestibule, located posteroinferior to the glans clitoridis and anterior to the orifice of the vagina. Usually it has raised margins and it is very distensible. Also called *orificium urethrae externum muliebris* (outmoded), *external orifice of female urethra.*

ostium urethrae externum masculinae [NA] A vertical slit-like opening at the tip of the glans penis that is the narrowest part of the urethra. It is bounded on each side by a small elevated lip. Also called *external orifice of male urethra, orificium urethrae externum virilis* (outmoded), *cutaneous opening of male urethra.*

ostium urethrae internum The crescentic internal orifice of the urethra, situated at the apex of the trigone of the bladder. Also called *orificium urethrae internum, internal orifice of urethra, internal urethral opening, vesicourethral orifice, vesicourethral opening.*

ostium uteri [NA] The opening in the center of the vaginal part of the cervix uteri through which the cavity of the uterus communicates with that of the vagina. It is placed transversely, with thick anterior and posterior lips. Also called *external orifice of uterus, orificium externum uteri* (outmoded), *os uteri externum, external os of uterus, orificium externum isthmi* (outmoded).

ostium uterinum tubae uterinae [NA] The small opening of the uterine tube in the anterolateral part of the uterine cavity. Also called *uterine orifice of uterine tube, ostium internum uteri* (outmoded), *uterine opening of uterine tube.*

ostium vaginae [NA] The external orifice of the vagina, partly or totally closed in the virgin by the hymen and located in the midline below and behind the external orifice of the urethra in the vestibule. Also called *orificium vaginae, hymenal orifice, aditus vaginae* (outmoded), *introitus vaginae, vaginal orifice.*

ostium venae cavae inferioris [NA] The orifice of the inferior vena cava in the lowest part of the right atrium of the heart near the interatrial septum. It is partly protected by a valve. Also called *opening of inferior vena cava.*

ostium venae cavae superioris [NA] The orifice of the superior vena cava in the posterosuperior part of the right atrium of the heart. It has no valve.

ostia venarum pulmonalium [NA] The openings of the pulmonary veins in the upper part of the posterior surface of the

left atrium of the heart, two on each side of the midline and devoid of valves. The two on the left often open into a single orifice.

ostium venosum cordis An outmoded term for OSTIUM ATRIOVENTRICULARE DEXTRUM.

ostomate An individual who has had an ostomy.

ostomy [Clipped form from *(col)ostomy.* See COLOSTOMY.] **1** The surgical creation of an artificial opening through which a body fluid may flow. **2** The opening surgically created for the purpose of fluid passage.

ostosis [OST- + -OSIS] **1** OSTEOGENESIS. **2** OSTEOSIS.

ostraceous Shaped like or resembling the appearance of an oyster shell.

ostracoderms [Gk *ostrako(n)* shell, potsherd + -DERM + s] The oldest and most primitive fossil vertebrates; the jawless fishes of the Ordovician and Silurian periods.

ostracosis An abnormal bone formation and deposition that resembles oyster shell in appearance.

ostreotoxism [Gk *ostreo(n)* oyster + TOX- + -ISM] Poisoning from ingestion of contaminated oysters.

Ostrum [Herman William *Ostrum,* Russian-born U.S. roentgenologist, born 1893] Ostrum-Furst syndrome. See under KLIPPEL-FEIL SYNDROME.

Ostwald [Wilhelm *Ostwald,* German chemist, 1853–1932] See under COEFFICIENT.

Oswaldocruzia [after *Oswaldo Cruz,* Brazilian physician, 1871–1917 + -IA] A genus of trichostrongylid nematodes parasitic in the intestines and lungs of amphibians and reptiles.

OT **1** old tuberculin. **2** original tuberculin (new tuberculin). **3** old term (in anatomy). **4** occupational therapy.

ot- OTO-.

Ota [Masao T. *Ota,* Japanese dermatopathologist, 1885–1945] See under NEVUS.

otalgia [OT- + -ALGIA] Pain in the ear. Also called *otodynia* (seldom used). Adjective: otalgic. ● In some parts of the world, the term is taken to mean only neuralgic pain, either trigeminal or referred.

otalgia dentalis Pain referred to the ear from a focus of disease in the teeth. A rarely used term.

geniculate otalgia Pain in the ear as a feature of the Ramsay Hunt syndrome.

otalgia intermittens Intermittent pain in the ear.

referred otalgia Pain referred to the ear from some site of disease elsewhere but within the areas innervated by the fifth, ninth, and tenth cranial nerves and the second and third cervical nerves. Also called *reflex otalgia, secondary otalgia.*

reflex otalgia REFERRED OTALGIA.

secondary otalgia REFERRED OTALGIA.

tabetic otalgia Otalgia in tabes dorsalis due to involvement of the nervus intermedius root of the facial nerve.

otalgic **1** Referring to or resembling otalgia. **2** An earache remedy.

otantritis [OT- + *antr(o)-* + -ITIS] Inflammation of the mastoid antrum. A rarely used term.

otaphone **1** An obsolete term for AUSCULTATION TUBE. **2** An obsolete term for HEARING AID.

OTC over the counter (designating drugs that may be purchased from stores without a prescription from a physician).

othelcosis [OT- + HELCOSIS] Ulceration of the ear. An obsolete term.

othematoma A rarely used term for HEMATOMA AURIS.

othemorrhagia [OT- + HEMO- + -RRHAGIA] Bleeding from the ear. A rarely used term. Also called *otorrhagia* (obsolete).

othemorrhea [OT- + HEMO- + -RRHEA] Blood-stained discharge from the ear. A rarely used term.

otiatrics [OT- + -IATRICS]   A rarely used term for OTOLOGY.

otiatry   A rarely used term for OTOLOGY. Adjective: otiatric.

otic [OT- + -IC]   Relating to the ear.

-otic[1] [adjectival suffix formed from noun suffix -OSIS]   A suffix meaning (1) of the nature of a state, condition, or process; (2) of or characterized by a diseased or abnormal condition; (3) marked by formation, production, or increase.

-otic[2] [Gk *ōtikos* (from *ous*, gen. *ōtos*, the ear) pertaining to the ear]   A combining form meaning of or relating to the ear.

oticodinia [OTIC + *o* + Gk *ōdis*, gen. *ōdinos*, pain, distress + -IA]   An obsolete term for AURAL VERTIGO.

oticodinosis [OTIC + *o* + Gk *ōdis*, gen. *ōdinos*, pain, distress + -OSIS]   An obsolete term for AURAL VERTIGO.

otitic   Pertaining to otitis.

otitis [OT- + -ITIS]   Inflammation of the ear. Adjective: otitic.

adhesive otitis   A popular term for ADHESIVE OTITIS MEDIA.

adhesive otitis media   A condition of the middle ear in which fibrous adhesions have formed as the result of past inflammation. Also called *adhesive otitis* (popular).   • The term is inaccurate because the inflammation is no longer active.

aviation otitis   AEROTITIS.

barotraumatic otitis   OTITIC BAROTRAUMA.

barotraumatic otitis media   Otitic barotrauma as it affects the middle ear. Also called *barotitis media*.

catarrhal otitis   SECRETORY OTITIS MEDIA.

catarrhal otitis media   An older term for SECRETORY OTITIS MEDIA.

otitis crouposa   An obsolete term for OTITIS DIPHTHERITICA.

otitis desquamativa   **1** A variety of external otitis in which the principal feature is desquamation. An older term.   **2** An older term for KERATOSIS OBTURANS.

otitis diphtheritica   Diphtheritic infection of the ear, usually involving the external ear. Nowadays it is a rare occurrence. An older term. Also called *otitis crouposa* (obsolete).

otitis externa   Inflammation of the external ear. The auricle or the external auditory meatus or both may be involved.

otitis externa circumscripta   Otitis externa where the inflammation of the external auditory meatus is circumscribed, as in the case of a furuncle.

otitis externa diffusa   Otitis externa where the whole external auditory meatus is diffusely inflamed. An outmoded term.

otitis externa furunculosa   FURUNCULAR OTITIS EXTERNA.

otitis externa hemorrhagica   A painful variety of otitis externa in which bullae or blisters, containing blood-stained fluid, appear in the external auditory meatus, on the surface of the tympanic membrane, or in both localities. It is thought to be due to virus infection, particularly influenza. Also called *influenzal otitis*.

otitis externa mycotica   MYCOTIC OTITIS EXTERNA.

exudative otitis   SECRETORY OTITIS MEDIA.

exudative otitis media   SECRETORY OTITIS MEDIA.

furuncular otitis   FURUNCULAR OTITIS EXTERNA.

furuncular otitis externa   Circumscribed inflammation of the external ear characterized by the presence of a furuncle or furuncles. Also called *furuncular otitis, otitis externa furunculosa*.

influenzal otitis   OTITIS EXTERNA HEMORRHAGICA.

otitis interna   A rarely used term for LABYRINTHITIS.

otitis intima   An outmoded term for LABYRINTHITIS.

otitis labyrinthica   An obsolete term for LABYRINTHITIS.

malignant otitis externa   A grave, frequently fatal variety of external otitis occurring in elderly diabetics and due to infection with *Pseudomonas aeruginosa*. Commencing with pain and purulent otorrhea, the condition spreads rapidly to involve cartilage and bone and even cranial nerves, particularly the facial

nerve. Treatment includes the intravenous use of the appropriate antibiotic and sometimes radical surgery. Also called *necrotizing otitis externa*.

otitis mastoidea   An obsolete term for MASTOIDITIS.

otitis media   Inflammation of the middle ear.

otitis media catarrhalis sicca   DRY CATARRH OF THE EAR.

otitis media with effusion   SECRETORY OTITIS MEDIA.

otitis media sclerotica   An older term for TYMPANOSCLEROSIS.

otitis media vasomotorica   Otitis media considered to be of vasomotor origin. An outmoded term.

mucosus otitis   An obsolete term for PNEUMOCOCCAL OTITIS MEDIA.   • This name was used when the causitive organism was classified as *Streptococcus mucosus*.

otitis mycotica   An older term for OTOMYCOSIS.

mycotic otitis externa   Otomycosis confined to the skin of the external ear, a common variety of external otitis in tropical climates and increasingly seen in temperate climates since the introduction of topical antibiotic treatment for external otitis. *Aspergillus niger* and *Candida albicans* are most frequently responsible. Also called *otitis externa mycotica*.

necrotizing otitis   NECROTIZING OTITIS MEDIA.

necrotizing otitis externa   MALIGNANT OTITIS EXTERNA.

necrotizing otitis media   A variety of severe otitis media in which the whole or a major part of the pars tensa of the tympanic membrane is destroyed. It was once common as a complication of the exanthematous fevers of childhood and still occurs where these diseases coincide with malnutrition. Also called *necrotizing otitis*.

parasitic otitis   Inflammation of the ear caused by a parasite. Such disease is almost unknown in man although infestation of the external ear of certain animals with mites (otoacariasis) is not rare. Also called *otitis parasitica*.   • In older texts, the fungus diseases of the ear will be found included as examples of parasitic otitis.

otitis parasitica   PARASITIC OTITIS.

pneumococcal otitis media   Otitis media caused by the pneumococcus (*Streptococcus pneumoniae*) recognized, prior to the advent of antibiotics, as a deceptively silent disease in which middle ear suppuration would sometimes exist in the presence of an intact and relatively normal tympanic membrane, or abscess formation would occur in the mastoid process in the course of acute otitis media after discharge had dried up and the tympanic membrane healed. Also called *mucosus otitis* (obsolete).

otitis sclerotica   An ambiguous term for TYMPANOSCLEROSIS.

secretory otitis   SECRETORY OTITIS MEDIA.

secretory otitis media   Nonsuppurative otitis media in which seromucous secretions collect in the middle ear probably as the result of malfunction of the eustachian tube. Most of the cases occur in children, in whom it is a common disease. It is widely treated by the insertion of ventilation tubes to correct negative pressure in the middle ear. Also called *secretory otitis, serous otitis, exudative otitis, seromucous otitis, catarrhal otitis, serous otitis media, exudative otitis media, seromucous otitis media, catarrhal otitis media* (older term), *tympanic hydrops, hydrotympanum, middle-ear effusion, glue ear* (popular), *hydrotis* (seldom used), *otitis media with effusion*.

seromucous otitis   SECRETORY OTITIS MEDIA.

seromucous otitis media   SECRETORY OTITIS MEDIA.

serous otitis   SECRETORY OTITIS MEDIA.

serous otitis media   SECRETORY OTITIS MEDIA.

traumatic otitis   Otitis following an injury to the ear. This includes both traumatic external otitis and traumatic otitis media but is usually taken to mean traumatic otitis media.

tuberculous otitis   TUBERCULOUS OTITIS MEDIA.

tuberculous otitis media   Otitis media due to infection with species of *Mycobacterium*, especially *M. tuberculosis*. In almost every case, it presents secondary to pulmonary tuberculosis. Also called *tuberculous otitis.*

oto- [Gk *ous* (genitive *ōtos*) ear]   A combining form denoting the ear. Also *ot-.*

otoacariasis   Infection in the auditory canal of cats, dogs, foxes, and ferrets due to the psoroptid mite *Otodectes cynotis*. The mites swarm in the ears of animals, causing tenderness and, in heavy infestations, wasting, loss of appetite, and convulsions. Also called *otocariasis.*

otoantritis [OTO- + *antr(o)-* + -ITIS]   In otitis media, inflammation of the tympanic cavity and the mastoid antrum. An imprecise and seldom used term.

otobiosis [*Otobi(us)* + -OSIS]   Infestation by larvae and nymphs of ticks of the genus *Otobius,* particularly *O. megnini.* They are found in the auditory canal of cats, dogs, horses, cattle, deer, coyotes, and other animals. The larvae may remain for several months before they drop out, pupate, and mature. Human infections have been reported.

Otobius [OTO- + Gk *bios* life, manner of life]   A genus of argasid ticks, the spinose ear ticks, marked by the absence of eyes and the presence of a hood, a vestigial hypostome in the adult but one well developed in nymphs, which are also spiny. In the adult there is a granulated integument.

Otobius lagophilus   The face tick of rabbits and hares in the western United States and Canada.

Otobius megnini   A species, the ear tick, or spinose ear tick, that causes otobiosis in dogs, horses, cattle, sheep, and many wild animals. The distribution is worldwide. It is a particularly important pest of animals in the southwestern United States. The larval and nymphal stages only are parasitic. Heavy infestation cause considerable irritation.

otoblennorrhea   Mucinous discharge from the ear.

otocariasis   OTOACARIASIS.

Otocentor nitens   See under *ANOCENTOR.*

otocephalic   Characterized by otocephaly.

otocephalus   An embryo, fetus, or newborn individual with otocephaly.

otocephaly [OTO- + CEPHAL- + -Y]   A developmental defect characterized by extreme underdevelopment of the lower jaw (agnathia), permitting close approximation or union of the ears on the anterior aspect of the neck (synotia).

otocerebritis   A seldom used term for OTOENCEPHALITIS.

otocleisis [OTO- + -CLEISIS]   Occlusion of the ear, usually the external ear, from whatever cause. A rarely used and ambiguous term.

otoconia   STATOCONIA.

otoconites   STATOCONIA.

otoconium   Singular of OTOCONIA.

otocrane   OTOCRANIUM.

otocranial   Pertaining to the otocranium.

otocranium   **1** The portion of the petrous part of the temporal bone that houses the internal ear.   **2** The petrous part and the mastoid process of the temporal bone, containing the hearing apparatus. Also called *petromastoid, otocrane.*

otocyst   The precursor of the membranous labyrinth of the internal ear. It is formed when the otic placode invaginates and closes off. It then becomes surrounded by mesoderm which forms the otic capsule. Also called *otic vesicle, acoustic vesicle, auditory vesicle.*

Otodectes   A genus of mites of the family Psoroptidae that are ectoparasitic in the ears of animals. The single species is *O. cynotis.*

Otodectes cynotis   The auricular mite, which causes otodectic

mange and otoacariasis in dogs, cats, and other small carnivores. The mite is parasitic in the ear and is rarely found on other parts of the host's body. It causes considerable irritation.

otodynia   A seldom used term for OTALGIA.

otoencephalitis   Encephalitis due to otitis media. Also called *otocerebritis* (seldom used).

otoganglion   A seldom used term for GANGLION OTICUM.

otogenic   OTOGENOUS.

otogenous   Originating in the ear; in particular, caused by ear disease. Also *otogenic.*

otolaryngologist   OTORHINOLARYNGOLOGIST.

otolaryngology   OTORHINOLARYNGOLOGY.

otolites   STATOCONIA.

otolith   See under STATOCONIA.

otologic   Pertaining to otology.

otologist [OTO- + -LOGIST]   A specialist in otology, usually a medical practitioner trained in otorhinolaryngology with a special interest in otology. Also called *aurist* (older term).

otology [OTO- + -LOGY]   The study of the ears, in particular their diseases and disorders and their treatment. Otology is a branch of otorhinolaryngology. Also called *otiatry* (rarely used), *otiatrics* (rarely used).

otomastoiditis   Inflammation of the middle-ear cleft including the mastoid process. A seldom used term.

otomucormycosis   Mycotic otitis externa caused by species of *Mucor,* a rare infection.

otomyasthenia   Weakness of the tympanic muscles sufficient to impair hearing, an outmoded concept.

Otomyces [OTO- + Gk *mykēs* mushroom, fungus]   An invalid genus of fungi implicated in outer ear infections. It is currently included in the genus *Aspergillus.*

Otomyces hageni   An obsolete species of uncertain taxonomic affinity, but probably an *Aspergillus* species.

Otomyces purpureus   An obsolete term for *ASPERGILLUS NIGER.*

otomycosis   Infection of the ear, usually the external ear, with a fungus though not necessarily a pathogenic fungus. Frequently the fungus is a saprophyte growing on the dead wax-keratin shed into the external auditory meatus. Also called *otitis mycotica* (older term).

otomycosis aspergillina   Mycotic otitis externa caused by any fungus of the genus *Aspergillus,* usually the species *A. niger,* in which case the black conidiophores produce a characteristic appearance. A seldom used term.

otomyiasis [OTO- + MYIASIS]   Infestation of the ear by the larvae of any myiasis-producing fly.

otoncus [OT- + -ONCUS]   A tumor of the ear. An obsolete term.

otoneuralgia   Neuralgic pain in the ear. It is a variety of otalgia.

otoneurology   NEURO-OTOLOGY.

otopathy [OTO- + -PATHY]   Any disease of the ear. A rarely used term.

otophone   **1** An obsolete term for AUSCULTATION TUBE.   **2** HEARING AID.

otopiesis [OTO- + Gk *piesis* a pressing, squeezing]   Retraction or collapse of the tympanic membrane or membranes. A rarely used term.

otoplasty [OTO- + -PLASTY]   Any plastic operation on the ear.

otopolypus   A seldom used term for AURAL POLYP.

otopyorrhea   Purulent otorrhea. An older term. Also called *pyotorrhea.*

otopyosis   Suppurative otitis. A rarely used term.

otorhinolaryngologist   A practitioner of otorhinolaryngology. Also called *otolaryngologist.*

otorhinolaryngology The study of the ears, nose, and throat, in particular the diseases and disorders of these parts and their treatment. Also called *ENT, otolaryngology*.

otorhinology The branch of otorhinolaryngology concerned particularly with the ear and nose and their interrelationship.

otorrhagia [OTO- + -RRHAGIA] An obsolete term for OTHEMORRHAGIA.

otorrhea [OTO- + -RRHEA] Discharge from the ear.

cerebrospinal fluid otorrhea Drainage of cerebrospinal fluid from the ear, usually evidence of fracture of the petrous bone with laceration of the dura-archnoid and perforation of the tympanic membrane, but also, rarely, of injury to the dura-arachnoid in the course of surgery on the ear.

otorrhoea A British spelling for OTORRHEA.

otosalpinx An outmoded term for TUBA AUDITIVA.

otosclerosis [OTO- + SCLEROSIS] A disease of the bone surrounding the inner ear, leading in approximately 15% of affected cases to impaired hearing, usually of the conductive kind. The hereditary pattern, probably autosomal dominant, is obscured by the high incidence of symptomless cases. The usual lesion, responsible for the characteristic slow deterioration of hearing, is ankylosis of the stapes. It is common among Caucasian peoples but rare among the Negro races. Surgery on the stapes has been used to improve the hearing of an increasing proportion of patients. Also called *otospongiosis*.

clinical otosclerosis Otosclerosis when it causes hearing impairment, either as the result of ankylosis of the stapes or, less commonly, cochlear involvement.

cochlear otosclerosis Otosclerosis producing sensorineural deafness as a result of involvement of the endosteal bone adjacent to the spiral ligament and, eventually, degenerative changes in the cochlear hair cells.

obliterative otosclerosis Otosclerosis at an advanced stage with otosclerotic bone obliterating the oval window and involving the crura, so that the margins of the footplate are no longer discernible. It is associated with a relatively severe degree of hearing loss.

otoscope [OTO- + -SCOPE] An instrument for examining parts of the external and middle ear by way of the external auditory meatus. Also called *auriscope*. See also AUSCULTATION TUBE.

Siegle's otoscope An otoscope for observing the effect on the tympanic membrane of air-pressure changes induced in the external ear. It consists of an ear speculum closed at the broad end by a lens and connected to a rubber bulb for producing the pressure changes. Also called *Siegle's pneumatic ear speculum*.

Toynbee's otoscope AUSCULTATION TUBE.

otoscopy [OTO- + -SCOPY] Examination of the ear by means of an otoscope.

otosis [OTO- + -SIS] Incorrect hearing of words or the sounds of speech resulting in errors of speech perception and of verbal comprehension.

otospongiosis OTOSCLEROSIS.

otosteons STATOCONIA.

ototomy [OTO- + -TOMY] Incision or dissection of some part of the ear. A rarely used term.

ototoxic [OTO- + TOXIC] Poisonous to the ear: applied particularly to drugs liable to be so. See also OTOTOXIC DRUG.

ototoxicity The quality of being ototoxic.

Otrivin A proprietary name for xylometazoline hydrochloride.

Otten [Max *Otten*, German physician, born 1877] See under VACCINE.

Otto [Adolph Wilhelm *Otto*, German surgeon, 1786–1845] Otto's disease, Otto pelvis. See under PROTRUSIO ACETABULI.

OU 1 oculi unitas (both eyes together). 2 oculus uterque (each eye).

ouabain $C_{29}H_{44}O_{12}$. 3-[(6-Deoxy-α-L-mannopyranosyl)oxy]-1,5,11α,14,19-pentahydroxycard-20(22)-enolide, a cardiac glycoside obtained from the seeds of *Strophanthus gratus* or the wood or root of *Acocanthera schimperi*. It is a crystalline solid, soluble in water and alcohol and slightly soluble in ether. The pharmacological action of ouabain is similar to that of digitalis but it acts more rapidly and has shorter duration. It is used in the treatment of congestive heart failure. Also called *G-strophanthin, acocantherin, acokantherin, ouabaio*.

ouabaio OUABAIN.

Ouchterlony [Orjan Thomas Gunnarsson *Ouchterlony*, Swedish bacteriologist, born 1914] 1 See under LINE. 2 Ouchterlony test. See under TECHNIQUE.

Oudin [Paul *Oudin*, French physician, 1851–1923] See under RESONATOR, CURRENT.

oula An outmoded term for GINGIVA.

oulectomy ULECTOMY.

oulhemorrhagia [Gk *oul(on)* gum + HEMO- + -RRHAGIA] An outmoded term for BLEEDING OF THE GINGIVA.

oulitis An outmoded term for GINGIVITIS.

ouloid [Gk *oul(ē)* a healed wound, scar + -OID] Resembling a scar. Also *uloid*.

oulonitis [Gk *oulon* a gum + -ITIS] An outmoded term for PULPITIS.

oulorrhagia ULORRHAGIA.

oulotomy ULOTOMY.

ounce [L *unica* the twelfth part of any whole, an ounce, inch] 1 A unit of mass or weight equal to 0.0625 pound avoirdupois and 0.0833 pound troy. See under OUNCE AVOIRDUPOIS, OUNCE TROY. • When *ounce* is used without qualification it is usually taken to mean *ounce avoirdupois*. 2 See under FLUID OUNCE.

apothecaries' ounce A unit of mass or weight, used especially in pharmacy, equal to 480 grains 31.1035 grams. Also called *ounce apothecary*. Symbol: oz ap (in the United States), oz apoth (in Great Britain)

ounce apothecary APOTHECARIES' OUNCE.

ounce avoirdupois A avoirdupois unit of mass or weight equal to 1/16 or 0.0625 pound; 437.5 grains; 28.3495 grams. Symbol: oz

fluid ounce 1 In the United States, a unit of capacity equal to 1/128 (US) gallon, 1/16 (US) pint or 29.5735 milliliters. Also called *liquid ounce*. Symbol: fl oz 2 In Great Britain, a unit of capacity equal to 1/160 (UK) gallon, 1/20 (UK) pint, or 28.4131 milliliters. Symbol: fl oz

imperial ounce A unit of mass or weight equal to 1/16 imperial pound; 28.3495 grams, approximately.

liquid ounce FLUID OUNCE. Symbol: liq oz

metric ounce MOUNCE.

ounce troy A troy unit of mass or weight equal to 1/12 or 0.0833 pound troy; 480 grains; 31.103 grams. Symbol: oz t (in the United States), oz tr (in Great Britain)

-ous [L *-osus*, adjectival suffix partly from termination *-us* of masc. adjectives] A suffix meaning possessing or characterized by.

outbreak The sudden appearance or increased incidence of a disease in a community. An outbreak may or may not spread more broadly to become an epidemic. • The term is usually restricted to infectious diseases but may apply to disease or injury due to other causes such as drug abuse or industrial or other toxins.

outbreeding 1 The mating of individuals who are less closely related than the average mating pair from the population. Compare INBREEDING. 2 In experimental genetics or animal or plant breeding, the purposeful mating of individuals who share as few alleles as possible, or who are different at selected loci, for the purpose of improving fitness or growth in the offspring through genetic diversity.

outcross **1** The product of outbreeding. **2** To engage in outbreeding.

outflow / craniosacral outflow Preganglionic parasympathetic fibers in the oculomotor (III), facial (VII), glossopharyngeal (IX) and vagus (X) cranial nerves and in the second, third, and fourth sacral spinal nerves.

thoracolumbar outflow SYSTEMA NERVOSUM AUTONOMICUM, PARS SYMPATHICA.

outfracture The surgical repositioning of a medially displaced nasal bone.

outgrowth / spore outgrowth The final stage in germination, in which the vegetative genes of the spore are selectively activated, their products convert the spore into a vegetative cell, and the disrupted spore integument is discarded.

outlay ONLAY GRAFT.

epithelial outlay EPITHELIAL ONLAY.

outlet In anatomy, an opening that permits escape or outward movement of some of the contents of a walled area or space, such as the pelvis and thorax.

pelvic outlet APERTURA PELVIS INFERIOR.

outlet of pelvis APERTURA PELVIS INFERIOR.

thoracic outlet APERTURA THORACIS INFERIOR.

outlet of thorax APERTURA THORACIS INFERIOR.

outlier [*out* + *li(e)* + -ER] An observation so far removed from the others in a set of observations as to suggest that it belongs to a different population or is the result of faulty technique of sampling or measurement.

outlimb The distal part of a limb.

outpatient A patient receiving care from a health care institution but not admitted for a stay in a facility of that institution. Compare INPATIENT.

clinic outpatient A patient treated or under continuing care at an ambulatory care clinic.

emergency outpatient A patient treated for emergency care needs entirely on an outpatient basis.

hospital outpatient A patient treated in a hospital ambulatory care facility or under continuing care by such a facility.

referred outpatient A patient referred from one provider to another for ambulatory care.

outpocket The protuberance of a tissue or organ as a result of evagination.

outpocketing EVAGINATION.

outpouching EVAGINATION.

output **1** The quantity produced by a system. **2** The power delivered by a mechanical machine or an electric circuit. **3** In digital computers, the computed results delivered by the computer. **4** In a computer or a circuit, the terminals which deliver the output.

average acoustic power output The acoustic power emitted, as from an ultrasound transducer, averaged over the pulse repetition period.

cardiac output The volume of blood ejected by the heart in a unit of time, usually one minute. Also called *kinemia* (outmoded).

energy output The quantity of energy that is produced by the body.

stroke output The volume of blood ejected in each ventricular systole.

urinary output The amount of water or solutes excreted by the kidneys per unit of time.

ov- OVO-.

ova Plural of OVUM.

oval **1** Having the shape of an egg. **2** Of or relating to an ovum.

ovalbumin A major protein of egg white. It is a glycoprotein, carrying one oligosaccharide chain, and has a molecular mass of about 44 kDa.

ovalocytary ELLIPTOCYTIC.

ovalocyte ELLIPTOCYTE.

ovalocytosis ELLIPTOCYTOSIS.

ovarialgia [*ovari(o)*- + -ALGIA] Pain in an ovary. Also called *oophoralgia*.

ovarian Of, relating to, or having the characteristics of an ovary or ovaries.

ovariectomy [*ovari(o)*- + -ECTOMY] OOPHORECTOMY.

ovario- [L *ovarium* ovary] A combining form denoting the ovary.

ovariocele [OVARIO- + -CELE¹] A hernia of an ovary, usually into the inguinal canal.

vaginal ovariocele Hernia of the ovary into the vagina. The condition is usually seen after hysterectomy.

ovariocentesis [OVARIO- + -CENTESIS] Puncture of an ovarian cyst or follicle in order to aspirate follicular fluid or oocytes. Also called *paracentesis ovarii*.

ovariocyesis [OVARIO- + CYESIS] OVARIAN PREGNANCY.

ovariodysneuria [OVARIO- + DYS- + NEUR- + -IA] Neuralgic pain in an ovary.

ovarioepilepsy [OVARIO- + EPILEPSY] CATAMENIAL EPILEPSY.

ovariogenic Emanating from the ovary. Also *oophorogenous*.

ovariohysterectomy [OVARIO- + HYSTERECTOMY] OOPHOROHYSTERECTOMY.

ovariolytic [OVARIO- + LYTIC] Having the property of destroying the ovary. A seldom used term.

ovariopathy [OVARIO- + -PATHY] OOPHOROPATHY.

ovariopexy OOPHOROPEXY.

ovariorrhexis [OVARIO- + -RRHEXIS] Rupture of an ovary.

ovariosalpingectomy [OVARIO- + SALPINGECTOMY] Removal of a uterine tube and ovary.

ovariosteresis [OVARIO- + Gk *sterēsis* (from *sterein* to deprive) privation, loss] OOPHORECTOMY.

ovariostomy [OVARIO- + -STOMY] OOPHOROSTOMY.

ovariotestis OVOTESTIS.

ovariotherapy OOTHERAPY.

ovariotomy [OVARIO- + -TOMY] OOPHOROTOMY.

ovariotubal Pertaining to both the oviduct and ovary.

ovaritis [*ovari(o)*- + -ITIS] OOPHORITIS.

ovarium [New L (from L *ov(um)* egg + -ARIUM -*ary*), ovary] (*plural* ovaria) [NA] One of the paired internal genital organs of the female, pearly-white, almond-shaped, and measuring about $3 \times 1.5 \times 1$ cm in the adult and located on each side of the uterus near the lateral wall of the pelvis, attached by the mesovarium to the posterosuperior surface of the broad ligament of the uterus usually posteroinferior to the uterine tube. Its position, however, changes with pregnancy and is influenced by the state of the intestines. Attached to it are the ovarian fimbria, the suspensory ligament of the ovary, and the ovarian ligament. It is covered by peritoneum adhering to a layer of germinal epithelium deep to which is a thick cortex which, after puberty, contains the follicles and corpora lutea and encloses a vascular medulla. Mature follicles rupture onto the surface each month, expelling a secondary oocyte that enters the uterine tube, which carries it to the uterus where it is either fertilized or becomes degenerate, to be expelled during the next menstrual period. The organ produces hormones including estrogens and progesterone, and it may interact with the hypophyseal gonadotrophic hormones and others. With increasing age it becomes more fibrotic and after the menopause most of its activities, such as forming follicles and corpora lutea, cease; ovary. Also called *female gonad, testis muliebris* (outmoded), *oophoron.*

ovarium bipartitum   An ovary whose shape is such that it resembles two connecting structures. Also called *ovarium disjunctum, ovarium lobatum.*

ovarium disjunctum   OVARIUM BIPARTITUM.

ovarium gyratum   An ovary whose surface has irregular convolutions or grooves.

ovarium lobatum   OVARIUM BIPARTITUM.

ovarium masculinum   An outmoded term for APPENDIX TESTIS.

ovarotherapy   OOTHERAPY.

ovary   [New L *ovarium.* See OVARIUM.]   One of the paired internal genital organs of the female; ovarium.

adenocystic ovary   An ovary which has numerous small cysts, thus resembling a glandular structure.

embryonic ovary   An ovary located in an embryo.

inferior ovary   The ovary of an epigynous flower, which is below the attachment of the stamens and perianth and adnate to the calyx.

mulberry ovary   An ovary of an immature rat in which changes have been induced by administration of anterior pituitary extracts (gonadotropins). Such ovaries contain multiple Graafian follicles of diverse sizes and many superficially located corpora lutea, so that the ovary looks somewhat like a mulberry. It has been used in a test for pregnancy.

oyster ovaries   Large, edematous ovaries containing multiple theca-lutein cysts, often associated with gestational trophoblastic disease.

polycystic ovary   An ovary containing multiple follicular cysts and often excessive fibrous tissue, sometimes associated with excessive secretion of androgenic hormone and varying degrees of virilization and ovarian dysfunction. Also called *sclerocystic disease of the ovary.*

undescended ovaries   Ovaries lying in the upper abdominal cavity.

OVD   occlusal vertical dimension.

overachiever   One whose actual performance exceeds, in a positive way, the predictions made about his behavior on the basis of psychological tests of aptitude or ability.

overbite   VERTICAL OVERLAP.

deep overbite   Excessive vertical overlap.

horizontal overbite   HORIZONTAL OVERLAP.

incomplete overbite   An incisor relationship in centric occlusion in which the lower incisors fail to occlude with either the upper incisors or the mucoperiosteum of the palate.

vertical overbite   VERTICAL OVERLAP.

overbreathing   A popular term for HYPERVENTILATION.

overclosure   An abnormally small vertical relation with the teeth, natural or artificial, in occlusion. It is often accompanied by an abnormally large interocclusal distance. Also called *closed bite.*

overcompensation   A pathologic striving for power and dominance as a way to compensate for an inferiority complex or feelings of inadequacy. Also called *hypercompensation.*

overcorrection   The prescription of a larger amount of dioptric strength than the refractive error.

overcrowding   1 The continual presence of an excess number of inhabitants in a specified dwelling such that a hazard to health or unacceptable quality of life results.   2 The presence of a population in an area, town, region, or country that exceeds the limits of available services to maintain an adequate standard of

life.   3 The presence in a defined area of too many animals, thus rendering the area incapable of sustaining healthful conditions.

overdenture   A denture constructed over deliberately retained roots which may be either exposed or covered with mucous membrane. If exposed the roots are root-filled and sometimes capped. Compare OVERLAY DENTURE.

overdependency   An excessive need for mothering, love, affection, security, or other types of support from others.

overdetermination   In psychiatry, the state of having a multiplicity of factors, motives, causes, or reasons upon which the final form of a symptom or neurosis depends. Also called *multidetermination.*

overdominance   A property of a phenotype by which, when the genotype at a locus is heterozygous, the quality or fitness of the phenotype is superior to that present when either allele is homozygous. Also called *monohybrid heterosis.*

overdrive   The device of purposely increasing heart rate, as by an artificial pacemaker, in order to eliminate undesirable rhythms.

overeruption   The vertical extrusion of a tooth beyond its normal position in the dental arch. It occurs when there is no opposing tooth at the time of eruption. At other times, overeruption is caused by periodontitis and in extreme cases it can prevent proper closure of the jaws. Artificial overeruption, by means of springs, may be used in the treatment of periodontitis to reduce pocket depth.

overextend   1 To project an instrument or filling material beyond the apical foramen of a tooth.   2 To extend a denture base beyond the usual limits.

overfill   1 To place more restorative material than necessary in a tooth cavity, usually with the intention of trimming the surplus away to create a contoured surface.   2 To overextend a root filling.

overflexion   HYPERFLEXION.

overgraft   1 To reinforce (a skin graft or other area from which epithelium has been stripped) by overgrafting.   2 A graft so reinforced.

overgrafting   A method of reinforcing a skin graft that has already taken or an area subjected to dermabrasion, by placing another graft over it. The epidermis from the first graft or area is removed and then the second graft, a split-thickness skin graft, is applied.

overgrowth   An increase in size of a body part due to either hypertrophy or hyperplasia.

overhang   The spread of surplus restorative material over the surface of a tooth adjacent to the gingival margin of a dental restoration.

overhydration   A state of excessive water content, as of the body.

overinclusiveness   A failure to observe boundaries or limits in thinking and speech. When it is a prominent feature, as in schizophrenic speech, irrelevant or distantly related elements adulterate the flow of thought, which becomes unfocused, vague, and meaninglessly abstract.

overinflation   Excessive inflation; hyperinflation.

nonobstructive pulmonary overinflation   Overinflation of the whole or a part of a lung which is not due to obstruction of a bronchus.

obstructive pulmonary overinflation   Overinflation of the lung due to air trapped beyond an obstruction to a bronchus.

overjet   HORIZONTAL OVERLAP.

overjut   HORIZONTAL OVERLAP.

overlap   The relation between the upper incisors and the opposing teeth. In normal arrangement of the teeth there is a slight overlap of the upper incisors over the lowers when all the teeth are in contact, with the jaws in centric occlusion.

horizontal overlap   The projection in the horizontal plane of the upper incisor teeth beyond the lowers so that there is a space between the upper and lower incisors when the jaws are in centric occlusion. Also called *horizontal overbite, overjet, overjut.*

vertical overlap   The overlap in the vertical plane of the upper incisors over the lowers with the jaws in centric occlusion. The opposing incisor teeth may be in contact with each other or there may also be a horizontal overlap. Also called *overbite, vertical overbite.*

overlay   **1** An additional component to an existing condition. **2** In digital computing, the technique of transferring segments of a large program from mass storage into temporary storage, where they execute instructions for different stages of a problem. **3** A cast inlay or crown that covers one or more cusps of a tooth. See also OVERLAY DENTURE.

emotional overlay   PSYCHOGENIC OVERLAY.

psychogenic overlay   The exaggeration of complaints or symptoms beyond what is usually produced by the organic condition and therefore assumed to be functional in origin. Also called *emotional overlay.*

overload   A load greater than the rated load of an electronic device and which can cause damage or waveform distortion.

aortic overload   Increased or excessive requirement of left ventricular work resulting from conditions in the aorta such as hypertension.

circulatory overload in renal failure   CIRCULATORY CONGESTION IN RENAL FAILURE.

iron overload   An excessive accumulation of iron in the body due to a greater than normal absorption of iron from the gastrointestinal tract or from parenteral injection. This may arise from idiopathic hemochromatosis, excessive iron intake, chronic alcoholism, certain types of refractory anemia, or transfusional hemosiderosis. The excess iron is deposited as hemosiderin in reticuloendothelial cells or parenchymal cells of various organs. Plasma iron and transferrin saturation are increased. Total iron-binding capacity is depressed. This disorder can lead to cirrhosis, diabetes, hyperpigmentation of the skin, cardiac failure, and hypofunction of the endocrine glands.

stimulus overload   The condition caused by excessive sensory stimulation resulting in an individual's inability to process and to respond to environmental stimuli and cues.

overloading   The condition resulting from excessive sensory stimulation, in which the stimuli are too intense or too rapid for an individual to respond appropriately.

overlying   Accidental asphyxiation of an infant sharing a bed with its mother or another adult, who while asleep lies upon the infant. Sudden death in infants was at one time often attributed to this accident.

overmaturity   POSTMATURITY.

overnutrition   The consumption of more food than is required by the body to sustain normal functions and maintain body weight. It is often used in reference to obesity (overconsumption of calories) and other pathologic states arising from overeating.

overproductivity   A mental state, occurring in mania, characterized by excessive speaking and thinking.

overprotection   Oversolicitousness and inhibition of independence in the guise of preventing harm or evil.

maternal overprotection   SMOTHER LOVE.

overriding   **1** A malposition of toes in which one digit lies wholly or in part on another. Also called *overtoe.* **2** The slipping of one fragment of a fractured bone over the other fragment.

overstain   To apply an excess of histologic stain such that sub-

sequent removal of the excess provides maximal differentiation of structural detail.

overstimulation   Traumatization occurring when there is a flooding of the organism with more stimuli than it can master, either because its coping mechanisms are not adequate or because the stimulus intensity is so great that it would constitute a significant stressor to anyone.

Overstreet   [Edmund William *Overstreet*, U.S. gynecologist and obstetrician, born 1908]   Gordan-Overstreet syndrome. See under SYNDROME.

overt   Apparent, as a sign of an illness; plainly demonstrable.

overtoe   OVERRIDING.

Overton   [Charles Ernst *Overton*, German anesthesiologist, born 1865]   Meyer-Overton theory. See under LIPOID THEORY OF NARCOSIS.

overtone   An additional tone emitted by a resonant musical instrument, the voice, and other sound-producing devices, which is higher in frequency than the fundamental tone and to which it bears a simple numerical relationship. It is usually one of a series of overtones or harmonics.

psychic overtone   The associations that enter consciousness when any image is presented to the mind. An older term.

overtransfusion   The introduction of excessive quantities of fluid into the circulation.

overventilation   HYPERVENTILATION.

overweight   Having a body weight in excess of that stipulated by standard height-weight tables, which may be due to an excess accumulation of adipose tissue or of lean body mass.

ovi   Of an ovum, as *vitellus ovi.*

ovi-   OVO-.

ovicide   [OVI- + -CIDE]   An agent or substance capable of destroying ova.

oviducal   OVIDUCTAL.

oviduct   **1** TUBA UTERINA.   **2** In zoology, the duct along which ova pass to the exterior of the body of the female.

oviductal   Relating to the oviducts. Also *oviducal.*

oviferous   Bearing ova.

ovification   OVULATION.

oviform   [OVI- + -FORM]   OVOID.

ovigenesis   [OVI- + GENESIS]   OOGENESIS.

ovigenetic   OOGENETIC.

ovigenic   [OVI- + -GENIC]   OOGENIC.

ovigenous   OOGENIC.

ovigerm   **1** OOGONIUM.   **2** OOCYTE.

ovination   [New L *ovin(ia)* (from Late L *ovin(us)* pertaining to sheep, from L *ov(is)* a sheep + *-inus* -INE; + New L *-ia* -IA) sheep pox + -ATION]   Inoculation with sheep pox virus.

ovine   [Late L *ovin(us)* (from L *ov(is)* sheep + *-inus* -INE) pertaining to sheep]   Of, relating to, or characteristic of sheep.

ovinia   [Late L *ovin(us)* pertaining to a sheep + -IA]   SHEEP-POX.

oviparous   [L *oviparus* (from *ov(um)* egg + *i* + *par(ere)* to bear young + *-us* -OUS) egg-laying]   Producing eggs that hatch outside the body. Compare OVOVIVIPAROUS, VIVIPAROUS.

oviposit   [OVI- + L *posit(us),* past part. of *ponere* to place, set, lay]   To lay eggs, especially if associated with specialized organs or behavior, as in many insects, such as the grasshoppers and cockroaches.

oviposition   The deposition or laying of eggs, as by insects.

ovipositor   [OVIPOSIT + -OR]   A specialized structure on the posterior abdomen of many female insects, which serves to deposit eggs in a substratum.

ovisac   VESICULAR OVARIAN FOLLICLE.

ovitesticular Pertaining to ovotestis.

ovium [New L, from L *ov(um)* egg + *-ium*, New L noun suffix] The mature female germ cell, or ovum.

ovo- [L *ovum* egg] A combining form denoting egg or ovum. Also *ovi-*.

ovoblast [OVO- + -BLAST] OOGONIUM.

ovocenter OOCENTER.

Ovocylin A proprietary name for estradiol.

ovocyte OOCYTE.

ovoflavin Riboflavin extracted from eggs.

ovogenesis [OVO- + GENESIS] OOGENESIS.

ovoglobulin The globulin portion of egg white.

ovogonium OOGONIUM.

ovoid [OV- + -OID] Resembling a hen's egg in shape. Also *oviform*.

fetal ovoid The ovoid intrauterine shape of the fetus.

Manchester ovoid An egg-shaped radium applicator with a diameter of 23 cm, used in the treatment of cancer of the cervix.

ovolarviparous [OVO- + *larv(a)* + *i* + *-parous*, combining form from L *par(ere)* to beget or bear young + -OUS] Producing eggs that hatch within the female, the larvae being held within the uterus and later deposited in the host organism: said of certain myiasis flies, nematodes, and other invertebrates.

ovomucin A glycoprotein precipitated when egg white is diluted with water.

ovomucoid A glycoprotein of the white of birds' eggs, having a molecular mass of about 28 kDa. It is an inhibitor of trypsin.

ovoplasm [OVO- + -PLASM] OOPLASM.

ovoserum Animal serum following injection of egg white. The serum precipitates egg albumin in another member of the same species.

ovotestis [OVO- + TESTIS] A gonad containing both ovarian and testicular elements, as seen in one form of true hermaphroditism. Also called *ovariotestis*.

ovotherapy OOTHERAPY.

ovotransferrin CONALBUMIN.

ovovitellin [OVO- + L *vitell(us)* the yolk of an egg + -IN] A protein in the yolk, or vitellus, of an ovum.

ovoviviparous [OVO- + VIVIPAROUS] Characterized by the production of large, yolky, shell-protected eggs which are retained and develop within the reproductive tract of the female. The young receive nourishment only from the yolk. Hatching is internal, and the young are then released to the outside. Some insects, sharks, fish, snakes, and lizards are ovoviviparous. Compare OVIPAROUS, VIVIPAROUS.

ovula Plural of OVULUM.

ovular [*ovul(e)* + -AR] Relating to an ovum or an ovule.

ovulation [New L *ovul(um)* (dim. of L *ovum* an egg) a little egg + -ATION] The expulsion of a secondary oocyte from a mature graafian follicle. Also called *ovification*.

amenstrual ovulation Ovulation in the absence of menstrual bleeding.

anestrous ovulation Ovulation in animals in the absence of other features of the estrous cycle.

paracyclic ovulation An additional ovulation during an estrous cycle, occurring at a time different from that of the regular ovulation in that cycle. Also called *supplementary ovulation*.

supplementary ovulation PARACYCLIC OVULATION.

ovulatory Relating to ovulation.

ovule [New L *ovul(um)*, dim. of *ovum* egg] **1** An ovum lying within a follicle. **2** A structure in seed plants that contains the female gametophyte with an egg cell. When mature, the ovule becomes a seed.

Naboth's ovules NABOTHIAN CYSTS.

primitive ovule An anlage of an ovum contained within the ovary. Also called *primordial ovule*.

primordial ovule PRIMITIVE OVULE.

ovulo- [New L *ovulum* (dim. of L *ovum* egg) a small egg, ovule] A combining form denoting ovule or ovum.

ovulum [New L (dim. of L *ovum* egg), a little egg] **1** OVUM. **2** Any small egglike structure resembling an ovum.

ovula nabothi NABOTHIAN CYSTS.

ovum [L, an egg] (*plural* ova) The unfertilized reproductive cell produced by the ovary in the female, appearing initially as an oogonium, then as a primary oocyte in the ovarian follicle where it matures into the secondary oocyte, which is surrounded by the zona pellucida or cells of the cumulus. When the follicle ruptures, the liberated oocyte enters the uterine tube and reaches the uterus surrounded by the cells of the corona radiata in a matrix containing hyaluronic acid, where it is either fertilized by a sperm or discharged during the next menstrual period. The oocyte undergoes a number of changes during maturation and when it is discharged from the ovarian follicle it contains half the number of chromosomes originally present in the primary oocyte. The term is applied to any or all of the above stages. Also called *ovulum*.

alecithal ovum MIOLECITHAL OVUM.

amniotic ovum An amniotic sac expelled intact in the form of a balloon, after an abortion, and looking like a complete conceptus.

blighted ovum An ovum whose development is arrested. Frequently, all that is seen is a fluid-filled sac either without a trace of a fetus or with a small amount of amorphous tissue where the fetus is usually located.

centrolecithal ovum An egg in which the relatively abundant yolk is concentrated in the interior with the cytoplasm distributed as a thin coat on the external surface. An island of cytoplasm is also present in the center of the egg. It occurs in arthropods, especially insects.

cleidoic ovum An ovum that contains all the nutrients, except oxygen, required to produce an embryo. An example is a hen's egg.

dropsical ovum A conceptus in which the embryo has died and where hydramnios is present.

ectolecithal ovum An egg in which the yolk is distributed around the periphery with the cytoplasm in the center. It occurs in Platyhelminthes.

fertilized ovum ZYGOTE.

Hertig-Rock ova A series of specimens of fertilized human ova and embryos ranging in estimated age from one to 17 days. Some were abnormal or blighted, but over 20 were considered normal and were described in detail. The series is unique in size and range.

holoblastic ovum An ovum that has undergone holoblastic cleavage.

homolecithal ovum MIOLECITHAL OVUM.

isolecithal ovum MIOLECITHAL OVUM.

lecithal ovum MEDIALECITHAL OVUM.

macrolecithal ovum MEGALECITHAL OVUM.

medialecithal ovum An ovum possessing a moderate amount of yolk or deutoplasm, as in amphibians. Also called *lecithal ovum, mesolecithal ovum*.

megalecithal ovum An ovum containing much yolk or deutoplasm, as in bony fishes, reptiles, and birds. Also called *macrolethical ovum, polylecithal ovum*.

meroblastic ovum An ovum rich in yolk (megalecithal), with partial segmentation, of which the part richest in yolk, having little or no contribution to make in segmentation, does not participate in the constitution of the embryo and only provides nutritive material. The other part, poor in yolk and rich in cytoplasm, and which contains the nucleus, is alone segmented into blastomeres, then in cells. It is the only region which participates in the formation of the embryo.

mesolecithal ovum   MEDIALECITHAL OVUM.

microlecithal ovum   MIOLECITHAL OVUM.

Miller ovum   An early human embryo, considered to have been slightly over ten days of age, recovered in 1899.

miolecithal ovum   An ovum having a small quantity of yoke evenly distributed throughout its cytoplasm, as found in many invertebrates, mammals, and man. Also called *alecithal ovum, homolecithal ovum, isolecithal ovum, microlecithal ovum, oligolecithal ovum.*

oligolecithal ovum   MIOLECITHAL OVUM.

permanent ovum   An ovum which has matured to a stage where fertilization is possible.

Peters ovum   An early human embryo estimated to have been some two weeks old, recovered in 1899.

polylecithal ovum   MEGALECITHAL OVUM.

primitive ovum   An ovum at an early stage of its development, either as an oogonium or an oocyte. Also called *primordial ovum.*

primordial ovum   PRIMITIVE OVUM.

telolecithal ovum   An ovum possessing moderate or much yolk. • The term has been used for both medialecithal and megalecithal eggs, and thus some authorities suggest it should not be used except as a synonym.

unfertilized ovum   The haploid female germ cell which has not been fertilized.

Owen [Edmund Blackett *Owen*, English surgeon, 1847–1915] See under OPERATION.

Owen [Sir Richard *Owen*, English anatomist, 1804–1892]   Lines of Owen. See under LINE.

Owren [Paul A. *Owren*, Norwegian hematologist, born 1905] Owren's disease. See under FACTOR V DEFICIENCY.

oxacillin $C_{19}H_{18}N_3O_5S$. An antibiotic with actions and uses similar to those of nafcillin. Its sodium salt is used for treatment of infections from staphylococci that are resistant to penicillin G or for mixed infections in which resistant staphylococci are present.

Oxaine   A proprietary name for oxethazaine.

oxalate   An ion, salt, or ester derived from oxalic acid. The dianion binds calcium ions strongly and precipitates them.

balanced oxalate   A mixture of two parts potassium oxalate, which causes erythrocytes to shrink, and three parts ammonium oxalate, which causes erythrocytes to swell. It is used as an anticoagulant for blood specimens that are to be subjected to hematologic examination. Also called *double oxalate.*

double oxalate   BALANCED OXALATE.

oxalated   Having oxalate dianion added, usually in order to remove calcium ions. This treatment inhibits the clotting of blood.

oxalemia   The presence of abnormally large amounts of oxalates in the blood.

oxalic acid   HOOC—COOH. Ethanedioic acid. It occurs in some plants and is toxic because it binds calcium ions tightly.

oxalism   Poisoning by oxalic acid or its salts. Ingestion of oxalic acid (about 5 g) can be fatal. It causes corrosive damage to the gastrointestinal tract, shock, convulsions, and renal damage. Kidney damage results from the formation of insoluble calcium oxalate deposited in the kidney.

oxaloacetate $^-$OOC—CO—CH$_2$—COO$^-$. The dianion of oxaloacetic acid, the form in which it exists in neutral solution. In the tricarboxylic acid cycle, it reacts with acetyl-CoA to form citrate; this is oxidized ultimately to regenerate oxaloacetate, the final step being the dehydrogenation of malate. It is also

formed reversibly from aspartate by transamination and decarboxylated, both enzymically and spontaneously, to pyruvate.

oxaloacetic acid   The acid corresponding to oxaloacetate.

oxalosis   The deposition of calcium oxalate crystals in many tissues and organs. The condition is associated with hyperoxaluria, but tests for oxalates in the urine are difficult. The diagnosis may be established by demonstration of birefractile crystals in polarized light that do not take up von Kossa's stain. The crystals have characteristic appearances on polarography and x-ray diffraction. On crystallographic analysis, renal oxalate calculi consist mostly of calcium oxalate monohydrate.

oxalosis I   A heritable error of oxalic acid metabolism that results in markedly increased urinary excretion of the salts of oxalic, glycolic, and glyoxylic acids. The basic defect is deficient activity of alphaketoglutarate:glyoxylate carboligase. The clinical syndrome is autosomal recessive and consists of progressive nephrocalcinosis and kidney accumulation of oxalate stones. Renal failure occurs in the second to third decades. Also called *primary hyperoxaluria type I, glycolic aciduria.*

oxalosis II   A heritable error of oxalic acid metabolism that results in increased urinary excretion of oxalate but normal amounts of glyoxylic and glycolic acids. The basic defect is a deficiency of D-glycerate dehydrogenase. Also called *primary hyperoxaluria type II, glyceric aciduria.*

oxalosuccinate   An enzyme-bound intermediate in the oxidative decarboxylation of isocitrate by isocitrate dehydrogenase to give 2-oxoglutarate. The enzyme can bind and decarboxylate free oxalosuccinate.

oxalosuccinic acid   HOOC—CH$_2$—CH(COOH)—CO—COOH. The undissociated form of oxalosuccinate.

oxaluria [*oxal(ate)* (from French *acide oxalique* oxalic acid) a salt or ester of oxalic acid + -URIA]   The excretion of oxalates in the urine. See also OXALOSIS.

oxamic acid   NH$_2$—CO—COOH. The half amide of oxalic acid.

oxamide $C_2H_4N_2O_2$, the diamide of oxalic acid. It is a white crystalline material that reacts with copper sulfate to form the violet biuret complex.

oxamniquine $C_{14}H_{21}N_3O_3$. A tetrahydroquinoline compound effective against *Schistosoma mansoni*. It is well absorbed from the gastrointestinal tract and its metabolites are excreted in the urine. The mechanism of action on the adult parasite is unknown.

oxanamide $C_8H_{15}NO_2$.   2,3-Epoxy-2-ethyl-hexanamide.   A tasteless, odorless, white crystalline compound used as a tranquilizer and sedative.

oxandrolone   A cyclic and rogenic steroid 17β-hydroxy-17α-methyl-2oxa-5α-androstan-3-one, an anabolic steroid.

oxazepam $C_{15}H_{11}ClN_2O_2$. An anxiolytic sedative or minor tranquilizer of the benzodiazepine class.

oxazolidine   Any heterocyclic compound with a saturated five-membered ring containing one oxygen and one nitrogen atom.

oxazolone   A compound whose molecule consists of a five-membered ring of three carbon atoms, one as a carbonyl group, one nitrogen atom, and an oxygen atom, and containing one double bond. N-Acyl derivatives of amino acids easily form such compounds when their carboxyl groups are activated for peptide synthesis. Since such oxazolones racemize easily, the product may contain diastereoisomers. Peptide synthesis has to be designed to avoid this danger.

oxethazaine $C_{28}H_{41}N_3O_3$. 2,2'-[(2-Hydroxyethyl)imino]bis[N-(1,1-dimethyl-2-phenylethyl)-N-methylacetamide]. A crystalline white powder with a bitter taste. It is a surface anesthetic that is poorly absorbed from mucous membranes. It has been given with antacids by mouth to relieve indigestion and gastric discomfort.

oxgall The bile of an ox. See under OX BILE EXTRACT.

oxicephaly OXYCEPHALY.

oxidant [French (now *oxydant*; pres. part. of *oxider*, now *oxyder*, to become oxidized, from Gk *oxys* sharp), having the property of being oxidized] A reactant that oxidizes another and is thereby reduced.

oxidase Any enzyme that uses dioxygen as an oxidant, reducing it to hydrogen peroxide, superoxide, or water. Also called *aerobic dehydrogenase* (obsolete).

xanthine oxidase The enzyme (EC 1.2.3.2) that catalyzes the oxidation of xanthine to uric acid, using dioxygen as second substrate. The other product is superoxide, which decomposes, enzymatically or spontaneously, to hydrogen peroxide. The enzyme also acts on hypoxanthine, and is important in purine catabolism. It is a flavoprotein. Also called *hypoxanthine oxidase* (outmoded), *Schardinger enzyme*.

oxidation [French (now *oxydation*; from *oxider*, now *oxyder*, to become oxidized, from Gk *oxys* sharp, + -*ation* -ATION), a combining with oxygen] The addition of oxygen in a chemical reaction, or any other process deemed to be equivalent, such as addition of an electronegative element, removal of hydrogen or of an electropositive element, removal of electrons.

aerobic oxidation Oxidation in the presence of air, usually with dioxygen of the air as oxidant.

anaerobic oxidation Oxidation in the absence of air, often with nitrate, sulfate, or other inorganic anion as electron acceptor. The process is of importance to many obligate and facultative anaerobic microorganisms.

anodic oxidation Oxidation at the anode of an electrolytic cell by removal of electrons at the electrode surface.

beta-oxidation The process of degradation of fatty acids, so called because C-3 of the fatty acid, its β-carbon, is the point of oxidation in the sense that 3-hydroxy and 3-oxo acids are formed as their coenzyme-A derivatives.

omega-oxidation A pathway of metabolism, of some importance in plants, by which a fatty acid is converted into a molecule with a carboxyl group at each end. The ω-carbon is the carbon atom furthest from the original carboxyl group.

oxide A compound with oxygen, usually a binary compound.

oxidizable Capable of being oxidized.

oxidize To bring about the oxidation of.

oxidoreductase Any enzyme that catalyzes the oxidation of one substrate and the reduction of another.

oxidoreduction A chemical reaction in which oxidation and reduction occurs. Such reactions are more commonly called oxidations or reductions, according to whether it is the oxidation of one reactant or the reduction of another that is to be emphasized. This term is used to emphasize the fact that both processes are occurring. See also OXIDATION-REDUCTION POTENTIAL.

oxime A compound of the type RR'C=N—OH, the imine formed between a carbonyl compound and hydroxylamine. Oximes are much more stable than most imines; i.e, hydroxylamine has a high affinity for carbonyl groups.

oximeter [*ox(ygen)* + *i* + -METER] A photoelectric instrument used to measure the oxygen saturation of blood. Also called *whole blood oximeter*.

whole blood oximeter OXIMETER.

oximetry The determination of oxygen saturation of blood by measuring the transmission of light through translucent tissue, especially the pinna of the ear. Also *oxymetry*.

oxo- [French *ox(ygène)* oxygen + *o*] **1** The prefix used in organic nomenclature to indicate replacement of a methylene group, —CH₂—, by the carbonyl group, —CO—, as in 2-oxo-

glutarate. **2** In inorganic nomenclature, a prefix indicating the binding of oxygen.

oxoacid **1** In organic chemistry, an acid, usually carboxylic, containing a carbonyl group. **2** In inorganic chemistry an acid with one or more oxygen atoms bound to a central atom, e.g. phosphooric acid, (HO—)₃P=O.

3-oxoacyl-ACP reductase The enzyme (EC 1.1.1.100), 3-oxoacyl-[acyl-carrier-protein] reductase, responsible for one step in fatty-acid biosynthesis in bacteria. A similar enzyme, which also reduces the carbonyl group to —CHOH—, is present in other organisms, but the carrier of the acyl group differs. Also called *β-ketoacyl-ACP reductase*.

3-oxoacyl-ACP synthase The enzyme (EC 2.3.1.41) that catalyzes the transfer of an acyl group from acyl-carrier protein onto a malonyl group that is also an acyl-carrier protein, with formation of a 2-oxoacyl group and release of carbon dioxide. This is the chain-lengthening reaction in fatty-acid biosynthesis.

oxogestone phenpropionate 20β-Hydroxy-19-norpregn-4-en-3-one, a progestin.

oxoglutarate dehydrogenase The first component of the multienzyme complex by which 2-oxoglutarate is oxidized to carbon dioxide and succinyl-CoA, with concomitant uptake of coenzyme A and reduction of NAD⁺ to NAD + H⁺. It is the component (EC 1.2.4.2) that catalyzes the decarboxylation of 2-oxoglutarate with combination of the residual 4-carbon compound, at the oxidation level of succinic semialdehyde, to the thiamin diphosphate molecule the enzyme contains. Also called *α-ketoglutarate dehydrogenase* (outmoded).

2-oxoglutaric acid HOOC—CH₂—CH₂—CO—COOH. An intermediate in the citric acid cycle, formed by the oxidative decarboxylation of isocitrate, and converted into succinyl-CoA by the action of the multienzyme oxoglutarate dehydrogenase complex. It may also be formed reversibly from glutamate, either by the action of glutamate dehydrogenase, which uses NADP⁺ or NAD⁺ as cosubstrate, or by the action of an aminotransferase, which uses another 2-oxoacid as cosubstrate. Also called *α-ketoglutaric acid*.

oxoisomerase An outmoded term for GLUCOSEPHOSPHATE ISOMERASE.

oxolinic acid C₁₃H₁₁NO₅. 5-Ethyl-5,8-dihydro-8-oxo-1,3-dioxolo-[4,5-g]quinoline-7-carboxylic acid. A synthetic antibiotic specific for Gram-negative organisms and used mainly in the treatment of urinary-tract infections.

oxonium The ion H₃O⁺. Since the name still applies to this ion when substituted, it generally means any compound containing a tervalent, positively charged, oxygen atom, e.g. triethyloxonium, Et₃O⁺. Also called *hydronium* (outmoded).

oxonuria A seldom used term for KETONURIA.

oxophenarsine C₆H₆AsNO₂·HCl. An odorless white hygroscopic powder, the hydrochloride of 2-amino-4-arsenosophenol. It is employed as an antitrypanosomal compound.

Oxsoralen A proprietary name for methoxsalen.

oxtriphylline C₁₂H₂₁N₅O₃. 1-Hydroxy-N,N,N-trimethylethanaminium salt with 3,7-dihydro-1,3-dimethyl-1H purine,2,6-dione. A compound of choline and theophylline used orally as a bronchodilator. Also called *theophylline cholinate*.

oxy-¹ [French *oxy(gène)* (from Gk *oxy(s)* sharp, pointed + *gen(nan)* to beget or bear, generate) oxygen] A combining form denoting the presence of oxygen in a compound.

oxy-² [Gk *oxys* sharp, pointed] A combining form meaning quick, sharp, keen.

oxyacanthine C₃₇H₄₀N₂O₆. A bitter white crystalline powder extracted from the root of *Berberis vulgaris* of the Berberidaceae family. It can cause central nervous system paralysis. Also called *oxycanthine, vinetine*.

oxyachrestia [OXY[1] + Gk *a*- priv. + *chrēst(os)* useful + -IA] Impaired delivery of glucose to neurons in hypoglycemia, presumably related to the pathogenesis of hypoglycemic coma.

oxyacoia   HYPERACUSIS.

oxyaphia [OXY-[2] + Gk *(h)aph(ē)* a touch, touching + -IA] HYPERAPHIA.

oxybenzoic acid   SALICYLIC ACID.

oxyblepsia [OXY-[2] + Gk *bleps(is)* sight + -*ia* -Y] Very good vision. Also called *oxyopia*.

oxybutyria   OXYBUTYRICACIDEMIA.

oxybutyricacidemia   A condition in which oxybutyric acid is found in urine or in blood, as in diabetic ketoacidosis. Also called *oxybutyria*.

oxycalorimeter   An apparatus in which food is burned in the presence of oxygen, the carbon dioxide produced is absorbed, and the oxygen consumed is measured to enable the indirect determination of the calorific value of the food.

oxycanthine   OXYACANTHINE.

Oxycel   A proprietary name for oxidized cellulose.

oxycephalia   OXYCEPHALY.

oxycephalic   Exhibiting oxycephaly. Also *acrocephalic, acrocephalous, oxycephalous, turricephalic*.

oxycephalous   OXYCEPHALIC.

oxycephaly [OXY-[2] + CEPHAL- + -Y] A form of craniostenosis characterized by an abnormally peaked or conical configuration of the cranium, resulting from premature closure of the lambdoidal and coronal sutures. Also called *acrocephaly, turricephaly, tower skull, acrocephalia, oxycephalia, oxicephaly, steeple head, tower head, steeple skull.*

oxychloride   Denoting a double salt of O^{2-} and Cl^- ions, e.g. *bismuth oxychloride* (bismuth chloride oxide), BiOCl. An obsolete term.

oxychromatic   Pertaining to a tissue or an organelle which has an affinity for, and is colored by, acid stains.

oxychromatin   The chromatin which has an affinity for acid stains.

oxyesthesia   HYPERESTHESIA.

oxyetherotherapy   An obsolete treatment for lung conditions by the inhalation of a mixture of ether vapor with oxygen.

oxygen [French *oxygène*. See OXY-[1].] Element number 8, having atomic weight 15.9994. It is a colorless, odorless, tasteless gas making up about 21% of the volume of the atmosphere and, in various compounds (water is the most familiar), comprising about 49% by weight of the lithosphere. It is obtained in pure form by fractional distillation of liquid air. An allotropic form of oxygen, ozone, is formed by the action on ordinary oxygen of ultraviolet light or by an electric discharge. Ordinary oxygen combines with most elements. The valence is 2. It is a component of countless organic compounds. Roughly one fourth of the atoms in the human body are oxygen atoms. Oxygen is required for respiration in plants and animals. Besides the three naturally occurring stable isotopes, there are five short-lived radioactive isotopes, the least unstable having a half-life of 122 seconds. Symbol: O

oxygen carrier   Any substance that carries oxygen, usually in the bloodstream of animals. It combines with oxygen at relatively high oxygen pressures and releases it at relatively low ones. Hemoglobin is the mammalian oxygen carrier.

excess oxygen   The oxygen used by the body in excess of basal metabolic requirements.

heavy oxygen   Oxygen 17 or oxygen 18, two of the natural stable isotopes of oxygen, as distinguished from oxygen 16, the third and most abundant stable isotope.

singlet oxygen   Dioxygen in an electronically excited state, in which its electrons are paired in spin. Dioxygen is unusual in that its lowest triplet state is lower in energy that its lowest singlet state. Singlet oxygen may be formed in chemical reactions, e.g. between hydrogen peroxide and hypochlorite, or by reaction of dioxygen in its ground (triplet) state with a dye molecule excited by illumination. It shows orange-red luminescence, and reverts to triplet oxygen with a half-life of a few microseconds in water. It is used for a variety of chemical reactions, e.g. to form hydroperoxides from olefins. Biologically occurring carotenes are efficient quenchers of singlet oxygen.

oxygen 15   One of the five radioactive isotopes of oxygen with a half-life of 122 seconds. It decays by beta emission of 1.74 MeV. It emits 512 keV photons by annihilation radiation and is an important radiotracer for positron imaging. Symbol: ^{15}O

oxygenase   Any enzyme that catalyzes the incorporation of oxygen from dioxygen into a single substrate. Oxygenases are divided into dioxygenases, which incorporate both atoms from the dioxygen, and monooxygenases, with which one atom is incorporated, and the other accepts hydrogen to form water.

oxygenate [French *oxygène* oxygen + English suffix -*ate*] To add or supply oxygen to. This may be done to a solution, by dissolving oxygen in it from a stream of air bubbles, or to substances, e.g., by reversible binding of a dioxygen molecule, as with hemoglobin.

oxygenated   **1** Containing oxygen or capable of yielding it.   **2** Treated with oxygen or with a substance that can yield it.

oxygenation   **1** A reversible addition of molecular oxygen to a compound, in contrast with oxidation by oxygen in which the oxygen molecule is more profoundly changed, as by reduction to water.   **2** Treatment of a substance with oxygen, especially passage of oxygen gas through a liquid to achieve a solution of oxygen.

apneic oxygenation   DIFFUSION RESPIRATION.

hyperbaric oxygenation   Administration of oxygen at pressure greater than one atmosphere.

oxygenator [*oxygenat(e)* + -OR] A mechanical device for oxygenating venous blood extracorporeally during cardiopulmonary bypass.

bubble oxygenator   A type of oxygenator that bubbles oxygen directly through the blood.

film oxygenator   An oxygenator in which a thin film of blood is produced to facilitate oxygenation.

membrane oxygenator   A device, generally consisting of a semipermeable silicone rubber or cellophane membrane encased in a container of oxygen, used for oxygenization of blood during cardiopulmonary bypass.

pump oxygenator   See under PUMP-OXYGENATOR.

rotating disk oxygenator   A device in which parallel disks are rotated through an extracorporeal pool of venous blood in an atmosphere of oxygen. Oxygenization is accomplished through the thin films of blood adhering to the disks.

screen oxygenator   A film oxygenator in which the blood is passed over a series of screens.

oxygeusia [OXY-[2] + Gk *geus(is)* a tasting, sense of taste + -IA] **1** Exceptionally keen taste perception.   **2** A variety of dysgeusia in which everything tastes sour.

oxyhaemoglobin   A British spelling for OXYHEMOGLOBIN.

oxyhematin   HEME.

oxyheme   HEME.

oxyhemochromogen   HEME.

oxyhemocyanin   The oxygenated form of hemocyanin.

oxyhemoglobin   The oxygenated form of hemoglobin, in which the iron atom has reversibly bound a molecule of dioxygen. It is bright scarlet. Also called *oxidized hemoglobin*.

oxyhydrocephalus [OXY-[2] + HYDROCEPHALUS] Hydrocephalus in which the enlarged cranium assumes a peaked or conical configuration instead of the usual spheroidal contour.

oxyiodopyridone-acetic acid $C_5H_3ONICH_2COOH$. An acid which, in the form of its sodium salt, was formerly used as a contrast medium for intravenous urography.

oxykrinin An obsolete term for SECRETIN.

oxylalia [OXY-^{2} + -LALIA] Fast speech, usually excessively fast.

Oxylone A proprietary name for fluorometholone.

oxyluciferin The oxidized form of any luciferin. It is produced by enzymic oxidation of a luciferin, the enzyme being a luciferase. This oxidation forms a molecule of oxyluciferin in an electronically excited state, and the molecule can fall to its ground state on emission of a quantum of light. The wavelength of the light emitted is determined by the nature of both the oxyluciferin and the luciferase to which it is bound.

oxymetazoline hydrochloride $C_{16}H_{24}N_2O$. 6-tert-Butyl-3-(2-imidazolin-2-ylmethyl)-2,4-dimethylphenol hydrochloride. A drug that is used as a nasal decongestant.

oxymetholone $C_{21}H_{32}O_3$. 17β-Hydroxy-2-(hydroxymethylene)-17-methyl-5α-androstan-3-one. An anabolic steroid used as an androgen and to ameliorate cachexia in chronic illness.

oxymetry OXIMETRY.

oxymorphone hydrochloride $C_{17}H_{20}ClNO_4$. 4,5-Epoxy-3,14-dihydroxy-17-methylmorphinan-6-one hydrochloride, a semisynthetic derivative of morphine with actions and properties like morphine, except that is has no significant antitussive activity. It is used for relief of severe pain and it is given parenterally.

oxymyoglobin The oxygenated form of myoglobin, in which the iron atom has reversibly bound a molecule of dioxygen.

oxyntic [Gk oxyn(ein) to sharpen, make acid + t + -IC] Acid-producing: used primarily in reference to the parietal cells of the stomach.

oxyopia OXYBLEPSIA.

oxyopter [OXY-^{2} + OPT- + -ER] The reciprocal of the visual angle, used as a measure of visual acuity.

oxyosis An obsolete term for ACIDOSIS.

oxyosmia [OXY-^{2} + osm(o)-^{2} + -IA] Heightened olfactory acuity. Also called *oxyosphresia* (seldom used).

oxyosphresia A seldom used term for OXYOSMIA.

oxypathia [OXY-^{2} + -PATHIA] HYPERPATHIA.

oxypathic HYPERPATHIC.

oxypathy [OXY-^{2} + -PATHY] HYPERPATHIA.

oxypertine $C_{23}H_{29}N_3O_2$. 5,6-Dimethoxy-2-methyl-3-[2-(4-phenyl-1-piperazinyl)ethyl]indole. An antidepressant drug of the indole family with psychotropic activity.

oxyphenbutazone $C_{19}H_{20}N_2O_3$. 4-Butyl-1-(4-hydroxyphenyl)-2-phenyl-3,5-pyrazolidinedione. A metabolite of phenylbutazone, occurring as a water-soluble sodium salt, also soluble in alcohol and organic solvents. It is an anti-inflammatory drug often used in the treatment of acute forms of arthritis, such as gout.

oxyphencyclimine $C_{20}H_{28}N_2O_3$. α-Cyclohexyl-α-hydroxybenzeneacetic acid (1,4,5,6-tetrahydro-1-methyl-2-pyrimidinyl)-methyl ester, an anticholinergic agent with antispasmodic, antisecretory, and antimotility activities on the gastrointestinal tract. It is used orally to treat peptic ulcer and spasms of the gastrointestinal tract.

oxyphenisatin A laxative drug, no longer marketed because of harmful side effects.

oxyphil ACIDOPHILIC.

oxyphilic ACIDOPHILIC.

oxyphilous ACIDOPHILIC.

oxyphonia [OXY-^{2} + PHON- + -IA] Abnormal sharpness of voice.

oxyplasm The portion of the cytoplasm which has an affinity for acid stains.

oxyquinoline sulfate 8-HYDROXYQUINOLINE SULFATE.

oxyrhine [OXY-^{2} + Gk *rhis*, gen. *rhinos*, nose] Having a pointed nose.

oxyrygmia [OXY-^{2} + Gk *(e)rygm(os)* a belching + -IA] Acidic belching. An obsolete term.

Oxyspirura A genus of nematodes of the family Thelaziidae, superfamily Spiruroidea, that infect eyes, chiefly of birds though one of the 47 species has been reported from mammals.

Oxyspirura mansoni A cosmopolitan species, Manson's eye worm, parasitic under the nictitating membrane in the eyes of chickens, turkeys, quail, geese, and peafowl. The cockroach *Psychoscellus surinamensis* serves as the intermediate host. When an infected roach is eaten by the fowl, the larvae are freed in the crop, migrate up the esophagus to the mouth and through the nasopharynx into the tear ducts, sometimes arriving there within 15 minutes after the roach is ingested.

oxyspore [OXY-^{2} + SPORE] SPOROZOITE.

oxytalan A periodontal fiber found in man and some other animals. After oxidation, it can be stained with aldehyde fuchsin.

oxytalanolysis [*oxytalan* + *o* + LYSIS] The destruction of oxytalan fibers.

oxytetracycline $C_{22}H_{24}N_2O_9$. 4-(Dimethylamino)-1,4,4α,5,5α,6,11,12α-octahydro-3,5,6,10,12,12α-hexahydro-6-methyl-1,11-dioxo-2-naphthacenecarboxamide. An antibiotic substance obtained from *Streptomyces rimosus*. It is a broad-spectrum antibiotic, acting by the inhibition of protein synthesis in a wide range of Gram-negative and Gram-positive organisms. Susceptible organisms include rickettsiae, mycoplasmas, and species of *Pasteurella* and *Vibrio*. It is usually given intramuscularly. Also called *hydroxytetracycline, riomitsin*.

oxytetracycline hydrochloride The monohydrochloride salt of oxytetracycline. It has the same properties and uses as the parent drug, and it is given orally or by intravenous injection.

oxytocia [OXY-^{2} + *toc(o)*- + -IA] Labor that is very rapid.

oxytocic 1 Inducing or stimulating uterine contractions. Also called *ecbolic, ocyodinic, parurifacient*. 2 An oxytocic agent, as oxytocin, prostaglandins, or ergot compounds. 3 Relating to oxytocia.

oxytocin One of the two major neurohormones secreted by the supraoptic nuclei of the hypothalamus and stored in the neurohypophysis. The other is vasopressin. Oxytocin is an octapeptide with an essential pentapeptide ring and a terminal glycine amide, differing structurally from vasopressin only in positions 3 and 8. Stimuli for release of the two hormones, such as sucking by the newborn, are similar. Actions are to stimulate milk ejection, uterine contraction, and vasodepression, antidiuretic and vasopressor actions being minimal. Its exact role in mammalian parturition is not known. It is used in man and animals to induce parturition and postpartum contraction of the uterus and in veterinary medicine to promote milk let-down in sows with agalactia and in cows and bitches in which environmental stress may have caused failure of release of oxytocin. Also called *oxytocic hormone, α-hypophamine* (seldom used).

oxytocinase A glycoprotein aminopeptidase, probably of uterine and placental origin, that appears in plasma during pregnancy, reaching greatest concentration before term and decreasing after parturition. The enzyme cleaves the 1-cysteine to 2-tyrosine peptide bonds of oxytocin and vasopressin, inactivating both hormones. Also called *vasopressinase*.

oxytoxin [OXY-^{1} + TOXIN] A toxin that has undergone oxidation.

oxytuberculin A tuberculin prepared from particularly virulent strains of *Mycobacterium tuberculosis* and modified by oxidation. It is no longer in use. Also called *Hirschfelder's tuberculin*.

oxyuria OXYURIASIS.

oxyuriasis [*oxyur(id worms)* + -IASIS] Infection with oxyurid worms, especially *Enterobius vermicularis*; enterobiasis. Also called *oxyurosis, oyxuria, oxyuriosis*.

oxyuricide [*oxyuri(d)* + -CIDE] An agent destructive to oxyurids.

oxyurid [OXY-² + Gk *our(a)* tail + -ID¹] 1 Of or belonging to the family Oxyuridae. 2 A member of the family Oxyuridae.

Oxyuridae [OXY-² + Gk *our(a)* tail + -IDAE] A large family of pinworms (superfamily Oxyuroidea) that are parasitic in the large intestine and cecum of many mammals, especially rodents. Among the important genera are *Aspicularis* (in rodents), *Enterobius* (primates and rodents), *Oxyuris* (equids, ruminants, rodents, and primates), *Passalurus* (rabbits and rodents), and *Syphacia* (rodents). *Enterobius vermicularis* is the only species normally found in humans.

oxyurifuge [*oxyuri(d)* + -FUGE] An agent that expels oxyurids from a host.

oxyuriosis OXYURIASIS.

Oxyuris [OXY-² + Gk *oura* the tail of an animal, the hinder parts] A genus of nematodes (family Oxyuridae) parasitic in the large intestine. The genus includes a number of nonpathogenic parasites of ungulates, all with a direct, or monoxenous, life cycle, in which maturation occurs in the intestinal lumen with no parenteral migration of the larvae.

Oxyuris equi A species of pinworm found in the large intestine of horses throughout the world. Infestation is associated with perianal pruritus and loss of hair around the base of the tail because of rubbing the area. The gravid female worms deposit their eggs on the perineum around the anus.

Oxyuris incognita HETERODERA RADICICOLA.

Oxyuris vermicularis An older term for *ENTEROBIUS VERMICULARIS*.

Oxyuris vivipara A former name for *PROBSTMAYRIA VIVIPARA*.

oxyuroid 1 Of or belonging to the superfamily Oxyuroidea. 2 A member of the superfamily Oxyuroidea.

Oxyuroidea [OXY-² + Gk *our(a)* tail + New L *-oidea*, from L *-oides* -OID + *-ea*, neut. pl. of *-eus* English *-eous*] A superfamily of secernentean (phasmidian) nematodes, the pinworms, usually parasitic in the intestine of vertebrates, but insects and other invertebrates may also be infected. They are characterized by a bulbous, muscular, valved posterior end of the esophagus. The female has a long, pointed tail.

oxyurosis OXYURIASIS.

oyster drill A predatory marine gastropod capable of drilling a hole through the shell of oysters and other mollusks to feed on the contents.

oz Symbol for the unit, ounce.

ozaena A British spelling for OZENA.

ozamin BENZOPURPURINE.

oz ap In the United States, symbol for the unit, apothecaries' ounce.

oz apoth In Great Britain, symbol for the unit apothecaries' ounce.

ozena [Gk *ozaina* (from *ozein* to have a smell) a fetid polyp in the nose] 1 Rhinitis of whatever kind that imparts a foul smell to the breath. Also called *coryza foetida*. 2 ATROPHIC RHINITIS. Adjective: ozenous.

ozena laryngis Advanced atrophic laryngitis, with foul-smelling crusting, secondary to ozena of the nose. It was once regarded as a separate clinical entity. Nowadays its occurrence is extremely rare.

ozenous Pertaining to or resembling ozena, particularly by virtue of the characteristic foul smell.

ozochrotia BROMHIDROSIS.

ozochrotous [Gk *oz(ein)* to smell + *o* + *chrōs*, gen. *chrōtos*, the skin + -OUS] Pertaining to an offensive skin odor.

ozone O_3. The triatomic allotrope of oxygen, formed from dioxygen subjected to an electric discharge. It is used for chemical oxidations, particularly that of carbon-carbon double bonds to form ozonides. Since ozonides react with water to form two carbonyl groups, the molecule attacked is normally split into two, so that analysis of the products allows the original double bond to be located. Ozone is toxic, but is removed by reaction fairly rapidly from air. It may be concentrated by liquefaction to a blue, explosive liquid. Oxygen containing ozone has been used as a disinfectant. The presence of ozone in the stratosphere sustains life by stopping ultraviolet radiation from the sun and preventing it from reaching the earth in lethal amounts.

ozone-ether A mixture of ethyl ether, ethanol, and hydrogen peroxide. It is used as an antiseptic.

ozonide The compound formed by addition of ozone to a carbon-carbon double bond. It contains a five-membered ring, with oxygen atoms at positions 1, 2, and 4, and it is formed by rearrangement, which involves breaking of the carbon-carbon bond, of the initial product with oxygen atoms at positions 1, 2, and 3. It is hydrolyzed by water to give two carbonyl groups and hydrogen peroxide.

ozonize To produce ozone in (oxygen). This is normally done by silent electric discharge through a stream of oxygen gas.

ozonized Containing ozone, or treated with ozone.

ozonizer An apparatus in which a stream of oxygen may be ozonized by a high-voltage electric field.

ozonolysis [*ozon(e)* + *o* + LYSIS] The process of breaking a molecule RR′C=CR″R‴ into RR′CO and R″R‴ CO, by treatment first with ozone, usually contained in a stream of oxygen gas from an ozonizer, and then with water to decompose the ozonide.

ozonometer An apparatus for determining the quantity of ozone in the atmosphere.

ozonometry The measurement of atmospheric ozone by means of special ozonoscopic papers impregnated with substances that change color according to the ozone concentration in the air.

ozonophore 1 CYTOPLASMIC GRANULE. 2 A seldom used term for ERYTHROCYTE.

ozonoscope [*ozon(e)* + *o* + -SCOPE] An apparatus for revealing the presence of ozone.

ozonoscopic Serving to detect atmospheric ozone, as *ozonoscopic paper*.

ozonosphere OZONE LAYER.

ozostomia [Gk *ozostom(os)* (from *ozein* to have a smell + *stoma* mouth) having a bad breath + -IA] FETOR ORIS.

oz t In the United States, symbol for the unit, ounce troy.

oz tr In Great Britain, symbol for the unit, ounce troy.